Appendices From CVT XIII on Evolve Website

KIRK'S
CURRENT VETERINARY THERAPY XIV

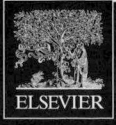

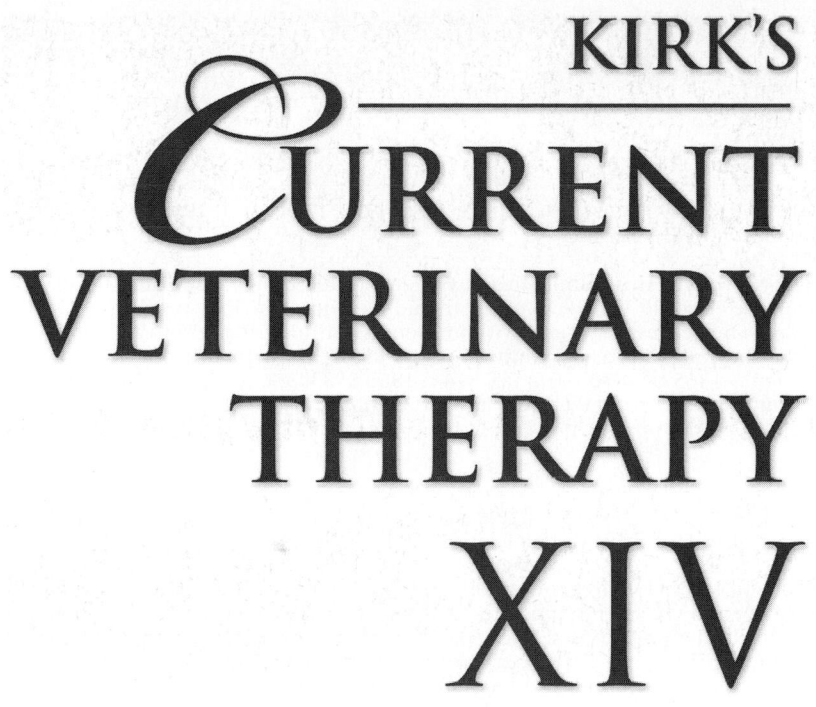

KIRK'S CURRENT VETERINARY THERAPY XIV

Editor

John D. Bonagura, DVM, MS, DACVIM
(Cardiology, Internal Medicine)
Professor
Department of Veterinary Clinical Sciences
College of Veterinary Medicine
The Ohio State University
Columbus, Ohio

Associate Editor

David C. Twedt, DVM, DACVIM
(Internal Medicine)
Professor
Department of Clinical Sciences
College of Veterinary Medicine and Biomedical Sciences
Colorado State University
Fort Collins, Colorado

with more than 325 illustrations

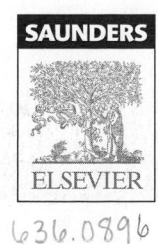

SAUNDERS

ELSEVIER

SAUNDERS
ELSEVIER

11830 Westline Industrial Drive
St. Louis, Missouri 63146

KIRK'S CURRENT VETERINARY THERAPY XIV   ISBN 978-0-7216-9497-9

Notice

Knowledge and best practice in this field are constantly changing. As new research and experience broaden our knowledge, changes in practice, treatment and drug therapy may become necessary or appropriate. Readers are advised to check the most current information provided (i) on procedures featured or (ii) by the manufacturer of each product to be administered, to verify the recommended dose or formula, the method and duration of administration, and contraindications. It is the responsibility of practitioners, relying on their own experience and knowledge of the patient, to make diagnoses, to determine dosages and the best treatment for each individual patient, and to take all appropriate safety precautions. To the fullest extent of the law, neither the Publisher nor the Editors assumes any liability for any injury and/or damage to persons or property arising out of or related to any use of the material contained in this book.

The Publisher

ISBN 978-0-7216-9497-9

Vice President and Publisher: Linda Duncan
Publisher: Penny Rudolph
Managing Editor: Jolynn Gower
Publishing Services Manager: Pat Joiner-Myers
Senior Project Manager: Karen M. Rehwinkel
Designers: Julia Dummitt, Charles J. Seibel

Printed in the United States of America

Last digit is the print number: 9 8 7 6 5 4 3 2 1

Consulting Editors

SECTION I CRITICAL CARE

Nishi Dhupa, BVM, DACVIM (Internal Medicine), DACVECC

SECTION II TOXICOLOGIC DISEASES

Michael J. Murphy, DVM, PhD, DACT

SECTION III ENDOCRINE AND METABOLIC DISEASES

Mark E. Peterson, DVM, DACVIM

SECTION IV ONCOLOGY AND HEMATOLOGY

Douglas H. Thamm, VMD, DACVIM (Oncology)

SECTION V DERMATOLOGIC DISEASES

Craig E. Griffin, DVM, DACVD
Wayne S. Rosenkrantz, DVM, DACVD

SECTION VI GASTROINTESTINAL DISEASES

David C. Twedt, DVM, DACVIM (Internal Medicine)

SECTION VII RESPIRATORY DISEASES

Eleanor C. Hawkins, DVM, DACVIM

SECTION VIII CARDIOVASCULAR DISEASES

John D. Bonagura, DVM, MS, DACVIM (Cardiology, Internal Medicine)

SECTION IX URINARY DISEASES

India F. Lane, DVM, MS, DACVIM

SECTION X REPRODUCTIVE DISEASES

Margaret V. Root Kustritz, DVM, PhD, DACT

SECTION XI NEUROLOGIC AND MUSCULOSKELETAL DISEASES

Rodney S. Bagley, DVM, DACVIM (Neurology, Internal Medicine)

SECTION XII OPHTHALMIC DISEASES

David J. Maggs, BVSc, DACVO

SECTION XIII INFECTIOUS DISEASES

Rance K. Sellon, DVM, PhD, DACVIM

APPENDIX I TABLE OF COMMON DRUGS: APPROXIMATE DOSAGES

Mark G. Papich, DVM, MS, DACVCP

Contributors

Jonathan A. Abbott, DVM
Associate Professor of Cardiology
Department of Small Animal Clinical Sciences
Virginia-Maryland Regional College of Veterinary Medicine
Virginia Polytechnic Institute and State University
Blacksburg, Virginia
Subaortic Stenosis

Mark J. Acierno, DVM, DACVIM
Assistant Professor
School of Veterinary Medicine
The Louisiana State University
Baton Rouge, Louisiana
Systemic Hypertension in Renal Disease

Larry G. Adams, DVM, PhD, DACVIM (SAIM)
Associate Professor, Small Animal Internal Medicine
Department of Veterinary Clinical Sciences
Purdue University
West Lafayette, Indiana
Laser Lithotripsy for Uroliths

Diane D. Addie, PhD, BVMS, MRCVS
Feline Institute Pyrenees
Etchebar, France;
Honorary Senior Research Fellow
Institute of Comparative Medicine
University of Glasgow Veterinary School
Glasgow, Scotland
United Kingdom
Control of Viral Diseases in Catteries
Feline Infectious Peritonitis: Therapy and Prevention

Christopher A. Adin, DVM, DACVS
Courtesy Faculty Appointment
Small Animal Clinical Sciences
College of Veterinary Medicine
University of Florida
Gainesville, Florida;
Small Animal Surgeon
Veterinary Specialists of Rochester
Rochester, New York
Renal Transplantation

Darcy B. Adin, DVM, DACVIM (Cardiology)
Veterinary Specialists of Rochester
Rochester, New York
Tricuspid Valve Dysplasia

Verena K. Affolter, DVM, PhD
Associate Professor for Clinical Dermatopathology
Department of Pathology, Microbiology, and Immunology
School of Veterinary Medicine
University of California
Davis, California
Histiocytic Disease Complex
Nonneoplastic Nodular Histiocytic Diseases of the Skin

P. Jane Armstrong, DVM, MS, MBA, DACVIM (SAIM)
Professor, Internal Medicine/Clinical Nutrition
Department of Veterinary Clinical Sciences
College of Veterinary Medicine
University of Minnesota
St. Paul, Minnesota
Feline Inflammatory Liver Disease

Clarke E. Atkins, DVM, DACVIM (Internal Medicine, Cardiology)
Professor of Medicine and Cardiology
Veterinary Teaching Hospital
College of Veterinary Medicine
North Carolina State University
Raleigh, North Carolina
Feline Heartworm Disease

Anne Avery, VMD, PhD
Assistant Professor
Director Clinical Immunopathology Service
Department of Microbiology, Immunology, and Pathology
College of Veterinary Medicine and Biomedical Sciences
Colorado State University
Fort Collins, Colorado
Canine Lymphoma

Sandra M. Axiak, DVM
Veterinary Specialists of North Texas and Animal Care Center
Dallas, Texas
Pulmonary Neoplasia

Todd W. Axlund, DVM, MS, DACVIM (Neurology)
Director
Metropolitan Veterinary Hospital
Akron, Ohio
Treatment of Intracranial Tumors

Rodney S. Bagley, DVM, DACVIM (Neurology, Internal Medicine)
Professor, Neurology and Neurosurgery
Department of Veterinary Clinical Sciences
Washington State University
Pullman, Washington
Treatment of Canine Cervical Spondylomyelopathy: A Critical Review
Treatment of Degenerative Lumbosacral Stenosis
Vestibular Disease of Dogs and Cats

Claudia J. Baldwin, DVM, MS, DACVIM (Internal Medicine)
Associate Professor, Veterinary Clinical Sciences
College of Veterinary Medicine
Iowa State University
Ames, Iowa
Pregnancy Loss in the Queen

Tania A. Banks, BVSc, FACVSc
Brisbane Veterinary Specialist Centre
Albany Creek, Queensland
Australia
Canine Soft-Tissue Sarcomas

Jeanne A. Barsanti, DVM, MS, DACVIM (SAIM)
Josiah Meigs Distinguished Teaching Professor
Department of Small Animal Medicine and Surgery
College of Veterinary Medicine
The University of Georgia
Athens, Georgia
Multidrug-Resistant Urinary Tract Infection

Joseph W. Bartges, DVM, PhD, DACVIM, DACVN
Professor of Medicine and Nutrition
The Acree Endowed Chair of Small Animal Research
Department of Small Animal Clinical Sciences
College of Veterinary Medicine
The University of Tennessee
Knoxville, Tennessee
Interpreting and Managing Crystalluria

Shane W. Bateman, DVM, DVSC, DACVECC
Associate Professor, Clinical
Department of Veterinary Clinical Sciences
College of Veterinary Medicine
The Ohio State University
Columbus, Ohio
Fluid Therapy
Ventilator Therapy

Karin M. Beale, DVM, DACVD
Staff Dermatologist
Gulf Coast Veterinary Dermatology & Allergy
Houston, Texas
Feline Demodicosis

Ellen N. Behrend, DVM, DACVIM
Associate Professor
Department of Clinical Sciences
College of Veterinary Medicine
Auburn University
Auburn, Alabama
Interpretation of Endocrine Diagnostic Test Results for Adrenal and Thyroid Disease

Adrienne Bentley, DVM
Resident in Surgery
School of Veterinary Medicine
University of Pennsylvania
Philadelphia, Pennsylvania
Drainage Techniques for the Septic Abdomen

Ellison Bentley, DVM, DACVO
Clinical Associate Professor
Comparative Ophthalmology
Department of Surgical Sciences
School of Veterinary Medicine
University of Wisconsin
Madison, Wisconsin
Nonhealing Corneal Erosions in Dogs

Allyson C. Berent, DVM, DACVIM
Staff Veterinarian in Small Animal Internal Medicine and Interventional Radiology
Waltham Lecturer: Minimally Invasive Diagnostics/Therapeutics
Matthew J. Ryan Veterinary Teaching Hospital
School of Veterinary Medicine
University of Pennsylvania
Philadelphia, Pennsylvania
Interventional Radiology in Urinary Diseases

Philip J. Bergman, DVM, MS, PhD, DACVIM (Oncology)
Chief Medical Officer
Bright Heart Veterinary Centers
Armonk, New York
Malignant Melanoma

Adam J. Birkenheuer, DVM, DACVIM (Internal Medicine)
Assistant Professor of Internal Medicine
Department of Clinical Sciences
College of Veterinary Medicine
North Carolina State University
Raleigh, North Carolina
Babesiosis
Thrombocytopenia

Karyn Bischoff, DVM, MS, DABVT
Diagnostic Toxicologist
Animal Health Diagnostic Center
Assistant Professor
College of Veterinary Medicine
Cornell University
Ithaca, New York
Aflatoxicosis in Dogs
Automotive Toxins

Dana R. Bleifer, DVM
Warner Center Pet Clinic
Woodland Hills, California
False Pregnancy in the Bitch

John D. Bonagura, DVM, MS, DACVIM (Cardiology, Internal Medicine)
Professor
Department of Veterinary Clinical Sciences
College of Veterinary Medicine
The Ohio State University
Columbus, Ohio
Management of Heart Failure in Dogs
Ventricular Septal Defect

Dino M. Bradley, DVM, MS
Research Associate
Scott-Ritchey Research Center
College of Veterinary Medicine
Auburn University
Auburn, Alabama
Acral Lick Dermatitis

Edward B. Breitschwerdt, DVM, DACVIM
Professor of Medicine and Infectious Diseases
Director, NCSU-CVM Biosafety Laboratory
Adjunct Associate Professor of Medicine
Duke University Medical Center
Department of Clinical Sciences
College of Veterinary Medicine
North Carolina State University
Raleigh, North Carolina
Bartonellosis

Janice M. Bright, BSN, MS, DVM, DACVIM (Internal Medicine, Cardiology)
Professor of Cardiology
Department of Clinical Sciences
College of Veterinary Medicine and Biomedical Sciences
Colorado State University
Fort Collins, Colorado
Cardioversion

Marjory B. Brooks, DVM, DACVIM
Associate Director, Comparative Coagulation Laboratory
Department of Population Medicine and Diagnostic
    Sciences
College of Veterinary Medicine
Cornell University
Ithaca, New York
Antiplatelet and Anticoagulant Therapy
Platelet Dysfunction

Cathy A. Brown, VMD, PhD, DACVP
Professor, Pathology
Athens Diagnostic Laboratory
College of Veterinary Medicine
University of Georgia
Athens, Georgia
Glomerular Disease

Barret J. Bulmer, DVM, MS, DACVIM (Cardiology)
Assistant Professor
Veterinary Clinical Sciences
College of Veterinary Medicine
Oregon State University
Corvallis, Oregon
Mitral Valve Dysplasia

Amanda Burrows, BSc, BVMS, FACVSc (Veterinary Dermatology)
Veterinary Hospital
Murdoch University
Murdoch
Western Australia
Avermectins in Dermatology

Julie K. Byron, DVM, MS, DACVIM
Assistant Professor, Small Animal Medicine
Department of Clinical Medicine
University of Illinois at Urbana-Champaign
Urbana, Illinois
Urinary Incontinence: Treatment With Injectable Bulking Agents

Clay A. Calvert, DVM, DACVIM (Internal Medicine)
Professor
Department of Small Animal Medicine
College of Veterinary Medicine
University of Georgia
Athens, Georgia
Cardiomyopathy in Doberman Pinschers
Syncope

Anthony P. Carr, DrMedVet, DACIM
Associate Professor
Western College of Veterinary Medicine
University of Saskatchewan
Saskatoon, Saskatchewan
Canada
von Willebrand's Disease and Other Hereditary Coagulopathies

Elizabeth W. Carsten, DVM, DACVIM
Internal Medicine Consultant
IDEXX Laboratories, Inc.
Oro Valley, Arizona
Esophagitis

James L. Catalfamo, MS, PhD
Director, Comparative Coagulation Laboratory
Department of Population Medicine and Diagnostic
    Sciences
College of Veterinary Medicine
Cornell University
Ithaca, New York
Platelet Dysfunction

Daniel L. Chan, DVM, MRCVS, DACVECC, DACVN
Lecturer in Emergency and Critical Care
Department of Veterinary Clinical Sciences
The Royal Veterinary College
University of London
London, England
United Kingdom
Nutrition in Critical Care

Annie V. Chen, DVM
Department of Veterinary Clinical Sciences
College of Veterinary Medicine
Washington State University
Pullman, Washington
Treatment of Canine Cervical Spondylomyelopathy:
    A Critical Review

Dennis J. Chew, DVM, DACVIM (Internal Medicine)
Professor
College of Veterinary Medicine
The Ohio State University
Columbus, Ohio
Idiopathic Feline Hypercalcemia
Treatment of Hypoparathyroidism
Urinary Incontinence: Treatment With Injectable Bulking Agents

Ruthanne Chun, DVM, DACVIM (Oncology)
Clinical Associate Professor
Member, University of Wisconsin Comprehensive Cancer Center
School of Veterinary Medicine
University of Wisconsin
Madison, Wisconsin
Anal Sac Tumors

Julie Churchill, DVM, PhD
Assistant Clinical Professor
Veterinary Clinical Sciences
College of Veterinary Medicine
University of Minnesota
St. Paul, Minnesota
Food Toxicoses in Small Animals

Craig A. Clifford, DVM, MS, DACVIM (Oncology)
Staff Oncologist
Red Bank Veterinary Hospital
Tinton Falls, New Jersey
Canine Hemangiosarcoma

Joan R. Coates, DVM, MS, DACVIM (Neurology)
Associate Professor
Veterinary Medicine and Surgery
Neurology/Neurosurgery Service Leader
Veterinary Medical Teaching Hospital
Department of Veterinary Medicine and Surgery
College of Veterinary Medicine
University of Missouri
Columbia, Missouri
Treatment of Animals With Spinal and Musculoskeletal Pain

Leah A. Cohn, DVM, PhD, DACVIM (SAIM)
Associate Professor of Veterinary Internal Medicine
Department of Veterinary Medicine and Surgery
College of Veterinary Medicine
University of Missouri
Columbia, Missouri
Canine Anaplasma Infection

Lynette K. Cole, DVM, MS, DACVD
Assistant Professor
Department of Veterinary Clinical Sciences
College of Veterinary Medicine
The Ohio State University
Columbus, Ohio
Systemic Therapy for Otitis Externa and Media

Patrick Concannon, MS, PhD, DACT (Honorary)
Visiting Fellow, Department of Clinical Sciences
Director
Laboratory for Comparative Reproduction Studies
Department of Biomedical Sciences
College of Veterinary Medicine
Cornell University
Ithaca, New York
Estrus Suppression in the Bitch

Gheorge M. Constantinescu, DVM, PhD, Drhc
Professor of Veterinary Anatomy
College of Veterinary Medicine
University of Missouri
Columbia, Missouri
Brachycephalic Upper Airway Syndrome in Dogs

Johanna C. Cooper, BSc, DVM, DACVIM
Cape Cod Veterinary Specialists
Buzzards Bay, Massachusetts
Diagnostic Approach to Hepatobiliary Disease

Brendan M. Corcoran, MVB, DipPharm, PhD, MRCVS
Senior Lecturer
Hospital for Small Animals
Division of Veterinary Clinical Studies
The University of Edinburgh
Easterbush Veterinary Centre
Edinburgh, Scotland
United Kingdom
Interstitial Lung Diseases

Etienne Côté, DVM, DACVIM (Cardiology, SAIM)
Assistant Professor
Department of Companion Animals
Atlantic Veterinary College
University of Prince Edward Island
Charlottetown, Prince Edward Island
Canada
Feline Cardiac Arrhythmias

Nancy B. Cottrill, DVM, MS, DACVO
Staff Ophthalmologist
Angell Animal Medical Center, Western New England
Woburn, Massachusetts
Differential Diagnosis of Anisocoria

Dennis T. Crowe, Jr., DVM, NREMT-I, PI, CFF, DACVS, DACVECC
President
Veterinary Surgery, Emergency and Critical Care Services and Consulting
Bogart, Georgia
Oxygen Therapy

Autumn P. Davidson, DVM, MS, DACVIM (Internal Medicine)
Clinical Professor
School of Veterinary Medicine
University of California
Davis, California
Canine Brucellosis
Dystocia Management

Thomas K. Day, DVM, MS, DACVECC, DACVA
Owner
Louisville Veterinary Specialty & Emergency Services
Louisville, Kentucky
Intravenous Anesthetic and Analgesic Techniques

Douglas J. DeBoer, DVM, DACVD
Professor
Department of Medical Sciences
School of Veterinary Medicine
University of Wisconsin
Madison, Wisconsin
Treatment of Dermatophytosis

Linda J. DeBowes, DVM, MS, DACVIM, DAVDC
Shoreline Veterinary Dental Clinic
Seattle, Washington
Feline Caudal Stomatitis

Louis-Philippe de Lorimier, DVM, DACVIM (Oncology)
Staff Medical Oncologist
Hôpital Vétérinaire Rive-Sud
Brossard, Québec
Canada
Canine Hemangiosarcoma

Helio Autran de Morais, DVM, PhD, DACVIM (SAIM, Cardiology)
Clinical Associate Professor
Department of Medical Sciences
University of Wisconsin
Madison, Wisconsin
Acid-Base Disorders

Robert C. DeNovo, DVM, MS, DACVIM
Professor and Head
Department of Small Animal Clinical Sciences
College of Veterinary Medicine
University of Tennessee
Knoxville, Tennessee
Canine Megaesophagus

Curtis W. Dewey, DVM, MS, DACVIM (Neurology), DACVS
Associate Professor, Neurology/Neurosurgery
Neurology/Neurosurgery Service Chief
Cornell University Hospital for Animals
Cornell University
Ithaca, New York
New Maintenance Anticonvulsant Therapies for Dogs and Cats
Traumatic Brain Injury
Treatment of Canine Chiari-Like Malformation and Syringomyelia

Anna R. Deykin, BSc, BVMS, FACVSc (Ophthalmology)
Veterinary Ophthalmologist
Brisbane Veterinary Specialist Centre
Brisbane, Queensland
Australia
Episcleritis and Scleritis in Dogs

Stephen P. DiBartola, DVM, DACVIM (SAIM)
Professor
Department of Veterinary Clinical Sciences
College of Veterinary Medicine
The Ohio State University
Columbus, Ohio
Acid-Base Disorders
Fluid Therapy

Patricia M. Dowling, DVM, MSc, DACVIM, DACVCP
Professor, Veterinary Clinical Pharmacology
Western College of Veterinary Medicine
University of Saskatchewan
Veterinary Biomedical Sciences
Saskatoon, Saskatchewan
Canada
Rational Empiric Antimicrobial Therapy

Kenneth J. Drobatz, DVM, MS, DACVIM, DACVECC
Director of the Emergency Service
Chief of Critical Care Section
Matthew J. Ryan Veterinary Hospital
School of Veterinary Medicine
University of Pennsylvania
Philadelphia, Pennsylvania
Noncardiogenic Pulmonary Edema
Urethral Obstruction in Cats

†Robert B. Duncan, DVM, PhD, DACVP
Associate Professor, Pathology
Department of Pathobiology and Biomedical Sciences
Virginia-Maryland Regional College of Veterinary Medicine
Virginia Polytechnic Institute and State University
Blacksburg, Virginia
Gastric Helicobacter *spp. and Chronic Vomiting in Dogs*

Marilyn Dunn, DMV, MVSc, DACVIM (SAIM)
Assistant Professor
Clinical Sciences
University of Montreal
Small Animal Clinic
Faculty of Veterinary Medicine
University of Montreal
Saint-Hyacinthe, Quebec
Canada
Antiplatelet and Anticoagulant Therapy

†Deceased.

David A. Dzanis, DVM, PhD, DACVN
Owner
Dzanis Consulting & Collaborations
Santa Clarita, California
Nutrition in the Bitch During Pregnancy and Lactation
Appendix III: AAFCO Dog and Cat Food Nutrient Profiles

Nicole P. Ehrhart, VMD, DACVS
Associate Professor
Department of Clinical Sciences
College of Veterinary Medicine and Biomedical Sciences
Colorado State University
Fort Collins, Colorado
Osteosarcoma

Bruce E. Eilts, DVM, MS, DACT
Professor of Theriogenology
Department of Veterinary Clinical Sciences
School of Veterinary Medicine
Louisiana State University
Baton Rouge, Louisiana
Canine Pregnancy Termination

Denise A. Elliott, BVSc (Hons), PhD, DACVIM, DACVN
Director of Scientific Affairs
Royal Canin
St. Charles, Missouri
Gastrostomy Tube Feeding in Kidney Disease

Jonathan Elliott, MA, Vet MB, PhD, Cert SAC, DECVPT, MRCVS
Department of Veterinary Basic Sciences
Royal Veterinary College
University of London
London, England
United Kingdom
Chronic Kidney Disease: Staging and Management

Gary C.W. England, BVetMed, PhD, DVR, DVRep, DECAR, DACT, ILTM, FRCVS
Foundation Dean
School of Veterinary Medicine and Science
University of Nottingham
Nottingham, England
United Kingdom
Breeding Management of the Bitch

Amara Estrada, DVM, DACVIM (Cardiology)
Assistant Professor
Small Animal Clinical Sciences
College of Veterinary Medicine
University of Florida
Gainesville, Florida
Pulmonic Stenosis

Timothy M. Fan, DVM, DACVIM
Assistant Professor, Medical Oncology
Veterinary Clinical Medicine
University of Illinois at Urbana-Champaign
Urbana, Illinois
Osteosarcoma

James P. Farese, DVM, DACVS
Associate Professor, Surgical Oncology
Small Animal Clinical Sciences
College of Veterinary Medicine
University of Florida
Gainesville, Florida
Surgical Oncology Principles

Edward C. Feldman, DVM, DACVIM
Professor
Department of Medicine and Epidemiology
School of Veterinary Medicine
University of California
Davis, California
Canine Hypercalcemia and Primary Hyperparathyroidism

Deborah M. Fine, DVM, MS, DACVIM (Cardiology)
Assistant Professor
Department of Veterinary Medicine and Surgery
University of Missouri
Columbia, Missouri
Arterial Thromboembolism in Cats

Bente Flatland, DVM, MS, DACVIM (Internal Medicine)
Resident, Clinical Pathology
Department of Pathobiology
College of Veterinary Medicine
University of Tennessee
Knoxville, Tennessee
Hepatic Support Therapy

Daniel J. Fletcher, DVM, PhD, DACVECC
Lecturer, Emergency and Critical Care
Cornell University Hospital for Animals
Cornell University
Ithaca, New York
Traumatic Brain Injury

Richard B. Ford, DVM, MS, DACVIM
Professor of Medicine
College of Veterinary Medicine
North Carolina State University
Raleigh, North Carolina
Bacterial Pneumonia
Bordetella bronchiseptica: Beyond Kennel Cough
Canine Vaccination Guidelines
Feline Vaccination Guidelines

Lisa J. Forrest, VMD, DACVR
Associate Professor
Surgical Sciences
University of Wisconsin
Madison, Wisconsin
Nasal Tumors

Theresa W. Fossum, DVM, MS, PhD, DACVS
Tom and Joan Read Chair in Veterinary Surgery
Associate Director Cardiothoracic Surgery and
    Biomedical Devices, Michael E. DeBakey Institute
Professor of Surgery
College of Veterinary Medicine
Texas A&M University
College Station, Texas
Pleural Effusion

**Susan F. Foster, BVSc, MVetClinStud, FACVSc,
    (Feline Medicine)**
Adjunct Senior Lecturer in Small Animal Medicine
Murdoch University
Murdoch, Australia
Nasopharyngeal Disorders

**Philip R. Fox, DVM, MSc, DACVIM (Cardiology),
    DACVECC**
Cardiologist
Bobst Hospital of the Animal Medical Center
Director, Caspary Research Institute
The Animal Medical Center
New York, New York
Right Ventricular Cardiomyopathy in Cats

Boel A. Fransson, DVM, MSc, PhD, DACVS
Assistant Professor, Small Animal Surgery
Department of Veterinary Clinical Sciences
Washington State University
Pullman, Washington
Treatment of Supraspinatus Tendon Disorders in Dogs

Lisa M. Freeman, DVM, PhD, DACVN
Associate Professor
Department of Clinical Sciences
Cummings School of Veterinary Medicine
Tufts University
North Grafton, Massachusetts
Nutritional Management of Heart Disease

Joni L. Freshman, DVM, MS, DACVIM
Owner
Canine Consultations
Colorado Springs, Colorado
Pregnancy Loss in the Bitch

**Angela E. Frimberger, VMD, DACVIM
    (Oncology)**
Director, Veterinary Oncology Consultants
Wauchope, New South Wales
Australia
Anticancer Drugs and Protocols: Traditional Drugs

**Virginia Luis Fuentes, MA VetMB, PhD, CertVR,
    DVC, MRCVS, DACVIM (Cardiology),
    DECVIM (Cardiology)**
Senior Lecturer
Veterinary Clinical Sciences
Royal Veterinary College
Hatfield, Hertfordshire
United Kingdom
Management of Feline Myocardial Disease

Tam Garland, DVM
Program Manager for Agricultural Security
Director for the Joint Agro Defense Office
Science and Technology Directorate
Department of Homeland Security
Washington, District of Columbia
Aflatoxicosis in Dogs

**Laurent S. Garosi, DVM, MRCVS, DECVN,
    RCVS**
European Specialist in Veterinary Neurology
Neurology/Neurosurgery Service Head
Davies Veterinary Specialists
Manor Farm Business Park
Higham Gobion, England
United Kingdom
Treatment of Cerebrovascular Disease

Anthony T. Gary, DVM, DACVIM
Arkansas Veterinary Internal Medicine
North Little Rock, Arkansas
*Evaluation of Elevated Serum Alkaline Phosphatase
    in the Dog*

**Anna R.M. Gelzer, Dr Med Vet, DACVIM
    (Cardiology), DECVIM (Cardiology)**
Assistant Professor of Veterinary Cardiology
College of Veterinary Medicine
Cornell University
Ithaca, New York
Pacing in the Critical Care Setting
Ventricular Arrhythmias in Dogs

**Alexander J. German, BVSc, PhD, DECVIM-CA
    (Internal Medicine)**
Senior Lecturer, Department of Veterinary Clinical
    Sciences
Small Animal Hospital
The University of Liverpool
Liverpool, England
United Kingdom
Inflammatory Bowel Disease

Rudayna Ghubash, DVM, DACVD
Staff Dermatologist
Animal Dermatology Clinic
Marina del Rey, California
Feline Viral Skin Disease

**Urs Giger, PD, Dr Med Vet, MS, FVH, DACVIM,
    DECVIM, DECVCP**
Charlotte Newton Sheppard Professor of Medicine
Chief of Medical Genetics
Department of Clinical Studies
School of Veterinary Medicine
University of Pennsylvania
Philadelphia, Pennsylvania
Blood-Typing and Crossmatching

Sophie Gilbert, DVM, PhD, DACVD
New York City Veterinary Specialists
New York, New York
Feline Pruritus Therapy

Rebecca E. Gompf, DVM, MS, DACVIM (Cardiology)
Associate Professor
Small Animal Clinical Sciences
College of Veterinary Medicine
University of Tennessee
Knoxville, Tennessee
Ventricular Septal Defect

Jody L. Gookin, DVM, PhD, DACVIM (Internal Medicine)
Assistant Professor, Molecular Biomedical Sciences
College of Veterinary Medicine
North Carolina State University
Raleigh, North Carolina
Tritrichicomonas

Sonya G. Gordon, DVM, DVSc, DACVIM (Cardiology)
Assistant Professor
Department of Small Animal Clinical Sciences
College of Veterinary Medicine and Biomedical Sciences
Texas A&M University
College Station, Texas
Canine Heartworm Disease
Patent Ductus Arteriosus

Gregory F. Grauer, DVM, MS, DACVIM (Internal Medicine)
Professor
Department of Clinical Sciences
Kansas State University
Manhattan, Kansas
Proteinuria: Implications for Management

Deborah S. Greco, DVM, PhD, DACVIM
Nestle Purina Petcare
St. Louis, Missouri
Complicated Diabetes Mellitus

Eric M. Green, DVM, DACVR (Radiology, Radiation Oncology)
Associate Professor
Veterinary Clinical Sciences
College of Veterinary Medicine
The Ohio State University
Columbus, Ohio
Radiotherapy: Basic Principles and Indications

Henry W. Green, III, DVM, DACVIM (Cardiology)
Assistant Professor, Cardiology
Veterinary Clinical Sciences
School of Veterinary Medicine
Purdue University
West Lafayette, Indiana
Dilated Cardiomyopathy in Dogs

Clare R. Gregory, DVM, DACVS
Professor
Department of Surgical and Radiological Sciences
Director, Comparative Transplantation Laboratory
School of Veterinary Medicine
University of California
Davis, California
Immunosuppressive Agents

Joel D. Griffies, DVM, DACVD
Animal Dermatology Clinic
Tustin, California
Topical Immunomodulators

Craig E. Griffin, DVM, DACVD
Animal Dermatology Clinic and Animal Allergy Specialists
San Diego, California
Allergen-Specific Immunotherapy
Cyclosporine Use in Dermatology

Carol B. Grindem, DVM, DACVP (Clinical Pathology)
Professor
College of Veterinary Medicine
North Carolina State University
Raleigh, North Carolina
Thrombocytopenia

Amy M. Grooters, DVM, DACVIM (SAIM)
Associate Professor and Chief
Companion Animal Medicine
Veterinary Clinical Sciences
Louisiana State University;
Chief of Staff
Small Animal Clinic
Veterinary Teaching Hospital
Baton Rouge, Louisiana
Pythiosis and Lagenidiosis

Sharon M. Gwaltney-Brant, DVM, PhD, DABVT, DABT
ASPCA Animal Poison Control Center
Urbana, Illinois
Lead Toxicosis in Small Animals
Recently Recognized Animal Toxicants

Susan G. Hackner, BVSc, MRCVS, DACVIM, DACVECC
Department Chair
Critical Care and Emergency Services
The Animal Medical Center
New York, New York
Pulmonary Thromboembolism

Kevin A. Hahn, DVM, PhD, DACVIM (Oncology)
Gulf Coast Veterinary Specialists
Houston, Texas
Pulmonary Neoplasia

Kelly Hall, DVM
Assistant Clinical Professor
Veterinary Clinical Sciences
University of Minnesota
St. Paul, Minnesota
Toxicosis Treatments
Toxin Exposures and Treatments:
  A Survey of Practicing Veterinarians

Holly L. Hamilton, DVM, MS, DACVO
Ophthalmologist
Animal Eye Center
Loveland, Colorado
Differential Diagnosis of Blindness

William R. Hare, DVM, MS, PhD, DABVT,
  DABT
Veterinary Medical Officer
United States Department of Agriculture
Agricultural Research Service
Animal and Natural Resources Institute
Beltsville Agricultural Research Center
Beltsville, Maryland
Urban Legends of Toxicology: Facts and Fiction

Kenneth R. Harkin, DVM, DACVIM (SAIM)
Associate Professor
Veterinary Clinical Sciences
College of Veterinary Medicine
Kansas State University
Manhattan, Kansas
Leptospirosis

Neil K. Harpster, VMD, DACVIM (Cardiology)
Department of Cardiology
Angell Memorial Animal Hospital
Boston, Massachusetts
Feline Cardiac Arrhythmias

Katrin Hartmann, Dr Med Vet, Dr Habil,
  DECVIM-CA
Professor of Internal Medicine
Head of Small Animal Internal Medicine Clinic
University of Munich
Munich, Germany
Feline Leukemia Virus and Feline Immunodeficiency
  Virus

Elizabeth A. Hausner, DVM, DABT, DABVT
Division of Cardio-Renal Drug Products
Center for Drug Evaluation and Research
U.S. Food and Drug Administration
Beltsville, Maryland
Herbal Hazards

Eleanor C. Hawkins, DVM, DACVIM
Professor, Internal Medicine
Department of Clinical Sciences
College of Veterinary Medicine
North Carolina State University
Raleigh, North Carolina
Pleural Effusion

Mattie J. Hendrick, VMD, DACVP
Staff Pathologist and Adjunct Full Professor
  of Pathology
School of Veterinary Medicine
University of Pennsylvania
Philadelphia, Pennsylvania
Feline Vaccine-Associated Sarcomas

Diane V.H. Hendrix, DVM, DACVO
Associate Professor, Ophthalmology
Department of Small Animal Clinical Sciences
College of Veterinary Medicine
University of Tennessee
Knoxville, Tennessee
Differential Diagnosis of the Red Eye

Rosemary A. Henik, DVM, MS, DACVIM
  (Internal Medicine)
Clinical Associate Professor
Department of Medical Sciences
School of Veterinary Medicine
University of Wisconsin
Madison, Wisconsin
Pulmonary Hypertension
Systemic Hypertension

Carolyn J. Henry, DVM, MS, DACVIM
  (Oncology)
Associate Professor of Oncology
Department of Veterinary Medicine and Surgery
College of Veterinary Medicine
Department of Internal Medicine
Division of Hematology/Oncology
School of Medicine
University of Missouri
Columbia, Missouri
Mammary Cancer

Michael E. Herrtage, MA, BVSc, DVSc, DVR,
  DVD, DSAM, MRCVS, DECVIM, DECVDI
Reader in Small Animal Medicine
Department of Veterinary Medicine
University of Cambridge
Cambridge, England
United Kingdom
Medical Management of Tracheal Collapse

A. Elizabeth Hershey, DVM, DACVIM (Oncology)
Integrative Veterinary Oncology
Phoenix, Arizona
Feline Vaccine-Associated Sarcomas

Daniel G. Hicks, DVM
Resident, Neurology and Neurosurgery
Department of Veterinary Clinical Sciences
Washington State University
Pullman, Washington
Treatment of Degenerative Lumbosacral Stenosis

Mark E. Hitt, DVM, MS, DACVIM (Internal Medicine)
Chief of Medicine
Atlantic Veterinary Internal Medicine, LLC
Annapolis, Maryland
Drug-Associated Liver Disease

Gaby Hoffmann, DVM, Dr Med Vet, DACVIM
Junior Lecturer, Clinical Genetics
Clinical Sciences of Companion Animals
Faculty of Veterinary Medicine
Utrecht University
Utrecht, The Netherlands
Copper-Associated Chronic Hepatitis

Daniel F. Hogan, DVM, DACVIM (Cardiology)
Associate Professor
Chief of Comparative Cardiovascular Medicine
Purdue University
West Lafayette, Indiana
Dilated Cardiomyopathy in Dogs

Kathleen M. Holan, DVM, DACVIM (Internal Medicine)
Assistant Professor
Department of Small Animal Clinical Sciences
College of Veterinary Medicine
Michigan State University
East Lansing, Michigan
Feline Hepatic Lipidosis

Steven R. Hollingsworth, DVM, DACVO
Assistant Professor of Clinical Ophthalmology
Department of Surgical and Radiological Sciences
School of Veterinary Medicine
University of California
Davis, California
Diseases of the Eyelids and Periocular Skin
Ocular Immunotherapy

Bradford J. Holmberg, DVM, MS, PhD, DACVO
Staff Ophthalmologist
Veterinary Referral Centre
Little Falls, New Jersey
Ocular Neoplasia

David E. Holt, BVSc, DACVS
Professor of Surgery
School of Veterinary Medicine
University of Pennsylvania
Philadelphia, Pennsylvania
Drainage Techniques for the Septic Abdomen

Heidi A. Hottinger, DVM, DACVS
Department of Surgery
Gulf Coast Veterinary Specialists
Gulf Coast Veterinary Surgery
Houston, Texas
Canine Biliary Mucocele

Lynn R. Hovda, RPh, DVM, MS, DACVIM
Director, Veterinary Services
Safety Call International
Bloomington, Minnesota
Toxin Exposures in Small Animals

Lisa M. Howe, DVM, PhD, DACVS
Associate Professor
Department of Small Animal Medicine and Surgery
College of Veterinary Medicine
Texas A&M University
College Station, Texas
Early-Age Neutering in the Dog and Cat

Geraldine B. Hunt, BVSc, MvetClinStud, PhD, FACVSc
Associate Professor
University Veterinary Centre
University of Sydney
Sydney, New South Wales
Australia
Nasopharyngeal Disorders

Takuo Ishida, DVM
Medical Director
Akasaka Animal Hospital
Tokyo, Japan
Feline Infectious Peritonitis: Therapy and Prevention

Toshiroh Iwasaki, DVM, PhD, DACVIM
Professor
Department of Veterinary Internal Medicine
Tokyo University of Agriculture & Technology
Tokyo, Japan
Interferons

Hilary A. Jackson, DVD, DACVD
Dermatology Referral Services
Glasgow, Scotland
United Kingdom
Hypoallergenic Diets: Principles in Therapy

Beth M. Johnson, DVM
Resident, Internal Medicine
Department of Small Animal Clinical Sciences
College of Veterinary Medicine
University of Tennessee
Knoxville, Tennessee
Canine Megaesophagus

Lynelle R. Johnson, DVM, PhD, DACVIM (SAIM)
Assistant Professor
Department of Medicine and Epidemiology
School of Veterinary Medicine
University of California
Davis, California
Chronic Bronchitis in Dogs
Rhinitis in the Cat

Boyd R. Jones, BVSc, FACVSc, DECVIM, MRCVS
Faculty of Veterinary Medicine
University College Dublin
Belfield, Dublin
Ireland
Hypokalemic Myopathy in Cats

Bruce W. Keene, DVM, MSc, DACVIM (Cardiology)
Professor
Department of Clinical Sciences
College of Veterinary Medicine
North Carolina State University
Raleigh, North Carolina
Management of Heart Failure in Dogs

Robert J. Kemppainen, DVM
Professor
Department of Anatomy, Physiology, and Pharmacology
College of Veterinary Medicine
Auburn University
Auburn, Alabama
Interpretation of Endocrine Diagnostic Test Results for Adrenal and Thyroid Disease

Michael S. Kent, MAS, DVM
Assistant Professor
Surgical and Radiological Sciences
College of Veterinary Medicine
University of California
Davis, California
Ocular Neoplasia

Marie E. Kerl, DVM, DACVIM (SAIM), DACVECC
Clinical Associate Professor
Department of Veterinary Medicine and Surgery
University of Missouri
Small Animal Medicine Section Head
Veterinary Medical Teaching Hospital
Columbia, Missouri
Treatment of Anemia in Renal Failure

Safdar A. Khan, DVM, MS, PhD, DABVT
Director of Toxicology Research
ASPCA Animal Poison Control Center
Urbana, Illinois
Recently Recognized Animal Toxicants

Chand Khanna, DVM, PhD
Director, Comparative Oncology Program
Center for Cancer Research
National Cancer Institute
National Institutes of Health
Bethesda, Maryland
Clinical Trials in Veterinary Oncology

Peter P. Kintzer, DVM, DACVIM
Staff Internist
Department of Medicine
Boston Road Animal Hospital
Springfield, Massachusetts
Hypoadrenocorticism

Rebecca Kirby, DVM, DACVIM (Internal Medicine), DACVECC
Animal Emergency Center
Glendale, Wisconsin
Colloid Fluid Therapy
Disseminated Intravascular Coagulation: Diagnosis and Management

Claudia A. Kirk, DVM, PhD, DACVN, DACVIM
Associate Professor of Medicine and Nutrition
Department of Small Animal Clinical Sciences
College of Veterinary Medicine
The University of Tennessee
Knoxville, Tennessee
Interpreting and Managing Crystalluria
Obesity

Deborah W. Knapp, DVM, MS, DACVIM (Oncology)
Dolores L. McCall Professor of Veterinary Medicine (Comparative Oncology)
Department of Veterinary Clinical Sciences
Purdue University
West Lafayette, Indiana
Urinary Bladder Cancer

Stephanie J. Kottler, DVM
Resident, Small Animal Internal Medicine
Department of Veterinary Medicine and Surgery
College of Veterinary Medicine
University of Missouri
Columbia, Missouri
Canine Anaplasma Infection

Marc S. Kraus, DVM, DACVIM (Cardiology, Internal Medicine)
Faculty
Department of Clinical Sciences
College of Veterinary Medicine
Cornell University
Ithaca, New York
Pacing in the Critical Care Setting
Syncope
Ventricular Arrhythmias in Dogs

John M. Kruger, DVM, PhD, DACVIM
Associate Professor
Department of Small Animal Clinical Sciences
College of Veterinary Medicine
Michigan State University
East Lansing, Michigan
Management of Feline Nonobstructive Idiopathic Cystitis

Ned F. Kuehn, DVM, MS, DACVIM (SAIM)
Chief of Internal Medicine
Michigan Veterinary Specialists
Southfield, Michigan
Rhinitis in the Dog

Michelle Anne Kutzler, DVM, PhD, DACT
Assistant Professor
Department of Clinical Sciences
College of Veterinary Medicine
Oregon State University
Corvallis, Oregon
Canine Postpartum Disorders

Andrew E. Kyles, BVMS, PhD, DACVS
Professor, Small Animal Surgery
Department of Surgical and Radiological Sciences,
School of Veterinary Medicine,
University of California
Davis, California
Management of Feline Ureteroliths

Mary Anna Labato, DVM, DACVIM
Clinical Associate Professor
Section Head, Small Animal Medicine
Department of Clinical Sciences
Foster Hospital for Small Animals
Cummings School of Veterinary Medicine
Tufts University
North Grafton, Massachusetts
Uncomplicated Urinary Tract Infection

Susan E. Lana, DVM, MS, DACVIM (Oncology)
Associate Professor
Oncology Section Head
Animal Cancer Center
Department of Clinical Sciences
Colorado State University
Fort Collins, Colorado
Canine Lymphoma

Gabriele A. Landolt, Dr Med Vet, MS, PhD
Assistant Professor
Department of Clinical Sciences
College of Veterinary Medicine and Biomedical
   Sciences
Colorado State University
Fort Collins, Colorado
Canine Influenza

India F. Lane, DVM, MS, DACVIM
Associate Professor and Director of Educational
   Enhancement
Department of Small Animal Clinical Sciences
College of Veterinary Medicine
The University of Tennessee
Knoxville, Tennessee
*Urinary Incontinence and Micturition Disorders:
   Pharmacologic Management*

**Catherine E. Langston, DVM, DACVIM
   (SAIM)**
Section Head, Nephrology, Endocrinology, Urology,
   and Hemodialysis
Animal Medical Center
New York, New York
Hemodialysis
Treatment of Anemia in Renal Failure

**Michael R. Lappin, DVM, PhD, DACVIM
   (Internal Medicine)**
Assistant Department Head for Research
The Kenneth Smith Professor in Small Animal Clinical
   Veterinary Medicine
Department of Clinical Sciences
College of Veterinary Medicine and Biomedical Sciences
Colorado State University
Fort Collins, Colorado
Toxoplasmosis

Alfred M. Legendre, DVM, MS, DACVIM
Assistant Department Chair
Department of Small Animal Clinical Sciences
College of Veterinary Medicine
The University of Tennessee
Knoxville, Tennessee
Systemic Fungal Infections

Michael S. Leib, DVM, MS, DACVIM (SAIM)
C.R. Roberts Professor of Small Animal Medicine
Department of Small Animal Clinical Sciences
College of Veterinary Medicine
Virginia Polytechnic Institute and State University
Blacksburg, Virginia
Gastric Helicobacter *spp. and Chronic Vomiting in Dogs*

Christine C. Lim, DVM
Resident, Comparative Ophthalmology
Veterinary Medical Teaching Hospital
University of California
Davis, California
Qualitative Tear Film Disturbances of Dogs and Cats

**Julius M. Liptak, BVSc, MvetClinStud, FACVSc,
   DECVS, DACVS**
Assistant Professor in Small Animal Surgery
Department of Clinical Studies
Ontario Veterinary College
University of Guelph
Guelph, Ontario
Canada
Canine Soft-Tissue Sarcomas

**Remo Lobetti, BVSc (Hons), MMedVet (Med),
   PhD, DECVIM (Internal Medicine)**
Bryanston Veterinary Hospital
Bryanston, South Africa
Pneumocystosis

Dawn Logas, DVM, DACVD
Staff Dermatologist
Veterinary Dermatology Center
Maitland, Florida
Ear-Flushing Techniques

**Cheryl A. London, DVM, PhD, DACVIM
   (Oncology)**
Associate Professor
College of Veterinary Medicine
The Ohio State University
Columbus, Ohio
Mast Cell Tumor

Andrea L. Looney, DVM, DACVA
Senior Lecturer, Department of Clinical Sciences
Section of Anesthesiology and Pain Management
Cornell University
Ithaca, New York
Acute Pain Management

Jody P. Lulich, DVM, PhD, DACVIM (SAIM)
Professor, Small Animal Medicine
Department of Small Animal Clinical Sciences
University of Minnesota
St. Paul, Minnesota
Laser Lithotripsy for Uroliths
*Incomplete Urolith Removal: Prevention, Detection, and
    Correction*

**Katharine F. Lunn, BVMS, MS, PhD, MRCVS,
    DACVIM (Internal Medicine), MRCVS**
Assistant Professor
Department of Clinical Sciences
College of Veterinary Medicine and Biomedical Sciences
Colorado State University
Fort Collins, Colorado
Canine Influenza
Managing the Patient With Polyuria and Polydipsia

Angela L. Lusby, DVM
Resident in Clinical Nutrition and Graduate Research
    Assistant
Department of Small Animal Clinical Sciences
College of Veterinary Medicine
The University of Tennessee
Knoxville, Tennessee
Obesity

John M. MacDonald, DVM, DACVD
Associate Professor
Department of Small Animal Surgery and Medicine
College of Veterinary Medicine
Auburn University
Auburn, Alabama
Acral Lick Dermatitis
Allergen-Specific Immunotherapy

**Kristin A. MacDonald, DVM, PhD, DACVIM
    (Cardiology)**
Staff Veterinary Cardiologist
Medicine and Epidemiology
University of California
Davis, California
Infective Endocarditis

Catriona M. MacPhail, DVM, PhD, DACVS
Assistant Professor, Small Animal Surgery
Department of Clinical Sciences
College of Veterinary Medicine and Biomedical Sciences
Colorado State University
Fort Collins, Colorado
Laryngeal Diseases

David J. Maggs, BVSc, DACVO
Associate Professor
Department of Surgical and Radiological Sciences
School of Veterinary Medicine
University of California
Davis, California
Antiviral Therapy for Feline Herpesvirus
Corneal Colors as a Diagnostic Aid
Pearls of the Ophthalmic Examination

Giovanni Majolino, DVM
Majolino and Ranieri Veterinary Clinic
Collecchio, Italy
*Aspermia/Oligozoospermia Caused by Retrograde Ejaculation
    in the Dog*

Annie Malouin, DVM, DACVECC
Metropolitan Veterinary Associates
Norristown, Pennsylvania
Shock

**F. Anthony Mann, DVM, MS, DACVS,
    DACVECC**
Professor
Department of Veterinary Medicine and Surgery
College of Veterinary Medicine
Director of Small Animal Emergency and Critical Care
    Services
Small Animal Soft Tissue Surgery Service Chief
Veterinary Medical Teaching Hospital
University of Missouri
Columbia, Missouri
Acute Abdomen: Evaluation and Emergency Treatment

Denis J. Marcellin-Little, DEDV, DACVS, DECVS
Associate Professor, Orthopedic Surgery
College of Veterinary Medicine
North Carolina State University
Raleigh, North Carolina
Medical Treatment of Coxofemoral Joint Disease

Rosanna Marsella, DVM, DACVD
Associate Professor in Veterinary Dermatology
Department of Small Animal Clinical Sciences
College of Veterinary Medicine
University of Florida
Gainesville, Florida
Pentoxifylline

Julie Martin, DVM, MS, DACVIM (Cardiology)
Cardiologist
Veterinary Heart and Lung Specialists
Englewood, Colorado
Cardioversion

Jocelyn A. Mason, DVM
Consulting Veterinarian in Clinical Toxicology
ASPCA Animal Poison Control Center
Québec, Canada
Recently Recognized Animal Toxicants

Karol A. Mathews, DVM, DVSc, DACVECC
Professor
Department of Clinical Studies
Ontario Veterinary College
University of Guelph
Guelph, Ontario
Canada
Gastric Dilation-Volvulus

Robert J. McCarthy, DVM, MS, DACVS
Staff Veterinarian
Department of Clinical Sciences
Foster Hospital for Small Animals
Cummings School of Veterinary Medicine
Tufts University
North Grafton, Massachusetts
Emergency Management of Open Fractures

Susan A. McLaughlin, DVM, MS, DACVO
Clinical Associate Professor
Veterinary Administration
School of Veterinary Medicine
Purdue University
West Lafayette, Indiana
Differential Diagnosis of Blindness

Mary A. McLoughlin, DVM, MS, DACVS
Associate Professor, Small Animal Surgery
Department of Veterinary Clinical Sciences
College of Veterinary Medicine
The Ohio State University
Columbus, Ohio
*Urinary Incontinence: Treatment With Injectable Bulking
    Agents*

Erick A. Mears, DVM, DACVIM
Medical Director
Florida Veterinary Specialists and Cancer Treatment Center
Tampa, Florida
Canine Megaesophagus

Colleen Mendelsohn, DVM, DACVD
Animal Dermatology Clinic
Tustin, California
Topical Therapy of Otitis Externa

**Kathryn M. Meurs, DVM, PhD, DACVIM
    (Cardiology)**
Professor
Department of Veterinary Clinical Sciences
Washington State University
Pullman, Washington
Cardiomyopathy in Boxer Dogs
Cardiomyopathy in Doberman Pinschers

Vicki N. Meyers-Wallen, VMD, PhD, DACT
Associate Professor
Baker Institute for Animal Health
College of Veterinary Medicine
Cornell University
Ithaca, New York
*Inherited Disorders of the Reproductive Tract in Dogs
    and Cats*

Ellen Miller, DVM, MS, DACVIM
Peak Veterinary Internists PC
Longmont, Colorado
Immune-Mediated Hemolytic Anemia

**Matthew W. Miller, DVM, MS, DACVIM
    (Cardiology)**
Professor
Department of Small Animal Clinical Sciences
College of Veterinary Medicine and Biomedical Sciences
Texas A&M University
College Station, Texas
Canine Heartworm Disease
Patent Ductus Arteriosus

Paul E. Miller, DVM, DACVO
Clinical Professor of Comparative Ophthalmology
Department of Surgical Sciences
School of Veterinary Medicine
University of Wisconsin
Madison, Wisconsin
Feline Glaucoma

Darryl L. Millis, DVM, MS, DACVS
Professor of Orthopedic Surgery
Small Animal Clinical Sciences
College of Veterinary Medicine
University of Tennessee
Knoxville, Tennessee
Physical Therapy and Rehabilitation of Neurologic Patients

**N. Sydney Moïse, DVM, MS, DACVIM
    (Cardiology, Internal Medicine)**
Professor
Department of Clinical Sciences
Chief of Cardiology Section
College of Veterinary Medicine
Cornell University
Ithaca, New York
Ventricular Arrhythmias in Dogs

Cliff Monahan, DVM, PhD
Parasitologist
Department of Veterinary Preventive Medicine
College of Veterinary Medicine
The Ohio State University
Columbus, Ohio
Appendix II: Treatment of Parasites

Eric Monnet, DVM, PhD, DACVS, DECVS
Associate Professor, Small Animal Surgery
Department of Clinical Sciences
College of Veterinary Medicine and Biomedical Sciences
Colorado State University
Fort Collins, Colorado
Laryngeal Diseases

William E. Monroe, DVM, MS, DACVIM (SAIM)
Professor, Small Animal Internal Medicine
Department of Small Animal Clinical Sciences
Virginia-Maryland Regional College of Veterinary Medicine
Virginia Polytechnic Institute and State University
Blacksburg, Virginia
Canine Diabetes Mellitus

Antony S. Moore, BVSc, MVSc, DACVIM (Oncology)
Veterinary Oncology Consultants
Wauchope, New South Wales
Australia
Anticancer Drugs and Protocols: Traditional Drugs

Lisa E. Moore, DVM, DACVIM (SAIM)
Staff Internist
Affiliated Veterinary Specialists
Maitland, Florida
Protein-Losing Enteropathy

Peter F. Moore, BVSc, PhD
Professor
Department of Pathology, Microbiology, and Immunology
College of Veterinary Medicine
University of California
Davis, California
Histiocytic Disease Complex

Adam Mordecai, DVM, DACVIM
Veterinary Medical Referral Service
Veterinary Specialty Center
Buffalo Grove, Illinois
Rational Use of Glucocorticoids in Infectious Disease

Karen A. Moriello, DVM, DACVD
Professor
Clinical Professor of Dermatology
Department of Medical Sciences
School of Veterinary Medicine
University of Wisconsin
Madison, Wisconsin
Treatment of Dermatophytosis

Daniel O. Morris, DVM, DACVD
Associate Professor of Dermatology
College of Veterinary Medicine
University of Pennsylvania
Philadelphia, Pennsylvania
Feline Demodicosis
Therapy of Malassezia *Infections and* Malassezia *Hypersensitivity*

Michael J. Murphy, DVM, PhD, DACT
Professor in Veterinary Population Medicine
Veterinary Diagnostic Labs
University of Minnesota
St. Paul, Minnesota
Food Toxicoses in Small Animals
Nephrotoxicants
Rodenticide Toxicoses
Small Animal Poisoning: Additional Considerations Related to Legal Claims
Sources of Help for Toxicosis

Rusty Muse, DVM, DACVD
Animal Dermatology Clinic
Tustin, California
Diseases of the Anal Sac

Masahiko Nagata, DVM, PhD, DAICVD (Asian College of Veterinary Dermatology)
Animal Dermatology Center
Tokyo, Japan
Canine Papillomaviruses

Larry A. Nagode, DVM, PhD
Department of Veterinary Biosciences
Goss Laboratory
The Ohio State University
Columbus, Ohio
Treatment of Hypoparathyroidism

Jill Narak, DVM
Neurology/Neurosurgery Resident
Department of Clinical Sciences
College of Veterinary Medicine
Auburn University
Auburn, Alabama
Treatment of Intracranial Tumors

Jennifer A. Neel, DVM, DACVP (Clinical Pathology)
Assistant Professor
College of Veterinary Medicine
North Carolina State University
Raleigh, North Carolina
Thrombocytopenia

Reto Neiger, Dr Med Vet, PhD, DACVIM, DECVIM (CA)
Professor in Small Animal Medicine
Veterinärmedizinische Fakultät,
Klinik für Kleintiere (Innere Medizin & Chirurgie)
Giessen, Germany
Canine Hyperadrenocorticism
Gastric Ulceration

O. Lynne Nelson, DVM, MS, DACVIM (Internal Medicine, Cardiology)
Associate Professor
Veterinary Clinical Sciences
College of Veterinary Medicine
Washington State University
Pullman, Washington
Pericardial Effusion

Richard W. Nelson, DVM, DACVIM
Professor, Internal Medicine
Department of Medicine and Epidemiology
School of Veterinary Medicine
University of California
Davis, California
Canine Hypercalcemia and Primary Hyperparathyroidism

Belle M. Nibblett, DVM
Resident, Small Animal Medicine
Department of Small Animal Clinical Sciences
Western College of Veterinary Medicine
University of Saskatchewan
Saskatoon, Saskatchewan
Canada
von Willebrand's Disease and Other Hereditary
Coagulopathies

Roberto E. Novo, DVM, DACVS
University of Minnesota
College of Veterinary Medicine
St. Paul, Minnesota
Surgical Repair of Vaginal Anomalies in the Bitch

Frederick W. Oehme, DVM, MS, PhD, DABVT,
DABT, DATS
Professor of Toxicology, Pathobiology, Medicine, and
    Physiology
Department of Diagnostic Medicine/Pathobiology
Comparative Toxicology Laboratories
Kansas State University
Manhattan, Kansas
Urban Legends of Toxicology: Facts and Fiction

Carl A. Osborne, DVM, PhD, DACVIM
Veterinary Clinical Sciences Department
College of Veterinary Medicine
University of Minnesota
St. Paul, Minnesota
Calcitriol
Evidence-Based Management of Chronic Kidney Disease
Incomplete Urolith Removal: Prevention, Detection, and
    Correction
Management of Feline Nonobstructive Idiopathic Cystitis

Elizabeth O'Toole, BSc, DVM, DVSc, DACVECC
Advanced Care Unit
Mississauga/Oakville Veterinary Emergency Hospital and
    Referral Group
Oakville, Ontario
Canada
Ventilator Therapy

Catherine A. Outerbridge, DVM, MVSC, DACVIM
Dermatology Service
Veterinary Medical Teaching Hospital
University of California
Davis, California
Diseases of the Eyelids and Periocular Skin
Nonneoplastic Nodular Histiocytic Diseases of the Skin

Mark A. Oyama, DVM, DACVIM
Department of Clinical Studies
School of Veterinary Medicine
University of Pennsylvania
Philadelphia, Pennsylvania
Permanent Cardiac Pacing in Dogs

Philip Padrid, RN, DVM, DACVIM
Adjunct Associate Professor
Small Animal Medicine
College of Veterinary Medicine
The Ohio State University
Columbus, Ohio;
Committee on Molecular Medicine
Pritzker School of Medicine
The University of Chicago
Chicago, Illinois
Chronic Bronchitis and Asthma in Cats

David L. Panciera, DVM, MS, DACVIM (SAIM)
Professor
Department of Small Animal Clinical Sciences
Virginia-Maryland Regional College of Veterinary
    Medicine
Virginia Polytechnic Institute and State University
Blacksburg, Virginia
von Willebrand's Disease and Other Hereditary Coagulopathies

Melissa Paoloni, DVM, DACVIM (Oncology)
Comparative Oncology Program
National Cancer Institute
National Institutes of Health
Bethesda, Maryland
Clinical Trials in Veterinary Oncology

Mark G. Papich, DVM, MS, DACVCP
Professor of Clinical Pharmacology
College of Veterinary Medicine
North Carolina State University
Raleigh, North Carolina
Appendix I: Table of Common Drugs: Approximate Dosages

Nolie K. Parnell, DVM, DACVIM
Clinical Assistant Professor
Small Animal Internal Medicine
Veterinary Clinical Sciences
Purdue University
West Lafayette, Indiana
Chronic Colitis

Edward E. (Ned) Patterson, DVM, PhD, DACVIM
Assistant Professor, Medicine, Genetics, and Epilepsy
Department of Veterinary Clinical Sciences
College of Veterinary Medicine
University of Minnesota
St. Paul, Minnesota
Methods and Availability of Tests for Hereditary Disorders
    of Dogs

Mark E. Peterson, DVM, DACVIM
Head of Endocrinology
Department of Medicine, Bobst Hospital
Associate Director, Caspary Research Institute
Chairman, Institute of Postgraduate Education
The Animal Medical Center
New York, New York
Hypoadrenocorticism
Radioiodine for Feline Hyperthyroidism

Simon R. Platt, BVM&S, MRCVS, DECVN, DACVIM (Neurology)
RCVS and European Specialist in Veterinary Neurology
Neurology/Neurosurgery Service Head
Animal Health Trust
Centre for Small Animal Studies
Suffolk, England
United Kingdom
Treatment of Cerebrovascular Disease

Michael Podell, MSc, DVM, DACVIM (Neurology)
Neurology and Neurosurgery Service
Animal Emergency and Referral Center
Northbrook, Illinois
Adjunct Professor
Department of Clinical Sciences
College of Veterinary Medicine
University of Illinois at Urbana-Champaign
Urbana, Illinois
Treatment of Status Epilepticus

David J. Polzin, DVM, PhD, DACVIM (Internal Medicine)
Professor
Department of Veterinary Clinical Sciences
College of Veterinary Medicine
University of Minnesota
St. Paul, Minnesota
Calcitriol
Evidence-Based Management of Chronic Kidney Disease

Eric R. Pope, DVM, MS, DACVS
Professor, Small Animal Surgery
Ross University School of Veterinary Medicine
Basseterre, St. Kitts
West Indies
Brachycephalic Upper Airway Syndrome in Dogs

Robert H. Poppenga, DVM, PhD, DABT
CAHFS Toxicology Laboratory
School of Veterinary Medicine
University of California
Davis, California
Herbal Hazards

Lynn O. Post, DVM, PhD, DABVT
Director, Division of Surveillance
Office of Surveillance and Compliance
Rockville, Maryland
Reporting an Adverse Drug Reaction to the Food and Drug Administration

Cynthia C. Powell, DVM, MS, DACVO
Associate Professor, Veterinary Ophthalmology
Department of Clinical Sciences
College of Veterinary Medicine and Biomedical Sciences
Colorado State University
Fort Collins, Colorado
Anterior Uveitis in Dogs and Cats

Barrak M. Pressler, DVM, DACVIM (SAIM)
Assistant Professor of Internal Medicine
Department of Veterinary Clinical Sciences
Purdue University
West Lafayette, Indiana
Cancer and the Kidney

Jennifer E. Prittie, DVM, DACVIM (Internal Medicine), DACVECC
Criticalist
Department of Emergency Medicine and Critical Care
The Animal Medical Center
New York, New York
Adrenal Insufficiency in Critical Illness

Beverly J. Purswell, DVM, PhD, DACT
Professor of Theriogenology
Virginia-Maryland Regional College of Veterinary Medicine
Virginia Polytechnic Institute and State University
Blacksburg, Virginia
Use of Vaginal Cytology and Vaginal Cultures for Breeding Management and Diagnosis of Reproductive Tract Disease

R. Lee Pyle, VMD, MS, DACVIM (Cardiology)
Professor Emeritus
Department of Small Animal Clinical Sciences
Virginia-Maryland College of Veterinary Medicine
Virginia Polytechnic Institute and State University
Blacksburg, Virginia
Subaortic Stenosis

Ian Ramsey, BVSc, PhD, DSAM Dip, ECVIM-CA, MRCVS
Senior Lecturer in Small Animal Medicine
Faculty of Veterinary Medicine
University of Glasgow
Glasgow, Scotland
United Kingdom
Canine Hyperadrenocorticism

Jacquie S. Rand, BVSc(Hons), DVSc, DACVIM (SAIM)
Professor of Companion Animal Health
Director, Centre for Companion Animal Health
School of Veterinary Science
Faculty of Natural Resources, Agriculture, and Veterinary Science
The University of Queensland
Brisbane, Queensland
Australia
Feline Diabetes Mellitus

Claudia E. Reusch, DVM, DECVIM-CA
Professor
Clinic of Small Animal Internal Medicine
Vetsuisse Faculty
University of Zurich
Zurich, Switzerland
Diabetic Monitoring

Keith P. Richter, DVM, DACVIM (SAIM)
Hospital Director and Internal Medicine Staff
Department of Internal Medicine
Veterinary Specialty Hospital of San Diego
San Diego, California
Feline Gastrointestinal Lymphoma

**Kenita S. Rogers, DVM, MS, DACVIM (Internal
    Medicine, Oncology)**
Professor and Associate Department Head
Small Animal Clinical Sciences
College of Veterinary and Biomedical Sciences
Texas A&M University
College Station, Texas
Collection of Specimens for Cytology

**Stefano Romagnoli, DVM, MS, PhD, DECAR
    (European College of Animal Reproduction)**
Professor, Clinical Veterinary Reproduction
University of Padova
Legnaro, Italy
*Aspermia/Oligozoospermia Caused by Retrograde Ejaculation
    in the Dog*

Margaret V. Root Kustritz, DVM, PhD, DACT
Assistant Clinical Specialist, Small Animal Reproduction
College of Veterinary Medicine
University of Minnesota
St. Paul, Minnesota
*Intermittent Erection of the Penis in
    Castrated Male Dogs*
Ovarian Remnant Syndrome in Cats
*Toxicology of Veterinary and Human Estrogen and
    Progesterone Formulations in Dogs*
Vaginitis

Wayne S. Rosenkrantz, DVM, DACVD
Partner
Animal Dermatology Clinics
Tustin, Marina del Rey, and San Diego, California
House Dust Mites and Their Control
Pyotraumatic Dermatitis ("Hot Spots")
Shampoo Therapy

Linda Ross, DVM, MS, DACVIM (SAIM)
Associate Professor
Department of Clinical Sciences
Cummings School of Veterinary Medicine
Tufts University
North Grafton, Massachusetts
Acute Renal Failure

**Sheri Ross, BSc, DVM, PhD, DACVIM (Internal
    Medicine)**
Hemodialysis/Nephrology Service
University of California Medical Center
San Diego, California
Calcitriol
Evidence-Based Management of Chronic Kidney Disease

Edmund J. Rosser, Jr., DVM, DACVD
Professor and Head of Dermatology
Department of Small Animal Clinical Sciences
College of Veterinary Medicine
Michigan State University
East Lansing, Michigan
Sebaceous Adenitis

Jan Rothuizen, DVM, PhD, DECVIM-CA
Professor of Internal Medicine
Chair, Department of Clinical Sciences of Companion
    Animals
Faculty of Veterinary Medicine
University of Utrecht
Utrecht, The Netherlands
Copper-Associated Chronic Hepatitis

Philip Roudebush, DVM, DACVIM (SAIM)
Director, Scientific Affairs
Hill's Pet Nutrition, Inc.
Topeka, Kansas
Flatulence

Elke Rudloff, DVM, DACVECC
Director of Education
Animal Emergency Center
Glendale, Wisconsin
Colloid Fluid Therapy
*Disseminated Intravascular Coagulation: Diagnosis and
    Management*

**Wilson K. Rumbeiha, DVM, PhD, DABVT,
    DABT**
Associate Professor, Pathobiology and Diagnostic
    Investigation
Section Chief, Toxicology
Diagnostic Center for Population and Animal Health
College of Veterinary Medicine
Michigan State University
Lansing, Michigan
Nephrotoxicants
Parasiticide Toxicoses: Avermectins

Clare Rusbridge, BVMS, PhD, MRCVS, DECVN
Stone Lion Veterinary Centre
Wimbledon Village
London, England
United Kingdom
*Treatment of Canine Chiari-Like Malformation and
    Syringomyelia*

**John E. Rush, DVM, MS, DACVIM (Cardiology),
    DACVECC**
Professor and Associate Department Chair
Department of Clinical Sciences
Cummings School of Veterinary Medicine
Tufts University
North Grafton, Massachusetts
Chronic Valvular Disease in Dogs

Marco Russo, DVM, PhD
Lecturer
Veterinary Clinical Sciences
Veterinary School of Naples "Federico II"
University of Naples
Naples, Italy
Breeding Management of the Bitch

Sherry Lynn Sanderson, DVM, PhD, DACVIM, DACVN
Associate Professor
Department of Physiology and Pharmacology
College of Veterinary Medicine
University of Georgia
Athens, Georgia
Measuring Glomerular Filtration Rate: Practical Use of Clearance Tests

H. Mark Saunders, VMD, MS, DACVR
Partner
Lynks Group PLC—Veterinary Imaging
Shelburne, Vermont
Noncardiogenic Pulmonary Edema

Patricia A. Schenck, DVM, PhD
Endocrine Diagnostic Section Chief
Assistant Professor
Department of Pathobiology and Diagnostic Investigation
Diagnostic Center for Population and Animal Health
Michigan State University
Lansing, Michigan
Idiopathic Feline Hypercalcemia
Treatment of Hypoparathyroidism

Karsten E. Schober, DVM, PhD, DECVIM (Cardiology)
Assistant Professor
Department of Veterinary Clinical Sciences
College of Veterinary Medicine
The Ohio State University
Columbus, Ohio
Myocarditis

Gretchen L. Schoeffler, DVM, DACVECC
Chief, Section of Veterinary Emergency and Critical Care
Cornell University Hospital for Animals
Cornell University
Ithaca, New York
Cardiopulmonary Cerebral Resuscitation

J. Catharine R. Scott-Moncrieff, MA, Vet MB, MS, MRCVS, DACVIM (SAIM), DECVIM (Companion Animal)
Professor
Department of Veterinary Clinical Sciences
School of Veterinary Medicine
Purdue University
West Lafayette, Indiana
Atypical and Subclinical Hyperadrenocorticism
Hypothyroidism

Howard B. Seim, III, DVM, DACVS
Professor
Department of Clinical Sciences
College of Veterinary Medicine and Biomedical Sciences
Colorado State University
Fort Collins, Colorado
Esophageal Feeding Tubes

Rance K. Sellon, DVM, PhD, DACVIM
Associate Professor
Department of Small Animal Medicine
College of Veterinary Medicine
Washington State University
Pullman, Washington
Rational Use of Glucocorticoids in Infectious Disease
Systemic Fungal Infections

Scott P. Shaw, DVM, DACVECC
Assistant Professor
Section of Emergency and Critical Care
Department of Clinical Sciences
Cummings School of Veterinary Medicine
Tufts University
North Grafton, Massachusetts
Hospital-Acquired Bacterial Infections
Thoracic Trauma

G. Diane Shelton, DVM, PhD, DACVIM (Internal Medicine)
Professor, Department of Pathology
Director, Comparative Neuromuscular Laboratory
School of Medicine
University of California
San Diego and La Jolla, California
Oropharyngeal Dysphagia
Treatment of Autoimmune Myasthenia Gravis
Treatment of Myopathies and Neuropathies

Robert G. Sherding, DVM, DACVIM (Internal Medicine)
Professor of Internal Medicine
Department of Veterinary Clinical Sciences
College of Veterinary Medicine
The Ohio State University
Columbus, Ohio
Respiratory Parasites

Deborah Silverstein, DVM, DACVECC
Assistant Professor, Critical Care
Department of Clinical Studies
School of Veterinary Medicine
University of Pennsylvania
Philadelphia, Pennsylvania
Shock

Kenneth W. Simpson, BVM&S, PhD, DACVIM, DECVIM-CA
Associate Professor of Medicine
College of Veterinary Medicine
Cornell University
Ithaca, New York
Canine Ulcerative Colitis

Kaitkanoke Sirinarumitr, DVM, MS, PhD
Assistant Professor, Faculty of Veterinary Medicine
Department of Obstetrics, Gynaecology, and Animal
    Reproduction
Veterinary Teaching Hospital
Kasetsart University
Bangkok, Thailand
*Medical Treatment of Benign Prostatic Hypertrophy and
    Prostatitis in Dogs*

D. David Sisson, DVM, DACVIM (Cardiology)
Department of Clinical Sciences
College of Veterinary Medicine
Oregon State University
Corvallis, Oregon
Permanent Cardiac Pacing in Dogs

Daniel D. Smeak, DVM, DACVS
Professor
Department of Veterinary Clinical Sciences
College of Veterinary Medicine
The Ohio State University
Columbus, Ohio
Pneumothorax

**Annette N. Smith, DVM, MS, DACVIM
    (Oncology, SAIM)**
Associate Professor
Department of Clinical Sciences
College of Veterinary Medicine
Auburn University
Auburn, Alabama
Treatment of Intracranial Tumors

Frances O. Smith, DVM, PhD, DACT
President, Orthopedic Foundation for Animals
Smith Veterinary Hospital
Burnsville, Minnesota
Pyometra

Patricia J. Smith, DVM, MS, PhD, DACVO
Animal Eye Care
Fremont, California
Retinal Detachment

**Candace A. Sousa, DVM, DABVP (Canine and
    Feline Practice), DACVD**
Senior Veterinary Specialist, Veterinary Specialty Team
Pfizer Animal Health
El Dorado Hills, California
Glucocorticoids in Veterinary Dermatology

Alan W. Spier, DVM, PhD, DACVIM (Cardiology)
Florida Veterinary Specialists
Tampa, Florida
Cardiomyopathy in Boxer Dogs

Wayne Spoo, DVM, DABVT, DABT
Master Toxicologist
Scientific and Regulatory Affairs
RJ Reynolds Tobacco Co.
Winston-Salem, North Carolina
Nicotine Toxicosis

**Jörg M. Steiner, Dr Med Vet, PhD, DACVIM,
    DECIVM-CA**
Associate Professor and Director of the GI Lab
Small Animal Clinical Sciences
Texas A&M University
College Station, Texas
Canine Pancreatic Disease

**Rebecca L. Stepien, DVM, MS, DACVIM
    (Cardiology)**
Clinical Associate Professor, Cardiology
Department of Medical Sciences
Cardiology Service Head
Veterinary Teaching Hospital
School of Veterinary Medicine
University of Wisconsin
Madison, Wisconsin
Systemic Hypertension

**Jennifer E. Stokes, DVM, DACVIM (Internal
    Medicine)**
Clinical Assistant Professor
Department of Small Animal Clinical Sciences
University of Tennessee
Knoxville, Tennessee
Diagnostic Approach to Acute Azotemia

Beverly K. Sturges, DVM, DACVIM (Neurology)
Assistant Clinical Professor, Neurology/Neurosurgery
Department of Surgery and Radiology
University of California
Davis, California
Diagnosis and Treatment of Atlantoaxial Subluxation

**Jane E. Sykes, BVSc(Hons), PhD, DACVIM
    (Internal Medicine)**
Assistant Professor of Small Animal Internal Medicine
Department of Medicine and Epidemiology
University of California
Davis, California
Feline Calicivirus Infection
Feline Chlamydiosis

Patricia A. Talcott, DVM, MS, PhD, DABVT
Associate Professor
Department of Veterinary Comparative Anatomy,
    Pharmacology, and Physiology
College of Veterinary Medicine
Washington State University;
Veterinary Diagnostic Toxicologist
Washington Animal Disease Diagnostic Laboratory
Pullman, Washington
Insecticide Toxicosis

**Séverine Tasker, BSc, BVSc, PhD, DSAM,
    DECVIM-CA, MRCVS**
Lecturer in Small Animal Medicine
School of Clinical Veterinary Science
University of Bristol
Bristol, England
United Kingdom
Canine and Feline Hemotropic Mycoplasmosis

Marion B. Tefend, RVT
Clinical Instructor
ICU Nursing Supervisor
Department of Clinical Sciences
College of Veterinary Medicine
Auburn University
Auburn, Alabama
Vascular Access Techniques

Douglas H. Thamm, VMD, DACVIM (Oncology)
Assistant Professor, Oncology
Department of Clinical Sciences
College of Veterinary Medicine and Biomedical Sciences
Colorado State University
Fort Collins, Colorado
Anticancer Drugs: New Drugs

Andrea Tipold, Dr Med Vet, DECVN
Professor of Neurology
Department Small Animal Medicine and Surgery
University of Veterinary Medicine
Hannover, Germany
Treatment of Primary Central Nervous System Inflammation (Encephalitis and Meningitis)

Anthony H. Tobias, DVM, DACVIM (Cardiology)
Associate Professor
Veterinary Clinical Sciences
University of Minnesota
St. Paul, Minnesota
Arterial Thromboembolism in Cats

Karen M. Tobias, DVM, MS, DACVS
Professor
Department of Small Animal Clinical Sciences
College of Veterinary Medicine
University of Tennessee
Knoxville, Tennessee
Portosystemic Shunts

Lauren A. Trepanier, DVM, PhD, DACVIM, DACVCP
Associate Professor
Department of Medical Sciences
School of Veterinary Medicine
University of Wisconsin
Madison, Wisconsin
Medical Treatment of Feline Hyperthyroidism

Gregory C. Troy, DVM, MS, DACVIM (Internal Medicine)
Professor and Department Head
Dr. and Mrs. Dorsey Taylor Mahin Endowed Professor
Department of Small Animal Clinical Sciences
Virginia-Maryland Regional College of Veterinary Medicine
Virginia Polytechnic Institute and State University
Blacksburg, Virginia
American Leishmaniasis

David C. Twedt, DVM, DACVIM (Internal Medicine)
Professor
Department of Clinical Sciences
College of Veterinary Medicine and Biomedical Sciences
Colorado State University
Fort Collins, Colorado
Evaluation of Elevated Serum Alkaline Phosphatase in the Dog
Feline Inflammatory Liver Disease

Shelly L. Vaden, DVM, PhD, DACVIM
Professor, Internal Medicine
Department of Clinical Sciences
College of Veterinary Medicine
North Carolina State University
Raleigh, North Carolina
Glomerular Disease

David M. Vail, DVM, DACVIM (Oncology)
Professor of Oncology
Director, Center for Clinical Trials and Research
Department of Medical Sciences
School of Veterinary Medicine
University of Wisconsin
Madison, Wisconsin
Anticancer Drugs: New Drugs
Paraneoplastic Hypercalcemia

Amy K. Valentine, DVM, MS
Private Specialty Practitioner
Oregon Veterinary Referral Associates
Springfield, Oregon
Pneumothorax

Carlo Vitale, DVM, DACVD
Staff Dermatologist
San Francisco Veterinary Specialists, Inc.
San Francisco, California
Methicillin-Resistant Canine Pyoderma

Petra A. Volmer, DVM, MS, DABVT, DABT
Assistant Professor of Toxicology
Departments of Veterinary Biosciences and Veterinary Diagnostic Laboratory
College of Veterinary Medicine
University of Illinois at Urbana-Champaign
Urbana, Illinois
Human Drugs of Abuse

Daniel A. Ward, DVM, PhD, DACVO
Professor of Ophthalmology
College of Veterinary Medicine
University of Tennessee
Knoxville, Tennessee
Ocular Pharmacology

Wendy A. Ware, DVM, MS, DACVIM (Cardiology)
Professor
Departments of Veterinary Clinical Sciences and Biomedical Sciences
Staff Cardiologist
Veterinary Teaching Hospital
Iowa State University
Ames, Iowa
Pericardial Effusion

A.D.J. Watson, BVSc, PhD, FRCVS, MACVSc, DECVPT
Glebe, New South Wales
Australia
Chronic Kidney Disease: Staging and Management

Craig B. Webb, DVM, PhD, DACVIM (SAIM)
Assistant Professor
Department of Clinical Sciences
College of Veterinary Medicine and Biomedical Sciences
Colorado State University
Fort Collins, Colorado
Anal-Rectal Disease

Cynthia R.L. Webster, DVM, DACVIM (Internal Medicine)
Associate Professor
Department of Clinical Sciences
Cummings School of Veterinary Medicine
Tufts University
North Grafton, Massachusetts
Diagnostic Approach to Hepatobiliary Disease
Ursodeoxycholic Acid Therapy

Douglas J. Weiss, DVM, DACVP
Professor, Veterinary and Biomedical Sciences
University of Minnesota
St. Paul, Minnesota
Nonregenerative Anemias

Chick W.C. Weisse, VMD, DACVS
Assistant Professor of Surgery
Director of Interventional Radiology Services
Veterinary Hospital of the University of Pennsylvania
Philadelphia, Pennsylvania
Interventional Radiology in Urinary Diseases
Intraluminal Stenting for Tracheal Collapse

Elias Westermarck, DVM, PhD, DECVIM
Emeritus Professor of Medicine
Department of Clinical Veterinary Sciences
University of Helsinki,
Helsinki, Finland
Tylosin-Responsive Diarrhea

Jodi L. Westropp, DVM, PhD, DACVIM
Assistant Professor
Department of Medicine and Epidemiology
College of Veterinary Medicine
University of California
Davis, California
Management of Feline Ureteroliths
Urinary Incontinence and Micturition Disorders: Pharmacologic Management

Maria Wiberg, DVM, PhD
Member of the Gastrointestinal Research Group
Department of Clinical Veterinary Sciences
Faculty of Veterinary Medicine
University of Helsinki
Helsinki, Finland
Exocrine Pancreatic Insufficiency in Dogs

Michael D. Willard, DVM, MS, DACVIM (Internal Medicine)
Professor
Department of Small Animal Medicine and Surgery
College of Veterinary Medicine and Biomedical Sciences
Texas A&M University
College Station, Texas
Esophagitis

David A. Williams, MA, VetMB, PhD, DACVIM, DECVIM-CA
Professor and Head
Department of Veterinary Clinical Medicine
University of Illinois at Urbana-Champaign
Urbana, Illinois
Feline Exocrine Pancreatic Disease

Marion S. Wilson, BVMS, MVSc MRCVS
Director, TCI Ltd
Te Kuiti, New Zealand
Endoscopic Transcervical Insemination

James S. Wohl, DVM, DACVIM, DACVECC
Professor
Department of Clinical Sciences
College of Veterinary Medicine
Auburn University
Auburn, Alabama
Vascular Access Techniques

J. Paul Woods, DVM, MS, DACVIM (Oncology, Internal Medicine), CVMA
Associate Professor
Department of Clinical Studies
Ontario Veterinary Teaching Hospital
University of Guelph
Guelph, Ontario
Canada
Feline Cytauxzoonosis

Kathy N. Wright, DVM, DACVIM (Cardiology, Internal Medicine)
Director of Cardiovascular Medicine
Internal Medicine
The CARE Center
Cincinnati, Ohio
Assessment and Treatment of Supraventricular Tachyarrhythmias

Debra L. Zoran, DVM, PhD, DACVIM (SAIM)
Associate Professor of Internal Medicine
Small Animal Clinical Sciences
College of Veterinary Medicine and Biomedical Sciences
Texas A&M University
College Station, Texas
Diet and Diabetes

Contributors to Evolve

Chapters by the following contributors were published in *CVT XIII* and are now available on Evolve at http://evolve.elsevier.com/Bonagura/Kirks/.

Verena K. Affolter, DVM, PhD
Associate Professor for Clinical Dermatopathology
Department of Pathology, Microbiology, and
    Immunology
School of Veterinary Medicine
University of California
Davis, California
Immunophenotyping in the Dog

F. J. Allan, BVSc, MVSc
Lecturer
Companion Animal Medicine
Centre for Companion Animal Health
Institute of Veterinary, Animal, and Biomedical
    Sciences
Massey University
Palmerston North, New Zealand
Assessment of Gastrointestinal Motility

**Philip J. Bergman, DVM, MS, PhD, DACVIM
    (Oncology)**
Chief Medical Officer
Bright Heart Veterinary Centers
Armonk, New York
Multidrug Resistance

G. Daniel Boon, DVM, MS, DACVP
President and Director of Pathology
United Veterinary Laboratories
Garden Grove, California
*Interpretation of Cytograms and Histograms of Erythrocytes,
    Leukocytes, and Platelets*

Edward B. Breitschwerdt, DVM, DACVIM
Professor of Medicine and Infectious Diseases
Director, NCSU-CVM Biosafety Laboratory
Adjunct Associate Professor of Medicine
Duke University Medical Center
Department of Clinical Sciences
College of Veterinary Medicine
North Carolina State University
Raleigh, North Carolina
Why Are Infectious Diseases Emerging?

Scott A. Brown, VMD, PhD, DACVIM
Josiah Meigs Distinguished Teaching Professor and
    Department Head
Small Animal Medicine and Surgery
College of Veterinary Medicine
University of Georgia
Athens, Georgia
The Kidney and Hyperthyroidism

Elaine R. Caplan, DVM, DABVP
Surgery Instructor
Veterinary Teaching Hospital
Iowa State University
Ames, Iowa
Treatment of Insulinoma in the Dog, Cat, and Ferret

Sharon A. Center, DVM, DACVIM
Professor, Internal Medicine
College of Veterinary Medicine
Cornell University
Ithaca, New York
Hepatoportal Microvascular Dysplasia

Mary M. Christopher, DVM, PhD, DACVP
Department of Pathology, Microbiology, and Immunology
School of Veterinary Medicine
Clinician, Veterinary Teaching Hospital
University of California
Davis, California
Disorders of Feline Red Blood Cells

Leah A. Cohn, DVM, PhD, DACVIM (SAIM)
Associate Professor of Veterinary Internal Medicine
Department of Veterinary Medicine and Surgery
College of Veterinary Medicine
University of Missouri
Columbia, Missouri
Diagnosis and Treatment of Parvovirus

Gheorge M. Constantinescu, DVM, PhD, Drhc
Professor of Veterinary Anatomy
College of Veterinary Medicine
University of Missouri
Columbia, Missouri
Feline Respiratory Tract Polyps

Laine A. Cowan, DVM, DACVIM
Associate Professor
Department of Clinical Sciences
College of Veterinary Medicine
Kansas State University
Manhattan, Kansas
Cutaneous and Renal Glomerulopathy of Greyhound Dogs

Dennis T. Crowe, Jr., DVM, NREMT-I, PI, CFF, DACVS, DACVECC
President
Veterinary Surgery, Emergency and Critical Care Services and Consulting
Bogart, Georgia
Microenteral Nutrition

Deborah J. Davenport, DVM, MS, DACVIM
Hill's Pet Nutrition, Inc.
Topeka, Kansas
Small Intestinal Bacterial Overgrowth

Helio Autran de Morais, DVM, PhD, DACVIM (SAIM, Cardiology)
Clinical Associate Professor
Department of Medical Sciences
University of Wisconsin
Madison, Wisconsin
Feline Congenital Heart Disease

Jennifer J. Devey, DVM, DACVECC
Head of Emergency and Critical Care Services
California Animal Hospital
Los Angeles, California
Microenteral Nutrition

Nishi Dhupa, BVM, DACVIM (Internal Medicine), DACVECC
Director of Emergency and Critical Care
Department of Clinical Sciences
College of Veterinary Medicine
Cornell University
Ithaca, New York
Sodium Nitroprusside: Uses and Precautions

Stephen P. DiBartola, DVM, DACVIM (SAIM)
Professor
Department of Veterinary Clinical Sciences
College of Veterinary Medicine
The Ohio State University
Columbus, Ohio
The Kidney and Hyperthyroidism

Steven W. Dow, DVM, PhD
Professor
Department of Microbiology, Immunology, and Pathology
College of Veterinary Medicine and Biomedical Sciences
Colorado State University
Fort Collins, Colorado
Why Are Infectious Diseases Emerging?

Cherie L. Drenzek, DVM, MS
Chief, Notifiable Diseases Epidemiology Section
Georgia Division of Public Health
Atlanta, Georgia
The Rabies Pandemic

Lisa A. Dzyban, DVM, DACVIM
Phoenix Central Laboratory
Everett, Washington
Peritoneal Dialysis

Sidney A. Ewing, DVM, PhD
Wendell H. & Nellie G. Krull Professor Emeritus of Veterinary Parasitology
Oklahoma State University
Stillwater, Oklahoma
Ticks as Vectors of Companion Animal Diseases

Leah S. Faudskar, DVM, DACVECC
Prairie Pet Clinic
Fosston Valley, Minnesota
Point-of-Care Laboratory Testing in the Intensive Care Unit

Edward C. Feldman, DVM, DACVIM
Professor
Department of Medicine and Epidemiology
School of Veterinary Medicine
University of California
Davis, California
Diagnosis and Management of Large Pituitary Tumors in Dogs With Pituitary-Dependent Hyperadrenocorticism

Peter J. Felsburg, VMD, PhD
Trustee Professor of Immunology
Department of Clinical Studies
Veterinary School of Medicine
University of Pennsylvania
Philadelphia, Pennsylvania
Hereditary and Acquired Immunodeficiency Diseases

Urs Giger, PD, Dr Med Vet, MS, FVH, DACVIM, DECVIM, DECVCP
Charlotte Newton Sheppard Professor of Medicine
Chief of Medical Genetics
Department of Clinical Studies
School of Veterinary Medicine
University of Pennsylvania
Philadelphia, Pennsylvania
Hereditary Erythrocyte Disorders

Brian C. Gilger, DVM, MS, DACVO
Professor of Ophthalmology
Department of Clinical Sciences
North Carolina State University
Raleigh, North Carolina
Diagnosis and Treatment of Canine Conjunctivitis
Ocular Manifestations of Systemic Diseases

Elizabeth A. Giuliano, DVM, MS, DACVO
Assistant Professor
Department of Veterinary Medicine and Surgery
University of Missouri
Columbia, Missouri
Keratoconjunctivitis Sicca

Tony Glover, DVM, MS, DACVO
College of Veterinary Medicine
The Ohio State University
Columbus, Ohio
Ocular Emergencies

**Jody L. Gookin, DVM, PhD, DACVIM
   (Internal Medicine)**
Assistant Professor, Molecular Biomedical Sciences
College of Veterinary Medicine
North Carolina State University
Raleigh, North Carolina
Indications for Nephrectomy and Nephrotomy

Marielle Goossens, DVM, DACVIM
East Bay Veterinary Specialists
Walnut Creek, California
*Diagnosis and Management of Large Pituitary Tumors in
   Dogs With Pituitary-Dependent Hyperadrenocorticism*

Deborah S. Greco, DVM, PhD, DACVIM
Nestle Purina Petcare
St. Louis, Missouri
*Treatment of Non–Insulin-Dependent Diabetes Mellitus in
   Cats Using Oral Hypoglycemic Agents*

**W. Grant Guilford, BVSc, BPhil, PhD,
   FACVSc, DACVIM**
Institute of Veterinary, Animal, and Biomedical Sciences
Massey University
Palmerston North, New Zealand
Assessment of Gastrointestinal Motility

Edward J. Hall, MA, VetMB, PhD
Professor
Division of Companion Animal Studies
University of Bristol
Bristol, England
United Kingdom
Dietary Sensitivity

Jean A. Hall, DVM, PhD, DACVIM
Associate Professor
Department of Biomedical Sciences
College of Veterinary Medicine
Oregon State University
Corvallis, Oregon
Gastric Prokinetic Agents

Bernie Hansen, DVM
Associate Professor, ICU Critical Care
School of Veterinary Medicine
Purdue University
West Lafayette, Indiana
Epidural Analgesia

**Stuart C. Helfand, DVM, DACVIM
   (Oncology, Internal Medicine)**
Oregon Cancer Center for Animals
Oregon State University
Corvallis, Oregon
Hematopoietic Cytokines: The Interleukin Array

Joan C. Hendricks, VMD, PhD, DACVIM
The Gilbert S. Kahn Dean of Veterinary Medicine
School of Veterinary Medicine
University of Pennsylvania
Philadelphia, Pennsylvania
Airway Management

Donna M. Hertzke, DVM, PhD, DACVP
Assistant Director
Veterinary Diagnostic Services
Marshfield Laboratories
Marshfield, Wisconsin
Cutaneous and Renal Glomerulopathy of Greyhound Dogs

David E. Holt, BVSc, DACVS
Section Chief, Surgery
Professor of Surgery, Clinical Educator
Department of Clinical Studies
School of Veterinary Medicine
University of Pennsylvania
Philadelphia, Pennsylvania
Feline Constipation and Idiopathic Megacolon

Dez Hughes, BVSc, MRCVS, DACVECC
Senior Lecturer in Emergency and Critical Care
Royal Veterinary College
University of London
London, England
United Kingdom
*Lactate Measurement: Diagnostic, Therapeutic, and
   Prognostic Implications*

Victoria G. Jones, DVM, MS, DACVO
Northwest Animal Eye Specialists
Kirkland, Washington
Nonulcerative Corneal Disease

Andrew J. Kaplan, DVM, DACVIM
City Veterinary Care
New York, New York
*Effects of Nonadrenal Disease on Adrenal Function Tests
   in Dogs*

**Charlotte B. Keller, DrMedVet, DACVO,
   DECVO**
Formerly Assistant Professor
Department of Clinical Studies
Ontario Veterinary College
University of Guelph
Guelph, Ontario
Canada
Epiphora

**Lesley G. King, MVB, MRCVS, DACVECC,
   DACVIM**
School of Veterinary Medicine
University of Pennsylvania
Philadelphia, Pennsylvania
Airway Management
Colloid Osmometry

Peter P. Kintzer, DVM, DACVIM
Staff Internist
Department of Medicine
Boston Road Animal Hospital
Springfield, Massachusetts
*Differential Diagnosis of Hyperkalemia and Hyponatremia
   in Dogs and Cats*

Rebecca Kirby, DVM, DACVIM (Internal Medicine), DACVECC
Animal Emergency Center
Glendale, Wisconsin
Cats Are Not Dogs in Critical Care

Mary Anna Labato, DVM, DACVIM
Clinical Associate Professor
Section Head, Small Animal Medicine
Department of Clinical Sciences
Foster Hospital for Small Animals
Cummings School of Veterinary Medicine
Tufts University
North Grafton, Massachusetts
Peritoneal Dialysis

Kenneth S. Latimer, DVM, PhD, DACVP
Professor
Department of Veterinary Pathology
College of Veterinary Medicine
University of Georgia
Athens, Georgia
Overview of Neutrophil Dysfunction in Dogs and Cats

Cheryl A. London, DVM, PhD, DACVIM (Oncology)
Associate Professor
College of Veterinary Medicine
The Ohio State University
Columbus, Ohio
Hematopoietic Cytokines: The Myelopoietic Factors

Chris L. Ludlow, DVM, MS, DACVIM
Staff Veterinarian
Veterinary Internal Medicine
Specialists of Kansas City
Overland Park, Kansas
Small Intestinal Bacterial Overgrowth

Marilena Lupu, DVM, PhD
Resident in Veterinary Oncology
Oregon Cancer Center for Animals
Department of Clinical Sciences
Oregon State University
Corvallis, Oregon
Hematopoietic Cytokines: The Interleukin Array

Douglass K. Macintire, DVM, MS, DACVIM, DACVECC
Professor of Acute Medicine and Critical Care
Department of Clinical Sciences
College of Veterinary Medicine
Auburn University
Auburn, Alabama
Bacterial Translocation: Clinical Implications and Prevention
Canine Hepatozoonosis

Ruth Marrion, DVM, PhD, DACVO
Staff Ophthalmologist
Essex County Veterinary Specialists
North Andover, Massachusetts
Ulcerative Keratitis

Glenna E. Mauldin, DVM, MS, DACVIM
Assistant Professor of Veterinary Oncology and Companion Animal Medicine
School of Veterinary Medicine
Louisiana State University
Baton Rouge, Louisiana
Nutritional Support of the Cancer Patient

Karrelle A. Meleo, DVM, DACVIM
Senior Oncologist
Veterinary Oncology Services
Redmond, Washington
Treatment of Insulinoma in the Dog, Cat, and Ferret

Carlos Melián, DVM, PhD
Director
Clinica Veterinaria Atlantico
Las Palmas de Gran Canaria
Spain
The Incidentally Discovered Adrenal Mass

†E. Phillip Miller, DVM, MS, DABVT, DABT
Formerly Director of Product Safety and Efficacy
Hill's Pet Nutrition, Inc.
Topeka, Kansas
Pet Food Safety

Eric Monnet, DVM, PhD, DACVS, DECVS
Associate Professor, Small Animal Surgery
Department of Clinical Sciences
College of Veterinary Medicine and Biomedical Sciences
Colorado State University
Fort Collins, Colorado
Thoracoscopy

Cecil P. Moore, DVM, MS, DACVO
Interim Dean and Professor
Department of Veterinary Medicine and Surgery
College of Veterinary Medicine
University of Missouri
Columbia, Missouri
Keratoconjunctivitis Sicca

Peter F. Moore, BVSc, PhD
Professor
Department of Pathology, Microbiology, and Immunology
College of Veterinary Medicine
University of California
Davis, California
Immunophenotyping in the Dog

Mark P. Nasisse, DVM, DACVO
Carolina Veterinary Specialists
Greensboro, North Carolina
Ocular Feline Herpesvirus-1 Infection

Rhett Nichols, DVM, DACVIM
Internal Medicine Consultant
Antech Diagnostics
Farmingdale, New York
Clinical Use of the Vasopressin Analogue DDAVP for the Diagnosis and Treatment of Diabetes Insipidus

---

†Deceased.

E. Christopher Orton, DVM, PhD, DACVS
Professor
Department of Clinical Sciences
Veterinary Teaching Hospital
Colorado State University
Fort Collins, Colorado
Current Indications and Outcomes for Cardiac Surgery

David L. Panciera, DVM, MS, DACVIM (SAIM)
Professor
Department of Small Animal Clinical Sciences
Virginia-Maryland Regional College of Veterinary
    Medicine
Virginia Polytechnic Institute and State University
Blacksburg, Virginia
Cardiovascular Complications of Thyroid Disease
Complications and Concurrent Conditions Associated With
    Hypothyroidism in Dogs

Mark G. Papich, DVM, MS
Professor of Clinical Pharmacology
College of Veterinary Medicine
North Carolina State University
Raleigh, North Carolina
Bacterial Resistance

Jennifer M. Pearson, DVM, MS, DACVIM
Staff Internist
Internal Medicine Department
Animal Hospital Center
Highlands Ranch, Colorado
Diagnosis and Treatment of Parvovirus

Mark E. Peterson, DVM, DACVIM
Head of Endocrinology
Department of Medicine, Bobst Hospital
Associate Director, Caspary Research Institute
Chairman, Institute of Postgraduate Education
The Animal Medical Center
New York, New York
Effects of Nonadrenal Disease on Adrenal Function Tests
    in Dogs
Growth Hormone Therapy in the Dog
Hyperadrenocorticism in the Ferret
The Incidentally Discovered Adrenal Mass

Eric R. Pope, DVM, MS, DACVS
Professor, Small Animal Surgery
Ross University School of Veterinary Medicine
Basseterre, St. Kitts
West Indies
Feline Respiratory Tract Polyps

†Jeffrey Proulx, DVM
Formerly Resident in Emergency and Critical Care
Cummings School of Veterinary Medicine
Tufts University
North Grafton, Massachusetts
Sodium Nitroprusside: Uses and Precautions

Marc R. Raffe, DVM, MS, DACVA, DACVECC
Adjunct Professor
Department of Clinical Sciences
Colorado State University
Fort Collins, Colorado
Point-of-Care Laboratory Testing in the Intensive Care Unit

David T. Ramsey, DVM, DACVO
Owner
The Animal Ophthalmology Center
Williamston, Michigan
Exophthalmos

John F. Randolph, DVM, DACVIM
Professor of Medicine
Department of Clinical Sciences
College of Veterinary Medicine
Cornell University
Ithaca, New York
Growth Hormone Therapy in the Dog

Karen L. Rosenthal, DVM, MS
Director of Special Species Medicine
Associate Professor
Abaxis Chair of Special Species Medicine
Department of Clinical Studies
School of Veterinary Medicine
University of Pennsylvania
Philadelphia, Pennsylvania
Hyperadrenocorticism in the Ferret

Linda A. Ross, DVM, MS, DACVIM (SAIM)
Associate Professor
Department of Clinical Sciences
Cummings School of Veterinary Medicine
Tufts University
North Grafton, Massachusetts
Peritoneal Dialysis

Philip Roudebush, DVM, DACVIM (SAIM)
Director, Scientific Affairs
Hill's Pet Nutrition, Inc.
Topeka, Kansas
Hypoallergenic Diets for Dogs and Cats

Charles E. Rupprecht, VMD, MS, PhD
Chief, Rabies Section
Centers for Disease Control and Prevention
Atlanta, Georgia
The Rabies Pandemic

Michael Scott, DVM, PhD, DACVP
Assistant Professor
College of Veterinary Medicine
University of Missouri
Columbia, Missouri
Interpretation of Cytograms and Histograms of
    Erythrocytes, Leukocytes, and Platelets

---

†Deceased.

Kenneth W. Simpson, BVM&S, PhD, DACVIM, DECVIM-CA
Associate Professor of Medicine
College of Veterinary Medicine
Cornell University
Ithaca, New York
Gastrinoma in Dogs

Patricia J. Smith, DVM, MS, PhD, DACVO
Animal Eye Care
Fremont, California
Hypertensive Retinopathy

Rebecca L. Stepien, DVM, MS, DACVIM (Cardiology)
Clinical Associate Professor, Cardiology
Department of Medical Sciences
Cardiology Service Head
Veterinary Teaching Hospital
School of Veterinary Medicine
University of Wisconsin
Madison, Wisconsin
Feline Congenital Heart Disease

Elizabeth A. Stone, DVM, MS, DACVS
Professor and Head
Department of Companion Animal and Special
    Species Medicine
College of Veterinary Medicine
North Carolina State University
Raleigh, North Carolina
Indications for Nephrectomy and Nephrotomy

Alain Théon, DrMedVet, MS, DACVR
Associate Professor
Department of Veterinary Medicine
Surgery and Radiological Science
School of Veterinary Medicine
University of California,
Davis, California
*Diagnosis and Management of Large Pituitary
    Tumors in Dogs With Pituitary-Dependent
    Hyperadrenocorticism*

Amy S. Tidwell, DVM, DACVR
Associate Professor
Department of Clinical Sciences
Cummings School of Veterinary Medicine
Tufts University
North Grafton, Massachusetts
*Use of Computed Tomography in Cardiopulmonary
    Disease*

Harold Tvedten, DVM, MS, PhD, DACVP
Professor of Pathology and Chief of Veterinary Clinical
    Pathology Section
Veterinary Teaching Hospital
Michigan State University
East Lansing, Michigan
*Interpretation of Cytograms and Histograms of Erythrocytes,
    Leukocytes, and Platelets*

Shelly L. Vaden, DVM, PhD, Diplomate ACVIM
Professor, Internal Medicine
Department of Clinical Sciences
College of Veterinary Medicine
North Carolina State University
Raleigh, North Carolina
Differentiation of Acute From Chronic Renal Failure

William Vernau, BSc, BVMS, DVSc, DACVP
Clinical Pathologist
Veterinary Medicine Pathology, Microbiology, and
    Immunology
School of Veterinary Medicine
University of California
Davis, California
Immunophenotyping in the Dog

Nancy Vincent-Johnson, DVM, MS, DACVIM
Major, US Army Veterinary Command
94th Medical Detachment (VM)
Fort Sam Houston
San Antonio, Texas
Canine Hepatozoonosis

Don R. Waldron, BS, DVM, DACVS
Professor of Surgery
Section Chief of Small Animal Surgery and Anesthesiology
Virginia-Maryland Regional College of Veterinary
    Medicine
Virginia Polytechnic Institute and State University
Blacksburg, Virginia
Urine Diversion by Tube Cystostomy

Ronald S. Walton, DVM, MS, DACVIM, DACVECC
US Army
Rocky Mountain District Veterinary Command
Fort Carson, Colorado
Thoracoscopy

Robert J. Washabau, VMD, PhD, DACVIM
Associate Professor and Section Chief of Medicine
Department of Clinical Studies
School of Veterinary Medicine
University of Pennsylvania
Philadelphia, Pennsylvania
Feline Constipation and Idiopathic Megacolon
Gastric Prokinetic Agents

In memory of Hazel Young Bonagura, my best teacher.

JDB

To my wife Liz and my son Ryan for their love and support.
To my parents for helping me achieve my dreams.

David C. Twedt

Preface

This new edition of *Kirk's Current Veterinary Therapy* is the fourteenth version of a textbook used by generations of practicing veterinarians and veterinary students. The general format and chapter presentation of this edition should be familiar to long-time users of "*CVT*". For our new readers it is my hope that you find the information in this textbook (and the related *CVT* website) both informative and accessible. Foremost, I hope *CVT* will help you provide the best possible care for your canine and feline patients. Whereas the overall format of this new edition follows the original formula outlined by Dr. Robert W. Kirk, there are also changes and enhancements.

As the title suggests, the focus of most chapters is therapy of important medical diseases of dogs and cats. *Current Veterinary Therapy* is divided into thirteen sections and three appendices. The sections are organized by organ system, including cardiovascular, dermatologic, gastrointestinal, hematologic, neurologic and musculoskeletal, ophthalmologic, reproductive, respiratory, and urinary diseases. Multisystemic diseases are detailed in the sections covering critical care medicine, infectious diseases, oncology and hematology, and toxicology. Appendix I, *Table of Common Drugs: Approximate Dosages,* and the tables in Appendix II, *Treatment of Parasites,* have been completely revised for this edition. Of great importance is the oversight provided by one or more specialists who served as Consulting Editor for each of these sections. I am most grateful to these outstanding clinicians for their guidance and editorial input.

It is worthwhile to highlight some of the changes adopted for this edition. Foremost has been the inclusion of an Associate Editor, Dr. David Twedt. Dave is recognized worldwide as an outstanding internist, gastroenterologist, and educator. I am most appreciative of his excellent editorial work, and have benefitted greatly from the perspective he brought to this volume. We also recruited some outstanding new Consulting Editors for this edition, while retaining the services of some of the most respected authorities in small animal medicine. Another change involved rearranging sections. Gone is the section on *Diseases of Birds and Exotic Pets*. In recent years these areas have exploded in terms of knowledge and practices, as demonstrated by the proliferation of complete textbooks covering these subjects. After some discussion, it was decided that *CVT* should now concentrate on canine and feline patients. Additionally, the *Special Therapy* section has been eliminated and its topics moved into the most relevant sections for those treatments. The former *Cardiopulmonary Diseases* section has been reasonably divided into two sections: *Cardiovascular Diseases* and *Respiratory Diseases*.

In keeping with current and still-evolving publishing practices, we have made one major change to the fourteenth edition in the guise of a *Current Veterinary Therapy* website. Owners of this textbook will have password access to this electronic content, which resides on the Elsevier Evolve website (http://evolve.elsevier.com/ Bonagura/Kirks/). We have included on this site chapters from the thirteenth edition that we believe are still useful to our readers. A number of these chapters have been updated by the original authors. These "still-current" chapters are organized by section along the same lines as the textbook. Additionally, the website contains an image library of figures printed in this new edition, with additional images also available in color. Website users can access an online, searchable index (citing chapters in both the current edition and *CVT XIII*). Appendices I-III from the textbook will also be provided in a searchable format on Evolve. Finally, we have made the decision to free up more pages for published chapters by moving some of the appendices to the Evolve website. Many of these tables relate to reference values, which we realize are often instrument and laboratory specific. Nevertheless, the interested reader will find a number of useful tables of laboratory results and values in the appendices on the website. The development of a *CVT* website also provides an avenue for disseminating information to readers between editions, for example, should issues arise related to drug use or dosage (a real concern with many extra-label uses of drugs in veterinary practice).

Current Veterinary Therapy XIV contains 286 published chapters and three appendices, with contributions by hundreds of authors active in their respective clinical specialties. I am indebted to these individuals for providing concise and clinically useful chapters for the current edition. We have tried to maintain the historical format of Kirk's chapters that considers the salient clinical features of a disease or disorder, the basis for rational therapy, and clear and practical pointers for treatment, while also addressing pending innovations in therapy. As stated above, most chapters are directed toward management of a specific condition. Others concentrate on important principles of therapy or general management approaches to diseases of dogs and cats. With the rapid development of knowledge across our diverse profession, we have undoubtedly omitted some topics. Treatment of some of these may have changed little in the past 5 years. Others are simply beyond our scope (or page allotment) or may be better covered elsewhere. This is especially true of specific surgical procedures, a subject area in which *CVT* provides only limited guidance.

The fastest way to find information in *Current Veterinary Therapy* is through the index. The index is organized to emphasize diseases based on anatomic and physiologic disorders and is extensively cross-referenced. Using either the index printed in the textbook or the online version on the website, the reader should be able to locate a concise chapter detailing the most important medical problems of dogs and cats. Many readers familiar with the *CVT* format will probably head straight for the individual sections' tables of content to peruse the section contents. Related chapters located on the Evolve website are also listed there. As some subjects "overlap" individual sections, we have made every attempt to cross-index information in chapters throughout the book.

Current Veterinary Therapy is written for both the veterinary practitioner and the veterinary student. It is my hope that *CVT* will be discovered by students who will later find its contents an asset to their professional work. I am always grateful to receive comments from readers, including any concerns about possible errors or omissions. Ideas designed to improve this textbook are most welcome. As I have written previously, I have tried to maintain *CVT* on the course first set by Dr. Kirk. I remain most appreciative of your acceptance of previous editions and this new one.

ACKNOWLEDGMENTS

I would like to acknowledge a number of individuals. I am most thankful to the veterinarians and scientists who have contributed to this edition and to the expertise and oversight of our Consulting Editors. Bringing Dr. David Twedt on board has been very helpful, and the book is far better for his efforts. I am especially appreciative of Jolynn Gower, Managing Editor at Elsevier. Without Jolynn's sustained efforts and encouragement, this edition would still be on my desktop (real and electronic). Publisher Penny Rudolph has provided helpful oversight and counsel throughout this endeavor, and I appreciate her patient support. Karen Rehwinkel, Senior Project Manager at Elsevier, has most ably handled the hundreds of manuscripts, electronic documents, authors' information, and page proofs to somehow create this volume. Liz Fathman, my former editor at Elsevier, was most helpful in getting this project started. Others at Elsevier, with whom I have not worked directly, have been important in creating this textbook, and I extend my deepest appreciation to them. Special thanks are extended to Debra Primovic, DVM, for indexing this and the previous volume of *CVT*.

John D. Bonagura, DVM
Columbus, Ohio

Contents

SECTION XI   NEUROLOGIC AND MUSCULOSKELETAL DISEASES

Rodney S. Bagley

CVT XIII Content on Evolve

†Deceased

†Deceased.

*Appendices I-III in this book are also available on Evolve. Appendices IV-XL were originally edited by Robert M. Jacobs, DVM, PhD, DACVP; Professor, Department of Pathobiology, Ontario Veterinary College, University of Guelph, Guelph, Ontario, Canada.

SECTION I

Critical Care

Nishi Dhupa

VOLUME XIII CONTENT ON EVOLVE: http://evolve.elsevier.com/Bonagura/Kirks/

Bacterial Translocation: Clinical Implications and Prevention

Cats Are Not Dogs in Critical Care

Collid Osmometry

Epidural Analgesia

Lactate Measurement: Diagnostic, Therapeutic, and Prognostic Implications

Microenteral Nutrition

Point-of-Care Laboratory Testing in the Intensive Care Unit

CHAPTER 1

Shock

ANNIE MALOUIN, *Philadelphia, Pennsylvania*
DEBORAH SILVERSTEIN, *Philadelphia, Pennsylvania*

Shock is a state of severe hemodynamic and metabolic derangements. It is characterized by poor tissue perfusion from low or unevenly distributed blood flow that leads to a critical decrease in oxygen delivery (DO_2) in relation to oxygen consumption (VO_2) (Fig. 1-1) and/or inadequate cellular energy production. If the shock state is not promptly recognized and treated, neurohormonal compensatory mechanisms will lead to stimulation of the renin-angiotensin-aldosterone system, as well as baroreceptor and chemoreceptor-mediated release of catecholamines and subsequent production of counterregulatory hormones (glucagon, adrenocorticotropic hormone [ACTH], and cortisol). These changes will increase cardiovascular tone, activate a variety of biochemical mediators, and stimulate inflammatory responses that contribute to the shock syndrome. This progression can cause or exacerbate uneven microcirculatory flow, poor tissue perfusion, tissue hypoxia, altered cellular metabolism, cellular death, and vital organ dysfunction or failure.

Box 1-1 lists the different types of shock, but this classification can be overly simplistic. Critically ill patients are subject to complex etiologic and pathophysiologic events and therefore may suffer from more than one type of shock simultaneously. The rationale for the functional classification of shock is the presumption that each underlying illness identified can be associated with a specific pathophysiologic process and rapid, appropriate therapy can be administered.

CLINICAL PRESENTATION

Dogs in compensatory shock demonstrate mild-to-moderate mental depression, increased heart rate, increased respiratory rate, peripheral vasoconstriction with cold extremities and pale mucous membranes, and a shortened capillary refill time with normal blood pressure. As compensatory mechanisms fail, they may develop severe mental depression, prolonged capillary refill time, increased heart rate, poor pulse quality, and decreased arterial blood pressure.

Dogs with sepsis or a systemic inflammatory response syndrome (SIRS) can show clinical signs of hyperdynamic or hypodynamic shock. The initial hyperdynamic phase of sepsis is characterized by tachycardia, fever, bounding peripheral pulse quality, and hyperemic mucous membranes secondary to peripheral vasodilation. If septic shock or SIRS progresses unchecked, a decreased cardiac output and signs of hypoperfusion may ensue as a result of cytokine effects on the myocardium or myocardial ischemia. Clinical alterations may then include tachycardia, pale (and possibly icteric) mucous membranes with a prolonged capillary refill time, hypothermia, poor pulse quality and dull mentation. Hypodynamic septic shock is the decompensatory stage of sepsis and without intervention will result in organ damage and death. Finally, the gastrointestinal (GI) tract is the shock organ in dogs and often leads to ileus, diarrhea, or melena.

In cats the hyperdynamic phase of shock is rarely recognized. Also, in contrast to dogs, changes in heart rate in cats with shock are unpredictable; they may exhibit tachycardia or bradycardia. In general, cats typically present with pale mucous membranes (and possibly icterus), weak pulses, cool extremities, hypothermia, and generalized weakness or collapse. In cats the lungs seem to be the organ most vulnerable to damage during shock or sepsis, and signs of respiratory dysfunction are common (Schutzer et al., 1993; Brady et al., 2000; Costello et al., 2004).

MANAGEMENT

General Diagnostics

For all patients in shock, basic diagnostic tests should be completed to assess the extent of organ injury and identify the etiology of the shock state. Venous or arterial blood gases, a complete blood cell count, blood chemistry panel, coagulation panel, blood typing, and urine analysis should be performed in all shock patients. Thoracic and abdominal radiographs, abdominal ultrasound, and echocardiography may be indicated once the patient is stabilized. Thoracic imaging can help distinguish cardiogenic forms of shock.

Monitoring Perfusion and Oxygen Delivery

The magnitude of oxygen deficit is a key predictor in determining outcome in patients with shock. Therefore optimizing tissue perfusion and DO_2 is the goal of effective therapy, and thorough monitoring is necessary to achieve this objective. An optimally perfused patient maintains the following characteristics: central venous pressure between 5 and 10 cm H_2O (2 to 5 cm H_2O in cats); urine production of at least 1 ml/kg/hour; a mean arterial pressure (MAP) between 70 and 120 mm Hg; normal body

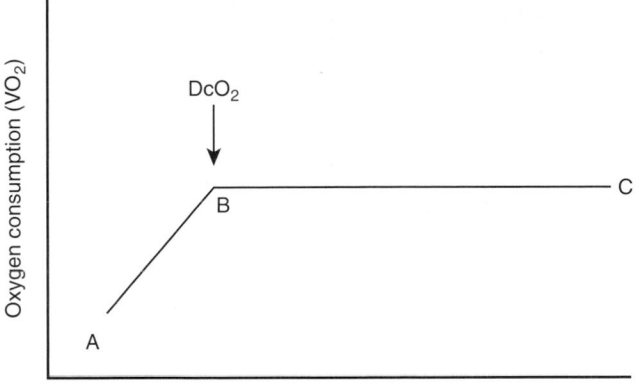

Fig. 1-1 The relationship between oxygen delivery and oxygen consumption. In region B-C the oxygen consumption remains constant as oxygen delivery is increased. The oxygen supply is in excess of consumption, and VO_2 is termed *supply independent*. During shock, as metabolic demand (VO_2) increases or DO_2 diminishes (C-B), Oxygen extraction ratio rises to maintain aerobic metabolism; thus consumption can remain independent of delivery. However, at point B, called *critical DO_2 (DcO_2)*, the maximum OER is reached. This is believed to be 60% to 70%, and beyond this point any further increase in VO_2 or decline in DO_2 must lead to tissue hypoxia.

Box 1-1

Functional Classifications and Examples of Shock

Hypovolemic: A Decrease in Circulating Blood Volume
- Hemorrhage
- Severe dehydration
- Trauma

Cardiogenic: A Decrease in Forward Flow From the Heart
- Congestive heart failure
- Cardiac arrhythmia
- Cardiac tamponade
- Drug overdose (e.g., anesthetics, β-blockers, calcium channel blockers)

Distributive: A Loss of Systemic Vascular Resistance
- Sepsis
- Obstruction (heartworm disease, saddle thrombosis)
- Anaphylaxis

Metabolic: Deranged Cellular Metabolic Machinery
- Hypoglycemia
- Cyanide toxicity
- Mitochondrial dysfunction
- Cytopathic hypoxia of sepsis

Hypoxemic: A Decrease in Oxygen Content in Arterial Blood
- Anemia
- Severe pulmonary disease
- Carbon monoxide toxicity
- Methemoglobinemia

---

temperature, heart rate, heart rhythm, and respiratory rate; and moist, pink mucous membranes with a capillary refill time of less than 2 seconds. Monitoring these parameters becomes the baseline of patient assessment. Additional monitoring elements that may prove beneficial include measuring blood lactate, indices of systemic oxygenation transport, and mixed venous oxygen saturation.

Blood Lactate Levels

Critically ill patients with inadequate tissue perfusion, DO_2, or oxygen uptake, often have a hyperlactatemia and acidemia that reflect the severity of tissue hypoxia. Humans with lactic acidosis are at greater risk of developing multiple organ failure and demonstrate a higher mortality rate than patients without an elevated lactate concentration (Nguyen et al., 2004). High blood lactate levels may also help to prognosticate mortality in dogs (Boag and Hughes, 2005; de Papp E et al., 1999; Nel et al., 2004; Lagutchik et al., 1998). The normal lactate level in adult dogs and cats is reported to be less than 2.5 mmol/L; lactate concentrations greater than 7 mmol/L are considered severely elevated (Boag et al., 2005). However, normal neonatal and pediatric patients may have higher lactate concentrations (McMichael et al., 2005). In addition, sample collection and handling techniques can affect lactate concentration (Hughes et al., 1999). Serial lactate measurements can be taken during the resuscitation period to gauge response to treatment and evaluate the resuscitation end points; the trends in lactate concentrations are a better predictor of outcome than are single measurements. It is well documented that the ability of the body to correct an elevated lactate concentration is directly correlated to survival.

Cardiac Output Monitoring and Indices of Oxygen Transport

The most direct way to assess the progress of resuscitation in shock patients is to measure indices of systemic oxygen transport. Measurement and monitoring of these values requires right-sided cardiac catheterization, which is performed using a specialized pulmonary artery catheter (PAC, also termed *Swan-Ganz catheter* or *balloon-directed thermodilution catheter*). The PAC allows access for the measurement of central venous and pulmonary arterial pressure, mixed venous blood gases (PvO_2 and SvO_2), pulmonary capillary wedge pressure (PCWP), and cardiac output. With these data additional information regarding the function of the circulatory and respiratory systems can be derived (i.e., stroke volume, end-diastolic volume numbers, systemic vascular resistance index, pulmonary vascular resistance index, arterial oxygen content, mixed venous oxygen content, DO_2 index, VO_2 index and the oxygen extraction ratio). The cardiac output is most commonly determined using thermodilution methods, although other techniques are available, including noninvasive Doppler-based methods.

A PAC can provide the clinician with useful information to assess and monitor the cardiovascular and pulmonary function of shock patients. It may also help the clinician evaluate the response to therapeutic interventions and allow titration of fluid therapy, vasopressors, and inotropic agents. Cardiac output and systemic DO_2 should be optimized by intravascular volume loading until the PCWP approaches 18 to 20 mm Hg. A higher PCWP (>18-20 mm Hg) promotes the formation of pulmonary edema; further impairing oxygenation and overall oxygen transport. In critically ill humans the cardiac index (CI), DO_2, and VO_2 have been found to be higher in survivors. Finally, the use of a PAC does not necessarily translate into reduced mortality in the critically ill shock patient; it is an invasive monitoring technique that is not without risk. Despite the fact that a tremendous amount of information can be obtained from the PAC, it is important to recognize that the accuracy of the measurements provided by the PAC rely on catheter placement, calibration of transducers, coexisting cardiac or pericardial disease, and interpretation of waveforms and measurements or calculations. PAC placement should be performed by experienced individuals, and interpretation of the data should be systematic. In humans the most common complications that occur during or after PAC insertion include arrhythmias, pulmonary injuries, thromboembolism, and sepsis.

Mixed Venous Oxygen Saturation and Central Venous Oxygen Saturation

Mixed venous oxygen saturation (SvO_2) can be used clinically to assess changes in the global tissue oxygenation (oxygen supply-to-demand). If VO_2 is constant, SvO_2 is determined by cardiac output, hemoglobin concentration, and systemic arterial oxygen tension. The SvO_2 is decreased if DO_2 is decreased (low cardiac output, hypoxia, severe anemia) or if VO_2 is increased (fever). SvO_2 is increased in hyperdynamic stages of sepsis and cytotoxic tissue hypoxia (e.g., cyanide poisoning). A reduction in SvO_2 may be an early sign that the patient's clinical condition is deteriorating. Also, SvO_2 may be a surrogate for measuring the CI during resuscitative efforts.

Ideally SvO_2 is measured in a blood sample from the pulmonary artery. However, in cases in which the insertion of a PAC is not possible or desirable, SvO_2 can be determined in the central circulation, using a central venous catheter in the cranial vena cava. SvO_2 is then termed *central venous oxygen saturation ($ScvO_2$)*. In critically ill patients with circulatory failure of any origin, $ScvO_2$ values generally are higher than SvO_2, but the two measurements closely parallel one another. Therefore the presence of a pathologically low $ScvO_2$ likely indicates an even lower SvO_2. The difference between the two values is usually about 5%; this is caused by the effect of blood flow redistribution and differences in oxygen consumption across the hepatosplanchnic, coronary, and cerebral circulations during shock states. Finally, a recent prospective randomized study comparing two algorithms for early goal-directed therapy in patients with severe sepsis and septic shock showed that maintenance of a continuously measured $ScvO_2$ above 70% (in addition to maintaining central venous pressure above 8 to 12 mm Hg, MAP above 65 mm Hg, and urine output above 0.5 ml/kg/hour) resulted in a 15% absolute reduction in mortality compared to the same treatment without $ScvO_2$ monitoring (see following paragraphs for further details) (Rivers et al., 2001).

THERAPY

If the animal is not breathing or displays signs of impending fatigue, immediate intubation and positive-pressure ventilation should be instituted. If the animal is breathing spontaneously, oxygen is administered. This can involve flow-by methods (50 to 150 ml/kg/minute) such as simply holding the oxygen tubing up to the nose or administration of oxygen into a mask, hood, or bag. Nasal catheter(s) are effective methods of oxygen administration (using rates of 50 to 100 ml/kg/minute per catheter). Once the vital signs are obtained, vascular access is established, and fluid administration is initiated if indicated. It is of utmost importance that preliminary diagnostics and appropriate treatment are rapidly initiated to maximize DO_2 to the tissues and prevent irreversible shock.

Fluid Therapy

Vascular Access

The first and most important therapeutic goal for noncardiogenic shock is to restore the effective circulatory volume. Appropriate vascular access is essential for rapid administration of large volumes of fluid (see Chapter 7 for further details). Poiseuille's law of flow states that resistance to flow through a catheter is directly proportional to the length of the catheter and inversely related to the fourth power of the radius. Thus large-bore, short intravenous catheters should be placed for resuscitation. For cats and small dogs 18- or 20-gauge catheters should be used; for larger dogs multiple venous catheters (14- to 18-gauge) should be placed. Faster intravenous fluid administration can be further facilitated by applying pressure around the fluid bag with a commercial pressure device or a blood pressure cuff.

Crystalloids

Isotonic crystalloids remain the cornerstone of treatment for noncardiogenic shock. Examples include 0.9% sodium chloride, lactated Ringer's solution, Normosol-R, and Plasmalyte-148. A shock dose of isotonic crystalloid solution is approximately one blood volume (i.e., 90 ml/kg in the dog and 50 ml/kg in the cat). The fluid administered rapidly distributes into the extracellular fluid compartment so that only ≈25% of the delivered volume remains in the intravascular space by 30 minutes after infusion (Silverstein et al., 2005). Although theoretically this increase in interstitial fluid volume might predispose to interstitial edema and deranged oxygen transfer to the cells, this has not been proven in human clinical trials. However, it is important that excessive fluid volumes are not administered to avoid volume overload. It is generally recommended that one third to one half of the shock dose be administered as quickly as possible, followed by additional boluses as indicated by clinical parameters and repeated physical examination. In patients that are bleeding it may even be advantageous to perform "hypotensive resuscitation" (to a MAP of ≈60 mm Hg) until the hemorrhage is controlled since aggressive fluid therapy in this setting can worsen bleeding and outcome. For animals with coexisting head trauma, the isotonic crystalloid of choice is 0.9% NaCl since it contains the highest concentration of sodium and is least likely to contribute to cerebral edema.

Hypertonic Solutions

Hypertonic (7% to 7.5%) sodium chloride administration causes a transient osmotic shift of water from the extravascular to the intravascular compartment. It is administered in small volumes (5 ml/kg) intravenously (IV) over 5 to 10 minutes. In addition to the fluid compartment shift caused by hypertonic saline, there is evidence that it may also be beneficial to reduce endothelial swelling, increase cardiac contractility, cause mild peripheral vasodilation, and decrease intracranial pressure. Because of the osmotic diuresis and rapid redistribution of the sodium cations that ensue following the administration of hypertonic saline, the intravascular volume expansion is transient (<30 minutes), and additional fluid therapy must be used with hypertonic saline (Silverstein et al., 2005). Hypertonic saline may be administered in conjunction with synthetic colloids.

Synthetic Colloids

Colloids are large molecules (molecular weight >20,000 daltons) that do not readily sieve across the vascular membrane. The colloidal particles in the most commonly used synthetic colloids (dextran 70 and hydroxyethyl starch) are suspended in 0.9% NaCl. They are hyperoncotic to the normal animal and therefore pull fluid into the vascular space. They cause an increase in blood volume that is greater than that of the infused volume and help to retain this fluid in the intravascular space in animals with normal capillary permeability. Dextran 70 is a 6% colloidal solution with particles that range from 15,000 to 3,400,000 daltons, a number average molecular weight of 41,000, and a colloid osmotic pressure of 60 mm Hg. Hetastarch is also a 6% solution with particles ranging from 10,000 to 1,000,000 daltons in molecular weight, a number average molecular weight of 69,000 daltons, and a colloid osmotic pressure of 34 mm Hg. The recommended dose of synthetic colloids for the treatment of shock is up to 20 ml/kg in the dog and up to 10 ml/kg in the cat (note that rapid administration of hydroxyethyl starch in the cat has been reported to cause vomiting). Excessive volumes can lead to volume overload, coagulopathies, and hemodilution. These fluids are appropriately used for shock therapy in acutely hypoproteinemic animals (total protein less than 3.5 g/dl) with a decreased colloid osmotic pressure. They can also be used with isotonic or hypertonic crystalloids to maintain adequate plasma volume expansion with lower interstitial fluid volume expansion and to expand the intravascular space with smaller volumes over a shorter time period. Despite multiple clinical studies in humans, there is no definitive documentation that the use of colloids is superior to the use of crystalloids for resuscitation, and the price of colloids is significantly greater than that of crystalloids (for further details, see Chapter 11).

Hypertonic Saline Plus Synthetic Colloid Solutions

To prolong the effect of the resuscitation fluids, a hypertonic saline/synthetic colloid (dextran 70 or hydroxyethyl starch) mixture can be administered for the treatment of shock. A 1:2.5 ratio of 23.4% NaCl with dextran 70 or hetastarch makes an ≈7.5% saline mixture (44 ml of 23.4% NaCl in 106 ml of dextran 70 or hydroxyethyl starch).

Blood Component Therapy

The need for blood products during resuscitation relates to the patient's disease process. Most fluid-responsive shock patients tolerate acute hemodilution to a hematocrit of less than 20%. In animals with acute blood loss that are unresponsive to fluid therapy alone, the hematocrit should be maintained at more than 25% to 30% to maximize oxygen-carrying capacity. Excessive increases in hematocrit should be avoided since this will increase blood viscosity. Most animals can tolerate an acute loss of 10% to 15% of blood volume without requiring a blood transfusion. Acute hemorrhage exceeding 20% of the blood volume often requires transfusion therapy in addition to the initial fluid resuscitation discussed previously. In animals with acute blood loss requiring transfusion therapy, fresh whole blood or packed red blood cells and fresh frozen plasma should be used in an attempt to stabilize clinical signs of shock and maintain the hematocrit above 25% and clotting times within the normal range.

Packed red blood cells and fresh frozen plasma are administered at a dose of 10 to 15 ml/kg, and fresh whole blood at a dose of 20 to 25 ml/kg. Refrigerator-stored plasma or frozen plasma that is more than 1 year old no longer contains platelets or the labile coagulation factors (V, VIII, and von Willebrand). Platelets are only present in fresh blood within 6 hours of collection, and their use is indicated in animals with thrombocytopenia/thrombocytopathia–induced bleeding disorders or massive hemorrhage. Plasma products are most commonly used in animals with profound blood loss, a coagulopathy, or severe hypoalbuminemia. The ability of these products to increase colloid osmotic pressure is limited compared to the hyperoncotic synthetic colloids. However, blood products do supply albumin, an important carrier of certain drugs, hormones, metals, chemicals, toxins, and enzymes. Blood products generally should be administered over at least 1 to 2 hours to monitor for a transfusion reaction and avoid volume overload, but it may be necessary to bolus these products in life-threatening situations. A blood type should be determined in all animals, especially cats, before transfusions are given. Crossmatching also helps to decrease the incidence of transfusion reactions.

Human Serum Albumin Solution

Animals with severe hypoalbuminemia may benefit from treatment with 25% human albumin. Albumin is crucial in the transport of drugs, hormones, chemicals, toxins, and enzymes. Preliminary studies in dogs show that human albumin administration in dogs increases circulating albumin concentrations, total solids, and colloid osmotic pressure, although the effect on mortality remains unknown. Current and future studies will provide more information regarding the use of this product. Potential risks are similar to those for any blood transfusion (i.e., fever, vomiting, increased respiratory effort) in addition to the potential for increasing clotting times.

Recent reports of albumin-induced anaphylaxis in normal dogs require further investigation (Mathews and Barry, 2005).

Vasopressors and Positive Inotropes

Shock patients that remain hypotensive despite intravascular volume resuscitation often require vasopressor and/or inotrope therapy. Since both cardiac output and systemic vascular resistance affect DO_2 to the tissues, therapy for hypotensive patients includes maximizing cardiac function with fluid therapy and inotropic drugs and/or modifying vascular tone with vasopressor agents. This is particularly important in cardiogenic shock (see Chapter 171). Commonly used vasopressors include catecholamines (epinephrine, norepinephrine, and dopamine) and the sympathomimetic drug phenylephrine. In addition, vasopressin, corticosteroids, and glucagon have been used as adjunctive pressor agents.

Different sympathomimetics cause various changes in the cardiovascular system, depending on the specific receptor stimulation caused by the drug. Conventionally adrenergic receptor location and function involve the α-1 and β-2 receptors located on the vascular smooth muscle cells that lead to vasoconstriction and vasodilation, respectively, whereas β-1 receptors in the myocardium primarily modulate inotropic and chronotropic activity. In addition, there are dopaminergic-1 receptors in the renal, coronary, and mesenteric microvasculature that mediate vasodilation and dopaminergic-2 receptors in the synaptic nerve terminals that inhibit the release of norepinephrine.

Dopamine has various potential actions on adrenergic and dopaminergic receptors. Primarily dopaminergic effects are seen at low intravenous dosages (1 to 5 mcg/kg/minute); mainly β-adrenergic effects are seen at moderate dosages (5 to 10 mcg/kg/minute); mixed α- and β-adrenergic effects are present at high dosages (10 to 15 mcg/kg/minute); and primarily α-adrenergic effects are seen at very high dosages (15 to 20 mcg/kg/minute). The actual dose-response relationship is unpredictable in a given patient because it depends on individual variability in enzymatic dopamine inactivation, receptor down-regulation, and the degree of autonomic derangement. Dopamine can be used as a single-agent therapy to provide both inotropic and pressor support in animals with vasodilation and decreased cardiac contractility. In comparison to other pressor drugs, dopamine is a less potent inotrope than epinephrine (or dobutamine) and less vasoconstricting than norepinephrine. The cardiovascular effects of dopamine may dissipate after several days of therapy, perhaps because of receptor down-regulation and/or induction of increased postsynaptic norepinephrine release. Despite the beneficial effects of dopamine on cardiac output and blood pressure, it may have deleterious effects on renal, mesenteric, and skeletal blood flow.

Norepinephrine (NE) has mixed α- and β-adrenergic receptor agonist effects with preferential α- receptor activity. Therefore the effects on heart rate and contractility are mild, and NE is commonly used as a pressor agent in animals with normal or increased cardiac output states. Canine septic shock models have demonstrated that the effects of NE on cardiac function are diminished compared to those of nonseptic controls. In septic patients with cardiac insufficiency and vasodilation, it may be desirable to use NE in conjunction with dobutamine (a potent β-agonist) to prevent the deleterious effects of increasing afterload in the face of a diseased heart. Renal blood flow may improve in animals with septic shock so long as arterial blood pressure is normalized. Conversely, NE administration to dogs with hypovolemic shock induces deleterious renal vasoconstriction. NE was also shown to improve urine output and creatinine clearance when added to dopamine or dobutamine in human patients with septic shock. Enhanced splanchnic DO_2 and increases in gastric mucosal pH are evident in humans who receive NE therapy for the treatment of hypotensive septic shock. The vasopressor dosage of NE in humans (and extrapolated to dogs) is 0.05 to 3.3 mcg/kg/minute IV.

Epinephrine (Epi) is a potent pressor with mixed α- and β-agonist activity. Although Epi is thought to have more potent β-agonist effects than NE, individual response is quite variable in patients with systemic inflammatory diseases and hypotension. Epi may significantly impair splanchnic blood flow compared to norepinephrine and dobutamine (in combination). This is most likely because of the strong α-adrenergic activity of Epi with subsequent vasoconstriction in regional vascular beds, although Epi also activates vasodilatory β-receptors. The vasopressor dosage of intravenous Epi is 0.01 to 0.1 mcg/kg/minute and for primarily β-agonist effects 0.005 to 0.02 mcg/kg/minute. Epi is rarely used as a sole first-line vasopressor agent because of its potential side effects, but it may be necessary in critically ill animals. Epi also inhibits mast cell and basophil degranulation and therefore is the drug of choice in patients suffering from anaphylactic shock. It is also commonly used for the treatment of cardiac arrest.

Phenylephrine is a pure α-agonist drug that causes profound vasoconstriction. It has been shown to cause an increase in cardiac output and blood pressure, presumably as a result of increased venous return to the heart and activation of α-1 receptors in the myocardium. Typically phenylephrine is used in patients that are unresponsive to other sympathomimetics, although it can be used as a sole first-line agent in vasodilated, hypotensive animals. Since phenylephrine has no β-agonist activity, it is the least arrhythmogenic of the sympathomimetic pressor drugs and therefore is desirable in animals that develop tachyarrhythmias in response to other pressor agents. The intravenous dosage range is 0.5 to 3 mcg/kg/minute.

Dobutamine is a β-agonist with weaker, dose-dependent α-effects. It increases cardiac output, DO_2, and VO_2 without causing vasoconstriction at lower doses. Therefore it is useful in animals with shock caused by cardiac insufficiency. Dobutamine may worsen or precipitate tachyarrhythmias and may precipitate seizure activity in cats. The intravenous dosage range is 1 to 5 mcg/kg/minute in cats and 2.5 to 20 mcg/kg/minute in dogs.

Vasopressin is a nonadrenergic vasopressor agent. It has both direct and indirect effects on the vascular smooth muscle via the V1 receptors and induces vasoconstriction in most vascular beds. In vitro vasopressin is a more potent vasoconstrictor than phenylephrine or NE. At low doses this drug causes vasodilation in renal, pulmonary, mesenteric, and cerebral vasculature in an attempt to maintain perfusion to these vital organs. Low flow states secondary to hypovolemia or septic shock are associated with a biphasic response in endogenous serum vasopressin levels. There is an early increase in the release of vasopressin from the neurohypophysis in response to hypoxia, hypotension, and/or acidosis, which leads to high levels of serum vasopressin. This plays a role in the stabilization of arterial pressure and organ perfusion in the initial stages of shock. There appears to be a subsequent decrease in circulating vasopressin levels, most likely a result of a depletion of hypothalamic stores. Therefore the use of vasopressin in animals in the later stages of shock, especially those that exhibit vasodilation and are refractory to catecholamine therapy, may be beneficial. The drug also enhances sensitivity to catecholamines and therefore may allow the dose of concurrent catecholamine therapy to be lowered. Experimental studies in dogs have demonstrated an increase in blood pressure and cardiac output with minimal side effects. A clinical case series using vasopressin at 0.5 to 4 mU/kg/minute found an increase in blood pressure following vasopressin therapy as well. This drug will require further investigation but may be considered in animals with catecholamine-resistant vasodilatory shock.

Glucagon typically is secreted from the pancreas and is classified as a counterregulatory hormone. It activates adenylate cyclase independent of β-adrenergic receptor stimulation. Exogenously administered glucagon causes a positive inotropic effect that leads to an increase in cardiac output and blood pressure. This drug may be useful in critically ill patients that are unresponsive to β-agonist drugs or those receiving sympathomimetic therapy that is complicated by β-blocker agents. Further research is needed.

Antimicrobials

Early antibiotic therapy is important in shock patients with proven or suspected sepsis. If possible, properly collected cultures of blood, urine, respiratory secretions (collected by endotracheal wash, transtracheal wash, or bronchoscopy) and other available body fluids (i.e., pleural, peritoneal, or cerebrospinal fluid) should be sampled carefully before antimicrobial therapy is begun. Broad-spectrum antibiotic therapy should be initiated pending culture and sensitivity results. Empiric antibiotic choices should be effective against gram-positive and gram-negative organisms and anaerobes. Initial combinations might include ampicillin (22 mg/kg IV q6-8h) and enrofloxacin (15 mg/kg IV q24h in dogs, 5 mg/kg IV q24h in cats); ampicillin and amikacin (15 mg/kg IV q24h); cefazolin (22 mg/kg IV q8h) and amikacin, ampicillin, and ceftazidime (22 mg/kg IV q8h); or clindamycin (10 mg/kg IV q8-12h) and enrofloxacin. Single agents such as ticarcillin/clavulanic acid (50 mg/kg IV q6h), cefoxitin (15 to 30 mg/kg IV q4-6h), or imipenem (5-10 mg/kg IV q6-8h, if bacterial resistance is suspected) could be used initially as well.

Gastrointestinal Protection

Stress-related mucosal disease (SRMD) and subsequent upper GI bleeding are frequently seen in critically ill humans and may also occur in dogs and cats. Clinical signs of hematemesis, hematochezia, or melena should alert the clinician to potentially serious GI hemorrhage. Hypoperfusion of the upper GI mucosa during shock, excessive gastric acid secretion, and impaired mucosal defense mechanisms (mucus secretion, production of growth factors) contribute to the development of SRMD. Furthermore, in humans factors thought to increase the risk of stress-related GI hemorrhage include prolonged mechanical ventilation, extensive burns, hepatic failure, renal failure, coagulopathy, head injuries, multiple trauma, high-dose corticosteroids, nonsteroidal antiinflammatory use, and absence of enteral nutrition. In veterinary patients the incidence of SRMD and clinically significant bleeding is unknown; therefore no guidelines exist for their management.

The initial strategy in critically ill dogs and cats should be to ensure adequate GI perfusion and use early enteral nutrition. High-risk patients should receive pharmacologic prophylaxis for stress-related GI hemorrhage. Based on the currently available evidence in human medicine, it appears that proton pump inhibitors (PPIs) are superior to histamine-2 receptor antagonists (H_2RAs), which are superior to sucralfate in the prevention of SRMD in adult critical-care patients. Drugs available include omeprazole (PPI) 0.7 to 1 mg/kg PO q24h, pantoprazole (PPI) 0.7 to 1 mg/kg IV q24h, famotidine (H_2RA) 0.5 to 1 mg/kg IV q12-24h PO, ranitidine (H_2RA) 0.5 to 4 mg/kg IV q8-12h, and sucralfate (protectant) 0.25 1 g/25 kg PO q6-8h. Recent evidence suggests that ranitidine does not decrease acid production in dogs at clinically recommended doses (Bersenas et al., 2005; Cook et al., 1999).

Nutrition

Following initial stabilization of the shock patient, nutritional status should be addressed (see Chapter 3). Adequate nutrition is critical in patients with secondary hypermetabolic states such as sepsis. The enteral route (orally or via nasoesophageal, esophagostomy, gastrostomy, or jejunostomy tube) is preferable if the animal is normotensive, not vomiting, and alert. Parenteral nutrition should be administered if the enteral route is not feasible or contraindicated. If the blood glucose falls below 60 g/dl, 0.5 ml/kg of 50% dextrose should be diluted 1:1 with sterile water and administered IV over 1 to 2 minutes. The fluids should also be supplemented with dextrose as needed (2.5% to 7.5%). Hyperglycemia should be avoided since it has been associated with an increased likelihood of infection and a poorer prognosis.

Novel Therapeutic Strategies

Early Goal-Directed Therapy

For many years it has been recognized that critically ill patients in shock benefit from rapid normalization of abnormal physiologic functions. Many therapeutic strategies have been studied, including reestablishing normal or even supranormal hemodynamics values to improve the outcome of patients in shock. Although the use of supranormal resuscitation has not proven beneficial, the use of early goal-directed therapy has shown early promise (Kern and Shoemaker, 2002).

Early goal-directed therapy is performed using a series of predefined resuscitation end points to help clinicians resuscitate shock patients as soon as the syndrome is recognized. The aim of these specific end points is to adjust cardiac preload, contractility, and afterload to balance systemic DO_2 with demand. Recently the effect of early goal-directed therapy was evaluated in a prospective, randomized clinical trial that included humans who presented to an emergency room with severe sepsis, septic shock, or sepsis syndrome (Rivers et al., 2001). During the first 6 hours of resuscitation from sepsis-induced hypoperfusion, patients treated with early goal-directed therapy received, in a sequential fashion, fluid resuscitation, vasopressors or dilator agents, red-cell transfusions, and inotropic medications to achieve target levels of central venous pressure (8 to 12 mm Hg), MAP (65 to 90 mm Hg), urine output (as least 0.5 ml/kg of body weight), and $ScvO_2$ (at least 70%). The other group of patients was treated following a standard therapy at their clinician's discretion. Ultimately patients resuscitated following the early goal-directed therapy plan had higher survival rates. In dogs and cats initiating a similar goal-directed therapy strategy immediately after recognition of a shock syndrome might be beneficial. The use of $ScvO_2$ monitoring requires further research in veterinary patients.

Relative Adrenal Insufficiency and Use of Steroids

Adrenal insufficiency of critical illness is a well-recognized clinical entity in humans, especially those suffering from sepsis (Cooper and Stewart, 2003). These patients have an increased morbidity and mortality, and the use of physiologic doses of steroids has been shown to improve outcome. Adrenal insufficiency may be secondary to both a decrease in glucocorticoid synthesis (i.e., adrenal insufficiency) and peripheral resistance to glucocorticoids. The diagnosis of the dysfunction relies on assessment of plasma cortisol before and after exogenous corticotropin administration (ACTH stimulation test). A relative adrenal insufficiency may lead to refractory hypotension in shock patients or those with critical illness since steroids normally suppress endogenous vasodilators such as the kallikrein-kinin system, prostacyclin, and nitric oxide. Glucocorticoids also modify the renin-angiotensin system and up-regulate angiotensin II receptors in the vasculature. The use of physiologic doses of steroids in people with refractory hypotension has been well studied (Annane et al., 2004). Critically ill, hypotensive animals may also benefit from physiologic doses of corticosteroids, but further research is required to confirm this. There is controversy regarding the definition of an "adequate" response, the dose of ACTH that should be administered, and the constituents of "replacement" therapy.

In specific situations critically ill patients might benefit from glucocorticoid supplementation. The use of etomidate, which blocks the synthesis of cortisol by reversible inhibition of 11-β-hydroxylase, has an inhibitory effect on adrenal function in critically ill patients and has been associated with an increase in intensive care unit mortality. Patients receiving treatment with corticosteroids for chronic autoimmune or inflammatory diseases and those receiving replacement therapy for hypoadrenocorticism should receive at least physiologic doses of prednisone or dexamethasone during severe illness.

References and Suggested Reading

Annane D et al: Corticosteroids for treating severe sepsis and septic shock, *Cochrane Database Syst Rev* 1:CD002243, 2004.

Bersenas AM et al: Effects of ranitidine, famotidine, pantoprazole, and omeprazole on intragastric pH in dogs, *Am J Vet Res* 66(3):425, 2005.

Boag A, Hughes D: Assessment and treatment of perfusion abnormalities in the emergency patient, *Vet Clin North Am Small Anim Pract* 35(2):319, 2005.

Brady CA et al: Severe sepsis in cats: 29 cases (1986-1998), *J Am Vet Med Assoc* 217(4):531, 2000.

Cook D et al: Risk factors for clinically important upper gastrointestinal bleeding in patients requiring mechanical ventilation, *Crit Care Med* 27(12):2812, 1999.

Cooper MS, Stewart PM: Corticosteroids insufficiency in acutely ill patients, *N Engl J Med* 348:727, 2003.

Costello MF et al: Underlying cause, pathophysiologic abnormalities, and response to treatment in cats with septic peritonitis: 51 cases (1990-2001), *J Am Vet Med Assoc* 225(6):897, 2004.

dePapp E et al: Plasma lactate concentration as a predictor of gastric necrosis and survival among dogs with gastric-volvulus: 102 cases (1995-1998), *J Am Vet Med Assoc* 215(1):49, 1999.

Hughes D et al: Effect of sampling site, repeated sampling, pH and Pco_2, on plasma lactate concentration in healthy dogs, *Am J Vet Res* 60(4):521, 1999.

Kern JW, Shoemaker WC: Meta-analysis of hemodynamic optimization in high-risk patients, *Crit Care Med* 30(8):1686, 2002.

Lagutchik MS et al: Increased lactate concentrations in ill and injured dogs, *J Vet Emerg Crit Care* 8(2):117, 1998.

Mathews KA, Barry M: The use of 25% human serum albumin: outcome and efficacy in raising serum albumin and systemic blood pressure in critically ill dogs and cats, *J Vet Emerg Crit Care* 15(2):110, 2005.

McMichael MA et al: Serial plasma lactate concentration in 68 puppies aged 4 to 80 days, *J Vet Emerg Crit Care* 15(1):17, 2005.

Nel M et al: Prognostic value of blood lactate, blood glucose and hematocrit in canine babesiosis, *J Vet Intern Med* 18(4):471, 2004.

Nguyen HB et al: Early lactate clearance is associated with improved outcome in severe sepsis and septic shock, *Crit Care Med* 32 (8):1637, 2004.

Rivers E et al: Early goal directed therapy in the treatment of severe sepsis and septic shock, *N Engl J Med* 345:1368, 2001.

Schutzer KM et al: Lung protein leakage in feline septic shock, *Am Rev Respir Dis* 147:1380, 1993.

Silverstein DC et al: Assessment of changes in blood volume in response to resuscitative fluid administration in dog, *J Vet Emerg Crit Care* 15(3):185, 2005.

CHAPTER 2

Acute Pain Management

ANDREA L. LOONEY, *Ithaca, New York*

Acute pain has many causes in the small animal population, from vehicular injury, myocardial damage, and musculoskeletal pain, through crush or fall injuries, pancreatitis, and gastric distention, to quill migration, disk injury, and surgical pain. Regardless of injury type, all patients share at least one common pathology—pain. Yet, despite this universality, there appears to be no clear definition across patients. However, we do know that pain induces many physiologic changes that can be acutely detrimental to patients. Among these are increased sympathetic tone, decreased or shunted gastrointestinal (GI) or urinary blood flow, increased blood viscosity, prolonged clotting time, and platelet aggregation. Long-term effects of uncontrolled pain include thromboembolism, ventilation perfusion mismatch, hypoxemia, hypercapnia, increased myocardial work and oxygen consumption, immunosuppression, decreased wound healing, and increased incidence of postsurgical complications. Because pain had surpassed the definition of "detriment" and was becoming recognized as an actual disease, the Joint Commission on Accreditation of Healthcare Organizations (JCAHO) announced standards for the regular assessment and management of pain in humans in 1999. The American Animal Hospital Association (AAHA) followed suit in 2003, releasing its Pain Management Standards, established to define pain in both preventable and treatable terms for all small animal patients. The American Pain Society has declared pain the "fifth vital sign." Accordingly, pain should now be assessed both subjectively and objectively in all veterinary inpatients and outpatients along with other vital parameters. This chapter describes assessment, prevention, and treatment of acute pain in these types of critical patients, cognizant of the emergent nature of many diseases, but striving toward appropriate analgesic management.

PAIN SCORING IN CRITICALLY ILL ANIMALS

The importance of assessing pain is magnified when caring for critically ill, intensive care, acutely traumatized, or surgical patients. Recent literature in emergency medicine suggests that intubated patients near or after code receive inadequate analgesia, likely because of initial misconceptions regarding autonomic signs. In one study intubated patients with hypertension received analgesia; those with hypotension did not. Higher mortality rates were seen in the latter group. Retrospective analysis demonstrated both groups to have shown subtle yet unequivocal behavioral signs of pain. Slower regular administration of analgesics (such as continuous-rate infusions [CRIs]), choosing analgesics with less effect on cardiac output (opioids, nonsteroidals), and using simple nonpharmacologic methods

of analgesia (e.g., local blockade, ice) would have been appropriate for these patients despite their hypotension. Animals with systemic inflammatory response syndrome demonstrate pain-induced dysfunction of neurons, vasculature, and many major organs; however, it is particularly difficult even for well-trained nurses, technicians, and clinicians to evaluate these patients regarding pain.

Although acute pain is associated with objective physiologic signs caused by autonomic nervous system activity, the critical or emergent patient may already be experiencing signs such as tachycardia, tachypnea, hypertension, and changes in blood glucose secondary to the surgical, traumatic, or acute-on-chronic conditions. Critical patients also have iatrogenically induced pain from recumbency, venipuncture, bandages or wraps, turning, wound care, catheterization, and suctioning. A recent study undertaken by the American Association of Critical Care Nurses identified positional turning alone as one of the most distressful and painful procedures for recent surgical and traumatized adult humans. Pain in these patients is also amplified as a result of stress, altered sleep, urination and defecation cycles, dietary changes, fear, anxiety, and polypharmacy interactions. Also unfortunate is the fact that pain may be unappreciated in the heavily sedated, paralyzed, or ventilated patient.

Pain scoring is the repetitive process whereby pain status is assessed regularly. More important than choosing one scoring system over another are a few simple facts: (1) serial assessment using both behavioral and physiologic parameters should be used; (2) *pain should be included as a cause of changes in physiologic parameters such as hypercapnia, tachycardia, or changes in blood sugar;* (3) individual behaviors suggestive of pain should override any "scoring"; and (4) the gold standard for determining if pain is the cause of a physiologic or behavioral change is administration of an analgesic drug or technique and observation of its effect. Although recent veterinary literature has stressed attention to both physiologic and behavioral characteristics of pain, it can be challenging to differentiate among the possible etiologies within critical patient populations. As such, behavioral "scoring" often takes precedence; appreciation of both overt and subtle changes in demeanor, responsiveness, and interaction qualities is needed.

In noncomatose patients, if objective characteristics of pain are not convincing, the patient should be examined for overt behavioral signs of pain. These include panting, shaking, increased respiratory effort, inability to position or move appropriately, pain on palpation near or distant from the wounds, licking, chewing, inappetence, crying, barking, and anxiety. The University of Melbourne Pain Scale and the Glasgow Composite Measures Pain Scale short form offer two well-established pain-scoring systems for

Simple Pain Scoring System for Noncomatose Patients

Technicians, nursing staff and clinicians ask these seven questions regularly (q2-6h in critical, emergent, or trauma patients). Answers to the questions guide assignment of a "score" based on a scale of 0 to 5, denoted on the line below. Final scoring is subjective but should be relative to the patient's previous score. Any obvious behavioral or physiologic sign indicative of pain automatically places the score at more than 3.

1. Is the patient's heart rate and respiratory rate comparable to its preinsult or species normal values?
2. Is the patient willing to get up, walk unassisted, and move without discomfort?
3. Is the patient's anxiousness, nervousness, aggravation, restlessness controlled?
4. Is the patient vocally quiet at rest and during interaction?
5. Is the patient appetent or interested in eating?
6. Can you palpate on or near the surgical site without the patient reacting?
7. Are your interactions with the patient pleasing to you and to him or her?

More "yes" answers to the above questions indicate lower pain scores (better-controlled pain). More "no" answers to the above questions indicate higher pain scores (animals need additional analgesia).

```
*                                                      *
0          1          2          3          4          5
Comfortable                                  Very painful
```

Pain Scoring System for Comatose, Heavily Sedated, Anesthetized, Intubated, Paralyzed, or Mechanically Ventilated Patients

Technicians, nursing staff, and clinicians ask these questions regularly (q2-6h). Answers to the questions guide assignment of a "score" based on a scale of 0 to 5, denoted on the line below. Final scoring is subjective but should be relative to the patient's previous score. Any obvious behavioral or physiologic sign indicative of pain automatically places the score at more than 3.

1. Is the patient's heart rate and respiratory rate comparable to its preinsult or species normal values?
2. Has pain been ruled out as a differential for vital parameter changes? (Test dose of fentanyl 3 to 5 mcg/kg and midazolam 0.1 to 0.3 mg/kg can be used to determine if pain is cause of parameter changes.)
3. Is the patient quiet at rest? (Listen for subtle moaning, crying, whining, or grunting. Mechanical ventilation may need to be silenced momentarily to perceive subtle vocalizations, especially in cats.)
4. Subtle muscle twitches or contractions; tremors; or fasciculations, including grimacing, squinting, whisker movement, lip, or muzzle changes; are not seen during interaction or observation. Is this true?
5. Overt stiffening of axial or appendicular muscles, splinting, opisthotonos or ventriflexion - is not seen during interaction. Is this true?
6. Palpation at or near the insult, injury, or surgical site is not painful. Is this true?
7. Defecation or urination is not seen during interaction. Is this true?
8. Urinary or anal sphincter tone does not change with interaction near or distant to the insult or injury site. Is this true?
9. There is an *absence* of teeth chattering, grinding, or temporomandibular and oropharyngeal activity during interaction or observation. Is this true?
10. There is no lacrimation or salivation seen with interaction or palpation of surgical/injury site. Is this true?
11. Increased or abdominal effort on inspiration is not observed, and respirations appear easy and uninhibited, not impeding mechanical ventilation if present. Is this true?

More "yes" answers to the above questions indicate lower pain scores (better-controlled pain). More "no" answers to the above questions indicate higher pain scores (animals need additional analgesia).

```
*                                                      *
0          1          2          3          4          5
Comfortable                                  Very painful
```

use in noncomatose patients. My own simple pain-scoring system for noncomatose patients is included in Box 2-1. In addition, within this population, some experts believe anxiety and pain should be scored and treated independently.

However, in the *comatose patient* pain is still present but with less overtly apparent expressions. Recent critical-care nursing literature shows that, no matter the level of consciousness, comatose and near-comatose adult patients react to a noxious stimulus by expressing subtle behavioral signs associated with pain. In veterinary patients I recommend close attention to subtle subjective assessment (presence or absence of squinting, grimacing, minor muscle twitching, papillary dilation, sphincter tone changes, body temperature changes, teeth grinding or chattering, ear pinning, photophobia), especially during nursing care or wound palpation, as a means of pain scoring. My pain-scoring system designed for comatose, mentally obtunded, sedated, or ventilated patients is summarized in Box 2-2.

THERAPY

Systemically administered opioids, α-2 adrenergic agonists, local anesthetics, and nonsteroidal antiinflammatory drugs (NSAIDs) are most widely used for acute pain therapy. Recently anticonvulsants, channel blocking agents, reuptake inhibitors, calcitonin, magnesium, β-blockade agents, bisphosphonates, and ketamine (classically labeled adjunctive agents) have been used to treat acute pain. Using a combination of drugs and techniques with different pain control mechanisms (known as *multimodal therapy*) improves analgesia and allows for a lower dosage of each single drug (supraadditive or synergistic effect), minimizing adverse drug effects of individual drugs. Ideally both nonpharmacologic and pharmacologic analgesia therapies should be directed at any or all of the four major steps in the nociceptive pathway: transduction at the periphery, transmission along neuronal axons to the dorsal horn of the spinal cord (peripheral nerves) or brainstem (cranial nerves), modulation at the dorsal horn of the spinal cord, and perception at the cerebrum.

Major Pharmacologic Agents

Opioid Analgesics

Opioids that interact with the mu receptor (fentanyl, morphine, oxymorphone, and hydromorphone) are noted for their ability to produce profound analgesia with mild if any sedation and little cardiovascular change. These are considered major analgesics and constitute the first line of pain control for critical, emergent, and acutely ill patients. Fentanyl, hydromorphone, and oxymorphone are my choices for acute pain management. Slow (over 2- to 5-minute) boluses constitute first-line analgesia, especially for the critical or acutely injured patient; CRIs of morphine, remifentanil, and fentanyl or, alternatively, intermittent injections of hydromorphone or oxymorphone allow continued analgesia in the same patient. Remifentanil is a potent analgesic requiring close attention to ventilatory status, but it is extremely useful because of its short half-life and metabolism via plasma esterases. Butorphanol, a mixed agonist-antagonist opioid, and buprenorphine, a partial agonist opioid, are *not* candidates for acute pain therapy because of their short-lived analgesic effect, profound sedative effect (masking pain), potent receptor adhesion, and ability to even potentiate (versus treat) pain.

A common "cocktail" used to treat patients in acute pain is the combination of an opioid (hydromorphone or oxymorphone 0.1 mg/kg, or fentanyl 3 to 5 mcg/kg) with a benzodiazepine (midazolam or diazepam 0.3 mg/kg) intravenously. Ketamine can also be added to these agents to provide analgesia along with immobilization. In most patients (except the animal with hypertension, hyperthyroidism, or overt cardiac failure), doses of 1 to 2 mg/kg of ketamine are usually well tolerated as an addition to the above cocktail. Transdermal opioids such as the fentanyl patch can be used as part of multimodal management. However, systemic uptake is very unreliable, especially in patients with circulatory and heat discrepancies. Furthermore, these agents are not capable of producing the immediate and profound analgesia necessary in traumatic, acute, or emergent situations. Transdermal systems are best used out of the emergent period or as adjunct methods of analgesia combined with more potent narcotics (intravenous [IV] opioids) and other agents initially. Fentanyl patches are best used in chronic, low-level pain states.

Of the major side effects seen with opioids, foremost is dose-related respiratory depression reflecting diminished response to carbon dioxide levels. Nausea, vomiting, and dysphoria are commonly observed in animals that are not in pain. The vast majority of injured patients either do not show or can tolerate these side effects. Outside of mild bradycardia, narcotics produce few if any clinically significant cardiovascular effects in dogs and cats. Bradycardia alone should not be contraindications to opioid use, especially in acute, emergent, or critical patients. Because opioids increase intracranial and intraocular pressure, they should be used more cautiously in patients with severe cranial trauma and/or ocular lesions. However, even in these patients opioids can be used with slow initial IV boluses, titratable CRI or intermittent low-dose intramuscular (IM) or partial IV/IM dosing. These approaches minimize vomiting and potent respiratory depression in ocular and head trauma patients. Most opioids depress the cough reflex via a central mechanism; this may be an advantage in intubated patients but may occasionally predispose to aspiration pneumonia.

Certain of the opioids are capable of causing intense histamine release (morphine/meperidine), which precludes them from being administered intravenously, at least in high dosages. Hydromorphone may cause panting but, more important, seems to cause consistent vomiting in small animals and frequent, sometimes dangerous, hyperthermia in cats. Repetitive use of opioids as solo analgesics often results in two complications: urinary retention and GI ileus (with inappetence, nausea, and constipation). Treatment of these complications involves multimodal therapy (using another form of analgesic concomitantly with the opioid), using a more titratable opioid (fentanyl or remifentanil), using antiemetic and prokinetic drugs, and instituting minor physical therapy (massage, passive range of motion [PROM], walking) if the patient's injury affords. Although analgesics are given intravenously whenever possible to ensure distribution of the drug and to avoid the need for painful IM injections, use of split IV and IM/ subcutaneous dosing at regular intervals (q6-8h) can reduce GI and urinary side effects, dysphoria, and agitation/panting, especially in feline patients.

A key characteristic of opioids that makes them desirable for use in emergency and critica-care situations is their reversibility. All reversal agents such as naloxone and naltrexone should be administered slowly (over 10 minutes) if given intravenously, in diluted form, and to effect. Many of the opiate reversal agents are stimulatory to the central nervous and cardiovascular systems if given quickly. Hypertension, tachycardias, and seizures may be seen with rapid administration. Antagonism of narcotics is very short-lived. As such it is common for these drugs to wane and for renarcotization to occur. All opioids are controlled substances; their strict regulations for ordering, storage, and record keeping may make them problematic. Yet these drugs are essential for pain control and constitute the most effective drug therapies for acute, critical, emergent, and perioperative pain (Table 2-1). Fig. 2-1 illustrates a reasonable first approach for using opioids for acute pain management in emergent patients.

Table **2-1**

Opioids for Critical Patient Management

Opioid	Dosage
Fentanyl	0.005-0.02 mg/kg q2h IM, IV, SQ or in CRI 0.1-0.2 mcg/kg/min
Remifentanil	1-3 mcg/kg IV, followed by 3-10 mcg/kg/h CRI because of extremely short initial bolus half-life
Morphine	0.1-0.5 mg/kg q4-8h IM, SQ in dogs; 0.1-0.3 mg/kg q12-24h in cats; or in CRI 0.02-0.1 mg/kg/hr in both species
Oxymorphone	0.02-0.1 mg/kg q4-12h IV, IM, SQ
Hydromorphone	0.02-0.2 mg/kg q4-12 h IV, IM, SQ
Meperidine	5-10 mg/kg IM, SC q2-4h

CRI, Continuous-rate infusion; *IM,* intramuscularly; *IV,* intravenously; *SQ,* subcutaneously.

Emergency case arrives

System triage
Venous access
Nova/Big 4

↓

Stabilization (airway, oxygen, volume, pressure, ventilator status, temperature, electrolyte, CNS status

↓

Injury, insult, or wound (SPICE)
(**S**tabilization, **P**rotection and Pressure, **I**ce and Immobilization, **C**ompression, **E**levation)

↓

Baseline pain score

Pain yes ←   → **Pain no**

Administer pure Mu agonist opioid +/− benzodiazepine[1]   Reassess in 15-30 min

Reassess pain score and stabilization within 1/2-1 hr   and

Pain yes ─────────────→ **Pain no** → Anxiety score → Microdose Acep[2]
                                                          → Benzodiazepine[2]
                                                          Microdose Alpha-two agent[2]

Moderate pain   **Severe pain**

Repeat pure Mu agonist opioid   Repeat pure Mu agonist opioid

Reassess for other sources of pain; reassess circulatory (pressure and volume), respiratory, CNS status

**And choose one or more of
the following agents listed below**

Mild pain   ***STABLE***   ***UNSTABLE***   ***STABLE***   ***UNSTABLE***
Choose one from
each category

TOPICAL AGENTS: **NSAIDS:**   **NMDA ANTAGONIST:**   **NSAIDS:**   **OPIOIDS:**
Lidocaine in sterile lube   Meloxicam 0.1 mg/kg IV   Ketamine 1-2 mg/kg IV,   Meloxicam 0.1 mg/kg IV   Fentanyl CRI[3]
Lidocaine patch   Carprofen 2.2 mg/kg SQ   IM, SQ q. 1-3 hr   Carprofen 2.2 mg/kg SQ   Remifentanil CRI[4]
Pramoxine 1%   ***ALPHA AGONISTS:***   **OPIOIDS:**   ***ALPHA AGONISTS:***   ***NMDA ANTAGONIST:***
Silver sulfadiazine   Medetomidine 2 mcg/kg IV   Fentanyl CRI[3]   Medetomidine CRI[5]   Ketamine CRI[6]
2% Diphenhydramine   ***Na CHANNEL BLOCK:***   ***Na CHANNEL BLOCK:***   ***COMBO INFUSIONS:***
                        Lidocaine CRI[7]   Lidocaine CRI[7]   MLK CRI[8]
                                                                                              FLK CRI[9]

OPIOIDS:
Buprenorphine 0.02 mg/kg IV, IM
or SQ q. 6-8 hr

Fentanyl patch application with   Would a ***Locoregional Block*** be possible and appropriate?
   repeat original opioid q. 4-8 hr

ADJUNCT ORAL MEDICATIONS:
Gabapentin 3-5 mg/kg PO q. 12 hr   ***Moderate pain***   ***Severe pain***
Tramadol 2-4 mg/kg PO q. 12 hr (dogs)   Epidural   Epidural catheter
   1-2 mg/kg PO q. 24 hr (cats)   Localized nerve or plexus blockade   Nerve or plexus catheter
Amantadine 3-5 mg/kg PO SID   Cavitary (e.g., intrapleural) or wound block   Wound soaker catheter
Acetaminophen 5 mg/kg PO (dogs only)   ↪
                                                                                Bupivicaine/Lidocaine/Morphine[10]
                                                                                   via catheter q. 4-8 hr or
IF STABLE:
Meloxicam 0.2 mg/kg PO, IV, SQ q. 24 hr   Lidocaine or Bupivicaine CRI
   (dogs), q. 48-72 hr (cats)   via catheter[11]
Carprofen 2.2 mg/kg PO, SQ q. 12 hr (dogs),
   q. 48-72 hr (cats)   Reassess critical system status and pain score q. 1-4 hr

α-2 Agonist Analgesics

This class of drug warrants special attention because of its potent analgesic power at doses that are also capable of inducing profound sedation and cardiovascular changes. α-2 Agonists have quickly attained "sedative analgesic" status in veterinary medicine. Used at ultra-low doses (often called microdoses), these are useful adjunct analgesics, especially when combined with narcotics. Medetomidine has proven to be equal to or better as a short-term analgesic than buprenorphine, hydromorphone, or oxymorphone for control of pain in dogs. Sedative and analgesic effects are the result of activation of presynaptic and postsynaptic α-2 receptors, which decrease pain-related norepinephrine transmission.

Most notable of α-2 agonist side effects are changes in heart rate and rhythm. Atrioventricular blocks, bradyarrhythmia, and sinus bradycardia are caused by vasoconstriction, decreased sympathetic output, and reflex increases in parasympathetic tone. These changes are even noticeable after microdosing. Arterial blood pressure usually increases transiently and then decreases to normal or mildly decreased levels. Cardiac output decreases drastically as a result of lowered cardiac contractile force and stroke volume, which precludes the use of α-2 agents as first-line analgesics for acute pain, even though myocardial circulation may actually improve in some species. Since α-2 receptors modulate the release of insulin by the pancreas, hyperglycemia and resultant glycosuria are produced. Diuresis is also caused by an antiadrenocorticotropic hormone effect on the renal tubules.

The coadministration of an opioid with medetomidine appears quite useful for enhanced sedation and analgesia well beyond that achieved with either drug alone. *Medetomidine and dexmedetomidine should be used after volume and pressure stabilization, perisurgically, and always as microdose adjunct agents in the acute pain care setting (see Fig 2-1).* Especially beneficial is the microdose of medetomidine (1 to 3 mcg/kg intravenously or intramuscularly, canine and feline) used to supplement pain relief provided by morphine, hydromorphone, or oxymorphone. Medetomidine brings a great benefit not appreciable with narcotic analgesics (i.e., stress reduction). Sympathetic stimulation is useful in the very peracute initial stages of injury but quickly (within 12 hours) becomes detrimental. Since systemic effects of the stress response add not only to difficulty in controlling pain via any method but also to increased chances of chronic pain states through central hypersensitization and "wind-up," blunting of this stress response can be extremely useful *in poststabilization* multimodal pain therapy. An added benefit of the α-2 agonists is the potential for rapid reversal in emergency or even titratable reversal with antagonist drugs such as atipamezole. Unlike reversal of the opioids, reversal of an α-2 agent is both complete and long lasting.

Contraindications for α-2 agonists include untreated shock, hypotension, hypertension, overt bleeding, clinical bradyarrhythmias, Addison's disease, and syncope. I use medetomidine as an adjunct agent with the following generalities: longer than 12 to 24 hours after initial insult (animal stabilized), in microdose form (Table 2-2) alternating between intermittent doses of narcotic or as a CRI, and, finally, only in patients capable of tolerating mild-to-moderate reduction of cardiac output. These drugs should not be used in patients experiencing shock or cardiovascular collapse.

Table **2-2**

Commonly Used α-2 Agonists

α-2 Agonist	Dosage
Dexmedetomidine	Dog: 0.001-0.003 mg/kg q4-6 h SQ, IM, IV
	Cat: 0.003-0.01 mg/kg q4-6 h SQ, IM, IV
	Both species: continuous-rate infusion of 0.2-2 mcg/kg/hr
Medetomidine	Dog: 0.001-0.005 mg/kg q 4-6 hr SQ, IM, IV
	Cat: 0.003-0.01 mg/kg q.4-6 hr SQ, IM, IV
	Both species: continuous rate infusion of 0.2-2 mcg/kg/hr

Fig. 2-1 Flow chart for acute pain management in the emergent patient. [1]Pure Mu agonists: Hydromorphone 0.05 to 0.1 mg/kg IV, IM, SQ; oxymorphone 0.1 to 0.2 mg/kg IV, IM, SQ; morphine 0.1 to 0.5 mg/kg IM; fentanyl 3 to 10 mcg/kg IV, IM, SQ. Benzodiazepines: Midazolam 0.3 to 0.5 mg/kg IV, IM, SQ; diazepam 0.2 to 0.5 mg/kg IV. SQ administration should be avoided in emergent, acute, and critical-care patients.
[2]Microdose anxiolytics: Acepromazine 0.01 to 0.05 mg/kg IV, IM, SQ not to exceed 0.3 mg in cats and 1 mg in dogs; diazepam and midazolam at doses noted in footnote 1; medetomidine or dexmedetomidine 1 to 3 mcg/kg IV, IM, SQ.
[3]Fentanyl continuous-rate infusion (CRI): 0.02 to 0.2 mcg/kg/min.
[4]Remifentanil CRI: 1 to 2 mcg/kg/hr; monitor ventilatory status cautiously in patients on remifentanil CRI. (MM Flores, personal communication.)
[5]Medetomidine CRI: 0.02 to 2 mcg/kg/hr.
[6]Ketamine CRI: 5 to 20 mcg/kg/min.
[7]Lidocaine CRI: dog: 50 to 100 mcg/kg/min.
[8]MLK CRI: see Table 2-4, drug calculator located at http://www.vasg.org/constant_rate_infusions.htm, or morphine 0.1 mg/kg/hr, lidocaine 50 mcg/kg/min, ketamine 10 mcg/kg/min (for cats delete lidocaine). (Courtesy of Dr. Robert Stein, DVM, DAAPM and Dr. David Thompson, DVM.)
[9]FLK CRI: Fentanyl 0.1 mcg/kg/min; lidocaine 50 mcg/kg/min; ketamine 10 mcg/kg/min (for cats, delete lidocaine).
[10]Intermittent injections via epidural catheter: 0.1 mg/kg morphine in 0.2 mg/kg bupivacaine with or without saline not to exceed 0.2 ml/kg total volume; intermittent injections via peripheral nerve catheters: 0.1 to 0.2 mg/kg bupivacaine with or without 0.2 to 1 mg/kg lidocaine with or without 0.01 mg/kg morphine with or without saline to expand for plexus coverage.
[11]CRIs via epidural catheter 0.05 mg/kg/hr bupivacaine or ropivacaine in 0.05 mg/kg/hr morphine.

Nonsteroidal Antiinflammatory Drugs

NSAIDs, classically used to treat chronic pain and inflammation, have taken on a new role in treatment of perioperative and acute pain. Potent oral and parenteral forms of these drugs compare favorably with opioids for treatment of acute inflammation and pain. Although multiple modes of action are proposed, most NSAIDs act by inhibiting the enzyme system cyclooxygenase (COX), an enzyme found in at least three forms (-1, -2, -3), prostanoids such as thromboxane, prostacyclin, prostaglandin (PG)E_2, PGF_2, and PGD_2. These prostanoids serve as mediators of inflammation and amplifiers of nociceptive input and transmission. They also affect homeostatic functions such as platelet adhesion, gastric epithelium turnover, renal vasodilation, and bronchodilation. Lipoxygenase (LOX), another enzyme inhibited by some NSAIDs, also acts on arachidonic acid to form eicosatetranoic acids and leukotrienes. All NSAIDs currently available inhibit COX-2, some avoid inhibition of COX-1 (coxibs), and some also act on LOX (tepoxalin). No single NSAID is substantially more effective than another at treating either acute or chronic pain. COX-1–sparing drugs are not inherently more effective than COX-1–inhibiting drugs.

There are definite and relative contraindications for the use of NSAIDs similar to those directed against the α-2 agents. NSAIDs should not be administered to patients with renal or hepatic insufficiency, dehydration, hypotension, conditions associated with low circulating volume (congestive heart failure, *unregulated anesthesia*, shock), or evidence of ulcerative GI disease. *The vascular volume, tone, and pressure of trauma patients should be completely stabilized before the use of NSAIDs.* Patients receiving concurrent administration of other NSAIDs or corticosteroids or those considered to be cushingoid should not receive parenteral NSAIDs, especially in emergent or acute situations. In addition, NSAIDs should not be used for patients with coagulopathies, particularly those that are caused by platelet number or function defects, or factor deficiencies, or for those with asthma or other bronchial disease.

Where does this leave us in terms of the acutely injured, traumatized, and emergent patient? *The administration of NSAIDs should ONLY be considered in the well-hydrated, normotensive dog or cat with normal renal or hepatic function, no hemostatic abnormalities, and no concurrent steroid administration.* Furthermore, although opioids and α-2 agonists seem to have an immediate analgesic effect, most NSAIDs take up to 30 minutes for a more subtle effect to be recognized. Thus NSAIDs are not first-line analgesics. However, their importance as part of the multimodal regimen should not be understated. NSAIDs are devoid of many of the side effects of narcotic administration and, compared to corticosteroids, do not suppress the pituitary-adrenal axis. NSAIDs are useful in treating initial tissue injury and suppressing central hypersensitization within the dorsal horn of the spinal cord, a phenomenon known to perpetuate chronic pain states. *These drugs are most useful in cases of orthopedic trauma, skin trauma, and appendicular soft-tissue bruising once stabilization of volume status and assessment of coagulation and renal function have occurred (see Fig 2-1).*

Cats are susceptible to the toxic effects of many NSAIDs because of slow clearance and dose-dependent

---

Table 2-3

Commonly Used NSAIDs

NSAID	Dosage
Carprofen	Dogs: 2-4 mg/kg PO, IM, IV, SQ q12h; cats: q48-72h
Flunixin meglumine	Dogs and cats: 0.5-1 mg/kg IM, SQ, IV q24-48h for three doses
Ketoprofen	Dogs: 0.5-1 mg/kg PO, IM, IV, SQ q12h; cats: q48-72h
Meloxicam	Dogs: 0.1-0.2 mg/kg q24h; cats 0.1 mg/kg q48-72h

IM, Intramuscularly; *IV,* intravenously; *SQ,* subcutaneously; *NSAID,* nonsteroidal antiinflammatory drug.

---

elimination secondary to deficient glucuronidation in this species. However, this species difference is not a contraindication to NSAID administration, especially when dealing with acute pain. Simply, both the dose and the dosing interval of most commonly used NSAIDs needs to be altered for these drugs to be used safely in cats.

In both canine and feline patients carprofen and meloxicam have impressive safety records compared to older injectable NSAIDs such as flunixin meglumine and ketoprofen. Nonloading (nonlabel) doses of either agent (Table 2-3) are preferred for acute multimodal therapy. Unlike opioids or α-2 agents, NSAIDs can be continued in the postacute care setting in oral forms.

Local and Regional Techniques of Pain Relief for the Acutely Painful Patient

Local anesthetics may be administered epidurally, intrathoracically, intraperitoneally, and intraarticularly. Lidocaine and bupivacaine are the most commonly administered local anesthetics. Lidocaine provides for quick, short-acting sensory and motor impairment. Bupivacaine provides for later-onset, longer-lasting desensitization without motor impairment. Combinations of the two agents diluted with saline are frequently used to provide for quick-onset analgesia with little motor impairment that lasts between 4 and 6 hours in most patients. Epinephrine-free solutions are recommended, especially in emergent patients. Placement of anesthetic close to nerves, roots, or a plexus is improved with the use of a stimulating nerve locator. Excellent reference to nerve localization for locoregional blockade is provided at www.ivis.org (see references). Cats seem to be more sensitive to the effects of local anesthetics, and the lower ends of most dosage ranges are safest for blockade in this species. Local and regional techniques block the initiation of noxious signals, thereby effectively "preventing" pain from entering the central nervous system. Frequently the neurohormonal response that is stimulated in both pain and stress is blunted as well. Overall the patient has less local and systemic adverse effects of pain, disease processes are minimized, chronic pain states are unlikely, and outcome is improved. Regional techniques are best applied as part of an analgesic regimen that consists of continuous administration, narcotics (with or without α-agonists), NSAIDs, anxiolytics, and good nursing (see Fig. 2-1). Extended-release (lipid-encapsulated) local anesthetics and opioids, recently available in human pain medicine, may make neuraxial and perineural catheterization unnecessary for long-term regional blockade.

Topical and Infiltrative Blockade

Lidocaine can be added to sterile lubricant in a one-to-one concentration to provide decreased sensation for urinary catheterization, nasal catheter insertion, minor road burn analgesia, and pyotraumatic dermatitis analgesia. Proparacaine is a topical anesthetic useful for corneal or scleral injuries. Local anesthetics can be infiltrated into areas of tissue trauma by using long-term continuous drainage catheters and small portable infusion pumps (www.milaint.com, www.bbraunusa.com). This is a very effective method of providing days of analgesia for massive surgical or traumatic soft-tissue injury. Even without the catheter, incisional or regional soft-tissue blocking using a combination of 1 to 2 mg/kg of lidocaine and 0.5 to 2 mg/kg of bupivacaine diluted with equal volume of saline is effective for infiltrating or "splash" blockading large areas of injury for 3 to 6 hours of analgesia.

Cranial Nerve Blockade

Administration of local anesthetic drugs around the infra-orbital, maxillary, ophthalmic, mental, and alveolar nerves can provide excellent analgesia for dental, orofacial, and ophthalmic trauma and surgical procedures. Each nerve may be desensitized by injecting 0.1 to 0.3 ml of a 2% lidocaine hydrochloride solution and 0.1 to 0.3 ml of a 0.5% bupivacaine solution using a 1.2- to 2.5-cm, 22- to 25-gauge needle. Precise placement (perineurally versus intraneurally with painful neuroma formation common with the latter) is enhanced by using catheters in the foramen versus simple needle administration. Aspiration should always be performed before administration of local agents to rule out intravascular injection.

Intrapleural Blockade

This block is used to provide analgesia for thoracic, lower cervical, cranial abdominal (gastric, hepatic, and pancreatic pain), and diaphragmatic pain. Following aseptic preparation, a small through-the-needle 20- to 22-gauge catheter is placed in the thoracic cavity between the seventh and ninth intercostal space on the midlateral aspect of the thorax. A 0.5- to 1-mg/kg dose of lidocaine and a 0.2- to 0.5-mg/kg dose of bupivacaine dose are aseptically mixed with a volume of saline equal to the volume of bupivacaine and slowly injected over a period of 2 to 5 minutes following aspiration to ensure no intravascular injection. Depending on the lesion, the patient should be positioned to allow the intrapleural infusion to "coat" the area. Most effective is positioning the patient in dorsal recumbency (if injury allows) for several minutes following the block to make sure that local anesthetic occupies the paravertebral gutters and thus the spinal nerve roots. The block should be repeated every 3 hours in dogs and every 8 to 12 hours in cats. The catheter is secured to the skin surface and capped for repetitive administration.

Brachial Plexus Blockade

Administration of local anesthetic around the brachial plexus provides excellent analgesia for forelimb surgery, particularly that distal to the shoulder, and for amputations. Nerve-locator guided techniques are much more accurate and successful than "blind" placement of local anesthetic; however, even the latter is very useful for forelimb injuries. Aseptic preparation is performed over a small area of skin near the point of the shoulder. A 22-gauge, 1.5- to 3-inch spinal needle is inserted medial to the shoulder joint, axial to the lesser tubercle, and advanced caudally, medial to the body of the scapula and toward the costochondral junction of the first rib. Aspiration ensures avascular injection of one third of the volume of local anesthetic mix. The needle is withdrawn slightly and then "fanned" dorsally and ventrally while the remaining solution is injected. Local anesthetic doses are similar to those for intrapleural blockade.

Epidural Anesthesia and Analgesia

Epidural analgesia refers to the injection of an opioid, a phencyclidine, an α-agonist, or an NSAID into the epidural space, whereas *epidural anesthesia* refers to the injection of only local anesthetic. In most patients a combination of the two is used. Epidurals are used for a variety of acute and chronic painful conditions, including surgery or trauma in the pelvis, hind limbs, abdomen, and thorax; amputations of forelimbs and hind limbs; tail or perineal procedures; C-sections; diaphragmatic hernia repairs; pancreatitis; peritonitis; and disk disease. Epidurals performed using opioids or less than 0.25% bupivacaine will not result in hind limb paresis or decreased urinary or anal tone (incontinence). Lidocaine or mepivacaine epidurals are prone to these side effects. Morphine is also one of the most useful opioids for administration in the epidural space because of its slow systemic absorption. Epidural catheters used for the instillation of drugs either through CRI or intermittent injection can be placed in both dogs and cats. Routinely placed through the lumbosacral space, these catheters are used with cocktails, including preservative-free morphine, bupivacaine, medetomidine, and ketamine. This therapy is effective for preventing "wind-up" pain in the peritoneal cavity or the caudal half of the body. Catheters may be maintained for 7 to 14 days if placed aseptically.

The animal is positioned in lateral or sternal recumbency. Sterile preparation is performed over the lumbosacral site. A 20- to 22-gauge 1.5- to 3-inch spinal or epidural needle is advanced through the skin caudal to the spine of L7. The skin penetration site is found by palpating the craniodorsal-most extent of the wings of the ilium bilaterally and drawing an imaginary line between them. The spine of L7 is located immediately behind this line. The site of entry is caudal to the spine. Entry into the epidural space is noted by loss of resistance or observing a drop of saline meniscus being pulled into the space. I prefer bupivacaine 0.1- to 0.3-mg/kg (motor sparing is less than 0.3%) with morphine 0.1 mg/kg for canine patients. This can be diluted to a total volume of 0.1 to 0.15 ml/kg with saline if advancement of the solution into the thoracic area is needed (e.g., thoracotomy, forelimb amputation, diaphragmatic repair). Total volume rarely exceeds 6 ml of saline, local and opioid combined for *dogs*. This calculation is appropriate for an injection made from the lumbosacral space. Injections made more cranial are reduced in volume by 25% per four to five vertebral bodies.

For cats 0.1 mg/kg of morphine is diluted with saline to a total volume of 0.1 to 0.2 ml/kg. Local anesthetic is rarely used because of the propensity to administer it into the subarachnoid space and the increased toxicity potential in this species.

Adjunct Agents and Techniques for Acute Pain

Over the past decade scores of other medications have been used to assist with analgesia in both critical and emergent patients. *Ketamine* was classically considered a dissociative anesthetic, but it also has potent activity as an N-methyl-D-aspartate receptor antagonist. This receptor located in the central nervous system mediates wind-up and central sensitization (a pathway from acute to chronic pain). Blockade of this receptor with microdoses of ketamine results in the ability to provide body surface, somatic, and skin analgesia and to potentially lower doses of opioids and α-agonists. Loading doses of 0.5 to 2 mg/kg are used intravenously initially and continued with CRIs of 2 to 20 mcg/kg/minute. High doses can aggravate, sensitize, or excite the animal in subacute or acute pain. *Tramadol* is an analgesic that possesses both weak mu opioid agonist activity and norepinephrine and serotonin reuptake inhibition. It is useful for mild-to-moderate pain when given orally at doses of 1 to 10 mg/kg PO SID/TID. Cats appear to require only once-a-day dosing, and some are intolerant of doses over 1 to 2 mg/kg/day. Regardless of its affinity for the opioid receptors, its true mechanism of action in companion animals remains largely unknown. *Gabapentin* is a synthetic analog of γ-aminobutyric acid. Originally introduced as an antiepileptic drug, its mechanism of action appears to be modulation of calcium channels. It is among a number of commonly used antiepileptic medications, including pregabalin, carbamazepine, and lamotrigine, that are used to treat central pain in humans. The rationale is their ability to suppress discharge in pathologically altered neurons. Chronic, burning, neuropathic, and lancinating pain (neuropathic pain) in small animals responds well to 3 to 10 mg/kg PO daily.

Ever since the introduction of local anesthetics, it has been common for clinicians to use drugs that block ion channels control pain. Sodium channels in particular are overexpressed in certain chronically inflamed tissues, particularly nervous tissue. *Lidocaine* is a local anesthetic. When given intravenously at a CRI, it is also effective in the treatment of acute and chronic pain. Side effects are minimal at a rate of 1 to 10 mcg/kg/minute for cats and 50 to 75 mcg/kg/minute in dogs. Pain relief in humans after even a brief IV infusion lasts many hours and sometimes even days. Acute pain is commonly treated in many postsurgical care units with *MLK infusions* (i.e., infusions containing standard amounts and rates of morphine, lidocaine, and ketamine). An example of one such infusion is included in Table 2-4. *Lidocaine patches* have been used for body surface, somatic, and skin pain in both cats and dogs. Patches come in 5% pliable, easily applicable, and moldable form; however, there is some concern about their adhesiveness in small animals, partially on haired skin. They are best applied to appendages and bandaged in place because of their inconsistent adhesive nature. In humans they appear to have a 12-hour life span, and recommendation is for removal before placement of another patch. Blood levels of lidocaine and by-products are not appreciated in either cats or dogs at this time. Likewise, potential for toxicity is low even in cats. Unlike fentanyl, there is little concern for respiratory depression, narcosis, or sedation in the patient or if human exposure occurs. These patches can also be cut and molded to fit an area of pain. I have used them on axial and appendicular structures for soft-tissue and bone pain, burns, road rash, hot spots, sprains, and strains at the following dosing scale (cats: ¼ to ½ 5% lidocaine patch q24 h; dogs: ¼ to 15% lidocaine patch q12 h). The patch should be removed for a minimum of 12 hours before application

---

Table 2-4

Morphine, Lidocaine, Ketamine (MLK) Continuous-Rate Infusion Formula for Perisurgical Analgesia

All milliliters of solution noted below are added to a 500-ml bag of balanced isotonic crystalloid fluids (avoid fluids containing lactate) after equal volumes of original solution are removed from the bag. If rate of delivery of final solution is maintenance rate of 60 ml/kg/day or 2.5 ml/kg/hour, the following analgesic rates will be administered: morphine 0.12 mg/kg/hour, lidocaine 50 mcg/kg/minute, and ketamine 10 mcg/kg/minute. If higher rates of intravenous fluids are required, additional nonadditive bags should be used to avoid overadministration or toxicity of constituent analgesics.

For cats, avoid lidocaine as part of continuous-rate infusion (CRI). I prefer reduction of each analgesic by half (milligram and milliliter amount) per 24 hours to avoid rebound pain from sudden CRI cessation.

	Concentration (mg/ml)	Milliliters of Analgesic to Add to 500 ml of Crystalloid Fluids	Total Milligrams of Analgesic Used (ml × concentration)	Total Milliliters of Crystalloid To Remove From 500-ml Bag Before Addition of Analgesics
Morphine	15	1.6	24	32.8 ml total = (1.6 ml + 30 ml + 1.2 ml)
Lidocaine	20	30	600	
Ketamine	100	1.2	120	

of a second patch. *Mexiletine* (4 to 10 mg/kg PO), an oral sodium channel blocker, can be used as an alternative to IV lidocaine for this background provision of analgesia.

Many physical therapy modalities are safe and can provide excellent analgesia for the patient in acute pain. The acronym of *PRICE* (protection, rest, ice, compression, and elevation), which applies to many acute musculotendinous injuries in human athletes, likely also fits many of our patients in acute pain. Patients in acute pain treated with both immobilization of the injured area (modified Robert Jones's bandage or a temporary splint) and cold compression have greater analgesia and less long-term inflammatory damage. Primary physiologic benefits of cold therapy are decreased local circulation, decreased pain, and decreased tissue extensibility. *Cold therapy compressed onto the injury site is one of the single most frugal means of providing immediate analgesia for acute injury.*

Analgesia goes hand-in-hand with solid nutrition, basic nursing care, attention to anxiety and stress, GI function, movement and motion, bladder and bowel control, and emotional state. Analgesia is also provided by getting an animal to its home environment as soon as possible, allowing family interaction and housemate socialization, and appropriate exercise and stimulation. These simple techniques and care concepts can prevent and reduce pain in the acute and chronically ill patient.

References and Suggested Reading

American College of Veterinary Anesthesiology: American College of Veterinary Anesthesiologists' position paper on the treatment of pain in animal, *J Am Vet Med Assoc* 213:628, 1998.

Campoy LC: Fundamentals of regional anesthesia using nerve stimulation in the dog. In Gleed RD, Ludders JW, editors: *Recent advances in veterinary anesthesia and analgesia*: companion animals, available at www.ivis.org.

Clark MR: Antidepressants. In Wallace MS, Staats PS, editors: *Pain medicine and management*, New York, 2005, McGraw Hill, p 52.

Gambling D et al: A comparison of DepoDur, a novel, single-dose extended-release epidural morphine, with standard epidural morphine for pain relief after lower abdominal surgery, *Anesth Analg* 100:1065, 2005.

Gelinas C et al: Validation of the critical care pain observation tool in adult patients, *Am J Crit Care* 15:420, 2006.

Granholm M et al: Evaluation of the clinical efficacy and safety of dexmedetomidine or medetomidine in cats and their reversal with atipamezole, *Vet Anaesth Analg* 33:214, 2006.

Hansen BD: Analgesia and sedation in the critically ill, *J Vet Emerg Crit Care* 15:285, 2005.

Hellebrekers LJ, Murrell JC: *Post-operative analgesia in dog*, *Proceedings from the 8th World Congress of Veterinary Anesthesia*, Knoxville, Tennessee, 2003, p 21.

Hellyer P: Objective, categoric methods for assessing pain and analgesia. In Gaynor JS, Muir WW, editors: *Handbook of veterinary pain management*, St Louis, 2002, Mosby, p. 82.

Holton LL et al: Development of a behaviour-based scale to measure acute pain in dogs, *Vet Rec* 148:525, 2001.

Holton LL et al: Comparison of three methods used for assessment of pain in dogs, *J Am Vet Med Assoc* 212:61, 1998.

Lomc B: Acute pain and the critically ill trauma patient, *Crit Care Nurs Q* 28:200, 2005.

Marino PL: *The ICU book*, ed 2, Baltimore, 1998, Williams & Wilkins.

Matthews KA: *Pain management for the critically ill parts I and II*, *Proceedings from the Western Veterinary Conference*, 2004, *Las Vegas*, NV.

Melzack R, Wall PD: *Handbook of pain management*, Philadelphia, 2003, Elsevier, p11.

Quandt JE, Lee JA, Powell LL: Analgesia in critically ill patient, *Compend Cont Educ Pract Vet* 23: 433, 2005.

Smith LJ et al: A single dose of liposome-encapsulated oxymorphone or morphine provides long-term analgesia in an animal model of neuropathic pain, *Comp Med* 53:280, 2003.

Stanik-Hutt JA et al: Pain experiences of traumatically injured patients in a critical care setting, *Am J Crit Care* 10:252, 2001.

Visser EJ: A review of calcitonin and its use in the treatment of acute pain, *Acute Pain* 7:185, 2005.

Resources on the Web

International Veterinary Academy of Pain Management: www.ivapm.org

International Veterinary Information Society: www.ivis.org

Veterinary Anesthesia Support Group: www.vasg.org

CHAPTER 3

Nutrition in Critical Care

DANIEL L. CHAN, *Hertfordshire, United Kingdom*

RATIONALE FOR NUTRITIONAL SUPPORT IN CRITICAL ILLNESS

Critical illness induces unique metabolic changes in animals that put them at high risk for malnutrition and its deleterious effects. In diseased states the inflammatory response triggers alterations in cytokines and hormone concentrations and shifts metabolism toward a catabolic state. In the absence of adequate food intake, the predominant energy source for the host is derived from accelerated proteolysis. Thus these animals may preserve fat deposits in the face of lean muscle tissue loss. Consequences of malnutrition include negative effects on wound healing, immune function, strength (both skeletal and respiratory), and ultimately overall prognosis. An important point in regard to nutritional support of hospitalized patients is that the immediate goal is not to achieve "weight gain," per se, which mostly likely reflects shift in water balance, but rather to minimize further loss of lean body mass. Reversal of malnutrition hinges on resolution of the primary underlying disease. Provision of nutritional support is aimed at restoring nutrient deficiencies and providing key substrates for healing and repair.

PATIENT SELECTION

As with any intervention in critically ill animals, nutritional support carries some risk of complications. The risk of complications most likely increases with the severity of the disease, and the clinician must consider many factors in deciding when to institute nutritional support. Of utmost importance, the patient must be cardiovascularly stable before any nutritional support is initiated. With reduced perfusion, processes such as gastrointestinal motility, digestion, and nutrient assimilation are altered; and feeding under such circumstances is likely to result in complications. Other factors that should be addressed before nutritional support include hydration status, electrolytes imbalances, and abnormalities in acid-base status.

In animals that have been stabilized, careful consideration must be given to the appropriate time to start nutritional support. A previously held notion that nutritional support is unnecessary until 10 days of inadequate nutrition have elapsed is certainly outdated and unjustified. Commencing nutritional support within 3 days of hospitalization, even before determining the diagnosis of the underlying disease, is a more appropriate goal in most cases; however, other factors should also be considered and are discussed in the next section.

NUTRITIONAL ASSESSMENT

Proposed indicators of malnutrition in animals include unintentional weight loss (typically greater than 10%), poor hair coat quality, muscle wasting, signs of inadequate wound healing, and hypoalbuminemia. However, these abnormalities are not specific to malnutrition and often occur late in the disease process. A greater emphasis is placed on evaluating overall body condition rather than simply noting body weight. The use of body condition scores (BCSs) has been shown to be reproducible and reliable and a clinically useful measure in nutritional assessment. Fluid shifts may significantly impact body weight, but BCSs are not affected by fluid shifts and therefore are helpful in assessing critically ill animals.

In light of the limitations of assessing nutritional status, it is crucial to identify early risk factors that may predispose patients to malnutrition such as anorexia of greater than 5 days' duration, serious underlying disease (e.g., severe trauma, sepsis, peritonitis, acute pancreatitis), and large protein losses (e.g., protracted diarrhea, draining wounds, or burns). Nutritional assessment also identifies factors that can impact the nutritional plan such as specific electrolyte abnormalities; the presence of hyperglycemia, hypertriglyceridemia, or hyperammonemia; or comorbid illnesses such as renal, cardiac or hepatic disease. In the presence of such abnormalities the nutritional plan should be adjusted accordingly to limit acute exacerbations of any preexisting condition.

Finally, since many of the techniques required for implementation of nutritional support (e.g., placement of most feeding tubes, intravenous catheters for parenteral nutrition) necessitate anesthesia, the patient must be properly evaluated and stabilized before induction of anesthesia. When the patient is deemed too unstable for general anesthesia, temporary measures of nutritional support that do not require anesthesia (e.g., nasoesophageal tube placement, placement of peripheral catheters for partial parenteral nutrition) should be considered.

NUTRITIONAL PLAN

Providing nutrition should occur as soon as it is feasible, with careful consideration for the most appropriate route of nutritional support. Providing nutrition via a functional digestive system is the preferred route of feeding, and particular care should be taken to evaluate if the patient can tolerate enteral feedings. Even if the patient can only tolerate small amounts of enteral nutrition, this route of feeding should be pursued and supplemented with parenteral nutrition (PN) as necessary to meet the patient's nutritional needs. However, if an animal demonstrates complete intolerance to being fed enterally, some form of PN should be provided. Implementation of the devised nutritional plan should also be gradual, with the goal of reaching target level of nutrient delivery in 48 to 72 hours. Adjustments to the nutritional plan are made on the basis of reassessment and the development of any complications.

CALCULATING NUTRITIONAL REQUIREMENTS

Based on indirect calorimetry studies in dogs, there has been a recent trend of formulating nutritional support simply to meet resting energy requirements (RERs) rather than more generous illness energy requirements (IERs). For many years clinicians used to multiply the RER by an illness factor between 1.1 and 2 to account for purported increases in metabolism associated with different disease states. However, less emphasis is now being placed on these extrapolated factors, and the current recommendation is to use more conservative energy estimates (i.e., start with the animal's RER) to avoid overfeeding and its associated complications. Examples of complications resulting from overfeeding include gastrointestinal intolerance, hepatic dysfunction, and increased carbon dioxide production. Although several formulas are proposed to calculate the RER, a widely used allometric formula can be applied to both dogs and cats of all weights. The formula most commonly used by the author is:

$$RER = 70 \times (\text{current body weight in kilograms})^{0.75}$$

Alternatively, for animals weighing between 3 and 25 kg, the following may be used:

$$RER = (30 \times \text{current body weight in kilograms}) + 70$$

In regard to protein requirements, hospitalized dogs should be supported with 4 to 6 g of protein per 100 kcal (15% to 25% of total energy requirements), whereas cats are usually supported with 6 or more g of protein per 100 kcal (25% to 35% of total energy requirements). In most cases estimation of protein requirements is based on clinical judgment and recognition that in certain disease states (e.g., peritonitis and draining wounds) protein requirements are markedly increased.

PARENTERAL NUTRITIONAL SUPPORT

PN can be delivered via a central vein (total PN [TPN]) or a peripheral vein (peripheral or partial PN [PPN]). TPN commonly refers to providing all of the animal's calorie and protein requirements via the intravenous route. PPN is reserved when the PN supplies only part of the animal's energy, protein, and other nutrient requirements. Because TPN supplies all of the animal's calorie and protein requirements, it is often the modality of choice for animals that cannot tolerate enteral feeding. The disadvantages are that it requires a jugular venous catheter, it is more expensive (typically about 15% to 25% more for a TPN solution compared to a PPN solution for the same-size animal), and it may be associated with more metabolic complications.

PPN may be an alternative to TPN in selected cases, but it is important to be aware that it will not provide all of the animal's requirements. Both TPN and PPN are typically a combination of dextrose, an amino acid solution, and a lipid solution. However, the concentration of some components (i.e., dextrose) varies, depending on whether TPN or PPN is chosen.

Crystalline amino acid solutions are an essential component of PN. The importance of supplying amino acids relates to the maintenance of positive nitrogen balance and repletion of lean body tissue, which may be vital in the recovery of critically ill patients. Supplementation of amino acids may support protein synthesis and spare tissue proteins from being catabolized via gluconeogenesis. The most commonly used amino acid solutions (e.g., Travasol, Clintec Nutrition, Deerfield, IL; Aminosyn II, Abbott Laboratories, North Chicago, IL) contain most of the essential amino acids for dogs and cats, with the exception of taurine. However, as PN is typically not used beyond 10 days, the lack of taurine does not become a problem in most circumstances. Amino acid solutions are available in different concentrations from 4% to 15%, but the most commonly used concentration is 8.5%. Amino acid solutions are also available with and without electrolytes.

Lipid emulsions are the calorically dense component of PN and a source of essential fatty acids. Lipid emulsions are isotonic and available in 10% to 30% solutions (e.g., Intralipid, Clintec Nutrition, Deerfield, IL; Liposyn III, Abbott Laboratories, North Chicago, IL). These commercially available lipid emulsions are made primarily of soybean and safflower oil and provide predominantly long-chain polyunsaturated fatty acids, including linoleic, oleic, palmitic, and stearic acids. The emulsified fat particles are comparable in size to chylomicrons and are removed from the circulation via the action of peripheral lipoprotein lipase. A common misconception exists in regard to the use of lipids in cases of pancreatitis. Although hypertriglyceridemia may be a risk factor for pancreatitis, infusions of lipids have not been shown to increase pancreatic secretion or worsen pancreatitis and therefore are considered safe. However, the one exception is in cases in which serum triglycerides are elevated, indicating a clear failure of triglyceride clearance. Although specific data regarding the maximal safe level of lipid administration in veterinary patients is not available, it would seem prudent to maintain normal serum triglyceride levels in patients receiving PN. Another concern surrounding the use of lipids in PN is their purported immunosuppressive effects via impairment of the reticuloendothelial system, particularly in PN solutions containing a high percentage of lipids. Despite in vitro evidence supporting the notion that lipid infusions can also suppress neutrophil and lymphocyte function, studies have not yet correlated lipid use and increased rates of infectious complications.

Electrolytes, vitamins, and trace elements also may be added to the PN formulation. Depending on the hospital and the individual patient, electrolytes can be added to the admixture, included as part of the amino acid solution, or left out altogether and managed separately. As B vitamins are water soluble, they are more likely to become deficient in patients with high-volume diuresis (e.g., renal failure, diabetes mellitus), and supplementation could be considered. Since most animals receive PN for only a short duration, fat-soluble vitamins usually are not limiting; therefore supplementation is not usually required. The exception is in obviously malnourished animals in which supplementation may be necessary. Trace elements serve as cofactors in a variety of enzyme systems and can become deficient in malnourished patients as well. In humans receiving PN, zinc, copper, manganese, and chromium are routinely included in the PN admixture. These are sometimes added to PN admixtures for malnourished animals, but their compatibility with the solution must be verified.

The addition of other parenteral medications to the PN admixture is possible; however, their compatibility must also be verified. Drugs that are known to be compatible and sometimes added to PN include heparin, insulin, potassium chloride, and metoclopramide. Although the addition of insulin to PN is often necessary in humans receiving PN, the hyperglycemia seen in veterinary patients with PN usually does not require insulin administration, except for diabetic patients that will require adjustments to their insulin regimen.

PARENTERAL NUTRITION COMPOUNDING

Based on the nutritional assessment and plan, PN can be formulated according to the worksheets found in Boxes 3-1 and 3-2. For TPN (Box 3-1) the first step is the calculation of the patient's RER. Protein requirements (grams of protein required per day) are then calculated, taking into consideration factors such as excessive protein losses or severe hepatic or renal disease. The energy provided from amino acids is accounted for in the energy calculations and subtracted from the daily RER to estimate the total nonprotein calories required. Some protocols do not account for the energy provided by amino acids in the calculations, which may lead to overfeeding in critically ill animals. The nonprotein calories are then usually provided as a 50:50 mixture of lipids and dextrose; however, this ratio can be adjusted in cases of persistent hyperglycemia or hypertriglyceridemia (e.g., a higher proportion of calories would be given from lipids in an animal with hyperglycemia). The calories provided from each component (amino acids, lipids, and dextrose) are then divided by their respective caloric densities, and the exact amounts of each component are added to the PN bags in an aseptic fashion. The amount of TPN delivered often will provide less than the patient's daily fluid requirement. Additional fluids can either be added to the PN bag at the time of compounding or be provided as a separate infusion.

For formulation of PPN, Box 3-2 provides a step-by-step protocol in which patients of various sizes can receive 70% of their RER and approximately meet their daily maintenance fluid requirement. In very small animals (≤3 kg), the amount of PPN will exceed the maintenance fluid requirement and increase the risk for fluid overload; thus adjustments may need to be made. Also, in animals requiring conservative fluid administration (e.g., congestive heart failure), these calculations for PPN may provide more fluid than would be safe. This formulation has been designed so that the proportion of each PN component depends on the weight of the patient, such that a smaller animal (between 3 and 5 kg) receives proportionally more calories from lipids compared to a large dog (>30 kg) that receives more calories in the form of carbohydrates. This allows the resulting formulation to approximate the patient's daily fluid requirement.

Ideally compounding of PN should be done aseptically under a laminar flow hood using a semiautomated, closed-system, PN compounder (e.g., Automix compounder, Clintec Nutrition, Deerfield, IL). If the appropriate facilities and equipment are not available, it may be preferable to have a local human hospital, compounding pharmacy, or human home health care company compound PN solutions using the formulations listed in Boxes 3-1 and 3-2. Alternatively, commercial ready-to-use preparations of glucose or glycerol and amino acids suitable for (peripheral) intravenous administration are available (e.g., ProcalAmine B, Braun Medical Inc., Irvine, CA). Although ready-to-use preparations are convenient, they provide only 30% to 50% of caloric requirements when administered at maintenance fluid rates and as a result should only be used for interim nutritional support or to supplement low-dose enteral feedings.

PARENTERAL NUTRITION ADMINISTRATION

The administration of any PN requires a dedicated catheter used solely for PN administration that is placed using aseptic technique. In most cases this requires placement of additional catheters since PN should not be administered through existing catheters that were placed for reasons other than PN. Long catheters composed of silicone, polyurethane, or tetrafluoroethylene are recommended for use with any type of PN to reduce the risk of thrombophlebitis. Multilumen catheters are often recommended for TPN because they can remain in place for long periods and separate ports can also be used for blood sampling and administration of additional fluids and intravenous medications without the need for separate catheters placed at other sites. Injections into the PN catheter infusion port or administration lines should be strictly prohibited. The high osmolarity of TPN solutions (often 1200 mOsm/L) requires its administration through a central venous (jugular) catheter, whereas PPN solutions can be administered through either a jugular catheter or catheters placed in peripheral veins. The concern with high osmolarity is that it may increase the incidence of thrombophlebitis, although this has not been well characterized in veterinary patients.

Because of the various metabolic derangements associated with critical illness, TPN should be instituted gradually over 48 hours. Administration of TPN is typically initiated at 50% of the RER on the first day and increased to the targeted amount by the second day. In most cases PPN can be started without gradual increase. It is also important to adjust the rates of other fluids being concurrently administered. For both TPN and PPN, the animal's catheter and infusion lines must be handled aseptically at all times to reduce the risk of PN-related infections.

Box **3-1**

Worksheet for Calculating a Total Parenteral Nutrition Formulation

1. Resting energy requirement (RER)

$$70 \times \text{(current body weight in kg)}^{0.75} = \text{kcal/day}$$

or for animals 3-25 kg, can also use:

$$30 \times \text{(current body weight in kg)} + 70 = \text{kcal/day} \quad \text{RER} = \underline{\hspace{2cm}} \text{kcal/day}$$

2. Protein requirements

	Canine	Feline
Standard*	4-5 g/100 kcal	6 g/100 kcal
Decreased requirements* (hepatic/renal failure)	2-3 g/100 kcal	3-4 g/100 kcal
Increased requirements* (protein-losing conditions)	6 g/100 kcal	6 g/100 kcal

$$(\text{RER} \div 100) \times \underline{\hspace{3cm}} \text{g/100 kcal} = \underline{\hspace{3cm}} \text{g of protein required per day (protein req)}$$

3. Volumes of nutrient solutions required each day

a. 8.5% amino acid solution = 0.085 g of protein per milliliter

$\underline{\hspace{3cm}}$ g of protein per day required ÷ 0.085 g/ml = $\underline{\hspace{3cm}}$ ml of amino acids per day

b. Nonprotein calories:

The calories supplied by protein (4 kcal/g) are subtracted from the RER to get total nonprotein calories needed:

$\underline{\hspace{3cm}}$ g of protein required per /day × 4 kcal/g = $\underline{\hspace{3cm}}$ kcal provided by protein

RER − kcal provided by protein = $\underline{\hspace{3cm}}$ nonprotein kcal needed per day

c. Nonprotein calories are usually provided as a 50:50 mixture of lipid and dextrose. However, if the patient has a preexisting condition (e.g., diabetes, hypertriglyceridemia), this ratio may need to be adjusted.

*20% lipid solution = 2 kcal/ml

To supply 50% of nonprotein kcal

$\underline{\hspace{3cm}}$ lipid kcal required ÷ 2 kcal/ml = $\underline{\hspace{3cm}}$ ml of lipid

*50% dextrose solution = 1.7 kcal/ml

To supply 50% of nonprotein kcal

$\underline{\hspace{3cm}}$ dextrose kcal required ÷ 1.7 kcal/ml = $\underline{\hspace{3cm}}$ ml of dextrose

4. Total daily requirements

$\underline{\hspace{3cm}}$ ml of 8.5% amino acid solution

$\underline{\hspace{3cm}}$ ml of 20% lipid solution

$\underline{\hspace{3cm}}$ ml of 50% dextrose solution

$\underline{\hspace{3cm}}$ ml total volume of total parenteral nutrition solution

5. Administration rate

Day 1: $\underline{\hspace{3cm}}$ ml/hr

Day 2: $\underline{\hspace{3cm}}$ ml/hr

Day 3: $\underline{\hspace{3cm}}$ ml/hr

*Be sure to adjust the patient's other fluids accordingly!

PN should be administered as continuous-rate infusions over 24 hours via fluid infusion pumps. Inadvertent delivery of massive amounts of PN can result if administration is not regulated properly. Once a bag of PN is set up for administration, it is not disconnected from the patient even for walks or diagnostic procedures—the drip regulator is decreased to a slow drip and accompanies the patient throughout the hospital. Administration of PN through a 1.2-micron in-line filter (e.g., 1.2-micron downstream filter, Baxter Healthcare Corp., Deerfield, IL) is also recommended and is attached at the time of setup. This setup process is performed daily with each new bag of PN. Each bag should only hold 1 day's worth of PN, and the accompanying fluid administration sets and in-line filter are changed at the same time using aseptic technique. PN should be discontinued when the animal resumes consuming an adequate amount of calories of at least 50% of RER. TPN should be discontinued gradually over a 6- to 12-hour period, but PPN can be discontinued without weaning.

Box **3-2**

Worksheet for Calculating a Partial Parenteral Nutrition Formulation

1. Resting energy requirement (RER)

$$70 \times \text{(current body weight in kg)}^{0.75} = \text{kcal/day}$$

or for animals 3-25 kg, can also use:

$$30 \times \text{(current body weight in kg)} + 70 = \text{kcal/day} \quad \text{RER} = \underline{\hspace{2cm}} \text{kcal/day}$$

2. Partial energy requirement (PER)

Plan to supply 70% of the animal's RER with partial parenteral nutrition (PPN):

$$\text{PER} = \text{RER} \times 0.70 = \underline{\hspace{2cm}} \text{kcal/day}$$

3. Nutrient composition

(NOTE: For animals ≤3 kg, the formulation will provide a fluid rate higher than maintenance fluid requirements. Be sure that the animal can tolerate this volume of fluids)

a. Cats and dogs 3-5 kg:

PER × 0.20 = _____ kcal/day from carbohydrate

PER × 0.20 = _____ kcal/day from protein

PER × 0.60 = _____ kcal/day from lipid

b. Cats and dogs 6-10 kg:

PER × 0.25 = _____ kcal/day from carbohydrate

PER × 0.25 = _____ kcal/day from protein

PER × 0.50 = _____ kcal/day from lipid

c. Dogs 11-30 kg:

PER × 0.33 = _____ kcal/day from carbohydrate

PER × 0.33 = _____ kcal/day from protein

PER × 0.33 = _____ kcal/day from lipid

d. Dogs >30 kg:

PER × 0.50 = _____ kcal/day from carbohydrate

PER × 0.25 = _____ kcal/day from protein

PER × 0.25 = _____ kcal/day from lipid

4. Volumes of nutrient solutions required each day

a. 5% dextrose solution = 0.17 kcal/ml

_____ kcal from carbohydrate ÷ 0.17 kcal/ml = _____ ml of dextrose per day

b. 8.5% amino acid solution = 0.085 g/ml = 0.34 kcal/ml

_____ kcal from protein ÷ 0.34 kcal/ml = _____ ml of amino acids per day

c. 20% lipid solution = 2 kcal/ml

_____ kcal from lipid ÷ 2 kcal/ml = _____ ml of lipid per day

5. Total daily requirements

_____ ml of 5% dextrose solution

_____ ml of 8.5% amino acid solution

_____ ml of 20% lipid solution

_____ ml of total volume of PPN solution

6. Administration rate

This formulation provides an approximate maintenance fluid rate.

_____ ml/hour of PPN solution

*Be sure to adjust the patient's other fluids accordingly!

ENTERAL NUTRITIONAL SUPPORT

In critically ill animals with a functional gastrointestinal tract, the use of feeding tubes is the standard mode of nutritional support. As discussed previously, a key decision is determining whether the patient can undergo general anesthesia for placement of feeding tubes. In animals with surgical disease requiring laparotomy, placement of gastrostomy or jejunostomy feeding tubes should receive particular consideration. Feeding tubes commonly used in critically ill animals are nasoesophageal, esophagostomy, gastrostomy, and jejunostomy. The decision to choose one tube over another is based on the anticipated duration of nutritional support (e.g., days versus months), the need to circumvent certain segments of the gastrointestinal tract (e.g., oropharyngeal injury, esophagitis, pancreatitis), clinician experience, and suitability of patient to withstand anesthesia (very critical animals may only tolerate placement of nasoesophageal feeding tubes). More in-depth information of the various feeding tube options is discussed elsewhere in this text (see Chapter 136).

MONITORING FOR COMPLICATIONS

Because the development of complications in critically ill animals can have serious consequences, an important aspect of nutritional support involves close monitoring. With implementation of enteral nutrition, possible complications include vomiting, diarrhea, fluid overload, electrolyte imbalances, feeding tube malfunction, and infectious complications associated with insertion sites of feeding tubes. Metabolic complications are more common with PN and include the development of hyperglycemia, lipemia, azotemia, hyperammonemia, as well as electrolyte abnormalities. Rarely nutritional support can be associated with severe abnormalities that are sometimes referred to as the refeeding syndrome. Strategies to reduce risk of complications include observing aseptic techniques when placing feeding tubes and intravenous catheters, using conservative estimates of energy requirements (i.e., RER), and careful patient monitoring. Parameters that should be monitored during nutritional support include body temperature; respiratory rate and effort; signs of fluid overload (e.g., chemosis, increased body weight); and serum concentrations of glucose, triglycerides, electrolytes, blood urea nitrogen, and creatinine. Detection of any abnormality should prompt full reassessment.

PHARMACOLOGIC AGENTS IN NUTRITIONAL SUPPORT

Since critically ill animals are often anorexic, there is the temptation to use appetite stimulants to increase food intake. Unfortunately appetite stimulants are generally unreliable and seldom result in adequate food intake in critically ill animals. Pharmacologic stimulation of appetite is often short-lived and only delays true nutritional support. I do not believe that appetite stimulants have a place in the management of hospitalized animals when more effective measures of nutritional support such as placement of feeding tubes are more appropriate. The use of appetite stimulants may be considered in recovering animals once they are home in their own environment, since ideally the primary reason for loss of appetite should be reversed by time of hospital discharge.

FUTURE DIRECTIONS IN CRITICAL CARE NUTRITION

The current state of veterinary critical-care nutrition revolves around proper recognition of animals in need of nutritional support and implementation of strategies to best provide nutritional therapies. Important areas that need further evaluation in critically ill animals include the optimal composition and caloric target of nutritional support, strategies to minimize complications, and optimize outcome. Recent findings implicating development of hyperglycemia with poor outcome in critically ill humans have led to more vigilant monitoring and stricter control of blood glucose, with obvious implications for nutritional support. Evidence of a similar relationship in dogs and cats is mounting, and ongoing studies are focusing on the possible consequences of hyperglycemia. Until further studies suggest otherwise, efforts to reduce the incidence of hyperglycemia in critically ill animals, especially those receiving nutritional support, should be strongly pursued.

Other exciting areas of clinical nutrition in critically ill humans include the use of special nutrients that possess immunomodulatory properties such as glutamine, arginine, and n-3 fatty acids. In specific populations these agents used singly or in combination have demonstrated promising results, even in severely affected people. However, results have not been consistent, and ongoing trials continue to evaluate their efficacy. To date there is limited information on the use of these nutrients to specifically modulate disease in clinically affected animals. Future studies should focus on whether manipulation of such nutrients offer any benefit in animals.

References and Suggested Reading

Buffington T, Holloway C, Abood A: Nutritional assessment. In Buffington T, Holloway C, Abood S, editors: *Manual of veterinary dietetics*, St Louis, 2004, Saunders, p 1.

Chan DL: Nutritional requirements of the critically ill patient, *Clin Tech Small Anim Pract* 19:1, 2004.

Freeman LM, Chan DL: Total parenteral nutrition. In DiBartola SP, editor: *Fluid, electrolyte, and acid-base disorders in small animal practice*, ed 3, St. Louis, 2006, Saunders, p 584.

Novak F et al: Glutamine supplementation in serious illness: a systematic review of the evidence, *Crit Care Med* 30:2022, 2002.

Pyle SC, Marks SL, Kass PH: Evaluation of complications and prognostic factors associated with administration of total parenteral nutrition in cats: 75 cases (1994-2001), *J Am Vet Med Assoc* 255:242, 2004.

Torre DM, deLaforcade AM, Chan DL: Incidence and significance of hyperglycemia in critically ill dogs, *J Vet Intern Med* 21:971, 2007.

Van den Berghe G et al: Intensive insulin therapy in critically ill patients, *N Engl J Med* 345:1359, 2001.

Walton RS, Wingfield WE, Ogilvie GK: Energy expenditure in 104 postoperative and traumatically injured dogs with indirect calorimetry, *J Vet Emerg Crit Care* 6:71, 1998.

CHAPTER 4

Antiplatelet and Anticoagulant Therapy

MARILYN DUNN, *Quebec, Canada*
MARJORY B. BROOKS, *Ithaca, New York*

Thrombosis is a major cause of mortality for humans with heart disease, cancer, and stroke—the three most common causes of death in developed countries. Hereditary defects of coagulation inhibitors, referred to as *thrombophilias*, further increase the burden of thrombus formation in humans. Aspirin, heparin, and warfarin have long been the mainstays of antithrombotic therapy in medicine. However, limitations in drug safety and efficacy have prompted the development of new antiplatelet and anticoagulant drugs to supplement or replace traditional drug regimens.

Although hereditary thrombophilias have not been identified in dogs or cats, thrombosis is recognized as a common complication of many acquired diseases, including cardiac, endocrine, inflammatory, and neoplastic disorders. Advances in our understanding of pathologic thrombus formation and recent pharmacokinetic studies of antithrombotic drugs in dogs and cats hold promise for the development of effective thromboprophylactic regimens in small animal practice.

PATHOGENESIS OF THROMBOSIS

Normal hemostasis is maintained through an intricate balance between endogenous anticoagulants and procoagulants. The net effect is preservation of blood flow in the systemic vasculature with localized coagulation at sites of vessel injury. Perturbations in this balance can tip the scales to either excessive bleeding or widespread thrombus formation (hypercoagulability). The concept of *Virchow's triad* (endothelial damage, alterations in blood flow, and hypercoagulability) refers to underlying factors that act singly or in concert to promote thrombus formation in various disease states. The primary disorder influences the site of thrombus formation (arterial or venous vasculature), the composition of the occluding thrombus, and the approach to antithrombotic therapy. The relative proportions of platelets and fibrin in the clot depend on the shear of the injured vessel. Arterial thrombi form under high shear forces and therefore tend to contain a large number of platelets held together by fibrin strands. Venous thrombi form under low shear forces and consist primarily of fibrin and red blood cells. Strategies to inhibit arterial thrombogenesis typically include the use of antiplatelet drugs, whereas anticoagulants are the mainstay of venous thromboprophylaxis. Ultimately clinical trials are required for optimization of drug dosages and drug combinations for specific thrombotic syndromes.

DIAGNOSIS OF HYPERCOAGULABILITY

Identification of hypercoagulability is a great challenge in veterinary medicine. Routine coagulation tests (prothrombin time [PT], partial thromboplastin time [PTT]) are designed to detect "hypocoagulability," and assays that measure consumption of anticoagulant proteins and fibrinogen are generally insensitive indicators of subclinical thrombosis. Nevertheless, low plasma antithrombin (AT) activity and high fibrin degradation product, D-dimer, and fibrinogen levels provide laboratory evidence of hypercoagulability. In human studies platelet hyperaggregability and expression of platelet activation markers such as P-selectin have been observed in patients with thrombotic tendencies. Thromboelastography (TEG) is a technique that depicts global hemostasis, beginning with clot formation and ending with clot lysis. Characteristic changes in the TEG profile have been associated with hypercoagulability in people. Evaluation of platelet function and TEG has been done and may prove useful in veterinary practice to detect hypercoagulability and monitor antiplatelet and anticoagulant therapy.

ANTIPLATELET DRUGS

Antiplatelet agents act through inhibition of platelet activation pathways or interference with membrane receptors. The three classes of antiplatelet drugs in current use include nonsteroidal antiinflammatory drugs (NSAIDs) (cyclooxygenase inhibitors), thienopyridines (adenosine diphosphate [ADP] receptor antagonists), and glycoprotein (GP)IIb/IIIa blockers (fibrinogen receptor antagonists).

Nonsteroidal Antiinflammatory Drugs

Aspirin is recommended as the first-line antiplatelet drug in human cardiac syndromes and is the most commonly used antiplatelet drug in veterinary medicine. Aspirin causes irreversible acetylation of the platelet cyclooxygenase active site, leading to decreased thromboxane A_2 synthesis. The effects of aspirin are permanent and last for the life span of the platelet (7 to 10 days). In contrast, other NSAIDs compete with arachidonic acid binding to cyclooxygenase, thereby producing a reversible inhibition. Despite its widespread use, prospective studies confirming the clinical efficacy of aspirin in thrombosis prevention in dogs and cats are lacking. In a retrospective study of immune-mediated hemolytic anemia (IMHA) in dogs, improved survival was attributed in part to low-dose (0.5 mg/kg PO) aspirin administration (Weinkle et al., 2005). A retrospective study of cats with arterial thromboembolism demonstrated no difference in survival for cats treated with low-dose aspirin (5 mg/cat PO every 72h) compared with standard-dose aspirin (≥40 mg/cat q24-72h) or warfarin (Smith et al., 2003). Cats receiving standard-dose aspirin had a greater risk of gastrointestinal hemorrhage than those receiving the low dose. Given the retrospective nature of the study, it was not possible to determine whether aspirin prophylaxis could prevent initial thrombus formation.

Thienopyridines

Thienopyridines irreversibly inhibit the binding of ADP to specific platelet ADP receptors (P2Y12). ADP receptor blockade impairs platelet release reaction and ADP-mediated activation of GPIIb/IIIa, thereby reducing primary and secondary aggregation response. These drugs must be metabolized by hepatic cytochrome p450, with platelet inhibition occurring by 3 days after initiation of therapy. Clopidogrel (Plavix, Sanofi-Aventis) and ticlopidine (Ticlid, Novopharm) are the two available thienopyridines. These drugs have been evaluated in healthy cats. Ticlopidine effectively decreased platelet aggregation but was associated with unacceptable gastrointestinal side effects. Clopidogrel at dosages of 18.75 to 75 mg PO every 24 hours was well tolerated and resulted in significant antiplatelet effects (Hogan et al., 2004). An ongoing prospective study (FATCAT) comparing clopidogrel to aspirin may help define the more effective agent for secondary prevention of feline aortic thrombosis. Plavix has been used empirically in dogs at a dosage of 1 to 2 mg/kg daily.

Glycoprotein IIb/IIIa Antagonists

Activation of GPIIb/IIIa is the final common pathway of platelet aggregation, regardless of the initiating stimulus. Therefore drugs capable of inhibiting fibrinogen binding to GPIIb/IIIa are potent antiplatelet agents. Three intravenous GPIIb/IIIa antagonist drugs have been developed for clinical use in humans: monoclonal antibodies that bind to the receptor (abciximab [ReoPro], Lilly), and competitive mimetics of fibrinogen (eptifibatide [Integrilin, Schering and tirofiban [Aggrastat], Merck). In a study of cats with induced arterial injury, abciximab combined with aspirin reduced thrombus formation compared with aspirin alone (Bright, Dowers, and Powers, 2003). Administration of eptifibatide to cats caused circulatory failure and death and therefore is contraindicated. Although dogs have been used in pharmacokinetic and pharmacologic studies of GPIIb/IIIa antagonists, clinical studies have not been performed.

ANTICOAGULANTS

Anticoagulants inhibit the generation of fibrin but do not dissolve preexisting fibrin clots (only thrombolytics can do this). Anticoagulants are used for thromboprophylaxis in patients considered at risk for a first thrombotic event and to limit fibrin formation in patients with documented thromboembolic disease.

Warfarin

Warfarin (Coumadin, DuPont) is a vitamin-K antagonist that alters the synthesis of vitamin K–dependent clotting proteins (factors II, VII, IX, and X) and the anticoagulants, proteins C and S. Warfarin interferes with hepatic reductase activity, leading to impaired posttranslational carboxylation. The resultant des-carboxy vitamin K–dependent clotting factors have greatly reduced or absent activity. The anticoagulant activity of warfarin is delayed (4 to 5 days) as the newly synthesized inactive clotting proteins gradually replace their functional counterparts. Rapid inhibition of proteins C and S results in a transient period of hypercoagulability in humans, but this phenomenon has not been documented in dogs or cats.

Warfarin is administered orally at an initial dosage of 0.2 mg/kg PO every 12 hours in dogs and 0.1 to 0.2 mg/kg PO every 24 hours in cats (Smith et al., 2000). Close monitoring for dosage adjustment is essential because the anticoagulant effect of warfarin is highly variable from one patient to another. Therapy is monitored based on PT, with a target prolongation to 1.5 times baseline. Because of the variability in PT reagent sensitivity, the World Health Organization has recommended that the PT be expressed as a ratio (International Normalized Ratio [INR]). The INR formula incorporates a factor (ISI) specific to each thromboplastin reagent and is calculated as follows: INR = (patient PT/control PT)^{ISI}. An INR target range of 2 to 3 is considered optimal, without causing excessive bleeding, for most human thrombotic syndromes. INR or PT monitoring is recommended daily for the first week of warfarin therapy, twice weekly for 3 weeks, then once a week for 2 months, and then every 2 months. Dose adjustments should be based on the total weekly dosage. Warfarin is available in 1-mg tablets that should not be divided because of uneven drug distribution throughout the tablet. Since most cats will receive 0.25 to 0.5 mg of warfarin, accurate dosing requires drug compounding. The most common veterinary use for warfarin is thromboprophylaxis for cats with cardiac disease; however, frequent monitoring to ensure optimal dosing is difficult in this patient population. Despite close monitoring, bleeding complications may occur. In one study between 13% and 20% of cats suffered bleeding complications, and 13% of cats had a fatal hemorrhage (Harpster and Baty, 1995). Clients must be informed of the risk of warfarin-induced hemorrhage and the requirement for intensive monitoring before warfarin therapy is initiated.

Heparin

Unfractionated heparin (UH) is a glycosaminoglycan consisting of alternating residues of D-glucosamine and uronic acid. It is a heterogeneous mixture of chains ranging in molecular weight from 5,000 to 30,000 daltons with a mean length of 50 saccharides. Approximately one third of UH molecules possess a pentasaccharide sequence that binds to AT and accelerates its interaction with activated factors IIa (thrombin), IXa, Xa, XIa, and XIIa.

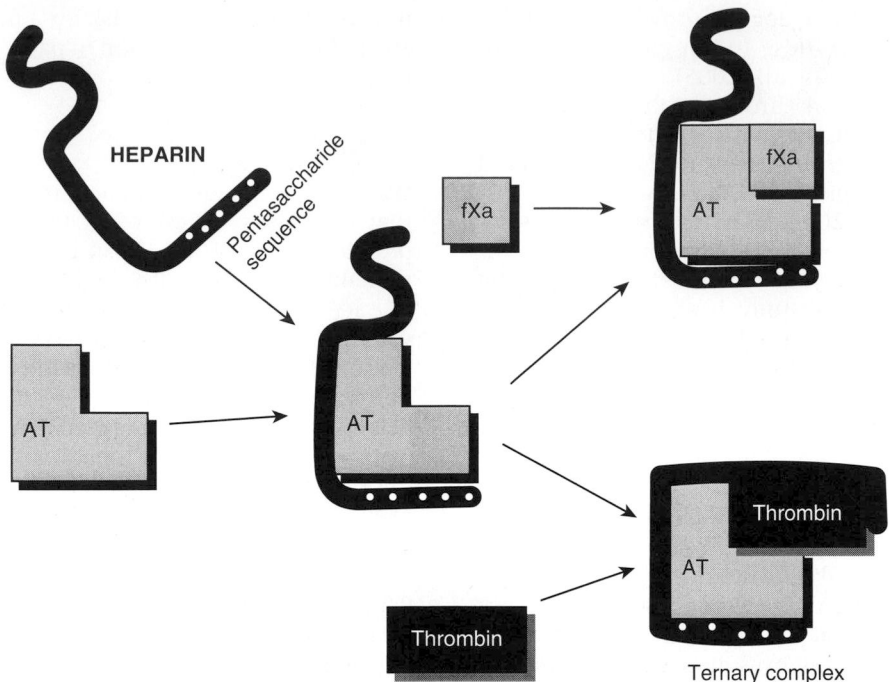

Fig. 4-1   Heparin binds antithrombin through the high-affinity pentasaccharide sequence and inactivates factor Xa. Inactivation of thrombin also occurs but necessitates an additional 13 saccharides. (Modified from Hirsh J, Levine MN: Low-molecular-weight heparin, *Blood* 79:1, 1992.)

Thrombin and factor Xa are most responsive to inhibition by AT. Thrombin inactivation requires formation of a ternary complex involving heparin, AT, and thrombin (Fig. 4-1). Heparin is an indirect anticoagulant, exerting most of its effect through potentiation of AT activity. The drug is administered either intravenously or subcutaneously since it is very poorly absorbed orally.

Heparin has been the anticoagulant of choice for thromboprophylaxis and treatment of thrombosis in human and veterinary medicine. Despite its widespread use, UH has a complex pharmacokinetic profile that produces an unpredictable anticoagulant effect. UH binds to numerous plasma proteins (lipoproteins, von Willebrand's factor, fibrinogen, acute-phase proteins, and AT) and to endothelial cells, macrophages, and platelets. Because of its extensive binding to macrophages and endothelial cells, low-dose subcutaneous UH has poor bioavailability.

For treatment of thrombosis in humans, UH typically is initiated with a bolus dose of 60 to 80 units/kg, followed by infusion of 12 to 15 units/kg/hour. Heparin therapy is then monitored by measurement of the PTT, with dosage adjustment to prolong values to 1.5 to 2.5 times the control value. In addition to PTT, heparin dosage has recently been based on measurement of plasma factor Xa inhibition, to the target range of 0.35 to 0.7 U/ml. Unlike PTT, anti-Xa activity is also suitable for monitoring low–molecular weight heparin (LMWH) therapy.

Empiric UH therapy in veterinary medicine varies widely, encompassing a subcutaneous dosage range of 50 to 500 units/kg every 6 to 12 hours. Pharmacokinetic studies in healthy dogs have shown that dosages of 250 to 500 units/kg will result in target-range anti-Xa activities; however, hematoma formation occurred in some dogs treated with 500 units/kg SQ at 8-hour intervals (Mischke, Schuttert, and Grebe, 2001). Little clinical data regarding UH monitoring exist in the veterinary literature; however, preliminary reports in IMHA dogs indicate that relatively high dosages (>300 units/kg SQ q6h) will be required to attain target anti-Xa levels (Breuhl, Scott-Moncrieff, and Brooks, 2005).

Low–Molecular Weight Heparin

LMWHs are produced by depolymerization of UH, yielding chains with a mean molecular weight of 5000 daltons and chain lengths of less than 18 saccharides. Like UH, LMWHs possess a pentasaccharide region that binds to AT and accelerates its inhibition of factor Xa. The majority of LMWH molecules are too short to form a ternary complex with thrombin and AT; therefore their ratio of factor Xa to factor IIa inhibitory activity is approximately 4:1. In comparison, UH has a ratio of anti-Xa to anti-IIa activity of 1:1 (Fig 4-2).

LMWHs bind poorly to plasma proteins and cells and undergo first-order renal clearance. In humans the subcutaneous bioavailability of LMWHs approaches 100%, and their elimination half-life allows once- or twice-a-day administration with no need for individual patient monitoring to adjust dosage. Although UH and LMWH demonstrate similar efficacy in most human trials, LMWH is gradually replacing UH because of its more favorable pharmacokinetic properties.

The pharmacokinetics of two LMWHs (dalteparin [Fragmin], Pfizer) and enoxaparin (Lovenox, Sanofi-Aventis) have been investigated in healthy dogs and cats, using anti-Xa activity to monitor anticoagulant effect. In dogs dalteparin has a half-life of 123 minutes, a vol-

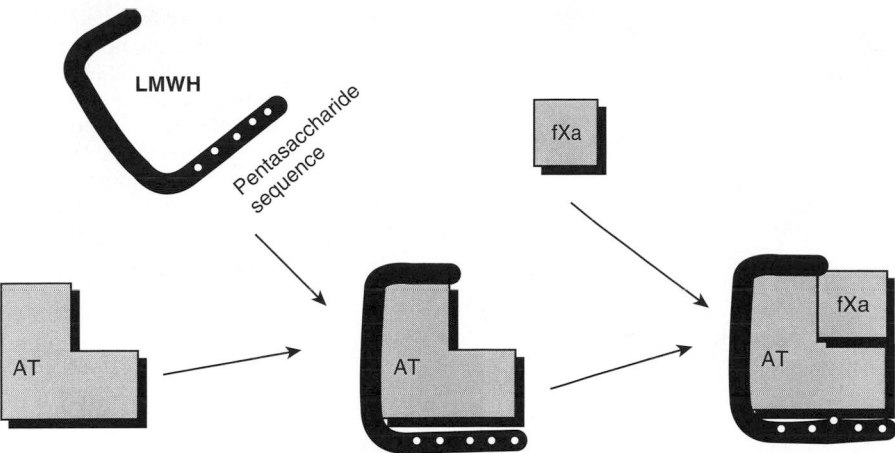

Fig. 4-2 LMWH binds antithrombin through the high-affinity pentasaccharide sequence and inactivates factor Xa. LMWH containing less than 18 saccharides cannot bind to thrombin. (Modified from Hirsh J, Levine MN: Low-molecular-weight heparin, *Blood* 79:1, 1992.)

ume of distribution of 50 to 70 ml/kg of body weight, and an absolute bioavailability of 104% when administered subcutaneously (Grebe et al., 2000). Enoxaparin given to dogs at 0.8 mg/kg every 6 hours produced sustained anti-Xa activity in the range of 0.5 to 2 U/ml (Lunsford et al., 2005). Dalteparin given to dogs at 150 U/kg every 8 hours resulted in anti-Xa activity in the range of 0.2 to 1 U/ml (Mischke et al., 2001). A number of other LMWHs have been used experimentally in dogs (tinzaparin, nadroparin) and appear to have pharmacokinetic properties similar to those in people. In contrast, pharmacokinetic studies of dalteparin and enoxaparin in healthy cats revealed rapid absorption and elimination of the drugs, with peak effects 2 to 3 hours after drug administration. The predicted dosages required to maintain anti-Xa activity equal to or greater than 0.5 U/ml were 150 units/kg every 4 hours for dalteparin and 1.5 mg/kg every 6 hours for enoxaparin (Alwood et al., 2007).

Although anti-Xa activity values are useful for defining UH and LMWH pharmacokinetics and comparing different dosage regimens in clinical trials, the in vivo anticoagulant effects of heparin are complex and not limited solely to factor Xa inhibition. A meta-analysis of human trials found that once-daily dosing of LMWHs was as effective in thromboprevention as 12-hour dosing (Dolovich et al., 2000), although once-daily dosing resulted in 12- to 14-hour periods with a subtherapeutic (defined as <0.4 U/ml) anti-Xa level. In humans peak anti-Xa activity appears to correlate more closely to efficacy; however, the relationship between target anti-Xa activity and clinical outcome remains to be fully defined.

Species differences in LMWH pharmacokinetics and anticoagulant effect will complicate the direct extrapolation of data from human trials. In a study of six ill dogs receiving dalteparin at 150 U/kg every 12 hours, results showed that anti-Xa activity peaked predictably 3 hours following administration and fell below therapeutic range 12 hours after the dose (Charland, Thorneloe, and Dunn, 2006). Mestre and colleagues (1985) reported a thrombosis-protective effect in dogs with an anti-Xa activity of 0.55 U/ml. A retrospective study of 57 cats

with cardiac disease treated with 100 units/kg of dalteparin once or twice daily showed that the drug was well tolerated and infrequently caused clinical bleeding (Smith et al., 2004). This study was not designed to test the efficacy of dalteparin, however, and anti-Xa activity was not measured. Ultimately clinical trials to optimize LMWH therapy for specific canine and feline thrombotic disorders will require drug monitoring with anti-Xa activity or other tests such as TEG and defined clinical outcome measures.

New Anticoagulants

Many new anticoagulant drugs are in various stages of development to further improve safety, efficacy, and/or ease of administration beyond that of LMWH. Fondaparinux (Arixtra, GlaxoSmithKline) is an ultra LMWH (consisting only of an AT-binding pentasaccharide sequence) currently approved for treatment and prophylaxis of venous thrombosis.

Direct thrombin inhibitors comprise a new class of anticoagulants that bind to distinct domains on thrombin and block its interaction with substrate. Unlike indirect anticoagulants, the direct thrombin inhibitors neutralize fibrin-bound thrombin. Parenteral drugs in this class include hirudin, bivalirudin, and argatroban. New drugs that inhibit novel procoagulants are in phase I or II trials. These drugs include recombinant TFPI (targeting tissue factor) nNAPC2 (targeting factors X and Xa), and TTP889 (targeting factor IXa).

References and Suggested Reading

Alwood AJ et al: Anticoagulant effects of low molecular weight heparins in healthy cats, *J Vet Intern Med* 21(3):378, 2007.

Breuhl EL, Scott-Moncrieff C, Brooks M: A prospective study of unfractionated heparin therapy to prevent thrombosis in canine immune-mediated haemolytic anemia, *J Vet Intern Med* 19(abstr):399, 2005.

Bright JM, Dowers K, Powers BE: Effects of the glycoprotein IIb-IIIa antagonist abciximab on thrombus formation and platelet function in cats with arterial injury, *Vet Ther* 4:35, 2003.

Charland C, Thorneloe C, Dunn M: L'utilisation d'héparine de faible poids moléculaire chez 6 chiens, *Méd Vét du Québec* 35:86, 2006.

Dolovich LR et al: A meta-analysis comparing low-molecular-weight-heparins with unfractionated heparin in the treatment of venous thromboembolism, *Arch Intern Med* 160:181, 2000.

Grebe S et al: Pharmakokinetik des niedermolkularen heparins fragmin D beim hund, *Berl Muench Tieraerztl Wochenschr* 113:103, 2000.

Harpster NK, Baty CJ: Warfarin therapy of the cat at risk of thromboembolism. In Bonagura JD: *Current veterinary therapy XII*, Philadelphia, 1995, Saunders, p 868.

Hogan DF et al: Antiplatelet effects and pharmacodynamics of clopidogrel in cats, *J Am Vet Med Assoc* 225:1406, 2004.

Lunsford K et al: *Pharmacokinetics of the biological effects of subcutaneous enoxaparin in dogs, Proceedings of the 23rd ACVIM Conference*, Baltimore, Md, 2005, p 830(abstr).

Mestre M et al: Comparative effects of heparin and PK 10169, a low-molecular-weight fraction, in a canine model of arterial thrombosis, *Thromb Res* 38:389, 1985.

Mischke RH, Schuttert C, Grebe SI: Anticoagulant effects of repeated subcutaneous injections of high doses of unfractionated heparin in healthy dogs, *Am J Vet Res* 62:1887, 2001.

Smith CE et al: Use of a low-molecular-weight heparin in cats: 57 cases (1999-2003), *J Am Vet Med Assoc* 225:237, 2004.

Smith SA et al: Plasma pharmacokinetics of warfarin enantiomers in cats, *J Vet Pharmacol Ther* 23:329, 2000.

Smith SA et al: Arterial thromboembolism in cats: acute crisis in 127 cases (1992-2001) and long-term management with low-dose aspirin in 24 cases, *J Vet Intern Med* 17:73, 2003.

Weinkle TK et al: Evaluation of prognostic factors, survival rates, and treatment protocols for immune-mediated hemolytic anemia in dogs: 151 cases (1993-2002), *J Am Vet Med Assoc* 226:1869, 2005.

CHAPTER 5

Cardiopulmonary Cerebral Resuscitation

GRETCHEN L. SCHOEFFLER, *Ithaca, New York*

Cardiopulmonary cerebral resuscitation (CPCR) describes a combination of rescue breathing, chest compressions, and other advanced support measures delivered to patients in cardiopulmonary arrest. The techniques consist of basic life support, advanced life support, and integration of postresuscitation care. In veterinary patients basic life support protocols continue to follow the *ABCs* (*A*irway, *B*reathing, and *C*irculation). Advanced life support measures include electrocardiographic evaluation of cardiac rhythms, administration of drugs, and defibrillation when necessary. These techniques aim to maintain adequate tissue oxygenation and preserve organ viability during the low-flow "arrest" state to improve the chances of survival, as well as the return of acceptable cerebral and motor functions. Like any other treatment, CPCR *should be administered only if it is expected to confer lasting benefit to the patient*. Patients that suffer cardiopulmonary arrest and have potentially reversible disease are much more likely to survive. Resuscitation of patients with chronic, debilitating illness is more likely to result in prolongation of death. When possible, the decision to not resuscitate should be made in advance, on the merits of each individual case, and in consultation with the owner.

BASIC LIFE SUPPORT

Airway and Breathing

When a patient in cardiopulmonary arrest is identified, it is important to first secure the airway. When orotracheal intubation is impossible, an emergency tracheostomy should be performed. Once an airway is secured, intermittent positive-pressure ventilation using 100% oxygen with either an Ambu bag or anesthesia machine equipped with a rebreathing bag is easily accomplished. It is not necessary to interrupt chest compressions to deliver positive-pressure breaths; breaths and compressions can be delivered simultaneously. It is reasonable to give each breath within a 1-second inspiratory time at a rate of 8 to 10 ventilations per minute. Hyperventilation must be avoided because it is associated with increased intrathoracic pressure, decreased coronary and cerebral perfusion, and in some studies decreased restoration of spontaneous circulation (ROSC). Positive-pressure breaths should achieve a relatively normal chest rise, and, unless lung compliance is very poor, peak airway pressure should not exceed 20 cm of H_2O. Excessively high airway pressures (greater than 20 cm of H_2O) or inadequate chest wall excursion should lead to a search for potential underlying causes such as tube malposition, occlusion, or pleural space disease. Overaggressive ventilation with high airway pressures can result in iatrogenic pneumothorax, thereby necessitating open-chest resuscitation.

Circulation

The goal of circulatory support during CPCR is to generate adequate forward flow of well-oxygenated blood to the heart and brain until spontaneous and effective circulation can be restored. For resuscitative efforts to be effective it is imperative that the technique be optimized in each patient. If the initial technique is not generating an improvement in mucous membrane color or measurable end-tidal carbon dioxide ($ETCO_2$) levels, an alternate technique should be tried. The compression force or rate could be altered, the position of the animal or the compressor's hands could be changed, or the compressor itself might be relieved. When optimizing the technique in an individual patient, it is not uncommon to try multiple variations.

Closed-Chest Cardiopulmonary Cerebral Resuscitation
The patient is placed in either lateral or dorsal recumbency on a firm flat surface or in a stable V-trough. It is important to stabilize the patient since excessive movement decreases the force of thoracic compressions. If the patient is in lateral recumbency, pressure should be applied over the lateral thoracic wall directly above the heart. If the patient is in dorsal recumbency, the pressure is applied to the caudal aspect of the sternum. The amount of pressure applied should be appropriate to the size of the patient. For example, the resuscitator might place his or her thumb on one side of the chest and the fingers on the other when resuscitating a cat, whereas a two-handed technique would be more appropriate for a large-breed dog. In general, the height of the chest cavity should be reduced by approximately 30% during compression. The resuscitator should maintain a minimum of 100 compressions per minute, with equal time for compression and decompression. Experimental studies have shown that faster compression rates result in improved hemodynamics over slower compression rates. It is also essential that the resuscitator allow for complete recoil of the chest after each compression. Incomplete chest recoil is associated with significantly increased intrathoracic pressure, decreased venous return, and decreased coronary and cerebral perfusion. When feasible, rescuers should frequently alternate compressor duties to ensure that fatigue does not interfere with delivery of high-quality chest compressions or adequate chest recoil. This switch should be made quickly to minimize interruption of cardiac compressions. Interruptions are associated with reduced ROSC and survival, as well as increased postresuscitation myocardial dysfunction.

A variety of alternatives to standard manual closed-chest CPCR, including interposed abdominal compressions; active compression-decompression; and the use of impedance threshold valves, mechanical pistons, and load-distributing band devices have been proposed to increase blood flow during closed-chest CPCR. Compared with standard CPCR, these techniques and devices typically require more personnel, training, or equipment. The only ancillary procedure readily applicable to the clinical veterinary cardiopulmonary-arrest patient is the interposed abdominal compression technique. When performing interposed abdominal compressions, the abdomen is compressed during the relaxation phase of chest compression. The force of abdominal compression is similar to that needed to palpate the abdominal aortic pulse. Although no significant complications have been reported in experimental models, blunt injuries to parenchymal organs have been witnessed when this technique has been used in dogs. Abdominal compressions may be contraindicated in patients with significant abdominal organomegaly, disease, trauma, or hemorrhage. When applied correctly, interposed abdominal compressions can augment blood pressure, cardiac output, and myocardial and cerebral blood flow. For this reason interposed abdominal compressions might be considered as an adjunct to closed-chest CPCR in veterinary patients without evidence of significant intraabdominal disease.

Open-Chest Cardiopulmonary Cerebral Resuscitation
An emergency thoracotomy is indicated in patients who develop cardiopulmonary arrest with penetrating chest or abdominal trauma; chest wall deformity; pericardial tamponade; hemoperitoneum; and significant pleural disease such as pleural effusion, tension pneumothorax, and diaphragmatic hernia. Other recommendations for open-chest CPCR include patients that weigh more than 20 kg or arrest during surgery. Open-chest CPCR should also be considered in any patient with cardiopulmonary arrest in which external chest compressions with advanced life support fail to restore spontaneous circulation within 5 minutes. Time is the single most important variable in the treatment of cardiopulmonary arrest. Successful resuscitation cannot be expected when instituting open-chest CPCR after a prolonged period of ineffective closed-chest CPCR. The timing of switching from closed-chest CPCR to open-chest CPCR will influence the outcome and prognosis of a patient in cardiopulmonary arrest.

Open-chest CPCR with internal cardiac massage has been shown to be hemodynamically superior to closed-chest CPCR because it increases arterial pressure, cardiac output, coronary perfusion pressure, ROSC, and cerebral blood flow. This technique has additional advantages, including direct visualization of the heart and palpable assessment of diastolic filling. If the heart does not fill rapidly following each individual compression, a lack of venous return is evident, and intravenous fluid bolus or α-adrenergic drug therapy is indicated. Moreover, cardiac fibrillation can be observed directly, and internal defibrillation performed rapidly. In hypovolemic patients or patients with uncontrolled hemorrhage, the descending aorta can be visualized, isolated, and compressed with a finger or cross-clamped with a Penrose drain or a Rumel tourniquet. Occluding the descending aorta directs blood flow to the brain and heart, buying time until adequate volume can be administered or active hemorrhage controlled. If the descending aorta is compressed, it should remain compressed until the resuscitation effort is discontinued. Once the resuscitation effort is discontinued and spontaneous circulation deemed stable, the tourniquet or compression can be released slowly over 15 to 20 minutes. Experimental studies have demonstrated improved neurologic and cardiovascular outcome and an increase in survival rate when compared to closed-chest CPCR.

The most common approach for performing an emergency thoracotomy for resuscitative purposes is a left lateral thoracotomy at the fifth or sixth intercostal space. The intended surgical site should be prepared rapidly by clipping the hair and quickly swabbing the area with antiseptic solution. The incision is performed midway between the ribs down to but not through the pleura. To minimize the risk of lung laceration the pleura should be penetrated between positive-pressure ventilations with a blunt instrument. The incision should be extended with scissors, taking care not to incise the large epaxial muscles dorsally or the internal thoracic artery ventrally. Incising through the large epaxial muscles or the internal thoracic artery (longitudinal to the sternum) can result in significant blood loss and negatively impact the chance for successful resuscitation. Better exposure of the chest cavity and its contents can be achieved by introducing a rib spreader or similar instrument. Once the pericardium is encountered, it is opened ventral to the phrenic nerve, and manual compressions begun. Small hearts may need to be compressed between two fingers; however, large hearts are best compressed between both hands. If the patient is too small to get both hands into the chest cavity, the right hand should be used to compress the heart against the body wall. Care must be taken not to perforate the heart with fingertips or to rotate or displace the heart in a way that may result in occlusion or tearing of the great vessels. The rate of compression should be coordinated to the rate of ventricular filling and, if preload is adequate, should be able to be performed at a minimum rate of 100 compressions per minute. If the open-chest resuscitation effort is successful and spontaneous circulation becomes stable, the thorax should be lavaged with warm, sterile, isotonic saline, and a routine closure achieved. Given the increased chance of survival combined with a very low incidence of complication, it is clear that open-chest CPCR should be the resuscitation method of choice in many of our veterinary patients.

ADVANCED LIFE SUPPORT

After initiating effective artificial ventilation and circulation, rescuers should institute advanced life support, including assessment of the electrocardiogram (ECG), establishment of intravenous access, and administration of appropriate therapy. The four most common ECGs associated with cardiopulmonary arrest in small animal patients include pulseless electrical activity, asystole, ventricular fibrillation, and sinus bradycardia. Unfortunately there is no specific treatment for pulseless electrical activity, asystole, or sinus bradycardia; and the only effective method for converting ventricular fibrillation to a perfusing rhythm is the application of electrical defibrillation.

Electrical Defibrillation

The most critical intervention during the first 1 to 2 minutes of ventricular fibrillation is immediate electrical defibrillation. When ventricular fibrillation persists for more than a few minutes, the myocardium becomes depleted of

oxygen and metabolic substrates. In this instance a brief period of compressions can deliver oxygen and energy substrates, increasing the likelihood that a perfusing rhythm will return following shock therapy. It is imperative that basic life support measures continue until the defibrillator is charged and it is time to "clear" the patient for shock delivery. In closed-chest CPCR standard handheld defibrillator paddles should be painted with a copious amount of conductive electrode paste and applied to each side of the chest. To maximize current flow through the myocardium, the defibrillator operator should maintain full paddle contact with the skin and reduce the space within the thoracic cavity by applying inward pressure with the paddles. In open-chest CPCR special paddles designed for internal defibrillation are wrapped in saline-soaked gauze and held firmly against either side of the heart. Initial energy guidelines for a *monophasic waveform* defibrillator are 1-2 J/kg for internal defibrillation and 8-10 J/kg for external defibrillation. Initial energy guidelines for a *biphasic waveform* defibrillator are 0.3-0.4 J/kg for internal defibrillation and 3-4 J/kg for external defibrillation. Immediately following the shock, basic life support measures are resumed for approximately 2 minutes before reassessing the ECG. The goal is to minimize the time between compressions and shock delivery and between shock delivery and the resumption of compressions. Frequent or long interruptions in compressions are associated with increased postresuscitation myocardial dysfunction and reduced survival rates. This fact suggests that a one-shock strategy may be preferable to the three shocks "stacked" sequence previously recommended for ventricular fibrillation. After successful defibrillation normal electrical impulse generation is established, and myocardial contraction follows. Drug therapy to modulate and support cardiac performance may be necessary during the postresuscitation period since myocardial dysfunction is common and the time to recovery may vary from minutes to hours.

Intravenous and Alternate Routes of Access

A large-bore venous catheter should be placed preferentially in either the external jugular vein (central) or the cephalic vein (peripheral). Catheterization should be accomplished in a vessel cranial to the diaphragm where cephalad blood flow is more pronounced. If percutaneous catheter placement is not rapidly achieved, surgical cutdown of the vessel or intraosseous cannulation should be performed.

Although atropine, epinephrine, vasopressin, naloxone, and lidocaine can be administered by the endotracheal route, plasma concentrations are variable and substantially lower than those achieved when the same drug is given by the intravenous or intraosseous routes. Because the optimal endotracheal dose of most drugs is unknown, these medications are typically administered at 2 to 2.5 times the recommended intravenous dose and diluted in 5 to 10 ml of sterile water to facilitate absorption. Animal studies suggest that high doses of endotracheal epinephrine combined with reduced pulmonary blood flow and absorption can result in the formation of a pulmonary epinephrine depot. During the low-flow state that occurs during CPCR the lower plasma epinephrine concentrations achieved when the drug is delivered by the endotracheal route may produce transient β-adrenergic effects. These effects are detrimental, causing hypotension, lower coronary artery perfusion pressure and flow, and reduced potential for ROSC. On the other hand, if spontaneous circulation does return and cardiac output and pulmonary blood flow are restored, the resulting rapid resorption of high doses of pulmonary epinephrine can result in arterial hypertension, malignant arrhythmias, and ventricular fibrillation. These detrimental results reinforce the fact that, although endotracheal administration of some resuscitation drugs is possible, intravenous or intraosseous drug administration is preferred because it will provide more predictable drug delivery and pharmacologic effect.

Although administering drugs directly into the heart reduces concerns about drug delivery, intracardiac injection may be associated with a number of risks and complications. Blind intracardiac injections should be avoided in closed-chest CPCR because of the inaccuracy in aiming at the cavity of the left ventricle and the inevitable interruption of cardiac compressions. Blind intracardiac injections may result in lung, coronary artery, and atrial or ventricular laceration. Accidental intramyocardial deposition of epinephrine may lead to refractory ventricular fibrillation. Many potential complications of blind intracardiac injections may be avoided when the technique is used during open-chest CPCR. During open-chest CPCR the left ventricle can be visualized, and an accurate injection performed. Regrettably intracardiac injections require an interruption to compressions, and multiple injections cause trauma, which may predispose to ventricular ectopic beats or ventricular fibrillation.

Drug Therapy

During cardiopulmonary arrest basic life support measures and early defibrillation (when indicated) are of primary importance, and drug administration is of secondary importance. Drugs and fluids for cardiopulmonary arrest are categorized as vasopressors, vagolytic agents, antiarrhythmics, other drugs, and fluids.

Vasopressors

Epinephrine remains the vasopressor of choice in patients with cardiopulmonary arrest. Although epinephrine possesses both α and β-adrenergic activity, it is the α-adrenergic (vasoconstrictor) effects that increase coronary and cerebral perfusion pressure and are of primary importance during cardiopulmonary resuscitation. The value and safety of the β-adrenergic effects are controversial because they may increase myocardial work and oxygen demand.

There has been much controversy about and research into the appropriate dose of epinephrine. Two separate doses, high-dose (0.1 to 0.2 mg/kg every 3 to 5 minutes) and low-dose (0.01 to 0.02 mg/kg every 3 to 5 minutes) of intravenous epinephrine are recognized. Current recommendations are to start with the low-dose and titrate up with higher doses if the desired effect is not achieved. The high-dose regimen should be reserved for patients that are refractory to the lower dosages. Many authors recommend ten times this dose when epinephrine is administered via the tracheal tube route. This route should be avoided if at all possible because evidence shows that there may be a paradoxic effect (see the section on endotracheal instillation). In all cases subsequent doses of epinephrine, if needed, should be given every 3 to 5 minutes.

Vasopressin is a nonadrenergic peripheral vasoconstrictor that achieves its effects via direct stimulation of specific vasopressin (V_1) receptors in vascular smooth muscle. Like epinephrine these vasoconstrictor effects increase coronary and cerebral perfusion pressure. However, vasopressin has several advantages over epinephrine and other catecholamines. For example, the vasoconstrictor effects of vasopressin are not blunted in the presence of acidosis; nor is its use associated with increased myocardial work or oxygen demand. Because the effects of vasopressin have not been shown to differ from those of epinephrine in cardiac arrest, it seems reasonable to use one intravenous dose of vasopressin (0.8 U/kg once intravenously) in place of a second dose of epinephrine in the treatment of pulseless arrest.

Vagolytic Agents

Atropine sulfate reverses cholinergic-mediated (parasympathetic) decreases in heart rate, systemic vascular resistance, and blood pressure. The development of sinus bradycardia, pulseless electrical activity, and asystole can be precipitated or exacerbated by excessive vagal (parasympathetic) tone. Atropine is inexpensive and easy to administer and has few side effects; therefore it should be considered for cardiopulmonary-arrest patients exhibiting these rhythms. The full vagolytic dose of atropine (0.04 mg/kg once intravenously) is reserved solely for patients with pulseless electrical activity or asystolic cardiac arrest. This dose of atropine is best avoided in patients with sinus bradycardia because it may result in a sustained tachycardia and increased myocardial oxygen demand. Although low-dose atropine (0.004 to 0.01 mg/kg once intravenously) may be associated with a transient centrally mediated exacerbation of bradycardia, it is the preferred dose in patients with sinus bradycardia.

Antiarrhythmics

Amiodarone is a membrane-stabilizing antiarrhythmic drug that increases the duration of the action potential and refractory period in atrial and ventricular myocardium. Atrioventricular conduction is slowed, and a similar effect is seen with accessory pathways. Although amiodarone (5 mg/kg once intravenously) is associated with a multitude of side effects, when used in conjunction with epinephrine it may prove useful in patients with refractory ventricular fibrillation.

Lidocaine is a class 1B antiarrhythmic that works by inhibiting the fast sodium current and shortening the time to repolarization. Although lidocaine has become the standard intravenous agent for suppression of serious ventricular arrhythmias (2 to 4 mg/kg intravenous bolus followed by continuous-rate infusion (CRI) of 25 to 80 mcg/kg/min intravenously), it has limited use during CPCR. Studies have shown that lidocaine can actually raise the defibrillation threshold, making it more difficult to defibrillate a fibrillating heart. As a result, lidocaine is recommended only in postcardiopulmonary-arrest patients that have persistent multifocal or hemodynamically unstable ventricular tachycardia. In addition, it is important to recognize that many patients with ROSC actually have stable idioventricular or ventricular escape rhythms and suppression of those rhythms with lidocaine or other antiarrhythmic agents may prove fatal.

Magnesium is a major intracellular cation and serves as a cofactor in a number of enzymatic reactions. Magnesium treatment (25 to 40 mg/kg or 0.15 to 0.3 mEq/kg slow bolus over 5 to 10 minutes intravenously followed by CRI of 1 to 2 mEq/kg/day intravenously) is indicated in patients with documented hypomagnesemia or with torsades de pointes regardless of cause; however, there are insufficient data to recommend for or against its routine use in cardiac arrest.

Other Drugs

Calcium plays a vital role in the cellular mechanisms underlying myocardial contraction, but there are very few data supporting any beneficial action of therapeutic calcium following most cases of cardiac arrest. High plasma concentration achieved after injection may have detrimental effects on the ischemic myocardium and may impair cerebral recovery. Thus calcium is given during resuscitation only when specifically indicated (e.g., in hyperkalemia, hypocalcemia, and clinically severe overdose of calcium channel blocking drugs). In cardiac arrest calcium gluconate (50 to 150 mg/kg every 15 to 20 minutes intravenously) may be given by rapid intravenous injection. In the presence of a spontaneous circulation it should be given slowly since it can slow the heart rate and precipitate arrhythmias.

Sodium bicarbonate to treat metabolic acidosis during cardiopulmonary arrest is controversial. Cardiopulmonary arrest results in combined respiratory and metabolic acidosis caused by cessation of pulmonary gas exchange and the development of anaerobic cellular metabolism. Data suggest that buffer administration not only lacks benefits but may also be deleterious. Although the routine use of sodium bicarbonate (1 to 2 mEq/kg every 10 to 15 minutes intravenously) in cardiac arrest is not recommended, it has a specific role in hyperkalemia and may be considered in patients with severe preexisting metabolic acidosis or prolonged cardiopulmonary arrest (>15 minutes).

Fluid Therapy

Although there is little evidence supporting intravenous fluid therapy during cardiopulmonary arrest, it has long been advocated as a standard practice in veterinary CPCR. Although high fluid rates are appropriate for animals with preexisting hypovolemia or significant ongoing losses, experimental studies indicate that volume loading of euvolemic patients my actually cause a decrease in myocardial and cerebral perfusion. These findings have prompted investigation into small-volume resuscitation protocols using colloidal solutions and hypertonic saline. Although there is not enough evidence to make a standard recommendation, small-volume resuscitation using hypertonic saline may have a positive effect on resuscitation success and recovery after cardiopulmonary arrest.

CPCR MONITORING

Once CPCR has been instituted, it becomes necessary to evaluate the effectiveness of the procedure. ECG monitors should be attached to all CPCR patients. Unfortunately *reading* the ECG requires cessation of chest compressions and therefore has an adverse effect on ROSC. To minimize

the interruption of chest compressions, additional methods of monitoring are recommended. Clinicians frequently try to palpate arterial pulses during chest compression. Unfortunately retrograde blood flow into the venous system may produce femoral vein pulsations. Thus generation of a palpable pulse is not a reliable indicator of adequate compression and is not indicative of effective arterial flow. Doppler ultrasonography may be used to assess blood flow, but it is frequently affected by movement artifact. Although assessment of coronary artery perfusion might be helpful, it is technically difficult to measure and not routinely available. During cardiopulmonary arrest pulse oximetry will not function because pulsatile blood flow is inadequate in peripheral tissue beds. Arterial blood gas monitoring enables estimation of the degree of hypoxemia and the adequacy of ventilation during CPCR but is not a reliable indicator of the extent of tissue acidosis. In low-flow states such as cardiopulmonary arrest venous blood gas measurements are more reflective of intracellular events in the peripheral tissue beds than are arterial measurements.

$ETCO_2$ monitoring is a safe and effective noninvasive indicator of cardiac output during CPCR. The $ETCO_2$ reading can be useful in monitoring the progression of CPCR because $ETCO_2$ is linearly related to stroke volume when ventilation is controlled. In low-flow states many of the alveoli are not perfused; thus carbon dioxide (CO_2) is unable to diffuse from the bloodstream into expired gas, and $ETCO_2$ measurements are low. As blood flow improves, more alveoli are perfused, and more CO_2 is excreted. Success of CPCR has been correlated with higher $ETCO_2$ values in human and porcine models.

References and Suggested Reading

2005 American Heart Association guidelines for cardiopulmonary resuscitation and emergency cardiovascular care, *Circulation* 112(24 suppl):IV1, 2005.

Alzaga-Fernandez AG, Varon J: Open-chest cardiopulmonary resuscitation: past, present and future, *Resuscitation* 64:149, 2005.

Cole SG, Otto CM, Hughes D: Cardiopulmonary cerebral resuscitation in small animals—a clinical practice review (part I), *J Vet Emerg Care* 12(4):261, 2002.

Cole SG, Otto CM, Hughes D: Cardiopulmonary cerebral resuscitation in small animals—a clinical practice review (part II), *J Vet Emerg Care* 13(1):13, 2003.

Haldane S, Marks SL: Cardiopulmonary cerebral resuscitation: emergency drugs and postresuscitative care, *Compend Cont Educ Pract Vet* 26(10):791, 2004.

Haldane S, Marks SL: Cardiopulmonary cerebral resuscitation: techniques, *Compend Cont Educ Pract Vet* 26(10):780, 2004.

Holowaychuk MK, Martin LG: Misconceptions about emergency and critical care: cardiopulmonary cerebral resuscitation, fluid therapy, shock, and trauma, *Compend Cont Educ Pract Vet* 28(6):420, 2006.

Rieser TM: Cardiopulmonary resuscitation, *Clin Tech Small Anim Pract* 15(2):76, 2000.

Varon J, Marik PE, Fromm RE: Cardiopulmonary resuscitation: a review for clinicians, *Resuscitation* 36:133, 1998.

Waldrop JE et al: Causes of cardiopulmonary arrest, resuscitation management, and functional outcome in dogs and cats surviving cardiopulmonary arrest, *J Vet Emerg Care* 14(1):22, 2004.

CHAPTER 6
Traumatic Brain Injury

DANIEL J. FLETCHER, *Ithaca, New York*
CURTIS W. DEWEY, *Ithaca, New York*

Trauma is a common presenting complaint in small animal veterinary emergency services, and traumatic brain injury (TBI) occurs in a high proportion of these animals. Common causes of TBI in dogs and cats include motor vehicle accidents, animal interactions, falls from heights, blunt trauma, gunshot wounds, and other malicious human behaviors. A global view of the patient is critical when treating TBI, and both extracranial and intracranial priorities must be addressed. Life-threatening extracranial issues such as penetrating thoracic and abdominal wounds or airway obstruction, as well as compromise of oxygenation, ventilation, or volume status must be identified and treated appropriately. Once extracranial factors have been addressed, the focus shifts to intracranial priorities such as maintenance of adequate cerebral perfusion pressure (CPP), oxygen delivery to the brain, and treatment of acute intracranial hypertension.

PATHOPHYSIOLOGY

The pathophysiology of head trauma can be separated into two categories: primary injury and secondary injury. Primary injury is the immediate result of the traumatic event, whereas secondary injury is comprised of a cascade of physiologic and biochemical events that occur in the subsequent hours to days.

Primary Injury

The major types of primary injury that occur after head trauma include concussion, cerebral contusion, cerebral laceration, intraaxial and extraaxial hematomas, and skull fractures. Concussion is characterized by a brief loss of consciousness and is not associated with underlying histopathologic lesions. Hemorrhage into the brain parenchyma and secondary edema comprises cerebral contusion, which can lead to variable severity of clinical signs. Although mild contusion can be difficult to differentiate from concussion, unconsciousness for more than several minutes is most consistent with contusion. Laceration is characterized by physical disruption of the brain parenchyma and can lead to intraaxial hematomas within the brain parenchyma, as well as extraaxial hematomas in the subarachnoid, subdural, and epidural spaces. These space-occupying lesions cause compression of the brain, leading to severe localizing neurologic signs or diffuse dysfunction.

Secondary Injury

TBI triggers a series of events that result in perpetuation of neuronal tissue damage, with both systemic and intracranial insults occurring independently and in combination. Systemic perfusion derangements contributing to secondary brain injury include hypotension and hypoxemia. Disorders of ventilation contribute to secondary brain injury as well, with hypoventilation causing increased cerebral blood volume (CBV) and hypoxemia, and hyperventilation leading to cerebral vasoconstriction and reduced perfusion. Metabolic abnormalities such as hyperglycemia, hypoglycemia, electrolyte imbalances, and acid-base disturbances further perpetuate secondary brain injury. Intracranial insults include increased intracranial pressure (ICP), compromise of the blood-brain barrier (BBB), mass lesions, cerebral edema, infection, vasospasm, and seizures. All of these factors ultimately lead to neuronal cell death.

Neuronal tissue is especially sensitive to oxidative damage because of its high lipid content. Many mechanisms favor production of reactive oxygen species after TBI, including local hemorrhage, catecholamine production, perfusion deficits, and local acidosis. Local biochemical processes in hypoperfused tissues lead to a milieu primed for generation of reactive oxygen species. Once perfusion is reestablished, these oxidized lipids, proteins, and deoxyribonucleic acids, result in further destruction of neurons.

Damaged neurons inappropriately release excitatory neurotransmitters, causing sodium and calcium influx and depolarization and increasing cellular metabolic activity, depleting adenosine triphosphate stores. Nitric oxide (NO) has been associated with secondary brain injury after trauma, likely because of vasodilatory effects and production of free radicals. Production of other inflammatory mediators has been associated with TBI, leading to secondary injury, including BBB disruption, induction of NO production, mononuclear and polymorphonuclear cell chemotaxis, and activation of the arachidonic acid cascade.

Compromise of Cerebral Perfusion

CPP is the net driving pressure leading to blood flow to the brain. It is defined as the difference between systemic mean arterial pressure (MAP) and ICP.

$$CPP = MAP - ICP$$

Primary and secondary brain injuries leading to increases in ICP, in combination with systemic sequelae of the trauma such as hypovolemia leading to decreases in MAP, ultimately result in worsening of cerebral injury as a result of decreased CPP.

Blood flow to the brain per unit time (cerebral blood flow [CBF]) is a function of CPP and cerebrovascular resistance (CVR). Autoregulatory mechanisms, dependent largely on local alterations in CVR, allow the normal brain to maintain a constant CBF over a wide range of MAP (50 mm Hg to 150 mm Hg). These autoregulatory mechanisms are commonly compromised in patients with TBI, making them more susceptible to ischemic injury with decreases in MAP.

Acute increases in ICP often trigger the "Cushing's reflex," a characteristic combination of systemic hypertension and sinus bradycardia. The initial drop in CPP resulting from increased ICP leads to a dramatic increase of sympathetic tone, causing systemic vasoconstriction and increased cardiac output, ultimately leading to significant increases in MAP. Stimulation of baroreceptors in the aorta and carotid sinus by the increase in MAP triggers a reflex sinus bradycardia. The presence of the Cushing's reflex in a patient with head trauma is a sign of a potentially life-threatening increase in ICP and should be treated promptly.

ASSESSMENT, DIAGNOSTICS, AND MONITORING

Neurologic Assessment

The modified Glasgow Coma Scale (MGCS) score is a quantitative measure that has been shown to be associated with survival to 48 hours in dogs with TBI and provides a score that can be used to assess both initial neurologic status and progression of signs (Platt, Radaelli, and McDonnell, 2001). This scale incorporates three domains: level of consciousness, posture, and pupillary size/response to light, with a score of 1 to 6 assigned to each domain. The final score ranges from 3 to 18, with lower scores indicating more severe neurologic deficits. The initial neurologic examination should be interpreted in light of the cardiovascular and respiratory systems since shock can have a significant effect on neurologic status.

Initial Diagnostics

Because of the likelihood of multisystemic injury associated with head trauma, initial diagnostics and patient monitoring should focus on a global assessment of patient stability. An initial emergency database should consist of a packed cell volume and total solids to assess for hemorrhage; blood glucose to assess severity of injury; and a blood gas (venous or arterial) to assess perfusion, ventilation, oxygenation, and acid-base status. If possible, samples for a complete blood count and blood chemistry should be obtained before therapy to assess renal and hepatic function and to screen for other systemic disease. In general, occlusion of the jugular vein is contraindicated in patients with TBI because this can lead to increased ICP caused by decreased venous outflow from the brain; therefore samples should be obtained peripherally or via peripherally inserted central catheters.

Imaging of the head is indicated in patients with localizing signs of brain dysfunction, those with moderate-to-severe neurologic deficits that do not respond to aggressive extracranial and intracranial stabilization, and those with progressive neurologic signs. These studies can yield information about targets of potential surgical intervention such as intraaxial or extraaxial hemorrhage, skull fractures, or cerebrospinal fluid leaks. Skull radiographs have low sensitivity in the assessment of patients with TBI and rarely yield useful diagnostic information. Computed tomography is a sensitive imaging modality that yields excellent detail for assessment of skull fracture, acute hemorrhage, and brain edema.

Monitoring

The overall duration and frequency of episodes of hypoperfusion and tissue oxygenation deficits have been associated with poorer outcomes in people with TBI. Therefore serial monitoring of these parameters is essential for successful management of these patients. Frequent qualitative assessment of tissue perfusion via mucous membrane color; capillary refill time; heart rate and pulse quality; and quantitative assessment of blood pressure, oxygenation, and ventilation is crucial. A minimal MAP of 80 mm Hg should be targeted to decrease the risk of inadequate CPP. If the Doppler technique is used for monitoring, a minimum systolic pressure of 100 mm Hg should be the target. Continuous electrocardiograph monitoring should also be used if possible; if episodes of sinus bradycardia are noted, blood pressure should be assessed for evidence of the Cushing's reflex, which warrants aggressive therapy directed at lowering ICP.

Techniques have been described for continuous or intermittent direct monitoring of ICP. These techniques are invasive and can lead to complications but yield valuable information for the management of patients with TBI and allow calculation of CPP, the most important of the parameters determining CBF. General guidelines are to maintain ICP below 20 mm Hg and to maintain a CPP of at least 60 mm Hg.

TREATMENT

Treatment priorities for patients with TBI can be divided into two broad categories: extracranial and intracranial. Successful management of patients with TBI depends on addressing both categories.

Extracranial Priorities

Because of the high likelihood of multisystem trauma in patients with TBI, assessment of potential extracranial injuries is an essential part of the initial diagnostic workup. As with any severely injured patient, the basics of *Airway*, *Breathing*, and *Circulation* (i.e., the ABCs) should be evaluated and addressed as necessary. Airway patency should be assessed as soon as possible. Endotracheal intubation or tracheostomy should be considered if complete or partial obstruction is present. Even mild hypercapnia can significantly increase ICP and should not be tolerated. Conversely, hyperventilation leading to hypocapnia can cause cerebral vasoconstriction, decreasing CBF and leading to cerebral ischemia. Therefore manual or mechanical ventilation should be used if necessary to maintain CO_2 at the low end of the normal range (i.e., venous PCO_2, 40 to 45 mm Hg; arterial PCO_2, 35 to 40 mm Hg). The pharynx and larynx should be suctioned as needed to maintain airway patency.

Because hypoxia is common in patients with traumatic injury, supplemental oxygen is indicated in the initial management of all patients with TBI. Patients with pulmonary contusions or other pulmonary parenchymal disease may require mechanical ventilation with positive end-expiratory pressure to maintain adequate oxygenation.

Patients with TBI commonly present in hypovolemic shock, and volume resuscitation goals should be aggressive (MAP of 80 to 100 mm Hg). For patients without electrolyte disturbances normal saline (0.9%) is the best choice of the isotonic crystalloids since it contains the smallest amount of free water and is least likely to contribute to cerebral edema. Synthetic colloids can have a more rapid and long-lasting effect in hydrated patients but are not effective in dehydrated patients. Patients with hypotension caused by hypovolemia and concurrent increased ICP will benefit from a combination of a synthetic colloid (see Chapter 11) (hetastarch or dextran 70) and hyperosmotic (hypertonic saline [HTS]) solution. See Table 6-1 for recommended doses. Patients who do not respond to volume resuscitation require vasopressor support. Because CPP is dependent on MAP, systemic hypotension must not be tolerated.

Intracranial Priorities

The main goals of intracranial stabilization are maintaining adequate cerebral perfusion by controlling ICP, reducing cerebral metabolism, and maintaining adequate systemic blood pressure.

Hyperosmotic Agents

Mannitol is an effective therapy for patients with increased ICP and has been shown to reduce cerebral edema, increase CPP and CBF, and improve neurologic outcome in TBI. It has a rapid onset of action, with clinical improvement occurring within minutes of administration, and these effects can last as long as 1.5 to 6 hours. Mannitol boluses of 0.5 to 1.5 g/kg have been recommended for treatment of increased ICP in dogs and cats. High-dose mannitol boluses (1.4 g/kg versus 0.7 g/kg) were shown to result in improved neurologic outcome in humans in a recent clinical trial (Cruz et al., 2004). Mannitol may increase the permeability of the BBB, an effect that is most pronounced when the BBB is exposed to the drug for prolonged periods of time. The increased permeability can allow mannitol to leak into the brain parenchyma, where it can exacerbate edema. To reduce the risk of this effect, the drug should be administered in repeated boluses rather than as a continuous-rate infusion. The diuretic effect of mannitol can be profound and can cause severe volume depletion. Therefore treatment must be followed with isotonic crystalloid solutions and/or colloids to maintain intravascular volume. In humans mannitol may induce acute renal failure if serum osmolarity exceeds 320 mOsm/L; therefore, if possible, serum osmolality should be measured when repeated doses are administered.

HTS is a hyperosmotic solution that may be used as an alternative to mannitol in patients with head injury. Because sodium does not freely cross the intact BBB, HTS

Table **6-1**

Drugs and Doses for Patients With Traumatic Brain Injury

Indication	Drug	Dose	Comments
Intracranial Hypertension			
Euvolemic, normotensive, or hypertensive patients	Mannitol 25%	0.5-1.5 g/kg IV over 15 minutes; may repeat	Potent osmotic diuretic. Follow with crystalloids and/or colloids to maintain intravascular volume. Monitor osmolality with repeat dosing.
Hypovolemic patients	HTS (7%)* + dextran-70 or hetastarch	3-5 ml/kg over 15 minutes; may repeat	Contraindicated in hyponatremic patients. Monitor serum sodium concentrations with repeat dosing.
Hypovolemic or euvolemic patients	HTS (7-7.8%)	3-5 ml/kg over 15 minutes; may repeat	Contraindicated in hyponatremic patients. Monitor serum sodium concentrations with repeat dosing. If using 23.4% solution, dilute 1 part HTS with 2 parts 0.9% saline or sterile water.
Anticonvulsant Therapy			
Actively seizing patients	Diazepam or midazolam	0.5 mg/kg IV or rectal bolus; may repeat; 0.2-0.5 mg/kg/hr IV CRI	Do not administer diazepam CRI into peripheral catheters because of the risk of phlebitis.
Prophylaxis for immediate or early seizures, status epilepticus, or cluster seizures	Phenobarbital	16 mg/kg loading dose (divided into 4 doses q2-4h); 2 mg/kg q12h maintenance dosage	Evaluate chemistry for evidence of hepatic dysfunction. Monitor ventilation and blood pressure during loading.
	Potassium bromide	120 mg/kg/day PO for 5 days, then 30 mg/kg/day PO	Sodium bromide can be substituted at the same dose and given IV.

CRI, Continuous-rate infusion; *HTS,* hypertonic saline; *IV,* intravenously.
*23.4% HTS: dilute 1 part HTS with 2 parts dextran-70 or hetastarch.
7% to 7.5% HTS: administer separate doses of HTS and dextran-70 or hetastarch (3-5 ml/kg each).

has osmotic effects similar to those of mannitol. Other beneficial effects of HTS include improved hemodynamic status via volume expansion and positive inotropic effects, as well as beneficial vasoregulatory and immunomodulatory effects (Ware et al., 2005). Rebound hypotension is uncommon with HTS administration because, unlike mannitol, sodium is actively resorbed in the kidneys, especially in hypovolemic patients. This makes it preferable to mannitol for treating patients with increased ICP and systemic hypotension caused by hypovolemia. Combining HTS with a synthetic colloid can prolong this volume expansion effect (see Table 6-1). HTS is contraindicated in patients with hyponatremia because it can cause rapid rises in serum sodium concentrations, leading to central pontine myelinolysis and delayed neurologic signs. In euvolemic patients with evidence of intracranial hypertension, both mannitol and HTS can have beneficial effects. If an individual patient is not responding to one drug, the other may yield a beneficial response.

Corticosteroids
Corticosteroids are potent antiinflammatory medications and have been recommended in human and veterinary medicine to treat TBI. A recent clinical trial evaluating over 10,000 human adults with head injury showed that treatment with corticosteroids was associated with worse outcome at 2 weeks and 6 months after injury (Edwards et al., 2005). Because of the lack of evidence of any beneficial effect of corticosteroids after TBI and strong evidence from the human literature showing a detrimental effect on neurologic outcome, corticosteroids should *not* be administered to dogs and cats with TBI.

Furosemide
Furosemide has been used to treat cerebral edema either as a sole agent or in combination with mannitol. This use has been called into question because of the potential for intravascular volume depletion and systemic hypotension, ultimately leading to decreased CPP (Chesnut et al., 1998). It should be reserved for patients in whom it is indicated for other reasons such as those with pulmonary edema or oligoanuric renal failure.

Decreasing Cerebral Blood Volume
Cerebral vasodilation and blood pooling can cause increases in the total volume of blood within the calvaria or in the CBV and can contribute to increased ICP. Several techniques to decrease CBV have been described and have been shown to be effective in people with increased ICP. Hypercapnia caused by hypoventilation can cause cerebral vasodilation and increased CBV. Ventilatory support should be targeted at maintenance of normocapnia (arterial CO_2 of 35 to 40 mm Hg). In cases of severe, acute intracranial hypertension, short-term hyperventilation to an arterial CO_2 of 25 to 35 mm Hg may be used to reduce CBV and ICP. However, chronic hyperventilation is not recommended because the decrease in CBF can lead to cerebral ischemia.

Elevation of the head by 15 to 30 degrees reduces CBV by increasing venous drainage, decreasing ICP, and increasing CPP without deleterious changes in cerebral oxygenation (Ng and Wong, 2004). It is imperative that occlusion of the jugular veins be avoided by using a slant board to prevent bending the neck. Angles greater than 30 degrees may cause a detrimental decrease in CPP.

Anticonvulsant Therapy
Seizures are common after TBI in humans, with reported incidence rates of up to 54% (Frey, 2003). Posttraumatic seizures are divided into three groups: immediate, occurring within 24 hours of the trauma; early, occurring 24 hours to 7 days after trauma; and late, occurring longer than 7 days after trauma. Several controlled clinical trials have been undertaken in human medicine to investigate the efficacy of prophylactic anticonvulsant therapy after TBI, and a meta-analysis showed an overall reduction in the risk of immediate and early seizures with prophylactic anticonvulsant therapy (Schierhout and Roberts, 1998). Given these data, short-term prophylactic therapy for 7 days after trauma may be indicated in patients with TBI, and anticonvulsant therapy should always be instituted for patients with TBI who develop immediate or early seizures, but there is little evidence to support the use of long-term anticonvulsant therapy to prevent late seizures in these patients. Suggested traditional anticonvulsant drugs and doses are listed in Table 6-1. In addition, several newer anticonvulsant medications have become available in recent years (see Chapter 232). These may prove to be useful alternatives by allowing more thorough neurologic evaluation than traditional anticonvulsants, which have significant sedative effects.

Control of Hyperglycemia
Presence and persistence of hyperglycemia have been associated with worse outcome in numerous clinical studies in human children and adults with TBI. Only one retrospective veterinary study has evaluated the association between hyperglycemia and TBI; and, although an association between admission hyperglycemia and severity of neurologic injury was noted, there was no association between hyperglycemia at admission and survival (Syring, Otto, and Drobatz, 2001). A recent small trial comparing 14 humans with TBI treated with intensive insulin therapy to maintain strict control of blood glucose levels to 33 humans treated with a less strict protocol found significantly lower brain glucose levels in the intensive therapy group but no significant difference in neurologic outcome between the groups (Vespa et al., 2006). This is an active area of research, but, until larger outcome studies are available, there is little evidence to support the use of insulin therapy in patients with TBI.

Decreasing Cerebral Metabolic Rate
TBI can lead to increased cerebral metabolic rate (CMR) and can result in cerebral ischemia and cellular swelling. Therefore therapies targeted at decreasing CMR can reduce secondary brain injury. Induction of barbiturate coma and hypothermia have been used in experimental studies and clinical trials in humans to reduce CMR. Barbiturate coma can effectively decrease ICP via reductions in CMR and has been shown to improve outcome in humans with refractory intracranial hypertension, but hypothermia has not been associated with improved outcome and is not recommended.

Decompressive Craniectomy

Several surgical procedures to address increased ICP have been described in human medicine, including CSF drainage and decompressive craniectomy. The goal of these therapies is to allow expansion of the various intracranial compartments without a subsequent increase in ICP. The use of decompressive craniectomy in human patients with TBI is controversial, and a large-scale, randomized human clinical trial is currently underway (the RESCUEicp Trial), which will compare aggressive medical management with decompressive craniectomy in 500 patients with TBI (Hutchinson et al., 2006). Pending results of this trial, we recommend adoption of current recommendations in the human literature; consider decompressive craniectomy within 12 hours in patients with sustained, increasing ICP that is refractory to medical therapy.

PROGNOSIS

Prognosis following TBI is difficult to predict, and only the MGCS has been shown to be correlated with outcome in small animal patients (Platt et al., 2001). However, our clinical experience would suggest that even patients with severe neurologic deficits at presentation can show marked improvement over the subsequent 24 to 48 hours. Therefore serial neurologic examinations are recommended. Client education is also of paramount importance since persistent or permanent neurologic deficits in patients with TBI are common.

References and Suggested Reading

Chesnut RM et al: Neurogenic hypotension in patients with severe head injuries, *J Trauma* 44:958, 1998.

Cruz J et al: Successful use of the new high-dose mannitol treatment in patients with Glasgow Coma Scale scores of 3 and bilateral abnormal pupillary widening: a randomized trial, *J Neurosurg* 100:376, 2004.

Edwards P et al: Final results of MRC CRASH, a randomised placebo-controlled trial of intravenous corticosteroid in adults with head injury-outcomes at 6 months, *Lancet* 365:1957, 2005.

Frey LC: Epidemiology of posttraumatic epilepsy: a critical review, *Epilepsia* 10(suppl):11, 2003.

Hutchinson PJ et al: Decompressive craniectomy in traumatic brain injury: the randomized multicenter RESCUEicp study (www.RESCUEicp.com), *Acta Neurochir* 96(suppl):17, 2006.

Ng I, Lim J, Wong HB: Effects of head posture on cerebral hemodynamics: its influences on intracranial pressure, cerebral perfusion pressure, and cerebral oxygenation, *Neurosurgery* 54:593, 2004.

Platt SR, Radaelli ST, McDonnell JJ: The prognostic value of the modified Glasgow Coma Scale in head trauma in dogs, *J Vet Intern Med* 15:581, 2001.

Schierhout G, Roberts I: Prophylactic antiepileptic agents after head injury: a systematic review. *J Neurol Neurosurg Psychiatry* 64:108, 1998.

Syring RS, Otto CM, Drobatz KJ: Hyperglycemia in dogs and cats with head trauma: 122 cases (1997-1999), *J Am Vet Med Assoc* 218:1124, 2001.

Vespa P et al: Intensive insulin therapy reduces microdialysis glucose values without altering glucose utilization or improving the lactate/pyruvate ratio after traumatic brain injury, *Crit Care Med* 34:850, 2006.

Ware ML et al: Effects of 23.4% sodium chloride solution in reducing intracranial pressure in patients with traumatic brain injury: a preliminary study, *Neurosurgery* 57:727, 2005.

CHAPTER 7
Vascular Access Techniques

JAMES S. WOHL, *Auburn, Alabama*
MARION B. TEFEND, *Auburn, Alabama*

Percutaneous placement of intravascular catheters is the most common method of achieving access to the vasculature for fluid therapy, frequent blood collection, and physiologic monitoring. In emergency patients large-bore peripheral catheters typically are indicated for rapid fluid resuscitation, but they can be problematic because of hypotension, hypovolemia, vascular collapse, trauma, and skin stiffness. Central line catheters are indicated in all severely hypovolemic patients or if central venous pressure monitoring or serial blood sampling is indicated.

In some instances emergency venous or arterial access requires a cutdown procedure. Knowledge of reliable anatomic landmarks and proper surgical technique facilitate successful placement of vascular catheters in the critically ill patient. Cutdowns help ensure that the vessel is cannulated on the first attempt and can allow placement of a larger catheter than what can normally be placed percutaneously. Intraosseous access can be used for all small patients, as well as small birds and reptiles. Intraosseous cannulation (Bonagura, 1992) provides a route for fluid and drug administration but is inadequate for blood collection and cardiovascular monitoring. Percutaneous placement of arterial catheters (Bonagura, 1995) is indicated in patients requiring repeated arterial blood gas analysis or direct arterial blood pressure measurement.

CATHETER SELECTION

Access to the vasculature in the critically ill or traumatized patient allows for the delivery of lifesaving medications, fluid therapy, blood products, or nutrition, all of which can be accomplished through a wide range of specialty catheters. Proper nursing care to patients harboring such devices is critical because any indwelling catheter or tube represents a focus for microbial colonization. Incorrect placement or positioning can cause patient discomfort or compromise. Appropriate selection as to the catheter or tube type, in combination with proper management techniques, is paramount to patient care. Recognizing the advantages and disadvantages of the different types of specialty tubes and the care necessary for maintaining patency of such tubes will benefit patient outcome and prevent unnecessary complications.

Peripheral venous catheters such as the over-the-needle type are the most commonly used method of obtaining *vascular access* in the small animal patient. Advantages of this catheter type include ease and speed of insertion, low cost, and versatility of access in different anatomic locations. Flow rates are greatly enhanced by placement of short (2-inch) large-bore (12 to 16 g) catheters placed intravenously. Anatomic location for the peripheral catheter is best used in the cephalic, accessory cephalic, or jugular vein during triage. Other sites of placement of the peripheral over-the-needle catheter can include the saphenous or medial saphenous vein, dorsal common digital vein, or articular or lingual vein. Other uses of the over-the-needle catheter type include pericardiocentesis, abdominocentesis, or thoracocentesis. Another advantage of the over-the-needle catheter is the variety of both the gauge and length available to the practitioner, ranging from 25 g to 12 g and from 2 inches up to 12 inches in length.

Central venous access catheters are advantageous for monitoring central venous pressure, obtaining serial blood sampling with minimal stress to the patient, long-term patient use, and administrating of hyperosmolar solutions. The central venous catheter is most commonly placed in the jugular vein but can be readily inserted into the caudal vena cava via the lateral or medial saphenous veins. Other advantages of the central venous catheter are the wide variety of styles available to the veterinarian. Some central venous catheters contain multiple lumens for the simultaneous delivery of incompatible fluid types. Such multilumen catheters are also advantageous to the critical patient in need of fluid therapy, central venous pressure monitoring, intravenous (IV) nutrition, or continuous-rate infusions of medications, all of which can be done through one catheter. Disadvantages of the central venous catheter include a longer placement time, expense, slight patient discomfort during placement, and the relatively narrow diameter of the catheter itself. Since most central venous catheters are long and narrow, rapid fluid administration is not recommended as the primary delivery route, particularly during resuscitation. In addition, since most central venous catheters are placed into a jugular vein, patients with coagulation deficiencies may have complications with association of such devices. Monitoring for extravasations in the central venous catheter is a little more difficult than in the peripheral over-the-needle catheter. Caregivers should monitor the patient for edema of the neck, shoulder, or face; pain with insertion of medication; sluggish flow through the catheter; or inability to aspirate blood back from the catheter.

Long over-the-needle types of central venous catheters are inexpensive and come in a variety of lengths and diameters, ranging from 22 to 16 gauge and from 6 to 12 inches in length. Disadvantages of these catheter types include patient discomfort since they tend to be stiff and are prone to kinking. In addition, most over-the-needle long catheters are made of Vialon or

Teflon material, and should be changed after 5 to 7 days. Central venous catheters placed by the Seldinger technique include the single-to-multilumen devices, which are soft and flexible, made of an antithrombogenic polyurethane material, and can be maintained for longer periods. In addition, some Seldinger central venous catheters are impregnated with antimicrobial solutions that may result in a reduction of catheter-related sepsis. Disadvantages to the Seldinger central venous catheter types are expense, increased risk of local hemorrhage during insertion, and procedure time needed for placement. However, it is our opinion that the advantages of such central venous catheters far outweigh the risks and expense in critical patient use.

Arterial catheters provide an important means by which to monitor a patient's status. Inserted primarily into the dorsal pedal artery, catheterization can also be accomplished in the femoral, brachial, or even the auricular artery. Advantages to arterial catheterization include monitoring patient ventilation, acid-base equilibrium, and direct blood pressure monitoring. Over-the-needle peripheral catheters can be used for such procedures, although arterial catheter kits are now available using the Seldinger technique for ease of placement and long-term use. Percutaneous arterial catheterization is technically difficult because arteries are surrounded by a dense adventitia, are located deeper in fascial tissues than veins, and are not visible through the skin. Arterial catheterization can be further complicated by hypotension or hypovolemia. Medications should not be administered through arterial catheters.

Vascular access ports, or implantable vascular access systems, are subcutaneous delivery systems that allow serial blood sampling or IV administration of medications or fluid. Such devices are advantageous to chronically ill patients that can be treated intermittently on an outpatient basis. Surgically implanted, the catheter and port are subdermal and can be accessed without patient discomfort. Complications associated with such systems are similar to those of other types of IV catheters, including topical infection, sepsis, thrombosis, or extravasations. Nursing care required for vascular ports include daily insertion site inspection, mild antiseptic cleansing, and intermittent heparinized flushes to prevent clogging or occlusion.

CATHETER PLACEMENT TECHNIQUES

Seldinger Technique

Catheters using the Seldinger technique can be placed percutaneously or following exposure of the vessel after mini cutdown or cutdown. Commercially available in single-, double-, or triple- lumen (Arrow, Cook, Beckon-Dickinson, Baxter, or Abbott catheter systems), sizes range from 22 to 16 gauge for peripheral use to 14 gauge to 24 gauge for central use. Lengths range from 16 to 30 cm. Most central catheters are made of polyurethane to help prevent thrombosis and can also be purchased with silver sulfadiazine and chlorhexidine (Arrow International) heparin coating. See Box 7-1 for venous access procedure and Box 7-2 for arterial access procedure.

Box **7-1**

Venous Access Procedure

1. Place patient in sternal recumbency with neck hyperextended.
2. Shave a wide area to avoid contamination of insertion site.
3. Perform surgical preparation with solutions containing povidine and isopropyl alcohol.
4. Apply sterile drape to area cranial to insertion site.
5. Premeasure guidewire; tip of guidewire should not exceed apex of heart.
6. *Premeasure central catheter length; tip of catheter should be located in cranial vena cava just outside of the right atrium for central venous pressure monitoring.*
7. Place large-bore, short cephalic catheter.
8. Insert straight end of wire into the vessel via the cephalic catheter to predetermined length.
9. Remove cephalic catheter; ensure that the wire does not inadvertently back out.
10. Insert the plastic dilator into the vessel by placing the wire through it and guiding it to the vessel. Passage of dilator may be facilitated by "tenting" the skin and gently rotating the dilator into the vessel; a cut into the skin with a No. 11 blade next to the wire may ease insertion. Insert one-half length of dilator into the vessel; then remove the dilator.
11. Insert the catheter over the wire and guide it into the vessel to predetermined length. Ensure that the end of the wire is projecting out the distal end of the catheter before advancement; the wire should be held as the catheter is advanced into the vessel. If double-lumen catheters are used, the wire should come out the distal (or colored) port.
12. Remove the wire, leaving the catheter in place
13. *Aspirate catheter* with small syringe; blood should easily flow into syringe. Flush the catheter with sterile saline and cap.
14. Secure the catheter in place with skin/fascia sutures, apply antiseptic/antibiotic ointment, and place under a sterile dressing. If entire length of catheter is not used, secure excess catheter with plastic catheter holders provided.

VENOUS CUTDOWN TECHNIQUES

Patient Preparation

Except in the most emergent situations, aseptic technique should be maintained during catheter placement. Clipping and surgical preparation of the skin 180 degrees around the cutdown site allow aseptic handling of a limb. Infusion of lidocaine into the skin and subcutis of the proposed cutdown site facilitates placement in awake or sedated patients. Final preparation includes a last surgical scrub and the maintenance of a sterile field containing the necessary instruments, catheters, syringes filled with heparinized saline, injection plugs, stopcocks, and fluid tubing. Sterile latex gloves should be worn when attempting invasive vascular access techniques. Since the focus of the surgeon is on the cutdown site, it is essential that nongloved assistants be present to monitor the patient's vital signs during the procedure.

Box 7-2

Arterial Access Procedure

Materials Needed
- Clippers
- Surgical scrub
- Suture material
- Heparinized saline flush
- Catheter cap
- Arterial catheter kit or cephalic catheter
- Bandage material
- Saline for infusion if continuous direct blood pressure monitoring is used

Procedure
1. Lay patient in lateral recumbency.
2. Give oxygen if body position compromises respiratory effort.
3. Clip and prep dorsal pedal area (down leg).
4. Palpate pulse with single digit.
5. Stab incision for cutdown at 45-degree angle and at least 1 inch away from palpable pulse.
6. Hold catheter like a dart; insert catheter with bevel up through tunneled area.
7. Insert catheter gently toward pulse (superficial); back out and redirect if no flash.
8. Once flash is obtained, be careful not to move catheter; slide entire length of wire via black tab-handle.
9. "Pop" catheter off the wire and into arterial space.
10. Remove wire and ensure blood flow (should be fast and in spurting or jet motion).
11. Cap and flush catheter; aspirate back to ensure blood flow and reflush.
12. Suture in place (three spots total).
13. Place small amount antibiotic cream over insertion site.
14. Cover with sterile gauze square.
15. Place one layer gauze bandage.
16. Cover catheter with light, stiff bandage and label catheter.

cutdown incisions should be made in the middle-to-cranial portion of the jugular groove. The maxillary vein is a branch of the external jugular vein and is located half the distance between the wing of the atlas and the mandibular salivary gland. For cephalic and lateral saphenous vein cutdowns, incisions are made over their expected locations on the dorsal antebrachium and lateral aspect of the distal tibia, respectively.

The surgical technique is similar for all venous sites. A scalpel blade is used to incise the skin directly over or adjacent to the vein. Either a transverse or a parallel skin incision can be made. Care should be taken to incise only the full thickness of the skin. Blunt dissection (e.g., with mosquito forceps) may be required to visualize the vein as a blue-to-purple tubular structure within the subcutaneous tissue. Minimal dissection is usually required for the placement of an over-the-needle or through-the-needle catheter.

In some instances it may be necessary to isolate the vein. Isolation is accomplished by blunt dissection parallel to the vein. Subcutaneous or adventitial tissue adjacent to the vein is retracted with atraumatic thumb forceps, exposing the vessel. Dissection with the use of sharp-ended scissors is then performed dorsally and ventrally to the vein. Dissecting in a parallel fashion minimizes the chances of rupturing or traumatizing the vessel. After freeing the vein from the subcutaneous tissue, a hemostat is advanced beneath the vein. A silk suture is then clasped by the hemostat and drawn beneath the vessel (Fig. 7-1). The vein can be briefly occluded proximally to enhance filling. The suture can then be used to retract the vein distally and provide adequate tension for the catheterization of the vessel (Fig. 7-2). Alternatively, the vessel may be sacrificed by ligating the vein distally and using the ligature to retract the vessel.

Mini Cutdown

The mini cutdown technique is used for gaining access to the cephalic and lateral saphenous veins. With the bevel facing the operator, a sterile 20- or 22-gauge hypodermic needle is scraped across the skin directly over and parallel to the underlying vein in a proximal-to-distal direction. Tearing skin in this fashion releases skin tension without damaging the underlying vessel. Alternatively a small incision can be made over the vein with a scalpel blade. Although an incision causes a less traumatic defect to the skin, care must be taken to avoid incising the vessel and subcutaneous tissue. A mini cutdown can be used to visualize a collapsed vein but is more commonly used to avoid tissue drag during catheter placement. This technique is most useful in cats with thick skin or when burring of an over-the-needle catheter is prohibiting percutaneous placement. Infusion of lidocaine before mini cutdown is rarely needed, especially in very sick patients.

Surgical Cutdown

Surgical cutdowns can be used over the external jugular, maxillary, cephalic, or lateral saphenous vein. If attempting catheterization of the external jugular vein,

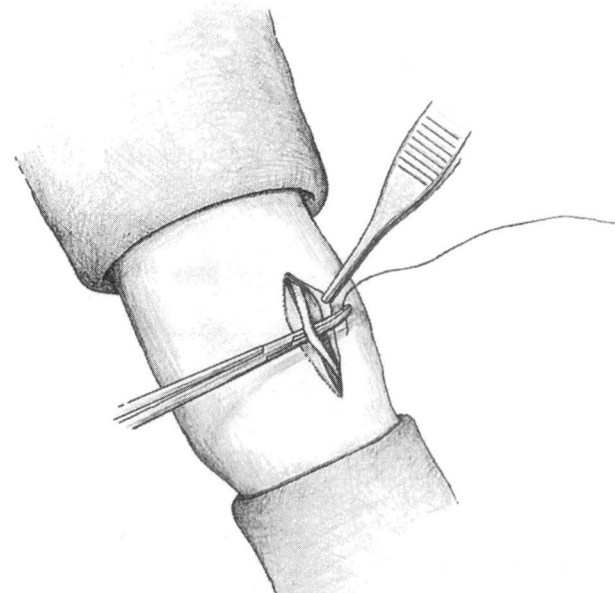

Fig. 7-1 Following isolation of the blood vessel, a hemostat is used to pass a silk suture beneath the vessel. (Art by Lisa Makarchuk; courtesy Auburn University, School of Veterinary Medicine, Auburn, Alabama.)

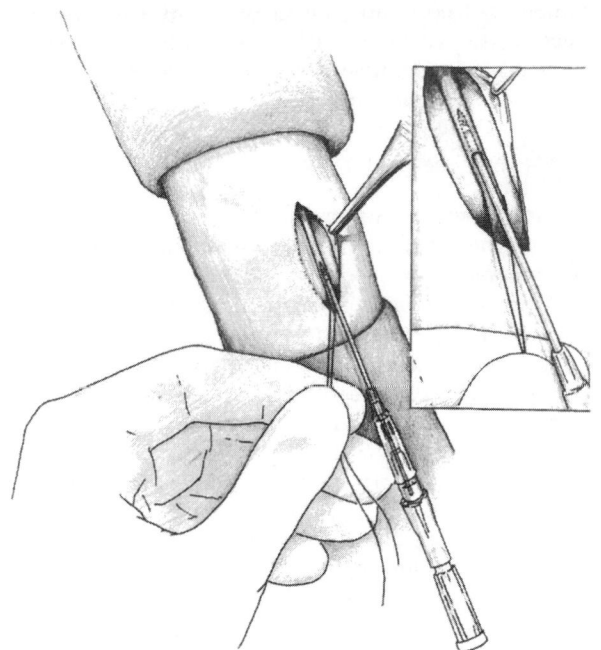

Fig. 7-2 Retraction of the vessel with a suture applies tension to the vessel, allowing introduction of an over-the-needle catheter. (Art by Lisa Makarchuk; courtesy Auburn University, School of Veterinary Medicine, Auburn, Alabama.)

A second suture is placed beneath the vessel proximally. The vein is then cannulated through a venotomy (or by venipuncture) between the two ligatures. Following catheterization, the proximal suture is ligated, securing the catheter in the vein.

ARTERIAL CUTDOWN TECHNIQUES

The most common site for arterial catheterization is the dorsal metatarsal artery. This artery is most superficial in the proximal metatarsus, medial to the extensor tendons, between the second and third metatarsal bones. A second arterial site is the dorsal pedal artery, which courses medial to the long digital extensor tendon at the level of the proximal tarsus. The femoral artery is less commonly used because of its location and the risk of hemorrhage, the potential danger of puncturing the external iliac artery, and retroperitoneal bleeding.

When a surgical cutdown is performed for arterial catheterization, a technique should be used that preserves vascular sufficiency. An incision is made over the pulsation of the dorsal metatarsal artery in the proximal metatarsus. When isolating the dorsal pedal artery, the incision is made medial and parallel to the long digital extensor in the proximal tarsus. Dissection is performed parallel to the direction of the artery, as described earlier for isolating a vein. The artery is identified as a white tubular structure. A pulse may be palpated, which will distinguish the artery from a nerve or tendon. A silk suture is placed beneath the artery and retracted distally to expose and place tension on the vessel.

An over-the-needle catheter, primed with heparinized saline, is recommended for arterial cannulation. Through-the-needle catheters have a smaller diameter than the penetrating needle and puncture wound; consequently, leakage of blood can result at the catheter insertion site. A more expensive alternative to an over-the-needle catheter is to use the modified Seldinger technique. This method uses a guidewire over which the catheter is advanced into the artery. A vessel dilator is sometimes used before introducing the catheter. Although the Seldinger technique is thought to be the least traumatic method of catheter placement, arterial cannulation usually can be achieved with over-the-needle catheters.

Topical administration of a few drops of 2% lidocaine onto the artery may prevent arterial spasm and facilitate cannulation. Retracting the artery with silk suture, the needle catheter assembly is inserted into the artery until rapid flow of red arterial blood fills the needle hub. The assembly is then repositioned in line with the artery and advanced an additional few millimeters. The catheter is then advanced off the needle and into the artery. The needle is discarded, and a sterile Luer-Lok injection plug is attached to the catheter. The catheter is flushed with a small volume of heparinized saline. Aspiration of arterial blood through the plugged catheter with a needle and syringe confirms the appropriate placement within the artery. It is important to keep the artery retracted during this procedure to prevent slippage of the artery off the unsecured catheter. In anesthetized patients venous blood may be superoxygenated and have the appearance of arterial blood. Observing pulsatile, rapid blood flow through the open catheter before the insertion of an injection cap indicates that the cannulated vessel is an artery. Blood gas analysis revealing an oxygen tension compatible with arterial blood or connection to a pressure-monitoring system will further confirm proper placement.

Securing the Catheter Without Sacrificing the Artery

The silk retraction suture is removed from beneath the artery. A silk suture with a swaged-on needle is placed above the artery but beneath the hub of the catheter. A finger trap suture is tied around the catheter hub, leaving excess suture on both ends of the second knot. The catheter is allowed to lie in a stationary position, and the remaining length of suture is used to anchor the catheter through the skin, placing minimal tension on the catheter. This method secures the catheter in place without sacrificing the artery and allows withdrawal of the catheter after cutting the anchoring skin suture. One or two interrupted skin sutures may be required proximal to the anchor suture to close the incision site.

Following suturing of the catheter and the incision site, a sterile dressing is applied, and the catheter is bandaged routinely. In awake patients, a soft, padded bandage can be used to inhibit movement of the tarsus. Patency of the catheter is maintained by periodic flushing with small volumes (1 to 2 ml) of heparinized saline injected through the injection cap with a 25-gauge needle or a low-dose saline continuous-rate infusion from a pressurized fluid bag if the catheter is used for continuous blood pressure monitoring. Manual flushing of larger volumes of fluid with a syringe can cause retrograde blood flow and embolization of particulate matter or air. Most transducer systems used for direct blood pressure monitoring use a squeeze clamp or pigtail flushing device. Attaching a multiport stopcock to the catheter allows connections to a blood pressure monitor and a flushing system and provides an additional site for blood collection. When not in use, stopcock ports should be attached to sterile injection plugs.

Blood Collection

With the stopcock to the designated collection port turned off, the sterile injection plug is removed and protected from contamination by placing it on a sterile gauze square or other sterile field. A sterile 3-ml syringe containing 1 ml of heparinized saline is then attached to the collection port. The stopcock to the flushing system is turned off, and 1 ml of blood is drawn through the catheter into the flush syringe. The stopcock to the patient is turned off, and the sample port and the flush syringe are discarded. The flushed blood mixture should *not* be reinfused following arterial blood collection. A new sterile syringe that has been purged with heparin (if obtaining a blood gas sample) is then attached, the stopcock closed to the flushing system, and the desired amount of blood is drawn *slowly* into the syringe. Rapid, forced withdrawal may injure the artery. After sample collection the stopcock is closed to the sample port, the sample syringe is removed, and the system is flushed for 1 second via the flushing system. To minimize thrombus formation and bacterial contamination, the sample stopcock should be flushed following blood collection. This is achieved by turning the stopcock to the patient off and allowing irrigation solution to flow through the open sample port. Sterile gauze can be used to collect the expelled solution. Following this procedure, the sterile injection plug is returned to the sample port.

Complications and Removal of Arterial Catheters

An arterial catheter should be removed as soon as it is no longer essential for proper patient management. In humans arterial catheters are associated with a higher rate of thrombus formation after a 3- or 4-day dwell time. Evidence of vasculitis, skin discoloration, hemorrhage, or an unexplained fever should prompt evaluation of the catheter site. Cooler-than-normal skin temperature distal to the catheter insertion site may indicate developing catheter-related insufficiency in blood supply and impending ischemic necrosis. Administration of medications through the arterial catheter is not recommended.

When an arterial catheter is removed, all bandage and dressing material should be removed. The anchoring suture is then cut. Firm pressure is applied proximal and distal to the insertion site while the catheter is removed with mild continuous suction applied by a syringe. This method facilitates aspiration of clots surrounding and within the catheter. On catheter removal firm manual pressure is applied over the insertion site for 5 to 10 minutes. After the application of manual pressure, a pressure dressing is applied for several hours. The insertion site is monitored periodically for internal or external hemorrhage.

MAINTENANCE OF VENOUS AND ARTERIAL CATHETERS

Any indwelling venous or arterial catheter predisposes a patient to the possibility of nosocomial infection. All personnel involved with placing the catheter or monitoring the patient must be aware of such risk and use caution when changing bandages, administering fluids or medications, withdrawing blood, or manipulating three-way stopcocks on monitoring devices attached to the catheter. Infection will occur as a result of contaminated IV solutions, failure to maintain a strict protocol for skin preparation, poor insertion technique, failure to clean equipment between patients, or failure to routinely change the catheter bandage. Insertion sites should be monitored routinely for thrombosis, patient discomfort, catheter migration, and extravasation.

Phlebitis is a commonly encountered complication of indwelling vascular catheterization. Phlebitis can occur as a result of inflammation associated with movement of a stiff catheter in a vein or artery or from bacterial infection that can lead to sepsis. Aseptic technique should be used whenever possible to minimize infection. Catheters should also be routinely changed according to type (e.g., changing over-the-needle peripheral catheters every 72 hours and long over-the-needle central catheters every 120 hours into new anatomic site). Minimizing tape use and anchoring with suture to secure catheters aid in insertion site inspection and patient comfort. Polyurethane Seldinger-type central catheters (Arrow International) may stay in for the length of patient hospitalization but still need daily insertion site cleaning, inspection for signs of thrombosis or leakage, and daily bandage changes.

Bacterial contamination of catheter sites can result from caregiver handling, heparinized flush syringes, blood left inside an injection port, and even tops of medication bottles. Caregivers should practice proper hygiene protocols, including washing hands frequently, swabbing ports and medication bottles with antiseptics, and frequently changing bandages to any catheter in any anatomic location. Flush solution should also be changed every 48 hours to avoid microbial contamination.

Sterile technique and catheter care should be maintained for *any* type of fluid administration. However, nursing management of catheters used for parenteral nutrition warrants special focus because nutritional formulas are excellent mediums for bacterial colonization. Catheter care includes strict sterile technique during insertion, including proper skin preparation, placement of a sterile underwrap over insertion site, and strict aseptic technique in care of IV tubing and administration bags. The IV lines should not be disconnected; if diagnostic testing or frequent walking is necessary, the IV lines and administration bags should accompany the patient. Intravenous injections should follow sterilization of the port. If a multilumen catheter is placed, proper identification to each port is necessary, with one line dedicated to the total parenteral nutrition solution only (usually the proximal port).

CATHETER CARE

Arterial and cephalic catheter care should be performed every 24 hours. All supportive bandages should be removed, and the insertion site inspected for signs of phlebitis or thrombosis (i.e., redness, swelling, or ropelike vein). The catheter should be flushed with a small amount of heparinized saline (1 to 2 ml) using a pulsing movement while palpating tip of catheter. If any swelling or pain results from the flush, the catheter should be removed. If the patient is not on IV fluids, the catheter should be flushed every 4 hours (cephalic or jugular). Arterial catheters used for blood pressure monitoring should be flushed with heparinized saline every 2 hours or alternatively attached to a pressurized continuous-rate infusion which will maintain patency. When using the latter approach, it is important to maintain sufficient pressure in the cuff surrounding the fluid bag.

If the catheter is patent, the area should be cleaned with dilute povidone scrub or alcohol wipe and then dried. A small amount of povidone or antibiotic ointment can be placed over the insertion site before rebandaging the catheter. Recommended bandaging material is 2-inch tape (one piece to secure the catheter, and one piece to anchor a T-port, if used), cast padding in a single layer, followed by Kling gauze and vet wrap for the final layer. The date of placement of the catheter should be recorded, as well as the date of the rewrap. Catheters should be checked routinely every 2 hours for leakage or swelling. Swelling distal to the catheter usually indicates a tight bandage. Swelling proximal to the catheter could indicate extravasation of the administering fluid or medication.

Jugular catheter care also requires daily inspection as indicated previously. The insertion site should be cleaned with povidone solution and/or alcohol. Since the jugular catheter is significantly longer in length than the cephalic catheter, signs of extravasation may not be as apparent. The midsternal region should be examined for edema related to jugular venous catheter placement, and the proximal aspect of the medial hind limb should be examined for edema related to lateral or medial saphenous venous catheter placement. Bandaging material needed includes a 4×4 gauze pad with antibiotic ointment, followed by a single layer of casting padding, followed by Kling gauze and vet wrap. No tape is necessary to anchor a jugular catheter if it has been sutured in place. Note that neck bandages should have the "two-finger rule" (i.e., the bandage should be loose enough to slide two fingers under for patient comfort). If the jugular catheter is made of polyurethane material (i.e., Arrow International), it does not need to be changed out within a 90-day period. Other catheter types made from polypropylene material (MILA, Intracath) can be changed on the fifth day.

References and Suggested Reading

Bonagura JD, editor: *Kirk's current veterinary therapy XI (small animal practice)*, Philadelphia, 1992, Saunders, p 107.
Bonagura JD, editor: *Kirk's current veterinary therapy XII (small animal practice)*, Philadelphia, 1995, Saunders, p 110.

CHAPTER 8

Pacing in the Critical Care Setting

ANNA R.M. GELZER, *Ithaca, New York*
MARC S. KRAUS, *Ithaca, New York*

Temporary cardiac pacing is a potentially lifesaving procedure for patients with severe bradyarrhythmias or those that are at a high risk of asystole in the emergency setting. Temporary cardiac pacing depends on rate support from an external pulse generator via electrodes that can be placed in a timely fashion and removed easily after a short period of pacing. Most situations requiring temporary pacing in veterinary medicine necessitate permanent pacing therapy, which will need to be initiated before removal of the temporary system (see Chapter 160).

This chapter focuses on two commonly used techniques in veterinary medicine: transcutaneous external pacing (DiFrancesco et al., 2003) and transvenous external pacing, procedures for which there are a number of clinical indications (Box 8-1). Transesophageal pacing may be used for atrial pacing, but ventricular capture is inconsistent. Because it has limited applicability to the veterinary critical care setting, it will not be discussed further.

Once the decision is made to support the heart rate by external pacing, pharmacologic interventions aimed at

Box **8-1**

Indications for Temporary Pacing in the Critical Care Setting

- Asystole during cardiopulmonary arrest
- High grade second- or third-degree atrioventricular (AV) block with slow ventricular escape rhythm and secondary hemodynamic compromise or syncope
- Symptomatic sick sinus syndrome: frequent episodes of sinus arrest resulting in syncope
- Sinus bradycardia or second-degree AV block with hypotension not responsive to atropine or isoproterenol
- Ventricular tachyarrhythmias secondary to bradycardia
- Overdrive suppression of tachyarrhythmias
- Causes of transient medically refractory sinus bradycardia or AV block resulting in hemodynamic instability (i.e., drug toxicities):
  - Calcium channel blockers
  - β-Blocker
  - Digoxin

rate support (anticholinergics, sympathomimetics) should be discontinued. These drugs tend to be proarrhythmic and can sensitize the myocardium to stimulation from catheter manipulations, causing ventricular arrhythmias.

EXTERNAL TRANSCUTANEOUS TEMPORARY PACING

External transcutaneous pacing (TCP) generators come as stand-alone units or incorporated into a defibrillator. Both Zoll Medical Corp., Chelmsford, MA (M SERIES models) and Medtronic Inc., Minneapolis, MN (Lifepak models) feature user-friendly pacemaker/defibrillator units. Pacing can be achieved rapidly with very limited training and without a need to move a patient to fluoroscopy. However, TCP creates significant skin and muscle pain, necessitating general anesthesia for the duration of temporary pacing.

Materials and Technique Required for Transcutaneous Pacing

The materials required to provide TCP include airway and anesthetic equipment and the external pacing unit with two sets of electrodes. Electrocardiograph (ECG) electrodes are used for rhythm monitoring, and larger pacing electrode pads for cardiac stimulation. (Lifepak, Medtronic and Zoll Medical provide proprietary pads, but other companies also offer pacing pads that can be used with adaptors.) Pacing electrode pads come in pediatric and adult sizes. Pediatric pads should be used for animals less than 10 kg. If the animal is conscious but hemodynamically unstable because of a bradyarrhythmia, the TCP should be planned by first establishing intravenous access and ensuring that airway management can be provided once the patient is anesthetized. The animal's chest needs to be clipped over at least as large an area as the pacing pads will cover. The pads are placed over the right and left precordia. The caudal edge of the pad should be positioned where the apex beat is felt strongest under the operator's hand; this "sandwiches" the heart between the pads. The ECG lead cables of the pacing unit need to be attached for the pacing system to monitor the inherent heart rhythm properly, including sensing of native electrical activity. While most units will also record the ECG from the thoracic electrode patches, rhythm monitoring during external pacing is best done from standard limb leads to reduce the confusion of local twitch artifact. It is important to place the ECG electrodes as far away from the pacing pads as possible to obtain a clear ECG signal on the pacing unit monitor. Set the pacing rate at 60 to 90 beats/min. The target heart rate is selected to maintain cardiac output and improve the blood pressure. For hemodynamically compromising bradycardia without cardiac arrest, start the pacing output at 0 mA, and increase the output by 10 mA until capture is achieved. In the asystole cardiac arrest setting, start at the maximum current setting and decrease the output to a value above where capture is lost. To achieve external pacing capture, a relatively high current output is required in dogs. Less than 70 or 80 mA does not usually result in successful capture, and most cases appear to require equal to or higher than 90 mA. The ECG generated by TCP should only be interpreted on the pacing unit monitor. A built-in filter and blanking protection change the high-output pacing stimulus to a smaller spike, preventing distortion of the ECG waveform. In contrast, regular ECG systems may display a huge pacing spike with no clearly identifiable ECG. In addition, chest thumping produced by TCP contributes to the artifactual appearance of the recordings from a regular ECG machine. To assess capture, look at the ECG tracing on the monitor for pacer spikes that are followed by both a QRS complex and a distinct T-wave. Electrical capture is manifest as a wide QRS complex, with a prominent T wave with opposite polarity of the QRS complex (Fig. 8-1). Both electrical and mechanical capture must be achieved to ensure cardiac output. Mechanical capture is only evidenced by a concurrent pulse (Fig. 8-2). Arterial pressure can be monitored with a direct arterial line, a Doppler sphygmomanometer system, or an oxygen saturation monitor displaying a pulse waveform. In the emergency setting palpation of a femoral pulse may be used. Skeletal muscle contractions occur with pacemaker current output as low as 10 mA and are not an indicator of electrical or mechanical capture. These become more intense as the current output is increased.

TCP is likely the least invasive and quickest means to achieve rate support in the course of cardiopulmonary resuscitation (CPR). It is safe to touch the patient or the pacing patches and perform CPR while TCP is ongoing. Since the patient is already unconscious, considerations regarding anesthesia for TCP are not applicable at that instant. However, it should be remembered that, if successful pacing is instituted, patients that were unconscious at the outset may regain consciousness, in which case general anesthesia must be readily available.

If surgery for a permanent pacemaker therapy is required following institution of TCP, it may be necessary to paralyze the animal during part of the surgery. The muscle stimulation of TCP can create so much body motion that surgical exposure of the jugular vein for

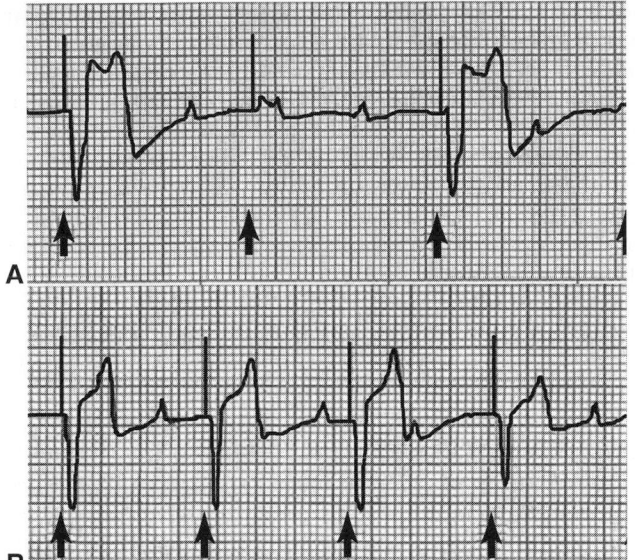

Fig. 8-1 **A,** ECG tracing of transcutaneous pacer unit with non-capture; the trace shows intermittent electrical capture. *Arrows* indicate paced beats. However, the second and fourth pacing stimuli do not result in capture (no QRS following the spike). The current output is set too low (60 mA) and should be increased. **B,** ECG tracing of transcutaneous pacer unit with capture. The trace shows continuous electrical capture. Each pacing spike is followed by a QRS complex. The current output was increased to 90 mA.

permanent pacemaker placement is impaired. In our experience large-breed dogs do not exhibit excessive twitching, but small-breed dogs and cats demonstrate significant whole-body thumping. To reduce muscle contractions, neuromuscular blockade with atracuronium (0.1 to 0.2 mg/kg intravenously [IV] for 20 minutes' duration) is

very effective but requires manual or mechanical ventilation because of paralysis of the diaphragm.

If a permanent pacemaker is placed during TCP, one should be aware that the pacing stimulus is sensed as a far-field signal by the permanent pacemaker (if it is programmed VVI or demand-mode) even at currents as low as 1 mA. This means that the permanent pacemaker is inhibited to pace, even after the output of the transcutaneous pacer is reduced to loose capture. Blood pressure monitoring will reveal loss of pacing instantly. To avoid this, the heart rate of the transcutaneous pacer should be set lower than the permanent pacemaker so as to not inhibit pacing.

TRANSVENOUS TEMPORARY PACING

Transvenous pacing (TVP) is effective, comfortable once in place for the awake patient, and fairly stable if correctly positioned. Therefore it is the treatment of choice for prolonged temporary pacing. Several companies provide external-demand pacing units. Medtronic (model 5348) and Oscor Inc. (model Pace 101H) both feature user-friendly, stand-alone, and economical external pacers. Several types of catheters can be used for TVP. We use regular bipolar pacing catheters (No. 4 or 5 Fr) that can be connected directly to the external pacing generator. Alternatively, easy-to-advance balloon-tipped pacing leads are available (Balloon Flotation Bipolar Pacing Catheter, Arrow International Inc.).

Sedation for Placement of Transvenous Pacing Catheter

Transvenous pacing is most commonly used to bridge the time until permanent pacemaker implantation can be

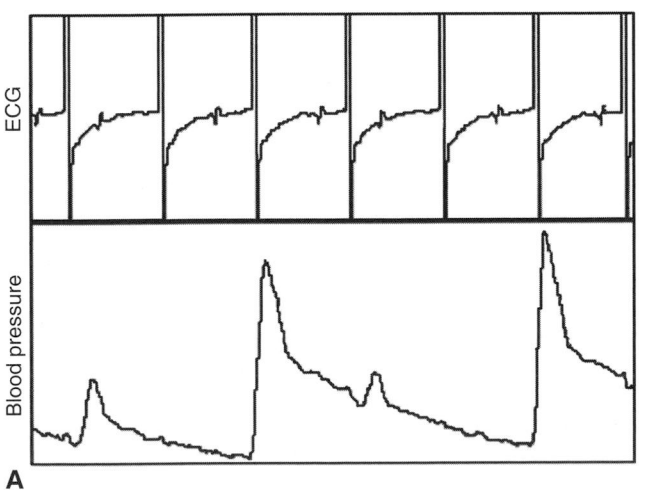
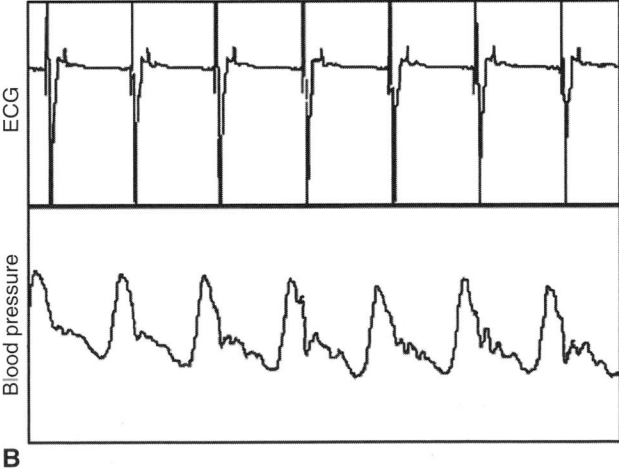

Fig. 8-2 **A,** Transthoracic pacing at 60 mA with no capture. Note that the surface ECG recorded with a regular physiorecorder shows large pacing spikes, obscuring the inherent ECG of the dog. Interpretation of the ECG alone would lead one to believe that there is adequate pacing. However, the blood pressure tracing reveals a discrepancy of heart rate between the ECG trace and the pressure trace because of lack of electrical and mechanical capture. The blood pressure trace shows the rate of the ventricular escape rhythm, displaying an irregular slow pulse. **B,** Transthoracic pacing at 90 mA with capture. Note that the surface ECG looks very similar to the example in panel A. The small positive deflection after the large pacing spike represents the QRS complex of electrical capture. However, only the concurrent blood pressure tracing confirms definitively that both electrical and mechanical capture is achieved.

performed. Since general anesthesia usually exacerbates bradyarrhythmias, the temporary pacing should be instituted before induction of general anesthesia. Light-to-heavy sedation and local anesthesia are usually required to insert the introducer sheath percutaneously. A combination of a sedative with a pain-relieving drug and an immobilizing agent is very effective. We like to use midazolam (0.3 to 0.5 mg/kg IV) with fentanyl (3 mcg/kg IV) and ketamine (1 to 2 mg/kg IV). If the animal needs to be even quieter, propofol (1 mg/kg IV) can be added. At the site of catheter insertion a local lidocaine block (2%, 0.5 ml SQ) should be infused to reduce pain. This protocol provides 10 to 20 minutes of sedation. The introducer sheath (No. 5 Fr, 6Fr, or 7 Fr Critical Care Arrow-Flex Polyurethane Sheath with Integral Hemostasis Valve/Side Port, Arrow International) is placed percutaneously using the modified Seldinger technique.

Placement of Transvenous Pacing Catheter

The proper choice of the insertion site is essential for success. If the temporary pacing lead is placed only to bridge a short time frame until permanent pacemaker surgery can be performed, we prefer to gain access via the femoral vein for TVP. This allows for a clean approach later to at least one or possibly both external jugular veins for the permanent pacing lead. However, if temporary pacing needs to last for several hours in the intensive care unit, the groin is not an optimal site for access. In an awake or only mildly sedated animal movement of the rear limb may displace the introducer sheath enough to pull out the pacing lead or result in local hemorrhage. If longer-term pacing is anticipated, a technically easier approach is cannulation of the external jugular vein. The right jugular vein is the shortest and most direct route, providing the most stable lead position. The introducer sheath can be secured safely to the skin and is subject to little movement if the neck is properly wrapped. The lateral saphenous vein may also be used for percutaneous access; however, we found that this approach can be impeded by the long distance and indirect route (i.e. navigating the catheter past the stifle joint is difficult because of the bend).

Except for sick sinus syndrome, in which right atrial pacing will suffice, most conditions requiring emergency pacing involve advanced atrioventricular (AV) block or asystole, requiring ventricular pacing. Blind advancement of temporary pacing leads from the introducer sheath to the right ventricular apex is challenging. Monitoring the ECG for signs of capture of the pacing spike may be helpful, but frequently blind advancement results in catheter malposition. The catheter could enter the internal thoracic vein, the azygos vein, or the caudal vena cava or potentially curl up in the right ventricle. As a consequence of curling, pacing capture is poor or intermittent as a result of improper contact of the lead tip with the endomyocardial surface. Some balloon-tipped pacing catheters feature a lumen for pressure monitoring, which is helpful for blind placement. However, in our experience by far the fastest method is to use fluoroscopic guidance.

Optimally a pacing catheter is placed with fluoroscopic guidance. For ease of handling, we only connect to the external pacer once the lead is positioned properly in the right ventricular apex. However, if the lead has to be advanced blindly, it must be connected to the external pacer during the placement to use the continuous ECG for guidance. A small pacing spike can be visualized once the wire tip is near the heart, and capture of the atrial myocardium (P wave) may occur while the catheter is advanced toward the tricuspid valve. The pacing spike will be followed by a wide QRS complex once ventricular capture is established (Fig. 8-3).

In a true emergency situation such as during CPR, pacing has to be achieved without fluoroscopy. Since blind transvenous placement is almost impossible during chest compression, it may become inevitable to proceed to open-chest resuscitation to provide external rate support. In such instances the tip of the pacing lead can be held directly on the epicardial surface of the heart to achieve capture until the patient is stabilized, and fluoroscopic imaging can be used to place a lead transvenously.

EXTERNAL PACER PROGRAMMING

The external pacer should be set on demand-pacing, or VVI, mode. This means that it will pace the ventricle when needed but also sense the patient's intrinsic ventricular activity, which inhibits the pacer. This avoids stimulation during the vulnerable period (T wave) of the intrinsic beats to prevent induction of ventricular arrhythmias. The heart rate should be set to the minimum rate to achieve an adequate blood pressure. It is not advised to pace much faster

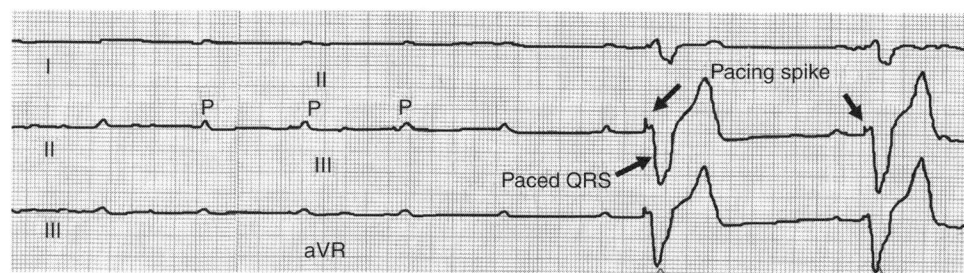

Fig. 8-3 Transvenous pacing. Surface ECG of a dog with third-degree atrioventricular block. The patient is being instrumented with a transvenous pacing catheter. After a long episode of asystole, a bipolar pacing spike is visualized, followed by a wide QRS complex, indicating successful ventricular capture.

than 80 to 90 beats/min unless absolutely necessary. In the case of sudden loss of capture, long episodes of sinus arrest may ensue as a result of overdrive suppression of the escape focus (the length of the pause is positively correlated to the preceding pacing rate). Typically ventricular capture by endocardial pacing can be achieved using between 1 to 5 V. Many temporary pacemakers do not indicate voltage but instead milliamperes of current output. If pacing resistance is low, capture is often obtained between 2 and 5 mA. The current threshold to achieve capture should be determined for each patient individually by gradually decreasing the voltage until loss of capture occurs. Twice threshold provides an adequate margin of safety. If the paced heart rate is less than the set rate, possible causes include: (1) poor lead position, (2) insufficient pacing voltage/current, (3) competing native rhythm (sinus capture, premature beats), and (4) T-wave sensing. T-wave sensing can be unmasked by briefly moving the selector switch to the full VOO (asynchronous) mode. If the paced rate is now correct, T-wave sensing is likely.

MONITORING OF PROLONGED TEMPORARY TRANSVENOUS PACING

Temporary TVP can be maintained for several days in an awake animal. Medically refractory drug toxicities such as overdose with a calcium channel blocker is an indication for longer-term temporary pacing. Aseptic technique during placement of the introducer sheath and pacing lead is imperative, and antibiotic coverage is recommended to prevent infection. The part of the lead extruding from the introducer sheath should be aseptically covered inside the neck wrap. Since the temporary pacing leads have a smooth profile with no fixation mechanism, spontaneous displacement is likely. We suture a clip right outside the introducer sheet, which fits tight around the catheter and seems to fix it in place fairly well. The external pacing unit needs to be attached securely to the patient to avoid accidental traction on the pacing lead, and the generator batteries should be checked regularly. If ventricular capture becomes intermittent or requires greater than 5 V, lead displacement may have occurred, and a chest x-ray is indicated.

References and Suggested Reading

Bocka JJ: *External pacemakers*, accessed 11/2005 from http://www.emedicine.com/emerg/topic699.htm.

Bocka JJ: External transcutaneous pacemakers, *Ann Emerg Med* 18:1280, 1989.

DeFrancesco TC, et al: Noninvasive transthoracic temporary cardiac pacing in dog, *J Vet Intern Med* 17:663, 2003.

Fitzpatrick A, Sutton R: A guide to temporary pacing, *Br Med J* 304:365, 1992.

Gammageer MD: Temporary cardiac pacing, *Heart* 83:715, 2000.

Seldinger SI: Catheter replacement of the needle in percutaneous arteriography; a new technique, *Acta Radiol* 39:368, 1953.

Trigano JA, Birkui PJ, Mugica J: Noninvasive transcutaneous cardiac pacing: modern instrumentation and new perspectives, *PACE* 15:1937, 1992.

Zoll PM et al: External noninvasive temporary cardiac pacing: clinical trials, *Circulation* 71:937, 1985.

CHAPTER 9
Fluid Therapy

STEPHEN P. DIBARTOLA, *Columbus, Ohio*
SHANE W. BATEMAN, *Columbus, Ohio*

Fluid therapy is supportive. The underlying disease process that caused the fluid, electrolyte, and acid-base disturbances must be diagnosed and treated appropriately. Normal homeostatic mechanisms allow considerable margin for error in fluid therapy, provided that the heart and kidneys are normal. This is fortunate because clinical estimation of dehydration may be quite inaccurate. Fluid therapy potentially consists of three phases: resuscitation, rehydration, and maintenance. Most patients in shock require rapid administration of a large volume of crystalloid or colloid to expand the intravascular space and correct perfusion deficits. Dehydrated patients require sustained administration of crystalloid fluids for 12 to 36 hours to replace fluid losses from interstitial and intracellular spaces. Normally hydrated patients unable to consume sufficient water require maintenance fluid therapy with crystalloid solutions. In formulating a fluid therapy plan, eight questions should be considered:

1. Is the patient suffering from a shock syndrome that requires immediate fluid administration?
2. Is the patient dehydrated?
3. Can the patient consume an adequate volume of water to sustain normal fluid balance?
4. What type of fluid should be given?
5. By what route should the fluid be given?
6. How rapidly should the fluid be given?
7. How much fluid should be given?
8. When should fluid therapy be discontinued?

IS THE PATIENT SUFFERING FROM A SHOCK SYNDROME THAT REQUIRES IMMEDIATE FLUID ADMINISTRATION?

Shock patients urgently require fluid therapy. The presence of altered mental status and cool extremities in association with tachycardia or severe bradycardia, mucous membrane pallor, prolonged or absent capillary refill time, reduced or absent peripheral pulses, and hypotension are among the most common physical examination findings in patients in shock. Such physical examination findings and a compatible clinical history are the basis for the decision to institute a resuscitation phase of fluid therapy. Hypovolemic and distributive shock states are most likely to respond to intravascular volume expansion. Obstructive forms of shock often respond favorably to moderate volume expansion. Fluid administration is contraindicated in patients with cardiogenic forms of shock.

Regardless of their underlying disease, severely dehydrated patients can be in shock and require a resuscitation phase of fluid therapy before initiating the rehydration phase. However, not all patients in shock are dehydrated, and some may not require a rehydration phase of therapy. The rapidity and volume of loss from both the intravascular and extravascular fluid compartments in conjunction with the extent of any compensatory response will determine whether the patient is in shock or is dehydrated.

IS THE PATIENT DEHYDRATED?

The need for a rehydration phase depends on the underlying condition of the patient and an assessment of the animal's state of hydration. The hydration status of the animal is estimated by careful evaluation of the history, physical examination findings, and the results of a few simple laboratory tests. In its most narrow sense dehydration refers to loss of pure water. However, the term *dehydration* usually is used to include hypotonic, isotonic, and hypertonic fluid losses. The type of dehydration is classified by the tonicity of the fluid remaining in the body (e.g., a hypotonic loss would result in hypertonic dehydration). Isotonic and hypotonic losses are most common in small animal practice. Severe volume depletion can result in nonosmotic stimulation of antidiuretic hormone (ADH) release, thus preventing effective excretion of consumed water and contributing to hypotonic dehydration.

Fluid Balance

Normally fluid input consists of water consumed in food, water that is drunk, and water produced metabolically in the body. Maintenance water and electrolyte needs parallel caloric expenditure; and normal daily losses of water and electrolytes include respiratory, fecal, and urinary losses. Respiratory loss of fluid can be important in dogs because panting has been adapted for thermoregulation in this species. Pyretic patients also can lose fluid by this route. Normally cutaneous losses are unimportant in dogs and cats because eccrine sweat glands are limited to the foot pads and do not play an important role in thermoregulation in these species.

In disease states decreased fluid intake results from anorexia, and increased fluid loss may occur by urinary (e.g., polyuria) and gastrointestinal (e.g., vomiting, diarrhea) routes. Less common routes of loss include skin (e.g., extensive burns), respiratory tract, and salivary secretions. Third-space loss of fluid occurs when effective circulating volume is decreased but the fluid lost remains in the body. Examples include intestinal obstruction, peritonitis, pancreatitis, and effusions or hemorrhage into body cavities. Decreased fluid intake and increased loss often coexist (e.g., anorexia, vomiting, and polyuria in a uremic animal).

History

The history may suggest the affected fluid compartment or compartments, as well as the patient's electrolyte and acid-base derangements. The time period over which fluid losses have occurred and an estimate of their magnitude should be determined. Information about food and water consumption, gastrointestinal losses (e.g., vomiting, diarrhea), urinary losses (i.e., polyuria), and traumatic losses (e.g., blood loss, extensive burns) should be obtained. Excessive insensible water losses (e.g., increased panting, pyrexia) and third-space losses may be determined from the history and physical examination. The clinician's knowledge of the suspected disease can aid in predicting the composition of the fluid lost (e.g., vomiting caused by pyloric obstruction leads to loss of hydrogen, chloride, potassium, and sodium ions and development of metabolic alkalosis; small-bowel diarrhea typically leads to loss of bicarbonate, chloride, sodium, and potassium ions and development of metabolic acidosis).

Physical Examination

Physical findings associated with fluid losses of 5% to 15% of body weight vary from no clinically detectable changes (5%) to signs of hypovolemic shock and impending death (15%). The hydration deficit is estimated by evaluating skin turgor, moistness of the mucous membranes, position of the eyes in their orbits, heart rate, character of peripheral pulses, capillary refill time, and extent of peripheral venous distention (i.e., inspection of jugular veins). A decrease in the interstitial compartment volume leads to decreased skin turgor and dryness of the mucous membranes. A decrease in plasma volume leads to tachycardia, alterations in peripheral pulses, and collapse of peripheral veins. When these cardiovascular signs are present, the patient is in shock and should be resuscitated promptly before correction of the hydration deficit. Typically such signs of hypovolemic shock appear with fluid loss that amounts to 10% to 12% of the patient's body weight. The fluid deficit in a given patient is difficult to determine with accuracy because of the subjectivity of skin turgor evaluation and the possibility of undetected ongoing (contemporary) losses. When evaluated by skin turgor, obese animals may appear well hydrated as a result of excessive subcutaneous fat despite being dehydrated. Conversely, emaciated and older animals may appear more dehydrated than they actually are because of lack of subcutaneous fat and elastin. Thus a crude clinical estimate of hydration status and the patient's response to fluid administration become important tools in evaluating the extent of dehydration and planning fluid therapy. The urinary bladder should be small in a dehydrated animal with normal renal function. In the absence of urinary obstruction, a large bladder in a severely dehydrated patient indicates failure of the normal renal concentrating mechanism.

Body weight recorded on a serial basis traditionally has been considered a good indicator of hydration status, especially when fluid loss has been acute and previous body weight has been recorded (i.e., 1-kg loss of body weight equals a 1-L fluid deficit). However, in one study clinician estimates of hydration in dogs and cats admitted to a veterinary teaching hospital intensive care unit did not reliably predict changes in weight after 24 to 48 hours of fluid therapy. In chronically ill animals loss of weight also includes loss of muscle mass. Anorexic animals have been estimated to lose 0.1 to 0.3 kg of body weight per day per 1000 kcal energy requirement. Losses in excess of this amount indicate fluid loss. Another factor that must be considered in evaluating body weight is the possibility of third-space loss. Fluid lost into a third space does not decrease body weight.

Laboratory Findings

Packed cell volume (PCV), total plasma protein concentration (TPP), and urine specific gravity (USG) are simple laboratory tests that aid in the evaluation of hydration. These results should be obtained before initiating fluid therapy. PCV and TPP should be evaluated together to minimize errors in interpretation. PCV and TPP increase with all types of fluid losses excluding hemorrhage; whereas serum sodium concentration increases, decreases, or remains unchanged, depending on the type of loss (e.g., hypotonic, hypertonic, isotonic) and the presence or absence of nonosmotic stimulation of ADH release. The USG before fluid therapy is helpful in the preliminary evaluation of renal function. It should be high (>1.045) in a dehydrated dog or cat if renal function is normal. This may not be true if other disorders affecting renal concentrating ability such as medullary washout of solute are present. Furthermore, previous administration of corticosteroids or furosemide can decrease urinary concentrating ability.

CAN THE PATIENT CONSUME AN ADEQUATE VOLUME OF WATER TO SUSTAIN NORMAL FLUID BALANCE?

Volume-resuscitated and rehydrated patients may not have recovered sufficiently to eat and drink normally. Such patients require ongoing fluid therapy. Maintenance fluid requirements have been determined from studies of normal animals, and the needs of partially or completely anorexic dogs and cats are not well understood. Also, absorption and metabolism of nutrients produce solutes that must be excreted in urine. Sensible fluid losses and urine production are decreased during fasting in normal animals because less solute requires excretion. Typically fluids are administered to veterinary patients in volumes predicated on the needs of animals that are not anorexic. Careful observation of urine production in such patients is warranted. If the patient has normal renal concentrating ability but is producing large volumes of dilute urine, excessive fluid administration likely is a contributing factor. Reduction of fluid administration and careful observation are warranted in such patients.

WHAT TYPE OF FLUID SHOULD BE GIVEN?

The composition of a *balanced* fluid (e.g., lactated Ringer's solution, Normosol-R, Plasma-Lyte 148) resembles that of extracellular fluid (ECF); whereas that of an *unbalanced* solution (e.g., normal saline) does not. Fluid preparations may be further classified as *crystalloids* or *colloids*. Crystalloids (e.g., 5% dextrose, 0.9% saline, lactated Ringer's solution) are solutions containing electrolyte and nonelectrolyte solutes capable of entering all body fluid compartments. Colloids are large–molecular weight substances that normally are restricted to the plasma compartment and include plasma, dextrans, hydroxyethyl starch (hetastarch), and hemoglobin-based oxygen-carrying fluids.

Crystalloid solutions expand the plasma compartment with equal effectiveness, but 2.5 to 3 times as much crystalloid solution must be given (compared with a colloid solution) because the crystalloid is distributed to other sites (e.g., interstitial compartment, intracellular compartment). Pulmonary capillaries normally are more permeable to protein, resulting in a higher interstitial concentration of protein and more resistance to leakage of fluid from capillaries. Peripheral edema is more likely to occur after crystalloid administration than pulmonary edema because muscle and subcutaneous capillaries are less permeable to protein.

Crystalloid solutions also can be classified as *replacement* or *maintenance* solutions. The composition of replacement solutions (e.g., lactated Ringer's, Normosol-R, Plasma-Lyte 148) resembles that of ECF. Maintenance solutions (e.g., Normosol-M, Plasma-Lyte 56) contain less sodium (40 to 60 mEq/L) and more potassium (15 to 30 mEq/L) than replacement fluids. Administering 5% dextrose (another commonly used crystalloid) is equivalent to giving water because the glucose is oxidized to CO_2 and water. In fact, the main reason for giving 5% dextrose is to correct a pure-water deficit. Except in very small animals, 5% dextrose cannot be relied on to maintain daily caloric needs because it provides only 200 kcal/L. Most animals that require fluid therapy can be managed with a limited number of crystalloid and additive solutions. The most useful crystalloid solutions for routine use are a balanced replacement solution (e.g., lactated Ringer's solution, Normosol-R, Plasma-Lyte 148), 0.9% saline, and 5% dextrose in water. Supplementation of crystalloid solutions with KCl may be necessary when body fluid losses have included large amounts of potassium. An empiric scale can be used to estimate the amount of potassium to add to parenterally administered fluids (Table 9-1). Other additive solutions include 50% dextrose, calcium chloride, calcium gluconate, potassium phosphate, 8.4% sodium bicarbonate, and water-soluble B vitamins.

The choice of fluid to administer depends on the nature of the disease process and the composition of the fluid lost. The patient's acid-base and electrolyte disturbances should be considered when choosing a fluid, and losses should be replaced with a fluid similar in volume and electrolyte composition to the fluid that has been lost. If clinical assessment of the patient suggests a fluid-responsive type of shock, the resuscitation phase of fluid therapy should be instituted. If the patient has abnormally low oncotic pressure or a disease that would benefit from low-volume resuscitation, synthetic colloids should be con-

Table 9-1

Sliding Scale for Potassium Supplementation

Serum Potassium Concentration (mEq/L)	mEq KCl to Add to 250 ml Fluid	Maximal Fluid Infusion Rate (ml/kg/hr)*
<2.0	20	6
2.1-2.5	15	8
2.6-3.0	10	12
3.1-3.5	7	16

* So as not to exceed 0.5 mEq/kg/hr.

sidered for resuscitation. If neither of these considerations applies, resuscitation with a balanced crystalloid solution is sufficient. If clinical signs of hypovolemia are not present, the hydration deficit and maintenance needs may be combined and administered during the next 24 hours.

Persistent vomiting caused by pyloric obstruction results in losses of hydrochloric acid, potassium, sodium, and water, potentially producing hypokalemia, hypochloremia, and metabolic alkalosis. The initial fluid of choice in this setting is 0.9% NaCl with 20 to 30 mEq of KCl per liter. Except in the case of vomiting of stomach contents, lactated Ringer's is a good first choice for fluid therapy while awaiting laboratory results. Normal saline (0.9% NaCl) is less ideal because it is not a balanced solution. It has a high chloride concentration relative to ECF (154 mEq/L versus 110 mEq/L in dogs and 120 mEq/L in cats) and is mildly acidifying because the chloride displaces bicarbonate in ECF.

Anions such as acetate, gluconate, and lactate are added to crystalloid solutions as a source of base because their oxidative metabolism in the body yields bicarbonate. For example, in the case of lactate:

$$NaC_3H_5O_3 + 3O_2 \rightarrow 2CO_2 + 2H_2O + Na^+HCO_3^-$$

Most lactate is produced in muscle and gut and metabolized to either glucose (via cytosolic gluconeogenesis) or CO_2 and water (via mitochondrial oxidation) in the liver. Normally gluconeogenesis predominates. Acetate is metabolized primarily in muscle. The alkalinizing effect of these anions is delayed because of the requirement for metabolism. Most patients treated with lactate-containing replacement solutions respond well, probably as a result of ECF volume expansion and improved tissue perfusion.

Whether converted to glucose or oxidized to CO_2 and water, lactate metabolism consumes hydrogen ions and has an alkalinizing effect:

Gluconeogenesis: $2CH_3CHOHCOO^- + 2H^+ \rightarrow C_6H_{12}O_6$

Oxidative metabolism: $CH_3CHOHCOO^- + H^+ + 3O_2 \rightarrow 3CO_2 + H_2O$

Concern sometimes is expressed that the lactate in lactated Ringer's solution may be harmful to patients with poor tissue perfusion and severe metabolic acidosis (pH <7.1 to 7.2).

Administration of lactate as a salt cannot contribute directly to metabolic acidosis. Rather, the ability of the liver to metabolize lactate and the potentially detrimental effect of lactate on myocardial contractility are debated. During severe hypoxia increased lactate production in gut and muscle and decreased hepatic extraction of lactate may lead to progressive lactic acidosis. In moderate metabolic acidosis administration of lactated Ringer's solution probably is beneficial because any tendency toward lactate accumulation likely is offset by improved hepatic perfusion and oxygen delivery as a result of ECF volume expansion. Some balanced crystalloid solutions (e.g., Plasma-Lyte 148, Normosol-R) contain approximately twice the amount of bicarbonate precursors when compared with lactated Ringer's solution. As a result, these solutions generally are thought to be more efficient than lactated Ringer's solution in treatment of metabolic acidosis, provided that metabolic conversion of the precursors to bicarbonate occurs quickly.

BY WHAT ROUTE SHOULD FLUIDS BE GIVEN?

The route of fluid therapy depends on the nature of the clinical disorder, its severity, and its duration. The *intravenous* route is preferred when the patient is very ill, when fluid loss is severe, or when fluid loss is acute. The intravenous route provides rapid dispersion of water and electrolytes and allows precise dosage. A large volume can be given rapidly, and hypertonic fluids can be given safely via a large vein. Vascular access is required, and close monitoring is necessary to avoid complications such as overhydration, thromboembolism, phlebitis, and infection. Veins available for vascular access include the jugular, cephalic, lateral saphenous, and femoral veins. There are advantages and disadvantages of each, but the jugular vein is useful because it allows delivery of large volumes, administration of hypertonic or potentially irritating solutions, measurement of central venous pressure (CVP), and repeated venous blood sampling. The cephalic vein also is commonly used, but fluid delivery can be hindered by flexion of the elbow, and extremely hypertonic or irritating solutions should not be used. Intravenous catheter function and the catheter-skin interface should be monitored routinely to detect complications. Catheters that remain clean and free of complications need not be replaced at a routine interval.

The *subcutaneous* route is convenient for maintenance fluid therapy in small dogs and cats. The subcutaneous space in dogs and cats can accommodate relatively large volumes of fluid, and potassium can be used in concentrations up to 30 mEq/L without irritation. Approximately 10 ml/kg or 50 to 200 ml may be administered per site. Volume overload is unlikely to occur when fluids are administered subcutaneously in patients with no underlying cardiac insufficiency. Furthermore, some owners can use subcutaneous administration to give fluids at home to animals with chronic disease problems. The subcutaneous route is not adequate for patients with acute and severe losses (e.g., shock) and is not recommended for extremely dehydrated or hypothermic animals because peripheral vasoconstriction may reduce absorption and dispersion of the administered fluid in these settings. The volume that may be given is limited by skin elasticity, and this route is not useful in larger animals requiring large volumes of fluids. Irritating or hypertonic solutions should not be used subcutaneously; only isotonic fluids are recommended. Isotonic fluids containing bicarbonate precursors other than lactate also are not recommended for subcutaneous administration. Although not harmful, they may cause mild local discomfort. Subcutaneous administration of 5% dextrose in water should be avoided because equilibration of ECF with a pool of electrolyte-free solution may lead to temporary aggravation of electrolyte imbalance.

The *oral* route is most physiologic, and fluids with a wide variety of compositions may be given. Oral fluid therapy is useful for administering hypertonic fluids with high caloric density. Fluid can be administered rapidly with minimal adverse effects, and caloric needs can be met. However, this route cannot be used in the presence of gastrointestinal dysfunction (e.g., vomiting, diarrhea). The oral route also is inadequate in animals with acute or extensive fluid losses because the administered fluid and electrolytes are not dispersed rapidly enough. In anorexic animals without vomiting or diarrhea, fluid can be administered orally using a number of different techniques (e.g., nasogastric, esophagostomy, or gastrostomy tube). Other uncommonly used routes of fluid administration include the *intraperitoneal* and *intramedullary* routes.

HOW FAST MAY FLUIDS BE GIVEN?

The rate of fluid administration is dictated by the magnitude and rapidity of the fluid loss. The patient with fluid-responsive shock syndrome requires aggressive fluid administration. Fluid administration rates may vary, depending on the type of fluid that has been chosen. One approach is to calculate a "shock fluid dose" and administer it as rapidly as possible in divided aliquots until a stable and sustainable cardiovascular end point has been achieved. Clinical evaluation of the patient should occur after administration of each aliquot using a "titrate to effect" approach. The shock dosage of synthetic colloids is 20 ml/kg for dogs and 10 to 15 ml/kg for cats. The shock dosage of isotonic crystalloids is 80 to 90 ml/kg for dogs and 40 to 60 ml/kg for cats. Contemporary losses also must be considered when adjusting the rate of fluid administration. Severe ongoing losses (e.g., vomiting and diarrhea in a patient with acute gastroenteritis) may necessitate rapid administration to keep pace with contemporary fluid loss. When fluids are given rapidly, cardiovascular and renal function should be monitored.

It usually is not necessary or desirable to replace the hydration deficit rapidly in chronic disease states. Instead, the hydration deficit may be calculated, the daily maintenance requirement of fluid added to this amount, and the total volume administered over 24 hours. Ongoing or contemporary losses also must be taken into consideration when estimating the patient's fluid requirements for a 24-hour period.

Infusion pumps are available for clinical use and provide a highly accurate record of the volume infused. Widespread availability of affordable electronic fluid pumps has facilitated fluid therapy in veterinary practice. Although use of infusion pumps makes fluid administration safer and more accurate, the equipment must be used appropriately, maintained in good working order, and tested regularly for accuracy. Mistakes in fluid administration still can occur as a consequence of human error or equipment failure.

HOW MUCH FLUID SHOULD BE GIVEN?

The purpose of fluid therapy is to increase tissue perfusion, repair fluid deficits, supply daily fluid needs, and replace ongoing losses.

Components of Fluid Therapy

The volume requirements of patients with fluid-responsive shock syndromes can vary widely. The goal of reestablishing widespread effective tissue perfusion dictates the volume of fluid administered. In general, the cardiovascular parameters used to characterize the patient's shock syndrome should return to normal (or to the extent they are able to do so considering the limitations of the patient's underlying disease). For example, a severely dehydrated dog with tachycardia, pale mucous membranes, prolonged capillary refill time, and hypotension should receive a volume of fluid sufficient to return these cardiovascular parameters to normal; and these parameters should not deviate from normal when the rate of fluid administration is decreased and rehydration of the patient begun. In patients without ongoing loss of fluid from the intravascular compartment or other more complex cardiovascular derangements, response to fluid resuscitation should be rapid and complete.

The initial assessment of hydration determines the volume of fluid needed to correct the hydration deficit (*replacement requirement*). The hydration deficit is calculated as the percentage of dehydration (estimated by physical examination) times the patient's body weight in kilograms. The resultant value is the fluid deficit in liters. During the rehydration phase of therapy this volume is administered over 24 hours in conjunction with maintenance fluid requirements and replacement of ongoing or contemporary losses.

Coincident with or after replacement of the animal's hydration deficit, the *maintenance requirement* must be administered. The maintenance fluid requirement is the volume needed each day to keep the animal in balance (i.e., no net change in body water). The maintenance fluid requirement for dogs and cats can be determined from reference charts that use formulas based on energy expenditure to calculate accurate daily fluid requirements. Although estimates of 40 to 60 ml/kg/day frequently are used to calculate maintenance fluid requirements, such estimates are only accurate for some animals. Cats, very small dogs, and very large dogs are not well served by the use of such estimates; these patients may benefit from more accurate assessment of their fluid requirements. Approximately two thirds of the maintenance require-

ment represents sensible (i.e., easy to measure) losses of fluid (i.e., urine output), and one third represents insensible (i.e., difficult to measure) losses (i.e., primarily fecal and respiratory water loss). Thus daily maintenance for a 10-kg dog may be 600 ml, with 400 ml representing sensible loss and 200 ml representing insensible loss. Some clinicians multiply maintenance fluid requirements by some factor between 1 and 3 to estimate the patient's 24-hour fluid needs. Assuming 60 ml/kg/day for maintenance, the information in Table 9-2 can be used to quickly estimate the implied hydration deficit and actual rate of fluid administration using this approach.

In addition to the hydration deficit (replacement requirement) and maintenance requirement, *contemporary (ongoing) losses* must be considered. These are not always easily determined but can be very important. Ongoing losses (including those caused by vomiting, diarrhea, polyuria, large wounds, drains, peritoneal or pleural losses, panting, fever, and blood loss) should be estimated and carefully replaced along with the maintenance volume of fluid. Box 9-1 summarizes the components of fluid therapy and their calculation.

Table **9-2**

Maintenance and Dehydration Fluid Volume Requirements

Maintenance (M) + Dehydration (%)	ml/kg/day	Factor × Maintenance
M	60	1.00
M + 1	70	1.17
M + 2	80	1.33
M + 3	90	1.50
M + 4	100	1.67
M + 5	110	1.83
M + 6	120	2.00
M + 7	130	2.17
M + 8	140	2.33
M + 9	150	2.50
M + 10	160	2.67
M + 11	170	2.83
M + 12	180	3.00

Box **9-1**

Components of Fluid Therapy

Hydration Deficit (Replacement Requirement)
Body weight (kg) × % dehydration as a decimal = deficit in liters

Maintenance Requirement (40-60 ml/kg/day)
Sensible losses (urine output): 27-40 ml/kg/day
Insensible losses (fecal, cutaneous, respiratory): 13-20 ml/kg/day

Contemporary (Ongoing) Losses (e.g., Vomiting, Diarrhea, Polyuria)

Failure to Achieve Rehydration

Repeated assessment of the patient by observation of clinical signs and determinations of body weight, urine output, PCV, TPP, and USG is necessary to make appropriate adjustments in fluid therapy. Reasons for failure to achieve satisfactory rehydration include calculation errors, underestimation of the initial hydration deficit, contemporary losses larger than appreciated, excessively rapid infusion of fluid with diuresis and urinary loss of fluid and electrolytes, administered fluid not reaching the ECF (e.g., technical problems, third-space loss), sensible losses larger than appreciated (i.e., polyuria), and insensible losses larger than appreciated (e.g., panting, fever). Failure to achieve successful hydration is an indication to increase the volume of fluid administered if the heart and kidneys are functioning adequately. As a rule the daily fluid volume may be increased by an amount equivalent to 5% of body weight if the initial infusion fails to restore hydration. Finally, if the animal does not gain weight despite several days of fluid therapy, the possibility must be considered that the animal was not dehydrated at presentation (e.g., abnormal skin turgor related to old age or emaciation).

MONITORING FLUID THERAPY

The hydration deficit determined by history and physical examination is only an estimate, and fluid therapy must be tailored to physical (e.g., body weight) and laboratory (e.g., PCV, TPP) findings during the first few days of fluid therapy.

Physical and Laboratory Findings

Physical examination, including evaluation of skin turgor and thoracic auscultation, should be performed once or twice daily on animals receiving fluids. PCV, TPP, and body weight should be monitored. Serial body weight is an important variable to follow, and animals receiving fluids should be weighed daily using the same scale. A gain or loss of 1 kg can be considered an excess or deficit of 1 L of fluid because lean body mass is not gained or lost quickly. A dehydrated patient should gain weight as rehydration is achieved, and afterward weight should remain relatively constant. However, weight may increase without restoration of effective circulating volume in patients with severe third-space losses. Despite these principles, clinical estimates of dehydration did not reliably predict changes in body weight after 24 to 48 hours of fluid therapy in one study.

Urine Output

The animal's urine output should be observed carefully after fluid therapy has begun. Oliguria should be suspected in patients with acute renal failure, especially those with possible ethylene glycol ingestion. Urine output (normal, 1 to 2 ml/kg/hour) should be monitored when fluids are administered intravenously at a rapid rate and renal function is in question. As the patient becomes rehydrated, physiologic oliguria should resolve, and urine output should increase. If oliguria present at admission persists after the hydration deficit has been corrected, daily fluid therapy should be divided into six 4-hour intervals if the status of renal function is uncertain. The calculated insensible volume plus a volume equal to the urine output of the previous 4 hours is administered during each 4-hour period (known as measuring "ins and outs"). The risk of overhydration is minimized, and fluid therapy keeps pace with urine output even if oliguria is present when this technique is used. If oliguria persists, increasing the daily fluid volume by an amount equal to 5% of body weight is justified on the assumption that the initial estimate of dehydration was inaccurate. If oliguria does not respond to mild volume expansion, administration of increased volumes of fluid may result in pulmonary edema.

Central Venous Pressure

Measurement of CVP (normal, 0 to 3 cm H_2O) with a jugular catheter positioned at the level of the right atrium allows the cardiovascular response to fluid administration to be monitored. CVP increases from below normal into the normal range when fluids are administered to a dehydrated animal. A progressive increase in CVP above normal during fluid therapy is an indication to decrease the rate of fluid administration or to stop fluid therapy temporarily. A sudden and sustained increase in CVP may indicate failure of the cardiovascular system to handle the fluid load effectively and could result in pulmonary edema caused by left-sided heart failure. In addition to the volume of fluid administered, other factors that may affect CVP include heart rate, vascular capacity, and cardiac contractility. A reduction in any of these three parameters could cause an increase in CVP.

Complications of Fluid Therapy

Signs of overhydration occur when fluid is administered too rapidly. These may include serous nasal discharge, chemosis, restlessness, shivering, tachycardia, cough, tachypnea, dyspnea, pulmonary crackles and edema, ascites, polyuria, exophthalmos, diarrhea, and vomiting. Expected laboratory abnormalities include a reduction in PCV and TPP and an increase in body weight.

When the intravenous route is chosen for fluid therapy, the clinician has made a commitment to careful, aseptic catheter placement and proper maintenance. The animal should be checked daily for cleanliness of the catheter site, local pain or swelling, fever, or cardiac murmurs. If any of these signs are observed, the catheter should be removed, its tip cultured, the patient started on appropriate antibiotic therapy, and a new catheter placed in another vein. Complications related to catheter placement include bacterial endocarditis, thrombophlebitis, and thromboembolism. When not in use, the catheter should be irrigated with a small volume (<1 ml) of a solution containing 1 to 5 U of heparin per milliliter of 0.9% NaCl ("heparinized saline").

WHEN SHOULD FLUID THERAPY BE DISCONTINUED?

Ideally fluid therapy is discontinued when hydration is restored and the animal can maintain fluid balance on its own by eating and drinking. As the animal recovers, fluid therapy usually is tapered by decreasing the volume of fluid administered by 25% to 50% per day. If an animal remains anorexic for more than 3 to 5 days, enteral or parenteral nutritional therapy must be considered.

References and Suggested Reading

Cornelius LM: Fluid therapy in small animal practice, *J Am Vet Med Assoc* 176:110, 1980.

Cornelius LM, Finco DR, Culver DH: Physiologic effects of rapid infusion of Ringer's lactate solution into dogs, *Am J Vet Res* 39:1185, 1978.

Hansen B, DeFrancesco T: Relationship between hydration estimate and body weight change after fluid therapy in critically ill dogs and cats, *J Vet Emerg Crit Care* 12:235, 2002.

Rose RJ: Some physiological and biochemical effects of the intravenous administration of five different electrolyte solutions in the dog, *J Vet Pharmacol Ther* 2:279, 1979.

Schaer M: General principles of fluid therapy in small animal medicine, *Vet Clin North Am Small Anim Pract* 19:203, 1989.

CHAPTER 10

Acid-Base Disorders

HELIO AUTRAN DE MORAIS, *Madison, Wisconsin*
STEPHEN P. DIBARTOLA, *Columbus, Ohio*

Acid-base disorders are often encountered in critical care and outpatient settings in association with several conditions. A clear understanding of metabolic-respiratory interactions and a systematic approach aimed at identifying the separate components of acid-base disorders not only serve as a diagnostic tool, but also help in formulating therapeutic interventions. For example, abnormal acid-base balance may be harmful in part because of the patient's response to the abnormality, as when a spontaneously breathing patient with metabolic acidosis attempts to compensate by increasing minute ventilation. Such a response may lead to respiratory muscle fatigue with respiratory failure or diversion of blood flow from vital organs to the respiratory muscles, eventually resulting in organ injury. Thus it is important to understand both the causes of acid-base disorders and the limitations of various treatment strategies.

Blood pH and bicarbonate concentration can change secondary to changes in carbon dioxide tension (Pco_2), strong ion difference (SID), or total plasma concentration of nonvolatile weak buffers (A_{tot}). Respiratory acid-base disorders occur whenever there is a primary change in Pco_2, whereas metabolic acid-base disorders occur whenever SID or A_{tot} is changing primarily. Changes in SID or A_{tot} can be identified clinically by alterations in HCO_3^- concentration or base excess (BE). The SID is the difference between all strong cations and all strong anions. Strong ions are fully dissociated at physiologic pH and therefore exert no buffering effect. However, strong ions do exert an electrical effect because the sum of completely dissociated cations does not equal the sum of completely dissociated anions. Because strong ions do not participate in chemical reactions in plasma at physiologic pH, they act as a collective positive unit of charge, the SID. The quantitatively most important strong ions in plasma are Na^+, K^+, Ca^{2+}, Mg^{2+}, Cl^-, lactate, β-hydroxybutyrate, acetoacetate, and SO_4^{2-}. The influence of strong ions on pH and HCO_3^- concentration can always be summarized in terms of the SID. Changes in SID of a magnitude capable of altering acid-base balance usually occur as a result of increasing concentrations of Na^+, Cl^-, SO_4^{2-}, or organic anions or decreasing concentrations of Na^+ or Cl^-. An increase in SID (by decreasing Cl^- or increasing Na^+) causes a strong ion (metabolic) alkalosis, whereas a decrease in SID (by decreasing Na^+ or increasing Cl^-, SO_4^{2-}, or organic anions) causes a strong ion (metabolic) acidosis. The main nonvolatile plasma buffers that constitute A_{tot} act as weak acids at physiologic pH (e.g., phosphate, imidazole [histidine] groups on plasma proteins). An increase in the total concentration of phosphate leads to A_{tot} (metabolic) acidosis, whereas a decrease in albumin concentration causes A_{tot} (metabolic) alkalosis.

STEPWISE APPROACH

A routine methodic approach to interpretation of blood gas data facilitates the clinician's assessment of the patient. The first step is a careful history to search for clues that may lead the clinician to suspect the presence of acid-base disorders, followed by a complete physical examination.

Obtain Simultaneous Blood Gas Measurement and Chemistry Profile

Blood pH can vary as a result of changes in P_{CO_2}, SID, and weak and strong acid concentration. Some strong ions (Na^+, Cl^-, and K^+) and the most important weak acids (albumin and inorganic phosphates) are part of the chemistry profile and help understand why pH is changing.

Identify the Primary Disturbance

The clinician should first consider the patient's blood pH. The primary disturbance (respiratory or metabolic) can be identified by determining if P_{CO_2} or HCO_3^- is changing in the same direction that pH changed. There are four classic primary acid-base disorders: respiratory alkalosis, respiratory acidosis, metabolic alkalosis, and metabolic acidosis. Metabolic acid-base disorders can be divided further based on changes in SID or A_{tot}.

Calculate the Expected Compensation

Any alteration in acid-base equilibrium sets into motion a compensatory response by either the lungs or the kidneys. The compensatory response attempts to return the ratio between P_{CO_2} and HCO_3^- to normal and thereby minimize the pH change. A primary increase or decrease in one component is associated with a predictable compensatory change in the same direction in the other component (Table 10-1). Adaptive changes in plasma HCO_3^- in respiratory disorders occur in two phases: acute and chronic. In respiratory acidosis the first phase represents titration of nonbicarbonate buffers, whereas in respiratory alkalosis the first phase represents release of H^+ from nonbicarbonate buffers within cells. This response is completed within 15 minutes. The second phase reflects renal adaptation and consists of increased net acid excretion and increased HCO_3^- resorption (decreased Cl^- resorption) in respiratory acidosis and a decrease in net acid excretion in respiratory alkalosis. Adaptive respiratory response to metabolic disorders begins immediately and is complete within hours. Some guidelines for use of compensatory rules from Table 10-1 are presented in Box 10-1.

The definition of a simple acid-base disturbance includes both the primary process causing changes in P_{CO_2} or HCO_3^- and the compensatory mechanisms affecting these measurements. Lack of appropriate compensation is evidence of a mixed acid-base disorder. Compensation is said to be inappropriate if a patient's P_{CO_2} differs from expected P_{CO_2} by more than 2 mm Hg in a primary metabolic process or if a patient's HCO_3^- differs from the expected HCO_3^- by more than 2 mEq/L in a respiratory acid-base disorder.

Calculate Gaps and Gradients

Calculating the various gaps and gradients can be useful in evaluation of acid-base disorders (Box 10-2).

Strong Ion Gap and Anion Gap
Increase in the *anion gap* (AG) and *strong ion gap* (SIG) are associated with increase in concentration of unmeasured anions, both strong (e.g., lactate, acetoacetate,

Table **10-1**

Compensatory Response in Simple Acid-Base Disturbances in Dogs and Cats*

	CLINICAL GUIDE FOR COMPENSATION	
Disturbance	**Dogs**	**Cats**
Metabolic acidosis	↓ in P_{CO_2} = 0.7 × ↓ in HCO_3^-	P_{CO_2} does not change
Metabolic alkalosis	↑ in P_{CO_2} = 0.7 × ↑ in HCO_3^-	↑ in P_{CO_2} = 0.7 × ↑ in HCO_3^-
Respiratory Acidosis		
Acute	↑ in HCO_3^- = 0.15 × ↑ in P_{CO_2}	↑ in HCO_3^- = 0.15 × ↑ in P_{CO_2}
Chronic	↑ in HCO_3^- = 0.35 × ↑ in P_{CO_2}	Unknown
Long-standing (> 30 days)	↑ in HCO_3^- = 0.55 × ↑ in P_{CO_2}	Unknown
Respiratory Alkalosis		
Acute	↓ in HCO_3^- = 0.25 × ↓ in P_{CO_2}	↓ in HCO_3^- = 0.25 × ↓ in P_{CO_2}
Chronic	↓ in HCO_3^- = 0.55 × ↓ in P_{CO_2}	Similar to dogs

*Modified from de Morais HSA, DiBartola SP: Ventilatory and metabolic compensation in dogs with acid-base disorders, *J Vet Emerg Crit Care* 1(2):39, 1991; and de Morais HSA, Leisewitz A: Mixed acid-base disorders. In DiBartola SP, editor: *Fluid, electrolyte, and acid-base disorders,* ed 3, Philadelphia, 2006, Elsevier, p 296.

Box **10-1**

Guidelines for Adequate Use of Compensatory Rules From Table 10-1

Time
Sufficient time must elapse for compensation to reach a steady state:

Acute respiratory disorders:	15 minutes
Chronic respiratory disorders:	7 days
Long-standing respiratory acidosis:	30 days
Metabolic disorders:	24 hours

pH
• Compensation does not return the pH to normal*
• Overcompensation does not occur

Values in the expected compensatory range:
• Do not prove that there is only one disturbance
• Provide support for a simple acid-base disturbance, if consistent with the remaining clinical data

From de Morais HSA, Leisewitz A: Mixed acid-base disorders. In DiBartola SP, editor: *Fluid, electrolyte, and acid-base disorders,* ed 3, Philadelphia, 2006, Elsevier, p 296.
*Exceptions: Chronic respiratory alkalosis (>14 days), and potentially long-standing respiratory acidosis (>30 days).

Box 10-2

Gaps and Gradients in Acid-Base Disorders

Estimation of Unmeasured Anions During Metabolic Acidosis
Anion gap (AG)
$AG = (Na^+ + K^+) - (HCO_3^- + Cl^-)$

Strong ion gap (SIG)
$SIG = [albumin] \times 4.9 - AG$ (for dogs)
$SIG = [albumin] \times 4.58 - AG + 9$ (for cats)

Interpretation
Increased in
- Acidosis caused by addition of unmeasured anions (lactic acidosis, ketoacidosis, renal failure, poisonings)
- Hyperphosphatemia (hyperphosphatemic acidosis)

Normal in
- Hyperchloremic acidosis

Decreased in
- Hypoalbuminemia (hypoalbuminemic alkalosis)
- SIG is not affected by changes in albumin concentration

Estimation of Severity of Strong Ion Difference Alkalosis and Acidosis Caused by Chloride changes
Chloride gap
$[Cl^-]gap = 110 - [Cl^-] \times 146 / [Na^+]$ (for dogs)
$[Cl^-]gap = 120 - [Cl^-] \times 156 / [Na^+]$ (for cats)

Sodium-chloride difference
$Na- Cl = [Na^+] - [Cl^-]$
Only valid if $[Na^+]$ is normal

Interpretation
Increased in
- Hypochloremic alkalosis

Normal in
- Hypoalbuminemic alkalosis

Decreased in
- Hyperchloremic acidosis

Identifying the Origin of Hypoxemia in Respiratory Acid-Base Disorders
Alveolar-arterial oxygen gradient
$(A-a) O_2 gradient = 150 - 1.25 PCO_2 - PO_2$

Interpretation (in hypoxemic patients)
Increased in
- Pulmonary disease (e.g.; ventilation-perfusion inequality, right-to-left shunt)

Normal in
Alveolar hypoventilation (e.g.; central alveolar hypoventilation, abnormality in chest wall or respiratory muscles)

β-hydroxybutyrate, strong anions of renal failure) and weak (e.g., phosphate). The AG also is used to differentiate between hyperchloremic (normal AG) and high-AG metabolic acidoses. The AG in normal dogs and cats is mostly a result of the net negative charge of proteins and thus is heavily influenced by protein concentration, especially albumin. At plasma pH of 7.4 in dogs, each decrease of 1 g/dl in albumin concentration is associated with a decrease of 4.1 mEq/L in the AG (Constable and Stämpfli, 2005). The SIG is not affected by changes in albumin concentration, and an increase in unmeasured strong anions is suspected whenever SIG is less than −5 mEq/L. The SIG has not been clinically tested in dogs and cats, but its derivation is sound, and it is superior to the AG to detect increases in unmeasured strong anions in other species.

Chloride Gap

Chloride is the most important extracellular strong anion. Increases in chloride lead to metabolic acidosis by decreasing SID, whereas decreases in chloride cause metabolic alkalosis by increasing SID. Therefore plasma Cl^- and HCO_3^- have a tendency to change in opposite directions in hypochloremic alkalosis and hyperchloremic acidosis. The contribution of Cl^- to changes in BE and HCO_3^- can be estimated by calculating the *chloride gap* (see Box 10-2). Chloride gap values greater than 4 mEq/L are associated with hypochloremic alkalosis, whereas values less than −4 mEq/L are associated with hyperchloremic acidosis. Whenever sodium concentration is normal, the *difference between the sodium and chloride concentrations* ($[Na^+] - [Cl^-]$) can be used. Normally $[Na^+] - [Cl^-]$ is approximately 36 mEq/L in dogs and cats. Values greater than 40 mEq/L are an indication of hypochloremic alkalosis, whereas values less than 32 mEq/L are associated with hyperchloremic acidosis.

Alveolar-Arterial Oxygen Gradient

Frequently patients with respiratory acidosis or alkalosis are also hypoxemic. When determining management options, it is important to differentiate between hypoxia from primary lung disease (e.g., ventilation-perfusion mismatching) and alveolar hypoventilation by calculating the alveolar-arterial oxygen gradient, or $(A-a) O_2$ gradient. Values less than 15 mm Hg generally are considered normal. If the $(A-a) O_2$ gradient is increased, a component of the hypoxemia results from ventilation-perfusion mismatching, although it may be increased in some patients with extrapulmonary disorders. Clinically a normal gradient excludes pulmonary disease and suggests some form of central alveolar hypoventilation or an abnormality of the chest wall or inspiratory muscles. To increase the specificity of the test to diagnose ventilation-perfusion mismatch, only patients with $(A-a) O_2$ gradient values more than 25 mm Hg should be considered abnormal (Johnson and de Morais, 2006). These patients are likely to have primary pulmonary disease, but extrapulmonary disorders cannot be ruled out completely.

RESPIRATORY ACID-BASE DISORDERS

Disorders of P_{CO_2}

Respiratory acid-base disorders are abnormalities in acid-base equilibrium initiated by a change in P_{CO_2}. The P_{CO_2} is regulated by respiration: a primary increase in P_{CO_2} acidifies body fluids and initiates the acid-base disturbance called respiratory acidosis, whereas a decrease in P_{CO_2} alkalinizes body fluids and is known as respiratory alkalosis.

Respiratory Alkalosis

Respiratory alkalosis or primary hypocapnia is characterized by decreased P_{CO_2}, increased pH, and a compensatory decrease in HCO_3^- concentration in the blood. Respiratory alkalosis occurs whenever the magnitude of alveolar ventilation exceeds that required to eliminate the CO_2 produced by metabolic processes in the tissues. Common causes of respiratory alkalosis include stimulation of peripheral chemoreceptors by hypoxemia; primary pulmonary disease; direct activation of the brainstem respiratory centers; overzealous mechanical ventilation; and situations that cause pain, anxiety, or fear (Box 10-3). It is difficult to attribute specific clinical signs to respiratory alkalosis in the dog and cat. The clinical signs usually are caused by the underlying disease process and not by the respiratory alkalosis itself. However, in humans headache, lightheadedness, confusion, paresthesias of the extremities, tightness of the chest, and circumoral numbness have been reported in acute respiratory alkalosis. If the pH exceeds 7.6 in respiratory alkalosis, neurologic, cardiopulmonary, and metabolic consequences may arise. Such a pH only can be achieved in acute respiratory alkalosis before renal compensation ensues. Alkalemia results in arteriolar vasoconstriction that can decrease cerebral and myocardial perfusion. In addition, hyperventilation (P_{CO_2} < 25 mm Hg) causes decreased cerebral blood flow, potentially resulting in clinical signs such as confusion and seizures. Treatment of respiratory alkalosis should be directed at relieving the underlying cause of the hypocapnia; no other treatment is effective. Respiratory alkalosis severe enough to cause clinical consequences for the animal is uncommon. Hypocapnia itself is not a major threat to the well-being of the patient. Thus the underlying disease responsible for hypocapnia should receive primary therapeutic attention.

Respiratory Acidosis

Respiratory acidosis, or primary hypercapnia, results when carbon dioxide production exceeds elimination via the lungs. Respiratory acidosis almost always is a result of respiratory failure with resultant alveolar hypoventilation and is characterized by an increase in P_{CO_2}, decreased pH, and a compensatory increase in blood HCO_3^- concentration. Respiratory acidosis and hypercapnia can occur with any disease process involving the neural control of ventilation, mechanics of ventilation, or alveolar gas exchange resulting in hypoventilation, ventilation-perfusion mismatch, or both. Acute respiratory acidosis usually results from sudden and severe primary parenchymal (e.g., fulminant pulmonary edema), airway, pleural, chest wall, neurologic (e.g., spinal cord injury), or neuromuscular (e.g., botulism) disease. Chronic respiratory acidosis results in sustained hypercapnia and has many etiologies, including alveolar hypoventilation, abnormal respiratory drive, abnormalities of the chest wall and respiratory muscles, and increased dead space (Box 10-4).

Most clinical signs in animals with respiratory acidosis reflect the underlying disease process responsible for hypercapnia rather than the hypercapnia itself, and subjective clinical evaluation of the patient alone is not reliable in making a diagnosis of respiratory acidosis. In fact, patients with chronic, compensated respiratory acidosis may have very mild clinical signs. Neurologic signs may develop, particularly in acute hypercapnia, and seem to depend on the magnitude of hypercapnia, rapidity of change in CO_2 and pH, and amount of concurrent hypoxemia. Acute hypercapnia causes cerebral vasodilation, subsequently increasing cerebral blood flow and intracranial pressure. Clinically the CNS effects of hypercapnia can result in signs ranging from anxiety, restlessness, and disorientation to somnolence and coma, especially when P_{CO_2} approaches 70 to 100 mm Hg.

The most effective treatment of respiratory acidosis consists of rapid diagnosis and elimination of the underlying cause of alveolar hypoventilation. For example, airway obstruction should be identified and relieved, and medications that depress ventilation should be discontinued if possible. A patient breathing room air at sea level will develop life-threatening hypoxia (PO_2 < 55 to 60 mm Hg) before life-threatening hypercapnia. Thus supplemental oxygen and assisted ventilation are needed in treating acute respiratory acidosis. Although oxygen

---

Box **10-3**

Principal Causes of Respiratory Alkalosis*

Hypoxemia (Stimulation of Peripheral Chemoreceptors by Decreased Oxygen Delivery)
- Right-to-left shunting
- Decreased P_{IO_2} (e.g., high altitude)
- Congestive heart failure
- Severe anemia
- Pulmonary diseases with ventilation-perfusion mismatch
  - Pneumonia
  - Pulmonary thromboembolism
  - Pulmonary fibrosis
  - Pulmonary edema
  - Acute respiratory distress syndrome

Pulmonary Disease (Stimulation of Stretch/Nociceptors Independent of Hypoxemia)
- Pneumonia
- Pulmonary thromboembolism
- Interstitial lung disease
- Pulmonary edema
- Acute respiratory distress syndrome

Centrally Mediated Hyperventilation
- Liver disease
- Hyperadrenocorticism
- Gram-negative sepsis
- Drugs
  - Corticosteroids
- Central neurologic disease
- Heatstroke

Overzealous Mechanical Ventilation

Situations Causing Pain, Fear, Anxiety

*Modified from Johnson RA, de Morais HSA: Respiratory acid-base disorders. In DiBartola SP, editor: *Fluid, electrolyte, and acid-base disorders,* ed 3, Philadelphia, 2006, Elsevier, p 283.

mechanical or assisted ventilation is begun, care must be taken to decrease Pa_{CO_2} slowly. A sudden decrease in P_{CO_2} can result in cardiac arrhythmias, decreased cardiac output, and reduced cerebral blood flow. It can also lead to posthypercapnic metabolic alkalosis and rapid diffusion of CO_2 from cerebrospinal fluid into blood, thus quickly increasing cerebrospinal pH.

METABOLIC ACID-BASE DISORDERS

Disorders of A_{tot}

Albumin, globulins, and inorganic phosphate are nonvolatile weak acids and collectively are the major contributors to A_{tot}. Changes in their concentrations directly change pH and HCO_3^-. Common causes of A_{tot} acidosis and alkalosis are presented in Box 10-5.

Nonvolatile Buffer Ion Alkalosis

Hypoalbuminemic alkalosis. Hypoalbuminemic alkalosis is common in the critical care setting. In vitro a 1-g/dl decrease in albumin concentration is associated with an increase in pH of 0.093 in cats and 0.047 in dogs (Constable and Stämpfli, 2005). Presence of hypoalbuminemia complicates identification of increased

---

> ### Box 10-4
>
> ## Causes of Respiratory Acidosis
>
> **Large Airway Obstruction**
> - Aspiration (e.g., foreign body, vomitus)
> - Mass (e.g., neoplasia, abscess)
> - Tracheal collapse
> - Asthma
> - Obstructed endotracheal tube
> - Brachycephalic syndrome
> - Laryngeal paralysis/laryngospasm
>
> **Respiratory Center Depression**
> - Drug-induced (e.g., narcotics, barbiturates, inhalant anesthesia)
> - Neurologic disease (e.g., brainstem or high cervical cord lesion)
>
> **Increased CO_2 Production With Impaired Alveolar Ventilation**
> - Cardiopulmonary arrest
> - Heatstroke
>
> **Neuromuscular Disease**
> - Myasthenia gravis
> - Tetanus
> - Botulism
> - Polyradiculoneuritis
> - Tick paralysis
> - Drug-induced (e.g., neuromuscular blocking agents, organophosphates, aminoglycosides with anesthetics)
>
> **Restrictive Extrapulmonary Disorders**
> - Diaphragmatic hernia
> - Pleural space disease (e.g., pneumothorax, pleural effusion)
> - Chest wall trauma/flail chest
>
> **Intrinsic Pulmonary and Small Airway Diseases**
> - Acute respiratory distress syndrome
> - Chronic bronchitis and asthma
> - Severe pulmonary edema
> - Pulmonary thromboembolism
> - Pneumonia
> - Pulmonary fibrosis
> - Smoke inhalation
>
> **Ineffective Mechanical Ventilation (e.g., Inadequate Minute Ventilation, Improper CO_2 Removal)**

*Modified from Johnson RA, de Morais HSA. Respiratory acid-base disorders. In: DiBartola SP, editor: *Fluid, electrolyte, and acid-base disorders*, ed 3, Philadelphia, 2006, Elsevier, p 283.

> ### Box 10-5
>
> ## Principal Causes of Nonvolatile Ion Buffer (A_{tot}) Acid-Base Abnormalities*
>
> **Nonvolatile Ion Buffer Alkalosis (Decreased A_{tot})**
> *Hypoalbuminemia*
> - Decreased production
>   - Chronic liver disease
> - Acute-phase response to inflammation
> - Malnutrition/starvation
> - Extracorporeal loss
>   - Protein-losing nephropathy
>   - Protein-losing enteropathy
> - Sequestration
>   - Inflammatory effusions
>   - Vasculitis
>
> **Nonvolatile ion buffer acidosis (increased A_{tot})**
> *Hyperalbuminemia*
> - Water deprivation
>
> *Hyperphosphatemia*
> - Translocation
>   - Tumor cell lysis
>   - Tissue trauma or rhabdomyolysis
> - Increased intake
>   - Phosphate-containing enemas
>   - Intravenous phosphate
> - Decreased loss
>   - Renal failure
>   - Urethral obstruction
>   - Uroabdomen

*From de Morais HSA, Constable PD: Strong ion approach to acid-base disorders. In DiBartola SP, editor: *Fluid, electrolyte, and acid-base disorders*, ed 3, Philadelphia, 2006, Elsevier, p 310.

---

therapy may aid in the treatment of acute respiratory acidosis, oxygen may suppress the drive for breathing in patients with chronic hypercapnia. In chronic hypercapnia the central chemoreceptors become progressively insensitive to the effects of CO_2, and O_2 becomes the primary stimulus for ventilation. As a result, oxygen therapy may further suppress ventilation, worsening respiratory acidosis. If oxygen is administered, PO_2 should be kept between 60 and 65 mm Hg because the hypoxic drive to breathing remains adequate up to this level. When unmeasured anions (e.g., lactate, ketoanions) because hypoproteinemia not only increases pH but also decreases AG. Thus the severity of the underlying disease leading to metabolic acidosis may be underestimated if the effects of hypoalbuminemia on pH, HCO_3^-, and AG are not considered. Treatment for hypoalbuminemic alkalosis should be directed at the underlying cause and the decreased colloid oncotic pressure.

Nonvolatile Buffer Ion Acidosis

Hyperphosphatemic acidosis. Hyperphosphatemia, especially if severe, can cause a large increase in A_{tot}, leading to metabolic acidosis. The contribution of phosphate to A_{tot} (and AG) can be estimated by multiplying the phosphate concentration in milligrams per deciliter by 0.58. Thus a phosphorus concentration of 5 mg/dl is equivalent to 2.88 mEq/L at a pH of 7.4. The most important cause of hyperphosphatemic acidosis is renal failure. Metabolic acidosis in patients with renal failure is multifactorial but mostly is caused by hyperphosphatemia and increases in unmeasured strong anions. Treatment for hyperphosphatemic acidosis should be directed at the underlying cause. Sodium bicarbonate administered intravenously shifts phosphate inside cells and may be used as adjunctive therapy in patients with severe hyperphosphatemic acidosis.

Disorders of Strong Ion Difference

Changes in SID usually are recognized by changes in HCO_3^- or BE from their reference values. It is important to understand that the change in SID from normal is equivalent to the change in HCO_3^- or BE from normal whenever the plasma concentrations of nonvolatile buffer ions (e.g., albumin, phosphate, globulin) are normal. A decrease in SID is associated with metabolic acidosis, whereas an increase in SID is associated with metabolic alkalosis. There are three general mechanisms by which SID can change (Table 10-2): (1) a change in the free water content of plasma; (2) a change in Cl⁻; and (3) an increase in the concentration of other strong anions.

Strong Ion Difference Alkalosis

There are two general mechanisms by which SID can increase, leading to metabolic alkalosis: an increase in Na⁺ or a decrease in Cl⁻. Strong cations other than sodium are tightly regulated, and changes of a magnitude that could affect SID clinically either are not compatible with life or do not occur. Conversely, chloride is the only strong anion present in sufficient concentration to cause an increase in SID when its concentration is decreased. Common causes of SID alkalosis are presented in Box 10-6.

Concentration alkalosis. Concentration alkalosis develops whenever a deficit of water in plasma occurs and is recognized clinically by the presence of hypernatremia or hyperalbuminemia. Solely decreasing the content of water increases the plasma concentration of all strong cations and strong anions and thus increases SID. Therapy for concentration alkalosis should be directed at treating the underlying cause responsible for the change in Na⁺. If necessary, serum Na⁺ concentration and osmolality should be corrected.

Hypochloremic alkalosis. When water content is normal, SID changes only as a result of changes in strong anions and can only increase with a decrease in Cl⁻. Hypochloremic alkalosis may be caused by an excessive loss of chloride relative to sodium or by administration of substances containing more sodium than chloride compared with normal extracellular fluid composition (see Box 10-6). The goal of treatment of metabolic alkalosis is to replace the chloride deficit while providing sufficient potassium and sodium to replace existing deficits, thus correcting the SID. Renal Cl⁻ conservation is enhanced in hypochloremic states, and renal Cl⁻ resorption does not return to normal until plasma Cl⁻ concentration is restored to normal or near normal. Dehydrated patients should be rehydrated accordingly. The SID can be corrected with a solution containing adequate amounts

---

Table **10-2**

Mechanisms for Strong Ion Difference Changes*

Disorder	Mechanism	Clinical Recognition
SID Acidosis		
↓ In strong cations	↑ Free water (↓ sodium)	Dilutional acidosis
↑ In strong anions ↑ Unmeasured strong anions	↑ Chloride	Hyperchloremic acidosis Organic acidosis
SID Alkalosis		
↑ In strong cations	↓ Free water (↑ sodium)	Concentration alkalosis
↓ In strong anions	↓ Chloride	Hypochloremic alkalosis

*From de Morais HSA, Constable PD: Strong ion approach to acid-base disorders. In DiBartola SP, editor: *Fluid, electrolyte, and acid-base disorders,* ed 3, Philadelphia, 2006, Elsevier, p 310.

Box **10-6**

Principal Causes of Strong Ion Difference Alkalosis in Dogs and Cats

Concentration Alkalosis (↓ in Free Water: Recognizable by ↑ Na⁺)
- Pure water loss
  - Inadequate access to water (water deprivation)
  - Diabetes insipidus
- Hypotonic fluid loss
  - Vomiting
  - Nonoliguric renal failure
  - Postobstructive diuresis

Hypochloremic Alkalosis (↓ Cl⁻ corrected)
- Excessive gain of sodium relative to chloride
  - Sodium bicarbonate administration
- Excessive loss of chloride relative to sodium
  - Vomiting of stomach contents
  - Therapy with thiazides or loop diuretics

*From de Morais HSA, Constable PD: Strong ion approach to acid-base disorders. In DiBartola SP, editor: *Fluid, electrolyte, and acid-base disorders,* ed 3, Philadelphia, 2006, Elsevier, p 310.

of chloride (e.g., 0.9% NaCl, lactated Ringer's solution, KCl-supplemented fluids). In cases in which expansion of extracellular volume is desired, intravenous infusion of 0.9% NaCl is the treatment of choice.

SID Acidosis

Three general mechanisms can cause SID to decrease, resulting in SID acidosis: (1) a decrease in Na^+; (2) an increase in Cl^-; and (3) an increased concentration of other strong anions (e.g., L-lactate, β-hydroxybutyrate). Common causes of SID acidosis are presented in Box 10-7.

Dilutional acidosis. Dilutional acidosis occurs whenever there is an excess of water in plasma and is recognized clinically by the presence of hyponatremia. Increasing the water content of plasma decreases the concentration of all strong cations and strong anions and thus SID. Large increases in free water are necessary to cause an appreciable decrease in SID. It has been estimated that in dogs and cats a decrease in serum Na^+ concentration by 20 mEq/L is associated with a 5 mEq/L decrease in BE (de Morais and Leisewitz, 2006). Therapy for dilutional acidosis should be directed at the underlying cause of the change in Na^+. If necessary, serum Na^+ concentration and osmolality should be corrected.

Hyperchloremic acidosis. Increases in $[Cl^-]$ can decrease SID substantially, leading to so-called hyperchloremic acidosis. Hyperchloremic acidosis may be caused by chloride retention (e.g., early renal failure, renal tubular acidosis), excessive loss of sodium relative to chloride (e.g., diarrhea), or administration of substances containing more chloride than sodium compared with normal extracellular fluid composition (e.g., administration of KCl, 0.9% NaCl). Treatment of hyperchloremic acidosis should be directed at correction of the underlying disease process. Special attention should be given to plasma pH. Bicarbonate therapy can be instituted whenever plasma pH is less than 7.2.

Organic acidosis. Accumulation of metabolically produced organic anions (e.g., L-lactate, acetoacetate, citrate, β-hydroxybutyrate) or addition of exogenous organic anions (e.g., salicylate, glycolate from ethylene glycol poisoning, formate from methanol poisoning) causes metabolic acidosis because these strong anions decrease SID. Accumulation of some inorganic strong anions (e.g., SO_4^{2-} in renal failure) will resemble organic acidosis because these substances decrease SID. The most frequently encountered causes of organic acidosis in dogs and cats are renal failure (uremic acidosis), diabetic ketoacidosis, lactic acidosis, and ethylene glycol toxicity. Management of organic acidosis should be directed at stabilization of the patient and treatment of the primary disorder. Patients with severe acidosis (pH <7.1) and *renal failure* may benefit from small, titrated doses of $NaHCO_3$. The efficacy of $NaHCO_3$ therapy in renal failure is related partly to the shift of phosphate inside the cell with consequent amelioration of the hyperphosphatemic acidosis. Sodium bicarbonate should be used cautiously because metabolism of accumulated organic anions normalizes SID and increases HCO_3^-. Treatment of *lactic acidosis* is controversial, and sodium bicarbonate administration is not likely to help patients with lactic acidosis. Tissue hypoxia is considered to be the most likely underlying problem in lactic acidosis. Thus therapeutic measures should be taken to augment oxygen delivery to the tissues and reestablish cardiac output. Sodium bicarbonate also is not indicated in *ketoacidotic* diabetic patients even if pH is less than 7.0 because $NaHCO_3$ administration is associated with deleterious effects in humans with ketoacidosis (Okuda et al., 1996; Viallon et al., 1999). Sodium bicarbonate is usually not necessary in such settings because the acidosis improves rapidly with appropriate management using fluid resuscitation, insulin, and correction of potassium deficits (Gauthier and Szerlip, 2002).

Box 10-7

Principal Causes of Strong Ion Difference Acidosis in Dogs and Cats

Dilution Acidosis (↑ in Free Water: Recognizable by ↓ [Na⁺])
- With hypervolemia (gain of hypotonic fluid)
  - Severe liver disease
  - Congestive heart failure
  - Nephrotic syndrome
- With normovolemia (gain of water)
  - Psychogenic polydipsia
  - Hypotonic fluid infusion
- With hypovolemia (loss of hypertonic fluid)
  - Vomiting
  - Diarrhea
  - Hypoadrenocorticism
  - Third-space loss
  - Diuretic administration

Hyperchloremic Acidosis (↑ [Cl⁻] Corrected)
- Excessive loss of sodium relative to chloride
  - Diarrhea
- Excessive gain of chloride relative to sodium
  - Fluid therapy (e.g., 0.9% NaCl, 7.2% NaCl, KCl-supplemented fluids)
  - Total parenteral nutrition
- Chloride retention
  - Renal failure
  - Hypoadrenocorticism

Organic Acidosis (↑ Unmeasured Strong Anions)
- Uremic acidosis
- Diabetic ketoacidosis
- Lactic acidosis
- Toxicities
  - Ethylene glycol
  - Salicylate

*From de Morais HSA, Constable PD: Strong ion approach to acid-base disorders. In DiBartola SP, editor: *Fluid, electrolyte, and acid-base disorders*, ed 3, Philadelphia, 2006, Elsevier, p 310.

References and Suggested Reading

Constable PD, Stämpfli HR: Experimental determination of net protein charge and A$_{tot}$ and Ka of nonvolatile buffers in canine plasma, *J Vet Intern Med* 19:507, 2005.

de Morais HSA, Constable PD: Strong ion approach to acid-base disorders. In: DiBartola SP, ed. *Fluid, Electrolyte, and Acid-Base Disorders*. 3rd ed., Philadelphia, Elsevier: 2006, p 310.

de Morais HSA, DiBartola SP: Ventilatory and metabolic compensation in dogs with acid-base disorders. *J Vet Emerg Crit Care.* 1:39, 1991.

de Morais HSA, Leisewitz A: Mixed acid-base disorders. In DiBartola SP, editor: *Fluid, electrolyte, and acid-base disorders,* ed 3, Philadelphia, 2006, Elsevier, p 296.

DiBartola SP: Introduction to acid-base disorders. In DiBartola SP, editor: *Fluid, electrolyte, and acid-base disorders,* ed 3, Philadelphia, 2006, Elsevier, p 229.

Gauthier PM, Szerlip HM: Metabolic acidosis in the intensive care unit, *Crit Care Clin* 18:298, 2002.

Johnson RA, de Morais HSA: Respiratory acid-base disorders. In DiBartola SP, editor. *Fluid, electrolyte, and acid-base disorders,* ed 3, Philadelphia, 2006, Elsevier, p 283.

Okuda Y et al: Counterproductive effects of sodium bicarbonate in diabetic ketoacidosis, *J Clin Endocrinol Metab* 81:314, 1996.

Viallon A et al: Does bicarbonate therapy improve the management of severe diabetic ketoacidosis? *Crit Care Med* 27:2690, 1999.

CHAPTER **11**

Colloid Fluid Therapy

ELKE RUDLOFF, *Glendale, Wisconsin*
REBECCA KIRBY, *Glendale, Wisconsin*

Severe intravascular volume depletion associated with conditions such as hemorrhage, trauma, systemic inflammatory response syndrome (SIRS) diseases, and various metabolic diseases ultimately results in poor tissue perfusion, tissue hypoxia, and cellular energy depletion. Loss of vascular tone and increased capillary permeability can be a consequence and cause maldistribution of fluid between the fluid compartments. Timely and appropriate intravascular fluid resuscitation becomes the mainstay of treatment.

The goals of resuscitation and maintenance fluid therapy in the critically ill animal are to restore and maintain perfusion and hydration without causing volume overload and complications caused by pulmonary, peripheral, and brain edema. By using colloid fluids in conjunction with crystalloid fluids, goal-driven resuscitation (also known as end-point resuscitation) can be achieved more rapidly and with less fluid volume. Maintaining an effective circulating volume can be challenging when there is vascular leakage, vasodilation, excessive vasoconstriction, inadequate cardiac function, hypoalbuminemia, or ongoing fluid loss. Whether a fluid administered intravenously remains in the intravascular compartment or moves into the interstitial or intracellular spaces depends on the dynamic forces that affect fluid movement between body fluid compartments.

FLUID DYNAMICS

The body fluids are distributed between three major compartments (intracellular, interstitial, and intravascular). The cellular membrane defines the intracellular space and is freely permeable only to water. Most ions must enter the cell by specific mechanisms such as channels, solvent drag, carriers, or pumps. Intracellular ions help retain water within the cell by osmosis. The intravascular space is contained within a vascular semipermeable "membrane" composed of a single thin layer of endothelium resting on collagen and fibrin. Fluid and nutrient exchanges between the blood and the tissues occur primarily at the level of the capillary membrane. Larger molecules such as the plasma proteins (albumin, fibrinogen, and globulins) are too large to freely cross this semipermeable membrane.

The Starling-Landis equation defines the forces that control the rate of the flow of fluid between the capillary and interstitium:

$$V = k \, [(HPc\text{-}HPi) - sigma \, (COPc\text{-}COPi)] - Q$$

where V = filtered volume, k = filtration coefficient, HP = hydrostatic pressure, c = capillary, i = interstitial fluid, sigma = membrane pore size, COP = colloid osmotic pressure, and Q = lymph flow

The main components that control intravascular fluid volume include intravascular colloid osmotic pressure (COP) and hydrostatic pressure (HP) (Fig. 11-1). Eighty percent of the COP is produced by albumin, which is the most abundant extracellular protein. The pressure generated by albumin is augmented by its negative charge, which attracts cations (e.g., sodium) and water. This unique property is termed the *Donnan effect.* Capillary membrane pore size and the filtration coefficient control

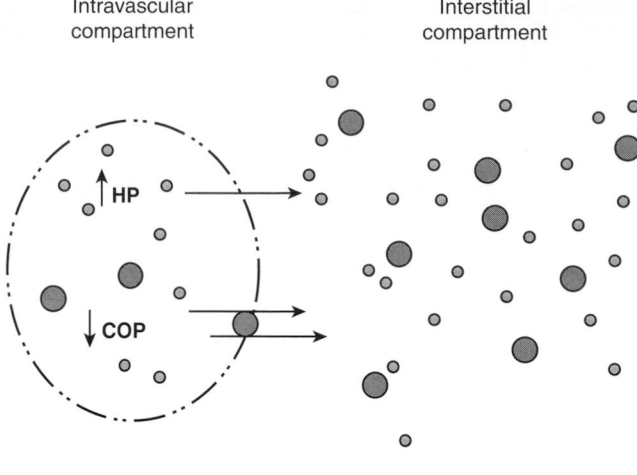

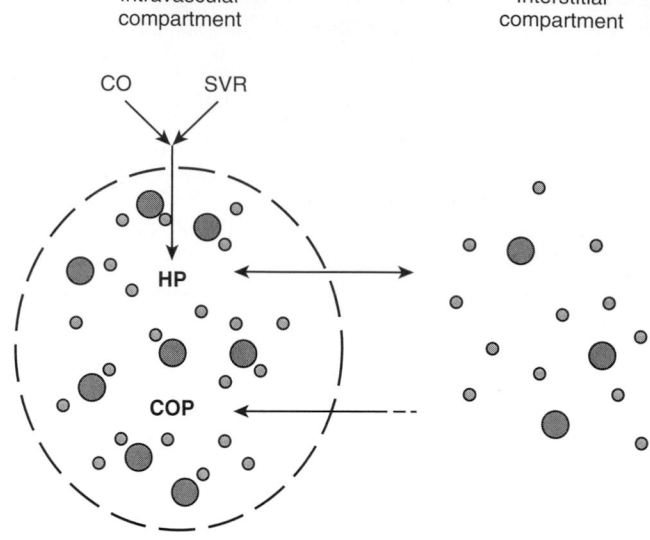

● Colloid molecule

○ Cations and water molecule

Fig. 11-1 The main components of the Starling-Landis equation that affect intravascular water content include intravascular hydrostatic pressure (HP) and colloid osmotic pressure (COP). The intravascular HP is a result of intravascular volume, cardiac output (CO), and systemic vascular resistance (SVR). Under normal conditions the HP favors the movement of fluid from the vessel into the interstitium. The COP is the force that opposes intravascular hydrostatic pressure, supporting intravascular water retention. The COP is generated by the presence of large molecules (primarily proteins) that do not readily pass the capillary membrane and create an osmotic effect.

● Colloid molecule

○ Cations and water molecule

Fig. 11-2 Fluid can pass out of the intravascular space under several conditions listed in Table 11-1: increased hydrostatic pressure (HP), increased capillary permeability, decreased filtration coefficient, and decreased colloid osmotic pressure (COP). These conditions lead to the consequences of peripheral edema and hypovolemia.

the ease with which these larger molecules leave the intravascular space. The size of the pore varies from tissue to tissue (e.g., tight junctions in the brain and large intercellular gaps in the liver). The filtration coefficient has been found to be variable and partly dependent on the amount of albumin in the intravascular space.

The dynamics of normal fluid movement across the capillary membrane can change with certain diseases. Fluid will move from the intravascular into the interstitial or third-space compartment under certain conditions (Fig. 11-2, Table 11-1). Plasma COP can increase with water loss (hemoconcentration), remain the same when there is acute volume depletion, or decrease with protein loss. In addition to capillary dynamics, the composition of intravenously administered fluids will determine how these fluids are distributed between fluid compartments.

BASIC COLLOID FLUID PHARMACOLOGY

The composition of intravenous fluids determines how these fluids are distributed between interstitial and intravascular fluid compartments. The two major categories of intravenous fluids are crystalloids and colloids. A crystalloid fluid is a water-based solution with small molecules permeable to the capillary membrane. A colloid fluid is a crystalloid-based solution containing large molecules that are impermeable to normal capillary membranes. When large volumes are needed for intravascular fluid resuscitation, crystalloids alone may fail to provide effective

Table 11-1

Examples of Conditions That Result in Movement of Fluid Out of the Intravascular Space

Condition	Example
Plasma to interstitial HP gradient increases over the COP gradient	Hypertension Fluid overload
Capillary membrane pore size becomes larger	SIRS-associated diseases • Pancreatitis • Peritonitis • Pyometra • Sepsis • Severe gastroenteritis • Burns • Multitrauma • Vasculitis
The filtration coefficient changes	Burns Hypoalbuminemia
Intravascular COP falls below interstitial COP	Hypoalbuminemia • SIRS disease • Liver dysfunction • Protein-losing nephropathy/enteropathy

COP, Colloid osmotic pressure; *HP,* hydrostatic pressure; *SIRS,* systemic inflammatory response syndrome.

intravascular volume support without causing interstitial volume overload with edema.

Ultimately the selection of a colloid or a combination of colloids for intravenous resuscitation and maintenance is based on the pharmacology of the fluid and the disorder requiring treatment. Each colloid solution is unique, and knowledge of the composition and pharmacology of the fluid is needed to make an appropriate colloid selection for a specific patient (see Table 11-2). It is the difference in macromolecular structure and weight that dictates the colloid osmotic effect, method of excretion, and half-life of the colloid solution. The more small molecules per unit volume of colloid, the greater is the initial colloid osmotic effect and plasma volume expansion. When the number of large molecules per unit volume of colloid is high, the colloid is retained longer within the vascular space.

Solutions that contain naturally produced proteins such as albumin (whole blood, plasma products, and concentrated human albumin solutions) or hemoglobin (hemoglobin-based oxygen carriers [HBOCs]) are referred to as natural colloids. Solutions that contain synthetically derived colloid particles such as dextrans (dextran 70) and hydroxyethyl starches (HESs) (hetastarch and pentastarch) are referred to as synthetic colloids.

Large-volume fluid resuscitation decreases the concentration of coagulation proteins in the plasma and can cause a dilutional coagulopathy. Synthetic colloids are not a substitute for blood products when albumin, hemoglobin, antithrombin, or coagulation proteins are needed.

ALBUMIN

Albumin, the most abundant colloid molecule in plasma, can be administered through plasma transfusions or concentrated (25%) human albumin. Frozen plasma and fresh frozen plasma contain approximately 5% albumin, whereas whole blood contains approximately 2.5% albumin. The size of the albumin molecule is constant, and the higher the concentration of albumin, the greater is the colloid osmotic effect per milliliter of solution. Plasma transfusions have an albumin concentration equal to that of plasma and may not add significantly to the intravascular COP when administered as the sole colloid. Because of its high concentration of albumin and high COP (200 mm Hg), 25% human albumin has the greatest capability of increasing plasma COP. When capillary permeability is normal, 25% albumin can be an effective colloid for rapid intravascular volume expansion. It can also be used to minimize interstitial edema in animals with hypoalbuminemia caused by inadequate albumin production or renal and gastrointestinal albumin loss. However, when increased capillary permeability allows plasma albumin to pass into the interstitium, the initial intravascular COP benefits of albumin infusion will be temporary and will likely lead to increased interstitial COP and edema.

Immunologic reactions are a risk with allogenic blood product transfusions. Human albumin has physiochemical properties that differ from canine and feline albumin, and complications appear to occur at a higher rate (about 20%) with human albumin administration in dogs than

Table **11-2**

Characteristics of Colloid Fluids

Colloid	Osmolarity (mOsm/L)	pH	Na+ (mEq/L)	Cl- (mEq/L)	K+ (mEq/L)	Mg++ (mEq/L)	Ca++ (mEq/L)	Dextrose (g/L)	Buffer	COP (mm Hg)	Miscellaneous
Natural											
Whole blood	300	Variable	140	100	4	0	0	0-4	None	20	
Frozen plasma	300	Variable	140	110	4	0	0	0-4	None	20	
25% Human albumin			0	0	0	0	0	0	None	200	
Oxyglobin	300	7.8	150	118	4	0	0	0	Lactate	40	
Synthetic											
6% Hetastarch 450/0.7 (Hespan)	310	5.5	154	154	0	0	0	0	None	32	C2:C6 = 4.6:1
6% Hetastarch 670/0.75 (Hextend)	307	5.9	143	124	3	0.9	5	0.99	Lactate	31	C2:C6 = 4.5:1
10% Pentastarch 260/0.45 (Pentaspan)	326	5.0	154	154	0	0	0	0	None	30	
Dextran 70	310	5.1-5.7	154	154	0	0	0	0	None	60	

COP, Colloid osmotic pressure.

with allogenic transfusions. Acute and delayed immune-mediated reactions have been reported after the administration of both human albumin and allogenic plasma and blood transfusions, requiring vigilant monitoring for allergic reactions. These colloids are administered slowly for the first hour, with careful monitoring for adverse reactions, before increasing to standard recommended rates of infusion.

HEMOGLOBIN-BASED OXYGEN CARRIERS

HBOC solutions bind with oxygen and transport it to the tissues where it is distributed to the cells. Because the solution is stroma free, it is able to pass through the microcirculation that might not allow the passage of red blood cells. The colloidal properties, oxygen-carrying capacity, and low antigenicity may make HBOC solutions an ideal fluid to administer to animals with severe anemia, hypotension, and/or hypovolemia.

Oxyglobin (Biopure), a stroma-free hemoglobin, is an ultrapure bovine-origin polymerized hemoglobin solution approved by the Food and Drug Administration for therapeutic use in dogs with anemia. Oxygen is bound to hemoglobin by a chloride-dependent process, facilitating its release at the capillary. In addition to acting as a temporary oxygen-carrying substitute for red blood cells, it maintains osmotic pressure and has a vasoconstricting effect that can reduce the volume required for resuscitation. It can be stored at room temperature with a 3-year shelf life if unopened, making it more easily available and transportable than blood transfusions. It has universal compatibility and is unlikely to transmit hematogenous diseases. It is excreted in the urine and bile. Its limitations include a short half-life (40 hours) once administered, interference with enzyme-based chemistry analyses, and requirements for red blood cell replacement if significant anemia is present. Side effects occur most commonly in euvolemic patients and include pulmonary edema, vomiting and diarrhea, and hypertension, requiring slow administration in small quantities, titrated to effect.

DEXTRAN 70

Dextrans are polysaccharides composed of linear glucose residues. These compounds are produced by the enzyme dextran sucrase during the growth of various strains of the bacterium *Leuconostoc* in media containing sucrose. Different molecular-weight dextrans can be produced by acid hydrolysis of the parent macromolecule. The development of acute renal failure is rare with dextran 70 in contrast to dextran 40.

Retained dextran 70 molecules are enzymatically metabolized by dextrinase to glucose in the liver and may increase serum glucose values. Having a molecular weight similar to albumin, dextran 70 molecules will diffuse into the interstitium when there is increased capillary permeability. At recommended doses dextran 70 can interfere with fibrin clot strength, reduce factor VIII and von Willebrand's factor, and affect platelet function. Partial thromboplastin and prothrombin times were prolonged in dogs reported to have received therapeutic doses of dextran 70. Its use

in animals undergoing surgery or with coagulation abnormalities should be with extreme caution.

Allergic reactions have not been reported in the dog or cat. Serum bilirubin concentration can be increased for unknown reasons. The presence of dextran 70 in the circulation may cause a change in the total solids value obtained via refractometry, not reflecting actual protein content (Bonagura, 1995). In addition, red blood cell cross-linking occurs with dextran 70 and appears as rouleaux formation, potentially interfering with blood typing and crossmatching.

HYDROXYETHYL STARCH

HES, the parent name of a synthetic polymer of glucose (98% amylopectin), is made from a waxy species of either plant starch maize or sorghum. It is a highly branched polysaccharide closely resembling glycogen, formed by the reaction between ethylene oxide and amylopectin in the presence of an alkaline catalyst. The molecular weight and molar substitution can be adjusted by the degree of substitution of hydroxyl groups with hydroxyethyl groups at the C2, C3, and C6 positions on the glucose molecule. The greater the substitution on position C2 in relation to C6 (C2:C6 ratio), the slower the degradation of the molecule by amylase. Renal function has been shown to decline after infusion of hetastarch with molar substitutions greater than 0.62 in humans undergoing surgery, a characteristic that has not been identified in animals. Renal effects of lower molar substitution solutions have not been evaluated.

The number-averaged molecular weight (M_n) is the arithmetic mean of the molecular weights of the polymers in solution. Weight-averaged molecular weight (M_w) is the sum of the number of molecules at each M_n divided by the total of all molecules. This weight is generally larger when larger polymers are present in solution.

The classification of different HES products includes the ratio of the M_w to the proportion of substitution. There are two HES products clinically available in the United States at this time: hetastarch and pentastarch. Hetastarch can be purchased in 0.9% sodium chloride (Hespan, Baxter; M_w of 450 kD and 0.7 degree of substitution) or in lactated Ringer's solution (Hextend, BioTime, Inc; a M_w of 670 kD and 0.75 degree of substitution). The use of Hextend may be associated with fewer coagulation abnormalities when compared to 6% hetastarch in saline because it contains calcium, which can become depleted in coagulopathic states. The electrolyte and buffer compositions of Hextend may reduce the incidence of hyperchloremic acidosis. Hextend also contains 0.45 mmol/L of magnesium and 99 mg/dl (0.99%) of dextrose. Pentastarch (Pentaspan, B. Braun McGaw) is a 10% solution that has a lower molecular weight than hetastarch (M_w of 264 kD and 0.7 degree of substitution).

Although HES can affect von Willebrand's factor and factor VIII function, it is not as significant as with dextran 70. Clinical evidence of bleeding has not been reported in animals receiving HES 450/0.7 at doses up to 20 ml/kg/day. However, we have experienced prolongation in activated clotting times (ACTs) less than 50% above normal at this dosage. An elevation in ACT above 50% of the normal reference range warrants investigation for concurrent coagulation problems. An HES product available in Europe,

Voluven (Fresenine Kabi), has a M_w of 130 kD and a 0.4 degree of substitution. The reduced M_w and molar substitution reduce the risk of coagulation side effects, and an increased C2:C6 ratio prolongs half-life. HES 130/0.4 doses have been recommended up to 50 ml/kg.

A differential charge may exist between administered HES molecules and the capillary pore, blocking the passage of HES molecules into the interstitium. This property is independent of molecular size. HES may also down-regulate and decrease expression of endothelial surface adhesion molecules, which has been reported to decrease inflammation, endothelial injury, and leukocyte migration into the interstitium. HES has been shown to reverse changes in microvascular permeability caused by oxygen-free radicals during reperfusion injury. This can explain why HES molecules remain in the vascular space in the septic patient when albumin does not (Marx et al., 2002).

Smaller HES molecules are filtered through the glomerulus and excreted in the urine, excreted through the bile, or passed into the interstitium and ingested by macrophages. Larger molecules are degraded by α-amylase into smaller HES molecules. Hetastarch has been reported as nontoxic and nonallergenic in doses up to 100 ml/kg in dogs (Ballinger, Solanke, and Thompson, 1966). The authors have observed signs of nausea, occasional vomiting, and hypotension with rapid infusion of hetastarch in the cat. Slow administration of small-volume increments has eliminated these side effects in cats.

CLINICAL USE

Goals for colloid administration are to improve intravascular volume and systemic blood flow while maintaining intravascular COP. Selection of a specific colloid or colloids is based on individual traits of the colloid and the disease process of the animal (Tables 11-2 and 11-3).

When capillary permeability is normal, hetastarch, dextran 70, and 25% human albumin are effective for expanding intravascular volume while minimizing interstitial edema. However, perfusion problems caused by SIRS are associated with increased capillary pore size and hypovolemia (see Fig. 11-2). An intravenous colloid solution should be administered that is larger than the pore size in the capillary membrane. When hypoalbuminemia is a prominent feature, HES is the colloid of choice. Human albumin is usually reserved for use in severely hypoalbuminemic animals with normal capillary permeability.

Dextran 70 is used with extreme caution in animals with coagulation abnormalities. If large volumes of HES are required to restore perfusion, plasma or whole blood transfusions may be required to supplement coagulation proteins and restore clotting times. Oxyglobin is selected when there is a need to improve tissue oxygenation associated with maldistribution of blood flow or anemia. Blood component transfusions are an option when anemia and/or coagulopathies exist.

Based on the disease process and resuscitation needs, a single colloid or a combination of colloids is selected to obtain the desired benefits. Colloids are typically administered in combination with isotonic crystalloids, allowing the crystalloid volume for intravascular volume replacement to be decreased by 40% to 60% of the amount calculated for crystalloid resuscitation alone. When more than one type of colloid is needed, the colloids are usually administered consecutively rather than simultaneously. Dogs can tolerate rapid intravenous infusion of synthetic colloids for immediate intravascular resuscitation. In the cat all forms of colloid are administered more slowly (over 5 to 15 minutes).

The volume of fluids to administer for resuscitation is directed toward achieving desired clinical end-point parameters (heart rate, blood pressure, central venous pressure, pulmonary capillary wedge pressure, pulses, and capillary refill time), described as early goal-directed therapy in humans and end-point or goal-oriented resuscitation in animals. The objective is to infuse the least amount of fluids necessary to achieve and maintain end-point perfusion

Table **11-3**

Colloid Choices and Resuscitation Goals Used Based on Hypovolemic Condition in the Dog*

Condition	Resuscitation Colloid	Resuscitation Goal
Hypovolemic and/or traumatic shock	HES Dextran 70 Oxyglobin	MAP 60–80 mm Hg[†] HR normal CVP 8-10 cm H_2O
Trauma or edema in the brain or lungs	HES Dextran 70 Oxyglobin	MAP 60 mm Hg HR <140 beats/min CVP 5-8 cm H_2O
Hypovolemic shock with hemorrhage	Oxyglobin Whole blood pRBC + HES/dextran 70	MAP 60 mm Hg HR <140 beats/min CVP 5-8 cm H_2O
Hypovolemic heart failure in a critically hypotensive animal	HES	MAP 60 mm Hg HR < 180 beats/min
Hypovolemia in the chronically hypoalbuminemic animal	HES 25% Human albumin	MAP 60–80 mm Hg HR normal CVP 8-10 cm H_2O

HES, Hetastarch; *HR,* heart rate; *MAP,* mean arterial pressure; *pRBC,* packed red blood cell transfusion.
*Colloid fluids are always used in conjunction with crystalloid fluids and appropriate analgesia.
[†]Systolic arterial pressure >90 mm Hg.

parameters for the condition being treated. End-point perfusion parameters to achieve with most clinical conditions will be within high normal or supranormal ranges. When the patient is at risk for heart failure, hemorrhage, or brain or lung edema, low normal end points are selected to avoid exacerbation of hemorrhage or edema.

When low normal resuscitation end points are the goal, replacement isotonic crystalloids are administered initially (10 to 15 ml/kg) with HES or dextran 70 (3- to 5-ml/kg increments) titrated to effect (up to 20 ml/kg). When high normal or supranormal end points are desired, larger volumes of replacement isotonic crystalloids can be administered initially (20 to 40 ml/kg) with HES or dextran 70 at larger volumes (10 to 15 ml/kg) titrated as needed (up to 30 ml/kg). If 25% human albumin is used for acute volume resuscitation, up to 4 ml/kg has been used as a slow bolus infusion (Mathews and Barry, 2005).

Hypothermia, hypotension, and bradycardia are typical clinical findings in the cat in hypovolemic shock. Hypothermia perpetuates hypotension and must be rapidly corrected as part of the resuscitation plan to prevent fluid overload. Initially replacement isotonic crystalloids are administered (10 to 15 ml/kg), and HES or dextran 70 (3 to 5 ml/kg) titrated to reach a systolic indirect peripheral blood pressure higher than 40 mm Hg. Maintenance crystalloids and colloids are given at this time while aggressive external warming is provided to bring the rectal temperature above 98° F (within 30 minutes). It is common for the arterial blood pressure and heart rate to reach desired end points after warming is achieved without the administration of additional resuscitation fluids. However, additional crystalloid and colloid doses can be administered if blood pressure remains suboptimal despite warming, assuming the underlying disorder is volume related and not the result of cardiogenic shock.

Bolus infusions of colloids are titrated in succession, and clinical parameters assessed in between boluses until end-point parameters are achieved. When large volumes are required to reach resuscitation end points, coagulation parameters are closely monitored, and coagulation factors replaced as needed. Once the resuscitation goal has been achieved, a continuous-rate infusion (CRI) of HES or dextran 70 (20 to 30 ml/kg/day) or Oxyglobin (cat: 10 ml/kg/day; dog: 30 ml/kg/day) can be used to maintain the intravascular COP until the capillaries restore their integrity and recovery is eminent. Crystalloids are administered simultaneously to restore and maintain hydration and replacement of ongoing losses.

When end-point parameters have not been reached despite adequate fluid replacement, causes of nonresponsive shock need to be examined for, and vasoactive agents considered. Oxyglobin has a vasoconstricting effect and can be used in situations resulting in persistent vasodilation. When Oxyglobin is used in the dog for its vasoconstricting properties, 5-ml/kg incremental infusions are given to reach desired end points (to a total of 30 ml/kg). We have used Oxyglobin, 1- to 3-ml incremental infusions in hypertensive cats, administered slowly to effect (up to 10 ml/kg) and have found that this slow titration reduces the risk of acute volume overload and pulmonary edema. An Oxyglobin CRI is then initiated to maintain the blood pressure along with crystalloids for maintenance of hydration and ongoing losses.

A critical animal that is receiving crystalloids may benefit from intravascular colloid support but does not require aggressive intravascular volume resuscitation. The daily dose of HES or dextran 70 (20 ml/kg) can then be administered over 2 to 4 hours by CRI, decreasing the amount of crystalloid infused during this period. When there is normal capillary permeability and albumin replacement is desired, 25% human albumin can be infused as a CRI (1 to 4 ml/kg over 12 to 72 hours). Plasma is administered when there is need for albumin, coagulation factors, and/or antithrombin. The dose of plasma is variable, with an end-point goal of maintaining and/or improving albumin, coagulation factor, and antithrombin concentrations. The rate of plasma infusion is calculated to maximize volume infusion without causing fluid overload.

Perfusion and hydration parameters are closely monitored during and after colloid infusion. Early clinical signs of fluid intolerance include serous nasal discharge, chemosis, tachypnea, dull lung sounds (pleural effusion), "moist" lung sounds or crackles (pulmonary edema), and gelatinous subcutaneous swelling (peripheral edema). Signs of allergic reaction include facial swelling, urticaria, abrupt hypotension, tachycardia, nausea, vomiting, fever, and hyperemia. Monitoring for acute allergic reaction and anaphylaxis is more important in patients receiving transfusions and concentrated albumin.

References and Suggested Reading

Ballinger WF II, Solanke TF, Thompson WL: Effect of hydroxyethyl starch upon survival of dogs subjected to hemorrhagic shock, *Surg Gynecol Obstet* 122:33, 1966.

Barron M, Wilkes M, Navickis R: A systemic review of the comparative safely of colloids, *Arch Surg* 139:552, 2004.

Boldt J et al: Effects of a new modified, balanced hydroxyethyl starch preparation (Hextend) on measures of coagulation, *Br J Anaesth* 89:722, 2002.

Boldt J et al: Influence of different volume therapies and pentoxifylline infusion on circulating soluble adhesion molecules in critically ill patients, *Crit Care Med* 24:385, 1996.

Bonagura JD, editor: *Kirk's current veterinary therapy XII (small animal practice)*, Philadelphia, 1995, Saunders, p 116.

Concannon KT, Haskins SC, Feldman BF: Hemostatic defects associated with two infusion rates of dextran 70 in dogs, *Am J Vet Res* 53:1369, 1992.

Gold MS et al: Comparison of hetastarch to albumin for perioperative bleeding in patients undergoing abdominal aortic aneurysm repair: a prospective, randomized study, *Ann Surg* 211:482, 1990.

Kirby R, Rudloff E: Crystalloid and colloid fluid therapy. In Ettinger S, Feldman E, *Textbook of veterinary internal medicine*, ed 4, St. Louis, 2005; Elsevier, p 412.

Marx G et al: Hydroxyethyl starch and modified fluid gelatin maintain plasma volume in a porcine model of septic shock with capillary leakage, *Intensive Care Med* 28:629, 2002.

Marx G et al. Resuscitation from septic shock with capillary leakage: hydroxyethyl starch (130 kD), but not Ringer's solution maintains plasma volume and systemic oxygenation, *Shock* 21:336, 2004.

Mathews K, Barry M: The use of 25% human serum albumin: outcome and efficacy in raising serum albumin and systemic blood pressure in critically ill dogs and cats, *J Vet Emerg Crit Care* 15(2):110, 2005.

Molnar Z et al: Fluid resuscitation with colloids of different molecular weight in septic shock, *Intensive Care Med* 30:1356, 2004.

Muir W, Wellman M: Hemoglobin solutions and tissue oxygenation, *J Vet Intern Med* 17:127, 2003.

Prittie J: Optimal end points of resuscitation and early goal-directed therapy, *J Vet Emerg Crit Care* 16:329, 2006.

Zikria BA et al: Macromolecules reduce abnormal microvascular permeability in rat limb ischemia-reperfusion injury, *Crit Care Med* 17:1306, 1989.

CHAPTER 12

Acute Abdomen: Evaluation and Emergency Treatment

F. ANTHONY MANN, *Columbia, Missouri*

Acute abdomen may be defined as the acute onset of abdominal pain necessitating prompt diagnosis and immediate medical or surgical intervention to prevent deterioration of the patient. Because many of the conditions responsible for acute abdomen may progress to a state of shock, abdominal pain may not be evident at the time the animal is presented for medical attention.

CLINICAL SIGNS

Abdominal pain may be manifested as peculiar posture such as the praying position. In the praying position the animal lies in sternal recumbence with the pelvic limbs in standing position to elevate the pelvis and caudal abdomen. Animals may also exhibit abdominal pain by a reluctance to move; by ambulating in a stilted gait; or by taking short, careful steps. Abdominal tenderness may be noted by an avoidance reaction, vocalization, or guarding ("splinting") when the abdomen is touched. Some animals with acute abdomen may become apprehensive in anticipation of abdominal contact. Nausea exhibited through hypersalivation may be apparent as a result of abdominal pain. Other clinical signs are related to the underlying cause of the acute abdomen, such as protracted vomiting from pancreatitis, fever caused by septic peritonitis, hemorrhagic diarrhea resulting from canine parvoviral enteritis, and pale mucous membranes caused by traumatic hemoabdomen.

DIFFERENTIAL DIAGNOSES

Differential diagnoses of disorders that may lead to the development of acute abdomen are listed in Table 12-1.

Some of these causes have obvious surgical or medical indications, whereas others require some decision making based on the individual situation. Many patients with acute abdomen have serious diseases that require prompt attention to patient status and appropriate stabilization measures before a definitive diagnosis can be achieved and specific therapy implemented.

INITIAL PATIENT MANAGEMENT

On presentation the patient with an acute abdomen should have a rapid primary survey to ascertain immediate needs and determine priorities in diagnostics and therapeutics. The primary survey should include an abbreviated physical examination with emphasis on mental, respiratory, and cardiovascular status. Severely depressed animals with abnormal breathing and altered (weak or bounding) peripheral pulses should be interpreted to be in (or progressing toward) shock and should have appropriate resuscitative measures before detailed diagnostics and definitive therapy (see other chapters in this section). Immediately before emergency treatment procedures (such as shock doses of intravenous fluids), blood and urine samples should be obtained for a minimal database.

DIAGNOSTIC TESTS

Signalment and History

Signalment and history can be helpful in shortening the list of differential diagnoses and arranging those remaining according to likelihood. For example, a miniature

Table 12-1

Differential Diagnosis for the Acute Abdomen

Body System Cause of Acute Abdomen	Treatment	Body System Cause of Acute Abdomen	Treatment
Gastrointestinal Digestive System		**Reproductive System**	
Gastric dilation	DS, PE	**Female**	
Gastric dilation-volvulus	DS, DE	Acute metritis	PS, PE
Gastroduodenal ulceration	NS	Pyometra	DS, DE
Gastroduodenal perforation	DS, PE	Uterine torsion	DS, DE
Gastroduodenal rupture	DS, DE	Dystocia	PS, PE
Gastroduodenal dehiscence	DS, DE	Uterine rupture	DS, DE
Gastroenteritis (viral, bacterial, toxic [i.e., garbage])	NS	Ovarian cyst	PS, PE
		Ovarian neoplasia	DS, PE
Hemorrhagic gastroenteritis	NS		
Intestinal obstruction (foreign body, intussusception, neoplasia)	DS, PE	**Male**	
		Acute prostatitis	NS
Functional intestinal obstruction: ileus	NS	Prostatic abscess	DS, PE
Intestinal ulceration	NS	Prostatic cysts	DS, PE
Intestinal perforation	DS, DE	Prostatic neoplasia	DS, PE
Intestinal rupture	DS, DE	Testicular torsion	DS, DE
Intestinal dehiscence	DS, DE		
Intestinal volvulus	DS, DE	**Hematopoietic System: Spleen**	
Cecal inversion	DS, PE	Splenic mass (hematoma, extramedullary hematopoiesis, neoplasia, nodular hyperplasia, abscess)	DS, PE
Obstipation	NS		
Colitis	NS		
Colonic obstruction	NS	Splenic rupture (mass)	DS, DE
Colonic perforation	DS, DE	Splenic rupture (trauma)	PS, PE
Colonic rupture	DS, DE	Splenic torsion	DS, DE
Colonic dehiscence	DS, DE		
		Peritoneum and Mesentery	
Hepatobiliary Digestive System		Peritonitis: septic	DS, DE
Acute hepatitis (toxic, infectious)	NS	Peritonitis: chemical (bile, urine, pancreatic enzymes)	PS, PE
Hepatic abscess	DS, PE	Parietal peritoneal trauma: blunt	NS
Hepatic trauma	PS, PE	Parietal peritoneal trauma: penetrating	DS, DE
Hepatic rupture	PS, PE	Mesenteric traction: large masses	DS, PE
Hepatobiliary neoplasia	PS, PE	Mesenteric lymphadenopathy	PS, PE
Biliary obstruction (calculi, neoplasia, pancreatitis, abscess)	PS, PE	Mesenteric lymphadenitis	NS
		Mesenteric volvulus	DS, DE
Biliary rupture	DS, DE	Mesenteric avulsion	DS, DE
Cholecystitis	PS, PE	Mesenteric artery thrombosis	DS, DE
Cholangiohepatitis	NS	Adhesions with organ entrapment, internal hernias	DS, PE
Pancreatic Digestive System		**Abdominal Wall**	
Acute pancreatitis	NS	Trauma	PS, PE
Pancreatic abscess	DS, PE	Abscess	DS, PE
		Hematoma	PS, PE
Urinary System		Strangulated hernias	DS, DE
Acute nephrosis (toxicosis)	NS		PS, PE
Acute nephritis-pyelonephritis	NS	**Extraabdominal**	
Urinary calculi: renal	PS, PE	Intervertebral disk disease	PS, PE
Urinary calculi: ureteral	PS, PE	Diskospondylitis	PS, PE
Urinary calculi: cystic	PS, PE	Toxicities (heavy metal)	NS
Urinary calculi: urethral	PS, PE	Thoracic wall disease	PS, PE
Trauma-avulsion-rupture (renal, ureteral, cystic, urethral)	DS, PE	Steatitis	NS
		Myositis	NS
Obstruction (neoplasia, stricture): ureter	DS, PE	Hypoadrenocorticism	NS
Obstruction (neoplasia, stricture): urethra	DS, PE		
Renal artery thrombosis	PS, PE		
Renal neoplasia	PS, PE		

DE, Definitely requires emergent surgery; *DS,* definitely surgical; *NS,* nonsurgical (the urgency of medical treatment depends on the specific problem and the condition of the animal; some nonsurgical acute abdomen cases may eventually require surgery on a nonemergent basis); *PE,* potentially requires emergent surgery (some conditions designated as PE may require surgery, although not on an emergent basis); *PS,* potentially surgical.

Box **12-1**

Historical Information to be Included in Cases of Acute Abdomen

- Diet
- Appetite
- Weight change
- Water consumption
- Urination: characterize polyuria, anuria, pollakiuria
- Defecation, diarrhea: characterize frequency, presence of blood, color, volume, relation to meals
- Vomiting: characterize frequency, presence of blood, color, volume, relation to meals
- Exposure to toxins, trauma (blunt, penetrating), foreign body ingestion
- Previous disease
- Previous abdominal surgery
- Length of illness
- How quickly signs develop

schnauzer with acute abdominal pain is more likely to have acute pancreatitis than gastric dilation-volvulus. A history of dietary indiscretion in a well-vaccinated dog with no exposure to other dogs would prioritize garbage intoxication over parvoviral enteritis. A complete history should be taken, but certain questions should be emphasized in cases of acute abdomen as listed in Box 12-1.

Physical Examination

A complete body systems review is important for a full understanding of the patient's condition, but the patient's initial status may dictate that some aspects of the physical examination receive a low priority. Physical evaluation not directly related to the patient's immediate status can be postponed. The abdominal portion of the physical examination should be performed in each case of acute abdomen. However, the abdominal evaluation should be the last part of the physical examination for two reasons: (1) serious extraabdominal abnormalities may otherwise be overlooked; and (2) manipulation of a tender abdomen may elicit pain and apprehension that could interfere with further evaluation.

Physical examination of the abdomen should include visual inspection, auscultation, percussion, ballottement, superficial and deep palpation, and digital rectal palpation. The examination should proceed from the least to most likely technique to elicit a pain response. Abnormalities that may be detected on visual inspection include distention (such as with abdominal effusion), deformity (caused by a large abdominal mass or hernia), swelling (such as with cellulitis associated with urine leakage), and bruising (associated with coagulopathy or blunt trauma). Bluish-red discoloration around the umbilicus (Cullen's sign) is indicative of intraabdominal hemorrhage. Visual inspection may also reveal puncture wounds (associated with penetrating trauma such as animal bites or projectiles), but the wounds may not be evident without clipping of abdominal hair.

Abdominal auscultation is performed to characterize gut sounds. Increased gut sounds may be evident in acute cases of enteritis, intestinal obstruction, and toxin ingestion. Absence of gut sounds suggests ileus, chronic intestinal obstruction, peritonitis, or abdominal effusion. Anorexia causes decreased intestinal motility, necessitating a long period (2 to 3 minutes) of auscultation before ascertaining that gut sounds are absent. Failure to auscult abnormal (increased or absent) gut sounds does not mean that the abdomen is normal; normal gut motility may be maintained in the early posttraumatic period and in early peritoneal effusion.

Percussion can be performed with or without the aid of a stethoscope to detect hyperresonance (indicating intraabdominal air, usually a gas-filled viscus) or hyporesonance (indicating intraabdominal fluid). If the animal is standing, a fluid line may be percussed between areas of hyperresonance and hyporesonance. Ballottement can be performed in standing and recumbent animals by tapping the abdomen and looking for a ripple effect to confirm the presence of intraabdominal fluid. Animals with a large amount of intraabdominal or extraabdominal fat can appear to ripple on ballottement, yielding a false-positive diagnosis of abdominal effusion.

The abdomen is palpated to detect pain; masses; and enlargement, displacement, or other abnormalities of abdominal organs. Superficial palpation is used to detect, characterize, and potentially localize pain and should be performed before deep palpation. Reproducible abdominal guarding ("splinting") in response to superficial palpation indicates abdominal pain. Stimulation of irritated parietal peritoneum by superficial abdominal palpation is a major reason for the pain response. Another potential response to parietal peritoneum stimulation is nausea and vomiting. Deep palpation should be performed to characterize the structures and abnormal findings in each of three regions: cranial, middle, and caudal abdomen. The final evaluation of the caudal abdomen should include digital examination per rectum to assess the prostate, pelvis, pelvic urethra, sublumbar lymph nodes (if enlarged), and rectum and to evaluate the character and color of the stool.

The physical examination will not necessarily provide a definitive diagnosis, nor will it necessarily dictate a particular therapeutic measure. However, it will help the clinician select the most appropriate diagnostic tests and, if performed serially, will keep the clinician abreast of changes in patient status.

Clinical Pathology

Laboratory testing of blood and urine is useful in providing confirmatory data, sometimes leading to a definitive diagnosis and, probably most important, providing a current picture of the patient's hematologic and metabolic status. A complete blood count provides information regarding anemia, platelet numbers, and hydration status (packed cell volume and total serum solids), which are important influences on treatment decisions. The leukogram provides information regarding the inflammatory status of the condition. A biochemistry profile may help localize the underlying disease to a specific organ and gives important information about the patient's acid-base balance and electrolyte status. Urinalysis, especially when interpreted in conjunction with biochemistry panels, provides essential information regarding renal function and other urinary tract abnormalities. In emergency situations such as when contemplating emergent celiotomy, waiting for laboratory test results can be detrimental to the patient's well-being. In such circumstances an emergency minimal database should include determinations of packed cell volume, total serum solids, serum creatinine or blood urea nitrogen, serum glucose, serum electrolytes, and urine specific gravity, as well as urine reagent strip test results. The remaining tests can be done later on pretreatment samples.

Diagnostic Imaging

Abdominal radiography, ultrasonography, and contrast studies may provide valuable directions to patient management. Abdominal radiographs should be taken as part of the standard evaluation in most cases of acute abdomen. Notable exceptions include (1) evisceration, (2) penetrating trauma (unless there is need to locate projectiles), (3) postoperative abdomen with peritonitis confirmed on abdominal fluid analysis, and (4) suspected cases of gastric dilation-volvulus in which the patient is in respiratory distress. In the latter example, once the animal is stable and the stomach is decompressed, a right lateral abdominal radiograph may be obtained to confirm the diagnosis. Standing lateral views may be used in cases of abdominal effusion that would otherwise have little abdominal detail. Notable positive radiographic findings in cases of acute abdomen include the presence of fluid (abdominal effusion), gas-distended intestines (obstruction or ileus), free abdominal air (ruptured viscus), masses, organomegaly, foreign bodies, urinary calculi, and signs of pancreatitis (loss of detail in the right cranial quadrant and lateral displacement of a gas-filled descending duodenum).

Abdominal ultrasonography is helpful in defining masses and enlarged organs, especially when abdominal effusion causes loss of radiographic detail. Ultrasonography is particularly helpful in the identification of fluid-filled lesions (such as abscesses) and the characterization of abnormalities of the liver, spleen, prostate, and kidneys. Fine-needle aspiration or needle biopsy of abnormal structures or both can be guided by ultrasonographic examination.

Contrast radiography of the gastrointestinal and urinary systems is sometimes necessary in acute abdomen if survey radiographs fail to define a suspected abnormality. Barium studies can be used to confirm and localize gastrointestinal obstruction. Water-soluble contrast agents should be used when gastrointestinal perforation is suspected. Intravenous urography and urethrocystography are used to confirm and localize discontinuity, obstruction, and other physical abnormalities of the urinary system. When diagnostic imaging fails to clearly define the diagnosis and course of therapy, sampling of abdominal fluid is necessary.

Abdominocentesis and Diagnostic Peritoneal Lavage

Sampling of abdominal fluid is most commonly performed to determine if the patient requires exploratory celiotomy, particularly emergent celiotomy. Abdominocentesis may result in a diagnostic sample if the abdominal fluid is of sufficient volume (approximately 20 ml/kg). Typically each of four abdominal quadrants is aseptically tapped using a hypodermic needle in an open drop technique or by attaching a syringe for gentle aspiration. Alternately a multiholed catheter may be used. A standard over-the-needle intravenous catheter can be modified for abdominocentesis by making side holes with a scalpel blade. Care should be exercised to make the side holes small and smooth to prevent kinking and tearing of the catheter within the abdomen. The four-quadrant tap is performed with the animal in a standing position if it can stand voluntarily. If all four sites fail to yield fluid or are otherwise nondiagnostic, diagnostic peritoneal lavage is the next step.

Diagnostic peritoneal lavage is performed with a multiholed catheter. Commercially available peritoneal lavage catheters can be used, or standard intravenous catheters can be modified as described for abdominocentesis. I prefer to use a commercially available thoracocentesis catheter (Kendall Turkel Safety Thoracentesis System, Covidien Animal Health and Dental Division, Mansfield, MA) that has a protected needle-stylet and four offset side holes. The ventral midline just caudal to the umbilicus has been recommended for diagnostic peritoneal lavage catheter placement (Crowe, 1988). However, I prefer to enter the abdomen just to the right (2 to 3 cm in midsize dogs) of the umbilicus to avoid interference with the falciform ligament and median ligament of the bladder. The right side is used to minimize the chance of iatrogenic damage to the spleen and descending colon. A subcutaneous bleb of local anesthetic is placed at the proposed entry site, and a tiny stab incision is made in the skin with a No. 11 scalpel blade. The catheter is advanced through the skin stab and into the abdomen. Once the catheter is in the abdomen, a syringe is attached, and gentle aspiration is applied. If a diagnostic sample is obtained, there is no need to progress with the lavage. In the absence of an adequate sample, 22 ml/kg of warmed, sterile isotonic saline is infused into the catheter via an intravenous infusion set with rapid gravity flow or by applying moderate pressure to the bag of saline. After completing the infusion, the patient is rolled gently from side to side, and the abdomen is gently ballotted to disperse the saline, taking care not to dislodge the catheter. Careful, slow aspiration of the catheter with a syringe is performed to collect a 10- to 20-ml sample. Ideally all the infused fluid should be removed, but typically only a small portion is retrievable. The catheter can be retained temporarily for serial evaluation of abdominal fluid in some instances, such as for assessing whether hemoabdomen is ongoing.

Fluid from abdominocentesis or diagnostic peritoneal lavage should be evaluated for color, packed cell volume, white blood cell count, and cytologic features. Occasionally bacterial cultures and chemistry panels should be performed. Red color suggests hemoabdomen. More definitively, a packed cell volume of diagnostic peritoneal lavage fluid that is 5% or greater indicates significant hemorrhage. Cloudiness suggests peritonitis. An elevated abdominal fluid white blood cell count is diagnostic of peritonitis, but the normally reactive response of the peritoneum to insult (such as surgical manipulation) limits the usefulness of cell counts for determining sepsis (Kirby, 2003). Cytologic characteristics are more meaningful than are cell counts in differentiating septic from nonseptic peritonitis. Toxic changes in neutrophils and the presence of intracellular or extracellular bacteria indicate septic peritonitis. In such cases aerobic and anaerobic bacterial cultures are appropriate, particularly if antibiotic therapy is to be initiated before surgical samples can be obtained. However, intraoperative culture samples are preferred.

In cases of suspected urinary system disruption, the most useful chemistry evaluation for abdominal fluid is creatinine. Urea nitrogen could also be used but is less desirable than creatinine because it is a smaller molecule and rapidly diffuses across the peritoneum and equilibrates with plasma. Diagnostic peritoneal lavage creatinine that is greater (usually two times greater) than serum creatinine indicates uroabdomen. Alternately potassium concentrations can be used to detect uroabdomen. A ratio of abdominal fluid potassium to peripheral blood potassium greater than 1.9:1 indicates uroabdomen (Aumann, Worth, and Drobatz, 1998). Three other chemistry analytes that are occasionally helpful are bilirubin, amylase, and glucose. Bilirubin test reagents can detect intraperitoneal bile, indicating disruption of the biliary system or duodenum. Elevated abdominal fluid amylase compared with serum amylase indicates pancreatitis or intestinal ischemia (Davenport and Martin, 1992). Abdominal fluid glucose can be helpful in differentiating septic from nonseptic peritoneal effusion. An abdominal fluid glucose concentration that is more than 20 mg/dl lower than the blood glucose concentration indicates septic peritonitis (Bonczynski et al., 2003).

Exploratory Celiotomy

When exploratory celiotomy is necessary in acute abdomen, the initial diagnostics should prepare the surgeon to anticipate certain findings. An acute abdomen condition for which surgery is indicated (see Table 12-1) should be on the differential diagnosis list for the patient in question. Exploratory celiotomy should be performed as soon as possible after the need for it is determined. A decision to delay surgery can be justified when the delay will decrease morbidity or the chance of mortality and when it is necessary for additional stabilization that will make the patient a better surgical candidate. Intraoperatively the surgeon should perform a complete systematic exploratory celiotomy to detect and correct all significant abnormalities. Occasionally during emergent celiotomy, life-threatening problems (such as ongoing hemorrhage) will require immediate attention; systematic exploration can be performed later in the procedure. Only rarely should systematic exploration be abandoned altogether (e.g., in patients judged to be at risk of death or severe disability if recovery from anesthesia does not take place soon).

THERAPY

Specific medical and surgical therapeutic measures for animals experiencing acute abdomen are dictated by the clinical status of the patient and the specific cause of the acute abdomen. Each patient should be considered at risk for deterioration; appropriate resuscitative measures are necessary in some cases before a definitive diagnosis can be achieved. Once the definitive cause is ascertained, specific medical or surgical treatments can be used. It is difficult to identify any common therapy for all cases of acute abdomen other than perhaps fluid therapy. However, there is one treatment that should not be overlooked—analgesic therapy.

If one considers that abdominal pain is present at some point in each case of acute abdomen and that definitive therapy is not necessarily going to immediately resolve the pain, analgesics become important. Analgesics should be administered to both medical and surgical patients. Various analgesic regimens are acceptable, but most patients can be managed with either buprenorphine (dogs and cats) if the major source of pain is visceral (such as a distended organ) or morphine (dogs) if the major source of pain is musculoskeletal (such as abdominal wall trauma). Although morphine would likely be effective for visceral pain, potential side effects (nausea, emesis, urine retention, constipation, and greater chance of respiratory depression than buprenorphine) make morphine a less desirable analgesic for most cases of acute abdomen. Buprenorphine can be given as a continuous-rate intravenous infusion (0.04 mg/kg/day) for the first 12 to 36 hours until a switch can be made to an oral opioid (or nonsteroidal antiinflammatory drug if there are no gastrointestinal concerns). When used, morphine can be given as a continuous-rate intravenous infusion (0.1 mg/kg/hour). As an adjunct to opioid analgesia or to minimize the amount of opioids used, lidocaine (20 mcg/kg/min) may be used (dogs only) as a continuous-rate intravenous infusion for the first 12 to 24 hours. When given together for infusion, buprenorphine (or morphine) and lidocaine may be mixed in the same bag of fluids, typically normal saline or the maintenance crystalloid solution being used for fluid therapy. Analgesics should be given as early in the course of treatment as possible. In surgical patients it is preferable to include analgesic administration as part of the preanesthetic medication and repeat administration as necessary before recovery from anesthesia. In nonsurgical patients and patients who undergo lengthy delays before surgery, analgesics are recommended as soon as it is ascertained that the drug effects will not interfere with the diagnostic evaluation. In most cases of acute abdomen, this means as soon as the physical examination is complete. Withholding analgesics for fear of masking important clinical signs should be the exception rather than the rule. Analgesics are not administered immediately to animals presented in shock but should be initiated soon after the shock state is reversed using the same guidelines discussed earlier. The duration of analgesic administration varies with the individual animal but should be at least 24 hours in both postoperative and nonsurgical patients.

References and Suggested Reading

Aumann M, Worth LT, Drobatz KJ: Uroperitoneum in cats: 26 cases (1986-1995), *J Am Anim Hosp Assoc* 34:315, 1998.

Bonczynski JJ et al: Comparison of peritoneal fluid and peripheral blood pH, bicarbonate, glucose, and lactate concentration as a diagnostic tool for septic peritonitis in dogs and cats, *Vet Surg* 32:161, 2003.

Crowe DT: The first steps in handling the acute abdomen patient, *Vet Med* 83:654, 1988.

Davenport DJ, Martin RA: Acute abdomen. In Murtaugh RJ, Kaplan PM, editors: *Veterinary emergency and critical care medicine*, St Louis, 1992, Mosby, p 153.

Kirby BM: Peritoneum and peritoneal cavity. In Slatter DH, editor: *Textbook of small animal surgery*, ed 3, Philadelphia, 2003, Saunders, p 414.

Saxon WD: The acute abdomen, *Vet Clin North Am Small Anim Pract* 24:1207, 1994.

CHAPTER 13

Drainage Techniques for the Septic Abdomen

ADRIENNE BENTLEY, *Philadelphia, Pennsylvania*
DAVID E. HOLT, *Philadelphia, Pennsylvania*

"There is probably no detail in modern surgical pathology that deserves more thorough comprehension, but which is less definitively understood.... than the nature of the reaction of the peritoneum to drainage."   John L. Yates, 1905

Since Yates's classic paper, there has been substantial investigation into the indications for and best methods of peritoneal drainage. However, universal guidelines for techniques of peritoneal drainage and consistent indications for their application have not emerged. Prophylactic drainage following routine, uncontaminated intraabdominal procedures has been largely abandoned in human surgery. In veterinary medicine, postoperative abdominal drainage is now generally reserved for cases with generalized septic peritonitis.

Septic peritonitis is a severe, life-threatening condition that poses many challenges for the small animal veterinarian. Obtaining an accurate and timely diagnosis; understanding peritoneal fluid and protein loss, hypovolemia, and the systemic inflammatory response syndrome/sepsis; and effective resuscitation are vital to successful treatment of peritonitis. Control of the source of peritoneal contamination remains the primary goal of exploratory laparotomy in cases of generalized septic peritonitis. More recently the benefits of copious intraoperative peritoneal lavage and the need for postoperative peritoneal drainage have been questioned. Although a detailed discussion of peritoneal lavage is beyond the scope of this chapter,

current recommendations include the judicious use of lavage to remove gross contamination and aspiration of the lavage fluid from the peritoneal cavity before closure (Platell, Papadimitriou, and Hall, 2000). This chapter focuses on the indications for and use of various drainage techniques in septic peritonitis.

Effective drainage of the peritoneal cavity in generalized septic peritonitis requires an understanding of intraperitoneal fluid circulation, normal intraperitoneal pressures, and the response of the peritoneal cavity to insertion of a foreign body such as a drain. Fluid injected into the peritoneal cavity disperses throughout the cavity within 15 minutes to 2 hours, depending on the site of injection (Hosgood et al., 1989). The clinical implication is that although fibrin, the omentum, the viscera, and the mesentery may try to localize a focus of contamination, it is likely that contaminated fluid can spread rapidly throughout the peritoneal cavity. Within the peritoneal cavity the gastrointestinal tract has a luminal pressure exceeding atmospheric pressure, whereas the pressure within the peritoneal space is subatmospheric. Even with experimental insufflation of air, the intraperitoneal pressure never exceeds atmospheric pressure (Gold, 1956). Unless either the intraperitoneal pressure becomes higher than atmospheric pressure or air can enter the peritoneal cavity after surgery through a vent, drainage from the peritoneal cavity will not occur without the use of a vacuum system.

Drains inserted into the peritoneal cavity are rapidly encased by the omentum and viscera (Yates, 1905). Thus in some studies it is not clear if drainage occurs from the peritoneal cavity or, more likely, from the encased area around the drain. In a previous experimental study in dogs, sump-Penrose drains were found to be encapsulated and isolated from the peritoneal cavity at necropsy after 48 hours (Hosgood et al., 1989). Despite this isolation, the drains continued to remove radiopaque contrast material from the peritoneal cavity. The use of closed-suction silicone drains for septic peritonitis has been reported (Mueller, Ludwig, and Barton, 2001). Drains in the cases described continued to accumulate fluid for up to 8 days, seeming to indicate adequate function. However, it is not clear if closed-suction drains are encased to the same extent as sump-Penrose drains and are draining a localized area, or if they retain functional drainage of the peritoneal cavity despite being encased.

INDICATIONS FOR POSTOPERATIVE DRAINAGE

The anticipation of significant postoperative fluid production caused by inability to control the source of contamination, generalized peritonitis, or severe local peritonitis is an indication for postoperative drainage. The efficacy of the peritoneal defense mechanisms may be limited by a large volume of fluid, either ongoing effusion or residual lavage. Phagocytosis of bacteria within fluid depends on the presence of opsonins in the fluid, which can become depleted. Therefore the presence of fluid may allow rapid bacterial proliferation. A large volume of fluid may also limit the localization of the contamination and speed the systemic absorption of bacteria and endotoxins (Platell, Papadimitriou, and Hall, 2000). A large volume of effusion also increases intraabdominal pressure. In some cases intraabdominal hypertension is sufficient to cause cardiopulmonary dysfunction, anuria or oliguria, and intestinal ischemia (abdominal compartment syndrome) (Drellich, 2000; Conzemius et al., 1995).

LOCAL PERITONITIS

In some cases peritonitis may not be generalized at the time of exploratory surgery. The two most common examples of localized peritonitis in small animal surgery are prostatic and pancreatic abscesses. Local peritoneal drainage has been used to treat these conditions and generally involved placement of one or more Penrose drains in the abscess cavity once débridement and local lavage were completed. These techniques have largely been replaced by omentalization. The abscess cavity is located by palpation, intraoperative ultrasound, or aspiration. It is opened, drained, and gently débrided with a moistened gauze sponge. After thorough local lavage with a warm, balanced electrolyte solution, the omentum is packed loosely into the cavity, and the abdominal incision is closed. The immunologic and angiogenic properties of the omentum promote local infection control and healing. The technique has been associated with long-term

success in 19 of 20 dogs with prostatic abscesses (White and Williams, 1995) and 6 of 12 dogs with pancreatic abscesses (Johnson and Mann, 2006).

GENERALIZED PERITONITIS

Primary Abdominal Closure Without Drainage

The decision to close the peritoneal cavity without drainage is based on control of the source of contamination and adequate decontamination of the peritoneal cavity. The clinician then relies on the body's peritoneal drainage and immune defense systems. Fluid absorption occurs primarily by passing through gaps (stomata) in the mesothelial cells into lymphatics and thereby the circulation. More microvilli are present on the mesothelial cells of the visceral peritoneum than the parietal peritoneum to promote movement of fluid toward the diaphragm for absorption. The number of mesothelial microvilli increases and lymphatics dilate in response to peritoneal inflammation. In addition to mesothelial cells, numerous immune cells are present in the peritoneal membrane and omentum, including macrophages, lymphocytes, and mast cells. The immune cells function in bacterial phagocytosis, antigen presentation, and antibody and cytokine production in cases of peritonitis. Finally, production of plasminogen activator inhibitor 1 by peritoneal mesothelial cells promotes the organization of fibrous adhesions, which facilitate phagocytosis and localize contamination (Yao, Platell, and Hall, 2003).

Lanz and colleagues (2001) reported 54% survival in a cohort of 28 cases of canine septic peritonitis managed with source control, intraoperative lavage, and closure of the peritoneal cavity without a means of additional postoperative drainage. As discussed, this method of surgical management relies on peritoneal drainage and may be appropriate when the source of contamination can be controlled definitively and peritonitis is not severe.

Open Peritoneal Drainage

Historically open peritoneal drainage has been reserved for the most severe cases of generalized septic peritonitis, which are anecdotally associated with a large volume of effusion after surgery. Assessment of the severity of peritonitis is largely subjective and based on individual experience but may include evaluation of factors shown in Box 13-1. Clear indications for open peritoneal drainage include the need for relaparotomy and anaerobic infection. Relaparotomy may be necessary in cases of ineffective source control or when additional débridement is required. Although the type of infection may not be definitively known at the time of initial laparotomy, an anaerobic infection may be suspected when the colon is the source of contamination. Although intraabdominal pressure is not routinely measured in the clinical setting, open peritoneal drainage is indicated when intraabdominal hypertension results in clinical signs such as anuria or oliguria (Conzemius et al., 1995).

Open peritoneal drainage is established through a long abdominal incision, extending from the xiphoid

Box 13-1

Factors Evaluated In Determining the Severity of Peritonitis

- Volume of effusion
- Character of effusion: opacity, color, odor
- Presence of gross contamination: fecal matter, food, hair
- Serosal changes of abdominal organs: erythema, encasement with fibrous adhesions
- Distribution of contamination and peritonitis: localized or generalized

process to the pubis and including the most dependent portion of the abdomen. The falciform fat should be excised according to standard exploratory laparotomy technique, but omentectomy is not necessary. The linea alba is closed with nonabsorbable suture in a simple continuous pattern with a gap of 1 to 6 cm between the edges, depending on the patient's size (Fig. 13-1). The subcutaneous tissues and skin are not closed. A sterile bandage consisting of laparotomy sponges and surgery towels underneath routine bandage material is applied and changed at least daily. If the bandage becomes wet from peritoneal effusion or urine or if it becomes displaced, it should be replaced as soon as possible. A urinary catheter helps to maintain the integrity of the bandage, especially in male dogs. Although early reports (Woolfson and Dulisch, 1986; Greenfield and Walshaw, 1987) describe performing bandage changes outside of the operating room with the patient standing, current recommendations include changing the bandage in the operating room with the patient sedated or anesthetized. During each bandage change, adhesions at the incision

are digitally disrupted; the incision is checked for organ evisceration; and additional surgical procedures such as peritoneal lavage, débridement, and feeding tube placement are performed as needed. The decision to close the peritoneal cavity is based on reassessment of the same factors used in selecting open peritoneal drainage. Clinical studies report a mean duration of open peritoneal drainage of 4 to 5 days, with a range of less than 1 day to as long as 2 weeks (Woolfson and Dulisch, 1986; Greenfield and Walshaw, 1987; Winkler and Greenfield, 2000).

Open peritoneal drainage is regarded as an efficient means of drainage, although evidence supporting this claim is limited. In an experimental study of five normal dogs, open peritoneal drainage resulted in rapid, equal, and relatively complete drainage of radiopaque contrast from the peritoneal cavity. Drainage occurred despite the fact that the laparotomy incisions were partially occluded by omentum in all five dogs at necropsy (48 hours after open drainage was established) (Hosgood et al., 1989). In another experimental study of six normal dogs, extreme variability in the volume of injected saline recovered through open peritoneal drainage precluded conclusions regarding drainage efficiency. Drainage occurred in these dogs despite omental adhesions along the entire length of the laparotomy incisions at necropsy (96 hours after open drainage was established) (Hosgood, Salisbury, and De Nicola, 1991). Similar to omental encasement of drains, the effect of omental adhesions to the laparotomy incision on the volume and distribution of fluid drained is unclear. Experimental studies evaluating the efficiency of open peritoneal drainage are limited by the lack of peritonitis, small number of dogs, and small volume of peritoneal fluid (Hosgood et al., 1989 and Hosgood, Salisbury, and DeNicola, 1991). The presence of peritonitis may help maintain the patency of laparotomy incisions and drains by resulting in a larger volume of effusion and omental adhesions to areas of the peritoneal cavity other than the incision or drain (Hosgood, Salisbury, and DeNicola, 1991). Finally, the minimum efficiency of peritoneal drainage necessary in clinical cases of peritonitis is unknown and likely case dependent.

Hypoproteinemia and nosocomial infection are reported complications of open peritoneal drainage, the clinical significance of which is not well established. Clinical reports have documented a relatively small number of patients with different bacterial culture results at the time of exploratory laparotomy and peritoneal closure. Moreover, the presence of a different bacterium at the time of closure does not appear to impact survival (Winkler and Greenfield, 2000; Greenfield and Walshaw, 1987; Woolfson and Dulisch, 1986). Hypoproteinemia is likely a consequence of septic peritonitis, regardless of drainage technique. Total protein concentration was not different between animals managed by peritoneal closure and open drainage 48 hours after surgery. Although a similar number of animals in each group received hetastarch, more animals in the open-drainage group received blood, plasma, and a jejunostomy tube. Animals in the open-drainage group also stayed in the intensive care unit longer than animals in the closed-peritoneal group (Staatz, Monnet, and Seim, 2002).

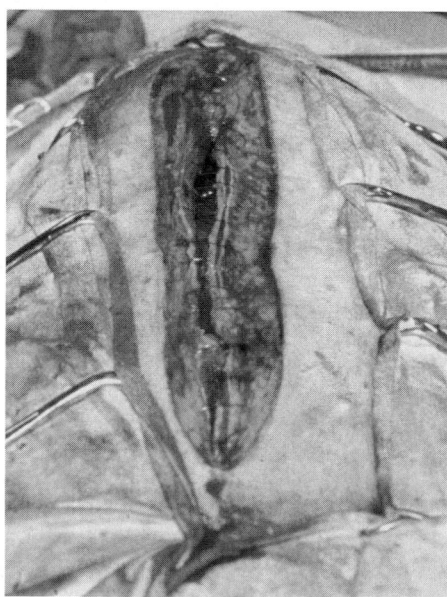

Fig. 13-1 Open peritoneal drainage is established by leaving a gap between the edges of the linea alba.

Vacuum-Assisted Closure

Originally designed for use in a variety of chronic wounds, the use of the vacuum-assisted closure (VAC) device in human medicine has simplified the management of patients with open peritoneal drainage. The VAC device (Kinetic Concepts, Inc., San Antonio, TX) consists of a polyurethane ether foam sponge that is cut to fit the wound. An adherent layer is placed over the sponge, and fenestrated evacuation tubing is placed under the adherent layer and connected to a vacuum pump through a drainage canister (Fig. 13-2). Intermittent subatmospheric pressure is applied to the wound through the VAC device (Venturi et al., 2005). Application of the VAC device to the open peritoneal cavity necessitates the addition of a fenestrated nonadherent layer (polyethylene) between the sponge and the peritoneal contents. The device is changed in the operating room as needed (Scott, Feanny, and Hirshberg, 2005). Use of the VAC device promotes wound healing by increasing blood flow, decreasing tissue edema, and removing excess fluid. As a result, bacterial counts are also decreased in the wound (Venturi et al., 2005). The VAC device may provide advantages over traditional open peritoneal drainage in veterinary patients by allowing the volume of effusion to be quantified and decreasing the frequency of labor-intensive bandage changes.

Closed-Suction Drainage

Closed-suction drainage is likely the most commonly used technique for the management of septic peritonitis in veterinary patients. Commercially available closed-suction drains consist of a fenestrated silicone drain connected to an external reservoir by a nonfenestrated tube such as the Jackson-Pratt drain (Cardinal Health [Fig. 13-3]). The drain is typically positioned near the diaphragm and liver in the most dependent portion of the peritoneal cavity, although a more caudal position may be appropriate, depending on the source of the contamination. The nonfenestrated portion of the drain is exited through a small paramedian incision in the body wall and secured with a purse string and

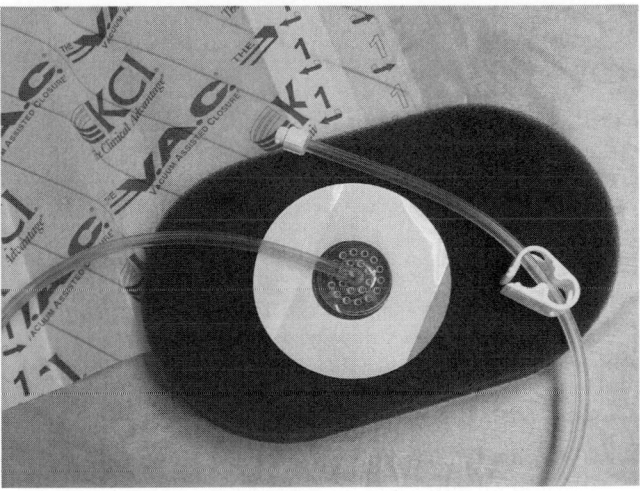

Fig. 13-3 Components of the vacuum-assisted closure (VAC) device include a foam sponge, fenestrated evacuation tubing, and an adherent layer. (Courtesy Kinetic Concepts, Inc.)

finger trap of nonabsorbable suture. Compression of the bulb reservoir creates negative pressure within the peritoneal cavity. A bandage is typically applied to cover the exit site of the drain and to provide a means of attaching the bulb reservoir to the patient. The contents of the reservoir are easily emptied, typically every 6 hours.

Mueller, Ludwig, and Barton (2001) reported 70% survival in a cohort of 30 dogs and 10 cats with septic peritonitis managed with closed-suction drains. Drains were in place for a mean of 3.6 days with a range of 2 to 8 days. The volume of fluid produced was variable but decreased with time. The drains remained patent until removal as evidenced by ongoing fluid collection. However, it is unclear if the closed-suction drains removed fluid from the entire peritoneal cavity and what percentage of the total peritoneal fluid volume they drained. No significant complications were reported with use of the closed-suction drains. Only five patients had bacterial cultures of peritoneal fluid performed both at the time of surgery and drain removal. In the two patients with a positive culture at drain removal, different bacteria were isolated compared to the intraoperative cultures, and both patients survived.

Closed-suction drains are relatively inexpensive and easy to place and seem to be free of significant complications. Advantages of closed-suction drainage over open peritoneal drainage include the ability to quantify the volume of effusion and decreased cost and labor. Closed-suction drains have an advantage over physiologic peritoneal drainage in their apparent ability to drain a large volume of effusion rapidly. In addition, closed-suction drains provide readily available peritoneal fluid samples after surgery for cytologic and biochemical analysis. Their use is indicated in most cases of septic peritonitis when the need for postoperative drainage is anticipated but the severity of the peritonitis or volume of effusion does not warrant open peritoneal drainage.

Summary

Postoperative drainage is indicated in septic peritonitis because a large volume of effusion has detrimental effects

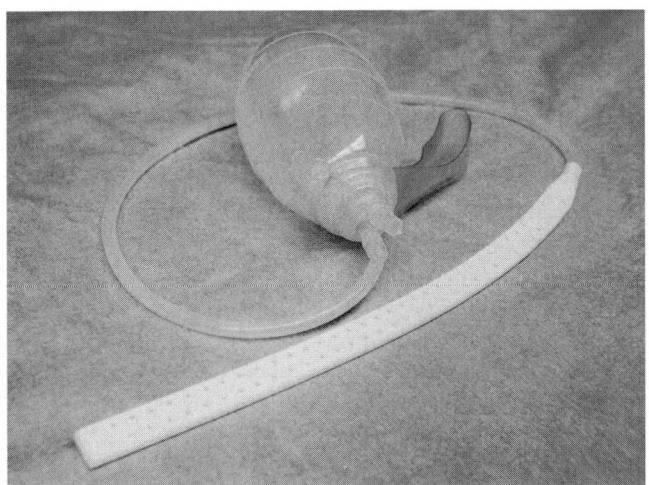

Fig. 13-2 Components of a closed-suction drain include a bulb reservoir connected to the fenestrated intraabdominal portion of the drain. (Jackson-Pratt drain courtesy Cardinal Health.)

Table 13-1

Comparison of Common Peritoneal Drainage Techniques

	Closure Without Additional Drainage	Open Peritoneal Drainage	Closed-Suction Drainage
Efficiency/efficacy	Relies on host peritoneal mechanisms	Uncertain	Uncertain
Labor/nursing care	Minimal	Extensive	Moderate
Cost	Minimal	Expensive	Moderate
Other		Allows relaparotomy	Volume of effusion quantified

Table 13-2

Suggested Criteria for Selecting a Method of Peritoneal Drainage

Peritoneal closure without additional drainage	Definitive control of the source of contamination Minimal peritonitis
Open peritoneal drainage	Inability to control the source at first laparotomy Need for additional débridement at second laparotomy Suspected anaerobic infection such as colonic source Severe peritonitis Abdominal compartment syndrome
Closed-suction drainage	Definitive control of the source of contamination Moderate peritonitis

on peritoneal defense mechanisms and organ function. Table 13-1 shows a comparison of the most commonly used peritoneal drainage techniques, including closure of the peritoneal cavity without additional drainage, open peritoneal drainage, and closed-suction drainage. Patient factors to consider in selecting a method of peritoneal drainage include the success of source control and the severity of the peritonitis (Table 13-2). Cost and the availability of intensive nursing care may also influence the technique selected.

References and Suggested Reading

Conzemius MG et al: Clinical determination of preoperative and post-operative intra-abdominal pressures in dogs, *Vet Surg* 24:195, 1995.

Drellich S: Intraabdominal pressure and abdominal compartment syndrome, *Compend Cont Educ Pract Vet* 22:764, 2000.

Gold E: The physics of the abdominal cavity and the problem of peritoneal drainage, *Am J Surg* 91:415, 1956.

Greenfield CL, Walshaw R: Open peritoneal drainage for treatment of contaminated peritoneal cavity and septic peritonitis in dogs and cats: 24 cases (1980-1986). *J Am Vet Med Assoc* 191:100, 1987.

Hosgood G, Salisbury SK, DeNicola DB: Open peritoneal drainage versus sump-Penrose drainage: clinicopathological effects in normal dogs, *J Am Anim Hosp Assoc* 27:115, 1991.

Hosgood G et al: Intraperitoneal circulation and drainage in the dog, *Vet Surg* 18:261, 1989.

Johnson MD, Mann FA: Treatment for pancreatic abscesses via omentalization with abdominal closure versus open peritoneal drainage in dogs: 15 cases (1994-2004), *J Am Vet Med Assoc* 228:397, 2006.

Lanz OI et al: Surgical treatment of septic peritonitis without abdominal drainage in 28 dogs, *J Am Anim Hosp Assoc* 37:87, 2001.

Mueller MG, Ludwig LL, Barton LJ: Use of closed-suction drains to treat generalized peritonitis in dogs and cats: 40 cases (1997-1999), *J Am Vet Med Assoc* 219:789, 2001.

Platell C, Papadimitriou JM, Hall JC: The influence of lavage on peritonitis, *J Am Coll Surg* 191:672, 2000.

Scott BG, Feanny MA, Hirshberg A: Early definitive closure of the open abdomen: a quiet revolution, *Scand J Surg* 94:9, 2005.

Staatz AJ, Monnet E, Seim HB: Open peritoneal drainage versus primary closure for the treatment of septic peritonitis in dogs and cats: 42 cases (1993-1999), *Vet Surg* 31:174, 2002.

Venturi ML et al: Mechanisms and clinical applications of the vacuum-assisted closure device, *Am J Clin Dermatol* 6:185, 2005.

White RA, Williams JM: Intracapsular prostatic omentalization: a new technique for management of prostatic abscesses in dogs, *Vet Surg* 24:390, 1995.

Winkler KP, Greenfield CL: Potential prognostic indicators in diffuse peritonitis treated with open peritoneal drainage in the canine patient, *J Vet Emerg Crit Care* 10:259, 2000.

Woolfson JM, Dulisch ML: Open abdominal drainage in the treatment of generalized peritonitis in 25 dogs and cats, *Vet Surg* 15:27, 1986.

Yao V, Platell C, Hall JC: Role of peritoneal mesothelial cells in peritonitis, *Br J Surg* 90:1187, 2003.

Yates JL: An experimental study of the local effects of peritoneal drainage, *Surg Gynecol Obstet* 1:473, 1905.

CHAPTER 14

Gastric Dilation-Volvulus

KAROL A. MATHEWS, *Ontario, Canada*

Gastric dilation-volvulus (GDV) is a complex medical and surgical emergency. Potentially it can occur in any size or breed of dog, as well as in cats, but typically it is problematic in large and giant breeds of dogs. In smaller breeds the dachshund is overrepresented. Deep-chested conformation may increase the susceptibility to GDV. The prevalence of GDV increases with increasing age, with the greatest occurrence between 7 and 10 years of age. The frequency of occurrence has been reported at 2.4 to 7.6 per 1000 canine hospital admissions (Glickman et al., 1994). The cause of GDV has not been fully elucidated. Delayed gastric emptying, pyloric obstruction, aerophagia, and engorgement contribute to gastric dilation (GD), with volvulus possibly occurring secondarily. Gastric volvulus can occur without prior dilation. Exercise after consuming a large meal may predispose to GDV. Splenic torsion has also been causally implicated because malposition of the spleen frequently occurs with GDV; however, GDV can occur in splenectomized dogs. Inhibition of gastric motility by pharmacologic agents, blunt abdominal trauma, spinal cord injuries, prolonged surgical procedures, or prolonged recumbency can predispose dogs to GD. Cereal diets have been suggested as a cause for GD; however, studies have not been able to confirm this finding. Recently a study specifically investigating the potential risk of GDV in predisposed dogs consuming dry dog foods with an increasing number of plant protein ingredients such as soy, wheat, corn and rice among the first four label ingredients determined that there was a 2.4–fold increased risk of GDV when an oil or fat ingredient was among the first four ingredients (Raghavan, Glickman, and Glickman, 2006). This discussion focuses on the initial and postoperative treatment of the animal with GDV. A detailed description of the pathophysiology of GD and GDV is covered elsewhere (Leib, 1987) and is only briefly outlined here as a basis for treatment rationale. The various techniques used for surgical correction of GDV can be obtained from standard surgical texts.

As a consequence of GDV, local and systemic effects occur to varying degrees. Gastric ischemia results in gastritis progressing to necrosis, with possible perforation and peritonitis. Compression of the caudal vena cava and portal vein results in decreased venous return to the heart, with subsequent reduction in cardiac output and systemic arterial blood pressure and perfusion of the myocardium and gastrointestinal tract. With gastrointestinal mucosal injury and subsequent translocation of bacteria and endotoxins, the patient is predisposed to sepsis and septic shock. Avulsion of the short gastric and right gastroepiploic vessels may occur, causing intraabdominal hemorrhage. The splenic veins may also become thrombosed. The effects of these events are hypotension, hypovolemia (blood loss, plasma loss, increased production and sequestration of gastric secretions), hypoxemia, acid-base and electrolyte abnormalities, sepsis, myocardial dysfunction, and disseminated intravascular coagulation (DIC). Prognosis for recovery may be associated with severity of systemic effects. Plasma/blood lactate measurements greater than 6 mmol/L have been associated with a 39% incidence of gastric necrosis (De Papp, Drobatz, and Hughes, 1999). Twenty-eight percent to 38% postoperative mortality has been associated with gastric resection, and 32% to 38% with the requirement for splenectomy. Although this information may be an indicator of prognosis, caution is required when imparting this information to clients since most dogs recover with optimal preoperative and postoperative management.

PRESENTATION

The clinical signs vary with the extent of GD or GDV and may not parallel the degree of gastric or splenic injury. Owners aware of the clinical signs associated with GDV may seek veterinary assistance at the onset of GD, whereas dogs left alone for several hours may present moribund. Typically dogs with GD or GDV have varying degrees of distention of the cranial abdomen with hypersalivation and unproductive retching. These animals are restless, dyspneic, or tachypneic and may or may not be depressed or moribund. In the early stages of GD, physical examination may reveal increased heart rate with strong pulses, normal capillary refill time, and mucous membrane color. In animals with advanced GDV, weak, rapid pulses—possibly associated with pulse deficits—are present; mucous membranes may be pale pink to pale gray with prolonged capillary refill time and the presence of petechiae, and the cranial abdomen may be tympanic with splenomegaly or free abdominal fluid present.

DIAGNOSIS

The diagnosis of GDV is often obvious from the presenting clinical signs. Radiographic examination is necessary and useful if the diagnosis is equivocal or, if after decompression, surgical management may not be an option (differentiation of dilation from volvulus will direct further management). The ability to pass an orogastric tube does not rule out the presence of volvulus.

When necessary, abdominal radiographs with the dog in right lateral recumbency are usually diagnostic. Evaluation of this radiographic view initially may minimize the patient stress associated with obtaining multiple radiographic views. When volvulus is present, the pylorus is visualized on a right lateral survey radiograph as a gas-filled structure dorsal and cranial to the gastric fundus. A compartmentalization line is frequently observed between the pylorus and fundus. This line represents the pyloric antral wall folding back and contacting the fundic wall. The pylorus cannot be clearly identified in a left lateral projection. Free air within the abdomen may indicate gastric rupture or air leakage after gastrocentesis.

Electrocardiographic monitoring is essential in the patient with GDV and evidence of cardiac arrhythmias. Ventricular arrhythmias are the most common (Muir, 1982). In addition, sinus tachycardia is almost always present in animals presenting with GDV.

The minimal database required for assessing the patient and diagnosing complications associated with the GDV syndrome includes evaluation of systemic arterial blood pressure; packed cell volume (PCV), total plasma solids (TS), activated clotting time (ACT) or activated partial thromboplastin time (aPTT), platelet count, white blood cell count and differential; blood urea nitrogen and glucose concentrations; venous blood gases or total serum carbon dioxide (these patients are frequently alkalemic in the early stage of GD but eventually become acidemic as the disease advances); and serum electrolytes, including lactate. This information is essential to manage the patient adequately and optimize outcome. A complete serum biochemical profile and complete hemostatic profile should be submitted to detect other potential organ dysfunction when appropriate and affordable.

INITIAL TREATMENT

Initial treatment should be considered in light of the presenting clinical signs and the consequences of the known pathophysiologic events. The primary objectives are to (1) prevent or reverse circulatory collapse (fluid and colloid resuscitation), (2) prevent or reduce the local and systemic events associated with GD or GDV by removing the inciting cause (gastric decompression and lavage), (3) treat associated complications (electrolyte and acid-base abnormalities, pain, cardiac arrhythmias, sepsis), and (4) prepare the animal for surgical treatment. For the rare patient that presents with dilation alone without evidence of circulatory compromise, orogastric decompression is the initial treatment. For the typical patient with GDV, circulatory compromise or collapse is present, and reversal of the shock state should be addressed before gastric decompression. In seriously compromised patients it may be necessary to partially decompress the stomach immediately to avoid impending respiratory or circulatory arrest. Gastrocentesis (see section on gastric decompression) is recommended in these situations to avoid the stress of orogastric intubation. In these patients complete decompression should be avoided until rapid fluid resuscitation is well under way. All patients with GDV require surgical correction as soon as possible because medical management alone results in a 75% recurrence rate.

Circulatory Resuscitation

A 14- or 16-gauge 2- to 4-inch catheter is placed into the jugular or cephalic vein or veins—not the saphenous vein. An alkalinizing (lactate or acetate) isotonic, balanced electrolyte solution (or acidifying if alkalemic (e.g., 0.9%) NaCl solution is administered at 90 to 120 ml/kg/hour initially, with continual monitoring and subsequent adjustment to effect. The crystalloid volume can be reduced by up to 40% if pentastarch (Pentaspan, DuPont Pharma, Canada), hetastarch (Hespan, DuPont Pharma United States) or dextran 70 (Gentran, Baxter) is administered at 10 to 20 ml/kg over 15 to 30 minutes (see Chapter 11). If shock is severe, 4 ml/kg of 5% or 7.5% hypertonic saline is administered over 5 to 10 minutes, followed by the aforementioned infusions of isotonic crystalloid or synthetic colloid solution until clinical signs of shock are reversed (Table 14-1). TS and PCV should be measured every 30 minutes. If the PCV decreases to less than 25% or the TS decrease to less than 45 g/L, whole blood, packed red blood cell, or plasma transfusion should be considered. Blood or plasma is administered at a rate of 20 ml/kg over 1 to 2 hours, depending on the resuscitative needs of the patient. Hemoglobin-based oxygen-carrying products (Oxyglobin) have been reported to improve cardiovascular parameters.

If hypotension persists, one should consider intravenous continuous-rate infusions (CRIs) of dopamine (Intropin, DuPont Pharma) or dobutamine (Dobutrex, Eli Lilly) at 2 to 20 mcg/kg per minute. Adjustment in administration rates should be made as needed to achieve a satisfactory hemodynamic end point (see Table 14-1). Norepinephrine (Levophed, Sanofi Winthrop), 0.05 to 0.3 mcg/kg/minute intravenously (IV), or higher doses to effect, can be administered if dopamine or dobutamine infusions fail to achieve the desired effect.

The most common acid-base abnormality in animals with GDV is nonrespiratory (metabolic) acidosis. This abnormality is frequently corrected by treating the underlying cause (shock) with aggressive resuscitative fluid therapy and gastric decompression. Bicarbonate (HCO_3) administration is not routinely necessary but may be

Table 14-1

Parameters to Assess and Goals to Achieve With Fluid and Colloid Resuscitation

Parameter	Goal
Mean arterial pressure	70-80 mm Hg
Systolic blood pressure	100-120 mm Hg
Central venous pressure	3-5 cm H_2O
Mucous membrane color	Pink
Capillary refill time	1-2 sec
Heart rate	120-140 beats/min
Peripheral pulse (dorsal pedal) pressure	Moderate to normal strength
Mentation	Improved to normal for the situation
Urine output	1-2 ml/kg/hr

indicated if serum [HCO$_3^-$] or total carbon dioxide is less than 12 mEq/L after fluid resuscitation. A suggested dose for HCO$_3$ administration (in milliequivalents) can be calculated using the following formula:

$$\text{Body weight (kg)} \times (12 - \text{patient } [\text{HCO}_3^-]) \times 0.3$$

The calculated dose can be administered intravenously over 30 to 60 minutes. Occasionally a patient may have a normal or increased blood pH, and empiric therapy with HCO$_3^-$ may be deleterious. When lacticemia is present, this rapidly resolves with fluid therapy and correction of the dilation-volvulus. In most instances reperfusion restores the acid-base status to normal without treatment with sodium bicarbonate therapy.

Ventricular arrhythmias frequently improve after circulatory resuscitation and gastric decompression; however, treatment is advised by some if the arrhythmia is sustained, paroxysmal, or polymorphic at an instantaneous rate greater than or equal to 170 beats/min (120 beats/min under general anesthesia), greater than or equal to 140 beats/min with mean arterial pressure (MAP) less than 70 mm Hg, when preexisting cardiac disease is present, or when an R-on-T phenomenon or torsades de pointes is observed on the electrocardiogram (see Chapter 162). Initial treatment for ventricular tachyarrhythmias is lidocaine (Xylocaine, Astra) administration at 2 mg/kg intravenously. If the initial bolus is ineffective, one or two additional boluses can be administered within 5 to 10 minutes of the initial bolus. If the arrhythmia is lidocaine-responsive, a CRI of lidocaine at 30 to 80 mcg/kg/minute is established. Failure of the rhythm to improve with lidocaine administration (reduction in rate to 120 to 140 beats/min and a reduction in abnormal complex morphologic features) requires reassessment of the electrocardiographic diagnosis and overall status of the patient (e.g., electrolyte, acid-base, sepsis, and pain) with consideration of alternative antiarrhythmic therapy. One should not expect to totally abolish the arrhythmia and should not feel compelled to treat the ventricular rhythms that are neither very fast nor causing hypotension. If there is uncertainty as to whether the arrhythmia is ventricular or supraventricular in origin or if the ventricular arrhythmia is not lidocaine responsive, procainamide (Pronestyl, Squibb) is administered intravenously at 6 to 10 mg/kg (rarely up to 20 mg/kg) by 2 mg/kg-increments every 5 minutes (to avoid hypotension). If procainamide administration is effective, it is continued at 6 to 10 mg/kg intramuscularly every 6 hours or as an intravenous CRI of 25 to 40 mcg/kg/minute. The administration of 20% magnesium sulfate solution at 0.15 to 0.3 mEq/kg (12.5 to 35 mg/kg) via 2- to 4-hour intravenous CRI three times in 24 hours may abolish or enhance the treatment response of patients with ventricular arrhythmias. For life-threatening arrhythmia, a magnesium sulfate dose of 0.15 to 0.3 mEq/kg could be administered over 15 to 20 minutes. Caution must be used with magnesium sulfate administration in patients with renal insufficiency (Bonagura, 1995, p. 132). Sinus tachycardia frequently resolves with resuscitative treatment and analgesic support. If sinus tachycardia persists, one should consider hypotension, hypovolemia (i.e., if not hypotensive, the possibility of

maximal patient compensation requiring continuation of resuscitative treatment), hypoxemia, anemia, hypercarbia, inadequate control of pain, gastric perforation, splenic infarction, or other major organ complication that requires immediate exploratory celiotomy.

Potassium-supplemented fluids, delivered through an intravenous line separate from the rapid infusion of crystalloids, should be administered at a dosage of 30 to 80 mEq/L delivered at a maintenance fluid rate when serum potassium concentrations are 3.5 mEq/L to less than 2 mEq/L, respectively. If the animal is acidemic, the serum potassium concentration may decrease during treatment with alkalinizing solutions. This possibility should be anticipated, assessed, and addressed by an increase in the rate of potassium infusion. Potassium infusions can be delivered at a maximal rate of 0.5 to 1 mEq/kg/hour when serum potassium levels are less than 3 mEq/L, ventricular arrhythmias are present, and continuous electrocardiography and serial serum potassium monitoring are possible every 2 hours.

Antibiotics with a spectrum of activity directed against gram-negative and anaerobic bacteria should be administered slowly intravenously during fluid resuscitation (cefoxitin, 20 mg/kg IV q6h, or ampicillin, 20 mg/kg IV q6h). Translocation of gut bacteria into the systemic circulation is a common complication of GDV and gastrointestinal hypoperfusion.

Administration of corticosteroids to patients with GDV is controversial. However, because of the potential for gastric hemorrhage, corticosteroids are not administered to patients with GDV at our hospital. Furthermore, the administration of nonsteroidal antiinflammatory analgesics is not recommended. Deferoxamine (Desferal, Ciba-Geigy Pharmaceutical Inc.), 50 mg/kg slowly intravenously, administered 10 minutes before gastric decompression, has shown promise in prevention of reperfusion injury when administered to dogs with experimentally induced GDV. However, this drug can cause significant hypotension when administered at 50 mg/kg; therefore 20 to 25 mg/kg is suggested, given over 10 minutes to avoid hypotension. Clinical trials are needed to demonstrate its efficacy and limitations.

Gastric Decompression

After resuscitative fluid administration, gastric decompression is initiated. If the animal requires sedation, butorphanol (Torbugesic, Ayerst), 0.2 to 0.4 mg/kg IV, fentanyl 2 to 5 mcg/kg, hydromorphone (Dilaudid, DuPont Pharma), or oxymorphone (Numorphan, DuPont Pharma) 0.02 to 0.05 mg/kg IV, is administered cautiously (to avoid vomiting) to effect. The addition of diazepam (Valium, Roche), 0.2 to 0.5 mg/kg IV, can be used concomitantly if needed in noncompliant dogs before decompression. If surgical correction is planned, hydromorphone or oxymorphone administration is preferred since these drugs reduce the inhalant anesthetic requirements, have greater analgesic effect, and produce a better sedative effect that facilitates tracheal intubation.

To perform orogastric decompression, the dog is placed in sternal or lateral recumbency or in an upright sitting position. A large-bore tube is premeasured from the chin to the xiphoid, and the distance is marked on the tube with tape. The tube is lubricated with water-soluble jelly and passed carefully through an oral speculum (or 2-inch roll of tape) through the esophagus and into the stomach (the mark on the tube is at the level of the incisor teeth). Rupture of compromised areas of the lower esophagus or stomach can occur if excessive force is used in orogastric intubation. If resistance to passage of the orogastric tube is experienced, the tube should be rotated gently while reattempting passage, or the position of the dog changed to facilitate passage.

Gastrocentesis should be performed immediately in patients with severe gastric distention and incipient cardiopulmonary arrest or in patients in which attempts at orogastric intubation have been unsuccessful and delay in partial decompression with further repositioning will be detrimental to the patient. A 10- × 10-cm area is aseptically prepared caudal to the right costal arch. The area is percussed to identify the tympanic stomach and to avoid needle puncture of the spleen. An 18-gauge needle or needle-styleted catheter is placed through the abdominal wall into the lumen of the stomach to allow gas to escape. Further decompression is often not necessary if the patient is to undergo surgical correction immediately. However, if surgical correction may be delayed, orogastric decompression should be repeated after gastrocentesis to reduce the rapid accumulation of gas. Orogastric decompression is more easily performed at this time because release of pressure on the cardia usually facilitates passage of the tube. After orogastric decompression, the stomach is lavaged with warm tap water to remove residual food. The absence of blood or coffee ground material in the lavage fluid does not rule out the presence of gastric necrosis.

If surgical correction cannot be performed immediately, decompression may be maintained by placement of a weighted nasogastric tube with stylet (EN-tube, Entech Inc., Lebanon, NJ), a pharyngostomy tube, or a temporary gastrostomy. Intermittent orogastric intubation is not recommended because this procedure is stressful and iatrogenic gastric rupture is a potential concern with repeated orogastric tube placement. The indications for maintaining temporary gastric decompression in these patients include (1) maintenance of gastric decompression for patient transportation to a referral facility, and (2) unavailability of a surgeon to perform immediate surgical intervention. Preparation for the placement of a temporary gastrostomy is as described for gastrocentesis but should only be considered when definitive correction is not possible for several hours. Anesthesia of the area to be incised can be obtained by infiltration of 4 to 6 ml of 1% lidocaine through the skin and subcutaneous and muscle layers, including the peritoneum, in an inverted L pattern. A 6-cm incision is made through the skin, and the approach to the peritoneum is made through muscle separation. The peritoneum is incised with caution since the stomach is adjacent to it. A circumferential, simple, continuous suture pattern is placed through the skin, abdominal wall, serosa, and muscles of the stomach. The stomach is then incised. Gastric emptying and lavage are then performed. Any temporary gastrostomy is closed and locally irrigated during the subsequent surgical approach

for definitive surgical correction. In general, the recommendation would be for definitive surgical correction for GDV within 1 to 2 hours after presentation in the majority of cases. Early intervention, after an initial period of circulatory resuscitation, has been shown to reduce postoperative fatality rates (Brockman, Washabau, and Drobatz, 1995). The disadvantages of postponing surgical intervention are (1) the increased prevalence of cardiac arrhythmias by 12 to 72 hours, (2) an increased risk of splenic and gastric infarction resulting from continuing malposition, and (3) the increasing risk with time of gastric perforation with consequent peritonitis (Bonagura, 2000).

SURGICAL TREATMENT

Preinduction oxygenation is recommended. Before inducing general anesthesia, lidocaine, 2 mg/kg IV, should be administered, followed with an infusion of 50 to 120 mcg/kg/minute (dose is dependent on presence or absence of ventricular arrhythmias) to reduce isoflurane requirements (Valverde). Anesthesia regimens to be considered in patients with GDV include hydromorphone, 0.02 to 0.05 mg/kg, or fentanyl, 5 to 10 mcg/kg, and mask administration of isoflurane (Forane, Ohmeda) for the severely compromised patient; and ketamine (Ketaset, Ayerst), 2 to 5 mg/kg, combined with diazepam, 0.1 to 0.3 mg/kg, and isoflurane for the stable but moderately depressed patient. Consider a fentanyl infusion of 5 to 20 mcg/kg/hour to reduce the inhalant further. Crystalloid, colloid, blood, or blood component administration; antiarrhythmic and electrolyte therapy; and continuous electrocardiography, along with serial blood pressure monitoring, should continue throughout the intraoperative period.

When early presentation is with dilation alone and no involvement of other organs or metabolic abnormality of importance, the laparoscopic gastropexy may be an alternative to laparotomy (Rawlings et al., 2002). The permanent incisional gastropexy technique is fast and not technically challenging; it is now the preferred technique for definitive correction of GDV in our hospital because of ease of performance and efficacy and has replaced the previously used belt loop gastropexy technique. The tube gastropexy was the preferred technique described in one report (Brockman, Washabau, and Drobatz, 1995). Regardless of the gastropexy used, during definitive surgical correction it is recommended that areas of gastric necrosis or questionably viable stomach be removed. Invagination into the gastric lumen of nonviable or potentially nonviable tissue, as suggested in some texts, can potentially predispose to postoperative DIC. Similarly, if there are questionable areas of necrosis in the spleen or if the spleen does not return to a normal size after derotation (performed before gastropexy to allow time for venous drainage), it should be removed. Unless pyloric outflow obstruction can be clearly demonstrated, pyloroplasty is not necessary, and the extended surgical time required to perform this procedure may contribute to patient morbidity. If there is a concern about pancreatitis or if any extended (>24 hours) restriction of oral food intake is anticipated, a jejunostomy tube should be placed for nutritional support.

POSTOPERATIVE MANAGEMENT

Recent studies in patients with GDV and surgical intervention reported mortality rates as low as 15% (Brockman, Washabau, and Drobatz, 1995) to 18% (Brourman et al., 1996). Of the nonsurvivors, postoperative mortality associated with gastric resection was 28% (Brockman, Washabau, and Drobatz, 1995) to 35% (Brourman et al., 1996); with splenectomy, it was 32% (Brourman et al., 1996) to 38% (Brockman, Washabau, and Drobatz, 1995); and with cardiac arrhythmias that were present on admission, postoperative mortality was 38% (Brourman et al., 1996). Cardiac arrhythmias developing *after surgery* did not influence outcome (Brourman et al., 1996; Brockman, Washabau, and Drobatz, 1995). With current standards of critical care management in the patients, survival rates appear to be higher than those reported.

Complications to be anticipated in patients after surgical correction of GDV include cardiac arrhythmias; fluid overload; gastroparesis and ileus; vomiting; pancreatitis; DIC; gastric and incisional dehiscence; gastric ulceration; ischemic necrosis of stomach, spleen, or gallbladder with peritonitis; incarceration of small bowel dorsal to the gastropexy site; or the development of acute renal failure. The intensity of postoperative care will vary, depending on the severity of illness and surgical intervention. To provide optimal care, for the first 24 hours the clinician should (1) continuously or serially observe the electrocardiogram and measure hemodynamics (goals are MAP >70 mm Hg, systolic pressure >110 mm Hg, central venous pressure (CVP) of 3 to 5 cm H_2O), provide pain assessment and treatment (hydromorphone 0.05 to 0.2 mg/kg q4h or to effect), and measure urine output (1 to 2 ml/kg/hour); (2) assess at least every 8 hours serum electrolytes (goals are electrolytes within normal limits, with K^+ >4.5 mmol/L), lactate (<2.5mmol/L) nonrespiratory acid-base status (venous pH 7.28 to 7.4, [HCO_3^-] 16 to 24 mmol/L, base excess ±5), PCV (25 to 45%), and TS (45 to 70 g/L); (3) measure every 12 hours ACT (normal range 70 to 100 seconds) and blood glucose concentration; and (4) assess each day serum magnesium, creatinine, albumin concentrations and complete blood count, and antithrombin levels (when DIC is suspected). Treatment approaches for abnormalities detected on serial postoperative testing need to be individualized to the patient.

The major electrolyte disturbance seen after surgery in almost all postoperative GDV patients is hypokalemia. Hypokalemia potentiates cardiac arrhythmias, and hypokalemia is potentiated by hypomagnesemia. In severely hypokalemic patients potassium supplementation in intravenous fluids may exceed 80 mEq/L even though crystalloids are being delivered at two to three times the normal requirement for maintenance. Magnesium sulfate 20% can be administered by intravenous CRI at 0.25 mEq/kg (30 mg/kg) divided over 4 hours and repeated at 8-hour intervals for 24 hours or as an intravenous CRI of 1 mEq/kg/day (125 mg/kg/day). Magnesium levels must be measured daily at this infusion rate. Serum potassium levels require frequent (q8-12h) monitoring during potassium and magnesium infusions.

Sinus tachycardia should not be present after surgery in patients without primary cardiac disease recovering from GDV. The presence of sinus tachycardia in these patients does not require antiarrhythmic therapy since this rhythm often represents a physiologic response to heart failure, pain, hypoxia, anemia, hypotension, sepsis, and other potential problems previously mentioned. These primary abnormalities should be identified and treated. However, if a primary supraventricular tachyarrhythmia has been identified, appropriate antiarrhythmic therapy is administered based on the specific rhythm problem (see Chapters 161 and 162). Ventricular tachyarrhythmias are treated as described in the section on initial treatment.

In the postoperative patient with GDV, isotonic crystalloid fluids and synthetic colloids are administered at a rate that maintains normal hydration, acid-base status, and urine output. Synthetic colloids, 20 to 30 ml/kg/day, should be administered when large-volume crystalloids are required to maintain the MAP at greater than 70 mm Hg, systolic arterial blood pressure at greater than 110 mm Hg, and urine output at greater than 1 ml/kg/hour or to prevent the development of interstitial or pulmonary edema in patients with decreased TS or colloidal osmotic pressure.

Antibiotic therapy as recommended in the section on initial treatment should be continued intravenously for 72 hours in patients requiring gastric resection or when gastric mucosal injury is highly suspect. Patients with simple GD or GDV without notable mucosal injury do not require antibiotic therapy after surgery.

It is not uncommon for patients with GDV or GD to acquire gastric atony and ileus after surgery. This occurrence predisposes animals to recurrence of GD and vomiting. If a gastrostomy tube is not in place, maintenance of gastric decompression may require the placement of a nasogastric tube. Metoclopramide administration (Reglan, Wyeth-Ayerst), 0.2 to 0.5 mg/kg every 8 hours subcutaneously or 1 to 2 mg/kg per day by intravenous CRI, is recommended as a promotility drug to enhance gastric emptying and as an antiemetic. To enhance gastric mucosal healing, reduce the possibility of gastric ulceration with hemorrhage, and prevent esophageal stricture secondary to reflux esophagitis, famotidine 0.5 mg/kg q12h IV, and sucralfate (200 mg/ml suspension) (Sulcrate or Carafate, Nordic), 5 ml/dog q8h PO, are recommended. Therapy may range from 2 to 5 days.

Gastric necrosis has been associated with abnormal hemostatic profiles (Millis, Hauptman, and Fulton, 1993). Therefore, when gastric or splenic necrosis is apparent at surgical correction, it should be assumed that DIC is present, especially if associated with prolonged ACT. These patients may benefit from at least one fresh frozen plasma transfusion. Heparin therapy is not routinely recommended; however, if thrombosis is a concern, the current suggestions are 100 to 150 U/kg SC q8h of unfractionated heparin or alternatively, after loading with this dose, a CRI of 12 to 15 U/kg/hour, although a dosing regimen is not established. The CRI 12 U/kg/hour via jugular catheter is recommended when jugular catheters are in use. aPTT or ACT should be monitored before each subcutaneous heparin dose or twice daily with the CRI. The goal of heparin therapy is to achieve a PTT or ACT of 1.5 to 2 times normal before the next dose. At our hospital normal ACT (human axillary incubation) is 75 to 100 seconds, and the target value with heparin therapy is 150 to 180 seconds.

The continued "bedside" assessment of these patients includes serial assessment of ACT, TS, PCV, and platelet count and physical examination (incisional oozing, petechial hemorrhages, and deterioration in attitude). If further abnormalities develop in any of the assessed parameters, another unit of fresh frozen plasma or fresh whole blood (to raise the PCV to 25% to 30%) should be administered, and consideration given to the possibility of an ongoing problem (progression of gastric or splenic necrosis) or another complication such as sepsis that may require further surgical treatment.

In most patients with uncomplicated surgical correction of GDV or GD, water should be offered at 12 hours after surgery, and a low-fat, good-quality protein canned dog food slurry should be offered soon after if the patient is alert and not vomiting. Oral feeding of patients with gastric resection should be started at the discretion of the surgeon based on the extent of, or surgical complications associated with, the resection and the presence or absence of a jejunostomy feeding tube. However, in general, feedings do not differ from noncomplicated cases.

If a jejunostomy feeding tube is in place, a CRI of an electrolyte solution with 5% dextrose (Plasma-Lyte, 56 with 5% dextrose, Baxter) is delivered at 0.5 ml/kg via the tube for the initial 12 hours after surgery. If this is tolerated by the patient, the addition of a prepared liquid diet (Canine Clinicare, PetAg) at one half the daily nonprotein caloric requirements (see equation) diluted 50:50 with the aforementioned crystalloid solution is delivered at 0.5 ml/kg/hour for the subsequent 24 hours. If no signs of discomfort or nausea are noted after this 24-hour infusion, the infusion should be increased to meet full nutritional requirements. Peripheral intravenous fluid therapy should be reduced by the appropriate amount once oral intake occurs or enteral nutritional support is instituted. The duration of jejunostomy feeding is individualized to each patient. A goal for daily caloric requirement to achieve over a 1- to 3-day period, depending on extent of gastric injury. is:

$$1.5 \times [70 \text{ (body weight in kg}^{0.75})]$$

Parenteral nutritional support is recommended for patients unable to eat, drink, or receive enteral nutrition for more than 36 hours after surgery (see Chapter 36). A common nutritional support technique used in our hospital is the administration of a partial parenteral nutritional (PPN) solution. In 1 L there is a 3.3% concentration of amino acids (Travasol, Baxter) and a 3.3% concentration of dextrose in an electrolyte solution (Plasma-Lyte 56 with 5% dextrose, Baxter). This can be prepared by removing 330 ml of the electrolyte solution from a 1-L bag and replacing it with 330 ml of Travasol under sterile conditions. Lipids (20% Intralipid, Clintec) can be piggy-backed into the administration set and delivered at a volume up to 50% of the patient's nonprotein caloric requirements. Both can be delivered through a peripheral intravenous catheter. Although strict aseptic technique is used in preparing and delivering this solution, a dedicated peripheral line offers ease of PPN administration without compromising the patient through administration via a common central venous access that may be used for CVP monitoring, blood sampling, and delivery of crystalloid fluids or medications. The amino acid–glucose solution is delivered as an intravenous CRI at a rate of 1 to 1½ normal daily fluid maintenance requirements. If further glucose supplementation appears necessary, it can be administered with the remaining replacement-maintenance crystalloid fluids. The hourly rate of administration for crystalloid fluid support should be reduced by an amount equal to that delivered via PPN to avoid overhydration.

The length of hospital stay will depend on the severity of illness but is expected to be 2 to 7 days. All dogs that have recovered from GDV or GD should be fed a good-quality canned dog food in small amounts (based on their normal daily nutritional requirements) four or five times daily initially and no less than three times daily in the future to avoid engorgement. Exercise after eating should be avoided. Owners should be made aware that gastropexy is not a guarantee against future episodes of GD or GDV in the patient.

References and Suggested Reading

Bersenas AME, Mathews KA, Allen DG, Conlon PD. The efficacy of gastric-acid lowering therapy in the dog, *Am J Vet Res* 66(3):425, 2005.

Bonagura JD, editor: *Kirk's current veterinary therapy XII (small animal practice)*, Philadelphia, 1995, Saunders.

Bonagura JD, editor: *Kirk's current veterinary therapy XIII (small animal practice)*, Philadelphia, 2000, Saunders, p 764.

Brockman DJ, Washabau RJ, Drobatz KJ: Canine gastric dilation/volvulus syndrome in a veterinary critical care unit: 295 cases (1986-1992), *J Am Vet Med Assoc* 207:460, 1995.

Brourman JD et al: Factors associated with perioperative mortality in dogs with surgically managed gastric dilatation-volvulus: 137 cases (1988-1993), *J Am Vet Med Assoc* 208:1855, 1996.

De Papp E, Drobatz KJ, Hughes D: Plasma lactate concentration as a predictor of gastric necrosis and survival among dogs with gastric dilation-volvulus: 102 cases (1995-1998), *J Am Vet Med Assoc* 215(1):49, 1999.

Glickman LT et al: Analysis of risk factors for gastric dilatation and dilatation-volvulus in dogs, *J Am Vet Med Assoc* 204:1465, 1994.

Leib MS: Therapy of gastric dilatation-volvulus in dogs, *Compend Cont Educ Pract Vet* 9:1155, 1987.

Matthiesen DT: Gastric dilation-volvulus syndrome. In Slatter D, editor: *Textbook of small animal surgery*, ed 2, Philadelphia, 1993, Saunders, 1993, p 580.

Millis DL, Hauptman JG, Fulton RB: Abnormal hemostatic profiles and gastric necrosis in canine gastric dilatation-volvulus, *Vet Surg* 22:93, 1993.

Muir WW: Gastric dilatation-volvulus in the dog, with emphasis on cardiac arrhythmias, *J Am Vet Med Assoc* 180:739, 1982.

Raghavan M, Glickman NW, Glickman LT: The effect of ingredients in dry dog foods on the risk of gastric dilatation-volvulus in dogs, *J Am Anim Hosp Assoc* 42:28, 2006.

Rawlings CA et al: Prospective evaluation of laparoscopic-assisted gastropexy in dogs susceptible to gastric dilatation, *J Am Vet Med Assoc* 221:1576, 2002.

Valverde A, Doherty TJ, Hernandez J, Davies W. Effect of lidocaine on the minimum alveolar concentration of isoflurane in dogs. *Vet Anaesth Analg* 4:264, 2004.

CHAPTER 15

Emergency Management of Open Fractures

ROBERT J. McCARTHY, *North Grafton, Massachusetts*

Open fractures, defined as those in which fractured bone has been exposed to the external environment, represent between 5% and 10% of all fracture cases seen in small animal practice. Any open fracture must be considered contaminated and a source of potential infection. These fractures require immediate intervention and should be treated as surgical emergencies.

Open fractures have been classified into three types, based on the wounding mechanism and the degree of hard- and soft-tissue damage (Table 15-1). Type I open fractures are the result of the lowest energy trauma and are frequently associated with the sharp point of a fractured bone penetrating the skin from the inside. Wound size is generally less than 1 cm in length. There is little soft-tissue injury, wounds are often relatively clean, and there is no crushing component. The bone end may remain exposed but more commonly returns to lie beneath the skin. Fractures are usually transverse or oblique, with minimal if any comminution. The tibia and radius are common sites of type I open fractures in small animals because of the close proximity of bone to the skin in the antebrachium and crus.

In a type II open fracture an external force produces a penetrating wound that communicates with the fracture from the outside. Wounds are usually greater than 1 cm in length. These fractures have more severe soft-tissue injury and contamination. There is a minimal-to-moderate crushing component to skin and musculature, and fractures may be comminuted. These fractures are about twice as likely to become infected as type I open fractures. Common examples include bite wounds and certain low-velocity gunshot fractures.

Type III open fractures are caused by high-energy trauma from an external source and are characterized by severe soft-tissue damage and contamination. There is often soft tissue or bone loss, and bone may be stripped of soft-tissue attachments. There is generally a severe crushing component. Fractures are usually highly comminuted, and repair may result in cortical defects. Risk of infection is considered about four times that in a type I open fracture. Examples are degloving injuries with underlying fracture and high-velocity gunshot injuries.

INITIAL ASSESSMENT AND EMERGENCY MANAGEMENT

Treatment of an open fracture should be started at home. Owners are instructed to minimize all limb manipulation and to cover the wound and exposed bone with a sterile dressing if possible. A clean cloth or diaper is an appropriate alternative if bandage materials are not available. Owners should be warned that injured animals may bite, and they should consider placing a muzzle if necessary. Compression is usually sufficient to control hemorrhage during transport to the hospital. Initial veterinary management is directed toward evaluation and treatment of other potentially life-threatening injuries unless the wound is inadequately covered or is hemorrhaging profusely (Box 15-1). In this situation a sterile dressing and pressure wrap should be applied. Ligation of actively bleeding vessels is occasionally required. Bone protruding from the wound should not be reduced into the wound at this time since this allows additional contamination of the fracture site.

Evaluation of the stabilized patient is begun with a thorough case history. Owners are questioned regarding the cause of the injury and the environment in which the injury occurred. It is significant whether the animal was "run into" or "run over" because in the latter situation a significant crushing component is more likely. The environment where the injury occurred may help determine potential wound contaminants and dictate the choice of future antibiotic therapy.

Initial wound evaluation should be directed toward a careful assessment of the neurologic and vascular status of the limb since they may alter treatment options. Simple diagnostic tests include clipping a toenail short to check for active bleeding, evaluation of extremity pulses distal to the wound, limb temperature assessment, and patient recognition of extremity sensation. Although the degree of wound contamination and apparent soft- and bony-tissue trauma should be determined, limb manipulation must be minimized, and wound probing avoided because they increase contamination, cause vascular damage, and result in pain. Potential problems associated with small puncture wounds should not be underestimated because debris may be under the skin, deep in the wound and medullary cavity. Preliminary deep wound cultures should be obtained at the time of initial wound evaluation. In humans 50% to 70% of open fractures produce positive results when cultured at presentation, and in 66% of cases the bacteria cultured at presentation are the same as those isolated later in infected wounds.

After the wound is assessed and cultured, radiographs are obtained, and a more functional immobilization dressing is applied. The purpose of this bandage is to prevent additional contamination, preserve vasculature, and decrease pain. Most organisms that are recovered from the

Table 15-1

Classification of Open Fractures

Classification	Wounding Mechanism	Soft Tissue and Bony Damage	Common Fracture Configuration	Relative Risk of Infection
Type I	Bone fragment protrudes outward from within	Minimal	Transverse, oblique	1
Type II	Penetrating external wound contacts bone	Moderate	Some comminution	2
Type III	Severe external force causes wound	Severe	Severe comminution	4

wound after the development of an orthopedic infection can be traced to the hospital; thus early protection of the wound is critical. Sterile dressings should be used in all cases, and strict asepsis maintained. A splint is generally applied to support open fractures below the elbow or stifle, whereas a spica-type bandage is required to immobilize fractures more proximal on the limb. Fractures proximal to the elbow or stifle are frequently difficult to immobilize properly, and in many cases it may be preferable simply to cover the wound and confine the animal to a small cage.

Antibiotics are always indicated for animals with open fractures because all wounds are contaminated and wounds that occurred longer than 6 to 8 hours before definitive surgical débridement and lavage are infected. In humans antibiotics administered within 3 hours of injury significantly decrease the rate of future wound infection. Risk of infection may be greater in animals with open fractures because of decreased host defense mechanisms caused by stress, or vascular compromise. Choice of antibiotic is based on the cause of injury, nature of the wound, likely bacterial contaminants, and knowledge of commonly isolated bacteria from patients with osteomyelitis. *Staphylococcus* spp. cause between 50% and 60% of bone infections in dogs, and many of these infections are monomicrobial. In general, concerns about penetration of antibiotics into bone interstitial fluid are unfounded.

First-generation cephalosporins such as cefazolin (Kefzol, Lilly, 20 mg/kg q8h) are often the initial drugs of choice because they are broad spectrum, can be given intravenously, are usually effective against β-lactamase–producing *Staphylococcus* spp., and are relatively inexpensive. If contamination with a gram-negative organism is expected, a

fluoroquinolone antibiotic such as enrofloxacin (Baytril, Bayer, 5 mg/kg SQ q24h) or a penicillin-derivative such as imipenem (Primaxin, Merck, 5 to 10 mg/kg IV q6-8h) may be added. Anaerobic infections are more common than previously thought, and clindamycin (Antirobe, Upjohn, 5 to 10 mg/kg PO q12h) or metronidazole (Flagyl, Searle, 25 to 40 mg/kg PO q12h) should be considered in addition to first-generation cephalosporins in animals with severely necrotic, avascular wounds. The initial choice of antibiotic is altered when culture and sensitivity test results become available. In type I and II open fractures that are not infected, antibiotic use can be discontinued immediately after fracture repair. In any type III open fracture or in type I or II open fractures that are infected, more prolonged use is indicated. In general, antibiotic therapy is continued for about 1 month in these cases. Antibiotics can be discontinued at that time if there is no clinical or radiographic evidence of infection.

Recognition of pain is difficult in dogs and cats because even animals with severe pain may show no overt clinical signs. Open fractures are associated with extensive pain and anxiety in humans, and a similar situation is expected in animals. Pain should be treated with narcotic analgesics. In general, pure opioid agonists such as hydromorphone (Dilaudid, Abbott, 0.05 to 0.1 mg/kg IV q6h) or oxymorphone (Numorphan, Dupont, 0.05 to 0.1 mg/kg IV or IM q6h) should be used to treat the severe pain associated with an open fracture (see also Chapter 2). A dermal fentanyl patch may be an adjunct for providing longer-term analgesia.

SURGICAL DÉBRIDEMENT

Patients with open fractures frequently require long hospitalization, multiple surgical procedures, and expensive medications; thus, before initiating definitive wound management and fracture repair, owners should be apprised carefully of the potential prognosis and cost. It is essential that the veterinarian communicate treatment options and prognosis in a manner that allows clients to understand the situation and then make rational, realistic decisions for themselves and their pets. An estimate in writing of the anticipated expense and treatment should be provided. Limb amputation may be a necessary alternative in some cases. Definitive surgical débridement of the open fracture wound should be performed as soon as safely possible, preferably within 6 to 8 hours after injury. This period is considered the "golden period" in which the wound is contaminated but bacteria have not had the opportunity to multiply and spread through adjacent tissues. If the patient is not yet stable for anesthesia, initial débridement can be attempted with a

---

Box 15-1

Treatment Protocol for Management of Patients With Open Fracture

1. Evaluate patient status and treat life-threatening injuries.
2. Control hemorrhage.
3. Place sterile dressing and bandage during patient stabilization.
4. Assess vascular and neurologic status of limb.
5. Obtain preliminary deep wound culture.
6. Start antibiotic therapy.
7. Manage pain.
8. Obtain radiographs.
9. Perform definitive surgical débridement and fracture fixation within 6-8 hours if possible.

local anesthetic or a regional anesthesia technique such as an epidural. Neuroleptanalgesia can also be considered.

Surgical preparation and removal of gross debris may be performed in the surgical preparation area, but definitive débridement is performed in the operating room. Most orthopedic infections originate from hospital organisms, thus strict aseptic technique is important. Sterile water-soluble gel can be placed in the wound to avoid contamination with hair while clipping. A water-impermeable barrier is placed between the limb and the rest of the body and surgery table during débridement to prevent wicking of contaminated fluids from the environment into the operative field.

The goal of surgical débridement is to convert a contaminated wound to a clean one. All foreign material and contaminated or dead tissue is removed, but undermining wound edges and extensive soft tissue dissection are avoided. Sharp dissection technique is preferred. Dependable features for predicting viability of muscle are ability to bleed, consistency, and contractility. Although commonly used, color is actually a relatively poor criterion because it depends greatly on the available light. If viability is questionable, it is better to leave tissue in place and remove it if necessary during a second procedure. As a guideline for débriding bone, if the bone has no soft-tissue attachment and is not critical for reconstruction of the fracture, it is excised. Bone that has no soft-tissue attachment but is critical for fracture reconstruction should be saved. Any bone that has good soft-tissue attachment is saved in the fracture site.

Wounds are irrigated with liters of isotonic saline or 0.05% chlorhexidine. Tap water has been used for wound irrigation but is not recommended because the hypotonicity of tap water may potentiate cellular damage. There is little evidence for incorporation of antibiotics into lavage fluids in dogs and cats. A pulsating irrigation delivery system is helpful, or lavage can be accomplished with a 35-ml syringe and an 18-gauge needle. Bullets retrieved from gunshot fracture wounds should be saved because of the potential for future litigation. A deep wound culture is obtained at the end rather than the beginning of surgery because this has been shown to correlate better with later infection.

FRACTURE REPAIR

Fracture fixation is performed as soon as safely possible, preferably during the initial wound débridement. If immediate fixation is planned, the operative field, the equipment, and the surgeon's gown and gloves should all be changed after the wound débridement. Rigid stabilization of the fracture increases patient comfort, improves blood supply to the tissues, facilitates wound healing, and promotes resistance to infection.

A number of techniques can be used for fracture repair. In general, after surgical débridement type I open fractures can be treated in the same manner as a closed fracture. Higher-grade open fractures require special consideration when planning repair. External coaptation with splints and casts is rarely appropriate since wound care is difficult and stabilization is generally inadequate. Use of intramedullary pins is avoided if possible, because they impede medullary circulation, may spread bacteria through the medullary cavity, and when used alone do not provide rigid stabilization. Bone screw and plate fixation can be used, but placement of a large metallic foreign body at the fracture site is a disadvantage. Implants potentiate bacterial proliferation because the surfaces become covered with glycolipid, which allows *Staphylococcus* spp. and other gram-positive organisms to adhere. The extensive open surgical approach required for bone plating also further compromises vascularity. Despite these limitations, rigid fixation with a bone plate and screws is generally acceptable and usually results in uncomplicated healing.

External skeletal fixation is generally the fixation technique of choice, since fixation pins can be placed away from damaged tissue and rigid stabilization is possible. External skeletal fixation is economical, readily available, and does not require specialized equipment. The wound can be visualized and treated as needed. The Ilizarov ring external skeletal fixator may be particularly useful in these patients because very small fixation pins under tension are used.

Autogenous cancellous bone grafts are indicated in many open fractures, since cortical defects are common and these fractures may heal slowly because of vascular and soft-tissue damage. Transplanted cancellous bone facilitates bone healing by means of osteoconductive, osteoinductive, and osteogenic properties. Cancellous bone grafts rarely become infected, and, when they do, they undergo harmless liquefactive necrosis. The graft should be collected with a separate set of equipment and gloves to avoid contamination of the graft site. Alternately a combination of cancellous allograft and demineralized bone matrix providing osteoconductive and osteoinductive properties can be obtained commercially (Osteo-Allograft Mix, Veterinary Transplant Services). In severely avascular wounds bone grafting should be delayed 1 to 2 weeks to allow sufficient proliferation of granulation tissue to provide vascular support for the graft. If delayed grafting is performed, the incision should be through previously undamaged tissue if possible. Although cortical allografts have been used successfully in open fractures, they are not recommended, because the risk of sequestration and resorption is high. Autogenous vascular bone grafts transplanted by microsurgery may prove beneficial in the future.

WOUND CLOSURE

Wound closure can be performed if débridement results in a surgically clean wound with adequate vascularity that can be closed without tension. Dead space drainage should be accomplished with aseptically placed closed suction drains. In general, more severe type II and all type III open fractures should be handled as open wounds with delayed primary or secondary closure. If there is any doubt, it is always better to leave the wound open.

References and Suggested Reading

Grant GR, Olds RB: Treatment of open fractures. In Slatter D, editor: *Textbook of small animal surgery*, Philadelphia, 2003, Saunders, p 1793.

Piermattei DL, Flo GL, DeCamp CE: Open fractures. In Piermattei DL, Flo GL, DeCamp CE: *Small animal orthopedics and fracture repair*, Philadelphia, 2006, Saunders, p 145.

CHAPTER 16

Thoracic Trauma

SCOTT P. SHAW, *North Grafton, Massachusetts*

Thoracic injury is common in dogs and cats following trauma. Thoracic trauma rarely occurs in isolation; patients frequently have other significant injuries that must be assessed. It has been estimated that 10% of all dogs presenting to the emergency room suffer from thoracic trauma severe enough to result in respiratory compromise. Common causes of thoracic injury include both blunt trauma, most commonly the result of a motor vehicle collision, and penetrating trauma, most commonly the result of bite wounds or projectile injury. Regardless of the cause of the injury, the clinician must be sure to perform a complete and thorough physical examination to ensure that no significant injuries are overlooked.

INITIAL APPROACH TO PATIENTS WITH THORACIC TRAUMA

One of the most challenging aspects of addressing patients with severe respiratory distress is their limited tolerance for stress. In some cases this may limit the clinician's ability to complete a thorough assessment until the patient's condition stabilizes. During the initial or primary survey the clinician should visually assess the patient from a distance. The observer should note the degree of distress, as well as the patient's respiratory rate and pattern and any noise. Changes in the respiratory pattern may signal further deterioration in patient condition, particularly if a breathing pattern characterized by an extended neck and short shallow breaths develops.

The observer should continue to assess the patient by auscultating and palpating the thorax. Lung and heart sounds should be auscultated bilaterally. Muffled heart and/or lung sounds may be heard in patients with pneumothorax, hemothorax, or diaphragmatic hernia. Crackles or increased adventitial sounds may indicate the presence of pulmonary contusions. The thorax should then be palpated. The clinician should look for injuries to the skin over the thorax and cranial abdomen, the presence of subcutaneous emphysema, and the loss of chest wall integrity caused by rib fractures.

Initial treatment for any patient with signs of respiratory distress should include oxygen supplementation. Options for oxygen supplementation include flow-by/face mask, the placement of nasal oxygen lines, the use of an oxygen cage, and in the most severe cases intubation and mechanical ventilation.

RADIOGRAPHIC ASSESSMENT OF THE ANIMAL WITH THORACIC TRAUMA

Survey thoracic radiographs are indicated in all patients with a history of moderate-to-severe trauma. However, thoracic radiographs should not be performed as part of the initial survey because many animals with respiratory impairment cannot handle the stress associated with radiography.

Once the patient is deemed stable for radiographs, two views should always be obtained. The clinician should evaluate the radiographs for diaphragmatic integrity, pulmonary infiltrates, the presence of pneumothorax, and rib and/or spinal fractures.

PULMONARY CONTUSIONS

Pulmonary contusions consist of hemorrhage and high-protein edema fluid that fill the alveoli. These are perhaps best thought of as bruises of the lung parenchyma. When the thoracic wall is struck, it initially absorbs the force of the impact. As the thoracic cage is compressed, the underlying lung parenchyma collapses and compresses. Once the compressive force is removed, the elastic recoil of the thoracic cage results in decompression of the parenchyma. This rapid compression-decompression results in rupture of the alveoli and alveolar capillaries. Subsequently hemorrhage and edema fluid fill the alveoli.

Clinical signs of pulmonary contusions include respiratory distress, hemoptysis, orthopnea, and cyanosis. Radiographically pulmonary contusions manifest themselves as a patchy interstitial-to-alveolar pattern that is generally worse on the side of impact and may be surrounded by pneumothorax. The radiographic changes associated with pulmonary contusions tend to worsen over the first 24 hours after injury, regardless of the patient's clinical course. In general, patients with life-threatening pulmonary contusion will present with moderate-to-severe respiratory distress.

Treatment of animals with pulmonary contusion is mainly supportive. The majority of animals with pulmonary contusions improve with oxygen supplementation and supportive care while other injuries are evaluated and treated. The most severe cases may require mechanical ventilation. Only 1% of dogs with pulmonary contusion go on to develop bronchopneumonia. Therefore prophylactic antimicrobial therapy is not indicated.

There is ongoing controversy concerning the optimal fluid therapy for patients with pulmonary contusions. There is considerable experimental evidence that overhydration results in worsening of pulmonary contusions. There is also some evidence that colloids may remain in the pulmonary interstitium for prolonged periods of time, leading to slower resolution of the contusions. As a result of these concerns, *judicious use of crystalloid fluids* seems most appropriate. It is also important that the clinician not underresuscitate the patient because of fear of worsening the pulmonary contusions.

The prognosis for dogs with pulmonary contusions varies widely. Animals that present with mild-to-moderate respiratory distress are very likely to recover. Patients with severe respiratory distress, particularly those requiring mechanical ventilation, warrant a more guarded prognosis.

PNEUMOTHORAX

Pneumothorax is the accumulation of air in the space between the lung parenchyma and muscles of the thoracic wall. Pneumothorax can be classified as either open or closed. Open pneumothorax is characterized by a disruption of the thoracic wall, which allows air to enter into the pleural space. Small-volume pneumothorax may result in no clinical signs and require no treatment, whereas large-volume pneumothorax may require rapid identification and treatment to save the patient.

Pneumothorax from thoracic trauma results from a sudden increase in airway pressure. This, combined with shear forces applied to the lung parenchyma, results in alveolar rupture and leaking of air into the pleural space. In cases of sharp, penetrating trauma direct disruption of the pulmonary parenchyma may result in the development of pneumothorax.

Given the relatively fixed volume within the thoracic cage, patients with pneumothorax have a decrease in tidal volume. Generally minute ventilation is maintained by an increase in the respiratory rate. In severe cases of pneumothorax minute ventilation falls to the point that hypoxemia develops. The most severe form of pneumothorax is a tension pneumothorax. A tension pneumothorax results when there is an increase in the volume of pneumothorax with each inspiration through a one-way flap. When intrapleural pressure exceeds alveolar pressure, the lung lobes on that side of the thorax collapse. There is a rapid decline is respiratory status, and respiratory arrest will develop if emergency therapy is not initiated.

Treatment of pneumothorax requires either percutaneous needle thoracocentesis or the placement of a thoracostomy tube (also see Chapter 154). Patients with a history of trauma and physical examination findings consistent with a pneumothorax frequently benefit from thoracocentesis before obtaining thoracic radiographs. In these patients the potential benefit far outweighs the minimal risk posed by percutaneous needle thoracocentesis in trauma patients. A thoracostomy tube should be considered in animals in which multiple needle thoracocentesis fail to achieve resolution, no end point is reached during needle thoracocentesis, or the patient requires positive-pressure ventilation.

DIAPHRAGMATIC HERNIA

A diaphragmatic hernia occurs when intraabdominal pressure exceeds abdominal pressure, such as might occur during blunt trauma. Many patients with a diaphragmatic hernia have paradoxic abdominal motion during respiration (abdomen is sucked in on inspiration). In addition, the abdomen may feel "empty" on palpation. Thoracic radiographs may provide evidence supportive of the diagnosis.

Gastric or bowel gas patterns crossing the plane of the diaphragm make the diagnosis simple, but gastrointestinal structures are not always misplaced. Pleural fluid or tissue can impair the ability to see the diaphragm completely; therefore additional techniques such as thoracic ultrasound may be required to confirm the diagnosis. Ultrasonography may be able to define borders of soft-tissue structures such as spleen or liver traversing the diaphragm.

Initial treatment of a patient with a diaphragmatic hernia involves stabilization of its cardiovascular and respiratory status. Patients with severe respiratory distress frequently have a large percentage of their abdominal contents within the thorax. In these cases mechanical ventilation may be needed to correct hypoxemia.

Correction of a diaphragmatic hernia requires surgery. In general, surgical intervention should be pursued as soon as the patient is stable. Historically it had been recommended that intervention be postponed for at least 24 hours; however, more recent investigation has supported intervention once the patient is stable.

FLAIL CHEST

Flail chest is defined as the paradoxic movement of a floating thoracic segment. This occurs when there is a fracture of two or more consecutive ribs in two places (ventral and dorsal). Paradoxic movement results from the changes in intrapleural pressures. On inspiration intrapleural pressure decreases, and the lungs and thoracic cage expand. Because of the instability of the flail segment, it does not move outward with the rest of the thoracic wall; instead the flail segment moves inward (toward the more negative pressure). The reverse is true on expiration. The combination of concurrent pulmonary contusion and pain can predispose to hypoxemia and hypoventilation.

Treatment should initially focus on relieving the pain caused by the flail segment. Placing the flail segment down helps to limit the motion, thus decreasing pain. Intercostal nerve blocks can be very effective at limiting the pain. Mechanical stabilization of the flail segment is rarely needed and only indicated in the most severe cases.

Suggested Reading

Campbell VL et al: Pulmonary function, ventilator management, and outcome of dogs with thoracic trauma and pulmonary contusions: 10 cases (1994-1998), *J Am Vet Med Assoc* 217:1505, 2000.

Gibson TW et al: Perioperative survival rates after surgery for diaphragmatic hernia in dogs and cats: 92 cases (1990-2002), *J Am Vet Med Assoc* 227:105, 2005.

Mazzaferro EM: Respiratory injury. In Wingfield WE, Raffe MR, editors: *The veterinary ICU book*, Jackson Hole, WY, 2002, Teton NewMedia, p 935.

Olsen D et al: Clinical management of flail chest in dogs and cats: a retrospective study of 24 cases (1989-1999), *J Am Anim Hosp Assoc* 38:315, 2002.

Powell LL et al: A retrospective analysis of pulmonary contusion secondary to motor vehicular accidents in 143 dogs: 1994-1997, *J Vet Emerg Crit Care* 9:127, 1999.

Sigrist EN, Doherr MG, Spreng DE: Clinical findings and diagnostic value of post-traumatic thoracic radiographs in dogs and cats with blunt trauma, *J Vet Emerg Crit Care* 14:259, 2004.

CHAPTER 17

Intravenous Anesthetic and Analgesic Techniques

THOMAS K. DAY, *Louisville, Kentucky*

Intravenous continuous (constant)–rate infusions (CRIs) are commonly used in dogs and cats to maintain anesthesia after induction. The CRI is optimal for all-injectable anesthesia techniques and also is applicable to the continuous administration of analgesic drugs. When using a CRI for an all-injectable anesthesia, several anesthetic drug combinations are likely to be needed and are more likely to maintain anesthesia safely when compared to a single agent. Furthermore, species differences between dogs and cats warrant special mention when administering all-injectable anesthesia.

Choices of anesthetic drugs applicable to critically ill dogs and cats are limited. Long-acting sedatives such as acepromazine should be avoided in most instances. However, if the dog or cat is hemodynamically stable, small doses of acepromazine (0.025 to 0.05 mg/kg IV) can be administered to control excessive excitement or dysphoria. Although useful for analgesia (see Chapter 2) in general the α-2 agonists should be avoided in critically ill dogs and cats since these drugs can cause further cardiopulmonary compromise.

Opioids alone or in combination with the local anesthetic lidocaine and the dissociative drug ketamine can be used to provide anesthesia and analgesia in many critically ill dogs and cats. Many combinations are available, and it is the decision of the clinician as to which CRI to administer. Decisions generally can be made based on severity of postoperative pain, species, procedure to be performed, and experience of the clinician.

The choice of drugs used in a CRI depends on many factors, including species, age, the procedure to be performed; and the physical status of the dog or cat. A "cook book" plan for administration of anesthetics and analgesics to critically ill dogs and cats is discouraged. The clinician should individualize the anesthetic protocol to maximize efficacy and safety. This chapter describes a number of proven CRI methods applicable to dogs and cats in the critical care setting.

CONTINUOUS-RATE INFUSIONS FOR DOGS

Morphine

Morphine is the prototype opioid used for analgesia. A morphine CRI (0.1 mg/kg/hour) provides excellent continuous analgesia in dogs. However, a morphine CRI used alone will likely not provide a level of sedation that is adequate. Appropriate preanesthetic medication (opioids or

neuroleptanalgesia) and induction of anesthesia with any agent followed by a morphine CRI may provide adequate short-term anesthesia in dogs.

Morphine-Lidocaine-Ketamine

This morphine-lidocaine-ketamine (MLK) "cocktail" works very well in dogs and minimizes some of the effects of high dosing of just one or two of these drugs. The local anesthetic lidocaine results in moderate central nervous system (CNS) depression. which, when combined with morphine, results in more reliable sedation than morphine alone. The amount of ketamine added in this combination does not stimulate the CNS but is very helpful for the prevention of wind-up pain. As with a morphine CRI, appropriate preanesthetic medication (opioids or neuroleptanalgesia) and induction of anesthesia with an intravenous agent, followed by an MLK CRI, provides reliable short-term anesthesia in dogs. To create an MLK infusion, the following drugs are added to a 1-L bag of lactated Ringer's solution (LRS): morphine (1.8 ml of a 15-mg/ml concentration), lidocaine (15 ml of 2% or 20-mg/ml concentration); ketamine (0.6 ml of a 100-mg/ml concentration). The initial administration rate is typically the usual anesthesia rate of crystalloid fluids (10 ml/kg/hour). The administration rate for analgesia following the surgical procedure is 2.5 ml/kg/hour.

Fentanyl

Fentanyl is approximately 100 times more potent than morphine and provides more reliable CNS depression. A fentanyl CRI (5 to 10 mcg/kg/hour) can provide excellent analgesia. A higher infusion rate (10 to 40 mcg/kg/hour) can result in surgical analgesia. The critically ill dog requires much less than a normal dog. Fentanyl has a very short half-life (minutes) and is ideal for inclusion as a CRI.

Fentanyl-Lidocaine-Ketamine

The addition of lidocaine to fentanyl, as with MLK, can result in profound CNS depression and more reliable sedation and anesthesia. The amount of ketamine does not create CNS side effects. To create a fentanyl-lidocaine-ketamine (FLK) infusion, the following drugs are added to a 1-L bag of LRS: lidocaine (15 ml of 2% or 20-mg/ml concentration); ketamine (0.6 ml of a 100-mg/ml concentration), and fentanyl. The volume of fentanyl (50 mcg/ml concentration) varies based on the rate of fluid administration. In general, a CRI of 3 to 5 mcg/kg/hour should be prepared for administration. The fluid rates are similar to those used for MLK preparations. Adjusting a prepared bag of FLK can be difficult. Alternatively the lidocaine and ketamine can be delivered as previously described, and fentanyl can be delivered via a syringe pump. The clinician can make the desired concentration of fentanyl and change the rate of fentanyl infusion with ease.

Propofol

Propofol is classified as a phenolic compound and is unrelated to opioids, barbiturates, or steroid anesthetics. Propofol induction is characterized as a very rapid and smooth induction with a very rapid and smooth recovery. Noncumulative effects make propofol an ideal drug for CRIs, provided the patient is not suffering from severe cardiovascular depression since propofol is a negative inotrope. Use of preanesthetic medication greatly reduces the dose of propofol required for induction and maintenance of anesthesia. Induction with propofol (1 to 5 mg/kg IV) followed by a CRI (0.14 to 0.4 mg/kg/minute IV) can result in long-term sedation for minimally invasive procedures. The level of sedation achieved depends on the preanesthetic medication and the achieved effect. Higher infusion rates are required to maintain a surgical plane of anesthesia and to maintain an endotracheal tube since propofol can result in significant respiratory depression. Another drawback is cost; a propofol CRI can become very expensive in a larger dog.

CONTINUOUS-RATE INFUSIONS FOR CATS

CRIs of opioid combinations for cats are prepared and administered differently than for dogs. Cats are more likely to have adverse effects from lidocaine, including seizures and hypotension. Therefore lidocaine is not used in these combinations. Furthermore, cats can become excited or dysphoric from opioid combinations and are less likely to become overtly sedated when compared to dogs. A tranquilizer such as acepromazine (0.025 mg/kg IV) or a sedative such as diazepam (0.2 mg/kg IV) can be useful to minimize side effects caused by opioids. Acepromazine must be used with caution if at all in cats that are hypotensive, bradycardic, or hypothermic.

Morphine

A morphine CRI in cats produces minimal sedation unless the cat is severely depressed. The infusion rate (0.1 mg/kg/hour) is similar to that for dogs, and neuroleptanalgesia or sedation is required to maintain the desired level of anesthesia.

Morphine-Ketamine

Morphine (1.8 ml of a 15-mg/ml concentration) and ketamine (0.6 ml of a 100-mg/ml concentration) (MK) are added to a 1-L bag of LRS. Alternatively one fourth of each drug can be added to a 250-ml bag of LRS. The initial administration rate is typically the anesthesia rate of fluids (10 ml/kg/hour) after induction of anesthesia. An administration rate of 2.5 ml/kg/hour is typical following the procedure.

Fentanyl-Ketamine (FK)

Ketamine (0.6 ml of a 100-mg/ml concentration) is added to a 1-L bag of LRS. The volume of fentanyl (50-mcg/ml concentration) will vary based on the rate of fluid administration. A volume to provide a CRI of 3 mcg/kg/hour should be prepared for use during the procedure following induction of anesthesia. The fluid rates are similar to those used for MK preparations, and the amount of fentanyl will be different for each rate. Alternatively the ketamine can be administered alone, and the fentanyl can be administered via syringe pump for ease and safety.

Propofol

Propofol can be administered in a similar fashion as described above for dogs. The induction and maintenance dosage will vary based on the drugs used for preanesthetic medication and induction. A common practice would be to induce anesthesia with propofol (1 to 3 mg/kg slow IV bolus) followed by a CRI (0.1 to 0.3 mg/kg/minute). The amount of propofol used will likely be much less than for larger dogs and should be more economical. Infusions lasting more than 30 minutes can result in a longer recovery than the same infusion time in dogs because cats metabolize propofol slower. The airway should be controlled when procedures are long. Consecutive-day infusions of propofol (for radiation therapy, wound management) can result in Heinz body production and possibly Heinz body anemia in cats.

Suggested Reading

Andress JL, Day TK: TThe effects of consecutive day propofol anesthesia on feline red blood cells, *Vet Surg* 24:277, 1995.

Day TK: Injectable anesthetic techniques for emergency and critical care procedures. In Bonagura JD, editor: *Kirk's current veterinary therapy XI (small animal practice)*, Philadelphia, 2000, Saunders, p 122.

Day TK: Anesthesia for the cardiac patient. In Tilley LP, Smith FKW, Oyama MA, and Sleeper MM, editors: *Manual of canine and feline cardiology*, ed 4, Philadelphia, 2008, Saunders, p 356.

Wagner AE: Opioids. In Gaynor JS, Muir WW: *Handbook of veterinary pain management*, St Louis, 2002, Mosby, p 164.

SECTION II

Toxicologic Diseases

Michael J. Murphy

VOLUME XIII CONTENT ON EVOLVE: http://evolve.elsevier.com/Bonagura/Kirks/

Pet Food Safety

CHAPTER 18

Toxin Exposures in Small Animals

LYNN R. HOVDA, *Bloomington, Minnesota*

The Pet Poison Helpline (PPH) is a division of SafetyCall International that began fee-for-service animal toxicology and poison information in 2004. The helpline is available to animal owners, veterinarians, veterinary students, veterinary technicians, pesticide control officers, and others 24 hours a day, 7 days a week for a one-time fee. The line is staffed by veterinarians, certified veterinary technicians, veterinary students, pharmacists, pharmacy students and technicians, medical doctors, zoologists, and others with specialized knowledge in fields such as reptiles and snakes.

During the 12-month period beginning July 1, 2005 and ending June 30, 2006, the PPH received over 9000 animal toxicology calls. The distribution of these calls is presented as a sampling of animal toxicology questions posed to small animal practitioners. The source of these calls, species affected, age of animals, and toxin types are briefly summarized.

About 70% of calls originated from pet owners, and 20% from veterinarians or veterinary hospitals or clinics. The remaining calls came from a myriad of sources, including zoological gardens, farms and ranches, restaurants, and stores.

Dog exposures accounted for about 88% of the calls, with cats accounting for 10%, and other species the remaining 2%. Animals included as other species were primarily caged birds and pocket pets (sugar gliders, rabbits, and small rodents) with a few potbellied pigs, goats, and horses.

Most of the calls involved animals in the younger age-group. Of canine-related calls, 79% were in the 5 years and under age-group, with 17% in the 6- to 12-year age range. Very few calls involved dogs in the 13- to 19-year age range. Cat-related calls involved 62% in the 0- to 5-year age range, and 23% in the 6- to 12-year age range. No age-related data were retrieved for the other animal calls.

There were 1831 calls pertaining to mixed breeds, followed in decreasing order by these breeds: the Labrador retriever (884), golden retriever (291), Yorkshire terrier (234), Chihuahua (232), and boxer (196). Cats were split between domestic shorthair, domestic longhair, and mixed breed or unknown.

Twenty-two deaths were recorded during the 12-month period (Table 18-1). This number may be falsely low because some cases had an unknown or undocumented outcome. Fifteen dogs, three cats, two birds, one pocket pet, and one horse died or were humanely euthanized. Two calls originated from offices or hospitals, and the rest from homes or farms. The most common cause of death in all species was from pesticides or other products used around the house and garden to eliminate insects, rodents, or weeds (8), followed by human drugs (4), and unknown toxins (4).

For the purpose of investigating the specific call type, calls were divided into eight general categories (Table 18-2) Subdivisions were used in each category as needed to further classify information.

Almost all of the calls involving plants and mushrooms (563 total calls) originated from the caller's home or personal residence. When corrected for increasing monthly volume, the number of calls per month was relatively steady across the calendar year. Two small spikes occurred: one in December when the number of poinsettia calls increased and one in April associated with an increase in Easter lily calls. Other common plant calls included azalea, sago palm, marijuana, cyclamen, lilies of all varieties, and all varieties of oxalate-containing plants. Over 60% of the plant ingestions involved symptomatic cats and were primarily associated with some form of lily or oxalate-containing plant. Sago palm and marijuana exposures were limited to the dog population.

Over 4000 human drugs and herbal supplements were identified as potential toxins. This number does not reflect the actual call volume because multidrug ingestions occurred with some frequency and were generally associated with the most serious and life-threatening ingestions. Within this category human prescription dugs constituted about 66% of calls, while exposure to over-the-counter (OTC) drugs and nutraceuticals constituted about 33% of the calls. Oral products accounted for almost all of the human prescription drug exposures, with ingestion of very few topical, patch, suppository, lollipop, or inhaled substances. Within the human prescription drug division, antidepressant drugs, antianxiety drugs, newer sleep-inducing drugs, drugs for attention-deficit disorder, and cholesterol-lowering drugs were overrepresented. Despite the large number of calls generated by these drugs, few serious outcomes occurred. Three of the drug-related deaths were from ingestion of topical products (5-fluorouracil and calcifediol) that were reported less than 14 times in the 12-month period. OTC drugs and nutraceuticals showed a slightly different picture, with about 10% of the ingestions involving topical medications and ophthalmic solutions. Within this category pain medications such as acetaminophen (APAP), aspirin, ibuprofen, and naproxen were the drugs most commonly ingested, followed by

Table **18-1**

Category of Deaths

Category	Number of Calls
House and garden	8
Insecticide (4)	
Zinc phosphide (2)	
Rodenticide (1)	
Herbicide (1)	
Unknown	4
Human drugs (prescription and over-the-counter)	4
Household products	2
Foreign bodies	2
Other	2

cough and cold products, multivitamins, herbal supplements, and calcium-containing supplements. With the exception of pain medications, clinical signs in this group were generally mild and self-limiting. One drug-related death occurred from a massive dose of ibuprofen.

Surprisingly, silica gel packets made up over 50% of the calls falling into the foreign body category. With the exception of one cat that ate a dryer sheet, all of the calls involved dogs, in particular Labrador retrievers and golden retrievers. Other common foreign body ingestions included batteries of all types, pens, pencils, fireplace starter logs, coins, and glues. Some of the more interesting items ingested included a stuffed alligator head, three forks, 40 pennies, a safety razor, a light bulb, and a lead x-ray glove.

Exposures involving household products were equally split between dogs and cats. The exposures were easily divided into those involving laundry products, general cleaning products, toilet products, and carpet-cleaning or carpet-freshening products. When further analyzed, cat exposures occurred most often in the laundry and bathroom area, whereas dogs ingested carpet-freshening agents and general cleaning products more often. Clinical signs in this category for all species were usually mild and self-limiting.

Of the 531 food-related calls, over half of them involved dogs ingesting some form of chocolate. This was con-

Table **18-2**

Classifications of Call Type

Call Type	Yearly Call Volume
Human drugs and nutraceuticals	4108
Pesticides: insecticides, rodenticides, fertilizers, herbicides, others	1793
Plants and mushrooms	563
Food	531
Veterinary products	513
Foreign bodies	437
Household products	420
Other	1302

sistent for each and every month. Other food products included nuts (almonds, macadamia nuts, and hazelnuts), onions, grapes and raisins, and xylitol-containing gums. When corrected for increasing call volume, a distinct increase occurred in December and again in late March and early April. Butter, gravy, meat products, and eggnog ingestions all increased in December, presumably because of increased availability and decreased surveillance. The number of chocolate and candy ingestions increased around Easter, again presumably because of the increased availability.

Almost 1800 calls involved exposures to house, lawn, and garden products. Included were products meant to eliminate insects and other pests or rodents, herbicides, and fertilizers. Pyrethrin-based insecticides accounted for over 80% of the insecticide calls, followed by avamectin or ivermectin, imidacloprid, and boric acid. Outcomes in this group varied from none to severe, with cats having the most severe symptoms. Calls regarding a carbamate, organophosphate, or arsenic compound occurred much less frequently, but the outcome was generally much more severe. Deaths in the insecticide group (three dogs, one pocket pet) were from exposure to either a concentrated product or very large amounts of a more dilute product. A genuine seasonal occurrence occurred with these calls, with the incidence highest in summer and lowest in winter.

All of the rodenticide calls concerning ingestion of long-acting anticoagulant agents occurred in dogs. Most of the calls originated from the caller's home and were managed with no clinical signs. Calls originating from a health care facility were often associated with more severe clinical signs and required prolonged care and treatment. Despite aggressive medical care, one dog died from a brodifacoum overdose. Brodifacoum ingestions occurred with the most regularity, and the call number varied little from month to month. The remainder of the long-acting anticoagulant calls included difethialone, diphacinone, bromethalin, and bromadiolone. Three or four calls each month involved some form of sticky board exposure and typically involved cats or small dogs.

Household herbicide and fertilizer calls were almost always of low toxicity and involved a taste, touch, or lick of a product or ingestion of treated grass. Rarely did any clinical effects develop, and signs that occurred involved primarily vomiting and other gastrointestinal signs. One cat death did occur from the ingestion of a liquid herbicide. There was a distinct seasonal occurrence to these calls, with lowest call volume in December and January and the highest in early spring and summer.

Zinc phosphide, although technically a pesticide, was counted separately because calls related to this product were almost always associated with a moderate-to-severe clinical outcome. This product is placed below ground in gopher or other small rodent holes, under mobile homes, or in other below-ground areas. In addition to the inherent toxicity, the product is often placed and forgotten until dug up and ingested by a curious dog. Two documented deaths occurred. Although primarily a problem in dogs, one horse died from eating a large amount of product from a bucket in the back of a pesticide control officer's truck.

Dogs and cats were equally represented in calls involving veterinary products. Topical flea and tick products, including pyrethrin-based products, showed a seasonal occurrence, whereas nonsteroidal antiinflammatory drug ingestion was steady from month to month. Clinical signs and outcomes were worse with pyrethrin-based flea products, especially in cats. Other calls, primarily dog calls, included heartworm medication, prescription animal drugs, anthelmintics, and nutraceuticals. Clinical effects for almost all of these categories were mild and self-limiting.

The remainder of the calls were lumped into a large "other" category. Within this group several subdivisions emerged. Automotive products were the most prevalent, with more than 150 exposures in the 12-month period. Of these, 16 were known exposures to ethylene glycol. Fortunately no reported deaths occurred. This may be the result of early and aggressive care, the introduction of easy-to-use in-house ethylene glycol testing kits, or the availability of an antidote. Personal care products such as shampoos, nail polish remover, deodorants, and other items accounted for numerous calls but were all of low toxicity and generally resulted in few clinical effects. Oddly, animal and insect bites or stings occurred year-round, with two to three calls occurring each month. The outcome was generally good, and clinical signs were mild to moderate.

It is interesting to note that, even though dog exposures made up the vast majority of calls, clinical effects were usually mild, and the outcome was excellent. Despite the smaller number of calls, cats seemed to have a more difficult time with ingestions, and the outcome often was not as good. This may be because of their environment and their ability to crawl into smaller places, as well as their inquisitive nature, relatively smaller body size, longer life span, or simple differences in metabolic pathways.

In summary, the PPH handled over 9000 calls, with 22 reported and documented deaths. The majority of calls originated from the caller's home, generally had no-to-few clinical signs, and were treated at home with no referral to a health care facility. Abut 88% of the calls involved young dogs, followed by cats and a variety of other species. The most common reported exposure was to human pharmaceuticals and OTC drugs/nutraceuticals, followed by pesticides and other agents used in the lawn and garden.

References and Suggested Readings

Barton J, Oehme FW: The incidence and characteristics of animal poisonings seen at Kansas State University from 1975-1980, *Vet Hum Toxicol* 23(2):101, 1981.

Buck WB: A poison control center for animals: liability and standard of care, *J Am Vet Med Assoc* 302(8):1118, 1993.

Forrester MB, Stanley SK: Patterns of animal poisonings reported to the Texas Poison Center Network: 1998-2002, *J Am Vet Med Assoc* 46(2):96, 2004.

Haliburton JC, Buck WB: Animal poison control center: summary of telephone inquiries during first three years of service, *J AM Vet Med Assoc* 182(5):514, 1983.

Hornfeldt CS, Murphy MJ: Poisonings in animals: a 1990 report of the American Association of Poison Control Centers, *Vet Hum Toxicol* 34(3):248, 1992.

Hornfeldt CS, Jacobs MR: A poison information service for small animals offered by a regional poison center, *Vet Hum Toxicol* 33(4):339, 1991.

Hornfeldt CS, Borys DJ: Review of veterinary cases received by the Hennepin Poison Center in 1984, *Vet Hum Toxicol* 27(6):525, 1985.

CHAPTER 19

Toxin Exposures and Treatments: A Survey of Practicing Veterinarians

KELLY HALL, *St. Paul, Minnesota*

A survey to gather information from veterinarians on common small animal toxin exposures and treatments was created via a collaborative effort between the University of Minnesota (Drs. K. Hall and M. Murphy) and the Veterinary Information Network (VIN) (Dr. M. Rishniw and colleagues). The survey was available online for VIN members to respond to for approximately 2 weeks in September 2006. There were 160 responses representing veterinarians from the United States (81.3%), Canada (8.1%), Australia (5%), United Kingdom (1.2%), and other countries (4.4%). Table 19-1 indicates the geographic distribution of respondents from the United States and Canada. Respondents selected the type of practice in which they work (Fig. 19-1). Responses included general practice (71%); emergency-only practice (13%); referral practice with emergency service (12%); general practice with emergency service (1%); university hospital (1%); and one respondent each for house call/acupuncture, 95% feline practice, relief veterinarian, and referral/general practice (2%). Respondents' qualifications (156 respondents) included DVM (83%), ABVP (5%), ACVECC diplomats (3%), MS or PhD (3%), non-ACVECC diplomats (2%), and other (4%, internship and residency trained, RN, MPVM).

The survey questions are listed in Box 19-1. Survey results are available for VIN members to view on the Internet at http://www.vin.com/Members/Library/.

COMMON EXPOSURES

Dogs

More that 50% of respondents selected anticoagulant rodenticide, ingestion of chocolate, and animal envenomation as the most common exposures seen in dogs. The top 10 selected toxins are listed in Table 19-2. Additional toxins that were chosen less frequently included bromethalin (12%), acetaminophen (9%), cholecalciferol (4%), cholinesterase inhibitors (4%), zinc (3%), grapes/raisins (2%), Gorilla Glue (2%), ethanol (2%), lead (1%), methanol (1%), gasoline (1%), soap/detergent (1%) and bleach (0). Toxins not included on the list that were mentioned by respondents included coffee, blue-green algae, ivermectin, strychnine, xylitol, and tremorgenic mycotoxin.

Of the 51% of respondents who chose animal envenomation as a most common exposure in dogs, bee or wasp (82%), snake (69%), and spider (38%) were most commonly selected; toad (9%) and scorpion (8%) were selected less frequently. Tick paralysis and ant swarms were each written in twice by respondents for the "other" category.

Of the 22% respondents who chose plant intoxication as a most common exposure, lily (66%), garlic/onion (32%), azalea (29%), and dieffenbachia (dumbcane) (24%) were most commonly selected from plants listed. Approximately 37% of respondents selected "other," including sago palm, mushroom, and oleander. Answers listed on the survey chosen least frequently included nightshade (5%), Japanese yew (5%), and bleeding heart (0).

Cats

More than 50% of respondents selected pyrethrin/permethrin and plant intoxication as the most common exposures seen in cats. The top 10 selected toxins are listed in Table 19-3. Toxins not included on the list included potpourri, oils (petrol, tea tree, lamp), macadamia nut, and paint/paint thinner. Additional toxins that were available for respondents to select from but were chosen less frequently included drugs of abuse (5%), soap/detergent (5%), bromethalin (3%), methaldehyde (3%), ethanol (2%), cholecalciferol (1%), bleach (1%), chocolate (1%), zinc (1%), lead (1%), methanol (gasoline 1%), gasoline (1%), grapes/raisins (0), and Gorilla Glue (0).

Of the 40% respondents who chose animal envenomation as a most common exposure in cats, bee or wasp (69%) and snake (61%) were most commonly selected; spider (18%), scorpion (2%), and toad (1%) were selected less frequently. Tick paralysis and skink/small lizard were each written in by respondents for the "other" category.

Of the 66% of respondents who chose plant intoxication as a most common exposure, lily ingestion far outweighed all other answers (90%). Additional answers included azalea (22%), dumbcane (21%), and garlic/onion (12%). Approximately 7% of respondents selected "other" and most frequently listed houseplants with oral and gastrointestinal topical effects (e.g., oxalates). Answers listed on the survey that were chosen least frequently included nightshade (3%), bleeding heart (2%), and Japanese yew (1%).

Table **19-1**

Regional Data From Question 2: "If you live in the United States or Canada, please enter your ZIP code."

Region	Respondents
United States (119 of 130 Respondents)	
Northeast (21)	New York (8), Pennsylvania (5), Ohio (5), Maryland (3)
Southeast (22)	North Carolina (6), Virginia (5), Florida (5), Georgia (4), West Virginia (1), South Carolina (1)
South (17)	Texas (7), Tennessee (2), Alabama (2), Mississippi (2), Louisiana (2), Arkansas (1), Oklahoma (1)
Midwest (18)	Wisconsin (5), Iowa (5), Minnesota (3), Michigan (2), Illinois (2), Missouri (1)
West (40)	California (23), Oregon (5), Colorado (5), Washington (2), Idaho (2), Utah (2), Arizona (1)
Noncontinental (1)	Alaska (1)
Canada (11 of 13 Respondents)	
East (7)	Ontario (6), Prince Edward Island (1)
West (4)	British Columbia (2), Alberta (2)

DECONTAMINATION

Dogs

Apomorphine was selected overwhelmingly (69%) as the method of choice for inducing emesis when clinically indicated in dogs (Fig. 19-2). Hydrogen peroxide (26%) was selected second most frequently. Xylazine, syrup of ipecac, morphine, and "I don't induce vomiting" were each selected less that 2% of the time. Of the options listed in the survey, medetomidine was never selected.

Cats

Fig. 19-3 illustrates respondents' selection for method of choice for inducing emesis when clinically indicated in cats. Hydrogen peroxide (29%), xylazine (24%), and apomorphine (22%) were selected most frequently. "I don't induce vomiting in cats" was selected by 14% of respondents. Medetomidine (5%), morphine (4%), and syrup of ipecac (2%) were selected by the fewest respondents.

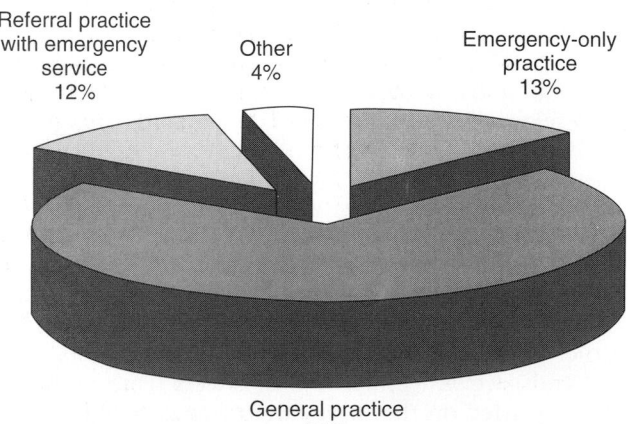

Fig. 19-1 Respondent's answer to question 3, *"In what type of practice do you primarily work?"*

Referral practice with emergency service 12%

Other 4%

Emergency-only practice 13%

General practice 71%

HOSPITAL SUPPLIES

Decontamination

A majority of respondents stocked activated charcoal (98%), saline eye flush (86%), hydrogen peroxide (84%), apomorphine (79%), mineral oil (60%), and mild soap/detergent (59%) in their practice for decontamination purposes. Many respondents selected xylazine (44%) as supplied in their hospitals. Syrup of ipecac (9%) and sodium sulfate (3%) were selected least frequently (Fig. 19-4). Many respondents wrote in decontamination supplies

Box **19-1**

Survey Questions Posted on Veterinary Information Network for 2 Weeks

1. In which country do you live?
2. If you live in the United States or Canada, please enter your zip code.
3. In what type of practice do you primarily work?
4. The FIVE (5) most common toxin exposures in DOGS that present to my practice are:
5. If you chose "Animal Envenomation" in question 4, please specify.
6. If you chose "Plant Intoxication" in question 4, please specify.
7. The FIVE (5) most common toxin exposures in CATS that present to my practice are:
8. If you chose "animal envenomation" in question 7, please specify.
9. If you chose "plant intoxication" in question 7, please specify.
10. What is your method of choice for inducing emesis when clinically indicated? Which of the following do you keep stocked in your practice for toxin exposure decontamination?
11. Which of the following toxin antidotes do you keep stocked in your practice?
12. Which of the following supportive care/symptomatic therapy products do you keep stocked in your practice for uses including care of toxicity patients?
13. What equipment do you have for dealing with toxin exposure?
14. What is your highest level of veterinary training?
15. Additional comments about animal intoxication and this survey.

Table 19-2

Top 10 Responses for Question 4: "The FIVE (5) most common toxin exposures in DOGS that present to my practice are:"

Toxin	Percent Respondents
1. Anticoagulant rodenticide	89
2. Chocolate	54
3. Animal envenomation (e.g., insects, reptiles)	51
4. Nonsteroidal antiinflammatory drugs (e.g., carprofen, aspirin)	45
5. Human prescription medication	45
6. Ethylene glycol	32
7. Plant intoxication	22
8. Pyrethrin/Permethrin	22
9. Drugs of abuse (e.g., marijuana, cocaine)	18
10. Methaldehyde (snail bait)	16

Table 19-3

Top 10 Responses for Question 7: "The FIVE (5) most common toxin exposures in CATS that present to my practice are:"

Toxin	Percent Respondents
1. Pyrethrin/permethrin	86
2. Plant intoxication	66
3. Ethylene glycol	47
4. Acetaminophen	42
5. Animal envenomation (e.g., insects, reptiles)	40
6. Nonsteroidal antiinflammatory drugs (e.g., carprofen, aspirin)	39
7. Human prescription medication	34
8. Anticoagulant rodenticide	27
9. Cholinesterase inhibitors	9
10. Other	7

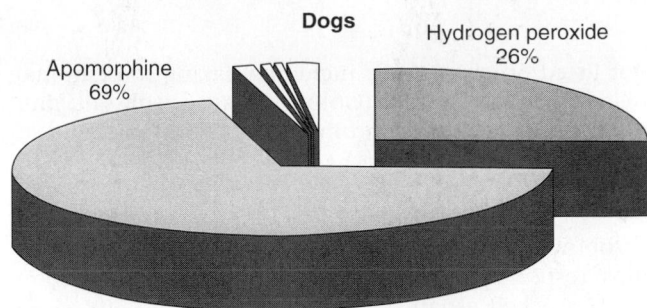

Fig. 19-2 Respondent's answer to question 10 (dogs), *"What is your method of choice for inducing emesis when clinically indicated?"*

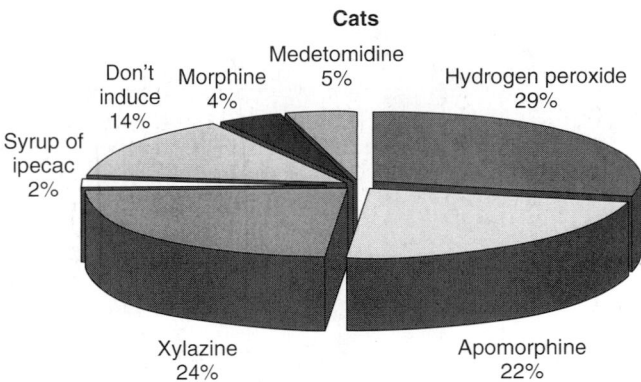

Fig. 19-3 Respondent's answer to question 10 (cats), *"What is your method of choice for inducing emesis when clinically indicated?"*

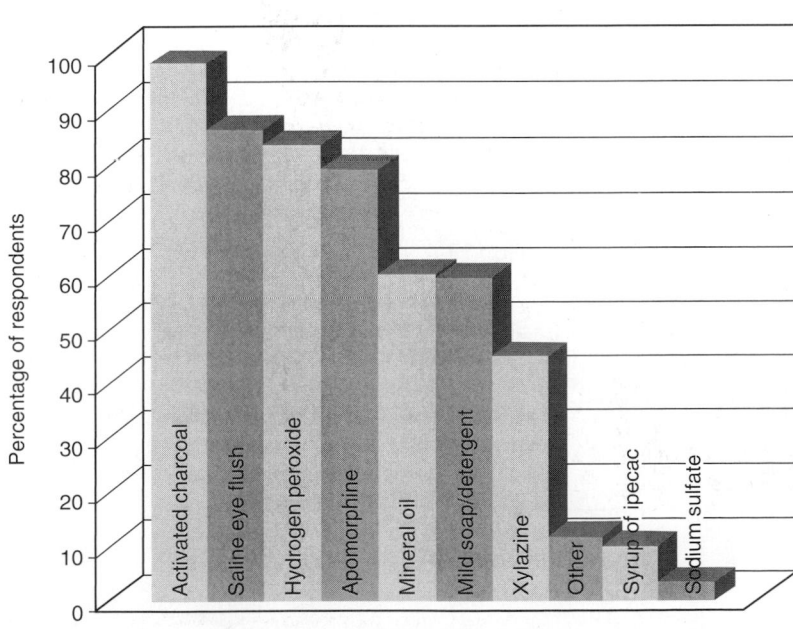

Fig. 19-4 Respondent's answers to question 11, *"Which of the following do you keep stocked in your practice for toxin exposure decontamination?"* Respondents were able to select all that applied.

not listed on the survey, including baking soda, human oiling removal products (GoJo, Swarfega), table salt, morphine, medetomidine, sorbitol, and milk of magnesia.

Specific Therapies (Antidotes)

Atropine (95%) and vitamin K (91%) were stocked by most respondent's clinics. Approximately half of respondents stocked ethanol (53%) and acetylcysteine (46%) (Fig. 19-5). Antidotes that were stocked less frequently included antivenin (27%), calcium ethylenediaminetetraacetic acid (EDTA) (23%), fomepazole (21%), 2-PAM (15%), calcitonin (10%), D-penicillamine (6%), and deferoxamine (2%). Other specific therapies not available on the survey that were written in by respondents included methocarbamol, yohimbine, and naloxone.

General Therapies (Supportive Care)

A majority of respondents indicated that their practice stocked diazepam, atropine, furosemide, acepromazine, oxygen, dextrose, crystalloids, opioids, calcium, mannitol, cimetidine, cyproheptadine, β-blockers, phenobarbital, doxapram, naloxone, potassium chloride, and dopamine for uses that included supportive care of toxicity cases. Sodium bicarbonate, sucralfate, pentobarbital, oxyglobin, packed red blood cells, milk of magnesia, plasma, and vitamin C were stocked less frequently.

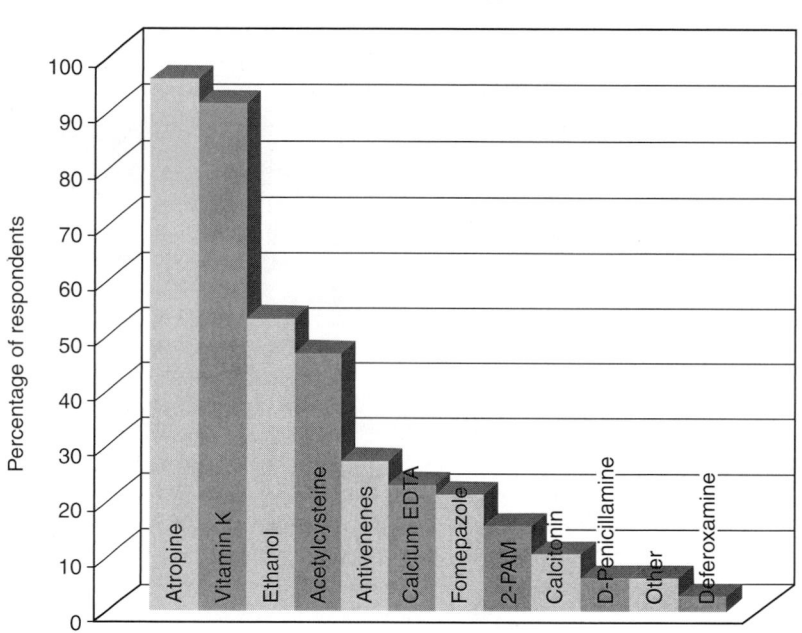

Fig. 19-5 Respondent's answers to question 12, *"Which of the following toxin antidotes do you keep stocked in your practice?"* Respondents were able to select all that applied.

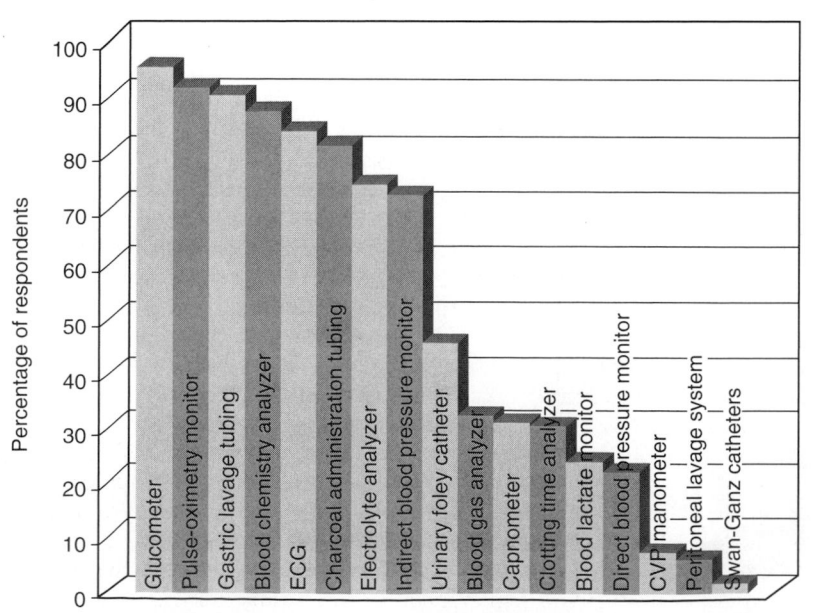

Fig. 19-6 Respondent's answers to question 14, *"What equipment do you have for dealing with toxin exposure?"* Respondents were able to select all that applied.

Ammonium chloride was not selected by any respondents. Other general therapies not included on the survey list but written in by respondents included methocarbamol (also listed frequently in specific therapies for tremorgenic toxins, oral or topical), midazolam, whole blood, and misoprostol.

Monitoring and Treatment Equipment

Most respondents had glucometers (95%), pulse-oximeters (92%), gastric lavage tubing (90%), blood chemistry analyzers (87%), electrocardiographs (84%), charcoal administration sets (81%), electrolyte analyzers (74%), and indirect blood pressure monitoring (72%) available in their clinics. Fewer respondents listed urinary Foley catheters (45%), blood gas analyzers (32%), capnometers (31%), clotting time analyzers (30%), blood lactate monitors (24%) and direct blood pressure monitors (22%) as being available in their clinics. Central venous pressure manometry (7%), peritoneal lavage systems (6%), and

Swan-Ganz catheters (1%) were rarely selected as being available in their practice by respondents. Equipment not included on the survey list but written in by respondents included ventilators, warm blankets/cage floors, enema delivery systems, and endoscopy (Fig. 19-6).

OTHER RESOURCES

Numerous comments at the end of the survey included information on where practitioners liked to find toxicology information or the need for the availability of more concise/immediate information. Multiple excellent resources are available to help veterinarians and owners deal with toxin exposure in pets, including SafetyCall International's Pet Poison Helpline (1-800-213-6680), the ASPCA Animal Poison Control Center (1-888-4ANI-HELP), emergency clinics, veterinary schools, veterinary diagnostic laboratories (www.aavld.org), and veterinarians who are board certified in emergency and critical care (ACVECCS) or as toxicologists (www.abvt.org).

CHAPTER **20**

Reporting an Adverse Drug Reaction to the Food and Drug Administration

LYNN O. POST, *Rockville, Maryland*

A great deal of time and expense is invested by industry and regulators to test the safety and efficacy of animal drug products before marketing an approved drug. The concern for the safety and effectiveness of a drug does not end at drug approval. Veterinarians and consumers must have some assurance that the products they administer to pets and livestock are also safe and effective in the postapproval period. *Pharmacovigilance* is defined as the science and activities relating to the detection and interpretation of safety concerns to minimize risk and allow for appropriate regulatory action. The results of adverse drug event (ADE) monitoring and risk assessment must be made available to veterinarians and consumers as quickly as possible. The Food and Drug Administration (FDA) relies on spontaneous reports, (i.e., reports that are voluntary from veterinarians and consumers) to accomplish its pharmacovigilance tasks.

Making sense of ADEs is a "fuzzy world" (Edwards, 1997). Separating a true adverse reaction, known as a *signal,* from background noise is difficult. The evaluation of ADE data does not achieve the criteria imposed on traditional scientific studies involving less than 50 animals per sample. There are usually many confounding factors, a clearly defined control group is often lacking, and it is more difficult to test the hypothesis of a cause-and-effect relationship (Avorn, 2004). Rather the fuzzy world of ADEs is characterized by observational data in which associations are derived from hundreds-to-thousands of animals and dozens of confounding factors, including weight, age, sex, preexisting medical conditions, administration of other drugs, and the lack of a definitive control group or baseline. Absolute cause and effect cannot be determined in the ambiguous world of ADEs. On the other hand, the limitations of observational studies do not mean that proper enforceable inferences cannot be drawn from ADE data.

ADVERSE DRUG EVENT REPORTING SYSTEM FOR APPROVED ANIMAL DRUGS

Adverse Drug Event Regulations

An *adverse drug experience (ADE)* is defined as an association of a clinical sign with the use of a new animal drug, whether or not the sign is considered to be drug related and whether or not the new animal drug was used in accordance with the approved labeling (i.e., the product may have been used according to label directions or in an extralabel manner, including but not limited to a different route of administration, different species, different indications, or other than labeled dosage) (21 Code of Federal Regulations [CFR] 514.3). Adverse drug experience includes but is not limited to:

- An adverse event occurring in animals in the course of the use of an animal drug product by a veterinarian or a livestock producer or other animal owner or caretaker.
- Failure of a new animal drug to produce its expected pharmacologic or clinical effect (lack of expected effectiveness).
- An adverse event occurring in humans from exposure during manufacture, testing, handling, or use of a new animal drug.

The regulations that specifically address the spontaneous reporting obligations of the drug sponsors of FDA-approved animal drugs are contained in "Records and reports concerning experience with new animal drugs for which an approved application is in effect" (21 CFR 514.80). Approved animal drugs are codified in the Federal Register and the CFR with a new animal drug application number. Reporting of ADEs for approved animal drugs is mandatory for the animal pharmaceutical industry. Once the veterinarian or consumer reports the ADE to the company, it is mandatory for the company to forward the information to the FDA. It is voluntary for veterinarians and consumers to report the ADE to the company or directly to the FDA. Companies report the ADE on Form FDA1932. Animal ADEs can be reported directly to the FDA by the veterinarian or consumer by using Form FDA 1932a, which is a shortened version of Form FDA1932 (available on the Center for Veterinary Medicine [CVM] website: http://www.fda.gov/cvm/adetoc.htm).

Reporting Adverse Drug Events to the FDA, USDA, and EPA

ADE submission is required only from companies marketing FDA-approved animal drugs. There are no requirements for submitting ADEs for human drugs used in animals or unapproved products labeled for animals. The FDA, Center for Drug Evaluation and Research, will not accept ADEs pertaining to extralabel use of human drugs in animals. The CVM accepts reports directly from consumers and veterinarians regarding extralabel use of human drugs and unapproved animal drug products. The CVM has limited resources to monitor the performance of these drugs in animals.

ADE reporting to CVM has significantly increased over the last decade. During the early 1990s the CVM received approximately 1000 ADEs each year. The CVM received about 33,000 ADE reports for the year 2005. Reasons for the increase are numerous but include the new types of drugs approved for use in companion animals, label information provided for contacting drug companies, and the interest of the public in reporting perceived product problems.

Veterinarians are encouraged to report ADEs directly to the sponsor* who will fill out Form FDA 1932 for submission to the CVM. About 99% of the ADEs received by the CVM are submitted by the sponsor on Form FDA 1932. Less than 1% of reported ADEs are submitted directly to the CVM by the veterinarian or consumer (Form FDA 1932a). Another reporting option is to call the CVM ADE hotline (1-888-FDA-VETS) to report an ADE. An FDA veterinarian will return the phone call. The reporter can also either call or write the CVM to obtain a prepostage-paid reporting form. If the ADE is not a drug, the following contacts may be useful: United States Department of Agriculture (animal biologics), 800-752-6255, http://www.aphis.usda.gov/vs/cvb/html/adverseeventreport.html; Environmental Protection Agency (topical insecticides), 800-858-7378, http://www.epa.gov/opp00001/health/pets.htm.

ADE Reports From Animal Pharmaceutical Companies

For industry reporting the ADEs are divided into three categories: (1) significant product defect reports that should be submitted to an FDA District Office within 3 days (21 CFR 514.80 [b] [1]); (2) ADEs involving unexpected animal injury and unexpected product ineffectiveness that should be submitted within 15 working days to the CVM (21 CFR 514.80 [b] [2]); and (3) the remaining types of ADEs and product defects that should be submitted at periodic intervals to the CVM (21 CFR 514.80 [a] [4]). All categories of complaints are required to be submitted by the drug sponsor on the Office of Management and Budget (OMB)-approved Form FDA 1932 ("Veterinary Adverse Drug Reaction, Lack of Effectiveness, and Product Defect Report").

Significant product defects are those involving either label mix-ups or a significant departure of the product from approved specifications in which the product defect may result in immediate harm to animals. Product defects that may result in a serious ADE are reported by the manufacturer to the FDA field office within 3 days. Corrective action is accomplished through the FDA Field Office responsible for the manufacturing site. More benign product defects that do not have the potential for serious ADEs are reported in the annual report directly to the CVM.

ADEs requiring 15-day submissions are serious and unexpected (21 CFR 514.3 and 514.80). A serious ADE:

- Is fatal or life threatening,
- Requires professional intervention,

---

*Sponsor: owner of the approved new animal drug.

- Causes an abortion, stillbirth, infertility, or permanent disability disfigurement, or
- Is an unexpected ADE that is not on the current label or may be pathophysiologically related to an ADE on the label.

Unexpected refers to information that is not contained either on product labeling or as part of the approved FDA application. Regulations further require reporting of unexpected adverse events that are associated with clinical use, studies, investigations, or tests, whether or not determined to be attributable to the suspected drug. These regulations also apply to extralabel use of the drug. A key phrase is "whether or not determined to be attributable to the suspected drug." The CVM expects the drug sponsor to submit all ADEs rather than only the reports that the firm believes to be associated with the ADE. The CVM considers selective report submission or filtering to introduce a bias that confounds the evaluation of submitted ADEs.

EVALUATION OF ADVERSE DRUG EVENT REPORTS

Adverse Drug Event Evaluation Algorithm

The CVM uses the modified Kramer algorithm to assign a causality score to each clinical sign in an ADE report (Hutchinson et al., 1979a, 1979b; Keller, Bataller, and Oeller, 1998). The causality assessment is a measure of an association and not cause and effect. The algorithm has six standardized criteria: (1) information from the scientific literature; (2) previous documentation of the clinical sign; (3) alternative explanations for the clinical sign; (4) timing of events and amount of the drug administered; (5) *dechallenge,* lessening of the clinical sign when the influence of the drug passes; and (6) *rechallenge,* reappearance of the clinical sign when the drug is given again.

This method uses a procedure that lends some objectivity to an otherwise very subjective process. The algorithm is applied to each clinical sign in an adverse event report. The numeric scores for each of the six criteria are summed to arrive at a causality assessment score. The numeric score is matched to one of the four general categories of drug-related associations consisting of: "Probable, Possible, Unlikely, and Unknown," as outlined in Box 20-1 (EMEA, 2004). All clinical signs with positive causality assessment scores in the "Possible and Probable" drug-related categories are transferred to the cumulative summary on the FDA CVM website. Clinical signs with negative causality assessment scores ("Unknown and Unlikely") are not transferred to the CVM web site.

An ADE becomes an adverse drug reaction when one or more clinical signs in the ADE report are scored with a positive causality assessment. This means that there may be some association or relationship between the ADE and the drug. A positive causality score for one clinical sign from a single ADE report does not generate an instant label change or regulatory action by the CVM. A limitation of the modified Kramer algorithm is the skewing to a lower causality assessment to the level of "Unlikely" or

---

Box 20-1

Causality Assessment Categories*

Probable: All of the following should apply for probable:

- There should be a reasonable association in time between the administration of the animal drug product and the onset and duration of the reported event.
- The description of the clinical signs should be consistent with an adverse drug reaction, or at least plausible, given the known pharmacology and toxicology of the product.
- There should be no other equally plausible explanation of the case. In particular, concurrent use of other products and possible interactions or preexisting medical conditions should be taken into account in the assessment.

When any of the above criteria cannot be satisfied because of conflicting data or lack of information, such reports can only be classified as "possible, unlikely, or not applicable."

- *Possible:* When the information suggests another possible explanation or plausible cause for the described event but the data do not meet the criteria for inclusion in the "Probable" category.
- *Unlikely:* When sufficient information exists to establish beyond a reasonable doubt that an animal drug product was not likely to be the cause of the event.
- *Unknown:* Unclassifiable or not assessable for cases in which insufficient information was not available to draw a conclusion to include all cases in which reliable data are unavailable or are insufficient to make an assessment of causality. The ADE could be related to the drug, but present data are not adequate to draw a conclusion. The category includes (1) inconclusive: cases in which other factors prevent a conclusion from being drawn but a product association cannot be discounted; and (2) unclassified: cases in which insufficient information did not allow a conclusion to be drawn.

*These definitions are not a substitute for a causality assessment process such as the modified Kramer algorithm. Each definition characterizes the level of certainty or uncertainty of the association between a drug and an adverse event.

"Possibly" drug-related from a more appropriate category of "Possibly or Probably." This results from the difficulty of assigning a positive number (placing a clinical sign in the "Possible" or "Probable" category) (see Table 20-1) to an event that occurs a long time after rechallenge or dechallenge. Thus a low frequency of a specific clinical sign could be overlooked as background noise rather than a signal. This is especially true in regard to long-acting drugs such as heartworm preventives.

Advantages of Adverse Drug Event Reports

The main advantage of ADE reporting is that large, heterogeneous animal populations are available compared to small, homogeneous populations in preapproval studies. Drugs are evaluated under actual conditions of use as opposed to a controlled laboratory setting. Signal detection often depends on confounding factors or conditions of use. Once a signal has been detected and discussed by industry and regulators, risk can be identified early in the marketing history of a product. The alternative would be to use thousands of animals in classical controlled studies, which would be cost prohibitive. It is unlikely that ADEs occurring at low frequencies would be manifested even in massive classical studies; in addition, these studies rarely duplicate actual conditions of use. On the other hand, signals generated by evaluation of ADE reports can be used to design classical studies to test hypotheses. The classical studies can corroborate or refute the observational studies that depend on ADE data.

Disadvantages of Adverse Drug Event Reports

It is difficult to calculate a true incidence for spontaneous ADE data. The numerator is underreported*; and the denominator, usually the number of doses administered, is almost never known. More severe clinical signs such as blindness and death are probably reported more often by veterinarians and consumers. A reporting rate can be calculated using the total number or frequency of clinical signs divided by the total number of ADE reports, but this is not a very useful number. Prospective epidemiologic studies could be designed with a more precise handle on the actual number of ADEs or clinical signs as the numerator divided by the total number of doses administered as the denominator. The resulting number would give a better estimate of incidence, but this could also be very expensive.

The length of time that a product has been on the market is also a factor. Generally ADEs for products that have been on the market for over 2 years are underreported. Pharmaceutical companies, veterinarians, and consumers become complacent about reporting ADEs on products that have been in use for many years. Veterinarians may be especially reluctant to report ADEs on well-known products that have been marketed for several years with few instances of side effects.

Report quality is a problem because veterinarians, lay staff at veterinary hospitals, and consumers do not always report all of the information (e.g., laboratory tests, concomitant drugs and preexisting medical conditions). Economics may be a factor because of some clients' reluctance to spend money on laboratory tests. Veterinarians simply may not want to take the extra time to evaluate and communicate laboratory results to the sponsor.

Regulatory Actions

The ADE database contains several thousand reports from 1987 to the present consisting of companion and food animal species. Safety reviewers manually enter relevant medical data such as the suspect drug, species, breed, weight, age, sex, and clinical signs into the database. At the same time, safety reviewers evaluate the clinical signs in the ADE report using the modified Kramer algorithm.

Presently safety reviewers identify trends and alert the product manager. Safety reviewers are veterinarians who are trained to evaluate ADE data and recognize trends. Product managers are veterinarians who are assigned to monitor the safety and effectiveness of specific products.

A group of similar clinical signs submitted in several ADE reports in a short period of time may be interpreted as a signal for further investigation by the CVM and the drug company. In the event that a potential problem is identified, the Monitored Adverse Reaction Committee (MARC) is convened by the product manager and the ADE coordinator to assist in evaluating information related to the potential problem. The MARC consists of experts from throughout the CVM to include the Office of New Animal Drug Evaluation (ONADE), the Office of Research (OR), and the Office of Surveillance and Compliance (OSC). There is a standing invitation for ONADE experts from the Divisions of Manufacturing and Chemistry, Food Animals, Companion Animals, or Human Food Safety, depending on the particular drug and needs of the MARC. Scientists from the OR are invited on an ad hoc basis. In the OSC product managers and ADE safety reviewers from the Division of Surveillance serve as the lead in presenting ADE data for review by the MARC. Subsequently the MARC recommends appropriate regulatory action if the problem is considered significant. This investigation may result in product recall of the affected lot(s) or a label change. The label change includes new information from the ADE reports containing clinical signs with a positive causality assessment. "Dear Doctor" letters are often issued by the company in conjunction with label changes at the request of the CVM. The "Dear Doctor" letters inform veterinarians about the label changes or other actions taken by the CVM and the industry. On rare occasions a drug may be removed from the market through voluntary recall by the company or withdrawal by FDA of the approval because the new evidence shows that the drug is no longer safe for its intended use. ADE information is released to the public by means of summary report publication on the CVM website. Additional requests for ADE information can be made through the Center's Freedom-of-Information Officer (HFV-12, 7519 Standish Place, Rockville, MD 20855, 240-276-9017).

Most Frequent Adverse Drug Reactions in Dogs and Cats

The thirty most frequent clinical signs in descending order for dogs and cats are summarized in Box 20-2. The clinical signs become adverse drug reactions when they receive positive causality assessment scores. For dogs the summarized list represents about 80,000 adverse reactions out of about 100,000 exposures across all animal drugs in the database during the period 1987 to the present. For cats the summarized list represents about 19,000 adverse reactions out of about 33,000 exposures across all animal drugs in the database during the period 1987 to the present. Specific drugs can be found on the CVM website.

The three most frequent signs for dogs and cats are depression/lethargy, vomiting, and anorexia. Overall this may be an accurate reflection of the entire population of dogs and cats in the United States, but it is mainly to the result of clinical signs that can be readily visualized by veterinarians versus specific laboratory results in the ADE database. Similarly, pet owners tend to report only clinical signs that are easily observed. This is to be expected because consumers usually do not report the results of

---

*Only about 10% of some ADEs or clinical signs are reported.

Box 20-2	

The 30 Most Frequent Adverse Drug Reactions in Dogs and Cats*

Dogs	Cats
Vomiting	Depression/lethargy
Depression/lethargy	Vomiting
Anorexia	Anorexia
Ineffective for heartworm larvae	Death
High alkaline phosphatase	Application site alopecia
Diarrhea	Ataxia
High SGPT/ALT	Diarrhea
Death	High BUN
Convulsions	Mydriasis
Ataxia	High creatinine
High BUN	Fever
High total bilirubin	Ineffective anesthesia
Death (euthanized)	Convulsions
Anemia	Hypersalivation
High creatinine	Dyspnea
Anaphylaxis/anaphylactoid	Apnea
Fever	Blindness
Pruritus	Prolonged anesthesia recovery
High WBC	Trembling
Bloody diarrhea	Death (euthanized)
Polydipsia	Cardiac arrest
Trembling	Application site lesions
Weight loss	Pruritus
Low platelets	Ineffective for ear mites
High SGOT/AST	Alopecia
Icterus	Dehydration
Polypnea	Anemia
Drug interaction	Ineffective for fleas
Weakness	Vocalization
High liver enzymes	Weight loss

BUN, Blood urea nitrogen; *SGOT/ALT,* serum glutamic oxaloacetic transaminase/aspartate aminotransferase; *SGPT/AST,* serum glutamic pyruvic transaminase; *WBC,* white blood cell count.

*The thirty most frequent clinical signs with positive causality assessment scores are listed in descending order across all approved drugs in the CVM database during the period 1987 to the present.

laboratory results and necropsy reports to the company or the CVM. In addition, many owners are more reluctant to pay for laboratory tests than for the forensic tests that are done much more routinely in human medicine. Therefore it is imperative that the practitioner gather as much information as possible when reporting an ADE to the sponsor. Laboratory results can make a difference between establishing a stronger association between an ADE and the drug and not having enough information to make any determination. Conversely, laboratory tests can cause a clinical sign to be placed in the "Unlikely" category.

Benefits of ADE Reporting

Practitioners should be able to depend on the label information to make professional decisions about the risks and benefits of the associated drug. The purpose of pharmacovigilance is to give some assurance that the animal drug labeling is accurate beyond the initial product launch. One ADE report does not provide enough information for a label change. A reliable safety profile emerges only after a product is marketed and administered to a relatively large population of animals. The pharmacovigilance network involves veterinarians, industry, and regulators. Practicing veterinarians play a pivotal role as observers and reporters of ADEs. Despite the scrutiny of drugs that undergo FDA approval, it is impossible to know everything about a drug before approval. Animal drug pharmacovigilance remains the best tool available to communicate risk to veterinarians and consumers in spite of the limitations of ADE reporting and evaluation.

GLOBAL PHARMACOVIGILANCE REPORTING

The U.S. Department of Agriculture and the FDA are participants in the construction of a global adverse event reporting platform. The reporting format for ADEs will be standardized; but the causality assessment, the evaluation of risk for each ADE, and the pharmacoepidemiologic approach that may include mathematic analyses will not be. Global harmonization of reporting requirements for ADEs is no small task. It must be kept in mind that, unlike human ADEs, veterinary medicine deals with multiple species, which adds more complexity to an already complicated process. In addition, reporting requirements differ substantially from country to country because missions, goals, resources, administrative procedures, and ADE sources vary considerably. The variations reflect the fundamental differences in the worldwide agencies and the laws they administer.

The International Cooperation on Harmonization of Technical Requirements for Registration of Veterinary Medicinal Products (VICH), is a trilateral organization (EU-Japan-USA) with two observer countries (Australia and Canada) whose aim is to harmonize technical requirements for animal medicinal product registration to include preapproval review and postapproval monitoring. In 1996, at the inception of VICH, one goal was the harmonization of pharmacovigilance reporting requirements: definitions, data elements, electronic submission protocols, and medical dictionaries.

Successful efforts of VICH will lead to the timely transmission of ADE information among all parties and organizations involved in animal pharmacovigilance. Electronic reporting standards will also available to consumers and veterinarians who could report directly to the regulatory agency rather than the company. The standardized ADE information will be disseminated worldwide for examination and analysis by all interested parties.

References and Suggested Reading

Avorn J: Powerful Medicines: *The benefits and, risks, and costs of prescription drugs,* ed 1, New York, 2004, Random House, p 39.
Bataller N, Keller WC: Monitoring adverse reactions to veterinary drugs: pharmacovigilance, *Vet Clin North Am Food Anim Pract*15(1):13, 1999.

Edwards RE: Adverse drug reactions: finding the needle in the haystack, *Br Med J* 315:500, 1997.

European Agency for the Evaluation of Medicinal Products (EMEA), Veterinary Medicine and Inspections, Committee for Veterinary Medicinal Products: *Guideline on pharmacovigilance for veterinary medicinal products—guidance on procedures for marketing authorization holders*, London, UK, 2004, available at http://www.emea.eu.int.

Hampshire VA, Brown, MA: Adverse drug reactions at the US Food and Drug Administration Center for Veterinary Medicine. In Papich M, editor: *Pharmacology and therapeutics,* ed 9, Ames, Ia, in press, Blackwell Publishing.

Hutchinson TA et al: An algorithm for the operational assessment of adverse drug reactions. I. Background, description, and instructions for use, *J Am Med Assoc* 242:623, 1979a.

Hutchinson TA et al: An algorithm for the operational assessment of adverse drug reactions. II. Demonstration of reproducibility and validity, *J Am Med Assoc* 242:633, 1979b.

International Cooperation on Harmonization of Technical Requirements for Registration of Veterinary Medicinal Products, VICH (2006): http://vich.eudra.org/.

Keller WC, Bataller N, Oeller DS: Processing and evaluation of adverse drug experience reports at the Food and Drug Administration Center for Veterinary Medicine, *J Am Vet Med Assoc* 213:208, 1998.

United States Code of Federal Regulations, 21, Part 500-599. Office of the Federal Register, National Archives and Records Administration, Washington, DC, 2005, US Government Printing Office, 21 CFR 514.3 and 514.80.

CHAPTER 21

Sources of Help for Toxicosis

MICHAEL J. MURPHY, *St. Paul, Minnesota*

Practitioners faced with questions about toxicoses can access a number of resources. These include specialists in veterinary toxicology, veterinary diagnostic laboratories, colleges of veterinary medicine, textbooks, on-line references, and poison control centers.

Perhaps the best source of veterinary toxicology information comes from veterinarians certified by the American Board of Veterinary Toxicology (ABVT) as specialists. The ABVT is one of the most established specialty groups recognized by the American Veterinary Medical Association's Board of Veterinary Specialties. A listing of ABVT Diplomates is available at www.abvt.org. Consultation with an ABVT toxicologist can be particularly helpful in complicated or obscure cases of toxicosis.

Many veterinary diagnostic laboratories and Colleges of Veterinary Medicine (CVMs) include ABVT Diplomates on staff. The veterinary diagnostic laboratory accredited by the American Association of Veterinary Laboratory Diagnosticians nearest to your practice can be identified by checking accreditation at http://www.aavld.org; colleges of veterinary medicine can be found at http://www.avma.org/education/cvea/colleges_accredited/colleges_accredited.asp.

Many practicing veterinarians have reference texts available in their clinic. Most veterinary toxicology texts are authored by ABVT Diplomates. A partial list of such reference texts that I recommend beyond this textbook includes the textbook series *A Field Guide to Common Animal Poisons*, by Murphy (www.blackwellprofessional.com); *Clinical Veterinary Toxicology* by Plumlee (Mosby, www.us.elsevierhealth.com/Veterinary); *Small Animal Toxicology* by Peterson and Talcott (Saunders, www.us.elsevierhealth.com/Veterinary); and *Toxicology* by Osweiler (Williams & Wilkins, www.lww.com.).

Poison control centers are another leading source of toxicology information. Some centers specialize in animals. Even though most poison control centers specialize in human exposures, about 135,000 animal exposure calls were recorded by human centers in 2004. Animal poison control centers include the American Association for the Prevention of Cruelty to Animals Animal Poison Control Center (www.aspca.org/apcc), the Pet Poison Helpline (www.petpoisonhelpline.com), and human poison control centers. Animal poison control centers may charge for services and information. The telephone number for the human poison control center in many areas is 1-800-Poison-1.

The practicing veterinarian should consider in advance the various sources available for information regarding animal toxicoses. Depending on the situation, a textbook reference or direct consultation with a toxicology specialist, veterinary diagnostic laboratory, college of veterinary medicine, or a poison control center may provide the information needed to appropriately manage toxicosis in the veterinary patient.

Website Resources

American Association for the Prevention of Cruelty to Animals Animal Poison Control Center: www.aspca.org/apcc.
American Association of Veterinary Laboratory Diagnosticians: www.aavld.org.
American Board of Veterinary Toxicology Diplomates: www.abvt.org.
American Veterinary Medical Association (accredited colleges): www.avma.org/education/cvea/colleges_accredited/colleges_accredited.asp.
Pet Poison Helpline: www.petpoisonhelpline.com.

CHAPTER **22**

Small Animal Poisoning: Additional Considerations Related to Legal Claims

MICHAEL J. MURPHY, *St. Paul, Minnesota*

"I think the neighbor is poisoning my pet."

Most practitioners hear this history many times in a career. Often the pertinent clinical signs are unrelated to any toxin; however, at other times toxicosis is the source of signs. Other chapters in this section are devoted to specific toxins or reporting of adverse events. This chapter considers situations when a pet toxicosis may involve the legal system.

Pet poisoning cases may involve the legal system through a variety of avenues, including insurance claims, product liability claims, civil claims, or criminal prosecution. As an example a criminal case is presented to highlight some of the issues that may arise when an animal toxicosis involves the legal system.

Celinski v. State

The criminal application of the Texas animal cruelty statute was reviewed in the case of *Celinski v. State*. Mr. Celinski was found guilty of cruelty to animals in part for poisoning two cats with acetaminophen. He appealed the conviction. The conviction was upheld by the Texas Court of Appeals based on the evidence.

The evidence cited by the Texas Court of Appeals in upholding Mr. Celinski's conviction was:

"(1) The cats were in good health when Jones [the owner] left; they were very sick when she returned the following day. They had diarrhea, were foaming at the mouth, and were too weak to stand.
(2) The veterinarian who treated the cats concluded that they were suffering from acetaminophen poisoning, based upon his observation of their physical symptoms and upon the results of a blood test.
(3) The veterinarian was unable to reverse the results of the poisoning with an antidote. He estimated that the cats had ingested the equivalent of five to six tablets apiece some time during the afternoon of February 21, 1994.
(4) Texas A&M laboratory results confirmed that Sugar Ray and Bonnie died of acetaminophen poisoning.
(5) The veterinarian had seen a dozen cases of feline acetaminophen poisoning in his 14 years of practice, but had never heard of a cat voluntarily ingesting Tylenol, nor had he ever seen a case of multiple cats simultaneously ingesting Tylenol.
(6) Appellant testified there were no pills lying about the apartment the day the cats became sick—pills they could have accidentally ingested. He was the only person present in the apartment with the cats on that day." (*Celinski v. State*)

NOTE: Criminal cases are commonly cited as *State v. Doe*, since the state is prosecutor and the individual accused of doing the poisoning is the defendant in the initial trial. In this case, Mr. Celinski appealed the initial court ruling to the Texas court of appeals; thus the case is *Celinski v. State*.

Other Signs

Mr. Celinski was also convicted of putting the cats in the microwave and turning it on. The cats had blistered feet, and some of their other signs could be related to the microwave.

The interest of the legal and medical professions is generally quite similar in these cases. That interest is to determine whether exposure to the suspect chemical caused the disease present in the animal. Both professions gather and analyze facts to determine whether such a conclusion can be reached.

This case illustrates a number of points regarding the importance of medical records in legal cases. The first four points listed by the Court of Appeals may be used to determine whether the cats had a previous illness, whether they were exposed to a potentially toxic dose of acetaminophen, and whether the previously known adverse effects of acetaminophen were observed in the cats. The last two points reviewed by the court of appeals were more directly aimed at determining whether the exposure was accidental or intentional.

The first point noted by the Court of Appeals was that the cats were previously healthy and then became acutely ill. A *preexisting medical condition* that could explain the clinical signs or other adverse effects observed in the animal is likely to be considered in a legal setting. This analysis would consider whether the clinical signs of the animal could be caused by the preexisting condition, exposure to the purported toxin, or both.

The second point noted by the Texas Court of Appeals was the cats were exposed to a dose of acetaminophen known to be toxic. Acetaminophen was detected in the cats, confirming exposure. Analytic chemistry confirmation of the presence of the chemical in the animal is very useful in a legal setting to confirm that the chemical was actually absorbed into the animal. Analysis of blood and urine is most commonly used to support an argument of systemic exposure to the chemical. All of this information presumably assisted the veterinarian in estimating that the cats had received five to six acetaminophen-containing tablets apiece.

The fourth point noted by the Court of Appeals was the cats died of acetaminophen poisoning. The "physical symptoms" observed by the veterinarian included "dark chocolate color of a blood sample." This blood color led the veterinarian to suspect acetaminophen toxicosis. Acetaminophen was confirmed as the cause of death by the laboratory at Texas A&M University. A thorough necropsy with appropriate supportive testing also can be very useful both to rule in the suspect toxin and rule out other possible causes of the animal's clinical condition.

The veterinarian's medical record is likely to be an important source of facts in a legal case. Consequently, the more facts present in the medical record, the stronger the support for an argument that the suspect chemical, and not another etiology, caused the disease.

The last two points (5 and 6) were used to find that death from acetaminophen was intentional and not accidental. The distinction between accidental and intentional poisoning is important in animal cruelty statutes as discussed in the following paragraphs.

This criminal case raises important questions that may be considered in other toxicosis cases, specifically:

- What should be included in veterinary medical records?
- When is animal poisoning considered animal cruelty?
- Are drugs of abuse considered poisons?
- How is client confidentiality balanced with reporting animal poisoning?

What Should Be Included in Medical Records?

The veterinarian's medical records will likely be thoroughly reviewed if a medical case becomes a legal case. The pet's medical record may be broader than sometimes appreciated. For example, "registration forms, consent forms, radiographs, estimate sheets, billing records, telephone consultations, controlled drug logs, laboratory results, surgery reports, discharge records, imaging recordings, patient history, treatment records, and consultation reports" may all be considered a part of a pet's medical record (Scott, 2006). Specific suggestions of facts to include in the medical record when animal cruelty is suspected are:

> "[w]henever nonaccidental injury is suspected, the attending veterinarian should obtain a minimum database, including estimated age, an accurate body weight, and a body condition score, and should perform a complete physical examination, a thorough oral examination to establish the condition of the teeth, otoscopic and ophthalmic examinations to identify potential head trauma, radiographic examinations to rule out occult injuries, and other species-specific examinations as necessary" (Babcock and Neihsl, 2006).

Despite these suggestions, the requirements for a veterinary medical record may be defined by the state in which one practices. This requirement, if it exists, should be considered. For example, the Minnesota Board of Veterinary Medicine has established, by Rule, the minimum standards for medical records for veterinary practice in Minnesota. Some of these record keeping requirements are:

> "A. A veterinarian performing treatment or surgery on an animal or group of animals, whether in the veterinarians's custody at an animal treatment facility or remaining on the owner's or caretaker's premises, shall prepare a written record or computer record concerning the animals containing, at a minimum, the following information:
>
> (1) name, address, and telephone number of owner;
> (2) identity of the animals, including age, sex, and breed;
> (3) dates of examination, treatment, and surgery;
> (4) brief history of the condition of each animal, herd, or flock;
> (5) examination findings;

(6) laboratory and radiographic reports;
(7) tentative diagnosis;
(8) treatment plan; and
(9) medication and treatment, including amount and frequency."

Minnesota Rule 9100.800 sub. 4, A

Practitioners may choose to consult their state licensing board to determine if guidelines exist in that state for minimal data to include in veterinary medical records. One should consider including more than the minimal requirement if litigation is anticipated. Information to consider documenting in the record of suspected poisoning cases includes telephone consultations, laboratory test results, and consultation reports. Referral or consultation may not be required.

The increase in the number of veterinary specialty practices has raised the question of when a practitioner has a "duty to refer" a case (Rollin, 2006; Block and Toss, 2006). I am aware of no such obligation in pet poisoning cases. Rather the timely treatment of an animal that has been poisoned may argue against such a referral.

I also am not aware of a "duty to consult" on poisoning cases. However, such consultation may be wise in some cases. Several sources of information for poisoning cases are summarized in Chapter 21. The practitioner may consider consulting a veterinary toxicologist (www.abvt.org), a veterinary diagnostic laboratory (www.aavld.org), or both to receive advice on which samples and what testing may be desirable to confirm a suspected toxicosis to the "reasonable degree of medical certainty" normally required in a legal setting. Documenting in the medical record telephone consultations, including the results of specific toxin testing, the owner's decision to decline such testing, and any consultation reports obtained may strengthen the final diagnosis reached in a specific case. Notation of the rationale used to rule in the toxicosis and rule out other differential diagnoses also may be useful.

Sometimes the legal aspects of a case are unknown or not recognized at the time of patient presentation. Updating a medical record certainly can be proper. Subsequent reflection may suggest a need to update the record with the facts remembered but not initially recorded. However, the record should be amended only in a way that allows the original record to be read. "Entries that are completely blacked out or obliterated always raise suspicion when records are viewed by a third party.... The corrected entry should be signed and dated by the person making the correction" (Scott, 2006).

When is Animal Poisoning Considered Animal Cruelty?

Most toxic exposures in animals are accidental. Sometimes pets may ingest plants, pesticides, automotive products, and over-the-counter or prescription drugs available in or around the home despite the owner's best efforts to prevent them from doing so. Accidental adulteration of pet food has also occurred in the United States during the past several years.

These accidental exposures may require testing that specifically identifies the chemical causing the disease and rules out other reasonable etiologies whenever a claim against a property owner, pesticide applicator, product manufacturer, or other third party arises. The medical records and diagnostic considerations discussed in the previous paragraphs apply to these cases as well.

Rarely, animals are intentionally poisoned. In some states this element of intent may support an argument that a crime of animal cruelty has been committed. Animal cruelty statutes that include a version of the term "poison" are found in Arkansas, California, Hawaii, Maine, Michigan, Minnesota, North Carolina, New Mexico, Nevada, Ohio, Pennsylvania, Texas, Utah, and Vermont at the time of this writing. (see list in references). Most of these statutes indicate that the act be "knowingly," "willfully," "intentionally," or "maliciously" committed.

Animal cruelty may be a misdemeanor or a felony. For example, in Minnesota:

"[a]ny person who unjustifiably administers any poisonous, or noxious drug or substance to any animal, or procures or permits it to be done, or unjustifiably exposes that drug or substance with intent that the drug be taken by any animal, whether the animal is the property of the person or another, is guilty of a gross misdemeanor" (Minnesota Statutes 2005, Chapter 343.27).

In the United States animal cruelty may rise to the level of a felony in 43 states (Babcock and Niehsl, 2006). For example, in Texas a person may be found guilty of a state jail offense if the person intentionally or knowingly: ...

"(5) kills, seriously injures, or administers poison to an animal, other than cattle, horses, sheep, swine, or goats, belonging to another without legal authority or the owner's effective consent..." (Tex. Penal Code Ann. § 42.09).

Presumably most cases of accidental unintentional animal poisoning would not satisfy the "intent" requirement of animal cruelty statutes. Consequently most pet poisoning cases would not likely rise to the level of animal cruelty, even in states where poisoning is recognized as one form of animal cruelty. Veterinarians should consider checking with their state licensing board to know the law in their state.

Are Drugs of Abuse Considered Poisons?

Alcohol, marijuana, cocaine, or other human drugs of abuse occasionally are encountered by veterinarians in emergency clinics or practices. Animals may certainly experience adverse effects after exposure to alcohol or these drugs (see Chapter 32). Many practitioners may not equate alcohol with "poison" in the routine veterinary practice. The Maine animal cruelty statute includes the phrase "gives poison or alcohol to an animal," apparently distinguishing alcohol from poison.

Screening pet's urine can be done to detect drugs of abuse using over-the-counter kits (Box 22-1). The kits are often used as a practical way to indicate to a concerned pet owner that such drugs are not detected in the urine of their animal when the test gives a negative result. Any positive results should probably be confirmed by analytic chemistry testing since most human kits have not been validated for use in animal urine. See www.aavld.org for laboratories that may be able to perform such analytical chemistry testing. It may be wise to consult the state licensing board to determine if positive findings for alcohol or human drugs of abuse identified in the urine of pets requires reporting to anyone not the client.

Balancing Client Confidentiality With Reporting

The question of client confidentiality should be considered whenever one considers reporting an animal's condition to someone who is not the client. For poisoning cases confidentiality is generally not an issue if the person or entity responsible for poisoning the pet is not the client. Clients may certainly disclose their pet's medical records to others at their discretion. Diagnostic laboratory reports confirming toxicosis have often been used to initiate investigations by a sheriff or humane officer when warranted. Presumably routine accidental animal toxicoses do not require reporting under animal cruelty statutes in most states because they do not meet the "intent" element, as discussed previously.

Balancing client confidentiality with reporting may be more difficult if the veterinarian suspects that the animal was intentionally poisoned by the client. See *Requirements for Mandatory Reporting of Animal Cruelty* for an expanded discussion of this issue (Babcock, 2006). Briefly, some states have mandatory animal cruelty reporting requirements or immunity from liability if animal cruelty is reported. Specifically Arizona, California, Illinois, Kansas, Minnesota, Oregon, West Virginia, and Wisconsin have a law requiring the reporting of animal cruelty (Babcock, 2006). Arizona, California, Colorado, Georgia, Idaho, Illinois, Florida, Kansas, Maine, Maryland, Massachusetts, Michigan, Mississippi, New Hampshire, New York, Oregon, Rhode Island, South Carolina, Vermont, Virginia, and West Virginia offer some immunity from liability for reporting suspected animal cruelty (Babcock, 2006). Veterinarians should consult their state licensing board for guidance before concluding that animal poisoning is animal cruelty that requires reporting to entities other than the client.

Some practice acts include very strong client confidentiality components. For example, the Texas Practice Act states:

> "Confidential relationship between the veterinarian and a client:
> Except as provided in subsection (c) of this section, a veterinarian shall not disclose any information concerning the veterinarian's care for an animal except:

> (A) on written or oral authorization or other form of waiver executed by the client; or
> (B) on receipt by the veterinarian of an appropriate court order or subpoena.
> (C) A veterinarian may, without authorization by the client, disclose information contained in a rabies certificate to a governmental entity only for purposes related to the protection of public health and safety." (Texas Board of Veterinary Medical Examiners Rule 573.27 See also Tex Atty Gen Op JM-656. 1987 WL 269439).

In summary, the veterinarian's medical records undergo close scrutiny when cases of pet toxicoses involve the legal system. These cases may involve insurance claims, civil or criminal action in your state. Veterinary medical records are most useful in each of these legal settings when the differential diagnoses is outlined and the results of examination, laboratory testing, consultation, and specific diagnosis are laboratory documented in the medical record.

It may be wise for veterinarians to consult their state licensing board to determine if (1) minimal standards for medical records exist in their state, (2) detection of alcohol or drugs of abuse in a pet requires reporting to anyone other than the client, (3) poisoning an animal could be considered animal cruelty, and (4) their state requires the reporting of animal cruelty.

References and Suggested Reading

Arkansas Code, Annotated § 5-62-102

Babcock SL, Neihsl A: Requirements for mandatory reporting of animal cruelty, *J Am Vet Med Assoc* 228(5):685, 2006.

Block G, Toss J: The relationship between general practitioners and board-certified specialists in veterinary medicine, *J Am Vet Med Assoc* 228(8):1188, 2006.

California Penal Code § 596

Celinski v. State 911 S.W.2d 177 (Tex. App. 1995)

Hawaii Statute § 711-1109

Hawaii Statute § 711-1109.5

Maine Citation: ME ST Tit. 7 § 4011-4018; ME ST Tit. 17 § 1011-1046

Maine Statute Tit. 7 § 4011-4018

Maine Statute Tit. § 1011-1046

Michigan Comp. Laws 750.50b

Minnesota Statutes 2005, Chapter 343.27

North Carolina ST § 14-360-363.2

Nevada ST 574.010-510

New Mexico ST § 30-18-1-15

Ohio ST § 959.01-99

Pennsylvania ST 18 Pa.C.S.A. § 5511

Rollin B: The ethics of referral, *Can Vet J* 47:717, 2006.

Scott JF: Veterinary Medical Records, Proceedings of the American Veterinary Medical Law Association *AVMLA*, 2006 CE Program.

Texas Attorney General Op JM-656. 1987 WL 269439

Texas Board of Veterinary Medical Examiners Rule 573.27

Texas Penal Code Ann. § 42.09

Utah ST § 76-9-301-307

Vermont ST T 13 § 351-400

CHAPTER 23

Urban Legends of Toxicology: Facts and Fiction

FREDERICK W. OEHME, *Manhattan, Kansas*
WILLIAM R. HARE, *Beltsville, Maryland*

Tens of thousands of potentially toxic exposures are reported to United States animal poison control centers annually. Many of these exposures are not life threatening. Understanding the realistic significance of these exposures depends on knowledge of the animal species, the actual toxicity of the chemical to which the animal was exposed, and the circumstances surrounding the exposure.

All substances must be considered potentially toxic; but whether clinical toxicity occurs is simply a matter of the dose delivered to the most sensitive biologic receptor. Given the numerous chemical and biologic variables involved in any exposure instance, it is not surprising that not all exposures to toxic substances result in clinical toxicosis. The role of the clinician is to review the case-by-case circumstances and offer appropriate judgment and recommendations. Favorable outcomes depend on prompt veterinary action in cases of true hazardous exposure.

All too frequently, however, individuals with emotional concerns and limited chemical and medical knowledge become vocal in news and electronic media—AKA the Internet—in declaring toxicologic problems inappropriately. These are often blanket statements incriminating products or situations as being the absolute causes of animal illnesses and deaths. Once these statements become ingrained in the media and are circulated widely, they become "urban legends." Such *urban legends* may be repeatedly presented to veterinary practitioners as inquiries, concerns, or even *facts*.

The truth is that almost all are exaggerations of potentially risky situations or misinterpretations of related information that are erroneously applied to everyday events or behaviors. It then becomes the responsibility of veterinarians to apply their knowledge and people skills to clarify the concerns and hopefully place the urban legend in its appropriate category.

Following are a selected number of statements of toxicosis exposure situations that have commonly been reported to veterinarians. In some cases the concerns are quite valid, whereas in others there is no evidence for significant toxic risk. Many are rumors spread through Internet communications. It almost goes without stating to be careful of Internet misinformation. As much as we all appreciate information, to quote former President Ronald Reagan, "Information is good information only if it can be verified."

Consider how you would respond to the following statements. Are they true, false, or possible? Remember that often it depends on those variables that ultimately come together to affect the outcome of every chemical exposure!

- **Ingestion of Swiffer WetJets kills dogs by liver failure.**
  False: This product contains water (80% to 90%), propylene glycol (1% to 4%), isopropyl alcohol (1% to 4%), and preservatives (0.1%). Propylene glycol is much less toxic than ethylene glycol found in antifreeze, and this concentration of propylene glycol should not be problematic. If there is a problem following ingestion, most likely a foreign body has been introduced, or it is the result of a preexisting condition.

- **Macadamia nuts produce muscle weakness in dogs.**
  True: Weakness, depression, and vomiting usually occur 6 or more hours after ingestion of a moderate quantity. About 1 nut per kilogram of body weight is usually enough to induce adverse clinical signs. Weakness and depression gradually improve after 24 hours in dogs without significant preexisting medical conditions.

- **Ingestion of grapes and raisins may result in acute renal failure in dogs.**
  True: Vomiting, polydipsia, and lethargy can occur 5 to 6 hours after ingestion, followed by anorexia, anuria, tremors, and diarrhea. One to two grapes per kilogram of body weight may be enough to induce adverse clinical signs. Significant ingestion warrants prompt decontamination (emesis) followed by oral dosing with activated charcoal. In addition, aggressive fluid therapy within 48 hours may prevent acute renal failure from developing. Interestingly, this syndrome has not been reported in cats and not in all dogs ingesting these products.

- **Ingestion of sugarless candy/gum containing xylitol is poisonous to dogs.**
  True: Weakness, ataxia, and total collapse may occur 30 to 60 minutes following ingestion of significant amounts of sugarless candy, gum, or breath-mints. Xylitol promotes insulin release by the pancreas, which results in profound hypoglycemia. Absorption is rapid, and activated charcoal is not efficacious in most instances. Acute hypoglycemia is best treated with intravenous dextrose—an initial bolus followed by continuous intravenous drip, with blood glucose concentrations being monitored over the next 12 to 24 hours.

- **Ingestion of Easter lilies (Lilium longiflorum) is highly poisonous to cats.**

  True: Vomiting, hypersalivation, depression, and anorexia usually occur within to 1 to 2 hours after ingestion, followed by anuria and severe renal failure 2 to 4 days later. All parts of the plant should be considered poisonous, and almost all species of *Lilium* should be considered toxic. Dogs only appear to be affected with gastrointestinal upset. The sooner treatment is begun, the better the prognosis.

- **Tea is a good poisoning antidote for cats and dogs.**

  False: Tea may contain 300 to 1200 mg/oz of caffeine, whereas semisweet chocolate contains 22 to 138 mg/oz, making tea on average 5 to 10 times more toxic than chocolate. Tea does have other beneficial actions, but for cats and dogs the bad effects from the high caffeine usually outweigh any potential good.

- **Ingestion of pennies and other coins are of little hazard for household pets.**

  False: United States' pennies minted since 1982 are copper coated, weigh 2.5 g, and contain 97.5% zinc. Although the adverse clinical signs of zinc poisoning, characterized by severe gastroenteritis and marked intravascular hemolysis, may be delayed following the ingestion of pennies, significant lodging of pennies in the acid media of the stomach increases the risk of zinc poisoning. Coins of other value do not contain zinc but can serve as foreign bodies.

- **Ingestion of chocolate can poison cats and dogs.**

  True: All chocolates contain the methylxanthines caffeine and theobromine, which are toxic. Unsweetened baking chocolate (40 and 390 mg/oz) contains the most methylxanthines, and white chocolate (0.8 and 0.2 mg/oz) has the least. Hyperactivity, polydipsia, vomiting, diuresis, diarrhea, restlessness, tachycardia, cardiac arrhythmia, and seizures usually occur in a progressive fashion beginning shortly after significant ingestions. Treatment should be directed at decontamination, control of anxiety and seizures, and the support of renal elimination through fluid diuresis.

- **Centipedes, if eaten by pets, can cause harm to the ingesting animal.**

  True: All species of the order Scolopendromorpha (i.e., centipedes having 21 or 23 pairs of legs) are venomous and can inflict harm by their bites or because they have been ingested. These centipedes have a stinging apparatus connected to their first pair of legs. Little is really known of their venom; however, various proteins, endopeptidase and cardiotoxin (toxin-S), as well as the nonprotein constituents serotonin, histamine, lipids, and various polysaccharides have been identified. No fatalities have been reported; but ingestion can produce vomiting, anxiety, and an irregular heartbeat or may simply induce a mild digestive upset.

- **Pot-scrubbing sponges contain dangerous amounts of Agent Orange (2,4-D + 2,4,5-T).**

  False: Packages of these commercially available sponges are moist inside because a liquid antimicrobial is included to ensure that no fungal growth develops. The antimicrobial agent is a nontoxic disinfectant and even has some perfume added. Now our hands will smell nice after "doing pots and pans." However, if the sponges become grease filled and are ingested, they could lead to gastrointestinal obstruction. It is best to properly dispose of these products following their use.

- **Cocoa beans, coca hulls, cola, coffee, and tea leaves should all be considered emergency ingestions in dogs.**

  True: All contain variable but potentially toxic concentrations of methylxanthines (caffeine, theobromine, and theophylline). Depending on the dose ingested, acute vomiting, excitement, cardiac irregularities, tremors, and seizures may result. Treatment includes early digestive tract evacuation plus activated charcoal/cathartics, diazepam for seizures, and lidocaine or atropine for life-threatening cardiac effects.

- **Febreze, the odor elimination product, is dangerous for household pets.**

  False: Zinc chloride, present in the pre-1998 formulation, was removed, and the product is now sold as a pump spray rather than as an aerosol that could be hazardous for birds in confined spaces. Febreze contains water, alcohol, a corn-derived odor eliminator, and fragrance. Toxicity is not expected with routine use, even with exaggerated exposure.

- **Onions and garlic can be bad for dogs.**

  True: Although *bad* is a relative term, too much acute or lesser-but-frequent dietary onion or garlic produces depression, rapid heart and respiratory rates, and pale mucous membranes. The anemia results from free radicals that cause Heinz bodies to be formed, damage to red blood cells, hemolysis, and methemoglobinemia. Effects persist for several days after exposure stops. Vitamin C and/or administration of other antioxidants may have therapeutic benefits.

- **Herbal products can harm cats and dogs.**

  True: When left open and available, potpourri, garden herbs, cooking powders, perfumes, and various odorants and similar scent products are attractive to cats. The essential oils in such materials are irritants, which cause damage to sensitive respiratory cells, skin epithelium, and mucous membranes in general. Herbal supplements may also contain steroids, benzodiazepines, heavy metals, analgesics, nonsteroidal antiinflammatory drugs, caffeine, atropine, and other constituents that are hazardous to pets that ingest or contact them.

- **Resolve spot and stain carpet cleaner is lethal when ingested by dogs and cats.**

  False: The formulation for this product contains soap, sodium bicarbonate, alcohols 1.5% (ethanol, 2-propanol, and carbinol), glycols 1% (propylene glycol, methyl ether), citrus/pine scent, and water. It is not a lethal formulation. It can cause temporary minor eye irritation and a mild gastrointestinal upset if ingested. It is best to keep all household products out of the reach of pets.

- **Ingestion of caterpillars and butterflies by cats and dogs can be harmful.**

  True: Several types of hair, setae, or bristles cover the bodies of butterflies, moths, and their caterpillars. These hairs are irritants and sometimes are associated with venomous glands. No less than 200 varieties of these insects are known to be poisonous. Harm may result as a dermatologic syndrome, an ophthalmic injury, or respiratory and digestive syndromes. Mild gastrointestinal upset appears to be the most common hazard.

- **Ingestion of poinsettia flowers or leaves can make cats and dogs sick.**

  True: *Native* poinsettia *(Euphorbia pulcherrima)* belongs to the large *Euphorbia* genus of flowering plants. This genus may contain a milkylike sap that contains diterpinoid esters. These compounds can act as irritants. On the other hand, cats or dogs chewing or ingesting the cultivated *ornamental* poinsettia flower or leaves rarely exhibit more than mild gastrointestinal upset or simply drool from the plant's taste. Serious consequences are rarely seen. Treatment usually consists of washing away the sap with a drink of water or milk.

- **Parenteral administration of penicillin G procaine can cause spinal cord damage.**

  False: Penicillin G procaine is an equimolar salt of procaine and penicillin G in sterile solution. Penicillin G is one of the safest parenteral antimicrobial drugs available for use in animals. It has been used successfully for over 50 years. However, there are always exceptions. A significant amount of penicillin G procaine injected directly into the spinal cord or even injected epidurally could cause spinal cord damage. Likewise, use of penicillin in animals known to be hypersensitive to penicillin is problematic. Use is contraindicated in guinea pigs and chinchillas, as well as in certain species of birds, snakes, turtles, and lizards.

- **Vitamins A and D have toxic potential for most animals.**

  True: Excessive amounts of vitamin A promote bone lesions with potential development of exostoses, which in turn may cause pressure on spinal nerves, resulting in paresis or other nerve deficits. Excessive amounts of vitamin D lead to hypercalcemia and calcium deposition of soft tissues, resulting in gastrointestinal, cardiopulmonary, and renal pathophysiology.

- **Ingestion of lipstick by your cat or dog will result in lead poisoning.**

  False: The formulation of lipstick and other cosmetics is closely regulated and does not include lead as a constituent. However, many of the paints used in arts and crafts still do contain potentially dangerous levels of heavy metals (including lead, barium, cadmium, and mercury). Red, yellow, orange, green, violet, vermillion, white, and black paints may contain toxic heavy-metal pigments and may also be potentially carcinogenic.

- **Ultra Clorox contains lye and therefore is potentially dangerous for your dog.**

  False: Both ultra Clorox and regular Clorox bleach formulations contain 5.25% aqueous sodium hypochlorite but not sodium hydroxide (AKA lye). However, sodium hypochlorite is still corrosive and may cause harm from eye or skin contact, ingestion, or inhalation. It is often used as a good premise disinfectant, but it is best to keep it away from pets.

- **Ingestion of Greenies treats is enjoyable but not risk free for cats and dogs.**

  True: Greenies are hard, green, molded bone-shaped treats that contain wheat gluten, glycerin, cellulose, and other additives that are both enjoyable and nutritious for pets. Greenies are intended to be chewed before ingestion to help prevent oral odors, tartar buildup, and gingivitis. Unfortunately pets occasionally will swallow large pieces of these hard treats rather than chewing them into smaller pieces. Ingestion of large pieces of Greenies has the potential of creating an esophageal or intestinal obstruction and fails to accomplish the intended use.

- **DEET Mosquito repellent products are safe for use on cats and dogs.**

  False: All DEET (N,N-diethyl-m-toluamide)–containing mosquito repellent products are potentially toxic to cats and dogs. Hypersalivation, vomiting, anxiety, tremors, ataxia, and seizures may occur within 6 hours following excessive exposure. Animals need to be decontaminated (dermal washing, oral-activated charcoal), their hydration monitored, and supportive therapy initiated as soon as possible following exposure. There is no antidote.

- **Ingestion of environmental mosquito larvicides containing Bacillus thuringiensis israelensis (Bti) is deadly to cats and dogs.**

  False: All mosquito prevention products containing BTI for use around the home (e.g., floating donuts, granules, liquids, briquettes) are generally safe. They may potentially cause a gastrointestinal upset 3 to 6 hours following ingestion, and on rare occasions ingestion of floating donuts could result in formation of a gastrointestinal obstruction. However, they do help eliminate mosquito pests.

- **Anything and everything can be potentially toxic for a companion animal.**

  True: DOSE ALONE MAKES ALL THE DIFFERENCE !

As may be seen from the previous examples of urban legends taken from various Internet sites, some have selected validity, some are clearly erroneous, and others are half-truths and depend on the circumstances of exposure. Veterinarians called on to respond to clients' concerns about such electronic postings or related neighborhood rumors must use their knowledge, experience, and common sense to provide appropriate, realistic, and professional clarifying information.

In some instances questions about the real toxicologic facts may develop, and other professional resources may be researched. Colleagues certified by the American Board of Veterinary Toxicologists are widely available and can be contacted at nearby universities or animal poison centers. Clarification of related chemical details and the expertise of veterinary toxicologists are usually no more than a telephone call or computer keyboard click away; once the networking has been initiated, keep the phone number or online address in a readily available and visible place. Misconceived or erroneous urban legends fade away slowly!

Suggested Reading

Material Safety Data Sheet (MSDS): For commercial products that are available from manufacturers.

Peterson ME, Talcott PA: *Small animal toxicology*, ed 2, St Louis, 2006, Elsevier.

CHAPTER 24

Toxicosis Treatments

KELLY HALL, *St. Paul, Minnesota*

Small animal cases presenting to veterinarians after known or suspected toxin exposure can be both challenging and rewarding. Unfortunately, important information, including the type of toxin, dose ingested, potential co-exposures, or the time frame in which the patient was exposed may not be readily available at the time of presentation. Consequently attention should be directed toward treating the patient rather than the toxin and to primum non nocere (first, do no harm). Many excellent resources are available to help veterinarians and owners deal with toxin exposure in pets, including SafetyCall International's Pet Poison Helpline (1-800-213-6680), the ASPCA Animal Poison Control Center (1-888-4ANI-HELP), emergency clinics, veterinary schools, veterinary diagnostic laboratories (www.aavld.org), and veterinarians who are board certified in emergency and critical care (ACVECCS) or toxicology (www.abvt.org), among others. This chapter considers decontamination, specific antidotes, and supportive or symptomatic care in small animal patients exposed to toxins and makes suggestions for stocking therapies indicated to treat these patients.

DECONTAMINATION

Exposure to poisonous substances may not always result in toxicity. Toxicity requires both exposure and the adverse effect associated with that toxin. Toxicity is avoided when animals are exposed to subtoxic doses of chemicals. Decontamination and treatment to reduce absorption are indicated when the dose of toxin exposure is unknown or greater than the amount expected to cause clinical signs. Exposures in small animals may include surface or skin, ocular, airway, and most commonly oral.

Surface Exposure

Surface exposure in animals primarily occurs on the skin or eyes. Patients with dermal toxin exposures such as dermal permethrin exposure in cats should be bathed with a mild detergent, rinsed thoroughly, then towel dried. Body temperature should be monitored closely to prevent overcooling with bathing or overheating with dryer use, particularly in patients showing clinical signs or those without a controlled airway. Ocular exposure requires irrigation for 10 to 20 minutes with appropriate saline or other eyewash solutions. Contact lens cleaning solutions should be avoided because they contain agents that can further irritate the eye. A thorough ocular examination (including fluorescein staining for the presence of corneal ulcers and Schirmer tear testing) should be performed after irrigation to evaluate for corneal lesions. If present, these should be treated appropriately.

Oral Exposure

Because of the curious nature of animals (particularly dogs), most toxicities are caused by oral exposure. In these cases inducing vomiting is often useful or curative. When clinically appropriate, emesis can be induced within 2 to 3 hours of toxin ingestion or when the timeline is unknown (unless medically contraindicated). For example, if an owner returns home after longer than 3 hours to find evidence of toxin ingestion, he or she does not know if the toxin was ingested 3 hours earlier (at which point it may be too late to decontaminate via emesis induction) or 30 minutes before the owner's return. A small moist meal may be offered before inducing vomiting to increase the likelihood of the toxin being included in the vomitus. Emetics and dosages used in dogs and cats are listed in Table 24-1.

However, inducing vomiting is contraindicated in seven instances.

1. Species that do not vomit such as some pocket pets, rodents, and rabbits
2. In patients already vomiting (there is no added benefit of emesis induction)
3. Following ingestion of a corrosive agent (emesis induction may further damage the esophagus and oral mucosa during vomiting, potentially leading to esophageal perforation); NOTE: If the agent is corrosive (i.e., bleach, battery acid), administration of water or milk at ≈1 ml/kg orally may be used to help dilute the substance
4. In the patient with epilepsy following ingestion of a stimulant that may induce seizures or in an animal that is already seizing (aspiration hazard)
5. In the patient with cardiovascular disease (emesis induction may be contraindicated because of stimulation of vagal reflexes leading to hypotension, bradycardia, and even cardiac arrest)
6. The comatose or otherwise debilitated patient that may have a reduced gag reflex, predisposing to aspiration pneumonia.
7. When patients have undergone recent abdominal surgery (the increased abdominal pressure may compromise sutures/abdominal wall healing)

When clinically appropriate, activated charcoal (AC) at a dose of 1 to 3 g/kg may be administered after the last vomiting episode via elective eating, orogastric tube administration, or force feeding (if swallowing). A brief delay of 15 to 45 minutes after vomiting is useful to minimize the risk

Table **24-1**

Emetics Used in Dogs and Cats

Emetic	Dose	Side Effects	Comment
3% Hydrogen peroxide	6.5 ml/kg (1 teaspoon/5 cc) Can repeat once after 10 minutes Max: 44 ml per animal (3 tbsp, 9 tsp) Anecdotally, not useful in cats	Severe esophagitis, pharyngitis, or gastritis, especially when overdosed	Readily available Owner can administer at home
Apomorphine	0.04 mg/kg IV or 0.25 mg/kg conjunctiva Reversal agent: naloxone 0.04 mg/kg IM, IV, or SC Use in cats is controversial	Excitement, restlessness, central nervous system or respiratory depression, bradycardia	
Xylazine	Cat: 0.44 mg/kg IM Dog: 1.1 mg/kg SQ or IM Reversal agent: Yohimbine 0.1 mg/kg IV* should be readily available to reverse effects if profound	Cardiovascular and respiratory depression, hypotension, respiratory arrest	
Syrup of ipecac	Cat: 2.2 ml/kg: dilute 50:50 in water Dog: 2.2 ml/kg (not more than 15 ml) Value questioned in human medicine	Increase in lacrimation, salivation, bronchial secretions, and rarely cardiotoxicity, arrhythmias, hypotension, or fatal myocarditis	Owner can administer at home Unpalatable: may need nasogastric or orogastric tube to deliver in cats

IM, Intramuscularly; *IV*, intravenously; *SQ*, subcutaneously.

of charcoal aspiration or charcoal vomiting. However, too long of a delay in administrating AC may result in more toxin being absorbed in the small intestine. A benefit of using apomorphine for emesis induction is that the effects can be reversed once the subconjunctival sac is flushed (or reversed with naloxone). If hydrogen peroxide is used to induce vomiting, there is always a risk the dog may vomit up the AC that was just delivered. Repeating half of the initial AC dose every 4 to 8 hours is useful in patients that have ingested toxins that have enterohepatic recirculation such as marijuana, nonsteroidal antiinflammatory drugs, ivermectin, and bromethalin. Finally the use of AC should be avoided when caustic material has been ingested because AC may potentially mask the ability to endoscopically evaluate the esophagus and gastrointestinal tract for damage.

Cathartics are included in many AC formulations to decrease gastrointestinal transit time. Specific cathartics include sodium sulfate (1 g/kg of body weight) and mineral oil (2 to 10 ml for cats and 5 to 30 ml for dogs). Extreme caution should be used with administration of mineral oil because aspiration into the airways from vomiting or misplacement of the orogastric tube can have catastrophic consequences.

SPECIFIC ANTIDOTES

A small number of toxins have antidotes that are indicated when clinical signs of toxicity occur despite decontamination measures. An antidote is an agent that counteracts a poison and neutralizes its effects. Table 24-2 lists these antidotes, their indications, the appropriate dose, and recommendations for stocking in practice. Antidotes are discussed in the following paragraphs based on toxin.

Acetaminophen Toxicity

The combined use of *N*-acetylcysteine, cimetidine (Tagamet), and ascorbic acid is more effective in treating acetaminophen toxicity than any of the therapies used alone. Stocking *N*-acetylcysteine and *S*-adenosylmethionine (SAM-e) or having readily available access to a 24-hour pharmacy is suggested for veterinary practices because of the short period of time available for intervention in acetaminophen toxicosis. Cimetidine (intravenously) and ascorbic acid (oral or intramuscularly, as labeled) are over-the-counter medications that can be added to the therapy regimen as soon as accessible if not stocked.

N-Acetylcysteine increases the synthesis and availability of glutathione, which binds and inactivates hepatotoxic metabolites of acetaminophen. Cimetidine may slow metabolism of acetaminophen into toxic metabolites by inhibiting the p-450 system in the liver. Ascorbic acid (vitamin C) enhances reduction of methemoglobin back to hemoglobin. SAM-e may be useful based on recent evidence suggesting that administration within 1 hour of acetaminophen ingestion to cats at a dose of 180 mg every 12 hours for 3 days and then 90 mg every 12 hours for 11 days improves clinical outcome (Webb et al., 2003). SAM-e use in a dog with acetaminophen toxicity has also been reported at an initial dose of 40 mg/kg of body weight orally followed by 20 mg/kg of body weight orally every 24 hours for 7 days (Wallace et al., 2002).

Anticoagulant Rodenticide Toxicity

Active vitamin K_1 enables the liver to produce clotting factors II, VII, IX, and X when their production is inhibited

Table 24-2

Antidotes Used in Dogs and Cats

Toxin	Antidote	Dose*	Recommended Practice Holdings (General, Emergency or Both)
Acetaminophen	Acetylcysteine (e.g., Mucomyst)	140 mg/kg PO initially, then 70 mg/kg q4h PO for at least 3-5 more treatments	Both
	Cimetidine (e.g., Tagamet)	5-10 mg/kg q6-8h PO or IV	Emergency
	Ascorbic acid (vitamin C)	20-30 mg/kg q6h PO	Neither
	S-adenosylmethionine (SAM-e)	<10 kg: 200-225 mg q24h PO 10 kg: 20 mg/kg (minimum dose) q24h PO	Both
Anticoagulant rodenticides	Vitamin K_1	2.5-5 mg/kg q24h PO, SC × 2-6 weeks (depends on specific anticoagulant) Oral absorption is more rapid (with a meal) than SC; intramuscular injection is contraindicated in coagulopathic animals	Injectable: both Oral: emergency
Cholinesterase inhibitors	Pralidoxime chloride (2-PAM) *Organophosphate toxicity only: DO NOT use in carbamate toxicity*	10-20 mg/kg q8-12h IV (slowly) or SQ for at least 36 h	Emergency
Organophosphate or carbamate toxicity	Atropine	0.1-0.5 mg/kg, ¼ given IV with the remainder given IM or SQ; administered as needed	Both
Ethylene glycol (antifreeze)	Ethanol 20%	Dog: 5.5 ml/kg q4h × 5 doses, then q6h × 4; dosed IV as CRI over 1 h Cat: 5 ml/kg q6h × 5, then q8h × 4; dosed IV as CRI over 1 h	Both
	Fomepizole (4- methylpyrazole)	Dog: 20 mg/kg initially, 15 mg/kg at 12 and 24 hr, 5 mg/kg at 36 hr IV Cat: 125 mg/kg initially, 31.25 mg/kg at 24, 48 and 72 h IV	Both
Metals *Lead, zinc, copper, iron*	Calcium EDTA	25 mg/kg q6h for 2-5 days SQ (dilute with D_5W solution to 10 mg/ml)	Both
Lead, mercury, arsenic	Meso-2.3 dimercaptosuccinic acid (DMSA, succimer)	10 mg/kg q8h for 5 days, then 10 mg/kg q12h for 2 weeks PO	Emergency
Iron	Deferoxamine	10 mg/kg q8h for 24 h IM or IV	Emergency
Metronidazole	Diazepam	Dog: 0.2-0.7 mg/kg initially IV, then q8h PO Cat: unknown (oral diazepam can be associated with hepatic necrosis in cats)	Both
Serotonin syndrome	Cyproheptadine	Dog: 1.1 mg/kg, q4-6 h PO Cat: 2-4 mg/cat, q4-6 h PO Can crush, dilute in saline, and give rectally; can administer until signs resolve	Emergency

*Dog and cat dose if not further specified.
CRI, Continuous-rate infusion; *DMSA*, dimercaptosuccinic acid (DMSA, succimer); *D_5W*, 5% dextrose in water; *EDTA*, ethylenediaminetetraacetic acid; *IM*, Intramuscularly; *IV*, intravenously; *SQ*, subcutaneously; *NE*, nasoesophageal; *PO*, orally.

by anticoagulant rodenticides. Vitamin K_1 therapy takes approximately 6 to 12 hours after oral or subcutaneous administration to clinically improve circulating clotting factor activity. It is best absorbed orally when given with a small fatty meal that stimulates bile salt secretion. Therapy needs to continue as long as anticoagulant rodenticide is in the body. This may be 2 to 4 weeks for the newer compounds. See Chapter 25 for more detail. Prothrombin time should be evaluated 48 to 72 hours after therapy has ended to ensure appropriate efficacy of therapy. Oral dosing can be initiated in eating, asymptomatic patients; however, the subcutaneous injectable form may be necessary in patients symptomatic for blood loss associated with toxicity. Intramuscular injections are not recommended in animals with a coagulopathy or thrombocytopenia. Finally, intravenous vitamin K_1 can result in acute anaphylactoid reactions. The injectable form of vitamin K_1 should be available in all practices.

Cholinesterase Inhibitor Toxicity

Organophosphate and carbamate insecticides are termed cholinesterase inhibitors. These chemicals inhibit the cholinesterase enzyme and reduce the normal breakdown of acetylcholine. Acetylcholine is a transmitter for both the nicotinic and muscarinic systems. Clinical signs are associated with overstimulation of these pathways.

Pralidoxime chloride (2-PAM) may relieve the nicotinic signs of muscle fasciculation and the muscarinic signs of salivation, bronchospasm, lacrimation, urination, or defecation in cholinesterase inhibitor toxicosis. It is most effective when given within 24 hours of exposure; thus it should be stocked or otherwise readily available. A greater time delay between exposure and 2-PAM treatment allows for stronger binding of some organophosphates with the cholinesterase enzyme. This binding makes 2-PAM therapy ineffective. 2-PAM is not indicated in cases of carbamate carbaryl toxicosis because it also inhibits the cholinesterase enzyme to some degree.

Atropine is typically stocked in most practices for multiple purposes and can be used in cholinesterase inhibitor toxicity to assist with resolution of muscarinic signs. Glycopyrrolate can also be used but has a slower onset and a longer duration of action and can be used in lieu of atropine.

Ethylene Glycol (Antifreeze) Toxicity

Acute renal failure in ethylene glycol (EG) toxicity is caused by oxalate and other products formed by metabolism of the EG molecule. Fomepizole and ethanol competitively inhibit alcohol and aldehyde dehydrogenase to prevent formation of these nephrotoxic metabolites. Initiation of therapy within 6 to 8 hours in dogs and 2 to 3 hours in cats of EG exposure is paramount for a successful outcome. Consequently, one or both of these products should be stocked in all practices.

Fomepizole (4-methylpyrazole) used at high doses has been successful in cats if initiated within 3 hours of exposure (Connally, Thrall, and Hamar, 2002). Fomepizole is quite expensive, which may be a factor in stocking for some practices.

Ethanol (20% concentration) may be beneficial if adverse effects are appreciated. Addition of 250 ml of 100% ethanol (e.g., Everclear) to 1-L bag of crystalloid fluid creates a 20% solution. Although profound central nervous system depression and increased serum osmolality side effects can be observed, the time frame of therapy overrides these factors. Ethanol should still be given judiciously, with cessation if any of the clinical signs are observed: lateral nystagmus, respiratory depression, or if the patient becomes too obtunded.

Metals

Therapies for lead, zinc, iron, copper, and other metal toxicosis include chelating agents that "trap" the metal to form a water-soluble product that enhances urinary excretion. Deferoxamine is the most effective chelator of iron. Deferoxamine therapy works best if administered within 12 hours of ingestion or exposure. Supportive care alone may not prevent mortality. Calcium ethylenediaminetetraacetic acid is a chelator useful in lead and zinc toxicity, although it is only available in injectable form. Meso-2,3 dimercaptosuccinic acid is another chelator useful in lead toxicosis. Lead should be removed from the gastrointestinal tract before initiating oral therapy to prevent chelation and enhancing lead absorption from the gastrointestinal tract. D-penicillamine can be effective for long-term oral therapy of lead toxicity.

Metronidazole Toxicity

Diazepam is useful for management of neurologic toxicity associated with dogs that are receiving metronidazole (especially at dosages greater than 30 mg of metronidazole per kilogram per day for 3 to 14 days). Evans and colleagues (2003) documented significantly decreased recovery times in metronidazole toxicity when patients were treated with diazepam and supportive care for 3 days versus supportive care alone. Immediate improvement (which may be mild) can be seen when intravenous diazepam (Valium) is given as a one-time dose. Because injectable valium is an important therapy for seizure activity, it is recommended for virtually all causes of seizures and should be stocked in all small animal practices.

Serotonin Syndrome Toxicity

Serotonin is a neurotransmitter that acts centrally as an excitatory inhibitor and peripherally to stimulate smooth muscle. Many medications affect the amount of serotonin present in the synaptic space; these include the monoamine oxidase inhibitors, selective serotonin reuptake inhibitors, and tricyclic antidepressants. Serotonin syndrome is caused by excessive serotonin in the synaptic space and was originally defined in humans as a constellation of symptoms, including at least three of the following: myoclonus, mental aberration, agitation, hyperreflexia, tremors, diarrhea, ataxia, and hyperthermia.

Cyproheptadine is a nonselective serotonin antagonist. If a positive clinical response is noted, it can be repeated every 4 to 6 hours orally or crushed and dissolved in saline and administered rectally until resolution of signs.

GENERAL THERAPIES

There is no specific antidote for most toxins. Furthermore, many sick veterinary patients have undiagnosed disease, with toxin exposure considered on their rule-out list. Accordingly, supportive and symptomatic care is the cornerstone for therapy in many patients—with and without known toxin ingestion. Table 24-3 lists therapies that are useful to stock in any practice, particularly for supportive care of toxicity patients. Determination of which items to stock is accomplished by reviewing frequency of use, shelf life, and availability from suppliers and local hospitals.

Table 24-3

General Therapies Useful in Supportive and Symptomatic Treatment of Poisonings

Drug	Use
Acepromazine	Sedation, anxiolytic
Ammonium chloride	Urinary acidification
Atropine	Bradycardia
β-blockers	Tachycardia
Calcium gluconate	Hypocalcemia
Dextrose solution	Hypoglycemia, hyperkalemia
Diazepam	Sedation/anticonvulsant
Dobutamine	Blood pressure support
Dopamine	Renal perfusion, blood pressure support
Doxapram	Respiratory stimulant
Fluids (e.g., crystalloid and colloid)	Volume expansion, rehydration, etc.
Furosemide	Hypercalcemia, diuresis
Mannitol	Cerebral edema, anuric renal failure
Naloxone	Opioid reversal
Opioids	Sedation, pain relief
Oxygen	Hypoxemia, CNS disease, carbon monoxide toxicity
Pentobarbital	Heavy sedation, anticonvulsant
Phenobarbital	Heavy sedation, anticonvulsant
Potassium chloride	Hypokalemia
Propofol	Anesthesia, heavy sedation
Sodium bicarbonate	Metabolic acidosis, hyperkalemia
Sucralfate	Esophageal and gastrointestinal protectant

CNS, Central nervous system.

References and Suggested Reading

Bonagura JD: *Kirk's Current veterinary therapy XIII*, Philadelphia, 2000, Saunders.

Connally HE, Thrall MA, Hamar DW: *Safety and efficacy of high-dose fomepizole as therapy for ethylene glycol intoxication in cats*, Abstracts from the 8th International Veterinary Emergency and Critical Care Symposium, 2002.

Evans J: Diazepam as a treatment for metronidazole toxicosis in dogs: a retrospective study of 21 cases, *J Vet Intern Med* 17:304, 2003.

Plumb DC: *Veterinary drug handbook*, ed 5, Ames, 2005, Blackwell Publishing.

Plunkett SJ: *Emergency procedures for the small animal veterinarians*, ed 2, Philadelphia, 2001, Saunders.

Wallace et al KP: *S-adenosyl-L-methionine (SAM-e) for the treatment of acetaminophen toxicity in a dog*, *J Am Anim Hosp Assoc* 38(3):246, 2002.

Webb CB et al: *S-adenosylmethionine (SAM-e) in a feline acetaminophen model of oxidative injury*, *J Feline Med Surg* 5:69, 2003.

Wingfield WE: *Veterinary emergency medicine secrets*, ed 2, Philadelphia, 2001, Hanley & Belfus.

CHAPTER 25
Rodenticide Toxicoses

MICHAEL J. MURPHY, *St. Paul, Minnesota*

Pesticides account for about 25% of toxin exposures in pets. Insecticides (see Chapter 26) and rodenticides are the majority of these pesticide exposures. The rodenticides most frequently encountered by dogs and cats are anticoagulant rodenticides, cholecalciferol, strychnine, zinc phosphide, and bromethalin. Cholecalciferol is discussed in Chapter 36. The key aspects of toxicosis associated with anticoagulant rodenticides, bromethalin, strychnine, and zinc phosphide follow.

ANTICOAGULANT RODENTICIDES

The anticoagulant rodenticides continue to be the pesticide most commonly inquired about by animal owners. These compounds (including warfarin, brodifacoum, bromadiolone, diphacenone, and chlorophacinone) represent a substantial proportion of actual toxicoses treated in veterinary and emergency clinics. All anticoagulant rodenticides act by inhibiting the recycling of vitamin K_1 from vitamin K_1 epoxide reductase. This inhibition leads to a reduction in the active forms of clotting factors II, VII, IX, and X in circulation, with factor VII and the extrinsic pathway affected initially. The reduction in the active forms of these factors leads to prolonged clotting times. Prolonged clotting time is most commonly measured by activated clotting time (ACT), one-stage prothrombin time (PT), activated partial thromboplastin time (APTT), or a combination of these tests in the clinic. Prolongation of these times to 15% to 25% above the upper end of the normal range is commonly interpreted as a coagulopathy. Toxic doses of anticoagulant rodenticides induce a coagulopathy. The coagulopathy is not always apparent on clinical presentation and typically is delayed for a number of days following ingestion. The so-called *second-generation* anticoagulant rodenticides have a much longer duration of action when compared to warfarin. The toxic dose and LD_{50} for various anticoagulant rodenticides in dogs and cats is quite variable. Data for specific compounds can be found in consultation with toxicologists.

Anticoagulant rodenticide toxicosis should be considered in dogs or cats with dyspnea or exercise intolerance related to intrathoracic or intrapulmonary hemorrhage. Intrapulmonary hemorrhage occurs commonly in anticoagulant redactive toxicosis. Large pleural effusions and marked intrapulmonary hemorrhage (seen as a coarse, alveolar lung pattern) may be evident on thoracic radiography. Prolonged bleeding from venipuncture sites may be observed. Hematomas, hematemesis, melena, hemoptysis, hematuria, and pallor of mucous membranes are other relatively common clinical signs observed in animals with anticoagulant rodenticide toxicosis. Bleeding may occur in unusual locations such as the pericardial space or into the spinal cord. Of course, anticoagulant rodenticides represent just one cause of coagulopathies in dogs and cats (see Chapters 59 to 62), and other bleeding disorders must be considered.

Detection of the specific anticoagulant rodenticide in serum is the most definitive means of confirming exposure to an anticoagulant rodenticide in a live animal. Liver is the specimen of choice for a dead animal. This testing is now available in many veterinary diagnostic laboratories throughout the United States (see www.aavld.org).

Anticoagulant rodenticide-induced coagulopathies are commonly distinguished from other causes of coagulopathy in the clinic by a relatively rapid response to vitamin K_1 treatment. ACT, PT, and APTT are each dramatically shortened within 24 hours of initiating daily therapy with 2.5 to 5 mg/kg of vitamin K_1 administered orally or subcutaneously (but *not* intravenously or intramuscularly) with a small-gauge needle. Anaphylaxis can occur with parenteral administration of K_1 by any route. Failure to see an initial response may suggest that the coagulopathy is not caused by anticoagulant rodenticide exposure. *Oral* therapy is very effective; some clinicians divide the daily dose into two or three treatments and aim to enhance absorption of the vitamin by administration with a fatty meal.

In certain cases of recent ingestion (within 2 to 4 hours of presentation), general measures for treatment of toxicosis should be considered, including induction of emesis and administration of activated charcoal (see Chapter 24). Clotting tests are often normal in these cases so they should be monitored for at least 3 days. Vitamin K_1 treatment should be administered if the clotting time is prolonged.

A severe coagulopathy may call for more than simple vitamin K_1 treatment, and the clinician must appreciate that effects of vitamin K_1 are not immediate. Animals with a packed cell volume less than 15 or those demonstrating complications of anemia may need fresh whole blood immediately. Furthermore, vitamin K_1 alone may be insufficient when results of coagulation tests show rapidly progressing prolongation in clotting times. In these cases, administration of fresh or frozen plasma may be needed to provide clotting factors. Blood product therapy may be required for 12 to 36 hours after initiating vitamin K_1 therapy to allow time for the synthesis of new functional clotting factors. Thoracocentesis may be needed if there is significant dyspnea related to bleeding within the pleural space. Rest and oxygen are appropriate for intrapulmonary hemorrhage.

The dose and duration indicated for vitamin K_1 varies with the specific anticoagulant rodenticide responsible for the coagulopathy. Dosages of 1 to 2.5 mg/kg daily for 3 to 5 days were often effective in treating toxicoses caused by warfarin and other first-generation anticoagulant rodenticides. The second-generation compounds, including brodifacoum, diphacenone, and chlorophacinone, now comprise the majority of the market share; thus many practices treat with vitamin K_1 at 2.5 to 5 mg/kg daily for 2 to 4 weeks, especially if the specific anticoagulant rodenticide is not identified with certainty. Tests of clotting function can be useful guides for the duration of therapy. The bioavailability of vitamin K_1 is greatest when given orally; thus this route is preferred unless contraindicated because of vomiting. Vitamin K_1 may be given subcutaneously but should not be given intramuscularly or intravenously because of the increased risk of massive hemorrhage or anaphylaxis, respectively. Vitamin K_3 therapy is contraindicated because it is not efficacious and may induce oxidative damage to red cells.

Clients should be educated to remove all anticoagulant rodenticide bait from the pet's environment. Unfortunately pets occasionally are reexposed to rodenticide bait following discharge from the clinic. The long-acting anticoagulant rodenticides may be present in the serum and liver of the pet for weeks following successful treatment and recovery. Accordingly some anticoagulant rodenticides may be detected by analytic chemistry techniques in animals with no demonstrable coagulopathy and consequently no toxicosis.

BROMETHALIN

Bromethalin is the active ingredient in rodenticide baits marked under the trade names Assault (Agrisel) and Terminator (Syngenta). This compound acts by uncoupling oxidative phosphorylation and leads to hyperexcitability in the acute phase of toxicosis followed by depression in the chronic phase. Muscle tremors, seizures, hind limb hyperreflexia, and death may be observed within approximately 10 hours after exposure to 5 mg/kg. These signs may progress to depression, recumbency, coma, and death. Clinical signs of toxicosis may persist for up to 12 days after exposure to 2.5 mg/kg of bromethalin.

With analysis of bait, stomach contents, or vomitus it is possible to confirm exposure to bromethalin in a veterinary patient. Analysis of tissues, including fat, may be used to confirm exposure at postmortem examination. Routine complete blood count, serum biochemistries, and urinalysis generally do not assist in the diagnosis of exposure to bromethalin.

No specific antidote exists. Aggressive charcoal therapy (see Chapter 24) is aimed at reducing absorption and possible enterohepatic circulation of bromethalin. Mannitol and glucocorticoids have been used to reduce cerebral fluid pressure, but they may not reliably reverse clinical signs.

STRYCHNINE

Strychnine distribution has been restricted in many areas of the United States. It has been replaced by zinc phos-

phide in many areas. Nevertheless, strychnine toxicosis is seen occasionally in clinical practice. Strychnine inhibits the postsynaptic buffering effects of glycine on sensory stimulation of motor neurons and interneurons. Consequently strychnine-poisoned animals appear apprehensive, tense, and stiff within minutes to hours of exposure. Rectal temperature may be increased from muscular hyperactivity. Clinical signs progress to tonic extensor rigidity, especially after sensory stimulation by light, sound, or touch. Animals often die in opisthotonus because of paralysis of respiratory muscles.

Urine samples obtained from a live animal and stomach contents retrieved from a dead animal are the samples of choice for analytic confirmation of exposure to strychnine. Other toxins can result in musculoskeletal stimulation, including mycotoxins, nicotine (Chapter 30), insecticides (Chapter 26), and zinc phosphide (see next section). Tetanus and hypocalcemia are other considerations.

Therapy is centered on sedating the patient to prevent seizures. This allows time for strychnine metabolism. Pentobarbital (2 to 15 mg/kg intravenously for dogs), administered to effect, is the most often used sedative/anticonvulsant. Methocarbamol may be administered for muscle relaxation at doses of 55 to 220 mg/kg intravenously. One half of the dose can be given as a bolus, with the rest administered slowly to effect. Daily dose should not exceed 330 mg/kg. Although diazepam normally is the initial drug of choice for seizing animals, efficacy for strychnine-induced seizures is variable. Activated charcoal may be administered to reduce further absorption as long as precipitation of seizures is avoided. Stimulation should be avoided, and a quiet, darkened hospital kennel may be beneficial. The patient should be given good nursing care, with attention to clinical and vital signs, as well as rectal temperature. Other treatments may include intravenous fluids and urinary acidification (ammonium chloride) to assist with urinary excretion.

ZINC PHOSPHIDE

Zinc phosphide is used for rodent and mole control and marketed under an increasing number of trade names, including Bartlett Waxed Mouse-Bait, Burrow Oat Bait, Rodent Bait, Rodent Pellets, ZIP RTU Bait, ZP Rodent Bait, and ZP Tracking Powder. This compound is more and more prevalent since it has replaced strychnine in many areas of the United States.

Animals exposed to zinc phosphide have a rapid course of clinical signs. These can progress through anorexia, lethargy, dyspnea, vomiting (occasionally with hematemesis), ataxia, agitation, muscle tremors, weakness, recumbency, and death. Signs develop within minutes to hours of ingestion of a toxic dose of zinc phosphide. Detection of zinc phosphide in the vomitus of a live animal or stomach contents of a dead animal supports the animal's exposure to it. Unfortunately this compound is volatile; freezing contents in air-tight receptacles may enhance the likelihood of detection in an analytic laboratory.

There is no specific antidote for zinc phosphide. Treatment is mainly supportive. Methods aimed at moving zinc phosphide from the stomach in known cases of ingestion, including emetics, can be used. Increasing gastric pH may be helpful by reducing phosgene liberation. Milk of magnesia has been used as a home remedy; in the hospital gastric lavage with 5% sodium bicarbonate (take care to prevent bloat) may be used. Diazepam or pentobarbital may be needed for excessive musculoskel-etal activity or seizures. In addition to intravenous fluid therapy, liver-supportive agents may be considered.

Suggested Reading

Murphy MJ: Rodenticides. *Vet Clin North Am Small Anim Pract,* 32:469, 2002.

CHAPTER **26**

Insecticide Toxicoses

PATRICIA A. TALCOTT, *Pullman, Washington*

Insecticides used in the United States to which small animals may be exposed include the organophosphate and carbamate cholinesterase inhibitor insecticides, the pyrethrin and pyrethroid groups of insecticides, the triazapentadiene compound amitraz, botanical insecticides, and miscellaneous insecticides that do not fit in any of these aforementioned groups. Each of these groups is discussed in turn.

ORGANOPHOSPHATE AND CARBAMATE INSECTICIDES

Organophosphate and carbamate insecticide poisonings are still one of the most commonly encountered toxicoses in small animals because of their widespread use on animals, around the house, and in agriculture (Hansen, 1995a, p. 245; Bonagura, 2000, p. 231). These insecticides may be used on animals intentionally or accidentally. Many exposures are accidental, caused by either inappropriate use by the applicator or accidental access to the product by the pet because of inappropriate storage or disposal of these compounds. Many insecticide products are intended to be applied to the premises or other property, but some are components of pet products including shampoos, flea and tick collars, and insecticide dips.

These products are generally formulated with oily vehicles or solvents to increase contact time and enhance stability. Literally hundreds of formulations are marketed in the form of sprays, dips, shampoos, collars, foggers, or bombs. These marketed products are sometimes mixed with food items to intentionally or maliciously expose pets.

Hundreds of cholinesterase inhibitor insecticides are marketed in the United States. See Box 26-1 for a list of some of the more commonly used chemicals. The toxicity of these chemicals varies widely. Unfortunately there are few well-established toxic or lethal doses for dogs or cats reported in the literature. Dermal or oral exposures are commonly encountered by dogs or cats. The inhalation route of exposure is more common in humans. Most of the organophosphate and carbamate insecticides are rapidly metabolized by hepatic enzymes; then both the parent compound and its metabolites are rapidly eliminated in the urine. However, a few lipophilic compounds have longer half-lives, giving them a greater potential to cause central nervous system effects.

Both the organophosphate and carbamate insecticides inhibit the acetylcholinesterase (AChE) and pseudocholinesterase enzymes. AChE is responsible for breaking down acetylcholine released at cholinergic sites. Thus animals poisoned with cholinesterase inhibitors often exhibit a mixture of clinical signs as a result of overstimulation of the nicotinic receptors of the somatic nervous system (skeletal muscle), sympathetic and parasympathetic preganglionic junctions, all parasympathetic postganglionic junctions (few sympathetic postganglionic junctions), and some neurons within the central nervous system.

The onset of clinical signs can vary between a few minutes to several hours, depending on the dose, the route of exposure, and the specific chemical involved. Commonly reported muscarinic signs include excessive salivation, anorexia, emesis, diarrhea, excessive lacrimation, miosis or mydriasis, dyspnea, excessive urination, and bradycardia or tachycardia. The mnemonics SLUD (i.e., salivation, lacrimation, urination, defecation) and DUMBBELS (i.e., diarrhea, urination, miosis, bronchospasm, bradycardia, emesis, lacrimation, salivation) are often used in the classroom

Box 26-1

Examples of Insecticides

Cholinesterase Inhibitors
Organophosphates
- Chlorpyrifos
- Coumaphos
- Cythioate
- Diazinon
- Dichlorvos
- Dimethoate
- Disulfoton
- Ethoprop
- Famphur
- Fenthion
- Malathion
- Mevinphos
- Parathion
- Phorate
- Phosmet
- Terbufos
- Tetrachlorvinphos

Carbamates
- Aldicarb
- Carbaryl
- Carbofuran
- Methiocarb
- Methomyl
- Oxamyl
- Propoxur

Pyrethrins, Pyrethroids
- Allethrin,
- Bifenthrin
- Bioallethrin
- Cismethrin
- Cyfluthrin
- Cyhalothrin
- Cypermethrin
- Deltamethrin
- Esfenvalerate
- Fenfluthrin
- Fenvalerate
- Flumethrin
- Fluvalinate
- Permethrin
- Phenothrin
- Pyrethrin
- Pyrethrum
- Resmethrin
- Sumethrin
- Tetramethrin
- Tralomethrin

Triazapentadiene Compounds
- Amitraz

Botanicals
- d-Limonene
- Linalool
- Melaleuca oil
- Pennyroyal oil
- Rotenone

Miscellaneous
- Fipronil
- Imidacloprid
- Lufenuron
- Methoprene
- Methoxychlor
- Nitenpyram
- Pyriproxifen
- DEET
- Avermectins

---

as a device to remember these changes. Prominent nicotinic signs include ataxia, weakness, and muscle twitching. In acute high-dose oral exposures, seizures can occur within 10 to 20 minutes. It is important to note that not all signs are seen in every poisoning case. Death is generally the result of respiratory failure and tissue hypoxia caused by excessive respiratory secretions, bronchoconstriction, paralysis of the respiratory muscles, and direct depression of the respiratory center in the medulla. Cats appear to be particularly sensitive to chlorpyrifos; anorexia, muscle weakness, ataxia, and depression are the predominant features. Exposure to these more lipophilic compounds has been referred to as the intermediate syndrome; additional clinical features may include muscle tremors, abnormal mentation, and abnormal posturing with hyperesthesia.

A clinical diagnosis of organophosphate or carbamate poisoning relies heavily on observing compatible clinical signs and a history of known exposure. Inhibition of whole blood, plasma, serum, retinal, or brain cholinesterase activity (at least 25% to 50% of normal) suggests an exposure to these compounds and toxicosis if the clinical signs are compatible. Cholinesterase testing can still be performed after the administration of atropine and may still be useful several days after pesticide exposure. Lack of inhibition cannot rule out exposure to carbamate compounds because of the reversibility of their binding to the cholinesterase enzyme. In addition, because of the acuteness in onset of signs and possible death and the lack of some compounds to readily traverse the blood-brain barrier, brain cholinesterase may be normal in the acutely poisoned patient. Lower red blood cell counts may also lower true AChE activity; this is one reason to check the packed cell volume before running the assay. Therefore cholinesterase testing should be regarded as a screening tool, and false negatives and positives may occur. Tissue analysis for the organophosphate or carbamate insecticide is primarily reserved for confirming an exposure following a postmortem examination. Stomach and intestinal contents, liver, kidney, fat, and skin (in cases of suspect dermal exposures) should be collected, individually bagged and labeled, and kept frozen during shipment to a laboratory.

Changes observed on a complete blood count, serum chemistry panel, and urinalyses are typically very nonspecific and highly variable. Pancreatitis accompanied by significant elevations in amylase and lipase has been reported following exposures to certain organophosphate insecticides.

Treatment should be aimed at preventing further absorption through aggressive decontamination procedures and controlling the muscarinic and nicotinic clinical signs. Many dermal exposures lead to subsequent oral exposures, particularly in cats; thus multiple decontamination procedures may be needed. In the asymptomatic orally exposed patient, emetics such as 3% hydrogen peroxide [a dose of 1 ml/pound; do not exceed a total dose of 10 ml in the cat or 50 ml in the dog, regardless of body weight; this volume has been routinely exceeded in dogs, and I have observed few serious complications; it can be used shortly after feeding a small amount of food] or apomorphine are generally recommended. If emesis is contraindicated, a gastric lavage can be performed after inducing light anesthesia, followed by the placement of a cuffed endotracheal tube. Induction of emesis and gastric lavage should always be followed with the use of activated charcoal and a cathartic. Administration of multiple activated charcoal doses may be warranted; care should be taken to reduce the subsequent cathartic doses and monitor the patient for the rare occurrence of hypernatremia or hypermagnesemia. A mild detergent bath and thorough rinsing are recommended in cases of dermal exposure. In the topically exposed patients, particularly cats, exposure may be both dermal and oral because of excessive grooming. In these cases both dermal and oral decontamination procedures may be beneficial.

Atropine sulfate, 0.20 to 0.50 mg/kg (one fourth intravenously [IV], the remainder subcutaneously [SC] or intramuscularly [IM]; some individuals administer the entire dosage IV), is used to control the muscarinic signs (e.g., miosis, salivation, diarrhea, bradycardia, bronchoconstriction). The dosage selected should be just enough to provide adequate atropinization, and atropine may be repeated at half the initial dose if signs return. Hypersalivation is often the most useful clinical sign for monitoring atropine therapy. Oxygen therapy with or without artificial respiration may be required until the patient is breathing normally on its own.

Seizures, muscle tremors, or agitation can be controlled with intravenous diazepam, methocarbamol, or phenobarbital. Pralidoxime chloride (2-PAM; 10 to 20 mg/kg IM or SC BID or TID) can help reduce muscle tremors resulting from nicotinic receptor stimulation by an organophosphate. A clinical effect should be observed within the first 3 to 4 days, and treatment should be continued as long as improvement is observed. 2-PAM has its best effect if administered within 24 hours of exposure; but some benefits may occur, particularly in cases involving large toxin exposures, if given within 36 to 48 hours. Rapid intravenous injection may cause tachycardia, muscle rigidity, transient neuromuscular blockage, and laryngospasm. The use of oximes in cases of carbamate poisonings is somewhat controversial (particularly since the carbamate binding is reversible); one should weigh the benefits and risks of its use in each case. It is impossible to tell based on clinical signs alone whether the exposure was caused by an organophosphate or a carbamate insecticide.

Diphenhydramine use is also controversial in the treatment of organophosphate and carbamate poisonings; I do not recommend it. One suggested dose of diphenhydramine in dogs is 2 to 4 mg/kg orally every 6 to 8 hours. However, there have been reports of excessive sedation or excitement and anorexia when used in dogs and cats.

Good supportive and nursing care, including intravenous fluid therapy, adequate nutritional management, and maintenance of normal body temperature and electrolyte balance, should also be considered in the acutely poisoned patient. Chlorpyrifos poisoning in cats requires special attention; these cats often show signs of ataxia, anorexia, depression, and muscle tremors for several days or weeks after initial exposure.

PYRETHRINS/PYRETHROIDS

Pyrethrins are organic esters extracted with fat solvents from flower heads of the pyrethrum plant, *Chrysanthemum cinerariifolium*. Pyrethroids are their synthetic cohorts that vary in both structure and potency. Pyrethroids generally are more toxic to insects and mammals and persist longer in the environment than pyrethrins (Hansen, 1995b; Bonagura, 2000, p. 233). A number of commonly used pyrethrin and pyrethroid chemicals are listed in Box 26-1. Many of these pesticide formulations are registered for topical use on dogs and cats for flea and tick control. Other formulations are marketed for household use, and still others can be used in agriculture. These products can be purchased through many readily available outlets and packaged as sprays, dips, shampoos, and spot-on formulations. The percentages of active ingredient can range from less than 1% to as much as 65% or greater; therefore it is crucial to read the label thoroughly when using them.

There are hundreds of pyrethrin- and pyrethroid-containing formulations, sometimes combined in mixtures along with insect growth regulators, insect repellents, and various synergists. Piperonyl butoxide is a common additive to pyrethrin products. Although it possesses limited insecticidal activity, it acts as a synergist to extend the killing duration of the pyrethrin. The mode of synergistic activity is not conclusively known. Hypothesized mechanisms of the synergistic effect of piperonyl butoxide include (a) prolongation of the action of pyrethrins by preventing rapid oxidation; (b) formation of complexes with the pyrethrins that lead to higher insecticidal activity; or (c) delay of pyrethrin detoxification by the insect's tissue enzymes. A number of pyrethroid products also contain insect repellents.

N-octyl bicycloheptene dicarboximide, di-n-propyl isocinchomeronate, and butoxypolypropylene glycol are insect repellents that are often present in pyrethrin/pyrethroid–containing products at concentrations ranging from 0.34% to 15%. Toxicity of these mixtures may be attributed solely to the pyrethrins and pyrethroids or be caused by the combined effects of the insecticides plus the additives, synergists, and solvents.

Pyrethrins work by stimulating the insect's central nervous system. This action results in muscular excitation, convulsions, and paralysis. When dissolved in thin oils, pyrethrins readily penetrate through the hard, chitinous covering of the insect, and their insecticidal action is rapid. Both pyrethrins and pyrethroids affect nervous tissue in mammals by reversibly prolonging sodium conductance, producing increased depolarizing afterpotentials that result in repetitive nerve firing. Their toxicity to mammals is low and, when used according to label instructions, should not induce deleterious effects in mammals. Toxicoses in mammals can be observed when these products are ingested or where there is overzealous heavy topical application, particularly in cats and small dogs. Many poisonings in clinical practice are the result of products labeled "for use in dogs only" being used on cats. There are also many anecdotal instances in which cats exhibited adverse effects following topical exposure to appropriately applied formulations. Clinical signs are normally observed within minutes to a few hours after exposure.

Clinical signs usually include excessive salivation (as a result of oral sensory stimulation), muscle tremors, depression, ataxia, anorexia, and vomiting. Less commonly reported adverse effects include weakness, dyspnea, diarrhea, hyperthermia or hypothermia, hyperesthesia (ear flicking, paw shaking; repeated contractions of the superficial cutaneous muscles), and recumbency. Occasionally one can see a topical allergic reaction characterized by urticaria, pruritus, and alopecia at the site of application. Death is rarely reported but can occur, typically following severe, uncontrollable seizure activity.

A clinical diagnosis of pyrethroid poisoning most commonly heavily relies on obtaining a history of recent use and access to these products. The clinical signs closely mimic other poisonings (e.g., organophosphate and carbamate poisonings), and there are no specific clinicopathologic abnormalities routinely observed in affected animals. Laboratory methods for analyzing pyrethrin/pyrethroid residues are not routinely available but can be done to confirm exposure if necessary. Since clinical signs often mimic organophosphate or carbamate poisonings, assessing blood or brain cholinesterase is recommended to rule out these differentials. Cholinesterase activity will not be inhibited in cases of pyrethrin/pyrethroid poisonings, whereas it may be in organophosphate or carbamate exposures and poisonings.

There is no specific antidote for pyrethrin/pyrethroid poisonings. Consequently treatment should be aimed at decontaminating the animal to prevent further absorption and addressing the clinical presentation. Bathing the animal in warm soapy water followed by a thorough rinsing is recommended for topical exposures. Long-haired dogs and cats may require multiple bathings-dryings-brushings or clipping to remove residues from the hair.

Oral ingestions can be treated with emetics, activated charcoal, and cathartics and more aggressively with light sedation and gastric lavage. Muscle tremors can usually be controlled with diazepam (0.5 to 1 mg/kg IV or to effect) or methocarbamol (55 to 220 mg/kg IV); it should be administered half rapidly, not to exceed 2 ml/minute, and the rest to effect. Continuous monitoring of body temperature for hypothermia or hyperthermia is essential. Providing adequate hydration and electrolyte status is also important in achieving a positive outcome. The oral cavity can be rinsed to help control hypersalivation. The prognosis for the majority of pyrethrin/pyrethroid poisonings is excellent, with most animals recovering within 24 to 72 hours.

AMITRAZ

Amitraz is a formamidine pesticide that is present in some tick collars used on dogs. It is often present at a concentration of 9%. The collars are designed to kill ticks for 4 months. Toxicosis can occur in dogs that ingest a substantial portion of, or the entire, collar. The entire collar weighs 27.5 g, so each gram of collar contains approximately 90 mg of amitraz. However, the collar is a controlled-release device that releases amitraz in first-order kinetics over an effective period of more than 90 days. Therefore release is much higher when the collar is new than after it has been used for 4 months. Mitaban liquid concentrate contains 19.9% amitraz. It is used topically for the control and treatment of generalized demodicosis. Several different treatment protocols have been suggested, depending on the location and severity of the disease and the age of the affected animal. The use of amitraz is not recommended in lactating or pregnant animals or in animals that weigh less than 5 kg.

The lethal dose of amitraz is estimated to be about 100 mg/kg orally in dogs, although toxic doses as low as 10 to 20 mg/kg have been reported. Amitraz is well absorbed by the gastrointestinal tract. Clinical signs of toxicosis usually begin within 1 hour of ingestion, sometimes as early as 30 minutes.

Amitraz is a monoamine oxidase inhibitor, an α_2-adrenergic agonist, and an inhibitor of prostaglandin synthesis. Ocular exposure to this compound can lead to mild irritation. The clinical signs can be severe but often transient and rarely fatal. Most clinical signs are associated with the α_2-adrenergic properties of amitraz and include depression, sedation, ataxia, bradycardia, mydriasis, hypothermia, vomiting, polyuria, and gastrointestinal stasis or diarrhea. Other signs that have been reported include hyperthermia, gastric dilation, hypersalivation, dyspnea, anorexia, shock, tachycardia, urinary incontinence, disorientation, tremors, and coma (Duncan, 1993; Grossman, 1993; Hovda and McManus, 1993). Clinical

laboratory data often reveal a hyperglycemia. Most signs, whether in mild exposures or excessive exposures followed by aggressive treatment, usually last no longer than 24 to 48 hours.

Treatment is aimed at decontamination to prevent further absorption and reversal of the adrenergic agonist effects. In the asymptomatic patient emesis should be induced with 3% hydrogen peroxide or apomorphine. Administering a nonoily laxative such as activated charcoal with a cathartic is recommended as long as no diarrhea is present. An enema to evacuate the colon may be administered 12 to 18 hours after ingestion if diarrhea has not occurred or the laxative does not produce the desired effect. Abdominal radiography is recommended if a length of collar is the suspected source of the amitraz or if the depression/sedation is severe and prolonged. Retrieval of the collar or pieces of collar can be performed by endoscopy, gastrotomy, or enterotomy. Xylazine should be avoided because of the possibility of exacerbating hypotension. All surgical procedures and anesthesia protocols should be considered carefully because of the potential to exacerbate preexisting problems of gastric dilation or bradycardia. The probability of requiring these more invasive decontamination procedures is rare.

Since amitraz is not a cholinesterase inhibitor, atropine and 2-PAM are contraindicated in the treatment of amitraz poisoning. In moderately or severely affected patients who cannot be aroused, yohimbine or atipamezole (both α_2-antagonists) may be administered at 0.1 mg/kg IV or 50 mcg/kg IM, respectively (Hsu, Lu, and Hembrough, 1986; Hugnet et al., 1996). Both compounds should reverse amitraz-induced changes within 20 to 30 minutes. Since the action of yohimbine is of short duration (half-life = 1.5 to 2 hours), it may need to be repeated until the dog's clinical condition improves significantly. Body temperature should be monitored following yohimbine use to avoid hyperthermia. Fluid therapy is also warranted in the bradycardic, dehydrated patient.

BOTANICAL OIL EXTRACTS

Various fragrant volatile oils that are currently marketed as having parasiticidal properties have been isolated from a number of plants. The most popular of these oils include d-limonene and linalool. These oils are sold as shampoos, sprays, and dips for flea and tick control on dogs and cats or for premise control. Some citrus oil extracts are also found in household cleaners. These oils are considered to be relatively nontoxic and are generally regarded as safe by the Food and Drug Administration. Both d-limonene and linalool are present in oils extracted from the skins of citrus fruits and are typically associated with poisonings in dogs and cats when used at excessive concentrations. Cats are more sensitive to developing clinical signs after exposures than dogs.

With normal use these compounds may cause temporary irritation to the eyes, skin, nose, throat, or respiratory tract. Adverse reaction to these compounds can occur following inhalation, dermal, or oral exposure. Clinical effects are often observed within 15 to 30 minutes after exposure. Typical signs after oral exposure include salivation, vomiting, diarrhea, and central nervous system depression. Other signs reported with higher exposures include muscle tremors, hypothermia, hypotension, ataxia, and mydriasis. Ataxia, weakness, depression, and dermal irritation (e.g., scrotal, perianal) have been seen following topical applications. Seizures and death are rare and are presumed to be secondary to severe hypotension and hypothermia. There has been one report of erythema multiforme major and disseminated intravascular coagulation in a dog following a dermal application of a d-limonene–containing dip (Rosenbaum and Kerlin, 1995). An acute necrotizing dermatitis and subsequent septicemia was reported in a 2-year-old cat following application of a d-limonene–containing insecticidal shampoo (Lee, Budgin, and Mauldin, 2002). Other signs reported included lethargy, inappetence, vocalization, and abnormal aggressive behavior.

Treatment is aimed at decontamination, with supportive care based on the clinical signs. Repeated bathings with warm, soapy water followed by thorough rinsing are recommended following topical applications. Gastric lavage with activated charcoal and a cathartic is recommended following oral ingestions. Body temperature and blood pressure should be monitored to prevent hypotension and hypothermia. Diazepam has been used to control the muscle tremors, and fluid therapy is generally recommended to prevent dehydration. Most affected animals recover within 24 hours.

Pennyroyal oil has long been used as a flea repellent and is sold as a shampoo, powder, or the pure oil itself. Pennyroyal is an herb consisting mainly of leaves from two different plants, *Mentha pulegium* and *Hedeoma pulegioides*. The oil is derived from the leaves and flowering tops of these plants. Pulegone constitutes approximately 85% of the pennyroyal oil and is metabolized to the toxic metabolite menthofuran by the liver. Toxicoses have been described in both animals and humans following dermal application and oral ingestion. Clinical signs are associated primarily with gastrointestinal upset, liver failure, and severe neurologic injury. Clinical signs include lethargy, vomiting, diarrhea, hemoptysis, epistaxis, dyspnea, miosis or mydriasis, seizures, and death (Anderson et al., 1996). Massive hepatic necrosis has been reported in the dog following topical application of the oil (Sudekum et al., 1992).

Pennyroyal oil ingestion is treated by decontaminating the stomach by gastric lavage and activated charcoal. Emesis is generally not suggested because of the rapid absorption of pennyroyal oil, the risk for developing aspiration pneumonia, and the potential for rapid onset of central nervous system depression. Repeated bathing with a mild detergent followed by thorough rinsings is recommended following topical applications. N-acetylcysteine has been suggested in cases in which there is a high risk of inducing a toxicosis, starting with a loading dose of 140 mg/kg and following with 70 mg/kg every 4 hours. N-acetylcysteine therapy should be beneficial within the first few hours of poisoning and should continue for at least 24 to 48 hours. The use of cimetidine has also been recommended in the treatment of this poisoning; mice pretreated with the cytochrome P-450 inhibitor cimetidine exhibited less liver disease associated with intraperitoneal pulegone administration than

the controls (Sztajnkrycer et al., 2003). Any additional therapy is supportive only and should be based on clinical signs; this may include the use of antiemetics and fluid therapy. Basic support for liver failure may include plasma transfusions, antibiotics, vitamin K_1, S-adenosylmethionine, vitamin E, and gastric protectants (sucralfate). A complete blood count, serum chemistry and coagulation profile, and urinalysis should be performed to monitor organ function.

Another essential oil, Melaleuca oil or tea tree oil, is obtained from the leaves of the Australian tea tree *(Melaleuca alternifolia)*. Melaleuca oil products are sold in products to be used topically for skin infections, as insect repellents, as antipruritics, or as household cleaners. Melaleuca oil is known to contain as much as 60% terpenes; thus the clinical signs in poisoned patients strongly resemble those described for the essential oils d-limonene and linalool.

Toxicities with these products have been reported in cats, dogs, rats, and humans, after either oral ingestion or topical application. Most reports of poisoning in pets occur after misuse of high topical doses of the product. The lipophilic terpenes are readily and rapidly absorbed across the skin and mucosal lining of the gastrointestinal tract. Cats are thought to be more sensitive than dogs, and toxicities might be observed more frequently in this species because of their fastidious grooming habits.

The onset of clinical signs may occur within minutes to 8 hours after topical application. The time interval is highly dependent on dose and the extent of oral exposure following grooming behavior. The most common adverse signs include ataxia, incoordination, weakness, tremors, depression, hypothermia, and behavior abnormalities (Villar et al., 1994). Elevation in liver enzymes (alanine aminotransferase, aspartate aminotransferase) has been reported in cats following topical exposure (Bischoff and Guale, 1998).

Treatment is directed toward symptomatic and supportive care. Topical exposures warrant bathing with a mild detergent followed by a thorough rinsing. Long-haired pets may benefit from having their hair cut or trimmed. Activated charcoal and a cathartic can be administered in orally exposed pets. Monitoring basic life support measures and correcting any temperature, fluid, and electrolyte abnormalities may be indicated. Prognoses are generally favorable, and most affected animals recover over a 2- to 3-day interval.

MISCELLANEOUS INSECTICIDES (METHOPRENE, LUFENURON, FIPRONIL, IMIDACLOPRID, PYRIPROXIFEN, NITENPYRAM)

Many of the insecticides described in this section are used topically. When an adverse effect related to topical/oral exposure to these products is suspected, it is essential to read the label ingredients carefully. Many of the insecticides listed in the following paragraphs can occur as a single ingredient or in combination with other insecticides, mainly pyrethrins and pyrethroids. In addition, several adverse reactions reported such as salivation or skin irritation following dermal or oral exposures may be caused by the carriers present in the formulation. Typically these signs are mild and self-limiting.

Insect growth regulators are a relatively new category in the war against fleas and ticks. All act as analogs of juvenile growth hormones, thereby interrupting the normal growth patterns of the insect. Methoprene preferentially kills fleas and ticks in the larval stage by binding to and activating juvenile hormone receptors. It thereby prevents larvae from developing into adult fleas. Methoprene can be absorbed from the gastrointestinal tract, through the intact skin, or by inhalation. However, it is considered to be virtually nontoxic when ingested or inhaled and only slightly toxic after dermal absorption. Methoprene is not considered an eye or skin irritant.

Lufenuron, a benzoylphenyl urea, inhibits the synthesis, polymerization, and deposition of chitin in the eggs or exoskeleton of fleas. Lufenuron is highly lipophilic and readily accumulates in adipose tissue. Lufenuron has shown no synergistic or additive effects when combined with other insecticides. It has proven to be safe at recommended dosage regimens in puppies and kittens as young as 6 weeks of age, as well as lactating dogs and cats and their offspring. Various studies in dogs and cats using up to 10 times the normal dosage have shown no serious health effects over an exposure period of 1 to 9 months. No adverse effects were seen in cats orally exposed to up to 17 times the recommended dosage. A mild decrease in food consumption was reported in puppies exposed from 8 weeks to 10 months of age to 18 to 30 times the recommended dosage. However, the majority of studies have shown no significant adverse effects on food consumption, body weight, hematology, clinical chemistries, and urinalyses following excessive exposures. Few effects on fertility and reproduction have been reported. Administration of lufenuron to breeding male and female dogs at 90 times the recommended dosage of 10 mg/kg resulted in a reduced pregnancy rate compared to controls. Pups born to treated females exhibited nasal discharge, pulmonary congestion, diarrhea, dehydration, and sluggishness. It appears that lufenuron concentrates in the milk at a 60:1 milk:blood concentration ratio (Ciba-Geigy Corp.).

Lufenuron, 90 mg/kg, was administered to breeding cats before mating and through gestation and lactation. Kittens born to these cats exhibited no adverse effects on health, growth, and survival (Ciba-Geigy Corp., 1996; Shipstone and Mason, 1995). Plumb (2005) lists vomiting, lethargy, depression, urticaria, diarrhea, dyspnea, anorexia, and reddened skin as rare adverse effects.

Fipronil is a phenylpyrazole flea and tick adulticide currently marketed as a spray and topical liquid that boasts a wide margin of safety. It can be used on dogs, cats, puppies, or kittens greater than 8 weeks old. No adverse effects were noted in studies in which dogs or cats were fed five times the maximum dose. Fipronil acts on the γ-aminobutyric acid–mediated chloride channels of invertebrates, thereby interrupting nervous transmission and leading to rapid death of the fleas and ticks. Mammals reportedly have receptors inside the chloride channel that are shaped differently than the invertebrate receptors, and fipronil is not thought to be able to bind them for a long period of time. Following dermal application, it is not considered systemically active and is thought to be sequestered in the pet's sebaceous glands. Mild skin irritation may occur following topical applications of these products.

Imidacloprid is another topically used adulticide that reportedly binds specifically to postsynaptic nicotinic acetylcholine receptors of insects and both kills adult fleas and exhibits some larvicidal action. Toxicity testing of imidacloprid has shown no adverse effects when used at five times the maximum dosage in dogs and cats. A few reports of alopecia and erythema have been observed following dermal application. Theoretically poisoning could occur by the oral route if the dosage or concentration were excessive. The most common complaint following ingestion is excessive salivation that is self-limiting. There is no specific antidote, and all treatment should be based on observed clinical problems. Topically exposed pets should be bathed and rinsed; orally exposed patients should be decontaminated by either emesis or lavage, followed by the use of activated charcoal and a cathartic.

Pyriproxifen and nitenpyram are two of the relatively newer products that have entered the marketplace. Nitenpyram in a neonicotinoid derivative that binds and inhibits specific nicotinic acetylcholine receptors. It does not inhibit AChE activity. Pyriproxifen is an insect growth regulator used topically to control insects. No significant adverse effects have been reported with either of these products.

References and Suggested Reading

Anderson IB: Pennyroyal toxicity: Measurement of toxic metabolite levels in two cases and review of the literature, *Ann Intern Med* 124:726, 1996.

Bishcoff K, Guale F: Australian tea tree (*Melaleuca alternifolia*) oil poisoning in three purebred cats, *J Vet Diagn Invest* 10:208, 1998.

Blagburn BL, et al: Efficacy dosage titration of lufenuron against developmental stages of fleas in cats, *Am J Vet Res* 55:98, 1994.

Blagburn BL, et al: Efficacy of lufenuron against developmental stages of fleas in dogs housed in simulated home environments, *Am J Vet Res* 56:464, 1995.

Blodgett DJ: Organophosphate and carbamate insecticides. In Peterson ME, Talcott PA, editors: *Small animal toxicology*, St Louis, 2006, Elsevier, p 941.

Bonagura JD, editor: *Kirk's current veterinary therapy XIII (small animal practice)*, Philadelphia, 2000, Saunders, pp 231, 233.

Campbell WR, Lynn RC: Tolerability of lufenuron (CGA-184699) in normal dogs and cats, *J Vet Intern Med* 3:2, 1992.

Ciba-Geigy Corporation: Program (lufenuron) for control of existing flea infestations. *Adv Pract Vet*, 1, 1996.

Ciba–Geigy Corporation: Summary of studies submitted as part of the new animal drug application, No 41-035, for lufenuron tablets, Ciba-Geigy Corp, Greensboro, NC, 800-637-0281.

Ciba-Geigy Corporation: Program (lufenuron): A radical breakthrough in flea control. Ciba Animal Health, Ciba-Geigy Animal Health, Greensboro, NC 27419.

Duncan KL: Treatment of amitraz toxicosis, *J Am Vet Med Assoc* 208(8):1115, 1993.

Fikes JD: Organophosphorus and carbamate insecticides, *Vet Clin North Am* 20(2):353, 1990.

Fikes JD: Feline chlorpyrifos toxicosis. In Kirk RW, Bonagura JD, editors: *Current veterinary therapy XI: small animal practice*, Philadelphia, 1992, Saunders, p 188.

Grossman MR: Amitraz toxicosis associated with ingestion of an acaricide collar in a dog, *J Am Vet Med Assoc* 203(1):55, 1993.

Hansen SR: Management of adverse reactions to pyrethrin and pyrethroid insecticides. In Bonagura JD, Kirk RW, editors: *Current veterinary therapy XII: small animal practice*, Philadelphia, 1995a, Saunders, p 242.

Hansen SR: Management of organophosphate and carbamate insecticide toxicoses. In Bonagura JD, Kirk RW, editors: *Current veterinary therapy XII: small animal practice*, Philadelphia, 1995b, Saunders, pp. 245.

Hansen SR: Pyrethrins and pyrethroids. In Peterson ME, Talcott PA, editors: *Small animal toxicology*, St Louis, 2006, Elsevier, p 1002.

Hansen SR, Buck WB: Treatment of adverse reactions in cats to flea control products containing pyrethrin/pyrethroid insecticides, *Feline Pract* 20(5):25, 1992.

Hink WF et al: Evaluation of a single oral dose of lufenuron to control flea infestations in dogs, *Am J Vet Res* 55:822, 1995.

Hooser SB: d-Limonene, linalool, and crude citrus oil extracts, *Vet Clin North Am Small Anim Pract* 20(2):383, 1990.

Hovda LR, McManus AC: Yohimbine for treatment of amitraz poisoning in dogs, *Vet Hum Toxicol* 35(4):329, 1993.

Hsu WH, Lu ZX, Hembrough FB: Effect of amitraz on heart rate and aortic blood pressure in conscious dogs: influence of atropine, prazosin, tolazoline, and yohimbine, *Toxicol Appl Pharmacol* 84:418, 1986.

Hugnet C et al: Toxicity and kinetics of amitraz in dogs, *Am J Vet Res* 57(10):1506, 1996.

Kanzler K, editor: *Veterinary pharmaceuticals and biologicals, 1995/1996*, ed 9, Lenexa, KS, Veterinary Medicine Publishing, p 841.

Lee JA, Budgin JB, Mauldin EA: Acute narcotizing dermatitis and septicemia after application of a d-limonene–based insecticidal shampoo in a cat, *J Am Vet Med Assoc* 221(2):258, 2002.

Miller TA: Personal communication, Virbac, Inc, 3200 Meacham Blvd, Fort Worth, TX 76137.

Plumb DC: *Plumb's veterinary drug handbook*, ed 5, Ames, Ia, 2005, Blackwell Publishing.

Rosenbaum MR, Kerlin RL: Erythema multiforme major and disseminated intravascular coagulation in a dog following application of a d-limonene–based insecticidal dip, *J Am Vet Med Assoc* 207(10):1315, 1995.

Shipstone MA, Mason KV: Review article: The use of insect development inhibitors as an oral medication for the control of the fleas *Ctenocephalides felis, C. canis* in the dog and cat, *Vet Dermatol* 6:131, 1995.

Sudekum M et al: Pennyroyal oil toxicosis in a dog, *J Am Vet Med Assoc* 200(6):817, 1992.

Sztajnkrycer MD : Mitigation of pennyroyal oil hepatotoxicity in the mouse, *Acad Emerg Med* 10(10):1024, 2003.

Valentine WM: Pyrethrin and pyrethroid insecticides, *Vet Clin North Am* 20(2):375, 1990.

Villar D et al: Toxicity of melaleuca oil and related essential oils applied topically on dogs and cats, *Vet Hum Toxicol* 36(2):139, 1994.

Whittem T: Pyrethrin and pyrethroid insecticide intoxication in cats, *Compendium* 17(4):489, 1995.

CHAPTER 27

Parasiticide Toxicoses: Avermectins

WILSON K. RUMBEIHA, *Lansing, Michigan*

Avermectins are a group of parasiticidal drugs derived from soil *Streptomyces* microorganisms. Biochemically they belong to a group of compounds known as macrocyclic lactones and are related to milbemycins. These drugs are widely used for their parasiticidal properties. Representative drugs include ivermectin (Heartgard), selamectin (Revolution), doramectin (Dectomax), eprinomectin (Eprinex), moxidectin (Proheart), milbemycin (Interceptor), and abamectin. In general these drugs have a substantial margin of safety in dogs and cats and are very active against a wide range of parasites, including nematodes and arthropods. Practically they are highly effective at very low doses such as micrograms per kilogram of body weight basis. These drugs are not active against trematodes or cestodes. As such, they may be combined with other drugs that are active against cestodes and trematodes in some formulations. They are available for oral, topical, and parenteral formulations for use in different domesticated species and humans.

TOXICITY OF AVERMECTINS AND MILBEMYCINS

Because of their wide safety margin, avermectins and milbemycins are used safely in the majority of dogs and cats. However, some specific breeds of dogs are more sensitive to this group of drugs (i.e., collies, Australian shepherds, Shetland sheepdogs, Old English sheepdogs, German shepherds, long-haired whippets, and silken windhounds). Recent findings have determined that these breeds possess a mutation in the multidrug resistance (MDR-1) gene. This gene regulates the synthesis of P-glycoprotein, a 170-kDa transmembrane protein, which plays a key role in regulating movement of xenobiotics across the blood-brain barrier and other tissues of the body. P-glycoprotein is responsible for extruding drugs and other xenobiotics from the brain across the blood-brain barrier. A mutation in the MDR-1 gene causes synthesis of a truncated P-glycoprotein molecule that is unable to perform this regulatory role. The result is that breeds of dogs with this mutation cannot efficiently extrude xenobiotics such as avermectins and milbemycins from brain tissue. Studies have demonstrated higher concentrations of ivermectin in brain tissues of dogs with the mutated MDR-1 gene than naïve control dogs that have normal functioning P-glycoprotein.

Collies as a breed have the highest prevalence of the MDR-1 mutation. Research from United States, Europe, and Japan indicates that 75% of all collies carry this genetic mutation and explains why avermectin toxicosis is more commonly observed in this breed. This statistic includes dogs that are either heterozygous carriers or homozygous for the mutant allele, making the animal sensitive. Note that collies not holding this mutation (i.e., homozygous for the normal allele) have the same sensitivity to avermectin and milbemycin toxicity as other normal breeds of dogs.

It is worth noting that some mixed breeds of dogs carry a single recessive gene mutation, making them heterozygous carriers. These dogs have sensitivity to avermectin toxicosis, which is between that of double recessive–sensitive mutants and naïve dogs with normal alleles.

Toxic Dose and Sources of Exposure

The monthly oral dose of ivermectin for prevention of heartworms in dogs and cats is 0.006 to 0.024 mg/kg (6 to 24 mcg/kg of body weight), respectively. The LD_{50} of ivermectin in beagle dogs is 80 mg/kg body weight. Most dogs with a normal MDR-1 gene tolerate oral dosages as high as 2.5 mg/kg body weight before they start to exhibit toxicity to this drug. However, dogs with a double recessive MDR-1 gene can only tolerate up to 0.1 mg/kg (100 mcg/kg of body weight) of ivermectin. Sensitive collies tolerated doses of 28 to 35.5 mcg/kg of body weight over a period of 1 year when administered oral chewable formulations of ivermectin. The highest observed nontoxic dose in cats is 1.3 mg/kg of body weight. However, toxicity in cats has been reported after as low as 0.3 mg/kg of body weight subcutaneously. Toxicosis to moxidexin was observed in a collie that received a dose 30 times higher than the recommended dose of 0.003 mg/kg of body weight. Toxicosis to milbemycin has been observed in collies at doses that are 10 times higher than the recommended therapeutic dose of 0.5 mg/kg orally. In one study collie sensitivity to milbemycin oxime at 10 mg/kg of body weight was judged to be clinically equivalent to that of ivermectin at 120 mcg/kg of body weight. Selamectin is potentially toxic to sensitive collies at oral doses greater than 15 mg/kg of body weight. For the other avermectins, the minimum toxic doses in sensitive breeds of dogs are not well established.

Typically toxicosis to avermectins and milbemycins is observed in the more sensitive breeds of dogs when dosage errors occur at >5 to 10 times recommended doses, depending on a specific drug; when dogs are accidentally given formulations for large animals; or when they eat a large number of drug tablets.

Clinical Signs of Toxicosis

Following acute exposure, clinical signs are seen within a few hours. However, clinical signs may also become evident after several days of topical exposure. Typically clinical signs of avermectin and milbemycin toxicity are associated with depression of the central nervous system. The animals develop ataxia, weakness, and recumbency; if the dose is severe, coma is evident. Some dogs exhibit signs of blindness and muscle tremors; in some cases seizures have been reported. These clinical signs result from avermectins acting as agonists of the γ-aminobutyric acid (GABA) in the central nervous system. Other non-GABA–related effects include mydriasis, hypothermia, vomiting, salivation, and shallow breathing. Avermectin toxicosis is a protracted disease that may last *days or weeks*. Treatment should be given with this in mind.

DIAGNOSIS AND THERAPY OF TOXICOSIS

Diagnosis of avermectin toxicosis consists of a history consistent with exposure to large amounts of these drugs, clinical signs consistent with avermectin intoxication, and chemical analysis of serum or blood plasma in live animals. In deceased animals adipose tissue, brain, and liver have been used for chemical analysis to confirm exposure to avermectins. However, there are no well-established concentrations of avermectins in these matrices that can be regarded as "diagnostic marker concentrations." As such, history of excessive exposure and clinical signs consistent with avermectin toxicosis remain the two most important diagnostic criteria to date. There is a molecular genetics test for the presence of a mutant gene (it is available at Washington State University Veterinary Clinical Pharmacology Laboratory). This test, which uses cheek brush samples, is helpful in determining whether an individual dog is sensitive to avermectins and other drugs with toxicokinetics that are regulated by the MDR-1 gene.

Therapy of avermectin toxicosis is symptomatic with no specific antidote. As such, prevention of absorption resulting from topical or oral exposure is key to successful therapy in cases of acute exposure. Animals exposed topically should be washed with mild dishwashing detergents and plenty of water. In cases of acute oral exposure, patients should be induced to vomit if exposure is within 1 to 2 hours. Apomorphine is recommended in dogs, and xylazine in cats as emetic drugs (see Chapter 24). Following emesis, activated charcoal can be given to bind the unexpelled drug. Avermectins are excreted largely unchanged through the feces. Activated charcoal may also be beneficial in binding these compounds that are normally excreted unmetabolized through bile and feces. Treatments with physostigmine, neostigmine, or picrotoxin have resulted in either temporary relief or mixed results.

Thus supportive care that includes fluid therapy, respiratory support, parenteral alimentation, and maintenance of normal body temperature is vital to a successful treatment outcome. Treatment of avermectin toxicosis is likely to be protracted since these drugs have prolonged half-lives in dogs of at least 2 days for ivermectin, 11 days for selamectin, and 19 days for moxidectin. The effective half-life is likely longer in MDR-1 double recessive dogs, which are more likely to accumulate higher brain tissue concentrations.

Suggested Reading

Griffin J et al: Selamectin is a potent substrate and inhibitor of human canine P-glycoprotein, *J Vet Pharmacol Ther* 28: 257, 2005.

Kawabata A, et al: Canine MDR-1 gene mutation in Japan, *J Vet Med Sci* 67(11):1103, 2005.

Mealy KL: Ivermectin: macrolide antiparasitic agents. In Peterson ME, Talcott PA, editors: *Small animal toxicology*, Philadelphia, 2006, Saunders, p 785.

Mealy KL: Therapeutic implications of the MDR-1 gene, *J Vet Pharmacol Ther* 27:257, 2004.

Mealy KL, Bentjen SA, Waiting DK: Frequency of mutant MDR-1 allele associated with ivermectin sensitivity in a sample population of collies from northwestern United States, *Am J Vet Res* 63(4):479, 2002.

Nelson OL et al: Ivermectin toxicity in an Australian Shepherd dog with the MDR-1 mutation associated with ivermectin sensitivity in collies, *J Vet Intern Med* 17(3):354, 2003.

Paul AJ et al: Evaluating the safety of administering high doses of chewable ivermectin tablets to collies, *Vet Med* 86(6):623, 1991.

Pawde AM et al: Ivermectin toxicity in dogs, *Indian Ass Vet Res* 1(2):51, 1992.

Shoop WL, Mrozik H, Fisher MH: Structure and activity of avermectins and milbemycins in animal health, *Vet Parasitol* 59:139, 1995.

Tranquilli WJ, Paul AJ, Todd KS: Assessment of toxicosis induced by high-dose administration of milbemycin oxime in collies, *Am J Vet Res* 52(7):1170, 1991.

CHAPTER **28**

Lead Toxicosis in Small Animals

SHARON M. GWALTNEY-BRANT, *Urbana, Illinois*

Lead contamination of residential environments has decreased through removal of lead from residential paints, gasoline, and other household items. Accordingly, the incidence of lead poisoning in small animals has decreased over the last 30 years, and lead now accounts for less than 1% of reported accidental poisonings in pets. Nevertheless, lead intoxication in pets does occur, and the vagueness of clinical signs that frequently accompany lead poisoning can create diagnostic challenges.

SOURCES OF LEAD TOXICOSIS

Lead may be found in a wide variety of man-made products, including paints, linoleum, caulking and putty compounds, solders, wire shielding, old metal tubing, certain weights (e.g., fishing sinkers, curtain weights), linoleum, roofing felt, golf balls, ammunition, computer equipment, wine cork covers, pottery glazing, lead-containing toys, and lead arsenate pesticides. In addition, contamination of soil or water can be a potential source of lead. The potential for exposure to organoleads from leaded

petroleum products has decreased considerably following legislation restricting the use of leaded gasoline and oil in the United States.

The most common source of lead in cases of small animal poisoning is leaded paints from buildings built before passage of the 1977 legislation requiring that residential paints contain no more than 0.06% (600 ppm) lead. In many cases older leaded paints have been painted over with unleaded paints, and it is estimated that 74% of privately owned homes built before 1980 still contain hazardous amounts of leaded paint. Renovation of these homes results in the generation of paint chips or dust that, if ingested by pets, can result in clinical lead intoxication. Cats may be at increased risk for toxicosis during these situations because of their grooming habits, which can result in significant ingestion of lead-containing particulates that collect in their fur.

Kinetics

The degree to which ingested lead will be absorbed depends on variables such as the physical form of lead, particle size, and matrix association. In addition, patient variables that influence the degree of lead absorption from the gastrointestinal (GI) tract include age, diet, and preexisting disease. The acidic environment of the stomach favors ionization of the lead, which is then absorbed from the duodenum. Lead shot embedded in soft tissues such as skeletal muscle is not appreciably absorbed and is not an important source of lead toxicosis. Conversely, lead shot that enters areas capable of active inflammation (e.g., joint cavities) may become solubilized by the enzymatic activity of the inflammatory reaction and could subsequently be absorbed.

Once absorbed, lead is carried primarily on the red blood cells, with less than 1% to 2% bound to albumin or free in the plasma. Unbound lead distributes widely through tissues, with the highest concentrations found in bone, teeth, liver, lung, kidney, brain, and spleen. Bone serves as a storage depot for lead, which substitutes for calcium in the bone matrix. During times of increased activity of bone remodeling such as fracture repair or lactation, stored lead may be released from the bone, resulting in toxicosis. Lead crosses the blood-brain barrier and concentrates in the gray matter of the brain. This passage of lead into the brain occurs to a greater extent in the young than in mature animals. Unbound lead crosses the placenta and is passed through the milk in lactating animals.

Most ingested lead is excreted in the feces unabsorbed. Lead in the blood passes through the glomerulus and accumulates in the renal tubular epithelium. During the natural process of sloughing of tubular epithelial cells, the lead is slowly eliminated from the body. Chelation therapy can greatly increase the rate of urinary excretion of lead by allowing the chelated lead to be passed in the urine without entering the tubular epithelium. Lead has a multiphasic half-life because of its distribution into depot areas such as bone and brain. In dogs intravenously administered lead has triphasic half-lives of 12 days, 184 days, and 4591 days.

Mechanism of Action

Lead has a wide variety of effects within the body, including interfering and competing with calcium ions, binding to cellular and enzymatic sulfhydryl groups, altering vitamin D metabolism, and inhibiting membrane-associated enzymes. Inactivation of the enzymes ferrochelatase and δ-aminolevulinic acid dehydratase results in impairment in heme synthesis, causing red blood cell abnormalities and, chronically, anemia. GI signs in lead-intoxicated patients may be caused in part by alteration of smooth muscle contractility as a result of interference of lead on intracellular calcium-dependent mechanisms. Lead decreases cerebral blood flow and alters neuronal energy metabolism and neurotransmission within the central nervous system (CNS).

Lead Toxicity

Toxic dosages of lead reported for dogs range from 191 to 1000 mg/kg, depending on the form of lead; 3 mg/kg/day caused vomiting and behavioral changes in cats. However, these dosages have little clinical relevance in most cases of lead toxicosis in small animals since the amount of lead ingested is rarely determined.

Young animals are at greater risk than mature animals because they absorb up to five times more lead following ingestion. Lead absorption is enhanced in animals deficient in calcium, zinc, iron, and/or vitamin D. Younger cats are thought to be at higher risk for development of lead-induced seizures.

CLINICAL SIGNS

The primary signs seen with lead intoxication in dogs and cats are related to GI upset. Anorexia, vomiting, diarrhea, weight loss, lethargy, and abdominal discomfort have been reported. In cats the most common signs are lethargy and anorexia. Neurologic signs may also occur but are less common than GI signs. Neurologic effects can include behavior changes, ataxia, tremors, seizures, and agitation. Less commonly other signs such as polyuria, polydipsia, blindness, aggression, dementia, pica, vestibular signs, coma, and megaesophagus (cats) have been reported.

LABORATORY AND RADIOGRAPHIC FINDINGS

In acute lead intoxication very few changes in clinical pathology parameters would be expected. Anemia, basophilic stippling, and elevations in nucleated red blood cells have been reported as indicative of lead toxicosis; but these abnormalities are not consistently found, nor are they pathognomonic for lead toxicosis. Basophilic stippling and nucleated red blood cells (>40 NRBCs per 100 white blood cells) are considered to be more likely to occur in dogs and less likely to occur in cats with lead toxicosis.

Radiography may be helpful in identifying lead opacities within the GI tract. *Lead lines,* linear opacities in the epiphyses of long bones used to aid in diagnosis of lead toxicosis in humans, are not commonly found in domestic animals.

PATHOLOGIC FINDINGS

Few gross lesions have been described in dogs and cats with lead toxicosis. Necropsy may reveal the presence of lead objects especially in the GI tract. Histopathologic findings may include degenerative changes within the white matter of the brain and spongiosus of the cerebrum. In dogs degenerative changes in the kidney and liver may be seen, occasionally associated with intranuclear inclusion bodies.

Diagnosis

The diagnosis of lead toxicosis can be difficult because the signs most commonly associated with this disease (anorexia, lethargy, vomiting) are nonspecific. Blood lead levels can be measured in a timely fashion and, when evaluated in light of compatible clinical signs, can be helpful in making a diagnosis. The widespread distribution of lead throughout the body can result in fluctuating blood levels, and the level of lead in the blood may not be indicative of the total body burden. Some animals may have fairly high blood lead levels without significant clinical signs, whereas other animals may have significant clinical signs with only moderately elevated blood lead levels. Most animals have a background lead level of 10 to 15 mcg/dl (0.1 to 0.15 ppm); blood lead levels exceeding 30 to 35 mcg/dl (0.3 to 0.35 ppm) along with appropriate clinical signs are suggestive for lead toxicosis. Levels greater than 60 mcg/dl are generally considered diagnostic for lead toxicosis.

TREATMENT

Management of lead toxicosis entails control of immediate clinical signs, removal of the source of lead, chelation therapy, supportive care, and removal of lead from the animal's environment. Seizures should be managed with anticonvulsants such as diazepam or barbiturates (see Chapter 231). Similarly, vomiting and diarrhea should be managed, and any fluid and electrolyte abnormalities should be corrected as needed.

GI decontamination must occur before chelation therapy since most chelators, with the exception of succimer, will actually enhance the absorption of lead from the GI tract. Sulfate-containing cathartics (magnesium sulfate, sodium sulfate) may be administered to aid in emptying the GI tract and to precipitate the lead as lead sulfate, which is poorly absorbed. Large lead-containing objects (e.g., lead sinkers, lead weights) may require removal via endoscopy or gastrotomy/enterotomy if they are too large to pass using bulking cathartics. When cats are suspected of exposure through grooming, thorough bathing should be performed.

Chelation therapy is intended to bind lead into a soluble complex that will be excreted via the urine. Because of the nephrotoxic nature of most chelators, as well as the lead chelate, it is imperative that renal parameters be assessed before and during chelation and that adequate hydration be maintained during chelation. Chelation of asymptomatic animals that have elevated blood lead levels is not recommended because the chelator may increase the blood lead level and precipitate clinical signs. In cases of asymptomatic animals with elevated blood lead levels, decontamination and removal from the source of lead will allow the animal to eliminate the lead at its own pace.

Available chelators include calcium disodium ethylene diamine tetracetate (Ca-EDTA), British anti-Lewisite (BAL), penicillamine, and succimer (meso-2,3-dimercaptosuccinic acid). Ca-EDTA was the first chelator agent used for lead toxicosis, and it has an established track record in veterinary and human medicine. Sodium EDTA should not be used for chelation because it will bind serum calcium and cause hypocalcemia. Ca-EDTA is administered parenterally and may cause pain at the injection site. The dosage for dogs is 100 mg/kg/day for 2 to 5 days (not to exceed 2 g per dog per day), with each dose divided every 8 hours, diluted to a final concentration of 10 mg of Ca-EDTA per milliliter of 5% dextrose and administered subcutaneously at different sites. Expect clinical improvement within 24 to 48 hours. If further treatment

is required after the first 5 days of therapy, a 5-day hiatus is recommended between treatments. Oral zinc supplementation may minimize the GI side effects of Ca-EDTA. The dose of calcium EDTA for cats is 27.5 mg/kg in 15 ml of 5% dextrose subcutaneously every 8 hours for 5 days.

BAL is occasionally used in combination with Ca-EDTA, especially when significant CNS signs are present. BAL increases both urinary and biliary excretion of lead. BAL is contraindicated in animals with hepatic dysfunction, is nephrotoxic, and causes pain on injection. Other potential side effects of BAL include vomiting, hypertension, sulfur odor of breath, and seizures. The dosage of BAL is 2 to 5 mg/kg intramuscularly every 4 hours for 2 days, then every 8 hours for 1 day, and then every 12 hours until recovery.

Penicillamine is an oral medication that eliminates the need for painful injections of BAL and Ca-EDTA. Penicillamine will bind essential nutrients such as zinc, iron, and copper; and its chelates may be nephrotoxic. Side effects reported with penicillamine include vomiting, fever, lymphadenopathy, and blood dyscrasias. Reported dosages for dogs are 30 to 110 mg/kg/day orally, divided every 8 hours for 7 days, and followed by a 7-day hiatus before reinstitution. Feline dosage is 125 mg per cat orally every 12 hours for 5 days.

Succimer is an analog to BAL, and it has several advantages over BAL, Ca-EDTA, and penicillamine. Succimer can be administered orally or in vomiting animals rectally. Succimer is much less likely to cause nephrotoxicosis than the other three chelators; and it does not bind essential minerals such as copper, zinc, calcium, and iron. Succimer does not enhance absorption of lead from the GI tract as do the other chelators, and it has been shown to decrease lead absorption in studies with rats. Succimer also has a lower incidence of GI side effects. It does impart a mercaptan odor to the breath, similar to BAL. The dose is 10 mg/kg orally or rectally every 8 hours for 10 days.

Following chelation therapy, blood lead levels may show a rebound within 2 to 3 weeks as a result of redistribution of lead from bone and tissue stores. Provided that this rebound is not associated with significant clinical signs, further chelation is not indicated. However, it is prudent to have the animal's environment evaluated to be sure the rebound is not caused by re-exposure to lead.

Supportive care involves providing adequate nutritional support since many animals with chronic lead toxicosis may be in a negative nutritional state because of chronic anorexia and vomiting. Hydration should be maintained, and force- or hand-feeding provided as needed.

Examination of the animal's environment is important to identify and remove any additional sources of lead so the animal does not become reexposed when reintroduced to its environment.

PROGNOSIS

Provided that prompt and appropriate care is pursued, including removing the source of lead from the animal's environment, the prognosis for animals showing mild-to-moderate signs is favorable. Animals showing severe CNS signs or with repeated exposure to lead may merit a more guarded prognosis.

PUBLIC HEALTH

The relative susceptibility of household pets makes them good sentinel animals for the potential for human exposure to lead. Veterinarians treating lead-intoxicated pets should ensure that pet owners are aware of the potential risk to family members, especially young children, from lead in the environment. Pet owners should be directed to their own health care professionals or public health officials for more information. Information on the risks of lead to human health can be found on the website of the Environmental Protection Agency (www.epa.gov).

Bibliography

Casteel SW: Lead. In Peterson ME, Talcott PA, editors: *Small animal toxicology*, ed 2, St Louis, 2006, Elsevier Saunders, p 795.

Gwaltney-Brant SM: Lead. In Plumlee KH, editor: *Clinical veterinary toxicology*, St Louis, 2004, Mosby, p 204.

Gwaltney-Brant SM, Rumbeiha WK: Newer antidotal therapies, *Vet Clin Small Anim* 32:323, 2002.

Knight TE, Kent M, Junk JE: Succimer for treatment of lead toxicosis in two cats, *J Am Vet Med Assoc* 218:1946, 2001.

Knight TE, Kumar MSA: Lead toxicosis in cats—a review, *J Feline Med Surg* 5:249, 2003.

CHAPTER 29

Automotive Toxins

KARYN BISCHOFF, *Ithaca, New York*

Various compounds for use in vehicle maintenance that are stored around the home have known toxic properties. An incomplete list of such chemicals includes ethylene glycol (EG), propylene glycol (PG), diethylene glycol (DEG), petroleum products, and methanol. EG is the most common component of antifreeze and unfortunately is the most common automotive product associated with poisoning in small animals. PG has been substituted for EG in antifreeze brands that are advertised as "safe" or "nontoxic." In fact, PG is much less toxic to companion animals than EG but is not without adverse effects.

ETHYLENE GLYCOL

EG is the most common cause of fatal poisoning in small animals (Thrall et al., 2006). EG is readily available in most households, is toxic in low doses, and is palatable. Toxicosis is most common in the late autumn or early spring, when radiators have been drained or open containers may be available to pets. Dogs occasionally chew through closed containers. Denatonium benzoate has been added to antifreeze to make it less palatable. California, New Mexico, and Oregon require addition of bittering agents to commercial antifreeze at the time of this writing.

EG, or 1,2-dihydroxyethane, is a colorless, sweet-tasting liquid with a density of 1.113, a high boiling point (197.2°C), a low freezing point (−12.3°C) and miscibility with water and alcohol. Other sources of EG include deicer, hydraulic brake and transmission fluids, additives in motor oils, paints, inks, wood stains and polishes, photographic solutions, and solvents used in the plastic industry.

Toxicity and Toxicokinetics

The minimum lethal dose for EG in dogs is about 4.4 ml/kg. Cats are more sensitive, with a minimum lethal dose around 1.4 ml/kg. Dogs are more frequently affected than cats, although cats may be more likely to become intoxicated through grooming activity after dermal contamination. Intact animals are more frequently affected.

EG is absorbed rapidly from the gastrointestinal tract, particularly on an empty stomach. Absorption of injected or inhaled EG is also rapid. Peak plasma concentrations occur within 3 hours of ingestion. Metabolism of EG begins within hours of ingestion and occurs predominantly in the liver, with minor renal and gastric metabolism. The metabolic pathway of EG is illustrated in Fig. 29-1. The metabolism of EG to glycoaldehyde and then glycolic acid to glyoxylic acid are both rate-limiting steps. Oxalic acid is the most important final metabolite of EG. The plasma half-life of EG is approximately 3 hours, and elimination is almost complete within 24 hours. The parent compound— EG—and its metabolites, including glycolic acid and oxalic acid, are eliminated in the urine.

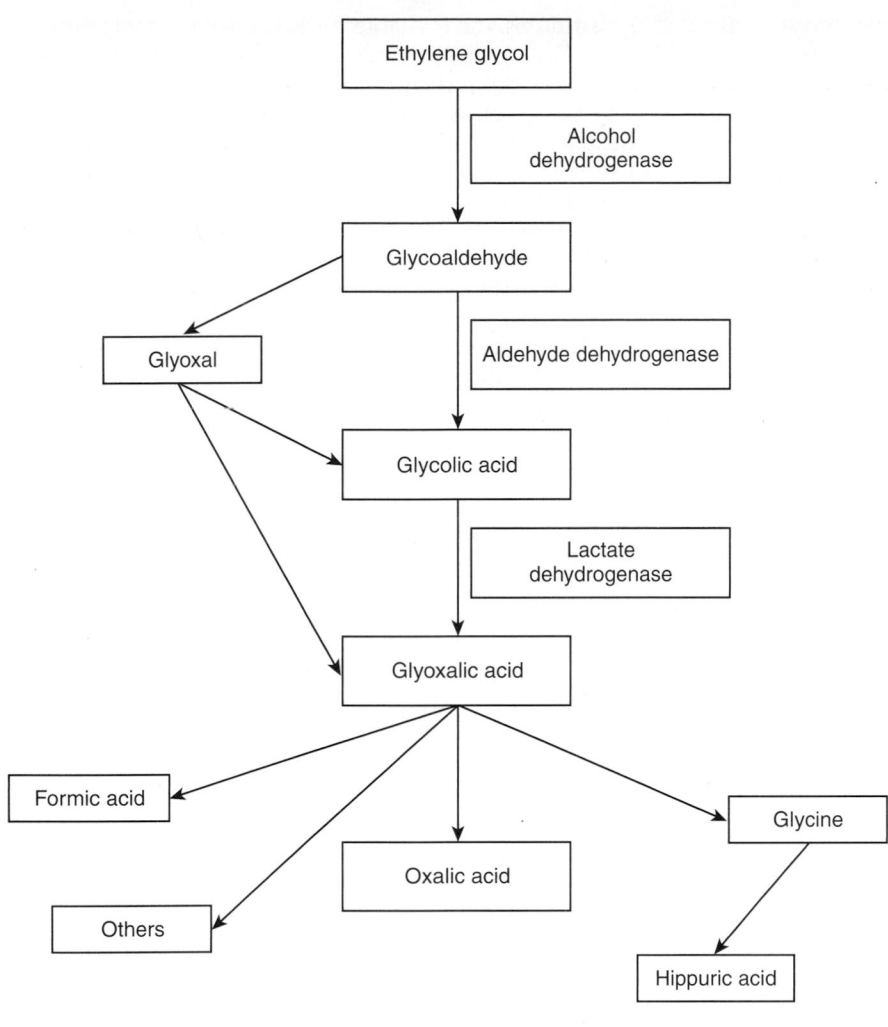

Fig. 29-1 Hepatic metabolism of ethylene glycol.

Mechanism of Action

In itself EG acts as a direct gastric irritant, causes central nervous system (CNS) depression, and may depress respiration. EG may increase serum osmolality, which may contribute to osmotic diuresis. The more severe effects associated with EG ingestion are caused by production of toxic metabolites. Acidosis is produced by such metabolic products of EG as glycolic acid and increased lactic acid production caused by nicotinamide adenine dinucleotide depletion during EG metabolism. Renal tubular damage is the most common cause of death in small animals poisoned with EG. Metabolites of EG are directly cytotoxic to renal tubular epithelium. Oxalic acid binds to calcium ions (Ca++) in the renal tubules (and other tissues) to form calcium oxalate crystals, leading to obstruction of tubules, epithelial damage, and hypocalcemia. Renal blood flow may be compromised in acidosis.

Clinical Signs

EG toxicosis is described as having three stages, although early stages may be missed and stages may overlap. The first stage usually occurs within 30 minutes of exposure and usually lasts for 2 to 12 hours. Animals may vomit early. Polyuria and polydipsia are described in dogs, and cats are frequently polyuric. Ataxia and hyporeflexia may

be apparent, and animals are sometimes described as "inebriated" at this stage. Dogs may show apparent recovery from CNS depressive effects, but cats typically do not.

The second stage usually occurs 8 to 24 hours after exposure and is related to acidosis. Clinical signs at this stage include CNS depression, changes in heart rate, hypothermia, muscle fasciculations, and sometimes coma. Cats may lose coordination in the pelvic limbs.

Small animals that survive the first two stages enter the third stage, acute renal failure. This stage begins within 1 to 3 days of EG ingestion. Animals progress through oliguria to anuria. Signs of uremia may include oral ulcerations, salivation, vomiting, anorexia, and seizures. Palpation of cats often reveals large, painful kidneys.

Serum chemistries often reveal an increased osmolal gap about an hour after EG ingestion, which may decline by 18 hours after exposure. The anion gap increases a few hours after exposure and can remain elevated for 48 hours in animals with acidosis. Phosphorus may be elevated early as a result of the phosphate additives in antifreeze and during renal failure. Hypocalcemia is reported in some patients. Serum urea nitrogen and creatinine are elevated 1 to 2 days after exposure in dogs and often within 12 hours in cats. Hyperkalemia occurs with the onset of renal failure. Urinalysis reveals isosthenuria as early as 3 hours after exposure as a result of osmotic diuresis and low urine pH. Calcium oxalate crystals are evident within the first 8 hours, although crystalluria may be evident in healthy animals. Other findings may include hematuria, proteinuria, glycosuria, and granular and cellular casts.

Diagnosis

Speed is of the essence in the diagnosis of EG toxicosis. The prognosis decreases precipitously with time if treatment is not instigated. EG concentrations begin to decline within 6 hours of exposure and may no longer be detectable in blood or urine by the time the animal presents to the veterinarian, which complicates the diagnosis.

Various analytic tests have been used to confirm exposure to EG. Commercial test kits are available, but these may cross-react with certain compounds, including PG and glycerol from pet foods and pharmaceuticals. It is best to collect samples for testing before treatment begins. Test kits are unable to detect EG at concentrations below 50 mg/dl and thus may not be sensitive enough to use on cats or on dogs exposed more than 12 hours previously. Gas chromatography (GC) is frequently used to assay blood, urine, or kidney tissue for EG at diagnostic laboratories; but results are delayed by sample shipping and processing.

Concurrent increase in the anionic and osmolal gap with the appropriate history and clinical signs is highly suggestive of EG toxicosis but does not always occur. Calcium oxalate monohydrate crystals are commonly found in the urine. Fluorescent dye is *sometimes* added to commercial antifreeze and may be seen with a Wood's lamp in the urine or around the oral cavity or vomitus of exposed animals. However, other components of urine and some plastic containers may fluoresce.

Finding the "halo effect" on renal ultrasound has been used to support an EG diagnosis. This is described as increased echogenicity in the cortex and medulla with decreased echogenicity at the corticomedullary junction and central medulla and occurs near the onset of anuria.

Postmortem findings typical of EG exposure may include gastric hemorrhage; pulmonary edema; and pale, firm kidneys. Histologic changes include degeneration and necrosis of the epithelium of proximal convoluted tubules with intraluminal birefringent crystals. Chronicity is indicated by evidence of tubular regeneration, interstitial fibrosis, and glomerular atrophy and synechia. Oxalate crystals may be found in other tissues, including the liver and CNS.

Management

The prognosis for EG toxicosis depends on the time of presentation. Animals treated early (stage 1) have an excellent prognosis, but the prognosis is poor for animals that present in renal failure (stage 3).

Gastrointestinal decontamination, including emetics or gastric lavage and activated charcoal orally, has been recommended for animals within a few hours of EG ingestion. The benefit of such treatment is questionable because of the rapid absorption of EG.

Antidotes are available for EG. They act by inhibiting metabolism of EG by alcohol dehydrogenase (Bonagura, 2000). Antidotal treatment is most effective when started early but recommended if exposure has occurred within the past 32 hours. Fomepizole, or 4-methyl pyrazole, is preferred. This product is used in dogs at an initial dose of 20 mg/kg intravenously (IV); then 15 mg/kg IV is given at 12 and 24 hours, and 5 mg/kg is given IV at 36 hours. Cats require much higher doses of fomepizole than dogs. The recommended dose for cats is 125 mg/kg IV initially and then 31.25 mg/kg every 12 hours for three more doses. Benefits of fomepizole include its lack of CNS depressant effects and the rarity of adverse effects. Fomepizole should never be used concurrently with ethanol therapy. Doing so will exacerbate clinical signs of ethanol toxicosis. Hemodialysis removes fomepizole from circulation. The prognosis is good if fomepizole therapy is started within 8 to 12 hours of EG ingestion for dogs or within 3 hours for cats. Fomepizole may not be immediately available; thus ethanol is still used therapeutically.

Ethanol competitively inhibits metabolism of EG because of its affinity for alcohol dehydrogenase. It has been used for many years to treat EG toxicosis. Ethanol enhances CNS depression, and bolus dosing may cause respiratory suppression. Animals remain stuporous during treatment, requiring close monitoring and supportive care. Ethanol is usually given IV to maintain blood concentrations of 50 to 100 mg/dl. A 5.5-ml/kg dose of 20% ethanol is given every 4 hours for the first five treatments and then every 6 hours for the next four treatments in dogs, or dogs may be given a bolus dose of 1.3 ml of 30% ethanol followed by a constant infusion rate of 0.42 ml/kg/hour for 48 hours. Cats are given 5 ml/kg of 20% ethanol IV every 6 hours for five treatments and then every 8 hours for four treatments.

Patients should be monitored for hydration, urine production, acid-base status, serum urea nitrogen, creatinine, electrolytes, and body temperature at least daily. Bladder catheterization may be needed to monitor urine production. Fluid therapy is used to correct dehydration and electrolyte imbalances and promote diuresis. Saline is used to establish urine flow in anuric patients before potassium is added. Slow infusion of bicarbonate solution is required to correct acidosis. B vitamins (pyridoxine and thiamine) are routinely added to fluid therapy regimens in humans to promote glyoxylic acid metabolism.

Peritoneal dialysis and hemodialysis have been used in veterinary and human medicine to treat renal failure, although fomepizole therapy must be adjusted. Tubular regeneration requires weeks or months, and the animal's urine concentrating ability may be lost for more than a year.

PROPYLENE GLYCOL

PG, or 1,2 propandiol, is used in commercial antifreeze as an alternative to the more toxic EG. PG is also used as a deicer, hydraulic fluid, industrial solvent, humectant, and plasticizer, as well as in pharmaceuticals, cosmetics, and foods. It is commonly used as antifreeze in recreational vehicles. PG may be kept in large barrels in veterinary clinics as a treatment for ketosis in ruminants. PG is classified as "Generally Recognized As Safe (GRAS)" by the U. S. Food and Drug Administration but is no longer used in cat food.

PG has a density of 1.036 and is colorless, odorless, and almost flavorless. Like other antifreeze compounds, it has a high boiling point (189°C) and a low freezing point (−60°C) and is freely miscible with water and alcohol.

Toxicity, Toxicokinetics, and Mechanism of Action

PG is less toxic than other glycols. Laboratory animal LD_{50}s tend to fall near 20 ml/kg. The median lethal dose in experimental dogs is 9 ml/kg. Dogs tolerate a diet containing up to 20% PG with minimal clinical effects; however, 5% to 6% PG in the diet causes increased Heinz body formation in kittens and cats. High doses (approximately 40% of the diet) have been associated with mild neurologic signs, including ataxia and depression in cats. Toxicosis has been reported in humans, horses, and cattle and experimentally produced in cats, dogs, laboratory animals, goats, and chickens. I have seen apparently malicious poisoning in dogs using PG.

PG is absorbed rapidly from the gastrointestinal tract and lungs, after injection, and through damaged skin. The volume of distribution is 0.5 L/kg in humans. About one third of PG is excreted unchanged in the urine; the rest is metabolized mostly in the liver and kidneys. Lactic acid is one major metabolite. PG may be conjugated to glucuronide in some species, but this metabolic pathway is inadequate in cats. Metabolites usually appear in the blood within 4 hours of exposure. PG may be excreted completely within a day in dogs.

PG causes osmotic diuresis and a direct narcotic effect similar to ethanol but at about one third the potency. Lactic acid, the metabolic product, is formed in 2 isomers. The L- isomer enters the citric acid cycle and is metabolized. D-lactic acid is not readily metabolized and contributes to lactic acidosis. The mechanism of PG-mediated Heinz body formation and the dose-dependent decrease in survival time for feline erythrocytes are not completely understood.

Clinical Signs and Diagnosis

Clinical signs in cats given high doses of PG include polyuria, polydipsia, and mild-to-moderate ataxia. Cats exposed to low dietary concentrations of PG may be asymptomatic but frequently have increased numbers of Heinz bodies, reticulocytes, and low red blood cell counts. Increased blood concentrations of D-lactic acid occur at higher dietary levels of PG.

Clinical signs of acute PG toxicosis are referable to acidosis. Osmotic diuresis is present in animals after oral or parenteral administration of PG. Hypotension and circulatory collapse have been reported in cats and other species after parenteral overdosing. Pure PG is hyperosmolar and is likely to cause hemolysis if given undiluted IV. Postmortem lesions are nonspecific but may include a foul, garliclike odor to gastrointestinal contents after PG ingestion.

Diagnosis is based on history and clinical signs. Serum, urine, tissues, or the suspected source of PG may be analyzed using GC.

Management

The prognosis for cats with chronic dietary exposure to PG is excellent. The number of Heinz bodies decreases once the source of PG is removed. The prognosis for acute toxicosis is fair to guarded, depending on the status of the animal. Decontamination using gastric lavage and activated charcoal may be effective if implemented very early, but gastrointestinal absorption is quite rapid. Dehydration, acidosis, and hypoglycemia are treated routinely as needed. Antioxidants such as vitamin E and vitamin C have been given to prevent erythrocyte damage without satisfactory results. *N*-acetylcysteine therapy has shown minimal benefit.

DIETHYLENE GLYCOL

DEG is an industrial solvent that may be present in brake fluid, hydraulic fluid, lubricants, and canned cooking fuels. High mortality is reported in epidemic human poisonings. DEG has a specific gravity of 1.118 and is a colorless, nearly odorless, palatable liquid.

Toxicity, Toxicokinetics, and Mechanism of Action

The median lethal dose of DEG in laboratory animals ranges from 3.6 to 11.6 ml/kg; thus it is more toxic than PG but less so than EG. DEG is rapidly absorbed through the gastrointestinal tract or damaged skin. Peak plasma levels occur within an hour or two. DEG is metabolized primarily in the liver by alcohol dehydrogenase and aldehyde dehydrogenase. DEG and metabolites are excreted in the urine, and excretion is almost complete within 36 hours. The mechanism of action of DEG is not understood. There is a direct narcotic effect and renal damage, but oxalate crystals are not produced.

Clinical Signs and Diagnosis

Clinical signs of DEG toxicosis are similar in most species. CNS depression and vomiting are reported early. These clinical signs appear to resolve but are followed by renal failure after 1 or more days. Cardiac abnormalities have been reported in some species. Serum chemistry findings include elevated urea nitrogen, creatinine, potassium, and evidence of lactic acidosis.

Findings at necropsy usually include pale, swollen, mottled kidneys that bulge on cut surface. There is necrosis and degeneration of proximal convoluted tubular epithelium and tubular ectasia. Hepatic lipidosis and centrilobular necrosis have been reported in some species. Hemorrhage involving the pericardium, adrenal medulla, lungs, and pleura has been reported in humans, and I have seen similar lesions in one dog.

Diagnosis is based on a history of exposure, clinical signs, and lesions. Tissues or suspected sources of DEG can be tested using GC, keeping in mind that elimination of DEG from the body is very rapid.

Management

Animals presenting soon after exposure to DEG have a fair- to-guarded prognosis; but, once animals have evidence of renal failure, the prognosis is poor. Therapy includes symptomatic and antidotal treatments similar to those described for EG toxicosis.

PETROLEUM COMPOUNDS

Petroleum compounds include a wide variety of products with variable physical and chemical characteristics. Such compounds include fuels such as propane, gasoline, kerosene, and diesel; solvents such as paint thinner and degreasers; lubricants such as motor oil; and carriers for pesticides, paints, and drugs. Animals may ingest spilled hydrocarbons or drink from open containers. Material spilled on the skin may be absorbed. Animals are occasionally given petroleum products intentionally.

Toxicity, Toxicokinetics, and Mechanism of Action

Toxicity for petroleum products is highly variable and dependent on such factors as volatility, viscosity, and surface tension. Highly volatile compounds are associated with more morbidity and mortality because they are more readily aspirated into the lungs or absorbed into systemic circulation. Aspirated products having low viscosity penetrate deeper airways, and low surface tension further enhances spread within the pulmonary parenchyma.

Absorption occurs through the gastrointestinal tract, skin, and lungs. Low–molecular weight compounds such as gasoline are better absorbed; whereas high–molecular weight compounds such as greases, mineral oils, and waxes are not well absorbed. Hydrocarbons are distributed to all major organs. Aliphatic hydrocarbons are oxidized in the liver to polar compounds that are more readily excreted. Respiratory excretion is important for volatile compounds, and highly volatile hydrocarbons may be excreted completely within 24 hours.

Aspirated hydrocarbons dissolve lipids in cell membranes and cause degeneration and necrosis of the respiratory epithelium. Bacterial pneumonia may occur secondarily. Direct irritation of the skin and eyes is caused by the solvent effects of volatile hydrocarbons on cell membranes. Absorbed compound may interact with neuronal cell membranes to cause CNS depression.

Clinical Signs and Diagnosis

Early clinical signs of ingestion include increased salivation, head shaking, and pawing at the muzzle. Vomiting and colic are typically seen with more volatile compounds, and diarrhea with heavier compounds such as mineral oil. Absence of emesis does not ensure that aspiration has not occurred. Signs of aspiration pneumonia may include choking, coughing, gagging, dyspnea, or cyanosis. Signs of CNS involvement include ataxia, confusion, depression, narcosis, and coma. Tremors and convulsions have been reported in a few cases. Cardiac arrhythmia and cardiovascular collapse have also been reported.

Animals that die after hydrocarbon ingestion frequently have gross lesions typical of aspiration pneumonia. Oily material may be visible in small airways. Secondary bacterial infection may be evident in animals that die late in the course of the disease. Centrilobular hepatic necrosis, myocardial necrosis, and renal tubular necrosis have been reported in animals surviving more than 24 hours according to Raisebeck and Daily (2006).

If vomitus or stomach contents from an animal that has ingested hydrocarbons are mixed with warm water, the petroleum compounds float to the top. If skimmed with a paper towel, these compounds evaporate quickly and have a characteristic odor. This odor may be detectable on the breath or skin of the affected animal. Confirmation of exposure involves analysis of the gastrointestinal content or material on the skin and suspected source material via GC. Samples should be collected quickly and placed in glass containers or wrapped in foil to avoid contact with plastic and frozen until analysis can be performed.

Management

The prognosis for animals that have ingested low-volatility compounds such as mineral oil or motor oil is good, assuming these products were not contaminated with other toxins such as pesticides or heavy metals. Management involves cage rest and observation. Animals that have no evidence of aspiration pneumonia 12 to 24 hours after ingestion have a good prognosis. Uncomplicated aspiration pneumonia is usually resolved after 2 weeks. However, the prognosis is poor if animals have extensive pulmonary lesions or present in a comatose state.

Early management involves identification of the compound involved. The owner should bring the container or label of the suspected source of exposure. If contamination is dermal, a mild detergent bath and clipping of long or matted hair are useful. Animals should be kept warm during this process. Use of mechanic's hand cleaner, lard, or similar substances may be required for removal of very viscous products such as tar. If the animal has ingested the material, gastrointestinal detoxification must be pursued with care. Emetics are usually contraindicated because of the risk of aspiration. Gastric lavage in the sedated, intubated animal and dosing with activated charcoal have been recommended. Instillation of mineral oil or vegetable oil to induce catharsis may increase the risk of aspiration pneumonia; thus it should be avoided.

Monitoring of the exposed animal should include auscultation and thoracic radiography to assess pulmonary function. Aspiration pneumonia is treated symptomatically with cage rest, supplemental oxygen, and β_2-agonists if needed for bronchospasm. Corticosteroids increase the risk of bacterial infection and should not be used. Prophylactic antibiotics should be considered. Cardiac function should be monitored, and arrhythmia treated as needed.

METHANOL

Methanol is used in automotive window washer fluids, gasoline antifreezes, canned cooking fuels, and various solvents. It is highly toxic to humans and other primates, causing formic acidosis, CNS disturbances, and retinal damage. Methanol is much less toxic to dogs and cats because they have an improved ability to metabolize formic acid using an enzyme system dependent on folate. In fact, it is less toxic in small animals than ethanol. Clinical signs of methanol toxicosis in dogs and cats are similar to those of ethanol inebriation. Treatment is based on monitoring and symptomatic and supportive care. Treatment with ethanol or fomepizole to inhibit alcohol dehydrogenase is discouraged.

References and Suggested Reading

Bischoff K: Diethylene glycol. In Peterson ME, Talcott PA, editors: *Small animal toxicology*, ed 2, St Louis, 2006a, Elsevier Saunders, p 693.

Bischoff K: Methanol. In Peterson ME, Talcott PA, editors: *Small animal toxicology*, ed 2, St Louis, 2006b, Elsevier Saunders, p 840.

Bischoff K: Propylene glycol. In Peterson ME, Talcott PA, editors: *Small animal toxicology*, ed 2, St Louis, 2006c, Elsevier Saunders, p 996.

Bonagura JD, editor: *Kirk's current veterinary therapy XIII (small animal practice)*, Philadelphia, 2000, Saunders, p 212.

Dalefield R: Propylene glycol. In Plumlee KH, editor: *Clinical veterinary toxicology*, St Louis, 2004a, Mosby, p 168.

Dalefield R: Ethylene Glycol. In Plumlee KH, editor: *Clinical veterinary toxicology*, St Louis, 2004b, Mosby, p 150.

Hill AS: Antioxidant prevention of Heinz body formation and oxidative injury in cats, *Am J Vet Res* 62:370, 2001.

Raisebeck MF, Dailey RN: Petroleum hydrocarbons. In Peterson ME, Talcott PA, editors: *Small animal toxicology*, ed 2, St Louis, 2006, Elsevier Saunders, p 986.

Ruble GR: The effect of commonly used vehicles on canine hematology and clinical chemistry values, *J Am Assoc Lab Anim Sci* 45:21, 2006.

Thrall MA: Ethylene glycol. In Peterson ME, Talcott PA, editors: *Small animal toxicology*, ed 2, St Louis, 2006, Elsevier Saunders, p 986.

Valentine WM: Short-chain alcohols, *Vet Clin North Am Small Anim Pract* 20:515, 1990.

CHAPTER **30**

Nicotine Toxicosis

WAYNE SPOO, *Winston-Salem, North Carolina*

Nicotine toxicosis is encountered occasionally in small animals, including dogs and cats. Toxic exposure is likely when a nicotine source is available and ingested in sufficient amounts or when dermal/oral membrane exposure occurs. Nicotine can become available to animals from a variety of sources. This chapter focuses on nicotine toxicosis as it relates to consumption of nicotine replacement products (NRPs) and smoked/unsmoked tobacco products.

SOURCES OF NICOTINE

There are many potential sources of nicotine in nature. Table 30-1 lists possible sources of nicotine in the home. The tobacco plant *Nicotiana* spp. contains significant amounts of nicotine (1% to 6% by dry weight) both during the growing and harvesting cycles and after it has been dried and processed for inclusion in cigarettes, cigars, and other tobacco products. However, dietary plant sources also exist. Davis and colleagues (1991) and Domino, Hornbach, and Demana (1993) found that a number of common food items, principally found in the family Solanaceae (among others), contained varying amounts of nicotine but no cotinine (one metabolite of nicotine).

Others have reported that a number of plants other than tobacco contain nicotine, with estimates reported from 12 families and 24 genera, but at levels substantially lower than those found in tobacco.

Why nicotine is present in plants is not known, but it is speculated to be a natural defense mechanism against bacteria, insects, and some animals. Dietary sources of nicotine are mentioned here as a potential source of exposure from homemade pet foods. Pet foods made with these products may provide an exposure mechanism to nicotine; however, there are no known reports of nicotine toxicosis in animals resulting from such exposures. No reports were identified that specifically linked toxicity related to inhalation of nicotine from cigarette smoke, although literature is available that describes the potential adverse health effects of cigarette smoke in pets.

Nicotine Replacement Products

Food and Drug Administration (FDA)–approved NRPs are used by humans as an aid to quit smoking. The products come in a number of forms and delivery methods, are used to replace nicotine normally inhaled during

Table 30-1

Sources of Nicotine

Source	Form	Specifics
Diet	Homemade pet foods, scraps, garbage	Tomatoes (canned or fresh), green peppers, potatoes, eggplant, cauliflower
Tobacco	Smoke	Environmental tobacco smoke or "second-hand" smoke
Tobacco	Unsmoked tobacco products	Cigars, cigarettes, snuff, chewing tobacco
Cigarette structural materials	Smoked and unsmoked tobacco products	Cigarette butts (i.e., filter, plug wrap, tipping paper from smoked cigarettes)
Smoking cessation products	Transdermal patches, gum, lozenges, etc.	FDA-approved nicotine replacement products (see Table 30-2)

FDA, Food and Drug Administration.

Table 30-2

Typical Nicotine Replacement Products Available in the United States

Product Type	Product Name	Approximate Nicotine Content*	Availability
Patch	Habitrol, Nicoderm, Prostep, store brand or generic	7, 14, and 21 mg delivered dose/24 hr	Over-the-counter
Gum	Nicorette, store brand or generic	2-4 mg/stick	Over-the-counter
Nasal spray	Nicotrol	0.5 mg/spray	Prescription
Inhaler	Nicotrol	4 mg/cartridge	Prescription
Lozenge	Commit, store brand or generic	4 mg/lozenge	Over-the-counter

*Nicotine levels reported here are estimates for comparison only and may vary with brand and delivery method.

smoking, and are intended for short-term use. Table 30-2 is a partial list of some NRPs available in the United States and can be used by clinicians as a guideline to determine potential exposure to nicotine via the devices. A complete list of FDA-approved NRPs can be found at the FDA's website.

Nicotine dosage can be estimated when the number of gums, lozenges, or sprays/inhaler exposures are known. With respect to NRP patch products, the manufacturer label typically reports the dosage of nicotine delivered transdermally in humans over a 24-hour period. In the case of oral exposure in animals, the total amount of nicotine contained in each patch is of most relevance; however, dosage estimation can be a challenge. This information is not reported on the label and is known to vary between manufacturers. For example, Habitrol (Novartis) delivers 7, 14, and 21 mg of nicotine per 24 hours in humans; however, the patches contain total amounts of 17.5, 35, and 52.5 mg of nicotine, respectively. Nicoderm CQ (Glaxo-Smith-Kline) reports to deliver the same 7, 14, and 21 mg of nicotine per 24 hours in humans as well; however, the patches contain total amounts of 36, 78, and 114 mg of nicotine, respectively. Practitioners should consider calling the manufacturer directly to help determine the approximate ingested dose of nicotine or contact a poison control center to obtain information about total nicotine content of an ingested product.

Tobacco

Whole cigarettes or cigarette butts are available sources of nicotine for pets within the household; tobacco products such as cigars, snuff, plug, and pipe tobacco are also potential sources. Nicotine content in tobaccos varies considerably among the types and brands of tobacco, and the list is too extensive to show here. Table 30-3 lists some general values for each of these types of tobacco and should be used as a guideline only. Other alkaloids in addition to nicotine are also found in tobacco at much lower levels,

Table 30-3

Guideline Values for Nicotine Content by Type of Tobacco

Product Type	Nicotine Content (Dry Weight Value)
Cigarette butt	1.4-1.7 mg
Plug	8 mg/g
Loose-leaf snuff	7-12 mg/g
Cigarettes	10-16 mg/rod*
Moist snuff	3-11 mg/g

*Rod weights vary by brand and style. For comparison purposes, 0.78 g of cut filler tobacco/rod was assumed.

including nornicotine, anabasine, myosmine, nicotyrine, and anatabine, and are not thought to be of toxicologic concern.

NICOTINE TOXICITY

Mechanism of Action, Kinetics, and Clinical Signs

Nicotine is a weak base, which initially inhibits its absorption when ingested. Little absorption occurs in the stomach because of low pH but likely increases as the nicotine enters the less acidic intestines. Despite these considerations, substantial amounts of nicotine are systemically absorbed after ingestion. Relatively better absorption is obtained from dermal and oral mucosa exposure. Nicotine is metabolized in the liver. Nicotine mimics acetylcholine, acting at the parasympathetic and sympathetic ganglia and the neuromuscular junctions. Clinical signs of toxicity at less than lethal doses include hyperactivity, vomiting, and salivation. As the dose increases, tremors, dyspnea, tachycardia, muscle weakness/paralysis, and death from respiratory paralysis ensue.

CLINICAL NICOTINE TOXICITY

Reports of clinical toxicity related to nicotine in animals are few, mainly limited to dogs. Less information is available for cats and birds. The median lethal dose (LD_{50}) in dogs is reported to be 9.2 mg/kg (Franke and Thomas, 1932). Clinical signs of toxicity have been reported to begin in the 1- to 2-mg/kg range (Osweiler, 1990), and a minimum LD in dogs and cats was reported to be 20 to 100 mg. Using these data, a 40-lb dog would need to ingest approximately 11 cigarettes to reach the LD_{50} dose (assuming 100% absorption) or one cigarette to achieve signs of clinical toxicity.

Vig (1990) reported nicotine toxicosis in a 12-week-old toy poodle that ingested approximately 1 tbsp of liquid from a spittoon. The dog presented with constricted pupils, central nervous system dysfunction (incoordination, trembling, opisthotonus), salivation, and increased heart rate. Blood nicotine and cotinine levels were not reported. Nicotine toxicosis was the most likely diagnosis; however, further characterization of the liquid that was ingested for nicotine content or other potentially toxic components was not reported. Treatment was symptomatic with oral activated charcoal, intravenous diazepam, and sodium bicarbonate. Fourteen hours after admission, the dog's clinical appearance was normal.

Matsushima, Prevo, and Gorsline (1995) reported on the adverse effects of nicotine after topical and oral administration of three transdermal nicotine products. Nicotine doses ranged from 1 to 2 mg/kg/day when dosed topically, resulting in plasma nicotine levels as high as 43 ng/ml. Two of 12 dogs exposed via this route exhibited mild clinical signs consisting of excessive salivation and emesis. When the patches were administered orally (2.8 mg/kg for one patch; 13.4 mg/kg for two patches) over 25 to 57 hours, mean plasma nicotine levels peaked within 1 to 2 hours after administration, with plasma nicotine levels roughly similar to that of the dermal route.

Two of the 12 dogs receiving two patches orally vomited. Other physiologic observations (e.g., heart rate, blood pressure) were not reported.

Cardiovascular effects related to nicotine have also been reported. Huckabee and associates (1993) reported increased regional blood flow in anesthetized dogs dosed with 3 to 100 mg/kg of moist snuff placed in the right buccal space. The nicotine content on the moist snuff on a per gram basis was not reported; thus the exact dose was unknown (see Table 30-3 for an estimated value). Moist snuff increased blood in the buccal tissue at the site of application, with a decrease in blood flow in the opposite (undosed) buccal space. In contrast to oral exposure scenarios, increases in aortic blood pressure, central venous pressure, and left ventricular diastolic and systolic pressure tended to increase as the dose of snuff increased. Similar cardiovascular findings in dogs were reported by Herman and colleagues (2001) using various nicotine patches and Skoal Bandits (moist snuff in a small pouch) placed in the buccal cavity. Nicotine has also been reported to alter renal function in dogs (Pawlik, Jacobson, and Banks, 1985) and elevations in serum angiotensin-converting enzyme (Sugiyama, Yotsumoto, and Takaku, 1986).

It is difficult to describe a typical toxicity scenario associated with nicotine-containing products related to household pets because of a lack of specific poisoning cases and dose information. It is reasonable to conclude that clinical signs related to nicotine toxicosis are likely to be less severe when ingesting cigarettes and/or cigarette butt(s) if treated quickly after ingestion. Signs manifested after ingestion of NRPs are likely to be more overt if the products are damaged and more nicotine is available for absorption versus the intact product (see Table 30-2) or if treatment is delayed. Animals that chew on tobacco products and do not swallow or are otherwise exposed via the oral mucosa only (i.e., puncturing a nasal inhaler) may also exhibit more severe clinical signs, which again depends on the product form.

TREATMENT OF NICOTINE TOXICOSIS

There is no specific treatment for nicotine poisoning; thus therapy is symptom specific. Given the basic nature of nicotine, oral absorption for the stomach is expected to be low, increasing as the nicotine reaches the intestinal tract. If ingestion of nicotine-containing products is suspected/known, evacuation of the gastric contents (if not contraindicated) should be instituted as soon after exposure as possible (see Chapter 24). Gastric lavage, activated charcoal therapy, and supportive care (e.g., fluid therapy, respiratory support) should also be considered. Atropine and benzodiazepines can also be used to counter parasympathetic stimulation. In cases of dermal exposure the nicotine source should be removed, the skin thoroughly washed with soap and water, supportive care administered, and the animal observed for signs of nicotine toxicosis.

Overall, consumption of nicotine from tobacco or NRPs is an occasional poisoning scenario in household pets. Clinical signs related to nicotine toxicity are dose, product, and route dependent. A thorough history related to intoxication, including identification of the specific nicotine form, estimation of nicotine dose, and time since exposure, is useful in determining treatment protocols and prognosis. Clinicians are encouraged to use Table 30-2 as a guide in determining how much nicotine the animal potentially received. Treatment should be implemented as quickly as possible, and supportive therapy instituted as appropriate.

References and Suggested Reading

Centers for Disease Control and Prevention: Determination of nicotine, pH, and moisture content of six US commercial moist snuff products—Florida, *MMWR* 48(19):398, 1999.

Davis RA et al: Dietary nicotine: a source of urinary cotinine, *Food Chem Toxicol* 29(12):821, 1991.

Domino EF, Hornbach E, Demana T: Relevance of nicotine content of common vegetable to the identification of passive tobacco smokers, *Med Sci Res* 21:571, 1993.

Food and Drug Administration website: http://www.accessdata. fda.gov/scripts/cder/drugsatfda/index.cfm.

Franke JE et al: Determination of nicotine in tobacco: collaborative study, *Beitrage Zur Tabakforschung International Contributions To Tobacco Research* 19:251, 2001.

Franke FE, Thomas JE: A note on the minimal fatal dose of nicotine for unanesthetized dogs, *Proc Soc Exp Biol Med* 29:1177, 1932.

Herman EH et al: Cardiovascular effects of buccal exposure to dermal nicotine patches in the dog: a comparative evaluation, *Clin Toxicol* 39:135, 2001.

Huckabee KD et al: Effects of snuff on regional blood flow to the cheek and tongue of anesthetized dogs, *Oral Surg Med Oral Pathol* 76:729, 1993.

Matsushima D, Prevo ME, Gorsline J: Absorption and adverse effect following topical and oral administration of three transdermal nicotine products to dogs, *J Pharm Sci* 84: 365, 1995.

Osweiler GD: *Toxicology*, Media, Pa, 1996, Williams & Wilkins.

Osweiler GD et al: *Clinical and diagnostic veterinary toxicology*, ed 3, Dubuque, Ia, 1976, Kendall Hunt Publishing.

Pawlik WW, Jacobson ED, Banks RO: Actions of nicotine on renal function in dogs, *Proc Soc Exp Biol Med* 178 585, 1985.

Richter P, Spierto FW: Surveillance of smokeless tobacco nicotine, ph, moisture, and unprotonated nicotine content, *Nicotine Tob Res* 5:885, 2003.

Sugiyama Y, Yotsumoto H, Takaku F: Increase in serum angiotensin-converting enzyme level after exposure to cigarette smoke and nicotine infusion in dogs, *Respiration* 49:292, 1986.

Vig MM: Nicotine poisoning in a dog, *Vet Hum Toxicol* 32:573, 1990.

CHAPTER **31**

Recently Recognized Animal Toxicants

JOCELYN A. MASON, *Chambly, Québec, Canada*
SAFDAR A. KHAN, *Urbana, Illinois*
SHARON M. GWALTNEY-BRANT, *Urbana, Illinois*

MINOXIDIL

Minoxidil, a hypotensive agent, has been used as a vasodilator and as a topical solution to enhance localized hair growth in humans. Minoxidil alters potassium channels in vascular smooth muscle, resulting in vasodilation and hypotension. The mechanism of enhanced hair growth is not entirely understood, but minoxidil may increase epithelial cell proliferation at the follicular base or vasodilation of scalp vasculature or both.

Oral formulations of minoxidil are well absorbed orally, with peak plasma concentrations within 2 hours in dogs. When applied topically, 0.3% to 4.5% of the dose is absorbed systemically. Kinetic information regarding ingestion of the topical product is not available. Although the plasma concentration declines rapidly after peak concentrations, the peak hypotensive effect is delayed by several hours and persists for at least 24 hours after exposure. In humans a large percentage of oral minoxidil is metabolized by conjugation with glucuronic acid. Consequently minoxidil elimination may be delayed in cats if cats eliminate minoxidil in the same way.

In experimental studies in dogs, short-term oral administration of minoxidil resulted in a variety of hemorrhagic and necrotic myocardial lesions, but dermal application of the topical product did not cause cardiac lesions or hypotension. To date significant hypotension in clinical canine cases of minoxidil exposure has only occurred through ingestion of tablets. Oral exposures to topical products have primarily produced vomiting and lethargy in dogs.

Two cats that had minoxidil solution applied topically showed lethargy and dyspnea within 36 hours of exposure, and pulmonary edema and pleural effusion were identified on radiography. Both cats died in spite of aggressive supportive care. Histopathology confirmed acute myocardial ischemia and edema resulting in severe cardiac compromise, pulmonary edema, and pleural effusion. Whether the minoxidil was absorbed dermally or ingested via grooming behavior is not clear. At least two instances of cats developing hypotension (one with pleural effusion) after licking the treated hair of their owners have been reported to the ASPCA Animal Poison Control Center (ASPCA Animal Poison Control Center, unpublished data). One of these cats died, and the other was lost to follow-up.

Because of the potential for serious cardiovascular compromise, exposures to minoxidil should be managed aggressively. Oral exposures to minoxidil should be managed with gastric emptying followed by activated charcoal. Rinsing the oral cavity with water may bring some relief because the topical solution may be irritating to oral mucous membranes.

Dermal exposures should be decontaminated with bathing in a liquid dishwashing detergent. Bathing may be effective as long as 48 hours after topical exposure because of delayed absorption of topical products. Cardiovascular and respiratory systems should be monitored closely for 36 to 48 hours. Pulmonary edema should be managed using furosemide or other standard treatment. Thoracocentesis may be required to remove pleural effusion and improve respiration. Intravenous fluid therapy is indicated if hypotension develops, although care must be used in managing fluid rates in cats with pulmonary edema. Pressor agents may be useful in hypotensive animals that do not respond to fluid administration alone. The use of colloids (Hetastarch, Gensia Sicor Pharm) at a 5-ml/kg bolus along with dopamine, intravenous crystalloids, and thoracocentesis resulted in successful resolution of pleural effusion and hypotension in one severely affected cat (ASPCA Animal Poison Control Center, unpublished data). The prognosis for animals exposed to minoxidil depends on the extent of exposure, severity of clinical signs, and promptness and aggressiveness of treatment. Animals showing significant cardiac or respiratory signs should be considered to have a guarded prognosis.

XYLITOL

Xylitol is a 5-carbon sugar-alcohol sweetener that is increasingly used in sugar-free products such as gums, baked goods, and candies. In humans xylitol does not cause significant increases in blood insulin or glucose levels. However, in dogs oral xylitol can cause a rapid and dose-dependent increase in blood insulin concentrations, with a concurrent drop in blood glucose concentration. Some dogs that have ingested larger amounts of xylitol-containing products have subsequently developed hepatic necrosis. The mechanistic cause of hepatic lesions has not

been established; however, a theory of interference with hepatocellular adenosine triphosphate production has been raised. The toxicity of xylitol to cats is not known.

Chewing gums with xylitol as the primary or sole sweetener contain about 0.3 to 0.4 g of xylitol per piece. Xylitol doses greater than 100 mg/kg (0.1 g/kg) have been associated with hypoglycemia; and doses greater than 1000 mg/kg of body weight have been associated with hepatic necrosis in dogs.

Clinical signs of hypoglycemia in dogs may occur within 30 minutes of ingesting xylitol-containing products. These signs may include vomiting, lethargy, disorientation, ataxia, tremors, collapse, and seizures. Other signs that may occur include weakness, diarrhea, abdominal pain, vocalization, tachypnea and fasciculation.

Clinical pathologic findings reported in dogs ingesting xylitol include hypoglycemia, hypokalemia, and mild hypophosphatemia. Occasionally hypoglycemia may be prolonged beyond 12 hours, especially in cases of xylitol-containing gum ingestion. Evidence of hepatic insufficiency may be seen by 8 to 12 hours after exposure, characterized by elevations in hepatic enzyme levels. Some dogs develop transient elevations of liver enzymes; whereas others progress to acute liver failure, hemorrhage, dissemination, and death. Not all dogs that develop acute hepatic failure after xylitol ingestion show signs of hypoglycemia. Some simply become acutely ill 48 hours after ingestion of xylitol. Serum chemistry reveals extreme elevations in alanine aminotransferase, elevated bilirubin, and prolonged prothrombin times (PTs) and partial thromboplastin times (PTTs). Some cases show initial hypophosphatemia with terminal hyperphosphatemia.

Management of xylitol exposures in dogs includes gastrointestinal (GI) emptying in asymptomatic dogs. The use of activated charcoal is debatable since results of one in vitro study have indicated that adsorption of xylitol by activated charcoal is limited and unreliable. Because of the potential for significant clinical signs to develop within 30 minutes, emesis and activated charcoal administration must be performed with care to avoid the risk of aspiration. Frequent small meals in asymptomatic animals with frequent monitoring of serum glucose levels for at least 6 to 12 hours are important. Administration of 5% dextrose intravenously (IV) may be needed to maintain normal blood glucose concentrations. Potassium supplementation may be required if potassium levels drop below 2.5 mEq/L.

In dogs ingesting potentially hepatotoxic doses of xylitol (>1000 mg/kg), an initial bolus of intravenous dextrose should be considered, followed by continuous-rate infusion of dextrose for 24 hours, with monitoring of liver enzymes and PT/PTT for 48 to 72 hours. The use of hepatoprotectants (e.g., S-adenosylmethionine) should be considered in dogs developing evidence of injury; although evidence of efficacy of these products in preventing liver injury is lacking, their antioxidant effects may help minimize secondary oxidative hepatic injury. Other standard treatments for hepatic injury (e.g., lactulose, antibiotics) may be required to manage liver injury.

The prognosis for xylitol toxicosis depends on the dose ingested, clinical signs, and the response to therapy. Hypoglycemia generally responds well to dextrose treatment, but prolonged seizure activity may result in hyperthermia and disseminated intravascular coagulopathy. The development of hepatic necrosis and coagulopathy warrants a guarded prognosis; hyperphosphatemia may be associated with poorer prognosis in dogs.

EXPANDABLE POLYURETHANE GLUE TOXICITY

Expandable polyurethane glues are available as industrial-strength wood glues marketed as Gorilla Glue, Elmer's ProBond Polyurethane Glue, or insulating foam sealants. These products contain diphenylmethane diisocyanate or polymethylene polyphenol isocyanate in various concentrations. The terms *isocyanate* and *diisocyanate* are usually listed in the active ingredient section of most expandable polyurethane glues.

Most glue or adhesive exposures in animals are acute and accidental. All animal species are susceptible; however, dogs are more likely to be involved, presumably because of their chewing habits. Dermal exposure in cats can lead to significant oral exposure after grooming.

Ingestion of expandable polyurethane glues (isocyanates) can form an expanding gastric foreign body. This is more likely to occur in dogs that chew the bottle of glue rather than lick or ingest products covered with the glue. An animal that ingests already polymerized and dried glue is not likely to experience foreign body obstruction.

Most clinical signs develop within 12 hours of exposure but may range from 15 minutes to 20 hours. Radiographic evidence of gastric outflow obstruction can be evident within 24 hours of exposure. The most commonly reported clinical signs of expandable polyurethane toxicosis include vomiting, retching, anorexia, lethargy, visible abdominal distention or presence of a large firm mass on palpation, diarrhea, tachypnea, and dehydration. Following ingestion, the glue polymerizes into a large, friable, black-to–dark brown foreign body. The foreign body may resemble kibble filling the entire stomach. Radiographic findings seen 4 to 5 hours after exposure include a large radiopaque, mottled density in the stomach; gastric dilation; or both. It has been suggested that the expandable polyurethane glue is hygroscopic in nature and absorbs water from the stomach. Warm body temperature may also play a role in glue expansion.

Diagnosis is made based on history of exposure, types of clinical signs present, and endoscopic or radiographic evidence of a foreign body. Before instituting any treatment, it is important to confirm that the patient has been exposed to expandable polyurethane glue versus nonexpandable glue. Cyanoacrylates (Superglue, Krazy glue) that contain ethyl-2-cyanoacrylate or poly (methylmethacrylate) and white glues containing polyvinyl acetate in various concentrations are not known to cause foreign body obstruction following ingestion. Reading the label of the product can be extremely helpful in determining the type of the glue involved. Most expandable glues have the word *isocyanate* or *diisocyanate* written in the active ingredient section.

The treatment of expandable polyurethane glue toxicosis involves (1) decontamination with the aim of preventing formation of a foreign body; (2) determination of the nature and severity of the foreign body; (3) surgical removal of the foreign body if necessary; and (4) supportive care.

With dermal exposure, the area should be washed thoroughly with a mild dishwashing detergent. The hair is clipped, or the glue manually removed using a toenail clipper. Once the glue dries, it is not normally irritating to the skin.

Induction of emesis with hydrogen peroxide or apomorphine in dogs following oral exposure is debatable. The fear is that, if part of the glue is lodged in the esophagus, it could lead to esophageal obstruction. In our opinion emesis could be tried cautiously under veterinary supervision only if exposure has been within 1 hour. The animal should be given a small amount of water or food after vomiting to clear the esophagus. Dilution with milk or activated charcoal is not recommended because it may enhance both the potential of foreign body formation by providing liquid for the adhesive to absorb and the risk of aspiration from vomiting.

It may be necessary to perform a gastrotomy to remove a gastric foreign body. Abdominal radiographs or endoscopic examination of the stomach may help determine the presence of a foreign body and esophageal and gastric mucosal damage (irritation, ulcers, rupture). Excellent results (100% recovery) have been achieved in dogs with appropriate medical and surgical intervention. Systemic toxic effects other than foreign body obstruction have not been described.

Anesthesia for performing gastrotomy can be induced with propofol (4 mg/kg IV) and maintained with isoflurane. Atropine sulfate is used as a preanesthetic agent (0.02 mg/kg IV). After removal of the foreign body, any damage to the stomach mucosa (i.e., presence of adhesions, ulcers, or rupture) is assessed. Sucralfate, an H_2 antagonist such as famotidine or cimetidine, and broad-spectrum antibiotics are administered after gastrotomy for 10 days or longer, as needed. Metoclopramide can be used for controlling vomiting. Food and water intake should be restricted for the first 12 to 24 hours after surgery. Pain should be controlled, and supportive care given, including intravenous fluids as needed. Several days may be needed for complete recovery after the surgery. Stomach rupture, torsion, and peritonitis are some possible complications following surgery.

BRUNFELSIA SPP. TOXICOSIS

The genus *Brunfelsia* belongs to the Solanaceae family. This plant is an erect, compact, evergreen shrub that grows to about 1.5 to 2 feet in height and diameter. *Brunfelsia* is native to South and Central America and the West Indies. The genus has about 40 different species. All species of *Brunfelsia* in the United States are ornamentals; consequently they are found outside in gardens in warmer regions and inside as potted plants in colder states. The showy flowers appear in clusters. The deep purple flowers gradually change to lavender and then to white over a 3-day period. One plant may have all three flower colors (purple, lavender, and white) at the same time. Brown-green berries can be found in summer and autumn. Each seed pod may possess about 20 small hard seeds.

Although only a few *Brunfelsia* species (*B. calcyina var. floribunda*, commonly known as *yesterday-today-and-tomorrow; B. pauciflora; B. australis; B. bondora*) have been implicated in animal poisoning cases, all species of this genus should be considered toxic to all animals. All parts (flowers, leaves, berries, and seeds) are toxic. Dogs appear to be particularly attracted to the berries.

There are a few case reports of *Brunfelsia* toxicosis reported in cattle, dogs, rats, and mice. Because of the increased popularity and availably of *Brunfelsia* species in the United States, the numbers of poisoning cases from *Brunfelsia* in the dog appear to be increasing. For example, in 2005 alone, nine *Brunfelsia* toxicity cases were reported to the ASPCA Animal Poison Control Center. Seven of these cases were reported from California, one was from Oregon, and one was from Texas. Most commonly reported clinical signs included seizures, hypersalivation, ataxia, tremors, head shaking, diarrhea, and lethargy. Death was reported in one dog.

The onset time of clinical signs in *Brunfelsia* toxicosis in dogs may occur within 15 minutes to several hours after the exposure. Clinical signs may start with agitation, nervousness, or excitement followed by tremors, shaking, muscular rigidity, paddling, and tonic-clonic seizures. The tonic-clonic seizures and other clinical signs such as muscular rigidity or sawhorse stance may resemble those caused by strychnine poisoning. Clinical signs may last from a few hours up to several days. *Brunfelsia* poisoning does not seem to cause any significant hematologic, chemistry, or pathologic changes in animals.

Although several biologically active compounds have been isolated from *Brunfelsia* species, two compounds of interest are hopeanine and brunfelsamidine. Hopeanine causes decreased activity, paralysis, seizures, and hypersensitivity in rodents; brunfelsamidine produces excitement, tonic and clonic seizures, and death. Brunfelsamidine may prove to be the toxin responsible for neurotoxicity in animals. Other unidentified toxins from *B. calcyina var. floribunda* are water soluble and maintain toxicity for 4 months.

Diagnosis of *Brunfelsia* toxicosis in dogs may be made based on a history or evidence of exposure to the plant (flowers, leaves, berries, or seeds present in the vomitus, or stool) and presence of characteristic central nervous system (CNS) signs (muscular rigidity, paddling, tonic-clonic seizures). Differential diagnosis list should include strychnine, metaldehyde, methylxanthine, organochlorine pesticides, lead, and illicit drug toxicosis.

The objectives of treatment are decontamination, seizure control, and supportive care. If the animal is presented with CNS signs, the first step should be to stabilize it (control seizures as described later in this paragraph) before starting decontamination or supportive care. Emesis can be induced when no clinical signs are present and exposure is known to have been within 2 hours. Emesis can be induced with hydrogen peroxide or apomorphine and should be followed by administration of activated charcoal. Repeated doses of charcoal every 6 to 8 hours can be useful if seeds or fruit have been ingested. Gastric or enterogastric lavage followed by charcoal administration can be considered when large amounts of seeds or berries have been consumed. Seizures can be controlled

with pentobarbital sodium IV; it should be given to effect and repeated as needed or with methocarbamol (100 to 200 mg/kg IV; maximum dosage of 330 mg/kg/day). Propofol (4-6 mg/kg IV) or diazepam (with variable success) may be used at 1 to 2 mg/kg IV. Isoflurane gas anesthesia should be tried if seizures are not controlled with the preceding treatment measures. Severely affected animals should be intubated, and artificial respiration provided; they should be kept in a dark and quiet place. The animal should be monitored for hyperthermia and treated as needed with cooling bath or fans. Intravenous fluid diuresis may be required for 1 to 2 days or longer. Complete recovery may take several days or a week or longer.

PAINTBALL TOXICOSIS

Dogs seem to be attracted to paintballs. They have been known to eat as many as 500 paintballs at one time. Paintballs are available in different colors, and one box may contain more than 1000 paintballs. Active ingredients vary, depending on the manufacturer, but often include polyethylene glycol, glycerol (glycerin), gelatin, sorbitol, dipropylene glycol, water, dye, titanium dioxide (found in most acrylic paints), and food coloring. Some paintballs have polyethylene glycol available as 94% and dipropylene glycol as 64%; however, concentrations of most ingredients are not listed on the label.

The most commonly reported clinical signs associated with paintball ingestion in dogs include vomiting with or without paint, ataxia, diarrhea, and tremors. Other less frequently seen clinical signs may include tachycardia, weakness, hyperactivity, hyperthermia, blindness, and seizures. Most commonly reported electrolyte changes include hypernatremia (22%), occasionally hyperchloremia, and hypokalemia. Clinical signs can develop within 1 hour to several hours after exposure, and ingestion of as little as 15 paintballs has led to development of clinical signs.

The exact mechanism of hypernatremia or other electrolyte changes following paintball ingestion is not known. It has been suggested that the presence of osmotically active agents such as polyethylene glycol, glycerol, and sorbitol in paintballs can cause fluid shifts, moving the water from the body tissues into the bowel lumen. Clinical signs of hypernatremia, including tremors, ataxia, and seizures, usually start when serum sodium concentration exceeds 160 mEq/L. Sometimes rapid change in serum sodium concentration may be more responsible for clinical signs than the absolute change in serum sodium concentration.

A clinical diagnosis may be based on history or evidence of exposure such as presence of paintballs in the vomitus or stool and presence of clinical signs, including vomiting, ataxia, tremors, and serum electrolyte changes (hypernatremia). Other causes of hypernatremia include salt (sodium chloride) toxicosis, excessive water loss caused by nephrogenic diabetes insipidus, inadequate water intake, heat stroke, and acute or chronic renal failure.

Treatment objectives are decontamination, correction of electrolytes, seizure control, and supportive care. The animal should first be stabilized by controlling seizures before starting decontamination or supportive care if animal is presented with CNS signs. Emesis can be induced with hydrogen peroxide or apomorphine if the exposure is within 2 hours and if no clinical signs are present. *Do not give activated charcoal* as it does not adsorb sorbitol or most glycols very well. Charcoal administration can also lead to development of hypernatremia in some dogs. After emesis a warm-water enema should be administered at 20 ml/kg to help move the paintballs out of the GI tract. Electrolytes are monitored; and hypernatremia is treated with 5% dextrose, 0.45% or 0.9% saline IV, or lactated Ringer's solution with 5% dextrose. Serum sodium concentration must not be decreased faster than 0.5 to 1 mEq/L/hour since a rapid drop in serum sodium concentrations can cause water influx into the brain and cerebral edema. Other electrolytes should be corrected as needed. Seizures should be controlled with diazepam (0.5 to 2 mg/kg IV as needed). Complete recovery may occur in 24 hours or longer.

GRAPE AND RAISIN TOXICOSIS

Etiopathogenesis

The link between grape or raisin ingestion and nephrotoxicosis in dogs is relatively new. A recent report from the ASPCA Animal Poison Control Center has described the development of acute renal failure (ARF) in 43 dogs following ingestion of fresh or desiccated fruits of the *Vitis* spp. Although the exact nephrotoxic principle found in grapes and raisins currently remains unknown, several theories have been proposed, including the possible presence of pesticide residues, heavy metals, or various molds producing mycotoxins.

Toxicity

Not all dogs ingesting grapes or raisins develop renal failure. The lowest documented grape and raisin dose associated with the development of ARF in dogs is 0.7 oz/kg and 0.11 oz/kg, respectively. A 10-kg dog ingesting 7 oz of grapes would have potential for developing ARF. However, one cannot conclude that these are in fact the lowest doses leading to ARF in dogs.

In terms of exposure, one grape is equal to one raisin, although there are more raisins per unit weight. Although grape and raisin toxicosis has been most commonly described in dogs, there are unconfirmed reports of ferrets and cats developing ARF following ingestion of fruits of the *Vitis* spp.

Clinical Features

In dogs clinical signs occur within a few hours of exposure or can be delayed for up to 24 hours. Commonly reported signs include vomiting (100%), lethargy (77%), anorexia (72%), diarrhea 51%), decreased urine output (49%), abdominal pain (28%), ataxia (23%), and weakness (23%). Clinical signs are quickly followed by characteristic changes in serum chemistry profile.

Clinical chemistry changes observed within 24 hours generally include elevations in serum creatinine and phosphorus and a higher $Ca \times P$ product. By 48 hours after exposure, the blood urea nitrogen (BUN) begins to climb; serum calcium elevations are observed approximately 48 to 72 hours later. A urinalysis may reveal presence of isosthenuria, casts, protein, and glucose. Anuria or oliguria are common sequelae in severe cases and, together with the development of neurologic signs such as ataxia and weakness, generally predict a poor prognosis. Hyperkalemia commonly accompanies oliguria and is associated with metabolic acidosis.

Pathologic Findings

Acute tubular necrosis, particularly of proximal tubules, and dystrophic mineralization of soft tissue may be observed histologically.

Differential Diagnoses

The differential diagnosis for raisin toxicosis includes ethylene glycol toxicity, nonsteroidal antiinflammatory drug (NSAID) toxicity, lily toxicity in cats, infectious diseases such as leptospirosis, bacterial pyelonephritis, hypoadrenocorticism (Addison's), vitamin D/analog ingestion, and chronic renal failure.

Treatment

If ingestion is less than 12 hours and the dog is asymptomatic, removal of the agent from the GI tract is the primary goal. Emesis induction followed by one to two doses of activated charcoal is recommended. In addition, if any grapes or raisins are found in the stool, an enema could be performed to further remove the agent from GI tract.

Intravenous crystalloid fluid diuresis at twice the maintenance rate is recommended to prevent or minimize renal tubular damage for 48 hours or longer. Patients with decreased urine production may require the administration of a loop diuretic such as furosemide, central venous pressure and urine output monitoring, and weighing regularly.

Baseline blood work evaluating renal function should be performed and repeated daily for 2 to 3 days or until the resolution of clinical signs. Monitor serum BUN, creatinine, calcium, phosphorus, electrolytes, bicarbonates, total protein, and a complete blood count. A urinalysis may show the presence of isosthenuria, casts, proteinuria, or glucosuria.

Vomiting can be controlled with an antiemetic such as metoclopramide, and GI protectants such as an H_2-blocker (famotidine) or a proton pump inhibitor (omeprazole) and sucralfate administered. Hyperphosphatemia can be treated with phosphate binders such as aluminum hydroxide at 30 to 90 mg/kg/day. Magnesium-containing phosphate binders are to be avoided since the renal elimination of magnesium may be impaired with decreased renal function. Placing the patient on a low-protein diet may also be beneficial. If diuresis-refractory oliguria or anuria develops, peritoneal dialysis can be performed and may aid in allowing time for the regeneration of renal tubules to occur.

The prognosis depends on various factors such as severity of exposure; individual susceptibility; preexposure renal function; and, most important, how quickly the condition is recognized and therapy is instituted. Hospitalization and supportive therapy may be required for days to several weeks. Mortality rate can be high; as nearly 50% of the 43 dogs reported in a recent retrospective study died or were euthanized.

LILY TOXICOSIS IN CATS

Etiopathogenesis

Members of the *Lilium* and *Hemerocallis* genera are considered nephrotoxic to cats, leading to ARF. Implicated species include Easter lilies (*Lilium longiflorum*), tiger lilies (*L. tigrinum*), stargazer lilies (*L. auratum*), rubrum lilies (*L. speciosum*), Japanese show lilies (*L. lancifolimu*), as well as daylilies (*Hemerocallis spp.*). Exposure to any part of the plant, including pollen, can lead to toxicosis. Consuming less than one leaf can lead to severe toxicosis. Thus far only cats are known to develop renal failure from lilies. Although the exact mechanism of action for lily toxicity remains elusive, studies suggest that the toxin is water soluble and is more concentrated in flowers than in leaves or other parts of the plant.

Not all plants containing the name *lily* are considered true lilies. As such, neither lily-of-the-valley (*Convallaria* spp.) nor the peace lily (*Spathiphyllum* spp.) belongs to the above-mentioned genera, but they can nevertheless be toxic by a different means. Peace lilies and calla lilies (*Zantedeschia* spp.) contain insoluble calcium oxalate crystals, which can lead to oral irritation and swelling.

Clinical Findings

Signs of lily toxicosis usually develop within 12 hours following exposure, although signs may develop within hours or be delayed for up to 5 days after exposure. Commonly reported signs include vomiting, anorexia, and depression, which typically occur in the hours following ingestion. BUN, creatinine, potassium, and phosphorus concentrations begin rising within 24 to 72 hours after exposure. The creatinine concentration is usually disproportionately elevated when compared to the BUN, with values as high as 53 mg/dl. A urinalysis is helpful in determining if renal tubular damage has occurred and typically reveals isosthenuria, presence of casts, protein, and glucose. Epithelial casts may be seen in the urine by 18 hours after exposure.

Differential Diagnoses

The differential diagnosis of lily toxicosis in cats includes ethylene glycol toxicity, NSAID toxicity, infectious diseases such as leptospirosis, bacterial pyelonephritis, lymphosarcoma and chronic renal failure.

Treatment

Renal failure may be permanent if not treated early. The therapeutic goal is to prevent renal tubular damage and obstruction secondary to necrosis and sloughing of epithelial cells. The most important first step is to remove plant material from the GI tract. If ingestion is less than 2 hours and the animal is asymptomatic, emesis can be induced. Emesis should be followed with one to two doses of activated charcoal (6 to 8 hours apart) with a cathartic for the first dose and without a cathartic for subsequent administrations. Baseline blood work should be obtained, especially serum BUN and creatinine. Obtaining a urine-specific gravity before treatment is also recommended. Renal function should be monitored daily for a minimum of 2 to 3 days or for as long as needed. Diuresis with lactated Ringer's solution should be initiated at twice maintenance rate of ≈130 ml/kg/day for a minimum of 48 hours. Intravenous fluid therapy should be continued longer if symptoms persist. Placing the animal on a low-protein diet is also recommended in the presence of ARF.

Prognosis

Delaying treatment by 18 to 24 hours may result in irreversible renal failure leading to death (or euthanasia) within the following few days. However, with prompt and aggressive treatment renal injury may be prevented. The prognosis is poor when anuria or oliguria develops, but renal function may be restored if peritoneal dialysis is performed. Treatment may be needed for days to weeks for complete recovery.

References and Suggested Reading

Burrows GE, Tyrl RJ: Toxic plants of North America, Ames, Ia, 2001, Iowa State University Press, p 1107.

DeClementi CD et al: Suspected toxicosis after topical administration of minoxidil in 2 cats, *J Vet Emerg Crit Care* 14:287, 2004.

Donaldson C: Paintball toxicosis in dogs, *Vet Med* 98:995, 2003.

Dunayer EK: Hypoglycemia following canine ingestion of xylitol-containing gum, *Vet Hum Toxicol* 46:87, 2004.

Eubig PA et al: Acute renal failure in dogs subsequent to the ingestion of grapes or raisins: a retrospective evaluation of 43 dogs (1992-2002), *J Vet Intern Med* 19:663, 2005.

Hall JO: Lily nephrotoxicity. In August JR, editor: *Consultations in feline internal medicine 4*, Philadelphia, 2001, Saunders, p 308.

Hortman CL et al: Gastric outflow obstruction after ingestion of wood glue in a dog, *J Am Anim Hosp Assoc* 39:4751, 2003.

Khan SA: Brunfelsia species: beautiful but deadly, *Vet Med* 3:138, 2008.

Milewski LM, Khan SA: An overview of potentially life threatening poisonous plants in dogs and cats, *J Vet Emerg Crit Care* 16(1):25, 2006.

Morrow CK et al: Canine renal pathology associated with grape or raisin ingestion: 10 cases, *J Vet Diagn Invest* 17(3):223, 2005.

Spainhour Jr.CB et al: A toxicologic investigation of the garden shrub *Brunfelsia calcyina var. floribunda* (yesterday-today-and-tomorrow) in three species, *J Vet Diagn Invest* 2:3, 1990.

Volmer PA: Easter lily toxicosis in cats, *Vet Med* 94(4):331, 1999.

CHAPTER 32

Human Drugs of Abuse

PETRA A. VOLMER, *Urbana, Illinois*

Animal exposures to human "drugs of abuse" occur periodically in veterinary medicine. In many cases the owners are reluctant to admit that the animal was exposed until it is in severe distress. Often illicit drugs are contaminated with other compounds that may possess pharmacologic activity, causing unique combinations of clinical signs. Diagnosis of a toxicosis is often based on characteristic clinical signs and history of exposure. There has been a recent introduction of over-the-counter drug testing kits available at most pharmacies. These kits are designed for rapid determination of drug presence in urine and, although designed for in-home human use, may provide useful diagnostic information in the veterinary clinical setting. Some kits may test for as many as 12 drugs.

AMPHETAMINES

This class of compounds includes a number of prescription and illicit products, all derivatives of the parent compound amphetamine. Most animal exposures are a result of the accidental ingestion of human prescription products used for the treatment of obesity, narcolepsy, and attention-deficit hyperactivity disorder. Exposure to unlawful amphetamine compounds can also occur. Street names for amphetamine can include *speed, uppers, dex or dexies,* and *bennies.* Methamphetamine production is on the rise in clandestine laboratories in many areas of the United States. Street names for methamphetamine can include *ice* and *glass* for the clear, translucent crystals; and *crystal, crank,* and *meth* for the white or yellow powder form. Designer amphetamines include 4-methylaminorex *(ice, U4EUh),* methcathinone *(cat),* 3,4-methylenedioxy-N-methyl-amphetamine (MDMA [*ecstasy, XTC, Adam, MDA*]) and 3,4-methylenedixoy-N-ethylamphetamine (MDEA *[Eve]*) (Volmer, 2006; Llera and Volmer, 2006)

The amphetamines as a class are well absorbed orally, with peak plasma levels occurring by 1 to 3 hours; thus clinical signs can develop rapidly. Some pharmaceutical products are extended-release preparations, with the result of prolonging absorption and delaying the onset of signs. Amphetamine and its metabolites are excreted in the urine in a pH-dependent manner, with a lower pH-enhancing excretion (Baggot and Davis, 1972). Amphetamines have a stimulant effect on the cerebral cortex through release of catecholamines, acting as a dopamine excitatory receptor agonist and enhancing release of serotonin. Toxic dosages of amphetamine products are low: the oral median lethal dosage for amphetamine sulfate in the dog is 20 to 27 mg/kg; for methamphetamine hydrochloride it is 9 to 11 mg/kg (Zalis et al., 1965). Signs in field cases can be seen at dosages much lower than experimental lethal dosages.

Exposed animals exhibit signs associated with stimulation. Behavioral effects can include initial restlessness, pacing, panting, and an inability to sit still. These signs can progress to pronounced hyperactivity, hypersalivation, vocalization, tachypnea, tachycardia, tremors, hyperthermia, seizures, and potentially death. In some cases animals may exhibit depression, weakness, and bradycardia.

Diagnosis is based on clinical signs and history of exposure. Amphetamines can be detected in urine. Over-the-counter drug testing kits may be of use in diagnosing an exposure in the acute clinical setting.

Animals should be stabilized and then decontaminated. Animals with known ingestions of amphetamine products less than 30 minutes prior can undergo induction of emesis followed by administration of activated charcoal and a cathartic. Animals already exhibiting signs of stimulation such as restlessness or worse should not be induced to vomit because of the risk of aspiration. Similarly, if the product is rapidly absorbed with the possible rapid onset of signs, emesis is not recommended. For those cases gastric lavage followed by the instillation of activated charcoal and a cathartic is a safer approach. Sustained-release medications may require repeated doses of activated charcoal.

Excitability, tremors, seizures, and other stimulant signs associated with amphetamine intoxication can be treated with acepromazine (0.5 to 1 mg/kg slowly intravenously [IV]; allow 15 minutes for onset of action; repeat as needed) or chlorpromazine (10 to 18 mg/kg IV repeated as needed). Phenothiazine tranquilizers have been shown to have a protective effect when used to treat amphetamine toxicoses (Catravas et al., 1977). Diazepam is not recommended because it can exacerbate the stimulatory signs in some animals. Phenobarbital, pentobarbital, and propofol may also be used to effect to prevent severe central nervous system (CNS) signs. In addition, cyproheptadine, a serotonin antagonist, may be useful to reduce the CNS signs. It has been used successfully to dampen the excessive stimulation from overexposure to antidepressant medications designed to increase serotonin in nerve synapses. Cyproheptadine is dosed at 1.1 mg/kg rectally in dogs.

Tachyarrhythmias should be treated with a β-blocker such as propranolol or metoprolol. Hyperthermia should be corrected using a water mist and fans. Animals should be monitored to prevent subsequent hypothermia. The animal should be housed in a dark, quiet environment to avoid external stimulation.

Intravenous fluids act to protect the kidneys and enhance elimination. Tremendous muscle stimulation can result in rhabdomyolysis and subsequent myoglobinuria, as well as a metabolic acidosis. Urinary acidification can promote elimination of amphetamines but must not be undertaken if the animal has compromised renal function or if acidosis is already present.

COCAINE

There are two main forms of cocaine: the hydrochloride salt and the pure cocaine alkaloid or *freebase*. The hydrochloride salt is the powdered form. It readily dissolves in water and is usually self-administered by humans either intravenously or intranasally. Some street names for cocaine powder include *coke, girl, gold or star dust, snow, blow, nose candy,* and *white lady*. Free base is the conversion of the hydrochloride form to the pure cocaine alkaloid. The pure alkaloid thus created exists as a flake, crystal, or rock form that vaporizes when heated, making a popping or cracking sound (i.e., *crack, rock, or flake*). Freebase is usually smoked but is sometimes taken orally (Volmer, 2006).

Cocaine is rapidly and well absorbed from all mucosal surfaces. Inflamed or irritated surfaces may promote absorption. Cocaine is rapidly and extensively metabolized in the liver and excreted in the urine. Cocaine is a strong CNS stimulant. It acts to block the reuptake of serotonin and norepinephrine and has the ability to block cardiac sodium channels (Parker et al., 1999).

The overall effect of cocaine intoxication is one of stimulation. Animals initially become restless and hyperactive. Signs can progress rapidly to tremors, tachycardia, hypotension, prolongation of QRS intervals, tachypnea, and seizures.

Diagnosis is usually based on clinical signs and history of exposure. Over-the counter drug test kits may be helpful in diagnosing a cocaine toxicosis.

Treatment is aimed at stabilizing the patient followed by decontamination. Because clinical signs can develop rapidly, increasing the risk of aspiration, caution should be used if inducing emesis. A safer approach may be to perform gastric lavage with administration of activated charcoal and a cathartic. Tremors and seizures can be controlled with diazepam, chlorpromazine, or a barbiturate. Pretreatment with chlorpromazine effectively antagonized the effects of cocaine in experimentally dosed dogs (Catravas amd Waters, 1981). Administration of sodium bicarbonate decreases the likelihood of development of ventricular arrhythmias, shortens the prolonged QRS complex duration, counteracts the reduction in mean arterial blood pressure, and reverses cocaine-induced sodium channel blockade (Llera and Volmer, 2006). Severe tachyarrhythmias can be treated with a β-blocker such as propranolol. Intravenous fluids should be administered to maintain renal blood flow and promote excretion. Acid-base and electrolyte status should be monitored and corrected. Hyperthermia can be severe in cocaine intoxications. Correction of body temperature can be achieved with evaporative cooling measures such as misting the animal with cool water and placing in front of a fan until normal body temperature is reached or by immersing in a tepid water bath while monitoring body temperature.

MARIJUANA

Tetrahydrocannabinol (THC), the major active cannabinoid in marijuana, can be found in all parts of the marijuana plant. Street names include *pot, Mary Jane, MJ, weed, grass, puff,* and *hemp*. Hashish is the dried resin from flower tops and can contain up to 10% THC. Hashish oil can contain up to 20% THC. Sinsemilla is seedless marijuana (Volmer, 2006).

THC is highly lipophilic, is highly protein bound, has a large volume of distribution, and is enterohepatically recirculated. All of these characteristics result in slow elimination from the body (Otten, 2002). Only 10% to 15% of THC or its metabolites are excreted in the urine, with the remainder through the feces via the bile. Marijuana has a wide margin of safety, with a minimum oral lethal dose in the dog of greater than 3 g/kg. However, clinical signs can occur at 1000 times less than this dose (Thompson et al., 1973).

Onset of clinical signs can occur within 30 to 60 minutes and can include depression, disorientation, lethargy, ataxia, bradycardia, vomiting, tremor, mydriasis, hypothermia, and urine dribbling. Analysis for THC can be performed on stomach contents and urine.

Treatment is primarily symptomatic and supportive. The cannabinoids have a wide margin of safety, and toxicoses are rarely fatal. If the animal is not exhibiting any clinical signs and no other contraindications exist, emesis should be induced following an ingestion. Because enterohepatic recirculation may prolong the residence time of the cannabinoids in the body, repeated doses of activated charcoal are recommended. Body temperature should be monitored for hypothermia and corrected. In most cases recovery should occur within 24 to 72 hours.

OPIOIDS

Opium, the dried milky exudate of the poppy plant, contains 24 alkaloids, including morphine, codeine, and thebaine. The opioids are synthetic compounds that bind to the opioid receptor and are classed as agonists, partial agonists, or antagonists. They differ in their specificity and efficacy at different types of receptors. Four major opioid receptors have been identified, with most of the clinically useful opioids binding to μ (mu) receptors. Naloxone is a pure competitive antagonist with no agonist activity and has a high affinity for the μ (mu) receptor (Volmer, 2006).

Most animal exposures involve ingestion of pharmaceutical preparations. The opioids are well absorbed from the gastrointestinal tract and rapidly metabolized in the liver. Morphine is glucuronidated, and the glucuronide is then excreted by the kidney. Clinical signs can include vomiting, defecation, salivation, lethargy and depression, and ataxia. In severe cases respiratory depression, constipation, hypothermia, coma and seizures, and pulmonary edema are possible.

Emesis is recommended for recent ingestions in animals that are not exhibiting clinical signs. Pylorospasm produced by the opioid may cause much of the drug to remain in the stomach; thus gastric lavage, activated charcoal, and a cathartic may be effective even several hours after ingestion. Respiratory depression is the most common cause of death with opioid overexposure and should be treated by establishment of a patent airway, assisted ventilation, and oxygen. Naloxone (0.01 to 0.02 mg/kg IV, intramuscularly, or subcutaneously) reverses respiratory depression but does not restore full consciousness. Naloxone may need to be repeated as clinical signs indicate.

BARBITURATES

Members in this class of compounds are all derivatives of barbituric acid. The barbiturates are used therapeutically as sedatives and anticonvulsants. Animal exposures can result from iatrogenic overdose, ingestion of illicit preparations, accidental administration of euthanasia solutions, and ingestion of euthanized carcasses. Illicit products are known as *downers, reds, Christmas trees,* and *dolls* (Volmer, 2006).

The barbiturates are well absorbed orally or following intramuscular injection. Lipid solubility of the drug determines the distribution of the barbiturate in the body and the duration of effect. The barbiturates are metabolized in the liver by hepatic microsomal enzymes and excreted in the urine. Acutely the barbiturates may interfere with metabolism of other compounds by binding to hepatic P-450 enzymes, preventing them from acting on other compounds. Chronically barbiturates act to increase microsomal enzyme activity (enzyme induction), thus enhancing the biotransformation of both exogenous and some endogenous substances. Approximately 25% of phenobarbital is excreted unchanged in the urine. It can be ion trapped in the urine by urinary alkalinization, increasing excretion fivefold to tenfold (Haddad and Winchester, 1998). The efficacy of ion trapping for other barbiturates is not as distinct.

Barbiturates activate γ-aminobutyric acid-a receptors and inhibit excitatory glutamate receptors. Clinical signs can include depression, ataxia, incoordination, weakness, disorientation, recumbency, coma, hypothermia, tachycardia or bradycardia, and death. Barbiturates can be detected in stomach contents, blood, urine, liver, and feces.

For recent ingestions in animals exhibiting no other clinical signs, emesis followed by repeated dosages of activated charcoal and a cathartic is recommended. Activated charcoal acts as a "sink," encouraging the drug to diffuse back into the intestine from the circulation, even for compounds administered parenterally (Plumb, 2005). Gastric lavage followed by activated charcoal and a cathartic is a safer alternative for animals exhibiting clinical signs (and risking aspiration from induction of emesis). Death is usually the result of respiratory depression; therefore intubation, administration of oxygen, and assisted ventilation may be required. Body temperature should be monitored and corrected. Ventricular fibrillation and cardiac arrest can result from some barbiturates and be exacerbated by profound hypothermia (Haddad and Winchester, 1998). Supportive care, including intravenous fluids, is recommended. Forced alkaline diuresis may facilitate the excretion of some barbiturates, especially phenobarbital.

References and Suggested Reading

Baggot JD, Davis LE: Pharmacokinetic study of amphetamine elimination in dogs and swine, *Biochem Pharmacol* 21:1967, 1972.

Catravas JD et al: The effects of haloperidol, chlorpromazine and propranolol on acute amphetamine poisoning in the conscious dog, *J Pharmacol Exp Ther* 202:230, 1977.

Catravas JD, Waters IW: Acute cocaine intoxication in the conscious dog: studies on the mechanism of lethality, *J Pharmacol Exp Ther* 217:350, 1981.

Haddad LM, Winchester JF: Barbiturates. In Haddad LM, Shannon MW, Winchester JF: *Clinical management of poisoning and drug overdose,* ed 3, Philadelphia, 1998, Saunders, 521.

Llera RM, Volmer PA: Hazards faced by police dogs used for drug detection, *J Am Vet Med Assoc* 228:1028, 2006.

Otten EJ: Marijuana. In Goldfrank LR et al: *Toxicologic emergencies,* ed 7, New York, 2002, McGraw-Hill, p 1055.

Parker RB et al: Comparative effects of sodium bicarbonate and sodium chloride on reversing cocaine-induced changes in the electrocardiogram, *J Cardiovasc Pharmacol* 34:864, 1999.

Plumb DC: Phenobarbital. In Plumb DC, editor: *Plumb's veterinary drug handbook,* ed 5, Ames, Ia, 2005, Blackwell Publishing, p 620.

Thompson GR et al: Comparison of acute oral toxicity of cannabinoids in rats, dogs, and monkeys, *Toxicol Appl Pharmacol* 25:363, 1973.

Volmer PA: Recreational Drugs. In Peterson M, Talcott P: *Small animal toxicology,* ed 2, Philadelphia, 2006, Saunders, p. 273.

Zalis EG et al: Acute lethality of the amphetamines in dogs and its antagonism by curare, *Proc Soc Exp Biol Med* 118:557, 1965.

CHAPTER 33

Toxicology of Veterinary and Human Estrogen and Progesterone Formulations in Dogs

MARGARET V. ROOT KUSTRITZ, *St. Paul, Minnesota*

Estrogens and progestins are naturally occurring synthetic hormones that are used therapeutically for a variety of problems affecting the reproductive and other body systems. The use of these hormones can be associated with toxicosis.

ESTROGENS

Estrogen formulations are used in small animal veterinary practice for treatment of urethral sphincter mechanism incontinence and pregnancy termination. Other uses of estrogen include estrus induction in bitches and treatment of prostate disease in dogs (although I have achieved only equivocal success with the former and do not recommend the latter).

The most commonly used forms of estrogen in clinical practice are estradiol cypionate (22 to 44 mcg/kg intramuscularly for pregnancy termination) and diethylstilbestrol (DES; 1 to 5 mg once daily orally for 5 days and then every 4 to 7 days as needed for urethral sphincter mechanism incompetence). Estradiol is the most active endogenous estrogen and is typically administered parenterally. It is metabolized by the liver and eliminated mostly in the urine and to a lesser extent in bile. The half-life of injectable estradiol in humans is 4 days. DES is a synthetic nonsteroidal compound with estrogenic activity. It is usually administered orally, metabolized by the liver, and finally eliminated in urine and bile. The half-life of oral DES in humans is 3 to 4 days.

Acute Overdose/Short-Term Effects

There are no reported studies describing acute toxicity of estrogens in dogs. In humans acute overdose is accompanied by nausea and vomiting. In rats toxicity studies demonstrated kidney or liver failure as the cause of death, with premonitory signs of depression, abnormal gait, and convulsions. The most serious short-term effect of estrogen administration in dogs is pancytopenia. This toxic effect of estrogen is reported to occur more commonly in older animals exposed to high doses of estrogen. However, I am unaware of studies quantifying the term *high* or differentiating a single exposure from chronic administration. Dogs are reported to be more sensitive to toxic effects of estrogen than humans or other animal species.

Estrogen may express a toxic effect on bone marrow directly through receptors for estradiol-1-β. The highest expression of receptors to endogenous estrogen in dogs may be present in canine bone marrow. Estrogen also may induce secretion of a myelopoiesis-inhibitory factor that suppresses replication of granulocyte and macrophage progenitor cells in the bone marrow. Clinically myeloid hyperplasia, evidenced by leukocytosis and thrombocytosis, is followed by myeloid hypoplasia, evidenced by leukopenia; thrombocytopenia; and later normocytic, normochromic, nonregenerative anemia.

In a review of 51 cases of pancytopenia in dogs (Weiss, Evanson, and Sykes, 1999), two (3.9%) were caused by estrogen toxicity. Other causes of pancytopenia in that report were exposure to chemotherapeutic drugs (43.1%), parvovirus infection (9.8%), malignant histiocytosis (9.8%), sepsis (5.9%), immune-mediated hemolytic disease (5.9%), lymphoblastic leukemia (3.9%), and ehrlichiosis (3.9%). Bone marrow suppression also has been reported in dogs with estrogen-secreting tumors of the testes.

Clinical signs of pancytopenia may include lethargy, pale mucous membranes, petechial or ecchymotic hemorrhages, hematuria, hemoptysis, melena, recurrent infections, and fever. Clinical signs and changes in the peripheral blood smear may not develop until up to 3 weeks after estrogen exposure. Definitive diagnosis of estrogen toxicity as a cause of pancytopenia requires knowledge of estrogen exposure. Determination of prognosis may require submission of aspirates or core biopsy specimens from the bone marrow.

Long-Term Effects

Chronic administration of estrogen to bitches in diestrus is associated with increased incidence of pyometra. Exposure to estrogen during pregnancy is contraindicated since estrogen is teratogenic and may be embryotoxic. In humans prenatal exposure to DES is associated with increased incidence of vaginal and cervical clear cell adenocarcinomas and possible increased incidence of testicular neoplasia. In one canine study long-term estrogen therapy was associated with development of ovarian papillary carcinomas. Finally, exposure to estrogen causes transformation of cuboidal or columnar epithelium to squamous epithelium in the genitourinary tract, including the renal cortex, and the thyroid gland. This squamous metaplasia is associated with secretory stasis and predisposition to prostatitis in dogs but has not been associated with changes in renal or thyroid function.

Therapy for Pancytopenia

Treatment for pancytopenia includes supportive therapy with intravenous fluids and antibiotics. Transfusion of whole blood or specific blood products such as platelet-rich plasma may be required, depending on the animal's clinical presentation. Potential sources of infectious disease should be avoided. Glucocorticoids are contraindicated in these immunosuppressed patients. It may be helpful to consult with a hematologist in difficult-to-manage patients. Resolution may occur within 30 to 40 days but may take several months. An undefined percentage of animals will die.

PROGESTINS

Progestins are used most commonly in small animal veterinary practice for estrus suppression. Other reported uses include treatment of false pregnancy in bitches and paraphimosis in neutered male dogs.

Many progestins are available worldwide since elective ovariohysterectomy is not performed in many countries, leaving medical estrus suppression as the standard of care. Compounds most commonly used in the United States are megestrol acetate (Ovaban, Schering) and medroxyprogesterone acetate. Both are synthetic progestins. Only megestrol acetate is approved for use in dogs in the United States. Megestrol acetate is administered orally and is metabolized slowly by the liver, with a half-life of 8 days. For estrus suppression megestrol acetate is administered at a dose of 0.55 mg/kg once daily orally for 32 days in anestrus or at a dose of 2.2 mg/kg once daily orally for 8 days in early proestrus; note that total dosage is the same.

Acute Overdose/Short-Term Effects

There are no reported studies describing acute toxicity of progestins in dogs. Short-term effects are not life threatening and are reversible on withdrawal of the drug. These changes include lethargy, polyphagia and weight gain, and altered personality.

Long-Term Effects

Progestins administered chronically to dogs can induce adrenocortical atrophy and iatrogenic hypoadrenocorticism. Serum cortisol concentrations are reported to return to normal within several weeks of drug withdrawal. Progestins also may induce insulin resistance and diabetes mellitus in dogs, which may or may not reverse on withdrawal of progestin therapy. Progestins are reported to induce cystic endometrial hyperplasia and pyometra in bitches, although the manufacturer of megestrol acetate claims the prevalence of pyometra to be less than 1% when the product is administered as directed. Finally, dogs are unique in the sensitivity of their mammary tissue to neoplastic change after long-term exposure to progesterone. This effect may be mediated by growth hormone. Experimental attempts to induce mammary neoplasia in dogs with progestin administration required very long-term exposure to high doses of the compounds used.

Management of progestin toxicosis involves withdrawal of the offending hormone and treatment of any related complications (e.g., pyometra, diabetes mellitus) when possible.

HUMAN ESTROGEN AND ESTROGEN/PROGESTIN MEDICATIONS

Dogs may be exposed to human hormone replacement or contraceptive preparations. Most hormone replacement therapies contain estrogen, and most contraceptives contain either progestins alone or a combination of estrogen and progesterone (Table 33-1). The ratio of estrogen to progesterone in human contraceptive preparation is such that dogs ingesting these medications tend to be overexposed to estrogen. Most human contraceptive pills or tablets contain 20 to 50 mcg of estrogen per unit. Dogs may also be exposed by ingestion of vaginal rings; skin patches; and topical creams or gels containing estrogen, progestin,

Table 33-1

Human Hormone Replacement and Contraceptive Preparations

Brand Name(S)	Progestin	Estrogen
Cenestin (Duramed)		X
Climara (Berlex)		X
Enjuvia (Duramed)		X
Estrace (Warner Chilcott/Bristol-Myers Squibb)		X
Estraderm (Novartis)		X
Estrasorb (Novavax)		X
Estrogel (Solvay)		X
Femring (Warner Chilcott)		X
Premarin (Wyeth-Ayerst)		X
Exluton (Organon)	X	
Femulen (Pharmacia)	X	
Microlut (Schering)	X	
MicroNovum (Schering)	X	
Microval (Wyeth-Ayerst)	X	
Neogest (Schering)	X	
Noregeston (Schering)	X	
Noriday (Pharmacia)	X	
NOR-QD (Watson)	X	
Ovrette (Wyeth-Ayerst)	X	
Alesse (Wyeth-Ayerst)	X	X
Brevicon (Searle)	X	X
Demulen (Searle)	X	X
Desogen (Organon)	X	X
Estrostep (Parke-Davis)	X	X
Jenest (Organon)	X	X
Levlen (Berlex)	X	X
Levlite (Berlex)	X	X
Levora (Watson)	X	X
Lo/Ovral (Wyeth-Ayerst)	X	X
Loestrin (Parke-Davis)	X	X

(Continued)

Table **33-1**		
Human Hormone Replacement and Contraceptive Preparations—(Cont'd)		
Brand Name(S)	**Progestin**	**Estrogen**
Mircette (Organon)	X	X
Modicon (Ortho-McNeil)	X	X
Necon (Watson)	X	X
Nordette (Wyeth-Ayerst)	X	X
Norethin (Roberts)	X	X
Norinyl (Watson)	X	X
Ortho-Cept (Ortho-McNeil)	X	X
Ortho-Cyclen (Ortho-McNeil)	X	X
Ortho-Novum (Ortho-McNeil)	X	X
Ortho-Tri-Cyclen (Ortho-McNeil)	X	X
Ovcon (Bristol-Myers Squibb)	X	X
Ovral (Wyeth-Ayerst)	X	X
Tri-Norinyl (Watson)	X	X
Triphasil (Wyeth-Ayerst)	X	X
Trivora (Watson)	X	X
Zovia (Watson)	X	X

X, Present.

or a combination of the two. As with any intoxication, information from the owner regarding the product and amount ingested is invaluable for determination of likelihood of adverse effects. An emetic such as apomorphine may be administered if the ingestion has occurred within 30 minutes.

Short- and long-term effects are as expected for the individual hormones described previously. Adverse effects and complications of long-term use of combination estrogen-progesterone therapies in humans include venous thrombosis, ischemic stroke, and heart disease. There are no reported studies evaluating such effects in dogs.

References and Suggested Reading

Mahony OM: Estrogen toxicity. In: Tilley LP, Smith FWK, editors: *The five-minute veterinary consult*, Philadelphia, 2004, Lippincott, Williams & Wilkins, p 430.

Maier WE, Herman JR: Pharmacology and toxicology of ethinyl estradiol and norethindrone acetate in experimental animals, *Regul Toxicol Pharmacol* 34:53, 2001.

Plumb DC: *Veterinary drug handbook*,. Ames IA, 2005, Blackwell Publishing, pp 357, 447, 694, 697.

Weiss DJ, Evanson O, Sykes J: A retrospective study of canine pancytopenia, *Vet Clin Pathol* 28:83, 1999.

CHAPTER **34**

Herbal Hazards

ELIZABETH A. HAUSNER, *Beltsville, Maryland*
ROBERT H. POPPENGA, *Davis, California*

The increased use of herbal preparations and the potential for intoxication or adverse events following their use obligate the clinician to consider these substances in cases of suspected poisonings. The incidence of animal toxicoses or adverse events following the use of natural remedies has not been specifically determined in veterinary medicine; however, it is not likely to be higher than the incidence of these effects from many conventional pharmaceuticals.

REGULATIONS

In 1994 Congress passed the Dietary Supplement and Health Education Act (DSHEA) creating a new category of substances termed *dietary supplements*. Dietary supplements include minerals, vitamins, amino acids, herbs, and any product sold as a "dietary supplement" before October 15, 1994. The Food and Drug Administration (FDA) Center for Veterinary Medicine interpreted the DSHEA as not applying to substances used in animals, leaving veterinary herbals and dietary supplements regulated as foods, food additives, or new animal drugs, depending on the ingredients and their intended use. Herbal products can be marketed as dietary supplements for humans without premarket testing for safety or efficacy, and they can be manufactured without regard to quality control. Consequently variation in the concentration of active ingredient and accuracy of the herbal material used are just two of the potential problems with current herbal or natural products. These problems can alter the efficacy of or potential toxicosis from these products. In contrast, proof of safety and efficacy are required by the FDA before marketing prescription and over-the-counter (OTC) drugs. In addition, their manufacture is regulated to ensure a consistent product. Of course, nothing prevents a product intended for use in or on humans from being used in or on animals.

INTOXICATION SCENARIOS

Unfortunately, there is almost no information regarding the overall incidence of adverse drug reactions (ADRs) to conventional drugs or herbal remedies in veterinary medicine, and it is likely that ADRs are underreported for both. It is worth noting that in several cases the reported incidence of animal intoxication from an herb, herbal preparation, or dietary supplement seems to parallel its popularity (Ooms, Khan, and Means, 2001; Gwaltney-Brant, Albretsen, and Khan, 2000).

There are a number of scenarios in which animals may experience an adverse reaction to or toxicosis from an herbal preparation.

1. A preparation may contain a known toxicant. For example, the dried rootstocks of *Aconitum* spp. contain several constituents that are acutely cardiotoxic (Lin, Chan, and Means, 2005). Pennyroyal oil containing the putative toxin pulegone was responsible for the death of a dog after dermal application to control fleas (Sudekum et al., 1992).
2. A remedy may contain a toxicant that is not acutely toxic but may be toxic when given chronically. Pyrrolizidine alkaloids are found in many plant species and, when ingested over time, cause severe liver disease (Prakash et al., 1999; Stedman, 2002).
3. Errors may be made when preparing a remedy. For example, an anise seed preparation was contaminated with the highly toxic *Conium maculatum* (poison hemlock) seed (deSmet, 1991). An outbreak of renal interstitial fibrosis in women taking Chinese herbs for weight loss was attributed to the use of *Aristolochia fangchi* instead of *Stephania tetranda* in imported powdered extracts (Vanderweghem, 1998).
4. Herbal preparations can be intentionally adulterated with chemical contaminants. Many Chinese herbal patent medicines contain drugs such as nonsteroidal antiinflammatory drugs (NSAIDs) or sedatives (Ko, 1998). Also, heavy metal and pesticide contamination has been reported (Ernst, 2002b; Saper et al., 2004). Salmonellosis has been reported in humans taking rattlesnake capsules contaminated with *Salmonella Arizona* (Fleischman, Haake, and Lovett, 1989).
5. The active constituents in herbal preparations can interact with other concurrently administered drugs, resulting in adverse interactions. For example, buckthorn bark and berries taken chronically can increase the loss of potassium, thus potentiating the action of cardiac glycosides and antiarrhythmic agents (DerMarderosian, 2001). Potassium loss may be exacerbated by simultaneous use of thiazide diuretics, corticosteroids, and licorice root (DerMarderosian, 2001). In addition, active constituents in herbal preparations can induce liver-metabolizing enzymes, which can alter the metabolism and kinetics of coadministered conventional drugs. For example, eucalyptus oil induces liver enzyme activity (DerMarderosian, 2001). This scenario of adverse pharmacologic interactions may occur when the owner does not inform the veterinarian of the intentional use of herbal preparations.
6. Finally, pets may consume improperly stored remedies, resulting in ingestion of a large quantity of a product. Ultimately of equal or greater concern than intoxication from herbal remedies is the potential delay in seeking treatment for otherwise treatable diseases.

ACTIVE HERBAL CONSTITUENTS

The following broad classes of active chemical constituents occur in plants: volatile oils, resins, alkaloids, polysaccharides, phenols, glycosides, and fixed oils (Hung, Lewin, and Howland, 1998). Volatile oils are odorous plant ingredients (e.g., catnip, garlic, and citrus). Resins are complex chemical mixtures that can be strong gastrointestinal irritants. Alkaloids are a heterogeneous group of alkaline, organic, and nitrogenous compounds. Glycosides are sugar esters containing a sugar (glycol) and a nonsugar (aglycone). In some cases the glycosides are not toxic. However, hydrolysis of the glycosides after ingestion can release toxic aglycones. Fixed oils are esters of long-chain fatty acids and alcohols. Herbs containing fixed oils are often used as emollients, demulcents, and bases for other agents; in general these are the least toxic of the plant constituents.

There is a misperception that preparations from plants are inherently safe and nonchemical in nature. Many plant-derived chemicals are biologically active and therefore potentially toxic. Concentrated extracts of a number of herbs have proven to be toxic even if the entire plant may be used with relative safety. Although green tea is consumed by many people with apparent safety, an extract of green tea marketed in Europe caused a significant number of adverse hepatic events, including fulminant hepatitis. The extract was withdrawn from the market (Gloro et al., 2005).

TOXICITY OF SPECIFIC HERBS OR OTHER NATURAL PRODUCTS

Some of the most commonly encountered herbals are discussed in the following paragraphs; others are listed in Table 34-1.

Blue-Green Algae

Blue-green (BG) algae are single-celled organisms that have been promoted for their nutritional properties. Several BG algal species produce potent toxins. *Microcystis aeruginosa* produces the hepatotoxic microcystins. *Anabaena flos-aquae* produce the neurotoxins anatoxin-a and anatoxin a$_s$. *Aphanizomenon flos-aquae* produce the neurotoxins saxitoxin and neosaxitoxin. Efforts are underway to better define the risks associated with ingestion of potentially toxigenic BG algae and to establish safe concentrations of

Table **34-1**

Additional Herbs of Toxicologic Concern

Scientific Name	Common Names	Active Constituents	Target Organs
Acorus calamus	*Acorus,* calamus, sweet flag, sweet root, sweet cane, sweet cinnamon	β-Asarone (procarcinogen)	Liver: potent hepatocarcinogen
Aesculus hippocasteranum	Horse chestnut, buckeye	Esculin, nicotine, quercetin, rutin, saponins, shikimic acid	Gastrointestinal, nervous
Arnica montana and *A. latifolia*	Arnica, wolf's bane, leopard's bane	Sesquiterpene lactones	Skin: dermatitis
Atropa belladonna	Belladonna, deadly nightshade	Atropine	Nervous: anticholinergic syndrome
Conium maculatum	Poison hemlock	Coniine, other similar alkaloids	Nervous: nicotine-like toxicosis
Convallaria majalis	Lily-of-the-valley, mayflower, conval lily	Cardiac glycosides	Cardiovascular
Cytisus scoparius	Scotch broom, broom, broom tops	l-sparteine	Nervous: nicotinic-like toxicosis
Datura stramonium	Jimsonweed, thorn apple	Atropine, scopolamine, hyoscyamine	Nervous: anticholinergic syndrome
Dipteryx odorata	Tonka, tonka bean	Coumarin	Hematologic: anticoagulant
Euonymus europaeus; E. atropurpureus	European spindle tree; wahoo, eastern burning bush	Cardiac glycosides	Cardiovascular
Eupatorium perfoliatum; E. purpureum	Boneset, thoroughwort; joe pye weed, gravel root, queen-of-the-meadow	Pyrrolizidine alkaloids	Liver
Heliotropium europaeum	Heliotrope	Pyrrolizidine alkaloids	Liver
Hyoscyamus niger	Henbane, fetid nightshade, poison tobacco, insane root, stinky nightshade	Hyoscyamine, yoscine	Nervous: anticholinergic syndrome
Ipomoea purga	Jalap	Convolvulin	Gastrointestinal
Mandragora officinarum	Mandrake	Scopolamine, hyoscyamine	Nervous: anticholinergic syndrome
Podophyllum peltatum	Mayapple, mandrake	Podophyllin	Gastrointestinal: gastroenteritis
Sanguinaris canadensis	Bloodroot, red puccoon, red root	Berberine	Gastrointestinal
Solanum dulcamara, other *Solanum* spp.	Woody, bittersweet, or climbing nightshade	Numerous glycoalkaloids including solanine and chaconine	Gastrointestinal, nervous, cardiovascular
Tussilago farfara	Coltsfoot	PA alkaloid, senkirkine	Liver
Vinca major and *V. minor*	Common periwinkle, periwinkle	Vincamine	Immune system

total microcystins in marketed products. *Spirulina* has also been promoted as a nutritional supplement and is not considered a toxigenic BG algae genus. However, some products have been found to be contaminated with mercury. Microbial contamination could possibly be a concern if harvested algae grow in water contaminated with human or animal wastes.

Ephedra or Ma Huang

The dried young branches of ephedra (*Ephedra* spp.) have been used for their stimulating and vasoactive effects. In addition, ephedra has been used in several products promoted for weight loss. The plant constituents responsible for biologic activity are the sympathomimetic alkaloids ephedrine and pseudoephedrine. A case series involving intoxication of dogs following ingestion of a weight-loss product containing guarana (caffeine) and ma huang (ephedrine) was recently reported (Ooms, Khan, and Means, 2001). Estimated doses of the respective plants associated with adverse effects were 4.4 to 296.2 mg/kg for guarana and 1.3 to 88.9 mg/kg for ma huang. Symptomatology included hyperactivity, tremors, seizures, behavioral changes, emesis, tachycardia, and hyperthermia. Ingestion was associated with mortality in 17% of the cases. North American species of ephedra (also called Mormon tea) have not been shown to contain the sympathomimetic alkaloids.

Citrus aurantium ("bitter orange" or "Seville orange") has appeared in many products labeled as "ephedrine-free" and is also combined with caffeine and/or guarana. The primary active components of *C. aurantium* are synephrine (structurally similar to epinephrine), octopamine (structurally similar to norepinephrine), and N-methyltyramine. The overall effect is that of stimulation (Fugh-Berman and Myers, 2004). Studies in humans have shown that bitter orange–containing preparations cause tachycardia and increases in systolic and diastolic pressure (Halle, Benowitz, and Jacob, 2005). Signs of intoxication can be expected to be similar to those seen with ephedra.

Guarana

Guarana is the dried paste made from the crushed seeds of *Paullinia cupana* or *P. sorbilis,* a fast-growing shrub native to South America. The primary active component in the plant is caffeine, with concentrations that range from

3% to 5%, which compares to 1% to 2% for coffee beans. Currently the most common forms of guarana include syrups, extracts, and distillates used as flavoring agents and as a source of caffeine for the soft-drink industry. More recently it has been added to weight-loss formulations in combination with ephedra. Oral lethal doses of caffeine in dogs and cats range from 110 to 200 mg/kg of body weight and 80 to 150 mg/kg of body weight, respectively (Carson, 2001). See Ephedra earlier in the chapter for a discussion of a case series involving dogs ingesting a product containing guarana and ephedra (Ooms, Khan, and Means, 2001).

White Willow

The active constituents in willow (*Salix* spp.) include salicylates (primarily in the form of glycosides salicortin and salicin) and tannins. Current indications for plant use include for fever and rheumatism and as an antiinflammatory. Both therapeutic and adverse effects occur through inhibition of prostaglandin synthesis. In addition, salicylates inhibit oxidative phosphorylation and Krebs cycle enzymes. In cats acetylsalicylic (AS) acid is toxic at 80 to 120 mg/kg given orally for 10 to 12 days. In dogs AS at 50 mg/kg given orally twice a day is associated with emesis; higher doses can cause depression, anorexia, diarrhea, bloody stool, melena, and metabolic acidosis. A dose of 100 to 300 mg/kg orally once daily for 1 to 4 weeks is associated with gastric ulceration; more prolonged dosing is potentially fatal (Osweiler, 1996). Cats are particularly vulnerable to overdose because of an inability to rapidly metabolize salicylates. A number of other plants contain salicylates, including *Betula* spp. (birch), *Filipendula ulmaria* (meadowsweet), and *Populus* spp. See Oil of Wintergreen later in the chapter.

ESSENTIAL OILS

Essential oils are the volatile, organic constituents of fragrant plant matter and contribute to plant fragrance and taste. They are extracted from plant material by distillation or cold-pressing. A number of essential oils are not recommended for use (e.g., aromatherapy, dermal or oral use) because of their toxicity or potential for toxicity (Tisserand and Balacs, 1999). They are listed in Table 34-2. These oils have unknown or oral LD_{50} values in animals of 1 g/kg or less. Most toxicity information has been derived using laboratory rodents or mice. Such data should only be used as a rough guide since they cannot always be extrapolated to other species. *Essential oil safety: a guide for health care professionals* is an excellent reference for in-depth discussions of general and specific essential oil toxicity. The following essential oils are of particular concern.

Camphor

Camphor is an aromatic, volatile, terpene ketone derived from the wood of *Cinnamomum camphora* or synthesized from turpentine. Camphor oil is separated into four distinct fractions: white, brown, yellow, and blue camphor (Tisserand and Balacs, 1999). White camphor is the form used in aromatherapy and in OTC products (brown and yellow fractions contain the carcinogen safrole and are not normally available). OTC products vary in form and camphor content; external products contain 10% to 20% in semisolid forms or 1% to 10% in camphor spirits. It is used as a topical rubefacient and antipruritic agent. Camphor is rapidly absorbed from the skin and gastrointestinal tract, and toxic effects can occur within minutes of exposure. In humans signs of intoxication include emesis, abdominal distress, excitement, tremors, and seizures followed by central nervous system (CNS)

Table 34-2

Most Toxic Essential Oils

Oil	Genus/Species	Oral LD$_{50}$ (g/kg)	Toxic Component (%)
Boldo leaf	*Peumus boldus*	0.13	Ascaridole: 16
Wormseed	*Chenopodium ambrosioides*	0.25	Ascaridole: 60-80
Mustard	*Brassica nigra*	0.34	Allyl isothiocyanate: 99
Armoise	*Artemisia herba-alba*	0.37	Thujone: 35
Pennyroyal (Eur.)	*Mentha pulegium*	0.40	Pulegone: 55-95
Tansy	*Tnacetum vulgare*	0.73	Thujone: 66-81
Thuja	*Thuja occidentalis*	0.83	Thujone: 30-80
Calamus	*Acorus calamus var angustatus*	0.84	Asarone: 45-80
Wormwood	*Artemesia absinthium*	0.96	Thujone: 34-71
Bitter Almond	*Prunus amygdalus var amara*	0.96	Prussic acid: 3
	Artemisia arborescens	?	Iso-thujone: 30-45
Buchu	*Barosma betulina; B. crenulata*	?	Pulegone: 50
Horseradish	*Cochlearia armoracia*	?	Allyl isocyanate: 50
Lanyana	*Artemiesia afra*	?	Thujone: 4-66
Pennyroyal (N. Am.)	*Hedeoma pulegoides*	?	Pulegone: 60-80
Southernwood	*Artemesia abrotanum*	?	Thujone: ##
Western red cedar	*Thuja plicata*	?	Thujone: 85

Data from Tisserand R and Balacs T, 1999.

depression characterized by apnea and coma. Fatalities have occurred in humans ingesting 1 to 2 g of camphor-containing products, although the adult human lethal dose has been reported to be 5 to 20 g (Tisserand and Balacs, 1999; Emery and Corban, 1999). A 1-tsp amount of camphorated oil (≈1 ml of camphor) was lethal to 16-month-old and 19-month-old children.

Citrus Oil

Citrus oil and citrus oil constituents such as D-limonene and linalool have been shown to have insecticidal activity. Although D-limonene has been used safely as an insecticide on dogs and cats, some citrus oil formulations or use of pure citrus oil may pose a poisoning hazard (Powers et al., 1988). Fatal adverse reactions have been reported in cats following the use of an "organic" citrus oil dip (Hooser, Beasley, and Everitt, 1986). Hypersalivation, muscle tremors, ataxia, lateral recumbency, coma, and death were noted experimentally in three cats following use of the dip according to label directions.

Melaleuca Oil

Melaleuca is derived from the leaves of the Australian tea tree (*Melaleuca alternifolia*); it is often referred to as tea tree oil. The oil contains terpenes, sesquiterpenes, and hydrocarbons. A variety of commercially available products contain the oil; shampoos and the pure oil have been sold for use on dogs, cats, ferrets, and horses. Tea tree oil toxicosis has been reported in dogs and cats (Villar et al., 1994; Bischoff and Guale, 1998). A recent case report describes the illness of three cats exposed dermally to pure *melaleuca* oil for flea control (Bischoff and Guale, 1998). Clinical signs in one or more of the cats included hypothermia, ataxia, dehydration, nervousness, trembling, and coma. There were moderate increases in serum alanine aminotransferase and aspartate aminotransferase concentrations. Two cats recovered within 48 hours following decontamination and supportive care. However, one cat died ≈3 days after exposure. The primary constituent of the oil, terpinen-4-ol, was detected in the urine of the cats. Another case involved the dermal application of 7 to 8 drops of oil along the backs of two dogs as a flea repellent (Kaluzienski, 2000). Within ≈12 hours one dog developed partial paralysis of the hind limbs, ataxia, and depression. The other dog only displayed depression. Decontamination (bathing) and symptomatic and supportive care resulted in rapid recovery within 24 hours.

Pennyroyal Oil

This volatile oil is derived from *Mentha pulegium* and *Hedeoma pulegoides*. Pennyroyal oil has a long history of use as a flea repellent. There is one case report of pennyroyal oil toxicosis in the veterinary literature in which a dog was dermally exposed to pennyroyal oil at ≈2 g/kg (Sudekum et al., 1992). Within 1 hour of application, the dog became listless, and within 2 hours it began vomiting. Thirty hours after exposure the dog exhibited diarrhea, hemoptysis, and epistaxis. Soon thereafter it developed seizures and died. Histopathologic examination of liver tissue showed massive hepatocellular necrosis.

Oil of Wintergreen

Wintergreen oil is derived from *Gaultheria procumbens*. The oil contains a glycoside that, when hydrolyzed, releases methyl salicylate. The oil is readily absorbed through skin and is used to treat muscle aches and pains. Salicylates are toxic to dogs and cats. Since cats metabolize salicylates much more slowly than other species, they are more likely to be overdosed. Intoxicated cats may present with depression, anorexia, emesis, gastric hemorrhage, toxic hepatitis, anemia, bone marrow hypoplasia, hypernea, and hyperpyrexia (see Willow earlier in the chapter).

PRODUCT ADULTERATION

There is a long history of Chinese patent medicines being adulterated with metals and conventional pharmaceuticals or containing natural toxins (Ko, 1998; Au et al., 2000; Ernst, 2002a; Dolan et al., 2003). Sedatives, stimulants, and NSAIDs are common pharmaceuticals added to patent medicines with no labeling to indicate their presence. Commonly found natural toxins in Chinese patent medicines include borneol (reduced camphor), aconite, toad secretions (*Bufo* spp., Ch'an Su), mylabris, scorpion-derived toxins, borax, *Acorus,* and strychnine (*Strychnos nux-vomica*) (Ko, 1998).

Chinese patent medicines often contain cinnabar (mercuric sulfide), realgar (arsenic sulfide), or litharge (lead oxide) as part of the traditional formula. Recently dietary supplements purchased largely from retail stores were tested for arsenic, cadmium, lead, and mercury (Dolan et al., 2003). Eighty-four of the 95 products tested contained botanicals as a major component of the formulation. Eleven of the 95 products contained lead at concentrations that would have caused lead intake to exceed recommended maximum levels in children and pregnant women had the products been used according to label directions.

Serious adverse health effects have been documented in humans using adulterated Chinese herbal medicines (Ernst, 2002a). There are no published cases in the veterinary literature, although we are aware of one case in which a small dog ingested a number of herbal tea "balls" that were prescribed to its owner for arthritis. The dog presented to a veterinary clinic in acute renal failure several days after the ingestion. Analysis of the formulation revealed low-level heavy metal contamination (mercury and lead) and large concentrations of caffeine and the NSAID indomethacin. The acute renal failure was most likely to the result of NSAID-induced renal damage.

DRUG-HERB INTERACTIONS

Drug-herb interactions refer to the possibility that an herbal constituent may alter the pharmacologic effects of a conventional drug given concurrently or vice versa. The result may be either enhanced or diminished drug or herb effects or the appearance of a new effect that is not anticipated from the use of the drug or herb alone.

Possible interactions include those that alter the absorption, metabolism, distribution, and/or elimination of a drug or herbal constituent and result in an increase or decrease in the concentration of active agent at the site of action.

For example, herbs that contain dietary fiber, mucilage, or tannins might alter the absorption of another drug or herbal constituent. Herbs containing constituents that induce liver enzymes might be expected to affect drug metabolism and/or elimination (Blumenthal, 2000). Induction of live metabolizing enzymes can increase the toxicity of drugs and other chemicals via increased production of reactive metabolites. The production of more toxic reactive metabolites is termed *bioactivation* (Zhou et al., 2004). Alternatively enhanced detoxification of drugs and other chemicals can decrease their toxicity or their therapeutic efficacy. Long-term use of herbs and other dietary supplements can induce enzymes associated with procarcinogen activation, thus increasing the risk of some cancers (Ryu and Chung, 2003; Zhou et al., 2004). The displacement of one drug from protein-binding sites by another agent increases the concentration of unbound drug available to target tissues. Pharmacodynamic interactions or interactions at receptor sites can be agonistic or antagonistic.

DIAGNOSIS OF HERBAL INTOXICATION

Because of the nonspecific signs associated with most intoxications, the diagnosis of a causative agent is extremely difficult without a history of exposure or administration. Such information may not be forthcoming from clients since they may not equate use of an alternative therapy with conventional drug use and therefore may not volunteer such information when queried about prior medication history. Also, clients may not volunteer such information because of embarrassment or belief that the veterinarian will not approve of such therapy. Therefore it is important to specifically question clients regarding use of natural products. An added complication is that, even with a history of exposure and a product package, the animal may have been exposed to adulterating or contaminating agents that are not listed on the package label.

Clinical pathologic or postmortem findings are rarely specific for intoxication from natural products but will assist in determining affected organ systems and thus will help formulate a differential list. It may be possible to detect specific herbal constituents in biologic specimens. For example, pulegone was detected in tissues from a dog intoxicated by pennyroyal oil (Sudekum et al., 1992). Currently however, analyses for organic natural products

Table 34-3

Drug Dosages for Treatment of Intoxications

Agent	Indication	Dosage
Activated charcoal	Adsorption of toxins	Loading dose of 1-2 g/kg. If multiple doses are given, follow with 0.25-0.5 g/kg q1-6h. Some preparations of activated charcoal contain a cathartic.
Syrup of ipecac	Emesis	Dogs: 1-2 ml/kg PO Cats: 3.3 ml/kg PO diluted 50:50 with water
3% hydrogen peroxide	Emesis	1-2 ml/kg PO; if emesis does not occur, may repeat once more
Apomorphine	Emesis	Do not use in cats. Dogs: 0.03 mg/kg IV or 0.04 mg/kg IM May also place 0.25- to 1.6-mg tablet in the conjunctival sac and dissolve with an ophthalmic irrigating solution. When emesis begins, thoroughly flush remaining material from the sac.
Sodium bicarbonate	Urine alkalinization	1 to 2 mEq/kg administered q3-4h to achieve a urine pH of 7.0 or greater
Digoxin Fab fragments	Cardiac glycosides (plants such as *Digitalis, Nerium* spp. and *Bufo* spp. toads)	Dosing is empiric. In humans it is suggested that 1.7 ml (of Digibind) be administered IV per milliliter of digoxin ingested. If dose is unknown, then 400 mg Digibind is given IV. Digibind is given over 30 minutes unless cardiac arrest is imminent, in which case a bolus is given. Monitor for anaphylaxis and hypokalemia.
Cimetidine	Gastric protection (H₂ blocker)	5-10 mg/kg IV or PO q8h
Sucralfate	Gastrointestinal protection	Small dogs: 0.5 g q8h Large dogs: 1 g q8h Cats: not recommended
Omeprazole	Treatment and prevention of ulcers	Dogs: 20 mg/dog q24h (or 0.7 mg/kg, q24h, PO)[†]
Diazepam	Antiseizure	Dogs: 0.5-2 mg/kg IV or 1 mg/kg rectally[2] Cats: 0.5 mg/kg IV or 1 mg/kg rectally
Lidocaine	Premature ventricular contractions	Loading dose of 1-2 mg/kg IV followed by maintenance IV drip of 40-60 mg/kg/min infusion rate to effect Should not be used in cats*
Metoprolol	Tachyarrhythmias	0.1-0.3 mg/kg TID
Misoprostol	GI protection	Dogs: 2-5 mcg/kg q6-8h, PO

Data from Poppenga, 2004 unless otherwise noted.
GI, Gastrointestinal; *IM*, intramuscularly; *IV*, intravenously; *PO*, Orally.
*Carson, 2001.
[†]From Papich MG: *Saunders handbook of veterinary drugs*, Philadelphia, 2002, Saunders, pp 352, 376.

in tissues are not widely available, although analytic methods may improve as their use continues to increase.

TREATMENT OF HERBAL INTOXICATION

The adage "treat the patient and not the poison" is appropriate in most suspected poisonings caused by herbal preparations. Treatment consists of decontamination followed by general supportive care. Indications and contraindications for decontamination procedures should be followed (Poppenga, 2004). Inducing emesis is contraindicated when there is high risk of aspiration (the patient is unconscious or there is neurologic depression) or the patient is having or is likely to have a seizure.

Generally dermal preparations can be removed by washing with a mild soap or detergent. Care should be exercised that the personnel performing this do not themselves become contaminated. Gloves, aprons, and good ventilation are necessary. It is also important to avoid hypothermia in the patient. Supportive care is based on the clinical signs exhibited by the patient. Body temperature, status of the major organ systems, hydration, acid-base balance, urine output, neurologic status, and cardiac function require regular monitoring and evaluation.

In rare cases an antidote might be available (e.g., digoxin Fab fragments for cardiac glycosides). There are also specific considerations for several botanical agents. Intoxication with salicylates frequently results in acidosis. Urinary alkalinization using sodium bicarbonate may increase the elimination by trapping the ionized salicylate molecules in the urine. It is also important to protect the gastrointestinal tract against the ulcerogenic potential of the salicylates. Treatment may include a protectant such as sucralfate, a histamine H_2-receptor antagonist (cimetidine, ranitidine or famotidine), a proton pump inhibitor (omeprazole), and misoprostol (a PGE_1 analog).

In cases of poisoning from caffeine/guarana, ephedra, *Citrus aurantium*, and other materials causing CNS stimulation, the animal should be monitored for hyperthermia, dehydration, acidosis, cardiac arrhythmias, and seizures. Along with decontamination, fluid therapy increases urinary excretion and helps to correct electrolyte imbalances. Frequent premature ventricular contractions should be treated with lidocaine (without epinephrine). Tachyarrhythmias may require the use of a β-blocker. It must be remembered that β-blockers may also mask the early signs of shock. Drug dosages are summarized in Table 34-3.

References and Suggested Reading

Au AM et al: Screening methods for drugs and heavy metals in Chinese patent medicines, *Bull Environ Contam Toxicol* 65:112, 2000.

Bent S et al: The relative safety of ephedra compared to other herbal products, *Ann Intern Med* 138(6):468, 2003.

Birdsall TC: 5-hyrdoxytryptophan: a clinically effective serotonin precursor, *Altern Med Rev* 3:271, 1998.

Bischoff K, Guale F: Australian tea tree (*Melaleuca alternifolia*) oil poisoning in three purebred cats, *J Vet Diagn Invest* 10:208, 1998.

Blumenthal M: Interactions between herbs and conventional drugs: introductory considerations, *Herbal Gram* 49:52, 2000.

Carson TL: Methylxanthines. In Peterson ME, Talcott PA, editors: *Small animal toxicology*, Philadelphia, 2001, Saunders, p 563.

DerMarderosian A, editor: *Review of natural products*, St Louis, 2001, Facts and Comparisons.

DeSmet PAGM: Toxicological outlook on the quality assurance of herbal remedies In De Smet PAGM et al, editors: *Adverse effects of herbal drugs 1*, Berlin, 1991, Springer-Verlag, p 1.

Dolan SP et al: Analysis of dietary supplements for arsenic, cadmium, mercury, and lead using inductively coupled plasma mass spectrometry, *J Agric Food Chem* 51:1307, 2003.

Emery DP, Corban JG: Camphor toxicity, *J Paediatr Child Health* 35:105, 1999.

Ernst E: Adulteration of Chinese herbal medicines with synthetic drugs: a systematic review, *J Intern Med* 252:107, 2002a.

Ernst E: Toxic heavy metals and undeclared drugs in Asian herbal medicines, *Trends Pharmacol Sci* 23(3):136, 2002b.

Fleischman S, Haake DA, Lovett MA: *Salmonella Arizona* infections associated with ingestion of rattlesnake capsules, *Arch Intern Med* 149:705, 1989.

Fugh-Berman A, Ernst E: Herb-drug interactions: a review and assessment of report reliability, *J Clin Pharmacol* 52:587, 2001.

Fugh-Berman A, Myers A: Citrus aurantium, an ingredient of dietary supplements marketed for weight loss: current status of clinical and basic research, *Exp Biol Med* 229:698, 2004.

Gloro R et al: Fulminant hepatitis during self-medication with hydroalcoholic extract of green tea, *Eur J Gastroeterol Hepatol* 17:1135, 2005.

Grande GA, Dannewitz SR: Symptomatic sassafras oil ingestion, *Vet Hum Toxicol* 29:447, 1987.

Gwaltney-Brant SM, Albretsen JC, Khan SA: 5-Hydroxytryptophan toxicosis in dogs: 21 cases (1989-1999), *J Am Vet Med Assoc* 216:1937, 2000.

Haller CA et al: An evaluation of selected herbal reference texts and comparison to published reports of adverse herbal events, *Adverse Drug React Toxicol Rev* 21(3):143, 2002.

Haller CA, Benowitz NL, Jacob PIII: Hemodynamic effects of ephedra-free weight-loss supplements in humans, *Am J Med* 118(9):998, 2005.

Hooser SB, Beasley VR, Everitt JI: Effects of an insecticidal dip containing D-limonene in the cat, *J Am Vet Med Assoc* 189:905, 1986.

Hung OL, Lewin NA, Howland MA: Herbal preparations. In Goldfrank LR et al, editors: *Goldfrank's toxicologic emergencies*, ed 6, Stamford, Ct, 1998, Appelton and Lange, p 1221.

Kaluzienski M: Partial paralysis and altered behavior in dogs treated with *Melaleuca oil J Toxicol Clin Toxicol* 38:518, 2000

Ko RJ: Herbal products information. In *Poisoning and toxicology compendium*, Cleveland, 1998, Lexi-Comp, p 834.

Lazarou J, Pomeranz BH, Corey PN: Incidence of adverse drug reactions in hospitalized patients: a meta-analysis of prospective studies, *JAMA* 279(15):1200, 1998.

Lin CC, Chan TYK, Deng JF: Clinical features and management of herb-induced aconitine poisoning, *Ann Emerg Med* 43:574, 2005.

Ooms TG, Khan SA, Means C: Suspected caffeine and ephedrine toxicosis resulting from ingestion of an herbal supplement containing guarana and ma huang in dogs: 47 cases (1997-1999), *J Am Vet Med Assoc* 218:225, 2001.

Osweiler GD: Over-the-counter drugs and illicit drugs of abuse. In *The national veterinary medical series: toxicology*, Philadelphia, Williams & Wilkins, pp 303, 1996.

Pirmohamed M et al: Adverse drug reactions as a cause of admission to hospital: prospective analysis of 18 820 patients, *Br Med J* 329:15, 2004.

Poppenga R: Treatment. In Plumlee KH, editor: *Clinical veterinary toxicology*, St. Louis, 2004, Mosby, p 13.

Powers KA et al: An evaluation of the acute toxicity of an insecticidal spray containing linalool, d-limonene, and piperonyl butoxide applied topically to domestic cats, *Vet Hum Toxicol* 30(3):206, 1988.

Prakash AS et al: Pyrrolizidine alkaloids in human diet, *Mutat Res* 443:53, 1999.

Ryu S, Chung W: Induction of the procarcinogen-activating CYP1A2 by a herbal dietary supplement in rats and humans, *Food Cosmet Toxicol* 41:861, 2003.

Saper RB et al: Heavy metal content of ayurvedic herbal medicine products, *JAMA* 292(23):2868, 2004.

Segelman AB et al: Sassafras and herb tea: potential health hazards, *JAMA* 236:477, 1976.

Stedman C: Herbal hepatotoxicity, *Semin Liver Dis* 22(2): 195-206, 2002.

Sudekum M et al: Pennyroyal oil toxicosis in a dog, *J Am Vet Med Assoc* 200:817, 1992.

Tisserand R, Balacs T: *Essential oil safety: a guide for health care professionals;* Edinburgh, UK, 1999, Churchill Livingstone.

Vanherweghem LJ: Misuse of herbal remedies: the case of an outbreak of terminal renal failure in Belgium (Chinese herbs nephropathy), *J Altern Complement Med* 4:9, 1998.

Villar D et al: Toxicity of *Melaleuca* oil and related essential oils applied topically on dogs and cats, *Vet Hum Toxicol* 36:139, 1994.

Yang S, Dennehy CE, Tsourounis C: Characterizing adverse events reported to the California poison control system on herbal remedies and dietary supplements: a pilot study, *J Herb Pharmacother* 2(3):1, 2003.

Zhou S et al: Herbal bioactivation: the good, the bad and the ugly, *Life Sci* 74:935, 2004.

CHAPTER 35

Aflatoxicosis in Dogs

KARYN BISCHOFF, *Ithaca, New York*
TAM GARLAND, *Washington, DC*

Aflatoxicosis in dogs was first described as *hepatitis X* in 1952. The disease was experimentally reproduced in 1955 using contaminated feed and again in 1966 using purified aflatoxin B₁. Moldy corn poisoning of swine and turkey X disease were reported in the 1940s. Turkey X disease was linked to aflatoxin in 1961.

Aflatoxins are a group of related compounds produced as secondary metabolites of various fungi, including *Aspergillus parasiticus, A. flavus, A. nomius,* and some *Penicillium* spp. Aflatoxins are not produced by all strains of these fungi. The most common aflatoxins in grains are named, in part, for their fluorescent color: aflatoxins B₁ and B₂, fluoresce blue; and aflatoxins G₁ and G₂, fluoresce green. Aflatoxin B₁ is the most common and most toxicologically potent of the aflatoxins.

High-energy agricultural crops are most often affected. Corn, peanuts, and cottonseed are frequently implicated; but rice, wheat, oats, sweet potatoes, potatoes, barley, millet, sesame, sorghum, cacao beans, almonds, soy, coconut, safflower, sunflower, palm kernel, cassava, cowpeas, peas, and various spices have been affected. Mold may grow on crops in the field or during storage. Factors that influence mold growth include temperature, humidity, drought stress, insect damage, and handling techniques.

Ingestion of homemade pet foods, moldy garbage, and improperly stored dog foods all have been implicated in aflatoxicosis.

Commercial grain is screened routinely for aflatoxins, but sampling error has been implicated in contamination of commercial dog food. Uneven distribution of mold growth within the grain (by analogy, one moldy orange in a large bag of fruit or blue veins in a block of blue cheese) increases the risk of sampling error. A simple black light at 366 nm induces fluorescence of kojic acid—a chemical also produced by many aflatoxin-producing fungi. Kojic acid fluoresces blue-green. Its presence neither confirms nor eliminates the presence of aflatoxins. More sensitive analyses use enzyme-linked immunosorbent assays, high-performance liquid chromatography (HPLC), and liquid chromatography/mass spectrometry. HPLC is both more sensitive and more specific. Many pet food companies currently sample each lot of grain before using it in food production and then sample batches of pet food after production to minimize the problem of sampling error.

TOXICITY

Dogs and cats are considered very sensitive to aflatoxin (Newbern and Butler, 1969). The oral median lethal dose

(LD$_{50}$) for aflatoxins in dogs has ranged from 0.5 to 1.8 mg/kg. It has been difficult to determine the total dose of aflatoxin received in field cases when the amount ingested and period of exposure may not be available. Although dog foods containing as low as 60 ppb of aflatoxin have been implicated in aflatoxicosis cases, it is rarely possible to know the actual aflatoxin exposure from food consumed before presentation. The experimental oral LD$_{50}$ for aflatoxin in cats is 0.55 mg/kg. No clinical cases of aflatoxicosis have been reported in cats.

Factors such as dose received, genetic predisposition, and concurrent disease may influence the course of aflatoxin poisoning. Generally younger animals, particularly males, may be more susceptible. Aflatoxin-related deaths in pups sucking a clinically healthy dam have been reported (Garland and Reagor, 2007). Pregnant and whelping bitches may be more susceptible to aflatoxicosis. Early castration decreases mortality in males of some species (Meerdink, 2004). Low dietary protein may enhance hepatocyte damage, whereas nutritional antioxidants, vitamin A, and carotene may decrease it.

TOXICOKINETICS

Aflatoxins are highly lipophilic and are absorbed rapidly and almost completely in the duodenum. Aflatoxins enter the portal circulation and are highly protein bound in blood. The unbound fraction is distributed to the tissues, with the highest concentration occurring in the liver.

The liver is the primary metabolic site for aflatoxins. Sites of secondary metabolic interest include the liver, kidneys, and small intestine. Phase I metabolism of aflatoxin B$_1$ by cytochrome P-450 enzymes produces the reactive intermediate aflatoxin B$_1$ 8,9-epoxide. Some aflatoxin B$_1$ is metabolized to aflatoxin M. During phase II metabolism aflatoxin B$_1$ 8,9-epoxide is conjugated to glutathione in a reaction catalyzed by glutathione *S*-transferase.

Metabolites of aflatoxin are excreted in both urine and bile. Dogs excrete primarily aflatoxin M$_1$ in the urine. More than 90% of aflatoxin metabolites are excreted in the urine within the first 12 hours after dosing in the dog, and urine aflatoxin is below detectable levels within 48 hours. Conjugated aflatoxin is excreted predominantly in the bile. Approximately 1% of a dose of aflatoxin is excreted as aflatoxin M$_1$ in the milk in dairy cattle.

MECHANISM OF ACTION

Phase I metabolism of aflatoxin B$_1$ produces the highly reactive electrophile aflatoxin B$_1$ 8,9-epoxide, which binds readily to other molecules within the cell, including nucleic acids, proteins, and other constituents of subcellular organelles. Formation of deoxyribonucleic acid (DNA) adducts modifies the DNA template; thus binding of DNA polymerase may be altered, which in turn affects cellular replication. Binding to ribosomal translocase affects protein production. These changes may lead to necrosis of hepatocytes and other metabolically active cells such as renal tubular epithelium. Coagulopathy may result from decreased prothrombin and fibrinogen production. Excretion kinetics of adducts is slower than the parent compound and the aforementioned metabolites.

Aflatoxin is a known carcinogen in rats, ferrets, ducks, trout, swine, sheep, and rats. *It is not known to be carcinogenic in dogs.* Aflatoxins are classified by the International Agency for Research on Cancer as class I human carcinogens. Hepatocellular carcinoma has been associated with chronic aflatoxin exposure and concurrent infection with hepatitis B virus.

CLINICAL SIGNS

Although aflatoxicosis is usually caused by prolonged exposure to contaminated feed, the presentation in small animals is usually acute. Dogs in recent cases involving contaminated commercial dog foods may have been ingesting the foods for weeks or months before becoming clinically ill. For example, adulterated pet food may have entered the market in October, but the first reported cases were not observed until December. Some dogs did not become symptomatic until up to 3 weeks after the diet was changed.

Clinical signs of aflatoxicosis in dogs usually occur within a few days of death but may be protracted for up to 2 weeks. If the concentration of aflatoxin is very high, this is usual; but animals can, and do, survive when the concentration is low or exposure is limited. Experimentally poisoned cats that died of aflatoxicosis survived only a few days after the onset of clinical signs. Conversely, some cats have been known to survive after clinical signs of aflatoxicosis following exposure to adulterated food.

The most commonly reported early clinical signs of aflatoxicosis in dogs include feed refusal or anorexia, weakness and obtundation, vomiting, and diarrhea. A few animals may die unexpectedly without showing clinical signs. Later in the course of the disease, dogs become icteric. Bilirubinuria was prominent in recent cases. Evidence of coagulopathy may include melena or frank blood in the feces, hematemesis, petechial hemorrhages, and epistaxis.

DIAGNOSIS

The primary differential diagnosis for dogs in recent food contamination–related cases of aflatoxicosis was leptospirosis, as was reported by Stenske and colleagues (2006). Other differential diagnoses that have been considered include parvovirus and anticoagulant rodenticide toxicosis based on the severe gastrointestinal hemorrhage and a variety of hepatotoxic agents, including acetaminophen; microcystin from cyanobacteria; amanitine from mushrooms; and toxins associated with cycad palms, phosphine, and iron.

Diagnosis of aflatoxicosis is often based on history, clinical signs, clinical pathology findings and postmortem changes. Laboratory testing of dog food or other implicated material may be helpful in confirming the diagnosis, but sometimes this material is no longer available. Often all of the contaminated food has been consumed by the time the animal presents to the veterinarian. During a recent dog food contamination incident, three groups of dogs with similar dietary histories and clinical signs were identified by a veterinarian. Dog food was submitted to the laboratory from each of the three households, but only one sample contained aflatoxin in toxicologically significant concentrations. If the dog food bags or codes from the bags are maintained, it is possible to learn what lot of food may have been contaminated.

Some laboratories test for aflatoxin M_1 in the urine, but urinary excretion is very rapid in dogs. There has been some success with testing serum or liver for aflatoxin, but, again because of the rapid metabolism and excretion of aflatoxin, we have found these tests to be of limited usefulness.

Clinical Chemistry

Complete blood count, serum chemistry, including bile acids, and urinalysis have been recommended to support the diagnosis of aflatoxin poisoning and rule out other causes of liver failure. Total bilirubin is increased in aflatoxicosis. Changes in hepatic enzyme concentrations are variable. Serum alanine aminotransferase was elevated consistently in one report and may increase progressively (Garland and Reagor, 2007). Other liver enzymes, including aspartate aminotransferase, alanine phosphatase, and γ-glutamyltransferase (GGT) may be elevated. Elevated GGT is high on the scale but when it was exceedingly high, it was more often an indication of undiagnosed Cushing's disease.

Other liver function tests have been used to support the diagnosis of aflatoxicosis. Serum albumin is often decreased, and prothrombin time is often increased. Serum protein C, antithrombin III, and cholesterol are often decreased in aflatoxicosis.

Postmortem Findings

Necropsy is helpful in confirming the diagnosis of aflatoxicosis and ruling out other conditions. Common gross pathology findings include icterus, hepatomegaly that may be mild, ascites, gastrointestinal hemorrhage, and multifocal petechia and ecchymosis. Pigmentary nephrosis has been reported.

The primary histologic changes of canine aflatoxicosis are associated with the liver, although necrosis of the proximal convoluted renal tubules has been reported (Hooser and Talcott, 2006). Liver lesions associated with acute aflatoxicosis include fatty degeneration of hepatocytes, which may contain one or many lipid vacuoles. Centrilobular necrosis and canalicular cholestasis are commonly reported. Inflammation is mild.

Dogs with subacute toxicosis still have hepatocytic fatty degeneration, canalicular cholestasis, and multifocal-to–locally extensive hepatic necrosis that may be associated with neutrophilic inflammation and hepatocyte regeneration. Fibrosis becomes more prominent, with bridging of portal triads and proliferation of bile ductules. The central vein may become obscured and replaced with dilated sinusoids. Chronic aflatoxicosis is characterized by less fatty degeneration of hepatocytes but marked disruption of the normal hepatic architecture by fibrosis. Regenerative nodules may be evident grossly.

Hepatic lesions reported in cats with aflatoxicosis are somewhat different. Experimentally affected cats had hepatomegaly with petechiation. Hepatocytes contained mostly glycogen with minimal lipid. There was bile duct hyperplasia in cats that had clinical signs for more than 72 hours before death.

MANAGEMENT

The prognosis for small animals with clinical signs of aflatoxicosis is guarded. Animals with severe clinical signs often respond poorly to treatment, although early intervention may improve the chances of survival.

As with most other conditions, patient assessment and stabilization are the first steps in management of aflatoxicosis. Toxin exposure should be limited. This may mean removing contaminated food after chronic ingestion and replacing it with a diet containing high-quality protein or giving activated charcoal orally for a recent high-dose exposure such as moldy garbage.

Supportive care includes correcting hydration and electrolyte imbalances with intravenous fluids. Vitamins B and K_1 and dextrose may be added to fluids. Vitamin K_1 therapy decreased clinical coagulopathy after 72 hours of therapy in one clinical case (Garland and Reagor, 2007). Parenteral nutrition may be needed in animals with severe gastroenteric signs. Sucralfate and famotidine have been used to treat these animals. Plasma transfusions have been used to improve clotting profiles.

Liver protectants such as extracts of milk thistle (*Silybum marianum*) have been used clinically and experimentally to treat aflatoxicosis. Silymarin is a mix of flavonolignans from milk thistle, including silybin. When given to chickens fed a diet containing aflatoxin B_1, changes in liver enzyme profiles and histologic lesions were decreased compared to controls. Various mechanisms of action for silybin have been proposed, such as inhibition of phase I metabolism of aflatoxin B_1, thus decreasing epoxide production. Although milk thistle products are believed to be liver supportive, when combined with S-adenosylmethionine (SAM-e) in the face of canine chronic aflatoxicosis presenting acutely, these products may prevent the aflatoxin adducts from forming, thus preventing the aflatoxin from leaving the body. (SAM-e) has also been used clinically as a hepatoprotectant in the treatment of aflatoxicosis (Stenske et al., 2006). Sulfhydryl groups on SAM-e may bind aflatoxin B_1 8,9-epoxide.

N-acetylcysteine may be given parenterally and has been used in severely intoxicated dogs. N-acetylcysteine is known to increase cytosolic and mitochondrial glutathione and may act directly as a free-radical scavenger. Experimentally N-acetylcysteine has been shown to enhance elimination of aflatoxin B_1 and prevent liver damage in poultry.

The antischistosomal drug oltripaz has been used to treat aflatoxicosis in humans and experimental animals. Oltipraz inhibits phase I enzymes, CYP1A2 in particular, that metabolize aflatoxin B_1 to the epoxide form. It also induces phase II enzymes, including glutathione S-transferase, to facilitate conjugation of aflatoxin B_1 8,9-epoxide. This drug protects against hepatocarcinogenesis in rats. Oltipraz has not been used in veterinary medicine to our knowledge.

References and Suggested Readings

Bastianello SS et al: Pathological finding in a natural outbreak of aflatoxicosis in dogs, *Onderstepoort J Vet Res* 64:635, 1987.

Bingham AK et al: Identification and reduction of urinary aflatoxin metabolites in dogs, *Food Chem Toxicol* 42:1851, 2004.

Garland Reagor T: Chronic canine aflatoxin and management of an epidemic. In Panter KE, Wierenga TL, Pfister JA, editors: *Poisonous plants: global research and solutions*, Wallingford, Oxon, UK, 2007, CABI Publishing.

Hooser SB, Talcott PA: Mycotoxins. In Peterson ME, Talcott PA, editors: *Small animal toxicology*, ed 2, St Louis, 2006, Elsevier Saunders, p 888.

Meerdink GL: Mycotoxins. In Plumlee KH, editor: *Clinical veterinary toxicology*, St Louis, 2004, Mosby, p 231.

Newbern PM, Butler WH: Acute and chronic effects of aflatoxin on the liver of domestic and laboratory animals: a review, *Cancer Res* 29:236, 1969.

Stenske KA et al: Aflatoxicosis in dogs and dealing with suspected contaminated commercial foods, *J Am Vet Med Assoc* 228:1686, 2006.

Tedesco D et al: Efficacy of silymarin-phospholipid complex in reducing the toxicity of aflatoxin B_1 in broiler chickens, *Poult Sci* 83:1839, 2004.

Valdivia AG et al: Efficacy of N-acetylcysteine to reduce the effects of aflatoxin B_1 intoxication in broiler chickens, *Poult Sci* 80:727, 2001.

Wang JS et al: Protective alterations in phase 1 and 2 metabolism of aflatoxin B_1 by oltipraz in residents of Qidong, People's Republic of China, *J Natl Cancer Inst* 91:347, 1999.

CHAPTER 36

Nephrotoxicants

WILSON K. RUMBEIHA, *East Lansing, Michigan*
MICHAEL J. MURPHY, *St. Paul, Minnesota*

The kidney is a frequent target for toxic chemicals (Box 36-1). The recent pet food recall associated renal damage has prompted further consideration of nephrotoxicity in dogs and cats. This chapter provides an overview of the more common nephrotoxicants and includes diagnostic considerations for nephrotoxicosis in veterinary patients at the clinic or at the time of postmortem evaluation. Issues related to pet food safety are addressed in Chapter 37.

PATHOPHYSIOLOGIC CONSIDERATIONS

Renal failure is common, and only a small percent of cases of renal insufficiency are the result of chemical toxins. The kidney constitutes only 1% of body weight in most mammals but receives about 25% of total cardiac output. This high cardiac output exposes the kidney to many substances foreign to the body, including food additives and drugs (i.e., xenobiotics). These chemicals often reach relatively high concentrations in the renal ultrafiltrate. In many instances a high concentration of xenobiotics is associated with nephrotoxicity, but other factors may also play a role.

The kidneys also conduct substantial metabolism of endogenous and exogenous chemicals. Bioactivation of some chemicals can lead to nephrotoxicity, although metabolism of most chemicals leads to detoxification.

Animals may be predisposed to nephrotoxicity. Young and geriatric animals generally are believed to be more susceptible to the nephrotoxic effects of xenobiotics. Young animals may not have fully developed detoxifying enzyme systems, and these systems may be diminished in geriatric animals. Malnutrition, dehydration, preexisting renal conditions, and concurrent exposure to multiple nephrotoxins are some of the factors that may influence the potential for nephrotoxicity.

Causes of acute renal failure in dogs and cats generally can be classified as hemodynamic-related, infectious, or toxic. Toxin-induced acute renal failure is commonly encountered in small animals. Younger animals are the most frequently involved. In dogs the most common causes of nephrotoxicosis are ethylene glycol (EG), nonsteroidal antiinflammatory drugs, cholecalciferol (CCF), and aminoglycoside antibiotics. In cats the most common causes of nephrotoxicity are EG, CCF, and lilies. An expanded list of known nephrotoxins is presented in Box 36-1. Only the most common causes of nephrotoxicosis are discussed here, with additional comments directed to the recent pet food–related toxicosis.

Box **36-1**

Known Nephrotoxins and Other Causes in the Differential Diagnosis of Acute and Chronic Renal Failure in Dogs and Cats

Household Products and Pesticides
- Cholecalciferol (see text)
- Sodium fluoride, superphosphate fertilizer
- Rodenticides (e.g., phosphorus, thallium)
- Herbicides (e.g., paraquat)

Industrial Compounds
- Ethylene glycol (see text)
- Chlorinated hydrocarbons (e.g., carbon tetrachloride, chloroform, hexachlorobutadiene)

Heavy Metals
- Mercury, cadmium, lead, arsenic, chromium

Pharmaceuticals, Diagnostic Aids, and Anesthetics
- Aminoglycoside antibiotics (see text)
- Cephalosporins (e.g., cephaloridine, cefazolin, cephalothin)
- Polymyxins
- Sulfonamides (e.g., sulfapyridine, sulfathiazole, sulfadiazine)
- Amphotericin B
- Nonsteroidal antiinflammatory drugs (see text)
- Lithium
- Phosphorus-containing urinary acidifiers
- Cyclosporine
- Antineoplastics (e.g., methotrexate, cisplatin)
- Methoxyflurane
- Chelating agents (e.g., D-penicillamine, ethylenediaminetetraacetic acid [EDTA])
- Radiologic contrast media
- Gold salts
- Diuretics (e.g., thiazides, furosemide)
- Vitamin D_3 analog (psoriasis medications)

Natural Toxins
- Easter lily (*Lilium longiflorum*; see text)
- Mycotoxins (e.g., ochratoxin A, citrinin)
- Snake venom
- Mushrooms (e.g., amatoxins)

Ischemic Renal Injury
- Severe volume depletion
- Hemolytic compounds (e.g., zinc toxicosis, acetaminophen toxicosis in cats)
- Thromboembolism of renal arteries in cats

Infectious Conditions
- Acute nephritis (e.g., leptospirosis) or pyelonephritis
- Chronic tubulointerstitial nephritis

Primary Renal Diseases
- Chronic renal disease (idiopathic)
- Amyloidosis
- Familial renal disease

Obstructive Uropathy
- Melamine cyanurate crystals

Ruptured Urinary Conduit

ETHYLENE GLYCOL AND DIETHYLENE GLYCOL

EG is a sweet-tasting liquid that is widely used as a solvent in several commercial products such as antifreeze, paints, and polishes. Antifreeze is the most common source of EG exposure in pets. Commercial antifreeze contains about 50% to 95% EG. EG toxicosis is reported all year round but is more prevalent in late fall and early spring.

Toxicosis most commonly occurs within hours of ingestion. EG is rapidly absorbed from the gastrointestinal tract, with peak plasma concentrations occurring about 2 to 3 hours after ingestion. The plasma half-life of EG in small animals is about 3 hours; thus about eight elimination half-lives occur in a day. Diethylene glycol (DEG) is also a widely used organic solvent in commercial products. Antifreeze is the most common source of EG exposure in pets.

EG is metabolized predominantly in the liver. It is metabolized from EG to glycoaldehyde by alcohol dehydrogenase. Glycoaldehyde is metabolized to glyoxalate by aldehyde dehydrogenase. Glyoxalate is finally converted to oxalate, glycine, and formate. The conversion of EG to glycoaldehyde and of glycoaldehyde to glycolate requires nicotinamide adenine dinucleotide (NAD) as a cofactor. Lactate dehydrogenase and glycolic acid oxidase catalyze the conversion of glycolate to glyoxylate. The conversion of EG to glycoaldehyde and of glycolate to glyoxalate are the rate-limiting steps in the metabolism of EG. EG itself is mildly toxic, but its metabolite products, especially glycoaldehyde, glyoxalate, and oxalate, are potentially lethal; thus treatment is aimed at preventing this metabolism.

Toxicity and Signs

Cats are more sensitive to EG toxicity than dogs. The minimum lethal dose of undiluted EG is 1.4 ml/kg in cats and 4.4 ml/kg in dogs. The clinical presentation of EG toxicosis in dogs and cats is often divided into three phases. The first phase generally is 0.5 to 8 hours after ingestion of a toxic doss. The predominant clinical signs in phase 1 are vomiting, depression, and ataxia (an almost "drunken" appearance). These signs are attributed to EG and glycoaldehyde. The latter reaches a peak plasma concentration 6 to 12 hours after EG ingestion. The second phase is generally 8 to 24 hours after ingestion. The predominant clinical signs in phase 2 are depression, anorexia, tachycardia, and pulmonary congestion. If the animal survives these two phases, the third phase begins about 25 to 72 hours after ingestion. The predominant signs during the third phase include vomiting, anuria or oliguria, and uremia, reflecting acute renal failure. Neurologic signs, including seizures, may be observed in some severe cases of intoxication. Laboratory tests are altered during these phases.

An increased anion gap, hyperosmolality, elevated blood urea nitrogen (BUN) and creatinine, hypocalcemia, isosthenuria, and calcium oxalate monohydrate crystals are the biochemical hallmarks of EG toxicosis in small animals. Glycolic and lactic acids are the main causes of acidosis in EG toxicosis. Lactic acid formation is favored by the increase in the ratio of NADH to NAD, which drives the lactate dehydrogenase reaction. Acidosis can be detected as early as 3 to 4 hours after EG ingestion. Acute renal failure is the consequence of the direct toxic effects of EG metabolism on renal epithelial cells and on the tubular obstructive effects of calcium oxalate crystals. Hyperechoic renal cortices may be evident on ultrasound examination of the kidneys. Bladder size may be small, indicating reduced urine formation.

Treatment of Ethylene Glycol Toxicosis

Treatment of EG toxicosis is most successful if initiated within 12 hours of ingestion (also see Chapters 24 and 29). Gastric decontamination should be initiated by inducing emesis, followed by administration of activated charcoal, provided the patient is presented within 4 to 6 hours of ingestion. Previously intravenous ethanol was the treatment of choice for EG toxicosis, but with approval of 4-methylpyrazole (4-MP) for EG toxicosis in dogs the situation has changed. However, ethanol is still the drug of choice for cats. Ethanol is a preferred substrate of alcohol dehydrogenase; thus it is used to inhibit EG metabolism. However, ethanol is normally of little use if the patient is presented more than 12 hours after ingestion. A 20% ethanol solution is given at 5.5 ml/kg intravenously every 4 hours for 24 hours or in a constant-rate infusion of 1.4 ml/kg/hour for dogs or 1.25 ml/kg/hour for cats. Maintaining ethanol therapy for up to 72 hours normally ensures complete EG elimination. The benefit of ethanol treatment has been questioned, especially in high-exposure situations and comatose animals.

Currently other alcohol dehydrogenase inhibitors may be used to inhibit conversion of EG. The drug 4-MP or Fomepizole (Orphan Medical) is approved for use in dogs (Kirk and Bonagura, 1995). The first dose is given as a 5% solution at 20 ml/kg intravenously. The second dose is given at 15 mg/kg 12 to 24 hours after the first dose. The third dose, if necessary, is given at 5 mg/kg 36 hours after the first one. Unfortunately 4-MP is not recommended in cats, partly because of poor efficacy in this species when using canine doses and the need to administer the drug almost concurrently with ingestion of EG.

Hemodialysis is a referral option in some areas and may be beneficial if started up to 24 hours after EG ingestion. However, dialysis is most effective when initiated within 3 to 4 hours of exposure. Further studies are needed to determine if hemodialysis removes the more toxic metabolites of EG, the time frame over which this therapy is beneficial, and whether or not 4-MP can be used in conjunction with hemodialysis.

Because most patients are presented for treatment late in the course of the disease, the mortality rate of EG toxicosis is higher than 70%. Treatment procedures for EG-induced nephrotoxicosis are summarized in Box 36-2 and Chapter 191.

DEG is also rapidly absorbed from the gut, with peak plasma concentrations reached in 1 to 2 hours.

Box 36-2

Summary of General and Supportive Treatment of Toxic-Induced Acute Renal Failure

Keep the Patient Alive
If Presented Less than 6 hours After Ingestion
- Emesis
  Apomorphine hydrochloride, 0.02-0.04 mg/kg IV or IM (if available)
  Syrup of ipecac, 2-6 ml PO
  or
  3% hydrogen peroxide, 5 ml/dog or cat
- Activated charcoal
  Acta-Char, 1-4 g/kg
  or
  Charcodote, 6-12 ml/kg
- Cathartics
  Mineral oil, 10-50 ml/dog, 10-25 ml/cat q12h PO
  or
  Sodium sulfate, 1 g/kg

Supportive Treatment
- Hyperkalemia and acidosis
  Sodium bicarbonate, 10 mg/kg q8-12h PO or BW (kg) × 0.3 × base deficit
  or
  (20 − TCO$_2$) in mEq; half of this dose is given slowly IV in 15-30 min
- Fluid therapy
  Ideal fluid is 0.9% normal saline, or 2.5% dextrose in 0.45% saline; to enhance urinary excretion of toxin, correct electrolyte imbalances, manage moderate acidosis, dilute waste products normally excreted by the kidneys
- Diuretics to enhance toxin and metabolic waste products excretion
  Furosemide (avoid in gentamicin nephrotoxicity), 2-4 mg/kg as needed IV, IM, SC
  Mannitol, 1 g/kg of 5%-25% solution IV (avoid in pulmonary edema)
- Antiemetics or H$_2$ blockers to correct uremia-induced vomiting
  Metoclopramide, 0.2-0.5 mg/kg IV, IM, q6-8h
  or
  Cimetidine, 2.5-5 mg/kg IV q8-12h
- Give proper nutrition: glucose supplementation, low-quantity but high-quality protein
- Peritoneal dialysis or hemodialysis if azotemia is progressive despite fluid therapy

Run Toxicology Tests to Identify and Remove Specific Underlying Causes
- Withdraw offending drug; eliminate sources (e.g., feed); give chelation therapy in cases such as exposure to heavy metals

BW, Body weight; IM, intramuscularly; IV, intravenously; PO, orally; SC, subcutaneously.

It is metabolized in the liver to its sole metabolite, 2-hydroxyethoxyacetic acid. Oxalate is not a metabolite of pure DEG. DEG is excreted in urine as both parent compound and metabolite. Toxicosis of DEG is characterized by renal failure, acidosis, and cardiac irregularities. The diagnosis of DEG nephrotoxicosis is difficult and can be supported by its presence or that of its metabolite in blood or urine. Ethers of EG such as EG butyl ether, a component of glass cleaners, may also cause oxalate-induced renal failure.

AMINOGLYCOSIDE ANTIBIOTICS

Aminoglycoside antibiotics are the most frequent class of drugs associated with nephrotoxicosis in dogs and cats. Gentamicin, tobramycin, amikacin, kanamycin, and netilmicin are used for the treatment of gram-negative infections but have a narrow therapeutic index and should be used with caution in animals at high risk for nephrotoxicity, especially those suffering from dehydration or receiving diuretic (furosemide) therapy.

Aminoglycosides are not metabolized in vivo and, because of their low molecular weights and high water solubility, are excreted almost exclusively through the urine. In vivo these antibiotics easily ionize to cationic complexes that bind to anionic sites on the epithelial cells of the proximal tubules. Following binding, the drugs are internalized by pinocytosis. Renal cortical concentrations of aminoglycoside antibiotics may exceed plasma concentration by tenfold. In general, the toxicity of aminoglycoside antibiotics correlates positively with the number of ionizable groups on the drug. For example, neomycin with six ionizable groups is extremely nephrotoxic and is not used systemically. Gentamicin, tobramycin, amikacin, kanamycin, and netilmicin all have five ionizable groups and a high potential for renal toxicity when used systemically. Aminoglycoside antibiotics can cause acute tubular necrosis through a variety of mechanisms.

Aminoglycoside-induced renal failure is most commonly iatrogenic in origin. Animals receiving aminoglycoside therapy should be monitored for renal injury with periodic urinalyses (specifically evaluation for protein and casts) and with serial determinations of serum urea nitrogen and creatinine. The mortality rate in monitored animals is low. Clinically affected animals may have polyuria, proteinuria, azotemia, and high urinary N-acetyl-B-D-glucosaminidase activity. Nephrotoxicity often can be prevented by increasing the dosage interval by a factor related to the serum creatinine concentration. For example, if the recommended dosing interval is 8 hours and the serum creatinine concentration is 3 mg/dl, the dosing interval should be extended by 3 × 8 hours = 24 hours.

The treatment of aminoglycoside-induced nephrotoxicosis consists of withdrawing aminoglycoside therapy and then initiating other nonspecific measures, as summarized in Box 36-2 and Chapter 191.

NONSTEROIDAL ANTIINFLAMMATORY DRUGS

Nonsteroidal antiinflammatory drugs (NSAIDs) have diverse chemical structures but similar pharmacologic effects. These drugs are broadly classified into two groups: the carboxylic acids and the enolic acids. Aspirin, indomethacin, tolmetin, sulindac, naproxen, ibuprofen, and flunixin meglumine belong to the carboxylic acid group. Phenylbutazone and piroxicam belong to the enolic acid group. Additional classification is based on inhibition of specific enzymes (e.g., COX-1 or COX-2 inhibition).

Many NSAIDs are sold over the counter and are widely available in homes. Because of their wide availability, the accidental ingestion of these medications is encountered commonly in small animal practice. Dogs are more involved frequently than cats with acute toxicosis. Iatrogenic NSAID toxicosis is encountered occasionally, is often chronic, and may be to the result of the higher sensitivity of some animals than others to these drugs. Dehydration, poor renal perfusion (as in heart failure), and concurrent treatment with corticosteroids may increase the likelihood of toxicosis.

The NSAIDs are a diverse group of compounds. In general, NSAIDs are well absorbed orally and predominantly metabolized in the liver. Some NSAIDs such as aspirin require glucuronidation. Cats are especially sensitive to the toxicosis of NSAIDs because they have a reduced glucuronic acid conjugating capacity. Nephrotoxicity is certainly not the only adverse effect of NSAIDs. In particular, hepatopathy and gastrointestinal erosions and ulceration pose serious risks to veterinary patients. Gastric and intestinal toxicity often creates signs of anorexia, vomiting, diarrhea, and anemia. Furthermore, these drugs can enhance bleeding tendencies and, especially in cats, predispose to methemoglobinemia. The nephrotoxic effects of these compounds are discussed in the following paragraphs.

The nephrotoxic and antiinflammatory effects of NSAIDs pertain to the ability of these drugs to inhibit prostaglandin production. Most NSAIDs inhibit cyclooxygenase, the enzyme responsible for conversion of arachidonic acid to endoperoxides. Endoperoxides are intermediates in prostaglandin synthesis. Ibuprofen, mefenamic acid, and indomethacin reversibly inhibit cyclooxygenase, whereas aspirin and phenylbutazone inhibit it irreversibly. Some NSAIDs may block prostaglandin receptors.

Ingestion of large doses of NSAIDs may induce acute renal failure. Chronic exposure to toxic doses of NSAIDs may cause renal papillary necrosis. Dehydrated animals, animals in shock, and those with preexisting renal disease are most vulnerable to NSAID-induced nephrotoxicity. Diagnostic tests of value include a careful history, examination of the stool for melena, urinalysis, tests of renal function, serum biochemistries reflecting liver injury, and a complete blood count.

The treatment of acute NSAID toxicosis should involve gastrointestinal decontamination with emetics and activated charcoal (see Chapter 24), intravenous fluid therapy to correct acidosis and maintain urine output, and other life-support measures as needed (see Box 36-2.) The gastrointestinal tract should be treated for potential ulceration and protected from further injury with drugs such as famotidine, omeprazole, sucralfate, or misoprostol (see Chapter 114). In chronic toxicosis the offending drug should be withdrawn. The prognosis is generally good in acute renal injury but is guarded to poor in chronic exposure situations when renal papillary necrosis has occurred.

CHOLECALCIFEROL

CCF (vitamin D$_3$) is marketed as a rodenticide as well as a nutritional supplement and a treatment for psoriasis. Toxicosis from this compound is related to disruption of calcium homeostasis. CCF toxicosis should always be considered whenever acute renal failure is observed in pets.

Rat baits containing CCF are sold over the counter as Quintox (Bell Laboratories), Rampage (Motomco Ltd.), Rat-B-Gon (The Ortho Group), and other trade names. Poisoning in pets occurs after accidental or intentional bait ingestion. Ingestion (including licking) of human psoriasis medications that contain synthetic vitamin D, analogs such as calcipotriol and calcipotriene, can lead to vitamin D toxicosis. These creams are dispensed under trade names that include Dovonex (Westwood Squibb Pharmaceutical Corp), Taclonex (Warner-Chilcott Company Inc.), or Psorcutan (Intendis).

Although the median lethal dose (LD$_{50}$) of CCF in dogs is widely reported to be 43 to 88 mg/kg, the experience in my laboratory is that as little as 10 mg/kg given once orally can be lethal. Normal dogs that ingest as little as 4 to 6 mg/kg of CCF once may become sick. Clinically normal dogs that ingest single doses of 2 mg/kg of CCF may develop serum calcium concentrations greater than 12.5 mg/dl.

CCF is rapidly absorbed after ingestion and then transported to the liver. CCF is stored and then slowly metabolized to 25-hydroxy-vitamin D$_3$ (25-OH-D$_3$). Then 25-OH-D$_3$ is metabolized to calcitriol (1,25-dihydroxyvitamin D$_3$), the active metabolite of CCF in the kidney. Calcitriol stimulates calcium uptake from the gut. In conjunction with parathyroid hormone, calcitriol mobilizes calcium from bone tissue and conserves calcium by enhancing calcium resorption from distal tubules. It is known that high serum concentrations of 25-OH-D$_3$ stimulate the 1,25-OH-D$_3$ receptors and trigger similar events. The combined result of these effects is hypercalcemia and hyperphosphatemia, an important point in the differential diagnosis of hypercalcemia or recent onset. Calcification of soft tissues, especially the kidneys, occurs when the calcium and phosphorous product (in milligrams per deciliter) exceeds 60. Renal calcification starts 12 to 18 hours after ingestion, but peak elevation may not be observed until 48 to 72 hours after CCF exposure, coinciding with elevations in serum BUN and creatinine. Early signs of CCF toxicosis include anorexia, vomiting, melena, and depression.

If there is no known history of ingesting bait or psoriasis cream, the clinical signs of toxicosis may be relatively nonspecific. Signs of hypercalcemia, including polydipsia, polyuria, vomiting, and constitutional illness, may be evident. Isosthenuria is typical. Hypercalcemia and hyperphosphatemia should prompt consideration of vitamin D toxicosis, especially if renal function is still normal. However, other causes of hypercalcemia must be considered, including malignancies (lymphoma, perianal adenocarcinoma, parathyroid tumors), renal failure, and hypoadrenocorticism.

Treatment of CCF Toxicosis

Treatment of hypercalcemia related to CCF toxicosis can be challenging (see also Chapter 54). Mortality rate is high because animals are often presented late in the course of disease after substantial renal injury has already occurred. Nonspecific gastrointestinal tract decontamination procedures should be attempted if the animal is presented within 6 to 8 hours of known ingestion (see Chapter 24). Specific therapy is aimed at lowering blood calcium to 8 to 11 mg/dl with the use of salmon calcitonin or another drug. The recommended dosage of calcitonin is 4 to 6 units subcutaneously every 4 to 6 hours until the calcium stabilizes (at least 3 weeks). Pamidronate disodium given at 1.2 mg/kg by a slow saline infusion over 2 hours has been shown to be an effective *alternative* therapy to calcitonin. Two intravenous infusions of pamidronate given 8 days apart have been shown to reverse hypercalcemia of 16 mg/dl to normal for 28 days. Other biphosphonate drugs have been used successfully for treatment of vitamin D–related toxicosis and hypercalcemias of different etiologies but should only be used after consulting an internal medicine specialist or toxicologist.

Nonspecific treatment (see Box 36-2) is frequently used in conjunction with specific calcium-lowering therapies, including furosemide at 2.5 to 4.5 mg/kg every 8 to 16 hours, prednisone at 2 to 6 mg/kg intravenously, intramuscularly, or orally every 24 hours or until blood calcium concentrations return to normal. Fluid therapy with normal saline (0.9% NaCl) is recommended to enhance urine flow and calcium excretion and to correct dehydration.

TOXIC ORNAMENTAL PLANTS

Ingestion of leaves, flowers, or both of the Easter lily (*Lilium longiflorum*) may cause nephrotoxicity in cats. Lily toxicosis in cats was first reported in 1992 and has subsequently been reproduced experimentally. Shortly after eating leaves or flowers, cats develop signs of gastrointestinal upset and become depressed. Acute renal failure characterized by polyuria, dehydration, proteinuria, and glucosuria may be observed 48 to 96 hours after exposure. The toxic agent and mechanism of toxicity have not been established.

The recommended nonspecific therapy includes gastrointestinal decontamination with the use of emetics, activated charcoal, sodium sulfate, and fluid therapy to correct dehydration (also see Chapter 191). This treatment approach is most likely to be beneficial when performed within 6 hours of plant exposure.

DIAGNOSTIC APPROACH TO SUSPECTED NEPHROTOXICITY

Nephrotoxicosis associated with consumption of pet food is quite rare. Yet several million pouches, cans, and bags of pet food were recalled during the spring of 2007 following calls into Regional Offices of the Food and Drug Administration after reports of possible pet food–related nephrotoxicity. Distal renal tubular degeneration and necrosis with crystals deposition were reported in most dogs and cats ingesting pet foods associated with this recall. At the conclusion of the episode, about 300 cats and dogs died and about an equal number were clinically affected but recovered with treatment. This extensive recall included the United States and Canada.

Diagnostic laboratories and the Food and Drug Administration (FDA) have identified the presence of melamine, ammelide, ammeline, and cyanuric acid in some recalled products. The presence of melamine and its analogs is unprecedented in the feed industry. Experimental studies in cats and pigs have revealed that crystal formation was a result of melamine cyanurate crystals. These crystals caused tubular blockage and distal tubular epithelial necrosis. Aspects of pet food safety are discussed in more detail in Chapter 37. The following discussion considers general concepts of diagnosis in terms of nephrotoxicity.

Critical Issues in Establishing Diagnosis of Food-Related Nephrotoxicity

A fundamental part of medicine is consideration of the differential diagnosis. As can be seen from Box 36-1, the causes of acute renal failure in dogs and cats are extensive. Refinement of a diagnosis usually relies on the history, clinical signs, physical examination, and results of laboratory testing. The goal in toxicology cases is establishing an etiology. Often the facts necessary for such a conclusion are not evident; and morphologic, presumptive, or clinical diagnoses are made.

The nephrotoxins EG, CCF, NSAIDs, aminoglycoside antibiotics, and *Lilium* spp. are further examined here to illustrate the point.

Two tenants of toxicology are exposure and dose response. Pets must be exposed to a toxin for it to cause a toxicosis. Further, they must be exposed to a potentially toxic dose and have the adverse effect previously demonstrated for that toxin before a clinician can reach a conclusion of a toxicosis.

In veterinary patients the history and specific laboratory tests are normally used to determine whether an animal has been exposed to a nephrotoxin. The history is often the less reliable of the two methods. For example, does the owner know if his or her pet was exposed to a potentially toxic dose of a drug (NSAIDs, aminoglycosides) with demonstrated nephrotoxicity? Specifically one might inquire if EG, CCF, NSAIDs, aminoglycosides, or *Lilium* spp. plants are present in or around the home. If so, the next step is to confirm or rule out exposure by specific laboratory testing when available. Tests should identify the parent compound or its metabolites.

Quick screening tests are often used to make treatment decisions, but analytic laboratory tests may be required to confirm an etiologic diagnosis. The availability of such confirmatory tests may be investigated by contacting a veterinary diagnostic laboratory (see www.aavld.org or www.abvt.org). Serum or urine is usually the specimen of choice in live animals. For example, although calcium oxalate crystals in urine might be present in toxicosis in a dog or cat with renal failure, this finding is nonspecific; so serum, urine glycolic acid, or EG concentrations would better support a diagnosis of EG exposure. Similarly serum concentrations of 25-hydroxycholecalciferol are used to indicate exposure to CCF; serum or urine concentrations of NSAIDs and aminoglycosides may be used for the same purpose.

The clinical signs, physical examination findings, and routine laboratory tests may be instructive. Clinical signs of renal toxicosis often include gastrointestinal upset, central nervous system depression, cardiopulmonary involvement, and acute renal failure, as observed with EG toxicosis. Ultrasound may show renal cortical damage. Involvement of other organ systems may provide diagnostic leads. For example, NSAID toxicosis causes often may include gastrointestinal bleeding and ulceration, acidosis, and mild elevations of hepatic enzymes. Clinical signs of CCF toxicosis include dark bloody feces, oliguria, or polyuria.

Laboratory testing often is required to establish the adverse effects of toxicity. Obviously serum urea nitrogen and creatinine along with urinalysis are used clinically to indicate renal injury. Calcium abnormalities are common with EG and with CCF toxicosis. Values within the normal range for all of these tests would be interpreted as arguing against a diagnosis of nephrotoxicity. Such findings may not exclude exposure to a subtoxic dose of a nephrotoxic chemical.

When a patient dies or is euthanatized, necropsy and histopathology findings can in some instances support an argument of exposure to a toxin. For example, the finding of antifreeze solution, CCF rodenticide bait, drug products, or lily plant parts supports exposure to the respective compounds. The observation of birefringent crystals histologically is very suggestive of EG exposure, but even in this case the findings are not specific. For example, such crystals can occur following exposure to soluble oxalates (*Oxalis* spp. plants). Similarly renal mineralization is compatible with, but not specific for, CCF exposure.

In conclusion, the diagnosis of nephrotoxicity must rely on evidence of exposure to a sufficient quantity of a toxic chemical, clinical or analytic laboratory findings that confirm or strongly suggest toxicosis, and clinical or necropsy findings of compatible illness. These same principles should be applied to the diagnosis of new toxicities, including those implied by the recent pet food recall.

Reference and Suggested Reading

Kirk RW, Bonagura JD, editors: *Kirk's current veterinary therapy XII (small animal practice)*, Philadelphia, 1995, Saunders, p 232.

CHAPTER 37

Food Toxicoses in Small Animals

MICHAEL J. MURPHY, *St. Paul, Minnesota*
JULIE CHURCHILL, *St. Paul, Minnesota*

"On March 15, FDA learned that certain pet foods were sickening and killing cats and dogs. FDA found contaminants in vegetable proteins imported into the United States from China and used as ingredients in pet food." (http://www.fda.gov/oc/opacom/hottopics/petfood.html)

This announcement marked the beginning of one of the most significant recalls of pet food in the United States and Canada. The chemicals melamine, ammiline, ammilide, and cyanuric acid were identified in pet food within weeks of the initial Food and Drug Administration (FDA) announcement. The presence of these chemicals in pet food was unprecedented and judged to be adulteration.

A number of dogs and cats known to have eaten these foods were also treated for clinical signs associated with a laboratory finding of acute renal failure. Questions related to the disease associated with foods subjected to this recall remain. Certainly the demonstration of nephrotoxicity from any chemical requires consideration of both diagnostic and toxicologic principles.

Since this recall many pet owners have become wary of commercial pet foods. Some are seeking nutritional advice and considering alternative diets such as raw meat diets or home-prepared diets. This chapter is designed to complement the general chapter on "Pet Food Safety" by the late Dr. Phillip Miller (see Section II on Evolve). Herein we consider the pet food recall, commercial pet food regulation, and some issues related to homemade pet food diets. The diagnosis and management of chemical nephrotoxicity is detailed in Chapter 36, and the treatment of acute renal failure outlined in Chapter 191.

PET FOOD RECALL

Many United States pet food companies voluntarily recalled some of their product after the FDA's March 15, 2007 announcement. Investigations by the FDA, veterinary diagnostic laboratories, and the pet food industry led to the identification of melamine and its analogs in some lots of pet food. The presence of melamine in some pet food led the FDA and pet food companies to consider the melamine-containing pet food as adulterated. Consequently several pet food companies voluntarily recalled millions of pounds of potentially adulterated product. The recalls proceeded under established FDA regulations.

The unprecedented adulteration of some pet food with melamine led to the widespread pet food recall.

Since widespread product recalls are not common, a brief summary of the regulatory basis for recalls is presented. "Food," "adulterated," and "recall" all have FDA definitions.

"The term "food" means (1) articles used for food or drink for man or other animals, ... and (3) articles used for components of any such article." *21 United States Code, Section. 321 (f)*

Pet food is an article used for food for animals; thus it fits the FDA legal definition of "food." Pet food is comprised of many components. Some of these components may also meet the FDA's legal definition of "food." Wheat gluten is an example of such a component. Some of the recalled pet food was judged to be adulterated.

"A food shall be deemed to be adulterated– ...
(4) if any substance has been added thereto or mixed or packed therewith so as to ... make it appear better or of greater value than it is." *21 United States Code, Section. 342 (b)(4).*

Adding a substance to a food component to "make it appear better or of greater value than it is" is commonly referred to as "economic adulteration." One theory proposed is that melamine was added to wheat flour as an economic adulterant.

The economic adulterant theory proposes that melamine was added to wheat flour to increase the measured concentration of protein in the wheat flour to that of wheat gluten. Wheat flour is generally lower in protein than wheat gluten. Generally the protein concentration is calculated by testing the product for its total nitrogen concentration and then multiplying the total nitrogen concentration by 6.25 to determine the total protein concentration. Melamine contains six nitrogen molecules per molecule. Addition of melamine to wheat flour apparently increased the calculated protein concentration from that of flour to that of wheat gluten. Because wheat gluten is purchased in large part based on its protein concentration, the price for wheat gluten is higher than the price for wheat flour. Consequently the addition of melamine to wheat flour made the flour "appear better or of greater value" than the flour would have been without the addition of the melamine, thereby satisfying the definition of adulteration.

The melamine-adulterated wheat flour was used as a component in the manufacture of a number of pet food products. One means of removing an adulterated product from the marketplace is a product recall.

"Recall means a firm's removal or correction of a marketed product that the Food and Drug Administration considers to be in violation of the laws it administers and against which the agency would initiate legal action, e.g., seizure. ..." *21 CFR 7.3 (g)*

The company frequently initiates the recall of a marketed product.

"A firm may decide of its own volition and under any circumstances to remove or correct a distributed product. A firm that does so because it believes the product to be violative is requested to notify immediately the appropriate Food and Drug Administration district office listed in § 5.115 of this chapter. ..." *21 CFR 7.46(a)*

Many pet food companies chose to recall pet food products that had been distributed and to notify the FDA of their recall. A list of these recalled products was posted on the FDA website at http://www.accessdata.fda.gov/scripts/petfoodrecall/.

It should be emphasized that not all adulterated products are poisonous. Adulteration is not equivalent to intoxication. Apparently melamine was an economic adulterant in some finished pet food, and this chemical also was detected in the kidneys and urine of some cats that died of renal failure. However, at the time of this writing, the FDA was not "fully certain that melamine is the causative agent" of the cats' death (FAQ, 2007). Investigations are ongoing regarding links between adulteration, specific toxins, and the clinical consequences of toxicosis.

PET FOOD REGULATION

The pet food recall has given rise to questions of regulation of the pet food industry. The widespread pet food recall demonstrates that considerable regulatory authority over the pet food industry exists. The FDA and American Association of Feed Control Officials (AAFCO) are the two major sources of pet food regulation in the United States.

The FDA administers the Federal Food, Drug, and Cosmetic Act (FFDCA). The FFDCA requires that "pet foods, like human foods, be pure and wholesome, safe to eat, produced under sanitary conditions, contain no harmful substances, and be truthfully labeled." (FAQ, 2007). The FDA also "ensures that the ingredients used in pet food are safe and have an appropriate function in the pet food." The "mineral and vitamin sources, colorings, flavorings, and preservatives may be generally recognized as safe or must have approval as food additives" (FAQ, 2007). For example, the FDA monitors bacteria, mycotoxins, pesticides, and metals in commercial pet food products.

The FDA and many states require the listing of food ingredients on the label. Specifically the FDA requires "proper identification of the product, net quantity statement, name and place of business of the manufacturer or distributor, and a proper listing of all the ingredients in order from most to least, based on weight" (FAQ, 2007).

Most states also have pet food labeling requirements. These state requirements generally are based on AAFCO standards. AAFCO is an association of state and federal officials with the basic goal of providing "a mechanism for developing and implementing uniform and equitable laws, regulations, standards and enforcement policies for regulating the manufacture, distribution and sale of animal feeds; resulting in safe, effective, and useful feeds" (AAFCO website). Although AAFCO provides nutritional guidelines related to feeds, complaints about a pet food product are generally directed to the state Department of Agriculture or to the FDA. Complaints to the FDA are normally made to the district office consumer complaint coordinator. The contact information for the district offices can be found at: http://www.fda.gov/opacom/backgrounders/complain.html (also see Chapter 20).

SOME ISSUES RELEVANT TO HOMEMADE PET FOODS

As with any feed, home-prepared pet diets are also subject to consideration for a number of health and stability factors. Among these are microbial content, aerobic stability, unsafe ingredients, and nutritional imbalances.

Microbial Content

A great many recipes for homemade pet food have been posted on the Internet since the pet food recall. Bacterial contamination is a critically important issue in the preparation of homemade pet foods. Generally speaking, microorganisms may grow in an environment in which the pH is greater than 4.6 and the water activity is greater than 0.85 (21 CFR 113.3[n]). The FDA requires that canned pet foods be processed under regulations to ensure the contents are free of viable microorganisms.

Many microorganisms of concern are found in human foods. These organisms include *Clostridium perfringens*, *Clostridium botulinum*, *Staphylococcus aureus*, *Bacillus cereus*, *Salmonella* spp., *Listeria* spp., Yersinia spp., *Aeromonas* spp., *Campylobacter* spp., *Escherichia coli*, *Vibrio* spp., *Enterococcus faecalis*, *Enterobacter cloacae*, and *Klebsiella ozaenae*. Other microorganisms to consider in raw meat include *Neorickettsia* spp., *Toxoplasma gondii*, *Neospora canis*, *Echinococcus* spp., and *Trichinella spiralis*.

The presence of microorganisms in uncooked meat may serve as a primary source of disease in pets. Similarly the growth of microorganisms on food during or after preparation should be considered, particularly if the food is not prepared daily. Disease in dogs from *Clostridium botulinum*, *Escherichia coli* 0157:H7, and *Salmonella* spp. in both dogs and cats has been reported (Barsanti, Walser, and Hatheway, 1978; Fenwick, Hertzke, and Cowan, 1995; Chengappa et al., 1993; Stiver et al., 2003).

Feeding raw meat can be dangerous not only to pets but also the people who care for them. Pathogenic bacteria from raw meat can contaminate work surfaces in the kitchen, utensils, dishes, the floor where the dog eats, and food and water bowls. This exposure poses an even greater risk in households with children, the elderly, or immunocompromised individuals.

Aerobic Stability

The aerobic stability of home-prepared food may also be an issue. Antioxidants are added to many prepared human food and commercial pet food products to reduce oxidative decomposition. Foods demonstrating oxidative decomposition are commonly referred to as *rancid*. Diets high in fat are particularly prone to rancidity, which can include destruction of fat-soluble vitamins. Rancidity and microbial growth are two causes of the "garbage gut" syndrome so often seen by practitioners in dogs and cats that have eaten improperly stored food. A similar situation may occur if home-prepared pet foods are not safely constituted or stored before feeding.

Toxic Human Foods

Many animal owners are unaware of the potential adverse effects of "human foods" on their pets. Although not specifically contaminated or rancid, these foods may contain chemicals or natural substances that are toxic to dogs and cats. For example, some human foods worth avoiding in homemade pet food recipes are *Alliuim* species (chives, onions, garlic), *Brassica* species (kale, Brussels sprouts), kelp, avocado, methylxanthine-containing products (chocolate), rhubarb, grapes, raisins, macadamia nuts, green potatoes, or tomatoes. A number of herbal products should also be avoided (see Chapters 23 and Chapter 34).

Nutritional Imbalances

Nutritional balance is a pivotal aspect of commercially prepared pet foods. A commercial product labeled as dog or cat "food" is by definition a complete and balanced product for that species and requires a nutritional adequacy statement on the product label. Of course there is no requirement or assurance of nutritional adequacy or nutritional balance in recipes published in books or downloaded from the Internet. The nutrient requirements of dogs and cats have recently been reviewed (NRC, 2006). Energy, carbohydrate and fiber, fat and fatty acid, protein and amino acid, mineral, vitamin, and water requirements of dogs and cats are known (NRC, 2006). Although energy, carbohydrate, fat, and protein may be considered by individuals making pet foods, over time vitamin or mineral imbalances may be difficult to avoid.

Nutritional imbalance is more likely to occur with high-protein diets based on meat or raw meaty bones. For example, calcium deficiencies have been documented to occur in meat diets. Diets with high meat content have very high concentrations of dietary phosphorus and low concentrations of calcium. Although it seems that the bones should offer a rich supply of calcium, larger pieces of bones do not appear to be digested and absorbed efficiently. This may result in nutritional deficiency even though bone is intended to serve as the calcium source. The availability of calcium to the dog is highly variable, depending on the size and amount of bones and the age and health of the animal. For example, if the diet contains a very high amount of ground bone, it could be potentially high in calcium, which can be especially harmful to large-breed puppies. High dietary calcium is also believed to contribute to a number of developmental bone diseases such as hip dysplasia, angular limb deformities, and cartilage abnormalities, including osteochondritis desiccans.

Mineral imbalances have also been associated with anemia, goiter, rickets, and secondary hyperparathyroidism.

Vitamin imbalances may also occur in homemade diets. Homemade diets based on meats using offal or high amounts of liver can result in vitamin A excesses and potential toxicity. Raw-meat diets tend to be high in fat, which can lead to either excessive or deficient absorption of the other fat-soluble vitamins. Vitamin imbalances have been associated with anemia, anorexia, dystrophic mineralization, hyperesthesia, myelin degeneration, osteoporosis, reduced growth, and a number of other diseases. Amino acid deficiencies may also occur in homemade diets.

A number of amino acids are classified as being indispensable or *essential*: 11 for cats and 10 for dogs. These essential amino acids must be supplied in the diet because they cannot be synthesized in the body. Most meat-based diets provide adequate amounts of essential amino acids. However, with the new trend toward vegetarian pet diets and with homemade feline diets, careful attention to the amino acid composition is needed to ensure nutritional adequacy.

Because most nutritional problems do not cause noticeable abnormalities until the nutritional imbalance has been present for many months, the link to diet may be hard to identify. Perhaps the best advice for the client insisting on home-prepared pet diets is the following: Question the credentials and training of those advocating the diets and select a recipe that has been formulated by a board-certified veterinary nutritionist.

These issues associated with pet food safety should encourage veterinarians to record a detailed and accurate diet history in the medical record. It is uncertain if pet food changes made by clients in response to the recall in 2007 will result in an increased prevalence of nutrition-based diseases, but veterinarians should be on the lookout for problems related to bacterial contamination, spoiled or rancid food, human food toxicity, or nutritional imbalances.

References and Suggested Reading

American Association of Feed Control Officials: http://www.aafco.org/

Barsanti JA, Walser M, Hatheway CL: Type C botulism in American foxhounds, *J Am Vet Med Assoc* 172:809, 1978.

Chengappa MM et al: Prevalence of *Salmonella* in raw meat used in diets of racing greyhounds, *J Vet Diagn Invest* 5:372, 1993.

Delay J, Laing J: Nutritional osteodystrophy in puppies fed BARF diet, Animal Health Laboratory Newsletter, vol 6, no 2, 2002, Ontario, University of Guelph.

FAQ: accessed 10 July 2007 from http://www.fda.gov/cvm/MenuFoodRecallFAQ.htm. See also 21 CFR, Parts 73, 74, 81, 573 and 582; FDA Regulation of Pet Food and Information on Marketing a Pet Food Product; and Interpreting Pet Food Labels and Interpreting Pet Food Labels—Special Use Foods.

Fenwick B, Hertzke DM, Cowan LA: Alabama rot: almost the complete story, Proceedings of the Eleventh Annual International Convention Canine Sports Medicine Symposium, Gainsville, Fla, 1995, p 15.

Freeman LM, Michel KE: Evaluation of raw food diets for dogs, *J Am Vet Med Assoc* 218:705, 2001.

Joffe DJ, Schlesinger DP: Preliminary assessment of the risk of *Salmonella* infection in dogs fed raw chicken diets, *Can Vet J* 43:441, 2002.

LeJeune JT, Hancock DD: Public health concerns associated with feeding raw meat diets to dogs, *J Am Vet Med Assoc* 219:1222, 2001.

Miller EP: Pet food safety. In Bonagura JD, editor: *Kirk's current veterinary therapy XIII (small animal practice)*, Philadelphia, 2000, Saunders, p 236.

National Research Council: Nutrient requirements of dogs and cats. National Academy of Science, Government Printing Office, 2006.

Stiver SL et al: Septicemic salmonellosis in two cats fed a raw-meat diet, *J Am Anim Hosp Assoc* 39:538, 2003.

Stogdale L, Diehl G: In support of bones and raw food diets, *Can Vet J* 44(10):783, 2003.

Stone GG et al. Application of polymerase chain reaction for the correlation of *Salmonella* serovars recovered from Greyhound feces with their diet, *J Vet Diagn Invest* 5:378, 1993.

SECTION III

Endocrine and Metabolic Diseases

Mark E. Peterson

VOLUME XIII CONTENT ON EVOLVE: http://evolve.elsevier.com/Bonagura/Kirks/

Interpretation of Endocrine Diagnostic Test Results for Adrenal and Thyroid Disease

ROBERT J. KEMPPAINEN, *Auburn, Alabama*
ELLEN N. BEHREND, *Auburn, Alabama*

The following questions represent frequent inquiries received by our endocrine diagnostic laboratory. In previous editions of this book (Kemppainen and Zerbe, 1989; Kemppainen and Clark, 1995) protocols and interpretation of common endocrine tests were described. Reference ranges mentioned are used by the Auburn University Endocrine Diagnostic Service. Refer to the Table "Systeme International (SI) Units in Clinical Chemistry" in the Appendices for conversions between SI (e.g., nmol/L) and mass units (e.g., g/100 ml).

ADRENOCORTICOTROPIC HORMONE STIMULATION TEST

I am having difficulty locating a source for adrenocorticotropic hormone (ACTH) gel. What should I do?

We recommend the use of Cortrosyn (synthetic ACTH or cosyntropin, Amphastar Pharmaceuticals, Rancho Cucamonga, CA). Cortrosyn is sold in packs of 10 or as a single vial of 0.25 mg (250 mcg). The dose for dogs is 5 mcg/kg intravenously (IV) (maximal dose, 250 mcg; Kerl et al., 1999); for cats the dose is 125 mcg IV. In dogs and cats a pre-ACTH sample is collected, ACTH is injected, and one post-ACTH sample is collected 1 hour later. Recent work indicates that the 5 mcg/kg dose is equally effective in dogs when given intramuscularly (IM), using the same sampling times (Behrend et al., 2006). Once a Cortrosyn vial is reconstituted, it can be stored in the refrigerator for up to 4 months and reused. We recently tested four ACTH formulations compounded by pharmacies and sold to veterinarians (Kemppainen, Behrend, and Busch, 2005). This study, performed using healthy laboratory dogs, showed that each of these products stimulated serum cortisol to an equivalent extent, as did Cortrosyn when samples were collected at 1 hour after ACTH injection; but values at 2 hours after ACTH varied considerably. Therefore we recommend that users of compounded ACTH products collect two post-ACTH samples (at 1 and 2 hours after ACTH). To our knowledge no studies have yet assessed responses to various forms of compounded ACTH in dogs with adrenal disease, nor have possible variations in responses related to lot-to-lot differences been conducted.

I performed an ACTH stimulation test to evaluate a dog for Addison's disease, and the post-ACTH cortisol value was greater than normal. Could this dog actually have hyperadrenocorticism?

It's unlikely. It is not uncommon to find a mildly-to-moderately elevated post-ACTH cortisol concentration in dogs tested for Addison's disease (in dogs not affected by the disease). Presumably a normal physiologic response to recent (or chronic) stress is the cause of the elevation; thus we consider this response to be indicative of a normal pituitary-adrenal axis. In true cases of Addison's disease, cortisol concentrations both before and after ACTH are usually very low (both less than 10 nmol/L).

Can recent steroid therapy affect the ACTH stimulation test?

Yes, glucocorticoids can affect the results in two ways. First, some glucocorticoids cross-react in the cortisol assay and can be detected as immunoreactive cortisol. In our assay, cross-reacting steroids include hydrocortisone, prednisone, and prednisolone. In general, we recommend waiting at least 12 hours after (oral) administration to allow these drugs to clear. Second, glucocorticoid therapy may suppress the pituitary-adrenal axis, causing reduced cortisol concentrations before and after ACTH administration. The severity and duration of this suppression is related to dose, potency, frequency of use, and chemical form (e.g., repositol versus oral) of the glucocorticoid therapy.

I treated a dog suspected of having Addison's disease with steroids yesterday, and now I want to perform an ACTH stimulation test. Will the results be meaningful?

Yes, they probably will be useful. A single injection (or infusion) of glucocorticoids may lower the cortisol values in the ACTH stimulation test. However, this type of short-term, nonrepositol treatment will only moderately lower the cortisol values (about 25%) relative to the normal range. Most dogs with Addison's disease have very low plasma cortisol concentrations and fail to show any increase in cortisol in response to ACTH.

How do I monitor the efficacy of mitotane therapy?

Periodic ACTH stimulation testing is recommended in all dogs with hyperadrenocorticism treated with mitotane. "Ideal" cortisol concentrations in a dog receiving treatment are between 30 and 150 nmol/L in both pre- and post-ACTH samples. If values are below ideal, mitotane should be discontinued, and the dog rechecked with ACTH stimulation periodically (i.e., about every 2 to 3 weeks at first). Once values rise into the ideal range, maintenance therapy can be instituted. If values are mildly-to-moderately greater than 150 nmol/L (e.g., in the 150- to 300-nmol/L range), one should consider increasing the dose (approximately 25%) if maintenance therapy is being given or continuing daily loading therapy for a few additional days. If values are higher, it is likely that 5 to 7 days of daily mitotane will be necessary to reduce the adrenal cortical mass to the target level. Clinical condition and recurrence of signs must be considered in the choice of therapy.

How long should I wait between performing a dexamethasone suppression test and an ACTH stimulation test?

We suggest waiting at least 48 hours after a low dose of dexamethasone (0.01 to 0.015 mg/kg) and 5 days after a high dose of dexamethasone (0.1 to 1.0 mg/kg). No delay is necessary when performing the combined dexamethasone suppression–ACTH stimulation test (Kemppainen and Zerbe, 1989). Dexamethasone suppression tests can be performed the day after ACTH stimulation testing.

DEXAMETHASONE SUPPRESSION TESTING

What form of dexamethasone should I use for a dexamethasone suppression test?

Dexamethasone in polyethylene glycol or dexamethasone sodium phosphate can be used, but the dose is based on the amount of active dexamethasone in solution. For example, a 4-mg/ml solution of dexamethasone sodium phosphate provides about 3 mg/ml of active dexamethasone. The dexamethasone can be given IV or IM, although we prefer the IV route.

I think I injected the dexamethasone outside the vein. What should I do?

It is best to wait 48 hours (low dose) or 72 hours (high dose) and repeat the test.

The calculated (low) dose of dexamethasone is only 0.03 ml for this poodle. How do I accurately administer such a small volume of dexamethasone?

It is important to administer the correct dose. Dilute the dexamethasone (e.g., make a 1:20 dilution by mixing 0.2 ml of dexamethasone with 3.8 ml of sterile saline or sterile water) so that a reasonable volume is given. (For Azium, a 1:20 dilution will make the solution 0.1 mg/ml.)

Can I use the results of the low-dose dexamethasone suppression test to both diagnose and differentiate hyperadrenocorticism in dogs?

Sometimes the results can strongly indicate a diagnosis of pituitary-dependent hyperadrenocorticism (but never adrenal-dependent hyperadrenocorticism). If the concentration in the 8-hour sample is greater than 30 nmol/L, the results are consistent with hyperadrenocorticism. If in addition the 4-hour postdexamethasone cortisol concentration is less than 30 nmol/L and/or the concentration in the 4- and/or 8-hour sample is less than 50% of the predexamethasone cortisol concentration, pituitary-dependent hyperadrenocorticism is likely.

GENERAL QUESTIONS CONCERNING THE DIAGNOSIS OF HYPERADRENOCORTICISM

Do normal results on an ACTH stimulation test or a low-dose dexamethasone suppression test rule out hyperadrenocorticism? Conversely, do abnormal results definitely diagnose the disease?

Results of the ACTH stimulation test will be in the normal range in at least 20% of dogs with hyperadrenocorticism, whereas the false-negative rate with the low-dose dexamethasone test is approximately 5%. If results of one test are normal but clinical suspicion for the disease is high, one should consider performing the other screening test. It is important to recognize that each test also has false-positives, particularly when dogs with nonadrenal disease are tested. Interestingly, of the two screening procedures the low-dose dexamethasone suppression test seems more prone to this potential error. About 50% of dogs in one study with nonadrenal illness had abnormal results (inadequate suppression of plasma cortisol) when tested with a low dose of dexamethasone (Kaplan, Peterson, and Kemppainen, 1995). None of the dogs in that study had a clinical presentation or signs consistent with hyperadrenocorticism. Assessment of test results in dogs with nonadrenal illness in which a clinical suspicion of hyperadrenocorticism is also present is challenging. The predictive value for hyperadrenocorticism of a positive screening test result increases in direct proportion to the number and severity of clinical signs and biochemical changes typically occurring in the disease.

What is the best test for hyperadrenocorticism in cats?

We recommend the high-dose dexamethasone suppression test, administering the steroid at a dose of 0.1 mg/kg IV and collecting a predexamethasone sample and two samples after dexamethasone administration (at 4 and 8 hours).

How and why should I try to differentiate pituitary- from adrenal-dependent hyperadrenocorticism in dogs?

Unless results of the low-dose dexamethasone suppression test support pituitary-dependent hyperadrenocorticism, a differentiating test is recommended. Results of ACTH stimulation testing cannot differentiate the types. The two endocrine tests for this purpose are the high-dose dexamethasone suppression test (0.1 or 1.0 mg/kg in dogs and 1 mg/kg in cats) and endogenous ACTH measurement. Timing of sample collection in the high-dose–dexamethasone suppression test is the same as for the low-dose test. If cortisol concentrations at 4 and/or

8 hours post dexamethasone suppress (>50% decline from baseline or decline to <30 nmol/L), a diagnosis of pituitary-dependent disease is made. However, in about 15% to 20% of dogs with pituitary-dependent hyperadrenocorticism, cortisol is not suppressed by dexamethasone. Considering that cortisol is not suppressed by dexamethasone in dogs with adrenal-dependent disease, and that pituitary-dependent disease is the most common form, a failure to suppress in response to dexamethasone means that the odds of having either form is about 50%. In other words, failure of cortisol concentrations to suppress in response to high-dose dexamethasone does not mean that a patient has an adrenal tumor. Endogenous ACTH measurement can positively differentiate the forms, since circulating ACTH concentrations are low to nondetectable in adrenal-dependent disease and normal to high in pituitary-dependent disease. Unfortunately there is also a grey zone relative to the interpretation of endogenous ACTH measurements, and values that fall into this range are nondiagnostic. Accurate measurement of ACTH in plasma requires special sample handling (Kemppainen and Clark, 1995). Other means to differentiate hyperadrenocorticism include ultrasonography and other imaging modalities and surgical exploration. It is important to distinguish the forms because of differences in therapy and prognosis. Surgical removal of an adrenal tumor can be curative. If mitotane is used for medical management, the therapeutic approach is different, depending on the type of disease. In general, adrenal-dependent disease requires higher dosages and a longer induction phase (Kintzer and Peterson, 1989). Overall the prognosis varies between the two forms.

What is the value in measuring a urinary cortisol:creatinine ratio (UCCR)?

This test is best used to determine if a dog does *not* have hyperadrenocorticism. Nearly 100% of dogs with spontaneous hyperadrenocorticism have an elevated UCCR. Unfortunately many dogs with an elevated UCCR do not have hyperadrenocorticism. Consequently a high ratio means that hyperadrenocorticism is possible, and a more definitive screening test (ACTH stimulation, low-dose dexamethasone suppression test) is indicated. Therefore a normal UCCR is valuable in ruling out hyperadrenocorticism.

CANINE HYPOTHYROIDISM

What is the value of measuring total thyroxine (T_4)?
Total T_4 can best be used to rule out the diagnosis of hypothyroidism. If the total T_4 is well into the normal reference range (i.e., >25 nmol/L), it is unlikely that the dog is hypothyroid. If the T_4 is less than normal, the dog may or may not be hypothyroid. Numerous nonthyroidal factors such as medications and chronic illness (i.e., euthyroid sick syndrome) can suppress T_4 to less than the normal range (also see Chapter 41 for additional details about thyroid testing).

What is the value of measuring free T_4?

Free T_4 (FT_4) is the portion of total T_4 not bound to protein and represents about 0.1% of total T_4. The pituitary-thyroid axis functions to maintain free, not total, T_4 within a certain range; thus measurement of FT_4 is a better test of thyroid function. Two methods are used to measure FT_4: analog radioimmunoassay and equilibrium dialysis. Analog radioimmunoassay is less expensive but is not reliable in dogs with euthyroid sick syndrome; it provides no additional diagnostic value over measurement of total T_4 (Nelson et al., 1991). Equilibrium dialysis gives more reliable estimates of true FT_4 concentrations. Measurement of FT_4 can be the initial test for the diagnosis of hypothyroidism, or it can be used in dogs that have been found to have borderline-low total T_4 concentrations. However, it has been demonstrated that nonthyroidal disease and therapy with certain drugs (e.g., phenobarbital, glucocorticoids) are associated with reduced FT_4, even when measured using the dialysis method (Ferguson and Peterson, 1992; Kantrowitz et al, 1999, 2001). Measurement of FT_4 by dialysis is more effective than total T_4 in distinguishing euthyroidism from hypothyroidism. However, all of the current tests for diagnosing hypothyroidism in dogs can be influenced by nonthyroidal factors.

How would I know if autoantibodies to thyroid hormones are present, and what is their significance?

Autoantibodies are usually suspected when total T_3 or T_4 concentrations are high in a sample from a dog evaluated for hypothyroidism. With procedures used by most diagnostic laboratories, the presence of autoantibodies causes false elevations in the apparent concentration. Total T_3 is most often affected; however, autoantibodies to T_3 are present in less than 1% of samples submitted to our laboratory. The exact clinical and prognostic significance of autoantibodies to thyroid hormones is unknown (Kemppainen and Young, 1992). Presence of autoantibodies to T_4 or T_3 does not mean that a dog is hypothyroid. If autoantibodies are present, it is best to measure FT_4 by equilibrium dialysis and thyroid-stimulating hormone (TSH) to better evaluate thyroid function. If the FT_4 and TSH concentrations are normal, the patient should be scheduled for periodic (every 4 to 6 months) FT_4 determination. If the FT_4 level is low and TSH is elevated, hypothyroidism is likely.

How valuable is measurement of endogenous canine TSH?

In dogs with primary hypothyroidism, TSH concentrations are expected to be elevated because of the loss of negative feedback by thyroid hormones on the pituitary. Since about 95% of canine hypothyroidism is caused by primary thyroid failure (and not deficiency of pituitary TSH), measurement of TSH should be a useful test. Indeed, thyroidectomized dogs had TSH levels approximately 30 times greater than normal (Williams et al., 1996). Data obtained using the assay so far are somewhat discouraging, at least in terms of the test providing an unequivocal diagnosis of the disease. In one study of 62 normal dogs, 3 showed elevated TSH concentrations; and, although 7 of 16 spontaneously hypothyroid dogs had clearly elevated TSH levels, 3 had only marginal increases, and 6 had TSH concentrations within the normal range (Scott-Moncrieff et al., 1998).

Another concern was that 4 of 33 dogs with euthyroid sick syndrome had elevated TSH concentrations. Thus data so far suggest that concentrations of TSH are elevated in most but not all dogs with primary hypothyroidism and that approximately 10% of healthy dogs and dogs with euthyroid sick syndrome have TSH concentrations greater than currently established normal ranges. More commonly it appears that a significant number (approximately 25% to 30%) of hypothyroid dogs have normal TSH concentrations. A sole determination of endogenous TSH concentration should not be used to diagnose hypothyroidism. The test should be used to supplement historical data and clinical examination findings in conjunction with measurement of total or FT_4 concentrations or both. Interestingly, concentrations of TSH appear less affected, compared with total T_4, total T_3, and FT_4 concentrations, by nonthyroidal illness in dogs (Kantrowitz et al., 2001).

The total T_4 concentration in a dog suspected of having hypothyroidism is less than normal. How certain can I be that this dog is hypothyroid?

A low total T_4 means that the dog may be hypothyroid; alternatively a nonthyroidal factor could be depressing T_4, or this dog could simply have a lower than "normal" circulating total T_4 concentration (and be euthyroid). Some options available for evaluating these patients are summarized below:

- FT_4 (dialysis method) and TSH can be measured. These tests are more definitive than total T_4. This is the best option.
- Total T_4 can be retested in 6 to 8 weeks. If the dog is hypothyroid, the T_4 should continue to decline, and clinical signs should become more profound.
- Trial thyroid hormone replacement therapy can be attempted. The dog should be reevaluated after 5 and 10 weeks of T_4 therapy using objective criteria (e.g., regrowth of hair) to assess recovery. A postpill T_4 level should be evaluated after 5 weeks to ensure that therapeutic and not elevated blood levels of the hormone are present. Trial therapy is complicated by partial responders and the fact that T_4 may have a pharmacologic effect to induce hair growth in some euthyroid dogs. Incorrect diagnosis can consign the owner to providing lifelong therapy; thus the first two options are strongly recommended in preference to the third.

How do I test for hypothyroidism when a dog is on thyroid supplementation?

Trying to confirm a diagnosis of hypothyroidism after thyroid replacement therapy has been initiated can be difficult. Therapy should be withdrawn, and the pituitary-thyroid axis allowed to recover. A total T_4 or better FT_4 by equilibrium dialysis should be measured after 1 month. If the result is borderline, therapy should be withheld for an additional 4 weeks, and the measurement repeated to see if there is continuing recovery. The time needed to allow full recovery of thyroid gland function after chronic suppression by exogenous T_4 is unknown.

FELINE HYPERTHYROIDISM

Does the finding of a normal T_4 level in a cat rule out hyperthyroidism?

No. Cats with early or mild hyperthyroidism may have a T_4 concentration within the upper half of the normal range (i.e., 25 to 50 nmol/L). The T_4 level can fluctuate in and out of the normal range in such cats. Alternatively nonthyroidal factors (illness) can suppress the T_4 level in a hyperthyroid cat into the upper half of the reference range.

If the T_4 level is normal but I am still suspicious of hyperthyroidism, what can I do?

If the T_4 level is less than 25 nmol/L, it is unlikely that the cat is hyperthyroid. If the T_4 level is in the upper normal range (25 to 50 nmol/L), further evaluation is warranted. In sick, older cats with a normal thyroid function, low total T_4 concentrations are typically measured (Peterson and Gamble, 1990). Options to consider in hyperthyroid-suspect cats with T_4 values in the upper normal range follow:

- FT_4 should be measured by equilibrium dialysis (Peterson et al., 2001).
- The total T_4 measurement should be repeated; sometimes T_4 will fluctuate into and out of the normal range in hyperthyroid cats. Alternatively tests such as T_3 suppression or thyrotropin-releasing hormone stimulation can be used.

What is the value of measuring FT_4 in cats suspected of being hyperthyroid?

The rationale of using the FT_4 to diagnose hyperthyroidism in cats is the same as that for using this measurement in dogs—that the concentration of FT_4 is less affected by nonthyroidal factors. In this instance FT_4 should be high in hyperthyroidism. Its use seems most appropriate for cats with mild or early hyperthyroidism or in cats suspected of being hyperthyroid with nonthyroidal illness that have total T_4 concentrations in the upper normal range (see earlier). In one study FT_4 was elevated in 191 of 205 mildly hyperthyroid cats (93%) as compared with finding an elevated total T_4 in 125 of these cats (61%) (Peterson et al., 2001). However, FT_4 may also be elevated in up to 12% of sick, euthyroid cats (Mooney, Little, and Macrae, 1996). To help discriminate between hyperthyroidism and euthyroid sick syndrome in cats, a total T_4 should be measured along with the FT_4. Hyperthyroid cats tend to have total T_4 concentrations in the upper half of the normal range; whereas sick, euthyroid cats have total T_4 values in the lower half of the normal range, even if they show elevated FT_4 (Mooney et al., 1996).

The total T_4 concentration in a cat I was testing for hyperthyroidism came back less than normal. Is the cat hypothyroid?

It is unlikely. It is most likely that the cat has the euthyroid sick syndrome since hypothyroidism is rare in cats. Measurement of FT_4 will help differentiate hypothyroidism from the euthyroid sick syndrome.

References and Suggested Reading

Behrend EN et al: Intramuscular administration of low-dose ACTH for ACTH stimulation testing in dogs, *J Am Vet Med Assoc*, 229:528, 2006.

Ferguson DC, Peterson ME: Serum-free and total iodothyronine concentrations in dogs with spontaneous hyperadrenocorticism, *Am J Vet Res* 53:1636, 1992.

Graves TK, Peterson ME: Diagnostic tests for feline hyperthyroidism, *Vet Clin North Am Small Anim Pract* 24:567, 1994

Kantrowitz LB et al: Serum total thyroxine, total triiodothyronine, free thyroxine, and thyrotropin concentrations in epileptic dogs treated with anticonvulsants, *J Am Vet Med Assoc* 214:1804, 1999.

Kantrowitz LB et al: Serum total thyroxine, total triiodothyronine, free thyroxine, and thyrotropin concentrations in dogs with nonthyroidal disease, *J Am Vet Med Assoc* 219:765, 2001.

Kaplan AJ, Peterson ME, Kemppainen RJ: Effects of disease on the results of diagnostic tests for use in detecting hyperadrenocorticism in dogs, *J Am Vet Med Assoc* 207:445, 1995.

Kemppainen RJ, Clark TP: CVT update: sample collection and testing protocols in endocrinology. In Bonagura JD, Kirk RW, editors: *Kirk's current veterinary therapy XII: small animal practice*, Philadelphia, 1995, Saunders, p 335.

Kemppainen RJ, Young DW: Canine triiodothyronine autoantibodies. In Kirk RW, Bonagura JD, editors: *Current veterinary therapy XI: small animal practice*, Philadelphia, 1992, Saunders, p 327.

Kemppainen RJ, Zerbe CA: Common endocrine diagnostic tests: normal values and interpretation. In Kirk RW, Bonagura JD, editors: *Current veterinary therapy X: small animal practice*, Philadelphia, 1989, Saunders, p 961.

Kemppainen RJ, Behrend EN, Busch KA: Use of compounded adrenocorticotropic hormone (ACTH) for adrenal function testing in dogs, *J Am Anim Hosp Assoc* 41:368, 2005.

Kerl ME et al: Evaluation of a low-dose synthetic adrenocorticotropic hormone stimulation test in clinically normal dogs and dogs with naturally developing hyperadrenocorticism, *J Am Vet Med Assoc* 214:1497, 1999.

Kintzer PP, Peterson ME: Mitotane (o,p'-DDD) treatment of cortisol-secreting adrenocortical neoplasia. In Kirk RW, Bonagura JD, editors: *Current veterinary therapy X: small animal practice*, Philadelphia, 1989, Saunders, p 1034.

Mooney CT, Little CJL, Macrae AW: Effect of illness not associated with the thyroid gland on serum total and free thyroxine concentrations in cats, *J Am Vet Med Assoc* 208:2004, 1996.

Nelson RW et al: Serum free thyroxine concentration in healthy dogs, dogs with hypothyroidism, and euthyroid dogs with concurrent illness, *J Am Vet Med Assoc* 198:1401, 1991.

Peterson ME, Gamble DA: Effect of nonthyroidal illness on serum thyroxine concentrations in cats: 494 cases (1988), *J Am Vet Med Assoc* 197:1203, 1990.

Peterson ME, Melian C, Nichols R: Measurement of serum concentrations of free thyroxine, total thyroxine, and total triiodothyronine in cats with hyperthyroidism and cats with nonthyroidal disease, *J Am Vet Med Assoc* 218:529, 2001.

Scott-Moncrieff JC et al: Comparison of serum concentrations of thyroid-stimulating hormone in healthy dogs, hypothyroid dogs, and euthyroid dogs with concurrent disease, *J Am Vet Med Assoc* 212:387, 1998.

Williams DA et al: Validation of an immunoassay for canine thyroid-stimulating hormone and changes in serum concentration following induction of hypothyroidism, *J Am Vet Med Assoc* 209:1730, 1996.

CHAPTER 39

Medical Treatment of Feline Hyperthyroidism*

LAUREN A. TREPANIER, *Madison, Wisconsin*

Hyperthyroidism is the most common endocrine disorder in cats, affecting approximately 2% of all cats presenting to veterinary teaching hospitals. Management options include radioiodine therapy, thyroidectomy, or medical treatment with antithyroid drugs such as methimazole. Radioiodine is considered the treatment of choice for hyperthyroidism based on its high efficacy and relative lack of complications (Table 39-1) (see Chapter 40). However, there are some situations in which methimazole therapy may be preferred over radioiodine. Methimazole is useful before thyroidectomy to normalize serum thyroxine (T_4) concentrations and reduce the risk of tachyarrhythmias during anesthesia. Methimazole, which is reversible, is similarly indicated in cats with renal insufficiency, either for long-term therapy or as a "clinical test" to determine whether serum T_4 can be safely lowered without causing renal decompensation. Practical considerations such as lack of a convenient referral center with a radiation license, client fears about radiation or quarantine, or initial cost to the client may also drive the use of methimazole.

METHIMAZOLE ACTIONS, DOSING, AND EFFICACY

Methimazole blocks thyroid hormone synthesis by inhibiting thyroid peroxidase, the enzyme involved in the oxidation of iodide to iodine, incorporation of iodine into thyroglobulin, and coupling of tyrosine residues to form T_4 and triiodothyronine (T_3). Methimazole does not block the release of preformed thyroid hormone, which explains the delay of 2 to 4 weeks before serum T_4 concentrations fully normalize after beginning treatment in cats. Methimazole does not decrease goiter size; in fact, goiters may become larger over time despite therapy.

Typical starting doses of methimazole range from 1.25 to 2.5 mg per cat twice daily (Table 39-2). More frequent dosing (three times daily) is rarely necessary. Higher doses of 5 mg two to three times daily, used in original cases of cats with relatively high serum T_4 concentrations, are probably not needed for initial therapy of cats with mild-to-moderate hyperthyroidism and could potentially increase the risk of renal decompensation from a rapid fall in serum T_4. Starting dosages can be titrated upward if there is an inadequate initial response to lower doses of methimazole over 2 to 4 weeks. In cats that tolerate methimazole without side effects, efficacy is greater than 90%.

In humans methimazole has a long residence time in the thyroid gland and can exert antithyroid effects for 24 hours or more. Because of this, methimazole can be given once daily in humans with remission rates that are comparable to divided daily dosing. However, when our group studied 40 hyperthyroid cats we found that once-daily dosing (5 mg) was less effective than divided dosing (2.5 mg twice daily), with only 54% of cats achieving a euthyroid state after 2 weeks of once-daily treatment compared to 87% of cats treated with divided dosing (Trepanier et al., 2003). Therefore, unless clients are unable to dose more frequently than once daily, divided twice-daily dosing of methimazole is preferred to maximize efficacy. Dosing less frequently than once daily is unlikely to be effective because serum T_4 concentrations rise to pretreatment hyperthyroid values within 48 hours after discontinuing methimazole.

METHIMAZOLE SIDE EFFECTS

Blood Dyscrasias

Methimazole can lead to neutropenia and/or thrombocytopenia in 3% to 9% of treated cats. Cats with methimazole-induced blood dyscrasias usually recover within a week of drug discontinuation. Continuing methimazole in the face of thrombocytopenia has led to clinically significant hemorrhage, including epistaxis and oral bleeding. Rechallenge with methimazole in cats with neutropenia can lead to a recurrent severe neutropenia within 1 week. Although the mechanisms for these blood dyscrasias in cats have not been established, methimazole-induced neutropenia in humans is associated with an arrest of myeloid progenitors in the bone marrow. Treatment with granulocyte-macrophage colony-stimulating factor has been advocated in human patients, but does not appear to hasten recovery in most people.

Facial Excoriation

Approximately 2% to 3% of cats treated with methimazole develop excoriations of the face and neck, leading to characteristic scabbed lesions in front of the pinnae. Generalized erythema and pruritus may also occur. These excoriations are only partially responsive to glucocorticoids, and drug discontinuation is almost always required.

*Supported in part by grants from the Winn Feline Foundation and the University of Wisconsin-Madison Companion Animal Fund.

Table 39-1

Advantages and Disadvantages of Major Therapies for Feline Hyperthyroidism

Treatment	Advantages	Disadvantages
Radioiodine	>90% efficacy Single injection Few side effects (rare dysphagia) Curative	High initial expense Somewhat limited availability Irreversible
Thyroidectomy	≈90% efficacy Curative	High initial expense Anesthetic risks Risk of hypoparathyroidism Risk of recurrent laryngeal nerve damage Irreversible
Methimazole	Low initial expense ≈90% efficacy in cats that do not have side effects Reversible	Daily drug administration Drug side effects

Table 39-2

Drugs Useful in the Medical Management of Hyperthyroidism

Drug	Indications	Dosage	Side effects	Comments
Methimazole	Hyperthyroid cats with azotemia or for clients declining radioiodine	1.25-5 mg per cat twice daily (start at lower end)	GI upset Facial excoriation Blood dyscrasias Hepatopathy	Transdermal route has fewer GI side effects
Carbimazole	Prodrug of methimazole	2.5-5 mg per cat twice daily	GI upset Facial excoriation Blood dyscrasias Hepatopathy	Not recommended in cats intolerant of methimazole
Iopanoic acid or calcium ipodate	Adjunct control of T_3 in cats intolerant of methimazole	100-200 mg per day (empiric)		Inhibits conversion of T_4 to T_3 Effects may be transient
Propylthiouracil	Unclear if useful for cats intolerant of methimazole	25 mg per cat twice daily (empiric)	Hemolytic anemia Thrombocytopenia Bleeding diathesis	
Propranolol	Control of tachyarrhythmias or hyperactivity Adjunct control of T_3 in cats intolerant of full dosages of methimazole	2.5-5 mg per cat three times daily	Bronchoconstriction in cats with prior lower airway disease	Inhibits conversion of T_4 to T_3
Atenolol	Control of tachyarrhythmias or hyperactivity	3.125-6.25 mg per cat twice daily	Sinus bradycardia AV block in susceptible cats	Selective β_1- blocker
Enalapril or benazepril	Control of hypertension	0.5 mg/kg once or twice daily	Lethargy Inappetence	Potential effect of limiting glomerulosclerosis in cats with renal disease Benazepril does not accumulate in renal failure
Amlodipine	Control of moderate-to-severe hypertension	0.625 mg per cat once daily	Lethargy Inappetence	Drug of choice for severe hypertension

GI, Gastrointestinal; T_3, triiodothyronine; T_4, thyroxine.

Pruritus has also been reported in human patients treated with methimazole, but the mechanisms for these reactions have not been explored.

Hepatotoxicity

Increases in serum alkaline phosphatase (SAP) and bilirubin, or alanine aminotransferase (ALT), are observed in approximately 2% of cats treated with methimazole (Peterson, Kintzer, and Hurvitz, 1988); liver biopsy may show hepatic necrosis and degeneration. Liver enzyme elevations are usually reversible over several weeks following drug discontinuation, although nutritional and fluid support may be required. Rechallenge can lead to recurrent hepatopathy, and future drug avoidance is generally recommended. In rodent models methimazole hepatotoxicity is exacerbated by glutathione depletion (Mizutani et al., 1999). The role of glutathione depletion, or supplementation, in methimazole-associated hepatotoxicity in cats has not been evaluated.

Simple Gastrointestinal Upset

Anorexia, vomiting, and lethargy are seen in approximately 10% of cats treated with methimazole. Simple gastrointestinal (GI) upset is most common in the first 4 weeks of treatment and can resolve with a dosage reduction. These signs may be caused in part by direct gastric irritation from the drug, since transdermal administration of methimazole is associated with significantly fewer GI side effects than the oral route (Sartor et al., 2004).

Renal Decompensation

Cats with hyperthyroidism have abnormally high glomerular filtration rates (GFRs), and treating hyperthyroidism by any method leads to decreases in GFR in most hyperthyroid cats. New onset azotemia is observed in 15% to 20% of hyperthyroid cats after normalization of serum T_4. Although these biochemical changes are generally clinically silent, occasional cats develop signs of illness referable to underlying renal disease. Because methimazole treatment is reversible, it is the preferred approach for initial treatment of hyperthyroid cats with preexisting azotemia to determine whether normalization of serum T_4 will lead to unacceptable renal decompensation.

Coagulation Abnormalities

Methimazole and to a lesser extent propylthiouracil (PTU) inhibit vitamin K–dependent clotting factor activation (γ-carboxylation) and epoxide reductase (necessary for vitamin K recycling, and the same enzyme targeted by warfarin) at high concentrations. In a study of 20 hyperthyroid cats treated with methimazole, there were no significant changes in prothrombin time or activated partial thromboplastin time, but one cat developed a prolonged protein-induced by vitamin K antagonism (PIVKA) clotting time (Randolph et al., 2000). No cats had clinically significant bleeding. This suggests a possible but apparently uncommon "warfarin-like" effect of methimazole in cats. This reaction is rare enough not to warrant routine monitoring but should be considered in any cat presenting with hemorrhage that is also being treated with methimazole.

Acquired Myasthenia Gravis

Another apparently rare side effect of methimazole in cats is the development of acquired myasthenia gravis. Neuromuscular weakness, along with antibodies to the acetylcholine receptor, has rarely been reported in cats treated with methimazole. Cats have responded to either drug discontinuation or the addition of prednisone to the methimazole treatment regimen. Although this does not appear to be a side effect of methimazole in humans, hyperthyroidism itself can copresent with myasthenia in humans; in one human patient methimazole therapy was thought to worsen the clinical signs of myasthenia.

CLINICAL MONITORING

Based on the spectrum of possible adverse reactions to methimazole, clinical monitoring at 2 to 3 and 4 to 6 weeks of treatment should include a complete blood count, ALT and SAP, and blood urea nitrogen and creatinine, in addition to serum T_4. In a cat with an apparent adverse reaction to methimazole, it is important to differentiate simple GI upset (for which a lower dose or a switch to transdermal methimazole may be curative) from blood dyscrasias or hepatopathy, for which methimazole should be discontinued. Therefore this same workup should also be performed if a cat becomes clinically ill during methimazole treatment.

It is also important to measure renal function and T_4 simultaneously during methimazole therapy to determine whether a cat's kidneys can tolerate the level of GFR associated with normal thyroid function. If a cat becomes newly azotemic with clinical signs, the dosage of methimazole can be titrated to maintain the serum T_4 in the high high-normal range, with additional use of drugs to control hypertension and tachyarrhythmias (see Management of Hypertension).

TRANSDERMAL METHIMAZOLE

Methimazole is available through custom compounding pharmacies in a transdermal formulation in pluronic lecithin organogel (PLO). PLO acts as a permeation enhancer to allow drug absorption across the stratum corneum. Although methimazole in PLO has been shown to have poor absorption in cats after a single dose, chronic dosing in hyperthyroid cats is effective in lowering serum T_4 concentrations. Methimazole in PLO is applied to the cat's inner pinna, alternating ears with each dose. Owners wear examination gloves or finger cots during administration and are instructed to remove crusted material with a moistened cotton ball before the next dose.

Transdermal methimazole had significantly fewer GI side effects (4% of cats) compared to oral methimazole (Sartor et al., 2004). When our group compared these methods, there were no differences between routes in the incidence of facial excoriation, neutropenia, thrombocytopenia, or hepatotoxicity. However, transdermal methimazole was associated with somewhat lower efficacy by 4 weeks (only 67% euthyroid) compared to oral methimazole (82% euthyroid). This may be due to the result of lower bioavailability of the transdermal formulation. Drawbacks of methimazole in PLO include erythema at the dosing site in some cats, increased formulation costs, and unproven drug stability beyond 2 weeks. However, methimazole in PLO appears to be effective (anecdotally) beyond 2 weeks. I recommend that serum T_4 values be checked toward the end of a 2-month prescription of the transdermal formulation to confirm that thyroid control persists.

ADMINISTRATION OF METHIMAZOLE BEFORE PERTECHNETATE SCANNING OR RADIOIODINE THERAPY

Because methimazole does not inhibit iodide uptake by the thyroid, concurrent methimazole therapy does not impair technetium 99m (^{99m}TC)–pertechnetate thyroid scanning in hyperthyroid cats and in fact may enhance imaging (Fischetti et al., 2005, Nieckarz and Daniel, 2001). However, methimazole does inhibit iodine organification, which may decrease the contact time of radioiodine within the thyroid. Humans given methimazole up to 4 days before radioiodine show no differences in outcome, but administration of methimazole immediately before or after radioiodine has been associated with poorer responses. In hyperthyroid cats retrospective studies have found no association between the time of methimazole discontinuation before radioiodine and long-term radioiodine efficacy (Chun et al., 2002, Forrest et al., 1996). However, without data from a prospective randomized study, discontinuation of methimazole before radioiodine therapy is still recommended. The 1- to 2-week washout period for methimazole recommended by many radioiodine facilities may be longer than necessary but is based on efficacy data from the largest case series published (Peterson and Becker, 1995).

MANAGEMENT OF HYPERTENSION

The prevalence of hypertension in hyperthyroid cats is reported to be 5% to 22%, and many cats with hypertension have concurrent azotemia. Normalizing serum T_4 may not significantly control blood pressure in the first weeks of therapy. Therefore direct management of moderate-to-severe hypertension is indicated along with antithyroid treatment. Commonly used antihypertensive agents include amlodipine, β-blockers, and the angiotensin-converting enzyme (ACE) inhibitors. There is one small clinical trial that has demonstrated a relatively poor response to atenolol in cats in terms of achieving blood pressure control. In cases of moderate to severe hypertension, or when hypertension is associated with target organ injury, amlodipine (starting dose of 0.625 mg PO per cat once or twice daily) is most likely to lower blood pressure effectively. β-blockers such as atenolol are useful if signs of hyperactivity or tachyarrhythmias are present (see Table 39-2). ACE inhibitors such as enalapril or benazepril (0.5 mg/kg once daily) have the potential benefit of reducing intraglomerular pressure in patients with renal disease. However, ACE inhibitors are inferior to amlodipine in control of moderate to severe hypertension.

In those cats in which renoprotective effects of an ACE inhibitor are desired, combination therapy with an ACE inhibitor should be considered (see Chapter 197). In cats with overt azotemia, benazepril, which does not accumulate in renal insufficiency, is preferred by the author over enalapril. In some hyperthyroid cats without initial hypertension, hypertension can actually develop several months after treatment for hyperthyroidism, possibly as a result of unmasking of underlying renal insufficiency. Therefore rechecking cats for hypertension 2 to 3 months after restoration of a euthyroid state is indicated.

OTHER ANTITHYROID DRUG OPTIONS

Propylthiouracil

PTU was the first drug used in the management of hyperthyroid cats in the early 1980s. This drug required high dosages (e.g., 50 mg two to three times daily) to normalize serum T_4 concentrations. PTU was associated with an unacceptably high incidence of adverse events, including positive ANA, Coombs'-positive hemolytic anemia, and thrombocytopenia with bleeding diathesis. Methimazole and PTU share structural similarities; and patients with blood dyscrasias, hepatopathy, or facial excoriation during methimazole treatment may well have similar adverse reactions to PTU. However, the degree of cross-reactivity has not been critically examined in cats.

Carbimazole

Carbimazole is a substituted derivative of methimazole that is a prodrug of methimazole. Carbimazole is used in the United Kingdom for treating cats with hyperthyroidism, and there are anecdotal reports that side effects are less common with carbimazole than with methimazole. This may be related to the fact that plasma methimazole concentrations are approximately 50% lower with carbimazole compared to an identical dose of methimazole. There are no definitive studies comparing the side effect rates of methimazole to carbimazole; and, because carbimazole is converted into methimazole, its use in cats with adverse reactions to methimazole is probably ill advised.

β-Blockers

β-Blockers can reduce the "sympathetic overdrive" characteristic of hyperthyroidism, including tachycardia, arrhythmias, hyperactivity, and aggression. Propranolol has the additional potential benefit of inhibiting the conversion of T_4 to T_3 (see Table 39-2) and may be useful for the short-term management of cats intolerant of methimazole before radioiodine or thyroidectomy. However, as a nonselective β-blocker propranolol can lead to bronchospasm in susceptible cats, and may require three-times daily dosing. Atenolol, a selective β_1-blocker, is not associated with bronchospasm and is preferred for β_1-blockade in cats with a prior history of reactive airway disease. Because neither of these treatments normalizes serum T_4 or prevents weight loss, these drugs alone are not appropriate for long-term management of hyperthyroidism. It should be noted that some cats develop a relatively slow sinus rhythm or even sinus bradycardia after a euthyroid state is achieved, and the dosage of the beta blocker may need to be reduced or the drug discontinued. Some old cats also have atrioventricular conduction disease as a comorbid condition (likely from conduction system degeneration), and beta blockers can result in AV block in susceptible cats. Since atenolol is water soluble and therefore eliminated by renal mechanisms, both heart rate and daily dosage should be reevaluated in cats that develop renal failure following a reduction of serum T_4.

Iodinated Contrast Agents

Iodinated contrast agents such as ipodate and iopanoic acid inhibit conversion of T_4 to T_3 and have been advocated for use in hyperthyroid cats that do not tolerate methimazole (Murray and Peterson, 1997). Ipodate (Oragrafin; 308 mg of iodine per 500 mg of calcium ipodate) is no longer marketed, but iopanoic acid (Telepaque; 333 mg of iodine per 500 mg of iopanoic acid) and diatrizoate meglumine (Gastrografin; 370 mg of iodine per milliliter) have been used anecdotally in hyperthyroid cats at comparable doses. Cats may respond initially with decreases in serum T_3 and clinical improvement. However, long-term control is likely to be poor since the effects of these agents are often transient. All iodine-containing agents interfere with thyroid scanning and radioiodine therapy. In humans iopanoic acid must be discontinued 2 weeks before radioiodine therapy, with most patients having a normalized thyroid scan and response to radioiodine by then. Similar data are not available for cats.

References and Suggested Reading

Becker T et al: Effects of methimazole on renal function in cats with hyperthyroidism, *J Am Anim Hosp Assoc* 36:215, 2000.

Chun R et al: Predictors of response to radioiodine therapy in hyperthyroid cats, *Vet Radiol Ultrasound* 43:587, 2002.

Fischetti AJ et al: Effects of methimazole on thyroid gland uptake of 99mTC-pertechnetate in 19 hyperthyroid cats, *Vet Radiol Ultrasound* 46:267, 2005.

Forrest L et al: Feline hyperthyroidism: efficacy of treatment using volumetric analysis for radioiodine dose calculation, *Vet Radiol Ultrasound* 37:141, 1996.

Hoffmann G et al: Transdermal methimazole treatment in cats with hyperthyroidism, *J Feline Med Surg* 5:77, 2003.

Mizutani T et al: Metabolism-dependent hepatotoxicity of methimazole in mice depleted of glutathione, *J Appl Toxicol* 19:193, 1999.

Murray LA, Peterson ME: Ipodate treatment of hyperthyroidism in cats, *J Am Vet Med Assoc* 211:63, 1997.

Nieckarz JA, Daniel GB: The effect of methimazole on thyroid uptake of pertechnetate and radioiodine in normal cats, *Vet Radiol Ultrasound* 42:448, 2001.

Peterson ME, Becker DV: Radioiodine treatment of 524 cats with hyperthyroidism, *J Am Vet Med Assoc* 207:1422, 1995.

Peterson ME, Kintzer PP, Hurvitz AI: Methimazole treatment of 262 cats with hyperthyroidism, *J Vet Intern Med* 2:150, 1988.

Randolph JF et al: Prothrombin, activated partial thromboplastin, and proteins induced by vitamin K absence or antagonists' clotting times in 20 hyperthyroid cats before and after methimazole treatment, *J Vet Intern Med* 14:56, 2000.

Sartor LL et al: Efficacy and safety of transdermal methimazole in the treatment of cats with hyperthyroidism, *J Vet Intern Med* 18:651, 2004.

Trepanier LA et al: Efficacy and safety of once versus twice daily administration of methimazole in cats with hyperthyroidism, *J Am Vet Med Assoc* 222:954, 2003.

CHAPTER 40

Radioiodine for Feline Hyperthyroidism

MARK E. PETERSON, *Bedford Hills, New York*

Hyperthyroidism is the most common endocrine disorder in cats, most frequently associated with adenomatous hyperplasia (or adenoma) involving one or both thyroid lobes. Because the pathogenesis of hyperthyroidism in cats is not known, treatment of the condition is directed at controlling the excessive secretion of thyroid hormone from the adenomatous thyroid gland. Treatment options include administration of antithyroid drugs (see Chapter 39), surgical removal of adenomatous thyroid tissue, and administration of radioiodine. Although each of these treatment options has its advantages and disadvantages, the use of radioiodine is considered by most authorities to be the treatment of choice for most hyperthyroid cats.

Radioactive iodine provides a simple, effective, and safe treatment for cats with hyperthyroidism. It is a particularly useful treatment for cats with bilateral thyroid involvement (found in approximately 70% of cats), cats with ectopic (intrathoracic) thyroid tissue, and the rare feline patient with thyroid carcinoma. Treatment with radioiodine avoids the inconvenience of daily oral administration and side effects associated with antithyroid drugs, as well as the risks and postoperative complications associated with anesthesia and surgical thyroidectomy. Although the therapy is simple and relatively stress free for cats, it does require special licensing and hospitalization facilities, nuclear medicine equipment, and extensive compliance with local and state radiation safety laws. The purpose of this chapter is to give an overview of aspects of radioiodine treatment germane to the practicing veterinarian who is referring hyperthyroid cats for this treatment.

ADVANTAGES OF RADIOIODINE FOR TREATMENT OF HYPERTHYROIDISM

Medical treatment with methimazole is effective in controlling hyperthyroidism in most cats, but for several reasons it may not be the best choice. First, some cats are difficult or impossible to medicate (antithyroid drugs must be administered orally or transdermally, generally one to three times daily). Second, mild reactions (e.g., loss of appetite, vomiting) are common, and a few cats develop serious untoward reactions to the antithyroid drugs (e.g., thrombocytopenia, leukopenia, hepatopathy). Because of the potential for these side effects, periodic blood tests (including complete blood and platelet counts) are necessary to monitor the cat's condition (see Chapter 39). Finally, some owners may not want to have to medicate

their cat on a daily basis for the rest of the cat's life, especially if the cat is only middle-aged.

Surgery is an effective treatment for hyperthyroidism in most cats but may have disadvantages. Many cats with hyperthyroidism have secondary cardiomyopathy and are higher surgical and anesthetic risks; therefore preoperative preparation of hyperthyroid cats with antithyroid drugs or β–adrenergic blocking agent (or concurrent administration of both drugs) is generally recommended. There is also a risk that there will be damage to the adjacent parathyroid glands during thyroid surgery, resulting in transient or, less commonly, permanent hypoparathyroidism and hypocalcemia. This complication can be life threatening and results in extra hospitalization and cost. After surgery cats may occasionally develop hypothyroidism (usually transient), necessitating treatment with thyroid hormone replacement. Finally, there is always the potential that the hyperthyroidism will not be cured with surgical treatment or that the condition will recur a few months to years after successful thyroidectomy. The prevalence that hyperthyroidism will persist or recur is higher among cats that have only one thyroid lobe removed at time of surgery because most cats have adenomatous hyperplasia involving both thyroid lobes. In addition, there is always a chance that one or both of the cat's adenomatous thyroid lobes has descended ventrally below the thoracic inlet or that the cat has hyperfunctional thyroid tissue at ectopic sites. In either case such intrathoracic or ectopic thyroid tissue may be difficult to resect surgically.

Radioiodine therapy has some distinct advantages over use of medical or surgical treatment. Overall, radioiodine provides a simple, effective, and safe treatment for cats with hyperthyroidism. With radioiodine the need for anesthesia and the risk of hypoparathyroidism (the major disadvantages with surgery) are eliminated. Antithyroid drug treatment is not needed; in fact, many treatment centers recommend that drug treatment must be discontinued for a short time (usually 1 to 2 weeks) *before* radioiodine is administered to the cats because lower doses of radioiodine may be needed. The administered radioactive iodine concentrates in and destroys hyperactive thyroid tissue within the cat's body, whether in the normal cervical area or in ectopic sites.

DISADVANTAGES OF RADIOIODINE TREATMENT

As with other major forms of treatment, there are a few disadvantages to the use of radioiodine in cats with hyperthyroidism. This treatment is not universally available and requires complete knowledge of radiation safety and the use of expensive and sophisticated equipment. The major drawback is that, after administration of radioiodine, the cat must be kept hospitalized for a specified period (7 to 10 days in most treatment centers) and visitation is not allowed. Because of the relatively long isolation period away from the owner, some cats do become depressed; however, it is much more common for the owners to complain of their emotional distress. Most cats tend to do well during the boarding period.

As with any therapy, radioiodine treatment is not perfect. A few cats (< 5%) may not respond adequately to a single treatment, thus requiring retreatment at a later time. Although the reason for such initial treatment failures is not always clear, most of these cats respond well to the second treatment with resolution of their hyperthyroidism.

MECHANISM OF ACTION OF RADIOIODINE TREATMENT

Thyroid hormones are the only iodinated organic compounds in the body. Therefore the only function of ingested iodine is for thyroid hormone synthesis. Ingested stable iodine (^{127}I) is converted to iodide in the gastrointestinal tract and absorbed into the circulation. In the thyroid gland iodide is concentrated or trapped by active transport mechanisms of the thyroid follicular cell, resulting in intracellular iodide concentrations that are 10 to 200 times that of serum. Once inside the thyroid cell, iodide is oxidized to iodine, which is incorporated into tyrosine residues of thyroglobulin (organification) to form the thyroid hormones thyroxine (T_4) and 3,5,3′ triiodothyronine.

The radioisotope used to treat hyperthyroidism is radioiodine-131 (^{131}I). The basic principle behind treatment of hyperthyroidism with ^{131}I is that thyroid cells do not differentiate between stable and radioactive iodine; therefore radioiodine, like stable iodine, is concentrated by the thyroid gland after administration. In cats with hyperthyroidism, radioiodine is concentrated primarily in the hyperplastic or neoplastic thyroid cells, where it irradiates and destroys the hyperfunctioning tissue. Normal thyroid tissue tends to be protected from the effects of radioiodine since the uninvolved thyroid tissue is suppressed and receives only a small dose of radiation (unless very large doses are administered).

When administered to a cat with hyperthyroidism, a large percentage of radioiodine accumulates in the thyroid gland (i.e., most cats extract between 20% to 60% of the administered radioiodine dose from the circulation). The remainder of the administered ^{131}I is excreted primarily in the urine and to a lesser degree the feces. ^{131}-I has a half-life of 8 days and emits both β-particles and γ-radiation. The β-particles, which cause 80% of the tissue damage, travel a maximum of 2 mm in tissue and have an average path length of 400 μm. Therefore β-particles are locally destructive but spare adjacent hypoplastic thyroid tissue, parathyroid glands, and other cervical structures.

PATIENT SELECTION AND PREPARATION BEFORE RADIOIODINE TREATMENT

Routine diagnostic testing generally should be performed by the referring veterinarian before referral for radioiodine treatment to determine if the cat is an appropriate candidate for this treatment. This is very important, inasmuch as these cats tend to be middle- to old-aged and therefore may have other geriatric problems unrelated to the cat's hyperthyroidism. Cats should be relatively stable before being considered for radioiodine therapy. Cats that have clinically significant cardiovascular, renal, gastrointestinal, endocrine (e.g., diabetes), or neurologic disease may not be very good candidates for this treatment, especially because of the length of boarding required after the ^{131}I treatment is administered.

The recommended pretreatment workup generally should include the following tests:

- Routine database, including a complete blood count, serum chemistry panel, and urinalysis
- Pretreatment or untreated serum total T_4 concentration (not on antithyroid drug treatment); if the cat has been treated antithyroid for longer than 1 to 2 months, the antithyroid medication might have be discontinued for 5 to 7 days, and another serum total T_4 determined to determine the true severity of the cat's hyperthyroidism
- Chest radiography or cardiac ultrasonography or both should be performed if cat has evidence of any clinically significant cardiac disease (especially pronounced heart murmur, arrhythmia, dyspnea, or jugular venous distension)

Determination of a pretreatment free T_4 concentration alone (without a total T_4 concentration) is generally not acceptable for referral for radioiodine treatment. It is clear that determination of free T_4 concentrations can be very useful in diagnosis of hyperthyroidism, especially in cats in which the disease is suspected but the total T_4 concentration remains within normal range. However, because a high free T_4 concentration also develops in some sick cats that do not have hyperthyroidism and certainly would not benefit from radioiodine treatment, the diagnosis of hyperthyroidism should never be based solely on the finding of a high free T_4 concentration alone. When a free T_4 determination is performed as a diagnostic test for hyperthyroidism, it must always be performed together with a total T_4 concentration.

If concurrent renal disease is suspected or known to be present, many recommend evaluating medical management before a more definitive means of treatment such as radioiodine. In these cats a low starting dose (i.e., 1.25 mg orally once daily) of methimazole with gradual dosage escalation is prudent, with monitoring (e.g., biochemical profile and total serum T_4 determination) and dose adjustments done every 2 weeks. Based on studies regarding changes in glomerular filtration rate (GFR) associated with treatment of hyperthyroidism, it appears that maintenance of euthyroidism for 1 month without azotemia should be sufficient to decide whether to proceed with definitive therapy. Once a cat has stabilized, radioactive iodine could be considered.

The veterinarian may choose to stabilize some cats for a few weeks or months before time of referral for radioiodine treatment by administering cardiovascular medications, β-blocking agents, or antithyroid drugs (see Chapter 39). Although concurrent administration of β–blocking agents does not interfere with radioiodine treatment, one should realize that prior or concurrent antithyroid drug treatment may influence the effectiveness of the radioiodine treatment, resulting in treatment failure. The effect of prior methimazole treatment on eventual outcome of radioactive iodine therapy in cats is controversial, however; and it has been variably suggested to worsen, enhance, or have no effect on radioiodine treatment. The thyroidal uptake of radioiodine is enhanced in healthy cats after recent methimazole withdrawal, and this short-term rebound effect may be potentially beneficial when treating hyperthyroidism in cats with radioactive iodine. Some have theorized that this enhanced thyroidal uptake of radioiodine therapy may lead to a higher incidence of radioiodine-induced hypothyroidism. However, other studies have shown that discontinuing methimazole for less than or greater than 5 days before radioactive iodine therapy has no effect on treatment outcome.

Overall, if antithyroid drugs have been administered, most treatment centers recommend that they be discontinued for at least 1 week before treatment with radioiodine. In some cats with severe, life-threatening hyperthyroidism or concurrent disease (e.g., renal failure), one may decide that is not wise to stop antithyroid drug treatment but to treat with antithyroidal drugs while the cat is still receiving the radioiodine administration. Such cases must be discussed with the radioiodine treatment center before the referral.

ESTIMATION OF THE RADIOIODINE DOSE TO ADMINISTER

Ideally administration of radioiodine restores euthyroidism with a *single* dose without inducing hypothyroidism. Numerous methods to calculate the administered radioiodine dose to cats with hyperthyroidism have been described, but the optimal method for determining the amount of radioactivity required for effective treatment in cats remains somewhat controversial. The reported methods used to calculate the radioiodine dose are quite variable but can be divided into three different methodologies.

The first method of determining the proper dose is to use tracer kinetic studies to estimate the percentage of iodine uptake and rate of disappearance from the gland and thyroid imaging to estimate the weight of the gland; the dose of radioiodine is then calculated from these measurements. Although this method of dose determination theoretically should produce the best results, measurement of the biologic half-life of iodine in hyperthyroid cats using tracer techniques has been shown to be a poor predictor of the biologic half-life of iodine following radioiodine therapy. Presumably this discrepancy originates with the changes in thyroid physiology that develop following the delivery of large doses of radiation to the thyroid gland. As a result, there can be a marked difference between the calculated dose of radioiodine and the actual dose delivered to the cat's thyroid tissue. Because of this poor correlation, most centers that treat hyperthyroid cats with radioiodine no longer calculate the cats' radioiodine doses based on measurements of the biologic half-life and uptake of iodine.

A second method of treating hyperthyroid cats is to administer a fixed, relatively high dose of radioiodine to all cats (i.e., 4 mCi or 5 mCi), regardless of the severity of hyperthyroidism or size of the thyroid tumor. To accomplish a reasonable success rate, the fixed dose method uses a radioiodine dose (4 to 5 mCi) that is above the median dose reported (3 mCi) for individualized dosing methods. As a result, a large number of cats treated using this method receive excessive amounts of radioiodine exposing both the patient and veterinary personnel to unnecessary levels of radiation. Although this method is the simplest, use of this approach results in undertreatment of a few cats with severe disease but more commonly overtreatment of a number of cats with mild disease.

In the third method of dose determination the dose of radioiodine administered to hyperthyroid cats is determined on the basis of a scoring system that takes into consideration the severity of clinical signs, the size of the cat's thyroid gland (based on either physical palpation or results of thyroid imaging, and the serum T_4 concentration. Using this scoring system, a low, medium, or relatively high ^{131}I dose is selected without determining thyroid gland kinetics. For example, cats with mild clinical signs, small thyroid tumors, and only slightly high serum T_4 concentrations would receive smaller doses of radioiodine (e.g., 3 mCi); cats with severe clinical signs, very large thyroid tumors, and markedly high serum T_4 concentrations would receive high doses of radioiodine (i.e., 5-6 mCi); and cats that lie between these extremes would receive intermediate doses of radioiodine (e.g., 4 mCi). This approach has been shown to provide treatment results comparable to those obtained when thyroid kinetics were determined (i.e., the first method of dose determination). The major advantage of this method is that nuclear medicine equipment is not needed, the time required to determine thyroid kinetics is eliminated, and sedation of the cat is not required. In addition, in contrast to the fixed dose method, the total radiation dosage delivered to the cats with mild hyperthyroidism was minimized since lower doses are given to these cats.

Radioiodine can be administered to cats intravenously or orally, but the subcutaneous route is preferred. The subcutaneous route has been shown to be equally as effective as the other routes of administration, not associated with gastrointestinal side effects, and safer for personnel, In addition, the dose can usually be administered with no or only light sedation, thereby avoiding anesthesia.

In cats with thyroid carcinoma (incidence <2.5% of all hyperthyroid cats), radioiodine offers the best chance for successful cure of the tumor because it concentrates in all hyperactive thyroid cells (i.e., carcinomatous tissue, as well as metastasis). However, thyroid carcinomas concentrate and retain iodine less efficiently than thyroid adenomas (adenomatous hyperplasia), and the size of carcinomas is usually much larger; therefore extremely high doses of radioiodine (10 to 30 mCi) are almost always needed for destruction of all malignant tissue. The combination of surgical debulking followed by administration of high-dose radioactive iodine also has been reported to be successful in cats with thyroid carcinoma. Longer periods of hospitalization are required with use of such high-dose radioiodine administration because of the prolonged radioiodine excretion.

RADIATION SAFETY PRECAUTIONS DURING THE HOSPITALIZATION PERIOD

Regardless of the method of dose determination selected, certain radiation safety restrictions and procedures must be followed after the radioiodine dose has been administered. The cats must be confined to a restricted and shielded area of the hospital (e.g., nuclear medicine isolation ward) that has minimal traffic. Also, the cats should be housed in appropriate cages so that urine and feces can be collected safely.

Personnel are restricted in the ward housing the cats, and only those properly trained in radiation safety and closely monitored are allowed into the ward. All personnel handling the cats, cages, food dishes, and excreta are required to wear protective clothing (e.g., long laboratory coats), disposable plastic gloves, and dosimeter monitors (film badges). All material removed from the cage must be handled as radioactive waste and stored until disposed of accordingly.

If the cat becomes ill during the quarantine period (a very rare occurrence when cats are selected carefully), it should be remembered that contact of veterinary personnel with the cat also should be limited, and special arrangements may be required for hospitalization. Clinical laboratories may decline to accept samples from patients during the quarantine period.

The cats are discharged from the hospital when the radiation dose rate has decreased to a safe level that has been determined by the radiation control office. Cats are hospitalized to protect people from radiation exposure, not because the cats require medical care. The hospitalization period varies from cat to cat and usually is approximately 7 to 10 days in most treatment centers for cats treated with typical radioiodine dosages. Cats treated with higher dosages (e.g., for functional thyroid carcinoma) may require longer hospitalization periods.

RADIATION SAFETY PRECAUTIONS AFTER DISCHARGE FROM THE HOSPITAL

On discharge the cats still excrete a small amount of radioiodine in their urine and feces. The remaining radioactivity is eliminated gradually from the cat over the next 2 to 4 weeks through radioactive decay and excretion into the urine and feces. However, until this is complete, the cat continues to emit low levels of radiation.

Owners must obey some safety precautions after their cat is discharged following ^{131}I treatment. These precautions are dictated by federal, state, and local laws and are designed to protect humans from excessive radiation exposure. These laws usually require keeping the cat strictly indoors for a period of time after treatment (e.g., 2 weeks), spell out the amount of contact time each person should have with the cat daily during this period

(10 to 20 minutes per person), and dictate how the owner should dispose of or store the cat's waste. Contact with children and pregnant woman during the first 2 weeks is usually prohibited.

In general, if the owner cannot avoid close, prolonged contact with the cat, it is generally recommended that the cat be boarded during this period. Additional information concerning handling of the cat on release to the owners and related radiation safety issues should be discussed with the veterinarian in charge of the radioiodine therapy.

ADVERSE EFFECTS/COMPLICATIONS ASSOCIATED WITH RADIOIODINE TREATMENT

Overall, side effects associated with radioiodine treatment of cats are extremely rare. Because radioiodine is relatively specific in its site of action, there is no hair loss or increase in skin pigmentation, as may be seen with external radiation therapy (cobalt radiation). In rare instances cats develop transient dysphagia (i.e., difficult swallowing) and fever during the first few days after treatment (probably as a result of radiation thyroiditis), but this condition is self-limited and resolves spontaneously. Rarely, they can develop a voice change after treatment, which may be permanent in some cases. A more serious problem directly caused by radioiodine treatment in cats is permanent hypothyroidism (see following paragraphs), which develops a few months after treatment with radioiodine in a small percentage of cats.

Most consider the development or worsening of renal disease to be the most serious complication of radioiodine treatment. However, if renal disease does develop, it is not caused by the radioiodine itself but rather because, by correcting the hyperthyroid state, the GFR and renal blood flow fall as the cat's cardiovascular status returns to normal. One must remember that hyperthyroidism itself may contribute to the development of renal disease in cats. Systemic hypertension, relatively common in cats with hyperthyroidism, can lead to an increase in glomerular capillary pressure and proteinuria, which may contribute to glomerular sclerosis and progression of renal disease.

In some cats untreated hyperthyroidism can mask preexisting, "hidden" renal disease by increasing the blood flow to the kidneys, which may become clinically apparent *only* after return of normal thyroid function. High renal blood flow associated with the hyperdynamic circulation that accompanies untreated hyperthyroidism may be beneficial in maintaining sustainable renal function, as well as in delaying the clinical and biochemical consequences of severe renal failure in some cats with chronic renal failure.

This development of azotemia occurs independently of treatment modality (i.e., it occurs with methimazole, surgical thyroidectomy, or radioiodine). Although the exact incidence of such deterioration in renal function is still under investigation, it is my estimate that some worsening in serum urea nitrogen or creatinine concentrations occurs in about 25% of treated cats. Such azotemia typically develops within 30 days after treatment of hyperthyroidism, but the azotemia tends to remain stable in most cats.

Other than the possible association between treatment of hyperthyroidism and the acute development of overt T_4 renal disease in a few cats, the long-term risk associated with administration of radioiodine to cats appears to be minimal. Therapeutic doses of radioiodine irradiate not only the thyroid gland but the whole body to some degree; this raises concerns about possible long-term effects such as carcinogenesis, genetic damage, and fetal damage. However, a number of recent studies of large populations of humans treated with radioiodine have failed to demonstrate increased risk of death from thyroid cancer, leukemia, or cancer in general. Likewise, increased risk of genetic abnormality in offspring of humans administered radioiodine has not been identified. Obviously this is less of a concern in cats with hyperthyroidism because most are usually neutered before hyperthyroidism develops.

FOLLOW-UP THYROID FUNCTION TESTING AFTER RADIOACTIVE IODINE TREATMENT

The ideal goal of ^{131}I therapy is to restore euthyroidism with a single dose of radiation without producing hypothyroidism. Indeed, most hyperthyroid cats treated with radioactive iodine are cured by a single dose. Thyroid hormone concentrations in the blood are normal within 2 weeks of therapy in approximately 85% of cats and in 95% of cats by 3 months. Although cats appear to feel better within days after treatment, the owner will notice gradual clinical improvement and resolution of the signs of hyperthyroidism over a 1- or 3-month period.

Approximately 5% of cats fail to respond completely and remain hyperthyroid after treatment with radioiodine. In studies from our institution, most cats with persistent hyperthyroidism had large thyroid tumors, severe hyperthyroidism, and very high serum T_4 concentrations. One explanation for persistent hyperthyroidism in these cats with large tumors and severe hyperthyroidism is that a greater number of adenomatous cells must be destroyed compared to cats with small tumors and mild disease. If these cats are not retreated, their signs of hyperthyroidism usually return a few months later. Therefore, if the hyperthyroid state persists for longer than 3 months after initial treatment, the referring veterinarian should discuss the possibility of again treating the cat with radioiodine with the veterinarian in charge of the radioiodine facility. In such cats retreatment is generally recommended because virtually all cats that remain hyperthyroid after the first treatment can be cured by a second treatment.

After treatment with radioiodine, it is common to see a transient fall in serum T_4 concentrations for a few weeks; but associate clinical signs of hypothyroidism do not develop, and treatment is almost never required. In most of those cats, free T_4 and thyroid-stimulating hormone (TSH) concentrations remain within reference range limits. In contrast, a few (less than 5%) of cats treated with radioiodine develop permanent hypothyroidism, with clinical signs developing 2 to 4 months after treatment. Clinical signs associated with iatrogenic hypothyroidism in these cats may include lethargy, nonpruritic seborrhea sicca, matting of hair, and marked weight gain; bilateral symmetric alopecia does not develop. Diagnosis is based on the cat's clinical signs, findings of low serum total and free T_4 concentrations (especially in combination with a high serum TSH concentration), and the response to replacement therapy. If hypothyroidism does develop, lifelong thyroid hormone supplementation is generally needed (i.e., 0.1 mg of L-T_4 per day).

After administration of radioiodine to cats, cure of hyperthyroidism is generally permanent, but recent studies have demonstrated that the disorder can reoccur. However, relapse is very uncommon, with a prevalence of less than 5%; and the time between treatment with radioiodine and relapse is generally 3 or more years. Therefore such relapse might indicate the development of new hyperplastic or neoplastic nodules arising from any remaining normal thyroid tissue rather than recurrence of the first adenomatous thyroid tumor that was treated with radioiodine. Nevertheless, the fact that both hypothyroidism and relapse can occur after treatment of cats with radioiodine indicates that continued, periodic monitoring of thyroid function (e.g., at least once yearly) is advisable once euthyroidism is restored.

The ongoing treatment of comorbid conditions such as systemic hypertension (see Chapters 30 and 197), cardiomyopathy (see Chapter 178), and renal failure requires clinical judgment and is approached on a case-by-case basis. Since geriatric cats are affected by a number of renal, cardiovascular, and gastrointestinal diseases, the clinician must appreciate that resolution of hyperthyroidism may not always resolve unrelated medical disorders. However, the vast majority of treated cats are improved clinically and appear to achieve a better quality of life.

References and Suggested Reading

Chun R et al: Predictors of response to radioiodine therapy in hyperthyroid cats, *Vet Radiol Ultrasound* 43:587, 2005.

DiBartola SP, Brown SA: The kidney and hyperthyroidism. In Bonagura JD, editor: *Kirk's current veterinary therapy XIII*, Philadelphia, 2000, Saunders, pp 337.

Fischetti AJ et al: Effects of methimazole on thyroid gland uptake of ^{99m}Tc-pertechnetate in 19 hyperthyroid cats, *Vet Radiol Ultrasound* 46:267, 2005.

Guptill L et al: Response to high-dose radioactive iodine administration in cats with thyroid carcinoma that had previously undergone surgery, *J Am Vet Med Assoc* 207:1055, 1995.

Nieckarz JA, Daniel GB: The effect of methimazole on thyroid uptake of pertechnetate and radioiodine in normal cats, *Vet Radiol Ultrasound* 42:448, 2001.

Peterson ME, Becker DV: Radioiodine treatment of 524 cats with hyperthyroidism, *J Am Vet Med Assoc* 207:1422, 1995.

Peterson ME, Melian C, Nichols R: Measurement of serum concentrations of free thyroxine, total thyroxine, and total triiodothyronine in cats with hyperthyroidism and cats with nonthyroidal disease, *J Am Vet Med Assoc* 218:529, 2001.

Slater MR et al: Long-term follow up of hyperthyroid cats treated with iodine-131, *Vet Radiol Ultrasound* 35:204, 1994.

Syme HM, Elliott J: Evaluation of proteinuria in hyperthyroid cats, *J Vet Intern Med* 15(3):299, 2001.

Theon AP, Van Vechten MK, Feldman E: Prospective randomized comparison of intravenous versus subcutaneous administration of radioiodine for treatment of hyperthyroidism in cats, *Am J Vet Res* 55:1734, 1994.

CHAPTER 41

Hypothyroidism

J. CATHARINE R. SCOTT-MONCRIEFF, *West Lafayette, Indiana*

Clinical signs of hypothyroidism result from decreased production of the thyroid hormones thyroxine (T_4) and triiodothyronine (T_3) by the thyroid gland. Acquired primary hypothyroidism is the most common form of the disease and usually is caused by either lymphocytic thyroiditis or idiopathic thyroid atrophy. Secondary hypothyroidism (deficiency of thyroid-stimulating hormone [TSH]) is less commonly recognized in the dog.

ETIOLOGY

Approximately 50% of cases of primary hypothyroidism are caused by lymphocytic thyroiditis. Grossly the thyroid gland may be normal or atrophic; whereas histologically there is multifocal or diffuse infiltration of the thyroid gland by lymphocytes, plasma cells, and macrophages. As thyroiditis progresses, the parenchyma is destroyed and replaced by fibrous connective tissue. Initially thyroiditis may be subclinical but usually progresses over time to cause overt hypothyroidism. Idiopathic thyroid atrophy, in which there is loss of thyroid parenchyma and replacement by adipose and connective tissue, may be caused by end-stage thyroiditis. Canine thyroiditis is believed to be immune mediated, and antithyroglobulin antibodies (ATAs) are a sensitive marker of thyroid inflammation. Approximately 50% of hypothyroid dogs have ATAs; however, the prevalence varies widely among breeds, which reflects a familial tendency for thyroiditis and resultant hypothyroidism.

SIGNALMENT

Any breed may develop hypothyroidism; however, some breeds such as the golden retriever and the Doberman pin scher have been reported to be at higher risk. Thyroiditis is clearly heritable in the beagle; the borzoi; and many other common breeds such as the golden retriever, Great Dane, Irish setter, Doberman pinscher, and Old English sheepdog have a high prevalence of ATAs (Nachreiner et al., 2002). The rate of clinical progression of thyroiditis also varies among breeds. In beagles the prevalence of thyroiditis is as high as 40%, but if the progression to hypothyroidism occurs at all, it occurs in middle age or later (Scott-Moncrieff et al., 2006). In other breeds such as the golden retriever, thyroiditis appears to progress more rapidly, with peak onset of hypothyroidism at 5 years of age but with some dogs diagnosed as young as 2 years of age. Overall middle-aged dogs are at increased risk of hypothyroidism. In one study mean age at diagnosis was

7 years with a range of 0.5 to 15 years. Spayed females and neutered male dogs are at increased risk for developing hypothyroidism compared with sexually intact animals.

CLINICAL SIGNS

Clinical signs of hypothyroidism are usually nonspecific and insidious in onset, and hypothyroidism is commonly misdiagnosed. Clinical signs that occur as a result of decreased metabolic rate include lethargy, mental dullness, weight gain, unwillingness to exercise, and cold intolerance. Dermatologic findings include dry scaly skin, changes in hair coat quality or color, symmetric alopecia, seborrhea, and superficial pyoderma. Hyperkeratosis, hyperpigmentation, comedone formation, hypertrichosis, ceruminous otitis, poor wound healing, increased bruising, and myxedema may also occur. Alopecia is usually bilaterally symmetric and is first evident in areas of wear, whereas the head and extremities tend to be spared. The hair may be brittle and easily epilated, and loss of undercoat or primary guard hairs may result in a coarse appearance or a puppylike hair coat. Fading of coat color may also occur, and failure of hair regrowth after clipping is common. Hypothyroid dogs are also predisposed to recurrent bacterial infections of the skin. Myxedema (cutaneous mucinosis) is a rare dermatologic manifestation of hypothyroidism, caused by deposition of hyaluronic acid in the dermis and characterized by nonpitting thickening of the skin, especially of the eyelids, cheeks, and forehead. A rare complication of myxedema is cutaneous mucinous vesiculation.

Reproductive dysfunction has been attributed to hypothyroidism. In male dogs low libido, testicular atrophy, hypospermia, and azoospermia have been reported; whereas hypothyroid bitches may develop prolonged interestrous interval, silent estrus, failure to cycle, spontaneous abortion, small or low–birth weight litters, uterine inertia, and weak or stillborn puppies. However, in both sexes evidence for an association between reproductive signs and hypothyroidism is weak. Inappropriate galactorrhea, apparently caused by hyperprolactinemia, has been reported in sexually intact hypothyroid bitches.

Both the peripheral and central nervous systems may be affected by hypothyroidism. Peripheral neuropathy is the best documented neurologic manifestation. Affected dogs have exercise intolerance, weakness, ataxia, quadriparesis or paralysis, deficits of conscious proprioception, and decreased spinal reflexes. Clinical signs resolve with levothyroxine (L–thyroxine) supplementation. A subclinical myopathy also occurs in hypothyroid dogs. Unilateral

185

lameness reported in hypothyroid dogs may be a manifestation of generalized neuromyopathy.

Dysfunction of multiple cranial nerves (facial, trigeminal, vestibulocochlear) and abnormal gait and postural reactions are also reported in hypothyroidism. Hypothyroid dogs with vestibular deficits have abnormal brainstem auditory–evoked responses, and some dogs also have electromyographic abnormalities in appendicular muscles. Clinical signs resolve with L-thyroxine supplementation. Although laryngeal paralysis and megaesophagus have been reported in association with hypothyroidism, treatment of hypothyroidism does not consistently result in resolution of clinical signs, and a causal relationship has not been confirmed. Myasthenia gravis has been reported in association with hypothyroidism. Concurrent hypothyroidism may exacerbate clinical signs of myasthenia gravis such as muscle weakness and megaesophagus.

In rare instances cerebral dysfunction occurs in hypothyroidism as a result of myxedema coma, atherosclerosis, or the presence of a pituitary tumor causing secondary hypothyroidism. Seizures, disorientation, and circling may occur as a result of severe hyperlipidemia or cerebral atherosclerosis; however, there is little evidence to suggest that hypothyroidism is a common cause of seizure disorders in dogs. In myxedema coma profound mental dullness or stupor may be accompanied by nonpitting edema, hypothermia with a lack of shivering, bradycardia, weakness, and inappetence. Concurrent disease, especially infection, is a common precipitating factor.

Behavioral abnormalities that have been attributed to canine hypothyroidism include aggression and cognitive dysfunction. Myxedema coma and atherosclerosis clearly can cause cognitive dysfunction in some individuals; however, these manifestations of hypothyroidism are rare. Evidence for a causal association between common behavioral problems and hypothyroidism is lacking.

Abnormalities of the cardiovascular system such as sinus bradycardia, weak apex beat, low QRS voltage, and inverted T waves occur in hypothyroid dogs. Reduced left ventricular pump function has also been documented, and hypothyroidism may exacerbate clinical signs in dogs with underlying cardiac disease. Although hypothyroidism rarely causes clinically significant myocardial failure in dogs, dilated cardiomyopathy and hypothyroidism may occur concurrently. Long-term improvement in cardiac function was reported after treatment with L-thyroxine in two Great Danes with concurrent dilated cardiomyopathy and hypothyroidism.

Ocular abnormalities reported in canine hypothyroidism include corneal lipidosis, corneal ulceration, uveitis, lipid effusion into the aqueous humor, secondary glaucoma, lipemia retinalis, retinal detachment, and keratoconjunctivitis sicca. However, a definite causal relationship has not been proven.

Congenital hypothyroidism results in mental retardation and stunted disproportionate growth caused by epiphyseal dysgenesis and delayed skeletal maturation. Affected dogs are mentally dull and have large broad heads, short thick necks, short limbs, macroglossia, hypothermia, delayed dental eruption, ataxia, and abdominal distention. A palpably enlarged thyroid gland may also be present, depending on the cause of the congenital defect. Other clinical signs include gait abnormalities, stenotic ear canals, sealed eyelids, and constipation. Affected puppies are often the largest in the litter at birth but start to lag behind their littermates within 3 to 8 weeks of age. Many severely affected puppies likely die without a diagnosis in the first few weeks of life. Congenital hypothyroidism with goiter caused by thyroid peroxidase deficiency has been recognized in toy fox terriers and rat terriers (Fyfe et al., 2003). The defect is an autosomal-recessive trait, and a nonsense mutation in the thyroid peroxidase gene of affected dogs has been identified. A deoxyribonucleic acid test that will detect carriers of the defect is available to screen breeding animals through the laboratory of comparative medical genetics at Michigan State University.

DIAGNOSIS OF HYPOTHYROIDISM

A clinical suspicion of hypothyroidism should be obtained by evaluation of the signalment; history and physical examination; and results of a hemogram, biochemical panel, and urinalysis. Measurement of total T_4 concentration is a sensitive initial screening test for hypothyroidism. Tests to confirm the diagnosis include measurement of free T_4 and TSH concentration, provocative thyroid function tests, and antibody tests for thyroiditis. In some equivocal cases evaluation of response to thyroid hormone supplementation is necessary to confirm the diagnosis.

Clinical Pathology

Clinicopathologic changes that are commonly observed in dogs with hypothyroidism are normocytic, normochromi, nonregenerative anemia, fasting hypertriglyceridemia, and hypercholesterolemia.

Basal Thyroid Hormone Concentrations

T_4 is the major secretory product of the thyroid gland, whereas the majority of serum T_3 is derived from the extrathyroidal deiodination of T_4. Both T_3 and T_4 are highly protein bound to serum carrier proteins. Only unbound (free) hormone penetrates cell membranes, binds to receptors, and has biologic activity. Protein-bound hormone acts as a reservoir and buffer to maintain a steady concentration of free hormone in the plasma despite rapid alterations in release and metabolism of T_3 and T_4 and changes in plasma protein concentrations. Free T_4 is mono-deiodinated within cells to T_3, which binds to receptors and induces the cellular effects of thyroid hormone. Diagnostic performance of basal thyroid hormone measurements in the diagnosis of canine hypothyroidism is shown in Table 41-1.

Total Thyroxine Concentration

Total T_4 concentration is the most commonly performed static thyroid hormone measurement and is a good initial screening test for canine hypothyroidism. In general a dog with a T_4 concentration well within the normal range may be assumed to have normal thyroid function; however, a basal T_4 concentration below the normal

Table **41-1**

Performance of Various Diagnostic Tests for Hypothyroidism in Dogs

	Sensitivity (%)	Specificity (%)	Accuracy (%)
Total T$_4$	89-100	75-82	85
Free T$_4$	80-98	93-94	95
TSH	63-87	82-93	80-84
TSH/T$_4$*	63-67	98-100	82-88
TSH/free T$_4$*	74	98	86

The data are compiled from three published studies of a total of 100 hypothyroid dogs and 164 euthyroid dogs. Not all studies evaluated all diagnostic tests listed.
T_4, Thyroxine; *TSH,* thyroid-stimulating hormone.
*A dog was considered to have hypothyroidism only if the T$_4$ or free T$_4$ was low and the TSH was high.

range is not diagnostic for hypothyroidism. In this case the dog may be normal, hypothyroid, or suffering from a nonthyroidal illness with a secondary decrease in the basal T$_4$ concentration (sick euthyroid syndrome). Factors such as time of day, age, breed, and ambient temperature may affect the total T$_4$ concentration without altering metabolically active free thyroid hormone concentrations. Not only does the T$_4$ concentration in *normal* dogs commonly fluctuate out of the reference range, but a number of breeds (e.g., Greyhounds, conditioned sled dogs) have been identified as having T$_4$ concentrations lower than established laboratory reference ranges (Evason et al., 2004; Lee et al., 2004). A significant decline in basal T$_4$ concentration with age adds yet another variable; estrus, pregnancy, obesity, and malnutrition also influence the basal T$_4$. There may also be a marked effect of some drugs on the thyroid axis (Table 41-2) (Daminet et al., 2003). Systemic illnesses that may decrease basal T$_4$ concentrations include hyperadrenocorticism, diabetes mellitus, hypoadrenocorticism, renal failure, hepatic failure, and infection. Interference by anti-T$_4$ antibodies can cause a spurious increase in the measured T$_4$ concentration, but this is usually to a value above the reference range.

Free Thyroxine Concentration
Because only the unbound fraction of serum T$_4$ is biologically active, measurement of free T$_4$ is more sensitive and specific than total T$_4$ in differentiation of euthyroid dogs from hypothyroid dogs, providing free T$_4$ assays that use equilibrium dialysis (ED) rather than analog methods. Free T$_4$ measured by ED is unaffected by antibody interference. Although the free T$_4$ concentration is a more accurate stand-alone test than the basal T$_4$, significant concurrent disease can cause a decrease in free T$_4$, and the assay is approximately twice as expensive in most commercial laboratories as the total T$_4$.

Total Triiodothyronine Concentration
In euthyroid dogs T$_3$ concentration fluctuates in and out of the normal range even more than T$_4$ concentration; therefore T$_3$ concentrations are less accurate in distinguishing euthyroid from hypothyroid dogs. Spurious T$_3$ measurements may also occur because of the presence of anti-T$_3$ antibodies that interfere with the T$_3$ assay.

Thyroid-Stimulating Hormone Concentration
Measurement of canine TSH concentration is helpful in dogs with a low total T$_4$ concentration because a low

Table **41-2**

Effect of Drug Treatment on Thyroid Function Testing in Dogs

Drug	TT$_4$ ($\downarrow$ or N)	Free T$_4$ ($\downarrow$ or N)	TSH ($\uparrow$ or N)	Clinical signs of hypothyroidism? (Y/N)*	Notes
Glucocorticoids	$\downarrow$	($\downarrow$ or N)	N	N	Effect dose and duration dependent
Phenobarbital	$\downarrow$	$\downarrow$	Slight $\uparrow$	N	Thyroid-stimulating hormone not increased outside reference range
Trimethoprim/sulfonamides	$\downarrow$	$\downarrow$	$\uparrow$	Y	Effect dose and duration dependent
Nonsteroidal antiinflammatory drugs	$\downarrow$	N	N or $\downarrow$	N	Effect varies, depending on specific drug used
Tricyclic antidepressants (TADs) (clomipramine)	$\downarrow$	$\downarrow$	N	N	Effect of other TAD drugs unknown in dog
Propranolol	N	N	N	N	
Potassium bromide	N	N	N	N	

From Daminet S, Ferguson DC: Influence of drugs on thyroid function in dogs, *J AM Vet Intern Med* 17:463, 2003.
N, No change; *TSH,* thyroid stimulating hormone; *TT$_4$,* thyroxine; $\uparrow$, increased; $\downarrow$, decreased.
*N, No; Y, yes.

T_4 in conjunction with a high TSH is highly specific for diagnosis of hypothyroidism (Table 41-3). The main disadvantage of measuring TSH is the lack of sensitivity of this assay because, for reasons that are unclear, approximately 30% of hypothyroid dogs have a TSH concentration within the reference range.

Thyroid-Stimulating Hormone Stimulation Test

The TSH stimulation test is a test of thyroid reserve. It is considered the gold standard test of thyroid function in dogs, but its use is limited by the expense and availability of TSH. The protocol requires collection of a serum sample for measuring T_4, administration of bovine TSH intravenously (IV) at a dose of 0.1 units/kg (maximum dose 5 units), followed by collection of a second sample for measurement of T_4 6 hours later. Alternatively human recombinant TSH (Thyrogen, Genzyme Corp.) may be used at a dose of 50 to 100 mcg IV with collection of 0- and 4 to 6-hour samples. One vial contains 1.1 mg of lyophilized TSH; after reconstitution it may be frozen for at least 8 weeks with no loss of potency. Current cost is approximately $1800 and contains enough TSH for 10 to 20 dogs. Bovine TSH currently is only available as the chemical grade preparation, and there have been reports of adverse effects after administration of this product.

Results of the TSH stimulation test may reveal a normal response, a blunted response (sick euthyroid syndrome), or no response (hypothyroidism). A diagnosis of hypothyroidism can be confirmed if both the basal and the post-T_4 samples are below the reference range for basal total T_4 concentration. A euthyroid state is confirmed if the post-T_4 concentration is greater than 2.5 to 3 mcg/dl. Interpretation of intermediate results is more difficult and should take into consideration the clinical signs and severity of concurrent systemic disease.

Thyroid-Releasing Hormone Stimulation Test

In dogs this test has been used predominantly to evaluate thyroid gland function by measuring a change in T_4 concentration after thyroid-releasing hormone (TRH) administration. Unfortunately the change is not as large as after TSH administration, and some dogs with normal thyroid function have a decreased response to TRH. For this reason the test is of limited clinical use. Current protocols recommend a fixed dose of 100 to 600 mcg TRH IV, with samples collected at 0 and 4 hours.

Thyroid Ultrasound

Measurement of thyroid gland size by ultrasound is a useful adjunctive test for differentiating between hypothyroid and euthyroid dogs (Brömel et al., 2005; Reese et al., 2005). Identification of both decreased thyroid volume and maximal cross-sectional area have high specificity for diagnosis of hypothyroidism; however, because some hypothyroid dogs have thyroid volumes within the reference range, ultrasonography lacks sensitivity for diagnosis of hypothyroidism. It is important that thyroid ultrasonography is performed by an operator with experience in performing and interpreting ultrasound studies of the cervical region.

Therapeutic Trial

In some cases the most practical approach to confirming a diagnosis of hypothyroidism is a therapeutic trial. Every attempt should be made to rule out nonthyroidal illness before starting a therapeutic trial. Supplementation with L-thyroxine should be initiated at a dose of 20 mcg/kg (0.1 mg/10 lb) every 12 hours. Few studies in dogs document the comparative efficacy of available T_4 supplements; however, the impact of differences in product bioavailability can be minimized if therapeutic monitoring is used to guide the final dose administered (Fig. 41-1). If possible, objective criteria should be used to assess response to treatment. If a positive response to treatment occurs, the clinician should be prepared to withdraw therapy to confirm that clinical signs return. This ensures that dogs with thyroid-responsive diseases (diseases in which the clinical signs improve because of the nonspecific effects of thyroid hormone or unrelated to therapy) do not remain on thyroid supplementation for life. If there is no response to treatment after 2 to 3 months of appropriate therapy

---

Table 41-3

Interpretation of Basal Thyroid Hormone Concentrations (T_4, Free T_4, TSH)

	Normal T_4/Free T_4	Low/Borderline T_4/Free T_4
Normal TSH	Normal dog Only consider further thyroid testing if strong clinical suspicion of hypothyroidism	Hypothyroid, normal variation, or concurrent illness Consider further diagnostic evaluation of thyroid function (thyroid autoantibodies, provocative testing) or therapeutic trial.
High TSH	Early subclinical hypothyroidism or recovery from concurrent illness Consider reevaluation of thyroid function in 1-3 months; if strong clinical suspicion for hypothyroidism, evaluate for thyroiditis	Hypothyroid Lifelong therapy with L-thyroxine is indicated; use therapeutic monitoring to adjust dose

T_4, Thyroxine; *TSH*, thyroid-stimulating hormone.

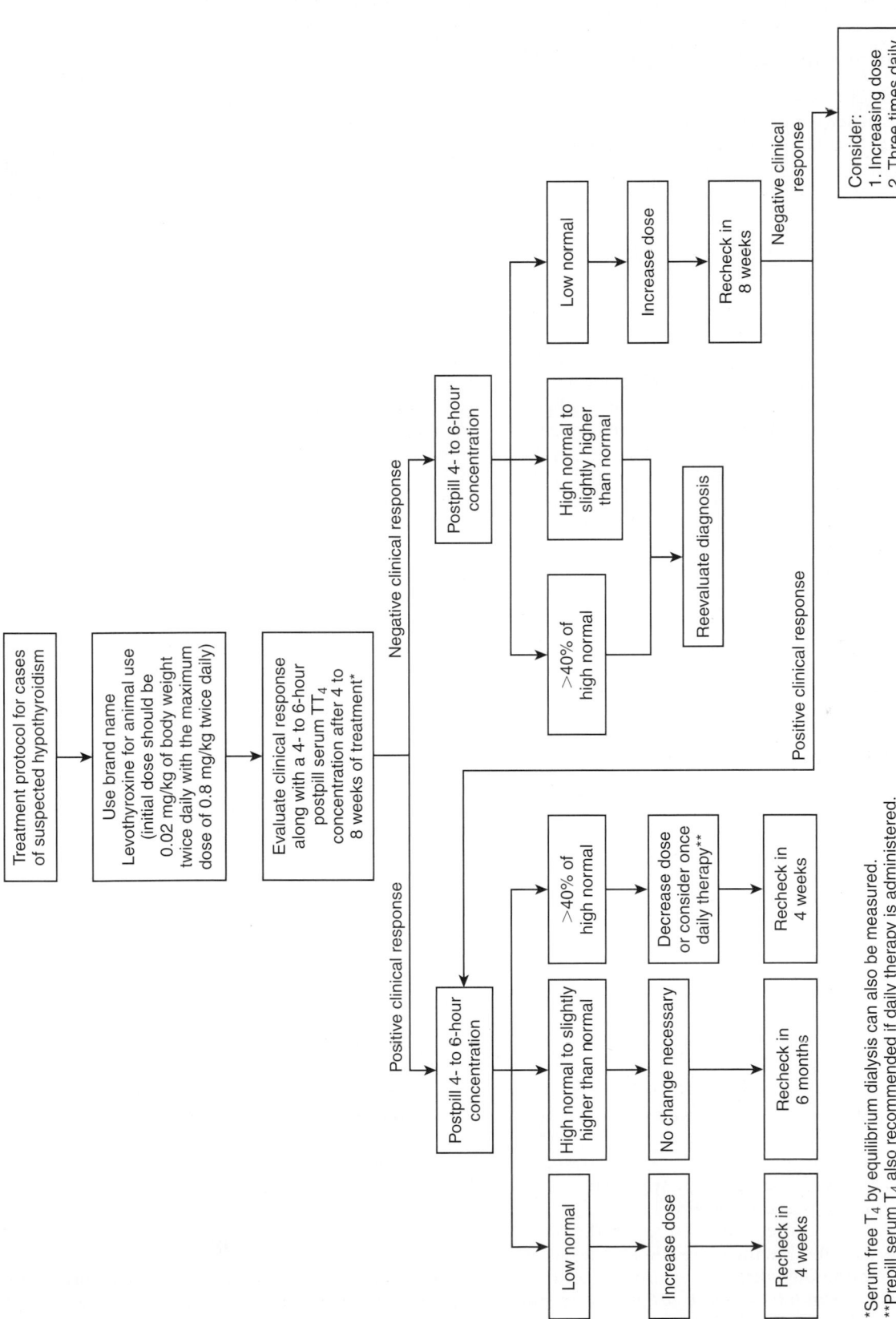

Fig 41-1 Algorithm outlining approach to treatment of canine hypothyroidism. (From Scott-Moncrief JCR, Guptill-Yoran L: Hypothyroidism. In Ettinger SJ, Feldman EC: *Textbook of veterinary internal medicine: diseases of the dog and cat,* ed 6, 2005, Elsevier.)

*Serum free T$_4$ by equilibrium dialysis can also be measured.
**Prepill serum T$_4$ also recommended if daily therapy is administered.

in the face of adequate serum T$_4$ concentrations, the clinician should be prepared to withdraw therapy and pursue other diagnoses.

Recommendations for Thyroid Testing

Initial evaluation of thyroid function is best made by measurement of either total T$_4$ or ideally free T$_4$ in conjunction with TSH. Further testing should be pursued when initial testing results are equivocal (see Table 41-3 and Chapter 38).

DIAGNOSIS OF THYROIDITIS

Antithyroglobulin Antibodies

ATAs are found in approximately 50% of hypothyroid dogs and are believed to be the result of leakage of thyroglobulin into circulation caused by lymphocytic thyroiditis. A commercially available enzyme-linked immunosorbent assay for ATAs appears to be a fairly sensitive and specific indicator of thyroiditis, although false-positive results do occur. Because ATAs are more common in hypothyroid dogs than euthyroid dogs, their presence may be useful in assessing thyroid function in dogs when other tests of thyroid function are equivocal. However, it is important to recognize that a positive ATA titer can occur in euthyroid dogs. The proportion of euthyroid dogs with ATAs that ultimately develop hypothyroidism is unknown. In one study approximately 20% of euthyroid dogs with thyroiditis developed some evidence of thyroid dysfunction within a year. A small percentage of dogs (15%) became ATA negative after 12 months. Possible causes for a transient increase in ATAs include recent vaccination, drug therapy, or viral infection.

Measurement of ATAs has been advocated for screening breeding stock with the aim of ultimately eliminating heritable forms of thyroiditis. The Orthopedic Foundation for Animals (OFA) maintains a thyroid registry and issues a breed database number to all dogs found to have normal thyroid function at 12 months of age (based on measurement of free T4, TSH, and ATAs by an OFA-approved laboratory). Each dog must also be examined by a veterinarian. It is recommended that reexamination and retesting occur at 2, 3, 4, 6, and 8 years of age.

Anti-T$_3$ and T$_4$ Antibodies
Antibodies directed against T$_3$ and T$_4$ also occur in canine thyroiditis, although they are less prevalent than ATAs. Anti-T$_3$ antibodies are identified in approximately 30% of hypothyroid dogs, whereas anti-T$_4$ antibodies are reported in 15% of hypothyroid dogs. Although some euthyroid dogs may be positive for anti-T$_3$ and T$_4$ antibodies, in the presence of other equivocal results the presence of antithyroid antibodies increases the likelihood of hypothyroidism. Antibodies directed against T$_3$ and T$_4$ may interfere with hormone assays, leading to a spurious increase or decrease in the measured hormone concentration. In theory these antibodies could also increase a low T$_4$ concentration into the normal range and result in a false diagnosis of euthyroidism, although typically the measured T$_4$ concentration is above reference range.

Anti-thyroid antibodies do not interfere with response to L-thyroxine supplementation.

TREATMENT

Synthetic sodium L-thyroxine is the initial thyroid supplement of choice in canine hypothyroidism. Synthetic products (salts of T$_3$ or T$_4$) are more stable and better standardized for potency. Liquid formulations are now available and have similar bioavailability to tablets. L-thyroxine has a serum half-life of 12 to 16 hours, and peak concentrations are achieved at 4 to 12 hours after administration; however, there is wide interdog variability. Recommendations for therapy are to administer L-thyroxine initially at a dose of 20 mcg/kg twice a day (see Fig. 41-1). Many dogs will ultimately only require supplementation once a day; however, starting at a twice-daily dosage maximizes the chance of a good response. Once a clinical response is achieved, a trial with once-a-day therapy can be instituted. In dogs with concurrent heart disease, a sudden increase in the basal metabolic rate may lead to cardiac destabilization; thus the starting dose should be decreased by 50% and then adjusted on the basis of therapeutic monitoring. This is especially important for dogs with congestive heart failure in which hypothyroidism could reduce myocardial function but hyperthyroidism will increase cardiac demands.

Synthetic T$_3$ administration is only indicated in the few situations when T$_4$ supplementation has failed to achieve a response in a dog with confirmed hypothyroidism. This may occur because of impaired T$_4$ absorption from the gastrointestinal tract. T$_3$ supplementation is not recommended for initial therapy. Dogs receiving T$_3$ supplementation are more susceptible to iatrogenic thyrotoxicosis. Combination products that contain both T$_3$ and T$_4$ should be avoided for similar reasons. The plasma half-life of synthetic T$_3$ is 5 to 6 hours; thus it needs to be administered three times a day. The initial starting dose is 4 to 6 mcg/kg every 8 hours. Intravenous L-thyroxine at a dose of 4 to 5 mcg/kg every 8 to 12 hours appears to be safe and effective for treatment of dogs in thyroid crisis caused by myxedema coma (Pullen and Hess, 2006). Other aspects of treatment in affected dogs include passive rewarming, supportive care, and treatment of concurrent disease.

Improvement in activity level in dogs treated for hypothyroidism should occur within 1 week. Improvement in other clinical signs should be observed 4 to 6 weeks after initiation of therapy, although dermatologic abnormalities may take several months to completely resolve. Initially the appearance of the hair coat may worsen as hair in the telogen phase is shed.

Therapeutic Monitoring

Monitoring of serum T$_4$ concentration during therapy allows individualization of the dose and dosing frequency and is also useful in evaluating dogs that fail to respond to thyroid supplementation. Measurement of serum T$_4$ concentration should be performed after at least 1 month of therapy. A serum sample is taken *before and 4 to 6 hours after treatment* and submitted for measurement of T_4 concentrations. Dosage and frequency of thyroid supplementation can then be adjusted appropriately (see Fig. 41-1). The trough sample concentration should be at the low end of the normal reference range, and the peak T_4 concentration should be within the upper end of the reference range or slightly above it (up to 6 mcg/dl is considered acceptable). If it is only possible to collect one sample, a post-pill sample should be collected. Concurrent measurement of TSH concentration during therapeutic monitoring may also be useful in dogs in which TSH was increased before treatment. Documentation of a normal TSH is evidence of adequate supplementation; however, because of poor sensitivity of canine TSH assays, detection of oversupplementation is not possible.

Poor Response to Therapy

An absent or inadequate response to therapy may be the result of incorrect diagnosis, poor owner compliance, inadequate dose of thyroid supplementation, poor oral absorption of thyroid supplement, or use of inappropriate formulation. Therapeutic monitoring allows differentiation of all these causes except incorrect diagnosis. Defective conversion of T_4 to T_3 and resistance of peripheral tissues to the action of thyroid hormone are theoretic causes of treatment failure that have not been documented in dogs.

References and Suggested Reading

Brömel C et al: Ultrasonographic evaluation of the thyroid gland in healthy, hypothyroid, and euthyroid golden retrievers with nonthyroidal illness, *J Vet Intern Med* 19:499, 2005.

Daminet S, Ferguson DC: Influence of drugs on thyroid function in dogs, *J Vet Intern Med* 17:463, 2003.

Evason MD et al: Alterations in thyroid hormone concentrations in healthy sled dogs before and after athletic conditioning, *Am J Vet Res* 65:333, 2004.

Ferguson DC: Small animal practice testing for hypothyroidism in dogs, *Vet Clin North Am* 37:647, 2007.

Fyfe JC et al: Congenital hypothyroidism with goiter in toy fox terriers, *J Vet Intern Med* 17:50, 2003.

Graham PA et al: Etiopathologic findings of Canine hypothyroidism, *Vet Clin North Am Small Anim Pract* 37:617, 2007.

Pullen WH, Hess RS: Hypothyroid dogs treated with intravenous levothyroxine, *J Vet Intern Med* 20:32, 2006.

Lee JA et al: Effects of racing and nontraining on plasma thyroid hormone concentrations in sled dogs, *J Am Vet Med Assoc* 224:226, 2004.

Nachreiner RF et al: Prevalence of serum thyroid hormone autoantibodies in dogs with clinical signs of hypothyroidism, *J Am Vet Med Assoc* 220:466, 2002.

Reese S et al: Thyroid sonography as an effective tool to discriminate between euthyroid sick and hypothyroid dogs, *J Vet Intern Med* 19:491, 2005.

Scott-Moncrieff JC et al: Lack of association between repeated vaccination and thyroiditis in laboratory beagles, *J Vet Intern Med* 20:818, 2006.

CHAPTER **42**

Obesity

ANGELA L. LUSBY, *Knoxville, Tennessee*
CLAUDIA A. KIRK, *Knoxville, Tennessee*

PREVALENCE AND RISK FACTORS FOR OBESITY

The incidence of obesity is reaching epidemic proportions worldwide, and the consequences of excessive body fat on overall health is a topic at the forefront of human medicine. Obesity in companion animal medicine has similar health impacts and should receive the same attention from practitioners as other chronic diseases. In dogs and cats a general definition for obesity is exceeding ideal body weight by 15% to 20% because of excess adipose tissue. Based on recent studies, approximately 35% to 40% and 25% to 35% of adult dogs and cats, respectively, are either overweight or obese, with informal surveys indicating that this number exceeds 50% in 2006. The percentage is even higher for middle-aged animals, reaching over 40% in both species.

Several risk factors are associated with obesity in dogs and cats. In both species the peak incidence occurs at middle age and is highly associated with gonadectomy. Several studies in cats suggest that weight gain after spaying or neutering is a combination of slower metabolic rate and increased food intake. The metabolic changes caused by gonadectomy in dogs are not clear, but increased food consumption with decreased activity levels are suggested mechanisms for weight gain. Gender can also influence weight gain, with spayed female dogs and neutered male cats having an increased risk for excess body fat. Breed also has a significant role in the development of obesity in dogs. In particular, the golden retriever, dachshund, Shetland sheepdog, Labrador retriever, cocker spaniel, and dalmatian are more likely to become overweight. Finally, environmental factors such as sedentary lifestyles and ad libitum feeding regimens contribute to both canine and feline obesity.

PHYSIOLOGY

Weight gain occurs when energy intake exceeds energy output. Certain diseases such as hypothyroidism can contribute to weight gain by decreasing the metabolic rate and energy output. However, most overweight dogs and cats do not have underlying thyroid disease, and weight gain is caused by excessive caloric intake with inadequate physical activity.

Until recently adipose tissue was thought to be passive and involved only in energy storage and insulation. However, the role of adipose tissue as an endocrine organ has since been established. Hormones and proteins secreted from adipose cells, termed *adipokines,* appear to have roles in appetite, inflammation, insulin sensitivity, and metabolism. To date over 50 adipokines have been identified; some of the most intensely studied examples are leptin, resistin, and adiponectin. Leptin levels increase with obesity, and leptin is thought to have an important role in maintaining satiety. Resistin also rises with obesity, but the role of resistin remains controversial. Unlike leptin and resistin, adiponectin decreases with fat deposition and appears to have beneficial effects on the cardiovascular system and insulin sensitivity.

Excessive adipose tissue has a myriad of effects on the body. The deleterious effects can be mechanical by compression of organs and excessive strain on joints or physiologic with alterations in metabolism and organ function. Obesity has also been implicated in the cause or progression of neoplasia, cardiorespiratory disease, urogenital disease, endocrinopathies, metabolic derangements, dermatologic disease, and orthopedic disorders (Box 42-1).

DIAGNOSIS OF BODY CONDITION

A variety of methods are available to evaluate the body condition of dogs and cat, but not all are practical or cost effective. Body condition scoring is a simple method for assessing a patient's body condition and correlates strongly with other techniques used to estimate body fat. Using visual observation and palpation, a body condition score is assigned using either a five- or a nine-point scale (Fig. 42-1). The choice of scale is based on personal preference since the scoring criteria are similar. The goal of assessing body condition is to estimate proportion of body fat, irrespective of weight; to help assess risk for obesity-related disease or physical dysfunction; and to monitor changes in body fat over time. Body condition scores can also be used to estimate a patient's percent body fat, which is useful for determining weight-loss goals (see Fig. 42-1).

TREATMENT

The concept behind the treatment of obesity is simple: decrease caloric intake and increase physical activity. However, management of real-life cases is rarely so straightforward. Practical issues such as dietary restrictions, owner compliance, and multiple-animal households can make the process of weight loss more challenging. It is important to take a thorough history before prescribing a weight-loss strategy to address issues early and minimize owner frustration. It is also important to have an accurate description of the current diet, including table scraps, to determine current caloric intake and to understand

Box 42-1

Diseases Associated With Obesity in Dogs and Cats

Endocrinopathies
- Hypothyroidism
- Hyperadrenocorticism
- Diabetes mellitus
- Insulinoma

Orthopedic disorders
- Osteoarthritis
- Cranial cruciate ligament rupture
- Intervertebral disk disease
- Humeral condylar fractures

Metabolic alterations
- Insulin resistance
- Glucose intolerance
- Hepatic lipidosis (cats)
- Hyperlipidemia/dyslipidemia

Cardiorespiratory disease
- Tracheal collapse
- Laryngeal paralysis
- Brachycephalic airway obstruction syndrome
- Dyspnea
- Hypertension

Dermatologic abnormalities
- Dry, flaky skin
- Feline acne
- Alopecia
- Seborrhea

Neoplasia
- Mammary
- Transitional cell carcinoma

Urogenital system
- Urolithiasis (calcium oxalate)
- Urethral sphincter mechanism incompetence
- Dystocia
- Urinary tract infection

Functional alterations
- Decreased immune function
- Increased anesthetic risk
- Heat intolerance
- Decreased life span

owners' perceptions and beliefs about food. Planning a weight-loss strategy has five main steps:

1. Estimate current body condition and body fat percentage (see Fig. 42-1)
2. Estimate ideal body weight; this estimation is often based on clinical experience; a weight history can also be useful to determine ideal weight since most animals are close to ideal at the onset of maturity (approximately 1 year of age).
3. Determine the current caloric intake through dietary history
4. Calculate desired caloric intake
5. Implement an exercise plan

5 pt scale	9 pt scale	% body fat	Body condition scoring	Dogs	Cats
1	1	≤5	**Emaciated**—ribs and bony prominences are visible from a distance. No palpable body fat. Obvious abdominal tuck and loss of muscle mass.	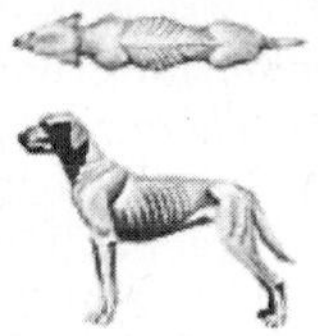	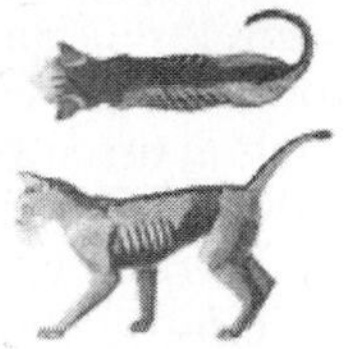
2	2	6-9	**Very thin**—ribs and bony prominences visible. Minimal loss of muscle mass, but no palpable fat.	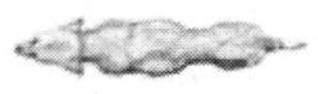	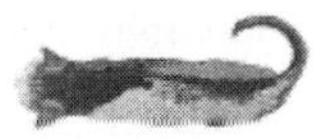
	3	10-14	**Thin**—ribs easily palpable, tops of lumbar are visible. Obvious waist and abdominal tuck.	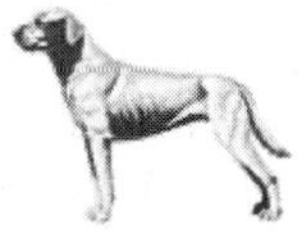	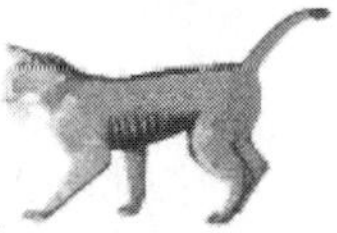
3	4	15-19	**Lean**—ribs easily palpable, waist visible from above. Abdominal tuck present. Abdominal fat pad is absent in cats.	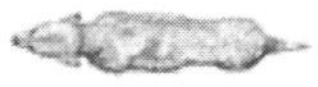	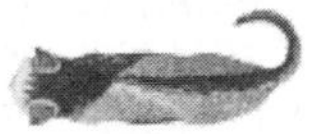
	5	20-24	**Ideal**—ribs palpable without excess fat covering. Waist and abdominal tuck present in dogs. Cats have a waist and a minimal abdominal fat pad.	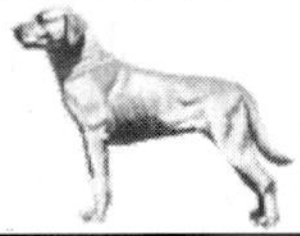	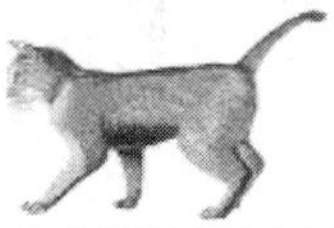
4	6	25-29	**Slightly overweight**—ribs have slight excess fat covering. Waist is discernible from above, but not obvious. Abdominal tuck still present in dogs. Abdominal fat pad is apparent, but not obvious in cats.	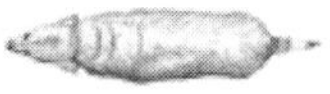	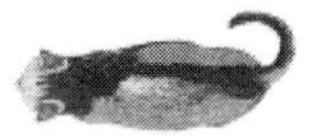
	7	30-34	**Overweight**—difficult to palpate ribs. **Dogs:** fat deposits over lumbar area and tail base. Abdominal tuck may be present, but waist is absent. **Cats:** moderate abdominal fat pad and rounding of the abdomen.	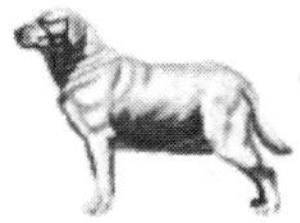	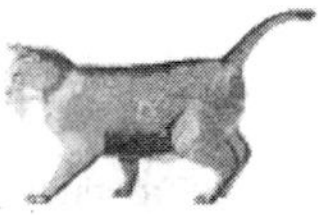
5	8	35-39	**Obese**—ribs not palpable and abdomen may be rounded. **Dogs:** heavy fat deposits over lumbar and base of tail. No abdominal tuck or waist. **Cats:** prominent abdominal fat pad and lumbar fat deposits.	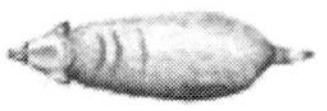	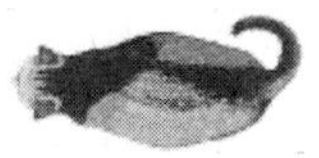
	9	40-45+	**Morbidly obese**—**Dogs:** large fat deposits over thorax, tail base, and spine with abdominal distension. **Cats:** heavy fat deposits over lumbar area, face, and limbs. Large abdominal fat pad and rounded abdomen.	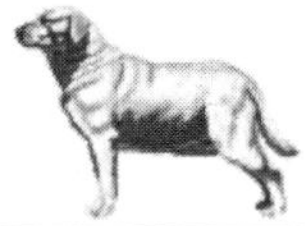	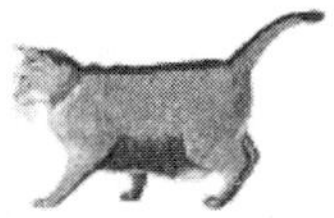

Fig 42-1 Description of body condition scoring systems and their relationship to body fat percentage. (Illustrations from Drs. Foster and Smith, Inc.)

Choosing an Appropriate Diet

Weight-loss diets for dogs and cats typically fall into two categories: over-the-counter light and lean products or prescription weight-loss diets. Although over-the-counter products may be sufficient in animals that are mildly overweight, prescription weight-loss diets are recommended for substantial weight loss. Owners often ask if they can simply reduce the amount fed of the animal's current diet. Switching to a diet designed for weight loss is more desirable. Maintenance diets are calorically denser, with higher levels of fat than calorie-restricted diets. In addition, the components of maintenance foods are balanced to provide adequate amounts of nutrients when standard feeding guidelines are followed. When the amount of a maintenance diet is significantly reduced below feeding recommendations, deficiencies in protein and other nutrients can occur. Diets formulated for weight loss are balanced to provide both adequate nutrients and energy restriction. In cases in which the diet cannot be changed because of medical conditions, the quantity of the current diet can be reduced, but review of total intake should ensure adequate nutrient intake.

Most canine weight-reduction diets rely on high levels of fiber, air, or moisture to reduce energy density. It has been proposed that high levels of fiber increase satiety by allowing the dog to ingest more food while receiving fewer calories. Although some evidence suggests that high levels of fiber do not affect satiety in dogs, other studies support the effect of diet bulk (i.e., fiber) in lowering total energy intake.

Following the trend in human dieting, low-carbohydrate, high-protein diets have also been proposed for use in dogs. Current evidence suggests limited benefit to using these diets for weight loss in dogs. In general, it appears that weight loss occurs with caloric restriction, regardless of the protein or fiber content. However, the proportion of fat loss over lean tissue loss is greater in dogs when fed high-protein foods compared to maintenance levels.

In recent years there has been much debate about the most appropriate diets for feline weight control. Cats are strict carnivores and naturally consume very high-protein diets. Therefore, many are advocating high-protein weight-loss diets for cats instead of more traditional high-fiber diets. Studies have shown that high-protein diets do appear to have beneficial effects on insulin sensitivity and diabetic control. However, a study evaluating only weight loss in cats did not detect any differences between high-protein and high-fiber diets, whereas the partitioning of weight loss, as in dogs, favored fat tissue loss when feeding low carbohydrate and high protein. For now, using high-protein, low carbohydrate or high-fiber diets for feline weight loss is a matter of personal preference. Further studies will be needed to truly determine if one diet is superior to another.

Estimating Desired Caloric Intake

As stated previously, obesity is the consequence of energy intake exceeding energy output. Energy output can also be called the daily energy requirement (DER). DER is made up of several components, but the resting energy requirement (RER) and the exercise energy requirement (EER) are the two largest contributors. The RER is the energy needed to maintain normal metabolic functions (e.g., blood flow, cellular metabolism, respiration) and is closely correlated with lean body mass. The RER typically accounts for 60% to 80% of the total DER. EER is the energy exerted through muscular activity and exercise and accounts for roughly 10% to 20% of DER in nonactive humans. Compared to lean mass, fat mass is metabolically inactive and contributes little to the RER. Therefore estimations of RERs should be based on ideal rather than current weight. RER can be estimated using the following formula:

$$RER = 70(BW_{kg}^{*0.75})$$

If a scientific calculator is not available, the linear equation achieves similar results in animals over 2 kg: RER = $(30 \times BW_{kg}) + 70$. The DERs needed to achieve weight loss are then estimated using the RER. The result is the total number of calories that should be fed in a 24-hour period.

Canine DER for weight loss = 1 to 1.2 × RER
Feline DER for weight loss = 0.8 × RER

Careful monitoring of patients should occur during any weight loss program. The goal is to achieve 1% to 2% loss of body weight per week. Although the formulas above

*Body weight at estimated ideal.

are useful for initial estimations, some animals, especially cats, may require further restriction to achieve weight loss. Reducing energy by 10% of calories every 2 weeks until adequate weight loss is achieved may be required.

Role of Exercise

Increasing physical activity is an intuitive part of any weight loss program, yet exercise is often overlooked in companion animals. In dogs a 20- to 30-minute walk 3 to 4 days a week is a good method for burning calories. It may be necessary to address limiting medical issues such as joint disease or osteoarthritis in some dogs (see Section XII). Having owners play games such as fetch or hide-and-seek with toys or treats can also increase activity. It is important to discuss any limitations the owners have in exercising their pets and then offer creative, helpful suggestions. Creativity becomes even more important when trying to increase the physical activity levels of cats. Indoor cats lead more sedentary lives than outdoor cats, and special efforts must be made to increase their activity. Owners can begin by changing the cat's environment by providing more vertical space to explore with items such as window hammocks, platforms, and cat furniture. Barriers such as baby gates can also be used to force cats to exert more effort while moving around the house. Meals can be served on top of surfaces that require the cat to climb. Toys that hide kibble and require effort to extract the treat can occupy some cats. In addition, owner interaction in the form of play can be very effective. Even increasing play or exercise for just 10 minutes a day can be highly effective in promoting weight loss.

Future Role of Pharmacotherapy in Veterinary Obesity Management

Pharmacologic therapies for the treatment of obesity can target several areas. They can decrease energy consumption through modulation of satiety signals or blocking intestinal absorption, increase energy expenditure by increasing metabolic rates, or redistribute stored energy in adipose tissue to more metabolically active tissue such as muscle. Currently only two drugs are approved for weight loss in humans. Sibutramine (Meridia, Abbott) exerts anorectic effects by inhibiting serotonin/norepinephrine reuptake, and orlistat (Xenical, Roche Pharmaceuticals) increases fecal fat excretion. In dogs and cats drugs such as sibutramine that increase serotonin availability are associated with significant adverse side effects. Orlistat has not been studied in cats, but in dogs only modest weight loss was achieved and treatment complications included leakage of colonic contents with perianal soiling.

The control of satiety is a complex process. The hypothalamus is the main center of the brain that mediates satiety. Factors that signal the hypothalamus to increase or decrease food intake include nutrients, hormones, and intestinal peptides found in circulation and neurologic impulses from vagal and sensory nerves. The complexity surrounding the regulation of food intake provides many potential targets for increasing satiety. In the early 1990s an endogenous cannabinoid system was discovered that regulates synaptic neurotransmission and exerts effects on many diseases and physiologic processes, including satiety, psychiatric disorders, and multiple sclerosis. A specific receptor in the cannabinoid system, cannabinoid-1 (CB-1) has been targeted for obesity treatment by the new drug rimonabant (Acomplia, Sanofi-Aventis), which is a CB-1 receptor antagonist. Rimonabant is currently in phase III clinical trials for humans. Unfortunately results in dogs and cats are not promising. Dogs appear to have transient weight loss that subsides after several weeks of therapy. In addition, side effects such as vomiting, diarrhea, and pruritus are significant at therapeutic doses. In cats CB-1 antagonists do not result in weight loss at tolerated doses.

Pharmaceutical induction of canine weight loss is now possible following the 2007 introduction of Slentrol (dirlotapide; Pfizer Animal Health) and Yarvitan (mitratapide; Janssen Animal Health). These drugs are classified as microsomal triglyceride transfer protein (MTP) inhibitors. Microsomal triglyceride transfer proteins are endoplasmic reticulum proteins expressed predominantly in intestinal and liver tissue where they play a pivotal role in the assembly of lipids to apoprotein B (apoB). Lipid assembly is required for export of lipoproteins across cell membranes and transport of lipids in the circulation. The MTP inhibitors for canine weight loss are selective for the intestine, thereby blocking MTP activity and the intraluminal transport of fat across the enterocyte. Turnover of lipid-laden enterocytes result in loss of fat (and calories) into the feces. More imortantly, intestinal lipid accumulation appears to increase release of potent satiety signals from the gut (e.g., pancreatic peptide YY; PYY) and inhibition of voluntary food intake. Up to 90% of the canine weight loss has been attributed to appetite control. These drugs are an effective tool for canine weight loss. However, if feeding and exercise plans are not initiated, dogs will regain weight when treatment is stopped. The selectivity of MTP inhibitors varies by species. Dirlotapide

and mitratapide are not to be used in humans or cats due to the possible risk of hepatic lipid accumulation.

References and Suggested Reading

Bennett N et al: Comparison of a low-carbohydrate–low-fiber diet and a moderate carbohydrate–high-fiber diet in the management of feline diabetes mellitus, *J Feline Med Surg* 8:73, 2006.

Butterwick RF, Markwell PJ: Effect of amount and type of dietary fiber on food intake in energy-restricted dogs, *Am J Vet Res* 58:272, 1997.

Diez M et al: Weight loss in obese dogs: evaluation of a high-protein, low-carbohydrate diet, *J Nutr* 132:1685S, 2002.

Fettman MJ: Effects of neutering on body weight, metabolic rate and glucose tolerance of domestic cats, *Res Vet Sci* 62:131, 1997.

Jeusette I et al: Effect of ovariectomy and ad libitum feeding on body composition, thyroid status, ghrelin, and leptin plasma concentrations in female dogs, *J Anim Physiol Anim Nutr* 90:12, 2006.

Kirk CA et al: Influence of dirlotapide, a microsomal triglyceride transfer protein inhibitor, on the digestibility of a dry expanded diet in adult dogs, *J Vet Pharmacol Ther* 30s1:66, 2007.

Koerner A, Kratzsch J, Kiess W: Adipocytokines: leptin—the classical, resistin—the controversial, adiponectin—the promising, and more to come, *Best Pract Res Clin Endocrinol Metab* 19:525, 2005.

Li J et al: Discovery of potent and orally active MTP inhibitors as potential anti-obesity agents, *Bioorg Med Chem Lett* 16:3039, 2006.

Lund EM et al: Prevalence and risk factors for obesity in adult cats from private US veterinary practices, *Intern J Appl Res Vet Med* 3:88, 2005.

Lund EM et al: Prevalence and risk factors for obesity in adult dogs from private US veterinary practices, *Intern J App Res Vet Med* 4:177, 2006.

Michel KE et al: Impact of time-limited feeding and dietary carbohydrate content on weight loss in group-housed cats, *J Feline Med Surg* 7:349, 2005.

CHAPTER 43

Canine Diabetes Mellitus

WILLIAM E. MONROE, *Blacksburg, Virginia*

DEFINITION, EPIDEMIOLOGY, AND PATHOPHYSIOLOGY

Diabetes mellitus in dogs is a persistent defect of carbohydrate metabolism associated with an absolute deficiency of insulin in nearly all cases. Therefore almost every affected dog will require administration of exogenous insulin for management of the disease. The underlying cause in dogs is poorly understood, but is likely multifactorial, including genetic predisposition; infectious, toxic, or inflammatory damage of the pancreatic islets with progressive immune-mediated destruction; or predisposing conditions such as natural or iatrogenic endocrine disorders, obesity, and hyperlipidemia that cause insulin resistance with subsequent β-cell exhaustion. The hospital prevalence in North American teaching hospitals seems to have increased between 1970 (19 dogs per 10,000) and 1999 (64 dogs per 10,000). Part but perhaps not all of this increase may be explained by a general increase in the age of hospital populations. Females, neutered or intact, and neutered males are overrepresented, although female predisposition may be declining. The peak age of occurrence is 7 to 11 years, with 70% of patients older than 7 years at the time of diagnosis. Diabetes occurs rarely in dogs younger than 1 year of age.

Absolute insulin deficiency associated with canine diabetes mellitus is also associated with an increase in glucagon concentration. Together these changes lead to hyperglycemia, both from increased hepatic production and lack of peripheral use. When blood glucose concentration exceeds the renal threshold (180 to 220 mg/dl), osmotic diuresis occurs, leading to secondary polydipsia. There is also fatty acid mobilization with consequent increased production of ketoacids by the liver because the peripheral tissues become energy starved. In addition, ketoacid production is increased because of the lack of the effects of insulin on lipoprotein lipase and hormone-sensitive lipase to facilitate the storage of fatty acids in adipocytes. As ketoacid production exceeds the quantity used for energy metabolism, acidemia occurs, and spillover of ketones into the urine contributes to polyuria. Without insulin the ability of cells to use glucose is markedly diminished. Furthermore insulin deficiency reduces fatty acid deposition in adipocytes and decreases the incorporation of amino acids to form protein. These metabolic abnormalities create a catabolic state with resultant weight loss despite adequate or excessive food consumption.

DIAGNOSIS AND MANAGEMENT PLAN

The diagnosis of diabetes mellitus is based initially on a combination of clinical signs that generally include polyuria and polydipsia, weight loss in spite of a good appetite, and the demonstration of persistent hyperglycemia with glucosuria. It is not necessary to repeat blood and urine glucose testing to confirm the persistence of hyperglycemia if the clinical signs of polyuria, polydipsia, and or polyphagia have been noted. Ketonuria may be present in 66% of dogs with uncomplicated diabetes mellitus. Increased serum alkaline phosphatase, alanine transaminase, and hypertriglyceridemia are also common.

Once the diagnosis of diabetes mellitus has been established, it is important to determine if the dog has *complicated* diabetes (see Chapter 47). This is critical as diabetic ketoacidosis or hyperosmolar, nonketotic diabetes are complications that require aggressive in-hospital management. Conversely, uncomplicated cases are better managed as outpatients. The major clinical criteria for determining if a dog requires aggressive management relates to clinical findings; in other words, is the patient ill, anorexic, or vomiting or, conversely, is the dog eating and drinking well and exhibiting a generally healthy attitude. The dog that appears generally well and shows a good appetite can be managed as an uncomplicated diabetic even in the presence of ketonuria. Morbidity in these patients is rarely severe enough to require hospitalization and intensive care.

Before initiating therapy, it is also important to discuss the effort and cost of management of a diabetic dog with the owner and identify comorbid conditions. Lifestyle or financial circumstances may prevent some owners from successfully managing a diabetic pet. Foremost, it is important that the clinician have a clear understanding of the owner's lifestyle and daily schedule so that a feasible treatment and monitoring protocol can be developed. Additionally, many of these older dogs manifest concurrent disease that can affect control of the diabetes and also may influence the owner's decision to treat or not. Accordingly, a thorough medical evaluation should be conducted to identify concurrent diseases. In addition to the history and physical examination recommended studies include a complete blood count, serum chemistries (including canine pancreatic lipase immunoreactivity [cPLI]), urinalysis, urine culture, thoracic radiographs, and abdominal ultrasonography or radiography. It is not unusual for diabetic dogs to have clinically silent urinary tract infections, including a lack of pyuria in the sediment examination; thus it is important to culture the urine of all patients even if urinalysis results are unremarkable.

DIET, FEEDING SCHEDULE, AND EXCERCISE

Diets that are high in fiber, low in simple sugars, and moderately restricted in fat and protein are recommended for diabetic dogs (also see Chapter 45). However, the most important aspect of diet for diabetic dogs is that it be a balanced diet that the dog will eat consistently.

If dogs receive insulin twice daily, it is recommended to feed two equal meals at the time of insulin administration. Some clinicians recommend that the dog be fed before injecting insulin and withholding the insulin injection anytime the dog does not eat its entire meal. Although this may work well for a dog that is a gluttonous eater, it is less effective for finicky eaters or those dogs that eat small amounts throughout the day.

Even when insulin is given just once daily, it is still recommended that the dog be fed twice daily. The second meal should coincide with the glucose nadir (depending on when the owner can be home to feed) or alternatively should be presented 12 hours after the insulin injection. Feeding a larger portion of the daily diet around the time of the glucose nadir may lead to a less fluctuating glucose curve. However, if lente insulin given once daily provides adequate control, the glucose response can be improved in some cases by feeding the larger meal at the time of the insulin injection. This is because lente insulin contains 30% short acting-insulin (Semilente) and 70% long-acting insulin (Ultralente) and is absorbed in many dogs in a manner such that there are two peaks of insulin activity, with the earlier peak leading to the higher insulin concentration.

Exercise affects both the absorption of insulin and the metabolic use of glucose. Consequently, exercise levels should be kept constant with activity provided at the same times every day.

INSULIN THERAPY

As stated above, virtually all diabetic dogs require insulin therapy. Only one insulin product has recently been approved in the United States for use in dogs. Therefore in the past, veterinarians by necessity have relied on products labeled for human use. Current trends toward the use of recombinant human insulin and insulin analogs have further limited the number of products appropriate for canine diabetics. Additionally, many insulin products commonly used to manage diabetic dogs in the past have been removed from the market. Both recombinant human insulin (with one amino acid difference from canine insulin) and porcine insulin (with an identical amino acid sequence to canine insulin) have been advocated for canine diabetes because they may be less antigenic in dogs. The use of compounded insulin products is not recommended because of a lack of consistency and stringent control of the formulation.

The general recommendation for insulin treatment in dogs involves administration of an intermediate-duration-of-action insulin twice daily, or a long-duration-of-action insulin once daily. The only intermediate-duration products that are available currently are recombinant human neutral protamine Hagedorn (NPH) insulin and porcine lente insulin (Vetsulin, Intervet, Inc). An advantage of Vetsulin is that it is approved by the Food and Drug Administration for the dog. Since this product is produced and marketed by a veterinary company primarily for treatment of dogs, it should be available for many years. There is some experience with this product as it has been used in Canada and many European countries under the brand name Caninsulin for many years. Although it is not the identical product as the previously utilized pure porcine lente insulin (previously marketed for humans by Eli Lilly), it is very similar, and likely can be used in a similar manner in dogs.

In a recent study of 53 diabetic dogs designed to determine the safety and efficacy of Vetsulin (Monroe et al., 2005), 66% of the dogs required injections every 12 hours for adequate control of blood glucose. Sixty days after the appropriate dose and schedule were determined, the median Vetsulin dose was between 0.75 and 0.78 U/kg per injection (range 0.28 to 1.4 U/kg) for dogs receiving insulin every 12 hours and 1.09 U/kg (range 0.43 to 2.18 U/kg) for dogs receiving insulin once daily. All 53 dogs were adequately controlled at the end of the dose determination period, and 75% remained adequately controlled 60 days later.

There is a long-acting protamine zinc insulin available for veterinary use (PZI VET, IDEXX Pharmaceuticals). This insulin product contains 90% beef and 10% porcine insulin. Currently this preparation is not recommended for use in dogs because beef insulin is more antigenic than human or porcine insulin. This may increase the production of antiinsulin antibodies, which can lead to poor glucose control in some dogs. However, it should be noted that beef:pork (90:10) insulins were used for years to manage diabetic dogs with few reported problems.

Insulin glargine (Lantus, Aventis) is a human insulin analog in which the amino acid asparagine has been replaced by glycine within the α-chain and two arginine molecules have been added to the C-terminus of the β-chain. In the vial it is in solution at a pH of 4.0, but the insulin solution forms crystals that are absorbed slowly when injected subcutaneously (SQ) into an environment with a pH close to 7.0. It cannot be mixed with any other insulin products. In humans it is intended to provide basal insulin levels over an extended period when administered once daily. Although there is very little information about the use of this product in dogs, it may be useful as a longer-acting insulin in patients for which NPH or lente insulins have too short a duration to provide adequate glycemic control with two daily injections.

Determining Insulin Dose and Frequency of Administration

In dogs with uncomplicated diabetes it is recommended to initiate treatment with an intermediate–duration-of-action insulin product such as recombinant human NPH or porcine lente (Vetsulin) at a dose of 0.25 U/kg every 12 hours SQ starting at time in the morning that will fit the client's schedule. Blood glucose is measured two or three times at 3-hour intervals during the first day to ensure that the dose is not so high as to create hypoglycemia. If the blood glucose drops below 100 mg/dl at any time during the first day, the dose should be reduced by 25%. Because it can take several days for the dog to adjust to any change of insulin dose or product type, it is sent home to receive insulin injections for 5 to 7 days before the first recheck to monitor the response to the insulin. In an attempt to prevent tissue irritation from injecting insulin at the same site while maintaining consistent absorption of insulin from each injection, it is recommended to alternate injections at approximately 1 to 2 inches on either side of the midline. The suggested level is over the thorax from just caudal to the scapulae to the last rib, alternating from side to side. This allows for an injection site with similar blood supply, skin thickness, and muscular activity.

Since each dog may react uniquely to any insulin product, the appropriate dose and number of injections per day must be determined by monitoring the blood glucose response to the product (also see Chapter 46). This is accomplished by taking a careful history and performing a thorough physical examination, including body weight, to determine if clinical signs have resolved or are resolving. In addition, one should perform a glucose curve at 5- to 7-day intervals until the appropriate protocol is determined, which often takes 4 to 6 weeks. Performing one or two blood glucose measurements after the morning injection to titrate the insulin dose is inadequate and often leads to poor glucose control and hypoglycemia. To provide adequate information, the glucose curve should be performed after feeding the same food and giving the same insulin product and dosage at the usual times on the morning of the test. Blood glucose is determined every 2 hours for 10 to 12 hours, beginning either just before the dog is fed and given insulin or within 1 hour of doing so. Deciding to feed and give insulin to the dog at home before coming to the hospital depends on some practical factors: 1) the time in the morning that the dog is usually fed and treated, and 2) whether or not the dog is likely to eat normally in the hospital setting. It is best to keep feeding and insulin administration within 1 hour of the usual schedule while beginning the curve at a time that is practical for the owner and veterinarian.

Glucose concentration can be determined using a point-of-care analyzer or handheld glucose meter to reduce the amount of blood drawn and the associated trauma to the patient. Handheld glucose meters generally underestimate the serum or plasma glucose concentration by 10% to 15% compared to a reference laboratory.

Based on the results of the clinical response of the patient and the blood glucose curves, the insulin dose is adjusted by 1 to 5 U per injection, depending on the size of the dog and blood glucose concentrations measured every 5 to 7 days. The dose is adjusted to obtain a blood glucose nadir concentration of 80 to 150 mg/dl and to attempt to maintain the blood glucose concentration less than 250 to 300 mg/dl. It is important to determine the duration of insulin activity based on glucose curve results. To determine the duration of insulin activity, the blood glucose nadir must fall sufficiently (to the range of 80 to 150 mg/dl) so that glucose concentrations of greater than 250 mg/dl can be considered as representing near complete loss of the administered insulin effect. In addition, it is important that the blood glucose nadir concentration remain above 65 mg/dl; otherwise counterregulatory hormonal responses may stimulate blood glucose concentrations exceeding 250 mg/dl prematurely, before the true duration of insulin activity has been exceeded. If the blood glucose concentration just before the next scheduled insulin injection is less than 150 mg/dl and the glucose nadir was appropriate, the dog should be fed without giving the next injection of insulin, and the glucose curve continued until the blood glucose exceeds 250 mg/dl to determine if the duration of activity of the insulin product is longer than 12 hours. If the blood glucose exceeds 250 mg/dl within 1 to 2 hours of feeding without giving insulin, the duration of insulin activity is likely very close to 12 hours. Some dogs do not have an increase in blood glucose for some time after the injected insulin has been completely metabolized unless they are fed to provide a glucose source. If the glucose rises after feeding without giving insulin, it is generally safe to continue giving the same dose of insulin every 12 hours.

If the duration of insulin activity is longer than 14 but shorter than 16 hours and an extended glucose curve and or clinical signs indicate blood glucose concentration drops too low overnight, then administering a dose of the intermediate-duration insulin in the evening that is lower than the morning dose provides safe and adequate control in most cases. If the duration of insulin activity is longer than 16 hours, the dog may be adequately controlled with one daily injection of the product.

If the duration of action of an intermediate-duration insulin is longer than 16 hours but the dog continues to have clinical signs of polyuria and polydipsia, particularly during the night, a different intermediate-acting preparation could be tried every 12 hours, or a longer-acting product such as PZI or insulin glargine could be given once or twice daily. It cannot be overemphasized that when starting a diabetic dog on any insulin once daily, the duration of the response to that product must be determined by means of an adequate glucose curve. There is great variation among dogs in the duration of action of insulin products; for example, an insulin that is considered of long duration may have an effect of less than 12 hours in certain dogs. Treating with once daily insulin, but without adequate glucose monitoring, often leads to hypoglycemia. This is explained by the tendency to continue to increase the daily insulin dose in response to continued polyuria and polydipsia when the actual problem is not an inadequate dose but an inadequate duration of activity.

Longer-Term Monitoring of Insulin Therapy

Once the appropriate insulin preparation, dose, and dosing interval have been determined, it is appropriate to reevaluate the dog in 30 days. At that examination a history and physical examination should be conducted, and urine ketones, blood glucose curve, and perhaps fructosamine concentration measured. Thereafter rechecks every 3 to 6 months are appropriate unless the dog develops problems such as recurrence of polyuria or polydipsia, weight loss, signs of hypoglycemia, or another disease. The owner may be asked to check urine glucose and ketones periodically, but the dose of insulin should not be altered on the basis of urine glucose determinations alone. The presence of ketonuria, or of consistently high urine glucose, particularly if checked in the afternoon, should prompt reevaluation by the veterinarian.

Once an appropriate dose and schedule have been determined, it must remain consistent. Alternatively, the dose may be changed by the owner within a narrow, acceptable range set by the veterinarian. The client must understand that, as with humans, the true insulin need is likely to vary from day to day but the goal is to identify a dosage and schedule that will prevent clinical signs without episodes of hypoglycemia on most days. Realistic therapeutic goals are first to maintain the dog as an acceptable companion and pet and second to attempt to prevent formation of diabetic cataracts.

It has been well documented that fructosamine values in dogs that are well controlled can overlap with those that are poorly controlled and glucose curve values can vary from day to day. Therefore it is important not to rely on just one parameter to determine adequacy of glucose control or to change the insulin dose. If the glucose curve values do not seem to coincide with the history and physical examination results, the glucose curve should be repeated at the hospital, by the owner at home, or using a continuous glucose monitoring device while the dog is in the home setting. The clinical history and physical examination demonstrating resolution of polyuria and polydipsia; maintenance of body weight; normal appetite; and lack of clinical signs of hypoglycemia are generally the most reliable parameters for determining adequacy of glycemic control.

COMPLICATIONS AND PROGNOSIS

Hypoglycemia is one of the most serious complications of insulin therapy in diabetic dogs. Owners should be educated about the clinical signs of hypoglycemia, and should be instructed to feed a meal when signs of low blood glucose develop, assuming the dog is sufficiently aware to consume food safely. For dogs that are not fully conscious, the owner should be instructed to rub syrup or honey on the gingival mucosa in an attempt to revive the dog before calling the veterinarian.

Most dogs live for a few years with diabetes. The average survival may be approximately 3 years, but survival likely depends on the age of onset, concurrent disease, ease of management, and owner commitment. Most dogs develop cataracts within 5 to 6 months of the diagnosis, and 80% develop cataracts by 16 months after diagnosis.

References and Suggested Reading

Beam S, Correa MT, Davidson MG: A retrospective-cohort study on the development of cataracts in dogs with diabetes mellitus: 200 cases, *Vet Ophthalmol* 2:169, 1999.

Briggs C et al: Reliability of history and physical examination findings for assessing control of glycemia in dogs with diabetes mellitus: 53 cases (1995-1998), *J Am Vet Med Assoc* 217:48, 2000.

Fleeman LM, Rand JS: Evaluation of day-to-day variability of serial blood glucose concentration curves in diabetic dogs, *J Am Vet Med Assoc* 222:317, 2003.

Graham PA, Nash AS, McKellar QA: Pharmacokinetics of a porcine insulin zinc suspension in diabetic dogs, *J Small Anim Pract* 38:434, 1997.

Guptill L, Glickman L, Glickman N: Time trends and risk factors for diabetes mellitus in dogs: analysis of veterinary medical data base records (1970-1999), *Vet J* 165:240, 2003.

Hess R, Ward C: Effect of insulin dosage on glycemic response in dogs with diabetes mellitus: 221 cases (1993-1998), *J Am Vet Med Assoc* 216:217, 2000.

Ling GV: Diabetes mellitus in dogs: a review of initial evaluation, immediate and long-term management, and outcome, *J Am Vet Med Assoc* 170:521, 1977.

Monroe WE: Efficacy and safety of a purified porcine insulin zinc suspension for managing diabetes mellitus in dogs, *J Vet Intern Med* 19:675, 2005.

CHAPTER 44

Feline Diabetes Mellitus

JACQUIE S. RAND, *Queensland, Australia*

Diabetes mellitus is the second most common endocrinopathy in cats and affects approximately 1 in 50 to 1 in 400, depending on the population studied. Diagnosis of diabetes mellitus is based on finding persistently increased blood glucose concentration.

Management of diabetic cats depends on the stage of β-cell failure. In most cats diabetes is usually not diagnosed until relatively late in the disease process when extensive β-cell function has been lost. Diagnosis is typically made once blood glucose concentration is above the renal threshold and signs of polyuria, polydipsia, and weight loss are apparent. In contrast, in humans with type 2 diabetes, diagnosis is made earlier in the disease process. Cats and humans have a very similar range for normal blood glucose concentration. However, in humans diabetes is defined as persistent blood glucose concentration above 126 mg/dl (7 mmol/L) because of the proven microvascular complications associated with higher blood glucose concentrations. Because of this difference in diagnosis and extent of β-cell failure, the majority of humans and the minority of cats can be managed satisfactorily with oral hypoglycemic drugs.

Based on data in other species, blood glucose concentrations below the renal threshold but persistently above normal (e.g., 180-216 mg/dl [10-12 mmol/L]) are likely associated with adverse effects such as glucotoxic damage to β-cells and in cats should be classed as diabetes. With the current availability of low-carbohydrate feline diets, research is urgently needed to determine the most appropriate blood glucose concentration for institution of dietary management. Logically, if there are no contraindications such as azotemia, cats should be changed to a low-carbohydrate, high-protein diet whenever there is persistently increased blood glucose concentration (e.g., above 144 mg/dl [8 mmol/L]). These diets significantly reduce blood glucose concentrations compared with high-carbohydrate diets. Cats should then be monitored on a regular basis (e.g., every 3 to 6 months), and strategies introduced to limit weight gain and maintain optimum body condition.

PATHOGENESIS OF DIABETES IN CATS

To effectively manage diabetic cats, an understanding of the pathogenesis and main features of feline diabetes is required. The majority of owned cats in developed countries that develop diabetes likely have type 2 diabetes, which is characterized by a relative lack of insulin secretion and insulin resistance. Insulin resistance reduces the glucose-lowering effect of insulin. Diabetic cats are on average six times less sensitive to insulin than healthy cats, representing a similar magnitude of insulin resistance to that identified in humans with type 2 diabetes. Insulin resistance results from a number of mechanisms, and in most diabetic cats more than one mechanism is likely operating. A small percentage of cats have other specific types of diabetes resulting from B-cell destruction associated with pancreatitis and neoplasia, or have marked insulin resistance from excess growth hormone or corticosteroids.

Insulin Resistance

In humans the most important causes of insulin resistance are genotype, obesity, and physical inactivity. These same factors are also the most likely causes of insulin resistance in cats. It is important to be aware of these predisposing factors so that they are appropriately managed. This is vital in cats at risk of diabetes and also in cats in diabetic remission to ensure that they have the best chance of remaining in remission. Obesity markedly decreases insulin sensitivity in cats. An increase in body weight from an ideal weight of 4 kg to 6 kg halves insulin sensitivity in cats. Therefore management of body condition is an important part of therapy for prevention and management of feline diabetes. Physically inactive cats have been shown to be at risk of diabetes, and increasing physical activity improves insulin sensitivity in other species. One study in cats also found that active play for 10 minutes daily produced the same rate of weight loss as calorie restriction.

Genetic predisposition is likely a risk factor for insulin resistance and diabetes in cats. Lean cats with insulin sensitivity values below the median for the population were at three times greater risk of developing impaired glucose tolerance when they gained weight than cats with higher insulin sensitivity. Impaired glucose tolerance is the glycemic state between normal and diabetic. It is likely that these cats had underlying insulin resistance associated with genotype and, with time, obesity would result in diabetes in some. Burmese cats are at increased risk of diabetes in Australia, New Zealand, and the United Kingdom and appear to have underlying insulin resistance.

High blood glucose concentration also contributes to insulin resistance. In dogs it has been shown that this effect has a relatively short-term influence, with insulin resistance related more closely to glycemia over the previous 48 hours rather than over longer periods. This is relevant especially in the initial phases of treatment, and clinicians need to be aware that with decreasing blood glucose concentration insulin sensitivity is increased.

Impaired Insulin Secretion

Insulin secretion is decreased in feline diabetes through a number of mechanisms, some of which are reversible. Loss of β-cells in type 2 diabetes is thought to result from apoptosis triggered by chronic hyperfunction secondary to insulin resistance. β-cell loss also occurs as a result of islet amyloid deposition. Reversible suppression of insulin secretion occurs when blood glucose or lipid concentrations are high. This is called *glucotoxicity* and *lipotoxicity*, and both may act through similar intracellular mechanisms in the β-cell. With time chronic hyperglycemia irreversibly damages β-cells, and they are permanently lost, which can lead to insulin-dependent diabetes. Loss of β-cells also occurs through pancreatitis, and approximately 50% of diabetic cats have histologic evidence of pancreatitis. In most cats the severity of the lesion is not sufficient by itself to cause diabetes but potentially contributes to loss of β-cells. When insulin resistance is not involved, clinical signs of diabetes ensue once approximately 80% to 90% of β- cells are lost. If insulin sensitivity is reduced, clinical signs of diabetes occur earlier. If insulin sensitivity is reduced, clinical signs of diabetes occur earlier with smaller loss of B-cells. For example, with obesity-induced insulin resistance, cats need 30% more insulin to maintain fasting glucose concentration than when they were lean, and develop diabetes earlier with less B-cell loss. Veterinarians need to impress on owners the importance of attaining an ideal body condition in their diabetic cats or cats at risk of diabetes.

Diabetic Remission

Within days to months of beginning treatment with insulin, a proportion of diabetic cats are able to maintain euglycemia without therapy. This is called *diabetic remission*. The proportion of cats that achieve diabetic remission depends on how early tight glycemic control is instituted, on the type of therapy, and the underlying cause of their diabetes. Cats require functioning β-cells to attain remission. It is believed that reversal of glucotoxicity and lipotoxicity leads to diabetic remission. Therapies that provide the best glycemic control are likely to lead to the highest remission rates. Cats in remission may relapse in weeks to months, and it is important that they are carefully monitored and managed in remission. With early reinstitution of insulin therapy, many cats can again achieve remission.

MANAGEMENT OF DIABETES

The most important goals of therapy are to resolve clinical signs and avoid clinical hypoglycemia, which can be life threatening. The best way to resolve clinical signs is to achieve diabetic remission. Treatments available for management of feline diabetes include dietary modification, insulin, and oral hypoglycemic drugs. The prevalence of diabetes is increasing as risk factors such as obesity and physical inactivity become more common. Management and prevention of diabetes need to also address these risk factors. Maintaining ideal body weight and avoiding drugs such as corticosteroids and progestins are important for maintaining remission.

Diet

Diet is an important component of therapy, and a low-carbohydrate diet is vital for cats achieving diabetic remission (also see Chapter 45). A high-carbohydrate diet (50% of energy from carbohydrate) can increase mean blood glucose concentrations from 4 to 18 hours after eating by 20% to 25% and peak glucose concentrations by more than 30% compared with a moderate-carbohydrate diet (25% energy from carbohydrate). Cats eating an ultra-low–carbohydrate diet (5% of energy) have even greater reduction in blood glucose concentration. Reducing carbohydrate content of the diet also decreases the demand on β-cells to secrete insulin. Cats in diabetic remission likely have reduced β-cell mass, and, from the limited testing reported, approximately 50% have impaired glucose tolerance. It is vital that these cats be fed diets that spare β-cell function. Feeding a low-carbohydrate diet once diabetic remission is achieved will likely prolong remission. To achieve and maintain remission, it is important to achieve an ideal body weight because of the negative impact of obesity on insulin resistance. Diet is also important for achieving weight loss. A minority of cats fed canned low-carbohydrate, high-protein diets self-restrict energy intake and lose weight spontaneously after their diet is changed. For the majority of cats, energy intake needs to be restricted to achieve weight loss. Physical activity promotes weight loss and improves insulin sensitivity in other species, independent of body weight. Encouraging owners to engage in active play with their cat is likely beneficial.

Insulin Therapy

Insulin therapy is the mainstay of therapy in diabetic cats. Veterinary insulin preparations available for maintenance treatment of diabetic cats include porcine lente insulin (40 U/ml; Caninsulin/Vetsulin, Intervet, Inc.), and protamine zinc insulin (PZI, 100 U/ml Shering-Plough and PZI Vet 40 U/ml IDEXX Pharmaceuticals). Human insulin preparations used for long-term maintenance of diabetic cats include neutral protamine Hagedorn (NPH), glargine, and detemir. Human lente and Ultralente insulin preparations have been removed from the market in most countries.

Glargine

Glargine and detemir are long-acting insulins with different mechanisms of action. Both insulins have been used in cats, but only glargine has been subject to a controlled trial. Anecdotal information in cats suggests that detemir and glargine have similar effects. Anecdotal information in cats suggests that detemir and glargine have similar

clinical effects. In a trial of 24 cats, eight of eight newly diagnosed diabetic cats treated with glargine and an ultra-low–carbohydrate diet (5% of energy from carbohydrate; Purina DM canned) achieved remission compared with three of eight for PZI and two of eight for porcine lente. Remission rates of greater than 80% to 90% often can be achieved using glargine combined with a low- or ultra-low–carbohydrate diet in newly diagnosed diabetic cats. This compares with 20% to 30% using other insulin preparations and a standard feline maintenance diet. One study reported 60% remission rates using PZI or lente insulin and a low-carbohydrate diet. Lower remission rates occur in long-term diabetic cats changed to glargine therapy. Diabetic remission is unlikely in cats that have been diabetic for more than 2 years.

Because of the huge advantage to the client and the cat in achieving diabetic remission, it is strongly recommended that the *first choice of insulin for diabetic cats be glargine*. If there is a legal requirement to first use a veterinary insulin product, PZI would be the first choice because it has longer duration of action than lente insulin. lente insulin has too short a duration of action for optimal blood glucose control in cats. Using lente insulin, there is a period of at least 4 hours twice daily when there is no exogenous insulin action and high blood glucose concentrations ensue, often 360 mg/dl (20 mmol/L) or higher. Because the blood glucose concentration is very high, administering a potent insulin such as lente results in a rapid drop in blood glucose concentration. The hypothalamic neurons detect a falling blood glucose concentration and trigger counterregulatory mechanisms before hypoglycemia occurs. This is because these neurones control their intracellular glucose concentration by limiting glucose uptake when plasma glucose concentration is high. With a rapidly dropping blood glucose concentration, the hypothalamic neurons become hypoglycemic at relatively high blood glucose concentration. The resultant counterregulatory mechanisms are often triggered when blood glucose concentration is still above the normal range. Cortisol, epinephrine, and glucagon are released, producing insulin resistance and increasing blood glucose concentrations. The end result is further shortening of insulin action, which for some cats treated with lente insulin is only about 3 hours. It also results in insulin resistance, and the following insulin injections may result in little appreciable glucose lowering effect.

Recommendations for Using Glargine

Glargine is a long-acting insulin designed to provide basal insulin concentrations in humans with type 1 and 2 diabetes. Administration in humans is coupled with prandial administration of an ultra-short–acting insulin or oral hypoglycemic drug. In cats, because the postprandial period is so prolonged (12 to 24 hours) compared with humans, administration of an ultra-rapid–acting insulin at the time of eating is unlikely to be useful.

Glargine is produced by recombinant deoxyribonucleic acid technology using *Escherichia coli*. It is supplied as a clear, colorless solution of monomeric insulin with a pH of 4.0. When injected into the subcutaneous tissues with a pH of 7.0, glargine forms hexamers, and microprecipitates deposit in the tissues. These slowly break down, releasing monomeric glargine into solution, which gives glargine its long duration of action. It is because of this mechanism of action that glargine cannot be diluted or mixed with other insulins. Glargine is available only at a concentration of 100 U/ml, which makes accurate dosing a problem in cats, particularly when very low doses are being administered close to remission. Insulin syringes with 0.25-U or ¼-U gradations, which are very useful for cats, are available in the United States.

Glargine has been used successfully in cats with a starting dose of 0.5 U/kg BID if blood glucose is ≥360 mg/dl (≥20 mmol/L). The initial starting dose should not exceed 3 U/cat BID. It is strongly recommended that glargine be administered twice daily in the first 4 months of therapy to maximize glycemic control and diabetic remission. Glargine administered once daily has been shown to be similar in effectiveness to lente insulin twice daily. In general the dose should not be increased in the first week, except if little or no glucose-lowering effect is still evident after the third day. In many cats the dose needs to be reduced in the first 7 days. It is important that if the dose is increased after the third day there is intensive glucose monitoring. Increasing the dose without monitoring can result in clinical hypoglycemia. It is recommended that close monitoring and adjustment of dose occur in the first month of treatment because many cats achieve diabetic remission within this time. It is prudent to keep the cat in the hospital and check blood glucose concentration for the first 3 days after institution of treatment to check for evidence of hypoglycemia. If this is not possible, closely monitor urine glucose concentration and water drunk as indicators of glycemic control. If a marked decrease in water drunk occurs in the first week or urine glucose becomes negative, recheck the cat because a lower insulin dose is likely indicated. If no monitoring of glucose, water drunk, or urine glucose concentration is possible, it is safer to begin with 1 U/cat BID and increase dose weekly. Poor monitoring and inadequate tailoring of the dose to control hyperglycemia will delay or prevent diabetic remission.

It is recommended that cats be checked weekly in the first 4 to 8 weeks after institution of therapy and the dose be adjusted appropriately (Box 44-1). Glargine can be used in combination with regular insulin in treating ketoacidosis. Administer the usual starting dose of glargine subcutaneously twice daily and regular insulin intramuscularly at 1 U every 2 to 4 hours, aiming to keep glucose between 145 and 250 mg/dL (8 and 14 mmol/L). Regular insulin is required until appetite returns or dehydration is resolved, which is 24 to 48 hours in most cats.

Occasionally the dose of glargine needs to be increased to 5 or 6 U/cat and rarely 10 U/cat twice daily over the first 1 to 2 months. In the majority of these cats, once glycemic control is achieved, the dose then needs to be reduced. Careful monitoring is required to prevent hypoglycemia. Rarely is hyperadrenocortism or acromegaly a cause for treatment failure. When they are present, high doses of insulin are often required, especially with acromegaly, which may require extreme doses (>25 U/cat BID) to control blood glucose concentration. Do not delay insulin therapy and wait to determine if blood glucose normalizes after instituting therapy for underlying conditions contributing to insulin resistance. If blood glucose

concentrations are elevated (≥270 mg/dl; ≥15 mmol/L), insulin therapy should be instituted immediately to preserve β-cells and not be delayed until after other specific therapy.

Determining If Diabetic Remission Is Present

Many cats achieve diabetic remission within 2 to 4 weeks. It is strongly recommended that insulin therapy not be withdrawn prematurely. Cats with almost normal β-cell

---

Box 44-1

Current Recommendations For Adjusting Dose of Glargine in Diabetic Cats

1. **Indications for increasing the dose of glargine**
   - If pre-insulin glucose concentration is ≥216 mg/dL (12 mmol/L), then increase dose by 0.25-1 U/injection, depending on the degree of hyperglycemia.
   and/or
   - If nadir (lowest) glucose concentration is ≥180 mg/dL (≥10 mmol/L), then increase dose by 0.5-1 U/injection.
   - Only for well well-controlled cats after several weeks of therapy, increase dose if nadir ≥145 mg/dL (≥8 mmol/L).
2. **Indications for maintaining the same dose**
   - If pre-insulin glucose concentration is ≥180-<216 mg/dL (≥10-<12 mmol/L)
   and/or
   - If nadir glucose concentration is 90-160 mg/dL (5-9 mmol/L).
   - For well-controlled cats after several weeks of therapy, aim for a nadir of 72-145 mg/dL (4-8 mmol/L).
3. **Indications for decreasing dose of glargine**
   - If pre-insulin glucose concentration is ≤180 mg/dL (≤10 mmol/L), decrease by 0.5-1 U/injection.
   - If nadir glucose concentration is <54 mg/dL (<3 mmol/L), decrease by 1 U/injection.
   - If clinical signs of hypoglycemia develop, administer 50% glucose IV bolus followed by 2.5% glucose infusion; then reduce dose by 50% and check for remission.
   - If clinical hypoglycemia develops and is not severe, it often can often be managed by feeding the cat, preferably food containing a higher carbohydrate level, such as some dry foods. However, it must be palatable enough to eat. Most weight-reducing and renal diets are high-carbohydrate diets, as are many grocery lines of dry food.
   - For cats with unexpected biochemical hypoglycemia (not clinical signs), some owners find that they can manage the hypoglycemia by delaying the insulin injection until blood glucose increases to 180 mg/dL (10 mmol/L) and then giving the same dose (the following dose of insulin may need to be reduced) whereas; others find it best to reduce the dose once glucose is 180 mg/dL (10 mmol/L), although this may result in subsequent hyperglycemia.
4. **Insulin dose may be maintained or decreased, depending on the water drunk, urine glucose, clinical signs, and length of time the cat has been treated with insulin**
   - If nadir is 54-72 mg/dL (3-4 mmol/L)

Modified from Rand and Marshall: *Vet Clinics of North America* 2004. Reprinted with permission. Updated recommendations can be found at www.uq.edu.au/vetschool/centrecah.

function can tolerate 0.5 to 1U once or twice daily and rarely develop clinical hypoglycaemia. If insulin therapy is stopped prematurely and hyperglycemia recurs, once insulin is reinstituted it can take weeks or months to achieve the same level of glycemic control. It is not recommended that insulin therapy be stopped within a minimum of 2 weeks of initiating treatment to facilitate β-cell recovery from glucotoxicity. Insulin dose should be decreased gradually based on dosing guidelines in Box 44-1. Once preinsulin blood glucose concentration is ≤180mg/dl (≤10mmol/L) and total dose is decreased to 0.5 to 1U BID, reduce the dosing frequency to once daily. If after 1 week preinsulin blood glucose is still ≤180mg/dl (≤10mmol/L) and nadir glucose concentration is in the normal range (72 to 126mg/dl; 4 to 7mmol/L), discontinue insulin therapy and monitor blood glucose concentration during the day. If blood glucose rises above 180mg/dl (10mmol/L) within 12 to 24 hours, immediately reinstitute insulin at 1U once daily and wait a minimum of 2 weeks before again attempting withdrawal of insulin. If blood glucose concentration is less than 180mg/dl (10mmol/L), continue to withhold insulin, checking blood glucose every 3 to 7 days for several weeks, and carefully monitor the cat for signs of hyperglycemia (increasing thirst and glycosuria). Owners should diligently measure water drunk and monitor urine glucose concentration because increased thirst or glycosuria likely indicates relapse. If blood glucose is ≥180mg/dl (10mmol/L), insulin therapy should be reinstituted immediately. Some cats regain substantial β-cell function but require 0.5 to 1U of insulin every 2 to 3 days to maintain normoglycemia.

In general, blood glucose concentration following glargine administration does not change as quickly as with shorter-acting insulins such as lente; therefore monitoring every 4 hours is usually adequate. Critical time points to monitor are the blood glucose concentration just before each glargine injection (i.e., the preinsulin morning and evening glucose concentrations). For many cats the evening blood glucose concentration is lower than the morning concentration and is often the nadir glucose concentration. It is important to understand that occasionally blood glucose concentration can change rapidly, especially during the night, and can increase from 54 to 324mg/dl (3 to 18mmol/L) in 2 hours. It is not clear whether this rapid increase in blood glucose is mediated by counterregulatory hormones (Somogyi phenomenon) or reflects marked hepatic gluconeogenesis associated with negligible insulin concentrations. A rapid increase in blood glucose is more common when glargine is given once daily. Cats with low normal glucose concentration when last monitored in the evening may have very high blood glucose concentrations the next morning. In some cats decreasing the dose of glargine decreases morning blood glucose concentration, suggesting that the morning hyperglycemia may be the result of a Somogyi response. Somogyi phenomenon appears to be very rare in cats treated with glargine compared with shorter-acting insulins such as lente insulin. Cats treated with glargine appear quite susceptible to stress-induced hyperglycemia associated with hospital monitoring of blood glucose. If marked hyperglycemia is occurring in the hospital, it is critical that information be obtained on glycemic control at home before the hyperglycemia is attributed to treatment failure. Measurement of water drunk, urine glucose concentration, or home monitoring of blood glucose concentration helps to clarify the level of glycemic control.

Biochemical Hypoglycemia

Cats treated with glargine often have biochemical hypoglycemia without clinical signs of hypoglycemia. Humans treated with glargine have significantly lower frequency of clinical hypoglycemia compared to those treated with NPH insulin. In cats clinical hypoglycemia also appears to be less common than when lente insulin is used. For cats with biochemical hypoglycemia (without clinical signs), some owners who are monitoring at home find that they can manage the hypoglycemia by feeding the cat and delaying the insulin injection until blood glucose increases to 180mg/dl (10mmol/L) and then giving the same dose; whereas others find it best to reduce the dose once glucose is 180mg/dl (10mmol/L), although this may result in subsequent hyperglycemia. If the first dose after biochemical hypoglycemia is not reduced, the second dose should be reduced unless the preinsulin blood glucose concentration is unusually high for that cat. Most cats showing signs of clinical hypoglycemia with glargine are in diabetic remission or will achieve remission within a few weeks.

Monitoring Glycemic Control

In addition to blood glucose measurements, water drunk and urine glucose concentration are invaluable indicators of glycemic control. Diabetic cats with exemplary glycemic control drink volumes similar to those of nondiabetic cats (<10ml/kg/24 hour if eating canned food and <60ml/kg/24 hour with dry food). When using glargine, in contrast to lente insulin, monitoring urine glucose concentration is less useful for detecting diabetic remission. This is because well-controlled diabetic cats that still require glargine to control blood glucose concentrations have negative or trace urine glucose concentration. However, urine glucose concentration is more useful for indicating a need for an increase in dose when using glargine. Fractious cats can be stabilized using urine glucose concentrations and water drunk alone, although glycemic control is usually not as good as when combined with blood glucose monitoring; therefore diabetic remission may be delayed or not achieved.

Storage of Glargine

Although the manufacturer recommends discarding glargine within 4 weeks of opening, an open vial of glargine can usually be kept for 6 months or more if *refrigerated*. The manufacturer's recommendation is based on the risk of bacterial contamination with multiple-use vials. Vials that develop any cloudy discoloration should be discarded immediately. This may represent precipitation or bacterial contamination.

Oral Hypoglycemic Agents

Oral hypoglycemic drugs act either by stimulating β-cells to secrete insulin, increasing insulin sensitivity, or by reducing glucose absorption from the gastrointestinal tract. Glipizide is the most commonly used oral hypoglycemic drug in cats and acts by stimulating β-cells. It should not be offered as a first line of therapy because of the poorer control of blood glucose concentration and the subsequently lower rate of diabetic remission. However, it can be lifesaving for cats when the owner would elect for euthanasia if insulin injections were the only available treatment. Glipizide may be used instead of insulin in cats that have insufficient β-cell function to achieve remission but require only minimal doses of insulin to control hyperglycemia.

Acarbose inhibits brush-border glycosidase activity in the intestine and reduces postprandial blood glucose concentrations. Changing to an ultra-low–carbohydrate diet has a greater glucose-lowering effect than administering acarbose. However, cats that need a reduced-protein diet (high-carbohydrate) for control of azotemia might benefit from the addition of acarbose at 12 to 25 mg/cat twice daily at the time of eating. It is minimally effective if the cat is eating multiple meals daily. Acarbose should be administered twice daily, even if the cat is only fed once daily.

In summary, management of diabetic cats is optimized by using glargine administered subcutaneously twice daily, combined with a low-carbohydrate, high-protein, feline diabetes diet and obesity management. Using this protocol to keep maximum blood glucose <200 mg/dL (<11 mmol/L). can result in diabetic remission in approximately 90% of newly diagnosed diabetic cats.

References and Suggested Reading

Lepore M et al: Pharmacokinetics and pharmacodynamics of subcutaneous injection of long-acting human insulin analog glargine, NPH insulin, and ultralente human insulin and continuous subcutaneous infusion of insulin lispro, *Diabetes* 49:2142, 2000.

Marshall R, Rand J: Treatment with insulin glargine results in higher remission rates than lente or protamine zinc insulins in newly diagnosed diabetic cats, *J Vet Intern Med* 19:425, 2005.

Marshall R, Rand J: Comparison of the pharmacokinetics and pharmacodynamics of once- versus twice-daily administration of insulin glargine in normal cats, *J Vet Intern Med* 16:373, 2002.

Rand JS, Marshall RD: Diabetes mellitus in cats, *Vet Clin North Am Small Anim Pract* 35:211, 2005.

Weaver KE: Use of glargine and lente insulins in cats with diabetes mellitus, *J Vet Intern Med* 20:234, 2006.

CHAPTER 45

Diet and Diabetes

DEBRA L. ZORAN, *College Station, Texas*

Diabetes mellitus in dogs and cats is a complex, multifactorial disease that results in insulin deficiency or a dysfunctional response to insulin. The disease affecting dogs is primarily one that results in the complete loss of β-cell function caused by destruction of these cells. In contrast, the disease in cats is quite different and is similar to the obesity-related diabetes associated with glucose toxicity and insulin resistance that is seen in adult humans. Nevertheless the end result in both forms of diabetes is hyperglycemia with associated abnormal lipid and protein metabolism, resulting in a catabolic state sometimes termed *starvation in the face of plenty*.

Insulin therapy is the mainstay of treatment for both diabetic dogs and cats (see previous chapters), but, because diabetes is a disease of disordered metabolism, nutritional therapy is a key component of the management of these patients. The goals of dietary therapy in any diabetic dog or cat are broad based and include the following: (1) to achieve and maintain optimal body condition; (2) to provide a nutritionally complete, balanced, and palatable food that is readily consumed (so intake is predictable); (3) to provide nutritional support for any concurrent diseases requiring nutritional modification; (4) to maintain consistency in the timing and type (e.g., ingredients and calories) of food to assist in achieving optimal glycemic control; and finally (5) because the primary determinant of postprandial glycemia is starch, to control the amount and types of dietary starch present in the diet. Unfortunately, because of the paucity of well-designed dietary studies in diabetic dogs and cats, dietary recommendations cannot be based on research alone. Further, recent work has uncovered some important differences between dogs and cats in the most effective dietary management strategies for this disease. This chapter reviews the most relevant aspects of nutritional management of diabetes, the major differences between dogs and cats, and the role of specific nutrients and supplements in the management of diabetes.

DIETARY MANAGEMENT OF CANINE DIABETES MELLITUS

Dogs with diabetes typically are presented for examination because of polyuria, polydipsia, polyphagia, and/or weight loss; and many diabetic dogs have a thin body condition at the time of diagnosis. Thus the goal of achieving optimal body condition in a diabetic dog requires a dietary strategy that will not only assist in the control of postprandial glycemia but will also allow the dog to regain its normal body weight (BW). However, some diabetic dogs will be obese or of normal body condition; in these dogs the dietary strategy is still focused on achieving optimal body condition, but the type and amount of diet may be somewhat different than that for a dog that is very thin and needs to gain weight. One key point is that there is no single dietary strategy that works for all canine diabetics; thus clinicians must tailor their dietary recommendations to fit the specific needs of the individual dog.

Dietary Fiber

For many years diets containing increased amounts of dietary fiber have been recommended for dogs with diabetes because they improve postprandial glycemia presumably by delaying gastric emptying, slowing carbohydrate digestion and absorption, and altering gut hormones. However, dietary fiber is a term that encompasses a wide variety of complex carbohydrates that have widely varying effects in the gastrointestinal (GI) tract. Thus it is necessary to understand how dietary fiber is characterized and how these characterizations affect the ability of the fiber to affect glycemia in dogs.

Generally fiber is characterized by its degree of solubility, which also generally reflects its degree of fermentability (i.e., how completely the intestinal bacteria can break it down) and its properties in water (e.g., intestinal juice). Highly soluble fibers such as guar gum have a great water-holding capacity and form a viscous gellike solution in the lumen of the intestine. Normal dogs fed diets high in soluble fibers have more rapid glucose absorption because of increased intestinal glucose transport, increased glucagon-like peptide-1, and increased insulin secretion. In normal dogs this type of fiber lowers circulating glucose levels in glucose tolerance tests, but it is unknown whether these same effects occur in diabetic dogs.

Studies in nondiabetic dogs have evaluated the effects of diets containing different fiber types (highly fermentable, poorly fermentable or insoluble, and mixed-fiber types) to further clarify these issues. In these reports there was no significant difference between the effects of diets on oral glucose tolerance testing; serum triglyceride levels; or the cholesterol content of high-density lipoproteins, low-density lipoproteins, or very low–density lipoproteins. The only significant difference created by the diets was that total serum cholesterol concentrations were lower in dogs fed the diets containing mixed fiber.

Studies in diabetic dogs suggest that diets high in insoluble or mixed fiber may be associated with improved glycemic control. Insoluble-fiber diets appear to exert little physiologic effect on the canine GI tract compared to soluble-fiber diets and are not fermented by the bacterial flora; therefore these diets are tolerated in higher levels with fewer side effects (e.g., diarrhea, flatulence). In studies comparing a mixed-fiber diet to a lower-fiber maintenance diet, there was significantly improved glycemic control in the group of diabetic dogs fed the mixed-fiber diet. However, regardless of the type or concentration of high-fiber diet fed or the duration of time over which the dogs were monitored, there was no significant difference in the daily insulin requirement or fasting triglyceride levels in diabetic dogs.

Finally there is a highly variable difference between dogs in their response to dietary fiber—in other words, there does not appear to be a uniform effect of fiber in all diabetics, and the effect of a type or amount of fiber in a diabetic dog is not predictable. A recent investigation in diabetic dogs compared a canned, high-fiber, moderate-starch diet to one that contained a moderate amount of fiber and starch but an increase in dietary fat. In these stable diabetic dogs there was no significant difference between the diets in insulin requirements or glycemic response.

Thus the decision to use a diet with increased dietary fiber in the therapy of a diabetic dog should be based on individual circumstances since there is no clear indication that these diets are beneficial in all cases. However, in dogs that may need to lose weight or those that are having poor glycemic control with a normal maintenance diet, diets containing increased insoluble or mixed fiber are reasonable choices. If the dog does not tolerate or will not eat a diet with increased amounts of fiber, the clinician should choose a maintenance or weigh-reduction diet containing lower fat and high complex carbohydrates. Table 45-1 illustrates different diets, both fiber-containing veterinary diets and non-fiber-containing diets that may be used in diabetic dogs.

Dietary Carbohydrates, Fat, and Protein

The glycemic index classifies food based on its potential to increase blood glucose following absorption from the GI tract. To make diets that result in a more manageable postprandial blood glucose concentration, the glycemic index of the starch must be considered in diabetic dogs. In healthy dogs the amount of starch in the diet is a major determinant of the glycemic index, no matter what type of dog food is tested. In one study of healthy dogs, rice-based diets resulted in significantly higher postprandial glucose levels, while sorghum-based diets (especially barley) resulted in the lowest glycemic response. However, predicting the glycemic index of food is not based solely on the type of starch present in a diet, but on the matrix in which the carbohydrate is found, the type of processing the carbohydrate has undergone, and the total amount of carbohydrate consumed. Unfortunately, there are little data about the responses of diabetic dogs to different diets and different types of carbohydrates; thus it is difficult to make specific evidence-based recommendations for these dogs with diabetes. However, because highly digestible diets designed for GI disease often contain rice-based carbohydrate sources, these diets may not be ideally suited for diabetic dogs.

Diabetic dogs also have abnormalities in lipid metabolism secondary to the lack of insulin production. These changes include hypertriglyceridemia; hypercholesterolemia; and increases in lipoproteins, chylomicrons, and free fatty acids. In contrast to humans, who have

Table 45-1

Canine Selected Diabetic Diet Comparisons of Prescription and Nonprescription Products*

Diet	Protein (% As Fed)	CHO type	CHO (% As Fed)	Fat (% As Fed)	Fiber Type and Amount (% As Fed)	Calories (kcal/ Cup or Can)
Hill's prescription diets w/d dry	17.2	Corn meal	44.7	8.1	Peanut hulls	243
Hill's prescription diets w/d canned	4.5	Corn meal, barley	13.2	3.2	Cellulose	372
Hill's Science Diet adult dry	23.3	Corn meal, sorghum, wheat	48.1	14.3	Mixed 1.9	365
Hill's Science Diet adult canned	5.7	Corn meal, barley	13.2	3.9	Mixed 0.2	408
Purina veterinary diet DCO	23.0	Corn, barley	43.5	11.3	Mixed 6.95	320
Purina Pro Plan small breed adult dry	31.7	Brewers rice, corn	32.2	19.1	Mixed 2.0	460
Purina Pro Plan weight management canned	9.5	Potatoes	5.10	3.1	Mixed 0.20	279
Purina Pro Plan weight management dry	27.9	Brewers rice, corn	44.6	9.3	Mixed 2.5	337
Royal Canin diabetic HF 18 dry	20.0	Rice, ground corn	44.2	9.0	Mixed 11.0	186
Royal Canin Hifactor formula dry	24.2	Corn, Brewers rice	33.4	11.5	Mixed 13.0	233

*Based on current product guides.

increased risk of cardiovascular disease and stroke, the major consequence of hypertriglyceridemia in dogs is the increased risk of pancreatitis, which clearly complicates the management of diabetes and increases the risk for secondary complications and morbidity. In most diabetic dogs the lipid values improve with the administration of insulin and by feeding a diet containing lower fat and higher fiber content. Current recommendations by nutritionists suggest feeding a diet that contains less than 30% of metabolizable energy from fat; however, there are very little published data on the influence of dietary fat or the optimal level of fat in dogs with diabetes.

In humans with diabetes, omega-3 fatty-acid supplementation has been recommended to reduce serum lipid levels, blood pressure, and platelet aggregation—all benefits that are important to reduce the risk of stroke and cardiovascular disease. However, in some humans with diabetes, consumption of increased amounts of omega-3 fatty acids results in increased blood glucose and an overall reduction in glycemic control. The effects of omega-3 fatty acids have not been adequately evaluated in dogs with diabetes; thus whether or not these same effects occur in dogs is not known.

Finally, L-carnitine is a conditionally essential vitamin-like nutrient that has an essential role in fatty acid metabolism. Dog with poorly controlled diabetes are prone to ketogenesis, weight loss, and altered fat metabolism—all factors that can be attenuated by improved lipid metabolism that may occur with supplementation of carnitine. The amount of carnitine that is needed to achieve this effect in dogs with diabetes is not clear, but in one report as little as 50 ppm added to a canine diet improved lipid parameters in normal dogs.

Protein catabolism occurs when insulin concentrations are low or ineffective. Catabolism of muscle proteins is a protective mechanism designed to supply substrate (amino acids) that can be used for gluconeogenesis. Thus in unregulated diabetics, in diabetics that are not eating well, or in those being fed inadequate protein in the diet, muscle proteins are used. To prevent this loss of essential tissue, it is necessary that both an adequate quality and quantity of protein be supplied in the diet of diabetic dogs. In general, diets for diabetic dogs should contain a highly digestible (85% to 90%), high-quality protein (18% to 25% on a dry-matter basis) to reduce muscle catabolism. Such diets also provide adequate protein for maintenance and repair but do not appear to increase the risk of diabetic nephropathy.

Micronutrients

When a complete and balanced diet is fed in appropriate quantities for a dog's BW and condition, there is no need for additional vitamin and mineral supplementation in the majority of diabetic dogs. However, in many diabetic dogs that are not consuming a balanced diet (e.g., those consuming homemade or single-item diets) or in those that have uncontrolled diabetes, the risk of development of a micronutrient imbalance is increased.

The macrominerals most likely to be affected in diabetic dogs are potassium, magnesium, and phosphorus. In most dogs with adequate glycemic control that are consuming appropriate amounts of an adult maintenance food, either no macromineral imbalance occurs, or it self-corrects. Appropriate monitoring of electrolytes is an important aspect of clinical evaluation of any diabetic, but especially in any dog that is not well controlled or is ill.

The importance of micronutrients in diabetics has been a topic of considerable interest in a variety of species for many years. The most important micronutrients in diabetes are zinc, chromium, selenium, copper, and manganese. Of these nutrients the essential role of zinc in the synthesis, storage, and secretion of insulin is clearly established; however, the exact mechanisms underlying altered zinc metabolism in diabetes in dogs have not been identified; thus specific recommendations for supplementation are difficult. Further, excesses of zinc can be quite detrimental and can cause complications such as gastritis and gastric ulceration, copper deficiency, and hemolytic anemia. The same ambiguity exists for the use of chromium in diabetic dogs. Chromium is essential for normal carbohydrate and lipid metabolism, and supplementation in humans with diabetes improves insulin sensitivity and overall control; but few studies have been performed in dogs with diabetes, and in one study no increase in glycemic control was observed.

Currently the best approach in diabetics is to feed a diet that has microminerals supplied according to the AAFCO recommendations for adult maintenance (see Appendix), and, if the dog is unwilling to eat this type of diet, a standard adult human vitamin-mineral supplement (1 tablet/dog/day) containing a United States Pharmacopeia (USP) label can be administered safely to prevent development of a micronutrient deficiency.

Food Type and Feeding Plans

As a general rule, most diabetic dogs, regardless of diet chosen, can be well managed with feeding a consistent diet at consistent times with concurrent administration of an appropriate amount of exogenous insulin. And, because there is no clear evidence that specific diets in diabetic dogs are essential to good glycemic control, the first rule of thumb is that the nutritional requirements of any concurrent disease in the diabetic dog should take precedence when choosing a diet. The next most important issue of diet selection is palatability to ensure that the dog will consistently and predictably consume the diet.

Both canned and dry foods are acceptable food types for diabetic dogs; however, because dry foods empty the slowest from the stomach, they have a somewhat greater effect in decreasing postprandial hyperglycemia than canned foods. Nevertheless, if the dog will more consistently consume the diet if it contains some canned food or if the dog needs the added water in its diet, canned foods are a completely acceptable diet for diabetics. Soft, moist foods should be avoided entirely because they contain large amounts of simple sugars (e.g., dextrose, fructose, sucrose, cane molasses) that are highly digestible and result in a large increase in blood sugar. In general, highly digestible foods (diets with greater than 90% digestibility) designed for GI disease may result in greater postprandial hyperglycemia; thus they are likely not the best diets for diabetic dogs. Conversely, diets with less than 80% nutrient digestibility and low fat concentrations may not be sufficient to help a thin diabetic regain lost BW.

Finally, it is ideal to choose a diet that has a fixed formula (as opposed to an open formula) so that there are fewer variations in the diet formulation that can affect the individual

Table 45-2

Calculating Calories

	Equations for Calculating Caloric Intake
Canine RER: ideal BW	$70(BW_{kg})^{0.75}$ or $45\text{-}50 \times BW_{kg}$
Canine MER: ideal BW	$125(BW_{kg})^{0.75}$ or $BW_{kg} \times 60\text{-}70$
Feline RER: ideal BW	$70(BW_{kg})^{0.75}$ or $40\text{-}45 \times BW_{kg}$
Feline MER: ideal BW	$90(BW_{kg})^{0.75}$ or $BW_{kg} \times 50\text{-}60$
Weight loss	Calculate calories for ideal BW (or a target below obese weight); if the number of calories is not less than what is currently being consumed, reduce intake by 10%-20%; assess in 2-4 weeks and readjust so that weight loss of 1%-2% per week is achieved

BW, Body weight; *MER,* maintenance energy requirement; *RER,* resting energy requirement.

response. Open-formula diets are those found in a typical grocery store or pet specialty supply stores, the formulation of which changes with market prices. Thus the glycemic index changes as the formulation of the open formula diet changes over time, which may result in a variable insulin response.

Once the diet is chosen, the next most important aspect of dietary management is to impress on the owner the importance of feeding consistent amounts of food at consistent times. Ideally diabetic dogs should be fed one half of their total daily energy requirement at a specified time in the morning at time of insulin administration. Then the second half of the dog's energy requirements should be given at the evening meal, approximately 12 hours later, coinciding with the evening insulin administration.

Calculation of energy requirements for diabetic dogs should be based on maintenance energy needs of the dog's ideal BW (Table 45-2). However, if the dog fails to gain weight despite an appropriate amount of insulin and food, an increase in the energy density of the food or increased daily caloric intake will be required. A final key point for a successful dietary management strategy in the dog is simply to monitor the BW and glycemic control and adjust the diet as needed but to maintain as much consistency as possible not only in the food type but also in the timing and amount.

DIETARY MANAGEMENT OF FELINE DIABETES

As in diabetic dogs, dietary therapy is a very important aspect of successful management of the diabetic cat. However, unlike the dietary therapy of dogs in which a diet containing increased dietary fiber and complex carbohydrate is recommended, management of feline diabetics requires a completely different strategy. There is now strong evidence showing that a diet containing high protein and low concentrations of carbohydrate is the most effective approach. In addition, because many feline diabetics are obese and have obesity-induced insulin resistance as part of their disease, dietary management of obesity is an essential aspect of therapy of this disease.

Thus, although dietary therapy of feline diabetes has similar goals to that in dogs, the approach is quite different.

Dietary therapy of feline diabetes has three major goals: (1) to correct or normalize BW (e.g., for the majority of cats that means to achieve weight loss); (2) to minimize the stimulation of pancreatic β-cells by glucose; and (3) to stimulate endogenous insulin secretion by feeding a diet high in arginine (a potent insulin secretagogue) and other amino acids.

Obesity is a major medical problem in the domestic feline population, with as many as 25% to 35% of cats in the United States being either overweight (15% to 20% over ideal BW) or obese (>20% over ideal BW). Obesity-induced diabetes currently is believed to be the most common form of diabetes in cats; thus both from the perspective of prevention as well as therapy, weight management is the first and possibly the most key aspect of dietary therapy. To induce weight loss in cats, a dietary strategy must be embraced that includes the following: (1) feed a diet high in protein to reduce muscle wasting and prevent the lipid and protein metabolic derangements that occur during calorie restriction; (2) feed a diet that is reduced in energy (both fat and carbohydrates) to stimulate fat mobilization; (3) adjust the food consumption to BW and response to food reduction; and finally, (4) consider supplementation with L-carnitine (a vitamin-like supplement that increases fat oxidation and maintenance of lean muscle tissue). A number of diets may be acceptable for this purpose, but the goal should be to have fat less than 4 g/100 kcal, starch less than 5 g/100 kcal, and protein content greater than 10 g/100 kcal. Diets with this profile stimulate loss of fat tissue and at the same time preserve lean muscle tissue (which is lost in cats fed lower-protein diets that are highly energy restricted).

The other essential aspect of achieving weight loss is to control energy intake. In most obese cats this means that meal feeding will be required to be able to provide the specified calories needed to achieve restriction. Maintenance energy needs for most indoor neutered cats are estimated to be 45 to 50 kcal/kg/day. However, to achieve weight loss the caloric intake may have to be more restricted, with a reduction in calories from the target goal of 10% to 40% being required in some cats. However, weight loss must be monitored carefully so that the loss does not exceed 1% to 2% per week or hepatic lipidosis will occur. Many canned diets have a high-protein, low- to moderate-fat, low-carbohydrate profile and provide a way to control calories by volume; thus they are a good dietary choice for a feline weight-loss program. One of the most difficult aspects of

any weight-loss program is controlling intake while feeding both protein and volume to provide satiety. Because caloric intake can be easily and specifically controlled, protein levels are often high, and the added water increases volume, canned foods are a highly desirable option for weight loss. Table 45-3 illustrates the caloric differences among several high-protein, low-carbohydrate canned and dry diets and other diets that are fed to cats for weight loss.

The second goal of dietary therapy of feline diabetes is to control systemic blood glucose levels and reduce the perpetuation of the phenomenon of glucose toxicity occurring in the pancreatic β-cells. Before our understanding of the importance of high-protein, low-carbohydrate diets in cats with diabetes, diets high in fiber and carbohydrates were recommended for dietary management. However, feeding these diets led to high postprandial blood glucose concentrations, glucose toxicity, and ultimately reduced insulin secretion by the β-cells. Because the overall strategy in feline diabetics is unique (i.e., to achieve clinical diabetic remission and normalization of β-cell production and release of insulin), the dietary strategy first has to be aimed at reduction of postprandial blood glucose levels by feeding low-carbohydrate diets. In one study of newly diagnosed diabetic cats, cats placed on insulin and a high-protein, low-carbohydrate diet were four times more likely to achieve clinical remission; and, in cats that did not achieve remission, the amount of insulin required to control their diabetes was reduced by half. In addition to the amount of carbohydrate present in the diet, the type of carbohydrate source also appears to be important in cats, as it is in dogs. However, studies in diabetic cats comparing these diets to low-carbohydrate diets are lacking.

The third major aspect of dietary therapy of feline diabetes, which is to stimulate insulin secretion, is also achieved by feeding a high-protein, low-carbohydrate diet. In cats arginine and other amino acids are potent insulin secretagogues. Even in cats with glucose-induced hyposecretion of insulin, insulin secretion in response to the presence of arginine is normal to increased. Feline diets that are rich in animal source proteins contain abundant arginine, which contributes to endogenous insulin secretion in the diabetic cat and subsequently may help lead to diabetic remission.

In addition to high-protein, low-carbohydrate diets, dietary management of diabetic cats requires some consideration of their eating habits and the potential for hypoglycemia as a result of return of β-cell function. Unlike dogs, cats with diabetes on high-protein, low-carbohydrate diets do not need to match feeding with insulin admin-

Table 45-3

Feline Diabetic Diet Comparisons*

	Protein (% As Fed)	CHO (% As Fed)	Fat (% As Fed)	Calories (kcal/Cup or Can)
Hill's prescription diet m/d dry	48.9	14.6	20.7	480
Hill's prescription diet m/d canned	13.1	3.9	4.8	156
Purina veterinary diets DM dry	53.3	13.8	16.5	592
Purina veterinary diets DM canned	12.9	3.4	4.0	194
Royal Canin diabetic DS 44 dry	46.0	23.8	12.0	239

*Based on product guides.

istration, especially if the insulin glargine is being used. This is because postprandial hyperglycemia is minimal and instead blood glucose is prolonged after a meal because of the cats' unique glucose metabolism. Blood glucose levels in both normal and diabetic cats rises slowly and steadily after a meal and stays elevated for several hours, making timing of insulin administration to coincide with a postprandial glucose peak unnecessary. Diabetic cats that are not obese may be fed ad libitum to mimic the natural feeding pattern of the cat, which also reduces the risk of hypoglycemia should their own insulin secretion resume. However, an obese diabetic cat must be meal fed; preferably these cats are fed several small meals spread over 24 hours to provide calorie control to initiate weight loss and to provide an energy source should the cat attain diabetic remission. Calorie restriction is necessary in an obese diabetic cat to achieve weight loss; however, it is also important to be cautious because an increase in caloric needs for the diabetes may result in too rapid weight loss.

Because diabetic remission is an important goal, especially in newly diagnosed obese or previously obese cats, frequent monitoring (both of weight loss and glycemic control) and access to small amounts of food is the best strategy. The specific techniques used to monitor successful control of blood glucose in feline diabetics are beyond the scope of this paper but represent an essential aspect of diabetic management in cats (see Chapter 44). However, with appropriate use of diet in the management of feline diabetes, the goal of successful control, which may include clinical remission of the diabetes, can be achieved.

References and Suggested Reading

Benner N et al: Use of a low-carbohydrate versus high-fiber diet in cats with diabetes mellitus, *J Vet Intern Med* 15:297, 2001.

Biourge VC: Feline diabetes mellitus: nutritional management, *Waltham Focus* 15:36, 2005.

Farrow HA, Rand JS, Sunvold GD: The effect of high-protein, high-fat, or high-carbohydrate diets on postprandial glycemia and insulin concentrations in normal cats, *J Vet Intern Med* 16:360, 2002.

Fleeman LM, Rand JS: Beyond insulin therapy: achieving optimal control in diabetic dogs, *Waltham Focus* 15:12, 2005.

Frank G et al: Use of a high-protein diet in the management of feline diabetes mellitus, *Vet Ther* 2:238, 2001.

Kimmel SE et al: Effects of insoluble and soluble dietary fiber on glycemic control in dogs with naturally occurring insulin-dependent diabetes mellitus, *J Am Vet Med Assoc* 216:1076, 2000.

Marshall R, Rand JS: Insulin glargine and high-protein low-carbohydrate diet are associated with high remission rates in newly diagnosed diabetic cats, *J Vet Intern Med* 18:401, 2004.

Mazzaferro EM et al: Treatment of feline diabetes mellitus using an alpha glucosidase inhibitor and a low-carbohydrate diet, *J Feline Med Surg* 53:183, 2003.

Nelson RW et al: Effect of dietary insoluble fiber on control of glycemia in dogs with naturally occurring diabetes mellitus, *J Am Vet Med Assoc* 212:380, 1998.

Rand JS, Marshall R: Understanding feline diabetes mellitus: pathogenesis and management, *Waltham Focus* 15:5, 2005.

Remillard RL: Nutritional management of diabetic dogs, *Compend Contin Educ* 21:699, 1999.

CHAPTER **46**

Diabetic Monitoring

CLAUDIA E. REUSCH, *Zurich, Switzerland*

The aim of therapy in diabetic pets is to eliminate the clinical signs of diabetes mellitus, prevent short-term complications (e.g., hypoglycemia and ketoacidosis) and enable a good quality of life. It is not necessary to establish normal or near-normal blood glucose levels as it is in humans, for whom it is well known that good glycemic control significantly reduces the risk of life-threatening chronic complications (e.g., nephropathy and cardiovascular disease). These complications require many years to develop and are considered rare in diabetic dogs and cats. Most diabetic pets are doing well if the blood glucose concentrations (BGCs) are kept between 5 and 15 mmol/L (90 to 270 mg/dl) throughout 24 hours.

Management of diabetic dogs and cats relies on the owner's observations of clinical signs and on periodic evaluation by a veterinarian. The latter includes assessment of the owner's observations, measurement of body weight, and determination of blood glucose and serum fructosamine concentrations. Traditionally blood glucose measurements and generation of serial blood glucose curves were almost always performed in veterinary hospitals because most owners were unable to collect venous blood samples. Recently methods have been developed to collect capillary blood samples from the pet's ear that allows owners to measure BGCs at home. Home monitoring of blood glucose has displaced the measurement of urine glucose nearly completely in the clientele in our practice.

MONITORING IN THE HOSPITAL

Frequency of Reevaluations

After diagnosis of diabetes mellitus, the owner should be informed that it usually takes 2 to 3 months until stable glycemic control is achieved (see Chapter 43) and that lifelong regular reevaluations in the hospital are required. The exception to this guideline is animals (usually cats) that develop remission of their diabetes (see Chapter 44). Initially frequent reevaluations should be scheduled. With time, intervals between rechecks can be extended. In our hospital reevaluations are suggested at 1, 3, 8, and 12 weeks after diagnosis and then at intervals of approximately every 4 months.

Serum Fructosamine

Fructosamine measurements are widely used as an indicator of glycemic control in diabetic dogs and cats. Measurement is done in serum using commercially available test kits adapted to autoanalysis. Storage at 25° C for 5 days does not cause a significant change in fructosamine concentrations, allowing shipping of serum samples. Since fructosamine is the product of an irreversible reaction between glucose and the amino groups of plasma proteins, it is assumed that its concentration reflects the mean BGC of the preceding 1 to 2 weeks. Serum fructosamine concentration is not affected by short-term increases of blood glucose (approximately less than 4 days); therefore it is also a valuable tool to differentiate between diabetic and stress hyperglycemia in cats. Reference ranges differ slightly among laboratories but usually are somewhere around 200 to 360 µmol/L.

In the vast majority of newly diagnosed diabetic dogs and cats, fructosamine levels are greater than 400 µmol/L, but they may be as high as 1500 µmol/L. Normal fructosamine levels may be seen in animals with very short duration of diabetes mellitus. Fructosamine may also be normal in animals suffering from certain concurrent diseases. It has been shown that hypoproteinemia, hyperlipidemia, and azotemia in dogs and hypoproteinemia and hyperthyroidism in cats can decrease the fructosamine concentration. In these cases fructosamine measurements should not be used for the diagnosis or the long-term management of diabetes mellitus.

In all other cases it is helpful to measure fructosamine concentrations during routine reevaluations. The parameter is independent of stress and lack of food intake, which are both major influencing factors for blood glucose measurements in the hospital. Fructosamine concentrations increase when glycemic control worsens and decrease when glycemic control improves. It should be noticed that differences between two consecutive measurements have to exceed 50 µmol/L to reflect a clinically significant difference in glycemic control.

As mentioned earlier, normoglycemia is not a treatment goal in veterinary medicine, and even well-controlled diabetic dogs and cats are slightly-to-moderately hyperglycemic throughout the day. Consequently fructosamine usually does not become completely normal during therapy. In contrast, the finding of a normal fructosamine level (in particular fructosamine levels in the lower half of the reference range) should raise concern for prolonged periods of hypoglycemia caused by insulin overdose. In cats in which fructosamine levels decrease into the normal range during therapy, the possibility of diabetic remission has to be considered. Fructosamine levels between 360 and 450 µmol/L usually suggest good control, levels between 450 and 550 µmol/L suggest moderate control, and levels greater than 600 µmol/L suggest poor metabolic control. In the latter situation fructosamine measurement does not help to identify the underlying problem. All reasons for poor regulation have to be considered, including insulin underdosage, too short duration of insulin effect, diseases causing insulin resistance, and the Somogyi phenomenon.

Over the years, we and others have sometimes seen discrepancies between fructosamine on one hand and clinical sign and blood glucose on the other hand. Although high fructosamine levels suggested poor control, the lack of clinical signs and glucose level within the desired range pointed to good control. The reason for the discrepancy remains ambiguous in most instances, but it is possible that there are individual differences with regard to the extent of protein glycation. In those cases the assessment based on clinical signs should be given priority over assessment of fructosamine.

In animals with diabetic ketoacidosis, dehydration, acidosis, and other unidentified factors may influence fructosamine concentrations. Therefore fructosamine levels measured at the time of admission may differ considerably from the fructosamine concentration measured a few days later after successful therapy. It is advisable to repeat the measurement at the time of discharge and to use this level as a reference point for future measurements.

Glycated Hemoglobin

Glycated (glycosylated) hemoglobin has been used in human medicine since the 1970s and is regarded as the cornerstone of assessment of glycemic control in all major clinical trials. Comparable to fructosamine, it is formed by nonenzymatic, irreversible attachment of glucose to a protein amino group. Glucose first enters red blood cells and then interacts with amino groups of the globin chain of the hemoglobin. Although glycation kinetics is relatively complicated, it is commonly assumed that glycated hemoglobin reflects the average BGC over the life span of the erythrocytes, which is 100 to 120 days in dogs and 70 days in cats. Currently glycated hemoglobin is only rarely used as a long-term parameter in veterinary medicine. The main explanation for this situation pertains to the numerous assays available each measuring different components of hemoglobin; therefore results may not be comparable among laboratories. Furthermore, many of those assays do not provide valid results in dogs and cats.

Blood Glucose Measurements and Serial Blood Glucose Curves

Single blood glucose measurements are usually insufficient to assess glycemic control. Exceptions to this rule are dogs and cats with unremarkable history and physical examination and a serum fructosamine between 360 and 450 µmol/L. In these cases the finding of a BGC between

180 and 270 mg/dl around the time of insulin injection would support the assumption of good glycemic control and may render further blood glucose measurements unnecessary. Evaluation of a serial blood glucose curve (BGC) is mandatory in the initial phases of diabetic regulation and in animals with persistence of clinical signs, ongoing weight loss, and fructosamine greater than 500 µmol/L. It is the BGC that provides guidelines for making rational adjustments in insulin therapy.

We usually recommend that feeding and insulin injection be done at home and that the animal be presented to the hospital as soon as possible thereafter. If technical difficulties are suspected, owners are asked to bring the animal to the hospital before the insulin application and to perform the whole administration procedure under the supervision of a veterinarian or a technician. Blood samples are then taken every 1 to 2 hours throughout the day until the next insulin injection in both cases.

BGCs enable the assessment of insulin efficacy, the glucose nadir, the time of peak insulin effect, the duration of the effect of insulin, and the degree of fluctuation in BGC. The most important parameters are insulin efficacy, glucose nadir, and duration of effect. Insulin efficacy, which is the difference between the highest and the lowest glucose concentration, has to be interpreted in the light of the highest BGC and the insulin dosage. A relatively small difference (e.g., 50 mg/dl) is acceptable in an animal in which the highest glucose concentration is less than 200 mg/dl; however, the same difference is not acceptable if the highest glucose level is greater than 300 mg/dl. Similarly the same difference (e.g., 100 mg/dl) may indicate insulin efficacy in an animal receiving a small dose of insulin (< 0.5 U/kg) but may point to insulin resistance if the insulin dose is high (>1.5 U/kg). In addition to insulin resistance, technical problems with the insulin administration procedure, stress hyperglycemia in the cat, and the counterregulatory phase of the Somogyi phenomenon also have to be considered.

After insulin effectiveness is confirmed, the glucose nadir should be interpreted and should ideally be between 90 and 140 mg/dl. A nadir less than 80 to 90 mg/dl can be seen with insulin overdosage, excessive overlap of insulin actions, lack of food intake, and strenuous exercise. In cases in which overdosage is identified, the insulin dosage should be reduced by 10% to 50%, and excessive overlap of insulin action may require a change to an insulin with shorter duration of action. If the nadir is greater than 160 to 180 mg/dl, insulin underdosage, stress hyperglycemia, the counterregulatory phase of the Somogyi phenomenon, and technical problems of the owners have to be considered. If the animal is already treated with high insulin doses, insulin resistance also may be possible. It is very important to identify the exact cause because treatment decisions differ and may be completely opposite of one another. For example, insulin underdosage should be treated by increasing the insulin dose by 10% to 25%, whereas the Somogyi phenomenon would be treated by decreasing the dosage by at least 50%.

Careful evaluation of the other parameters of glycemic control such as clinical signs and serum fructosamine is mandatory. In addition, it may be necessary to assess the owner's insulin administration technique. It should be remembered that the counterregulatory phase of the Somogyi phenomenon may last up to 72 hours. Therefore several BGCs may be required to demonstrate a decrease of blood glucose to less than 60 mg/dl (or a very rapid decrease regardless of the nadir), followed by an increase in blood glucose to a concentration greater than 300 mg/dl within a 12-hour period following insulin administration.

Duration of insulin effect is evaluated if the glucose nadir lies in the desired range of 90 and 140 mg/dl and if there has not been a very rapid decrease of blood glucose after insulin injection. The duration is defined as the time from insulin injection through the glucose nadir until the BGC exceeds 250 to 270 mg/dl. If the duration of insulin effect is less than 8 to 10 hours, animals usually show clinical signs of diabetes mellitus. In contrast, if the duration is longer than 14 hours, the risk of developing hypoglycemia or the Somogyi phenomenon increases.

Problems Encountered With Monitoring Blood Glucose in the Hospital

Interpretation of BGCs generated in hospitalized animals may be difficult because of the potential influence of stress, abnormal housing conditions (e.g., lack of exercise), and decreased food intake on BGCs. A recent study by Fleeman and Rand (2003) showed that there is a large day-to-day variability when BGCs were performed on consecutive days in diabetic dogs. In addition, BGCs are time-consuming and expensive; therefore they are often not performed as frequently as required. Many patients would benefit from more frequent blood glucose determinations. For example, short-notice adjustments of the insulin dosage are necessary in diabetic patients with infections (increased dose) or at times of increased physical activity (mostly decreased dose). Close monitoring of BGC is also indicated in diabetic patients that are treated for a concomitant disease such as hyperadrenocorticism or hypothyroidism. Similarly, intact bitches may require adjustments of the insulin dosage at the transition from one stage of the cycle to another. Because of the abolition of the resistance to insulin associated with these conditions, the required insulin dosage may have to be reduced drastically to prevent life-threatening hypoglycemia. It is difficult to manage these cases without frequent blood glucose determinations.

MONITORING AT HOME BY THE OWNER

Frequency of Monitoring

Owners should assess their animals with regard to the clinical signs of diabetes mellitus on a daily basis. Body weight should be taken at least once a week. It is important that the owner be familiar with the clinical signs of the most important complications of diabetes mellitus (i.e., hypoglycemia and diabetic ketoacidosis). Today measurement of blood glucose is also feasible for owners and may be recommended for many owners.

Home Monitoring of Blood Glucose

Problems with diabetic control in people are similar in principle to those encountered in veterinary medicine.

Many of these issues have been largely eradicated since the late 1970s with the introduction of self-monitoring of blood glucose (SMBG) concentration. For SMBG humans obtain a drop of capillary blood by pricking a fingertip with a lancing device. The drop is then placed on a test strip, and the glucose concentration is measured using a portable glucose meter (PBGM). During the last few years similar methods for monitoring BGC have been developed for dogs and cats. The method used in Zurich is performed with a lancing device creating a negative pressure (Microlet Vaculance, Bayer Diagnostics, Zurich, Switzerland). Capillary blood is obtained from the inner aspect of the pinna, and BGC is determined with a PBGM. The method is relatively inexpensive, fast and easy to perform, and can be used by owners of diabetic dogs and cats to determine BGC and to generate BGC at home. Other techniques for blood sampling such as the marginal ear vein technique have also been described by Thompson and colleagues (2002).

Since their introduction, the quality control of PBGMs has been a frequent topic of discussion in human medicine. Studies have shown that accuracy can vary greatly but in general tends to be poor for very low as well as for very high glucose concentrations. Factors with a possible effect on the results of glucose measurements include variation in hematocrit, altitude, environmental temperature and humidity, hypotension, hypoxia, and triglyceride concentrations. It has become difficult to maintain the overview for the accuracy of all available PBGMs because new devices are frequently being developed by various companies, all of which claim to be smaller in size, faster in action, and easier to handle than their predecessors. Because PBGMs are usually made for use in humans and accuracies differ, quality control studies before their use in dogs and cats are extremely important. However, overall performance of these systems depends not only on analytic performance of the meter and quality of the test strips but also on the skills of the user.

For pet owners, home monitoring (HM) of blood glucose can constitute a challenge; therefore it is important to minimize technical difficulties as much as possible. Owners should be provided with a PBGM that is simple to operate. In our experience, the Ascensia Elite or the latest generation Ascensia Contour (both made by Bayer Diagnostics) are very easy to operate. Both meters have no buttons to press, turn on automatically when the test strip is inserted, and require a very small amount of blood, which is automatically aspirated into the reaction chamber after contacting the test strip. For the Ascensia Contour the measurement range is 10 to 600 mg/dl, the results are displayed within 15 seconds, and the last 240 measurements are stored. An additional advantage is the very low amount of blood (0.6 µl) required for blood glucose measurement. For more than 6 years, we have been involved in HM of diabetic dogs and cats, and the results have been extremely positive. The majority of owners are very interested in measuring blood glucose in their pets, and about 70% have been capable and willing to perform HM on a long-term basis.

A number of steps should precede the introduction of HM. The first step is a definitive diagnosis of diabetes mellitus. Additional tests to diagnose concurrent diseases may be indicated at this point. The owner then receives detailed information about various aspects of diabetes mellitus and careful instruction on injection technique, and the concept of HM is mentioned for the first time. This consultation takes approximately 45 minutes. The second step consists of reevaluation of the patient after 1 week. Observations made by the owner are discussed, a clinical examination is performed, and fructosamine concentration and a 12-hour BGC are generated in the hospital. Treatment is adjusted if necessary. At the time of discharge, the importance of the BGC in the control of the disease is emphasized. In addition, the advantages of HM for owner and pet are discussed, and the owner is informed that this procedure can be started after the next reevaluation.

The third step follows approximately 3 weeks after the diagnosis has been made. The owner is now provided the opportunity to learn the technique of HM. This requires a minimum of 30 minutes and consists of repeated demonstrations of the use of the lancing device and the PBGM. The owner then performs the technique several times in the pet. He or she is also taught how to calibrate the PBGM (if needed), how to check the meter's accuracy using the control strips, and how to record the blood glucose values on forms prepared by our clinic. HM is not started before the third week after a diagnosis of diabetes mellitus. This allows the owner to become familiar with the disease and to gain experience with the injection of insulin. However, introduction of HM is delayed to a later date if the owner does not seem ready for it.

Once the owner is comfortable with the procedure, we request that a fasting BGC be determined twice weekly and a BGC once monthly. The former serves to detect morning hypoglycemia, in which case the owner is instructed to call us. For determination of a BGC, the BGC is measured before the insulin injection (fasting) and every 2 hours thereafter. Since all our diabetic animals receive insulin BID, the BGC is performed over a 12-hour period. The owner sends the results of the BGC, and appropriate changes in treatment are discussed, if necessary, on the telephone. The assessment of the BGC generated at home follows the same rules as for the BGC generated in the hospital. Periodic reassessments of the entire procedure in the hospital are mandatory. For the first 2 months the patient is reassessed at least once a month; after that time, the frequency of rechecks is reduced to approximately every 4 months.

It is important that owners have ready access to veterinary support, if required. The majority of our clients call for advice one or more times, especially after the start of HM. Sometimes support via telephone is not sufficient, and additional explanation or demonstration of the technique must be provided. By watching an owner perform the procedure, a veterinarian can identify and correct errors immediately. The most frequently encountered technical problems included inadequate formation of a blood drop caused by excessive pressure of the finger behind the ear while lancing the ear, repeated depression of the plunger instead of allowing the negative pressure to slowly build up, and failure to fill the test strip to the mark. Therefore these procedural steps require explicit explanation and demonstration. Handling the PBGM usually is not a problem for owners, and most report that their pet tolerates blood collection well. The skin puncture does not seem to be painful, and the puncture sites are barely visible, even after numerous blood collections.

Recently Casella and colleagues (2003) and Casella, Hässig, and Reusch (2005) compared BGCs generated at home with those generated in the hospital with regard to treatment decisions. In about 60% of cases treatment decisions would have been the same; in about 40% treatment decisions would have been different. In the 40% in which treatment decisions would have differed, only 3% of dogs and 8% of cats would have had treatment decisions that would have been contrary (e.g., increase versus decrease of insulin dosage); in the others, although the decisions would have been different, they would have had little clinical consequence. Our most recent studies indicate that there also is a lot of variability if BGCs are performed at home on consecutive days. Therefore single curves may not reflect the true glycemic situation regardless of whether they are generated in the hospital or at home. However, one of the major advantages of HM is that it enables frequent generation of BGCs, which may be of particular importance in animals that are difficult to regulate. In those cases more than one BGC can be performed at home before a decision is made concerning therapy.

Long-term compliance of pet owners is good; many perform HM for several years. According to a recent retrospective survey in cat owners, only a minority adjusted insulin doses independently, and most of them called the hospital for advice. All cat owners believed that HM provides major advantages over in-hospital monitoring.

It has been argued that pet owners who are able to perform HM would visit the hospital less frequently. However, our observations over the last years do not support this. Frequency of reevaluation does not differ among pets with or without HM.

HM is a valuable additional tool in the management of dogs and cats with diabetes mellitus. One of its major advantages is that blood glucose can be measured more frequently than when it has to be done in the hospital. In animals that are difficult to regulate, several BGCs generated at home can be interpreted before a treatment decision is made.

Monitoring of Urine Glucose

Until blood glucose measurement became possible, urine glucose testing was the main method of assessing glycemic control at home. Glucose is freely filtered at the glomerulus and actively resorbed at the proximal tubule. The resorption capacity for glucose is limited; and, when the BGC exceeds the so-called renal threshold (approximately 180 mg/dl in dogs and approximately 300 mg/dl in cats), urine glucose excretion is roughly proportional to hyperglycemia. However, measurement of urine glucose may be misleading for several reasons: (1) the result does not reflect the actual blood glucose but is an average over the time of urine accumulation in the bladder; (2) a negative urine test does not differentiate between hypoglycemia, normoglycemia, or mild hyperglycemia;

and (3) hydration status and urine concentration may affect the result. It is also possible that in individual dogs and cats the renal threshold may increase or decrease as is known to occur in humans. Therefore severe hyperglycemia may exist without glucosuria, and glucosuria may occur with a normal BGC.

We do not adjust insulin dosages on urine glucose measurements, nor do we allow owners to do this. Owners who are unable to measure blood glucose but still want monitor may be advised to use urine glucose measurements in all urine samples voided throughout 1 day per week. Persistent glucosuria would suggest inadequate glycemic control and the need for thorough evaluation in the hospital. In susceptible animals (repeated bouts of diabetic ketoacidosis), we recommend that owners check the urine for ketone bodies on a regular basis to detect impending or actual ketoacidosis.

References and Suggested Reading

Casella M et al: Home monitoring of blood glucose concentration by owners of diabetic dogs, *J Small Anim Pract* 44:298, 2003.

Casella M, Hässig M, Reusch CE: Home-monitoring of blood glucose in cats with diabetes mellitus: evaluation over a 4-month period, *J Feline Med Surg* 7:163, 2005.

Crenshaw KL et al: Serum fructosamine concentration as an index of glycemia in cats with diabetes mellitus and stress hyperglycemia, *J Vet Intern Med* 10:360, 1996.

Feldman EC, Nelson RW: Canine and feline endocrinology and reproduction, ed 3, St Louis, 2004, Saunders, pp 486, 539.

Fleeman LM, Rand JS: Evaluation of day-to-day variability of serial blood glucose concentration curves in diabetic dogs, *J Am Vet Med Assoc* 222:317, 2003.

Graham PA, Mooney CT, Murray M: Serum fructosamine concentrations in hyperthyroid cats, *Res Vet Sci* 67:171, 1999.

Jensen AL: Serum fructosamine in canine diabetes mellitus: an initial study, *Vet Res Commun* 16:1, 1992.

Kley S, Casella M, Reusch CE: Evaluation of long-term home monitoring of blood glucose concentrations in cats with diabetes mellitus: 26 cases (1999-2002), *J Am Vet Med Assoc* 225:261, 2004.

Lutz TA, Rand JS, Ryan E: Fructosamine concentrations in hyperglycemic cats, *Can Vet J* 36:155, 1995.

Reusch CE et al: Fructosamine: a new parameter for diagnosis and metabolic control in diabetic dogs and cats, *J Vet Intern Med* 7:177, 1993.

Reusch CE, Tomsa K: Serum fructosamine concentration in cats with overt hyperthyroidism, *J Am Vet Med Assoc* 215:1297, 1999.

Reusch CE, Haberer B: Evaluation of fructosamine in dogs and cats with hypo- or hyperproteinaemia, azotaemia, hyperlipidaemia and hyperbilirubinaemia, *Vet Rec* 148:370, 2001.

Reusch CE, Gerber B, Boretti FS: Serum fructosamine concentrations in dogs with hypothyroidism, *Vet Res Commun* 26:531, 2002.

Thompson MD et al: Comparison of glucose concentrations in blood samples obtained with a marginal ear vein nick technique versus from a peripheral vein in healthy cats and cats with diabetes mellitus, *J Am Vet Med Assoc* 221:389, 2002.

Wess G, Reusch C: Capillary blood sampling from the ear of dogs and cats and use of portable meters to measure glucose concentration, *J Small Anim Pract* 41:60, 2000.

CHAPTER 47

Complicated Diabetes Mellitus

DEBORAH S. GRECO, *St. Louis, Missouri*

Complications arising from the diabetic state are the most common reason for mortality from diabetes mellitus; the majority of diabetic animals die of renal failure, infections, or hepatic/pancreatic disease rather than from diabetes mellitus itself. Most cats presented for diabetic ketoacidosis (DKA) have concurrent diseases, including hepatic lipidosis, cholangiohepatitis, pancreatitis, chronic renal failure, urinary tract infection, and neoplasia. Many diabetic dogs exhibit elevated liver enzymes, lipemia, and bacteriuria. Diabetic dogs often suffer from conditions such as dermatitis or otitis externa, hyperadrenocorticism, acute pancreatitis, tumors, and hypothyroidism

Frequently there is an underlying stressful event that precipitates the shift from diabetes mellitus to DKA or nonketotic hyperosmolar diabetes mellitus. The precipitating event may be a urinary tract infection; other viral or bacterial infection; or an inflammatory disorder such as pancreatitis, pyelonephritis, cholangiohepatitis, inflammatory bowel disease (IBD), eosinophilic granuloma complex, prostatitis, pyometra, upper respiratory infection, or pneumonia. Other concurrent diseases may include renal insufficiency or failure, hepatic lipidosis, neoplasia, or congestive heart failure. Recent drug therapy may also precipitate a crisis, especially administration of corticosteroids or progestagens. Therefore further diagnostic testing of the diabetic patient that presents in a crisis is essential, particularly use of abdominal radiography and/or ultrasonography, as well as thoracic radiography and/or echocardiography, if indicated. Additional testing for concurrent endocrine diseases such as hyperthyroidism in cats and hypothyroidism and hyperadrenocorticism in dogs may also be indicated but should be postponed until some control of the diabetes mellitus is achieved, inasmuch as uncontrolled disease may affect the results of the tests.

Concurrent conditions may be difficult to distinguish from complications of diabetes mellitus. Generally diabetic complications fall into the following six major categories: (1) diabetic nephropathy, (2) diabetic neuropathy (peripheral and autonomic), (3) susceptibility to infections (e.g., urinary, pulmonary), (4) hepatic and pancreatic disease, (5) diabetic ocular problems (cataracts), and (6) hypoglycemic complications.

DIABETIC NEPHROPATHY

Diabetic nephropathy occurs in approximately 40% to 50% of insulin-dependent humans with diabetes; however, the complication develops over a long period of time, often as long as 20 years. Although dogs may suffer from diabetic nephropathy, as evidenced by proteinuria and systemic hypertension, cats are more likely to suffer the long-term consequences of diabetic nephropathy because of a longer life span. However, the exact incidence of diabetic nephropathy in cats remains unknown. Diabetic nephropathy, like other diabetic complications, is associated with poor glucose regulation.

The earliest sign of diabetic nephropathy is microalbuminuria followed by increases in urine protein-to-creatinine ratio. Systemic hypertension, caused by activation of the renin-angiotensin system, may contribute to glomerulosclerosis and further renal damage. Azotemia is a late consequence of diabetic nephropathy but may be partially or completely reversible with good diabetic regulation. Hyperglycemia increases glomerular filtration rate and renal plasma flow and may increase binding of plasma proteins to glomerular basement membranes. Elevation of tissue polyol concentrations, a sequelae of hyperglycemia, contributes to renal dysfunction. Thickening of the glomerular basement membranes and glomerular hypertension may also contribute to renal problems. Early identification of diabetic nephropathy may result in reversal of glomerular damage if glycemic control improves.

Diabetic nephropathy occurs in some cats with type 2 diabetes mellitus, as evidenced by increased presence of microalbuminuria. Poorly regulated diabetic cats are more likely to exhibit proteinuria than well-regulated diabetic cats, and a significant relationship of systolic pressure to microalbuminuria has been noted in cats with diabetes.

Early identification of diabetic nephropathy may allow for proper treatment and potential reversal of glomerular damage. Improvement of glycemic control is the key therapeutic intervention; however, wide swings in blood glucose should be avoided. Equally as important in controlling hyperglycemia is minimizing the insulin dosage. Large fluctuations of blood glucose contribute to glycosylation of tissues, including glomerular tissue. Proper treatment of type 2 diabetes mellitus in cats using a low-carbohydrate diet, oral hypoglycemic agents, and basal insulin (e.g., glargine) may help prevent progression of diabetic nephropathy. Dietary protein should not be restricted until significant azotemia is present. High-protein diets have been associated with improved diabetic regulation; therefore restriction of protein leads to loss of diabetic regulation in cats with advanced renal disease and diabetes.

DIABETIC NEUROPATHY

Because of the difficulty in achieving adequate glycemic control with insulin therapy in cats with type 2 diabetes mellitus, diabetic neuropathy is a common attending condition in diabetic cats. Most diabetic cats suffer from a clinical or subclinical form of diabetic neuropathy, as can be shown via neurologic examination, impaired motor and sensory peripheral nerve studies, and nerve biopsy (e.g., myelin degeneration in the Schwann cell).

Clinical signs include severe manifestations such as plantigrade stance when standing and walking. Cats are unable to communicate sensory deficits or abnormalities; however, sensorimotor neuropathy, characterized by conduction deficits and increased F wave and cord dorsum potential latencies in both pelvic and thoracic limbs, has been documented in diabetic cats. Furthermore, nerve structural abnormalities such as splitting and ballooning of myelin and demyelination, indicative of Schwann cell injury, is common in cats with neuropathy. Axonal degeneration is less common, developing in severely affected cats.

INFECTION

Impaired immune function secondary to diabetes mellitus increases the risk of infections. In one study half of diabetic dogs had occult urinary tract infections without evidence of pyuria. Urine from diabetic animals should always be cultured to determine the presence or absence of infection. If infections are detected, a long course (i.e., 6 to 8 weeks) of an appropriate bacteriocidal antibiotic is indicated. Good choices for antibiotic therapy that penetrate into the urinary tract include the penicillins, cephalosporins, quinolones, and potentiated sulfas. The latter two antibiotics should be used in male dogs to ensure penetration into the prostate.

Other common sites of infection in diabetic animals include the liver (e.g., infectious cholangiohepatitis); lung, skin, and ears (e.g., yeast and bacterial infections); small intestine (e.g., bacterial overgrowth); and teeth (e.g., dental abscesses). In cats the stress of a condition as common as dental disease can lead to the release of counterregulatory factors. With resolution of the disease, insulin requirements may decline to the point at which the patient is no longer diabetic. Therefore dental prophylaxis should be considered standard treatment in diabetic cats.

HEPATIC DISEASE

Concurrent gastrointestinal disease is very common in diabetics, particularly diabetic cats. In the study by Crenshaw and Peterson (1996), 39 of 42 cats presented for DKA had concurrent diseases, including hepatic lipidosis, cholangiohepatitis, pancreatitis, chronic renal failure, urinary tract infection, and neoplasia. In another survey of concurrent disorders in 221 diabetic dogs, over 70% had elevated liver enzymes (Hess and Ward, 2000). Alanine aminotransferase and aspartate aminotransferase are most commonly affected; these increase secondary to hypovolemia and poor hepatic blood flow and subsequent hepatocellular damage. Further increases in serum alkaline phosphatase concentration may occur if pancreatitis and secondary cholestasis ensue. Concurrent hepatopathies are often present in patients with DKA, but evaluation is complicated by the effect of both the diabetes mellitus and DKA on liver enzymes and liver function tests.

Ultrasonography and biopsy may be useful in these cases to differentiate primary hepatic disease from secondary complications of diabetes mellitus such as hepatic lipidosis and cholangiohepatitis.

PANCREATIC DISEASE

Pancreatitis is a common concurrent disease with diabetes mellitus (also see Chapters 148 and 149). As such, it is not necessarily a complication of diabetes, but the two occur concurrently in about 40% of dogs and 50% of cats.

Cats and dogs with acute necrotizing pancreatitis usually present with vomiting, abdominal pain, and concurrent DKA. Physical examination findings include icterus, cranial abdominal pain, and abdominal effusion. Radiographs may reveal a "ground glass" appearance of the abdomen, and abdominal ultrasound usually shows enlargement and hypoechogenecity of the pancreas. Diagnostic peritoneal lavage is usually necessary to demonstrate inflammatory, nonseptic peritonitis; abdominal lipase is usually increased dramatically in affected cats and dogs.

If serum amylase and lipase are determined on presentation, they may be elevated in the absence of pancreatitis, secondary to severe dehydration, or renal insufficiency. Therefore demonstration of a high circulating concentration of pancreatic lipase immunoreactivity (PLI) may be a more reliable means of diagnosis.

OCULAR COMPLICATIONS OF DIABETES

The classical ocular complication of diabetes mellitus in dogs is the formation of diabetic cataracts. The incidence of cataracts in newly diagnosed diabetic dogs is about 40%; however, after a year of insulin therapy, the incidence of cataracts rises to about 80%. In contrast, cataracts are rare in cats with diabetes.

Polyol pathways in the eye rapidly convert glucose to sorbitol via aldose reductase and slowly to fructose via polyol dehydrodrenase. In dogs this accumulation of sorbitol within the lens fibers may lead to imbibing water and eventual swelling and opacity of the lens. Older cats have lower aldose reductase activity. Since diabetes mellitus occurs in older cats more often than younger cats, this may explain the lack of cataracts in most diabetic cats compared with diabetic dogs.

Other complications of diabetes, more common in dogs than cats, include decreased corneal sensitivity, lens-induced uveitis, and keratoconjunctivitis sicca.

HYPOGLYCEMIA

Recent studies have suggested that as many as 25% of diabetic cats and approximately 10% of diabetic dogs experienced hypoglycemic episodes that required hospitalization. The dose of insulin prescribed for a newly diagnosed diabetic patient should be conservative (<2 U per cat BID and <0.5 U/kg for dogs). One large survey found that the majority of dogs presented for hypoglycemia were receiving insulin injections of greater than 1.5 U/kg. Overdosing, double-dosing, and persistent dosing in the face of anorexia or reduced food intake are common iatrogenic causes of hypoglycemia.

Common causes of noniatrogenic hypoglycemia in previously well-regulated diabetics frequently involve reversal of glucose toxicity in cats. Because cats are often type 2 diabetics, their insulin requirements can be extremely labile. With a change to a low-carbohydrate, high-protein diet, an increase in activity level, and a shift from body fat to body muscle, a cat's insulin requirement can change quickly and dramatically. To complicate matters further, the administration of insulin or oral hypoglycemic agents may reverse pancreatic islet cell resistance (glucose toxicity), resulting in a restoration of insulin secretory capability; this may result in hypoglycemia. For either dogs or cats, concurrent disease usually increases insulin requirements; thus, if the concurrent disease is controlled or resolved, insulin requirement may decline significantly.

To avoid hypoglycemia in diabetic patients, both written and verbal instructions should be given the owner. Common early warning signs of hypoglycemia such as nervousness and hyperexcitability in dogs and extreme lethargy in cats should be communicated to the owner.

The home remedy for a hypoglycemic crisis involves the application of glucose (i.e., Karo syrup) to the animal's mucous membranes; however, there is no evidence to suggest that this raises blood glucose concentrations significantly. If possible, the animal should be fed and transported to a veterinary facility for more aggressive intravenous glucose therapy. Prevention of hypoglycemia via client education is the best therapy.

DIABETIC KETOACIDOSIS

Frequently an underlying stressful event precipitates the shift from diabetes mellitus to DKA or nonketotic hyperosmolar diabetes mellitus. The precipitating event may be a urinary tract infection or other viral or bacterial infection or inflammatory disorder such as pancreatitis, pyelonephritis, cholangiohepatitis, IBD, eosinophilic granuloma complex, prostatitis, pyometra, upper respiratory infection, or pneumonia. Other concurrent diseases may include renal insufficiency or failure, hepatic lipidosis, neoplasia, or congestive heart failure. Recent drug therapy may also precipitate a crisis, especially administration of corticosteroids or progestagens.

Therefore further diagnostic testing of the diabetic patient that presents in a ketoacidotic crisis is essential. Abdominal radiography and/or ultrasonography, thoracic radiography, and echocardiography may be indicated. Additional testing for concurrent endocrine diseases such as hyperthyroidism in cats and hypothyroidism and hyperadrenocorticism in dogs may also be indicated; however, tests for hyperadrenocorticism should be postponed until some control of the diabetes mellitus is achieved because uncontrolled disease may affect the results of the tests.

DKA is the culmination of diabetes mellitus that results in unrestrained ketone body formation in the liver, metabolic acidosis, severe dehydration, shock, and possibly death. Hepatic lipid metabolism becomes deranged with insulin deficiency, and nonesterified fatty acids are converted to acetyl coenzyme A (acetyl CoA) rather than being incorporated into triglycerides. Acetyl CoA accumulates in the liver and is converted first to acetoacetyl

CoA and ultimately to acetoacetic acid, β-hydroxybutyrate (primary ketone body in dogs and cats), and acetone. As insulin deficiency culminates in DKA, accumulation of ketones and lactic acid in the blood and loss of electrolytes and water in the urine result in profound dehydration, hypovolemia, metabolic acidosis, and shock. Ketonuria and osmotic diuresis caused by glycosuria causes sodium and potassium loss in the urine, exacerbating hypovolemia and dehydration. Nausea, anorexia, and vomiting caused by stimulation of the chemoreceptor trigger zone via ketonemia and hyperglycemia contribute to the dehydration caused by osmotic diuresis. Dehydration leads to further accumulation of glucose and ketones in the blood. Stress hormones such as cortisol and epinephrine contribute to the hyperglycemia in a vicious cycle. Eventually severe dehydration may result in hyperviscosity, thromboembolism, severe metabolic acidosis, renal failure, and finally death.

Treatment of DKA includes the following steps in order of importance: (1) fluid therapy using 0.9% saline initially, followed by 2.5% or 5% dextrose as serum glucose falls; (2) insulin therapy (low-dose intramuscular or intravenous insulin); (3) electrolyte supplementation (i.e., potassium, phosphorus, magnesium); and (4) reversal of metabolic acidosis (Box 47-1).

Fluid therapy should consist of 0.9% NaCl supplemented with potassium when insulin therapy is initiated; however, hypernatremic patients may be rehydrated with lactated Ringer's solution to limit sodium load. Placement of a large central venous catheter is preferred for intravenous access because central venous pressure may be monitored, thereby providing the means to avoid overhydration. In addition, the need for repeated venipuncture necessary for frequent monitoring of glucose, electrolytes, and blood gases is eliminated. Rapid initiation of fluid therapy is the key for successful treatment of the DKA patient. Fluid rates vary, depending on degree of dehydration, maintenance requirements, continuing losses such as vomiting and diarrhea, and presence of diseases such as congestive heart failure and renal disease. Extreme caution should be exercised when considering initiating fluid therapy with a hypotonic solution because this increases the risk of cerebral edema. Fluids containing dextrose may be required to maintain blood glucose concentrations as insulin treatment for the DKA is continued.

In dogs insulin therapy should be initiated as soon as possible using either intravenous insulin or low-dose intramuscular methods (see Box 47-1). Intravenous continuous-rate infusion of regular insulin therapy is accomplished by placement of two catheters: a peripheral catheter for the insulin infusion and a central catheter for sampling blood and administering drugs and other fluids. A dosage of 2.2 U/kg for dogs or 1.1 U/kg for cats of regular (neutral, soluble) insulin is diluted in 250 ml of saline. Approximately 50 ml of fluid and insulin is allowed to run through the intravenous drip set and is discarded because insulin binds to the plastic tubing. The species of regular insulin (beef, pork, or human) does not affect response; however, the type of insulin given is very important. Regular insulin must be used; lente, isophane, and protamine zinc insulins should never be given intravenously. Using intravenous insulin administration, blood

Box **47-1**

Stepwise Treatment of Diabetic Ketoacidosis

Step One: Fluid Therapy
- Place IV catheter, preferably central venous.

Administration rate:
- Estimate dehydration deficit (ml):
  Deficit (ml) = Dehydration (%) × body weight (kg) × 1000 ml

- Estimate maintenance needs:
  2 ml/kg/hr × hours required to rehydrate (24 hours)
- Estimate losses (vomiting, diarrhea)

Fluid dose = Dehydration deficit + maintenance needs + losses
Hourly fluid administration rate (ml/hr) = Fluid dose (ml) ÷ 24 hours

Fluid Composition:

Blood Glucose (mg/dl)	Fluids	Rate	Route	Monitor	Frequency
>250	0.9% saline	Up to 90 ml/kg/hr to rehydrate	IV	PCV, TS, sodium, potassium, osmolality	Every 4 hr
200-250	0.45% saline plus 2.5% dextrose	Up to 90 ml/kg/hr to rehydrate	IV	PCV, TS, sodium, potassium, osmolality	Every 4 hr
150-200	0.45% saline plus 2.5% dextrose	Up to 90 ml/kg/hr to rehydrate	IV	CVP, urine output	Every 2 hr
100-150	0.45% saline plus 2.5% dextrose	Up to 90 ml/kg/hr to rehydrate	IV	CVP, urine output	Every 2 hr
<100	0.45% saline plus 5% dextrose	Up to 90 ml/kg/hr to rehydrate	IV	CVP, urine output	Every 2 hr

Step Two: Insulin
Intravenous insulin (regular only) is mixed in 250 ml of 0.9% saline; 50 ml is allowed to run through the administration set.

Blood Glucose (mg/dl)	Rate	Route	Dose (U/kg)	Monitor	Frequency
Intravenous (regular only)					
>250	10 ml/hr	IV	C: 1.1 D: 2.2	Blood glucose	Every 1-2 hr
200-250	7 ml/hr	IV	C: 1.1 D: 2.2	Blood glucose	Every 1-2 hr
150-200	5 ml/hr	IV	C: 1.1 D: 2.2	Blood glucose	Every 4 hr
100-150	5 ml/hr	IV	C: 1.1 D: 2.2	Blood glucose	Every 4 hr
<100	Stop intravenous insulin; begin subcutaneous insulin every 4 hours	SQ	0.1-0.4	Blood glucose	Every 2 hr
Intramuscular (regular only)					
>250 mg/dl	Initial dose	IM	0.2	Blood glucose	Hourly
	Every hour	IM	0.1	Blood glucose	Hourly
<250 mg/dl	Every 4-6 hr	IM	0.1	Blood glucose	Every 4-6 hr
	Every 6-8 hr	SQ	0.1-0.4	Blood glucose	Every 6-8 hr

Step Three: Electrolytes

Electrolyte Concentration	Amount Added to Fluid (mEq/L)	Maximum Fluid Administration Rate (ml/kg/hr)
Potassium		
3.6-5.0 mEq/L	20	26
2.6-3.5 mEq/L	40	12
2.1-2.5 mEq/L	60	9
<2.0 mEq/L	80	7
Phosphorus		
1-2 mg/dl	0.03 mmol/kg/hr	Monitor serum phosphorus every 6 hr
<1.0 mg/dl	0.1 mmol/kg/hr	Monitor serum phosphorus every 6 hr

(Continued)

Box 47-1—Cont'd

Stepwise Treatment of Diabetic Ketoacidosis

Magnesium

| <1.2 mg/dl | 0.75-1 mEq/kg/day (magnesium chloride or sulfate) in a constant-rate infusion | Use 5% dextrose; magnesium is incompatible with calcium and sodium bicarbonate solutions |

Step four: Acid-Base Balance

pH	Bicarbonate Concentration	Dose of Bicarbonate (ml)	Rate
<7.1	<12 mEq/L	0.1 × body weight (kg) × (4 – bicarbonate [mEq/L])	Over 2 hr

From Greco DS: Endocrine pancreatic emergencies, *Compend Cont Educ Pract Vet* 19(1):23, 1997 (with permission).
C, Cat; *CRI*, continuous-rate infusion; *CVP*, central venous pressure; *D*, dog; *IM*, intramuscular; *IV*, intravenous; *PCV*, packed cell volume; *SQ*, subcutaneous; *TS*, total solids.

glucose decreases to below 250 mg/dl by approximately 10 and 16 hours in dogs and cats, respectively. Once this has been achieved, the animal is maintained on subcutaneous regular insulin (0.1 to 0.4 U/kg subcutaneously every 4 to 6 hours) until it starts to eat and/or the ketosis has resolved. Often the transition from hospital to home maintenance therapy can be made by using a low dose (1 to 2 U) of regular insulin combined with the intermediate or long-acting maintenance insulin at the recommended dosages.

Potassium should be supplemented as soon as insulin therapy is initiated (see Box 47-1). Although serum potassium may be normal or elevated in DKA, the animal actually suffers from total body depletion of potassium. Correction of the metabolic acidosis tends to drive potassium intracellularly in exchange for hydrogen ions. Insulin facilitates this exchange, and the net effect is a dramatic decrease in serum potassium, which must be attenuated with appropriate potassium supplementation in fluids. Refractory hypokalemia may be complicated by hypomagnesemia. Supplementation of magnesium along with potassium may be indicated in cats or dogs with hypokalemia that is unresponsive to potassium chloride supplementation.

Serum and tissue phosphorus may also be depleted during a ketoacidotic crisis, and some of the potassium supplementation should consist of potassium phosphate (one third of the potassium dose as potassium phosphate), particularly in small dogs and cats that are most susceptible to hemolysis caused by hypophosphatemia. Caution should be used since oversupplementation of phosphorus can result in metastatic calcification and hypocalcemia.

Bicarbonate therapy may be necessary in some patients with a blood pH less than 7.1 or if serum HCO_3 is less than 12 mmol/L. Caution is recommended as metabolic alkalosis may be difficult to reverse.

NONKETOTIC HYPEROSMOLAR DIABETES

Nonketotic hyperosmolar diabetes is defined by extreme hyperglycemia (>600 mg/dL), hyperosmolality (>350 mOsm/L), severe dehydration, and central nervous system (CNS) depression without ketone formation and with no or only mild metabolic acidosis. Affected animals commonly have underlying renal or cardiovascular disease and are more likely to be noninsulin dependent.

Although this specific syndrome, as defined in humans, is uncommonly encountered in veterinary medicine, it is not uncommon to have ketotic or nonketotic diabetic cats with significant hyperosmolality and CNS alterations. Treatment consists of slow rehydration with isotonic or hypotonic fluids and postponement of insulin therapy for 24 hours.

References and Suggested Reading

Bashor AWP, Roberts SM: Ocular manifestations of diabetes mellitus: diabetic cataracts in dogs, *Vet Clin North Am* 25:661, 1995.

Crenshaw KL, Peterson ME: Pretreatment clinical and laboratory evaluation of cats with diabetes mellitus: 104 cases (1992-1994), *J Am Vet Med Assoc* 209:943, 1996.

Diehl KJ: Long-term complications of diabetes mellitus. Part II: Gastrointestinal and infectious, *Vet Clin North Am* 25:731, 1995.

Hess RS, Ward CR: Effect of insulin dosage on glycemic response in dogs with diabetes mellitus: 221 cases (1993-1998), *J Am Vet Med Assoc* 216:217, 2000.

Kern TS, Engerman RL: Arrest of glomerulopathy in diabetic dogs by improved glycaemic control, *Diabetologia* 33:522, 1990.

Mizisin AP et al: Neurological complications associated with spontaneously occurring feline diabetes mellitus, *J Neuropathol Exp Neurol* 61, 872, 2002.

Munana KR: Long-term complications of diabetes mellitus. Part I: Retinopathy, nephropathy, neuropathy, *Vet Clin North Am* 25:715, 1995.

Nichols R, Crenshaw KL: Complications and concurrent disease associated with diabetic ketoacidosis and other severe forms of diabetes mellitus, *Vet Clin North Am* 25:617, 1995.

Richter M, Guscetti F, Spiess B: Aldose reductase activity and glucose-related opacities in incubated lenses from dogs and cats, *Am J Vet Res* 63:1591, 2002.

Struble AL et al: Systemic hypertension and proteinuria in dogs with diabetes mellitus, *J Am Vet Med Assoc* 213:822, 1998.

Whitley NT, Drobatz KJ, Panciera DL: Insulin overdose in dogs and cats: 28 cases (1986-1993), *J Am Vet Med Assoc* 211:326, 1997.

CHAPTER 48

Atypical and Subclinical Hyperadrenocorticism

J. CATHARINE R. SCOTT-MONCRIEFF, *West Lafayette, Indiana*

Classical hyperadrenocorticism is a syndrome caused by excess secretion of cortisol from the adrenal gland(s). Approximately 80% to 85% of cases of spontaneous hyperadrenocorticism in both dogs and cats are caused by pituitary-dependent hyperadrenocorticism, with the remainder the result of a functional adrenocortical tumor. Although cortisol is the major product of the adrenal gland, which is typically oversecreted in hyperadrenocorticism, excessive secretion of other adrenocortical hormones (i.e., sex hormones and mineralocorticoids) has also been documented. In some dogs with signs of hyperadrenocorticism, cortisol excess cannot be demonstrated, but increased concentrations of adrenal sex steroids are found. In these situations measurement of sex hormones may provide useful additional diagnostic information to support a diagnosis of hyperadrenocorticism.

ADRENAL STEROID HORMONE PRODUCTION IN THE ADRENAL CORTEX

Adrenal steroids are derived from cholesterol. Four cytochrome P-450 enzymes present in the adrenal cortex (side chain cleavage enzyme, 17α-hydroxylase, 21β-hydroxylase, and 11β-hydroxylase), and one noncytochrome enzyme (3β-dehydrogenase) catalyze formation of the different adrenal steroids (Fig. 48-1).

The adrenal cortex is composed of three zones: the zona glomerulosa, the zona fasciculata, and the zona reticularis. The zona glomerulosa is deficient in 17α- hydroxylase activity; thus it is incapable of synthesizing cortisol or androgens. The zona glomerulosa does contain aldosterone synthase, which catalyzes the synthesis of aldosterone from corticosterone. The major secretory products of the zona fasciculata and zona reticularis in normal animals are cortisol and the adrenal androgens dehydroepiandrosterone and androstenedione. The zona fasciculata and zona reticularis cannot synthesize aldosterone. Although progesterone is synthesized in the adrenal gland as a precursor to androgens in healthy dogs, very little progesterone is normally secreted into the circulation. Similarly in normal animals only very small amounts of testosterone and estrogen are synthesized by the adrenal cortex; however, adrenal androgens serve as substrates for synthesis of testosterone and estrogen in peripheral tissues.

Cortisol production from the adrenal gland is regulated by the hypothalamic-pituitary-adrenal axis. Aldosterone production is regulated by the renin-angiotensin system, the plasma potassium concentration, and to a lesser extent the hypothalamic-pituitary-adrenal axis. Regulation of secretion of other adrenal steroid hormones is poorly understood but likely involves both adrenocorticotropic hormone (ACTH) and other non-ACTH factors.

CLINICAL SIGNS OF HYPERADRENOCORTICISM

Clinical signs of hyperadrenocorticism include polydipsia, polyuria, polyphagia, abdominal enlargement, hepatomegaly, cutaneous changes (e.g., alopecia, cutaneous atrophy, calcinosis cutis, hyperpigmentation), muscle weakness, decreased exercise tolerance, excessive panting, truncal obesity, lethargy, weight gain, immunosuppression, insulin resistance, and decreased sexual function. Although excessive circulating concentrations of cortisol are the primary cause of clinical signs in dogs with spontaneous hyperadrenocorticism, increased circulating concentrations of other adrenal steroid hormones such as progesterone or 17-hydroxyprogesterone may also cause clinical signs that are indistinguishable from those caused by glucocorticoid excess. This is hypothesized to be caused by the marked intrinsic glucocorticoid activity of progestagens. In addition, progestins may increase availability of cortisol by displacing it from its binding proteins. In rare cases of hyperadrenocorticism, increased concentrations of adrenal androgens, estrogens, and mineralocorticoids may cause virilization, feminization, or hypertension, respectively.

DIAGNOSIS OF HYPERADRENOCORTICISM

Diagnosis of hyperadrenocorticism is made by consideration of historical findings, physical examination, review of a laboratory minimum database (i.e., complete blood count, serum biochemical profile, urinalysis), and pituitary-adrenal endocrine function testing. Commonly performed screening endocrine tests include the ACTH stimulation test, the low-dose dexamethasone suppression test, and the urine cortisol:creatinine ratio.

ACTH Stimulation Test

This test relies on the assumption that hyperplastic or neoplastic adrenals have abnormally large reserves of cortisol and therefore hyperrespond to ACTH administration with maximal stimulation. The ACTH stimulation test is abnormal in 85% to 90% of dogs with

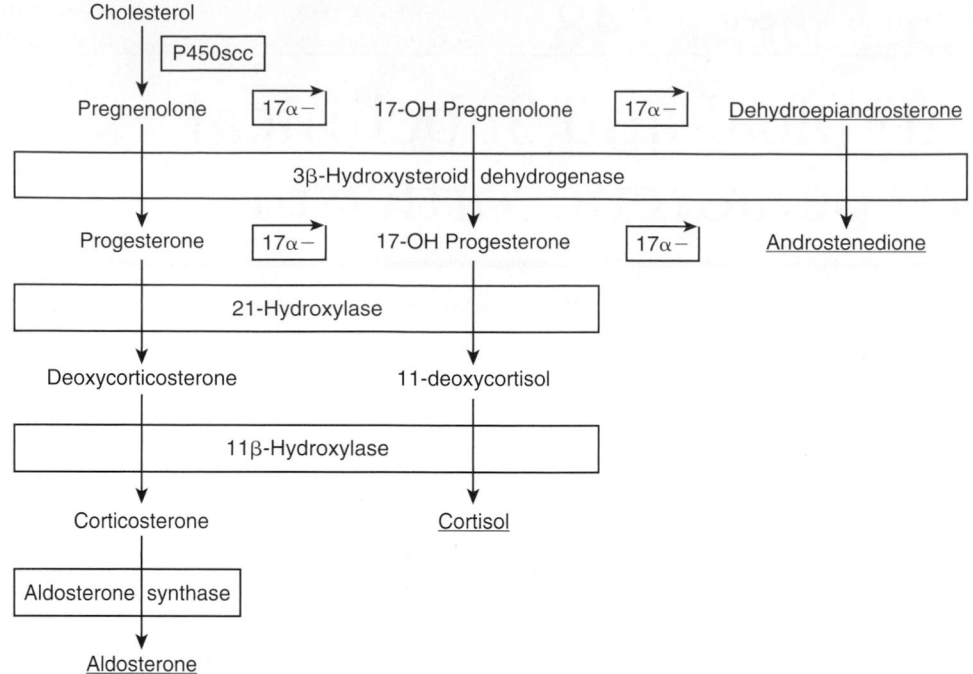

Fig. 48-1 Pathway for adrenal steroid hormone synthesis within the adrenal gland.

pituitary-dependent hyperadrenocorticism and in 50% of dogs with functional adrenocortical tumors. Advantages of the ACTH stimulation test are that it allows differentiation of iatrogenic from spontaneous hyperadrenocorticism and is less affected by stress and concurrent disease than the low-dose dexamethasone suppression test. However, the ACTH stimulation test cannot distinguish between dogs with adrenocortical tumors or pituitary-dependent hyperadrenocorticism. Because of the low sensitivity of this test, a diagnosis of hyperadrenocorticism should not be excluded based on a normal ACTH stimulation.

Low-Dose Dexamethasone Suppression Test

The low-dose dexamethasone suppression test is a better screening test for hyperadrenocorticism since it is more sensitive (95%) than the ACTH stimulation test. However, it does not allow detection of iatrogenic hyperadrenocorticism. Administration of an adequate dose of exogenous glucocorticoids suppresses the secretion of ACTH from the normal pituitary and therefore the production of cortisol from the normal adrenal gland. This suppression persists in the normal dog for 24 to 48 hours. Since dexamethasone is not detected by the assay for cortisol, a decrease in cortisol secretion can be measured after dexamethasone administration. Adrenal tumors function independently of ACTH control, whereas a hyperplastic or neoplastic pituitary gland is relatively resistant to negative-feedback inhibition from circulating steroids; therefore cortisol suppression fails to occur in dogs with either type of hyperadrenocorticism.

Urinary Cortisol:Creatinine Ratio

The urine cortisol:creatinine ratio is an estimate of 24-hour cortisol production by the adrenal gland. The measurement is made on a voided morning urine sample collected at home; thus it is a very convenient initial screening test. The urine cortisol:creatinine ratio is an extremely sensitive test for diagnosis of hyperadrenocorticism but has *low specificity*. A urine cortisol:creatinine ratio within the reference range is helpful in ruling out hyperadrenocorticism as a differential diagnosis; however, many nonadrenal diseases also increase the urine cortisol:creatinine ratio; thus further testing is necessary for confirmation.

Differentiation of Pituitary-Dependent Hyperadrenocorticism From Adrenal Tumors

Clinical and routine laboratory findings are not useful in distinguishing pituitary-dependent hyperadrenocorticism from functional adrenal tumors. The ACTH stimulation test and urine cortisol:creatinine ratio do not differentiate adrenal tumors from pituitary-dependent hyperadrenocorticism.

The low- and high-dose dexamethasone suppression tests and measurement of the endogenous ACTH concentration are the most useful endocrine tests for distinguishing adrenocortical tumor from pituitary-dependent hyperadrenocorticism. Additional tests that may be necessary to differentiate dogs with pituitary-dependent hyperadrenocorticism from those with adrenocortical tumors include abdominal radiography, abdominal ultrasound, and computed tomography (abdomen and brain).

Problems in Diagnosis: Atypical Hyperadrenocorticism

Although in most dogs with hyperadrenocorticism the diagnosis is straightforward, there are some dogs with clinical signs suggestive of hyperadrenocorticism that have normal ACTH stimulation and low-dose dexamethasone suppression test results. In many of these dogs other causes for the clinical signs have been ruled out, and in some repeated cortisol testing over a period of several months confirms diagnosis of hyperadrenocorticism. Dogs with overt clinical signs of hyperadrenocorticism, lack of evidence for cortisol excess by routine endocrine testing, and positive response to treatment for hyperadrenocorticism have been described as having atypical hyperadrenocorticism. Measurement of serum concentrations of other adrenal steroid hormones may assist in diagnosis of such cases.

ADRENAL STEROID HORMONE SECRETION PATTERNS IN DOGS AND CATS

Normal Dogs

Concentrations of many of the adrenal steroid hormones vary, depending on the dog's sex and neuter status; therefore reference ranges must be established for each sexual category. Most hormones increase after administration of ACTH, and evaluation of both pre-ACTH and post-ACTH samples is recommended.

Dogs With Classical Hyperadrenocorticism

Most dogs with classic hyperadrenocorticism (confirmed by use of ACTH stimulation or low-dose dexamethasone suppression tests) also have elevations of other steroid adrenal hormones both before and after stimulation with ACTH. Hormones that are commonly increased include dehydroepiandrosterone, androstenedione, progesterone, and 17-hydroxyprogesterone. Although testosterone and estradiol concentrations are evaluated as part of some adrenal steroid hormone panels, they are less commonly abnormal. Profiles observed in dogs with hyperadrenocorticism vary from dog to dog, but most dogs with classical hyperadrenocorticism have at least one steroid hormone (in addition to cortisol) that is increased. Typically two-to-three hormone concentrations are abnormal; however, it is unusual for all hormones in the profile to be increased.

Adrenal steroid hormone concentrations may be increased in dogs with either pituitary-dependent hyperadrenocorticism or adrenocortical tumor. Although the highest concentrations are typically found in dogs with adrenocortical carcinomas, there is extensive overlap between dogs with pituitary-dependent hyperadrenocorticism and adrenocortical tumor.

Concentration of 17-hydroxyprogesterone has been evaluated most extensively in dogs with hyperadrenocorticism. The percentage of dogs with hyperadrenocorticism that have an increase in 17-hydroxyprogesterone after stimulation with ACTH ranges from 55% to 85% (Benitah et al., 2005; Hill et al., 2005). Thus sensitivity of 17-hydroxyprogesterone for diagnosis of classical hyperadrenocorticism is lower than that reported for measurement of cortisol after ACTH stimulation.

Dogs With Nonadrenal Illness

Some dogs with nonadrenal illness also have increases in 17-hydroxyprogesterone secretion. In a group of dogs with nonadrenal neoplasia that did not have clinical signs of hyperadrenocorticism, 11 of 35 (31%) had high post-ACTH 17-hydroxyprogesterone concentrations, whereas only 3 of 35 (9%) had high cortisol concentrations after ACTH stimulation (Behrend et al., 2005). This suggests that the specificity of 17-hydroxyprogesterone for diagnosis of hyperadrenocorticism is lower than that of serum cortisol. Similar results were reported for measurement of corticosterone concentration.

Specificity of other adrenal steroid hormone measurement for diagnosis of hyperadrenocorticism has not been reported. However, four of six dogs with noncortisol secreting adrenal tumors (five of which were pheochromocytomas) had one or more abnormalities on an adrenal steroid hormone profile in one study (Hill et al., 2005).

Dogs With Atypical Hyperadrenocorticism

In dogs with atypical hyperadrenocorticism, serum cortisol concentrations measured during routine endocrine function testing (with ACTH stimulation, low-dose dexamethasone suppression, or urine cortisol:creatinine ratio) are within or below the reference range, whereas other adrenal steroid hormone concentrations may be increased. The reason for lack of hypercortisolemia in dogs with atypical hyperadrenocorticism is poorly understood. In those with adrenocortical tumor, mutations within neoplastic adrenal tissue may lead to a blockade of cortisol synthesis (see Noncortisol-Secreting Adrenal Tumors later in the chapter), but atypical hyperadrenocorticism has also been well documented in dogs with pituitary-dependent hyperadrenocorticism. It is likely that these dogs have increased adrenal steroid hormone concentrations as a result of adrenal gland hyperplasia and increased secretion of all adrenal gland products. It is possible that 24-hour production of cortisol is abnormal in these dogs, even though random circulating cortisol concentration is within reference range limits. Further studies are necessary to investigate the cause of atypical hyperadrenocorticism, especially in dogs with pituitary-dependent hyperadrenocorticism.

In dogs with clinical signs supportive of hyperadrenocorticism that have normal or borderline results on routine cortisol testing, marked increases in two or three adrenal steroid hormone concentrations are very supportive of a diagnosis of atypical hyperadrenocorticism. An example of an adrenal steroid hormone panel in a dog with clinical signs of hyperadrenocorticism in which a diagnosis of atypical pituitary-dependent hyperadrenocorticism was made is shown in Table 48-1.

Table 48-1

Adrenal Steroid Hormone Profile in a 13-year-old Male Castrated Terrier With Pituitary-Dependent Atypical Hyperadrenocorticism*

Adrenal Hormone	Basal Concentration	Reference Range	Post ACTH	Reference Range
Cortisol (mcg/dl)	1.8	1-6	18.3	7-17
Androstenedione (ng/ml)	3.7	0.1-3.6	87.6	2.4-29
Estradiol (pg/ml)	95.7	23-85	93.4	23-89
Progesterone (ng/ml)	0.06	0.01-0.17	3.66	0.22-1.45
17-hydroxyprogesterone (ng/ml)	0.17	0.01-0.24	6.59	0.02-0.42

ACTH, Adrenocorticotropic hormone.
*Low-dose dexamethasone suppression test was normal. All clinical signs resolved after treatment with mitotane.

Dogs and Cats With Non-cortisol–Secreting Adrenal Tumors

In some dogs and cats with functional adrenocortical tumors, adrenal steroid hormones other than cortisol are the major secretory product of the tumor, and serum cortisol concentrations are low. Increased production of adrenal steroids other than cortisol may be caused by deficiencies of one or more enzymes involved in normal steroidogenic pathways, possibly the result of mutations in neoplastic adrenal tissue. Deficiency of these enzymes causes accumulation of precursor steroids proximal to the blocked step, with shunting of precursors into other metabolic pathways (see Fig. 48-1). Increases in enzyme activity may also play a role in steroid hypersecretion. Circulating cortisol concentrations in these dogs are hypothesized to be low because of suppression of the hypothalamic-pituitary axis by high circulating concentrations of progestins or other adrenal sex hormones.

All reported cases of non-cortisol–secreting adrenal tumors in dogs and cats have been carcinomas. This is similar to the situation in humans in which adrenal carcinomas are usually inefficient in conversion of cholesterol to cortisol and production of cortisol precursors is disproportionately high. In contrast, adrenal adenomas generally exhibit very efficient steroidogenesis, and production of precursors is low or normal in relation to cortisol production.

In dogs and cats with non-cortisol–secreting adrenocortical carcinomas, clinical signs are generally consistent with those of hyperadrenocorticism, and adrenal tumors are identified by imaging studies. However, endocrine function tests do not demonstrate hypercortisolemia, and results of ACTH stimulation testing typically show low cortisol concentrations that do not increase normally after ACTH administration. Hormones that have been reported to be increased in different combinations are 17-hydroxyprogesterone, progesterone, estradiol, testosterone, and androstenedione. Increased concentrations of corticosterone and aldosterone have also been reported in dogs and cats with non-cortisol–secreting adrenocortical carcinomas. An example of an adrenal steroid hormone panel in a dog with clinical signs of hyperadrenocorticism in which a non-cortisol–secreting carcinoma was diagnosed is shown in Table 48-2. The clinical syndrome of non-cortisol–secreting adrenocortical tumors in dogs and cats appears to be a distinctly different entity from dogs with classical hyperadrenocorticism that secrete sex hormones in conjunction with normal-to-increased cortisol concentrations.

Dogs With Alopecia X

Alopecia X is a form of canine adult-onset alopecia that may be caused by mild hyperadrenocorticism. The problem affects Nordic breeds (Alaskan malamute, chow-chow,

Table 48-2

Adrenal Steroid Hormone Profile in a 9-year-old Male Castrated Poodle With Adrenocortical Carcinoma*

Adrenal Hormone	Basal Concentration	Reference Range	Post ACTH	Reference Range
Cortisol (mcg/dl)	3.0	1-6	3.6	7-17
Androstenedione (ng/ml)	24.7	2.7-8.0	83.7	3-10
Estradiol (pg/ml)	80.7	28-63	79.1	30-69
Progesterone (ng/ml)	2.1	<0.1	16.1	<1.2
17-hydroxyprogesterone (ng/ml)	0.9	<0.1	16.4	0.4-1.2

ACTH, Adrenocorticotropic hormone.
*All hormone concentrations normalized following resection of the tumor.

keeshond, Pomeranian, Samoyed, Siberian husky) and also the miniature poodle. Affected dogs have no other clinical signs of systemic illness; some studies have demonstrated borderline ACTH stimulation and low-dose dexamethasone suppression test results and mild increases in the cortisol: creatinine ratios in affected dogs. A mild form of hyperadrenocorticism is suspected in at least some affected dogs.

Many dogs with alopecia X have increased serum sex hormone concentrations, both basally and following ACTH stimulation testing. The most frequent abnormalities detected include increased concentrations of progesterone, androstenedione, and 17-hydroxyprogesterone, although not all dogs have values outside the reference range.

CLINICAL INDICATIONS FOR ADRENAL STEROID HORMONE PANEL

At this time it is not recommended that adrenal steroid hormone measurement be used for routine diagnosis of hyperadrenocorticism. However, measurement of a panel of adrenal steroid hormones before and after ACTH stimulation should be considered in dogs that have clinical signs and clinical laboratory evidence for hyperadrenocorticism, no evidence of another cause for their clinical signs, and normal or borderline cortisol testing on routine endocrine testing. Adrenal steroid hormone measurement should also be considered in dogs and cats with clinical signs of hyperadrenocorticism and suppressed cortisol concentrations after ACTH stimulation if treatment with exogenous steroids or mitotane is ruled out; this is particularly true if an adrenal mass is visualized with ultrasound or computed tomography. Measurement of an adrenal steroid hormone profile may also be useful in dogs with suspected alopecia X. Because of the paucity of information about the specificity of these measurements, every effort should be made to rule out other causes for the observed clinical signs before running an adrenal steroid hormone panel.

A number of laboratories offer individual adrenal steroid hormone assays. The most extensive adrenal steroid hormone profile is offered by the Clinical Endocrinology Service at the University of Tennessee. Their profile includes androstenedione, estradiol, progesterone, 17-hydroxyprogesterone, and aldosterone. The protocol for running the test is identical to that for a standard ACTH stimulation test, but the profile requires a larger sample (2 ml) of serum. In a dog with clinical signs of hyperadrenocorticism, marked increases (1.5 to 2 times greater than the high end of the reference range) of at least two and preferably three adrenal steroid hormone concentrations is consistent with a diagnosis of atypical hyperadrenocorticism.

TREATMENT OF ATYPICAL HYPERADRENOCORTICISM

Dogs with pituitary-dependent atypical hyperadrenocorticism respond well to routine therapy for hyperadrenocorticism (see Chapter 49). Good clinical responses have been reported with both mitotane and trilostane. No advantage of trilostane treatment over mitotane has been documented.

Although most dogs with atypical pituitary-dependent hyperadrenocorticism have borderline or normal cortisol responses to ACTH stimulation, routine ACTH stimulation tests with measurement of cortisol alone are adequate for monitoring therapy. The reason for this is that the goal of treatment is suppression of cortisol concentration below the reference range for post-ACTH cortisol (2 to 6 mcg/dl).

Monitoring adrenal steroid hormone profiles during treatment is not currently recommended because of expense and limited usefulness. For example, in dogs with atypical hyperadrenocorticism successfully treated with mitotane, 17-hydroxyprogesterone concentrations decrease; in those treated with trilostane, 17-hydroxyprogesterone concentrations increase despite a positive clinical response to therapy. Since trilostane inhibits the 3β-dehydrogenase enzyme, 17-hydroxyprogesterone would be predicted to decrease, not increase. It is possible that trilostane acts at additional steps in the synthetic cascade or that there is cross-reactivity of the assay for 17-hydroxprogesterone with precursors such as pregnenolone and hydroxypregnenolone.

Although melatonin has been demonstrated to decrease sex hormone concentrations in normal dogs, there is no evidence to suggest that this is an effective therapy in dogs with atypical hyperadrenocorticism. Mitotane, trilostane, and melatonin have all been reported to be effective in the treatment of some dogs with alopecia X; however, dogs that responded to melatonin did not have decreases in adrenal steroid hormone concentrations during treatment.

In dogs with adrenocortical tumors, whether typical or atypical, the treatment of choice is usually surgical resection. Although some cortisol-secreting adrenal tumors do respond well to medical therapy with mitotane or trilostane, noncortisol-secreting adrenocortical tumors tend to respond poorly to medical management with either mitotane or trilostane.

References and Suggested Reading

Behrend EN et al: Serum 17-a-hydroxyprogesterone and corticosterone concentrations in dogs with nonadrenal neoplasia and dogs with suspected hyperadrenocorticism, *J Am Vet Med Assoc* 227:1762, 2005.

Benitah N et al: Evaluation of serum 17-hydroxyprogesterone concentrations after administration of ACTH in dogs with hyperadrenocorticism, *J Am Vet Med Assoc* 227:1095, 2005.

Cerundolo RC et al: Treatment of canine alopecia X with trilostane, *Vet Dermatol* 15:285, 2004.

Chapman PS et al: Evaluation of the basal and post-adrenocorticotrophic hormone serum concentrations of 17-hydroxyprogesterone for the diagnosis of hyperadrenocorticism in dogs, *Vet Rec* 153:771, 2003.

Frank LA, Schmeitzel LP, Oliver JW: Steroidogenic response of adrenal tissues after administration of ACTH to dogs with hypercortisolemia, *J Am Vet Med Assoc* 218:214, 2001.

Frank LA, Hnilica KA, Oliver JW: Adrenal steroid hormone concentrations in dogs with hair cycle arrest (alopecia X) before and after treatment with melatonin and mitotane, *Vet Dermatol* 15:278, 2004.

Hill KE et al: Secretion of sex hormones in dogs with adrenal dysfunction, *J Am Vet Med Assoc* 226:556, 2005.

Norman EJ, Thompson H, Mooney CT: Dynamic adrenal function testing in eight dogs with hyperadrenocorticism associated with adrenocortical neoplasia, *Vet Rec* 144:551, 1999.

Ristic JME et al: The use of 17-hydroxyprogesterone in the diagnosis of canine hyperadrenocorticism, *J Vet Intern Med* 16:433, 2002.

Syme HM et al: Hyperadrenocorticism associated with excessive sex hormone production by an adrenocortical tumor in two dogs, *J Am Vet Med Assoc* 219:1725, 2001.

CHAPTER 49

Canine Hyperadrenocorticism

IAN RAMSEY, *Glasgow, United Kingdom*
RETO NEIGER, *Giessen, Germany*

Hyperadrenocorticism, or Cushing's syndrome, results from a chronic excess of glucocorticoids and is one of the most common canine endocrinopathies. This chapter summarizes the current knowledge of the treatment of this syndrome. Attention is focused on recent developments such as the use of trilostane. For a detailed description of the more well-known aspects of this disease, readers should consult one of the standard textbooks.

Hyperadrenocorticism has two spontaneous forms and may also be produced iatrogenically by the administration of steroids. The most common cause of hyperadrenocorticism is the overproduction of adrenocorticotropic hormone (ACTH) by a small, benign pituitary microadenoma (pituitary-dependent hyperadrenocorticism). A less common cause of hyperadrenocorticism, accounting for about 15% of cases, is the overproduction of cortisol by an adrenal tumor (adrenal-dependent hyperadrenocorticism).

It is useful, but not always essential, to distinguish between pituitary-dependent-hyperadrenocorticism and adrenal-dependent hyperadrenocorticism. Differentiating between the two causes of hyperadrenocorticism helps improve the treatment that can be offered and provides information on the likely prognosis and progression of the condition. Interested readers should consult Chapter 38 and other texts for a full discussion of the various methods of achieving this distinction (e.g., low-dose dexamethasone suppression test, endogenous ACTH assay, and abdominal ultrasonography).

TREATMENT OF PITUITARY-DEPENDENT HYPERADRENOCORTICISM

In general, all dogs with pituitary-dependent hyperadrenocorticism should be treated. However, cases identified fortuitously during routine health checks may not require immediate treatment. The risks of not treating hyperadrenocorticism, especially when more advanced, include the development of pulmonary thromboembolism, diabetes mellitus, and calcium oxalate urolithiasis.

Treatment of pituitary-dependent hyperadrenocorticism may be associated with the unmasking of steroid-responsive diseases, including arthritis and atopic dermatitis. The sudden reduction in cortisol concentrations may result in rapid growth of a pituitary tumor, leading to neurologic signs such as ataxia, depression, apparent blindness, inappetence, aimless walking, seizures, and alteration in normal behavior patterns. Treatment may also be associated with a unilateral facial nerve paralysis; it is often unclear if this is a result of the disease or the treatment, but it is seen with both trilostane and mitotane therapy.

Owners of dogs with pituitary-dependent hyperadrenocorticism often ask for the "best" treatment. The answer to this question is now more complicated than it has ever been, and there are at least three effective treatments. No one regimen is perfect for all cases. Local laws and personal experience are important factors in determining the advice that is offered.

Surgical Options

Transsphenoidal hypophysectomy has been described for the treatment of pituitary tumors in dogs with pituitary-dependent hyperadrenocorticism. Only specialists working in suitable facilities should perform such surgery. The success rate in experienced hands is acceptable, but serious complications may occur. Currently only one institution in Europe performs this procedure on a regular basis.

Medical Options

Mitotane

This drug is the mainstay of medical management of hyperadrenocorticism in many countries and is reviewed in detail elsewhere (Kintzer and Peterson, 1991). It is a cytotoxic agent that principally causes necrosis of the zona fasciculata and zona reticularis of the adrenal glands. It is slightly more efficacious than trilostane (see next section) but is reported to have a higher incidence of side effects (Kintzer and Peterson, 1991). Because it can be absorbed through the skin and is cytotoxic to humans, it should be handled carefully with gloves. Splitting tablets should be avoided when possible.

Mitotane is given initially as an induction course (50 mg/kg orally) administered once daily or divided twice daily, as required. Since it is a drug that has a narrow therapeutic index, stabilization in a hospital should be considered in some cases (e.g., dogs with concurrent diabetes) during the induction phase. The drug should be administered either in or immediately following a meal since this enhances its absorption. The induction course is monitored by carefully measuring the dog's water intake and observing its feeding behavior. Concomitant prednisolone administration is generally not recommended. Mitotane can also be used at higher doses in a protocol designed to permanently destroy the adrenal gland. This protocol is no longer in widespread use, and readers are advised to consult relevant texts for further details.

Treatment is stopped when the water consumption or the appetite starts to decrease. Once these end points are reached, if the animal is unusually listless, begins vomiting, or has diarrhea or 7 days of treatment have elapsed, an ACTH stimulation test is performed. A response indicative of mild adrenal cortex suppression indicates satisfactory control. For most laboratories this means a post-ACTH cortisol less than 120 nmol/L (<4.3 mcg/dl).

Most induction courses last 5 to 10 days. Almost all dogs with pituitary-dependent hyperadrenocorticism respond by day 14. Maintenance therapy (25 to 50 mg/kg orally every 7 days) is then given and checked by ACTH stimulation tests, initially every month and then every 3 months.

Many dogs show relapses at some stage and require adjustments to the dose of mitotane. Responses to ACTH stimulation tests that suggest a failure of adrenal suppression (post-ACTH cortisol greater than 250 nmol/L (>9 mcg/dl)) should be treated with a 3-day reinduction course and the effects of this monitored with further ACTH stimulation tests.

Dogs that are treated with mitotane, particularly those that have been treated for several months, may develop acute signs of hypoadrenocorticism (e.g., severe depression, anorexia, vomiting, and diarrhea). Intravenous fluids, glucocorticoids, and rest are usually effective.

Occasionally there may be evidence of hyperkalemia and hyponatremia. If these occur, an ACTH stimulation test should be performed; post-ACTH cortisol should be expected to be less than 20 nmol/L or (<0.7 mcg/dl). Mineralocorticoids should be given if hyperkalemia has been documented (see Chapters 50 and 51). Pancreatitis and hemorrhagic gastroenteritis are potential complications of the acute iatrogenic hypoadrenocorticism. Oral prednisolone (0.2 to 0.4 mg/kg orally every 24 hours) is given once the vomiting has subsided. Some dogs require this for life, but others may revert to their original state of hyperadrenocorticism.

Routine monitoring with ACTH stimulation tests is recommended; the frequency of monitoring largely depends on the clinical progression of the case. Some dogs receiving long-term prednisolone as a result of mitotane-induced hyperadrenocorticism only require ACTH stimulation tests annually.

Some animals become intolerant of mitotane and show signs of gastrointestinal upset without a reduction in post-ACTH cortisol concentrations. These dogs should be treated by other means.

Trilostane

Trilostane is a synthetic steroid that competitively inhibits steroid synthesis by blocking 3β-hydroxysteroid dehydrogenase. The adrenal glands and in particular the synthesis of glucocorticoids are more susceptible to its action than other steroid-producing tissues. The reasons for this are not known. Trilostane is now licensed in most European countries for the treatment of canine hyperadrenocorticism, and it can be obtained in the United States from the European manufacturer (Dechra Ltd, UK) by completing a letter with all the necessary information (form sent to the Division of Compliance HFA-230, Centre of Veterinary FDA, Metro Park North, 7500 Standish Place, Rockville MD 20855).

Trilostane has been found to be well tolerated by almost all dogs with pituitary-dependent hyperadrenocorticism in several published trials (totaling more than 120 dogs) and also two unpublished large multicenter studies performed for licensing purposes. Very few dogs develop signs of hypoadrenocorticism when treated with trilostane, although mild asymptomatic hyperkalemia is quite common. When hypoadrenocorticism does occur, dogs usually rapidly recover with appropriate therapy. A very few dogs have died despite withdrawal of trilostane and administration of appropriate therapy. A few sudden deaths without signs of hypoadrenocorticism while on trilostane therapy have also occurred; the role of trilostane in these cases has not been determined. The low prevalence of side effects compares favorably to those reported with mitotane.

Trilostane is safer for owners to handle when compared to mitotane. However, pregnant women are advised to wear gloves when handling the drug since it has been shown to cause abortion in monkeys given large doses.

Although few pharmacokinetic studies have been performed, trilostane is known to be short acting. The recommended starting dose is 2 to 5 mg/kg orally once daily, using the lower dosage range in small dogs. Trilostane is absorbed better if given with food. It is effective in resolving the signs of pituitary-dependent hyperadrenocorticism in about 75% of cases (Neiger and colleagues, 2002; Ruckstuhl, Nett, and Reusch, 2002). Polyuria, polydipsia, and polyphagia should dissipate within 4 weeks after starting trilostane. If this has not happened, the dose should be increased. Skin changes should resolve within 4 months of starting treatment. All these improvements should be maintained as long as the dogs remain on adequate doses of trilostane.

The efficacy of the drug and the required dosages are assessed using ACTH stimulation tests carried out 7 to 14 days, 30 days, and 90 days after starting therapy. ACTH stimulation tests should be started 4 hours after dosing; however, it is probably acceptable to start as early as 2 hours after dosing and as late as 5 hours (such that the last sample is then taken at 6 hours). There are significant differences between the cortisol responses to ACTH if stimulation tests are performed at other times (Bell and colleagues, 2006). Many dogs require a change in dose (increase or decrease), and much higher doses may be required in some cases. Doses up to 40 to 50 mg/kg (divided twice daily) have been given with no unwanted side effects (Braddock and associates, 2003).

Post-ACTH cortisol concentrations should be between 40 nmol/L (1.5 mcg/dl) and 150 nmol/L (5.6 mcg/dl). If the post-ACTH cortisol concentration is lower, trilostane is stopped for 5 to 7 days and reintroduced at a lower dose. If the post-ACTH cortisol concentration is higher, the dose of trilostane may need to be increased, depending on the resolution of clinical signs. However, if the post-ACTH cortisol concentration is between these two values and the patient appears not to be clinically well controlled, the trilostane may need to be given twice daily. If an ACTH stimulation test is performed inadvertently at times other than 2 to 6 hours after dosing with trilostane, the post-ACTH cortisol concentration should be greater than 20 nmol/L (0.7 mcg/dl) and less than 250 nmol/L (9 mcg/dl).

Once the clinical condition of the animal and the dosage rate have been stabilized, the dog should be examined, and an ACTH stimulation test performed every 3 months. Serum biochemistry (especially potassium measurement) can be performed periodically to check for hyperkalemia, but with increasing clinical experience this becomes less important. Many dogs show relapses at some stage and require adjustments to the dosage of trilostane.

Care should be exercised when using trilostane with aldosterone antagonists (such as spironolactone), and the effects of angiotensin-converting enzyme inhibitors may be potentiated. The drug should be used with greater caution in animals with preexisting renal or cardiac disease. No specific data on drug interactions exist, and these comments are purely precautionary. No unwanted drug interactions have been seen in dogs receiving trilostane and various nonsteroidal antiinflammatory drugs, antibiotics, insulin preparations, and levothyroxine.

Minor side effects are sometimes seen, such as mild lethargy, decreased appetite, and slight electrolyte abnormalities. These may occur from 2 to 4 days after the start of the therapy and are often transient and respond to dose reduction. If more serious signs of vomiting, diarrhea, or lethargy develop, trilostane should be stopped, and prednisolone given for 1 or 2 days. In some cases dogs may require very much lower doses for the remainder of their lives. This has been linked to acute adrenal necrosis, the cause of which remains unknown.

Long-term adverse effects have not been documented, but it has been suggested that adrenal glands increase in size in response to therapy, probably as a result of chronic overstimulation with endogenous ACTH. There have been no documented instances of adrenal tumors developing in trilostane treated dogs.

The survival of dogs with pituitary-dependent hyperadrenocorticism treated with trilostane or mitotane was recently compared (Barker and colleagues, 2005). There was no significant difference between the 123 trilostane-treated dogs, surviving a median of 662 days (range 8 to 1971 days), and the 25 mitotane-treated dogs, surviving a median of 708 days (range 33 to 1339 days). A comparison of twice-daily trilostane with mitotane-induced adrenocorticolysis also did not demonstrate a significant difference.

It is important to note that many aspects of trilostane use in canine hyperadrenocorticism are still under investigation; therefore the above recommendations may change. Veterinarians who are unfamiliar with the use of the drug should consult the manufacturer or recognized specialist for up-to-date information.

Other Medical Treatments

Ketoconazole at high serum concentrations inhibits steroid synthesis and therefore exerts effects similar to those of trilostane. In those countries where trilostane is unavailable, ketoconazole is indicated for the treatment of pituitary-dependent hyperadrenocorticism, particularly in dogs that cannot tolerate mitotane. Ketoconazole is hepatotoxic at high doses. The initial dose is 5 mg/kg orally every 12 hours for 7 days. If there are no problems, the dose may be increased by 5 mg /kg orally every 12 hours until control is achieved or a maximum dose of 30 mg/kg is being given. An ACTH stimulation test is performed 1 week later. The same target range as for trilostane and mitotane is used, with a goal of post-ACTH cortisol concentrations between 20 and 120 nmol/L (0.7 to 4.3 mcg/dl).

In the United States and some other countries, *selegiline* (L-Deprenyl) is licensed for the treatment of pituitary-dependent hyperadrenocorticism. It is thought to increase dopamine concentrations in the brain and thereby decrease ACTH production. The dose is 1 mg/kg orally every 24 hours for 60 days, increasing to 2 mg/kg after this time if there is no response. If there is no response after a further month, alternative therapy should be considered. The current evidence indicates that there is minimal endocrinologic but some clinical improvement with selegiline therapy (Reusch, Steffen, and Hoerauf, 1999).

Various other drugs have been suggested for the treatment of hyperadrenocorticism, including phosphatidylserine, cyproheptadine, metapyrone, and aminoglutethimide. Some of these drugs have been found to be ineffectual; others have not been investigated. None are currently regarded as useful treatments for canine hyperadrenocorticism.

TREATMENT OF DOGS WITH PITUITARY-DEPENDENT HYPERADRENOCORTICISM AND NEUROLOGIC SIGNS

Neurologic signs may develop during any stage of treatment; these usually indicate an expanding pituitary tumor. Magnetic resonance imaging and to a lesser extent computed tomography can diagnose such a tumor in dogs that have pituitary-dependent hyperadrenocorticism and neurologic signs. The presence of a large intracranial tumor should not be regarded as a poor prognostic sign per se, although the chance of intracranial hemorrhage (pituitary apoplexy) or the sudden expansion of the tumor following treatment is increased with larger tumors. The severity of the neurologic deficits associated with the pituitary tumor is the clinically most relevant prognostic indicator.

External beam radiotherapy has been used for pituitary tumors associated with pituitary-dependent hyperadrenocorticism. In general the neurologic signs improve more rapidly than the endocrinologic signs. There can be dramatic reduction in tumor size, but no long-term survival studies have been reported. With the availability of effective drugs to treat hypercortisolemia, radiotherapy should probably be considered only in cases of hyperadrenocorticism with neurologic signs. Treatment protocols vary among centers and need to be tailored to the individual patient.

TREATMENT OF ADRENAL-DEPENDENT HYPERADRENOCORTICISM

When treating adrenal-dependent hyperadrenocorticism, owners can opt for a high-risk surgical strategy with a potentially excellent but possibly disastrous outcome or a low-risk medical strategy with a more predictable but less positive outcome. Accurate imaging is essential in informing this decision. Good communication between the veterinarian and client is essential when owners of dogs with hyperadrenocorticism are deciding which strategy is the most appropriate for them and their animal.

Surgical Options

Unilateral adrenalectomy is indicated for adrenal-dependent hyperadrenocorticism, but careful owner counseling is important since this form of hyperadrenocorticism may also be managed medically. The extent of any local invasion or metastatic spread should be investigated before surgery is performed.

Preoperative stabilization probably improves survival, but this has not been clearly demonstrated. Mitotane may be less useful than trilostane or ketoconazole in this respect because it may make the tumor more friable.

Medical Options

Mitotane

The cytotoxic properties of mitotane make it the logical choice for the long-term medical management of canine adrenal-dependent hyperadrenocorticism. Tumor regression has been demonstrated in some cases; however, most adrenal tumors are relatively resistant to the cytotoxic effects. This means that, when compared to dogs with pituitary-dependent hyperadrenocorticism, dogs with adrenal-dependent hyperadrenocorticism are more variable in their response to mitotane. They may respond very quickly to normal doses, or they may require prolonged induction courses of mitotane at increased

doses. Therefore careful patient monitoring is essential. Even if the response to an ACTH stimulation test was normal at the onset of treatment, the test can still be used to monitor mitotane therapy since the aim is to reduce the post-ACTH cortisol to less than 120 nmol/L (4.3 mcg/ml). A starting dosage of 50 mg/kg orally every 24 hours should be given. However, if there is no improvement in clinical signs or if the ACTH stimulation test results have not been suppressed after 10 days, the dosage can be increased to 75 mg/kg orally every 24 hours.

Relapses are common during maintenance therapy. Furthermore, dogs may develop signs of mitotane toxicity (such as vomiting, anorexia and diarrhea) without control of cortisol production having been achieved.

Trilostane

Only one case of long-term trilostane treatment of a dog with adrenal-dependent hyperadrenocorticism has been reported. However, amelioration of clinical signs, a reduction in post-ACTH cortisol concentrations, and improvement of clinical pathologic parameters, as well as extended survival times (more than 2 years) have been achieved in several cases (our and others' unpublished observations). Furthermore, median survival of dogs with adrenal-dependent hyperadrenocorticism treated with trilostane seems comparable to that of dogs treated with mitotane (our unpublished studies). Although trilostane is not cytotoxic and thus has no effect on the growth of the tumor or of metastases, experience has shown that the same recommendations in dogs with adrenal-dependent hyperadrenocorticism are valid as for dogs with pituitary-dependent hyperadrenocorticism. Interestingly, the doses required to achieve clinical stabilization do not seem to increase significantly with time in dogs that do respond to the initial therapy.

References and Suggested Reading

Barker E et al: A comparison of the survival times of dogs treated for hyperadrenocorticism with trilostane or mitotane, *J Vet Intern Med* 19: 810, 2005.

Bell R et al: Effects of once daily trilostane administration on cortisol concentrations and ACTH responsiveness in hyperadrenocorticoid dogs, *Vet Rec* 159:277, 2006.

Braddock JA et al: Trilostane treatment in dogs with pituitary-dependent hyperadrenocorticism, *Aust Vet J* 81:600, 2003.

Kintzer PP, Peterson ME: Mitotane (o,p'-DDD) treatment of 200 dogs with pituitary-dependent hyperadrenocorticism, *J Vet Intern Med* 5:182, 1991.

Neiger R et al: Trilostane treatment of 78 dogs with pituitary-dependent hyperadrenocorticism *Vet Rec* 150:799, 2002.

Reusch CE, Steffen T, Hoerauf A: The efficacy of l-Deprenyl in dogs with pituitary-dependent hyperadrenocorticism, *J Vet Intern Med* 13: 291, 1999.

Ruckstuhl NS, Nett CS, Reusch CE: Results of clinical examinations, laboratory tests, and ultrasonography in dogs with pituitary-dependent hyperadrenocorticism treated with trilostane, *Am J Vet Res* 63:506, 2002.

Wenger M et al: Effect of trilostane on serum concentrations of aldosterone, cortisol, and potassium in dogs with pituitary-dependent hyperadrenocorticism, *Am J Vet Res* 65:1245, 2004.

CHAPTER 50

Adrenal Insufficiency in Critical Illness

JENNIFER E. PRITTIE, *New York, New York*

Relative adrenal insufficiency is a transient inability of the adrenal glands to mount an appropriate cortisol response to severe stress or illness. This syndrome has been well documented in septic human patients, contributing to the development of refractory hypotension and death. Administration of supraphysiologic steroids in affected patients leads to rapid shock reversal and decreased mortality. This chapter reviews the incidence, characteristics, diagnosis, and treatment of adrenal insufficiency in critically ill humans and provides a brief overview of available comparative data concerning pituitary-adrenal function in critically ill dogs or cats.

THE ROLE OF CORTISOL IN HEALTH AND DISEASE

Activation of the hypothalamic-pituitary-adrenal (HPA) axis in response to acute illness or injury is paramount for maintenance of homeostasis and adaptation during periods of severe stress. Cortisol, the predominant glucocorticoid produced by the adrenal cortex, plays an important role in maintenance of normal endothelial integrity, vascular permeability, and distribution of total body water. This hormone affects vascular tone by increasing the number and improving the function of α_1-and β-adrenergic receptors as well as via inhibition of nitric oxide production. Cortisol improves myocardial contractility and attenuates the down-regulation of adrenergic receptors that occurs secondary to catecholamine therapy in septic shock. In addition, cortisol modulates immune-mediated inflammation via inhibition of leukocyte migration, neutrophil and endothelial adhesion, and macrophage and endothelial function.

Among other physiologic stressors, severe illness, trauma, and surgery result in profound activation of the HPA axis with a resultant increase in circulating corticotropin (ACTH) and cortisol concentrations. The magnitude of the increase in serum cortisol concentration has been correlated positively with both illness severity and mortality.

ADRENAL INSUFFICIENCY IN HUMANS WITH CRITICAL ILLNESS

Absolute Adrenal Insufficiency

Absolute adrenal insufficiency can be primary, resulting from destruction of the adrenal glands (Chapter 51), or secondary to disorders affecting the hypothalamus or pituitary gland. Patients suffering from absolute adrenal insufficiency demonstrate a low basal cortisol concentration that responds minimally or not at all to stimulation with ACTH. This syndrome is rare in humans with critical illness, affecting approximately 2% to 5% of intensive care unit (ICU) patients.

Relative Adrenal Insufficiency

In a subset of critically ill patients, normal or increased basal cortisol concentrations are inadequate *relative* to the increased demand during periods of extreme stress. These patients have limited adrenal reserve, with an insufficient cortisol response to combat ongoing inflammation or infection, and they exhibit blunted responses to exogenous ACTH stimulation *independent* of basal cortisol values (which are often high in absolute terms at the onset of the septic episode). This "relative adrenal insufficiency" is functional as opposed to structural and is transient in nature, resolving following recovery from illness. Depending on the criteria used for diagnosis, relative adrenal insufficiency affects approximately 10% to 50% of all critically ill humans with sepsis.

Causes of Relative Adrenal Insufficiency in Critical Illness

The cause of relative adrenal insufficiency is unknown, but the development of this syndrome in septic patients is most likely multifactorial, involving a complex interaction between endocrine and immune systems. Various cytokines circulating during systemic infection (e.g., tumor necrosis factor–α) inhibit ACTH-releasing hormone and ACTH and directly impair adrenal function. Leptin and corticostatin, peptides produced by adipocytes and immune cells, respectively, also circulate in high concentrations in septic patients. These peptides impair adrenocortical function and may contribute to the development of relative adrenal insufficiency.

Clinical and Laboratory Features of Relative Adrenal Insufficiency in Critical Illness

Impairment of the normal cortisol response during critical illness can result in hypotension that mimics either hypovolemic shock (characterized by decreased preload and increased systemic vascular resistance) or septic/hyperdynamic shock (characterized by increased cardiac output and decreased systemic vascular resistance). Hemodynamic instability with hypotension refractory to fluid and vasopressor therapy is common in humans with relative adrenal insufficiency. Additional clinical features suggestive of this syndrome include weakness, fatigue, gastrointestinal disturbances (nausea, vomiting, and anorexia), and fever. Compatible laboratory findings include hypoglycemia, hyponatremia, and hyperkalemia (infrequently reported in relative adrenal insufficiency). Absolute or relative eosinophilia has also been reported.

Because clinical signs are vague and nonspecific, relative adrenal insufficiency can be challenging to diagnose clinically. Index of suspicion should be particularly high in critically ill patients who exhibit refractory hypotension, who are unable to be weaned from mechanical ventilation, or who have ongoing inflammation with no obvious source.

Definitive Diagnosis of Relative Adrenal Insufficiency in Critical Illness

Biochemical evaluation of adrenal function typically involves administration of the ACTH stimulation test. This test bypasses the hypothalamic-pituitary axis and assesses only the integrity of the adrenal gland. Traditionally a total dosage of 250 mcg of synthetic ACTH is administered intravenously (IV) to a human or dog, whereas cats received a total dosage of 125 mcg. Serum or plasma cortisol concentration is measured before, 30 minutes after, and/or 60 minutes after ACTH administration. Low basal and ACTH-stimulated cortisol concentrations are consistent with a diagnosis of absolute adrenal insufficiency. A blunted response to ACTH stimulation, irrespective of basal cortisol concentration (which is typically high), is suggestive of relative adrenal insufficiency.

Several factors complicate the evaluation of adrenal function in critically ill patients. First, there is marked heterogeneity in basal and ACTH-stimulated cortisol concentrations in sick patients. Reference ranges for the standard ACTH stimulation test in both humans and animals were established by use of healthy control subjects, and it is likely that inaccuracy will be introduced if these normal values are applied to ICU patients.

Second, laboratory criteria that are used to diagnose relative adrenal insufficiency are controversial. To improve the usefulness of the ACTH stimulation test in humans with critical illness, it has been recommended that defining threshold cortisol levels below which relative adrenal insufficiency is likely and above which relative adrenal insufficiency is unlikely may be more appropriate in this patient population (Cooper and Stewart, 2005). For patients with random cortisol measurements between such low and high values, response to ACTH stimulation can be used to assess adrenal reserve and identify patients who may benefit from corticosteroid administration.

Other investigators advocate the change in serum cortisol following ACTH stimulation (i.e., the delta cortisol) as the primary diagnostic criterion for this syndrome of relative adrenal insufficiency. Using a cortisol response of less than or equal to 9 mcg/dl, over half of humans with sepsis had relative adrenal insufficiency in one study (Annane et al., 2000). As with basal cortisol, the incremental cortisol response following ACTH administration, or the delta cortisol, has been shown to vary inversely with illness severity and mortality in humans. A third factor that may confound the diagnosis of relative adrenal

insufficiency in critically ill patients is the dose of ACTH used in test subjects. The standard ACTH stimulation test (250 mcg total dosage per patient) involves administration of supraphysiologic doses of ACTH, far surpassing the endogenous ACTH level achieved following normal stress-induced release. This large dose of ACTH may result in a normal cortisol response despite adrenal ACTH resistance and lack of adequate adrenal reserve. Use of a low-dose (1-mcg) ACTH stimulation test may be more sensitive than the 250-mcg test in documentation of relative adrenal insufficiency, but further validation is warranted before acceptance of this test in the clinical setting.

Treatment of Relative Adrenal Insufficiency in Patients With Critical Illness

Prompt recognition of relative adrenal insufficiency in critically ill patients can have dramatic effects on patient morbidity and mortality. High basal cortisol concentration and a blunted response to ACTH stimulation identify not only patients with a higher risk of death but also those who might benefit from corticosteroid therapy. Additional therapies for relative adrenal insufficiency include underlying disease eradication and general supportive measures designed to optimize end-organ perfusion.

There are several randomized, controlled trials of glucocorticoid replacement in human septic shock patients suspected of having relative adrenal insufficiency. Most clinical trials have demonstrated more rapid shock reversal (i.e., ability to wean from vasopressor support) in patients administered supraphysiologic steroids versus placebo. In addition, a recent trial evaluating 300 humans with septic shock showed a survival advantage associated with concurrent administration of glucocorticoids and mineralocorticoids versus placebo (Annane, 2002). Mineralocorticoid deficiency in critically ill humans has been documented in several studies, but the value of aldosterone replacement in these patients is unclear at this time.

Supraphysiologic glucocorticoid administration in patients suspected of having relative adrenal insufficiency has also been efficacious in critically ill human trauma and surgical patients. Steroid administration in these patients was associated with rapid cessation of vasopressor therapy, ability to wean from ventilatory support, and fever resolution.

The role of glucocorticoids in treatment of septic shock has long been debated. Most investigators have reported that short-term administration of pharmacologic steroids (methylprednisolone, 30 mg/kg IV) is of no benefit and may be harmful (because of pronounced immunosuppressive effects) in septic humans. Therefore it is currently strongly recommended that high-dose steroids not be administered to these patients. Conversely, a more prolonged course of "low-dose" glucocorticoids (100 mg, or approximately 1.5 mg/kg, of hydrocortisone every 6 to 8 hours IV) can be recommended for humans suffering from refractory septic shock. The recommendation was included in the 2004 Surviving Sepsis Campaign guidelines.

The glucocorticoid dose currently recommended for relative adrenal insufficiency is supraphysiologic, resulting in a plasma cortisol concentration several times higher than that achieved via ACTH stimulation. This regimen of therapy was initially based on the maximum secretory rate of cortisol found in humans following major surgery (i.e., 300 mg of hydrocortisone per day). However, the optimal dose and duration of treatment with steroids has yet to be determined.

Which patients may benefit from supraphysiologic steroid administration and when to initiate this therapy are also unclear. Clinical signs of relative adrenal insufficiency may be subtle and vague, and definitive diagnosis is difficult to achieve with available biochemical tests. The question remains: does response to ACTH stimulation in critically ill patients predict response to steroid therapy? Debate persists regarding the appropriateness of steroid administration without laboratory confirmation of adrenal dysfunction.

A recent clinical trial documented a trend, albeit insignificant, toward increased mortality in "responders" to ACTH stimulation who received supplemental steroids during the study period (Annane, 2002). This finding may refute the argument that response to treatment is an appropriate diagnostic test for relative adrenal insufficiency. The current recommendation in humans is to initiate steroid treatment in patients suffering from refractory shock pending diagnostic confirmation of adrenal dysfunction. This treatment is withdrawn if there is no laboratory evidence of adrenal insufficiency (absolute or relative).

RELATIVE ADRENAL INSUFFICIENCY IN DOGS AND CATS

To date there are limited data evaluating the HPA axis in critically ill animals, and the incidence of relative adrenal insufficiency in these patients is largely unknown. Investigators have documented adrenal dysfunction in experimental rat models of severe hemorrhage and sepsis, suggesting the presence of relative adrenal insufficiency in these subjects. Prittie and colleagues (2003) evaluated adrenocortical function in 20 critically ill cats. Basal cortisol concentrations were higher in sick versus healthy cats but did not correlate with outcome in this population. Similarly, ACTH-stimulated and delta cortisol had no prognostic value in these cats. Cats with neoplasia, but not cats with sepsis, demonstrated lower delta cortisols than did other patients in this study population, suggesting that relative adrenal insufficiency may occur in this subset of critically ill cats. Farrelly and associates (1999) similarly documented adrenal dysfunction in cats with lymphosarcoma, based on blunted cortisol responses to ACTH stimulation. None of these cats had cytologic or histopathologic confirmation of normal adrenal structure, but ultrasound measurements of adrenal size were within normal limits. Relative adrenal insufficiency has recently been reported in a cat recovering from polytrauma and being treated for suspected sepsis (Durkan, 2007). This patient exhibited vasopressor-dependent hypotension that resolved following supraphysiologic steroid administration, and a blunted response to ACTH stimulation (i.e., a delta cortisol of 3.2 mcg/dl).

The occurrence of relative adrenal insufficiency in dogs remains to be determined. One study evaluated pituitary-adrenal function in critically ill dogs through daily ACTH stimulation tests during ICU hospitalization (Prittie and colleagues, 2002). No dog developed relative adrenal insufficiency during the study period; basal cortisol and ACTH-stimulated cortisol concentrations remained within or above the reference range established for healthy dogs. Basal cortisol concentration did not correlate with illness severity or outcome in these dogs, unlike the case in many human studies. Delta cortisol was not evaluated. More recently adrenal function was examined retrospectively in 42 sick dogs (Shaw and associates, 2005). Four dogs demonstrated adrenal dysfunction characterized by low basal and delta cortisol levels, and all were nonsurvivors. However, there was not a clear delineation between absolute and relative adrenal insufficiency in that study population.

Given the paucity of information available regarding the occurrence of relative adrenal insufficiency in critically ill small animals, currently there are no guidelines for diagnosis and treatment of this disorder. As is the case with human ICU patients, a high index of suspicion of relative adrenal insufficiency is warranted in critically ill veterinary patients that are volume loaded and remain vasopressor dependent. This is especially the case in cats with cancer that have been shown to have evidence of adrenal dysfunction. Relative adrenal insufficiency in these cats may explain the dramatic clinical response to glucocorticoid administration that precedes implementation of chemotherapy. If clinical suspicion of relative adrenal insufficiency is high, supraphysiologic glucocorticoid replacement pending results of confirmatory laboratory tests seems prudent.

References and Suggested Reading

Annane D et al: A 3-level prognostic classification in septic shock based on cortisol levels and cortisol response to corticotropin, *J Am Med Assoc* 283:1038, 2000.

Annane D et al: Effect of treatment with low doses of hydrocortisone and fludrocortisone on mortality in patients with septic shock, *J Am Med Assoc* 288:862, 2002.

Cooper MS, Stewart PM: Corticosteroid insufficiency in acutely ill patients, *N Engl J Med* 348:727, 2005.

Durkan S et al: Suspected relative adrenal insufficiency in a critically ill cat, *J Vet Emerg Crit Care* 17:197, 2007.

Farrelly J et al: Evaluation of pituitary-adrenal function in cats with lymphoma. In Proceedings of the 19th Annual Veterinary Cancer Society Conference, 1999, p 33.

Lefering R, Neugebauer EAM: Steroid controversy in sepsis and septic shock: a meta-analysis, *Crit Care Med* 23:1294, 1995.

Martin L, Groman R: State of the art review: relative adrenal insufficiency in critical illness, *J Vet Emerg Crit Care* 14:149, 2004.

Prittie JE et al: Hypothalamopituitary adrenal (HPA) axis function in critically ill cats. In *Proceedings of the 9th International Veterinary Emergency and Critical Care Symposium*, 2003, p 771.

Prittie JE et al: Pituitary ACTH and adrenocortical secretion in critically ill dogs, *J Am Vet Med Assoc* 200:615, 2002.

Shaw SP et al: Relative adrenal insufficiency in critically ill dogs. *In Proceedings of the 11th International Veterinary Emergency and Critical Care Symposium*, 2005, p 1050.

CHAPTER 51

Hypoadrenocorticism

PETER P. KINTZER, *Springfield, Massachusetts*
MARK E. PETERSON, *Bedford Hills, New York*

Spontaneous canine hypoadrenocorticism is a well-recognized but uncommon endocrine disorder. Hypoadrenocorticism is characterized by a deficiency of glucocorticoid and/or mineralocorticoid production by the adrenal cortices. Although mild destruction or atrophy of adrenocortical tissue can impair adrenocortical reserve, typically at least 90% of the adrenal cortex needs to be nonfunctional before clinical signs of hypoadrenocorticism are observed under nonstressful conditions.

ETIOLOGY

Primary hypoadrenocorticism results from destruction or atrophy of the adrenal cortices and usually results in a deficiency of both glucocorticoid and mineralocorticoid secretion. Causes include idiopathic spontaneous (probably immune-mediated) primary hypoadrenocorticism (Addison's disease), iatrogenic disease resulting from mitotane or trilostane therapy, and very rare cases of adrenocortical destruction resulting from granulomatous disease, metastatic neoplasia, or hemorrhage.

A subset of dogs with primary hypoadrenocorticism appear to develop a selective glucocorticoid deficiency with apparently normal mineralocorticoid secretion, based on the findings of low basal and adrenocorticotropin hormone (ACTH)–stimulated serum cortisol values with normal concentrations of serum electrolytes. This type of hypoadrenocorticism is commonly referred to as "atypical" hypoadrenocorticism. In most of these dogs mineralocorticoid deficiency eventually develops, but a few dogs do not develop deficient mineralocorticoid secretion or serum electrolyte changes when followed for many months or years.

Secondary hypoadrenocorticism is caused by insufficient pituitary ACTH production and the resultant atrophy of the portion of the adrenal cortices responsible for glucocorticoid production. The result is deficient glucocorticoid secretion; mineralocorticoid secretion is preserved. Causes include iatrogenic disease resulting from overly rapid discontinuation of long-term and/or high-dose glucocorticoid therapy, pituitary or hypothalamic lesions, or idiopathic isolated ACTH deficiency.

DIAGNOSIS

Although most affected dogs present in young to middle age, naturally occurring hypoadrenocorticism has been reported in dogs ranging from 2 months to 14 years of age. A genetic predilection has been confirmed in standard poodles and bearded collies and suggested in certain breeds such as Nova Scotia duck tolling retrievers, Leonbergers, Portuguese water spaniels, Great Danes, rottweilers, and wheaten and West Highland white terriers. Female dogs are about twice as likely to develop naturally occurring hypoadrenocorticism as males.

The historical findings, clinical signs, and laboratory abnormalities associated with spontaneous hypoadrenocorticism are well described (Tables 51-1 and 51-2). The severity and duration of clinical signs vary greatly among cases, from the acute life-threatening addisonian crisis to the chronic intermittent signs seen in some dogs with chronic hypoadrenocorticism. Many of the historical and clinical findings are nonspecific and also occur in many more common diseases, particularly gastrointestinal and renal disorders. No set of findings is pathognomonic for canine hypoadrenocorticism. A high index of suspicion is needed to recognize some cases. Findings that should heighten this suspicion include a waxing/waning course, previous response to fluid or glucocorticoid therapy, and exacerbation of clinical signs in stressful situations.

The classic electrolyte abnormalities associated with spontaneous primary hypoadrenocorticism are hyperkalemia and hyponatremia. In our experience one or both are present in 90% to 95% of affected dogs. Prior treatment with fluids, steroids, or both may mask serum electrolyte changes. Therefore one should never exclude a diagnosis of primary hypoadrenocorticism in a dog suspected of having hypoadrenocorticism on a basis of normal serum electrolyte concentrations alone. Also, some dogs with secondary hypoadrenocorticism caused by isolated pituitary ACTH deficiency are hyponatremic with normal potassium concentrations. Although Addison's disease is often the first disorder thought of when these electrolyte abnormalities are found, the presence of hyperkalemia and hyponatremia cannot be relied on for the diagnosis of canine hypoadrenocorticism. Indeed these electrolyte abnormalities may be associated with a wide variety of diseases more common than hypoadrenocorticism, including gastrointestinal disorders, renal disease, effusive disorders, and acidosis.

Definitive diagnosis of hypoadrenocorticism requires demonstration of inadequate adrenal reserve. This is done by performing an ACTH stimulation test, considered the gold standard for diagnosis of hypoadrenocorticism. The preferred method is to determine serum cortisol concentrations before and 1 hour after the intravenous administration of 5 mcg/kg of cosyntropin (Cortrosyn, Amphastar Pharmaceuticals, Rancho Cucamonga, CA). Following reconstitution, the solution, when refrigerated, is stable

Table 51-1

Clinical Findings in Dogs With Hypoadrenocorticism

Finding	Percent
Lethargy/depression	95
Anorexia	90
Vomiting	75
Weakness	75
Weight loss	50
Dehydration	45
Diarrhea	40
Waxing/waning course	40
Collapse	35
Previous response to therapy	35
Hypothermia	35
Slow capillary refill (perfusion) time	30
Shaking	25
Polydipsia/Polyuria	25
Melena	20
Weak pulse	20
Bradycardia	18
Painful abdomen	8
Hair loss	5

Table 51-2

Laboratory Findings in Canine Hypoadrenocorticism

Finding	Percent
Hyperkalemia	90
Hyponatremia	80
Na/K ratio <27	95
Hypochloremia	40
Hypercalcemia	30
Azotemia	85
Acidosis	40
Elevated ALT or AST	30
Hyperbilirubinemia	20
Hypoglycemia	15
Anemia	25
Eosinophilia	20
Lymphocytosis	10
Urine specific gravity <1.030	60

ALT, Alanine aminotransferase; *AST,* aspartate aminotransferase

for at least 4 weeks. Otherwise the remaining solution can be divided into aliquots and frozen.

If cosyntropin is not available, the ACTH stimulation test can also be performed by determining the serum cortisol concentration before and after the intramuscular injection of 2.2 U/kg of ACTH gel. Acthar Gel (80 U/ml; Questor Pharmaceuticals, Union City, CA) is available but very expensive. If this product is used, the post-ACTH sample is collected at 2 hours. Alternatively ACTH gel (usually 40 U/ml) is available from several compounding pharmacies. The bioavailability and reproducibility of all of these formulations have yet to be carefully evaluated. A recent study in dogs by Kemppainen, Behrend, and Busch (2005) using four compounded ACTH gels demonstrated increases in serum cortisol concentrations comparable to cosyntropin injection 1 hour after intramuscular injection of each of the four formulations but considerable variation at 2 hours after injection. The investigators recommended determining serum cortisol concentrations at both 1 and 2 hours post-ACTH administration when using a compounded ACTH gel. The determination of a third cortisol level would likely offset any presumed cost saving derived from using the compounded product. The potential for lot-to-lot variability in compounded ACTH gel formulations has not been evaluated. Therefore one should consider assessing the activity of each new vial by performing an ACTH stimulation test on a normal dog.

In normal dogs administration of a supraphysiologic dose of ACTH produces a rise in serum cortisol to values usually above 10 mcg/dl. In contrast, dogs with hypoadrenocorticism have an absent or blunted response to ACTH administration. Basal and post-ACTH serum cortisol concentrations are less than 1 mcg/dl in over 75% of dogs and less than 2 mcg/dl in virtually all dogs with primary hypoadrenocorticism. Although the post-ACTH serum cortisol concentration may be as high as 2 to 3 mcg/dl in a few dogs with secondary hypoadrenocorticism, the great majority of these dogs also have ACTH-stimulated cortisol concentrations of less than 2 mcg/dl.

The ACTH stimulation test using intravenous cosyntropin can be performed during institution of initial treatment if dexamethasone is used for glucocorticoid replacement since dexamethasone does not interfere with the cortisol assay. If prednisone, prednisolone, or hydrocortisone have been administered, these treatments must be discontinued, and glucocorticoid supplementation changed to dexamethasone for at least 24 hours before ACTH stimulation testing. ACTH gel cannot be used in dehydrated or hypovolemic patients since impaired absorption may lead to inaccurate results. Alternatively, testing can be delayed until after the patient is stabilized.

A recent study in dogs comparing an in-house cortisol assay (SNAP Cortisol, IDEXX Laboratories, Westbrook, ME) with a reference laboratory chemiluminescent assay showed very positive correlation between the two assays. The in-house assay is particularly useful when a rapid determination of the presence of hypoadrenocorticism is desired, such as differentiating in an emergency patient between an addisonian crisis and a disease with a poorer prognosis such as acute renal failure.

Secondary hypoadrenocorticism can be differentiated from atypical primary hypoadrenocorticism by measurement of a plasma ACTH level. Plasma ACTH is high (>500 pg/ml) with primary hypoadrenocorticism and undetectable-to-low with secondary hypoadrenocorticism. ACTH is labile; therefore the diagnostic laboratory performing the assay should be consulted for appropriate sample handling instructions. Plasma for ACTH determination must be collected before instituting therapy, especially glucocorticoid treatment. Even a relatively low dose of glucocorticoid may reduce previously-high ACTH concentrations into the normal-to-low reference range; thus the results must be interpreted in conjunction with a careful drug history. To properly evaluate the endogenous ACTH test result, the dog ideally should not have received any form of steroid treatment in the preceding weeks. If plasma ACTH is measured in a dog that has received recent glucocorticoid treatment, a false-positive diagnosis of secondary hypoadrenocorticism may be entertained.

Recently an alternate approach was proposed in dogs for assessing the pituitary-glucocorticoid axis by measuring basal cortisol and plasma ACTH concentrations and then calculating a cortisol-to-ACTH ratio (Javadi and colleagues, 2006). Similarly the renin-angiotensin-aldosterone system was assessed by determining the basal plasma concentrations of aldosterone and plasma renin activity and then calculating an aldosterone-to-renin ratio.

Dogs with primary hypoadrenocorticism have low basal concentrations of cortisol with high plasma ACTH concentrations. In contrast, dogs with secondary hypoadrenocorticism have low plasma cortisol concentrations with low plasma ACTH concentrations. Therefore dogs with primary hypoadrenocorticism have much lower cortisol-to-ACTH ratios than do normal dogs or dogs with secondary hypoadrenocorticism, with little to no overlap in ratio values.

In states of aldosterone deficiency such as primary hypoadrenocorticism, the inability to retain sodium leads to hypovolemia, which subsequently stimulates renin release. Thus dogs with primary hypoadrenocorticism have low basal concentrations of aldosterone with high plasma renin activity. In secondary hypoadrenocorticism aldosterone secretion is not decreased; therefore plasma renin activity remains relatively normal. Accordingly, dogs with primary hypoadrenocorticism have much lower aldosterone-to-renin ratios than do normal dogs or dogs with secondary hypoadrenocorticism, again with little to no overlap in ratio values.

The advantage of the use of cortisol-to-ACTH and aldosterone-to-renin ratios is that such measurement of endogenous hormone variables in a single blood sample allows for the specific diagnosis of primary hypocortisolism and primary hypoaldosteronism. A dynamic stimulation test is not required. The use of these paired-hormone ratios generally allows for clear differentiation between primary and secondary hypoadrenocorticism; this dual assessment is particularly relevant when isolated hormone deficiency is suspected (i.e., isolated glucocorticoid deficiency or isolated mineralocorticoid deficiency).

Disadvantages of this approach to diagnosis include the considerable expense to measure plasma concentrations of cortisol, ACTH, aldosterone, and renin activity, as well as sample handling, including the absolute necessity of collecting blood for measurement of hormone and renin concentrations before any fluid or steroid treatment. Furthermore, it may be difficult to find a laboratory that can accurately measure plasma renin activity in dogs.

TREATMENT

The intensiveness of therapeutic intervention depends on the individual patient's condition. Acute hypoadrenocorticism (addisonian crisis) is a medical emergency requiring prompt treatment, whereas dogs with chronic hypoadrenocorticism generally do not need aggressive therapy, although many may benefit from hospitalization for parenteral fluids and glucocorticoids.

Acute Hypoadrenocorticism

If the clinical presentation is consistent with an addisonian crisis, treatment must be instituted immediately once blood is collected for a complete blood count, chemistry profile, and other indicated laboratory work and urine obtained for urinalysis. Definitive diagnostic workup is begun while initial treatment and stabilization is in progress. Goals of therapy are to restore plasma volume status, correct electrolyte and acid-base disturbances, improve vascular integrity, and provide an immediate source of rapid-acting glucocorticoid.

Of primary importance in therapy for acute hypoadrenocorticism is the rapid infusion of large volumes of intravenous fluids, preferably 0.9% NaCl, at an initial rate of 60 to 80 ml/kg/hour for 1 to 2 hours. This initial rate of infusion helps to address hypotension and hypovolemia. In addition, serum potassium concentration is reduced by dilution, increased renal perfusion, and thereby potassium excretion. A colloid also can be administered to address hypotension and hypovolemia, but this is rarely needed. The rate of saline infusion is then gradually reduced to a maintenance rate and eventually discontinued over a few days based on the dog's clinical response and laboratory parameters, including serial blood pressure, renal function, and electrolyte measurements. Urine output should be quantified to assess its adequacy and to help guide fluid therapy. If severe hyponatremia is present on initial evaluation, it should be corrected no faster than 10 to 12 mEq/dl per day over the first 48 hours of therapy. Overly rapid correction of hyponatremia can result in neurologic damage (myelinosis).

Also critically important to the therapy of acute hypoadrenocorticism is the intravenous administration of a rapid-acting glucocorticoid. Dexamethasone sodium phosphate (2 to 4 mg/kg) or prednisolone sodium succinate (15 to 20 mg/kg) is preferred; dexamethasone sodium phosphate must be used if the ACTH stimulation test is in progress. This initial dose of dexamethasone can be repeated in 2 to 6 hours if needed. Glucocorticoid supplementation is then gradually tapered to a maintenance dose of prednisone (0.2 mg/kg) over the next several days as dictated by clinical response. The maintenance dose of prednisone may not be reached until after the patient is at home. Parenteral supplementation is indicated until vomiting has ceased and oral intake has begun.

Hyperkalemia is often successfully corrected by parenteral fluid therapy alone. However, for severe hyperkalemia causing life-threatening myocardial toxicity manifested by significant arrhythmias (including atrial standstill, abnormal ST-T waves, and widening of the QRS complex), more aggressive therapy is necessary. Our preferred treatment is intravenous insulin and dextrose. Regular insulin (0.5 U/kg) is given intravenously. Glucose (2 to 3 g/U of insulin) is given half as an intravenous bolus and half in the intravenous fluids over the next 6 to 8 hours. These dogs must be closely monitored for hypoglycemia, with hourly blood glucose determinations. Dogs with hypoadrenocorticism are very sensitive to the glucose-lowering action of insulin; however, the administration of the rapid-acting glucocorticoid as described previously before or concurrent with insulin administration would be expected to counteract this tendency. Alternatively slow intravenous administration of 10% calcium chloride (0.1 ml/kg over 10 to 20 minutes) or $NaHCO_3$ (1-2 mEq/kg over 10-15 minutes) can be considered to treat advanced hyperkalemic myocardial toxicity.

Hypoglycemia and metabolic acidosis may demand treatment in some cases. Dextrose (2.5% to 5%) is added to the intravenous fluids as needed. Symptomatic hypoglycemia is treated with a slow intravenous bolus of 0.5 to 1.5 ml/kg of 50% dextrose. Mild-to-moderate acidosis is usually corrected with parenteral fluid therapy. Severe metabolic acidosis (pH < 7.1) is treated with sodium bicarbonate. The total dosage is calculated as follows:

$$\text{Deficit in mEq} = (\text{body weight in kilograms})\,(0.5)\,(\text{base deficit})$$

One fourth of the calculated dosage is administered in the intravenous fluids over the next 6 to 8 hours, and the acid-base status then reassessed. It is unusual for additional bicarbonate therapy to be needed.

No rapid-acting parenteral mineralocorticoid preparation is currently available for treatment of acute hypoadrenocorticism. This does not constitute a significant clinical problem because prompt aggressive treatment as described previously is sufficient to stabilize a dog suffering an addisonian crisis. Nonetheless we typically give a desoxycorticosterone pivalate (DOCP; Percorten-V, Novartis Animal Health, Greensboro, NC) injection as soon as the diagnosis of primary hypoadrenocorticism is confirmed. Alternatively, fludrocortisone acetate (Florinef, Bristol-Myers Squibb) can be used. Such mineralocorticoid supplementation is not harmful and may help correct serum electrolyte abnormalities.

Chronic Hypoadrenocorticism

Dogs with chronic hypoadrenocorticism present with clinical signs of varying severity and duration and do not require the aggressive therapy described previously for cases of acute hypoadrenocorticism. However, fluid therapy and parenteral glucocorticoid supplementation may be indicated in some cases, particularly if azotemia, dehydration, hypotension, or significant vomiting or diarrhea is present. In these dogs parenteral therapy is continued until these abnormalities have resolved and maintenance therapy can be instituted. Similarly, in dogs recovering from an addisonian crisis, maintenance therapy is instituted once the dog is stable and oral medication can be tolerated.

Dogs with naturally occurring primary hypoadrenocorticism typically require both glucocorticoid and mineralocorticoid replacement therapy for life. The few dogs with atypical primary hypoadrenocorticism can be started on glucocorticoid replacement therapy alone but must have serum electrolyte concentrations frequently monitored since most of these dogs will develop the typical electrolyte abnormalities after weeks to months and require mineralocorticoid supplementation as well.

Either DOCP or fludrocortisone can be used for chronic mineralocorticoid replacement. We typically institute treatment with DOCP given at 2.2 mg/g subcutaneously or intramuscularly every 4 weeks. Side effects associated with DOCP therapy are rare. A dosage interval of 3 to 4 weeks is effective in almost all cases, and most are controlled with an injection every 4 weeks. After the first one or two injections of DOCP, electrolyte and creatinine levels are monitored at 2, 3, and 4 weeks following injection to determine the duration of action and help make dosage adjustments if necessary. Once stabilized, serum electrolyte and creatinine concentrations are checked every 3 to 6 months.

Although a DOCP dose of less than 2.2 mg/kg would be sufficient in some cases, a dose of 2.2 mg/kg is still recommended at least for the initial treatment. Less than 10% of dogs require a DOCP dose greater than 2.2 mg/kg, and a starting dose of 2.2 mg/kg eliminates the need for the clinician to incrementally increase the DOCP dosage over the first several months of therapy, which often happens in dogs started on a lower initial DOCP dose. However, if financial constraints are a factor, one can attempt to gradually reduce the monthly dose of DOCP to the lowest effective dose based on close monitoring of serum electrolyte concentrations. Alternatively, the interval between DOCP injections can be incrementally lengthened (typically in 1-week intervals) as dictated by monitoring of serum electrolyte concentrations. Dogs with hypoadrenocorticism and congestive heart failure (such as some Rottweilers with dilated cardiomyopathy) may require higher doses of furosemide the first 2 weeks following DOCP administration to prevent pulmonary edema (fludrocortisone represents an alternative treatment for this group).

Fludrocortisone acetate is given at an initial oral dosage of 0.01 to 0.02 mg/kg/day, and the dosage is adjusted by 0.05 to 0.1 mg/day as determined by serial serum electrolyte concentrations. After initiation of fludrocortisone therapy, serum electrolyte and creatinine levels should be monitored until stabilized within the normal range. Once this is achieved, the dogs should be reevaluated monthly for the first 3 to 6 months of therapy and then every 3 to 6 months thereafter. In many dogs in which fludrocortisone is used as long-term mineralocorticoid replacement, the daily dose required to control the disorder gradually increases; this is most evident in the first 6 to 24 months of treatment. In most dogs the final fludrocortisone dosage needed is 0.02 to 0.03 mg/kg/day. Very few dogs can be controlled on a dosage of 0.01 mg/kg/day or less. Adverse effects (usually polyuria and polydipsia), development of a relative resistance to the effects of fludrocortisone, or financial considerations (especially when treating large- or giant-breed dogs) may necessitate a change to DOCP therapy in some dogs.

Many dogs with primary hypoadrenocorticism, particularly those receiving DOCP, require chronic glucocorticoid supplementation in addition to mineralocorticoid supplementation to prevent signs of glucocorticoid deficiency. In general, all dogs with primary hypoadrenocorticism are started on glucocorticoid replacement with prednisone or prednisolone (0.2 mg/kg/day) in conjunction with mineralocorticoid replacement (usually DOCP). If warranted because of the development of side effects, the glucocorticoid dosage can be tapered to alternate days and then discontinued if necessary to evaluate if glucocorticoids are needed as part of maintenance therapy. The fact that glucocorticoids can be discontinued without the recurrence of significant clinical signs in some dogs with hypoadrenocorticism is especially important in dogs that have developed signs of intolerance of glucocorticoid administration (e.g., polyuria/polydipsia) after treatment. In many of these dogs cessation of glucocorticoids reverses signs of iatrogenic hyperadrenocorticism, and mineralocorticoid replacement alone controls signs of hypoadrenocorticism. Nevertheless, additional glucocorticoid supplementation (2 to 10 times normal recommended replacement dosage) may be necessary during periods of stress such as illness, trauma, or surgery; therefore the owner should always have some glucocorticoid on hand and be informed of situations in which the dog might require glucocorticoid supplementation. Dogs with documented secondary hypoadrenocorticism (isolated pituitary ACTH deficiency) require only glucocorticoid replacement therapy. Oral administration of prednisone or prednisolone at a dosage of 0.2 mg/kg/day usually suffices, except during periods of stress or illness when higher doses are necessary. If secondary hypoadrenocorticism has not been documented by the presence of undetectable-to-low plasma ACTH concentrations in hypoadrenal patients with normal serum electrolyte concentrations, one must continue to determine serum electrolyte concentrations on a regular

(e.g., monthly) basis. As mentioned previously, many dogs with atypical primary hypoadrenocorticism originally presenting with normal serum electrolyte concentrations and suspected of having secondary hypoadrenocorticism and being managed with only glucocorticoid supplementation will subsequently develop the typical electrolyte abnormalities of primary hypoadrenocorticism and require mineralocorticoid replacement therapy.

References and Suggested Reading

Church DB: Canine hypoadrenocorticism. In Mooney CT, Peterson ME, editors: *BSAVA Manual of canine and feline endocrinology*, ed 3, Quedgeley, Gloucester, 2004, British Small Animal Veterinary Association, p 172.

Feldman EC, Nelson RW: Hypoadrenocorticism (Addison's disease). In Canine and feline endocrinology and reproduction, ed 3, Philadelphia, 2004, Saunders, p 394.

Javadi S et al: Aldosterone-to-renin and cortisol-to-adrenocorticotropic hormone ratios in healthy dogs and dogs with primary hypoadrenocorticism, *J Vet Intern Med* 20:556, 2006.

Kemppainen RJ, Behrend EN, Busch KA: Use of compounded adrenocorticotropic hormone (ACTH) for adrenal function testing in dogs, *J Am Anim Hosp Assoc* 41:368, 2005.

Kintzer PP, Peterson ME: Diseases of the adrenal gland. In Birchard SJ, Sherding RG, editors: *Saunders Manual of small animal practice*, ed 3, St. Louis, 2006, Saunders, p 357.

Kintzer PP, Peterson ME: Treatment and long-term follow-up of 205 dogs with hypoadrenocorticism, *J Vet Intern Med* 11:43, 1997.

Peterson ME, Kintzer PP, Kass PH: Pretreatment clinical and laboratory findings in dogs with hypoadrenocorticism: 225 cases (1979-1993), *J Am Vet Med Assoc* 208:85, 1995.

CHAPTER 52

Idiopathic Feline Hypercalcemia

DENNIS J. CHEW, *Columbus, Ohio*
PATRICIA A. SCHENCK, *Lansing, Michigan*

Since the early 1990s unexplained hypercalcemia has been recognized increasingly as an incidental finding in cats and has been termed *idiopathic. Idiopathic hypercalcemia (IHC)* is defined as abnormally elevated serum ionized calcium (iCa) concentration, the cause of which remains unknown after extensive medical evaluation to rule out known causes of hypercalcemia. Little is known about this syndrome, even though it appears to be the most common cause of hypercalcemia in cats. Although once thought to be a local geographic phenomenon, it is widespread across the United States, and anecdotal reports are emerging from other parts of the world (England, Scandinavia, Switzerland).

DIFFERENTIAL DIAGNOSIS

Hypercalcemia is typically noted on an initial analysis of serum total calcium (tCa) and is often a fortuitous discovery when a blood sample is taken for other reasons (e.g., wellness examinations, preanesthesia screening, evaluation of urolithiasis, evaluation of gastrointestinal signs). When a mild increase in serum tCa is noted, a second sample collected after a 12-hour fast should be submitted to verify the increase. If this mild increase in tCa is repeatable, an iCa measurement should be obtained. If a moderate or severe elevation in tCa is noted initially, iCa concentration should be measured as soon as possible. Serum iCa concentration needs to be measured because the prediction of iCa status from tCa measurement is not accurate.

Hypercalcemia may be parathyroid independent or parathyroid dependent (primary hyperparathyroidism). In parathyroid-independent hypercalcemia, the elevation of iCa results in *suppression* of parathyroid hormone (PTH) production. In cats with IHC, PTH values are usually normal to low normal (see below).

There are many potential causes of hypercalcemia in the cat (Box 52-1). A differential diagnostic list ensures that all possibilities for the development of hypercalcemia have been considered. However, such a list does not give any indication as to the frequency of the diagnoses. The most common diagnoses in cats with persistent elevations in iCa are idiopathic hypercalcemia (IHC) and malignancy. Renal failure often is accompanied by elevations in serum tCa, but iCa is rarely elevated in this condition. In many cases the diagnosis is obvious on analysis of history and physical examination. In others the cause may not be evident; and further workup, including hematology, serum biochemistry, body cavity imaging, cytology, and histopathology is necessary. A diagnosis of IHC is made when all other causes of hypercalcemia are excluded. It should be noted that while IHC is the most frequent diagnosis in cats with hypercalcemia, it is an exceedingly uncommon finding in dogs following adequate diagnostic workup (see Chapter 54).

The magnitude of elevation of serum tCa cannot be used to make a diagnosis since there is considerable overlap in the degree of hypercalcemia in cats with IHC or other conditions. IHC may present with mild increases in tCa concentration (11 to 12 mg/dl; 2.75 to 3.00 mmol/L), whereas some cats may have tCa concentrations greater than 15 to 20 mg/dl (3.75 to 5 mmol/L).

CLINICAL PRESENTATION

Cats with IHC may have persistent elevations in iCa for months without apparent clinical signs, and no relationship has been noted between the magnitude of elevation and occurrence of clinical signs. In a review of 427 cats with IHC, the mean age at presentation was 9.8 years (range 0.5 to 20 years old), and long-haired cats were overrepresented (27% of cases). Both genders were equally represented. Almost half of the cats had no clinical signs (46%), 18% had mild weight loss, 6% had inflammatory bowel disease, 5% had chronic constipation, 4% presented with vomiting, and 1% were anorectic. Uroliths were reported in 15% of cats with IHC, and calcium oxalate stones were specifically present in 10% of cases.

Serum iCa was increased, and PTH concentration was in the lower half of the reference range (reference range 0 to 4 mmol/L) in our study. Concentrations of both ionized magnesium and 25-hydroxyvitamin D were within the reference range in most cats. In a small number of cats with IHC in which calcitriol (1,25-dihydroxyvitamin D) was measured, the calcitriol concentration was suppressed in most. Some cats with IHC develop chronic renal failure (CRF) secondary to the persistent hypercalcemia, and cats with CRF may develop IHC over time. A few cats may have both CRF and IHC on initial presentation. Serum phosphorus is usually in the normal range in cats with IHC unless it is increased as a result of concurrent CRF. Urinary specific gravity typically is within the reference range, and it appears that many cats with hypercalcemia can still maximally concentrate their urine if they do not have concurrent CRF.

TREATMENT

The treatment of hypercalcemia usually targets the dysregulated mechanisms that are responsible; however, in IHC these mechanisms remain unknown. Thus treatments at this time are empiric.

Differential Diagnosis of Hypercalcemia: HARDIONS Eponym

H: Hyperparathyroidism (1°, 3°, hyperplasia), HHM, houseplants, hyperthyroid

A: Addison's disease, aluminum toxicity, vitamin A, milk-alkali

R: Renal disease, raisins (grapes)—dogs

D: Vitamin D toxicosis (granulomatous Dz), drugs, calcipotriene (Dovonex), dehydration, DMSO (calcinosis cutis), diet

I: Idiopathic (cats), infectious, inflammatory, immobilization

O: Osteolytic (osteomyelitis, immobilization, local osteolytic hypercalcemia, bone infarct)

N: Neoplasia (HHM and LOH), nutritional

S: Spurious, schistosomiasis, salts of calcium, supplements

DMSO, Dimethylsulfoxide; *HHM,* humoral hypercalcemia of malignancy; *LOH,* local osteolytic hypercalcemia.

Should All Cats With IHC Receive Treatment?

Minor elevations in serum iCa concentrations are often ignored since many of these cats have mild or no apparent clinical signs. This mild elevation of calcium may increase gradually or remain at the initial increased level for long periods of time. Excess calcium is toxic to cells, particularly in the central nervous system, gastrointestinal tract, heart, and kidneys. Mineralization of soft tissues is an important complication, and the serum phosphorus concentration when hypercalcemia develops is important in determining the extent of mineralization. When the calcium (mg/dl) times phosphorus (mg/dl) product is greater than 60, soft-tissue mineralization is most severe. The need for therapy in IHC increases when iCa continues to elevate or clinical signs become more obvious (weight loss, depression, vomiting, constipation, urinary stones, emergence of CRF, development of less concentrated urine). The consequences of longstanding hypercalcemia can be devastating in those that develop CRF or urolithiasis, and aggressive treatment for hypercalcemia is warranted in these cases. Continued elevation of iCa leads to further development of renal lesions and development of new stones. An algorithm for decision to treat is presented in Fig. 52-1. Treatment plans for hypercalcemia that is increasing are presented in Figs. 52-2 and 52-3.

Diet Therapy

Normocalcemia may be restored after a change to a different diet. High-fiber diets (e.g., Hill's W/D, Royal Canin HiFactor Formula, Purina One Advanced Nutrition Hairball, Eukanuba/Iams Optimum Weight Control) have been noted to restore normocalcemia in some cats with IHC and calcium oxalate urolithiasis. In five cats with IHC and calcium oxalate uroliths, normocalcemia returned when a higher-fiber diet that was similar to the original diet in terms of urinary acidification and magnesium restriction was fed. However, in another study

there was no beneficial effect of high-fiber diets in cats with IHC. The effects of fiber on intestinal absorption are complex and depend on the type and amount of fiber in the diet and the interactions with other nutrients in the diet. High-fiber diets may decrease intestinal transit time; however, most manufacturers increase the quantity of calcium in high-fiber diets to offset the potential for decreased absorption.

Veterinary diets designed for cats in renal failure (e.g., Eukanuba/Iams Multi-Stage Renal, Hills Science Diet K/D, Purina NF Formula, Royal Canin Renal LP, Royal Canin Modified Formula) have very different compositions than maintenance diets designed for feeding healthy cats; the feeding of a renal failure diet may result in normocalcemia in some cats with IHC. Most renal diets are less acidifying than maintenance diets and are low in calcium and phosphorus. Canned diets are generally more restricted in calcium than dry diets. The decreased consumption of calcium leads to a decrease in the amount of calcium absorbed, and the effects of alkalinization may decrease the release of calcium from bone. However, veterinary renal diets may also enhance renal calcitriol synthesis caused by the dietary restriction of phosphorus. This increase in calcitriol synthesis could offset the advantage of the decreased calcium absorption in cats with IHC.

Veterinary diets developed to prevent calcium oxalate urolithiasis (e.g., Eukanuba/Iams Moderate pH/O, Hill's Science Diet X/D, Royal Canin/IVD Urinary SO, Purina Veterinary Diets UR Urinary St/Ox) may be beneficial in the treatment of cats with IHC. These diets are restricted in calcium and have less urinary acidification (neutral pH urine production). Some are also restricted in oxalic acid and sodium and have increased moisture in the canned formulation. In two of three cats with IHC and calcium oxalate uroliths, hypercalcemia resolved after feeding a calcium oxalate–prevention diet. One cat did not become normocalcemic but did have a reduction in the magnitude of hypercalcemia.

The addition of sodium chloride may be useful in cats with IHC as long as the added salt enhances calcium excretion without an increased risk of calcium oxalate uroliths. Increased dietary sodium chloride increases urine volume but does not increase calcium oxalate relative supersaturation in healthy cats. However, an increase in urinary excretion of calcium does not always correlate to the development of calcium urolithiasis, since the concentration of calcium in the urine also depends on the degree of water excreted at the same time. At this time the effects of additional dietary sodium chloride have not been examined in cats with IHC.

It is doubtful that IHC is the result of excess vitamin D intake since concentrations of 25-hydroxyvitamin D have been within the reference range in most cats with IHC. However, the minimal requirement for vitamin D in cats is debatable since reference ranges have been established in cats fed vitamin D–supplemented diets. Normal concentrations of 25-hydroxyvitamin D could still potentially be associated with IHC in cats if there are mutations in the vitamin D or calcitriol receptors. These possibilities have not yet been investigated. Since the amount of vitamin D supplied in most diets is not listed on the diet label, it is difficult to choose a diet that is lower in vitamin D.

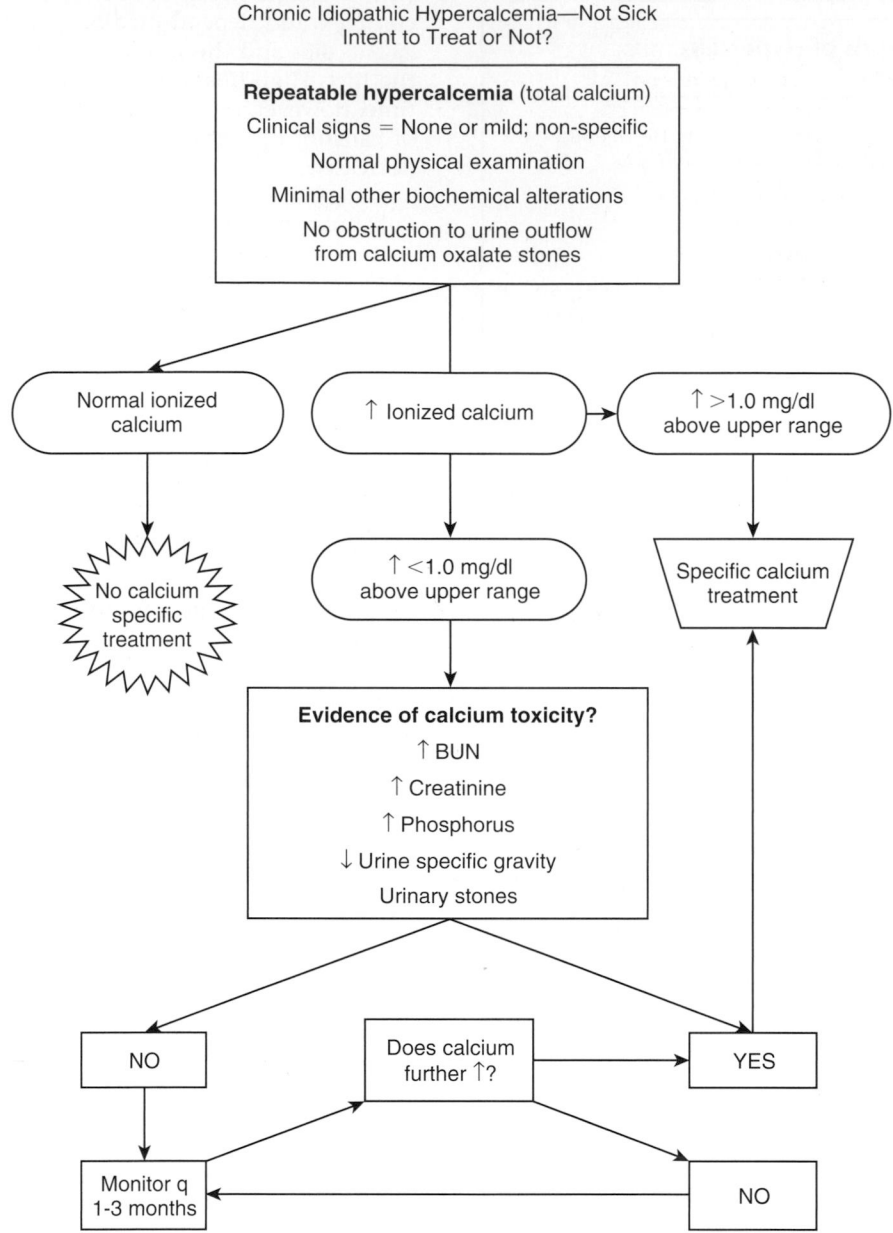

Chronic Idiopathic Hypercalcemia—Not Sick
Intent to Treat or Not?

Repeatable hypercalcemia (total calcium)

Clinical signs = None or mild; non-specific

Normal physical examination

Minimal other biochemical alterations

No obstruction to urine outflow
from calcium oxalate stones

Normal ionized calcium

↑ Ionized calcium

↑ >1.0 mg/dl above upper range

No calcium specific treatment

↑ <1.0 mg/dl above upper range

Specific calcium treatment

Evidence of calcium toxicity?

↑ BUN

↑ Creatinine

↑ Phosphorus

↓ Urine specific gravity

Urinary stones

NO

Does calcium further ↑?

YES

Monitor q 1-3 months

NO

Fig. 52-1 Diagnostic plan for initiation of treatment in hypercalcemic cats.

Hypercalcemia may return in some cats with IHC that previously have been successfully treated with a dietary change. In these cases changing to another diet or medical therapy should be considered.

Glucocorticosteroids

If normocalcemia has not been restored after a dietary feeding trial of 6 to 8 weeks, treatment with glucocorticosteroids should be considered. Administration of glucocorticosteroids can decrease serum calcium concentration by decreased intestinal absorption of calcium, decreased renal tubular calcium resorption, and

decreased skeletal mobilization of calcium. Cats usually do not exhibit serious side effects from glucocorticosteroid treatment as do dogs. Prednisone is given orally at 5 mg/cat/day for 1 month before reevaluation. If iCa concentration is normal, this dose is continued for several months. If serum iCa concentration is still increased, the dose is increased to 10 mg/cat/day. Some cats may require as much as 15 to 20 mg of prednisone per day to restore normocalcemia. Approximately 50% of cats with IHC become normocalcemic with 5 or 10 mg of prednisone per day, but some may require increasing doses to remain normocalcemic over time.

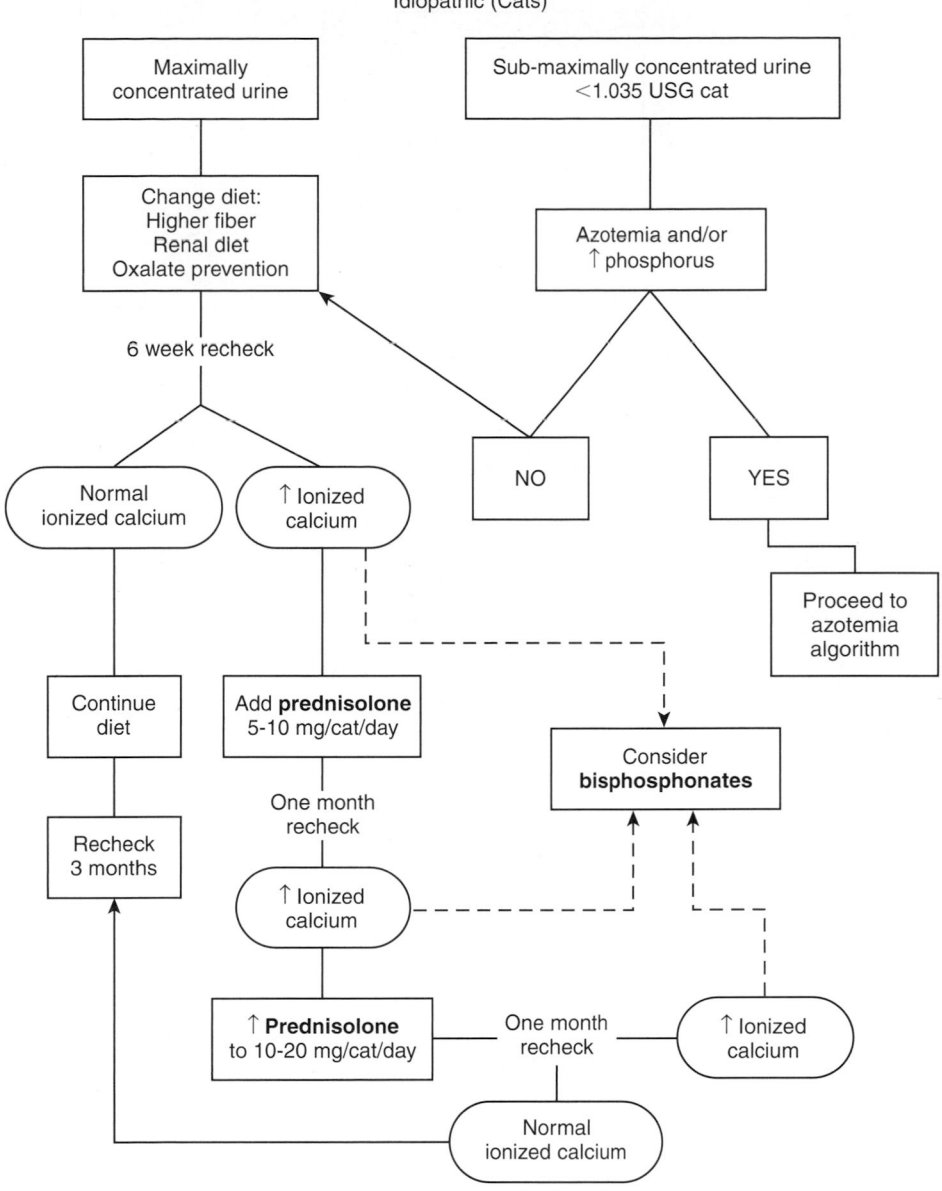

Fig. 52-2   Treatment of minimally symptomatic ionized hypercalcemia in cats.

There is some concern that glucocorticosteroids may increase urinary excretion of calcium, contributing to calcium oxalate urolith formation. However, little is known regarding the effects of glucocorticosteroids on filtration and tubular resorption of calcium in the cat. In a few healthy cats that have been studied, oral prednisolone treatment did not result in diuresis or an increase in calcium oxalate excretion.

Bisphosphonates

Bisphosphonates reduce the activity and number of osteoclasts following binding to hydroxyapatite. Treatment with bisphosphonates may be useful for hypercalcemia in IHC if there is increased osteoclastic bone resorption.

Bisphosphonate therapy may be an alternative to glucocorticosteroid use in cats that failed dietary intervention. The safety and efficacy of pamidronate given intravenously to two cats with hypercalcemia have been reported. Adequate hydration is essential when treating with bisphosphonates since these drugs may cause nephrotoxicity, especially at higher doses. A small number of cats with IHC have been treated successfully with 10 mg of alendronate orally once weekly for up to 1 year. Erosive esophagitis is noted as a possibility in women receiving oral bisphosphonates; although the risk for development of esophagitis in cats is unknown, it is recommended to follow the weekly pill with 6 ml of water given with a dosing syringe and then to dab a small amount of butter on the cat's lips to increase licking and salivation, which

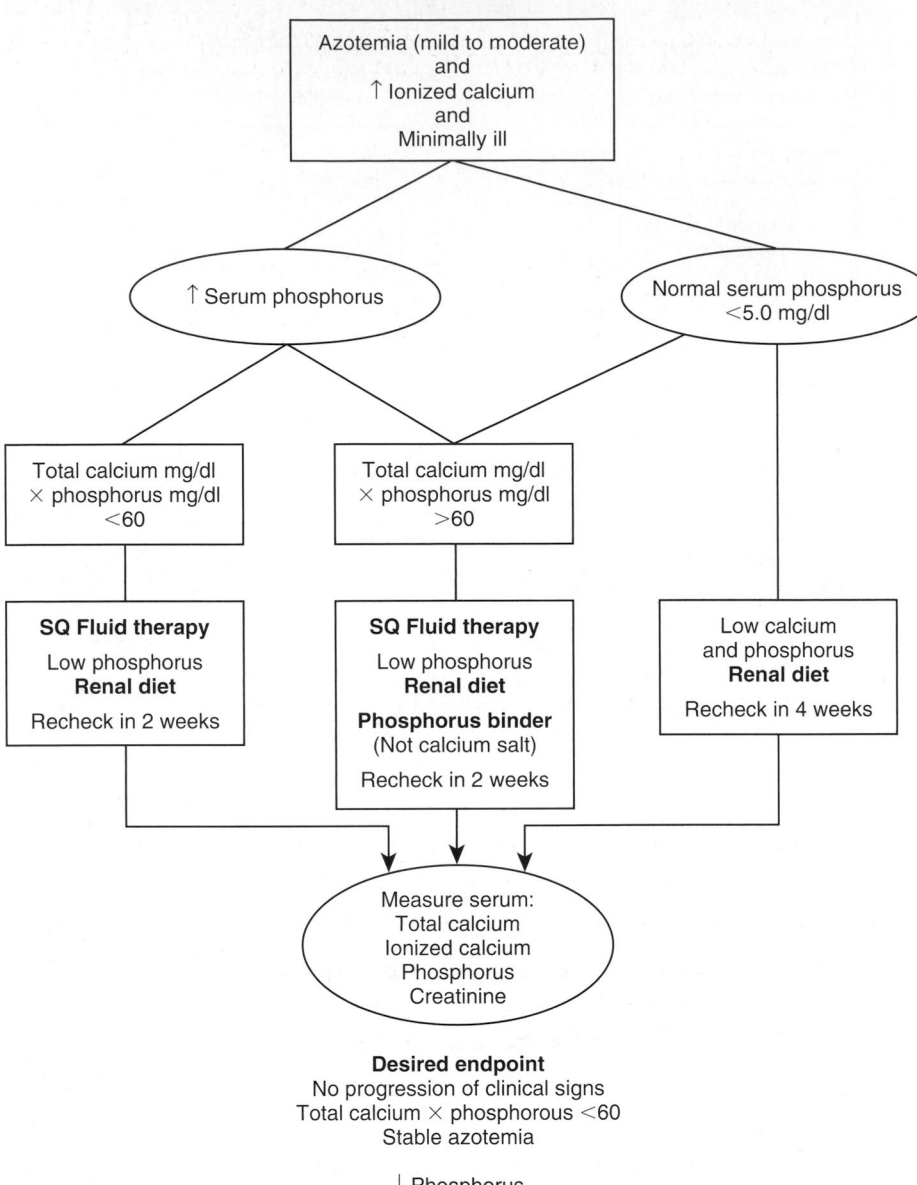

Treatment of Cats with Idiopathic Hypercalcemia and Azotemia

Fig. 52-3 Treatment plan for mild-to-moderate chronic ionized hypercalcemia.

further promotes the transit of the pill to the stomach. As seen with other therapies, hypercalcemia may return after a period of normocalcemia, requiring an increase in dose. Unfortunately the long-term safety and efficacy of oral bisphosphonates in cats is unknown.

Miscellaneous Treatments

Fluid therapy is a possible treatment option in cats with IHC but has not been evaluated. The administration of subcutaneous fluids on a daily or every-other-day basis potentially could expand the extracellular fluid and promote calciuresis. Diuretics such as furosemide have been used effectively to decrease serum iCa during acute rescue

protocols for hypercalcemia, usually in combination with intravenous fluids. Little is known about the effects of chronic furosemide administration regarding calcium status and the development of dehydration. It is a concern that cats receiving chronic diuretics will undergo diuresis but will not increase their water intake, leading to dehydration.

Calcimimetics are a new class of drug that has emerged in human medicine. Calcimimetics interact with the calcium receptor directly and have been proven effective in lowering iCa, phosphorus, and PTH concentrations in human dialysis patients. The potential future use of calcimimetics in the treatment of IHC is an interesting possibility.

References and Suggested Reading

Chew DJ et al: Utility of diagnostic assays in the evaluation of hypercalcemia and hypocalcemia: parathyroid hormone, vitamin D metabolites, parathyroid hormone–related protein, and ionized calcium. In Bonagura JD, editor: *Kirk's current veterinary therapy XII: small animal practice*, Philadelphia, 1995, Saunders, p 378.

Hostutler RA et al: Uses and effectiveness of pamidronate disodium for treatment of dogs and cats with hypercalcemia, *J Vet Intern Med* 19:29, 2005.

Lulich JP et al: Effects of diet on urine composition of cats with calcium oxalate urolithiasis, *J Am Anim Hosp Assoc* 40:185, 2004.

McClain HM, Barsanti JA, Bartges JW: Hypercalcemia and calcium oxalate urolithiasis in cats: a report of five cases, *J Am Anim Hosp Assoc* 35:297, 1995.

Midkiff AM et al: Idiopathic hypercalcemia in cats, *J Vet Intern Med* 14:619, 2000.

Schenck PA, Chew DJ: Idiopathic hypercalcemia in cats, *Waltham Focus* 15:20, 2005.

Schenck PA, Chew DJ, Behrend EN: Updates of hypercalcemic disorders. In August J, editor: *Consultations in feline internal medicine*, St Louis, 2005 Elsevier, p 157.

Schenck PA: Calcium metabolic hormones in feline idiopathic hypercalcemia, *J Vet Intern Med* 18:442, 2004.

Schenck PA: Disorders of calcium: hypercalcemia and hypocalcemia. In DiBartola SP, editor: *Fluid therapy in small animal practice*, St. Louis, 2005, Elsevier, p 122.

CHAPTER 53

Treatment of Hypoparathyroidism

DENNIS J. CHEW, *Columbus, Ohio*
LARRY A. NAGODE, *Columbus, Ohio*
PATRICIA A. SCHENCK, *Lansing, Michigan*

PATHOPHYSIOLOGY AND DIFFERENTIAL DIAGNOSIS

Hypoparathyroidism is a state of absolute or relative deficit of parathyroid hormone (PTH) secretion that can be permanent or transient. Hypocalcemia and clinical signs referable to low ionized calcium are the hallmarks of advanced hypoparathyroidism. This endocrine disorder is an uncommon cause of hypocalcemia in dogs and cats (Box 53-1), but it is the only condition requiring acute and chronic treatment to alleviate clinical signs associated with hypocalcemia. Hypoparathyroidism in dogs is most commonly an idiopathic or primary condition, whereas surgical removal or injury during thyroidectomy to correct hyperthyroidism is the most common cause in cats. In humans with idiopathic hypoparathyroidism, a variety of mutations have been identified that affect PTH production or PTH receptors (pseudohypoparathyroidism), but these conditions have not yet been described in dogs or cats. The treatment for hypoparathyroidism is the same, regardless of cause or genetic defect.

Inappropriately low levels of PTH cause hypocalcemia, hyperphosphatemia, and decreased levels of 1, 25-dihydroxycholecalciferol (calcitriol). Hypocalcemia is explained by increased urinary loss (hypercalciuria), reduced bone mobilization, and decreased intestinal absorption as a result of decreased calcitriol formation during periods of low PTH levels. Hyperphosphatemia results from the decreased urinary loss of phosphorus (hypophosphaturia), which overcomes decreased bone mobilization and low intestinal absorption of phosphorus during periods of decreased PTH levels. PTH is a potent stimulator, and phosphorus is a potent inhibitor of the 25(OH)-cholecalciferol–1α-hydroxylase system in the renal tubules; consequently, the absence of PTH and the presence of hyperphosphatemia work together to decrease renal synthesis of calcitriol. Decreased levels of calcitriol contribute to hypocalcemia largely through decreased intestinal calcium absorption. A component of hypocalcemia that is unrelated to low PTH levels may arise from increased uptake of calcium into bone following rapid correction of long-standing hyperparathyroidism or hyperthyroidism, both of which are associated with loss of bone calcium before treatment (hungry bone syndrome).

Box 53-1

Conditions Associated With Hypocalcemia Based on Total Serum Calcium

Common
- Hypoalbuminemia (ionized calcium is normal)
- Chronic renal failure
- Puerperal tetany (eclampsia)
- Acute renal failure
- Acute pancreatitis
- Undefined cause (mild hypocalcemia)

Occasional
Hypoparathyroidism
- Primary
- Absent or destruction of parathyroid glands
- Idiopathic-spontaneous/immune
- Bilateral thyroidectomy
- Following sudden reversal of chronic hypercalcemia (atrophy of remaining parathyroid glands)
- Suppressed PTH secretion (without destruction of gland)
- Magnesium depletion or excess
- After sudden reversal of hypercalcemia
- Ethylene glycol intoxication
- Phosphate enema
- Following NaHCO$_3$ administration
- Soft-tissue trauma/rhabdomyolysis

Uncommon
- Laboratory error
- Improper sample anticoagulant (ethylenediaminetetraacetic acid)
- Rapid intravenous infusion of phosphates
- Acute calcium-free intravenous infusion (dilutional)
- Intestinal malabsorption/severe starvation
- Hypovitaminosis D
- Blood transfusion (citrated anticoagulant)
- Nutritional secondary hyperparathyroidism
- Infarction of parathyroid gland adenoma (dog)
- Hypomagnesemia
- Tumor lysis syndrome
- Canine distemper virus affecting parathyroid gland

Human
- Sepsis/critical illness
- Drug-induced hypoparathyroidism (aluminum, asparaginase, doxorubicin, cytosine arabinoside, cimetidine, ethanol)
- Antiresorptive agents (estrogen, plicamycin, calcitonin, bisphosphonates)
- Pseudohypoparathyroidism
- Parathyroid gland agenesis
- Osteoblastic bone neoplasia (prostate cancer)
- Hypercalcitonism
- ^{131}I radiation damage

Magnesium also plays a role in PTH production. Severe magnesium depletion blunts maximal PTH secretion, increases end-organ resistance to PTH, and may also impair calcitriol synthesis.

Veterinary patients with hypoparathyroidism can be divided into three categories: (1) those with absence or destruction of parathyroid glands, (2) those with sudden correction of chronic hypercalcemia, or (3) those with suppressed secretion of or responsiveness to PTH without parathyroid gland destruction. The most common category of hypoparathyroidism in dogs and cats is that associated with the absence or destruction of the parathyroid glands.

CLINICAL SIGNS

Clinical signs related to hypocalcemia are identical, regardless of the underlying cause. Decreased serum ionized calcium concentration increases excitability of neuromuscular tissue, which accounts for many of the clinical signs of hypoparathyroidism. Mild decreases in serum ionized calcium may result in no obvious clinical signs. The duration and magnitude of the decrease in serum calcium, as well as the rate of decrease, interact to determine the severity of clinical signs. In its most severe forms, hypocalcemia can cause death from harmful circulatory effects (hypotension and decreased myocardial contractility) and respiratory arrest from paralysis of respiratory muscles. Serum total calcium concentration below 4 mg/dl can cause death especially if the decline was rapid. Other electrolyte and acid-base abnormalities can either magnify or diminish the signs of hypocalcemia. Correction of hypokalemia may precipitate the onset of clinical signs of hypocalcemia when hypocalcemia is present concurrently. Respiratory alkalosis following exercise or excitement may also increase the clinical signs of hypocalcemia as ionized calcium shifts to the protein-bound fraction.

Clinical signs of primary hypoparathyroidism from hypocalcemia include seizures, muscle tremors or fasciculations, muscle cramping, stiff gait, and behavioral changes (restlessness, excitation, aggression, hypersensitivity to stimuli, disorientation) (Box 53-2). Most seizures resolve without treatment but often recur despite treatment with anticonvulsants. Growling attributable to pain or behavior change and intense rubbing of the face with the paws or on the ground are commonly observed. These signs are attributed to either paresthesias or pain from facial muscle spasms. Pyrexia may be caused by increased muscular activity; lethargy, anorexia, and weakness may be noted, especially in cats. Polyuria and polydipsia occur in some cases as a result of psychogenic mechanisms or renal injury from hypercalciuria. Anterior and posterior lenticular cataracts occur in some affected dogs and cats, and prolapse of the third eyelid is sometimes seen with acute hypocalcemia in cats.

Seizures caused by hypocalcemia appear different than those associated with idiopathic epilepsy. With hypocalcemia, seizures are often preceded by apprehension or nervousness, and affected animals may remain partially conscious and retain urinary continence during the seizure. Clinical signs caused by acute postoperative hypocalcemia are similar in dogs and cats relating to excitation of neuromuscular tissue. Focal twitching of facial muscles and whiskers may be noticed before more generalized muscle tremors or seizures.

Box 53-2

Clinical Signs Associated With Severe Ionized Hypocalcemia

Common
- Muscle tremors/fasciculations
- Seizures/status epilepticus
- Facial rubbing
- Muscle cramping
- Stiff gait
- Behavioral change
- Restlessness/excitation
- Aggression
- Hypersensitivity to stimuli
- Disorientation
- Growling

Occasional
- Panting
- Pyrexia
- Lethargy/depression
- Anorexia
- Prolapse of third eyelid (cats)
- Posterior lenticular cataracts
- Tachycardia/electrocardiogram arrhythmia, prolonged QT interval

Uncommon/None
- Polyuria/polydipsia
- Hypotension
- Respiratory arrest/death

DIAGNOSIS

There are numerous causes of hypocalcemia (see Box 53-1). However, primary hypoparathyroidism is the only disorder characterized by hypocalcemia, elevated serum phosphorus, and low PTH concentration, along with normal renal function. Decreased serum calcium with increased serum phosphorus may be seen in nutritional or renal secondary hyperparathyroidism, following phosphate-containing enema administration, and in tumor lysis syndrome; however PTH concentration is increased in all of these conditions. A presumptive diagnosis of hypoparathyroidism can be made on the basis of decreased serum calcium, high serum phosphorus, normal renal function, and the absence of an obvious alternative diagnosis. The definitive diagnosis of hypoparathyroidism requires the finding of an inappropriately low or reference range PTH level concurrently with hypocalcemia since hypocalcemia should provide a strong stimulus to the normal parathyroid gland to secrete PTH at a high level. Primary hypoparathyroidism requires lifelong treatment; thus confirmation of the diagnosis with PTH measurement is highly recommended. Since magnesium depletion can cause functional hypoparathyroidism, measurement of serum ionized magnesium concentration is also recommended since over 75% of dogs and cats with primary hypoparathyroidism have marginal or low serum ionized magnesium concentrations.

TREATMENT

Treatment is individualized based on the severity of calcium-specific signs, the magnitude of the hypocalcemia, the rapidity of the decline in serum calcium levels, and trends toward a further decrease or stability in the serum calcium concentration. More aggressive treatment is prescribed for patients with severe signs of hypocalcemia, patients with severe ionized hypocalcemia with or without signs, and patients in which the serum calcium level appears to be steadily or rapidly declining. Acute, subacute, and chronic rescue treatment regimens are available using supplementation with calcium salts and calcitriol (the active vitamin D metabolite). The goal of therapy is to predictably and smoothly increase the serum calcium concentration to a level that alleviates the signs of hypocalcemia, lessens the likelihood of hypercalcemia developing later, and reduces the magnitude of hypercalciuria. For suspected temporary postsurgical hypoparathyroidism, it is desirable to keep serum calcium levels on the low side to maximize compensatory hypertrophy of remaining parathyroid glands.

No treatment regimen completely compensates for the full physiologic actions of absent PTH. Calcitriol treatment corrects the low intestinal absorption of calcium but does not completely protect the kidneys from hypercalciuria as would occur when working in concert with PTH. Similarly, calcitriol does not exert as powerful an effect on bone in the absence of PTH. Replacement therapy with once-daily subcutaneous injections of human PTH-(1-34) is highly effective in humans and provides good 24-hour calcemic control with better control of serum phosphorus and less hypercalciuria. Use of synthetic human PTH amino terminal compounds for treatment of veterinary patients is conceivable but has not been used because of its cost and the rate of success of oral calcitriol and calcium supplementation.

Hypocalcemia that is severe enough to create clinical signs should be anticipated in dogs undergoing parathyroidectomy as treatment for hypercalcemia resulting from a parathyroid gland tumor (see chapter 54). Those with very high levels of serum calcium, PTH, and serum bone alkaline phosphatase (BALP) may be at greater risk for developing postoperative hypocalcemia. In these cases, postoperative hypocalcemia is the consequence of acute hypoparathyroidism from chronic suppression of the remaining parathyroid glands, as well as calcium uptake into "hungry bones." One should anticipate hypocalcemia in cats that undergo bilateral thyroidectomy since as many as 30% of patients can be expected to demonstrate a lower serum calcium level transiently.

We do not agree with the recommendation of others to wait for signs of tetany before instituting calcium-specific therapy to increase serum calcium. Preemptive therapy to increase serum calcium levels may be a good choice for patients with marked hypocalcemia despite an absence of clinical signs or for those in which calcium is steadily or rapidly declining. Prophylactic therapy to prevent hypocalcemia in dogs undergoing surgery for hyperparathyroidism should be considered, especially in those with more severe levels of hypercalcemia. Calcitriol should be started before surgery in these instances because there is a lag until maximal effect; calcitriol given at the time of surgery or after surgery fails to prevent the development of hypocalcemia.

Acute Management of Hypocalcemia Causing Tetany or Seizures

Tetany or seizures caused by hypocalcemia requires treatment with intravenous calcium salts. Calcium is given to effect at 5 to 15 mg/kg of elemental calcium (0.5 to 1.5 ml/kg of 10% calcium gluconate) over a 10- to 20-minute period. The percentage of calcium varies widely with the specific calcium salt (Table 53-1). There is no difference in the effectiveness of intravenous calcium salts to correct hypocalcemia when the dose is based on elemental calcium content. Calcium gluconate is often chosen as the calcium salt of choice because it is nonirritating if the solution is injected outside a vessel; calcium chloride is extremely irritating to tissues but provides more elemental calcium in each milliliter of solution (see Table 53-1).

The heart rate and electrocardiogram should be monitored during acute infusion of calcium salts. Bradycardia may signal the onset of cardiotoxicity from infusing calcium at too rapid a rate; sudden elevation of the ST segment, shortening of the QT interval, or premature ventricular complexes may also indicate cardiotoxicity from the calcium infusion. Not all clinical signs immediately abate following acute correction of hypocalcemia because resolution of some signs may lag by as much as 30 to 60 minutes. Nervousness, panting, and behavioral changes may persist despite the return of normocalcemia during this period, perhaps reflecting a lag in cerebrospinal fluid equilibration with the calcium in extracellular water (since there is slow equilibration between calcium in extracellular water and that in cerebrospinal fluid). Hyperthermia that results from increased muscle tremor activity or seizures may also take some time to dissipate.

Subacute Management of Hypocalcemia

The initial bolus injection of elemental calcium can be expected to decrease signs of hypocalcemia for a limited time, for as little as 1 hour to as long as 12 hours if the initial cause of the hypocalcemia persists. Calcitriol therapy should be started as soon as possible because 24 hours to a few days of treatment are required before the effects to enhance intestinal calcium transport are maximized.

Additional parenteral calcium salt administration is necessary to maintain a required degree of calcemia until therapy with calcitriol is effective in maintaining serum calcium at acceptable levels.

Multiple intermittent intravenous injections of calcium salts can be given to control clinical signs, but this method is not recommended because wide fluctuations in serum calcium concentrations are likely to be encountered. Continuous intravenous infusion of calcium is recommended at 60 to 90 mg/kg/day of elemental calcium (2.5 to 3.75 mg/kg/hour) until oral medications provide calcemic control. Initial doses in the higher range are administered to patients with more severe hypocalcemia, and the dose is decreased according to the level of calcemia achieved. The dose of intravenous calcium is tapered further as oral calcium salts and calcitriol therapy become more effective.

Ten milliliters of 10% calcium gluconate provides 93 mg of elemental calcium. A convenient method to infuse calcium is available when intravenous fluids are given at a maintenance volume of 60 ml/kg/day (2.5 ml/kg/hour). Approximately 1 mg/kg/hour, 2 mg/kg/hour, or 3 mg/kg/hour of elemental calcium is provided by adding 10, 20, or 30 ml of 10% calcium gluconate, respectively, to each 250-ml fluid bag. Obviously the same rate of calcium infusion is provided by adding 20, 40, or 60 ml of 10% calcium gluconate to each 500 ml fluid bag to be infused at maintenance rates.

Calcium salts should not be added to fluid therapy preparations that contain lactate, acetate, bicarbonate, or phosphates because calcium salt precipitates can occur. Alkalinizing fluid therapy containing sodium bicarbonate decreases ionized calcium and may expose clinical signs of hypocalcemia in animals with borderline hypocalcemia; consequently they should not be used.

Subcutaneous administration of calcium gluconate has been regarded as safe for use in hypocalcemia when diluted to at least 1:1 by volume. However, there are reports of adverse reactions when subcutaneous calcium gluconate has been administered, resulting in calcinosis cutis, pyogranulomatous dermatitis, dermoepidermal separation, skin ulceration, and severe pyogranulomatous panniculitis. Most animals are euthanized because of the severity of the skin reaction. Because of the severity of adverse reactions that have recently been observed, the administration of subcutaneous fluids containing calcium gluconate is no longer recommended.

Table **53-1**

Treatment of Hypocalcemia With Parenteral Calcium*

Drug	Preparation	Available Elemental Calcium	Dose	Comment
Calcium (Ca) gluconate	10% solution	9.3 mg of elemental Ca/ml	a. Slow IV to effect (0.5-1.5 ml/kg) b. 5-15 mg/kg/hr elemental Ca IV	Stop if bradycardia or shortened QT interval occurs Infusion to maintain normal Ca
Calcium chloride	10% solution	27.2 mg of elemental Ca/ml	5-15 mg/kg/hr IV	Extremely caustic perivascularly

IV, Intravenously.
*Do not mix calcium solution with bicarbonate containing fluids because precipitation may occur.

Table 53-2

Treatment of Hypocalcemia With Oral Calcium Salts*

Drug	% Elemental Calcium Available	Preparation	Dose (Elemental) (mg/kg/day)	Comment
Calcium carbonate	40 (tablet)	Many sizes	25-50	Most common calcium supplement
Calcium chloride	27	Powder	25-50	May cause gastric irritation
Calcium citrate	21	Many sizes	25-50	
Calcium lactate	13 (tablet)	325, 650 mg tablets	25-50	
Calcium gluconate	10	Many sizes	25-50	

*Oral calcium: Calculate dose on elemental calcium content.

Subacute and Chronic Maintenance Therapy

Supplemental elemental calcium is administered orally (Table 53-2) to guarantee adequate available calcium for intestinal absorption following activating effects from vitamin D metabolites. Oral calcium administered by pill or slurry is most important during initial treatment, especially if the animal is not eating. Active intestinal transport mechanisms of calcium uptake are under the control of calcitriol when calcium intake is low, but vitamin D–independent passive intestinal absorption of calcium occurs when calcium intake is high. One can take advantage of the passive mechanisms for intestinal calcium transport before vitamin D actions are effected in the intestine. Normal dietary intake contains sufficient calcium to maintain adequate calcium levels in the presence of vitamin D metabolite treatment for most patients. Consequently oral calcium salt supplementation can be tapered and discontinued in many instances as vitamin D compounds reach maximal effect.

Calcium carbonate is the most widely used oral preparation of the commonly prescribed calcium salts because it contains the greatest percentage of elemental calcium, and this translates into fewer pills administered. The degree of calcium ionization and bioavailability for absorption vary by the specific calcium salt and the conditions within the intestine; consequently it is not simply a matter of determining the elemental calcium content of a specific oral calcium salt. Oral calcium is usually given at 25 to 50 mg/kg/day of elemental calcium divided over the day. Oral calcium carbonate serves as an intestinal phosphate binder in addition to providing additional calcium for intestinal absorption. It is advisable to continue oral calcium carbonate therapy for its intestinal phosphate-binding effects if serum phosphorus levels remain increased. Lower serum phosphorus concentrations may allow increased endogenous synthesis of calcitriol as the phosphate-mediated inhibition of the renal tubular 1α-hydroxylase system in the renal tubules is relieved.

Vitamin D preparations (Table 53-3) include ergocalciferol, cholecalciferol, 25(OH)-cholecalciferol (calcidiol), 1α-hydroxycholecalciferol, and 1,25-dihydroxycholecalciferol (calcitriol). Ergocalciferol and calcitriol are the preparations most commonly used in veterinary medicine. Dihydrotachysterol (DHT) has been used in the past but is no longer available. Lifelong treatment with some form of vitamin D metabolite is necessary for patients with primary hypoparathyroidism or in those with postoperative hypocalcemia that fails to resolve.

Ergocalciferol is favored by some because of its low cost, but it has several features that make it the least attractive agent for treatment. Ergocalciferol and its immediate metabolite 25-hydroxyergocalciferol have minimal vitamin D receptor avidity; consequently high doses are used to increase interactions with the vitamin D receptor. Calcitriol is about 1000 times as effective as the parent vitamin D compound and 500 times as effective as its precursor calcidiol (25-hydroxyvitamin D) in binding to the natural calcitriol receptor. Ergocalciferol is highly lipid soluble, requiring weeks to saturate body stores to achieve maximal effect; it also has a long half-life. Consequently prolonged periods of hypercalcemia occur after any overdose with ergocalciferol. In addition, there is extreme individual variation in the dose of ergocalciferol required to achieve the target level of serum calcium. Loading doses reduce the time required to achieve maximal calcemic effect (see Table 53-1).

Table 53-3

Vitamin D Compounds

Preparation	Daily Dose	Time for Maximal Effect To occur	Time for Toxicity Effect To Resolve
Vitamin D$_2$ (ergocalciferol)	Initial: 4000-6000 U/kg/day Maintenance: 1000-2000 U/kg once daily to once weekly	5-21 days	1-18 weeks
1,25-Dihydroxyvitamin D$_3$ (Calcitriol)	Initial: 20-30 ng/kg/day × 3-4 days Maintenance: 5-15 ng/kg/day	1-4 days	2-7 days

Calcitriol is the vitamin D metabolite of choice to provide calcemic actions because it has the most rapid onset to maximal action and the shortest biologic half-life. The dose of calcitriol can be adjusted more frequently because of more "real-time" effects on serum calcium. Should hypercalcemia occur, it is likely to abate quickly following dose reduction. The half-life of calcitriol in blood is 4 to 6 hours, whereas its biologic half-life is 2 to 4 days, which facilitates the rapid correction of hypercalcemia should it occur. A loading protocol for calcitriol use is used when more rapid calcium correction is desirable. A loading dose of calcitriol of 20 to 30 ng/kg/day for the initial 3 to 4 days, followed by a maintenance dosage of 5 to 15 ng/kg/day, is effective in most patients. Calcitriol only programs undifferentiated cells in the intestinal crypts of Lieberkühn, and the turnover of crypt cells is complete every 24 hours. For this reason the dose of calcitriol is divided twice daily to ensure sustained priming effects on intestinal epithelium for calcium transport. Calcitriol is available commercially in 0.25- and 0.50-mcg capsules (250 and 500 ng per respective capsule; Rocaltrol, Hoffman-LaRoche) and in a liquid form at 1 mcg/ml (1000 ng/ml). Reformulation of calcitriol capsules in doses suitable for a variety of animal sizes is necessary. It may be useful to prescribe calcitriol in liquid formulation so that small adjustments in dosage can be made accurately. A number of specialty pharmacies reformulate human drugs for veterinary use and can create any calcitriol doses needed. If there is documented low serum ionized magnesium concentration, supplementation with magnesium should also be considered (magnesium sulfate, 1 to 2 mEq/kg/day). In some cases correction of serum ionized magnesium deficiency may lead to a decrease in required doses of calcium and calcitriol.

Thiazide diuretics are sometimes used to treat humans with primary hypoparathyroidism as a maneuver to reduce hypercalciuria. This is especially useful when hypercalciuria continues despite a serum calcium level that is within the low normal range. It is likely that further reduction of the calcitriol dose would be necessary after starting thiazides since calcium levels would be higher because of more reclaimed calcium by the kidney. The effects of thiazide diuretics on urinary calcium excretion are debatable in dogs and unknown in cats.

Following the Patient and Managing Complications

Periods of hypocalcemia and hypercalcemia occur sporadically in patients during initial efforts to manage serum calcium levels. Daily measurement of total serum calcium during the initial stabilization of serum calcium is necessary; then weekly calcium measurements suffice during maintenance therapy until the target level of calcium has been achieved and maintained. Quarterly measurement of total serum calcium is recommended thereafter in animals with permanent hypoparathyroidism. The target level for serum calcium ideally should be just below the reference range rather than the middle or upper range of normal calcium concentrations. This not only lessens the likelihood that hypercalcemia will develop but also reduces the level of hypercalciuria

that occurs in patients missing the renal effects of PTH. Maintaining a mildly decreased level of serum calcium also ensures an ongoing stimulus for hypertrophy of any remaining parathyroid tissue in patients with postoperative hypoparathyroidism.

It is important to change the dose of calcitriol gradually following evaluation of serum calcium values and to make sure that enough time has elapsed to observe its maximal effect before the dose is changed. The time lag for this effect varies with the vitamin D metabolite used (see Table 53-1). Dosage increases of 10% to 20% are recommended for most cases that are still below the desired calcium target level. Vitamin D metabolites and calcium salt supplementation should be discontinued temporarily in patients with hypercalcemia. Doses should be reduced until the serum calcium level falls to just less than the reference range.

Hypercalcemia is a serious side effect that can result in the death of the animal or chronic renal damage severe enough to cause both acute and chronic renal failure. Owners should be taught the early signs of hypercalcemia and instructed to seek veterinary attention so that serum calcium can be measured if signs suggest hypercalcemia. Signs of hypercalcemia that clients are likely to recognize include polydipsia and polyuria, anorexia, vomiting, and depression. Animals with severe hypercalcemia require a combination of hospitalization, intravenous fluids, furosemide, steroids, and perhaps bisphosphonates or calcitonin initially. All patients with symptomatic vitamin D metabolite–induced hypercalcemia should be placed on a calcium-restricted diet because hypervitaminosis D is a form of hypercalcemia in which intestinal hyperabsorption of calcium contributes substantially to the development of hypercalcemia.

The long-term prognosis for quality and length of life has not been reported for dogs and cats during treatment of chronic hypoparathyroidism. Patients that have frequent episodes or long duration of hypercalcemia during treatment have poor prognoses. Patients that maintain calcium levels in the target zone are often managed successfully for years. In our experience patient management with calcitriol is easier and more successful in inducing and maintaining target zone calcium levels than are older therapeutic approaches.

Hypercalciuria, nephrocalcinosis, urolithiasis, and reduced renal function have all been noted in humans treated for chronic hypoparathyroidism. As many as 80% of humans treated for 2 years or longer have decreased creatinine clearance. These abnormalities can be attributed to episodes of hypercalcemia and hyperphosphatemia, as well as hypercalciuria that occurs in the absence of the full calcium-retaining actions of PTH at the level of the renal tubule. In the absence of PTH, hypercalciuria occurs more readily at all levels of serum calcium concentration and is especially severe as calcium concentrations approach the normal level, which increases the filtered load of calcium. Nephrocalcinosis, reduced renal function, and chronic renal failure have also been suspected in veterinary patients receiving long-term treatment for hypoparathyroidism, but the risk for these disorders has not been critically evaluated.

Great care is given to tailor the dosage of vitamin D metabolites in humans to both the level of serum calcium and the degree of hypercalciuria achieved during treatment. Maintaining a mildly decreased serum calcium level does not guarantee that hypercalciuria will not occur. Hypercalciuria is monitored by measuring 24-hour millimolar urinary calcium excretion or by determination of the urinary calcium:urinary creatinine ratio. Guidelines to assess the magnitude of hypercalciuria in veterinary patients have not yet been developed.

Calcitriol treatment is gradually tapered and then discontinued in patients with postsurgical hypoparathyroidism because hypocalcemia is usually transient. Most cats are able to maintain normal levels of serum calcium 2 weeks after thyroidectomy, although some may take as long as 3 months. Dogs with hypocalcemia usually require 6 to 12 weeks of treatment following removal of a parathyroid gland tumor. We usually start tapering calcitriol 1 month into therapy. If serum calcium declines substantially, the previous dose is resumed, and a taper attempted once again 1 or 2 months later. Permanent hypoparathyroidism is likely if failure to maintain reasonable levels of serum calcium occur following a taper of calcitriol at 3 months.

References and Suggested Reading

Feldman EC, Nelson RW: Hypocalcemia and primary hypoparathyroidism. In Feldman EC, editor: *Canine and feline endocrinology and reproduction*, Philadelphia, 2004, Saunders, p 716.

Hazewinkel HA, Tryfonidou MA: Vitamin D3 metabolism in dogs, *Mol Cell Endocrinol* 197:23, 2002.

Naan EC et al: Results of thyroidectomy in 101 cats with hyperthyroidism, *Vet Surg* 35:287, 2006.

Peterson ME: Hypoparathyroidism. In: Kirk RW, editor: *Current veterinary therapy IX: small animal practice*, Philadelphia, 1986, Saunders, p 1039.

Schenck PA: Serum ionized magnesium concentrations in dogs and cats with hypoparathyroidism, 23rd Annual Forum of the American College of Veterinary Internal Medicine (ACVIM), 2005, p 913.

Schenck PA, Chew DJ: Diseases of the parathyroid gland and calcium metabolism. In Birchard SJ, Sherding RG, editors: *Manual of small animal practice*, ed 3, St Louis, 2006, Elsevier, p 343.

Schenck PA: Disorders of calcium : hypercalcemia and hypocalcemia. In DiBartola SP, editor: *Fluid therapy in small animal practice*, ed 3, St. Louis, 2005, Elsevier, p 122.

Welches CD et al: Occurrence of problems after three techniques of bilateral thyroidectomy in cats, *Vet Surg* 18:392, 1989.

CHAPTER 54

Canine Hypercalcemia and Primary Hyperparathyroidism

EDWARD C. FELDMAN, *Davis, California*
RICHARD W. NELSON, *Davis, California*

DIFFERENTIAL DIAGNOSIS AND DIAGNOSTIC APPROACH TO HYPERCALCEMIA

Hypercalcemia is an abnormality that is usually serendipitously identified on serum biochemical analysis. Disorders associated with hypercalcemia in dogs, in an approximate incidence order as seen at our hospital, include lymphosarcoma, acute and chronic renal failure, hypoadrenocorticism, primary hyperparathyroidism (PHP), vitamin D toxicosis, apocrine gland carcinoma of the anal sac, multiple myeloma, uncommonly in association with a variety of carcinomas (lung, mammary, nasal, pancreas, thymus, thyroid, vaginal, and testicular), and uncommonly in association with certain granulomatous diseases (blastomycosis, histoplasmosis, schistosomiasis). Information from the history, physical examination, complete blood count (CBC), urinalysis, serum biochemistry analysis, thoracic and abdominal radiographs, abdominal ultrasound, and examination of cytology and biopsy specimens usually provide adequate information to establish the diagnosis in dogs.

History and Physical Examination

Since hypercalcemia is almost always an unsuspected finding, it is never a mistake to obtain a second blood sample to be certain that laboratory error has been ruled out. In our experience laboratory error is extremely rare. With confirmation of hypercalcemia, the veterinarian should review the signalment and history with the owner to identify clues to a definitive diagnosis that may not have been noted initially. From the history one can attempt to identify a tentative explanation for the hypercalcemia such as possible exposure to toxins containing vitamin D (e.g., rodenticides, inappropriate supplementation of food), evidence of pain from a lytic bone lesion (multiple myeloma or mammary tumor), difficulty eating because of oral lesions associated with renal failure, or a waxing/waning course of illness sometimes noted with hypoadrenocorticism. The physical examination should also be repeated in an attempt to identify a tentative explanation for hypercalcemia. The spine, ribs, and long bones should be palpated to identify bone pain caused by a lytic lesion, the mammary chain evaluated for neoplasia, the oral cavity for "rubber jaw" or lesions consistent with renal failure, the rectal and perineal area for apocrine gland carcinoma of the anal sac or other tumor, the heart rate and pulse for abnormalities consistent with hypoadrenocorticism, and the peripheral lymph nodes for enlargement suggestive of lymphoma (most hypercalcemic lymphoma dogs have a mediastinal mass and unremarkable peripheral nodes). Dogs with PHP have unremarkable physical examinations, and parathyroid masses are rarely palpable.

Routine Database

A thorough review of the CBC, serum biochemistry profile, and urinalysis should be completed. The urine specific gravity is commonly less than 1.020 in hypercalcemic dogs with renal disease, hypoadrenocorticism, and primary hyperparathyroidism. Urinary tract infection is common in these disorders. The CBC may demonstrate a normocytic, normochromic, nonregenerative anemia that is relatively common in renal failure, hypoadrenocorticism, and various neoplasias. The serum biochemistry profile should also be reviewed to assess the blood urea nitrogen (BUN), creatinine, and serum phosphate for increases consistent with renal failure; hyperkalemia and hyponatremia consistent with hypoadrenocorticism; hyperglobulinemia consistent with myeloma; and abnormal liver enzyme activities in association with a variety of malignancies. To this point the only "new" expense has been the repeated serum calcium concentration since all we have done is talk with the owner, repeat a physical examination, and review the laboratory results that were already obtained to identify the hypercalcemia in the first place.

Radiographs and Ultrasonography

Assuming that the review of the history, physical examination, and database has not defined the cause for hypercalcemia, thoracic radiographs are the next diagnostic step. The primary purpose for this study is to assess the cranial mediastinum for a mass consistent with lymphoma. If present, fine-needle aspiration or tissue obtained via biopsy should be evaluated. Radiographs also provide an opportunity to evaluate the perihilar area and lungs for neoplasia or systemic mycoses, the spine and ribs for lytic lesions caused by neoplasia, and the heart for microcardia of hypoadrenocorticism. Abdominal radiographs can also be assessed, although ultrasound examination of the abdomen is preferred. The size and consistency of the liver, spleen, and mesenteric and sublumbar lymph nodes can be evaluated for abnormalities suggestive of malignancy (lymphoma) or other conditions. Diagnostic imaging to evaluate for malignancy (lymphoma) applies to a variety of tumors located in other organs, but tumors other than lymphoma are an uncommon cause of hypercalcemia. When possible, abnormal areas should be aspirated or biopsied to determine the presence or absence of neoplasia. The size and consistency of the kidneys can be assessed, although renal failure should have been ruled in or out on the initial blood test results. The bladder should be evaluated for the presence of cystic calculi, which develop in about 30% of dogs with PHP and can develop in any hypercalcemic dog. If these studies fail to indicate a diagnosis other than PHP, the index of suspicion for PHP increases. Until a specific cause for hypercalcemia is confirmed, lymphoma should never be ruled out. Cervical ultrasonography, which is discussed in a later section, has become an extremely valuable screening test in dogs with hypercalcemia.

SIGNALMENT, HISTORY, AND PHYSICAL EXAMINATION IN DOGS WITH PRIMARY HYPERPARATHYROIDISM

Dogs with PHP are usually 6 years of age or older. The mean age from our series of 210 dogs with PHP was 11.2 years. Dogs of both genders are almost equally affected, and about 20% of affected dogs are keeshonds. Dogs with PHP, unlike those afflicted with most other diseases that cause hypercalcemia, are usually not ill or not as ill. Owners of 88 of 210 PHP dogs had observed no abnormalities in their pet related to hypercalcemia. The reason that blood had been obtained from these dogs was as part of a routine geriatric evaluation or as part of a preanesthesia screen before a dentistry procedure.

The most common owner-observed abnormalities in dogs with PHP (~50%) were those suggestive of urolithiasis or urinary tract infection (i.e., straining to urinate, increased frequency of urination, and hematuria), both relatively common in PHP. Other clinical signs reported by owners of 210 dogs with PHP included polyuria and polydipsia (48% of dogs), weakness (46%), decreased activity (43%), decreased appetite (37%), weight loss or muscle wasting (18%), vomiting (13%), and shivering or trembling (10%). It is important to remember that, even when clinical signs are observed, they are often relatively mild. When observed, signs were present for as long as 2 years. Few abnormalities are detected on physical examination. In 149 of 210 dogs with PHP (71%), the medical record stated that no abnormalities were noted on physical examination. When noted, abnormalities included muscle wasting, slow to rise, obesity in some, and thin body condition in others. Each of these problems was seen in less than 10% of dogs with PHP.

CLINICOPATHOLOGIC ABNORMALITIES IN DOGS WITH PHP

Hypercalcemia (i.e., serum total calcium concentrations greater than 12 mg/dl; reference range of 9.9 to 11.6 mg/dl) was identified in all 210 dogs. This degree of "sensitivity" (100%) may be slightly misleading since we do not evaluate dogs for hypercalcemia unless this criterion is met. The mean total serum calcium concentration was 14.5 mg/dl with a range of 12.1 to 23.4 mg/dl. About 50% of these dogs had serum total calcium concentrations greater than 12 and less than 14 mg/dl; about 30% had values greater than 14 and less than 16 mg/dl, about 10% had values greater than 16 and less than 18 mg/dl, and slightly more than 5% had values greater than 18 mg/dl. The mean plasma ionized calcium concentration in the 210 dogs with PHP was 1.71 mmol/L (range 1.22 to 2.41; normal reference range 1.12 to 1.41 mmol/L). Just under 10% of the dogs with PHP had a serum ionized calcium concentration within the reference range, almost 30% had values between 1.42 and 1.65 mmol/L, and almost 50% had concentrations between 1.66 and 1.90 mmol/L, with the remaining 16% having concentrations greater than 1.91 mmol/L.

It may be of interest to point out the most common reason for *referral* of dogs ultimately diagnosed with PHP: concern on the part of the referring veterinarian that, if not treated, these dogs would develop renal failure. However, this is not the case. Of 210 dogs with PHP, their mean BUN concentration (<17 mg/dl) was less than the reference range of 18 to 30 mg/dl; their mean serum creatinine concentration (0.8 mg/dl) was well within the reference range; and their mean serum phosphate concentration (2.8 mg/dl) was less than the reference range of 3 to 6.5 mg/dl. All of these values were significantly less than values from 200 dogs of similar ages that were randomly reviewed from our hospital population. In other words, PHP actually seems to protect these dogs from renal failure rather than predisposing to this condition. Duration of hypercalcemia also was not a factor since some PHP dogs went as long as 2 to 3 years without treatment. The polyuria and polydipsia were well supported by finding a mean urine specific gravity of 1.012 in 210 dogs with PHP. Of the dogs with PHP, 30% had urinary tract infection, and about 30% had cystic calculi. Although impending renal failure is rare and not a reason for treating a dog that has PHP, infection and calculi are common and certainly would be reason for recommending therapy.

CONFIRMATION OF PRIMARY HYPERPARATHYROIDISM (Use of Serum Parathyroid Hormone and Parathyroid Hormone–Related Protein Concentrations)

Are Parathyroid Hormone Assay Results Vital?

Veterinarians value a logical, practical, and cost-effective approach to problem solving. One can rest assured that the differential diagnosis for hypercalcemia is relatively small and veterinarians should be able to rule in or rule out most of the possibilities based on the diagnostic approach recommended at the beginning of this chapter. The need for sophisticated and relatively expensive studies such as assaying serum parathyroid hormone (PTH) and parathyroid hormone–related protein (PTHrP) concentrations take on less importance in this context. We have assayed serum PTH concentrations on every dog with PHP that we have diagnosed since the early 1980s. However, to be fair, a majority of these results are seen days to weeks *after* treatment has been completed. In other words, diagnosis was made without evaluating these assay results because a logical approach to the potential causes of hypercalcemia was used. This is not to suggest that the assays have no value; rather it is to suggest that in many dogs the assay results are not vital.

Serum Parathyroid Hormone Concentrations

Serum PTH concentrations are commercially available, and normal–to–increased concentrations confirm the diagnosis of PHP in nonrenal failure hypercalcemic dogs. Dogs with renal failure may also have increased serum PTH concentrations; therefore, within the context of the renal parameters, the serum phosphate concentration, the ionized serum calcium concentration, and other pertinent information, PHP should be distinguished from renal failure.

One must remember that, as serum calcium concentrations rise in healthy dogs, serum PTH concentrations should become undetectable. Therefore the term *normal range* can be misleading since the average dog with PHP has a serum PTH concentration that is "normal." This seems counterintuitive. The term *reference range* makes more sense since increasing serum calcium concentrations should drop the serum PTH concentration below the reference range, whereas values within the reference range are physiologically abnormal when an individual is hypercalcemic. The reference range for serum PTH concentrations is 2 to 13 pmol/L, and 135 of 185 (73%) dogs with PHP had serum PTH concentrations within that range: 45% had results of 2.3 to 7.9 pmol/L, 28% had results of 8 to 13 pmol/L, 11% had results between 13 and 20 pmol/L, and 16% had results >20 pmol/L.

Serum Parathyroid Hormone–Related Protein Concentrations

Increased serum PTHrP concentrations in hypercalcemic dogs would be most consistent with lymphoma or apocrine gland carcinoma of the anal sac. If a specific explanation for hypercalcemia remains elusive, we recommend that "response to treatment" be a *last resort*. Before any medication is given, aspiration or biopsy of lymph nodes, spleen, and/or liver should be considered in an attempt to rule out lymphoma. Lymphoma is emphasized here because in some dogs it can be quite difficult to confirm, even more difficult if glucocorticoids have been administered.

LOCALIZING PARATHYROID TISSUE CAUSING HYPERPARATHYROIDISM

Surgery

Once the diagnosis of PHP has been confirmed, the most cost-effective and expedient approach to patient management is surgical exploration of the neck. Abnormal, autonomously secreting parathyroid masses may not always be obvious at surgery, although experienced surgeons rarely have difficulty in identifying the parathyroid tissue causing hypercalcemia. The abnormal parathyroid adenoma, carcinoma, or adenomatous hyperplastic tissue is typically larger and a different color than normal parathyroid glands. Surgeons may benefit from knowing which side of the neck or specific location within one side of the neck that a tumor or abnormal parathyroid tissue is likely to be found.

Cervical Ultrasound

Ultrasound examination of the cervical area has recently received attention because it is available, noninvasive, and relatively cost efficient. Ultrasonography, as much as any diagnostic tool used in veterinary medicine, is "operator dependent." The skill of the individual performing the examination is a major factor in assessing the value of ultrasound. As facilities, use of various transducers, and the experience of radiologists and internists improve, this diagnostic tool holds great potential. Parathyroid tumors are typically round-to-oval hypoechoic masses that measure 4 to 8 mm in greatest diameter. Some are as large as 20 mm in greatest diameter. Most masses are 4 to 6 mm in greatest diameter. Cervical ultrasound was performed in 130 of 210 dogs with PHP in our series. In 116 of these 130 dogs, a solitary parathyroid mass was visualized. In 13 dogs two distinct parathyroid masses were seen. In one dog no parathyroid mass was visualized. Ultrasonography correctly identified 142 of 143 parathyroid tumors. This level of success is impressive, but it is a direct reflection of the experience of the individuals performing the ultrasound examinations and the quality of the imaging equipment used. Less experienced radiologists or internists may not visualize a parathyroid mass that a more experienced person would identify and ultrasound systems and transducers with insufficient imaging resolution may also lead to false negative or positive diagnoses.

Other Tests

Abnormal parathyroid tissue has been localized in humans using technetium 99 sestamibi nuclear scintigraphy. Results in dogs with PHP have been inconsistent at best, and the procedure is not recommended. Recent attempts to localize abnormal parathyroid tissue using selective venous sampling to measure the serum concentrations of PTH have not been satisfactory.

TREATMENT OF PRIMARY HYPERPARATHYROIDISM

Pretreatment Considerations—Candidates for Percutaneous Treatment

Treatment options for PHP include surgical removal and percutaneous heat or ethanol ablation. Several factors should be considered before suggesting a treatment recommendation. First, if a dog has cystic calculi, especially a male dog, surgery is recommended to remove the calculi; surgery on the neck to remove the parathyroid tumor is performed under the same anesthesia. Second, percutaneous treatment candidates must have a tumor large enough to have a needle placed percutaneously, and the mass cannot be too close to the carotid artery. Masses larger than 15 mm in greatest diameter are uncommon and often are managed surgically since we do not have much experience percutaneously ablating masses this large. If a dog has two parathyroid masses and one is located on each side of the neck, surgery is recommended; alternatively the percutaneous treatment can be "staged" at least 30 days apart to avoid iatrogenic laryngeal paralysis, an uncommon but possible problem.

Pretreatment Considerations—Serum Calcium Concentrations

If the pretreatment serum calcium concentration is ≥12 but ≤14 or fewer mg/dl, we simply monitor serum calcium or ionized calcium concentrations twice daily for 5 to 7 days after surgery or percutaneous therapy. Typically dogs are not at risk for developing hypocalcemia in the first 24 to 48 hours after treatment. Vitamin D therapy is only instituted if the serum calcium concentration decreases below 8 mg/dl, the ionized calcium decreases below 0.85 mmol/L, or clinical signs of tetany are observed. This level of decrease usually takes 3 to 7 days. If the serum calcium concentration before therapy is ≥15 mg/dl or if a dog has more than one parathyroid mass, the incidence of postsurgical hypocalcemia is greater, and we initiate vitamin D therapy (calcitriol; 2 to 10 ng/kg BID) the morning of or immediately after treatment. Vitamin D is then tapered to ever-decreasing dosages over a 2- to 6-month time period. Monitoring of serum calcium is carried forth as described, and parenteral calcium is only administered if tetany occurs or is thought to be imminent.

Percutaneous Ultrasound-Guided Heat Ablation

This procedure has become the recommended treatment of dogs with PHP at our hospital if the previously mentioned criteria are met. Dogs are placed under anesthesia, and with ultrasound guidance a needle is placed into the parathyroid mass. The needle is attached to a radiofrequency unit (radio frequency waves are naturally converted to heat at the needle tip). The wattage is started at a low level and increased based on observation of a "bubbling" appearance to the tissue. The needle tip is repositioned several times to ensure that the entire parathyroid mass has been ablated. Percutaneous ultrasound-guided heat ablation requires 15 to 30 minutes of anesthesia and is usually about one half the cost of surgery. Post-heat ablation management of the dog is identical to the management following surgical removal of a parathyroid mass. Of the first 48 dogs so treated, 44 (92%) had resolution of their PHP: 43 with one treatment, and one dog required a second procedure.

Percutaneous Ultrasound-Guided Ethanol Ablation

Percutaneous ethanol ablation is no longer recommended. The procedure used was similar to that described for the heat ablation except that the needle is connected to a syringe containing a volume of ethanol similar to the calculated volume of the parathyroid nodule. Ethanol was infused slowly in an effort to expose all tissue to ethanol, and the needle tip was repositioned several times to aid in accomplishing this goal. The reason that ethanol was abandoned was that leakage of this caustic material invariably occurred following the procedure. Such leakage could cause nerve damage and secondary laryngeal paralysis.

Surgery

Complete exploratory surgery of both thyroid lobe areas is recommended for dogs with PHP that do not meet the criteria for percutaneous ultrasound-guided heat ablation. An effort should be made to evaluate both sides of the neck and both the ventral and dorsal surfaces of the thyroid lobes. In most dogs with PHP the abnormal parathyroid tissue is solitary, off-color, and larger-than-normal; easily recognized; and easily extirpated. Only the abnormal parathyroid tissue is removed if possible; although, when a parathyroid tumor lies within a thyroid lobe, both are usually removed. If no parathyroid mass is observed and the diagnosis is thought to be correct, one thyroid/parathyroid complex should be removed and examined histologically. If two abnormal parathyroids are observed, both should be removed.

Since we began performing percutaneous treatment, 52 dogs have been treated at our hospital with surgery. Fifty of these 52 dogs (96%) had complete resolution of their PHP. One of these 52 dogs required a second procedure. Thus percutaneous and surgical treatments are both efficacious.

POSTTREATMENT CARE

Dogs are kept in the hospital for 5 to 7 days after treatment to monitor serum calcium concentrations and, more important, to keep the dog quiet. Since most dogs are quiet in the hospital, it can be appreciated that the quiet hypocalcemic dog is less prone to clinical tetany than would be the case if the dog is active. For this reason, dogs that are unusually active in the hospital are sent home. We usually monitor serum total calcium concentrations twice daily until release from the hospital.

Histology

Parathyroid tumors have been classified histologically as adenoma, carcinoma, or hyperplasia. These classifications have not had use clinically since all parathyroid masses are biologically similar. We have not experienced a dog with local tumor invasion or distant metastasis. Recurrence rate is about 10% regardless of the histology.

References and Suggested Reading

Feldman EC, Hoar B, Pollard R, et al: Pretreatment clinical and laboratory findings in dogs with primary hyperparathyroidism: 210 cases (1987-2004). *J Am Vet Med Assoc* 227:756, 2005.

Long CD, Goldstein RE, Hornof WJ, et al: Percutaneous ultrasound-guided chemical parathyroid ablation for treatment of primary hyperparathyroidism in dogs. *J Am Vet Med Assoc* 215:217, 1999.

Pollard RE, Long CD, Nelson RW, et al: Percutaneous ultrasonographically guided heat ablation for treatment of primary hyperparathyroidism in dogs. *J Am Vet Med Assoc* 218:1106, 2001.

Wisner ER, Penninck D, Biller DS, et al: High-resolution parathyroid sonograph. *Vet Radiol Ultrasound* 38:462, 1997.

SECTION IV

Oncology and Hematology

Douglas H. Thamm

VOLUME XIII CONTENT ON EVOLVE: http://evolve.elsevier.com/Bonagura/Kirks/

CHAPTER 55

Immunosuppressive Agents

CLARE R. GREGORY, *Davis, California*

Over the last half of the 20th century immuno-suppressive agents have evolved from nonspecific, myelotoxic drugs to agents that target specific enzymes catalyzing reactions required for normal immune function. Much of our current understanding of T-cell function has been provided by research performed to understand the mechanism of action of cyclosporine. As each element of antigen recognition, T-cell activation, cytokine synthesis, and T cell–dependent cytolysis is unraveled, investigators are devising specific, less toxic, and more efficacious agents for interrupting the immune response. This process, termed *rational drug development,* replaces the selection of potential immunosuppressive agents based on their ability to lyse or inhibit the activation of T and B cells in vitro. Although specific immunosuppression with the use of naturally induced and genetically engineered antibodies, soluble receptor fragments, and other biologic methods is available for the treatment of human diseases, most of these therapies are either inapplicable or unavailable for treatment of animal diseases. For the foreseeable future in veterinary medicine, immunosuppression will rely on chemotherapies. As new immunosuppressive agents become more available and clinicians familiar with their indications, effects, and adverse effects, immunosuppressive therapy should become more specific, effective, and safe.

MYELOTOXIC AGENTS

Cyclophosphamide

The major effect of cyclophosphamide results from alkylation of deoxyribonucleic acid (DNA) during the S phase of the cell cycle. The alterations in DNA structure can be lethal to the cell or may produce miscoding errors that inhibit cell replication or DNA transcription. Cyclophosphamide produces T- and B-cell lymphopenia and suppresses both T-cell activity and antibody production. Cyclophosphamide is administered to dogs for the treatment of corticosteroid-resistant immune-mediated hemolytic anemia (IMHA), corticosteroid-resistant immune-mediated thrombocytopenia (IMTP), rheumatoid arthritis (RA), and polymyositis (in conjunction with corticosteroids). Cyclophosphamide is administered to cats for the treatment of IMHA and RA. Myelosuppression, gastroenteritis, alopecia, and hemorrhagic cystitis are the major complications associated with cyclophosphamide therapy.

Azathioprine

Azathioprine is a purine analog that is metabolized to ribonucleotide monophosphates. Poor conversion to diphosphates and triphosphates leads to an intracellular accumulation of monophosphates that produces a feedback inhibition of the enzymes required for the biosynthesis of purine nucleotides. The triphosphate analogs that do form become incorporated into DNA and result in ribonucleic acid miscoding and faulty transcription. Azathioprine has a greater effect on humoral than on cell-mediated immunity. For the treatment of immune-mediated diseases in dogs, azathioprine is generally administered in conjunction with a corticosteroid and/or cyclophosphamide.

Azathioprine has been used for the treatment of IMTP, IMHA, autoimmune skin diseases, chronic hepatitis, myasthenia gravis, immune-mediated glomerulopathy, chronic atrophic gastritis, systemic lupus erythematosus, and inflammatory bowel disease. Although very myelotoxic in cats, azathioprine has been used for the treatment of feline autoimmune skin diseases. Azathioprine and prednisolone, when administered at maximally tolerated levels, do not effectively suppress the rejection response against canine major histocompatibility complex (MHC)–nonmatched renal allografts. However, when administered on an every-other-day schedule (1 to 3 mg/kg orally [PO]) with cyclosporine, azathioprine has been used to successfully maintain canine MHC-matched renal allografts. In feline renal transplantation patients with suspected inflammatory bowel disease or following an allograft rejection episode, azathioprine is administered with cyclosporine at a dose of 0.3 mg/kg every 3 days PO. The dose is decreased if the total white blood cell count falls below 3000 cells/μl or there is biochemical evidence of hepatotoxicity. The primary complication encountered with the administration of azathioprine is bone marrow suppression that can result in leukopenia, anemia, and thrombocytopenia. Acute pancreatitis and hepatotoxicity may also occur.

Methotrexate

Methotrexate competitively inhibits folic acid reductase, which is necessary for the reduction of dihydrofolate to tetrahydrofolate and affects the production of both purines and pyrimidines. The effects of methotrexate manifest during the S phase of the cell cycle. Methotrexate is used occasionally as an antineoplastic agent in dogs and cats for lymphomas, carcinomas, and sarcomas. In human medicine methotrexate is administered for the treatment of RA and psoriasis. Gastrointestinal toxicity is the most common complication encountered with the administration of methotrexate.

GLUCOCORTICOIDS

Prednisolone

Glucocorticoids and in particular prednisolone have both direct and indirect effects on the immune response. Glucocorticoids stabilize the cell membrane of endothelial cells and inhibit the production of local chemotactic factors, thus decreasing infiltration of neutrophils, monocytes, and lymphocytes. In allogeneic tissues the secretion of destructive proteolytic enzymes such as collagenase, elastase, and plasminogen activator is inhibited. Glucocorticoids also inhibit the release of arachidonic acid from membrane phospholipids. This inhibition prevents the synthesis of prostaglandins, thromboxanes, and leukotrienes, which are major mediators of inflammation. Glucocorticoids redistribute monocytes and lymphocytes from the peripheral circulation to the lymphatics and bone marrow. This redistribution affects primarily T cells. T-cell activation and cytotoxicity are also reduced. Glucocorticoids suppress cytokine activity and alter macrophage function. Prednisolone and prednisone are considered to be the first-line immunosuppressive agents for the treatment of immune-mediated and chronic inflammatory diseases in dogs and cats because of their general efficacy and low cost.

Immune-mediated hemolytic anemia and IMTP, autoimmune and allergic skin diseases, myasthenia gravis, allergic pneumonitis and bronchitis, immune-mediated arthritis, and systemic lupus erythematosus are just some of the indications for corticosteroid therapy in animals. Prednisolone has been used in both dogs and cats to slow allograft rejection; however, when administered as a single agent, prednisolone is not capable of preventing allograft rejection. For the prevention of allograft rejection in cats, prednisolone is administered with cyclosporine at an initial dose of 2.5 to 5 mg PO every 12 hours. This dose is generally reduced to 2.5 to 5 mg PO every 24 hours 30 days following transplantation. Over the next several months, following serum creatinine and blood urea nitrogen concentrations, the prednisolone dose is reduced to 2.5 mg PO every 24 hours or discontinued.

Although inexpensive and often effective, the chronic use of corticosteroids can result in severe complications, usually manifested as signs of iatrogenic hyperadrenocorticism. This complication, in addition to the fact that corticosteroids suppress multiple elements of the immune response, has led to the search for *steroid-sparing* immunosuppressive protocols.

CALCINEURIN INHIBITORS

Cyclosporine

Cyclosporine is bound in the cytosol of lymphocytes by cyclophilins (cyclosporine-binding proteins). The cyclosporine-cyclophilin complexes associate with calcium-dependent calcineurin-calmodulin complexes to impede calcium-dependent signal transduction. Transcription factors that promote cytokine gene activation are either direct or indirect substrates of the serine-threonine phosphatase activity of calcineurin. This enzymatic activity is reduced by association of the cyclosporine-cyclophilin bimolecular complex with calcineurin. Via this mechanism of action, cyclosporine inhibits early T-cell activation (G_0 phase of the cell cycle) and prevents synthesis of several cytokines, in particular interleukin-2 (IL-2). Without stimulation by IL-2, further T-cell proliferation is inhibited, and T-cell cytotoxic activity is reduced. Cyclosporine may also exert an immunosuppressive effect as it stimulates mammalian cells to secrete transforming growth factor–β (TGF-β) protein. TGF-β is a potent inhibitor of IL-2–stimulated T-cell proliferation and generation of antigen-specific cytotoxic lymphocytes. Cyclosporine is not cytotoxic or myelotoxic and is specific for lymphocytes. This specificity spares other rapidly dividing cells and allows nonspecific host defense mechanisms to continue to function.

Cyclosporine has gained widespread use in veterinary medicine. Combination cyclosporine and prednisolone immunosuppression has maintained normal function of MHC-nonmatched feline renal allografts for more than 12 years. Cyclosporine in combination with azathioprine, prednisolone, and antithymocyte serum has been used to maintain MHC-nonmatched canine renal allografts. Bone marrow transplantation has been performed successfully in cats with the use of cyclosporine immunosuppression. Cyclosporine has also been used to control corticosteroid-resistant IMHA and IMTP in dogs. Cyclosporine is available in an ophthalmic preparation (Optimmune, Schering-Plough, Kenilworth, NJ) for the control of keratoconjunctivitis sicca in dogs. Cyclosporine (10 to 20 mg/kg q24h PO) was found to significantly reduce the size and depth of perianal fistulas in dogs (Mathews and Sukhiani, 1997). Most dogs did not require further therapy, either medical or surgical, after 6 to 8 weeks of therapy. In a more recent study (Hardie et al., 2005) cyclosporine resolved or reduced the lesions in 25 of 26 dogs. However, residual or recurrent lesions were encountered that required long-term medical therapy or surgical resection. Cyclosporine (5 mg/kg q24h PO induction dose, reduced by 50% to 75% over weeks to months, depending on response) has been shown to be effective in the reduction of skin lesions and pruritus in dogs with atopic dermatitis (Steffan, Favrot, and Mueller, 2006). The use of cyclosporine for the treatment of other dermatologic diseases such as pemphigus foliaceus is under investigation (Guaguere, Steffan, and Olivry, 2004). There are reports that cyclosporine may be effective for the treatment of granulomatous meningoencephalitis (Adamo and O'Brien, 2004) and steroid-refractory inflammatory bowel disease (5 mg/kg q24h PO for 10 weeks; Allenspach et al., 2006).

Cyclosporine is available in two oral formulations: Sandimmune and Neoral (Sandoz). Both contain cyclosporine in a concentration of 100 mg/ml, but the two solutions are not biologically equivalent. Sandimmune consists of an olive oil base, and adsorption of cyclosporine requires emulsification of the agent by bile salts and digestion by pancreatic enzymes. The absorption percentage can be as little as 4%, and there is a tremendous variation in dose-trough whole-blood levels among individuals of the same species. Neoral is a microemulsion preconcentrate of cyclosporine that becomes a microemulsion when in contact with gastrointestinal fluids. The micro-emulsion is directly absorbed through the gut epithelium, resulting in more sustained and consistent blood levels of the drug. When Neoral replaces Sandimmune as treatment, most feline renal transplant recipients have had a reduction in the dosage level necessary to maintain the same trough whole-blood levels. In addition, feline renal transplant patients have been administered Sandimmune at a dose of 10 to 15 mg/kg over 24 hours to initiate immunosuppression at the time of surgery. To achieve the same trough whole-blood levels of cyclosporine (approximately 500 ng/ml), Neoral is administered at a dose of 1 to 4 mg/kg over 24 hours. Neoral appears be a more effective immunosuppressant than Sandimmune because of a more complete absorption, which results in a more sustained and predictable blood level. In addition, it is more economical to use.

To achieve immunosuppression with cyclosporine in dogs, I recommend attaining a 12-hour whole-blood trough level (measured just before the next oral dose) of at least 500 ng/ml. With Sandimmune, achieving this level requires an oral dosage of 10 to 25 mg/kg over 24 hours divided into two doses. Neoral can be initiated at 5 to 10 mg/kg over 24 hours divided into two doses. With either formulation gastrointestinal inflammation increases the dosage requirements, and blood levels of the agent must be measured starting 24 to 48 hours after initiation of therapy to ensure that adequate blood levels are achieved. Blood levels of cyclosporine should be measured at periodic intervals during the time of therapy. To reduce the cost of the cyclosporine necessary to treat medium-size– to large-dogs, I administer ketoconazole at a dose of 10 mg/kg over 24 hours in addition to the cyclosporine. Ketoconazole interferes with the hepatic metabolism of cyclosporine, and it reduces the dosage requirement of cyclosporine by as much as 60%. I have not encountered toxic effects with the coadministration of these agents, but it has been reported that the chronic administration of ketoconazole to dogs may result in cataract formation.

To achieve immunosuppression with cyclosporine in cats, I recommend attaining a 12-hour whole blood trough level of 250 to 500 ng/ml. With Sandimmune, obtaining this level requires an oral dosage of 4 to 15 mg/kg over 24 hours divided into two doses. Neoral can be initiated at 1 to 5 mg/kg over 24 hours divided into two doses. Again it is imperative to measure blood levels 24 to 48 hours after initiation of therapy to ensure that adequate blood levels have been achieved. Blood levels must also be measured periodically during the course of therapy. Based on recent pharmacokinetic studies in the cat, trough whole-blood concentrations of cyclosporine may not correlate well with drug exposure (Mehl et al., 2003). The whole-blood concentrations measured at 2 hours after administration of the drug may correlate better with drug exposure and give a better index for drug dosage and change in dose. The blood concentration of cyclosporine measured 2 hours after administration is recommended for therapeutic drug monitoring in human renal transplant patients.

Whole blood or plasma levels of cyclosporine can be determined by high-pressure liquid chromatography, fluorescence polarization immunoassay, and specific monoclonal antibody radioimmunoassay. Most medical centers that serve humans perform cyclosporine assays and will serve veterinary needs.

Unlike the situation in humans, cyclosporine does not appear to be hepatotoxic in dogs and cats unless extremely high blood levels are maintained (>3000 ng/ml). Although not as frequently encountered in humans, cyclosporine can be nephrotoxic in the cat. Nephrotoxicity in the cat does not seem to be related to the level of the drug in whole blood and can occur at relatively low plasma concentrations. Cats with extremely high cyclosporine whole-blood concentrations (>4000 ng/ml) often show no toxicity at all. In my experience cyclosporine nephrotoxicity has only developed in one dog. This dog had a chylothorax that resulted in trough whole-blood concentrations of cyclosporine of greater than 3000 ng/ml. Levels higher than 1000 ng/ml can cause inappetence in cats. If levels of 1000 ng/ml are maintained for several weeks or months, opportunistic bacterial and fungal infections can occur. As in humans, cyclosporine could promote the development of neoplasia, particularly lymphomas, in cats and dogs. The administration of high levels (1 to 2 mg/kg over 24 hours) of prednisolone with cyclosporine increases the likelihood of tumor formation. As in humans, cyclosporine has resulted in a marked increase in hair growth in several of my feline renal transplant recipients. When administered to dogs, cyclosporine can result in severe gingival hyperplasia, fibropapillomatosis, and severe or fatal pyodermas, especially when combined with azathioprine (Gregory et al., 2006).

Cyclosporine has a distinctly unpleasant taste to both humans and animals, necessitating administration in gelatin capsules. Novartis supplies capsules containing 25 or 100 mg of cyclosporine. For most cats these capsules are too large. I place the oral solution in No. 0 or No. 1 gelatin capsules. Some cats need only a very small dose of cyclosporin: (1- to 3-mg/dose). Measuring and administering this small amount (0.01 to 0.03 ml) of a drug is very difficult and imprecise. Sandimmune can be diluted and stored in olive oil; I usually make a 1-to-10 dilution. Neoral can be diluted in any oral solution, but it must be administered immediately after it is diluted because it is a microemulsion concentrate. I dilute Neoral in tap water.

Cyclosporine is also available in an intravenous solution (Sandimmune IV) that must be diluted in 0.9% sodium chloride or 5% dextrose in water. For the treatment of acute renal allograft rejection, I administer a dose of 6 mg/kg over 4 hours in the calculated maintenance fluid requirement. Intravenous cyclosporine is administered to control organ rejection episodes, for an acute hemolytic crisis, or during periods when a patient cannot tolerate oral medications.

Tacrolimus

Although tacrolimus, or FK-506 (Prograf, Fujisaw), is structurally different from cyclosporine, it shares a similar mechanism of action. Tacrolimus binds in the cytosol of lymphocytes with an immunophilin,

FK-binding protein (FKBP). As with the cyclosporine-cyclophilin complex, the tacrolimus-FKBP complex binds to calcineurin and inhibits its phosphatase activity. This inhibition directly and indirectly inhibits de novo expression of nuclear regulatory proteins and T-cell activation genes. The transcription of cytokines (IL-2, IL-3, IL-4, IL-5, interferon-γ, tumor necrosis factor-α [TNF-α], and granulocyte-macrophage colony-stimulating factor) responsible for lymphocyte activation is suppressed, as is the expression of IL-2 and IL-7 receptors. Tacrolimus in vitro is 50 to 100 times more potent as an inhibitor of lymphocyte activation than cyclosporine. Tacrolimus also inhibits B-cell proliferation and production of antibody by unknown mechanisms. Tacrolimus decreases the hepatic damage associated with ischemia-reperfusion injury, perhaps by inhibiting production of TNF-α and IL-6 by hepatocytes, and stimulates hepatic regeneration following liver injury. Experimentally allograft recipients from many species have been treated successfully with tacrolimus at doses several times less than those for cyclosporine. Tacrolimus has prolonged the survival of renal, liver, pancreas, heart, lung, and vascularized limb grafts in rodents, dogs, and nonhuman primates. In human organ recipients tacrolimus is superior to cyclosporine for the reversal of ongoing rejection. Also the steroid-sparing effect of tacrolimus seems to be greater than that of Sandimmune, but it may not be superior to that of Neoral. The toxicity of tacrolimus is similar to that of cyclosporine in humans.

Little if any use of tacrolimus has been applied to veterinary patients, but based on its effectiveness in experimental animal trials, it could be very useful in controlling a wide range of immune-mediated conditions. Tacrolimus may be particularly effective in controlling IMHA, IMTP, and immune-mediated arthritis because of its inhibition of antibody synthesis T-cell proliferation. Despite the potential benefits of tacrolimus for treating diseases in dogs, a major concern is the possible toxicity of the drug. A dose of 0.16 mg/kg every 24 hours intramuscularly or 1 mg/kg every 24 hours PO has been reported to be effective in prolonging renal allograft survival in beagle dogs. The side effects included anorexia, vasculitis, and intestinal intussusception. In a study using mongrel dogs the same doses were not effective in prolonging renal allograft survival, and most of the dogs developed severe vasculitis leading to fatal myocardial infarction, hepatic failure, and intussusception. Combination therapy with cyclosporine appears to have an additive effect with less toxicity. Blood levels of tacrolimus are assayed at human medical centers with the use of monoclonal immunoassays. The effective serum trough level of tacrolimus in dogs is approximately 0.1 to 0.4 ng/ml, about 100 times lower than that of cyclosporine. Trough levels of 2 ng/ml or greater can result in death. Used topically in a 0.1% solution, tacrolimus has safely controlled the lesions of discoid lupus erythematosus and pemphigus foliaceus in dogs (Rosenkrantz et al., 2004). Tacrolimus is also available in a topical 0.02% aqueous suspension for the effective treatment of dogs with keratoconjunctivitis sicca (Berdoulay, English, and Nadelstein, 2005).

INHIBITORS OF CYTOKINE AND GROWTH FACTOR ACTION

Sirolimus

Sirolimus, or rapamycin (Rapamune, Wyeth-Ayerst) is a macrocyclic antibiotic with a structure similar to that of tacrolimus that also binds in the cell cytosol to FKBP. However, sirolimus and tacrolimus affect different and distinct sites in the signal transduction pathway. The immunosuppressive activity of sirolimus appears to be a consequence in part of the sirolimus-FKBP complex blocking the activation of the mammalian target of rapamycin, (mTOR). mTOR is a serine/threonine protein kinase and is involved in the regulation of cell proliferation through the initiation of gene translation in response to amino acids, growth factors, cytokines, and mitogens. The kinase activity of additional cell cycle regulatory proteins cyclin-dependent kinase-2 and cyclin-dependent kinase-4 is also inhibited by sirolimus. Sirolimus blocks IL-2 and other growth factor–mediated signal transduction (signal 3 of the allograft rejection response) and the calcium-independent CD28/B7 (CD80/CD86) costimulatory pathway. Cyclosporine and tacrolimus block T-cell cell cycle progression at the G_O to G_1 stage; sirolimus prevents cells from progressing from G_1 to the S phase. Sirolimus blocks T-cell activation by IL-2, IL-4, and IL-6 and stimulation of B-cell proliferation by lipopolysaccharide. Sirolimus directly inhibits B-cell immunoglobulin synthesis caused by interleukins.

Sirolimus has been shown to prevent acute, accelerated, and chronic rejection of skin, heart, renal, islet, and small bowel allografts in rodent, rabbit, dog, pig, and nonhuman primate graft recipients. It has also been shown to be efficacious in models of autoimmunity; insulin-dependent diabetes, and systemic lupus erythematosus. The antagonism of cytokine and growth factor action by sirolimus is not limited to cells of the immune system. It inhibits the proliferation of fibroblasts, endothelial cells, hepatocytes, and smooth muscle cells induced by growth factors such as platelet-derived growth factor and fibroblast growth factor. Sirolimus has been very effective in preventing intimal smooth muscle proliferation (arteriosclerosis) following mechanical or immune-mediated arterial injury. In human clinical trials supplementation of cyclosporine-based protocols is associated with a reduction in acute allograft rejection; however, the combination of the two drugs increases the risk for nephrotoxicity, hemolytic-uremic syndrome, and hypertension. Other reported side effects include hyperlipidemia, thrombocytopenia, delayed wound healing, delayed graft function, mouth ulcers, pneumonitis, and interstitial lung disease. Everolimus, another inhibitor of mTOR, is a derivative of sirolimus.

Mycophenolate Mofetil

Mycophenolate mofetil (MMF), also known as RS-61443 or mycophenolic acid (Cellcept, Roche), is a prodrug hydrolyzed by liver esterases to mycophenolic acid. MMF is cytostatic for lymphocytes, owing to its inhibition of inosine monophosphate dehydrogenase, an enzyme necessary for de novo purine biosynthesis. MMF is a relatively selective inhibitor of T- and B-cell proliferation during the S phase of the cell cycle via its ability to prevent guanosine and deoxyguanosine biosynthesis. MMF has been shown to reduce allograft rejection in multiple animal models, demonstrating the most effect when combined with cyclosporine, tacrolimus, and/or sirolimus. MMF was developed in part as a nonmyelotoxic replacement for azathioprine in human allograft patients. Early clinical trials in human renal allograft recipients showed a decrease in biopsy-proven acute rejection episodes in patients receiving MMF in place of azathioprine. At therapeutic doses MMF can be toxic to animals. The primary dose-limiting effects are anemia and weight loss in rats; leukopenia, diarrhea, and anorexia in monkeys; and gastrointestinal hemorrhage, anorexia, and diarrhea in dogs. To reduce the toxic effects, the dose can be lowered, or mycophenolic acid can be given in combination with other immunosuppressive agents. MMF (10 mg/kg q12h PO) has been used in combination therapy in veterinary medicine to control renal allograft rejection in dogs (Broaddus et al., 2006).

There are anecdotal reports of the use of MMF for the treatment of RA, myasthenia gravis, and renal allograft rejection in the dog. In humans MMF has been used to treat scleroderma lung disease and Evans syndrome. MMF can also inhibit growth factor–induced smooth muscle and fibroblast proliferation. Sirolimus and MMF in combination are extremely effective in preventing arterial intimal smooth muscle proliferation following mechanical injury. This has marked implications for the control of chronic allograft rejection in humans.

Leflunomide and Leflunomide Analogs

Leflunomide is a synthetic organic isoxazole that the intestinal mucosa metabolizes to the active form, A77 1726. Leflunomide mediates at least part of its antiproliferative activity during the S phase of the cell cycle by inhibiting the de novo pathway of pyrimidine biosynthesis. The target of A77 1726 in this pathway is the enzyme dihydroorotate dehydrogenase. At higher concentrations leflunomide is also an inhibitor of tyrosine kinases associated with growth factor receptors. In addition to T and B lymphocytes, leflunomide also has an antiproliferative effect on smooth muscle cells and fibroblasts, which is also caused by the result of inhibition of the pyrimidine biosynthetic pathway in these cells. Leflunomide is currently approved for the treatment of RA in humans. It has been shown to be an effective disease-modifying antirheumatic drug free from the side effects commonly associated with currently approved immunosuppressants.

In addition to its efficacy in humans and animal models with autoimmune diseases, leflunomide has been found to control acute, ongoing, and chronic allograft rejection of the kidney, skin, heart, vessels, and lung in small- and large-animal models. I have used leflunomide to successfully treat steroid-resistant autoimmune hemolytic anemia and systemic histiocytosis in dogs. In combination with cyclosporine, leflunomide has completely prevented the rejection of canine MHC-

nonmatched renal allografts in both experimental and clinical studies. At doses used in humans, leflunomide causes gastrointestinal toxicity in dogs as a result of the accumulation of a metabolite trimethylfluoroanaline (TMFA). Fortunately the canine lymphocyte is far more sensitive than the human lymphocyte to the effects of the active agent A77 172, and much lower oral doses are equally effective in achieving immunosuppression. I currently use a dose of 4 mg/kg PO over 24 hours and adjust the dose as needed to obtain a 24-hour serum trough level of 20 mg/ml. Early studies in the cat suggest that TMFA does not present the toxicity problem encountered in dogs; cats metabolize the drug much more slowly and may only require 2 mg/kg/day once or twice a week to maintain effective blood concentrations. Leflunomide (70 mg/cat once weekly PO) in combination with methotrexate (7.5 mg/cat once weekly PO) has been used to treat feline RA (Hanna, 2005). Both cats and dogs with diminished renal function may be subject to TFMA toxicity since it is excreted by the kidneys. Leflunomide is marketed under the trade name Arava (Aventis Pharmaceuticals). The use of leflunomide in dogs has been very expensive; however, a generic form of the drug is now available, reducing the cost of therapy by approximately 80%.

Leflunomide analogs currently are under development for transplantation applications. A combination of cyclosporine and FK778, a leflunomide analog, significantly prolonged MHC-mismatched canine renal allograft survival.

INVESTIGATIONAL COMPOUNDS

FTY 720 is derived from myriocin, a fungus-derived sphingosine analog. After phosphorylation, FTY 720 engages lymphocyte sphingosine-1-phosphate receptors and profoundly alters lymphocyte trafficking, acting as a functional sphingosine-1-phosphate antagonist. FTY 720 sequesters naïve and activated CD4+ and CD8+ T and B cells from the blood into lymph nodes and Peyer's patches without affecting their functional properties. It is important to note that FTY 720 does not impair cellular or humoral immunity to systemic viral infection nor does it affect T-cell activation, expansion/proliferation, or immunologic memory.

FTY 720 synergizes effectively with inhibitors of T-cell activation and proliferation to prevent allograft rejection in a wide range of animal models. In combination with subtherapeutic concentrations of cyclosporine, FTY 720 has been shown to delay or prevent the rejection of skin, heart, small bowel, liver, and kidney allografts in rats, dogs, and nonhuman primates. Similar results have been seen when FTY 720 is combined with sirolimus and tacrolimus. FTY 720 is metabolized extensively in the liver via cytochrome enzymes that are not involved in the metabolism of cyclosporine, sirolimus, or tacrolimus; therefore variations in drug concentrations when these agents are coadministered are unlikely to occur. The pharmacokinetic profile of FTY 720 is characterized by linear dose-proportional exposure over a wide range of doses, only moderate interpatient variability, and a prolonged elimination half-life (89 to

150 hours). These factors suggest that FTY 720 will be administered once daily without the need for monitoring blood concentrations or dose titration. Human renal transplant patients experienced a significant reduction in peripheral blood lymphocyte counts by up to 85%. In the initial clinical trials in human renal transplant patients, FTY 720 was well tolerated and did not cause any significant toxicity, allograft loss, increase in infection rates, or other complications such as diabetes. However, when administered in combination with cyclosporine in later studies, possible toxic side effects were revealed that may negate the development of the drug for transplantation in humans. Pharmacokinetic and pharmacodynamic studies are currently under way in cats.

COMBINATION THERAPY

Most of the currently used or soon-to-be-available immunosuppressive agents have differing mechanisms of action and are effective at different stages of the cell cycle. Experimentally and clinically, combining agents often results in more effective immunosuppression with fewer drug-induced side effects. In human transplant patients cyclosporine or tacrolimus is currently considered to be the first line of immunosuppressive agents. To increase their effectiveness and decrease toxicity, azathioprine, sirolimus, prednisolone, and/or MMF are added to antirejection protocols. Few of the new nonmyelotoxic agents have been used in veterinary patients, but many published experimental animal trials investigating autoimmune disease and organ transplantation provide indications and insight into their use. Based on experimental and clinical experience in canine MHC-nonmatched organ transplantation, the combination of cyclosporine and leflunomide or cyclosporine and azathioprine is extremely effective in preventing renal allograft rejection.

References and Suggested Reading

Adamo FP, O'Brien RT: Use of cyclosporine to treat granulomatous meningoencephalitis in three dogs, *J Am Vet Med Assoc* 225:1211, 2004.

Allenspach K et al: Pharmacokinetics and clinical efficacy of cyclosporine treatment of dogs with steroid-refractory inflammatory bowel disease, *J Vet Intern Med* 20:239, 2006.

Berdoulay A, English RV, Nadelstein B: Effect of topical 0.02% tacrolimus aqueous suspension on tear production in dogs with keratoconjunctivitis sicca, *Vet Ophthalmol* 8:225, 2005.

Broaddus KD et al: Renal allograft histopathology in dog leukocyte antigen mismatched dogs after renal transplantation, *Vet Surg* 35:125, 2006.

Chiba K et al: Immunosuppressive activity of FTY720, sphingosine 1-phosphate receptor agonist. 1. Prevention of allograft rejection in rats and dogs by FTY720 and FTY720-phosphate, *Transplant Proc* 37:102, 2005.

Gregory CR et al: Results of clinical renal transplantation in 15 dogs using triple drug immunosuppressive therapy, *Vet Surg* 35:105, 2006.

Gregory CR, Bernsteen L: Organ transplantation in clinical veterinary practice. In Slatter D, editor: *Textbook of small animal surgery*, ed 3, Philadelphia, 2003, Saunders, p 122.

Guaguere E, Steffan J, Olivry T: Cyclosporin A: a new drug in the field of canine dermatology, *Vet Dermatol* 15:61, 2004.

Halloran PF: Immunosuppressive drugs for kidney transplantation, *N Engl J Med* 351:2515, 2004.

Hanna FY: Disease modifying treatment for feline rheumatoid arthritis, *Vet Comp Orthop Traumatol* 18:94, 2005.

Hardie RJ et al: Cyclosporine treatment of anal furunculosis in 26 dogs, *J Small Anim Pract* 46:3, 2005.

Kyles AE et al: Immunosuppression with a combination of the leflunomide analog, FK778, and microemulsified cyclosporine for renal transplantation in mongrel dogs, *Transplantation* 75:1128, 2003.

Mathews KA, Sukhiani HR: Randomized controlled trial of cyclosporine for the treatment of perianal fistulas in dogs, *J Am Vet Med Asso* 211:1249,1997.

Mehl ML et al: Disposition of cyclosporine after intravenous and multi-dose oral administration in cats, *J Vet Pharmacol Ther* 26:349, 2003.

Rosenkrantz WS: Pemphigus: current therapy, *Vet Dermatol* 15:90, 2004.

Steffan J, Favrot C, Mueller R: A systematic review and meta-analysis of the efficacy and safety of cyclosporin for the treatment of atopic dermatitis in dogs, *Vet Dermatol* 17:3, 2006.

CHAPTER 56

Blood-Typing and Crossmatching

URS GIGER, *Philadelphia, Pennsylvania*

Transfusion therapy has assumed an increasingly important role in the life support of companion animals since the early 1980s. The use of blood products in treating critically ill animals and supporting those undergoing surgical and other procedures has increased tremendously. Despite this trend, blood products represent a limited and sometimes unavailable resource. Since these products are biologicals from donor animals, transfusion also carries the inherent risks of transmitting infectious agents and causing adverse reactions. Accordingly, the need for blood-typing, crossmatching, and testing of donors for transmittable diseases is pivotal to insuring safe and efficacious transfusions. The Association of Veterinary Hematology and Transfusion Medicine and American Association of Veterinary Blood Banking have been established towards these ends, and these groups are developing blood-banking and transfusion therapy standards. Veterinary clinicians play a key role in the provision of safe and effective transfusion; therefore they must be aware of transfusion principles. This chapter summarizes some of the advances in blood compatibility testing in dogs and cats and offers practical recommendations for transfusion therapy.

CANINE BLOOD TYPES

Blood types are genetic markers on erythrocyte surfaces that are antigenic and species specific. A set of blood types of two or more alleles makes up a blood group system. More than a dozen blood group systems have been described in dogs. The various systems are generally referred to as dog erythrocyte antigens (DEAs), with the abbreviation DEA followed by a number (note: there is no DEA 2 system). No reagents are currently available for many antigens, and additional blood types continue to be recognized. For all blood group systems other than the DEA 1 system, red blood cells from a dog can be either positive or negative for that blood type. For instance, for the DEA 7 system, a dog's red blood cells can be DEA 7 positive or DEA 7 negative, and these blood types appear to be codominantly inherited. In the DEA 1 system, which represents an exception, DEA 1.1 (A_1) and 1.2 (A_2) are allelic, and there may even be a DEA 1.3 (A_3). Thus a dog can be DEA 1.1 positive or negative, and DEA 1.1–negative dogs can be DEA 1.2 positive or negative.

Only very limited surveys report on the frequency of these blood types with some suggestions of geographic and breed-associated differences. Some of the blood types are seen rarely (e.g., DEA 3), whereas others occur very commonly (DEA 4). In Japan additional blood-group systems have been proposed, but their associations to the DEA systems and their clinical importance have not been documented. Most recently an apparently new common red cell antigen that seems to be missing in some dalmatians, hence named *Dal* red cell antigen, has been identified.

Strongly antigenic blood types are of great clinical importance because they can elicit a potent alloantibody response. These alloantibodies may be of the immunoglobulin (Ig)G or IgM class and may be hemagglutinins or hemolysins. Clinically the most antigenic blood type in dogs appears to be DEA 1.1. Based on experimental and clinical data, dogs can become sensitized after receiving a mismatched transfusion (i.e., a blood unit positive for one or more blood types not found on the recipient's red blood cell). Sensitizing dogs in experimental studies in the 1950s led to the documentation of some transfusion reactions caused by blood-group incompatibilities and to the characterization of new blood types.

There are no clinically important naturally occurring alloantibodies (also known as isoantibodies) present before sensitization of a dog with a transfusion. Furthermore, pregnancy does not cause sensitization because of a complete placenta in dogs and thus does not induce alloantibody production. Transfusion of DEA 1.1–positive cells to a DEA 1.1–negative dog invariably elicits a strong alloantibody response. After a first transfusion, anti–DEA 1.1 antibodies develop after more than 4 days and may cause a delayed transfusion reaction. However, a previously sensitized DEA 1.1–negative dog will develop an acute hemolytic reaction after transfusion of DEA 1.1–positive blood. Transfusion reactions may also occur after a sensitized dog receives blood that is mismatched for a red blood cell antigen other than DEA 1.1. For instance, a whippet developed an alloantibody against a common red blood cell antigen, resulting in a general incompatibility with any donor except a littermate. Similarly a dog with DEA 4–negative blood, another common antigen, showed an acute hemolytic transfusion reaction after receiving a second DEA 4–positive blood transfusion. Because administration of a small (<1 ml) amount of incompatible blood can result in life-threatening reactions, the practice of giving small "test volumes" of donor blood to assess blood-type compatibilities is unacceptable.

CANINE BLOOD-TYPING PROCEDURE

To ensure efficacious and safe transfusions, blood donor and recipient should be blood typed. Canine blood-typing is generally based on serologic identification by agglutination reactions. Originally serum from sensitized dogs was used for typing, but such polyvalent alloantibodies vary from batch to batch and therefore are not optimal. Recently monoclonal antibodies against DEA 1.1 have been developed at Kansas State University and at the University of Lyon. Because of the strong antigenicity of DEA 1.1, typing of *donors* for DEA 1.1 is strongly recommended. Whenever possible, the *recipient* should also be typed to allow the use of DEA 1.1–positive blood for DEA 1.1–positive recipients. A blood-typing card has been available for a decade as a simple standardized in-practice kit (DMS Laboratories, Flemington, NJ) to classify dogs as DEA 1.1 positive or negative. This assay requires a small amount of anticoagulated blood (0.1 ml) and is based on an agglutination reaction that occurs within 2 minutes when DEA 1.1–positive erythrocytes interact with a murine monoclonal DEA 1.1 alloantibody. Based on limited data, it appears possible that this card may give a weak positive agglutination reaction with DEA 1.2–positive red cells. A new point-of-care cartridge for DEA 1.1 typing has recently been introduced (Alvedia, Lyon, France), which may make interpretation simpler.

Typing for DEA 1.1 is also available through most commercial and veterinary school laboratories. These laboratories had employed either the card method or a tube assay using reagents from Midwest Animal Blood Services, which requires the addition of a Coombs' reagent. Furthermore, a unique gel column technology, widely used in human blood banking, recently has been adopted for DEA 1.1 typing and found to be an excellent laboratory technique. This method uses a 4% red cell suspension in a standardized method with a monoclonal alloantibody for DEA 1.1 typing (which does not cross-react with DEA 1.2–positive cells) and gel columns, in which the agglutinating DEA 1.1–positive cells are retained on top of (or within) the gel by the reagent-induced hemagglutination. These cells are readily separated from the nonagglutinating (DEA 1.1–negative) cells, which pass through the gel after centrifugation (DiaMed, Cressier, Switzerland).

Dogs that are DEA 1.1 negative are considered universal blood donors for a previously untransfused dog. However such donors can still sensitize a recipient against other red cell antigens. Pregnancy does not sensitize a dog to develop alloantibodies.

Caution should be exercised during blood-typing whenever the patient's blood is autoagglutinating or has a very low hematocrit (<10%).

It is recommended to check for autoagglutination of blood with either buffer/saline on a slide or using the card test. Furthermore, with autoagglutination the control gel column may become positive, which negates interpretation of any typing results. Autoagglutinating blood first may be washed three times with (phosphate-buffered) physiologic saline. This procedure will help overcome apparent autoagglutination when performing the Coombs' test or crossmatch tests within tubes in a laboratory setting. However, if autoagglutination after three washes persists at greater than 1+, it is considered to reflect true autoagglutination. True autoagglutination precludes blood-typing (as well as crossmatching and Coombs' testing), because the sample will always appear as DEA 1.1–positive blood. In such circumstances DEA 1.1–negative blood should be used for transfusion until the patient no longer agglutinates and after the transfused cells are eliminated. At that point the patient's blood can be retyped.

DEA 1.1–positive blood from very anemic animals may not agglutinate when exposed to the DEA 1.1 or other reagents because of the prozone effect. In these cases some of the patient's plasma may be discarded before applying a drop of blood onto the card.

Finally recently transfused dogs may also create practical problems in blood-typing. Samples may display a mixed field reaction with only the transfused or recipient cells agglutinating.

Some veterinarians recommend using only canine donors that are negative for all testable DEAs except DEA 4 (as >98% of dogs are DEA 4–positive) to prevent sensitization against these blood types. Typing services and polyclonal antisera are available for DEA 1.1, 1.2, 3, 4, 5, and 7 (Midwest Animal Blood Services, Michigan) for extended typing. However, the clinical relevance of these and other blood groups to any given canine patient is usually identified following crossmatching of a previously-transfused dog. The use of these more extensive blood-typing products requires some expertise and experience. For these and other reasons the author does not support routine typing for blood types other than DEA 1.1. Additional typing unnecessarily removes many active and potential canine donors, is cost prohibitive, and does not eliminate the need for crossmatching following the first transfusion. There are no supporting published clinical studies demonstrating that transfusion reactions can be reduced substantially by extended blood-typing. Similarly, human patients are only typed for the ABO and Rh blood group systems, although greater than two dozen other blood group systems are known.

FELINE BLOOD TYPES

Although the feline AB blood group system remains the most clinically relevant and best recognized system, additional feline blood groups have recently been described. These systems may contribute to blood incompatibility reactions. Cats lacking a certain antigen on the red cell surface may have naturally occurring or induced alloantibodies (also known as *isoantibodies*) against the missing blood antigen (type). These alloantibodies can be responsible for acute hemolytic transfusion reactions and anti-A–mediated hemolysis of the newborn, a condition known as neonatal isoerythrolysis (NI).

The AB blood group system is recognized as the major blood group system and contains three types: type A, type B, and the rare type AB. The "a" allele is dominant over the "b" allele. Thus cats with type A blood have the genotype a/a or a/b, and only homozygous b/b cats express the type B antigen on their erythrocytes. A third allele is recessive to "a" and codominant to "b" and leads to the expression of both A and B substances on erythrocytes in the extremely rare AB cats. Thus AB cats are not produced by mating a type A to a type B cat unless the A cat carries the rare AB allele. Type AB blood has been seen in many purebred and domestic short-hair (DSH) cat breeds known to have type B blood. No type O or null type cats have been recognized. The molecular basis of the feline AB blood group has recently been determined and DNA testing is now available, which may be helpful for breeding purposes (Vet Gen Lab, UC, Davis).

An extensive survey of more than 20,000 DSH and purebred cats in the United States has been done at my institution over the past two decades, and many additional smaller studies have screened the blood types of cats in certain geographic areas, including DSH and purebred cats. Although type A is the most common blood type, the frequency of types A and B in DSH cats varies worldwide and even among regions. However, in purebred cats the frequency of A and B blood types varies greatly, although not as much geographically, probably because of the international exchange of breeding cats. The type B frequency may vary from none, as in the Siamese and related breeds, to 40%, as in the British shorthair and Devon rex breeds. In contrast, type AB is extremely rare, with a frequency of less than 1% in DSH and some purebred cats. Furthermore, kitten losses caused by A-B incompatibility and the resultant changes in breeding practices influence the frequency of A and B in various breeds. Indeed A-B incompatibility results in an unusual selection against heterozygous kittens and thereby an allele disequilibrium.

Most blood donors have type A blood, but some institutions also keep cats with the rare type B and type AB as donors. All blood donors must be typed, as there are no universal donor cats. Table 56-1 denotes the frequency of A and B blood types in various geographic locations and various cat breeds.

Additional feline blood groups have been suspected despite A-B compatibility. This conclusion is based on incompatible blood crossmatching results or the recognition of hemolytic reactions following transfusion in A-B compatible cats. Some cats develop blood incompatibilities to practically all potential donors, making safe and effective transfusion nearly impossible. These cats likely lack a high frequency or common red cell antigen. Very recently the author's laboratory documented a novel *Mik* antigen in most but not all DSH cats. Blood transfusions of *Mik*-positive blood to cats lacking the *Mik* antigen resulted in acute hemolytic transfusion reactions. The presence of naturally occurring anti-*Mik* alloantibodies has been documented in several additional *Mik*-negative cats since our initial report. The clinical relevance of the *Mik* antigen and corresponding alloantibody underlie our concern for potential hemolytic transfusion reactions in cats. Recent unpublished studies by the author's laboratory suggest other feline blood types along with the presence of naturally-occurring or induced alloantibodies.

BLOOD-TYPING PROCEDURES

Blood typing is recommended for both donor and recipient cats to allow for an appropriately matched transfusion, and for breeding cats to ensure blood-compatible mates and prevent isoerythrolysis in newborn kittens. Feline blood-typing generally is based on serologic identification by agglutination reactions. Originally serum from sensitized cats was used for A and B typing; but the lectin *Triticum vulgaris* has replaced the anti-B serum. Monoclonal anti-A and anti-B antibodies have been developed at Kansas State University and Lyon, France and are used in the

Table 56-1

Selected Blood Type A and B Frequencies in Cats*

Domestic Shorthair Cats	PERCENTAGE (%)		Purebred Cats	PERCENTAGE (%)	
	Type A	Type B		Type A	Type B
U.S. Northeast	99.7	0.3	Abyssinian	84	16
U.S. North Central	99.6	0.4	American shorthair	100	0
U.S. Southeast	98.5	1.5	Birman	82	18
U.S. Southwest	97.5	2.5	British shorthair	64	36
U.S. West Coast	95.3	4.7	Burmese	100	0
Argentina	97.0	3.0	Cornish rex	67	33
Australia (Brisbane)	73.7	26.3	Devon rex	59	41
India (Bombay)	88.0	12.0	Exotic shorthair	73	27
Europe			Himalayan	94	6
Austria	97.0	3.0	Japanese bobtail	84	16
England	97.1	2.9	Maine coon	97	3
Finland	100	0	Norwegian forest	93	7
France	85.1	14.9	Oriental shorthair	100	0
Germany	94.0	6.0	Persian	86	14
Hungary	100	0	Scottish fold	81	19
Italy	88.8	11.2	Siamese	100	0
Netherlands	96.1	3.9	Somali	82	18
Scotland	97.1	2.9	Sphinx	83	17
Switzerland	99.6	0.4	Tonkinese	100	0
Turkey	75.4	24.6	Turkish angora/van	50	50

* Ignoring the rare AB type.

blood-typing gel column and cartridge kits. Several AB typing techniques have been developed for use in practice or in the laboratory setting.

For the tube assay for feline blood-typing, washed red cell suspensions are mixed with anti-A serum from type B cats or antiserum from *T. vulgaris*, as anti-A and anti-B, respectively. Although this is the gold standard, currently it is only performed in the author's reference laboratory and at a few other sites. The same reagents at higher concentrations can also be used with whole blood in a simple slide agglutination screening test, but autoagglutination may preclude correct interpretation. A novel tube assay has become available using a red cell suspension (Shigeta Pharmaceutical,) but this test is not commercially available in the United States and appears to be somewhat cumbersome for use in private practice.

For over a decade, a commercial feline AB blood-typing card test has been available for in-practice use (DMS Laboratories), although the A reagent has been switched from anti-A serum to two anti-A monoclonal antibodies. This assay requires a small amount of anticoagulated blood (0.1 ml) and is based on an agglutination reaction that occurs within 2 minutes when type A- and/or B-positive erythrocytes interact with two murine monoclonal anti-A alloantibodies and/or lectin in the respective wells. While simple to perform in the practice setting, complications similar to those observed with canine typing cards have been observed. Occasionally no agglutination in either well occurs, suggesting a faulty card; or slight agglutination occurs in both wells, suggesting an AB blood type when in fact the cat has autoagglutination. This seems to be of particular concern on cards in which lectin and anti-A serum were replaced with monoclonal antibodies. Autoagglutination should be revealed by agglutination in the autocontrol well; and, if noted, the red cells can be washed three times with saline and the blood retested. There are other rare misinterpretations that occur using blood-typing cards. Sometimes type AB cats are not recognized by the card kit and are erroneously typed as either A or B. Blood from severely anemic cats may not agglutinate because there might be an excess of antibody present compared to the number of red cells (i.e., prozone effect).

In addition to card tests, other technologies have been used for feline blood-typing. A point-of-care typing cartridge with monoclonal anti-A and Anti-B antibodies has recently been introduced (Alvedia, Lyon, France). Most recently the gel column technology has been introduced for feline AB typing (DiaMed, Switzerland). This method originally used dilute unwashed red cell suspensions and a gel column with either a polyclonal anti-A alloantibody and the lectin *T. vulgaris* as anti-B. Now this test uses anti-A and anti-B monoclonal antibodies. This provides clear differentiation among type A-, type B-, and type AB-positive blood (if the autoagglutination control column using saline is negative). This test is restricted to larger laboratories because a special centrifuge is needed for the gel columns. In various surveys and comparative studies in the author's laboratory, this technique was found to be a highly reliable and easily standardized method. The same gel column technique has also been effectively used with anti-DEA 1.1 monoclonal antibodies to screen for DEA 1.1–positive and DEA 1.1–negative dogs. Finally, molecular genetic typing methods have become available (Vet Gen Labs, UC, Davis).

Typing for other feline blood types is not commercially available at the time of this writing, but is offered at the University of Pennsylvania laboratory (www.vet.upenn.edu/penngen). More studies are required to develop simple, widely-available typing tests. There is also a need to evaluate the clinical indications for screening for additional blood types before these are included in every compatibility workup.

In contrast to dogs, cats possess naturally occurring alloantibodies against the blood type antigen they lack. In particular, all type B cats develop very strong anti-A antibodies with high hemolysin and agglutinin titers (>1:32) after a few weeks of age. These anti-A antibodies are responsible for the life-threatening incompatibility reactions such as NI and acute hemolytic transfusion reactions.

A mismatched transfusion with type A blood given to a type B cat (but also type B blood given to a type A cat) results in a very serious acute hemolytic transfusion reaction. A *first* transfusion of as little as *1 ml of incompatible blood* may cause a fatal reaction without prior sensitization. Affected cats may show anaphylactic signs of hypotension, bradycardia, vomiting, and convulsions followed by hemolytic signs of pigmenturia and icterus without a transfusion-associated rise of the hematocrit. Thus mismatched transfusions are dangerous, as well as ineffective.

Kittens of blood types A and AB, receiving anti-A alloantibodies through the colostrum from type B queens (including primiparous queens), during the first 16 hours of life are at risk for NI. Hemolysis of the newborn is characterized by dark pigmenturia, anemia, icterus, anorexia, and sudden death within the first week of life. Survivors may develop tail tip necrosis.

In contrast to type B cats, type A cats have generally weak anti-B alloantibodies with low anti-B titers of 1:2. These antibodies cause shortened survival of transfused B cells in type A cats with signs of acute hemolytic anemia. Anti-B antibodies have not been associated with NI in type B kittens born to type A queens.

BLOOD CROSSMATCHING TEST

Blood-typing tests reveal the *blood group antigens* on the red blood cell surface, and blood crossmatching tests indicate the *serologic* compatibility or incompatibility between donor and recipient. Thus the crossmatching tests check for the presence or absence of naturally occurring and induced alloantibodies in serum (or plasma). These antibodies may be hemolysins and/or hemagglutins and can be directed against known blood groups or other red blood cell surface antigens. The *major crossmatch* tests for alloantibodies in the recipient's plasma against donor cells, whereas the *minor crossmatch* looks for alloantibodies in the donor's plasma against the recipient's red blood cells. Generally tube segments from collection bags are used for this purpose in dogs. Blood in a small EDTA tube is saved at the time of the blood collection by a small open or specially prepared closed system in cats.

Clearly, collecting and storing even small quantities of blood units for compatibility testing are technically difficult and further reduce the amount of blood to be transfused. Several crossmatch techniques are used in clinics and laboratories to screen for alloantibodies. For reference laboratories, a standardized tube crossmatching procedure has been proposed and is in use at many sites. This crossmatching test requires considerable technical expertise and experience, and is usually accomplished through a veterinary laboratory along with blood typing. The test is performed on EDTA-anticoagulated blood from the recipient and potential donor. Dilute red cell suspensions and plasma (or serum) are used, and some protocols include Coombs' reagents to enhance the reaction. Furthermore the author has evaluated the novel (DiaMed) gel column technique and found it in studies to be a simple, sensitive, and standardized laboratory method to crossmatch dogs and cats. The saline gel tests can be used for crossmatching in any species, but gel columns containing species-specific Coombs' (canine or feline antiglobulin) reagents may be more sensitive in recognizing blood incompatibilities, particularly in cats. This test is also applicable for the diagnosis of immune-mediated hemolytic anemias in cats and dogs. Persistent autoagglutination or severe hemolysis may preclude crossmatch testing. Initial studies performed in our laboratory used the saline gel column system and we were able to readily detect any A-B and also *Mik*-related incompatibilities. In more recent investigations we introduced a feline-specific antiglobulin gel column, which seems to be a sensitive but still simple and specific test. These methods hold promise for detecting both known and additional blood incompatibilities in laboratories. Most recently a gel-based tube major crossmatch assay for in-practice use has been introduced (DMS Laboratories, Flemington, NJ), but no studies have been published regarding use of this test. A simple slide test is sometimes used in clinical practice prior to feline transfusions and is described below.

A major crossmatch incompatibility is of greatest importance because it predicts that the transfused donor cells will be attacked by antibodies in the patient's plasma, thereby causing an acute hemolytic transfusion reaction that could become life threatening. As stated previously, fatal reactions may occur with less than 1 ml of incompatible blood, and therefore compatibility testing by administering a small amount of blood is inappropriate. Animals with an incompatible crossmatch should not be transfused with blood from that particular donor; instead, another potential donor should be tested for blood compatibility. The diligent application of appropriate blood-typing and crossmatching tests can ensure that blood is effectively and safely transfused in dogs and cats. A minor crossmatch incompatibility may be of lesser concern because the donor's plasma volume is small, particularly in packed red blood cell products, and the plasma is markedly diluted in the patient. The presence of autoagglutination or severe hemolysis may preclude crossmatch testing. There are some important differences in expected crossmatch test results between dogs and cats.

Dogs

The initial blood crossmatch between two dogs that have never before received a transfusion should be compatible because dogs do not have clinically important naturally occurring alloantibodies. Therefore one might omit a crossmatch before the first transfusion of a patient if the donor has not been transfused previously. Because the crossmatch does not determine the blood type of the patient and donor, a compatible crossmatch does not prevent sensitization of the patient against donor cells within 1 to 2 weeks. Therefore previously transfused dogs should *always* be crossmatched, even when they receive blood from the same donor, and should never be used as blood donors. The time span between the initial transfusion and incompatibility reactions may be as short as 4 days, and the risk of a reaction lasts for many years (i.e., years after the last transfusion, as alloantibodies may be present). Obviously a blood donor should never have received a blood transfusion to avoid sensitization.

Cats

Since cats have naturally occurring A or B alloantibodies (unless the cat has blood type AB), a blood crossmatch test will detect an A-B mismatch. In fact, mixing a drop of donor/recipient blood with donor/recipient plasma, respectively, will detect any A-B incompatibility in a patient over 3 months of age because by that time the cat will have developed its naturally occurring alloantibodies. Any previously transfused (>4 days earlier) cat needs to be crossmatched before receiving additional blood, even when getting it from the same donor, and a major and minor crossmatch should be performed. Because of the recent discovery of additional feline blood groups such as *Mik* with naturally occurring alloantibodies present in many cats, crossmatching of any cat to be transfused with AB-matched blood may be the proper recommendation in the near future. This is particularly likely to occur once standardized Coombs'-based tests are more available.

Unlike the situation in dogs, the first crossmatching test between cats may demonstrate transfusion incompatibility, even before the first transfusion, due to naturally-occurring alloantibodies. This result may be caused by anti-A alloantibodies, anti-B alloantibodies, *Mik* alloantibodies, or reactions to some other common red cell antigens. Thus, if blood-typing is unavailable in an urgent clinical setting or if the results from a point of care typing test are difficult to interpret, at least a crossmatch test can be done. Because of strong anti-A agglutinins in any cat older than 3 months, these blood type incompatibilities in cats often can be recognized by a simplified crossmatch procedure. This is done by mixing 2 drops of plasma with 1 drop of blood from either the recipient or the donor on a slide at room temperature.

The issue of naturally occurring alloantibodies in cats also impacts plasma transfusions. For this reason, only AB plasma can be safely transfused to cats; in fact, since additional naturally occurring alloantibodies may exist in a plasma unit, plasma crossmatching may need to be considered.

ALTERNATIVES TO BLOOD TRANSFUSIONS

Since blood is a scarce resource and may cause various transfusion reactions, alternatives should be considered before administrating a transfusion. Indeed, in many cases specific treatment of the underlying disease and other supportive care are all that is needed. Crystalloid and colloid fluids are appropriate in cases in which hypovolemia and low oncotic pressure are the major concerns. Oxygen therapy adds little to oxygen delivery in an anemic patient and therefore should only be considered when there is concomitant pulmonary-induced hypoxemia, as is sometimes observed in patients with lung injury associated with immune-mediated hemolytic anemia. Human recombinant erythropoietin may have a place in the management of some anemias, as with the anemia associated with chronic renal failure. However, the effects of erythropoietin are not evident for weeks, and it is therefore an ineffective therapy in emergency situations. This therapy has also induced cross-reacting antibodies against erythropoietin resulting in aplastic anemia.

In case of tissue hypoxia caused by a lack of red cells (hemoglobin), bovine ultrapurified hemoglobin solution (Oxyglobin, Biopure, MA) can be used as a blood substitute in place of packed red blood cells. Oxyglobin is approved for dogs and has been shown to be effective and safe as a transient oxygen carrier in various clinical case series; however, because of its strong oncotic properties at higher doses, hypervolemia and pulmonary edema are of particular concern in cats and any patient with a compromised cardiovascular system. Furthermore, the benefit of reaching capillaries with oxygen transported by free hemoglobin rather than red cells may be countered by some of the other compromising cardiovascular effects of Oxyglobin.

Although in human medicine various recombinant human products are available as alternatives for plasma transfusion, these options have not been evaluated completely and may be unsafe or cost prohibitive in dogs and cats. Human albumin has been used in cases of severe hypoalbuminemia, but major concerns have been raised about the development of reactions against this human product in animals. Recombinant coagulation factors have dramatically reduced the use of fresh frozen plasma in humans. Recombinant human factor VIIa (FVIIa) has been evaluated in dogs with factor VII deficiency as well as some other conditions. While there is no commercial canine or feline Ig concentrate, human intravenous Ig has been used successfully in the acute management of dermal and systemic toxic drug reactions in some veterinary situations. Again these are human products that carry the risk for reactions, particularly after repeated use.

In conclusion, to ensure safe and effective transfusions, every blood donor and recipient should be blood typed and in dogs (if previously transfused) also crossmatched. Crossmatching may be indicated at the time of the first feline transfusion. Small volume test transfusions are dangerous and the practice is unacceptable. Simple and standardized typing and crossmatching techniques have become available and will avoid most hemolytic transfusion reactions caused by blood-type incompat-

ibilities. Appropriate controls must be performed to exclude autoagglutination and typing and compatibility misinterpretation. True (persistent) autoagglutination precludes blood-typing, crossmatching, and Coombs' testing. Unlike the situation in dogs, major and minor crossmatching tests can show incompatibilities before any transfusion in cats. Transfusion of blood that is crossmatch incompatible is unsafe and ineffective.

*Original studies by the author were supported in part by the National Institutes of Health (RR02512).

References and Suggested Reading

Bell K: Blood groups of domestic animals. In Agar NS, Board DG, editors: Red blood cells of domestic mammals, Amsterdam, 1983 Elsevier, p 137.

Bighignoli B et al: Cytidine monophospho-N-acetylneuraminic acid hydroxylase (CMAH) mutations associated with the domestic cat AB blood group, BMC Genet 8:27, 2007.

Blais MC et al: Canine Dal blood type: a red cell antigen lacking in some Dalmatians, J Vet Intern Med 21:281, 2007.

Bücheler J, Giger U: Alloantibodies against A and B blood types in cats, J Vet Immunol Immunopathol 38:283, 1993.

Callan MB, Jones LT, Giger U: Hemolytic transfusion reactions in a dog with an alloantibody to a common antigen, J Vet Intern Med 9:277, 1995.

Giger U, Bücheler J, Patterson DF: Frequency and inheritance of A and B blood types in feline breeds of the United States, J Hered 82:15, 1991a.

Giger U, Bücheler J: Transfusion of type A and type B blood to cats, J Am Vet Med Assoc 198:41, 1991b.

Giger U, Stieger K, Palos H: Comparison of various canine blood-typing methods, Am J Vet Res 66:1386, 2005.

Giger U et al: An acute hemolytic transfusion reaction caused by dog erythrocyte antigen 1.1 incompatibility in a previously sensitized dog, J Am Vet Med Assoc 206:9, 1995.

Griot-Wenk M et al: Biochemical characterization of the feline AB blood group system, Anim Genet 24:401, 1993.

Griot-Wenk ME et al: Blood type AB in the feline AB blood group system, Am J Vet Res 57:1438, 1996.

Hohenhaus AE: Importance of blood groups and blood group antibodies in companion animals, Transfus Med Rev 18:117, 2004.

Jackson KV, Withnall E, Giger U: Initial assessment of a novel gel column Coombs' test to detect auto- and alloantibodies in dogs. J Vet Intern Med 21:623, 2007.

Melzer KJ et al: A hemolytic transfusion reaction due to DEA 4 alloantibodies in a dog, J Vet Intern Med 17:931, 2003.

Stieger K, Palos H, Giger U: Comparison of various blood-typing methods for the feline AB blood group system, Am J Vet Res 66:1393, 2005.

Weinstein NM et al: A newly recognized blood group in domestic shorthair cats: the Mik red cell antigen, J Vet Intern Med 21:287, 2007.

CHAPTER 57

Immune-Mediated Hemolytic Anemia

ELLEN MILLER, *Longmount, Colorado*

PATHOPHYSIOLOGY

Immune-mediated hemolytic anemia (IMHA) is a life-threatening hematologic disease of dogs and cats. Erythrocytes are destroyed by a type II hypersensitivity reaction that results in extravascular or intravascular hemolysis. Extravascular hemolysis occurs when immunoglobulin (Ig)– or complement-coated erythrocytes are removed by phagocytic cells of the mononuclear phagocyte system. If the red blood cells (RBCs) are coated with enough IgG or IgM molecules to fix complement, intravascular hemolysis also may result. Ten to twenty percent of dogs with IMHA have the intravascular form.

Primary IMHA is a true autoimmune reaction against RBCs. The majority of dogs with IMHA (60% to 75%) are thought to have this form of the disease since no underlying etiology can be identified. In secondary IMHA erythrocytes are destroyed as "innocent bystanders" in an immune reaction against some foreign protein that may be adherent to the erythrocyte surface. Usually the triggering protein is a result of viral or bacterial infection, drug administration, or neoplastic processes. Secondary IMHA is the more common form in cats.

It is important to realize that hemolytic anemia is not caused only by immunologic mechanisms. Other diseases, drugs, or toxins associated with hemolytic anemia are listed in Box 57-1. In the diagnostic approach to the patient with hemolytic anemia one should consider all the other potential etiologies.

DIAGNOSIS OF IMMUNE-MEDIATED HEMOLYTIC ANEMIA IN DOGS

Clinical Presentation

Signalment

Immune-mediated hemolytic anemia is a disease of middle-age dogs (median age of affected dogs is 6 to 7 years). Although any breed may be affected, cocker spaniels, English springer spaniels, collies, poodles, Old English sheepdogs, and Irish setters are overrepresented. Most reports of canine IMHA have noted a predominance of female dogs. A recent study of cats with primary IMHA reported a median age of 2 years (Kohn et al., 2006). No single breed was shown to be at risk. Eleven male and eight female cats were diagnosed with the disease.

Clinical Signs

Box 57-2 summarizes the historical and physical examination abnormalities in dogs with IMHA. The clinical signs associated with IMHA are a reflection of the inflammatory reaction and the resultant anemia. The onset of IMHA can be acute or insidious. Lethargy, depression, and anorexia are the most common signs. Vomiting and diarrhea are reported occasionally. Sudden collapse and syncope are less common signs. The owner may note discolored urine. Most often discoloration is caused by bilirubin content, but occasionally port wine–colored urine is seen, consistent with intravascular hemolysis. The relationship of vaccination to the development of IMHA is controversial. The most common signs in cats with primary IMHA are anorexia and lethargy. Other signs (pica, vomiting, pruritus, dyspnea, epistaxis, polydipsia, and obstipation) are less common (Kohn et al., 2006).

Physical examination findings in dogs include pallor, icterus, depression, and weakness. Tachycardia is present in approximately one third of dogs. Occasionally cardiac murmurs are noted secondary to severe anemia or underlying heart disease. Hepatosplenomegaly can often be noted on abdominal palpation. The hair in the perineal area or around the penis may be discolored by the bilirubin or hemoglobin in the urine. Petechial hemorrhages may be evident in mucous membranes and in the skin of animals that have a concurrent thrombocytopenia or vasculitis. Fever and lymphadenopathy are sometimes present. Cats were reported to have pale and sometimes icteric (2 of 19) mucous membranes, lymphadenopathy, and heart murmurs (Kohn et al., 2006). Respiratory distress in animals with IMHA may be consequent to pulmonary thromboembolism.

Laboratory Results

The typical results of laboratory evaluation in dogs are listed in Table 57-1. Anemia can be moderate to severe. Packed cell volume (PCV) can be as low as 6%. As many as 50% of dogs with IMHA have nonregenerative or poorly regenerative anemia based on reticulocyte index. Eleven of 19 cats with IMHA had anemia categorized as nonregenerative (Kohn et al., 2006). Spherocytosis is a common but nonspecific finding in dogs with IMHA. Spherocytosis implies an underlying immune mechanism but does not indicate whether the etiology is primary or secondary. Spherocytosis may also be hereditary in certain breeds of dogs. Because of small erythrocyte size in cats, spherocytes are difficult to detect. Polychromasia, anisocytosis, and nucleated RBCs are present

Box 57-1

Causes of Hemolytic Anemia in Dogs and Cats

Inherited Causes
- Pyruvate kinase deficiency
- Phosphofructokinase deficiency
- Chondrodysplasia/anemia
- Nonspherocytic hemolytic anemia

Immune-Mediated Causes (Primary)
- Primary (idiopathic) immune-mediated hemolytic anemia (IMHA)
- IMHA associated with systemic lupus erythematosus
- Neonatal isoerythrolysis
- Incompatible transfusions

Metabolic Causes
- Hypophosphatemia

Neoplastic Causes
- Microangiopathic anemia associated with hemangiosarcoma or lymphoma

Infectious Causes
- *Babesia canis*
- *Babesia gibsoni*
- *Mycoplasma haemominutum*
- *Mycoplasma haemofelis*
- *Mycoplasma haemocanis*
- *Dirofilaria immitis*
- *Bacterial endocarditis*
- *Feline leukemia virus*
- *Leptospirosis*
- *Cytauxzoon felis*
- *Ehrlichia canis*

Toxin- or Drug-Related Causes
- Onion toxicity
- Zinc toxicity
- Methylene blue
- Copper toxicity
- Propylthiouracil
- Methimazole
- Sulfa drugs
- Penicillins and cephalosporins
- Quinidine

Box 57-2

Most Common Clinical Signs in Dogs With Immune-Mediated Hemolytic Anemia

- Anorexia
- Lethargy
- Pallor
- Weakness
- Icterus
- Tachycardia
- Hepatosplenomegaly

Table 57-1

Laboratory Findings in 17 Dogs With IMHA

Laboratory Parameter	Mean (SD)	Range
Packed cell volume (%)	15.7 (6.3)	6-35
MCV (fl)	78.4 (11.9)	60-129
Reticulocyte count ($\times 10^3/\mu l$)	173.7 (188.6)	0-1,102.5
WBC ($\times 10^3/\mu l$)	31.0 (21.1)	5.4-109.5
Platelet count ($\times 10^3/\mu l$)	185 (170)	1-922
Bilirubin (mg/dl)	7.2 (13.2)	0.01-63.6
BUN (mg/dl)	31.5 (23.4)	8-85
Creatinine (mg/dl)	0.78 (0.36)	0.3-1.6
Glucose (mg/dl)	94.5 (26.2)	37-128
Calcium (mg/dl)	9.0 (0.6)	8.1-10.4
Phosphorous (mg/dl)	5.0 (1.6)	3.2-9.0
ALP (units/L)	92.2 (1344.2)	21-5570
ALT (units/L)	132.2 (251.8)	20-1072
Albumin (g/dl)	3.03 (0.48)	2.3-3.8
Globulin (g/dl)	2.99 (0.86)	2.1-6
TCO_2 (mEq/L)	14.7 (4.1)	7.2-21.8

ALP, Alanine phosphatase; *ALT,* alanine aminotransferase; *BUN,* blood urea nitrogen; *MCV,* mean corpuscular volume; *TCO_2,* total carbon dioxide; *WBC,* white blood cell.

on blood smears from dogs with an appropriate regenerative response. Macrocytosis is common in dogs with strongly regenerative anemias. Microscopic autoagglutination is noted in blood smears from some dogs with IMHA.

Leukopenia is uncommon and may result from antibody-mediated neutropenia, sepsis, or decreased bone marrow production. Very high white blood cell counts (up to 100,000/µl) have been attributed to the inflammatory reaction, cytokines that act as colony-stimulating factors for various cell lines, and general activation of the bone marrow secondary to anemia. One study (McManus and Craig, 2001) found a correlation between leukocytosis in dogs with IMHA and tissue necrosis, specifically centrilobular hepatic necrosis, presumably secondary to hypoxemia. Cats with primary IMHA generally have normal leukocyte counts but can demonstrate a mild leukocytosis.

Thrombocytopenia is a concurrent finding in approximately 70% of dogs and 42% of cats with IMHA. Thrombocytopenia can be a result of immune-mediated platelet destruction or consumptive processes such as sepsis or disseminated intravascular coagulation (DIC).

Autoagglutination is considered the hallmark of class I IMHA and negates the need for direct Coombs' testing. In my retrospective study of 105 cases of canine IMHA, 70 of the 73 dogs tested had blood samples that were positive for autoagglutination. In 19 cats with primary IMHA, all had macroscopic slide agglutination. Erythrocytes coated with high titers of warm antibody and complement can spontaneously agglutinate. To ensure that the agglutination is real autoagglutination and not the result of rouleaux formation, 1 drop of ethylenediaminetetraacetic acid–anticoagulated (EDTA) blood is placed with 1 to 2 drops of saline on a glass microscope slide. The slide is gently rocked to mix the blood and saline, and if agglutination is still present a presumptive diagnosis of IMHA can be made.

There are no consistent serum biochemical abnormalities that aid in the diagnosis of IMHA. Serum biochemical parameters often reflect hemolysis, dehydration, and hypoxic damage to organs. More than two thirds of dogs with IMHA exhibit hyperbilirubinemia. Prerenal azotemia can be noted in patients that are severely affected. Azotemia secondary to acute renal failure is rare but can result from renal ischemia, DIC, sepsis, and hemoglobin (pigment) nephropathy. Mild-to-moderate elevations in serum hepatic transaminases have been attributed to hepatocyte hypoxia. Serum alkaline phosphatase may be increased because of cholestasis from mononuclear phagocyte system hyperplasia or extramedullary hematopoiesis within the liver. Low total carbon dioxide (TCO_2) or serum bicarbonate concentration may reflect probable lactic acidosis associated with decreased tissue oxygen delivery. Hyperglobulinemia is noted occasionally and may be indicative of the inflammatory response. Cats with IMHA have hyperbilirubinemia as the primary biochemical abnormality. Liver enzymes were normal in 9 of 19 cats and were variably increased in the remainder of the cats studied. Six of 19 cats were azotemic.

Bilirubinuria is the most common finding on urinalysis. In dogs with intravascular hemolysis, hemoglobinuria is evident as a dark red color, which persists following centrifugation. Additional abnormalities may include proteinuria, hematuria, and cylinduria. Bacteriuria and pyuria are indicative of concurrent urinary tract infection. Any signs of urinary tract infection warrant further workup because bacterial endocarditis can cause urinary tract infection and a secondary IMHA. The urine is usually concentrated if the dog is dehydrated; however, the urine specific gravity can be isosthenuric if acute or chronic renal failure is present.

Direct Coombs' Test

The direct Coombs' test detects the presence of antibodies and/or complement on the erythrocyte surface. The Coombs' test result is positive in 35% to 60% of dogs with IMHA. False-positive test results can be produced by concurrent disease states such as neoplasia, mycoplasmosis, babesiosis, bacterial infections, administration of certain drugs, previous transfusion, improper antisera preparation, and nonspecific adsorption of serum proteins on damaged RBCs. It is important to interpret the test results in light of the individual patient and realize that a positive test result is consistent with but not diagnostic for IMHA. A positive Coombs' test in cats can occur with feline leukemia virus infection, *Mycoplasma haemofelis* infection, feline infectious peritonitis virus infection, myeloproliferative diseases, other neoplastic diseases, and chronic bacterial infections. A direct-flow cytometric erythrocyte immunofluorescence assay for dogs may be more sensitive and cost effective when it becomes more widely available (Quigley et al., 2001). The authors showed a sensitivity of 92% with flow cytometry compared to 53% for the Coombs' test and a specificity of 100% for both tests.

Additional Diagnostic Tests

Arterial blood gas analysis is indicated in the dyspneic dog. Profound hypoxemia with normocapnia and normal acid-base balance is consistent with pulmonary thromboembolism (PTE) (see Chapter 155). The calculated alveolar arterial oxygen gradient is markedly increased in these dogs. Hypoxemia also can be caused by pulmonary edema or pleural effusion consequent to infusion of crystalloids.

Coagulation parameters in dogs and cats with IMHA have been the subject of recent interest. A hypercoagulable state in dogs with IMHA has been suspected and was supported by studies of Mischke (1998). Scott-Moncrieff and associates (2001) prospectively studied 20 dogs with IMHA and showed that the activated partial thromboplastin time (aPTT) was prolonged in nine dogs and the one-stage prothrombin time (OSPT) was prolonged in two dogs. Fibrinogen concentration was increased in 17 dogs, fibrin degradation products were increased in 12 dogs, and D-dimer concentration was increased in 16 dogs. Antithrombin activity was decreased in 10 dogs. Nine dogs (45%) were diagnosed with DIC based on the authors' criteria. Cats with primary IMHA also demonstrate coagulation abnormalities. Three of 10 cats in one study had prolongation of aPTT and OSPT. Two of these cats also had thrombocytopenia.

Bone marrow examination may be useful, especially in cases in which the regenerative response is poor. Evaluation of bone marrow aspirates from the majority of dogs with IMHA shows erythroid or generalized marrow hyperplasia. Erythrophagocytosis is seen occasionally and may be indicative of immune-mediated red cell destruction within the bone marrow. Erythrocyte hypoplasia or erythroid maturation arrest can also be seen, implying targeting of common antigens expressed both on mature RBCs and RBC precursors. The bone marrow in cats with IMHA has been described by Weiss (2006). Bone marrow from these cats was normal-to-hypercellular with predominant changes in the erythroid line, including maturation defects, binucleation, fragmented nuclei, and mild megaloblastosis. There was also an increase in small lymphocytes in the marrow of affected cats.

Imaging of the thorax and abdomen is warranted in some animals with IMHA. Thoracic radiographs aid in ruling out underlying diseases such as neoplasia and infection that may be associated with secondary IMHA. Routine radiography may also detect evidence of PTE in dogs. A pronounced interstitial pattern is most commonly noted; however, a patchy alveolar pattern and pleural effusion can also be seen (Klein, Dow, and Rosychuk, 1989). Other considerations for increased lung density in IMHA patients include secondary bronchopneumonia, congestive heart failure, noncardiogenic pulmonary edema, and circulatory overload from fluid therapy. Hepatosplenomegaly can be detected by abdominal radiography. In addition, evidence of abdominal neoplasia, gastric foreign bodies, or other intraabdominal abnormalities may be detectable by radiography or ultrasonography.

Pulmonary perfusion can be assessed with nuclear scintigraphy in dogs with IMHA and suspected PTE. This modality is the most accurate, although generally unavailable, method of detecting thromboembolism, and carries practical difficulties related to the radiopharmaceutical. Irregular distribution of radiolabeled macroaggregated albumin is consistent with vascular obstruction by thromboemboli.

THERAPY FOR IMMUNE-MEDIATED HEMOLYTIC ANEMIA

The therapy for dogs with IMHA is both supportive and specific for the disease. Supportive care is necessary for patients with severe IMHA such as the intravascular or autoagglutinating forms of the disease. There have been few controlled clinical studies supporting the use of specific therapeutic regimens.

Supportive Care

Supportive care primarily involves maintenance of hydration, acid-base balance, and organ perfusion. In addition, diuresis is indicated in patients with intravascular hemolysis to prevent hemoglobin nephrosis. Although the role of free hemoglobin as a nephrotoxin is controversial, in my experience a significant portion of dogs with intravascular IMHA have clinical laboratory data suggestive of acute renal failure and necropsy evidence of hemoglobin (pigment) nephrosis. Subcutaneous fluid administration may be adequate; however, this route is contraindicated in dogs that are severely thrombocytopenic because of the risk of subcutaneous hemorrhage. Intravenous catheter placement in a peripheral vein is recommended but has been identified as a risk factor for the development of PTE. Jugular vein catheterization may not be advisable because of the potential for coagulopathy, both hemorrhagic and hypercoagulable states. Vigorous volume expansion can lead to pulmonary edema or pleural effusion. Such patients often demonstrate jugular venous distension or pulses. Noncardiogenic pulmonary edema may develop possibly related to injury to the alveolar capillary membrane. Congestive heart failure may be precipitated by acute anemia and crystalloid therapy in dogs or cats with preexistent heart disease.

Attention to aseptic technique and the use of latex gloves when handling patients with IMHA are extremely important. Immunosuppressive therapy increases the risk of sepsis in these patients. Although prophylactic antibiotic therapy is not necessary, routine monitoring for sepsis is mandatory. A dog that is being treated with immunosuppressive doses of glucocorticoids may not be able to generate a fever; thus body temperature is not an accurate means of identifying sepsis.

Dogs should be walked outside to urinate several times daily, if possible, to minimize urine retention and the potential for urinary tract infections. Cages should be well padded to aid in the prevention of decubital ulcers.

Specific treatment may be indicated in patients with vomiting related to IMHA or to the immunosuppressive therapy. Gastrointestinal ulceration may be prevented by the early use of histamine H_2 blockers, proton pump blockers, or prostaglandin analogs. Antiemetics such as metoclopramide may be necessary for controlling vomiting.

Blood Transfusion

Unique risks are associated with transfusions in dogs with IMHA. The presence of autoantibodies in the patient may shorten the survival of the transfused RBC,

reducing the benefit of the transfusion. Transfusion may suppress the erythropoietic response of the patient, prolonging the time to erythroid recovery. Transfusions have been suspected of increasing the risk of PTE in dogs with IMHA (Klein, Dow, and Rosychuk, 1989).

Individual patient selection is important; there is no exact PCV that indicates transfusion. The patient's need for transfusion is determined by evaluation of laboratory parameters and the clinical signs associated with the anemia. Frequent assessment of the PCV is important in determining the trend (up or down) and the rate of the change. Patients undergoing severe, rapid hemolysis should be monitored more frequently. If the PCV is stable, transfusion may not be warranted. Clinical parameters, including patient attitude, exercise tolerance, respiratory rate, and heart rate, may indicate the need for a transfusion. In general, if the dog is stable and comfortable at rest, transfusion is not necessary.

If blood transfusion is indicated, the clinical status of the dog must be taken into consideration in choosing the best blood product for the animal (also see Chapter 56). In general, if the patient has not been typed, blood from universal donors (i.e., DEA 1-7 negative, except DEA 4 can be positive) should be used. If RBCs are the only component needed by the patient, fresh packed RBCs may be given to reduce the risk of transfusion reactions to plasma proteins present in whole blood. The recipient gains the most benefit from a fresh unit. If the dog has a coagulopathy such as DIC in conjunction with anemia, fresh whole blood or packed RBCs and fresh-frozen plasma may be needed. Administration of blood products should be initiated cautiously (0.5 to 1 ml/kg/hour for the first 30 minutes), and the patient monitored closely for signs of transfusion reactions. If no reactions are noted, the rate can be increased so that the full unit is completely administered within the next 4 hours. Blood can be administered at a rate of 20 to 80 ml/kg/hour in life-threatening situations. If the patient has reduced cardiovascular function, transfusion rates should not exceed 4 ml/kg/hour. Hemoglobin solutions (Oxyglobin, Biopure) may also be considered in patients requiring increased oxygen delivery to tissues. Survival rates in one study were not different for dogs with IMHA that received Oxyglobin/blood, blood/Oxyglobin, or Oxyglobin alone (Rentko, Hasndler, and Hanson, 2000).

Immunosuppressive Therapy

Glucocorticoids

Glucocorticoids are the mainstay of therapy in the majority of dogs and cats with IMHA. The major therapeutic effect of glucocorticoids in IMHA is to decrease Fc receptor–mediated RBC destruction within the mononuclear phagocyte system. Glucocorticoids also inhibit complement activation and reduce circulating levels of cytokines, thereby diminishing the amplification of the immune response. Prednisone/prednisolone or prednisolone acetate is recommended at immunosuppressive doses of 2 mg/kg twice daily orally or by injection, respectively. This dosage is maintained until the patient shows clinical improvement (rising PCV) for at least 5 to 7 days. At this point the dosage can be reduced by 25% to 50% every 3 to 4 weeks if the complete blood count supports the view that remission is maintained. If at any time there is any indication of relapse such as return of autoagglutination or a reduction in PCV, the dose of prednisone is increased to the next higher dose, and future dosage tapering is slowed. In severe relapses initial immunosuppressive doses may need to be reinstituted. When the dose of prednisone is reduced to 0.5 mg/kg/day, alternate-day therapy may be initiated at the next monthly recheck evaluation if remission has been maintained. Although no clinical trials have been completed to assess the need for lifelong therapy, relapse of IMHA does occur.

Cytotoxic Drugs

In severe cases of IMHA (intravascular or autoagglutinating) or in cases unresponsive to glucocorticoids alone, the addition of cytotoxic or immunosuppressive drugs may be necessary (see Chapter 55 for more information regarding immunosuppressive drugs). Cyclophosphamide and azathioprine have been used individually or together in these situations.

Azathioprine. The recommended dose of azathioprine (Imuran, Glaxo Wellcome) is 2 mg/kg given daily or on alternate days. I use azathioprine daily for 4 days and then on alternate days. When the prednisone dose is reduced to alternate-day administration, azathioprine can be given on the days when prednisone is not given. If after 4 weeks remission is maintained, the azathioprine can be discontinued. In dogs that are sensitive to the side effects of glucocorticoids, azathioprine can be used on alternate days to maintain remission. The side effects of azathioprine include gastrointestinal upset, bone marrow suppression, poor hair growth, and pancreatitis. The study of Mason and colleagues (2003) demonstrated no benefit to combination cyclophosphamide-prednisone therapy when compared to simple prednisone therapy in the treatment of extravascular IMHA.

Cyclosporine A. Cyclosporine A (CsA, Neoral, Sandoz Pharmaceuticals) is a potent immunosuppressive drug directed at cell-mediated immune responses. CsA blocks the expression of the interleukin-2 and interferon-γ genes within T lymphocytes, thereby blocking the amplification of the immune response at a crucial step in T-cell activation. It has been used effectively alone or in combination with other immunosuppressive therapies in dogs with IMHA. Because of variability in gastrointestinal absorption, predictable blood levels are difficult to attain, necessitating the determination of serum drug concentrations for accurate dosing. In dogs the most common side effects include vomiting, diarrhea, and anorexia. Therapy with CsA is initiated at a dosage of 5 mg/kg PO every 12 to 24 hours. Ideally therapeutic drug monitoring is recommended at 2- to 4-week intervals. A trough concentration of 100 to 300 ng/ml as measured by high-performance liquid chromatography is recommended (Vaden et al., 1995).

Mycophenolate Mofetil. Mycophenolate mofetil (Cell-Cept, Roche Pharmaceuticals) is an immunosuppressive medication that has been used to treat myasthenia gravis, another immune-mediated disease in dogs. Mycophenolate mofetil is converted to mycophenolic acid, which inhibits purine synthesis primarily in B and T lymphocytes, thus reducing autoantibody production. Mycophenolate mofetil is used at a dosage of 10 to 20 mg/kg every 12 hours orally. Side effects are minimal and are usually nausea, vomiting, or diarrhea. In refractory cases of IMHA in dogs, mycophenolate mofetil is used to aid in inducing remission and then may be discontinued. Studies need to be completed to identify the role of mycophenolate mofetil in the treatment of IMHA.

Intravenous γ-Globulin

Intravenous γ-globulin (IVGG) administration has been used to treat several immune-mediated diseases in people, specifically IMHA, immune-mediated thrombocytopenia, and immune-mediated neutropenia. The mechanism by which IVGG suppresses the immune destruction of RBCs is thought to be blockade of macrophage Fc receptors and possibly antiidiotypic downregulation of autoantibody production. When given at a dose of 1 g/kg intravenously over 6 to 12 hours, a profound reticulocytosis occurs, followed by a more slowly rising PCV. In a recent study of IVGG in dogs with IMHA, 8 of 11 dogs survived and attained a remission, although long-term follow-up data were not available (White et al., 2003). No adverse side effects of IVGG treatment were noted.

Liposome-Encapsulated Clodronate

The use of liposome-encapsulated clodronate (dichloromethylene diphosphonate) to deplete splenic macrophages and block clearance of Ig-coated RBCs has been evaluated in a mouse model of IMHA and more recently in dogs with IMHA (Mathes, Jordan, and Dow, 2006). It appears to be well tolerated in dogs, and preliminary evidence suggests its ability to rapidly block the clearance of opsonized RBCs in normal dogs and dogs with IMHA, resulting in improved survival.

COMPLICATIONS OF IMMUNE-MEDIATED HEMOLYTIC ANEMIA IN DOGS

Complications of IMHA can be severe and life threatening. They include refractory anemia, hemorrhage, bacterial or fungal infections, acute renal failure, and PTE. It is difficult to glean from the literature the proportion of dogs that die from specific causes. In my retrospective study at a referral institution 40% of the dogs with IMHA responded to treatment and survived. Sixty percent died or were euthanized because of refractory anemia, relapse of anemia, or other complications of the disease or its treatment. The cause of death as determined by necropsy was available in 25 dogs. Three dogs with intravascular hemolysis had evidence of acute renal failure secondary to hemoglobin nephrosis. One dog died of sepsis. PTE was found in 22 dogs.

Refractory anemia is common in dogs with IMHA. Failure of the dog to respond to immunosuppressive agents often leads to death or euthanasia.

Complications of IMHA also include hemorrhage, which may result from the disease itself or its treatment. Gastrointestinal hemorrhage is commonly seen and can result from the combined effects of ischemia, thrombocytopenia, DIC, and drug-associated alterations in epithelial cell turnover and gastric acid and mucus production.

Therapy for IMHA is still crude and nonspecific. Unfortunately immunosuppressive drugs inhibit not only aberrant immune responses but also immune responses necessary to protect the host from infection. Disseminated bacterial, fungal, and protozoal infections have contributed to the deaths of dogs with IMHA.

PTE is a common cause of death in dogs with IMHA. In a study by Klein, Dow, and Rosychuk (1989), 32% of 31 dogs with IMHA died of PTE based on findings at necropsy. The authors postulated that hypercoagulability is most probably responsible for thrombus formation. Potential causes of hypercoagulability may include an imbalance in procoagulant and naturally occurring anticoagulant factors, DIC, endothelial cell–mediated coagulation triggered by antierythrocyte antibodies, and procoagulant factors released from damaged erythrocytes. Hyperbilirubinemia, hypoalbuminemia, intravenous catheter placement, and severe thrombocytopenia (<50,000/µl) have been identified as risk factors for the development of PTE (Klein et al., 1989; Carr, Panciera, and Kidd, 2002). The clinical signs of acute dyspnea, orthopnea, and profound anorexia should prompt further evaluation (Chapter 155). Sudden death without prior clinical signs also occurs.

Prophylactic therapy to prevent thrombosis has been recommended in dogs with IMHA. As stated previously, DIC is common in dogs with IMHA. Plasma has been used to treat DIC initiated by other disorders such as sepsis, but plasma did not decrease mortality of dogs with IMHA and PTE in one study (Thompson, Scott-Moncrieff, and Brooks, 2004). Heparin has not consistently prevented the development of PTE. Two recent studies of heparin in dogs with IMHA failed to show a benefit on survival (Fryer, McMichael, and Slater, 2005; Breuhl, Scott-Moncrieff, and Brooks, 2005). In one of these studies doses of up to 300 units of unfractionated heparin per kilogram every 6 hours were not successful in attaining target anti-Xa activity. The addition of aspirin at a dose of 1 to 2 mg/kg every 24 hours may be of benefit. A study of aspirin in dogs with IMHA showed a significantly improved survival rate in dogs receiving azathioprine and aspirin in conjunction with glucocorticoids compared to those receiving azathioprine and glucocorticoids or azathioprine, heparin, and glucocorticoids (Weinkle et al., 2005). Until the underlying mechanisms promoting thrombus formation are identified, it is unlikely that an effective antithrombotic protocol will be developed.

References

Breuhl EL, Scott-Moncrieff C, Brooks M: *A prospective study of unfractionated heparin therapy to prevent thrombosis in canine immune-mediated hemolytic anemia*, Proceedings of the ACVIM Forum, Baltimore, 2005.

Carr AP, Panciera DL, Kidd L: Prognostic factors for mortality and thromboembolism in canine immune-mediated hemolytic anemia: a retrospective study of 72 dogs, *J Vet Intern Med* 16:504, 2002.

Fryer JS, McMichael MA, Slater MR: *Effect of heparin use on survival to discharge of dogs with immune-mediated hemolytic anemia*, Proceedings of the ACVIM Forum, Baltimore, 2005.

Klein MK, Dow SW, Rosychuk RAW: Pulmonary thromboembolism associated with immune-mediated hemolytic anemia in dogs: ten cases (1982-1987), *J Am Vet Med Assoc* 195:246, 1989.

Kohn BV et al: Primary immune-mediated hemolytic anemia in 19 cats: diagnosis, therapy and outcome, (1998-2004), *J Vet Intern Med* 20:159, 2006.

Mason N et al: Cyclophosphamide exerts no beneficial effect over prednisone alone in the initial treatment of acute immune-mediated hemolytic anemia in dogs: a randomized controlled clinical trial, *J Vet Intern Med* 17:206, 2003.

Mathes M, Jordan M, Dow S: Evaluation of liposomal clodronate in a spontaneous canine model of autoimmune hemolytic anemia, *Exp Hematol*, 34:1393, 2006.

McManus PM, Craig LE: Correlation between leukocytosis and necropsy findings in dogs with immune-mediated hemolytic anemia: 34 cases (1994-1999), *J Am Vet Med Assoc* 218:1308, 2001.

Mischke VR: Haemostatic disorders as a complication of autoimmune haemolytic anemia in dogs, *Dtsch Tierartzl Wschr* 105:13, 1998.

Quigley KA et al: Application of a direct flow cytometric erythrocyte immunofluorescence assay in dogs with immune-mediated hemolytic anemia and comparison to the direct antiglobulin test, *J Vet Diagn Invest* 13:297, 2001.

Reimer ME, Troy GC, Warnick LD: Immune-mediated hemolytic anemia: 70 cases (1988-1996), *J Am Anim Hosp Assoc* 35:384, 1999.

Rentko VT, Hasndler SR, Hanson BJ: *Influence of oxygen-carrying support on survival in dogs with immune-mediated hemolytic anemia: 143 cases, (1999)*, Proceedings of the International Veterinary Emergency Critical Care Society, Orlando, 2000.

Scott-Moncrieff JC et al: Hemostatic abnormalities in dogs with primary immune-mediated hemolytic anemia, *J Am Anim Hosp Assoc* 37:220, 2001.

Thompson MF, Scott-Moncrieff C, Brooks M: Effect of a single plasma transfusion on thromboembolism in 13 dogs with primary immune-mediated hemolytic anemia, *J Am Anim Hosp Assoc* 40(6):446, 2004.

Vaden SL et al: Effects of cyclosporine versus standard care in naturally occurring glomerulonephritis in dogs, *J Vet Intern Med* 9:259, 1995.

Weinkle TR et al: Evaluation of prognostic, survival rates, and treatment protocols for immune-mediated hemolytic anemia in dogs: 151 cases (1993-2002), *J Am Vet Med Assoc* 226(11):1869, 2005.

Weiss DJ: Evaluation of dysmyelopoiesis in cats: 34 cases, *J Am Vet Med Assoc* 228:893, 2006.

White HL et al: Intravenous immunoglobulin studied as potential immune-mediated hemolytic anemia treatment, *Vet Pract News* 15(2):31, 2003.

CHAPTER 58

Nonregenerative Anemias

DOUGLAS J. WEISS, *St. Paul, Minnesota*

EVALUATION OF NONREGENERATIVE ANEMIAS

Nonregenerative anemias are caused by a broad spectrum of primary and secondary disease processes that must be differentiated before determining a prognosis or instituting a therapeutic plan. A diagnostic plan for evaluation of anemic disorders is outlined in Box 58-1. Initial evaluation should include a careful history to exclude drug or toxin exposure that may have caused the hematologic dyscrasia. In addition, immune-mediated and infectious causes of anemia should be evaluated with appropriate diagnostic testing (see Chapter 57). Mild-to-moderate nonregenerative anemias frequently occur secondary to inflammatory neoplastic, renal, hepatic, and certain endocrine disorders. Appropriate testing should be performed to detect these conditions. Once this initial evaluation has been completed, bone marrow aspiration cytology and core biopsy are indicated. The combination of bone marrow aspiration cytology and core biopsy is essential to fully evaluate both cytologic details and histopathologic alterations.

DRUG-INDUCED HEMATOLOGIC DYSCRASIAS

A growing number of drugs are associated with hematologic disorders in animals. Some drugs, most notably chemotherapeutic agents, consistently cause hematologic disorders at or near the therapeutic doses. Other drugs induce idiosyncratic hematologic dyscrasias. The most frequent types of idiosyncratic drug reactions are immune-mediated hematologic reactions and toxic injury to bone marrow. Drugs most frequently reported to induce hematologic dyscrasias include chemotherapeutic agents, estrogenic compounds (dogs), phenylbutazone, acetaminophen, aspirin, trimethoprim/sulfadiazine, phenobarbital (dogs), propylthiouracil (cats), methimazole (cats), and griseofulvin. Other drugs associated with hematologic dyscrasias include cephalosporins, carprofen, meclofenamic acid, chloramphenicol, primidone, phenytoin, metronidazole, levamisole, albendazole, fenbendazole, thiacetarsemide, amiodarone, captopril, quinidine, colchicine, and mitotane.

HEMATOLOGIC DISORDERS SECONDARY TO OTHER DISEASE PROCESSES

Inflammatory diseases are consistently accompanied by a mild-to-moderate normocytic, normochromic, nonregenerative anemia, a condition termed *anemia of inflammatory disease (AID)*. The hematocrit drops within the first few days after onset of inflammation and then stabilizes. Hematologic alterations also commonly accompany large or metastatic malignancy. Disseminated malignancy is generally accompanied by AID, although acute or chronic blood loss also may be involved. Chronic blood loss can cause an iron deficiency that further impairs erythropoiesis. Microangiopathic hemolytic anemia can result from damage to vascular endothelium or from fibrin deposition within the vessels. The hallmark of this process is the presence of schistocytes and keratocytes in the blood of affected animals. In most animals with AID or anemia of malignancy, the anemia is mild and does not require treatment. The anemia usually resolves with successful treatment of the underlying disease and usually responds to erythropoietin (EPO) therapy.

Chronic renal disease/renal failure consistently results in normocytic, normochromic, nonregenerative anemia. The anemia, although complex, is primarily the result of decreased EPO production by the kidney and is responsive to EPO replacement therapy. Alternatively some dogs and cats with late-stage renal failure develop pancytopenia associated with an aplastic bone marrow.

INFECTIOUS DISEASES

Ehrlichia and *Anaplasma* Infections

Acute monocytic and granulocytic ehrlichiosis are well-recognized disease conditions in dogs but have also been identified in cats. In dogs thrombocytopenia is the most consistent hematologic alteration. Although dogs with granulocytic ehrlichiosis readily respond to doxycycline therapy, dogs with monocytic ehrlichiosis frequently develop subclinical and chronic phases of the disease after an initial response to doxycycline. In chronic canine monocytic ehrlichiosis, pancytopenia is the result of decreased bone marrow production. In feline monocytic ehrlichiosis, nonregenerative anemia is a consistent finding, with neutropenia and thrombocytopenia present in some cats. Because some *ehrlichia*-infected cats test positive for antinuclear antibodies, feline ehrlichiosis can be confused with immune-mediated disease processes. A polymerase chain reaction test is available for detection of ehrlichiosis.

Parvovirus Infection

Parvovirus invades and destroys rapidly proliferating intestinal epithelium and bone marrow precursor cells in dog and cats. This results in diarrhea and panleukopenia. Bone marrow injury can also occur secondary to septicemia or

Diagnostic Approach to Evaluation of Nonregenerative Anemias and Multiple Cytopenias

Initial Evaluation
A. Establish the presence and severity of anemia
  1. Complete blood count
  2. Blood smear examination
  3. Reticulocyte count
B. Evaluate history for drug-induced hematologic disorders
C. Test for diseases causing secondary suppression of erythropoiesis
  1. Infectious/inflammatory diseases
  2. Neoplasia
  3. Chronic renal disease
  4. Chronic liver disease
  5. Hypothyroidism
  6. Hypoadrenocorticism
D. Test for infectious diseases
  1. *Ehrlichia*
  2. *Anaplasma phagocytophilum*
  3. *Parvovirus*
  4. Feline leukemia virus
  5. Feline immunodeficiency virus
E. Test for immune-mediated diseases
  1. Direct Coombs' test
  2. Antinuclear antibody test

Secondary Evaluation
A. Bone marrow aspirate and core biopsy
  1. Nonregenerative immune-mediated anemia
    a. Erythroid hyperplasia
    b. Maturation arrest
    c. Pure red cell aplasia
  2. Aplastic anemia
    a. Infectious (*Ehrlichia*, *Parvovirus*, feline leukemia virus)
    b. Drugs
    c. Chronic renal failure
    d. Idiopathic
  3. Myelonecrosis
  4. Myelofibrosis
  5. Inflammation
    a. Acute
    b. Pyogranulomatous
    c. Granulomatous
  6. Hemophagocytic syndrome
  7. Dysmyelopoiesis
    a. Myelodysplastic syndromes (MDS-RC, MDS-SD, MDS-EB)
    b. Secondary dysmyelopoiesis
  8. Neoplastic conditions
    a. Acute leukemia
    b. Chronic leukemia
    c. Malignant lymphoma
    d. Multiple myeloma
    e. Malignant histiocytosis

MDS-EB, MDSs with excess myeloblasts; *MDS-RC,* MDSs with refractory cytopenias; *MSD-SD,* MDSs with sideroblastic differentiation

endotoxemia. The bone marrow is characterized by severe degenerative changes in hematopoietic precursor cells, multifocal areas of necrosis, and many phagocytic macrophages. Broad-spectrum antibiotic therapy and supportive care is essential to recovery. Hematologic recovery is usually rapid if the animals survive the secondary bacterial infection.

Feline Leukemia Virus Infection

In cats infected with feline leukemia virus (FeLV), anemia and granulocytopenia frequently develop early and predispose to bacterial infections. The anemia is frequently macrocytic and nonregenerative. Either thrombocytosis with increased mean platelet volume or thrombocytopenia can be seen. Bone marrow of infected cats is characterized by granulocyte hypoplasia or by a maturation arrest at the myelocyte or metamyelocyte stage. Other hematologic dyscrasias that have been documented in FeLV-infected cats include hemolytic anemia, pure red cell aplasia (PRCA), aplastic anemia, and myelofibrosis.

Feline Immunodeficiency Virus Infection

Feline immunodeficiency virus (FIV)–infected cats have transient neutropenia and persistent lymphopenia. Thrombocytopenia is a less frequent finding. Bone marrow alterations in symptomatic cats include granulocyte and erythroid hyperplasia and dysplastic changes in erythroid and megakaryocyte cell lines. When coinfected with FeLV, FIV-infected cats are frequently anemic and leukopenic.

NONREGENERATIVE IMMUNE-MEDIATED ANEMIAS/PURE RED CELL APLASIA

Several studies indicate that a high percentage of dogs and cats with immune-mediated hemolytic anemia (IMHA) have a nonregenerative anemia when initially diagnosed. Associated bone marrow changes include erythroid hyperplasia with few polychromatophilic erythrocytes, erythroid maturation arrest, or PRCA. In addition, dysmyelopoiesis, myelofibrosis, myelonecrosis, and acute inflammation may be present. Plasma cell hyperplasia is a consistent finding in dog bone marrow, and lymphocytosis is a frequent finding in cat bone marrow.

Diagnosis of IMHA can be problematic. If the diagnosis is restricted to a positive direct Coombs' test or autoagglutination (or spherocytosis in dogs), some cases of IMHA will be missed. Therefore IMHA sometimes becomes a diagnosis of exclusion. Differential diagnosis in cats includes FeLV and FIV infections, feline infectious peritonitis, feline infectious anemia, hemolytic drugs/toxins, and myelodysplastic syndromes. In dogs ehrlichiosis, babesiosis, leishmaniasis, and hemolytic drugs/toxins should be excluded. Immune-mediated hemolytic anemia also can develop as a secondary condition. Associated disorders include lymphoma, a variety of drug treatments and vaccinations, ehrlichiosis, and bee stings.

PRCA is defined as the presence of a severe nonregenerative, normocytic, normochromic anemia and a marked erythroid hypoplasia in bone marrow. Total leukocyte and platelet counts are within or above reference intervals. It occurs in both dogs and cats and is thought to result from an immune response that attacks early erythroid precursor cells in the bone marrow. However, in cats PRCA also can be caused by FeLV subgroup C infection. Although affected dogs tend to be middle aged, cats tend to be younger. In cats the percentage of lymphocytes in bone marrow is invariably increased, and a slight lymphocytosis may be present in the blood.

The approach to treatment of nonregenerative IMHA and PRCA is similar to that of regenerative IMHA, and in my experience the response rate is similar. Prednisone (2.2-4.4 mg/kg q24h orally [PO] as a single or divided dose) has been the mainstay in treatment of IMHA. Because of the high rate of thromboembolism and evidence of circulating activated platelets in dogs, ultralow-dose aspirin (0.5 mg/kg q24h PO) is recommended for all patients. Concurrent azathioprine therapy (2 mg/kg q24h PO tapering to 0.5 to 1 mg/kg q48h) has resulted in improved survival times (see Chapters 19 and 20).

APLASTIC ANEMIA

Aplastic anemia is defined as the presence of a bicytopenia or pancytopenia in the blood and a marrow in which more than 95% of the hematopoietic space is occupied by adipose tissue. Causes of aplastic anemia in dogs include infectious agents (*Ehrlichia canis*, *Parvovirus*) drug toxicities (estrogen, phenylbutazone, trimethoprim-sulfadiazine, quinidine, chemotherapeutic agents, thiacetarsemide, albendazole, captopril, griseofulvin), ionizing radiation, and idiopathic causes. Dogs with idiopathic aplastic anemia are usually less than 3 years old. The anemia is moderate to severe, and neutropenia and thrombocytopenia are usually severe. Although the prognosis for idiopathic aplastic anemia is guarded to poor, some dogs do recover with supportive care. No specific therapy short of bone marrow transplantation is available at this time.

Disease conditions associated with aplastic anemia in cats include chronic renal failure, FeLV infection, and methimazole and griseofulvin toxicities. Idiopathic aplastic anemia also occurs in cats. In some cats starvation may play a role in the development of marrow aplasia.

MYELONECROSIS

Myelonecrosis in the dog consists of focal or multifocal areas of coagulative necrosis or individual cell necrosis. In cats individual cell necrosis is seen, but coagulative necrosis is rarely seen. Chronic necrosis is frequently accompanied by variable degrees of myelofibrosis. Associated disease conditions in dogs include sepsis, lymphoma, IMHA, and systemic lupus erythematosus. Drug treatments associated with bone marrow necrosis include phenobarbital, carprofen, metronidazole, mitotane, cyclophosphamide, vincristine, colchicine, and fenbendazole. Although there is no specific treatment for canine myelonecrosis, the prognosis appears to be quite good, with complete hematologic recovery seen in most cases. Diseases associated with myelonecrosis in cats include nonregenerative IMHA, FeLV infection, myelodysplastic syndromes, and acute leukemia. The prognosis for myelonecrosis in cats depends on the associated disease process.

SECONDARY MYELOFIBROSIS

Myelofibrosis is defined as proliferation of fibroblasts, collagen, or reticulin fibers in bone marrow. Myelofibrosis (i.e., secondary myelofibrosis) occurs most frequently secondary to bone marrow injury. Therefore it is a frequent sequela of myelonecrosis. Myelofibrosis also occurs as a rare chronic myeloproliferative condition termed *idiopathic myelofibrosis*. In dogs secondary myelofibrosis is associated with IMHA; neoplasia; and drug treatments, including phenobarbital, phenytoin, phenylbutazone, and colchicine. Diseases associated with secondary myelofibrosis in cats include IMHA, myelodysplastic syndromes, acute myelogenous leukemia and chronic renal failure. The most frequent hematologic finding in both dogs and cats is moderate-to-severe nonregenerative anemia, with relatively few animals being neutropenic or thrombocytopenic. Other frequent blood findings in dogs included ovalocytosis, dacryocytosis, and metarubricytosis. No specific treatment for myelofibrosis is available. Although the prognosis for secondary myelofibrosis is guarded, approximately half of affected dogs recover.

INFLAMMATION

Acute, pyogranulomatous, and granulomatous inflammation has been documented in bone marrow. Acute inflammatory lesions have been associated with nonregenerative IMHA, bacterial sepsis, and feline infectious peritonitis. Some affected dogs have a history of acute onset of lameness or bone pain. Neutrophilia, left shift, and toxic change may be seen in the blood. Bone marrow core biopsies are characterized by dilation of sinusoids, fibrin deposits, multifocal accumulations of neutrophils, and necrosis. Affected dogs and cats tend to have moderate-to-severe anemia. Pyogranulomatous inflammation has been observed in dogs and cats with disseminated histoplasmosis, and anemia may be quite prominent in some animals. Granulomatous inflammation has been seen in dogs with systemic fungal infections. Approach to treatment of inflammatory bone marrow disorders is based on treatment of the associated disease condition.

HEMOPHAGOCYTIC SYNDROME

Hemophagocytic syndrome is a benign proliferative disorder of macrophages and must be differentiated from a malignant proliferation of histiocytes (i.e., malignant histiocytosis). Criteria for diagnosis of hemophagocytic syndrome include the presence of bicytopenia or pancytopenia in the blood and greater than 2% hemophagocytic macrophages in bone marrow. Cases that have concurrent myelonecrosis, myelofibrosis, or marrow inflammation should be excluded because the hemophagocytic macrophages are probably the result of these conditions and not a primary disorder. Disease conditions associated with hemophagocytic syndrome in dogs include IMHA, systemic lupus erythematosus, sepsis, *E. canis* infection, blastomycosis, lymphoma, and myelodysplastic syndromes. Approximately 20% of canine cases are idiopathic. These cases are characterized by acute onset of weakness, lethargy, fever, and splenomegaly.

Survival appears to depend on the associated disease condition. Records from the University of Minnesota Veterinary Medical Center indicate that nine of nine dogs with immune-associated hemophagocytic syndrome died within 1 month, whereas four of five dogs with infection-associated hemophagocytic syndrome survived. Therapy of hemophagocytic syndrome should be directed at treating associated disease conditions and administering immunosuppressive doses of prednisone (2.2 to 4.4 mg/kg q24h PO as a single or divided dose) to suppress macrophage activity.

DYSMYELOPOIESIS

Dysmyelopoiesis is defined as a hematologic disorder characterized by the presence of morphologic abnormalities (i.e., dysplasia) in one or more hematologic cell line in the blood or bone marrow. Dysmyelopoiesis has been classified in several ways but has most recently been divided into myelodysplastic syndromes (MDSs), secondary dysmyelopoiesis, and congenital dysmyelopoiesis.

Myelodysplastic Syndromes

MDSs are acquired clonal proliferative disorders that are thought to result from a genetic mutation in hematopoietic stem cells. Differentiating an MDS from acute leukemia is based on the percentage of myeloblasts in the bone marrow. Historically leukemias were defined as more than 30% myeloblasts, and MDS as fewer than 30% myeloblasts. More recently some pathologists prefer to use 20% as the cutoff. Myelodysplastic syndromes have been divided into two major categories: MDS with refractory cytopenias (MDS-RC) and MDS with excess myeloblasts (MDS-EB); and one minor category, MDS with sideroblastic differentiation (MSD-SD). In both dogs and cats MDS-RC and MDS-EB are differentiated based on the percentage of myeloblasts in the bone marrow. MDS-RC has less than 6% myeloblasts, whereas MDS-EB has 6% to 30% myeloblasts.

Hematologic alterations in dogs with MDS-RC consist of moderate-to-severe normocytic, normochromic, nonregenerative anemia. Dysplastic features in bone marrow are usually restricted to the erythroid series. Alternatively cats with MDS-RC have a macrocytic normochromic anemia, and many are pancytopenic. The presence of metarubricytosis and autoagglutination is a frequent finding in blood smears of cat, making it easy to confuse MDS-RC with IMHA. Unlike dogs, dysplasia is seen frequently in all cells lines in the bone marrow of cats. Both dogs and cats with MDS-RC tend to be less severely ill when initially evaluated, tend to have substantially better response to supportive therapy, and have much longer survival times when compared to MDS-EB. The anemia in dogs with MDS-RC is frequently responsive to EPO therapy (50 to 2000 units/kg subcutaneously three times/week).

Dogs and cats with MDS-EB have bicytopenia or pancytopenia. Bone marrow has dysplastic features in all cell lines, and 6% to 30% myeloblasts are present. Survival for both dogs and cats is short. Treatment is mostly supportive. EPO and other hematopoietic growth factors have been used, but they do not appear to prolong survival. Chemotherapeutic agents, including hydroxyurea, low-dose cytosine arabinoside, and low-dose aclarubicin have been tried with limited success.

MDS-SD is seen infrequently in dogs and cats. It is characterized by a microcytic or hypochromic nonregenerative anemia with siderocytes or sideroblasts in the blood and ringed sideroblasts in bone marrow. Because of the microcytic and hypochromic nature of the anemia, MDS-SD can be confused with chronic iron deficiency anemia.

Secondary Dysmyelopoiesis

Secondary dysmyelopoiesis is associated with a variety of hematologic disorders and drug treatments. Secondary dysmyelopoiesis in dogs has been associated with IMHA, immune-mediated thrombocytopenia, lymphoma, myelofibrosis, and multiple myeloma. Drugs that have been associated with dysmyelopoiesis in dogs include chemotherapeutic agents, estrogen, cephalosporins, chloramphenicol, phenobarbital, and colchicine. Secondary dysmyelopoiesis in cats has been associated with IMHA, immune-mediated thrombocytopenia, lymphoma, and chemotherapy. Cytologic features of MDS and secondary dyserythropoiesis are difficult to differentiate. Features that can be used to differentiate the two disorders include the presence of increased numbers of myeloblasts or rubriblasts in bone marrow in most animals with MDS and the presence of associated disease conditions in secondary dysmyelopoiesis.

BONE MARROW NEOPLASIA

Leukemia

Most dogs and cats with acute and chronic leukemias have a nonregenerative anemia at the time of diagnosis, and some are thrombocytopenic. If leukemic cells extensively displace normal hematopoietic cells in the bone marrow (myelophthisis), pancytopenia can develop. Approximately half of the acute leukemias diagnosed at the University of Minnesota are "aleukemic" (e.g., do not have circulating atypical cells); therefore bone marrow evaluation is critical to establish a diagnosis. Alternatively chronic leukemias usually have moderate-to-marked leukocytosis at the time of diagnosis.

Lymphoma

Unlike in cats, lymphoma is the most frequently diagnosed neoplastic condition in canine bone marrow. Disseminated lymphoma must be differentiated from acute lymphoblastic leukemia. This distinction is based on identification of lymphoblasts in multiple lymph nodes or organs, relatively low numbers of lymphoblasts in the blood, and lack of severe cytopenias. The most consistent hematologic finding in disseminated lymphosarcoma is a mild-to-moderate nonregenerative anemia (see Chapter 72).

Multiple Myeloma

Multiple myeloma is the second most frequently diagnosed neoplastic condition in the bone marrow of dogs and cats. Diagnosis of multiple myeloma depends on finding large numbers of atypical plasma cells in bone marrow with or without the presence of hypercalcemia, osteolytic lesions, a monoclonal gammopathy, or light-chain proteinuria. Features most helpful in differentiating malignant plasma cells from reactive plasma cell hyperplasia include anisocytosis, anisokaryosis, high nuclear-to-cytoplasmic ratio, binucleation, and clustering of plasma cells. These anaplastic features are important in differentiating multiple myeloma from plasma cell hyperplasia associated with immune-mediated diseases, ehrlichiosis, and feline infectious peritonitis infection. Dogs and cats with multiple myeloma frequently have a nonregenerative anemia and may be concurrently thrombocytopenic or neutropenic.

Malignant Histiocytosis

Malignant histiocytosis (MH) appears to occur relatively frequently in dogs with distinct breed predilections, but is diagnosed infrequently in cats. Organs frequently involved include the liver, spleen, lungs, and bone marrow. Affected dogs can have multiple cytopenias, whereas cats may only be anemic. Both dogs ands cats have large numbers of histiocytic cells in bone marrow, but features of malignancy are variable. Features of MH that are useful in differentiating it from hemophagocytic syndrome include greater than 30% histiocytic cells in bone marrow, high nuclear-to-cytoplasmic ratio, and multinuclearity. In addition, MH is rarely confined to the bone marrow. At present disease progression is usually rapid, and disease outcome is invariably fatal (see Chapter 75).

Suggested Reading

Harvey JW: Canine bone marrow, normal hematopoiesis, biopsy techniques, and cell identification and evaluation, *Compend Contin Educ Pract Vet* 6:909, 1984.

Kohn B et al: Primary immune-mediated hemolytic anemia in 19 cats: diagnosis, therapy, and outcome (1998-2004), *J Vet Intern Med* 20:159, 2006.

Rentko VT, Cotter SM: Feline anemia: the classifications, causes, and diagnostic procedures, *Vet Med* 85:584, 1990.

Stokol T, Blue JT: Pure red cell aplasia in cats: 9 cases (1987-1997), *J Am Vet Med Assoc* 214:75, 1999.

Stokol T, Blue JT, French TW: Idiopathic pure red cell aplasia and nonregenerative immune-mediated anemia in dogs: 43 cases (1988-1999), *J Am Vet Med Assoc* 216:1429, 2000.

Weiss DJ: Recognition and classification of dysmyelopoiesis in the dog: a review, *J Vet Intern Med* 19:147, 2005.

Weiss DJ: A retrospective study of the incidence and classification of bone marrow disorders in cats (1996-2004), *Comp Clin Pathol* 14:179, 2006.

von Willebrand's Disease and Other Hereditary Coagulopathies

ANTHONY P. CARR, *Saskatoon, Saskatchewan, Canada*
BELLE M. NIBBLETT, *Saskatoon, Saskatchewan, Canada*
DAVID L. PANCIERA, *Blacksburg, Virginia*

A number of bleeding disorders demonstrate a genetic basis. The inheritance patterns of hereditary bleeding disorders have been a focus of much attention, but in many instances the genetic basis in dogs and cats is still unknown. However, a variety of genetic tests have recently become available, and these assessments promise to increase accuracy of diagnosis and also reduce the frequency of some of hereditary bleeding disorders. Genetic testing is especially attractive since it often can determine if a dog is affected, a carrier, or free of the offending gene. In contrast, when factor assays are used to determine disease status, the distinction between carrier and free individuals is often difficult. However, even genetic testing will be unable to diagnose all canine and feline bleeding disorders since new mutations can arise. In some cases different mutations are responsible for the same bleeding disorder. Thrombocytopenia, disseminated intravascular coagulation, and platelet function disorders are also discussed in the following three chapters.

VON WILLEBRAND'S DISEASE

von Willebrand's disease (vWD) is the most common inherited bleeding disorder in dogs. It is caused by a lack of von Willebrand's factor (vWF). vWF is an adhesive glycoprotein that is produced by endothelial cells and megakaryocytes. Unlike platelets in other species, canine platelets do not contain large amounts of vWF in their α-granules. Extracellular vWF is found in the subendothelium and circulating in plasma in multimeric form. The multimers vary in size from 0.5 to 20 million daltons (D), with the larger multimers being more hemostatically active. The multimers are composed of identical 270,000-D subunits joined by disulfide bonds.

The predominant function of vWF is to promote the adhesion of platelets to exposed subendothelium, especially in areas of high shear stress. vWF is produced by the endothelium, with 95% secreted constitutively and the other 5% stored in Weibel-Palade bodies (as well as a small amount in platelets). The predominant function of vWF is to promote the adhesion of platelets to exposed subendothelium via binding to the glycoprotein (GP)Ib α-receptor on platelets. This is especially vital in areas of high shear stress such as arteries. vWF also plays a role in platelet-to-platelet aggregation in conjunction with the GPIIb/IIIa complex (integrin αIIbβ3) and fibrinogen. The other major function of vWF is to form a tightly bound complex with factor VIII, thereby prolonging the half-life of factor VIII, although this is of lesser importance in dogs.

Three types of vWD occur in dogs. In type I vWD all multimers are present but in considerably reduced quantity. This form of vWD is most common. It has been identified in more than 50 breeds of dogs. Breeds associated with type I vWD and a hemorrhagic tendency include the Doberman pinscher, standard poodle, Shetland sheepdog, and German shepherd. The hemorrhagic tendency, although variable, often manifests as increased bleeding associated with surgical procedures or after trauma. Spontaneous mucosal bleeding (epistaxis, urogenital bleeding) can be seen occasionally. Other stressors that suppress hemostasis, such as the transient thrombocytopenia noted to occur after vaccination with a modified-live vaccine or the administration of nonsteroidal antiinflammatory agents that inhibit platelet activity can precipitate bleeding. In severely affected animals spontaneous hemorrhage may be seen and can be protracted. In some dogs decreased vWF has been documented, but a bleeding tendency does not seem to exist. Type I vWD probably represents a heterogeneous group of diseases with marked breed variation. In type II vWD the larger, more effective multimers are absent, and bleeding can be severe. This form of the disease has been identified in German shorthaired and German wirehaired pointers. The most severe form of vWD is type III, in which all multimers are absent. This form of the disease is associated with life-threatening hemorrhagic episodes. It has been reported to occur in Scottish terriers, Chesapeake Bay retrievers, Dutch kooikers, and Shetland sheepdogs.

The mode of inheritance of vWD remains largely unknown, although some of the mutations leading to the disease are recognized. Type I vWD can occur through a large number of defects that typically involve a substitution or deletion of a single nucleotide, resulting in abnormal splicing or a frame shift. This mutation can be autosomal recessive or autosomal dominant, possibly depending on the amount of incorrect splicing that occurs. Males and females are equally affected. Expression of type I vWD is complex in Doberman pinchers and may or may not be related to homozygosity or heterozygosity of the mutation, but it is not explained by a simple autosomal-recessive inheritance pattern (Brooks, Erb, and Foureman, 2001). It has been proposed that the disease in Doberman pinschers may be produced by a single gene defect (Moser, Meyers, and Russon, 1996), with each allele being responsible for 50% of the vWF level the dog has. A defective allele would result in less than 15% of normal vWF production. The mutation leading to type II vWD is unknown. Inheritance of type III vWD is autosomal recessive and results when the mutation results in a severe change in the intended protein. Variable expression of vWD is related to heterozygosity, inheritance of dominant negative mutations, and other inherited and noninherited extragenic influences (i.e., posttranslational modification) and physiologic factors.

Diagnostic Testing

Determination of vWF levels still remains central to diagnosis of vWD; although, with the sequencing of the canine vWF gene, the underlying genetic abnormalities associated with vWD have been determined for certain breeds of dogs. The validity of many of these assays has not yet been published, and test results should not be interpreted without vWF levels. The deoxyribonucleic acid analysis has the advantage of allowing improved detection of carriers. However, without simultaneously measuring vWF there is risk of false negatives as the individual may have a different mutation leading to vWD than the one that is currently being tested. An individual may have a unique mutation, or there may be multiple mutations leading to disease in certain breeds.

When vWF is analyzed, the patient's vWF is reported as a percentage of a control canine pool. The pool is considered to represent 100%, often expressed as 100 units. Blood for analysis should be anticoagulated with citrate at a 9:1 ratio of blood to anticoagulant or with 15% ethylenediaminetetraacetic acid at a ratio of 1:100. Hemolyzed samples are not to be used since hemolysis causes a significant decrease in vWF levels (Moser et al., 1996). The blood is centrifuged immediately and is then frozen for storage before analysis. The sample should be shipped frozen on dry ice to prevent thawing. In the process of thawing, some proteolysis may occur. This breakdown of protein would tend to elevate vWF artificially when an antigenic assay is used because breaking up large multimers into smaller subunits exposes more antigenic sites (Stokol and Parry, 1995).

Testing of vWF is usually by means of an enzyme-linked immunosorbent assay (ELISA) with the concentration expressed as vWF:antigen (Ag). Using an ELISA, workers at the Comparative Hematology Laboratory at Cornell University established the following ranges: normal range, 70% to 180% vWF:Ag; borderline range, 50% to 69% vWF:Ag; abnormal range, 0% to 49% vWF:Ag (Brooks, 1992). These assays do not determine biologic activity or multimeric distribution. When this system is used, dogs in the normal range are considered free from vWD and are unlikely to transmit the disease. Dogs in the abnormal range are diagnosed as carriers of vWD and can transmit

the trait to offspring. Results can be ambiguous, and dogs in the borderline range cannot be classified definitively. Daily variation in vWF:Ag concentration can be high; thus multiple measurements may be necessary to establish the von Willebrand status of a dog. In cases in which vWF is in the normal range but unexplained bleeding is occurring, electrophoresis can be useful to diagnose type II vWD.

Multimeric distribution can be determined with the use of electrophoresis. This modality is of value in that the larger multimers are thought to be more hemostatically active. It is also possible to measure functional capacity of vWF using vWF collagen-binding activity. Bleeding times can be measured in patients to determine whether a defect of primary hemostasis is present. Both the cuticle bleeding time (CBT; duration of hemorrhage from a toenail that is cut short enough to bleed) and the buccal mucosal bleeding time (BMBT) are prolonged in vWD. The BMBT is the preferred test since the CBT is also prolonged in coagulopathies such as hemophilia A and B. The BMBT is measured by determining the duration of hemorrhage from small standardized cuts in the upper lip (Johnson, Turrentine, and Kraus, 1988). Normal dogs have a BMBT of less than 4 minutes. When one evaluates BMBT results, it is important to remember that BMBT is a global test of primary hemostasis. Not only vWD, but also thrombocytopenia, platelet function defects, and vasculitis result in a prolonged BMBT. The accuracy of BMBT is limited by the finding of up to a 2-minute interobserver and intraobserver variability in test results (Sato, Anderson, and Parry, 2000).

Physiologic Factors Affecting vWF:Ag

A variety of factors are known to affect measured vWF:Ag levels. Within individuals, levels can vary substantially over time, making classification into affected, carrier, or disease-free categories very difficult if based on a single sample. When blood is drawn from a cephalic vein, vWF:Ag levels are greater than when it is drawn from a jugular vein. Strenuous exercise, epinephrine, and pregnancy raise vWF levels (Moser et al., 1996). The effect of thyroid status has been debated; however, studies show no association between hypothyroidism and acquired vWD (Panciera and Johnson, 1996). It also has been shown that thyroid hormone supplementation to euthyroid Dobermans with vWD does not increase vWF concentration or activity (Heseltine, Panciera, and Troy, 2005). Blood type remains to be investigated but is known to have an effect in human vWD.

Therapy

The mode of therapy used to treat vWD depends on the presenting situation, although blood products generally are indicated in cases of ongoing or anticipated hemorrhage. If anemia is not present or mild, the use of fresh plasma, fresh-frozen plasma, or cryoprecipitate (CP) is recommended. CP is especially valuable since the clinician can give larger quantities of vWF without having to be concerned about volume overload. Administration of CP significantly increases vWF levels within 30 minutes of administration in Doberman pinschers with type I vWD, an effect that remains apparent for at least 4 hours (Ching et al., 1994). Similarly the BMBT was rapidly improved, but by 4 hours it was at the same level as before treatment. In animals given fresh plasma the vWF level increased in a manner similar to that of patients given CP, but no improvement in BMBT occurred. The significance of this observation is unclear since clinical experience suggests that fresh plasma is effective in the treatment of vWD. Human recombinant vWF has been used experimentally in dogs with minimal effect and no change in observed bleeding times (Turecek et al., 1997).

Desmopressin acetate can also be useful in the treatment of vWD, especially in situations in which therapy is initiated to prevent or control hemorrhage in association with surgery. Desmopressin is used extensively in humans with vWD and appears to have a variety of effects that promote hemostasis, including the release of stored vWF from endothelial cells. In many dogs with vWD the increase in vWF is slight, although the BMBT decreases (Kraus et al., 1989). The onset of activity occurs in 30 minutes, and the duration of effect is approximately 2 hours. Since desmopressin releases stored vWF, repeating the injection has significantly less effect than the initial treatment. Desmopressin can be given to donor dogs to maximize vWF levels before phlebotomy. Although an intravenous product is available, its cost has led to the successful use of an intranasal product given subcutaneously at 1 to 4mcg/kg.

HEMOPHILIA A

Hemophilia A is the most common inherited coagulation factor deficiency in dogs and is an X-linked recessive disease caused by factor VIII deficiency. Generally the female is the carrier, and only males express signs of the disease. However, a mating between a carrier female and an affected male would result in affected females. The disease has been diagnosed in more than 40 breeds and also in mixed-breed dogs. A higher prevalence is observed in German shepherd dogs. The clinical manifestations vary, depending on the degree of deficiency. As with most coagulopathies, body cavity hemorrhages (abdomen, thorax, and joints) and extensive bruising are the most common manifestations. In severely affected individuals death at birth can result from umbilical cord hemorrhage. In others the first clinical manifestations may be evident during teething. Since factor VIII is involved in the intrinsic coagulation pathway, prolongations of activated clotting time (ACT) and activated partial thromboplastin time (APTT) are seen. The diagnosis is verified by specific factor analysis. Factor VIII activity varies from 0% to 25% in affected animals, with disease being classified as mild (>5% factor activity), moderate (1% to 5% factor activity), and severe (<1% factor activity). Therapy for hemophilia A consists of administration of blood products. If red blood cells are needed because of anemia, whole blood can be given. Fresh-frozen plasma or CP is preferred if anemia is not present.

HEMOPHILIA B

Hemophilia B (Christmas disease) results from factor IX deficiency. The disease has an X–linked recessive mode of inheritance and has been identified in 19 breeds and mixed-breed dogs. Factor IX is a vitamin K–dependent protein produced in the liver. The clinical signs of hemophilia B mimic those encountered with hemophilia A.

The clinical manifestations vary in severity from mild to fatal hemorrhages. Unlike dogs with hemophilia A, dogs with factor IX deficiency invariably have less than 1% of normal factor activity detected. Both ACT and APTT are prolonged in dogs with this disease because factor IX is a part of the intrinsic coagulation pathway. The final diagnosis depends on specific factor analysis.

Therapy for factor IX deficiency consists of the administration of blood products. Fresh-frozen plasma or cryosupernatant is indicated when anemia is not marked. Factor IX is also found in serum, so it could also be given. Gene therapy with a liver-directed adenoviral vector holds promise.

Genetic Basis of Hemophilia A and B

The molecular basis of hemophilia A is not described. There have been five mutations described so far that result in hemophilia B. The genes coding for factors VIII and IX are highly mutable, allowing for a large number of mutations. Hemophilia frequently can result from spontaneous or new mutations.

Other Less Common Hereditary Coagulopathies

A variety of other coagulopathies have been identified in dogs (Fogh and Fogh, 1988). In some the only clinical manifestation is an alteration of routine hemostatic tests without an associated bleeding tendency. Definitive diagnosis requires testing by reference laboratories involved in research on coagulation disorders in animals. Hypofibrinogenemia (factor I deficiency) has been identified in Saint Bernard dogs associated with a prolongation of one-step prothrombin time (OSPT; extrinsic pathway of coagulation) and marked bleeding diathesis in severely affected animals. An autosomal-recessive factor II (prothrombin) deficiency has been identified in a family of boxer dogs with prolongation of OSPT. Bleeding was severe in some pups but was generally mild in adults. Factor VII deficiency has been identified as an autosomal-dominant disease in beagle dogs. Bleeding is rarely reported, although OSPT values are prolonged. In cocker spaniels factor X deficiency has been reported as an autosomal-dominant trait with a variable expression of the hemorrhagic tendency. Both APTT and OSPT are prolonged in this disease. Severely affected animals generally do not survive. Factor XI deficiency has been seen in Kerry blue terriers, Great Pyrenees, and English springer spaniels as an autosomal-recessive trait. The disease manifests as a prolongation of APTT and a variable bleeding tendency. Factor XII (Hageman factor) deficiency has been identified in miniature poodles but is much more commonly identified in cats. Deficiency of this factor causes a prolongation of APTT, but it is not associated with a bleeding tendency. Prekallikrein deficiency has been seen in a variety of breeds. It causes a prolongation of APTT, apparently without an associated tendency toward hemorrhage.

BLOOD PRODUCTS FOR COAGULOPATHY

Whole Blood

In cases in which anemia is a significant problem, fresh whole blood (less than 6 hours since collection) is the product of choice. Factor VIII, vWF, and factor V are inactive when blood has been stored, but the vitamin K–dependent factors (factor II, VII, IX, and X) retain their activity. Canine donors should be negative for canine red cell antigens DEA 1.1, 1.2, and 7 (see Chapter 56). The volume of transfusion depends on the severity of the anemia, but a general guide is 12 to 24 ml/kg, which would be expected to raise the packed cell volume by 5% to 10%. The major drawback in treating a coagulopathy with blood is the volume overload that can occur, even though the quantity of coagulation factors given is small. Blood products containing red blood cells should be reserved for animals with significant anemia because transfusion can lead to sensitization to red cell antigens. Such sensitization could preclude safe administration of red cells at a later date, when they may be vitally needed. Local control of hemorrhage with bandages, pressure, and topical adhesives should always be used maximally to minimize need for transfusion therapy.

Fresh and Fresh-Frozen Plasma

Plasma harvested from whole blood within 6 hours of collection is termed *fresh plasma*. If this plasma is transfused within the 6-hour time frame, all vital coagulation protein activity is retained. Rapid separation from whole blood preserves the activity of factors V and VIII and vWF. Fresh plasma also contains albumin, complement proteins, antithrombin III, and immunoglobulins. Plasma frozen within 6 hours of the blood collection is termed *fresh-frozen plasma* and can be stored frozen (preferably at –70° C) and retain its coagulation activity for as long as 1 year. Usually 6 to 10 ml/kg is transfused, and this amount can be administered every 8 hours as needed. Volume overload is a consideration with plasma administration, especially when an animal is severely affected with vWD and needs multiple transfusions.

Stored or Frozen Plasma

Stored plasma results when plasma is separated from red blood cells more than 6 hours after collection. When frozen, this plasma is termed *frozen plasma*. It is deficient in factors V and VIII and vWF activity but does have the other coagulation factors present (including factor IX). It is generally not used in the treatment of coagulopathies.

Cryoprecipitate

When fresh-frozen plasma is slowly thawed (at 4°C), a precipitate is formed, called *CP*. Most of the factor VIII, fibrinogen, and vWF in the plasma is contained in the CP. It generally is only one tenth of the volume of the original plasma. The remainder of the plasma is called cryo-free plasma or cryosupernatant. Cryosupernatant still contains most of the other active coagulation factors and plasma proteins. CP and cryosupernatant can be frozen again and stored for as long as 1 year. The reported

concentration of vWF in CP varies from approximately four times that in the original plasma (Stokol and Parry, 1995) to twenty times the original (Ching et al., 1994). The larger multimers appear to preferentially precipitate (Ching et al., 1994). A dose of 1 unit of CP (CP produced from 150 ml of plasma) per 10 kilograms of body weight has been recommended. CP can be obtained from commercial animal blood banks.

References and Suggested Reading

Brooks M: Management of canine von Willebrand's disease, *Probl Vet Med* 4:636, 1992.

Brooks M, Barnas J, Fremont J: Cosegregation of factor VIII microsatellite marker with mild hemophilia A in golden retriever dogs, *J Vet Intern Med* 19:205 2005.

Brooks M, Erb J, Foureman P: von Willebrand disease phenotype and von Willebrand factor marker genotype in Doberman pinchers, *Am J Vet Res* 62:364, 2001.

Brooks M, Raymond S, Catalfamo J: Severe, recessive von Willebrand's disease in German wirehaired pointers, *J Am Vet Med Assoc* 209:926, 1996.

Callan M, Giger U, Catalfamo J: Effect of desmopressin on von Willebrand factor multimers in Doberman pinchers with type I von Willebrand disease, *Am J Vet Res* 66:861, 2005.

Ching YN et al: Effect of cryoprecipitate and plasma on plasma von Willebrand factor multimers and bleeding time in Doberman pinchers with type-I von Willebrand's disease, *Am J Vet Res* 55:102, 1994.

Fogh JM, Fogh IT: Inherited coagulation disorders, *Vet Clin North Am Small Anim Pract* 18:231, 1988.

Heseltine J, Panciera D, Troy G: Effect of levothyroxine administration on hemostatic analytes in doberman pinchers with von Willebrand disease, *J Vet Intern Med* 19:523, 2005.

Johnson GS, Turrentine MA, Kraus KH: Canine von Willebrand's disease: A heterogeneous group of bleeding disorders, *Vet Clin North Am Small Anim Pract* 18:195, 1988.

Kraus KH et al: Effect of desmopressin acetate on bleeding times and plasma von Willebrand factor in Doberman Pinscher dogs with von Willebrand's disease, *Vet Surg* 18:103, 1989.

Moser J, Meyers KM, Russon RH: Inheritance of von Willebrand factor deficiency in Doberman pinschers, *J Am Vet Med Assoc* 209:1103, 1996.

Moser J et al: Temporal variation and factors affecting measurement of canine von Willebrand factor, *Am J Vet Res* 57:1288, 1996.

Panciera DL, Johnson GS: Plasma von Willebrand factor antigen concentration and buccal mucosal bleeding time in dogs with experimental hypothyroidism, *J Vet Intern Med* 10:60, 1996.

Sato I, Anderson GA, Parry BW: An interobserver and intraobserver study of buccal mucosal bleeding time in greyhounds, *Res Vet Sci* 68:41, 2000.

Stokol T, Parry BW: Stability of von Willebrand factor and factor VIII in canine cryoprecipitate under various conditions of storage, *Res Vet Sci* 59:152, 1995.

Turecek PL et al: In vivo characterization of recombinant von Willebrand factor in dogs with von Willebrand disease, *Blood* 90:3555, 1997.

van Oost B, Versteeg S, Slappendel R: DNA testing for type III von Willebrand disease in Dutch kooiker dogs, *J Vet Intern Med* 18:282, 2004.

Venta P, Li J, Yuzbasiyan-Gurkan V: Mutation causing von Willebrand's disease in Scottish terriers, *J Vet Intern Med* 14:10, 2000.

CHAPTER 60

Thrombocytopenia

JENNIFER A. NEEL, *Raleigh, North Carolina*
ADAM J. BIRKENHEUER, *Raleigh, North Carolina*
CAROL B. GRINDEM, *Raleigh, North Carolina*

Thrombocytopenia is the most common platelet disorder observed in dogs and cats. At our institution thrombocytopenia was found in approximately 5% of dogs presenting from 1996 to 2006 and 3.6% of cats presenting from 2004 to 2006. Previous studies at this university have shown that in dogs the etiology of thrombocytopenia is 5% primary immune mediated, 13% neoplasia, 23% infectious or inflammatory disease, and 59% miscellaneous or multifactoral causes (Grindem et al., 1991). In cats causes of thrombocytopenia included 2% primary immune mediated, 20% neoplasia, 29% infectious diseases, 7% cardiac diseases, 22% multiple etiologies, and 20% unknown causes (Jordan, Grindem, and Breitschwerdt, 1993).

Pseudothrombocytopenia occurs when platelets present in a specimen are not counted. This must be eliminated as the cause of a low platelet count. Platelet aggregation caused by activation during blood sampling is a major cause of falsely decreased counts and occurs commonly in cats; one study found low automated platelet counts in 71% of feline samples (Norman et al., 2001). Large platelets are also a cause of low platelet counts on some automated hematology analyzers when the size of the platelets overlaps with the size of red blood cells (RBCs). Ethylenediaminetetraacetic acid (EDTA)–induced platelet clumping has rarely been reported. Some breeds such as cavalier King Charles spaniels and greyhounds normally have lower platelet counts than most dogs or established platelet reference intervals.

MECHANISMS OF THROMBOCYTOPENIA

Thrombocytopenia occurs by one of four general mechanisms: decreased production, increased consumption/destruction, sequestration, and excessive loss. Often more than one mechanism occurs in any single disease or disorder. Decreased production is seen with suppression or destruction of megakaryocytes caused by immune-mediated disease, drugs, infectious agents, whole body irradiation, and myelophthisic disorders. Increased consumption or destruction is a common cause of thrombocytopenia in dogs and cats; etiologies include primary or secondary immune-mediated disease, drugs, disseminated intravascular coagulation (DIC) (vascular damage, septicemia, endotoxemia, massive tissue necrosis/damage, or release of procoagulant substances), disseminated neoplasia, and infectious diseases. Thrombocytopenia resulting from sequestration or abnormal distribution of platelets can be caused by splenic congestion/splenomegaly, hepatomegaly, neoplasia, severe hypothermia in dogs, and experimentally induced endotoxemia. Marked thrombocytopenia is not typically noted, and the effect is often transient. Excessive loss can occur with massive blood loss and is observed in some cases of hemorrhage associated with rodenticide toxicity, but often platelet counts are normal to increased in these patients. This article focuses on causes and treatment of immune-mediated and infectious thrombocytopenia.

IMMUNE-MEDIATED THROMBOCYTOPENIA

Immune-mediated thrombocytopenia (IMTP) can be primary, secondary, vaccine induced, or posttransfusion. *Primary, or idiopathic, IMTP* is reported most commonly in dogs but has also been reported in cats. This is a disease of exclusion; other potential causes of secondary IMTP must be eliminated before a diagnosis of primary IMTP can be made. Acquired amegakaryocytic thrombocytopenia is a rare form of immune-mediated disease resulting from autoantibodies directed towards megakaryocytes. In a case series of four dogs, two had no evidence of concurrent disease (presumed idiopathic IMTP), and two had evidence of infectious disease (presumed secondary IMTP) (Lachowicz et al., 2004).

Secondary IMTP occurs when antibody targets nonself antigens adsorbed onto the surface of platelets or when immune complexes become bound to platelet surfaces. Underlying mechanisms include systemic autoimmune diseases (systemic lupus erythematosus), neoplasia, infectious agents, and drugs; but occasionally additional causes are identified. One report documents the presence of thrombocytopenia in 2.5% of dogs with idiopathic inflammatory bowel disease. Known causes of thrombocytopenia were eliminated, and the authors postulated that the thrombocytopenia was secondary to the primary disease (Ridgway, Jergens, and Niyo, 2001).

Thrombocytopenia associated with neoplasia is often multifactorial, with secondary immune-mediated destruction representing one potential component. Lymphoma in dogs has been associated most commonly with secondary IMTP, but it can occur with any neoplasm. In one study 10% of dogs with neoplasia had concurrent thrombocytopenia, and of this group 61% did not have identifiable factors known to cause secondary IMTP (Grindem et al., 1994). As with neoplasia, thrombocytopenia in infectious diseases is often multifactorial and can include a secondary immune-mediated component. Antiplatelet antibodies have been detected in various infectious diseases, including *Ehrlichia canis* infections and Rocky Mountain spotted fever (RMSF). Drugs are rarely reported to cause a true primary IMTP; more typically it is secondary in nature (Kristensen, 2000). With this mechanism the drug acts as a hapten, allowing immune-mediated targeting of the platelets. A few drugs are capable of causing a secondary immune-mediated reaction without a history of prior exposure (heparin in horses), but most occur following extended use or prior exposure. Several documented cases involving trimethoprim sulfonamide/sulfamethoxazole have been reported in dogs, but it could potentially be caused any number of drugs. Vaccine-induced thrombocytopenia has been reported in dogs following immunization with modified live vaccines (canine distemper). Typically thrombocytopenia is mild and develops within 3 to 10 days after vaccination, but marked thrombocytopenia can occur. Posttransfusional thrombocytopenia has been reported occasionally in dogs.

INFECTIOUS ETIOLOGIES ASSOCIATED WITH THROMBOCYTOPENIA

See Table 60-1 for a list of infectious agents associated with thrombocytopenia in dogs and cats (Greene, 2006). Thrombocytopenia associated with infectious etiologies is often multifactorial, involving increased consumption, destruction, vasculitis, or sequestration; and in many cases the pathogenesis is incompletely understood. As mentioned previously, a number of agents are associated with secondary IMTP. Some are known to cause bone marrow suppression, including feline leukemia virus (FeLV) infection, feline immunodeficiency virus (FIV) infection, feline panleukopenia (parvovirus), canine parvovirus, and chronic monocytotrophic ehrlichiosis (*Ehrlichia canis, Ehrlichia chaffeensis*). FeLV and FIV are of particular importance in feline thrombocytopenia. In one study 30% and 15% of thrombocytopenic cats tested positive for FeLV and FIV, respectively, indicating that these diseases are major causes of or contributing factors to the development of thrombocytopenia (Jordan, Grindem, and Breitschwerdt, 1993).

Table **60-1**

Infectious Causes of Thrombocytopenia in Dogs and Cats

Disease	Species	Mechanism	Diagnostic Tests*	Therapy
Viral				
Canine distemper	C	U	Ag detection, PCR, serology	Supportive
Canine herpesvirus	C	V	Ag detection, serology, VI	Supportive
Canine parvovirus infection: canine parvovirus 2	C	P, U	Ag detection, EM feces, PCR, serology	Supportive
Infectious canine hepatitis: canine adenovirus 1	C	U, V	Serology, PCR, VI	Supportive
Feline immunodeficiency virus	F	P	Serology, PCR	Supportive
Feline infectious peritonitis: feline corona virus	F	U, V	Ag detection, histopathology, PCR, serology,	Supportive
Feline leukemia virus	F	P	Ag detection, PCR, serology	Supportive
Feline panleukopenia/feline parvovirus	F	P, U	Ag detection, EM, fecal VI, PCR, serology	Supportive
Rickettsial, neorickettsial, anaplasmal, mycoplasmal				
Canine granulocytotropic anaplasmosis: *Anaplasma phagocytophilum*	C	D, U	Blood smear, PCR, serology	Doxycycline (10mg/kg PO q24h for 21 days)
Canine granulocytotropic ehrlichiosis: *Ehrlichia ewingii*	C	D, U	Blood smear, PCR, serology	Doxycycline (10mg/kg PO q24h for 21 days)
Canine monocytotrophic ehrlichiosis: *Ehrlichia canis, Ehrlichia chaffeensis*	C	D, P, U	Blood smear, PCR, serology	Doxycycline (10mg/kg PO q24h for 21 days)
Feline granulocytotropic anaplasmosis: *A. phagocytophilum*	F	D?	PCR, serology	Doxycycline (10mg/kg PO q24h for 21 days)
Feline mononuclear ehrlichiosis *E. canis, Neorickettsia ristici* (?)	F	D?	PCR, serology	Doxycycline (10mg/kg PO q24h for 21 days)
Hemotropic mycoplasmosis: *Mycoplasma haemofelis, Mycoplasma haemominutum, Mycoplasma haemocanis*	C, F	D, S	Ag detection, blood smear, PCR	Doxycycline (10mg/kg PO q24h for 21 days), Enrofloxacin (5mg/kg PO q24h for 14 days)
Rocky mountain spotted fever: *Rickettsia rickettsii*	C	D, V	Ag detection (skin), PCR, serology,	Doxycycline (10mg/kg PO q24h for 21 days)
Salmon poisoning disease: *Neorickettsia helminthoeca*	C	D, U	Cytology, fecal examination	Doxycycline (10mg/kg PO q24h for 21 days)
Thrombocytotropic ehrlichiosis: *Anaplasma platys*	C	D, U	Ag detection, blood smear, PCR, serology	Doxycycline (10mg/kg PO q24h for 21 days)

Table **60-1—Cont'd**

Disease	Species	Mechanism	Diagnostic Tests*	Therapy
Bacterial				
Bacteremia/septicemia	C, F	D, U, V	Blood, urine, body fluid culture	Ampicillin sulbactam (30 mg/kg IV q8h) and Enrofloxacin (10 mg/kg IV q24h)
Bartonellosis: *Bartonella vinsonii*	C	D, V	Culture, PCR, serology	Optimal treatment is unknown. Azithromycin (5 mg/kg PO q24h for 5 days, then EOD for 45 days) has been recommended
Endotoxemia: most often *Escherichia, Klebsiella, Enterobacter, Proteus, Pseudomonas*	C, F	S	Blood, urine, wound culture, often presumptive	Ampicillin sulbactam (30 mg/kg IV q8h) and Enrofloxacin (10 mg/kg IV q24h)
Leptospirosis	C	D, U, V	Ag detection, histopathology, PCR, serology, urine dark-field microscopy, urine or blood culture	Ampicillin (22 mg/kg IV q8h for 2 weeks) followed by Doxycycline (5 mg/kg PO q12h for 3 weeks). Some recommend Doxycycline for initial therapy
Plague: *Yersinia pestis*	F	S, U	Ag detection, culture, PCR, serology	Doxycycline (10 mg/kg PO q24h for 21 days), Enrofloxacin (5 mg/kg PO q24h for 14 days)
Salmonellosis	C, F	D, S, U, V	Culture, PCR	Enrofloxacin (5-10 mg/kg IV q24h) reserved for patients with septicemia
Tularemia: *Francisella tularensis*	C, F	D, U, V	Ag detection, culture, PCR, serology	Doxycycline (5 mg/kg PO q12h)
Protozoal				
Babesiosis: *Babesia canis, Babesia gibsoni*	C	U, S	Blood smear, PCR, serology	Imidocarb dipropionate (6.6 mg/kg IM twice, 2 weeks apart) for *B. canis*, Atovaquone (13.5 mg/kg PO q8h for 10 days) and azithromycin 10 mg/kg PO q24h for 10 days) for *B. gibsoni*
Cytauxzoonosis: *Cytauxzoon felis*	F	U, S	Blood smear, cytology, PCR†	Imidocarb dipropionate (2-3 mg/kg IM twice one week apart) or Atovaquone (15 mg/kg PO q8h for 10 days) and azithromycin 10 mg/kg PO q24h for 10 days
Leishmaniasis	C	U	Ag detection, cytology, PCR, serology, western blot analysis	Meglumine antimonite (100 mg/kg SQ q24h) and allopurinol (15 mg/kg PO q12h) for 3-4 months, allopurinol indefinitely
Toxoplasmosis: *Toxoplasma gondii*	C, F	U	Fecal (cats), serology, cytology	Clindamycin (12.5-25 mg/kg PO q12h)
Nemotodal				
Heartworm disease: *Dirofilaria immitis*	C	D, U, V	Ag detection, blood smear, Knott's test, serology	Melarsomine (2. 5 mg/kg IM)
Fungal				
Disseminated candidiasis	C, F	U	Culture, cytology,	Itraconazole (5-10 mg/kg PO q12h)
Histoplasmosis: *Histoplasma capsulatum*	C, F	U	Ag detection, culture, cytology, serology	Itraconazole (5-10 mg/kg PO q12h)

Ag, antigen; *C,* canine; *D,* destruction; *EM,* electron microscopy; *F,* feline; *PCR,* polymerase chain reaction; *S,* sequestration; *U,* utilization; *V,* vasculitis; *VI,* virus isolation.

* Refer to Greene CE: *Infectious diseases of the dog and cat,* ed 3, for more information on diagnostic tests, available test kits, specimens and commercial diagnostic laboratories.

† Available at the North Carolina State University, Tick-Borne Disease Laboratory, Raleigh, NC.

? Uncertain.

DIC is commonly seen in gram-negative sepsis, infectious canine hepatitis (ICH), leptospirosis, salmonellosis, babesiosis (virulent strains), canine and feline parvovirus, cytauxzoonosis, and plague. Vascular damage occurs in endotoxemia, septicemia, heartworm disease, feline infectious peritonitis (FIP), ICH, RMSF and bartonellosis. Platelet sequestration within the spleen, liver, or lungs is noted in endotoxemia; plague; salmonellosis;

babesiosis; cytauxzoonosis; and in hemolytic crisis secondary to babesiosis, hemotrophic mycoplasmosis (formerly hemobartonellosis), or cytauxzoonosis. Etiologic agents vary with geographic location and may be limited by the vector, intermediate host, or environmental requirements of the organism.

The degree of thrombocytopenia can vary. Although thrombocytopenia is most severe in IMTP and overwhelming sepsis (counts of less than 50,000/μl and often fewer than 10,000/μl), it can be moderate to severe in canine monocytotrophic ehrlichiosis. In one report on prevalence of *E. canis* infection in thrombocytopenic dogs in an endemic region, infection was found in 63.1% of dogs with a platelet count of less than 100,000/μl but in only 21% of dogs with platelet counts between 100,000 and 200,000/μl; nonthrombocytopenic dogs had an infection rate of 1.4% (Bulla et al., 2004). Severe, cyclic thrombocytopenia is also seen with thrombocytotropic ehrlichiosis, but dogs are not systemically sick; clinically ill dogs with this disease should be evaluated for concurrent tick-borne diseases such as monocytotrophic ehrlichiosis.

Tests used to diagnose infectious diseases include serology, polymerase chain reaction (PCR), antigen detection in fluids or tissues, cytology, blood smear evaluation, culture, virus isolation, electron microscopy, and histopathology (see Table 60-1; Greene, 2006).

CLINICAL EVALUATION OF THROMBOCYTOPENIA

Because thrombocytopenia typically is secondary to another disease or condition, signalment, history, and physical examination findings are extremely important. Primary IMTP is more commonly reported in middle-aged female dogs, especially cocker spaniels, German shepherds, poodles, and Old English sheepdogs, but can occur in any breed at any age. Most animals present for signs relating to the underlying disease, or the thrombocytopenia is found serendipitously on routine blood work. Risk of bleeding increases as platelet counts decrease below 20,000/μl, although spontaneous bleeding typically does not occur, even with marked thrombocytopenia. We have seen primary IMTP in dogs with platelet counts of fewer than 5000/μl that have no bleeding tendencies or clinical signs.

When present, signs directly related to thrombocytopenia can include petechiae, ecchymoses, prolonged bleeding after trauma, venipuncture, whelping or surgical procedures, prolonged estrus, bruising, melena, hematemesis, intraocular hemorrhage or blindness, hematuria, oral bleeding, neurologic signs associated with cerebral bleeding, and epistaxis. Petechiae and ecchymoses are easiest to identify on mucous membranes or thin-skinned regions such as the abdomen. Other signs related to the underlying cause of thrombocytopenia may include fever, weight loss, enlarged lymph nodes, splenomegaly, hepatomegaly, abdominal masses, stiffness, joint pain, neurologic signs, or edema.

A careful and thorough history can provide valuable clues to the etiology of thrombocytopenia. Vaccination history; FeLV and FIV status; exposure to drugs or toxins; travel history; exposure to infectious agents, ticks, or other animals; history of previous illnesses; tick/flea/heartworm preventive use; indoor/outdoor status; and clinical signs or changes noted by the owner should all be ascertained.

DIAGNOSTIC APPROACH TO INFECTIOUS OR IMMUNE-MEDIATED THROMBOCYTOPENIA

The first step is to confirm the presence of thrombocytopenia by performing a complete blood count with an automated platelet count and examining a peripheral blood smear. Extremely high or low platelet counts may not be assessed accurately by automated instruments if they are outside instrument linearity, and platelet clumps or large platelets can result in spuriously low counts. For these reasons abnormal automated platelet counts must always be confirmed by examination of a blood smear. Platelet clumping is best appreciated along the feathered edge of the smear and, if present, indicates that a new sample must be collected. If repeated samples yield clumped platelets, blood can be collected into a syringe rinsed with EDTA. Alternatively a needle can be inserted into a peripheral vein, and blood collected directly from the hub into the capillary tube of a Unopette manual white blood cell and platelet count system (Becton Dickinson) for a manual platelet count. When clumps are found, platelets typically are present in sufficient numbers to prevent spontaneous hemorrhage. If clumps are not present, the platelet count can be estimated by multiplying the mean platelet count in ten 100× fields within the monolayer of the blood film by 15,000 to give the total platelet count per microliters. A patient with a normal or increased platelet count with signs of a primary hemostatic defect (petechia, ecchymosis) should be evaluated for platelet function defects or vascular disorders.

Platelet size and morphology should also be evaluated in the thrombocytopenic patient. Large platelets are an indication of increased platelet production and support a regenerative response by the bone marrow. Normal-size platelets may be seen in acute disorders in which the bone marrow has not had time to respond, or they can indicate a hyporesponsive or unresponsive marrow. Small platelets or platelet fragments can be associated with early or nonregenerative IMTP. *Anaplasma platys* may be identified as stippled blue morulae within platelets during clinical episodes.

Evaluation of the erythrogram, leukogram, and a peripheral blood smear can help distinguish decreased platelet production from increased use or destruction. Decreased production or suppression of only the megakaryocytic line is rare; most etiologies are associated with decreased production or suppression of the myeloid and erythroid series as well. Typically a peripheral neutropenia without a left shift is seen. A nonregenerative anemia may be present in long-standing conditions but is not expected in acute conditions or conditions of short duration because of the long life span of RBCs (110 days in dogs, 68 days in cats). Conditions or diseases causing increased platelet destruction or consumption are often associated with an inflammatory leukogram characterized by a neutrophilia or neutropenia with a left shift. Toxic change may also be seen in a variety of inflammatory conditions; when moderate to marked, it is most indicative of a bacterial infection. A mild, nonregenerative anemia (anemia of inflammatory disease) often accompanies inflammatory conditions. Although classically associated with chronic conditions, this anemia can develop within a week of the onset of significant inflammation. Evidence of hemolytic disease may be seen with some etiologic agents such as *Babesia*, *Cytauxzoon*, and *Mycoplasma*; these agents may also be identified in RBCs on a peripheral blood smear. Morulae may be found within neutrophils in acute canine granulocytotropic ehrlichiosis and anaplasmosis or in monocytes in monocytotrophic ehrlichiosis. IMTP can also accompany primary or secondary immune-mediated hemolytic anemia, which is classically characterized by a regenerative anemia with spherocytosis and an inflammatory leukogram. Vasculitis and DIC often result in circulating schistocytes.

Examination of the bone marrow may be indicated if the cause of the thrombocytopenia is not apparent from the routine clinical evaluation. Other indications for bone marrow examination include suspicion of leukemia, multiple myeloma, lymphoma or other myeloproliferative disorder, or the presence of multiple cytopenias of unknown etiology. Collection of a bone marrow aspirate for cytology and a bone marrow core biopsy for histopathology is ideal; these provide the greatest amount of information when interpreted together. Even when thrombocytopenia is severe, it is not a contraindication for performing a bone marrow biopsy. Patients rarely have significant hemorrhage from the procedure; however, it is wise to choose a site without significant muscle mass such as the proximal humerus where hemorrhage can be more easily controlled. Transfusion may be necessary before performing the biopsy if the patient is bleeding actively. Increased numbers and immaturity of megakaryocytes indicate a regenerative response; decreased numbers indicate an unresponsive or preregenerative marrow (a regenerative response should occur within 3 to 5 days of acute thrombocytopenia).

A coagulation profile consisting of prothrombin time (PT), activated partial thromboplastin time (APTT), and fibrin degradation products (FDPs) should ideally be performed in all animals with thrombocytopenia. D-dimer levels may also be useful in dogs. Fulminant DIC is classically characterized by a prolonged PT and APTT with significantly increased FDPs and D-dimer levels, but peracute or chronic DIC should not be ruled out if coagulation parameters are within reference intervals and clinical suspicion of DIC is high. DIC is a common secondary condition in a variety of infectious, inflammatory, and neoplastic diseases and is triggered by vascular damage, massive tissue damage, or release of activating substances (see Chapter 61 for more information). Hemorrhage caused by rodenticide toxicity is characterized by markedly prolonged PT and APTT with normal FDPs or D-dimer levels. The proteins inhibited by vitamin K antagonism or absence (PIVKA) test can confirm rodenticide poisoning.

Selection of additional diagnostic tests is based on information provided by the patient's history, signalment, physical examination findings, and initial blood work. EDTA anticoagulated blood and a serum sample should be collected and saved for serology, PCR, and culture and antiplatelet antibody assays; it is important to collect these specimens before initiating therapy. Culture of blood or other fluids/tissues should be performed on any animal with suspected septicemia. Survey radiographs or ultrasonography may be indicated. Enlarged lymph nodes or organs, masses, and effusions should be examined via cytology or histopathology. Joint fluid should be collected and examined cytologically in animals with joint pain or swelling, and cerebrospinal fluid (CSF) collection and cytologic evaluation may be indicated in animals with neurologic disease. Titers for infectious diseases, PCR, and culture can also be performed on joint fluid or CSF. For animals with suspected systemic immune-mediated disease, antinuclear antibody testing, antierthrocytic antibody testing (Coombs' test), and potentially histopathologic and immunohistochemical examination of dermal lesions should be performed.

Tests to confirm IMTP are available, but it is important to remember that no test can distinguish primary from secondary disease; thus all causes of secondary immune-mediated disease must be ruled out before a diagnosis of primary IMTP can be made. Tests can detect platelet-bindable autoantibodies in patient serum or plasma (indirect assays) or antibody present on the surface of platelets or megakaryocytes (direct assays). Direct assays are preferred because they are more specific; indirect assays fail to differentiate autoimmune antibodies from alloantibodies, circulating immune complexes, or nonspecific immunoglobulin G aggregates formed in stored serum. Shipping and handling potentially can be problematic for direct antiplatelet antibody assays; thus it is advisable to contact the reference laboratory regarding sample handling before collection and shipping. The direct megakaryocytic immunofluorescence assay (D-MIFA) circumvents sample handling issues by using unstained, air-dried bone marrow smears. When using this assay, it is important to remember that poorly cellular specimens or specimens with inadequate numbers of megakaryocytes preclude adequate evaluation. In addition, autoantibodies targeting platelets may not target megakaryocytes; thus a negative result cannot be used to rule out immune-mediated disease. Low sensitivity has been reported with this test (Kristensen, 2000).

THERAPY

The goals of treatment are to stop hemorrhage, halt ongoing platelet destruction, and treat any underlying disorders. Treatment usually consists of a combination of both specific and supportive measures. Supportive measures include the use of blood products (whole blood or packed red blood cells) or purified polymerized bovine hemoglobin solutions to maintain oxygen delivery to tissues and crystalloid fluids to maintain hydration in patients that are anorexic and not drinking. Venous access may not be necessary in patients that are stable. When intravenous access is needed, catheterization of the jugular vein is contraindicated in patients with severe thrombocytopenia because of the difficulty in controlling hemorrhage at this site. The use of fresh-frozen plasma is limited to patients with concurrent coagulopathies associated with decreased clotting factors such as rodenticide intoxication or DIC. Platelet transfusions have limited use because of difficultly in transfusing a large enough number of platelets to exert a clinical benefit combined with the short circulating half-life of transfused platelets in patients with destructive platelet disorders. Platelet transfusions may provide transient improvement in hemostasis but typically do not increase detectable platelet counts. They can be performed using platelet concentrates, platelet-rich plasma, or whole blood and should be reserved for patients with life-threatening hemorrhage. Since the gastrointestinal tract is the most common site of significant bleeding secondary to thrombocytopenia, gastroprotectants (sucralfate, H_2 blockers, proton-pump inhibitors) are frequently used. However, since true ulceration is rarely present in dogs with IMTP, the use of these drugs for gastrointestinal bleeding secondary to thrombocytopenia is questionable.

If an underlying infectious cause of thrombocytopenia is identified or highly suspected, specific therapy should be instituted. Treatments for selected infectious causes of thrombocytopenia are listed in Table 60-1. In patients that are stable and not experiencing life-threatening hemorrhage, antimicrobial therapy alone may be sufficient to resolve the thrombocytopenia. However, specific therapy against infectious agents may not be sufficient to halt the immune-mediated destructive process, and concurrent immunosuppressive therapy may be indicated. When immunosuppressive and antimicrobial therapy are started concurrently, worsening of infection from the immunosuppressive therapy is rare, except with systemic fungal infections or cases in which immunosuppression has been ongoing for weeks to months before antimicrobial therapy. When instituted simultaneously in cases with IMTP secondary to infectious diseases, immunosuppressive therapy frequently can be weaned more quickly (i.e., 25% dose reductions every 2 weeks) than in dogs with primary IMTP.

When no underlying cause of IMTP can be identified, immunosuppressive therapy is the treatment of choice. Corticosteroids remain the backbone of therapy for the treatment of primary IMTP. Prednisone is usually administered at a dose of 1 to 2 mg/kg every 12 hours orally for a minimum of 3 to 4 weeks or at least until the platelet count is greater than 200,000/μl. Vincristine (0.02 mg/kg intravenously once) has been used in patients with IMTP and was associated with shorter hospitalization times (Rosanski EA et al., 2002). If treatment with corticosteroids and vincristine do not result in increased platelet counts within 7 to 10 days, one or more adjunctive immunosuppressive drugs should be used (Table 60-2; see Chapter 55).

Long-term immunosuppressive therapy (≥6 months) is necessary for most cases of primary IMTP, and client expectations should be set accordingly. Some patients may require lifelong therapy to maintain normal platelet counts. The main cause for the relapse of thrombocytopenia in our experience is rapid corticosteroid taper (i.e., dose reductions at intervals equal to or less than 2 weeks) and/or failure to document the platelet count before each dose reduction. Tapering of the corticosteroid dose by approximately 25% of the current dosage every 3 to 4 weeks should only be attempted *after*

Table 60-2

Adjunctive Immune Suppressive Therapies

Drug	Dose	Side Effects/Monitoring
Azathioprine	2 mg/kg PO q24h for 2 weeks, then 2 mg/kg PO every other day	Bone marrow suppression, hepatotoxicity, pancreatitis, complete blood counts, serum biochemical profiles
Cyclosporine	5-10 mg/kg PO q12h	Vomiting, diarrhea, therapeutic drug monitoring
Human γ-globulin	0.5-1 g/kg IV over 6-12 hours once	Anaphylaxis, thromboembolism
Mycophenolate mofetil	10-20 mg/kg PO q12h	Vomiting, diarrhea, pyoderma

IV, Intravenously; *PO,* orally.

the platelet count has returned to, and remained within, the reference interval. Steroids can usually be discontinued completely when the dose administered is similar to the physiologic amount of cortisol produced in a normal patient (0.2 mg/kg/day of prednisone). If thrombocytopenia recurs during the tapering of the corticosteroids, the dose should be increased to the *original* dose, and adjunctive immunosuppressive drugs should be added if not already in use (see Table 60-2). Corticosteroids should then be tapered as before, down to the last dose at which a normal platelet count was detected. This dose is often maintained indefinitely or for a minimum of several months before tapering of corticosteroids is attempted again.

Splenectomy has been recommended as an adjunctive treatment for thrombocytopenia. This should typically be considered as a last resort; and thorough screening for infectious diseases, particularly babesiosis, should be performed before the procedure. Splenectomy can exacerbate hemoparasite infections and is associated with resistance to antiprotozoal treatments.

The prognosis for IMTP is guarded to good. In some university studies mortality rates have been 25% to 30%, but these often represent the most severe cases. Although formal studies of prognostic indicators for survival are minimal, most clinicians agree that clinically significant bleeding with anemia and intracranial hemorrhage are the worst prognostic indicators. The severity of the thrombocytopenia does not appear to be a significant prognostic indicator.

References

Bulla C et al: The relationship between the degree of thrombocytopenia and infection with *Ehrlichia canis* in an endemic region, *Vet Res* 35:141, 2004.

Garon CL et al: Idiopathic thrombocytopenic purpura in a cat, *J Am Anim Hosp Assoc* 35:464, 1999.

Greene CE: *Infectious diseases of the dog and cat*, ed 3, St. Louis, 2006, Elsevier.

Grindem CB et al: Epidemiologic survey of thrombocytopenia in dogs: a report on 987 cases, *Vet Clin Pathol* 20:38, 1991.

Grindem CB et al: Thrombocytopenia associated with neoplasia in dogs, *J Vet Intern Med* 8:400, 1994.

Jordan HL, Grindem CB, Breitschwerdt EB: Thrombocytopenia in cats: a retrospective study of 41 cases, *J Vet Intern Med* 7:261, 1993.

Kristensen AT: Platelets—Clinical platelet disorders. In Feldman BF, Zinkl JG, Jain NC, editors: *Schalm's veterinary hematology*, ed 5, Baltimore, 2000, Lippincott Williams & Wilkins, p 467.

Lachowicz JL et al: Acquired amegakaryocytic thrombocytopenia—four cases and a literature review, *J Small Anim Pract* 45:507, 2004.

Lewis DC, Meyers KM: Canine idiopathic thrombocytopenic purpura, *J Vet Intern Med* 10:207, 1996.

Norman EJ et al: Prevalence of low automated platelet counts in cats: comparison with prevalence of thrombocytopenia based on blood smear estimation, *Vet Clin Pathol* 30:137, 2001.

Ridgway J, Jergens AE, Niyo Y: Possible causal association of idiopathic inflammatory bowel disease with thrombocytopenia in the dog, *J Am Anim Hosp Assoc* 37:65, 2001.

Rosanski EA et al: Comparison of platelet count recovery with use of vincristine and prednisone or prednisone alone for treatment for severe immune-mediated thrombocytopenia in dogs, *J Am Vet Med Assoc* 220:477, 2002.

CHAPTER 61

Disseminated Intravascular Coagulation: Diagnosis and Management

ELKE RUDLOFF, *Glendale, Wisconsin*
REBECCA KIRBY, *Glendale, Wisconsin*

Disseminated intravascular coagulation (DIC) is a syndrome characterized by systemic microthrombosis, which can progress to life-threatening hemorrhage. DIC is reported in dogs but is less commonly recognized in cats. The DIC syndrome occurs secondary to an underlying acute or chronic condition associated with one or more of the following: systemic inflammation, tissue necrosis, capillary stasis, loss of vascular integrity, red cell hemolysis, and particulate matter in the blood.

PATHOGENESIS

The pathogenesis of DIC is characterized by: (1) increased thrombin production, (2) suppression of physiologic anticoagulant pathways, (3) impaired fibrinolysis, and (4) activation of inflammatory pathways (Fig. 61-1). Tissue factor (TF) is expressed on monocytes and endothelial cells within the circulation during inflammation and on malignant cells in cancer patients. The tissue factor: factor VIIa complex (extrinsic pathway), the main stimulus for thrombin formation in DIC, activates factor IX (intrinsic pathway) and factor X (common pathway) (Fig. 61-2). In human cancer patients DIC can also involve the

expression of a specific cancer procoagulant, a cysteine protease that has factor X–activating properties.

Impaired function of the normal physiologic anticoagulant pathways (see Fig. 61-2; Fig. 61-3) during DIC allows thrombin generation and the resultant fibrin formation to become exaggerated. Antithrombin (AT), a natural anticoagulant, binds to thrombin; inactivating thrombin; and factors IXa, Xa, XIa, and TF:FVIIa. During DIC AT levels are reduced as a result of increased AT consumption by AT-thrombin complex formation, AT degradation by neutrophil elastase, impaired hepatic synthesis of AT, and loss of AT because of increased capillary permeability. Depression of endogenous anticoagulant protein C:protein S activity results from enhanced consumption, impaired hepatic synthesis, and capillary leakage. In addition, proinflammatory cytokines (tumor necrosis factor [TNF]-α and interleukin [IL]-1β) can cause down-regulation of protein C–thrombomodulin expression on endothelial cell surfaces.

During DIC fibrin deposition typically surpasses fibrinolysis. The release of plasminogen activators from endothelial cells rapidly initially increases fibrinolytic activity during sepsis. However, this is usually followed

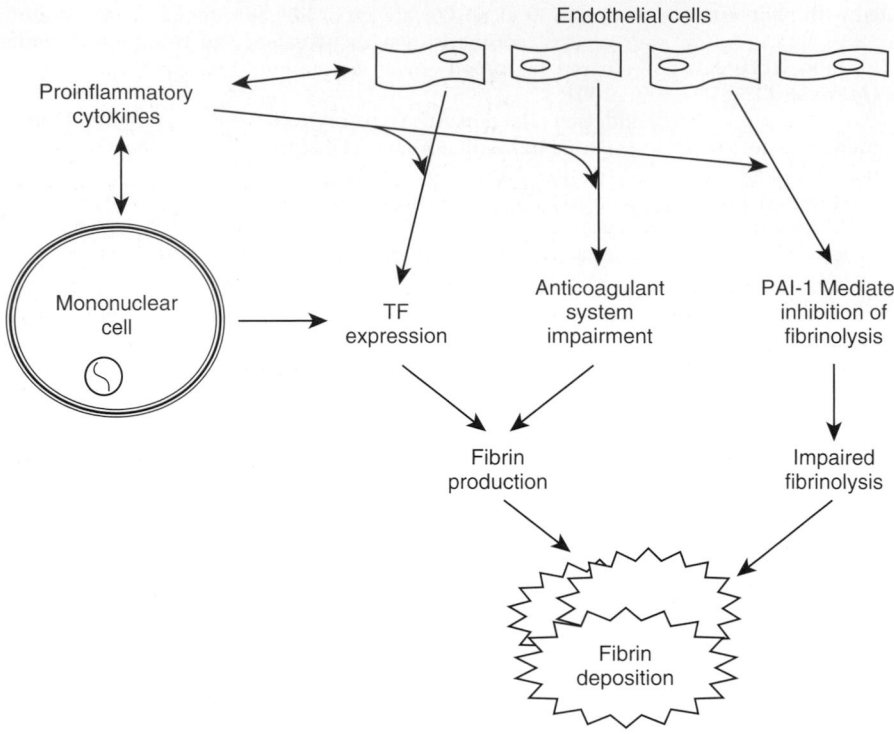

Fig. 61-1 Alterations in coagulation and anticoagulation during systemic inflammation and DIC. Fibrin deposition exceeds fibrinolysis when tissue factor (TF) expression is enhanced, the anticoagulation system is impaired, and levels of plasminogen activator inhibitor, type-1 (PAI-1) are increased.

by a prompt suppression of fibrinolytic activity caused by endothelial release of plasminogen activators and increased plasma levels of plasminogen activator inhibitor, type-1. In contrast, people with acute promyelocytic leukemia may exhibit a severe hyperfibrinolytic state associated with systemic coagulation activation.

The "cross talk" between the coagulation system and the inflammatory reaction is an important factor contributing to DIC pathogenesis (see Fig. 61-1). Activated coagulation proteins stimulate the endothelial cells to release inflammatory cytokines. Recruited white blood cells release TNF-α (activating factor VII), IL-1, and IL-6 (activating factors VII and XII). Platelet-activating factor,

a strong promoter of platelet aggregation, is also released from inflammatory cells. Additional activation of the inflammatory cascade is promoted by thrombin and other serine proteases interacting with protease-activated receptors on cell surfaces. The typical antiinflammatory effect of activated protein C is lost with depression of the protein C system during DIC, thereby enhancing the proinflammatory state of DIC.

It is important to recognize that the hypercoagulable condition occurs early in the course of DIC and bleeding associated with prolongation of coagulation times occurs later in the course of DIC. As a consequence of coagulation activation, platelets, coagulation factors,

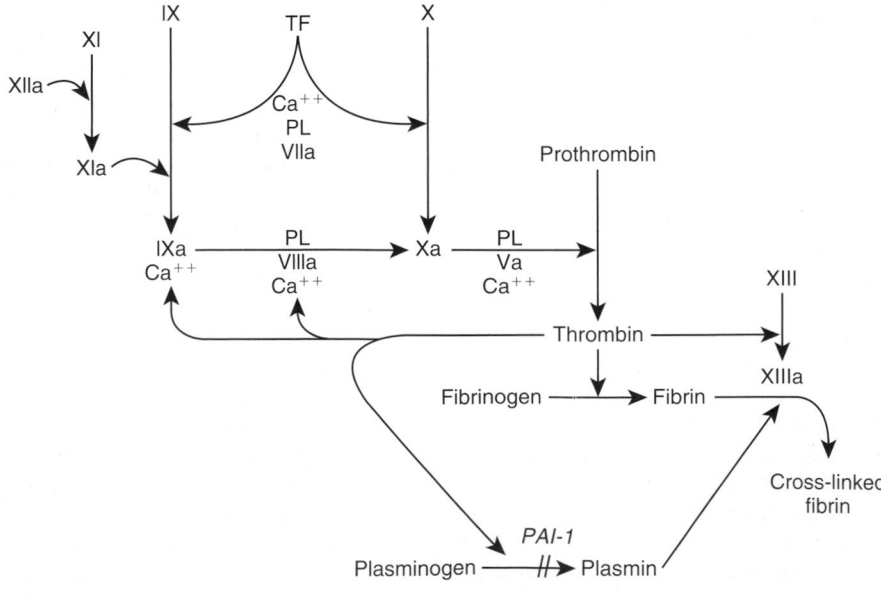

Fig. 61-2 Coagulation during inflammation promoting thrombin and fibrin production. Tissue factor (TF) is the prime initiator of coagulation. Amplification of the coagulation scheme during DIC occurs by activation of factor IX (cross talk) and continued activation of factors VIII and IX and platelet surfaces by thrombin (feedback). Plasminogen activator inhibitor-type 1 (PAI-1) prevents plasmin activation and fibrinolysis. During inflammation there is inhibition of fibrinolysis when PAI-1 is upregulated and promotion of fibrin deposition. *Ca++*, Calcium; *PL*, phospholipase.

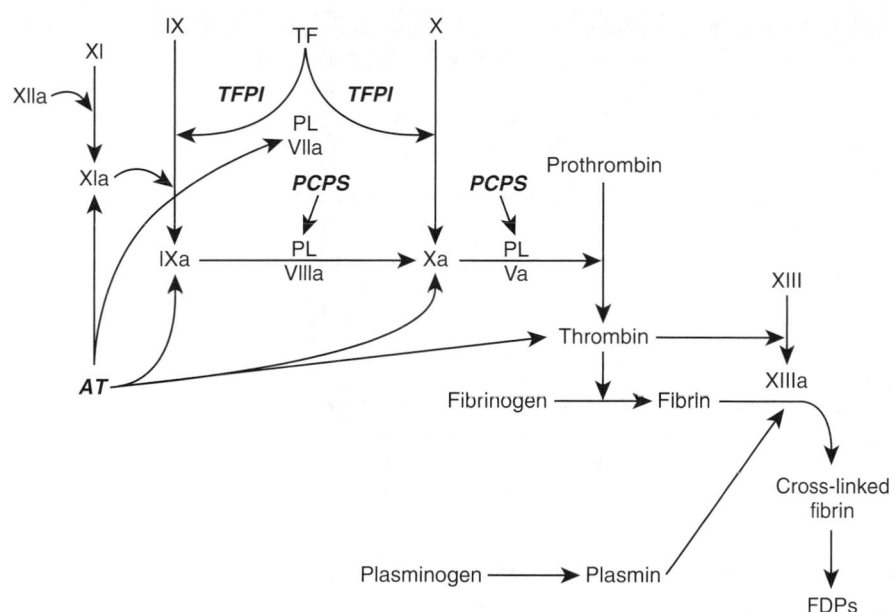

Fig. 61-3 This scheme depicts anticoagulation, which should normally balance coagulation. Tissue factor pathway inhibitor (TFPI) is a protease inhibitor of tissue factor complex. Bound to thrombin, antithrombin (AT) inactivates thrombin and factors IXa, Xa, XIa, and TF:FVIIa. Protein-C:Protein-S (PCPS) system irreversibly inactivates factors Va and VIIIa. Activation of plasminogen produces plasmin, which lysis fibrin and fibrinogen into fibrin degradation products and fibrin monomers. During inflammation there is consumption and inhibition of the anticoagulants and promotion of fibrin deposition.

and anticoagulants are consumed, degraded, and/or inhibited. A transition from accelerated coagulation to consumption of coagulants and anticoagulants corresponds with the clinical consequences of microthrombosis and vascular occlusion followed by uncontrolled hemorrhage. Therefore variations and combinations of the coagulation-anticoagulation-fibrinolytic-inflammatory derangements exist, depending on the underlying cause and coexisting disease processes. Diagnosis of an active DIC process is made through clinical findings and laboratory testing.

CLINICAL FINDINGS

DIC should be an anticipated complication in any animal experiencing one or more of the following: hypotensive crisis, impaired blood flow to a major organ, systemic inflammatory response syndrome, and/or release of vasoactive agents into the vasculature (Box 61-1). The severity of clinical signs associated with DIC can range from no signs to life-threatening complications of vascular microthrombosis reflected by organ dysfunction and/or evidence of systemic bleeding. Clinical signs can vary as DIC progresses.

The earliest (peracute) phase of DIC typically is characterized by subtle abnormal laboratory findings (Table 61-1) without obvious clinical signs. Clinical signs more compatible with the acute (days to weeks) phase of DIC include evidence of organ dysfunction from microthrombosis and/or hemorrhage with laboratory findings suggestive of alterations in hemostasis. Animals experiencing consumption of endogenous coagulation proteins during this phase can demonstrate bleeding from venipuncture sites, bleeding along the gum line, petechiae, ecchymosis, purpura, hematomas, and/or hemarthrosis.

The chronic phase (weeks to months) of DIC can develop from low-grade or intermittent procoagulant release (see Box 61-1). In the compensated state of chronic DIC, time exists for replenishment of coagulation factors, anticoagulation proteins, and platelets. There may

be abnormal laboratory findings without obvious clinical signs (see Table 61-1). Stress, concurrent disease, and disease progression can cause decompensation, abnormal laboratory findings, and clinical signs associated with microthrombosis and/or hemorrhage.

Box 61-1

Disease States Associated With Disseminated Intravascular Coagulation

Peracute
- Sepsis (bacterial, viral, fungal, protozoal)
- Severe gastroenteritis
- Vascular disorders
- Immune-mediated disorders
- Severe toxic or immunologic reactions (e.g., viper envenomation)
- Transfusion reaction
- Severe hepatic failure

Acute
- Sepsis (bacterial, viral, fungal, protozoal)
- Trauma/crush injuries
- Pancreatitis
- Burns/heatstroke
- Severe gastroenteritis
- Vascular disorders
- Immune-mediated disorders
- Severe toxic or immunologic reactions (e.g., viper envenomation)
- Transfusion reaction
- Severe hepatic failure
- Neoplasia

Chronic
- Neoplasia
- Protein-losing nephropathy
- Protein-losing enteropathy
- Heartworm disease
- Chronic hepatic disease
- Vascular disorders
- Hyperadrenocorticism

Table 61-1

Laboratory Values Supporting a Diagnosis of DIC

Test	Peracute	Acute	Chronic
Prothrombin time	N or ↓	N or ↑	N
Partial thromboplastin time	N or ↓	N or ↑	N
Activated clotting time	N or ↓	N or ↑	N
Platelets	N or ↓	↓	N
Fibrinogen	N or ↓	N or ↓ or ↑	N or ↓ or ↑
Fibrin degradation products	N or ↑	↑	N or ↑
D-dimer	N or ↑	↑	↑
Antithrombin	N or ↓	↓	N or ↓

N, Normal.

LABORATORY FINDINGS

No single laboratory test is sufficiently sensitive or specific to confirm a diagnosis of DIC. A diagnosis of DIC can be made when a clinical condition known to be associated with DIC and a combination of the following laboratory findings is present (also see Table 61-1):

1. Prolongation of coagulation times
2. Reduction in platelet numbers
3. Elevation of D-dimer or soluble fibrin
4. Decrease in AT activity
5. Clinical or postmortem evidence of thrombosis.

Stokol and colleagues (2001) report that a negative D-dimer test in dogs excludes DIC as a diagnosis with a confidence interval of 95%.

A scoring algorithm is used in humans with an underlying condition known to be associated with DIC. The scoring system incorporates a decreased platelet count, prolongation of prothrombin time, decreased fibrinogen, and increasing plasma levels of a fibrin-related marker (D-dimer, soluble fibrin or fibrin degradation products [FDPs]) as predictive of DIC. The use of fibrinogen to predict DIC can be questioned because fibrinogen levels are influenced by many factors other than DIC. An alternate scoring system in humans evaluates a dynamic coagulopathy score in which changes in AT, prothrombin time, and D-dimers are used. A similar scoring system is under investigation in veterinary medicine to assist in the diagnosis of DIC and the categorization of DIC to predict mortality.

THERAPY

Once a disease process associated with DIC has been identified, early recognition and aggressive therapy can improve outcome. Therapy is focused on promoting capillary blood flow, eliminating the underlying cause, supporting target organs, replacement therapy, and anticoagulants.

Promoting Capillary Blood Flow

Restoring capillary blood flow and tissue oxygenation requires rapid intravascular volume resuscitation of perfusion deficits. Administering a combination of crystalloids with synthetic colloids (see Chapter 11 for more information on colloid therapy) increases capillary fluid volume and improves microvascular flow. Dextran-70 and hetastarch may improve flow dynamics and reduce platelet aggregation during hypercoagulable states. Red blood cell transfusions are used when hemoglobin levels have dropped precipitously (<8 to 10 g/dl). Oxyglobin (Biopure), a hemoglobin-based oxygen carrier approved for use in dogs, provides colloid osmotic pressure and oxygen-carrying molecules for the transport of oxygen to tissue beds experiencing maldistribution of blood flow. The vasoconstricting property of Oxyglobin can aid in reversing hypotension that is refractory to standard crystalloid and synthetic colloid infusion. Maintaining capillary flow depends on meeting ongoing fluid needs through continuous crystalloid and colloid infusions.

Eliminating Underlying Cause

Identification and treatment of the underlying disease process is crucial to the elimination of DIC. When a septic process is suspected, tissue and fluid samples are collected for histopathology, cytology, culture and sensitivity, and serology testing. Antimicrobial therapy for bacterial, protozoal, or fungal etiologies is initiated as early in the disease course as deemed appropriate. Removal and/or drainage of infected, torsed, ischemic, or necrotic tissue may be necessary. Antivenom and specific antidotes are used when indicated. Immune-mediated diseases require immunosuppressive medications. Neoplastic conditions may require surgical or medical treatment. Animals with medical conditions such as pancreatitis, severe gastroenteritis, or liver failure require aggressive cardiovascular support throughout hospitalization to minimize the effects of DIC during medical management.

Supporting Target Organs

Organs with high blood flow or high oxygen requirements are more susceptible to microthrombosis, hemorrhage, or tissue hypoxia secondary to DIC. Oxygen therapy, either with or without ventilatory support, may be necessary when hypoxemia or hypoventilation results from pulmonary pathology. Renal insufficiency and oliguria may require administration of diuretics and low-dose dopamine infusion (1 to 3 mcg/kg/minute) to promote afferent arteriolar dilation and renal blood flow. Early enteral nutrition supports gastrointestinal mucosal integrity.

Replacement Therapy

Blood Products

Correction of coagulation times (prothrombin and partial thromboplastin time) to normal is usually not possible when DIC is ongoing. The volume of blood products required varies among patients. Factors used to determine type and dose of transfusion include degree of factor deficiency, degree of anemia, and the patient's volume status.

Plasma transfusion can be administered to rebalance coagulant and anticoagulant proteins. Fresh whole blood and fresh frozen plasma contain all coagulation factors and AT. Stored whole blood and frozen plasma lack factors V and VIII. Fresh whole blood, platelet-rich plasma, or platelet concentrate are needed to provide platelets if bleeding attributed to thrombocytopenia is causing organ malfunction (e.g., ocular hemorrhage, myocardial arrhythmias, increased intracranial pressure). When significant anemia is present, fresh or stored whole blood, packed red blood cells, or Oxyglobin is given to improve oxygen-carrying capacity (see Chapter 58).

Antithrombin

AT activity accelerated by heparin inactivates thrombin and factors IXa, Xa, XIa, and TF:VIIa. In addition, AT binds to heparin sulfate proteoglycan receptors on the endothelial surface, stimulating the production of the antiinflammatory and antiplatelet cytokine prostacyclin. AT binds directly to cellular receptors on neutrophils and monocytes, limiting proinflammatory signaling. In phase III clinical trials high-dose recombinant AT has not been associated with a significant improvement in mortality in humans unless it is used without heparin (Warren et al., 2001). Recombinant human AT concentrate has not been investigated clinically in animal patients with DIC. Allogeneic AT can be infused in the form of plasma products when AT replacement is desired. The use of heparin in conjunction with AT supplementation is controversial (see section on Heparin later in the chapter).

Activated Protein C

Recent large-scale phase III clinical trials in humans with severe sepsis have shown a reduction in organ damage and mortality when recombinant human activated protein C (APC) was administered early in the course of disease. Additional benefits included a decrease in inflammatory cytokines and improved clotting times. The use of recombinant human APC or allogenic plasma transfusion for APC replacement has not yet been investigated clinically in veterinary patients.

Anticoagulant Therapy

Aspirin

Aspirin is a nonreversible thromboxane-2 inhibitor that reduces platelet aggregation and adhesion. Aspirin is used for reducing thrombotic events in people with coronary artery disease. Low-dose aspirin administration (0.05 mg/ kg q24h orally) has been associated with reduced mortality in dogs with immune-mediated hemolytic anemia (a disease associated with DIC) receiving azathioprine and prednisone. Further studies still need to be performed to determine its use for other forms of DIC.

Heparin

Heparin is a glycosaminoglycan that exerts an antithrombotic effect by binding to and potentiating the inhibitory actions of AT on thrombin and factors IXa, Xa, XIa, and TF:VIIa. Heparin administration has been established as beneficial for the prevention of venous thrombosis in people. Heparin therapy has been a long-standing mainstay of DIC therapy, but its use has become controversial. A beneficial effect of heparin on DIC has not been demonstrated in controlled clinical trials in humans and can be detrimental when overt bleeding is occurring. Heparin is ineffective in patients with reduced plasma levels of AT. In critically ill dogs heparin administration has been shown to further decrease AT levels (Rozanski et al., 2001). Binding of heparin to AT can reduce AT antiinflammatory effects (see section on Antithrombin earlier in the chapter).

Heparin cannot eliminate existing thrombi but can help prevent the formation of new thrombi or expansion of established thrombi. At this time there is insufficient information to advocate the use of heparin in any phase of DIC. Heparin therapy may be most useful for patients with chronic DIC conditions in which there is predominantly a prothrombotic stage of DIC and no significant inflammatory stimulus.

Tissue Factor Pathway Inhibitors

A number of agents targeting the TF pathway are currently under study, including TF pathway inhibitor (TFPI), recombinant nematode anticoagulant protein C2 (NAPc2), recombinant hyrudin, and inactivated factor VIIa. Phase III clinical trials in humans are lacking, and use in veterinary medicine has not at this time been investigated.

References and Suggested Reading

Bateman S: Disseminated intravascular coagulation in dogs: review of the literature, *J Vet Emerg Crit Care* 8:29, 1998.

Bateman S et al: Diagnosis of disseminated intravascular coagulation in dogs admitted to an intensive care unit, *J Am Vet Med Assoc* 215:798, 1999.

Feldman B, Madewell B, O'Neill M: Disseminated intravascular coagulation: antithrombin, plasminogen, and coagulation abnormalities in 41 dogs, *J Vet Med Assoc* 179:151, 1981.

Maruyama H et al: The incidence of disseminated intravascular coagulation in dogs with malignant tumor, *J Vet Med Sci* 66:573, 2004.

Rozanski EA et al: The effect of heparin and fresh frozen plasma on plasma antithrombin III activity, prothrombin time and activated partial thromboplastin time in critically ill dogs, *J Vet Emerg Crit Care* 11:15, 2001.

Stokol T et al: D-dimer concentrations in healthy dogs and dogs with disseminated intravascular coagulation, *Am J Vet Res* 61:393, 2000.

Vincent J et al: Drotrecogin alfa (activated) treatment in severe sepsis from global open-label trial ENHANCE: further evidence for survival and safety and implications for early treatment, *Crit Care Med* 33:2266, 2005.

Warren BL et al: High-dose antithrombin III in severe sepsis: a randomized controlled trial, *J Am Med Assoc* 286:1869, 2001.

CHAPTER 62

Platelet Dysfunction

MARJORY B. BROOKS, *Ithaca, New York*
JAMES L. CATALFAMO, *Ithaca, New York*

Platelets are small, anucleated cell fragments, yet their active participation is crucial for initiating and regulating hemostasis. This chapter describes the clinical management of bleeding diatheses caused by thrombopathia, or platelet dysfunction.

NORMAL PLATELET FUNCTION

Platelets circulate in the vascular compartment as discrete, nonadhesive, smooth disks. When a blood vessel is injured, platelets are rapidly transformed into adhesive spiny spheres that attach to the damaged subendothelial surface and to each other. The adherent platelets release numerous substances from platelet storage organelles. These substances accumulate locally and recruit additional platelets to the injury site. As local platelet numbers increase, platelet aggregates accumulate and bridge the zone of vascular damage to form a hemostatic plug. The plug is stabilized by the generation of a thrombin-mediated platelet fibrin meshwork that traps platelets and red blood cells. The growing clot is later consolidated by the action of platelet contractile proteins that retract the clot (Colman et al, 1994).

The ability of platelets to respond to injury-induced stimuli is central to their role in maintaining vascular integrity (Fig. 62-1). These stimuli initiate platelet activation by mediating a change in concentration of intracellular second messengers such as ionized calcium, inositol triphosphate, diacylglycerol, and arachidonic acid metabolites. Prostacyclin (PGI_2) and prostaglandin E_2 (PGE_2) and D_2 (PGD_2) are endoperoxides synthesized by endothelial cells and released into the vascular space. PGI_2 inhibits platelet reactivity by elevating intraplatelet cyclic adenosine monophosphate (cAMP) and decreasing free ionized calcium and inositol phosphate formation. Prostaglandin E_2 and PGD_2 modulate expression of endothelial cell adhesion molecules. Endothelium-derived nitric oxide can also reduce platelet responsiveness by raising the level of intracellular cyclic guanosine monophosphate (cGMP).

The rapid transition from nonadhesive disk to adhesive sphere requires that platelets recognize cell adhesion molecules in the plasma and subendothelial matrix. Adhesion (platelet-subendothelial matrix interactions) and aggregation (platelet-platelet association) depend on integrin and other platelet glycoprotein (GP) receptors. Integrin receptors (GPs) are composed of α- and β-subunits. The GPIIb/IIIa ($\alpha_{IIb}\beta_3$) complex is the most abundant platelet integrin and functions as the activation-dependent receptor for fibrinogen, fibronectin, and von Willebrand's factor (vWF). The binding of fibrinogen to this receptor is essential for normal platelet aggregation. Platelet adhesion and aggregation at high shear rates depends on vWF binding to GPIb-IX-V. Platelet adhesion to collagen is supported by its binding to the integrin receptor GPIa/IIa ($\alpha_2\beta_1$). This receptor and GPVI are also involved in signaling collagen-induced platelet activation.

CLINICAL SIGNS OF PLATELET DYSFUNCTION

The characteristic signs of platelet dysfunction include cutaneous ecchymoses, bleeding from mucosal surfaces (gingival hemorrhage, epistaxis, melena, hematuria), and prolonged or excessive bleeding at the sites of surgery or trauma. Pinpoint hemorrhage or petechiae are more commonly seen in thrombocytopenic patients, but there are no pathognomonic signs to differentiate platelet dysfunction from other primary hemostatic disorders. The systemic diseases that cause acquired platelet dysfunction often cause concurrent deficiency or inhibition of the coagulation cascade. In these cases the bleeding diathesis is more severe than that caused by platelet dysfunction alone and may include hematoma formation or spontaneous hemorrhage into the central nervous system (CNS) or pleural or peritoneal spaces. Frequently the most obvious findings on initial examination are signs of acute or chronic blood loss anemia. Therefore identification of an underlying defect of platelet function requires an index of suspicion that a bleeding diathesis is present and a diagnostic plan for evaluating hemostatic pathways.

DIAGNOSTIC APPROACH

The initial evaluation of bleeding in dogs and cats should be directed at differentiating blood loss caused by injury to a local or focal group of vessels from a systemic bleeding diathesis. A thorough history and physical examination, in some cases including ancillary diagnostics (radiography, ultrasonography, endoscopy), is usually sufficient for locating the source and underlying cause of hemorrhage from large vessels. A history of repeated episodes of hemorrhage, bleeding at multiple sites, and concurrent disease known to affect hemostasis suggests the presence of a systemic bleeding diathesis. Preliminary screening tests should then be performed to rule out the more common bleeding disorders before one pursues detailed studies of platelet function. Table 62-1 lists screening tests of hemostasis and definitive tests for identifying platelet dysfunction.

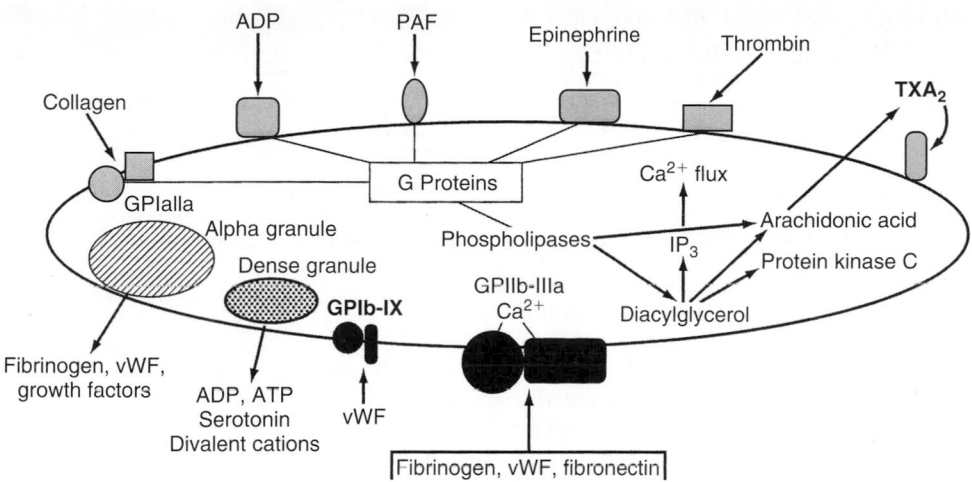

Fig. 62-1 Receptors and second messengers involved in platelet activation. Platelet stimuli bind to specific cell surface receptors activating phospholipase C via coupled G proteins, including the integrin receptor for collagen, GPIa/IIa. Activated phospholipase C hydrolyzes phosphoinositides to generate inositol 1,4,5-triphosphate (IP_3), and diacylglycerol (DAG) and to mobilize ionized calcium from platelet storage sites. Ca^{2+} also activates phospholipase A_2 to release arachidonic acid, which is converted to thromboxane A_2 (TXA_2). TX is released and activates other platelets via its surface receptor. DAG stimulates protein kinase C to phosphorylate intraplatelet proteins critical for platelet function, including dense and α-granule release. von Willebrand factor binds to either GPIb-IX or GPIIb/IIIa to support platelet adhesion to damaged subendothelium. Platelet aggregation is mediated by bound fibrinogen bridging GPIIb/IIIa receptors on adjacent platelets. The release of dense granule constituents amplifies platelet reactivity. α-Granules secrete hemostatic proteins and other factors to support platelet adhesion and wound healing. The elevation of intraplatelet cyclic adenosine monophosphate blocks ionized calcium mobilization and phosphoinositide hydrolysis. *PAF*, platelet-activating factor.

Table **62-1**

Diagnosis of Platelet Dysfunction

Initial Screening Tests	Ruleout
Platelet count	Thrombocytopenia
Coagulation assays aPTT, PT, TCT, fibrinogen	Coagulation factor deficiency or coagulation inhibitor
vWF:Ag	vWD
Buccal mucosal bleeding time	Thrombocytopenia, platelet dysfunction, vWD
PFA-100 closure time	Thrombocytopenia, platelet dysfunction, vWD
Antithrombin	Thrombotic syndromes, DIC
FDP, D-dimer	Thrombotic syndromes, DIC

Platelet Function Studies	Specific Parameters
Clot retraction	
Platelet aggregation studies	Response to ADP, collagen, other agonists
Platelet secretion studies	Serotonin, ADP, ATP release
Flow cytometric detection of membrane receptors and ligands	CD42 (GPIb), CD61 (GPIIIa), CD62P (P-selectin), phosphatidylserine, fibrinogen
Platelet ultrastructure (EM)	

ADP, Adenosine diphosphate; *ATP,* adenosine triphosphate; *APTT,* activated partial thromboplastin time; *DIC,* disseminated intravascular coagulation; *EM,* electron microscopy; *FDP,* fibrin/fibrinogen degradation products; *GP,* glycoprotein; *PT,* prothrombin time; *TCT,* thrombin time; *vWD,* von Willebrand's disease; *vWF:Ag,* von Willebrand's factor antigen.

Preliminary Evaluation

Thrombocytopenia and coagulation factor deficiencies are the most common bleeding diatheses in dogs and cats. Therefore a platelet estimate from a blood smear and/or platelet count and coagulation screening tests are performed as the first step in evaluating any patient suspected of having a bleeding disorder. Determination of plasma vWF concentration provides a rapid screening test for von Willebrand's disease (vWD). This defect of primary hemostasis is indistinguishable clinically from platelet dysfunction and should be ruled out in dogs and cats before one moves on to platelet function studies. A complete drug history and metabolic profile are included in the preliminary evaluation to identify disease processes likely to impair platelet function and to direct therapy. Platelet dysfunction commonly accompanies the disseminated intravascular coagulation (DIC) process. Tests for defining or characterizing DIC complete the initial laboratory screening process (see Chapter 61). In vivo assessment of primary hemostasis is performed by measuring buccal mucosa bleeding time (BMBT; Forsythe and Willis, 1989). The finding of a prolonged bleeding time, normal platelet count, and normal vWF concentration is compatible with either acquired or inherited platelet dysfunction. However, the clinical severity of bleeding caused by platelet dysfunction does not always correlate with prolongation of bleeding time. The PFA-100 (Dade Behring, Newark, DE) is a tabletop platelet function analyzer that measures platelet adhesion and aggregation based on platelet plug occlusion of an agonist-treated membrane (closure time). Although prolonged PFA-100 closure time is compatible with platelet dysfunction or vWD, nonspecific prolongation of closure time also occurs in patients with thrombocytopenia, anemia, drug therapy, and disorders that affect blood viscosity (Mischke and Keidel, 2002).

Specific Platelet Function Testing

Platelet response and specific platelet defects are characterized by performing a series of in vitro tests to evaluate platelet structure and function (see Table 62-1). Test procedures and reagents must be adapted and validated for use in dogs and cats to accommodate species-specific differences. Accurate measurement of platelet function in aggregation and release studies requires that samples be analyzed within 3 hours of collection to ensure the viability of patient platelets. This requirement necessitates patient referral to the clinic or center where testing is performed. Platelet aggregation in response to different agonist compounds is measured by detecting changes in light transmission of platelet-rich plasma samples or changes in electrical impedance of whole blood samples. Whole-blood aggregation studies use small sample volume and are simple to perform, features useful for detecting dysfunction in patients that have acquired disorders secondary to disease or drug administration. Aggregation studies that use platelet-rich plasma (PRP) are difficult to perform, but they provide more detailed information for characterizing and defining platelet response in patients having inherited platelet function defects. Flow cytometry can be used to assess platelet membrane GP composition and activation response, with the potential advantage of small sample volumes. Special platelet function testing is available at our laboratory and at other veterinary teaching hospitals (including Auburn University and the University of Pennsylvania).

SPECIFIC DISORDERS

Acquired Platelet Dysfunction

Platelet dysfunction occurs in association with many common disease conditions and drug therapies. The clinical significance of impaired platelet function is highly variable under these conditions. The clinician should be prepared to closely monitor and, if needed, treat patients with hemorrhagic complications. Conversely, if hemorrhage caused by platelet dysfunction is suspected, a thorough search to identify underlying disorders or drug administration is indicated.

Platelet Dysfunction Secondary to Disease
The disorders most commonly associated with platelet dysfunction are listed in Box 62-1. Complex and variable patterns of abnormalities are often seen in platelet function studies of these patients, and the mechanisms underlying platelet dysfunction are likely to be multifactorial. Factors extrinsic to the platelet may predominate, such as impairment of platelet adhesion caused by changes in blood viscosity in anemic patients or the presence of paraproteinemia. Uremia is believed to cause an intrinsic platelet function defect by altering PG

Box 62-1

Diseases Associated With Acquired Platelet Dysfunction

- Anemia
  - Chronic regenerative or nonregenerative
- Disseminated intravascular coagulation
- Liver disease
  - Cholestasis and acquired or inherited shunts
- Paraproteinemias
  - Lymphocytic leukemia, multiple myeloma, benign macroglobulinemia, polyclonal gammopathies
- Uremia

---

metabolism, in addition to an extrinsic defect related to an increase in plasma levels of dialyzable metabolites.

Platelet Dysfunction Secondary to Drug Administration
Many drugs demonstrate platelet inhibitory effects in vitro; however, clinically significant impairment of hemostasis has been reported for relatively few of these products. Aspirin and other nonsteroidal antiinflammatory drugs (NSAIDs) are most commonly implicated in cases of drug-induced platelet dysfunction in dogs and cats. These drugs block production of thromboxane, a potent platelet agonist, by inactivating platelet cyclooxygenase. The effects of aspirin on platelet function are irreversible, lasting as long as 7 days; whereas inhibition caused by NSAIDs is transient, lasting for only a few hours (Grauer et al, 1992). The drugs listed in Table 62-2 have proven or

Table 62-2

Drug-Induced Platelet Dysfunction

Category	Drug	Mode of Action
Antibiotics	Carbenicillin	Unknown
	Cephalothin	Membrane*
	Moxalactam	Membrane
	Sulfonamides	Membrane
Antiinflammatory drugs	Aspirin	Prostaglandin inhibition[†]
	Ibuprofen	Prostaglandin inhibition[‡]
	Naproxen	Prostaglandin inhibition[‡]
	Phenylbutazone	Prostaglandin inhibition[‡]
Cardiac or respiratory drugs	Aminophylline	Phosphodiesterase[§]
	Isoproterenol	Membrane
	Propranolol	Membrane
	Theophylline	Phosphodiesterase
	Verapamil	Prostaglandin inhibition[‡]
Miscellaneous	Barbiturates	Signal transduction[¶]
	Dextran	Membrane
	Heparin	Unknown
	Hydroxyethyl starch	Membrane

* Interacts or interferes with platelet membrane receptors.
[†] Irreversible acetylation of platelet cyclooxygenase.
[‡] Reversible inhibition of prostaglandin metabolites.
[§] Inhibitor of phosphodiesterase causing increased intraplatelet cyclic adenosine monophosphate.
[¶] Interferes with the rise of intraplatelet calcium levels.

potential platelet inhibitory effects and should be used cautiously, if at all, in patients undergoing surgery or demonstrating signs of abnormal hemostasis.

Inherited Platelet Dysfunction

Inherited disorders of platelet function can be classified broadly into disorders of platelet membrane GPs, defects involving platelet storage granules, defects of intracellular signaling, or lack of platelet procoagulant activity (Kottke-Marchant and Corcoran, 2002). Inherited platelet defects are rare and often breed specific (Table 62-3). Affected dogs and cats may be maintained as pets provided that they are managed carefully, with transfusion therapy as needed for bleeding crises.

TREATMENT OF PLATELET DYSFUNCTION

Effective treatment of platelet dysfunction includes control of hemorrhage from the sites of active bleeding, stabilization of the patient to ameliorate signs of hypovolemia or blood loss, and correction of any underlying disease that may cause or exacerbate the hemostatic defect. Acquired platelet dysfunction is far more common than inherited platelet disorders, and the long-term management of dogs and cats with acquired disorders is dictated by the specific primary disease process (see Box 62-1). Initial treatment for both acquired and inherited disorders can be divided into transfusion and nontransfusion support.

Transfusion Therapy

In contrast to management of thrombocytopenic patients, limited transfusion support is often effective in controlling hemorrhage caused by platelet dysfunction. The physical presence and any residual function of thrombopathic platelets enable them to participate in the formation of hemostatic plugs initiated by the normal, transfused platelets.

Blood Collection and Processing for Platelet Transfusions

Blood products that supply active platelets include fresh whole blood (FWB), PRP, and platelet concentrates (PCs). Special collection and processing techniques are needed to maintain maximal platelet viability and prevent the formation of platelet aggregates (Mooney, 1992). The most important of these include (1) maintenance of blood products at room temperature throughout collection, processing, and storage; (2) use of plastic bags or syringes and citrate-based anticoagulants rather than glass receptacles and heparin anticoagulant; and (3) transfusion within 24 hours of collection (FWB) or within 3 days (PRP, PCs). Special care is given to aseptic collection technique because platelet transfusions are maintained at room temperature. It is ideal to administer these products as soon as possible after collection.

PRP is prepared by centrifugation of FWB for less time and at a lower speed (soft spin) than routinely used for separation of fresh plasma. Platelets remain suspended in the supernatant plasma, with an expected yield of about 80% of the platelets in whole blood. Platelet concentrates are prepared by centrifugation of PRP using a high speed (hard spin) to form a platelet pellet and then suspending the pellet in a small volume (50 to 75 ml) of plasma (Abrams-Ogg et al., 1993). The PRP and PCs prepared in this manner have some contamination with donor red and white blood cells, albeit at a much lower concentration than that of the whole blood from which they are prepared. The equipment and supplies for production of PRP and PCs are readily adapted for dogs, but the short storage life of these products limits their use primarily to the referral centers where they are prepared. Transfusion of platelet components in feline medicine has been reported only in research rather than clinical settings.

Guidelines for Platelet Transfusion

Donor selection. Donors should be blood-type compatible with recipients because all platelet replacement

---

Table **62-3**

Hereditary Platelet Function Defects*

Type Defect	Reported Breeds	Laboratory Features
Thrombasthenia	Otter hound, Great Pyrenees	Abnormal adhesion and clot retraction, aggregation failure, reduced or absent GPIIb/IIIa
Storage pool	Persian cat	Associated with Chédiak Higashi syndrome; lack of dense granules, secretion failure, abnormal aggregation, normal clot retraction
	American cocker spaniel	Dense granule number normal, abnormal ADP storage and secretion, abnormal aggregation, normal clot retraction
Signal Transduction	Basset hound	Abnormal adhesion and aggregation, abnormal cAMP metabolism, normal clot retraction
	Spitz	Abnormal adhesion and aggregation, abnormal signaling pathway, normal clot retraction
Platelet procoagulant activity	German shepherd	Normal aggregation and secretion, normal clot retraction, abnormal prothrombinase activity, abnormal PS externalization and microvesiculation
Complex or Undefined Defects	Collie	Associated with cyclic neutropenia, partial aggregation defect, abnormal uptake and storage of serotonin, abnormal protein phosphorylation
	Boxer	Abnormal aggregation to ADP and collagen

ADP, Adenosine diphosphate; *cAMP,* cyclic adenosine monophosphate; *PS,* phosphatidylserine.
* Clinical severity ranges from mild-to-severe bleeding tendency.

products (FWB, PRP, PCs) contain red cells. Feline donors and recipients should be matched for blood type A or B, whereas dogs negative for DEA 1.1 and DEA 1.2 (see Chapter 56) can be used as universal donors for platelets. Greyhounds are not recommended as donors for production of PRP because it is difficult to obtain high yields of their platelets with the use of routine centrifugation protocols. Recipients likely to need repeated transfusions over long periods of time (months) are at risk for developing alloantibodies to foreign platelet antigens. Sequential donations from a single donor rather than pooled platelet donations are likely to delay the immunization process (Slichter et al., 1986).

Platelet administration. Intravenous catheters should be placed in peripheral veins of thrombopathic patients because catheterization of the jugular vein might cause perivascular hemorrhage and interfere with respiration. If intravenous catheter placement is impossible, transfusion via the intraosseous route is an acceptable alternative for platelet replacement. Intraperitoneal transfusion and intraoperative salvage of blood are not effective means of supplying active platelets. In-line blood filters should be used for FWB and platelet component transfusions. An appropriate rate for transfusion is 6 ml/min for dogs, with the transfusion completed over the period of 1 to 2 hours for both dogs and cats. Routine pretreatment with corticosteroid or antihistamine is not required.

Clinical indications. Platelet transfusion is always indicated to provide rapid control of hemorrhage in critical functional sites such as the CNS or respiratory tract. A single transfusion is often sufficient to control epistaxis or other mucosal hemorrhage, whereas transfusion support for patients undergoing surgery is more intensive. A first transfusion is given before surgery, within 1 to 2 hours of the procedure. A second dose is given after surgery for major surgery or if any excess hemorrhage is noted. Close monitoring of the surgical site and serial determinations of hematocrit should be performed for the first 24 hours after surgery, and an additional platelet transfusion given if required. It is unusual for rebleeding to occur if hemostasis is adequate at 24 hours after surgery. The BMBT is not an accurate predictor of perioperative bleeding complications.

FWB is the optimal product for treating thrombopathic dogs or cats having signs of acute blood loss anemia and active hemorrhage. Platelet components (PRP, PCs) are ideal for preoperative prophylaxis and for thrombopathic patients requiring repeated transfusion within a 24-hour period. Platelet concentrates provide most of the active platelets, in less than one half the volume, of the PRP from which they are prepared. Nevertheless, transfusion of PRP is usually sufficient to supply effective numbers of platelets without volume overload, and the extra time and expense in preparing PCs is rarely worthwhile when one treats acquired or inherited platelet dysfunction. Table 62-4 presents general dosage guidelines for platelet replacement. The most successful transfusion strategy is to treat with an initial high dose of blood products to supply enough active platelets for hemostatic plug formation.

Table 62-4

Guidelines for Platelet Transfusion

Product	Dose	Frequency
Fresh whole blood	12 to 20 ml/kg	q24h (volume overload limits interval)
Platelet-rich plasma	5 to 10 ml/kg	q6-12hr
Platelet concentrate	1 unit */15 kg	q6-12hr

*One unit is defined as the platelet concentrate produced from 450 ml of fresh whole blood.

Transfusion Reactions

Transfusion of platelet products may be complicated by any of the acute, chronic, immune, or nonimmune reactions associated with transfusion of whole blood. Acute reactions are treated by stopping the transfusion and administering symptomatic or supportive care. Febrile reactions are the most common complication. These reactions tend to be self-limiting and are probably mediated by white blood cells in the platelet products. Procedures for removing contaminant white blood cells (special centrifugation techniques, leukocyte filters) also reduce platelet yield. Urticaria and anaphylaxis are uncommon acute immune transfusion reactions. Urticaria may be a reaction to plasma proteins; this condition is treated with administration of antihistamine and short-acting corticosteroid. Anaphylaxis may result from transfusion of incompatible red blood cells or transfusion of large aggregates of activated platelets. These complications are prevented with the use of only type- and crossmatch-compatible platelet donors, careful collection techniques, and transfusion through blood filters. Dogs that receive repeated transfusions throughout their lives are at greatest risk for alloimmunization, causing shortened survival of transfused donor platelets. Posttransfusion purpura refers to an immune thrombocytopenia in a recipient caused by the development of high titer alloantibodies that cross-react with the recipients' platelet antigens.

Nontransfusion Therapy and Supportive Care

No drug or hormonal therapy can substitute for the structural and metabolic roles of platelets in initiating primary hemostasis. In human medicine desmopressin acetate (DDAVP; 1-deamino[8-D-arginine] vasopressin) is used as adjuvant therapy for patients with mild or nonspecific signs of defective primary hemostasis. This drug may be applicable for the treatment of dogs and cats, but there are no controlled studies demonstrating clinical efficacy.

For secondary or drug-induced platelet dysfunction, treatment of the underlying disorder or discontinuation of the suspected drug may be sufficient to prevent or control hemorrhage and obviate the need for transfusion. In these cases invasive procedures should be avoided or delayed, pending the response to specific treatment.

Local treatment of surgical or traumatic wounds can eliminate or reduce the transfusion requirements of thrombopathic patients. Procedures for improving local hemostasis include electrocautery, ligation of small vessels, multilayer closure of incisions, and application of pressure wraps. Topical tissue adhesives are very effective in controlling hemorrhage from small wounds on cutaneous or mucosal surfaces, provided that bleeding is first controlled with direct pressure and the tissues are dry. Oral tissues are rich in fibrinolysins and are likely to bleed. To minimize hemorrhage from gingival injuries and tooth extraction sites, these wounds can be packed with absorbable sponges and sutured.

References

Abrams-Ogg ACG et al: Preparation and transfusion of canine platelet concentrates, *Am J Vet Res* 54:635, 1993.

Boudreaux MK et al: Type I Glanzmann's thrombasthenia in a Great Pyrenees dog, *Vet Pathol* 33:503, 1996.

Colman RW et al: Overview of hemostasis. In Colman RW, Hirsh J, Marder VJ, et al, eds: *Hemostasis and thrombosis*, Philadelphia, Lippincott-Raven, 1994, p3.

Forsythe LT, Willis SE: Evaluating oral mucosa bleeding times in healthy dogs using a spring-loaded device, *Can Vet J* 30:344, 1989.

Grauer GF et al: Effects of low dose aspirin and specific thromboxane synthetase inhibition on whole blood platelet aggregation and adenosine triphosphate secretion in healthy dogs, *Am J Vet Res* 53:1631, 1992.

Kottke-Marchant K, Corcoran G: The laboratory diagnosis of platelet disorders, *Arch Pathol Lab Med* 126:133, 2002

Mooney SA: Preparation of blood components. In Hohenhaus AE, editor: *Problems in veterinary medicine, transfusion medicine*, Philadelphia, 1992, Lippincott-Raven, p 594.

Mischke R, Keidel A: Influence of platelet count, acetylsalicylic acid, von Willebrand disease, coagulopathies, and hematocrit on results obtained using a platelet function analyzer in dogs, *Vet J* 165:43, 2002.

Slichter SJ et al: Canine platelet alloimmunization: the role of donor selection, *Br J Haematol* 63:713, 1986.

CHAPTER 63

Clinical Trials in Veterinary Oncology

CHAND KHANNA, *Bethesda, Maryland*
MELISSA PAOLONI, *Bethesda, Maryland*

Clinical trials in veterinary oncology are growing in scope and importance. Trials that evaluate novel therapies for dogs and cats with cancer have the opportunity to improve the outcome and quality of life for veterinary patients, as well as human patients with cancer. The demand for clinical trials has been fueled by the rapid increase in the number of pet animals treated for cancer and the pet-owning public's interest in effective and well-tolerated treatments for their companions. Interest from the human cancer drug development industry is based on a need for more reliable ways to evaluate new cancer drugs and the strong similarities established between veterinary and human cancers. Accordingly, well-designed clinical trials in veterinary oncology offer the opportunity to develop new drugs in both species. Interestingly the clinical outcome for patients who are managed within a clinical trial has consistently been shown to be superior to use of the same agents outside the setting of a clinical study. This suggests the value of clinical trials not only to future patient care but also to the actual patient involved in a study. Through the conduct of clinical trials our opportunities to prevent, diagnose, and treat cancer will continue to improve. This requires greater direct and indirect participation from both primary care veterinarians and veterinary specialists.

TRIAL DESIGNS

Clinical trials aim to answer specific scientific questions to find better ways to improve care for patients with cancer. The first step in the design of a clinical trial is to articulate the questions that the trial should address. Generally this is done by asking: what is the primary study objective? Based on a combination of primary and secondary objectives, investigators define the optimal trial design for a specific study. There are three general types of clinical trials: therapeutic, prevention, and screening. Irrespective of the intent of the trial, clinical trials are prospectively conducted.

Therapeutic Trials

Therapeutic trials test new therapies such as new drugs, radiation protocols, combination therapies, or novel modalities such as gene therapy or cancer vaccines.

Prevention Trials

Prevention trials assess new approaches to reduce the risk of developing certain types of cancer. These are less common in veterinary medicine but can be thought of as those that involve lifestyle changes for pets such as diet changes or supplement administration. In the future these trials may assess the ability of an intervention to reduce the risk of cancer development in a high-risk animal (i.e., breeds at high risk for specific cancers).

Screening Trials

Screening trials evaluate novel tests that diagnose or define the stage of a cancer. These tests may involve new imaging techniques such as positron emission tomography, magnetic resonance imaging, or new molecular tests such as polymerase chain reaction to confirm a diagnosis of leukemia in a patient with lymphocytosis.

Retrospective Studies

Trial designs described below are distinctly different from retrospective studies that are commonly seen in the veterinary literature. Retrospective studies are those in which patients have already received a specified treatment or undergone a specific test from which data in their medical records are collected for analysis. Retrospective trials are particularly inferior when assessing the benefits of one therapy over another.

Prospective Trials

Prospective trials involve the deliberate design of a clinical trial intended to answer a specific objective or question. Patients are entered into this trial and managed within the constraints of a carefully designed study protocol. A protocol provides the background, specifies the objectives, and describes the design/organization of the trial. The value of this careful protocol design ensures the accuracy and consistency of results that come from clinical studies and provides an opportunity to verify and validate results. In general, the results from prospective clinical trials are considered to be more valuable than results from retrospective studies. Prospective trials are those most likely to make inferences about effectiveness of a new treatment. It is these trials that will be the basis of subsequent discussion.

PHASES OF CLINICAL TRIALS

Most clinical research in human oncology is very well defined, and the testing of new therapies proceeds in a stepwise process. Clinical trials are broken up into three phases so that the questions they answer are distinct. Table 63-1 outlines the most traditional phases. Although the named phases of clinical trials are not always used in veterinary oncology trials, many veterinary studies aim to answer the same questions of safety, efficacy, and comparison to conventional therapy.

RANDOMIZATION AND STRATIFICATION

Randomization is the process of assigning patients to a treatment group within a clinical trial by chance instead of choice. Treatment groups may include the standard of care, the standard of care plus a new therapy, a new therapy alone, or in some cases a placebo. The goal of randomization is to reduce bias (i.e., influence) for known and unknown characteristics (e.g., age, stage of disease, previous treatments) that may influence a response to the study therapy. Randomization tends to produce comparable treatment groups in terms of factors (i.e., confounders), not necessarily part of a study, that may affect a treatment outcome. Depending on the study, group randomization may be balanced 1:1, in which a patient has an equal chance of assignment to one study group over another, or skewed. Skewed or weighted randomization strategies can allow more patients to enter one group versus another. This strategy is most often used in placebo-

Table 63-1

Phases of Clinical Trials

	Phase I	Phase II	Phase III
Aim	Toxicity Dose finding	Efficacy/Responding histologies	Comparison to standard of care
Patient Number	Small	Large	Large
Dose	Escalating in cohorts	Fixed	Fixed
Single therapy	Yes	Yes or No*	Yes or no*
Randomization	No	Yes or No	Yes

*Can be combination therapy.

Phase I trials define a maximally tolerated dose of a new drug/regimen through dose escalation. In this trial toxicities associated with the new therapy can be defined. If a phase 1 trial is successful, its discovered dose moves into a phase II trial to assess efficacy and identify responding histologies. Phase III trials enroll larger number of patients to compare the dose of the new therapy to standard-of-care treatment. Phase III trials can also assess if a new treatment is less toxic or less expensive with equal/improved efficacy to current standards.

controlled studies in which a 4:1 randomization structure would result in four dogs randomized to receive the active treatment for every one dog that receives a placebo. During treatment, assessment, or follow-up it is common for the randomization of patients to be *"blinded"* or left unknown to participants, investigators, and statisticians. Historical controls are confounded by many variables that cannot be balanced between groups. These confounding variables may include differences in patient diagnosis, selection for a treatment, or the type of follow-up provided to patients. These variables may influence outcome to a greater extent than the treatment itself.

In some cases a patient characteristic (e.g., age, breed, past treatment, stage) is known or suspected to have an effect on the outcome of patients included in a clinical trial. For example, dogs with T-cell lymphoma are known to have a poorer outcome compared to dogs with B-cell lymphoma. To ensure that this variable is equally distributed across treatment groups, the strategy of *stratification* of dogs for these known prognostic variables occurs before randomization (Fig. 63-1).

END POINTS

Common end points in clinical trials include safety/toxicity and efficacy. Criteria for *safety* and *toxicity* have recently been established for veterinary patients through the Veterinary Cooperative Oncology Group. These published guidelines list a number of adverse events that may be noted in the evaluation of an animal in a clinical trial and allow the categorization of the severity of these events on a grade from I (least severe) to V (most severe—related

to death). These guidelines allow consistency in the reporting of safety/toxicity end points in clinical trials. Activity of a new cancer agent can be measured in several ways, including *response rate* in measurable/macroscopic disease, *disease or progression free interval* (DFI/PFI), *overall survival*, and *quality of life* (QOL). Biologic end points such as pharmacokinetic and pharmacodynamic assessments are also becoming increasingly important in veterinary oncology clinical trials. These biologic end points have been incorporated into study designs to better understand the mechanism of novel therapies/interventions. End points differ, depending on the type and objectives of a study, and are defined prospectively in the study protocol.

POWER

The *power* of a study is a measure of its ability to identify statistically significant differences between treatment groups. If the difference between treatment groups is small, the number of patients needed to be included in a trial needs to be large. The size of the patient population is a primary determinant of the power of a study. The calculation of sample size using a power analysis should be conducted before the initiation of a study. Increasing the statistical power in a study strengthens the chance of finding a statistically significant result when there is one. Veterinary trials are commonly underpowered and may be reported as "non-significant" even when there is a clear "trend" towards efficacy. Sometimes, simply increasing the number of study animals in each treatment group can lead to demonstration of both statistical and clinical significance of a treatment.

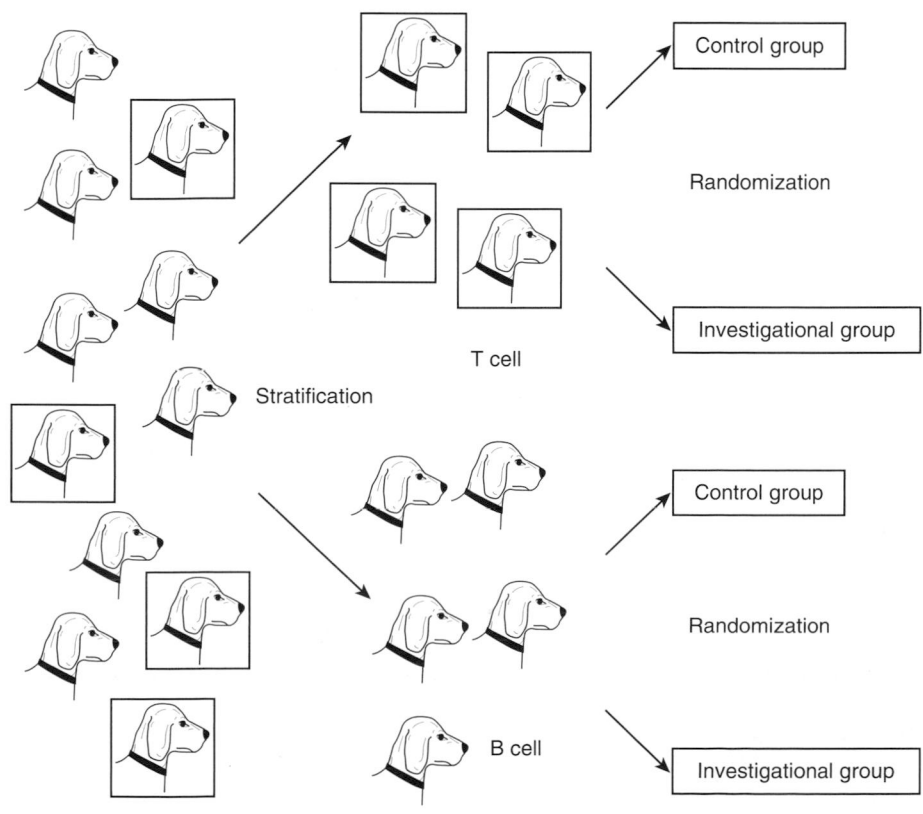

Fig. 63-1 Stratification can prevent potential bias from known prognostic factors such as immunophenotype in canine lymphoma. For example, it may appear that a treatment arm is doing poorly, thus concluding that the treatment is ineffective. But this cohort had a majority of dogs with T-cell lymphoma. Therefore the immunophenotype effect could mask the would-be positive benefits of the new therapy. Stratifying dogs by immunophenotype before randomization would allow researchers to look at separate subgroups and see if differences exist between "equal" treatment and control arms.

ETHICAL CONSIDERATIONS

There are key ethical standards used in clinical trial design, and it is the goal of all clinicians to ensure that these standards are met when presenting the option of a trial to a client or enrolling a patient in a clinical trial. The motivation for clients to enter clinical trials includes the lack of treatments currently effective for their pet's cancer, side effects that may limit their interest in pursuing conventional treatments, and the high costs of many cancer therapies. For the most part, clinical trials are provided at no or limited cost to clients. It is increasingly important to include the option of clinical trials when presenting the medical options available for a specific patient. In many cases owners' motivation to choose a clinical trial is influenced by their desire to help their pet and to improve outcomes for future pets or people with cancer.

Informed consent is required for all patients to enroll in a clinical trial. This is a written acknowledgement created by a trial's principal investigators, signed by a client, of the possible positive benefit and conversely the *adverse effects* of participating in a clinical trial. This informed consent defines the purpose of the trial and the requirements of the client to return with the pet for future follow-up procedures/appointments. Adverse events outside of those described are always possible; informed consent ensures that clients understand that in many trials the outcome/adverse effects are yet unknown.

It is important to protect all patients that enter clinical trials from expected and unexpected harm. *Stopping rules* within a trial protocol are used to remove participants in a trial if severe side effects are seen or if there is evidence that the patient's cancer is progressing in the face of treatment. If a patient fails to respond or progresses while in one treatment arm, it can be possible to *cross over* into another treatment arm. In addition to stopping rules for patients in a trial, the entire trial might also be stopped prematurely if there is strong evidence that the new intervention/agent is very effective or if the overall incidence of side effects is higher than expected. More recent innovative trial designs, referred to as Bayesian or outcome-adaptive randomization trials, assign more patients to the treatment arm that appears to be most effective. The increased use of such adaptive trials increases the benefit and reduces side effects for all participants in a trial. *Compassionate use* of an investigational agent is a mechanism for patients to continue on a therapy or have access to a therapy outside of the original clinical trial objectives or design. Collectively these measures ensure that a patient's best interests are maintained during their participation in a trial.

PRACTITIONER INVOLVEMENT IN CLINICAL TRIALS

The active engagement of veterinary general practitioners in conducting oncology clinical trials is integral to their success. These clinicians are the first to recognize and diagnose cancer in companion animals, and can act as the front line for education of clients regarding the availability of clinical trials. This information should be one of the options available to a family. Reassuring clients about the myriad of treatment options available today to pets with cancer and removing the mystery surrounding clinical trials is one of the most important concepts in developing new techniques to fight cancer in companion animals. It is also proven that involving patients in clinical trials provides the best care to patients in both the short and long term.

Clinical trials are often conducted through academic veterinary teaching hospitals or referral centers and increasingly include direct involvement from private practitioners. Patients may not be able to return to tertiary care centers for recheck examinations; thus these are often handled locally by their referring veterinarians. The timely reporting of these rechecks to the study center site and accurate record keeping are necessary for the reporting of clinical trial results, which include all possible long-term adverse events (side effects) from a new therapy, as well as outcome data.

Suggested Reading

Bell, JG, Brady M, Copeland LJ: The ethics of reporting and disseminating results of clinical research trials, *Cancer* 100:1107, 2004.

Giacinti L, Lopez M, Giordano A: Clinical trials, *Front Biosci* 11:8, 2006.

Green SJ, Pauler DK: Statistics in clinical trials, *Curr Oncol Rep* 6:36, 2004.

Hansen K, Khanna C: Spontaneous and genetically engineered animal models: use in preclinical cancer drug development, *Eur J Cancer* 40:858, 2004.

Ma BB, Britten CD, Siu LL: Clinical trial designs for targeted agents, *Hematol Oncol Clin North Am* 16:1287, 2002.

Porrello A, Cardelli P, Spugnini EP: Oncology of companion animals as a model for humans: an overview of tumor histotypes, *J Exp Clin Cancer Res* 25:97, 2006.

Trotti A, Bentzen SM: The need for adverse effects reporting standards in oncology clinical trials, *J Clin Oncol* 22:19, 2004.

Vail DM: Veterinary Cooperative Oncology Group—common terminology criteria for adverse events following chemotherapy or biologic antineoplastic therapy, *Vet Comp Oncol* 2:194, 2004.

CHAPTER 64

Collection of Specimens for Cytology

KENITA S. ROGERS, *College Station, Texas*

The usefulness of cytology as a diagnostic tool is well established. Evaluation of high-quality cytology preparations can provide a definitive diagnosis in many cases and may at least provide powerful supportive evidence of a disease process in others. Cytology can play an important role in establishing a prognosis, as well as guiding further diagnostic and therapeutic decisions. Collection of representative cells from a lesion or organ remains the quality-limiting step of this important technique. Poor-quality samples even have the potential to be quite misleading in the diagnostic workup and can prompt inappropriate therapy. This chapter focuses on cellular collection techniques, necessary supplies, appropriate slide preparation methods, and problems that may arise during this process.

Indications for cytologic evaluation include a palpable external mass, swelling, or ulceration; mass lesions arising from an internal organ; irregularity in an organ within the thoracic or abdominal cavity noted by physical examination or imaging techniques; organomegaly, including lymph nodes, liver, spleen, prostate, or kidneys; or fluid accumulation in body cavities, including joints, peritoneum, pleura, or pericardium. Cytology can also be used to assess for inflammation or tumor infiltration in organs that are grossly normal on examination. Because of its immediacy, cytology can be used effectively to help with decision making in the intraoperative setting.

The basic supplies required for sample collection are listed in Box 64-1. Whereas 1- to 1.5-inch needles are adequate for many clinical cases, longer spinal needles are often required for intracavitary aspirates to access deeper tissues. The recommended needle size varies with the tissue type and expected exfoliation. Large 18- to 20-gauge needles may be needed for lesions that are unlikely to exfoliate well such as bone aspirates, whereas most lesions and organs can be aspirated adequately with 21- to 25-gauge needles. The recommended syringe size is typically between 6 and 12 cc, which provides adequate suction and also is a comfortable fit for the operator's hands.

METHODS OF CELL COLLECTION

The technique recommended for collecting cytologic specimens varies, depending on lesion location, expected tissue characteristics, and patient restraint issues. No skin preparation is needed for external lesions or lymph nodes; but, if a body cavity is to be penetrated, surgical preparation of the skin is required. The area to be penetrated by the needle is small; thus extensive shaving is not necessary.

Imprints

The simplest method to collect cells is to directly imprint tissues onto a glass slide. This is an effective technique for biopsy specimens from organs or masses that exfoliate well. Blood and tissue fluid is blotted from the cut surface of the specimen, which is subsequently touched to the surface of a clean glass slide. Depending on the size of the specimen, several imprints may be made per slide. If the biopsy was retrieved as a small core, the specimen can be gently rolled down the slide with a small-gauge needle, avoiding crushing or fragmenting the biopsy. Imprinting may also be used to collect cells from discharges, typically from the nasal or vaginal cavities or external ulcers. Although easily accomplished, imprinting discharge fluid or an ulcerated surface often collects superficial inflammation, dysplastic cells, and contaminating bacteria, which may not be representative of the underlying disease process. For a superficial lesion or discharge, a glass slide is impressed directly to the lesion to collect material. If the material appears to be too thick, horizontal or vertical pull-apart smears can be made to ensure that some areas are thin enough for evaluation (see section on Slide Preparation later in the chapter). Swabs may be used to collect cells from fistulous tracts; ear canals; or the vaginal, nasal, or respiratory tracts. A sterile cotton swab or biopsy brush is used to collect cells from these sites and is then rolled down the length of the slide.

Fine-Needle Aspiration

Fine-needle aspiration (FNA) is preferred for cell collection from mass lesions and organs. It avoids superficial contamination and is more likely than imprinted specimens to be representative since several adjacent areas can be aspirated. The classic method of cellular collection involves piercing a mass or organ with a needle (21- to 25-gauge) that is attached to an empty syringe (6 to 12 cc). A 4- to 8-cc amount of suction is placed on the syringe to create a pressure vacuum that encourages cells to dislodge and move into the needle. With pressure held, the needle can be moved in different directions within the mass. If the aspirated site is intraabdominal, the risk of hemorrhage may be slightly increased with repeated needle redirection, and it is often recommended that the area be examined with ultrasound following the procedure to note any evidence of continued bleeding from the site. Redirection of the needle is not recommended with lung aspirates because of the risk of developing clinically

Box 64-1

List of Supplies Required for Basic Cytologic Collection Techniques

- Clean, dust-free glass slides
- 6- to 12-cc syringes
- Variety of 1- to 1.5-inch needles (20- to 25-gauge needles)
- 2.5- to 3.5-inch spinal needle with stylet
- Scalpel blades (Nos. 10 and 11)
- Romanowsky-type stain: Diff-Quik
- Slide dryer
- Marker for identifying slides
- Ethylenediaminetetraacetic acid (purple top) and serum (red top) tubes

significant pneumothorax. When aspiration has been completed, pressure is released, and the needle and syringe are withdrawn from the lesion. The cells collected typically are within the needle, and there may be no visible material within the syringe. Indeed, if material or blood is noted within the syringe, suction should be released, and the aspiration technique stopped. The needle is disconnected from the syringe, which is subsequently filled with air. After reattaching the air-filled syringe to the needle and holding the tip close to the slide, air is expelled through the needle to push material onto an appropriate area of the glass slide. Aspiration is facilitated by immobilization of the mass while the aspiration occurs. One helpful method is to hold a palpable mass between the thumb and index finger of the left hand with the palm up (for the right-handed clinician). This leaves the remaining fingers and palm free to grasp the barrel of the syringe while the right hand is used to apply suction.

Coring Technique

To avoid the cellular disruption that can be caused by the pressure of aspiration, the coring technique uses only a needle to collect cells. The needle is advanced through the mass or organ and is redirected several times for the purpose of dislodging cells and causing them to be driven into the hollow shaft of the needle. After the needle has been removed from the lesion, an air-filled syringe is used to expel the contents of the needle onto a slide similar to FNA. Alternatively, an air-filled syringe can already be attached to the needle, expediting the process. The coring technique diminishes blood contamination of the specimen in vascular tissues; and there is better control of needle placement, which is particularly useful for ultrasound-guided collections.

Scraping

Although FNA and coring are excellent methods for collecting cells from masses that exfoliate well, some types of tissue are very compact and do not readily release cells by these techniques. For these situations a scalpel blade or spatula can be used on the lesion or biopsy specimen to scrape across the surface several times and remove a small portion of the tissue. This fragment is placed on the proximal end of the slide and then spread as thinly as possible over the remainder of the slide by the blade or a second slide. There remain some tissues such as tumors of fibrous connective tissue origin that have cellular adhesion characteristics that do not allow the cells to be spread adequately over the slide for cytologic evaluation; for these specimens histopathology is required for definitive diagnosis. For superficial ulcerative lesions such as squamous cell carcinoma (SCC), a scraping may be used to collect cells below the ulcerated surface. In this case representative cells may have been difficult to collect with FNA because of the thin layer of tumor cells that characterizes some SCCs. Scraping collects a large amount of material; but, like imprints, if the collected cells are too superficial, they may not be representative of the underlying disease process.

Intracavitary Collection

FNA and the coring technique can be performed on mass lesions within the thoracic, peritoneal, or pericardial cavities. Differences in technique include the need to clip a small area of hair and perform a surgical preparation of the area. In addition, the animal must be well restrained, and in some cases sedation is necessary. Additional risks may be encountered with intracavitary aspirates. These include hemorrhage, which is usually minor and self-limiting, and the risk of rupturing an abscess or neoplasm that may spill into and contaminate a body cavity. Pneumothorax is an important potential complication when performing lung FNA. Use of small-gauge needles and appropriate patient selection can diminish this risk. Patients that are significantly tachypneic or in respiratory distress have a higher complication rate with this procedure, and fractious animals should be sedated to avoid unnecessary movement. The risk of pneumothorax is small when aspirating cranial mediastinal masses because the lungs are pushed caudally. Lung aspirates are most rewarding with diffuse infiltrative disease or large focal lesions. Many primary lung tumors have necrotic centers; thus recovery of only inflammatory material from a lung mass does not rule out neoplasia. Although intracavitary lesions can be aspirated based on triangulation techniques or mass palpation, ultrasound guidance improves the accuracy of cellular recovery. Blood contamination is a particularly common problem with joint aspirates. The use of small-gauge needles, gentle aspiration with no redirection of the needle, and patience as the viscous fluid is collected are helpful. If the disease process appears multifocal, multiple joints should be aspirated.

SLIDE PREPARATION

The quality of the slide depends not only on the number of cells collected but the percentage of cells that remain intact and available for microscopic evaluation. Artifactual cell rupturing and cellular distribution on the slides can be affected greatly by the techniques used in slide preparation. Smears should be made immediately after the material has been placed on the slide. If a large amount of material is collected, placing a portion on more than one slide helps avoid preparations that are too thick.

Having too much material on a slide initially greatly diminishes the chance of spreading it into a monolayer that can be easily assessed microscopically. Making multiple slides increases the chance of obtaining a diagnostic sample. In addition, material that is placed near the end or edges of a slide may be difficult to bring into focus at different magnifications. The ultimate goal is to have a well-prepared slide with many intact, representative cells. A description of the two most common slide preparation techniques follows.

Making Smears

Cells from lesions or organs that are deemed to be fragile can best be prepared using the *vertical pull-apart* technique (Fig. 64-1). The cells collected within the needle are pushed onto the center of the first slide. The center of the second slide is gently placed at right angles directly down on the cellular material, which then spreads between the slides. If the material is too thick, very gentle compression of the slides may be necessary. With as little rotational motion or shear force as possible, the two slides should be separated vertically; the material is likely to be fairly evenly distributed between the two slides, providing mirror images of the cytology preparation. This technique is often required for fragile tissues such as lymph nodes, and it is particularly useful when lymphoma is suspected since malignant lymphocytes are often even more fragile than healthy normal lymphocytes. A potential negative outcome of preparing a vertical pull-apart slide is that cells are not allowed to separate as well as with other methods and many areas may be too thick to evaluate properly. This can result in particular difficulty in differentiating cells that are truly clustering (epithelial origin) from cells that are simply very close together because of the method of slide preparation, thereby leading to confusion regarding the type of tumor represented on the slide.

Most tissues have cells that can withstand some degree of shear force and trauma in preparation without causing widespread cellular disruption. These samples and materials collected by scraping or other thick preparations should be prepared by *horizontal pull-apart* techniques (Fig. 64-2). In this case cells are pushed from the needle

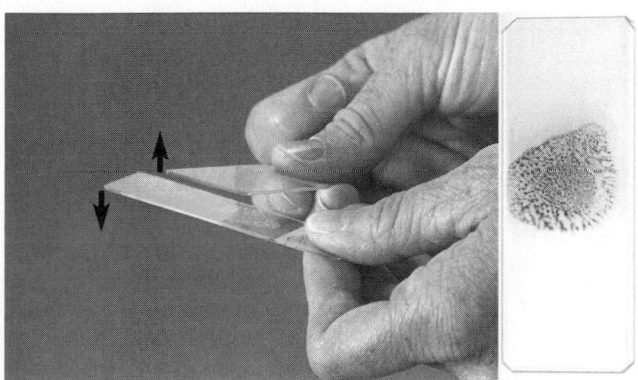

Fig. 64-1 Technique for making vertical pull-apart slides. The stained specimen on the right represents a properly prepared vertical pull-apart slide.

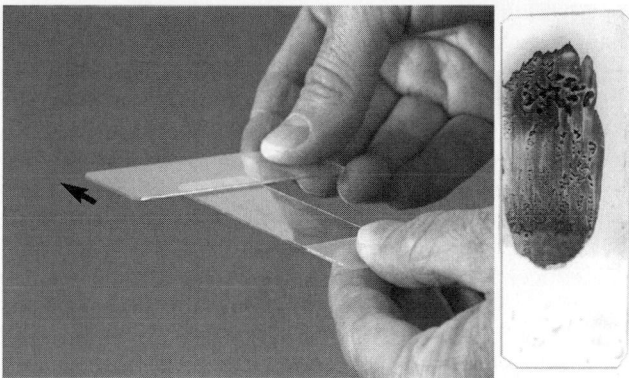

Fig. 64-2 Technique for making horizontal pull-apart slides. The stained specimen on the right represents a properly prepared horizontal pull-apart slide.

onto one end of the slide. The second slide is used to smear the cellular material along the length of the first slide in a continuous motion, with the flat surfaces of the slides remaining parallel to one another. In most cases the majority of the cellular material remains with the first slide. One form of a horizontal preparation is the technique used to make a blood smear. A small drop of thin fluid is placed at one end of the slide while a second slide is pulled backward at a 45-degree angle to touch the drop, which spreads along the surface of contact. The second slide is advanced immediately, spreading the cellular material along the length of the first slide. The advantage of a horizontal preparation is that the cells are spread more thinly over the length of the slide and there is less confusion regarding the spatial relationship of the cells to one another. The most important disadvantage is a greater risk of cellular rupture.

After collection of a fluid sample (pleural, pericardial, peritoneal, or joint effusions; transtracheal wash; bronchoalveolar lavage; peritoneal lavage; prostatic or bladder wash), aliquots should immediately be placed in ethylenediaminetetraacetic acid tubes to prevent clotting and appropriately collected for culture and sensitivity testing if indicated. Cytologic smears should be made quickly after fluid collection. Direct smears are made from well-mixed fluid or alternatively from the spun pellet of cells after centrifugation. The slide made from a drop of the fluid or sediment can be prepared vertically, horizontally, or similar to blood smear preparation.

Fixation and Staining

Ideally, when several slides are made, a few should remain unstained in the event that special procedures are required at a later time. The most common cytologic stains used in the practice setting are Romanowsky-type stains such as Diff-Quik and occasionally new methylene blue. Although new methylene blue provides wonderful nuclear detail, the visual aesthetics, practicality, and permanence of the Romanowsky-type stains make them the most useful agents for routine cytology. They are inexpensive, easily obtained, and simple to use. These polychromatic stains highlight organisms and cytoplasm very well, and nuclear and nucleolar detail is usually adequate for assessing inflammation, neoplasia, and characteristics of malignancy. Smears must first be air dried, which allows the cells to adhere to the slide. With most staining kits there are typically four individual steps. The first is fixation of the cells; lipid droplets from ruptured lipocytes often dissolve in this step. The red and blue stains follow, and then the slides are rinsed. Each manufacturer recommends specific staining procedures, but in general the thinner the smear and the lower the total protein concentration on the slide, the less time required for staining. Conversely, the thicker the preparation and the higher the total protein concentration, the more time the slide needs to remain in contact with the stain. Therefore, based on the perceived cellularity and thickness of the preparation, the clinician must adjust the amount of time used in the staining procedure. Drying the slides is important before evaluating them microscopically with oil immersion lenses. A nail dryer can be modified for use if several slides need to dry simultaneously. The patient and the site of cell collection should be clearly identified on all slides.

If cytology specimens will be submitted to an outside laboratory, all glass slides should be packaged in such a way that breakage is avoided. Steps should be taken to prevent motion of the slides, even within commercially available slide holders; a box within a box is a common approach. It is important to remember that, if cytology slides are packaged with samples for histopathology, formalin fumes can inhibit the cells from adequately taking up stain. Ideally two to three air-dried, unfixed slides and two to three stained slides should be submitted to the cytologist for evaluation.

COMMONLY ENCOUNTERED PROBLEMS

The clinician must feel comfortable that the submitted material is representative of the disease process, thus it is important for the individual collecting the material to look at slides before submission to ensure that adequate, representative material has been collected before the patient leaves the hospital. There are a variety of reasons why a slide may not contain adequate diagnostic material. Some lesions, particularly mesenchymal tumors, do not typically exfoliate well; the needle can miss the lesion, or an area of central necrosis within a tumor can be aspirated. Making several slides from multiple locations can be helpful in obtaining a representative diagnostic specimen. Excessive blood contamination can dilute tissue cells and cause clotting of the sample, make diagnosis more difficult. Using smaller-gauge needles, less aggressive aspiration, or the coring technique can help diminish blood contamination.

Poorly stained specimens can result from inadequate staining times or weakened stain from overuse or dilution. The stains may need to be changed at different intervals based on frequency of use and thickness of the specimens. In addition, the stains should be changed when unexpected contaminating organisms or cells appear on slides. It is helpful to have two separate sets of stain available, one for cytology and one for "contaminated" samples such as ear or fecal swabs. Typically the blue stain and the rinse need to be changed most frequently. If a slide needs to be restained, skip the fixative step, dip the slide a few more times in the red and blue stains, and then rinse again.

One criticism of Diff-Quik stain is that, since it does not undergo the metachromatic reaction, granules from some mast cell tumors do not stain. I have only rarely found this to be a problem in the clinical setting. However, if mast cell tumor is suspected, new methylene blue or Giemsa stain can be used to demonstrate the presence of mast cell granules.

Cellular collection and slide preparation are the first steps in using cytology as a diagnostic tool; the ability to accurately interpret what is on the slide becomes the next limiting factor. Many clinicians are extremely capable of slide interpretation, and with practice every clinician can continue to improve. One simple method of practicing these skills is to make a cytology preparation each time a biopsy specimen is submitted to the laboratory. When the histopathology report returns, results are compared, and the cytology slide reviewed again. If most cytologies are sent to a diagnostic laboratory for interpretation, developing a good working relationship with the cytologist is critical. The clinician's role is to provide high-quality specimens with accurate clinical information so that the cytologist has every opportunity to be an effective part of the diagnostic team.

Suggested Reading

Meyer DJ: The acquisition and management of cytology specimens. In Raskin RE, Meyer DJ, editors: *Atlas of canine and feline cytology*, Philadelphia, 2001, Saunders, p 1.

Meyer DJ: The essentials of diagnostic cytology in clinical oncology. In Withrow SJ, MacEwen EG, editors: *Small animal clinical oncology*, Philadelphia, 2001, Saunders, p 54.

Morrison WB, editor: *Cancer in dogs and cats: medical and surgical management*, Jackson, WY, 2002, Teton New Media.

Rogers KS, Barton CL, Habron JM: Cytology during surgery, *Compend Cont Educ Pract Vet* 18:153, 1996.

Tyler RD et al: Introduction. In Cowell RL, Tyler RD, Meinkoth JH, editors: *Diagnostic cytology and hematology of the dog and cat*, St. Louis, 1999, Mosby, p 1.

CHAPTER 65

Anticancer Drugs and Protocols: Traditional Drugs

ANTONY S. MOORE, *Wauchope, New South Wales, Australia*
ANGELA E. FRIMBERGER, *Wauchope, New South Wales, Australia*

INTRODUCTION TO CHEMOTHERAPY

As the only major cancer treatment modality to exert systemic effects, chemotherapy is the principal approach for treatment of systemic or metastatic malignancies. In managing chemotherapy, effective communication between the veterinarian and the pet owner is essential. Clients should understand that quality of life is the primary goal in most veterinary chemotherapy situations, and that adverse effects of chemotherapy are less severe than those seen in human patients. In veterinary chemotherapy, dose intensity is modified to avoid most unacceptable adverse effects. Of course, the definition of "unacceptable" is subjective. For some owners it may be *any* loss of quality of life, whereas for others it may be the need for hospitalization. Because quality of life for humans depends largely on preservation of body image as well as organ function, owners may interpret their pet's well-being in similar terms. The veterinarian can help clients understand that these benchmarks are not necessarily valid for animals. When proposing chemotherapy, all therapeutic options should be presented, and the clients should be encouraged to ask questions and communicate their concerns. A continuing, open dialogue allows the client to make an informed decision and will ultimately create a "team" approach to treatment of the pet's cancer. Supplementing verbal instructions with written information about the disease and the treatment to be used will greatly assist owners in making decisions and retaining information.

It is important to determine the goal of treatment at the outset because it often determines the course of therapy. *Cure*, the permanent eradication of all tumor cells, is an ideal outcome although not always realistic in veterinary oncology. If treatment is to be undertaken with curative intent, a greater likelihood of adverse effects may be accepted because of greater potential long-term benefit. *Palliation* is designed to improve quality of life but without expectation of cure; therefore the drug dosages and schedules used are less likely to result in adverse effects. In veterinary medicine this may result in prolonged survival because euthanasia is delayed.

Staging and Health

Before undertaking any treatment, it is important to establish the definitive diagnosis, the clinical stage of disease, and the patient's overall health. The histologic diagnosis and stage are important both in establishing a prognosis and prescribing a treatment plan, and prognostic information assists the client in choosing a goal of treatment. The general health screen is necessary to determine if other conditions are present that may affect the patient's life expectancy (e.g., other systemic disease), that need to be resolved before starting chemotherapy (e.g., subclinical urinary tract infection), or that need to be taken into account in planning chemotherapy (e.g., subclinical cardiac or renal disease).

The likelihood of a successful outcome for a patient treated with chemotherapy is as dependent on drug metabolism and elimination (and drug absorption for orally administered chemotherapy) as it is on the sensitivity of the tumor. Consequently information gained during staging may identify problems that will impact the type and dosage of chemotherapy to optimize efficacy while limiting toxicity. For example, hepatic dysfunction may lead to delayed drug elimination (e.g., vinca alkaloids, doxorubicin [DOX]) and therefore greater toxicity such as myelosuppression. In contrast, cyclophosphamide is activated in the liver; thus hepatic dysfunction may result in poor efficacy. Similarly, preexisting renal dysfunction predisposes to increased toxicity of nephrotoxic drugs, whereas reduced renal excretion of carboplatin exacerbates myelosuppression.

Drug Choice

There are no strictly veterinary chemotherapy drugs. However, there is an established track record for most of the older human drugs, particularly those that have been used for the treatment of lymphoma and osteosarcoma (OSA). The body of literature available means that veterinarians should feel secure in using dosages and schedules provided in published protocols. Treatment using most veterinary drugs is expected to result in less than 20% need for dose reductions (hospitalization, severe neutropenia) and less than 5% risk of life-threatening toxicity when established dosages are used, with less than 1% risk of treatment-related mortality.

Because the costs of drug development are high, newer chemotherapeutic drugs may be quite costly. However, generic versions of many older drugs are available (vincristine, DOX, cisplatin). Some pharmacies supply small quantities of injectable drugs to veterinarians, and compounding pharmacies reformulate smaller dosages of oral medications (e.g., lomustine [CCNU], procarbazine) for cats and small dogs.

Clinical veterinary chemotherapy research is advancing at a great rate. However, even when clinical trials are completed, it may be a year or more until the results are published. The best resources for veterinary practitioners are veterinary oncologists, the Veterinary Cancer Society (www.vetcancersociety.org), and Internet literature databases such as Medline (www.ncbi.nlm.nih.gov/entrez).

Timing of Chemotherapy

Veterinary chemotherapy protocols are often very simple, consisting of one or two agents given at an interval that minimizes the risk of toxicity but maintains the highest possible dose intensity (e.g., cisplatin as an adjuvant to surgery for dogs with OSA). In contrast, lymphoma protocols are often more complex, with many agents scheduled in combination (Table 65-1).

Primary Treatment

In veterinary oncology primary chemotherapy is usually reserved for hematopoietic tumors (LSA, leukemias, multiple myeloma). The use of chemotherapy alone for solid tumors (carcinomas and sarcomas) is rarely successful and is better considered to be palliative. The stages of a primary chemotherapy protocol can include:

Induction: Often intensely scheduled initial treatments during which a patient has a relatively higher risk of toxicity but usually also the greatest chance of response (e.g., the first 12 weeks of VELCAP).

Consolidation: Sometimes used at the end of induction using unrelated, effective drugs to further reduce the proportion of surviving cancer cells (e.g.,

mechlorethamine, Oncovin, procarbazine, prednisone [MOPP] and CCNU in VELCAP-SC).

Maintenance: A less intense (usually decreased frequency of administration) phase using drugs already used during induction. Maintenance therapy probably has little influence on whether an animal is cured or not but may prolong survival in animals by slowing the time to relapse.

Rescue: Therapy given when drugs used during the other three phases are no longer effective. Unrelated drugs, often alkylating agents because they are less likely to show cross-resistance, are used in the rescue setting.

Adjuvant Treatment

Chemotherapy can be used in combination with other modalities, including surgery, radiation therapy, or both. Adjuvant chemotherapy is used following resection of a primary tumor with significant metastatic risk to delay or prevent the progression of metastatic disease. The optimum time to administer adjuvant chemotherapy is when the metastatic disease is microscopic rather than when there are gross metastases. An example of successful adjuvant veterinary chemotherapy is the use of platinum compounds and/or DOX following surgery for canine OSA.

Chemotherapy Dosing

Most chemotherapy drugs have narrow therapeutic margins (i.e., the host toxic dose is very close to the effective dose). Therefore it is important to calculate doses as accurately as possible. Although imperfect, current dosage recommendations for most chemotherapy drugs are based on "metabolic body size" (body surface area [BSA], m^2). This scheme implies that smaller animals have a higher metabolic rate and therefore should receive a higher dosage

Table 65-1

Schedule of Chemotherapy Administration for Tufts VELCAP-SC for Canine Lymphoma

Week	VCR	L-Asp	CTX	DOX	Must	Procarb	Pred	CCNU
1	X	X					X	
2	X						X	
3				X			X	
4		X					X	
5	X		X				X	
6								
7				X				
8								
9	X		X					
11				X				
13	X				X	X	X	
14	X				X	X	X	
17								X
18								
20								X

CTX, Cyclophosphamide; *DOX,* doxorubicin; *L-Asp,* L-asparaginase; *Must,* mechlorethamine; *Pred,* prednisone; *Procarb,* procarbazine; *VCR,* vincristine.
Remission is induced over 11 weeks with a combination of VCR (0.75 mg/m² IV), L-asp (10,000 units/m² SQ, maximum dose 10,000 units), DOX (<1 m² = 1 mg/kg IV, >1 m² = 30 mg/m²), *CTX,* (200 mg/m² IV plus furosemide 2 mg/kg IV once) and a tapering dose of Pred starting at 40 mg/m² PO daily. Dogs in remission at week 13 receive consolidation treatments of MOPP (Must [3 mg/m² IV], VCR [0.5 mg/ m² IV], Procarb [50 mg/m² PO daily × 14 days], and Pred [40 mg/ m² PO daily ×14 days]) at weeks 13 and 14, followed by lomustine (CCNU) (60-90 mg/m² PO once) at weeks 17 and 20. Dogs that are in complete remission (CR) by week 21 discontinue chemotherapy.

on a body weight basis. For some drugs (e.g., DOX), dosage based on BSA is imperfect, and small dogs and cats should be dosed at a lower rate than large dogs. For other drugs (e.g., ifosfamide) the dosage for cats is entirely different, whereas yet other drugs (e.g., cisplatin) should be avoided altogether in cats. Until further guidelines are available, the veterinarian should check the species- and body size specific dosing basis for any drug to be used, become familiar with the individual drugs that require a lower dosage for small pets, and use a BSA conversion table when metabolic dosing is indicated.

When oral chemotherapeutics are used, the need for accurate dosing can be confounded by the available tablet or capsule sizes, particularly in cats and small dogs. It is important to use a compounding pharmacy to reformulate oral chemotherapeutics to maintain accurate dosing for smaller pets. Tablets and capsules should never be split or opened by veterinarians or pet caregivers because it results in both inaccurate dosing and drug exposure.

The concept of *dose intensity* is an important principle of chemotherapy. It is defined as milligrams per square meter of drug per week of therapy and should be the highest tolerated by the animal with minimal toxicity. For example, in dosing of myelosuppressive drugs, because there will be variation in individual metabolism of drugs and in the sensitivity of normal tissues, the aim should be to deliver doses that produce a neutrophil nadir of between 1000 and 1500 cells per microliter. There is ample evidence in both human and veterinary oncology that optimal dose intensity improves the outcome for chemotherapy.

Drug Combinations and Drug Resistance

Combination chemotherapy has two major aims. The first is to slow the onset of drug resistance in tumor cells. The use of agents that have differing targets and mechanisms of action is most likely to provide long-term tumor control. The use of alkylating agents in combination protocols for lymphoma may slow the development of multiple drug resistance (see Section IV on Evolve). The second aim of combination chemotherapy is to maximize tumor cell kill while minimizing toxicity. Combinations that include myelosuppressive drugs with drugs that are minimally myelosuppressive may fulfill this aim (e.g., cyclophosphamide and vincristine; DOX and cisplatin). It is important that combinations use *effective* drugs; there is little point in using a nontoxic combination when one drug is not efficacious against the tumor. Therefore combinations use drugs that have activity as single agents. Some combinations may result in altered toxicity because of changes in the way a drug is metabolized or excreted. For example, L-asparaginase is thought to slow hepatic metabolism of drugs such as vincristine and DOX, thereby increasing the risk of myelosuppression. The practitioner is wise to use only combinations for which published efficacy and toxicity data are available.

Toxicity, Monitoring, and Support

Chemotherapy toxicity is usually dose related; and, because most chemotherapy drugs are effective in the active phases of the cell cycle, renewing tissues are most commonly affected.

Hematologic

Myelosuppression is a general term applied to the toxic effects of chemotherapy on the bone marrow. In veterinary clinical practice the dose-limiting aspect of myelosuppression is usually *neutropenia*. In general the prognosis for uncomplicated myelosuppression is good, and most veterinary patients recover within a few days. Most myelosuppressed dogs and cats have no clinical signs at all. The nadir (low point) of peripheral neutrophil counts occurs between 5 and 10 days after a myelosuppressive insult. Thus the usual timing for myelosuppressive drug administration is every 2 to 3 weeks. Some drugs (e.g., CCNU and carboplatin) may have delayed or prolonged nadirs, and dosing intervals may be longer for these drugs.

A complete blood count (CBC), including a platelet count, should be collected at the expected neutrophil nadir, usually 1 week after chemotherapy administration. The absolute neutrophil count (not the total leukocyte count) should be evaluated. Neutrophil recovery is usually rapid; however, a nadir of less than 1000 neutrophils per microliter should prompt a 20% to 25% dosage reduction for all subsequent administrations of that drug. It is not necessary to reduce the dosage of other myelosuppressive drugs since they may not cause the same degree of suppression. Each drug should be assessed individually. If the dose is reduced, CBC should be repeated after the next dose.

A CBC should also be assessed immediately before the next chemotherapy treatment; neutropenia is a reason to delay administration of a myelosuppressive drug (but not a nonmyelosuppressive drug such as L-asparaginase or prednisone). In general a neutrophil count of less than 3000/μL requires a chemotherapy delay of several days to 1 week before rechecking the CBC. If recovery is prolonged (e.g., many cats and some dogs after receiving carboplatin), it may be necessary to reduce the dosage so that the optimal intertreatment interval and dose intensity may be maintained.

Occasionally neutropenia may be severe (<500 cells per microliter) at the nadir. The risk of sepsis is low in animals that are receiving concurrent antibiotics because the nadir rarely persists for more than 2 to 3 days. Many oncologists recommend use of a prophylactic broad-spectrum, oral antibiotic (such as trimethoprim-sulfa [TMS], 15 mg/kg q12h orally [PO]) for patients receiving a myelosuppressive agent for the first time. If the nadir is more than 1500 neutrophils per microliter, subsequent administrations may be given without prophylactic antibiotics. Administration of TMS to dogs for 14 days from the day of treatment with DOX reduces the risk of gastrointestinal toxicity (vomiting or diarrhea) and hospitalization and improves quality of life. The effect is most marked in dogs with lymphoma and may be caused by reduced bacterial translocation in damaged intestinal epithelium.

When a patient is severely neutropenic, it is tempting to use recombinant granulocyte colony-stimulating factor (G-CSF). Dogs that are neutropenic have high endogenous G-CSF and are unlikely to benefit from exogenous administration. In addition, the available human recombinant product (hr-G-CSF; Neupogen, Amgen) carries a risk of inducing neutralizing and cross-reacting anticanine G-CSF antibodies. Appropriate use of hr-G-CSF would be when an inadvertent and potentially lethal chemotherapy overdose has been delivered. For such a patient, hr-G-CSF from 24 hours after chemotherapy administration and beyond the neutrophil nadir has the best chance of preventing sepsis and death (see Section IV on Evolve for additional information about hematopoietic growth factors in oncology).

Thrombocytopenia may be dose limiting for select chemotherapy agents (carboplatin, cumulative for CCNU) but is rarely clinically significant for other drugs. Thrombocytopenia infrequently causes clinical signs; however, at counts less than 50,000/μL the risk of bleeding increases, and the veterinarian should be alert to petechiation, ecchymoses, or mucosal bleeding. Platelet nadirs occur later than neutrophil nadirs but are rarely as severe, and recovery is slower but usually complete. Significant thrombocytopenia in a patient scheduled to receive CCNU should prompt discontinuation.

Gastrointestinal

The gastrointestinal mucosa is another site of renewing tissue, and clinical signs include inappetence, anorexia, nausea, vomiting, or diarrhea, usually occurring 3 to 5 days following treatment. Supportive care is important in prophylaxis and treatment. In general the use of antiemetics and appetite stimulants can prevent mild toxicities. Diarrhea may be treated with dietary management, sulfasalazine, or metronidazole once specific causes have been eliminated. Chemotherapy doses should be reduced if the pet requires hospitalization for gastrointestinal signs or if such signs are unacceptable to the owner. With a 20% to 25% dosage reduction it is very unlikely that subsequent chemotherapy administration will be associated with toxicity.

Anorexia is a common side effect of chemotherapy in cats (particularly DOX or vincristine). Cyproheptadine (0.35 to 1 mg/kg PO q12-24h in cats and 0.3 to 2 mg/kg PO q12h in dogs) may stimulate appetite. Megestrol acetate is an effective appetite stimulant in cats at a dosage of 0.25 to 0.5 mg/kg daily for 3 to 5 days and then every 2 to 3 days. In humans megestrol acetate not only improves appetite but also enhances enjoyment of food. It should be used with caution in cats as it may induce diabetes mellitus.

Vincristine may result in intestinal ileus in cats and less commonly in dogs. Prokinetic drugs such as metoclopramide may prevent or reverse this toxicity. The use of prophylactic metoclopramide is recommended by some practitioners to reduce the risk of inappetence caused by vincristine and also DOX (perhaps by central action to reduce nausea). In the prophylactic setting treatment is started at the time of chemotherapy and continued for 4 to 5 days. Before administering strong emetogens such as cisplatin, owners should withhold food since this reduces the risk of vomiting and may prevent future "aversion" to that food.

The recent introduction of serotonin antagonists such as ondansetron and dolasetron has dramatically reduced gastrointestinal toxicity for animals treated with many drugs. Nausea and vomiting leading to inappetence, dehydration, and weight loss are possible following treatment with drugs such as cisplatin (in dogs) and DOX (in cats and dogs). Dolasetron (0.5 to 1 mg/kg intravenously [IV] or PO given once 20 to 30 minutes before treatment) may

markedly reduce the risk of this toxicity. A recently released veterinary product, maropitant citrate (Cerenia™, 1 mg/kg SQ q 24h) up to 5 days, a neurokinin 1(NK1) antagonist, appears to be very effective in the prevention and treatment of nausea and vomiting in dogs given chemotherapy.

Diet should be appropriate and consistent. Prophylactic use of absorbents such as kaolin may reduce the risk of diarrhea. If diarrhea occurs, a bland diet should be offered; if it persists and other causes such as parasitism in immunocompromised patients have been eliminated, sulfasalazine or metronidazole may reduce the severity. Prophylactic TMS should be considered (see earlier discussion).

Cardiac

In veterinary oncology cardiotoxicity is only a problem clinically with DOX in dogs. Chronic cardiotoxicity is one of the few irreversible chemotherapy toxicities and carries a poor to grave prognosis. The end result resembles dilated cardiomyopathy and congestive heart failure. Injury to the conduction system also may develop. The occurrence of cardiotoxicity is related to the total cumulative dose of DOX rather than the amount of each individual dosage. Although cardiotoxicity in dogs can occur at any cumulative dosage, it is most frequent above 180 mg/m^2, and DOX should not be given above this level without echocardiographic monitoring. As DOX cardiotoxicity is usually progressive, treatment should be discontinued if contractility is below normal while the patient is still asymptomatic rather than waiting for signs of early cardiac failure.

Breeds susceptible to cardiomyopathy, such as the Doberman pinscher, are more susceptible to this toxicity at lower cumulative doses and should be treated with caution if at all. In dogs with valvular dysfunction, mild changes in cardiac muscle function caused by early DOX cardiotoxicity may exacerbate the clinical signs of the valvular disease. In these patients echocardiography should be performed periodically through treatment, ideally before each treatment.

The cardioprotective beta-blocker carvedilol has strong antioxidant properties and in experimental studies protects cardiomyocytes from doxorubicin-induced injury. Whether or not this treatment has clinical merit in veterinary practice requires appropriate clinical study.

Urinary Tract

Nephrotoxicity is the primary dose-limiting toxicity of cisplatin and also carries a poor prognosis. Its occurrence depends on both the individual and cumulative dosage and is dramatically reduced by pretreatment and posttreatment fluid diuresis. DOX has been anecdotally associated with nephrotoxicity in cats. Renal function should be assessed by serum creatinine and urine specific gravity before administration of nephrotoxic drugs or renally excreted drugs (carboplatin).

Urothelial toxicity (sterile hemorrhagic cystitis) is associated with cyclophosphamide and ifosfamide administration in dogs. Cyclophosphamide and ifosfamide are hepatically metabolized to their active forms and other metabolites, including acrolein. Prolonged contact between the bladder wall and acrolein results in hemorrhagic cystitis. Severity of clinical signs varies; but stranguria, dysuria, and hematuria can be severe and prolonged over many weeks. Furosemide (2 mg/kg) given once at the time of cyclophosphamide administration almost completely abrogates this toxicity and is recommended even in dogs receiving concurrent prednisone. Allowing ample opportunity for the dog to void urine is also important, and cyclophosphamide preferably is administered in the morning rather than late in the day. This toxicity should be distinguished from infectious cystitis by bacterial culture; however, even if bacteria are isolated and signs resolve with antibiotic administration, the drug should not be administered again because infectious cystitis could have been secondary to chemical irritation. Symptomatic treatment includes antiinflammatory drugs (e.g., piroxicam 0.3 mg/kg once daily in dogs, not concurrent with corticosteroids). For prolonged cases intravesicular dimethylsulfoxide may accelerate recovery.

Hepatotoxicity

Liver enzyme serum activities (alanine aminotransferase [ALT]) should be assessed before CCNU administration. Irreversible hepatic toxicity can result if CCNU therapy is continued in the face of rising serum ALT concentrations. Elevations in serum bilirubin should also prompt dose reductions in hepatically metabolized drugs.

Soft Tissue

Whenever chemotherapy is given IV, a catheter should be used rather than a needle. Extravasation is rarely a problem if chemotherapy is administered carefully through an over-the-needle catheter placed as the first puncture in an intact vein. The catheter should be tested with a saline flush both before the drug is administered and after infusion is complete. If any drug is extravasated, as much drug as possible should be aspirated before removing the catheter. For vinca alkaloids warm compresses should be applied; for anthracyclines ice should be applied.

Hypersensitivity

Hypersensitivity reactions may occur during DOX administration as a result of histamine release from mast cells. This effect only occurs with rapid administration and is not a problem if the drug is given slowly. True anaphylaxis may occur following L-asparaginase administration, particularly by the IV or intraperitoneal route. This toxicity is rare if L-asparaginase is administered intramuscularly (IM) or subcutaneously (SQ).

Felines

Specific cat toxicities may occur with chemotherapy. Cisplatin causes a fatal, acute pulmonary edema in cats and should not be administered systemically. Any administration of 5-fluorouracil causes acute fatal neurotoxicity in cats, and products containing this drug should not be used.

SPECIFIC CHEMOTHERAPEUTIC AGENTS

Alkylating Agents

Alkylating agents create cross-links in deoxyribonucleic acid (DNA), causing strand breaks. An interesting feature of this class of drugs is the apparent lack of cross-resistance between different alkylating agents or with other classes of drugs.

Cyclophosphamide

Used primarily for treatment of lymphoma in dogs and cats
Route: PO or IV
Dosage: Dogs 200-250 mg/m^2; cats 250-300 mg/m^2 (see specific protocol)
Monitor: CBC

Chlorambucil

Used primarily for treatment of chronic lymphocytic leukemia or low-grade lymphoma in dogs and cats; also as a substitute for cyclophosphamide if hemorrhagic cystitis occurs
Route: PO
Dosage: Dogs and cats: 6-8 mg/m^2 daily for 14 days and then every other day *or* 15 mg/m^2 for 4 consecutive days repeated every 3 weeks
Monitor: Neutropenia and thrombocytopenia can occur; however, severe myelosuppression is rare at doses used in animals. Monitor CBC every 2 weeks for first 6 weeks and then every 3 months. Monitor liver enzymes (ALT) on same schedule.

Melphalan

Used primarily for treatment of multiple myeloma in dogs and cats
Route: PO
Dosage: Dogs and cats: 1.5 mg/m^2 alternate days or 10 days on, 10 days off (see individual protocol)
Monitor: CBC

Mechlorethamine

Used in MOPP protocol for LSA in dogs and cats
Route: IV (caution for extravasation)
Dosage: Dogs and cats: in MOPP, 3 mg/m^2
Monitor: CBC

Procarbazine

Used in MOPP protocol for LSA in dogs and cats
Route: PO
Dosage: Dogs and cats: 50 mg/m^2 daily for 14 days *or* 10 mg/cat daily for 14 days
Monitor: CBC. In humans myelosuppression may occur 2-3 weeks after cessation of therapy. There is limited information for dogs and cats.

Lomustine (CCNU)

Used for treatment of lymphoma, mast cell tumors, brain tumors (responses in gliomas and meningiomas), and malignant histiocytosis
Route: PO
Dosage: Dogs: 60-90 mg/m^2 every 3-4 weeks or according to protocol (lower doses for small dogs); cats: 50-60 mg/m^2 every 4-6 weeks (reformulated)
Monitor: CBC and platelet counts immediately before and 7 days after each treatment. Leukopenia and thrombocytopenia are expected, it is dose limiting, and it may be cumulative. Platelet counts are obtained immediately before CCNU treatments because of the potential hazard of delayed, irreversible

thrombocytopenia. Serum ALT and creatinine are obtained before each treatment because of potential hepatic and renal toxicities.

Antitumor Antibiotics

These drugs act by DNA intercalation, interfering with topoisomerases and other mechanisms. They can exhibit cross-resistance with other drugs, mediated by the MDR drug efflux pump.

Doxorubicin

The most active single agent in treatment of lymphoma in dogs and highly effective in combinations for lymphoma in dogs and cats; broad-spectrum efficacy in treatment of solid tumors, particularly OSA, and in combinations with cyclophosphamide

Route: IV with caution for extravasation: slowly inject into the injection port on the line of a running infusion of 0.9% saline over 20 minutes; wait for the color to clear before giving next small amount. NOTE: may be associated with histamine release and anaphylactoid reaction. Use plain normal saline for flushing—heparin may cause a precipitate to form.
Dosage: Large dogs: 30 mg/m²; small dogs: 1 mg/kg; cats: 1 mg/kg or 25 mg/m²; given every 2 to 3 weeks or according to protocol
Monitor: CBC, gastrointestinal signs (colitis, vomiting), liver function, electrocardiogram/echocardiogram; cats: monitor renal function

Mitoxantrone

Efficacious in combination with piroxicam for transitional cell carcinoma in dogs; moderate efficacy for lymphoma in dogs, low in cats; used as substitute for DOX in dogs at risk for cardiotoxicity and cats at risk for nephrotoxicity
Route: IV: slowly inject (with caution to prevent extravasation) into the injection port on the line of a running infusion of 0.9% saline over 10 minutes; wait for the color to clear before giving next small amount.
Dosage: Dogs: 5-6 mg/m² (5.5 mg/m² if less than 15 kg of body weight) every 3 weeks; cats: 5-6.5 mg/m² every 3 weeks
Monitor: CBC

Actinomycin-D

Alternative to DOX for canine lymphoma
Route: IV over 10 minutes with caution for extravasation: slowly inject into the injection port on the line of a running infusion of 0.9% saline over 10 minutes; wait for the color to clear before giving next small amount; discard unused solution.
Dosage: In protocol; 0.5 to 0.8 mg/m² IV every 1 to 3 weeks
Monitor: CBC and gastrointestinal signs

Platinum Drugs

Platinum compounds create cross-links in DNA. These drugs are similar to alkylating agents, and there is no cross-resistance with other classes of chemotherapeutic drugs.

Cisplatin

Efficacious in treatment of canine OSA and many carcinomas; not to be used in cats because of high risk of fatal pulmonary edema
Route: IV, intracavitary or intralesional, according to protocol
Dosage: *DO NOT USE IN CATS.*
Cisplatin *must* be preceded and followed by a diuresis period. Dogs (every 3-4 weeks):
<5 kg: 50 mg/m²; 5-20 kg: 60 mg/m², >20 kg: 70 mg/m²
Administration: Needles or intravenous sets containing aluminum parts that may come in contact with solution should not be used for preparation or administration. Aluminum reacts with cisplatin, causing precipitate formation and loss of potency.

1. Pretreatment fluid diuresis: 4 hours at 18.3 ml/kg/hour using 0.9% NaCl
2. Antiemetic administration (e.g., dolasetron 0.6-1 mg/kg slowly IV) 15 minutes before cisplatin
3. Cisplatin: diluted in 6.1 ml/kg 0.9% NaCl to be given at same fluid rate over 20 minutes
4. Posttreatment diuresis: 2 hours at 18.3 ml/kg/hr using 0.9% NaCl

Monitor: Vomiting immediately after treatment (may need intravenous fluid support); CBC day 7 and 14 after treatment; renal function (serum creatinine and urine specific gravity) before each treatment
Cisplatin is excreted primarily in the urine over 48 hours following administration. *Avoid contact with urine* and discard rather than wash soiled bedding.

Carboplatin

Has efficacy similar to cisplatin without apparent renal toxicity; safe for use in cats
Route: IV, according to protocol; intracavitary or intralesional has been reported; 10 mg/ml diluted to a total dosage volume of 50 ml with *5% dextrose*: slowly inject into the injection port in the line of a running infusion of *5% dextrose* over 15-20 minutes
Dosage: Dogs (every 3-4 weeks): <15 kg: 250 mg/m²; >15 kg: 300 mg/m²; cats: 210 mg/m² for cats every 4 weeks (individual variability: see protocol)
In azotemic animals ideally calculate dose based on glomerular filtration rate if possible; otherwise arbitrarily reduce dose by 50% to 75%.
Monitoring: Creatinine before each treatment; reduce dose if creatinine is elevated; CBC at 7, 14, *and* 21 day

Enzymes

L-Asparaginase

Used in combination for lymphoma in dogs (not as single agent because of rapid resistance)
Route: SQ or IM *(can cause an anaphylactic reaction if given IV)*
Dosage: Dogs and cats: 10,000 units/m² (maximum dose at any one time is 10,000 units)
Reconstitute with 2 ml 0.9% NaCl slowly (will form bubbles if mixed too fast) to final concentration of 5000 units/ml.

Mitotic Inhibitors: Plant Alkaloids

Vinca alkaloids inhibit assembly of the mitotic spindle.

Vincristine

Curative for canine transmissible venereal tumor;
effective for lymphoma in dogs and cats; included in
some combinations for treatment of sarcomas; not
effective for mast cell tumor
Route: IV bolus with caution for extravasation
Dosage: 0.5-0.75 mg/m² or according to protocol
Monitor: CBC

Vinblastine

Effective for lymphoma in dogs and cats but less used
because of myelosuppression (making it harder than
vincristine to include with other drugs); efficacious
for mast cell tumors in dogs
Route: IV bolus with caution for extravasation
Dosage: 2 mg/m² every 7-14 days (but see individual
protocol)
Monitor: CBC 7 days after administration

Antimetabolites

Antimetabolites are analogs of normal metabolites and
are incorporated into DNA where they interfere with
enzyme activity or transcription or translation. These
drugs often have significant toxicity with low efficacy at
veterinary dosages; thus they are not in frequent use in veterinary oncology.

Suggested Reading

Frimberger AE: Anticancer drugs: new drugs or applications for
veterinary medicine. In Bonagura JD, editor: *Kirk's current vet-
erinary therapy XIII*, Philadelphia, Saunders, 2000, p 474.
Frimberger AE: Principles of chemotherapy. In Ettinger SJ,
Feldman EC, editors: *Textbook of veterinary internal medicine*, ed
6, Philadelphia, 2005, Elsevier, p 708.
Moore AS: Practical chemotherapy. In Ettinger SJ, Feldman
EC, editors: *Textbook of veterinary internal medicine*, ed 6,
Philadelphia, 2005, Elsevier, p 713.
Morrison-Collister KE et al: A combination chemotherapy proto-
col with MOPP and CCNU consolidation (Tufts VELCAP-SC)
for the treatment of canine lymphoma, *Vet Com Oncol* 1:180,
2004.
Ogilvie GK, Moore AS: *Feline oncology: a comprehensive guide to
compassionate care*, Trenton, NJ, 2001, Veterinary Learning
Systems.
Ogilvie GK, Moore AS: *Managing the canine cancer patient: a
comprehensive guide to compassionate care*, Trenton, NJ, 2006,
Veterinary Learning Systems.

CHAPTER 66
Anticancer Drugs: New Drugs

DOUGLAS H. THAMM, *Fort Collins, Colorado*
DAVID M. VAIL, *Madison, Wisconsin*

Of the treatment modalities available in veterinary
oncology, surgery remains the most commonly
applied and the most likely to effect cure. However,
local recurrence and/or distant metastasis result in the
majority of cancer-related deaths. The use of antineoplastic chemotherapy has increased greatly in the last decade
in both general and specialty veterinary practice. Well-
designed clinical trials are constantly being performed to
determine the appropriate dose, tolerability, and efficacy of
novel antineoplastic drugs. General practitioners should be
aware of this expanding knowledge base, whether they will
be using these drugs in their practice or referring clientele to
centers elsewhere to receive them. There is ever-increasing
information regarding optimal doses, schedules, combinations, and routes of delivery of "established" chemotherapeutic agents in veterinary practice (see Chapter 65).
This chapter focuses on newer classical cytotoxic agents
(rather than "targeted" agents, monoclonal antibodies, or
antiangiogenic or immunomodulatory compounds) that
have U.S. Food and Drug Administration approval for use
in humans. A summary is provided in Table 66-1. For additional information, the reader is referred to other reviews
(Chun et al., 2004; Moore and Kitchell, 2003).

IFOSFAMIDE (IFEX)

Ifosfamide is an alkylating agent and has been evaluated in tumor-bearing dogs and cats (Payne et al., 2003;
Rassnick et al., 2000; Rassnick et al., 2006a, 2006b).
It must be given during a diuresis and with a thiol
compound, sodium 2-mercaptoethane sulfonate (mesna),
to prevent sterile hemorrhagic cystitis induced by acrolein, a metabolite that is toxic to bladder urothelium.
Mesna and ifosfamide are sold and packaged together.

Table **66-1**

Newer Cytotoxic Agents in Veterinary Oncology

Agent	Reported Dose	Documented Toxicity	Reported Efficacy
Docetaxel	*Dogs:* 20-30 mg/m² slow IV infusion, q2-3 weeks (anecdotal); requires antihypersensitivity premedication *Cats:* Not established	Hypersensitivity (less severe than paclitaxel) Neutropenia likely to be dose limiting	Various carcinomas, some sarcomas (humans)
Gemcitabine	*Dogs:* 675 mg/m² slow IV infusion q2 weeks *Cats:* Not established; anecdotally 250 mg/m²	Neutropenia is dose limiting Gastrointestinal toxicity is generally mild and self-limiting Retinal detachment reported	Minimal activity reported; lymphoma, malignant melanoma, squamous cell carcinoma
Ifosfamide	*Dogs:* 375 mg/m² slow IV infusion with mesna, q 2-3 weeks *Cats:* 900 mg/m² slow IV infusion with mesna q3 weeks	Neutropenia is dose limiting Gastrointestinal toxicity is generally mild and self-limiting Urothelial toxicity avoided with concurrent use of mesna Nephrotoxicity reported in cats	Cutaneous hemangiosarcoma, leiomyosarcoma, vaccine-associated sarcoma
Paclitaxel	*Dogs:* 132 mg/m² slow IV infusion q3 weeks; requires antihypersensitivity premedication *Cats:* Not established	Hypersensitivity Neutropenia is dose limiting Alopecia Gastrointestinal toxicity is generally mild and self-limiting	Osteosarcoma, various carcinomas, malignant histiocytosis
Pegylated liposomal doxorubicin	*Dogs:* 1 mg/kg IV q3 weeks *Cats:* 1 mg/kg IV q3 weeks	Cutaneous toxicity (PPES) is dose limiting in dogs—may be ameliorated by concurrent pyridoxine administration Nephrotoxicity is dose limiting in cats	Lymphoma, including doxorubicin-refractory cases; various sarcomas; various carcinomas; malignant histiocytosis; vaccine-associated sarcoma
Vinorelbine	*Dogs:* 15-18 mg/m² IV weekly *Cats:* Not established	Neutropenia is dose limiting Gastrointestinal toxicity is uncommon	Pulmonary carcinoma, mast cell tumor (anecdotal)

IV, Intravenous; *PPES,* palmar-plantar erythrodysesthesia syndrome.

The recommended dose and delivery schedule in dogs is to give mesna (reconstituted in 0.9% NaCl to a concentration of 20 mg/ml) at 20% of the calculated ifosfamide dose. Mesna is first given as an intravenous bolus, and then the patient is diuresed with 0.9% NaCl at 18.3 ml/kg/hour for 30 minutes. Ifosfamide (375 mg/m² reconstituted in 0.9% NaCl to a volume of 9.15 ml/kg of body weight) is then given over 30 minutes, followed by an additional 5 hours of saline diuresis (18.3 ml/kg/hour). Two additional mesna doses are given at 2 and 5 hours during the postifosfamide diuresis. Ifosfamide can be dosed at either 2- or 3-week intervals in dogs. Phase I and subsequent phase II studies suggest that ifosfamide can safely be given at doses of 900 mg/m² every 3 weeks in cats using a similar administration protocol.

When given with mesna, the dose-limiting toxicity (DLT) of ifosfamide is myelosuppression, manifested primarily by neutropenia. Mild, self-limiting gastrointestinal toxicity (inappetence, vomiting, diarrhea) also can be seen. Nephrotoxicity has been reported infrequently in cats.

In one study of 72 tumor-bearing dogs, an overall response rate of 6% was reported. Responses were noted in dogs with sarcomas, including cutaneous hemangiosarcoma (HSA) and leiomyosarcoma (Rassnick et al., 2000). Only one of 40 dogs with lymphoma (LSA) responded. A protocol of alternating doxorubicin (DOX) and ifosfamide has been evaluated in dogs with HSA; when compared retrospectively to dogs treated with single-agent DOX, there

was no apparent improvement in outcome (Payne et al., 2003). Based on the published data, it is possible that the canine dose may be escalated further, which may improve antitumor activity. Ifosfamide appears to be an active drug for the treatment of feline vaccine-associated sarcoma (VAS); an overall response rate of 41% was reported in a recent phase II study (Rassnick et al., 2006b).

PEGYLATED LIPOSOMAL DOXORUBICIN (DOXIL, CAELYX)

Liposomes are closed vesicular structures that consist of one or more lipid bilayers. Several different types of liposome can be engineered with different physical properties that can dramatically alter drug pharmacokinetics and/or pharmacodynamics. Most liposomal formulations are designed to enhance antitumor efficacy, decrease normal tissue toxicity, or a combination of the two. Doxil, a liposomal formulation of DOX, has been used effectively in dogs and cats (Vail et al., 1997; Poirier et al., 2002). Unlike free (unencapsulated) DOX, myelosuppression and cardiotoxicity are not dose limiting. This makes it a suitable drug for use in dogs with preexisting cardiac disease or in dogs that have received cumulative doses of free DOX that are approaching cardiotoxic levels. The DLT in dogs is a cutaneous toxicity called palmar-plantar erythrodysesthesia syndrome (PPES), characterized by lesions ranging from mild erythema and alopecia to severe crusting and ulceration primarily in the axilla, inguinal region, and skin surrounding the footpads. The severity of PPES can be diminished with concurrent use of vitamin B_6 (pyridoxine, 25 to 50 mg q8h orally [PO]) throughout treatment. The DLT of Doxil in cats is a delayed nephrotoxicity, although it is rare at the recommended dose; as with native DOX, adequate renal function is imperative in cats receiving the drug. The recommended dosage for Doxil in both dogs and cats is 1 mg/kg intravenously [IV] every 3 weeks as a 10-minute bolus.

Canine tumors reported to respond to Doxil include LSA, malignant histiocytosis, soft-tissue sarcomas, mammary adenocarcinoma, anal sac adenocarcinoma, and squamous cell carcinoma. In addition, dogs with LSA resistant to native DOX have responded to Doxil, implying some mechanism of abrogating drug resistance. Feline VASs have been reported to respond to Doxil; however, native DOX appears as effective as the more expensive liposomal formulation. Anecdotal responses have also been seen in cats with various carcinomas and cutaneous HSA.

PACLITAXEL (TAXOL; GENERICS ALSO EXIST)

Paclitaxel, originally extracted from the bark of the Pacific yew tree, is an inhibitor of microtubule depolymerization that results in mitotic arrest. It has significant activity in several types of human epithelial cancers and has recently been evaluated in veterinary practice (Poirier et al., 2004a). The recommended dosage in dogs is 132 mg/m² by slow intravenous infusion once every 3 weeks. The most difficult aspect of paclitaxel administration is a result of the carrier, Cremophor EL, which is used to solubilize the drug. Cremophor EL is highly allergenic in most species, including dogs and cats. In the dog treatment with antihistamines and corticosteroids is required both before and during paclitaxel delivery. A premedication and infusion protocol has been devised to prevent or minimize hypersensitivity reactions (Box 66-1).

Box 66-1

Paclitaxel Premedication and Administration Protocol in Dogs

Day before treatment:	Prednisone 1 mg/kg PO
30-60 minutes before treatment:	Diphenhydramine 4 mg/kg IM Cimetidine 4 mg/kg IV Dexamethasone sodium phosphate 2 mg/kg IV

Paclitaxel delivery protocol:
- Suspend paclitaxel (132 mg/m²) in a 10× volume of 0.9% NaCl for injection.
- Start IV infusion at 30 ml/hour for 10 min.
- If no hypersensitivity reaction noted, increase infusion rate to 60 ml/hour for 10 min.
- If no hypersensitivity reaction noted, increase infusion rate to 90 ml/hour until complete.
- If hypersensitivity reaction is noted, premedication is repeated and infusion rate reduced as necessary.

IM, Intramuscularly; *IV,* intravenously; *PO,* orally.

Other than hypersensitivity-related side effects during infusion, the DLT in dogs is neutropenia. Hair loss, vomiting, and diarrhea (usually self-limiting) are also observed. Antitumor responses have been observed in dogs with metastatic osteosarcoma, mammary adenocarcinoma, and malignant histiocytosis. Stabilization of disease has been observed in dogs with various carcinomas. Further evaluations in larger patient populations are currently under way; and, although paclitaxel can be difficult to administer, a subset of patients will benefit from its use. In our experience paclitaxel is extremely difficult to administer to cats; the hypersensitivity reactions are usually too severe to allow delivery of a therapeutic dose. Formulations of paclitaxel that do not use Cremophor EL are under development.

DOCETAXEL (TAXOTERE)

A drug related to paclitaxel, docetaxel (Taxotere, Sanofi-Aventis) is currently being evaluated in veterinary patients. It has antitumor activity in a variety of human carcinomas and some sarcomas. In humans and in dogs treated to date the incidence of severe hypersensitivity reactions appears less than with paclitaxel because of to the absence of the Cremophor EL emulsifier. Patients are premedicated using a protocol identical to that used for paclitaxel. Docetaxel is then administered IV as a 2-hour infusion. Preliminary information suggests that a dosage of 20 to 30 mg/m² every 2 to 3 weeks is usually well tolerated by dogs and that neutropenia is likely to be dose limiting. There is no information regarding the use of docetaxel in cats.

VINORELBINE (NAVELBINE; GENERICS ALSO AVAILABLE)

Vinorelbine is a semisynthetic molecule in the vinca alkaloid class of drugs. Its mechanism of action is similar to that of other members of the group in that they disrupt polymerization of microtubules, especially those comprising the mitotic spindle apparatus, ultimately inducing metaphase arrest in dividing cells. In a recent phase I study in dogs, vinorelbine was well tolerated and, although efficacy was not a primary end point, preliminary evidence of antitumor effect was observed (Poirier et al., 2004b). The maximum tolerated dose was found to be between 15 and 18 mg/m² once weekly. It is recommended that treatment in dogs be initiated at 15 mg/m²; if toxicity is acceptable, escalation to 18 mg/m² should be considered. Neutropenia was the DLT. Anorexia, vomiting, diarrhea and one case of a cutaneous rash were also observed; but these generally were self-limiting and did not require hospitalization. Although no phase II trials have yet been reported for vinorelbine in canine cancer, the phase I trial suggested activity in dogs with primary lung tumors, and there is anecdotal evidence of efficacy against canine mast cell tumors, including those that have failed prior therapy with the related vinca alkaloid vinblastine. At present no published information exists for vinorelbine use in cats.

GEMCITABINE (GEMZAR)

Gemcitabine is an antimetabolite nucleoside (pyrimidine) analog that has been used in veterinary medicine, both as a direct cytotoxic agent and as a radiation sensitizer (Kosarek et al., 2005; LeBlanc et al., 2004). As with other nucleoside analogs, the mechanism of action of gemcitabine is attributed to its incorporation into deoxyribonucleic acid (DNA) and ultimate inhibition of DNA replication. Several anecdotal dosing regimens have been suggested; a biweekly (every 2 weeks) dosage of $675\,mg/m^2$ as a 30-minute intravenous infusion appears to be well tolerated in dogs. The drug is diluted in $10\,ml/kg$ of body weight of 0.9% NaCl immediately before delivery. A safe dose in cats has not been published; however, anecdotally $250\,mg/m^2$ has been used. It appears that the biologic effect of gemcitabine may be influenced heavily by its duration of infusion: longer infusion times may result in increased intracellular conversion of gemcitabine to its active metabolite, resulting in increased toxicity or a necessity for dose reduction.

Gemcitabine has not been evaluated extensively in veterinary patients, but very limited antitumor efficacy has been reported in tumor-bearing dogs to date. Responses have been observed in a small number of dogs with LSA, malignant melanoma, and squamous cell carcinoma. Short-term (2 to 5 months) disease stabilization was also observed for some other canine tumor types and a small number of cats with oral squamous cell carcinoma.

Hematologic and gastrointestinal toxicity in dogs at the suggested dose appears mild and self-limiting in most cases. One case of retinal detachment in a dog receiving gemcitabine has been reported. Twice weekly "radiosensitizing" doses of $50\,mg/m^2$ in the dog and $25\,mg/m^2$ in the cat were found to have unacceptable hematologic and local tissue toxicity in one study (LeBlanc et al., 2004).

Given their apparent synergy in human studies, combinations of gemcitabine and carboplatin currently are being evaluated in veterinary patients.

References and Suggested Reading

Chun R et al: Cancer chemotherapy. In Withrow SJ, MacEwen EG, editors: *Small animal clinical oncology*, ed 3, Philadelphia, 2001, Saunders, p 92.

Kosarek CE et al: Clinical evaluation of gemcitabine in dogs with spontaneously occurring malignancies; *J Vet Intern Med* 19:81, 2005.

LeBlanc AK et al: Unexpected toxicity following use of gemcitabine as a radiosensitizer in head and neck carcinomas: a Veterinary Radiation Therapy Oncology Group pilot study, *Vet Radiol Ultrasound* 45:466, 2004.

Moore AS, Kitchell BE: New chemotherapy agents in veterinary medicine, *Vet Clin North Am Small Anim Pract* 33:629, 2003.

Payne SE et al: Treatment of vascular and soft-tissue sarcomas in dogs using an alternating protocol of ifosfamide and doxorubicin, *Vet Comp Oncol* 1:171, 2003.

Poirier VJ et al: Liposome-encapsulated doxorubicin (Doxil) and doxorubicin in the treatment of vaccine-associated sarcoma in cats, *J Vet Intern Med* 16:726, 2002.

Poirier VJ et al: Efficacy and toxicity of paclitaxel (Taxol) for the treatment of canine malignant tumors, *J Vet Intern Med* 18:219, 2004a.

Poirier VJ et al: Toxicity, dose, and efficacy of vinorelbine (Navelbine) in dogs with spontaneous neoplasia, *J Vet Intern Med* 18:536, 2004b.

Rassnick KM et al: Evaluation of ifosfamide for treatment of various canine neoplasms, *J Vet Intern Med* 14:271, 2000.

Rassnick KM et al: Phase I trial and pharmacokinetic analysis of ifosfamide in cats with sarcomas, *Am J Vet Res* 67:510, 2006a.

Rassnick KM et al: Results of a phase II clinical trial on the use of ifosfamide for treatment of cats with vaccine-associated sarcomas, *Am J Vet Res* 67:517, 2006b.

Vail DM et al: Preclinical trial of doxorubicin entrapped in sterically stabilized liposomes in dogs with spontaneously arising malignant tumors, *Cancer Chemother Pharmacol* 39:410, 1997.

CHAPTER 67

Radiotherapy: Basic Principles and Indications

ERIC M. GREEN, *Columbus, Ohio*

Radiotherapy (RT) is the treatment of disease using ionizing radiation. Just over a year after the discovery of x-rays by Wilhelm Konrad Röntgen in 1895, Wilhelm Alexander Freund, a German surgeon, reported the disappearance of a hairy mole in a human patient after treatment with x-rays. Years later in 1906 Richard Eberlein, a German physician and veterinarian, first reported the use of RT in animals. Today veterinary RT is a growing field with roughly 63 radiation oncologists worldwide certified by the American College of Veterinary Radiology. There are now 65 private veterinary practices and universities in the United States that offer RT as part of a comprehensive approach to cancer care listed on the Veterinary Cancer Society's website (www.vetcancersociety.org).

This chapter provides a basic understanding of the principles of RT, reviews the indications for RT, and discusses some of the common side effects of treatment.

PRINCIPLES OF RADIOTHERAPY

Radiation is classified as either particulate or electromagnetic. Particulate radiations are those that have mass and may have a charge and include electrons (also known as β-particles), protons, neutrons, and α-particles (a helium nucleus). Electromagnetic radiations are those that have no mass and no charge. These are merely packets of energy (photons) and include x-rays and γ-rays. These two differ only in their method of creation. X-rays are created through the interaction of fast-moving electrons with a heavy metal target as in an x-ray tube or linear accelerator, whereas γ-rays arise from the nucleus of radioactive elements. All of the listed particulate and electromagnetic radiations can be used for the purposes of RT. Most often photons from a linear accelerator are used for RT; thus from this point forward it will be assumed that irradiation will be performed using photons.

To be useful for therapeutic purposes, the radiation used must be energetic enough to ionize atoms within the patient. It is this ionization process that begins the cascade of cellular damage. Ionizing radiation is capable of causing cellular damage through either a direct or an indirect action of the radiation within tissue. One third of the time when a photon enters a patient, that photon strikes an electron within an atom, giving it enough energy to knock it out of its orbit (creating a positive ion—the remaining atom without its electron). This free electron then goes on to cause damage to the cellular deoxyribonucleic acid (DNA). This is termed *direct action*. The other two thirds of the time the free electron liberated by the photon interaction interacts with water molecules near the DNA, creating free radicals, which damage the DNA. This is termed *indirect action*. Oxygen must be present at the time of irradiation for the effects of the indirect action to be most damaging. This is because oxygen binds to the DNA/free radical combination, fixing (making permanent) this free radical damage.

The resulting damage to the DNA is the same whether it is a result of direct or indirect action and is in the form of single- and double-strand breaks. Single-strand breaks occur with great frequency but are often of little consequence. Given enough time, cells can repair much of this type of damage. Double-strand breaks occur at the rate of 4 for every 100 single-strand breaks but are of greater significance. They are more difficult for the cell to repair and therefore often result in the death of the cell, by either initiating the apoptotic pathway or creating chromosomal aberrations that result in cell death at a subsequent mitosis. Since radiation kills cells, RT is potentially useful for the treatment of cancer. However, radiation does not discriminate between neoplastic cells and normal cells, and the death of the normal cells in the treatment field results in radiation side effects. This collateral injury is minimized by careful therapy planning.

Repair and Fractionation

As previously mentioned, both normal and tumor cells often can repair some of the DNA damage caused by ionizing radiation. Generally only the single-strand breaks can be repaired. To repair all the single-strand breaks, the cell must have enough time. It is generally believed that about 6 hours is required for normal tissues to repair most radiation-induced single-strand breaks. The repair that occurs in the normal tissues is advantageous since it allows these tissues to tolerate a subsequent dose of radiation without experiencing the same amount of cell death as the tumor tissues. The other advantage relates to the fact that tumors repair DNA inefficiently. This very important fact allows RT to be successful. If normal and neoplastic tissues had the same response to radiation, it would be impossible to treat tumors effectively without inducing significant, life-threatening side effects in the normal tissues. The goal of the radiation oncologist is to deliver enough radiation in a way that allows the normal tissues to best tolerate the damage while killing the tumor cells. This is achieved through *fractionation,* the delivery of multiple doses of radiation at intervals that allow the normal tissues time to repair DNA damage. During the interval between radiation treatments, the tumor cells repair some of the single-strand breaks. At the next irradiation additional single-strand breaks are created that may be in close proximity to unrepaired breaks so that they effectively act as a double-strand break.

Each single dose of radiation kills the same percent of cells each time. Therefore it is unlikely that one large dose of radiation is sufficient to kill all the cells in a tumor. By fractionating the therapy, many smaller doses of radiation are delivered to the patient, killing a percentage of the remaining cells each time. If enough doses are delivered, the number of tumor cells remaining is very small, and the likelihood of recurrence is minimal.

Dose and Fractions

The term *dose* is used to refer to the amount of radiation absorbed by the patient. It is a measure of the amount of energy deposited in a known mass of tissue. The accepted International System of Units (SI) unit is the gray (Gy), which represents 1 J of energy deposited in 1 kg of mass. Older literature may refer to radiation dose in units of the rad, where 100 rad are equal to 1 Gy.

The term *fraction* is used to refer to an individual treatment of radiation. Radiotherapy protocols are designed to deliver a given total dose in a given number of fractions. Fractions are usually given daily (Monday through Friday) or once weekly, depending on the goal of therapy. Typical protocols may range from several weekly fractions of 8 to 10 Gy to daily fractions of 2.5 to 4.2 Gy for 2 to 4 weeks.

Sensitivity to Radiation

Both normal and tumor cells vary in their sensitivity to the effects of radiation. Some characteristics of cells increase sensitivity to radiation damage. In 1906 French radiobiologists Bergonié and Tribondeau stated,

> "...X-rays are more effective on cells which have a greater reproductive activity; the effectiveness is greater on those cells which have a longer dividing future ahead, on those cells the morphology and the function of which are least fixed..."

This means that sensitive cells are those that are mitotically active, undergo many divisions, and are undifferentiated. In general this would mean that most tumors and rapidly dividing normal tissue stem cells are the most radiosensitive. This is good in the sense that tumor cells die when irradiated and at the same time bad because the sensitive normal tissues suffer the same fate. One can rank normal tissues by their relative radiosensitivity in the following order from most sensitive to least sensitive: rapidly dividing stem cells (bone marrow, skin, mucosa, conjunctiva); intermediate stages in the hematopoietic series; connective tissue cells (endothelium); most parenchymal organs and glands; and granulocytes, myocytes, and neurons. It is the sensitive normal tissues in the radiation treatment field that need to be considered when planning RT because the death of these tissues leads to side effects.

INDICATIONS FOR RADIOTHERAPY

The decision to include RT in a patient's course of cancer therapy is based on several factors. RT can be used in several circumstances, depending on the desired outcome. Often the first choice that needs to be made is whether to offer definitive or palliative RT. Definitive therapy usually involves a protocol of several weeks of daily fractions and is intended to result in long-term tumor control. Typically one can expect some acute side effects with definitive protocols, but usually the risk of late side effects is low because of the smaller fraction sizes. Palliative therapy usually involves a protocol of once-weekly treatments for 3 to 4 weeks and is intended to result in the alleviation of pain or clinical signs and/or to achieve short-term tumor control. Acute side effects generally are not observed with palliative protocols since the goal is to improve the patient's quality of life with the treatment; but the risk of late side effects is far greater because of the large dose per fraction. One needs to weigh the risks of both acute and late side effects against the length of tumor control or improved quality of life that is expected with each protocol. In determining the appropriate treatment protocol for each patient, one can look at several factors: tumor type, tumor grade and stage, and tumor location.

Tumor Type

It is well established that different tumor types have different inherent radiosensitivities. Higher doses of radiation are required to control some types (sarcomas), whereas others may require a lower dose (carcinomas). Some tumors respond better to higher doses per fraction given weekly (melanoma), whereas most others require smaller doses per fraction delivered daily.

Tumor Grade and Stage

These are often prognostic, and it is important to understand the implications of each. The histologic grade may predict a more aggressive behavior that may require a more aggressive radiation protocol. The clinical stage may suggest that a definitive protocol may not be appropriate or that regional lymph nodes may need to be included in the same or separate treatment field. It may also be inappropriate to use a definitive protocol on a patient that has a poor long-term prognosis as predicted by the tumor grade and stage or serious concurrent illness.

Tumor Location

Because the normal tissues around the tumor experience side effects from the radiation, it is important to use a protocol that these tissues can tolerate without experiencing life-threatening damage. Most RT protocols are designed to treat to the tolerance of the normal tissues in the treatment field such that the acute side effects in those tissues are acceptable. Occasionally the protocol must be modified to account for larger treatment fields that may include large volumes of normal tissue.

The previous factors merely allow one to select the most appropriate RT protocol based solely on tumor-related factors. One also needs to consider the owner's expectations, as well as whether the patient has concurrent disease or can tolerate the daily or weekly anesthesia required to undergo RT. Financial issues may also be of concern for owners; and, whereas a definitive RT protocol may be the treatment of choice, it is often expensive. A less expensive palliative protocol may be a reasonable option for owners who want to do what they can but do not have the financial means. In addition, the factors listed previously more often than not will demonstrate the need for a multimodality approach that may involve surgery and/or chemotherapy in conjunction with RT.

Combination Therapy: Surgery and Chemotherapy

Frequently more than one modality is necessary to affect the greatest tumor control in a patient. For many tumors surgery is used to remove the gross tumor, and RT used to treat the remaining microscopic disease. Systemic chemotherapy may also be used to address the potential for metastatic disease in the same patient; and in some circumstances, particularly when the tumor is very large, surgery may be used after RT. There are advantages and disadvantages to both preoperative and postoperative RT; these need to be considered on an individual patient basis.

The primary advantage of preoperative RT is that a smaller treatment field can be used, thus minimizing the normal tissue side effects. The gross tumor can be treated most effectively because its exact location is known, either by palpation or imaging. To account for microscopic extension, a margin of normal tissue around the gross tumor is included in the treatment field. The resulting radiation field is smaller before surgery because a postoperative field would need to include any surgical scar (always larger than the original tumor) and a margin around it. Radiotherapy has the potential to improve the resectability of tumors by shrinking them before surgery. In addition, because of the tumor cell death, the risk of metastatic spread at the time of surgery theoretically is reduced with preoperative RT. The major disadvantage of RT before surgery is the potential for surgical complications such as delayed wound healing. Theoretically the entire radiation field should be removed surgically, and the wound closed with unirradiated tissue opposing itself. Realistically this is unlikely to be the case; thus care must be taken to close the wound securely and avoid excessive tension. One other disadvantage is that surgery must wait until the acute side effects of the radiation have healed. During this time the tumor continues to grow and may have more opportunity to metastasize.

The primary advantage of postoperative RT relates to the concept that radiation is more effective at eradicating smaller number of cells left behind after surgery than large number of cells present in the gross tumor. Additional advantages include the immediate removal of the tumor and therefore a lower risk of metastasis. Furthermore, critical information may be gained at surgery that may influence further therapy (i.e., regional lymph node status or the presence of disease not detected by prior imaging studies). Disadvantages of postoperative RT include

the larger treatment field needed (increasing the normal tissue side effects) and the fact that the RT must wait until any surgical complications have healed (e.g., seroma, hematoma). Important also is the issue that without accurate original tumor information (size and location), the radiation oncologist must increase the field size because the surgical scar may not relate well to the original tumor site, particularly if the tumor was not in the skin. This is a particular problem for cases that are referred for RT to another hospital after surgery. To minimize this disadvantage, surgeons are encouraged to take photographs of the tumor before surgery and place hemoclips at all margins of the surgical bed. Radiographs or computed tomography images can then be obtained of the tumor site to aid in RT planning.

The decision to combine chemotherapy with radiation should be based on the metastatic potential of the tumor. Also, chemotherapy may act synergistically with the radiation to result in a greater tumor cell kill than either modality alone. However, care should be taken when combining chemotherapeutics that are known radiosensitizers since the acute side effects in the normal tissues are likely to be more severe. A true radiosensitizing chemotherapeutic could be used at a dose much lower than the conventional systemic dose to enhance the cell-killing effects of the radiation while avoiding normal tissue acute side effects. In that case the agent would not be as effective at controlling metastatic disease with the lower dose.

Very little is published in the veterinary literature describing appropriate radiosensitizing doses. It may be prudent to delay chemotherapy until after the RT protocol is complete when using radiosensitizing agents at systemic doses. A short list of agents known to be radiosensitizers includes: 5-fluorouracil, cisplatin, carboplatin, etopiside, gemcitabine, and paclitaxel. Another consideration when using chemotherapy after RT is radiation recall. This is the manifestation of acute side effects within the radiation field well after the conclusion of RT when certain chemotherapeutics are given. Although not yet reported in the veterinary literature, this is a well-established phenomenon in human patients subsequent to the administration of actinomycin, doxorubicin, methotrexate, 5-fluorouracil, hydroxyurea, and paclitaxel.

SPECIFIC TUMOR APPLICATIONS

Many veterinary tumors may benefit from treatment with radiation. What follows is not meant to be all-inclusive, but represents the most common applications for RT in veterinary medicine.

Brain Tumors

The exact histologic type of brain tumor in a dog or cat is rarely known, although inferences can be made from the imaging characteristics and epidemiologic data. Regardless, RT is the treatment of choice for inoperable or incompletely resected brain tumors. A recent review suggests survival times of 700 days in patients who received definitive RT (Bley et al., 2005). Stereotactic radiosurgery (a technique that pinpoints radiation in the tumor and spares more normal brain tissue) holds great promise with a few reported survival times of 56, 66, and 227 weeks (Lester et al., 2001). This technique requires advanced equipment not readily available to all radiation oncologists.

Nasal Tumors

Radiotherapy is *essential* in the treatment of most nasal tumors and results in survival times of 12 to 19 months with definitive protocols. Palliative protocols have been described and result in a modest survival time of 7 months (Mellanby et al., 2002). Recently post-RT nasal exenteration has been described as an option for select patients with mid-to-rostral nasal cavity tumors and has resulted in an overall median survival time of 48 months (Adams et al., 2005).

Oral Tumors

Surgery is often the treatment of choice for most oral tumors; thus cosmetic and functional outcome following resection is an important consideration. Patients with small, rostrally located tumors fair far better after surgery because resection is often curative. In cases in which aggressive surgery may be associated with unacceptable morbidity, a less aggressive surgery followed by RT may prove most beneficial for the patient. This approach using a definitive RT protocol is reasonable for most carcinomas and sarcomas of the oral cavity. Acanthomatous epulides are a special case in which definitive RT alone often results in long-term durable tumor control. Oral melanomas present a different dilemma in that they are highly metastatic, but local control is often necessary for preservation of quality of life. A palliative protocol combined with platinum-based chemotherapy as a radiosensitizer resulted in a median survival time of 1 year (Freeman et al., 2003).

Soft-Tissue Sarcomas

As with oral tumors, surgery provides the greatest chance for tumor control, but many tumor locations prevent wide excisions (head or extremities). Again RT can control the residual microscopic disease left after incomplete excision. For many well-differentiated soft-tissue sarcomas (fibrosarcoma and peripheral nerve sheath tumor), tumor control rates at 1 and 2 years following surgery and definitive RT are 95% and 91%. Vaccine-associated sarcomas in cats require a more aggressive approach. Radiation, either before or after surgery, followed by chemotherapy provides the longest survival times, about 500 to 600 days.

Mast Cell Tumors

The different grades of mast cell tumors present a unique challenge when deciding how best to treat them. For tumors of any grade, complete surgical excision with wide margins should be attempted. When resection is incomplete, RT and chemotherapy provide options for follow-up treatment. The 3-year recurrence rate for moderately differentiated mast cell tumors treated with surgery and

RT is only 7% (Frimberger et al., 1997). When the regional lymph node is positive, RT of both the primary site and the lymph node combined with prednisone can result in good long-term control approximating 41 months (Chaffin and Thrall, 2002). Incompletely resected grade III mast cell tumors or other grades with visceral metastasis may still benefit from a palliative RT protocol combined with chemotherapy. Radiotherapy for multiple cutaneous mast cell tumors is often impractical.

SIDE EFFECTS OF RADIOTHERAPY

Normal cells in the treatment field die as a result of irradiation. This often results in clinical side effects. These side effects of RT can be divided into two categories based on when they occur. *Acute effects* occur during or shortly after RT in rapidly dividing normal tissues (epithelium, mucosa, conjunctiva) in the treatment field. They are the result of the death of the stem cell population in these tissues. Acute effects occur after a threshold dose is received and become more severe as the dose is increased beyond that threshold. They typically result in inflammation and ulceration of the tissues and specifically include oral mucositis and desquamation. They often begin within the final week of treatment. Because these tissues are rapidly dividing, they replenish themselves, provided all of the stem cells are not destroyed, and the acute effects resolve 2 to 3 weeks after therapy is complete.

Oral mucositis is often a consequence of irradiation of nasal or oral tumors. It usually begins as erythema and inflammation of the oral mucosa and may progress to ulceration with sloughing of the superficial layers of oral epithelium. Excessive salivation often accompanies the mucositis. The patients frequently become inappetent because of pain. The medical management of oral mucositis consists of antibiotics to combat secondary infection of the damaged mucosa and analgesics. Maintaining appropriate hydration and caloric intake is essential while the patient is experiencing mucositis. Owners are encouraged to feed soft food and provide plenty of fresh water for their pets while the mucositis heals over 2 to 3 weeks. Occasionally esophagostomy or gastrostomy tubes are placed as a temporary measure to allow adequate hydration and nutrition until mucositis subsides.

Desquamation results after irradiation of the skin exceeds a threshold dose. Like mucositis, desquamation begins as erythema but can progress to dry desquamation (flaking of epithelium) or even moist desquamation (loss of superficial epithelium and oozing of serum onto skin). Hair loss (temporary or permanent) and changes in skin or hair color may also occur but are usually only a cosmetic issue. Management of desquamation focuses on limiting self-trauma and keeping the area clean and dry. Topical creams or ointments generally are avoided, and there is little support in the literature for their use. Elizabethan collars are essential to prevent the patient from licking the site because this exacerbates the wound. Nonadherent light dressings may be used, but only to keep the area clean, and should be changed frequently to prevent the treatment area from staying too moist. Oral antibiotics may be used in patients with moist desquamation to prevent a secondary infection because the epithelial barrier to bacterial invasion is destroyed. Oral analgesics often are necessary since desquamation can be quite uncomfortable.

The likelihood of experiencing acute effects is related to the total dose of radiation delivered and the total time of the entire treatment protocol. If one delivers a high dose of radiation in a short period of time, the acute effects are severe and cause significant morbidity. However, this situation is best for tumor cell kill and ultimately tumor control. Radiotherapy protocols must carefully balance an acceptable level of acute side effects with an acceptable duration of tumor control to be most effective and useful.

Late effects are those that occur several months after RT in slowly proliferating normal tissues (often endothelium or parenchymal cells) in the treatment field. The cells in these tissues eventually die when they undergo mitosis. Because there are no stem cells to replace these lost cells, late effects are permanent changes. Late effects can be a consequence of endothelial cell death that results in areas of ischemia and subsequent tissue fibrosis. Specific examples of late effects include bowel stricture, cataracts, demyelinating myelopathy, osteoradionecrosis, keratoconjunctivitis sicca, and skin fibrosis. Frequently little can be done once late effects manifest themselves clinically, and management of these side effects focuses on controlling the clinical signs that are associated with the late effect. Surgery may be required to correct a bowel stricture or repair an oronasal fistula secondary to osteoradionecrosis. Certainly some late effects can be catastrophic and may result in the euthanasia of the patient because of quality-of-life concerns. This situation is avoided as best as is possible by choosing an appropriate RT protocol.

The likelihood of experiencing late effects is related to the dose per fraction. The larger the dose per fraction, the more likely it is that late effects will occur. It is important to be aware of the expected life span after treatment with RT protocols that use large doses per fraction. Typically palliative protocols designed to relieve pain or gain short-term tumor control have large doses per fraction. These protocols are carefully reserved for patients that are not expected to live a very long time after therapy; thus the potential risk of experiencing a late effect is minimized. With most definitive RT protocols, the risk of late effects is very low, which is important as long-term tumor control is expected.

References and Suggested Reading

Adams WM et al: Outcome of accelerated radiotherapy alone or accelerated radiotherapy followed by exenteration of the nasal cavity in dogs with intranasal neoplasia: 53 cases, *J Am Vet Med Assoc* 227:936, 2005.

Bergonié J, Tribondeau L: De quelques resultats de la radiotherapie et essai de fixation d'une technique rationnelle, *Comptes rendus des séances de l'académie des sciences*, 143:983, 1906.

Bley CR et al: Irradiation of brain tumors in dogs with neurologic disease, *J Vet Intern Med* 19:849, 2005.

Burk RL, King GL, editors: Radiation oncology, *Vet Clin North Am Small Anim Pract* 27:1, 1997.

Chaffin K, Thrall DE: Results of radiation therapy in 19 dogs with cutaneous mast cell tumor and regional lymph node metastasis, *Vet Radiol Ultrasound* 43:392, 2002.

Freeman KP et al: Treatment of dogs with oral melanoma by hypofractionated radiation therapy and platinum-based chemotherapy (1987-1997), *J Vet Intern Med* 17:96, 2003.

Frimberger AE et al: Radiotherapy of incompletely resected moderately differentiated mast cell tumors in the dog: 37 cases (1989-1993), *J Am Anim Hosp Assoc* 33:320, 1997.

Kobayashi T et al: Preoperative radiotherapy for vaccine associated sarcoma in 92 cats, *J Am Vet Med Assoc* 43:473, 2002.

Larue SM, Gilette EL: Radiation therapy. In Withrow SJ, MacEwen EG, editors: *Small animal clinical oncology*, ed 3, Philadelphia, 2001, Saunders, p 119.

LeBlanc AK: Unexpected toxicity following use of gemcitabine as a radiosensitizer in head and neck carcinomas: a veterinary radiation therapy oncology group pilot study, *Vet Radiol Ultrasound* 45:466, 2004.

Lester NV et al: Radiosurgery using a stereotactic head frame system for irradiation of brain tumors in dogs, *J Am Vet Med Assoc* 219:1562, 2001.

McEntee MC: A survey of veterinary radiation facilities in the United States during 2001, *Vet Radiol Ultrasound* 45:476, 2004.

Mellanby RJ et al: Long-term outcome of 56 dogs with nasal tumours treated with four doses of radiation at intervals of seven days, *Vet Rec* 151:253, 2002.

CHAPTER 68

Surgical Oncology Principles

JAMES P. FARESE, *Gainesville, Florida*

Animals with cancer often have very advanced (locally invasive or metastatic) disease. It is imperative that veterinarians consulting with owners have a strong knowledge base regarding the behavior of the tumors that commonly occur in dogs and cats. Insufficient knowledge may preclude the appropriate diagnostic testing and procedures commonly performed by oncologic specialists. Many tumors demand an aggressive surgical approach that can only be delivered effectively by an experienced operator. In these cases referral to a specialist should be considered because *the best chance to remove a tumor is the first attempt.* In addition to knowing when tumor resection is possible, it is equally important to realize when the extent of disease has become too advanced to recommend surgical treatment. Veterinarians must always be mindful of the impact of any intervention on the quality of their patients' lives. Convincing owners of the importance of quality of life can be a difficult task when owners struggle to accept the limitations of the therapies that are currently available.

TUMOR EXCISION

One fundamental of oncologic surgery is an understanding of the classification scheme that describes different types of tumor excision. This nomenclature, published by Enneking (1983), serves as an important means of communication between oncologists.

Intracapsular

The intracapsular approach involves piecemeal removal of a mass with the dissection plane interior to the tumor capsule. It is a debulking or cytoreductive surgery that leaves behind macroscopic disease, making local recurrence almost guaranteed if the tumor is malignant. This approach is commonly used to treat benign diseases such as bone cysts, select malignancies (such as invasive thymoma reduction to alleviate clinical signs) or to improve the probability of radiation therapy controlling local disease.

Marginal

A marginal excision is immediately outside the tumor pseudocapsule with the dissection plane through the reactive zone (a layer of reactive tissue consisting of proliferating mesenchymal cells, inflammatory cells, and neovascularization). This technique generally is used for benign tumors (e.g., lipoma); when used for malignant tumors, it often results in residual microscopic disease. When used for malignancies, this approach is often combined with adjunctive radiation therapy (RT). For example, a low-grade soft-tissue sarcoma (STS) of the extremity could be removed with a marginal excision followed by postoperative RT to address the potential for local recurrence if the margins are incomplete.

Wide

A wide excision is removal of the mass; pseudocapsule; reactive zone; and a wide margin of normal tissue (e.g., 2 to 3 cm) or an anatomic mesodermal barrier to tumor cell migration such as fascia, cartilage, or bone. Because the entire tissue compartment (e.g., entire bone or muscle belly) is not removed, it is possible that "skip" metastases (satellite tumor colonies nearby but separate from the primary mass) could be left behind. There is some controversy regarding the necessary margin width for curative surgery. However, most surgeons accept the 3-cm rule in all directions for tumors such as mast cell tumors (MCTs) and STSs. It has also been suggested that 2-cm margins may be satisfactory for grades I and II MCTs (Simpson et al., 2004). Tumor identity and grade impact margin width. For example, low-grade STSs may require smaller margins, whereas other tumors such as vaccine-associated sarcomas call for maximal margin width because of the fingerlike extensions along fascial planes.

Radical

A radical excision is an en bloc removal (removal of the primary mass, draining lymphatic vessels, and lymph nodes [LNs] with a single incision) of a mass and the entire tissue compartment that contains it. The dissection plane is extracompartmental (the compartment refers to the tissue planes that act as natural barriers to tumor invasion). This technique is often used during limb amputations for appendicular osteosarcoma and radical mastectomy for mammary neoplasia.

UNDERSTANDING TUMOR BIOLOGY

All tumors are not created equal, and even within the benign and malignant categories there is wide variation in tumor behavior. It is critical that the surgeon be familiar with the individual tumor types since tumor identity impacts many aspects of case management. In general carcinomas metastasize via the lymphatic system, and sarcomas via the hematogenous route. However, the two vascular systems are connected by lymphovenous communications, and there are exceptions to these patterns. A strong knowledge base enables the surgeon to perform thorough physical examinations and educate the client about tumor behavior (i.e., degree of local invasion, patterns of metastasis), important staging tests, the type of resection required for cure, and long-term prognosis. Perhaps the best example of the importance of understanding tumor behavior is illustrated by the behavior of appendicular osteosarcoma. In these cases it is critical that the client understands that, despite "clean" chest radiographs, dormant micrometastasis in the lungs likely is present and that the possibility of cure is extremely low. Knowing tumor behavior helps guide these preoperative staging evaluations.

CLIENT COMMUNICATION

It is essential that the surgeon develop a good relationship with the client and communicate effectively. Owners of pets with cancer are often anxious and overwhelmed about the condition of their pet, making effective communication challenging. Given the aggressive nature of some surgical resections (e.g., nasal planum resection), it is important that the surgeon prepare clients for the expected postoperative appearance of their pet. This is best done by creating a library of images and videos depicting immediate postoperative and follow-up appearance from other cases. It is imperative that the client have a good understanding about the patterns of the disease, the likelihood of local recurrence, and the overall prognosis.

Almost as important as knowing when to recommend surgery is knowing when the disease state is too advanced to warrant surgery or will cause the patient to have a poor quality of life because of the extent of the resection. For example, resection of a large thyroid carcinoma that is fixed and invading underlying tissues would likely be incomplete and associated with significant hemorrhage and high morbidity. Furthermore, this surgery would not likely be curative because of local tumor thrombi and/or metastatic disease. The value of this determination cannot be overemphasized, and the ability to communicate this effectively to clients takes experience. Reactions from clients vary greatly as to what they view as acceptable surgical procedures. Some clients may be comfortable with radical laryngectomy and a permanent tracheostomy for a laryngeal neoplasm; others will not consider limb amputation because they cannot bear the thought of seeing their pet with such an altered appearance. Clients who initially are reluctant to have a certain procedure performed often change their minds once they have had a chance to reconsider the information and encouragement provided by the surgeon. At the same time, the surgeon must not impose a decision on clients who are undecided about surgery and must ensure the client is comfortable with the plan. Many veterinary cancer centers use mental health professionals to assist with the surgeon-client communication and provide support to clients during the decision making and/or treatment process.

TUMOR STAGING

In the approach to case management there are two important considerations: (1) whether to obtain a preoperative biopsy, and (2) the extent of preoperative staging. These questions are usually easy to answer in hindsight. Staging varies, depending on tumor type, but typically consists of thoracic radiographs and aspiration of regional LNs, with or without abdominal imaging. It is important to understand that a lack of LN enlargement does not mean that nodal metastasis has not occurred.

The value of knowing the tumor identity before surgical excision cannot be disputed since tumor behavior can influence case management in many ways: degree of local invasion, metastatic potential, and biologic activity (e.g., release of histamine, heparin with manipulation of an MCT). However, the decision of whether to obtain a preoperative (versus postoperative) biopsy is not always straightforward. A major consideration is whether the information obtained will affect case management. A good example of this is the handling of oral tumors. The types of oral tumors vary widely in their behavior. For example, the treatment of a fibromatous epulis differs drastically from that of a fibrosarcoma. Aside from melanomas, many oral tumors have a similar gross appearance. Thus it is essential in this scenario that veterinarians perform preoperative biopsy and properly stage the disease if they are to educate the client and help them make an informed decision.

Regarding biopsy techniques for tumor diagnosis, consideration also should be given to the invasiveness of the procedure and the potential for causing hemorrhage into a body cavity (e.g., a large, cavitated splenic mass) or the seeding of tumor cells into a body cavity or along a needle tract (e.g., a transitional cell carcinoma of the urinary bladder). If the need for surgery is clear, as with a staged-clean cavitated splenic mass that is hemorrhaging, it may be in the patient's best interest to forego additional diagnostic efforts. The surgeon must decide whether the risks of the diagnostic tests are justified.

Incisional versus Excisional Biopsy

Incisional biopsy is the removal of a portion of a tumor by sharp incision. This technique is usually performed in cases in which knowing the specific behavior of a tumor may affect an owner's willingness to treat the pet surgically or when knowing the identity of the tumor would alter the treatment plan. Common methods include the following:

Wedge incision: Small, wedge-shaped section of tumor tissue removed with a scalpel blade or biopsy punch. For deeper subcutaneous tumors or those under superficial muscle bellies, a short skin incision is necessary to approach the mass.

Needle core biopsies: Large-bore needles used to sample deeper tumors or tumors of bone (e.g., Tru-cut for soft tissue, Jamshidi needle for bone). This type of tissue sampling can usually be performed with sedation and local anesthesia.

Disadvantages of the incisional biopsy approach are that it often requires a second surgical procedure to be performed and it creates a direct communication between the tumor tissue and the surrounding normal tissue, possibly increasing the chance of local recurrence. The approach for incisional biopsy must be planned such that the incision site and entire dissection tract can be easily excised during the definitive resection. For example, for a mandibular oral tumor the biopsy should be performed through the overlying oral mucosa rather than through skin that is intended to be preserved.

In contrast, excisional biopsy is the removal of the entire tumor (usually a small mass) with a surrounding barrier of normal tissue. The main advantage is that biopsy and gross tumor removal are performed in a single procedure. The main disadvantage is that, if the tumor is highly invasive and the surgeon does not know the identity of the tumor, he or she may not plan a wide enough resection to completely remove the tumor. Cytology results and the anatomic location are important factors in deciding which approach to use. For example, cytology results may be diagnostic for an MCT, obviating the need for a tissue biopsy. Tumors in the flank region may allow an excisional biopsy to be performed with wide (i.e., 3-cm) margins, whereas the same approach on a distal extremity would result in a large open wound that would not allow primary closure. Other instances in which excisional biopsy is almost exclusively performed include intrathoracic and intraabdominal masses, since the invasiveness of the biopsy procedure may involve too much risk or equal the morbidity of the definitive resection if an open biopsy is performed.

When performing an incisional or excisional biopsy on a tumor of unknown histotype, it is important to forewarn the owner that the main purpose of the biopsy is to *establish a diagnosis*; additional diagnostic tests, additional surgery, or other forms of therapy may be necessary following receipt of the histopathology results.

ROLE OF REGIONAL LYMPH NODES

Palpation (or ultrasonographic evaluation in deeper locations such as the sublumbar area) of regional LNs should become a reflex for clinicians evaluating tumors; and whenever needle aspirates can be safely performed, cytology should be done. There is still some controversy as to the role of the LN in tumor biology. The older Halstedian theory stated that tumor cells disseminate in an orderly anatomic manner of ever-larger circles (e.g., from the primary tumor to the closest draining LN and so on). An alternative theory is that cancer cells do not spread in an orderly manner and that regional LNs are largely ineffective barriers to cancer spread. Experimentally tumor cells have been shown to pass through LNs and appear in the efferent lymph within hours. Regardless of the role of the LN, there is some value in removal of LNs along with excision of the primary tumor. First, staging of the tumor can be performed if it was not possible via cytology before surgery. The other advantage to LN removal is that of cytoreduction since the tumor burden may be reduced to a microscopic level, making adjunctive chemotherapy and RT more effective. On the other hand, if preoperative LN cytology shows the node to be negative for metastatic cells, the LN should probably left in place.

It has not been shown definitively that histopathology is superior to cytology for staging, and some important local immune function may be lost with removal of a normal LN.

PALLIATIVE SURGERY

When surgery is performed in an effort to make a patient more comfortable or improve quality of life and the surgeon knows that the procedure will not cure the patient of the disease, the treatment is considered palliative in intent. A good example of palliative surgery is limb amputation for canine osteosarcoma; although pulmonary metastasis has almost invariably occurred by the time of diagnosis, surgery can alleviate the pain associated with the primary bone tumor and dramatically improve the quality of life that remains.

CURATIVE-INTENT RESECTION

A thorough knowledge of anatomy is necessary when palpating the extent of a primary tumor and planning the resection. Aside from tumor size, factors that influence resectability include proximity to nonexpendable anatomic structures, degree of local tissue invasion, and tumor grade. Advanced imaging modalities such as computed tomography and magnetic resonance imaging provide a great deal of preoperative information; however, there are still instances in which it is not clear whether a given tumor is excisable until it is approached surgically. The final preoperative physical evaluation typically is done just after induction of anesthesia. In planning the resection it is essential that the surgeon appreciate the limits of various resection procedures. Consideration must be given to surrounding normal anatomic structures that can be sacrificed to achieve a complete excision yet not cause unacceptable postoperative morbidity or complications. For most cutaneous malignancies the general rule is to make a plan that will allow the surgeon to excise all tissue necessary for complete removal and consider wound closure secondarily. If an aggressive, curative-intent resection is performed and the wound cannot be closed routinely, the defect may be closed with a reconstructive surgical technique such as a skin flap or graft. Alternatively the wound can be left to heal by second intention. Skin flaps should be used with some caution because they usually increase the size of the surgical field and thereby complicate postoperative RT planning.

In some cases it may be prudent to plan a more conservative resection and accept that the surgical plan may result in microscopic residual disease. For example, a low-grade subcutaneous STS of moderate size on the extremity in a 14-year-old dog that is owned by a client who is opposed to the thought of postoperative wound management could be removed via a marginal excision. Although this approach alone would not likely result in a cure, the owner may prefer the possibility of local recurrence over a protracted course of wound management or limb amputation. However, this surgical approach should be questioned if the same patient is entirely asymptomatic and the tumor is slow growing.

There are several technical aspects to consider when performing tumor resections.

1. Perioperative antibiotics should be considered, and strict aseptic technique adhered to since some cancer patients can be immunosuppressed.
2. An open incisional biopsy creates a communication between the tumor tissue and the edges of the normal tissues in the dissection path. Thus excision of the biopsy tract is indicated to ensure removal of all tumor cells. Adequate excision of the biopsy tract is facilitated by well-planned biopsy approaches. Biopsy incisions should be oriented in a direction that is *parallel to the tension lines* to facilitate closure of the surgical wound following definitive resection of the mass and associated biopsy tract.
3. In some procedures such as nephrectomy for a renal neoplasm or lung lobectomy, it has been advocated to ligate the venous side first to minimize embolization of tumor cells into the venous circulation that may occur as a result of tumor manipulation.
4. Manipulation and handling of the tumor should be minimized. In addition to possibly causing more cells to gain access to systemic circulation, rupture of the tumor capsule might occur and allow tumor cells to seed the surgical field. Moistened laparotomy sponges wrapped around large tumors (such as a splenic mass) can be used to minimize the possibility of tumor rupture and glove contamination during the procedure. Excessive manipulation of MCTs can cause degranulation of mast cells and profound hypotension. For this reason patients with MCTs are often pretreated with diphenhydramine prior to surgery.
5. Once the tumor has been excised and removed from the surgical field, gloves and instruments should be changed, and a new pack of surgical towels should be placed over the original surgical drape to help prevent seeding of the wound. The wound should also be lavaged to wash away exfoliated tumor cells. Consideration should be given to the order of procedures if more than one mass resection or some other unrelated procedure (such as on ovariohysterectomy) is planned during the same anesthetic episode. For example, it would be best to remove a subcutaneous lipoma before performing a cystotomy to excise a transitional cell carcinoma because of fear of seeding the incision with tumor cells.

HISTOPATHOLOGY

All excised tumors should be evaluated histologically. When submitting the specimen, the surgeon should provide the pathologist with a concise but accurate history and help the pathologist maintain proper orientation of the tissue. This orientation may be communicated by making a drawing and placement of a suture on a specified margin of the specimen. Knowing the orientation can be very helpful if tumor cells are observed extending to one of the tissue margins and further local therapy is indicated. Alternatively small tumor bed samples (i.e.,

small incisional biopsies of the wound bed following resection) can be harvested from areas of higher concern just before closure. Following removal of the mass the surgical margins of the excised specimen should be marked with ink to document the original plane of dissection. Inking the margins can very valuable, particularly when it is necessary to reevaluate the submitted specimen after the initial sectioning has been performed. The ink is "painted" on with cotton-tipped applicators by the surgeon and should be allowed to dry for 5 to 10 minutes before the specimen is placed in formalin. Multiple colors are available; however, some pathologists prefer black or yellow since these colors cannot be confused with the hematoxylin and eosin tissue stains (blue and red). Like suture tags, different ink colors can be used to direct the pathologist to areas of greater concern. The volume ratio of formalin to tumor mass should be 10:1 to ensure proper fixing of tissue. With large tumors fixative incisions should be made 1 cm apart throughout the tumor parenchyma (similar to slicing bread) to allow proper fixation. However, it is critical that the surgeon not allow fixative incisions to connect to the surgical margins since that will lead to confusion when the pathologist examines the tissue.

INCOMPLETE RESECTION AND LOCAL RECURRENCE

Local recurrence often can be predicted with a good histologic assessment of the surgical margins. When "dirty margins" are not treated, a mass may appear along or beneath the line of incision weeks to months after the initial surgery, depending on the tumor histotype. In this scenario location, tumor histotype, and the results of restaging dictate the course of action. For example, a local recurrence of a synovial cell sarcoma of the tarsal joint previously excised in an aggressive manner is best treated by limb amputation provided there is no evidence of LN or pulmonary metastasis. In other cases additional surgery on the same operative site might be possible to remove the remaining neoplastic cells. In general, this approach is more likely to be effective soon after the initial surgery (i.e., when cells are still present at microscopic levels). Failing to include a fascial plane in the resection is one of the most common reasons for incomplete excision of subcutaneous masses. Although it is best to advise the client against taking the "wait-and-see" approach when incomplete margins have been documented histologically, a small percentage of these cases may never develop local recurrence.

ADJUNCTIVE RADIATION THERAPY

Alternative therapies such as RT and chemotherapy should also be considered in cases with incomplete excision, especially if an aggressive attempt at surgery was made during the initial procedure by an experienced surgeon and there is insufficient tissue to allow reexcision. Although adjunctive chemotherapy is rarely effective in "cleaning up" dirty margins after surgery, adjunctive RT can be a very useful tool for this purpose. For example, postoperative RT is often successful in treating incompletely resected MCTs and STSs of the extremity treated by marginal excision. In some instances RT is more advantageous before surgery. The advantages and disadvantages of the two approaches follow:

Preoperative Radiation Therapy

The advantages of preoperative RT are that a smaller field is required, there is less tumor hypoxia (hypoxic cells are more resistant to radiation), and the extent of the surgical procedure potentially is reduced if the mass decreases in size. Although surgeons prefer not to operate through irradiated tissues, in some instances this approach may have its advantages (e.g., for feline vaccine-associated sarcomas because of their fingerlike extensions along fascial planes). The main disadvantage of this approach is that irradiated skin is more likely to develop incisional complications, especially if there is tension on the closure. Anecdotally some oncologists believe that feline skin is less sensitive to the effects of radiation than canine skin.

Postoperative Radiation Therapy

The advantages of postoperative RT are that there is no delay in surgery and there are no adverse effects on wound healing (if the incision is already healed at the time RT is initiated). The main disadvantages are that a larger radiation treatment field is required and that hypoxia from microvessel surgical trauma may lower sensitivity of remaining tumor cells to radiation. When the surgeon is anticipating the need for postoperative RT, the incision should be oriented in a manner that optimizes the radiation treatment field. In addition, to facilitate radiation planning, metal hemoclips can be placed within the wound just before closure to mark the cranial, caudal, dorsal, and ventral extents of the surgical field (see Chapter 67 for more information).

References and Suggested Reading

Berg J: Surgical therapy. In Slatter D, editor: *Textbook of small animal surgery*, ed 3, Philadelphia, 2002, Saunders.

Enneking WF: Surgical procedures. In Enneking EF, editor: *Musculoskeletal tumor surgery*, New York, 1983, Churchill Livingstone, p 89.

Gilson SD, Stone EA: Principles of oncologic surgery, *Compend Contin Educ Pract Vet* 6:827, 1990.

Gilson SD: Clinical management of the regional lymph node, *Vet Clin North Am Small Anim Pract* 25:149, 1995.

Simpson AM et al: Evaluation of surgical margins required for complete excision of cutaneous mast cell tumors, *J Am Vet Med Assoc* 224:236, 2004.

Withrow SJ: Surgical oncology. In Withrow SJ, Vail DM: *Small animal clinical oncology*, ed 4, Philadelphia, 2007, Saunders, p 157.

CHAPTER 69

Canine Soft-Tissue Sarcomas

TANIA A. BANKS, *Albany Creek, Queensland, Australia*
JULIUS M. LIPTAK, *Guelph, Ontario, Canada*

TERMINOLOGY

Sarcoma is a broad term for a malignant tumor of mesenchymal origin. Soft-tissue sarcomas (STSs) are a particular subgroup of sarcoma. Specific histotypes falling under the STS classification include malignant peripheral nerve sheath tumor, hemangiopericytoma, malignant schwannoma, neurofibrosarcoma, fibrosarcoma, undifferentiated sarcoma, liposarcoma, leiomyosarcoma, myxosarcoma, myxofibrosarcoma, and rhabdomyosarcoma. They are grouped together because they possess similar biologic behavior and histologic features. The behaviors common to all STSs are:

- An ability to arise from any anatomic site in the body, although skin and subcutaneous tissues are most common.
- A tendency to appear as pseudoencapsulated soft-to-firm tumors.
- Exceptional local invasion of tissues and poorly defined histologic margins, with tumor cells infiltrating through and along fascial planes.
- A known potential for local recurrence after conservative or incomplete surgical resection (and recurrent tumors are notoriously more difficult to treat).

- A low-to-moderate metastatic rate.
- A tendency to metastasize hematogenously (e.g., to lungs).
- Regional lymph node metastasis unusual (except for synovial cell sarcomas and histiocytic sarcomas).
- A similar histologic appearance.
- Histologic grade predictive of metastasis and surgical margins predictive of local tumor recurrence.
- Measurable or bulky tumors (>5 cm in diameter) generally have a poor response to chemotherapy and radiation therapy (RT).

Some sarcomas are not included in the traditional STS classification because of more aggressive biologic behavior (e.g., higher metastatic rates) and different histologic features. These include osteosarcoma, chondrosarcoma, histiocytic sarcoma, hemangiosarcoma (HSA), synovial cell sarcoma, mesothelioma, lymphangiosarcoma, oral sarcoma, and malignant peripheral nerve root tumors.

INCIDENCE AND RISK FACTORS

STSs account for 15% and 7% of all skin and subcutaneous tissues in the dog and cat, respectively. The annual incidence of STSs is 35 per 100,000 dogs and 17 per 100,000 cats. The etiology is generally unknown; however, in dogs sarcomas occasionally have been associated with RT, trauma, foreign bodies, orthopedic implants, and the parasite *Spirocerca lupi*. In cats sarcomas have been associated with feline sarcoma virus, vaccines and other subcutaneous injections, and trauma (e.g., intraocular sarcoma). This discussion is limited to spontaneous, nonvaccine-associated STSs in dogs and cats (see Chapter 71 for feline vaccine-associated sarcomas).

CLINICAL FEATURES

Most STSs are solitary and occur in middle-aged–to-older dogs and cats. They are more common in medium- to large-breed dogs but can occur in any age or breed. STS often presents as a soft to firm, spherical, nonpainful cutaneous or subcutaneous mass over the trunk or extremities and can be fixed to the underlying tissue. They can originate in visceral or nonvisceral sites. Generally they are slow growing, and clinical signs are related to the site of involvement and degree of invasion.

DIAGNOSIS AND CLINICAL WORKUP

A complete physical examination of the animal is the first diagnostic step. The mass is palpated to give an idea of site, size, fixation to underlying or adjacent structures, and an initial assessment of the extent of local disease. The regional lymph nodes also should be palpated for enlargement and fixation to underlying tissues.

Fine-needle aspirates are recommended to exclude other differential diagnoses but are often insufficient for obtaining a definitive diagnosis of STS. In one study in which fine-needle aspirates were performed on STSs from 40 dogs, 15% were incorrectly diagnosed, a further 23% were nondiagnostic, and only 62% were correctly diagnosed (Baker-Gabb et al., 2003).

A definitive preoperative diagnosis of STS requires a needle core, punch, incisional, or excisional biopsy. The biopsy should be planned so that the biopsy tract can be included in the curative-intent treatment, whether it be surgery and/or RT, without increasing the surgical dose or size of the RT field. Excisional biopsies are not recommended since they are rarely curative and subsequent surgery required to achieve complete histologic margins is often more aggressive than surgery following core or incisional biopsies, resulting in additional morbidity and expense. Furthermore, multiple attempts at resection, including excisional biopsy, before definitive therapy have a negative impact on survival time in dogs with STSs.

Histopathologic grading (low, intermediate, high or I, II, III) is ascertained from large biopsy specimens and should always be requested from the pathologist. Tumor grade is predictive of behavior and prognosis and is critical to treatment planning. Less than 10% of grade I, 20% of grade II, and 50% of grade III STSs will undergo eventual metastasis. Higher-grade lesions also tend to grow more rapidly and are more locally invasive.

The tests performed for workup and clinical staging depend on the type and location of the STS but usually include routine hematologic and serum biochemical blood tests, urinalysis, three-view thoracic radiographs, and regional tumor imaging. Blood tests are usually within the normal reference range for most dogs with STSs; however, anemia and thrombocytopenia are relatively common in dogs with disseminated histiocytic sarcoma and HSA. Paraneoplastic hypoglycemia is reported with intraabdominal leiomyosarcomas or leiomyomas.

Further imaging of the local tumor may be required for planning the surgical approach or RT if the mass is very large, within a body cavity, fixed to underlying bone, or impinging on or in close proximity to vital structures. Three-dimensional imaging techniques such as computed tomography and magnetic resonance imaging are particularly useful for staging local disease. The surgeon may then better assess the feasibility of and more accurately plan an aggressive surgical resection. Other imaging modalities for staging the local tumor include survey radiographs, ultrasonography, angiography, and nuclear scintigraphy.

The most important diagnostic test for staging of metastatic disease is three-view thoracic radiographs since the lungs are the most common metastatic site for STS. Lymph node metastasis is uncommon with typical STS. Fine-needle aspiration or biopsy of regional lymph nodes should be performed in dogs with clinically abnormal lymph nodes or atypical STS with a high rate of metastasis to regional lymph nodes such as HSA, histiocytic sarcoma, lymphangiosarcoma, synovial cell sarcoma, leiomyosarcoma, and possibly rhabdomyosarcoma. Abdominal imaging (e.g., ultrasonography or advanced imaging) may also be used to assist in further staging in selected cases.

TREATMENT OPTIONS

Local tumor control is the most important consideration for optimal management of nonmetastatic STSs because of their locally aggressive behavior. On gross examination

STSs appear to be well encapsulated. This is not the case because microscopically the pseudocapsule is composed of compressed tumor cells. These peripheral cells are more aggressive and responsible for the invasion into adjacent normal tissues. "Shelling out" the tumor leaves behind the more aggressive subpopulation of these peripheral, invasive cells. Consequently recurrent lesions are often behaviorally more aggressive or of a higher grade than the initial lesion and may compromise the optimal treatment and long-term outcome for the animal.

Incomplete surgical excision for canine STS has been reported to result in a 60% probability of local recurrence within the first 12 months (Bostock and Dye, 1980), increasing in subsequent years. In one study 28% of dogs with incomplete surgical margins had local recurrence and were over 10 times more likely to have local recurrence than dogs with completely excised STSs (Kuntz et al., 1997).

Surgical Resection With Wide Margins

Surgical resection with wide margins provides the best chance for a cure for cats and dogs with STS. Proper preoperative staging and diagnosis provides essential information to formulate a surgical plan. Excision of the STS, with associated biopsy tracts and any areas of fixation (e.g., bone, fascia), with wide margins is the recommended treatment. The minimum recommended surgical margins are 3 cm of grossly normal tissue lateral to the tumor and one uninvolved fascial layer deep to the tumor.

In two different studies surgical resection with wide, histologically complete margins resulted in 90% to 100% local disease control and a 90% to 93% 1-year disease-free survival. In these studies resected specimens were processed and fixed to emulate their in situ dimensions as closely as possible, and surgical margins were evaluated using a standardized protocol. Resected specimens were pinned to cardboard to prevent shrinkage during fixation and processing, painted with tissue-marking ink to mark the entire surgical margin, and fixed in formalin for 24 hours. The deep margin was always the closest margin in cases of clean resection, or the dirty margin in cases of incomplete resection and therefore more likely to be a site of treatment failure than either lateral margin. In all but one dog, tumors resected with deep margins greater than 1 mm did not develop local recurrence because all had a layer of fascia resected as part of the deep margin. These studies showed margins of 11 to 30 mm may be acceptable for grades I and II STSs, especially when a deep uninvolved fascial layer is removed en bloc with the lesion. Another study reported that canine STSs removed with attempted wide margins, regardless of completeness of excision, had an 85% rate of local tumor control with a median time to recurrence of 368 days. In another study 79% of canine STSs resected with wide, complete histologic margins were controlled for 2 years. The extent of surgery was the only factor significantly associated with survival time in a series of 56 dogs with liposarcomas. Resection of liposarcomas with wide margins resulted in a median survival time of 1188 days, compared to 649 days for marginal excision and 183 days for incisional biopsy (see Chapter 68 for additional information regarding surgical oncology principles).

Marginal Resection and Adjuvant Radiation Therapy

If the tumor or previous scar cannot be excised with wide margins, particularly for STS of the extremity, marginal resection followed by adjuvant RT is recommended to prolong disease-free interval and preserve limb function. This treatment regimen ideally involves a radiation oncologist from the outset rather than use of RT as a rescue procedure. In two studies marginal resection followed with alternate-day megavoltage RT resulted in 16% local recurrence rate with a median time to recurrence of 700 to more than 798 days (Forrest et al., 2003; McKnight et al., 2000). The optimal fractionation scheme and total radiation doses for canine STS have not been determined; but cumulative dosages greater than 50 Gy are recommended, and local tumor control is better with higher cumulative doses. In some cases RT can be used before surgery to decrease tumor volume so that the tumor is more amenable to wide surgical excision. Ideally the use of RT should involve a team approach with the surgical oncologist and the radiation oncologist. (See Chapter 67 for additional information about radiation therapy.)

Radiation Therapy Alone

RT alone achieves local control in 48% to 67% of tumors in the first 12 months, with higher cumulative radiation doses resulting in better control rates; however, this reduces to 20% to 33% at 2 years. Thus RT is not considered adequate as sole therapy but is generally considered palliative. Hyperthermia alone (100% recurrence rate) or with adjunctive RT (65% to 91% response rate with a 1-year recurrence rate of 30% to 64%) has also been used for treatment of canine STS.

Chemotherapy

Candidates for chemotherapy include animals with distant metastasis, inoperable tumors (because of size or location), recurrent tumors not amenable to further surgical treatment or RT, and grade III STS. However, chemotherapy has a limited role (if any) in the management of canine and feline STS in any of these situations, based on the failure of any study to date to document a positive effect.

Three chemotherapy drugs are active in adult human STS: anthracyclines (doxorubicin [DOX] and epirubicin), ifosfamide, and dacarbazine. In dogs DOX is considered the most active single agent to treat STS with objective response rates of up to 23%. Mitoxantrone has a variable effect in canine STS with a 0% to 33% response rate; a response rate of 21% has been reported in cats, with better response rates in lower-grade tumors. Ifosfamide conferred a complete response rate of 15% in 13 dogs with sarcomas of skin, bladder, and spleen. However, in dogs the combination of DOX with either ifosfamide or cyclophosphamide does not appear to be more efficacious than DOX alone. Antitumor responses observed following chemotherapy are usually incomplete and of short duration. The response of humans with extremity STS to preoperative DOX was prognostic in one study, with responders having a significantly improved overall and disease-free survival compared to nonresponders (Pezzi et al., 1989). The role of neoadjuvant chemotherapy in the management of cats and dogs with STS has not been investigated.

Postoperative Chemotherapy

Grade III cutaneous STSs are associated with an increased risk of metastasis (41% to 50%) and decreased survival times. Chemotherapy may have a role in these cases to delay or prevent the development of metastatic disease. However, metastasis usually occurs late in the course of disease (median time to metastasis of 365 days), and this may minimize the beneficial effects of postoperative chemotherapy in such cases. Studies investigating DOX-based protocols, single-agent ifosfamide and mitoxantrone, and dual agent DOX-ifosfamide in canine STSs have demonstrated no difference in disease-free interval or survival time between dogs receiving surgery alone and those receiving surgery and chemotherapy. In humans chemotherapy also does not affect overall survival time but may improve local tumor control. In one study postoperative DOX was not beneficial in increasing the metastasis-free interval or overall survival time in dogs with high-grade STSs of various locations (Selting et al., 2005). Situations in which postoperative chemotherapy should be considered include intraabdominal STSs (e.g., splenic sarcomas), metastatic disease, and dogs with histologic subtypes with a higher rate of metastasis (e.g., histiocytic sarcoma, hypodermal HSA [stage II or III], synovial cell sarcoma, rhabdomyosarcoma, and lymphangiosarcoma).

Intracavitary Chemotherapy

Marginal resection with implantation of an intracavitary biodegradable polymer of open-cell polylactic acid containing cisplatin has been reported with a 31% local tumor recurrence rate and a median time to recurrence of 640 days. This product is not available commercially, and local toxicity is common.

Metastatic Disease

Animals with metastatic disease should be managed palliatively rather than being treated with more aggressive curative-intent techniques such as surgery and/or RT. Pulmonary metastasectomy has not been evaluated for metastatic STS.

PROGNOSIS

Prognostic Factors for Local Tumor Recurrence

Prognostic factors for local tumor recurrence include tumor size, tumor location, tumor grade, and completeness of surgical excision. Tumors larger than 5 cm in diameter are more likely to develop local tumor recurrence. Site is also prognostic, with STSs located in superficial sites or the extremities having a better prognosis than tumors that are deep, truncal, invasive, or close to the spinal cord. This is probably because location can affect ability to achieve complete surgical resection. Dogs with incomplete resection are over 10 times more likely to develop local disease recurrence. Tumor grade (low or intermediate grade are more favorable) and thickness of deep margin (>10 mm or at least one fascial plane nonadherent to the tumor) are prognostic factors for local recurrence. Tumors that are freely movable have a more favorable prognosis than those fixed to underlying tissues.

Prognostic Factors for Metastasis

The absence of metastatic disease at diagnosis is a positive prognostic factor. Mitotic rate has been shown to be significantly associated with the development of metastasis at a distant site. In one study dogs with 20 or more mitotic figures per 10 high-power fields were five times more likely to develop metastasis than dogs with less than 20 mitotic figures per 10 high-power fields. Degree of differentiation, tumor grade, and histologic type also significantly affected the likelihood of metastasis. Dogs with high-grade tumors have a higher risk of metastasis and death compared to dogs with low-grade tumors. Fewer than 10% of grade I STSs, 20% of grade II STSs, and 50% of grade III STSs undergo metastasis to the regional lymph nodes and lungs.

Prognostic Factors for Survival

Tumor-related deaths in animals with STS are usually caused by uncontrolled local disease. The median survival times for dogs with nonoral STSs treated with wide surgical resection or marginal surgical resection combined with adjuvant megavoltage RT are 1416 and 2270 days, respectively. Mitotic rate and percent tumor necrosis were significantly associated with survival time. Dogs with more than 10% necrosis are 2.8 times more likely to die of tumor-related causes than dogs with less than 10% necrosis. Dogs with 20 mitotic figures or more per 10 high-power fields were 2.6 times more likely to die of tumor-related causes than dogs with less than 20 mitotic figures per 10 high-power fields. Other prognostic factors for overall survival include tumor size, completeness of surgical resection, degree of differentiation, histologic tumor grade, and local tumor control.

References and Suggested Reading

Baez JL et al: Liposarcomas in dogs: 56 cases (1989-2000), *J Am Vet Med Assoc* 224:887, 2004.

Baker-Gabb M, Hunt GB, France MP: Soft tissue sarcomas and mast cell tumors in dogs: clinical behavior and response to surgery, *Aust Vet J* 81:732, 2003.

Banks TA et al: Prospective study of canine soft tissue sarcoma treated by wide surgical excision: quantitative evaluation of surgical margins, *Vet Cancer Soc Newsletter* 23:21, 2003.

Banks TA et al: Soft-tissue sarcomas in dogs: a study assessing surgical margin, tumour grade and clinical outcome, *Aust Vet Pract* 34:158, 2004.

Bostock DE, Dye MT: Prognosis after surgical resection of canine fibrous connective tissue sarcomas, *Vet Pathol* 17:581, 1980.

Graves GM, Bjorling DE, Mahaffey E: Canine haemangiopericy-toma: 23 cases (1067-1984), *J Am Vet Med Assoc* 192:99, 1998.

Kuntz CA et al: Prognostic factors for surgical treatment of soft-tissue sarcomas in dogs: 75 cases (1986-1996), *J Am Vet Med Assoc* 211:1147, 1997.

Liptak JM, Forrest LJ: Soft-tissue sarcomas. In Withrow SJ, Vail DM, editors: *Small animal clinical oncology*, ed 4, Philadelphia, 2007, Saunders, p 425.

McChesney SL et al: Radiotherapy of soft-tissue sarcomas in dogs, *J Am Vet Med Assoc* 194:60, 1989.

McKnight JA et al: Radiation treatment for incompletely resected soft tissue sarcomas in dogs, *J Am Vet Med Assoc* 217:205, 2000.

Pezzi CM et al: Preoperative chemotherapy for soft tissue sarcomas of the extremities, *Ann Surg* 211:47, 1989.

Postorino NC et al: Prognostic variables for canine haeman-giopericytoma: 50 cases (1979-1984), *J Am Anim Hosp Assoc* 24:501, 1988.

Sarcoma meta-analysis collaboration. Adjuvant chemotherapy for localized, resectable soft-tissue sarcoma of adults: meta-analysis of individual data, *Lancet* 350:1647, 1997.

Selting KA et al: Outcome of dogs with high-grade soft-tissue sarcomas treated with and without adjuvant doxorubicin chemotherapy: 39 cases (1996-2004), *J Am Vet Med Assoc* 227:1442, 2005.

CHAPTER 70

Canine Hemangiosarcoma

CRAIG A. CLIFFORD, *Tinton Falls, New Jersey*
LOUIS-PHILIPPE de LORIMIER, *Brossard, Québec, Canada*

A highly malignant tumor originating from endo-thelial cells, hemangiosarcoma (HSA) is diagnosed more frequently in dogs than in any other domestic species and has a high mortality rate. Representing approximately 2% of all canine tumors, HSA tends to affect older dogs of either sex, with a median age of 10 years at diagnosis. Although any breed can be affected, German shepherds, golden retrievers, and Labrador retrievers appear predisposed.

ETIOLOGY

The definitive etiology of canine HSA remains uncertain, although the strong breed association suggests a genetic predisposition. Chronic ultraviolet light exposure is a known risk factor for superficial (dermal) HSA in lightly pigmented short-haired breeds of dogs and similarly may be a risk factor for the conjunctival location according to a recently published retrospective study.

Research has shown overexpression of the oncopro-tein STAT3 to be common in canine vascular tumors, with 100% of 22 HSA samples determined to be positive and with a higher percentage of positive cells in HSA than benign hemangiomas. Mutations in p53 and PTEN, two important tumor suppressor genes, were recently dem-onstrated in canine HSA and may also contribute in the malignant transformation of vascular endothelial cells.

Angiogenesis, the formation of new blood vessels, is a tightly regulated process involving both proangiogenic and antiangiogenic factors. This pathway is often dysregu-lated in neoplasia via up-regulation of angiogenic factors and down-regulation of antiangiogenic factors. When com-pared to healthy dogs, vascular endothelial growth factor (VEGF), one of the most potent angiogenic factors, was shown to be elevated in the plasma and effusions of dogs with HSA. Angiopoietins, proteins playing a central role in the regulation of angiogenesis, were shown to be overex-pressed in a canine splenic HSA sample when compared to normal spleen. Interestingly endostatin, a negative modu-lator of angiogenesis, was also recently found to be elevated in the serum of dogs with HSA. Evidence derived from in vitro research suggests that HSA cells are capable of pro-ducing a plethora of angiogenic factors such as VEGF, basic fibroblastic growth factor (bFGF), and the angiopoietins.

With the help of multiparameter flow cytometry, recently it was demonstrated that canine HSA originates from hema-topoietic precursors with commitment to the endothelial lineage rather than from the malignant transformation of mature endothelial cells in the peripheral vasculature. The expression patterns of cell-surface markers observed in those multipotential bone marrow–derived stem cells with differentiation arrest at the hemangioblast stage may help in confirming the diagnosis of HSA, monitoring minimal residual disease, and obtaining an early diagnosis.

Ongoing research on the etiology of the disease, through collaborative efforts of the Dog Disease Mapping Project at the Broad Institute of the Massachusetts Institute of Technology, Harvard University, and a num-ber of veterinary investigators aims to identify genetic mutations that increase susceptibility to development of HSA. Identification of the genetic basis of HSA will allow for a better understanding of the biology of the disease and development of a deoxyribonucleic acid (DNA) test that eventually may advance preventative measures and novel targeted therapies.

BIOLOGIC BEHAVIOR AND PROGNOSIS

As an endothelial-derived tumor, HSA can develop anywhere in the body. The spleen, heart (right atrium or auricle), skin or subcutaneous tissues, and liver are the four most common primary sites. Other reported primary sites include kidney, muscle, bone, oral cavity, bladder, and lung. Metastatic dissemination and local infiltration occur early in disease, either hematogenously or via local seeding following tumor rupture. The lungs, liver, and omentum are the most frequent sites of dissemination. Hemangiosarcoma is recognized as the most common sarcoma to metastasize to the central nervous system (CNS). Certain primary tumor locations may be associated with a better prognosis; dermal, conjunctival and possibly subcutaneous HSA tend to have a lower metastatic rate than visceral tumors. Studies have demonstrated that higher clinical stage (Box 70-1) results in earlier metastasis and shorter survival time for splenic and subcutaneous HSA. When advanced metastatic disease is present, it is often impossible to identify the primary site, and the prognosis is unsurprisingly poor to grave, although occasional responses to therapy have been observed.

DIAGNOSIS AND STAGING

Since clinical stage affects prognosis and HSA is a highly metastatic cancer, complete clinical staging is highly recommended at diagnosis when the patient is sufficiently stable. In cases in which emergency surgical intervention

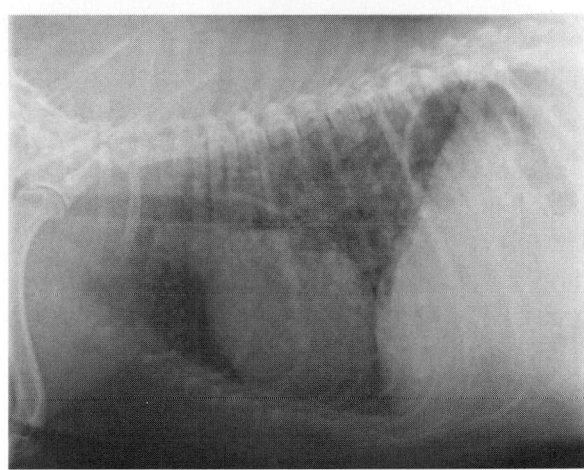

Fig. 70-1 Left lateral digital radiograph of a dog with pulmonary metastasis from splenic hemangiosarcoma, demonstrating the typical interstitial miliary pattern.

must be performed to save the patient's life, certain staging procedures may have to be postponed temporarily. As previously mentioned, metastatic disease frequently affects the lungs; liver; omental surfaces; and occasionally soft tissues, adrenal glands, and the CNS. Although it is not considered metastatic dissemination, it is known that approximately 25% of dogs with HSA in one location (e.g., spleen) also have another primary HSA in a second site (e.g., right atrium), a process described as metachronous disease.

As a result, complete clinical staging should include three-view thoracic radiographs, abdominal ultrasonographic study, and multiple image-plane echocardiography, in addition to standard blood work. Although the typical appearance of measurable pulmonary metastatic disease is that of a coalescing miliary pattern, either nodular or generalized miliary interstitial patterns also can be observed on occasion (Fig. 70-1). Abdominal ultrasonography is a fairly sensitive routine imaging technique permitting the detection of splenic or hepatic lesions, occasionally of omental nodules as well, and in most cases identifies free abdominal fluid when present. Echocardiography remains the method of choice to identify right atrial masses; these are more easily identified when at least some degree of pericardial effusion is present and when multiple right and left-sided image planes are obtained by experienced examiners. Although urinalysis and serum biochemistry rarely help in the diagnosis of HSA, the complete blood cell count typically has changes that may suggest a microangiopathic process, including the presence of regenerative anemia, thrombocytopenia, and fragmented red blood cells (schistocytes). In addition, when the spleen is severely affected, a deficient reticuloendothelial system will permit higher numbers of metarubricytes (nucleated red blood cells) to appear in the peripheral blood.

In select cases additional imaging techniques may be required for identification of suspect metastasis based on physical examination findings (e.g., suspect bone or CNS metastasis). Advanced imaging in the form of computed tomography (CT) or magnetic resonance imaging (MRI) is recommended for invasive subcutaneous or

---

Box **70-1**

Clinical Staging System for Hemangiosarcoma

Primary Tumor (T)
- T0: No measurable tumor
- T1: Tumor less than 5 cm in diameter, confined to primary site; does not invade beyond dermis (cutaneous HSA)
- T2: Tumor 5 cm or greater in diameter, or ruptured; invades subcutaneous tissues (cutaneous HSA)
- T3: Tumor invades adjacent structures; invades into the underlying muscle (cutaneous HSA)

Regional Lymph Nodes (N)
- N0: No regional lymph node involvement
- N1: Regional lymph node involvement
- N2: Distant lymph node involvement

Distant Metastasis (M)
- M0: No measurable distant metastasis
- M1: Detectable distant metastasis
- Stage I: T0 or T1, N0, M0
- Stage II: T1 N1 or T2 N0, M0
- Stage III: T2 N1 or T3 N0, or N2, M1

HSA, Hemangiosarcoma.

intramuscular HSA to assess invasiveness and plan surgical resection and/or radiation therapy, if indicated. In addition, recent work has shown that imaging modalities such as MRI and CT carry a high sensitivity and specificity in discriminating benign from malignant splenic and hepatic lesions. Furthermore, recently published and ongoing studies are confirming the increased sensitivity of thoracic CT for early pulmonary metastasis detection. As the routine use of such diagnostic techniques increases in veterinary medicine, these studies may be incorporated more routinely in the thorough staging of dogs with HSA.

The definitive diagnosis of HSA is only confirmed with histopathology. It is crucial to remember that no imaging technique can confirm with certainty that the observed lesion is in fact HSA. Therefore no patient with hemoabdomen should be euthanized based on a splenic mass that "is consistent with HSA," especially since nonmalignant splenic lesions, including hematomas and hemangiomas, appear identical in many cases, bear a very good prognosis with splenectomy alone, and are often diagnosed in breeds known to be overrepresented for HSA. The precise number of patients with hemoabdomen and associated malignancy has varied in different reports. Several retrospective studies have shown that for splenic nodules a third to 50% are benign and curable with a sole splenectomy. However, a recent study of patients presenting with a nontraumatic hemoabdomen noted that 80% were secondary to visceral neoplasia, of which 70% were confirmed as HSA. Although cytology is a noninvasive and clinically valuable technique for the diagnosis of cancer in general, the diagnostic yield for HSA is reported to be low (25%).

One possible way to improve the prognosis of canine HSA may come in the form of earlier detection. The current standard for diagnosing HSA remains histopathology of measurable lesions usually after metastatic dissemination has already occurred; however, new detection methods eventually may help obtain an early diagnosis for high-risk dogs. One such method involves flow cytometry of peripheral blood to identify cells of primitive endothelial lineage, coexpressing certain cell surface markers, detected in higher numbers in dogs harboring HSA than in healthy controls or dogs rendered free of measurable HSA following surgical excision.

The current research aiming to identify causative mutations of certain genes eventually may enable the development of DNA tests capable of identifying susceptible individuals and those that may pass these genes to their progeny. Such tests would allow owners and veterinarians to follow susceptible dogs more closely for tumor occurrence, possibly before life-threatening complications occur.

TRADITIONAL THERAPY

Traditional therapy for HSA, as for other cancers, involves surgery, radiation therapy, and systemic cytotoxic chemotherapy, alone or in a multimodality setting.

Surgery

Splenectomy, liver lobectomy, excision of dermal or subcutaneous masses, and right auriculectomy all have been reported. Such surgeries are performed to remove all macroscopic tumors and prevent further risk of acute hemorrhage, establishment of disseminated intravascular coagulation, or death. Surgery alone for splenic, cardiac, subcutaneous, or hepatic HSA has yielded unsatisfactory results and is generally considered purely palliative, with median survival times (MSTs) generally averaging 1 to 3 months. A recent study of 23 dogs with cardiac HSA reported a MST of 43 days (n=8) and 118 days (n=15) following resection of right atrial or auricular HSA, respectively. The MST was significantly prolonged in eight dogs receiving chemotherapy (175 days) when compared to 15 dogs treated with surgery alone (42 days). Pericardiectomy via thoracotomy or thoracoscopy can alleviate life-threatening cardiac tamponade, but alone it is unlikely to significantly prolong survival. Surgical resection of superficial dermal or conjunctival HSA often results in prolonged survival times because of the lower metastatic rate observed with these primary locations.

Chemotherapy

Doxorubicin (DOX)-based adjuvant chemotherapy, with or without the addition of cyclophosphamide or vincristine, has provided the best survival times to date. Common protocols include single-agent DOX; DOX and cyclophosphamide (AC protocol); and vincristine, DOX, and cyclophosphamide (VAC protocol). Survival times ranging from 140 to 202 days have been reported for the various DOX-based protocols; however, no protocol is regarded as clearly superior. In an attempt to improve on the MST, a dosage-intense protocol with every-other-week DOX administration and intracavitary chemotherapy administration with the liposome-encapsulated form of DOX (Doxil) were investigated. Unfortunately these did not result in significant survival benefit. Ifosfamide, an alkylating agent with therapeutic activity in human sarcomas, was administered following splenectomy in six dogs with HSA, resulting in a MST of 147 days. When a combination of ifosfamide and DOX was recently evaluated in the adjuvant setting on 27 dogs with HSA, a disappointing MST of 149 days was obtained. Although the benefits of adjuvant chemotherapy on survival times are well recognized, additional or novel therapeutic modalities are clearly needed.

Radiation Therapy

There is a paucity of published information regarding the use of radiation therapy for canine HSA. However, anecdotal clinical responses and quality-of-life improvements have been observed when coarse fractions of megavoltage radiation therapy are delivered (once or twice weekly) to invasive and nonresectable subcutaneous or intramuscular HSA lesions. In such cases radiation therapy is considered palliative, decreasing pain and bruising and occasionally resulting in tumor shrinkage, and generally is combined with systemic DOX-based chemotherapy.

NOVEL THERAPY

Since the combination of traditional therapeutic modalities has reached a plateau unlikely to be surpassed, with

MSTs averaging 6 to 7 months, new therapies are awaited impatiently. The growing body of knowledge on the molecular alterations observed in canine HSA cells may hopefully unveil numerous novel targets.

Immunotherapy has long been a field of active research, and an aggressive and rapidly progressing cancer such as HSA provides a great opportunity for even small improvements to be detected. Although initial studies evaluating nonspecific immunotherapy had failed to provide similarly positive outcomes, a randomized, prospective evaluation in canine HSA patients combining the AC protocol with liposomal muramyl tripeptide phosphatidylethanolamine (L-MTP-PE), a synthetic macrophage activator derived from mycobacterial cell wall, resulted in the only published study reporting a MST significantly superior to traditional chemotherapy alone (273 days). Although this study firmly established a role for immunotherapy in treating canine HSA, L-MTP-PE is not commercially available. Recently an unpublished pilot study using an intraperitoneally administered allogeneic HSA vaccine demonstrated encouraging results, conferring an MST greater than 7 months in seven dogs with stage III HSA receiving the vaccine in combination with standard chemotherapy. Further studies are ongoing.

Antiangiogenic therapy is an important field of investigational cancer therapy in humans and is the subject of numerous ongoing clinical studies on canine HSA. Systemic administration of interleukin-12 (IL-12), a cytokine known to possess potent antiangiogenic properties, inhibited the growth of canine HSA in a murine model. Studies in dogs evaluating IL-12, interferon-α-2a, thrombospondin-1, protease inhibitors, and thalidomide eventually may demonstrate benefits in terms of improved MST, and the results are highly anticipated. Although novel humanized monoclonal antibodies directed against certain angiogenic proteins (e.g., bevacizumab targeting VEGF) may not be practical for use in dogs because of the induction of neutralizing canine antihuman antibodies, the ongoing research on small-molecule inhibitors targeting the same signaling pathways (VEGF, bFGF, integrins) raises cautious optimism for eventual application in the veterinary field.

In contrast to most canine carcinomas evaluated to date, it appears that canine HSA typically does not overexpress COX-2. However, because nonsteroidal drugs have also demonstrated clinical efficacy in certain non-COX-2 overexpressing tumors, it is conceivable that incorporating a COX-2 inhibitor to standard therapy might prolong the survival time of dogs with HSA. However, a recently completed but unpublished prospective study found no overall improvement in survival when a COX-2 selective inhibitor was coadministered with adjuvant DOX therapy in dogs with splenic HSA.

As previously stated, mutated tumor suppressor genes may contribute to malignant transformation. Interestingly it is also possible for such genes to be transiently silenced through epigenetic changes, opening the way for therapy targeting such reversible alterations. Although occasional reports of long-term survival following surgery alone have been reported, a published case report described a dog surviving in excess of 1000 days following splenectomy for HSA after receiving a histone deacetylase (HDAC) inhibitor as the sole adjuvant therapy. This encouraging outcome and further large-scale prospective in vivo studies with HDAC inhibitors hold promise for dogs with aggressive malignancies such as HSA.

Finally the use of traditional chemotherapy agents can also be revisited through novel methods or schedules of administration. A study evaluating concurrent systemic and inhalational therapy with DOX demonstrated encouraging results in diminishing pulmonary metastasis from HSA. "Metronomic" (continuous, low-dose) dosing of traditional cytotoxic chemotherapy agents is another new approach. The therapeutic target is then shifted from the cancer cells to the endothelial cells by administering frequent low doses of chemotherapy. By so doing, the common problems of toxicities and drug resistance can largely be avoided. Ongoing clinical studies aim to evaluate the potential benefit of low-dose metronomic chemotherapy on measurable HSA and in the adjuvant setting.

References and Suggested Reading

Clifford CA et al: Plasma vascular endothelial growth factor concentrations in healthy dogs and dogs with hemangiosarcoma, *J Vet Intern Med* 15:131, 2001.

Fosmire SP et al: Canine malignant hemangiosarcoma as a model of primitive angiogenic endothelium, *Lab Invest* 84:562, 2004.

Heller DA et al: Assessment of cyclooxygenase-2 expression in canine hemangiosarcoma, histiocytic sarcoma, and mast cell tumor, *Vet Pathol* 42:350, 2005.

Lamerato-Kozicki AR et al: Canine hemangiosarcoma originates from hematopoietic precursors with potential for endothelial differentiation, *Exp Hematol* 34:870, 2006.

Payne SE et al: Treatment of vascular and soft-tissue sarcomas in dogs using an alternating protocol of ifosfamide and doxorubicin, *Vet Comp Oncol* 1:171, 2003.

Pirie CG et al: Canine conjunctival hemangioma and hemangiosarcoma: a retrospective evaluation of 108 cases (1989-2004), *Vet Ophthalmol* 9:215, 2006.

Rossmeisl Jr JH et al: Endostatin concentrations in healthy dogs and dogs with selected neoplasms, *J Vet Intern Med* 16:565, 2002.

Sorenmo KU et al: Efficacy and toxicity of a dose-intensified doxorubicin protocol in canine hemangiosarcoma, *J Vet Intern Med* 18:209, 2004.

Thamm DH et al: Biological and molecular characterization of a canine hemangiosarcoma-derived cell line, *Res Vet Sci* 81:76, 2006.

Weisse C et al: Survival times in dogs with right atrial hemangiosarcoma treated by means of surgical resection with or without adjuvant chemotherapy: 23 cases (1986-2000), *J Am Vet Med Assoc* 226:575, 2005.

CHAPTER 71

Feline Vaccine-Associated Sarcomas

MATTIE J. HENDRICK, *Philadelphia, Pennsylvania*
A. ELIZABETH HERSHEY, *Phoenix, Arizona*

Since 1991 there have been several reports supporting a strong association between the administration of vaccines, particularly feline leukemia and rabies, and the subsequent development of sarcomas in cats at the site of vaccination. Although these sarcomas are uncommon, with estimates of their occurrence ranging from 1 in 1,000 to 1 in 10,000 cats receiving vaccinations, they are aggressive, resulting in significant morbidity and mortality. Most tumors have proved resistant to standard treatment modalities, and many cats have multiple recurrences, with euthanasia as the final outcome. Despite many years of epidemiologic and investigational research, feline vaccine-associated sarcomas (VASs) remain a significant problem in veterinary medicine.

CLINICAL APPEARANCE AND BEHAVIOR

Most VASs arise in the interscapular subcutis, along the dorsal and lateral thorax and flank, and in the musculature of the thigh or more distal limb, reflecting common vaccination sites. Recommendations by the Vaccine-Associated Feline Sarcoma Task Force (VAFSTF)* and other veterinary organizations to use the distal limbs rather than the interscapular region for vaccination have been followed by practicing veterinarians with mixed success. Typical tumors are grayish-white, firm, well demarcated, and partially encapsulated. Most tumors are larger than 4 cm in diameter when found by the owner or veterinarian and have a necrotic center, giving them a cystic appearance. Despite the circumscribed gross appearance of the tumor, there are often "tongues" of tumor extending away from the mass along fascial planes, most clearly seen by computed tomography or magnetic resonance imaging. The majority of VASs are fibrosarcomas, but malignant fibrous histiocytomas (also called myofibrosarcomas or myofibroblastic sarcomas), osteosarcomas,

chondrosarcomas, rhabdomyosarcomas, myxosarcomas, and liposarcomas have also been reported. Histologically most VASs have a high degree of nuclear pleomorphism, cellular atypia, and multinucleated giant cells. Many but not all have peripheral aggregates of lymphocytes and macrophages. In some the macrophages contain a globular grayish-brown material that has been shown to be aluminum, a common adjuvant used in feline vaccines.

In one retrospective study (Hendrick et al., 1994), 62% of the tumors recurred following excisional biopsy, most within 6 months. A total of 22% of cats had VASs recur two, three, or four times. Based on published reports, the metastatic rate of VAS is variable, ranging from 0% to 28%, the higher rates occurring in cats that had repeated recurrences or radiation therapy (RT).

PATHOGENESIS

Based on morphologic and immunohistochemical evidence, VASs appear to arise from primitive mesenchymal cells that have features of fibroblasts and myofibroblasts. The exact origin of myofibroblasts is controversial, but many believe they represent a "transitional stage" through which fibroblasts or some other primitive mesenchymal cells pass during the process of wound healing. Injection of vaccines commonly results in a localized granulomatous and lymphocytic reaction that varies in severity and duration, depending on the vaccine and adjuvant.

The increased incidence of fibrosarcomas in cats began in the late 1980s, shortly following the introduction and widespread use of killed aluminum-adjuvanted rabies and leukemia virus vaccines not previously used in the cat. Macy (1999) has documented that these vaccines consistently produce palpable inflammatory masses at the site of injection in cats. Hypothetically VASs may arise from inappropriate or overzealous inflammatory or immunologic reactions associated with the presence of vaccine components in vaccination sites that lead to uncontrolled proliferation of fibroblasts and myofibroblasts. Despite the importance of feline leukemia virus (FeLV) and feline sarcoma virus (FeSV) in many diseases and neoplasms in cats, these viruses do not appear to play a role in the pathogenesis of VASs (Ellis et al., 1996).

Research in the senior author's laboratory and by other investigators has focused on growth factors and oncogenes as likely players in this neoplastic transformation. Many studies and animal models support the hypothesis that growth factors promote neoplastic transformation.

---

* The Vaccine-Associated Feline Sarcoma Task Force is a combined effort of the American Veterinary Medical Association, the American Animal Hospital Association, the American Association of Feline Practitioners, and the Veterinary Cancer Society. Its membership is composed of representatives from the aforementioned groups, veterinary researchers and clinicians, and representatives from the U.S. Department of Agriculture and the Animal Health Institute. The guidelines are based on discussions and materials provided by this group, the Academy of Feline Medicine, and the California Veterinary Medical Association.

A large percentage of human tumors have been shown to have receptors for growth factors that they themselves produce in an abnormal or autonomous fashion. Termed *autocrine stimulation,* I and others have documented this phenomenon in feline VAS, using immunohistochemical and molecular methods. Specifically platelet-derived growth factor (PDGF) and its receptor are overexpressed in feline VAS and in cultured cell lines from these tumors. McEwen and later Vail and associates (Katayama et al., 2004) showed that the use of a tyrosine kinase inhibitor blocks signaling through the PDGF receptor, resulting in decreased viability of the cultured sarcoma cells, inhibition of tumor growth in nude mice, and enhancement of the sensitivity of the cultured cells to chemotherapeutic agents. Last, dysregulation of p53, a tumor suppressor protein, appears to be a feature of many feline fibrosarcomas, including those associated with vaccination (Hershey et al., 2005). Clearly differences in host genome and alterations in p53 and growth factor expression play a role in the pathogenesis of these tumors and should be the focus of continuing research.

TREATMENT

Effective treatment of VAS resulting in long-term control remains challenging. Although surgery remains the mainstay of treatment, by itself it rarely achieves long-term tumor control. Completeness of surgical excision does not always guarantee tumor control because tumors can recur in the face of histologically "complete" surgical excision. Whether this tumor recurrence represents true local recurrence or the effect of "field cancerization" remains unclear. More aggressive or radical first excision of VAS is an important first step in achieving long-term tumor control (Hershey et al., 2000). In one study radical first excision of VAS yielded a longer median disease-free interval (DFI) (325 days) when compared with marginal first excision (79 days). In addition, cats with tumors located on the limbs had a longer DFI (325 days) than cats with tumors located in other sites (66 days). This reflects the ability of radical excision (i.e., amputation) to be achieved should a VAS occur. However, few cats (13.8%) that received only surgical treatment had long-term control of greater than 2 years. In multiple studies the recurrence rate was higher for cats with multiple surgeries than cats that had only one surgery (Hershey et al., 2000, Cohen et al., 2001). In addition, tumors have been noted to recur in shorter intervals with each successive surgery. Thus adjuvant treatments with RT and/or chemotherapy are warranted in most patients.

Chemotherapy with doxorubicin (DOX) and Doxil (liposome-encapsulated doxorubicin) has been evaluated objectively as an adjuvant to surgery in cats with VASs (Poirier et al., 2002). Cats receiving either DOX or Doxil after surgery had a significantly longer DFI compared to historical controls receiving surgery alone (388 versus 94 days). Cats with complete excision had a longer DFI (449 days) than cats with incomplete excision (281 days). No significant difference was noted in the outcomes between the two chemotherapy agents. DOX with or without cyclophosphamide may also be beneficial in treating macroscopic disease, providing palliation, or making some nonresectable tumors amenable to surgery (Poirier et al., 2002, Barber et al., 2000).

Carboplatin may also be a useful agent in the treatment of VAS. Six of 16 cats with measurable VASs treated with carboplatin experienced a partial response. In addition, cats treated with carboplatin concomitant with preoperative RT in one study had a longer median DFI compared to other chemotherapy treatments (Kobayashi et al., 2002). This may be caused by the effect of carboplatin as a radiation sensitizer when given in conjunction with RT. Other potentially effective drugs include mitoxantrone, ifosfamide, and lomustine.

Several studies have reported treatment outcomes of multimodality therapy combining surgery, RT, and chemotherapy. Outcomes have been similar between the studies for preoperative and postoperative RT; advantages can be argued for both. With no clear improvement in DFI, the decision for preoperative or postoperative RT should be made on a patient-by-patient basis. The use of chemotherapy concomitant with RT did not significantly influence DFI in any study. However, in one study overall survival times were longer with use of carboplatin in conjunction with RT than with other chemotherapies (Kobayashi et al., 2002). No direct comparisons have been made between combined surgery and RT versus combined surgery and chemotherapy. A comparison of treatment outcomes is reported in Table 71-1.

The efficacy of RT without chemotherapy in the treatment of VAS is unclear. Given the potential for metastasis in VASs, systemic therapy in conjunction with local therapy is warranted.

In summary, surgery as a sole therapy results in a high rate of local recurrence, except in tumors of the distal limb in which amputation is performed. The high frequency of recurrence in cats with histologically complete surgical resection indicates that adjuvant therapy should be considered in all cats with VASs. Combined therapy with RT and/or chemotherapy results in an improved DFI over surgery alone. However, in spite of combined therapies, long-term control is difficult to achieve, and attention must be directed at prevention of these tumors.

PREVENTION

The most important recommendation in the prevention of VAS is not to overvaccinate. One study clearly shows an increased incidence of VASs with increased number of vaccines administered (Kass et al., 1993). Vaccination should be viewed as a medical procedure similar to any other medical procedure and performed based on the medical needs of the individual patient. Veterinarians and cat owners must decide the relative risk of disease for individual cats and make appropriate decisions regarding vaccination. FeLV vaccine should not be administered indiscriminately since the epidemiologic data suggest it may be the most common cause of VAS in cats. There is an age-related susceptibility to FeLV, with kittens being at most risk of persistent infection. The risk of infection with FeLV decreases with age, with fewer than 15% of cats over 1 year of age becoming infected when challenged. The decision to vaccinate for FeLV should be based

Table 71-1

Treatment Outcomes For Vaccine-Associated Sarcomas

Study	Treatment	No. of Cats	DFI	OST	RR (%)	RM (%)	Comments
Cronin, Page, and Thrall 1998	Preop RT, sx ± DOX	33	398	600	45	24	Outcome influenced by completeness of excision; use of chemo did not influence outcome
Hershey et al., 2000	Surgical excision	61	94	576	86.2	22.5	Radical excision (i.e., amputation) improves DFI
Bregazzi et al., 2001	Sx, postop RT ±DOX	25	661 (+ chemo) NR (– chemo)	674 (+ chemo) 842 (– chemo)	28	0	No significant difference in outcome with use of chemo
Cohen et al., 2001	Sx, postop RT ± DOX/ cyclophosphamide	78	405	730	41	12	Use of chemo not associated with RR, RM, OST; extent of excision not associated with RR
Kobayashi et al., 2002	Preop RT, sx ± carboplatin	92	584	Not evaluated	37	21.7	Completeness of excision related to DFI
Poirier et al., 2002	Sx + DOX or Doxil	75	388	846	44	5	No difference between Doxil and DOX; renal toxicity noted with Doxil when dose escalated
Martano et al., 2005	Preop DOX + sx sx alone	49 20	NR NR	NR NR	40.8 35	12 10	No significant difference between groups

Chemo, Chemotherapy; *DFI,* disease-free interval (in days); *NR,* median not reached; *OST,* overall survival time in days; *RM,* rate of metastases; *RR,* rate of recurrence; *RT,* radiation therapy; *Sx,* surgery.

on the lifestyle of the cat, and few clinicians currently recommend FeLV vaccine for strictly indoor cats in a closed household. Rabies vaccination recommendations should follow state and local regulations.

It must be stressed that individual cats be vaccinated no more frequently than necessary and only against infectious diseases to which the individual has a realistic risk of exposure. Annual revaccination may not always be needed and may increase the risk that sarcomas will develop at vaccination sites. In one study many of the commercial vaccines had a duration of immunity longer than 1 year (Scott and Geissinger, 1997), supporting an every–3-year–program of vaccination.

The use of monovalent versus polyvalent vaccines is controversial. In one study (Kass, 1993) there was a significant increase in the risk of sarcoma development with increasing numbers of vaccines. However, Hendrick and associates (1994) found no association between vaccine site tumors and the number of vaccines administered simultaneously. Although conflicting results exist, it seems prudent that vaccines be injected at different sites and that polyvalent vaccines not be used.

The use of vaccines containing aluminum adjuvants is controversial. Aluminum-adjuvanted vaccines are the most consistent producers of vaccine site inflammation, a key factor in the development of VAS. The canary pox vectored recombinant feline rabies vaccine creates virtually no cellular infiltrate at the site of injection (Macy and Chretin, 1999). However, this vaccine must be administered annually rather than every 3 years. It seems logical to think there would be less risk if a less inflammatory product were administered less frequently. However, it is still not known whether other vaccine components contribute to the formation of VAS.

Current recommendations are for administration of vaccine as distally on the limb as possible. The site of administration does not likely affect the development of a sarcoma. However, if the sarcoma is located on the distal limb, the tumor may be identified at a smaller size, and amputation may allow better tumor control. In one study (Hershey et al., 2000) cats that had sarcomas in the distal portion of the limb treated by amputation had a longer median DFI than cats with sarcomas excised from other sites.

The following are guidelines based on the recommendations of the VAFSTF and the American Association of Feline Practitioners:

1. Veterinarians should adopt a standardized protocol for vaccination sites and document the locations of each injection, type of vaccine, and manufacturer or serial number.
2. Vaccines containing antigens limited to panleukopenia virus, feline herpesvirus type-1, and feline calicivirus with or without *Chlamydia* antigens should be administered on the right shoulder.
3. Vaccines containing rabies virus antigen, with or without any other antigen, should be administered on the right hind limb as distally as possible.
4. Vaccines containing FeLV antigen, with or without any other antigen except rabies virus antigen, should be administered on the left hind limb as distally as possible.

OWNER EDUCATION

Although the risk of VAS occurrence is real, owners should be educated as to the relative risk of VAS development versus the risk of serious, preventable infectious disease, allowing them to make informed decisions about vaccination administration and frequency. Furthermore, as with most tumors, early detection and appropriate therapy have the potential to lead to improved outcomes. As previously mentioned, almost all cats develop some degree of inflammatory reaction at the site where a vaccine is administered. It is useful to have criteria for when a lump at a vaccine site is a cause for concern. A helpful mnemonic for owners is the so-called "3-2-1 rule." The veterinarian should be notified if the lump persists for more than 3 months following vaccination, if it exceeds 2 cm in diameter at any time, or if it is continuing to enlarge 1 month after vaccination. Vaccine-site lumps meeting any of these criteria should be investigated by incisional or excisional biopsy.

References and Suggested Reading

Barber LG et al: Combined doxorubicin and cyclophosphamide chemotherapy for nonresectable feline fibrosarcoma, *J Am Anim Hosp Assoc* 36:416, 2000.

Bregazzi VS et al: Treatment with a combination of doxorubicin, surgery, and radiation versus surgery and radiation alone for cats with vaccine-associated sarcomas: 25 cases (1995-2000), *J Am Vet Med Assoc* 218:547, 2001.

Cohen M et al: Use of surgery and electron beam irradiation, with or without chemotherapy, for treatment of vaccine-associated sarcomas in cats: 78 cases (1996-2000), *J Am Vet Med Assoc* 219:1582, 2001.

Cronin KL, Page RL, Thrall DE: Radiation and surgery for fibrosarcoma in 33 cats, *Vet Radiol Ultrasound* 39:51, 1998.

Davidson EB, Gregory CR, Kass PH: Surgical excision of soft tissue fibrosarcomas in cats, *Vet Surg* 26:265, 1997.

Ellis JA et al: Use of immunohistochemistry and polymerase chain-reaction for detection of oncornaviruses in formalin-fixed, paraffin-embedded fibrosarcomas from cats, *J Am Vet Med Assoc* 209:767, 1996.

Hendrick MJ et al: Comparison of fibrosarcomas that developed at vaccination sites and at nonvaccination sites in cats: 239 cases (1991-1992), *J Am Vet Med Assoc* 205:1425, 1994.

Hershey AE et al: Prognosis for presumed feline vaccine-associated sarcoma after excision: 61 cases (1986-1996), *J Am Vet Med Assoc* 216:58, 2000.

Hershey AE et al: Aberrant p53 expression in feline vaccine-associated sarcomas and correlation with prognosis, *Vet Pathol* 42:805, 2005.

Kass PH et al: Epidemiologic evidence for a causal relation between vaccination and fibrosarcoma tumorigenesis in cats, *J Am Vet Med Assoc* 203:396, 1993.

Katayama R et al: Imatinib mesylate inhibits platelet-derived growth factor activity and increases chemosensitivity in feline vaccine-associated sarcoma, *Cancer Chemother Pharmacol* 54:25, 2004.

Kobayashi T et al: Preoperative radiotherapy for vaccine-associated sarcoma in 92 cats, *Vet Radiol Ultrasound* 43:473, 2002.

Macy DW, Chretin J: Local postvaccinal reactions of a recombinant rabies vaccine, *Vet Forum* 16:44, 1999.

Martano M et al: Surgery alone versus surgery and doxorubicin for the treatment of feline injection-site sarcomas: a report on 69 cases, *Vet J* 170:84, 2005.

Poirier VJ et al: Liposome-encapsulated doxorubicin (Doxil) and doxorubicin in the treatment of vaccine-associated sarcomas in cats, *J Vet Intern Med* 16:726, 2002.

Scott FW, Geissinger C: Duration of immunity in cats vaccinated with an inactivated feline panleukopenia, herpesvirus, and calicivirus vaccine, *Feline Pract* 25:12, 1997.

CHAPTER 72

Canine Lymphoma

SUSAN E. LANA, *Fort Collins, Colorado*
ANNE AVERY, *Fort Collins, Colorado*

Canine lymphoma is the most common hematologic malignancy encountered in both the specialty and general practice setting. Treatment with chemotherapy is the standard of care for this disease, with multidrug protocols providing 80% to 90% remission rates. In spite of this high response rate, canine lymphoma is not considered curable; average reported survival times are in the 12- to 14-month range (Vail, 2001). Over the last several years relatively little progress has been made in improving these outcomes; although, as we learn more about the genetic and molecular basis of canine lymphoma, there is hope that this will change. The purpose of this chapter is to discuss recent trends and possible advancements in the treatment, diagnosis, and prognosis for canine lymphoma. Extensive reviews about specific drug protocols, rescue strategies, and atypical variants of canine lymphoma can be found elsewhere in the literature (Vail, MacEwen, and Young, 2001).

VARIATIONS ON A THEME: THE CHOP PROTOCOL

Most veterinary oncologists agree that the best response rates and most durable remissions are achieved with a combination of drugs given in sequence over a period of weeks. Currently the drugs most commonly used are vincristine (Oncovin), cyclophosphamide (Cytoxan), doxorubicin (Adriamycin), and prednisone. This combination of drugs has been the mainstay of treatment for human non Hodgkin's lymphoma in a protocol commonly referred to as CHOP (*C*, cyclophosphamide; *H*, hydroxydaunorubicin [the initial name for doxorubicin hydrochloride]; *O*, Oncovin, *P*, prednisone). The CHOP-based protocol commonly used at our institution can be found in Table 72-1. Attempts have been made to vary drug sequence and dose to improve outcome, but no clear clinical benefit has been seen with these strategies. L-asparaginase (L-asp) is also included in many published veterinary protocols. Because of unforeseen drug availability problems, the benefit of using L-asp in combination with CHOP has been called into question. In one large case study evaluating 115 dogs with lymphoma, no increase in first remission duration, overall response rates, overall survival times, or toxicity was seen with the addition of L-asp to the treatment protocol (MacDonald et al., 2005). Because of this, many oncologists now reserve the use of L-asp for a rescue or salvage setting. Recent studies evaluating the CHOP protocol have focused on specific aspects, including

adding radiation therapy, increasing dose intensity, and investigating discontinuous protocols that do not involve long-term maintenance therapy. These are discussed in the following paragraphs.

Maintenance versus No Maintenance

Traditionally treatment of lymphoma in both humans and dogs has at one time or another involved induction protocols followed by a less intense, protracted maintenance schedule lasting in some cases for years. Many original CHOP-based protocols described for the treatment of canine lymphoma continued for as long as 104 weeks. Current trends have shown that shortened, discontinuous protocols without a maintenance phase have resulted in similar overall remission rates and survival times. The advantages of the shortened treatment schedule include decreased time in the veterinary clinic; decreased cost to the owner; and possibly a decrease in potential late effects of long-term chemotherapy exposure, although the risk of this in veterinary medicine is low because of the poor cure rate and shortened life span. Garrett and associates (2002) showed that a 25-week protocol resulted in no significant difference in disease-free interval (DFI) or survival when compared to a 104-week protocol with a maintenance phase. Median DFI and survival of the study group compared to the maintenance group were 282 and 397 versus 220 and 303 day, respectively. In another study a 12-week CHOP-based protocol was evaluated in 77 dogs, and a median first complete remission of 243 days reported (Simon et al., 2006).

Dose Intensification and Bone Marrow Transplantation

Dose intensification is another strategy used in an attempt to improve outcome for canine lymphoma. With an increased dose an increase in toxicity is also expected. In one study a CHOP-based protocol was dose intensified by increasing the dose of both cyclophosphamide ($250\,mg/m^2$ vs. $200\,mg/m^2$) and doxorubicin ($37.5\,mg/m^2$ vs. $30\,mg/m^2$). No DFI or survival benefit was found compared to a longer maintenance protocol, and the number of patients that died of toxicity in the dose-intensified group was 13 of 49 (27%) compared to 2 of 55 (4%) of dogs treated with traditional doses (Chun, Garrett, and Vail, 2000). Without a benefit in outcome the increase in toxicity is unacceptable to most pet owners. Another approach used successfully in humans is high-dose ablative chemotherapy

Table 72-1

Example of a CHOP-Based Protocol

DRUG	DOSE	WEEK															
		1	2	3	4	6	7	8	9	11	12	13	14	16	17	18	19
Vincristine	0.5-0.7 mg/m² IV	X		X		X		X		X		X		X		X	
Cyclophosphamide	250 mg/m² IV* or PO		X				X				X				X		
Doxorubicin†	30 mg/m² IV				X				X				X				X
Prednisone‡	2 mg/kg PO q24h	X	X	X	X												

IV, Intravenously; *PO*, orally.

* Furosemide (1 mg/kg IV) is given concurrently with IV cyclophosphamide
† Decrease dose to 1 mg/kg in dogs < 15 kg in body weight
‡ Week 1: 2 mg/kg PO q24h; week 2: 1.5 mg/kg PO q24h; week 3: 1 mg/kg PO q24h; week 4: 0.5 mg/kg PO q24h, then discontinue.

followed by some form of bone marrow transplant as a rescue from toxic side effects. Although this type of approach currently is not feasible for general practice, a variant has been reported in a small number of canine lymphoma patients with variable outcomes. Twenty-eight dogs with lymphoma underwent nonmyeloablative but dose-intense (up to 500 mg of cyclophosphamide per square meter) chemotherapy following a standard CHOP-based induction. They then received autologous bone marrow rescue. Toxicity from this approach was manageable and acceptable, and some patients achieved a long-term remission (Frimberger et al., 2006). Further investigation is needed to determine the subgroup of patients that might benefit from this approach.

Radiation Therapy

Lymphoid tissue is very sensitive to the effects of radiation therapy (RT). In the past RT generally has been used in a regional or local fashion to augment systemic chemotherapy (see Chapter 67). Recent studies have explored using a whole-body RT approach given in half-body increments to take advantage of the fact that relatively low doses of radiation are effective against lymphoma and can have minimal negative effect on the patient. A pilot study and a larger case series (Gustafson et al., 2004; Williams et al., 2004) have explored an approach combining CHOP-based chemotherapy with whole-body RT using two consecutive 4-Gy fractions to the cranial half of the body followed 3 to 4 weeks later by the same treatment to the caudal half of the body. Preliminary data from these studies have shown that toxicity associated with the addition of RT has been minimal and that remission and overall survival may be improved. One caveat to these results is that the patients who seem to benefit most are those that have already achieved a complete response with chemotherapy and perhaps would have done well in spite of additional treatment. Further investigation combining these two modalities is definitely needed to show sustained benefit of this combination approach.

DIAGNOSIS AND PROGNOSIS

The diagnosis of lymphoma often can be made by aspiration cytology alone, but in relying solely on cytology a significant amount of prognostic information may be lost. For the most prognostic power, the diagnosis ideally is made using the combination of biopsy and immunophenotyping. Clonality testing, which detects as few as 1 malignant cell in 100 normal cells, can be used as an aid to the diagnosis when histology or cytology is equivocal (Avery and Avery, 2004).

Multiple studies at different institutions spanning many years have demonstrated that, when taken as a whole, T cell lymphomas have a significantly worse prognosis than B cell lymphomas. However, recently increasing attention has been devoted to using combination of histology and immunophenotype in determining prognosis. When both are considered, indolent lymphomas of both B and T cell immunophenotypes have a comparatively favorable prognosis, with some evidence that indolent T cell lymphomas (referred to as "T zone" or "small clear cell" lymphomas) may have a better prognosis (Valli et al., 2006). Thus, if prognosis is an important consideration in the decision of whether or not to treat, it may be important to determine both immunophenotype and histologic classification.

Dogs with indolent forms of lymphoma may have a long history (up to a year and longer) of lymphadenopathy, which is classified as lymphoid hyperplasia or atypical lymphoid hyperplasia by cytology and/or histology. When such equivocal results are obtained, there are several ways to distinguish reactive hyperplasia from neoplasia. All rely on the general principle that neoplasia involves expansion of a single clone and therefore manifests as a homogeneous population of lymphocytes, whereas reactive hyperplasia generally involves multiple lymphocyte subsets. Immunophenotyping on formalin-fixed, paraffin-embedded tissue sections, using anti-CD3 (to stain T cells) and anti-CD79a (to stain B cells), is one widely available technique that may in some cases help pathologists recognize neoplasia in equivocal samples.

Box 72-1

Laboratories accepting samples from outside clients for flow cytometry at the time of this writing are listed. All laboratories request that clients contact them for information before sending samples.

Colorado State University
Clinical Immunopathology
Anne Avery, VMD, PhD
200 West Lake Street, Fort Collins, CO 80523
Ph: 970-491-1170
Fax: 970-491-0603
anne.avery@colostate.edu
http://www.dlab.colostate.edu/webdocs/general/forms.html

Kansas State University
Melinda J. Wilkerson, DVM, PhD
Diplomate, ACVP
1800 Denison Ave.
Dept. Diagnostic Medicine/Pathobiology
Kansas State University CVM
Manhattan, KS 66506
Ph: 785-532-4818
Fax: 785-532-4851
Wilkersn@vet.k-state.edu
http://www.vet.ksu.edu/depts/dmp/service/immunology/index.htm

North Carolina State University
Attn: Linda English
Clinical Immunology Laboratory College of Veterinary Medicine, NCSU
4700 Hillsborough St
Raleigh, NC 27606
Ph: 919-513-6364

University of Tennessee
Stephen Kania, PhD
University of Tennessee College of Veterinary Medicine
Department of Comparative Medicine
Clinical Immunology Service, RM A-239
2407 River Drive
Knoxville, TN 37996-4500
skania@utk.edu
Ph: 865-974-5643
http://www.vet.utk.edu/diagnostic/immunology.shtml

Laboratory accepting samples for the PARR assay:

Colorado State University
Clinical Immunopathology
Anne Avery, VMD, PhD
200 West Lake Street, Fort Collins, CO 80523
Ph: 970-491-1170
Fax: 970-491-0603
anne.avery@colostate.edu
http://www.dlab.colostate.edu/webdocs/general/forms.html

Alternatively fresh lymph node aspirates may be analyzed by flow cytometry. Box 72-1 lists laboratories that currently offer flow cytometry as a commercial service. This technique establishes if the lymphocyte population is dominated by a single lymphocyte phenotype (neoplasia) or heterogenous expansion (reactive hyperplasia). It has the advantage that a large panel of antibodies can be used on freshly aspirated samples but the disadvantage of not being able to examine cells within the context of the lymph node architecture. Clonality assessment is the most sensitive way to detect neoplastic lymphocytes

within a lymph node (see Box 72-1 for the laboratory that currently offers this test commercially). This is a polymerase chain reaction (PCR)-based assay (PCR for antigen receptor rearrangements [PARR]) that is best carried out on deoxyribonucleic acid from any source other than paraffin-embedded samples (fresh aspirates, stained or unstained cytology preparations, peripheral blood, effusions). Detection of neoplastic cells relies on the observation that the genes for antigen receptors (immunoglobulin and T cell receptor genes for B and T cells, respectively) are different in length and sequence in each lymphocyte. PCR amplification of gene segments from these antigen receptor genes results in a single-sized product if the lymphocytes present are derived from the same clone (neoplasia). Multiple PCR products are amplified if the lymphocytes are heterogeneous (reactive). In practice the kinetics of the PCR reaction allow for the detection of as few as 1 in 100 neoplastic cells in cases of early neoplasia (Burnett et al., 2003). This makes the assay useful for detecting neoplasia before it is evident histologically or cytologically. It is important to note that the conditions for the assay have a profound effect on the sensitivity and specificity of the results; therefore each laboratory conducting the assay should report these numbers when they report results to allow proper interpretation of the findings.

In addition to immunophenotype and histologic subtype, clinical stage has consistently been demonstrated to correlate with outcome. Multicentric lymphoma is the most common form in dogs, and these cases usually present as stage III or higher. Perhaps the most consistent prognostic factor associated with staging is the substage; patients with substage a disease (no systemic signs) have considerably better survival times than patients with substage b disease (systemic signs).

Although clinical staging, histology, and immunophenotyping should be used routinely for determining diagnosis and prognosis, a host of other factors have been investigated for their ability to contribute to prognosis and in the future may be used more routinely. These include various markers of proliferation, including argyrophilic nucleolar organizer region (AgNOR) staining, serum levels of thymidine kinase, expression of the Ki-67 marker, serum levels of circulating endothelial markers and matrix metalloproteases, and additional immunophenotypic markers. It seems likely that these will be most useful when applied within a particular histologic and immunophenotypic subclassification of lymphoma.

Although many of these methods may be useful for the diagnosis and prognosis of lymphoma, at present there are no objective tests beyond clinical measures of disease burden that allow clinicians to follow patients in remission or to determine when a patient has come out of remission. Flow cytometry does not appear to be useful, and cytology often can be equivocal and subjective. The assessment of remission currently is based primarily on physical examination findings and cytology. The PARR assay may prove to be useful in this regard because it can give a quantitative determination of tumor burden and can detect relatively small numbers of tumor cells in the blood and lymph nodes. The use of this assay to monitor patients after treatment is currently under investigation.

GENETIC DISCOVERIES IN CANINE LYMPHOMA

In human oncology lymphomas are further categorized by cytogenetic abnormalities and the expression of oncogenes. Histologically and immunophenotypically homogeneous groups of human lymphomas have been shown to be remarkably heterogeneous in the nature of the chromosomal rearrangements they harbor, and these in turn can be used to further subdivide this tumor into prognostically meaningful subsets. For example, human diffuse large B cell lymphoma is considered to be analogous to the most common form of canine lymphoma. Within this tumor type a combination of cytogenetic studies to identify chromosomal translocations and gene expression profiling to characterize the expression of groups of genes involved in specific functions (such as proliferation and apoptosis) has been used to subdivide patients into those with good prognosis and poor prognosis. Similar investigations have begun in canine lymphomas but have not yet been used to determine diagnosis or prognosis. Currently investigators have developed the tools to carry out large-scale analysis of chromosomal duplications and deletions using comparative genomic hybridization arrays (Thomas et al., 2003). One early finding from this work is that particular breeds may be predisposed to particular types of chromosomal changes, raising the possibility that such studies may ultimately be able to uncover the genetic basis for a predisposition to developing lymphoma (Modiano et al., 2005). Such information would have implications beyond veterinary medicine since few genes linked to a predisposition to human lymphoma have been discovered.

In spite of better characterization of canine lymphoid malignancies into distinct histologic or genetic subgroups, this information has yet to make a routine impact on the day-to-day treatment options presented to pet owners. Additional studies are needed to better define the clinical characteristics of patients in each subgroup so that more individualized treatment can be pursued.

References and Suggested Reading

Avery PR, Avery AC: Molecular methods to distinguish reactive and neoplastic lymphocyte expansions and their importance in transitional neoplastic states, *Vet Clin Pathol* 33:196, 2004.

Burnett RC et al: Diagnosis of canine lymphoid neoplasia using clonal rearrangements of antigen receptor genes, *Vet Pathol* 40:32, 2003.

Chun R, Garrett LD, Vail DM: Evaluation of a high-dose chemotherapy protocol with no maintenance therapy for dogs with lymphoma, *J Vet Intern Med* 14:120, 2000.

Frimberger AE et al: A combination chemotherapy protocol with dose intensification and autologous bone marrow transplant (VELCAP-HDC) for canine lymphoma, *J Vet Intern Med* 20:355, 2006.

Garrett LD et al: Evaluation of a 6-month chemotherapy protocol with no maintenance therapy for dogs with lymphoma, *J Vet Intern Med* 16:704, 2002.

Gustafson NR et al: A preliminary assessment of whole-body radiotherapy interposed within a chemotherapy protocol for canine lymphoma, *Vet Comp Oncol* 2:125, 2004.

MacDonald VS et al: Does L-asparaginase influence efficacy ortoxicity when added to a standard CHOP protocol for dogs with lymphoma? *J Vet Intern Med* 19:732, 2005.

Modiano JF et al: Distinct B-cell and T-cell lymphoproliferative disease prevalence among dog breeds indicates heritable risk, *Cancer Res* 65:5654, 2005.

Simon D et al: Treatment of dogs with lymphoma using a 12-week maintenance-free combination chemotherapy protocol, *J Vet Intern Med* 20:948, 2006.

Thomas R et al: Chromosome aberrations in canine multicentric lymphomas detected with comparative genomic hybridization and a panel of single locus probes, *Br J Cancer* 89:1530, 2003.

Vail DM, MacEwen EG, Young KM: Canine lymphoma and lymphoid leukemias. In Withrow SJ, MacEwen EG, editors: *Small animal clinical oncology*, ed 3, Philadelphia, 2001, Saunders, p 558.

Valli VE et al: Canine indolent nodular lymphoma, *Vet Pathol* 43:241, 2006.

Williams LE et al: Chemotherapy followed by half-body radiation therapy for canine lymphoma, *J Vet Intern Med* 18:703, 2004.

CHAPTER 73

Feline Gastrointestinal Lymphoma

KEITH P. RICHTER, *San Diego, California*

EPIDEMIOLOGY

Lymphoma is the most frequently diagnosed feline cancer and the most common gastrointestinal (GI) neoplasm in cats. There are several anatomic locations for lymphoma; the GI tract is the most common site, accounting for 32% to 72% of total cases. Discrepancies in the reported incidence of the various forms of lymphoma may be the result of the differences in classification schemes used, a change in incidence over time, differences in feline leukemia virus (FeLV) subtypes in various geographic areas, and a decreased incidence of non-GI forms since the introduction of an FeLV vaccine. An increase in the proportion of GI lymphomas over time is apparent by comparing incidences in the same institutions over different time periods. For example, in the New England area the proportion of GI lymphomas in cats increased from 8% in 1979 to 18% in 1983 and to 32% in 1996. Likewise, in the New York City area the proportion of GI lymphomas in cats increased from 27% in 1989 to 72% in 1995.

The association between FeLV and lymphoma in cats is well established. The incidence of FeLV antigenemia in cats with GI lymphoma ranges from 0% to 38%. However, such estimation of FeLV infection rate is significantly influenced by the method of testing. Underestimation of FeLV incidence with immunohistochemistry (IHC) versus polymerase chain reaction (PCR) has been suggested. In one study PCR testing detected FeLV viral nucleic acid sequences in up to 63% of cats with GI lymphoma, whereas only 38% of cats were positive by IHC (Jackson et al., 1993). Generally cats with leukemia or mediastinal lymphoma tend to be young and FeLV positive, whereas those with GI lymphoma typically are older and FeLV antigen negative. An association between lymphoma and feline immunodeficiency virus also has been proposed, especially when coinfected with FeLV.

GROSS PATHOLOGIC FINDINGS

The gross appearance of feline GI lymphoma varies with the specific anatomic location. Many segments of the GI tract, including the liver, may be involved. There can be a focal mass or diffuse infiltration. In some cases, especially with low-grade lymphocytic lymphoma, the gross appearance may be normal. When a focal alimentary tract mass is present, there is usually transmural thickening with or without mucosal ulceration. Mural thickening is often eccentric, resulting in preservation of the lumen, although a functional obstruction may develop. This contrasts with

intestinal carcinoma, which often results in a mechanical obstruction from decreased luminal diameter, often appearing as a "napkin ring". With diffuse infiltration the intestinal wall may be visibly and/or palpably thickened. Mesenteric lymphadenopathy is often obvious grossly or on ultrasonographic examination. Intussusception can develop secondary to intestinal lymphoma, with the jejunum being the most common location. Hepatic involvement can have a variable appearance. In some cases the liver appears to be grossly normal, whereas in others there may be an enhanced lobular pattern, a mottled appearance, or a gross nodular appearance.

In summary, the appearance of lymphoma is extremely variable in all regions of the GI tract. In light of how commonly this neoplasm develops in cats, lymphoma should be considered as a differential diagnosis for GI illness with normal or grossly abnormal organ appearance.

HISTOPATHOLOGY AND IMMUNOHISTOCHEMISTRY

There are different grades of GI lymphoma, commonly referred to as low grade (lymphocytic or small cell), high grade (lymphoblastic, immunoblastic, or large cell), and intermediate grade. Less common descriptions such as large granular lymphocytic lymphoma also exist. Most published reports are either of undetermined grade or predominately high-grade lymphomas, although low-grade lymphocytic lymphoma was described in a large case series (Fondacaro et al., 1999). In this study 50 of 67 cats (75%) diagnosed with GI lymphomas had low-grade lymphocytic lymphoma. Criteria used to classify lymphoma as lymphocytic have been described (Fondacaro et al., 1999). In marked contrast to palpable masses of lymphoblastic lymphoma, masses formed by lymphocytic lymphoma are not distinct microscopically because the mucosa beyond the apparent mass is also involved.

The use of a standard grading scheme for GI lymphoma may lead to a greater recognition of low-grade lymphocytic lymphoma. However, criteria have been difficult to establish because of the difficulty in interpreting small endoscopic biopsies, differences in pathologists' opinions, and a lack of characterization using IHC. Consequently further studies are needed to define specific criteria for differentiating lymphocytic lymphoma, lymphocytic inflammation, and T-cell infiltrative disease and to correlate such classifications with clinical outcome.

In addition, the role of endoscopic biopsies versus full-thickness biopsies needs to be better defined. Many pathologists are comfortable making the diagnosis on endoscopic biopsy analysis, whereas others believe that full-thickness biopsies are necessary. In my practice I rely heavily on the analyses of endoscopic biopsies. Although it is customary to consider that there is a continuum from inflammatory bowel disease to lymphoma, there are little supporting data.

Recently IHC has been used to better characterize feline lymphoma. In some studies GI lymphomas were more likely to be of B cell rather than T cell phenotype, whereas other studies describe a predominantly T cell phenotype. Furthermore, in a limited number of studies immunophenotype did not appear to correlate with response to chemotherapy treatment or survival. Thus further study is necessary to determine the clinical value of immunophenotyping.

CLINICAL FINDINGS

Signalment

Males appear to be predisposed to GI lymphoma. Although a breed predilection is not apparent, most cats are domestic shorthair. The median age ranges from 9 to 13 years in different studies, with an age range spanning from 1 to 18 years.

Clinical Signs and Physical Examination Findings

Irrespective of the histologic grade, clinical signs include weight loss, anorexia, vomiting, diarrhea, lethargy, and polydipsia/polyuria. Importantly, many cats have minimal or no vomiting and/or diarrhea, with anorexia, weight loss, or both as the only historical findings. Therefore, when confronted with these signs in a geriatric cat with an otherwise unrewarding initial evaluation, GI lymphoma should be considered as a differential diagnosis. Physical findings may include poor body condition, thickened intestinal loops, and/or a palpable abdominal mass. The presence of an abdominal mass is more suggestive of high-grade lymphoma. Notably many cats may have a normal abdominal palpation.

Ancillary Test Findings

Laboratory findings generally are noncontributory, with mild anemia and/or hypoalbuminemia most commonly seen. Abnormalities on plain abdominal and thoracic radiographs are also uncommon and usually nonspecific. An abdominal ultrasound examination may be helpful in many cases and is considered more sensitive than radiography. Lesions can be nodular (focal or multifocal) or diffuse. Although the most common ultrasonographic abnormality observed is thickening of the gastric or intestinal wall, other important findings include loss of normal intestinal wall layering, localized mass effects associated with the intestine, decreased intestinal wall echogenicity, regional hypomotility, regional lymphadenopathy, and rarely ascites. Since ultrasonography provides information about the specific site of involvement of the lesion, as well as other abdominal organs, it assists in staging the regional extent of disease and in screening for concurrent disorders. It also allows for precise guidance of fine-needle aspiration or biopsy for cytologic or histopathologic sampling, and it can be used to noninvasively and objectively assess response to therapy. A limitation of ultrasonography would be the difficulty in assessing the exact anatomic location and extent of certain lesions, possibly because of the inability of ultrasound waves to penetrate gas-filled structures such as the bowel and lack of distinct fixed anatomic landmarks. Furthermore ultrasonography is very operator, experience, and ultrasound-system dependent. Findings may also be normal, especially in cases of low-grade lymphoma.

Endoscopy can be an effective tool for diagnosing GI mucosal lymphoma when involved areas are within reach of an endoscope. Most gross endoscopic findings are nonspecific, with considerable overlap with inflammatory bowel disease and other GI diseases. In many cases the endoscopic appearance can be grossly normal.

TREATMENT

Reports of treatment strategies for feline GI lymphoma are fairly limited, and only a few of these reports give detailed results in cats specifically with GI lymphoma. In addition, the outcome in different forms of GI lymphoma remains ill-defined because many reports do not describe histologic grade or results of complete anatomic staging and different combinations of chemotherapeutic agents were used.

A summary of reported treatments and outcomes in cats with GI lymphoma is provided in Table 73-1. In general, response rates are in the 50% to 67% range, with reported median survival times (MSTs) of 3 to 9 months. Few studies have evaluated outcome by histologic grade; however, those evaluating high-grade lymphomas only generally report poor outcomes (Mahoney et al. 1995; Fondacaro et al., 1999).

These findings contrast with those of cats having low-grade lymphoma. Fondacaro and associates (1999) described 50 cats with low-grade GI lymphoma, 36 of which were treated with chemotherapy. Twenty-nine cats with lymphocytic lymphoma were treated with prednisone (10 mg/cat PO q24 h) and high-dose pulse chlorambucil (Leukeran, Glaxo SmithKline; 15 mg/m^2 of body surface area PO q24h for 4 days, repeated every 3 weeks). Sixty-nine percent of the cats achieved a clinical complete remission (CR), with a median disease-free interval for cats that achieved a CR of 20.5 months (range: 5.8 to 49 months). The MST for all cats was 17 months (range: 0.33 to 50 months), with an MST of 22.8 months for cats that achieved a CR (range: 10 to 50 months). Twelve of the 20 cats that achieved a CR were "rescued" with cyclophosphamide at a dosage of 225 mg/m^2 of body surface area PO every three weeks. These cats had a cumulative median disease-free interval of 24 months (including first and second remissions) and an MST of 29 months (cumulative). Seven cats were alive at the time of data collection; all but one of these cats had received rescue treatment with cyclophosphamide. Adverse reactions

Table 73-1

Reported Outcomes Following Treatment for Cats With Gastrointestinal Lymphoma

Authors	No. of Cats (No. of GI Lymphoma Cases)	Protocol	% CR	Median ST	Comments
Cotter, 1983	7 (7)	COP	86	26 weeks	Grade not reported
Jeglum, Whereat, and Young, 1987	14 (14)	COP + M	NR	12 weeks	Grade not reported
Mooney et al., 1989	103 (28)	COP + M + LA	62	30 weeks if CR	Outcome in GI LSA not reported separately; grade not reported
Mauldin et al., 1995	132 (95)	COP + M + DOX + LA	67	30 weeks	Outcome in GI LSA not reported separately but location did not affect outcome; grade not reported
Zwahlen et al., 1998	21 (21)	COP + M + DOX + LA	38	40 weeks (41.5 weeks if CR)	Grade not reported
Malik et al., 2001	60 (14)	COP + M + DOX + LA	80	17 weeks (27 weeks if CR)	Outcome in GI LSA not reported separately; grade not reported
Kristal et al., 2001	19 (7)	DOX	26	12 weeks (64 weeks if CR)	Outcome in GI LSA not reported separately; grade not reported
Mahoney et al., 1995	28 (28)	COP	32	7 weeks (30 weeks DFI if CR)	25 High grade; 3 low grade
Fondacaro et al., 1999	11 (11)	COP or COP + DOX + LA	18	11 weeks	All high-grade
Fondacaro et al., 1999	29 (29)	Chlorambucil, prednisone	69	74 weeks (99 weeks if CR)	All low-grade

COP, Cyclophosphamide/vincristine/prednisone; *CR,* complete response; *DFI,* disease-free interval; *DOX,* doxorubicin; *GI,* gastrointestinal; *LA,* L-asparaginase; *LSA, lymphosarcoma; M,* methotrexate; *NR,* not reported; *ST,* survival time.

to chlorambucil were rare but included vomiting, diarrhea, anorexia, lethargy, and neutropenia. No cats required hospitalization or discontinuation of therapy. Subsequently neurologic side effects (including myoclonus and seizures) have been described in cats receiving chlorambucil.

Some conclusions and recommendations can be made from these studies. In general, response to chemotherapy for high-grade GI lymphoma is poor, whereas the clinical response for low-grade lymphoma is good. For cats with high-grade GI lymphoma, combining doxorubicin with other agents in a multiagent protocol such as cyclophosphamide/Oncovin (vincristine)/prednisone (COP) and L-asparaginase is associated with longer remission and survival times when compared with single-agent doxorubicin or COP alone. For cats with low-grade lymphoma, excellent results can be achieved with oral prednisone and high-dose pulse chlorambucil therapy. However, it is unknown whether these cats would do better with a more aggressive multiagent protocol or even with a low, every-other-day dose of chlorambucil. For example, some institutions use 1 mg of chlorambucil orally every other day. Finally, chemotherapy generally is well tolerated by cats. Self-limiting anorexia, vomiting, diarrhea, and myelosuppression may be observed in some patients. It may be difficult to distinguish some of these chemotherapy-related side effects from active or progressive lymphoma.

The role of surgery in the treatment of GI lymphoma has been evaluated. Studies have shown either no effect or a negative effect of surgical intervention on disease-free interval and survival. However, this effect is most likely not caused by the surgical intervention itself but is more likely because cats requiring surgery (i.e., those with GI obstruc-

tion) have shorter survival periods because of the severity of their disease. The main indications for surgery are partial or complete intestinal obstruction, intestinal perforation, or to obtain biopsy specimens for definitive diagnosis. It should be noted that some patients with solitary masses that are surgically resected and subsequently receive chemotherapy can have long survival times.

It is believed that some patients with transmural focal disease are at risk for perforation when treated with cytotoxic chemotherapy that induces a rapid response, although this is rare in my experience. Surgery may result in dehiscence at intestinal anastomosis sites and may require a delay in initiation of chemotherapy to allow proper wound healing. Following resection of a focal GI or mesenteric mass, chemotherapy is still warranted since most cases have diffuse or multifocal microscopic involvement, and lymphoma should be considered a systemic disease in most cases.

PROGNOSTIC FACTORS

Few prognostic factors have been defined for cats with GI lymphoma. Histologic grade is a strong indicator of outcome. Compared to cats with high-grade lymphoma treated with a multiagent chemotherapy regimen, cats with low-grade lymphoma treated with oral prednisone and chlorambucil have a significantly better remission rate and survival time. Therefore low- and high-grade GI lymphomas in many ways represent different disease entities and must be considered separately.

In a majority of studies the most significant prognostic indicator for a positive outcome is initial response to chemotherapy. In general cats that survive the initial induction period and achieve remission generally also have a better long-term outcome. Although this may seem intuitively obvious, it may give clinicians and owners encouragement to continue chemotherapy treatment in cats that attain a CR. Otherwise there is no consistent association with any patient or tumor characteristic that is predictive of outcome (including sex, immunophenotype, clinical stage, age, and body weight). In most recent studies, FeLV virus antigenemia was not a negative prognostic factor. Some studies also showed little benefit of an exhaustive "staging evaluation" since very few factors have enough impact on prognosis to make their determination helpful. Investigators have looked at molecular markers as prognostic factors. However, argyrophilic nucleolar organizer region (AgNOR) frequency and proliferating cell nuclear antigen labeling index (PCNA-LI) showed no correlation with response to chemotherapy or survival (Rassnick et al., 1999; Vail et al., 1998). Similarly the immunophenotype of tumor cells also does not seem to correlate with outcome in cats. This is in contrast to dogs, in which a T cell phenotype has long been recognized as a negative prognostic factor for response to therapy and survival. Concentration of serum α_1-acid glycoprotein, an acute-phase protein, has recently been evaluated in cats with lymphoma and was not shown to be useful in predicting response to treatment or survival. Limitations of many studies published include incomplete staging, inconsistent grading, multiple unsampled GI locations, lack of prospective randomization to different chemotherapy protocols, lack of control (untreated) patients, and lack of confirmation of remission through follow-up biopsies. Prospective, controlled, and randomized cohort studies with large numbers of cats aimed at investigating the response of each grade of GI lymphoma to uniform chemotherapeutic regimens seem warranted. Furthermore, additional studies to correlate clinical outcome with immunophenotype and molecular markers are needed.

References and Suggested Reading

Cotter SM: Treatment of lymphoma and leukemia with cyclophosphamide, vincristine, and prednisone. II. Treatment of cats, *J Am Anim Hosp Assoc* 19:166, 1983.

Fondacaro JV et al: Feline gastrointestinal lymphoma: 67 cases (1988-1996), *Eur J Comp Gastroenterol* 4:5, 1999.

Jackson ML et al: Feline leukemia virus detection by immunohistochemistry and polymerase chain reaction in formalin-fixed, paraffin-embedded tumor tissue from cats with lymphosarcoma, *Can J Vet Res* 57:169, 1993.

Jeglum KA, Whereat A, Young K: Chemotherapy of lymphoma in 75 cats, *J Am Vet Med Assoc* 190:174, 1987.

Kristal O et al: Simple agent chemotherapy with doxorubicin for feline lymphoma: a retrospective study of 19 cases (1994-1997), *J Vet Intern Med* 15:125, 2001.

Mahony OM et al: Alimentary lymphoma in cats: 28 cases (1988-1993), *J Am Vet Med Assoc* 207:1593, 1995.

Malik R et al: Therapy for Australian cats with lymphosarcoma, *Aust Vet J* 79:808, 2001.

Mauldin GE et al: Chemotherapy in 132 cats with lymphoma: 1988-1994, Proceedings of the 15th Annual Conference of the Veterinary Cancer Society, Tucson, Ariz, 1995, p 35.

Mooney SC et al: Treatment and prognostic factors in lymphoma in cats: 103 Cases (1977-1981), *J Am Vet Med Assoc* 194:696, 1989.

Rassnick KM et al: Prognostic value of argyrophilic nucleolar organizer region (AgNOR) staining in feline intestinal lymphoma, *J Vet Intern Med* 13:187, 1999.

Vail DM et al: Feline lymphoma (145 cases): proliferation indices, cluster of differentiation 3 immunoreactivity, and their association with prognosis in 90 cats, *J Vet Intern Med* 12:349, 1998.

Zwahlen CH et al: Results of chemotherapy for cats with alimentary malignant lymphoma: 21 Cases (1993-1997), *J Am Vet Med Assoc* 213:1144, 1998.

CHAPTER **74**

Paraneoplastic Hypercalcemia

DAVID M. VAIL, *Madison, Wisconsin*

Hypercalcemia of malignancy (HCM) is one of the most commonly recognized systemic manifestations of cancer (i.e., paraneoplastic syndrome) in veterinary and human medicine. The clinical recognition of HCM is important for several reasons: it may represent the first clinical sign of disease (presenting complaint); it may aid the search for distant or metastatic disease beyond the primary site; it may help quantify and monitor response to therapy; it may aid in the evaluation of recurrence; and its management may take precedence over treating the primary disease. These points combined with the ability of HCM to mimic other disease conditions make a working knowledge of the diagnostic and management steps involved in HCM important.

TUMORS IMPLICATED IN HYPERCALCEMIA OF MALIGNANCY

Any tumor histotype can be associated with HCM; however, several are much more commonly implicated, including lymphoma (15% of all forms and nearly 40% of cranial mediastinal forms), apocrine gland (anal sac) adenocarcinomas, multiple myeloma, and feline head and neck squamous cell carcinoma. The mechanisms by which these tumors result in HCM vary and will be considered subsequently. Although parathyroid adenomas can result in profound hypercalcemia, these tumors are often not included in a discussion of HCM because the cell of origin is normally involved in parathyroid hormone (PTH) production and the result is characterized as primary hyperparathyroidism (see Chapter 54).

CALCIUM HOMEOSTASIS

To understand both the mechanisms by which tumors can alter blood calcium levels and the means by which the clinician can intervene, knowledge of the normal calcium homeostatic machinery is necessary. Three organs, the gut, kidney, and bone, under the control of a complex set of hormones and cytokines are primarily responsible for serum calcium regulation. These three organs can exchange calcium across the extracellular fluid space; however, under normal conditions the net effect is a zero balance (Clines and Guise, 2005). Although several known (and unknown) humoral factors are involved in this complex interplay, PTH and vitamin D (in particular calcitriol, $1,25-(OH)_2D_3$) are by far the most important. Calcitonin also receives attention for calcium homeostasis, but its actual role is poorly understood and likely limited to short-term regulation. Table 74-1 outlines the effects of these humoral regulators on their target organs. Systemic PTH concentrations are regulated primarily by serum calcium levels through a simple feedback loop involving calcium-sensing receptors on parathyroid cells. Renal hydroxylation of vitamin D to the most active $1,25-(OH)_2D_3$ is regulated primarily through stimulation by PTH, hyperphosphatemia, and inhibition by calcitriol through a negative feedback loop via renal tubule receptors.

As our understanding of molecular cell signaling advances, it is becoming apparent that many of the aforementioned humoral factors involved in calcium homeostasis ultimately interact with these signaling pathways, which could serve as potential therapeutic targets and therefore are germane to the topic of HCM. The receptor activator of nuclear factor-KB (RANK)/RANK ligand (RANKL)/osteoprotegerin (OPG) pathway is the most well-known PTH-signaling pathway controlling osteoclastogenesis. Briefly RANKL, largely under the control of PTH, leads to osteoclast activation, bone resorption, and hypercalcemia. OPG competes with RANKL for binding to RANK and has an opposite effect (i.e., counterregulatory to PTH).

ETIOLOGY OF HYPERCALCEMIA OF MALIGNANCY

Tumors typically produce hypercalcemia by one or a combination of two major mechanisms. The first and most common in veterinary oncology is indirectly through the production of systemically active humoral factors that unbalance normal calcium homeostasis. The second less common mechanism is secondary to direct effects on bone subsequent to tumor spread to bone by local extension or distant metastasis and the ensuing production of locally acting (and possibly systemically acting) mediators of bone resorption. In human patients, the second mechanism is actually the more common etiology because of the higher incidence of metastatic epithelial cancers (e.g., breast, prostate) in people. Regardless of which mechanism is most responsible, the calciotropic factors that unbalance normal calcium homeostasis in each case may be the same.

Parathyroid Hormone–Related Peptide (PTHrP)

The most commonly involved mediator of HCM is parathyroid hormone–related peptide (PTHrP). This protein, produced normally by a variety of cells, shares close sequence homology with PTH at the N-terminus and as such binds and activates the PTH receptor, resulting in similar but not identical effects as PTH. When it is produced at normal physiologic levels in the nontumor-bearing host, PTHrP has a wide variety of normal regulatory actions on several organ systems, including the skin, placenta, heart, bladder, and intestine. However, when

Table 74-1

Simplified Overview of Humoral Control of Calcium Homeostasis

Humoral Signal	ORGAN EFFECT				Net Effect
	Kidney	Gastrointestinal Tract	Bone	Parathyroid Gland	
PTH/PTH-rP	More Ca^{++} resorption	Indirectly more Ca^{++} absorption secondary to more vitamin D activation	More osteoclastic bone resorption		Increased serum Ca^{++}
	Less PO_4^{2-} resorption				Lower serum PO_4^{2-}
	More renal activation of vitamin D				
Vitamin D $(1,25-(OH)_2D_3$	Potentiates PTH mediated renal Ca^{++} resorption	More Ca^{++} absorption	More osteoclast bone resorption	Less PTH production	Increased serum Ca^{++}
		More PO_4^{2-} absorption			Increased serum PO_4^{2-}
Calcitonin			Rapidly less osteoclast bone resorption		Lower serum Ca^{++}
					Lower serum PO_4^{2-}

produced in supraphysiologic levels in HCM, PTHrP mediates hypercalcemia and has several significant progrowth, survival, and metastatic effects on the tumor itself. This is the primary mechanism by which apocrine gland adenocarcinoma of the anal sac in dogs produces HCM (Rosol et al., 1990, 1992).

Vitamin D (or Vitamin D Analogs)

Likely the second most important mediator of HCM is $1,25\text{-}(OH)_2D_3$ or other active vitamin D analogs that can be produced directly by the tumor cells or indirectly by the renal parenchyma secondary to PTHrP elevations. This appears to be the most common etiology for HCM in human diffuse large cell non-Hodgkin's lymphoma. A significant percentage of dogs with lymphoma have also been shown to have high circulating levels of $1,25\text{-}(OH)_2D_3$; and, although some may be secondary to increased production secondary to PTHrP expression (also occurring in a significant percentage of dogs with lymphoma), the concentrations present appear to support tumor-derived $1,25\text{-}(OH)_2D_3$ production (Rosol et al., 1992; Meuten et al., 1983a, 1983b).

Other Potential Calciotropic Factors

Several other factors may be involved in HCM, either alone in limited cases or in combination with PTHrP or $1,25\text{-}(OH)_2D_3$. These include PTH, interleukin-1β (IL-1β, formerly osteoclast-activating factor [OAF]), IL-6, prostaglandins of the E series, transforming growth factor–α (TGF-α), and tumor necrosis factor–α (TNF-α).

DIFFERENTIAL DIAGNOSIS FOR HYPERCALCEMIA

It is important to note that nearly half of elevated total calcium concentrations appearing on standard serum biochemistry profile reports are caused by laboratory error or interference secondary to hyperalbuminemia, lipemia, hemolysis, or acidosis. If the reported hypercalcemia does not fit the clinical picture, steps to confirm the value should be taken (i.e., with regard to hyperalbuminemia, performing an ionized calcium to confirm or using a simple mathematical correction for dogs):

$$\text{Corrected calcium} - [\text{Lab Ca}^{++} - \text{Albumin}] + 3.5$$

It should be emphasized that this "correction" is the "average" correction based on serum albumin and the 3.5 constant is the "best fit" relationship for dogs based on one study. The mathematical calculation based on albumin concentration is less accurate in confirming true hypercalcemia than the measured ionized Ca^{++}.

Beyond laboratory error, the differential diagnoses for hypercalcemia include HCM, primary hyperparathyroidism (parathyroid adenoma), hypoadrenocorticism, vitamin D toxicosis, renal secondary hyperparathyroidism, nutritional secondary hyperparathyroidism, granulomatous disease, and widespread bony disease. In addition, young growing animals may have a mild, transient hypercalcemia.

DIAGNOSTIC PLAN FOR HYPERCALCEMIA OF MALIGNANCY

The diagnostic plan for hypercalcemia of unknown origin should be performed, with consideration of the differential diagnoses, in a stepwise fashion, performing the most cost-effective and least invasive tests first. First diagnostic steps include performing a confirmatory ionized calcium, considering and "correcting" nonionized serum calcium for albumin if appropriate, and completing a careful complete physical examination (including rectal examination and lymph node palpation). Furthermore, a complete blood count, serum biochemistry profile, electrolytes, urinalysis, and tests of adrenal function should be obtained. In HCM secondary to PTHrP or primary hyperparathyroidism (parathyroid adenoma), serum phosphorous is typically low (unless significant renal disease is also present), whereas with vitamin D toxicosis serum phosphorous usually rises concurrently with serum calcium. The clinician must also be reminded that, in the face of hypercalcemia, renal concentrating ability is impaired because of interference with normal antidiuretic hormone function. Therefore isosthenuria and azotemia in the face of hypercalcemia should not be interpreted as being consistent with renal azotemia; rather prerenal azotemia is still very likely.

If the diagnosis is still uncertain at this point, the clinician begins a "tumor hunt," including aspiration of a few representative lymph nodes (even if they are of normal size), thoracic and abdominal radiographs, a bone marrow aspirate, and an abdominal/parathyroid ultrasound. Serum PTH and PTH-rP concentrations are also very helpful. In most cases of HCM resulting from a PTHrP-expressing tumor, PTHrP is detectable, whereas PTH is well below the normal range. Importantly, if the PTH concentration is in the normal range in the face of hypercalcemia, primary hyperparathyroidism (parathyroid adenoma) becomes the most likely possibility since nearly three fourths of these cases have PTH concentrations within the normal range (Feldman et al., 2005; see Chapter 54). In *cats* with elevated serum calcium the possibility of "idiopathic hypercalcemia" should be considered (Chapter 52) if other causes have been excluded.

In rare cases in which this thorough diagnostic approach still does not reveal the cause of hypercalcemia, surgical exploration of the parathyroid glands and/or the abdomen, or so-called *provocative testing*, may become necessary. Provocative testing makes the assumption that the hypercalcemia is caused by HCM secondary to either occult lymphoma or myeloma and involves a short course of chemotherapy (e.g., cyclophosphamide or vincristine) to see if the calcium levels normalize. If successful, then a full course of combination chemotherapy is instituted. It is important to note that corticosteroids should not be a part of the provocative protocol because they can lower, albeit modestly, serum calcium levels resulting from several non-HCM disease processes. A third option in animals with mild hypercalcemia that have mild clinical signs and are not azotemic is to pursue no therapy but to recheck the patient after 4 to 6 weeks. Occasionally an occult lymphoid neoplasm may become clinically apparent after this waiting period, or inconclusive test results may become more definitive with time.

CLINICAL CONSEQUENCES OF HYPERCALCEMIA OF MALIGNANCY

The severity of the observed clinical consequences of hypercalcemia varies with the degree and the rate of rise of serum calcium elevations. If the rise in serum calcium is slow and long-standing, the signs tend to be more subtle and nonspecific. Adverse effects include reversible and potentially irreversible renal effects, neuromuscular dysfunction (e.g., weakness, cardiac arrhythmias [QT shortening, bradycardia], GI hypertonicity, or constipation), anorexia, weight loss, nausea, and dehydration. Dehydration can lead to further declines in GFR and exacerbate the hypercalcemia. Most renal consequences of HCM are reversible and secondary to dehydration (i.e., prerenal azotemia); however, renal tubular calcification and necrosis can occur if the hypercalcemia is long-standing and marked. Weakness or nonresponsiveness secondary to the neuromuscular effects of hypercalcemia can progress to coma. In primary hyperparathyroidism (parathyroid adenoma), the most common clinical signs are attributable to urolithiasis or urinary tract infection (Feldman et al, 2005).

MANAGEMENT OF HYPERCALCEMIA OF MALIGNANCY

As with any paraneoplastic syndrome, the paramount goal should be removal of the inciting malignancy. Whether the initial therapy should be aimed at removing the tumor or at normalizing the calcium is based on the severity of clinical signs attributable to hypercalcemia, the degree of renal impairment, and the ease by which remission of the primary tumor can be achieved. I find the algorithm presented in Fig. 74-1 to be helpful for creating a therapeutic plan. As stated previously, removal of the inciting tumor is ideal, and this may be relatively easy in the case of hematopoietic tumors such as lymphoma or multiple myeloma; however, if this is not possible initially (e.g., metastatic anal gland adenocarcinoma), therapies directed at lowering serum calcium should be instituted. Replacement of fluid deficits and diuresis with high sodium crystalloids (e.g., 0.9% NaCl), beginning at twice maintenance level volume expands the patient and promotes renal ionic exchange of Ca^{++} for Na^+. It is important to monitor for signs of overhydration and semiquantitate urinary output in the event that hypercalcemic nephrosis is already present. Some also advocate the addition of the loop diuretic furosemide at this point to further enhance ionic exchange of Ca^{++} for Na^+; however, if given before volume expansion, this can result in further decline in glomerular filtration rate and can actually exacerbate the hypercalcemia. In addition, fluid diuresis alone is usually as effective; therefore I do not advocate the addition of furosemide. Other means of lowering serum calcium include the use of glucocorticoids, calcitonin, bisphosphonates, mithramycin, and gallium nitrate.

Glucocorticoids inhibit the action of vitamin D, counteract prostaglandins of the E series, decrease gastrointestinal uptake, and increase the urinary excretion of calcium. It is imperative that glucocorticoid use be reserved until a diagnosis has been confirmed for the cause of the HCM.

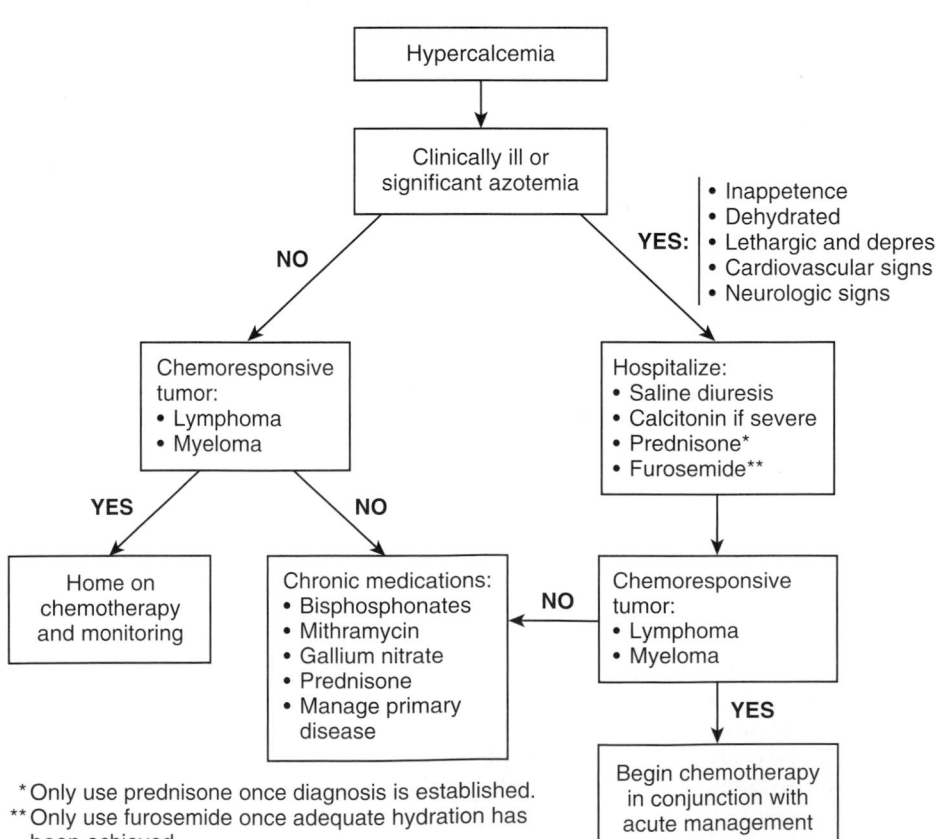

Fig. 74-1 Algorithm for management of hypercalcemia of malignancy.

* Only use prednisone once diagnosis is established.
** Only use furosemide once adequate hydration has been achieved.

Initiating glucocorticoids before diagnosis can result in short-lived remissions of lymphoma and myeloma, precluding a timely diagnosis and appropriate initiation of therapy. In addition, lymphoma that recrudesces following single-agent corticosteroid therapy can be less responsive to subsequent chemotherapy because of a selection for multidrug resistance.

Calcitonin is reserved for those cases in which the absolute serum concentration of calcium is extremely high and the clinical signs are marked (e.g., coma, cardiovascular emergency), necessitating intervention that will rapidly normalize serum calcium. Calcitonin (4 to 6 units/kg SQ BID) often normalizes serum calcium within 2 to 3 hours; however, "overshoot" hypocalcemia can occur, and the clinician should watch for signs of acute hypocalcemia (i.e., tremors, irritability, rubbing, and scratching at the face). Calcitonin is not for long-term use since tachyphylaxis (i.e., nonresponsiveness to subsequent treatments) can occur within a few days.

The bisphosphonate classes of drugs (e.g., pamidronate, zoledronate), although moderately expensive, have become the standard of care in human oncology for HCM and are rapidly becoming so in veterinary oncology (Clines and Guise, 2005; Fan et al., 2005; Hostutler et al., 2005; Milner et al., 2004; Pecherstorfer et al., 2003). They act by several mechanisms; however, the most important is to inhibit osteoclast function, thereby inhibiting normal and abnormal bone resorption. They do not act as quickly as calcitonin, taking a few days to normalize serum calcium; however, for long-term use they are superior. I use these agents primarily for cases in which the primary tumor is unlikely to be resolved and the patient is likely to experience long-term hypercalcemia (e.g., anal sac adenocarcinoma). Pamidronate has been used most frequently at a dose of 1 mg/kg in both dogs and cats (given intravenously along with 30 ml [cat] or 250 ml [dog] of normal saline as a 2-hour infusion), once every 4 to 6 weeks, to effect. The primary adverse effect of the bisphosphonates is renal tubular toxicity; thus appropriate hydration and periodic monitoring of renal parameters are important. A newer-generation bisphosphonate, zoledronate, has been used effectively in dogs (0.2 to 0.25 mg/kg in 200 ml of normal saline, infused intravenously over 30 minutes) with HCM. The calcium normalizing effects typically last approximately 4 to 6 weeks following a single dose (Fig. 74-2).

Mithramycin and gallium nitrate are mentioned more for historical importance, although the latter is enjoying a moderate resurgence in physician-based oncology in refractory cases and those cases with widespread metastatic disease.

INVESTIGATIONAL THERAPIES

The investigation of novel therapies for HCM is actively ongoing in human oncology because of the significance of the problem and the impact on quality of life for a large proportion of the tumor-bearing population (Clines and Guise, 2005). Disruption of the PTH-signaling pathway at the level of bone resorption (RANK/RANKL) through

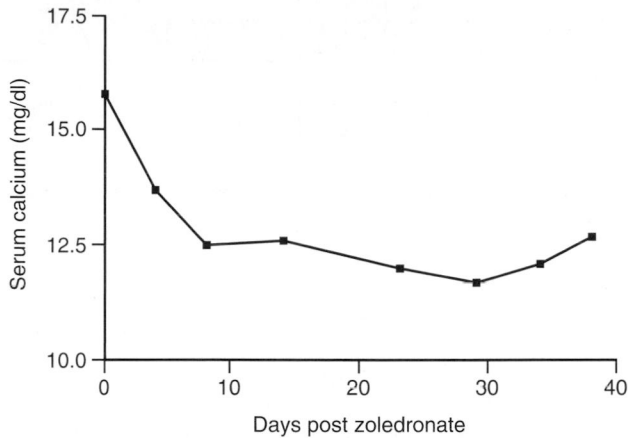

Fig. 74-2 Serum calcium concentrations in a dog with hypercalcemia of malignancy secondary to an apocrine gland adenocarcinoma of the anal sac. At day 0 intravenous zoledronate at 0.2 mg/kg was given. Note that calcium decreased to normal by Day 8 and the effect was maintained for approximately 5 weeks.

the use of recombinant OPG or anti-RANKL antibodies is showing early promise. In addition, clinical trials evaluating anti-PTHrP antibodies are currently underway for women with metastatic breast cancer. Other potential targets to be modulated include the calciotropic factors involved in hypercalcemia, including IL-1β, IL-6, TGFα, and TNF-α.

References and Suggested Reading

Clines GA, Guise TA: Hypercalcemia of malignancy and basic research on mechanisms responsible osteolytic and osteoblastic metastasis to bone, *Endocr Relat Cancer* 12:549, 2005.

Fan TM et al: Evaluation of intravenous pamidronate administration in 33 cancer-bearing dogs with primary or secondary bone involvement, *J Vet Intern Med* 19:74, 2005.

Feldman EC et al: Pretreatment clinical and laboratory findings in dogs with primary hyperparathyroidism: 210 cases (1987-2004), *J Am Vet Med Assoc* 227:756, 2005.

Hostutler RA et al: Uses and effectiveness of pamidronate disodium for treatment of dogs and cats with hypercalcemia, *J Vet Intern Med* 19:29, 2005.

Meuten DJ et al: Hypercalcemia in dogs with adenocarcinoma derived from apocrine glands of the anal sac, *Lab Invest* 48:428, 1983a.

Meuten DJ et al: Hypercalcemia in dogs with lymphosarcoma, *Lab Invest* 49:553, 1983b.

Milner RJ et al: Bisphosphonates and cancer, *J Vet Intern Med* 18:597, 2004.

Pecherstorfer M, Brenner K, Zojer N: Current management strategies for hypercalcemia, *Treat Endocrinol* 2:273, 2003.

Rosol TJ et al: Parathyroid hormone (PTH)–related protein, PTH, and 1,25-dihydroxyvitamin D in dogs with cancer-associated hypercalcemia, *Endocrinology* 131:1157, 1992.

Rosol TJ et al: Identification of parathyroid hormone–related protein in canine apocrine adenocarcinoma of the anal sac, *Vet Pathol* 27:89, 1990.

CHAPTER 75

Histiocytic Disease Complex

PETER F. MOORE, *Davis, California*
VERENA K. AFFOLTER, *Davis, California*

HISTIOCYTIC DIFFERENTIATION AND CANINE HISTIOCYTOSIS

The development of canine-specific monoclonal antibodies for many of the functionally important molecules of macrophages and dendritic antigen-presenting cells (DCs) has enabled the identification of the cell lineages involved in canine and feline histiocytic disorders. Despite the large variation of clinical and pathologic features of histiocytic diseases, the majority represent proliferations of cells of various DC lineages.

Histiocytes differentiate from CD34+-committed stem cell precursors into *macrophages* and several DC lineages, which include *intraepithelial DCs* or *Langerhans cells* (LCs), *interstitial DCs* in many organs (e.g., dermal DCs in skin), and *interdigitating DCs* of T cell domains in peripheral lymphoid organs. DCs are the most potent *antigen-presenting cells* (APCs) for induction of immune responses in naïve T cells. Canine DCs occur in skin within the epidermis (LCs) and within the dermis, especially adjacent to postcapillary venules (interstitial DCs or dermal DCs). Canine DCs abundantly express CD1 molecules, which together with major histocompatibility complex (MHC) class I and MHC class II molecules are responsible for presentation of peptides, lipids, and glycolipids to T cells. Thus DCs are best defined by their abundant expression of molecules essential to their function as APCs. DCs also use adhesion molecules such as the β2 integrins (CD11/CD18) in their function as APCs. CD11/CD18 expression is highly regulated in normal canine macrophages and DCs. CD11c is frequently expressed by DCs, whereas macrophages predominately express CD11b (or CD11d in the splenic red pulp and bone marrow).

Successful interaction of DCs and T cells in response to antigenic challenge also involves the orderly appearance of costimulatory molecules (B7 family—CD80 and CD86) on DCs and their ligands (CD28 and CTLA-4) on T cells. The defective interaction of DCs and T cells appears to contribute to the development of reactive histiocytic proliferative diseases, cutaneous histiocytosis (CH), and systemic histiocytosis (SH), which are related DC disorders arising out of disordered immune regulation (see following paragraphs).

Lineage distinctions among histiocytes (LCs, interstitial DCs, and macrophages) are best made via immunohistochemistry (IHC) performed on frozen sections with extensive panels of leukocyte markers (monoclonal antibodies). These analyses are only performed by specialized laboratories by prior arrangement since the fresh, unfixed biopsy specimen must be shipped overnight for optimum results. Less definitive but useful distinctions can also be attained via IHC on routine formalin-fixed paraffin sections with panels of leukocyte markers developed for use in this format and more widely available in commercial and academic pathology services.

AN OVERVIEW OF CANINE HISTIOCYTIC DISEASES

Histiocytic disorders of dogs include histiocytoma and the related disorder LC histiocytosis (LCH), localized histiocytic sarcoma (HS), disseminated HS (malignant histiocytosis [MH]), and the reactive histiocytoses: CH and SH. These are a frustrating group of diseases because they may be difficult to differentiate from granulomatous inflammation, reactive inflammatory diseases, or lymphoproliferative diseases by examination of regular paraffin sections. The clinical presentation, behavior, and responsiveness to therapy vary tremendously among the syndromes. Clinical and pathologic images of canine histiocytic diseases and details of histiocytic lineages are available on a website that we maintain (http://www.histiocytosis.ucdavis.edu).

CANINE CUTANEOUS HISTIOCYTOMA COMPLEX

Histiocytoma

Histiocytoma is a common, benign, cutaneous neoplasm of the dog. Histiocytomas usually occur as solitary lesions that undergo spontaneous regression. The age-specific incidence rate for histiocytomas drops precipitously after 3 years, although histiocytomas do occur in dogs of all ages. Reports of local or distant recurrence of histiocytomas are rare, and multiple tumors are unusual. Epidermal invasion by cells of histiocytoma frequently occurs, and intraepidermal nests of histiocytes resemble Pautrier's aggregates, which are characteristically found in epidermotropic T cell lymphoma (mycosis fungoides [MF]). Epidermal invasion in histiocytoma, especially in aged dogs, can present a diagnostic dilemma; and distinction from MF is difficult on purely morphologic grounds.

Histiocytoma is readily distinguished from other histiocytic disorders and cutaneous lymphoma with the aid of IHC. Our work has shown clearly that histiocytomas have the phenotype of epidermal LCs; thus cutaneous histiocytoma is a localized epidermal LC tumor. Tumor histiocytes express CD1, MHC class II, CD11c, and E-cadherin. Among skin leukocytes, E-cadherin expression is unique to LCs. Histiocytomas lack expression of CD4 and Thy-1, which are consistently expressed by histiocytes in CH and SH. Cutaneous T cell lymphomas are readily detected by the demonstration of CD3 expression.

Multiple Histiocytomas

Although rare, multiple histiocytomas occur more frequently in shar-peis. Multiple histiocytomas are also readily confused with CH on clinical appearance, although morphologically histiocytomas are consistently epidermotropic and commonly epidermally invasive, which are not features of CH. Delayed regression of multiple histiocytomas may occur, and lesions can persist for many months. We have a cohort of 35 dogs with multiple histiocytomas limited to skin; 11 dogs were shar-peis. Outcomes were available for 19 dogs; regression of histiocytomas occurred in 9 dogs. The remaining 10 dogs were euthanized, with survival times from days to 6 months. Another cohort of 12 dogs had multiple histiocytomas with concurrent lymphadenopathy caused by metastasis. Outcomes were available for 10 dogs; all were euthanized, with survival times from days to 9 months. Curiously, we have a cohort of four dogs with solitary histiocytomas, which metastasized to lymph nodes. Regression occurred in three dogs, and only one dog was euthanized.

Canine Langerhans Cell Histiocytosis

Canine LCH is a rare disease characterized by extensive regional cutaneous infiltration by histiocytes, which otherwise resemble those in histiocytoma, although rapid systemic metastasis is observed. LCH is also recognized as a rare disease of humans, in which marked variation in clinical behavior is recognized. We have a cohort of 11 dogs with LCH, occurring over an 11-year period. Outcomes were available for 10 dogs, which were all euthanized within days to 3 months.

Therapy

There is no effective medical treatment for LCH or the aggressive histiocytoma syndromes described in the previous paragraphs. Surgical management is indicated if the number of tumors allows. Treatment with corticosteroids or other immunosuppressive drugs (e.g., cyclosporine A) is contraindicated since regression of histiocytomas consistently occurs via activation of cytotoxic T cells, which would be inhibited by immunosuppression. Treatment with lomustine (chloroethylcyclohexylnitrosourea [CCNU]), which has been used widely in the treatment of HS, has not been successful. Radiation therapy may be efficacious but has not been widely used because of the extensive topographic involvement commonly encountered in these aggressive syndromes.

CANINE REACTIVE HISTIOCYTOSES

The reactive histiocytoses traditionally have included CH and SH. We believe that the continued distinction of SH and CH as entirely separate entities is probably no longer justifiable. It would be preferable to consider them within the spectrum of reactive histiocytoses of interstitial DC origin, in which clinical outcome is predictable more by the distant migratory potential of the proliferating histiocytes beyond the skin. In this view CH and SH would be regarded as skin-limited and systemic interstitial DC proliferations, respectively. A wide range of clinical behavior is to be expected within each grouping, with SH usually exhibiting more aggressive disease. CH and SH should not be confused with malignant DC disorders (HS and MH), which can occur in the same locations. Cytologic and immunophenotypic differences can distinguish these diseases in most instances.

Systemic Histiocytosis

SH was originally recognized in related Bernese mountain dogs. SH is a generalized histiocytic proliferative disease with a marked tendency to involve skin, ocular, and nasal mucosae and peripheral lymph nodes. The disease predominantly affects young to middle-aged dogs (2 to 8 years). It has been observed in other breeds (e.g., Irish wolfhounds, basset hounds) less commonly. Clinical signs vary with the severity and extent of the disease and include anorexia, marked weight loss, stertorous respiration, and conjunctivitis with marked chemosis. Multiple cutaneous nodules may be distributed over the entire body but are especially prevalent on the scrotum, nasal apex, nasal planum, and eyelids. Ulceration of the skin overlying the nodules is common. Peripheral lymph nodes often are palpably enlarged. The disease course may be punctuated by remissions and relapses, which may occur spontaneously, especially early in the disease course. In severe disease lesions become persistent and do not respond to immunosuppressive doses of corticosteroids.

Cutaneous Histiocytosis

CH is a histiocytic proliferative disorder that primarily involves skin and subcutis and does not extend beyond the local draining lymph nodes. CH occurs in a number of breeds. Evidence of spread beyond the skin and draining lymph nodes would invoke the diagnosis of SH, a closely related disorder. Lymphadenopathy has not been emphasized in published reports and has only been documented in a small number of our cases. The lesions occur as multiple cutaneous and subcutaneous nodules up to 4 cm in diameter. Overlying skin ulceration is common. Lesions may disappear spontaneously or regress and appear at new sites simultaneously. Lesions commonly are found on the face, ears, nose, neck, trunk, extremities (including foot pads), perineum, and scrotum.

Histiocytes in CH and SH express markers expected of DCs such as CD1, C11c, and MHC II. However, the lack of consistent epidermotropism in SH and CH lesions and the expression of Thy-1 (expressed by dermal DC) and CD4 (a marker of DC activation) suggest that histiocytes in these diseases are activated interstitial type DCs rather than LCs. In skin dermal DCs are mostly of interstitial DC type. The clinical behavior and consistent clinical response to immunosuppressive therapy with agents capable of inhibiting T cell activation have reinforced the concept that SH and CH occur in the context of disordered immune regulation arising from defective interaction between DCs and T cells. The end result of this dysregulated immune interaction is chronic proliferation of DCs and T cells. The initiation of the process is probably antigen driven, although studies to identify the nature of the antigens involved have been unrewarding. Thus it is important to perform tests to rule out infectious agents in the initial workup of a reactive histiocytosis case (culture and/or special stains for microorganisms in tissue).

Therapy

Lesions of CH and SH may wax and wane and even spontaneously resolve without treatment in the initial presentation. If lesions are not in sensitive sites and are not bothersome, it is worth waiting a few weeks to see if spontaneous resolution will occur. Some cases of CH respond well to immunosuppressive doses of corticosteroids, but the majority of CH and SH cases do not respond to corticosteroid treatment. SH in particular is a progressive disease that eventually requires continuous immunosuppression (for details see Chapter 55). The current therapeutic agent of choice for reactive histiocytoses is cyclosporine A coupled with ketoconazole to reduce the necessary dose of cyclosporine A. Leflunomide is also highly efficacious, but until recently it was prohibitively expensive for use in large dogs. The recent availability of generic leflunomide has lowered the cost significantly. Dogs on these potent immunosuppressive drugs are susceptible to infections. Risk of exposure to infectious agents should be minimized (e.g., avoidance of events in which many dogs are in attendance). Routine vaccinations should also be suspended while dogs are immunosuppressed.

HISTIOCYTIC SARCOMA COMPLEX

HS and the related disorder MH occur with greatest frequency in Bernese mountain dogs, rottweilers, flat-coated retrievers, golden retrievers, and sporadically in many other breeds. HS occurs as solitary lesions in spleen, lymph nodes, lung, bone marrow, skin and subcutis, brain, and periarticular tissue of large appendicular joints. HS can also occur as multiple lesions in single organs (especially spleen) and rapidly disseminate to involve multiple organs. Thus disseminated HS is difficult to distinguish from MH, which is a multisystem, rapidly progressive disease in which there is simultaneous involvement of multiple organs such as spleen, lymph nodes, lung, bone marrow, skin, and subcutis.

Clinical signs of HS/MH include anorexia, weight loss, and lethargy. Other signs depend on the organs involved and are a consequence of destructive mass formation. Accordingly pulmonary symptoms such as cough and dyspnea have been seen. Central nervous system involvement (primary or secondary) can lead to seizures, incoordination, and paralysis. Lameness is often observed in periarticular HS.

The clinical, clinicopathologic, and pathologic features of the distinctive *hemophagocytic HS* were the subjects of a recent publication (Moore, Affolter, and Vernau, 2006). This disease is frequently confused with immune-mediated hemolytic anemia/thrombocytopenia by clinicians and clinical pathologists despite negative Coombs' tests in all cases. Regenerative anemia and thrombocytopenia have been documented consistently in hemophagocytic

HS. Affected dogs also frequently demonstrate hypoalbuminemia and hypocholesterolemia. Histiocytes expand the splenic red pulp, which leads to diffuse splenomegaly. Simultaneous involvement of bone marrow is observed consistently. Extensive invasion of hepatic sinuses without mass formation occurs via the portal vein; this lesion is often missed by pathologists in the early stages. Hemophagocytic HS is associated with rapid demise (mean survival is about 7 weeks). Severe anemia and attendant coagulopathy complicates clinical management.

Histiocytes in HS/MH lesions express leukocyte surface molecules characteristic of DCs (CD1, CD11c and MHC II). The exact sublineages of DCs involved in HS/MH have not been determined in most instances. The most likely candidates include interdigitating DCs in lymphoid tissues and perivascular interstitial DCs in other involved tissues. Diffuse expression of E-cadherin, Thy-1, and CD4 has not been observed in HS or MH in skin or other sites; this together with cytomorphology assists in the distinction of HS/MH from histiocytoma and reactive histiocytosis (CH and SH). In hemophagocytic HS histiocytes express CD11d instead of CD11c, and MHC II. Expression of CD1 molecules is inconsistent. This phenotype is consistent with macrophage differentiation rather than DC differentiation, in which abundant expression of CD1 and CD11c is expected. This phenotype may explain the aggressive erythrophagocytosis, which is prevalent in this disease.

Immunophenotyping and careful morphologic assessment should also avoid confusion of HS and MH with the large cell form of T cell lymphoma (CD3+), pleomorphic large B cell lymphoma (CD20+, CD79a+), plasmacytoma (usually CD45+, CD45RA+, CD79a+), and poorly differentiated mast cell tumors (CD18+ variable, CD45+, CD45RA+, Tryptase+, c-kit+).

Therapy

Localized HS affecting skin and subcutis has been cured by early surgical excision, which in some instances apparently has been successfully supplemented by local radiation therapy. In the case of periarticular HS, which occurs in the subsynovial tissues of the extremities, amputation of the affected limb is required as a result of the inoperable nature of the primary lesion, which usually ensnares structures vital to limb function. It is important to establish absence of gross metastasis via thoracic radiographs, abdominal ultrasound, and regional lymph node aspiration cytology before embarking on limb amputation. Even despite due diligence, early undetected dissemination may have occurred, and the dog may develop widespread metastatic disease. *Disseminated HS* (including MH) is not readily treated surgically since even in the splenic form early metastasis to the liver has often occurred. Response to chemotherapy has been at best brief, and the disease progresses rapidly (weeks to months) to death or euthanasia. Lomustine is the chemotherapeutic agent most commonly used to treat HS. Response to lomustine reportedly is better if the tumor burden is low. Hemophagocytic HS has been treated by splenectomy followed by lomustine chemotherapy. The rationale for this approach is that the major tumor burden is within the spleen; hence splenectomy is the most expeditious approach to reducing tumor burden before lomustine treatment. However, in the few cases we've followed the survival time was not clearly prolonged by this protocol. The dogs did well initially, but the existence of prior micrometastatic foci resulted in clinical disease progression.

FELINE HISTIOCYTIC DISEASES

Cats have a narrower range of histiocytic proliferative diseases than dogs. Clear feline equivalents of cutaneous histiocytoma and the reactive histiocytoses (CH and SH) have not been described. Cats are afflicted by the HS complex and present with many of the same clinical syndromes as in dogs, including hemophagocytic HS. However, the incidence is much lower. The most common histiocytic disorder of cats is feline progressive histiocytosis (FPH), which has no canine equivalent. Two previous reports of cutaneous histiocytoma in the cat were likely examples of FPH.

Feline Progressive Histiocytosis

FPH is a disease of adult cats (mean 8.8 years; range 2 to 17 years; n=30). Cats present with skin lesions, which are solitary or multiple nonpruritic, firm papules, nodules, and plaques. Lesions have a predilection for feet, legs, and face. Lesions consist of poorly circumscribed epitheliotropic and nonepitheliotropic histiocytic infiltrates of the superficial and deep dermis, with variable extension into the subcutis. The histiocytic population is relatively monomorphic and well differentiated early in the clinical course. With disease progression, cellular pleomorphism is more frequently encountered, and the lesions are then indistinguishable from HS. Histiocytes express CD1a, CD1c, CD18, and MHC class II molecules. This immunophenotype suggests an interstitial DC origin of these lesions. Coexpression of E-cadherin, a feature of cutaneous LCs, was only observed in three cats. FPH followed a progressive clinical course; however, the lesions were limited to the skin for an extended period of time (mean 13.4 months; range 1 to 36 months).

Extracutaneous involvement was documented in all cats that were euthanized and evaluated (7/15 cats). The etiology of FPH remains unknown. FPH is best considered an initially indolent cutaneous neoplasm, which is mostly slowly progressive and may spread beyond the skin in the terminal stage.

Therapy

Chemotherapy or immunosuppressive or immunomodulatory therapy was not successful in any of the cats. Agents used included vincristine and vinblastine (two cats), lomustine (two cats), L-asparaginase (one cat), corticosteroids (11 cats), cyclosporine A (one cat), leflunomide (one cat), interferon-γ (one cat), retinoids (one cat), and antibiotics (three cats). Surgical removal of the lesions was not successful largely because of the appearance of new lesions at distant sites in all cats (n=8).

Suggested Reading

Affolter VK, Moore PF: Canine cutaneous and systemic histiocytosis: reactive histiocytosis of dermal dendritic cells, *Am J Dermatopathol* 22:40, 2000.

Affolter VK, Moore PF: Localized and disseminated histiocytic sarcoma of dendritic cell origin in dogs, *Vet Pathol* 39:74, 2002.

Affolter VK, Moore PF: Feline progressive histiocytosis, *Vet Pathol* 43:646, 2006.

Mays MB, Bergeron JA: Cutaneous histiocytosis in dogs, *J Am Vet Med Assoc* 188:377, 1986.

Moore PF: Systemic histiocytosis of Bernese mountain dogs, *Vet Pathol* 21:554, 1984.

Moore PF, Rosin A: Malignant histiocytosis of Bernese mountain dogs, *Vet Pathol* 23:1, 1986.

Moore PF, Affolter VK, Vernau W: Canine hemophagocytic histiocytic sarcoma: a proliferative disorder of CD11d+ macrophages, *Vet Pathol* 43:632, 2006.

Moore PF et al: Canine cutaneous histiocytoma is an epidermotropic Langerhans cell histiocytosis which expresses CD1 and specific beta-2 integrin molecules, *Am J Pathol* 148:1699, 1996.

Shortman K, Liu YJ: Mouse and human dendritic cell subtypes, *Nat Rev Immunol* 2:151, 2002.

CHAPTER 76

Nasal Tumors

LISA J. FORREST, *Madison, Wisconsin*

PATHOLOGY AND CLINICAL PRESENTATION

Tumors of the nasal passage and paranasal sinuses in dogs account for approximately 1% to 2% of all canine neoplasms, with the majority being carcinoma (60%) and sarcoma (30%) histologies. Further breakdown of histology includes adenocarcinoma, squamous cell carcinoma, fibrosarcoma, chondrosarcoma, and osteosarcoma. Dolichocephalic breeds and dogs with exposure to indoor coal or kerosene heaters are at increased risk for development of nasal tumors. Most dogs presenting with nasal tumors are middle to older age, with reported median ages of 7.6 to 11.3 years. Nasal tumors generally are locally invasive and slow to metastasize but can metastasize to local lymph nodes (mandibular/retropharyngeal and less often to lung, abdominal organs, bone, and brain). Clinical signs in dogs with nasal tumors include nasal obstruction/respiratory stridor, sneezing, reverse sneezing, epistaxis, facial deformity, and exophthalmos. Initially signs may respond partially to antibiotics or antiinflammatory treatments because of the concurrent inflammation and secondary bacterial infection that is inevitably present. These tumors often are quite locally advanced when diagnosed, and occasionally patients can present with neurologic signs (seizures, altered mentation, behavior change) secondary to destruction of the cribriform plate and extension into the brain.

STAGING AND DIAGNOSIS

Imaging

Thoracic radiographs to evaluate for pulmonary metastases and as a general cardiac and geriatric evaluation should be obtained. Nasal radiographs can be used to image animals with nasal disease and should include the following:

1. Straight lateral to medial view
2. Open-mouth ventrodorsal maxillary view, angled 10 degrees rostral-caudal
3. Intraoral dorsoventral maxillary view
4. Frontal sinus view (rostral-caudal oblique)

However, cross-sectional imaging is preferred. Computed tomography (CT) is the most commonly used imaging modality for evaluating dogs and cats with nasal disease, but magnetic resonance imaging (MRI) is also used. Both imaging modalities have advantages and disadvantages in the imaging of nasal disease in cats and dogs. Bone destruction is easier to identify on CT (Fig. 76-1), and soft-tissue changes are better delineated on MRI. Generally MRI studies are more expensive, and imaging time is

longer than CT studies. Because computer-based radiation therapy (RT) plans are commonly generated using CT images, CT may be the preferred imaging modality if RT is contemplated.

Biopsy

Biopsy and histology of the nasal tumor are needed for definitive diagnosis. Before the biopsy procedure, additional evaluation should include complete blood count and blood chemistry along with a clotting profile. Fine-needle aspiration cytology of mandibular lymph nodes should also be performed as part of tumor staging. A transnostril biopsy technique using a closed suction technique, a bone curette, or cup-type biopsy forceps should be performed under general anesthesia to collect a sample. Whenever a transnostril biopsy technique is used, it is important to measure and mark the biopsy instrument so as to penetrate no farther than the distance from the tip of the nose to the medial canthus of the eye. This prevents penetration of the cribriform plate. Tumor tissue generally is white in color; mild-to-moderate hemorrhage is expected and usually subsides within a few minutes. Cytology of nasal swabs or expectorated material is rarely rewarding. Some large nasal tumors protrude into the nasopharynx and can be sampled using retrograde rhinoscopy. When obtaining biopsy samples with smaller endoscopic instruments, there is also a risk of sampling surrounding inflammation as opposed to the tumor.

TREATMENT AND PROGNOSIS

A variety of treatments for nasal tumors are reported in the literature, including RT, surgery, cryosurgery, chemotherapy, or a combination of these modalities. Unfortunately long-term survival for dogs with nasal tumors generally has been poor, with median survival times ranging from 5 to 23 months, depending on the treatment used. Generally surgery is considered ineffectual as a sole treatment modality.

At this time external-beam RT alone (see Chapter 67) or in combination with surgery or chemotherapy is the most effective treatment available, and the clinician is encouraged to speak with a radiation oncologist or oncologist with experience in managing nasal tumors. Because of the close proximity of the eyes to the nasal cavity, there is unavoidable acute and late toxicity of RT to ocular structures. Most dogs develop keratoconjunctivitis sicca (KSC) and cataracts in at least one eye. Dogs may also develop retinal hemorrhage and corneal ulcers. Chronic ocular toxicities are seen in approximately 45% of dogs. Lower-energy orthovoltage RT has been used alone and after surgical exenteration of the nasal tumor with reported

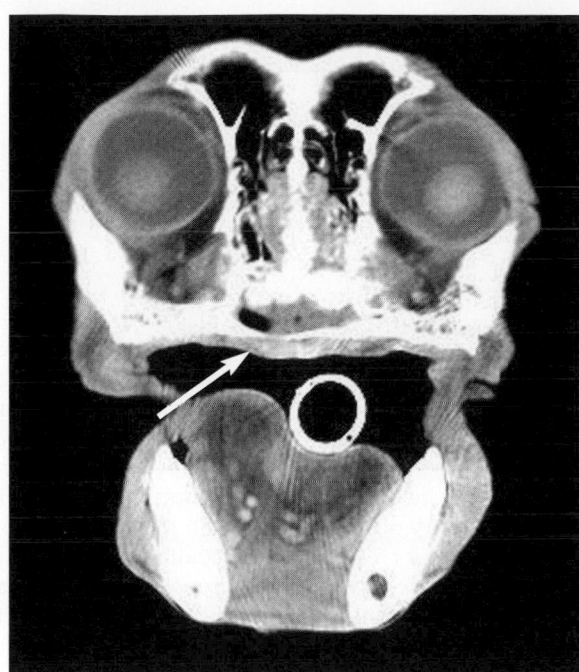

Fig. 76-1 Computed tomographic axial slice of a dog with a nasal tumor at the level of the eyes. Note the soft-tissue attenuating material (tumor) in both caudal nasal passages and the nasopharynx. Tumor destruction of the hard palate *(white arrow)* is seen as thinning of palatine bone.

survival times of 7.4 to 23 months, respectively. Currently megavoltage external-beam RT, delivered via linear accelerator or Cobalt machines, is commonly used to treat nasal tumors, with reported median survival times of 5.9 to 19 months. The course of treatment varies among institutions and practices; treatments can be delivered on a daily Monday-to-Friday schedule for 2 to 4 weeks or on a Monday, Wednesday, Friday schedule for 4 to 6 weeks.

Cisplatin and other chemotherapy agents have been used in some dogs with nasal tumors because of their radiosensitizing properties. A recent study of 51 dogs treated with external-beam RT in combination with slow-release cisplatin chemotherapy reported a median survival time of 15.8 months. Recently a small study of eight dogs receiving chemotherapy alone reported a good outcome using a protocol of alternating doses of doxorubicin, carboplatin, and oral piroxicam.

Use of an accelerated fractionated RT protocol (4.2 Gy × 10 fractions = 42 Gy) results in similar median survival times of 14 to 19 months, compared to more conventional fractionation schemes. Surgical exenteration following accelerated RT increased overall survival to 47.7 months in a small study of 13 dogs. However, the dogs reported in this study had significant morbidity associated with surgery; 69% of dogs had rhinitis, 31% had osteomyelitis, and 2/10 had significant hemorrhage during surgery that required a transfusion. Attempts at increasing the RT dose to the tumor by using a boost technique (additional dose delivered to a smaller tumor volume) resulted in increased normal tissue morbidity and no improvement in tumor control. With current methods, increasing total tumor dose is impossible without increasing normal tissue toxicity.

Feline Tumors

Nasal lymphoma is the most common nasal tumor in the cat followed by carcinoma and least often sarcoma. Clinical signs in cats include nasal discharge, dyspnea, epistaxis, stertor, facial deformity, and anorexia. Nasal lymphoma often extends into the nasopharynx. Treatment approaches for cats with nasal lymphoma include external-beam RT alone, chemotherapy alone, or combination RT and chemotherapy. As with dogs, treatment of choice for nasal carcinoma and sarcomas is external-beam RT. Many cats with nasal lymphoma eventually will have systemic spread of disease, although long-term local disease control is often reported following local therapy alone.

FUTURE DIRECTIONS

There is clearly room for advancement in the treatment of tumors of the nasal and paranasal sinuses. Use of CT and MR imaging has improved the ability to accurately delineate the tumors. The use of three-dimensional computerized treatment plans has also increased the accuracy of the delivered RT dose. More and more radiation oncology centers are installing linear accelerators with multileaf collimators, allowing the radiation oncologist to shape the treatment beam to the tumor and avoid critical ocular tissues. A multileaf collimator and appropriate software allow intensity-modulated radiotherapy (IMRT) in which the treatment beam intensity and the treatment field shape can be conformed. Helical tomotherapy, which is image-guided IMRT, was used in a small trial of dogs in which the goal was to treat the nasal tumor and avoid ocular structures. None of the dogs has experienced significant ocular side effects, and all dogs are visual with no signs of KCS or other uncomfortable ocular toxicity. Tumor response in the trial is similar to that previously reported. These results would indicate that the future of treating canine nasal tumors lies with IMRT technology and early diagnosis when tumor burden is smaller.

References and Suggested Reading

Adams WM et al: Outcome of accelerated radiotherapy alone or accelerated radiotherapy followed by exenteration of the nasal cavity in dogs with intranasal neoplasia 53 cases (1990-2002), *J Am Vet Med Assoc* 227:936, 2005.

Hahn KA et al: Clinical response of nasal adenocarcinoma to cisplatin chemotherapy in 11 dogs, *J Am Vet Med Assoc* 200:355, 1992.

Klein MK: Multimodality therapy for head and neck cancer, *Vet Clin Small Anim Pract* 33:615, 2003.

Lana SE, Withrow SJ: Tumors of the respiratory system—nasal tumors. In Withrow SJ, MacEwen EG, editors: *Small animal clinical oncology*, ed 3, Philadelphia, 2001, Saunders, p 370.

Langova V et al: Treatment of eight dogs with nasal tumours with alternating doses of doxorubicin and carboplatin in conjunction with oral piroxicam, *Aust Vet J* 82:676, 2004.

Malinowski C: Canine and feline nasal neoplasia, *Clin Tech Small Anim Pract* 21:89, 2006.

Park RD, Beck ER, LeCouteur RA: Comparison of computed tomography and radiography for detecting changes induced by malignant nasal neoplasia in dogs, *J Am Vet Med Assoc* 201:1720, 1992.

CHAPTER 77

Pulmonary Neoplasia

KEVIN A. HAHN, *Topeka, Kansas*
SANDRA M. AXIAK, *Dallas, Texas*

LUNG

Pathology and Natural Behavior

The incidence of primary lung tumors in the dog and cat is low. The majority of tumors are malignant, and the most frequently reported tumor type is adenocarcinoma in both the dog and cat. The average age at presentation is 9 to 10 years in dogs and 11 to 12 years in cats. There is no breed or sex predisposition and no proven etiology. Clinical signs tend to occur late in disease and vary at presentation. Often a chronic nonproductive cough is present; however, lung tumors may be diagnosed incidentally during radiography for another indication. Other signs are lethargy, dyspnea, weight loss, and tachypnea. Lameness is seen in cats with musculoskeletal metastasis (lung-digit syndrome seen with pulmonary adenocarcinoma, bronchial carcinoma, and squamous cell carcinoma), and in dogs with hypertrophic osteopathy (rare in the cat).

Diagnostic Approach

Thoracic radiographs are the most important diagnostic test. Common findings are soft-tissue density mass(es) (discrete or ill-defined); lobar consolidation; and diffuse interstitial, alveolar, peribronchial, or mixed patterns. The appearance of pulmonary neoplasia in cats can vary dramatically, ranging from solitary lesions that may be cavitated to diffuse mixed patterns of disease. Differential diagnoses for discrete soft-tissue opacity masses are abscess, hematoma, cyst, and granuloma; for other patterns they are pneumonia, metastasis, hemorrhage, edema, and fibrosis. Thoracic ultrasonography and cytologic examination of needle aspirates, pleural fluid, or bronchoalveolar lavage washes can aid in diagnosis. However, it is important to note that sensitivity of detecting neoplasia in pleural effusions is as low as 60% in both the dog and cat; thus biopsy may be required for definitive diagnosis (Hirshbeger et al, 1999). Computed tomography (CT) may be used to better determine the extent of disease before surgery if this information will alter the owner's decision with regard to treatment (Paoloni et al., 2006).

Treatment and Prognosis

Surgical removal is the treatment of choice for primary lung tumors. Reported median survival times following lung lobectomy are in the 10- to 13-month range. Positive prognostic indicators are: absence of clinical signs at presentation, solitary nodule, peripheral location, and less than 5 cm in diameter. Negative prognostic indicators are lymph node involvement, more than one nodule, central location, greater than 5 cm in diameter, and high histologic grade (Hahn and McEntee, 1998: McNiel et al., 1997). Small case series of chemotherapy with vindesine/cisplatin or vinorelbine have been reported in dogs, with antitumor activity observed with both protocols (Melhaff et al., 1984; Poirier et al., 2004). Radiation therapy for solitary lung masses has not been reported in veterinary medicine. Hypertrophic osteopathy in dogs, if present, usually resolves after removal of the primary mass. There is no information regarding the efficacy of postoperative chemotherapy for dogs or cats with lung tumors.

PLEURAL SPACE

Pathology and Natural Behavior

Primary cancer of the pleura is called mesothelioma. Exposure to asbestos, especially amphibole fibers (long and thin), is considered a risk factor in humans. The mechanism by which it causes malignant transformation is unknown. Mesothelioma is highly metastatic and can invade the diaphragm and implant on abdominal structures. Neoplastic differentials include metastatic tumors of the pleural space, which in both dogs and cats most commonly occur from carcinomas. The most common clinical sign is respiratory distress caused by pleural effusion (pericardial effusion can also occur with mesothelioma of the pericardium). Reactive mesothelial cells may be interpreted as malignant mesotheliomas based on cytology. However, a true mesothelioma in veterinary medicine is rare.

Diagnostic Approach

Fluid collected from the pleural space can range in appearance from hemorrhagic to chylous. Fine-needle aspiration can be obtained with ultrasound guidance, but cytologic diagnosis of pleural disease is problematic. Reactive mesothelial cells can appear malignant; thus cytology of fluid does not usually give a definitive diagnosis. Diagnosis usually requires a biopsy of the pleura via thoracotomy or thoracoscopy. Differentials include tumor seeding from cardiac hemangiosarcoma (HSA), chemodectoma, or metastatic carcinoma. Imaging of the thoracic and abdominal cavities is indicated to rule out primary tumors.

Treatment and Prognosis

Prognosis is poor for primary mesothelioma or for disease metastatic to the pleura. Since no successful definitive treatments have been reported, the goal of treatment is palliation of clinical signs. Intracavitary cisplatin has been described in six dogs to reduce pleural effusion of various causes. The survival of three dogs with pleural mesothelioma ranged from 129 to 410 days, and duration of response lasted 129 to 306 days (Moore, Kirk, and Cadona, 1991). Intracavitary mitoxantrone and carboplatin, with or without intravenous chemotherapy, has been described in 12 dogs, with a median survival time of 332 days (Charney et al., 2005). Intracavitary carboplatin has been reported in one cat with suspected mesothelioma, with reduction of pleural fluid and a survival time of 121 days (Sparkes et al., 2005). Systemic chemotherapy has not been effective in either dogs or cats. Cytoreductive surgery may be used for larger masses before intracavitary therapy. Similar therapeutic approaches may be considered for animals with pleural carcinomatosis.

MEDIASTINUM

Pathology and Natural Behavior

The incidence of mediastinal masses is low in both dogs and cats. The two most common differentials for a mediastinal mass are thymoma and lymphoma (LSA). Branchial cyst, ectopic thyroid carcinoma, and chemodectoma can also occur but are less common. The mean age at presentation is 9 years in dogs and 10 years in cats. Benign mediastinal cysts are also recognized in cats, and carry a good prognosis with transthoracic needle drainage.

Thymomas originate from thymic epithelium and are infiltrated with lymphocytes (making differentiation from LSA difficult). It is the epithelial portion of the thymic tissue that is considered neoplastic. Benign thymomas are noninvasive and well encapsulated, whereas malignant thymomas are locally invasive and aggressive. Thymomas rarely metastasize.

LSA is considered a systemic disease in both dogs and cats. Cats presenting with mediastinal LSA usually are young (mean age of 2 years) and positive for feline leukemia virus (FeLV). Clinical signs for mediastinal masses include coughing, tachypnea, dyspnea, anterior caval syndrome, muscle weakness, or megaesophagus caused by myasthenia gravis (a paraneoplastic syndrome associated with thymoma).

Diagnostic Approach

History may include cough, respiratory distress, or signs of esophageal disease. Physical examination findings include pitting edema of the head, neck, or forelimbs if precaval (cranial vena caval) syndrome is present. Lung sounds may be decreased because of compression of lung lobes by the mass or associated pleural effusion. Infrequently, Horner's syndrome is identified from compression of ascending sympathetic nerves. Peripheral lymphadenopathy may be present in dogs with LSA. Hypercalcemia in association with mediastinal LSA is common, with a 25% to 50% incidence rate in dogs; but it has also been reported with thymomas and thus cannot be used to distinguish between the two diseases. Thoracic radiographs reveal a cranial mediastinal mass, pleural effusion, and/or megaesophagus (Fig. 77-1). Ultrasonography of the medi-

astinal mass may be instructive, and can help distinguish solid tumors from cysts (especially in older cats). Fine-needle aspiration and cytology of thymomas generally reveal mature lymphocytes and sometimes mast cells, whereas fine-needle aspiration of LSA often reveals lymphoblasts. These procedures are optimally guided by ultrasound or CT. However, obtaining a definitive diagnosis with cytology is often difficult, and a biopsy should be considered to distinguish between LSA and thymoma. A CT scan can provide information for staging and surgical removal of thymomas but cannot differentiate between tumor types.

Treatment and Prognosis

Surgical excision is the treatment of choice for thymomas and can be curative. Radiation therapy is used if surgical incision is incomplete or not possible. With radiation therapy alone for the treatment of thymomas in both

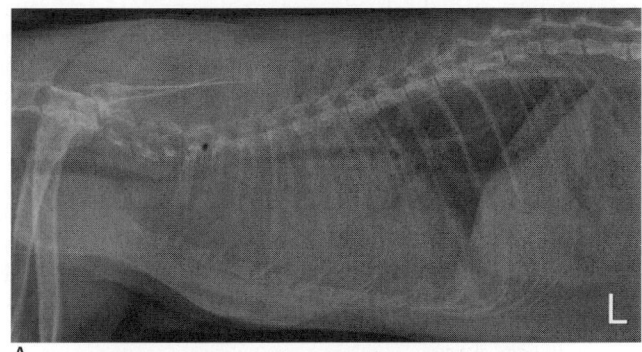

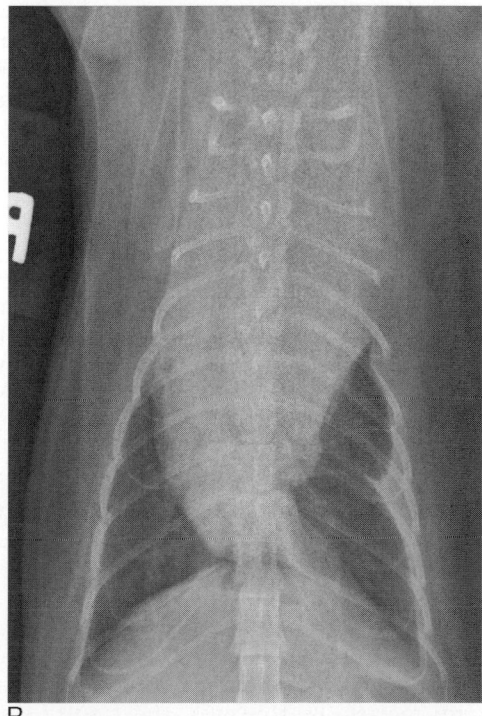

Fig. 77-1 Thoracic radiographs (left lateral) **(A)** and ventrodorsal view **(B)** in an FeLV-positive cat with lymphoma, showing mild pleural effusion and large mediastinal mass. *FeLV,* Feline leukemia virus.

dogs and cats the response rate is 75%, and the median survival time is 248 days in dogs and 720 days in cats (Smith et al., 2001). The prognosis for surgically resected benign thymomas without myasthenia gravis is good, with an 83% 1-year survival reported in dogs and 2-year median survival reported in cats. Chemotherapy targeting the malignant (epithelial) component of thymoma has not been shown to be effective in dogs or cats.

Systemic combination chemotherapy is recommended for the treatment of mediastinal LSA, with radiation therapy if needed to alleviate clinical signs. With an aggressive chemotherapy protocol, median survival times range from 6 to 12 months for dogs and 6 to 9 months (if FeLV negative) or 3 to 6 months (if FeLV positive) for cats. See Chapter 72 for further discussion of LSA treatment.

HEART

Pathology and Natural Behavior

Primary myocardial tumors are rare in both dogs and cats. The majority of tumor types are malignant. The most common tumor type in dogs is HSA, with the German shepherd dog being predisposed (Chapters 70 and 181). In cats the most common primary heart tumor is LSA. Other differentials for both the dog and cat include aortic body tumor (chemodectoma), ectopic thyroid carcinoma, and rhabdomyosarcoma. Dogs and cats are middle-aged to older at presentation. Most cardiac masses are located intrapericardially (intracavitary heart masses are rare) and can cause pericardial effusion. Mesothelioma of the pericardium can also lead to pericardial effusion.

Clinical signs vary and depend on tumor location and invasiveness. Clinical signs are variable. In acute intrapericardial hemorrhage, signs can be acute with collapse and features of hypotension and cardiogenic shock. Chronic pericardial effusion generally leads to congestive heart failure with jugular venous distension, ascites, and often pleural effusion. Syncope may be caused by cardiac arrhythmias, heart failure, obstruction to venous return, or ventricular outflow obstruction. Respiratory distress may also develop from pleural effusion, pulmonary thromboembolism, or metastatic lung disease. Acute death from tumor rupture and blood loss can occur. Major differentials for these clinical signs are idiopathic pericardial effusion, pericarditis, cardiomyopathy, congestive heart failure, and valvular insufficiency.

Diagnostic Approach

Electrocardiographic (ECG) findings may correlate with the mass location or be secondary to myocardial ischemia or pericardial effusion. Possible abnormalities include low amplitude QRS complexes, electrical alternans, ST-segment changes, and cardiac arrhythmias. Thoracic radiographs may show a globoid-shaped heart (as a result of pericardial effusion), cardiomegaly, heart base mass, or pulmonary metastasis. However, the cardiac silhouette may be just modestly increased in size making recognition of pericardial effusion difficult. Cytology of pericardial fluid occasionally may help to distinguish between neoplastic and nonneoplastic causes, especially with LSA.

Echocardiography is the test of choice to identify and determining tumor location and size, as well as the presence of pericardial effusion.

Treatment and Prognosis

Medical treatment is aimed at palliating signs of heart failure and arrhythmias. Pericardiocentesis is the initial treatment of choice to stabilize patients with cardiac tamponade (see Chapter 181). Surgical resection of accessible masses can be successful (consult an experienced thoracic surgeon). Palliation of signs of pericardial effusion can also be achieved by a pericardial window or pericardiectomy.

However, prognosis depends largely on the tumor type. For example, the prognosis for atrial or pericardial HSA in both dogs and cats is poor (see Chapter 70). Although surgical excision of right atrial HSA is feasible and associated with a relatively low rate of complication, metastasis generally occurs rapidly, and postoperative chemotherapy is indicated. The prognosis for most primary cardiac tumors is poor, and in general they do not respond well to medical management. Conversely, long-term survival exceeding one year is not uncommon with aortic body tumors (chemodectoma) palliated by a large pericardial window is much better (see below). The outcomes with pericardial mesothelioma are quite variable, and some long-surviving cases have likely been misdiagnosed due to pronounced mesothelial reaction.

MAJOR VESSELS

Pathology and Natural Behavior

Tumors arising from the carotid or aortic body are most commonly chemodectomas (arising from the chemoreceptor organs). Chemoreceptor organs are part of the parasympathetic nervous system and initiate changes in blood pressure, respiration depth and rate, and heart rate. Chemodectomas are nonfunctional, and clinical signs are caused by space occupation and mechanical disturbances. These tumors are more common in the dog than in the cat. Other differentials for heart base masses include thymoma, HSA, ectopic thyroid carcinoma, abscess, and granuloma. Dogs are middle aged to older at presentation, with males being at a higher risk for developing aortic body tumors. Brachycephalic breeds are at a higher risk of developing chemodectomas; this is thought to be caused by chronic hypoxia. Clinical signs are those associated with right-sided heart failure (aortic body mass: dyspnea, arrhythmia, ascites, pericardial or pleural effusion, coughing, cyanosis) or space-occupying mass in the neck (carotid body mass, dyspnea, Horner's syndrome, laryngeal paralysis). Concurrent endocrine neoplasia (testicular, ovarian, thyroid, parathyroid, adrenal, pituitary, and pancreatic) is a common finding, with an incidence of up to 50% in dogs.

Diagnostic Approach

Thoracic radiographs often show dorsal deviation of the trachea, a mass at the base of the heart, and right-sided heart enlargement. Metastasis can also be seen in some cases. ECG can be normal; or electrical alternans, low amplitude QRS complexes, or arrhythmias (premature ventricular contractions or ventricular tachycardia) may be seen. Abdominal radiographs and ultrasound can be performed to check for involvement of the liver, spleen, or lymph nodes and the presence of ascites. Echocardiography can identify a mass at the base of the heart and pericardial effusion and can also aid in the determination of surgical resectability. Chemodectomas do not exfoliate well; thus cytology of pericardial or pleural fluid usually is not helpful. Definitive diagnosis requires histopathology from surgery or necropsy.

Treatment and Prognosis

Early surgical excision is the treatment of choice. However, chemodectomas tend to be highly invasive and also have the moderate potential to metastasize. Pericardiectomy can be performed at the time of biopsy and has been shown to extend survival time (whether or not pericardial effusion is present). In dogs with aortic body tumors, those that have a pericardiectomy have a median survival time of 730 days, whereas those without a pericardectomy have a median survival time of 42 days (Ehrhart et al., 2002). Even when the mass is not respectable, pericardial windows may be beneficial to prevent accumulation of pericardial effusion. This treatment may often be accomplished using minimally invasive "mini"-thoracotomy approaches or thorascopic methods.

Radiation therapy has not been well studied as an adjuvant therapy in dogs and cats, although chemodectoma is considered a radiation-sensitive neoplasm in humans. The prognosis for both dogs and cats is guarded because of the metastatic potential and locally aggressive nature. The median survival time for dogs after surgical resection is 25 months.

References

Charney SC et al: Evaluation of intracavitary mitoxantrone and carboplatin for treatment of carcinomatosis, sarcomatosis, and mesothelioma, with or without malignant effusions: a retrospective analysis of 12 cases (1997-2002), *Vet Comp Oncol* 3(4):71, 2005.

Ehrhart N et al: Analysis of factors affecting survival in dogs with aortic body tumors, *Vet Surg* 31:44, 2002.

Hahn KA, McEntee MF: Prognosis factors for survival in cats after removal of a primary lung tumor: 21 cases (1979-1994), *Vet Surg* 27:307, 1998.

Hirshberger J et al: Sensitivity and specificity of cytologic evaluation in the diagnosis of neoplasia in body fluids from dogs and cats, *Vet Clin Pathol* 28:142, 1999.

McNiel EA et al: Evaluation of prognostic factors for dogs with primary lung tumors: 67 cases (1985-1992), *J Am Vet Med Assoc* 211:1422, 1997.

Mehlhaff CJ et al: Surgical treatment of pulmonary neoplasia in 15 dogs, *J Am Anim Hosp Assoc* 20: 799, 1984.

Moore AS, Kirk C, Cadona A: Intracavitary cisplatin chemotherapy experience with six dogs, *J Vet Intern Med* 5:227, 1991.

Paoloni MC et al: Comparison of results of computed tomography and radiography with histopathologic findings in tracheobronchial lymph nodes in dogs with primary lung tumors: 14 cases (1999-2002), *J Am Vet Med Assoc* 228: 1718, 2006.

Poirier VJ et al: Toxicity, dosage, and efficacy of vinorelbine (Navelbine) in dogs with spontaneous neoplasia, *J Vet Intern Med*, 18:536, 2004.

Smith AN et al: Radiation therapy in the treatment of canine and feline thymomas: a retrospective case study (1985-1999), *J Am Anim Hosp Assoc* 37: 489, 2001.

Sparkes A et al: Palliative intracavitary carboplatin therapy in a cat with suspected pleural mesothelioma, *J Feline Med Surg* 7:313, 2005.

CHAPTER 78

Osteosarcoma

NICOLE P. EHRHART, *Fort Collins, Colorado*
TIMOTHY M. FAN, *Urbana, Illinois*

Appendicular osteosarcoma (OSA) is the most common primary bone tumor diagnosed in dogs, accounting for ≈75% to 80% of focal, malignant bone lesions. Arising from malignantly transformed osteoblasts, OSA frequently develops within the metaphyseal regions of long bones. Similar to most neoplastic processes, OSA tends to affect middle-aged to older dogs (7 to 10 years); however, some reports demonstrate an additional incidence peak at 2 years of age. Unlike some tumor histologies that clearly demonstrate strong sex predilections, the incidence of OSA only subtly favors development in males, with a reported male-to-female ratio of 1.5:1. Specific breeds with large skeletal mass, including Saint Bernards, rottweilers, Great Danes, greyhounds, and Labrador retrievers, appear to be at increased risk for OSA development.

DIAGNOSIS

History and Physical Examination

The most common sites of OSA development include the distal radius, proximal humerus, and proximal tibia. Given these anatomic sites, dogs with appendicular OSA commonly present for acute-to-chronic lameness and limb swelling. Clinical signs of lameness are often temporally associated with perceived traumatic events such as running, jumping, or rough play with other dogs. In addition to varying degrees of lameness, dogs may also present with significant peritumoral soft-tissue swelling. Following the onset of lameness, some canine patients partially improve with symptomatic therapy, including rest, nonsteroidal antiinflammatory drugs, or other analgesics; however, recurrent and progressive bone pain refractory to conservative therapy is the most common clinical disease course. Subsequent to long-standing chronic pain, dogs with OSA may demonstrate significant discomfort of the affected limb even following minimal or light manipulation; these are clinical signs suggesting the establishment of hyperalgesia and allodynia.

Imaging Modalities

In dogs with OSA radiography remains an important and valuable diagnostic tool for determining the extent of disease. Given the biologic behavior of appendicular OSA, every canine patient should have radiographs of not only the primary tumor site but also the thoracic cavity. At presentation, radiographs of the primary lesion typically reveal bony proliferation and lysis in the metaphyseal region of long bones, whereas thoracic radiographs demonstrate gross metastatic disease in fewer than 10% of dogs. Despite the low incidence of overt metastatic disease at diagnosis, it is well established that the vast majority (>90%) of canine patients affected by OSA eventually develop radiographically evident pulmonary metastatic disease. In addition to determining the extent of disease at diagnosis, thoracic radiographs can also provide valuable prognostic information since dogs with visible pulmonary metastases typically have considerably worse long-term outcomes than dogs radiographically free of pulmonary metastases at presentation.

Additional advanced imaging modalities may be appropriate for patients being considered for less conventional, yet extremely effective treatment options such as limb-spare surgeries. In such patients it is critical to ensure that additional skeletal metastases or metachronous primary lesions are not present before limb-spare procedures. For such global skeletal assessments the acquisition of whole-body radiographs is feasible; however, this methodology can be cumbersome and inefficient. Thus nuclear scintigraphy is the imaging modality of choice for assessing global skeletal health. Nuclear scintigraphy is more sensitive than plain radiographs for imaging skeletal metastases because it readily identifies alterations in bone remodeling dynamics, which develop before structural changes can be detected radiographically. Although scintigraphy to screen OSA patients for occult skeletal disease may be very sensitive, this methodology lacks specificity, and any scintigraphic "hot spot" should be verified by high-detail radiographs and subsequent biopsy.

DIFFERENTIAL DIAGNOSES

Differential diagnoses for OSA include other primary bone tumors, bacterial or fungal osteomyelitis, metastatic bone tumors, and systemic diseases that affect bone such as multiple myeloma or lymphoma. Benign processes such as bone cysts and degenerative or active remodeling can also be considered. It is important to obtain a complete history (including a travel history to areas of endemic mycotic infection) so that the clinician can take into account all factors when making a diagnosis. Radiographic appearance is helpful, especially when there is a classic appearance in a classic location. However, the classic radiographic appearance of OSA (metaphyseal location, mixed lytic and blastic pattern, loss of trabecular pattern, cortical lysis, Codman's triangle, sunburst periosteal pattern, and soft-tissue swelling) is not present in every case. In addition, other primary bone tumors may have a similar radiographic appearance. Multiple affected bones are uncommon in OSA; however, synchronous primary OSA occasionally can occur. Metastatic disease affecting bone is usually in a diaphyseal location rather than in the metaphysis but can be either lytic or proliferative. Multiple punched-out lesions in several bones suggest multiple myeloma.

The most accurate means to differentiate OSA from other bone diseases is through a bone biopsy. However, because bone biopsy is an invasive procedure and the results are not always immediately available, fine-needle aspiration cytology can be helpful initially to help rule out other differential diagnoses. Most bone tumors have a soft-tissue component that yields cells on needle aspirate. A cytologic specimen devoid of inflammation and yielding a population of malignant mesenchymal cells supports the diagnosis of a primary bone malignancy. OSA cannot be differentiated from chondrosarcoma, synovial cell sarcoma, and fibrosarcoma on a cytologic specimen with standard staining methods. Staining for alkaline phosphatase activity has been reported to be helpful to further characterize malignant mesenchymal cells as OSA from bone tumor aspirates. Presumably only mesenchymal cells of osteoblastic origin (OSA cells) should stain positive for alkaline phosphatase. In one study alkaline phosphatase staining of 61 bone lesion aspirates provided an accurate diagnosis of OSA with 100% sensitivity and 89% specificity (Barger et al., 2005)

The gold standard for diagnosis remains the biopsy. There are several methods for obtaining bone tissue for biopsy. The two most common techniques are either closed biopsy using a Jamshidi bone marrow biopsy needle (American Pharmaceal Company) or open biopsy using a trephine or curette. Both methods require general anesthesia, and regional radiographs should be available to aid the clinician in selecting an appropriate area within the tumor to collect the biopsy. Attempts should be made to obtain a sample from the center of the radiographic lesion. Advantages of needle biopsy are that the procedure can be done through a single tiny stab incision without a surgical approach. The resulting bone defect is small, typically involving a single cortex, and therefore is unlikely to initiate a pathologic fracture. The disadvantage of the closed technique is the relatively small sample size obtained. An open biopsy using a trephine requires a surgical approach and creates a bigger defect through both cortices; however, the sample obtained is larger. A larger sample may provide more representative tissue, thereby allowing a more accurate diagnosis. The down side of this is that there is a higher potential risk for pathologic fracture. Regardless of the method used to obtain the biopsy, it is important to send the tissue to an experienced pathologist with expertise in bone pathology.

It must be emphasized to clients that no diagnostic test is 100% accurate. A diagnosis of reactive bone is not uncommon on preoperative biopsy of an OSA, whether obtained by needle core or trephine. In cases in which the histopathologic interpretation does not match the clinical picture, OSA should not be ruled out. A histologic report of reactive bone from a lesion with classic OSA appearance on radiographs may simply be a function of the fact that the relatively small sample was not representative of the true underlying pathology. In some cases repeat larger biopsies still yield reactive bone; yet, when the entire lesion is submitted following definitive surgery, the pathologist can readily make a diagnosis of OSA. Similarly, one should be cautious when interpreting bone biopsy results indicating the presence of primary bone fibrosarcoma, chondrosarcoma, or hemangiosarcoma. Although these other primary tumors do occur on occasion, OSA is far more common. In fact, OSA has various histologic subtypes, including fibroblastic, chondroblastic, and telangiectatic (hemangiosarcoma-like), that can be interpreted incorrectly on small biopsy samples where there is little-to-no osteoid present.

BIOLOGIC BEHAVIOR

Appendicular OSA is a locally invasive, highly metastatic neoplasm. Although arising from the medullary canal, OSA is rapidly invasive, with most patients demonstrating significant cortical bone destruction early in the course of disease. Osteosarcoma typically possesses the cellular machinery required for successful metastasis. The pulmonary parenchyma is the most common metastatic site, whereas involvement of regional lymph nodes appears relatively uncommon. Pulmonary metastatic lesions usually appear as discrete soft-tissue nodules, and multiple lesions are common. Additional sites of metastases include bone, skin, and other extraskeletal sites. Supporting the observed clinical behavior of canine OSA, several studies have identified key proteins associated with tissue invasion, metastasis, and angiogenesis in spontaneously arising OSA samples.

CLIENT EDUCATION AND TREATMENT OPTIONS

There are many treatment options available for OSA. Treatment choices fall into two major categories based on the pet owner's goals: palliative-intent treatments or curative-intent treatments. Palliative-intent treatments have as their main goal the relief of symptoms associated with OSA. With palliative treatment it is accepted that the disease will continue to progress during treatment. Curative-intent treatments have as their main goal prolonged symptom-free survival or cure. Although a true cure occurs in less than 10% of canine patients with OSA, survival can be greatly increased with the use of curative-intent therapy. Owners need to have an accurate understanding of a given treatment goal, possible side effects, benefits, costs, and lifestyle changes expected with each category (palliative- or curative-intent) of treatment and each treatment within a category.

It is important to emphasize that there are no "right" or "wrong" treatments; rather there are simply choices that must be made based on current published information, known tumor biology, and the individual patient's circumstances and co-morbidities. Because OSA is an aggressive disease and can be considered to be systemic at the time of diagnosis, curative-intent therapy must be multimodal (including both local and systemic therapy) to improve survival. At minimum, curative-intent therapy involves surgical removal of the tumor by amputation or limb salvage surgery and adjuvant chemotherapy. If no treatment is given, most owners seek euthanasia within 2 months after diagnosis.

Surgical Options

Amputation

Amputation remains the gold standard of surgical therapy for OSA. Amputation is by far the simplest, least expensive surgical solution with the fewest complications. In addition, for most common OSA locations, amputation affords generous bone and soft-tissue margins, making the risk of local recurrence very low, and requires no special surgical training to perform. Forequarter amputation (removal of the scapula en bloc with the limb) for forelimb tumors and disarticulation at the level of the coxofemoral joint for hind limb tumors is recommended. Removal of the scapula for forelimb amputations results in a cosmetic outcome superior to disarticulation at the scapulohumeral joint. In patients with hind limb OSA, disarticulation at the coxofemoral joint provides a larger margin of normal tissue between the tumor and the amputation site. OSA may invade locally along fascial planes, making amputation using a midfemoral or proximal femoral osteotomy risky, especially for tumors located in the distal femur or proximal tibia. For OSA located in the proximal femur, partial hemipelvectomy (acetabulectomy) is required to prevent local recurrence.

Function, cosmesis, and patient acceptance following amputation have been excellent even in very large- and giant-breed dogs. Although deciding to move forward with an amputation in a large- or giant-breed dog with OSA is often difficult for owners, most are satisfied with the functional outcome. It is important to point out that in many cases amputation provides an improved quality of life that would not have been possible otherwise. Keeping amputation patients comfortable during the immediate postoperative phase is very important for a rapid recovery. To this end, preemptive analgesia is recommended before surgery, and amputation patients should remain hospitalized on injectable pain medications for at least 15 to 24 hours following surgery to ensure comfort. If effective analgesia is administered, most dogs are ready for discharge the day after surgery. Oral analgesics can be administered by the owner at home for the next 5 to 7 days following discharge. Owners should be instructed to keep early postoperative amputees away from slippery surfaces unless they can provide support using a sling. Most dogs are able to go up stairs immediately following discharge yet have some apprehension and difficulty going down stairs. Weight control and controlled physical activity are important for long-term mobility. Many large-breed OSA patients have concurrent preexisting degenerative joint disease in other limbs that will require lifelong management for the best functional outcome.

Limb Salvage Surgery

Several alternatives to amputation are available to salvage the OSA-affected limb. Limb salvage is a more costly and complicated option than amputation, and there is no survival advantage associated with limb salvage per se. The only advantage of limb salvage is that the patient retains the affected limb. Some dogs with severe concurrent arthritis or neurologic conditions are not able to ambulate on three limbs and therefore require limb salvage if curative-intent treatment is pursued. However, more commonly owners choose limb salvage because an amputation seems like a less desirable option. Disadvantages of limb salvage are that it is a more complex surgery to perform, often requires specialized training and equipment, involves dissection very near the tumor (and therefore is associated with a higher risk of local recurrence), and has a high complication rate. Limb salvage surgery involves removal of the portion of bone affected by the tumor along with a margin of normal bone. Candidates for limb salvage surgery should have no known metastatic disease, no serious intercurrent health issues other than the OSA, no pathologic fractures, and a tumor involving less than 50% of the length of the affected bone with a small soft-tissue component. The most suitable cases for limb salvage are those with tumors in the distal radius. Except for rare circumstances, limb salvage requires arthrodesis of an adjacent joint. Dogs with carpal arthrodeses have excellent function, but arthrodesis of high-motion joints such as the knee and shoulder results in poorer limb function. As a result, limb salvage for tumors near the stifle or shoulder typically is not recommended.

Methods of limb salvage include allograft reconstruction, metal endoprosthesis reconstruction, and bone transport osteogenesis (BTO). BTO is a method of creating new bone in a defect by distraction using an external fixator. Choice of procedure depends on surgeon experience, case selection, and owner preference. All limb salvage procedures require an experienced surgical team and intensive aftercare. The most common complications associated with allograft and metal endoprosthesis reconstruction are infection and hardware failure (screw failure or backout). Interestingly there seems to be a survival advantage in canine OSA patients that develop infection. Several retrospective studies have confirmed this observation. Limb salvage patients with OSA that develop infection survive 1.5 to 2 times longer than limb salvage patients that do not develop infection. Infection may be associated with an immunomodulatory effect that results in longer survival, although this has not been proven. Most infections in limb salvage patients can be managed with lifelong antibiotic therapy; however, periodic flare-ups occur, and occasionally amputation is necessary. Infection has not been reported as a complication with BTO limb salvage; however, these patients must have a circular external fixator on the limb for an extended period (several months), and the owner must be comfortable with adjusting the frame multiple times daily to create distraction osteogenesis for several weeks after surgery. Not every owner or dog is a good candidate for BTO limb salvage, and the number of surgeons experienced with the technique and postoperative management is limited. Overall limb use is good in 80% of all limb salvage patients. Local recurrence rates are 10% to 20% and do not differ between techniques. Local recurrence does not automatically require amputation since revision surgeries can be performed. Local recurrence does not negatively impact overall survival or metastatic rates. Therefore limb salvage is a viable surgical alternative to amputation for curative-intent treatment of canine OSA.

Other Ablative Surgery

Osteosarcoma located in the pelvis, maxilla, mandible, or scapula is often amenable to ablative surgery. Scapulectomy, hemipelvectomy, maxillectomy, or mandibulectomy can be used to successfully treat OSA and obtain clean margins in many cases. Advanced imaging such as magnetic resonance imaging and computed tomography is often necessary to discern appropriate candidacy for these types of procedures. Owners should seek the services of a surgical oncologist or board-certified surgeon who has specific experience with advanced oncologic surgeries such as these. Function and cosmesis can be excellent following scapulectomy, hemipelvectomy, maxillectomy, or mandibulectomy.

Systemic Chemotherapy

The adjuvant use of systemic chemotherapy for extending the survival time of dogs diagnosed with appendicular OSA subsequent to limb amputation or limb-spare procedures has been firmly established and demonstrated by multiple studies. Although a definitive consensus exists for the added survival benefit that chemotherapy provides, there remains some controversy as to which anticancer agents, used alone or in combination, are most effective. A simple answer for this fundamental question does not exist because response to systemic chemotherapy is not solely dictated by the anticancer agent used but equally influenced by the tumor population being treated. Given the heterogeneity of most canine OSAs, very large prospective studies would be necessary to determine the superiority of one chemotherapeutic regimen over another. Until such massive prospective studies are conducted, information regarding effective adjuvant treatment options will have to be based on more limited sample populations. In general effective adjuvant chemotherapy protocols are based around doxorubicin, platinum-based chemotherapy drugs, or combinations of the two. Results from select studies are included in Table 78-1.

NEW DEVELOPMENTS

Survival times for dogs and humans with OSA undergoing standard surgery and chemotherapy have reached a plateau over the last 10 to 20 years. The biologic behavior, metastatic pattern, and response to chemotherapy of canine OSA are remarkably similar to their human counterpart. Recognition of this fact has led to collaborative relationships between human and veterinary cancer researchers who study OSA. As new agents and therapies become available, clinical trials involving these novel treatments are taking place in many veterinary cancer centers, often at much reduced costs to owners. Several of these treatments show promise for the future for both dogs and humans. Immunotherapy, therapeutic radiopharmaceutical agents, and γ-knife radiation therapy are some of the active areas of research in veterinary cancer centers. Many of these trials have led to pivotal clinical trials in human medicine and are shaping the way both humans and dogs with OSA will be treated in the future. Veterinarians should contact the major veterinary cancer centers in their area for up-to-date trial availability for their clients who are seeking new therapies for their pets with OSA (see Chapter 63).

PALLIATIVE THERAPIES

Reported survival times for canine patients treated with palliative-intent therapy range from 3 to 10 months. As stated earlier, it remains paramount that pet owners fully understand that the intent of palliative treatment is to improve quality of life, not cure the disease process. As such palliative treatment options center around controlling cancer-induced bone pain, a debilitating consequence of malignant osteolysis.

Palliative radiation therapy is effective for the management of malignant bone pain and typically involves administering coarse fractions of 8 to 10 Gy of megavoltage irradiation in 2 to 4 consecutive weekly treatments. Palliative radiation therapy reportedly improves limb function and quality of life in the majority of patients treated (74% to 92%), providing clinical pain relief for several months in responding patients (Ramirez et al., 1999; Green, Adams, and Forrest, 2002). The concurrent administration of systemic chemotherapy along with palliative radiation therapy appears to enhance analgesic response rates and durations and should be recommended.

Table 78-1

Select Postoperative Chemotherapy Regimens for the Treatment of Canine Appendicular Osteosarcoma

Surgery and Chemotherapy Protocol	Investigators	Median Survival Time
DOX (30 mg/m² day 1) + cDDP (60 mg/m² day 21) × 2 doses	Mauldin et al., 1988	300 days
cDDP 70 mg/m² q21d × 2 doses	Straw et al., 1991	262-282 days
cDDP 60 mg/m² q21d × 1-6 doses	Berg et al., 1992	325 days
DOX 30 mg/m² q2wks × 5 doses	Berg et al., 1995	366 days
Carbo 300 mg/m² q21d × up to 4 doses	Bergman et al., 1996	321 days
cDDP (50 mg/m² day 1) + DOX (15 mg/m² day 2) × 4 doses	Chun et al., 2005	300 days
Carbo (175 mg/m² day 1) + DOX (15 mg/m² day 2) × 4 doses	Bailey et al., 2003	235 days
Alternating carbo (300 mg/m²) + DOX (30 mg/m²) every 21 days × 3 doses	Kent et al., 2004	227 days

cDD, Cisplatin; *DOX,* doxorubicin; *carbo,* carboplatin.

The systemic administration of a bone-seeking radionuclide called [153]Samarium-EDTMP has been described for appendicular OSA in dogs and provides pain relief in many treated patients. By delivering concentrated radiation doses to the site of active bone remodeling, [153]Samarium-EDTMP administration is capable of providing significant and meaningful palliation of bone pain in dogs suffering from appendicular OSA (Lattimer et al., 1990). The main toxicity is myelosuppression, which may continue for up to 4 weeks after therapy.

Stereotactic radiosurgery involves the precise delivery of a single large dose of radiation to a designated tumor target and has been used for the treatment of brain tumors, as well as canine appendicular OSA. The use of stereotactic radiosurgery in dogs with OSA can provide pain alleviation, long-term local tumor control, and improvement in limb function (Farese et al., 2004). Similar to palliative radiation therapy, combining systemic chemotherapy with stereotactic radiosurgery appears to enhance response rates and durations.

The pharmaceutical use of bisphosphonates is accepted for the treatment of neoplastic bone disorders in human cancer patients. At low concentrations bisphosphonates inhibit bone resorption without inhibiting the process of bone mineralization. This results in stabilization and even enhancement of bone mineral density. Bisphosphonates directly inhibit bone resorption by binding to hydroxyapatite crystals and inducing osteoclast apoptosis. In part, pain associated with bone cancers is a direct consequence of malignant bone resorption. Therefore inhibiting pathologic bone resorption with bisphosphonates theoretically would decrease the likelihood of pathologic fracture, as well as alleviate intense bone pain. Intravenous pamidronate for the management of osteolytic pain in dogs with appendicular OSA has recently been described (Fan et al., 2005). Treatment with pamidronate at a dosage of 1 mg/kg or 2 mg/kg administered as an intravenous infusion every 28 days resulted in a clinical response rate of 40%, with responding patients demonstrating increased bone mineral density.

TREATING METASTATIC DISEASE

Approximately 90% of dogs with OSA ultimately succumb to metastatic disease despite treatment. Pulmonary metastasis is the most common form of treatment failure, although metastasis to bone is being observed more and more frequently. Dogs with metastatic disease have a wide range of reported survival times. In a recent study dogs with metastatic disease to any anatomic site had a median survival of 76 days with a range of 0 to 1583 days (Boston et al., 2006). In another recent study dogs with metastasis to the regional lymph nodes had a median survival time of 59 days with a range of 19 to 365 days (Hillers et al., 2005). Given the negative impact on survival time

for dogs diagnosed with regional nodal involvement, lymph node status should be evaluated routinely in dogs with OSA.

In some cases surgical removal of pulmonary metastases can improve survival. This requires either thoracotomy or thoracoscopy. Case selection is critical. As a rule, candidates for pulmonary metastasectomy should: (1) have no evidence of tumor elsewhere; (2) be at least 300 days from initial diagnosis (indicating that their particular tumor is no more aggressive than the average OSA); (3) have fewer than three detectable pulmonary nodules; and (4) have slowly progressive disease (a greater than 30-day doubling time of nodules). In one study dogs that underwent metastasectomy that met these criteria had a median disease-free interval of 128 days (O'Brien et al., 1993). Computed tomography is more sensitive than standard three-view radiographs for detection of small metastatic lesions and is recommended before surgery to ensure candidacy for pulmonary metastasectomy. Measurable metastatic disease is often resistant to standard chemotherapy. Some institutions have anecdotally reported responses using a combination of low-dose cyclophosphamide, nonsteroidal antiinflammatory agents, and doxycycline given daily (metronomic therapy). This combination is theorized to inhibit angiogenesis, thereby slowing the growth of metastatic lesions. Its efficacy in a large number of patients with metastatic OSA has not yet been studied.

References

Barger A et al: Use of alkaline phosphatase staining to differentiate canine osteosarcoma from other vimentin-positive tumors, *Vet Pathol* 42:161, 2005.

Boston SE et al: Evaluation of survival time in dogs with stage III osteosarcoma that undergo treatment: 90 cases (1985-2004), *J Am Vet Med Assoc* 228:1905, 2006.

Fan TM et al: Evaluation of intravenous pamidronate administration in 33 cancer-bearing dogs with primary or secondary bone involvement, *J Vet Intern Med* 19:74, 2005.

Farese JP et al: Stereotactic radiosurgery for treatment of osteosarcomas involving the distal portions of the limbs in dogs, *J Am Vet Med Assoc* 225:1567, 2004.

Green EM, Adams WM, Forrest LJ: Four fraction palliative radiotherapy for osteosarcoma in 24 dogs, *J Am Anim Hosp Assoc* 38:445, 2002.

Hillers KR et al: Incidence and prognostic importance of lymph node metastases in dogs with appendicular osteosarcoma: 228 cases (1986-2003), *J Am Vet Med Assoc* 226:1364, 2005.

Lattimer JC et al: Clinical and clinicopathologic response of canine bone tumor patients to treatment with samarium-153-EDTMP, *J Nucl Med* 31:1316, 1990.

O'Brien MG et al: Resection of pulmonary metastases in canine osteosarcoma: 36 cases (1983-1992), *Vet Surg* 22:105, 1993.

Ramirez O III et al: Palliative radiotherapy of appendicular osteosarcoma in 95 dogs, *Vet Radiol Ultrasound* 40:517, 1999.

CHAPTER 79

Mammary Cancer

CAROLYN J. HENRY, *Columbia, Missouri*

Mammary tumors are among the most commonly encountered neoplasms in dogs and cats, consistently reported as one of the top three tumors in both species. Compared to their human counterparts, dogs are three times more likely to develop mammary tumors. Despite steady improvement in the survival rates for women with breast cancer over the past 30 years, there have been relatively few advances in the treatment of canine and feline mammary tumors. Perhaps the greatest progress has been in the area of public education regarding measures to prevent tumor development in both species. It has long been established that spaying dogs before the age of 2½ years is protective against the development of mammary cancer, and recent work suggests that ovariectomy at a young age (<1 year) has a similar protective effect in cats. Beyond educating clients regarding the potential benefits of ovariectomy, practitioners should alert clients to the relative frequency of mammary cancer development and the need for early detection and appropriate case management. This chapter summarizes what is known regarding the natural behavior and prognosis associated with canine and feline mammary tumors and provides guidelines for case management in both species.

CANINE MAMMARY TUMORS

Incidence, Etiology, and Pathogenesis

The incidence of mammary tumor development in dogs is difficult to determine since many small or benign-appearing tumors may go untreated and thus unreported. However, a recent insurance population study of female dogs in Sweden reported 111 mammary tumor claims per 10,000 dog-years at risk. Prior reports indicated that the annual incidence of canine mammary tumors (CMTs) in the United States approximates 200 per 100,000 dogs at risk. Breeds reported to be at increased risk include English springer, Brittany, and cocker spaniels, toy and miniature poodles, English setters, pointers, German shepherds, Maltese, Yorkshire terriers, and dachshunds. Mammary tumors most commonly affect middle-aged (9 to 11 years) female dogs, with an increased incidence beginning at approximately 6 years of age. The influence of hormones on CMT development is supported by the early work showing that the risk of developing mammary tumors rises to 26% for dogs spayed after their second estrus, compared to 0.5% and 8% for dogs spayed before their first or second estrus, respectively (Schneider, Dorn, and Taylor, 1969). It is thought that sex steroid hormones have their primary effect on target cells during the early stages of mammary carcinogenesis, thus accounting for the lack of protective effect with spaying beyond two estrous cycles. The use of products containing medroxyprogesterone acetate (progestin and estrogen combination) for the prevention of estrus or to treat pseudopregnancy has also been linked to an increased incidence of CMTs. Although primarily a disease of female dogs, approximately 1% of CMTs affect males and can be associated with hormonal abnormalities such as estrogen secretion by a Sertoli cell tumor. Other factors reportedly associated with an increased risk of CMT development include obesity at a young age and feeding homemade diets as opposed to commercial foods. Compared to controls, dogs with CMTs in one study had lower serum retinol concentrations. However, additional research is needed to elucidate the impact of retinol concentration and other dietary components on CMT development.

Clinical Presentation

Mammary tumors are often detected during routine wellness examinations in older female dogs or are discovered by conscientious owners. In over half of all cases of CMT, dogs present with more than one mammary mass; these may either be simultaneous primary masses or may reflect one primary lesion with regional extension or metastasis. Although some studies have suggested that the caudal mammary glands are the most commonly affected in the dog, other reports have not confirmed this. Either the axillary or inguinal lymph nodes may be palpably enlarged in dogs with nodal metastases, given the complex pattern of lymphatic drainage for canine mammary tissue. Of the five pairs of mammary glands in the dog (two cranial/thoracic, two abdominal, and one caudal/inguinal), the thoracic glands generally drain to the axillary or sternal nodes, the inguinal glands are drained by the inguinal nodes, and the two abdominal glands may drain to either site. The presence of lymph node enlargement, lymphedema, skin ulceration, and fixation to underlying tissue is a characteristic that suggests malignancy.

Inflammatory mammary carcinoma (IMC) is a unique clinical entity that warrants an altered approach to diagnosis and case management. This tumor type may be mistaken for mastitis since dogs classically present with warm, erythematous mammary tissue and associated lymphedema; ulceration and vesicles; and significant pain on any manipulation of the tissue. Alternatively the diagnosis of IMC may become apparent when wound dehiscence occurs secondary to what was anticipated to be a routine mammary mass excision (referred to as secondary IMC).

Diagnostics and Staging

The diagnosis of CMTs relies on histologic examination of incisional or excisional biopsy samples. It is vital to bear in mind that benign and malignant nodules may coexist in canine mammary tissue. Thus it is necessary to confirm the histologic diagnosis independently for each nodule rather than assume that one nodule is representative of all tumors present. Estimates vary in the literature, but a simple rule of thumb for CMTs is that approximately 50% are malignant and approximately 50% of the malignant tumors metastasize. Tumor types reported in the dog and their relative frequency are detailed in Table 79-1. Of these, sarcomas and IMCs are associated with the worst prognosis. Mixed malignant tumors and squamous cell carcinomas are also associated with poor survival times. Of the carcinomas, solid carcinomas are reported to have worse survival times than either tubular or papillary carcinomas. Carcinomas that warrant a better prognosis include carcinoma in situ and adenocarcinomas.

The original clinical staging for CMTs was based on a four-stage system developed by the World Health Organization (WHO) and reported in 1980 (Owen, 1980). Since that time a modified staging system has been reported and is described in Table 79-2, with the primary difference being the addition of a stage V for dogs with distant metastatic disease and the designation of a stage IV (rather than stage II or III) for those with nodal metastasis. Either staging system necessitates evaluation of regional lymph nodes and assessment of potential distant sites of metastasis, especially distant lymph nodes and lungs. Preoperative cytology of any palpable lymph nodes may aid in determining disease extent before surgery. Regardless of preoperative assessment, lymph node tissue removed at the time of surgery should be submitted for histologic examination. Although standard hematoxylin and eosin (H&E) staining of slides from nodal tissue permits accurate identification of micrometastasis in most cases, cytokeratin immunostaining using an antipancytokeratin antibody AE1/AE3 was reported to detect occult micrometastasis in 12 of 131 (9.2%) lymph nodes from dogs judged

to have node-negative disease based on H&E results. The impact of micrometastatic disease on prognosis for CMTs is unknown at this time. Three-view thoracic radiographs are essential before surgery because pulmonary metastases warrant a poor prognosis and may dictate therapy decisions.

In addition to clinical staging, a histologic staging system is outlined in Table 79-3. In this system stages 0, I, and II are based on histologic assessment, whereas stage III is based on clinical assessment of distant metastasis. This system is not to be confused with the clinical staging systems proposed in Table 79-2. Although the histologic staging system is not universally applied in veterinary medicine, it is highlighted in this chapter based on its correlation with clinical outcome in a report of 232 dogs undergoing mastectomy for CMTs (Gilbertson et al., 1983).

Table 79-1

Frequency of Various Histologic Types of Mammary Tumors in Dogs

Tumor Type	Relative Frequency
Benign (51%)	
Fibroadenomas (benign mixed tumor)	45.5
Simple adenomas	5.0
Benign mesenchymal tumors	0.5
Malignant (49%)	
Solid carcinomas	16.9
Tubular adenocarcinomas	15.4
Papillary adenocarcinomas	8.6
Anaplastic carcinomas	4.0
Sarcomas	3.1
Carcinosarcoma (malignant mixed tumors)	1.0

Figures were obtained from an unselected series of 1625 canine mammary tumors submitted by general practitioners to the Department of Clinical Veterinary medicine, Cambridge, England, for diagnosis. Reproduced with permission from Bostock R: Neoplasia of the skin and mammary glands in dogs and cats. In Bonagura JD, editor: *Kirk's current veterinary therapy VI: small animal practice,* Philadelphia, Saunders, 1977, p. 493.

Table 79-2

Comparison of the Original and Modified Staging Systems for the Classification of Canine Mammary Tumors

Stage	Original WHO Staging	Modified WHO Staging
I	T1 (<3 cm) $N_0 M_0$	T1 (<3 cm) $N_0 M_0$
II	$\leq$T2 (<5 cm) $N_1 M_0$ (histologically positive node, but not fixed to underlying tissues)	T2 (3-5 cm) $N_0 M_0$
III	Any T3 or any with fixed nodal involvement	T3 (>5 cm) $N_0 M_0$
IV	Distant metastasis (any T, any N, M_1)	Regional node metastasis (any T, $N_1 M_0$)
V	No stage V	Distant metastasis (any T, any N, M_1)

TNM system: *T*, size of primary tumor; *N*, regional lymph node involvement; *M*, distant metastasis. For example, N_0 is without lymph node involvement, and N_1 is confirmed lymph node involvement. *WHO*, World Health Organization.

| Table 79-3 |

Histologic Staging System for Canine Mammary Tumors

Stage	Features	Frequency of de Novo or Recurrent CMT 2 Years After Surgery
0	Tumor cells are limited to ductal tissue	25%
I	Tumor cells invade stromal tissue	72%
II	Vascular/lymphatic invasion and/or regional lymph node metastasis	95%
III	Systemic metastasis	Not reported; dogs with Stage III disease by definition have no disease-free interval

Gilbertson SR et al: Canine mammary epithelial neoplasms: biologic implications of morphologic characteristics assessed in 232 dogs, *Vet Pathol* 20:127, 1983.

Treatment

Surgery

Surgery is the mainstay of therapy for most CMTs, with the exception of IMC (see following paragraphs). In their pivotal study published in 1985, MacEwen and associates demonstrated that type of surgery is not a major prognostic factor for CMTs, provided resection is complete as assessed by histologic examination. Thus they established the surgical standard of care for CMTs that remains in place to this day to include minimal but adequate tumor excision, usually via lumpectomy or partial mastectomy. This has been supported by more recent studies, as well (Chang et al., 2005). The issue of whether or not to perform ovariohysterectomy (OHE) at the time of mammary tumor excision has long been debated in the veterinary literature. Given the high rate of estrogen-positive tumors in dogs, it is reasonable to consider hormone ablation via OHE as an adjunctive therapy for treatment of CMT. However, early reports suggested that no benefit was derived from spaying dogs at the time of tumor excision. Data from two more recent studies suggest that there is a survival advantage for dogs that undergo OHE. In the first report, dogs undergoing OHE within 2 years before or at the time of CMT removal survived 45% longer than intact dogs or dogs spayed more than 2 years before CMT excision (Sorenmo, Shofer, and Goldschmidt, 2000). In a subsequent study dogs undergoing OHE were more likely to survive at least 2 years after surgery than dogs that remained intact. This was especially true for dogs with complex carcinomas (Chang et al., 2005). Although one may not know the underlying diagnosis (malignant versus benign) at the time of surgery, these two latter studies certainly support a recommendation for OHE as an adjunct to complete tumor excision when feasible if malignant CMT is suspected.

Chemotherapy

Chemotherapy has not been clearly documented to provide a survival advantage for dogs with CMT. However, based on responses in women with breast cancer, various chemotherapy agents, including paclitaxel, fluorouracil (5-FU), cyclophosphamide, doxorubicin, mitoxantrone, and carboplatin have been used for treatment of high-grade or metastatic mammary carcinoma in dogs. In one prospective study comparing outcome for eight dogs with

CMT treated with 5-FU (150 mg/m^2 intravenously [IV]) and cyclophosphamide (100 mg/m^2 IV) once weekly for 4 weeks to that of eight dogs treated with surgery alone, a significant improvement in survival was demonstrated for the dogs receiving chemotherapy. Dogs in the chemotherapy group had a median survival time of 24 months compared to 6 months for dogs in the surgery only group. A more recent prospective study of postoperative doxorubicin or docetaxel (n=12) versus surgery alone (n=19) for dogs with invasive mammary cancer failed to demonstrate a significant impact of chemotherapy on recurrence-free interval, time to metastasis, or overall survival. Additional randomized prospective studies are necessary to determine the role of chemotherapy in the clinical management of dogs with mammary cancer.

Radiation Therapy

Although it is an important component of breast cancer treatment in women, radiation therapy remains largely unexplored for the treatment of CMTs. Anecdotal reports of palliation for nonresectable lesions or for IMC serve as the only current evidence to support radiation therapy for CMTs. Given the efficacy of radiation therapy in women with breast cancer, further evaluation of this treatment modality for CMTs is warranted.

Hormonal Therapy

Because of the relative difficulty of performing routine estrogen and progesterone receptor assays on CMTs, the use of hormonal therapy in dogs with mammary tumors has lagged behind that in human oncology. In addition to the efforts at hormone ablation via ovariectomy described previously, tamoxifen is a drug that has been evaluated as hormonal therapy for CMTs. Tamoxifen has both estrogenic and antiestrogenic effects and has been advocated for many years for the treatment of estrogen receptor–positive human breast cancer patients. A pilot study evaluated outcome for 16 dogs with mammary carcinoma treated with 2.5 to 10 mg (mean dose 0.42 mg/kg q12h PO) of tamoxifen. Five of seven dogs with either metastatic or nonresectable mammary carcinoma experienced a decrease in tumor burden. In another report of 10 dogs with advanced mammary cancer treated with 0.7 mg/kg of tamoxifen every 24 hours, no measurable responses were noted. Adverse effects, including vaginal discharge, vulvar swelling, urinary incontinence, urinary tract infection, mental dullness, signs of estrus, and partial alopecia have been seen in dogs undergoing tamoxifen therapy. One quarter of the treated dogs in the former study developed pyometra (one closed-cervix pyometra and three stump pyometras). An identical rate of pyometra (20%) induction was also seen in a 1988 report of 20 bitches treated with 1 mg/kg of tamoxifen every 12 hours orally for 10 days for prevention or termination of pregnancy. Thus clients must be counseled regarding this potential side effect if tamoxifen therapy is to be considered.

Various nonspecific immunomodulatory approaches have been investigated for the treatment of CMTs, including *Corynebacterium parvum*, bacillus Calmette-Guérin (BCG), levamisole, and liposome-encapsulated muramyl tripeptide phosphatidylethanolamine. However, none have been clearly demonstrated to be of clinical benefit for dogs with CMT.

Therapy for Inflammatory Mammary Carcinoma

Although no therapy option has been shown to be of significant benefit for dogs with IMC, there is general agreement among veterinary oncologists that surgery is contraindicated. Wound dehiscence, ventral and limb edema, and disseminated intravascular coagulation are all potential complications of IMC, which is unlikely to be amenable to complete surgical excision. There are anecdotal reports of disease palliation with radiation therapy, nonsteroidal antiinflammatory drugs, and doxorubicin-based chemotherapy protocols, but the prognosis remains poor despite all treatment attempts reported to date.

Prognosis

Prognostic factors for CMTs have been examined in multiple prospective and retrospective studies. Factors determined to correlate with prognosis in multivariate analysis are the most compelling since the interdependent effects of multiple factors are considered in such analyses. Although conflicting reports exist regarding the impact of many factors on prognosis, those generally accepted to have a negative impact on prognosis are listed in Table 79-4.

FELINE MAMMARY CANCER

Incidence, Etiology, and Pathogenesis

Mammary cancer is the third most common feline tumor after skin tumors and lymphoma. As in dogs, mammary

Table 79-4

Comparative Aspect of Canine and Feline Mammary Tumors

	Dog	Cat
Estimated annual incidence in the United States	199/100,000	25/100,000
Percent of tumors that are benign	50-70	10-20
Most common malignancy	Complex carcinoma	Tubulopapillary carcinoma
Hormone receptor expression in invasive carcinomas	Majority (62.5%) are ER-α+ and PR–	Majority (57%) are ER-α– and PR+
Genetic mutations — BRCA1 and BRCA2	Unknown	Unknown
Genetic mutations — HER-2/neu	Protein overexpressed in 17.6%	Protein overexpressed in 59.6%
Genetic mutations — p53	15%-75%	19%-33%
Metastatic behavior	32%-77%, depending on histologic type	>50% Metastatic
Poor prognostic factors	Diagnosis of ductal carcinoma, Inflammatory mammary carcinoma or sarcoma Ulceration of skin Invasive growth; fixed to adjacent tissue Increased age at diagnosis Estrogen receptor negative German shepherd breed Heat shock protein expression Advanced stage Large tumor size >3 cm High histologic grade Nodal or pulmonary metastasis Nonovariectomized	High AgNOR count Tumor size >3 cm Ki-67 index >25.2 Lymphatic invasion Increased WHO stage
Overall prognosis	Reported mean survival time (MST): 439 days MST: 70 weeks after surgery for malignant vs. 114 weeks for benign tumors	1-year survival noted for ≈1/3 to ½ of cats treated with surgery alone; up to 59% with adjuvant chemotherapy 2-year survival is ≈15%-20% with surgery alone; improves to ≈37% with addition of chemotherapy

tumors may affect both male and female cats. Both estrogen and progesterone are thought to play important roles in feline mammary cancer (FMC) development, although the underlying mechanisms are less clear than for CMTs. Intact females and cats exposed regularly to progestins have been shown to be at an increased risk for mammary cancer development. The literature also suggests that, as in dogs, early ovariectomy may lower the risk of developing FMC. One published report demonstrated that cats ovariectomized at 6 months of age had an approximately sevenfold reduction in risk of FMC compared to intact cats (Dorn et al., 1968). A more recent study compared a population of 308 cats with biopsy-proven FMC to a control population of 400 female cats that were not diagnosed with mammary tumors (Overley et al., 2005). There was a statistically significant reduction in risk of FMC development reported for cats spayed before 1 year of age compared to intact cats. Specifically a 91% reduction in risk was reported for those spayed before 6 months of age, and an 86% reduction was demonstrated in those spayed before 1 year of age. Parity was not significantly related to risk of developing FMC. Thus there is some justification for recommending ovariohysterectomy before 1 year of age in cats.

Clinical Presentation

As is the case in dogs, the presentation associated with FMC generally relates to a palpable nodule detected by the owner or veterinarian. However, in contrast to dogs the majority (80% to 96%) of mammary tumors in cats are malignant. Ulceration of lesions is not uncommon and is suggestive of malignancy. As in the dog, multiple lesions are often present at the time of diagnosis, although cats are less likely to have a combination of benign and malignant lesions.

Diagnostics and Staging

Complete evaluation of a cat with suspected mammary carcinoma should include an assessment of general health with a urinalysis, complete blood count, and serum biochemical evaluation in anticipation of anesthesia and surgery. Thoracic radiographs (right lateral, left lateral, and ventrodorsal views) and regional lymph node palpation/aspiration are critical, given that the reported metastatic rate for FMC ranges from 25% to as high as 100%, with the most common sites being the lymph nodes and lungs. In a review of the literature between 1952 and 1996, Waters and associates (1998) found 338 cases of extraskeletal metastases in 799 cats with malignant mammary tumors. Interestingly, cats have a very low rate of skeletal metastasis from mammary carcinoma compared to people and dogs.

Histopathologic examination is necessary to confirm a diagnosis of FMC. Often biopsy specimens are obtained at the time of definitive surgery rather than as a presurgical evaluation. The majority of mammary tumors in cats are diagnosed as adenocarcinomas, specifically of tubular, papillary, solid, or cribriform type. Less common malignant lesions include squamous cell carcinomas, sarcomas, and mucinous carcinomas. IMC was first described in cats in 2004, with three cats having lesions typical in gross appearance to that of human and canine IMC and with a similar poor prognosis. Features in the feline IMC that differed from those typical of human or canine IMC included positive immunohistochemical staining for ER-α, occurrence only after prior mastectomy, and severe inflammation of the dermis and subcutaneous tissue.

As described for dogs, fine-needle aspiration and cytology of mammary lesions is seldom of clinical use but may be considered if cutaneous or subcutaneous lesions of nonmammary tissue origin such as mast cell tumors are suspected. Cytologic evaluation of pleural effusion fluid or of aspirates from enlarged lymph nodes is warranted when these conditions are present. As with dogs, the staging system for FMC has been modified from the original system proposed by Owen in 1980. The modified system limits nodal metastasis to stage III or IV, whereas the original system placed those with histologically confirmed nodal metastasis but without fixation of nodes to surrounding tissue into stage II. A comparison of the staging systems is outlined in Table 79-5.

Table 79-5

Comparison of the Original and Modified Staging Systems for the Classification of Feline Mammary Carcinoma

Stage	Original WHO Staging	Modified WHO Tumor Staging
I	T1 (<1 cm) $N_0 M_0$	T_1 (<2 cm) $N_0 M_0$
II	≦T2 (<3 cm) $N_{1+} M_0$ (histologically positive node, but not fixed to underlying tissues)	T_2 (2 to 3 cm) $N_0 M_0$
III	Any T3 or any with fixed nodal involvement	Regional node metastasis or T3 (>3 cm) lesion or both, but no distant metastasis
IV	Distant metastasis (any T, any N, M_1)	Distant metastasis (any T, any N, M_1)

TNM system: *T*, size of primary tumor; *N*, regional lymph node involvement; *M*, distant metastasis. For example, N_0 is without lymph node involvement, and N_1 is confirmed lymph node involvement. *WHO*, World Health Organization.

Treatment

Surgery

Surgery is the primary treatment for FMC, often with adjuvant chemotherapy. Unlike the recommendations for CMT, unilateral or bilateral mastectomy is generally considered the preferred surgical method in cats. There are conflicting reports regarding whether radical mastectomy provides a survival advantage, although the procedure has been shown to significantly decrease the recurrence rate of FMC. When bilateral radical mastectomy is performed, it may be done as one surgical procedure or as a staged procedure, with the second unilateral mastectomy 2 to 6 weeks after the first. The inguinal lymph node is removed with the caudal mammary glands; however, axillary node excision is not a routine part of the radical mastectomy. Removal of the axillary node is only recommended if it is known to have metastatic disease since prophylactic axillary node excision is unlikely to benefit the patient.

Chemotherapy

Few studies have assessed the role of chemotherapy for the primary or adjuvant treatment of FMC. Doxorubicin-based protocols have been evaluated most frequently, with approximately one third to one half of cats with stage III or IV disease (see Table 79-5 for staging criteria) having measurable responses to the combination of doxorubicin and cyclophosphamide. In a recent retrospective study of 67 cats with mammary adenocarcinoma receiving adjuvant doxorubicin chemotherapy (1 mg/kg q21d IV for an intended five treatments) beginning at the time of suture removal, the median survival time was 448 days, and the 1- and 2-year survival rates were 58.9% and 37.2%, respectively (Novosad et al., 2006). I and others have recently completed a randomized, prospective clinical trial comparing mitoxantrone (5 mg/m^2 q21d IV for four total doses) to doxorubicin (four doses at 20 mg/m^2 q21d IV) for adjuvant therapy of FMC after radical mastectomy. Data analysis indicates no significant difference in survival times between the two groups, with median survival times of 747 days for the mitoxantrone group and 484 days for the doxorubicin group. The literature supports use of adjuvant chemotherapy for advanced-stage FMC, although its role for treatment of Stage I tumors is less clear.

Prognosis

Size of a mammary tumor and therefore T stage according to the WHO staging system is the single most reliable prognostic indicator in cats. In one report the median survival time for cats with tumors larger than 3 cm was 12 months compared to 21 months for cats with lesions less than 3 cm. Other prognostic factors and a summary of the literature regarding survival times are shown in Table 79-4.

References and Suggested Reading

Bostock DE: Neoplasia of the skin and mammary glands in dogs and cats. In Bonagura JD, editor: *Kirk's current veterinary therapy VI: small animal practice,* Philadelphia, Saunders, 1977, p 493.

Chang, et al: Prognostic factors associated with survival two years after surgery in dogs with malignant mammary tumors: 79 cases (1998-2002), *J Am Vet Med Assoc* 227:1625, 2005.

Dorn et al: Survey of animal neoplasms in Alameda and Contra Costa Counties, California. II. Cancer morbitity in dogs and cats from Alameda County, *J Natl Cancer Inst* 40:307, 1968.

Gilbertson SR et al: Canine mammary epithelial neoplasms: biologic implications of morphologic characteristics assessed in 232 dogs, *Vet Pathol* 20:127, 1983.

MacEwen EG et al: Evaluation of the effect of levamisole and surgery on canine mammary cancer, *J Biol Resp Mod* 25:540, 1985.

Novosad CA et al : Retrospective evaluation of adjunctive doxorubicin for the treatment of feline mammary gland adenocarcinoma: 67 cases, *J Am Anim Hosp Assoc* 42:110, 2006.

Owen LN: *TNM* Classification of tumors in domestic animals, Ed VPH/CMO.80.2, Geneva, 1980, World Health Organization.

Overley B, Shofer FS, Goldschmidt MH: Association between ovariohysterectomy and feline mammary carcinoma, *J Vet Intern Med* 19:560, 2005.

Schneider R, Dorn CR, Taylor DON: Factors influencing canine mammary cancer development and postsurgical survival, *J Natl Cancer Inst* 43:1249, 1969.

Sorenmo KU, Shofer FS, Goldschmidt MH: Effect of spaying and timing of spaying on survival of dogs with mammary carcinoma, *J Vet Intern Med* 14:266, 2000.

Waters DJ et al: Skeletal metastasis in feline mammary carcinoma: case report and literature review, *J Am Anim Hosp Assoc* 34:103, 1998.

CHAPTER 80

Urinary Bladder Cancer

DEBORAH W. KNAPP, *West Lafayette, Indiana*

CANINE URINARY BLADDER TUMORS

Urinary bladder cancer comprises approximately 2% of all reported malignancies in the dog. With the pet dog population in the United States exceeding 65 million, this translates into several thousand cases of urinary bladder cancer annually. The hospital prevalence or proportionate morbidity of bladder cancer at university-based veterinary hospitals is also increasing (Knapp et al., 2000a; Mutsaers, Widmer, and Knapp, 2003).

Transitional cell carcinoma (TCC) is the most common form of canine urinary bladder cancer (Knapp et al., 2000a; Mutsaers et al., 2003; Valli et al., 1995). The majority of dogs that develop TCC have papillary infiltrative cancer of intermediate- to high-grade TCC, with only a small percentage of dogs having low-grade, superficial TCC (Norris et al., 1992; Valli et al., 1995). TCC is most often located in the trigone region of the bladder. Papillary lesions and bladder wall thickening can lead to partial or complete urinary tract obstruction. In a series of 102 dogs with TCC, the tumor involved the urethra (as well as the bladder) in 57 of 102 dogs (56%) and the prostate in 11 of 38 (29%) male dogs (Knapp et al., 2000a). In addition to causing urinary tract problems, TCC has the propensity to metastasize to other organs. The most common sites of TCC metastases are regional lymph nodes and lung. Less common sites of metastases include liver, kidney, spleen, prescapular lymph node, heart, uterus, cecum, bone, ilium, colon, abdominal wall, diaphragm, eye, and oral mucosa.

The clinician should not assume that all bladder masses are TCC. Mass effects in the bladder can occur with benign conditions, such as polyps and inflammatory lesions, or with other tumors. The latter can include squamous cell carcinoma, adenocarcinoma, undifferentiated carcinoma, lymphoma, rhabdomyosarcoma, hemangiosarcoma, fibroma, and other mesenchymal tumors (Norris et al., 1992; Valli et al., 1995).

Etiology and Possible Prevention Strategies

The etiology of canine bladder cancer is not completely known but is most likely multifactorial. Risk factors identified include exposure to older-generation flea control products (dips, powders, sprays), herbicides, and insecticides; obesity; possibly cyclophosphamide administration; female gender (female:male ratio 1.7:1); and breed (Glickman et al., 2004; Knapp et al., 2000a; Mutsaers et al., 2003; Raghavan et al., 2004). Breeds at increased risk of TCC are listed in Table 80-1.

It is appropriate to educate dog owners of high-risk breeds regarding the predisposition for TCC in their pets, especially with advancing age. Pet owners should be aware of notable clinical signs of disease (hematuria, stranguria, inappropriate urination). Some form of disease screening can be considered in older at-risk dogs (such as urinalysis with sediment examination, urine antigen test, abdominal ultrasound, more frequent physical examination), although the most effective and appropriate methods of TCC screening approaches have not been determined.

The development of TCC is thought to represent a combination of genetic factors and environmental exposures. An association between herbicide exposure and TCC in dogs was identified in a case control study in 166 Scottish terrier dogs (Glickman et al., 2004). Exposure to herbicides was compared between TCC cases (n = 83) and control dogs (n = 83; Scottish terriers at least 6 years of age with no evidence of TCC and no history of urinary tract disease in the 2 years before entry into the study). TCC risk was significantly increased in dogs exposed to lawns or gardens treated with herbicides alone or gardens treated with herbicides and insecticides, although not with insecticides alone. It is likely that important gene-environment interactions were involved in the TCC development. Results of this study indicate the importance of limiting dogs' exposure to herbicides, especially in breeds of dogs at increased risk for TCC.

An earlier case-control study revealed an association between TCC and exposure to topical application of flea and tick dips (summarized in Knapp et al., 2000). In the highest-risk group (overweight female dogs), the risk for TCC was 28 times that of normal-weight male dogs not exposed to the insecticides. The authors speculated that the "inert" ingredients (solvents and petroleum distillates), which accounted for more than 95% of the product, were the probable carcinogens. Newer, spot-on types of flea control products appear safer. In a recent case control study in Scottish terriers, spot-on products containing fipronil were not associated with increased risk for TCC (Raghavan et al., 2004).

Recently ingestion of vegetables has been reported to be associated with a lower risk of TCC (Raghavan et al., 2005). In a case control study, Scottish terriers that consumed vegetables at least three times per week along with their normal diet had reduced risk for TCC.

Presentation, Diagnosis, and Clinical Staging

Typically canine TCC is a disease of older dogs. The reported mean age at diagnosis is 11 years. The mean body weight in a series of 102 dogs with TCC was 15.67

Table 80-1

Breed and Risk of Urinary Bladder Cancer in Pet Dogs (Summary Data From Veterinary Medical Data Base)*

Breed	Odds Ratio	95% Confidence Interval
Mixed breed	1.0[†]	
All pure breeds	0.74	0.62- 0.88
Scottish terrier	19.89	7.74-55.72
West Highland white terrier	5.31	2.51-11.63
Shetland sheepdog	4.46	2.48-8.03
Beagle	4.15	2.14-8.05
Wirehaired terrier	3.20	1.19-8.63
Miniature poodle	0.86	0.55-1.35
Miniature schnauzer	0.92	0.54-1.57
Doberman pinscher	0.51	0.30-0.87
Labrador retriever	0.46	0.30-0.69
Golden retriever	0.46	0.30-0.69
German shepherd	0.40	0.26-0.63

* Initially reported in 2000 (Knapp et al., 2000a) with updated information (Knapp and Glickman, unpublished data) added in 2006.
[†]Reference category.

± 10.25 kg (range 3 to 51 kg), and the female-to-male ratio was 1.7:1 (Knapp et al., 2000a). Common clinical signs in dogs with TCC include hematuria, dysuria, pollakiuria (often of chronic or recurrent nature), and less commonly lameness caused by bone metastasis or hypertrophic osteopathy. It is important to note that the lower urinary tract signs observed with TCC are not distinguishable from those that occur with urinary tract infection or calculi. Factors that raise suspicion for TCC include persistent or recurrent lower urinary tract signs or infection (especially after appropriate dose and duration of antibiotic therapy based on culture and sensitivity), older age, and high-risk breed.

The physical examination of a dog with possible TCC should include a thorough rectal examination. The extent of findings may depend somewhat on the size of the dog, but findings could include thickening of the urethra, prostatic enlargement, a trigonal mass, and/or enlarged lymph nodes. Abdominal palpation may reveal a distended bladder. Bladder masses often are not detected on abdominal palpation, and normal physical examination does not rule out TCC.

When TCC is suspected, the clinician should pursue tests to (1) make a definitive diagnosis, (2) determine the stage of the cancer if present, and (3) assess the overall health of the patient. This evaluation could include complete blood count, serum biochemistry profile, urinalysis, urine culture, thoracic radiography, abdominal ultrasonography, and bladder imaging (contrast cystography or cystosonography). Urine should be obtained by free catch or catheter sample and not by cystocentesis, which may seed the TCC along the needle track.

A diagnosis of TCC requires histopathologic confirmation. Although neoplastic cells may be present in the urine of 30% of dogs with TCC, cancer cells are often indistinguishable from reactive epithelial cells associated with inflammation. Urine antigen tests for TCC have been found to be sensitive for TCC, but high numbers of false-positive results limit the value of these tests. It is essential to perform histopathologic examination of the abnormal tissues to determine if TCC is present. Methods for obtaining tissue for histopathologic diagnosis include cystotomy, cystoscopy, and traumatic catheterization. If surgery is performed, *great care must be taken to avoid TCC seeding.* Similarly percutaneous biopsy methods (e.g., transabdominal ultrasound-guided needle core biopsies or fine-needle aspirates) should be avoided because these can lead to tumor seeding.

Thoracic radiography and abdominal ultrasonography are recommended to evaluate for metastases. Lymph node and distant metastases were present in 16% and 14% of 102 dogs, respectively, at the time of diagnosis of TCC in one study (Knapp et al., 2000a). Distant metastases were detected in 50% of dogs at the time of death. Tumor stage can be assigned following the World Health Organization clinical staging system for canine bladder tumors (Box 80-1). In addition to detecting enlarged lymph nodes or other organ metastases, abdominal ultrasound is useful for detecting ureteral obstruction and hydronephrosis. This could be an indication for the placement of ureteral stent(s), especially if other therapies do not relieve the urinary obstruction (see Chapter 209).

Bladder imaging is recommended to determine the location of the tumor within the urinary tract and to obtain baseline measurements to monitor response to subsequent therapy. Cystography has been the traditional method of bladder imaging. It is best performed with the patient anesthetized, with air (4 to 9 ml/kg, depending on bladder capacity) and positive contrast (0.1 to 0.2 ml/kg) instilled in the bladder and with images made in right lateral, left lateral, and ventrodorsal recumbency. Caution must be taken when passing a urinary catheter during

Box 80-1

World Health Organization Clinical Stage (TNM) of Canine Urinary Bladder Cancer

T: Primary tumor
Tis: Carcinoma in situ
- T0 No evidence of primary tumor
- T1 Superficial papillary tumor
- T2 Tumor invading the bladder wall, with induration
- T3 Tumor invading neighboring organs (prostate, uterus, vagina, and pelvic canal)
N: Regional lymph node (internal and external iliac lymph node)
- N0 No regional lymph node involved
- N1 Regional lymph node involved
- N2 Regional lymph node and juxta regional lymph node involved
M: Distant metastases
- M0 No evidence of metastasis
- M1 Distant metastasis present

TNM, Tumor, node, metastasis.

diagnostic procedures to avoid penetration of the diseased bladder or urethral wall.

Ultrasonography has also been used to image the bladder. As with cystography, the degree of bladder distention is important when performing ultrasonography. When the bladder is empty or minimally distended, it may be difficult to visualize some lesions, and it is not possible to determine if evident lesions are invading or remote to the trigone (where surgical resection may be possible). When using ultrasonography to monitor tumor size during therapy, consistent bladder distention (on repeated visits) is important. Some bladder masses appear smaller in a well-distended bladder than in a less-distended bladder. When multiple lesions are present, lesions can become superimposed within the less-distended bladder, making comparison of tumor burden between studies difficult. For the most accurate comparison of bladder mass size between visits, a urinary catheter should be passed, and the bladder distended with the same volume of sterile saline for each examination. The amount of saline needed to distend the bladder varies from case to case, depending on bladder capacity (which could be lessened by tumor or previous surgery) but is typically 4 to 9 ml/kg. Measuring the bladder masses in at least two consistent planes (e.g., dorsal, transverse) and having the same examiner each time fosters a more accurate assessment of mass volume change over time.

Urinary cystoscopy, using either rigid or flexible cystoscopes, provides a means of visualizing the mucosal surface of the urinary bladder and urethra. The tumor location and involvement of the ureteral stomas may be determined by this imaging. Often, urethral involvement of bladder tumors that is not readily appreciated using ultrasound or contrast studies can be identified with cystoscopy. Most small endoscopes used for cystoscopy have ports that allow the operator to biopsy tumor tissue.

TCC can infrequently metastasize to bone. Radiographs or bone scan may be considered if lameness is present that is not easily explained by other orthopedic or neurologic disease.

Treatment

Surgery
Surgical excision of TCC should be considered for lesions in the bladder apex in which 3-cm margins of grossly normal bladder can be removed around the tumor mass. Unfortunately most TCCs are trigonal and many involve the urethra, precluding surgical excision. In addition, many dogs appear to develop multifocal TCC in the bladder. This is consistent with the "field effect" proposed in human bladder cancer patients, in which the entire bladder lining is thought to undergo malignant change in response to exposure to carcinogens in urine. In a series of 67 dogs with TCC that underwent surgery for biopsy or for therapeutic intent at Purdue University, complete surgical excision of the tumor with tumor-free margins was only possible in two dogs. One of these two dogs had relapse in the bladder 8 months later, and the second dog developed metastatic disease. Transurethral resection of bladder and urethral tumors has been attempted in a small number of dogs but has been limited by complications of

the procedure and local disease recurrence. Carbon dioxide laser ablation of bladder tumor tissue combined with medical therapy also has been reported, but it is not currently known if this approach offers an advantage over traditional surgery and medical therapy.

Surgery has also been used as an emergency palliative procedure to debulk nonresectable tumors in dogs with urinary tract obstruction. Other procedures to bypass urinary obstruction such as the placement of ureteral and urethral stents (Chapter 209) and prepubic cystostomy tubes (see Section IV on Evolve) have also been used.

Radiation Therapy
Studies of the effects of radiation therapy on TCC are very limited. Whole-bladder intraoperative radiation therapy was evaluated in 11 dogs with TCC and 2 dogs with other bladder tumors several years ago (Walker, 1987). Although 1- and 2-year survival rates were encouraging at 69% and 23%, respectively, complications of therapy (urinary incontinence and cystitis with accompanying pollakiuria and stranguria) detracted from quality of life. Other studies have confirmed the complications associated with pelvic radiation.

Medical Therapy of TCC
Medical management of TCC is indicated in dogs with nonresectable or metastatic tumors. Medical therapy of TCC has consisted of chemotherapy, cyclooxygenase (COX) inhibitors (also referred to as nonsteroidal antiinflammatory drugs), and combinations of these two types of treatment (Henry et al., 2003; Knapp et al., 2000a; Knapp et al., 2000b; Mutsaers et al., 2003). Study results support at least three options for the medical therapy of dogs with TCC: (1) COX inhibitor alone, (2) mitoxantrone combined with a COX inhibitor, or (3) referral for participation in clinical trials of other therapy.

COX inhibitor treatment. The non-selective COX inhibitor that has been used the most in dogs with TCC is piroxicam. Piroxicam as a single agent provides a useful palliative treatment for dogs with TCC (Knapp et al., 2000a; Mutsaers et al., 2003). The quality of life in most dogs receiving piroxicam is excellent. Tumor responses in 62 dogs with TCC receiving piroxicam as a single agent included 2 complete responses (CRs), 9 partial responses (PRs, 50% or greater reduction in tumor volume), 35 stable disease (SD, <50% change in tumor volume), and 16 progressive disease (PD). The two dogs that had CR died of nontumor-related causes more than 2 years after beginning piroxicam therapy and were free of tumor on postmortem examination. The survival time in piroxicam-treated dogs (median 195 days) compares favorably to that of 55 dogs in the Purdue Comparative Oncology Program Tumor Registry treated with debulking surgery alone (median survival 109 days). Piroxicam has been used at a dosage of 0.3 mg/kg orally every 24 hours in dogs. It is necessary to have a compounding pharmacy prepare piroxicam for use in small to medium-sized dogs because the commercially available 10-mg capsules are too large for dogs of this size.

Although the majority of dogs tolerate piroxicam well, care must be taken to detect any *gastrointestinal toxicity* that may occur. If vomiting, melena, or anorexia occurs, it is important to withdraw piroxicam and give supportive care as needed until the toxicity resolves. If piroxicam is to be reinstituted, misoprostol may be given along with the piroxicam to reduce the risk of gastrointestinal irritation.

It is not currently known if selective COX-2 inhibitors have the same antitumor activity as nonselective COX inhibitors. Because COX-2 is overexpressed in the majority of canine TCC and COX-2 is considered a major target of COX inhibitor therapy, selective COX-2 inhibitors may have similar antitumor activity. Selective COX-2 inhibitors have an advantage of causing fewer gastrointestinal side effects than nonselective COX inhibitors.

Chemotherapy combined with COX inhibitor. The results of single-agent chemotherapy for TCC have been disappointing, with remission rates typically less than 20%. However, studies of cisplatin combined with piroxicam have demonstrated an additive to synergistic effect (Knapp et al., 2000b). Although the antitumor activity of cisplatin combined with piroxicam has been impressive (50% to 70% remission rate), renal toxicity has been frequent, and this combination of drugs is not recommended. Other attempts to combine platinum chemotherapy and piroxicam have been less rewarding. Reducing the dose of cisplatin did not prevent renal toxicity of cisplatin/piroxicam. Carboplatin/piroxicam induced remission in 38% of dogs, but the duration of remission and survival times were relatively short. Encouraging results have been published when another chemotherapeutic agent, mitoxantrone, was combined with piroxicam. Mitoxantrone (5 mg/m^2 intravenously q21d) combined with piroxicam induced remission in 35% of dogs with TCC with minimal toxicity, and resulted in a median survival time of 291 days (Henry et al., 2003). Specific information regarding the various chemotherapy agents discussed is provided in Chapters 65 and 66.

Regardless of the treatment regimen pursued, basic concepts apply in tailoring the therapy to the individual dog with TCC. Complete staging of the TCC defining the extent of the disease and size of lesions should be performed before and after approximately 6 weeks of treatment. After the 6 weeks of treatment, if the tumor is smaller or is stable in size and if the treatment is acceptable in regard to any adverse effects, the same treatment should be continued. Restaging should be performed at 6-week intervals, and therapy adjusted as appropriate. If a CR occurs, then treatment should be continued for an additional 6 weeks to address residual microscopic disease. Therapy would also be continued if PR or SD was noted. A particular treatment should be discontinued if PD (≥50% increase in tumor volume or development of new tumor lesions) or unacceptable toxicity is noted. A different therapy could then be considered.

Other therapies for TCC. Although substantial progress has been made in the treatment of canine TCC, much room for improvement exists. Clinical trials of new approaches are important to define better treatment approaches for this deadly disease. By participating in a clinical trial, the pet dog with TCC may gain access to a therapy that will be better than current "standard" medical therapies for TCC, and information gained from that canine patient will be useful in developing better therapy approaches for other dogs and potentially for humans. Websites posted by veterinary schools, the Veterinary Cancer Society, and veterinary oncologists can provide information to help veterinarians and pet owners learn about TCC trials being performed. See Chapter 63 for additional information about clinical trials.

In addition to new drugs under study, different types of therapy approaches are also being studied. Photodynamic therapy (PDT) is under study as a treatment for TCC. Following promising in vitro studies and studies in normal dogs, PDT with 5-aminolevulinic acid was given to five dogs with TCC, resulting in tumor progression–free intervals ranging from 4 to 34 weeks (median 6 weeks). Because of the possibility of posttreatment swelling of diseased tissues (possibly leading to reduced urine flow), dogs with TCC must be selected carefully for PDT.

Supportive care. Dogs with TCC are at high risk for secondary bacterial infections. Urinalysis and urine culture should be performed regularly, and antibiotics prescribed as needed. Antibiotic therapy should be based on results of urine culture and sensitivity testing, and the appropriate antibiotic should be given for 3 weeks or more. Urination should be monitored closely. If urinary tract obstruction occurs, catheterization, definitive anticancer therapy, antibiotics to reduce inflammation associated with secondary bacterial infection, surgical debulking, or placement of stents or a cystotomy tube to relieve obstruction could be considered.

Prognosis

Unfortunately most dogs that develop TCC ultimately die or are euthanized related to the disease. However, it is possible for many dogs with TCC to live several months or longer with a good quality of life, especially with favorable response to therapy. Median survival times in several studies have exceeded 6 months. Even with piroxicam treatment alone, approximately 20% of dogs survive more than 1 year. Survival has been strongly associated with tumor, node, metastasis (TNM) stage at diagnosis. Using data from 102 dogs with TCC at Purdue University, factors associated with more advanced TNM stage at diagnosis included younger age (increased risk of nodal metastasis), prostate involvement (increased risk of distant metastasis), and higher T stage (increased risk for nodal and distant metastasis) (Knapp et al., 2000). More advanced T stage at diagnosis and glandular differentiation in histopathologic examination were associated with poor response to medical therapy. Recently urethral involvement has also been associated with greater probability of the development of metastatic disease.

FELINE URINARY BLADDER TUMORS

Information concerning urinary bladder cancer in cats is very limited. A report of a series of 27 feline bladder tumors included 15 carcinomas, 5 benign mesenchymal tumors, 5 malignant mesenchymal tumors, and 2 cats with lymphoma (Schwarz, Greene, and Patnaik, 1985). There were 20 male and 7 female cats, and most were elderly. The treatment of feline bladder tumors has not been defined. Results of partial cystectomy were reported in nine cats, and four cats (two with leiomyoma, one with hemangiosarcoma, and one with leiomyosarcoma) survived longer than 6 months.

References and Suggested Reading

Glickman LT et al: Herbicide exposure and the risk of transitional cell carcinoma of the urinary bladder in Scottish terrier dogs, *J Am Vet Med Assoc* 224:1290, 2004.

Henry CJ et al: Clinical evaluation of mitoxantrone and piroxicam in a canine model of human invasive urinary bladder carcinoma, *Clin Cancer Res* 9:906, 2003.

Knapp DW et al: Naturally-occurring canine transitional cell carcinoma of the urinary bladder: a relevant model of human invasive bladder cancer, *Urol Oncol* 5:47, 2000a.

Knapp DW et al: Cisplatin versus cisplatin combined with piroxicam in a canine model of human invasive urinary bladder cancer, *Cancer Chemother Pharmacol* 46:221, 2000b.

Mutsaers AJ, Widmer WR, Knapp DW: Canine transitional cell carcinoma, *J Vet Intern Med* 17:136, 2003.

Norris AM et al: Canine bladder and urethral tumors: a retrospective study of 115 cases (1980-1985), *J Vet Intern Med* 6:145, 1992.

Raghavan M et al: Topical spot-on flea and tick products and the risk of transitional cell carcinoma of the urinary bladder in Scottish terrier dogs, *J Am Vet Med Assoc* 225:389, 2004.

Raghavan M et al: Evaluation of the effect of dietary vegetable consumption on reducing risk of transitional cell carcinoma of the urinary bladder in Scottish terriers, *J Am Vet Med Assoc* 227:94, 2005.

Schwarz PD, Greene RW, Patnaik AK: Urinary bladder tumors in the cat: a review of 27 cases, *J Am Anim Hosp Assoc* 21:237, 1985.

Valli VEO et al: Pathology of canine bladder and urethral cancer and correlation with tumour progression and survival, *J Comp Pathol* 113:113, 1995.

Walker M, Breider M: Intraoperative radiotherapy of canine bladder cancer, *Vet Radiol* 28:200, 1987.

CHAPTER 81
Mast Cell Tumor

CHERYL A. LONDON, *Columbus, Ohio*

BIOLOGY AND FUNCTION OF MAST CELLS

Mast cells are derived from the bone marrow and migrate to tissues throughout the body where they undergo differentiation. They are discrete round cells possessing distinct cytoplasmic granules that stain with dyes such as toluidine blue, Giemsa, and methylene blue. These granules may not be visualized with stains such as Diff-Quik, precluding identification on some cytologic specimens. Mature mast cells bind immunoglobulin (Ig)E on their cell surface through expression of the high-affinity IgE receptor. Cross-linking of IgE results in the release and production of various mediators, including histamine; heparin; proteases; lipid mediators; and cytokines such as TNF-α, interleukin (IL)-4, IL-5, and IL-6. These mediators induce increased vascular permeability, vasodilation, smooth muscle spasm, pruritus, and anticoagulation and activate eosinophils and neutrophils. Collectively these effects can lead to local hypersensitivity reactions, or more seriously, systemic hypersensitivity (anaphylactic shock). As such, mast cells have primarily been associated with allergic reactions/disorders. However, it is now evident that they play an important role in the initiation of innate immune responses, particularly with respect to sustaining neutrophil migration and activation in response to bacteria (Galli, Maurer, and Lantz, 1999). Indeed, mast cells are often seen at sites of inflammation, as well as in reactive lymph nodes. Therefore, in addition to playing a role in the induction of pathologic allergic responses, mast cells are critical players in protective immune responses.

Kit is a tyrosine kinase receptor found on mast cells (as well as hematopoietic stem cells and melanocytes, among others), and its ligand, stem cell factor (SCF), is produced by stromal cells. Binding of Kit by SCF induces downstream signal transduction that promotes the differentiation, survival, and function of mast cells (Galli, Zsebo, and Geissler, 1994). Mutations in Kit have been demonstrated to occur in systemic mastocytosis in humans; these mutations lead to Kit signaling in the absence of SCF stimulation, resulting in loss of normal growth control (Longley, Reguera, and Ma, 2001). Several authors have identified the presence of Kit mutations in canine MCTs, and these also induce uncontrolled signaling (Downing et al., 2002, London et al., 1999). Although up to 30% of all canine MCTs may have Kit mutations, these are not germ line in nature (i.e., are not inherited) but occur during the process of tumor development. However, MCTs with Kit mutations exhibit higher rates of local recurrence and metastasis.

CANINE MAST CELL TUMORS

Incidence and Signalment

Mast cell tumors (MCTs) occur frequently in dogs, representing up to 20% of all cutaneous tumors (reviewed in London and Seguin, 2003). Several breeds appear to be at increased risk for the development of MCTs, including dogs of bulldog descent (boxer, Boston terrier, English bulldog), Labrador and golden retrievers, cocker spaniels, schnauzers, and shar-peis. The etiopathogenesis of MCTs in the dog is unknown, as is the reason for the extremely high incidence in this species. Although some studies have suggested the possibility of a viral cause, there is no epidemiologic evidence to indicate horizontal transmission of tumors. The increased incidence of MCTs in certain breeds suggests the possibility of an underlying genetic cause, and studies are ongoing to identify these putative genetic risk factors. Interestingly, although dogs of bulldog ancestry are at higher risk for MCT development, it is generally accepted that MCTs in these dogs are more likely to be behaviorally benign. In addition, it was demonstrated recently that pugs develop multiple MCTs that behave in a benign fashion (McNiel, Prink, and O'Brien, 2006). In contrast, anecdotal evidence suggests that shar-peis develop MCTs that are biologically aggressive.

History and Clinical Signs

The overwhelming majority of MCTs in the dog occur in the dermis and subcutaneous tissue (London and Seguin, 2003). Rarely primary MCTs may present in other sites such as the oral cavity, nasopharynx, larynx, and gastrointestinal tract. Visceral MCTs involving the spleen, liver, and/or bone marrow (often referred to as disseminated mastocytosis) are usually the result of systemic spread of an aggressive primary cutaneous MCT, athough this condition can occur as an independent syndrome. Cutaneous MCTs tend to occur as solitary nodules, although roughly 10% to 15% of dogs present with multiple tumors, with most found on the trunk, perineal region, and limbs. It is important to note that the clinical appearance of MCTs can vary widely from well circumscribed, raised, and firm to ulcerated and fixed to lipoma-like. They may be extremely slow growing, present for 6 months or more, or rapidly progressive. Clinical signs are often caused by the release of histamine, heparin, and other vasoactive amines. Mechanical manipulation of the tumor during physical examination can induce degranulation leading to erythema and wheal formation (Darier's sign), and occasionally an owner reports that the tumor appears to change in size over short periods of time. Gastrointestinal ulceration is also a potential complication of MCTs because of elevated levels of circulating histamine stimulating H_2 receptors on parietal cells causing increased acid secretion, resulting in vomiting, anorexia, melena, and abdominal pain.

Diagnosis and Staging

Cytologic evaluation of fine-needle aspirates is probably the easiest method to diagnose the presence of an MCT. As mentioned previously, mast cell granules may not stain with Diff-Quik, leading to difficulty in making a definitive diagnosis by cytology in some cases. In addition, poorly differentiated malignant mast cells may contain few, if any, granules, in which case special stains may be required. Other round cell tumors that should be included in the differential diagnosis include lymphoma, plasmacytoma, histiocytoma, transmissible venereal tumor, and occasionally melanoma. Although the diagnosis can almost always be made by fine-needle aspiration cytology, excisional biopsy is required for histologic grading of the tumor. It is important to note that, because wide surgical excision is the treatment most likely to cure the majority of MCTs, every effort should be made to obtain a definitive diagnosis via cytology before surgical intervention. Moreover, since any cutaneous tumor may potentially be an MCT and dogs with this disease may have multiple tumors, fine-needle aspiration should be performed on all masses before removal. If cytologic diagnosis proves difficult, a needle or punch biopsy of the tumor can be obtained before surgery.

Any MCT is capable of metastasis, and it is therefore recommended that dogs be staged to determine the extent of their disease and overall health. A minimum database (complete blood count [CBC], biochemical profile, urinalysis) should be part of the workup. Dogs with MCTs (especially those with systemic disease) may have eosinophilia as a result of chemotactic factors and IL-5 produced by the mast cells. Anemia may be present secondary to hypersplenism or gastrointestinal bleeding. Rarely mast cells may be seen on a routine CBC. For many years examination of the buffy coat for circulating mast cells was used to screen dogs with MCTs for the presence of systemic/metastatic disease. However, several studies have demonstrated that dogs with many syndromes, including pneumonia, parvovirus, pancreatitis, skin disease, and gastrointestinal diseases may have mast cells circulating in the periphery (McManus, 1999). Therefore, although easy to perform, the buffy coat is probably not a very useful diagnostic test. In the normal bone marrow mast cells are found infrequently, and as such the presence of mast cells in the marrow is indicative of systemic disease. Since it is usually easier to find evidence of systemic involvement in other organs (liver, spleen), routine bone marrow aspiration is not recommended on most patients.

All regional lymph nodes should be examined carefully for signs of enlargement, and any suspicious nodes should be aspirated for cytologic examination. In addition, since metastatic nodes may palpate within normal size, it is recommended that all accessible regional lymph nodes be examined by aspiration cytology. Mast cells may be present in normal lymph nodes, and they are often found in reactive lymph nodes; thus it may be difficult to determine if mast cells identified on cytologic examination are neoplastic or part of the normal immunologic cellular repertoire. However, malignant mast cells in metastatic lymph nodes are often found in clusters/aggregates rather than singly, aiding in a diagnosis of metastasis. If possible, lymph node aspiration should be performed before surgical removal of the MCT because postoperative inflammation can result in mast cell migration to local nodes and thus confuse the interpretation. If necessary, ultrasound can be used to identify the local lymph node of interest to facilitate needle aspiration.

Thoracic radiographs are always indicated as part of any staging procedure, although pulmonary involvement is uncommon in dogs with MCTs. Abnormalities reported include lymphadenopathy (sternal, hilar), pleural effusion, and anterior mediastinal masses. Evaluation of the abdominal cavity is important in dogs with MCTs because spread to the liver, spleen, and other abdominal structures may be noted. Ultrasound is a more sensitive diagnostic technique for evaluation of abdominal organs than radiography. It is recommended that fine-needle aspiration of the liver and spleen be performed if abnormalities are detected in these organs during ultrasound examination or if the dog possesses negative prognostic indicators (e.g., clinical signs, rapidly growing ulcerated tumor, evidence of lymph node metastasis, high-grade tumor).

Prognosis

Canine MCTs possess a wide range of biologic behaviors, from benign to extremely aggressive, leading to metastasis and eventual death from disease. Several prognostic factors have been identified that help to predict the biologic behavior of an MCT and direct the course of therapy. The histologic grade of an MCT is usually determined after excisional biopsy of the tumor and *cannot* be assessed simply by cytologic evaluation of fine-needle aspirates. The grade of an MCT is determined by the characteristics of the neoplastic cells (e.g., degree of granulation, cytologic and nuclear pleomorphism), number of mitotic figures, and the extent of tumor invasion into the underlying tissues. Histologic grade using the system described by Patnaik, Ehler, and MacEwen (1984) is the *most consistent prognostic factor* and correlates significantly with survival, but it does not predict the behavior of every tumor.

Grade 1 tumors are considered to behave in a benign manner, and complete surgical excision is usually curative. Historically these represented between 30% and 55% of all MCTs reported (London and Seguin 2003; Patnaik, Ehler, and MacEwen, 1984). However, recently there is a trend toward fewer tumors being classified as grade 1, with most being placed in the grade 2 category.

The grade 2 tumors represent between 25% and 45% of all MCTs reported, and their biologic behavior is more difficult to predict (London and Seguin 2003; Patnaik, Ehler, and MacEwen, 1984). On histopathology they exhibit invasion into the underlying subcutaneous tissue. As a result they may be more challenging to remove by surgical excision. Many grade 2 tumors are cured with wide surgical excision; furthermore, radiation therapy (RT) following incomplete excision of solitary grade 2 MCTs can cure more than 80% of affected patients (Frimberger et al.,1997). It is important to note that grade 2 MCTs have the ability to spread to local lymph nodes, as well as distant sites, and a proportion of dogs that undergo definitive therapy (surgery and radiation) may go on to develop metastatic disease. Furthermore, some dogs that present with grade 2 MCTs already have evidence of metastatic disease, making appropriate staging imperative for these dogs. Given the wide variation in biologic behavior among grade 2 tumors, there is now an effort to identify

subcategories of grade 2 tumors that may be more likely to behave in an aggressive manner using additional prognostic indicators described later.

Grade 3 tumors represent between 20% and 40% of all MCTs, and these often behave in a biologically aggressive manner, exhibiting metastasis early on in the course of disease. The mean survival time of dogs with grade 3 MCTs has been reported as 18 weeks when treated with surgery alone. In one study the percentage of dogs with grade 3 MCTs surviving at 1500 days was reported as 6%, and in another study the percentage of dogs surviving at 24 months was 7%, indicating that these tumors are particularly malignant (London and Seguin, 2003; Patnaik, Ehler, and MacEwen, 1984). With the recent addition of postoperative chemotherapy to the treatment regimen of grade 3 MCT patients, evidence suggests that survival times may be improved.

Although a clinical staging scheme has been developed for prognostic purposes, stage (0 to IV) has not necessarily been proven to correlate with prognosis. For example, two studies demonstrated that the presence of mast cells in the regional lymph node was a negative prognostic factor for survival and disease-free interval (LaDue et al., 1998; Thamm, Mauldin, and Vail, 1999). However, an additional study revealed that dogs with grade 2 tumors and lymph node metastasis treated with RT after surgery achieved long-term survival (Chaffin and Thrall 2002). Last, although it would seem intuitive that dogs with multiple cutaneous MCTs do not do well, two separate studies have demonstrated that this does not necessarily affect prognosis (Murphy et al., 2006; Thamm, Mauldin, and Vail, 1999).

MCTs that develop in the oral cavity, nail bed, inguinal, preputial, and perineal regions were originally reported to behave in a more malignant fashion regardless of histologic grade. Two recent reports now demonstrate that, at least for MCTs in the inguinal, preputial, and perineal regions, this is likely to be untrue because dogs with tumors in these locations do not necessarily fare poorly (Cahalane et al., 2004; Sfiligoi et al., 2005). MCTs that originate in the viscera (gastrointestinal tract, liver, spleen), bone marrow, or peripheral blood carry a grave prognosis. As previously mentioned, certain breeds (pugs, Boston terriers) are more likely to develop benign MCTs, whereas others such as shar-peis are more likely to develop malignant disease. Tumors present for long periods of time (months to years) may be more likely to behave in a benign manner. In one study 83% of dogs with tumors present for longer than 28 weeks before surgery survived for at least 30 weeks, compared to only 25% of dogs with tumors present for less than 28 weeks (Bostock, 1973). The same study demonstrated that most dogs surviving for longer than 30 weeks after surgery appeared to be cured.

Several proliferative indices have been evaluated in an attempt to predict the outcome of canine MCTs. Perhaps the most useful is Ki-67, a protein found in the nucleus, the levels of which appear to correlate with cell proliferation. In one study the mean number of Ki-67-positive nuclei was significantly higher for dogs that died of MCTs than for those that survived (Abadie, Amardielh, and Delverdier, 1999). For dogs with grade 2 tumors, the number of Ki-67 was significantly associated with outcome. This was confirmed recently by an additional study that demonstrated that the Ki-67 score can be used to divide grade 2 MCTs into two groups with markedly different expected survival times (Scase et al., 2006). The mitotic index (MI, number of mitoses per 10 high-power fields) is often used as a prognostic indicator in other tumor types. A recent study (Romanski et al., 2007) suggests that this may be extremely useful for predicting the biologic behavior of canine MCTs. When dogs presenting with metastatic disease were excluded from analysis, those with tumors possessing an MI of 5 or less had a median survival time of 80 months compared to 3 months for those possessing an MI more than 5, suggesting that MI is a strong predictor of overall survival for dogs with MCTs.

Treatment

The choice of treatment modalities used for a particular canine MCT depends heavily on the prognostic indicators discussed previously, especially the histologic grade and clinical stage; these are summarized in Box 81-1. Wide surgical excision is indicated for all canine MCTs because, although they may feel like discrete masses, microscopically most extend well beyond the palpable borders. Historically it has been recommended that the margins need to be at least 3 cm in each direction; deep margins are as important as the lateral margins. Recent work indicates that for grade 1 or "low-grade" grade 2 tumors, the margins do not need to be as large (Simpson et al., 2004). However, clinically the diagnosis of MCT is often reached cytologically, and tumor grade is rarely known before the surgery. Because of this, it appears prudent to still recommend a 3-cm lateral margin and one fascial plane for the deep margin when feasible. All of the excised tissue should be submitted; the lateral and deep margins should be labeled accurately so the pathologist is able to specifically identify any areas of incomplete excision (see Chapter 68). However, it is sometimes difficult for the pathologist to determine if a mast cell present at the tissue margin represents a malignant or a normal cell. This is reflected in

the finding that a substantial proportion of incompletely excised MCTs do not recur. For example, in a recent study the estimated proportions of grade 2 tumors that recurred locally following incomplete excision at 1, 2, and 5 years were 17.3%, 22.1%, and 33.3%, respectively. In this study the combination of Ki-67 and proliferating cell nuclear antigen (PCNA) scores was prognostic for local recurrence, and development of local recurrence was prognostic for decreased overall survival (Seguin et al., 2006). Therefore ancillary therapies may not always be indicated in the setting of incomplete excision of grade 2 tumors.

Substantial data suggest that radiation (Chapter 67) is extremely effective at eliminating remaining microscopic disease following incomplete excision of grades 1 and 2 MCTs (greater than 90% 3-year control rate) (Al-Sarraf et al., 1996; Frimberger et al., 1997). Unfortunately dogs with grade 3 tumors do not fare as well; although RT may be effective at preventing local recurrence of tumor, many dogs eventually develop metastasis; this may be less likely to occur if chemotherapy is included in the treatment plan (see following paragraphs). RT has also been used to treat gross MCTs (macroscopic disease) when surgery was not an option. Although varying degrees of success have been reported, RT should not be used as the primary therapeutic modality if surgical intervention is an option. Coarsely fractionated or "palliative" RT has also been used to treat dogs with nonresectable high-grade MCTs. This may result in an improvement in quality of life but is unlikely to significantly increase survival time. Moreover, systemic effects of mast cell degranulation following RT may lead to vomiting, hypotension, and gastrointestinal ulceration.

The use of adjuvant chemotherapy is indicated following excision of grade 3 MCTs, metastatic MCTs, or any other MCT with negative prognostic factors. Although RT is considered the treatment of choice for incompletely excised grades 1 and 2 MCTs, evidence now suggests that postoperative chemotherapy may help to delay or prevent local recurrence (unpublished results) and therefore should be considered for patients who are not candidates for RT or if such therapy is unavailable or declined by the owners. In general chemotherapy for bulky MCTs has for the most part been unrewarding, and long-term responses have not been demonstrated in well-controlled clinical trials. The following drugs are used to treat MCTs.

Corticosteroids
The exact mechanism explaining how corticosteroids kill malignant mast cells is unknown. The reported response rate of canine MCT to prednisone is 20%, with remission times of 10 to 20 weeks. Partial remissions are more common than complete remissions, and at least some of the observed response may be because of a decrease in tumor-associated edema. This decrease is likely caused by stabilization of mast cell granules and a reduction in mast cell mediator production.

Lomustine (CCNU)
An alkylating agent that has been used to treat lymphoma and brain tumors in dogs, lomustine was recently found to have activity against canine MCT. A response rate of approximately 42% was noted when dogs with grades 2 and 3 MCTs that had failed all other therapies were treated

---

Box 81-1

Postsurgical Treatment Recommendations for Canine Mast Cell Tumors

Grade 1: Complete excision; no further therapy
Grade 1: Incomplete excision; wider excision or radiation therapy if surgery not possible; may consider no further therapy

Grade 2: Complete excision; chemotherapy only if negative prognostic factors present
Grade 2: Incomplete excision; wider excision or radiation therapy if surgery not possible; may consider no further therapy if there are no negative prognostic indicators; chemotherapy if negative prognostic factors present

Grade 3: Complete excision; chemotherapy
Grade 3: Incomplete excision; chemotherapy ± wider excision or radiation therapy

with lomustine (Rassnick et al., 1999). As with prednisone, most of these were partial responses, and the median duration of response was only 3 months. Additional studies suggest that lomustine given in the adjuvant setting after surgery (either alone or with prednisone and vinblastine) can significantly prolong survival times of dogs with high-grade tumors or tumors with negative prognostic indicators. It should be noted that lomustine can produce both hematopoietic and hepatic toxicity, including severe neutropenia, irreversible thrombocytopenia, and liver failure. Patients receiving this drug should be monitored *very closely,* and the lomustine should be discontinued if there is evidence of either toxicity. In general lomustine is dosed at 50 to 90 mg/m^2 orally every 3 to 4 weeks, with small dogs receiving doses in the lower end of the range. A CBC and liver panel should be performed before each dose.

Vinblastine

Vinblastine has been reported to have efficacy against canine MCTs. A retrospective analysis of dogs with various forms of MCTs treated with a combination of vinblastine and prednisone revealed a 47% response rate (Thamm, Mauldin, and Vail, 1999). Recent data have confirmed the potential use of vinblastine in the adjuvant setting for high-risk grade 2 MCTs in which 100% of dogs treated with prednisone and vinblastine following surgical removal of the tumor were alive at 3 years (Thamm, Turek, and Vail, 2006). The dosage of vinblastine is 2 to 3 mg/m^2 given every 1 to 3 weeks. The major toxicity of this drug is neutropenia, and occasional gastrointestinal upset is noted. This drug is a vesicant and thus must be given through intravenous injection. In many cases lomustine and vinblastine are administered in an alternating fashion (i.e., every 2 to 3 weeks) in combination with prednisone (Box 81-2).

Miscellaneous drugs

In limited clinical reports both L-asparaginase and chlorambucil have been found to have activity against MCTs. Small-molecule inhibitors of Kit recently have been demonstrated to have clinical activity against canine MCTs in two separate studies. These inhibitors are administered orally and act by blocking Kit phosphorylation and subsequent signal transduction. In one study a response rate of 55% was observed in dogs with MCTs treated with an oral Kit inhibitor (London et al., 2003). As expected, most of these responses occurred in dogs with MCTs possessing Kit mutations. Additional clinical work with Kit inhibitors is ongoing, and evidence suggests that they may be particularly useful for dogs with tumors exhibiting Kit mutations.

Animals with large primary MCTs, evidence of metastatic disease, or systemic signs should be treated with medications to block some or all of the effects of histamine release. To prevent gastrointestinal ulceration, any of the standard H$_2$ antagonists may be used, including cimetidine, ranitidine, or famotidine. Alternatively proton pump inhibitors such as omeprazole may be used; these inhibitors are probably more useful in the setting of gross mast cell disease in which standard H$_2$ antagonists may be less effective. Mast cell degranulation can lead to hypotensive shock and death, consequently patients with gross mast cell disease should be placed on the H$_1$ antagonist diphenhydramine.

References and Suggested Reading

Abadie JJ, Amardeilh MA, Delverdier ME: Immunohistochemical detection of proliferating cell nuclear antigen and Ki-67 in mast cell tumors from dogs, *J Am Vet Med Assoc* 215:1629, 1999.

al-Sarraf R et al: A prospective study of radiation therapy for the treatment of grade 2 mast cell tumors in 32 dogs, *J Vet Intern Med* 10:376, 1996.

Bostock DE: The prognosis following surgical removal of mastocytomas in dogs, *J Small Anim Pract* 14:27, 1973.

Cahalane AK et al: Prognostic factors for survival of dogs with inguinal and perineal mast cell tumors treated surgically with or without adjunctive treatment: 68 cases (1994-2002), *J Am Vet Med Assoc* 225:401, 2004.

Chaffin K, Thrall DE: Results of radiation therapy in 19 dogs with cutaneous mast cell tumor and regional lymph node metastasis, *Vet Radiol Ultrasound* 43:392, 2002.

Downing S et al: Prevalence and importance of internal tandem duplications in exons 11 and 12 of c-*kit* in mast cell tumors of dogs, *Am J Vet Res* 63:1718, 2002.

Frimberger AE et al: Radiotherapy of incompletely resected, moderately differentiated mast cell tumors in the dog: 37 cases (1989-1993), *J Am Anim Hosp Assoc* 33: 320,1997.

Galli SJ, Maurer M, Lantz CS: Mast cells as sentinels of innate immunity, *Curr Opin Immunol* 11:53, 1999.

Galli SJ, Zsebo KM, Geissler EN: The kit ligand, stem cell factor, *Adv Immunol* 55:1, 1994.

LaDue T et al: Radiation therapy for incompletely resected canine mast cell tumors, *Vet Radiol Ultrasound* 39:57, 1998.

London CA, Seguin B: Mast cell tumors in the dog, *Vet Clin North Am Small Anim Pract* 33:473, 2003.

London CA et al: Spontaneous canine mast cell tumors express tandem duplications in the proto-oncogene c-*kit*, *Exp Hematol* 27:689, 1999.

London CA et al: Phase I dose-escalating study of SU11654, a small-molecule receptor tyrosine kinase inhibitor, in dogs with spontaneous malignancies, *Clin Cancer Res* 9:2755, 2003.

Longley BJ, Reguera MJ, Ma Y: Classes of c-KIT activating mutations: proposed mechanisms of action and implications for disease classification and therapy, *Leuk Res* 25:571, 2001.

McManus PM: Frequency and severity of mastocytemia in dogs with and without mast cell tumors: 120 cases (1995-1997), *J Am Vet Med Assoc* 215:355, 1999.

McNiel EA, Prink AL, O'Brien TD: Evaluation of risk and clinical outcomes of mast cell tumors in pug dogs, *Vet Comp Oncol* 4:2, 2006.

Box 81-2

Chemotherapy Protocol for Canine Mast Cell Tumors

Day 1: CBC; vinblastine 2 mg/m^2 IV; begin prednisone 1 mg/kg PO SID for 7 days, then EOD for maintenance (can reduce to 0.5 mg/kg EOD)

Day 14: CBC; chemistry panel; lomustine 50-70 mg/m^2 PO

Day 21: CBC at nadir; if no neutropenia noted, do not need to repeat after then next Lomustine

Day 28: CBC; Vinblastine 2 mg/m^2

Day 42: CBC; chemistry panel, lomustine 50-70 mg/m^2 PO; continue for a total of 6 months.

CBC, Complete blood count; *EOD,* every other day; *IV,* intravenously; *PO,* orally; *SID,* once a day.

Murphy S et al: Effects of stage and number of tumours on prognosis of dogs with cutaneous mast cell tumours, *Vet Rec* 158:287, 2006.

Patnaik AK, Ehler WJ, MacEwen EG: Canine cutaneous mast cell tumors: morphologic grading and survival time in 83 dogs, *Vet Pathol* 21:469, 1984.

Rassnick KM et al: Treatment of canine mast cell tumors with CCNU (lomustine), *J Vet Intern Med* 13:601, 1999.

Romanski EM et al: Mitotic index is predictive for survival in cutaneous mast cell tumors, *Vet Pathol* 44:335, 2007.

Scase TJ et al: Canine mast cell tumors: correlation of apoptosis and proliferation markers with prognosis, *J Vet Intern Med* 20:151, 2006.

Seguin B et al: Recurrence rate, clinical outcome, and cellular proliferation indices as prognostic indicators after incomplete surgical excision of cutaneous grade II mast cell tumors: 28 dogs (1994-2002), *J Vet Intern Med* 20:1933, 2006.

Sfiligoi G et al: Outcome of dogs with mast cell tumors in the inguinal or perineal region versus other cutaneous locations: 124 cases (1990-2001), *J Am Vet Med Assoc* 226:1368, 2005.

Simpson AM et al: Evaluation of surgical margins required for complete excision of cutaneous mast cell tumors in dogs, *J Am Vet Med Assoc* 224:236, 2004.

Thamm DH, Mauldin EA, Vail DM: Prednisone and vinblastine chemotherapy for canine mast cell tumor—41 cases (1992-1997), *J Vet Intern Med* 13:491, 1999.

Thamm DH, Turek MM, Vail DM: Outcome and prognostic factors following adjuvant prednisone/vinblastine chemotherapy for high-risk canine mast cell tumour: 61 cases, *J Vet Med Sci* 68:581, 2006.

CHAPTER 82

Malignant Melanoma*

PHILIP J. BERGMAN, *Armonk, New York*

Melanoma is a common tumor of dogs (≈4% of all canine tumors) and demonstrates extremely diverse biologic behavior related to a variety of identifiable factors. An understanding of these factors helps the clinician delineate the appropriate staging, prognosis, and treatment options for canine melanomas. The primary factors determining the biologic behavior of a melanoma in any given dog include site, size, stage, and histologic parameters. Unfortunately, even with an understanding of these variables, there are occasional melanomas that exhibit unreliable biologic behavior. Accordingly there is a desperate need for additional research into this relatively common, heterogeneous, but frequently malignant tumor. This chapter reviews management options for melanomas in dogs, and assumes that a diagnosis of melanoma has already been established (although this can be difficult at times). The discussion focuses on the aforementioned biologic behavior parameters, staging, and treatment of canine melanoma.

BIOLOGIC BEHAVIOR

The biologic behavior of canine melanoma is extremely variable and best characterized based on anatomic site,

size, stage, and histologic parameters. On divergent ends of the spectrum would be a 0.5-cm haired-skin melanoma with an extremely low grade, likely to be cured with simple surgical extirpation, versus a 5-cm high-grade malignant oral melanoma with a poor-to-grave prognosis. Similar to the development of a rational staging, prognostic, and therapeutic plan for any tumor, two primary questions must be answered: what is the local invasiveness of the tumor and what is the metastatic propensity? The answers to these questions will determine the prognosis, and to be discussed later, the treatment.

SITE

The anatomic site of melanoma is highly, although not completely, predictive of local invasiveness and metastatic propensity. Melanomas involving the haired skin that are not in proximity to mucosal margins often behave in a benign manner. Surgical extirpation through a lumpectomy is often curative, but histopathologic examination is imperative for delineation of margins as well as a description of cytologic features. In haired-skin melanomas exhibiting histopathologic criteria of malignancy, the reader is referred to the grade discussion that follows.

Oral and/or mucosal melanoma routinely has been considered an extremely malignant tumor with significant local invasiveness and high metastatic potential. This biologic behavior is very similar to human oral and/or mucosal melanoma. Melanoma is the most common

---

*The fields of veterinary tumor immunotherapy and veterinary oncology and I personally are greatly indebted to the tireless work and seeds laid by the late Dr. Greg MacEwen; he is greatly missed, and this chapter is dedicated to him.

oral tumor in the dog; additional common neoplastic differentials include squamous cell carcinoma, fibrosarcoma, and epulides/odontogenic tumors.

For canine oral/mucosal melanomas with histologic reporting suggestive of a benign lesion, the reader is referred to the grade discussion that follows. The anatomic sites that split the prognostic spectrum of generally benign-acting haired-skin versus typically malignant and metastatic oral/mucosal melanomas include those melanomas located on the digits or foot pads. Dogs with melanoma of the digits but without lymph node or further metastasis are reported to have median survival times of ≈12 months when treated with digit amputation. Of these 42% to 57% are alive at 1 year and 11% to 13% alive at 2 years. Unfortunately metastasis from digit melanoma at presentation is reported in 30% to 40% of cases, and the aforementioned outcomes even with surgery suggest that distant metastasis is common even when no metastasis is found at initial presentation. The prognosis for dogs with melanoma of the foot pad has not been reported previously. I have found this anatomic site to be similar in metastatic propensity and prognosis to digit melanoma. Interestingly, human acral lentiginous melanoma (plantar surface of the foot, palms of the hand, and digit) has an increased propensity for metastasis compared with cutaneous melanoma of other sites.

SIZE AND STAGE

For dogs with oral melanoma, primary tumor size has been found to be prognostic. The World Health Organization (WHO) staging scheme for dogs with oral melanoma is primarily based on size: stage I, less than 2 cm–diameter tumor; stage II, 2 cm– to less than 4 cm–diameter tumor; stage III, 4 cm or larger tumor and/or lymph node metastasis; and stage IV, distant metastasis. MacEwen and colleagues (1986) reported median survival times (MSTs) for dogs with oral melanoma treated with surgery to be approximately 17 to 18, 5 to 6, and 3 months with stages I, II, and III disease, respectively. More recent reports suggest that stage I oral melanoma treated with standardized therapies, including surgery, radiation, and/or chemotherapy, have an MST of approximately 12 to 14 months, with most dogs dying of distant metastatic disease, not local recurrence.

A number of limitations can be identified with the present WHO staging scheme for canine oral melanoma. First, the size of the tumor is not standardized to the size of the patient. Therefore a 1.8-cm oral melanoma without lymph node metastasis is a stage I melanoma in a rottweiler and in a Chihuahua. Further investigations with standardization to patient size are needed. In addition, the histologic appearance and other histologically based indices of melanomas are not accounted for in the present WHO staging scheme, and unfortunately proposed alternate schemes incorporating histologic criteria have not gained traction in management of canine melanoma. For these and other reasons, investigators have pursued other prognostic factors in canine oral melanoma with the intent of developing alternative staging systems. These investigations have substantiated that size is highly prognostic, but have also identified the following *negative*

prognostic factors: conservative extirpation and incomplete surgical margins; location (caudal mandibular and rostral maxillary do more poorly); tumor mitotic index higher than 3; and bone invasion/lysis. Prospective investigations, including these variables into an expanded WHO staging system, are needed.

The staging system for canine nonoral melanoma is remarkably less well defined to date. Henry and colleagues (2005) used the WHO tumor, node, metastasis (TNM) system for canine digital tumors, which defines T1 as a tumor smaller than 2 cm and superficial, T2 as a tumor 2 to 5 cm with minimum invasion, T3 as a tumor larger that 5 cm or invading subcutis, and T4 as a tumor invading fascia or bone. They reported that metastasis-free interval was inversely associated with T stage across all digit tumors. When specifically examining dogs with digit melanoma, there was one dog with T2, five dogs with T3, and four dogs with T4 tumors. Further studies defining staging schemes for canine nonoral melanoma with clinical variables and outcomes are also encouraged.

GRADE AND HISTOLOGIC PARAMETERS

Histopathologic grading of a tumor by the pathologist delineates degree of malignancy. Grading systems vary across tumor types. The histologic grade is commonly predictive of survival, metastatic rate, and other clinical variables in a wide variety of tumors across species, including canine melanoma. For example, in haired-skin melanomas exhibiting multiple histopathologic criteria of malignancy (high mitotic rate, invasiveness, or poor differentiation), metastatic propensity is increased, and the prognosis is worse. Bostock (1979) reported that 45% of dogs with malignant skin melanomas died within 1 year, whereas 8% of dogs with "benign" skin melanomas died from their disease. Furthermore, 10% of dogs with haired-skin melanoma with a mitotic index of 2 or less died from their tumor 2 years after surgery compared to more than 70% of dogs that died from a tumor with a mitotic index of 3 or more. Dogs with haired-skin melanomas within 1 cm of mucosal margins have been minimally investigated to date; I have seen multiple patients with histologically benign, haired-skin melanoma within 1 cm of a mucosal margin develop subsequent distant metastatic disease.

The most exhaustive review of histologic findings in canine melanocytic neoplasms was published by Spangler and Kass (2006). In this paper 384 dogs with melanoma or melanocytoma had their tumors comprehensively histologically examined and statistically tested for association with malignant behavior (recurrence and/or metastasis) and MSTs via follow-up provided by the veterinarians submitting the samples. Significant *negative* prognostic factors included metastasis (i.e., stage as discussed previously); size/tumor volume; and a variety of histologic criteria such as mitotic index, nuclear atypia, tumor score, presence of deep inflammation, intralesional necrosis, and junctional activity. As expected, these investigators also found three primary anatomic-location mortality groups: (1) oral (19% of samples), (2) feet and mucosal surface of lips (19% of samples), and (3) cutaneous (59%

of samples). Too few ocular melanomas were investigated to make recommendations.

An unexpected finding from this investigation was the presence of 32% of dogs with oral melanoma without malignant behavior according to their criteria (no recurrence, no metastasis, and alive at the end of study or dead from competing causes). I see no reason why oral melanomas may not occasionally behave in a benign fashion; however, 32% is a significantly different enough frequency from all previous reports (which report a very small proportion to benign oral melanomas) to warrant additional study. Similarly, the number of benign-acting oral melanomas was relatively small (n = 22); and a variety of factors, such as lack of necropsy, standardization of follow-up, lack of reporting of number of lost to follow-up cases, and, last, the large number of cases disqualified for inclusion because of poor differentiation, may have led to an increased frequency of benign-behaving cases. Similarly, I have seen in excess of 10 dogs in the last 4 years with a previous histopathologic diagnosis of "benign oral melanoma" presenting with florid distant metastasis. This is consistent with Bostock's report (1979) that three of seven dogs with "benign" oral melanomas eventually died of their disease.

Spangler and Kass (2006) also reported that 38% and 12% of foot/mucosal surface of lips and cutaneous melanocytic tumors, respectively, behaved in a malignant fashion. Four percent and 27% of the dogs that died of a foot/lip and cutaneous melanoma, respectively, had a tumor score that would have predicted benign behavior. On further review of those cases, no attributes were found that would allow for prediction of malignant behavior. This suggests that additional testing is needed beyond routine light microscopy for delineation of malignant versus benign behavior for canine cutaneous melanoma. Laprie and associates (2001) reported the use of Ki-67 expression via immunohistochemistry in 68 canine cutaneous melanomas. This group found that the predictive value of Ki-67 proliferative index (97%) was greater than the predictive value of classical histology (91%) for biologic behavior in canine cutaneous melanoma. This strongly suggests that the use of Ki-67 immunohistochemistry and possibly other proliferative markers (e.g., AgNOR and others) in canine cutaneous melanoma should be commonly performed after the histopathologic diagnosis is made.

STAGING

The staging of dogs with melanoma is relatively straightforward. A minimum database should include a thorough history and physical examination, complete blood count and platelet count, serum biochemical profile, urinalysis, three-view thoracic radiographs, and local lymph node aspiration cytology. Both ipsilateral and contralateral nodes should be sampled in cases of oral melanoma because of variability in draining patterns, whether lymphadenomegaly is present or not. Williams and Packer (2003) reported in dogs with oral melanoma that 70% had metastasis when lymphadenomegaly was present but, more importantly, ≈40% had metastasis when no lymphadenomegaly was present. Additional considerations should be made for abdominal compartment imaging (e.g., abdominal ultra-sound) in all cases of canine melanoma, especially in cases with potentially moderately-to–highly metastatic anatomic sites such as the oral cavity, feet, or mucosal surface of the lips since melanoma may metastasize to the abdominal lymph nodes, liver, adrenal glands, and other sites.

TREATMENT

The treatment for dogs with melanoma without distant metastatic disease on staging starts with local tumor control. This is generally best completed through surgical extirpation because of its speed, increased curative intent, and reduced cost compared to other modalities. The extent of surgery is generally based on the anatomic site of the melanoma, with cutaneous melanomas usually requiring lumpectomy and all other sites requiring more aggressive and wide excision. Although large resections such as partial mandibulectomy or maxillectomy carry an inherent level of morbidity, owner satisfaction rates are routinely 85% to 90% or greater. The importance of complete staging cannot be overstated when contemplating larger resections; the presence of distant metastatic disease would attenuate the use of more radical surgical procedures and convert the patient to medical and/or palliative care options.

Radiation therapy (RT, Chapter 67) plays a role in the treatment of canine melanoma when the tumor is not surgically resectable, the tumor has been removed with incomplete margins, and/or the melanoma has metastasized to local lymph nodes without further distant metastasis. The use of smaller fractions of RT (e.g., 3 to 4 Gy) given daily to every other day can allow for a greater total dosage and fewer chronic RT reactions; however, melanoma appears resistant to these types of fractionation schemes. Coarse fractionation schemes for canine melanoma using 6 to 9 Gy weekly to every other week to a total dosage of 24 to 36 Gy have been reported by a variety of investigators, with complete remission rates of 53% to 69% and partial remission rates of 25% to 30%. Unfortunately recurrence and/or distant metastasis were common in all of these studies. Other modalities reported for local tumor control as case reports and/or case series have included intralesional cisplatin implants, intralesional bleomycin with electronic pulsing, and many others; but widespread use has not been reported to date.

In dogs with melanoma in anatomic sites predicted to have a moderate-to-high metastatic propensity or dogs with cutaneous melanoma with a high tumor score and/or increased proliferation index through increased Ki-67 expression, the use of systemic therapies is warranted. Rassnick and colleagues (2001) reported an overall response rate of 28% using carboplatin for dogs with malignant melanoma. Unfortunately only one dog had a minimally durable complete response, and the rest were nondurable partial responses. Similarly Boria and colleagues (2004) reported an 18% response rate and an MST of 119 days with cisplatin and piroxicam in canine oral melanoma. Other reports using single-agent dacarbazine, melphalan, or doxorubicin suggest poor-to-dismal activity. More recently and importantly, two studies (Proulx et al., 2003; Murphy et al., 2005) suggest that chemotherapy plays an insignificant role in the adjuvant treatment of canine melanoma. It can be argued that the studies performed to date to evaluate the activity of chemotherapy in an adjuvant setting for canine melanoma have been suboptimal for a variety of reasons; however, the extensive human literature in this specific setting suggests that melanoma is an extremely chemotherapy-resistant tumor. It is clear that new approaches to the systemic treatment of this disease are desperately needed.

Immunotherapy represents one potential systemic therapeutic strategy for melanoma. A variety of immunotherapeutic strategies for the treatment of human melanoma have been reported previously, with typically poor outcomes because of a lack of breaking tolerance to the "self" antigens present on the tumor cells. Immunotherapy strategies to date in canine melanoma have used autologous tumor cell vaccines (with or without transfection with immunomodulatory cytokines and/or melanosomal differentiation antigens), allogeneic tumor cell vaccines transfected with interleukin 2 or GM-CSF, liposomal-encapsulated nonspecific immunostimulators (e.g., L-MTP-PE), intralesional Fas ligand deoxyribonucleic acid (DNA), bacterial super-antigen approaches with granulocyte macrophage colony-stimulating factor or interleukin 2 as immune adjuvants, and canine dendritic cell vaccines loaded with melanosomal differentiation antigens. Although these approaches have produced some clinical antitumor responses, the methodologies for the generation of these products are expensive; time consuming; sometimes dependent on patient tumor samples being established into cell lines; and fraught with the difficulties of consistency, reproducibility, and other quality control issues.

The advent of DNA vaccination circumvents some of the previously encountered hurdles in vaccine development. DNA is relatively inexpensive and simple to purify in large quantity. The antigen of interest is cloned into a bacterial expression plasmid with a constitutively active promoter. The plasmid is introduced into the skin or muscle with an intradermal or intramuscular injection. Once in the skin or muscle, professional antigen-presenting cells, particularly dendritic cells, are able to present the transcribed and translated antigen in the proper context of major histocompatibility complex and costimulatory molecules. Although DNA vaccines have induced immune responses to viral proteins, vaccinating against tissue-specific self-proteins on cancer cells is clearly a more difficult problem. One way to induce immunity against a tissue-specific differentiation antigen on cancer cells is to vaccinate with a xenogeneic (different species) antigen or DNA that is homologous to the cancer antigen. It has been shown that vaccination of mice with DNA-encoding cancer differentiation antigens is ineffective when self-DNA is used, but tumor immunity can be induced by orthologous DNA from another species.

At the Animal Medical Center in collaboration with human melanoma investigators at Memorial Sloan-Kettering Cancer Center (MSKCC), we have chosen to target defined melanoma differentiation antigens of the tyrosinase family. Tyrosinase is a melanosomal glycoprotein, essential in melanin synthesis. Immunization with xenogeneic human DNA–encoding tyrosinase family proteins induced antibodies and cytotoxic T-cells against syngeneic B16 melanoma cells in C57BL/6 mice, but immunization with mouse tyrosinase-related DNA did not induce detectable immunity. In particular, xenogeneic DNA vaccination induced tumor protection from syngeneic melanoma challenge and autoimmune hypopigmentation. Thus xenogeneic DNA vaccination could break tolerance against a self tumor differentiation antigen, inducing antibody, T-cell, and antitumor responses. We have investigated the use of human tyrosinase, murine gp75, murine tyrosinase, and murine tyrosinase with or without human GM-CSF in dogs with advanced malignant melanoma (Bergman et al., 2003 and 2006). The results of these trials demonstrate that xenogeneic DNA vaccination in canine malignant melanoma: (1) is safe, (2) leads to the development of antityrosinase antibodies (Liao et al., 2006), (3) is potentially therapeutic, and (4) is an attractive candidate for further evaluation in an adjuvant, minimal residual disease phase II setting. To this end our research group and industrial sponsor are presently completing a multisite U.S. Department of Agriculture safety trial of human tyrosinase DNA vaccination in dogs with locoregionally controlled stage II/III malignant melanoma and have received conditional licensure for commercial sale of this product in April 2007. The efficacy portion of this trial is ongoing and human trials of MSKCC using murine and human tyrosinase DNA vaccination are also ongoing.

At the time this chapter was written, there were three sites pursuing active immunotherapy trials for canine melanoma in North America: the Animal Medical Center, the University of Wisconsin-Madison (UW-Madison),* and the University of Florida.† Although a number of immunotherapy approaches for melanoma and other tumors have been investigated, the present UW-Madison approach for canine melanoma immunotherapy is with a whole-cell allogeneic tumor cell vaccine (ATCV). The canine melanoma cell line 17CM98, developed by G. Hogge and associates, is electroporated with human GM-CSF cDNA. Each ATCV aliquot is 2×10^7 transfected cells given intradermally once weekly ×4 and then every other week ×2 and monthly ×3. The present approach at the University of Florida is a GD3 ganglioside (tumor-associated carbohydrate antigen expressed on tumors of neuroectodermal origin such as melanoma and small-cell lung carcinoma) vaccine with MPL adjuvant and CpG motifs. There were no side effects with this vaccine in normal dogs and no side effects to date in the 13 dogs accrued with resectable gross melanoma receiving three monthly vaccines.

In summary, the future is looking brighter for canine melanoma on multiple fronts. We have a greater understanding of the prognostic aspects of this disease, and there is now a commercially available vaccine for treatment. It is hoped in the future that this same vaccine may also play roles in the treatment of melanoma in other species (e.g., horses, cats, humans) because of its xenogeneic origins and in melanoma prevention once the genetic determinants of melanoma risk in dogs are further defined. Veterinary oncologists are in a unique position to contribute to advances in both canine and human melanoma, in addition to other cancers with similar comparative aspects across species.

---

*The primary contact at UW-Madison is Dr. Ilene Kurzman (kurzmani@svm.vetmed.wisc.edu).

†The primary contact at the University of Florida is Dr. Rowan Milner (milnerr@mail.vetmed.ufl.edu).

References and Suggested Reading

Bergman PJ et al: Long-term survival of dogs with advanced malignant melanoma after DNA vaccination with xenogenic human tyrosinase: a phase I trial, *Clin Cancer Res* 9:1284, 2003.

Bergman PJ et al: Development of a xenogeneic DNA vaccine program for canine malignant melanoma at the Animal Medical Center, *Vaccine* 24:4582, 2006.

Boria PA et al: Evaluation of cisplatin combined with piroxicam for the treatment of oral malignant melanoma and oral squamous cell carcinoma in dogs, *J Am Vet Med Assoc* 224:388, 2004.

Bostock DE: Prognosis after surgical excision of canine melanomas, *Vet Pathol* 16:32, 1979.

Henry CJ et al: Canine digital tumors: a veterinary cooperative oncology group retrospective study of 64 dogs, *J Vet Intern Med* 19:720, 2005.

Laprie C et al: MIB-1 immunoreactivity correlates with biologic behaviour in canine cutaneous melanoma, *Vet Dermatol* 12:139, 2001.

Liao JC et al: Vaccination with human tyrosinase DNA induces antibody responses in dogs with advanced melanoma, *Cancer Immun* 6:8, 2006.

MacEwen EG et al: Canine oral melanoma: comparison of surgery versus surgery plus *Corynebacterium parvum, Cancer Invest* 4:397, 1986.

MacEwen EG et al: Adjuvant therapy for melanoma in dogs: results of randomized clinical trials using surgery, liposome-encapsulated muramyl tripeptide, and granulocyte macrophage colony-stimulating factor, *Clin Cancer Res* 5:4249, 1999.

Murphy S et al: Oral malignant melanoma—the effect of coarse fractionation radiotherapy alone or with adjuvant carboplatin therapy, *Vet Comp Oncol* 4:222, 2005.

Proulx DR et al: A retrospective analysis of 140 dogs with oral melanoma treated with external beam radiation, *Vet Radiol Ultrasound* 44:352, 2003.

Rassnick KM et al: Use of carboplatin for treatment of dogs with malignant melanoma: 27 cases, *J Am Vet Med Assoc* 218:1444, 2001.

Spangler WL, Kass PH: The histologic and epidemiologic bases for prognostic considerations in canine melanocytic neoplasia, *Vet Pathol* 43:136, 2006.

Williams LE, Packer RA: Association between lymph node size and metastasis in dogs with oral malignant melanoma: 100 cases (1987-2001), *J Am Vet Med Assoc* 222:1234, 2003.

CHAPTER 83

Anal Sac Tumors

RUTHANNE CHUN, *Madison, Wisconsin*

Anal sac adenocarcinomas (ASACs) are relatively rare tumors in dogs and extremely rare in cats. German shepherd dogs are consistently overrepresented in the literature, as are golden retrievers. Other canine breeds at risk for ASAC include cocker spaniels and English springer spaniels. Contrary to earlier reports, several recent studies identify a 1:1 male:female ratio. The single case report of a cat with ASAC involved a neutered male Siamese cat. Differential diagnoses for animals presenting with a suspected ASAC include anal sac abscess; other anal sac neoplasms such as squamous cell carcinoma; or other perineal neoplasia such as perianal adenoma, perianal adenocarcinoma, or occasionally mast cell tumor (see also Chapter 122 on Anal-Rectal Disease).

HISTORY AND CLINICAL SIGNS

The majority of dogs are presented for examination because of visible perianal swelling. Other client concerns include tenesmus, licking or biting at the perianal area, stranguria, scooting, or hind limb weakness. Tenesmus may be caused by a large primary tumor or because of large sublumbar or intrapelvic lymph nodes. Nonspecific complaints from owners of dogs with ASAC include polyuria and polydipsia (PU/PD), lethargy, and anorexia. The most common cause of PU/PD in this population is hypercalcemia of malignancy secondary to tumor production of parathyroid hormone–related peptide (see Chapter 74). Up to 50% of dogs may have no reported problems, and an anal sac mass is found on routine physical examination.

PHYSICAL EXAMINATION FINDINGS

Physical and careful rectal examinations reveal a mass in the anal sac. Tumor size varies at the time of presentation from $100 \, cm^2$ or larger to less than $1 \, cm^2$. Rarely bilateral ASAC may be detected. In addition to identifying the anal sac mass, rectal examination may allow for detection of enlarged intrapelvic lymph nodes. In small dogs or dogs with significant enlargement, sublumbar lymphadenomegaly may also be identified either on rectal examination or abdominal palpation. An interesting phenomenon reported in dogs with metastatic ASAC is the finding of a small primary tumor with very large metastatic regional lymph nodes. Animals may also have fecal impaction.

DIAGNOSTIC EVALUATION

Tissue Diagnosis

Fine-needle aspirate of the anal sac mass is well tolerated and easy to perform. The anal sac is isolated between the thumb and forefinger via rectal palpation, and the needle is introduced through the perineal tissues. Sedation is rarely required for this procedure. Cytologic findings compatible with malignancy include the finding of basophilic epithelial cells with a high nuclear-to-cytoplasmic ratio, anisokaryosis, and nuclear moulding. Specific criteria for the cytologic diagnosis of ASAC have not been described. However, this quick and inexpensive diagnostic test rules out anal sac abscess and supports further diagnostic testing.

A biopsy is required for definitive diagnosis of ASAC. For very large masses an incisional biopsy is appropriate. For smaller anal sac masses, anal sacculectomy may be performed. Owners should be cautioned that a second surgery may be recommended if adequate surgical margins are not achieved through excisional biopsy. The surgeon should have a complete understanding of the surgical anatomy, including regional innervation and blood supply.

Minimum Database

The majority of dogs with ASAC are older, and since treatment of these tumors involves surgery and possibly radiation and chemotherapy, a minimum database is important. This generally includes a complete blood count, serum chemistry profile, and urinalysis. In addition, paraneoplastic hypercalcemia is present in up to 30% of dogs with ASAC. If hypercalcemia is present, careful attention should be paid to the calcium:phosphorus product. If it is higher than 60, soft-tissue mineralization and renal failure may be an issue. Further, if the hypercalcemia exceeds 18 mg/dl or if the patient has muscle fasciculations, bradycardia, or other cardiac arrhythmias or neurologic signs such as lethargy, coma, or seizures, aggressive therapy should be initiated immediately. For information on management of hypercalcemia (see Chapters 52 and 54).

Staging Tests

Dogs with ASAC present with identifiable metastasis to regional lymph nodes in 36% to 96% of cases; lung metastases are recognized in 10% to 25% of cases. Thus staging should include three-view thoracic radiographs and abdominal ultrasound examination. Pulmonary nodules, as opposed to a more reticular pattern, are the typical radiographic pattern of lung metastasis with ASAC. Llabres-Diaz (2004) reported that increased size or number of detected lymph nodes or finding rounder or sonographically heterogeneous lymph nodes could differentiate normal lymph nodes from neoplastic lymph nodes. Even if these nodes are not enlarged, an attempt should be made to sample palpable or visible regional lymph nodes via needle aspirate. Because ASAC can also metastasize to bone, in particular the lumbar vertebrae, abdominal radiographs that include the vertebral column are also recommended.

BIOLOGIC BEHAVIOR

As indicated previously, ASAC are highly metastatic and locally invasive tumors. Small primary tumors can be associated with bulky metastatic lesions. The presence of hypercalcemia is a poor prognostic factor if it cannot be controlled pharmacologically or by resolution of the underlying tumor. Dogs can be managed relatively long term for obstructive rectal lesions; but, if they have uncontrollable hypercalcemia, their outlook is poor.

TREATMENT

Combination Therapy Is Ideal

Surgery Alone

As with any solid tumor, surgical resection is the mainstay of treatment. Because sublumbar or intrapelvic lymphadenomegaly can adversely impact quality of life, cytoreductive surgery of these nodes is appropriate when they are enlarged. Intrapelvic nodes are difficult to remove without splitting the pelvis; and clients should be informed of the additional morbidity associated with this procedure. Omentalization of a cystic metastatic sublumbar lymph node has been reported to prolong survival time in a dog that was significantly symptomatic for a caudal abdominal mass. Unfortunately the majority of metastatic lymph nodes are not cystic, and lymph node extirpation is required for effective palliation.

Large tumors that require 180-degree or greater anoplasty are associated with a higher postoperative complication rate. Postoperative infection and fecal incontinence are the most common complications. Tumors larger than $10\,cm^2$ are also associated with shorter survival times compared to dogs with smaller tumors. With surgery alone, recurrence rates of approximately 50% have been reported. Bennett and colleagues (2002) documented a median disease-free interval of 10 months in dogs treated with surgery alone. Median survival of dogs treated only with surgery ranges from 7.9 to 16.7 months. In a large retrospective study Williams and associates (2003) found that dogs treated with surgery (with or without radiation therapy or chemotherapy) had significantly longer survival than dogs that did not have surgery. Adjuvant therapy appears to prolong survival (see following paragraphs).

Surgery and Radiation Therapy

Postoperative radiation therapy has been evaluated to a limited degree. Turek and associates (2003) described 15 dogs treated with postoperative radiation therapy (15 fractions of 3.2-Gy delivered Monday through Friday for 3 weeks) and mitoxantrone chemotherapy ($5\,mg/m^2$ q21d intravenously [IV]). Both the sublumbar lymph nodes and the primary site were treated in 12 dogs; in 3 dogs only the perineal site was treated. Although the median survival time was 31.9 months, both acute and chronic radiation complications were common and contributed to euthanasia decisions in two cases. It is likely that smaller fractions over a longer time period would be better tolerated. Radiation therapy as the sole treatment modality has not been reported.

Surgery and Chemotherapy

Surgery combined with chemotherapy also has been reported. A retrospective study by Emms (2005) discussed the outcome of 14 dogs treated with cytoreductive surgery followed by melphalan chemotherapy ($7 \, mg/m^2 \times 5$ days, q3wks PO) for an indefinite number of cycles. All of the dogs had local excision of the anal sac with a 1-cm margin; seven dogs also had the sublumbar lymph nodes removed because of palpable lymphadenomegaly. Median survival time of these 14 dogs was 20 months, and there was no significant difference in survival time between dogs with and without lymph node metastasis. Median disease-free interval was not reported. Other reports of dogs treated with surgery and adjuvant chemotherapy are harder to interpret since chemotherapy protocols and extent of disease at the time chemotherapy was initiated varied significantly.

Chemotherapy Alone

Chemotherapy alone may be contemplated for palliation of patients when surgery is not possible because of location or extent of disease. Chemotherapy as the sole treatment modality is associated with a median survival time of 7 months. Although nothing more than short-lived partial remissions have been reported, agents with activity against ASAC include actinomycin-D (0.7 to $0.9 \, mg/m^2$ q3wks IV), cisplatin ($70 \, mg/m^2$ q3wks IV), carboplatin ($300 \, mg/m^2$ q3wks IV), and doxorubicin ($30 \, mg/m^2$ q2-3wks IV).

Palliative Treatments

Dogs with owners that decline definitive therapy may continue to have a reasonable quality of life for weeks to months, as long as hypercalcemia can be managed. I recommend pamidronate (1 to 2 mg/kg in 250 ml 0.9% NaCl IV over 2 hours q28d) as the most effective drug to manage chronic hypercalcemia. Although corticosteroids are less expensive, they are less effective and have more side effects than monthly pamidronate. After hypercalcemia, the main issue affecting quality of life is whether the animal can defecate. The stool can be kept soft through the judicious use of lactulose (1 ml/4.5 kg q8h orally) and/or psyllium (1 tsp to 2 Tbsp per day mixed into the food) titrated to effect and a low-residue diet. Owners must be instructed to monitor their pet's ability to defecate, urinate, and ambulate comfortably. Skeletal or pulmonary metastases may become more of an issue than rectal obstruction, and quality of life should be discussed.

References and Suggested Reading

Bennett PF et al: Canine anal sac adenocarcinomas: clinical presentation and response to therapy, *J Vet Intern Med* 16:100, 2002.

Emms SG: Anal sac tumours of the dog and their response to cytoreductive surgery and chemotherapy, *Aust Vet J* 83:340, 2005.

Esplin DG, Wilson SR, Hullinger GA: Squamous cell carcinoma of the anal sac in five dogs, *Vet Pathol* 40:332, 2003.

Hoelzer MG, Bellah JR, Donofro MC: Omentalization of cystic sublumbar lymph node metastases for long-term palliation of tenesmus and dysuria in a dog with anal sac adenocarcinoma, *J Am Vet Med Assoc* 219:1729, 2001.

Hostuttler RA et al: Uses and effectiveness of pamidronate disodium for treatment of dogs and cats with hypercalcemia, *J Vet Intern Med* 19:29, 2005.

Llabres-Diaz FJ: Ultrasonography of the medial iliac lymph nodes in the dog, *Vet Radiol Ultrasound* 45:156, 2004.

Mellanby RJ et al: Anal sac adenocarcinoma in a Siamese cat, *J Feline Med Surg* 4:205, 2002.

Ross JT et al: Adenocarcinoma of the apocrine glands of the anal sac in dogs: a review of 32 cases, *J Am Anim Hosp Assoc* 27:349, 1991.

Turek MM et al: Postoperative radiotherapy and mitoxantrone for anal sac adenocarcinoma in the dog: 15 cases (1991-2001), *Vet Comp Oncol* 1:94, 2003.

Williams LE et al: Carcinoma of the apocrine glands of the anal sac in dogs: 113 cases (1985-1995), *J Am Vet Med Assoc* 223:825, 2003.

SECTION V

Dermatologic Diseases

Craig E. Griffin, Wayne S. Rosenkrantz

VOLUME XIII CONTENT ON EVOLVE: http://evolve.elsevier.com/Bonagura/Kirks/

Hypoallergenic Diets for Dogs and Cats

CHAPTER 84

Cyclosporine Use in Dermatology

CRAIG E. GRIFFIN, *San Diego, California*

INTRODUCTION AND INDICATIONS

Cyclosporine has been evaluated in dogs and introduced into the veterinary field as the drug Atopica (Novartis). Atopica is approved for treating canine atopic dermatitis. The manufacturer has performed, supported, and published numerous and extensive studies in cyclosporine therapy in dogs. Many of these investigations have been summarized in several review articles (Guaguere et al., 2004 and Steffan et al., 2004). Cyclosporine is the first alternative therapy to glucocorticoids that has shown similar efficacy to prednisolone and methylprednisolone. Since its release cyclosporine has also been evaluated or anecdotally reported as effective for a variety of allergic and cutaneous diseases of dogs and cats (Table 84-1). This list continues to grow, and the drug has been tried in most glucocorticoid-responsive and idiopathic inflammatory disorders. A major drawback to its use is the cost, which many clients consider prohibitive, especially in medium- to large-sized dogs. For this reason, many practitioners do not stock Atopica, or they limit its use to small dogs and cats. Alternate dosing methods are suggested in this chapter. These regimens are designed to minimize the drug cost to clients. I believe practitioners should consider cyclosporine as an alternative treatment option in dogs and cats for the dermatologic conditions listed in Table 84-1.

CYCLOSPORINE FORMULATIONS

Different cyclosporine formulations are available and include both human brand name products and generic formulations. Two main types of formulations available are an emulsion and a microemulsified form. The microemulsified formulations generally are better absorbed. Atopica is a microemulsion concentrate that is absorbed quickly and more effectively through the gastrointestinal tract of dogs than nonmicroemulsified formulations. Although absorption is better with Atopica, it is still somewhat erratic, and bioavailability varies from 23% to 45%. Presence of food in the gastrointestinal tract increases the range of bioavailability and can reduce absorption by up to 20%; however, other dogs have increased absorption, especially when the diet is high in fat. Currently the only veterinary-approved product is Atopica, which may be more convenient than the human and generic formulations because it is available in a wider range of capsule sizes (10 mg, 25 mg, 50 mg, and 100 mg). Some generic formulations have a warning on the label stating a lack of bioequivalence; and it has been my experience that some

dogs do not respond as well to generic formulations or they only respond at a higher dose, which generally offsets any cost savings. My preference is to start initial therapy with Atopica and adjust to the lowest dosage to maintain a response. Then, if the maintenance cost is considered too expensive, a generic formulation is substituted at the same dosing regimen, and the treatment response determines if the generic product can be used long term.

DOSE AND USE OF CYCLOSPORINE

Cyclosporine is most commonly given at 5 mg/kg every 24 hours. For some diseases such as perianal fistula and atopic dermatitis in cats with concurrent asthma, initial dosages as high as 7.5 to 10 mg/kg every 24 hours or 4 mg/kg every 12 hours may be used. It may take 2 to 4 weeks to see a response, and generally a 4-week trial is the minimum. Dogs that show greater than 50% response in the first 4 weeks are more likely to be maintained long term. Once a response is obtained, the dosage may then be tapered. It is best to continue the induction dosage until clinical improvement is complete or a steady state of response is reached. Tapering is achieved by maintaining the dose at 5 mg/kg but changing the treatment interval to every 48 hours for 1 month. If symptoms return, the daily dose is reinstituted until a response is again achieved; then an alternate attempt at dose reduction is tried: 2 days on and 1 day off. This method results in a 33% reduction in cost. If a favorable response is maintained after 1 month at every-48-hours dosing, the dosing is again tapered to every 72 hours. As long as improvement and control are maintained, further tapering to every 4 to 7 days may be attempted.

The Radowicz 2003 study reported that some dogs with atopic dermatitis had complete responses (for over 6 months); even once cyclosporine was discontinued these dogs maintained long-term remissions. The frequency of this response rate requires further definition, but I find that some patients can discontinue cyclosporine for months before symptoms return. Another study (Steffan et al., 2004) also showed temporary remissions once the drug was stopped. In such responsive cases, going on and then off the drug for long intervals represents yet another way to manage some patients. This approach may also keep the cost within a client's comfort level. Some dogs can be maintained on relatively low levels of cyclosporine long term by first tapering the dose and the going off the drug for extended periods. In these cases, when it does become necessary to reintroduce cyclosporine, it is often possible to rapidly taper to a maintenance dosage.

Table **84-1**

Cyclosporine Cutaneous Indications

Specific Disease/Syndrome	Dog	Cat
Allergic Diseases		
Atopic dermatitis	X	X
Atopic otitis	X	
Contact allergy	X	
Adverse food reactions /allergy	X	X
Autoimmune		
Alopecia areata	X	
Bullous pemphigoid	X	
Cutaneous lupus erythematosus	X	
Discoid lupus erythematosus	X	
Pemphigus complex	X	X
Immune-Mediated Diseases		
Erythema multiforme	X	
Pseudopelade		X
Vasculitis	X	
Miscellaneous Inflammatory Disorders		
Chronic pedal furunculosis	X	
Eosinophilic granuloma complex		X
Granulomatous folliculitis	X	
Idiopathic facial dermatitis		X
Sterile granulomatous dermatitis	X	X
Plasmacytic stomatitis and pododermatitis		X
Some drug reactions	X	X
Miscellaneous Indications		
Alopecia, some forms referred to as alopecia x	X	
Lupoid onychodystrophy	X	
Metatarsal fistula of German shepherds	X	
Perianal fistula	X	
Proliferative otitis	X	
Sebaceous adenitis	X	
Sterile nodular panniculitis	X	
Ulcerative dermatosis of the philtrum of St. Bernard	X	
Urticaria pigmentosa		X

Another approach that may allow a dosage reduction is based on altering the metabolism of cyclosporine, which is predominantly metabolized by cytochrome P-450 3A12 enzyme primarily in the liver. Drugs that decrease this enzyme result in an increase in blood levels of cyclosporine. Ketoconazole specifically inhibits hepatic microsomal cytochrome P-450 3A12 enzyme and is the most common drug used to allow a reduction in cyclosporine dose. Ketoconazole, 5 mg/kg orally, is given as frequently as cyclosporine, approximately 8 to 12 hours before cyclosporine administration. This results in many dogs responding to a lower dose of cyclosporine in the range of 2 to 4 mg/kg. Since not all dogs respond to the cyclosporine/ketoconazole combination, it is still preferable to initiate therapy first with cyclosporine at 5 mg/kg. After a response is obtained and a maintenance dosage is established, ketoconazole is then added to allow further tapering of the drug dosing. When clients with large dogs are reluctant to use the recommended dose because of cost, the initial therapy can be a combination of ketoconazole and 2.5 mg/kg of cyclosporine. However, clients should be warned that the response rate could be poorer using this protocol.

CYCLOSPORINE ADVERSE REACTIONS

Adverse reactions have been reported in two large studies by Steffan, Parks, and Seewald (2005) and Steffan, Favrot, and Mueller (2006). Based on these studies, other reports, and my experience, the most commonly encountered side effects are vomiting and diarrhea, which occasionally can result in owners discontinuing therapy. In the 2006 Steffan, Favrot, and Mueller review of cyclosporine use in 672 atopic dogs, 25% had vomiting, and 15% had soft stools or diarrhea, which usually occurred within the first month. Dogs that vomit should have the drug administered with food, and often after several days the drug can then be administered on an empty stomach without problems. If vomiting recurs, cyclosporine should be given with a fatty meal on a long-term basis. However, this may interfere with drug absorption. Concurrent administration with ketoconazole in some dogs also induces vomiting when cyclosporine alone is tolerated. Sometimes concurrent use of metoclopramide, 0.2 to 1 mg/kg every 24 hours, may allow continued use of Atopica. Management of diarrhea involves temporarily stopping the drug and then treating again with the addition of metronidazole or fiber (such as pumpkin or psyllium husk) to the diet. In spite of these therapies, gastrointestinal signs are still the most common adverse reaction that causes cessation of therapy.

Other side effects seen with some frequency include hirsutism and gingival hyperplasia. Hirsutism is characterized by a generalized thickened dense hair coat often associated with increased shedding. In other cases there are patterns in which the hair growth is exceptionally long. The patterns most commonly seen or at least recognized include hirsutism of the paws, especially interdigital hair growth, as well involvement of the head or face. The gingival hyperplasia often requires discontinuation of therapy, although rare cases may have lesion regress by temporarily stopping the drug, followed by resuming it at a lower dose. Some cases of gingival hyperplasia are associated with bacterial overgrowth and respond to systemic antibiotic therapy. Papillomatous hyperplasia is infrequently seen, and usually the lesions are negative for papilloma virus. Cytology should be performed whenever lesions occur and when bacteria are seen; antibiotic therapy and cyclosporine dose reductions usually eliminate the lesions. Bacterial infections are always a concern and may also appear as atypical lesions. Bacteriuria may also be found, but a true relation to cyclosporine therapy has not been established. Bacteriuria occurs less commonly with dogs taking cyclosporine than in canine dermatologic cases treated with long-term glucocorticoids.

Infrequent or rare reactions may also be observed. Increased pruritus is uncommon, but cases have been observed in which the cyclosporine has been associated with moderate-to-intense pruritus on provocation testing. If pruritus increases after cyclosporine therapy is initiated, it may take some trials to determine if the cyclosporine is the cause, if the underlying disease is becoming more severe, or if secondary microbial infections are developing. There are anecdotal reports of upper respiratory infections in cats taking cyclosporine. Fatal toxoplasmosis has been reported in cats; this has led to some clinicians recommending that all cats being tested before beginning therapy. Atypical systemic fungal and aspergillosis infections have been seen in a limited number of cases and most commonly have occurred in dogs treated with concurrent high-dose glucocorticoids. A relatively high incidence of nephrotoxicity and hepatic toxicity is reported in humans but has not been observed in dogs and cats, although elevations in creatinine levels have been reported in dogs. When creatinine elevations occur, they do not typically progress into abnormal levels during the first year of therapy. Elevated liver enzymes are more prevalent when ketoconazole is given concurrently either for *Malassezia* or as a dose-sparing agent. While rare in dogs, elevated blood pressure is another major concern of cyclosporine therapy in humans. It is recommended that blood pressure should be monitored periodically in dogs and cats taking this drug. In humans there is also an increased risk for malignancy, especially skin neoplasia, with cyclosporine therapy; however, this relationship has yet not been documented in dogs.

MONITORING

Routine monitoring of serum levels of cyclosporine for therapy of skin disease is not recommended because serum levels generally do not correlate with clinical responses. However, there may be some value in monitoring levels when clinical responses are not observed. If serum levels are still in the low nontherapeutic range, dosages can be increased in an attempt to obtain a response. The most important indication for monitoring is when adverse effects such as skin lesions, hirsutism, and gingival hyperplasia occur. These adverse effects may be dose related, and follow-up evaluations are recommended. Baseline biochemistry and urine evaluations should be evaluated when cyclosporine is used as a long-term therapy.

Physical examinations initially at 3 months and then at least once every 6 months are recommended. One should pay close attention to the gingiva, skin, and hair coat. Even though organ dysfunction is uncommon, regular monitoring is prudent since long-term experience with cyclosporine is still limited. Complete blood counts, chemistry profiles, urinalyses, and blood pressure testing are indicated at a frequency of 4 to 12 months. In cases having increasing creatinine levels, monitoring every 4 months is warranted at least until values have stabilized.

References and Suggested Reading

Guaguere E, Steffan J, Olivry T: Cyclosporine A: a new drug in the field of canine dermatology, *Vet Dermatol* 15:61, 2004.

Radowicz S, Power H: Long-term use of cyclosporine therapy in the treatment of canine atopic dermatitis, *Vet Dermatol* 14:234, 2003.

Steffan J, Parks C, Seewald W: Clinical trial evaluating the efficacy and safety of cyclosporine in dogs with atopic dermatitis, *J Am Vet Med Assoc* 226:1855, 2005.

Steffan J, Favrot C, Mueller RS: A systematic review and meta-analysis of the efficacy and safety of cyclosporine for the treatment of atopic dermatitis in dogs, *Vet Dermatol* 17:3 2006.

Steffan J et al: Remission of the clinical signs of atopic dermatitis in dogs after cessation of treatment with cyclosporine A or methylprednisolone, *Vet Rec* 154:681 2004.

CHAPTER 85

Interferons

TOSHIROH IWASAKI, *Tokyo, Japan*

Interferons (IFNs) belong to the class of cellular proteins referred to as cytokines. These proteins are secreted by cells of the immune system in response to viral infection or neoplasia. IFNs exert inhibitory effects on viral and cell proliferation and affect the immune regulatory system and inflammatory reactions. Recently IFNs have been used in a number of trials for treatment of atopic dermatitis in dogs.

CLASSIFICATION

IFNs are classified as either type I or type II. Type I IFNs bind to the cell via the INFAR receptor. Type I IFNs are further classified as either α, β, or ω. IFN-γ is the only cytokine classified into type II IFN. Mature IFN-γ forms a homodimer that binds to the IFN γ-receptor complex by which it exerts its effect.

Recombinant feline IFN-ω and recombinant canine IFN-γ are only available in a few countries, but various types of recombinant human IFNs are more widely available. In Japan natural human IFN-α has been approved for the treatment of bovine diarrhea. There have been no clinical trials conducted to study IFN-α efficacy in treating small animal skin diseases.

MODE OF ACTION

IFNs are antiviral and also possess antioncogenic properties. IFNs are directly induced by the presence of viruses; and when large amounts of double-stranded ribonucleic acid (RNA) are found within the cell in association with Toll-like receptors, IFNs are synthesized and secreted to surrounding cells. IFNs are also induced by other cytokines such as interleukin (IL)1, IL2, IL12, and tumor necrosis factor.

IFN-α and IFN-β are produced by various types of cells, including lymphocytes, macrophages, and fibroblasts. They also activate macrophages and natural killer lymphocytes and directly inhibit tumor cell proliferation. IFN-γ is produced by activated Th1 cells and has an immunomodulating effect on Th1/Th2 cytokine balance.

CLINICAL APPLICATION OF INTERFERONS IN SMALL ANIMAL DERMATOLOGY

Interferon-α and Interferon-β

There are a number of anecdotal reports on the treatment of animal skin diseases using recombinant human IFN-α2b (rHuIFNα2b) and IFN-α2a (rHuIFNα2a). In one published report rHuIFNα2b was used for the management of idiopathic recurrent canine pyoderma at a dosage of 1000 units/ml/day and was found to provide transient benefits compared with placebo (Thompson et al., 2004). rHuIFNα was administered at a dosage of 1,000,000 units/kg subcutaneously three times a week for 2 weeks to treat canine papillomavirus–associated hamartoma and squamous cell carcinoma, but the efficacy of these therapies is uncertain (Callan, Preziosi, and Mauldin, 2005).

Interferon-γ

Recombinant canine IFN-γ (rCaIFNγ) is produced by silkworms via the transfer of canine full-length IFN-γ genes. It was launched on the Japanese market for the treatment of canine atopic dermatitis in 2005. Six subcutaneous injections of rCaIFNγ given in 2 consecutive weeks modified Th1 and Th2 cytokine messenger RNA profiles such as IL4 and IFN-γ toward Th1 cytokine predominance. Treatment showed improvement of clinical signs in 10 atopic dogs (Iwasaki et al., 2005). It also decreased total immunoglobulin (Ig)E in sera, although allergen-specific IgE was not determined.

Recently a randomized clinical trial for rCaIFNγ was performed in 92 atopic dogs by subcutaneous administration at a dosage of 10,000 units/kg three times a week for 2 weeks, followed by once-a-week administration for 2 weeks. The rCaIFNγ group showed 72% efficacy, whereas the control group given antihistamine spray showed 20% efficacy (Iwasaki and Hasegawa, 2006).

A placebo-controlled, double-blinded study was conducted by Hasegawa, Sakurai, and Iwasaki (2004) using the same protocol as the previous study used for treating atopic dogs. A 58% decrease in lesion size was determined using a computer-assisted imaging analyzer evaluation compared to the 38% decrease in the placebo group. Based on these clinical studies the manufacturer recommends a dosage of rCaIFNγ of 10,000 units/kg, given subcutaneously three times a week for the first 4 weeks, followed by once-a-week injections for the next 4 weeks. Although the mode of action of this drug has not yet been clarified, modification of the Th1 and Th2 cytokine profiles may play some role in the improvement of clinical signs in canine atopic dermatitis. Only a few side effects, including pain at the injection site, were noted.

Interferon-ω

Recombinant IFN-ω (rFeIFNω) produced by silkworms has been launched in Europe and Japan for the treatment of feline calicivirus and canine parvovirus infections. Recently Carlotti and associates (2004) reported the efficacy of rfIFNω against canine atopic dermatitis. They administered rFeIFNω to 20 atopic dogs at a dosage of 1,000,000 units/kg subcutaneously three times a week for 3 weeks and found a 60% decrease of clinical scores at day 42. Sieback and colleagues (2006) examined the effects of both rFeIFNω and recombinant human IFN-α (rHuIFNα) on in vitro replication of feline herpes virus 1. When given at a higher dosage, rFeIFNw showed stronger inhibition of viral replication than rHuIFNα, indicating the efficacy of rFeIFNω against feline herpes virus infection.

References and Suggested Reading

Callan MB, Preziosi D, Mauldin E: Multiple papillomavirus-associated epidermal hamartomas and squamous cell carcinomas in situ in a dog following chronic treatment with prednisolone and cyclosporine, *Vet Dermatol* 16:338, 2005.

Carlotti DN et al: Use of recombinant omega interferon therapy in canine atopic dermatitis: a pilot study, *Vet Dermatol* 15(suppl 1): 32, 2004.

Hasegawa A, Sakurai T, Iwasaki T: A placebo-controlled, double-blinded study of recombinant IFN-γ in dogs with atopic dermatitis, *Vet Dermatol* 15(suppl 1):55, 2004.

Iwasaki T, Hasegawa A: A randomized comparative clinical trial of recombinant canine interferon-gamma (KT-100) in atopic dogs using antihistamines as control, *Vet Dermatol* 17:195, 2006.

Iwasaki T et al: Effect of treatment with recombinant canine IFN-γ on the clinical signs, histopathology and Th1/Th2 cytokine mRNA profiles in Shih Tzu and a basset hound with atopic dermatitis, *Adv Vet Dermatol* 5:82, 2005.

Siebeck N et al: Effects of human recombinant alpha-2b interferon and feline recombinant omega interferon on in vitro replication of feline herpesvirus-1, *Am J Vet Res* 67:1406, 2006.

Thompson LA et al: Human recombinant interferon alpha-2b for management of idiopathic recurrent superficial pyoderma in dogs: a pilot study, *Vet Ther* 5:75, 2004.

CHAPTER 86

Avermectins in Dermatology

AMANDA BURROWS, *Murdoch, Western Australia*

AVERMECTINS IN DERMATOLOGY

The avermectin class of antiparasitic agents includes two distinct chemical families: avermectins (ivermectin, abamectin, doramectin, eprinomectin, salinomectin, and selamectin) and milbemycins (moxidectin and milbemycin oxime). These are important antiparasitic agents because of their wide spectrum of activity, high potency, safety margins, and unique mechanism of action. Each member exerts a similar mode of antiparasitic action, but there is variation in efficacy, which is presumed to relate to differences in the chemical structure. Avermectins and milbemycins are closely related macrocyclic lactones produced naturally as fermentation by-products of actinomycetes from the genus *Streptomyces*. In veterinary dermatology the avermectins and milbemycins of importance are ivermectin, selamectin, and doramectin and milbemycin oxime and moxidectin, respectively. There is a wide use of these compounds for management of parasitic diseases. Despite the clinical evidence for therapeutic efficacy and safety, many of the clinical indications and dosage regimens recommended for avermectins in dogs and cats are extra-label or unapproved. Accordingly, the veterinarian is wise to secure written owner informed consent before embarking on an extra-label course of therapy.

Mechanism of Action

Avermectins and milbemycins have two modes of action. The primary mode of action is selective, high-affinity binding to specific glutamate gated chloride channels in synapses between inhibitory interneurons and excitatory motor neurons in nematodes and in myoneural junctions in arthropods. These compounds also enhance the release of γ-aminobutyric acid (GABA) in presynaptic neurons, which in turn opens postsynaptic GABA-gated chloride channels. In either case the influx of chloride ions reduces cell membrane resistance, which prevents the potential hyperpolarisation of neural stimuli to muscles, resulting in flaccid paralysis and death. Mammals, unlike nematodes and arthropods, have GABA-mediated interneuronal inhibitors only in the central nervous system. It is believed that the mammalian blood-brain barrier is impermeable to the avermectin class drug; thus toxicity in mammals occurs at a much higher concentrations compared with nematodes and arthropods.

AVERMECTINS

Ivermectin

Ivermectin is a derivative of avermectin B1 and licensed in small animals only for the prevention of dirofilariasis at a dosage of 6 to 12 mcg/kg once a month orally. The ivermectin formulation most commonly used in dogs and cats for the extralabel treatment of ectoparasites in veterinary dermatology is available commercially as a 1% nonaqueous injectable solution formulated in 60% propylene glycol and 40% glycerol (Ivomec, Merial Animal Health). This can be diluted with sterile propylene glycol for accurate dosing for kittens and small dogs; however, propylene glycol can be irritating when administered subcutaneously and can cause bradycardia and respiratory and central nervous system depression. For this reason some veterinary dermatologists prefer to use the aqueous 0.8% oral drench approved for use in sheep and goats (Ivomec Liquid, Merial Animal Health), which can be administered undiluted or diluted with sterile water. The oral solution of ivermectin must be given by mouth, whereas the injectable propylene glycol–based formulation can be administered subcutaneously or orally. A 0.5%, alcohol-based pour-on ivermectin formulation (Ivomec Pour-on, Merial Animal Health) approved for use in cattle has been used in dogs and cats. Ivermectin is sensitive to ultraviolet light and should be stored in the dark or dispensed in an opaque bag to prolong its shelf life.

Ivermectin has a wide margin of safety in dogs and cats; however, an increased susceptibility to acute toxicity is evident in a subpopulation of collie and collie-type dogs. The oral dose of ivermectin shown to cause adverse effects in noncollie dog breeds is in the range of 2,500 to 10,000 mcg/kg. In contrast, clinical signs of toxicity develop after the administration of only 100 mcg/kg in the subpopulation of susceptible breeds. Clinical signs include mydriasis, depression, ataxia, hypersalivation, bradycardia, hyperthermia, apparent blindness, decreased menace response, muscle tremors, and disorientation, which may progress to weakness, recumbency, unresponsiveness, stupor, and coma. Acute ivermectin toxicity has been reported in other breeds, including Australian shepherds, Shetland sheepdogs, Old English sheepdogs, Dobermans, and their crossbreeds. This idiosyncratic toxicity is associated with the homozygous expression of a four-base pair deletion mutation of the multidrug resistant (MDR-1) gene in collies and Australian shepherds.

The MDR-1 gene encodes a large transmembrane protein forming an integral part of the blood-brain barrier, p-glycoprotein. P-glycoprotein plays an important role in integrity of the blood-brain barrier by limiting drug uptake into the brain. Altered expression or function of p-glycoprotein may allow elevated brain concentrations of ivermectin and thereby potentiate neurotoxicity. Whether other affected breeds have the same MDR-1 mutation is unknown. A commercial polymerase chain reaction (PCR)–based method for MDR-1 genotyping using canine

deoxyribonucleic acid (DNA) from mouth cells is available for detecting the mutation in dogs and should be considered if ivermectin must be used in potentially susceptible breeds. Information is available at the Washington State University Veterinary Clinical Pathology website: www.vetmed.wsu.edu/depts-vcpl/test.asp. Recently a rapid PCR-based method that can discriminate between homozygous and heterozygous alleles using a small amount of genomic DNA from a blood sample has been developed (Geyer et al., 2005). Further studies are awaited to clarify the reliability of this test for large-scale screening and to define the frequency of the MDR-1 mutation in dog breeds. Acute ivermectin toxicity in adult cats is rare, but kittens are susceptible to the toxic effects of ivermectin; and lethargy, ataxia, coma, and death have been reported after administration of a single 300 mcg/kg subcutaneous injection.

Safety in administering oral ivermectin may be improved but not ensured by beginning with a low test dose and increasing the amount administered over several days until the desired dose is reached. In our dermatology clinic we initially administer 100 mcg/kg orally, and then we increase the dosage to 200, 300 mcg/kg, etc., every 48 hours orally in an effort to identify ivermectin-sensitive dogs. Owners are instructed to observe the pet closely over this period and to cease administration if symptoms of lethargy, incoordination, or mydriasis develop. Because of the relatively long half-life of ivermectin, serum concentrations of ivermectin administered daily continue to increase before reaching equilibrium at much higher levels than with weekly therapy. Thus chronic toxicity caused by cumulative therapy may develop with prolonged daily ivermectin treatment. In this light it is recommended that dogs receiving ivermectin be checked regularly for evidence of clinical signs suggestive of chronic toxicity; in our dermatology clinic we reevaluate dogs every 4 weeks for the first 3 months of treatment and then every 3 months thereafter.

Adverse reactions to ivermectin have been encountered with the rapid destruction of the microfilariae of *Dirofilaria immitis* in dogs. Most reactions are mild; occur within 1 to 4 hours of administration; and manifest as ataxia, vomiting, and dyspnea. However, anaphylactic shock has been observed and is more likely to occur when the microfilaria counts are high. Dogs should be screened for heartworm infection before ivermectin administration, particularly in heartworm-endemic regions.

Selamectin

Selamectin is a derivative of the avermectin endectocide doramectin. It is available as a solution (6% or 12%) in an isopropyl alcohol and dipropylene glycol methyl-ether vehicle (Revolution, Pfizer Animal Health). It is licensed for topical application at a dose of 6 mg/kg for dogs and cats not less than 6 weeks of age for the treatment and prevention of fleas (*Ctenocephalides* spp.), sarcoptic (*Sarcoptes scabiei*) and otodectic (*Otodectes cynotis*) mites, ascarids (*Toxocara* spp.), hookworms (*Ancylostoma tubaeformis*) and the prevention of heartworm (*Dirofilaria immitis*). A single dorsal application on the skin at the base of the neck in front of the scapulae is recommended. If the volume of the total dose exceeds 3 ml, the manufacturer recommends that the dose be divided among multiple areas in the dorsal neck region.

Extensive safety studies have shown that selamectin has a wide margin of safety when administered to dogs and cats, including puppies and breeding animals. The drug is safe for topical administration in ivermectin-sensitive breeds and in dogs and cats with dirofilariasis. The likelihood of accidental oral ingestion is reduced by dorsal application at the base of the neck, but inadvertent oral consumption of selamectin causes only mild salivation and intermittent vomiting in cats and no reaction in dogs.

Doramectin

Doramectin is a relatively newer semisynthetic avermectin licensed as an endectocide for subcutaneous administration in cattle, sheep, and swine (Dectomax, Pfizer Animal Health). It is not licensed for use in dogs and cats, but its extralabel use as an endectocide in these species has been widely reported. It is available commercially as a 1% solution formulated in a 90:10 volume:volume sesame oil and ethyl oleate vehicle for subcutaneous injection in the lateral midline of the back as a single dose. It is well tolerated without pain or inflammatory reaction at the injection site. In ruminants and in equine species doramectin expresses higher bioavailability and persistent efficacy when compared with ivermectin; however, recent studies indicate that this is not the case in the dog. Doramectin generated a significantly lower plasma concentration when compared to ivermectin following oral administration in the dog, whereas no significant differences were observed following subcutaneous administration (Gokbulut et al., 2006). This suggests that different formulations of doramectin for oral and subcutaneous administration may need to be developed for the dog.

There is little reported information on the safety of doramectin in dogs and cats. Some avermectin-sensitive breeds in my dermatology referral practice have displayed clinical signs of salivation, mydriasis, vomiting, tremors, ataxia, and depression when doramectin was administered at doses between 200 and 400 mcg/kg by single subcutaneous injection. Recently similar toxicity was reported in a collie dog following the single subcutaneous administration of 200 mcg/kg (Yas-Natan et al., 2003). Caution should be exercised with the administration of doramectin to potentially avermectin-sensitive breeds. I recommend that clinicians take precautions similar to those for ivermectin administration (i.e., the dose of doramectin should be increased with each weekly injection, beginning at a test dose of 50 to 100 mcg/kg). No toxic reactions have been recorded in cats.

MILBEMYCINS

Milbemycin Oxime

Milbemycin oxime is a semisynthetic derivative of milbemycin A3/A4 and is licensed for use in dogs as a prophylactic against *D. immitis* and for control of gastrointestinal parasites (Interceptor Spectrum, Novartis) at a dosage of 500 mcg/kg administered every 30 days from 4 weeks of age orally. It is available in some countries as a tablet containing milbemycin oxime 23 mg in combination with praziquantel 228 mg. Milbemycin oxime used to be available as a single ingredient (Interceptor, Novartis), but unfortunately this product recently has been discontinued.

Milbemycin oxime has a very wide margin of safety in dogs. Mild signs of lethargy have been reported when the drug was administered at the extralabel dosage rate of 2 mg/kg every 24 hours orally, with transient, reversible signs of toxicity (stupor, trembling, and ataxia) observed at higher dosages of 3.8 mg/kg every 24 hours orally. Some avermectin-sensitive collies treated with 5 mg/kg of milbemycin oxime developed transient depression, and all collies treated with 10 mg/kg of milbemycin oxime exhibited ataxia and depression resolving within 24 hours of administration (Tranquilli, Paul, and Todd, 1991). These findings support the generally wide safety margin of milbemycin oxime. However, because occasional patients still develop neurologic adverse effects, particularly at higher doses, thorough client education and appropriate monitoring are indicated, especially in breeds at risk. Treatment of heartworm-infected dogs with milbemycin oxime is not recommended because of the development of mild transient hypersensitivity reactions. There are no reports of side effects using milbemycin oxime in cats.

Moxidectin

Moxidectin is a semi-synthetic milbemycin derivative of nemadectin. It is available as an oral tablet licensed for the prevention of canine heartworm at a dose of 3 mcg/kg once a month and a 1% or 2.5% topical spot on formulation combined with 1% or 10% imidacloprid (Advocate, Bayer Animal Health). This is licensed for application at the dosage of 0.1 ml/kg every 30 days for the treatment and prevention of gastrointestinal parasites and the prevention of heartworm (*Dirofilaria immitus*) in dogs and cats, sarcoptic (*Sarcoptes scabiei*) mites and biting and sucking lice (*Trichodectes canis*, *Linognathus setosus*) in dogs, otodectic (*Otodectes cynotis*) mites in cats and generalized demodicosis (*Demodex canis*) in dogs (*Europe and Australia*). A single dorsal application on the skin at the base of the neck in front of the scapulae is recommended. If the volume of the total dose exceeds 4 ml, then the manufacturer recommends the dose is divided among multiple areas in the dorsal neck region. The formulation used most commonly in dogs and cats for extralabel use in veterinary dermatology is a 1% injectable solution licensed for use in cattle (Cydectin, Fort Dodge Animal Health).

Evaluation of moxidectin has a wide margin of safety in dogs. The oral dose of moxidectin shown to cause adverse effects in noncollie dog breeds is in the range of 2000 to 4000 mcg/kg. There was no evidence of toxicity when ivermectin-sensitive collies were administered oral moxidectin doses up to five and 30 times the recommended dose of 3 mcg/kg for heartworm prevention (Paul, Tranquilli, and Hutchens, 2000); however, the safety of higher moxidectin dosages in ivermectin-sensitive collies has not been evaluated. Transient ataxia, lethargy, inappetence, and vomiting have been reported in noncollie breeds administered 200 to 400 mcg/kg every 24 hours orally for the treatment of generalized demodicosis. Recently severe neurotoxicity, including ataxia, crawling, acoustic, and tactile hyperexcitability was reported in an Australian shepherd with a homozygous MDR-1 mutation after the administration of a single dose of moxidectin 400 mcg/kg orally (Geyer et al., 2005). There are no reports of side effects or moxidectin toxicity in the cat.

COMMON USES OF AVERMECTINS IN VETERINARY DERMATOLOGY

Sarcoptic Mange

Sarcoptic mange is a highly contagious, nonseasonal, pruritic skin condition caused by infestation with the burrowing mite *Sarcoptes scabiei*. Several macrocyclic lactones (e.g., ivermectin, milbemycin oxime, oral and topical moxidectin, and selamectin) have been used successfully for the control of canine sarcoptic mange. With the exception of selamectin and topical moxidectin, these drugs are not licensed for this purpose, and the clinician should obtain informed consent from the client before beginning treatment.

Ivermectin can be administered by subcutaneous injection, orally, or topically. Although experimental reports indicate that a single subcutaneous dose of 200 mcg/kg is effective, 200 to 400 mcg/kg every 7 days (orally) to 14 days (subcutaneously) for 4 to 6 weeks is more reliable. Because the mite can be highly contagious, all dogs and cats in contact with known affected animals also should be treated. The 0.5% pour-on at a dosage of 500 mcg/kg twice at 14-day intervals may be a convenient and economical alternative when large numbers of animals are involved. Precautions should be taken with the use of the topical formulation in ivermectin-sensitive collies and collielike breeds.

Selamectin is licensed as a topical spot-on formulation for application at a dosage of 6 to 12 mg/kg every 30 days for the treatment and control of canine scabies. Field studies conducted by the manufacturers reported comparable efficacy rates to a reference positive-control product when the drug was applied at 6 to 12 mg/kg on two occasions 30 days apart. However, other dermatologists and I have observed a small number of treatment failures when using the drug according to the manufacturer's recommendations, and there is concern about the potential misinterpretation of a negative response to a therapeutic trial. Consequently many dermatologists recommend using the extralabel protocol of 6 to 12 mg/kg every 14 days for three applications. This regimen is also effective against feline *Sarcoptes scabiei* infestation, although the drug is not registered for this purpose in the cat.

Milbemycin oxime at a dosage of 2 mg/kg every 7 days orally for 3 or 5 weeks was effective in 71% or 100%, respectively, of treated cases of canine scabies. Although more expensive than ivermectin, milbemycin at these dosages is well tolerated in collie and related breeds and therefore is a safe alternative therapy in high-risk breeds.

Topical 2.5% moxidectin spot-on formulation is licensed for the treatment and control of canine sarcoptic mange. Field studies conducted by the manufacturers reported comparable efficacy rates to a reference positive-control product when the drug was applied at 0.1 mg/kg on two occasions 4 weeks apart. Currently there are no independent studies published to support these data. Using the 1% injectable moxidectin formulation, 90% of dogs given 0.2 to 0.25 mg/kg every 7 days for 3 to 6 weeks either orally or by subcutaneous injection were cured; but side effects such as urticaria, angioedema, and ataxia were observed in seven dogs. Side effects appeared to occur more frequently with subcutaneous administration, and this route of administration probably should be avoided.

Injectable doramectin, 1%, has been shown to be effective in the treatment of sarcoptic mange in cattle, sheep, pigs, and Angora rabbits; but published information on its efficacy for the treatment of canine sarcoptic mange is sparse. A single subcutaneous dose of 200 mcg/kg has been used without adverse effect to successfully treat notoedric mange in cats.

Otodectic Mange

Otoacariasis is caused by *Otodectes cynotis*, an obligate parasite that inhabits the ear canals of dogs and cats. Ivermectin is effective at a dosage of 0.2 to 0.4 mg/kg every 7 days when given orally. The same dosage can be administered every 14 days by the subcutaneous route. At least 3 to 4 weeks of therapy is needed. All dogs and cats in contact with affected animal should also be treated. Ivermectin solution, 1%, diluted to 1:9 with propylene glycol administered every 24 hours via the otic route for 3 weeks cured all cats in one study, although some authors suggest that topical otic application is less effective than the subcutaneous route. Topical 0.5% ivermectin pour-on at a dosage of 0.5 mg/kg (0.1 ml/kg) twice at 14-day intervals is also effective.

Selamectin is licensed at the registered dose rate for the treatment and control of *Otodectes cynotis* in cats based on the results of controlled field trials by the manufacturer. An independent, uncontrolled trial using selamectin to treat naturally acquired feline otoacariasis failed to detect any mites within 17 days of treatment, although some cats had residual erythema and/or pruritus after testing negative for mites. Most dermatologists recommend the use of selamectin at 6 ml/kg at 14-day intervals for three applications for the treatment of otoacariasis, although the drug is not registered at this dose.

Topical 1% moxidectin is licensed for the treatment and control of otoacariasis in cats and kittens, and field studies conducted by the manufacturers reported 100% efficacy when the drug was applied at 0.1 mg/kg on two occasions 4 weeks apart. Currently there are no independent studies available to verify these data. Oral or subcutaneous moxidectin at 0.2 mg/kg has been shown to be effective in dogs when given twice at 10-day intervals, but reinfestation occurred in cats when a single subcutaneous injection was administered.

Cheyletiellosis

Cheyletiellosis is caused by the surface dwelling parasites *Cheyletiella blakei*, *Cheyletiella parasitovorax*, and *Cheyletiella yasguri* in dogs and cats. Currently there are no veterinary products licensed for treatment of cheyletiellosis. Affected animals can be treated with oral or injectable ivermectin at 200 to 300 mcg/kg at 7- (orally) to 14- (subcutaneously) day intervals for 6 to 8 weeks, providing the owner gives informed consent. Topical pour-on 0.5% ivermectin resolved infestation when applied to cats at 14-day intervals for four treatments. Ivermectin applied by this route was generally well tolerated, but a few cats developed a transient, alopecic patch and mild scaling at the site of application.

Selamectin may provide a safer alternative for the treatment of canine and feline cheyletiellosis, although the drug is not licensed for this purpose. In one study selamectin was effective in resolving infestation in cats when applied topically at a dosage of 6 mg/kg once a month for three applications, whereas 6 to 12 mg/kg applied topically at 14-day intervals for four applications achieved a successful outcome in dogs (Mueller, 2002).

In dogs milbemycin oxime has been shown to be effective in the control of cheyletiellosis when given at 2 mg/kg every 7 days orally for 3 weeks. However, a relapse in several dogs necessitated repeating the course of treatment.

Demodicosis

Canine demodicosis is a common skin disease encountered in veterinary practice. Ivermectin at a dosage of 300 to 600 mcg/kg every 24 hours orally is recommended for the treatment of generalized demodicosis. Although there are anecdotal reports that weekly subcutaneous administration of ivermectin is effective, the reported evidence strongly suggests a lack of efficacy using this dosing regimen. Ivermectin administered at a reduced dosage interval of 450 to 600 mcg/kg every 48 hours orally can be effective in some dogs, but treatment is generally required for a longer time period. Topical 0.5% pour-on ivermectin solution is ineffective.

Milbemycin oxime administered at a dosage of 2 mg/kg every 24 hours orally is very effective for the treatment of generalized demodicosis, but unfortunately the current lack of a commercially available product that can be safely administered on a daily basis has made this therapeutic option less viable. Moxidectin at a dosage of 200 to 400 mcg/kg every 24 hours orally is another milbemycin that has been evaluated in several studies for the therapy of canine demodicosis. Side effects reported include reversible ataxia, lethargy, inappetence, and vomiting. Although more studies are required to identify the safety of moxidectin in ivermectin-sensitive breeds, I believe, particularly in the absence of milbemycin, that oral moxidectin is a useful option in some dogs that cannot tolerate ivermectin administration. Topical 2.5% moxidectin is registered for the treatment of demodicosis at a dose of 0.1 ml/kg at 4-week intervals applied for two to four treatments. Although the manufacturer data report a reduction in mite numbers of 98% in dogs treated with this dosage regimen, mites were present in a significant proportion of dogs at the end of the study. Many dermatologists believe that topical 2.5% moxidectin at the registered dosages is not effective for the treatment of canine generalized demodicosis, and further studies are needed to ascertain whether the extralabel application of this product may improve the efficacy of treatment.

Doramectin has been used successfully for therapy of canine and feline generalized demodicosis in one study at a dosage regimen of 600 mcg/kg every 7 days subcutaneously (Johnstone, 2002). None of the animals in this study showed any adverse effects. Further investigations are needed to evaluate the usefulness of doramectin, and in my opinion caution should be exercised with the use of doramectin in ivermectin-sensitive breeds.

Fleas

Selamectin has adulticidal, larvicidal, and ovicidal effects against *Ctenocephalides felis* and is the only avermectin or milbemycin with any activity against flea infestation. Selamectin administered at the registered dose rate eliminates fleas between 12 and 24 hours after application in cats and between 24 and 36 hours after application in dogs. In multicenter field trials conducted by the manufacturer, selamectin applied at the registered dosage rate for 3 months reduced flea counts on day 30, 60, and 90 by 92.1%, 99%, and 99.8% in dogs and by 92.5%, 98.3%, and 99.3% in cats.

Ticks

Ivermectin reportedly has been used to treat tick infestation with *Ixodes ricinus* in cats, but I do not find ivermectin useful for tick control in dogs. Selamectin is registered for the control of *Rhipicephalus sanguineus* and *Dermacentor variabilis* in dogs at 6 to 12 mg/kg every 30 days, but most dermatologists use selamectin applied at 14-day intervals for three applications and then once a month for tick control, despite the fact that the drug is not registered at this dosage.

Lice

A single injection of ivermectin at a dosage of 200 mcg/kg subcutaneously or a single application of topical selamectin at 6 mg/kg is effective at eliminating biting lice *Trichodectes canis* in dogs and *Felicola subrostratus* in cats. Neither drug is registered for this purpose.

Fur mites

A single injection of ivermectin at a dose of 300 mcg/kg subcutaneously is effective at eliminating *Lynxacarus radovskyi* infestation in cats.

References and Suggested Reading

Curtis CF: Current trends in the treatment of *Sarc optes, Cheyletiella* and *Otodectes* mite infestations in dogs and cats, *Vet Dermatol* 15:109, 2004.

Geyer J et al: Development of a PCR-based diagnostic test detecting a nt230(del4) MDR1 mutation in dogs: verification in a moxidectin-sensitive Australian shepherd, *J Vet Pharmacol Ther* 28:95, 2005.

Gokbulut C et al: Comparative plasma disposition of ivermectin and doramectin following subcutaneous and oral administration in dogs, *Vet Parasitol* 135:347, 2006.

Johnstone I: Doramectin as a treatment for canine and feline demodicosis, *Aust Vet Pract* 32:98, 2002.

Mueller RS: Efficacy of selamectin in the treatment of canine cheyletiellosis, *Vet Rec* 151:773, 2002.

Mueller RS: Treatment protocols for demodicosis: an evidence-based review, *Vet Dermatol* 15:75, 2004.

Paul AJ, Tranquilli WJ, Hutchens DE: Safety of moxidectin in avermectin-sensitive collies, *Am J Vet Res* 61:482, 2000.

Shoop WL, Mrozik H, Fisher MH: Structure and activity of avermectins and milbemycins in animal health, *Vet Parasitol* 59:139, 1995.

Tranquilli WJ, Paul AJ, Todd KS: Assessment of toxicosis induced by high-dose administration of milbemycin oxime in collies, *Am J Vet Res* 52:1170, 1991.

Yas Natan E et al: Doramectin toxicity in a collie, *Vet Rec* 718, 2003.

CHAPTER 87

Hypoallergenic Diets: Principles in Therapy

HILARY A. JACKSON, *Glasgow, Scotland*

INDICATIONS AND USE OF HYPOALLERGENIC DIETS

Hypoallergenic diets are designed primarily for the diagnosis and management of adverse reactions to food ingredients in dogs and cats. There are also additional indications for their use in the patient with dermatologic disease. The following definitions are used in this discussion.

- Adverse food reaction: Any clinically abnormal response attributable to the ingestion of food or food additive
- Food intolerance: An abnormal physiologic response to food with no immunologic basis
- Food allergy: An immunologically mediated adverse food reaction

The ideal hypoallergenic diet used in the diagnosis and management of adverse food reactions should contain a protein source that is either novel to the animal under treatment or in a form that does not incite an adverse immunologic, pharmacologic, or toxicologic response. Commercially available diets generally are designed for the management of true food allergy, although the incidence of immunologically mediated disease in the dog and cat is currently unknown. In humans most food allergies are mediated by immunoglobulin (Ig)E antibodies and are most common in infants and young children (Sampson, 2004). Many food allergens have been characterized at the molecular level in humans, whereas those inciting specific reactions in dogs and cats are unknown. Food allergens are generally glycoproteins with a molecular weight greater than 10,000 kD, and they are stable to digestive processes. Molecules smaller than this are less likely to bridge two IgE molecules on the mast cell surface and incite degranulation, one of the first events in type one hypersensitivity reactions (Taylor et al., 1987).

The currently available commercial hypoallergenic diets contain either novel or hydrolyzed proteins with added carbohydrate and nutrients to balance for long-term feeding. It is assumed that it is the dietary protein that is allergenic, although there is a report of dogs with spontaneous food allergy reacting to cornstarch (Jackson et al., 2003). Whether this was a reaction to the carbohydrate itself or to traces of protein from the carbohydrate source is unknown and a high percentage of infants allergic to cow's milk will have adverse immunological and clinical reactions. This chapter considers a number of key issues related to hypoallergenic diets (see Section V on Evolve).

HYDROLYZED PROTEIN DIETS

Hydrolyzed protein diets have been available for many years in the human field, specifically for the management of infants with milk allergy. They consist of hydrolyzed (digested) protein and are available in two forms: partial and complete hydrolysates. These formulations have been subject to rigorous study in infants with proven cow's milk allergy. Before a claim for hypoallergenicity can be made, the complete hydrolysate formula should be demonstrated to be tolerated by 90% or more infants with milk allergy in double-blinded placebo-controlled conditions (Baker et al., 2000). The protein in complete milk protein hydrolysates is in the form of free amino acids and peptides less than 1500 kD. In contrast, the milk proteins in partially hydrolyzed formulations are not as extensively hydrolyzed (Rugo, Wall, and Wahn, 1992).

The hydrolyzed veterinary diets available at the time of this writing would be classified as partial hydrolysates (Table 87-1). There are a number of published studies supporting the use of veterinary hydrolysate diets for diet trials in dogs. A limitation in the recommendation of their use in veterinary patients is a lack of data documenting whether dogs allergic to the parent protein can tolerate the hydrolyzed product. Nestle Purina Veterinary Diets HA HypoAllergenic brand Canine Formula (Nestle Purina PetCare) containing hydrolyzed soy protein and cornstarch has been evaluated in two small studies in dogs with pruritic skin conditions. A randomized blinded feeding study demonstrated a reduction in pruritus in soy- and corn-allergic individuals of 50% and 80%, respectively, when fed this diet (Beale and Laflamme, 2001). When HA Formula was fed to Maltese-beagle mixed breed dogs with food allergy at North Carolina State University, 11 of 14 dogs with soy and/or corn allergy showed no adverse reaction (Jackson et al., 2003). In neither of these studies was the nature of the adverse food reaction truly known, although there is evidence that the disease in the Maltese-beagle mixed breed dogs may be mediated in part by IgE. In addition, these diets are recommended for the treatment of canine and feline adverse food reactions based on the assumption that most adverse food reactions in these species are mediated by IgE, as they are in humans. Since this is not necessarily the case, the size of the protein hydrolysate may not be critical, or paradoxically hydrolysis could enhance uptake and presentation to the immune system.

Table 87-1

Currently Available Hydrolyzed Diets As of 2008*

Name of Diet	Protein Hydrolysate	Carbohydrate	Formulation	Species
Purina veterinary diets HA hypoallergenic brand canine formula[1]	Soy	Cornstarch	Dry kibble	Canine
Purina veterinary diets HA hypoallergenic brand feline formula[1]	Soy, chicken	Rice	Dry kibble	Feline
Royal Canin Hypoallergenic DR21[2]	Soy, poultry	Rice	Dry kibble	Canine
Royal Canin Hypoallergenic DR25	Soy, poultry liver	Rice	Dry kibble	Feline
Prescription diet canine z/d low allergen[2]	Chicken	Rice	Dry kibble	Canine
Prescription diet canine z/d ULTRA allergen free[3]	Chicken	Cornstarch	Dry kibble	Canine
Prescription diet feline z/d low allergen[3]	Chicken	Rice	Dry kibble	Feline
Prescription diet feline z/d ULTRA allergen free[3]	Chicken	Cornstarch	Canned	Feline
Prescription diet canine z/d ULTRA allergen free[3]	Chicken	Cornstarch	Canned	Canine

*The availability of diets may vary with geographic region and formulations may be subject to change.
[1]Nestle Purina Petcare Company, St. Louis, Missouri.
[2]Royal Canin, Aimargues, France.
[3]Hills Pet Nutrition, Topeka, Kansas.

HOME-COOKED DIETS

Home-cooked diets are often advocated when performing a diet trial, thus avoiding pet food additives that might have the potential to cause adverse reactions. Although additives are often incriminated as causing adverse reactions in pets, there are no well-documented reports to support this idea. Home-cooked diets usually include a single novel protein and a single carbohydrate source, which have been selected on the basis of a good dietary history. An analysis of home-cooked diets in use by members of the American Academy of Veterinary Dermatology showed that these invariably were nutritionally inadequate for maintenance or growth (Roudebush and Cowell, 1992). Balanced recipes for home-cooked diets are available in various veterinary textbooks (Roudebush 1994; Remillard et al., 2000). The use of home-cooked diets may lead to poor client compliance because of the added effort required in diet preparation. The importance of client education cannot be overemphasized. In one study 36% of clients preparing home-cooked food for their dogs discontinued the diet trial prematurely (Tapp et al., 2002). Another investigator documented a failure rate of 52% of cases when the clients were asked to prepare home-cooked diets for their dogs; the failure rate dropped to 27% after better client education was instituted (Chesney, 2002).

There are reports of animals tolerating home-cooked diets but not a commercial equivalent (White, 1986; White and Sequoia, 1989; Jeffers et al., 1991). The reasons for this are unknown but may be related to differences in the processing of the proteins that can change form when heated and render them more or less allergenic. Food additives or the presence of vasoactive amines in commercial diets might also be causative (Roudebush, 2000). There has been recent interest from the pet-owning public in the feeding of raw meat diets to their pets. There is no justification in the use of these diets from the standpoint of diagnosis or management of the pet with food allergies. Furthermore, the use of these diets raises significant public health concerns related to the high bacterial burden often present on raw meat (see Chapter 37).

Whichever type of diet is used, the diet selected should be based on a thorough dietary history. This should include details of the main diet but also any treats, table scraps, and flavored toothpaste or toys to which the animal is exposed on a regular basis. Clients often hide pills in food for ease of administration of medications to their pets; thus, if therapy concurrent with the diet trial is prescribed, this practice must be discontinued. Cost and palatability are also important factors to consider. The protein in the diet should be one to which the animal has had little or no previous exposure. Unfortunately many of the protein sources currently used in prescription diets are now used in generally available pet foods, making dietary selection more challenging. In this context the hydrolyzed diets may become more useful.

Dogs with suspected atopic dermatitis, in which a dietary component of their disease is under investigation, are often less than 1 year of age. In most cases the commercially available hypoallergenic foods support growth for the 6- to 8-week period of the diet trial. However, this may not be the case in the giant breeds, and advice from an experienced nutritionist should be sought in this situation. Hypoallergenic diets specially formulated for the growing dog are available, and these should be fed preferentially. The use of home-cooked diets in growing animals must be undertaken with great care unless balanced by an experienced veterinary nutritionist. Calcium-phosphorus ratios are often incorrect and could lead to pathologic skeletal development. In the feline patient an unbalanced home-cooked diet should not be fed for more than 3 to 4 weeks.

ADDITIONAL BENEFITS OF HYPOALLERGENIC DIETS

Since most of the commercially available hypoallergenic diets have an enhanced ω-3 and ω-6 essential fatty acid (EFA) content, they can be useful in the management of dogs with impaired epidermal barrier structure or function. Ceramide-1, which contains α-linoleic acid, is an important component of the lipid barrier in the cornified layer of the epidermis. Thus supplementation with this ω-6 fatty acid has the potential to enhance skin health.

There is evidence that dogs with atopic dermatitis triggered by environmental allergens have structural impairment of the epidermal barrier (Inman et al., 2001), the consequences of which might be enhanced transepidermal allergen penetration, increased transepidermal water loss, and/or establishment of microbial infections. In addition, dogs with atopic dermatitis may have impaired fat absorption or increased plasma triglyceride clearance (van den Broek and Simpson, 1990); thus increased EFA intake might be beneficial in these cases and account for the clinical improvement often noted after feeding a hypoallergenic diet in the absence of proven adverse food reaction. In addition, dogs with primary or secondary disorders of cornification often benefit from the feeding of hypoallergen diet. Presumably because of increased epidermal turnover time in these diseases causing a relative EFA deficiency.

References and Suggested Reading

Baker SS et al: Hypoallergenic infant formulas, *Pediatrics* 106:346, 2000.

Beale KM, Laflamme DP: Comparison of a hydrolyzed soy protein diet containing corn starch with a positive and negative control diet in corn- or soy-sensitive dogs, *Vet Dermatol* 12:237, 2001.

Chesney CJ: Food sensitivity in the dog, a quantitative study, *J Small Anim Pract* 43:203, 2002.

Inman AO et al: Electron microscopic observations of the stratum corneum intercellular lipids in normal and atopic dogs, *Vet Dermatol* 4:151, 2001.

Jackson HA et al: Evaluation of the clinical and allergen specific serum IgE responses to oral challenge with cornstarch, corn, soy and a soy hydrolysate in dogs with spontaneous food allergy, *Vet Dermatol* 14:181, 2003.

Jeffers JG, Shanley KJ, Meyer EK: Diagnostic testing of dogs for food hypersensitivity, *J Am Vet Med Assoc* 198:245, 1991.

Remillard RL et al: Making pet foods at home. In Hand MS et al, editors: *Small animal clinical nutrition*, Topeka, Ks, 2000, Mark Morris Institute, p 163.

Roudebush P: Nutritional management of the allergic patient. In August JR, editor: *Seminars in feline internal medicine*, Philadelphia, 1994, Saunders, p 201.

Roudebush P: Adverse reactions to food. In Hand MS et al, editors: *Small animal clinical nutrition*, Topeka, Ks, 2000, Mark Morris Institute, p 438.

Roudebush P, Cowell CS: Results of a hypoallergenic diet survey of home-made diet prescriptions, *Vet Dermatol* 3:23, 2000.

Rugo ER, Wahl R, Wahn U: How allergenic are hypoallergenic infant formulae, *Clin Exp Allergy* 22:635, 1992.

Sampson HA: Update on food allergy, *J Allergy Clin Immunol* 113:805, 2004.

Tapp TC et al: Comparison of a commercial limited-antigen diet versus home-prepared diets in the diagnosis of canine adverse food reaction, *Vet Therapeut* 3:244, 2002.

Taylor SR et al: Food allergens: structure and immunological properties, *Ann Allergy* 59:93, 1987.

Van den Broek AHM, Simpson JW: Fat absorption in dogs with atopic dermatitis. In Tscharner C, Halliwell REW, editors: *Advances in veterinary dermatology 1*, London, 1990, Baillière-Tindall, p 155.

White SD: Food hypersensitivity in 30 dogs, *J Am Vet Med Assoc* 188:695, 1986.

White SD, Sequoia D: Food hypersensitivity in cats: 14 cases, *J Am Vet Med Assoc* 194:692, 1989.

CHAPTER **88**

Pentoxifylline

ROSANNA MARSELLA, *Gainesville, Florida*

INTRODUCTION

Pentoxifylline (PTX) is a methylxanthine derivative with multiple hemorrheologic and immunomodulatory properties. PTX is available as a generic or a brand name (Trental, 400-mg tablets). This drug has been used for almost 30 years in humans with intermittent claudication caused by peripheral and cerebrovascular atherosclerotic disease; however, the interest in veterinary medicine for PTX is relatively recent. The list of conditions for which PTX has been found to be beneficial has grown rapidly. This chapter reviews the use of PTX in small animal dermatology.

PROPERTIES OF PENTOXIFYLLINE

PTX is a nonspecific phosphodiesterase (PDE) inhibitor. Through its hemorrheologic properties, PTX changes the conformation of red blood cells and improves microcirculatory blood flow and tissue oxygenation. Aged red blood cells have rigid membranes because of reduced adenosine triphosphate levels and increased calcium. By increasing cyclic adenosine monophosphate (cAMP, the second messenger of the beta-adrenergic system), and by modulating intracellular calcium, PTX increases red blood cell deformability. Besides its effect on red blood cells, PTX also exerts its beneficial effects on platelets by decreasing platelet aggregation and blood viscosity. Once again, this is caused by the inhibition of PDE and the decrease in cAMP degradation. It is interesting to note that PTX restores normal cAMP levels and has an effect on aggregation only in conditions in which the platelets are hyperaggregable and have altered levels of cAMP. PTX does not appear to effect normal platelets and therefore does not prolong bleeding.

PTX exerts multiple beneficial effects on the inflammatory cascade by increasing intracellular cAMP and decreasing TNF-α synthesis. Since TNF-α is a proinflammatory cytokine with a broad spectrum of actions, its decrease leads to multiple antiinflammatory effects. These include a decreased release of other proinflammatory cytokines such as interleukin (IL)-1 and IL-6, decreased leukocyte adhesion and aggregation, decreased neutrophil degranulation and superoxide release, inhibition of B cell activation (by suppressing IL-6 synthesis), and inhibition of T cell activation (through CD23 and CD26 pathway) (Bruynzee, 1995). Based on *in vitro* studies, the decrease of cytokine expression is dose dependent. The beneficial effects of PTX have been shown in numerous animal studies using models of ischemia-reperfusion and septic shock (Zhang, 1994). In these studies PTX significantly improved survival rates by both decreasing the inflammatory reaction and improving tissue oxygenation. Finally PTX also improves wound healing by increasing fibroblast collagenases and decreasing collagen production, fibronectin, glycosaminoglycans, and fibroblast response to TNF-α.

PHARMACOKINETICS

The pharmacokinetics and pharmacodynamic properties of PTX have been well characterized in human patients. PTX is rapidly and extensively absorbed after oral administration (Marsella et al., 1997). After absorption from the gastrointestinal tract, it binds to the red blood cells, where it is immediately reduced to metabolite 1 (M1). This transformation is reversible, and M1, which also binds to the erythrocyte membrane, serves as a reservoir for PTX. The other six metabolites are formed in the liver and appear in plasma soon after dosing. Extensive enterohepatic recycling occurs, and more than 90% of the absorbed drug is excreted in the urine in the form of metabolites. M1 and M5 are the major metabolites, and the plasma levels of these compounds are five and eight times greater, respectively, than the parental drug. Bioavailability in humans averages 20% to 30% and is affected by food. Excretion is almost completely urinary. M1 and M5 are present in the highest concentration in the urine, whereas no PTX is found in the urine.

Only a few studies have been done in dogs to evaluate the disposition of PTX and its active metabolites. In one study (Marsella et al., 2000) PTX was found to be rapidly absorbed and eliminated after oral administration. Peak plasma concentration for PTX (15 mg/kg) was achieved 30 minutes after oral administration. Concentrations rapidly declined, and no drug was detected after 4 hours. After intravenous administration (15 mg/kg), elimination proceeded rapidly, and no drug was detectable after 3 hours. Peak plasma concentration of M1 and M5 after intravenous and oral administration was achieved after 20 minutes and

60 minutes, respectively. Mean bioavailability after oral administration ranged from 15% to 32% among treatment groups and was not affected by the presence of food. Higher plasma PTX concentrations and apparent bioavailability were observed after oral administration of the first dose compared with the last dose during the 5-day treatment regimens. It was concluded that oral administration of PTX at 15 mg/kg resulted in plasma concentrations similar to those produced by therapeutic doses in humans and that a three-times-a-day dosing regimen was the most appropriate. No adverse effects were observed.

In another study (Rees et al., 2003) PTX was readily metabolized and bioavailable (50% ± 26%). Both active metabolites (M1 and M5) were detectable, with M5 predominating. Human drug therapeutic concentrations (1000 ng/ml) were present for 170 ± 24 minutes following intravenous administration and 510 ± 85 minutes after oral dosing. This study emphasized the large variability of absorption and disposition of PTX in dogs. None of the dogs experienced any adverse effects after PTX administration. No hematologic effects were detected.

ADVERSE EFFECTS OF PENTOXIFYLLINE

In contrast to other methylxanthines, PTX has few cardiac effects. PTX can be a gastric irritant, and in humans the main adverse effect is gastrointestinal upset (e.g., vomiting and diarrhea). Other reported adverse effects in humans include angina/chest pain, agitation, dizziness, headache, and tremors. Side effects are dose related and can be decreased by lowering the dose. Dogs appear to tolerate oral PTX very well, even on an empty stomach. Gastrointestinal upset can be seen, although it is not common. I have observed some short-coated dogs that develop transient flush and erythematous macules.

INDICATIONS FOR USE IN VETERINARY DERMATOLOGY

PTX has been used for a variety of dermatologic conditions with variable success. Since several of the conditions have a waxing and waning course and many of the studies done were open studies, a scientific evaluation of the efficacy of the drug was not always possible. Nevertheless the list of dermatologic diseases for which PTX has been reported to be beneficial is quite extensive.

Dermatomyositis

Canine familial dermatomyositis is an inflammatory disease in which microvascular vasculopathy is thought to play a role. Therefore dermatomyositis was one of the first dermatologic diseases in which PTX was tried and reported to have useful effects. In the management of dermatomyositis cases PTX is usually considered as a steroid-sparing agent and rarely as the only form of treatment (Jennette, 2003). The advantage of using PTX is the better safety profile and the lack of atrophogenic properties when compared to glucocorticoids. The response to treatment is variable and typically slow (2 to 3 months). Historically a large range of dosages and treatment regimens have been suggested. Recommended dosage ranges from 200 to 400 mg once daily or once every other day. Based on a study by Rees and colleagues (2003) it appears that 25 mg/kg twice daily resulted in positive clinical response (4/10 complete, 6/10 partial response). In that study the authors investigated whether a direct correlation could be established between concentrations of PTX and its metabolites and clinical response and concluded that, because of the variability in disposition and metabolite formation among individuals, monitoring of PTX did not offer a therapeutic advantage.

Contact Allergy

PTX has also been used with success for the prevention of clinical signs caused by contact allergy. The rationale behind the use of PTX for contact allergy is its ability to decrease the production of TNF-α, an important inflammatory mediator in this condition, to down-regulate the expression of adhesion molecules on keratinocytes, and to suppress T cell adherence to keratinocytes. PTX has been reported to suppress patch test reactions in human patients and, when taken 48 hours before exposure, either abolished or drastically decreased the development of clinical signs of contact allergy (Schwarz et al., 1993a, 1993b). The same observations appear to hold for dogs with contact allergy to plants of the Commelinenceae family. In that study PTX was able to prevent contact allergy at a dose of 10 mg/kg twice daily).

I have observed that the protective effect appears to be dose related. Clinical benefit seems to be evident after 2 days of oral therapy (10 mg/kg) and does not last for a prolonged period of time after discontinuation of therapy (1 week) (Marsella et al., 1997). Based on these clinical observations and the more recent information regarding the pharmacokinetic properties of this drug in dogs, I currently use PTX at 15 mg/kg two to three times daily to improve efficacy in severe cases.

PTX does not appear to have been studied as treatment of contact allergy once lesions have already developed. Because of the moderate antiinflammatory properties of this drug, it probably would be more effective to treat active lesions of contact allergy with glucocorticoids and use PTX as a preventive agent before exposure to the offending allergen.

Canine Atopic Dermatitis

PTX has also been used for the management of canine atopic dermatitis (AD). The rationale behind its use is that PTX is a PDE inhibitor; thus it stabilizes a variety of cells, including mast cells, and has the ability to suppress the synthesis of many proinflammatory cytokines that play a role in atopic dermatitis (e.g., TNF-α, IL-6), indirectly affecting the release of chemokines that would mediate the recruitment of leukocytes in the skin. Although we are still lacking a comprehensive understanding of the pathogenesis of this disease, all of the antiinflammatory properties of PTX have been proposed to be beneficial in patients suffering from AD.

There has been one randomized, double-blinded, placebo-controlled study that has evaluated the efficacy of PTX for the management of canine AD (Marsella and Nicklin, 2000). In that study the clinical efficacy and the effect of 4 weeks of PTX on intradermal skin test reactivity were evaluated. PTX decreased owners' and investigator's pruritus scores and investigator's erythema scores, although most dogs had residual clinical signs at the end of the trial. No suppression on immediate intradermal skin test reactivity was detected, whereas delayed reactions were decreased. It was concluded that PTX may be considered as an adjunctive treatment for canine AD, especially to reduce the frequency of administration of glucocorticoids.

Anecdotally it appears that older dogs and dogs with reactions mostly to grasses seem to have the best clinical response to PTX therapy. I tend to use this drug in geriatric dogs in which the use of glucocorticoids or cyclosporine is contraindicated. This is based on the large safety and tolerability profile of PTX in dogs, and a reported improvement in the overall cognitive function of these patients in conjunction with a beneficial effect on their skin condition. The better response in patients with mostly grass allergies is an interesting clinical observation in light of the recent observations on the importance of the epicutaneous route of allergen exposure in canine AD and the speculation that some individuals may suffer from a combination of both contact allergy and AD.

Vasculitis

PTX is commonly used as steroid-sparing agent for the treatment of vasculitis of various origins (Atzori, 1999; Milling, 1994). The most commonly used dosage is 10 to 15 mg/kg twice daily (Nichol, Morris, and Beale, 2001). This is because of the combination of its potent hemorheologic properties (which increase erythrocyte deformability, thus allowing the cells to more readily pass through compromised blood vessels) and its antiinflammatory effects. Unfortunately the onset of clinical benefit is slow, and several weeks to months may be required to observe clinical response. In human patients this time frame has been reported to range from 2 weeks to 14 months. Thus PTX is rarely used alone in the early phases of therapy. It is usually combined with glucocorticoids; this combination is hypothesized to have synergistic effect in the ability to decrease inflammation, possibly through the common ability to decrease TNF-α synthesis.

Because PTX is commonly used in combination in cases that show favorable response, it is sometimes difficult to assess the exact benefit of therapy. Nevertheless I have had several cases that were well controlled just on PTX after glucocorticoids were discontinued but would relapse if PTX were discontinued. Similarly I have seen cases that were well controlled on Trental that would relapse once switched to generic PTX. This clinical observation has raised concerns about whether generics can be considered equivalent to Trental. Unfortunately no studies have been done to investigate this question; thus no definitive recommendation can be made at this time other than to consider switching to Trental when generic formulations of PTX do not have clinical benefit.

Symmetric Lupoid Onychodystrophy

Symmetric lupoid onychodystrophy is a syndrome with multiple possible causes, including vasculitis and immune-mediated mechanisms. For this reason PTX has been used either as sole therapy or in conjunction with other immunomodulatory treatments. In one retrospective study (Mueller, Rosychuk, and Jonas, 2003) PTX was used in six dogs. Excellent response was observed in two dogs, and a good response in two others. The remaining two patients showed no improvement. One of the dogs with an excellent response had previously not responded to treatment with doxycycline, niacinamide, and fatty acids for 4 months and then underwent spontaneous remission for 6 months. When clinical signs recurred, this dog responded rapidly to PTX. As it is for other conditions, clinical benefit is slow; thus PTX should be tried for several months before improvement can be fully assessed.

Miscellaneous Conditions

There are anecdotal reports of PTX therapy of other vasculopathies, including thrombovascular necrosis, ear pinna dermatosis, rabies vaccine–related alopecia, greyhound vasculopathy, and metatarsal fistulae of German shepherds. Similarly PTX has been tried in diseases in which necrosis is a concern such as spider bites. Because of the role of TNF-α in erythema multiforme, PTX can be beneficial in cases in which an underlying cause for erythema multiforme cannot be identified, particularly in geriatric cases that have recurrent disease. Because of its combined antiinflammatory properties and the ability to decrease fibrosis, PTX also can be considered as adjunctive therapy for dogs with lick granulomas. Another potential use for PTX could be as adjunctive therapy in canine patients diagnosed with cancer and undergoing chemotherapy to possibly counteract the negative consequence of excessive release of TNF-α.

References and Suggested Reading

Atzori L, Ferreli C, Biggio P: Less common treatment in cutaneous vasculitis, *Clin Dermatol* 17:641, 1999.

Bruynzeel I, Liesbeth MH, Stoof TJ: Pentoxifylline inhibits T-cell adherence to keratinocytes, *J Invest Dermatol* 104:1004, 1995.

Hargis AM, Mundell AC: Familial canine dermatomyositis, *Compend Contin Educ* 14:855, 1992.

Jennette CJ, Rees CA, Boothe DM: Therapeutic response to pentoxifylline and its active metabolites in dogs with familial canine dermatomyositis, *Vet Ther* 4:234, 2003.

Marsella R, Nicklin CF: Double-blind placebo-controlled, crossover clinical trial on the efficacy of pentoxifylline in canine atopy, *Vet Dermatol* 11:255, 2000.

Marsella R, Kunkle GA, Lewis DT: Use of pentoxifylline in the treatment of allergic contact reactions to plants of the Commelinenceae family in dogs, *Vet Dermatol* 8:121, 1997.

Marsella R et al: Pharmacokinetics of pentoxifylline in dogs after oral and intravenous administration, *Am J Vet Res* 61:631, 2000.

Milling DM, Falk RJ: Vasculitis affecting the skin, *Arch Dermatol* 130:899, 1994.

Mueller RS, Rosychuk RA, Jonas LD: A retrospective study regarding the treatment of lupoid onychodystrophy in 30 dogs and literature review, *J Am Anim Hosp Assoc* 39:139, 2003.

Nichols PR, Morris DO, Beale KM: A retrospective study of canine and feline cutaneous vasculitis, *Vet Dermatol* 12:255, 2001.

Rees CA et al: Dosing regimen and hematologic effects of pentoxifylline and its active metabolites in normal dogs, *Vet Ther* 4:188, 2003.

Schwarz A et al: Pentoxifylline suppresses allergic patch test reactions in humans, *Arch Dermatol* 129:513, 1993a.

Schwarz A et al: Pentoxifylline suppresses irritant and contact hypersensitivity reactions, *J Invest Dermatol* 101:549, 1993b.

Zhang H et al: Pentoxifylline improves the tissue oxygen extraction capabilities during endotoxic shock, *Shock* 2 (2):90, 1994.

CHAPTER 89

Glucocorticoids in Veterinary Dermatology

CANDACE A. SOUSA, *El Dorado Hills, California*

WHAT ARE THEY?

Steroids are hormones that are manufactured from and resemble cholesterol. Structurally these hormones consist of three hexane rings and one pentane ring, which collectively are known as the steroid nucleus. Steroids are produced primarily in the cortex of the adrenal gland, but other organs such as the testicles and ovaries also contribute to their production. Some of the metabolically active substances included in this group are the sex hormones, bile acids, and cortisone.

Androgens such as testosterone and estrogens are *steroids that contain 19 carbon atoms. Corticosteroids* (or *corticoids*) *(CSs)* are 21-carbon steroid hormones that are produced by the adrenal cortex. Progesterone is secreted in minute amounts by the adrenal cortex and is also a 21-carbon hormone. The major stimulus for the adrenal cortex to synthesize and secrete steroids is *adrenocorticotropic hormone*

(*ACTH*), which in turn is synthesized in and released from the pituitary gland. ACTH release is stimulated by *cortico-tropin-releasing factor (CRF)*, produced by the hypothalamus. *Mineralocorticoids (MCs)* are CSs produced primarily in the zona glomerulosa of the adrenal cortex. They exert their greatest effect on electrolyte metabolism—sodium, potassium, and chloride in particular. The most potent naturally occurring member of this group is aldosterone. Its main actions are induction of renal tubular resorption of sodium and increased renal excretion of potassium. Its release is mediated through the renin-angiotensin feedback mechanism.

CSs that increase gluconeogenesis (i.e., cause an increase in blood sugars and liver glycogen) are called *glucocorticoids (GCs)*. These are products of the inner zones of the adrenal cortex, the zonac fasciculata, and reticularis. The primary physiologic CS is *cortisol*, also termed *hydrocortisone*. At least 95% of the GC activity of the adrenocortical secretions results from the secretion of cortisol. In humans cortisol is estimated to be produced at a rate of 10 mg/day. The daily production rate of cortisol can rise tenfold in response to severe stress. In dogs daily cortisol production is 0.2 to 1 mg/kg/day. No information is available for cats.

Cortisone is the synthetic inactive form of the hormone cortisol. The active form of the hormone cortisol is formed in the liver by the action of 11β-hydroxysteroid dehydrogenase (type 1). If an additional double bond is added to cortisone, the result is increased GC activity and a decreased rate of degradation. The product of this first synthetic change is *prednisone*, which is also an inactive GC and requires hydroxylation in the liver at the C-11 position by 11β-hydroxysteroid dehydrogenase, converting it to *prednisolone*, the biologically active form of the hormone (Fig. 89-1). There is positive evidence that cats and probably horses may not absorb prednisone well or convert it to prednisolone in the liver, making the latter a more appropriate therapeutic choice in these species.

Methylprednisolone (Medrol, Pfizer Animal Health) is formed by the addition of a methyl group to prednisolone at C-6. This tends to decrease the salt-retaining effects and slightly increases the GC effects. When a fluorine molecule is added to hydrocortisone at the C-9 position, this results in increased GC but also marked MC activity (fludrocortisone). Further modification by methylation at C-16 results

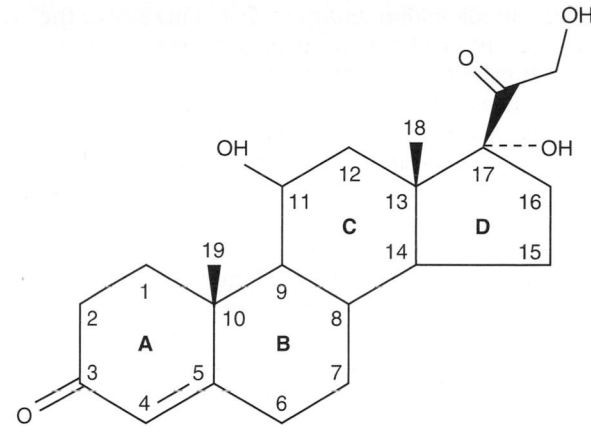

Hydrocortisone (cortisol)

Prednisone

Fig. 89-1 The chemical structure of naturally occurring hydrocortisone (cortisol, an active compound) compared with synthetic prednisone (an inactive compound) (the difference in the structure from hydrocortisone is circled).

in the synthesis of *dexamethasone* or *betamethasone*. These latter two molecules have high GC but low MC effects.

The duration of action of synthetic GCs is determined by the structure of the drug molecule. This in turn determines potency and the dose used. Generally the larger the dose and the more potent the GC, the longer the drug will have an effect (Table 89-1). However, in the clinical situation the

Table **89-1**

Comparison of Water-Soluble Glucocorticoids Used in Dogs and Cats

Generic Drug	Relative Mineralocorticoid Potency	Relative Glucocorticoid Potency (Antiinflammatory Potency)	Equivalent Dose (mg)	Plasma Half-life (hours)	Duration of Action (adrenal suppression) in Humans (hours)
Hydrocortisone	1	1	20	1	<12
Prednisone/prednisolone	0.8	4	5	(?) 1	12-36
Methylprednisolone	0.5	5	4	1.5	12-36
Triamcinolone*	0	3 - 5	4	(?) 4	24-48
Dexamethasone	0	25-30	0.75	2	>48
Betamethasone	0	25-30	0.6	(?) 5	>48
Flumethasone		30	1.5		>48

*Triamcinolone acetonide has a greater potency (approaching that of dexamethasone).

route of administration and the water solubility of the carrier substance usually are more important factors affecting the duration of action. Generally oral GCs are formulated as a free base or an ester that is digested to the free base and subsequently absorbed. Parenteral GCs (i.e., injectable) are usually esters of acetate, diacetate, sodium phosphate, or sodium succinate. The sodium phosphate and succinate esters are very water soluble and rapidly attain serum levels even when given intramuscularly (i.e., prednisolone sodium succinate, Solu-Delta-Cortef, Pfizer Animal Health). In contrast, the acetate or diacetate esters are poorly water soluble and are slowly absorbed, providing a continuous low level of GC for several days to weeks (i.e., methylprednisolone acetate, Depo-Medrol, Pfizer Animal Health). This slow absorption may greatly prolong the adrenal suppressive effects. Concern regarding adrenal suppression is the basis for the recommendation of alternate-day dosing of short-acting oral GCs when long-term treatment is needed.

HOW DO THEY WORK?

The primary role of endogenous CSs is the maintenance of homeostasis. GCs influence a variety of body functions because they affect nearly every cell in the body, altering the function of multiple systems. They exert most of their actions by binding to steroid receptors on the plasma membrane and in the cytoplasm of target cells. The complex is then transported to the nucleus, where it binds to cellular deoxyribonucleic acid and alters gene expression.

In general, GCs alter carbohydrate, fat, and protein metabolism; fibroblast proliferation (important for wound healing); the inflammatory response; electrolyte and water balance; synthesis of red blood cells; central nervous system function; gastric acid production; muscle strength and function; the immune system (especially the inate arm of the immune system); and a variety of other metabolic processes. As stated earlier, GCs seem to have some effect on almost every metabolic process.

One of the most important medical uses of CSs relates to their antiinflammatory effects. Inflammation comprises the changes in the tissue in response to injury. There are four classical signs of inflammation: pain (dolor), heat (color), redness (rubor), and swelling (tumor). When tissue injury occurs, whether it be by bacteria, trauma, chemicals, or any other phenomenon, histamine and other humoral substances are liberated by the damaged cells into the surrounding fluids. This causes an increase in local blood flow as well as the permeability of capillaries, allowing large quantities of fluid and cells to leak into the tissue. The exact mechanism of action by which GCs decrease inflammation is unknown, but they decrease or prevent tissue responses to inflammatory processes, thereby reducing the symptoms of inflammation without affecting the underlying cause.

GCs stabilize the membranes of lysosomes so they rupture with difficulty. This helps prevent the usual tissue damage and destruction that occurs when lysosomal enzymes are released. GCs also decrease the production of bradykinin, which is a potent vasodilator that also increases permeability of the capillary membrane during inflammation. GCs minimize the inflammatory response through

the action of lipomodulin, which inhibits phospholipase A_2, which normally converts membrane phospholipids into arachidonic acid (AA), a proinflammatory product. The decrease in AA limits available precursor molecules for lipoxygenase and cyclooxygenase to produce the AA-derived mediators of inflammation. Last, GCs inhibit the expression of adhesion molecules on the endothelial cells (particularly ELAM-1 and ICAM-1) and thereby interfere with the movement of leukocytes from the vasculature into inflamed tissues. This is the cause of the commonly noted leukocytosis seen with GC administration.

GCs block the inflammatory response to an allergic reaction exactly the same way that they block other types of inflammation. The basic allergic reaction between an antigen and antibody is not affected, and even some of the secondary effects of the allergic reaction such as the release of histamine still occur. However, because the subsequent inflammatory response is responsible for many of the serious and sometimes fatal effects of the allergic reaction, administration of GCs can be lifesaving.

Immunosuppression induced by CSs is not completely understood. CSs generally are considered less immunosuppressive than antiinflammatory. Prevention of inflammatory mediator release, inhibition of inflammatory cell migration to and response at the site, reduced capillary permeability, and the prevention of passage of immune complexes through endothelial and basement membranes all provide beneficial effect in treating immune-mediated diseases. The functional capacity of monocytes, macrophages, and eosinophils is decreased via inhibition of the formation of interleukins. The alteration of the movement and circulation of leukocytes may alter the immune response. The effect on the cellular arm of the immune system is more pronounced than the effect on the humoral arm. GCs have minimal effects on plasma immunoglobulin concentrations but can modulate immunoglobulin function. For example, opsonization of bacteria is inhibited.

At immunosuppressive doses (the exact dose has not been determined scientifically) GCs can induce decreased production of intracellular signaling cytokines such as interleukin (IL)-1, IL-6, tumor necrosis factor-α, interferon-γ, and granulocyte-macrophage colony-stimulating factor (GM-CSF). These are the signals that T and B lymphocytes use to communicate, and decreased production of intracellular signaling cytokines related to glucocorticoid therapy results in an alteration of the immune system at multiple stages. In general, there is a decline in the number of leukocytes at the site of infection or inflammation and an interference with their function.

GCs cause marked changes in leukocyte numbers and distribution. A mature neutrophilia is a characteristic component of a physiologic stress response as well as a response to exogenous GC treatment. Increases in circulating neutrophils occurs from a combination of an increased release of mature neutrophils from the bone marrow, decreased margination, and decreased migration of neutrophils out of the blood vessels, resulting in a prolonged circulatory half-life.

In contrast, the administration of GCs leads to a decreased number of circulating lymphocytes, eosinophils, and basophils. Lymphopenia results from a redistribution of circulating lymphocytes to nonvascular lymphatic compartments such as the lymph nodes. Since lymphopenia is not a marked or a consistent component of the feline stress leukogram, this species is considered relatively steroid resistant.

Systemic GCs are probably the most commonly used drugs in veterinary medicine and are undoubtedly the most commonly used and abused drugs in veterinary dermatology. Their intended and appropriate use in veterinary dermatology is for their antipruritic, antiinflammatory, and immunomodulatory properties. A beneficial response is seen in animals with pruritic diseases, allergic disorders, inflammatory skin diseases, and autoimmune or immune-mediated dermatoses.

The specific GC effects that occur with their therapeutic use are summarized in Box 89-1, and need be considered, particularly if ongoing therapy will be needed. The following sections consider adverse effects and specific uses of GCs in veterinary dermatology.

ADVERSE EFFECTS

As with any other class of drugs, CSs have clear value when used to treat a disorder for which they have proven therapeutic benefit and when administered at the appropriate dose, frequency, and duration of administration. Their recognized antiinflammatory and immunosuppressive effects make them a valuable addition to veterinary medicine. There is no question that side effects occur with GC therapy. However, excessive concern for these may prevent the appropriate use of this class of drugs when they are indeed indicated. The use of CSs tends to be shunned by some practitioners who worry about iatrogenic suppression of the hypothalamic-pituitary-adrenal (HPA) axis, immune suppression, and other side effects.

The benefits of any therapy must always be weighed against the possible and/or probable side effects. It is well recognized that the excessive use of GCs can be associated with many adverse effects. Although GCs are desired for their therapeutic effects, their antiinflammatory and immunosuppressive actions may facilitate the establishment or spread of other infectious or parasitic diseases. As a result, dogs treated with GCs have a tendency to develop secondary bacterial infections of the skin, urinary tract, or respiratory tract. Urinary tract infections have been documented in 18% (Torres et al., 2005) to 39% (Ihrke et al., 1985) of dogs treated with 0.28 to 0.8 mg/kg/ day of GCs for more than 6 months.

The most serious side effects of CS are related to prolonged use of large doses, which may suppress the HPA axis. The effects of chronic elevations in GC levels are readily seen with naturally occurring hyperadrenocorticism (Cushing's disease). Unfortunately the same problems can be created by overuse of GCs by the veterinarian and/or client, even when administered on an alternate-day basis. These high levels of exogenous steroids can result in a hyperglycemia, fat redistribution and a pendulous abdomen, decreased skin elasticity, atrophy of the skin, poor wound healing, poor-quality coarse hair, alopecia (e.g., hair loss from breakage and failure to regrow), comedones (e.g., follicular plugs or blackheads), a variety of bacterial infections (especially of the bladder and skin), and even calcinosis cutis (e.g., mineral deposits in the skin). Localized dermal and adnexal atrophy following subcutaneous and occasional intramuscular repositol GCs have also been reported. If the GC used also has low MC effects, polyuria (e.g., production of an increased amount of urine) and polydipsia (e.g., drinking an excessive amount) may also be present.

In addition, GCs have effects on other body systems. Through various feedback loops they can suppress the synthesis and secretion of thyroid-stimulating hormone, follicle-stimulating hormone, prolactin and luteinizing hormone, and growth hormone. GCs have direct positive chronotropic and inotropic actions on the heart. They enhance vasoconstriction and decrease capillary permeability (including that induced by inflammation.) Blood pressure is increased. GCs also enhance lipolysis, and fatty acids are mobilized from adipose tissue; however, they also enhance appetite, which stimulates hyperinsulinemia and results in lipogenesis.

Iatrogenic secondary adrenocortical insufficiency is a side effect that can be seen after withdrawal of the GC therapy. When an animal is treated with a GC, the adrenal glands, in natural response to the effect of the exogenous GCs on the HPA axis, stop producing steroid hormones for a period of time. The duration of this suppressive effect is known to be dependent on the type of steroid and duration of treatment. However, the precise degree and length of suppression in any individual dog cannot be predicted. One intravenous injection of dexamethasone at 0.1 mg/kg, which equals approximately 3 mg/kg of hydrocortisone (cortisol) or three times the highest daily natural production, can suppress the HPA axis for 32 hours in a healthy dog (Kemppainen and Sartin, 1984). In general, the longer the therapy and the higher the dose, the longer the time before natural production of steroid hormones by the adrenal gland returns. This resultant lack of endogenous (physiologic) GCs is the cause of weakness and possible circulatory collapse that can occur with cessation of exogenous GC therapy.

Box 89-1

Specific Cellular and Antiinflammatory Effects of Glucocorticoids

1. Suppress the release of CRF by the hypothalamus and ACTH by the pituitary gland (caused by negative feedback inhibition) and therefore suppress the release of CSs by the adrenal cortex
2. Reduce the number of circulating lymphocytes through redistribution and suppress T lymphocyte function
3. Reduce the number of circulating eosinophils
4. Help maintain cell membrane integrity
5. Inhibit macrophage function
6. Suppress antibody function
7. Inhibit the release of endogenous pyrogen (IL-1)
8. Depress prostaglandin and leukotriene synthesis
9. Alter the complement and kinin cascades
10. Interfere with leukocyte migration and adhesion
11. Suppress lysosomal release from neutrophils by stabilizing lysosomal membranes
12. Suppress phagocytosis
13. Reduce fibroblast activity that causes delayed healing and thinning of the skin
14. Effect enzyme actions and other cellular functions

CONTRAINDICATIONS TO THE USE OF CORTICOSTEROIDS

Because GCs cause an elevation in blood glucose, caution should be exercised when they are administered to animals with diabetes mellitus. Concurrent use with nonsteroidal antiinflammatory drugs should be minimized because of the increased risk of gastrointestinal ulceration. When used together, gastric protection should be strongly considered. The use of GCs should be avoided in pregnant animals since to avoid induction of parturition. Congestive heart failure has been reported in cats as a possible side effect, likely related to effects on cardiac muscle and stimulation of water retention.

USE OF CORTICOSTEROIDS IN VETERINARY DERMATOLOGY

Cortisone and ACTH were first used to treat a variety of inflammatory dermatoses in humans in the 1950s. The major indications for their use in veterinary dermatology include treatment of allergic or pruritic dermatoses, autoimmune dermatoses, and feline eosinophilic granulomas.

Because the GCs affect every cell in the body in often beneficial but also potentially negative ways, it is important to administer these medications to produce the maximum positive effect with the fewest side effects. The use of GCs is an art that requires the clinician to skillfully integrate knowledge of patient details, the owner's care and perceptions, and the disease so that an appropriate type and dose of GC can be used. Changes and adjustment in doses and even in the type of CS used may be needed depending on the response of the disease and the adverse effects that develop. Physiologic doses of GC are those that approximate the daily cortisol production by normal individuals. In dogs daily cortisol production has been reported to be 0.2 to 1 mg/kg/day. A pharmacologic dose of GC exceeds physiologic requirements. There is no optimal dose established in the veterinary literature, and each case should be treated individually. The primary guideline is to always use the lowest induction dose necessary to gain effective control of the clinical signs for the shortest amount of time and then to taper the amount even lower if possible to maintain control of the condition. There are guidelines that serve as a good starting point. Using oral prednisone or prednisolone (or methylprednisolone) in dogs as the drug of choice, the recommendations are:

Antipruritic dosages: 0.5 mg/kg/day for 3 to 10 days; then decreased to lowest effective dosage
Antiinflammatory doses: 1 to 1.5 mg/kg/day for 7 to 10 days; then decreased to the lowest effective dosage
Immunosuppressive doses: 2 to 6 mg/kg/day for induction; then decreased as possible to maintain control of the disease

Compared with dogs, cats seem to require about twice the dose of oral GCs to achieve the same effects.

LONG-TERM USAGE OF GLUCOCORTICOIDS

The use of alternate-day therapy has been recommended to minimize adrenocortical suppression and the other side/adverse effects of the prolonged administration of GCs. For alternate-day therapy to be successful, the administration of GCs with a duration of action of 12 to 36 hours (prednisone, prednisolone, or methylprednisolone) is necessary.

The following section presents my personal opinions regarding the generally safe dosages of GCs when used long term. There is no evidence-based formula regarding safe dosing in dogs and cats, and the disease as well as individual variation and adverse effects must be considered.

My formula for dogs is as follows. Starting with the concept that dogs manufacture 0.2 to 1 mg/kg/day of cortisol and need this to survive and using a 40-kg dog as an example:

$$40\,kg \times 0.4\,mg \times 365\,days = 5840\,mg\ of\ cortisol$$
produced/year (I chose 0.4 mg since it is on the lower side of the mid range for production)

Since prednisone (or prednisolone) is considered approximately four times as potent as hydrocortisone (cortisol), dividing 5840 by 4 equals 1460 mg of prednisone. Thus this 40-kg dog would "see" in a normal physiologic state approximately 1460 mg of prednisone (or prednisolone) per year.

From these calculations I have developed what I called my "safe annual steroid dose" formula:

$$Body\ weight\ (BW)(kg) \times 30 = milligrams\ of\ prednisone$$
per year
$$or\ BW\ (lb) \times 15 = milligrams\ of\ prednisone\ per\ year$$

365 Days times 0.4 equals 36.5; but, for the sake of ease of mathematics and to be even safer, I have chosen to use the number 30. This number (30) is based on a combination of several publications reporting the side effects of GCs as related to dose and on over 10 years of using this formula in my own practice and arriving at the safe use.

Again considering the 40-kg dog, I would calculate: $40 \times 30 = 1200\,mg$ of prednisone to be the "safe annual steroid dose". This value is less than the range of that considered physiologic for that dog (1460 mg).

If this dog required more than what I believed to be the "safe annual dose" of prednisone or prednisolone to control its dermatologic disease (i.e., pruritus from allergies or atopic dermatitis), I would either add a second medication in an effort to decrease the amount of GC needed or change medications (i.e., to cyclosporine). Steroid treatment protocols generally begin with higher doses and then are tapered, but again looking at these calculations in this way can be a helpful guide.

If the dog needs more than the "safe annual steroid dose" and the owner declines further diagnostic workup or other therapy, I recommend monitoring for weight gain and urinary tract infection since these are the most prevalent side effects with ongoing GC therapy. First, I would discuss in detail my recommendations for feeding and have the dog weighed regularly to monitor for weight gain. I would also perform a cystocentesis for urinalysis and urine culture and sensitivity test. It is critical that the urine in dogs receiving steroid therapy be cultured to identify an infection. Dilution of the urine and the antiinflammatory effects of the steroids reduce the likelihood of identifying bacteriuria or inflammatory changes suggestive of infection in the routine urinalysis. Although the urine specific gravity would be expected to be low (about 1.012), if there were protein or glucose in the dilute urine, a serum chemistry to assess for any early renal disease or diabetes would be indicated. I would expect the alkaline phosphatase and alanine aminotransferase to be elevated and for the complete blood count to reveal a stress leukogram.

In summary, the rational use of GCs in veterinary dermatology requires the clinician to be familiar with the pharmacologic, physiologic, and side effects of steroids as a class and the individual formulations used in their practice. GC use should be limited and kept to a minimum by using adjunctive therapies (e.g., antibiotics, antihistamines, fatty acids, topical therapies) whenever possible. A diagnosis should be made before determining the therapeutic regimen, and long-term therapy should be monitored with frequent examinations and laboratory testing as indicated.

References and Suggested Reading

Boothe DW: *Small animal clinical pharmacology and therapeutics*, Philadelphia, 2001, Saunders, p 313.

Ettinger SJ, Feldman EC, editors: *Textbook of veterinary internal medicine: diseases of the dog and cat*, ed 4, vol 1, Philadelphia, 1995, Saunders, p 284.

Feldman EC, Nelson RW: *Canine and feline endocrinology and reproduction*, ed 3, St Louis, 2004, Saunders, p 464.

Graham-Mize CA, Rosser EJ, Hauptman J: Absorption, bioavailability, and activity of prednisone and prednisolone in cats. In Hillier A, Foster AP, Kwochka KW, editors: *Advances in veterinary dermatology*, vol 5, Oxford, 2005, Blackwell Publishing, p 152.

Gubash R, Marsella R, Kunkle GA: Evaluation of adrenal function in small-breed dogs receiving otic glucocorticoids, *Vet Dermatol* 15:200, 2004.

Hardman JG, Limbird LE, Gilman AG: *Goodman & Gilman's the pharmacologic basis of therapeutics*, ed 10, St Louis, 2001, McGraw-Hill, p 1649.

Ihrke PJ et al: Urinary tract infection associated with long-term corticosteroid administration in dogs with chronic skin disease, *J Am Vet Med Assoc* 186:43, 1985.

Kemppainen RJ, Sartin JL: Effects of single intravenous doses of dexamethasone on baseline cortisol concentrations and response to synthetic ACTH in healthy dogs. *Am J Vet Res* 45:742, 1984.

McDonald RK, Langston VC: Use of corticosteroids and nonsteroidal anti-inflammatory agents. In Mueller R: *Dermatology for the small animal practitioner*, Jackson, Wy, 2000, Teton New Media, p 129.

Scott DW: Dermatologic therapy. In Scott DW, Miller Jr WH, Griffin CE, editors: *Muller & Kirks' small animal dermatology*, ed 6, Philadelphia, 2001, Saunders, p 244.

Torres SMF et al: Frequency of urinary tract infection among dogs with pruritic disorders receiving long-term glucocorticoid treatment, *J Am Vet Med Assoc* 227:239, 2005.

CHAPTER **90**

Feline Pruritus Therapy

SOPHIE GILBERT, *New York, New York*

INTRODUCTION

To maximize treating a pruritic cat, it is important to address the underlying cause. A complete signalment and history, along with a thorough physical examination and diagnostic procedures are required. Once the underlying cause is known, a specific treatment can be instituted. At his time, or during the diagnostic workup, some cats will require a short-term symptomatic treatment to increase their quality of life, as well as that of their owners. Because most underlying pruritic diseases in cats cannot be cured, most affected cats require a combination of specific and symptomatic therapy to control the condition and to provide them with a comfortable life.

SPECIFIC TREATMENTS

Once the underlying cause has been diagnosed, it may be possible to address the cause of the pruritus by giving a specific treatment. Many of these are discussed elsewhere in this section. Some examples of specific therapies are summarized below.

- Parasitic dermatitis (notoedric acariasis, otodectic acariasis, cheyletiellosis, pediculosis, trombiculiasis, and demodicosis): lime sulfur dips, selamectin, ivermectin, fipronil spray; treat all in contact animals (see Chapter 98)
- Dermatophytosis: topical and parenteral antifungal products; treat all in contact animals, as well as in the environment (see Chapter 105)
- Pyoderma/*Malassezia* dermatitis: appropriate oral antibiotic for 3 to 4 weeks for pyoderma and oral antifungal product for *malassezia* dermatitis (see following paragraph)
- Flea allergy dermatitis: strict flea control, which includes treating the cat with adulticidal and larvicidal products and treating the environment

- Food allergy: restrictive diet that does not include the offending food stuff (see Chapter 87 and Section V on Evolve).
- Atopic dermatitis (AT): avoidance of the offending allergens and allergen-specific immunotherapy (ASIT) (see discussion later in the chapter and in Chapter 92)
- Psychogenic alopecia: correction of the triggering factor with or without administration of behavior modification drugs (see discussion later in the chapter)

Treating the Secondary Infections (Pyoderma and *Malassezia* Dermatitis)

When evidence of pyoderma and/or *malassezia* dermatitis is evident from the cytologic examination, these should be treated because as infection may contribute considerably to the pruritus and in rare cases may be the only cause of the pruritus. Antibiotic or antifungal therapy may be given as sole therapy for 3 to 4 weeks to assess their efficacy. When a pyoderma is present, culture and antibiotic sensitivity may be recommended. However, because cytologic examination often reveals the presence of cocci, in many cases, empiric antibiotic therapy is usually tried first. Antibiotics that have been used successfully to treat pyoderma in cats include clavulanic acid/amoxicillin (15 mg/kg q12h orally [PO]), cefadroxil (22 mg/kg q12h PO), marbofloxacin (Zeniquin, Bayer, 3 to 5 mg/kg q24h PO), lincomycin (20 mg/kg q12h PO), and clindamycin (5.5 mg/kg q12h or 11 mg/kg q12h to 24h PO). Vomiting and diarrhea are common side effects of most of these drugs.

Malassezia dermatitis can be treated with oral itraconazole (Sporanox, Janssen Pharmaceutica, 5 mg/kg q24h PO). Intermittent ongoing therapy may be necessary to control recurrent infections. Terbinafine (Lamisil, Novartis) has been used successfully to treat secondary *malassezia* dermatitis in allergic dogs at a dosage of 30 mg/kg once daily (Rosales et al., 2005). Therefore terbinafine may also be considered as a treatment option for cats with *malassezia* dermatitis.

Treating Feline Atopic Dermatitis

The diagnosis of AD in the cat is based primarily on the history and clinical signs and by ruling out other pruritic diseases. It is important to explain to the owner that AD is not curable but only manageable and that both specific and symptomatic treatments will likely be required for life. Combining treatments helps to optimize the chance of controlling the pruritus in these patients. Specific treatments of AD include avoiding the offending allergen and allergen-specific immunotherapy or ASIT. These treatments require identification of the environmental allergens involved in the disease, which may be done by performing intradermal testing (IDT) and/or allergen-specific IgE serology (for more details, see *Kirk's Current Veterinary Therapy XIII*, p 564). Because nonrelevant positive reactions can be seen with both tests, special care should be taken when interpreting them and selecting the allergens to be included in the ASIT.

Although considered the gold standard, IDT is more difficult to perform and interpret in the cat than in the dog because of the thinner skin of the cat. This makes performing intradermal injections more difficult. Furthermore, positive tests in cats may be characterized by the formation of softer, nonerythematous wheals or by wheals that are very subtle and disappear rapidly when compared to dogs. Weak reactions also may be caused by the use of suboptimal allergen concentrations. Indeed, recently it was shown that allergen concentrations used in cats should be revised since most appear too low (Austel et al., 2006).

Allergen-specific IgE serology offers an alternative to IDT. Because of the difficulty of performing and interpreting IDT in the cat and because the benefits of successful ASIT may be comparable to those of IDT (Halliwell, 1997), many dermatologists prefer this test over IDT in this cats. Greer Laboratories (www.greerlabs.com), Heska Corporation (Allercept, www.heska.com), and VARL (Veterinary Allergy Reference Laboratory, www.varallergy.com,) offer allergen-specific IgE serology in cats in the United States.

Limiting contact with the offending allergen is often impossible or impractical, but avoidance may be possible with some allergens, including wool, kapok, tobacco, and feathers. It is also possible to decrease the level of dust mites in the environment (see Chapter 94); and although difficult, it may be possible to limit exposure to pollens.

ASIT is the treatment of choice for dogs with AD when it is not possible to avoid the offending allergen. Double-blinded, placebo-controlled studies demonstrating the efficacy of ASIT are still lacking in the cat. However, open studies have shown success rates that vary from 45% to 100% (O'Dair and Foster, 1995; Scott, Walton, and Slater, 1986). Accordingly, ASIT may represent the most appropriate long-term control method for a cat with nonseasonal AD. The success of ASIT depends on the accuracy of the diagnosis, the formulation of the vaccine (selection of the allergens), and the realization that each program must be tailored to the specific needs of the patient, relative to frequency of injections and number of allergens used. In addition, ASIT requires compliant owners and cooperative patients.

The recommended induction protocol of ASIT is the same in the cat as in the dog; however, the protocol may be varied, and I prefer to use a lower maintenance dosage of 0.5 ml every 1 to 2 weeks (rather than the canine protocol of 1 ml every 10 days to 3 weeks). Again, intervals between injections may be decreased or increased according to the response obtained, and the dose may be decreased to reduce the severity of potential side effects such as increase in pruritus. In addition, it may be helpful to premedicate the cat with an antihistamine before giving the injection. Some cats with severe pruritus may also require the administration of oral symptomatic therapy during the induction phase of ASIT while waiting for the benefits of ASIT to become clinically apparent (see following paragraphs). If improvement is not evident after 1 year, ASIT is considered a failure and should be discontinued. However, if improvement is noted, injections should be given for life. It is important to give positive reinforcement to the client such as handouts, phone communications, and rechecks to continue what can be a difficult task for some.

SYMPTOMATIC TREATMENTS FOR PRURITUS

It is important to make a point of understanding each client's tolerance for his or her cat's level of pruritus. The choice of symptomatic therapy may differ, depending on whether it will be used for short-term or long-term administration.

Concomitant short-term symptomatic therapy may be required during the time of the diagnostic procedures or during the induction phase of ASIT if the cat is severely pruritic and uncomfortable. In this case fast and satisfactory relief is required; therefore corticosteroids are often chosen over other antipruritic drugs. It is important to remember that symptomatic therapy is likely to interfere with the diagnostic procedures and may delay IDT. Therefore, to assess the effect of a treatment trial such as flea control, ectoparasite therapy, or elimination diet, the oral corticosteroid therapy should be discontinued, and the cat should be monitored closely for recurrence of the pruritus and clinical signs. In addition, to rule out food allergy, the elimination diet trial must be followed by challenging the cat with its original diet.

When long-term therapy is required, nonsteroidal therapy should be tried first because it may be successful and carries fewer potential side effects than corticosteroids. Although the success rate is much lower than with corticosteroids, I generally prescribe chlorpheniramine in conjunction with essential fatty acids (EFAs). Nonsteroidal therapy is also recommended in cats in which corticosteroids are contraindicated. However, some pruritic diseases or reaction patterns do not respond to nonsteroidal therapy, and many cats are still given corticosteroids as a long-term therapy.

Medicating may be a problem in some cats, and owners should be counseled about the techniques and "tricks" useful for oral treatment of cats. Administration of drugs may be limited to only once daily in difficult cats. If an elimination diet trial is not ongoing, tuna juice, butter, and petroleum jelly may be used to hide the medication; or the drug may be compounded with flavor added. Some drugs such as corticosteroids (methylprednisolone acetate [Depo Medrol, Pfizer]) may also be administered parenterally rather than orally.

Corticosteroid Therapy

Corticosteroids are the most consistently effective drugs in the management of pruritus in cats. Because corticosteroids usually provide fast and satisfactory relief, they represent a better option for short-term antipruritic therapy than nonsteroidal agents that have a lower success rate. Moreover, despite all diagnostic and therapeutic efforts, some cats may respond only to corticosteroid therapy. However, use of corticosteroids implies a compatible differential diagnosis, and they should not be administered to cats with suspicion of infectious diseases such as dermatophytosis, immunosuppressive viral infection, latent toxoplasmosis, or other bacterial or viral diseases. A number of systemic or organ-system based diseases can also constitute relative contraindications for corticosteroids, particularly repositol compounds. These include diabetes mellitus, pancreatitis, kidney failure, cardiomyopathy, and some liver diseases.

Oral short-acting corticosteroids are preferred over injectable long-acting (repositol) corticosteroids since they can be discontinued any time, which enables the efficacy of the treatment trial to be assessed or development of adverse effects to be limited. However, repositol corticosteroids may be used in cats unable to swallow pills or difficult to treat (e.g., aggressive cats, outside cats). Because prednisone must be converted into active prednisolone in the liver and cats may be deficient in this capacity, prednisolone is preferred over prednisone in this species (Graham-Mize and Rosser, 2005).

Cats may be relatively resistant to corticosteroids in comparison to dogs because of the rate of the metabolism of the corticosteroids, a difference in the extent of oral absorption, or a difference in the number and affinity of corticosteroid receptors in the skin and the liver (van den Broek and Stafford, 1992). Although cats tolerate corticosteroids fairly well, side effects may be seen, especially with long-term therapy. The possibility of developing diabetes mellitus is a serious concern in cats receiving long-term corticosteroid therapy. Iatrogenic hyperadrenocorticism, although rare in cats, may also occur.

When oral corticosteroids are used long term, tapering doses should be given according to the response observed. The initial dose is usually higher than in dogs and is given daily until remission is obtained (usually 1 week to 10 days). The dosage is gradually reduced to the lowest alternate-day schedule that controls the symptoms. Suggested corticosteroids and dosing schedules follow:

- *Prednisolone* or *methylprednisolone* 1 to 2 mg/kg q24h PO for 1 to 2 weeks; then switch to alternate-day basis at lowest possible dose
- *Dexamethasone* 0.1 to 0.2 mg/kg or 0.25 to 1 mg/cat q24h PO for 1 week; then gradually increase the interval between therapy to one to three times a week
- *Triamcinolone* 0.2 to 0.4 mg/kg q24h PO for 1 week; then gradually increase the interval between therapy from every week to every three weeks.
- *Methylprednisolone acetate injectable,* 4 mg/kg or 20 mg/cat intramuscularly. Cats should not receive more than four injections a year (and no more often than once, every 3 months). However, some cats with severe lesions of the eosinophilic disease complex may initially require up to three injections 2 weeks apart before showing a response.

When giving corticosteroid therapy, I usually start with prednisolone at the dosage of 1 mg/kg once daily and have found this dose to be generally successful in controlling the pruritus of atopic cats. Lesions of the eosinophilic disease complex such as eosinophilic granuloma and indolent ulcer may be more difficult to control and often require higher doses or more potent corticosteroids. If the expected result is not obtained or if the cat is showing undesirable effects (e.g., polyphagia, polyuria-polydipsia) with one type of corticosteroids, another type may be tried. Antihistamines and EFAs may potentiate the effects of corticosteroids, facilitating a decreased dose of corticosteroids. Tachyphylaxis may occur with long-term corticosteroid therapy. Some cats may require the use of oral corticosteroids only when they have a pruritic outbreak.

NONSTEROIDAL THERAPIES

Essential Fatty Acids

EFA supplements containing ω-3/ω-6 fatty acids are potent modulators of prostaglandin and leukotriene synthesis. These supplements have been shown to be effective in some pruritic cats. Formulations containing ω-3/ω-6 have been reported to be of help and to give positive response in 40% to 75% of cats with inflammatory skin disease (Miller, Scott, and Wellington, 1993; Harvey, 1993). However, I have not been able to reduce the pruritus level in cats with the administration of EFA as the only treatment. Because these studies did not take into consideration the EFA content of the diet and therefore the type of fatty acids, the ω-6/ω-3 ratio (5:1 to 10:1) and the dose of each fatty acid necessary to provide a maximum of efficacy are still unknown.

Many formulations composed of either ω-3 or combination of ω-6 and ω-3 at varying ratios can be found. Liquid formulation, capsule, or chewable tablets can be purchased (3V Caps, IVX Animal Health; Dermcaps, IVX Animal Health; Efavet, Efamol; Vetriderm, Bayer; Actis Omega, Sogeval). EFAs should not be administered during an elimination diet trial, and cats having allergy to fish should not be given fish oil.

EFAs should be given for at least 6 weeks to be able to assess their efficacy, and, if improvement is noted, they should be given for life. It is recommended to give the EFAs in combination with antihistamines for synergistic effects and as a supplement to long-term corticosteroid therapy for their sparing effect on the corticosteroids. Even when ineffective for decreasing pruritus, EFAs increase the skin and hair coat quality considerably. Adverse effects are uncommon but include vomiting, diarrhea, and weight gain.

Antihistamines

Antihistamines are most likely to be effective when the skin is minimally inflamed and therefore efficacy is likely to be increased after treating the complicating factors, underlying causes, and controlling inflammation with a short course of corticosteroid therapy. Conversely, antihistamines are believed to work best if given before histamine release and therefore should be administered without interruption in cats with chronic pruritus.

Chlorpheniramine was reported to be very effective in atopic cats, with improvement in 73% of cases (Miller and Scott, 1990). Chlorpheniramine (2 to 4 mg/cat q12h PO) is my recommended antihistamine in cats because it is often the most effective and is usually well tolerated. The 4-mg tablet makes it convenient to administer, although, once broken, it may have a bitter taste. Alternatively clemastine (0.67 mg/cat q12h PO) can also be used and was shown to give positive results in 50% of cases (Miller and Scott, 1994). Other antihistamines that have been used in cats with variable success are diphenhydramine 0.5 mg/kg q12h PO, cyproheptadine 2 mg/cat q12h PO,

hydroxyzine 1 to 2 mg/kg q12h PO, and oxatomide 10 to 30 mg/cat q12h PO.

Because response to antihistamines is notoriously individualized and unpredictable, an antihistamine trial with several antihistamines may be performed. Each antihistamine is given to the cat for 2 weeks to assess its effect and elicit which has the greatest efficacy. There may be a synergistic effect between the EFAs and antihistamines, and, like EFAs, antihistamines may also potentiate the effect of the corticosteroids. Adverse effects include lethargy, diarrhea, polyphagia, polyuria/polydipsia, and behavioral changes (vocalization). Some cats may experience hyperexcitability. Antihistamines must be used with caution in the presence of liver disease, glaucoma, urinary retention, gastrointestinal atony, seizures, and pregnancy.

Behavior Modification Drugs

Behavior modification drugs are mostly recommended in cats with behavior disorders but may also be helpful in cats in which excessive grooming is their primary clinical presentation. Their efficacy is the result of their specific effect on anxiety and stereotypic behavior and the antihistaminic properties that some of these agents have.

Clomipramine (Clomicalm, Novartis, 2 to 5 mg/cat q24h PO) and amitriptyline (5 mg/cat q12h to q24h PO) are tricyclic antidepressants. Tricyclic antidepressants exert their primary clinical effects by inhibiting the presynaptic reuptake of serotonin and norepinephrine. In addition, they have the ability to block H_1 and H_2 receptors. Adverse effects include sedation; increase in appetite; weight gain; and anticholinergic effects such as dry mouth, urine retention, and reduced tear production. Tricyclic antidepressants may be contraindicated in cats with heart or hepatic disease and history of urinary retention and in epileptic patients. Clomipramine comes in 20-mg tablets and has a bitter taste. For convenience, it may be compounded in 2- to 5-mg tablets with flavor added.

Fluoxetine (Prozac, Lilly, 1 to 5 mg/cat q24h PO) is a selective serotonin reuptake inhibitor (SSRI). Because of their specificity, SSRIs do not affect histamine or acetylcholine; however, they can still cause anorexia, irritability, nervousness, anxiety, sleep disturbance, and changes in elimination patterns.

Behavior modification drugs should be administered for a minimum of 4 weeks before evaluating the clinical response. They should not be discontinued abruptly but should be slowly tapered over a period of 3 weeks (clomipramine and amitriptyline) to 6 weeks (fluoxetine). Tricyclic antidepressants and SSRIs should not be used together or concurrently with monoamine oxidase inhibitors (MAOIs) (i.e., amitraz, selegiline) because MAOIs enhance their toxicity and can lead to the serotonin syndrome. Serotonin syndrome is characterized by a hyperserotonergic state resulting from elevations of central nervous system serotonin, which may reach potentially fatal levels. It usually occurs when drugs with different mechanisms of action are mixed together. Clinical signs may include agitation, drowsiness, myoclonus, hyperreflexia, tremor, hyperthermia, diarrhea, coma and death.

Cyclosporine

Cyclosporine is a calcineurin inhibitor with potent immunomodulatory activity. It is used in dogs with AD with success rates similar to those of corticosteroids (see Chapters 55 and 84). Because side effects that are reported with corticosteroids are not observed with cyclosporine, this drug represents a good option in atopic cats in which corticosteroids are contraindicated, when the dose of corticosteroids cannot be tapered to an acceptable dose, and when nonsteroidal therapy has failed. Infectious diseases, if present, should be cleared before starting cyclosporine therapy. Theoretically, cyclosporine may be used before IDT and at the beginning of ASIT since, unlike corticosteroids, it is believed not to interact with the results of the test and the therapy. However, this notion has been challenged by a recent study. Brazis and colleagues (2006) did show a significant inhibition of cutaneous histamine release and wheal formation following intradermal challenge in dogs sensitized to *Ascaris suum* that were treated with cyclosporine. The dogs were given 5 mg/kg of cyclosporine orally for 4 weeks. Inhibition of histamine release and wheal formation was already significant after 2 weeks of treatment. Based on these results, administration of cyclosporine may not be recommended before IDT in cats since IDT reactions in this species are already often weak and subtle.

In cats cyclosporine has been used with encouraging results to treat eosinophilic disease complex lesions, facial/neck pruritus, self-induced symmetric alopecia, plasmacytic stomatitis, and urticaria pigmentosa. The recommended dosage ranges from 5 to 8 mg/kg q24h orally. Lesions of eosinophilic disease complex may require higher dosages (up to 12.5 mg/kg q24h). It may be possible to start alternate-day regimen after 4 to 6 weeks if sufficient improvement of the clinical signs is seen. The lesions may stay in remission or be controlled with twice-weekly administrations in some cats. Corticosteroids may be given in conjunction with cyclosporine to provide a faster/better control of the lesion. Then corticosteroids are discontinued and cyclosporine is continued alone.

Cyclosporine is available in microemulsion designed to increase the drug intestinal absorption and bioavailability (Atopica, Neoral, Novartis). The possibility of food affecting the bioavailability of cyclosporine has not been studied in the cat; therefore it is unknown if the drug should be given on an empty stomach rather than with food. Oral solution and 10- and 25-mg capsules can be purchased for convenience in cats. The drug may be compounded with flavor added to increase compliance in difficult cats not receiving an elimination diet trial. My colleagues and I have used the injectable form of cyclosporine (Sandimmune) in some difficult cats that could not be given pills, with apparently similar success as when given orally. The initial dose used varied from 2.5 to 5 mg/kg daily subcutaneously, and it was possible to increase the interval between injections to once or twice weekly in some cats. Overall the injections were well tolerated, and adverse reactions were not observed.

The most common side effects reported in cats include anorexia, vomiting, and diarrhea, which usually resolve spontaneously or after discontinuing the medication for a few days. When vomiting is persistent, the administration of metoclopramide (2.5 mg/cat PO 30 minutes before administration of the cyclosporine two to three times a day) may help. Less common adverse effects are gingival hyperplasia, hypertrichosis, and modification in behavior.

Although cyclosporine appears to be a safe medication, it is only recently that this drug is being used as long-term therapy. Therefore long-term safety is still unknown, and cyclosporine must be used with caution. It may be wise to recommend monitoring the cat by performing semiannual complete blood count, chemistry panel, and urinalysis. Feline immunodeficiency virus and feline leukemia virus serology are recommended before starting cyclosporine therapy. Because fulminant and fatal newly acquired acute toxoplasmosis has occasionally been reported in cats (Last et al., 2004), a serologic test for toxoplasmosis is also recommended. The interpretation of the serology is still uncertain; however, it may be prudent to recommend that seronegative cats not be fed raw meat, poultry viscera, or bones and not be allowed to hunt and scavenge during cyclosporine therapy because they may be at risk for developing the disease. Seropositive cats may also be at risk for developing the disease. Nevertheless, and although not known, it is unlikely that reactivation would occur with the dose used to treat atopic cats (much lower than the dose given for renal transplant). Human patients who developed cutaneous lymphoma while being treated with cyclosporine therapy raised some concerns in animals. So far there are only anecdotal cases of dogs developing neoplasia, and this has not been reported in cats.

Adjunctive Therapy

Topical Therapy

Giving a bath to a cat may be a real challenge, and topical antipruritic therapy with cream and gel has little value because of licking and self-grooming. However, some antipruritic lotion and pump spray products containing hydrocortisone, triamcinolone, lidocaine, diphenhydramine, or pramoxine may be helpful as adjunctive therapy in cases of localized pruritus. Potent topical corticosteroids such as triamcinolone (Genesis Spray, Virbac), should be used with special care in cats because of their thin skin and the potential risk of inducing skin fragility.

I have used tacrolimus ointment (Protopic 0.1%, Astellas) in atopic cats with eosinophilic plaques or focal pruritus. Tacrolimus is a macrolide immunosuppressant that belongs to the same family as cyclosporine (see Chapter 55), but it is for topical dermatologic use only. A thin film of the ointment is applied to the lesion once or twice daily until resolution or significant improvement of the lesion and then as needed. The cat should wear an Elizabethan collar following application to prevent licking of the drug and systemic absorption. Secondary infections should be treated before starting tacrolimus therapy. Rare cases of malignancy (such as lymphoma) have been reported in humans treated with tacrolimus ointment. Therefore, even though a causal relationship has not been established in these patients, owners should wear gloves when using this ointment. Cases of malignancy have not been reported in dogs and cats; however, caution should be exercised.

Flea Control

Because of the high frequency of flea allergy dermatitis, any pruritic cats living in an area where fleas are seen should receive strict flea control. In addition, like dogs, cats with AD may also be predisposed to develop flea allergy dermatitis or flea bites may exacerbate the AD.

Elizabethan Collar, Bandannas/Neck Wraps, and Soft-Paws

An Elizabethan collar can be used to limit self-trauma during the initiation of the symptomatic treatment. The collar may also reduce licking of topical treatment, therefore reducing any systemic absorption of the drug or decreasing drug efficacy. Clear plastic or soft foamlike collars are preferred. Bandannas and neck wraps can prevent self-mutilation in the neck areas in cases of neck pruritus or idiopathic ulcerative dermatosis. Soft-paws (SmartPractice) are soft plastic covers that are glued onto the nail. They are marketed as an alternative to declawing but may be also useful in preventing self-induced trauma.

References and Suggested Reading

Austel M et al: Evaluation of three different histamine concentrations in intradermal testing of normal cats and attempted determination of "irritant" threshold concentrations for 48 allergens, *Vet Dermatol* 17:189, 2006.

Brazís P et al: Dermal microdialysis in the dog: in vivo assessment of the effect of cyclosporin A on cutaneous histamine and prostaglandin D2 release, *Vet Dermatol* 17:169, 2006.

Graham-Mize CA, Rosser EJ: Bioavailability and activity of prednisone and prednisolone in cats. In Hillier A, Foster AP, Kwochka KW, editors: *Advances in veterinary dermatology*, vol 5, Blackwell Publishing, 2005, Oxford, p 152.

Halliwell RW: Efficacy of hyposensitization in feline based upon results of in vitro testing for allergen-specific immunoglobulin E, *J Am Anim Hosp Assoc* 33:282, 1997.

Harvey RG: A comparison of evening primrose oil and sunflower oil for the management of papulocrustous dermatitis in cats, *Vet Rec* 133:571, 1993.

Last RD et al: A case of fatal systemic toxoplasmosis in a cat being treated with cyclosporine A for feline atopy, *Vet Dermatol* 15:194, 2004.

Miller WH, Scott DW: Efficacy of chlorpheniramine maleate for the management of pruritus in cats, *J Am Vet Med Assoc* 197:67, 1990.

Miller WH, Scott DW: Clemastine fumarate as an antipruritic agent in pruritic cats: results of an open clinical trial, *Can Vet J* 35:502, 1994.

Miller WH, Scott DW, Wellington JR: Efficacy of DVM derm caps liquid in the management of allergic and inflammatory dermatoses of the cat, *J Am Anim Hosp Assoc* 29:37, 1993.

O'Dair HA, Foster AP: Focal and generalized alopecia. In Kunkle G, editor: Feline dermatology, *Vet Clin North Am Small Anim Pract* 15:851, 1995.

Rosales MS et al: Comparison of the clinical efficacy of oral terbinafine and ketoconazole combined with cephalexin in the treatment of *Malassezia* dermatitis in dogs—a pilot study, *Vet Dermatol* 16:171, 2005.

Scott DW, Walton DK, Slater MR: Miliary dermatitis: a feline cutaneous reaction pattern, *Proc Annu Kal Kan Semin* 2:11, 1986.

van den Broek AHM, Stafford WL: Epidermal and hepatic glucocorticosteroid receptor in cats and dogs, *Res Vet Sci* 52:312, 1992.

CHAPTER 91

Shampoo Therapy

WAYNE S. ROSENKRANTZ, *Tustin, California*

INTRODUCTION TO SHAMPOO THERAPY

The use of topical therapeutics and in particular shampoo therapy has gained increasing popularity in veterinary dermatology. Shampoos are one of the easiest and most complete vehicles to use when applying topical therapeutics, and shampoo therapy can be highly beneficial in the management of many different types of skin disorders (Guaguere, 1996; Kwochka, 1993). This is particularly the case in allergic, seborrheic, and infectious diseases. In many patients shampoo therapy can be used as a sole treatment or as an adjunctive therapy that allows reduced dosages or reliance on systemic therapy (Scott et al., 2001). Owner compliance can sometimes be a problem with this type of therapy, as it can be difficult and time-consuming. However, it does allow many owners to actively participate in the management of their pets' skin condition.

Gaining familiarity with the shampoo products that are commercially available is very important. Many products are not closely regulated regarding their active ingredients or formulations; thus first-hand experience is necessary. By using the shampoos on his or her own pets and patients, the veterinarian can gain experience regarding the potency, efficacy, and safety of a product and be knowledgeable about recommending these products to clients for their pet's skin conditions. The recommended frequency of shampooing varies with the underlying condition. However, in most chronic skin diseases weekly shampooing with the proper product can be very helpful. Some products require adequate contact time for the best efficacy, but it is critical that complete rinsing be emphasized to avoid or reduce irritancy. In general cool water is recommended, especially in cases with allergic skin disease.

SHAMPOOS FOR ALLERGIC SKIN DISEASES

Topical therapy is extremely important in the management of allergic skin diseases. Many new products are available that contain better delivery systems and active ingredients that help to control pruritus and moisturize the skin. The use of these shampoos allows for reduced systemic absorption and increased activity. The main advantages are control of pruritus by removing allergens from the skin surface and having direct antipruritic effects. For this form of therapy to be most effective, frequent shampooing is often necessary; this may vary from case to case, but generally once to twice a week and occasionally more frequently. When combined with systemic therapy, even weekly bathing can have a synergistic effect.

Water is often overlooked as a therapeutic agent. It aids in hydrating and cooling the skin and can help remove crusts and soften and clean the skin. Water combined with a shampoo can be particularly effective. When combined with proper emollients and moisturizing agents it can help retain the moisture in the skin after hydration during bathing. On the other hand, if used repeatedly without proper emollients and moisturizing agents, water can dry out the skin by removing the skin's natural barriers that prevent xerosis.

Many different specific antipruritic and moisturizing agents can be incorporated into shampoos (Table 91-1). Because shampoos are not left on indefinitely and are rinsed off after a period of time, some active ingredients are not as effective or practical to use in shampoo delivery systems. Many companies offer leave-on rinses or sprays that contain the same active ingredients that can be used after or in-between shampooing to prolong their beneficial effects. Such rinses and sprays are more commonly incorporated into products used for allergy management but can also be found for other conditions. Short-term relief from pruritus can be achieved by using shampoos with specific antipruritics. The mechanism of action varies among different products. Some inactivate pruritic mediators (glucocorticoids and antihistamines); others act as topical anesthetics (pramoxine, benzoyl peroxide, and tars); still others function by moisturizing the skin. Moisturizing agents include oils (safflower, sesame, lanolin) and hygroscopic agents (propylene glycol, glycerin, colloidal oatmeal, urea, and lactic acid). Since there are so many products available on the market, it is important that the practitioner become familiar with specific products that contain these active ingredients to be able to make proper selections for specific cases.

One of the antipruritic topical agents that I use most commonly is the topical anesthetic pramoxine hydrochloride. It is available in a few commercial products (see Table 91-1). The duration of action is short and becomes even shorter when used frequently and repetitively. Pramoxine is used primarily in combination with colloidal oatmeal. Diphenhydramine is an antihistamine available for topical use and available in veterinary formulations: Histacalm, Resihist, and Histacalm spray (2% diphenhydramine) (Virbac). Topical antihistamines have limited value in controlling pruritus in veterinary dermatology, but an occasional case exhibits some benefits.

Other popular products that are useful in the management of allergic skin disease are moisturizing and hypoallergenic shampoos. Many times these products are followed with the same active agent as a leave-on spray or rinse. My favorites are Hy-Lyt-EFA and Relief (DVM Pharmaceuticals); Allermyl, Allergroom, and Epi-Soothe (Virbac); and Dermal Soothe Hydra-Pearls cream rinse (Vetoquinol). Allermyl shampoo (Virbac) is a relatively

Table **91-1**

Antipruritic and Moisturizing Products

Products	Ingredients	Formulation	Manufacturer
Allergroom	Moisturizing	Shampoo	Virbac
Allermyl	Moisturizing	Shampoo/rinse	Virbac
Hy-Lyt-EFA	Moisturizing	Shampoo/rinse	DVM Pharmaceuticals
Hydra Pearls	Moisturizing	Shampoo/rinse	Vétoquinol
DermaHypoCS	Moisturizing	Shampoo	DermaPet
EpiSoothe	Colloidal oatmeal	Shampoo	Virbac
Allay oatmeal	Colloidal oatmeal	Shampoo	DermaPet
Resisoothe	Colloidal oatmeal	Rinse	Virbac
Relief	1% Pramoxine	Shampoo/rinse	DVM Pharmaceuticals
Resiprox	1.5% Pramoxine	Rinse	Virbac
Histacalm	Diphenhydramine	Shampoo/rinse	Virbac
Fluocinolone acetonide	Triamcinolone 0.01%	Shampoo	Hill
Cortisoothe	Hydrocortisone 1%	Shampoo	Virbac
Douxo	Phytosphingosine	Shampoo/spray spot-on	Sogeval

new shampoo for atopic dermatitis and contains linoleic acid, vitamin E, and L-rhamnose in a microemulsion. L-rhamnose has been shown to inhibit some proinflammatory cytokines in vitro, and the formulation is meant to restore the barrier function of the stratum corneum, which may be impaired in atopic dermatitis. In a 3-week clinical trial greater then 50% improvement in pruritus in 35 dogs with atopic dermatitis was seen when shampooing with Allermyl and topical application of Allermyl rinse every 3 days (Reme et al., 2004).

A new group of products containing phytosphingosine (PS) has just been released (Douxo, Sogeval) that has been used primarily for seborrheic conditions; however, the active agent also has moisturizing and antiinflammatory properties and may be of value for allergic skin disease management as well. PS is a key molecule in the natural defense mechanism of the skin. It is a component of ceramides, 40% to 50% of the main lipids responsible for maintaining the cohesion of the stratum corneum and correct moisture balance of the skin. PS has antiinterleukin-1 activity, which impairs the production of prostaglandin E_2 and inhibits kinase protein C. This may be one of the mechanisms by which it may help with allergic skin disease management.

Another new area of interest is using topical therapy as a denaturing agent to inactivate percutaneous allergens before they can create disease. This has been recommended mostly for control of house dust mite allergens, which is the most common environmental allergen involved with canine atopic disease (see Chapter 94). The allergen denaturing agent is incorporated in a shampoo base (Allerase, Aveho Biosciences) and may help to control pruritus by lowering allergen levels on the skin. I and others have anecdotal reports of help with Allerase (shampoo and spray formulations) as a topical therapy in canine atopic dermatitis.

Shampoos with glucocorticoids can be tried for more generalized allergic conditions but often have no residual effects because they are rinsed off of the skin. One common product incorporates hydrocortisone (Cortisoothe, Virbac) and has no known detectable systemic absorption or side effects. A more potent fluorinated glucocorticoid shampoo is available (Fluocinolone acetonide, Hill) but is expensive. It carries minimal concerns regarding systemic absorption and side effects and appears safe to use as long as it is adequately rinsed off the skin.

SHAMPOOS FOR SEBORRHEIC DISORDERS

Antiseborrheic shampoos function by normalizing epithelialization or removing surface scale. A keratoplastic effect is optimal for an antiseborrheic shampoo to be effective. This is where the rate of division of the basal cells is reduced or "normalized". Most antiseborrheic shampoos also have a keratolytic effect, in which there is an elimination of excess corneal layers by increasing desquamation. This is thought to be caused by a softening and a reduction of the intercellular connection of the corneocytes, resulting in increased desquamation of the stratum corneum. Many keratoplastic and keratolytic agents are commercially available in shampoo formulations (Table 91-2). Also, many of the previously listed moisturizing shampoos that are used for allergic skin disease management can be used in mild, dryer forms of scaly skin disorders. These function primarily by increasing the moisture content of the skin; many products also have emollient effects.

Salicylic Acid and Sulfur Shampoos

Salicylic acid is a keratolytic agent. It causes a reduction in skin pH, which leads to an increase in the amount of water that the keratin of the stratum corneum is able to absorb. In the desquamation process it has a direct effect on intercellular cement and intercellular junction system (desmosomes). These actions help soften the corneal layer. Salicylic acid acts synergistically with sulfur and these two compounds are often present in equal quantities in shampoos. Its efficacy varies with concentration. Sulfur is mildly keratolytic. It forms hydrogen sulfide in the corneal layer and has numerous other antiseborrheic properties. The keratoplastic action is explained by a direct cytostatic effect and possibly because it interacts

Table 91-2

Antiseborrheic Shampoos

Product	Ingredients/Uses (Active Ingredients)	Formulation	Manufacturer
SebaLyt/SeboRx	Sulfur 2%/2%, salicylic acid 3%/2%, triclosan 0.5/0.5%	Shampoo	DVM Pharmaceuticals
Sebolux	Sulfur 2%, Na-salicylate 2.3%	Shampoo	Virbac
SebaMoist/ SebaHex	Sulfur 2%, salicylic acid 2%/chlorhexidine 2%	Shampoo	Vétoquinol
DermaSebS	Benzoyl peroxide 2.5%, sulfur 2%, salicylic acid 2%,	Shampoo	Dermapet
NuSal-T	Coal tar 2%, salicylic acid 3%, menthol 1%	Shampoo	DVM Pharmaceuticals
T-Lux	Coal tar 4%, sulfur 2%, Na-salicylate 2.3%	Shampoo	Virbac
LyTar	Juniper tar 3%, sulfur 2%, salicylic acid 2%	Shampoo	DVM Pharmaceuticals
Allerseb-T	Coal tar 4%, sulfur 2%, salicylic acid 2%	Shampoo	Virbac
Sulf OxyDex	Benzoyl peroxide 2.5%, sulfur 2%	Shampoo	DVM Pharmaceuticals
Selsun Blue	Selenium sulfide 1%	Shampoo	Ross
Keratolux	Salicylic acid 1%, zinc gluconate 0.5%, pyroxidine 0.5%	Shampoo	Virbac
Etiderm	Ethyl lactate 10%	Shampoo	Virbac
Douxo	Phytosphingosine	Shampoo/spray/spot-on	Sogeval

with epidermal cysteine to form cystine, an important component of the corneal layer. It is also antiseptic. Sulfur can be very drying, however, and it also can carry an odor, depending on the formulation. It exerts synergistic activity with salicylic acid most effectively when both substances are incorporated into the shampoo in equal concentrations. My favorite combination salicylic acid and sulfur products are: Sebolux (Virbac), Sebalyt and SeboRx (DVM Pharmaceuticals), and SebaMoist and SebaHex (Vetoquinol), and DermaSebS Shampoo (Dermapet). Sulfur and salicylic acid shampoos work best for light scaling and flaking keratinization defects.

Tar Shampoos

Tar is a keratoplastic agent. It reduces nuclear synthesis in the epidermal basal layers and creates antiseptic and antipruritic effects. There are many different sources and varieties of this active agent. Skin drying, discoloration of light-colored coats, and irritation can be seen with tar-based products but are more common when the concentration is above 3%. There is also some concern about coal tar–based products being carcinogenic; some products containing coal tar have a labeling warning about this concern. Tar shampoos are *contraindicated in the cat* because of a much higher degree of irritancy; in some cases they make cats systemically ill. Because of the increased effectiveness of other nontar products, I rarely use tar-based products. If necessary in more severe forms of seborrhea, particularly in some variants of idiopathic cocker seborrhea or severe forms of sebaceous adenitis, I use solubilized tar (T-lux [Virbac]), 2% tar and salicylic acid (NuSal-T [DVM Pharmaceuticals]), or even more potent tars (Lytar, [DVM Pharmaceuticals] and Allerseb-T [Virbac]). Because of their potency and potential side effects, it is critical to make sure that all tar shampoos are completely rinsed off the skin.

Selenium Disulfide Shampoos

Selenium disulfide is keratolytic and keratoplastic by reducing epidermal turnover and impairing disulfide bridge formation in keratin. It is also antiseborrheic but can have irritant and drying effects. It is contraindicated in the cat for the same reasons listed for tars. I rarely use this shampoo; but on occasion it can be of value in very greasy, oily keratinization defects with concurrent yeast dermatitis in which client finances are a concern because it is less expensive and available over the counter.

Benzoyl Peroxide Shampoos

Benzoyl peroxide is often thought of as being antibacterial, but it is also antiseborrheic by hydrolyzing sebum and reducing sebaceous gland activity. Benzoyl peroxide exerts a follicular flushing action, which is very useful when treating comedone disorders and/or follicular hyperkeratosis. Irritant side effects have been reported, especially in concentrations above 5%. The skin may become dry; thus applying emollients after using this ingredient may be helpful. Many of the newer benzoyl peroxide products have moisturizing agents added to prevent excessive drying. My favorite benzoyl peroxide product to use in seborrheic conditions is SulfOxyDex (DVM Pharmaceuticals) because of the additive or possibly synergistic effects that the sulfur adds to the benzoyl peroxide. The most common products used are listed in the antibacterial shampoo section.

Zinc Gluconate and Pyridoxine Shampoos

Zinc gluconate has antiseborrheic properties. Zinc is a type 1 5α-reductase inhibitor, down-regulates sebum production, and is used in human dermatology to treat acne vulgaris, both topically and orally. Vitamin B$_6$ (pyridoxine) also plays a role in sebum secretion, and there is a synergistic effect of unknown mechanism with zinc. Zinc gluconate and vitamin B$_6$ are combined with essential fatty acids in a newer shampoo that has both antiseborrheic and antibacterial properties (Keratolux [Virbac]).

Phytosphingosine Shampoos

Products containing PS have just been released (Douxo, Sogeval) and, as mentioned previously, have been used for both seborrheic and allergic skin disease conditions. PS is available in shampoo—spray-on and residual spot-on formulations. My preliminary clinical evaluation has shown great promise with these products in all forms of seborrheic skin conditions. In addition PS-based products also have antimicrobial activity, which can help many seborrheic skin disease conditions (see below).

SHAMPOOS FOR INFECTIOUS DISEASES

Pyoderma

Topical therapy can be used in all types of pyoderma. It usually decreases bacterial counts and reduces surface colonization of bacteria, thus helping to prevent or reduce the incidence of recurrences. There are many different topical antimicrobial vehicles; however, shampoos are the most practical and effective (Table 91-3).

The frequency of shampooing for pyoderma depends on the severity of the case and the owner's willingness to do the work. Deep pyoderma cases benefit from frequent bathing (every 2 to 3 days) initially, followed by a weekly maintenance. Most cases respond best if the overlying hair is clipped before bathing. The most common antibacterial agents found in shampoos include benzoyl peroxide with or without sulfur, chlorhexidine, ethyl lactate, and triclosan.

Benzoyl Peroxide

Benzoyl peroxide is considered the most effective for *Staphylococcus intermedius*. In addition to its antibacterial effects, it is an excellent follicular flushing agent, which promotes removal of inspissated debris and is comedolytic. It also has excellent keratolytic and degreasing effects. It is available in several different products: OxyDex and Sulf/OxyDex (DVM Pharmaceuticals), Pyoben (Virbac), Benzoyl Plus (Vetoquinol), DermaBenSs (DermaPet). It can be drying and irritating in some cases, but this is rare with the products listed since most have additional moisturizing agents to counteract this.

Table **91-3**

Antimicrobial Shampoos

Product	Ingredients/Uses (Active Ingredients)	Formulation	Manufacturer
Sulfoxydex, Oxydex	Benzoyl peroxide 2.5%/5%	Shampoo/gel	DVM Pharmaceuticals
Pyoben	Benzoyl peroxide 3%/5%	Shampoo/gel	Virbac
Benzoyl Plus	Benzoyl peroxide 2.5%	Shampoo	Vétoquinol
DermaBenSs	Benzoyl peroxide 2.5%, sulfur/salicylic acid 1%	Shampoo	DermaPet
ChlorhexiDerm	Chlorhexidine 2%/4%	Shampoo/rinse	DVM Pharmaceuticals
Hexadine	Chlorhexidine 3%	Shampoo	Virbac
SebaLyt and SeboRx	Triclosan 2%/3%	Shampoo	DVM Pharmaceuticals
Etiderm	Ethyl lactate 10%	Shampoo	Virbac
Keratolux	Salicylic acid and zinc gluconate	Shampoo	Virbac
Malaseb	Chlorhexidine and miconazole	Shampoo/rinse/towelettes/ pledgets	DVM Pharmaceuticals
Ketochlor	Chlorhexidine 2%, ketoconazole 1%	Shampoo	Virbac
Nizoral/Generics	Ketoconazole 1% and 2%	Shampoo	Janssen/Generics
Miconazole	Miconazole	Shampoo/lotion	Vétoquinol
Resichlor	Chlorhexidine 2%	Lotion	Virbac
Resizole	Miconazole 2%	Lotion	Virbac
Seba-hex	Chlorhexidine 2%, sulfur/salicylic acid	Shampoo	Vetoquinol
Malacetic	Boric acid 2%, acetic acid 2%	Shampoo/rinse/wipes	Dermapet
Douxo	Phytosphingosine/chlorhexidine 3%	Shampoo	Sogeval
Selsun Blue	Selenium sulfide 1%	Shampoo	Ross

Chlorhexidine

Another favorite antibacterial agent is chlorhexidine. It is less drying and irritating than benzoyl peroxide, but at the 2% concentration it is not as effective (Chlorhexiderm [DVM IVX Pharmaceuticals] and Hexadine [Virbac]). However, a 4% formulation has been quite impressive in clinical cases (4% ChlorhexiDerm, DVM Pharmaceuticals). Some formulations combine chlorhexidine with other products to give combined benefits. Sulfur and chlorhexidine (SebaHex, Vetoquinol), chlorhexidine and ketoconazole (Ketochlor, Virbac) and phytosphinogosine and 3% chlorhexidine (Doxuo, Sogeval).

Triclosan and Ethyl Lactate

Two other antimicrobial agents that have antibacterial effects are triclosan and ethyl lactate. Triclosan has less activity against *Staphylococcus* than the agents listed previously, and it is not effective against *Pseudomonas* spp. Ethyl lactate is liposoluble and penetrates hair follicles and sebaceous glands. It is hydrolyzed by bacterial lipases into lactic acid and ethanol. This lowers the skin pH, thereby inhibiting bacterial lipases, making it bactericidal and bacteriostatic. These products are considered nonirritating. However, they are not routinely selected for most *S. intermedius* pyoderma cases because of the superior effectiveness of the previously mentioned products. There are a few products that contain triclosan (SebaLyt and SeboRx, DVM Pharmaceuticals) and ethyl lactate (Etiderm, Virbac).

Salicylic Acid and Zinc Gluconate

A shampoo that has both antimicrobial and antiseborrheic effects is Keratolux (Virbac). Keratolux is a salicylic acid, zinc gluconate, and B_6 vitamin- and fatty acid–based shampoo. In a study comparing it to a salicylic tar-based shampoo, it had similar antimicrobial and antiseborrheic effects (Reme, 2005).

Phytosphingosine

The PS-containing products (Douxo, Sogeval) mentioned previously also have good antimicrobial properties in helping to control surface *S. intermedius, Escherichia coli,* and *Pseudomonas aeruginosa.* When combined with 3% chlorhexidine, there is an additive effect.

Malassezia Dermatitis

Malassezia dermatitis is frequently a recurrent skin infection associated with an underlying disease process. Topical therapy is useful in eliminating infection, but it may also be beneficial when used routinely to help prevent recurrence of infection. For generalized infections shampoo therapy is most useful, whereas localized infections may benefit from use of other vehicles such as creams, lotions, pledgets, towelettes, and sprays. Dogs with generalized infections show the most rapid response when topical therapy is used in conjunction with systemic therapy.

Chlorhexidine, Miconazole, Ketoconazole, Acetic Acid, and Selenium Sulfide

When chlorhexidine is being used to treat *Malassezia* dermatitis, a 2% to 4% formulation is required. Some of the more effective products combine chlorhexidine with other antiyeast or antimicrobial agents: chlorhexidine and miconazole (Malaseb [DVM Pharmaceuticals], chlorhexidine and ketoconazole (Ketochlor, Virbac), and chlorhexidine and phytosphinogosine (Douxo/chlorhexidine PS, Sogeval). Miconazole and ketoconazole are both available in shampoo formulations as only the active ingredient (miconazole shampoo [Vetoquinel] and ketoconazole [Janssen]). An alternative to these products for control of *Malassezia* dermatitis includes acetic acid–based products (Malacetic, DermaPet) and selenium sulfide shampoo (Selsun Blue, Ross).

Dermatophytosis

For generalized infections, topical shampoo therapy can be used as an adjunct to systemic therapy in the management of dermatophyte infections. The main goal of topical therapy is to decrease spread of infection and environmental contamination. Clipping the hair coat is recommended in generalized infections to decrease shedding of contaminated hairs into the environment; however, some studies have demonstrated that shaving infected cats with localized lesions can actually cause the lesions to spread. Although many specialists use shampoo therapy for dermatophytosis, others consider it controversial since there are anecdotal reports that it can cause lesions to spread because of vigorous rubbing. Most also advocate leave-on sprays or dips following shampooing for additional residual activity. All of the same products listed under the *Malassezia* section can be used for dermatophytosis. Most of these are shampoos or leave-on rinses or sprays that contain single active ingredients or combinations containing miconazole 1% to 2%, ketoconazole 1% to 2%, chlorhexidine 2% to 4%, clotrimazole 1% to 2%, enilconazole 0.2%, or lime sulfur 4%.

References and Suggested Reading

Guaguere E: Topical treatment of canine and feline pyoderma, *Vet Dermatol* 7:145–151 1996

Kwochka KW: Symptomatic topical therapy of scaling disorders. In Griffin CE, Kwochka KW, Mac Donald JM, editors: *Current veterinary dermatology*, Mosby, 1993, St Louis, p 191.

Reme CA et al: Efficacy of combined topical therapy with anti-allergic shampoo and lotion for the control of signs associated with atopic dermatitis in dogs, ESVD and ACVD *Vet Dermatol* 15(suppl 1):20, 2004.

Reme CA et al: Antimicrobial efficacy of tar and non-tar antiseborrheic shampoos in dogs. In Hillier A, Foster AP, and Kwochka KW, editors: *Advances in veterinary dermatology*, vol 5, Oxford, UK, 2005, Blackwell Publishing, p 383.

Scott DW, Miller WH, Griffin CE, editors: *Muller and Kirk's small animal dermatology*, ed 6, Philadelphia, 2001, Saunders, p 207.

CHAPTER **92**

Allergen-Specific Immunotherapy

CRAIG E. GRIFFIN, *San Diego, California*
JOHN M. MACDONALD, *Auburn, Alabama*

Allergen-specific immunotherapy (ASIT) is often used in the management of canine and feline atopic dermatitis. ASIT can be defined as the practice of administering gradually increasing quantities of an allergen extract to an allergic subject. The goal of ASIT therapy is to reduce or eliminate the clinical signs associated with subsequent exposures to the causative allergen. This mode of therapy carries potential advantages and some disadvantages compared to other forms of therapy for atopic skin disease. However, it is generally considered the treatment of choice before instituting lifelong continuous glucocorticoid or cyclosporine therapy since ASIT creates less adverse effects than systemic treatments.

The application of ASIT is predicated on the controlled delivery of clinically relevant allergens. These allergens are constituted within a sterile protein-containing liquid that is an extract of the allergenic material, referred to as the allergen solution. Since the actual allergen is part of this protein complex, the volume of allergen in solution is related to the amount of protein in the liquid extract. The protein content is commonly expressed (in the United States) as protein nitrogen units (PNU), with higher numbers ostensibly equated to a higher allergen protein concentration within the solution. Weight relative to volume is another method for reporting the level of protein. The majority of dermatologists and allergen supply companies in the United States treat with aqueous allergens, which is the basis of this discussion.

ASIT therapy is initiated by injecting the most dilute or lowest protein concentration allergens first and then gradually increasing the volume of injections through the relative concentrations of the protein within each solution until a maintenance dosage is reached. A treatment protocol detailing the amount and interval of injections to be administered from the respective concentration is followed until the maintenance dosage is reached. Many protocols call for initial injections given as frequently as every other day to weekly. Once a maintenance dosage is reached, the time between injections increases, with intervals of 7 to 21 days commonly used. Less allergen is generally administered when the interval between injections is shortened. Allergen supply and serum allergy testing laboratories usually provide an ASIT treatment protocol.

ALLERGEN-SPECIFIC IMMUNOTHERAPY PROTOCOLS

Currently a large number of protocols for aqueous ASIT are available. The schedules should emphasize what clients should watch for and report (Box 92-1), including scoring the degree of pruritus as an "Itch Score." Clients also need to be reminded of reevaluation schedules. I (CG) use one protocol for large dogs, a different one for small dogs (under 20 pounds of body weight), and a third protocol for cats (Boxes 92-2 to 92-4). Author JM uses a three-vial protocol for dogs over 20 pounds and a second protocol for dogs under 20 pounds and cats (Boxes 92-5 and 92-6). Whichever protocol is followed, the clinician must recognize that any protocol is simply a starting point and adjustments may and often should be made based on the patient's response to ASIT. The following guidelines apply to aqueous ASIT; the doses and injection intervals of nonaqueous ASIT differ, but the principles of when and how to adjust are similar.

ADJUSTING THE ALLERGEN-SPECIFIC IMMUNOTHERAPY SCHEDULE

ASIT can be adjusted in a number of ways. The volume of solution and therefore the total amount of protein injected can be changed. The interval between injections can be altered so that injections are given more or less frequently. A second individual set of allergens may be started along with (or combined with) with the original set of allergens. Finally, allergens can be remixed or reformulated, with the concentration of antigen (protein level/volume) increased or decreased or the allergen mixture modified. Modifying

Box 92-1

Allergen-Specific Immunotherapy Home Therapy: Information for Clients

- Grade itching on an "itch scale" of 0 (none) to 10 (severe scratching).*
- Call in 4 weeks and report the grade of itching.
- Call if itch score increases by more than two levels
- Call before giving any more shots if there are adverse reactions.
  - Vomiting, diarrhea, anxiousness, weakness are possible reactions.
  - NOTE: Reactions will usually occur within 1 to 2 hours after shot is given.
- Recheck appointments should be scheduled around day 60 and day 120 of therapy.
- Watch for the pattern of itching in relation to when shots are given.
  - Itch score increases before the next shot is due or after a shot is given.
  - Itch decreases after a shot is given.

*Baseline should be determined after control of any skin infection or control of any fleas

Box 92-2

Allergen-Specific Immunotherapy Administration Schedule for Dogs Over 20 lb of Body weight

Day	Date	Symptoms Itch Score	Volume (ml)
Vial No. 1			
1			0.1
3			0.2
5			0.3
7			0.4
9			0.6
11			0.8
13			1.0
Vial No. 2			
15			0.2
17			0.3
19			0.4
21			0.6
23			0.8
25			1.0
(Continue Vial No. 2)			
10-Day Interval			
35			1.0
45			1.0
55			1.0
14-Day Interval			
69			1.0
83			1.0
97			1.0
111			1.0

the volume or the interval is the simplest approach and does not require reformulation.

Clinical responses to ASIT therapy often dictate protocol adjustments. Reasons to adjust ASIT vary but mainly relate to improving efficacy or decreasing adverse reactions. In some instances the interval of therapy is modified because of convenience. A common reason to adjust ASIT is some clinical improvement after an injection followed by an exacerbation in symptoms "X" days later. In this situation we alter the injection schedule to the interval of "X" or "X" plus 1 or 2 days when "X" is less than 5 days. Alternatively, if the problem persists, the interval may be changed to exactly "X" days. The volume given is determined by the basic rules described in the following paragraphs; but in general, when the interval is shortened, the amount given is also decreased. It may be more convenient to choose a schedule of twice weekly such as every Wednesday and Saturday when the interval is less than 5 days. The animal may stay at this shortened interval long term; or, if preferred by the owner, once the animal has done well for 3 months, the interval between injections may again be lengthened since the response of some animals to ASIT continues to improve for a couple of years. Some animals also have seasonal exacerbations of their atopic disease that may result in a shorter interval during the bad season and longer intervals in the "good" season, with the maximum interval being 30 days.

Box 92-3

Allergen-Specific Immunotherapy Administration Schedule for Dogs Under 20lb of Body Weight

Day	Date	Symptoms Itch Score	Volume (ml)
Vial No. 1			
1			0.1
3			0.2
5			0.3
7			0.4
9			0.6
11			0.8
13			1.0
Vial No. 2			
15			0.1
17			0.2
19			0.3
21			0.5
23			0.5
25			0.5
(Continue Vial No. 2)			
5-Day Interval			
30			0.5
35			0.5
40			0.7
10-Day Interval			
50			0.7
60			0.7
70			0.7
80			0.7
14-Day Interval			
94			0.7
108			0.7
122			0.7
136			0.7
150			0.7

Box 92-4

Allergen-Specific Immunotherapy Administration Schedule for Cats

Day	Date	Symptoms Itch Score	Volume (ml)
Day			Volume
Vial No. 1			
1			0.1
3			0.2
5			0.3
7			0.4
9			0.6
11			0.8
13			1.0
Vial No. 2			
15			0.1
17			0.2
19			0.3
21			0.4
23			0.5
25			0.5
(Continue Vial No. 2)			
5-Day Interval			
30			0.5
35			0.5
40			0.5
7-Day Interval			
47			0.5
54			0.5
61			0.5
68			0.5
10-Day Interval			
78			0.5
88			0.5
98			0.5
108			0.5
118			0.5

Often adjustments are made based on adverse reactions; therefore it is essential that the owner be aware of potential adverse reactions.

Adverse Reactions

Adverse reactions in humans are observed and categorized as either local or systemic. Local reactions characterized by erythema and swelling at the injection site are reported as fairly common. Systemic reactions are much less common and are usually mild, with rapid response to medications. Symptoms may include increased allergy symptoms such as sneezing, nasal congestion, or urticaria. Anaphylaxis is referred to as rare. Most systemic reactions develop within 30 minutes of allergen administration. Fatal reactions are reported in humans but are considered even rarer. A report of one fatality per 63 million injections supports the infrequent occurrence (American College of Allergy, Asthma and Immunology, 1997). Risk factors associated with the fatalities include dose errors; seasonal exacerbation of allergic disease, especially symptomatic asthma; high degree of allergen sensitivity; injections from a new vial of allergen; and β-blocker use. Nonfatal systemic reactions are more common and have been reported at a rate

of 0.05 to 3.2 per 100 injections (mean of 0.5%) (Stewart and Lockey, 1992).

Adverse Reactions to Allergen-Specific Immunotherapy in Dogs and Cats

Unfortunately there are limited records of adverse reactions to ASIT, and much of the consensus is based on clinical observation and anecdotal reports. The most common reaction noted, particularly in the dog, is pruritus. The pattern of itching may be typical of the atopic distribution (face, ears, axillary, inguinal, feet, and extremities) or generalized. The pruritic event may be spontaneous and related to the allergen injection or more persistent without any noticeable relation to the allergen injection. The most common association is toward the conclusion of the induction schedule as the maintenance regimen is reached. The intensity of the pruritus may be greater: (1) at the phase of induction with the introduction of the vial containing the next level of concentration; (2) during the continuation of therapy with a new replacement vial of allergen solution; (3) during the time when a higher intensity of natural allergen load occurs; or (4) when

Box 92-5

Allergen-Specific Immunotherapy Administration Schedule for Dogs Over 20 lb of Body weight Using a Three-Vial System

Day	Vial No. 1 1:1000 (ml)	Vial No. 2 1:100 (ml)	Vial No. 3 Maintenance (ml)
0	0.2		
2	0.4		
4	0.6		
6	0.8		
8	1.0		
10		0.2	
12		0.4	
14		0.6	
16		0.8	
18		1.0	
20			0.1
22			0.2
24			0.4
26			0.6
28			0.8
35			1.0
45			1.0
65			1.0
85			1.0
105			0.75-1
	Continue every 21 days		0.75-1

Box 92-6

Allergen-Specific Immunotherapy Administration Schedule for Dogs Under 20 lb of Body Weight and Cats Using a Three-Vial System

Day	Vial No. 1 1:1000 (ml)	Vial No. 2 1:100 (ml)	Vial No. 3 (ml) Maintenance
0	0.1		
2	0.2		
4	0.4		
6	0.6		
8	0.8		
10		0.1	
12		0.2	
14		0.4	
16		0.6	
18		0.8	
20			0.1
22			0.2
24			0.3
26			0.4
28			0.5
35			0.5
42			0.5
49			0.5
63			0.5
70			0.5
	Continue weekly		0.3-0.5

concurrent annual infectious disease immunizations have been administered. Smaller dogs (less than 10 kg) may be at greater risk. It may be difficult to determine the contribution of the allergen therapy to the increasingly pruritic animal during its normal allergic season. In these cases temporary discontinuation of allergen injections usually results in improvement because the animal goes back to its baseline level of disease within several days. Routine annual immunization coincidental to the allergen therapy, particularly toward the end of the induction phase, may contribute to the elicitation of pruritus or other adversities. Exposure to other offensive allergens such as fleas or food may further confuse the association of allergen therapy with the clinical features. The incidence of pruritus as an adversity of allergen immunotherapy is not completely known but appears to be common. In Rosser's study (1998) of 52 dogs that were maintained on immunotherapy greater than 6 months, 26 (50%) had adverse reactions, 11 (21%) and 15 (29%) a persistent worsening of pruritus. Eight dogs (15%) definitely had pruritus as part of the adverse reaction. The number of dogs with persistent increasing pruritus was not determined. Well-designed prospective studies evaluating adverse reactions in dogs and cats have not been reported.

The therapeutic intervention in the event of speculated or substantiated adverse reaction is dictated by the extent of the clinical features observed. Conservative therapy in events of mild pruritus with relevant association to the injections may require only decreasing the volume of allergen injected. Reduction should be at least to the previous level at which no adversity was observed, or it may require an empiric reduction by 50% or more. Some

specialists recommend treatment with no dose change, dose changes in addition to the integration of antihistamine therapy, and/or low-dose alternate-day oral glucocorticoid therapy and topical antipruritic treatment. We prefer lowering the volume given to levels that do not stimulate an adverse reaction. In the event of reaction that occurs during the induction phase, it may be necessary to prepare a lower concentration or resort to the previous dilution for continued therapy, with the intent to continue a slow incremental increase to reach at least a low volume (0.1 ml) of the typical maintenance dosage of 10,000 to 20,000 PNU/ml. In rare cases this cannot be achieved because of persistent reactions; some animals remain on more dilute allergen doses and generally require injections more frequently, sometimes as often as every 2 to 4 days.

More substantial adverse reactions (i.e., urticaria, angioedema, vomiting, or diarrhea) may be observed. Some breeds seem to be more predisposed for these reactions. Our experience includes dachshunds, boxers, Boston terriers, schnauzers, and English Bulldogs in this higher-risk category. These reactions are cause for greater concern and should be taken seriously because they border on a systemic reaction. Allergen therapy should be discontinued temporarily, and systemic antihistamine and glucocorticoid therapy should be integrated in the treatment plan. Parenteral administration of drugs may be indicated for more urgent care or emergency therapy. Reinitiation of allergen therapy should be considered when the adversity has been resolved. Recurrence can be minimized by adjusting the allergen dosage to 50% of the volume causing the reaction; this injection should be given in the clinic or hospital with monitoring. Some specialists also pretreat

½ hour before future injections with an antihistamine with or without concurrent glucocorticoid therapy.

The most severe reaction is anaphylactic shock, which manifests as hyperventilation, collapse, or pale mucous membranes with weakness. The following protocols should be considered in the event of severe systemic or an anaphylactic reaction. For a peracute reaction epinephrine should be administered. The dose is 0.01 mg/kg or 0.1 ml/kg of a 1:10,000 concentration intravenously. The solution is made by diluting a 1:1000 concentration using 1 ml of epinephrine in 9 ml of saline. The volume of milliliters to be administered equals the body weight in kilograms divided by 10. A tongue vein may serve as a route if unable to obtain intravenous access, or injection directly in the tongue parenchyma may also be considered. Alternatively the epinephrine is administered via an endotracheal tube to the level of the carina, using a male urinary catheter. Transcutaneous injection into the trachea is another route but may require an increased dose (doubling). Fluid therapy should be initiated at 1.5 to 5 ml/kg/minute or 90 ml/kg/hour for a dog or 50 ml/kg/hour for a cat. If hypotension is unresponsive to this volume of fluids, a colloid may be added (either pentastarch or hetastarch, 5 ml/kg for dogs or 2.5 ml/kg for cats, in a bolus with as much as 20 ml/kg for dogs or 10 ml/kg for cats over 15 minutes). Blood pressure and physical response should be monitored. Antihistamine therapy may be integrated with parenteral administration in an anaphylactic patient. Diphenhydramine is suggested at 1 to 2 mg/kg with a maximal dose of 50 mg intramuscularly every 8 hours. Caution is expressed for intravenous administration because of hypotensive effect and vomiting. Tripelennamine HCl may be administered intravenously or intramuscularly at 1 mg/kg every 12 hours. Glucocorticoid therapy is routinely included in the treatment regimen for an allergic reaction. Prednisolone sodium succinate or methylprednisolone succinate at 2 mg/kg intravenously should be administered over 15 to 20 minutes. An intramuscular injection may be the alternate route in the event of inaccessible intravenous administration. Dexamethasone sodium phosphate may be administered slowly intravenously at 0.25 to 0.5 mg/kg. Alternatively intramuscular or subcutaneous administration may be necessary. Corticosteroid therapy may be useful in controlling ongoing anaphylaxis, but its benefit in reversing the life-threatening situations is questionable. Withholding glucocorticoid therapy until the intravenous volume has been reestablished is recommended since corticosteroids may cause hypotension. Dopamine is suggested for protracted hypotension by some emergency manuals, using an initial dose of 2-10 mcg/kg/minute. Referral to an emergency manual is recommended to obtain further information on infusion procedures with dopamine. Repeat therapy with epinephrine at 1 ml/kg/hour continuous-rate infusion is preferred by some emergency clinicians over dopamine, with the addition of 4 mg of epinephrine to 1 L of saline. Emergency situations should always include critical monitoring of hematocrit, total solids, and urinary output. Other emergency therapy may be indicated in the event of protracted respiratory distress (refer to appropriate emergency manual). Famotidine may be integrated at 0.5 mg/kg every 12 hours if gastric ulceration is suspected.

Strong consideration should be given to alternative therapy for the atopic problem in lieu of continuing with allergen immunotherapy.

Extreme caution should be exercised if allergen therapy is to be continued in cases with severe systemic reactions. It is advisable to conduct the treatment under the direct supervision of a veterinarian in a hospital environment equipped for handling allergic emergencies. Significant reduction of allergen must be considered to avoid recurrence of the anaphylaxis. Pretreatment with antihistamine and glucocorticoid is advisable. A well-established protocol should be determined if therapy is to be continued by the pet owner. Pretreatment with antihistamine and glucocorticoid is necessary until such time as it seems tolerance has been reached.

Determining the Maintenance Frequency

For many dogs and cats the maintenance dosage (volume of 10,000 to 20,000 PNU/ml) is reached by following the protocol; if no adverse reactions are seen, a final volume of 1 ml in large dogs, 0.7 ml in small dogs, and 0.5 ml in cats is attained. In others the maintenance dosage is determined based on adverse reactions as previously described. Further adjustments are then made to the intervals between injections. If the animal is doing well for the complete duration between shots, the time between injections is gradually lengthened, generally by 2 to 3 days. The new interval is used for three consecutive injections; if the animal is still doing well, more days are added to the interval between injections. The maximum interval is 30 days since longer intervals may allow the allergen solution to become outdated and adverse reactions become more of a concern if errors are made in doses given and intervals not accurately followed.

Determining the Maintenance Dosage

In general, the goal is to reach 1 ml of a 10,000 to 20,000 PNU/ml allergen solution or to find the highest injectate volume that will not aggravate clinical signs. The aim is for a maintenance volume to average about 0.05 ml/day; most dogs receive an average of 0.05 to 0.1 ml/day, with occasional cases going as low at 0.03 ml/day. Once the maintenance dose is identified, the frequency is then adjusted so that the improvement is maintained over the time between injections. If the patient is not responding, the maintenance dosage is given at shorter intervals; if the maintenance dosage is 1 ml, this is 10 days and if the maintenance dose is less than 1 ml, the interval is by the formula of 1 day for every 0.1 ml in the maintenance dose. In dogs that still show no response, 0.5 ml is given every 5 days for 1 month; if there is still no response, 0.7 ml is given every 5 days. If the above is unsuccessful the therapy will likely be ineffective.

Predicting Long-Term Maintenance Cost of Allergen-Specific Immunotherapy

Understanding this general dosage range makes it easy to predict the long-term cost of ASIT therapy because in most cases the volume will be 1 to 3 ml per month. The ASIT cost then includes the cost of the liquid, the cost for syringes based on ASIT frequency of injections per month, and the cost of reevaluations. There is no need to monitor any blood work or urinalysis in dogs on long-term ASIT since no known adverse reactions are detectable by these tests. When the pet has an excellent response to ASIT with total control (15% to 20% of cases), only the cost of 12 to 36 ml of allergen, the syringes, and one annual recheck is involved in controlling the pet's atopic disease. In many other cases (40%) the animals are much improved but still have an occasional exacerbation of their allergic signs, possibly inducing secondary infections that may require 2 to 4 weeks of therapy. In these cases the cost of this short-term therapy once or twice a year must also be considered in determining long-term management costs.

Concurrent Therapies

Generally if the pet's allergy symptoms are not severe, systemic antipruritic therapies are avoided in the initial induction until it is determined that the maximum volume and concentration of allergen solution that does not stimulate an adverse reaction has been reached. In cases with moderate-to-severe pruritus, compassionate use of concurrent medications is indicated. These are avoided in other cases so that mild adverse reactions and patterns of pruritus associated with injections may be observed. Although concurrent administration of systemic antihistamine is preferred during the period of dosage adjustment, systemic oral glucocorticoid therapy may also be used. Prednisone or prednisolone at 0.5 to 1 mg/kg (1 to 2 mg/kg in cats) every other day is a conventional regimen that in our experience does not pose a detrimental effect on the overall response to allergen treatment. Many times the use of glucocorticoid therapy is for a short term. The integration of oral methylprednisolone may be beneficial at a low dosage of 0.1 to 0.2 mg/kg every other day in combination with daily oral antihistamine therapy. Cyclosporine (5 mg/kg daily for 6 to 8 weeks and then every other day for maintenance) may also be used; although, if not previously used, there may be a 7- to 14-day period before it shows efficacy at controlling pruritus. There is no evidence that these therapies interfere with successful response to ASIT, and at least in humans bee venom immunotherapy with concurrent antihistamine therapy appears to improve the response.

The integration of therapeutic modalities is often a necessity for optimal control of atopic dermatitis in the dog or cat. ASIT continues to remain a mainstay in the choices of specific treatment, with the appeal of positive response rate and low observation of adversity. Providing injection therapy at a convenient interval is often an appealing alternative to more aggressive oral therapy for the treatment of a disease with a protracted course. The repetitive and intermittent evaluations of the animal are a prerequisite to maximal control. Responsiveness to treatment modification and observation for complicating problems (bacterial pyoderma, cutaneous *malassezia*, dermatophytosis, or demodicosis) with proper response accounts for an increase in the control of atopic animals.

References and Suggested Reading

American College of Allergy, *Asthma and immunology: fact sheet: efficacy and safety of immunotherapy*, www.accai.org, 1997.

Rosser E: Aqueous hyposensitization in the treatment of canine atopic dermatitis: a retrospective and prospective study of 100 cases. In Kwochka K, Willemse T, vonTscharner C, editors: *Advances in veterinary dermatology*, vol 3, Butterworth Heinemann, 1998, Boston p 169.

Stewart GE, Lockey RF: Systemic reactions from allergen immunotherapy, *J Allergy Clin Immunol* 90:567, 1992.

CHAPTER 93
Topical Immunomodulators

JOEL D. GRIFFIES, *Tustin, California*

TOPICAL IMMUNOMODULATORS

Immunomodulators have been defined as drugs used for their effect on the immune system. This effect may be immunosuppressant as in the case of corticosteroids and calcineurin inhibitors or immunostimulatory as occurs with the use of vaccines or drugs such as imiquimod. With topical application these drugs are allowed to have a focused effect at the site of disease with, in many cases, significantly decreased or no systemic effects. Although a large body of research has developed on the use of these compounds in humans, the indications for topical immunomodulators in animals is just emerging. However, the mechanism of activity, minimal absorption, and increased potency of these drugs, as well as early clinical and anecdotal evidence makes these drugs attractive, and suggest that a number of applications will likely be adapted to veterinary medicine and become useful tools for the practitioner.

Calcineurin Inhibitors

Calcineurin inhibitors, including drugs such as cyclosporine, tacrolimus, and pimecrolimus, are an important class of immunomodulators that have been at the forefront of this genre in the last few years (also see Chapter 55). Calcineurin is a key enzyme in the activation of T lymphocytes. It functions in the induction of gene transcription of a number of inflammatory mediators, including many interleukins (ILs) (e.g., IL-2, IL-3, IL-4), granulocyte-macrophage colony-stimulating factor (GM CSF), tumor necrosis factor-α (TNF-α), and interferon-γ (IFN-γ). Calcineurin *inhibitors* function by binding to a carrier protein with a high affinity for calcineurin, preventing its activity (Fig. 93-1). They have also been shown to inhibit the activation of mast cells, basophils, eosinophils, keratinocytes, and Langerhans cells. Both cyclosporine and tacrolimus decrease the number and activity of epidermal dendritic cells and down-regulate the expression of the high-affinity immunoglobulin E receptor ($F_{C\epsilon}RI$) on Langerhans cells. Calcineurin inhibitors have been used in both humans and animals for many years. Specifically the use of oral cyclosporine for atopic dermatitis (AD) has received much interest recently in veterinary medicine, whereas topical calcineurin inhibitors have been a hot topic in human dermatology literature.

Cyclosporine

Oral cyclosporine has been well studied for its role in managing AD and a number of other dermatologic diseases (see Chapter 84). It is a highly lipophilic cyclic polypeptide with a molecular weight of 1202 kd. Because of molecular size and structural and biologic differences from the other calcineurin inhibitors, its use as a topical treatment modality for inflammatory skin disease has been unrewarding and limited to only anecdotal reports of success.

Tacrolimus

Since its discovery in 1984, intravenous and oral formulations of tacrolimus have been used worldwide in the prevention of organ rejection following allogenic transplants in humans. Although similar to cyclosporine in its mechanism of activity, it is structurally different. Tacrolimus is a hydrophobic macrolide lactone with an atomic weight of 822 kd (smaller than cyclosporine) and is well absorbed into the epidermis via topical administration. The potency of tacrolimus has been estimated at 10 to 100 times greater than cyclosporine. It is currently approved in the United States for use in humans with moderate-to-severe AD. In numerous large multicenter studies it has been found to have significant benefit in the treatment of both pediatric and adult atopic patients. More recently additional applications, including treatment of actinic (solar) dermatosis, psoriasis, and early stages of cutaneous T cell lymphoma have been reported. In veterinary medicine data regarding the use of topical tacrolimus is much more limited but shows promising findings in a number of applications.

CANINE ATOPIC DERMATITIS

Marsella and colleagues performed early studies with topical tacrolimus for treatment of AD in dogs. In the initial

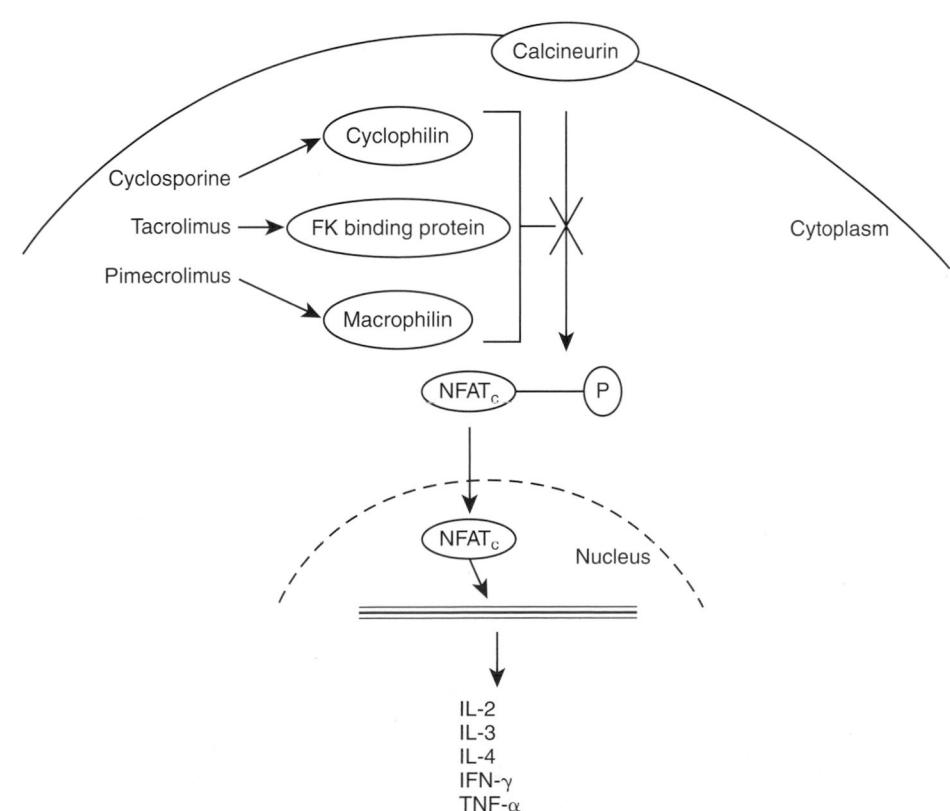

Fig 93-1 Mechanism of action of calcineurin inhibitors. *GM CSF,* granulocyte-macrophage colony-stimulating factor; *IL,* interleukin; *IFN,* interferon; *NFAT,* nuclear factor of activated T cells; *P,* phosphorylation; *TNF,* tumor necrosis factor.

pilot study, using a 0.3% lotion formulated from the oral product, investigator scores for erythema decreased over placebo, but owner scores for pruritus were not significantly different (Marsella and Nicklin, 2002). However, a later randomized, double-blinded placebo-controlled crossover study using commercially available 0.1% tacrolimus ointment (Protopic, Astellas Pharma Manufacturing) found more encouraging results (Marsella et al., 2004). In this study treatment with topical tacrolimus was evaluated in 12 dogs that were diagnosed with AD. After 4 weeks of once-daily application, investigator scores for the tacrolimus- treated group decreased (improved) significantly, whereas no significant differences were detected within the placebo group. When dogs were divided based on severity of disease, those with generalized disease had significantly greater improvement than those with localized disease in both owner and investigator assessments. In conclusion, this study found that tacrolimus ointment decreased clinical signs of AD over a 4-week period with minimal adverse effects or safety concerns. A third study investigated efficacy of 0.1% tacrolimus ointment in treatment of localized lesions of AD on the front paws (Bensignor and Olivry, 2005). All subjects had lesions at other sites, but these were not included in either treatment or evaluation. At the end of the 6-week study the primary investigator found that all dogs who completed the study had a greater than 50% decrease in lesions evaluated (erythema, lichenification, oozing, and excoriations). This study did not evaluate pruritus. Although the results of these studies show benefit from topical tacrolimus, especially in localized AD, I have noted only limited benefit in the treatment of this disease. My experience corresponds with the observation that localized lesions may improve but progress is generally limited to decreases in erythema with less effect on pruritus. As a result, owners have not perceived a benefit substantial enough to warrant continued administration in most cases. Tacrolimus remains a potential option for treatment of localized AD, especially when trying to minimize the use of other treatment modalities with greater concerns for adverse effects (i.e., topical or systemic glucocorticoids), but at least in my practice it is not used as a sole therapy.

IMMUNE-MEDIATED DISEASES

An open-label study was performed by my practice evaluating 0.1% topical tacrolimus in the management of immune-mediated diseases such as discoid lupus erythematosus (DLE) and pemphigus erythematosus (PE). In this study 10 dogs with DLE and two dogs with PE were treated with the commercially available 0.1% tacrolimus ointment (Griffies et al., 2004). All cases had lesions localized to the nasal planum and adjacent regions of the muzzle. Owners applied 0.1% tacrolimus ointment to the affected areas every 12 hours. Each dog's lesions were assessed for degree of erythema, crust, ulceration or erosion, depigmentation, and scarring and were evaluated 2, 4, and 8 weeks after starting therapy. Ten of 12 dogs exhibited improvement in clinical lesions associated with PE or DLE (five excellent response, five partial response) over the 8-week trial. Of the dogs that showed progress, eight of 10 were treated with tacrolimus

alone by the end of the study and remained in remission at 12 weeks. Two of these cases followed for an additional 2 years continued to do well with topical tacrolimus alone. In my practice 0.1% tacrolimus has become a first-line drug for mild-to-moderate DLE. In mild cases it is often used alone every 12 hours for the first 2 weeks and decreased to every 24 hours, depending on progress. Once clinical lesions are resolved, many cases allow tapering to every other day or twice weekly. In moderate-to-severe cases 0.1% tacrolimus ointment is often used as an adjunctive therapy combined with tetracycline and niacinamide, vitamin E, or oral corticosteroids. In these cases topical tacrolimus may allow reduction of systemic therapies and can become a part of the longer-term maintenance of this chronic disease. Similarly in my practice topical tacrolimus has become an adjunctive to managing localized lesions of pemphigus foliaceus, but it is not considered a successful primary or exclusive therapy for this disease. However, it may assist in managing localized lesions that remain on the nasal planum, for example, without necessitating an increase in or modification of systemic medications such as corticosteroids or azathioprine when the majority of other lesions have resolved.

CUTANEOUS VASCULITIS

Cutaneous vasculitis may be present in a variety of clinical manifestations, including purpura, wheals, edema, papules, plaques nodules alopecia scarring, necrosis, and ulceration, often involving the extremities. One of the most common presentations seen by general practitioners and veterinary dermatologists is an ischemic dermatopathy often linked to vaccine administration. Lesions observed are the results of loss of blood supply from vasculitis or a vasculopathy. The prototypical form is that seen following rabies vaccination, usually 1 to 5 months after administration. A classic postvaccinal lesion may occur characterized by an annular hypopigmented or hyperpigmented area of alopecia that may also be indurated, erythematous, or scaly. Multiple distal lesions may occur with or without the presence of an injection site reaction. These commonly include lesions at the apex and often concave aspect of the pinnae, especially at the margins; but other areas such as the paw pads, tip of the tail, periocular region, and junction of the nasal planum and haired skin may also be involved. Topical tacrolimus has been especially useful in managing the mild-to-moderate pinnal lesions associated with this disease. Twice-daily application of the 0.1% ointment to crusted, indurated, and erythematous lesions typically affects improvement in these lesions within 2 to 4 weeks. Because of the ischemic nature of the lesions seen, some scarring, alopecia, or hyperpigmentation may be expected to remain even after the lesions are no longer active. In more severe cases topical tacrolimus therapy is often combined with other systemic therapies. Similar benefit has been seen in decreasing edema and erythema associated with early lesions associated with rabies injection site reactions. Alopecia again is expected to persist. With the more aggressive proliferative thrombovascular necrosis of the pinnae, topical tacrolimus has been less effective since these cases typically need a more aggressive systemic therapeutic approach.

PERIANAL FISTULAS

Perianal fistulas are chronic, painful, often progressive inflammatory lesions of the perianal, anal, and perirectal tissues (see also Chapter 122). This condition has been reported most commonly in the German shepherd dog but have also been observed in Irish setters, Labrador retrievers, Old English sheepdogs, Border collies, bulldogs, and others. Lesions may vary from superficial microscopic fistulas to large ulcerations and sinus tracts and often are complicated by secondary bacterial infection. Although a specific etiopathogenesis has not been recognized, most recent efforts suggest an immune-mediated component. Clinical signs may include tenesmus, dyschezia, constipation, excessive perianal licking, and increased frequency of defecation. Previous therapies have included a variety of surgical methods, including excision, cryotherapy, chemical cauterization, and laser surgery. Reported remission rates from surgical therapy vary greatly (48% to 97%) along with complication rates (13% to 100%) and recurrences (13% to 56%). More recently medical therapies for this disease have produced more encouraging results. Most notably the use of cyclosporine with or without ketoconazole has shown substantial success in improving and resolving the lesions and clinical signs associated with perianal fistulas.

As reviewed earlier, the similar mechanism of action of topical tacrolimus makes it a good choice for this disease. Misseghers, Binnington, and Mathews (2000) reported clinical observations of 10 dogs treated with a 0.1% topical tacrolimus ointment formulated from the oral product before the release of the commercial ointment. As a sole therapy in this case series, five of 10 dogs had a complete response, and four of 10 had a partial response. In our practice we have found the 0.1% commercially available tacrolimus ointment to be a useful tool for perianal fistulas. However, because of the discomfort often associated with these lesions, the use of any topical medication as an initial therapy is less successful. A more practical protocol is to use oral cyclosporine alone (5 to 7 mg/kg daily) or oral cyclosporine (1 to 3 mg/kg daily) in combination with ketoconazole (5 to 10 mg/kg daily, respectively) initially. Once lesions are seen to improve, tacrolimus may be added once or twice daily. This allows reduction of cyclosporine, an often cost-prohibitive drug, while continuing to show progress. In my experience long-term maintenance has been possible using tacrolimus alone daily to two or three times per week.

EMERGING THERAPIES

Metatarsal Fistulation of German Shepherd Dogs

Metatarsal fistulation is an uncommon condition reported in German shepherd dogs. It has been suggested as a familial disorder of collagen caused by similar ancestry and antibodies against types I and II collagen found in dogs studied. Affected dogs develop fistulous tracts proxi-

mal to the metatarsal pads that typically have a serous or serosanguinous discharge. Therapies described for the management of this condition include antibiotic therapy along with oral immunomodulators such as corticosteroids. Researchers reported in a workshop that 0.1% topical tacrolimus was useful in these cases in an open clinical trial. At the end of 6 weeks of therapy, treated lesions in four of seven cases were in complete remission, and three had palpable but not visible lesions (Kwochka and Rosenkrantz, 2005). After following these cases for an additional 2 years I have been able to maintain them with intermittent topical tacrolimus therapy. Our success with this disease has been similar with positive results and an ability to improve and maintain plantar fistulas with intermittent topical tacrolimus therapy along with oral antibiotics for secondary bacterial infections when present.

OTHER APPLICATIONS

As a new topical tool for veterinary dermatologic conditions, tacrolimus has been used in a number of different types of cases. Anecdotal reports of success with topical tacrolimus include its use as an adjunctive in the treatment of acral pruritic nodules, combined with systemic antibiotics. I have found it only mildly useful in this application. Other areas may include assistance in management of actinic dermatosis and feline eosinophilic granuloma/plaque lesions.

Pimecrolimus

Although pimecrolimus (Elidel, Novartis Pharmaceuticals) has a virtually identical mechanism of action to tacrolimus and cyclosporine, no reports of its success in veterinary medicine have been published. It is produced commercially as a topical hydrophilic cream. In human literature side-by-side comparisons of pimecrolimus and tacrolimus found tacrolimus to be superior for the treatment of AD, although both drugs showed benefit. In my limited experience pimecrolimus has been less successful for the management of the diseases mentioned previously. Anecdotal reports suggest that the pimecrolimus molecule is not well absorbed when applied topically, which may explain these observations. Until more positive experience is obtained with this calcineurin inhibitor, I cannot recommend it.

Safety Concerns

In 2002 the Food and Drug Administration required a black box label to be applied to the packaging of topical calcineurin inhibitors, including tacrolimus and pimecrolimus. Unfortunately, based on a number of independent reviews, these concerns are largely unfounded. The potential risk of malignancies, especially lymphoma, with the use of systemic immunosuppressive drugs has been well studied. It has been noted with *oral* administration of cyclosporine, tacrolimus, azathioprine, and others. Studies supporting these concerns with topical immunomodulators have included the use of quantities overwhelmingly higher than those typically used in human medicine and than those suggested for animals in this and other papers. Although the future of this concern will be determined only by retrospective studies, the opinion of those at the forefront of research with these drugs is that their use stimulates only minor concern in this area.

In the handful of recent studies using topical tacrolimus for dermatoses, none have noted significant systemic or topical adverse effects. Absorption of tacrolimus has been confirmed in some studies by measurable blood levels in treated patients. However, these levels have remained far below previously established toxicity levels and have had no effect on routine complete blood count and biochemical parameters. This information suggests that use of topical calcineurin inhibitors is unlikely to predispose veterinary patients or their owners to lymphoma. However, I still recommend that they be applied with gloves and that owners wash their hands after handling them.

Imiquimod

In contrast to the calcineurin inhibitors, imiquimod is an immune response modifier that functions by *stimulating* or enhancing local innate immune response. An imidazoquinoline amine, imiquimod (Aldara, 3M Pharmaceuticals) has potent antiviral and antitumor activity in animal research models. It has been shown to be a ligand for toll-like receptor (TLR) 7. Activation of TLR 7 results in cell-mediated immunity facilitated by T helper lymphocytes and can result in tissue-specific apoptosis. It is approved for the topical treatment of external genital and perianal warts in humans (commonly caused by human papillomavirus), as well as superficial basal cell carcinoma and actinic keratosis. Topically applied imiquimod can induce cells, including keratinocytes, to synthesize and release cytokines, including IFN-α, IL-6, and TNF-α among others. Although not antiviral itself, the induction of these cytokines, specifically IFN-α, inhibits viral replication and promotes stronger cell-mediated immune responses. A component of the innate immune system, IFN-α helps infected cells and their neighbors eliminate virus without a specific cell-mediated immune response. The cells respond as though they have been infected and begin making IFN-γ and other cytokines, which help to clear viral pathogens and lesions caused by them. As a biologic response modifier and an agent fostering a cell-mediated immune response, imiquimod may also help treat other dermatologic disorders, infections, and neoplasms. To this end, imiquimod has been reported to aid in the treatment of a variety of human diseases, including squamous cell carcinoma in situ (Bowen's disease), basal cell carcinoma, molluscum contagiosum, actinic keratosis, and various forms of cutaneous lymphoma.

In animal models imiquimod also stimulates innate immune response by increasing natural killer cell activity, activating macrophages to secrete cytokines and nitric oxide, and inducing proliferation and differentiation of B lymphocytes (Sauder, 2000).

In veterinary patients reports of imiquimod are limited but again show promise. Similar to its use in humans, imiquimod has been a useful tool in managing localized disease associated with viral infection.

Squamous Cell Carcinoma In Situ (Bowen's Disease)

Squamous cell carcinoma in situ (Bowen's disease) is an uncommon disorder in cats linked to a papillomavirus. Lesions are often found on the head, neck, and forelimbs. Topical use of imiquimod has shown positive success in managing localized lesions. It has been my experience on occasion that sites distant to those treated may improve or resolve while other lesions are being treated. Because of concern for inflammation and irritation at the site of application, a protocol of intermittent application is typically used. This may include alternate-day or three times–a-week application or applications on 2 to 3 consecutive days followed by 2 to 4 days off. Limitations of this therapy include the high cost of imiquimod and small surface area that can be treated with the small volume of medication per packet. I commonly reseal an open packet and use it repetitively to treat smaller lesions. However, even with larger lesions, the cost of repeated topical application may be less than traditional or CO_2 laser surgery.

Feline Herpesvirus

Feline herpesvirus one (FHV-1) is a common cause of upper respiratory disease in domestic cats and an uncommon cause of cutaneous erosion and ulceration (see Chapter 99). The localized nature of cutaneous lesions when present makes this disease an excellent candidate for topical imiquimod. As seen with other conditions, application of imiquimod often incites an initial inflammatory response that appears to worsen clinical lesions. However, following the initial inflammation, lesions may heal and be replaced by localized scarring. In at least one case polymerase chain reaction for FHV-1 was positive from both the cutaneous lesion and the conjunctival sac (a known site of FHV-1 sequestration) before treatment and negative after treatment with imiquimod. This suggested that not only did lesions clear but that the immune response stimulated may have been able to clear the virus entirely. Whether this was a true finding or a temporary change is difficult to ascertain and warrants further investigation.

Canine Cutaneous Papillomatosis

Clinical syndromes associated with papillomavirus in the dog include oral papillomatosis, cutaneous papillomas, cutaneous inverted papillomas, and papillomavirus-associated canine pigmented plaques. Of these, cutaneous inverted papillomas and cutaneous papillomas have been managed successfully with imiquimod. In most cases seen, topical imiquimod has been used following recurrence after surgical excision of solitary lesions. Unlike the surgical procedures, when the recurrent lesions are cleared via topical imiquimod, further relapse has not been observed.

Other Potential Uses

Because of its innovative mechanism of action and the induction of an immune response by local cells, imiquimod is very likely to have a number of additional uses. Based on applications in human medicine, these may include management of actinic keratosis lesions in dogs and cats. Recent reports of success with topical imiquimod in treatment of equine sarcoid have also been published (Nogueira et al., 2006).

References and Suggested Reading

Beck LA: The efficacy and safety of tacrolimus ointment: a clinical review, *J Am Acad Dermatol* 53:S165, 2005.

Bensignor E, Olivry T: Treatment of localized lesions of canine atopic dermatitis with tacrolimus ointment: a blinded randomized controlled trial, *Vet Dermatol* 16:52, 2005.

Griffies JD et al: Topical 0.1% tacrolimus for the treatment of discoid lupus erythematosus and pemphigus erythematosus in dogs, *J Am Anim Hosp Assoc* 40:29, 2004.

Kwochka KW, Rosenkrantz WS: Shampoos and topical therapy. In Hillier A, Foster A, Kwoshka K, editors: *Advances in veterinary dermatology*, Oxford, UK, 2005, Blackwell Publishing, p 378.

Marsella R, Nicklin CF: Investigation on the use of 0.3% tacrolimus for atopic dermatitis, *Vet Derm* 13:203, 2002.

Marsella R et al. Investigation on the clinical efficacy and safety of 0.1% tacrolimus ointment (Protopic) in canine atopic dermatitis: a randomized, double-blinded, placebo-controlled, cross-over study, *Vet Dermatol* 15:294, 2004.

Misseghers BS, Binnington AG, Mathews KA: Clinical observations of the treatment of canine perianal fistulas with topical tacrolimus in 10 dogs, *Can Vet J* 41:623, 2000.

Nogueira SA et al: Efficacy of imiquimod 5% cream on the treatment of equine sarcoid: a pilot study, *Vet Derm* 17:259, 2006.

Patel GK et al: Imiquimod 5% cream monotherapy for cutaneous squamous cell carcinoma in situ (Bowen's disease): a randomized, double-blind, placebo-controlled trial, *J Am Acad Dermatol* 54:1025, 2006.

Sauder DN: Immunomodulatory and pharmacologic properties of imiquimod, *J Am Acad Dermatol* 43:S6, 2000.

CHAPTER 94

House Dust Mites and Their Control

WAYNE S. ROSENKRANTZ, *Tustin, California*

IMPORTANCE OF HOUSE DUST MITES IN ATOPIC DERMATITIS

House dust mite (HDM) hypersensitivities are extremely common throughout the world. In a review of 469 cases of atopic dermatitis (AD) at the Animal Dermatology Clinics of southern California, dust mites were the top reactors (*Dermatophagoides farinae* 55.2%, *Dermatophagoides pteronyssinus* 39.7%). In other reports positive skin tests or serum IgE specific for HDM allergens may be as high as 6% to 90% in canine AD cases. House dust allergy is common even in clean homes and is a major cause of year-round allergy symptoms for humans as well as pets. House dust is a mixture of many mites and their body part allergens. The most common HDMs belong to members of the family Pyroglyphidae and include *D. farinae, D. pteronyssinus,* and *Euroglyphus mayne.* Other mites of importance include some mites that have been classified as storage, mold, or grain mites belonging to the family Acaridae (*Acarus siro* and *Tryophagus putrescentia*) and mites belonging to the family Glycyphagidae *(Glycyphagus domesticus, Blomia tropicalis* and *Lepidoglyphus destructor).* Some of these can

be found in high levels outside food sources and are also considered environmental mites that could contribute to mite hypersensitivity reactions.

The concentration of dust mites in the home environment varies, depending on what part of the country or world in which one lives. Environmental factors such as moisture or humidity are very important. The most important antigen fractions come from *D. farinae* and *D. pteronyssinus* (Der f 1 and f 2, Der p 1 and p 2, and Der f 15, a high–molecular weight antigen). It is possible that some mites may be more resistant to dryer or less humid environments. *D. farinae* is considered more resistant to dryer climates and may still be found in desert climates such as Las Vegas, compared to its counter part *D. pteronyssinus.* In more humid or subtopical environments *B. tropicalis* may be found and in some cases may be the most prevalent. The HDM content varies from home to home as well as within areas of the home, depending on the type of furniture, building materials, and presence of pets. The highest allergen concentrations are found in pillows, mattresses, carpeting, and upholstered furniture. Levels have also been detected in automobiles and on the hair coats and bedding of dogs (Randal et al., 2005).

There may be as many as 19,000 HDMs in 1 g of dust, but more typically 100 to 500 mites live in each gram of dust. Each mite produces about 10 to 20 waste fecal particles per day and lives for about 30 days. Egg-laying females can add 25 to 30 new mites to the population during their brief lifetime.

ISOLATED ALLERGENS AND METHODS OF DETECTION

Allergens are divided according to their chemical properties and allergen cross-reactivity; they have cross-reacting and species-specific epitopes. Antigens are named by mite species and group antigen designations (e.g., Der p 1, Der f). Group 1 antigens Der p 1 and Der f 1 are the most allergenic for humans; they are associated with or found in mite feces and probably represent intestinal enzymes cysteine protease. Group 2 Der p 2 and Der f 2 are more stable than group I in the environment; they contain molecules associated with male reproductive tracts and have more species cross-reactivity. The other classified allergens include group 3: fecal trypsin; group 4: amylase; group 6: chymotrypsin; group 8: glutathione-S-transferase; group 9: another serine protease (an important human allergen); group 10: tropomyosin; group 11: paramyosin; group 13: fatty acid–binding protein; group 15: chitinase; group 16: gelsolin; group 17: calcium-binding protein; and group 18: chitinase. There are other as yet unclassified or identified allergenic epitopes considered less important or minor allergens.

The current information about which antigens dogs react to would indicate little reactivity with groups 1 and 2 antigens. There are higher–molecular weight (HMW) allergens recognized by atopic dog sera (Nuttal et al., 2006). One of the HMW antigens has been characterized as Der f 15, a digestive chitinase (McCall et al., 2001). Other HMW antigens that may be important in the canine include another chitinase (Der f 18) and tropomyosin (Der f 10). These allergens may be very difficult to denature and destroy, creating more difficulty in elimination from the environment.

Currently identifying HDM allergens in the environment or on the pet is rarely performed, and the association between mite levels and clinical disease has not been studied in the dog as it has in humans. Therefore when HDM sensitivity is detected, HDM control is generally recommended when feasible and especially when it is the only or primary allergen to which the dog reacts. When the owner or clinician wants to identify mites in the environment, the following techniques are available: mite counts/gram of dust, specific antigen assay (enzyme-linked immunosorbent assay [ELISA] or amplified ELISA), and measurement of mite fecal matter, with measurement of fecal guanine levels. Dust and mites are usually collected with dust by vacuum techniques. Fecal material can be sampled with a semiquantitative measurement of guanine (fecal product) by a commercially available test kit (Acarex); less than 0.6 mg of guanine per gram of dust can be detected and provides an estimate of dust mite fecal antigens. Antigens by ELISA using monoclonal antibody reagents for groups 1 and 2 Der p and Der f antigens are available. Amplified ELISA detection threshold (300 pg/ml) using MITE-T-Fast (AVEHO

Biosciences) is a validated wipe test. This technique uses a porous sampling pin in association with an immuno-chromatographic test system that detects Der p 2/f 2 with sensitivity 62%—specificity 94% when compared with ELISA assay. It can be used to identify dust mite allergen levels on textiles such as carpets, furniture, or bedding or on a pet's hair coat. Although species specificity exists, some cross-reactivity may exist between HDM allergens or related allergens such as storage mites or even scabies or otodectes. These tests need to be reviewed carefully and always interpreted in conjunction with clinical history and physical findings.

CONTROL OF HOUSE DUST MITES IN THE HOME AND ON PET

Mite antigens are difficult to remove from the environment. Commonly recommended techniques such as vacuuming, steam cleaning, and dry cleaning are often ineffective. Even using acardial products and reducing home humidity do not always work. All methods have variable effectiveness, and their benefits in clinical control of related HDM hypersensitivities in humans are controversial. However, there is one study (Swinnen and Vroom, 2004) and some anecdotal reports that suggest that there is clinical value in HDM control for canine atopic dermatitis.

Basic strategies include reducing carpeting, textile furniture, regular washing of bedding, vacuuming, reducing humidity, and using mattress and pillow encasements. Elimination of carpeting and switching to hardwood or tile floors can be helpful. Elimination of upholstery furniture and switching to wood, vinyl, or leather are also recommended. Washing bedding weekly in hot water (130° F) kills mites and removes most allergens. Dry cleaning kills mites but does not remove all allergens. Vacuuming weekly removes only surface mites and allergens and may be more effective if used in conjunction with other acardial agents (see following paragraphs). Dehumidifiers and air conditioning can be helpful in trying to maintain the relative humidity below 50%. However, even when the home environment is controlled, it may not be possible to completely control the microenvironment on a mattress or mattress pad because of the humidity created by body temperature. Mattress and pillow encasements lower mite levels but are controversial on their effectiveness in clinical control of related HDM hypersensitivities in humans. Mattress and pillow encasements are occlusive, vapor-permeable, nonwoven synthetic or tight-weave fabrics with certified pore size (5 to 9 micron) and are available commercially.

More intensive methods of HDM control include the use of specific acardial and mite allergen denaturing agents. Their effectiveness has been more controversial. One of the more classic agents is benzyl benzoate. In one study (Swinnen and Vroom, 2004) HDM detection and control with benzyl benzoate (Acarosan spray, Allergopharma) and changing the pets' bedding showed that after treatment 29 out of 60 dogs sensitive to HDMs or storage mites, 48% showed no skin lesions or pruritus. Moderate results were achieved in 22 dogs (36%) (i.e., reduced pruritus and minimal skin lesions but still requiring medication). This product has limited availability and is considered a potential carcinogen.

Borates have received a lot of attention for HDM control. In a noncontrolled pilot study I looked at sodium polyborates for HDM control in treated (six) and untreated (three) homes. HDMs and their antigens were assessed via direct counts and for guanine antigen levels via the (Acarex) test. Significant reduction in HDM levels occurred; however, allergen levels remained elevated but reduced. In another placebo-controlled study carpet pieces were inoculated with *D. farinae* and *D. pteronyssinus* and treated with disodium octaborate tetrahydrate (DOT). Pretreated and posttreated measurements at 2, 4, and 8 weeks showed marked reduction in total mite counts: 885 to 10, 17500 to 1100 mite/gram dust *D. farinae* and *D. pteronyssinus*, respectively (Arlian and Mills, 2001). A placebo-controlled 6-month study in 93 homes with active, placebo (water), and negative control groups showed promising results. Dust collected before and after every 2 months from carpets and sofas and live mites, total mites, and mite allergen levels were measured. DOT killed mites in carpets and sofas for up to 6 months; sofas were less affected. HDM allergen was significantly lower in the carpets and sofas at 6 months after treatment (Codina, et al., 2003).

Denaturing agents have also been evaluated to inactivate the protein moiety of the HDM allergen, and some have also been proposed to kill the live mites. Tannic acid is one such product that may perform both functions. However, it is very drying and has significant problems with staining of fabrics. Another denaturing agent (Allerase, Aveho Biosciences) contains a citric acid derivative with soybean-extracted fatty acids and fatty alcohol surfactants. The active ingredient in the Allerase product has been evaluated both clinically and in unpublished in vitro studies. One study evaluated the denaturing effects of this product on Der p 1 and p 2 and showed superior reduction of HDM allergens when compared to other denaturing agents, including tannic acid and benzyl benzoate (Williams, 2000). However, the same effectiveness on the more important canine allergens may not occur with this product because high–molecular weight allergens are more difficult to completely denature. This was supported by another canine in vitro study in which HDM allergen was exposed in a 1:2 and 1:4 dilution with Allerase overnight. Although there was a detectable reduction in immunoglobulin E reactivity, it was not considered significant (Esch, 2003). However, this study did not use full-strength concentration. Another study exposed HDM-allergic dogs to HDM extract applied to kennel floors and compared it to a placebo control. The results showed no statistical difference between the groups. However, the concentration and volume of the product were used at lower than would approximate clinical applications (Marsella, Nicklin, and Lopez, 2005). I have been evaluating the effects of Allerase (spray and shampoo formulations) as a topical therapy directly on the hair coat and skin as a means of eliminating or reducing percutaneous absorption of allergen on the skin surface. This seemed appropriate based on the work showing the presence of HDM allergens on dogs' coats and bedding (Jackson et al., 2005; Randall et al., 2005). I and others have anecdotal experience of some dogs responding to these products and I currently recommend its use in all primarily HDM-positive dogs.

Although many insecticides and growth regulators are ineffective for the control of environmental mites, one insect growth hormone regulator, pyriproxifen (Virbac), has been advocated as an environmental method of HDM control. Although I have not used this product, it is a recommended treatment in Europe and the United Kingdom.

References and Suggested Reading

Arlian LG, Platts-Mills TAE: The biology of dust mites and the remediation of mite allergens in allergic disease, *J Allergy Clin Immunol* 107:406, 2001.

Codina R et al: Disodium octaborate tetrahydrate (DOT) application and vacuum cleaning, a combined strategy to control HDM, *Allergy* 58:1, 2003.

Esch B: Allerase—ELISA inhibition potency assay, May 2003, Greer Labs, Lenoir, North Carolina.

Jackson AP et al: Prevalence of house dust mites and *Dermatophagoides* group 1 antigens collected from bedding, skin, and hair coat of dogs in southwest England, *Vet Dermatol* 16:32, 2005.

Marsella R, Nicklin C, Lopez, J: Evaluation of the effects of Allerase spray on clinical signs in HDM-allergic high-IgE beagle dogs using a randomized, double-blinded, placebo-controlled design, 20th Proceedings of North American Veterinary Dermatology Forum, Sarasota, Fla, 2005, p 211.

McCall C et al: Characterization and cloning of a major high molecular weight house dust mite allergen (Der f 15) for dogs, *Vet Immunol Immunopathol* 78:231, 2001.

Nuttall TJ et al: House dust and forage mite allergens and their role in human and canine atopic dermatitis, *Vet Dermatol* 17: 223, 2006.

Randall AJ et al: Quantitation of house dust mite allergens (Der f1 and group 2) on the skin and hair of dogs, *Am J Vet Res* 66:143, 2005.

Swinnen C, Vroom M: The clinical effect of environmental control of house dust mites in 60 house dust mite–sensitive dogs, *Vet Dermatol* 15:34, 2004.

Williams PB: *The ecology works anti-allergen solution products composition studies*, May 2000, IBT Reference Laboratory, Hobe Sound, Florida.

CHAPTER 95

Topical Therapy of Otitis Externa

COLLEEN MENDELSOHN, *Tustin, California*

Canine ear disease is a prevalent and persistent problem and accounts for up to 15% of all canine veterinary case presentations. The large variety and quantity of veterinary topical otic preparations available demonstrate the demand for a wide range of therapeutics for this condition. Primary causes of otitis externa include hypersensitivity disorders (e.g., atopy, food allergy), parasitic diseases, and metabolic disorders (e.g., primary keratinization defects, hypothyroidism, hyperadrenocorticism). Perpetuating and predisposing factors such as proliferative changes, excessive cleaning, or the use of inappropriate cleaning products also contribute to the prevalence of ear problems. Otitis externa can also be secondary to an infection of the ear canal. *Malassezia pachydermatis* is the most common isolate from diseased ears.

Identifying and managing the primary disease(s) are the goals of treating most cases of canine otitis externa and are often sufficient to prevent recurrence if no perpetuating factors are present. However, even when the primary cause is identified and addressed, cases occasionally require continuous topical and/or systemic therapy. On the other hand, in some cases of allergic otitis, as well as other chronic primary conditions, controlling secondary infections is sufficient to alleviate clinical signs. Otic preparations are designed to either address an immediate infection/infestation or prevent recurrence in chronic disease. Otic preparations that address bacterial and/or yeast infections are usually combinations of corticosteroids and antimicrobials. Preparations designed for long-term control are combinations of mild cleansers, drying agents, or disinfectants and may contain antimicrobial agents.

Overall the therapeutic approach to chronic ear disease is truly an art, and there is no "blanket" approach for treating this condition. Each case represents varying levels of proliferation and exudate with a different degree of infection versus inflammation. Therapy needs to be targeted at each aspect of the condition. Becoming familiar with the products available and their effects is essential to formulating the best therapeutic plan for each patient. Since new products are introduced into the market each month, it is important to have a good relationship with the various industry representatives who can keep the practitioner updated on what is newly available and the advantages the products may provide.

GENERAL PROPERTIES OF TOPICAL FORMULATIONS

The Vehicle

As with all forms of topical therapy, multiple formulations and vehicles are used in otic products. Each has specific properties that need to be considered when selecting an appropriate product. The various vehicles have different mechanisms for delivery of the active ingredients, as well as therapeutic, irritant, or cosmetic properties that determine their efficacy in practice. Various vehicles encountered in veterinary topical otic therapy include solutions/rinses, lotions, creams, emulsions, and ointments.

Rinses generally are formulated by diluting concentrated solutions or powders with water. These can be poured into the ear in large amounts and therefore are the most appropriate vehicle for cleansers. Lotions are liquids in which the active ingredient has been dissolved or suspended. Thus, when the liquid dries, a thin layer of powder is left in the ear. Lotions tend to be drying because of their alcohol or propylene glycol content. Generally a "cooling" lotion or solution tends to contain alcohol, whereas a "soothing" one does not. Creams, emulsions, and ointments are occlusive and prevent contact with the environment. Creams are least occlusive, and ointments are the most occlusive; emulsions have characteristics of both. In exudative cases, use of an ointment may be contraindicated since increased water loss and drying are desired.

Active Ingredients

Astringents, soothing agents, acidifiers, alkalinizing agents, keratolytic agents, keratoplastic agents, antibiotics, antifungals, and antiinflammatory and antiparasiticidal products all can be found in the enormous milieu of topical otic preparations. Often these products are combined. When a practitioner is choosing a topical otic product, the patient's specific condition, as well as the practitioner's familiarity with the product, must be taken into consideration. Practitioners and dermatologists occasionally prepare "in-house" otic remedies from injectable antibiotics or antifungal agents or mix a variety of available otic products to create a single mixture that targets their specific patient's need. This practice is a controversial and extralabel use of these drugs and is a topic beyond the scope of this chapter. However, if this approach is taken, it is important to remember that the stability and efficacy of the active ingredients may be affected, and the client must be clearly informed of the off-label formulation.

TREATMENT OF INFECTIONS

Initial Approach

Cytology: Cytology is an inexpensive procedure that can be performed easily in house, allowing the practitioner to make immediate decisions regarding treatments or further diagnostics; it should be performed with every reevaluation of the ear. Often the character of the infection or the degree of inflammation will change. Repeating cytology may reveal a change in the infectious organisms that indicates that a change in the topical antimicrobial is in order. In addition, the presence of various inflammatory cells could be a sign that an irritant or allergic/immune-mediated reaction might be present. If a practitioner is not comfortable making decisions based on his or her abilities, duplicate slides can be submitted to a commercial laboratory for corroboration.

Cleaning: Cleaning and removing purulent, ceruminous, or foreign debris from an ear canal before initiating therapy is imperative for effective management of otitis. In addition to being therapeutic, cleaning removes exudates that can not only prevent a thorough examination of the ear canal but also interfere (chemically and physically) with the therapeutic agents. Ceruminolytic agents used in the clinic can aid greatly in removing debris; however, use of the more potent ceruminolytic formulations is not generally recommended for home care by the client. Table 95-1 lists a variety of different cleansers that can be selected based on severity of debris in the ear canal and whether the product is to be used in the practice or at home by the owner. Numerous cleaning techniques are described in the literature (see Chapter 97).

Cleaning is imperative for successful therapy; however, excessive cleaning by clients is often a perpetuating factor in chronic recurrent otitis. It is generally found that the initial cleaning is best left to the clinician during the initial acute phase of therapy. Once the acute episode is resolved, clients can be given products and instructions to keep the ears from relapsing. Most cleansers should be used no more than two to three times weekly. In some cases of mild otitis secondary to mild seasonal allergies, regular cleaning should only be recommended during the offending season or not recommended at all. One of the exceptions to this rule is in cases of chronic ceruminous otitis (e.g., cocker seborrhea). In this case regular ear cleaning and maintenance by the client are extremely important if any kind of therapeutic success is to be achieved.

Antibacterial Therapy

Topical therapy of active infections is imperative to success. Systemic (oral or injectable) therapy is sometimes necessary but is unlikely to achieve therapeutic concentrations within the ear as a sole treatment modality (see Chapter 96). The antimicrobial agent best used is often chosen empirically based on cytologic examination of ear canal exudate and otoscopic evaluation of the ear canal. Bacterial culture and sensitivity results can be of value, especially when dealing with gram-negative organisms (e.g., *Pseudomonas* spp.) from the middle ear. However, sensitivity results of bacterial cultures may be misleading since topical antimicrobial concentrations are much higher than serum concentrations. Occasionally cultures need to be repeated because infected ear canals often contain numerous bacteria colonies with different resistant patterns that are not all represented with one single culture.

Several veterinary topical otic formulations contain antibacterial agents (Table 95-2). It is important to consider previous therapies the patient may have received for the infection, the type of bacteria encountered, and the degree of inflammation and amount of exudate in the ear canal. If the canals are severely inflamed, the patient will likely need to return on a weekly basis for cleaning and reevaluation until the bulk of the infection and inflammation is resolved. For more resistant bacterial infections, especially gram-negative infections such as *Pseudomonas aeruginosa*, pretreatment of the canal with a tromethamine ethylenediaminetetraacetic (Tris EDTA)–containing product before administration of a topical antibiotic is recommended. Tris EDTA has antibacterial properties but also acts synergistically with aminoglycosides and fluoroquinolones to increase their bactericidal activity. A product (T8 Keto) is available that contains both Tris EDTA and ketoconazole to help control mixed bacterial and yeast infections.

Antiyeast Therapy

Numerous products are available to address yeast otitis (Table 95-3). Many of these products contain potent, broad-spectrum antibiotics; however, the antifungal included is sometimes less potent against the commonly encountered yeast organism *M. pachydermatis*. On the other hand, in cases of mild allergic yeast otitis, decreasing the otic inflammation with a topical glucocorticoid alone can aid in the elimination of a yeast infection or overgrowth by controlling many of the inflammatory by-products on which yeast survive. In chronic recurrent yeast otitis the use of boric acid or acetic acid–containing products is often effective in preventing recurrence of infection. Acetic acid may be markedly irritating to the ear canal, especially at concentrations of 2% or higher (white vinegar has a concentration of 5%). It has generally been found that boric acid solution, without the presence of acetic acid (Zinc Otic) is effective at managing chronic recurrent yeast otitis and has been demonstrated effective in treatment of mild-to-moderate acute yeast otitis.

Antiinflammatory Therapy

The majority of antimicrobial topical formulations contain antiinflammatory agents (Table 95-4). These aid in decreasing inflammation of the canal associated with the primary ear disease and also reduce inflammation from secondary infections. In some situations products used to clean and treat the ear can have irritant effects, and the addition of glucocorticoids may counteract some of these effects. It is important to remember that the use of products containing more potent steroids such as dexamethasone or betamethasone can suppress the adrenal axis and that animals may exhibit systemic side effects when these are used on a long-term basis. A recently released formulation is a mixture of gentamicin, clotrimazole, and mometasone (Mometamax). Mometasone is a potent topical glucocorticoid, with minimal systemic effects in normal and laboratory animals. It also has longer residual effects, thus allowing for once-daily therapy, and is potentially less of a concern for adrenal axis suppression.

Table 95-1

Cleansers and Drying Agents

Products	Ingredients	Uses/Comments	Manufacturer
Alocetic	Acetic acid Aloe	Maintenance therapy for chronic recurrent otitis	DVM Pharmaceuticals
Bur-Otic	Burrow's solution Acetic acid 1% Hydrocortisone	Antipruritic Antiinflammatory Minor antiyeast and antibacterial effect (acetic acid)	Virbac
Cerulytic	Benzyl alcohol Butylated hydroxytoluene Propylene glycol base	Ceruminolytic: soften otic exudate Indicated in inflamed, highly exudative ear canals Used to loosen exudate before flushing the canal	Virbac
Cerumene	Cerumene (Squalane) 25% in petrolatum base	Ceruminolytic: soften otic exudate Indicated in inflamed, highly exudative ear canals Used to loosen exudate before flushing the canal	Evsco
Chlorhexiderm flush	2% Chlorhexidine gluconate	Mild cleanser Chlorhexidine can induce topical irritancy Not approved for otic use	DVM Pharmaceuticals
CleaRx cleansing solution Klearwax	Dioctyl sodium Sulfosuccinate 6.5% Urea peroxide 6%	Ceruminolytic: soften and emulsify wax and debris Ideal in highly exudative/proliferative ears without a lot of inflammation	CleaRx: DVM Pharmaceuticals Klearwax: Dermapet
Duoxo micellar solution	Phytosphingosine (0.02%) Polidocanol Rhamnosoft	Recommended for maintenance of seborrheic conditions Micellar solution that enables delivery of phytosphingosine and soothing agents Remove cellular debris and excess sebum Antiinflammatory and antimicrobial properties	Sogeval
Epi-Otic and Epi-Otic Advanced	2.7% Lactic acid 0.1% Salicylic acid Advanced: Antiadhesive Spherulites	Decrease pH of the ear canal (Epi-Otic only; Epi-Otic Advanced is neutral) Effective in maintenance of mild chronic recurrent otitis Advanced formulation has properties to prevent bacterial adherence and deodorizer	Virbac
MalAcetic Otic	2% Acetic acid 2% Boric acid	Effective as maintenance therapy in chronic recurrent yeast otitis	DermaPet
OtiCalm, OtiClens	Benzoic acid Malic acid Salicylic acid	Routine cleansing of mildly exudative ears	Oticalm: DVM Pharmaceuticals Oticlens: Pfizer Animal Health
OtiFoam	Cocamidopropyl Betaine Salicylic acid Oil of eucalyptus	Breakdown of large debris Can be used in ears with purulent exudate	DVM Pharmaceuticals
OtiRinse	Dioctyl sodium sulfosuccinate (DSS) Salicylic acid Lactic acid Benzoic acid Aloe vera	Routine cleansing of mildly exudative ears Deodorizer	DVM Pharmaceuticals
Otoclean	Salicylic acid (0.23%) Lactic acid Oleic acid Propylene glycol	Markedly ceruminolytic Shown an effective ceruminolytic in in vitro studies	Laboratorios Dr Esteve SA
Zinc Otic	Zinc gluconate Boric acid	Effective as maintenance therapy in chronic recurrent yeast otitis Effective for acute yeast infections	Addison Biological Laboratory, Inc.
Zymox otic	Enzymatic solution with lysozyme, lactoferrin, and lactoperoxidase	Some antibacterial and antiyeast product Can be used as maintenance as well as treatment of dirty "waxy" ears Some practitioners recommend cleaning after Zymox used to break up debris	Leclede, Inc.

Table 95-2

Selected Veterinary Topical Otic Products With Antibacterial Agents

Antibacterial Agent	Uses/Comments	Formulations	Products/Manufacturers
Enrofloxacin	Fluoroquinolone: Bactericidal Gram negative or gram positive bacteria	Emulsion containing silver sulfadiazine	Baytril otic/Bayer
Gentamicin	Aminoglycoside: Bactericidal Gram-negative or gram-positive bacteria	Ointment with betamethasone and clotrimazole Ointment with mometasone and clotrimazole Solution with betamethasone	Otomax/Schering-Plough DVMax/DVM Pharmaceuticals MalOtic/Vedco MometaMax/Schering-Plough Gentocin Otic/Schering-Plough
Marbofloxacin	Fluoroquinolone: bactericidal Gram negative or gram positive bacteria	Solution containing clotrimazole and dexamethasone	Aurizon/Vétoquinol
Neomycin	Aminoglycoside: bactericidal Similar to gentamicin, but less potent; often chosen for gram-positive bacteria Contact/irritant reactions reported	Ointment with nystatin, thiostrepton, and triamcinolone Solution with thiabendazole and dexamethasone Ointment with isoflupredone acetate and tetracaine hydrochloride	Panalog/Fort Dodge Tritip/Pharmacia Tresaderm/Merial TriTop/Pfizer
Silver sulfadiazine	Structural and metabolic cell disruption Mechanisms not completely understood Broad-spectrum antibacterial and some antiyeast activity	Cream emulsion containing enrofloxacin	Silvadene Cream/Monarch Pharmaceuticals Baytril Otic/Bayer
Tromethamine ethylenediaminetetraacetic (Tris EDTA)	Alkalinizing chelating agent Gram-negative infections Usually used synergistically with other antibiotic	Tris EDTA solution with ketoconazole Tris EDTA solution with chlorhexidine	T8/DVM Pharmaceuticals Triz-EDTA/DermaPet T8 Keto/DVM Pharmaceuticals TrizEDTA Plus/Dermapet

Table 95-3

Selected Veterinary Topical Otic Products With Antifungal Agents

Antifungal Agent	Uses/Comments	Formulation	Products/Manufacturers
Boric acid	Detergent with activity against yeast otic organisms	2% solution containing Zinc 2% solution containing 2% acetic acid	Zinc-Otic/Addison Biological Laboratory, Inc. Malacetic/Dermapet
Clotrimazole	Imidazole antifungal: disrupt ergosterol synthesis Mild-to-moderate potency against *M. pachydermatis*	Ointment containing gentamicin and betamethasone Ointment containing marbofloxacin and dexamethasone	Otomax/Schering-Plough; DVMax/DVM Pharmaceuticals; MalOtic/Vedco Aurizon/Vétoquinol
Ketoconazole	Imidazole antifungal: disrupts ergosterol synthesis	Solution containing Tris-EDTA 2% Cream	T8 Keto/DVM Pharmaceuticals Ketoconazole Cream/Taro Pharmaceuticals
Miconazole	Imidazole antifungal: disrupts ergosterol synthesis	1% Lotion or 2% cream Solution with chlorhexidine gluconate	Conofite/Schering-Plough Malaseb Flush/DVM Pharmaceuticals
Nystatin	Polyene antifungal: binds sterols in the fungal cell membrane Relatively weak activity against *Malassezia pachydermatis*	Ointment with neomycin, thiostrepton, and triamcinolone	Panalog/Fort Dodge
Terbinafine	Allylamine antifungal: inhibition of squalene epoxidase	Various 1% over-the-counter preparations	Lamisil/Novartis
Thiabendazole	Benzimidazole antifungal: disrupts ergosterol synthesis	Solution with neomycin and dexamethasone	Tresaderm/Merial

Table 95-4

Antiinflammatory Agents Available in Topical Products

Antiinflammatory Agent	Uses/Comments	Formulations	Products/Manufacturers
Betamethasone	25 times as potent as HC Even short-term use can result in suppression of the adrenal axis and systemic effects	Ointment with gentamicin and clotrimazole Solution with gentamicin	Otomax /Schering-Plough; DVMax/DVM Pharmaceuticals; MalOtic/Vedco Gentocin Otic/Schering-Plough
Dexamethasone	25 times as potent as HC Even short-term use can result in suppression of the adrenal axis and systemic effects	Solution with neomycin and thiabendazole Ointment with marbofloxaxin and clotrimazole	Tresaderm/Merial Aurizone/Vétoquinol
Dimethyl sulfoxide (DMSO)	Nonsteroidal antiinflammatory Possible reduction in fibroplasia	Solution with fluocinolone	Synotic/Fort-Dodge
Fluocinolone	100 times as potent as HC Even short-term use can result in suppression of the adrenal axis and systemic effects	Solution with DMSO (which will add to systemic absorption)	Synotic/Fort Dodge
Hydrocortisone (HC)	Mild steroidal antiinflammatory Use in mild chronic recurrent ceruminous otitis	Solution with Burrow's solution and acetic acid Solution with 2.5% acetic acid and 2% colloidal sulfur Enzymatic solution containing HC Solution with 2% acetic acid and 2% boric acid Lotion (not approved for otic use)	BurOtic/Virbac CleaRx Drying Agent/DVM Pharmaceuticals Zymox Otic/Laclede, Inc. Malacetic HC/DermaPet CortiCalm Lotion/DVM Pharmaceuticals
Mometasone	25 times as potent as HC Negligible systemic bioavailability, minimal systemic adverse effects	Ointment with gentamicin and clotrimazole Numerous human inhaled and topical products	Mometamax/Schering-Plough Nasonex/Schering-Plough; Elocon Cream/Schering-Plough
Triamcinolone	Five times as potent as HC	Ointment containing nystatin, neomycin, and thiostrepton	Panalog/Fort Dodge

Products containing hydrocortisone can potentially be used for chronic recurrent otitis secondary to mild allergies. However several of these products contain ingredients that are irritating, which can negate the mild antiinflammatory effect of hydrocortisone. Maintenance hydrocortisone products need to be selected on a case-by-case basis, depending on how effective they are in controlling the inflammation from the primary disease, usually allergic. They are not very beneficial in acute, exudative, or proliferative otitis.

Topical Ototoxicity

Patients with otitis commonly present with ruptured tympanic membranes. Certain formulations contain ingredients that have been shown to be ototoxic and are contraindicated when a ruptured tympanum is present. Ototoxicity is defined as the tendency of certain therapeutic agents to cause functional impairment and cellular degeneration of the inner ear and the eighth cranial nerve. It may be reversible or irreversible. Ototoxicity is differentiated from neurotoxicity, in which the site of action is central to the eighth cranial nerve. Most notable of the ototoxic drugs are the aminoglycoside antibiotics (especially gentamicin), but other numerous known ototoxic agents are listed below (Box 95-1). Products such as acetic acid that are not ototoxic but are irritating can also be a concern. At times culture and sensitivity testing directs clinicians to use ototoxic antibiotics if other options are not available. Dermatologists may recommend these products in resistant cases; however, the client must be informed of the risks and benefits of pursuing this therapy.

MAINTENANCE OF CHRONIC RECURRENT CONDITIONS

Cases of chronic, recurrent otitis are usually secondary to an inadequately controlled primary condition, permanent

Box 95-1

List of Known Ototoxic Substances

Antibiotics	Miscellaneous Drugs	Environmental Chemicals
Aminoglycoside antibiotics	**Salicylates**	Butyl nitrite
Streptomycin	Acetylsalicylic acid (aspirin)	Nicotine
Dihydrostreptomycin	Nicotine	Mercury
Kanamycin	Quinine	Carbon disulfide
Gentamicin	Loop diuretics	Styrene
Neomycin	Furosemide	Carbon monoxide
Tobramycin	Ethacrynic acid	Tin
Netilmicin	Bumetanide	Hexane
Amikacin	**Platinum-based antineoplastic agents**	Toluene
Macrolide antibiotics	Carboplatin	Lead
Erythromycin	Cisplatin	Trichloroethylene
Clindamycin		Manganese
Azithromycin		Xylene

damage to the ear canal, or undiagnosed/uncontrolled otitis media. Changes to the canal from chronic recurrent disease can destroy the physical and immunologic mechanisms of the ear canal that keep it free of pathogens and debris. This makes the ear even more susceptible to recurrent infections. Table 95-1 gives a list of products frequently used by veterinarians; however, scores of products are available over the counter through pet stores and on the Internet. It is important to know which products are being applied into the patient's ears and to understand their possible effects.

Maintenance therapy has the following goals:

1. To keep the ear clean and free of excess wax and ceruminous debris. This is achieved with cleaning and sometimes antiinflammatory agents that decrease excessive wax and cerumen production.
2. To decrease inflammation and pruritus, thus avoiding self-trauma and discomfort. This is achieved by addressing the primary disease and providing antiinflammatory therapy and/or by achieving the other goals listed and thus decreasing the inflammation.
3. To decrease the number of infectious organisms in the canal and maintain an "unfriendly" environment for their growth, by either decreasing the canal pH or adding detergents or other products that interfere with microorganism metabolism and growth.

4. To provide therapy that promotes regulation of epithelialization and wound healing. For example, products such as Alocetic or Otirinse contain aloe to help soothe and maintain the moisture barrier of the ear canal. Another product, Duoxo micellar solution contains phytosphingosine and other products to decrease excessive buildup in seborrheic conditions. In addition, Zinc Otic contains zinc gluconate with the goal of promoting normalization of canal epithlium and wound healing.

References and Suggested Reading

Gortel K: Otic flushing, *Vet Clin North Am* 34(2):557, 2004.

Mendelsohn CL et al: Efficacy of boric-complexed zinc and acetic-complexed zinc otic preparations for canine yeast otitis externa, *J Am Anim Hosp Assoc* 41(1):12, 2005.

Mendelsohn CL, Rosenkrantz WS, Griffin: Practical cytology for inflammatory skin diseases, *Clin Tech Small Anim Pract* 3:17, 2006.

Morris DO: Medical therapy of otitis externa and otitis media, *Vet Clin North Am* 34(2):591, 2004.

Rosser EJ: Causes of otitis externa, *Vet Clin North Am* 34(2):459, 2004.

Scott DW, Miller WHJ, Griffin CE: *Muller & Kirk's small animal dermatology*, ed 6, Philadelphia, 2001, Saunders, pp 207, 1185.

CHAPTER 96

Systemic Therapy for Otitis Externa and Media

LYNETTE K. COLE, *Columbus, Ohio*

Otitis externa is defined as inflammation of the external ear canal that may also involve the pinna. It is the most common disease of the external ear canal of the dog and cat. The reported prevalence in the dog ranges from 10% to 20% of the population; in the cat otitis externa is less common, ranging from 2% to 10%, and is usually caused by a parasitic etiology.

ETIOLOGIES OF OTITIS EXTERNA

The etiologies of otitis externa may be broken down into predisposing factors, primary causes, and perpetuating factors. If these factors and causes are not diagnosed, treated, and controlled, the otitis externa may become chronic and recurrent. Predisposing factors alone do not cause the otitis externa, but they increase the risk of development of the disease. These predisposing factors include otic conformation (stenotic canals, hair in canal, pendulous pinnae) excessive moisture (swimmer's ear), and treatment effects (trauma from cotton-tipped applicators, irritant topical solution, inappropriate use of combination topical therapy). Primary causes directly cause the otitis externa and include parasites (*Otodectes cynotis*, demodicosis, *Otobius megnini*), hypersensitivity disorders (atopic dermatitis, cutaneous adverse food reaction, allergic contact dermatitis), keratinization disorders (primary idiopathic seborrhea, hypothyroidism), neoplasms, polyps, and autoimmune diseases. Perpetuating factors are factors that prevent the resolution of the otitis externa and include bacteria, yeast, otitis media, and progressive pathologic changes.

OTITIS MEDIA

Otitis media is defined as inflammation of the middle ear cavity. The most common cause of otitis media is an extension of an infectious otitis externa into the middle ear cavity through a ruptured tympanic membrane. In dogs otitis media occurs in 16% of acute otitis cases, whereas in cases of chronic otitis externa 50% to 89% may have concurrent otitis media. An intact tympanic membrane does not rule out otitis media because the defect may heal over the infection.

MANAGEMENT OF OTITIS

Goals of Medical Management of Otitis

The goals of medical management of otitis externa and otitis media are to reduce inflammation and resolve infection. Successful long-term medical management of otitis externa and otitis media requires identification and control of the primary underlying disease and the predisposing and perpetuating factors. Topical therapy is recommended for all cases of otitis externa and otitis media and may include ear cleaning and drying agents, glucocorticoids, antibiotics, antifungals, or antiparasiticidals (see Chapter 95). Systemic therapies used for medical management of otitis externa and otitis media are similar and include glucocorticoids, antibiotics, antifungals, and antiparasiticidals. However, systemic therapy is not always required in the management of otitis.

Systemic Glucocorticoids

Systemic glucocorticoids are used to help alleviate the pain and inflammation associated with otitis externa. Glucocorticoids are antipruritic, antiinflammatory, and antiproliferative and decrease sebaceous and apocrine secretions in the ear. In addition, in patients with severe hyperplasia and stenosis of the ear canal, systemic glucocorticoids are warranted to reduce the inflammation to allow examination of the ear and otic flushing if required. If on reevaluation the hyperplasia and stenosis have not decreased to allow the otic examination, surgical management of the otitis may be indicated. Short-acting systemic glucocorticoids such as prednisone or prednisolone are administered orally at 0.05 to 1 mg/kg every 24 hours for up to 14 days. This treatment course may be extended if initial improvement is noted, but moderate proliferation of the ear canal is still present. The dosage remains the same, but the frequency is tapered to every other day. In cases with marked hyperplasia and stenosis, initial doses up to 2 mg/kg every 24 hours for the first 3 to 5 days, reduced to 1 mg/kg every 24 hours, may be required.

When there is only vertical ear canal stenosis, intralesional triamcinolone acetonide (Vetalog) may be effective. It is injected using a spinal needle or 25-gauge needle in a ring pattern around the vertical ear canal, injecting approximately three or four locations with a total dose of no more than 0.1 mg/kg. Short-term side effects of glucocorticoids include polyuria, polydipsia, polyphagia, and panting. Longer use of glucocorticoids may induce additional side effects such as iatrogenic hyperadrenocorticism, steroid hepatopathy, gastric ulcers, alopecia, cutaneous atrophy, hypertension, demodicosis, and urinary tract infections.

Systemic Antimicrobial Therapy

Indications for Systemic Treatment of Bacterial Otitis

Systemic antimicrobial therapy for infectious otitis externa and otitis media is controversial. In dogs with end-stage otitis externa and concurrent otitis media, bacterial organisms may be isolated from the exudate in the lumen of the vertical ear canal (Cole et al., 2005a) and middle ear cavity (Cole et al., 2005b), as well as from the tissue from these sites. Therefore most agree that systemic antibiotics are indicated in patients with otitis media, with severe proliferative chronic otitis externa, with ulcerative otitis externa, when inflammatory cells are seen cytologically (indicating deeper skin involvement), and when owners cannot administer topical therapy. The selection of a systemic antimicrobial agent must be made based on culture and susceptibility (C/S) testing from the external ear (for otitis externa) and middle ear (for otitis media). However, therapy may be initiated based on cytologic results while awaiting the C/S results.

Systemic Therapy for Staphylococcal Otitis

The most common coccoid bacteria isolated from dogs with otitis externa or otitis media is *Staphylococcus intermedius*. Good empiric choices while waiting on C/S results include cephalexin (22 mg/kg q12h, orally [PO]) or amoxicillin trihydrate-clavulanate potassium (Clavamox, Pfizer Animal Health, 13.75 to 22 mg/kg q12h, PO).

Systemic Therapy for *Pseudomonas* Otitis

Probably the most challenging bacterial otic infections are those infected with *Pseudomonas aeruginosa* (Table 96-1). Systemic treatment options may be limited because of antibiotic resistance. At the present time the fluoroquinolones are the only oral systemic antibiotic available for the treatment of *P. aeruginosa*. Most veterinary dermatologists recommend starting an oral fluoroquinolone while waiting on the C/S results. When using the fluoroquinolones in the dog, the upper end of the dose should be administered. Rare reports of blindness caused by retinal degeneration have been reported in cats administered enrofloxacin; therefore the low end of the dose of an oral fluoroquinolone should be administered in the cat.

In multidrug-resistant *P. aeruginosa* infections, systemic β-lactam antibiotics such as ticarcillin disodium-clavulanate potassium (Timentin, GlaxoSmithKline), imipenem (Primaxin, Merck), meropenem (Merrem, AstraZeneca LP), and ceftazidime sodium (Fortaz, GlaxoSmithKline) may be options but are very expensive, must be administered parenterally, and should only be considered after topical cleaning and antimicrobial agents have been ineffective. A potential side effect of imipenem and meropenem is seizures, and they should be used cautiously in patients prone to seizure disorders.

Aminoglycoside antibiotics such as gentamicin and amikacin are less commonly prescribed but remain potentially efficacious drugs for the treatment of *P. aeruginosa*

Table **96-1**

Systemic Drugs and Suggested Dosages for the Treatment of *Pseudomonas Aeruginosa* Otitis Externa/Otitis Media

Drug Name (Trade Name)	Dosage
Fluoroquinolone Antibiotics	
Marbofloxacin (Zeniquin, Pfizer Animal Health)	Dog: 5.5 mg/kg q24h, PO Cat: 2.75 mg/kg q24h, PO
Enrofloxacin (Baytril, Bayer Animal Health)	Dog: 20 mg/kg, q24h, PO Cat: 5 mg/kg q24h, PO
Ciprofloxacin	Dog: 20 mg/kg q24h, PO
β-Lactam Antibiotics	
Ticarcillin disodium-clavulanate potassium (Timentin, GlaxoSmithKline)	Dog: 15 to 25 mg/kg q8h, IV
Imipenem (Primaxin, Merck & Co)	Dog and cat: 10 mg/kg q8h, diluted in 100 ml suitable IV solution, administered IV over 30 to 60 minutes
Meropenem (Merrem, AstraZeneca LP)	Dog: 12 mg/kg q8h, SQ or 24 mg/kg q8h, IV
Ceftazidime sodium (Fortaz, GlaxoSmithKline)	Dog and cat: 30 mg/kg q6h, IV, IM Dogs only: 30 mg/kg q4h, SQ Dogs only: Constant IV infusion: loading dose of 4.4 mg/kg, followed by 4.1 mg/kg/hr, delivered in IV fluids
Aminoglycoside Antibiotics	
Gentamicin	Dog: 10 to 14 mg/kg q24h, IM, SQ, IV Cat: 5 to 8 mg/kg q24h, IM, SQ, IV
Amikacin	Dog: 15 to 30 mg/kg q24h, IM, SQ, IV Cat: 10 to 15 mg/kg q24h, IM, SQ, IV

otic infections. These drugs are also administered parenterally and have the potential for nephrotoxicity. Animals must be monitored with periodic urinalysis for increased protein or tubular casts and serum blood urea analysis and creatinine.

Indications for Systemic Treatment of Yeast Otitis

Indications for systemic antifungal agents are similar to those mentioned previously for bacterial infections and include patients with yeast otitis media, patients with severe yeast otitis externa, or owners who cannot administer topical therapy. In one study neither pulse-dose or daily-dose itraconazole alone significantly decreased yeast organisms identified cytologically from otic exudate in dogs with yeast otitis externa, suggesting that otic yeast infections may require topical therapy in addition to systemic therapy for resolution (Pinchbeck et al., 2002). Both ketoconazole (5 mg/kg q24h) and itraconazole ([Sporanox, Janssen Pharmaceutica Products, LP], 5 mg/kg PO q24h or pulse-dosed 2 days on and 5 days off) have been used in dogs, whereas itraconazole (5 mg/kg PO q24h) is recommended for use in the cat.

Systemic Antiparasiticidal Therapy

Treatment of *O. cynotis* in the dog or cat requires treatment of all in contact animals, as well as the affected animal. Selamectin (Revolution, Pfizer Animal Health) is a semisynthetic avermectin topical endectocide approved by the Food and Drug Administration for the treatment of *O. cynotis* in the dog and cat (two treatments at 30-day intervals). Even though selamectin is applied topically to the skin, it is quickly absorbed into the bloodstream, forming reservoirs in the sebaceous glands. Ivermectin (0.2 to 0.3 mg/kg q2weeks, subcutaneously for three treatments) is effective against *O. cynotis* in the dog and cat. Side effects from ivermectin may include ataxia, hypermetria, disorientation, hyperesthesia, tremors, hyperreflexia, mydriasis, hypersalivation, depression, blindness, coma, and death. Nonspecific signs include vomiting, diarrhea, and anorexia. Ivermectin should not be administered to collies and collie-crosses, Australian shepherds, Shetland sheepdogs, Old English sheepdogs, English shepherds, long-haired whippets, and silken windhounds due to profound adverse reactions or to heartworm-positive dogs. The use of ivermectin for the treatment of *O. cynotis* is off label; therefore a consent form should be signed by the owner before administration.

References and Suggested Reading

Cole LK et al: Comparison of bacterial organisms and their susceptibility patterns from otic exudate and ear tissue from the vertical ear canal of dogs undergoing a total ear canal ablation, *Vet Ther* 6:252, 2005a.

Cole LK et al: Comparison of bacterial organisms from otic exudate and ear tissue from the middle ear of untreated and enrofloxacin-treated dogs with end-stage otitis. In Hillier A, Foster AP, Kwochka KW, editors: *Advances in veterinary dermatology*, vol 5, Oxford, 2005b, Blackwell Publishing, p 147.

Moore KW, Trepanier LA, Lautzenhiser SJ: Pharmacokinetics of ceftazidime in dogs following subcutaneous administration and continuous infusion and the association with in vitro susceptibility of *Pseudomonas aeruginosa, Am J Vet Res* 61:1204, 2000.

Nuttal TJ: Use of ticarcillin in the management of canine otitis externa complicated by *Pseudomonas aeruginosa, J Small Anim Pract* 39:165, 1998.

Papich MG: *Saunders handbook of veterinary drugs*, Philadelphia, 2002, Saunders.

Papich MG: Solving problems in therapy: new drugs, new approaches. In *Just the FAQs: managing microbes/pain management*, Proceedings of North American Veterinary Conference, Orlando, Fla, 2005 and Western Veterinary Conference, New York, 2005, Pfizer Animal Health, p 15.

Pinchbeck LR et al: Comparison of pulse administration versus once-daily administration of itraconazole for the treatment of *Malassezia pachydermatis* dermatitis and otitis in dogs, *J Am Vet Med Assoc* 220:1807, 2002.

CHAPTER 97

Ear-Flushing Techniques

DAWN LOGAS, *Maitland, Florida*

EAR FLUSHING

The most important first step in the management of any case of otitis is to properly clean the external ear canal and flush the middle ear cavity if the tympanum is absent or diseased. The procedure should be performed at the initial visit after obtaining cytologic specimens and possibly a specimen for culture from the diseased ear. In mild cases of otitis, ear flushing may be performed with gentle restraint, but in most cases the ears are painful enough to warrant heavy sedation with propofol (Diprivan 1%, Zeneca) or ketamine and diazepam. In more severe cases of otitis externa and in most cases of otitis media, general anesthesia is necessary.

In some of the most severe cases, in which the canals are extremely inflamed and swollen, systemic and topical therapy is initiated first, and a 3- to 14-day delay is necessary before cleaning. This allows the canal to open and the tympanic membrane to be visualized more easily.

The flushing solution used depends on the degree of inflammation, the characteristics of the discharge, and the status of the tympanic membrane. Commonly used solutions are dioctyl sodium sulfosuccinate (DSS), CLEAR$_x$ ear cleansing solution (DVM Pharmaceuticals), or squalane (Cerumene, Evsco Pharmaceuticals) for waxy discharges; and Epi-Otic (Allerderm/Virbac), tromethamine ethylenediaminetetraacetic (Tris EDTA), 0.05%

to 0.2% chlorhexidine solutions, and 2.5% acetic acid (50:50 vinegar:water) or saline for purulent discharges. All of these solutions except saline have the potential to damage exposed middle-ear structures, although the caseous or purulent material being removed from the middle ear probably poses a greater threat. When the tympanum is known to be absent, a gentle solution such as 2.5% acetic acid or saline should be used if possible. Unfortunately many times these solutions alone do not remove the debris, and a more caustic cleaning solution must be used. At the end of the procedure it is important to flush the caustic solution out of the canal and middle ear completely with water or saline to minimize any damage the solution may cause.

In-Office Ear Flushing

A bulb syringe (Davol, Inc.) or a No. 3 to No. 12 Fr red rubber feeding tube attached to a 6- to 12-ml syringe is an excellent and relatively safe flushing apparatus for in-office use. The wide end of the tube must be trimmed to accommodate the syringe hub. The tip is then cut off the other end so the final length of the tube is 4 to 6 inches or one to two times the length of the ear canal. Both straight and curved dull buck ear curettes (Edward Week & Co) can be used to remove large pieces of wax and debris. Once the horizontal canal has been cleared, it is usually easier to assess the status of the tympanic membrane. In many cases of chronic otitis, the tympanum is still difficult to visualize because the canal is stenotic secondary to lichenification and fibrosis. If the tympanum cannot be visualized, its status can be assessed indirectly by observing the curette catching on any bony prominence, the tube tip disappearing from view, the use of excessive tubing and fluid in the canal, or the act of the patient swallowing after infusion of fluid. Any of these observations would indicate a false middle ear or imperforate tympanum. If the tympanum is visually intact but this is a case of chronic otitis (>3 months' duration), a myringotomy using a dull buck curette may be necessary. A culture should always be taken from the middle ear if there is any evidence of fluid behind the membrane or if there is membrane opacity and fibrosis.

The hazards of deep ear cleaning include inadvertent rupture of the tympanum, vestibular dysfunction, auditory dysfunction, contact irritant and allergy, and introduction of other pathogens. The most common hazard is the potential rupture of the tympanic membrane. A normal tympanum is difficult to rupture; therefore, if the membrane ruptures with gentle manipulation, it was probably weakened and diseased. The occurrence of vestibular auditory dysfunction is unpredictable. In the dog it is uncommon, usually mild, and most of the time lasts only a few hours to a couple of days. It occurs more frequently in the cat, and the signs are usually more pronounced and may be permanent. To avoid contact irritation, a gentle solution should be used whenever possible, or more caustic solutions must be rinsed out extremely well with water or saline. New pathogens can also be introduced into an already inflamed ear via unsterilized ear-cleaning equipment. Bulb syringes and feeding tubes should not be used for multiple patients. It is difficult to completely sterilize the rubber; therefore resistant strains of *Pseudomonas, Escherichia coli,* and *Proteus* can propagate.

At-Home Ear Flushing

Once the ear has been cleaned in the office, a home treatment plan for the owners must be designed according to the organism or organisms found on cytologic studies or culture, the chronicity of the ear disease, and the presence of a tympanum. In many cases a prepared solution in a squeeze bottle is all that is necessary. If there is a great deal of purulent material, a bulb syringe should be used, and the owners instructed in its appropriate use. After each use the bulb syringe should be rinsed out several times with 50:50 vinegar with isopropyl alcohol to minimize bacterial overgrowth in the bulb. The bulb syringe should be changed every 2 to 5 weeks, depending on the severity of the infection.

In the case of severe otitis or in a fractious patient, a flushing device may temporarily be affixed to the animal. Heavy sedation or general anesthesia should be used. The open end of a red rubber feeding tube is secured via sutures or glue to the dorsal skin of the neck and head. The tube is then placed into the ear canal rostrally through the area of the pretragic incisure and secured in place with glue or suture. The tip of the tube should be trimmed so that the end of the tube is one half to three quarters of the way down the horizontal canal but not touching the tympanum or the middle-ear cavity. The tube should be approximately one-half to three-fourths the diameter of the horizontal canal. This helps minimize tube movement and subsequently patient discomfort. There should be enough space around the tube for fluid to backwash out of the ear during flushing. This will prevent a buildup of water pressure and possible middle ear and vestibular damage. The tube usually remains in place for 5 to 10 days, but it can remain in place longer if needed. There should be an Elizabethan collar on the dog at all times. Owners should be instructed to flush the cleaning solution (i.e., chlorhexidine solution (0.05% to 0.2%), saline, or 50:50 vinegar with water) through the tube gently with a 6- to 12-ml syringe. Each time the canal is flushed, a total volume of 10 to 15 ml should be instilled. As much of the fluid as possible should be evacuated from the ear canal after each infusion. The ear should be flushed once to three times daily, depending on the severity of the infection. Antibiotic solutions can also be instilled into the horizontal canal through this apparatus by infusing 0.5 to 1 ml of medication into the tube and then flushing the medication through the tube into the canal using air.

The type of solution and frequency of flushing prescribed for home care depend on the severity of infection, consistency of the discharge, chronicity of the otitis, presence of yeast or bacteria, and presence or absence of a tympanum. For bacterial infections chlorhexidine solution (0.05 to 0.2%) and saline are good, gentle flushes. For *Pseudomonas aeruginosa* infections, a 5- to 10-minute contact time with Tris-EDTA, 50:50 vinegar:water or otic Domeboro solution (Bayer Pharmaceutical) is a better choice because these agents have bactericidal activity against *Pseudomonas*. It is important to remember that purulent discharge inactivates many topical antibiotics; accordingly the ear should be flushed before each application of antibiotic until the ear is producing little-to-no purulent material. Initially the frequency of flushing for severe cases, especially resistant *Pseudomonas* infections, can be three to four times daily. In most cases of less severe otitis, twice daily suffices. As therapy continues, the frequency should decrease to several times per week and then once weekly to every other week prophylactically.

As with bacterial otitis, flushing ears can be important in the treatment of yeast otitis. Flushing helps to remove the waxy organism-filled debris, acidify, and then dry the horizontal canal, making the microenvironment of the canal unsuitable for yeast growth. The frequency of application again depends on the severity of otitis and the chronicity of the disease. In severe cases flushing may be one to two times daily but should quickly drop to two to three times weekly. Over time it drops further to a maintenance level of once weekly to once every other week. The agents most commonly used are Epi-Otic, DSS, and 50:50 vinegar with alcohol.

It is particularly important that dogs with chronic histopathologic ear canal changes such as fibrosis, stenosis, and lichenification be placed on a maintenance flushing program. Ears with chronic changes usually have increased cerumen production, hyperplasia of the stratum corneum, and decreased epidermal migration (self-cleaning). This leads to an increased buildup of debris in the canal. Flushing the ears helps to remove the debris and acidify the canal, which helps prevent recurrence of active infections. The frequency of flushing ranges from two to three times weekly to once every other week. The solutions commonly used are Epi-Otic, chlorhexidine flush, Otic Domeboro, and vinegar with alcohol or water (50:50).

Although flushing is extremely important in the management of both chronic and acute otitis, it is imperative that the clinician remember that flushing too vigorously and too frequently can also be detrimental to the otic epidermis. The animal with severe otitis undergoing flushing numerous times per day should be checked frequently, and flushing should be varied, depending on the cytologic and otic examination. This prevents the ear flushes from doing more harm than good.

Suggested Reading

Griffin CE: Otitis externa and otitis media. In Griffin CE, Kwochka KW, MacDonald JM, editors: *Current veterinary dermatology*, St. Louis, 1993, Mosby, p 245.

Matousek, JL: Ear disease, *Vet Clin North Am Sm Anim Pract* 34(2):379, 2004.

Rosychuk RAW: Management of otitis externa, *Vet Clin North Am Small Anim Pract* 24:921, 1994.

CHAPTER **98**

Feline Demodicosis

KARIN M. BEALE, *Houston, Texas*
DANIEL O. MORRIS, *Philadelphia, Pennsylvania*

Feline demodicosis is considered a relatively "rare" parasitism; however, in certain regions this condition is endemic and is not uncommon. When compared to canine demodicosis, little is known about feline demodicosis. Infected cats may present with a wide variety of clinical signs and should be considered in the differential diagnosis of many feline skin disorders. Two species of mites have been recognized to cause feline skin disease.

DEMODEX GATOI

Clinical Signs and Differential Diagnosis

Demodex gatoi is a short, broad mite that inhabits the stratum corneum (the most superficial layer) of the epidermis. The mite is similar in appearance to *Demodex criceti*, the superficial dwelling mite causing skin disease in hamsters. The primary clinical sign resulting from infection with this mite is pruritus, and the intensity of the pruritus is suggestive of a hypersensitivity response. The most common clinical presentation is self-inflicted alopecia caused by overgrooming. The alopecia is often symmetric in nature and is typically quite extensive. Most commonly the ventral abdomen, flanks, and anterior forelimbs are affected. This is more likely because these areas are most easily reached with grooming rather than being related to areas most inhabited by the mites. Other clinical signs typical of the cutaneous reaction patterns most commonly associated with feline allergic dermatoses may be present: miliary dermatitis and the eosinophilic dermatitis complex (i.e., eosinophilic plaques, indolent lip ulcers, and eosinophilic granulomas).

Occult cases of *D. gatoi*, appear to be common. This is similar to canine scabies and further supports the presence of a hypersensitivity component. The scarcity of mites on many pruritic cats with *D. gatoi* can easily lead to a missed diagnosis (see following paragraphs). It is suspected that affected cats are physically removing the mites (by licking), making the mites difficult or impossible to find with routine skin scrapings. The difficulty in finding these mites with skin scrapings and the ease with which they can be overlooked is another important factor that can contribute to misdiagnoses.

It is very important to note that some infested cats demonstrate no clinical signs whatsoever, further supporting the possibility that the pruritus induced in affected cats may be associated with a hypersensitivity response to the parasite. In a multiple-cat household there may be a combination of cats demonstrating clinical signs and cats that are asymptomatic. The feline housemates of affected cats should always be screened for parasitism. The distribution pattern of clinical signs is variable, but most commonly the ventral abdominal and flank regions are affected. However, facial and acral lesions may also occur, as can otitis externa. The pattern of lesions may be a reflection more of areas that cats typically groom rather than the distribution of mites. The differential diagnosis for a cat presenting with the pattern of self-induced alopecia should include flea-allergic dermatitis, atopic dermatitis, adverse food reaction, Cheyletiellosis, *Otodectes cynotis*, and psychogenic alopecia; in the case of miliary or plaque lesions, dermatophytosis, pyoderma, and cutaneous neoplasia should be considered.

Transmission

A unique feature of *D. gatoi* infestation when compared to canine demodicosis is an apparent risk for contagion among cats via casual contact. Fomite transmission may occur as well. Most infested cats have a history of going outdoors, being boarded, or possibly having been adopted from a shelter. This is the only *Demodex* species of domestic mammals for which horizontal transmission through casual contact has been reported.

Pathogenesis

The pathophysiology of *D. gatoi* infestation is not well known. Some cases reported in the literature have had histories of glucocorticoid therapy, although it is unclear whether this is truly a risk factor for the development of disease. It is more likely that the cats were treated with glucocorticoids for the pruritus induced by the mite. Other sources of systemic or localized immunosuppression have been reported in conjunction with *D. gatoi* infestation, including retroviral infection, diabetes mellitus, and cancer chemotherapy. We have diagnosed *D. gatoi* infestation in cats that have no history of glucocorticoid therapy and no associated systemic disease. Cats often have a history of roaming or exposure to other cats. Introduction of an asymptomatic infected cat from a shelter to a household with other cats may lead to disease in previously unaffected cats.

It is unknown if *D. gatoi* is part of the normal microfauna of feline skin, but our suspicion is that it is not. There appears to be marked regional variability in the distribution of this parasite since the condition is commonly diagnosed in the Gulf Coast region of the United States and is less commonly reported in other areas.

DEMODEX CATI

Clinical Signs and Differential Diagnosis

Demodex cati is a long, slender mite that has a similar morphology to *Demodex canis*. Like *D. canis*, the habitat of *D. cati* is the hair follicle and sebaceous glands/ducts. The presence of the mite provokes follicular inflammation, leading to a combination of alopecia, follicular plugging (comedones), papules, pustules, scale, crusts, and even erosion/ulceration. The distribution of skin lesions is variable, but most commonly lesions are focal and involve the head/face and distal limbs. Generalized demodicosis with *D. cati* is uncommon. The mite may also inhabit the external ear canals, leading to a ceruminous otitis externa, which is variably pruritic. Otitis may be the only manifestation of disease or may be seen concurrently with skin disease.

Differentials for *D. cati* infestation include dermatophytosis, pemphigus foliaceus, bacterial folliculitis, *Notoedres cati* (feline sarcoptic mange), *O. cynotis* (ear mites), and bacterial and yeast otitis externa. Pruritus is commonly seen with infection; therefore allergic dermatitis (atopy, food allergy/intolerance, and flea allergy) would be differentials in the pruritic cat.

Pathophysiology

The mite is considered part of the naturally occurring microfauna of feline skin, and mite reproduction to the point of causing dermatitis may be associated with an underlying systemic disease (retroviral infection, diabetes mellitus, neoplasia) or iatrogenic immunosuppression (glucocorticoids, cancer chemotherapy). Localized immunosuppression (caused by squamous cell carcinoma in situ) has also been implicated as a predisposing cause. Some patients with *D. cati* infestations have no apparent underlying disease or predisposing drug use; therefore alterations in immune response may not be a prerequisite for developing disease. Studies evaluating the cell-mediated and humoral immune responses of cats to *D. cati* have not been performed.

Diagnosis of Demodicosis

The diagnosis of *D. cati* is usually straightforward since mites are typically found with scrapings. Since they reside in hair follicles, deep/concentrated scrapings (such as one might perform for canine *Demodex*) are necessary. The skin should be squeezed gently to express mites toward the surface in-between cycles of scraping, until a generous amount of blood and debris is collected. For areas more difficult to scrape (such as eyelids, toes, and interdigital spaces) evaluating trichograms may be useful since mites may be dislodged along with the hairs. In heavily crusted or ulcerated areas, skin biopsy may reveal the diagnosis and help rule out other differentials. In rare cases low numbers of mites can make diagnosis more difficult. Although *D. cati* is part of the normal cutaneous microfauna, even a single mite should be considered suspicious when collected from a compatible skin lesion. If no other explanation for the lesion is found, treatment should be instituted on a trial basis.

In cases involving *D. gatoi*, in which occult infestation is common, a single mite found from the composite of multiple scrapings is diagnostic. A scraping technique similar to that used for scabies is appropriate: broad, superficial scrapings of large surface areas. Areas that are not easily reached with grooming (i.e., dorsal neck, thorax) may be more likely to produce positive results since the mites can't be physically removed from these areas. Negative findings on scrapings can't be relied on to rule out this condition. This is particularly true in endemic areas. Alternative measures include fecal flotation (as pruritic cats appear to groom away and ingest the mites) and therapeutic trials (see following paragraphs). The mites may also be found on occasion using cellophane tape to collect samples from the surface of the skin. It is strongly recommended that all in-contact cats be screened for infestation since some asymptomatic cats may have positive results on skin scrapings.

Regardless of the mite species involved, cats with demodicosis should be screened for retroviral diseases (leukemia and immunodeficiency viruses) and for other systemic diseases if indicated by clinical signs. For pruritic cats that have previously received glucocorticoid therapy, a final diagnosis must be reserved until miticidal treatment is finished because some may have another primary pruritic dermatosis.

Treatment

The recommended treatment for infested cats is a series of six lime sulfur dips performed at weekly intervals. A concentration of 2% is effective, but failures with 1% solutions have been documented. The hair coat should be totally saturated, and cats should "soak" in the lime sulfur for a minimum of 5 minutes. The topical solution should not be rinsed off, and the cats should be allowed to air dry. An Elizabethan collar is recommended to prevent ingestion of the dip while drying. Lime sulfur causes a temporary discoloration of light-colored fur and is extremely malodorous while wet. Persons using the solution should be advised that it tarnishes jewelry. Cats typically demonstrate significant clinical improvement after three treatments; however, mites may still be found with skin scrapings at that time. After the third dip some cats may experience an increase in scaling and pruritus, which is most likely caused by the drying (or potentially irritating) effects of the dip itself. This usually resolves rapidly after dipping is discontinued.

Cats with negative findings on skin scrapings that have symmetric alopecia and are on appropriate flea control may have an occult infestation with *D. gatoi*. A therapeutic trial with three lime sulfur dips is recommended. If the cat demonstrates improvement after the third dip, a full series of six dips is recommended, and other household cats should be dipped as well. If the cat is not better by the third week, it is unlikely that the pruritus is caused by demodicosis.

Because of the aesthetically unappealing nature of lime sulfur dips, many owners are reluctant to use this treatment, and other options have been used. Treatment with once-weekly ivermectin has been ineffective for both species of mites. Treatment with topical selamectin on a weekly basis has also been ineffective. Once-daily or every-other-day ivermectin at 300mcg/kg is effective in treating both species of mites. For *D. cati* treatment should be continued until negative scrapings are obtained. For *D. gatoi* infestation, we recommend treatment for 2 weeks past resolution of clinical signs with a minimum of 6 weeks of treatment. Because of the potential for toxicity with ivermectin (including Heinz body anemia resulting from the propylene glycol vehicle), lime sulfur is preferred over daily or every-other-day ivermectin treatment.

Treatment of all cats in a household with an infected or potentially infected cat is recommended. In the case in which occult demodicosis is suspected in one cat and the owner is reluctant to treat all cats, the potentially infested individual should be isolated during the treatment period. If the cat improves with treatment, all the other cats in the household should be treated as well. If the owner is unwilling to treat all household cats, he or she should be aware that there is the possibility of reinfestation when treatment is stopped if the other cats happen to be harboring an occult infestation.

Suggested Reading

Beale KM: Contagion and occult demodicosis in a family of 2 cats, Proceedings of the 14th AAVD/ACVD meeting, San Antonio, Tex, 1999, p 99.

Beale KM, Rustemeyer-May E: Selamectin in the treatment of feline *Demodex*, *Vet Dermatol* 12:237, 2001.

Desch CE, Stewart TB: *Demodex gatoi*: new species of hair follicle mite from the domestic cat, *J Medical Entomology* 36:167, 1999.

Guaguere E et al: *Demodex cati* infestation in association with feline cutaneous squamous cell carcinoma in situ: a report of five cases, *Vet Dermatol* 10:61, 1999.

Morris DO: Contagious demodicosis in three cats residing in a common household, *J Am Anim Hosp Assoc* 32:350, 1996.

Morris DO, Beale KM: Feline demodicosis: a retrospective of 15 cases, Proceedings of the 13th AAVD/ACVD meeting, Nashville, Tenn, 1997, p 127.

Morris DO, Beale KM: *Feline demodicosis*. In Bonagura JD, editor: *Kirk's current veterinary therapy XIII*, Philadelphia, 2000, Saunders, 2000, p 580.

CHAPTER 99

Feline Viral Skin Disease

RUDAYNA GHUBASH, *Marina del Rey, California*

FELINE HERPESVIRUS-1

Feline herpesvirus-1, a virus in the Herpesviridae family, is a common cause of respiratory illness, conjunctivitis, stomatitis, and corneal ulceration in feline patients. The majority of cats who contract this virus become asymptomatic carriers that harbor the virus in the trigeminal ganglia. Symptoms commonly recur when these animals experience stress such as moving, entering multicat households, boarding, pregnancy, surgery, or receiving glucocorticoids. In the cases reported in the literature, there has not been a causal link between this condition and animals with feline leukemia virus (FeLV) or feline immunodeficiency virus (FIV).

It has been demonstrated that this virus can manifest itself with dermatologic lesions in the absence of concurrent ophthalmic or respiratory symptoms in domestic cats and in cheetahs. There does not appear to be an age, breed, or sex predilection. Skin lesions typically follow the path of the trigeminal nerve on the haired surface of the face and nasal planum, although the ears, feet and ventrum can also be affected. The lesions are characterized by an ulcerative, erosive crusting dermatitis that can also display marked erythema and swelling. Because of shedding of the virus, skin lesions are often noticed to be associated in the location of lacrimal and salivary secretions. Feline herpesvirus can also be an underlying trigger of erythema multiforme in the cat with the absence of the ulcerative, erosive lesions described here.

Differential diagnoses of this condition include allergic disease, mosquito bite hypersensitivity, squamous cell carcinoma, eosinophilic granulomas complex lesions, pemphigus foliaceus, and idiopathic ulcerative dermatitis of Persian cats.

Diagnosis of this condition is made with a combination of *histopathology and polymerase chain reaction (PCR) of skin* samples. Histopathology is characterized by necrosis and ulceration of the epidermis extending into the dermis. Hair follicles and the perivascular dermis are usually inundated with a mixed inflammatory cell dermatitis, with a significant eosinophilia. Although they can be difficult to find, intranuclear viral inclusions in the superficial and follicular epithelium can be appreciated. Immunohistochemistry and PCR can be done to confirm these inclusions as herpesvirus-1 inclusion bodies. Even if intranuclear inclusion bodies are not appreciated, PCR and immunohistochemistry can be used to detect feline herpesvirus in tissue, with PCR considered the more sensitive test. It is not useful to run PCR on serum or mucocutaneous samples alone, since many cats have been exposed to the virus and a positive result on serum may be an incidental finding and not confirmation of a diagnosis. Many diagnostic laboratories offer feline herpesvirus PCR on fresh-frozen biopsy samples.

Cutaneous manifestations of feline herpesvirus can be difficult to resolve, and the prognosis is guarded. Several treatment options are available that can manage, although not always cure, this condition. L-lysine, which inhibits herpesvirus replication by blocking the availability of the amino acid arginine, can be effective at a dosage of 200 to 500 mg/cat orally twice daily. Interferon-α (IFN-α), a cytokine with antiviral properties, has also been used to treat this virus, but the dosages reported in the literature vary wildly. Dosages ranging from 30 units/cat/day orally to 250 to 500 units/cat orally three times weekly and 10,000 units/kg subcutaneously twice daily have been reported, with the 30 units/day–dosage used most commonly for dermatologic conditions. Imiquimod (Aldara), a topical cream for treatment of human genital warts caused by papillomavirus whose exact mechanism is unknown although interaction with toll-like receptors is considered most likely, can be effective in these cats when applied every 48 to 72 hours. Topical and oral glucocorticoids are contraindicated.

FELINE CALICIVIRUS

Feline calicivirus (FCV), a virus in the Caliciviridae family, is a common cause of ocular discharge, nasal discharge, oral ulceration, and conjunctivitis in felines. It has been isolated from some cases of feline chin acne, although it is unknown whether this was an incidental finding. Twenty five percent of animals that are infected with this virus become chronic carriers and relapse with clinical symptoms when faced with stressful symptoms, as with feline herpesvirus.

Recently a severe hemorrhagic virulent form of FCV was reported that produced a mortality rate of 33% to 60% (Pesavento et al., 2004). Systemic signs exhibited by these cats included fever, anorexia, and diffuse edema. An ulcerative, crusting dermatitis of the face, ears, and feet was also a symptom in many symptomatic animals. Histopathology of skin lesions was characterized by necrosis of the epidermis and ballooning degeneration of the epidermis, with immunohistochemistry identifying the presence of FCV antigen.

Many affected cats in the literature were current on their calicivirus vaccine, but it appeared to not be protective against this viral strain. Treatment consisted of supportive care, and at this time no effective treatment has been developed in case of another outbreak.

FELINE LEUKEMIA VIRUS

FeLV is caused by a retrovirus typically transmitted by bite wounds, although it can also be transmitted by close contact with nasal and salivary excretions. It causes generalized immunosuppression.

In the early 1990s it was reported that some FeLV-positive cats can have a distinctive giant cell dermatoses, in which the FeLV antigen can be detected by immunohistochemistry in the epidermis (Gross, 2005). Common clinical signs include alopecia, crust, and an exfoliative dermatitis that typically involves the head and muzzle but can be diffuse. Pruritus has been a clinical feature in the majority of reported cases. Diagnosis is made with histopathology and immunohistochemistry, and no successful treatment has been reported to treat this disease.

Cutaneous horns (i.e., protruding growths of keratin) have been associated with several conditions, including squamous cell carcinoma, viral papillomas, dilated pores, and FeLV. Because the horns associated with all of these conditions appear similar, it is important to perform blood testing for FeLV and immunohistochemistry on feline cutaneous horns to evaluate for the possibility of FeLV or papillomavirus-induced horn formation. When the horns are secondary to FeLV, surgery or laser procedure can be performed to remove them, but these cases are prone to relapse because of the difficulty in controlling the underlying viral infection. Although its efficacy on FeLV-positive cats with dermatologic symptoms has not been specifically evaluated, feline IFN at a dosage of 1 million units/kg/day subcutaneously once daily for five consecutive days in three series at day 0, 14, and 60 improved clinical signs and decreased mortality levels in FeLV and feline immunodeficiency patients (de Mari et al., 2004). These findings were statistically significant, and this treatment should be considered as a way to alleviate dermatologic symptoms.

FELINE IMMUNODEFICIENCY VIRUS

FIV is a naturally occurring lentivirus predominantly transmitted between cats via bite wounds. Early stages of the disease can go unnoticed by the owner, but later stages are characterized by myeloid or lymphoid tumors, neurologic symptoms, and secondary infections caused by immunosuppression. At this time there is no effective treatment or prevention for this disease, although feline IFN can be used as described for FeLV skin disease since it has been shown to decrease clinical signs and improve mortality rates in cats coinfected with FeLV and FIV.

At this time, no unique dermatoses have been associated with this disease, but cats with FIV are prone to several conditions secondary to the immunosuppression caused by this disease. Bacterial folliculitis, dermatophytosis, demodectic mange, and notoedric mange are the more commonly occurring skin conditions secondary to FIV infection, although atypical mycobacteriosis, subcutaneous abscesses, cowpox infections, and cellulitis all have been reported.

FELINE PAPILLOMAVIRUS

Papillomaviruses are very species-specific viruses that tend to favor the stratified squamous epithelium. Papillomavirus infections have been reported in several wild cats such as the snow leopard, Florida panther, Asian lion, and domestic cat (Sundberg et al., 2000). There are few cases of domestic cats reported in the literature, but based on the small sample population, Persians appear to be overrepresented.

As discussed in the FeLV section, cats with papillomavirus can develop cutaneous horns on their paw pads; for this reason papillomavirus immunohistochemistry should be performed on horns.

Papillomavirus has been associated with flat viral plaques that appear as slightly scaly, irregular raised lesions typically under 8 mm in diameter. Diagnosis is made by detecting papillomavirus in samples with either immunohistochemistry or PCR. These lesions can be subtle to discover, and it has been postulated that they may be the early form of Bowen's disease or cutaneous squamous cell carcinomas in situ in some cats. It has been demonstrated that as many as 48% of cats with Bowen's disease can be positive for papillomavirus antigens (Friberg, 2006). Antiviral therapy has been an effective treatment in many of these cases.

Numerous treatment options are available for felines with papillomavirus-induced skin lesions resulting in cutaneous horns, viral plaques, and Bowen's disease. Depending on the lesion, laser ablation can be an effective treatment. Imiquimod can be used on all of these lesions every 48 to 72 hours, with clinical remission possible in many cases. Other protocols use imiquimod every 24 hours for 2 to 3 consecutive days of each week.

A fibroblastic proliferation triggered by papillomaviruses has been reported in the cat and is termed *fibropapilloma* or *feline sarcoid*. Affected cats typically present with singular or multiple firm nodules on the nose, lip, paws, ears, tail tip, and rarely the oral cavity. They have been mainly reported in domestic cats living in rural areas, especially "barn" cats. These lesions can be difficult to differentiate from spindle cell tumors with histopathology and immunohistochemistry. Although surgery is an option, recurrence at surgical site prompted cryosurgery, radiation therapy, and amputation to be previously recommended as the treatments of choice. However, a recent study found imiquimod cream to show 75% or greater improvement in 80% of equine sarcoid lesions (Nogueira et al., 2006). Although studies need to be conducted evaluating its efficacy on feline sarcoids, imiquimod may be a reasonable therapy to start with before progressing to more aggressive therapies.

FELINE COWPOX

Dermatologic lesions secondary to cowpox, a virus in the *Orthopoxvirus* genus, have been reported in cats in the United Kingdom and continental Europe but not the United States. Cats become infected by hunting and eating rodents, which are the reservoir of this virus. This condition is zoonotic, and animals suspected of having it should be handled accordingly.

Cats with cowpox can have mild upper respiratory symptoms, anorexia, and depression; but most display a primary dermatologic lesion of an ulcerating macule or plaque and secondary lesions 7 to 10 days later of disseminated macules, papules, and nodules.

Differential diagnoses of this condition include deep fungal infections, atypical mycobacteria, nocardia, and neoplastic conditions. Diagnosis is made by histopathologic presence of large epithelial eosinophilic intracytoplasmic inclusions (type A inclusion bodies), and by isolation of the cowpox virus using PCR or immunohistochemistry on dried crust lesions.

No definitive treatment is available, but L-lysine, IFN-α, and Imiquimod can be attempted as described for feline herpesvirus infections. Extreme care should be used when treating these cats topically because of the highly zoonotic nature of this disease.

References and Suggested Reading

de Mari K et al: Therapeutic effects of recombinant feline interferon-omega on feline leukemia virus (FeLV)-infected and FeLV/feline immunodeficiency virus (FIV)-coinfected symptomatic cats, *J Vet Intern Med* 18:477, 2004.

Friberg C: Feline facial dermatoses. In Campbell KL, editor: *Veterinary clinics of North America small animal practice: updates in dermatology*, Philadelphia, 2006, Saunders, p 115.

Gross TL et al: *Skin diseases of the dog and cat: clinical and histopathologic diagnosis*, ed 2, Oxford 2005, Blackwell Publishing, pp 124, 157, 710.

Hargis AM, Ginn PE: Feline herpesvirus 1-associated facial and nasal dermatitis and stomatitis in domestic cats. In: Campbell KL, editor: *Veterinary clinics of North America small animal practice: dermatology*, Philadelphia, 1999, Saunders, p 1281.

Hargis AM et al: Ulcerative facial and nasal dermatitis and stomatitis in cats associated with feline herpesvirus 1, *Vet Dermatol* 10:267, 1999.

Hawrenek T et al: Feline orthopoxvirus infection transmitted from cat to human, *J Am Acad Dermatol* 49:513, 2003.

Hurley KF et al: An outbreak of virulent systemic feline calicivirus disease, *J Am Vet Med Assoc* 224:241, 2004.

LeClerc SM, Clark EG, Haines DM: Papillomavirus infection in association with feline cutaneous squamous cell carcinoma in situ, Proceedings of the 13th AAVD/ACVD meeting, Nashville, Tenn, 1997, p 125.

Mansell JK, Rees CA: Cutaneous manifestations of viral disease. In August JR, editor: *Consultations in feline internal medicine*, vol 5, St Louis, 2006, Elsevier Saunders, p 11.

Nogueira S, et al: Efficacy if imiquimod 5% cream in the treatment of equine sarcoids: a pilot study, *Vet Dermatol* 17:259, 2006.

Pesavento PA et al: Pathologic, immunohistochemical, and electron microscopic findings in naturally occurring virulent systemic feline calicivirus infection in cats, *Vet Pathol* 41:257, 2004.

Sundberg JP et al: Feline papilloma and papillomaviruses, *Vet Pathol* 37:1, 2000.

van Vuuren M, Goosen T, Rogers P: Feline herpesvirus infection in a group of semi-captive cheetahs, *J S Afr Vet Assoc* 70:132, 1999.

CHAPTER **100**

Canine Papillomaviruses

MASAHIKO NAGATA, *Tokyo, Japan*

The papillomavirus (PV) was first described in 1933, when Shope recognized the causative agent responsible for cutaneous papilloma in the cottontail rabbit. Watrach (1969) first recognized the structural characterization of the canine PV (CPV) in 1969. Yet this group of viruses has been refractory to standard virologic study because all efforts to date that have been aimed at tissue culture propagation of any of the PVs have remained unsuccessful. Since the mid-1980s there has been a virtual explosion in research and interest in the PVs because differentiation of PV by cleavage patterns produced by treating viral deoxyribonucleic acid (DNA) has emphasized the heterogeneity of the PVs.

VIRAL PROPERTIES

The PVs are grouped together with the polyomaviruses to form the papovaviruses. The PV is a small, naked virus with double-stranded, circular DNA. The size of the CPV has been estimated at 33 to 49 nm; the particles form closely packed crystalline structures within the nuclei. The lack of a lipid envelope may account for the relative resistance of the virus to physical or chemical destruction. PV infections appear to be limited to the epidermis and epithelium. Epidermal DNA is present in the basal layer of the epidermis, and viral replication depends on epidermal cellular differentiation. The site of viral latency is in the basal layers, although complete viral particles are found at the granular level. The viral genome is divisible into several major early (E) and late (L) open reading frames. The early viral proteins E1 and E2 play a role in replication of the viral genome; and E5, E6, and E7 control cell growth and cell cycle to maximize viral DNA replication. The function of E3 and E4 is not well known, and E3 is expressed in only BPV1, whereas the late protein L1 and L2 genes encode for viral capsid proteins. More than 90 different strains of PVs have been identified in humans, but only three genetically distinct PV types have been sequenced thus far in dogs.

CLINICAL FEATURES

The clinical manifestation of PV depends on the host, the PV type, and the anatomic site infected, even though the most common outcome of PV infection may be asymptomatic infection. Clinical and histopathologic features, as well as the viral strains identified by transmission studies, immunohistochemistry, in situ hybridization methods, and polymerase chain reaction, have suggested that there are at least five or more distinct PV-associated skin disorders in dogs.

Canine Oral Papilloma

Canine oral papilloma (COP) is a self-limited infectious disease that is normally confined to mucosal tissue of the oral cavity or lips in young dogs, but it also can produce papillomas on the conjunctiva and external nares. The lesions begin as white, flat, smooth, shiny papules and plaques and progress to whitish-gray, pedunculated or cauliflower-like hyperkeratotic masses. Light microscopy revealed papillomatous proliferations of thick squamous epithelium, in which some cells are swollen with vesicular cytoplasm. Canine oral PV (COPV)–induced generalized papillomas occasionally may be the presenting sign in immunosuppressed and cyclosporine-administered dogs (Favrot et al., 2005). The lesions regress spontaneously in most cases, although malignant transformation into carcinomas has been reported.

Cutaneous Exophytic Papilloma

Cutaneous exophytic papilloma (CEP) occurs at any age but is most often seen in dogs less than 2 years of age. CEP lesions may be single or multiple and occur mainly on the head, eyelids, and feet. The lesions present as white, pink, or pigmented papillated masses that may be sessile or pedunculated. Lesions are typically less than 1 cm and have a fimbriated surface. Microscopically CEP consists of marked epithelial proliferations on numerous thin fibrovascular stalks. Many but not all CEPs spontaneously regress over a period of weeks to months.

Cutaneous Inverted Papilloma

Cutaneous inverted papilloma (CIP) was described by Campbell and associates (1988) as single or multiple nonpigmented, small, raised, firm masses covered by skin with a central pore opening to the surface. It is usually seen in dogs less than 3 years of age and occurs commonly on the ventral abdomen and groin. Lesions are less than 2 cm and

are supported by thin fibrovascular stalks. Light microscopy shows an inverted flasklike structure below the level of the normal epidermis. CIP usually does not undergo spontaneous regression, although a spontaneously regressed case has been reported (Shimada et al., 1993).

Canine Pigmented Plaques

PV-associated canine pigmented plaques (CPPLs) have been reported by Nagata and associates (1995) to occur in some pugs and miniature schnauzers during young adulthood. Boston terriers, French bulldogs, and shar-pei, as well as immunosuppressive individuals, are also suspected to have an increased incidence of this wart (Gross et al., 2005; Stokking et al., 2004). Lesions are multiple, scaly, deeply pigmented macules, plaques, and sometime papules commonly seen on the ventral neck, ventral trunk, and extremities. CPPLs develop progressively over time and never regress. The potential for transformation to squamous cell carcinoma (SCC) has also been reported. The presumed familial nature of CPPLs suggests that it is equivalent to epidermodysplasia verruciformis (EV) in humans. EV is considered to be genetically determined and is caused by unusual susceptibility to EV-specific human PV infection.

Canine Pigmented Papules

PV-associated canine pigmented papules (CPPAs) have been reported to occur in a boxer under long-term corticosteroid therapy by Le Net and colleagues in 1997. Multiple black, rounded papules up to 2 mm were recognized on the ventral skin. Histologically the lesions consisted of well-demarcated cup-shaped foci of epidermal endophytic hyperplasia with marked parakeratosis and no papillary proliferations. Spontaneous regression occurred within 3 weeks after cessation of corticosteroids.

Miscellaneous Forms Suggesting Different CPV Infestations

Canine Digital Papillomatosis
Multiple papillomas, strictly limited to the junction of the footpad and adjacent skin and not involving footpads on all four feet, was reported to occur in a 9-month-old intact male beagle (Debey et al., 2001). Histopathologic findings were similar to those of CPPAs, and immunohistochemical and electron microscopic study confirmed the presence of CPV particles. All of the papillomas had been completely resolved within 2 months after diagnosis. These distinctive clinical and histologic findings could be associated with a novel CPV, even though the PV has not been cloned yet.

Nail Bed Inverted Squamous Papillomas
Nail bed inverted squamous papilloma has been described as a single swollen digit, usually with a thickened, abnormally soft nail, which may be broken or absent (Gross et al., 2005). Histopathologic features show a well-circumscribed, cup-shaped, thick layer of squamous epithelial cells that form papillary projections extending into the keratin core. Occasional epithelial cells may exhibit cytoplasmic vacuolation resembling koilocytosis, even though neither papillomaviral DNA nor antigens have been demonstrated.

Canine Genital Papillomatosis

Canine genital papillomatosis is probably caused by a different CPV, since neither the oral nor the cutaneous CPV induces tumors of the lower genital tract. This form of CPV infection is less frequently reported and has yet to be given a properly detailed description.

Squamous Cell Carcinoma

PVs appear to be involved in the etiology of certain forms of SCC in dogs. Sundberg and O'Banion (1989) reported that some dogs treated with a live virus vaccine made from PV isolated from naturally occurring COP experienced SCCs at their vaccine inoculation sites. In naturally occurring SCC, COPV DNA was demonstrated in nests of the epithelial tumor cells surrounding horn pearls or disseminated in the carcinoma tissue (Teifke, Lohr, and Shirasawa, 1997). In addition, PV-associated SCC in situ following chronic administration of cyclosporine and prednisone and invasive SCC related to bone marrow–transplanted canine X-linked severe combined immunodeficiency have also been reported in dogs (Calla, Preziosi, and Mauldin, 2005; Goldschmidt et al., 2006). It was suggested that a progression of viral papillomas into carcinomas in dogs may occur and that a genetic variety of CPV exists.

TREATMENTS

The search for an effective treatment against PV-associated skin diseases has been frustrated by the nature of CPV immunity, which remains inadequately understood at this time. In addition, PVs are very resistant within the environment and are difficult to eliminate with disinfectants. Fortunately routine treatment of these lesions is not crucial. The majority of PV infections regress spontaneously after the development of a cell-mediated immune response, and older animals have developed solid immunity as a result of previous exposure to the virus. However, lack of regression of the papillomas, interference with function, cosmetic embarrassment, or risk of malignancy may indicate vigorous therapy. In humans no treatment has yet had a very high success rate (average 60% to 70% clearance in 3 months), and the highest clearance rates for various treatments are usually found in younger individuals who have a short duration of infection. The use of surgery and destructive therapies such as cryotherapy and laser therapy have been discussed in the previous edition of the text (Bonagura, 2000); antiviral treatments are the focus of this revised chapter and represent the most current therapies for PV-associated skin diseases.

Immunotherapy

Imiquimod (Aldara, 3M Pharmaceuticals), an imidazoquinoline amine, is an immune response modifier (see Chapter 93). Imiquimod differs in that it does not have direct antiviral properties but rather it induces a significant production of cytokines, including interferon (IFN)-α, IFN-γ, interleukin (IL)-6, IL-12, and tumor necrosis factor-α. These cytokines stimulate the helper T cell (Th) Th1 pathway and inhibit the Th2 pathway via stimulation of monocytes and dendritic cells. In addition, imiquimod activates immune cells via binding to cell surface receptors such as the toll-like receptors that play an important role in host defense by regulating both innate and adaptive immune responses. Moreover, imiquimod was found to be effective in human cutaneous premalignancies and malignancies. Since tumor development depends on blood vessel supply, the inhibition of angiogenesis could be responsible for the antitumor activity. In humans imiquimod is applied before bedtime and after washing areas to be treated once a day for 3 days a week. It is well tolerated; but occasional side effects include erosion, excoriation, flaking, edema, and erythema. No controlled studies have been reported in dogs, and the cost is fairly high.

Autogenous vaccines have been used especially for treatment of mucous membrane warts in humans and dogs. It has been demonstrated by Bell and associates (1994) that systemic administration of a formalin-inactivated COP vaccine can protect against mucosal infection with COPV. In this study 26 dogs received two doses of phosphate-buffered saline intradermally, and 99 dogs received two doses of the inactivated vaccine. One month after the second dose, all dogs were challenged with infectious COPV by scarification of the oral mucosa. All control dogs acquired papillomas 6 to 8 weeks after infection, whereas none of the vaccinated dogs did. Sundburg and associates (1994) reported that the vaccine might be protective against COPV epidermal infections that develop as a consequence of the spread of oral lesions to the skin in immunosuppressed dogs. In addition, the vaccination might play a role in protecting against the development of SCC in dogs infected with COPV.

Sensitization to dinitrochlorobenzene followed by an application of dinitrochlorobenzene to lesions and contact sensitization with diphenylcyclopropenone has proven to be a useful treatment of cutaneous malignancies and refractory warts in humans. However, such treatment has been tried in only a limited number of human studies, and no canine studies have been conducted.

Antiviral Therapy

IFN is produced in the body and exerts the biologic action to protect cells from any kind of virus infection. There are three main classes of human IFNs (i.e., IFN-α, IFN-β and IFN-γ, as well as a minor class called IFN-ω). IFN-α elicits broad activities inhibitory to virus replication (also see Chapter 85). An intracellular mechanism, by which IFN-α2a inhibits human papillomavirus (HPV)–transformed cell proliferation and presumably HPV-induced papillomas, operates through the suppression of viral oncoprotein expression and the cytostatic arrest of cycling at G1. In dogs it was reported that 1.5 to 2 million units/m² of IFN-α2a (Roferon-A, Hoffman-LaRoche) given subcutaneously three times a week is effective for the treatment of severe cases of oral or cutaneous viral papillomatosis or both. In addition, IFN-α2a therapy, 1000 units given orally on a 21-day on, 7-day off schedule was reported as an adjunctive therapy for CPPLs (Stokking et al., 2004). The effectiveness of IFN-α2b (Intron A, Schering-Plough), 30 units/ml given orally, has been reported anecdotally, but the recommended dose and frequency varied widely. In some instances combining IFN-α with other treatments could increase the likelihood of effective treatment.

Besides IFN-α the efficacy of IFN-γ therapy has been evaluated in several studies in humans, but it remains controversial. There are no reports on use of IFN-γ in dogs, although one report (Andre, 2004) indicated that IFN-ω could be useful as an alternative with the aim of reducing the size of papillomas. A 4½-month-old dog with papillomatosis on the mucocutaneous junctions was treated with 2 million units (MU) of intralesional IFN-ω (Virbagen Omega, Virbac; Intercat, Toray). The lesions regressed in both size and number without side effects and were removed surgically. Furthermore, my experience has suggested that IFN-ω, 1 MU/kg given subcutaneously three times a week for a month, could be helpful in the treatment of CPPL.

In humans the common side effects of IFN treatment are the influenza-like symptoms such as fever, chills, nausea, fatigue, myalgia, and loss of appetite. Such side effects usually show a tendency to be less severe with time and are usually tolerable. It should be emphasized that no properly controlled studies nor any safety studies on IFN therapy against canine papillomatosis have been conducted so far; thus IFN is best considered as a treatment of last resort because of its high cost and inconsistent effects.

References and Suggested Reading

Andre F: Juvenile papillomatosis in a female dog, *L'Action Veterinaire* 1668:11, 2004.

Bell JA et al: A formalin-inactivated vaccine protects against mucosal papillomavirus infection: a canine model, *Pathobiol* 62:194, 1994.

Bonagura JD, editor: *Kirk's current veterinary therapy XIII (small animal practice)*, Philadelphia, 2000, Saunders, p 569.

Callan MB, Preziosi D, Mauldin E: Multiple papillomavirus-associated epidermal hamartomas and squamous cell carcinomas in situ in a dog following chronic treatment with prednisone and cyclosporine *Vet Dermatol* 16:338, 2005.

Campbell KL et al: Cutaneous inverted papillomas in dogs, *Vet Patrol* 25:67, 1988.

Debey BM et al: Digital papillomatosis in a confined beagle, *J Vet Diagn Invest* 13:346, 2001.

Favrot C et al: Evaluation of papillomaviruses associated with cyclosporine-induced hyperplastic verrucous lesions in dogs, *Am J Vet Res* 66:1764, 2005.

Goldschmidt MH et al: Severe papillomavirus infection progressing to metastatic SCC in bone marrow-transplanted X-linked SCID dogs, *J Virol* 80:6621, 2006.

Gross TL et al: *Skin disease of the dog and cat: clinical and histopathologic diagnosis*, ed 2, Oxford, 2005, Blackwell Science, p 567.

Le Net JL et al: Multiple pigmented cutaneous papules associated with a novel canine papillomavirus in an immunosuppressed dog, *Vet Pathol* 34:8, 1997.

Nagata M et al: Pigmented plaques associated with papillomavirus infection in dogs: is this epidermodysplasia verruciformis? *Vet Dermatol* 6:179, 1995.

Shimada A et al: Cutaneous papillomatosis associated with papillomavirus infection in a dog, *J Comp Pathol* 108:103, 1993.

Stokking LB et al: Pigmented epidermal plaques in three dogs, *J Am Anim Hosp Assoc* 40:411, 2004.

Sundberg JP, O'Banion MK: Animal papillomaviruses associated with malignant tumors, *Adv Viral Oncol* 8:55, 1989.

Sundberg JP et al: Involvement of canine oral papillomavirus in generalized oral and cutaneous verrucosis in a Chinese Shar Pei dog, *Vet Patrol* 31:183, 1994.

Teifke JP, Lohr CV, Shirasawa H: Detection of canine oral papillomavirus-DNA in canine oral squamous cell carcinomas and p53 overexpressing skin papillomas of the dog using the polymerase chain reaction and non-radioactive in situ hybridization, *Vet Microbiol* 28:119, 1998.

Watrach AM: The ultrastructure of canine cutaneous papilloma, *Cancer Res* 29:2079, 1969.

Zaugg N et al: Detection of novel papillomaviruses in canine mucosal, cutaneous and in situ squamous cell carcinomas, *Vet Dermatol* 16:290, 2005.

CHAPTER 101

Pyotraumatic Dermatitis ("Hot Spots")

WAYNE S. ROSENKRANTZ, *Tustin, California*

Hot spots, more appropriately described as pyotraumatic dermatitis, are defined as a circumscribed, moist exudative area that is most commonly brought on by self-trauma. The self-trauma results from attempts to alleviate pain or pruritus associated with an underlying disease that is creating this sensation. Primary bacterial infections are very rare and in theory could create localized moist exudative lesions with minimal self-trauma.

The most common causes of hot spots are allergic conditions such as flea allergy, atopic dermatitis, adverse food reaction, scabies, and anal gland problems (Box 101-1). Clipping or grooming complications such as razor burn or trauma can also create localized inflammation that results in pruritus and hot spot formation. Occasionally other infectious conditions (*Staphylococcus* spp., *Pseudomonas* spp., demodicosis, or dermatophytosis) can result in localized multifocal

Box 101-1

Causes of Hot Spots

Common Causes	Uncommon Causes
Allergies: flea, atopy, food	Dermatophytosis
Parasitic: scabies, *Demodex*	Injection site reactions
Anal gland disease	Drug reactions
Clipping or grooming	Autoimmune disease
Result of deep pyoderma	Panniculitis
	Vasculitis

areas of pain and pruritus leading to hot spot–like lesions. Other less common causes of hot spots are listed in Box 101-1.

Although any breed of dog can experience hot spots, some consider certain breeds to be predisposed. These include the golden retriever, Labrador retriever, St. Bernard, collie, and German shepherd. However, many of these breeds are actually predisposed to the common underlying causes of hot spots such as allergies. Long-haired coat length has also been thought to be involved with a predisposition to hot spots. However, in a report on 40 dogs 50% had short hair, and 50% had long hair (Schroeder et al., 1996).

The role of *Staphylococcus* in the development of hot spots remains controversial. *Staphylococcus* can be isolated from the skin of normal dogs. Higher numbers of these organisms are found in allergic dogs, even in those without active skin disease. Therefore allergies may contribute to hot spots not only by the presence of pruritus but also by creating a favorable environment for larger numbers of staphylococci to flourish on the skin. One investigator proposes that hot spots are of two types based on histopathologic patterns (Reinke et al., 1987). One is a superficial lesion in which bacteria are considered surface colonizers. The other is a folliculitis that may be a deep lesion. Coagulase-positive *Staphylococcus* spp., particularly *Staphylococcus intermedius*, are most commonly cultured from these lesions. This same study showed a strong tendency for young dogs, golden retrievers, and St. Bernards to be predisposed to the deeper form of hot spots. In a more recent evaluation, 44 privately owned dogs in a flea scarce environment had their lesions separated histopathologically into four patterns by the presence or absence of eosinophils and/or folliculitis (Holm et al. 2004). Eosinophils have not previously been recorded in pyotraumatic dermatitis but were seen in 29 cases. Acute folliculitis was seen in 20 cases. However, no correlation was seen among age, sex, breed, underlying cause, or site of lesion and histopathology. Twenty-seven cases were cultured for bacteria, of which 25 grew *S. intermedius* and two were negative. In another study *Staphylococcus* was isolated from all lesions before topical treatment (Schroeder et al., 1996). The condition in placebo vehicle control groups cleared completely within 7 days without topical antimicrobial treatment. The role of *Staphylococcus* as a primary cause in hot spots is certainly unclear.

CLINICAL FEATURES

The historical hallmark of hot spots is intense pruritus, and it represents one of the situations in which clients are generally correct when reporting that the lesion "just happened." The intense self-trauma can produce large lesions in minutes.

Regardless of the cause, most hot spots look similar clinically. They are generally well circumscribed, moist, erosive-to-ulcerated, erythematous, and usually painful lesions. The overlying hair is matted and coated with a serous-to-suppurative exudative discharge. Variable amounts of crusted debris may be present. It is not uncommon to see peripheral smaller lesions adjacent to the primary site. Acute lesions tend to be edematous, whereas chronic lesions may be thickened with lichenified-to-scarred peripheral areas resembling acral lick dermatitis. The most common body locations for pyotraumatic dermatitis include the rump, lateral upper thigh, perineal-rectal area, and lateral aspect of the face below the ear. The rump and lateral upper thigh are the most common locations and can be associated with flea allergy, adverse food reactions, or atopic dermatitis. The perineal-rectal area lesions generally are caused by anal gland disease or adverse food reactions (see Chapter 87). The lateral cervical facial lesions can be caused by ear problems, atopic dermatitis, or adverse food reactions.

DIAGNOSIS

Diagnosis is generally made from the history and physical examination. The intensity of pruritus, body location, and physical appearance are often all that is necessary to make a diagnosis. Initially skin scrapings and cytologic studies should be considered to rule out *Demodex* infection and determine if cocci are present. In more chronic or relapsing conditions, fungal and bacterial cultures, biopsies, and allergy workups (allergy testing and elimination diets) should be performed. If these tests do not lead to a diagnosis, laboratory testing for underlying immune-mediated or systemic problems should be performed.

THERAPY

Topical Therapy

Regardless of the cause and independent of what is used either topically or systemically, shaving the hair and cleansing the hot spot is the initial form of therapy. To shave or clean the wound, a topical desensitizing agent or sedation may be necessary because of the pain and discomfort associated with the lesion. After the area is clipped, the full extent and nature of the lesion can be observed. An antimicrobial shampoo containing benzoyl peroxide (Oxydex, Sulf/Oxydex, Eliminate Ivax/DVM Pharmaceuticals; Pyoben, Virbac; Micro Pearls benzoyl peroxide, Vétoquinol; DermaBenSs, DermaPet) or chlorhexidine (ChlorhexiDerm, Eliminate Ivax/DVM Pharmaceuticals; Hexadene, Virbac; Nolvasan; and Douxo, Sogeval) are my favorites. Over-the-counter antimicrobial shampoos such as those containing benzalkonium chloride can also be effective.

After the site is clipped and washed appropriately, additional topical and, in some situations, systemic treatments are needed. Occlusive vehicles (ointments and creams) should be avoided. Nonocclusive vehicles (sprays, rinses, gels, and lotions) are preferable to allow exudation to occur and prevent occlusion of follicles and progression into a deeper folliculitis.

Many practitioners like to use an astringent for the first 24 to 48 hours on hot spots. Astringents precipitate proteins and usually do not penetrate deeply. These products do tend to dry out and decrease the exudation. An example of a currently used astringent is aluminum acetate solution (Burow's solution, Domeboro, Bayer) diluted 1:40 in cool water. Other less commonly used astringents include 5% tannic acid, 25% silver nitrate solution, and potassium permanganate 1:1000 to 1:30,000 solution. I prefer Domeboro because it is tolerated best and does not stain compared with the other astringents.

The most common topical products used on hot spots are antipruritic sprays, gels, and lotions. Some of these products substitute another sensation for the pruritus such as heat or cold. Cooling tends to decrease pruritus. Examples include 0.12 to 1% methol, 0.12 to 1% camphor, 0.5 to 1% thymol, or cold ice packs. Other products use local anesthetic or desensitizing agents such as benzocaine, tetracaine, lidocaine, 1% pramoxine (Relief, Eliminate Ivax/DVM Pharmaceuticals; Dermacool, Virbac), benzoyl peroxide (Oxydex Gel, Eliminate Ivax/DVM Pharmaceuticals; Pyoben Gel, Virbac), and tars. These agents are short acting. Topical antihistamines are considered effective in humans but in my experience have limited value in the dog. Anecdotal reports suggest that topical 2% diphenhydramine (Histacalm, Virbac) is effective in reducing pruritus in dogs with hot spots. Colloidal oatmeal rinses and shampoos can also give topical relief from pruritus. Commonly used products include Epi-Soothe (Virbac) and Aveeno (Rydelle). The most effective topical products in controlling the pruritus associated with hot spots are glucocorticoids. Hydrocortisone is the safest and is anecdotally effective. Hydrocortisone 1% is considered particularly safe and can be used long term with no adverse topical or systemic side effects. The most commonly used veterinary products include CortiSpray (Eliminate Ivax/DVM Pharmaceuticals), Dermacool-HC (Virbac), Cortisoothe (Virbac), and CortiCalm (Eliminate Ivax/DVM Pharmaceuticals). A newer low-dose 0.015% triamcinolone spray (Genesis, Virbac) also has been evaluated and appears to be much more effective than the hydrocortisone-based products; in controlled studies it appeared to have no significant systemic absorption. However, when applied to the flanks and medial thighs, localized cutaneous atrophy reactions have been seen.

Topical antimicrobial agents can be used alone or in combination with other ingredients. Alcohol-based products can be bactericidal and astringent but also can be irritating to ulcerated surfaces. The most commonly used alcohol product is 2% benzyl alcohol. Some of the active agents mentioned in the shampoo section are also available in gel and solution forms and can be used on focal lesions. Chlorhexidine diacetate or gluconate and 2.5 to 5% benzoyl peroxide gels (Oxydex, Eliminate Ivax/DVM Pharmaceuticals; Pyoben, Virbac) are examples. One of the oldest antimicrobials is iodine. The "tamed" iodines (povidone-iodine [Betadine] and polyhydroxydine [(Xenodine]) are less irritating and less staining than their precursors but generally are not as effective as some of the other antimicrobials mentioned. Surface-acting agents such as the quaternary ammonium compounds (e.g., benzalkonium chloride) are effective broad-spectrum antibacterial agents.

Many potent topical antibacterial agents are available. My favorite veterinary topical antibiotic is mupirocin because of its high efficacy for coagulase-positive staphylococci and its ability to penetrate deeper pyodermas. Veterinary products are no longer available but can be formulated by compounding pharmacies. Other products that can be helpful include neomycin, gentamicin, bacitracin, and polymyxin B.

Combination antibiotic and glucocorticoid products often produce the best results and quickest healing. One study (Schroeder et al, 1996) supported this when neomycin, prednisolone, and neomycin-prednisolone products were compared. The combination product produced the quickest recovery. The most commonly used veterinary products include Tresaderm (Merial), Gentocin topical spray (Schering-Plough) and generics, Panolog (Fort Dodge), and Otomax and Mometamax (Schering-Plough). Because these products contain potent glucocorticoids, their use should be limited and are not for the long term.

Systemic Therapy

The need for systemic therapy for hot spots varies on a case-by-case basis. Most dogs benefit from a course of systemic antibiotics, particularly if the hot spot represents a deeper folliculitis. Antibiotic selection should be based on proven efficacy for *S. intermedius* and should be used for a minimum of 14 days and generally continued 7 to 10 days beyond clinical cure. My personal favorites include cephalexin, 20 to 30 mg/kg every 12 hours; ormetoprim-sulfadimethoxine (Primor, Pfizer Animal Health), 55 mg/kg for the first 24 hours and then 27.5 mg/kg every 24 hours after that; amoxicillin-clavulanate (Clavamox, Pfizer Animal Health), 15 to 20 mg/kg every 12 hours; and enrofloxacin (Baytril, Bayer), 5 mg/kg every 24 hours, or marbofloxacin (Zeniquin, Pfizer Animal Health), 2.5 mg/kg every 24 hours.

The use of systemic glucocorticoid therapy is more controversial. Some dermatologists avoid glucocorticoids, especially for deeper pyotraumatic folliculitis, arguing the concern for immune depression. Certainly if the practitioner elects to use glucocorticoids, long-acting injectables should be avoided, and only short courses of oral prednisone or prednisolone should be used to break the pruritic cycle. Suggested dosages would include antiinflammatory dosages (1 mg/kg every 24 hours for 3 to 5 days).

The client should be warned about future lesions because this is commonly a recurring problem if the underlying disease is chronic. Therefore identifying, eliminating, or controlling the underlying disease is the long-term goal for prevention of hot spots. The client should be educated about the various differentials, and diagnostic tests should be performed accordingly. Attention to increased episodes of pruritus after grooming and bathing should be stressed.

Maintaining parasite control and routinely examining the ears and anal glands are also recommended.

References and Suggested Reading

Holm BR et al: A prospective study of the clinical findings, treatment, and histopathology of 44 cases of pyotraumatic dermatitis, *Vet Dermatol* 6:369, 2004.

Reinke SI et al: Histopathologic features of pyotraumatic dermatitis, *J Am Anim Hosp Assoc* 190:57, 1987.

Schroeder H et al: Efficacy of a topical antimicrobial-antiinflammatory combination in the treatment of pyotraumatic dermatitis in dogs, *Vet Dermatol* 7:163, 1996.

Scott DW, Miller WH, Griffin CE: *Muller and Kirk's, small animal dermatology*, ed 6, Philadelphia, 2001, Saunders, p 1104.

CHAPTER **102**

Methicillin-Resistant Canine Pyoderma

CARLO VITALE, *San Francisco, California*

The emergence of methicillin-resistant *Staphylococcus aureus* in humans in 1961 in the United Kingdom set the stage for the need of a more globally organized monitoring and surveillance program. This allowed the medical world to institute preventive programs, outline responsible antibiotic usage, and encourage research to adapt accordingly to the inevitable increase in resistance. In veterinary medicine there are very basic recommendations and guidelines for the judicious use of antibiotics. Unfortunately there is no specific guidance or systematic surveillance programs for veterinarians regarding the proper use of antibiotics.

Methicillin is a penicillin-type antibiotic that is no longer available in any form; thus oxacillin is used as a marker for methicillin resistance. On the basis of bacterial culture and susceptibility testing, resistance to oxacillin also proves resistance to all penicillins and cephalosporins (beta-lactams). Acquisition of an altered penicillin-binding protein 2a (PBP2a) renders species of *Staphylococcus* resistant to methicillin. This resistance occurs when a bacterial isolate carries and mobilizes PBP2a, encoded by the gene mecA. The terms *methicillin-resistant S. aureus (MRSA)* and *Staphylococcus intermedius (MRSI)*, are preferred over the term oxacillin-resistant *Staphylococcus*.

INCIDENCE

Historically, *S. intermedius* is the most common bacterial isolate from cases of canine pyoderma. It appears, however, that many strains previously identified as *S. intermedius* are *S. pseudintermedius*, as shown recently through multilocus sequence typing (Bannoehr et al., 2007). According to most commercial veterinary reference lab- oratories, methicillin-resistant strains of *Staphylococcus intermedius* are not uncommon. The clinical presentation of methicillin-resistant pyoderma generally does not differ from routine cases. Articles have been published documenting methicillin resistance in cases of *S. intermedius* (Cole et al., 2004; Gortel et al., 1999; Morris et al., 2006). Interestingly, in another study 2 of 57 *S. intermedius* isolates were resistant to methicillin; however, about half of the total expressed PBP2a, indicating that the genetic capability is present to be resistant under the right conditions (Kania et al., 2004).

Since most of the attention has been given to methicillin-resistant *S. aureus* in animals, it is clear that there has been a definite increase in the numbers of reports of MRSA infections in pets (Baptiste et al., 2005; Gortel et al., 1999; Kania et al., 2004; Loeffler et al., 2005; Morris et al., 2006). *Staphylococcus schleiferi* has recently been associated with cases of canine pyoderma and has demonstrated methicillin resistance (May et al., 2005; Morris et al., 2006). MRSA and methicillin-resistant *S. schleiferi* appear to be rare in dogs. Most strains of methicillin-resistant *Staphylococcus* are not multidrug resistant. However, the true incidence of methicillin-resistant *Staphylococcus* in dogs is not known because of the paucity of large-scale studies.

ZOONOSIS

MRSA is considered to be an emerging reverse zoonosis (human-to-animal transmission). There have been several documented cases of likely transmission of MRSA from humans to animals (Weese et al., 2006; O'Mahony et al., 2005; Tomlin et al., 1999; Manian 2003, van Duijkeren et al., 2004). Transmission of MRSA to pets via contact with infected humans likely results in colonization (primarily nasal and rectal), infection, or both. In addition, some of these reports have shown that pets can serve as a "reservoir," thus allowing transmission back to the owner. I have seen several cases of nasal colonization with MRSA in dogs that acted as a source for reinfection to individuals who had intimate contact with the affected pet. In these cases the exact same strain was isolated from the dog's and the owner's nares, and only after nasal clearance of the dog did the owner's lesions cease to recur. Apparently it is believed MRSA colonization in pets usually is a transient occurrence.

MANAGEMENT AND THERAPY

Overall practicing veterinarians have received little in the way of specific detailed guidelines regarding the proper use of antibiotics for the treatment of methicillin-resistant canine pyoderma. The following recommendations may be useful to establish treatment success and possibly reduce the risk of further antibiotic resistance.

The most common first-line antibiotic prescribed empirically for routine canine pyoderma is cephalexin. The American College of Veterinary Internal Medicine and several university teaching hospitals have guidelines for the general use of antibiotics. Some of these institutions have found it useful to separate antibiotic usage into three different categories: first-line, second-line, and third-line (Weese, 2006b). In all cases of chronic and/or recurrent canine pyoderma, bacterial culture and susceptibility testing is recommended, and treatment is based on the results. However, some veterinary reference laboratories may provide inadequate or poor results with regard to culture and identification or susceptability testing. When submitting bacterial culture and susceptibility testing, I suggest that veterinarians alert the laboratory that they are concerned about methicillin resistance, which could be supported clinically by a lack of response to cephalexin. In this situation the laboratory may subculture and repeat culture technique to reconfirm oxacillin resistance. Some laboratories are already offering this, but not all laboratories do; contacting your laboratory on their isolation techniques is a good idea. The National Committee for Clinical Laboratory Standards (NCCLS) for humans has new recommendations; we hope our veterinary reference laboratories would follow their advice when applicable. In addition, accurate identification of methicillin resistance can be difficult in some cases because of the presence of different clones (resistant and susceptible) coexisting within the same "pure" culture. This phenomenon is termed *heteroresistance* and occurs mostly with strains of methicillin-resistant *Staphylococci.* Consultation with a microbiologist may prove useful to properly interpret results of susceptibility tests. I have found chloramphenicol or clindamycin to be a superior alternative to cephalexin in cases of documented methicillin resistance. Treatment generally is recommended for

at least 3 weeks in cases of superficial pyoderma and up to 6 weeks in cases of deep pyoderma.

As in all cases of infectious disease, it is extraordinarily important to wash hands thoroughly and frequently after examining each patient. Proper hand hygiene (frequent warm water with soap or waterless alcohol-based rubs) is the single most important factor in preventing infections. Gloves are generally not recommended because most caretakers touch multiple sites and do not change them often enough between patients. In cases of MRSA, all patients suspected or proven to be infected should be managed in a proper isolation ward.

References and Suggested Reading

Bannoehr J et al: Population genetic structure of the *Staphylococcus intermedius* group: insights into *agr* diversification and the emergence of methicillin-resistant strains, *J Bacteriol* 189:8685, 2007.

Baptiste KE et al: Methicillin-resistant staphylococci in companion animals, *Emerg Infect Dis* 11:1942, 2005.

Cole LK et al: Methicillin-resistant *Staphylococcus intermedius* organisms from the vertical ear canal of dogs with end stage-otitis externa, *Vet Dermatol* 15:35, 2004.

Gortel K et al: Methicillin resistance among staphylococci isolated from dogs, *Am J Vet Res* 60:1526, 1999.

Kania SA et al: Methicillin resistance of staphylococci isolated from the skin of dogs with pyoderma, *Am J Vet Res* 65:1265, 2004.

Loeffler A et al: Prevalence of methicillin-resistant *Staphylococcus aureus* among staff and pets in a small animal referral hospital in the UK, *J Antimicrob Chemother* 56:692, 2005.

Manian FA: Asymptomatic nasal carriage of mupirocin-resistant, methicillin-resistant *Staphylococcus aureus* (MRSA) in a pet dog associated with MRSA infection in household contacts, *Clin Infect Dis* 36:e26, 2003.

Morris DO et al: Screening of *Staphylococcus aureus, Staphylococcus intermedius,* and *Staphylococcus schleiferi* isolates obtained from small companion animals for antimicrobial resistance: a retrospective review of 749 isolates (2003-04), *Vet Dermatol* 17:332, 2006.

May ER et al: Isolation of *Staphylococcus schleiferi* from healthly dogs and dogs with otitis, pyoderma, or both, *J Am Vet Med Assoc* 227:928, 2005.

O'Mahony R et al: Methicillin-resistant *Staphylococcus aureus* (MRSA) isolated from animals and veterinary personnel in Ireland, *Vet Microbiol* 109:285, 2005.

Tomlin J et al: Methicillin-resistant *Staphylococcus aureus* infections in 11 dogs, *Vet Rec* 144:60, 1999.

van Duijkeren E et al: Human-to-dog transmission of methicillin-resistant *Staphylococcus aureus,* *Emerg Infect Dis* 10: 2235, 2004.

Weese JS et al: Suspected transmission of methicillin-resistant *Staphylococcus aureus* between domestic pets and humans in veterinary clinics and in the household, *Vet Microbiol* 115:148, 2006.

Weese JS: Investigation of antimicrobial use and the impact of antimicrobial use guidelines in a small animal veterinary teaching hospital: 1995-2004, *J Am Vet Med Assoc* 228:553, 2006.

CHAPTER 103

Sebaceous Adenitis

EDMUND J. ROSSER, JR., *East Lansing, Michigan*

Sebaceous adenitis is an inflammatory disease process directed against the sebaceous glands of the skin and has an unknown etiology and pathogenesis (Rosser et al., 1987; Scott, 1986). In standard poodles the results of pedigree analyses and prospective breeding studies of affected animals suggest that sebaceous adenitis is a heritable, autosomal-recessive skin disease of variable expression (Dunstan and Hargis, 1995), and a similar mode of inheritance has been proposed for Akitas with sebaceous adenitis (Reichler et al., 2001).

CLINICAL FEATURES

Sebaceous adenitis occurs primarily in young adult to middle-aged dogs with no apparent sex predisposition. However, more recent reports have indicated the onset of this disease in older dogs, including those in the range of 7 to 11 years of age, and this has also been my experience with this disease (Linek et al., 2005; Reichler et al., 2001). Sebaceous adenitis can be divided into two major forms based on their differences in clinical presentation and histopathologic changes (Rosser, 1992).

The first form occurs in long-coated breeds and has been recognized most frequently in the standard poodle, Akita, and Samoyed. This form of the disease is characterized by a dull, brittle hair coat; alopecia; moderate-to-severe scaling; and the formation of follicular casts. Pruritus and malodor are variable; they tend to be mild or absent early in the course of the disease and may become moderate to severe in advanced cases or when a secondary bacterial folliculitis develops. In standard poodles the lesions most commonly affect the dorsal regions of the body, including the dorsal planum of the nose, top of the head, pinnae, dorsal trunk, and tail. When the disease is progressive, the affected areas develop tightly adherent scales (varying from silver-white to brown, depending on hair coat color) with small tufts of hair matted within the scales. The disease in standard poodles may present in several clinical forms: (1) a subclinical form (detectable only on histopathologic examination of skin biopsy specimens of apparently normal skin); (2) a localized, mild, and self-limiting form; (3) a progressive moderate-to-severe form; and (4) a cyclic form with periods of spontaneous improvement or worsening independent of any treatment. In Samoyeds the alopecia, scaling, and follicular casts most commonly affect the entire trunk and pinnae. The disease in the Akita may represent its own variant of sebaceous adenitis in long-coated breeds of dogs because it differs by the additional presence of greasiness of the skin and hair coat and the frequent presence of papules and pustules. Akitas may also show signs of systemic illness such as fever, malaise, and weight loss (Power and Ihrke, 1990).

However, a more recent study of 23 Akitas reported a progression of the disease similar to that observed in standard poodles, both clinically and histologically, and an absence of any systemic signs (Reichler et al., 2001). It was also reported that 16 of 23 owners of affected dogs in this study reported that an illness, glucocorticoid or progestagen treatment, general anesthesia, estrus, molting, neutering, or an environmental change preceded the onset of the disease.

The second form of sebaceous adenitis occurs in breeds of dogs with short coats and has been most frequently recognized in the vizsla. This form of the disease is characterized by "moth-eaten," annular, or diffuse areas of alopecia and mild scaling with occasional small firm nodules, affecting the trunk, head, and ears. Dogs usually do not have pruritus, and the development of secondary bacterial folliculitis is rare.

DIAGNOSIS

The breed affected, the historical development of the problem, and the physical findings first lead the clinician to suspect sebaceous adenitis. The diagnosis is confirmed by the histopathologic examination of several skin biopsy specimens that are representative of the different degrees of lesion severity noted during the physical examination. Sites selected for biopsy should include any apparently normal skin, mildly affected areas, and severely affected areas. The most common histologic finding is a nodular granulomatous-to-pyogranulomatous inflammatory reaction at the level of the sebaceous glands (Dunstan and Hargis, 1995; Gross et al, 2005).

In the chronic stages of the disease in long-coated breeds of dogs, there is often a complete absence of sebaceous glands with little or no inflammation, perifollicular fibrosis, and marked follicular and surface hyperkeratosis. This may easily be misinterpreted as being consistent with an underlying endocrine skin disease. For this reason it is suggested that such biopsy samples be submitted to individuals specifically trained in veterinary dermatohistopathology. In contrast, in short-coated breeds of dogs, the periadnexal nodular granulomatous to pyogranulomatous inflammatory reaction is usually present throughout the disease process, with occasional complete obliteration and loss of all adnexal structures.

TREATMENT AND MANAGEMENT

Long-term management of sebaceous adenitis can be a frustrating experience for owners and veterinarians because the response to therapy varies, depending on the severity of the disease at the time of diagnosis; in addition, there is a lack of a consistent response to any single treatment regimen. This problem has led to several treatment recommendations and much confusion about which treatments should be tried. For this reason, I recommend a systematic approach to the treatment of sebaceous adenitis in dogs.

The goal of therapy should be to remove the excess scales, improve the luster of the hair coat, and regrow hair whenever possible (in standard poodles the hair regrowth is usually straight rather than curled). When response to treatment is evident, some level of maintenance therapy is usually required to control the disease. In severe or chronic cases in which the sebaceous glands have been completely lost, the prognosis for accomplishing these goals is guarded. However, a successful response to treatment (White et al., 1995), as well as the reappearance of sebaceous glands (Dunstan, personal communication, 1997), can occur even when the initial histopathologic examination of skin biopsy specimens revealed follicular fibrosis and apparent loss of the sebaceous glands.

Specifically, a significant regeneration of sebaceous glands was observed in dogs with sebaceous adenitis while being treated with cyclosporine for 12 months (Linek et al., 2005). In this study, followup biopsies taken every 4 months over a 12-month time period indicated an increase from only 2% of hair follicles exhibiting sebaceous glands to 40% of hair follicles exhibiting sebaceous glands. However, the severity of the follicular keratosis did not change significantly.

In mildly affected dogs the regular use of antiseborrheic shampoos, conditioners, and emollients and essential fatty acid dietary supplements (Bonagura, 2000, p. 538) may be effective. If the response is inadequate, my first recommendation is the consistent use of a combination of essential fatty acid dietary supplements (Derm Caps ES, DVM Pharmaceuticals, Inc.), one capsule orally every 12 hours; and evening primrose oil, 500 mg orally every 12 hours per dog (Rosser, 1992). This treatment should be continued for 2 months before being considered ineffective. Occasionally observed side effects include vomiting, diarrhea, and flatulence. This treatment has been most effective in the standard poodle and Samoyed breeds and usually requires lifelong administration to control the disease. An alternative to this treatment is the use of vitamin A at an initial dosage of 8,000 to 10,000 units BID; if significant improvement is not observed within 3 months, the dosage may be increased to 20,000 to 30,000 units BID (DeManuelle and Rothstein, 2002; Sousa, 2006). When this is ineffective or in dogs with large areas of tightly adherent scales (as in standard poodles), a bath oil treatment can be recommended. This is carried out by mixing any light mineral oil–containing bath oil (e.g., Alpha Keri Bath Oil, Bristol-Myers Squibb Pharmaceuticals or generic bath oil) 50:50 with water and spraying over the entire coat (Blair, 1993). The bath oil is rubbed well into the hair coat and allowed to soak into the coat for 1 hour. The dog should be put in a crate or kennel during the 1-hour soak. The bath oil is then removed by several baths (usually three shampoos) with a liquid dishwashing detergent (e.g., Palmolive dish soap, Ivory dish soap) while the hair coat is scrubbed with a soft hair brush. A conditioner, humectant, or creme rinse (HyLyt, DVM Pharmaceuticals; Humilac, Virbac; Hydra-Pearls, Vetoquinol Pharmaceuticals) should be applied after the final bath. This process results in the removal of a significant amount of the excess scaling, and this treatment alone may control the scaling and allow the regrowth of hair. This procedure

is repeated every 7 days for the first month and then every 14 to 30 days as needed. It must be mentioned that this procedure is relatively labor intensive but can be effective. An alternative to this form of treatment is the use of a 50:50 or 75:25 mixture of propylene glycol and water applied once daily as a spray to the affected areas (Griffin, 1988).

When these treatments have been ineffective, the use of a synthetic retinoid may be considered (see Section V on Evolve). In the management of sebaceous adenitis in vizslas, isotretinoin (Accutane, Roche) has been shown to be a most effective retinoid (Stewart, White, and Carpenter, 1991; White et al, 1995). The recommended dosage of isotretinoin is 1 mg/kg orally every 12 to 24 hours, with improvement usually noticed within 6 weeks. If improvement is evident, an attempt can be made to decrease the dosage to 1 mg/kg orally every 24 to 48 hours for another 6 weeks. If improvement continues, the long-term goal is to control the disease with either 1 mg/kg orally every 48 hours or 0.5 mg/kg every 24 hours.

However, it is important to note that as of this writing, systemic retinoids have become unavailable for use by veterinarians in the treatment of diseases for animals. This is due to recent strict regulations regarding the release of the drug to only registered physicians, and the required use of a human patient consent form when prescribing systemic retinoids.

For management of refractory cases of sebaceous adenitis in long-coated breeds of dogs (primarily standard poodles and Akitas), either isotretinoin or acitretin (Soriatane, Connetics Corp.) can be recommended (Power and Ihrke, 2002). One study indicated that it could not be predicted whether isotretinoin or etretinate would be more effective in the treatment of sebaceous adenitis in any long-coated dog breeds (White et al., 1995). Therefore these dogs can be treated initially with either isotretinoin (1 mg/kg orally [PO] q12 to 24h) or etretinate (1 mg/kg PO q12 to 24h) for an observation period of 6 weeks. Since etretinate is no longer commercially available, acitretin is being considered as the alternative and similarly acting retinoid. If there is a poor response to therapy on the first chosen retinoid, the dog should be switched to the second retinoid for an observation period of 6 weeks. If improvement is noted using either of these retinoids, an attempt can be made to decrease the dosage to 1 mg/kg orally every 24 to 48 hours for another 6 weeks. If improvement continues, the long-term goal is to control the disease using retinoid either at a dosage of 1 mg/kg every 48 hours or 0.5 mg/kg orally every 24 hours.

A treatment option in the management of sebaceous adenitis that has been nonresponsive to retinoid therapy is the use of cyclosporine (Atopica, Novartis) at a dosage of 5 mg/kg orally every 12 hours (Carothers, Kwochka, and Rojko, 1991; Linek et al, 2005; see Chapter 84 for a discussion of the side effects and toxicities in the use of cyclosporine in dogs). Most recently cyclosporine has been applied as a topical solution, using a micro-emulsified cyclosporine oral solution (Neoral, Novartis; 100 mg/ml concentration) and mixing 25 ml of the oral solution with 250 ml of water (1:10 dilution), which is then sprayed over the alopecic areas once daily (Patterson, 2005). A response to treatment with evidence of hair regrowth usually occurs within 2 weeks if this regimen is to be effective. If hair regrowth is observed, the treatment may be decreased from a once-daily application to twice-weekly therapy as maintenance in some cases. In long-coated breeds of dogs the hair should be kept clipped short to facilitate the application of the spray down to the skin. The owners should be instructed to wear gloves during the application process; let the dogs dry for 10 minutes after each application before handling the dog; and apply the spray in the late evening to minimize the handling of the dogs. To date no adverse reactions or toxicities to this treatment have been reported. A conditioner or humectant in a spray form (HyLyt, DVM Pharmaceuticals; Humilac, Virbac; Hydra-Pearls, Vetoquinol Pharmaceuticals) should be used following each treatment with the topical cyclosporine.

Sebaceous adenitis appears to be relatively refractory to either antiinflammatory or immunosuppressive dosages of corticosteroids. When a secondary bacterial folliculitis is present, the treatment should include the use of an appropriate systemic antibiotic along with a keratolytic, antibacterial, and follicular flushing shampoo (Sulf Oxydex, DVM Pharmaceuticals, Inc.).

References and Suggested Reading

Blair GL: Home therapy of sebaceous adenitis, *Prog SA Research Genodermatosis Research Foundation, Inc.), Winter/Spring* Newsletter, 1993, p 4.

Carothers MA, Kwochka KW, Rojko JL: Cyclosporine-responsive granulomatous sebaceous adenitis in a dog, *J Am Vet Med Assoc* 198:1645, 1991.

DeManuelle T, Rothstein E: Food allergy and nutritionally related skin disease, *Adv Vet Dermatol* 4:224, 2002.

Dunstan DW, Hargis AM: The diagnosis of sebaceous adenitis in standard poodle dogs. In Bonagura JD, Kirk RW, editors: *Kirk's current veterinary therapy XII*, Philadelphia, 1995, Saunders, p 619.

Griffin CE: Common dermatoses of the Akita, shar-pei, and chow-chow. Proceedings of the annual meeting of the American Academy of Veterinary Dermatology, Washington DC, 1988, p 31.

Gross TL et al: *Skin diseases of the dog and cat: clinical and histopathologic diagnosis*, Oxford, 2005, Blackwell Publishing, p186.

Linek M et al: Effects of cyclosporine A on clinical and histologic abnormalities in dogs with sebaceous adenitis, *J Am Vet Med Assoc* 226:59, 2005.

Patterson S: Topical cyclosporine in sebaceous adenitis. In Kwochka KW, Rosenkrantz WS: *Shampoos and topical therapy*, Oxford, 2005, Blackwell Publishing, p 382.

Power IIT, Ihrke PJ: Synthetic retinoids in veterinary dermatology, *Vet Clin North Am Small Anim Pract* 20:1525, 1990.

Reichler IM: Sebaceous adenitis in the Akita: clinical observations, histopathology and heredity, *Vet Dermatol* 12:243, 2001.

Rosser EJ: Sebaceous adenitis. In Kirk RW, Bonagura JD, editors: *Current veterinary therapy XI*, Philadelphia, 1992, Saunders, 1992, p 534.

Rosser EJ et al: Sebaceous adenitis with hyperkeratosis in the standard poodle: a discussion of 10 cases, *J Am Anim Hosp Assoc* 23:341, 1987.

Scott DW: Granulomatous sebaceous adenitis in dogs, *J Am Anim Hosp Assoc* 22:631, 1986.

Sousa CA: Sebaceous adenitis, *Vet Clin North Am Small Anim Pract* 36:243, 2006.

Stewart LJ, White SD, Carpenter JL: Isotretinoin in the treatment of sebaceous adenitis in two vizslas, *J Am Anim Hosp Assoc* 27:65, 1991.

White SD et al: Sebaceous adenitis in dogs and results of treatment with isotretinoin and etretinate: 30 cases (1990-1994), *J Am Vet Med Assoc* 207:197, 1995.

CHAPTER 104

Therapy of *Malassezia* Infections and *Malassezia* Hypersensitivity

DANIEL O. MORRIS, *Philadelphia, Pennsylvania*

Malassezia dermatitis (MD) and *Malassezia* otitis (MO) are superficial fungal (yeast) infections occurring on and within the stratum corneum of the epidermis of many mammalian species. Canine *Malassezia* hypersensitivity (MH) is a type-1 (immediate) hypersensitivity reaction to soluble allergens produced by the yeast; these allergens are recognized by the host's immune system in a manner similar to aeroallergens and contribute to the pathology of atopic dermatitis (AD). In dogs and cats *Malassezia pachydermatis* colonizes the skin during the immediate perinatal period and is the primary yeast species associated with skin and ear canal disease.

PATHOGENESIS

Malassezia yeast colonizes the skin and external ear canals of animals in very low numbers. Overt "infection," sometimes referred to as "overgrowth," is defined by increased numbers of the yeast on the skin surface in conjunction with inflammation. In a diseased state alterations of the microclimate of the surface of the skin contribute to increased susceptibility to yeast infection. Primary diseases that cause increased moisture, altered surface lipids, and/or disruption of stratum corneum barrier function encourage secondary overgrowth of the organism. Pruritic inflammatory diseases (allergic and parasitic) result in microclimate changes caused by scratching (disruption of barrier function), licking (added moisture), and increased production of sebum. Endocrinopathies, especially hyperadrenocorticism, directly cause alterations in sebum characteristics and stratum corneum function. Metabolic diseases that result in hyperkeratosis (such as zinc-reponsive dermatosis, hepatocutaneous syndrome/superficial necrolytic dermatitis of dogs, and thymoma-associated dermatosis of cats) also appear to be risk factors. Secondary MD is also associated with primary (idiopathic) seborrhea of dogs and cats and paraneoplastic alopecia secondary to internal carcinomas in cats.

In some dogs with AD, antigens produced by *M. pachydermatis* may be recognized by the immune system as allergens (i.e., MH), in which case a highly inflammatory and pruritic response can be mounted to relatively low numbers of yeast organisms, blurring the line between cytologic definitions of "colonization" and "infection." However, many dogs with MH also have overt infection, as defined cytologically by overgrowth of yeast on the skin surface (see section on Cytology later in the chapter for guidelines). MH has not yet been studied or defined in cats with allergic skin disease, although MD does appear to contribute to the pruritic threshold of some cats with AD.

CLINICAL SIGNS

Several excellent reviews regarding the clinical presentations of MD and MO in dogs and cats are available (Matousek and Campbell, 2002; Moriss, 1999; Muse, 2000). Some key points are included here.

Although MD is usually intensely pruritic, the only primary lesion produced is erythema. Secondary lesions, including excoriations, seborrheic plaques, lichenification, maceration, and intertrigo, are common and cannot reliably be distinguished from staphylococcal pyoderma without cytologic examination. Therefore look for the yeast on the surface of any pruritic skin lesion.

The clinical appearance of the skin in cases of MD is highly variable. It may either be dry and flaky (seborrhea sicca) or tacky/greasy (seborrhea oleosa). In rare cases *M. pachydermatis* can cause a folliculitis that mimics staphylococcal folliculitis, dermatophytosis, and demodicosis.

The distribution pattern of canine MD is variable but most commonly affects some combination of the face (especially periocular and perioral skin), feet (interdigital spaces and claw folds), intertriginous areas (axillae, groin/inguinal area, facial folds, vulvar and mammary folds), and perineum. Generalized cases of MD may occur in chronic cases of allergic dermatitis. *Malassezia* overgrowth can provoke an overwhelming pruritic response in atopic dogs, which can occur acutely and be misconstrued as increased exposure to aeroallergens. Resolution of the yeast infection can reduce the pruritic threshold of an atopic dog by as much as 75% to 100% in some cases, depending on concurrent exposure to other allergens. Therefore undiagnosed MD is one of the most common reasons for perceived failure in the management of atopic dogs.

Malassezia pododermatitis may occur with or without more widespread MD. The feet are the most common single body area affected in allergic dogs. Patients with interdigital *Malassezia* pododermatitis are presented for the complaint of paw licking/chewing. Paronychia (inflammation of the claw beds) may also occur as the sole presenting sign of MD and often causes claw biting. Physical examination usually reveals a reddish-brown staining of the proximal claw or a waxy exudate in the claw fold, with inflammation of the surrounding soft tissue.

In any dog with a known endocrine or metabolic disease, MD must be ruled out (by surface cytology) if pruritus, cutaneous inflammation, or even noninflammatory seborrhea are present.

Malassezia yeast also play an important role in cases of ceruminous otitis externa, in which they are highly proinflammatory. Some cases appear to be primary and associated only with moisture trapping (especially in swimming dogs).

DIAGNOSIS

Diagnosis of MD and MO is made by microscopic examination of surface cytology specimens. Diagnosis of MH in dogs is made by intradermal testing with a commercial *M. pachydermatis* extract.

Cytology

Because of its unipolar budding process, *M. pachydermatis* appears as oval, peanut, or bowling pin-shaped organisms cytologically (depending on the state of budding), with sizes ranging from 2 to 2.5 × 4 to 5µm (Gueho, Midgley, and Guillot, 1996). Although this is the species most commonly isolated from normal and inflamed skin of dogs and cats, occasionally other species are identified. *Malassezia globosa*, which is sometimes associated with ceruminous otitis of cats (and less commonly in dogs), has a more spherical shape with tiny budding "heads." Methods for collection include dry skin scrapings, adhesive tape stripping, cotton-tipped swabs, and direct impression smears with glass slides.

For dry skin, scrapings and adhesive tape stripping (or direct skin impression with adhesive-coated slides [Duro-Tak, Dermatologic Lab & Supply] work best. Clear adhesive tape (Scotch Tear-By-Hand Tape, 3M), which is my favorite method, works well in tight spaces and is very economical. The slide or adhesive tape should be applied to the area of interest two to three times in succession. Impression smears and tape stripping allow quantification of yeast per each microscopic field. With scrapings it may be necessary to mix the material with saline and heat fix until dry (to adhere the material to the slide). For greasy skin direct impression smears (without adhesive) often work better. For paronychia (inflammation of the claw bed) a cotton-tipped swab, the broken end of its wooden handle, or a metal spatula is used to scrape the claw fold; exudate is pressed or rolled firmly onto a glass slide.

For examination of ear exudate in dogs with ceruminous or exudative otitis externa, rolling exudate in a thin layer on glass slides with a cotton-tipped swab is the preferred method. It is often useful to sample the skin of the concave pinna separately from the ear canal if pinnal dermatitis is present.

Preparing Samples for Microscopic Examination

When material is applied to a glass slide, a modified Wright's stain (such as Diff-Quik) is used. Heat fixing the slide before staining is performed by many dermatologists, but a study has shown it generally to be unnecessary. When adhesive tape is used, it may be dipped in the final stain only (no need to use a fixative), rinsed, and dried with a warm air dryer. The tape is applied to a glass slide while it is still warm and sticky for best adhesion. Some clinicians prefer wet mounts: a drop of new methylene blue stain is placed on a glass slide, and the tape strip is laid on top.

Cytologies should be examined under oil immersion (1000×) or high-dry (400×) for oval or budding yeast. I prefer oil immersion for more reliable identification of bacteria and yeast cells.

Interpretation of Cytologic Results: How Many Is Too Many?

For skin, 1 yeast per high-power (1000×) oil immersion field (hpoif) is a general guideline used by many dermatologists. For ear canals a study semiquantitatively evaluated the expected (commensal) populations of *Malassezia* spp. yeast residing in normal and diseased canals. It showed that normal dogs may routinely exhibit up to 5 organisms per high-dry (400×) field (roughly equivalent to ≤2 per hpoif), whereas cats may harbor up to 12 organisms per high-power dry field (roughly ≤5 per hpoif) (Ginel, 2002).

These numbers are guidelines only. Since dogs may mount a hypersensitivity response to *M. pachydermatis*, some individuals may suffer a pathologic effect from what would otherwise be considered a normal population of yeast colonizing the skin or ear canals. For example, a study examining yeast numbers on healthy and atopic canine skin suggested that 1 yeast per 27 hpoif may be sufficient to correlate with hypersensitivity (Morris, 1998). Since a threshold this low is almost impossible to quantify and appreciate clinically during routine practice, *I generally recommend antifungal chemotherapy when more than 1 yeast per 5 hpoif is identified on inflamed skin or more than 1 yeast per hpoif is identified from swabs of an inflamed ear canal.*

Intradermal Testing for *Malassezia* Hypersensitivity

A commercial *M. pachydermatis* extract is available for intradermal testing and subcutaneous immunotherapy (Greer Laboratories). This allergenic extract is available in 20,000 protein nitrogen units (pnu)/ml and 40,000 pnu/ml concentrations. A study conducted in healthy dogs with normal skin and dogs with AD (both with and without overt MD based on cytologic evaluation) has demonstrated a threshold concentration of 1000 pnu/ml for use in intradermal testing (Farver et al., 2005). The threshold concentration of an allergen is that to which 90% of the nonallergic population is nonreactive (i.e., ceases to develop an irritant reaction). Ideally the threshold concentration also should correctly identify at least 90% of sensitized individuals, although this is difficult to assess because of lack of a validated gold standard. This extract is now included in the battery of allergens used for intradermal testing in my group practice for evaluation of dogs with a clinical diagnosis of AD.

To date a validated in vitro commercial assay for anti-*Malassezia* immunoglobulin E has not been reported in the scientific literature. Because of great discrepancies in results reported by research laboratories, any commercial offering of an enzyme-linked immunosorbent assay for detection of anti-M*alassezia* antibodies in canine serum should be scrutinized carefully by sound scientific methods before it can be recommended for routine use.

TREATMENT

The antifungal regimen chosen for therapy of MD or MO should be based on the distribution of the infection, the general health status of the patient, and expectations of the pet owner concerning time and effort commitment (relevant to topical therapy) and side effects (most relevant to systemic therapy). Diagnosing and eliminating (or controlling) underlying diseases are also paramount to long-term prevention of recurrence. Since *M. pachydermatis* is part of the normal cutaneous microflora, complete elimination of the organism is likely to be impossible.

Systemic Therapy (Table 104-1)

Unless there is a specific contraindication to using an oral antifungal drug, I prefer to treat all cases of

Table **104-1**

Systemic Drugs for Treatment of *Malassezia* Dermatitis and Otitis Media

Drug	Supplied As	Dose/Frequency/Duration	Species
Ketoconazole	200-mg tablets	5-10 mg/kg qd × 21-28 days, or (low-dose regimen) 5 mg/kg qd × 10 days, then eod × 10	D
		Pulse dosage regimen for *prophylaxis*: 5-10 mg/kg 2 consecutive days/week	D
Itraconzole	100-mg capsules or 10 mg/ml elixir	5 mg/kg qd × 21-28 days, or 5 mg/kg 2 days/week × 3 weeks	D and C
Fluconazole	50-, 100-, 150-, 200-mg tablets and oral powder for 10 mg/ml suspension	2.5-5 mg/kg qd × 21-28 days	D and C
Terbinafine	200-mg tablets	30 mg/kg qd × 21-28 days	D
		30-40 mg/kg qd × 21-28 days	C

generalized and regional MD (e.g., pododermatitis) systemically. Otitis media also requires systemic therapy to (assumedly) achieve therapeutic drug levels within the tympanic cavity. Oral ketoconazole, itraconazole, or fluconazole is most commonly recommended. Griseofulvin is ineffective against *Malassezia* spp.

Ketoconazole (Nizoral, Janssen; and generics) is an imidazole antifungal with proven efficacy for canine MD. It undergoes extensive metabolism by the liver, and its use in patients with hepatic disease is contraindicated. It is also a known teratogen in dogs. Adverse effects include gastrointestinal upset (anorexia, vomiting, diarrhea), thrombocytopenia (rare), and hepatotoxicity, although none of these side effects is at all common. However, hepatotoxicity is a moderate risk in cats, and its use in feline MD is not recommended. In aged or debilitated dogs, liver enzymes should be evaluated before use of ketoconazole. I do not routinely perform screening tests in young/healthy dogs. For long-term or repeated use, monitoring of hepatic function is performed on a case-by-case basis as dictated by clinical signs (some dermatologists recommend monthly monitoring). This drug should always be administered with food for maximum absorption.

Itraconazole (Sporanox, Ortho Biotech) and *fluconazole* (Diflucan, Roerig; and generics) are triazole antifungals with less risk for hepatotoxicity than ketoconazole. Itraconazole is metabolized by the liver, whereas fluconazole is excreted via the kidneys. Because of cost, fluconazole is rarely chosen as a first-line treatment. Itraconazole is the treatment of choice in cats unless preexisting hepatopathy is known, in which case fluconazole should be used. Itraconazole should always be administered with food, whereas feeding does not influence the absorption of fluconazole.

Terbinafine (Lamisil, Novartis; and generics) is an allylamine antifungal with a high margin of safety for use in mammals. It is a less proven drug for MD but, based on its ability to reduce *Malassezia* colonization on healthy basset hounds, it is likely to be effective.

Lufenuron (Program, Novartis Animal Health) is a benzoylphenylurea drug that disrupts chitin synthesis in the cell wall of insects and perhaps some fungi. There is no evidence at this time to suggest that this drug is effective in the treatment of MD.

Topical Therapy

Topical antifungals are most useful for treatment of localized infections or as adjunctive therapy along with oral drugs. Topicals are also quite valuable in the prophylaxis of chronic or relapsing MD.

For regional or generalized disease, shampoos containing miconazole, ketoconazole, chlorhexidine, or selenium sulfide are available and have met with variable success, depending on client compliance, frequency and technique of application, and severity of disease. For frequently relapsing cases, shampoo therapy (once to twice weekly, 10 minutes' minimum contact time) may be adequate for prophylaxis. Leave-on conditioners containing miconazole or chlorhexidine are also available and provide for more residual action than shampoos. Rinses such as lime sulfur dip and enilconazole can be quite effective; however, lime sulfur dip is not available in the United Kingdom; enilconazole is available in Canada but not in the United States.

Miconazole, clotrimazole, or ketoconazole sprays, lotions, wipes, or creams may be used for "spot" therapy of the skin. Ointments and lotions containing nystatin, thiabendazole, miconazole, or clotrimazole are commonly used for otitis externa. Some products also contain glucocorticoids and antibacterials. An in vitro study comparing the efficacy of the azoles against *Malassezia* spp. yeast indicated that thiabendazole is the least effective, followed by clotrimazole (with efficacy comparable to nystatin), miconazole (with 10 times the potency of nystatin), ketoconazole, and itraconazole (Lorenzini, Mercantini, and De Bernardis, 1985). My clinical bias is that miconazole is the most effective topical therapy on a per-case basis, and poor clinical responses to nystatin, thiabendazole and clotrimazole have been common in my practice population.

Immunotherapy for *Malassezia* Hypersensitivity

The *M. pachydermatis* extract produced by Greer Laboratories has been evaluated in a multicenter study to determine its use as an immunotherapeutic extract. Atopic dogs that had been on allergen-specific immunotherapy for a minimum of 12 months but that continued to have chronic/recurrent MD and required antifungal prophylaxis were enrolled. A total dosage of 1000 pnu was administered weekly by subcutaneous injection, and cases were followed for 12 months. Although data from all member study sites have not been collated, it is clear from four cases enrolled at my practice that it can be effective. Two of four dogs had an excellent response with resolution of pruritus, discontinuation of maintenance antifungal therapy, and negative cytology, whereas the other two improved enough that the owners elected to continue with immunotherapy. Personal communication with clinicians at other study sites (A. Yu, Guelph, Ontario, Canada; L. Sauber, Tulsa, OK) suggests that this has also been the case elsewhere.

References and Suggested Reading

Farver K et al: Humoral measurement of type-1 hypersensitivity reactions to a commercial Malassezia pachydermatis allergen, *Vet Dermatol* 16:261, 2005.

Ginel PJ et al: A semiquantitative cytological evaluation of normal and pathological samples from the external ear canal of dogs and cats, *Vet Dermatol* 13:151, 2002.

Gueho E, Midgley G, Guillot J: The genus Malassezia with description of four new species, *Antonie van Leeuwenhoek* 69:337, 1996.

Lorenzini R, Mercantini R, De Bernardis F: In vitro sensitivity of Malassezia spp. to various antimycotics, *Drugs Exp Clin Res* 11 (6):393,1985.

Matousek JL, Campbell KL: Malassezia dermatitis, *Compend Contin Educ Small Anim Pract* 24:224, 2002.

Morris DO: *Malassezia* dermatitis and otitis. In Campbell KA, editor: *Veterinary clinics of North America: small animal practice,* Philadelphia, 1999, Saunders, p 1303.

Morris DO: *Malassezia* dermatitis. In Birchard SJ, Sherding RG, editors: *Saunders manual of small animal practice,* ed 3, St Louis, 2006, Saunders, 2006, p 445.

Morris DO, Olivier NB, Rosser EJ: Type-1 hypersensitivity reactions to *Malassezia* pachydermatis extracts in atopic dogs, *Am J Vet Res* 59:836, 1998.

Muse R: *Malassezia* dermatitis. In Bonagura JD, editor: *Kirk's current veterinary therapy XIII,* Philadelphia, 2000, Saunders, p 574.

CHAPTER 105

Treatment of Dermatophytosis

DOUGLAS J. DeBOER, *Madison, Wisconsin*
KAREN A. MORIELLO, *Madison, Wisconsin*

Dermatophytosis is a zoonotic disease caused by infection of the dead, keratinized portions of cutaneous tissues (hairs, claws, and/or stratum corneum) with a superficial fungus adapted to living on the skin. Approximately 90% of feline dermatophytosis is caused by *Microsporum canis*; dogs may be infected with *M. canis, M. gypseum,* or *Trichophyton mentagrophytes.* Recently cats infected with alternate species such as *Microsporum persicolor* or *Trichophyton* spp. have been reported. For an infection to become established, there must be contact with another infected animal or a contaminated environment, often coupled with some predisposing host factor such as youth, debilitating disease, compromised immunologic status, or poor husbandry.

Dermatophytosis is more common in cats than in dogs. The disease may be pruritic or nonpruritic. Hair loss, scaling, and crusting are common clinical findings. In cats the disease can mimic almost any reported skin disease or reaction pattern. The disease can even mimic pemphigus foliaceus; therefore fungal cultures should always be part of the core diagnostic evaluation of any cat with skin disease. Rarely long-haired cats can develop a subcutaneous nodular form of the disease called *pseudomycetoma.* In dogs what is often diagnosed as dermatophytosis is the typical circular lesions of bacterial pyoderma. Dermatophytic *kerion reactions* appear as nodular-to-draining lesions that may mimic deep bacterial pyoderma. Infections in both dogs and cats cat be very subtle, with lesions easily missed. This is most common in long-haired cats and long-haired small dogs, especially Yorkshire terrier dogs.

IMPORTANT POINTS TO REMEMBER ABOUT DIAGNOSTIC TESTS

Role of the Wood's Lamp, Direct Examination, and Biopsy

Wood's lamp (ultraviolet lamp) examination is a reasonable screening tool for *M. canis* infection, but a positive test is not diagnostic. It is most useful in animals with lesions to identify potentially infected hairs for culture or for direct examination. The fluorescence must be *bright "apple green"* and located along the hair shafts to be considered suspicious. Direct microscopic examination of hairs can confirm the presence of an infection. Examination of hairs for ectothrix spores is recommended only with Wood's lamp–positive hairs and if the clinician or technician has some expertise. Clearing agents or mineral oil can be used to examine hairs. Suspected fluorescing hairs or hairs with apparent ectothrix spores must be cultured to confirm presence of dermatophyte infection. It is rarely necessary to resort to a skin biopsy for diagnosis. Exceptions to this include confirmation of fungal kerion reactions or pseudomycetoma.

Fungal Culture

The standard of care for diagnosis or confirmation of infection is a fungal culture. Many commercial fungal culture media are available; work by one of the authors (KAM) has found little difference among routinely available media, provided that the culture plate has sufficient depth of medium to avoid premature drying. On a conventional 10-cm Petri dish, at least 15 ml of medium is necessary, and more if possible. Cultures should be incubated between 24° and 30°C (75° and 86°F); inexpensive digital aquarium thermometers can be used to ensure this temperature. Cultures incubated at lower temperatures (e.g., 18°C or 65°F) may not sporulate, or sporulation may be delayed by up to 10 days. The most widely used fungal culture medium is dermatophyte test medium (DTM), which contains inhibitors of bacterial and saprophyte growth and a color indicator. A toothbrush is ideal for obtaining a culture sample from most animals; the technique has been widely described. Animals with large amounts of debris on the hair coat should be wiped with a cloth first. If culture of the environment is desired, it can be sampled using small squares of Swiffer (Procter & Gamble) cloths brushed across the contaminated areas. Daily visual examination of inoculated plates allows for rapid identification of highly suspicious colonies. Suspect pathogenic colonies are pale or white with a red ring of color developing around them as they grow on DTM. Microscopic confirmation is required because some nonpathogenic fungi can turn DTM red immediately and all saprophytic fungi will eventually cause a red color change given sufficient time. Once the medium has turned completely red, the usefulness of the color indicator is lost. Microscopic examination is not difficult. The preferred fungal stain is lactophenol cotton blue; new methylene blue stain can also be used. Clear or frosted acetate tape is used to sample the colony by brushing the sticky side lightly across it. Clear tape is placed sticky side down over a drop of stain on a microscope slide; frosted tape is placed sticky side up on the slide. In either case a second drop of stain is placed on top of the tape followed by a glass coverslip. Examine at 100× and 400× total magnification. The reader is referred to a mycology textbook or websites such as www.doctor-fungus.com for additional information on identification of microscopic colonies. If dermatophyte colonies are not confirmed, it is important to be sure that the culture has been incubated at an appropriate temperature and wait 1 to 4 more days before resampling. In some cases subculturing may be needed. Most pathogens grow within 7 to 10 days; however, cultures from animals undergoing treatment should be held for 21 days because treatment slows growth of cultures.

TREATMENT PRINCIPLES AND OPTIONS

In most healthy animals dermatophytosis is a self-curing disease and eventually (in weeks to months) will resolve spontaneously. However, this zoonotic disease *should* always be treated to shorten the course of infection and minimize the chances of transmission to other animals or humans. The best treatment protocol is a combination of three elements: *environmental treatment*, *adjunct topical treatment*, and *systemic treatment*. Newer drugs coupled with increasing clinical studies on this disease now allow veterinarians to offer a variety of effective treatment options to clients.

Limiting and Controlling Contamination of the Environment

Limiting spread of the disease in the environment is often the last point discussed with clients. However, we recommend *starting* treatment discussion with this point because it is then easier for clients to understand and comply with treatment recommendations. In any dermatophyte infection, infective hairs and spores are always shed into the environment. The severity of environmental contamination is related to the host species (cats shed more material than dogs), the severity of lesions, and the number of animals. Environmental contamination studies by one of the authors (KAM) have shown that the more the animal is allowed to roam in the home, the more widespread the contamination. Confinement of animals restricted dissemination of spores; reasonable cleaning of the home and the confinement area minimized spore contamina-

tion. Once an infected animal was removed or cured, culture-positive homes could be returned to culture-negative status with appropriate cleaning procedures.

The key things owners can do to limit environmental contamination of the home (Box 105-1) include: (1) *confinement of the pet* to one room that can be cleaned easily twice weekly; (2) removal of infective hairs from the coat either by *clipping or bathing*; and (3) topical *whole body antifungal rinses*. Twice-weekly cleaning should include thorough vacuuming of the room, followed by use of Swiffer (Procter & Gamble) cloths to trap residual hairs and spores not collected by vacuuming. Also recommended are cleaning with a detergent safe for use on the surfaces in the room and use of a sporicidal disinfectant on nonporous surfaces. Pets should be provided with bedding (e.g., towels) that can be washed daily. Contamination is most severe in areas where the pet spends the most amount of time; thus these areas should receive special attention.

Many disinfectants labeled as effective for killing dermatophytes in the household or veterinary clinic are not practically effective for this purpose. Commercial disinfectants are tested for antifungal activity by observing their effects on suspensions of fungal spores or fungal mycelium in a test tube. However, in a house or a veterinary hospital the predominant contamination is not with spores or mycelium but rather with small fragments of infected hairs. It is possible that the hair shaft and associated organic debris protects the fungus from the actions of disinfectants. Studies that simulate actual conditions of use demonstrate that, of many different disinfectants tested, the only products that were safe and practical to use in the home were chlorine laundry bleach (sodium hypochlorite 5%) and enilconazole environmental spray. The latter is available and registered for animal facility use in some countries, including for use in ringworm-infested

---

Box 105-1

Recommended Environmental Control Measures in Treatment of Dermatophytosis

For Household Situations With One or a Few Animals

- Confine pets to easily cleaned room or rooms.
- Thoroughly vacuum floors and furniture (removes many infected hairs and spores). Discard or empty vacuum cleaner bag.
- Wash hard floor and other contact surfaces with detergent and water.
- Dust other surfaces with Swiffer cloths to remove spores.
- Launder (hot water wash and hot dryer) area rugs, animal bedding, and bed linens if pet is allowed on furniture.
- Launder, disinfect, or discard pet toys and grooming aids.
- If possible, carefully disinfect hard-floor surfacing with 1:128 bleach solution; allow 10 minutes' wetting time.
- Vacuum (and disinfect if possible) any vehicles and transport cages used for animals.
- Repeat cleaning and disinfection twice weekly.
- After cure or removal of animal, culture areas for contamination by wiping small squares of Swiffer cloths over exposed areas and inoculating soiled surface of cloth onto fungal culture plate.

animal shelters. In North America it is registered only for use in poultry house *Aspergillus* disinfection (Clinafarm, Sterwin). For bleach disinfection, the higher the concentration, the better the effectiveness; but the solution is also highly corrosive and toxic and damages carpets and fabrics. Bleach also is irritating to the mucous membranes of pets and humans. We find that a reasonable compromise is a 1:128 dilution of household chlorine laundry bleach (1 oz of bleach per gallon of water) that is sprayed on targeted surfaces after initial cleaning. It is important to note that a contact time of 10 minutes is needed. This concentration is effectively fungicidal yet not too overpowering for the owner to use. The owner should be advised to wear protective clothing and eyewear, and good ventilation should be provided for both the pets and people. It is most safely applied using a small spray bottle that allows for direct and controlled application.

Clipping of the Hair Coat

Removing infected hairs by clipping reduces the quantity of infective spores that could contaminate the environment, spread the infection to other animals, or spread the infection to other areas on the same animal. However, clipping the hair coat can temporarily worsen the infection by mechanical spread of the spores and microtrauma to the skin. Electric clippers are contaminated in the process, as is the area where the clipping is performed, creating need for additional environmental decontamination. One of the authors (KAM) has been a strong proponent of clipping the hair coat but, after encountering many situations in which clipping the hair coat resulted in "clipper burn" or true thermal burns to the patient, now advocates a more restrained case-by-case consideration. Whole-body clipping is advisable in long-haired cats and long-haired dogs, especially if they have failed therapy or are clinically recovered but still culture positive. Many pet animals are presented early in the disease state when it may be possible to clip hairs from around lesions gently with scissors or pluck individual glowing hairs, making whole-body clipping unnecessary. Mechanical removal of infected hairs is facilitated by bathing and combing the hair coat to remove loose hairs. If a glowing strain of *M. canis* is present, another strategy can be used: initiating antifungal therapy, allowing the hairs to grow out for a week or so, and then scissor-clipping the glowing tips of infected hairs.

Adjunct Topical Treatments

The goal of adjunct topical therapy is to help shorten the course of infection and limit the spread of infective material to people, other animals, and the environment. Localized topical therapy ("spot-treatment") with creams, lotions, and ointments *is not recommended* because subclinical areas of infection will be missed or induced. Whole-body treatment with an antifungal rinse or shampoo is strongly recommended. Various studies have shown that lime sulfur, enilconazole, and miconazole are effectively antifungal (Sparkes et al., 2000). Miconazole or ketoconazole plus chlorhexidine shampoos or rinses (Malaseb, DVM Pharmaceuticals; KetoChlor, Virbac) are more effective than the single ingredients; the combination of an azole drug and chlorhexidine is synergistic (Perrins and Bond, 2003). Currently favored topical whole-body rinses for dermatophytosis are summarized in Table 105-1. Lime sulfur solution is safe even for kittens or puppies as young as 1 week of age, although it is odiferous. Enilconazole (Imaverol, Janssen) is a topical antifungal rinse licensed in many countries (but not the United States) for dogs and horses. It has been used on cats (an off-label use; Hnilica and Medleau, 2002); some clinicians advocate the use of an Elizabethan collar after each rinse until the coat is dry, thus preventing ingestion of the solution.

Although controlled comparative studies are not available, we believe that lime-sulfur or enilconazole rinses are the most effective adjunct topical treatments; however, their disadvantages (odor, unavailability) may limit their use in some situations. A second-choice topical regimen is miconazole-chlorhexidine rinse after shampooing used twice weekly. Isolated infective spore studies have shown that this rinse is equally sporicidal as lime sulfur; however, in field studies animals treated with lime sulfur cured faster than animals treated with the miconazole-chlorhexidine rinse.

Table **105-1**

Summary of Recommended Adjunct Topical Products for Treatment of Dermatophytosis in Dogs or Cats

Treatment	Usage and Comments
Lime-sulfur rinse (sulfurated lime solution)	Per label, dilute in water at 4-8 oz/gallon (1:16 to 1:32 dilution); shake well before each use. Saturate entire hair coat by sponging or spraying twice weekly. Do not rinse, towel dry. May stain jewelry, light hair coats, or porous surfaces.
Enilconazole topical rinse (Imaverol)	Per label, dilute in water to a 0.2% solution. Apply as for lime sulfur, twice weekly. If used on cats, place Elizabethan collar until hair coat is dry. Not available in United States.
Miconazole-chlorhexidine rinse (Malaseb Concentrate Rinse)	Per label, dilute in water at 1 oz/quart. Apply as for lime sulfur, twice weekly. Efficacy is not as well established as for lime sulfur or enilconazole but is widely available and odor free.
Antifungal shampoos: Miconazole-chlorhexidine (Malaseb) Ketoconazole-chlorhexidine (KetoChlor)	Optional treatment; does not replace use of whole-body rinses above. Use twice weekly before antifungal rinse.

Whole-body rinses are easily applied using a garden watering can or small pressurized tank-type garden sprayer. It is important to apply the solution close to the skin and soak the hairs and skin thoroughly. The solution should not be rinsed from the coat; the animal should be towel dried.

Systemic Treatment Options

After discussing methods for limiting the spread of infective spores into the environment, deciding whether or not the hair coat or lesions will be clipped, and what adjunct topical therapy will be used, a systemic antifungal drug should be selected (Table 105-2). It is important to remember that dermatophytosis is an intrafollicular disease and that systemic treatment is responsible for actually shortening the course of infection in the individual animal.

Griseofulvin

Griseofulvin is becoming difficult to obtain and is being used less and less often. However, if it can be obtained, nearly all feline and canine patients with *Microsporum* infections and most with *Trichophyton* infections are cured by this drug. Griseofulvin is highly teratogenic and *must not be used in pregnant animals!* In cats bone marrow suppression is a severe and unpredictable side effect. It is not dependent on dose, breed, or length of therapy. Blood counts (especially white blood cell) are recommended *at least* monthly (some clinicians recommend every 1 to 2 weeks) when using this drug in cats. Cats should be tested for feline leukemia virus and feline immunodeficiency virus infection before use since there may be an association between infection and these adverse reactions. In one controlled study griseofulvin therapy alone required a mean of 70 days of treatment to cure experimentally infected cats (Moriello and DeBoer, 1995). Because of the pharmacokinetics of this drug, it is not suitable for pulse-therapy options. We do not recommend griseofulvin as a first choice in cats. In large dogs it may be more cost effective. *The dose is dependent on the formulation (microsize versus ultramicrosize).*

It is critically important to determine the exact preparation one is prescribing to prevent potentially lethal dosages of griseofulvin. Absorption is enhanced with a fatty meal. Vomiting, diarrhea, and inappetence are common adverse effects.

Ketoconazole

The true clinical efficacy of ketoconazole in dermatophytosis is unknown; there are limited anecdotal reports on its efficacy. Some strains of *M. canis* are resistant to ketoconazole. The drug is not well tolerated in cats and is not recommended for use in this species. Studies suggest a high prevalence ($\approx 25\%$) of hepatotoxicity in cats and occasionally at higher doses in dogs. Ketoconazole as a systemic antifungal is best reserved for infections in dogs, particularly *Trichophyton*. Ketoconazole has become inexpensive over the past few years, but other than this it has no advantage over other drugs in routine cases of dermatophytosis.

Itraconazole

In many areas of the world itraconazole is currently the most commonly used drug for the treatment of dermatophytosis in both dogs and cats. Itraconazole (Sporanox capsules or oral solution, Janssen) is a triazole antifungal that accumulates and persists in hair and epidermis dermatophytosis in pulse-therapy protocols. These schedules are easier for owners and more cost effective. In countries where itraconazole is licensed for veterinary use, the official label directions are 5 mg/kg once daily PO. Treatment is initiated with three "pulses" of 1 week on, 1 week off (i.e., 3 weeks of drug administration out of a total treatment length of 6 weeks). In working with infected catteries and shelters, one of the authors (KAM) has noted occasional need for higher dosages (up to 10 mg/kg/day) and/or need for daily (not pulsed) treatment in some cats before mycologic cure can be obtained. Pulse therapy is not ideal for animals that are ill or have limited body fat because the drug is stored in body fat. An alternative protocol that I have used is 21 to 28 days of once-daily treatment; it is important to note that this protocol is only recommended if adjunct topical therapy with lime sulfur is used.

Table 105-2

Summary of Recommended Systemic Products for Treatment of Dermatophytosis in Dogs or Cats

Treatment	Usage and Comments
Griseofulvin	Dogs or cats, effective but difficult to obtain; ultramicrosize form recommended if available; 5-10 mg/kg once daily or divided PO; for microsize form, 25-50 mg/kg once daily or divided PO; teratogenic; possible myelotoxicity in cats, monitor white blood cell counts
Ketoconazole	For use in dogs only; hepatotoxic in cats; may be useful for *Trichophyton* infections; less certain for *Microsporum*; 5-10 mg/kg once daily PO; inexpensive generic available in United States
Itraconazole (Sporanox or Itrafungol)	Dogs or cats; systemic drug of choice, but cost may limit its use to cats or small dogs; 5-10 mg/kg once daily PO on alternate weeks (e.g., administer for 7 days, then skip treatment for 7 days); manufacturer recommendation is 5 mg/kg/day, but we find occasional animals (especially stressed or ill animals in shelter situations) that clear very slowly on this dosage and require the higher dosage and/or continuous daily treatment
Terbinafine (Lamisil)	Most reported use is in cats for apparently azole-resistant infections; limited experience in dogs; very expensive; feline dosage: 30-40 mg/kg once daily PO; optimal canine dosage not established; possibly hepatotoxic, monitor liver enzymes

For cats the 100-mg capsules can be divided into smaller doses manually and repackaged in empty gelatin capsules or mixed with a small amount of food; alternatively one can use the 10-mg/ml oral solution. Both are marketed in North America for human use; the oral solution is marketed for cats in Europe (Itrafungol, Janssen). Toxicity problems are rare to nonexistent with this protocol, even in cats. As a note of caution, we are aware that some owners have obtained bulk itraconazole powder inexpensively in foreign countries, and anecdotally this treatment often fails. Itraconazole requires careful formulation in appropriate vehicles to ensure its absorption, and use of any material other than the "official" approved products is not recommended because it may result in treatment failure.

Fluconazole or Terbinafine

Fluconazole has received some recent attention from cattery breeders as an alternative drug. It is not well studied for animal use, and recent studies indicate that it is probably less active against animal dermatophytes than itraconazole. Current evidence and clinical anecdotes suggest that there is no advantage of this drug over the "more proven" itraconazole. Oral terbinafine (Lamisil, Novartis) in initial studies also seems to be effective in some situations. Again, this drug is much less studied, is very expensive, and currently appears to offer no advantages over itraconazole. Cats with *M. canis* infections apparently resistant to azole drugs can sometimes be treated successfully with terbinafine. Various dosages have been used (10 to 40 mg/kg once daily PO), but cats treated at the higher end of the dosage range cure significantly faster. Liver enzymes should be monitored; this drug may elevate ALT in cats, although no clinical toxicity is necessarily seen. We frequently see requests from owners for "the newest and best wonder drug" to eradicate an infection. However, it is important to note that systemic drug selection is invariably the *least* prevalent reason why control of an infection has failed!

Lufenuron

A published case series (Ben-Ziony and Arzi, 2000) caused speculation that lufenuron (Program, Novartis) may be beneficial in treatment of feline or canine dermatophytosis. Although there have been anecdotal reports of "cures" from lufenuron, controlled studies have shown consistently that lufenuron is ineffective as both a treatment and preventive drug. In controlled studies using feline experimental infection models (DeBoer et al., 2006), lufenuron did not prevent initial establishment of ringworm in cats, did not result in faster cure once the infections were established, and was not synergistic with terbinafine. With wide availability of proven, effective treatments for this zoonotic disease, we do not recommend use of lufenuron.

Endpoint of Therapy

Regardless of the combination of topical and systemic treatments selected, all infected animals should be treated until at least two negative fungal cultures are obtained 1 to 2 weeks apart. Toward the end of treatment, when visible lesions may no longer be present, sampling of the entire hair coat with the toothbrush method is greatly preferred. One of the authors (KAM) is a strong advocate of weekly fungal cultures to monitor response to therapy.

Treatment of Catteries and Animal Shelters

It is not within the scope of this chapter to discuss eradication of dermatophytosis from catteries and animal shelters. Such treatment involves many important details, and the reader is referred to the reading list for more information and complete treatment protocols (Moriello and Newbury, 2006). With respect to animal shelters, the reader is also encouraged to contact a regional veterinary school that has an active shelter medicine program.

References and Suggested Reading

Ben-Ziony Y, Arzi B: Use of lufenuron for treating fungal infections of dogs and cats: 297 cases (1997-1999), *J Am Vet Med Assoc* 217:1510, 2000.

DeBoer DJ et al: Lufenuron does not augment effectiveness of terbinafine for treatment of *Microsporum canis* infections in a feline model. In Hillier A, Foster AP, Kwochka KW, editors: *Advances in veterinary dermatology*, vol 5, Oxford, 2006, Blackwell, p 123.

Hnilica KA, Medleau L: Evaluation of topically applied enilconazole for the treatment of dermatophytosis in a Persian cattery, *Vet Dermatol* 13:23, 2002.

Moriello KA: Treatment of dermatophytosis in dogs and cats: review of published studies, *Vet Dermatol* 15:99, 2004.

Moriello KA, DeBoer DJ: Efficacy of griseofulvin and itraconazole in the treatment of experimental feline dermatophytosis, *J Am Vet Med Assoc* 207:439, 1995.

Moriello KA, DeBoer DJ: Recent research on dermatophytosis. In August JR, editor: *Consultations in feline internal medicine*, vol 5, St Louis, 2006, Saunders, p 291.

Moriello KA, Newbury S: Recommendations for the management and treatment of dermatophytosis in animal shelters, *Vet Clin North Am Small Anim Pract* 36:89, 2006.

Perrins N, Bond R: Synergistic inhibition of the growth in vitro of *Microsporum canis* by miconazole and chlorhexidine, *Vet Dermatol* 14:99, 2003

Sparkes AH et al: A study of the efficacy of topical and systemic therapy for the treatment of feline *Microsporum canis* infection, *J Feline Med Surg* 2:135, 2000.

CHAPTER 106

Nonneoplastic Nodular Histiocytic Diseases of the Skin

VERENA K. AFFOLTER, *Davis, California*
CATHERINE A. OUTERBRIDGE, *Davis, California*

Histiocytes include macrophages and dendritic antigen-presenting cells, both of which have different tissue distribution and function (see also Chapter 75). Macrophages are primarily involved with phagocytosis and intracellular digestion of foreign antigens, whereas dendritic antigen-presenting cells are poorly phagocytic but are specialized in processing and presenting antigens. Macrophages and dendritic cells cannot reliably be differentiated based on light microscopic features. However, they express different leukocyte antigens, which can be identified by immunohistochemistry on fresh, snap-frozen tissue.

Nodular granulomatous and pyogranulomatous dermatitis are of either infectious or sterile origin (Box 106-1). These lesions are characterized by numerous macrophages and dendritic cells accompanied by various numbers of neutrophils and lymphocytes. Canine reactive histiocytosis of dendritic cell origin may be limited to the skin—cutaneous histiocytosis—or affect skin and other organ systems (systemic histiocytosis). Canine reactive histiocytosis is discussed in detail in Chapter 75 together with the other proliferative histiocytic diseases, including canine cutaneous histiocytoma, Langerhans cell histiocytosis in dogs, and progressive histiocytosis in cats. Chapter 75 also discusses the histiocytic sarcomas of dendritic cell or macrophage origin.

This chapter focuses on the discussion of other noninfectious nodular skin diseases that are largely predominated by histiocytes (often referred to as histiocytic and/or granulomatous dermatitis). The diseases discussed include cutaneous xanthoma, foreign body reaction, palisading granuloma, canine sarcoidosis, and reactive fibrohistiocytic nodules.

Nodular granulomatous and histiocytic skin lesions may present with similar clinical features and can mimic cutaneous neoplasia or follicular cysts. Histopathology is required to achieve the correct diagnosis. Special stains, immunohistochemical evaluation (bacillus Calmette-Guérin stains), cultures, and polymerase chain reactions for identification of bacterial and fungal elements assist to rule out possible lesional infectious pathogens. However, the differentiation between macrophages and dendritic cells can only be achieved by immunohistochemistry on fresh, snap-frozen tissue (see previous paragraphs).

CUTANEOUS XANTHOMA

Etiology and Pathogenesis

Cutaneous xanthomas (xanthomatosis) are granulomatous skin lesions containing deposits of lipoprotein. In general, lipoproteins deposits occur secondary to elevated serum lipid levels induced by dyslipoproteinemias, usually a hyperlipidemia, hyperlipoproteinemia, or hypercholesterinemia. These lipid disturbances may be inherited (primary) or acquired (secondary). Exact mechanisms inducing lipid depositions in tissues in dogs and cats with a lipid metabolism disturbance are not known. Trauma has been suggested as a triggering factor. *Cats with primary disorders of lipid metabolism* present with exacerbation of any clinical signs if fed a fat-laden diet. Depending on the type of lipid disorder, cats may have elevated fasting triglycerides, cholesterol, or low-density lipoproteins (LDLs). Interestingly, cats with familial lipoprotein lipase (LDL) deficiency do not tend to develop xanthomas. Primary

---

Box 106-1

Nodular to Diffuse Granulomatous and Pyogranulomatous Dermatitis of Infectious and Noninfectious Etiology in Dogs and Cats

Infectious Etiology	Noninfectious etiology
Actinomycosis and nocardiosis	Sterile granuloma and pyogranuloma syndrome
Bacterial pseudomycetoma	Reactive histiocytosis*
Feline leprosy syndrome	Palisading granuloma*
Canine leproid granuloma	Cutaneous xanthoma*
Opportunistic mycobacterial infections	Canine sarcoidosis*
Dermatophyte pseudomycetoma	Foreign body reaction*
Cutaneous blastomycosis, coccidioidomycosis, histoplasmosis	Juvenile sterile granulomatous dermatitis and lymphadenitis
Cryptococcosis	Granulomatous drug reaction
Sporotrichosis	
Opportunistic fungal infections	
Pythiosis, lagenidiosis, entomophthoromycosis	
Prototheocosis	
Leishmaniosis	

*Sterile lesions predominated by histiocytes are discussed in this chapter.
From Gross TL et al: *Skin diseases of the dog and cat: clinical and histopathologic diagnosis*, ed 2, Oxford, 2005, Blackwell Publishing, p 320.

hypercholesterolemia is most commonly associated with the development of xanthomas. *Cats with secondary disorders of lipid metabolism* most commonly present with xanthomas as a result of megestrol acetate–induced diabetes mellitus with associated hypertriglyceridemia. A decreased LPL activity from insulin deficiency was documented in one cat. Alternatively, prolonged corticosteroid administration may result in hyperlipoproteinemia and thus may have contributed in a case of feline xanthomas and arteriosclerosis. *Xanthomas in dogs* have been reported in association with secondary disorders of lipid metabolism such as high cholesterol diet and hypertriglyceridemia with or without associated diabetes mellitus.

Clinical Features

Cutaneous xanthomas are rare in the cat and very rare in the dog. No breed or sex predilection is known. *In cats* pale, yellow-to-white, occasionally brown papules, nodules, or plaques are typically seen. The lesions tend to be friable and may have an erythematous border. Minor trauma often results in hemorrhage. The lesions are mostly found on the head—in particular symmetrically in the preauricular area and the pinna. Other locations are bony prominences on the legs and also on paw pads. *In dogs* yellow papules and nodules may develop in various locations. Face, ears, neck, legs and feet, tail, and ventrum are the most common sites. Fasting 24-hour lipid profiles and lipoprotein electrophoresis to evaluate for changes in triglycerides, cholesterol, and lipoproteins assist in making the diagnosis of xanthomas.

Histopathology

Sampling of ulcerated and traumatized lesions should be avoided since hemorrhage and secondary inflammation may be the overwhelming histologic features. Typically the normal tissue is disrupted by a nodular-to-diffuse infiltrate of large foamy histiocytes consistent with macrophages. The histiocytes may palisade along collagen bundles. Extracellular lakes of lipid, sometimes associated with cholesterol clefts, may separate the histiocytic infiltrate. Eosinophils are often present; whereas infiltration by lymphocytes, plasma cells, and neutrophils is less prominent.

Clinical Management

Dietary adjustments should be made, and the affected animal should be fed a low-fat and low-cholesterol diet since this hopefully will minimize the effects of a primary lipid disorder. If present, diabetes mellitus must be addressed as well, with appropriate management of the disease. Surgical removal of the skin nodules does not prevent development of new lesions but may ameliorate any discomfort from existing lesions.

FOREIGN BODY REACTIONS

Etiology and Pathogenesis

Penetrating foreign bodies commonly pass through the epidermis and eventually get trapped in the dermis, panniculus, or the subcutis, inducing a granulomatous response ("foreign body granuloma").

Exogenous Foreign Bodies
Some plant foreign bodies such as grass awns (foxtails, cactus spines, burdock burrs, seeds) and porcupine quills have regional distributions. Many foreign bodies occur worldwide (wood slivers, suture material, road gravel, fiberglass fibers, and air gun pellets). With exogenous foreign bodies it is not unusual to see secondary infectious processes, including bacterial infections (*Staphylococcus intermedius*, actinomycetes *Nocardia spp.*, opportunistic mycobacteria, anaerobic bacteria), saprophytic or systemic fungal infections, dermatophytes, saprophytic water molds (*Pythium insidiosum* and *Lagenidium* spp., Chapter 274), and algae (*Prototheca* spp).

Endogenous Foreign Bodies
Free hair shaft keratin and keratin lamellae within the dermis secondary to furunculosis or traumatic follicular damage can elicit a marked inflammatory reaction. Altered extracellular matrix, including amyloid deposition or poorly defined collagen alterations secondary to degranulation and degradation of eosinophils (previously referred to as "collagenolysis"), can solicit a marked granulomatous response.

Clinical Features

Clinical signs may present with a lag period because the inflammatory reaction around the foreign body takes time to develop. Localized erythema and swelling is observed, which progresses into firm dermal and subcutaneous nodules or abscesses, with or without fistulation. Seropurulent or serosanguineous exudates and occasionally parts of the foreign material may extrude from the draining tract. Migration of pointed foreign bodies and barbed plant awns (such as foxtails) may be enhanced by muscular movement.

Dogs
Cutaneous and subcutaneous foreign body reactions are common in outdoor dogs, in particular in young hunting and working dogs. Plant foreign bodies are more commonly seen in long-coated breeds with a higher incidence in late summer and autumn. Sex predilections have not been noted. The external ear canal and dorsal interdigital webs are common locations for grass awn entry.

Cats
Except for entrapped plant material, foreign bodies are uncommon in cats. Effective grooming behavior may help to avoid the entrance of penetrating foreign bodies in this species.

Histopathology

The usually chronic inflammatory process involves deep dermis, subcutis, and possibly skeletal muscle. The center may be cavitated. With secondary infectious processes lesions may contain a marked suppurative inflammation. Typically numerous histiocytes are present. The central cavitation may include the foreign material, in which case numerous large epithelioid macrophages palisade along the foreign material. In subacute-to-chronic lesions prominent fibrosis surrounds the process, and the periphery contains numerous plasma cells and lymphocytes. Occasionally there is a draining tract connecting the center of the lesions with the skin surface.

Clinical Management

Foreign bodies may have been eliminated via fistulation and formation of draining tracts. Subsequently the lesions heal. Secondary infectious processes have to be addressed with appropriate wound cleaning, drainage, and antibiotic therapy. Secondary endogenous foreign body reaction such as free hair shafts resulting from additional trauma may complicate the process and tend to cause persistent inflammatory response such as that seen in interdigital nodular pododermatitis.

PALISADING GRANULOMA

Etiology and Pathogenesis

Palisading granuloma can be observed in dogs. The exact etiology is unknown, but blunt trauma may be an initiating factor because many lesions occur over pressure points. Alternatively, local ischemia has been proposed as a triggering factor. The latter hypothesis is based on the description of a palisading granuloma in conjunction with an underlying arteriovenous malformation. Lesions resembling Churg-Strauss granuloma, a process associated with systemic immunoreactive or autoimmune diseases in humans, has been observed in a dog with altered secretion of antidiuretic hormone.

Clinical Features

Palisading granulomas are seen predominantly in larger-breed dogs. There is no sex or age predilection. Typically solitary dermal nodules are seen over pressure points such as zygomatic arch and hip or on the lips. Palisading granulomas also can develop on the tongue.

Histopathology

The nodules are located in the dermis and/or subcutis and may have an elongated shape. The diffuse granulomatous inflammation is composed of coalescing granulomas centered on collagen fibers, which often have an altered tinctorial, brightly eosinophilic appearance and are fragmented. A pale eosinophilic, amorphous material may encircle the collagen bundles; and numerous macrophages are aligned (i.e., palisade) along the collagen. Variable numbers of lymphocytes and plasma cells are present. If neutrophils are evident, they are usually observed in areas of cellular necrosis. The overlying epidermis is normal or atrophic.

Clinical Management

Palisading granulomas are most commonly solitary lesions, and surgical excision is curative.

REACTIVE FIBROHISTIOCYTIC NODULES

Etiology and Pathogenesis

The etiology of canine fibrohistiocytic nodules is unknown. This reflects the situation in humans. Various terms have been used to refer to this lesion: benign fibrous histiocytoma, juvenile xanthogranuloma, and fibroxanthoma. The exact origin of the histiocytic cells is not known, but the presence of lipid-type vacuoles in many of the lesional histiocytes suggests macrophage origin with phagocytic activity. The benign morphology of the histiocytes, presence of a mixed cell population, and biologic behavior suggest an inflammatory reactive process; but the possible triggering factor has not yet been identified.

Clinical Features

Canine reactive fibrohistiocytic nodules are uncommon and mostly affect dogs less than 3 years of age. The mostly solitary or occasionally multiple, firm cutaneous nodules measure less than 1 cm in diameter. They may be partially alopecic. Predilection sites are face, scrotum, and legs. There is no breed or sex predilection.

Histopathology

The nonencapsulated, wedge-shaped dermal nodules are predominated by a round-to-polygonal or plump spindle-shaped histiocytic infiltrate, which usually extends to the dermal-epidermal junction. The histiocytes contain variable numbers of delicate lipid vacuoles. The sparse collagenous matrix, which may be partially hyalinized, most likely represents residual dermal collagen. Mitotic figures are observed infrequently, and occasional multinucleated cells are present. Some elongated spindle cells consistent with fibrocytes may be interspersed with the histiocytes. Lymphocytes and fewer neutrophils and eosinophils may be present.

Clinical Management

Surgical excision is curative. Most reactive fibrohistiocytic nodules are solitary and diagnosed after surgical excision. Therefore it is not known if spontaneous regression occurs.

CANINE SARCOIDOSIS

Etiology and Pathogenesis

Sarcoidosis is a multisystemic granulomatous disorder of unknown etiology and has best been described in humans and horses. This disease mostly affects the skin, lungs, lymph nodes, and eyes. In humans an antigen-driven process supported by a $CD4^+$ helper-inducer T cell (TH_1) milieu is suggested. Recently mycobacterial deoxyribonucleic acid was identified in some cases of human cutaneous sarcoidosis, but no infectious pathogens have been found in equine lesions. Lesions consistent with canine sarcoidosis have been seen only in the skin; infectious pathogens have not been identified.

Clinical Features

The following clinical observations are based on a small number of cases; and sex, age, or breed predilections are not known at this point. Erythematous papules, plaques, and nodules are observed. The lesions have been described on the trunk, neck, face, and ears. Pruritus or pain is not observed.

Histopathology

Lesions typically seen in sarcoidosis are referred to as *naked granulomas* since associated lymphoid infiltrates are sparse. The nodules are mostly in the superficial and middermis, but subcutaneous involvement has been described. Epithelioid histiocytes and variably vacuolated macrophages predominate the lesions with little or no marginal lymphocytic infiltrates. Neutrophils are rare.

Clinical Management

Based on the small numbers of cases observed, no information about clinical management is available. Corticosteroid therapy and antihistamine administration were successful in some horses with sarcoidosis.

Suggested Reading

Affolter VK, Moore PF: Histocytes in skin disease. In Thoday K, Foil C, Bond R, editors: *Advances in veterinary dermatology*, vol 4, Oxford, 2002, Blackwell Publishing, p 111.

Bonenberger TE, Ihrke PJ, Affolter VK: Rapid identification of tissue microorganisms in skin biopsy specimens from domestic animals using polyclonal BCG antibody, *Vet Dermatol* 12:41, 2001.

Chastain CB, Graham CL: Xanthomatosis secondary to diabetes mellitus in a dog, *J Am Vet Med Assoc* 172:1209, 1978.

Lee MW et al: Cutaneous extravascular granuloma (Churg Strauss granuloma), *Clin Exp Dermatol* 24:193, 1999.

Li N et al: Identification of mycobacterial DNA in cutaneous lesions of sarcoidosis, *J Cutan Pathol* 26:271, 1999.

Spiegel IB et al: Retrospective study of cutaneous equine sarcoidosis and investigation of potential underlying infectious etiologies using polymerase chain reaction assay, *Vet Dermatol* 17:51, 2006.

Vitale CB, Ihrke PJ, Gross TL: Diet-induced alterations in lipid metabolism and associated cutaneous xanthoma formation in 5 cats. In Kwochka KW, Willemse T, von Tscharner C, editors: *Advances in veterinary dermatology*, vol 3, Oxford, 1998, Butterworth Heinemann, p 243.

Wisselink MA et al: Hyperlipoproteinaemia associated with atherosclerosis and cutaneous xanthomatosis in a cat, *Vet Q* 16:199, 1994.

CHAPTER **107**

Diseases of the Anal Sac

RUSTY MUSE, *Tustin, California*

Diseases and abnormalities of the anal sac are common concerns faced by pet owners and the general practitioner. Unfortunately the volume of research, literature, and information available about anal sac disease does not correspond to the frequency with which these problems occur. Knowledge of normal anal sac structure and function, and an appreciation of the various disorders that can involve these tissues, is critical to successful management of anal sac diseases.

Anal sacs are paired invaginations of the skin located between the internal and external sphincters of the anus. Each sac is connected to the surface by a duct that opens at the mucocutaneous junction of the anus in the dog. The anal duct of cats opens onto a prominence just lateral to the anus. The anal sacs are lined with stratified squamous epithelial cells and contain large apocrine glands with smaller numbers of sebaceous glands. In addition, the walls of the anal sac are lined with elastic and smooth muscle fibers. The duct is lined with both apocrine glands and large sebaceous glands.

The anal sacs provide a reservoir for the secretions of these glands admixed with desquamated epithelial cells. This forms the brown, oily-to-waxy secretion that is normally evacuated as a result of pressure from fecal excretions. However, change in character of the secretion or alteration in muscle tone or fecal form may cause overfilling and plugging of the sacs and resultant fermentation, inflammation, and infection. Because of the thinness of the anal sac and the ease with which it is normally evacuated, it is not distended in normal dogs. However, if enlarged, it can be palpated easily at the four and eight o'clock positions between the smooth muscle of the anal canal and the striated muscle of the external anal sphincter.

PHYSICAL CHARACTERISTICS

The normal characteristics of anal sac secretion and histologic evaluation have long been used to try to attempt to discern disease of the anal sac; however, these data also have been evaluated and reported only occasionally. Several recent studies have provided new sources of information regarding the gross, cytologic, and bacteriologic characteristics of normal anal sac secretions in the normal dog (Robson, Burton, and Lorimer, 2003; Lake et al., 2004) and in dogs with various dermatologic diseases (Pappalardo, Martino, and Noli, 2002).

Gross Characteristics

In one study (Robson, Burton, and Lorimer, 2003) the anal sac secretions in normal dogs were reported as a thin liquid exudate in 19 of 27 dogs, whereas 8 of 27 had either thick liquid or pasty discharge. Color of the discharge was reported as either light or dark brown in 21 of 27 dogs. Similar characteristics were noted between the right and left anal sac in most dogs (10 of 11 had similar consistency, whereas 9 of 11 had similar color). Another study (Lake et al., 2004) reported that of 41 pairs of anal sac evaluations in clinically normal dogs, the consistency of the discharge was reported as "watery" in 33 of 41 dogs in at least one of the sacs; however, the consistency was similar between the right and left sacs in only 18 of 41 dogs. Color of the discharge of one or both anal sacs in this study varied widely from creamy whitish-yellow in 15 of 41 dogs, grayish-tan in 13 of 41 dogs, orange-yellow in 11 of 41 dogs, and reddish-brown in 10 of 41 dogs. In another study that evaluated anal sac secretions in normal dogs and dogs with various dermatologic disorders (atopic dogs, dogs with pyoderma, and atopic dogs with *Malassezia* dermatitis) (Pappalardo, Martino, and Noli, 2002), significant differences were noted among the groups in anal sac size, color, or consistency or in the presence of granules in the content. However, an unpleasant odor was found significantly more frequently in dogs with *Malassezia* infection and in those with atopy. Pasty secretions were noted most commonly and were brown or dark brown in color; whereas in viscous or liquid secretions all colors were noted and evenly distributed among cream, beige, brown, dark brown, and red-brown.

Cellular Characteristics

Cellularity in normal dogs was somewhat similar and showed keratinocytes (Robson, Burton, and Lorimer, 2003), and parabasal epithelial cells (Lake et al., 2004). Neutrophils were noted in both studies, although degenerate neutrophils were predominant in one study (Robson, Burton, and Lorimer, 2003) and nondegenerate cells were noted in the other (Lake et al., 2004). In another study (Pappalardo, Martino, and Noli, 2002) neutrophils were noted in 12.5% of normal dogs and 30% of dogs with *Malassezia* and atopic dermatitis, in 70% of dogs with pyoderma, and in 80% of dogs with uncomplicated atopic dermatitis. Erythrocytes and eosinophils were not noted with any regularity in any study.

Bacterial Characteristics

Bacterial counts were also detailed in these studies. In one report (Robson, Burton, and Lorimer, 2002) indicated that coccoid bacterial counts were low, with 77.9% containing few coccoid organisms and only 2.4% demonstrating more than 319 organisms per oil immersion field. This is in contrast to a study by Lake (2004) that reported that 86% of anal sac secretions contained mostly gram-positive cocci; Pappalardo, Martino, and Noli (2002) reported that 48.75% of all normal dogs had "abundant" numbers of bacteria present. However, all dogs with various skin diseases had higher numbers of bacterial counts,

ranging from 60% in atopic dermatitis without complications to 90% in dogs with pyoderma. Each of these studies did find that intracellular bacteria and large numbers of *Malassezia* organisms appear to be a relatively uncommon finding. Previous studies have revealed the presence of various gram-positive coccoid and rod-shaped bacteria as a normal part of the flora of the anal sac and include *Streptococcus faecalis, Streptococcus faecium, Escherichia coli, Clostridium perfringens, Staphylococcus intermedius, Proteus* spp., and coagulase-negative staphylococci. In the most recent study to evaluate cultures of the anal sac secretions, Pappalardo, Martino, and Noli (2002) found the most common organisms to be *Proteus mirabilis, E. coli, Streptococcus intermedius*, β-hemolytic *Streptococcus* spp., *S. faecalis, Bacillus* spp., and *Pseudomonas aeruginosa*.

Thus, although these recent studies seem to indicate variability in the physical characteristics of anal sac secretions, they do add significant data to this field in helping to allow the clinician to use visual and microscopic evaluations to establish the presence or absence of disease of the anal sac.

DISORDERS OF THE ANAL SAC

Impaction

Diseases of the anal sac vary from impactions, infections (sacculitis) with or without abscessation, and neoplasia. Anal sac impactions have been reported to occur in 2% to 12% of dogs (Scott, Miller, and Griffin, 2001). Clinically these usually result in pruritus or the classic "scooting" that is noted by most owners. Although anal sac disease is a common cause of anal pruritus, the clinician should be alert to the fact that many other causes of pruritus to the anal or perianal area have been documented and may include any number of dermatologic, psychologic, metabolic, nutritional, and gastrointestinal diseases. Skin diseases such as atopy, food allergy, insect hypersensitivity, *Malassezia* or bacterial dermatitis, parasitic skin disease, and keratinization defects may all result in persistent pruritus of the anal or perianal areas. Diagnostic procedures such as cutaneous cytologic evaluations, skin scrapings, dermatophyte cultures, food trials, and allergy testing may be necessary to uncover the causes of any residual pruritus. However, if the pruritus completely resolves after expression of the anal sac, a true anal sac disorder is likely. In addition, I strongly advocate that the routine expression of anal sacs in dogs during grooming, bathing, and boarding processes by veterinarians, technicians, groomers, and others be discouraged. Chronic manipulation and inadvertent trauma may predispose normal dogs to chronic recurrent anal sac disease.

Increased incidence of impactions has been associated with smaller breeds (under 15 kg), especially miniature and toy poodles, Chihuahuas, American cockers, and English springer spaniels (Scott, Miller, and Griffin, 2001). The presence of dermatologic problems such as primary or secondary keratinization defects in the spaniels may also be an accentuating factor. Impaction of the anal sacs in cats is less common. Secretions of the cat anal sac are somewhat different in that the anal sacs of cats contain larger amounts of sebaceous glands, which may allow for more lipid production and subsequently easier expression. In addition, since the anal duct opens laterally to the anus in cats, it may be less susceptible to occlusion by fecal matter.

Impaction may be a result of alterations of glandular secretion. Loss of apocrine secretions may result in hard granular material that is unable to be expressed by the normal bowel movement of the dog. Glandular hypersecretions associated with generalized seborrhea may also cause plugging of the duct. Chronic loose stools or bouts of diarrhea may result in pasty secretions and subsequent impaction. Dietary manipulation with higher-fiber diets or endoscopic investigation for the possibility of gastrointestinal diseases causing chronic soft or loose stools may be of benefit. In addition, tapeworm segments have been identified in anal sacs and may cause impaction.

Impactions should be gently but thoroughly manually expressed. Complete expression of the anal sac is best accomplished via digital compression through the rectal canal. In addition, a complete palpation of the anal sac can be achieved. Expression should relieve the pruritus associated with a simple impaction. If pruritus is not resolved, additional causes of anal pruritus should be investigated as discussed previously. Sedation and irrigation of the anal sac with sterile saline may be required to soften firmer secretions or for more recurrent impactions. Every attempt should be made to elucidate and correct underlying causes for chronically recurrent impactions. If the pruritus is not relieved by manual expression, infection or inflammation of the anal sac may also be present.

Anal Sacculitis

Chronic or recurrent impactions may predispose to infection and abscesses of the anal sac. Prolonged retention may result in fermentation followed by inflammation and bacterial infection. Infection may stay confined to the anal sac or spread to surrounding subcutaneous tissues with resultant abscessation. Rupture of the anal sac may result in a cellulitis as well. Clinical signs of anal sac infections include pruritus, a hesitancy to sit or lift the tail, and pain that may be mild to severe with a swollen perineum in the cases of abscessation. Some animals may be unwilling to defecate, which may result in additional gastrointestinal concerns. When rupture of the perineum occurs, it is usually just lateral to the anus. Abscesses in cats must be differentiated clinically from cat bite abscesses, although, with the exception of the Siamese, infections of the anal sacs are rare in the cat (Scott, Miller, and Griffin, 2001). No studies have undertaken to quantify the physical characteristics of cat anal sacs. A greenish, and blood-tinged or purulent foul-smelling discharge with or without the presence of intracellular bacteria in the dog (and likely the cat) would be suspicious of infection.

Treatment options for infections vary with the severity. Routine expression with infusion of antibiotic-containing ointment may be curative in some cases; however, refractory or recurrent cases may need more aggressive therapy. Patients may need to be sedated or anesthetized, and the anal sacs infused via a tomcat catheter or lacrimal flush canula with ceruminolytic agents to break up thick secretion, followed by antibacterial lavage and ointment (otic or ophthalmic preparations). This may need to be repeated weekly to biweekly initially to resolve the infection.

Abscessed anal sacs may need to be drained surgically with an incision and curettage. Healing may be by granulation. Broad-spectrum oral antibiotics that have efficacy against most gram-positive cocci such as cephalosporins, macrolide antibiotics (clindamycin), or amoxicillin-clavulanate should be considered. Treatment should continue until no evidence of typical infectious discharge or intracellular bacteria is noted, likely 2 to 3 weeks. Last, surgical excision or marsupialization may be necessary for any chronically impacted or infected anal sac. Surgical techniques for both procedures are described in most surgical texts and are considered routine. However, caution should be exercised by the clinician in recommending anal sac removal as a resolution for anal pruritus. I routinely see cases in which chronic anal sac disease is attributed to chronic pruritus of the perianal area; however, the problem persists even after removal of the anal sacs.

Neoplasia

Adenocarcinoma is by far the most common neoplasm affecting the anal sac (also see Chapter 83). However, other neoplasms have been noted recently, including squamous cell carcinoma arising from the lining of the sac (Esplin, Wilson, and Hullinger, 2003) and at least one case of malignant melanoma has been noted (Emms, 2005). Most previous reports note a female predisposition for adenocarcinomas; however, a more recent review of 113 cases found an approximately equal distribution between male and female dogs (Williams et al., 2003). This same study reported the clinical signs at initial presentation to consist of perianal swelling (61% of dogs), tenesmus (34%), perianal pruritus (30%), perianal bleeding (24%), polyuria/polydipsia (22%), and scooting (21%). In addition, no clinical signs may be noted in some cases, and the masses found on routine palpation. Although the presence of hypercalcemia was not present in all dogs, it was identified as a significant predictor in survival time in treated dogs; dogs that exhibited hypercalcemia survived 256 days, and normocalcemic dogs survived 584 days. Other factors that resulted in significantly shorter survival times included treatment with chemotherapy alone, no surgical intervention, and a tumor size larger than $10 \, cm^2$.

Perianal Fistula

Perianal fistula (or anal furunculosis) is a disease characterized by deep fistulous tracts and ulcerating sinuses that occurs in the perianal tissue (also see Chapter 122). German shepherds are predisposed, although the pathogenesis of the disease is not well understood and likely involves a number of genetic and immune mechanisms. The pathophysiology and relationship to the anal sac proper are also unclear. Clinical signs generally involve significant anal discomfort, pruritus, and tenesmus with variable amounts of purulent discharge noted to the tracts and fistulae. These lesions often begin with small tracts that ultimately coalesce to form large connecting sinuses and ulcerative areas. These tracts may extend deep into the perianal tissues and involve the anal sacs themselves. Numerous therapies have been advocated over the years, and until recently surgical intervention to dissect the sinuses and remove anal sacs was the therapy most commonly used. However, a number of newer medical therapies have been used more recently with often better success and less risk of surgical complications.

In multiple studies cyclosporine, 5 mg/kg daily, has been shown to be quite effective at resolving fistulae and allowing for complete resolution of disease. Relapses do occur, however, and side effects (most notably vomiting and diarrhea) can be seen that limit the use of this drug in some dogs. Furthermore, the expense of cyclosporine can be a concern for clients. Recently a combination ketoconazole and low-dose cyclosporine has been advocated to reduce the dosage of the cyclosporine needed for remission and control of symptoms. In one study (Mouatt, 2002) 16 dogs were treated with 10 mg/kg of ketoconazole once daily in conjunction with cyclosporine at 1 mg/kg twice daily for 16 weeks. Complete resolution was noted to the perianal fistulae in 13 of 14 cases that competed the study. In addition, 7 of 14 of those had no recurrence after 12 months. The use of this combination therapy may create less concern for cyclosporine side effects and immune suppression and help to mitigate cost concerns in treating large dogs. Another therapeutic modality, tacrolimus ointment, which is a potent immunosuppressive medication, has also been evaluated in dogs with perianal fistulae. One published study (Misseghers, Binnington, and Mathews, 2000) evaluated 10 dogs with perianal fistulae that were treated with topical tacrolimus ointment once or twice daily for 16 weeks. Full resolutions of the fistulae were noted in 50% of the dogs, with noticeable improvement in 90%. I routinely use both therapies in conjunction when treating clinical cases of perianal fistulae. Topical therapy initially is often difficult in these dogs because of pain; therefore initial therapy with cyclosporine and ketoconazole or cyclosporine alone for the first 4 weeks aids in shrinking the lesions and minimizing pain. Once this is achieved, topical tacrolimus 0.1% ointment applied twice daily should be initiated. Once the lesions are resolved, discontinuation of the oral therapy and continued use of the topical tacrolimus have resulted in excellent results in managing and maintaining these cases in clinical remission. Additional studies with tacrolimus may provide further support for this less invasive and less expensive therapy as an alternative approach to perianal fistulae.

References and Suggested Reading

Bennett PF et al: Canine anal sac adenocarcinomas: clinical presentation and response to therapy, *J Vet Intern Med* 16:100, 2002.

Emms SG: Anal sac tumours of the dog and their response to cytoreductive surgery and chemotherapy, *Aust Vet J* 83:340, 2005.

Esplin DG, Wilson SR, Hullinger GA: Squamous cell carcinoma of the anal sac in five dogs, *Vet Pathol* 40:332, 2003.

Lake AM et al: Gross and cytological characteristics of normal canine anal-sac secretions, *J Vet Med Assoc* 51:249, 2004.

Misseghers BS, Binnington AG, Mathews KA: Clinical observations of the treatment of canine perianal fistulas with topical tacrolimus in 10 dogs, *Can Vet J* 41:623, 2000.

Mouatt JG: Cyclosporin and ketoconazole interaction for treatment of perianal fistulas in the dog, *Aust Vet J* 80:207, 2002.

Pappalardo E, Martino PA, Noli C: Macroscopic, cytological and bacteriological evaluation of anal sac content in normal dogs and in dogs with selected dermatological disease, *Vet Dermatol* 13:315, 2002.

Robson DC, Burton GG, Lorimer MF: Cytological examination and physical characteristics of the anal sacs in 17 clinically normal dogs, *Aust Vet J* 81:36, 2003.

Scott DW, Miller WH, Griffin, CE: *Muller and Kirk's small animal dermatology*, ed 6, Philadelphia, 2001, Saunders, p 1200.

van Duijkerern E: Disease conditions of canine anal sacs, *J Small Anim Pract* 36:12, 1995.

Williams LE et al: Carcinoma of the apocrine glands of the anal sac in dogs: 113 cases (1985-1995), *J Am Vet Med Assoc* 223:825, 2003.

CHAPTER **108**

Acral Lick Dermatitis

JOHN M. MacDONALD, *Auburn, Alabama*
DINO M. BRADLEY, *Skillman, New Jersey*

Acral lick dermatitis (ALD) is a multifactorial condition characterized by excessive, compulsive licking at an area of the extremities resulting in a firm, proliferative, ulcerative, alopecic plaque or plaques. This condition, also referred to as *lick granuloma* and *acral pruritic nodule*, remains one of the more challenging and frustrating problems seen by both the specialist and the private practicing veterinarian. One of the more difficult aspects of the treatment is related to the multifactorial etiology. Although environmental stress such as boredom, confinement, loneliness, or separation anxiety may contribute to the onset of the condition, it appears to be less important than other factors.

By definition the lesion is located on an extremity, and cases appear to be distributed equally between the front and rear legs, most noticeably on the dorsal aspect of the carpus, metacarpus, tarsus, or metatarsus. Lesions usually begin with a small area of self-trauma and alopecia and progress to more extensive lesions through persistent licking or chewing. The expansion of the lesions often produces tissue proliferation and scarring and may interfere with locomotion. In some situations this can result in deeper bony tissue alterations. This condition is more commonly seen in older (5 to 12 years old), large-breed dogs (Doberman pinscher, Great Dane, Golden retriever, Labrador retriever, German shepherd, and boxer), although it has also been observed in other breeds, including the dalmatian, English setter, shar-pei, and weimaraner, and may afflict any breed of dog.

The development of ALD may be related to numerous causes. Constant licking of the affected area results in hair loss, erosions, or ulcerations. Exposure of the sensory nerve endings can cause or intensify the site to be pruritic, and the dog licks the affected area to alleviate the pruritic sensation. This perpetuates a vicious cycle, resulting in the development of an ulcerated skin lesion, which does not heal because of the dog's constant self-trauma. This condition should be approached as are other dermatologic problems in which a *primary disease* becomes complicated by *perpetuating factors* and results in persistence of the problem. Since there may be a number of simultaneous diseases and factors causing ALD, it is apparent that no single treatment is effective in treating all cases. Symptomatic therapy may decrease the compulsive tendency of licking but is unlikely to resolve the lesion, particularly in a dog with a chronic history. Although conventional treatments such as intralesional injection with glucocorticoids (triamcinolone or methylprednisolone acetate) may produce an antiinflammatory effect, they actually may intensify the infection that is almost always present. History taking becomes an important part of the diagnostic approach to these cases, and identifying an underlying disorder is truly the key to successful management.

PRIMARY FACTORS

Although boredom and stress factors are often considered predominant causes of ALD, they seem to be less important than other *primary* factors (Box 108-1). There is some variability with regard to certain breeds. The Great Dane and Doberman pinscher often do not have an obvious coexisting problem or underlying disease associated with the ALD. In contrast, in many other breeds allergy is the primary cause of the initial compulsive licking. Secondary bacterial folliculitis further potentiates and perpetuates the development of the lesion, especially in the Labrador retriever, Golden retriever, German shepherd, shar-pei, and dalmatian. Allergic diseases to be considered include canine atopy (see Section V on Evolve), food allergy, and flea allergy. Historical information about early-onset pruritic disease may be helpful

---

Box 108-1

Primary Causes and Perpetuating Factors in Acral Lick Dermatitis

Primary Factors	Perpetuating Factors
Allergic dermatitis	Bacterial infection
Arthropathies	Osteomyelitis
Foreign bodies	Keratin foreign bodies
Neuropathies	Periostitis
Trauma	Secondary arthritis
Neoplasia	Learned behavior
Mycotic infection	
Parasitism (e.g., scabies)	
Psychogenic factors	

---

in defining the relationship of allergy to the evolution of these lesions. Food allergy has notably been related to the development of ALD and may result from an abrupt onset of aggressive pruritus and occur spontaneously in the older dog (>6 years).

PERPETUATING FACTORS

Perpetuating factors may be as important as the primary cause and, if left untreated, ultimately result in failure to control the problem (see Box 108-1). One of the most important of these factors is infection. The infectious agent most commonly isolated from lesions of ALD is *Staphylococcus intermedius*. Infection starts as an area of folliculitis and progresses further to furunculosis. Histologic and microbial assessments of ALD lesions almost always demonstrate infected tissue. Treatment for bacterial infection should routinely be included in the therapeutic regimen. Although lesions are not exudative, cultures of aseptically acquired tissue almost always reveal a staphylococcal species and in chronic cases may include a gram-negative organism (*Pseudomonas*, *Proteus*, *Escherichia coli*).

It is well recognized that licking or scratching incites a cycle of irritation and intensifies pruritus. A theory of potentiation of this behavior suggests that endorphin release as a consequence of chronic licking induces repetition of the activity. Regardless of the mechanisms involved, the learned behavior of chronic licking may present an obstacle as a perpetuating factor that will impede resolution of the problem even if the primary and other perpetuating factors are no longer present. Thus most ALD cases involve both primary factors and consequential perpetuating factors. If the problem were as simple as a psychogenic or obsessive-compulsive behavioral disorder, treatment with psychoactive drugs should demonstrate greater efficacy than is currently observed.

DIAGNOSTIC APPROACH

One of the common causes of failure in the treatment of ALD is the inability to identify either primary or perpetuating factors. The appearance of the lesion nearly always elicits a "knee-jerk" response with regard to the name of the problem and an oversimplistic approach.

Associated and underlying factors are often overlooked. Routine topical or systemic therapy is instituted before understanding the relationships involved with the disease evolution and progression. Although ALD may be considered a purely psychogenic phenomenon, the diagnostic plan must include tests to rule out underlying causes of chronic licking and self-mutilation. Initial appraisal of focal or multifocal lesions should include documentation of location and size. Calipers may be used to quantify the size and shape of the lesion. The use of acetate film or plastic kitchen wrap and an indelible felt-tip pen provides a convenient method for tracing the lesion. A permanent record may be kept for comparison during the treatment process. Routine blood work (complete blood count and survey profile), urinalysis, and a minimal database of skin scrapings, impression or aspiration cytology, and a dermatophyte test medium culture should be obtained. Suspicion of possible underlying disease should influence the direction of diagnostics for that individual animal. History of allergic episodes should direct the clinician toward pursuing allergic disease.

Skin Biopsy

Biopsy of lesions associated with ALD remains controversial among some dermatologists, although it is included as part of our diagnostic workup. This provides a relatively expedient way to rule out neoplasia or mycotic infection with a similar cutaneous presentation. Mast cell tumor, histiocytoma, and squamous cell carcinoma are examples of tumors that may be associated with compulsive licking of the area. Likewise, infectious diseases, including superficial keratinophilic fungi (dermatophytosis), deep mycoses (blastomycosis), or sporotrichosis, may all be ruled out by this procedure. Histopathologic features usually are not diagnostic but show characteristic features that include an ulcerative lesion surrounded by irregular epidermal hyperplasia; mild perivascular inflammation of neutrophils, mononuclear cells, and plasma cells; and dermal fibroplasia. Epitrichial sweat glands are often surrounded by plasma cells, and sebaceous glands are hyperplastic. A specific type of a dermal fibroplasia has been described, with ALD referred to as "vertical streaking" when there is perpendicular fibroplasia seen in the papillary dermis. Tissue may also be sent for microbiologic evaluation (bacterial culture and susceptibility testing or fungal culture) during this procedure. Impression smears made from biopsy specimens should be obtained routinely, with the expectation of aiding in the diagnosis of neoplasia or infectious diseases.

Radiography

Depending on the chronicity and progression of the lesions, radiography may or may not be included in the initial diagnostic approach. This is certainly indicated with chronic and larger lesions or if there is concern about an underlying arthropathy associated with the problem. Radiography is most helpful when evaluating the prognosis. Lesions with more extensive radiographic evidence of bony involvement are least likely to be satisfactorily resolved.

Fine-Needle Aspiration and Cytologic Studies

Fine-needle aspiration should be included in the initial phase of the diagnostic workup to provide early recognition of cutaneous neoplasia, especially if biopsy specimens are not going to be acquired, although lack of evidence does not rule it out. Cytologic examination of material acquired from the typical ALD lesion shows little cellularity aside from representative inflammatory cells. Impression smears of the surface exudate contain many different bacteria and white blood cells, demonstrating opportunistic colonization of an ulcerative lesion.

Bacterial Culture and Susceptibility Testing

Bacterial cultures are often included in the diagnostic workup but must be obtained from an aseptically acquired biopsy punch specimen to offer credible results. Punch biopsy samples from the center of a lesion are submitted for maceration and inoculation to a microbiology laboratory on culture medium for identification of microorganisms. Transport media must be used if specimens cannot be taken to the laboratory promptly. Several commercial products that contain Stuart's transport media are available and are appropriate for this purpose. Culture may be helpful in chronic lesions, particularly when gram-negative organisms may be present. Culturing the *surface* of the lesion offers little diagnostic help in either antibiotic selection or understanding the relationship of perpetuating factors. Some clinicians use a Culturette to sample the defect left by a punch biopsy, but in our experience this method is not reliable in identifying important microorganisms.

Electrodiagnostic Testing

Electrodiagnostic testing consisting of electromyography and motor-sensory nerve conduction velocities may be conducted to rule out the presence of an underlying neuropathy or nerve root lesion. Results of these studies are not generally useful, except in situations in which automobile accidents or other types of trauma may result in peripheral neuropathy.

Allergy Testing

Allergy testing should be considered a part of the diagnostic evaluation if canine atopy is suspected based on history and clinical symptoms. Intradermal allergy testing or in vitro allergy testing is desirable for identification of allergens with the anticipation of implementing antigen therapy (Bonagura, 2000, p. 560). Although this does not have an immediate effect on the active lesion, it may be helpful in preventing further lesions. Intradermal allergy testing may need to be deferred if repeated intralesional injection of glucocorticoids has been performed. Of course, treating the primary problem may not provide a measurable contribution if the perpetuating factors represent a large component. Food trials should be considered routinely in animals in which food allergy is suspected, particularly the Golden retriever, Labrador retriever, shar-pei, dalmatian, and German shepherd.

TREATMENT

There is no *one* specific treatment for ALD. Identifying and specifically treating the primary condition and the perpetuating factors are critical to satisfactory resolution. Chronic unresponsive lesions have an extremely poor prognosis for resolution. Preventing licking by introduction of mechanical barriers should be included in the initial phase of all therapy. Bandaging may have limited value because of rapid removal by the dog, but it may be helpful in certain cases. Wire muzzles and bandaging have proved a good combination for deterring continued licking. Elizabethan collars, although poorly accepted by most pet owners and their pets, can be effective. An alternative to the Elizabethan collar is the use of a plastic bucket with a hole cut in the bottom. This can be slipped over the head and secured to a collar. Some innovative pet owners and veterinarians have used modified polyvinyl chloride piping to cover lesions and provide sufficient air flow through perforations so as not to cause dermatitis. Intermittent examinations are critical to determine response to therapy. We strongly recommend the use of a measuring mechanism and digital pictures to record changes in the size of focal lesions so that their progression can be followed.

Antibiotics

Antibiotics are one of the most important treatments of ALD. These agents should be used systemically, and therapy may require a protracted period (4 to 6 months). The selection of antibiotics should be based on culture and susceptibility testing when available. Cephalosporins have been used commonly with more success than other antibiotics (e.g., cephalexin [Keflex, Lilly and generics] 30 mg/kg orally [PO] q12h; or sulfadimethoxine/orme-toprim [Primor, Pfizer] 55 mg/kg for the first day and then 27 mg/kg once daily thereafter). Fluoroquinolones, including enrofloxacin (Baytril, Bayer) 5 mg/kg once daily or marbofloxacin (Zeniquin, Pfizer) 2.5 mg/kg once daily, have been useful, particularly if there is significant scarring or if gram-negative organisms are present. Treatment of the animal should be carried out 3 to 4 weeks beyond regression of the lesion. Maintenance antibiotic therapy may be required in the event of incomplete resolution of the lesion or when the lesion recurs after the termination of antibiotic administration. Pulse therapy has been used successfully in some cases in which administration of antibiotics is alternated with periods of no antibiotics.

Treatment of Allergic Diseases

Allergen-specific immunotherapy (see Chapter 92) should always be considered when canine atopy has been determined to be one of the primary factors. The decreased use of systemic glucocorticoids is an objective of treatment in chronically infected lesions, and antigen therapy may help accomplish this goal. It is important with any allergic condition to consider avoidance as an optimal treatment, but practically this is limited to food or flea allergy. ALD predominantly affecting the rear legs with coexisting lesions over the pelvic area should be evaluated for flea allergy and treated with parasiticidal therapy regardless of gross observation of fleas. The products most helpful for this trial include "on-the-animal" adulticides such as imidacloprid and fipronil. Dietary trials and challenge should be used to identify the optimal food for routine feeding of the food-allergic or food-intolerant animal. Owners should be cautioned about deviating from the restricted food.

Cyclosporine (Atopica, Novartis) has also proved to be of substantial value in controlling ALD associated with allergic skin disease. Following protocols used for management of atopic dermatitis can be quite helpful (see Chapter 84).

Systemic Glucocorticoid Therapy

Although systemic glucocorticoid therapy is contraindicated in many cases of ALD because of the concurrent presence of bacterial infection, its judicious use after infection is addressed can be helpful in many cases. It can often break the licking and chewing cycle to allow healing to occur. It can reduce pain and inflammation and aid in the reduction of scar tissue formation. If used, oral formulations of prednisone, prednisolone, or methylprednisolone are first-choice selections at routine antiinflammatory dosages. In some situations the use of oral triamcinolone is selected since it may have more dramatic effects on reducing scar tissue formation than other glucocorticoids. The use of glucocorticoids should be short term, and tapering to the lowest effective alternative dosing is recommended within 2 weeks of initiation (see Chapter 89).

Surgery or Cryotherapy

Surgical intervention is often met with postoperative complications and incomplete resolution of the problem. This is a salvage procedure and indicated if underlying arthropathy is identified in a location where arthrodesis may be used for joint stability and pain reduction. Foreign bodies are also treated surgically. Surgical excision of the lesion does not prevent recurrence. The primary disease must be treated.

OTHER THERAPY

Some clinicians have reported laser therapy to be beneficial. Other reports suggest that this treatment can be partially helpful, depending on the underlying cause, but should be used cautiously. In a small number of cases acupuncture has been reported to be beneficial.

Radiation Therapy

Radiation therapy has been used for treatment of ALD with varying degrees of success. The earlier, less-pronounced lesions with minimal fibrosis and inflammation demonstrate the best response; whereas larger, chronic lesions with underlying bony involvement do not respond as well. The cost factors and unavailability of treatment centers make radiation therapy impractical in the vast majority of cases unless the underlying lesion is a radiosensitive tumor with a difficult surgical approach.

Topical Antipruritic and Antiinflammatory Treatment

The sole use of topical antiinflammatory drugs has a limited effect in the majority of cases in our experience. They may be prescribed after initial resolution has been observed with antibiotic therapy. A variety of choices are available, including Tresaderm (Merck Ag Vet), Otomax or Momentamax (Schering Plough Animal Health), or the Synotic-Banamine combination. Synotic-Banamine is preferred, and preparation is made by placing 3 ml of flunixin meglumine (Banamine, Schering Plough) in a vial of Synotic (Syntex) with application twice daily for 30 days. The use of capsaicin (Zostrix, GenDerm) has been helpful in some cases. This compound is a substance P inhibitor that is available as an antiarthralgic-myalgic preparation in ointment form for human application. The topical application on and around lesions may help decrease the reinforcing sensations but must be used consistently at a rate of three to four times per day. This drug is now available as a nonprescription item. It is formulated as a 0.025% and 0.075% ointment. A more concentrated formulation (Dolorac, GenDerm) contains 0.25% capsaicin. We have used this in combination with mupirocin antibiotic (compounded generics) in a 1:1 mixture applied three times daily. The use of bitter apple and Heet Liniment (Whitehall) in a ratio of two parts bitter apple to 1 part Heet has also been popular as a topical antipruritic therapy. Heet contains capsaicin (0.025%), methylsalicylate (15%), and camphor (3.6%) and has activity similar to that of the generic capsaicin or Zostrix. A substantial trial period is necessary (4 to 6 weeks) to evaluate these topical products. It must be stressed that this type of treatment by itself has little impact on chronic lesions. Specific treatments of the primary and perpetuating factors are critical for any hope of resolving the lesions.

Intralesional Injection

Intralesional injections of glucocorticoids are *not* recommended, particularly in the early stage of disease management, because the vast majority of lesions are infected with *Staphylococcus* spp. and possibly by gram-negative microorganisms. Many acute lesions become chronic in nature with progression of the infection. Acute lesions should be treated with a regimen of antibiotic therapy before consideration of intralesional steroid therapy. Topical antiinflammatory drugs are far more conservative and would be better used in lieu of intralesional steroid therapy. We have seen cases that require protracted treatment with antibiotics (>13 months) when the lesion had been treated with glucocorticoid therapy. Intralesional steroid injections should be withheld at least until a complete appraisal of the case has been made and a course of antibiotic therapy evaluated.

CANINE ACRAL LICK DERMATITIS AND OBSESSIVE-COMPULSIVE DISORDER

There may be similarities between the uncontrollable licking experienced by dogs suffering from ALD and the uncontrollable actions of humans suffering from obsessive-compulsive disorder (OCD). This condition in humans is characterized by recurrent, persistent thoughts or impulses (obsessions) or by repetitive, unnecessary behavior (compulsions). OCD, expressed by acts such as chronic hair pulling (trichotillomania), hand washing, or nail biting, has been considered an exaggeration of normal grooming habits. Some think that ALD is a manifestation of exaggerated grooming habits in animals.

Investigations into the etiology of OCD indicate that these patients have an abnormality in the pathway that links the frontal lobes of the cerebral cortex with the basal ganglia. The frontal lobes promote deliberation and judgment, with the basal ganglia serving as a relay station for planning and execution of movements. It is suspected that the caudate nucleus, a portion of the basal ganglia, is deficient in filtering messages from the frontal lobes to the rest of the brain.

Biochemically it appears that serotonin is linked directly with the presence of OCD. Simply stated, serotonin is a neuromodulator that plays a role in sensory perception, emotion, arousal, and higher cognitive functions. Serotonin-releasing fibers are distributed throughout the central nervous system, influencing the sleep cycle, sex drive, body temperature, appetite, respiration, cardiovascular activity, mood, and aggression.

After a meal serotonin (5-hydroxytryptamine [5-HT]) is made from the amino acid L-tryptophan after it reaches serotonin-releasing neurons in the brain. Once synthesized, serotonin is enclosed within vesicles at the presynaptic terminal. An action potential at the presynaptic terminal releases the serotonin into the synaptic gap, allowing binding to specialized receptors on the postsynaptic neuron. The serotonin is removed from its binding site and transported back to the presynaptic terminal, where it is reused or degraded to its primary metabolite, 5-hydroxyindoleacetic acid.

Experimentally it has been shown that the primary function of the brain serotonin system is to facilitate tonic motor actions and inhibit sensory information processing. In patients with OCD serotonin neuronal activity is low, resulting in impairment of these functions. It is thought that the repetitive motor activities of an OCD patient serve to increase serotonin neuronal activity. These repetitive acts are a means of self-medication. Since the pattern of exaggerated grooming behavior applies to canines, it would appear that the chronic licking of ALD may serve to increase serotonin neuronal activity as well.

Therapy Using Drugs That Modify Neurologic Activity

Recent clinical investigations indicate that certain medications effective in the treatment of OCD in humans have a similarly positive effect on dogs with ALD. The drugs that show the most promise are tricyclic antidepressants (TCAs) and selective serotonin reuptake inhibitors (SSRIs), which affect central serotonin neurotransmission. The specific mechanism of action is based on the prevention of removal of serotonin from the synaptic cleft, increasing the functional activity of the serotonin. TCAs block the reuptake of both norepinephrine and 5-HT by their presynaptic terminals. Adverse reactions in humans include cardiotoxicity, resulting in arrhythmias or heart block, or central nervous system toxicity. SSRIs are more specific in their mode of action, acting to block reuptake of 5-HT by presynaptic terminals. This eliminates many of the adverse effects noted with the use of TCAs.

Clomipramine (Anafranil, Ciba-Geigy), a TCA, administered orally at a dosage of 1 to 3 mg/kg once daily, has shown some efficacy in the treatment of ALD in some dogs (Bonagura, 2000, p. 90). Because of the transient side effects of vomiting or diarrhea, we recommend treating the dog with 1 mg/kg orally for the first 3 days of therapy, with a gradual increase in dosage based on clinical response. The SSRI, fluoxetine hydrochloride, (Reconcile, Eli Lilly and Co.), administered at a dosage of 1 mg/kg orally once daily, has also been an effective treatment for ALD. Other SSRIs currently available for treatment of OCD in humans are paroxetine HCl (Paxil, SmithKline Beecham Pharmaceuticals) and fluvoxamine maleate (Luvox, Solvay Pharmaceuticals). Hydrocodone has been used in the treatment of ALD. The dosage is variable, pending response and tolerance of the drug. The standard dosage is 5 mg/20 kg of body weight twice daily and has also been used at 10 mg/20 kg of body weight three times daily.

These drugs should also be efficacious in the management of ALD in dogs, but there are no publications evaluating their clinical application for this particular condition. In any event, one should anticipate a lag phase of at least 4 to 5 weeks before any change in excessive grooming behavior is seen.

References and Suggested Reading

Brignac MM: Hydrocodone treatment of acral lick dermatitis. Proceedings of the Second World Congress of Veterinary Dermatology, Montreal, Canada, 1992, p 50.

David Duclos: Lasers in veterinary dermatology, *Vet Clin Small Anim* 36:15, 2006.

Goldberger E, Rapoport JL: Canine acral lick dermatitis: response to the antiobsessional drug clomipramine, *J Am Anim Hosp Assoc* 27:179, 1991.

Jacobs BL: Serotonin, motor activity and depression-related disorders, *Am Sci* 82:456, 1994.

Looney AL, Rothstein E: Use of acupuncture to treat psychodermatosis in the dog, *Canine Pract* 23:18, 1998.

Luescher UA, McKeown DB, Halip J: Stereotypic or obsessive-compulsive disorders in dogs and cats, *Vet Clin North Am* 21:401, 1991.

Marder AR: Psychotropic drugs and behavioral therapy, *Vet Clin North Am* 21:329, 1991.

Rapoport JL, Rylord DH, Kriete M: Drug treatment of canine acral lick dermatitis: an animal model of obsessive compulsive disorder, *Arch Gen Psychiatry* 49:517, 1992.

Rivers B, Walter PA, McKeever PJ: Treatment of canine acral lick dermatitis with radiation therapy: 17 cases (1979-1991), *J Am Anim Hosp Assoc* 29:542, 1993.

Scott DW, Walton DK: Clinical evaluation of a topical treatment for canine acral lick dermatitis, *J Am Anim Hosp Assoc* 20:565, 1984.

Shanley K, Overall K: Psychogenic dermatoses. In Kirk RW, Bonagura JD, editors: *Current veterinary therapy XI*, Philadelphia, 1992, Saunders, p 552.

Shoulberg N: The efficacy of fluoxetine (Prozac) in the treatment of acral lick and allergic inhalant dermatitis in canines. Proceedings of the American Academy of Veterinary Dermatology and the American College of Veterinary Dermatology, Scottsdale, Az, 1991, vol 6, p 31.

White SD: Naltrexone for treatment of acral lick dermatitis in dogs, *J Am Vet Med Assoc* 196:1073, 1990.

SECTION VI

Gastrointestinal Diseases

David C. Twedt

VOLUME XIII CONTENT ON EVOLVE: http://evolve.elsevier.com/Bonagura/Kirks/

Assessment of Gastrointestinal Motility

Diagnosis and Treatment of Parvovirus

Dietary Sensitivity

Feline Constipation and Idiopathic
Megacolon

Gastric Prokinetic Agents

Gastrinoma in Dogs

Hepatoportal Microvascular Dysplasia

Small Intestinal Bacterial Overgrowth

CHAPTER 109

Feline Caudal Stomatitis

LINDA J. DeBOWES, *Seattle, Washington*

The most common cause of oral inflammation in cats is periodontal disease (gingivitis, periodontitis). Inflammation of the buccal mucosa (stomatitis) may also be associated with severe periodontal disease. Eosinophilic complex–related disorders, neoplasia, trauma, irritation caused by ingestion of noxious materials, immune-mediated diseases, and metabolic abnormalities are also potential causes of oral inflammation.

Infectious diseases have been related to oral inflammation. Cats with altered immune function from infection with feline leukemia virus or feline immunodeficiency virus may have more severe periodontal disease or oral inflammation. Chronic calicivirus infection has been implicated as a factor in severe oral inflammation, especially in cats with inflammation lateral to the palatoglossal fold (caudal stomatitis). In one study of 25 cats with gingivostomatitis, 81% were shedding both feline calicivirus and feline herpesvirus 1 compared to 21% in a similar number of cats with periodontal disease (Lommer and Verstraete, 2003). *Bartonella henselae* infection has been suggested as a possible factor in the development of feline chronic gingivostomatitis (Hardy, Zuckerman, and Corbishley, 2002). However, there is a high prevalence rate of *B. henselae* antibody-positive healthy cats, making it difficult to determine the significance of an antibody-positive test in a cat with chronic gingivostomatitis. A recent study of 34 cats with chronic stomatitis and 34 age-matched healthy control cats reported no significant differences in the prevalence rates of polymerase chain reaction-positive *(Bartonella* spp.) cats and antibody-positive *(B. henselae)* cats between the two groups (Dowers and Lappin, 2005).

Cats with chronic gingivostomatitis have decreased salivary IgA compared to healthy cats; however, the significance of this in the development of disease is unknown (Harley, Gruffydd-Jones, and Day, 2003). Cats with chronic gingivostomatitis also have higher serum immunoglobulin (Ig)G, IgM, and IgA concentrations compared to healthy cats.

Oral inflammatory disease of unknown cause is a common problem in cats. The degree of inflammation is variable and may be severe. These cats present a diagnostic and therapeutic challenge, and management is frequently frustrating for both the veterinarian and owner. Inflammation may involve the gingiva (gingivitis), buccal mucosa (stomatitis), or tissues of and adjacent to the palatoglossal fold (caudal stomatitis) or pharyngeal area (pharyngitis). Current knowledge about the cause of chronic gingivostomatitis unrelated to periodontal disease in cats is limited. The condition has been referred to as lymphocytic-plasmacytic stomatitis based on the major cellular infiltrate present on histologic examination.

The histologic description is compatible with a chronic inflammatory or immunologic response but does not provide a definitive diagnosis as to the primary cause. Cats with severe chronic gingivostomatitis are often grouped together as all having the same unknown problem; yet, based on clinical presentation and variable response to treatment, it is more likely that multiple factors are involved.

HISTORICAL AND CLINICAL SIGNS

Cats with chronic gingivostomatitis frequently present with a history of dysphagia, inappetence, or anorexia and pain when eating is attempted. The cat may appear interested in food but is unwilling to eat or may attempt to eat but drops the food from its mouth or paws at its muzzle. The affected cat is usually reluctant to eat hard food but may eat soft food. As the severity of the inflammation increases, the cat becomes pickier about what it will eat, or blood-tinged saliva may be noted after eating. In severe cases the cat may be in a great deal of pain, causing a reluctance to swallow and drooling (pseudoptyalism). Weight loss may be a significant problem, depending on the severity and duration of inflammation. Affected cats may exhibit altered behavior such as reduced activity, demonstrating aggressive behavior toward other pets or persons, or expressing an aversion to having their face or head touched. These cats may present with an unkempt appearance resulting from a reluctance to groom because of oral pain. Owners may notice that the cat no longer yawns.

ORAL EXAMINATION

Before examining the oral cavity, the regional lymph nodes should be palpated, and the mandible and maxilla examined for swelling or pain. It may not be possible to complete the initial oral examination if the cat has severe oral pain. In severe cases the inflamed tissues may be ulcerated and bleed readily. Proliferation of oral tissues may make it difficult to visualize the teeth. Cats with severe gingivostomatitis may have extreme pain on opening the mouth; thus the initial examination should be performed with the mouth closed while gently retracting the lips. This examination is performed slowly to minimize pain. The mouth is then opened gently if possible. Lesions of the oral cavity may include inflammation of the gingiva (gingivitis), oral buccal mucosa (stomatitis), and tissues lateral to the palatoglossal fold (caudal stomatitis). Often a complete oral examination is not possible without benefit of sedation or general anesthesia.

DIAGNOSTIC EVALUATION

A complete blood count, biochemical profile, and urinalysis are performed to identify concurrent or contributory diseases. The complete blood count is usually unremarkable. Hyperglobulinemia has been identified in some cats with chronic gingivostomatitis. Serologic evaluation for feline leukemia virus antigen and feline immunodeficiency virus antibody should be performed. It is ideal to include virus isolation studies on specimens obtained from oral swabs of inflamed tissues in cats with gingivostomatitis. Although bacterial cultures are not part of a basic evaluation in most cases, bacterial culture and sensitivity testing may be helpful in chronic cases that do not respond to the antibiotics commonly used for oral infections. A biopsy specimen of any lesion that appears neoplastic or of unknown cause should be obtained and submitted for histopathologic examination.

A complete oral and dental examination is performed with the cat under general anesthesia. The animal is evaluated for periodontal disease, tooth resorption, and other problems that may cause oral inflammation. Dental radiographs are obtained to evaluate for alveolar bone loss (indicating periodontitis), tooth resorption, and to identify retained roots.

MANAGEMENT

The goals of management are aimed at controlling plaque bacteria and decreasing the inflammatory and immunologic response. Controlling the plaque bacteria can be attempted by several methods, including scaling, topical antimicrobial application, systemic antimicrobial therapy, and tooth removal.

Cats that have generalized chronic gingivostomatitis, including caudal stomatitis, are best treated with extraction of all premolars and molars. This includes the extraction of any retained roots. Extraction of the teeth removes the surfaces that are available for plaque retention and consequently decreases plaque and the associated inflammation. Extractions are successful in decreasing inflammation when the plaque is initiating the excessive inflammatory response. Retained roots may be a source of residual bacteria and, if found in association with oral inflammation, should be extracted as well.

When an owner is not willing or able to proceed with extractions of premolars and molars, the cats should be managed with plaque removal, plaque control, and medications to suppress the inflammatory response. The first step is a complete scaling and polishing along with extraction of teeth that show evidence of periodontitis or tooth resorption. Oral antibiotic administration for 4 to 6 weeks following the dental surgery is recommended. In severe cases, when the patient is not eating, it is necessary to decrease the inflammation quickly so the patient will resume eating. To manage the inflammation and maintain appetite initially, most cats require methylprednisolone administration every 4 to 6 weeks and over time possibly as frequently as every 3 weeks. Alternatively other antiinflammatory or immunosuppressive drugs can be considered. Once the inflammation has decreased and the cat is eating, toothbrushing is instituted if the owners are able to adequately brush the teeth and the cat is cooperative. Many owners are not able to brush the teeth sufficiently to decrease plaque accumulation and prevent inflammation. A topical rinse, using a 0.12% chlorhexidine product, is an adjunctive treatment in managing plaque accumulation. I inform the owners on the initial visit that extractions of all premolars and molars provides the best long-term results. Medical management with antibiotics and glucocorticoids generally loses effectiveness over time, and severe clinical signs return, requiring more aggressive medical management or extractions. For these reasons, the author believes that extraction of all premolars and molars provides the best long-term management for the majority of affected cats.

Extractions

Extractions are indicated when there is severe periodontitis or when teeth have type 1 tooth resorption. In addition to extractions for treatment of related periodontal disease and tooth resorption, removing healthy teeth is an option for cats with chronic gingivostomatitis. Plaque bacteria attach to the tooth surfaces (crowns and roots), eliciting an inflammatory response. Oral hygiene directed at plaque control is difficult in cats with severe inflammation and oral pain. Extraction of the premolars and molars removes the surfaces to which plaque attaches and therefore decreases the plaque in the cat's mouth. Dental radiographs are needed to confirm removal of all premolar and molar roots in these cats.

When inflammation is present adjacent to the incisors, they should also be extracted. It is rarely necessary to extract the canine teeth unless they have severe periodontitis or resorptive lesions. The response to extractions is variable, ranging from complete resolution of the inflammation to no improvement, and clients should be so advised. Cats tolerate extractions, even full-mouth extractions, very well and can eat dry and moist cat food without teeth. After extractions some cats may show significant improvement, and medical management may not be required to keep the cat free of clinical signs. Other cats may exhibit a partial response, requiring less aggressive medical management than that required before extractions. Another group of cats appears to have minimal response to extractions, and medical management is continued as before the extractions. In my practice cats that responded poorly to full-mouth extractions often were those in which calicivirus was isolated from the oral cavity or cats that received long-term (months to years) medical management. In a report of 30 cats with gingivitis, stomatitis, and faucitis (caudal stomatitis), the response to periodontal treatment and extraction of selected teeth, including retained root tips, was generally favorable (Hennet, 1994). Oral inflammation resolved completely in 60% (18 of 30) of the cats, with an additional 20% (6 of 30) responding with minimal residual inflammation and no oral pain. None of these 24 cats required medical treatment to manage oral inflammation after the treatment. Initial improvement requiring continued medical therapy to control clinical signs was found in 13% (4 of 30), and no improvement occurred in 7% (2 of 30) of the cats.

When long-term medical management becomes ineffective, or when side effects of drug therapy are unacceptable, extractions of the premolars and molars offer the next option. The maximal clinical improvement may require several weeks in cats with severe and chronic inflammation. Some of these cats may benefit from enteral feeding to maintain an adequate caloric intake (Chapter 3) and balanced nutrition.

Appropriate pain management should also be administered (Chapter 2). Buprenorphine HCL at 0.01 mg/kg to 0.03 mg/kg administered in the cheek (buccal mucosal absorption) every 6 to 12 hours for 3 days is usually adequate for postoperative pain control. Buprenorphine may also be beneficial for pain control in cats with owners who have chosen medical management.

Scaling and Polishing

The teeth should be scaled to remove plaque, bacteria, and calculus. Plaque bacteria may be a factor in the excessive inflammatory response present in these cats. The teeth should be polished after any scaling to smooth the tooth surface. Plaque attaches and becomes established on the tooth surfaces within several hours after the scaling and polishing procedures; therefore continued control measures should be undertaken. Cats with severe oral inflammation are usually in too much pain for toothbrushing to be practical; thus plaque control must be maintained initially with topical or systemic antimicrobial therapy. Once the oral inflammation is well controlled, the owner may attempt plaque control with toothbrushing. A finger toothbrush or small toothbrush designed for cats is used with an acceptably flavored veterinary dentifrice.

Antimicrobial Therapy

Antimicrobial therapy is best accomplished with systemic antibiotic administration. A variable response is observed with antibiotic therapy, although therapy of 4 to 6 weeks may result in improvement of clinical signs in some cats. Antibiotics as a single treatment are rarely effective in the initial management of inflammation, and combined treatment with antibiotics and glucocorticoids is usually required. Amoxicillin–clavulanate acid (Clavamox, Pfizer), clindamycin (Antirobe, Pfizer), and metronidazole are useful antibiotics in managing these cats. Repeated treatment with antibiotics may be necessary. Complete resolution of clinical signs is unlikely, and relapses are common. Topical chlorhexidine may be used for adjunctive antimicrobial therapy.

Antiinflammatory and Immunosuppressive Therapy

Immunosuppressive doses of glucocorticoids are required in most cats to decrease the inflammation and reduce pain sufficiently so the cat will eat. Methylprednisolone acetate (Depo-Medrol, Pfizer) at 15 to 20 mg total dosage intramuscularly, subcutaneously is generally adequate, and cats usually demonstrate a decrease in the oral inflammation and a willingness to eat within 1 to 2 days. Satisfactory results are less common with oral prednisone administration in cats having severe inflammation. For cats demonstrating moderate improvement after extractions and requiring further control of residual inflammation, oral prednisone (1 to 2 mg/kg every other day) may be sufficient; however, higher doses may be required, with the ultimate dose being determined by the response. Clients should be cautioned about potential adverse effects of corticosteroids in cats, including diabetes mellitus and precipitation of congestive heart failure in cats with cardiomyopathy. Alternative immunosuppressive therapies such as gold salts or cyclosporine A (Chapter 55) have also been recommended as treatments, although I have limited experience with these drugs and little information currently available documenting the therapeutic effects of these drugs in affected cats.

Metacam (Merial) is an antiinflammatory that may provide an alternative for short-term control of inflammation before an extraction procedure. Long-term use of Metacam in cats with normal renal function to reduce clinically significant inflammation has had little success in my practice.

Miscellaneous Treatments

A trial treatment of coenzyme Q_{10} (CoQ_{10}) supplementation at 30 to 100 mg daily for 4 months is recommended in cats with residual inflammation following extractions or as a supplement to medical management. There is anecdotal evidence of improvement in cats with chronic gingivostomatitis and humans with chronic periodontitis after 3 to 4 months of supplementation with CoQ_{10}. Prospective studies are needed to prove efficacy.

References and Suggested Reading

Dowers KL, Lappin MR: The association of *Bartonella* spp infection with chronic stomatitis in cats, Proceedings of the American College of Veterinary Internal Medicine, Baltimore, 2005.

Hardy WD, Zuckerman E, Corbishley J: Serological evidence that *Bartonella* causes gingivitis and stomatitis in cats, Proceedings of the 16th Annual Veterinary Dental Forum, Savannah, Ga, October 3–6, 2002, p 79.

Harley R, Gruffydd-Jones TJ, Day MJ: Salivary and serum immunoglobulin levels in cats with chronic gingivostomatitis, *Vet Rec* 152:125, 2003.

Hennet P: Results of periodontal and extraction treatment in cats with gingivo-stomatitis, Proceedings of the World Veterinary Dental Congress, Philadelphia, 1994, p 49.

Lommer MJ, Verstraete FJ: Concurrent oral shedding of feline calicivirus and feline herpesvirus 1 in cats with chronic gingivostomatitis, *Oral Microbiol Immunol* 18:131, 2003.

CHAPTER 110

Oropharyngeal Dysphagia

G. DIANE SHELTON, *La Jolla, California*

Dysphagia, defined as an abnormality in swallowing, can be one of the most difficult diagnostic challenges encountered in clinical veterinary practice. Normal swallowing is a well-coordinated process involving the tongue, hard and soft palate, pharyngeal muscles, esophagus, and gastroesophageal junction. In addition to normally functioning striated muscle and neuromuscular transmission, the integrity of several cranial nerves, including sensory and motor fibers of the trigeminal nerve and facial nerves; the glossopharyngeal, vagus, and hypoglossal nerves; their nuclei in the brainstem; and the swallowing center in the brain reticular formation; are critical to the swallowing process. Difficulties in swallowing may be found in very young animals associated with congenital abnormalities or as an acquired condition in mature animals. Swallowing is a complex process, and abnormalities of this process have been classified functionally based on cineradiographic analysis as the oropharyngeal, esophageal, and gastroesophageal dysphagias (Suter and Watrous, 1980; Watrous and Suter, 1983). Because of the complexity, the diagnosis of swallowing disorders should be approached in a systematic manner. Esophageal and gastroesophageal dysphagias are described in Chapter 111.

As a clinical sign of oropharyngeal dysfunction, dysphagia is relatively common in dogs and less common in cats and can result from either morphologic or functional abnormalities. Structural changes that interfere with swallowing may include traumatic injury, strictures, foreign bodies, or neoplastic processes. Most functional abnormalities are caused by neurologic, peripheral nerve, neuromuscular junction, or primary muscle diseases. Dysphagia may be the sole presenting clinical sign or associated with multiple clinical abnormalities. A common misconception is that dysphagia is a specific disease. The term *cricopharyngeal achalasia* refers to a rare form of dysphagia characterized by inadequate relaxation of the cricopharyngeal muscle occurring in very young animals and surgically treated with a myotomy. Dysphagia may also be part of a generalized inherited myopathy in young dogs such as a muscular dystrophy. It is most commonly an acquired condition in adult dogs with weakness of the pharyngeal muscles, resulting in inadequate propulsion of the bolus from the mouth into the proximal esophagus. In this context dysphagia is a clinical sign of disease and not a specific disease.

FUNCTIONAL ANATOMY

Oropharyngeal dysphagia can be divided into three stages based on the site of dysfunction: the oral, pharyngeal, and cricopharyngeal stages. The oral stage is characterized by bolus accumulation at the base of the tongue. In oral dysphagia there is difficulty in prehending and transporting food to the oropharynx. Rostral-to-caudal pharyngeal constrictors act in concert with the plungerlike action of the tongue to propel the bolus from the base of the tongue to the cricopharyngeal passage in the second or pharyngeal stage. The inability to propel a bolus from the base of the tongue to the cricopharyngeal region is characteristic of pharyngeal dysphagia. The cricopharyngeal or third stage consists of relaxation of the cricopharyngeal muscles (also referred to as the upper esophageal sphincter) and passage of the bolus into the cranial esophagus. Synchrony between constriction of the pharyngeal muscles and relaxation of the cricopharyngeal muscle allows the passage of a bolus into the esophagus. Failure of a normally propelled bolus to pass through the cricopharyngeal region is termed *cricopharyngeal dysphagia*. Clinical signs of the three stages of oropharyngeal dysphagia are described in Table 110-1.

Table 110-1

Clinical Signs Associated With Dysfunction in the Three Stages of Oropharyngeal Dysphagia

Clinical Sign	Oral Stage	Pharyngeal Stage	Cricopharyngeal Stage
Respiratory involvement	No	Yes	Yes
Differential ability to handle liquids and solids	No	Yes	Yes
Reduced gag reflex	Yes	Yes	No
Excessive salivation and drooling	Yes	Yes	Yes
Difficulty prehending food	Yes	No	No
Repeated attempts to swallow	No	Yes	Yes
Excessive head movement	No	Yes	Yes
Dropping food from the mouth	Yes	Yes	Yes

PHYSICAL AND NEUROLOGIC EXAMINATION

An accurate identification of a swallowing disorder is critical to reaching a specific diagnosis and devising a therapeutic plan. Visual examination of the oropharynx under tranquilization or general anesthesia may allow the identification of many of the morphologic abnormalities that cause oral dysphagia, including oral foreign bodies, dental disease, and neoplasia. Evaluation of cranial nerves should be performed, including assessment of tongue and jaw tone and abduction of the arytenoid cartilages with inspiration. Complete physical and neurologic examinations may identify clinical signs of a generalized neuromuscular disorder, including muscle atrophy, stiffness, or depressed or absent spinal reflexes (Glass and Kent, 2000).

Observation of the animal eating and drinking may demonstrate repeated unsuccessful attempts to swallow, excessive head movements, dropping food from the mouth, reingestion of dropped food, and gagging. The gag reflex should be evaluated by placing a finger in the pharynx. The normal response is to repel the finger from the pharyngeal area. An animal with a depressed reflex or absent sensory response may move its head away without actively pushing away the stimulus. Clinical signs of aspiration pneumonia, a common complication, and of esophageal dilation and regurgitation may occur concurrently with pharyngeal dysphagia. The cervical region should be observed for a ballooning esophagus.

DIAGNOSTIC TESTING

Neuromuscular Minimum Database

Once dysphagia has been identified on physical and neurologic examination, whether as the only clinical sign or associated with signs of generalized neuromuscular disease, the following minimum database is suggested: a complete blood count, serum chemistries, including creatine kinase (CK) activity and electrolyte concentrations, urinalysis, evaluation of thyroid function, and the acetylcholine receptor (AChR) antibody titer for acquired myasthenia gravis (MG). A persistently elevated CK, even if only mildly elevated, could be an indication of an underlying inflammatory myopathy. Markedly elevated CK activity may suggest a necrotizing or dystrophic myopathy. Electrolyte abnormalities may be indicative of an endocrine disorder such as Addison's disease. Neuromuscular complications of hypothyroidism have also been described.

Acquired MG is the most commonly diagnosed neuromuscular disorder in my laboratory and should be high on the list of differential diagnoses in dogs with a recent onset of dysphagia, whether alone or as part of a generalized neuromuscular disorder (Shelton, 2002). In a study of a large group of dogs with acquired MG (Shelton, Schule, and Kass, 1997), focal signs, including pharyngeal, esophageal, and laryngeal weakness without clinically detectable limb muscle weakness, were described in 43% of dogs. Pharyngeal weakness, as the only clinical sign of MG, was described in 1% of the myasthenic dogs. Similarly focal signs, including megaesophagus and dysphagia, were described in 14% of cats in a similar study (Shelton, Ho, and Kass, 2000).

Imaging Modalities

Lateral survey radiographs of the neck are necessary to exclude radiodense foreign bodies or space-occupying lesions as causes of dysphagia. Thoracic radiographs may also demonstrate megaesophagus, a cranial mediastinal mass, or metastatic lung disease. Since swallowing is not a static process, motility should be evaluated fluoroscopically using both liquids and solids. All three phases of swallowing can be evaluated; the three stages of the oropharyngeal phase can also be separately evaluated.

Most recently magnetic resonance imaging (MRI) has been used to identify inflammatory lesions in difficult-to-diagnose cases of dysphagia (Fig. 110-1, Platt et al, 2006). In inflammatory myopathies, cellular infiltrates can have a patchy or multifocal distribution and be missed on individual biopsy specimens. The MRI examination can aid in locating lesions and guiding a diagnostic biopsy, or it can be used for follow-up examinations. Neoplasia involving cranial nerves may also be evident on MRI evaluations. Areas of hyperintensity may also be identified on screening examinations when the diagnosis is in question. Since dysphagia may be the primary clinical abnormality in dogs with inflammatory myopathies (Ryckman et al., 2005) without other clinically evident signs of generalized weakness, imaging studies should be performed as an early diagnostic procedure.

If a central cause of pharyngeal dysphagia is suspected based on the clinical signs and neurologic examination, evaluation of the brain by MRI should be performed along with concurrent evaluation of the cerebrospinal fluid. Evaluation of intracranial diseases is described in standard textbooks of veterinary neurology.

Electrodiagnostic Testing

Electrodiagnostic evaluation, including electromyography and measurement of motor and sensory nerve conduction velocities, can provide important information as to the severity, distribution, and character of a myopathic or neuropathic disease process. In addition to evaluation of limb muscles, testing should also include evaluation of the pharyngeal muscles and tongue. Results of these studies can help guide the direction of biopsy procedures. Electrodiagnostics are performed by specialists trained in the procedures, are generally available only at referral centers, and must be performed under general anesthesia. Since a lengthy anesthesia is required for these procedures, the health status of the animal must be taken into consideration, weighing the risks and benefits. In cases of suspected MG, evaluation of the serum AChR antibody titer should be performed before anesthesia. If the antibody titer is negative and a diagnosis of MG is still a consideration, electrodiagnostic testing can then be performed to measure the

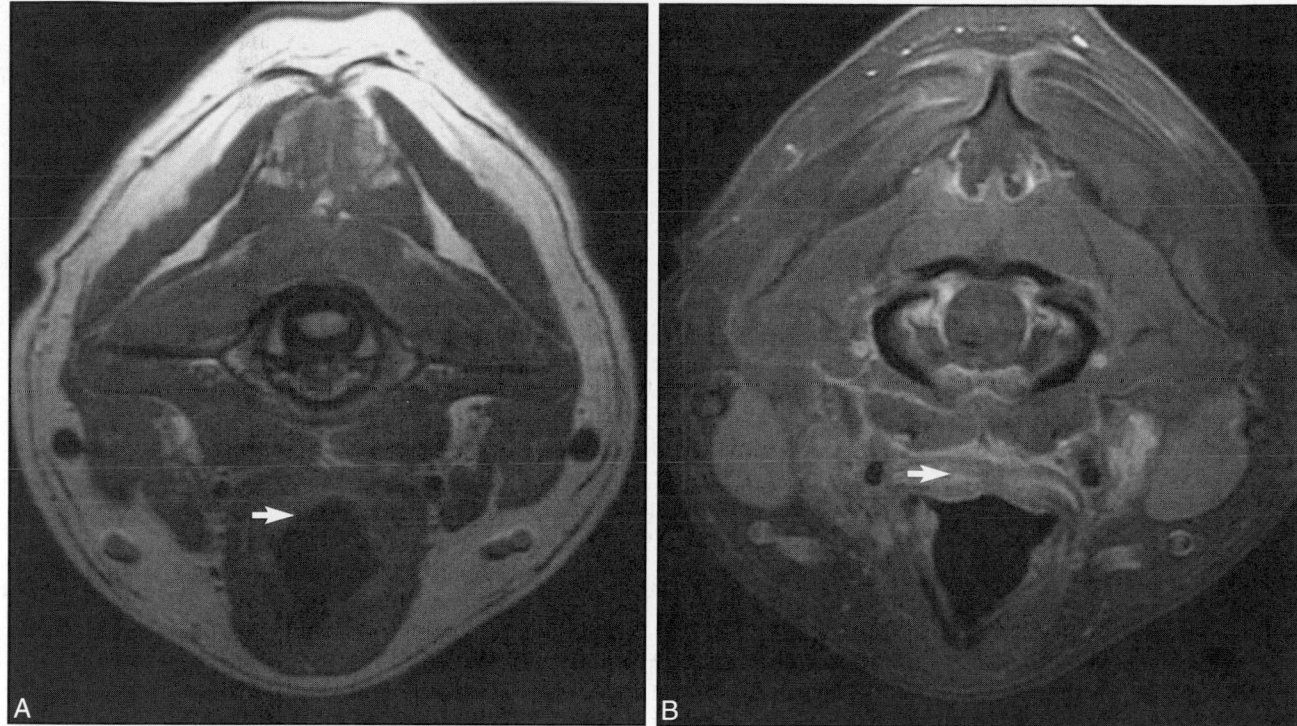

Fig. 110-1   A, Transverse T1-weighted image of the laryngeal and pharyngeal muscles in a 2.5-year-old female Briard with dysphagia. There is a mild isointense to hyperintense signal present compared to normal muscle. (*TR,* 500 ms; *TE,* 10 ms; *arrow head* is pharyngeal muscle, *arrow* is laryngeal muscle). **B,** Transverse T1-weighted image of the laryngeal and pharyngeal muscles post-contrast administration demonstrating a hyperintense signal in the associated musculature. (*TR,* 500 ms; *TE,* 10 ms; *arrow head* is pharyngeal muscle, *arrow* is laryngeal muscle). (Courtesy Dr. Simon Platt.)

decremental response to supramaximal repetitive nerve stimulation. This should be performed only if the dog is stable and aspiration pneumonia is under control. In most cases electrodiagnostics do not provide a specific diagnosis but can indicate whether the underlying disease process is myopathic or neuropathic and the pattern of muscle and peripheral nerve involvement. A complete discussion of electrodiagnostic testing is described elsewhere (Cuddon, 2002).

Muscle and Nerve Biopsies

The goal of diagnostic testing is to identify a specific disease and formulate a treatment plan. With the exception of MG, which is best diagnosed by the serum AChR antibody titer, and the congenital myotonias, which are identified by electromyography, the muscle biopsy and in some cases the peripheral nerve biopsy are the only ways to reach a specific diagnosis. If the problem is in the muscle or nerve, go to the source of the problem. As with most treatable neuromuscular diseases, the goal is to reach an accurate diagnosis early in the course of the disease, before fibrosis and myofiber loss is extensive and treatment options become few. In cases of pharyngeal dysphagia, a biopsy should be obtained from a pharyngeal muscle if possible, in addition to a biopsy from a large proximal pelvic limb muscle such as the vastus lateralis or a thoracic limb muscle such as the triceps muscle.

If a pharyngeal muscle biopsy is not possible, a limb muscle biopsy may provide the diagnosis. A complete discussion of how to correctly collect and prepare muscle and nerve biopsy specimens is described elsewhere (Dickinson and LeCouteur, 2002).

TREATMENT

The treatment of oropharyngeal dysphagias depends on the underlying cause and whether the condition is congenital or acquired and morphologic or functional. Unfortunately an underlying cause in cases of congenital dysphagia is only rarely found. Very little information is in the literature accurately describing these disorders, but most are likely neurogenic in origin. If a failure of relaxation of the cricopharyngeal muscle can be identified, a myotomy may be of benefit. If there is asynchrony between the pharyngeal constrictors and relaxation of the cricopharyngeal muscle, a myotomy is contraindicated. If a morphologic disorder is identified such as stricture, foreign body, neoplasia, or structural abnormality, treatment should be directed to the specific abnormality. In my experience the majority of cases of dysphagia occur in mature animals, are acquired, and are associated with an underlying neuromuscular disease. Many of the neuromuscular diseases such as MG and polymyositis are treatable; thus an early diagnosis and appropriate therapy should increase the chances of a positive clinical outcome. In inflammatory myopathies, once muscle mass is lost and fibrosis is significant, the chance of regaining normal muscle mass and function is poor. If severe aspiration pneumonia is present, the prognosis is also poor for recovery. Specific treatments for MG, inflammatory myopathies, and other neuromuscular diseases are covered in Chapters 241and 242.

In all cases supportive care is important, but particularly for the pharyngeal dysphagias in which aspiration pneumonia is a risk. If aspiration pneumonia is identified, specific respiratory therapy should be initiated (Chapter 149). Appropriate fluid and nutritional support should be provided, and a gastrostomy tube should be placed if necessary to provide adequate nutrition and lessen aspiration pneumonia.

PROGNOSIS

The prognosis depends on early recognition of dysphagia, identification of an underlying cause, and the presence of a treatable disease. Although the most common causes of acquired dysphagia such as MG, myositis, and possibly the endocrine myopathies associated with hypothyroidism and Addison's disease are treatable, they must be diagnosed early in the course of the disease for the best clinical outcome. Many neuromuscular diseases are not treatable, such as the muscular dystrophies and most of the peripheral neuropathies, and the prognosis for recovery is poor in these cases. Aspiration pneumonia and severe debilitation may present fatal complications.

References and Suggested Reading

Cuddon PA: Electrophysiology in neuromuscular disease, *Vet Clin North Am Small Anim Pract* 32:31, 2002.

Dickinson PJ, LeCouteur RA: Muscle and nerve biopsy, *Vet Clin North Am Small Anim Pract* 32:63, 2002.

Glass EN, Kent M: The clinical examination for neuromuscular disease, *Vet Clin North Am Small Anim Pract* 32:1, 2002.

Platt SR et al: Magnetic resonance imaging in the diagnosis of canine inflammatory myopathies: report of 3 cases, *Vet Radiol Ultrasound* 47:532, 2006.

Ryckman LR et al: Dysphagia as the primary clinical abnormality in two dogs with inflammatory myopathy, *J Am Med Vet Assoc* 226:1519, 2005.

Shelton GD, Myasthenia gravis and disorders of neuromuscular transmission, *Vet Clin North Am Small Anim Pract* 32:189, 2002.

Shelton GD, Schule A, Kass PH: Risk factors for acquired myasthenia gravis in dogs: 1,154 cases (1991-1995), *J Am Med Vet Assoc* 211:1428, 1997.

Shelton GD, Ho M, Kass PH: Risk factors for acquired myasthenia gravis in cats: 105 cases (1986-1998), *J Am Vet Med Assoc* 216:55, 2000.

Suter PF, Watrous BJ: Oropharyngeal dysphagias in the dog: a cinefluorographic analysis of experimentally induced and spontaneously occurring swallowing disorders. I. Oral stage and pharyngeal stage dysphagias, *Vet Radiol* 21:24, 1980.

Watrous BJ, Suter PF: Oropharyngeal dysphagias in the dog: a cinefluorographic analysis of experimentally induced and spontaneously occurring swallowing disorders. II. Cricopharyngeal stage and mixed oropharyngeal dysphagias, *Vet Radiol* 24:11, 1983.

CHAPTER **111**

Esophagitis

MICHAEL D. WILLARD, *College Station, Texas*
ELIZABETH W. CARSTEN, *Oro Valley, Arizona*

PATHOPHYSIOLOGY

Esophagitis (inflammation of the esophageal mucosa) is most often caused by gastric acid, other caustic substances, or trauma (e.g., foreign objects). Of these, gastric acid is probably the most common cause of clinically serious esophagitis. Esophagitis can develop when the esophageal mucosa is exposed to excessive acid because of gastroesophageal reflux (GER), frequent vomiting of gastric acid (e.g., parvoviral enteritis), or production of greater than normal amounts of acid (e.g., gastrinoma). In GER gastric contents move into the esophagus unrelated to vomiting. Normal animals experience occasional GER without harm because esophageal peristalsis quickly returns acid to the stomach. However, severe mucosal damage may ensue when acid persists in or repeatedly enters the esophagus. For example, chronic esophagitis caused by spontaneous GER is well reported in cats (Han, Broussard, and Baer, 2003; Gualtieri and Olivero, 2006), and it is usually the result of hiatal hernia or lower esophageal sphincter (LES) abnormalities.

Anesthetized animals are a special case because acid can linger in the esophagus for minutes to hours. Anesthesia-associated reflux appears to be an important cause of esophagitis and stricture formation, with approximately 65% of esophageal strictures being attributed to anesthetic-associated esophagitis in two studies (Melendez et al., 1998; Leib et al., 2001). The choice of preanesthetic and anesthetic agents, length of preoperative fasting, age, and intraabdominal versus extraabdominal procedures may influence the incidence of intraoperative GER (Wilson and Walshaw, 2004), but esophagitis caused by anesthesia-associated GER occurs erratically and unpredictably.

Nonacid damage may include drug-induced esophagitis, especially from doxycycline (Melendez, Twedt, and Wright, 2000). Cats occasionally lick caustics (e.g., benzalkonium chloride) off of their fur, sustaining oral and esophageal lesions. Bones and fishhooks are probably the most common canine esophageal foreign objects, but they seldom cause strictures because they typically produce only focal inflammation. Recently there have been anecdotal reports of chew treats causing circumferential damage in the canine esophagus, and cats occasionally have hairballs that can cause a similar lesion. Finally the esophagus may be infected primarily (e.g., pythiosis) or secondarily in immunodeficient patients (e.g., dogs being treated with steroids, azathioprine, or cyclosporin for immune-mediated disorders). Rarely an esophageal tumor causes mucosal inflammation.

When the esophagus becomes inflamed, motility can be impaired, allowing food to be retained and ultimately regurgitated. More important, poor esophageal motility allows acid refluxed into the esophagus to remain longer, worsening the esophagitis. LES dysfunction may occur secondary to esophagitis, allowing more GER. Chronic esophagitis caused by GER can be associated with severe histologic changes in the distal esophagus, including metaplastic changes somewhat comparable to Barrett's esophagus in humans (Gualtieri and Olivero, 2006; Han, Broussard, and Baer, 2003). If the mucosal damage is severe (e.g., penetrating to the muscularis), healing may be accompanied by cicatrix and esophageal stricture. Most strictures resulting from GER occur between the thoracic inlet and the diaphragm, where GER typically causes the most severe damage. Strictures cranial to the thoracic inlet are often secondary to foreign objects, but severe reflux can cause acid-induced injuries in this region.

CLINICAL SIGNS

The magnitude of clinical signs depends on the severity and depth of the esophageal inflammation and the presence and degree of stricture. Animals with esophagitis may regurgitate or be anorexic (ostensibly because of esophageal pain). The more severe the inflammation, the more severe is the anorexia. Blood is seldom present in regurgitated material. If a caustic agent was ingested, there might be contributory lingual and oral burns. Vomiting may be prominent in some patients, but in that case the esophagitis is usually secondary to the cause of the vomiting.

Signs of esophagitis secondary to anesthesia-associated GER often begin 1 to 3 days and occasionally up to 2 weeks after a causative anesthetic event (Wilson and Walshaw, 2004). Esophagitis may produce immediate (caused by inflammation) or delayed (caused by stricture) signs.

Animals with profuse vomiting may begin to regurgitate concurrently. Regurgitation in animals that were previously vomiting suggests that esophagitis has developed secondary to the vomiting and persistent exposure of the esophageal mucosa to excessive gastric acid. Animals with previously asymptomatic esophageal disease (e.g., mild esophageal dilation) that vomit (e.g., acute gastritis, foreign object) can retain substantial amounts of gastric acid in the dysfunctional esophagus. They may subsequently start regurgitating because of the resulting esophagitis.

Clinical signs of stricture depend on the degree of obstruction. In general, the narrower the stricture, the more pronounced is the regurgitation. Animals with mild-to-moderate obstruction often ingest and retain liquids (if not drunk too fast) and sometimes soft foods (if eaten slowly and in small amounts). Obstructions closer to the mouth usually cause more immediate regurgitation because of the smaller esophageal luminal reservoir proximal to the obstruction. Pain may occur if the esophagus is forcefully pushing a food bolus against a stricture. Modest obstructions may cause no signs until the patient attempts to swallow a large food bolus or foreign object. Sometimes there is obvious progression in severity as the stricture matures and contracts, causing greater obstruction.

DIAGNOSIS

Esophagitis or esophageal stricture may be suspected from the history (as described previously) or from clinical circumstances. Survey thoracic radiographs are seldom diagnostic; esophageal dilation is often minimal or absent. Mediastinal or pleural air or fluid may indicate perforation. Contrast radiographs are often diagnostic of strictures but are unreliable in detecting inflammation. If perforation seems likely (e.g., pneumothorax or septic pleural effusion), contrast films are seldom needed. But, if one is unsure and believes the contrast study is indicated, an iodinated contrast agent should be used instead of barium. Otherwise barium often provides a more definitive study.

Esophagitis is suggested by an irregular esophageal mucosa with some retention of barium. Liquid barium may quickly pass through a partial stricture, making it easy to miss the obstruction, even when using fluoroscopy. Nonetheless, liquid barium should be administered first so that any aspiration will produce minimal morbidity. If no lesions are detected using liquid barium, barium mixed with canned food (this should be a relatively solid consistency as opposed to a more liquid form) should be used next. Fluoroscopy is preferred over static images because it may reveal partial obstructions not seen with the latter (i.e., a bolus may "squeeze" through a partial stricture in the period between the bolus being eaten and the radiograph being obtained). Barium paste offers no substantive advantage and should be avoided.

Hiatal hernia can be easy or extremely difficult to diagnose. Some animals have obvious abnormalities on plain thoracic radiographs, whereas others have normal barium contrast studies, even when fluoroscopy is used. Diagnosis may require administering liquid barium and viewing the LES area fluoroscopically while applying pressure to the abdomen. This maneuver may force the gastric fundus through the hernia, confirming the diagnosis. This technique may also reveal GER; however, it can be difficult to distinguish "innocent" from clinically significant reflux. Sometimes endoscopy is the most sensitive way to diagnose hiatal hernia.

Endoscopy is the most *sensitive and specific* way to detect esophagitis. Erythema, friability, bleeding, erosions, and exudative pseudomembranes usually are obvious. The esophageal mucosa just aboral to the cricopharyngeal sphincter normally is a little rougher than the rest of the esophagus. Humans can have esophagitis that can only be diagnosed histopathologically, but such cases have not been well documented in dogs and cats. Nonneoplastic canine esophageal mucosa is difficult to biopsy adequately with flexible endoscopic biopsy forceps. Rigid forceps are often necessary to obtain a biopsy specimen of canine esophageal mucosa that is not obviously diseased. Distal feline esophageal mucosa is easier to sample with flexible forceps.

There are a few potential pitfalls when looking for strictures endoscopically. Although typically strictures are obvious at endoscopy, large dogs may have an esophageal stricture that decreases the luminal diameter by 50% or more and yet is missed by the endoscopist. The scope diameter can be so small when compared with the esophageal lumen of a larger-breed dog that the tip of the scope readily passes through a partial stricture without the operator noticing that the luminal diameter was diminished. This error is especially likely if the stricture is near the LES (i.e., the endoscopist believes that cicatrix is simply the normal LES). This is particularly significant because many strictures occur near the LES. When the tip of the endoscope cannot pass through a stricture, one cannot determine the extent of the stricture or if other strictures exist further aboral. Postanesthetic strictures in particular may be focal or extensive (up to 15 cm has been reported; Wilson and Walshaw, 2004), and there may be a poorer prognosis when attempting to dilate longer, more extensive strictures.

THERAPY

Inflamed esophageal mucosa usually heals if it is protected from further damage. Therefore it is important to eliminate predisposing factors (e.g., hiatal hernia), foreign objects, or predisposing drug therapy. Preventing further exposure to gastric acid is usually the crucial aspect. Esophageal mucosa is more easily damaged by acid than is gastric mucosa because the esophagus does not have a mucus-bicarbonate preepithelial barrier and does not heal by epithelial restitution (also see Chapter 114 on Gastric Ulceration). Furthermore, endogenous prostaglandins are not as effective in protecting the esophageal epithelial surface, and the esophagus does not produce a "mucus cap" after epithelial injury. Thus minute amounts of acid can severely damage the esophagus, and healing requires preventing additional vomiting or GER. Human esophagitis usually results from GER, and effective therapy requires prokinetic drugs to keep the stomach empty and/or drugs that lessen or eliminate acid secretion.

Metoclopramide (a prokinetic agent effective in the stomach) is minimally effective in preventing esophagitis caused by GER in humans, but cisapride (Propulsid, Janssen) was clearly beneficial before its use in humans was curtailed because of adverse cardiac effects. Cisapride was at least as effective as histamine-2 (H_2) receptor antagonists, and cisapride plus an H_2 receptor antagonist was more effective than the latter by itself. The main disadvantage of cisapride therapy is that it is administered orally (and hence may never reach the stomach in regurgitating patients), whereas metoclopramide may be given parenterally. Cisapride was particularly effective in preventing recurrence after esophagitis had been brought under control. We prefer cisapride at 0.25 mg/kg every 8 to 12 hours and use metoclopramide if cisapride cannot be administered successfully.

H_2 receptor antagonists inhibit gastric acid secretion, thus diminishing the volume that can be refluxed into the esophagus. These drugs are competitive inhibitors of gastric acid secretion (see Chapter 114). Although effective in treating milder forms of human esophagitis, they are not as useful in severe esophagitis. This is probably because H_2 receptor antagonists may increase the gastric pH only to between 4.0 and 5.0, which, although effective in treating gastric ulcers, may be inadequate for esophageal disease. Using larger and more frequent doses of more potent H_2 receptor antagonists is more effective in humans because of greater suppression of acid secretion. The same is probably true in dogs and cats, but objective data are lacking. In humans H_2 receptor antagonists that have gastric prokinetic activity (e.g., nizatidine) may be more effective than those that do not (e.g., cimetidine, famotidine) (Hamamoto et al., 2005).

Proton pump inhibitors are noncompetitive and diminish gastric acid secretion to a much greater degree for a much longer time than do the H_2 receptor antagonists. The two most commonly used proton pump inhibitors in the United States are omeprazole and lansoprazole. Therapy with omeprazole can produce near anacidity in the stomach and refluxed material. Consequently these drugs may be effective in patients that are resistant to H_2 receptor antagonists. We prefer omeprazole 0.7 to 2 mg/kg every 12 to 24 hours. Once- or twice-daily therapy lends itself to greater client compliance than does the schedule of every 6 to 8 hours required with some H_2 receptor antagonists. Omeprazole is recommended primarily when severe esophagitis occurs or is anticipated. The medical therapy that we prefer in severely affected patients has been a combination of cisapride and omeprazole. Unfortunately omeprazole is given orally and may be regurgitated before it reaches the stomach, and it requires 2 to 5 days to attain maximal gastric acid suppression. We generally use H_2 receptor antagonists if oral omeprazole cannot be administered successfully or if one cannot wait 2 to 5 days for maximal gastric acid suppression. Lansoprazole is at least as effective as omeprazole in humans, and there are anecdotal reports of its use in dogs (1 mg/kg, IV, every 24 hours) and cats.

A gastrostomy tube is recommended to ensure adequate nutrition while minimizing esophageal mucosal irritation. These tubes also allow administration of cisapride and omeprazole with confidence. Esophagostomy and pharyngostomy tubes may perpetuate esophageal inflammation (via continued contact between the tube and the ulcerated mucosa) and are not recommended. Aggressive medical management (i.e., cisapride, omeprazole, and gastrostomy feeding tube) is strongly recommended for patients with severe disease or inflamed strictures.

Orally administered sucralfate has been used for esophagitis. Although this therapy intuitively makes sense, studies in humans have usually demonstrated minimal or no benefit. One probably must time the sucralfate administration to coincide with high acid levels in the otherwise neutral esophagus if sucralfate is to function as desired. Therefore there is some rationale for administering sucralfate and hoping that, if GER occurs, the sucralfate will be carried back into the esophagus, where it will be effective because of the now acid esophageal environment.

Corticosteroids are often administered systemically to try to prevent stricture formation; however, they are of uncertain efficacy. Humans ingesting caustic agents such as sodium hydroxide (which causes an extremely severe lesion) are not clearly benefited by such therapy and might be at increased risk of infection. However, dogs and cats seldom have such a severe lesion, and they might benefit. Antibiotics are often used to protect denuded esophageal mucosa from bacterial infection. Although antibiotics intuitively seem indicated in these patients, they have not clearly aided the healing of esophagitis. If antibiotics are used, one should choose broad-spectrum drugs that are also effective against the anaerobic bacteria that are commonly found in the oral cavity (e.g., *Prevotella* spp., *Porphyromonas* spp., *Fusobacterium* spp., *Bacteroides* spp.).

Ballooning and bougienage are used to eliminate strictures. Surgical resection of esophageal strictures should be considered only as a last-ditch, salvage option because strictures commonly recur at the surgical site. Bougienage allows more force to be applied to the stricture than is possible with a balloon, which is important for patients with large amounts of thick, fibrous cicatrix that balloons cannot break down and for strictures so small that balloons cannot be inserted through them. Studies in humans suggest that bougienage is about as effective and safe as balloon dilation. Bougienage can be more traumatic and cause perforation; however, side effects and complications seem more operator dependent than technique dependent. Ballooning may be less likely to cause esophageal perforation, especially when bougienage is performed by an inexperienced operator. However, neither technique is completely safe. If ballooning is chosen over bougienage, the procedure is best performed by using over-the-wire or through-the-scope esophageal balloons. Flexible guidewires seem to reduce the risk of iatrogenic esophageal trauma from the tip of the catheter cutting into the esophagus during inflation.

The endoscopist should visualize the stricture site while it is being dilated. It is important to minimize the amount of trauma so as to minimize the likelihood of stricture recurrence. In particular one should avoid creating deep fissures and removing mucosa from the site (something that is easy to do when aspirating blood or moving the endoscope back and forth through the site). It is often better to plan on several less aggressive procedures in animals with extensive strictures, each causing minimal trauma, as opposed to attempting one aggressive dilation that ultimately causes more trauma, making stricture recurrence more likely. In general two-to-four dilation procedures are typically needed (Melendez et al.,

1998; Leib et al, 2001; Wilson and Walshaw, 2004), but 10 to 15 may be needed in some difficult cases. In some difficult cases mild dilation is performed two to three times weekly in an attempt to maintain patency of the stricture site while causing as little trauma as possible. Intralesional steroid injection and three or four quadrant notchings of the stricture before dilation may be considered in severe cases. Intralesional steroid injection seems to have a place in the treatment of difficult-to-resolve benign strictures in humans (Altintas et al, 2004). Finally, overinflation of the esophagus should be avoided lest tension pneumothorax develop from esophageal rupture.

The esophagus should be evaluated gently after the procedure to detect excessive iatrogenic trauma. The thorax should be radiographed after difficult procedures or if there is any hint of respiratory difficulty to detect pneumothorax secondary to esophageal rupture. Conservative medical care (which may include gastrostomy and/or chest tubes) often allows healing if the esophagus is excessively traumatized or if pneumothorax develops.

Patients with esophagitis caused by ongoing acid reflux should usually be reexamined by endoscopy again after 5 to 8 days of medical therapy, and oral feeding reinitiated if the esophagus has healed. After the patient is able to eat normally without regurgitating, medical therapy can be tapered or perhaps discontinued. If the esophagitis was the result of a nonrecurring cause (e.g., foreign body), repeat endoscopy is usually unnecessary unless signs of dysfunction persist. Animals in which strictures were dilated may be reexamined endoscopically 5 to 7 days after the procedure. However, if the patient is eating without difficulty, a repeat endoscopy is probably unnecessary, although rare patients have stricture recurrence weeks to months later. Patients with stricture plus severe esophagitis and those with very extensive, long strictures should be closely monitored because these are usually the most difficult to manage. Repeat endoscopic procedures are usually important in such patients. Occasionally additional strictures arise (usually close to the LES) while the first one is being treated. Patients that have severe strictures or ones that continually recur after ballooning might benefit from intralesional injection of steroids (Altintas et al., 2004). The goal is not necessarily to eliminate the stricture altogether but rather to achieve an esophageal lumen that is large enough to allow the animal to eat without regurgitating (although this sometimes means feeding softened foods).

PROGNOSIS

Prognosis typically depends in part on the underlying cause. Animals with GER secondary to congenital hiatal hernias often require surgical correction, but their prognosis is usually reasonably good. There is currently no evidence that animals experiencing anesthesia-induced GER and subsequent stricture are at increased risk for recurrence if reanesthetized. If the animal is treated before the inflammation is severe enough to cause a stricture, the prognosis is usually better. Strictures accompanied by substantial inflammation seem more difficult to resolve, and the owners should be prepared for multiple dilation procedures. Typically animals with severe inflammation are salvageable if the owner can afford the multiple procedures that may be necessary. Success rates of 77% to 88% have been reported in animals undergoing stricture dilation, depending on the definition of success (Melendez et al., 1998; Leib et al., 2001; Wilson and Walshaw, 2004). If the esophageal stricture cannot be resolved or if the stricture is caused by terminal malignancy, a permanent, low-profile gastrostomy device may palliate the patient. Esophageal stents can have more problems in dogs and cats than in humans because of the change in direction of the esophagus at the thoracic inlet.

References and Suggested Reading

Altintas E : Intralesional steroid injection in benign esophageal strictures resistant to bougie dilation, *J Gastroenterol Hepatol* 19:1388, 2004.

Gualtieri M, Olivero D: Reflux esophagitis in three cats associated with metaplastic columnar esophageal epithelium, *J Am Anim Hosp Assoc* 42:65, 2006.

Hamamoto N et al: Comparative study of nizatidine and famotidine for maintenance therapy of erosive esophagitis, *J Gastroenterol Hepatol* 20:281, 2005.

Han E, Broussard J, Baer KE: Feline esophagitis secondary to gastroesophageal reflux disease: clinical signs and radiographic, endoscopic, and histopathologic findings, *J Am Anim Hosp Assoc* 39:161, 2003.

Leib MS et al: Endoscopic balloon dilation of benign esophageal strictures in dogs and cats, *J Vet Intern Med* 15:547, 2001.

Melendez LD, Twedt DC, Wright M: Suspected doxycycline-induced esophagitis with esophageal stricture formation in three cats, *Feline Pract* 28:10, 2000.

Melendez LD et al: Conservative therapy using balloon dilation for intramural, inflammatory esophageal strictures in dogs and cats: a retrospective study of 23 cases (1987–1997), *Eur J Comp Gastroenterol* 3:31, 1998.

Sellon RK, Willard MD: Esophagitis and esophageal strictures, *Vet Clin North Am* 33:945, 2003.

Wilson DV, Walshaw R: Postanesthetic esophageal dysfunction in 13 dogs, *J Am Anim Hosp Assoc* 40:455, 2004.

Wilson D, Evans A, Miller R: Effects of preanesthetic administration of morphine on gastroesophageal reflux and regurgitation during anesthesia in dogs, *Am J Vet Res* 66:386, 2005.

CHAPTER 112
Canine Megaesophagus

BETH M. JOHNSON, *Knoxville, Tennessee*
ROBERT C. DeNOVO, *Knoxville, Tennessee*
ERICK A. MEARS, *Tampa, Florida*

Symptoms of esophageal disease occur when esophageal motility is disturbed or when there is obstruction to the movement of ingesta. Swallowing becomes difficult, even painful, and food will not go down. Regurgitation, dysphagia, and ptyalism are common signs; and aspiration pneumonia is a frequent complication. Typically both liquid and solid foods pass poorly with motility disturbances of the esophagus, whereas liquids often pass easily with obstruction of the esophagus. A thorough physical examination and often an extensive diagnostic workup are necessary for determining the cause of esophageal disease and designing a treatment plan. Box 112-1 lists the primary causes of esophageal dysfunction in the dog.

FUNCTIONAL ANATOMY

The esophagus is not simply a tube through which food passes. It is an organ with complex innervation and patterns of motility designed to transport fluid and food efficiently from the pharynx to the stomach. The esophagus begins at the pharyngoesophageal junction, commonly referred to as the upper esophageal sphincter (UES), which prevents reflux and aspiration of ingesta from the esophagus. The body of the canine esophagus consists of two layers of skeletal muscle that propel ingesta to the stomach. The gastroesophageal junction, referred to as the lower esophageal sphincter (LES), is the distal limit of the esophagus and prevents reflux of gastric content into the esophagus.

The UES separates the pharynx from the cervical portion of the esophagus and is formed by the cricopharyngeus and thyropharyngeus muscles dorsolaterally and the cricoid cartilage ventrally. These striated muscles are innervated by the glossopharyngeal, pharyngeal, and recurrent laryngeal branches of the vagus nerve that originate in the brainstem nucleus ambiguus. The muscles of the sphincter remain contracted at all times, except during a swallow, when they relax momentarily to allow passage of a bolus. The muscles contract promptly to maintain closure of the sphincter and protect against esophagopharyngeal reflux and aspiration.

Box **112-1**

Disorders of the Esophagus

Motility Disorders
- Megaesophagus
- Congenital
- Acquired
  - Primary (idiopathic)
  - Secondary (see Box 112-2)
- Dysautonomia
- Hiatal hernia?

Inflammatory Disease
- Esophagitis
- Gastroesophageal reflux
- Hiatal hernia

Obstructive Lesions
- Foreign body
- Stricture
- Vascular ring anomaly
- Neoplasia

Miscellaneous
- Diverticula
- Bronchoesophageal fistula

In contrast to the feline esophagus that is composed of smooth muscle in the distal one third, the canine esophageal body is composed entirely of two oblique layers of skeletal muscle and is innervated by the somatic branches of the vagus nerve. The LES is a physiologic sphincter rather than a true anatomic sphincter because it does not consist of a distinct muscle mass. It consists of an outer layer of longitudinal striated muscle and an inner layer of circular smooth muscle that merge with the smooth muscle of the stomach. The LES remains closed except to allow passage of a bolus. Competence of the LES is maintained by the gastric rugal folds, the muscular sling of the right crus of the diaphragm, the oblique angle of the gastroesophageal junction, and gastric compression on the esophagus. This sphincter separates the esophagus from the cardia of the stomach and allows ingesta to pass into the stomach while preventing reflux of stomach content into the esophagus. Cholinergic, nonadrenergic noncholinergic, and myogenic mechanisms all play a role in maintaining gastroesophageal sphincter tone. Increases in tone, which serve to protect the esophagus from gastroesophageal reflux, are mediated by moderately increased intragastric pressure; acid in the cardia; high-protein diet; and a number of hormones such as gastrin, histamine, and acetylcholine (ACh). Conversely, marked increases in intragastric pressure decrease sphincter tone to facilitate eructation and prevent gastric rupture.

Esophageal contraction occurs in response to swallowing (primary peristalsis) and esophageal distention (secondary peristalsis). The oropharyngeal phase of swallowing and the movement of food through the UES initiate primary peristalsis. Afferent vagal receptors in the pharynx and proximal esophagus are stimulated by the presence of food; solids are more effective than liquid in stimulating a swallowing reflex. The origin of the vagus nerve, the nucleus ambiguus for striated muscle, initiates an efferent response via the somatic nerve fibers of the vagus. This neuronal pathway ends at the myoneural junction with a coordinated contraction of the UES and propagation of a peristaltic wave aborally along the body of the esophagus, through the LES, and into the stomach. Remaining intraluminal ingesta within the esophagus stimulate esophageal afferent receptors to initiate a secondary peristaltic wave to clear the lumen. Any disease or lesion affecting any part of this neuromuscular pathway can alter normal esophageal motility and cause megaesophagus (Box 112-2).

Box **112-2**

Diseases Associated With and Causes of Megaesophagus in the Dog

Central Nervous System
- Distemper
- Cervical vertebral instability with leukomalacia
- Brainstem lesions
- Neoplasia
- Trauma

Peripheral Neuropathies
- Polyneuritis
- Polyradiculoneuritis
- Ganglioradiculitis
- Dysautonomia
- Giant cell axonal neuropathy
- Spinal muscular atrophy
- Toxicity
  - Lead
  - Thallium
  - Acrylamide
- Bilateral vagal damage

Neuromuscular Junction
- Myasthenia gravis
- Botulism
- Tetanus
- Anticholinesterase toxicity

Esophageal Musculature
- Esophagitis
- Systemic lupus erythematosus
- Glycogen storage disease
- Polymyositis
- Dermatomyositis
- Cachexia
- Trypanosomiasis
- Hypoadrenocorticism
- Hypothyroidism?

Miscellaneous
- Pyloric stenosis
- Gastric dilation volvulus
- Pituitary dwarfism
- Thymoma
- Mediastinitis

MEGAESOPHAGUS

Megaesophagus is a condition characterized by decreased or absent esophageal motility that usually results in diffuse dilation of the esophagus. Megaesophagus occurs as a congenital disorder that becomes clinically apparent at or shortly after weaning, or it can occur as an acquired disorder in a previously normal adult. Acquired megaesophagus can be secondary to a variety of diseases that cause neuromuscular dysfunction, or it can occur as a primary disorder for which the cause is unknown (idiopathic megaesophagus).

Congenital Megaesophagus

Congenital megaesophagus occurs in both pure and mixed-breed dogs. It is known to be inherited in the wire-haired fox terrier as an autosomal-recessive trait and in the miniature schnauzer as either an autosomal-dominant or autosomal-recessive trait with partial penetrance. Congenital megaesophagus occurs with increased prevalence in Great Danes, German shepherds, Labrador retrievers, Newfoundlands, Chinese shar-peis, and Irish setters. Although not proved, the predilection for megaesophagus in these breeds, in addition to reports of entire litters of German shepherds, Great Danes, Newfoundlands, and shar-peis being affected, suggests that a hereditary basis for megaesophagus exists. For this reason owners are best advised not to use affected dogs or those closely related to affected dogs for breeding. Clinical signs usually occur by 3 months of age; however, dogs with mild symptoms might not be presented until 1 year of age.

Although the pathogenesis of congenital megaesophagus is unclear, esophageal function studies of affected dogs indicate defects in the vagal afferent innervation of the esophagus. Other studies have confirmed that vagal efferent innervation in affected dogs is normal but that esophageal motor function is decreased, possibly secondary to abnormal biomechanical properties of the esophageal muscle.

Acquired Megaesophagus

Acquired megaesophagus can occur in any breed; however, it is worthy to note that the breeds at a significantly increased risk for developing the disease include some of the same breeds discussed previously (i.e., German shepherd dogs, golden retrievers, Irish setters, and Great Danes). Secondary megaesophagus can be caused by any disorder that inhibits esophageal peristalsis either by disrupting esophageal neural pathways or by causing esophageal muscular dysfunction. Numerous central and peripheral neuropathies, diseases of the neuromuscular junction, and myopathies have been reported to cause megaesophagus (see Box 112-2). Most of these diseases are uncommon, and an exhaustive search to rule out all is unrealistic. However, several diseases should routinely be considered.

Myasthenia gravis (MG) is the most common cause of acquired megaesophagus in the dog (also see Chapter 241). It occurs rarely as a congenital disease and more frequently as an acquired disease; both can cause megaesophagus. Acquired MG is an autoimmune disorder that interferes with normal neuromuscular transmission. Production of autoantibodies against nicotinic ACh receptors decreases the number of receptors available for normal neuromuscular transmission, resulting in skeletal muscle weakness. Two forms of acquired MG, generalized and focal, have been identified. Generalized MG causes exercise-related generalized muscle weakness that worsens after exercise and improves with rest. Most dogs with generalized MG also have megaesophagus. Focal MG causes weakness that predominantly affects esophageal, pharyngeal, or facial muscles. Affected dogs are usually presented to the clinician with symptoms of megaesophagus.

Diagnosis of MG is made by measuring increased antibody titers to ACh receptors, but it is important to be aware that serum ACh receptor antibody concentrations tend to be lower in focal MG than in the generalized form. ACh receptor antibodies are negative in up to 15% of generalized MG and up to 50% of focal MG in humans (Dewey, 1997). Seronegative myasthenics exist in the veterinary population as well. Approximately 2% of dogs with generalized myasthenia gravis are seronegative. The percentage of dogs with seronegative focal myasthenia gravis has not been determined (Shelton, 2002). Immunocytochemical staining, which localizes the immune complexes at the neuromuscular junction after incubation of patient serum with normal canine muscle, is a second diagnostic method that is also relatively inexpensive and easy to perform. This test is not specific for antibodies against the ACh receptors; thus a positive result is not definitive. However, it is a useful screening test.

Many dogs diagnosed as having "idiopathic" megaesophagus are likely to have focal MG. In a study by Shelton and associates (1990), serum samples from 152 dogs with idiopathic megaesophagus were tested for ACh receptor antibodies. Results confirmed that 40 of 152 (26%) had antibody titers diagnostic for MG. Another 17 cases (11%) that did not have positive titers had positive immunocytochemical staining of immune complexes. Of those affected, 48% had clinical improvement or remission of clinical signs with treatment.

Occasionally megaesophagus is observed in dogs with primary, secondary, or atypical hypoadrenocorticism. Impaired muscle carbohydrate metabolism and depletion of muscle glycogen stores resulting from glucocorticoid deficiency and decreased catecholamine activity have been suggested as possible causes. Megaesophagus has been reported to resolve with prednisone treatment in dogs with glucocorticoid-deficient hypoadrenocorticism (Bartges et al., 1992).

Hypothyroidism has historically been cited as a possible cause of megaesophagus. However, a definitive association between hypothyroidism and megaesophagus has not been proved. In a case-controlled study by Gaynor and associates (1997) of 136 dogs with acquired megaesophagus, 272 control dogs from the general hospital population, and 151 control dogs that underwent thyroid-stimulating hormone response tests, no association between megaesophagus and hypothyroidism was found. In one retrospective study of 29 hypothyroid dogs, four had megaesophagus; one dog showed clinical improvement in esophageal symptoms when treated with thyroid supplement. Radiographic evidence of a dilated esophagus persisted in all four dogs (Jaggy et al., 1994). There is an association between MG and hypothyroidism, most likely caused by a common immune-mediated disorder. Therefore thyroid function should still be evaluated in dogs with megaesophagus until MG has been definitively ruled out.

Dysautonomia, an idiopathic condition that results in clinical signs attributable to failure of the sympathetic and parasympathetic nervous systems, is becoming a more common cause of megaesophagus. Dysautonomia typically affects young dogs from rural environments with the freedom to roam. Clinical signs are consistent with autonomic dysfunction and include vomiting, regurgitation, weight loss, dysuria, decreased anal tone, mydriasis with absent pupillary light reflexes, decreased tear production, and dry mucous membranes. Greater than 60% of patients with dysautonomia have radiographic evidence of megaesophagus; 71% of those have concurrent lung disease (Detweiler, 2001). Radiographic evidence of megaesophagus with dysautonomia is indistinguishable from that seen with other causes of megaesophagus; however, gastric motility should be normal with causes other than dysautonomia.

Another condition that should prompt evaluation for megaesophagus is laryngeal paralysis. Laryngeal paralysis may be a risk factor for acquired megaesophagus because both diseases have a common pathogenesis involving the vagus nerve. The vagus nerve may be the only affected nerve, or it may be affected as part of a diffuse polyneuropathy. Similarly, dogs with histories of chronic or recurrent gastric dilation with or without volvulus should be evaluated for megaesophagus. In these cases LES obstruction or esophagitis secondary to vomiting is the proposed mechanism for acquired megaesophagus.

Idiopathic Megaesophagus

Idiopathic megaesophagus is a severe and often fatal disease characterized by a large dilated esophagus with no apparent motility. It occurs spontaneously, usually in large-breed adult dogs between 5 and 12 years of age. There appears to be no sex or breed predisposition. Unfortunately the majority of adult dogs with megaesophagus are diagnosed as having idiopathic megaesophagus. The etiopathogenesis of this disorder is unknown; however, recent studies have clarified that the abnormality appears to be neurogenic rather than myogenic. Manometric studies have shown that the function of the UES and LES is normal in response to a swallow, indicating that the efferent innervation is intact. However, when the esophagus is distended with an intraluminal balloon to initiate secondary peristalsis, compliance of the esophagus is increased compared to normal dogs, the UES and LES fail to relax as in normal dogs, and inhibition of diaphragmatic electromyographic activity does not occur as in normal dogs. These observations indicate a defect of either afferent sensory innervation of the esophagus or esophageal muscle function (Tan and Diamant, 1987; Holland et al., 1996).

Clinical Signs

Regurgitation is the most common clinical sign observed with megaesophagus. Most owners fail to recognize the difference between regurgitation and vomiting and report vomiting as the primary complaint. The clinician must differentiate between these clinical signs to ensure proper localization and diagnosis of the problem. Regurgitation is characterized as a passive evacuation of fluid, mucus, and undigested food from the esophagus. No consistent temporal relationship occurs between eating and regurgitation

caused by esophageal disease. Other signs observed with megaesophagus include ptyalism, halitosis, and vomiting. Cough, nasal discharge, and dyspnea caused by aspiration pneumonia are frequent presenting complaints, especially in young or debilitated dogs. Some dogs appear normal on physical examination, whereas others are underweight to cachectic from poor nutritional intake, depending on the duration and severity of disease. Puppies with congenital megaesophagus are usually smaller than their littermates. Swelling of the ventral neck near the thoracic inlet from esophageal distention with ingesta is present occasionally. Other clinical signs may reflect diseases causing secondary megaesophagus. Careful examination should be performed for neuromuscular disease such as muscle weakness, pain, or neurologic deficits.

Diagnosis

Diagnosis of megaesophagus is based on radiographic identification of a dilated or hypomotile esophagus. Survey thoracic radiographs confirm the presence of generalized megaesophagus in most cases and usually reveal an esophagus dilated with air, fluid, or ingesta. In equivocal cases with mild or segmental dilation or if hypomotility without dilation is suspected, a contrast esophagogram is indicated. Barium liquid and barium meal contrast studies must be performed to detect subtle hypomotility and to rule out a stricture, foreign body, or other obstructive lesion. Although the availability of fluoroscopy in practice is limited, esophageal motility can be assessed well with static contrast radiographs during and immediately after a swallow of contrast material. Esophageal retention of any contrast material in a dog that is symptomatic for esophageal disease is abnormal. Radiographic signs of aspiration pneumonia, even in the absence of clinical or radiographic signs of esophageal disease, should alert the clinician to the potential for esophageal disease and the need for a contrast esophagogram. Dogs that have significant retention of contrast material in the esophagus are at risk for severe aspiration. They should be held in a vertical position for 5 to 10 minutes after the procedure and closely observed for at least an additional 30 minutes.

Esophageal motility is best evaluated using fluoroscopic, manometric, or scintigraphic procedures, which are usually limited to referral practices and teaching hospitals. Fluoroscopy provides visualization of swallow dynamics and helps to identify anatomic abnormalities of the esophagus. Manometry and scintigraphy provide quantitative measures of esophageal motility. Manometry is most useful to evaluate subtle motility abnormalities that are not evident on fluoroscopy. Manometry uses a catheter passed into the esophageal lumen for dynamic measurement of esophageal pressures, transit rate, and lower esophageal pressures during a swallow. Scintigraphy is a newer quantitative technique used to measure the transit time of a radiolabeled food bolus as it moves through the esophagus. Scintigraphy has the advantage of evaluating the response of the esophagus to a normal bolus in an awake patient without the influence of foreign material such as barium or an esophageal catheter.

Once the presence of megaesophagus has been confirmed, the clinician must determine whether the disorder is primary (idiopathic) or secondary. Generally most dogs with idiopathic megaesophagus have a very large, dilated, aperistaltic esophagus. Contrast material is slow to move into the stomach and may not do so for hours. Dogs with secondary megaesophagus are often not as severely affected and have less dilation and some motility. A recent study to evaluate whether dogs with megaesophagus secondary to myasthenia gravis had less esophageal dilatation radiographically than dogs with other causes of megaesophagus documented a small, but significantly increased esophageal diameter in nonmyasthenic dogs. However, due to large overlap in values, the finding offers limited clinical utility (Wray and Sparkes, 2006).

Formulating a logical and economic diagnostic plan can be challenging. The initial diagnostic plan should be broad and include a complete blood count; a serum chemistry profile that includes a creatine kinase determination, electrolyte determination, and urinalysis; and a fecal examination. Results of these tests help determine which additional diagnostic tests should be considered. A complete blood count might provide a clue to the presence of hypoadrenocorticism, immune-mediated disease, lead toxicosis, or pneumonia. Serum chemistry profiles are useful to detect hypoadrenocorticism or myositis. Proteinuria is supportive of the diagnosis of systemic lupus erythematosus, and a fecal examination might identify *Spirocerca lupi* in dogs from endemic areas. Patients with congenital or idiopathic megaesophagus generally have few if any laboratory abnormalities.

If results of the initial diagnostic tests are inconclusive, an ACh receptor antibody test should be performed to rule out focal or generalized MG. The immunoprecipitation radioimmunoassay (Comparative Neuromuscular Laboratory, University of California at San Diego, La Jolla, CA) is a specific and sensitive test. When the index of suspicion for MG is high, but a diagnosis is not confirmed with ACh receptor antibody serology, a motor point muscle biopsy may be submitted to the aforementioned laboratory for immunocytochemical staining. This test is less specific for MG but is highly suggestive for diagnosing seronegative myasthenics. Although hypoadrenocorticism is infrequently associated with megaesophagus, this disease is a potentially treatable cause of megaesophagus. Dogs with unexplained acquired megaesophagus should have adrenal function (adrenocorticotropic hormone stimulation test) evaluated. Furthermore, because of an indirect association to megaesophagus through association with other polyneuropathies such as MG, hypothyroidism should be ruled out with thyroid hormone evaluation. If gastric hypomotility is also suspected on radiographs, several simple pharmacologic tests can aid in an antemortem diagnosis of dysautonomia. Affected dogs should develop miosis in response to ocular installation of dilute (0.1%) pilocarpine solution, have no change in heart rate after administration of atropine, and have no flare response to intradermally administered histamine (Berghaus, 2001; Harkin, 2002).

Esophagoscopy usually is not helpful in determining the cause of megaesophagus. It is indicated if an obstructive lesion or foreign body is suspected but not confirmed by radiographs and to confirm the presence of esophagitis.

Other tests should be considered for individual cases if specific clinical signs or results of preliminary laboratory tests or both indicate the presence of a toxic, neurologic, or muscular disease. Lead, thallium, and anticholinesterase toxicities can be diagnosed by history, clinical signs, and toxicologic assay. Serum creatine kinase determinations, electromyography, and muscle biopsy are used to confirm the presence of myopathy or myositis. Systemic lupus erythematosus is diagnosed by the presence of systemic signs and positive antinuclear antibody or lupus erythematosus tests or both. Laryngeal paralysis can be diagnosed with direct laryngeal examination. Symptoms of central nervous system disease can be evaluated with distemper titers, cerebrospinal fluid analysis, computed tomographic brain scans, or a combination of these methods. Such diseases are infrequent causes of megaesophagus.

Treatment

The goals in the management of megaesophagus are to identify and treat the primary cause, decrease the frequency of regurgitation, prevent overdistention of the esophagus, provide adequate nutrition, and treat complications such as aspiration pneumonia and esophagitis. Dogs with secondary megaesophagus that can be treated specifically for underlying disease may show improvement of esophageal motility with time; however, responses are variable. Treatment of dogs in which an underlying cause cannot be found is entirely symptomatic.

Cases of focal and generalized MG are treated with long-acting anticholinesterase drugs. Either pyridostigmine bromide, 1 to 3 mg/kg orally every 8 to 12 hours, or neostigmine, 0.04 mg/kg intramuscularly every 6 hours (if oral medication is not tolerated), is effective. If pyrodostigmine bromide is administered in the syrup form, it should be diluted at a 50:50 ratio in water to avoid gastric irritation (Shelton, 2002). Improvement of clinical signs accompanied by a decrease in ACh receptor antibody concentration indicates a positive response to treatment. Antibody concentrations should be checked every 4 to 6 weeks to determine the course of the disease and adjust therapy, since spontaneous remissions do occur in a large percentage of dogs. Treatment should be continued until serum antibody titers are within the normal range. If clinical remission does occur, esophageal dilation may completely resolve, and medication can be discontinued; however, relapses do occur. The time course until remission can vary from 1 month to longer than 1 year. Some dogs with focal MG progress to generalized MG, usually within several weeks of the initial onset of clinical signs. Myasthenia is an immune-mediated disease; thus in most cases immunosuppression with corticosteroid therapy or a steroid-sparing agent such as azathioprine may be warranted. A retrospective study by Bartges, Hansen and Hardy (1997) evaluated 30 dogs with acquired MG and megaesophagus and discovered that glucocorticoid therapy alone resulted in clinical remission in 67% of cases. Multiple case reports of myasthenics experiencing clinical remission and a decrease in ACh receptor antibody titer after therapy with azathioprine are also available (Dewey et al., 1999). Other immune-directed therapy includes plasmapheresis, the filtration of plasma to rid the body of circulating antibodies. Shelton and associates (1990) evaluated 53 dogs with MG and saw spontaneous clinical and immunologic remission in 89% of dogs treated with anticholinesterase therapy alone. Therefore the use of immunosuppressive therapy is somewhat controversial, and the decision must be made on a case-by-case basis. Aspiration pneumonia should be ruled out or treated before the use of immunosuppressants, and the patient monitored closely for signs of developing infection.

Megaesophagus associated with hypoadrenocorticism resolves with corticosteroid and mineralocorticoid replacement. Immune-mediated polymyositis and polyneuritis and systemic lupus erythematosus may respond to immune suppression. Toxic causes of megaesophagus are treated by removal of the offending agent or the use of specific antidotes or both. Treatment of dysautonomia is limited to symptomatic therapy, including cholinergic drugs to relieve some of the signs of parasympathetic dysfunction, such as bethanechol to improve bladder function and pilocarpine to relieve photophobia. Artificial tears and humidifying the air can help eliminate the dryness associated with eyes and oral and nasal mucous membranes. Symptomatic management of the associated megaesophagus is described in the following paragraphs. Despite supportive care, the prognosis for dysautonomia is poor.

The management of idiopathic megaesophagus, as well as most cases of megaesophagus resulting from neurologic disease, is entirely symptomatic and centers on special feeding techniques. A diet should be formulated using a high-calorie food to provide adequate nutritional intake. Meals should be fed in small portions several times daily and given to the dog in an upright position. This can be accomplished by placing the food on an elevated feeding platform or by simply holding the dog in a vertical position for several minutes after eating. Upright feeding provides surprisingly effective symptomatic control of regurgitation in many dogs. There is also an online support group (www.geocities.com/bailey_chair/) for megaesophagus dog owners as well as instructions on building a "Bailey chair" for upright feedings.

Because dogs with megaesophagus vary in their ability to swallow foods of various consistencies, the type of diet fed should be tailored for each patient. Liquefied foods tend to flow more easily with gravity than do solids, but liquids stimulate little peristaltic activity. Solids stimulate more peristalsis and perhaps pose less risk of aspiration. Barium contrast radiography using liquid, canned, and dry food might help determine the best consistency of food for a particular patient. Ultimately food trials are the best way of determining the consistency of food to be fed. In our experience, feeding small meatballs made of canned food provides the best symptomatic control.

Some dogs cannot tolerate oral feeding, especially if the esophagus is extremely distended, secondary esophagitis is present, or the patient is severely debilitated. Providing nutritional intake in these instances requires gastrostomy tubes for long-term feeding. Surgical, endoscopic, or nonendoscopic techniques for gastrostomy tube placement can be used. We have successfully managed the nutritional needs of large dogs with idiopathic megaesophagus for longer than 1 year using gastrostomy tube feeding. Esophagostomy tubes can exacerbate regurgitation and should not be used.

Aspiration pneumonia should be treated with broad-spectrum antibiotic therapy while culture and sensitivity results of a transtracheal wash are pending. Many dogs with megaesophagus appear to acquire esophagitis, which can worsen the clinical signs. Systemic antacid treatment with drugs such as ranitidine or omeprazole and protectant drugs such as sucralfate help control symptoms in some patients (see Chapter 111).

Many types of drugs have been used unsuccessfully in an attempt to improve motility and esophageal emptying in dogs with megaesophagus. Anticholinergic drugs and calcium channel blocking drugs such as nifedipine have been used to decrease LES pressure. Little if any response has been observed. Anecdotal observations indicate that some dogs with megaesophagus improve clinically when treated with prokinetic drugs such as metoclopramide or cisapride. These observations have been questioned because metoclopramide and cisapride both increase motility by binding 5-HT$_4$ (serotonin) receptors on enteric cholinergic neurons, resulting in depolarization and contraction of gastrointestinal smooth muscle; canine esophagus consists of striated muscle. In normal dogs cisapride has actually been shown to decrease or slow the rate of transit of a food bolus through the esophagus (Mears, 1996). Therefore cisapride and other prokinetic drugs cannot be recommended to improve esophageal motility in dogs with megaesophagus.

If reflux esophagitis is suspected as a cause of esophageal hypomotility or a complication of megaesophagus, a trial with prokinetic drugs should be considered. These drugs do increase LES pressure, potentially decreasing episodes of reflux and subsequent esophagitis. However, this decision must be made carefully since increasing LES pressure can actually diminish esophageal clearance and perpetuate clinical signs in dogs with megaesophagus.

Bethanechol is a drug that has shown some promise in stimulating esophageal propagating contractions in some dogs affected with megaesophagus by directly binding to and stimulating cholinergic (muscarinic) receptors (Diamant and Szezepanski, 1974). This study was performed before the availability of testing for MG; thus it is impossible to know whether the documented improved motility is the result of treating megaesophagus secondary to undiagnosed MG or an indication that cholinomimetics can improve some cases of acquired idiopathic megaesophagus. There is still a population of undiagnosed myasthenics composed of both dogs that have not yet seroconverted and seronegative myasthenics. Therefore it is our opinion that dogs with acquired idiopathic megaesophagus should be treated as myasthenics with acetylcholinesterase inhibitors and immunosuppression as previously described.

Surgical treatment of congenital and idiopathic megaesophagus has not proved beneficial. Myotomy of the LES and techniques to plicate or resect the redundant esophagus may actually worsen the clinical signs. If radiographic evaluation of a patient shows failure of the LES to open and manometric studies confirm elevated sphincter pressures that did not relax in response to a swallow, a modified Heller's esophageal myotomy might be indicated.

Prognosis

The prognosis for megaesophagus is variable and difficult to predict. Successful outcomes depends on early diagnosis and aggressive dietary management. Even with diligent care, owners should be warned that aspiration pneumonia is a frequent and often fatal complication.

Congenital megaesophagus has at best a guarded prognosis for the animal to become a healthy and functional pet. Reported recovery rates vary from 20% to 46%. Some dogs improve with maturity, especially if the condition is recognized early and dietary management is begun before severe and irreversible dilation occurs. For example, most miniature schnauzers acquire improved or normal esophageal function by 6 to 12 months of age (Cox, 1980). There is one report of hypertrophic osteoarthropathy (HO), congenital megaesophagus, and no other pulmonary or extrathoracic disease in a German shepherd (Watrous and Blumenfeld, 2002). This dog was euthanized at 6 years of age because of cachexia and HO, but in a single report of a human with achalasia and HO the bone changes regressed after successful surgical treatment of the achalasia. One proposed mechanism is a neurogenic basis in which chronic vagal dysfunction initiated a reflex arc leading to HO.

Adult-onset idiopathic megaesophagus has a poor prognosis. Some affected dogs respond to aggressive symptomatic management, but most die of aspiration pneumonia or are euthanized because of persistent regurgitation and debilitation within 5 months of the time of diagnosis. Spontaneous recovery rarely occurs.

The prognosis for dogs with secondary megaesophagus is good if the underlying disease can be treated successfully. This is especially true for MG in which clinical recovery can be expected to occur in at least 50% of the cases. Megaesophagus appears to respond well to corticosteroid therapy in dogs with hypoadrenocorticism. Megaesophagus secondary to dysautonomia carries a grave prognosis. Dogs with megaesophagus from polyradiculoneuritis, polymyositis, systemic lupus erythematosus, and botulism can recover esophageal function after successful treatment of the primary disease.

References and Suggested Reading

Bartges JW, Hansen D, Hardy RM: Outcome of 30 cases of acquired myasthenia gravis in dogs (1982-1992), Proceedings of the American College of Veterinary Internal Medicine, Lake Buena Vista, Fla, Forum 164 (Abstract), 1997.

Bartges JW, Nielson DL: Reversible megaesophagus associated with atypical primary hypoadrenocorticism in a dog, *J Am Vet Med Assoc* 201:889, 1992.

Berghaus RD et al: Risk factors for development of dysautonomia in dogs, *J Am Vet Med Assoc* 218:8, 2001.

Boudrieau RJ, Rogers WA: Megaesophagus in the dog: a review of 50 cases, *J Am Anim Hosp Assoc* 21:33, 1985.

Cox VS et al: Hereditary esophageal dysfunction in the miniature schnauzer dog, *Am J Vet Res* 41:326, 1980.

Detweiler DA et al: Radiographic findings of canine dysautonomia in twenty-fiour dogs, *Vet Radiol Ultrasound* 42:2, 2001.

Dewey CW et al: Azathioprine therapy for acquired myasthenia gravis in five dogs, *J Am Anim Hosp Assoc* 35:396, 1999.

Dewey CW: Acquired myasthenia gravis in dogs. Part I, *Compend Contin Educ Pract Vet* 19:12, 1997.

Diamant N, Szczepanski M: Idiopathic megaesophagus in the dog: reasons for spontaneous improvement and a possible method of medical therapy, *Can Vet J* 15:66, 1974.

Gaynor AR, Shofer FS, Washabau RJ. Risk factors for acquired megaesophagus in dogs, *J Am Vet Med Assoc* 211:11, 1997.

Harkin KR, Andrews GA, Nietfeld JC: Dysautonomia in dogs: 65 cases (1993-2000), *J Am Vet Med Assoc* 220:5, 2002.

Holland CT, Stachell PM, Farrow BRH: Vagal esophagomotor nerve function and esophageal motor performance in dogs with congenital idiopathic megaesophagus, *Am J Vet Res* 57:906, 1996.

Jaggy A et al: Neurological manifestations of hypothyroidism: a retrospective study of 29 dogs, *J Vet Intern Med* 8:328, 1994.

Mears, EA, Jenkins C, Daniel G et al: The effect of cisapride and metoclopramide on esophageal motility in normal beagles. Proceedings of the 14th American College of Veterinary Internal Medicine, San Antonio, Texas, Forum 738 (Abstract), 1996.

Shelton GD : Acquired myasthenia gravis: selective involvement of esophageal, pharyngeal, and facial muscles, *J Vet Intern Med* 4:281, 1990.

Shelton GD: Myasthenia gravis and disorders of neuromuscular transmission, *Vet Clin North Am Small Anim Pract* 32:1, 2002.

Tan BJ, Diamant, NE: Assessment of the neural defect in a dog with idiopathic megaesophagus, *Dig Dis Sci* 32:1, 1987.

Watrous BJ, Blumenfeld B: Congenital megaesophagus with hypertrophic osteopathy in a 6-year-old dog, *Vet Radiol Ultrasound* 43:6, 2002.

Wray JD, Sparkes AH: Use of radiographic measurements in distinguishing myasthenia gravis from other causes of canine megaesophagus, *J Small Anim Pract* 47, 2006.

CHAPTER 113

Gastric *Helicobacter* spp. and Chronic Vomiting in Dogs

MICHAEL S. LEIB, *Blacksburg, Virginia*
ROBERT B. DUNCAN, *Blacksburg, Virginia*

Spiral bacteria were identified in the stomachs of humans and animals in the late 1800s. However, it was not until the early 1980s that Warren and Marshall proposed a relationship between *Helicobacter pylori* and gastric disease in humans. Soon after, studies demonstrated that spiral bacteria were common in the stomachs of clinically normal dogs and cats, as well as those with signs of gastrointestinal (GI) disease. Experimental infection in both dogs and cats resulted in lymphoid follicular gastritis; however, clinical signs were absent or very mild.

Currently a direct causal relationship between spiral bacteria and chronic gastritis and vomiting has not been firmly established in dogs or cats. Based on several clinical studies evaluating dogs and cats treated for *Helicobacter* spp. and identifying improvement or resolution of clinical signs, we believe that gastric *Helicobacter* spp. can cause or contribute to the clinical signs in some dogs with chronic gastritis and vomiting. This is supported by two published studies on the effects of treatment in dogs with clinical signs and gastric *Helicobacter* spp. (Happonen, Linden, and Westermarck, 2000; Leib, Duncan, and Ward, 2007).

We routinely determine if gastric *Helicobacter* spp. are present in all dogs and cats with chronic vomiting that undergo upper GI endoscopy. In most instances dogs and cats with gastric *Helicobacter* spp. and gastritis, with and without inflammatory bowel disease (IBD), are initially treated for *Helicobacter* spp. If clinical signs continue, dietary or antiinflammatory therapies for gastritis and IBD are instituted. We emphasize that, although the potential pathogenic role of gastric *Helicobacter* spp. in dogs and cats is being investigated, a thorough diagnostic evaluation to search for other potential causes of vomiting should always be performed before considering *Helicobacter* spp. to be the primary etiologic agent. The purpose of this chapter is to describe the commonly used methods of identifying gastric spiral bacteria in dogs and cats and to review the evidence behind current treatment recommendations. Recommendations for humans with *H. pylori* have been modified by the results of hundreds of clinical studies. Treatment recommendations in dogs and cats no doubt will also change as further studies are performed.

Helicobacter spp. are gram-negative, microaerophilic, motile, curved-to-spiral bacteria with multiple terminal flagella. They contain large quantities of the enzyme urease, which results in the production of ammonia and bicarbonate when in contact with urea. This reaction alters the pH immediately surrounding the bacteria and helps colonize the acidic environment of the stomach.

More than 30 species currently have been identified in humans and animals. In addition to the gastric species, others have also been identified in the intestine and liver. *H. pylori* is the most common gastric species in humans. It has been shown to be a major cause of gastritis and peptic ulcers and to increase the risk of gastric cancer. Infection rates can approach 100% in developing countries and 25% to 60% in developed countries. Infection is usually acquired in childhood and most often persists for life; natural immunity does not clear the infection. Most infected humans remain asymptomatic, but peptic ulcers may occur in 10% of those infected, whereas gastric cancer may develop in 1% to 2% of infected humans. Eradication of *H. pylori* usually results in healing of gastric and duodenal ulcers and complete remission of low-grade gastric mucosa-associated lymphoid tissue (MALT) lymphoma.

Although *H. pylori* has been identified in a research colony of cats, infections in pet dogs and cats with other species of *Helicobacter* is more common. Gastric *Helicobacter* spp. usually found in dogs and cats are larger than *H. pylori* (1.5 to 3μm). Initially these large spiral bacteria (4 to 10μm) were called *Gastrospirillum hominis* but were later reclassified as *Helicobacter heilmannii*. Other large gastric spiral bacteria such as *Helicobacter felis*, *Helicobacter bizzozeronii*, and *Helicobacter salomonis* occur and are indistinguishable from *H. heilmannii* using rou-

tine light microscopy. Multiple species can also be present within an individual animal. Peptic ulceration associated with gastric *Helicobacter* spp. is rare in dogs and cats, demonstrating a pathophysiologic difference between *H. pylori* and the gastric spiral bacteria commonly found in dogs and cats.

In addition to the role of *Helicobacter* in the pathogenesis of gastritis and chronic vomiting in dogs and cats is the potential for zoonotic transmission. Most evidence indicates zoonotic transmission to be very low, but the potential is real. *H. heilmannii* is a rare cause of gastritis in humans, accounting for approximately 0.1% of cases. An epidemiologic survey of humans with *H. heilmannii* gastritis showed that contact with dogs and cats was a significant risk factor (Meining, Kroher, and Stolte, 1998). In addition, there was an association between *H. heilmannii* gastritis and gastric lymphoma, although this relationship could be coincidental (Stolte et al., 1997). *H. pylori* has also been identified in a research colony of cats, and other studies have identified cat ownership as a risk factor for *H. pylori* infection in humans. Other studies found contact with dogs or cats not to be a risk factor for *H. pylori* infection. Although the potential for zoonotic transmission appears slight, until this issue is conclusively resolved, it seems prudent to identify the presence of gastric *Helicobacter* spp. in dogs and cats during the diagnostic evaluation of chronic vomiting.

DIAGNOSTIC TESTS

Invasive methods of diagnosis of gastric *Helicobacter* infection in humans include bacterial culture, routine microscopic or ultrastructural examination, polymerase chain reaction, or rapid urease testing of gastric mucosal biopsy specimens, usually obtained via endoscopy. Noninvasive methods of diagnosis include urea breath testing, fecal antigen determination, and serology. Although many of these noninvasive tests have been investigated in dogs and cats, they are not routinely available. Presently the clinical diagnosis of gastric *Helicobacter* spp. in dogs and cats requires endoscopic examination or exploratory celiotomy for retrieval of gastric biopsy samples. In our clinic spiral bacteria are identified on gastric biopsy, from brush cytology specimens, or indirectly by a positive rapid urease test of a gastric mucosal sample. Results from a rapid urease test and gastric brush cytology are available much sooner than histopathology. For reasons discussed in the following paragraphs, we consider gastric brush cytology and histologic evaluation of biopsy samples to be the most practical diagnostic tests available for the practicing veterinarian.

Brush Cytology

Gastric brush cytology is the least expensive and most practical diagnostic method with the quickest turnaround time. After completion of an endoscopic examination and collection of biopsy samples from the duodenum and stomach, a brush cytology specimen is collected. A guarded cytology brush is passed through the biopsy channel of the endoscope into the gastric body along the greater curvature. The cytology brush is extended from the sheath and gently rubbed along the mucosa from the antrum toward the fundus, along the greater curvature. Hemorrhagic areas associated with previous biopsy sites should be avoided. The brush is retracted into the protective sheath and withdrawn from the endoscope. The brush is extended from the sheath, gently rubbed across several glass microscope slides, which are air dried, and stained with a rapid Wright stain (Dip Quick stain, Jorgensen Laboratories Inc.).

The slide is examined under 100× oil immersion. Areas with numerous epithelial cells and large amounts of mucus are examined initially for *Helicobacter* spp. If present, the spiral bacteria are easily seen. They are usually at least as long as the diameter of a red blood cell, and their classic spiral shape is obvious (Fig. 113-1). The number of spiral bacteria can be highly variable, from one every several fields to massive numbers in most fields. We examine at least 10 oil immersion fields on two slides before the specimen is considered negative. Unlike diagnostic tests that involve using a single or several small biopsy samples, brush cytology gathers surface mucus and epithelial cells from a much larger area, increasing the chances for identification of bacteria. Brush cytology was found to be more sensitive than urease testing or histopathologic examination of gastric tissues in identifying gastric *Helicobacter* spp. organisms in dogs and cats (Happonen et al., 1996).

Rapid Urease Test

The rapid urease test detects the presence of bacterial urease, produced by the *Helicobacter spp.*, in a gastric biopsy sample. A commercially available test, the CLOtest (Ballard Medical Products, Draper, UT 84020), is used in our clinic (Fig. 113-2). Individual tests cost approximately $7. An agar gel with urea and a pH indicator, phenol red, is placed within a small plastic well. The tests should be kept refrigerated before use. A routine microbiologic urea slant tube can also be used for this same purpose. An endoscopic biopsy sample obtained from the angularis incisura of the

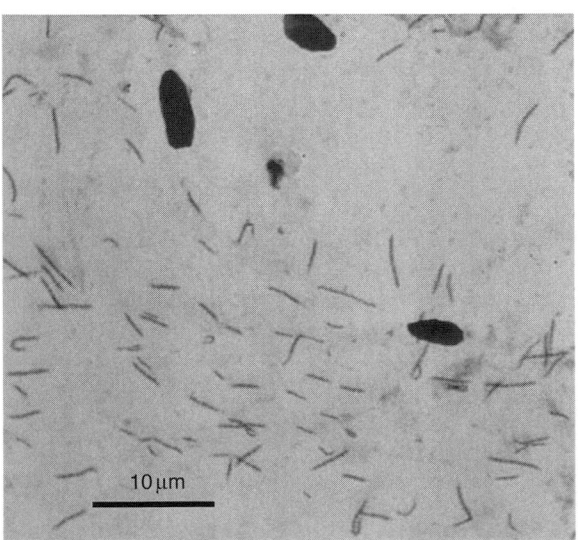

Fig. 113-1 Gastric brush cytology specimens stained with Dip Quick stain. Large numbers of spiral bacteria are visible. Cellular debris is scattered throughout the photograph. (With permission from Leib and Duncan: *Compend Contin Educ Pract Vet* 27:221, 2005.)

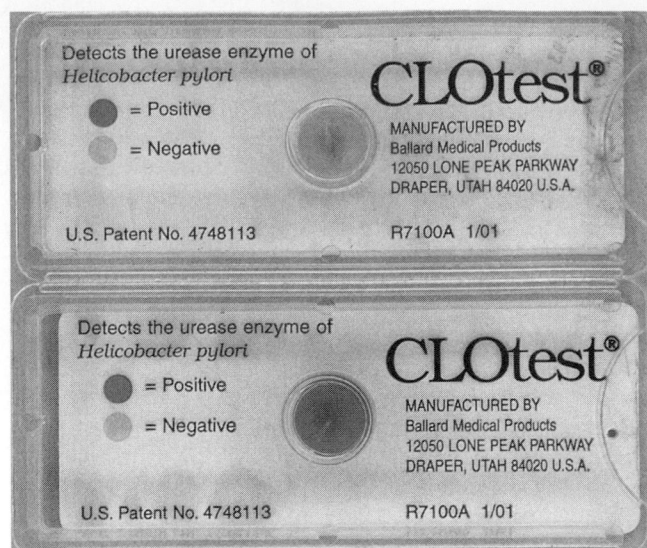

Fig. 113-2 CLOtest Top well is negative. Bottom well has changed color and is positive. (With permission from Leib and Duncan: *Compend Contin Educ Pract Vet* 27:221, 2005.)

stomach is pushed into the gel. The test is maintained at room temperature and examined frequently for a 24-hour period. If bacterial urease is present, urea is hydrolyzed to ammonia, which changes the pH of the gel. The color of the gel turns from yellow to magenta. The rate at which the gel changes color is proportional to the number of *Helicobacter* spp. present in the sample. When large numbers of bacteria are present in the biopsy sample, the rapid urease test quickly changes color, often within 15 to 30 minutes. If the color of the gel has not changed within 24 hours, the test is interpreted as negative.

Occasionally we have observed false-positive tests, perhaps because of contamination of other urease producing pharyngeal or intestinal bacteria, and false-negative tests because of the patchy distribution of bacteria within the stomach or the use of drugs that decrease acid secretion (increase in pH alters the activity of urease). Because of false positives and negatives, the cost of the tests, the turnaround time for results (especially if negative), and the ease and reliability of brush cytology, we find the rapid urease test to be a less valuable diagnostic method.

Histopathologic Identification

Histopathologic identification of *Helicobacter* spp. within gastric biopsy samples, using hematoxylin and eosin (H&E) or special stains, has a specificity of 100% and a sensitivity of greater than 90% in studies in humans. Because of the patchy distribution of organisms within the stomach, examination of samples from multiple gastric locations increases sensitivity. In our clinic samples from the pylorus, angularis incisura, gastric body along the greater curvature, and cardia are examined routinely. Spiral bacteria can be seen within the mucus covering the surface epithelium, the gastric pits, glandular lumen, and the parietal cells (Fig. 113-3). In cats bacteria have been identified submucosally within gastric lymphoid follicles. Spiral bacteria associated with the mucosal surface or within gastric pits are relatively easy to detect with

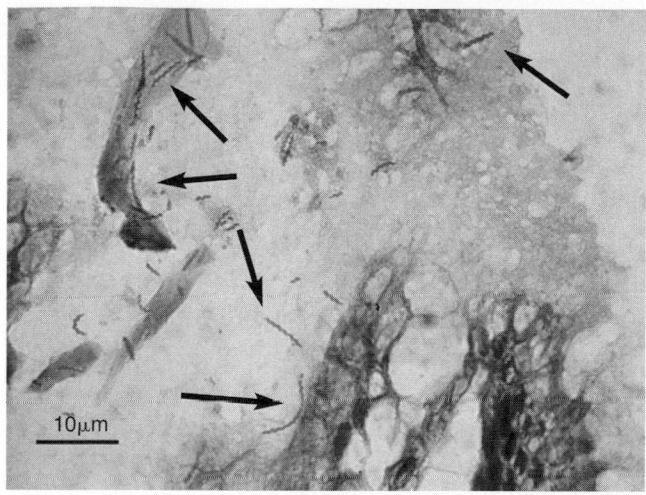

Fig. 113-3 Photomicrograph of gastric mucosal samples stained with H&E showing spiral bacteria along the mucosal surface *(arrows)*. (With permission from Leib and Duncan: *Compend Contin Educ Pract Vet* 27: 221, 2005.)

routine H&E staining of tissues. However, if the distribution of bacteria favors gastric glands and glandular epithelial cells, bacteria are much more readily detected with a modified Steiner's silver stain. Because of similarities in morphologic characteristics it is not possible to identify specific species using routine histologic staining techniques. Histopathologic evaluation of biopsy samples also allows assessment of inflammation in the stomach and duodenum or identification of neoplasia that may be the cause of the animal's clinical signs.

TREATMENT

Many studies evaluating therapy have been performed in humans with *H. pylori*. The most effective treatment regimens contain two or three antimicrobials combined with a proton pump antagonist given for 1 to 2 weeks.

Multiple antibiotics are used because treatment with a single antibiotic has resulted in eradication rates less than 20%. Studies in humans not only have demonstrated effective regimens but also have evaluated protocols associated with the highest treatment compliance: fewest side effects, the least number of tablets/day, and the shortest duration of therapy. Treatment protocols with eradication rates determined 4 weeks after completion of therapy that are higher than 80% to 90% are considered clinically effective. Reappearance rates after eradication of approximately 1% have been demonstrated, thought mostly to be the result of recrudescence. Successful treatment of bacteria within the gastric lumen is difficult. Antibiotics must penetrate the thick mucus layer within the gastric lumen and be active at an acid pH. The volume of gastric contents is constantly changing during a meal because of acid secretion and gastric emptying. In addition, metronidazole and clarithromycin, and rarely amoxicillin, resistance has been detected in strains of *H. pylori*.

Table 113-1 lists the treatment protocols described in the veterinary literature and used in our hospital. Our current treatment recommendations include either triple therapy with amoxicillin, metronidazole, and bismuth subsalicylate (Pepto Bismol) or dual therapy with clarithromycin and amoxicillin. All treatments are given BID for 2 weeks. Because gastric ulceration does not commonly occur in dogs with gastric spiral bacteria, acid suppression therapy may not be necessary. This may increase treatment compliance by reducing the number of daily medications. A similar benefit may occur with dual therapy, based on preliminary data shown to be as effective as triple therapy in dogs.

We (Leib, Duncan, and Ward, 2007) treated 24 pet dogs diagnosed with gastric *Helicobacter* spp. and chronic vomiting with either amoxicillin, metronidazole, and bismuth subsalicylate (triple therapy) or with triple therapy and famotidine (quadruple therapy). The median duration of vomiting before therapy was 19 weeks, and the median frequency of vomiting was 3.5 episodes per week. The presence of gastric *Helicobacter* spp. was determined by histologic assessment of gastric biopsy specimens

Table **113-1**

Treatment Protocols for Gastric *Helicobacter* spp. in Dogs

Protocol	Drugs	Dosage mg/kg	Frequency/day	Duration (days)
Happonen, Linden, and Westermarck, 2000	Amoxicillin	20	BID	10-14
	Metronidazole	10	BID	10-14
	Bismuth subcitrate	6	BID	14-28
Leib, Duncan, and Ward, 2007	Amoxicillin	15	BID	14
	Metronidazole	10	BID	14
	Bismuth subsalicylate	<5 kg-65.5 mg 5-9.9 kg-131 mg 10-24.9 kg-262 mg >25 kg-524 mg	BID	14
	Famotidine	0.5	BID	14
Leib and Duncan, 2005	Amoxicillin	15	BID	14
	Clarithromycin	7.5	BID	14
Cornetta et al, 1998; Simpson et al., 1999	Amoxicillin	20	BID	14
	Metronidazole	20	BID	14
	Famotidine	0.5	BID	14

obtained before therapy, 4 weeks, and 6 months after completion of therapy. Eradication rates were 70% and 78.5% 4 weeks after therapy for the triple and quadruple therapy respectively. Eradication rates decreased to 44.4% and 41.7% 6 months after therapy for the triple and quadruple therapy groups, respectively. Eight dogs that were negative at 4 weeks were positive at 6 months because of either reinfection or recrudescence of infection.

Both treatments reduced the vomiting frequency compared to the historical vomiting frequency. The median reduction in the frequency of vomiting episodes during the first 4-week period after therapy was 91.8% for triple-therapy dogs and 72% for quadruple-therapy dogs. After completion of therapy, the median reduction in the frequency of vomiting episodes for the entire 6-month period was approximately 86% for both groups. These data suggest that gastric *Helicobacter* spp. caused or contributed to clinical signs in some of the dogs in this study and treatment decreased the incidence of clinical signs.

Because it is often presumed that treatment compliance may decrease as the number of drugs administered increases, omitting acid suppressors in treatment protocols might improve client compliance and treatment success in some cases. Acid suppression may not be necessary in dogs and cats with gastric *Helicobacter* spp. because peptic ulceration is very uncommon when compared to its incidence in humans. However, the use of proton pump antagonists such as omeprazole have been demonstrated to have other potential benefits in humans with *H. pylori*, including bacteriostatic effects in vitro, facilitation of bacterial clearance from the stomach when combined with antibiotics, and inhibition of bacterial urease. Further study of the potential role of acid suppression in dogs and cats with gastric *Helicobacter* spp. is warranted.

The high infection rates 6 months after therapy in the Leib, Duncan, and Ward study (2007) were thought to be caused by initial treatment failure (25%), reinfection from the environment, or recrudescence of infection. High rates of treatment failure and potential recrudescence indicate that more effective treatment regimens should be developed to reach higher than 80% to 90% eradication rates. In our study it was not possible to differentiate between reinfection and recrudescence. It is possible that both treatments were effective initially and reinfection from the environment occurred. Because of canine social habits and the relatively unsanitary nature of the environment in which they live, reinfection after successful eradication therapy seems more likely to occur in dogs than in humans. If further research confirms that reinfection commonly occurs, treatment strategies should include minimizing environmental contamination and exposure, treatment of asymptomatic animals within the household, and possibly periodic retreatment if clinical signs recur.

We are aware of only one other published study that evaluated the effects of triple antimicrobial therapy on gastric *Helicobacter* spp. in pet dogs with upper GI signs (Happonen, Linden, and Westermarck, 2000). Seven of nine dogs that received amoxicillin, metronidazole, and bismuth subcitrate (see Table 113-1) became negative for *Helicobacter* spp. Clinical signs improved in all treated dogs, including two that remained positive. However, complete resolution of clinical signs required additional therapies. Four of these dogs were reevaluated a mean of 2.5 years after therapy, and all were found to be positive for gastric *Helicobacter* spp. However, these four dogs remained normal or only occasionally had mild clinical signs. The results of this study also suggested that gastric *Helicobacter* spp. contributed to the clinical signs in this group of dogs.

Two studies have evaluated the 2-week treatment of asymptomatic beagles naturally infected with gastric *Helicobacter* spp. with famotidine, amoxicillin, and metronidazole (see Table 113-1) (Cornetta et al., 1998; Simpson et al., 1999). In both reports all dogs were positive for gastric *Helicobacter* spp. 29 days after completion of therapy. It is difficult to compare the results of these two studies with our study because the beagles did not have clinical signs and our study included a third antimicrobial agent, bismuth. Besides its beneficial effects in healing peptic ulcers in humans, bismuth compounds have antimicrobial effects and can suppress but not eliminate *H. pylori* from humans. Bismuth compounds have been shown to decrease the adherence of *H. pylori* from the gastric epithelium, distort bacterial structure by causing vacuolization, and be present both within the cell wall and on the external surface of the bacteria.

Because of the need to identify more effective treatment protocols, we have recently investigated the effectiveness of a dual antibiotic protocol using clarithromycin and amoxicillin. The combination of clarithromycin and amoxicillin with a proton pump antagonist has been very effective in eradicating *H. pylori* in humans with peptic ulceration. Because famotidine did not improve results in our previous study and because of the additional cost of such therapy and the potential for decreased client compliance, a proton pump antagonist was not used. Preliminary results are available for the initial 4 weeks after therapy. The median duration of vomiting was 47 weeks, and the median frequency of vomiting was 1.6 episodes per week. Seventy percent (7 of 10) of dogs became negative 4 weeks after therapy, and the median reduction in the vomiting frequency was 95.5%, although there was considerable variation. More dogs need to be evaluated before conclusions about the effectiveness of this treatment protocol can be made.

In summary, the role of gastric *Helicobacter spp.* as a cause of chronic vomiting in dogs and cats remains speculative. It is our opinion that approximately 50% of dogs with chronic vomiting, chronic gastritis, and *Helicobacter* spp. dramatically improve after successful treatment. It is prudent to determine if gastric spiral bacteria are present in dogs and cats with chronic vomiting. This can be accomplished easily with brush gastric cytology specimens or routine histologic assessment of gastric biopsy samples. If other etiologies of chronic vomiting are not identified, a 2-week treatment protocol for gastric *Helicobacter* spp. is indicated. If clinical signs do not improve after treatment, dietary trials and/or antiinflammatory drugs should be considered. Additional studies will further define the potential pathogenic role of gastric *Helicobacter* spp. in dogs, and more effective treatment recommendations no doubt will emerge.

References and Suggested Reading

Cornetta AM : Use of [^{13}C] urea breath test for detection of gastric infection with *Helicobacter spp* in dogs, *Am J Vet Res* 59:1364, 1998.

Flatland B: *Helicobacter* infection in humans and animals, *Compend Contin Educ Pract Vet* 24:688, 2002.

Geyer C et al: Occurrence of spiral-shaped bacteria in gastric biopsies of dogs and cats, *Vet Rec* 133:18, 1993.

Happonen I et al: Comparison of diagnostic methods for detecting gastric *Helicobacter*-like organisms in dogs and cats, *J Comp Pathol* 115:117, 1996.

Happonen I, Linden J, Westermarck E: Effect of triple therapy on eradication of canine gastric *Helicobacters* and gastric disease, *J Small Anim Pract* 41:1, 2000.

Leib MS, Duncan RB: Diagnosing gastric *Helicobacter* infections in dogs and cat, *Compend Contin Educ Pract Vet* 27:221, 2005.

Leib MS, Duncan RB, Ward DL: Triple antimicrobial therapy and acid suppression in dogs with chronic vomiting and gastric *Helicobacter* spp, *Submitted J Vet Intern Med* 21:1185, 2007.

Meining A, Kroher G, Stolte M: Animal reservoirs in the transmission of *Helicobacter heilmannii*, *Scand J Gastroenterol* 33:795, 1998.

Neiger R, Simpson K: *Helicobacter* infection in dogs and cats: facts and fiction, *J Vet Intern Med* 14:125, 2000.

Simpson K et al: Gastric function in dogs with naturally acquired gastric *Helicobacter spp.* infection, *J Vet Intern Med* 13: 507, 1999.

Stolte M et al: A comparison of *Helicobacter pylori* and *H. heilmannii* gastritis: a matched control study involving 404 patients, *Scand J Gastroenterol* 32:28, 1997.

CHAPTER **114**

Gastric Ulceration

RETO NEIGER, *Giessen, Germany*

Ulcers in the stomach form when damage from acid and pepsin overcomes the ability of the mucosa to protect itself and replace damaged cells. Superficial injury of the mucosa results in hemorrhage and erosion; ulcer formation is only seen when the muscular layer is affected. The prevalence of gastric ulcers in dogs or cats is unknown; however, pets are regularly presented with hematemesis, and in these cases some breach of the gastric mucosa is likely.

PHYSIOLOGY

To understand the treatment and prevention of peptic ulcers, it is important to understand gastric secretion and mucosal protection. Acid is produced by the H$^+$-K$^+$-ATPase enzymes in parietal cells, which are located in the oxyntic glands. H$^+$-ions are pumped into the lumen in exchange for K$^+$; the latter accumulates in the cell and moves down the electrochemical gradient, leaking across the luminal and basolateral cell membranes. Stimulation of the parietal cell occurs via acetylcholine (M$_3$), gastrin (CCK$_B$) and/or histamine (H$_2$) receptors on the basolateral membrane via second messengers (Fig. 114-1). A further hormone, tentatively named *enterooxyntin*, seems to stimulate acid secretion as well (Johnson, 2001). There are several interactions between these secretagogues, and potentiation occurs if two or more stimulants act simultaneously, meaning that the sum of the response exceeds that of each individual response. Histamine is found in enterochromaffin-like (ECL) cells within the lamina

propria of the gastric glands. ECL cells have receptors for gastrin and acetylcholine.

Pepsinogen, produced by chief cells in the gastric mucosa, is converted to pepsin when the pH is below 5.0. Pepsin, which begins the digestion of protein by splitting interior peptide linkages, can itself catalyze the formation of pepsin from pepsinogen. The stimulation of pepsinogen secretion is through vagal activation (acetylcholine), acid-triggered local effects, and in dogs gastrin-induced acid secretion. Secretin, which is produced in the duodenum by secretin cells, also has a pepsinogen-secreting effect, albeit weaker than the other effects.

Three general stimuli or phases are known to initiate gastric secretion: cephalic, gastric, and intestinal. Cephalic stimuli such as tasting, smelling, chewing, and swallowing instigate nerve impulses through vagal efferent stimuli into the stomach. Besides direct activation on the parietal cell, the gastrin (G) cell is stimulated through gastrin-releasing peptide (GRP) or bombesin. In the gastric phase distention of the stomach initiates a vagovagal reflex, meaning that both afferent and efferent impulses are carried through the vagus nerve, which then causes acetylcholine release. Furthermore, peptides and amino acids in the stomach stimulate gastrin release from G cells. Finally, in the intestinal phase digested proteins in the duodenum stimulate acid secretion without increasing serum gastrin levels, potentially through enterooxyntin.

Several mechanisms underlie the remarkable abilities of normal gastroduodenal mucosa to defend itself against

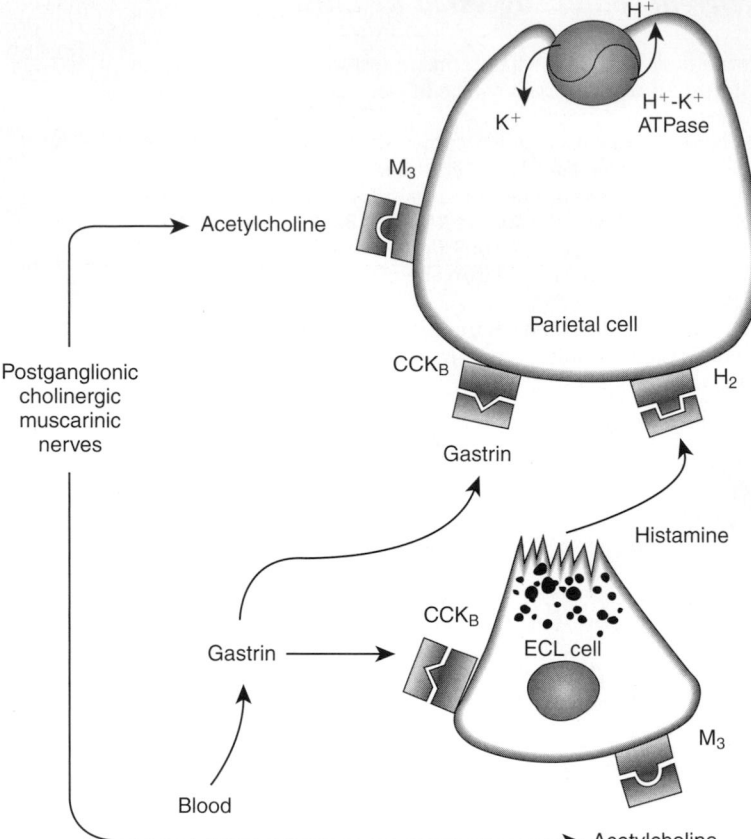

Fig. 114-1 Physiologic mechanism of gastric acid secretion. The parietal cell contains receptors for gastrin, acetylcholine, and histamine. In addition, gastrin and acetylcholine release histamine from the enterochromaffin-like cell (ECL-cell).

injury from acid/pepsin activity in gastric juice and to rapidly repair injury when it does occur. These mechanisms entail three lines of defense: preepithelial, epithelial, and subepithelial (Fig. 114-2). Factors that play a role in maintaining mucosal protection against the ulcerogenic effects of acid and pepsin are mucus; blood flow; bicarbonate secretion; cellular renewal; and chemical factors such as prostaglandins, gastrin, and epidermal growth factor. Surface mucus cells secrete mucoproteins in response to chemical or physical stimuli. This secreted gel entraps alkaline components, neutralizes a certain amount of acid, and prevents pepsin from coming into contact with the mucosa. Prostaglandins play a key role in protecting the gastric mucosa against injury caused by a variety of necrotizing agents. Prostaglandins exert two actions: inhibition of acid secretion and enhancement of mucosal resistance to injury by mechanisms independent of acid secretory inhibition, also called *cytoprotection*.

CAUSES

A variety of causes for peptic ulcers in dogs and cats have been reported. Although nonsteroidal antiinflammatory drugs (NSAIDs) are thought to be the most common cause, the true incidence of gastrointestinal side effects of NSAIDs in dogs is unknown. Only one case of NSAID-induced ulceration has been reported in a cat. NSAIDs are thought to cause gastrointestinal mucosal injury by several mechanisms. Primarily these drugs impair prostaglandin-dependent mucosal protective mechanisms by nonselective inhibition

of two isoforms of cyclooxygenase (COX), COX-1 and COX-2. However, a direct correlation is lacking between the extent of COX inhibition and NSAID-induced gastrointestinal damage (Fig. 114-3). COX-1 inhibition leads to reduced bicarbonate secretion, reduced mucus formation, and vascular actions. Other effects unrelated to prostaglandin synthesis include a "topical" action of NSAIDs on the gastric mucosa, involving mitochondrial injury ("uncoupling") by a direct toxic action. All commonly used NSAIDs, whether COX-2–specific or not, have been found to cause gastric lesions, although true ulcers with sufficient depth to reach or penetrate the muscularis mucosa seem to be rare. In the largest study of gastric ulcers in dogs, only 4 of 43 cases were thought to have peptic ulcers primarily caused by NSAIDs (Stanton and Bright, 1989). However, close temporal association of various NSAIDs and steroids must be avoided because an increased likelihood of gastric ulceration has been reported (Lascelles et al., 2005).

Corticosteroids alone are hardly ulcerogenic; however, this class of drugs enhances the damaging effect of NSAIDs, hypotension, and other factors causing peptic ulcers. Corticosteroids decrease mucosal cell growth, mucus production, and prostaglandin secretion and enhance gastric acidity. In general, only immunosuppressive doses of prednisolone, when used alone, may result in gastromucosal damage. However, in combination with NSAIDs or concurrent ulcerogenic factors, even antiinflammatory doses can cause *severe* problems; dexamethasone seems to have a higher ulcerogenic property, possibly because of its higher glucocorticoid effect.

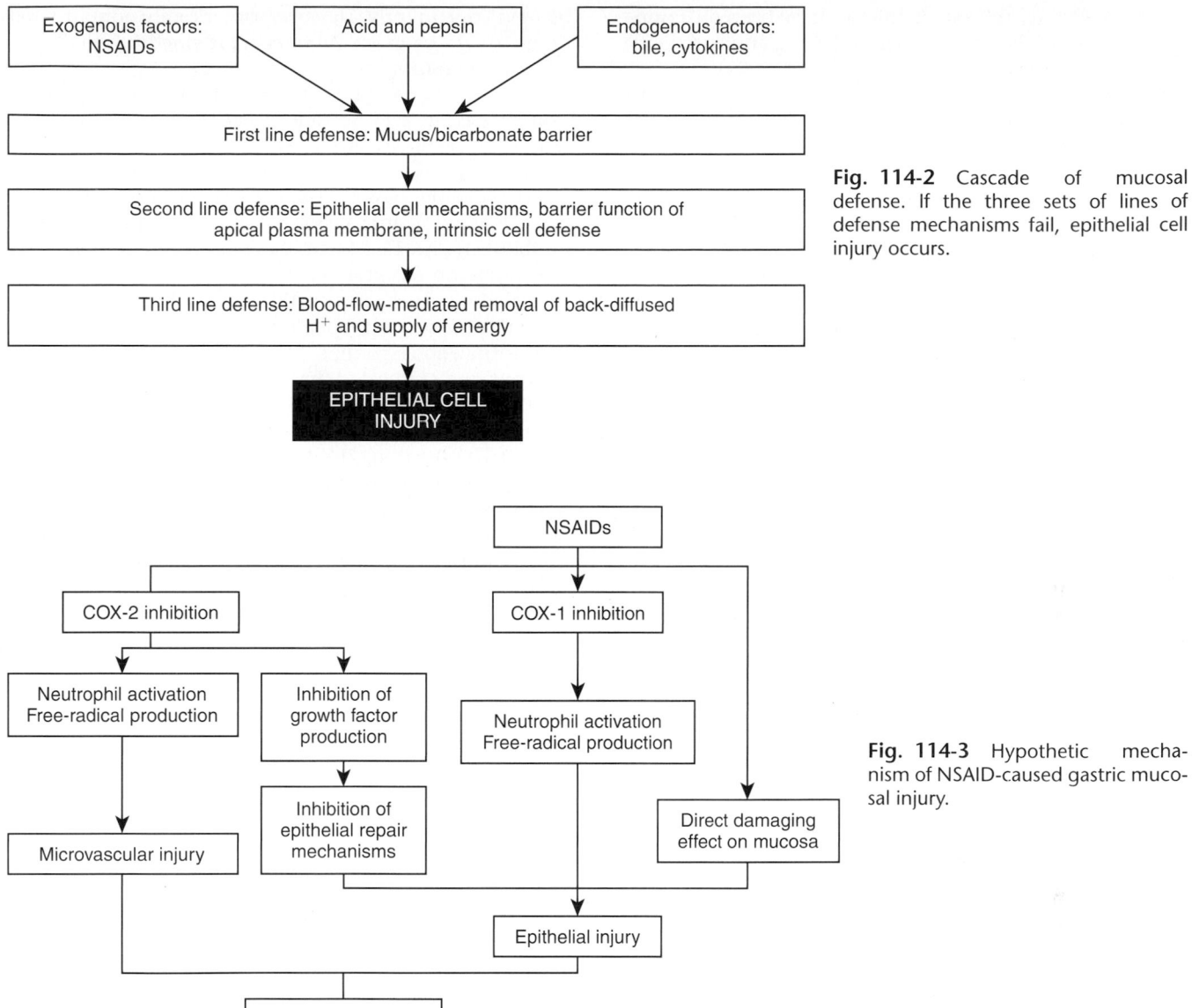

Fig. 114-2 Cascade of mucosal defense. If the three sets of lines of defense mechanisms fail, epithelial cell injury occurs.

Fig. 114-3 Hypothetic mechanism of NSAID-caused gastric mucosal injury.

One of the most important risk factors for peptic ulceration in dogs is decreased mucosal blood flow caused by hypotension, shock, sepsis, hypovolemia, intervertebral disk disease, or surgery. These factors seem to become even more important if they happen concomitantly or combined with NSAIDs or steroids (Hinton et al., 2002). Less common but still potential risk factors for peptic ulcers are infiltrative gastrointestinal disease, hepatic or renal disease, congestive heart failure, and gastric outflow obstruction.

Large ulcers in the pyloric antral region, often near the incisura, are commonly seen in dogs with gastric tumors. In cats 14 of 33 peptic ulcers were caused by a neoplasia, mostly lymphoma or adenocarcinoma (Liptak et al., 2002). Hyperacidity-induced peptic ulcers caused by a gastrinoma have been described both in dogs and cats; but these tumors are rare, and hyperacidity caused by mast cell tumors rarely develops gastric ulceration.

Although *Helicobacter pylori* is one of the most common causes of peptic ulceration in humans, the status of gastric *helicobacter*-like organisms causing ulcers or other lesions in the canine and feline stomach is unresolved (see Chapter 113). Gastric ulcers resulting from these spiral organisms have not been reported.

DIAGNOSTIC FEATURES

There are no common signs in animals with peptic ulcers. Vomiting, sometimes with blood, abdominal pain, and nonspecific symptoms such as lethargy and anorexia may be noted. Blood loss into the gastrointestinal tract results in melena, sometimes seen on rectal palpation, and pale mucous membranes if anemia is moderate to severe.

Laboratory tests are nonspecific; however, they are used to rule out other causes of vomiting. Chronic blood loss may result in anemia, sometimes nonregenerative and typical for iron deficiency (hypochromic, microcytic). Biochemistry results may show electrolyte abnormalities as a consequence of profound vomiting. Fecal occult blood tests are useful only if animals have been on a non-meat diet for at least 3 days before testing and specificity is rather low (Tuffli, Gaschen, and Neiger, 2001).

Survey radiographs are useful in the general workup of the patient; however, they are insensitive to abnormal gastric wall thickness or peptic ulcers. A pneumoperitoneum most often indicates a ruptured viscus such as a perforated gastric ulcer. Contrast radiographs with barium might outline ulceration of the mucosa. The low sensitivity and risk of aspiration pneumonia with barium, the fact that it is a time-consuming procedure, and the problem with a subsequent gastroscopy have made this technique less useful. Ultrasound showing abnormal wall thickness and loss of layers of the mucosa is suggestive of a gastric tumor.

Gastroscopy is the technique of choice to diagnose peptic ulcers. A caveat lies on the characterization of the mucosal damage. The critical characteristic of a true ulcer is that it has sufficient depth to reach or penetrate the muscularis mucosa (i.e., a depth that increases the risk of perforation). However, lesion depth cannot be measured at endoscopy. True ulcers are often confused with the very common and largely trivial erosive lesions found in gastroduodenal mucosa exposed to NSAIDs. That these "endoscopic ulcers" are largely erosive in nature and not true ulcers is borne out by the rarity of clinically relevant bleeding. It is important to inspect the entire stomach and take multiple biopsies from abnormal-looking areas. The rim of an ulcer should be biopsied because the center of the ulcer is usually necrotic tissue.

THERAPY

Treatment of peptic ulcer disease must first address predisposing causes; second, give supportive medications; and last, suppress further damage by suppressing gastric acid secretion. NSAIDs or glucocorticoids should be stopped if possible, and alternative drugs should be used. Tumors are excised surgically (adenocarcinoma, gastrinoma, mast cell tumor) or treated with chemotherapy (lymphoma). Other predisposing factors such as hypotension, stress, and renal or hepatic disease are addressed appropriately.

Fluid replacement for dehydration or a blood transfusion for anemia should be given as needed for gastric ulceration. In a vomiting animal antiemetics are useful to minimize fluid and electrolyte loss and reduce the risk of aspiration pneumonia. If indicated from clinical findings, abdominal ultrasound may be indicated to identify signs of peritonitis related to gastric perforation. Surgical consultation is indicated when perforation is suspected.

The ulcerated mucosa is vulnerable to further damage and mucosal protection with sucralfate (1g/10kg orally [PO] q8h) is indicated. Sucralfate is a sulphated disaccharide–aluminium hydroxide complex that adheres to ulcerated tissue and provides a barrier to acid and pepsin penetration. It also stimulates endogenous prostaglandin synthesis in the gastric mucosa. Since sucralfate is effective at acidic to almost neutral pH, antisecretory drugs can be used concurrently. However, other orally administered drugs should be given 2 hours apart since sucralfate can affect their absorption.

The cornerstone of peptic ulcer therapy is the reduction of gastric acid secretion; Schwartz's dictum from 1910, "no acid, no ulcer," remains valid today. A variety of drugs are available; the two most commonly prescribed drug classes in veterinary medicine are histamine-2 receptor antagonists (H_2-RAs) and proton pump inhibitors (PPIs). H_2-RAs act via competitive inhibition at the histamine receptor on parietal cells (see Fig. 114-1). Several drugs such as cimetidine, ranitidine, nizatidine, and famotidine are available in this group, both in oral and intravenous format, depending on the country. A recent study indicated that ranitidine at the regular dosage (2 mg/kg intravenously [IV] q12h) did not differ from saline in increasing the intragastric pH, whereas famotidine (0.5 mg/kg IV q12h) was significantly more effective than saline (Bersenas et al., 2005). It is the general belief that H_2-RAs are less effective than PPIs, and it seems that ranitidine might not increase intragastric pH sufficiently in dogs to treat peptic ulcers.

PPIs inhibit the final step of acid secretion, the gastric pump, and thus prevent histamine, acetylcholine, and gastrin-induced acid secretion (see Fig. 114-1). All currently available PPIs are substituted benzimidazoles. A 3- to 5-day lag-phase to achieve maximum acid inhibition has been reported in humans, but this seems not to be the case in dogs. Omeprazole (1 mg/kg PO q24h) and pantoprazole (1 mg/kg IV q24h) were both effective in increasing intragastric pH after 2 days (Bersenas et al., 2005). PPIs are the drug of choice for all hypersecretory states but are also indicated in animals with concurrent risk factors for peptic ulcers and when marked mucosal disruption is seen via endoscopy. It seems that all commercially available PPIs (omeprazole, lansoprazole, esomeprazole, pantoprazole, and rabeprazole) (tenatoprazole launch expected in 2008) are equally effective and safe and have minimal side effects in dogs.

Misoprostol, a synthetic prostaglandin analog, has effects similar to those of endogenous prostaglandins (i.e., stimulation of mucus secretion, increased bicarbonate secretion and gastric mucosal blood flow, and reduction of acid secretion). Because of these properties misoprostol is indicated in preventing NSAID-induced gastric damage. Misoprostol is not indicated when a peptic ulcer is already present since its capacity to reduce gastric acid is far less than that of H_2-RAs or PPIs. Side effects such as diarrhea and abdominal pain are quite common, and its marked abortifacient effects are a further drawback.

Several other means of decreasing gastric acid are available. Most are not sufficiently effective (e.g., antacids) or are not yet available (gastrin-receptor antagonists, gastrin-releasing peptide receptor antagonists). A class of drugs that might be of future interest is the potassium-competitive acid blocker (P-CAB); P-CABs block the action of the H^+-K^+-ATPase by competing with K^+. Soraprazan and revaprazan are currently under development, but no information in dogs or cats is yet available.

References and Suggested Reading

Bersenas AME et al: Effects of ranitidine, famotidine, pantoprazole, and omeprazole on intragastric pH in dogs, *Am J Vet Res* 66:425, 2005.

Hinton LE et al: Spontaneous gastroduodenal perforation in 16 dogs and seven cats (1982-1999), *J Am Anim Hosp Assoc* 38:176, 2002.

Johnson LR. *Gastrointestinal physiology*, ed 6, St. Louis 2001, Mosby.

Lascelles BDX et al: Gastrointestinal tract perforation in dogs treated with a selective cyclooygenase-2 inhibitor: 29 cases (2002-2003), *J Am Vet Med Assoc* 227:1112, 2005.

Liptak JM et al: Gastroduodenal ulceration in cats: eight cases and a review of the literature, *J Feline Med Surg* 4:27, 2002.

Mössner J, Caca K: Developments of the inhibition of gastric acid secretion, *Eur J Clin Invest* 35:469, 2005.

Stanton ME, Bright RM: Gastroduodenal ulceration in dogs: retrospective study of 43 cases and literature review, *J Vet Intern Med* 3:238, 1989.

Tuffli SP, Gaschen F, Neiger R: Effect of dietary factors on the detection of fecal occult blood in cats, *J Vet Diagn Invest* 13:177, 2001.

CHAPTER **115**

Inflammatory Bowel Disease

ALEXANDER J. GERMAN, *Liverpool, England, United Kingdom*

In companion animal gastroenterology, *inflammatory bowel disease (IBD)* is the term used to describe patients that are affected by persistent or recurrent gastrointestinal (GI) signs and have histopathologic evidence of inflammation in intestinal biopsy material. The condition can only be termed *idiopathic IBD* if no underlying cause for the inflammation can be found. Although there have been recent studies into pathogenesis, diagnosis, and treatment, much controversy remains. A diagnosis of IBD requires detailed investigations to exclude other potential causes of intestinal inflammation; however, it is likely that IBD represents a syndrome comprising a group of disorders with similar characteristics rather than a single disease entity. This chapter briefly reviews the current understanding of this enigmatic condition and then concentrates on current therapeutic practice, highlighting the most recent work in the field.

CLASSIFICATION

IBD is classified according to both the region of the intestine affected and the predominant cell type in the inflammatory infiltrate. Any region of the GI tract may be affected in any combination. The lymphocytic-plasmacytic variety is the most common form reported in both dogs and cats. Eosinophilic inflammation is the second most common type of IBD reported, and there are occasional reports of inflammation with a granulomatous pattern (e.g., regional enteritis). A neutrophilic predominance in the inflammatory infiltrate is rare. However, on many occasions a mixed pattern of cellular infiltrate is described. Despite these different varieties and the importance often placed on histologic classification, little is known of the significance of such differences in terms of differing etiology, pathogenesis, treatment, and prognosis. Finally certain unique IBD syndromes occur overwhelmingly more often in some breeds; examples include the protein-losing enteropathy (PLE)/protein-losing nephropathy complex in soft-coated wheaten terriers, the immunoproliferative enteropathy of basenjis, IBD in Norwegian lundehunds, and histiocytic ulcerative colitis in boxers.

ETIOPATHOGENESIS

IBD reportedly has an immune-mediated etiology; thus the GI lymphoid tissue (GALT) likely plays a critical part in pathogenesis (German, Hall, and Day, 2003). In brief, the intestinal mucosa has a barrier function (immune exclusion) and controls exposure of antigens to the GALT, which must generate protective immune responses against pathogens while remaining tolerant of harmless environmental antigens such as commensal bacteria and food. IBD develops when the normal decision-making process breaks down, leading to inappropriate immune responses and uncontrolled inflammation. Genetic factors are thought to play a part in disease expression, and examples in human IBD include certain human leukocyte antigen determinants and nucleotide-binding oligomerization domain 2 containing protein (NOD2).

Human Inflammatory Bowel Disease and Animal Models

Much of our understanding of IBD and chronic mucosal inflammation has come from genetically engineered animal models, which are characterized by a variety of spontaneously arising or induced disruptions of the mucosal barrier, the mucosal immune system, or the endogenous microflora. Critical to the development of inflammation in these models is a breakdown in tolerance to normal luminal antigens (particularly endogenous bacterial species). This loss of tolerance may result from disruption of the mucosal barrier, leading to excessive antigen exposure to the underlying immune system; from dysregulation of normal mucosal immune system function; or from a combination of these processes. The end effect of this tolerance breakdown is uncontrolled inflammation, which is the result of activation of the many effector pathways. The inflammation can then lead to architectural disruption, resulting in adverse effects on function, which depend on the part of the bowel affected.

Companion Animal Inflammatory Bowel Disease Pathogenesis

Although it has been suggested that the pathogenesis of canine IBD is similar to that of the human diseases (ulcerative colitis and Crohn's disease) and mouse models of intestinal inflammation, direct data in support of this supposition are limited. Despite the fact that numerous studies have been performed, many gaps in our understanding remain.

Many studies have used histochemical and immunohistochemical techniques to quantify immune cell populations within the intestinal mucosa with variable results (German, Hall, and Day, 2003). For canine IBD some have shown a decrease in certain lymphocyte populations (total T cells and immunoglobulin [Ig]G$^+$ plasma cells); whereas others have shown increases in $\alpha\beta$-T cells, CD4$^+$ T cells, IgG$^+$ plasma cells, and macrophage and granulocyte numbers. The confusion is compounded by the finding that in feline IBD, a disease with similar histopathologic changes to the canine form, the only reported difference from control samples was an increase in cells expressing major histocompatibility complex (MHC) class II.

Inconsistent results have also been seen with the studies conducted to date on mucosal cytokine gene expression. First, semiquantitative reverse transcriptase polymerase chain reaction (PCR) studies have suggested increased or decreased gene expression for canine chronic enteropathies. However, more reliable information comes from a recent study using real-time PCR techniques, and this work failed to demonstrate any alteration in cytokine gene expression (Peters et al., 2005). Unfortunately, like its predecessors, this study suffers from the critical flaw that gene expression alone has been assessed and not the functional protein. Nonetheless, even with this limitation in mind, it is odd that such a sensitive and powerful technique as real-time PCR did not detect any alteration in the expression of any cytokine gene. This concern, coupled with the histochemical and immunohistochemical studies that failed to detect immune cell alterations, questions our very understanding of IBD, leading some cynics to ask the question: "if this is IBD, then where is the inflammation?" It may be that the problem lies in the chosen gold standard, namely histopathology, which itself is variable and lacks consensus among pathologists

(see following paragraphs). However, we could actually be dealing with a syndrome in which *inflammation* is present in only a proportion of cases. Perhaps the syndrome would be better known as *idiopathic bowel disease*? Given these limitations to the understanding of companion animal IBD pathogenesis, veterinarians must currently be cautious about their approach to diagnosis and therapy.

An Infectious Etiology for Inflammatory Bowel Disease?

Histiocytic ulcerative colitis is a unique form of IBD, which predominantly affects boxer dogs (also see Chapter 120). The disease is characterized by accumulations of periodic acid-Schiff–positive macrophages, although a mixed inflammatory response with T cells, IgG plasma cells, and macrophages has been noted, together with up-regulation of epithelial MHC class II expression. An infectious etiology has long been hypothesized, but early attempts at disease transmission failed. However, recently the condition has been reported to be sensitive to enrofloxacin, and a recent study has demonstrated that the disease is associated with selective intramucosal colonization by *Escherichia coli* strains (Simpson et al., 2006). These strains have an adherent and invasive phenotype and similarities to similar organisms isolated from the mucosa of Crohn's disease patients.

DIAGNOSIS OF INFLAMMATORY BOWEL DISEASE

A detailed investigative workup usually is required for the IBD case. Given that IBD is largely diagnosed on histopathologic criteria, intestinal biopsy is an essential step in diagnosis. Often a staged approach is recommended that involves a combination of laboratory tests (blood tests, urinalysis, fecal analyses) and diagnostic imaging in addition to histopathologic assessment of intestinal tissue samples. Furthermore, given the current controversies over definition and diagnosis of IBD, well-conducted therapeutic trials have now become an important diagnostic tool. Thus not only can the condition be better defined (food-responsive, antibacterial-responsive), but a superior treatment plan is also put in place in which only those therapies truly required are used.

Recent Advances in Laboratory Testing

A recent innovation in assessment of intestinal protein loss is measurement of fecal α_1-proteinase inhibitor concentrations. This test correlates well with the gold standard for intestinal protein loss. Preliminary work has suggested that it is valuable for the diagnosis of PLE, and it may prove to be a more sensitive marker than serum albumin concentrations for the detection of early disease.

Although measurement of serum cobalamin concentrations is not novel, this test remains of critical importance when assessing cases of chronic GI disease. Deficiencies in either of these B vitamins are not pathognomonic for the presence of any particular GI condition, but they alert the clinician to the presence of intestinal malabsorption. Cobalamin deficiency may have systemic metabolic consequences, and response to specific therapy may be suboptimal if it remains unresolved. A recent study has also demonstrated that this is a common complication of feline GI disorders (Simpson et al., 2001).

Diagnostic Imaging

Although both radiographic and ultrasonographic studies can be used in investigation of patients with GI signs, ultrasonography has become the preferred imaging tool. It can be used to assess all abdominal organs and help eliminate the possibility of disease in other organs. The whole of the intestinal tract can also be examined directly, and wall thickness can be measured. It was suggested previously that increased wall thickness occurs in canine IBD, but recent work has suggested this measurement to be of no significant value in IBD diagnosis. Instead the power of ultrasonography is more for its ability to document focal intestinal disease and enable targeted cytologic analysis. In the future, Doppler may prove to be a useful tool for investigation of intestinal disease since a recent work has suggested that it may be useful to aid in the diagnosis of food sensitivity disorders (Kircher et al., 2004).

Intestinal Biopsy

Intestinal biopsy is essential to prove the presence of intestinal inflammation and confirm a diagnosis of IBD. Endoscopic biopsy is the simplest and least invasive method of specimen collection; limitations include small sample size, superficial samples, and limited sampling sites (stomach, proximal small intestine (SI), distal ileum [occasionally], and colon). In some cases exploratory celiotomy and full-thickness biopsy are necessary, although this procedure is more invasive and wound healing can be problematic if severe hypoproteinemia is present and corticosteroids need to be given urgently. However, it may be more suitable for cats, given the tendency for concurrent hepatic and pancreatic involvement and the small size of endoscopic biopsies achievable in this species.

Although the histopathologic assessment of intestinal biopsy material remains the gold standard for diagnosis of many intestinal diseases, it has marked limitations. The major problem is the poor agreement among pathologists (Willard et al., 2002). In this study overall agreement among pathologists was poor, and some even made a diagnosis of lymphoma after assessing tissues from healthy dogs. Histopathologic scoring schemes and standardized criteria have been suggested as a means of improving agreement, but marked variability in interpretation still exists. A World Small Animal Veterinary Association–sponsored Gastrointestinal Standardization Group has been established to try to resolve these inconsistencies, and it is hoped that a reliable grading scheme will be developed in the near future.

Ultimately the primary clinician must interpret histopathology results cautiously and try to relate them to the clinical presentation. Results should be questioned if the histopathologic diagnosis does not fit the clinical picture or the response to apparently appropriate therapy is poor. In some cases repeat biopsy (e.g., by exploratory celiotomy) may be required. Alternative methods of assessing biopsy tissue include immunohistochemical or flow cytometric characterization of mucosal immune cell populations and assessment of T-cell clonality. However, although such techniques may be useful in the diagnosis of alimentary lymphoma, they have not yet been shown to be of use in the diagnosis of IBD.

Two more recent markers with potential use in IBD are mucosal perinuclear antineutrophilic cytoplasmic antibody (pANCA) and lamina propria lymphocyte P-glycoprotein expression. High pretreatment pANCA expression has recently been shown to correlate with cases that respond principally to dietary therapy rather than those that ultimately respond to steroids (Luckschander et al., 2006). Thus assessment of pANCA expression pretreatment could help predict the most appropriate therapy for a particular case. P-glycoprotein is a transmembrane protein functioning as a drug-efflux pump in the intestinal epithelium. In human IBD cases high lymphocyte P-glycoprotein expression is seen in patients who fail to respond to treatment with steroids. Recent work in canine IBD demonstrated that low pretreatment mucosal lymphocyte P-glycoprotein expression correlated with a favorable response to treatment, suggesting that it may be a useful predictor of prognosis (Allenspach et al., 2006). However, the main limitation of this assay is the necessity for repeat endoscopy to monitor cases, given that many owners may be reluctant to allow their pet to undergo such procedures.

Treatment As a Diagnostic Tool

After the diagnostic investigations have been performed, a frequent mistake is to assume that the work of the clinician is done. In many cases clinicians can instigate an organized therapeutic plan that helps to confirm the diagnosis (based on the treatment to which the case responds) and tailor therapy to the individual case. Unless the animal is debilitated, I prefer to instigate single therapeutic modalities sequentially, and the owner is asked to record precisely in an event diary the frequency and nature of clinical signs. The clinician should review the diary on a regular basis to ascertain whether each treatment has led to a genuine improvement in clinical signs. My favored order of treatment trials is anthelmintic/antiparasitic medication (e.g., fenbendazole, 50 mg/kg q24h orally [PO] for 3 to 5 days), followed by dietary modification (preferably with an antigen-limited or hydrolyzed protein diet) for 3 to 4 weeks, followed by a 3- to 4-week antibacterial trial (usually tylosin, 10 mg/kg q8h PO, or metronidazole, 10 mg/kg q12h PO), and finally trial immunosuppressive therapy (initially prednisolone, 1 mg/kg q12h PO). Often partial responses to single agents are noted; in such cases the genuine need for multimodality therapy can be justified. The treatment trial approach is labor intensive but is the best way of achieving successful resolution of the clinical signs. Clients appreciate the interest shown by the clinician and are more accepting of the advice than when communication is poor following diagnosis.

MONITORING PROGRESSION OF INFLAMMATORY BOWEL DISEASE

In all species IBD is a condition that is most commonly controlled rather than cured with therapy. Currently the preferred approach to monitoring outcome is assessing for resolution of clinical signs. In humans activity indices are used to quantify IBD disease severity, aiding the assessment of the response to treatment and the prognosis and allowing comparisons among published studies in the literature. Recently an activity index has been suggested for canine IBD. Its use in the clinical setting provides a more objective measure of therapeutic response. However, clinicians must understand that increases in canine IBD activity index (CIBDAI) simply suggest an increase in severity of GI signs and that high values do not confirm the diagnosis of IBD. This was demonstrated in a recent paper in which increased CIBDAIs were seen in dogs with food-responsive conditions and values decreased on successful treatment (Spichiger et al., 2006). Thus perhaps CIBDAI should instead be known as chronic GI disease activity index.

Recent research has investigated novel methods of monitoring therapy in IBD; these include noninvasive (e.g., acute-phase proteins, insulin-like growth factor-1 [IGF-1]) and invasive (e.g., repeat histopathologic examination, P-glycoprotein) techniques. For example, C-reactive protein is an acute-phase protein that is elevated in dogs with IBD and reduces on resolution of therapy, correlating with a decrease in CIBDAI (Jergens et al., 2003). Plasma IGF-1 has recently been assessed in canine IBD and been shown to increase on successful therapy (Spichiger et al., 2006). Although such methods may prove to be useful for monitoring in the future, the main current limitation is the lack of commercial availability of the assays.

TREATMENT

Despite the fact that much has been written on therapy for companion animal IBD, most is opinion, and there remains little objective evidence of efficacy for any modality. Therefore this review focuses on my preferred approach, together with evidence that is available from peer-reviewed publications.

Approach to Therapy

The fact that IBD is usually controlled rather than cured is highlighted by a number of cases that have shown that mucosal inflammation remains despite resolution of clinical signs. In addition, most cases respond to combinations of therapy rather than single agents. The therapy used includes dietary modification, antibacterials, and immunosuppressive drugs. As described previously ("Treatment as a Diagnostic Tool"), I use a staged approach to therapy, except in seriously ill patients in which immediate intervention with immunosuppressive medication may be essential.

Dietary Management of IBD

Most clinicians would agree that dietary management is a key component in the successful treatment strategy for IBD cases, and in support of this dietary modification has recently been shown to play a critical part in long-term therapy for cats with chronic GI disease (Guilford et al., 2001). The main options for dietary management include switching to a highly digestible diet, an exclusion diet, and/or a diet high in fiber.

High digestibility ensures that components can be assimilated readily in the face of suboptimal digestive function. Efficient absorption also minimizes the substrate that is available to intestinal bacteria or for commanding an osmotic potential. Protein should be of high biologic value. Gluten is perceived to be a common food allergen, largely because of its known association with gluten-sensitive enteropathy in Irish setters. As a result, most formulated diets are now gluten free. However, although undoubtedly responsible for some adverse reactions to food, there is no evidence that gluten is any more antigenic than other commonly fed proteins. Fat restriction traditionally was recommended because of concerns over malabsorption, meaning that unassimilated fatty acids could be available for hydroxylation, thus stimulating electrolyte secretion. However, the need for fat restriction has recently been challenged since most cases can tolerate a higher dietary fat content and fat restriction may exacerbate existing weight loss. Supplementation with ω-3 fatty acids may also be of benefit in treating inflammatory diseases, although as yet there is no direct evidence confirming efficacy.

Exclusion diets are used when an adverse reaction to food is suspected; they are covered in more detail elsewhere. Most commercial exclusion diets are also highly digestible, enabling clinicians to choose the same diet for both purposes. The main recent advance in this field has been the advent of hydrolyzed protein diets, in which a native chicken or soy protein has undergone chemical or enzymatic treatment, producing low–molecular weight protein derivatives. In theory such diets should be less antigenic, and recent work has demonstrated reduced in vitro antigenicity compared with the native molecule. Their other main benefit is the improved digestibility of the protein components, which may be superior to traditional single-source protein-exclusion diets. Thus they are now the exclusion diet of choice for many clinicians, and recent clinical trials in both dogs and cats have been encouraging.

High-fiber diets are used most commonly in cases presenting predominantly with large intestinal signs. The clinician can either choose a purpose-formulated commercial diet or add a fiber supplement (e.g., Ispaghula husk) to the existing diet. Different fiber sources have different physiologic properties. Dietary fibers with a low solubility include cellulose and have their effect by increasing the bulk in the intestine, binding nonabsorbed fluid, and helping to regulate intestinal motility. Fibers with higher solubility include beet pulp, pectins from carrots or fruits, and gumlike fiber. These fiber sources can be easily fermented by intestinal bacteria, and the short-chain fatty acids (e.g., butyric acid) that are released can be partly used by the colonic mucosa. Further the addition of fermentable dietary fiber reduces the concentrations of some bacteria that are potentially harmful and increases the concentrations of some bacteria that are regarded as being beneficial. Thus a mix of insoluble and soluble fiber is usually chosen; either a purpose-formulated commercial ration can be used, or a fiber supplement can be added to the existing diet.

Whichever type of diet is chosen, it must be palatable and should be introduced in gradually increasing amounts over 4 to 7 days. It is best to feed the chosen diet exclusively in small, frequent meals (e.g., four to five per day). Finally, although enteral nutrition is usually preferred, parenteral nutrition may be beneficial in a case of severe, debilitating IBD.

Antibacterial Therapy

The use of antimicrobials in IBD can be justified in part by the potential to treat any undiagnosed enteropathogens and in part by the fact that it is bacterial antigens that are thought to drive the pathogenetic pathways. Currently metronidazole (10 mg/kg q12h PO) is the preferred antibacterial for most forms of IBD in small animals, and it has long been suggested to have immunomodulatory properties in addition to an antimicrobial action. Tylosin (10 mg/kg q8h PO) may also have immunomodulatory effects and may have some efficacy in canine IBD.

Although few studies demonstrate the efficacy of both of these drugs in companion animal IBD, a recent study in a rat model of IBD (colitis induced by 2,4,6-trinitrobenzene sulfonic acid) has suggested that tylosin is effective in decreasing inflammation (Menozzi et al., 2005). This work is particularly interesting in light of the recent report of a series of dogs with diarrhea that responded to tylosin therapy (see Chapter 116). However, the relationship between this condition and the IBD syndrome is not well understood. Finally, there are recent reports that histiocytic ulcerative colitis of boxers is responsive to enrofloxacin, supporting the hypothesis that this particular form of IBD is the consequence of an infection with a specific organism (see earlier discussion).

Antiinflammatory and Immunosuppressive Therapy

The mainstay of immunosuppressive therapy is prednisolone or prednisone (both 1 mg/kg q12h, PO initially, then tapering) with or without azathioprine in dogs (2 mg/kg q24h PO initially, then tapering) or chlorambucil (2 to 6 mg/m² q24h PO) in cats. However, controlled clinical trials on the use of these medications are lacking. A recent study in dogs has suggested that CIBDAI decreases on successful treatment with steroids (Spichiger et al., 2006), although neither mucosal permeability nor histopathologic abnormalities change significantly. This further supports the supposition that the condition is controlled rather than cured with such therapy. Hematologic parameters should be monitored regularly if azathioprine or chlorambucil is used. If cases respond, the medication can be tapered gradually, starting with the steroid, to an every-48-hour dosing regimen.

Budesonide is a glucocorticoid medication with high first-pass metabolism, and an enteric-coated formulation of this drug has been successful in maintaining remission in human IBD. A preliminary study showed apparent efficacy in dogs and cats, but limited information on the use of this drug is available. However, hypothalamic-pituitary-adrenal suppression and development of a steroid hepatopathy have been demonstrated in dogs. The optimal dosage has not yet been determined, although anecdotally a dosage of 1 mg/m² every 24 hours orally has been recommended. Sulfasalazine (and related drugs) are often used in dogs when IBD is limited to the large intestine. Side effects include keratoconjunctivitis sicca; therefore tear production should be monitored regularly.

A recent uncontrolled study has shown that cyclosporin (5 mg/kg q24h PO) may be effective in IBD that is refractory to steroid therapy (Allenspach et al., 2006). Cases responded to therapy based on improvement noted by CIBDAI. Biopsies taken after cyclosporin therapy showed a decrease in T cell numbers but no change in histopathology scores. A single case study recently reported response of severe IBD with concurrent hypoproteinemia and lymphangiectasia, to methotrexate after a combination of prednisolone and cyclosporin was ineffective (Yuki et al., 2006). This observation should be confirmed with larger case series and preferably evidence-based medicine before routine use of this drug can be recommended.

Treatment of Patients With Severe Protein-Losing Enteropathy

PLE is a recognized complication in a subset of IBD cases (Chapter 118), and the presence of low serum albumin concentrations (suggesting severe PLE) has been shown to be a poor prognostic marker in IBD. Patients with albumin concentrations of 1.5 g/dl (or below) are at risk of developing ascites, pleural effusion, and subcutaneous edema. They may also be at risk of complications associated with intestinal biopsy by celiotomy; plasma transfusion, human albumin infusion, or synthetic colloid (e.g., hydroxyl-ethyl starch) may be indicated during the perioperative period. Further, I usually hospitalize such cases for the initial treatment period, enabling cage rest (which may assist with the clearance of ascites fluid), and allowing use of glucocorticoids by the parenteral route (ideally using a prednisolone preparation designed for intramuscular injection). This approach is based on the potential for concurrent malabsorption, meaning that oral preparations may not be adequately absorbed. I favor an intramuscular preparation of prednisolone (Deltastab, Sovereign Medical; 2 mg/kg, q24h intramuscularly) and use both serum albumin concentrations and clinical signs to assess response. Once albumin concentrations begin to increase, oral glucocorticoid medications can be substituted; assuming that albumin concentrations continue to climb, the patient can be discharged from the hospital. Finally diuretics may be required for the management of effusions, and combinations of diuretics are preferred (e.g., furosemide and spironolactone) with monitoring of serum electrolytes and renal function.

Adjunctive Therapy

Hypocobalaminemia is common in both dogs and cats with IBD and should be corrected with parenteral supplementation if present. I use a dosage of 20 mcg/kg every 7 days subcutaneously for 4 weeks and then the same dosage every 28 days for a further 3 months. Reassessment of serum cobalamin concentration verifies the efficacy of therapy. Thromboembolism is a feature of some patients with PLE, and prophylactic low-dose aspirin has been advocated. A small cases series in canine IBD suggested an association with iron deficiency anemia and required iron supplementation to correct.

Probiotics have been suggested to be beneficial for human IBD, although no truly objective data (e.g., double-blind placebo-controlled trials) exist despite promising initial reports. More work is required before probiotic use becomes commonplace in companion animal IBD therapy.

PROGNOSIS

Many clinicians have the impression that treatment of companion animal IBD has a high success rate, but in published reports the actual response rate is variable. A recent retrospective paper suggested that only 26% of cases progress to complete remission, intermittent signs remain in approximately half of cases, 4% are completely uncontrolled, and 13% are euthanized because of poor response (Craven et al., 2004). This suggests that prognosis is guarded and quality of life of IBD patients can be poor. The main negative prognostic sign identified was that of hypoalbuminemia.

References and Suggested Reading

Allenspach K et al: P-glycoprotein expression in lamina propria lymphocytes of duodenal biopsy samples in dogs with chronic idiopathic enteropathies, *J Comp Pathol* 134:1, 2006.

Allenspach K et al: Pharmacokinetics and clinical efficacy of cyclosporine treatment of dogs with steroid-refractory inflammatory bowel disease, *J Vet Intern Med* 20:239, 2006.

Craven M et al: Canine inflammatory bowel disease: retrospective analysis of diagnosis and outcome in 80 cases (1995-2002), *J Small Anim Pract* 45:336, 2004.

German AJ, Hall EJ, Day N: Chronic intestinal inflammation and intestinal disease in dogs, *J Vet Intern Med* 17:8, 2003.

Guilford WG et al: Food sensitivity in cats with chronic idiopathic gastrointestinal problems, *J Vet Intern Med* 15:7, 2001.

Jergens AE et al: A scoring index for disease activity in canine inflammatory bowel disease, *J Vet Intern Med* 17:291, 2003.

Kircher PA et al: Doppler ultasonographic evaluation of gastrointestinal hemodynamics in food hypersensitivities: a canine model, *J Vet Intern Med* 18:605, 2004.

Luckschander N et al: Perinuclear antineutrophilic cytoplasmic antibody and response to treatment in diarrheic dogs with food responsive disease or inflammatory bowel disease, *J Vet Intern Med* 20:221, 2006.

Menozzi A et al: Effect of the macrolide antibacterial drug, tylosin, on TNBS-induced colitis in the rat, *Pharmacology* 74:135, 2005.

Peters IR et al: Cytokine mrna quantification in duodenal mucosa from dogs with chronic enteropathies by real-time reverse transcriptase polymerase chain reaction, *J Vet Intern Med* 19:644, 2005.

Simpson KW et al: Subnormal concentrations of serum cobalamin (vitamin b12) in cats with gastrointestinal disease, *J Vet Intern Med* 15:26, 2001.

Simpson KW et al: Adherent and invasive *Escherichia coli* is associated with granulomatous colitis of boxer dogs, *Infect Immun* 74:4778, 2006.

Spichiger AC et al: Plasma insulin-like growth factor-1 concentration in dogs with chronic enteropathies, *Vet Med* 51:35, 2006.

Willard MD et al: Interobserver variation among histopathologic evaluations of intestinal tissues from dogs and cats, *J Am Vet Med Assoc* 220:1177, 2002.

Yuki M et al: A case of protein-losing enteropathy treated with methotrexate in a do, *J Vet Med Sci* 68:397, 2006.

CHAPTER **116**

Tylosin-Responsive Diarrhea

ELIAS WESTERMARCK, *Helsinki, Finland*

Antibiotic treatment often leads to resolution of clinical gastrointestinal (GI) signs, and thus the term *antibiotic-responsive diarrhea* was coined for these cases. Recently trials have been published in which the antibiotic tylosin proved to be particularly effective in treating dogs with chronic or intermittent diarrhea, with the effect of tylosin differing from that of other antibiotics; thus it is referred to as tylosin-responsive diarrhea (TRD).

CLINICAL PHARMACOLOGY

Tylosin is a macrolide, bacteriostatic antibiotic that has activity against most gram-positive and gram-negative cocci, gram-positive rods, and *Mycoplasma*. However, the gram-negative bacteria *Escherichia coli* and *Salmonella* spp. are intrinsically tylosin resistant. Tylosin is used only in veterinary medicine, and the most common indications are for treating pigs with diarrhea or poultry with chronic respiratory diseases. Tylosin has also been used as a feed additive in food animal production, and it has been shown to increase weight gain and feed efficiency, especially in pigs. There is debate into the mechanisms underlying tylosin-mediated growth enhancement.

Tylosin is used in a powder form for pigs and poultry. For small animals tylosin powder is usually reconstituted in capsules or mixed with the food for administration. In some European countries tylosin is also available in tablet form, which facilitates its use in dogs.

THERAPEAUTIC USE

My experience with tylosin was first derived from studies in dogs having exocrine pancreatic insufficiency (EPI) and continued diarrhea following appropriate enzyme therapy. These studies found that tylosin had a favorable effect as a supportive therapy for dogs with EPI and diarrhea.

In recent years in Finland tylosin has become the most frequent antibiotic used in the treatment of nonspecific intermittent or chronic diarrhea in dogs. Anecdotal reports from veterinarians and dog owners reveal that many dogs with diarrhea respond quickly to tylosin treatment, generally within a few days of initiation of therapy. When tylosin is discontinued, the diarrhea often reappears within a matter of weeks or months. Some of these dogs require ongoing treatment for very long periods of time. It was also observed that the tylosin effect in controlling diarrhea signs does not appear to diminish with time and the need for an increased dosage is not required. No apparent tylosin-associated adverse effects have been reported.

My clinical experience finds that TRD affects dogs of all breeds and ages, but is most often observed in middle-aged, large-breed dogs. Signs often begin as intermittent diarrhea that becomes progressively more frequent and often persistent. Abnormal loose fecal consistency is the predominant sign. The majority of the owners describe their dogs' feces as watery and or of mucoid consistency, suggesting that TRD involves both small- and large-bowel diarrhea. Increased frequency of borborygmus and flatulence typically are also described, and vomiting is reported occasionally during the diarrheal outbreaks.

Diagnostic evaluation of TRD cases have failed to identify an underlying etiology. Routine blood parameters, fecal examinations, and diagnostic imaging studies are usually normal. When intestinal biopsies are obtained, the histologic findings are considered either to be normal or to have only mild inflammatory changes.

CLINICAL STUDIES USING TYLOSIN FOR CHRONIC DIARRHEA

Only a few studies treating diarrhea in dogs with tylosin have been published. Van Kruiningen (1976) reported over 30 years ago that tylosin was effective in the treatment of unspecific canine diarrhea. Recently our study group performed two prospective clinical trials to obtain more information on TRD (Westermarck E et al., 2005). The first study consisted of 14 adult client-owned dogs of 12 different breeds. Each dog's diet remained unchanged throughout the study. All dogs had chronic or intermittent diarrheal signs for a period of longer than 1 year. All dogs previously had been treated successfully with tylosin for at least 6 months. Tylosin had been discontinued at least twice, but the diarrhea had always recurred. These dogs were then considered to have TRD. When the study commenced, all dogs had been on tylosin for at least 1 month and were healthy and free of diarrhea. Tylosin was then discontinued, and the dogs were monitored for a period of up to 1 month to determine whether signs of diarrhea would reappear. Diarrhea reappeared in 12 of

14 dogs (85.7%) within 30 days. Tylosin, prednisone, or a probiotic treatment trial was initiated when diarrhea was present. Tylosin resulted in resolution of diarrhea in all dogs within 3 days of initiation of therapy, with most resolving within 24 hours. In contrast, prednisone did not completely resolve diarrheal signs, and the probiotic *Lactobacillus rhamnosus GG* did not prevent the relapse of diarrhea in any of the dogs.

In a second study seven beagles with chronic diarrhea for a duration of at least 1 month were identified from an experimental dog colony. Treatment trials of antibiotics, prednisone, and diet were used. Tylosin was administered for 10 days, and during that time the feces became significantly firmer, although they remained unacceptably loose. When the treatment was discontinued, diarrhea reappeared within 3 weeks. Next treatment trials with other antibiotics (metronidazole, trimethoprim-sulfadiazine, or doxycycline) and prednisone had almost no effect on fecal consistency in these dogs. The diet was then changed for a 10-day period from a highly digestible moist pet food to a dry food developed for normal adult dogs. The feces again became significantly firmer, although the fecal consistency remained loose in some dogs. The dry food feeding period was then extended to 3 months, and the fecal consistency continued to fluctuate from ideal to diarrhea. Since the consistency was not satisfactory on diet alone, tylosin was added to the therapy for 10 days. The fecal consistency became normal and remained so throughout the entire 3-month follow-up time of this study. The study demonstrated that, in this group of experimental dogs having chronic diarrhea, the fecal consistency became significantly firmer using tylosin in conjunction with dietary modification. Neither treatment alone was sufficient to obtain ideal fecal consistency; but, when the dogs were treated simultaneously with both regimens, ideal fecal consistency was achieved and maintained. The study suggests that tylosin and feeding regimens had a synergic effect.

PATHOPHYSIOLOGY

The etiology of TRD remains obscure. Since tylosin is an antimicrobial agent, it has been speculated that some pathogenic bacteria likely are responsible for the diarrheal signs. Based on negative fecal culture results and enzyme-linked immunoadsorbent assay testing for clostridial enterotoxin, we have excluded such common enteropathogenic bacteria as *Clostridium perfringens, Clostridium difficile, Salmonella* spp., *Campylobacter* spp., and *Yersinia* spp. as causative factors for the diarrheal signs occurring in TRD. Less well-defined species causing diarrhea in dogs such as *Plesiomonas shigelloides, Lawsoni intracellularis,* and *Brachyspira* spp. were also excluded.

Our ongoing studies have revealed that administration of tylosin leads to significant but transient changes in the composition of the small intestinal microflora. The results support the hypothesis that tylosin promotes the growth of beneficial commensal bacteria while suppressing deleterious bacteria.

In addition to antibacterial properties, tylosin may also possess antiinflammatory properties, contributing to its effectiveness in treating canine diarrhea. The mode of action is most likely different from the immunomodulatory effects of prednisone because prednisone treatment did not completely resolve diarrheal signs in the dogs that responded to tylosin.

DIAGNOSTIC PROTOCOL FOR CHRONIC DIARRHEA

The diagnostic protocol used for dogs with chronic diarrhea by the Faculty of Veterinary Medicine at the University of Helsinki is represented in Fig. 116-1. In patients with chronic diarrhea, every effort should be made to achieve a diagnosis to enable a specific therapy. Unfortunately this is not always possible, in which case empiric therapeutic trials are used in the workup of these patients. There are conflicting opinions about how long an empiric therapy should be attempted. We recommend 10 days if a dog has chronic diarrhea or if the interval between intermittent diarrheal episodes is only a few days. If signs of diarrhea disappear or resolve during this period, the treatment should be continued another 2 to 6 weeks. When the interval between episodes of intermittent diarrhea is long (i.e., more than 1 week), the length of the empiric treatment period should be prolonged. The workup protocol displayed in Figure 116-1 for patients with chronic or intermittent diarrhea is applicable for most veterinary

practices. It is also useful regardless of whether the clinical signs are typical of large or small intestinal disease.

The initial evaluation (A) comprises obtaining a thorough case history, conducting a physical examination, and taking the basic laboratory tests, including a complete blood count, a serum chemistry profile, fecal evaluation for parasites, and measurement of serum concentrations of trypsin-like immunoreactivity. According to the initial evaluation, the patients are then divided into one of two groups. The first group includes patients in which abnormal findings are identified (Group B), whereas the second group has no obvious abnormalities other than diarrhea (Group C).

Patients in group B identified with obvious abnormalities of systemic disorders (B1a) such as hepatic failure, renal failure, hypoadrenocorticism, or EPI (B1b) require specific therapy. Animals having hypoproteinemia (B1c), melena and or anemia (B1d), or abnormal palpation findings (B1e) require advanced diagnostics (D), including imaging studies, endoscopy, and or intestinal biopsy. Most often these animals have inflammatory bowel disease, lymphangiectasia, or GI neoplasia.

Dogs with diarrhea but no identified abnormalities (C) on the initial evaluation are first treated orally with fenbendazole 50 mg/kg for 3 days (C1) to rule out endoparasites as the causative factor for GI signs. When endoparasites have been ruled out, adverse food reactions (C2)

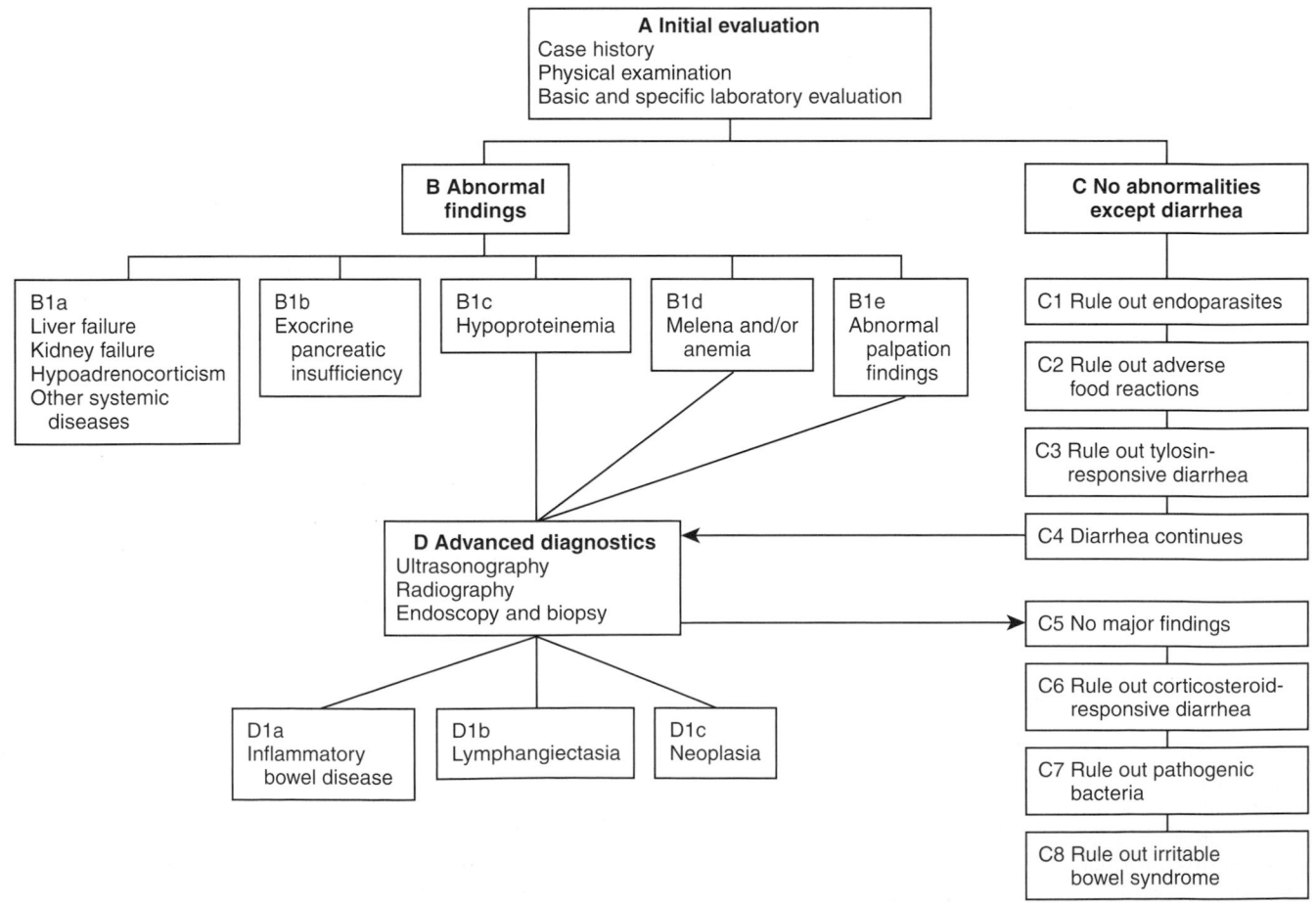

Fig. 116-1   Diagnostic approach to dogs presenting with chronic diarrhea at the Veterinary School in Helsinki, Finland.

should be investigated. Food is probably the most common cause of diarrhea, and adverse food reactions should always be excluded before empiric treatment trials with different drugs are initiated. Opinions vary widely on the type of diets used for a dietary treatment trial (see Section VI on the Evolve site). Unfortunately current recommendations are largely based on anecdotal evidence rather than on controlled trials. The most common recommendation is to use a diet with novel protein and carbohydrate sources, with the protein restricted to a single animal source.

If modifying the feeding regimen fails to produce a satisfactory fecal consistency, the next step is to treat the dog with tylosin 25 mg/kg of body weight every 24 hours (C3). Dogs responding to tylosin treatment usually do so within 3 to 5 days, and the stool remains normal as long as treatment continues. In many TRD cases the diarrhea reappears within weeks on discontinuation of treatment. If diarrheal signs reappear, further dietary trials should once again be initiated to make sure that an adverse food reaction is not involved in the etiology of the signs. If diarrheal signs continue, tylosin treatment is reinitiated. I have treated TRD in some dogs for years. The dose of tylosin for long-term use should be tapered to the lowest possible dose that controls the clinical signs. Many dogs may need only half of the recommended dose to be diarrhea

free. Although no adverse effects during tylosin treatment have been observed, efforts should be made to reduce or discontinue the use of tylosin if possible. Recently studies that I conducted identified that tylosin causes wide resistance to intestinal antibiotics (unpublished results).

Certain probiotic lactic acid bacteria (LAB) have been shown to be effective in the prevention and treatment of a variety of diarrheal disorders in humans and in experimental mouse models. Possibly a probiotic LAB can be used instead of tylosin to treat or prevent chronic diarrhea in dogs with TRD.

Dogs not responding positively to dietary modification or tylosin treatment require advanced diagnostic studies (D). The workup is continued and further diagnostic considerations as displayed in Figure 116-1.

References and Suggested Reading

Van Kruiningen HJ: Clinical efficacy of tylosin in canine inflammatory bowel disease, *J Am Anim Hosp Assoc* 12:498, 1976.

Westermarck E, Wiberg M: Exocrine pancreatic insufficiency in dogs, *Vet Clin North Am Small Anim Pract* 33:1165, 2003.

Westermarck E, Frias R, Skrzypczak T: Effect of diet and tylosin on chronic diarrhea in beagles, *J Vet Intern Med1* 9:822, 2005.

Westermarck E et al: Tylosin-responsive chronic diarrhea in dogs. *J Vet Intern Med* 19:177, 2005.

CHAPTER 117

Tritrichomonas

JODY L. GOOKIN, *Raleigh, North Carolina*

Trichomonads are flagellated protozoans characterized by an undulating membrane that courses along the length of a pear-shaped body. They are similar in size to *Giardia* spp. and obligate parasites of warm, moist, anaerobic areas within the gastrointestinal or genitourinary tract of their hosts. Trichomonads do not form cysts, they reproduce by binary fission, and they are transmitted directly from host to host in the form of trophozoites. Pathogenic and nonpathogenic species of trichomonads can be found in animals. *Pentatrichomonas hominis* inhabits the large intestine of a number of mammalian hosts and is considered to be a commensal, whereas *Tritrichomonas foetus* is recognized as an important venereal pathogen of naturally bred cattle. *T. foetus* was first identified as a cause of chronic large bowel diarrhea in cats in 2003; the duration of its existence in cats before that time is unknown (Levy et al., 2003). In cats *T. foetus* colonizes the distal ileum and

colon, resulting in lymphoplasmacytic and neutrophilic colitis and chronic foul-smelling diarrhea. The prevalence of *T. foetus* infection is high among densely housed cats, with 31% of 117 cats from 89 catteries sampled were positive at an international cat show (Gookin et al., 2004).

SIGNALMENT AND CLINICAL FINDINGS

Generally cats with diarrhea and *T. foetus* infection are young, but asymptomatic infection in older cats may also be common. Cats originating from a cattery (e.g., purebred) or shelter appear to be at increased risk for infection because of a history of dense housing. A true breed predisposition has not been shown (Gookin et al., 2004). Clinical signs are characterized by large bowel diarrhea occasionally containing fresh blood and mucus. Diarrhea is semiformed to cowpie in consistency and malodorous.

In very young cats and with poor housing conditions, the anus may appear inflamed and painful; involuntary dribbling of feces or rectal prolapse may be present. In general, cats maintain good health and normal appetite and body condition. Consistency of the diarrhea waxes and wanes and typically improves during antimicrobial treatment but quickly resumes when treatment is discontinued (Gookin et al., 1999). *T. foetus*–infected cats are often misdiagnosed as having *Giardia* spp. Cats diagnosed with *Giardia* spp. on the basis of a fecal smear that fail to respond to appropriate antimicrobial therapy should be closely reevaluated for the possibility that the observed trophozoites were *T. foetus*.

DIAGNOSIS

Feline *T. foetus* infection may be diagnosed by identifying the organism in feces by direct smear examination, selective protozoal culture, and polymerase chain reaction (PCR) using species-specific primers or by observation of trichomonads in colonic mucosal biopsy specimens.

Direct Fecal Smear Examination

Fecal samples should be diarrheic and *freshly* voided or obtained directly from the rectum using a fecal loop. Areas in which feces are particularly moist or contain mucus and blood are ideal locations to sample. A scant amount of feces should be mixed in a drop of saline and examined under a coverslip using a 40× objective. Lowering the microscope condenser to increase contrast enhances visualization. Trichomonads are approximately the size of *Giardia* spp. and highly motile. The key microscopic differences between trichomonads and *Giardia* spp. are a "falling leaf" motility characteristic of *Giardia* spp. and presence of an undulating membrane on trichomonads. Multiple smears should be examined for organisms. If necessary, survival of *T. foetus* in feces can be extended from 0 to 4 days by removing adherent litter and diluting the sample with normal saline to avoid desiccation (3 ml 0.9% saline per 2 g of feces)(Foster et al., 2004). Trichomonads do not survive refrigeration and are not typically observed using fecal flotation or sedimentation techniques. Concurrent antibiotic therapy decreases the number *T. foetus* present in feces. It is often prudent to discontinue antibiotics for a few days in such cases and repeat the examination if negative results were obtained initially. The sensitivity of direct fecal smear examination for diagnosis of *T. foetus* is low (2% in cats with experimentally induced infection and 14% in cats with spontaneous disease). It can be difficult to reliably distinguish *T. foetus* from nonpathogenic trichomonads such as *P. hominis* on the basis of light microscopic appearance, making this means of diagnosis presumptive.

Protozoal Culture of Feces

If repeated direct microscopic examination results are negative for *T. foetus*, feces may be cultured in commercially available pouches marketed for diagnosis of *T. foetus* infection in cattle (In Pouch TF, Biomed Diagnostics). Pouches should be inoculated with 0.05 g (about the size of a rice grain) of freshly voided or loop-collected feces. The pouch can be incubated either at 37° C for 48 hours or at room temperature (25° C) for up to 12 days. Bacterial overgrowth and gaseous distention of the pouch is a problem if overinoculated with feces and more common when incubated at 37° C. Pouches should be cultured upright and in the dark and examined daily (37° C) or every other day (25° C) for the presence of trichomonads. Before examination pouches should be tapped against the bench top to dislodge adherent organisms and then placed within a manufacturer-provided clamp that allows the pouch to be mounted onto the stage of a light microscope. Trichomonads are most easily found along the seams of the pouch using a 20× or 40× objective. Although feces may be shipped to some laboratories for cultivation, given the fragile nature of the organisms it is strongly recommended that this user-friendly culture technique be performed in-house for best results. Fecal culture using In Pouch TF has a detection limit of 1000 or more *T. foetus* organisms per 0.05 g of feces and is superior to direct fecal smear examination for diagnosis of *T. foetus* infection. Neither *Giardia* spp. nor *P. hominis* organisms survived in Pouch TF for longer than 24 hours in one study; thus positive cultures are strongly suggestive of *T. foetus* infection (Gookin et al., 2003). However, strictly speaking the types of trichomonads potentially hosted by cats and the specificity of In Pouch TF with regard to these other types of trichomonads are unknown. Positive In Pouch TF cultures do not preclude the possibility of coinfection with *P. hominis* or *Giardia* spp.

Polymerase Chain Reaction

A sensitive and specific single-tube nested PCR based on amplification of a conserved portion of the *T. foetus* internal transcribed spacer region (ITS1 and ITS2) and 5.8S rRNA gene from feline feces is commercially available and superior to fecal culture for diagnosis of infected cats. PCR requires approximately 180 to 220 mg of feces devoid of litter, and samples should be preserved in 3 to 5 ml of 70% isopropyl alcohol (rubbing alcohol) before shipment at room temperature. Sensitivity of the PCR is 10 trichomonads per 200-mg sample of feces (Gookin et al., 2002).

Histopathology

Colonic mucosal biopsy is often appropriate in cases of large bowel diarrhea in which less invasive diagnostics fail to identify a cause for diarrhea and appropriate empiric medical and dietary treatment trials have failed to result in a resolution of signs. Histopathology should not be relied on to make a diagnosis of *T. foetus* infection, although a diagnosis can be attained if organisms are identified. The diagnostic feature is the presence of trichomonads, which can be found in close proximity to the surface of the mucosa or in the lumen of colonic crypts. Less commonly subepithelial invasion of trichomonads may also be observed. Inflammatory infiltrates consist of plasma cells, lymphocytes, and neutrophils. Lesions can be segmental in distribution; therefore multiple sites should be biopsied. It is advisable to indicate that

T. foetus is a differential diagnosis because a minimum of six tissue sections should be examined to achieve 95% or greater confidence that trichomonads will be identified (Yaeger and Gookin, 2005).

TREATMENT

Coexisting Infectious Diseases

Any coexisting intestinal infection in a *T. foetus*–infected cat should be identified and treated if possible. Studies of experimental feline infection suggest that coexisting intestinal infection (e.g., cryptosporidiosis) worsens clinical signs of diarrhea and increases the shedding of *T. foetus* organisms. Coinfection with *Giardia* spp. is common in *T. foetus*–infected cats and, if present, should be treated (Gookin et al., 2004). If helminth parasites are not identified, empiric treatment with fenbendazole is recommended. Other infections to consider are *Cryptosporidium* spp. In most cases systemic disease or viral infections (feline leukemia virus/feline immunodeficiency virus) are not identified.

Spontaneous Resolution of Diarrhea

When left untreated, 88% of cats with *T. foetus* infection had spontaneous resolution of diarrhea within 2 years (median 9 months; range 5 months to 2 years). Time to resolution of diarrhea was significantly longer for cats from multiple-cat households and those receiving a variety of different diets and antimicrobial drugs in an attempt to treat the condition. Stressful events may be associated with a relapse in diarrhea (e.g., surgery, oral antimicrobial therapy, travel, or a change in diet). The wait-for-resolution approach to treatment of *T. foetus* infection is best suited for a stable household with a low number of cats where further spread of infection is of little concern and owners are willing to tolerate the long course of diarrhea. It is important to note that spontaneous resolution of diarrhea does not imply recovery from infection since 57% of these cats remain infected with *T. foetus* as determined by PCR when performed 2 to 5 years after diagnosis (Foster et al., 2004).

Medical Therapy

Dietary trials, homeopathic remedies, and antimicrobial drugs have not been consistently effective in ameliorating signs of diarrhea in *T. foetus*–infected cats, and studies suggest that these interventions may prolong the duration of clinical signs, perhaps by perturbing the balance of colonic microflora on which the trichomonads depend. Despite the presence of inflammatory colitis, diarrhea does not appear to be improved by treatment with corticosteroids. In vitro studies suggest that *T. foetus* is inherently resistant to many drugs or rapidly acquires resistance in vivo (Gookin et al., 2001). Trichomonads lack mitochondria and ferment pyruvate in reductive organelles called hydrogenosomes. Reduction of nitroimidazole antibiotics by hydrogenosomes results in formation of toxic anion radicals that serve as the basis for susceptibility of trichomonads to drugs such as

metronidazole. Unfortunately feline *T. foetus* infection is not responsive to metronidazole.

Ronidazole

Ronidazole (RDZ) is a 5-nitroimidazole relative of metronidazole that has been used for the treatment of *Histomonas meleagridis* (turkey blackhead), *Treponema hyodysenteriae* (swine dysentery), and *Treponema hyodysenteriae* infection (pigeon canker). RDZ has been demonstrated to be effective at killing feline isolates of *T. foetus* in vitro at concentrations greater than 0.1 mcg/ml and eradicated *T. foetus* from experimentally infected cats (on the basis of PCR) when administered at 30 mg/kg every 12 hours orally for 14 days (Gookin et al., 2006). RDZ is not registered for human or veterinary use in the United States and is currently banned from use in food-producing animals because of human hazards. Due diligence is required for protection of humans from exposure to RDZ, and veterinarians are advised to obtain informed consent before use of this drug in cats. Gloves should be worn when handling RDZ. Several pharmacies compound chemical grade RDZ for veterinary use. Because of its foul taste, compounding into gelatin capsules rather than flavored liquids is highly recommended. Storing the capsules in the freezer may improve drug stability. RDZ is popular in Europe for the treatment of *T. gallinae* in racing pigeons. Several 10% active-drug formulations for dilution in the drinking water of birds can be obtained without prescription from pigeon supply warehouses. Because of their undetermined quality, composition, and low active-drug concentration, these products are not recommended.

It is important to note that pharmacokinetic data have not been published for RDZ and that neurotoxicosis may be a common and serious side effect. Therefore treatment with RDZ should only be considered in cases of confirmed *T. foetus* infection in which informed consent has been obtained. Cats should be isolated during treatment to decrease the risk of reinfection. It is suspected that asymptomatic infections are common in multiple-cat colonies; thus isolation from cats with clinical signs alone may not be sufficient to avoid reinfection. A prolonged follow-up period is necessary to determine if infection has been eradicated. Testing by PCR at 1 to 2 weeks and 20+ weeks after completion of treatment is recommended. Negative results should be interpreted with caution since PCR cannot prove the absence of infection and prolonged asymptomatic carriage of the organism after antimicrobial therapy may be common. Until sufficient information about the pharmacokinetics and safety of RDZ is available or safer treatments are identified, isolation and treatment of individual cats rather than entire catteries is recommended if RDZ is prescribed.

References and Suggested Reading

Foster DM et al: Outcome of cats with diarrhea and *Tritrichomonas foetus* infection, *J Am Vet Med Assoc* 225:888, 2004.
Gookin JL et al: Diarrhea associated with trichomonosis in cats, *J Am Vet Med Assoc* 215:1450, 1999.

Gookin JL et al: Experimental infection of cats with *Tritrichomonas foetus*, *Am J Vet Res* 62:1690, 2001.

Gookin JL et al: Single-tube nested PCR for detection of *Tritrichomonas foetus* in feline feces, *J Clin Microbiol* 40:4126, 2002.

Gookin JL et al: Use of a commercially available culture system for diagnosis of *Tritrichomonas foetus* infection in cats, *J Am Vet Med Assoc* 222:1376, 2003.

Gookin JL et al: Prevalence of and risk factors for feline *Tritrichomonas foetus* and Giardia infection, *J Clin Microbiol* 42:2707, 2004.

Gookin JL et al: Efficacy of ronidazole for treatment of feline *Tritrichomonas foetus* infection, *J Vet Intern Med* 20:536, 2006.

Levy MG et al: *Tritrichomonas foetus* and not *Pentatrichomonas hominis* is the etiologic agent of feline trichomonal diarrhea, *J Parasitol* 89:99, 2003.

Yaeger MJ, Gookin JL: Histologic features associated with *Tritrichomonas foetus*–induced colitis in domestic cats, *Vet Pathol* 42:797, 2005.

CHAPTER 118

Protein-Losing Enteropathy

LISA E. MOORE, *Maitland, Florida*

Protein-losing enteropathy (PLE) is not a disease per se, but a term used to describe a disease that results in a nonselective loss of serum proteins into the intestinal tract. PLEs can be associated with a large number of intestinal and systemic disorders. The loss of proteins can be caused by a loss of mucosal barrier function that results in increased intestinal permeability such as inflammatory or erosive disorders or by malfunction or abnormalities of intestinal lymphatic drainage (Jeffries, 1983). PLEs are more common in the dog than in the cat. Many diseases have been reported to cause PLE in dogs, including intestinal lymphangiectasia (primary or secondary), inflammatory disorders (lymphoplasmacytic, eosinophilic, granulomatous enteritides, gluten-sensitive enteropathy), gastrointestinal ulceration, neoplasia (alimentary lymphoma, intestinal carcinoma), intestinal fungal or parasitic infections (histoplasmosis, pythiosis, trichuriasis, ancylostomiasis), foreign bodies, chronic intussusceptions, acute viral enteritis (parvovirus), acute or chronic bacterial enteritides, immune-mediated and allergic diseases (systemic lupus erythematosus), constrictive pericarditis, right-sided heart failure, and hypoadrenocorticism.

CAUSES OF PROTEIN-LOSING ENTEROPATHIES

Intestinal Lymphangiectasia

Intestinal lymphangiectasia (IL) is considered to be the most common disorder associated with PLE (Tams and Twedt, 1981; Melzer and Sellon, 2002). IL can be primary or secondary. Primary IL is a congenital disease in which insufficient or malformed lymphatic vessels result in poor intestinal lymphatic flow and drainage. Congenital IL is considered uncommon to rare in the dog and cat. The disease can also be associated with systemic abnormalities of the lymphatic system (Fossum, 1989). Secondary IL usually results from obstruction to lymphatic flow, either in the lymphatic system (inflammatory lesions of the intestinal wall, neoplastic disorders) or subsequent to venous hypertension (congestive heart failure, portal vein thrombosis, pericardial disease). When the pressure in the lymph vessels increases, the intestinal villous lacteals dilate, become fragile, rupture easily, and leak lymph into the intestinal tract. This lymph is high in lymphocytes, chylomicrons, and proteins. The underlying disease can also limit the resorptive ability of the intestinal mucosa (Melzer, 2002). Lipogranulomas are often observed around the lymphatics in inflammatory disorders (Van Kruiningen et al., 1984).

Inflammatory Bowel Disease

Inflammatory and immune diseases of the intestines include lymphoplasmacytic, eosinophilic, and granulomatous enteritides. Lymphoplasmacytic enteritis is the most common cause of PLE in this category (Tams and Twedt, 1981; Craven et al., 2004). This disease is characterized by a diffuse infiltration of lymphocytes and plasma cells in the lamina propria of the intestinal mucosa. Inflammatory bowel disease is a chronic disorder for which no cause can be determined, but current theories are concentrating on defining immunoregulation, dietary allergens, reactions to normal enteric bacterial flora, or other chronic antigenic stimuli (Guilford, 1996; also see chapter 115). Regardless of the cause or causes, the final pathway is inflammation that results in damage to the gastrointestinal tissue, which can result in protein loss.

Breed-Related Protein-Losing Enteropathy

Breeds with a higher incidence of PLE include basenjis, soft-coated wheaten terriers, and lundehunds (Breitschwerdt, 1992; Vaden et al., 2000). These breeds appear predisposed to lymphoplasmacytic enteritis, resulting in a significant PLE. The basenji enteropathy is associated with hypoalbuminemia and hyperglobulinemia (Breitschwerdt, 1992).

Miscellaneous Disorders

As mentioned previously, various other diseases can cause gastrointestinal protein loss (Tams and Twedt, 1981; Jeffries, 1983). Conditions resulting in erosion or bleeding of the intestinal mucosa, submucosa, or muscularis can result in loss of plasma or loss of blood if the lesion is more severe. Examples would include erosion or ulceration caused by foreign objects, drugs (most commonly nonsteroidal anti-inflammatory drugs), and intussusceptions. Infiltrative disorders such as histoplasmosis and lymphoma are also reported causes of PLE. Acute and chronic infectious diseases should be included. Parvoviral enteritis can result in severe hypoproteinemia because of destruction of the villus and subsequent plasma leakage into the intestines. Various bacterial diseases, including small intestinal bacterial overgrowth, and parasitic infections can cause PLE.

CLINICAL SIGNS

Clinical signs can be variable but almost always include weight loss (loss of muscle mass and body condition). Other signs can be those associated with the gastrointestinal tract such as vomiting and diarrhea. It should be noted that not all animals with PLE have diarrhea; weight loss may be the only clinical sign. Polyphagia is seen occasionally, but many dogs and cats have variable inappetence. Other signs are related to the hypoproteinemia. Ascites, peripheral edema, and dyspnea resulting from hydrothorax all can be seen. Uncommonly some animals present with clinical signs related to thromboembolic disease such as respiratory signs caused by a pulmonary thrombus or posterior paresis caused by a distal aortic thrombus. Abdominal palpation may reveal thickened intestinal loops, lymphadenopathy, or a mass. Thoracic auscultation may reveal cardiac abnormalities.

DIAGNOSIS

The hypoproteinemia seen in animals with PLE is nonselective; therefore serum albumin and globulin levels are both decreased. Two notable exceptions include the PLE of basenji dogs (see previous discussion) and intestinal histoplasmosis. Intestinal histoplasmosis has been associated with a normal or elevated globulin fraction, presumably caused by the inflammatory response (Williams, 1996). Other abnormalities that may be noted include lymphopenia, hypocalcemia, hypomagnesemia, hypocholesterolemia, decreased antithrombin (if measured), and variably elevated liver enzymes and electrolyte abnormalities (Bush et al., 2001; Mellanby et al., 2005).

Other causes of hypoalbuminemia should be ruled out. Urinalysis and urine protein:creatinine ratio are abnormal with renal protein loss. Decreased albumin production can be caused by severe hepatic disease, and hepatic function testing such as bilirubin and serum preprandial and postprandial bile acid analysis should be performed to eliminate this possibility. Protein loss can also occur with chronic blood loss, in which case anemia should also be present. Radiography is useful to rule out obstructive lesions (foreign objects), cardiac disease, and pulmonary metastatic or fungal lesions. Ultrasonography can be helpful to rule out mass lesions (e.g., neoplasia, pythiosis). Ultrasonographic abnormalities may be seen in animals with PLE and IL. Findings such as a corrugated small intestine and/or focal thickening of the small bowel with a loss of layering may be seen, but these changes are generally nonspecific (Moon, Biller, and Armrbrust, 2003; Louvet and Denis, 2004). Hyperechoic mucosal striations seen ultrasonographically have been associated with lacteal dilation (Sutherland-Smith et al., 2007).

If all initial results are normal, the intestinal tract should be evaluated. Multiple fecal examinations (flotations and direct smears) should be performed. If all results are negative, empiric use of a broad-spectrum anthelmintic such as fenbendazole can be used before more expensive and invasive testing is carried out.

Intestinal function testing can be performed to detect malabsorption or maldigestion. Sudan staining of fecal material can be used to detect steatorrhea, which can indicate fat malassimilation. Oral D-xylose testing can indicate poor carbohydrate absorption. Cytologic examination of fecal smears or colonic scrapings may reveal fungal or protozoal organisms or leukocytes. Determination of serum folate and cobalamin levels, along with breath hydrogen and intestinal permeability testing, can further document gastrointestinal disease.

The gold standard for documenting intestinal protein loss is to quantitate radiolabeled (chromium-51) albumin in the feces after intravenous administration (Williams, 1996). For many reasons the application of this test is limited in veterinary medicine. A test that is more readily available and useful is the measurement of α-1 proteinase inhibitor (α-1-PI) in the feces (Williams, 1996). α-1-PI has a molecular weight similar to that of albumin. This protein is present in the vascular and interstitial spaces, as well as in lymph. Therefore α-1-PI can be lost into the intestinal tract in cases with PLE and is excreted in the feces intact, unlike albumin, which is broken down by bacterial degradation. Fecal α-1-PI can then be measured using an immunoassay and to provide an indirect quantitation of intestinal protein loss (Murphy et al., 2003). The assay requires collection of three separate, freshly passed fecal samples into specific preweighed tubes provided by the laboratory. This can be of value in both diagnosis and monitoring treatment (Murphy et al., 2003).

Ultimately intestinal biopsies and histopathology usually are required to define the disease process causing PLE. Endoscopic or full-thickness biopsies via exploratory laparotomy can be performed. Laparotomy provides the advantages of being able to evaluate the entire intestinal tract since some diseases may be focal and of being able to evaluate extraintestinal structures. Dilated lymphatics may be visualized as a milky weblike pattern on the serosal surface of the intestines and throughout the mesentery. However, because animals with PLE generally are malnourished and hypoproteinemic, there is delayed wound healing that may lead to dehiscence of the intestinal anastomosis site. Accordingly, exploratory laparotomy carries a definite postoperative risk of peritonitis. In many cases endoscopic biopsies are adequate to diagnose diffuse mucosal diseases. Endoscopy allows visualization of the mucosa; dilated lacteals seen with lymphangiectasia often have the appearance of small, white pinpoint foci in the mucosa. Ileal biopsies also can be obtained endoscopically to increase the chances of finding lesions.

TREATMENT

Since hypoproteinemic animals tend to be hypovolemic because of reduced oncotic pressure, oncotic support with plasma or synthetic colloids (e.g., hetastarch, Hespan; American Critical Care) should be considered before administration of anesthesia to avoid hypotension (also see Chapter 111). Plasma also can be considered, but it is not a strong colloid unless a 20-ml/kg dose can be given, which is often not cost effective in medium- and large-breed dogs. However, plasma may be a better choice if the patient has a coagulopathy secondary to loss of antithrombin. Human albumin may also be an option if other colloids are not available, but there is a risk of allergic reaction since this is a foreign protein. The incidence of this type of reaction to human albumin in the dog is unknown.

Treatment should be aimed at any identifiable underlying disease. PLE from acute viral infections usually resolves with supportive care, and PLE caused by bacterial or parasitic infections resolves with appropriate specific therapy. Other diseases should be treated accordingly (e.g., antifungal agents for histoplasmosis, chemotherapy for lymphoma).

The mainstay of treatment for the two most common diseases causing PLE (IL and lymphoplasmacytic enteritis) is dietary control, along with antiinflammatory medication when indicated (Williams, 1996; Melzer and Sellon, 2002; also see Chapter 115). Enteral nutrition is optimal because this allows the enterocytes to repair and regenerate. Animals that cannot tolerate enteral nutrition may be fed via total parenteral nutrition or partial peripheral nutrition to stabilize them for diagnostic testing or as initial treatment for the PLE. Ultimately, though, enteral nutrition is required.

Options for enteral nutrition include elemental diets, commercially prepared foods, or home-cooked diets. Patients with severe PLE may require elemental diets initially. These diets are composed of nutrients in their elemental rather than polymeric form. They should not require significant digestion and can be easily absorbed. They usually do not contain enough protein for dogs and especially cats for long-term use, and they can be hypertonic. Several human products are available (Vivonex TEN, Sandoz Nutrition; Portagen, Mead Johnson).

Animals with less severe disease can be started on specific enteral nutrition immediately. The diet chosen should be low in triglycerides containing long-chain fatty acids, which must be transported into the circulation via the intestinal lymphatics. Short-chain triglycerides can be absorbed directly into the portal system. The diet should also be low in lactose, easily digestible, and low in fiber. Diets high in fiber may inhibit digestion and absorption of proteins and carbohydrates. Commercially available diets can be used, or a homemade diet can be prepared (Fossum, 1989). The caloric density of the diet can be increased by adding medium-chain triglyceride (MCT) oil (Mead Johnson) or high-quality protein to the diet if needed. MCT oil is used at a dosage of 1 to 2 ml/kg/day; it may be expensive, is unpalatable to some animals, does not provide essential fatty acids, and has become controversial in recent years. It has been shown in dogs that MCTs may not be absorbed directly but may actually require normal lymphatic flow (Newton, McLoughlin, and Brichard, 2000). High-quality protein can be added in the form of cooked egg whites or low-fat cottage cheese. Alternatively one of the elemental diets can be used as a supplement (Fossum, 1989). Hydrolyzed diets may also be an alternative because they are highly digestible and low in fat and contain smaller protein particles, which are more easily absorbed.

In addition to dietary therapy, corticosteroids can prove effective in secondary IL and the inflammatory enteritides. Prednisone at a dosage of 2 mg/kg/day can be used, followed by a slow taper once a response has been seen. A maintenance dosing schedule is usually required indefinitely, preferably on an alternate-day basis. If no response is seen with corticosteroids, immunosuppressive agents such as azathioprine, cyclosporine, or methotrexate can be used (Craven et al., 2004; Allenspach et al., 2006; Yuki et al., 2006). Antibiotics may also be needed in some cases to treat intestinal bacterial overgrowth. Metronidazole and tylosin are common choices. Cobalamin may need to be supplemented parenterally (see Chapter 115 for more information about these treatments). Various electrolytes and fat-soluble vitamins may also be supplemented as needed. Prognosis can be difficult to determine because few long-term studies have been performed in dogs and cats. In general the prognosis should be guarded until a response is seen. Indefinite therapy is usually required, and relapses may occur.

References and Suggested Reading

Allenspach K et al: Pharmacokinetics and clinical efficacy of cyclosporine treatment of dogs with steroid-refractory inflammatory bowel disease, *J Vet Intern Med* 20:2, 2006.

Breitschwerdt EB: Immunoproliferative enteropathy of basenjis, *Semin Vet Med Surg* 7:153, 1992.

Bush WW et al: Secondary hypoparathyroidism attributed to hypomagnesemia in a dog with protein-losing enteropathy, *J Am Vet Med Assoc* 219:12, 2001.

Craven M et al: Canine inflammatory bowel disease: retrospective analysis of diagnosis and outcome in 80 cases (1995–2002), *J Small Anim Pract* 45:7, 2004.

Fossum TW: Protein-losing enteropathy, *Semin Vet Med Surg* 4: 219, 1989.

Guilford WG: Idiopathic inflammatory bowel diseases. In Guilford WG, Strombeck DR: *Strombeck's small animal gastroenterology*, Philadelphia, 1996, Saunders, p 451.

Jeffries GH: Protein-losing gastroenteropathy. In Sleisenger MH, Fordtran JS, editors: *Gastrointestinal disease*, Philadelphia, 1983, Saunders, p 280.

Jergens AE et al: Idiopathic inflammatory bowel disease in dogs and cats: 84 cases (1987-1990), *J Am Vet Med Assoc* 201:1603, 1992.

Kull PA et al: Clinical, clinicopathological, radiographic, and ultrasonographic characteristics of intestinal lymphangiectasia in dogs: 17 cases (1996-1998), *J Am Vet Med Assoc* 219:2, 2001.

Louvet A, Denis B: Ultrasonographic diagnosis—small bowel lymphangiectasia in a dog, *Vet Radiol Ultrasound* 45:6, 2004.

Mellanby RJ et al: Hypocalcemia associated with low serum vitamin D metabolite concentrations in two dogs with protein-losing enteropathies, *J Small Anim Pract* 46:7, 2005.

Melzer KJ, Sellon RK: Canine intestinal lymphangiectasia, *Compend Contin Educ Pract Vet* 24: 12, 2002.

Moon ML, Biller DS, Armbrust LJ: Ultrasonographic appearance and etiology of corrugated small intestine, *Vet Radiol Ultrasound* 44:2, 2003.

Murphy KF et al: Fecal alpha-1-proteinase inhibitor concentration in dogs with chronic gastrointestinal disease, *Vet Clin Pathol* 32:2, 2003.

Newton JD, McLoughlin MA, Brichard SJ: Transport pathways of enterally administered medium-chain triglycerides in dogs. In Reinhart GA, Carey DP, editors: *Proceedings of the Iams Nutritional Symposium*, Orange Frazer Press, Inc., Willmington, OH, 2000, p 143.

Sherding RG: Intestinal lymphangiectasia In Kirk RW, editor: *Current veterinary therapy IX*, Philadelphia, 1986, Saunders, p 885.

Sutherland-Smith J et al: Ultrasonographic intestinal hyperechoic mucosal striations in dogs are associated with lacteal dilation, *Vet Radiol Ultrasound* 48:1, 2007.

Tams TR, Twedt DC: Canine protein-losing gastroenteropathy syndrome, *Compend Contin Educ Pract Vet* 3:105, 1981.

Vaden SL et al: Evaluation of intestinal permeability and gluten sensitivity in soft-coated wheaten terriers with familial protein losing enteropathy, protein-losing nephropathy, or both, *Am J Vet Res* 61:5, 2000.

Van Kruiningen HJ et al: Lipogranulomatous lymphangitis in canine lymphangiectasia, *Vet Pathol* 21:377, 1984.

Williams DA: Evaluation of fecal alpha-1-protease inhibitor concentration as a test for canine protein-losing enteropathy (PLE), *J Vet Intern Med* 5:133, 1991.

Williams DA: Malabsorption, small intestinal bacterial overgrowth, and protein-losing enteropathy. In Guilford WG, Strombeck DR: *Strombeck's small animal gastroenterology*, Philadelphia, 1996, Saunders, p 367.

Yuki M et al: A case of protein-losing enteropathy treated with methotrexate in a dog, *J Vet Med Sci* 68:4, 2006.

CHAPTER 119

Chronic Colitis

NOLIE K. PARNELL, *West Lafayette, Indiana*

The colon plays an important role in conservation of water and electrolytes, specifically sodium and chloride, and is the major site of fecal storage until expulsion is necessary. Not as well recognized is the role of the colon in digestion and metabolism. For example, the colonic bacterial flora play an important role in the fermentation of undigested carbohydrates with the primary substrate being dietary fiber. Disruptions to the normal homeostasis of the colon leads to changes in both absorption and motility, and clinically this is often manifested as large bowel diarrhea.

Chronic colitis is a common cause of large bowel diarrhea. Chronic colitis is defined as inflammation of the colon that is present for at least 2 weeks. This chapter reviews the pathophysiology of chronic colitis, the various histologic forms of colitis, and the clinical approach I use when evaluating patients with chronic large bowel disease. A discussion of therapy is also included, and throughout the chapter, differences between the dog and cat are noted.

PATHOPHYSIOLOGY

The pathophysiology of inflammatory bowel disease is extremely complex and mostly unknown. Evidence exists that a multifactorial process occurs that involves an abnormal immune response to an antigen, whether luminal or mucosal, the commensal bacteria, and a genetic susceptibility (also see Chapter 115). The activation of CD4+ cells within the intestinal epithelium without a concomitant activation of the suppressor cells, which creates tolerance, causes inflammation (German, Hall, Day, 2003). The mucosal immune response leading to inflammation involves B and T lymphocytes, plasma cells, macrophages, cytokines, interleukins, and several inflammatory mediators (e.g., tumor necrosis factor-α, interferon-γ, nitric oxide). Although the inflammatory responses of the small and large bowel are very similar, some differences occur. For example, the immunologic response of the canine colon seems to be primarily T helper cell (Th)1 mediated, but in the canine small bowel there is a mixed response of both Th1 and Th2. The colonic Th1 response leads to up-regulation of interferon-γ, tumor necrosis factor-α, interleukin-2, and interleukin-12. It is unknown if the feline colonic mucosal immunity acts in a similar fashion as the canine mucosal immunity.

Inflammation of the colon reduces the amount of water and electrolytes absorbed and changes colonic motility. Cytokines produced alter smooth muscle function, resulting in abnormal motor activity. Inflammation suppresses the normal colonic contractions that mix and knead, and stimulates giant migrating contractions (GMCs). GMCs are more powerful contractions that rapidly propel intestinal contents. In a normal animal these contractions only occur once to twice daily. Colonic inflammation increases the number of daily GMCs. It is believed that these GMCs are a major factor in producing the diarrhea, abdominal cramping, and increased urgency associated with colitis. Goblet cells respond to inflammation by producing increased amounts of mucus.

HISTOPATHOLOGIC TYPES OF COLITIS

Evaluation of chronic colitis histologically is difficult because of the lack of standardization and the influence of subjectivity. Colitis is usually defined histologically by the predominant inflammatory cell type present, the alterations of the normal colonic architecture (e.g., crypt collapse, goblet cell hyperplasia), and the severity of the disease process. The predominant cell types are lymphocytic-plasmacytic, eosinophilic, and granulomatous.

Lymphocytic-Plasmacytic Colitis

Lymphocytic-plasmacytic colitis is the most common form of colitis in both the dog and cat. Numerous studies have found that most dogs are middle-aged and there is no sex predilection. There may be an association between colitis in dogs and perianal fistulas, especially in the German shepherd dog. Cats with chronic colitis tend to be middle-aged, with the mean age at onset of clinical signs 5.1 years. Purebred cats were affected more often than nonpurebred cats. As with dogs, there was no sex predilection. Typically there are increased numbers of lymphocytes and plasma cells in the lamina propria, although occasionally they can be found in the submucosa and muscularis. Other inflammatory cells may also be evident histologically but not in the same numbers as lymphocytes and plasma cells. Crypt dilation, loss of surface epithelial cells, and decreased goblet cells are other histopathologic changes associated with chronic colitis.

Eosinophilic Colitis

Eosinophilic colitis is characterized by accumulations of eosinophils in the lamina propria. Diagnostics for eosinophilic colitis may reveal a peripheral eosinophilia. This finding also may be one component of feline hypereosinophilic syndrome. Compared to lymphocytic-plasmacytic colitis, eosinophilic colitis occurs uncommonly, and the animals affected tend to be younger. Endoparasites, infectious agents, and food allergy have all been incriminated in this form of colitis, but none have been proven.

Regardless, when a predominance of eosinophils is found histologically, it is prudent to investigate and eliminate these potential etiologies first since treatment of eosinophilic colitis tends to be more difficult than that of lymphocytic-plasmacytic colitis.

Granulomatous Colitis

Granulomatous colitis is characterized by the presence of macrophages and other inflammatory cells within the lamina propria. These macrophages are not periodic acid-Schiff positive, which is a discriminating feature of histiocytic ulcerative colitis (also see Chapter 120). Granulomatous colitis is rare and usually presents as a segmental, thickened, partially obstructed segment of bowel. The ileum and colon appear to be affected most commonly. Because of its histologic characteristics, it is important to eliminate inflammation secondary to fungal disease, intestinal parasites, feline infectious peritonitis, and foreign material. Treatment remains controversial, although most advocate surgical resection if possible. Medical management has variable results.

DIFFERENTIAL DIAGNOSIS

It is important to obtain a definitive diagnosis for any animal that has chronic large bowel diarrhea. Since the clinical signs of chronic colitis are similar to those of other diseases of the large bowel, it is imperative to perform diagnostics to establish a diagnosis. Although chronic colitis is a common diagnosis in a referral hospital, it is not the most common cause of large bowel diarrhea. Other more common causes of chronic large bowel diarrhea include *Trichuris vulpis* for dogs, *Clostridium perfringens*, and food hypersensitivity for both species. Other infectious agents to consider are *Histoplasma capsulatum* if geographically near the Mississippi, Ohio, or Missouri Rivers; and *Pythium insidiosum* for animals located in south and southeast. Idiopathic large bowel diarrhea is diagnosed if all test results are normal, including colonic histopathology. Neoplasia, particularly adenocarcinoma and lymphosarcoma, also causes chronic large bowel diarrhea. Both forms of neoplasia occur most commonly in older animals, although any age may be affected. Adenomatous polyps occur in dogs and are usually found on a thorough rectal examination.

Granulomatous colitis of boxer dogs, also known as histiocytic ulcerative colitis, was originally believed to be an inflammatory bowel disease of young boxer dogs (see Chapter 120). This disease differed histologically by demonstrating periodic acid Schiff–positive macrophages. Historically affected animals responded poorly to antiinflammatory and immunosuppressive therapies, and euthanasia was not uncommon. It is now believed that colonization of a selective strain of *Escherichia coli* is responsible for the inflammatory changes found on histopathology. This etiopathogenesis is further supported by the positive response these boxer dogs have to antibiotic therapy alone without the use of antiinflammatory or immunosuppressive drugs. Enrofloxacin is currently the treatment for choice for granulomatous colitis of boxer dogs.

Young cats with chronic large bowel diarrhea should be evaluated for trichomonosis (see Chapter 117). *Tritrichomonas foetus* is a flagellated protozoan parasite that causes clinical signs in a cat that is otherwise thriving. Trichomonosis is most commonly seen in purebred cats, especially Abyssinians and Bengal cats that are densely housed. *T. foetus* is frequently misdiagnosed as *Giarida* spp. Trichomonosis is histopathologically associated with mild-to-moderate lymphoplasmacytic and neutrophilic colitis. Clinical signs may resolve in some cats with no treatment, but for cases that do not, ronidazole is the current treatment of choice. Neurotoxicity has been reported in cats receiving ronidazole for the treatment of trichomonosis.

CLINICAL SIGNS AND PHYSICAL EXAMINATION

The most common clinical sign of chronic colitis is large bowel diarrhea. The characteristics of large bowel diarrhea include mucus, hematochezia (frank blood in the stool), tenesmus (straining to defecate), and occasionally pain when defecating. There is often an increased urgency and frequency of defecation, but the amount of feces per bowel movement is greatly reduced. In one study of cats with chronic colitis, hematochezia without diarrhea was the most common clinical sign. Vomiting and weight loss can occur in some cases of chronic colitis, but these tend to be the more severe cases or those that have concurrent disease that also affects the stomach or small intestine.

Historical findings may reveal a waxing or waning course of clinical signs. Initially the clinical signs may be sporadic, but progression usually occurs. The period of time during which there is large bowel diarrhea increases, and in many cases the diarrhea becomes persistent. In severe cases of chronic colitis owners may also complain that their pets are lethargic and inappetent.

The physical examination in cases of chronic colitis is usually within normal limits. In severe cases of chronic colitis or those that have concurrent disease of the small intestine, poor body conditioning suggestive of weight loss may be found. Every patient with signs of chronic colitis should have a rectal examination performed. Rectal examination may reveal an irregular or thickened mucosal surface, elicit pain, and demonstrate frank blood or mucus on the examination glove. In addition, a thorough rectal examination may discover a rectal polyp or malignant neoplasm, which can mimic the signs of chronic colitis.

DIAGNOSTIC PLAN

The diagnostic approach for chronic colitis should be systematic and thorough and include colonic biopsies. It is important to exclude all other diseases that can mimic the signs of chronic colitis. Multiple fecal examinations should always be part of the initial diagnostic plan since endoparasitism occurs more commonly than chronic colitis. Since the helminth *T. vulpis* commonly causes large bowel diarrhea in dogs, routine fecal flotations should be performed. For cats, evaluation for *T. foetus* should be performed using direct observation of trichomonads in feces that are suspended in physiologic saline solution, by culturing feces for *T. foetus*, or using polymerase chain reaction techniques (see Chapter 117).

Rectal cytology is an invaluable diagnostic tool to eliminate other causes of large bowel diarrhea. A specimen can be collected using a gloved finger, a moistened cotton swab, or conjunctival spatula. Epithelial cells exfoliate easily; thus only minimal force is necessary when scraping the rectum and transferring the specimen to a glass slide. Normal rectal cytology should contain colonic epithelial cells, a mixed population of bacteria and yeast, and some debris. Abnormal findings include inflammatory cells, neoplastic cells, and certain infectious organisms (e.g., *H. capsulatum*). Evaluation for *C. perfringens* colitis can begin by screening fecal cytology for the presence of a large number of clostridial endospores. It has been reported that greater than five endospores per high power field may suggest the presence of *C. perfringens* enterotoxicosis. However, there is a poor correlation between the number of endospores seen and the detection of *C. perfringens* enterotoxin (CPE) since not all endospores produce CPE. Cases of suspected clostridial colitis should be confirmed by identifying CPEs A and B in feces using a commercially available enzyme-linked immunosorbent assay after a fecal bacterial culture is performed.

I recommend a dietary trial before pursuing more advanced diagnostics such as colonoscopy. A highly digestible diet should be given exclusively for a 4- to 6-week period to determine response to the diet manipulation. Several commercially prepared prescription diets are available and include i/d (Hill's Prescription Diets), EN (Purina Veterinary Diets), Intestinal HE (Royal Canin Veterinary Diet), and Low Residue (Eukanuba Veterinary Diets). If a therapeutic diet trial does not eliminate clinical signs, supplementing the diet with soluble fiber should be attempted. It has been demonstrated that adding psyllium (Metamucil) at 1.33g/kg per day to a highly digestible diet resulted in a favorable response in greater than 85% of patients with chronic idiopathic large bowel diarrhea. Soluble fibers hold water, thereby improving the consistency of feces, stabilizing colonic motility, and altering colonic bacterial metabolism, which could manipulate the colonic flora (e.g., *C. perfringens*).

If the clinical signs persist despite these initial steps, further diagnostics are indicated. A complete blood count, biochemical profile, and urinalysis should be performed to rule out other diseases and in preparation for general anesthesia, but in the majority of cases with chronic colitis the results are normal. For cats, feline leukemia virus/feline immunodeficiency virus testing is also recommended, as well as a T_4 if it is age appropriate. Routine abdominal radiographs are also usually normal but occasionally demonstrate intraluminal narrowing, which could indicate an infiltrative disease process. In these cases the primary problem is luminal obstruction that manifests itself clinically as colitis because only a small amount of feces is able to pass through the narrowed lumen. In my practice the majority of these cases are cats with colonic lymphoma, although pathologic strictures have been seen with dogs.

Colonoscopy is indicated to visually inspect the colonic mucosal surface and obtain specimens for histopathology.

Patient preparation is essential in obtaining a reliable examination when small or subtle lesions could be missed by residual fecal material on the mucosal surface. Food should be withheld for 24 to 48 hours before the procedure. A combination of enemas and an oral colonic lavage solution, such as GoLYTELY, should adequately prepare the colon for the endoscopist. Multiple samples from the cecum, ascending, transverse, and descending colon should be obtained regardless of the gross morphologic appearance. The severity of lesions can vary at different locations, and the gross morphologic appearance of the colon does not always correlate with either the clinical signs or the histopathologic findings. A standardized system of evaluation has been proposed for both the gross morphologic findings and the histologic interpretation of colonic mucosal samples obtained endoscopically. Difficulty lies with differentiating normal colonic mucosa from mild colitis and severe lesions from lymphosarcoma.

TREATMENT

There is little evidence-based medicine in the veterinary literature regarding the management of chronic colitis. Most therapeutic protocols involve a combination of dietary and pharmacologic choices. Which diets and drugs are chosen is usually clinician dependent. Regardless of the therapy used, treatment should continue 2 to 4 weeks past resolution of clinical signs before commencing reduction of the medications given. In a study evaluating endoscopic biopsies before and after pharmacologic therapy in patients with inflammatory bowel disease of the small intestine, there were no significant changes histopathologically before or after therapy (García-Sancho et al., 2007). This study would suggest that repeating the endoscopy to obtain posttreatment biopsy samples is not necessary, although the need for posttreatment biopsy samples has not been evaluated in the colon.

Because of the intermittent shedding of ova by whipworms, therapeutic deworming should occur even if the results of the fecal examinations are negative. There are several safe and effective therapeutic options to eliminate whipworms, but my preference is fenbendazole (50mg/kg orally once daily for 3 days). If there is a positive clinical response, there is an indication to continue treatment, which includes repeating the fenbendazole treatment in 3 weeks and again in 3 months.

NUTRITIONAL MANAGEMENT

The therapeutic value of diet should not be overlooked. Loss of immunologic tolerance to either commensal luminal bacteria or food antigens potentially plays a significant role in the development of intestinal inflammation. Therefore it would be intuitive that alterations in the diet could significantly modulate inflammation. Multiple studies evaluating intestinal inflammation in both the cat and dog have shown clinical improvement with diet manipulation. Dietary therapy may also help reduce the amount of pharmacologic management used in these cases. In a study of 14 cats with colitis, six cats responded to dietary management alone, and four were treated successfully with dietary and pharmacologic management. Of the four

cats treated with a combination therapy, 60% eventually were able to be managed with diet alone. Which diet to choose is a difficult question to answer since no prospective studies comparing the different categories of diets have been performed.

Novel protein diets have been effective in controlling the clinical signs of colitis in both the dog and the cat. In a report of 13 dogs with colitis, clinical signs improved in all dogs following the introduction of a novel protein diet (Nelson, Stookey, and Kazacos, 1988). For a novel protein diet to be effective, a detailed, thorough dietary history must be obtained to determine which protein sources are indeed novel; and the chosen diet must be fed exclusively for 4 to 6 weeks without the introduction of other foods, including snacks. This may prove to be a difficult task for cats who tend to be more food selective than dogs.

Hydrolyzed diets also have been evaluated in the treatment of colitis and found to be effective. Hydrolyzed protein diets are specialized diets that disrupt the protein structure sufficiently to remove any allergens and allergenic epitopes and therefore prevent immune recognition. In one study of dogs with refractory inflammatory bowel disease, two thirds of dogs treated with a soy-based hydrolysate diet showed clinical improvement with the diet change alone. These dogs previously had failed to respond to a novel protein diet (Marks, Laflamme, and McCandish, 2002).

Other aspects of diet therapy with potential therapeutic benefit that should be considered in cases of chronic colitis include a highly digestible diet, the inclusion of ω-3 fatty acids, or soluble fiber. The benefits of soluble fiber have been discussed earlier in this chapter. ω-3 fatty acids reduce inflammation by competitively inhibiting formation of prostaglandins and leukotrienes derived from arachidonic acid.

PHARMACOLOGIC MANAGEMENT

Dietary management alone may ameliorate clinical signs in mild cases of chronic colitis, but pharmacologic therapy is usually required for the moderate-to-severe cases.

Pharmacologic management of colitis can be divided into several different categories: antiinflammatory (5-aminosalicylates), immunosuppressive (corticosteroids, cyclosporine), antimicrobial (metronidazole), and motility-modifying (loperamide). Commonly used dosages of the drugs discussed subsequently are summarized in Table 119-1.

5-Aminosalicylates

Sulfasalazine (Azulfidine; Pharmacia and Upjohn) is frequently the drug of choice for chronic colitis in dogs. Sulfasalazine is a prostaglandin synthetase inhibitor and also has antileukotriene activity. This drug consists of mesalamine linked to sulfapyridine in an azochemical bond. This linkage prevents absorption in the upper gastrointestinal tract and allows most of the drug to be transported to the large intestine. Once it has reached the large intestine, it is metabolized by cecal and colonic bacteria, releasing both components. Mesalamine acts locally on the colonic mucosa to reduce mucosal inflammation. Sulfapyridine is believed to be systemically

Table **119-1**

Drugs for Treating Chronic Colitis

Drug	Dosage
Azathioprine	2 mg/kg PO q24h (C)
	0.3 mg/kg PO q48h (F)
Budesonide	1 mg PO q24h (small C)
	2 mg PO q24h (large C)
	1 mg PO q24h (F)
Chlorambucil	2 mg/m² PO q48h (C)
	2 mg PO q48h (F)
Cyclosporine	5 mg/kg PO q24h (C)
Mesalamine	10-20 mg/kg PO TID (C)
Metronidazole	10-20 mg/kg PO BID (C, F)
Olsalazine	10-20 mg/kg PO TID (C)
Prednisone/Prednisolone	2 mg/kg PO BID (C, F)
	20 mg/m² PO BID for dogs >25 kg
Sulfasalazine	20-30 mg/kg PO TID (C)
	10-20 mg/kg PO q24h (F)
Tylosin	10-40 mg/kg PO BID (C, F)

BID, Twice a day; *C,* canine; *F,* feline; *PO,* orally; *TID,* three times a day.

absorbed and therefore does not have any therapeutic effect in colitis but is blamed for the side effects of sulfasalazine. Common side effects include vomiting and keratoconjunctivitis; thus tear production should be monitored closely during treatment. Treatment should be continued for approximately 2 weeks past resolution of clinical signs. At that time a reduction of the drug can begin. I prefer a reduction schedule of 25% of the dose every 2 to 4 weeks, depending on the severity of the case.

Because of the risk of salicylate toxicity in cats, sulfasalazine is *not* used as the drug of choice in feline colitis. Salicylates are metabolized in the liver by hepatic enzymatic processes involving glucuronyl transferase. Since cats are deficient in this enzymatic pathway, salicylates have prolonged half-lives in the cat. If sulfasalazine is used in cats, it has been recommended to decrease both the frequency and the dose that is accepted in the dog.

Efforts have been made to reduce the toxicity seen with sulfasalazine. The newer 5-aminosalicylate formulations have eliminated the sulfa moiety to reduce toxicity, although keratoconjunctivitis has still been reported in the dog. Other compounds have been substituted for the sulfa moiety as the delivery vehicle to the colon. Olsalazine (Dipentum; Pharmacia) links two mesalamine molecules via an azo bond to ensure delivery to the colon. Asacol (Norwich Eaton Pharmaceuticals) and Pentasa (Marion Merrell Dow) are both mesalamine compounds. Asacol is a compound that has a pH-sensitive polymer coating that is the delivery agent. Pentasa has a timed gradual release in the distal small intestine and colon. This release in the distal small intestine is advantageous in patients that have disease in both the colon and the distal small bowel. Rowasa (Solvay Pharmaceuticals) is a 5-aminosalicylic acid containing enema, which may bring patients with severe colitis of the descending colon

immediate relief. These products have not been evaluated in the cat and therefore should be used with caution.

Glucocorticoids

Glucocorticoids in combination with dietary management and metronidazole are the treatment of choice for chronic colitis in cats. In one study of 60 cats with enterocolitis, when prednisone alone or in combination with another drug was initiated, 80% of cats had a positive response (Hart et al., 1994). Glucocorticoids may be introduced into the therapeutic plan for dogs when the previously discussed therapies are not successful in ameliorating clinical signs or if there are unwanted side effects from the 5-aminosalicylates. Combination therapy with sulfasalazine or metronidazole may reduce the dosage of glucocorticoids needed to successfully eliminate the clinical signs of chronic colitis. Prednisone or prednisolone is used most frequently because it is widely available and economical. I use an initial dosage of 2 mg/kg/day orally (or 20 mg/m² PO BID for dogs >25 kg) for 2 weeks after resolution of clinical signs before commencing a tapering schedule. Reducing the dosage of glucocorticoids by 25% every 2 to 4 weeks is usually successful in maintaining remission. If clinical signs have not resolved in 4 weeks, a change in the therapeutic plan should occur. If immediate relief of colitis is needed and the disease is located primarily in the distal colon, Cortenema (Solvay Pharmaceuticals), a hydrocortisone enema, is available.

Cats generally are tolerant of glucocorticoids and generally do not develop many side effects. However, side effects are common with dogs and include polyuriapolydipsia, polyphagia, gastrointestinal bleeding, increased susceptibility to infection, iatrogenic hyperadrenocorticism, and pituitary-adrenocortical suppression. Budesonide is a nonhalogenated glucocorticoid that has been used in the treatment of Crohn's disease in humans secondary to the concentrated local effects on the intestinal mucosa. Budesonide undergoes significant first-pass metabolism in the liver, which theoretically should reduce the side effects often seen with traditional glucocorticoids since little of the active drug is systemically available. In one study of 10 healthy dogs, the pituitary-adrenocortical axis was suppressed, but no other adverse effects were seen (Stroup et al, 2006). An enteric-coated form of budesonide is available for treatment of patients with inflammatory bowel disease.

Antimicrobials

Metronidazole is considered one of the primary pharmacologic agents in feline chronic colitis. Although categorized as an antibiotic, the therapeutic effects of metronidazole are multiple: antiprotozoal, antimicrobial, and inhibition of some aspects of cell-mediated immunity. All of these therapeutic properties are thought to be beneficial in the treatment of chronic colitis in both dogs and cats. Metronidazole is not usually used as a sole therapeutic agent but is combined either with dietary management or in combination with other pharmacologic agents. Although generally well tolerated by both species, neurologic side effects (e.g., nystagmus, ataxia, seizures) have been reported in both the cat and dog. Most neurologic side effects are observed either with chronic therapy or at high doses. Neurotoxicosis should be reversible within 5 to 7 days after cessation of the drug.

Tylosin is a macrolide antibiotic that is used primarily in food animal production. Its spectrum of activity targets mainly facultative and obligate anaerobic gram-positive bacteria (see Chapter 116). It is also effective against some gram-negative bacteria, although *E. coli* and *Salmonella* spp. are resistant. Tylosin has been used effectively in chronic enteropathies. The reasons for its therapeutic effectiveness are most likely secondary to interference with bacterial adhesion to the mucosa and its antimicrobial and immunomodulating effects. In a study of 14 dogs with both small and large bowel clinical signs, seven of nine dogs had a rapid response to tylosin, although enteropathogenic bacteria, including *C. perfringens*, was concluded not to be the cause (Westermarck E et al, 2005). Tylosin is also well tolerated by both cats and dogs with minimal side effects. I use tylosin as a long-term alternative to metronidazole or when occasional outbreaks of diarrhea occur during treatment.

Immunosuppressive Agents

Several different immunosuppressive agents are available as adjunct therapeutics in the management of severe chronic colitis. Both azathioprine and chlorambucil are rarely used as single agents in the treatment of inflammatory bowel disease and are used mostly in combination with glucocorticoids. The serious side effects of azathioprine in cats (myelosuppression and hepatotoxicity) severely limit its use in feline colitis, but chlorambucil has been shown to be efficacious in refractory cases of feline inflammatory bowel disease. Cyclosporine has been shown to be an effective alternative drug in dogs with steroid-refractory inflammatory bowel disease. It has not been evaluated in the cat. Cyclosporine suppresses activated T cells in the intestinal mucosa by inhibition of interleukin-2, which ultimately reduces the amount of proinflammatory cytokines. In a study of 14 dogs with severe inflammatory bowel disease, 78% (11 out of 14) of the dogs positively responded to the drug, with 9 of the 11 dogs considered to be in complete remission of clinical signs (Allenspach et al., 2006). Side effects of cyclosporine include gastrointestinal disturbances, gingival disease, and alopecia.

PROGNOSIS

The short-term prognosis for chronic colitis is good for both the dog and the cat, although most reports indicate that cats have a slightly better overall response rate. Long-term prognosis for complete resolution, no relapses, and no chronic treatment seems to be poor. Most cases of inflammatory bowel disease are not curable, and the owner should be educated that most likely some form of treatment will be necessary long term. Fortunately for some animals, especially feline patients, dietary management alone may be a possibility for long-term management of chronic colitis.

References and Suggested Reading

Allenspach K et al: Pharmokinetics and clinical efficacy of cyclosporine treatment of dogs with steroid-refractory inflammatory bowel disease, *J Vet Intern Med* 20:239, 2007.

Craven M et al: Canine inflammatory bowel disease: retrospective analysis of diagnosis and outcome in 80 cases (1995-2002), *J Small Anim Pract* 45(7):336, 2004.

Dennis JS, Kruger JM, Mullaney TP: Lymphocytic/plasmacytic colitis in cats: 14 cases (1985-1990), *J Am Vet Med Assoc* 202(2):313, 1993.

García-Sancho M et al: Evaluation of clinical, macroscopic, and histopathologic response to treatment in nonhypoproteinemic dogs with lymphocytic-plasmacytic enteritis, *J Vet Intern Med* 21(1):11, 2007.

German AJ, Hall EJ, Day MJ: Chronic intestinal inflammation and intestinal disease in dogs, *J Vet Intern Med* 17:8, 2003.

Hart JR et al: Lymphocytic-plasmacytic enterocolitis in cats: 60 cases (1988-1990), *J Anim Hosp Assoc* 30:505, 1994.

Jergens AE et al: Idiopathic inflammatory bowel disease in dogs and cats: 84 cases (1987-1990), *J Am Vet Med Assoc* 201(10):1603, 1992.

Marks SL et al: Evaluation of methods to diagnose *Clostridium perfringens–associated* diarrhea in dogs, *J Am Vet Med Assoc* 214(3):357, 1999.

Marks SL, Laflamme DP, McCandish AP: Dietary trial using a commercial hypoallergenic diet containing hydrolyzed protein for dogs with inflammatory bowel disease, *Vet Ther* 104(2):109, 2002.

Nelson RW, Stookey LJ, Kazacos E: Nutritional management of idiopathic chronic colitis in the dog, *J Vet Intern Med* 2(3):133, 1998.

Simpson KW et al: Adherent and invasive *Escherichia coli* is associated with granulomatous colitis in boxer dogs, *Infect Immun* 74(8):4778, 2006.

Stroup ST et al: Effects of oral administration of controlled-ileal-release budesonide and assessment of pituitary-adrenocortical axis suppression in clinically normal dogs. *AM J Vet Res,* 67(7):1173, 2006.

Washabau RJ, Holt DE: Diseases of the large intestine. In Ettinger SJ, Feldman EC, editors: *Textbook of veterinary internal medicine,* Philadelphia, 2005, Saunders, p 1378.

Westermarck E et al: Tylosin-responsive chronic diarrhea in dogs. *J Vet Intern Med* 19:177, 2005.

Yaeger MJ, Gookin JL: Histologic features associated with *Tritrichomonas foetus–*induced colitis in domestic cats, *Vet Pathol* 42:797, 2005.

CHAPTER 120
Canine Ulcerative Colitis

KENNETH W. SIMPSON, *Ithaca, New York*

Histiocytic ulcerative colitis (HUC) (also known as granulomatous colitis) is a severe inflammatory disease of unknown etiology that typically affects boxer dogs under 4 years of age. Others breeds such as mastiff, Alaskan malamute, Doberman pinscher, and French bulldogs are affected sporadically.

PATHOPHYSIOLOGY

From a comparative perspective it is clear that HUC in dogs has features in common with spontaneous idiopathic inflammatory bowel diseases in humans, such as ulcerative colitis (macroscopic appearance, regional distribution, immunopathology), Crohn's disease (granulomatous inflammation, bacteria within macrophages, response to fluoroquinolones) and Whipple's disease (PAS-positive macrophages, bacteria within macrophages); but it is not identical to any one of these diseases.

Evidence is mounting that inflammatory bowel disease in humans is a consequence of an abnormal host response to the enteric bacteria that can be viewed as normal flora or opportunistic pathogens (Hanauer, 2006). With this thought in mind two studies have recently explored the possibility that an uncharacterized infectious agent such as *Trophyrema whippelii* (the causative agent of Whipple's disease) or an abnormal mucosa-associated flora is involved in the etiopathogenesis of HUC in boxer dogs. One of these studies used a combination of culture-independent molecular techniques (16srDNA sequencing and fluorescence in situ hybridization) to examine the mucosa-associated bacterial flora of colonic biopsies from healthy dogs, dogs with lymphoplasmacytic colitis, and boxer dogs with HUC. Those investigators demonstrated selective intramucosal colonization of HUC biopsies by *Escherichia coli* (Simpson et al., 2006). Another study described the immunolocalization of *E. coli, Lawsonia intracellularis, Campylobacter,* and *Salmonella* to macrophages in the colon of 10 of 10, 3 of 10, 2 of 10, and 1 of 10 boxer dogs with granulomatous colitis, respectively (dogs without colitis or other forms of colitis were not examined) (Van Kruiningen et al., 2005). These findings strongly suggest that HUC is a consequence of mucosal colonization by luminal *E. coli* in a susceptible individual (i.e., an undefined breed-specific abnormality in boxer dogs).

Interestingly, the *E. coli* strains isolated from the colonic mucosa of dogs with HUC adhered to, invaded, and persisted in cultured epithelial cells to the same degree as *E. coli* strains associated with Crohn's disease. Initial investigations of HUC and Crohn's-associated *E. coli* indicate that they are more similar in phylogeny and virulence gene profiles to extraintestinal pathogenic *E. coli* (e.g., uropathogenic *E. coli)* than diarrheagenic *E. coli* and point to the association of *E. coli* that resembles extraintestinal pathogenic strains in genotype with chronic intestinal inflammation (Simpson et al., 2006).

CLINICAL AND PATHOLOGIC FEATURES

Dogs are usually presented for the investigation of frequent bloody mucoid stools and weight loss. Clinicopathologic abnormalities generally are limited to anemia and hypoalbuminemia. Abdominal ultrasonography may show thickening of the colon and regional lymphadenopathy. Lymph node aspirates may contain histiocytes. Colonoscopy is frequently characterized by thickening and ulceration of the colon (Fig. 120-1, *A*).

The dominant histologic features of colonic biopsies are loss of colonic epithelium and goblet cells and the accumulation of large numbers of periodic acid-Schiff (PAS)–positive macrophages (Fig. 120-1, *B* and *C*). The PAS-positive material is thought to be derived from remnants of bacterial cell wall glycoprotein, and the accumulation of PAS-positive material in macrophages may be caused by defective phagocytosis. Immunopathologic studies describe an increase in immunoglobulin (Ig)G_3 and IgG_4 plasma cells, CD3 T cells, L1 and major histocompatibility complex (MHC)II–positive cells (German et al., 2000).

Several studies have described bacteria within the mucosa of affected dogs; but known enteropathogens such as *Salmonella, Campylobacter Yersinia,* and *Shigella* have not been isolated (Van Kruiningen et al., 1965). Ultrastructural studies suggest active phagocytosis of bacteria that in some instances resemble *Chlamydia.* An attempt to reproduce colitis in boxer dogs with *Mycoplasma* isolated from the colon and regional lymph nodes of four affected dogs was unsuccessful. The predilection for boxer dogs, with only sporadic cases of this type of colitis reported in non-boxer dogs, and absence of a causal infectious agent have led to HUC being considered a breed-specific, immune-mediated disease of unknown etiology.

TREATMENT

In contrast to the widely accepted view that HUC is an incurable immune-mediated disease, the original description by Van Kruiningen (1965) describes a favorable outcome in six of nine dogs treated with chloramphenicol. The results of three recent studies provide clear evidence of clinical and histologic remission in 12 boxer dogs and 1 English bulldog treated with antibiotic regimens containing fluroquinolones (Davies et al., 2004; Hostutleret al., 2004). Treatment with enrofloxacin

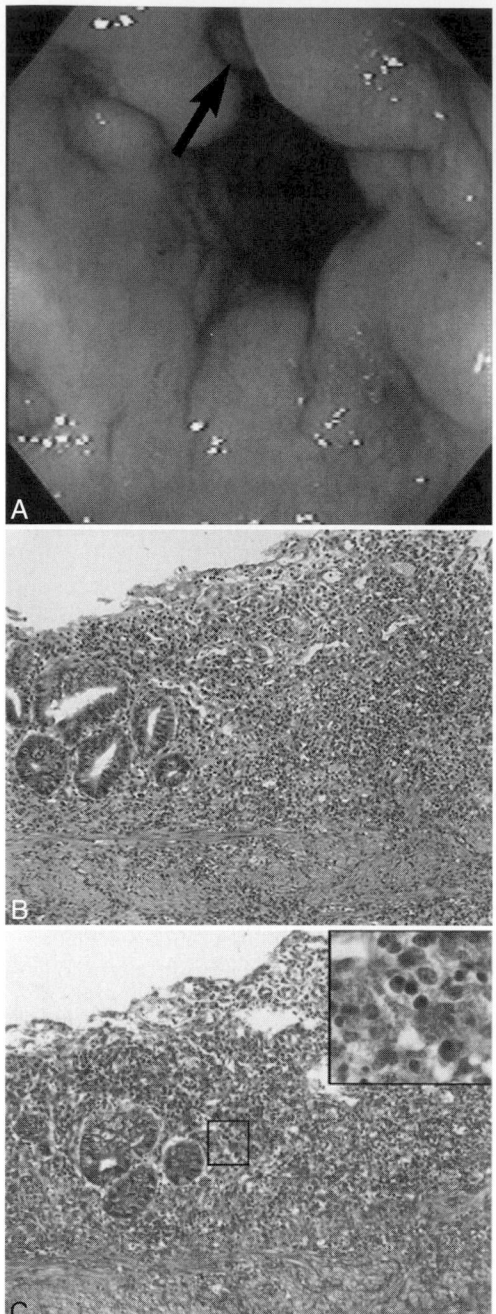

Fig. 120-1   Clinical and pathologic features of granulomatous colitis of boxer dogs. **A,** Colonoscopy shows a diffusely thickened and ulcerated mucosa *(arrow).* **B,** Histologically there is severe loss of glandular structure and cellular infiltration (H&E). **C,** Mucosal infiltration with PAS staining foamy macrophages *(inset)* is a dominant feature. (Reproduced from Simpson KW et al: Adherent and invasive *Escherichia coli* is associated with granulomatous colitis in boxer dogs, *Infect Immun* 74:4778, 2006.)

alone or in combination with metronidazole and/or amoxicillin was generally reported to induce resolution of clinical signs within 2 weeks. Approximately one third of dogs remained free of clinical signs during a 5- to 14-month follow-up after discontinuation of treatment. In the remaining dogs clinical remission was maintained by continuing enrofloxacin at dosages ranging from 68 mg

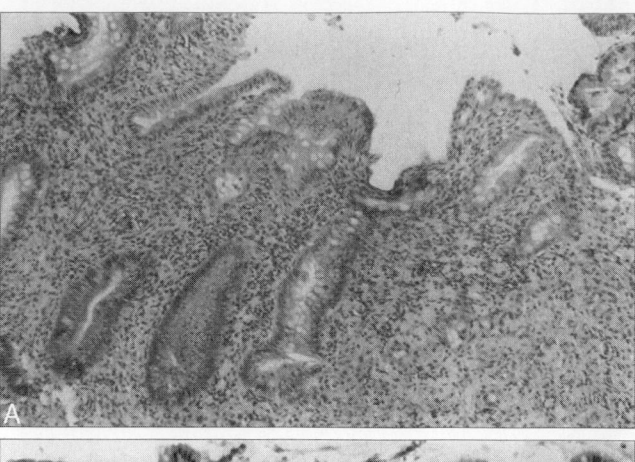

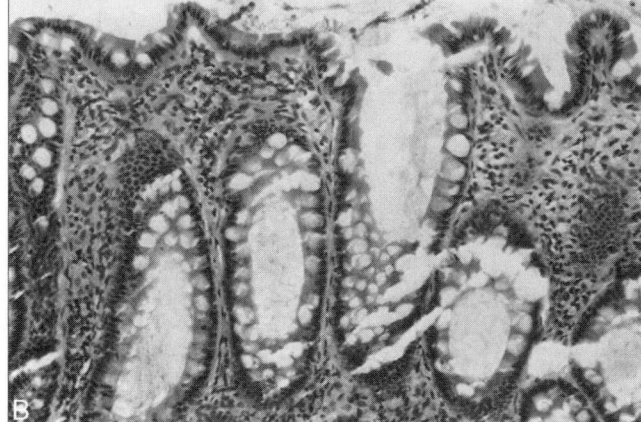

Fig. 120-2   Colonic biopsies of a boxer dog with granulomatous colitis before **(A)** and after **(B)** clinical remission induced by enrofloxacin.

orally every 24 hours to 68 mg orally every 72 hours for between 2 to 21 months. A few dogs relapsed, and remission was achieved by retreatment with enrofloxacin. Repeated biopsy specimens were obtained from eight dogs after treatment, and all showed marked histologic improvement (Fig. 120-2). Resolution of clinical signs and colitis was associated with eradication of intramucosal *E. coli* (Simpson et al., 2006).

It is noteworthy that one dog started on enrofloxacin at 6 months of age developed carpal lameness after approximately 1 year of therapy. Cartilage abnormalities have been described in young dogs receiving enrofloxacin, and this is clearly of concern. This dog continued to receive enrofloxacin 68 mg orally every 72 hours for 6 months after the diagnosis of lameness, and no other complications secondary to long-term therapy were noted. Alternative antibiotics have not been evaluated, but azithromycin and chloramphenicol are possible considerations.

References and Suggested Reading

Darfeuille-Michaudet AJ et al: High prevalence of adherent-invasive *Escherichia coli* associated with ileal mucosa in Crohn's disease, *Gastroenterology* 127:412, 2004.

Davies DR et al: Successful management of histiocytic ulcerative colitis with enrofloxacin in two boxer dogs, *Aust Vet J* 82:58, 2004.

German AJ et al: An immunohistochemical study of histiocytic ulcerative colitis in boxer dogs, *J Comp Pathol* 122(2-3):163, 2000.

Hanauer SB: Inflammatory bowel disease: epidemiology, pathogenesis, and therapeutic opportunities, *Inflamm Bowel Dis* 12(suppl 1):S3, 2006.

Hostutleret RA et al: Antibiotic-responsive histiocytic ulcerative colitis in 9 dogs, *J Vet Intern Med* 18:499, 2004.

Kleessen BA et al: Mucosal and invading bacteria in patients with inflammatory bowel disease compared with controls, *Scand J Gastroenterol* 37:1034, 2002.

Martin HM et al: Enhanced *Escherichia coli* adherence and invasion in Crohn's disease and colon cancer, *Gastroenterology* 127:80, 2004.

Relman DA et al: Identification of the uncultured bacillus of Whipple's disease, *N Engl J Med* 327:293, 1992.

Simpson KW et al: Adherent and invasive *Escherichia coli* is associated with granulomatous colitis in boxer dogs, *Infect Immun* 74:4778, 2006.

Van Kruiningen HJ et al: A granulomatous colitis of dogs with histologic resemblance to Whipple's disease, *Pathol Vet* 2:521, 1965.

Van Kruiningen HJ et al: The comparative importance of *E. coli* antigen in granulomatous colitis of boxer dogs, *Apmis* 113:420, 2005.

CHAPTER **121**

Flatulence

PHILIP ROUDEBUSH, *Topeka, Kansas*

Flatulence is defined as excessive formation of gases in the stomach or intestine and is usually associated with noticeable flatus, belching, borborygmus, abdominal distention, or a combination of these clinical signs. *Flatus,* rather than flatulence, is the term that should be used for gas expelled through the anus. *Belching* is the noisy voiding of gas from the stomach through the mouth, whereas *borborygmus* is a rumbling or gurgling noise caused by the propulsion of gas through the intestines.

Excessive flatus is a chronic objectionable problem that occurs often in dogs and less often in cats. Although belching, borborygmus, and abdominal distention are less common complaints of pet owners, routine questioning may elicit their presence. Flatus, belching, and borborygmus occur in normal pets but may also develop as a consequence of gastric, small intestinal, or colonic disorders. At times excessive flatus is the primary reason pet owners seek veterinary advice.

PRODUCTION OF INTESTINAL GAS

The tendency to treat flatus as a humorous topic has obscured appreciation of the complex physiology that underlies the formation of intestinal gas. The quantitatively important gases in the intestinal tract are nitrogen (N_2), oxygen (O_2), hydrogen (H_2), carbon dioxide (CO_2), and methane (CH_4). These odorless gases comprise more than 99% of the intestinal gas volume in people and pet animals (Table 121-1). The characteristic unpleasant odor of intestinal gas comes primarily from the presence of trace gases that contain volatile sulfur compounds such as hydrogen sulfide (H_2S), methanethiol (CH_3SH), and dimethylsulfide (CH_3SCH_3). The noxious odor of flatus in both humans and dogs correlates most strongly with the concentration of hydrogen sulfide.

Gas in the gastrointestinal (GI) tract is normal and is derived from four primary sources (see Table 121-1): aerophagia (O_2 and N_2); interaction of gastric acid and alkaline food, saliva, or pancreatic bicarbonate (CO_2); diffusion from the blood (CO_2, N_2 and O_2); and bacterial metabolism/fermentation (CO_2, H_2, CH_4 and a variety of trace gases, including volatile sulfur compounds). Gases can be removed from the gut via passage out the esophagus or anus, diffusion into the blood, and consumption by bacteria. The net of these processes proximal to a given site in the GI tract determines the volume and composition of gas passing that site.

Swallowed air is thought to contribute the most to gas in the digestive tract. Air can enter the stomach in association with the swallowing of liquids or solids. Studies using ultrafast computed tomography in humans show that a mean of 17 ml of air accompanies the swallowing of 10 ml of water. Given the quantity of food and fluid ingested each day, large amounts of air may normally enter the stomach. If not belched, swallowed air passes through the GI tract with minimal absorption and is often passed per rectum. Air can also be swallowed in the absence of food or water ingestion via the propulsion of a bolus of air into the pharynx. This may be the cause of excessive flatus commonly seen in many brachycephalic breeds. Vigorous exercise and rapid and competitive eating situations may exacerbate aerophagia. Intestinal transit time is considerably shorter for gases than for liquids or solids. Air introduced into the stomach can result in flatus within 15 to 35 minutes. It has been estimated that gases can move 10 cm per second through the GI tract. The interaction between hydrochloric acid and alkaline food, saliva, or bicarbonate

Table 121-1

Types and Sources of Intestinal Gas

Gases	Source
Quantitatively Important Intestinal Gases	
Nitrogen (N_2)	Swallowed air
	Diffusion from blood
Oxygen (O_2)	Swallowed air
	Diffusion from blood
Hydrogen (H_2)	Bacterial fermentation (large intestine)
Carbon dioxide (CO_2)	Diffusion from blood
	Bacterial fermentation (large intestine)
	Gastric acid + food, saliva or bicarbonate
Methane (CH_4)	Bacterial fermentation (large intestine)
Odoriferous Gases	
Volatile sulfur compounds (hydrogen sulfide, methanethiol, dimethylsulfide)	Bacterial fermentation (large intestine)

secreted by the pancreas produces carbon dioxide in the stomach and intestines. Belched gas is largely swallowed air plus variable quantities of carbon dioxide.

A large amount of gas is formed from bacterial fermentation in the colon. Substrates for bacterial gas production include dietary substances (fiber, poorly digestible protein, and carbohydrate), and endogenous sources (mucin, bile acids). Foods that contain large amounts of nonabsorbable oligosaccharides (e.g., raffinose, stachyose, verbacose) are likely to produce large amounts of intestinal gas. Dogs and cats lack the digestive enzymes needed to split oligosaccharides into absorbable monosaccharides. Therefore bacteria in the colon rapidly ferment these sugars, producing hydrogen and carbon dioxide. Soybeans, beans, peas, and other legumes contain large quantities of nonabsorbable oligosaccharides and are often associated with excessive flatus. Many fibers used in pet foods are fermented by colonic microflora and may contribute directly to flatus. Rapidly fermentable fibers in pet foods include pectins and most gums. Fiber-containing foods may contribute to flatus indirectly through reduced dry matter digestibility. Intestinal gas production is also increased by fresh or dried foods containing fructose, resistant starches, and fermentable fiber (e.g., apples, grapes, prunes, raisins, bananas).

Diseases that cause maldigestion or malabsorption are often associated with borborygmus, abdominal distention, and excessive flatus because large amounts of malassimilated substrates are available for bacterial fermentation. Flatus is also frequent in adult dogs and cats fed excessive amounts of lactose-containing foods.

Sulfur-containing gases are the major malodorous components of human and canine flatus. Dietary sources of sulfur (sulfates and sulfur-containing amino acids), and endogenous sulfur-containing compounds (e.g., mucin, taurocholate) are converted by sulfate-reducing bacteria to the odoriferous compounds hydrogen sulfide, methanethiol, and dimethylsulfide. Onions, nuts, spices, cruciferous vegetables (e.g., broccoli, cabbage, cauliflower, Brussels sprouts), and carrageenan contain high levels of sulfate and often increase production of malodorous gases. High-protein ingredients may also increase malodorous gas production.

ASSESSMENT OF PATIENTS WITH FLATULENCE

Pet owners often express concerns with clinical manifestations of flatulence and may describe an increase in frequency of belching, flatus, or borborygmus, objectionable odor of flatus, or abdominal distention. In one study 43% of dog owners reported flatus in their otherwise healthy pet dogs, and 13% of owners reported objectionable odor associated with the flatus episodes (Jones et al., 1998). Dogs housed indoors and less active dogs were more likely to have evidence of flatus. Temperament, frequency of feeding, specific diet, eating habits, age, gender, and history of previous GI disease were not found to be risk factors for flatulence in this particular study.

At times it may be possible to elicit a history of dietary change or dietary indiscretion in association with flatulence. Specific foods, major food ingredients, treats, supplements, and opportunities for dietary indiscretion should be evaluated. A thorough assessment should also include verification of the feeding method currently used. Items to consider include feeding frequency, amount fed, how the food is offered, access to other food (e.g., a dog eating food for cats in the same household), relationship of feeding to exercise, and who feeds the animal.

There is widespread belief that some individuals are consistently more flatulent than others. This is probably true since studies in humans have shown great variability in the frequency of flatus and such variation probably occurs in pet animals as well. Rectal gas excretion rates in humans range from 400 to 1500 ml/day (mean 705 ml/day). Humans eating their usual diet passed gas per rectum an average of eight to 10 times per day with an upper normal limit of 20 times per day. In general, frequency of flatus correlates with volume of intestinal gas; thus increases and decreases in episodes of flatus can be used to obtain a relative idea of changes in intestinal gas volume. Frequency of gas passed per rectum has not been evaluated in pets whose owners have complained of problems with flatus.

Belching, abdominal distention, and flatus may develop in conjunction with other GI signs, including weight loss, diarrhea, and steatorrhea. This type of history is very suggestive of an underlying small intestinal disorder. Examples of chronic intestinal disorders often associated with flatulence include exocrine pancreatic insufficiency, inflammatory bowel disease, small intestinal bacterial overgrowth, wheat-sensitive enteropathy, food sensitivity, and lymphangiectasia. In one study 26% of cats with chronic diarrhea and/or vomiting had flatus, and 11% of these cats had abdominal distention (Guildford, 2001). Cats with clinical evidence of flatulence should always be evaluated closely for underlying chronic GI problems such as inflammatory bowel disease or food sensitivity.

Excessive aerophagia is a risk factor for flatulence and is seen with brachycephalic working and sporting canine breeds and dogs with aggressive and competitive eating behaviors. Dietary indiscretion and ingestion of certain pet food ingredients may be risk factors for certain individuals. Excessive belching, rapid eating, and aerophagia have also been identified as risk factors for gastric dilation-volvulus (GDV) syndrome and should be considered important clinical findings in dogs at risk for GDV syndrome.

In many cases physical examination findings are unremarkable in dogs and cats with flatulence. Intestinal gas often can be detected during abdominal palpation, but it is difficult to assess the quantity of gas from palpation alone. Laboratory testing is usually not indicated. Animals may be in poor body condition if objectionable flatus occurs secondary to an underlying GI condition. Further evaluation is in order if concomitant vomiting, diarrhea, or weight loss is present.

FEEDING PLANS FOR PATIENTS WITH FLATULENCE

Dietary management of flatulence is primarily concerned with decreasing intestinal gas production by bacterial fermentation of undigested food (Box 121-1). In general, animals with excessive or objectionable flatus benefit from highly digestible foods (dry matter digestibility >90%) offered in small frequent meals. This protocol reduces food residues available for bacterial fermentation in the large intestine and should reduce gas production.

Box **121-1**

Summary of Feeding Plans for Patients With Flatulence

1. Control aerophagia.
   - Feed several small meals daily.
   - Discourage rapid or competitive eating.
   - Feed a mixture of moist and dry foods.
   - Surgically correct stenotic nares and elongated soft palate in brachycephalic dogs.
2. Decrease intestinal gas production.
   - Feed a highly digestible food (dry matter digestibility >90%).
   - Change to food(s) with rice as the sole or predominant carbohydrate source.
   - Avoid food(s) containing ingredients from legumes, such as soybean meal, soybean mill run, peas, pea fiber.
   - Eliminate vitamin, mineral, or fat supplements.
   - Avoid foods or treats containing lactose (e.g., cheese, milk, ice cream).
   - Avoid fresh or dried fruit.
3. Decrease substrates for noxious gas production.
   - Change the dietary protein source(s).
   - Decrease dietary protein levels.
   - Eliminate vitamin, mineral, or fat supplements.
   - Avoid onions, nuts, spices, or cruciferous vegetables (broccoli, cabbage, cauliflower, Brussels sprouts).
   - Avoid canned pet foods that contain carrageenan.
4. Walk dog outdoors within 30 minutes of meals to encourage defecation and elimination of intestinal gas. In general, more activity and exercise results in fewer problems with flatus.
5. If changes in the feeding plan do not result in significant improvement, consider use of carminitives.

Certain protein, carbohydrate, and fiber ingredients or levels may affect flatus production in individual animals. Of the numerous foods alleged to enhance flatus in people, baked beans are the only natural food that have been carefully studied. Flatulent animals may benefit from eating foods that do not contain a source of legumes such as soybean meal, soybean mill run, soy hulls, peas, pea fiber, or pinto beans.

Changing the sources of dietary protein or carbohydrate may benefit some flatulent individuals. In general, aerophagia and dietary carbohydrate contribute most to the volume of intestinal gas, whereas dietary protein sources contribute to odoriferous gases. Reports in humans confirm that a diet in which all carbohydrate is supplied by white rice reduces intestinal gas formation. Studies in dogs also suggest that intestinal gas production is lowest for foods containing rice as the carbohydrate source when compared to other carbohydrate sources such as wheat or corn. Therefore use of commercial or homemade foods containing rice as the major or sole carbohydrate source is a prudent recommendation for flatulent dogs and cats. For example, changing from a commercial dry food that contains corn, chicken meal, and soybean meal to a dry food that contains lamb meal and rice may be helpful.

In addition, vegetarian-based foods containing strongly flavored, sulfur-containing vegetables or legumes should be avoided in patients with flatulence. In some cases reducing dietary protein content alleviates odoriferous flatus. In most cases vitamin-mineral supplements should be avoided because these products may alter intestinal microbial activity. The lactose content of food and treats (e.g., cheese, ice cream, milk) may be a factor in adult animals, and lactose-containing foods should also be eliminated from the diet. Foods that are high in fructose, resistant starch, and/or fermentable fiber should be avoided. A series of dietary trials is often successful in finding a food that lessens excessive flatulence or objectionable flatus in individual pets.

Reducing aerophagia is important in the control of flatulence in dogs, especially in brachycephalic breeds. Several small meals should be fed daily in an effort to discourage rapid eating and gulping of air. Feeding in a quiet, isolated location eliminates competitive eating and reduces aerophagia. These same feeding methods plus feeding a mixture of moist and dry foods may be helpful in reducing the risk of GDV in dogs. Surgical correction of stenotic nares and overlong soft palates may help reduce aerophagia in some brachycephalic dogs.

Simple changes to feeding routines may also improve objectionable flatus. If possible, dogs should be walked outdoors within 30 minutes of meals. This will encourage defecation and elimination of intestinal gas and lessen indoor effects of unwanted flatus. As mentioned previously, less active dogs are at higher risk of having objectionable flatus.

CARMINITIVES

Carminitives are medicines or preparations that relieve flatulence. Various herbal and botanical preparations have been used for thousands of years as carminitives. More recently commercial products have been introduced that claim to reduce or control flatulence. These products can be used in conjunction with changes in the feeding plan and usually contain activated charcoal, bismuth subsalicylate (BSS), zinc acetate, simethicone, *Yucca schidigera* preparations, α-galactosidase, pancreatic enzyme supplements, probiotics, or various herbal/botanical preparations. Nonabsorbable antibiotics such as neomycin and rifaximin also have been shown to reduce flatulence and the number of flatus episodes in healthy people and dogs. However, routine use of nonabsorbable antibiotics in otherwise healthy pet animals with flatulence is not indicated.

Dry activated charcoal adsorbs virtually all odoriferous gases when mixed directly with feces and flatus gas. However, ingestion of activated charcoal by humans has not been effective in reducing the number of flatus events, volume of intestinal gas released, odor of feces, or breath hydrogen excretion after bean ingestion. In vitro studies suggest that the failure of ingested charcoal to reduce liberation of volatile sulfur compounds is because of the saturation of charcoal binding sites during passage through the gut. Uptake of sulfur-containing gases is slowed considerably by wetting of activated charcoal. Activated charcoal is found in a number of commercial canine treats purported to control flatulence.

BSS reduces fecal and flatus odor in humans when given frequently (four times daily). Bismuth is the active ingredient and avidly adsorbs hydrogen sulfide, forming insoluble bismuth sulfide. Bismuth sulfide imparts a characteristic black color to feces. Bismuth also has antibacterial activity, which may account for some of its effects. BSS is found in various commercial veterinary antidiarrheal-adsorbent products, as well as in over-the-counter antidiarrheal products for human use (e.g., Pepto-Bismol). BSS may be effective in controlling objectionable flatus in pet animals but probably needs to be given multiple times per day, which precludes its practical long-term use. BSS should be used with caution in cats because of concerns with salicylate toxicosis.

Similar to bismuth, zinc acetate binds sulphydral compounds and has also been shown to reduce volatile sulfur compounds when exposed directly to flatus gas. Addition of zinc acetate to food (1% total diet) decreased fecal hydrogen sulfide concentrations and improved flatus odor in rats. One report showed that an oral treat containing zinc acetate, activated charcoal, and *Yucca schidigera* extract reduced highly odoriferous episodes of flatus in dogs (Gifford et al., 2001).

Simethicone (dimethylpolysiloxane) is an antifoaming agent that reduces surface tension of gas bubbles and is found in commercial veterinary products and over-the-counter products for human use. Why simethicone would be beneficial in patients with flatulence is not obvious; however, one could speculate that altered gas bubbles might be more effectively eliminated. In general, simethicone has no effect on total daily flatus volume, number of flatus episodes, or average volume per flatus event in people. Simethicone may help reduce gastric accumulation of gas and alleviate upper GI symptoms. The effectiveness of simethicone in controlling flatulence in pet animals is unknown. It would not be expected to control objectionable flatus odors.

Extracts of the *Yucca schidigera* plant have been used to control fecal malodor in animal waste lagoon systems and may help decrease fecal aroma. The mechanisms of action are poorly understood and may include "binding" of ammonia or alterations in microbial activity. In the United States *Yucca* preparations are only approved as flavoring agents in pet foods, and it is unknown whether they effectively control flatulence or objectionable flatus odors when ingested by pet animals.

Products containing α-galactosidase are available as human (Beano) and veterinary (CurTail) products. They reduce flatus volume by improving digestion of nonabsorbable oligosaccharides found in soybeans, beans, pea, and other legumes. These products would not be expected to improve excessive flatus from other causes (e.g., aerophagia) or the odor of flatus. Anecdotal reports suggest that these products may be beneficial in some animals.

Pancreatic enzyme supplementation has been shown to decrease abnormal intestinal gas production in dogs with exocrine pancreatic insufficiency. Pancreatic enzyme preparations have also been widely used for bloating and abdominal distention in people. Because ingestion of these preparations should add little to the enzyme output of the pancreas in otherwise normal individuals, there is no solid rationale for their use in flatulent patients without pancreatic disease. Nevertheless, one study in humans showed that a microencapsulated pancreatic enzyme preparation significantly reduced postprandial symptoms of bloating and abdominal distention experienced by healthy humans ingesting a high-calorie, high-fat meal. This finding suggests that pancreatic enzyme supplements might benefit some patients with flatulence.

Use of probiotic supplements containing various live bacterial cultures has been shown to improve flatulence in some humans with irritable bowel syndrome or functional abdominal bloating (feeling of fullness or bloating without another functional GI disorder). No studies have evaluated use of probiotic preparations in animals with flatulence. More than 30 herbal and botanical preparations have also been listed as carminitives. The dosage, safety, and efficacy of herbal/botanical preparations in pets with flatulence have not been established.

To date the best evidence is available for short-term use of BSS, zinc acetate, and nonabsorbable antibiotics as carminitives. Less evidence can be found for use of activated charcoal, simethicone, digestive enzyme preparations, *Yucca* extract, probiotics, and herbal preparations. Changing the feeding plan (food and feeding method) rather than using carminitives offers the best opportunity for successful long-term management of flatulence in pet animals.

MONITORING PATIENTS WITH FLATULENCE

Patients should be evaluated for evidence of maldigestion or malabsorption if feeding methods and ancillary therapy outlined in this chapter are not successful in reducing or controlling flatulence. Relapses in animals that have been previously asymptomatic often indicate dietary indiscretion. The prognosis for control of flatulence is good in most cases. However, pet owners should be educated about normal intestinal gas production and not expect complete cessation of flatulence, especially in pets with excessive aerophagia. In some cases the following advice may still be necessary: "After trying empirical therapy for pets with chronic flatulence, sound advice for the client is to always stand upwind from the patient" (Lorenz, 1974).

References and Suggested Reading

Cho S. *The gas we pass: the story of farts*, Brooklyn, NY, 1994, Kane/Miller Book Publishers.

Giffard CJ et al: Administration of charcoal, *Yucca schidigera*, and zinc acetate to reduce malodorous flatulence in dogs, *J Am Vet Med Assoc* 218:892, 2001.

Guilford WG et al: Food sensitivity in cats with chronic idiopathic gastrointestinal problems, *J Vet Intern Med* 15:7, 2001.

Jones BR et al: Flatulence in pet dogs, *NZ Vet J* 46:191, 1998.

Lorenz MD: Flatulence in small animals. In Kirk RW, editor: *Current veterinary therapy V*, Philadelphia, 1974, Saunders, p 95.

Lowe JA, Kershaw SJ: The ameliorating effect of Yucca schidigera extract on canine and feline faecal aroma, *Res Vet Sci* 63:61, 1997.

Roudebush P: Flatulence: causes and management options, *Compend Contin Educ Pract Vet* 23:1075, 2001.

Suarez FL, Levitt MD: An understanding of excessive intestinal gas, *Curr Gastroenterol Rep* 2:413, 2000.

Washabau RJ et al: Evaluation of intestinal carbohydrate malabsorption in the dog by pulmonary hydrogen gas excretion, *Am J Vet Res* 47:1402, 1986.

Yamka RM et al: In vivo measurement of flatulence and nutrient digestibility in dogs fed poultry by-product meal, conventional soybean meal, and low-oligosaccharide low-phytate meal, *Am J Vet Res* 67:88, 2006.

CHAPTER **122**

Anal-Rectal Disease

CRAIG B. WEBB, *Fort Collins, Colorado*

Anal-rectal disorders of the dog and cat are rarely life threatening unless caused by malignancy. Diseases found in this area are often painful for the patient and difficult for the owner to manage; and they frequently result in secondary complications such as constipation, diarrhea, or fecal incontinence. The patient's quality of life can be severely affected and, because many of these conditions fail to respond adequately to attempts at intervention, could result in a decision to euthanize the pet.

ANATOMY

The rectum is a continuation of the colon that begins at the pelvic inlet and ends at the anal canal. Inflammation of the rectal mucosa results in an increase in goblet cell mucus secretion, tenesmus, and dyschezia. The anal canal extends from the rectum to the exterior anal opening. Surrounding the anal canal, the internal anal sphincter is composed of involuntary smooth muscle, and the external anal sphincter is composed of skeletal muscle. Innervation of this area is provided by both divisions of the autonomic nervous system: parasympathetic nerve fibers control defecation (contraction of the rectum, relaxation of the internal anal sphincter muscle), whereas sympathetic nerve fibers control storage of feces (relaxation of the rectum, contraction of the internal anal sphincter). Striated muscles of the external anal sphincter are innervated by a branch of the pudendal nerve. Damage to this nerve and loss of external anal sphincter function result in fecal incontinence. Muscles of the pelvic diaphragm (sacrococcygeal and levator ani) are also important in maintaining normal anal-rectal anatomy and function.

ANAL DISEASE

Atresia Ani

Atresia ani (anal agenesis) is a congenital condition that carries with it a grave prognosis. The absence of a normal anal opening may become apparent even before weaning; signs are associated with tenesmus, a bulging perineum, abdominal distention, and discomfort. The presence of an alternate route of evacuation from a rectovaginal, rectovestibular, or rectourethral fistula may lessen the clinical signs and delay the diagnosis. Surgical correction is the only therapeutic option and is often accompanied by complications such as dehiscence, fecal incontinence, or anal-rectal stricture formation. A surgical technique designed to preserve an existing fistula along with the sphincter musculature has shown promising long-term results in several dogs, but concurrent megacolon may become a limiting factor, even in patients that undergo successful surgical correction of the anal opening.

Although this condition is most often diagnosed in dogs, there is a report of atresia ani with concurrent rectovaginal fistula in three kittens, two of which were Manx littermates.

Anal Sacculitis

Anal sac disease is rare in cats but common in dogs and is usually diagnosed based on historical findings and a thorough physical examination of the area (see also Chapter 107). Affected dogs exhibit any number of behaviors that suggest that the anal area is painful such as scooting, licking, or painful defecation. Examination of the region may reveal anal sac contents that are resistant to manual expression; a palpable mass; obvious inflammation; or even abscessation, rupture, or draining fistulas. The chronicity of disease and presence of impaction or secondary infection may determine the degree of inflammation and dictate the treatment requirements. Manual extrusion of the anal sac contents, flushing with saline, and infusion with antibiotics and steroid ointments may suffice in simple cases, but systemic antibiotics are required for more involved or chronic cases. All patients benefit from proper nursing care, including frequent gentle expression of the anal sac contents, warm compresses, and attention to hygiene. Abscessed anal sacs should be addressed surgically, providing adequate drainage and abscess management. Recurrence of significant anal sacculitis may warrant complete surgical removal of the anal sacs.

Anal Sac and Perianal Neoplasia

Adenocarcinoma of the Apocrine Gland of the Anal Sac
Adenocarcinoma of the apocrine gland of the anal sac is a malignant, locally aggressive neoplasm that has metastasized frequently by the time of diagnosis (see also Chapter 83). It was previously thought that anal sac adenocarcinomas were most common in older spayed female dogs, although recent surveys suggest that neither gender nor reproductive status is a predisposing factor. These tumors have metastasized in over half of the cases at the time of diagnosis, most often to sublumbar lymph nodes. Common clinical signs include tenesmus, constipation, anorexia, and weight loss. Some patients exhibit polyuria/polydipsia secondary to tumor-induced hypercalcemia from the production of a parathormone-related protein (PTHrp). Because of this relationship, unexplained hypercalcemia in a case should initiate a rectal examination for the possibility of this tumor. A wide variety of treatment options have been investigated, including surgery, chemotherapy, radiation, and various combinations thereof. With surgery alone survival time appears to be between 10 and 20 months. The prognosis may be decreased if hypercalcemia or metastatic disease is present or if the tumor is greater than $10\,cm^2$ in size. Survival time is also shorter in dogs treated with only chemotherapy. One report suggests that combining tumor resection with iliac lymph node removal prolongs survival if the tumor is not locally invasive, whereas another survey concluded that there was no difference in median survival of dogs with sublumbar metastases compared to those without. Multiple sequential surgeries have also been used to prolong survival time. Combining surgical

excision of the anal sac with sublumbar lymph node removal and melphalan chemotherapy resulted in a modest increase in survival times; and the combination of surgery, radiation, and mitoxantrone appeared to increase survival time in a number of dogs.

There is one report of an anal sac adenocarcinoma in a 12-year-old male neutered Siamese cat (Mellanby et al., 2002). The cat presented with a history of inappetence, lethargy, and an enlarged left anal sac, which was surgically excised. The neoplasia returned 4 months later, and the cat was euthanized.

Perianal Adenomas
Perianal adenomas are the most common perianal tumor, appearing most often in intact male dogs, suggesting hormonally mediated growth. These tumors are not associated with paraneoplastic syndromes (i.e., the hypercalcemia seen with anal sac adenocarcinomas) or metastatic disease, nor are they considered a premalignant condition. Treatment includes castration and surgical removal and carries with it an excellent prognosis.

Other Tumors
Other tumor types reported in the anal and perianal region of dogs are rare and include benign cystadenoma, malignant melanoma, squamous cell carcinoma, and malignant perianal sebaceous gland adenocarcinoma in addition to soft-tissue sarcoma, leiomyoma, lymphoma, and mast cell tumor. Perianal tumors are rarely found in the cat.

Anal Furunculosis

Anal furunculosis, more commonly referred to as perianal fistula disease, is a progressive inflammatory condition characterized by perianal ulceration and sinus tract formation. As with most anal diseases, clinical signs include tenesmus; excessive licking of the area; tail chasing; or abnormal tail carriage, hematochezia, and dyschezia. The clinical condition may progress to include weight loss, lethargy, constipation, fecal incontinence, diarrhea, and purulent discharge and is usually associated with significant discomfort. German shepherds are predisposed; however, the condition has been described in other breeds, including Labrador retrievers, Irish setters, Old English sheepdogs, and collies. The etiology underlying perianal fistula disease is unknown; possible contributing factors include the anatomy of the area in certain breeds, infectious agents, and endocrine or hormonal influences. The disease is also likely to be a clinical manifestation of an underlying immune system dysfunction; whether that is an immunoglobulin A deficiency, abnormal antigen-presentation, or a specific T cell dysfunction remains to be determined. Historically perianal fistula disease has been considered very refractory to medical management, but recent therapeutic protocols appear more promising. A variety of surgical approaches have been reported, including 360-degree anoplasty, cryosurgery, tail amputation, the débridement of necrotic tissue followed by reconstruction, or bilateral anal sacculectomy. Postoperative complications include dehiscence, fecal incontinence, and stricture formation. Positive results are reported in a significant number of dogs when en bloc surgical resection of diseased tissue and primary wound closure were combined with bilateral anal sacculectomy and postoperative metronidazole. Using a carbon dioxide laser to surgically address perianal diseases, including fistulas, may also be a strategy for reducing postoperative morbidity.

Attempts to medically manage perianal fistula disease have included the use of prednisone (begin with 2 mg/kg q24h), cyclosporine, azathioprine, metronidazole, and topical tacrolimus ointment. A hypoallergenic or low-residue diet is often incorporated into the treatment regimen.

Azathioprine (50 mg orally [PO] q24h) and metronidazole (400 mg PO q24h) were used before surgery in a small number of dogs to effectively reduce the size and inflammation of the fistula disease. Following approximately 4 weeks of this therapy, the perianal area was surgically débrided, and the remaining anal sac tissue removed. The medications were continued, and these dogs remained disease free for at least 10 months. One potential advantage of this protocol is the cost of azathioprine and metronidazole compared to the more expensive cyclosporine.

Cyclosporine has been used as a single-agent therapy for anal furunculosis with positive results in many dogs, with treatment duration lasting up to 20 weeks and remission periods in excess of 14 months (also see Chapter 84). A starting dose of 7.5 mg/kg BID is used but adjusted based on blood trough levels 48 hours after initiating therapy. Blood levels should be somewhere between 100 to 600 ng/ml pending clinical response. The value of adjusting a patient's cyclosporine dosage based on blood levels is in question, and an alternative approach is to treat with a predetermined dosage (4 mg/kg BID to 7.5 mg/kg q24h for 13 to 24 weeks) until no further clinical improvement is observed. At that time any residual lesions may be addressed surgically. Gastrointestinal absorption of cyclosporine is improved when given with a fatty meal. Hair coat turnover, vomiting, anorexia, diarrhea, gingival hyperplasia, and papillomatosis are potential adverse effects of cyclosporine administration; and recurrence of fistula disease can be anticipated in 30% to 50% of patients. Because of the expense of cyclosporine, it is often combined with ketoconazole, which inhibits the hepatic metabolism of the drug and reduces the dose necessary to attain similar trough levels. The combination of cyclosporine (5 to 10 mg/kg BID initially with trough levels maintained above 200 ng/ml) and ketoconazole (5 to 10 mg/kg q24h) does not appear to be any more effective than cyclosporine alone but can be significantly less expensive. Remission times are similar, and recurrence should still be anticipated in at least 30% of patients.

Topical application of the immunosuppressive ointment tacrolimus (Protopic 0.1% ointment thin film applied q12-24h after gently cleaning the area) resulted in either resolution or significant improvement of perianal fistulas in a number of dogs treated for 16 weeks. The owner should wear gloves when applying the tacrolimus. Potential disadvantages of this treatment strategy include having to apply something topically to what is normally a painful area and the patient's tendency to lick at the area. Topical tacrolimus appears to be most effective in management of small lesions or as a less expensive option

following remission with cyclosporine. Treatment should continue for 4 weeks beyond clinical resolution.

Adjunct therapy involves the use of stool softeners and perianal hygiene. It is not uncommon to have fecal soiling in the perianal area, and I advise keeping the area clean and dry. Tucks Medicated Pads, topical astringent pads, are also helpful. Pain management (such as tramadol 2–5 mg/kg TID) and hot packing the area are used as needed.

Severe dyschezia secondary to perianal lesions has also been reported in dogs with cutaneous or discoid lupus erythematosus. The diagnosis is made based on histopathologic changes and therefore requires a biopsy of the area. Treatment involves immunomodulation, and response to therapy is usually good.

RECTAL DISEASE

Perineal Hernia

Perianal swelling and tenesmus are the most common presenting complaints in patents with a perineal hernia. In some animals the anatomic defect may lead to urinary bladder or prostate entrapment, and both the clinical signs and consequences quickly become more serious because of urinary obstruction. If left unattended the presence of a perineal hernia may lead to obstipation and megacolon. Perineal hernias occur most commonly in older, intact male dogs, with brachycephalic breeds predisposed to the condition. In these dogs there is an idiopathic weakening of the pelvic diaphragm. Castration appears to reduce the incidence of perineal hernias and the recurrence following surgical repair. The hormone relaxin, produced by the prostate, may be a factor in the connective tissue changes to predispose intact male dogs to herniation. Physical examination usually reveals a visible, easily reducible perineal swelling. Delineation of the defect requires a rectal examination finding a loss of the normal pelvic diaphragm laterally with a with an out pouching of the rectal wall. The herniation is generally unilateral, with the defect more commonly appearing in the right perianal region. Although it is usually rectal tissue alone that herniates, the defect may progress to include abdominal tissue such as retroperitoneal fat and/or pelvic organs such as the urinary bladder. A standard perineal herniorrhaphy, herniorrhaphy using an autogenous fascia lata graft, use of a semitendinosus muscle flap, or transposition of the internal obturator muscle has been used to surgically correct perineal hernias. In cases of bilateral herniation or in patients with prostatic disease or urinary bladder involvement, a two-step approach is used, starting with laparotomy and some combination of colopexy, vas deferens pexy, cystopexy, and prostatic omentalization. This is then followed by one of the standard surgical repair procedures. This approach appeared to be effective in a significant number of these complex cases, although urine dribbling and fecal straining were permanent conditions in a small number of dogs. Potential complications of the standard surgical repair techniques include wound infection and fecal incontinence. Recurrence following surgery appears to be rare, as does rectal prolapse or sciatic nerve injury. Urinary problems may persist following surgery if bladder entrapment occurred with the herniation. Preoperative antibiotics to cover enteric flora are followed by postoperative lactulose to soften the stool and feeding a highly digestible, low-residue diet.

Rectal Strictures

I performed a retrospective survey of benign rectal strictures in dogs and identified 19 cases over an 8-year period (Webb, McCord, and Twedt, 2007). The vast majority of patients presented with the complaint of tenesmus, and almost all of the strictures could be identified by digital rectal examination. An underlying etiology was identified in most cases: postoperative stricture formation following surgical rectal tumor resection; the presence of foreign material (wood or bone foreign body); or stricture secondary to a chronic, severe inflammatory condition such as perianal fistula disease, histoplasmosis, anal sacculitis, or inflammatory bowel disease. My standard treatment protocol involves general anesthesia with balloon dilation of the stricture combined with intralesional injections of triamcinolone (2- to 6-mg total dose) for local antiinflammatory effects. Lesional injection can be directed with digital palpation. Some patients were also treated with a variety of other medications, including lactulose, prednisone, tylosin, or other immunosuppressive drugs.

Stricture dilation involved placement of different-diameter balloons to dilate the lumen of the stricture. Based on the size of the patient and the severity of the stricture, the diameter of balloons (generally 10 to 25 mm) and number of separate dilation sessions varied with the majority of patients. Most required one or two separate procedures performed within 7 to 10 days of each other. In general the response to this treatment protocol was good.

A rectal stricture was identified in only two cats over the same time period. In one case the stricture appeared several weeks after manual deobstipation with towel forceps in a cat with megacolon. In the other cat the stricture appeared to be secondary to inflammatory bowel disease. The cat with inflammatory bowel disease eventually did well but required multiple dilations; the other cat responded well to a treatment protocol similar to that described for the dogs.

Rectal Neoplasia

Rectal neoplasia is rare in both dogs and cats, occurring most frequently in older animals. Adenomatous polyps and adenocarcinoma represent the most common benign and malignant canine rectal tumors, respectively. Colorectal lymphoma and rectal adenocarcinoma are the rectal tumors occurring most frequently in cats, although they are uncommon. Tumors of the smooth muscle, plasmacytomas, fibromas, fibrosarcomas, and a ganglioneuroma have also been reported in the rectum of small animals.

Adenomatous rectal polyps are focal, pedunculated growths of tissue that rarely metastasize. A locally invasive and often sessile form of polyp found in the dog is referred to as a *carcinoma in situ*. Most dogs present with single, solitary masses. Despite the lack of metastasis, recurrence can be seen in up to 40% of cases, and malignant transformation of these tumors has been reported. The likelihood of recurrence and malignant transformation is greatest in dogs that have multiple masses initially or diffuse disease and in those dogs diagnosed with carcinoma in situ.

The patient's presenting complaint and clinical signs are similar to those described for other forms of perianal disease, with hematochezia the most common sign, often accompanied by tenesmus and dyschezia. Anorexia, diarrhea, and weight loss may occur as the disease becomes more chronic or severe. Often the owner reports fresh bright-red blood that appears on the surface of otherwise normally formed stool toward the end of the bowel movement. Most rectal polyps and neoplasms can be palpated digitally during rectal examination, and fresh blood is frequently found on the examination glove afterwards. It is important to remember that palpation of an annular rectal ring or stricture may represent a benign response or may be primary malignant tissue. A tissue biopsy is required for a histopathologic diagnosis. Although tissue in the rectum can be obtained using a rigid proctoscopy or speculum and biopsy forceps, a more extensive examination of the colon using a flexible endoscope may better define the extent of the disease orad to the rectum or the presence of a concurrent disorder (i.e., inflammatory large bowel disease). Even with endoscopy, the mucosal biopsy may be superficial and underestimate the extent, degree, or severity of disease. Surgery is the initial treatment of choice for rectal tumors other than lymphosarcoma or plasma cell tumors. Rectal "pull-through" for the removal of a benign polyp is a relatively straightforward procedure with rare complications. Surgical removal of malignant neoplasia is more problematic, with complications that include dehiscence, infection, rectal stricture formation, or fecal incontinence. Because of this, a variety of surgical and nonsurgical treatment options continue to be explored, including radiation therapy, laser therapy, cryosurgery, electrocautery, incontinent end-on colostomy, and even piroxicam in oral or suppository forms.

Rectal Prolapse

Prolapse of the rectum, seen as a cylindric mass protruding from the anal orifice, usually results from chronic tenesmus. In dogs rectal prolapse is usually secondary to inflammation of the rectum or anus, a tumor, foreign body, perineal hernia, dystocia, proctitis, cystitis, or urethral obstruction. Rectal prolapse in the cat has been associated with chronic enteritis, dysautonomia, and rectal leiomyoma; although in most cases an etiology is not identified. Manx cats may also be predisposed to rectal prolapse. In one feline report the rectal prolapse was presumed to be secondary to tenesmus resulting from a urinary bladder transition cell carcinoma. In all cases rectal prolapse must be distinguished from the protrusion of an intestinal intussusception. In the case of rectal prolapse there is continuity between the prolapsed rectal tissue and the mucocutaneous junction of the anus. Differentiating a prolapsed intussusception from a rectal prolapse one can pass a probe in between the anus and prolapsed tissue in an intussusception.

Treatment of rectal prolapse involves removal of the underlying cause, if identified, or recurrence is highly likely. Manual reduction of a prolapsed rectum can be attempted following rehydration and reduction of the exposed edematous tissue. Water-soluble lubrication and gentle manipulation may be sufficient in some cases. Following successful reduction a nonconstricting purse-string suture should be placed in the anus, and stool softeners and a low-residue diet should be prescribed. The purse string may remain in place for a number of weeks while the underlying primary problem is addressed. Unfortunately recurrence is seen in a significant number of cases. Surgical colopexy is then the treatment of choice for recurring rectal prolapse and has been highly effective in both dogs and cats.

References and Suggested Reading

Brissot HN, Dupre GP, Bouvy BM: Use of laparotomy in a staged approach for resolution of bilateral or complicated perineal hernia in 41 dogs, *Vet Surg* 33:412, 2004.

Doust R, Griffiths LG, Sullivan M: Evaluation of once daily treatment with cyclosporine for anal furunculosis in dogs, *Vet Rec* 152:225, 2003.

Hardie RJ et al: Cyclosporine treatment of anal furunculosis in 26 dogs, *J Small Anim Pract* 46:3, 2005.

Mellanby RJ et al: Anal sac adenocarcinoma in a Siamese cat, *J Feline Med Surg* 4:205, 2002.

Milner HR: The role of surgery in the management of canine anal furunculosis: a review of the literature and retrospective evaluation of treatment by surgical resection in 51 dogs, *NZ Vet J* 54:1, 2006.

Mouatt JG: Cyclosporin and ketoconazole interaction for treatment of perianal fistulas in the dog, *Aust Vet J* 80:207, 2002.

O'Neill T, Edwards GA, Holloway S: Efficacy of combined cyclosporine A and ketoconazole treatment of anal furunculosis, *J Small Anim Pract* 45:238, 2004.

Popovitch CA, Holt D, Bright R: Colopexy as a treatment for rectal prolapse in dogs and cats: a retrospective study of 14 cases, *Vet Surg* 23:115, 1994.

Valerius KD et al: Adenomatous polyps and carcinoma in situ of the canine colon and rectum: 34 cases (1982-1994), *J Am Anim Hosp Assoc* 33:156, 1997.

Webb CB, McCord KW, Twedt DC: Rectal strictures in 19 dogs: 1997-2005, *J Am Anim Hosp Assoc* 43:332, 2007.

Williams LE et al: Carcinoma of the apocrine glands of the anal sac in dogs: 113 cases (1985-1995), *J Am Vet Med Assoc* 223:825, 2003.

Zoran DL: Rectoanal disease. In Ettinger SJ, Feldman EC, editors: *Textbook of veterinary internal medicine*, ed 6, St Louis, 2005, Elsevier, p 1408.

CHAPTER 123

Exocrine Pancreatic Insufficiency in Dogs

MARIA WIBERG, *Helsinki, Finland*

Chronic diseases of the exocrine pancreas may affect pancreatic function and lead to inadequate production of digestive enzymes with associated maldigestion signs of exocrine pancreatic insufficiency (EPI). The exocrine pancreas has a large reserve in terms of secretory capacity, and clinical signs do not occur until about 90% of secretory capacity is lost. EPI in dogs can be the result of pancreatic acinar atrophy, chronic pancreatitis, pancreatic hypoplasia, and pancreatic neoplasia.

ETIOPATHOGENESIS

Pancreatic acinar atrophy is by far the most common reason for the clinical signs of EPI. It has been reported in many different breeds, but the breeds most commonly affected are German shepherd dogs and rough-coated collies. Recent studies suggest that in German shepherd dogs and collies pancreatic atrophy is a result of *autoimmune-mediated atrophic lymphocytic pancreatitis*, which gradually may lead to almost total destruction of pancreatic acinar tissue (Wiberg, Saari, and Westermarck, 2000). Typically the endocrine part of the pancreas is unaffected. Genetic predisposition to the disease and the typical histologic findings during the progression of acinar atrophy have been taken as primary evidence of the autoimmune nature of the disease. In both German shepherd dogs and in collies, pedigree analyses have suggested an autosomal-recessive inheritance model. Thus far genetic studies have not been able to identify the genes involved (Moeller et al., 2002; Clark et al., 2005). Females and males usually are equally affected. Acinar atrophy is a progressive disease, as it was reported in one dog that was born with a histologically normal pancreas but developed atrophy later in life (Westermarck et al., 1993). Wiberg, Saari, and Westermarck (1999b) divided progression of acinar atrophy into a subclinical and clinical phases. The subclinical phase is characterized by marked lymphocytic inflammation into a partially atrophied acinar parenchyma. Cytotoxic T cells are predominant when the tissue destruction is in progress. When the disease progresses to end-stage atrophy, the clinical phase of EPI develops. An atrophied pancreas is thin and transparent, with no increase of fibrotic tissue.

Clinical signs of EPI usually appear at ages 1 to 5 years of age, but also can be seen in older dogs. The natural progression of the atrophic pancreatitis can vary markedly. Dogs may remain in the subclinical phase for years and sometimes for life (Wiberg and Westermarck, 2002). Markers that predict which dogs are likely to develop clinical disease or environmental factors that trigger disease have not been identified thus far.

Chronic pancreatitis is the most common cause of EPI in cats and humans. In dogs, even if chronic pancreatitis has been recognized as a cause of EPI, its prevalence and overall significance is still unclear. Unlike the situation of autoimmune atrophic pancreatitis, in chronic pancreatitis there is usually a progressive destruction of both the exocrine and endocrine pancreas accompanied by fibrosis. Clinical signs are nonspecific gastrointestinal signs and sometimes related to the development of diabetes mellitus. The congenital form of exocrine or exocrine and endocrine pancreatic hypoplasia is sometimes found in young puppies. EPI is rarely reported in association with pancreatic neoplasia.

CLINICAL SIGNS

Typical clinical signs of EPI include increased fecal volume and defecation frequency, yellow or gray feces, weight loss, and flatulence. Other common signs are polyphagia; poorly digested, loose, and pulpy feces; or coprophagia. Signs of nervousness or aggressiveness may occur possibly because of abdominal discomfort caused by increased intestinal gas. Severe watery diarrhea is usually only temporary. Skin disorders have also been reported. Although the signs of EPI are considered to be quite typical, they are not pathognomonic for pancreatic dysfunction since similar maldigestion signs may be observed in other small intestinal disorders.

DIAGNOSIS

Diagnosis of exocrine pancreatic dysfunction is based on typical clinical findings and confirmed with abnormal pancreatic function testing. Routine serum biochemistry profile and complete blood count often show unremarkable changes. Serum amylase and lipase activities are not useful in the diagnosis of EPI. Various pancreatic function tests that measure pancreatic enzymes in the blood and feces have been used in diagnosing canine EPI. The diagnostic value of the tests has relied mostly on their ability to distinguish whether the clinical maldigestion signs are caused by EPI or a disease of the small intestine.

Serum Trypsin-Like Immunoreactivity

The measurement of serum canine trypsin-like immunoreactivity (TLI) has become one of the most commonly used pancreatic function tests to diagnose canine EPI (Williams and Batt, 1988). Serum TLI measurement is both species and pancreas specific, with high sensitivity and specificity for diagnosing EPI. The reference range for canine TLI (cTLI) in healthy dogs is greater than 5.7 to 45.2 mcg/L (RIA). In dogs showing clinical maldigestion signs of EPI, cTLI concentrations are usually very low (< 2.5 mcg/L), indicating severe loss of digestive

enzyme–producing acinar tissue. However, the interpretation of cTLI values is not always straightforward. Pathologic processes affecting exocrine pancreatic function are gradually progressive, and cTLI levels can vary from normal to abnormal, depending of the degree of pancreatic tissue lost. Overlapping results between normal and affected dogs can be expected, and a normal cTLI greater than 5 mcg/L does not necessary exclude the possibility of mild-to-moderate pancreatic dysfunction. In general the lower the cTLI value, the more valuable a single measurement is in assessing the pancreatic dysfunction. Dogs with serum cTLI concentrations in the range of 2.5 to 5 mcg/L and gastrointestinal signs can be a diagnostic challenge. Whether the signs are caused by a decreased exocrine pancreatic function or disease of the small intestine may be difficult to assess, and further diagnostic procedures repeating the cTLI measurement or treatment trials are needed. In breeds predisposed to autoimmune atrophic pancreatitis, repeatedly subnormal cTLI values (2.5 to 5 mcg/L) in dogs showing no typical signs of EPI indicate subclinical EPI and suggest partial atrophy (Wiberg, Nurmi, and Westermarck, 1999a).

Fecal Enzyme Measurements

Fecal proteolytic activity measurement has been used previously for diagnosis of EPI. The problem with this test relates to the finding that at times normal dogs also show decreased proteolytic activity. To avoid this problem, fecal proteolytic activity has been measured from repeated fecal samples and after using pancreatic stimulation by giving raw soybean in the food during the test period.

Canine fecal elastase is a new species- and pancreas-specific test with high sensitivity but relatively low specificity. It has been shown that a single fecal elastase concentration greater than 20 mcg/g is valuable for excluding EPI in the dogs with chronic diarrhea. Values less than 20 mcg/g in association with typical clinical signs of EPI are suggestive of severe pancreatic dysfunction (Spillmann et al., 2000; Battersby et al., 2005).

TREATMENT

Enzyme Replacement Therapy

When clinical maldigestion signs of EPI appear, enzyme replacement therapy is indicated. Basic treatment involves supplementation of the dog's ordinary food with pancreatic enzyme extracts. Various pancreatic enzyme extracts are available. The highest enzyme activity in the duodenum has been achieved by using nonenteric-coated supplements such as powdered enzymes or raw chopped pancreas, and these supplements have proved to be equally effective in controlling clinical signs. The value of enteric-coated supplements was shown to be limited in dogs because of the delayed gastric emptying of the preparations. The maintenance dosage for the powdered enzyme depends on the preparation used (Viokase-V, Fort Dodge), 1 tsp/meal and raw frozen pancreas 50 to 100 g/meal for dogs that weigh 20 to 35 kg. The use of raw pig's pancreas is prohibited in many countries because of possibilities of zoonotic diseases.

Supportive Treatments

Supportive treatments should be considered when the treatment response to enzyme replacement therapy alone is not satisfactory. Orally administered enzymes may be largely destroyed by gastric acid; and, despite accurate enzyme administration, the digestive capacity does not return to normal. In some dogs the increase of enzyme dosage or change to another nonenteric-coated supplement may be beneficial. EPI also may be associated with secondary problems that may worsen the clinical signs. These include small intestinal bacterial overgrowth, malabsorption of cobalamin, and the coexistence of a small intestinal disease.

Antibiotics

Antibiotics are the most commonly used supportive treatment. An increased amount of substrates for bacteria in the small intestine, a lack of bacteriostatic factors of the pancreatic juice, and changes in intestinal motility and immune functions are possible reasons for accumulation of bacteria in the small intestine of dogs with EPI. Antibiotics have been used during the initial treatment when clinical signs such as diarrhea, increased intestinal gas, and flatulence have not resolved with enzyme therapy or when these signs have recurred during long-term treatment. Commonly used antibiotics are tylosin (10 to 20 mg/kg q12h) or metronidazole (10 to 15 mg/kg q12h) for 1 to 3 weeks (Wiberg, Lautala, and Westermarck, 1998).

Dietary Modification

Clinical feeding studies during long-term treatment of EPI have shown that the need for special diets is minimal and the dogs may continue to be fed with their original diet (Wiberg, Lautala, and Westermarck, 1998; Westermarck and Wiberg, 2006). However, radical dietary changes should be avoided, and special attention should be paid to individual needs since responses to different diets varied among dogs. Furthermore, it has been shown that the severity of some clinical signs of EPI can be decreased with dietary modification. A highly digestible, low-fiber, and moderate-fat diet can alleviate clinical signs such as defecation frequency, increased fecal volume, and flatulence. Highly digestible diets may be of particular value in the initial treatment until the nutritional status has improved and possible mucosal damage has been repaired. A low-fat diet has been recommended because enzyme supplements alone are incapable of restoring normal fat absorption. Fat absorption may also be affected by bacterial deconjugation of bile salts in a small intestinal disease, producing metabolites that in turn may result in diarrhea. Dietary sensitivities may be a consequence of EPI; therefore hypoallergic diets may benefit some dogs, especially those with concurrent skin problems.

Cobalamin

Cobalamin deficiency in dogs with EPI is partly the result of increased uptake of cobalamin by intestinal bacteria and partly because of the lack of the pancreatic intrinsic factor, shown to have a major role in the absorption of cobalamin. Because cobalamin deficiency is common in canine EPI, serum cobalamin should be measured in dogs that are clinically suspicious for EPI or do not respond satisfactorily to the enzyme treatment. Cobalamin is given subcutaneously, and the dosage currently recommended is 250 to 1000 mcg once a week, depending of the size of the dog. The treatment should be repeated based on the serum levels (Ruaux, 2002).

Other Supportive Treatments

Inhibition of gastric acid secretion by H_2-antagonist may be indicated, especially when clinical signs such as vomiting or inappetence appear. Malabsorption of fat-soluble vitamins may be expected with EPI; however, the clinical importance of vitamin A, D, E, or K deficiency has not been reported. When the treatment response to enzymes and supportive therapies is still unsatisfactory, concomitant disease of the small intestine should be suspected.

Treatment of Subclinical EPI

Dogs with partial acinar atrophy but no clinical signs of EPI do not require treatment. In autoimmune atrophic pancreatitis the value of early immunosuppressive treatment in slowing the progression of the autoimmune-mediated tissue destruction was found to be questionable; thus it is not recommended (Wiberg and Westermarck, 2002).

PROGNOSIS

When the clinical signs of EPI appear, the loss of pancreatic tissue is already almost total. The changes are considered to be irreversible, and lifelong enzyme treatment is usually required. Response to enzyme treatment is usually seen during the first weeks of treatment, with weight gain, cessation of diarrhea, and decrease in fecal volume. The level of treatment response achieved during the initial treatment period seems to remain fairly stable. Although some dogs experience short relapses with associated clinical signs, the permanent deterioration of the clinical condition during long-term treatment is uncommon. During long-term treatment with nonenteric-coated enzyme supplements the gastrointestinal signs considered typical for dogs with EPI were almost completely controlled in half of the dogs (Wiberg, Lautala, and Westermarck, 1998). Although it was not always possible to eliminate all signs, acceptable resolution of signs was achieved, especially in more serious signs. Poor response to treatment was observed in 20% of the dogs despite similar treatment regimens. Furthermore about 20% of dogs diagnosed with EPI were euthanized during the first year of diagnosis. The most common reason for euthanasia was poor treatment response. Another reason was owner reluctance for expensive and lifelong treatment. A rare but severe complication of EPI is mesenteric torsion. Today mesenteric torsion is seldom seen, probably because of the more efficient enzyme preparations now available.

References and Suggested Reading

Battersby IA et al: Effect of intestinal inflammation on fecal elastase concentration in dogs, *Vet Clin Pathol* 34:49, 2005.

Clark LA et al: Linkage analysis and gene expression profile of pancreatic acinar atrophy in the German shepherd dog, *Mamm Genome* 16:955, 2005.

Moeller EM et al: Inheritance of pancreatic acinar atrophy in German shepherd dogs, *Am J Vet Res* 10:1429, 2002.

Ruaux CG: Cobalamin and gastrointestinal disease, Proceedings of the 20th ACVIM Congress, Dallas, TX, 2002.

Spillmann T et al: Canine faecal pancreatic elastase (cE1) in dogs with clinical exocrine pancreatic insufficiency, normal dogs and dogs with chronic enteropathies, *Eur J Comp Gastroenterol* 2:5, 2000.

Westermarck E, Wiberg ME: Effects of diet on clinical signs of exocrine pancreatic insufficiency in dogs, *J Am Vet Med Assoc* 228:225, 2006.

Westermarck E et al: Sequential study of pancreatic structure and function during development of pancreatic acinar atrophy in a German shepherd dog, *Am J Vet Res* 54:1088, 1993.

Wiberg ME, Westermarck E: Subclinical exocrine pancreatic insufficiency in dogs, *J Am Vet Med Assoc* 220:1183, 2002.

Wiberg ME, Lautala H-M, Westermarck E: Response to long-term enzyme replacement treatment in dogs with exocrine pancreatic insufficiency, *J Am Vet Med Assoc* 1:86, 1998.

Wiberg ME, Nurmi A-K, Westermarck E: Serum trypsin-like immunoreactivity measurement for the diagnosis of subclinical exocrine pancreatic insufficiency in dogs, *J Vet Intern Med* 13:26, 1999a.

Wiberg ME, Saari SAM, Westermarck E: Exocrine pancreatic atrophy in German shepherds and rough-coated collies: an end-result of lymphocytic pancreatitis, *Vet Pathol* 36:530, 1999b.

Wiberg ME, Saari SAM, Westermarck E: Cellular and humoral immune responses in atrophic lymphocytic pancreatitis in German shepherd dogs and rough-coated collies, *Vet Immunol Immunopathol* 76:103-115, 2000.

Williams DA, Batt RM: Sensitivity and specificity of radioimmunoassay of serum trypsin-like immunoreactivity for the diagnosis of canine exocrine pancreatic insufficiency, *J Am Vet Med Assoc* 192:195, 1988.

CHAPTER 124

Canine Pancreatic Disease

JÖRG M. STEINER, *College Station, Texas*

Pancreatitis is a common disorder in dogs, but as in humans, it is believed that the majority of cases remain undiagnosed. Mild cases of pancreatitis that do not show classical clinical signs such as vomiting and abdominal pain may be very difficult to diagnose. Moreover, the treatment of canine patients with suspected or confirmed pancreatitis remains challenging. This is in part because of the variation in severity and unpredictable course of this disease. This chapter focuses on the diagnosis and treatment of canine pancreatitis.

DIAGNOSIS

Clinical Picture

Clinical signs in dogs with pancreatitis depend on the severity of the disease. Mild cases may remain subclinical. More severe cases may present with anorexia, vomiting, weakness, abdominal pain, dehydration, and diarrhea. Severe cases can present with systemic clinical signs such as fever or even cardiovascular shock. Clinical signs in patients with pancreatitis are caused by pancreatic inflammation or systemic effects of the pancreatic inflammation. Recent data suggest that the exocrine pancreas responds to several different noxious stimuli by a decrease in secretion of pancreatic enzymes. This is followed by the formation of giant cytoplasmic vacuoles within pancreatic acinar cells, visible only by electron microscopy. Biochemical studies have shown that these vacuoles are the product of colocalization of the zymogens of digestive enzymes and lysosomal enzymes, which are normally strictly segregated. The ensuing decrease in pH and/or the presence of the lysosomal enzymes such as cathepsin B lead to premature activation of trypsinogen. Trypsin in turn activates other zymogens, leading to local effects such as inflammation, pancreatic edema and hemorrhage, pancreatic necrosis, and parapancreatic fat necrosis. These local effects are associated with clinical signs such as vomiting and abdominal pain. Until recently it was believed that systemic signs commonly seen in pancreatitis patients, like local effects, are a direct result of circulating pancreatic enzymes. Although there is little doubt that some of these systemic effects such as systemic lipodystrophy are caused by circulating pancreatic enzymes, recent data would suggest that other systemic sequelae are a consequence of the release of inflammatory mediators in response to pancreatic inflammation. A systemic inflammatory response consisting of release of neutrophils from the bone marrow; chemotaxis of leukocytes; degranulation of mast cells, basophils, and eosinophils; and platelet aggregation occurs commonly in patients with severe forms of pancreatitis. This response can lead to fever. Other systemic effects seen in patients with severe pancreatitis are systemic vasodilation leading to hypotension and sometimes acute renal failure, pulmonary edema leading to respiratory failure, disseminated intravascular coagulation, and in some cases multiorgan failure. Neurologic signs such as disorientation have been seen in both human and canine patients with severe pancreatitis and are sometimes referred to as pancreatic encephalopathy. Although clinical signs are not specific for pancreatitis, vomiting and cranial abdominal pain are key clinical signs in dogs with pancreatitis; and a canine patient presenting with both of these signs should be evaluated carefully for the presence of pancreatitis.

Diagnostic Tests

Complete blood count and serum chemistry profile often show mild and nonspecific changes. More severe changes can be observed in patients with severe forms of pancreatitis. Serum amylase and lipase activities are of limited clinical use for the diagnosis of pancreatitis in the dog. The specificity of both of these tests is only about 50%, even when stringent criteria are applied. Thus serum amylase and lipase activities should be used only for the preliminary diagnosis of canine pancreatitis until more definitive diagnostic tests can be performed. Radiographic changes seen in some cases include a decreased contrast in the cranial abdomen and displacement of abdominal organs. However, these changes are rather subjective, and abdominal radiography is nonspecific for canine pancreatitis. Abdominal ultrasound is useful in the diagnosis of canine pancreatitis. The sensitivity of abdominal ultrasonography in dogs is up to 68%. However, this value is largely operator dependent. Changes identified include pancreatic swelling, changes in echogenicity of the pancreas (hypoechogenicity in cases of pancreatic necrosis and hyperechogenicity in cases of pancreatic fibrosis) and the peripancreatic fat (hyperechogenicity in cases of peripancreatic fat necrosis), fluid accumulation around the pancreas, and less frequently a mass effect in the area of the pancreas. Other findings that have been described are a dilated pancreatic duct or an enlarged duodenal papilla. Abdominal computed tomography is a routine procedure in humans suspected of having pancreatitis, but it appears to be very insensitive for the diagnosis of pancreatitis in veterinary species.

Trypsin-like immunoreactivity (TLI) is specific for exocrine pancreatic function. However, the sensitivity of serum canine TLI (cTLI) concentration for pancreatitis in dogs is only about 30% to 60%, making it a suboptimal diagnostic test for pancreatitis in this species. However, serum cTLI concentration remains the diagnostic test of choice for the diagnosis of EPI in dogs.

Recently an assay for measurement of canine pancreatic lipase immunoreactivity (cPLI, now measured as Spec cPL) has been developed and validated. Many different cell types in the body synthesize and secrete lipases. In contrast to catalytic assays for the measurement of lipase activity, use of immunoassays does allow for the specific measurement of lipase originating from the exocrine pancreas.

Factors that might influence cPLI have been evaluated in a number of reports. Serum cPLI was measured in a group of dogs with exocrine pancreatic insufficiency, and the median serum cPLI concentration was significantly decreased compared to that of clinically healthy dogs (Steiner et al., 2006). In addition serum cPLI concentration was nondetectable in most of the dogs, and minimal serum cPLI concentrations were observed in the rest of the dogs, indicating that serum cPLI concentration originates from the exocrine pancreas and is specific for exocrine pancreatic function. In another study serum cPLI was evaluated in dogs with experimentally induced chronic renal failure (Steiner et al., 2006). Although serum cPLI was significantly higher in dogs with experimentally induced chronic renal failure than in clinically healthy dogs, most dogs had serum cPLI concentrations within the reference range, and none of the dogs had serum cPLI concentrations that were above the currently recommended cutoff value for pancreatitis. These data suggest that the serum cPLI concentration can be used as a diagnostic test for pancreatitis even in dogs with renal failure. The long-term oral administration of prednisone has not demonstrated any effect on serum cPLI concentration. Finally, the sensitivity of different minimally invasive diagnostic tests was compared in dogs with proven pancreatitis. The sensitivity of serum TLI concentration was below 35%, and that of serum lipase activity was less than 55%. In contrast, the sensitivity for serum cPLI concentration for pancreatitis was above 80%.

Traditionally, a pancreatic biopsy has been viewed as the most definitive diagnostic tool for pancreatitis. Pancreatic biopsies can be collected during abdominal exploratory surgery or by laparoscopy. The presence of pancreatitis is easily diagnosed by gross appearance of the pancreas in many cases. However, the absence of pancreatitis can be difficult to prove. In a recent study histopathologic findings in dogs with pancreatitis were evaluated (Porterpan, Zoran, and Steiner, 2006). Pancreata were sectioned every 2 cm. In one half of all dogs with pancreatic inflammation and in two thirds of dogs with chronic pancreatitis, evidence of pancreatic inflammation was found in less than 25% of all sections. Thus, even if multiple biopsies are collected, pancreatic inflammation, especially in cases of chronic pancreatitis, may easily be missed. It should also be noted that, although a pancreatic biopsy in itself is not associated with many complications, many patients with pancreatitis are poor anesthetic risks.

TREATMENT OF SEVERE PANCREATITIS

Severe pancreatitis is characterized by extensive pancreatic necrosis and systemic complications and is often associated with a poor prognosis. Severe pancreatitis can occur in patients with acute disease or as an exacerbation of chronic pancreatitis.

Removal of Inciting Cause

Unfortunately the cause remains unknown in many dogs with pancreatitis. However, every possible effort should be made to identify a cause and remove it. Several causes and risk factors have been identified for pancreatitis in dogs (Hess et al., 1998).

Nutrition

There is much anecdotal but little scientific evidence that a fatty meal causes pancreatitis. Thus dogs with pancreatitis should be evaluated for the presence of hypertriglyceridemia. If hypertriglyceridemia is present, it may either be the cause or an effect of pancreatitis. Regardless, measures should taken to decrease serum triglyceride concentrations, initially by placing the patient on a low-fat diet or, if dietary management alone is insufficient in controlling hypertriglyceridemia, by also adding gemfibrozil or other lipid binders to the diet. It may be prudent to switch pancreatitis patients to a low-fat diet even if they do not have hypertriglyceridemia.

Toxins and Drugs

Many drugs and drug classes have been implicated in causing pancreatitis in humans. However, definitive proof of a cause-and-effect relationship is extremely rare. Drugs that have been implicated in causing pancreatitis in humans that are also used in veterinary medicine include calcium, potassium bromide, L-asparaginase, azathioprine, estrogen, organophosphates, and some less commonly used drugs. Corticosteroids do not appear to cause pancreatitis, although they can increase serum lipase activity in dogs without causing pancreatitis.

Trauma and Hypoperfusion

Several cases of pancreatitis after traffic accidents and similar traumatic injuries have been reported. Surgical trauma has also been implicated as a cause of pancreatitis. However, evidence from the human literature, as well as experimental data, would suggest that hypoperfusion of the gland secondary to hypotensive states such as may occur during anesthesia rather than trauma to the pancreas per se is responsible for pancreatitis in the majority of postsurgical cases of canine pancreatitis.

Other Causes

Hypercalcemia has been shown to cause pancreatitis in several species and should be corrected by appropriate management when identified. Pancreatitis can also occur in association with neoplastic infiltration by pancreatic adenocarcinoma.

Supportive Care

Aggressive fluid therapy is the mainstay of treatment for pancreatitis and must be individualized, depending on the needs of the patient. The fluid rate chosen depends on the estimated degree of dehydration, the estimated ongoing fluid losses, and the calculated daily maintenance rate. Careful attention to maintenance of a normal serum potassium concentration is particularly important because anorectic, vomiting patients with pancreatitis are particularly prone to hypokalemia. Although hypocalcemia is often noted, it is usually mild, and calcium supplementation should be reserved for the rare animals that manifest clinical signs in association with serum calcium concentrations less that 6.5 mg/dl. Acid-base imbalances are common in dogs with pancreatitis. Since either acidemia (most common) or alkalemia may develop, blind correction of suspected acid-base imbalance should not be attempted. Arterial blood pH, P_{CO_2}, and bicarbonate should be measured in patients with severe pancreatitis whenever possible.

Metabolic Support

It is still common practice to give nothing orally to patients with pancreatitis. This recommendation is sensible in patients that are vomiting. However, the importance of this therapeutic strategy remains scientifically unproven. I currently recommend withholding food and water only from patients that vomit and only for a maximum period of 2 to 4 days. When vomiting ceases, small amounts of water can be offered several times per day. If vomiting does not recur, small amounts of a diet that is low in fat and moderate in protein content (rice, pasta, potatoes, or a commercial diet) can be given. If vomiting does not subside and oral feeding is withheld for more than 2 to 4 days, the nutritional needs of the patient have to be met by alternative metabolic support such as jejunostomy tube or total or partial parenteral nutrition (see Chapter 3 and Section VI on Evolve).

Symptomatic Therapy

Analgesic Therapy

Many patients with pancreatitis do not show overt signs of abdominal pain. Regardless of clinical signs, patients with pancreatitis should be assumed to have abdominal pain and should be treated accordingly. There are many possible choices for antianalgesic therapy, including many opioids or lidocaine (see Chapter 2). Lidocaine can be added to the analgesic protocol by the intravenous or intraperitoneal route.

Antiemetics

The use of antiemetics used to be controversial. Metoclopramide was one of the most commonly used antiemetic agents. However, metoclopramide is a dopamine antagonist, and pancreatic blood flow is regulated via dopaminergic receptors. The advent of new antiemetics has dramatically changed the therapy of patients with pancreatitis. Dolasetron (Anzemet, given at 0.3 to 0.6 mg/kg once to twice daily IV, SQ, or PO) is a 5HT antagonist and a very potent antiemetic with few side effects. In many patients vomiting can be stopped altogether after therapy with dolasetron has been instituted. Another newer veterinary antiemetic, maropitant (Cerenia, Pfizer) given at 1 mg/kg once daily SQ), is a neurokinin 1(NK1) antagonist with broad spectrum action and appears to be very effective in the management of vomiting from pancreatitis.

Plasma Therapy

α_2-Macroglobulin, one of the scavenger proteins for activated proteases in plasma, is depleted rapidly in severe pancreatitis, with resultant uninhibited protease activity leading to acute disseminated intravascular coagulation, hypotensive shock, and death. Fresh frozen plasma not only replenishes α_2-macroglobulin but also supplies albumin and coagulation factors, which have several beneficial effects, including maintaining plasma oncotic pressure and preventing disseminated intravascular coagulation. Although there is no scientific evidence that plasma has beneficial effects in either human or canine patients with severe pancreatitis, I routinely give fresh frozen plasma (50 to 250 ml once a day) to patients with severe pancreatitis.

Antibiotic Therapy

There has been much debate about the use of antibiotics in humans with pancreatitis. Evidence is limited that humans with pancreatitis benefit from prophylactic antibiotic use, even though nearly 50% of all patients with fatal pancreatitis die of an infectious complication. Dogs with pancreatitis rarely have infectious complications; thus there is no evidence to support routine antibiotic therapy in canine patients with pancreatitis. Furthermore, inappropriate antibiotic therapy may increase the risk of antibiotic-resistant infections. If an infectious complication is suspected, efforts should be made to identify the causative organism before initiating treatment with an appropriate broad-spectrum antibiotic agent.

Other Treatment Strategies

Antiinflammatory Drugs

There is no evidence to support the use of corticosteroids or nonsteroidal antiinflammatory drugs in the treatment of canine pancreatitis. Treatment with corticosteroids should be reserved for use in cases of severe shock and should be used only for a short time in concert with other aggressive supportive measures.

Protease Inhibitors

Initial experimental data in dogs showed a benefit of protease inhibitors such as aprotinin in canine pancreatitis. However, clinical trials in humans led to disappointing results; and, given the new information concerning the pathogenesis of severe pancreatitis, this is not surprising. Once premature activation of pancreatic zymogens has occurred, a massive inflammatory response follows that is mediated by inflammatory cytokines. At that point further premature activation of pancreatic zymogens probably plays a very minor role in the progression of the disease; thus inhibition of pancreatic enzymes would not confer any medical benefit.

Antioxidants

Over the last two decades multiple studies have evaluated the use of antioxidants in humans with pancreatitis. Some noncontrolled studies found a benefit, whereas controlled studies did not identify any benefit of selenium or other antioxidants. Only one report is available about the use of antioxidants in dogs with pancreatitis. In this study the authors showed a significantly decreased mortality rate in dogs treated with standard care and selenium when compared to dogs treated with standard care alone. Unfortunately the control reference group consisted of historic control dogs, thus the results of this study leave many questions.

Miscellaneous Treatment Strategies

Many other treatment strategies have been evaluated in human or veterinary patients with pancreatitis. Antisecretory agents such as anticholinergics, calcitonin, or glucagon have all failed to show any beneficial effect in humans with pancreatitis and have not been evaluated systematically in dogs. Nasogastric suctioning and inhibition of gastric acid secretion also have not proved effective in human patients. Somatostatin has shown promise in reducing complications in humans with pancreatitis, but in some recent experimental studies in rats somatostatin administration led to deterioration of the experimental pancreatitis. Surgical management of pancreatitis has become uncommon in humans with pancreatitis. This is mainly because surgical management is not associated with improved outcome and many patients with acute pancreatitis are poor surgical risks.

TREATMENT OF MILD PANCREATITIS

Mild pancreatitis is associated with minimal pancreatic necrosis and few systemic effects and is usually followed by complete recovery. It is likely that many animals recover spontaneously without medical intervention after a few days of mild depression and inappetence. However, some animals present with repeated signs of vomiting, abdominal discomfort, and depression, with evidence of either recurrent acute or chronic pancreatitis. Such animals may ultimately develop diabetes mellitus or exocrine pancreatic insufficiency if enough pancreatic tissue has been destroyed. Unfortunately little is known about treatment of mild chronic pancreatitis and prevention of progression toward end-stage disease. As with acute pancreatitis, an effort should be made to identify the cause and rectify it if possible. Miniature schnauzers commonly exhibit hypertriglyceridemia. If serum triglyceride concentrations are increased, feeding a low-fat diet may help reduce triglyceride concentrations and improve clinical signs. Chronic abdominal pain is one of the most important problems in humans with chronic pancreatitis and may affect some canine patients as well. If pain is suspected, the animal can be given 0.5 to 2 tsp of dried pancreatic extract (Viokase; or Pancrezyme, Virbac) with each meal on a trial basis. Although these patients do not have exocrine pancreatic insufficiency and do not require enzyme replacement for digestive purposes, the feedback effect of digestive proteases within the gut lumen appears to reduce the drive on pancreatic secretion and perhaps reduce the pancreatitis-associated discomfort. Patients with chronic mild pancreatitis should also be evaluated for concurrent conditions such as inflammatory bowel disease, hepatitis, and diabetes mellitus.

Over the last decade the frequency of a diagnosis of autoimmune pancreatitis has increased dramatically in humans. Although autoimmune pancreatitis has not been diagnosed definitively in dogs, many dogs with chronic pancreatitis show a lymphocytic infiltration of the exocrine pancreas. Thus I have cautiously attempted treatment of mild chronic pancreatitis with glucocorticoids in cases that do not improve with a low-fat diet alone and do not have any concurrent diseases.

References and Suggested Reading

Heinrich S et al: Evidence-based treatment of acute pancreatitis. a look at established paradigms. *Ann Surg* 243:154, 2006.

Hess RS et al: Clinical, clinicopathologic, radiographic, and ultrasonographic abnormalities in dogs with fatal acute pancreatitis: 70 cases (1986-1995), *J Am Vet Med Assoc* 213:665, 1998.

Newman S et al: Localization of pancreatic inflammation and necrosis in dogs, *J Vet Int Med* 18:488, 2004.

Porterpan B, Zoran D, Steiner JM: Serial serum pancreatic lipase immunoreactivity concentrations in a dog with histologically confirmed pancreatitis, *Vet Med* 101:170, 2006.

Steiner JM: Diagnosis of pancreatitis, *Vet Clin North Am Small Anim Pract* 33:1181, 2003.

Steiner JM, Rutz GM, Williams DA: Serum lipase activities and pancreatic lipase immunoreactivity concentrations in dogs with exocrine pancreatic insufficiency, *Am J Vet Res* 67:84, 2006.

CHAPTER **125**

Feline Exocrine Pancreatic Disease

DAVID A. WILLIAMS, *Urbana, Illinois*

The incidence of exocrine pancreatic disorders has traditionally been considered to be low in the cat. However, a large retrospective study of necropsy findings showed 1.3% of 6504 feline pancreata to have pathologically significant lesions. In contrast, of 180,648 cats entered into the Veterinary Medical Data Base over a 10-year period, only 1027 (0.57%) were diagnosed with exocrine pancreatic disorders. Thus it appears that, although cats suffer from diseases of the exocrine pancreas quite frequently, these disorders often escape diagnosis.

PANCREATITIS

Classification

A simple classification system for pancreatitis has been established for human patients (Bradley, 1993), and, since no such system has been devised for veterinary medicine, the human classification system is applied when possible. Acute pancreatitis is an inflammatory condition of the pancreas, which is completely reversible after removal of the inciting cause. In contrast, chronic pancreatitis is characterized by irreversible histopathologic changes of exocrine pancreatic tissue, most notably fibrosis and atrophy. Both forms can be mild or severe. Mild forms of pancreatitis are associated with little or no pancreatic necrosis or systemic effects, and usually complete recovery is possible. In contrast, severe forms of pancreatitis are associated with extensive pancreatic necrosis and multiple organ involvement and often have a poor prognosis. Chronic forms of pancreatitis appear to be more common than the acute form in cats, whereas in dogs the diagnosis of chronic pancreatitis is uncommon.

Etiology and Pathogenesis

Extensive studies of experimental pancreatitis in cats and other species have led to the generally accepted hypothesis that pancreatic acinar cells ultimately respond in a common fashion to a variety of differing harmful stimuli. Briefly an initial decrease in secretion of pancreatic enzymes is followed by formation of abnormal cytoplasmic vacuoles in which the contents of lysosomes and zymogen granules colocalize. This leads to an inappropriate intracellular activation of trypsin and subsequently other digestive zymogens. These activated digestive enzymes lead to local effects, including inflammation, hemorrhage, acinar cell necrosis, and peripancreatic fat necrosis. Digestive enzymes released into the bloodstream may cause systemic effects, including systemic inflammatory changes, systemic vasodilation leading to hypotension, pulmonary edema, disseminated intravascular coagulation, central neurologic deficits, respiratory failure, renal failure, and even multiorgan failure.

Several diseases and risk factors have been associated with feline pancreatitis. Traumatic pancreatitis (caused by road traffic accidents or falling from heights) has been reported and probably develops secondary to pancreatic ischemia rather than from trauma per se. Infectious agents have been shown to cause feline pancreatitis, with the strongest evidence for a causal relationship for *Toxoplasma gondii* and rare cases of *Amphimerus pseudofelineus* fluke infestation. Weaker evidence has been presented for feline parvovirus infections in kittens, and infections with feline herpesvirus-1I and feline infectious peritonitis virus. Feline pancreatitis has been reported subsequent to topical use of fenthion, an organophosphate cholinesterase inhibitor. Many other pharmaceutic compounds have been implicated in causing pancreatitis in humans and dogs (including azathioprine, chlorothiazide, hydrochlorothiazide, estrogens, furosemide, tetracycline, sulfonamides, L-asparaginase, 6-mercaptopurine, methyldopa, pentamidine, nitrofurantoin, dideoxyinosine, valproic acid, and procainamide). However, no cases have yet been reported in the cat. Cholangitis and cholangiohepatitis may also coexist in feline patients with pancreatitis, but the significance of this relationship is unknown. Most cases of feline pancreatitis are idiopathic.

Clinical Picture and Diagnosis

Clinical signs of cats with pancreatitis are nonspecific. In one report of 40 cats with severe pancreatitis lethargy was reported in 100% of the cases, anorexia in 97%, dehydration in 92%, hypothermia in 68%, vomiting in 35%, abdominal pain in 25%, a palpable abdominal mass in 23%, dyspnea in 20%, ataxia in 15%, and diarrhea in 15% (Hill and Van Winkle, 1993). Especially remarkable is the low incidence of vomiting and abdominal pain, both of which are common clinical signs in human and canine patients with severe pancreatitis. Other clinical signs, such as polyphagia, constipation, fever, icterus, polyuria, polydipsia, and adipsia have also been reported. Concurrent conditions occur frequently, including hepatic lipidosis, inflammatory bowel disease, interstitial nephritis, diabetes mellitus, and cholangiohepatitis (Akol et al.,1993). Clinical signs in less severe cases are not documented, but many cases are associated with very vague signs such as poor body condition, and some cases can be subclinical.

Complete blood count and serum chemistry profile often show mild and nonspecific changes. Serum activities of lipase and amylase are within the reference ranges in most cases, and both tests are considered unreliable for the diagnosis of pancreatitis in the cat. Typical radiographic changes seen in some cases may include decreased contrast in the cranial abdomen with displacement of the duodenum laterally and dorsally, the stomach to the left, and the transverse colon caudally. Abdominal ultrasound is considered more useful in the diagnosis of feline pancreatitis than radiographs. Changes identified include pancreatic swelling, increased echogenicity of the pancreas, fluid accumulation around the pancreas, and less frequently a mass effect in the area of the pancreas. Abdominal computed tomography is reported to have low sensitivity (approx 33%) for detecting feline pancreatitis and is rarely used.

Immunoassay of serum feline trypsin-like immunoreactivity (fTLI) and more recently feline serum pancreatic lipase immunoreactivity (fPLI), currently only available through my former laboratory at Texas A&M University (the gastrointestinal laboratory), have both been evaluated as a diagnostic tool for feline pancreatitis. Available evidence found an increase in serum fTLI and fPLI in many cats with pancreatitis (Steiner and Williams, 1996). Subsequent studies in cats with experimental mild transient pancreatitis indicate that increases in serum fTLI, while often dramatic, are transient and return to normal within 2 to 3 days; whereas increases in serum fPLI in the same cats are far more prolonged, usually persisting for at least 7 to 10 days. Consequently fPLI appears to be a better clinical diagnostic test for acute and chronic pancreatitis in the cat, but large clinical studies are required to better support this observation.

A definitive diagnosis of feline pancreatitis may be made by examination of pancreatic biopsy samples obtained at exploratory laparotomy or laparoscopy. Several areas should be sampled because lesions often have a patchy distribution. Although pancreatic biopsy per se is safe, this intervention is obviously relatively expensive and may be contraindicated in some patients because of high anesthetic risk.

Therapy

Supportive Therapy
Whenever possible the inciting cause should be removed. Exposure to unnecessary drugs, especially those implicated in causing pancreatitis, should always be avoided. Aggressive fluid therapy is the mainstay of supportive therapy for acute pancreatitis and helps reverse and minimize pancreatic ischemia. Fluid, electrolyte, and acid-base imbalances need to be assessed and corrected as soon as possible. Plasma transfusions should be considered in any patients exhibiting severe clinical signs and in those with hypoalbuminemia.

Alimentation
The traditional recommendation for any patient with pancreatitis is to feed nothing by mouth for several days. This recommendation is justified in patients that vomit, but there is little evidence to substantiate this strategy in cats that will eat and do not vomit. This issue is complicated further by the fact that cats with pancreatitis may have concurrent hepatic lipidosis (Akol et al., 1993). Current clinical experience indicates that the benefit of nutritional support for cats with hepatic lipidosis overrides the conventional dogma that food should be withheld from patients with pancreatitis. Reassuringly, recent studies have failed to show any harmful effects resulting from feeding humans with pancreatitis. Theoretically the preferred route of alimentation is via a jejunostomy tube, but this is impractical in many cases; and both gastrostomy and nasogastric tubes appear to be well-tolerated alternatives, providing that the patient does not vomit. Cats do not seem to benefit from feeding of a specially formulated low-fat diet, and commercially available feline liquefied diets appear to be well tolerated despite their high fat contents. If there is no evidence to support concurrent hepatic lipidosis, cats should probably be held NPO for

3 to 4 days, especially if they are vomiting frequently. After this time oral water is slowly reintroduced, followed by trial feeding of small meals.

Analgesia

Even though abdominal pain is rarely appreciated in cats with pancreatitis, it is probably present frequently and may be a major contributing cause of anorexia. Routine analgesic administration is warranted in most patients with acute disease. Historical concerns that some analgesics such as morphine may exacerbate pancreatitis are now discounted, and any of the agents currently used in cats is suitable for use. Meperidine (Demerol HCl, Winthrop-Breon) at a dosage of 1 to 2 mg/kg every 2 to 4 hours can be given intramuscularly or subcutaneously. Butorphenol tartrate (Torbutrol or Torbugesic, Fort Dodge) at a dosage of 0.2 to 0.4 mg/kg every 6 hours subcutaneously can also be used, but there are also many other alternatives (see Chapter 2).

Plasma

Studies in dogs show that, when α_2-macroglobulin, one of the scavenger proteins for activated proteases in serum, is depleted, death ensues rapidly. Fresh frozen plasma (FFP) or fresh whole blood contains not only α_2-macroglobulin, but also albumin, which has many beneficial effects in patients with experimental pancreatitis. Clinical trials in humans have not shown enhanced survival, but, because of my experience and anecdotal reports of beneficial effects of FFP in canine patients with pancreatitis, I recommend the use of FFP or fresh whole blood in cats with severe acute pancreatitis.

Antibiotic Therapy

There is no evidence to recommend the routine use of antibiotic agents in cats with acute pancreatitis. Infectious complications of feline acute pancreatitis are very rare and are usually not the cause of death in fatal cases. Antibiotic therapy should be reserved for patients with known or suspected concurrent infectious diseases or complications such as infected catheters, and these patients should be treated aggressively after appropriate antibiotic sensitivity testing of the causative agent.

Cats having acute neutrophilic (suppurative) cholangitis, thought to be the result of an ascending bacterial infection of the biliary system, may also have a concurrent bacterial infection in the pancreatic duct system because of the direct communication of the common bile duct and pancreatic ducts in the cat. In these cases antibiotic therapy directed against enteric aerobes would be indicated.

Antiinflammatory Agents

There are no data on the use of antiinflammatory agents in cats with severe pancreatitis, and no benefit was found in humans. In cats having severe acute pancreatitis corticosteroids should only be used in cases of secondary cardiovascular shock. However, corticosteroids may be helpful when treating cats with chronic pancreatitis and concurrent inflammatory bowel disease or cholangitis. Corticosteroid therapy does not appear to have any adverse consequences, and improvement of clinical signs together with reductions in serum fTLI and fPLI are noted frequently.

Dopamine

Dopamine has been shown to have beneficial effects in experimental cases of feline acute pancreatitis when given in the first 12 hours after induction, but there was no beneficial effect when given after 12 hours. In addition, dopamine must be used carefully in patients with cardiac arrhythmias and may also cause nausea and vomiting. Therefore it cannot be recommended for routine use in feline patients with pancreatitis but may be of value in selected cases.

Other Therapeutic Strategies

Many other therapeutic strategies such as the administration of trypsin-inhibitors (e.g., Trasylol [recently taken off the market]), antacids, antisecretory agents (i.e., anticholinergics, calcitonin, glucagon, somatostatin), or selenium, as well as peritoneal lavage, have been evaluated in human and canine patients suffering from pancreatitis. None of these strategies has shown any beneficial effect at this point and therefore cannot be recommended until evidence for their usefulness is forthcoming.

It should also be remembered that many cats suffer from mild forms of chronic pancreatitis, which is almost certainly a distinct entity from severe acute pancreatitis. These cats often suffer from concurrent conditions, most notably inflammatory bowel disease, cholangitis, or both and, as mentioned previously, may benefit from corticosteroid therapy directed primarily to treat the intestinal or liver disease. In many of these cats the pancreatitis may be relatively or completely subclinical. Some cats with persistent elevations in pancreatic marker enzymes (fTLI and fPLI) often do not do as well as cats in which values decrease or become normal during therapy. This may reflect the persistence of clinically significant pancreatitis in these individuals, and unfortunately very little is known about appropriate therapy for these patients if corticosteroids are ineffective. Treatment should be directed at any concurrent conditions in the hope that the pancreatitis component is of minimal clinical significance, which in many patients appears to be the case, since they can do very well despite persistence of mild-to-severe increases in serum fTLI and fPLI.

Prognosis

The prognosis for cats suffering from severe acute pancreatitis depends on the severity of the disease, the extent of pancreatic necrosis, the occurrence of systemic and pancreatic complications, the duration of the condition, and the presence of concurrent disease. The prognosis for chronic pancreatitis is certainly better; in some cases the disease can be subclinical, and some cases respond positively to corticosteroid therapy given primarily to treat concurrent inflammatory bowel disease. In the long term some patients with chronic disease may develop diabetes mellitus and/or exocrine pancreatic insufficiency (EPI) if sufficient pancreatic tissue is irreversibly destroyed.

EXOCRINE PANCREATIC INSUFFICIENCY

EPI is a syndrome that is caused by insufficient synthesis and secretion of digestive enzymes by the exocrine portion of the pancreas, leading to insufficient activity of digestive enzymes in the lumen of the small intestine (Williams, 1994).

Etiology and Pathogenesis

As in humans, chronic pancreatitis is the most common cause of EPI in the cat, although pancreatic acinar atrophy resembling that seen in dogs also occurs. A rare cause is infestation with the fluke *Eurytrema procyonis*.

Almost all of the functional capacity of the exocrine portion of the pancreas must be lost before clinical signs develop. The lack of digestive enzymes in the duodenum leads to maldigestion, but secondary disturbances of intestinal mucosal transport mechanisms also contribute to nutrient malabsorption. These changes lead to variable diarrhea, weight loss, and malabsorption of selected nutrients, including cobalamin and some fat-soluble vitamins.

Clinical Picture and Diagnosis

Cats with EPI often present with a chronic history of polyphagia, diarrhea, and weight loss, each of which can vary markedly in severity. The hair coat can appear greasy, especially in the perineal and tail region, as a consequence of steatorrhea. The remainder of the hair coat can have an unkempt and wet appearance related to cobalamin deficiency. Results of a complete blood count, serum chemistry profile, and urinalysis are within the reference ranges in most cases; and there are no abnormalities on abdominal radiographic and ultrasonographic examination. The most reliable test for the diagnosis of EPI in the cat is radioimmunoassay of serum fTLI (Steiner, Medinger, and Williams, 1996), which reveals markedly subnormal values in affected cats (Steiner and Williams, 1996). Cats with EPI almost always have severely reduced serum cobalamin concentrations and less frequently folate concentrations. Therefore serum cobalamin and folate concentrations should be determined in all cats with suspected EPI.

Management

Pancreatic Enzyme Supplementation
Pancreatic enzyme supplementation using dried powdered extracts of porcine or bovine pancreas is the mainstay of therapy for cats with EPI. Initially ½ to 1 teaspoonful should be mixed into each meal immediately before feeding. It is rare for cats with EPI to refuse treated food; but, if this is a problem, the enzymes can be packed into gelatin capsules or raw pork or beef, or other pancreas can be given. Pancreas can be stored frozen for many months without losing activity, and 1 to 3 oz (30 to 90 g) of chopped raw pancreas is given per meal initially. Tablets, capsules, and enteric-coated products should be avoided. Preincubation of the food with pancreatic enzymes, supplementation with bile salts, or concurrent antacid therapy is unnecessary. Once clinical signs have resolved, the dose of pancreas extract can be decreased gradually until a minimal effective dose is determined. This dose differs among patients and may also change with different batches of the pancreatic supplement.

Dietary Considerations
There are no studies of the effect of differing diets on feline patients with EPI, and most cats do well on any high-quality commercial maintenance diet. Low-fat diets should be avoided because of their lower calorie density, as should diets containing unusually high amounts of fiber because some types of dietary fiber interfere with pancreatic enzyme activity. Unless an individual patient has a suboptimal response, routine feeding of a special diet is not necessary.

Vitamin Supplementation
Most cats with EPI are severely cobalamin deficient. Some of these cats do not respond well to enzyme supplementation until cobalamin is also supplemented. Initially 250 mcg of cobalamin (cyanocobalamin injection, Elkins-Sinn, Goldline, or others) are given subcutaneously once a week. The serum concentration of cobalamin should be rechecked immediately before the fifth or sixth injection. If serum cobalamin concentration has normalized, the dosing schedule can be changed to monthly maintenance injections. Although this prevents recurrence of deficiency, some owners report that their cats do better when receiving injections every 1 to 2 weeks. Supplementation is required for life; otherwise cobalamin deficiency will recur. Cats with subnormal serum folate should be treated with 200 mcg of folic acid daily added to the food for 1 month. The risk of recurrence of deficiency once folate supplementation is stopped is not known; thus serum folate should be retested at least annually. Deficiencies of fat soluble-vitamins are uncommon but have been reported and should be anticipated as potential complications. Vitamin K deficiency can lead to death from acute gastrointestinal hemorrhage, but patients at risk can be identified by evaluation of prothrombin and activated partial thromboplastin times, and deficiency is reversed by appropriate supplementation with vitamin K injections. Vitamin E deficiency may contribute to neurologic abnormalities and retinal atrophy and can be overcome by supplementation of the diet with 30 units of tocopherol daily.

Treatment of Concurrent Conditions
Some cats with EPI do not respond appropriately to enzyme and vitamin supplementation. Many of these cats have concurrent small intestinal disease (as often indicated by observation of subnormal serum folate concentration) and must be evaluated and treated appropriately for villous atrophy and inflammatory bowel disease. Finally some cats with EPI suffer from concurrent diabetes mellitus and must be managed accordingly.

Prognosis

EPI is associated with irreversible loss of pancreatic acinar tissue in most cases; therefore recovery is improbable. However, with appropriate management and monitoring these patients usually become clinically normal and should enjoy a normal life span.

EXOCRINE PANCREATIC NEOPLASIA

Pancreatic adenomas are benign tumors of the exocrine pancreas, whereas pancreatic adenocarcinoma is the most common malignant neoplastic condition of the exocrine pancreas in the cat (Andrews, 1987). Spindle cell sarcoma and lymphosarcoma have also been reported in feline patients.

Pathogenesis

Pancreatic adenomas are usually subclinical but, if large, may lead to clinical signs because of the transposition of other abdominal organs. Pancreatic adenocarcinomas can also lead to signs of EPI related to obstruction of the pancreatic duct and acinar atrophy or pancreatitis related to either tumor necrosis and/or local pancreatic ischemia. Metastatic disease may lead to clinical signs related to dysfunction of other organs.

Clinical Signs and Diagnosis

The presenting clinical signs of feline patients with exocrine pancreatic neoplasia are nonspecific. In a case series of 58 cases, clinical signs most commonly reported were anorexia, weight loss, lethargy, and vomiting (Andrews, 1987). Clinical signs reported in other cases are icterus, constipation, diarrhea, polyuria, fever, dehydration, and distended cranial abdomen. Finally, some reported clinical signs that are related to metastatic lesions, may include dyspnea, lameness, bone pain, or alopecia.

Results of routine blood tests are usually unremarkable. Serum lipase and amylase activities have been reported in few cases and have rarely been elevated. Radiographic findings are also nonspecific in most cases, but ultrasonographic examination of the abdomen is often very helpful, revealing a soft-tissue mass in the region of the pancreas. Even though most pancreatic adenocarcinomas exfoliate poorly into the peritoneal fluid, peritoneal effusion, if present, should be aspirated and evaluated cytologically. Tissue sampling by either fine-needle aspiration or transcutaneous biopsy under ultrasound guidance can be attempted when masses are identified, but in many cases definitive diagnosis is made at exploratory laparotomy or necropsy.

Therapy and Prognosis

Pancreatic adenomas are benign and theoretically do not need to be treated unless they are causing clinical signs. However, the final distinction between pancreatic adenoma and adenocarcinoma is often made at exploratory laparotomy, and a partial pancreatectomy should be performed at that time, even in cases of suspected pancreatic adenoma. The prognosis for pancreatic adenoma is excellent.

Pancreatic adenocarcinomas usually present at a late stage of the disease, and metastasis has been reported to occur in more than 80% of cats at the time of diagnosis. In the few cases when metastatic lesions are not identified at the time of diagnosis, surgical resection can be attempted. However, owners should be forewarned that clean surgical margins are rare. Total pancreatectomy and pancreaticoduodenectomy, although theoretically possible, have not been described in cats; and, given experiences in experimental animals and humans, both high morbidity and mortality are likely. Further the expense and complexity of lifelong management of concurrent postsurgical EPI and diabetes mellitus would make this option unacceptable for many owners. Chemotherapy and radiation therapy have shown little success in humans or veterinary patients with pancreatic adenocarcinomas. Overall the prognosis for cats with pancreatic adenocarcinoma is grave.

PANCREATIC BLADDER

A pancreatic bladder is an abnormal extension of the pancreatic duct, forming a sac. Only a few feline cases have been described in the literature. These cats presented with clinical signs compatible with biliary duct obstruction. Many cases are probably subclinical. Optimum management has not been described, but surgical reconstruction may be most suitable in cats presenting with clinical signs.

PANCREATIC PSEUDOCYST

Pancreatic pseudocyst, a collection of sterile pancreatic juice enclosed by fibrous or granulation tissue, is a recognized complication of pancreatitis in humans and has recently been reported in a cat (Hines et al.,1996). Clinical signs observed in the cat were similar to those in cats with pancreatitis. Abdominal ultrasound revealed a cystic structure in close proximity to the left lobe of the pancreas. Pancreatic pseudocysts in humans are treated by surgical correction when they enlarge or do not regress. Surgical intervention was also successful in the management of the cat reported.

PANCREATIC ABSCESS

A pancreatic abscess is a collection of pus with little or no pancreatic necrosis, most commonly in close proximity to the pancreas. Pancreatic abscess has been described as a complication of pancreatitis in humans and dogs but not in the cat. However, I am aware of one feline patient with pancreatic abscess confirmed by histopathology. Surgical intervention and aggressive antibiotic therapy are the treatments of choice in humans and dogs with pancreatic abscess and were successful in treating this cat.

PANCREATIC PARASITES

Eurytrema Procyonis

The pancreatic fluke of the cat, *Eurytrema procyonis*, has been found in pancreatic ducts of cats, foxes, and raccoons. The parasites can lead to ductular thickening and fibrosis of acinar tissue. A significant decrease of pancreatic secretions has been shown in some cases. However, clinical signs of EPI in cats with *E. procyonis* are rare. Diagnosis is made by identification of eggs in fresh feces. Fenbendazole (Panacur, Hoechst) at a dosage of 30 mg/kg orally once a day for 9 days has been recommended for therapy.

Amphimerus Pseudofelineus

The hepatic fluke of the cat, *Amphimerus pseudofelineus*, can also invade the pancreas and cause pancreatitis. Etiologic diagnosis is possible by identification of eggs on fecal examination by formalin-ethyl acetate sedimentation. In one clinical report treatment with praziquantel (Droncit, Miles), 40 mg/kg orally once daily for 3 consecutive days was successful.

References and Suggested Reading

Akol KG et al: Acute pancreatitis in cats with hepatic lipidosis, *J Vet Intern Med* 7:205, 1993.

Forman MA et al: Evaluation of feline pancreatic lipase immunoreactivity and helical computed tomography versus conventional testing for the diagnosis of feline pancreatitis, *J Vet Intern Med* 18(6): 807, 2004.

Hill RC, Van Winkle TJ: Acute necrotizing pancreatitis and acute suppurative pancreatitis in the cat: a retrospective study of 40 cases (1976-1989), *J Vet Intern Med* 7:25, 1993.

Hines BL et al: Pancreatic pseudocyst associated with chronic-active necrotizing pancreatitis in a cat, *J Am Anim Hosp Assoc* 32:147, 1996.

Steiner JM, Williams DA: Feline trypsin-like immunoreactivity in feline exocrine pancreatic disease, *Compend Contin Educ Pract Vet* 18:543, 1996.

Steiner JM, Medinger TL, Williams DA: Development and validation of a radioimmunoassay for feline trypsin-like immunoreactivity (fTLI), *Am J Vet Res* 1996.

Steiner JM, Wilson BG, Williams DA: Development and analytical validation of a radioimmunoassay for the measurement of feline pancreatic lipase immunoreactivity in serum, *Can J Vet Res* 68:309, 2004.

Williams DA: Feline exocrine pancreatic insufficiency. In Kirk RW, Bonagura JD, editor: *Current veterinary therapy XII*, Philadelphia, 1994, Saunders.

Williams DA: Exocrine pancreatic disease. In Strombeck DR, editors: *Small animal gastroenterology*, ed 3, Philadelphia, 1996, Saunders, p 381.

Zoran DL: Pancreatitis in cats: Diagnosis and management of a challenging disease, *J Am Anim Hosp Assoc* 42:1, 2006.

CHAPTER 126

Diagnostic Approach to Hepatobiliary Disease

CYNTHIA R.L. WEBSTER, Grafton, Massachusetts
JOHANNA C. COOPER, Plymouth, Massachusetts

Diagnosing primary hepatobiliary disease in small animals is often a challenge. The clinical signs of hepatobiliary disease generally reflect deficiencies in the varied functions of the liver. These diverse metabolic and biochemical activities include carbohydrate, lipid, and protein metabolism; fat digestion; detoxification of endogenous and exogenous substances; and immune surveillance. However, the clinical signs that develop with liver disease are seldom specific for that organ. Furthermore, the high blood flow of the liver, its dual blood supply (systemic and portal), and its role in detoxification render the liver sensitive to injury from both systemic disorders and diseases in organs drained by the portal circulation (Box 126-1). To complicate the situation, the tremendous hepatic reserve capacity almost assures that relatively specific signs of hepatobiliary dysfunction such as icterus, hypoglycemia, bleeding tendencies, hepatic encephalopathy (HE), and ascites occur only in late-stage disease. The purpose of this chapter is to provide a rational approach to the diagnosis of hepatobiliary disease in small animal patients.

The first step in the diagnosis of hepatobiliary disease is to obtain an accurate history. Pertinent information includes the use of potentially hepatotoxic drugs, supplements, or neutraceuticals; exposure to environmental toxins, infectious agents, or recent anesthetic events; and details on housing, supervision outdoors, and travel and vaccine status (leptospirosis, canine adenovirus). Recognition of an agent's hepatotoxic potential (Box 126-2) and prompt withdrawal can prevent further liver damage. Often a sequence of events may increase the suspicion for hepatobiliary disease. A history of inappetence and weight loss in a previously overconditioned feline is suggestive of hepatic lipidosis. Anesthetic intolerance, failure to thrive, and postprandial behavioral abnormalities in a predisposed canine breed should increase one's suspicion of a portosystemic vascular anomaly (PSVA) (Box 126-3). Primary hepatobiliary disease should always be considered in breeds predisposed to inflammatory/fibrotic hepatopathies (see Box 126-3).

Patients with hepatobiliary disease may exhibit nonspecific clinical signs referable to the gastrointestinal (intermittent anorexia, vomiting, diarrhea, and/or weight

Box **126-1**

Extrahepatic Disease Associated With Elevation in Serum Hepatobiliary Enzymes

- Gastrointestinal
  - Inflammatory bowel disease
  - Pancreatitis
- Vascular
  - Severe anemia
  - Congestive heart failure
  - Postcaval syndrome
- Cholestasis of Sepsis
- Systemic Infection
- Muscle Injury
- Endocrine
  - Hyperadrenocorticism
  - Adrenal hyperplasia syndromes
  - Diabetes mellitus
  - Hyperthyroidism
  - Hypothyroidism
- Paraneoplastic
- Bone Disorders

Box **126-2**

Agents Associated With Hepatotoxicity

Chemicals
- Arsenic
- Carbon tetrachloride
- Chlorinated hydrocarbon
- Dimethynitrosamine
- Heavy metals
- Pine oil
- Selenium
- Tannic acid

Food Additives
- Xylitol

Drugs
- Acetaminophen
- Amiodarone
- Asparaginase
- Carprofen
- Diazepam
- Griseofulvin
- Halothane
- Ketoconazole
- Lomustine
- Mebendazole
- Methotrexate
- Oxibendazole-DEC
- Phenobarbital
- Stanozolol
- Tetracyclines
- Thiacetarsemide
- Potentiated sulfonamides

Alternative Medicines
- Chaparral leaf
- Comfrey
- Germander
- Jin Bu Huan
- Kava
- Pennyroyal oil

Environmental Agents
- Aflatoxins
- Amanita mushroom
- Blue-green algae toxins
- Cycad seeds

loss), urinary (polyuria, polydipsia, stranguria, and dysuria), or central nervous systems (lethargy and depression). More specific signs of hepatobiliary disease include the diffuse cerebral signs that accompany HE (blindness, head pressing, stupor, coma, and ptyalism [cats]), jaundice, bleeding tendencies, or dermatologic abnormalities (superficial necrolytic dermatitis).

Physical examination in patients with primary hepatobiliary disease may reveal jaundice, hepatomegaly, a poor body condition score, abdominal pain, or a fluid wave. Additional findings may include abnormalities on fundic examination (iridocyclitis or chorioretinitis) from an infectious etiology or pyrexia from infectious or inflammatory disease.

LABORATORY EVALUATION OF HEPATOBILIARY DISEASE

Clinicopathologic evaluation helps to verify the presence of liver disease and determine the degree to which other organ systems are affected. The initial database should include a complete blood count (CBC), biochemical profile, and urinalysis.

The most consistent CBC abnormalities include changes in erythrocyte size and morphology, including microcytosis, target cells, poikilocytes, and Heinz body formation (cats). Microcytosis without anemia, most likely associated with impaired iron transport, occurs in dogs and cats with congenital PSVA and in dogs with acquired shunting secondary to portal hypertension. Target cells and poikilocytes result from alteration in the erythrocyte plasma membrane lipoprotein content, causing altered cell deformability. Anemia may accompany hepatic disease either from a bleeding gastric ulcer, a coagulopathy, or the anemia of chronic disease. Some dogs with hepatobiliary disease have a mild thrombocytopenia, reflecting a systemic infectious disorder or synthetic failure from decreased hepatic thrombopoietin production.

Alanine aminotransferase (ALT), aspartate aminotransferase (AST), alkaline phosphatase (ALP), and γ-glutamyl transferase (GGT) are serum enzymes used as screening tests for hepatobiliary disease. Increases occur as a result of: (1) leakage from damaged hepatobiliary cells (ALT, AST); (2) elution from damaged membranes (ALP, GGT); or (3) increased synthesis (ALP). Although elevations in these serum enzymes have a high sensitivity for the detection of hepatobiliary damage, increases also occur in the absence of clinically important primary hepatobiliary disease. There are several reasons for this discordance. First, increases in serum hepatobiliary enzymes can originate from nonhepatic tissues. Second, in the dog endogenous or exogenous corticosteroids and phenobarbital can

Box 126-3

Feline and Canine Breeds Predisposed to Hepatobiliary Disease

Congenital Portosystemic Vascular Anomalies
- Australian cattle dog
- Cairn terrier
- Dachshund
- Golden retriever
- Irish wolfhound
- Labrador retriever
- Maltese terrier
- Miniature schnauzer
- Yorkshire terrier
- Himalayan
- Persian

Hepatic Amyloidosis
- Chinese shar-pei
- Abyssinian
- Siamese

Copper-Associated Hepatopathy
- Bedlington terrier
- Dalmatian
- Skye terrier
- West Highland white terrier
- Siamese

Idiopathic Inflammatory
- American and English cocker spaniel
- Doberman pinscher
- Labrador retriever
- Standard poodle

induce the production of excess hepatobiliary enzymes in the absence of liver damage. Finally, the liver is uniquely susceptible to secondary injury from primary disease in other organs, particularly the pancreas and gastrointestinal tract (see Box 126-1).

Elevations in ALT and AST result secondary to leakage from damaged hepatocytes. ALT is a liver-specific cytosolic enzyme; however, increases may also occur with severe muscle necrosis in the dog. The half-life (T½) of ALT is 2.5 days in dogs. No published values are available for cats; however, the T½ is presumed to be much shorter (around 6 hours). The largest elevations in ALT occur with acute hepatocellular necrosis and inflammation. Mild-to-moderate elevations occur with primary hepatic neoplasia. AST, which is present in both the cytosol and mitochondria, is more sensitive but somewhat less specific for liver disease than ALT. Increases in AST typically parallel those of ALT but are of a smaller magnitude. AST elevations in excess of ALT indicate either a muscle source or the release of mitochondrial AST caused by severe irreversible hepatocellular injury. The T½ of AST is 22 hours in the dog and 77 minutes in the cat.

ALP is a membrane-bound enzyme (see Chapter 127). In dogs ALP has a high sensitivity (80%) but low specificity (51%) for hepatobiliary disease. Its low specificity is caused by the presence of several isoenzymes and its sensitivity to drug induction. In the dog three isoenzymes make up the total serum ALP (T-ALP), including a bone (B-ALP), liver (L-ALP), and corticosteroid (C-ALP) isoenzyme. B-ALP comprises one third of the T-ALP in dogs and is elevated in conditions with increased osteoblastic activity such as bone growth, osteomyelitis, osteosarcoma, and secondary renal hyperparathyroidism. L-ALP is present on the luminal surface of biliary epithelial cells and the hepatocyte canalicular membrane. L-ALP T½ is 70 hours in dogs and 6 hours in cats. Because of the cats' short T½ and the fact that feline hepatocytes contain less ALP, increases typically do not approach those seen

in canine patients. These characteristics and the fact that cats lack C-ALP make T-ALP less sensitive (50%) but more specific (93%) for liver disease than in the dog. The largest increases in L-ALP are associated with focal or diffuse cholestatic disorders and primary hepatic neoplasms. Less dramatic increases are found in chronic hepatitis, hepatic necrosis, and canine nodular hyperplasia. C-ALP is located on the hepatocyte canalicular membrane. C-ALP increases in dogs exposed to exogenous corticosteroids or in cases of spontaneous hyperadrenocorticism; however, increases are also associated with chronic illness, possibly secondary to increases in endogenous glucocorticoid secretion.

Hepatic GGT is located on the hepatocyte canalicular membrane. In dogs GGT has a lower sensitivity (50%) but higher specificity (87%) for hepatobiliary disease than T-ALP. If an elevated ALP is noted with a concurrent increase in serum GGT, specificity for liver disease increases to 94%. The most marked elevations in GGT result from diseases of the biliary epithelium such as bile duct obstruction, cholangiohepatitis, and cholecystitis. Moderate elevations accompany primary hepatic neoplasia, whereas mild elevations result from hepatic necrosis. In cats GGT has a higher sensitivity (86%) but lower specificity (67%) for hepatobiliary disease than T-ALP. Serum GGT may be considerably greater than ALP in some cats with cirrhosis, extrahepatic bile duct obstruction (EHBDO), or cholangitis. In feline idiopathic hepatic lipidosis GGT is typically only mildly elevated.

In dogs substantial increases in hepatobiliary enzymes can result secondary to corticosteroid and phenobarbital therapy. These increases may result from hepatobiliary enzyme induction and/or hepatocyte damage. Exogenous or endogenous excess of corticosteroids increases serum enzyme activity (L-ALP, C-ALP, ALT and GGT) secondary to induction. In general, the most marked increases occur in ALP and GGT, with lesser elevations in ALT. Typically induction of AST is minimal. Cessation of corticosteroid therapy in the absence of liver damage results in a gradual normalization of enzyme values over a period of 2 to 3 months. As corticosteroids induce morphologic vacuolar change in hepatocytes and have resulted in focal areas of hepatic necrosis in experimental studies, hepatocyte damage may be the cause of some of the increased enzyme activity.

Idiosyncratic hepatotoxic reactions to phenobarbital may occur in dogs, leading to chronic inflammatory disease or the hepatocutaneous syndrome. In both of these disorders moderate-to-marked increases in ALP, moderate increases in ALT, and mild increases in AST are typically seen. Phenobarbital therapy in the dog has been reported to induce the production of hepatobiliary enzymes (primarily ALP). Prospective studies to assess the relative role of induction versus damage in dogs on phenobarbital therapy have resulted in conflicting results. In one study there was no increase in ALT and ALP enzyme activity in whole-liver homogenates from phenobarbital-treated dogs, suggesting that induction was not occurring (Gaskill et al., 2005). However, another study found increased T-ALP activity in the liver of phenobarbital-treated dogs, supportive of induction (Unakami et al., 1987). Overall the available literature suggests that mild-to-moderate increases in ALP (up to five times the upper limit of normal) and ALT (usually less than two times the upper limit of normal) may reflect enzyme induction. However, increases in GGT and AST are seldom caused by induction and may be suggestive of primary liver disease.

The magnitude of serum hepatobiliary enzyme elevation is usually proportional to the severity of active hepatobiliary damage; however, the degree of elevation is not predictive of hepatobiliary functional capacity. Marked increases in these enzymes may indicate substantial hepatobiliary injury but are not necessarily indicative of a poor prognosis because of the tremendous regenerative capacity of the liver. Alternatively normal or only mildly increased serum hepatobiliary enzymes may be seen in end-stage chronic liver disease because of replacement of hepatocytes by fibrosis and/or prolonged enzyme leakage, resulting in depletion of hepatic stores. Thus a single determination of serum hepatobiliary enzyme values has little prognostic significance. Prognostic value increases with sequential evaluation in conjunction with liver function testing and biopsy.

Assessment of liver function requires evaluation of parameters that reflect the synthetic and excretory capacity of the liver. Several hepatic function tests are included on routine biochemical testing, including bilirubin, glucose, cholesterol, blood urea nitrogen (BUN), and albumin. Although these tests are not particularly sensitive or specific, they are easily obtained and may help build a case for primary hepatobiliary disease. Hyperbilirubinemia, the most sensitive and specific of these parameters, in the face of a normal hematocrit is caused by hepatic disease resulting in inadequate uptake, conjugation and/or excretion of bilirubin, posthepatic disease interfering with biliary excretion of bilirubin, or the cholestasis of sepsis. In cholestasis of sepsis cytokines released during sepsis inhibit the expression of hepatocyte transporters necessary for bilirubin transport. Cholestasis of sepsis may occur in the presence or absence of hepatobiliary damage and appears to be common in the septic cat.

Hypoglycemia occurs only when 75% of hepatic mass is nonfunctional as a result of decreased gluconeogenesis and clearance of insulin. Hypoglycemia also occurs periodically in dogs with congenital PSVA, possibly secondary to impaired glucose production, reduced glycogen stores, decreased responsiveness to glucagon, or a combination of these factors. Serum cholesterol levels in hepatobiliary disease are variable; cholestatic disease is frequently associated with hypercholesterolemia, whereas hypocholesterolemia is seen most often in end-stage liver disease. The BUN may be low in dogs with chronic liver disease or PSVA since the hepatic conversion of ammonia to urea decreases with decreasing hepatic mass or shunting of blood past the liver. Since the liver is responsible for the synthesis of albumin, hypoalbuminemia may accompany chronic hepatic disease. Synthetic failure occurs only when 70% of hepatic functional mass has been lost. However, serum hypoalbuminemia may also occur with protein-losing nephropathies or enteropathies, vasculitis, blood loss, or from third spacing in ascitic patients.

Urinalysis in cases of hepatobiliary disease may reveal bilirubinuria or ammonium biurate crystals. Since the canine renal threshold for bilirubin is low and dogsare capable of tubular secretion of bilirubin, bilirubinuria may be present in the absence of bilirubinemia.

However, cats have a high threshold for bilirubin and are not bilirubinuric unless also bilirubinemic. Freshly collected urine samples may reveal ammonia biurate crystalluria in dogs and cats with PSVA.

Ancillary Diagnostic Tests

Hepatobiliary disease may result in ascites formation secondary to portal hypertension. Portal hypertension occurs as a result of obstruction at the level of the right atrium/cranial vena cava, hepatic parenchyma, or portal vein. Portal hypertension from the latter two causes typically results in a low-protein ascites, whereas posthepatic portal hypertension is associated with a high-protein ascites. Generally ascitic fluid caused by hepatic disease is a pure transudate but with chronicity may have characteristics of a modified transudate. An effusion bilirubin value in excess of serum bilirubin is consistent with bile duct/gallbladder rupture. Ascites is rare even in cats with end-stage liver disease.

Other ancillary clinicopathologic tests that may be indicated include serology for infectious disease (leptospirosis, ehrlichiosis, Rocky Mountain spotted fever, toxoplasmosis, neosporosis, dirofilariasis, systemic mycosis), autoantibody testing (Coombs' or antinuclear antibody) and a coagulation profile (prothrombin time [PT], partial thromboplastin time [PTT], fibrinogen levels, and fibrinogen degradation products). Coagulation test abnormalities are quite common in dogs and cats with hepatobiliary disease, although spontaneous bleeding is rare. These abnormalities may be caused by hepatic synthetic failure, vitamin K deficiency, or the presence of a consumptive coagulopathy.

In cases in which secondary hepatobiliary disease is suspected, assessment for pancreatitis (serum lipase levels/pancreatic lipase immunoreactivity) and evaluation for an underlying endocrinopathy (hypothyroidism, hyperthyroidism, hyperadrenocorticism, and adrenal hyperplasia syndromes) or gastrointestinal disease (inflammatory bowel disease) may be pursued (see Box 126-1).

Hepatobiliary Function Tests

When a minimum database suggests the presence of hepatobiliary disease, the next step generally includes specific liver function tests and abdominal imaging. In many cases a definitive diagnosis requires hepatic biopsy.

Total serum bile acids (TSBAs) are common hepatic function tests. Bile acids are synthesized from cholesterol exclusively in the liver. Once conjugated to either glycine or taurine, they are secreted into the bile and subsequently stored and concentrated within the gallbladder. After a meal cholecystokinin (CCK) release initiates gallbladder contraction; and bile acids are transported to the intestine, where they aid in the emulsification and digestion of fats. At the terminal ileum bile acids are resorbed and returned to the liver via the blood (enterohepatic circulation), where they are reextracted by hepatocytes. Normally enterohepatic circulation of bile acids occurs with 95% to 98% efficiency. Disruption of this enterohepatic circulation results in increases in TSBAs and occurs in the presence of acquired or congenital PSVA or cholestatic hepatobiliary disease. An endogenous challenge to assess the enterohepatic circulation of bile acids is used clinically by determining TSBAs after a 12-hour fast (preprandial) and then 2 hours after a test meal (postprandial).

TSBAs have a high specificity for hepatobiliary disease. In dogs the specificity of fasting and postprandial TSBAs for hepatobiliary disease is 95% and 100% when cutoff values greater then 15 µmol/L and 25 µmol/L are used, respectively. In cats, using similar cutoff values, fasting and postprandial TSBAs have a specificity of 96% and 100%, respectively. The sensitivity of TSBAs for hepatobiliary disease (ranging from 54% to 74%) is not high enough to support the routine use of TSBAs as screening tests for hepatobiliary disease. The two exceptions are congenital PSVA in dogs and cats and cirrhosis in dogs in which the sensitivity of postprandial TSBAs at the above cutoff value is 100%.

A number of factors can influence the interpretation of TSBA testing. Higher fasting than postprandial values may result secondary to interdigestive gallbladder contraction or as a result of variations in gastric emptying, intestinal transit, or response to CCK release. Inaccurate postprandial values may occur because of failure of CCK release or gallbladder contraction if the test meal is inadequate in fat or amino acid content or if an insufficient amount is consumed. In addition, 2 hours may not represent the optimal time for postprandial sample collection in some animals. Finally severe ileal disease or resection can decrease the bile acid resorption, thereby decreasing postprandial TSBAs.

Interpretation of abnormal TSBAs must occur with an understanding of the test limitations. TSBAs cannot be used to discriminate one hepatobiliary disease from another or to predict the severity of the histologic lesion or degree of portosystemic shunting. When monitoring disease progression or response to therapy using sequential TSBAs, only a return to normal can be used to indicate clinical remission.

Urinary bile acids have been evaluated as a diagnostic test for hepatobiliary disease. The urinary excretion of water-soluble bile acids reflects the TSBA concentration during the period of urine formation such that persistently elevated TSBAs result in elevated urine bile acid levels. Normalized urine nonsulfated bile acids (UNSBAs): urine creatinine and combined normalized urine sulfated (USBAs) and UNSBAs: urine creatinine had a higher specificity (100% vs 67%) but lower sensitivity (62% vs 78%) than TSBAs for the diagnosis of hepatobiliary disease in dogs (Balkman et al., 2003). In the cat these urinary values were equivalent to TSBAs with respect to sensitivity (87%) and specificity (88%) for hepatobiliary disease (Trainor et al., 2003). However, in both species urine bile acids appear to have a lower sensitivity for the detection of PSVA then postprandial TSBAs.

The liver detoxifies ammonia, primarily from the gastrointestinal tract, to urea. Elevations in blood ammonia concentrations result secondary to: (1) portosystemic shunting, (2) greater than 70% reduction in liver parenchyma, and (3) inborn errors of metabolism in the urea cycle. Transient hyperammonemia has been reported in young Irish wolfhounds and with deficiencies of cobalamin and arginine in the dog and cat, respectively. Elevated fasting blood ammonia levels (>46 µmol/L) have been shown to be a sensitive (98%) and specific (89%) test for the detection of congenital or acquired PSVA in dogs (Gerritzen-Bruning, van den Ingh, and Rothuizen, 2006). Currently ammonia is the only toxin that can be measured clinically for the diagnosis of HE. The diagnostic use of blood ammonia is limited by the need for meticulous sample handling, including avoidance of hemolysis, use of cold heparinized tubes, transfer on ice, and refrigerated centrifugation and assay, all ideally within an hour of collection.

DIAGNOSTIC IMAGING IN THE EVALUATION OF HEPATOBILIARY DISEASE

The size, shape, position, opacity, and margins of the liver can be assessed on standard radiographs of the cranial abdomen. Hepatomegaly is associated with congestion (right-sided heart failure), vacuolar hepatopathy (glycogen, lipid, amyloid), infiltrative disease (neoplasia), extramedullary hematopoiesis, and inflammatory liver disease. Microhepatica may be seen with PSVA or chronic hepatitis/cirrhosis (dogs). Increased opacity may be noted secondary to mineralization within the biliary system (49% of choleliths) or hepatic parenchyma (granulomas, long-term hematomas, abscesses, neoplasia, chronic hepatopathies, or regenerative nodules). Gas may be within the biliary tree (emphysematous cholecystitis, cholangitis), portal vessels (severe necrotizing gastroenteritis), or hepatic parenchyma (hepatic abscesses).

Ultrasonography enables differentiation among focal, multifocal and diffuse disease; evaluation of the biliary system and portal vasculature; and procurement of tissue for hepatic histopathology. Focal hepatic diseases include cysts, hematomas, abscesses, granulomas, regenerative nodules, primary and metastatic neoplasms, infarcts, and biliary pseudocysts. Diffuse hyperechoic parenchyma may be noted because of fatty change (hepatic lipidosis), vacuolar hepatopathy, or cirrhosis. Diffuse hypoechoic parenchyma may be noted in cases of hepatic congestion and suppurative hepatitis. Evaluation of the biliary tree and gallbladder may reveal a gallbladder mucocele, choleliths, and intrahepatic or extrahepatic bile duct dilation. A normal ultrasound scan does not preclude a diagnosis of hepatobiliary disease.

In many cases of PSVA ultrasonography permits direct visualization of the shunting vessel. Ultrasonography is more sensitive for the detection of intrahepatic shunts (100%) than extrahepatic shunts (80% to 98%). The sensitivity of ultrasound for the diagnosis of PSVA is enhanced by duplex-Doppler or color-flow Doppler, although this requires a cooperative patient and operator patience for accurate interpretation. Reduced or reversed portal flow is seen with multiple acquired shunts secondary to portal hypertension. When combined, findings of a small liver, enlarged kidneys, and uroliths had a positive predictive value of a 100% for a congenital PSVA in dogs. Portal vein/aorta and portal vein/caudal vena cava values of greater or equal to 0.8 and 0.75, respectively, consistently ruled out an extrahepatic PSVA (d'Anjou et al., 2004).

Ultrasonography is currently the best imaging modality to evaluate for EHBDO. Ultrasonographic signs of EHBDO include dilation of the cystic duct, common bile duct

(>3 mm in dogs and >4 mm in cats), or intrahepatic bile ducts and identification of an intraluminal or extraluminal mass obstructing the biliary tract. The degree of gallbladder distention appears to be variable and thus should not be used as a sole criterion to diagnose EHBDO, particularly in cats.

Scintigraphy may be a useful adjunct in cases of suspected EHBDO or PSVA. In scintigraphic imaging of the biliary tract, an intravenous technetium 99m (^{99m}Tc)-iminodiacetic acid derivative is taken up by hepatocytes and subsequently undergoes biliary excretion. Using a cutoff of 180 minutes for the dye to enter the small intestine, the sensitivity of scintigraphy to identify complete EHBDO is high (83% to 100%), but the specificity is lower because partial bile duct obstruction may also slow dye excretion. Sensitivity remains similar, whereas specificity is markedly increased when the cutoff time is increased to 24 hours after injection. High serum bilirubin concentration did not reduce the diagnostic usefulness of scintigraphy.

Transcolonic pertechnate scintigraphy (TCPS) is used for the detection of PSVA. In TCPS ^{99m}Tc pertechnetate is administered rectally and is subsequently absorbed into the portal venous system. In normal animals radioisotope activity is detected in the liver before its detection in the heart. In animals with PSVA the radioisotope activity is detected in the heart before the liver. In dogs TCPS has a high positive predictive value for the diagnosis of PSVA and discriminates dogs with macroscopic PSVA from those with primary hypoplasia of the portal vein since TCPS is abnormal only in the former.

Transplenic portal scintigraphy (TSPS) can also be used to diagnose PSVA. Ultrasound-guided TSPS results in higher radioisotope count densities, more consistent splenic and portal venograms, and a significant decrease in radiation exposure when compared to TCPS. TSPS misses cases of PSVA when the shunt originates distal to the splenic vein.

The value of magnetic resonance imaging (MRI) and helical computed tomography in the diagnosis of hepatobiliary disease is currently under evaluation. MRI has shown promise in the differentiation of benign from malignant focal hepatic lesions in canine patients. Magnetic resonance angiography and helical computed tomography angiography have been used in dogs for the diagnosis of PSVA and offer the added advantage of accurate anatomic characterization of the shunt. The diagnostic use of these modalities is currently limited by both availability and cost.

HEPATIC BIOPSY ACQUISITION AND INTERPRETATION

Indications for hepatic biopsy include persistent serial increases in liver enzymes, abnormal hepatic function tests, hepatomegaly of undetermined cause, ultrasonographic abnormalities in hepatic parenchyma, and evaluation for the presence of a breed-specific hepatopathy. Hepatic biopsy can be obtained by ultrasound guidance (Tru-cut biopsy) or exploratory or laparoscopy (wedge biopsy). The advantages of the latter two methods are the ability to grossly evaluate the liver, acquire large tissue samples, and quickly identify and control postbiopsy hemorrhage. When wedge biopsy is used as the gold standard, discordance between wedge and Tru-cut biopsies may be as high as 48% (Cole et al., 2002). However, the true gold standard for any study evaluating the accuracy of hepatic biopsies is histopathologic assessment of the whole liver at necropsy. Thus any hepatic biopsy, no matter how it is obtained, must be interpreted in light of sampling error.

Prebiopsy considerations should include the patient's overall clinical status and the risk of hemorrhage. Acquisition of hepatic tissue is contraindicated in the presence of a hemodynamically unstable patient, coagulopathy, and encephalopathy. A PT, PTT, and platelet count should be performed. Tru-cut biopsy should be avoided with elevations in PT and PTT of greater than 1.5 times normal and a platelet count of less than 80,000. A buccal mucosal bleeding time may improve the sensitivity of detecting bleeding deficiencies in cases of mild thrombocytopenia. Vitamin K is routinely administered 24 hours before hepatic biopsy. Fresh frozen plasma may be considered before biopsy in cases in which mild elevations in PT and PTT are noted.

The method of biopsy acquisition is influenced by the size of the liver, the suspected diagnosis, and the clinical condition of the patient. Microhepatica and large-volume abdominal effusion are contraindications for percutaneous ultrasound-guided biopsy. In some conditions, such as primary hypoplasia of the portal vein and nodular hyperplasia, a wedge biopsy is often necessary to obtain a definitive diagnosis. In cases of diffuse vacuolar hepatopathy, inflammatory disease, or neoplasia, a diagnosis can be obtained with a percutaneous ultrasound-guided Tru-cut biopsy (a 16-gauge needle in dogs and an 18-gauge needle in cats). Multiple biopsy samples (three to five) should be taken from different areas of the liver.

In general hepatic biopsy is preferred over fine-needle aspiration (FNA) to characterize liver disorders. When compared to hepatic biopsy, discordance rates with FNA may be as high as 70%. However, in animals with bleeding disorders or large cavitary lesions or abscesses, ultrasound-guided FNA can be performed safely. In focal or diffuse hepatic disease (vacuolar or neoplastic) FNA may yield diagnostic samples. Occasionally FNA may identify an infectious agent that can be easily missed on histopathology. However, FNA cannot reliably diagnose necroinflammatory or vascular disease. Percutaneous cholecystocentesis has been shown to be a safe technique by which to obtain bile for cytology and culture.

It is important that the clinician understand the benefits and limitations of hepatic histopathology. The purposes of obtaining hepatic tissue are to: (1) determine the category of disease (inflammatory, neoplastic, vascular, or vacuolar); (2) define the extent of the disease; (3) assess the duration of illness, and (4) provide tissue for special stains and culture to aid in the diagnosis of metabolic and infectious causes. Although histopathology may result in a definitive diagnosis in the case of metabolic disease (hepatic lipidosis) and neoplasia, more often certain reaction patterns are described, which then provide clues as to the underlying etiology. Correct interpretation of the biopsy results requires dialogue with the pathologist and reevaluation of the patient's history and clinical picture.

Since a liver biopsy specimen represents only a small portion of the entire liver and frequently even diffuse disorders have an uneven distribution, the clinician should always be critical of whether the histopathologic diagnosis fits with the clinical picture.

References and Suggested Reading

Balkman CE et al: Evaluation of urine sulfated tand nonsulfated bile acids as a diagnostic test for liver disease in dogs, *J Am Vet Med Assoc* 222:1368, 2003.

Cole TL et al: Diagnostic comparison of needle and wedge biopsy specimens of the liver in dogs and cats, *J Am Vet Med Assoc* 220:1483, 2002.

d'Anjou MA et al: Ultrasonographic diagnosis of portosystemic shunting in dogs and cats, *Vet Radiol Ultrasound* 45:424, 2004.

Gaskill CL et al: Liver histopathology and liver and serum alanine aminotransferase and alkaline phosphatase activities in epileptic dogs receiving phenobarbital, *Vet Pathol* 42:147, 2005.

Gerritzen-Bruning MJ, van den Ingh TSGAM, Rothuizen J: Diagnostic value of fasting plasma ammonia and bile acid concentrations in the identification of portosystemic shunting in dogs, *J Vet Intern Med* 20:13, 2006.

Head LL, Daniel GB: Correlation between hepatobiliary scintigraphy and surgery or postmortem examination findings in dogs and cats with extrahepatic biliary obstruction, partial obstruction, or patency of the biliary system: 18 cases (1995–2004), *J Am Vet Med Assoc* 227:1618, 2005.

Trainor D et al: Urine sulfated and nonsulfated bile acids as a diagnostic test for liver disease in cats, *J Vet Intern Med* 17:145, 2003.

Unakami S et al: Molecular nature of three liver alkaline phosphatases detected by drug administration in vivo: differences between soluble and membranous enzymes, *Comp Biochem Physiol B* 88:111, 1987.

CHAPTER **127**

Evaluation of Elevated Serum Alkaline Phosphatase in the Dog

ANTHONY T. GARY, *Little Rock, Arkansas*
DAVID C. TWEDT, *Fort Collins, Colorado*

Increased serum alkaline phosphatase (ALP) is a common laboratory finding in canine patients. In one survey of consecutive blood samples submitted to a reference laboratory, 39% of all dogs and 51% of dogs older than 8 years of age had increased ALP levels (Comazzi et al., 2004). The high sensitivity (86%) of increased ALP for detection of liver disease is complicated by the poor specificity (49%) because numerous diseases outside of the liver, as well as drugs and glucocorticoids, may induce production of the enzyme. Often the evaluation of canine patients with increased ALP becomes a diagnostic dilemma.

PATHOPHYSIOLOGY

ALP is a heterogeneous group of enzymes with poorly defined biologic functions that catalyze the hydrolysis of phosphate from various organic compounds at an alkaline pH. Normally bound to cellular membranes, ALP has been isolated from the kidney, liver, bone, placenta, and intestine. Two genes encode for ALP: tissue nonspecific (TNS) and intestinal. The products of these genes are two isoenzyme proteins with different polypeptide sequences but similar enzymatic function. Products of the TNS gene include the isoforms of ALP that are found in the kidney, liver, bone, and placenta; and each differ only in degree of glycosylation. The intestinal gene encodes for the ALP found in the intestine (I-ALP), as well as corticosteroid ALP (C-ALP), a unique enzyme found only in the dog. Although several different isoenzymes/isoforms of ALP have been identified, only three are measured in serum because of their longer half-lives (approximately 70 hours): liver (L-ALP), bone (B-ALP), and C-ALP. The half-life of I-ALP, kidney, and placenta ALP are minutes.

Total serum ALP is the sum of L-ALP, B-ALP, and C-ALP. The proportion of each isoenzyme changes with age in normal dogs. B-ALP predominates in dogs less than 1 year of age, making up 96% of the total ALP; this proportion declines with age to approximately 25% in dogs older than 8 years of age. C-ALP comprises 10% to 30% of ALP in normal dogs, with higher proportions present in older dogs and smaller proportions in younger dogs. L-ALP is the predominant isoenzyme in dogs older than 1 year of age.

Liver Alkaline Phosphatase

L-ALP is located predominantly in the periportal zone of the liver associated with hepatocyte membranes that comprise the bile canaliculi and the sinusoidal membranes. Two mechanisms are responsible for increasing serum activity of this enzyme: cholestasis and drug induction. Induction is the increased synthesis of a protein or enzyme through modification of transcription, translation, or other processes involved in protein synthesis. Cholestasis leads to accumulation of bile salts from impaired bile flow and induces the production of L-ALP. The enzymes then accumulate on hepatocyte membranes, and solubilization of the membrane-bound enzyme occurs by the activity of glycosylphosphatidylinositol (GPI) phospholipase, an enzyme found in the plasma and on cellular membranes. Bile salts have been shown to play an important facilitory role by increasing activity of GPI phospholipase and thus releasing L-ALP into circulation.

For L-ALP induction also occurs secondary to various drugs, most notably phenobarbital and endogenous or exogenous glucocorticoids. The underlying pathophysiologic mechanisms are poorly understood. Elevated L-ALP, B-ALP, and C-ALP were found in one study after phenobarbital administration, a finding most consistent with induction because all isoenzymes were affected (Gaskill et al., 2004). However, total L-ALP was not different between treated and untreated dogs in a separate study, an unexpected finding if induction was the primary mechanism (Gaskill et al., 2005). It is also possible that increased serum levels may be secondary to increased activity of GPI phospholipase and subsequent release of ALP in serum or by direct liver injury, causing cholestasis. Glucocorticoids have been shown to increase serum C-ALP and L-ALP through induction by increasing levels of messenger ribonucleic acid (mRNA) within 24 to 48 hours of exposure.

Corticosteroid Alkaline Phosphatase

C-ALP is a product of the I-ALP gene that only differs from I-ALP in carbohydrate composition. I-ALP is devoid of carbohydrates, whereas C-ALP is heavily glycosylated with sialic acid and is thought to be responsible for the different half-lives of the two enzymes. The hepatocyte is the site of de novo synthesis of C-ALP after exposure to both endogenous and exogenous glucocorticoids (Wiedmeyer et al., 2002). Expression of the I-ALP gene in the liver is delayed after exposure to steroids, as shown by increased mRNA expression and elevated L-ALP and serum C-ALP approximately 10 days after initiation of prednisone in experimental dogs. C-ALP accumulates on hepatocyte membranes in the area that comprises the bile canaliculi and sinusoidal surfaces, and elevated serum levels occur through solubilization of C-ALP by activity of GPI phospholipase.

Total ALP can be further quantified by determining the percent of C-ALP isoenzyme in the serum using electrophoresis, selective inhibition (levamisole treatment), or a heat inactivation process in the laboratory. Measuring the isoenzymes of ALP is widely available in most diagnostic laboratories but often of little clinical use. For example, the high sensitivity (95%) of elevated C-ALP for detection of hyperadrenocorticism (HAC) is complicated by the poor specificity (18%). Elevations in C-ALP are often present with diabetes mellitus (DM), primary liver disease, or other chronic illness possibly because of stress and increases in endogenous cortisol. Although finding increased C-ALP cannot confirm the presence of HAC, it is generally accepted that low values of C-ALP decrease the likelihood of this disease. Progesterones are also thought to bind to the corticosteroid receptor on the hepatocyte and induce C-ALP production, and phenobarbital has been shown to induce production of the C-ALP isoenzyme through unknown mechanisms.

Bone Alkaline Phosphatase

B-ALP is attached to the external cellular membrane of osteoblasts. The function of the enzyme is unknown, but it likely plays a role in bone formation. Increased serum levels generally are associated with increased osteoblastic activity that occurs with bone growth in young animals, fracture healing, osteosarcoma, and less commonly nutritional osteopathies and renal secondary hyperparathyroidism. Elevations are typically mild (<4× normal) with osteosarcoma; however, they have been correlated to poor survival and are found only in tumors with increased osteoblastic activity (i.e., osteoblastic osteosarcoma). Benign familial hyperphosphatasemia has been reported in Siberian huskies and results from increases in B-ALP.

DIAGNOSTIC EVALUATION

History and Physical Examination

Evaluation of the patient with elevated ALP begins with a thorough history and physical examination (Fig. 127-1). The signalment may provide insight as to the underlying cause of ALP elevation. For instance, mild elevations in ALP (<2× normal) are often present in young growing animals because of increased B-ALP. The calcium and phosphorous are also often mildly increased in these dogs, and all three are expected findings in young dogs. Postsuckling puppies also have increases in ALP, possibly as a result of colostral ALP or induction of ALP after ingestion of colostrum. Values typically return to normal within 10 days.

Because elevated ALP may occur as a result of enzyme induction, a careful drug history should be obtained. Commonly identified drugs include glucocorticoids and phenobarbital. It is important to note that, in addition to oral steroids, topical and ocular forms may also be associated with increased ALP. Specific questioning is usually needed to ensure that other forms of steroids are not being given because topical therapy is often not considered a medication by owners and is frequently not disclosed without direct questioning. Exposure to phenobarbital or other anticonvulsants is often easily determined, but other drugs also have been associated with elevated liver enzymes and liver toxicity and are discussed elsewhere (see also Chapter 126). Various holistic herbal and nutritional supplements may also induce the production of ALP or cause liver damage. Discontinuation of the

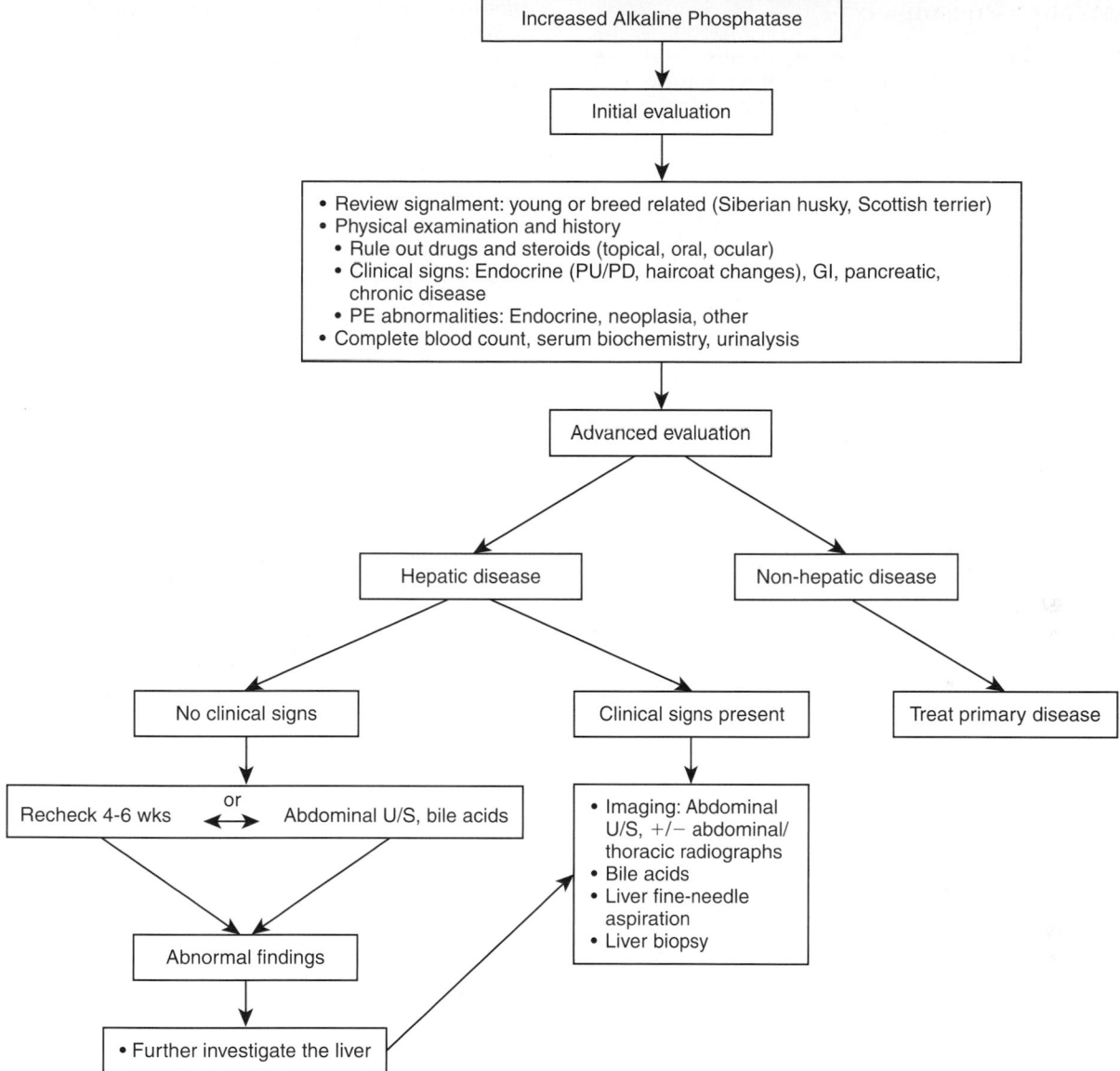

Fig. 127-1 Algorithm for evaluation of alanine phosphatase.

substance and subsequent resolution of ALP elevation over the following weeks is consistent with drug-induced abnormalities.

Endocrine diseases, including HAC, DM, and hypothyroidism, are frequently associated with elevations in ALP. The diagnosis is based on clinical findings and supportive laboratory testing. HAC is often suspected based on elevations in ALP that occur secondary to increased cortisol, as well as intrahepatic cholestasis caused by hepatocyte swelling from glycogen accumulation; this finding is present in 90% to 95% of dogs with HAC. The ALP concentrations are usually dramatically increased with HAC, whereas DM usually results in mild-to-moderate elevations in ALP (2 to 5× normal) and concurrent changes in ALT from intrahepatic cholestasis secondary to hepatocellular swelling from the metabolic derangements of the disease (hepatic lipidosis). Higher elevations in ALP may be seen from DM alone, but concurrent diseases also should be considered if this is the case (i.e.,

pancreatitis, neoplasia, primary liver disease, or HAC). Similarly ALP is occasionally increased in hypothyroid dogs, but this finding is inconsistent. Abnormal concentrations of progestins (progesterone or 17-hydroxyprogesterone) are also thought to cause increases in serum ALP in some dogs.

Preliminary Evaluation
When an elevation in serum ALP is identified, routine blood work, including complete blood count, a comprehensive serum biochemistry, and urinalysis, should be performed. Primary hepatic disease, secondary reactive hepatopathies, and induction caused by drugs are the most likely causes. Common causes are listed in Box 127-1. Nonhepatic disease is a common cause of ALP elevations, resulting from secondary reactive changes (reactive hepatopathies) occurring in the liver. Potential causes include enteritis, pancreatitis, or systemic inflammatory or infectious diseases. Histologic evidence of disease as indicated by

Box 127-1

Differentials for increased Alkaline Phosphatase

- Cholestasis
- Intrahepatic cholestasis
  - Nodular hyperplasia
  - Neoplasia (primary, metastatic)
  - Chronic hepatitis/cirrhosis
  - Vacuolar hepatopathy
  - Miscellaneous
    - Infectious/inflammatory
    - Toxic
- Extrahepatic cholestasis
  - Pancreatitis
  - Biliary disease
    - Mucocele
    - Cholangitis/cholangiohepatitis
  - Neoplasia (biliary, duodenum, pancreas)
  - Cholelithiasis
- Secondary/reactive
  - Chronic disease
    - Neoplasia, infection/inflammation, pancreatitis
  - Gastrointestinal disease
  - Endocrine (hypothyroid, diabetes mellitus, hypoadrenocorticism)
- Induction
  - Drugs (phenobarbital, other)
- C-ALP
  - Hyperadrenocorticism
  - Exogenous corticosteroids
- B-ALP
  - Young animals
  - Bone neoplasia
  - Nutritional osteopathy
  - Hyperparathyroidism
- Breed-related
  - Siberian huskies
  - Scottish terriers

B-ALP, Bone alkaline phosphatase; *C-ALP,* corticosteroid alkaline phosphatase.

a variety of nonspecific reactive changes (e.g., hydropic change and periportal inflammation) is often present. Typically ALP values are threefold to fourfold above normal. Elevations in C-ALP also can result from chronic illness and endogenous glucocorticoid release. Both conditions generally cause only mild ALP elevations.

The highest values of ALP are generally seen with focal or diffuse cholestatic disease, glucocorticoid exposure, chronic hepatitis, and hepatic neoplasia. Concurrent elevations in other liver parameters (alanine aminotransferase [ALT], alanine aspartate aminotransferase [AST], γ-glutamyltransferase [GGT], and total bilirubin) are often helpful in distinguishing a cholestatic disease process from hepatocellular injury. With cholestasis, elevations in ALP, GGT, and bilirubin are expected. Elevations in the leakage enzymes ALT and AST are often present but should be of smaller magnitude when compared to cholestatic enzymes. Liver enzyme elevations primarily caused by ALT or AST are most consistent with diseases causing hepatocellular injury (i.e., chronic hepatitis).

Advanced Evaluation

Symptomatic patients. For symptomatic patients further evaluation of increased ALP is often required if elevations cannot be explained by nonhepatic diseases, drugs, or endocrine disorders. In these cases primary hepatic or biliary disease is likely, and imaging is essential to further characterize the etiology.

Although abdominal radiographs are useful for determining liver size and the presence of other abdominal abnormalities, they lack specificity with regard to hepatobiliary disease. Thoracic radiographs are obtained routinely to screen for metastatic neoplasia or other concurrent disease, especially in older patients, before more invasive diagnostics directed toward the liver.

Ultrasound is required to more fully characterize abnormalities of the biliary system and hepatic parenchyma. However, one major limitation is the variability in sonographer experience and thus the quality of the imaging procedure. Ultrasound of the hepatic parenchyma may identify masses or nodules, whereas changes in the echogenicity of the liver may suggest the presence of diffuse or focal hepatic disease. The absence of ultrasonographic abnormalities does not rule out liver disease. For example, diffuse hepatic lymphoma can be associated with hyperechoic, hypoechoic, and isoechoic hepatic parenchyma on ultrasound. In addition, dogs with benign nodular hyperplasia may have either normal or abnormal ultrasonographic changes. Lesions of the biliary system often consist of dilation of the hepatic and common bile ducts, as well as gallbladder distention, wall thickening, calculi, and sludging. Mass lesions affecting the biliary system are also commonly identified.

Specific lesions in the liver should be sampled with fine-needle aspiration (FNA) or biopsy. Often FNA is performed initially if solitary masses or diffuse hepatic changes are observed because the technique is safe and requires minimal or no sedation. In addition, FNA is often adequate to diagnose neoplasia and is used if diffuse parenchymal disease is suspected. FNA cytology results consistent with neoplasia are generally trusted, but false-positive results are possible; other findings should be interpreted with caution because FNA and histopathology may have a poor correlation based on the disease involved. Lipidosis and vacuolar hepatopathies are examples of diffuse diseases in which FNA and histology generally correlate well; however, vacuolar hepatopathy may be seen with any number of diseases, including HAC, steroid exposure, and chronic illness (Sepesy et al., 2006). Wedge or laparoscopic liver biopsy is pursued if FNA results are questionable or a histologic diagnosis is required. In addition to biopsy, collection of bile for culture, Gram staining, and cytology is recommended in dogs with evidence of biliary disease.

Preprandial and postprandial bile acids are obtained routinely to further assess liver function if diagnostic evaluation has failed to reveal the underlying cause of ALP elevation. Abnormal bile acids generally are seen with decreased liver function, acquired or congenital portosystemic shunting, and cholestasis. If results are abnormal, a liver biopsy is warranted because there is strong evidence to support the presence of primary liver disease. However, normal bile acids do not rule out significant hepatobiliary disease; thus biopsy is also warranted in patients with or without clinical signs that have persistent or increasing ALP values that are unexplained for longer than 4 to 6 weeks.

Asymptomatic patients. Increased ALP is often found incidentally on preanesthetic or annual blood work. Initial evaluation in these patients should proceed as described previously by ruling out exposure to drugs or supplements and assessing for the possibility of nonhepatic disease, including endocrine, gastrointestinal, and neoplastic disorders. History and physical examination should be repeated to ensure that clinical abnormalities are truly absent.

Options for further evaluation include (1) monitoring ALP over time, and (2) pursuing additional diagnostics. For most cases it is appropriate to monitor ALP over 4 to 6 weeks. If progressive or persistent increases occur, further workup is indicated as described previously for symptomatic patients. Alternatively abdominal ultrasound and bile acid measurements are pursued initially to rule out obvious structural and functional abnormalities of the liver and biliary system because we have seen several cases of hepatic neoplasia in asymptomatic patients with ALP as the only clinical abnormality. The decision for additional monitoring or immediate evaluation may also be based somewhat on the degree of ALP elevation. Moderate-to-severe increases are more often associated with hepatobiliary disease or exposure to glucocorticoids and are unlikely to resolve over time.

Common hepatic causes of ALP elevation in asymptomatic patients include neoplasia, benign nodular hyperplasia, chronic hepatitis, idiopathic vacuolar hepatopathy, and breed-related conditions. Benign nodular hyperplasia, idiopathic vacuolar hepatopathy, and breed-related conditions often have ALP increases only, with little or no other liver enzyme involvement (Box 127-2). Idiopathic vacuolar hepatopathy is associated with vacuolated hepatocytes containing glycogen. In some of these cases abnormal adrenal production of progesterone or 17-hydroxyprogesterone is thought to be the cause. Adrenal steroids can be measured in conjunction with adrenocorticotropic hormone stimulation using specific diagnostic laboratories. Some also refer to this condition as atypical Cushing's disease because liver biopsy changes are identical to those of a steroid hepatopathy. These patients often do not progress, and therapy is controversial; however, some report that melatonin or typical HAC therapy resolves hepatic changes and the elevations in C-ALP.

A common finding in Scottish terriers is ALP elevation, often without other concurrent laboratory abnormalities.

Box 127-2

Common Conditions Resulting in Only Serum ALP Elevations

- Hyperadrenocorticism
- Idiopathic vacuolar hepatopathy
- Hepatic neoplasia
- Nodular hyperplasia
- Drug induction
- Breed-related

In a recent study Scottish terriers have been shown to have a higher incidence of increased ALP (Nestor et al., 2006). An additional report describes seven Scottish terriers evaluated for increased ALP with no identifiable cause after thorough imaging, adrenocortical testing, and liver biopsy, suggesting that a benign familial hyperphosphatasemia may be present (Gallagher et al., 2006). A study that we performed found the ALP to be predominately C-ALP but failed to reveal an association between elevated endogenous steroid hormone precursors (i.e., 17-hydroxyprogesterone) and elevations in ALP in affected Scottish terriers. In fact, similar abnormalities in 17-hydroxyprogesterone and progesterone were present in terriers with high ALP and those with normal ALP. Currently the underlying cause for elevations in ALP in Scottish terriers is unknown; however, the condition appears to be benign.

References and Suggested Reading

Comazzi SC et al: Haematological and biochemical abnormalities in canine blood: frequency and associations in 1022 samples, *J Small Anim Pract* 45(7):343, 2004.

Gallagher AE et al: Hyperphosphatasemia in Scottish terriers: 7 cases, *J Vet Intern Med* 20(2):418, 2006.

Gaskill CL et al: Serum alkaline phosphatase isoenzyme profiles in phenobarbital-treated epileptic dogs, *Vet Clin Pathol* 33(4):215, 2004.

Gaskill CL et al: Liver histopathology and liver and serum alanine aminotransferase and alkaline phosphatase activities in epileptic dogs receiving phenobarbital, *Vet Pathol* 42(2):147, 2005.

Nestor DD et al: Serum alkaline phosphatase activity in Scottish terriers versus dogs of other breeds, *J Am Vet Med Assoc* 228(2):222, 2006.

Sepesy LM et al: Vacuolar hepatopathy in dogs: 336 cases (1993–2005), *J Am Vet Med Assoc* 229(2):246, 2006.

Wiedmeyer CE et al: Kinetics of mRNA expression of alkaline phosphatase isoenzymes in hepatic tissues from glucocorticoid-treated dogs, *Am J Vet Res* 63(8):1089, 2002.

CHAPTER 128

Hepatic Support Therapy

BENTE FLATLAND, *Knoxville, Tennessee*

Supportive treatment of patients with hepatic disease addresses general pathophysiologic mechanisms common to many hepatic diseases. Although some treatments (e.g., antioxidants) apply to both acute and chronic disorders, supportive treatments are commonly discussed in the context of chronic inflammatory and neoplastic hepatic diseases. Some supportive treatments (e.g., antifibrotics) are by their very nature more applicable to chronic disease. Since most of these treatments are administered orally, their use in both acute and chronic cases may be limited by a patient's ability to take oral medication.

Ideally treatment of hepatic disease should be aimed at a specific underlying etiology. Given the enormous regenerative capacity of the liver, timely identification and elimination of any underlying cause offer the best hope for disease resolution in both acute and chronic cases. Evidence from human medicine suggests that fibrosis and even cirrhosis may be reversible in some cases when a specific etiology can be addressed (Rocky, 2005). In cases in which an underlying cause can be identified and eliminated, supportive care of hepatic disease may be finite. In chronic inflammatory disease, especially when the etiology is not known, or in advanced neoplastic disease when the etiology cannot be eliminated, supportive treatments are recommended indefinitely.

Our understanding of the causes of chronic inflammatory hepatobiliary disease is extremely limited, a fact that hampers research by limiting our ability to stratify patients and interpret results according to etiology. Lack of standardized supplement preparations with which to undertake clinical trials can also be a limiting factor in research. Recommendations for standardized clinical and histologic approaches to canine and feline hepatobiliary disease were recently published by the World Small Animal Veterinary Association Liver Standardization Group and, if widely adopted, should facilitate future research (Rothuizen J et al, 2006). Most recommendations for supportive care of small animal hepatic diseases, regardless of the etiology, are extrapolated from human medicine or are based on anecdotal experience and individual case reports rather than on evidence from prospective, randomized, placebo-controlled clinical trials involving large numbers of patients. The treatment recommendations in this chapter should be accepted with these limitations in mind.

Treatment of hepatic disease incorporates the following general principles:

- Address the underlying cause, if known (e.g., withdrawal of an hepatotoxic drug).
- Reduce and prevent inflammation.
- Reduce and prevent copper accumulation, if applicable.
- Reduce and prevent oxidative damage.
- Reduce and prevent fibrosis.
- Provide adequate nutrition.
- Treat complications as needed (e.g., hepatic encephalopathy, coagulopathy, gastric ulceration, fluid/electrolyte disturbances, ascites, and infection/endotoxemia)

This chapter reviews antioxidant and antifibrotic treatments commonly used for supportive care of hepatic disease and discusses treatment of hepatic disease–associated coagulopathy and ascites. For information concerning treatment of specific hepatic diseases, antiinflammatory treatments, treatment of copper accumulation, treatment of gastric ulceration, and management of hepatic encephalopathy, the reader is referred to the other chapters in this section.

ANTIOXIDANTS

It is well established that oxidative stress plays a role in the pathogenesis of liver disease in both humans and animals. Cats with hepatic lipidosis and both dogs and cats with obstructive biliary and inflammatory hepatic disorders exhibit reduced glutathione concentrations. This likely predisposes them to oxidative hepatic injury, given the ability of glutathione to detoxify reactive oxygen species. Accordingly, use of antioxidants and compounds that replenish hepatic glutathione stores seems warranted in the supportive treatment of canine and feline hepatobiliary disease (Center, Warner, and Erb, 2002). In addition to the substances discussed in the following paragraphs, zinc and ursodeoxycholate are proposed to benefit liver disease patients through antioxidant effects, although these are more often used for their copper-reducing and choleretic properties, respectively. Vitamin C (L-ascorbic acid) has also been recommended for its antioxidant and free-radical scavenging properties, but its use is less common than other antioxidants and therefore is not discussed.

Vitamin E

Vitamin E refers collectively to the antioxidant compounds known as tocopherols and tocotrienols. α-Tocopherol is the most biologically active form of vitamin E. The D stereoisomer is abundant in nature, where it is synthesized by plants. Synthetic vitamin E contains both D and L stereoisomers of α-tocopherol (Matthai, 1996). Food sources of vitamin E include vegetable oils, nuts, seeds, and grains. Because the various vitamin E isomers have differing biologic activities, preparations of vitamin E are standardized to international units (IU). One IU is equivalent to the activity of 1 mg of synthetically prepared dl-α-tocopherol. Vitamin E is fat soluble and requires bile and pancreatic juice for maximal intestinal absorption. High dosages of vitamin E may interfere with absorption of other fat-soluble vitamins and may predispose to development of vitamin K–dependent coagulopathy. Vitamin E supplementation traditionally has been thought harmless; however, a recent metaanalysis of vitamin E use in humans with various diseases revealed that supplementation at dosages above 150 units/day was associated with increased all-cause mortality. This finding led to recommendations against vitamin E supplementation, particularly at dosages above 400 units/day (Miller et al., 2005).

In veterinary hepatology vitamin E is a commonly used antioxidant. Dosage recommendations for dogs have been reported in conference proceedings and vary from 10 units/kg every 24 hours orally to 250 or 400 units/dog every 24 hours orally. I have used the 10-unit/kg every-24-hour oral dose most commonly. Dosing small patients can be problematic since commonly available vitamin E preparations contain 400 or 1000 units. Controlled clinical trials evaluating efficacy and safety of vitamin E supplementation in canine and feline liver disease patients are unavailable. I do not recommend vitamin E supplementation in liver disease patients with evidence of vitamin K deficiency. In such cases *S*-adenosylmethionine (SAMe) or milk thistle is a preferred antioxidant.

Milk Thistle (Silymarin)

The term *silymarin* refers collectively to the four flavonolignan isomers (silybin, isosilybin, silydianin, silychristine) that comprise the active ingredients of the herb milk thistle (*Silybum marianum*). Silybin is the most biologically active isomer and comprises 50% to 70% of silymarin. These flavonolignans are found throughout the milk thistle plant but are concentrated in its fruit and seeds. Commercially available preparations of silymarin vary in content and bioavailability, a fact that makes dosage recommendations difficult and hampers use of silymarin in carefully designed, prospective clinical trials. Accordingly in 2005 the National Center for Complementary and Alternative Medicine (NCCAM) issued a request for industry collaboration to develop a well-characterized, standardized formulation of silymarin that could be used in human liver disease clinical trials. If such a standardized formulation is developed, it has the potential to benefit veterinary medicine also.

The primary effect of silymarin is thought to be as an antioxidant and free-radical scavenger, but it is also proposed to have antifibrotic, antiinflammatory, and immunomodulatory actions. In humans silymarin is used primarily to treat alcoholic liver disease, viral hepatitis, and toxin-induced liver disease. Randomized controlled clinical trials using silymarin in specific human liver diseases have yet to be published.

In experimental animal models silymarin has been shown to ameliorate hepatic injury secondary to acetaminophen, carbon tetrachloride, radiation, iron overload, alcohol, cold ischemia, and the death cap mushroom (*Amanita phalloides*). Indeed, silymarin is so effective at reducing *A. phalloides* toxicosis by preventing hepatocyte uptake of mushroom toxins in both humans and dogs that an intravenous formulation has been developed specifically for the purpose of treating mushroom poisoning in humans (Seeff, 2001). In veterinary medicine, clinical trials evaluating efficacy of silymarin in dogs and cats with naturally occurring hepatic disease have not been published. Dosage recommendations reported in conference proceedings vary, but 20 to 50 mg/kg every 24 hours orally (dogs and cats) is commonly recommended. A veterinary product is now available containing silybin bound to phosphatidylcholine for improved gastrointestinal absorption (Marin, Nutramax Laboratories, Inc., 5 to 10 mg/kg every 24 hours orally).

S-Adenosylmethionine

SAMe is present in almost all bodily tissues and fluids and is a nucleotide-like molecule synthesized from the amino acid methionine and adenosine triphosphate. Of particular importance in the liver, SAMe plays a crucial role in transmethylation, transsulfuration, and aminopropylation pathways. These metabolic pathways are responsible for metabolism of various endogenous and xenobiotic compounds, generation of endogenous sulfur compounds, and production of molecules important in cell signaling and gene transcription, respectively (Center et al., 2005). Among sulfur compounds generated by the transsulfuration pathways is glutathione, an important component of the endogenous antioxidant system of the liver (Center, Warner, and Erb, 2002).

A commercial veterinary form of SAMe is available (Denosyl, Nutramax Laboratories, Inc.) and has been investigated. Oral administration of SAMe has been shown to significantly increase plasma SAMe concentrations in dogs and cats, with a peak effect occurring 1 to 4 hours after the dose in fasted animals. SAMe administration in dogs and cats increases hepatic glutathione concentrations and improves markers of red blood cell and hepatocyte redox status, justifying its use as a supportive treatment in canine and feline hepatobiliary disease (Center et al., 2005).

A recommended dosage of SAMe in dogs and cats is 20 mg/kg every 24 hours orally. Administering SAMe to fasted animals is recommended to maximize its absorption. Although numerous preparations of SAMe are available through health food stores and other sources, these may have varying bioavailability. Use of the commercially available veterinary preparations in dogs and cats is recommended for consistency.

SAMe has been shown to ameliorate oxidative stress induced by corticosteroid administration in dogs, although it does not prohibit corticosteroid-induced hepatic vacuolar change (Center et al., 2005). Clinical trials evaluating the role and efficacy of SAMe in specific canine and feline liver disorders are lacking and represent the next step in our understanding of the role of SAMe in the management of canine and feline hepatobiliary disease. The availability of a veterinary formulation of SAMe with proven bioavailability in dogs and cats will continue to facilitate research involving this compound.

ANTIFIBROTICS

Hepatic fibrogenesis is an active area of research in human medicine, and potential therapeutic targets continue to be revealed as mechanisms of fibrogenesis are elucidated. Current understanding of hepatic fibrogenesis emphasizes the importance of hepatic stellate cells (also known as Ito cells, lipocytes, or perisinusoidal cells) in the development and maintenance of fibrosis. Future antifibrotic treatments may include compounds that interfere with hepatic stellate cell activation and/or function (Rocky, 2005).

Colchicine

Colchicine is a plant alkaloid derived from *Colchicum autumnale* (autumn crocus, meadow saffron) and has been a mainstay of antifibrotic treatment in both human and veterinary medicine. Colchicine is purported to inhibit fibrosis by binding selectively and reversibly to microtubules, inhibiting their polymerization and thus collagen secretion. Aggregate data from numerous studies of various human liver diseases reveal that colchicine generally is safe and may improve biochemical markers of, and even mortality from, hepatic disease. However, the drug does not appear to decrease fibrosis in humans, making its recommendation as an antifibrotic drug problematic. Use of colchicine has been recommended for treatment of canine hepatic diseases with fibrosis based on a few individual case reports, but critical evaluation of its efficacy in a large number of dogs has not been published. The recommended dosage for colchicine in dogs is 0.014 to 0.03 mg/kg every 24 hours orally (Honeckman, 2003). Overdosage can be fatal, as demonstrated by a case report of accidental colchicine poisoning in a dog ingesting an unknown quantity of colchicine but calculated to be between 0.5 and 3.6 mg/kg (Wagenaar, 2004). To my knowledge colchicine has not been used for treatment of feline hepatic disease, and no cat dosage is present in the veterinary literature.

Other Antifibrotics

Other substances with proposed antifibrotic effects include interferon-γ, milk thistle, penicillamine, prednisone, ursodeoxycholic acid, and zinc. None of these compounds have been critically evaluated for their ability to inhibit fibrosis in dogs and cats with liver disease, and there is no evidence to support their use specifically for that purpose at this time. Nevertheless milk thistle, penicillamine, prednisone, ursodeoxycholic acid, and zinc are already used in veterinary hepatology for other reasons (e.g., copper reduction in the case of penicillamine); thus any potential antifibrotic effect would be a coincidental benefit. For further information concerning the use of penicillamine, ursodeoxycholate, and zinc, the reader is referred to Chapters 129 and 130 in this section.

TREATMENT OF HEPATIC DISEASE–ASSOCIATED COAGULOPATHY

Although coagulopathy is a common complication of hepatic disease, spontaneous bleeding in hepatic disease patients is uncommon. Bleeding is usually induced by a hemostatic challenge such as venipuncture, surgical procedures, or gastric ulceration. In hepatic disease mechanisms of coagulopathy include decreased synthesis of vitamin K–dependent coagulation factors (factors II, VII, IX, and X) and development of disseminated intravascular coagulation (DIC). Patients in which DIC is identified should be treated as needed with fresh frozen plasma and heparin.

Mechanisms of reduced vitamin K–dependent coagulation factor synthesis in hepatic disease include lack of dietary vitamin K intake, poor vitamin K absorption caused by cholestasis, altered bacterial flora associated with antibiotic usage, and/or hepatic dysfunction–associated impairment of the vitamin K epoxide cycle. Vitamin K–dependent coagulation abnormalities may be identified and should be monitored using prothrombin time (PT) or proteins induced by vitamin K absence or antagonism (PIVKA). Evaluation of clotting times should be performed routinely before hepatic biopsy. Parenteral vitamin K_1 (phytonadione) at a dosage of 0.5 to 2 mg/kg every 12 hours subcutaneously for two to three dosages (or until normalization of PT or PIVKA concentrations) is recommended for dogs and cats with hepatic disease (smaller patients should receive the lower end of this dosage range) (Honeckman, 2003). In affected patients vitamin K supplementation is recommended for 24 to 36 hours before invasive procedures such as hepatic biopsy or feeding tube placement.

TREATMENT OF HEPATIC DISEASE–ASSOCIATED ASCITES

Ascites caused by hepatic disease is most often caused by a combination of portal hypertension and low colloid osmotic pressure resulting from hypoalbuminemia. Patients having complete portal vein obstruction (e.g., from thrombosis) develop very high portal pressure and may develop ascites from this mechanism alone. Cats rarely develop ascites secondary to hepatic disease. Accumulation of ascites and the associated relative or absolute reductions in circulating blood volume activate the rennin-angiotensin-aldosterone system, causing sodium and water retention and potassium loss.

Apart from resolving the underlying mechanism, the mainstay of supportive care for ascites is the cautious use of diuretics. The goal of diuretic therapy is not complete elimination of ascites but rather to keep the patient comfortable. Furosemide, a loop diuretic, causes renal potassium loss; and high dosages of this drug should be avoided in liver disease patients. Spironolactone, an aldosterone receptor antagonist, spares potassium loss and is the preferred diuretic, although it is relatively weak in terms of diuretic effect. The dosage of spironolactone is 1 to 4 mg/kg every 12 hours orally (dogs) or 1 to 2 mg/kg every 12 to 24 hours orally (cats). Starting at the low end of the dosage range is recommended, and the dose may be titrated upward at weekly intervals if no affect is achieved. If the recommended dosage of spironolactone does not control ascites adequately, it may be used in combination with furosemide 1 to 2 mg/kg every 12 to 24 hours orally. Potential side effects of spironolactone and furosemide are dehydration and electrolyte imbalances. Skin lesions have been reported in cats receiving spironolactone chronically.

Other considerations when treating hepatic disease patients with ascites include addressing the underlying cause of hepatic disease if possible, feeding a sodium-restricted diet, and maintaining adequate hydration and a normal serum potassium concentration. Abdominocentesis should be considered only for diagnostic purposes and to relieve tense ascites that is causing discomfort and/or impaired respiration. Removing large volumes of ascitic fluid is discouraged since this may promote dehydration and exacerbate hypoproteinemia.

References and Suggested Reading

Center SA, Warner KL, Erb HN: Liver glutathione concentrations in dogs and cat with naturally occurring liver disease, *Am J Vet Res* 63:1187, 2002.

Center SA et al: Evaluation of the influence of S-adenosylmethionine on systemic and hepatic effects of prednisolone in dogs, *Am J Vet Res* 66:330, 2005.

Honeckman A: Current concepts in the treatment of canine chronic hepatitis, *Clin Tech Small Anim Pract* 18:239, 2003.

Matthai J: Vitamin E updated, *Indian J Pediatr* 63:242, 1996.

Miller ER et al: Meta-analysis: high-dosage vitamin E supplementation may increase all-cause mortality, *Ann Intern Med* 142:37, 2005.

Rocky DC: Antifibrotic therapy in chronic liver disease, *Clin Gastroenterol Hepatol* 3:95, 2005.

Rothuizen J, et al: editors. WSAVA standards for clinical and histological diagnosis of canine and feline liver diseases, Edinburgh, Saunders/Elsevier, 2006.

Rothuizen J: General principles in the treatment of liver disease. In Ettinger SJ, Feldman EC, editors: *Textbook of veterinary internal medicine*, ed 6, St Louis, 2005, Elsevier, p 1435.

Seeff LB et al.: Complementary and alternative medicine in chronic liver disease, *Hepatology* 34:595, 2001.

Wagenaar Z: Accidental colchicine poisoning in a dog, *Can Vet J* 45:55, 2004.

Webster CRL: History, clinical signs, and physical findings in hepatobiliary disease. In Ettinger SJ, Feldman EC, editors: *Textbook of veterinary internal medicine*, ed 6, St. Louis, 2005, Elsevier, p 1422.

CHAPTER **129**

Copper-Associated Chronic Hepatitis

GABY HOFFMANN, *Utrecht, The Netherlands*

JAN ROTHUIZEN, *Utrecht, The Netherlands*

Hepatic copper accumulation can result from increased uptake of copper, a primary defect in hepatic copper metabolism, or altered biliary excretion of copper. Copper toxicity depends on the molecular association and subcellular localization of the molecule, as well as the total concentration of copper in liver tissue. In inherited copper storage disorders copper accumulation is always localized centrolobularly (e.g., Bedlington terrier copper toxicosis, Wilson's disease in humans, liver disease in Long-Evans Cinnamon rats). In secondary copper loading of liver cells during cholestasis, copper is mainly restricted to the periportal parenchyma.

COPPER METABOLISM

Forty to 60% of the ingested copper is absorbed from the upper small intestine. Copper transporter 1 (CTR1) is responsible for hepatocellular uptake of copper. In the liver cell copper is immediately bound to the transport proteins COX17, ATOX1 and CCS, which deliver copper to their target destination in the cell. These targets include superoxide dismutase, which depends on copper for appropriate function, and mitochondrial enzymes of the respiratory chain. In the Golgi apparatus the ATPases ATP7A (Menkes disease protein) and ATP7B (Wilson's disease protein) are responsible for preparation of copper excretion. For excretion into the bloodstream copper is bound to ceruloplasmin. In conditions of copper excess excretion of the metal into bile occurs via interaction with copper metabolism murr1 domain-containing protein 1 (COMMD1). Metallothionein is responsible for copper storage. A summary of the proteins involved in copper metabolism is given in Fig. 129-1.

INHERITED COPPER-ASSOCIATED CHRONIC HEPATITIS

Inherited copper toxicosis is a well-described disease in the Bedlington terrier, in which a deletion of exon 2 in the COMMD1 gene (previously called *MURR1*) causes

Fig. 129-1 Hepatic copper metabolism. Normal hepatic copper metabolism involves several intracellular pathways. Free copper has a high potential for oxidative damage; therefore there is basically no free copper present in the cell. Copper is excreted into blood after incorporation in ceruloplasmin. Excessive copper is excreted into bile. *CTR1*, copper transporter 1; *COX17, CCS, ATOX1*, target specific copper transporters; *ATP7A*, Menkes disease protein; *ATP7B*, Wilson's disease protein; *SOD*, superoxide-dismutase1; *COX*, cytochrome-c-oxidase; *MURR1=COMMD1*, copper metabolism murr1 domain-containing protein 1.

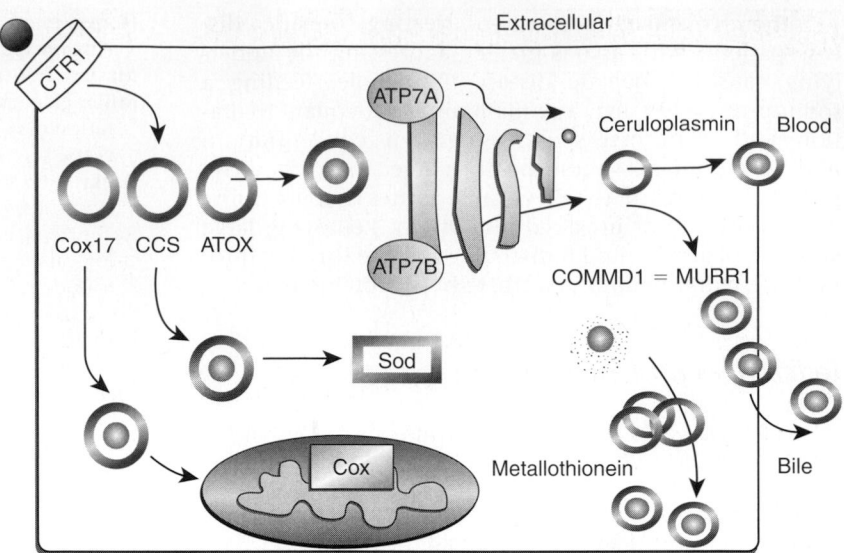

accumulation of copper in hepatocytes, resulting in chronic hepatitis. Hepatic copper storage and associated hepatitis are also breed associated in the West Highland white terrier, Skye terrier, Doberman, dalmatian, and Labrador retriever (Haywood, Rutgers, and Christian, 2006; Hoffmann et al., 2006; Mandigers et al., 2004; Thornburg et al., 1986; Webb, Twedt, and Meyer, 2002).

The average canine liver copper concentration is 200 to 400 ppm (ppm = mcg/g = mg/kg) per dry weight (DW) liver. Hepatic copper levels in breeds with primary copper storage disease vary among individual animals and among breeds from 600 to above 2200 ppm. Normal copper concentrations appear to vary little from breed to breed (Table 129-1).

Clinical Findings

Dogs with inherited copper-associated hepatitis may begin to accumulate copper at 5 to 6 months of age but may appear normal for years before they develop clinical signs late in the disease process. One investigator followed Bedlington terriers with the COMMD1 deletion from birth to 3 years of age. Copper accumulated in the liver by 1 year of age, but histologic signs of hepatitis did not occur before affected dogs were 2 years old. It appears

that dogs with inherited copper storage disorders may be subject to a prolonged initial delay period of several years between severe accumulation of copper and development of histologic evidence of inflammation and a second delay between histologic evidence of inflammation and recognition of clinical symptoms of disease.

With the exception of hemolysis from hepatic copper release into blood, which is only described for Bedlington terriers, symptoms of the disease are generally nonspecific and result from liver dysfunction. The clinical signs may start with a calmer behavior or loss of appetite. In most cases the owner only recognizes these intermittent signs retrospectively. Over weeks to months dogs may have days of decreased activity and long periods when they appear completely normal. After months to years the symptoms become more evident. The affected dogs may salivate and have intermittent vomiting and nausea. Polyuria and polydipsia, icterus, diarrhea, and ascites may develop in advanced disease (Box 129-1).

A clue to the diagnosis would be elevations in liver-specific enzymes or evidence of loss of liver function. Because copper-associated liver disease is a hepatocellular disorder, alanine aminotransferase (ALT) activity is relatively greater when compared to alkaline phosphatase

Table 129-1

Normal Range for Hepatic Copper in Liver Tissue of Dogs

Range (ppm per dw)	Normal Range	Breed	Method	Dogs
91-358	206 ± 56	Bedlington terriers	sp	22
94-270	190 ± 56	Mixed breed dogs	sp	15
60-270	155 ± 66	Mixed breed dogs	sp	13
38-650	156 ± 119	5 mixed breed dogs + 32 pure breeds	sp	37
100-700	197 ± 113	Doberman Pinscher	NAA	13
120-304	<400	Labrador retrievers	NAA	6

DW, Dry weight; *NAA,* neutron activation analysis; *sp,* spectroscopy.
Note that ppm equals mcg/g and mg/kg per dry weight.

Clinical Signs of Copper-Associated Chronic Hepatitis in Dogs

- Reduced endurance/depression
- Loss of appetite/anorexia
- Weight loss
- Nausea/salivation
- Vomiting
- Polyuria/polydipsia
- Diarrhea
- Icterus
- Ascites
- Seizures

A Histochemical Grading System for Assessment of Canine Liver Tissue Stained With Rhodanine or Rubeanic Acid*

0. No copper
1. Solitary liver cells with some copper-positive granules
2. Small groups of liver cells with small-to-moderate amounts of copper-positive granules
3. Larger groups or areas of liver cells with moderate amounts of copper-positive granules
4. Large areas of liver cells and RHS cells with many copper-positive granules
5. Diffuse presence of liver cells and RHS cells with many copper-positive granules

*Copper scores above 2 are abnormal (see Fig. 129-2 for photographs)
RHS, Reticulohistiocytosis.

activity. ALT elevation is the first and most consistent laboratory abnormality reported in Bedlington terriers with inherited copper toxicosis. Radiologic examination does not usually provide specific findings characteristic for chronic hepatitis. Ultrasound examination is helpful to exclude other diseases. Liver size is normal in most cases but may be decreased in cirrhosis. Echogenicity can be normal, increased, decreased, or irregular with a patchy appearance.

Diagnostic Criteria

Histology
Histopathologic evaluation of liver tissue is the only method for a definitive clinical diagnosis of the disease. Two or more liver biopsies, taken with a large-core needle (suggested 14 gauge), are a required minimum to evaluate liver tissue and to determine hepatic copper concentrations quantitatively or semiquantitatively.

The typical magnitude and localization of copper within zone 3 in the liver lobule is characteristic of primary copper storage diseases. As copper accumulates in hepatocytes, hepatocellular inflammation with copper-laden macrophages and chronic hepatitis result. Histology of chronic hepatitis is characterized by hepatocellular apoptosis, necrosis, regeneration, and fibrosis, as well as inflammatory infiltrates, which can be mononuclear or mixed. Cirrhosis results as the end stage of the disease. Fibrosis is part of the pathologic definition of chronic hepatitis but may appear very late in the disease process. Therefore early in the disease histology may not immediately reflect characteristic changes in chronic hepatitis and requires follow-up examinations.

Copper Assessment
Copper concentrations in liver tissue can be assessed quantitatively by irradiation of biopsies and measurement of the induced copper radioactivity in small amounts of tissue (2 mg of tissue) or by spectrophotometric methods on larger pieces of fresh frozen liver (1 to 2 g of tissue needed). For the latter method formalin-fixed tissue can be submitted, but measurement of copper concentrations in wet weight liver tissue is not recommended because the reference range for copper is established on a DW basis.

Alternatively histochemical stains, using rubeanic acid and rhodanine, can be used to assess liver tissue copper accumulation semiquantitatively. These stains consistently detect copper in liver specimens when amounts exceed the normal range of 400 mcg/g DW.

A histochemical grading system for evaluation of liver tissue stained with rhodanine was developed by Johnson (1984) for semiquantitative evaluation of hepatic copper concentrations in Bedlington terriers. The same grading system was applied for assessment of semiquantitative copper scores in rubeanic acid–stained liver tissue of Bedlington terriers, Doberman pinchers, and Labrador retrievers. A grading scale of 0 to 5 is used, with 0 having no copper. According to both staining methods copper scores above 2 are considered abnormal (Box 129-2). Fig. 129-2 shows histochemically stained samples in dogs with copper accumulation.

Specific Breeds

Bedlington Terrier
Hepatic copper toxicity was first identified in Bedlington terriers in 1975. It was subsequently shown that affected dogs have an inherited autosomal-recessive defect of the MURR1 gene, which was renamed to COMMD1. The extent of hepatic damage tends to parallel the increasing hepatic copper concentrations, which result from decreased copper excretion into bile in COMMD1-deficient liver cells. The accumulated copper in liver tissue is seen as dense granules in lysosomes and occurs mainly in the centrolobular region of the liver lobule. The histologic changes extend from focal necrosis to chronic hepatitis and cirrhosis. In some cases acute hepatic necrosis, copper-associated hemolytic anemia, and acute liver failure may occur. Female and male dogs are affected equally.

Copper toxicosis in Bedlington terriers can be divided into three stages clinically. In the first stage hepatic copper concentrations increase from 400 to 1500 ppm DW. Copper accumulation occurs in the centrolobular hepatocytes (zone 3). This stage remains clinically silent. A liver biopsy reveals increased concentrations of copper. The

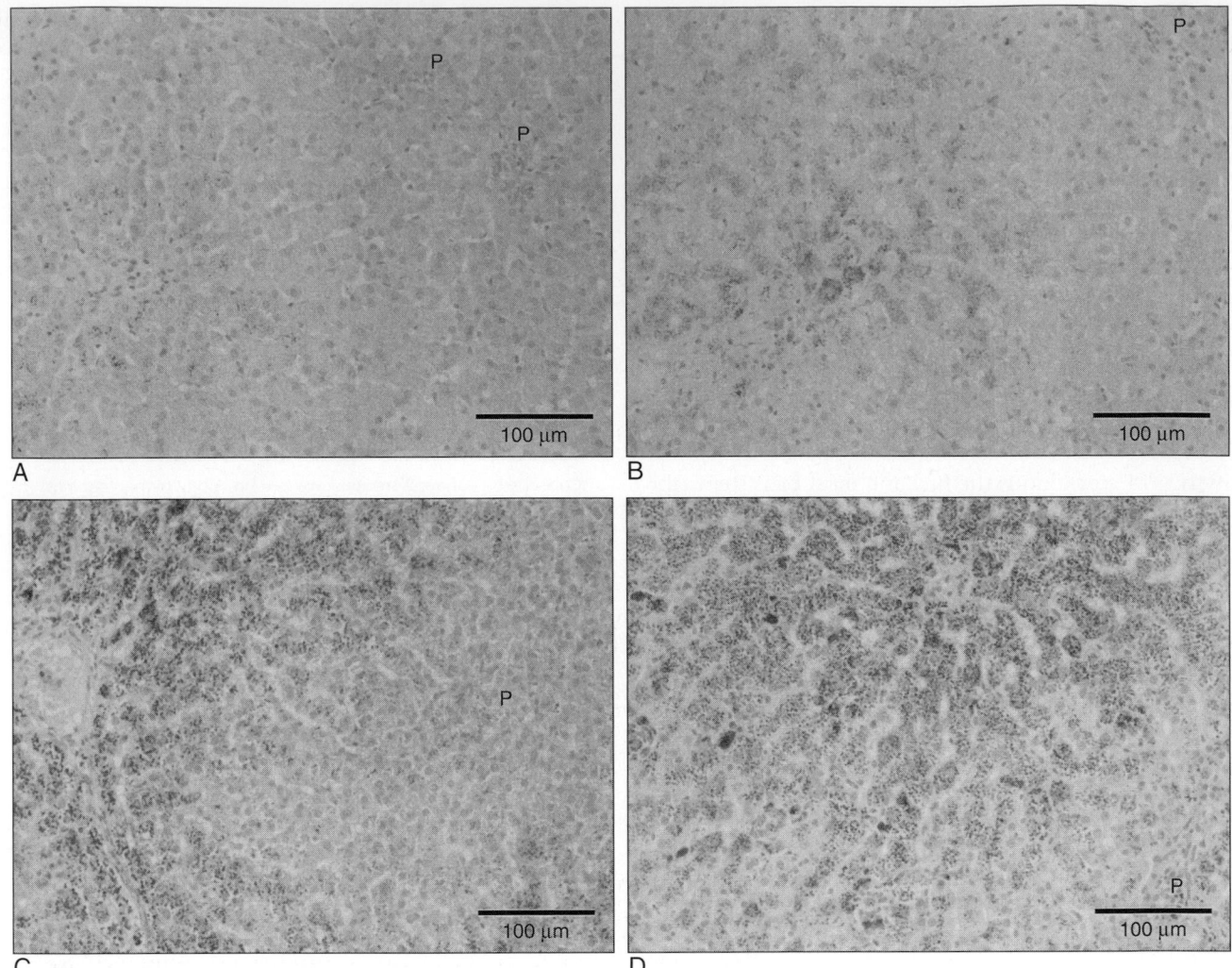

Fig. 129-2   Histology slides (3-μm thickness) of liver tissue from dogs stained with rubeanic acid stain for copper showing different histochemical grades. *P,* portal area; *A.* score 2+; *B,* score 3+; *C,* score 4+; *D,* score 5+ according to Box 129-2. (Courtesy Dr. T.S.G.A.M van den Ingh, TCCI Consultancy BV, Utrecht, The Netherlands.)

histologic liver structure is normal but stains positive for copper granules.

In the second stage copper concentrations increase further in a range of 1500 to 2000 ppm DW. Histologically copper accumulation is now also found in the midzonal and periportal hepatocytes (zones 2 and 1). A liver biopsy reveals inflammation. Mixed cell foci can be found centrolobular and contain necrotic hepatocytes, lymphocytes, plasma cells, neutrophils, and copper-laden macrophages. In the most advanced stage the dogs become clinically ill. Copper concentrations usually exceed 2000 ppm DW. Histology reveals hepatitis and cirrhosis. Cholestasis and bile duct proliferation occur along with fibrosis possibly because of the compression exerted on bile ducts in a distorted fibrotic liver and a cytokine-induced proliferation of bile ducts.

Heterozygous carrier dogs show increases of hepatic copper concentrations out of the normal range until around 6 to 9 months of age before concentrations fall back into the normal range. Liver biopsies in dogs under 1 year of age do not differentiate carrier dogs from those in affected dogs.

Affected dogs are diagnosed by either copper measurement in liver biopsies and/or genetic testing. Estimates of the incidence of copper toxicosis in Bedlington terriers varied between 34% and 66% before genetic testing became available. Genetic assays are commercially available that determine the presence of a particular microsatellite marker, which is in linkage disequilibrium with the COMMD1 mutation, or they detect the deletion of exon 2 of COMMD1 directly.

Doberman Pinscher

The disease almost exclusively affects female Dobermans, beginning in young dogs (1 to 3 years of age) with increased ALT concentrations, centrolobular copper accumulation, and subclinical hepatitis. Clinical evidence of liver disease usually begins around 4 to 7 years of age with chronic hepatitis and cirrhosis. Copper appears to be associated with the disease because recent studies found that copper was often increased before development of clinical hepatitis (Mandigers et al., 2004). Copper excretion studies also found decreased biliary excretion of copper in affected dogs. Copper chelator therapy with penicillamine in subclinical dogs normalized copper concentrations, with improvement in the grade of histologic damage.

Dalmatian

A retrospective study summarized 10 dalmatians with copper-associated chronic hepatitis (Webb, Twedt, and Meyer, 2002). Two of the dogs were related, and all presented for gastrointestinal clinical signs. Males and females were affected equally, and all dogs had elevated liver enzymes and necroinflammatory liver changes, as well as centrolobular copper accumulations. In five dogs hepatic copper concentrations exceeded 2000 mcg/g DW liver.

West Highland White Terrier

The described dogs ranged from 3 to 7 years of age. Some dogs had elevated hepatic copper concentrations (centrolobular) but no evidence of liver disease, which led to the suspicion that copper may later develop into chronic hepatitis or cirrhosis. Copper accumulation does not appear to increase with age in the West Highland white terrier, and there is no gender preference (Thornburg et al., 1986). Biliary excretion studies revealed a decreased excretion of radioactive copper in affected dogs.

Skye Terriers

Cholestasis was suspected as the etiology of copper-associated chronic hepatitis/cirrhosis in Skye terriers. The 10 described dogs were 1 to 10 years old. Female and male dogs were affected equally and presented with intermittent anorexia, vomiting, and ascites. At a terminal stage of the disease the animals developed jaundice and died (Haywood, Rutgers, and Christian, 1988). Further studies are required to better describe this syndrome in Skye terriers.

Labrador Retriever

Chronic hepatitis is reported to be common in this breed, and copper accumulation is associated with about 75% of the cases. Females are more commonly affected and generally present around 7 years of age (range 2 to 10 years). Clinical symptoms are nonspecific, including anorexia, vomiting, and weight loss. Hepatic copper concentrations generally range between 650 and 3000 mcg/g DW liver and a histochemical grade greater than 2+ using rubeanic acid staining. The histologic localization of copper in the centrolobular region of the liver lobule suggests primary copper accumulation (Hoffmann et al., 2006).

Other Breeds

An Anatolian shepherd, 6 German Shepherds, 11 keeshonds, a boxer, and 2 cats have been reported to have liver disease associated with hepatic copper accumulation.

Copper Accumulation Secondary to Cholestasis

Copper may accumulate in the liver secondary to cholestatic liver diseases. This is a result of defective copper excretion via bile. Cholestatic liver diseases often result in copper accumulation in the periportal areas. The magnitude of copper accumulation from cholestasis is not as high as in inherited copper storage disorders. In a review of 17 liver biopsies from breeds not yet identified to have inherited copper-associated liver disease, the mean copper concentration was 984 mcg/g DW liver. Another study found that a 3+ or higher histochemical grade for detection of copper in the central area of the liver lobule indicates a primary copper storage disease (Spee et al., 2006). In this study the authors were able to find clear distinction criteria to determine whether copper accumulation is primary or secondary to hepatitis by comparing liver biopsies from Bedlington terriers with copper toxicosis with noncopper-associated breeds and chronic extrahepatic cholestasis. Copper metabolism and oxidative stress were analyzed using histochemical staining and quantitative reverse transcriptase polymerase chain reaction to compare the expression of genes that are involved in copper metabolism and protection against oxidative stress. This approach allowed the authors to identify expression profiles of certain genes that are characteristic for primary hepatic copper storage disorders.

TREATMENT

Chelator Therapy

Penicillamine

Penicillamine chelates a variety of metals, including copper. The drug leads to mobilization of copper from tissues and promotes copper excretion in urine. Penicillamine may also increase the synthesis of metallothionein (a copper-binding protein) and has antiinflammatory, immunosuppressive, and antifibrotic effects. Because of potential teratogenic effects of penicillamine, owners should be informed about safe handling of the drug (gloves for breaking pills or opening capsules), and pregnant women should not come in contact with the drug. The recommended dosage of penicillamine for dogs is 10 to 15 mg/kg every 12 hours orally. Lifelong therapy may be required. Adverse effects such as anorexia, vomiting, and diarrhea occur frequently in dogs. Most of these adverse effects can be avoided by mixing the drug with food and dividing the dose to more frequent dosing intervals per day. Adverse effects from long-term therapy with penicillamine may include anemia (normocytic or microcytic) and glycogen storage of the liver. Patients should be monitored clinically, as well as by 6-month assessments of the complete blood count and an annual-to-biennial liver biopsy. Side effects reported in humans include vitamin B deficiency from increased urinary loss and lupus-like symptoms with lymphadenopathy, cytopenias, fever, cutaneous eruptions, and proteinuria. Penicillamine is teratogenic and may cross the placenta; thus use during pregnancy is not recommended.

Clinical improvement from penicillamine treatment takes weeks to months, and there are large interindividual variations with respect to the effectiveness of the drug. Therefore follow-up liver biopsies are required to determine the effectiveness of chelation. One author describes an average detoxification rate of around 900-ppm copper decrease per year during penicillamine treatment in Bedlington terriers (Rolfe and Twedt, 1995).

Penicillamine was effective for treatment of Doberman pinschers with copper-associated subclinical hepatitis.

We have also tested copper chelation therapy with penicillamine in Labrador retrievers in a randomized, double-blinded, placebo-controlled study and found the drug to be effective given 10 to 15 mg/kg every 12 hours orally for 3 to 6 months.

Trientine

Trientine hydrochloride (Syprine) is available in the United States for humans intolerant to penicillamine. Although clinical experience with the drug is limited, from current knowledge trientine may have fewer gastrointestinal effects than penicillamine in dogs. Trientine is a copper chelator that acts by increasing urinary excretion of copper. In addition, the drug may also help to decrease intestinal absorption of copper. One investigator described trientine as more potent than penicillamine for decreasing copper concentrations in plasma and concluded that the drug might be superior for treatment of acute hemolytic crisis (Twedt, Hunsaker, and Allen, 1988). Trientine has teratogenic effects in animals. Therefore owners need to be informed about safe handling. The recommended dosage is 10 to 15 mg/kg every 12 hours orally 1 to 2 hours before feeding.

Zinc

Oral zinc is given to reduce copper absorption from the diet. Recommended dosage is 100 mg of elemental zinc every 12 hours orally per dog. Zinc given orally induces the production of metallothionein in intestinal mucosal cells. Metallothionein binds copper from the diet and therefore prevents the uptake of copper into the circulation. Since the rate of removal of hepatic copper is relatively slow, dogs with severe or fulminant copper-induced hepatitis should not be treated with zinc therapy alone. Theoretically zinc given orally together with penicillamine may decrease the effectiveness of both drugs.

The type of zinc salt used does not influence efficacy of the drug but may affect tolerability. Gluconate may be more tolerable than sulfate and acetate. Theoretically zinc should be given apart from feeding because some food constituents (such as phytates) can bind zinc and diminish efficacy. Zinc is often a gastric mucosa irritant, leading to nausea and vomiting. Mixing the drug with small amounts of food has been recommended. Plasma zinc concentrations of normal dogs range between 90 and 120 mcg/dl. Plasma zinc concentrations above 200 mcg/dl are required during therapy to suppress copper uptake, but at plasma zinc concentrations above 1000 mcg/dl hemolysis may occur. Serum zinc concentrations should be monitored monthly for several months to ensure that concentrations are in the therapeutic range. In a study of three Bedlington terriers and three West Highland white terriers with copper toxicosis,

200 mg of elemental zinc was given daily to each dog to achieve therapeutic plasma concentrations of zinc above 200 mcg/dl. Effectiveness of zinc for prevention of copper uptake from the intestine was assessed by measurement of peak plasma concentrations of radioactive copper. A minimum of 3 months of zinc treatment was necessary before copper uptake from the intestine was blocked. Although zinc is currently reserved for maintenance treatment, it has been used as first-line therapy in asymptomatic humans.

Dietary Management

The goal of dietary medical therapy is to reduce the absorption of copper from the intestinal tract. Heavily copper-supplemented diets or copper-containing vitamin-mineral supplements should be avoided. Foods with excessive copper such as eggs, liver, shellfish, organ meats, beans, mushrooms, chocolate, nuts, and cereals should be excluded from the diet (Rolfe and Twedt, 1995).

Balanced low-copper diets are commercially available for dogs. Although the effectiveness of such diets to prevent further copper accumulation has not been tested in controlled studies, dietary management seems a reasonable choice as an auxiliary measure during treatment for copper-associated liver diseases.

References and Suggested Reading

Haywood S, Rutgers HC, Christian MK: Hepatitis and copper accumulation in Skye terriers, *Vet Pathol* 25:408, 1988.

Hoffmann G et al: Copper-associated chronic hepatitis in Labrador retrievers, *J Vet Intern Med* 20:856, 2006.

Johnson GF, et al: Cytochemical detection of inherited copper toxicosis of Bedlington terriers, *Vet Pathol* 21(1):57, 1984.

Mandigers PJ et al: Association between liver copper concentration and subclinical hepatitis in Doberman pinschers, *J Vet Internal Med* 18(5):647, 2004.

Rolfe DS, Twedt DC: Copper-associated hepatopathies in dogs, *Vet Clin North Am Small Anim Pract* 2:399, 1995.

Spee B et al: Copper metabolism and oxidative stress in chronic inflammatory and cholestatic liver diseases in dogs, *J Vet Intern Med* 20:1085, 2006.

Speeti M et al: Lesions of subclinical doberman hepatitis, *Vet Pathol* 35(5):361, 1998.

Thornburg CP et al: High liver copper levels in 2 Doberman pinschers with subacute hepatitis, *J Am Anim Hosp Assoc* 1003, 1983.

Thornburg CP et al: Hereditary copper toxicosis in West Highland white terriers, *Vet Pathol* 23:148, 1986.

Thornburg CP et al: The relationship between hepatic copper content and morphologic changes in the liver of West Highland white terriers, *Vet Pathol* 33:656, 1996.

Twedt DC, Hunsaker A: Use of 2,3,2-tetramine as hepatic copper chelating agent for treatment of copper hepatotoxicosis in Bedlington terriers, *JAVMA* 192:52, 1988.

Webb CB, Twedt DC, Meyer DJ: Copper-associated liver disease in dalmatians: a review of 10 dogs (1998–2001), *J Vet Intern Med* 16:665, 2002.

CHAPTER 130

Ursodeoxycholic Acid Therapy

CYNTHIA R.L. WEBSTER, *Grafton, Massachusetts*

For many years practitioners of Eastern medicine have known of the healing powers of Chinese black bear bile. The major bile acid in this bear's bile, ursodeoxycholic acid (UDCA), has been commercially synthesized and marketed as a hepatoprotective agent in Japan since the 1930s. It was not until the 1970s that Western medicine began to appreciate the medicinal value of UDCA when a synthetic version of this bile acid received approval (Actigall, Watson) to be marketed for the dissolution of cholesterol gallstones in humans. In the 1980s physicians noticed that UDCA therapy in patients with concurrent gallstones and chronic hepatic disease resulted in improvement in liver function test results. Since then numerous studies have demonstrated the beneficial action of UDCA in treating a variety of hepatopathies. In 1998 a second form of UDCA (URSO, Axcan Pharma) was approved to treat primary biliary cirrhosis (PBC), an autoimmune disease of the intrahepatic bile ducts in humans.

HEPATOPROTECTIVE ACTIONS OF URSODEOXYCHOLIC ACID

Mammalian bile acids are actually a family of amphipathic organic anions that share a steroid nucleus with hydroxylation at the 3 position. The primary bile acids synthesized from cholesterol in the liver, chenodeoxycholic acid and cholic acid, are characterized by additional hydroxylations at the 7 and the 7 and 12 positions, respectively. These primary bile acids are conjugated in the liver with either glycine or taurine. In humans the major circulating bile acid is the di-hydroxy bile acid glycochenodeoxycholate, whereas in the dog and cat it is the tri-hydroxy bile acid taurocholate. Bile acid conjugation and hydroxylation increase the aqueous solubility of bile acids and by doing so decrease their passive resorption in the biliary tract and intestine. This permits the accumulation of the high biliary and intestinal bile acid concentrations necessary for their role in maintaining bile flow and fat absorption. Although the exact mechanism(s) responsible for this hepatoprotective effect of UDCA have not been fully characterized, the following beneficial actions have been proposed: (1) replacement of the more hydrophobic hepatotoxic bile acids in the circulating pool, (2) induction of choleresis, (3) stabilization of mitochondrial function, and (4) immunomodulation.

Some members of the bile acid family are hepatotoxic and, depending on their concentration, lead to apoptosis (at 50 to 200 μM) or necrosis (at >500 μM). Since many hepatobiliary diseases are accompanied by increases in serum and hepatic concentration of bile acids of this mag-

nitude, it is likely that bile acids contribute to the pathologic progression of these disorders. The relative toxicity of bile acids is loosely correlated with their degree of hydrophobicity. Both bile acid conjugation and hydroxylation decrease hydrophobicity and thus toxicity. UDCA, a di-hydroxy bile acid, is a relatively hydrophilic, nonhepatotoxic bile acid even though it is almost structurally identical to the much more hepatotoxic bile acid, chenodeoxycholate. This discrepancy is in part explained by the orientation of the hydroxyl groups in the two molecules. In chenodeoxycholate the OH groups are oriented at the α-face of the steroid nucleus, leaving a large hydrophobic face. In UCDA the 7-OH group is oriented at the β-face of the steroid nucleus, rendering the molecule much more hydrophilic. Thus one mechanism by which UDCA may be hepatoprotective is by replacing more hydrophobic hepatotoxic bile acids such as chenodeoxycholate from the circulating bile acid pool. However, this view is overly simplistic, since in humans a correlation between enrichment of the bile acid pool with UDCA and its therapeutic effect has been hard to demonstrate. In addition, this effect would be of limited value in dogs and cats in which the major circulating bile acid is the relatively nontoxic tri-OH bile acid cholate.

UDCA is a potent choleretic agent. Induction of choleresis stimulates the biliary excretion of bile acids and other potentially toxic endogenous metabolites that are retained during cholestasis such as copper, leukotrienes, bilirubin, and cholesterol. UDCA-induced choleresis occurs by two mechanisms. The most important means is by increasing the plasma membrane expression of membrane transporter necessary to generate bile flow. This is accomplished by mobilizing intracellular stores of the transporters through activation of signal transduction molecules such as protein kinase C. A second mechanism whereby UDCA promotes choleresis is known as cholehepatic shunting. Unconjugated UDCA is secreted into bile, where it becomes protonated, leading to the generation of bicarbonate ion. Protonated UDCA is then passively absorbed by the biliary epithelial cells, leaving the net secretion of one bicarbonate ion. The bicarbonate then serves as an osmotic draw for biliary water secretion.

In hepatocytes UDCA prevents apoptosis caused by several important physiologic stimuli, including ethanol, Fas ligand, tumor necrosis factor (TNF), and bile acids. In addition, UDCA protects nonhepatic cells, most notably colonic epithelial cells, neurons, and cardiac myocytes, from apoptosis. Accumulating evidence suggests that UDCA mediates its antiapoptotic effect by stabilizing mitochondrial function. Mitochondria are key regulators of apoptotic pathways. When cells receive a death signal, whether from a death receptor (Fas, TNF) or from intracellular stress, small proteins of the Bcl-2 family such Bax and Bid translocate from the cytosol to the mitochondria. Together these proteins integrate into the mitochondrial membrane, disrupt membrane permeability, and lead to the release of apoptogenic factors that ultimately lead to cell death. UDCA protects mitochondria by decreasing the cellular expression of Bax and preventing Bax translocation to the mitochondria. UDCA can also directly interact with mitochondrial membranes to inhibit Bax-mediated membrane perturbations. As a result of its protective effects on mitochondria, UDCA prevents the loss of mitochondrial membrane potential during apoptosis and decreases the mitochondrial production of reactive oxygen species. UDCA also increases mitochondrial glutathione levels perhaps by stabilizing mitochondrial membrane transporters or by increasing the activity of methionine adenosyltransferase. The latter effect would lead to increased generation of *S*-adenosylmethionine, which can then be metabolized by transsulfuration to glutathione. Glutathione is the major antioxidant in the liver and an especially important free-radical scavenger in the mitochondria. The cellular basis for the antiapoptotic actions of UCDA on the mitochondria likely involves stimulation of cellular survival signaling. In hepatocytes, neurons, and cardiac myocytes, UDCA protection against cell death requires activation of the lipid kinase phosphoinositide-3-kinase and downstream activation of the serine/threonine kinase AKT. UDCA-mediated activation of mitogen-activated kinases has also been implicated in its protective effect in hepatocytes.

Several immunomodulating effects of UDCA have been reported. UDCA decreases the production of immunoglobulin by B lymphocytes and interleukin-1 and interleukin-2 by T lymphocytes in response to nonspecific stimuli. UDCA treatment also decreases expression of hepatocyte cell surface membrane HLA class I molecules. Several studies suggest that UDCA works as a biologic response modifier of the glucocorticoid receptor (GR). Glucocorticoids bind to cytosolic GRs, resulting in translocation of the receptor to the nucleus. In the nucleus the GR interacts with the glucocorticoid response element to modulate the transcription of genes involved in inflammation. The cortisol-GR complex also regulates the action of another proinflammatory transcription factor, nuclear factor-κ-β (NF-κ-β). Studies show that UDCA activates the GR by binding to a region distinct from that to which glucocorticoids bind. The UDCA-GR complex translocates to the nucleus and can block NF-κ-β–mediated transcription. The importance of GR binding in the cytoprotective effect of UDCA has been demonstrated in hepatocytes where small interfering RNAs that prevent the UDCA-GR interaction abolish the protective effect of UDCA in cytokine-mediated apoptosis. Clearly the study of the interaction between UDCA and the GR is still in its infancy; but, considering the clinical safety profile of UDCA, elucidation of the nature of this interaction may lead to the development of more selective and potent GR modifiers that promote the antiinflammatory and immunosuppressive effects of glucocorticoids without the negative biologic effects that so often limit their use.

THERAPEUTIC USE OF URSODEOXYCHOLIC ACID

In humans UCDA is used to treat a variety of chronic hepatopathies, including PBC, primary sclerosing cholangitis, pediatric cholestatic disorders, and intrahepatic cholestasis associated with pregnancy. The largest body of information on the clinical use of UDCA in humans is with PBC. Although most clinical trials with PBC show that UDCA improves serum liver tests and clinical signs, evidence that UDCA inhibits the progression of disease and improves long-term survival is conflicting. However, many studies are limited by the small number of patients; the short duration of treatment; and the long, unpredictable natural course of PBC in humans. More recent evidence suggests that UDCA therapy is most beneficial in early disease.

Following oral administration of UCDA in humans, 30% to 60% is absorbed primarily in the small intestine (80%) with smaller amounts in the colon (20%). Oral absorption is enhanced if the drug is taken with a meal. UDCA has high hepatic first-pass metabolism (70%). Once within hepatocytes, extracted UDCA becomes conjugated to taurine or glycine and then undergoes enterohepatic circulation. The bioavailability of UDCA may decrease with advance cholestasis because of decreased hepatic extraction and increased renal elimination. Thus in patients with severe cholestasis there may be some benefit to higher doses or twice-daily administration of UCDA. In humans UDCA given at 10 to 15 mg/kg/day results in 40% enrichment of bile; higher doses do no better. UDCA is metabolized to lithocholate in the colon and eliminated in the feces. In severe cholestasis renal clearance becomes more prominent. The safety profile of UDCA is outstanding in humans with only limited reports of mild diarrhea. Coadministration with aluminum hydroxide decreases bioavailability. UDCA may increase the bioavailability of lipophilic compounds such as vitamin E or cyclosporine.

There is little information in the literature to guide veterinarians in the proper use of UDCA in small animals. In a dog with chronic hepatitis, UDCA (15 mg/kg/day) resulted in enrichment of UDCA in the serum and was associated with biochemical and clinical improvement (Meyer et al., 1997). Another study has verified the choleretic properties of oral UDCA in healthy dogs (Yanaura and Ishikawa, 1978). Extensive toxicologic studies for Food and Drug Administration approval of UDCA performed in healthy dogs did not reveal any serious side effects of therapy. In normal cats UDCA (10 to 15 mg/kg/day) for 8 to 12 weeks was well tolerated with no changes seen in physical condition, serum liver enzymes, or hepatic histology. Both UDCA and tauroUDCA were detected in the serum of treated cats. A decrease in serum cholesterol was noted in some cats (Nicholson et al., 1996; Day et al., 1994). Anecdotal clinical impressions from veterinary hepatologists who frequently use URSO in feline and canine patients with hepatic disease corroborate these experimental findings. The only side effects reported with any frequency are rare instances of vomiting and diarrhea. In normal dogs and cats oral supplementation of UDCA can increase preprandial and postprandial total serum bile acids, but typically these increases are not above the reference range

It is currently unknown whether UDCA has any therapeutic benefit in treating canine or feline hepatobiliary disorders. The answer to this question awaits the results of prospective clinical trials. Extrapolation of information generated in the human literature and in experimental models of hepatotoxicity in several species suggests that UDCA should have beneficial effects in dogs and cats as well. The choleretic action of UDCA should be beneficial in acute and chronic hepatobiliary disorders marked by cholestasis. In addition, UDCA supplementation may reverse the loss of membrane transport function seen in cholestatic disorders. The possibility of extrahepatic biliary obstruction should always be ruled out before starting therapy because the use of choleretics is contraindicated in this instance. The long-term hepatoprotective and immunomodulating actions of UDCA should be of benefit in the treatment of chronic inflammatory hepatobiliary disease in both the dog and cat. It is my belief that UDCA is not a panacea for all chronic inflammatory hepatic disorders but may be of some benefit in slowing the progression of disease, especially when used at an early stage. Currently I incorporate UDCA in the therapy of most cases of inflammatory hepatobiliary disease in dogs and cats. In some asymptomatic animals with evidence of hepatobiliary disease discovered serendipitously having increases in serum liver enzymes or when corticosteroids are contraindicated in the therapy (e.g., diabetic animals), I often use UDCA as the only therapy. In addition, appropriate therapeutic measures to manage the complications of hepatobiliary disease (Bonagura, 1995, p. 749) are also instituted. The animals are monitored for 2 to 3 months by following body condition score, appetite, attitude, and the levels of serum hepatobiliary enzymes. If no response is seen during this time, the drug is discontinued or in cases of severe cholestasis the dose is doubled.

There has been some reluctance to use UDCA in the feline hepatic lipidosis (FHL) syndrome because increased bile flux can decrease hepatic production and egress of very low–density lipoproteins. This effect is likely mediated through the binding of bile acids to their nuclear receptor, farnesoid X (FXR). However, bile acids differ in their ability to activate FXR, with UDCA functioning as a very poor ligand. Thus UDCA-induced modification

of the bile acid pool in cats with FHL may actually be beneficial in this regard.

UDCA is available as a 300-mg capsule (Actigal, and also available generically) and a 250- and 500-mg pill (URSO) for oral administration. The two formulations are essentially equivalent, and I do not hesitate to prescribe the generic form since the medication is expensive. The recommended dosage for both dogs and cats, 10 to 15 mg/kg per day orally, is extrapolated from human medicine. The medication is best given with food. There are no known drug interactions between UDCA and other drugs used to treat hepatobiliary disease such as s-adenosylmethionine, corticosteroids, azathioprine, vitamin E, or silymarin.

References and Suggested Reading

Bellentani S: Immunomodulating and anti-apoptotic actions of ursodeoxycholic acid: where are we and where should we go, *Eur J Gastroenterol Hepatol* 17:137, 2005.
Beuers U: Drug insight: mechanisms and sites of action of ursodeoxycholic acid in cholestasis, *Nat Clin Pract Gastroenterol Idepatol* 3:318, 2006.
Bonagura JD, Kirk RW, editors: *Kirk's current veterinary therapy XII (small animal practice)*, Philadelphia, 19952, Saunders.
Day D, Meyer D, Johnson SE: Evaluation of total serum bile acids concentration and bile acid profiles in healthy cats after oral administration of ursodeoxycholic acid, *Am J Vet Res* 55:1474, 1994.
Lazarida KN, Gores G, Lindor K: Ursodeoxycholic acid mechanisms of action and clinical use in hepatobiliary disorders, *J Hepatol* 35:134, 2001.
Meyer D, Thompson MB, Senior D: Use of ursodeoxycholic acid in a dog with chronic hepatitis: effects on serum hepatic tests and endogenous bile acid composition, *J Vet Intern Med* 11:195, 1997.
Nicholson BT et al: Effects of oral ursodeoxycholic acid in healthy cats on clinicopathologic parameters, serum bile acids and light and ultrastructural features of the liver, *Res Vet Sci* 61:258, 1996.
Rodriques CM et al: Tauroursodeoxycholic acid prevents Bax-induced membrane perturbation and cytochrome C release in isolated mitochondria, *Biochemistry* 43:3070, 2003.
Serviddio G et al: Ursodeoxycholic acid protects against secondary biliary cirrhosis in rats by preventing mitochondrial oxidative stress, *Hepatology* 39:711, 2004.
Schoemaker MH et al: TUDCA protects rat hepatocytes from bile acid induced apoptosis via activation of survival pathways, *Hepatology* 39:1563, 2004.
Yanaura S, Ishikawa S: Choleretic properties of ursodeoxycholic acid and chenodeoxycholic acid in dogs, *Jpn J Pharmacol* 28:383, 1978.

CHAPTER 131

Drug-Associated Liver Disease

MARK E. HITT, *Annapolis, Maryland*

Drug-associated liver disease (DALD) is a relatively common diagnosis in veterinary practice. It may also be referred to in the human medical literature as drug-induced liver injury (DILI). Hepatoxicity is the most common clinical pathologic reason for discontinuation or alteration of medication treatment plans.

To recognize DALD, the veterinary clinician must have the possibility of an adverse drug reaction in mind when prescribing any drug. Familiarity of the clinician with the pharmacologic principles of a drug is critical to minimizing risks and early detection of adverse interactions and toxic effects in a specific patient. It is not uncommon for a case with DALD to also involve additional adverse drug reactions to that same product. The liver has many functions in the body, including recognition and detoxification of foreign substances (xenobiotics) and endogenous wastes, recognition and elimination of toxins, manufacturing of substances, storage of metabolic products, metabolic activations, and metabolite eliminations. DALD can develop as the result of a direct effect or consequent to a reactive metabolite of that drug. As practicing veterinarians we are treating ever more complicated medical problems that occur in ever more complex combinations. This leads to increasing numbers of drugs used in situations and in combinations that may not have been anticipated or tested. The more commonly reported drugs associated with liver disease in dogs and cats are listed in Table 131-1. Drugs that are less commonly used in dogs and cats, or that have fewer specific references are included in Box 131-1.

MECHANISMS AND PATHOPHYSIOLOGY

The principle mechanisms of DALD follow the same pathophysiologic mechanisms as those established for many nonpharmaceutical substances that can injure the liver. Hepatotoxins can be drugs, metabolites of drugs, xenobiotics, endogenous toxins, or exogenous toxins. The mechanisms of injury are broadly categorized as *direct* or *idiosyncratic*. DALD events cause dysfunction of liver metabolism or create overt pathology in the liver. If the adverse effect on the liver is considered predictable based on the dose of a medication, it is considered a *direct hepatotoxin*. If the development of liver injury appears random in nature, the pattern is considered to be an *idiosyncratic hepatotoxin*. In this situation it takes hundreds or thousands of uses of the drug in question in true clinical situations to discover a drug's potential for hepatotoxicity. There may be some degree of overlap in how idiosyncratic versus direct reactions are viewed as greater numbers of patients are exposed to a drug. Idiosyncratic DALD remains poorly understood.

Affected individuals may carry a rare combination of genetic and environmental host factors that, if identified, would greatly improve understanding of underlying mechanisms. The role of pharmacogenomics will have important future implications related to our understanding of hepatic drug reactions. One example is the finding of familial lines of herding dogs that are deficient in P-glycoprotein enzymes that limit their metabolism of certain drugs (e.g., azathioprine) through biliary cannulicular excretion as one of several mechanisms. Once thousands of doses of medication have been used, a relative prevalence is established even for idiosyncratic DALD events. This information blurs the concept of predictable versus nonpredictable hepatotoxicity.

The liver is in a central position in the body to be exposed to potentially toxic or metabolically stressful situations. Most pharmacologically active substances are lipophyllic. Elimination and/or enhancement of positive effect, or of toxicity, is increased by making them more hydrophyllic via the phase I and II enzymatic actions of the liver. Metabolism within the liver also depends on oxygen flow via both arterial and portal vessels. Potentially toxic substances can arrive at the liver via ingestion (portal flow) or parenteral administration (arterial delivery). The acinar zones within the hepatic lobules are affected variably by the route of delivery of toxin, the enzymatic concentrations of various metabolic processes in each acinar zone, and the relative degree of oxygenation (or hypoxia) for those zones.

Drugs can be associated with multiple mechanisms of hepatic injury. Hepatic injury can occur via *cytopathic change on hepatocytes* (e.g., hydropic change, lysis, necrosis), *induction of cholestasis* and metabolic dysfunctions, *induction of an immune system* activity against hepatocytes, and/or production of *subsequent proinflammatory responses* to the liver. Adverse hepatic effects of drugs can range from minimal changes in clinical pathologic values to death of the pet.

Overt *cytopathic hepatocellular* injury occurs via damage to cell membranes and injury to mitochondrial energy functions. This results in loss of membrane integrity and is represented by microscopic appearance of hydropic degeneration and necrosis. These changes can also be nonlethal or lethal to the cells. Changes lead to dysfunction of cellular energy systems, leakage of enzymes, retention of irritating wastes (e.g., bile acids), and even initiation of apoptosis. Cell death is furthered by the progressively cascading release of cytokines, superoxide radical formation, and stimulation of inflammatory responses. These inflammatory responses are part of the process of postnecrotic inflammation.

The second major pattern of hepatic toxicity that is seen via histopathology and clinical chemistries is a *cholestatic pattern*. This develops if the effects of the drug

Table 131-1

Drugs More Frequently Associated With Liver Disease in Dogs and Cats

Reported Drugs	Species
Acetaminophen	Dogs and cats
Amiodarone	Dogs
Amoxicillin/Ampicillin products	Dogs and cats
Azathioprine	Dogs
Azithromycin	Cats
CCNU (lomustine)	Dogs
Cephalosporins	Dogs
Cyclosporine	Dogs and cats
Diazepam	Cats
Diethylstilbestrol	Dogs
Enrofloxacin	Dogs
Kava kava	Dogs
Ketoconazole and azole antifungals	Dogs and cats
Glucocorticoids	Dogs (less commonly cats)
Halothane (particularly repeated exposures)	Dogs
Mebendazole	Dogs
Megesterol acetate	Dogs
Methimazole	Dogs and cats
NSAIDs: *carprofen may have increased awareness*	Dogs and cats
Oxibendazole	Dogs
Phenobarbital	Dogs and cats
Phenytoin	Dogs
Primidone	Dogs
Stanozolol	Cats
Sulfonamides	Dogs
Tetracycline antibiotics	Dogs and cats
Thiacetarsemide	Dogs and cats
Trimethoprim-sulfa combinations	Dogs
Ormetoprim-sulfadiazine	Dogs

NSAID, Nonsteroidal antiinflammatory drug.

Box 131-1

Drugs Known to Have Anecdotal or Rare Evidence of Causing Drug-Associated Liver Disease in Dogs or Cats*

- Acarbose
- Albendazole
- Allopurinol
- Amitraz
- Amlodipine
- Butorphanol
- Clomipramine
- Danazol
- Desoxycorticosterone
- Diethylcarbamazine
- Enalapril
- Ethanol
- Etodolac
- Febantel/praziquantel
- Fenbendazole
- Griseofulvin
- Iron
- Isoniazid
- Ivermectins
- Lufenuron
- Lisinopril
- Marbofloxaxin
- Macrolide antibiotics
- Meclofenamic acid
- Metronidazole
- Methotrexate
- Mexiletine
- Mibolerone
- Mitotane
- Ormetoprim
- Rifampin
- Tamoxifen
- Terbinafine
- Trilostane
- Trovafloxacin
- Valproic Acid

*Some of these are based on U.S. Food and Drug Administration: Cumulative Veterinary Adverse Drug Experience (ADE) Reports.

tend to be more intracellular, often resulting in abnormal storage of substrates (e.g., glycogen, bile acids, bilirubin, lipids, and other metabolites) or impaired Golgi complex activities. Stimulation of enzyme production (e.g., alkaline phosphatase, γ-glutamyl transpeptidase) follows.

Mixed patterns also develop in some patients with some drugs. These occurrences may be related to the offending drug, the degree or pattern of necrosis, repetitive exposures, or persistent chronic low-level exposures over time. In some situations, particularly with preexisting genetic make up (certain breed- and sex-related haplotypes), exposure of surface and internal cell membrane antigens may more likely result in formation of protein haptens that act as neoantigens to self. These then trigger autoimmune responses to cell membrane components in biliary epithelium and hepatocytes.

As a cascading series of events, DALD could be seen to include the initial drug-related cell membrane injury and then neoantigen formation via covalent protein binding of drug or drug metabolite, which then creates new adducts from the drug to which the immune system responds. Intracellular inhibition of mitochondrial function and reduced vesicle formation lead to decreased elimination of toxins, swelling of cells and retention of bile acids, and poor transport or production of bile, which are themselves toxic to hepatocytes. Further cell death is enhanced as apoptosis (programmed cell death) is triggered via Fas pathways and tumor necrosis factor. These also enhance reduced mitochondrial function and subsequent reactive oxygen radicals (superoxide radicals, lipid peroxidation). Fibrosis then may be an end result of postinflammatory stimuli. Some degree of postnecrotic cirrhosis is reported to occur in 30% to 40% of patients that have suffered severe hepatocellular injuries.

The susceptibility of an individual to DALD is affected by multiple factors. First is the drug and its pharmacologic profile. If it is a drug that has a predictable pattern of direct hepatotoxicity, clinicians are more likely to recognize DALD, providing they are familiar with the drug profile. The sex, species, breed, status of organ systems, concurrent disease, nutritional status, age, and concurrent use of other medications also influence the severity of DALD.

CLINICAL PRESENTATION AND DIAGNOSIS

Clinical presentations of DALD are diverse. No specific age, sex, breed, or other signalment would eliminate concern for a DALD. Liver enzyme elevations may be mild to severe. DALD may be discovered incidentally following review of a routine chemistry profile obtained for preanesthetic or geriatric screening. At the other end of the spectrum, a patient may die within days of a drug-induced insult with severe clinical signs. Common recognized symptoms of DALD include nausea, anorexia, vomiting, jaundice, lethargy, and weakness. Less common signs include hepatic encephalopathy, diarrhea, bleeding, increased urination, and other symptoms of liver disease. Jaundice is not a necessary indicator at the time of presentation. Icterus may only develop late in the course of disease. In most veterinary clinical situations, *acute liver failure* (ALF) is a rare sequela of DALD. However, fatal cases do occur, especially when high or repeated doses of medication have been used without monitoring of the patient. Most often the clinician detects some of the symptoms described previously or monitoring of a serum chemistry profile reveals changes in one or more values: alanine aminotransferase (ALT), alkaline phosphatase (ALP), γ-glutamyltransferase (GGT), or bilirubin. Evaluation should include routine tests such as a complete blood count, platelet count, serum chemistry profile, and urinalyses.

The distinction between liver injury and clinical loss of function is important. In most nonlife-threatening situations, hepatic function remains adequate. Often there is concern for use of drugs that require hepatic metabolism for their activation or that may induce enzyme functions of the liver. There should be a clinical decision as to whether to use another drug, adjust the dose, or avoid these products (e.g., cimetidine, phenobarbital, corticosteroids, enrofloxacin, propranolol). Monitoring of coagulation profiles, and prothrombin time in particular, as a reflection of degree of function for the liver and the possible development of disseminated intravascular coagulopathy is warranted. Use of prothrombin time assay may provide earlier warning of severity of injury. Other common tests used to assess functional hepatic impairment include albumin, blood urea nitrogen, and bilirubin. The clinical first indicators of DALD (at home or in the clinic) can be dark urine, abdominal discomfort, fatigue, anorexia, or nausea.

In veterinary medicine liver injury is often considered significant when values exceed normal reference ranges or increase in comparison to values obtained before the introduction of a drug. In human patients, liver injury is defined by a figure two times the upper limit of ALT or conjugated bilirubin; or by combining results of ALP, GGT, ALT and bilirubin testing, provided that one is greater than twice an upper normal range. Further, clinical pathology changes may appear to be more hepatocellular (predominant ALT) or cholestatic (primarily ALP) in nature. These patterns are not mutually exclusive as mixed or intermediate patterns occur. It is important to recognize that the magnitude of enzyme elevations, even with ALT, is not prognostic for survival. Certainly severe elevations are viewed with more concern in our clinical judgments and actions. But in my experience survival cannot be predicted proportionately to the level of enzyme elevations. Hepatocellular injury is often more defined by ALT elevations. Conceptually a very high value could be caused by the death of a few pockets of hepatocytes with a proportionately large release of enzyme or from large numbers of mildly injured cell membranes that leak a little ALT from each cell. With an acute DALD that is more direct in type, it is not uncommon to see the ALT rise first, followed by the ALP and then bilirubin. The presence of persistent elevations of liver enzymes in the course of chronic drug use (e.g., phenobarbital) requires investigation to prevent progressive damage to the liver. Ascites is not common at the time of initial presentation unless intrahepatic or portal venous thrombosis has occurred.

Routine radiographs of the abdomen should be taken because this remains the primary method of estimating liver size for a given patient. In acute DALD the liver may be swollen, whereas in chronic disease the liver may be atrophied or cirrhotic. Abdominal sonography is now commonly performed to help assess structural changes to the liver. This does not provide specific tissue information, but assists with the formation of the differential diagnoses, clinical assessment, and further treatment and diagnostic plans. Increasing availability of computerized tomography and magnetic resonance imaging may add further insight into determination of types of injury.

Fine-needle aspiration cytology or liver biopsy should only be done if there is a question of diagnosis related to the history or an inconsistent finding with imaging (see Chapter 126). Before invasive testing the patient should be stabilized, and coagulation testing performed. I believe that a buccal (oral) mucosal bleeding time test is very relevant when used in conjunction with the prothrombin time, partial thromboplastin time, and platelet numbers. When activated clotting time is done in a standardized manner, it may also be used to test for a severe coagulopathy.

Diagnosis is often made via the history, symptoms, and supportive findings in clinical pathology. *If a DALD event is suspected, rechallenge of the drug should not be pursued.* The differential diagnostic list for DALD often includes acute leptospirosis, fulminant toxoplasmosis, infectious canine hepatitis, feline infectious peritonitis, per acute Rocky Mountain spotted fever, per acute ehrlichiosis, trauma, septic ascending cholangiohepatitis, *Amanita* (mushroom) poisoning, aflatoxin ingestion, blue/green algae, disseminated intravascular coagulation, unknown drug ingestion, and acute necrotizing pancreatitis. Consideration of the patient's environment, medical history, drug exposures, and previously discussed testing all are needed to make a diagnosis. In some cases the process of elimination results in a "clinical or probable" diagnosis of DALD.

TREATMENT AND MONITORING

When a DALD event is diagnosed, the clinician's judgment determines the degree of intervention required and the need for hospitalization. There should be a strong emphasis on nursing care for patients with DALD. In mild cases removal from the suspect drug is the first and only step required. With moderate-to-severe presentations, emphasis switches to more intensive efforts. The maintenance of microvascular perfusion in the liver is essential. This is done via correction of hypovolemic situations using replacement crystalloid fluids. Assessment of acid base status is part of critical care monitoring; sodium bicarbonate solutions may be used in correction of acidosis. The reader should refer to specific guidelines in acid-base management (see Chapter 10). In severe cases, I place a central venous double-lumen catheter to provide flexibility in treatment and to give partial parenteral nutrition. I commonly use solutions containing 2.5% to 5% dextrose while monitoring blood glucose levels. Monitoring of electrolytes should be routine, and supplementation adjusted as needed, particularly potassium if using dextrose concurrently. If hypoalbuminemia is present, colloid therapy is advised (e.g., Hetastarch or frozen plasma). Vitamin K$_1$ is often administered (0.5 to 1 mg/kg q12–24h subcutaneously [SQ]) until coagulation status is clearly established. Nasal oxygen therapy is advised in severe cases to assist with likely hypoxia in the edematous, damaged liver. Glutathione is one of the most potent antioxidant substances on which the liver relies and has been shown to be depleted in cases of liver disease. Administration of thiol and glutathione precursors is advised in moderate-to-severe cases. Some severe situations of acute liver failure (e.g., acetaminophen toxicity) are treated as recommended with N-acetylcysteine. The dose is generally started at 140 mg/kg diluted in equal volume of saline and given by slow intravenous infusion. This is followed with 70 mg/kg diluted in saline, slow intravenous infusion, every 6 hours for five to eight treatments or until the patient can be given oral medications. I have found this treatment to be helpful for acetaminophen, thiacetarsemide, amanita, and undetermined and acute nonsteroidal antiinflammatory drug– related DALD. Because sepsis and septic enterotoxic shock are always possible in severely ill patients, coverage with antibiotics is generally advised. Use of intravenous ampicillin (20 mg/kg intravenously [IV] q8h) with enrofloxacin (5 mg/kg IV q24h) or use of ampicillin with sulbactam (10 to 20 mg/kg IV or intramuscularly [IM] q8h) are common initial regimens. Because B vitamins serve as cofactors to many metabolic processes within the liver and they can be depleted rapidly with fluid therapy, it is common to supplement vitamin B–complex preparations via parenteral administration but with no specific guidelines as to dose. I commonly administer 0.01 ml/kg subcutaneously every 24 hours. Prolonged inanition may require parenteral nutritional support. It is likely that 50% of calorie support is more realistic as a goal while the patient is critically ill. When a patient can take oral feedings again, this becomes the preferred route for nutrition and medications. Use of s-adenosylmethionine (SAMe) in an oral stable formulation (15 to 20 mg/kg orally [PO] q24h) is advised for support of metabolic function and replenishing glutathione stores (see Chapter 128). It should be given with at least a 2-hour separation from feedings, which may limit its use in some cases. Gastric hyperacidity has been reported to be present in humans with severe liver disease. Use of parenteral antacids initially should be with famotidine (0.5 mg/kg IV, PO, SQ q12h). Use of omeprazole at 0.7 to 1 mg/kg orally can be added as the patient becomes oral. I also introduce ursodiol (8 mg/kg PO q24h) as part of long-term management. Vitamin E (d-α-tocopherol) (100 to 400 units per patient per day) is given long term. Use of a well-trusted milk thistle component such as silybin is also thought to be helpful, but no specific dosages are documented for effectiveness in dogs or cats (see Chapter 128).

Management of hepatic encephalopathy (HE) generally is not indicated as part of initial therapy. As a caution, reintroduction of food is often with moderate protein diets until hepatic function is more clearly established. If HE is determined to be present based on clinical signs, standard care with lactulose orally and lactulose and cleansing enemas should be pursued.

If the patient is responding to treatment and withdrawal of the involved drug, the primary indicators may be the patient's vital signs and status. The ALT often decreases 30% to 40% in each 24-hour period; but the ALP and the total bilirubin to a lesser extent may continue to rise as secondary cholestatic effects become manifest. Consistently rising bilirubin without subjective patient improvement is a poor prognostic indicator in human cases of DALD. It may also be prognostic in veterinary medicine since it can suggest secondary fibrosis resulting from inflammatory events and hence partial or complete extrahepatic biliary obstruction or intracellular cholestasis.

Treatment is adjusted constantly via reassessment of the patient and monitoring of laboratory values as warranted to the situation. For a moderately to severely ill patient, it is not uncommon to be hospitalized for 3 to 10 days. As recovery progresses, it remains important to maintain supportive fluids and medications and to retest chemistries, prothrombin time, urinalyses, and blood counts every 24 to 48 hours initially and then spreading out the interval between laboratory testing based on patient assessment. For several months after apparent recovery, it is suggested to monitor these tests and occasionally use paired serum bile acids since post-necrotic cirrhosis can occur. In human medicine some drugs causing DALD (e.g., acetaminophen, dantrolene, isoniazid) have been demonstrated to initiate immune chronic hepatitis, and this may be the case in some veterinary cases as well.

The presentation for DALD is variable. The review of the history, signalment, and environment is critical along with the physical examination in making a diagnosis of DALD. In cases with significant symptoms, aggressive treatment and monitoring are advised. The degree of elevation of liver enzymes, although alarming, is not necessarily predictive of outcome. Aggressive treatment efforts should be pursued, with removal of suspected drugs being the first step. It is advised that the veterinary practitioner faced with a case of DALD review other involved topics dealing with the diagnosis and management of liver diseases in dogs and cats. Some of this information is available in other chapters within this section.

Suggested Reading

Mealey KL: Adverse drug reactions in herding-breed dogs: the role of P-glycoprotein, *Compend Contin Educ Pract Vet* 28(1):23, 2006.

Navaro VJ, Senior JR: Drug-related hepatotoxicity, *N Engl J Med* 354(7):731, 2006.

Trepanier LA: Idiosyncratic toxicity associated with potentiated sulfonamides in the dog, *J Vet Pharmacol Ther* 27(3):129, 2004.

Twedt DC et al: Association of hepatic necrosis with trimethoprim sulfonamide administration in 4 dogs, *J Vet Intern Med* 11(1):20, 1997.

US Food and Drug Administration: Cumulative Veterinary Adverse Drug Experience (ADE) Reports—1987 to Oct 3, 2006, US Food and Drug Administration, Center for Veterinary Medicine, www.fda.gov/cvm/ade_cum.htm.

CHAPTER 132

Feline Hepatic Lipidosis

KATHLEEN M. HOLAN, *East Lansing, Michigan*

Feline hepatic lipidosis (HL) is a commonly recognized clinical syndrome observed in debilitated domestic cats. By definition it is the excessive accumulation of lipid within hepatocytes. Ultimately in cats it has the potential to lead to severe hepatic dysfunction and even death. HL occurs either as an idiopathic (primary) condition or secondary to some other primary pathologic process. Development of this disease depends on the establishment of a catabolic state that leads to enhanced mobilization of peripheral fat stores to the liver in conjunction with impaired dissemination of lipid from hepatocytes. The exact physiologic mechanisms that lead to the development of HL are still incompletely understood and are likely multifactorial. A fact that is understood relates to the importance of early recognition along with the prompt initiation of appropriate nutritional therapy. These factors are pivotal to successful management and recovery in the great majority of our affected feline patients.

PATHOPHYSIOLOGY

There are many metabolic and hormonal mechanisms involved in normal feline lipid metabolism. Specifically these mechanisms include those that are responsible for the mobilization of peripheral fat from adipocytes to the liver, as well as those responsible for fatty acid metabolism within the liver and subsequent removal of lipid from hepatocytes. Aspects of protein metabolism unique to obligate carnivores add essential metabolic requirements to overall feline lipid metabolism. The adipocyte, under the influence of hormone-sensitive lipase and lipoprotein lipase and with its ability to contribute to hormonal control of lipid metabolism and appetite control, is increasingly appreciated as an important potential "player" in the development of feline HL syndrome. Prolonged protein malnutrition can have severe consequences, resulting in derangement in all aspects of normal feline lipid metabolism. Systemic oxidative injury, to which cats are particularly susceptible under normal conditions, is also greatly augmented. Better understanding of these mechanisms will undoubtedly improve our ability to treat and prevent HL.

HISTORY AND CLINICAL SIGNS

A majority of cats that develop HL are historically overweight, and most have experienced a period of anorexia before the onset of lipidosis (Barsanti et al., 1977; Center et al., 1993). Although the triggering event for the development of anorexia is often difficult to identify, a complete review of a cat's recent history may elucidate an acute illness or change in environment sufficient to instigate anorexia and subsequent lipidosis. Cats of any age can develop HL; however, most tend to be middle-aged or older and of either sex. There is no known breed predilection.

Affected cats can present with a variety of clinical signs, including anorexia, depression, weakness, vomiting, ptyalism, diarrhea or constipation, and weight loss. Weakness, depression, and ptyalism may also indicate concurrent hepatic encephalopathy (HE). Physical examination findings often include dehydration, an unkempt coat, icterus, hepatomegaly, and ventriflexion of the neck. Many systemic diseases have been associated with HL in cats, including but not limited to diabetes mellitus, pancreatitis, inflammatory bowel disease, cholangiohepatitis, and various neoplasias. Abnormal physical examination findings related to specific underlying disease processes may also be identified.

DIAGNOSTICS

The purpose of the diagnostic workup in cats with HL is twofold. One is to definitively diagnose the presence of lipidosis within the liver, and the second is to simultaneously rule in or out the presence of an underlying disease process. The diagnostic approach typically begins with a minimum database (complete blood count, biochemical profile, and urine analysis), coagulation profile, diagnostic imaging, and ultimately the procurement of hepatic samples for cytologic and/or histopathologic evaluation. Additional diagnostic tests to help rule out concurrent diseases or as dictated by a patient's clinical status may also be within the initial diagnostic plan. These frequently include a thyroid hormone profile, feline leukemia virus/feline immunodeficiency virus testing, feline pancreatic lipase immunoreactivity (fPLI), and thoracic radiographs.

Blood Work

The complete blood count of a lipidotic cat can be normal or may exhibit changes, including a stress leukogram, nonregenerative anemia, poikilocytosis, or the presence of Heinz bodies. The presence of an inflammatory leukogram should alert the clinician to an underlying disorder. It is important to note that, even if not present initially, anemia, poikilocytosis, and Heinz bodies all have the potential to develop during treatment and therefore warrant close monitoring of the hematocrit.

The biochemical profile of HL patients may reflect a variety of abnormalities as they relate specifically to cholestasis or to other processes occurring. Common liver enzyme abnormalities include elevated activities of alkaline phosphatase, alanine aminotransferase (ALT), and aspartate aminotransferase. Total bilirubin is usually elevated, and blood urea nitrogen may be normal or decreased. In contrast to other hepatobiliary diseases with a significant necroinflammatory component, HL is not usually associated with elevated γ-glutamyltranspeptidase activity (Center et al., 1986). Hypokalemia, hypochloremia, hypophosphatemia, and hypomagnesemia may be present as the consequence of anorexia or vomiting or may develop during treatment as a result of volume expansion or refeeding. Other biochemical alterations that might be observed include subnormal albumin, increased cholesterol, and hyperglycemia.

The urine analysis of lipidotic cats may reveal lipiduria. An abnormal finding may be bilirubinuria, which precedes the development of hyperbilirubinemia.

Coagulation abnormalities are common in cats with HL. In the largest retrospective study of cats with HL, 45% of cats tested had one or more present (Center et al., 1993). The most common coagulopathy was prolongation of the prothrombin time (PT) as a result of vitamin K deficiency. Vitamin K deficiency in cats with HL can be the result of anorexia, malabsorption caused by severe cholestasis, or decreased production by enteric bacteria secondary to antibiotic therapy. Interestingly, of the 45% of cats with coagulopathies (20 of 44 cats tested) only 3 of 20 had demonstrable bleeding tendencies (Center et al., 1993). This finding underscores the importance of screening for coagulopathies in cats with suspected HL. Hypofibrinogenemia, likely the result of decreased hepatic production, is another coagulopathy noted in cats with HL (Center et al., 1993). Clinical tests available for the assessment of coagulation status include a platelet count, PT, activated partial thromboplastin time (APTT), fibrinogen, fibrin degradation products, and the proteins invoked by vitamin K absence (PIVKA) clotting test (Thrombotest; Nycomed AS). Although PIVKA may be a more sensitive indicator of prolonged clotting times in clinically ill cats, including cats with HL, when compared to PT, APTT, fibrinogen, and thrombocytopenia (Center et al., 2000), it is not readily available in all laboratories. Cats with coagulation abnormalities should be treated with parenteral vitamin K_1 as described later in this chapter.

Liver function tests often considered in cats with HL include measurement of serum bile acids and/or measurement of fasting ammonia levels or tolerance. Most cats with HL are hyperbilirubinemic at the time of presentation, which precludes any additional diagnostic value of measuring serum bile acids. Measurement of serum bile acids may be indicated in the (rare) nonicteric, nonbilirubinuric patient suspected of having HL. Although HE is not a common metabolic consequence of HL, assessment of a fasting ammonia level may be used as a means of diagnosing its presence in cases in which there is a high clinical index of suspicion. However, not all animals with HE have an elevated fasting ammonia level, and there is poor correlation between the degree of elevation of ammonia and clinical HE. Patients with suspected encephalopathy should be fed a protein-restricted diet

such as Prescription Diet k/d (Hill's Pet Nutrition, Inc.) or Feline NF (Nestle Purina PetCare Co.). Lactulose (0.25 to 5 ml q8–12h orally [PO]) should also be administered. The dosage is adjusted until semiformed stools are produced. In moribund patients without enteral access, lactulose can be administered rectally as a retention enema using three parts lactulose to seven parts water. The solution (20 ml/kg q4–6h) should be left in place for 15 to 20 minutes. Antibiotic therapy may also be instituted to help reduce colonic bacteria responsible for ammonia production. Metronidazole (7.5 mg/kg q12h PO), ampicillin (22 mg/kg q8h PO), or neomycin sulfate (20 mg/kg q8–12h PO) can be used to help manage HE. Neomycin sulfate liquid in water (22 mg/kg) can also be used as a retention enema.

Diagnostic Imaging

Abdominal radiography and ultrasonography are commonly used to evaluate the liver and other organs of HL patients. Hepatobiliary scintigraphy and computed tomography are other modalities that have been evaluated for diagnosis of HL, but neither has proven to be clinically reliable. Radiographic changes observed in HL patients can include hepatomegaly and rarely an abdominal effusion. Ultrasonography offers the advantage of examination of other organs associated with diseases that are common predisposing conditions for the development of HL. In addition to the liver, the stomach, intestines, lymph nodes, biliary system, and pancreas can also be evaluated. Ultrasonographically the livers of cats with HL often appear diffusely hyperechoic relative to the falciform fat and may be mildly or moderately enlarged. Careful evaluation of associated organs should always be performed because abnormalities in any of these organs may alter the diagnostic recommendations if more invasive techniques necessitate adequate biopsy sampling.

Fine-Needle Aspiration

Although definitive diagnosis of HL requires histopathologic confirmation, ultrasound-guided fine-needle aspiration of the liver provides cytologic samples that in most cases are adequate for establishing a preliminary diagnosis of HL. Cytologic confirmation of HL is made when a representative sample of liver tissue demonstrates cytosolic vacuolization of at least 50% of the hepatocytes. However, it is important to remember that fine-needle aspiration is not a reliable means of diagnosing inflammatory liver diseases and may miss focal neoplasia. Therefore cytologic diagnosis must always be interpreted with caution and in accordance with hematologic and biochemical and clinical findings. Identification of inflammatory cells or any cells that are not expected hepatic parenchymal cells should prompt recommendation for hepatic biopsy.

Liver Biopsy

As previously stated, the definitive way to diagnose HL is via histopathologic evaluation. Liver biopsy also offers the ability to evaluate hepatic lobular architecture for the presence of inflammatory conditions such as cholangitis or cholangiohepatitis that fine-needle aspiration cannot determine. However, the clinician must make important clinical considerations before deciding whether to pursue a biopsy. These include the status of the patient, as well as the method used to get a biopsy sample. Because all biopsy procedures require the use of general anesthesia, many cats are not candidates for biopsy at the time of presentation. Existing coagulation abnormalities and metabolic disturbances must be corrected before anesthesia, given the potential for complications during biopsy procedures. Many HL patients must be stabilized for a period of days before they are good anesthetic candidates. For these reasons, along with the relative reliability of fine-needle cytologic findings, not all cats with HL need to have their livers biopsied. Often the decision to do so is reserved for cases that are not improving in response to supportive care or when other suspected diseases are present that warrant biopsy of other organs via laparoscopy or exploratory laparotomy.

TREATMENT

Treatment of HL centers on providing appropriate nutritional support to reverse the catabolic state that has developed while also providing adequate fluid therapy and managing any clinical complications such as vomiting, HE, or bleeding tendencies.

Feeding Methods

Most cats with HL are anorectic at the time of presentation. This almost always necessitates the placement of a feeding tube for enteral nutritional support. Force feeding is one method of delivering nutrition that is tolerated by some cats without the placement of a feeding tube, but in many cases tends to exacerbate preexisting nausea and vomiting. This method frequently does not deliver enough calories to metabolically reverse HL and may also cause a food aversion syndrome that can ultimately lead to a delay in the return to self-alimentation (Center, 2005). In my view this method is only recommended when financial limitations prevent placement of a feeding tube and is *not* an option in vomiting or moribund patients. The types of feeding tubes available for placement include nasogastric, esophagostomy, and gastrostomy tubes. See Bonagura (2000) and Chapter 136 for discussions regarding feeding tubes.

Dietary Considerations

Provision of a high-quality protein diet in amounts that deliver enough energy to reverse the progression of HL is the most important aspect of therapy for feline HL. Diets that derive the majority of their calories from protein or fat are preferable. Many commercially available diets meet these requirements, including Clinicare, Abbott Laboratories; Maximum Calorie, CNM Feline CV formula, Feline Nutritional Recovery Formula, The Iams Co.; and Prescription Diets a/d, m/d, c/d, or p/d, Hill's Pet Nutrition, Inc. The exception to feeding a high-quality protein diet is the encephalopathic patient, in which case this type of diet is contraindicated. In all situations the use of a specifically feline diet is recommended. Diets formulated for other species often lack essential nutrients required for feline metabolism. If such diets are used, supplementation with taurine (250 mg/day) and arginine (250 mg/100 kcal) is recommended. Cats with preexisting medical conditions may have dietary limitations that preclude the use of a high-protein diet. Usually these diets suffice during the recovery period and need not be changed.

Although the exact energy requirements for cats with liver disease are not known, there are formulas readily available for calculation of basal and recovery energy requirements. Bonagura (2000) lists these calculations along with feeding regimen recommendations.

Nutritional Supplementation

Over the years a large number of nutritional supplements have been advocated for the treatment of HL in cats. Most have been recommended based on their role in various aspects of lipid metabolism, the urea cycle, or because of their antioxidative effects. Unfortunately there are few controlled studies in cats with HL to either prove or disprove their beneficial effects. Some nutritional supplements appear to have good empiric and/or scientific evidence in cats or other species to imply a potential benefit, while other supplements have been reported to improve survival rates of cats with HL (Center, 2005). It also makes sense in many cases to prescribe other supplements to replace perceived metabolic deficits in patients not consuming adequate calories in spite of lacking scientific evidence. Most are safe when given at recommended dosages and do not to potentiate harmful consequences. It must be stated that there is no consensus among clinicians regarding the necessity of nutritional supplementation for cats with HL, and fortunately many of these patients are able to recover and survive without it. Ultimately the decision to use nutritional supplements is often based on clinician experience and supplement availability. In my hospital supplementation tends to depend mainly on clinician preference and experience. B vitamins, including cobalamin, are fairly routinely administered; antioxidant therapy is more variable. Amino acids are supplemented infrequently. Commonly considered supplements are categorized below.

Water-Soluble Vitamins
Anorectic cats are susceptible to depletion of B vitamins, especially thiamine (B_1) and cobalamin (B_{12}). Cats with underlying intestinal disease are especially prone to cobalamin deficiency. The addition of 1 to 2 ml of a fortified B-vitamin complex per liter of crystalloid fluids is recommended for thiamine deficiency. If added, the fluids should be protected from direct light. Plasma cobalamin (B_{12}) levels should be measured in any cat suspected of having HL or underlying intestinal disease. Often cats are given an empiric initial dose of 250 to 500 mcg subcutaneously, with subsequent therapy, if indicated, based on results of plasma levels.

Fat-Soluble Vitamins
Vitamin E (α-tocopherol) is a potent hepatic antioxidant, and depletion of vitamin E is suspected to occur in cats

with HL, thereby lessening the ability of the liver to protect itself against oxidative damage. Although not scientifically proven to be efficacious, dosage ranges between 10 units/kg/day orally and 100 units/cat every 12 hours orally have been recommended.

Vitamin K_1 is administered for treatment of coagulopathies. Dosages of 0.5 to 1.5 mg/kg every 12 hours subcutaneously for three treatments have been shown to be effective in correcting coagulation abnormalities in cats with HL based on PIVKA testing (Center et al., 2005). Because of cholestatic interference with normal absorption, oral administration should be avoided. Excessive or prolonged administration should also be avoided because oxidative injury to organs and red blood cells can ensue. Cats that continue to have coagulation abnormalities despite vitamin K_1 therapy may have more severe hemostatic derangements such as disseminated intravascular coagulopathy and may require transfusions of whole blood or fresh frozen plasma.

Amino Acids

L-carnitine is essential for hepatic lipid metabolism. Studies have suggested that cats with HL may develop a relative deficiency of L-carnitine and that supplementation in cats undergoing weight loss helps to increase fatty acid oxidation and decrease lipid accumulation within hepatocytes. Dosages of 250 to 500 mg per cat per day are recommended. Medical grade L-carnitine has better bioavailability than other commercial products and is recommended over other formulations. Taurine is an essential amino acid for cats, and cats with HL have lower plasma concentrations of taurine than healthy cats. Taurine is important in feline bile acid conjugation, as well as other normal metabolic processes that can become disrupted during the development of HL. A dosage of 250 to 500 mg/day either every 24 hours or divided every 12 hours can be added to the food.

Antioxidants

S-adenosylmethionine (SAMe) is essential for the hepatocellular production of glutathione (GSH), and GSH produced in the liver acts as a systemic antioxidant. As a result of protein malnutrition, decreased hepatic levels of SAMe and GSH during HL predispose the liver, other organs, and red blood cells to oxidative injury. SAMe, at an initial dosage of 35 to 60 mg/kg every 12 to 24 hours or a maintenance dosage of 20 mg/kg every 24 hours, is recommended to help reestablish normal liver GSH levels and prevent the formation of Heinz bodies. Because the bioavailability of SAMe is reduced in the presence of food, administration on an empty stomach is preferred. Ursodeoxycholic acid is a hydrophilic bile acid with many beneficial properties, including antiinflammatory and antioxidative effects. Ursodeoxycholic acid promotes bile flow and potentially lessens the noxious effects of more hydrophobic bile acids through alteration of their concentration. Its potential benefit in cats with HL is not known. The use of ursodeoxycholic acid is contraindicated in the presence of any obstruction of biliary outflow. It is well tolerated, and side effects are uncommon. The recommended dosage is 10 to 15 mg/kg every 24 hours.

Fluid Therapy

Cats with HL are usually dehydrated at the time of presentation and require fluid therapy to correct both existing and ongoing fluid losses from vomiting and diarrhea, if present. In most cases, intravenous fluid therapy is the preferred route of administration. Subcutaneous fluids can be administered in mild cases if owner objection because of cost or hospitalization prohibits placement of an indwelling intravenous catheter. Owners can be taught to administer subcutaneous fluids at home, which is helpful in situations in which intravenous fluids are not an option. In general, this method is not advisable for very debilitated patients or patients with profuse vomiting or diarrhea. A balanced, polyionic crystalloid fluid such as Ringer's or lactated Ringer's solution is recommended for initial support. In cases of severe HL, concern regarding the inability of the liver to properly metabolize lactate may make solutions without lactate a better choice if available. Dextrose-containing fluids should be avoided since carbohydrates tend to promote hepatic triglyceride accumulation, inhibit hepatocellular fatty acid oxidation, and may exacerbate hypokalemia and hypophosphatemia via insulin stimulation.

Electrolyte Therapy

Electrolyte imbalances are often identified in HL patients at the time of presentation or may develop during treatment as a result of fluid therapy or refeeding. Hypokalemia is the most common electrolyte abnormality in cats with HL and is significantly associated with failure to survive (Center et al., 1993). Lethargy, muscle weakness, ventriflexion of the neck, intestinal stasis, myocardial depression, and inability to concentrate urine can all start to develop when serum K^+ is 2.5 mEq/L or less. Supplementation in the form of potassium chloride (KCl) is added to the fluids. The amount of K^+ added to fluids depends mostly on the initial serum levels and the rate of administration of the intravenous fluids. The rate of administration of KCl should never exceed 0.5 mEq/kg/hour. Initially serum potassium levels should be monitored twice daily to ensure adequate supplementation, especially as refeeding begins. Serum potassium levels can worsen as a consequence of the insulin-mediated intracellular shift that occurs in response to alimentation and may necessitate more aggressive supplementation. Persistent hypokalemia in the face of otherwise appropriate therapy may be the result of concurrent hypomagnesemia and warrants assessment of serum magnesium levels. Hypomagnesemia-induced hypokalemia will not resolve until the hypomagnesemia is corrected. Magnesium is an important enzyme cofactor, and low serum levels can cause muscle weakness manifesting in many of the same clinical signs observed with hypokalemia and hypophosphatemia. Supplementation is in the form of intravenous administration of either magnesium sulfate or magnesium chloride, which are packaged as 50% solutions. They should be administered as 20% solutions in 5% dextrose and water (D_5W). An initial starting dosage of 0.75 to 1 mEq/kg/day continuous-rate infusion (CRI) is given the first day, after which the dosage is lowered to 0.3

to 0.5 mEq/kg/day for another 2 to 5 days. Serum levels should be monitored daily. Overdoses are treated with calcium gluconate given intravenously at a 50-mg bolus followed by a 10 mg/kg/hour CRI.

Hypophosphatemia is a potentially serious electrolyte abnormality that may be evident at the time of presentation or more likely develop as a result of refeeding. Cats with HL may be hypophosphatemic from low intake, decreased intestinal absorption, or increased renal loss. With the introduction of food, stimulation of insulin secretion promotes intracellular uptake of phosphorus and glucose, further lowering serum levels within 12 to 72 hours of the commencement of feeding (Justin and Hohenhaus, 1995). Manifestations of hypophosphatemia can include muscle weakness, hemolytic anemia, leukocyte dysfunction, platelet dysfunction, and decreased tissue oxygenation as a result of decreased levels of 2,3,-diphosphoglycerate. Phosphorus is supplemented when serum levels fall below 2 mg/dl. Intravenous administration of either potassium phosphate or sodium phosphate is recommended at 0.01 to 0.06 mmol/kg/hour. These need to be given in calcium-free solutions to prevent precipitation of calcium phosphate. If potassium phosphate is used, the potassium content needs to be taken into consideration when calculating overall potassium supplementation. During treatment, serum phosphorus and calcium levels should be monitored twice daily since hypocalcemia can be a consequence of intravenous phosphate therapy (Adams et al., 1993). Once phosphorus levels are above 2 mg/dl, the intravenous dosage can be reduced by 50% and tapered off shortly thereafter. Oral supplementation can continue until serum levels are within the normal range. The recommended oral dosage is 0.5 to 2 mmol/kg/day. Skim milk or commercial phosphate supplements can be offered orally or provided through a feeding tube. For patients with lactose intolerance, use of lactose-free products divided into multiple small servings can help prevent diarrhea from occurring. Phosphorus supplementation should always be closely monitored, especially in patients with concurrent renal disease. It is not recommended in cats that are oliguric or hypercalcemic (Griffin, 2000). Phosphate binders such as aluminum hydroxide or sucralfate should not be used in patients with low phosphorus levels.

Hypocalcemia, if present, may be secondary to acute pancreatitis or may develop as a result of phosphorus supplementation. This is an uncommon finding, and treatment usually is not necessary unless clinical signs of deficiency develop.

Additional Therapeutic Considerations

Control of Vomiting

Vomiting is a common clinical problem in cats with HL. Causes include electrolyte imbalances, gastric and intestinal stasis, excessive feeding, feeding tube complications, liver dysfunction, or underlying diseases such as inflammatory bowel disease or pancreatitis. The use of antiemetics is often necessary in the initial management of HL. However, in conjunction with antiemetic therapy, the clinician should always be sure to reevaluate aspects of intestinal health, as well as feeding and feeding tube issues. Constipation is a common sequela of dehydration, and evacuation of impacted fecal material can help to establish normal intestinal motility. Feeding tubes should be evaluated for any signs of irritation or infection at the site of placement. Concerns regarding tube placement or possible kinking can be addressed with radiography and are enhanced with the administration of a radiopaque iodinated contrast solution into the tube. Cats with HL frequently have gastric atony from prolonged anorexia, and even small meals can induce vomiting as a result of gastric distension. Alternatively many cats do very well initially, with food delivered as a CRI. This is best accomplished by providing a liquefied diet via an intravenous fluid line that is attached to the feeding tube. Fluid or syringe pumps are used to deliver a specified number of milliliters per hour. This method tends not to overdistend the stomach and is well tolerated. The rate of delivery of food can be increased slowly over a period of days to ensure tolerance while the frequency of vomiting is diminished. Once this is accomplished, a transition to individual meals can be made.

Despite these considerations, many cats still require medical antiemetic therapy. Metoclopramide is usually the initial drug of choice and can either be administered in fluids as a CRI (0.01 to 0.02 mg/kg/hour or 1 to 2 mg/kg/day) or given subcutaneously (0.2 to 0.5 mg/kg q8h SQ 30 minutes before feeding a meal). Metoclopramide has antiemetic and prokinetic effects, both of which are beneficial in HL patients. In cases in which vomiting is not controlled with metoclopramide, use of ondansetron (Zofran, Glaxo Wellcome; 0.1 mg/kg q12–24h PO or 0.1 to 0.3 mg/kg q8–12h intravenously [IV]) or dolasetron (Anzemet, Hoecht Marion Russel; 0.5 mg/kg q24h PO, SQ, IV) is usually effective. In my opinion these are the second antiemetics of choice. My hospital frequently uses dolasetron because of its decreased frequency of administration. These drugs are relatively expensive, which may prohibit their use. Phenothiazine derivatives are associated with marked side effects and are contraindicated in patients with hepatic insufficiency. Their use is not recommended in cats with HL.

Promotility agents are often used in HL patients, especially when significant gastric and intestinal stasis is suspected. As mentioned, metoclopramide at recommended dosages offers the advantage of promoting gastric emptying in addition to its antiemetic effects. For many cats this therapy alone is enough. Additional benefit, if needed, may be gained by the addition of cisapride to the treatment regimen. Cisapride (0.1 to 0.5 mg/kg q8–12h PO) is a more potent stimulator of intestinal motility than metoclopramide and can be helpful in patients that are refractory to metoclopramide or in those that have not produced a bowel movement despite several days of significant alimentation. Ranitidine (Zantac, Glaxo Wellcome), an H_2 receptor antagonist with some prokinetic activity may also be considered (0.5 to 2 mg/kg q8–12h PO, IV) but in my experience is not as effective as cisapride for increasing intestinal motility.

H_2 receptor blockers decrease gastric acid production and are considered beneficial because of their ability to help alleviate the symptoms of gastritis or gastric ulceration that can be associated with liver disease and inflammatory bowel disease. Famotidine (Pepcid, Merck Sharp Dohme), cimetidine (Tagamet, Smith Kline French), nizatidine (Axid, Eli Lily), and ranitidine are options. Famotidine (0.5 to 1 mg/kg q12–24 hr, PO, IV) is the most common H_2 receptor blocker used in our hospital. Advantages include once-daily dosing and the fact that it does not affect hepatic P-450 enzymes. Cimetidine should be avoided because of its effect on the hepatic P-450 enzymes.

Antibiotic Therapy

Prophylactic antibiotic therapy for HL is not recommended. However, complications might arise that warrant their use. These can include development of bacterial infections either at the site of the feeding tube or intravenous catheter placement or the presence of HE, discussed earlier in this chapter. Appropriate antibiotic therapy should be based on culture and sensitivity results whenever possible; otherwise broad-spectrum antimicrobial coverage should be considered. Tetracyclines should not be used in cats with HL because of their untoward effects on hepatocellular metabolism (Center, 2005).

Appetite Stimulation

For many reasons the use of appetite stimulants to encourage self-alimentation in cats with HL is not advised. Many of the commonly recommended drugs, including diazepam, oxazepam, clonazepam, and cyproheptadine, require hepatic metabolism and have been associated with hepatic failure. Benzodiazepines may act to activate the γ-aminobutyric acid/benzodiazepine receptor system, a theorized factor in the pathogenesis of HE. For reasons discussed in the following paragraph, propofol should also not be used for appetite stimulation in cats with HL.

Drugs Not Recommended

In general, steroids are not recommended for treatment of HL. Glucocorticoids are catabolic and can interfere with normal hepatocellular lipid metabolism. Stanozolol (Winstrol R, Winthrop), an anabolic steroid occasionally prescribed for use in cats, has been shown to produce hepatotoxicity (Harkin et al., 2000). Any drugs that are associated with increased risk of oxidative injury should also be avoided. In cats these include products with propylene glycol carriers and benzene derivatives. Vitamin K_1 therapy can be associated with the development of Heinz bodies and resultant hemolytic reactions that can occur with either excessive or prolonged dosing. Propofol toxicity can develop in cats with HL. Although the exact causes for this are not completely understood, proposed mechanisms include

an inability to properly metabolize the phenol component of the drug, as well as impaired mitochondrial fatty acid oxidation, a syndrome observed in critical human pediatric patients (Center, 2005).

MONITORING

The amount of monitoring necessary for successful management of cats with HL is somewhat case dependent. Cats that are not extremely debilitated or exhibit few complications at the time of presentation or cats that begin eating shortly after supportive measures have begun may not require a large degree of intensive monitoring before they are able to be managed at home. Others require intensive monitoring of their electrolytes, hematocrit, and coagulation status for many days before and after the placement of a feeding tube. Once a cat has been stabilized and a feeding tube placed, the immediate 72 hours tend to be the most critical time for the development of life-threatening electrolyte disturbances as a result of refeeding. After that, periodic checks of liver parameters, including total bilirubin, serum alkaline phosphatase, and ALT, are helpful to establish either a trend toward normalization or to raise suspicion for the need for further diagnostics. If metabolic imbalances can be managed and vomiting controlled, most cats are able to make a full recovery within weeks.

References and Suggested Reading

Adams LG et al: Hypophosphatemia and hemolytic anemia associated with diabetes mellitus and hepatic lipidosis in cats, *J Vet Intern Med* 7:266, 1993.

Barsanti JA et al: Prolonged anorexia associated with hepatic lipidosis in three cats, *Feline Pract* 7:52, 1977.

Bonagura JD, editor: *Kirk's current veterinary therapy XIII (small animal practice)*, Philadelphia, 2000, Saunders, pp 84, 597, 688.

Center SA et al: Diagnostic value of serum gamma-glutamyl transferase and alkaline phosphatase activities in hepatobiliary disease in the cat, *J Am Vet Med Assoc* 188:507, 1986.

Center SA et al: A retrospective study of 77 cats with severe hepatic lipidosis, *J Vet Intern Med* 7:349, 1993.

Center SA et al: Proteins invoked by vitamin K absence and clotting times in clinically ill cats, *J Vet Intern Med* 14:292, 2000.

Center SA: Feline hepatic lipidosis. In Richards JR, editor: *Veterinary clinics of North America small animal practice*, Philadelphia, 2005, Saunders, pp 246, 253, 256, 260.

Griffin B: Feline hepatic lipidosis: Treatment recommendations. *Compend Cont Educ Pract Vet* 22(10):910, 2000.

Justin RB, Hohenhaus AE: Hypophosphatemia associated with enteral alimentation in cats, *J Vet Intern Med* 9:228, 1995.

Harkin KR et al: Hepatotoxicity of stanozolol in cats, *J Am Vet Med Assoc* 217:681, 2000.

CHAPTER 133

Feline Inflammatory Liver Disease

DAVID C. TWEDT, *Fort Collins, Colorado*
P. JANE ARMSTRONG, *St. Paul, Minnesota*

Liver disease is a common clinical finding in the cat. The disorders described are most frequently hepatic lipidosis, chronic inflammatory disease, neoplasia, and hepatocellular necrosis (such as toxic or drug-related conditions). This chapter covers only the common inflammatory disorders. Based on a 10-year retrospective study of feline liver biopsy data from the University of Minnesota, inflammatory liver disease is the second most common category of liver disease in cats in the United States after hepatic lipidosis (Gagne, Weiss, and Armstrong, 1996). A smaller study at Colorado State University identified a similar prevalence of lipidosis followed by inflammatory liver disease in cats having total bilirubin concentrations greater than 3 mg/dl.

THE CHOLANGITIS COMPLEX

Inflammatory liver disease in cats is confusing with regard to both nomenclature and pathologic grouping of histologic lesions. The lack of consistency in terminology has hindered our ability to clarify the clinical syndromes as to the etiology, therapy, and prognosis for the various subtypes of this disorder. Recently the World Small Animal Veterinary Association (WSAVA) sponsored an international group of pathologists and clinicians given the charge to standardize the histologic classifications of small animal liver disease. The WSAVA Liver Standardization Group now proposes a simplified classification scheme for the different types of inflammatory liver disease in cats (van den Ingh et al., 2006). Collectively inflammatory liver diseases were grouped into different types of cholangitis (Box 133-1). The WSAVA Liver Standardization Group further recommends that the term *cholangitis* be used in preference to cholangiohepatitis in cats because, unlike in dogs, the primary inflammatory changes are centered on or surrounding bile ducts. In some cases of feline cholangitis, the inflammatory changes may extend into and involve the hepatic parenchyma; this has previously been referred to as cholangiohepatitis. It should be noted that primary chronic inflammatory parenchymal disease, unrelated to specific infectious diseases such as feline infectious peritonitis or toxoplasmosis, is rare in cats. This is in contrast to dogs, in which chronic hepatitis represents the major class of inflammatory liver disease diagnosed. Disruption of the limiting plate of the portal triad with extension of inflammation into hepatic parenchyma is not considered to be a consistent feature of the feline cholangitis syndrome.

The WSAVA Liver Standardization Group recognizes three distinct forms of cholangitis in cats: neutrophilic, lymphocytic, and cholangitis associated with liver flukes. However, the reader should be aware that in the cholangitis complex there is considerable overlap of the clinical syndromes. The neutrophilic form of cholangitis can also be clinically and pathologically subdivided into an acute neutrophilic form (ANF) and a chronic (and less suppurative) neutrophilic form (CNF). These two subclassifications are thought to likely represent different stages of a single disease process. Lymphocytic cholangitis and cholangitis associated with liver flukes are also discussed but appear to be less common in occurrence. A separate entity, referred to as lymphocytic portal hepatitis, is usually mild and may represent a nonspecific reactive or aging change. However, in some cats it can be associated with clinical and/or biochemical signs of liver disease. It remains an unanswered question as to whether lymphocytic portal hepatitis is a distinct clinical syndrome or simply a common histologic lesion found in many older cats.

NEUTROPHILIC CHOLANGITIS

Neutrophilic cholangitis, previously referred to as suppurative or exudative cholangitis/cholangiohepatitis, is the most common type of biliary tract disease observed in cats in North America. Neutrophilic cholangitis is thought to be the result of biliary tract infection ascending from the gastrointestinal tract. In the ANF, the lesions are exclusively neutrophilic or suppurative, but over time it is thought that cases may progress to a CNF having a mixed inflammatory pattern containing variable numbers of neutrophils, lymphocytes, and plasma cells.

Acute Neutrophilic Form

In the ANF of cholangitis, neutrophilic inflammation is centered on the bile ducts. Enteric bacteria, most often *Escherichia coli*, may be cultured from either the bile or liver. Other bacterial isolates reported in affected cases have included *Enterococcus* spp., *Bacteroides* spp., *Clostridia* spp., *Staphylococcus*, and α-hemolytic *Streptococcus*. Preliminary investigations using culture-independent methods have also resulted in identification of deoxyribonucleic acid (DNA) sequences of *Helicobacter* spp. from a few cats with inflammatory liver disease (both ANF and CNF). These DNA sequences were enteric *Helicobacter* spp. but distinct from the reported gastric species found in cats. Further support for the enteric bacteria theory of pathogenesis comes from unpublished data that the author (DT) obtained. Enteric bacteria were observed in or around bile ducts in approximately 25% of cats that

Classification of Feline Inflammatory Liver Disease

- Neutrophilic cholangitis
  - Acute neutrophilic form
  - Chronic neutrophilic form
- Lymphocytic cholangitis
- Cholangitis associated with liver flukes
- Lymphocytic portal hepatitis

had histologic evidence of cholangitis and were examined using a florescence in situ hybridization (FISH) assay. Some cats affected with cholangitis may also have related diseases, most often pancreatitis and inflammatory bowel disease (IBD). Since cats normally have high enteric bacterial concentrations in the upper gastrointestinal tract, it is speculated that, when concurrent IBD is present, the inflammation may alter distal common bile duct function or perhaps the vomiting from the IBD causes intestinal pressure changes predisposing to ascending bacterial infections. Anatomic abnormalities of the gallbladder or common bile duct or the formation of choleliths may also predispose cats to cholangitis.

The classical histologic description of the ANF of cholangitis is neutrophils within the walls and lumen of biliary ducts and surrounding the portal areas. Sometimes bacteria can be seen in the bile duct lumen or walls. There is bile duct epithelial degeneration and necrosis. Inflammation can also extend through the limiting plate to involve the periportal hepatic parenchyma. The intrahepatic and extrahepatic bile ducts may become dilated, but usually there is minimal biliary hyperplasia or periductal fibrosis in the acute cases. In some very acute conditions, inflammation may be confined to the larger bile ducts, with the gallbladder and hepatic parenchyma spared.

Clinical Findings

This disorder is observed primarily in young-to–middle-aged male cats (generally 3 to 5 years of age). Most cats present because of acute illness of one or several weeks' duration. Common clinical signs include acute vomiting, diarrhea, anorexia, and lethargy. Vomiting appears to be a very consistent clinical sign in most cats with biliary tract disease. Physical examination often reveals a fever, dehydration, icterus, abdominal pain or discomfort on cranial abdominal palpation, and hepatomegaly (<50% of cases). Laboratory findings with all types of cholangitis are quite variable, and the ANF of cholangitis is no exception. A mild-to-moderate leukocytosis is common in most cats having a fever. Typically there are mild-to-moderate increases in serum activities of alanine aminotransferase (ALT), alkaline phosphatase (ALP), γ-glutamyltransferase (GGT), total bilirubin, and bile acids. Because the inflammation is centered on bile ducts, increases in the cholestatic enzymes (GGT and ALP) are expected. Early in the course of disease, inflammation may be limited to the larger bile ducts or gallbladder sparing the liver resulting in normal liver enzymes. In these cases there is also often

minimal if any histologic change in the liver parenchyma. Rarely we have observed peracute cases of cholangitis in which only the total bilirubin was elevated. Inspissation of the bile is common in neutrophilic cholangitis and may cause partial or complete obstruction of the common or intrahepatic bile ducts.

Routine abdominal radiographs are rarely helpful in making a diagnosis, but ultrasound can be rewarding. Changes in bile ducts may sometimes be observed in the ANF. Ultrasonographic changes may include gallbladder or bile duct distention, cholelithiasis, cholecystitis, or sludging (hyperechoic) material in the biliary system. The bile ducts and gallbladder also may be thickened because of edema and inflammation. Occasionally biliary obstruction occurs. It is suggested by a dilated gallbladder and tortuous bile ducts and a common bile duct diameter of greater than 5 mm.

Definitive diagnosis requires a liver biopsy and/or biliary cytology and culture, but a tentative diagnosis is often made based on the clinical and laboratory findings coupled with a response to appropriate antibiotic therapy. Cytologic examination of fine-needle liver aspirates that shows suppurative inflammation helps support the diagnosis. It is important to be aware that liver aspirate cytology often has a poor correlation with histopathology. This is particularly a concern when peripheral neutrophilia is present and the inevitable blood contamination of the liver aspirate may be difficult to distinguish from neutrophilic inflammation in the liver. Whenever possible, a 22-gauge ultrasound-guided gallbladder aspirate for bile cytology and culture should also be performed. Bile aspirates are relatively safe if the needle is directed through the right medial liver lobe and into the gallbladder lumen. With this approach, any bile leakage drains back into the liver and not into the peritoneal cavity. Suppurative inflammation and bacteria may be observed in the bile cytology and is diagnostic for the ANF of cholangitis.

If a liver biopsy is performed, hepatic tissue should always be cultured for aerobic and anaerobic bacteria. Techniques for biopsy include ultrasound-guided needle biopsy, laparoscopy, or laparotomy. The latter two techniques also make it possible to examine the extrahepatic biliary system, pancreas, and other intraabdominal structures.

Treatment

The ANF of cholangitis requires prompt initiation of antibiotic therapy, ideally based on culture and sensitivity. If cultures are negative or empiric antibiotic selection becomes necessary, the clinician must make an educated guess as to an appropriate antibiotic to use based on the most common bacterial isolates from bile (Wagner, Hartmann, Trepanier, 2007). We suggest selecting an antibiotic that is effective against most enteric gram-negative aerobes and that has good hepatic and biliary penetration. We prefer cephalosporins, amoxicillin, or amoxicillin-clavulanic acid but some cases will require a fluoroquinolone. We recommend that cats be treated for at least 4 weeks even though most cats improve in approximately a week with appropriate antibiotics. Others suggest that an even longer duration of therapy (2 months or longer) is required to prevent relapse, but this has not been documented. Additional management includes appropriate fluid and electrolyte replacement.

Ensuring adequate intake of a high-energy, high-protein diet is a priority throughout treatment. Nutritional support, often by short-term use of a nasoesophageal tube, may be indicated in the anorexic cat because it is important to prevent the development of concurrent hepatic lipidosis. Protein restriction is rarely needed because it is unusual for biliary tract disease to result in sufficient parenchymal damage to cause encephalopathy. Protein is an important nutrient for liver repair and regeneration and should not be restricted unless hepatic encephalopathy is present.

Hepatobiliary disease can be painful, and pain management is indicated in these cases. Most acute pain control can be accomplished through the use of drugs such as hydromorphone or buprenorphine (the latter drug can be administered sublingually and is absorbed through the buccal mucous membranes). Meperidine or butorphanol can also be used, and for longer-duration pain control, a fentanyl patch is very effective.

Surgical therapy is uncommon but may be required for cholelith removal or bile duct decompression if biliary obstruction is present. Occasionally the bile becomes the consistency of a thick sludge to the point of obstruction, and this requires vigorous flushing of the extrahepatic biliary system. This is best accomplished by opening the gallbladder and flushing antegrade down the common bile duct. Sometimes it is also necessary to open the duodenum and flush retrograde from the duodenal papilla as well. We advise preserving the normal biliary anatomy and avoiding biliary bypass surgical techniques (cholecystoduodenostomy or cholecystojejunostomy) whenever possible. These surgical procedures should be performed only when necessary because they are often associated with chronic postoperative problems.

We believe that ursodeoxycholic acid (Actigall, Novartis, 10 to 15 mg/kg q24h orally [PO]) should be used in cats with cholangitis. This drug has been shown to have many positive benefits in cholestatic biliary tract disease in other species. Among its effects include amelioration of damage to cell membranes caused by retained toxic bile acids. Ursodeoxycholic acid improves biliary secretion of bile acids, may improve bile flow (choleresis), and has immunomodulatory properties that may reduce immune-mediated liver damage. Studies in cats have found minimal-to-no toxicity. Some clinicians avoid its use when there is the slightest potential for bile duct obstruction, fearing that ursodeoxycholic acid could make the damage worse or even potentiate rupture of the ducts or gallbladder from the choleretic action of the drug. This theory is unfounded and not supported in experimental studies. For example, one study in rats with surgical obstruction of the common bile duct treated with either placebo or ursodeoxycholic acid found that the ursodeoxycholic acid treated rats had less hepatocellular damage than the placebo group showing a protective effect (Frezza et al., 1993). However, if an obstruction is identified in a cat with cholestatic liver disease, surgery would be indicated.

Chronic Neutrophilic Form

The ANF of cholangitis is thought to progress in some cats to a more chronic form, but the time frame and factors for this progression are unknown. The condition has also been referred to as nonsuppurative or lymphocytic-plasmacytic cholangitis. In the CNF of cholangitis there is mild-to-marked infiltration of portal areas by plasma cells and lymphocytes with a variable number of neutrophils. As with the ANF, the inflammation is centered on the bile duct walls, and inflammatory cells may be observed within the bile duct lumen. Inflammation is associated with biliary epithelial degeneration and necrosis. The inflammatory process may also extend through the limiting plate to involve parenchyma. Biliary hyperplasia, a sign of chronicity, is common, and occasionally periductal (sclerosing) fibrosis and bridging fibrosis may develop. In very rare cases biliary cirrhosis can develop, resulting in liver failure.

The etiology for the CNF is unknown, but it is thought by some to be caused by persistent inflammation initiated by an inciting bacterial etiology. As mentioned previously, many enteric bacteria, *Helicobacter* spp., and even *Bartonella* spp. have been implicated as potential etiologic agents. Our yet unpublished study found enteric bacteria using a FISH assay in the biliary epithelium in some cats with the CNF of cholangitis that were cultured negative. Others have postulated immune-mediated mechanisms as factors for the chronic form, possibly triggered by persistent infection or inflammation.

It has been observed that many cats with cholangitis also have concurrent chronic pancreatitis and IBD. This is supported by a study that found that 83% of affected cats with chronic biliary tract disease also had histologic evidence of IBD and 50% had concurrent chronic pancreatitis (Gagne et al., 1999). The association of concurrent inflammation in the three different organs has been referred to as the *feline triaditis syndrome*. In most cases the IBD and pancreatitis are rather mild. When pancreatitis is present, it is generally chronic and described predominantly as ductal inflammation and fibrosis. Possibly the common channel theory, whereby the pancreatic ducts and bile ducts join as a common duct before entering the duodenum, may explain the relationship of biliary tract disease and chronic pancreatitis, whereby ascending bacterial infections in the biliary system are likely to involve the pancreatic ducts as well.

Clinical Findings

Cats having the chronic form of cholangitis tend to be older than those with the ANF at the time of the diagnosis. The clinical signs are often intermittent and can include vomiting, lethargy, anorexia, and weight loss. The signs often tend to wax and wane over months. The membranes on examination may be icteric; this is most easily observed in the sclera and hard palate. Laboratory abnormalities are quite variable. A leukocytosis is uncommon; but most cases have increases in GGT, ALP, total bilirubin, and bile acids, with variable increases in ALT and alanine aspartate aminotransferase. Ultrasound evaluation in cats with the CNF of cholangitis may show changes similar to those in the more acute cases. As fibrosis and bile duct replication take place, the portal areas become more hyperechoic, and the bile ducts can become more torturous. Because of the association with chronic pancreatitis and IBD, both of these organs should also be carefully examined. Chronic pancreatitis usually appears as a nodular irregular organ. Increases in serum amylase and lipase activities do not correlate with the diagnosis of pancreatitis in cats. Feline pancreatic lipase immunoreactivity concentration may be abnormal with concurrent ongoing chronic pancreatitis, and it is the better laboratory test to support the diagnosis of chronic pancreatitis.

A definitive diagnosis of the CNF of cholangitis requires a liver biopsy and possibly a gallbladder aspirate. Fineneedle hepatic aspirates with cytology are less helpful in making the diagnosis of this more chronic and less suppurative form. Liver biopsy tissue and bile should always be cultured for aerobes and anaerobes. When laparoscopic or surgical biopsies are performed, the pancreas and intestine should be evaluated and possibly biopsied.

Treatment

Since the etiology of the CNF of cholangitis is unknown, the role of bacteria in this condition is unclear, and no reported studies investigating therapy are available. This makes definitive therapeutic recommendations difficult to provide. We believe that an appropriate course of antibiotic therapy as described with the ANF of cholangitis is indicated, with or without a positive culture. The duration of therapy should extend for several weeks if not longer. If the biopsy sections contain relatively few neutrophils with a predominance of lymphocytic and plasmacytic inflammation, a combination of antimicrobial and corticosteroid therapy is often used, either concurrently with the antimicrobial therapy or starting after about 2 weeks of antibiotic therapy. Corticosteroids are given to control the inflammatory component of the disease. Alternatively corticosteroids may be added if cats fail to respond to antibiotic therapy after several weeks of therapy. A dosage of 1 to 2 mg/kg every 24 hours orally of prednisolone is used initially. If successful in improving clinical signs and biochemical changes, the dosage is slowly tapered to an alternate-day dose for long-term maintenance. A schedule commonly used is to start therapy at 1 mg/kg every 12 hours for 2 weeks and then progressively reduce the dosage to 1 mg/kg every 24 hours for 2 weeks, 0.5 mg/kg every 24 hours for 2 weeks, and finally 0.5 mg/kg every 48 hours for 4 weeks. Biochemical values and clinical response should be monitored before each reduction in dosage. If the clinical and biochemical responses are satisfactory, dosages as low as 0.5 mg/kg every 48 hours may be sufficient if long-term maintenance is required. Ideally treatment decisions would be based on repeat liver biopsies. Long-term corticosteroid treatment is tolerated well by most cats, and side effects are usually minimal. There are no reported studies using other types of immunosuppressive therapy. An additional therapeutic strategy includes dietary manipulation for documented or presumed concurrent IBD. It should be noted that corticosteroid therapy is not contraindicated in cats having current chronic pancreatitis and may actually be beneficial for the same reasons mentioned earlier.

If coagulation abnormalities are present, administer vitamin K_1 (0.5 to 1.5 mg q12h SQ or IM) (using a 25-gauge needle) for two doses and monitor coagulation profiles. Hepatic encephalopathy appears to be relatively uncommon in cats with acquired liver disease and is manifested most frequently by excessive salivation. Hepatic encephalopathy can be managed by giving lactulose orally (0.5 to 1 ml/kg q8h PO) with or without addition of enteric antibiotics (neomycin 20 mg/kg q8-12h PO). Anorexia must be managed promptly to prevent further deterioration in clinical condition and possible development of concurrent hepatic lipidosis. Assisted oral feeding should be attempted for 12 to 24 hours following beginning of therapy; after which, if the patient has inadequate food intake, a nasoesophageal, esophagostomy, or gastrostomy feeding tube should be placed. Ensuring adequate intake of a high-energy, high-protein diet is a high priority throughout treatment.

There is increasing interest in the use of neutraceuticals in the treatment of feline liver disease. They are generally given for their antioxidant effects. At this time controlled clinical trials are lacking, but their widespread use likely reflects clinician frustration in treating many forms of liver disease and the belief that they are relatively safe. Oxidative damage from free radical formation is one potential mechanism of cellular damage in liver disease. High concentrations of bile acids, accumulation of heavy metals, and inflammation cause free radical generation in the liver. Vitamin E and SAMe are commonly used; vitamin C and phosphatidylcholine may also be considered. The herb milk thistle has also recently attracted both human and veterinary attention for its reported hepatoprotective effects. Clinical trials on its use in veterinary patients have not yet been published. The author (DT) has studied pharmacokinetic properties of silybin (a potent isomer of milk thistle) and identified no toxicity in the cats studied. When bound to phosphatidylcholine, silybin improves drug absorption. A suggested dosage for silybin-phosphatidylcholine (Marin, Nutramax Labs) is 5 mg/kg every 24 hours orally.

LYMPHOCYTIC CHOLANGITIS

Lymphocytic cholangitis (severe lymphocytic portal hepatitis, progressive lymphocytic cholangitis, or nonsuppurative cholangitis) is described as a very chronic inflammatory biliary tract condition that progresses over months and years. This disorder appears to be more common in European than in North American cats and has many similarities to primary biliary cirrhosis in humans. The pathology of the liver is characterized by a consistent moderate-to-marked infiltration of small lymphocytes predominantly restricted to the portal areas, often associated with variable portal fibrosis and biliary proliferation. The lymphocytic infiltrates are centered on, and may infiltrate into, the walls of the bile ducts, but occasionally infiltrates extend into the hepatic parenchyma. There may be lymphoid aggregates, obliteration of bile ducts, bile duct dilation and biliary hyperplasia, and fibrosis or bridging portal fibrosis. A few plasma cells and eosinophils may be scattered in the portal areas. The chronic stage is characterized by predominant monolobular fibrosis, but with this there is also a reduction in the intensity of lymphocytic infiltration. This later stage results in considerable distortion of liver architecture. The bile ducts can also become irregular with dilation and fibrosis. In some cases, lymphocytic infiltrates in the portal areas may be confused with welldifferentiated lymphocytic lymphoma.

It is postulated that lymphocytic cholangitis could be the result of immune-mediated mechanisms based on preliminary immunologic studies, whereas Boomkens (2004) found DNA fragments of *Helicobacter pylori* in the bile of some cats, suggesting bacterial involvement in the pathogenesis of the disease. Recently *Helicobacter* spp. have also been implicated in human primary sclerosing cholangitis and primary biliary cirrhosis.

The European studies describe this condition as a slowly progressive chronic disease continuing over months and years. It is often first identified in cats under 4 years of age; and Persian cats appear to be overrepresented, suggesting a possible genetic predisposition. The most common clinical features observed late in the disease include ascites, jaundice, and hypergammaglobulinemia (in almost all cases). The elevation in globulins reflects ongoing chronic inflammatory changes but could lead the clinician to consider FIP or other differentials for hypergammaglobulinemia. Fever is generally not a feature of the disease. Cats with lymphocytic cholangitis initially present because of chronic weight loss and hyporexia. Because the disease develops slowly, there may be only mild or variable increases in liver enzymes. Increases in ALP, GGT, bilirubin, and bile acids are usual. Leukocytosis is an uncommon finding. In advanced cases ultrasonographic examination often demonstrates dramatic changes in intrahepatic and extrahepatic bile ducts, showing marked segmental dilations with areas of stenosis that may lead the operator to believe there is an obstruction. The liver has markedly hyperechoic portal areas and nodularity to the parenchyma. Liver aspirates may show increased numbers of small lymphocytes, but generally cytology is not helpful in the diagnosis. Ascites and hepatic encephalopathy occur late in the disease as a result of acquired portal hypertension and hepatic dysfunction. This syndrome is one of the few feline liver diseases in which ascites is a prominent feature.

The treatment for chronic lymphocytic cholangitis involves using antiinflammatory or immunosuppressive therapy in addition to supportive therapy as described for neutrophilic cholangitis. A European report evaluating cats with lymphocytic cholangitis treated with corticosteroids found no significant improvement in liver enzymes or biopsy, concluding that corticosteroids had no significant effect on the course of the disease (Rothuizen, 2006). This author theorized that an immune-mediated etiology was less likely. The author also reports that a second group of cats with lymphocytic cholangitis had a better response when treated with ursodeoxycholic acid. This finding is not completely unexpected because ursodeoxycholic acid has been shown to have a positive treatment effect in human patients with chronic primary biliary cirrhosis.

CHOLANGITIS ASSOCIATED WITH LIVER FLUKES

Liver fluke infestation is associated with chronic cholangitis in cats. The trematode *Platynosomum* spp. is the most common genus identified and is found in subtropical and tropical climates of the world. The life cycle of *Platynosomum* spp. includes two intermediate hosts, the first being a land snail. The second intermediate host is usually a lizard, gecko, or toad. Affected cats acquire the parasite by ingesting the second intermediate host. Immature

liver flukes then migrate from the intestine through the bile ducts to the liver. Liver fluke infections cause marked thickening and cystic dilation of the bile ducts. Severe ectasia of the bile ducts or bile duct obstruction can occur. Microscopically marked periductal and portal fibrosis with mild-to-severe chronic inflammation are characteristic. Adult flukes or operculated eggs may be observed within the bile ducts on histopathologic examination.

Affected clinical cases are generally adult outdoor cats that have contact with the second intermediate host of the liver fluke. The severity of clinical signs and liver biochemistry is usually proportional to the degree and duration of the parasitism. The clinical signs are varied and range from asymptomatic cases to hepatic failure and death. Episodes of vomiting, anorexia, and fever are common; and substantial increases in liver enzymes are observed. Icterus from severe cholestatic liver disease or bile duct obstruction can occur. Peripheral eosinophilia was reported early in the disease in experimental infections in cats.

The diagnosis is supported by ultrasonographic findings of bile duct enlargement and tortuosity. It is important to note that other causes of cholangitis can result in similar large ductular changes as well. A definitive diagnosis requires identification of operculated fluke eggs on fecal examination or the presence of eggs or flukes in bile ducts on liver biopsy. The recommended treatment is praziquantel (20 to 30 mg/kg PO q24h for 3 days).

LYMPHOCYTIC PORTAL HEPATITIS

A subset of cats has lymphocytic portal hepatitis on liver biopsy. This condition is generally associated with mild inflammatory liver disease described by small numbers of lymphocytes, with some neutrophils and plasma cells limited to the portal areas. As opposed to cats having cholangitis (inflammation centered on bile ducts), the lymphocytic portal hepatitis cases lack bile duct involvement, infiltration of inflammatory cells into hepatic parenchyma (characterized by disruption of the limiting plate), or periportal necrosis.

Lymphocytic portal hepatitis is thought to be a common histologic finding in liver biopsies of older cats. In a retrospective study 82% of cats older than 10 years had histopathologic changes consistent with lymphocytic portal hepatitis, whereas only 10% of cats younger than 10 had these histopathologic changes (Gagne et al., 1999). These observations suggest that this histologic finding is either a common aging change or possibly a subclinical form of a specific disease. The lymphocytic portal hepatitis appears to progress slowly with varying degrees of portal fibrosis and bile duct proliferation but without pseudolobule formation. Because of the presence of lymphocytes and plasma cells in portal areas and the lack of identifiable concurrent diseases, some have speculated that lymphocytic portal hepatitis may be an immune-mediated disease; but the WSAVA Liver Standardization Group considers the histologic diagnosis to be a nonspecific reactive change possibly reflecting extrahepatic disease. Liver enzymes are quite variable or normal, and icterus is uncommon. Most cats with this diagnosis have a prolonged survival, bringing speculation into the rationale for immunosuppressive therapy. There are no data on the role of immune mechanisms in the initiation and/or perpetuation of lymphocytic portal hepatitis, and controlled studies on therapy are also lacking. The mean survival for cats with lymphocytic portal hepatitis was reported to be 3 years, but the reader should note that most all of the cases were over 10 years of age at the time of diagnosis and death from other diseases becomes more common in cats over 10 years of age.

References and Suggested Reading

Boomkens SY et al: Detection of *Helicobacter pylor* in bile of cats, *Immunol Med Microbiol* 42:307, 2004.

Day DG: Feline cholangiohepatitis complex, *Vet Clin North Am Small Anim Pract* 25:375, 1995.

Frezza EE et al: Effect of ursodeoxycholic acid administration on bile duct proliferation and cholestasis in bile duct ligated rat, *Dig Dis Sci* 38:1291, 1993.

Gagne JM, Weiss DJ, Armstrong PJ: Histopathologic evaluation of feline inflammatory liver disease, *Vet Pathol* 33:521, 1996.

Gagne JM et al: Clinical features of inflammatory liver disease in cats: 41 cases (1983-1993), *J Am Vet Med Assoc* 214:513, 1999.

Haney DR, Christiansen JS, Toll J: Severe cholestatic liver disease secondary to liver fluke *(Platynosomum concinnum)* infection in three cats, *J Am Anim Hosp Assoc* 42:234, 2006.

Lucke VM, Davies JD: Progressive lymphocytic cholangitis in the cat, *J Small Anim Pract* 25:249, 1984.

Newell SM et al: Correlations between ultrasonographic findings and specific hepatic diseases in cats: 72 cases (1985-1997), *J Am Vet Med Assoc* 213:94, 1998.

Rothuizen J: Cholangitis in cats—a review, Proceedings of the 31st World Small Animal Congress, Prague, Czech Republic, 2006, p 47.

van den Ingh TSGAM et al: Morphological classification of biliary disorders of the canine and feline liver. In Rothuizen J et al, editors: *WSAVA standards for clinical and histological diagnosis of canine and feline liver diseases*, Edinburgh, 2006, Saunders/Elsevier, p 61.

Wagner KA, Hartmann FA, Trepanier LA: Bacterial culture results from liver, gallbladder, or bile in 248 dogs and cats evaluated for hepatobiliary disease: 1998-2003, *J Vet Intern Med* 21(3):417, 2007.

Weiss DJ, Armstrong PJ, Gagne J: Inflammatory liver disease, *Semin Vet Med Surg (Small Anim)* 12:22, 1997.

CHAPTER 134

Portosystemic Shunts

KAREN M. TOBIAS, *Knoxville, Tennessee*

Portosystemic shunts (PSSs) are vascular anomalies that divert blood from the abdominal to the systemic venous circulation while bypassing the hepatic sinusoids. Products absorbed from the intestines are delivered to the heart without undergoing the extraction and detoxification processes that are normally performed by hepatocytes. This reduction in hepatic blood flow and function leads to decreases in protein production and glycogen storage, reticuloendothelial dysfunction, and altered metabolism of ammonia and other toxins. PSSs can occur as congenital anomalies or may develop secondary to liver disease and portal hypertension. Although clinical signs from multiple acquired shunts must be managed medically, congenital PSSs have been treated successfully with surgery in many dogs and cats.

ANATOMY

In dogs the ductus venosus, which carries oxygenated placental blood to the fetal systemic circulation while bypassing the hepatic circulation, normally closes within 10 days of birth. Abnormal patency of this vessel, or abnormal communications between the fetal cardinal and vitelline venous systems, results in a congenital PSS. Congenital PSSs usually occur as single large vessels, although some animals have two or more shunts. Common types of congenital PSSs include intrahepatic portocaval shunts, such as a patent ductus venosus, and extrahepatic portocaval or portal-azygos shunts. In a small percentage of dogs with congenital PSSs, the prehepatic portal vein is absent.

ETIOLOGY

Congenital PSSs are reported in 0.18% of all dogs and 0.05% of mixed-breed dogs. Yorkshire terriers are the most commonly reported breed in the United States; risk of a congenital PSS in this breed is 59 times greater than in mixed-breed dogs and 36 times greater than in all other breeds combined. Increased risk has also been noted in a variety of other dog breeds and in Himalayan cats; thus an underlying hereditary cause is suspected. Familial relationships have been noted in Irish wolfhounds with PSS, and incidence of the disease has been reduced by breeding outside of these lines. In Yorkshire and cairn terriers, inheritance is not simple dominant, simple recessive, or sex linked. Breeding of dogs with congenital portal vein hypoplasia (hepatic microvascular dysplasia) can result in offspring with PSSs, suggesting that the diseases may be related.

SIGNALMENT, HISTORY, AND CLINICAL SIGNS

Congenital intrahepatic and extrahepatic PSSs are usually diagnosed in immature animals. No sex predilection is evident. Intrahepatic PSSs are found primarily in large-breed dogs such as Irish wolfhounds and in medium-sized breeds such as Australian shepherds and Australian cattle dogs. Extrahepatic PSSs occur primarily in small-breed dogs. In cats PSSs are most often extrahepatic.

Clinical signs associated with PSSs involve the nervous system, gastrointestinal tract, and urinary tract. General clinical signs include poor growth rate, weight loss, fever, polydipsia, and anesthetic or tranquilizer intolerance. Neurologic dysfunction is seen in most animals with PSSs and may include lethargy, ataxia, head pressing, circling, seizures, behavioral changes, and amaurotic blindness. Gastrointestinal clinical abnormalities may include anorexia, vomiting, and diarrhea. Some dogs have no apparent signs or present only with signs of cystitis or urinary tract obstruction. Many cats have hypersalivation and seizures, and some have unusual copper-colored irises.

Hepatic Encephalopathy

Hepatic encephalopathy has been recognized in animals with PSSs, end-stage liver disease, and congenital urea cycle enzyme deficiencies. Clinical signs include depression, dementia, stupor, and coma. Muscle tremors, motor abnormalities, and focal and generalized seizures have also been reported. Precipitating factors of hepatic encephalopathy include protein overload, zinc deficiency, arginine deficiency in cats, hypokalemia, alkalosis, hypovolemia, hypoxia, gastrointestinal hemorrhage, infection, azotemia, constipation, drugs, and transfusion of stored blood that is high in ammonia. Increased cerebral sensitivity to sedative, analgesic, and anesthetic agents may induce coma in animals with PSSs, even when normal dosages of the drugs are used.

DIAGNOSIS

Abnormalities found on hemograms of some animals with PSSs include leukocytosis, anemia, and microcytosis. In dogs severity of preoperative leukocytosis is correlated with postoperative outcome. Biochemical abnormalities associated with PSSs in dogs include decreases in blood urea nitrogen, protein, albumin, glucose, and cholesterol and increases in serum alanine aminotransferase and alkaline phosphatase. Increase in alkaline phosphatase is most likely from bone growth since cholestasis is not usually a problem in animals with PSSs. Albumin less than 1.3 g/dl usually indicates a poor prognosis. Cats with PSSs may have normal albumin and cholesterol concentrations but usually have increased liver enzymes. Up to half of dogs with congenital PSSs have prolonged partial thromboplastin times; however, this does not usually result in a clinically significant problem.

Urine abnormalities include low urine specific gravity and ammonium biurate crystalluria. At magnifications of 400× or more, ammonium biurate crystals often have a spiky shape and golden color. Abnormal urine sediment suggestive of cystitis (hematuria, pyuria, and proteinuria) in animals with PSSs is most likely associated with inflammation or infection secondary to crystalluria or urolithiasis (urate).

Hepatic histologic changes in animals with PSSs include generalized congestion of central veins and sinusoids, lobular collapse, bile duct proliferation, hypoplasia of intrahepatic portal tributaries, proliferation of small vessels and lymphatics, diffuse fatty infiltration, hepatocellular atrophy, and cytoplasmic vacuolization. These pathologic changes are variable and can also be seen in dogs with congenital portal vein hypoplasia (hepatic microvascular dysplasia) that do not have single congenital shunts and in dogs with other hepatic diseases; thus liver biopsy cannot be used for definitive diagnosis of a PSS.

Liver Function Tests

Although history, physical examination, and routine laboratory tests may be suggestive of portosystemic shunting, function tests such as the ammonia tolerance test (ATT) and measurement of fasting and postprandial serum bile acid concentrations are more reliable for diagnosing liver dysfunction.

Bile Acids

During food intake neurohumoral and hormonal factors such as cholecystokinin stimulate gallbladder contraction and excretion of bile acids into the small intestines, where they form micelles that enhance lipid emulsification and absorption. At least 95% of intestinal bile acids are actively resorbed in the ileum and transported by portal blood back to the liver via the enterohepatic cycle. In healthy animals bile acid concentrations are increased minimally after a meal because of rapid first-pass hepatic extraction.

Serum bile acid concentrations increase in conditions that affect hepatocellular uptake, such as cholestasis or primary hepatic disease, or those that alter vascular flow to the liver, such as PSSs. They are not significantly affected by dehydration, hypovolemia, or passive hepatic congestion, although results can be mildly affected by lipemia and hemolysis. No special techniques are required for handling and storage of serum for bile acid samples. Prolonged fasting may result in normal bile acid concentrations in animals with PSSs; therefore fasting and 2-hour postprandial samples should be analyzed. Most protein-restricted diets, particularly those used in animals with liver disease, have sufficient fat to stimulate gallbladder contraction.

Bile acid concentrations are usually very high ($\geq 100 \mu mol/L$) in dogs with PSSs, although in one report some dogs with PSSs had serum bile acids of 25 μmol per liter or less (Winkler et al., 2003). Falsely lowered results may occur with delayed absorption from prolonged intestinal transit time, lack of gallbladder contraction because of inadequate food intake or delayed gastric emptying, or malabsorption/maldigestion with subsequent decrease in enterohepatic recirculation. Postprandial bile acid concentrations are less than fasting in 20% of animals because of spontaneous interdigestive gallbladder contraction or with prolongation of gastric emptying or intestinal transit times. Measurement of urine bile acids is less sensitive than measurement of serum bile acids for detecting liver disease.

Bile acids may be increased falsely in some patients. Increases in postprandial bile acids that were mild (>31 μmol/L) or moderate to severe (>80 μmol/L) were reported in 79% and 34% of Maltese, respectively (Tisdall et al., 1995). Most of these dogs had normal ATT, and bile acids were significantly lower when measured by high-performance liquid chromatography, indicating that bile acids measured spectrophotometrically in Maltese may be increased by some other cross-reacting substance.

Ammonia

Increased resting ammonia concentration usually indicates decreased hepatic mass or shunting of portal blood. Concentrations of blood ammonia are not well correlated with severity of hepatic encephalopathy, and ammonia levels may be normal in up to 21% of dogs with PSSs, especially after prolonged fasting or with effective medical treatment. In dogs with PSSs, sensitivity of postprandial ammonia is 91% 6 hours after feeding compared to 81% before feeding. Since erythrocytes contain two to three times the amount of ammonia in plasma, improper sample cooling, hemolysis, incomplete plasma separation, or delays in sample analysis falsely increase ammonia values. Concentrations of ammonia measured with tabletop analyzers can be increased falsely if ammonia-based cleaners are used nearby or if ammonia-rich skin oils contaminate the apparatus.

The ammonia tolerance test was developed to provide a more accurate diagnosis of liver dysfunction. A heparinized baseline sample is taken after a 12-hour fast, and ammonium chloride is administered orally by stomach tube or in gelatin capsules (0.1 g/kg, maximum 3 g) or as an enema (2 ml/kg of a 5% solution inserted 20 to 35 cm into the colon). A second blood sample is obtained 30 minutes after ammonium chloride administration. Blood samples are transported on ice for immediate plasma separation and analysis. Results are invalid after oral ammonium chloride administration if vomiting occurs and after rectal administration if diarrhea or shallow rectal instillation occurs.

Diagnostic Imaging

Diagnosis of microhepatica from survey abdominal radiographs is usually based on an upright, more cranial stomach position. Renomegaly has been reported in dogs with PSSs; its etiology has not been determined. Urate calculi are normally radiolucent but occasionally are seen in the renal pelvis, ureter, or bladder on survey films. To definitively diagnose a portosystemic shunt and determine its location, imaging techniques such as angiography, ultrasonography, scintigraphy, computed tomography, and magnetic resonance angiography can be used.

Ultrasonography

Ultrasonographic evidence of PSSs includes microhepatica, decreased numbers of hepatic and portal veins, and detection of the anomalous vessel. Extrahepatic PSSs can be more difficult to diagnose with ultrasonography because the patient is usually small and structures such as ribs and intestines can obscure the vessel. Color flow Doppler imaging is useful for detecting changes in direction and rate of blood flow in the portal vein. The combination of small liver, large kidneys, and uroliths is highly suggestive of shunting in dogs, and dogs and cats with extrahepatic shunts have reduced portal vein to aorta ratios.

Nuclear Scintigraphy

In dogs technetium 99m (^{99m}Tc) is extracted from the circulation primarily by the liver. In animals with PSSs ^{99m}Tc rapidly circulates to the heart and lungs. Normal dogs have a shunt fraction of less than 15% on scintigraphy; most dogs with shunts have fractions greater than 60%. Rectal scintigraphy primarily provides a diagnosis of shunting or no shunting and may be inaccurate with shallow or incomplete instillation or in dogs with colonic fecal contents. Percutaneous splenic injection of ^{99m}Tc permits a reduction of up to 90% in the dosage of the radioactive material, reducing exposure of personnel. In addition, clearance is more rapid with this technique, so that animals are releasable within an hour of study completion. The technique may also provide more information regarding number (single versus multiple) and termination (portocaval versus portoazygos) of the PSSs; composite images frequently produce a portogram that guides the surgeon in shunt location. Nondiagnostic scans may occur in dogs with thin spleens if the ^{99m}Tc is accidentally injected outside of the splenic parenchyma.

Portography

Presence, number, and location of PSSs can be determined with intraoperative mesenteric portography (IOMP). Celiotomy is usually required unless the clinician has experience with transvenous retrograde portography. During IOMP water-soluble contrast medium (maximum total dose 2 ml/kg) is injected into a catheterized jejunal or splenic vein, and one or more radiographs are taken during completion of the injection. Alternatively the spleen can be injected directly and percutaneously in a sedated dog. However, there is a risk of splenic laceration with this technique, and images are often of poorer quality compared to direct intravascular injection. Catheterization of the abdominal arterial and venous systems can also provide diagnostic angiograms during the venous return phase of an arteriogram or consequent to selective venous injections of vessels drained by the shunt. Retrograde placement of two angiographic catheters via the jugular vein can permit simultaneous injections of contrast into the caudal vena cava and the distal portal vein (which is entered via the shunt). This delineation is typically performed during percutaneous stent and coil closure of an intrahepatic shunt (see below).

Differentiation of intrahepatic and extrahepatic PSSs may be made on most portograms. If the most caudal loop of the shunt or the point at which the shunt diverges from the portal vein is cranial to the T13 vertebra, the shunt location is probably intrahepatic. Shunt location varies by one half to three fourths of a vertebral length, depending on the phase of respiration.

DIFFERENTIAL DIAGNOSES

Single congenital portosystemic shunts must be differentiated from neurologic conditions such as hydrocephalus and epilepsy and from other primary hepatic diseases, including congenital portal vein hypoplasia (hepatic microvascular dysplasia) and multiple acquired shunts secondary to portal hypertension. Congenital portal vein hypoplasia is found in many small breeds predisposed to congenital PSSs and can cause similar biochemical, hematologic, histologic, and clinical changes, although gross shunting is not detectable by portography or scintigraphy. Protein C activity (100% being normal) may be helpful in differentiating congenital vascular diseases; protein C activity ≥70% in dogs with portal vein hypoplasia and <70% in dogs with PSS (Olivier et al., 2006).

MEDICAL MANAGEMENT OF PSS

Medical management of animals with PSSs includes correction of fluid, electrolyte, and glucose imbalances and prevention of hepatic encephalopathy by controlling precipitating factors. Dietary protein is restricted to reduce substrates for ammonia formation by colonic bacteria. Daily energy intake should be calculated based on ideal body weight, since patients with shunts may be thin or have poor muscle development. At least 30% to 50% of dietary calories should be provided as easily digested, complex soluble carbohydrates; and diets for dogs and cats should contain 15% to 30% and 20% to 40% of fat, respectively, on a dry matter (DM) basis. Protein requirements are approximately 2.11 g of crude protein per kilogram of body weight per day or approximately 15% to 20% DM and 30% to 35% DM for dogs and cats, respectively. Soybean meal and dairy proteins are often recommended because of their high digestibility and levels of soluble carbohydrates and fermentable fibers. If homemade diets are used, zinc, fat-soluble vitamins, and vitamins B and C should be supplemented.

Lactulose can be used to decrease intestinal transit time, acidify colonic contents, and reduce production and absorption of ammonia. Lactulose may be given orally or by enema; dosages should be regulated so that feces is soft but formed. Yogurt with active cultures can be substituted in place of lactulose to alter colonic flora.

Gastrointestinal hemorrhage (Chapter 114), intestinal parasites, and cystitis should be treated appropriately. Gastric ulcers may be observed even following partial successful closure of a shunt and may require long term management with proton-pump blockers. Urate uroliths may respond to low-protein diets; renal calculi reportedly have dissolved after shunt ligation. In severely encephalopathic animals oral antibiotics effective against urease-producing bacteria such as neomycin or metronidazole can be administered to decrease bacterial populations; however, clinicians should be aware of the potential toxicity of these drugs. Enemas with water and lactulose may be used to reduce colonic bacteria and substrates; intravenous fluids should be administered to obtunded animals. Fresh frozen plasma or hetastarch may be required in patients with coagulopathy or decreased oncotic pressure, respectively. Cats may require phenobarbital or other anticonvulsive medications to prevent and control seizures. For patients with severe neurologic signs,

a neurologist should be consulted about optimal antiseizure therapy prior to an interventional procedure.

Prognosis With Medical Management

With proper medical management, weight and quality of life stabilizes or improves with treatment in most animals. One third of dogs do well with medical management as the sole method of treatment, with many living to 7 years of age or older (Watson and Herrtage, 1998). Duration of survival with medical management alone has been correlated to age at initial signs and with blood urea nitrogen (BUN) concentration; dogs that are older at presentation or have a higher BUN live longer. Over half of dogs treated with medical management alone are euthanized, usually within 10 months of diagnosis, because of uncontrollable neurologic signs and in some cases progressive hepatic fibrosis and subsequent portal hypertension. In some older dogs with PSSs onset of clinical signs may be associated with other hepatic diseases, and the shunt may be an incidental finding. With medical management alone, survival time of cats with PSSs, particularly those that are neurologic, is usually less than 2 years.

SURGERY

Surgical treatment is recommended in most patients to improve long-term outcome. Options include acute ligation with suture; gradual occlusion with ameroid constrictors, cellophane banding, or hydraulic occluders; or embolization with coils. Prognosis for successful surgical treatment is best for dogs with extrahepatic shunts, for animals that undergo complete shunt occlusion, and for those that present with urinary tract signs and no hepatic encephalopathy. When suture ligation is performed, portal and central venous pressures are measured to determine the acceptable degree of attenuation since 30% to 60% of animals cannot tolerate complete acute occlusion. Compared to gradual attenuation, acute complete or partial ligation of a PSS with suture is associated with higher complication rates, including perioperative death in 14% to 22%, seizures in 7% to 11%, recurrence of clinical signs in 40%, and development of multiple PSSs.

Ameroid constrictors (Research Instruments N.W., Inc.) provide gradual, complete shunt occlusion over 2 to 3 weeks through device swelling and local inflammatory tissue reaction. Excellent outcomes are seen in 80% to 85% of dogs after ameroid constrictor placement, although persistent shunting may occur in 17% to 21%. Cellophane bands also cause gradual shunt occlusion secondary to fibrosis. Cellophane is obtained from candy and flower shops and is cut into strips and sterilized for use. Outcome after cellophane banding in dogs is similar to that after ameroid constrictor placement.

More recently a less invasive interventional radiology technique has been used for partial occlusion of intrahepatic PSSs. This approach involves placement of a self-expanding vascular stent within the segment of vena cava communicating with the shunt. A small catheter is advanced through the interstices of the stent into the shunt vessel. Thrombogenic coils are then delivered into the shunt and are contained by the stent (which prevents the coils from entering the caudal vena caval flow). The resultant clotting partially occludes the shunt vessel at the entry into the vena cava. If the shunt is later found to be insufficiently closed, additional coils can be added relatively easily using a percutaneous, minimally invasive approach. Clinical experience at a number of referral centers suggests this can be a safe and seemingly effective treatment. However, as yet there are no reports comparing outcomes of this procedure with the surgical methods described above.

With any surgical technique, postoperative complications, particularly blindness and seizures, are more common in cats. Shunts in cats may not close after cellophane banding or silk suture ligation because of inadequate fibrous tissue response. Glucocorticoids or use of narrow constricting bands may also reduce fibrous tissue formation and result in persistence of shunting in dogs and cats.

POSTOPERATIVE CARE

After surgery animals are monitored closely for hypothermia; hypoglycemia; seizures; and signs of portal hypertension, including shock, pain, and abdominal distention. Most animals need analgesics such as opioids. Sedation with a low dose (0.01 to 0.02 mg/kg IM) of acepromazine may be necessary if dogs are vocalizing or abdominal pressing since these activities increase portal pressure and hyperexcitability. Acepromazine does not appear to lower seizure threshold in PSS patients, but the effects may be prolonged so careful dosing is critical. About 25% of dogs develop hypoglycemia despite concurrent intravenous treatment with dextrose-containing fluids. Patients with nonresponsive hypoglycemia, poor anesthetic recovery, or signs of circulatory disturbances (decreased systolic pressure, increased capillary refill time, poor peripheral pulses, pale mucous membranes) may require treatment with one or more doses of steroids (0.02 to 0.1 mg/kg dexamethasone sodium phosphate IV).

As many as 18% of dogs may develop seizures after shunt ligation. Etiology is unknown; and affected animals usually do not respond to fluids, dextrose, lactulose, or enemas. Single seizures are treated with a bolus of diazepam, correction of any hypoglycemia, and administration of

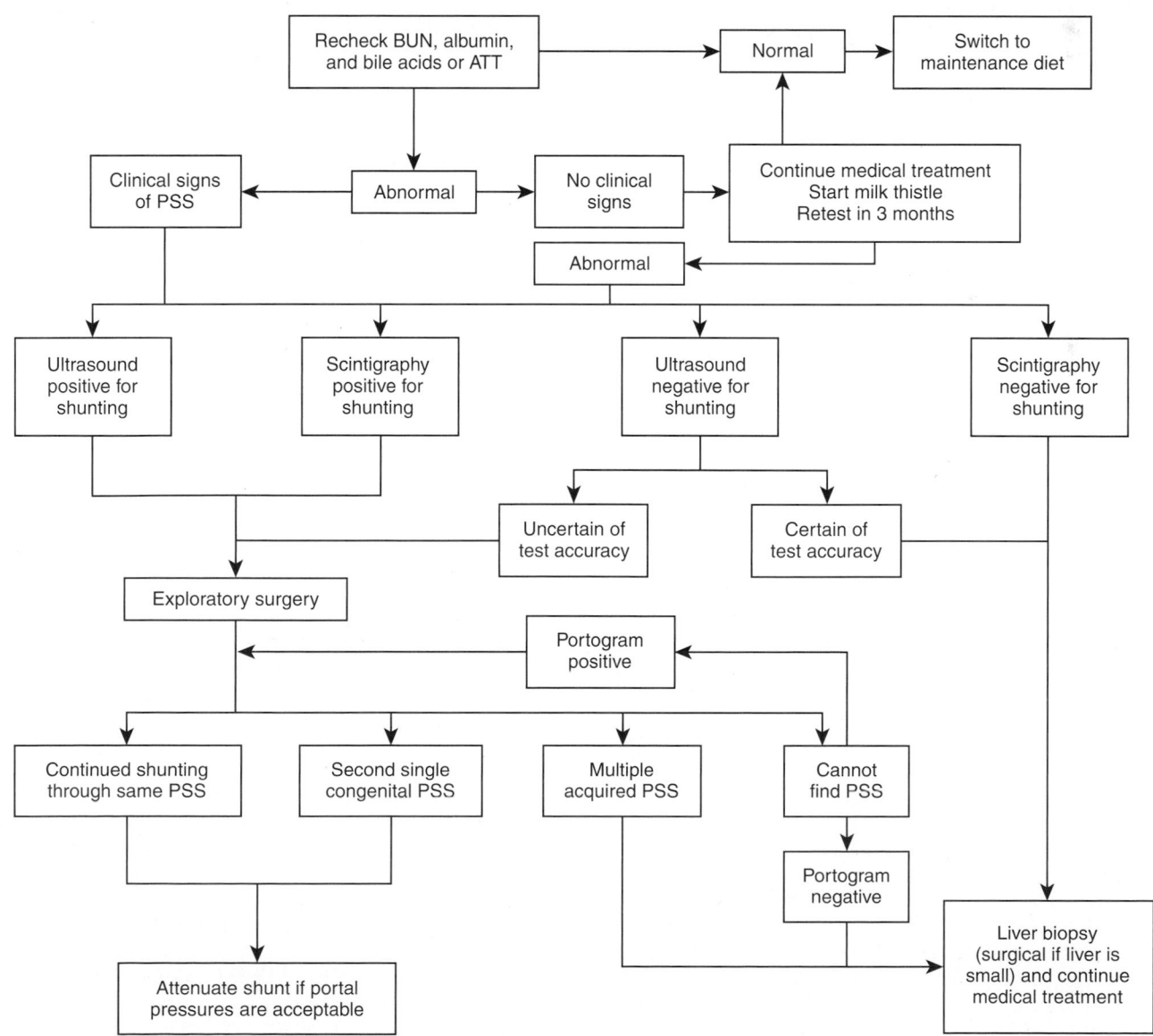

Fig. 134-1 Algorithm for evaluation of animals with single congenital shunts 3 months after surgery.

lactulose retention enemas in case there is an underlying encephalopathy. If seizures recur, animals can be treated with intravenous phenobarbital, a continuous rate infusion of diazepam in 0.9% saline or 3% sodium bromide in sterile water (dogs only), and later placed on a maintenance dose of oral phenobarbital (cats) or potassium bromide (dogs). Animals with uncontrollable seizures are treated with a continuous intravenous infusion of propofol (0.025 to 1 mg/kg/minute) over 12 to 24 hours and intravenous mannitol every 6 hours. Prognosis is poor for animals with postoperative seizures, and many that survive continue to have neurologic problems. At our clinic postoperative seizures are rare in dogs; most dogs receive intraoperative hetastarch for oncotic support, preoperative and postoperative acepromazine for tranquillization, and postoperative dexamethasone as needed for signs of functional hypocortisolemia. Surgery time is decreased by use of ameroid constrictor placement without jugular catheter placement or portal venous pressure measurements. It is unknown which of these factors plays the greatest role in reducing postoperative seizure rates in dogs.

Portal hypertension occurs most frequently after acute ligation. Treatment includes intravenous fluids, hetastarch, broad-spectrum systemic antibiotics, fresh frozen plasma and low–molecular weight heparin if coagulation times are prolonged, and usually surgery to remove the constrictor or ligature. Factors that may increase portal pressure after surgery include excessive intraoperative fluid administration, increased systemic blood pressure from anesthetic recovery, and increased intraabdominal pressure from bandages, pain, or vocalization. Portal hypertension occasionally resolves with intensive medical management without surgery.

Medical management is continued after surgery until liver function improves. Frequently animals can be gradually weaned off of lactulose 2 to 6 weeks after the surgery unless they are constipated or clinical signs recur. Bile acids and albumin are evaluated 3, 6, and 12 months after the surgery to assess liver function. Protein in the diet can be increased gradually once bile acids are nor-

mal. In dogs with mildly increased bile acids and normal albumin, it may be necessary to monitor clinical response to diet change to determine whether protein content can be gradually increased. Milk thistle may be used in animals with persistently increased bile acids or ammonia concentrations to improve hepatic function and regeneration. Animals with persistent clinicopathologic abnormalities may require further workup to determine the underlying cause (Figure 134-1). Yorkshire terriers commonly have increased bile acids 3 to 6 months after surgery despite clinical improvement; this may be secondary to underlying congenital portal vein hypoplasia.

References and Suggested Reading

Hunt GB et al: Outcomes of cellophane banding for congenital portosystemic shunts in 106 dogs and 5 cats, *Vet Surg* 33:25, 2004.

Mehl ML et al: Evaluation of ameroid ring constrictors for treatment for single extrahepatic portosystemic shunts in dogs: 168 cases (1995-2001), *J Am Vet Med Assoc* 226:2020, 2005.

Morandi F et al: Use of 99MTCO Trans-splenic portal scintigraphy for diagnosis of portosystemic shunts in 28 dogs, *Vet Radiol Ultrasound* 46:153, 2005.

Olivier T et al: Evaluation of plasma protein C activity for detection of hepatobiliary disease and portosystemic shunting in dogs, *J Am Vet Med Assoc* 229:1761, 2006.

Tisdall PLC et al: Post-prandial serum bile acid concentration and ammonia tolerance in Maltese dogs with and without hepatic vascular anomalies, *Aust Vet J* 72:121, 1995.

Tobias KM: Portosystemic shunts and other hepatic vascular anomalies. In Slatter D, editor: *Textbook of small animal surgery*, ed 3, Philadelphia, 2003, Saunders, p 727.

Tobias KM, Rohrbach BW: Proportional diagnosis of congenital portosystemic shunts in dogs accessed by veterinary teaching hospitals: 1980-2002, *J Am Vet Med Assoc* 223:1636, 2003.

Watson PJ, Herrtage ME: Medical management of congenital portosystemic shunts in 27 dogs—a retrospective study, *J Small Anim Pract* 39:62, 1998.

Winkler JT et al: Portosystemic shunts: diagnosis, prognosis, and treatment of 64 cases (1993-2001), *J Am Anim Hosp Assoc* 39:169, 2003.

CHAPTER 135

Canine Biliary Mucocele

HEIDI A. HOTTINGER, *Houston, Texas*

Biliary mucoceles were rarely reported in dogs before 1990 but have since become one of the most common causes of extrahepatic biliary disease in canine patients. Their distinct characteristics—grossly, histologically, and ultrasonographically—make it unlikely that mucoceles were previously misdiagnosed or missed altogether. Therefore it seems that this is a newly developing disease process in veterinary medicine for which an etiologic cause has not yet been determined.

PATHOGENESIS

A biliary mucocele is an accumulation of the mucus component of bile within the gallbladder. Grossly it appears as shiny green-black gelatinous material that has lamellar striations along fracture lines (Fig. 135-1). Functional or structural obstruction of the cystic or common bile duct is the usual cause in humans and has been proposed as a cause in the dog. Obstruction can lead to resorption of the liquid portion of bile, allowing the mucinous component to accumulate within the gallbladder. However, studies to date do not support this theory. Primary obstruction of the cystic or common bile ducts is rarely found on diagnostic tests or at the time of surgery, and histologically there is typically evidence of hyperplasia of the mucus-secreting glands of the gallbladder mucosa. An inflammatory or bacterial component is rarely present in reported cases. Therefore primary disease of the mucus-secreting glands of the gallbladder is the more likely cause of biliary mucoceles in dogs. Associated diseases such as underlying liver disease, chronic pancreatitis, and Cushing's disease have been suggested as predisposing factors for biliary mucoceles; but none have been proven to have a definitive cause-and-effect association. Even though these conditions have not been proven to be predisposing causes, no other predisposing factors have been identified; thus all patients should be evaluated carefully for other underlying diseases that may be predisposing or contributing conditions. The recent recognition of biliary mucoceles in veterinary medicine may also suggest a role for nutritional or environmental factors in the etiology. Genetics may also be relevant, as evidenced by the overrepresentation of a few breeds, in particular Shetland sheepdogs, cocker spaniels, dachshunds, and miniature schnauzers.

DIAGNOSTICS

As with any disease or disease process, the diagnosis of a biliary mucocele is achieved by assimilating data from the presentation and owner history, physical examination, laboratory data, imaging studies, and histopathology.

Patients typically present as middle-aged to older, small-to-medium breed dogs. Although no breed predispositions have been reported definitively, Shetland sheepdogs appear to be overrepresented, as do dachshunds, miniature Schnauzers, and cocker spaniels (Aguirre AL, et al, 2007). No sex predilection is evident.

Most dogs with clinical evidence of gallbladder mucoceles present to the veterinarian with a history of subacute-to-acute onset of nonspecific clinical signs. Signs of systemic illness typically include vomiting, inappetence or anorexia, lethargy, diarrhea, polydipsia and polyuria, and vague signs of discomfort. Any combination of these symptoms may be present, or the mucocele may be found as an incidental finding with no clinical symptoms of systemic disease. Physical examination findings are also vague in nature and may include abdominal pain, icterus, tachypnea, tachycardia, dehydration, pendulous abdomen or fluid wave, and fever. Patients may also present with no abnormal examination findings. Because historical and physical examination findings are vague and general, many animals are presumed to be suffering from other disease processes such as pancreatitis, necessitating careful examination and review of all available information to achieve an accurate and timely diagnosis.

The most common laboratory abnormalities include increases in serum liver enzyme activity (alkaline phosphatase, alanine aminotransferase, alanine aspartate aminotransferase, γ-glutamyltransferase, increased total bilirubin) and elevated white blood cell counts. Abdominal radiographs have limited usefulness in the diagnosis of a biliary

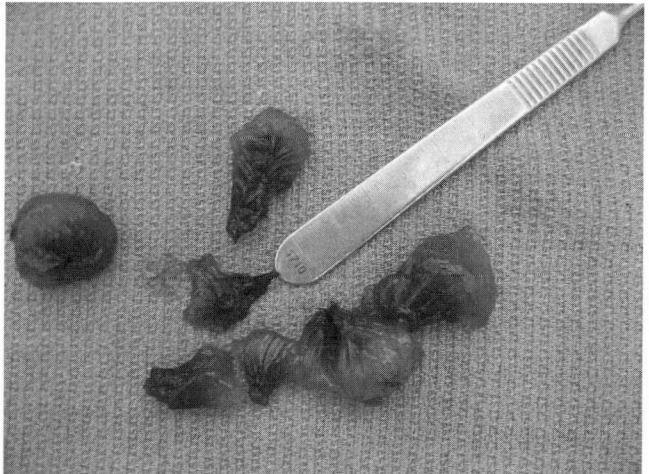

Fig. 135-1 A biliary mucocele with green-black gelatinous mucus material and lamellar striations along fracture lines.

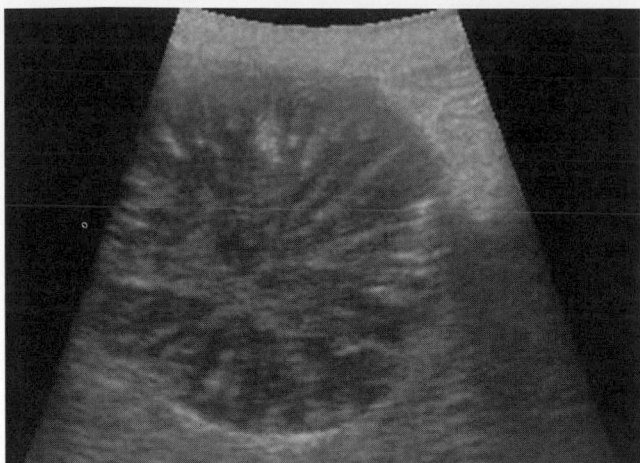

Fig. 135-2 Ultrasound view of a gallbladder mucocele demonstrating the characteristic striated or stellate (kiwi-shaped) pattern within the lumen of the gallbladder.

mucocele but may be critical in ruling out other causes of the historical or physical findings such as gastrointestinal obstruction, abdominal mass, or other causes of vomiting and lethargy. Although uncommon, choleliths may be visible on abdominal radiographs, and these occasionally may lead to biliary tract obstruction. Abdominal ultrasound is the diagnostic test of choice for gallbladder mucoceles, which have distinct characteristics on ultrasonographic images. The content of the gallbladder mucocele is echogenic and nongravity dependent when ballottement or repositioning of the patient is performed, and a striated or stellate (kiwi-shaped) pattern is noted within the lumen of the gallbladder. This kiwi appearance is very specific for biliary mucoceles (Fig. 135-2). Ultrasonography may also detect varying degrees of extrahepatic biliary obstruction caused by extension of the mucinous bile into the cystic, common, and hepatic ducts. Although the ultrasound examination can be very sensitive for the diagnosis of biliary mucoceles, it does not always correspond as favorably to the severity of disease assessed at surgery, in particular the presence of pressure necrosis of the gallbladder wall or cystic duct that can lead to eventual rupture.

TREATMENT

Medical and surgical treatments have been reported for the management of gallbladder mucoceles. Medical management typically involves the use of antibiotics, hepatosupportive supplements, and choleretics. It is not surprising that reports of medical management have shown limited success or failure since the mucocele content is typically a semisolid mass of mucoid material by the time of diagnosis, which is unlikely to dissolve and pass from the gallbladder. Hydrophobic bile salts have been demonstrated to be hepatotoxins, and increased exposure of the canine gallbladder epithelium to bile salts has produced documented increases in mucus secretion. These facts suggest that future research in the field of bile acids may reveal medical interventions that will be helpful in the prevention of biliary mucoceles and potentially even in the treatment of early mucoceles.

Surgical management with a cholecystectomy appears to be the preferred treatment for biliary mucoceles. This recommendation is based on the facts that histology consistently suggests that the gallbladder is the primary diseased component; the mucocele is usually semisolid to solid at the time of diagnosis and unlikely to dissolve; the expanding size of the mucocele typically leads to pressure necrosis of the gallbladder wall with a high risk of eventual rupture and development of bile peritonitis; and the risk that the mucocele can develop a secondary bacterial infection that results in a high mortality rate when associated with bile peritonitis.

At the time of surgery it is common to find localized peritonitis in the cranial abdomen, which presents as adhesions of the omentum, stomach, liver and diaphragm to the necrotic gallbladder wall. This localized peritonitis helps to contain rupture of the gallbladder or cystic duct, but occasionally rupture progresses to generalized bile peritonitis. The majority of reported mucoceles are sterile; thus the prognosis with rupture of the gallbladder wall is much more favorable than that associated with septic bile peritonitis. If adhesions are present, they should be gently broken down, and the gallbladder dissected from the hepatic fossa. Before removal of the gallbladder, the common and hepatic bile ducts should be carefully evaluated for patency. Digital manipulation can be used to express the common bile duct in many patients by gently manipulating the contents normograde into the duodenum. If mucocele contents are present in the common bile duct, digital expression may not be possible. Normograde and retrograde lavage is necessary in this scenario to establish patency. Normograde lavage is accomplished through a cholecystotomy incision and passage of a flexible catheter into the cystic duct. It is not usually possible to pass the catheter past the cystic duct because of the presence of a sharp bend and a valve at the junction of the cystic and common ducts. Retrograde lavage is achieved through an antimesenteric duodenotomy over the major duodenal papilla, allowing passage of a flexible catheter through the sphincter of Oddi. Once patency of the hepatic and common bile duct is verified, the gallbladder can be removed. Necrosis and/or rupture of the biliary tree in patients with mucoceles typically occur at the apex of the gallbladder but can also occur in the cystic duct. Care should be exercised to ensure that the site of ligation is distal to all necrotic tissue and sites of rupture that may be present in the cystic duct. If necrosis of the common bile duct is present, reconstruction techniques typically are unsuccessful, and the prognosis is grave. There is a very low incidence of infection associated with mucoceles, but it is still recommended to obtain culture samples at the time of surgery. Samples should be collected from bile, the gallbladder wall, and the liver. Biopsy samples of the liver and gallbladder should also be submitted.

Copious abdominal lavage is indicated if bile rupture is present or if spillage of bile occurred during surgery. Use of a closed suction drainage system is necessary only when generalized peritonitis is present.

PROGNOSIS

Long-term prognosis is very good for patients treated with cholecystectomy that survive the perioperative period.

Unfortunately perioperative mortality can be high (20% to 25%), and no predictors for survival have been identified. Reported preoperative serum biochemistry values and ultrasonographic findings have been similar in survival and nonsurvival groups. Likewise the presence of biliary tract rupture and bile peritonitis or the development of postoperative pancreatitis had no impact on survival. The immediate postoperative period is the most critical time for these patients. The reported causes of perioperative mortality include cardiopulmonary arrest, supposed thromboembolic disease, septic bile peritonitis, and pancreatitis. Preoperative and postoperative pancreatitis is a reported complication that seems to have a high enough incidence rate to warrant some simple preventive measures. Withholding food for 24 to 48 hours after surgery, keeping rich aromas away from the cage, and monitoring pain and comfort levels closely have the potential to improve the perioperative recovery period significantly. Many patients with biliary mucoceles also have abnormalities on liver biopsy with the typical histologic changes, including variable degrees of bile duct hyperplasia, portal fibrosis, bile stasis, cholangiohepatitis, nodular regeneration, and hepatocellular vacuolar change. Despite these changes, elevations in liver enzymes return to normal in many patients after surgery. Concurrent underlying liver disease does remain in some patients, which may require medical management for optimal long-term results.

The excellent long-term outcome of patients with biliary mucoceles treated with cholecystectomy indicates that the gallbladder is the primary diseased organ. Early intervention before the development of bile peritonitis is preferable in terms of patient morbidity but does not seem to have a detrimental effect on survival in reported studies. It is my opinion that perioperative mortality will continue to improve as this disease process is recognized in earlier stages and patients receive surgical treatment before debilitation of the hepatobiliary system. This can be a difficult recommendation to make for a nonsymptomatic dog in light of the reported perioperative mortality rate. However, only a few clinical reports exist in the literature, and they compile data from dogs in the early phases of recognition and treatment of this disease. Subsequent reports may find a higher success rate as this disease is diagnosed and managed earlier and more aggressively.

References and Suggested Reading

Aguirre AL et al: Gallbladder disease in Shetland Sheepdogs: 38 cases (1995-2005), *J Am Vet Med Assoc.* 231:79, 2007.

Besso JG et al: Ultrasonographic appearance and clinical findings in 14 dogs with gallbladder mucocele, *Vet Radiol Ultrasound* 41:261, 2000.

Bunch SE: Biliary tract disorder. In Nelson RW, Couto CG, editors: *Small animal internal medicine*, ed 3, St Louis, 2003, Mosby, p 538.

Fossum TW: Surgery of the extrahepatic biliary system. In Fossum TW, editor: *Small animal surgery*, ed 2, St Louis, 2002, Mosby, p 475.

Pike FS et al: Gallbladder mucocele in dogs: 30 cases (2000-2002), *J Am Vet Med Assoc* 224:1615, 2004.

Worley DR, Hottinger HA, Howard LJ: Surgical management of gallbladder mucoceles in dogs: 22 cases (1999-2003), *J Am Vet Med Assoc* 225:1418, 2004.

CHAPTER **136**

Esophageal Feeding Tubes

HOWARD B. SEIM, III, *Fort Collins, Colorado*

Feeding the inappetent patient has been shown to decrease both mortality and morbidity. Further, if the gastrointestinal tract is functional, feeding by the enteral route is preferred to a parenteral route. Enteral tube feeding is a more physiologic means of nutrition. It is easier and less expensive and has fewer complications than parenteral feeding. As a general rule, the closer feeding tubes are placed to the mouth, the more efficient the assimilation and digestion of nutrients and the greater the flexibility in formula composition. Conversely the further tube placement is from the mouth, the less efficient is the assimilation and digestion of nutrients, and greater care must be taken in choosing the type and composition of the diet. In addition, the location of gastrointestinal tube feeding dictates diameter of the feeding tube, and tube diameter in turn dictates usable feeding formulas based on viscosity and particulate matter size. The most common tube feeding routes of administration for enteral alimentation include oral, nasoesophageal, pharyngostomy, esophagostomy, gastrostomy, gastroduodenostomy, and jejunostomy. Each route has specific indications, contraindications, advantages, disadvantages, and complications.

This chapter focuses on the use of esophagostomy feeding tubes (E tubes) in dogs and cats. E tubes are easy to place, well accepted by the patient, and have few complications.

INDICATIONS

Nutritional support is indicated in patients unable to meet nutritional demands because of an inability or reluctance to consume a prescribed diet. E tube feeding is indicated in anorexic patients of any cause having a functional gastrointestinal tract distal to the site of tube placement. E tube feeding is particularly useful in anorexic cats with hepatic lipidosis, anorexic cancer patients, or patients having disorders of the oral cavity or pharynx. Surgical procedures that lend themselves to E tube placement include mandibulectomy, maxillectomy, or cleft palate repair.

CONTRAINDICATIONS

E tube placement is contraindicated in patients with esophageal dysfunction such as megaesophagus, esophagitis or esophageal stricture, gastrointestinal dysfunction or obstruction, and persistent vomiting or patients that are a poor anesthetic risk.

TECHNIQUE

Tube Placement

Patients require general anesthesia and endotracheal intubation for E tube placement. They are placed in right lateral recumbency with left side uppermost. Although the tube can be placed on either the right or left side of the midcervical region, the esophagus lies slightly left of midline, making left-sided placement more desirable. The tube entry site in the left lateral midcervical area is aseptically prepared. The head and neck are slightly extended, and the mouth is held open using a mouth speculum. Esophageal feeding tubes are generally polyvinyl chloride or Silastic in composition. In dogs a 20- to 24-Fr–diameter tube is used; in cats a 14-to 18-Fr tube is used. Before tube

placement it is suggested to enlarge the two lateral exit openings of the feeding tube or cut off the distal rounded end of the feeding tube to encourage smoother flow of blended diets through the tube (Fig. 136-1). The feeding tube is then measured from the level of the midcervical region entry point to the level of the seventh or eighth intercostal space; this point is marked on the tube for later reference during tube placement. This ensures that the tube extends only to the mid-distal esophagus and does not cross the lower esophageal sphincter (LES). Feeding tubes that cross the LES frequently cause LES incompetence and subsequent gastroesophageal reflux. Several techniques have been described to place E tubes: one method involves using an Eld percutaneous gastrostomy feeding tube placement device (Eld device) (Fig. 136-2); another method involves the use of curved Carmalt forceps; and a third method involves the use of a specialized esophageal feeding tube applicator (esophageal feeding tube applicator, Firma Fixomed). I have not used the third method and thus will not describe it in detail.

Eld Device Technique

An Eld device originally designed for gastric tube placement can be used to place an E tube (Fig. 136-3). This technique

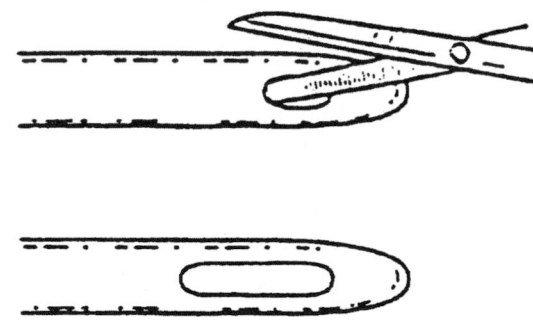

Fig. 136-1 Modifications of the distal orifice of the feeding tube with scissors. The orifice is elongated 3 to 4 cm without compromising the strength of the tube. (From Devitt CM, Seim HB III: Clinical evaluation of tube esophagostomy in small animals, *J Am Anim Hosp Assoc* 33:55, 1997, with permission.)

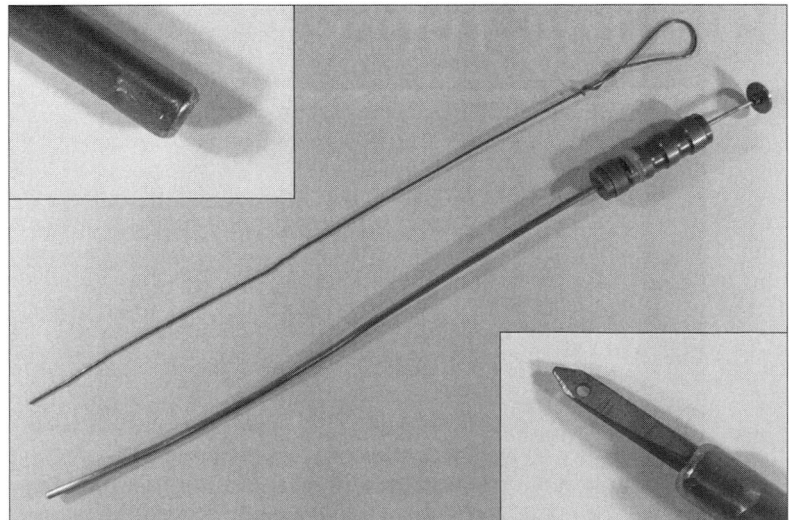

Fig. 136-2 ELD percutaneous feeding tube applicator and stylet. *Upper insert,* Close-up view to the distal tip of the applicator with the blade retracted. *Lower insert,* Close-up view of the distal end of the applicator with the blade extended. Note the eyelet for securing suture material to the blade.

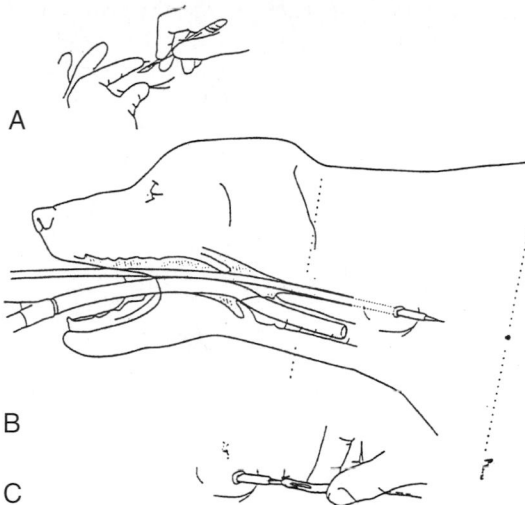

Fig. 136-3 Insertion of the Eld percutaneous feeding tube applicator to the midcervical esophagus. **A,** The distal tip is palpated, and an incision is made through the skin and subcutaneous tissue over the tip of the Eld. The trocar is advanced through the esophageal wall and directed through the incision. **B,** The remainder of the shaft is advanced through the esophageal wall. **C,** The distal end of the feeding tube is secured to the eyelet of the trocar with suture material. (From Devitt CM, Seim HB III: Clinical evaluation of tube esophagostomy in small animals, *J Am Anim Hosp* Assoc 33:55, 1997, with permission.)

works best in medium- to large-sized dogs. The oblique tip of the instrument shaft is placed through the oral cavity and into the esophagus to the level of the midcervical region (i.e., equal distance between the angle of the mandible and point of the shoulder), and the tip is palpated as it creates a bulge in the cervical skin. A small skin incision is made over the device tip. The spring-loaded instrument blade is activated until it penetrates the esophageal wall, cervical musculature, and subcutaneous tissue and is visible through the skin incision. The incision is carefully enlarged in the subcutaneous tissue, cervical musculature, and esophageal wall with the tip of a No. 15 scalpel blade to allow penetration of the instrument shaft through the tissues. A 2–0 nylon suture is placed through the previously enlarged side holes of the feeding tube and through the hole in the instrument blade. The suture is tightened until the tip of the instrument blade and the feeding tube tip are in close apposition. The instrument blade is retracted into the instrument shaft so the feeding tube tip just enters the instrument shaft (i.e., deactivating the instrument blade). Sterile water-soluble lubricant is placed on the tube and instrument shaft. The instrument is retracted, and the feeding tube is pulled into the oral cavity to its predetermined measurement. The 2–0 nylon suture is removed to free the feeding tube from the instrument. See Redirection of Tube for placement into the esophagus.

Curved Forceps Technique
Placement of an E tube using curved forceps is done in a manner similar to placement using the Eld device. The animal is positioned in right lateral recumbency. With the head and neck extended, the curved end of the forceps

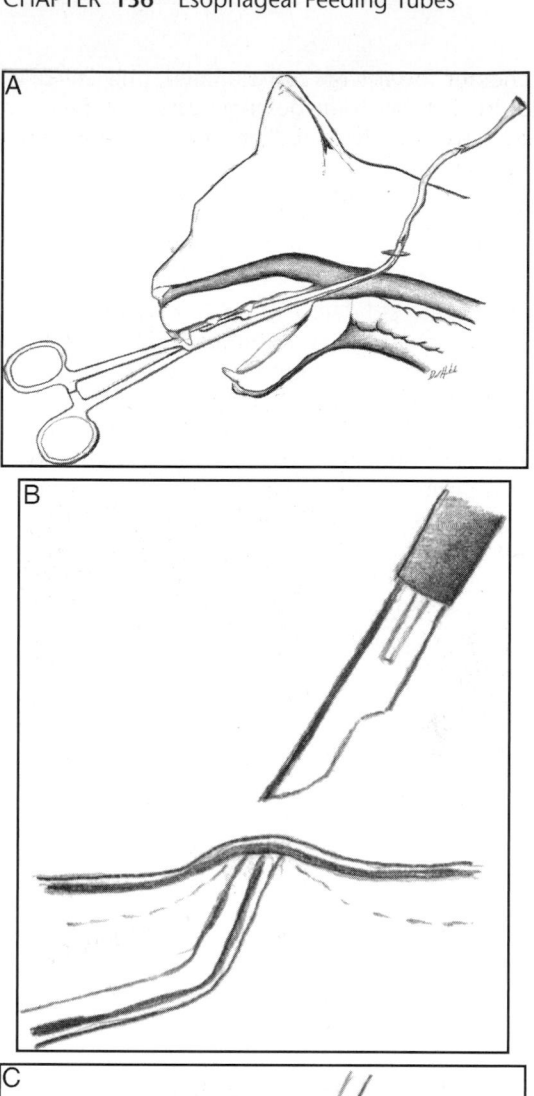

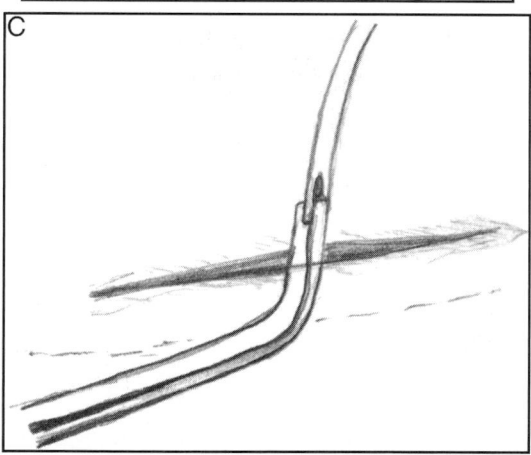

Fig. 136-4 A, For cats and small dogs the curved end of a Carmalt hemostat is passed through the oral cavity into the midcervical esophagus. **B,** The curved tip of the hemostat is then pushed up so the tip can be seen elevating the esophagus, subcutaneous tissues, and skin. The tip of the hemostat is palpated, and a skin incision is made until the tip of the hemostat is exteriorized. **C,** The distal end of the feeding tube is then grasped with the hemostat, and the hemostat is retracted, thus pulling the feeding tube into the oral cavity.

is passed through the oral cavity into the midcervical esophagus (Fig. 136-4). The curved tip of the forceps is then pushed up so the forceps tip is seen elevating the esophagus, subcutaneous tissues, and skin over the tip.

The ends of the forceps are palpated, and an incision is made through the skin down to the forceps tip so the forceps tip is exteriorized. The distal end of the feeding tube is then grasped with the forceps, and the forceps are retracted, thus pulling the feeding tube into the oral cavity.

Redirection of Tube

With either the Eld device or curved forceps method, the distal end of the tube exits the oral cavity, and the flared end of the feeding tube approaches the tube entry point. The next step is to redirect the distal end of the feeding tube back into the esophagus so that it terminates in the midthoracic esophagus. There are two methods to accomplish this: one involves using a hemostat to advance the distal tip of the catheter into the esophagus, and the second involves inserting a stylet through the side opening of the feeding tube and against its tip (Fig. 136-5).

Use of a stylet to redirect the feeding tube. In the dog a stylet (such as a rigid wire or stiff male urinary catheter) is placed through one of the side holes of the feeding tube and against the feeding tube tip. The feeding tube is lubricated and advanced into the esophagus until the entire oral portion of the tube disappears. The stylet is gently retracted from the oral cavity, taking care to ensure its release from the feeding tube. The tube must be placed to its premeasured mark. It is advised to take a radiograph to document tube location. *This technique is recommended*

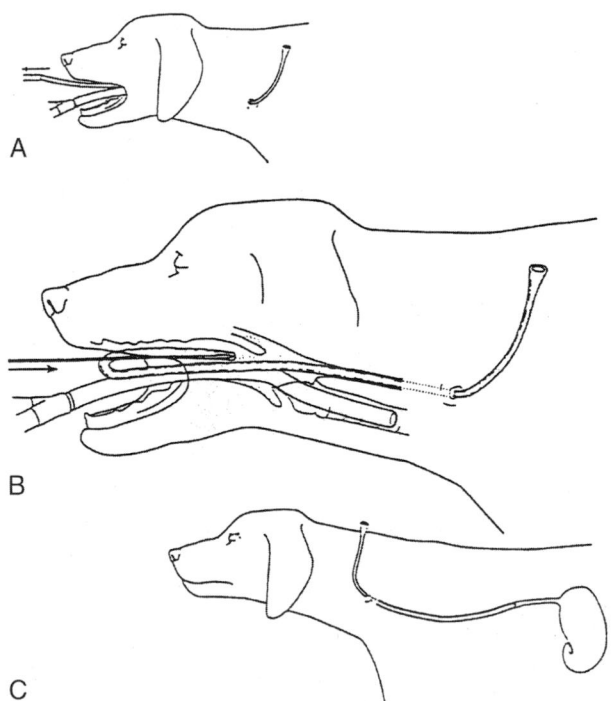

Fig. 136-5   A, The Eld and attached feeding tube are retracted into the esophagus and exteriorized out the oral cavity. **B,** The feeding tube is redirected into the esophagus by inserting a wire stylet (dogs only) into the enlarged orifice and resting against the distal tip of the feeding tube. **C,** The tube is directed into the midthoracic esophagus and retracted or advanced to the previously marked level on the tube. (From Devitt CM, Seim HB III: Clinical evaluation of tube esophagostomy in small animals, *J Am Anim Hosp Assoc* 33:55, 1997, with permission.)

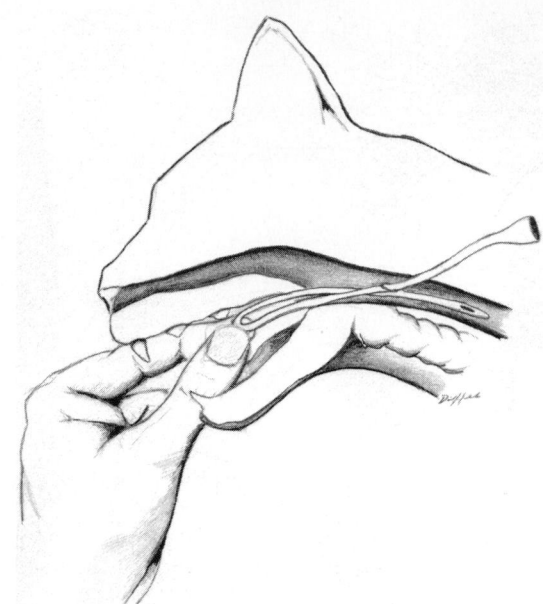

Fig. 136-6   The feeding tube is simply advanced into the esophagus using fingers (cat) or hemostats (dog).

for large- and medium- sized dogs. A metal stylet should never be used to redirect the feeding tube in a cat.

Use of forceps to redirect the feeding tube. In cats and small dogs the tube is advanced into the esophagus with fingers or hemostats until as much of the oral portion of the tube as possible is in the esophagus. It is advised to take a radiograph to document tube location (Fig. 136-6).

Esophageal Tube Applicator Technique

This technique described by von Werthern and Wess (2001) uses a specialized tube applicator. Essentially this is a large tube with a "shoe horn" bulb in the distal third of the tube. A groove 8 mm wide extends from the bulb to the distal end of the tube. With the bulb portion in the midcervical esophagus, one can cut through skin, subcutaneous tissues, and esophagus into the groove of the tube. A feeding tube is then placed into the esophagus and into the tube. Because of the shoe horn shape of the applicator tube, the feeding tube can be directly aborally, avoiding the need to bring the tube through the mouth and then to redirect it aborally.

Tube Management

The tube is secured to the cervical skin with a "Chinese finger-trap" friction suture using 0 or 1–0 monofilament nonabsorbable suture material (Fig. 136-7). The exit point of the tube can be left exposed or loosely bandaged. A column of water is placed in the tube after each feeding, and the end capped. A 20-gauge hypodermic needle cap or 3-ml syringe barrel works well for this purpose, thus preventing intake of air, reflux of esophageal contents, and occlusion of the tube by diet. Most patients tolerate the tube without the need of an Elizabethan collar. E tubes can be removed immediately

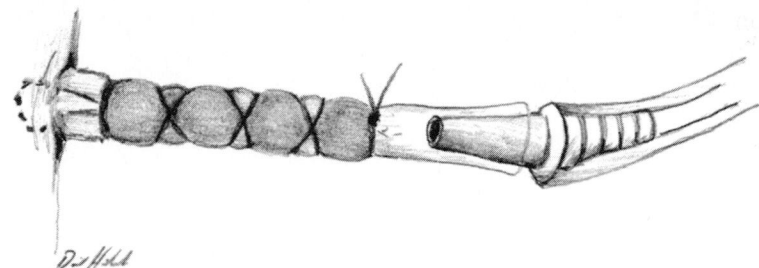

Fig. 136-7 The tube is secured to the cervical skin using a "Chinese finger-trap" friction suture with 0 or 1-0 monofilament nonabsorbable suture material.

after placement or left in place for weeks to months. The tube exit site should be cleaned periodically with an antiseptic solution.

Feeding can commence immediately through the feeding tube unless otherwise contraindicated. Diets available for use include a variety of blenderized canned diets, monomeric diets, and polymeric diets. The tube entrance site should be maintained with daily inspection and cleaning with antiseptic solution. When nutritional support is no longer necessary, the tube is removed by cutting the retaining suture and pulling the tube. No further exit wound care is necessary; the hole seals in 1 to 2 days and heals in 3 to 5 days.

ADVANTAGES

The technique of midcervical E tube placement is economical and simple to perform and provides a large-diameter feeding tube. E tube placement is suitable in nutritionally compromised small animals with a functional esophagus and gastrointestinal tract. E tubes should be placed from the midcervical esophagus to the midthoracic-to-distal esophagus but should not cross the LES. Feeding via E tube can commence immediately following tube placement. Long-term use of E tubes in dogs and cats is not associated with significant complications. Following tube removal, the esophagocutaneous fistula heals readily by second intention.

COMPLICATIONS

Complications associated with E tube placement include early removal by the patient, vomiting the tube, and tube removal or migration. Minor complications include scratching at the E tube entry site, local skin infection, and mechanical problems. The most frequent owner problems include feeding difficulty or clogging of the tube with food. Tube clogging can usually be avoided if the tube is flushed with water and capped after each feeding. I have observed two cases of esophageal perforation in cats having E tube placement. These perforations were believed to occur during tube redirection with a metal stylet. Esophageal perforation has not been observed by me in cats since eliminating the stylet from placement protocol. Esophageal perforation has not been reported in the dog. No significant long-term complications have been reported; but potential complications could include esophagi-

tis, esophageal stricture, esophageal diverticulum, or subcutaneous cervical cellulitis. Reflux esophagitis can occur from improper tube placement (i.e., through the LES) or esophageal irritation from the tube itself. Midesophageal placement of silicone rubber tubes greatly reduces the incidence of esophageal injury and eliminates reflux esophagitis.

CONCLUSION

Various methods are available for providing nutritional support in small animals, including nasogastric, nasoesophageal, pharyngostomy, gastrostomy, and jejunostomy tubes. Each method has advantages and disadvantages. Although general anesthesia is required for placement, the E tube has the advantage over the nasoesophageal or nasogastric tube because it provides a large-diameter feeding tube that eliminates the need for specialized diets. E tube placement has the advantage over nasogastric, nasoesophageal, and pharyngostomy tubes because it is placed further caudad, eliminating the risk of aspiration or upper airway obstruction. E tube placement has the advantage over gastrostomy and jejunostomy tubes because it eliminates the risk of peritonitis if the gastrostomy or jejunostomy tube is prematurely dislodged, and it has the advantage over a jejunostomy tube in that E tube placement does not require laparotomy or endoscopy for placement, specialized liquid diets, or expensive equipment for diet delivery.

References and Suggested Reading

Crowe DT Jr: Nutritional support for the hospitalized patient: an introduction to tube feeding. *Compend Contin Educ* 12:1711, 1990.

Devitt CM, Seim HB III: Clinical evaluation of tube esophagostomy in small animals, *J Am Anim Hosp Assoc* 33:55, 1997.

Ireland LM et al: A comparison of owner management and complications in 67 cats with esophagostomy and percutaneous endoscopic gastrostomy feeding tubes, *J Am Anim Hosp Assoc* 39:241, 2003.

Rawlings CA: Percutaneous placement of a mid-cervical tube esophagostomy: new technique and representative cases, *J Am Anim Hosp Assoc* 29:526, 1993.

von Werthern CJ, Wess G: A new technique for insertion of esophagostomy tubes in cats, *J Am Anim Hosp Assoc* 37:140, 2001.

SECTION VII

Respiratory Diseases

Eleanor C. Hawkins

VOLUME XIII CONTENT ON EVOLVE: http://evolve.elsevier.com/Bonagura/Kirks/

Airway Management
Feline Respiratory Tract Polyps
Thoracoscopy

CHAPTER 137

Oxygen Therapy

DENNIS T. CROWE, JR., *Bogart, Georgia*

This chapter considers: (1) basic principles of oxygen use within the body and factors that influence oxygen delivery (DO_2) to cells pertinent to supplemental oxygen therapy; (2) indications for delivering supplemental oxygen; (3) methods of providing supplemental oxygen and the effectiveness of each approach; (4) methods of determining effectiveness of oxygen supplementation; including interpretation of blood gases; (5) guidelines for managing dysoxic patients that do not respond favorably to oxygen supplementation; and (6) an overview of a special form of supplemental oxygen delivery involving the use hyperbaric chambers.

BASIC PRINCIPLES OF OXYGEN DELIVERY AND USE

Oxygen is necessary for all normal metabolic processes involving cellular function. If DO_2 is insufficient to meet the needs of cells, particularly those with high metabolic rates as indicated by high oxygen consumption (VO_2), the resultant *dysoxia* causes a measurable decrease in adenosine triphosphate (ATP) production within a matter of seconds. Over 90% of generated ATP is used to maintain plasma membrane function and integrity. Dysoxia begins affecting overall cell function immediately. If these cells are cerebral neurons or myocardial cells, severe dysoxia can lead to irreversible dysfunction and death within minutes. If the cells are enterocytes, dysfunction can lead to death within hours as a result of mucosal barrier dysfunction, the consequences of endotoxin and bacterial absorption. In wounds dysoxia is associated with an increase in infection rates and prolonged healing time.

FACTORS THAT INFLUENCE CELLULAR OXYGEN DELIVERY

Oxygen is delivered to the cells in two forms: that dissolved in the arterial blood (and responsible for the diffusion pressure driving oxygen to tissues), and the remaining 97% that is attached to hemoglobin.

The most important factors influencing this amount of oxygen in the blood are the amount or concentration (g%) of hemoglobin in the blood (Hb) and the percentage of the hemoglobin that is saturated with oxygen (SaO_2). The amount of oxygen dissolved in plasma can be measured as the partial pressure of oxygen (pO_2). It is this partial pressure of oxygen that provides the diffusion gradient responsible for movement of oxygen into the interstitial space and cells. The formula for the total content of oxygen in arterial blood (CaO_2) is

$$CaO_2 = (1.34 \times [Hb] \times SaO_2) + (PaO_2 \times 0.0031)$$

There is a direct although nonlinear relationship between the SaO_2 and the PaO_2 in the blood. Supplemental oxygen increases the partial pressure in the alveolus, which in turn raises the partial pressure of oxygen (PO_2) in the blood. A hemoglobin concentration of 10 g/dl (packed cell volume of 30%) is probably optional for most critical patients provided cardiac output (CC) and microcirculatory flow are adequate. Although the majority of oxygen is transported in the blood via hemoglobin, the PaO_2 in the plasma provides the diffusion gradient creating uptake (saturation) and downloading of oxygen onto the hemoglobin molecule. DO_2 is also determined by the PO_2 within the alveoli, pulmonary capillary blood flow, matching of ventilation and perfusion in the lungs, and delivery of blood to the microcirculation. Delivery of blood to the microcirculation is determined by cardiac output (CO) and functional capillary density and the amount of interstitial space present between the capillary and the cell. Functional capillary density is influenced by both precapillary and postcapillary tone and surrounding interstitial space pressure and distance. Interstitial space *distance* is that between the capillary and the tissue cells. This space or distance is increased with interstitial edema.

INDICATIONS FOR PROVIDING SUPPLEMENTAL OXYGEN

Any clinical condition that negatively affects oxygen intake, uptake across the pulmonary capillary, CO blood flow (pulmonary or systemic), microcirculatory flow, capillary density, and oxygen transport through the interstitial space can negatively influence DO_2. Any of these disorders may constitute an indication for supplemental oxygen.

The American College of Chest Physicians and the National Heart Lung and Blood Institute recommendations for instituting oxygen therapy are cardiac and respiratory arrest; hypoxemia ($PaO_2 < 7.8$ kPa, $SaO_2 < 90\%$), hypotension (systolic blood pressure <100 mm Hg); low cardiac output and metabolic acidosis (bicarbonate <18 mmol/L); and respiratory distress (respiratory rate >24/min). Their guidelines for initial oxygen dose are cardiac or respiratory arrest 100%, and hypoxemia 40% to 60%.

The SaO_2 and PaO_2 are the main clinical indicators for initiating, monitoring, and adjusting oxygen treatment. However, PaO_2 and SaO_2 can be normal when tissue hypoxia is caused by low output cardiac states, anemia, or failure of tissues to use oxygen. In these circumstances, mixed venous oxygen partial pressure (Pvo_2), which is measured in pulmonary artery blood, is a better measure of tissue oxygenation. A third choice is to sample blood from a central venous catheter. Even in the presence of a normal Pao_2 and Pvo_2, *severe hypoxia in a single organ may result in death. Supplemental oxygen may be a deciding factor in these cases.* Measurement of individual tissue oxygenation is difficult, requiring specialized techniques, including tonometry and oxygen probes.

Recent studies have proven that providing supplemental oxygen to animals in hemorrhagic shock *prior* to blood and fluid replacement decreases the amount of reperfusion injury over those not given supplemental oxygen beforehand (Meier et al., 2004). Elevating the fractional percent of inspired oxygen (FiO_2) from 0.2 to nearly 1 in hemorrhagic shock elevated brain oxygen tension ($PbrO_2$) from a baseline of 15 mm Hg to 36 mm Hg; when ventilation was added, $PbrO_2$ increased to 88 mm (Manley et al., 1999). Research also has proven that providing supplemental oxygen after major surgery is associated with a decrease in wound infection rate. In one study involving 500 humans who underwent colorectal resection, the wound infection rate had decreased from 11.2% to 5.2% when supplemental oxygen was added (Greif et al., 2000). Tissue oxygen tensions are 10 to 20 mm Hg higher when supplemental oxygen is provided (Whitney et al., 2001).

The need for supplemental oxygen treatment can induce: (1) *history and physical findings* indicating dysoxia (Box 137-1); (2) a *physical condition* that has been shown to benefit from supplemental oxygen (Box 137-2); (3)

monitoring abnormalities that develop because of the lack of oxygen in the tissues (Box 137-3), or (4) *laboratory abnormalities* that indicate either low oxygen tension or the consequence of such (Box 137-4). Although pulse oximetry is commonly used to determine the need for oxygen supplementation, it can be unreliable because there are times when this monitoring device yields false information. Blood gas determinations, especially arterial PO_2, are the gold standard used to determine the need for oxygen supplementation. Values below 80 mm Hg indicate the need for supplemental oxygen. Because arterial samples can be more difficult to obtain, venous samples also have been used in critical patients to assess oxygenation. Venous PO_2 values are influenced by the amount of oxygen in the arterial blood, tissue perfusion, and uptake of oxygen into the tissues (oxygen extraction ratio). If venous PO_2 is below 30 mm Hg, this indicates either that arterial oxygen levels were low or that the blood flow and tissue perfusion is inadequate (creating a high oxygen extraction ratio). In either case supplemental oxygen is indicated.

If arterial blood PO_2 is below 80 mm Hg and partial pressure of carbon dioxide (PCO_2) is greater than 50 mm Hg, there is a need to support the patient's ventilation

---

Box 137-1

Clinical Signs of Dysoxia

- Restlessness
- Anxiousness
- Increased breathing rate and effort
- Frantic behavior
- Increased breath sounds, adventitial sounds
- Use of accessory muscles with each breath
- Struggling efforts with breathing
- Light discoloration of mucous membranes
- Cyanosis
- Gasping
- Darkening cyanosis, poor refill time
- Unconsciousness
- Seizurelike activity

Box 137-2

Physical Conditions That May Benefit From Supplemental Oxygen

- Trauma
- Sepsis
- Heart disease (failure)
- Neurologic diseases
- Head injury (early supplemental oxygen decreases secondary brain injury, edema, neuronal death)
- Shock (all types)
- Pulmonary edema (all causes)
- Severe wounds
- Surgical wounds
- Pancreatitis
- Snake and spider bite

Box 137-3

Common Physiologic Monitoring Abnormalities That May Indicate Dysoxia

- Electrocardiogram (ST segment changes, arrhythmias, tachycardia, bradycardia)
- Arterial blood pressure (below 80 or above 150 systolic)
- Arterial pulse pressure (difference between systolic and diastolic less than 30)
- Doppler flow (weak, feeble sounds or very bounding sounds)
- Toe web temperature: rectal temperature differential (greater than 10°F)
- Rectal or aural temperature (above 104°F)
- Pulse oximetry (values below 92%)
- Central venous pressure (values below 3–4 cm H_2O)
- Urinary output (values below {1/4} ml/kg/hr for cats, below {1/2} ml/kg/hr for dogs)

Box 137-4

Common Laboratory Monitoring Abnormalities That May Indicate Dysoxia

- Reduced hematocrit (any acute drop of 10 or any value below 30)
- Low total plasma solids (any acute drop of 0.6 or greater, before fluid support)
- Low partial pressure of venous oxygen (any levels below 30 mm Hg)
- Low partial pressure of arterial oxygen (any levels below 80 mm Hg)
- Low partial pressure of capillary oxygen (any levels below 45 mm Hg)
- Base deficit (minus 6)
- Elevated, blood lactate (greater than 3 mmol/L)

in addition to providing supplemental oxygen. If the patient does not respond favorably to supplemental oxygen with a decrease in respiratory effort and rate, additional treatment may be useful. This is done using a "tight-fitting" mask, and providing positive-pressure ventilation (PPV) with the use of a bag-valve (AMBU bag). The reservoir is connected to a flow of oxygen (5-15 L/min) to keep the attached reservoir bag partially full (providing nearly 100% oxygen). The addition of a positive end-expiratory pressure (PEEP) valve on the exhalation port of the AMBU bag will increase pulmonary functional residual capacity (FRC) and decrease the work of breathing. This is recommended in patients with pulmonary edema, severe intrapulmonic hemorrhage, and any other lung parenchyma diseases that lead to ventilation:perfusion mismatching. Mild sedation may be required for the patient to accept a mask. A recommended sedative combination is intramuscular or intravenous acepromazine (0.005 to 0.01 mg/kg), butorphanol (0.1 to 0.2 mg/kg), and, if necessary, ketamine (1 to 4 mg/kg) starting at the lower dosages. If auscultation suggests a pneumothorax with decreased breath sounds, thoracentesis should be performed, and any free air removed. Insertion of a chest tube is necessary if a negative vacuum is not reached. In extreme cases a tracheotomy or the use of a neuromuscular blocker such as succinylcholine with deeper sedation and laryngoscopic-assisted tracheal intubation is needed to provide adequate ventilation and oxygenation. Cases that may need this care include acute aspiration, fulminate pulmonary edema from many etiologies, pneumonia, or severe intrapulmonary hemorrhage.

Common clinical conditions indicating the need for oxygen supplementation include the following:

- Pulmonary edema from any cause
- An acute drop in hemoglobin concentration to less than 9 g/dl with clinical signs of anemia
- An acute decrease in CO, including that due to cardiac tamponade
- Blood volume loss
- Significant localized interstitial space edema secondary to a severe wound, which causes a decrease in oxygen tension to tissues at the wound site
- Head and spinal cord injury

Any acutely ill or injured patient has an increased demand for oxygen and removal of carbon dioxide (CO_2) because of the higher metabolic rates of the cells. Clinical indications of increased oxygen demands include increases in respiratory rate, respiratory effort, heart rate, blood flow (assessed by Doppler), blood pressure, body temperature, decreased capillary refill time, and bright mucous membranes. When these are noted, it can be concluded that VO_2 and CO_2 production is greater than normal.

METHODS USED TO SUPPLY SUPPLEMENTAL OXYGEN

Supplemental oxygen can be provided by a number of delivery methods, both noninvasive and invasive.

Blow-By Oxygen

This is most easily provided by using small-diameter oxygen tubing that is connected directly to the oxygen source. The end of the tube is placed in front of the patient's nose or mouth. The flow rate generally varies from 3 to 15 L/minute. A small nozzle, such as a 14g IV catheter attached to the patient end of the oxygen tubing, creates a jet that will be especially effective in a patient with small restricted airways. It may also decrease the work of breathing. A mask can also be used but is usually not well tolerated, especially if the patient is panting.

Oxygen Hood

Many animals tolerate having their heads placed inside a plastic bag as a temporary treatment method. The oxygen tubing is placed through a small hole in the front of the bag, and the back of the bag is left open to allow gas to escape. This is particularly useful in the obtunded patient because high concentrations of oxygen can be provided (85% to 95%) (Engelhardt and Crowe, 2004), while allowing other procedures to be performed (e.g., blood drawing, placement of catheters, x-rays). Oxygen hoods may not be tolerated by the panting dog since the hood may become rapidly overheated and overhumidified. In these cases it is necessary to sedate the dog or use an oxygen collar. The temperature of the inside of the hood should be checked periodically.

Oxygen Collar

An oxygen canopy device can also be made by covering the ventral 50% to 75% of an Elizabethan collar with plastic wrap (Crowe, 2003a; Engelhardt and Crowe, 2004). This can be used for long-term therapy, but mild sedation may be required for some patients to tolerate it. The Elizabethan collar should be one size larger than would normally be used for the patient. The oxygen tubing is placed along the inside of the collar and taped in place ventrally. Oxygen concentrations of up to 80% generally can be achieved. Flow rates of approximately 1 L/10 kg of body weight usually provide an adequate inspired FiO_2. Flow rates should be adjusted based on clinical response to the oxygen supplementation and patient comfort. In heavily panting dogs, the plastic in the front of the collar may have to be decreased to only just above the nose. No humidification should be added in these situations. Use of a commercial collar that is zipped up in front, completely covering the opening, has been associated with over-heating, and if used, it should only cover a portion of the collar. Since oxygen is heavier than room air, the coverage should be started at the ventral aspect of the collar. To measure the amount of oxygen in the collar an oxygen analyzer (example: MiniOx-l Oxygen Analyzer, MSA Medical Products) is recommended. Minimum FiO_2 for chronic conditions is 35% to 40% and for acute or emergency conditions is 60% to 90% or above and by adding a small strip of plastic wrap over the ventral half of the collar, oxygen levels will be increased to greater than 60% (FiO_2 0.6).

Nasal Cannula

Most dogs and cats tolerate short human nasal cannulas. These have two sections of tubing extending from a small nose piece that is attached to flexible oxygen tubing shaped into a loop that can be slipped behind the patient's head. They come in three different sizes: infant, which is used for the cat and small dog (2 to 5 kg of body weight); pediatric, which is used for the medium-sized dog (11 to 24 kg); and adult, which is used for the large dog (>25 kg). A few drops of proparacaine or lidocaine are first placed into each nostril. If the patient objects significantly, stress and struggling should be reduced by sedation with a mixture of ketamine, butorphanol, and acepromazine (as described previously). After waiting a few minutes for the sedation and local anesthetic to take effect, the tips of the cannula are placed into the nostrils, and the tubing is brought to each side of the nose and secured with skin staples. The tubing is continued behind the patient's head, and the loop is tightened where the loop comes together. The continuation of the flexible oxygen tubing is secured with tape around the patient's neck or chest to prevent tension on the nostrils. The tubing is attached to a source of humidified oxygen. Oxygen is then delivered to the system at 50 to 100 ml/kg up to a maximum rate of 5 to 6 L/minute. This provides at least a 40% nasal oxygen concentration. As with other types of nasal tubes, these patients should have an Elizabethan collar in place if they start to bother the catheter.

Nasal Catheters

This is one of the most effective ways to provide oxygen (Fitzpatrick and Crowe, 1986). A narrow-bore red rubber tube (3.5 to 8 Fr) is placed in the ventral nasal meatus and sutured or glued to the patient's face. For small patients 3.5- to 5-Fr tubes are used. For medium-sized dogs 5- to 8-Fr tubes are used, and for larger dogs 8-Fr tubes are placed. Several drops of 0.5% proparacaine ophthalmic solution are instilled in the nose. Lidocaine also can be used. If lidocaine is being used in cats, the dose should be monitored to ensure that a toxic level is not reached. A small amount of sterile water-soluble gel or lidocaine gel placed on the outside of the tube facilitates passage of the tube. If the patient objects to placement, sedation (see prior section) should be considered.

The nasal catheter typically is measured from the tip of the nose to the lateral canthus (nasopharyngeal). In cats the tube readily passes into the nasal meatus. Pushing the nasal planum of the dog dorsally (not needed in cats) and directing the tube ventromedially should enable the tube to pass easily into the ventral meatus. The tube is sutured close to the nostril (maximum 0.5 cm from the nares). This suture is very important. A second suture is placed on the lateral aspect of the face or on the bridge of the nose between the eyes. Nasal oxygen should be avoided in the patient with severe nasal or pharyngeal disease or in the patient with severe thrombocytopenia, a bleeding disorder, or head trauma. Sneezing elevates intracranial pressure, and nasal tubes should be avoided if this is a concern.

At flow rates of 50 ml/kg/min in small dogs and cats and 100 ml/kg in larger dogs the FiO_2 is approximately 0.4 to 0.5. If higher flow rates are desired, a second tube can be placed in the other nostril, or the tube can be placed deeper as a nasotracheal oxygen catheter. For *nasal-nasal* catheters the nasal catheter tip ends with the tip in the middle of the nose. For *nasopharyngeal* catheters the catheter tip ends in the proximal pharynx, which corresponds to the angle of the mandible. The oxygen administered by this method typically provides 60% to 70% oxygen at the same flow rates as nasal catheters, which provide 40%. If the patient is swallowing a lot of air, providing oxygen in this manner may contribute to gastric overdistention; thus the patient should be monitored closely. For *nasotracheal* oxygen catheters the catheter tip ends in the proximal tracheal lumen. Oxygen provided by this method provides 80% to 90% oxygen at 50% of the same flow rates of those of nasal catheters. With nasotracheal catheters the tube is measured to the level of the thoracic inlet or further to the tracheal bifurcation or the fifth intercostal space if indicated. The patient's head should be held in an extended position to facilitate blind passage into the trachea. If coughing is noted, lidocaine can be infused via the tube to anesthetize the larynx. Nasotracheal oxygen is a very useful in the patient with laryngeal dysfunction or collapsing cervical trachea. Oxygen should be delivered into the trachea at rates of 50% of that used for nasal catheters. The oxygen should always be humidified, except under emergency conditions; then the duration of unhumidified oxygen should be as short as possible.

Transtracheal Catheters

In the patient who has an upper airway obstruction transtracheal oxygen can be provided on an emergent basis. This route also can be used as an alternative to nasal routes (Mann et al., 1992). A large-bore over-the-needle catheter or commercially available tracheal catheter can be placed between tracheal rings in the midcervical region. An adaptor is attached to the catheter and connected to oxygen. A 14-g intravenous catheter attached to a syringe can be inserted into the cricothyroid membrane or between tracheal rings and into the airway. The syringe plunger is then pulled back to verify that the tip of the catheter is in the airway (since air will be easily aspirated). The catheter is advanced, and the needle portion removed. Humidified oxygen can be delivered by an intravenous administration set improvised to attach to the catheter hub with the male end of the set. The "spike" end of the administration set is attached to the oxygen-humidifier system. A 3-mm endotracheal tube connector can then be inserted into the hub of the catheter, and oxygen and ventilation provided by the use of a resuscitator (AMBU) bag. Ventilating at a very rapid rate (150 breaths per minute) with oxygen attached and using the resuscitator bag with a reservoir attached provides adequate stop-gap ventilation and oxygenation (Crowe, 2003a).

Oxygen Cages

Oxygen cages are commonly used because it is very easy to deliver supplemental oxygen in this way. However, oxygen cages have several drawbacks. First is the length of time it takes to get the oxygen concentration up to a level that will help the patient (Engelhardt and Crowe, 2004). It can take 30 minutes to reach a 45% oxygen concentration at 15 L/minute and 45 minutes to reach a 60% concentration. The oxygen concentration may never exceed 30% at the 5-L/minute rate. The second problem with the use of oxygen cages is the inability to evaluate or physically treat the patient. Only visual observation is possible. The third problem occurs when the oxygen cage is opened to perform and evaluate treatment: the oxygen level within the cage drops substantially (generally from .4 to .2). This can lead to significant patient anxiety and respiratory compromise because the patient is now "back to room air," which occurs fairly suddenly. Animals that have been receiving significant relief of their dysoxia from the supplemental oxygen are at risk for cardiovascular collapse while they are being handled. The fourth problem is cost—of the cage itself and also of the oxygen. From my experience and those of many others, most oxygen cages require at least a 10 L/minute flow rate to maintain a 40% oxygen concentration. Even if the cage is door is not opened frequently, which is unlikely in critical cases, the oxygen cost is approximately 10 times that for the same patient with nasopharyngeal oxygen in place.

We have investigated the effectiveness of other noninvasive methods to provide supplemental oxygen (Engelhardt and Crowe, 2004). Oxygen flow rates of 5 and 15 L/minute were used to evaluate various methods of delivery (i.e., plastic sheeting place over a standard commercial cage, plastic sheeting placed over the top of a standard size "book box" cardboard box, clear plastic anesthesia "cat" box, a Crowe-oxygen collar [an E-collar one size too big fitted in front with a section of clear plastic wrap that covered the bottom half of the collar], blowby oxygen, and a plastic bag hood [allowing the oxygen to flow out from the bottom]). The hood and the Crowe collar reached maximum oxygen concentrations of 85% within 1 minute from the onset of oxygen flow of 5L/min. Other modalities of supplying supplemental oxygen also have been investigated, including the use of human nasal cannulas (infant, pediatric, and adult), nasal tubes (unilateral or bilateral), nasopharyngeal tubes, nasotracheal tubes, cricothyroid tubes, and tracheotomy tubes. The FiO_2 commonly obtained in the shortest period of time were nasal catheters (single) 45% in 2 minutes; nasal cannulas 60% in 1 minute; bilateral nasal catheters 85% within 2 minutes, nasopharyngeal catheter 85% in 2 minutes using 3-L flow rates; nasotracheal tube 85% in 30 seconds; transtracheal catheter nearly 100% within 30 seconds when 5-L/minute flow rates were used.

DETERMINING SUPPLEMENTAL OXYGEN EFFECTIVENESS

The effectiveness of supplemental oxygen is determined by clinical evaluation, pulse oximetry, and measurement of arterial blood gases.

Clinical Evaluation

This is the most common and most relied on approach. The amount of change in respiratory effort and the speed that it occurs once oxygen supplementation is begun are noted. It is hoped that both respiratory rate and effort are drastically reduced and that this reduction is observed within 20 minutes of starting oxygen supplementation. Other favorable responses may include restoration of calmness, a decrease in heart and pulse rate to normal, a return of normal blood flow (as determined by Doppler methods), and normalized blood pressure (as determined by either direct or indirect methods). Other methods of clinical evaluation include changes in blood lactate levels, strength of cardiac contractions or aortic velocity time integral as observed by echocardiography, and resolution of electrocardiographic abnormalities.

Pulse Oximetry

Pulse oximetry involves the measurement of the peak oxygen saturation of hemoglobin in capillary blood. Many factors can influence pulse oximeter accuracy; blood flow, probe contact, extraneous light, pigment, and movement are common causes for measurement inaccuracies. If these can be minimized, clinical studies have shown the methodology to be accurate and effective in the clinical detection of global dysoxia. Probes are usually placed on tissue beds that can be analyzed readily. Transmission probes include the tongue, toe webbing, ear pinna, and lip; reflectance probes include the esophagus and rectum. Units that provide a graph of the pulse contour are preferred over those that just provide a bar showing signal strength. Any saturation of peripheral oxygen (SpO_2) value below 92 mm Hg indicates an amount of oxygen desaturation that warrants oxygen supplementation; the lower the value, the greater the need for oxygen.

Arterial Blood Gas

This method hinges on the ability to obtain an arterial blood sample of sufficient volume to allow testing of the PO_2. Ventilation effectiveness can also be evaluated by analyzing the PCO_2. Arterial PO_2 should be at 65 mm Hg or above. A PaO_2 value below 65 mm Hg in spite of oxygen supplementation indicates a right-to-left shunt or severe pulmonary dysfunction and the need to consider positive-pressure ventilation. Other possible causes of unresponsive PaO_2 include pneumothorax, severe hypovolemic shock, cardiogenic shock, and obstructive airway disease.

CARE OF DYSOXIC PATIENTS NOT RESPONDING TO SUPPLEMENTAL OXYGEN

Response to supplemental oxygen therapy usually can be gauged by monitoring respiratory rate and effort, presence of cyanosis, and pulse oximetry readings. If the patient does not respond to supplemental oxygen, anesthesia, intubation, and ventilation should be strongly considered. As an intermediate step, assisted ventilation with the use of sedation followed by placement of a tight-fitting mask and positive-pressure support ventilation timed with each patient breath can be tried. It is important to recognize that patients who have been working hard to breathe for an extended period of time may die from ventilatory failure secondary to exhaustion. Simply sedating the patient generally allows the placement of a AMBU bag attached to a reservoir and oxygen supply, delivering oxygen at

5 to 15L/min. The mask is applied firmly with the patient's head and neck extended (with the tongue pulled out and the mouth closed over the extended tongue (if the patient allows). The bag is squeezed with inhalation, thus assisting the patient with positive-pressure breathing. Timing each squeeze of the bag with the beginning of each breath may relieve the patient's respiratory difficulty before anesthesia and intubation. Administration of a mixture of ketamine (5 mg/kg) and diazepam (0.25 mg/kg), given to effect, generally allows tracheal intubation. Other drugs can be used such as 2.5% thiopental (5 to 10 mg/kg) and propofol (3 to 8 mg/kg), but in my experience these produce more significant cardiovascular depression and are not my drugs of choice. Etomidate also can be used. It is especially useful as part of a rapid sequence induction anesthesia or for conscious sedation. It has a rapid onset of action and a low cardiovascular risk profile. The dose ranges from 0.025 mg/kg for sedation to 0.05 to 0.25 mg/kg for rapid anesthesia induction, with an average of 0.1 mg/kg for the moderately compromised patient. Neuromuscular blockers (succinylcholine 0.01 mg/kg intravenously [IV] or atracurium 0.25 mg/kg IV) can also be used after ketamine, diazepam, or an opioid are given (atracurium is preferred over succinylcholine because it does not cause muscular contractions). In the compromised patient doses should always be titrated because much less drug is generally required than is needed for the healthy patient. Once intubated (preferably with a laryngoscope since this provides for less laryngeal manipulation and reduced vasovagal response), positive-pressure ventilation is continued. Sedation for ventilatory support can be achieved with a continuous rate infusion of various drugs. These include sodium pentobarbital (1 mg/kg/hr), hydromorphone (0.1 mg/kg/hr with ketamine 2 mg/kg/hr, or 1 mg/kg/hr with the addition of lidocaine 3 mg/kg/hr). There are many other combinations that can be used. Institution of positive pressure ventilation is most often made very late in the stages of respiratory failure. I highly recommend positive pressure ventilatory support with PEEP early in the course of the disease.

Bag-Valve-Mask Continuous Positive Airway Pressure Ventilation

Continuous positive airway pressure (CPAP) is defined as maintaining the pressure above atmospheric pressure throughout the respiratory cycle. A modified form of CPAP can be provided to most awake (but sedated) dogs and cats using the interim method for patient support discussed previously. A tight-fitting mask attached to an anesthetic circuit or an AMBU bag is placed on the patient. The pop-off valve of the anesthetic machine is tightened down, and the oxygen flow rate is increased until the pressure on the circuit at end-exhalation registers 5 cm H_2O. Alternatively a positive end-expiratory pressure (PEEP) valve is added to the exhalation port of the AMBU bag. The patient breathes spontaneously while oxygen under pressure is delivered during inspiration by manual squeezing of the AMBU bag. This decreases the work of breathing and also improves gas exchange by increasing functional residual capacity. This also acts to mobilize edema fluid. It is one way to effectively treat acute respiratory failure secondary to pulmonary injury,

edema, and intrapulmonary hemorrhage. Applied more frequently at lower tidal volumes, it is helpful for patients with a diaphragmatic hernia and as a means of preoxygenating patients before attempting tracheal intubation and ventilation (Crowe, 2003b).

Ventilatory Support and Positive End-Expiratory Pressure

Ventilatory support is required for at least several hours (minimum) in most patients who remain hypoxemic despite oxygen supplementation or in patients who have an impaired ability to exhale CO_2 ($PaCO_2$ >50 mm Hg). As a rule of thumb patients should be ventilated at 10 to 20 breaths per minute at tidal volumes of 5 to 10 ml/kg (up to 15 to 20 ml/kg). Peak inspiratory pressures should try to be kept below 15 to 17 mm Hg whenever possible to reduce the likelihood of barotrauma. Ventilatory parameters (tidal volume and respiratory rate) should be adjusted based on capnometry and/or blood gases or, if these are unavailable, to the point of patient compliance at which the patient does not "fight" the positive-pressure breaths provided. When patients require high peak inspiratory pressures, PEEP should be added. Alveoli are prevented from collapsing when PEEP is used; use of PEEP increases the functional residual capacity, which leaves air in the lungs a little longer, increasing the time for gas exchange. This often allows peak inspiratory pressures to be decreased. As a rule of thumb it is recommended to begin PEEP at 5 to 10 cm H_2O. Excessive PEEP (>15) itself can cause barotrauma; thus this should be used only if necessary (continued PaO_2 below 60 mm Hg, SpO_2 below 80% or visible cyanosis). The major side effects of PEEP are an increase in intrathoracic pressure, which can decrease venous return to the heart and an increase in dead space. Once initiated, ventilation with PEEP is often needed for multiple hours to multiple days (see next chapter).

Patients Requiring Supplemental Oxygen That Must Be Transported

Patients needing oxygen may require 24-hour care. If a patient must be transported to another facility, it should be sent on oxygen. This is best provided with the use of a small oxygen cylinder attached to a flowmeter/regulator that can be purchased for approximately $80.00 from many emergency medical services suppliers (Galls)(Crowe, 2003a). If a tank and regulator are not available, most local home flowmeter/medical supply businesses or oxygen suppliers provide small oxygen tanks at very little cost. A regulator can be rented for minimal expense, although on occasion a deposit may be required. Many of these services have 24-hour availability.

HYPERBARIC OXYGEN: APPLICATION IN WOUNDS AND OTHER DYSOXIC CONDITIONS

Oxygen tension in wounds plays a significant role in healing and the potential for necrosis and infection (Crowe, 2002; Greif et al., 2000; Whitney et al., 2001). As measured by microelectrodes, the wound space is initially hypoxic

(PO$_2$ 0 to 15 mm Hg), hypoglycemic (2 to 4 mM), acidotic (pH 6.5 to 7.2), hyperkalemic (5.5 to 7.5 mM), hyperlactic (50 to 120 mM), and hypercarbic (60 to 90 mm Hg). Part of this unusual environment is caused by activated macrophages. A pH as low as 3.7 has been measured on the surface of activated macrophages. At the edge of a wound where there is viable circulation, PO$_2$ has been measured at 40 mm Hg. Oxygen is rapidly consumed as it diffuses from the edge of the viable capillaries into the wound space. Within 100 to 150 microns PO$_2$ can approach zero. Local tissue hypoxia has also been documented in surgical wounds when tight sutures impair local microcirculation. The tissue hypoxia is associated with a decreased oxidation-reduction potential, and this promotes tissue death and necrosis. The low pH also is associated with decreased polymorphonuclear (PMN) leukocyte function (Whitney et al., 2001). These conditions promote anaerobic and microaerophilic bacterial growth. The bacteria may be introduced by way of outside contamination or from an endogenous source (i.e., the gastrointestinal tract). In infections associated with an aerobic and anaerobic bacteria there may be bacterial synergism in which the growth of the aerophilic or microaerophilic bacteria further lowers the pH, allowing the growth of the more fastidious anaerobes to accelerate rapidly. The wound environment with bacterial growth involved becomes even more hypoxic. In bacterial osteomyelitis PO$_2$ of bone is lowered by 50%. One of the best ways to stop this vicious cycle is to provide oxygen to the wound, especially if it can be provided under hyperbaric conditions (pressures higher than sea level).

Oxygen given under hyperbaric conditions diffuses into the wound much more efficiently and may also be "stored" in the ground substance of the interstitial space. Treatments of hyperbaric oxygen are 1 to 2 hours in length and are done once or twice daily for a series of 3 to 15 days or more, depending on the wound condition. Chronic wounds or those involving an infection in the bone or dense connective tissues such as ligaments or tendons require the longer treatment times. In acute wounds even one treatment may be beneficial in preventing tissue death from ischemia or infection.

There are various ways of providing oxygen at hyperbaric conditions. One method is by simply placing the involved limb or area of the body into a pouch that becomes fairly airtight and then filling the pouch with oxygen. These "bags of oxygen" are mildly effective in raising oxygen tensions in wounds; however, problems with leakage and the need for sedation minimize potential value. If the wound is inflamed, the pressure may induce pain.

The second method, which I use very frequently, is to use a low-pressure monoplace chamber. The animal is placed into this chamber, which is made of a high-density flexible synthetic clothlike material. The chamber is filled with air using two compressors that increase the pressure to 1.25 to 1.3 atmospheres (3.5 to 4.5 pounds per square inch [PSI] greater than sea level). Most of the time the animal is mildly sedated. In some cases an oxygen Crowe collar is applied to increase oxygen concentrations to 60% to 80% as described previously.

The third method involves the placement of the animal in a chamber made of stainless steel, Plexiglas, or Mylar in which 100% oxygen is used to pressurize the chamber. Pressures are increased from 11 to 15 PSI, which corresponds to 1.8 to 2.1 atmospheres. In most chambers the amount of oxygen needed to produce a treatment of 1 hour at 15 PSI requires about 2300 L of oxygen. The higher-pressure chamber is able to elevate the PO$_2$ in tissues much higher than low-pressure chambers (i.e., 1560 mm Hg of oxygen with the high-pressure chamber verses 600 mm Hg of oxygen with the lower-pressure, lower-concentration [60%]) chamber). This appears clinically most important when infections involve anaerobic or microaerophilic organisms or when wounds or tissues have significant edema present (Crowe 2000, 2002a, b).

Experimental and clinical investigations of wounds that have been treated with hyperbaric oxygen reveal that wound infections are prevented. Antibiotic effectiveness in infected wounds is increased as PMN and macrophage function is also increased. Edema in wounds is lessened significantly, allowing for better blood flow and DO$_2$ that continues following the hyperbaric oxygen therapy (HBOT). Lymphatic flow is increased, and pain is lessened as the edema and dysoxia dissipate. Wound healing rates also speed up as the oxygen stimulates fibroplasia and osteon proliferation. Pain and inflammation are lessened with HBOTs. The wound bed is much more oxygenated, and tissue that is necrotic is defined quicker with the use of HBOTs. Pain is lessened from decreasing edema and hypoxia at nerve endings. Other potential indications include pancreatitis, aortic thrombosis, acute cortical blindness, fibrocartilaginous embolus, and acute intervertebral disk herniation. Further investigations are required to elucidate the clinical conditions that may benefit from the use of hyperbaric oxygen therapy. Box 137-5 is a summary of the various diseases that I have treated with hyperbaric oxygen with clinical benefits noted (Crowe 2000, 2002a).

Box 137-5

Possible Indications for Hyperbaric Oxygen Therapy

- Brain and spinal cord edema, injury, trauma
- Post intervertebral disk herniation, fibrocartilage embolus
- Pancreatitis
- Abdominal sepsis, bowel obstruction, postgastric dilation volvulus
- Pyothorax
- Posttraumatic or ischemic shock
- Postcardiopulmonary resuscitation neurologic impairment
- Acute cortical blindness
- Swollen limbs and joints following trauma, orthopedic surgery
- Severe sinusitis, septic rhinitis
- Aortic thromboembolism
- Vestibular syndrome
- Suspected stroke
- Severe wounds
- Infected wounds
- Chronic ulcers (gastrointestinal)
- Chronic delayed unions
- Bad complex fractures
- Postradiation necrosis
- Snake and spider bite

References and Suggested Reading

Crowe DT: Hyperbaric oxygen therapy in veterinary medicine: a case series at Carson-Tahoe Veterinary Hospital, *Hyperbaric Med Today* 1:13, 2000.

Crowe DT: Physiotherapy and hyperbaric oxygen therapy in the critical patient. Proceedings of the Annual Scientific Meeting European College of Veterinary Surgeons, University of Veterinary Medicine, Vienna, Austria, July 5-7, 2002a, p 324.

Crowe DT: Hyperbaric oxygen in wound healing. Proceedings of the American College of Veterinary Surgeons 12th Annual Veterinary Symposium, San Diego, Calif, October 17-20, 2002b, p 398.

Crowe DT: Supplemental oxygen therapy in critically ill or injured patients, *Vet Med* 98:935, 2003a.

Crowe DT: Rapid sequence intubation and surgical intervention in respiratory emergencies, *Vet Med* 98:954, 2003b.

Engelhardt MH, Crowe DT: Comparison of six non-invasive supplemental oxygen techniques in dogs and cats, Scientific Proceedings of the 10th International Veterinary Emergency and Critical Care Symposium, Sept 8-12, 2004, San Diego, Calif, p 983.

Fitzpatrick RK, Crowe DT: Nasal oxygen administration in dogs and cats: experimental and clinical investigations, *J Am Anim Hosp Assoc* 22:293, 1986.

Greif R et al: Supplemental oxygen to reduce the incidence of surgical-wound infection: Outcomes Research Group, *N Engl J Med* 342:161, 2000.

Manley GT et al: Brain tissue oxygenation during hemorrhagic shock, resuscitation, and alterations in ventilation, *J Trauma* 46:261, 1999.

Mann FA et al: Comparison of intranasal and transtracheal oxygen administration in healthy, awake dogs, *Am J Vet Res* 53:856, 1992.

Meier J et al: Hyperoxic ventilation reduces six-hour mortality after partial fluid resuscitation from hemorrhagic shock, *Shock* 22:240, 2004.

Whitney JD et al: Tissue and wound healing effects of shorts duration postoperative oxygen therapy, *Biol Res Nurs* 2:206, 2001.

CHAPTER 138
Ventilator Therapy

SHANE W. BATEMAN, *Columbus, Ohio*
ELIZABETH O'TOOLE, *Oakville, Ontario, Canada*

Patients with respiratory failure should receive assisted ventilation with a modern positive-pressure ventilator designed for that purpose. The aims of mechanical ventilation are to improve gas exchange and to decrease the work of breathing in patients with a reversible underlying disease process. Ventilators designed for use in anesthesia are not suitable for ventilating critically ill patients because they typically cannot regulate the oxygen concentration. Prolonged delivery of high oxygen concentrations can cause toxicity and worsen lung injury. Critical care ventilators are also more complex than ventilators designed for use in anesthesia and include a variety of modes for applying positive-pressure ventilation, allowing specifically tailored respiratory therapy.

It is a common fallacy that patients who require mechanical ventilation are doomed to die. Two factors have contributed to this fallacy: a previous lack of understanding of the special requirements for ventilating lung-injured patients and a tendency to initiate ventilation too late in the course of disease as a "last-ditch attempt" when patients typically have been hypoxemic and hypercarbic for some time. The pathophysiologic consequences of these two factors are significant and should not be underestimated. Ventilator care has an important place in the management of carefully selected critically ill patients.

DEFINITION OF RESPIRATORY FAILURE

Although a strict definition of respiratory failure, and thus the requirement for ventilatory care, is not universally agreed on, the following blood gas guidelines are appropriate to identify inadequate gas exchange or hypoventilation:

- Arterial partial pressure of carbon dioxide (PCO_2) above 50 mm Hg
- Arterial partial pressure of oxygen (PO_2) will not rise above 50 mm Hg on a test dose of 100% O_2, or arterial PO_2 cannot be maintained above 50 mm Hg with fractional percent of inspired oxygen (FiO_2) of 0.6 or less

In addition to these blood gas guidelines, the work of breathing needed to maintain current gas exchange must be critically assessed for each patient. This assessment is subjective and based on clinical judgment. Respiratory muscle exhaustion can occur rapidly and may precede respiratory failure and sudden death. The decision to initiate mechanical ventilation should be based on evidence of both the failure of gas exchange and the work of breathing.

INDICATIONS FOR MECHANICAL VENTILATION

In the past, many clinicians have associated the use of mechanical ventilation with certain death. Unfortunately this historic attitude is still prevalent, and mechanical ventilation is often undertaken too late. Mechanical ventilation may be unsuccessful in some cases simply because the opportunity to successfully treat the patient's condition has already passed. With the improvements in diagnostic, supportive, and monitoring technology in veterinary critical care, this attitude needs to be readdressed. Mechanical ventilation frequently is successful in treating veterinary patients with respiratory failure provided patients are chosen carefully, appropriate ventilation strategies are chosen, and the decision to initiate mechanical ventilation is made early in the course of disease.

Several authors have offered the following thoughts about the place of mechanical ventilation in critical care.

- The indication for intubation and mechanical ventilation is THINKING of it.
- Artificial airways are not a disease; ventilators are not an addiction.
- Intubation is not an act of weakness; it is an act of kindness.

Two classifications of patients benefit from mechanical ventilation: those with primary pulmonary pathology (lung-injured patients), and those with neuromuscular apparatus failure (nonlung-injured patient). Examples of primary respiratory pathology include noncardiogenic and cardiogenic pulmonary edema; pneumonia; pulmonary contusions; and acute lung injury, including acute respiratory distress syndrome (ARDS), upper and lower airway obstruction, and smoke inhalation. Examples of neuromuscular apparatus failure include polyradiculoneuritis (coonhound paralysis), myasthenia gravis, tick paralysis, botulism, tetanus, cranial cervical spinal cord lesions, brain injury, anesthetic complication, drug overdose, postcardiopulmonary resuscitation, respiratory muscle exhaustion caused by high work of breathing, diaphragmatic herniation, and chest wall trauma.

Mechanical ventilation can be used successfully to treat patients with various types of respiratory failure. However, it is an invasive procedure, requiring an artificial airway, heavy sedation, and intensive monitoring by trained professional caregivers. Potential complications such as ventilator-induced lung injury and nosocomial pneumonia may occur. There are also physiologic consequences secondary to the positive pressure applied to the lungs that may have a detrimental effect on cardiovascular, renal, hepatic and gastrointestinal functions.

CAUSES OF HYPOXEMIA

There are five main causes of hypoxemia: alveolar hypoventilation, ventilation-perfusion (V/Q) mismatch,

shunt, low inspired FiO_2 (high altitudes), and diffusion impairment. Clinically the first three causes are the most relevant.

Hypoventilation

Decreased alveolar minute ventilation *always* produces hypercarbia and hypoxia. The hypoxia can be abolished if the patient is breathing an increased FiO_2 (FiO_2 >0.21), but the hypercarbia persists until an increase in minute ventilation occurs.

Ventilation/Perfusion Mismatching

This is the most common cause of hypoxemia. Alterations in V/Q ratios occur in diseased lung units through changes in airway resistance (asthma, bronchoconstriction), airway or vascular obstruction (airway secretions, alveolar/interstitial edema, and thromboemboli), and perfusion changes (pressure, permeability, cardiac output). Abnormalities in V/Q matching tend to have a more significant effect on the oxygen (O_2) content of the blood rather than on the carbon dioxide (CO_2) content. This effect can be attributed to the sigmoidal shape of the oxyhemoglobin-dissociation curve when compared to the linear relationship between CO_2 and hemoglobin saturation.

Shunt

Shunting occurs when blood flow continues through unventilated alveoli (or bypasses the lungs completely as in the case of an anatomic shunt such as a cardiovascular anomaly). This is the *only* cause of hypoxemia resistant to oxygen supplementation, but it is rarely present in a pure form (i.e., not accompanied by other causes of hypoxemia).

CAUSES OF HYPERCAPNIA

Hypercapnia is always associated with an inability to adequately remove CO_2 from the venous blood. This is usually because of a failure of the ventilatory pump (i.e., the bellows motion of the lungs to move air in and out). This may occur either because of an overload of the pump (increased cellular CO_2 production, airway obstruction, and exhaustion from the work of breathing) or the inability to pump (central nervous system [CNS] disease, hypoventilation, and respiratory muscle dysfunction).

Theoretically both V/Q mismatch and shunt should cause hypercapnia, but the respiratory centers detect the elevation and increase minute ventilation to maintain CO_2 levels. Thus only when the injury is sufficiently severe, further increases in minute ventilation cannot be accomplished, and the work of breathing exhausts the patient does hypoventilation occur and elevate CO_2 levels.

VENTILATOR SETTINGS

Modern critical care ventilators are complex with multiple settings to optimize the breath delivery to the patient. The first decision is determining whether control is based on delivered gas volume per breath (volume-cycled) or the applied inspiratory pressure per breath (pressure-cycled). Volume-cycled ventilators deliver a predetermined tidal volume regardless of the airway pressure delivered volume creates. Pressure-cycled ventilators deliver a breath to a predetermined airway pressure; as a result tidal volumes may vary. Modern critical care ventilators are able to deliver both volume- and pressure-cycled ventilation. In patients with healthy lungs volume-cycled modes offer predictable minute ventilation without significant risk of creating ventilator-induced lung injury. In patients with lung injury limiting the inspiratory pressure (pressure-cycled ventilation) decreases the risk of damage to the diseased airways. The major disadvantage of this mode is the unpredictability of cycle-to-cycle tidal volumes because the volume of gas delivered is determined by the lung mechanics at any given moment in time.

The next decision is determining how much control the patient will exert over the breaths delivered by the ventilator. There are three types of patient breaths. *Controlled* breaths are delivered according to the respiratory rate and tidal volume settings of the ventilator. A controlled breath is delivered at a set time interval and ignores the patient's efforts to breathe. *Assisted* breaths are delivered according to the tidal volume settings of the ventilator, but the patient can, within some parameters, determine the rate of breath delivery. The patient is able to initiate an *assisted* breath; however, the ventilator then mechanically delivers the remainder of the breath to achieve the volume or pressure limits of tidal volume delivery. *Spontaneous* breaths can also occur in some ventilator modes. Spontaneous breaths occur when the patient is breathing faster than the rate settings of the ventilator in some modes (see following paragraphs). Traditionally the ventilator did not mechanically support spontaneous breaths, and the patient encountered high levels of resistance and dead space by having to breathe through an endotracheal tube and the ventilator circuit tubing. Modern ventilators frequently have several support options for spontaneous breaths designed to decrease the work of breathing associated with spontaneous breaths.

Two additional settings to consider in the initial ventilator setup include the *sensitivity* and the FiO_2. The responsiveness of the ventilator to patient efforts to initiate breathing (assisted or spontaneous breaths) is determined by the sensitivity setting. It should be set to maximize patient comfort and minimize patient-ventilator asynchrony. The FiO_2 of breath delivery determines the concentration of oxygen in the breath delivery and should be set to the lowest concentration possible to allow adequate blood oxygen content and delivery.

The breath delivery mode of the ventilator should be chosen to achieve maximal patient-ventilator synchrony. The available modes on most ventilators include assist/control (A/C), synchronized intermittent mandatory ventilation (SIMV), and spontaneous (SPONT). In *A/C* mode no spontaneous breaths are allowed. In this mode the ventilator assists patient inspiratory efforts faster than the rate setting of the ventilator (assisted breaths). If the patient makes no inspiratory efforts, controlled breaths are delivered at the rate set by the ventilator. This mode tends to be used most commonly when patients are under general anesthesia or have a poor respiratory drive. Patients capable of making significant inspiratory efforts are not likely to be comfortable in this mode of ventilation.

The *SIMV* mode allows both mechanical and spontaneous breaths to be delivered according to patient demand. The type of breath delivered depends on the rate setting of the ventilator and the inspiratory efforts made by the patient. If the ventilator detects no patient effort, controlled breaths are delivered according to the rate setting. If the patient is making some efforts, the ventilator attempts to synchronize assisted breaths with patient effort as often as possible. If the patient is making inspiratory efforts above the ventilator rate settings, spontaneous breaths are permitted. This mode allows more comfort for the patient and is less likely to result in ventilator-patient asynchrony. Patients with high respiratory drive and vigorous inspiratory efforts may not find this mode comfortable, depending on how many mandatory machine-delivered (assisted/controlled) breaths are set.

In *SPONT* mode the ventilator delivers no mandatory mechanical breaths. All breaths are spontaneous. If the ventilator permits spontaneous breath support, the amount and type of support can be titrated to the patient's needs. This mode is typically used for patients in which the underlying condition has improved significantly and those that have vigorous and strong inspiratory efforts. This mode is frequently a preweaning mode.

The final setting to determine concerns *positive end-expiratory pressure* (PEEP) and how much will be applied. After a positive-pressure breath, the patient's lung is allowed to return to normal atmospheric pressure at the end of expiration. In injured lungs this results in cyclic opening and collapse of small airways and alveoli, which contributes to further lung damage and worsening gas exchange. Application of PEEP prevents the lung from returning to normal atmospheric pressure at the end of expiration. PEEP acts as an airway splint at the end of expiration to prevent further airway injury and can also result in improved oxygenation as a result of: (1) increase in the functional residual capacity, (2) alveolar recruitment, (3) improved V/Q matching, and (4) redistribution of the extravascular lung water.

A clinician responsible for ventilator care must be familiar with the settings, modes of ventilation offered, and additional options for tailoring breath delivery of the ventilator in use. Such knowledge optimizes breath delivery to the patient while decreasing the risk of ventilator injury.

VENTILATOR-INDUCED LUNG INJURY

In past decades our understanding of acute lung injury and the pulmonary response to ventilation has increased dramatically. Patients with lung injury have edema, bleeding, or inflammation within the alveolus and connecting airways. These substances inactivate surfactant and lead to alveolar collapse and atelectasis. In severe disease only a fraction of the lung may be ventilating and perfusing normally, thus dramatically decreasing effective gas exchange. Experimental trials using traditional mechanical ventilation strategies have documented many types of ventilator-induced lung injury in these settings. High mean airway pressures and use of tidal volumes that are excessive to the amount of functional gas exchange tissue cause capillary fragmentation, tearing, and leakage of blood and plasma into the alveolus, setting the stage for further collapse and more functional loss. A second type of injury also occurs in marginal small airways and alveoli, which are partially collapsed. If the end-expiratory pressure is allowed to return to atmospheric pressure, these airways are repeatedly opened and closed, and a shear stress injury occurs to the airway/alveoli. Human clinical trials and experimental animal studies have demonstrated the increased production of proinflammatory cytokines in the lungs during these conditions. The increased production of cytokines may have a systemic effect, increasing the risk of multiple organ dysfunction in patients with ARDS.

A lung-protective strategy has been developed to lessen the ventilator-induced injury in lung-injured patients. This approach uses very low tidal volumes (4 to 6 ml/kg) and limits airway pressures (<35 cm of H_2O) to minimize pressure- and volume-induced injury and uses PEEP (8 to 14 cm of H_2O) to maintain marginal airways/alveoli open, prevent airway shear stress, and improve oxygenation. One cost of such lung protection is often hypoventilation. A lung-protective ventilation strategy permits mild-to-moderate hypercapnia (partial pressure of alveolar CO_2 [$PaCO_2$] of approximately 70 to 80 mm Hg) to occur.

VENTILATING THE NON–LUNG-INJURED PATIENT

When ventilating the patient that has not experienced lung injury, the following are the goals of therapy:

1. Restore respiratory function until resolution of the underlying problem occurs (i.e., neuromyopathy resolves or muscle strength returns).
2. Restore/maintain normal gas exchange. No lung pathology should exist; thus normal blood gas values should be achievable on or just above room air (21% oxygen).
3. Sedation should be titrated to prevent agitation associated with mechanical ventilation. Heart rate, blood pressure, oxygenation, and patient-ventilator synchrony (tolerance of endotracheal tube and ventilator breaths and general anxiety) should serve as guidelines of patient comfort.
4. If the duration of ventilation is expected to be longer than 24 hours, early consideration of a tracheostomy is appropriate (ideally within the first 12 hours).
5. Continuous monitoring of the electrocardiogram (ECG), blood pressure, urine output, end-tidal CO_2 (ETCO$_2$ using a capnograph), and oxygen saturation (SaO$_2$ using a pulse oximeter) should take place. Arterial blood gases should be measured twice daily and compared to noninvasive parameters to assess patient status and noninvasive monitoring efficacy. Deviations of ETCO$_2$ and SaO$_2$ out of normal ranges or worsening of clinical status also indicate a need for arterial blood gas analysis.

Initial recommended ventilator settings for these patients include the following:

Mode:	SIMV or A/C using volume-cycled breath delivery
Tidal volume:	10 to 12 ml/kg
Rate:	10 to 15 beats/min
FiO$_2$:	0.21 to 0.30
PEEP:	1 to 5 cm of H_2O
Sensitivity:	2 to 5 cm H_2O or 1 to 2 L/min (adjust for patient-ventilator synchrony)

Ventilation at these settings should continue for 20 minutes and then be assessed with blood gas analysis. Initial FiO$_2$ settings can be higher until the patient is stable but should then be decreased to the lowest value that permits adequate oxygenation. Fine tuning can then take place unless the patient appears distressed or bedside monitors indicate that earlier changes are required. Alarms should be adjusted to maintain reasonably safe zones but not so tight that frequent violation occurs (unless the patient is currently functioning in the edge of a safe zone).

VENTILATING THE LUNG-INJURED PATIENT

When ventilating the patient with pulmonary injury, the goals of therapy include the following:

1. Support ventilation and oxygenation until sufficient lung healing or respiratory muscle strength returns to allow weaning.
2. Because of lung injury and impaired gas exchange, blood gas values should not be expected to be ideal. Oxygen therapy should be adjusted to maintain arterial partial oxygen pressure at 60 to 80 mm Hg using the lowest possible concentration of oxygen to decrease the likelihood of oxygen toxicity. Levels above 60% for greater than 24 to 36 hours are thought to contribute to such toxicity.
3. PEEP should be used to recruit collapsed airways and increase compliance and oxygenation.
4. Patients with severe lung injury have decreased lung volumes available for gas exchange; thus ventilation with normal tidal volumes can induce volume and pressure injury to the healthy lung because of overdistention. Use of small tidal volumes, pressure-cycled ventilation and close trending of both peak and mean airway pressure in conjunction with PEEP therapy help to prevent further ventilator-induced lung injury. Use of such a lung-protective strategy may result in some CO_2 retention. Hypercapnia at mild-to-moderate levels (70 to 80 mm Hg) does not appear to have any detrimental effects on the patient.
5. Sedation should be titrated to the lowest level to prevent agitation associated with mechanical ventilation. Heart rate, blood pressure, oxygenation, and patient-ventilator synchrony (tolerance of endotracheal tube and ventilator breaths and general anxiety) should serve as guidelines of patient comfort. Lung-injured patients with permissive hypercapnia have strong respiratory efforts in response to CO_2 elevations and require deep sedation or anesthesia to achieve acceptable patient-ventilator synchrony.

6. If the duration of ventilation is expected to be longer than 24 hours, early consideration should be given to tracheostomy.
7. Continuous monitoring of $ETCO_2$, SaO_2, ECG, blood pressure, and urine output should take place. The accuracy of capnography and pulse oximetry is likely to be significantly less accurate in lung-injured, severely hypoxemic patients; thus a greater reliance should be placed on frequent arterial blood gas samples. Capnography and pulse oximetry can still be used for trending and can alert the caregiver of potential problems.

Initial ventilator settings for the lung-injured patient include the following:

Mode:	SIMV pressure-cycled breaths with spontaneous breath support
Tidal volume:	Dependent on pressure setting. Aim for lowest possible pressure setting that achieves tidal volumes of 4 to 6 ml/kg. Do not exceed mean airway pressures of 35 cm of H_2O if possible.
Rate:	18 to 30 beats/min
FiO_2:	0.30 to 1 (use the lowest possible fraction)
PEEP:	8 to 15 cm of H_2O
Sensitivity:	2 to 5 cm of H_2O or 1 to 2 L/minute (adjust for patient-ventilator synchrony)

Ventilation at these settings should continue for 20 minutes and should then be assessed with blood gas analysis. Fine-tuning can then proceed unless the patient appears distressed or bedside monitors indicate that earlier changes are required. Alarms should be adjusted to maintain reasonably safe zones but not so tight that frequent violation occurs (unless patient is currently functioning in the edge of a safe zone).

CARDIOVASCULAR IMPLICATIONS OF POSITIVE-PRESSURE VENTILATION

The interactions of positive-pressure ventilation and the cardiovascular system are complex and depend to a large extent on the mode of ventilation being used. Elevated intrathoracic pressure from positive-pressure ventilation can impede ventricular filling and decrease preload and cardiac output. Conversely high pressures can decrease afterload from elevation of transmural pressure on the ventricle, increasing cardiac output. Thus the end result of an increased or decreased cardiac output depends to a large extent on volume status of the patient, underlying myocardial function, and mean intrathoracic pressures produced by mechanical ventilation. Patients with impaired left ventricular function may have an increase in cardiac output, but patients with hypovolemia or in which higher levels of PEEP are necessary may experience a decline in cardiac output. Ultimately the goal of mechanical ventilation should be to improve oxygen delivery to the tissues, not to increase the oxygen content of the arterial blood; thus maintaining cardiac output is extremely important. At some point the cost of ventilation (in declining cardiac output and resultant decreasing oxygen delivery) outweighs the benefit of increasing arterial oxygen content.

Small decreases in cardiac output likely result in activation of the renin-angiotensin-aldosterone-vasopressin system, with retention of sodium and water. Thus mechanically ventilated patients may experience decreased urine output because of these effects. Peripheral edema also may occur.

PATIENT-VENTILATOR ASYNCHRONY

Patient agitation and distress can result in counterproductive fighting against the ventilator. The most common causes of this problem are incorrect ventilator setup for the patient's respiratory drive or psychologic comfort, an acute change in the clinical status of the patient, obstruction of the airway, development of pneumothorax, or malfunction of the ventilator. The correct response to patient-ventilator asynchrony should involve the following steps:

1. Auscultate both lung fields for breath sounds and observe chest wall motion for synchrony.
2. Assess depth of sedation (palpebral reflex, jaw tone).
3. Disconnect the patient and hand ventilate to assess compliance.
4. Suction the airway.
5. Consider reintubation of the patient.
6. Perform an arterial blood gas analysis to determine the patient's status.

If none of these activities reveal the problem, the patient should be repositioned to a more comfortable position, or if this is not possible the plane of sedation adjusted. As a final step consideration of a different mode of ventilation may be necessary (e.g., changing from A/C to SIMV may provide more patient comfort).

MAINTAINING SEDATION/ANALGESIA DURING MECHANICAL VENTILATION

Several combinations of drugs can maintain patient comfort during mechanical ventilation. Generally patients without lung injury can be maintained comfortably using combined continuous infusions of opioids and benzodiazepines. Morphine (0.1 to 0.3 mg/kg/hour), hydromorphone (0.015 to 0.03 mg/kg/hour), or fentanyl (1 to 5 mcg/kg/hour) and diazepam (0.1 to 0.5 mg/kg/hour) following loading doses are reliably safe and inexpensive and both drug classes can be reversed easily when weaning is attempted.

Lung-injured patients typically are more difficult to control because of high ventilatory drive from hypercarbia or hypoxemia. The use of lung-protective ventilation strategies may also increase the likelihood of hypercapnia, auto-PEEP at high respiratory rates (RR), decreased alveolar minute volume, and ventilator-patient asynchrony. To overcome these issues, more potent CNS-depressant drugs must be administered. Historically pentobarbital was the most commonly used agent for this purpose and was administered as a continuous infusion (1 to 5 mg/kg/hour) after induction of anesthesia at 5 to 15 mg/kg. However, pentobarbital appears to have immunosuppressive effects when used for several days and is no longer the first choice in maintaining sedation (particularly in infectious pneumonia). Combinations of medications seem to be a better choice. The combinations that are potentially beneficial are propofol with a benzodiazepine or opioid infusion (fentanyl, hydromorphone, or morphine) or ketamine (100 to 300 mcg/kg/minute) in combination with an opioid and benzodiazepine infusion. Propofol infusions are also helpful during weaning from the ventilator because of its superior ability to achieve rapid titration (25 to 600 mcg/kg/minute). In severe situations when these regimens are unable to control patient ventilator asynchrony, the addition of a neuromuscular blocking agent should be used. Continuous infusion of atracurium is associated with the least side effects but should not be used for longer than 12 to 24 hours because of the incidence of severe myopathy/myoparesis syndromes (0.3 to 0.5 mg/kg/hour after a loading dose of 0.2 to 0.4 mg/kg). Atracurium is metabolized by Hoffman elimination; thus reduced dosages are necessary in acidemic or hypothermic patients. It is *essential* to provide analgesia and sedation in addition to neuromuscular blockage. Monitoring of the blockade and adjustment of dosage should be based on neuromuscular stimulation (train of four). Neuromuscular blockade must be reversed completely before weaning attempts.

CARE AND COMFORT OF THE MECHANICALLY VENTILATED PATIENT

Pulmonary Toilet

Airway obstruction caused by excessive buildup of secretions in the airway results in inefficient ventilation and can be caused by loss of the cough reflex, abrogation of the mucociliary clearance apparatus, and bronchorrhea (in lung injury). However, frequent suctioning can inflict further injury to the trachea and the mucociliary clearance. Therefore suctioning of the airway should be performed only as needed. Sterile in-line suction catheters are commercially available for this purpose. *Strict aseptic techniques should be used at all times.* Advancing the suction catheter only to the end of the tube in place, applying suction only on the withdrawal phase, and withdrawing slowly so that only one cycle of suctioning gets most of the secretions aids in reducing iatrogenic airway damage. Secretions can be collected for culture and sensitivity from the suction catheter or via separate tracheal wash samples. The patient should be preoxygenated and hand ventilated during suctioning if required.

Humidification of the airway, gases, and secretions is vital to successful treatment. Use of a heat and moisture exchanger should be sufficient to accomplish this goal. Alternatively humidification and temperature adjustment of the inspired gas can be accomplished with specifically designed humidification devices. Medications (β-agonists, anticholinergics, and corticosteroids) can be delivered by metered-dose inhalers through the ventilator circuit if necessary.

Other measures are important. Corneal ulceration and conjunctivitis are also very common. Sterile eye lubricants should be applied when necessary to prevent drying. A urinary catheter should be placed to maintain patient comfort. Diligent assessment of urinalysis for signs of bacterial cystitis and culture and sensitivity should be performed on a regular basis. Regular position shifts, massage, and physical therapy are helpful to maintain patient comfort. Adequate padding and absorbent bedding that is kept clean and dry is a requirement for these patients. Use of enteral feeding methods is desirable to maintain good gut barrier health, prevent translocation of bacteria, and prevent colonization of the flora with more pathogenic microbial strains.

Ventilator-Associated Pneumonia

Ventilator-associated pneumonia (VAP) is a possible sequel to mechanical ventilation and increases the risk of mortality by 2 to 10 times in humans. Mechanically ventilated patients are at an increased risk of developing a nosocomial pneumonia for several reasons such as altered level of consciousness, decreased gag reflex, alteration in the normal host respiratory tract defenses, delayed gastric clearance, ileus, previous antimicrobial usage, days of hospitalization, and aspiration of oropharyngeal secretions. Endotracheal intubation increases the risk of this complication in humans by 6 to 21 times, and every day of ventilation raises this risk by 1% to 3%. The pathogenesis of VAP is associated with the colonization of the aerodigestive tract with pathogenic microbes early in the course of hospitalization and aspiration of the contaminated secretions. The patient may also become infected by direct inoculation from intubation or secondary to caregivers who act as fomites for resistant microbes in the intensive care unit (ICU) environment. Strict attention to aseptic technique helps to prevent this complication. Implementation of strict hand-washing polices, barrier protective clothing, and policies directing traffic patterns within the ICU unit are considered helpful preventive measures. However, to prevent this complication a multifaceted approach is required. Excellent oral care, enteric feedings, titration of sedation to the lowest levels to ensure patient comfort, use of ventilator modes that aid in patient-ventilator synchrony, and responsible stewardship of antimicrobial drugs may all contribute to a decreased incidence of VAP. Early recognition of this complication is important, along with prompt initiation (ideally less than 12 hours after clinical diagnosis) of appropriate broad-spectrum antibiotics with culture and sensitivity testing to confirm and narrow the choice of antimicrobials.

Oral lesions are also very common in ventilator-dependent patients because of pressure necrosis from the endotracheal tube and monitoring devices. Cleansing of the oral cavity four to six times daily with dilute chlorhexidine solution (include the oropharynx and subglottal regions) and use of glycerin-soaked gauze pads on pressure points help maintain a more desirable oral bacterial flora. A sterile endotracheal tube should be used initially, and this tube should not be replaced unless viscous secretions are occluding the lumen.

WEANING FROM THE VENTILATOR

Weaning from mechanical ventilation can be a difficult process in some patients. Ideally a gradual reduction in the amount of ventilatory support with a concomitant increase in the participation of the patient in the work of breathing should take place. No objective measurement determines weaning success in humans, and no standardized methods have been described in veterinary medicine. One recommended technique is to use daily trials of spontaneous breathing. Most patients who fail the weaning process rapidly develop an increased frequency and decreased tidal volume of breathing. Patients who fail a weaning process should be continued on the latest level of support with further decreases of ventilatory assistance at prescribed intervals. Daily trials of spontaneous breathing should continue until weaning is successful. During the weaning process sedation with agents that are rapidly reversible or with short half-lives is preferred.

Suggested Reading

Brower RG et al: Ventilation with lower tidal volumes as compared with traditional tidal volumes for acute lung injury and the acute respiratory distress syndrome, *N Engl J Med* 342:1301, 2000.

Chastre J: Conference summary: ventilator-associated pneumonia, *Respir Care* 50(7):975, 2005.
Esteban A et al: A comparison of four methods of weaning patients from mechanical ventilation, *N Engl J Med* 332:345, 1995.
Fudge M et al: Oral lesions associated with orotracheal administered mechanical ventilation in critically ill dogs, *Vet Emerg Crit Care* 7:79, 1997.
Gali B, Goyal DG: Positive pressure mechanical ventilation, *Emerg Med Clin North Am* 21(2):453, 2003.
Hopper K et al: Indications, management, and outcome of long-term positive-pressure ventilation in dogs and cats: 148 cases (1990-2001), *J Am Vet Med Assoc* 230:64, 2007.
Marini JJ, Arthur P: *Critical care medicine: the essentials*, ed 2, Baltimore, 1997, Lippincott Williams & Wilkins.
Marino PL: *The ICU book*, ed 2, Baltimore, 1998, p 421.
Shapiro BA: A historical perspective on ventilator management, *New Horiz* 2:8, 1994.
Wingfield WE, Raffe MR: *The veterinary ICU book,* Jackson Hole, 2002, Teton NewMedia, p 96.

CHAPTER **139**
Rhinitis in the Dog

NED F. KUEHN, *Southfield, Michigan*

Sneezing and nasal discharge usually are associated with diseases of the nose, paranasal sinuses, and nasopharynx. Sneezing frequently precedes the onset of notable nasal discharge. The severity and frequency of sneezing may diminish over time, whereas the nasal discharge frequently worsens in severity and changes in character. Therefore dogs with chronic rhinitis are frequently presented with chronic nasal discharge rather than persistent sneezing. The nature of sneezing may aid in localizing the region of the problem. Expiratory sneezing typically is associated with sinus or intranasal disease. Reverse or inspiratory sneezing (aspiration reflex) is a normal response to mechanical irritation of the dorsal nasopharyngeal mucosa. The presence of reverse sneezing is usually correlated with caudal nasal, nasopharyngeal, or sinus disease. Some dogs may have posterior rather than anterior nasal discharge, and the only indication for primary nasal disease may be obstructive nasal breathing.

The causes for nasal discharge in the dog are included in Box 139-1. The principle diseases associated with chronic rhinitis are sinonasal neoplasia, idiopathic lymphoplasmacytic rhinitis, and fungal rhinitis (Lefebvre et al., 2005). Nasal discharge is not limited to primary nasal disease but also may occur with systemic and extranasal disorders. Very often extranasal disorders have systemic signs (e.g., depression, pyrexia, hemorrhage) and a history of acute onset, whereas primary nasal disorders have a more chronic duration. Important extranasal disorders that may present with nasal discharge include coagulopathies, vasculitis, hypertension, hyperviscosity syndrome, and pneumonia.

The character and type of nasal discharge may be helpful in developing a list of potential causes, but they are not characteristic for specific diseases. Unilateral discharge is often associated with neoplasia, fungal and foreign body rhinitis, and dental disease. Bilateral discharge is typical of systemic disorders, advanced neoplasia or fungal rhinitis,

Box 139-1

Differential Diagnosis for Nasal Discharge

Nasal and Paranasal Sinus Disorders
- Allergic rhinitis
- Bacterial rhinitis (*Bordetella bronchiseptica,* *Pasteurella multocida*)
- Ciliary dyskinesia
- Dental disease
- Foreign body
- Fungal rhinitis (*Aspergillus fumigatus, Penicillium* spp., *Rhinosporidium seeberi, Cryptococcus neoformans*)
- Hyperplastic rhinitis (Irish wolfhounds)
- Idiopathic lymphoplasmacytic rhinitis
- Neoplasia
- Nasal parasites (*Pneumonyssus caninum, Eucoleus [Capillaria] boehmi*)
- Oronasal fistula
- Palatine defects
- Trauma

Viral infection or Extranasal Disorders
- Coagulopathies
- Cricopharyngeal disease
- Environmental agents (dusts, smoke)
- Esophageal stricture
- Hypertension
- Hyperviscosity syndrome
- Immunoglobulin A immunodeficiency
- Megaesophagus
- Oropharyngeal diseases
- Pneumonia
- Polycythemia
- Thrombocytopenia
- Vasculitis
- Vomiting

idiopathic lymphoplasmacytic rhinitis, and allergic rhinitis. However, it also is possible for systemic disorders and idiopathic lymphoplasmacytic rhinitis to present with only unilateral nasal discharge. Serous nasal discharge may be seen initially with a variety of nasal disease but often becomes mucopurulent as disease progresses and secondary bacterial invasion occurs. Mucopurulent nasal discharge is most common and indicates bacterial infection *secondary* to an underlying disorder that has damaged the nasal mucosa with resultant bacterial invasion. Primary bacterial infection is an exceedingly rare cause of rhinitis in dogs. Mucopurulent and serous discharges may be blood tinged as a result of mucosal erosion. Epistaxis usually results from an underlying nasal disorder causing erosion of a major blood vessel but also may be seen with systemic disorders such as coagulopathies, hypertension, vasculitis, or hyperviscosity syndrome.

DIAGNOSIS

Clinical history and physical examination findings generally offer an indication for primary nasal disease as opposed to systemic or extranasal disease. Routine laboratory tests (complete blood count, serum chemistries, urinalysis), coagulation profile, blood pressure, and thoracic radiographs are important to rule out most of the systemic or extranasal causes for nasal discharge. Cytologic evaluation of nasal discharge is rarely helpful other than possibly for identification of *Eucoleus [Capillaria] boehmi* parasitic ova. Bacterial and fungal cultures of nasal discharge are not recommended because they are nonspecific and simply represent resident bacteria and fungi. Serologic tests for aspergillosis and penicilliosis should be delayed because some normal dogs and some dogs with nasal neoplasia have positive results (Sharp, 1998). Empiric antimicrobial treatment is not advised and merely delays definitive diagnosis unless chronic *Bordetella bronchiseptica* or *Pasteurella multocida* rhinitis (both very rare) or pneumonia is present. Mucopurulent nasal discharge is almost always a result of secondary bacterial rhinitis caused by an underlying primary nasal disease.

Anesthesia is required for further evaluation of most dogs with rhinitis. A thorough oral examination with inspection of the hard palate, oropharynx, and dental structures should be performed. A periodontal probe should be used to inspect the gingival sulci of maxillary teeth. Oronasal fistulae are often associated with the maxillary third incisors, first and second premolars, and mesial root of the third premolar.

Diagnostic imaging studies are performed with the patient under anesthesia. Imaging studies often are essential in most dogs with chronic rhinitis to help achieve a diagnosis. It is critical that imaging studies be completed *before* rhinoscopy or collection of intranasal samples so that secondary hemorrhage does not obscure subtle lesions or affect the quality of diagnostic images. If dental disease is suspected, dental films are recommended to evaluate the questionable teeth and surrounding structures. Radiographic images of the nose and sinuses may provide some insight but often do not reveal a specific cause for the nasal disease. Radiographs often lack sufficient resolution to identify or localize early nasal disease. Computed tomography (CT) is vastly superior to plain radiographs of the nasal cavity (Lefebvre et al., 2005). Nasal CT provides a thorough assessment of the nasal cavities and paranasal sinuses and provides superior insight to the nature and extent of disease (Figs. 139-1 to 139-5). Nasal CT often can differentiate neoplasia, fungal rhinitis, and inflammatory rhinitis. Contrast-enhanced CT images are useful to distinguish between vascularized soft tissue and mucus accumulation. Because nasal CT clearly demonstrates the location and extent of nasal disease, it is often used to help guide postimaging rhinoscopic and biopsy procedures and delineate nasal tumors for radiation therapy. If routine diagnostics do not provide a cause for rhinitis, referral to an institution providing CT imaging is advised. Although magnetic resonance imaging (MRI) is often considered superior to CT for delineation of tumor borders, a recent study failed to document an advantage of MRI over CT in detecting intracalvarial changes in dogs with nasal neoplasia (Dhaliwal et al., 2004) CT images regularly provide valuable clinical information without the need for MRI.

Rhinoscopy should only be performed after all imaging studies are completed with the patient under anesthesia. The nasopharynx is examined before the nasal cavity because, if hemorrhage is induced by examination of the

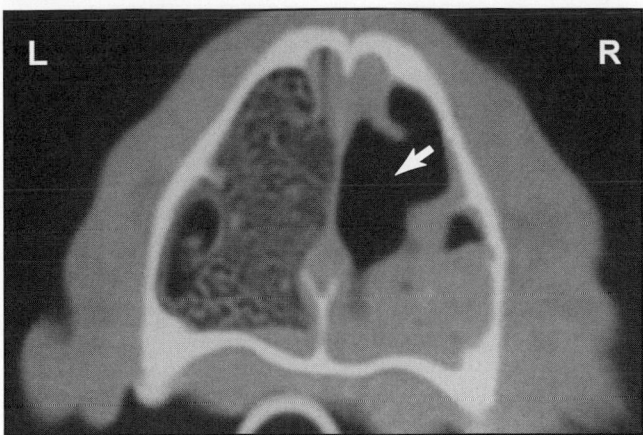

Fig. 139-1 Computed tomography scan from the middle region of the nasal cavity in a dog with nasal aspergillosis involving the right nasal cavity. The right nasal cavity is devoid of turbinate structures *(arrow)* with scattered regions of soft-tissue densities (mucopus) present. The left nasal cavity has normal turbinate structures.

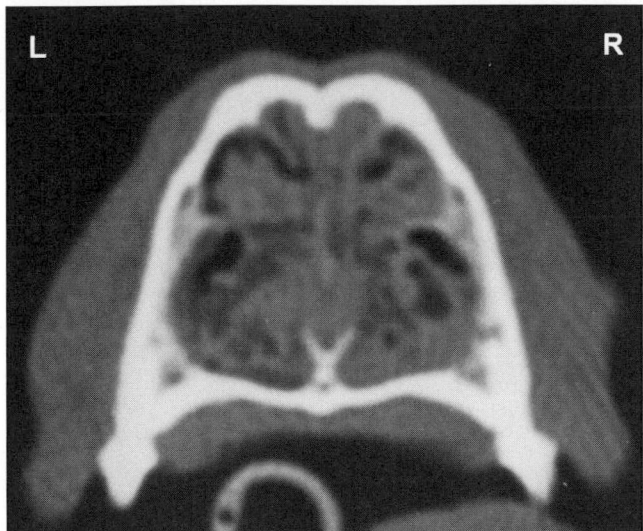

Fig. 139-2 Computed tomography scan within the midregion of the nose from a dog with lymphoplasmacytic rhinitis. Moderate turbinate destruction with scattered soft-tissue densities (mucopus) is present within both sides of the nasal cavity.

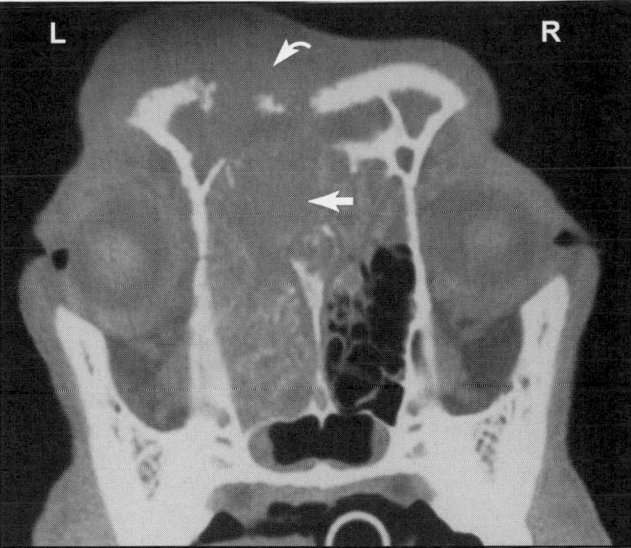

Fig. 139-3 Computed tomography scan within the caudal region of the nose from a dog with adenocarcinoma. Destruction of the dorsal nasal septum *(straight arrow)* and extensive destruction of the bones surrounding the left frontal sinus *(curved arrow)* are present. Facial deformity was present and can be appreciated by the soft-tissue swelling above the left frontal sinus.

nasal cavities, blood frequently pools in the nasopharynx and obscures visualization of this area. Retroflex nasopharyngoscopy is performed by turning a small flexible scope 180 degrees around the caudal margin of the soft palate to evaluate the caudal nares, dorsal soft palate, and nasopharynx. Tumors or foreign bodies lodged within the caudal nares or within the nasopharynx are occasional causes for rhinitis in dogs. Anterior rhinoscopy may be limited by the size of the nasal cavity compared to the size of the scope, lesion location, and impeded visualization of intranasal structures by mucus or hemorrhage. The convoluted nature of the nasal passages does not allow for evaluation of the entire nasal cavity; thus foreign bodies and neoplastic masses may be overlooked. The mucosa should be evaluated for color, vascularity, friability, edema, and presence of parasites or fungal plaques. Artifacts associated with close illumination of the mucosa should be

appreciated. The nasal passages should be evaluated for obstruction by tissue masses, foreign bodies, or secretions. A loss of normal nasal turbinates would indicate the presence of a destructive rhinitis secondary to fungal infection or severe idiopathic lymphoplasmacytic rhinitis. Rhinoscopy is especially helpful to aid in the diagnosis of fungal rhinitis and rostrally positioned nasal foreign bodies. Fungal rhinitis often is associated with widespread turbinate destruction, and rhinoscopy may reveal a cavernous nasal cavity with off-white–to grey-fungal plaques scattered across the surface of the nasal mucosa.

Procurement of nasal specimens and biopsies of nasal tissue should be performed only after imaging and visual examinations are completed and while the patient is still under anesthesia. Cytology of nasal secretions is rarely useful, but brush cytology from masses or fungal plaques may be useful. Stained direct smears of nasal tissue specimens also can be helpful for identifying fungal organisms. Tissue from lesions visualized during rhinoscopy may be obtained by direct biopsy with forceps passed either adjacent to or through the endoscope. Rhinoscopic-directed biopsies from masses identified within the nose can be limited by the size of tissue samples obtained and inflammation surrounding the mass. Lymphoplasmacytic inflammation often is present with intranasal neoplasms, whereas idiopathic lymphoplasmacytic rhinitis is not associated with mass lesions in the nose. I prefer to use nasal CT images to guide instrumentation for procurement of biopsy samples. Depending on the size of the nose, either small clam-shell or colonic biopsy forceps are advanced to the site of disease as identified from CT images, and multiple biopsies are then obtained. During the biopsy procedure it is recommended that the dog be in sternal recumbency with the rostral end of the nose directed downward to facilitate drainage of hemorrhage away from the nasopharynx and oropharynx. Following

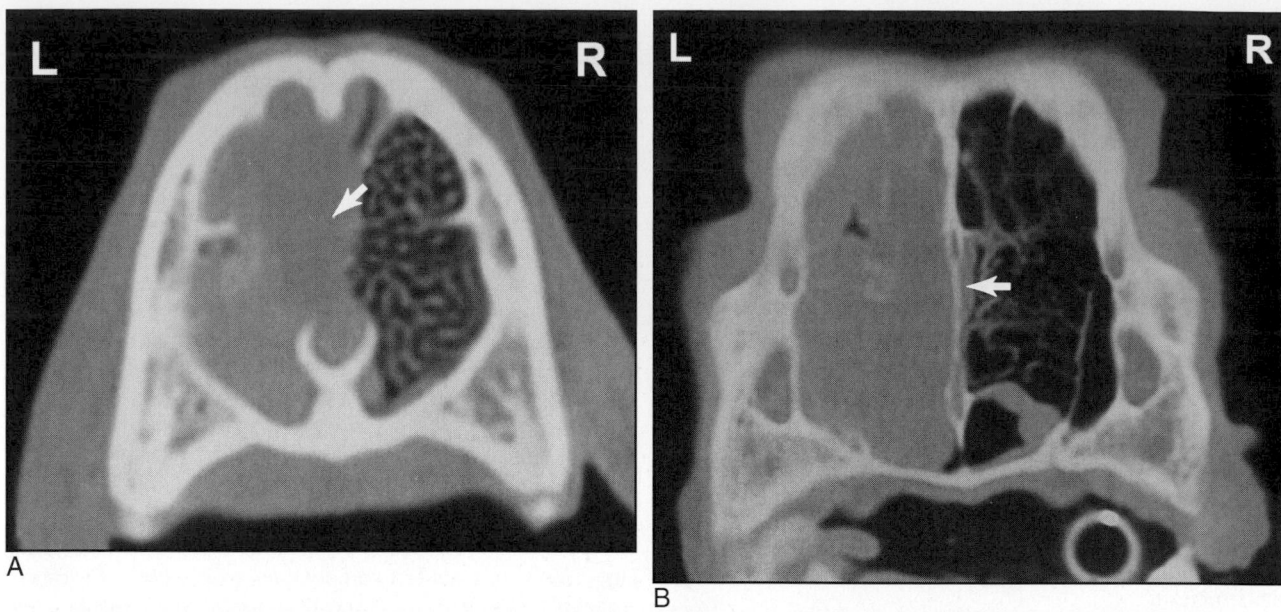

Fig. 139-4   Computed tomography scans from the midregion **(A)** and further caudal region **(B)** of the nose in a dog with adenocarcinoma. The nasal septum is destroyed rostrally *(arrow A)* by the neoplasm but intact caudally *(arrow B)*.

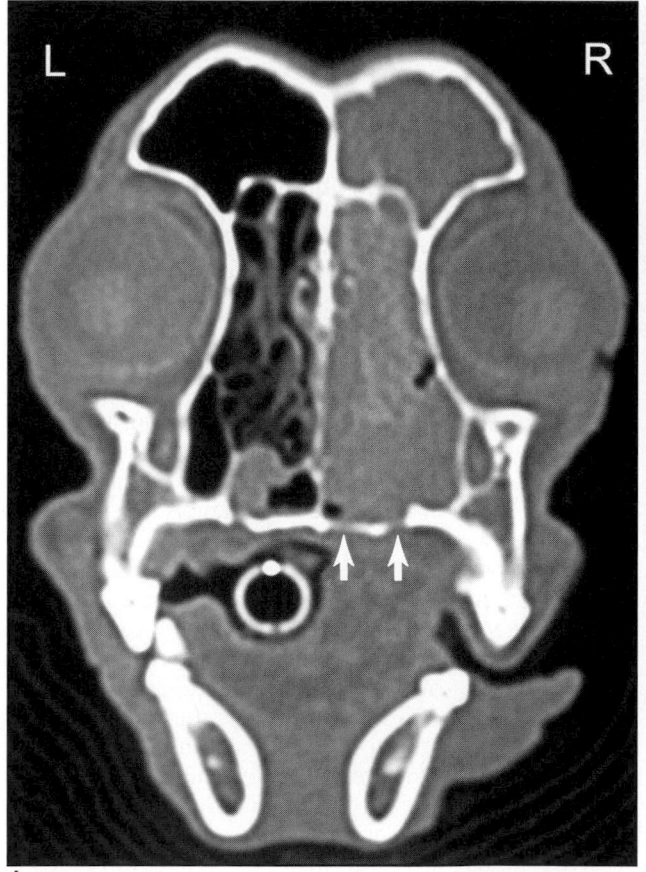

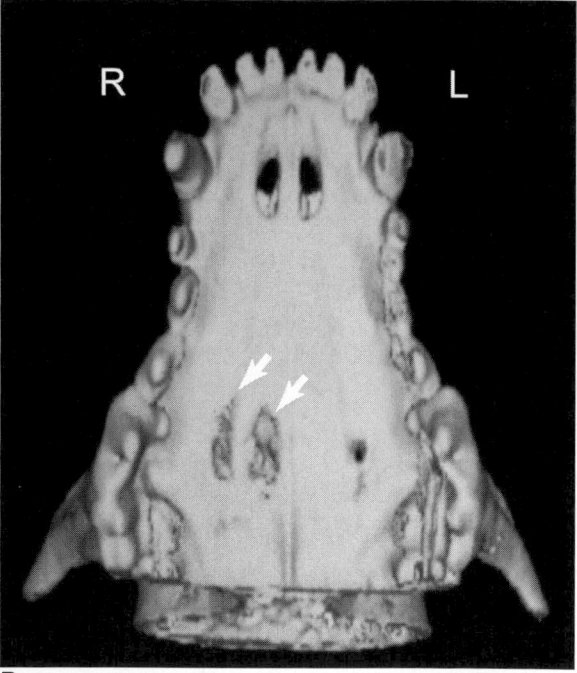

Fig. 139-5   **A** shows a computed tomography (CT) scan of nasal adenocarcinoma involving the right ventrocaudal nasal cavity. There appears to be subtle destruction of the caudal hard palate *(arrows)*. **B** is a three-dimensional reconstruction of the CT study with soft-tissue structures removed. The extent of boney destruction of the hard palate is clearly evident *(arrows)*.

biopsy, the tip of the nose remains positioned downward, and the oropharynx and cranial esophagus are suctioned to remove blood clots. Nasal lavage may be required to dislodge foreign material identified or suspected to be present within the nose. The rostral aspect of the nose should be directed downward while copious amounts of

saline are flushed vigorously through the nostrils. The endotracheal tube cuff should be inflated to prevent aspiration pneumonia. Some clinicians surround the glottis with surgical sponges or gauze.

Tissue samples are not submitted routinely for bacterial or fungal culture unless osteomyelitis is present. Nasal fungal and bacterial tissue cultures must be interpreted cautiously because fungal and bacterial isolates may be a consequence of nasal passage colonization rather than the cause of a given disease process. Primary bacterial rhinitis is exceedingly rare in the dog, and almost all bacterial infections develop secondary to underlying primary nasal disease. A heavy growth of even one or two bacterial isolates may merely be indicative of bacterial colonization; however, pure isolates of *B. bronchiseptica* and possibly *P. multocida* may be significant if the clinical history is supportive. Normal dogs and dogs with nasal neoplasia or foreign bodies may have positive fungal cultures for *Aspergillus* spp. A positive fungal culture should be supported by diagnostic imaging, cytologic, rhinoscopic, or histologic evidence of infection (Mathews, 2004). If tissue cultures are submitted, these must be interpreted carefully in light of histopathologic and other diagnostic information.

TREATMENT OF COMMON CAUSES OF RHINITIS

Geographic locality plays a role; but, excluding nasal foreign bodies (Aronson, 2004) and dental disease, the most common causes for chronic rhinitis in dogs are neoplasia, idiopathic chronic (lymphoplasmacytic) rhinitis, and fungal rhinitis. Parasitic rhinitis is uncommon. The treatment for nasal mites (*Pneumonyssus caninum*) is ivermectin 0.2 mg/kg orally, with the dose repeated in 2 to 3 weeks. The treatment for nasal nematodes (*E. [Capillaria] boehmi*) is not clearly defined, although ivermectin 0.2 mg/kg orally once reportedly has been effective. Allergic rhinitis is often mild; but, if severe, antihistamines such as diphenhydramine, chlorpheniramine, or trimeprazine-prednisone (Temaril-P, Pfizer Animal Health) may be prescribed to control symptomatology. In the rare situation of bacterial rhinitis caused by *B. bronchiseptica*, doxycycline 5 to 10 mg/kg every 12 hours orally for 2 weeks may be effective.

Fungal Rhinitis

Fungal rhinitis is a relatively common cause of chronic rhinitis in the dog in various geographic regions throughout the world. *Aspergillus fumigatus* is the most common cause of fungal rhinitis in dogs, but occasionally *Penicillium* spp., *Rhinosporidium seeberi*, and very rarely *Cryptococcus neoformans* may cause disease in dogs. *R. seeberi* is associated with the growth of a granulomatous mass within the rostral nasal cavity. Cytology of tissue from these granulomatous masses is often diagnostic. Treatment for rhinosporidiosis is best accomplished by aggressive surgical resection of the granulomatous mass.

Nasal aspergillosis is most commonly seen in young to middle-aged dolichocephalic dogs, with German shepherd and rottweiler breeds reported to be predisposed. Affected dogs present with copious unilateral or bilateral mucopurulent nasal discharge. Sneezing is common and may be accompanied by mild-to-severe epistaxis. Facial pain and depigmentation and ulceration of the nasal planum may be present. In contrast to nasal neoplasia, facial distortion is unusual in all but advanced cases of fungal rhinitis. Nasal CT (see Fig. 139-1) along with rhinoscopy is noteworthy for the presence of dramatic turbinate loss within the nasal cavity (Saunders, 2004). Sinus involvement may be present. Invasion through the maxillary or palatine bones with extension into surrounding soft-tissue structures is seen occasionally. Nasal CT scan is preferred over radiographs so that the integrity of the cribriform plate can be evaluated before local antifungal therapy. A noninvasive form of nasal aspergillosis infrequently occurs in the dog and is characterized by compact masses of mycelia ("fungal balls") filling larger airspaces or frontal sinuses.

Diagnosis of nasal aspergillosis is confirmed by visualization of fungal plaques on nasal mucosa and demonstration of branching septate hyphae on cytologic or histologic samples from affected regions within the nose. Serologic tests positive for aspergillosis also support the diagnosis, although negative results may occur even with extensive disease. Occasionally special staining methods for fungi may be useful for identifying fungal elements in tissue biopsy samples. Cultures of nasal discharge may be misleading in that 30% to 40% of cultures from normal dogs and those with nasal neoplasia can yield *Aspergillus* or *Penicillium* spp. Despite properly obtained samples some cases fail to demonstrate fungal organisms. Repeated sampling or a trial of antifungal drugs may well be indicated in dogs with a high index of suspicion for nasal aspergillosis.

The prognosis for treatment of nasal aspergillosis is fair to good, but relapses are possible necessitating retreatment (Schochet and Lappin, 2005). Treatment of nasal aspergillosis is best approached with topical infusion of either clotrimazole or enilconazole provided that the cribriform plate is intact. Topical therapy is more effective than orally administered antifungal agents. Clotrimazole (Lotrimin solution, Schering Plough Corp.) is available over the counter as a 1% solution, and enilconazole (Clinifarm-EC, Sterwin Labs, Inc.) is provided as 13.8% concentrate, which is diluted to a 1%, 2%, or 5% solution before instillation in the nasal cavity. Topical therapy with either drug alone is not effective in dogs in which the organism has invaded soft-tissue structures adjacent to the nose. In these cases it is recommended that topical therapy be combined with systemic antifungal agents. Rhinotomy and turbinectomy before topical treatment or oral antifungal therapy are often detrimental and not recommended.

The topical application of enilconazole through surgically placed catheters into the frontal sinuses and nasal chambers has a success rate as high as 90%. Catheters are implanted surgically into both nasal chambers and frontal sinuses via trephine holes in the sinuses. Enilconazole is flushed through the catheters twice daily at a dosage of 10 mg/kg for a total of 7 to 10 days. Unfortunately this procedure is quite distressing to most patients. Complications include premature removal of the catheters, subcutaneous emphysema, inappetence, and ptyalism. Some patients may become aggressive and intolerant of the procedure, necessitating premature abandonment of therapy. Because of these serious and frequent side effects, topical therapy with clotrimazole has become the treatment of choice. Clotrimazole is applied as a soak, with the solution maintained in the nasal cavities for 1 hour with the patient under anesthesia (Bonagura, 1995, 2000). A total volume of 60 ml of a 1% solution of clotrimazole is infused slowly through catheters placed into the right and left nares.

A nasopharyngeal Foley catheter and sponges placed in the caudal pharyngeal region are positioned before the procedure to minimize leakage of the infusate caudally, and the external nares are also obstructed with Foley catheters. The head is rotated every 15 minutes to ensure contact with all nasal surfaces. As many as 90% of patients may be cured with a single procedure, although some dogs require a second procedure 3 weeks later. Side effects of clotrimazole therapy include severe pharyngitis and pharyngeal edema.

Recently another approach with excellent success rate, shorter treatment time, and low patient morbidity has been reported using a combination of clotrimazole irrigation and depot therapy (Sissener et al., 2006). Frontal sinus trephination is followed by a short, 5-minute flushing of 1% topical clotrimazole solution followed by a 1% clotrimazole cream instilled as a depot agent into the frontal sinuses. The procedure includes a number of steps. The anesthetized dog is positioned in sternal recumbency with the pharynx packed with cotton gauze to prevent aspiration of fluid debris, and the head is tilted downward to allow fluid from the nasal sinuses to drain rostrally. The frontal bone is trephined to permit passage of a 10 Fr–gauge Jacques urethral catheter into each sinus. The sinuses are first irrigated with 500 ml of warm saline over 5 minutes to establish appropriate catheter placement and patency of the nasofrontal ostium (which communicates the frontal sinus with the nasal cavity). The sinuses are then irrigated with 1% clotrimazole solution. For dogs weighing more than 10 kg, a total of 500 mg is used (25 ml per side). Clotrimazole 1% cream is then introduced into the frontal sinuses. For dogs larger than 10 kg a total of 40 g (20 g per side) is used, and for dogs weighing less than 10 kg a total of 20 g (10 g per side) is applied. The catheters are then removed, the skin incisions are closed, and excess fluid is allowed to drain from the sinuses before the pharyngeal gauze is removed. With this treatment protocol, 86% of dogs with nasal aspergillosis or penicilliosis established a cure from infection. I suspect that cure rate might be greater if débridement and removal of diseased nasal turbinates through the rostral nares were to precede treatment using the combination of clotrimazole irrigation depot therapy.

Oral antifungal agents have relatively poor efficacy against *Aspergillus* infection but are recommended if imaging demonstrates that the cribriform plate is penetrated. Oral antifungal agents are used in combination with topical agents if invasion of local bone and soft-tissue structures is present. The newer azole derivatives offer the best results. Side effects of the azole antifungal agents include anorexia, vomiting, lethargy, elevated blood urea nitrogen, skin ulcerations, fever, and hepatotoxicity. Itraconazole (Sporanox, Janssen) is recommended because of its low toxicity. Itraconazole 5 mg/kg every 12 hours orally given for 3 to 6 months may cure up to 60% to 70% of dogs with aspergillosis, although some studies have shown marginal effects of the drug on this disease. Terbinafine (Lamisil, Novartis) is another option; it is well tolerated. Terbinafine 5 to 10 mg/kg every 12 hours orally appears to have similar efficacy to itraconazole when given for 3 to 6 months. Fluconazole (Diflucan, Pfizer) is another alternative with a cure rate up to 60% when given at a dose of 2.5 to 5 mg/kg every 12 hours orally for 3 to 6 months. Voriconazole (Vfend, Pfizer) is a new-generation broad-spectrum antifungal agent that shows activity against a wide range of yeasts and filamentous fungi. Voriconazole demonstrates both fungicidal and fungistatic activities in vitro against *Aspergillus* spp. superior to that of fluconazole. Voriconazole may prove to be an effective antifungal drug for treatment; however, clinical experience with this drug is limited in veterinary medicine. Initial clinical experience in dogs suggests an oral dose of 5 mg/kg every 12 hours for voriconazole.

Idiopathic Lymphoplasmacytic (Chronic) Rhinitis

Idiopathic lymphoplasmacytic rhinitis is a relatively common cause of chronic nasal disease in the dog. The definitive etiology of lymphoplasmacytic rhinitis remains undetermined; however, it is likely a stereotyped chronic inflammatory response to multiple precipitating factors (Windsor, 2004). Inhaled aeroallergens and irritants probably play a primary role in development of this disease. Hypersensitivity to native commensal fungal organisms within the nose also may play a role in some patients. Young to middle-aged dolichocephalic and mesaticephalic large-breed dogs and dachshunds typically are affected. Chronic unilateral-to-bilateral mucoid-to-mucopurulent nasal discharge is often present, although some dogs may have mucohemorrhagic discharge or epistaxis. Obstruction to airflow through the nose may result from excessive mucus within nasal passages and turbinate mucosal edema. Since lymphoplasmacytic inflammation may be present with nasal neoplasia, fungal rhinitis, or foreign body rhinitis, it is imperative that these diseases be thoroughly excluded before a diagnosis of idiopathic lymphoplasmacytic (chronic) rhinitis is entertained.

Nasal radiography is not sufficient to differentiate chronic inflammatory rhinitis from neoplasia or fungal rhinitis because similar changes such as turbinate destruction and soft-tissue opacification of the nasal passages and frontal sinus may be seen in each of these diseases. Nasal CT is recommended because it greatly enhances the ability to differentiate inflammatory from neoplastic diseases. Nasal CT lesions with idiopathic chronic rhinitis may be completely unremarkable or disclose unilateral or bilateral mild-to-moderate turbinate destruction with mucus accumulation within air passages and sinuses (see Fig. 139-2). Occasionally the turbinate destruction may be severe, mimicking that seen with fungal rhinitis. Destruction of the nasal septum, frontal sinuses, or cribriform plate or extension of soft-tissue density into the nasopharynx or periorbital region is not expected with idiopathic chronic rhinitis. These findings should prompt investigation into fungal rhinitis or neoplastic disease.

The most common rhinoscopic abnormalities seen are unilateral or bilateral erythema or hyperemia and edema of the nasal mucosa with the presence of mucopus within air passages. Turbinate atrophy or loss is appreciated occasionally. Nasal samples for microbial culture are neither informative nor recommended. Histologic changes include mild-to-severe lymphoplasmacytic inflammation with occasional infiltration of neutrophils or eosinophils. Turbinate remodeling or destruction may be absent or vary from mild to severe. The severity of histologic changes may show discordance between the right and left sides of the nasal cavity.

Treatment for idiopathic lymphoplasmacytic rhinitis is extremely frustrating, with cure rarely achieved. Although this is not a life-threatening disease, owners of dogs so affected are often distraught by their pet's nasal obstruction or the need to frequently clean up nasal discharge or nasal hemorrhage within the house. Allergen avoidance is rarely helpful; however, avoidance of secondhand smoke can substantially reduce signs in some dogs. Despite earlier reports in the literature, systemic or topical corticosteroids are seldom effective in controlling clinical signs and actually may worsen them. Antihistamine medications are rarely effective, but they occasionally slightly reduce the severity of nasal discharge. Long-term administration of antibiotics with immunomodulatory effects combined with nonsteroidal antiinflammatory agents can be helpful in some dogs. Doxycycline 3 to 5 mg/kg every 12 hours orally or azithromycin 5 mg/kg every 24 hours orally in combination with piroxicam 0.3 mg/kg every 24 hours orally is recommended. If distinct clinical improvement is observed in 4 to 8 weeks, daily piroxicam therapy is continued; but the frequency of administration of doxycycline is reduced to once daily or azithromycin reduced to twice weekly. Therapy likely will be required for a minimum of 6 months if not indefinitely.

I am currently investigating itraconazole therapy in dogs refractory to other therapeutic modalities. Nasal biopsies from dogs with lymphoplasmacytic rhinitis have been reported to display an elevated transcription of fungal genes compared to dogs with nasal neoplasia using polymerase chain reaction techniques. Whether hypersensitivity to commensal nasal fungal organisms is involved or molecular techniques are detecting entrapment of fungal organisms is unclear. Preliminary experience with the administration of itraconazole 5 mg/kg every 12 hours orally for a minimum of 3 to 6 months has shown dramatic beneficial improvement and even resolution of signs in some dogs with this disease.

Nasal Neoplasia and Nasal Polyps

Nasal neoplasia is an important cause of chronic nasal disease in middle-aged to older dolichocephalic and mesaticephalic dogs (McEntee, 2004). Nasal neoplasia accounts for approximately one third of all dogs with chronic nasal disease, and tumors of epithelial origin cause about two thirds of these neoplasms. The majority of nasal tumors are malignant and primarily arise within the nasal cavity, although occasionally they originate in the paranasal sinuses. Nasal tumors tend to be invasive with local- to widespread destruction of nasal turbinates seen initially and invasion of septal, cribriform, or facial bones observed later in the course of disease. Metastasis to regional lymph nodes or lung may occur, but this is rare and generally occurs in the very late stages of disease. Clinical signs are related primarily to obstruction of air flow through the nasal cavities, mucopurulent nasal discharge, epistaxis, sneezing, and sometimes reverse sneezing. Facial deformity or swelling, exophthalmia, or neurologic signs may stem from tumor destruction of facial bones or the cribriform plate. Facial pain and head shyness are rarely seen (unlike that with fungal rhinitis). In some patients initial clinical signs may be very subtle, with unexplained onset of snoring and occasional reverse sneeze reported.

For dogs presenting primarily for epistaxis, a coagulation profile, complete blood count with platelet count, blood pressure, and serum proteins should be evaluated initially to rule out coagulopathy, hypertension, and hyperviscosity syndromes as causes of epistaxis. Nasal radiographs frequently are insensitive for subtle lesions, and radiographic changes seen with nasal tumors often overlap with those of lymphoplasmacytic and fungal rhinitis. Nasal CT is a vastly superior imaging modality for differentiating neoplastic from nonneoplastic disease and detection of bone destruction and neoplastic extension into surrounding structures (see Figs. 139-3 and 139-4). Nasal CT also is needed for tumor staging, delineating tumor boundaries, and planning radiation therapy. Three-dimensional reconstructions of the CT study may clarify the extent of bone destruction in situations in which subtle boney lesions are present (see Fig. 139-5). Thoracic radiographs are recommended when nasal neoplasia is identified before radiation therapy to rule out metastatic lung disease. Retroflex nasopharyngoscopy is useful to evaluate the nasopharyngeal region and identify tumor extension through the caudal nares. Anterior rhinoscopy in dogs with nasal neoplasia may reveal a mass lesion protruding within and occluding nasal air passages. Multiple biopsies of masses should be obtained to increase the likelihood of diagnosis because severe inflammation often surrounds nasal tumors and can create a false-negative biopsy result. Frequently nasal tumors cannot be visualized during rhinoscopy because of hemorrhage or because the origin is inaccessible. In these situations nasal CT studies facilitate direction and location for blind biopsy sampling of the affected region of the nose.

Radiation therapy is the treatment of choice for most nasal tumors. Surgery alone is ineffective, with survival times similar to those observed in untreated dogs. Cytoreductive surgery is recommended before orthovoltage radiation therapy but not for cobalt or linear accelerator therapy. There is evidence suggesting that exenteration of the nasal cavity significantly prolongs the survival time in dogs with intranasal neoplasia that have previously undergone accelerated radiotherapy (Adams et al., 2005). However, exenteration after radiotherapy may increase the risk of chronic complications, including development of chronic or recurrent rhinitis and osteomyelitis. Cisplatin is used occasionally as a radiation sensitizer in radiotherapy protocols. Depending on the mode of radiation therapy available, approximate median survival times are between 16.5 to 23 months, and approximate 1-year survival rates are between 54% to 60% in dogs with nasal neoplasia. Results with cryosurgery, either alone or in combination with radiation therapy, have been disappointing; therefore it is not recommended. There is limited information on the response of nasal tumors to chemotherapy alone. The median survival in a very small group of dogs with nasal adenocarcinoma given cisplatin alone was 20 weeks, which is comparable to no treatment.

Polyps within the nasal cavity are very rare in dogs. These are usually unilateral, and rhinotomy is required for removal of the polypous tissue and surrounding conchae. Recurrence 1 to 2 years later is possible. To date in all dogs I have seen with an initial diagnosis of a polyp, careful review of nasal CT has demonstrated localized turbinate destruction, and the subsequent histologic diagnosis following surgical resection of the polypous tissue has been low-grade fibrosarcoma associated with moderate-to-severe chronic inflammation.

References and Suggested Reading

Adams WM et al: Outcome of accelerated radiotherapy alone or accelerated radiotherapy followed by exenteration of the nasal cavity in dogs with intranasal neoplasia: 53 cases (1990-2002), *J Am Vet Med Assoc* 227:936, 2005.

Aronson LR: Nasal foreign bodies. In King LG, editor: *Respiratory disease in dogs and cats,* Philadelphia, 2004, Saunders-Elsevier, p 302.

Bonagura JD, Kirk RW, editors: *Kirk's current veterinary therapy XII (small animal practice),* Philadelphia, 1995, Saunders, p 899.

Bonagura JD, editor: *Kirk's current veterinary therapy XIII (small animal practice),* Philadelphia, 2000, Saunders, p 315.

Dhaliwal RS: Subjective evaluation of computed tomography and magnetic resonance imaging for detecting intracalvarial changes in canine neoplasia, *Intern J Appl Res Vet Med* 2(3):201, 2004.

Lefebvre J, Kuehn NF, Wortinger A: Computed tomography as an aid in the diagnosis of chronic nasal disease in dogs, *J Small Anim Pract* 46:280, 2005.

Mathews KG: Fungal rhinitis. In King LG, editor: *Respiratory disease in dogs and cats,* Philadelphia, 2004, Saunders-Elsevier, p 284.

McEntee MC: Neoplasms of the nasal cavity. In King LG, editor: *Respiratory disease in dogs and cats,* Philadelphia, 2004, Saunders-Elsevier, p 293.

Saunders JH: Radiographic, magnetic resonance imaging, computed tomographic, and rhinoscopic features of nasal aspergillosis in dogs, *J Am Vet Med Assoc* 225:1703, 2004.

Schochet RA, Lappin MR: Delayed recurrence of nasal aspergillosis in a dog, *J Small Anim Pract* 46:27, 2005.

Sharp NJH: Canine nasal aspergillosis-penicilliosis. In Green CE, editor: *Infectious disease of the dog and cat,* ed 2, Philadelphia, 1998, Saunders, p 404.

Sissener TR et al: Combined clotrimazole irrigation and depot therapy for canine aspergillosis, *J Sm Anim Pract* 47:312, 2006.

Venker-van Haagen AJ: Diseases of the nose and nasal sinuses. In Ettinger SJ, Feldman EC, editors:*Textbook of veterinary internal medicine,* ed 6, Philadelphia, 2005, Saunders-Elsevier, p 1186.

Windsor RC: Idiopathic lymphoplasmacytic rhinitis in dogs: 37 cases (1997-2002), *J Am Vet Med Assoc* 224:1952, 2004.

CHAPTER   140

Rhinitis in the Cat

LYNELLE R. JOHNSON, *Davis, California*

Feline chronic rhinosinusitis (CRS) is a disease with high morbidity in the feline population. Despite the commonality of the syndrome, much remains unknown regarding the etiopathogenesis of disease. Multiple clinical reports have implicated involvement of feline herpesvirus type 1 (FHV-1) in CRS; however, the high prevalence of infection with this virus and the ability of the virus to cause latent infection in the feline population have made it difficult to demonstrate a causal relationship between the presence of virus and disease (Maggs et al., 1999; Johnson et al., 2005). In addition, cats with CRS often demonstrate improvement or lessening of clinical signs in response to antibiotics, suggesting that bacterial species or products of bacterial infection play a role in disease. It is possible that severe early viral infection, viral persistence within nasal epithelium, or chronic reactivation of FHV-1 into nasal tissues damages the respiratory epithelium and results in mucus accumulation, sneezing, and ultimately turbinate destruction. Viral damage might

allow bacterial invasion of nasal tissue, resulting in further turbinate destruction via bacterial and inflammatory products.

Management of cats with rhinosinusitis is challenging, and a clinically relevant question must be answered for individual affected animals: when in the course of disease should advanced diagnostic testing be performed? CRS should be considered a *disease of exclusion*, and some cats may have nasal disease requiring specific treatment. Nasal cryptococcosis or aspergillosis, foreign body disease, dental-related nasal disease, and nasal neoplasia can all result in chronic nasal discharge; and these diseases should not be overlooked. Immune suppression related to feline immunodeficiency virus infection should be ruled out. In addition, consideration should be given to the therapeutic value of nasal lavage in the management of affected cats, and this procedure is easily performed following imaging and rhinoscopy with biopsy. Therefore I recommend performing diagnostic testing within 6 to 12 months of unsuccessful therapeutic trials, even if idiopathic disease is the most likely diagnosis.

CLINICAL FINDINGS

Chronic rhinosinusitis affects all ages of cats, with clinical signs first apparent in cats anywhere from 6 months to 20 years of age. Stertor, mucopurulent or hemorrhagic nasal discharge, and sneezing are the most common historical complaints and clinical signs, although some cats exhibit only mucoid or serous discharge. Nasal discharge is often bilateral; however, some cases are remarkably unilateral. In acute upper respiratory tract disease, ocular signs are common; however, in the chronic syndrome these are usually absent. In addition, cats with chronic upper respiratory tract disease are systemically well compared to cats or kittens with the acute syndrome, which is often accompanied by fever, inappetence, and malaise.

Cats with CRS generally have preservation of nasal airflow compared to cats with neoplasia or nasal cryptococcosis in which airflow can be obstructed by a mass lesion. Airflow can be assessed by holding a wisp of cotton up to each nostril and noting movement by air or by alternately occluding each nostril and observing the cat for difficulty in respiration. The soft palate should be palpated for abnormalities because a nasopharyngeal mass often can be felt as a space-occupying lesion dorsal to the soft palate that provides resistance to dorsal compression. Lymph nodes generally are normal in cats with CRS, although rarely enlarged mandibular nodes are detected as a result of lymphoid reactivity. In these situations it is essential to aspirate the nodes to rule out fungal disease or neoplastic infiltration. Differential ocular retropulsion in a cat with unilateral nasal discharge should be considered suspicious for neoplasia rather than CRS.

DIAGNOSIS

The diagnosis of CRS is one of exclusion. The recommended diagnostic approach involves an assessment of the extent of systemic illness with a minimum database and cryptococcal antigen test. In cats with hemorrhagic nasal discharge, blood pressure evaluation and a coagulation panel should be performed before anesthesia. Evaluation of the nasal cavity is performed to rule out conditions that mimic rhinosinusitis such as nasal foreign body, neoplasia, or fungal infection.

In the cat with chronic rhinitis, skull radiographs or computed tomography should be performed under general anesthesia to ensure optimal positioning. These show variable degrees of turbinate lysis and increased fluid density within the nasal cavity. Disease is usually bilateral, but some cases are remarkably unilateral. The middle ear or the sinuses are sometimes involved in the disease process or may be fluid filled. In many cases the severity of radiographic or tomographic changes overlap with those typically found in nasal neoplasia, making biopsy differentiation crucial (Schoenborn et al., 2003).

Rhinoscopy with biopsy is performed after imaging has been completed to avoid causing hemorrhage that would alter the radiologic appearance of the nasal cavity. First nasopharyngoscopy is accomplished by retroflex of a flexible endoscope above the soft palate. This technique is recommended to rule out the possibility of nasopharyngeal stenosis, foreign body, or a mass lesion. Rhinoscopy of the nasal cavity is best performed using a small (2.8-mm) rigid telescope. The examiner should search for evidence of primary nasal disease, including fungal plaques or neoplasia. In general cats with CRS have hyperemic mucosa, large amounts of mucoid-to-purulent discharge, and irregular turbinate structures, although some affected cats have minimal visual changes. Destructive rhinitis is evident as increased space between the turbinates. Rhinoscopic appearance does not predict the presence or absence of substantial inflammation, and bilateral nasal biopsy is recommended to assess the type and severity of inflammation.

Cats with chronic rhinitis have potential pathogens isolated from nasal samples more commonly than do normal cats (Johnson et al., 2005). Deep nasal swabs or biopsy specimens for bacterial culture (aerobic, anaerobic, and *Mycoplasma*) are sometimes helpful in guiding antibiotic therapy for secondary bacterial rhinitis. Bordetellosis can be diagnosed when the organism is isolated from nasal secretions of a symptomatic cat. Some laboratories recommend transport of the sample in Amies medium for successful culture of *Bordetella* or *Mycoplasma*.

Histologic evidence of nasal inflammation is virtually always present in cats with CRS, with the majority of severe cases demonstrating neutrophilic inflammation. Lymphoplasmacytic inflammation is noted in some cats, whereas in my experience eosinophilic infiltrates are relatively uncommon. The significance of the varying types of inflammation has not been investigated, although it is tempting to relate eosinophilic inflammation to potential FHV-1 related disease, given the association between eosinophilic inflammation and herpesvirus infection in facial dermatitis of cats (Hargis et al., 1999).

After rhinoscopy, dental probing is performed to identify oronasal fistulae or large periodontal pockets that could be responsible for dental-related nasal disease.

THERAPY

Antibiotics

Chronic antibiotic therapy is usually prescribed in an attempt to control secondary bacterial rhinitis. Choice of antibiotics for the individual cat can be based on culture of a deep nasal flush or biopsy sample or may be made based on an understanding of potential pathogens that have been isolated previously from cats with rhinitis. These organisms include aerobes (*Pasteurella multocida, Escherichia coli, Corynebacterium ulcerans, Bordetella bronchiseptica, Streptococcus viridans, Pseudomonas aeruginosa, Actinomyces slackii*), anaerobes (*Peptostreptococcus anaerobius, Bacteroides fragilis, Bacteroides ureolyticus, Prevotella, Fusobacterium nucleatum*), and *Mycoplasma felis* (Johnson et al., 2005). I prefer doxycycline (approximately 50 mg/cat orally divided every 12 hours or given once daily) because it has efficacy against these bacteria, as well as in vitro efficacy for *Bordetella*. In addition, doxycycline may help control clinical signs through antiinflammatory or immunomodulatory effects. Doxycycline is readily available, well tolerated by most cats even when administered long term, and inexpensive. The primary caution with use of this drug is the potential for induction of an esophageal stricture if the pill lodges in the esophagus. Instruction labels should always contain the recommendation to follow administration of the pill with a small volume of water or food.

Most isolates of *Bordetella* are susceptible in vitro to tetracycline, doxycycline, and enrofloxacin; but resistance to tetracyclines has been reported. Oral antibiotic treatment generally reduces clinical signs, but it does not eliminate shedding of bacteria. Some cats remain as chronic carriers of the organism and are culture positive. It is unclear whether these cats are chronic or intermittent shedders of the organism into the environment. Improving cleanliness, ventilation, and husbandry in an affected cattery or shelter should help limit spread of disease. If *Bordetella* is documented in a cat and the animal does not respond to oral antibiotics, use of topical gentamicin (Gentocin, Schering-Plough) (intranasal drops or nebulization) should be considered since this method is more likely to reduce bacterial numbers.

Other commonly used antibiotics include azithro–mycin, cephalexin, and amoxicillin-clavulanic acid. Azithromycin is an appealing option because it is available in liquid form and can be given once daily for 3 to 5 days at 5 mg/kg and then twice weekly because of its ability to accumulate in tissue. Penicillin-like drugs are efficacious in many cats, although they lack efficacy against *Mycoplasma* spp., which are cell wall–deficient organisms. These drugs are also frequently associated with gastrointestinal side effects. Enrofloxacin (Baytril [Bayer], 2.5 mg/kg orally every 24 hours) generally is reserved for infections that are susceptible to this antibiotic, and high doses are to be avoided since they have been associated with a type of toxic retinopathy. Clindamycin can be efficacious in cases with extensive bony involvement because of its ability to penetrate bone. Antibiotic treatment usually is continued at the full dose for at least 3 to 6 weeks based on the assumption that turbinates are infected. In cats with recurrent clinical signs, intermittent treatment with antibiotics (1 week of each month) or suppressive antibiotic therapy (once daily administration of drug) may be required.

Antiinflammatory Agents

Control of nasal inflammation can sometimes be achieved with the use of piroxicam at 0.3 mg/kg orally daily or every other day. This drug is commercially available as a 10-mg tablet, and drug compounding is required. This nonsteroidal antiinflammatory causes subclinical gastric erosion, and caution is warranted in its use in older animals or in cats with renal insufficiency. Meloxicam is a tempting alternative to piroxicam because it is easier to dose and administer, although subjectively cats do not appear to respond as well to it.

Glucocorticoids are sometimes advocated for treatment of cats with CRS, and in severely affected animals with inspissated mucus in the nasal cavity administration of oral steroids may reduce mucus accumulation and promote appetite. Inhaled or topical steroids are sometimes used, although it would seem wise to clear all mucus from the nasal cavity before use to provide a mucosal surface area for local absorption and action. Liquid steroid medications are available in drop formulations or as nasal sprays. Metered-dose inhaler preparations containing steroids such as fluticasone require administration with a spacer chamber and face mask.

Antihistamine administration might improve clinical signs in some cats, although these drugs can also cause excessive drying of respiratory secretions. Multiple over-the-counter preparations are available, and individual cats can show variable response to different types of antihistamines.

Antiviral Therapy

The role of FHV-1 in induction or promotion of clinical signs in cats with CRS has not been clearly established, and specific antiviral therapy is not recommended in cats with chronic disease. A novel antiviral therapy that is unlikely to result in harmful side effects is dietary supplementation with lysine, an amino acid that competes with arginine for use by the viral machinery in replication. The recommended dose of lysine is 500 mg/cat orally twice daily; this dose does not result in a drop in serum arginine levels in the cat. Lysine can be purchased at most health food stores as a pill or a capsule containing granules, and veterinary paste formulations are also available. Trial therapy with lysine should be considered in any cat with CRS and is particularly indicated when intranuclear inclusions are detected or an eosinophilic inflammatory infiltrate is reported on histology.

ADDITIONAL THERAPY

Rigorous flushing of the nasal cavity when the animal is anesthetized for diagnostic testing undoubtedly improves the clinical demeanor of cats with CRS. Cats can also benefit from intermittent airway humidification via steam inhalation or nebulization.

PROGNOSIS

It seems unlikely that cats with CRS can be cured given the abnormalities that are often found in nasal anatomy by the time veterinary intervention is sought or diagnostics are typically performed. Owners should be aware that this disease can often be controlled but is rarely cured. Most cats have recurrent episodes of nasal discharge periodically, and a reasonable goal of therapy is to limit the severity and frequency of disease exacerbations.

References and Suggested Reading

Hargis M et al: Ulcerative facial and nasal dermatitis and stomatitis in cats associated with feline herpesvirus 1, *Vet Dermatol* 10:267, 1999.

Johnson LR et al: Assessment of infectious organisms associated with chronic rhinosinusitis in cats, *J Am Vet Med Assoc* 227:579, 2005.

Maggs DJ et al: Evaluation of serologic and viral detection methods for diagnosing feline herpesvirus-1 infection in cats with acute respiratory tract or chronic ocular disease, *J Am Vet Med Assoc* 214:502, 1999.

Schoenborn WC et al: Retrospective assessment of computed tomographic findings of feline sinonasal disease in 62 cats, *Vet Radiol Ultrasound* 44:185, 2003.

CHAPTER 141

Brachycephalic Upper Airway Syndrome in Dogs

ERIC R. POPE, *Bassesterre, St. Kitts, West Indies*
GHEORGE M. CONSTANTINESCU, *Columbia, Missouri*

The brachycephalic upper airway syndrome is a group of congenital and acquired abnormalities of the upper airway that results in signs of upper airway obstruction. Congenital anatomic abnormalities encountered include varying degrees of stenotic nares; shortening, widening, and flattening of the nasal cavity and pharynx, causing increased airway resistance; elongation, thickening, and flaccidity of the soft palate; and decreased glottic size. These animals may also have a hypoplastic trachea, which adds to the increased airway resistance. Acquired abnormalities resulting from the greatly increased inspiratory effort include edema and further thickening of the soft palate, eversion of the laryngeal saccules, edema of the pharyngeal and laryngeal mucosa, enlargement of the tonsils, and progressive laryngeal dysfunction ending with complete laryngeal collapse.

The English bulldog, pug, Boston terrier, chow-chow, Pekingese, Shih Tzu and shar-pei are commonly affected breeds. Stenotic nares may also occur in short-nosed breeds of cats such as the Persian and Himalayan. Progressively worsening inspiratory dyspnea, which is exacerbated by exercise, is the most common clinical sign. If stenotic nares are the primary pathology, the clinical signs are relieved by open-mouth breathing. Coughing, gagging, and stridor generally are associated with elongated soft palate and/or acquired abnormalities of the pharyngeal/laryngeal area.

A complete upper airway examination should be performed before undertaking surgical correction of any of these problems. The nares and soft palate usually can be evaluated in the awake patient, but adequate visualization of the pharynx and larynx typically requires sedation or anesthesia. If a light plane of anesthesia is maintained, stimulation of the laryngeal mucosa induces deep respiratory efforts, making assessment of the ability of the laryngeal cartilages to abduct easier. Deep respirations can also be induced by the administration of doxapram (1 mg/kg intravenously [IV]). In most instances surgical correction immediately follows the examination. The prognosis is largely determined by the severity of the secondary changes, especially laryngeal dysfunction. If the laryngeal changes are limited to eversion of the laryngeal saccules and edema of the mucosa, marked improvement is usually seen following correction of the underlying anatomic abnormalities and excision of the everted saccules.

Surgical treatment usually includes correction of the stenotic nares, resection of excessive soft palate, and amputation of the everted laryngeal saccules. If respiratory distress continues after surgery because of poor laryngeal function, partial arytenoidectomy and vocal fold resection can be performed, but the results are quite variable (see Chapter 143). Respiratory distress may continue because of further collapse of the weakened cartilages. Permanent tracheostomy is the best means of providing an adequate airway in animals with severe laryngeal collapse but can be challenging because of the loose, redundant skin on the neck and the small size of the trachea.

STENOTIC NARES

Stenotic nares greatly increase airway resistance. Surgical correction should be performed as soon as possible (i.e., 3 to 4 months of age) to reduce the development of the secondary changes previously described. Correction involves lateralization of the wing of the nostril (alar wing) and possibly resection of a portion of the alar fold to increase the size of the nares. Vertical, horizontal, and dorsolateral wedge resection techniques and amputation of a portion of the alar wing have been described. Recently an alapexy technique was described that might potentially maintain long-term lateralization better than other surgical methods. This method has been used by some surgeons for both primary reconstruction and when the other techniques have failed. Selection of specific technique is based on both manipulation of the alar wing once the patient has been anesthetized and surgeon preference.

The vertical and horizontal wedge techniques are performed using a No. 11 scalpel blade or CO_2 laser. The alar wing to be removed is grasped with Brown-Adson thumb forceps. The scalpel blade is used to remove a wedge (ellipse) of tissue sufficiently wide to relieve the obstruction. The cut must also be deep enough to allow rotation of the ventral (medial) portion of the alar wing. Since hemorrhage may be brisk, it is important to assess the amount of tissue that needs to be removed and then resect it with single bold strokes. Digital pressure and/or wound closure is usually sufficient to control bleeding. The use of electrocautery should be avoided. The edges are sutured with fine (4/0 to 5/0) monofilament suture material in an interrupted pattern. The sutures are tied only tight enough to appose the edges. Excessive tension may result in discomfort, causing the animal to rub the sutures. If bleeding continues after placing the sutures, digital pressure is applied for 5 to 10 minutes.

The dorsolateral wedge technique is preferred by many veterinary surgeons over the vertical and horizontal wedge techniques. An ellipse of tissue is removed at the junction of caudal alar wing adjacent to the haired skin. Most of the tissue is removed from the alar wing. Again it is important to make the wedge deep enough to allow lateralization of the alar wing. This generally means going down almost to the nasal mucosa. The alar wing is sutured to the adjacent skin with fine monofilament suture material. If the alar fold is prominent and restricts the opening into the nasal cavity, it can be excised as described in the following paragraphs.

A potential complication of the wedge techniques is collapse of the ala and recurrence of signs over time. The alapexy technique is suggested as a more effective technique for preventing this complication. Two approximately 5- to 10-mm long × 3-mm wide × 3-mm deep strips of skin are removed from the ventrolateral aspect of the alar wing and from the haired skin 3 to 5 mm lateral to the alar wing. The alar wing is lateralized to appose the wound edges. The adjacent deep wound edges are sutured with interrupted or continuous sutures using monofilament absorbable suture. The adjacent outer wound edges are sutured with interrupted or cruciate sutures using monofilament absorbable or nonabsorbable suture material.

The CO_2 laser also can be used to correct stenotic nares. Hemorrhage is reduced significantly, improving visualization. In small dogs and cats the ventromedial portion of the alar wing is amputated, and the wound is allowed to heal by second intention. In larger dogs wedge resection can be performed as described previously. Similar to the original amputation technique performed with a scalpel, the cosmetic result of amputation by laser resection may not be a good as with the other techniques but is generally very acceptable to the owner.

Some patients have a very prominent alar fold that compromises the opening of the nostril even when the alar wing is adequately lateralized or removed. This can cause significant resistance to airflow and should be addressed if present. The CO_2 laser is an excellent tool for excising a portion of the alar fold. The hemostasis provided improves visualization and control of the amount of tissue removed. The tissue can also be removed with a scalpel blade, but bleeding impairs visualization. Bleeding is controlled by applying pressure.

ELONGATED SOFT PALATE

In the normal animal the caudal border of the soft palate slightly covers the tip of the epiglottis. In patients with brachycephalic airway syndrome, the soft palate may become so elongated that it is sucked into the laryngeal aditus during inspiration. The goal of the surgery is to reestablish the normal anatomic relationship of the soft palate and epiglottis. Since the soft palate functions to occlude the nasopharynx during swallowing, excessive resection can result in nasal reflux, causing chronic rhinitis, and may also predispose the patient to aspiration pneumonia.

Because most patients have some edema of the pharyngeal structures and surgical manipulation of the soft palate induces more swelling, corticosteroids (e.g., prednisolone [0.5 to 1 mg/kg]) are usually given before surgery at induction. Following induction of general anesthesia, an oral speculum is placed. The base of the tongue is depressed with the blade of a laryngoscope; the tip must not cover the epiglottis. The point at which the tip of the epiglottis touches the palate is marked with a skin marker or pinched with a hemostat. A cuffed endotracheal tube is placed. Laterally the soft palate should extend to the caudal border of the tonsillar crypt. Palatectomy can be performed with clamps used to demarcate the amount of palate to be removed or the tissue can be cut freehand using cold steel or laser.

Surgeons without access to a laser and particularly those with minimal experience will likely be more comfortable performing the clamp technique described next. It is easier to perform than the freehand techniques because there is more control of the cut, particularly when the palate is thickened; but it is also the most traumatic technique. Curved hemostats or right-angle Meeker forceps are placed across the soft palate from the caudal border of the tonsillar crypt to the mark on the midline of the soft palate on each side so that tips oppose each other. The distal portion of the palate is excised along the clamp with a scalpel; or alternatively the clamp can be removed from one side, and the palate cut with scissors along the line of crushed tissue. When this technique is used, our preference is to excise all the excess palate with a scalpel, remove the clamp from one side, and then suture the oral and nasopharyngeal mucosa of the palate with a continuous pattern using fine (4/0 to 5/0) absorbable monofilament suture material. When the midpoint is reached, the clamp is removed from the other side, and suturing continued from the midline laterally. Although the clamp technique is more traumatic than the noncrush "cut and sew" technique described next, when the clamps are used it is much easier to control the amount of palate resected and to establish a smooth curve to the caudal border of the soft palate.

The freehand "cut and sew" technique is less traumatic than the clamp technique and is recommended if a laser is not available. A suture is placed at the caudal border of the tonsillar crypt on one side. The palate is grasped at the midpoint with forceps and retracted rostrally. The palate is cut with scissors from the lateral border to the midline. It is sutured with a continuous pattern (as described previously) to the midpoint. The other side of the palate is then excised and sutured. Performing the procedure in two steps facilitates tissue manipulation and reduces the amount of hemorrhage.

Resection of the soft palate using the CO_2 laser is the least traumatic technique. An advantage of the laser is that minimal manipulation of the palate is required. Saline-moistened sponges are placed in the pharynx and behind the palate after determining the amount of palate to be resected. The palate is then excised freehand beginning laterally on one side and then working across to the opposite side. A long-handled thumb forceps (e.g., DeBakey forceps) can be used to grasp the caudal edge of the palate while it is being cut with the laser. Some surgeons prefer to use a handpiece with a backstop to further minimize the risk of collateral damage. Because minimal manipulation of the soft palate is necessary, it is much easier to maintain orientation during the resection. Suturing is not necessary when the laser is used, and hemorrhage is usually negligible.

EVERTED LARYNGEAL SACCULES

The laryngeal ventricles are small pockets in the wall of the larynx just rostral and lateral to the vocal folds. With chronic increased respiratory effort, the mucosa of the ventricles can evert. As the tissues become edematous, they protrude into the laryngeal aditus and appear as small pea-shaped masses just in front of the vocal folds. The everted saccules can be grasped with forceps and then amputated at their base with long-handled scissors. Hemorrhage is usually minimal and controlled by pressure. Cotton swabs soaked with dilute epinephrine can also be used if bleeding occurs. The mucosal defects heal by second intention.

LARYNGEAL COLLAPSE

If the underlying conditions are not recognized and treated early, the chronically increased inspiratory effort ultimately can lead to progressive distortion and complete collapse of the laryngeal cartilages. Eversion of the laryngeal saccules is considered to be the first step in the pathogenesis of laryngeal collapse (stage 1). As the condition progresses to stage 2 the cuneiform processes rotate medially, and there may be only minimal or no abduction of the arytenoids when viewed during laryngoscopy. In stage 3 complete loss of support occurs so that the corniculate and cuneiform processes may abut each other medially or even overlap. The latter change carries a poor prognosis, and permanent tracheostomy is the most successful treatment.

If only minor laryngeal dysfunction is noted (stage 1), the other upper airway abnormalities are corrected as previously described, and the animal is allowed to recover. If respiratory distress persists or progresses, laryngeal surgery or permanent tracheostomy is indicated. All patients undergoing laryngeal surgery should receive corticosteroids before surgery unless temporary tracheostomy is performed. Everted laryngeal saccules are amputated if this has not been previously done.

Partial Arytenoidectomy and Vocal Fold Resection

Dogs with stage 2 collapse (cartilages are collapsing medially, but some glottic lumen remains) may improve following partial arytenoidectomy and vocal fold resection. Partial arytenoidectomy can be performed unilaterally or bilaterally. Partial arytenoidectomy is performed via an oral approach using long-handled instruments such as a uterine biopsy forceps to remove small bites from the medial wall of the corniculate processes. If bilateral partial arytenoidectomy is performed, the incidence of postoperative stricture can be reduced by not extending the arytenoidectomy to the dorsal midline. Excessive removal of tissue, particularly when done bilaterally, may predispose to aspiration pneumonia. Bilateral resection of the vocal folds is also performed using the uterine biopsy forceps. Postoperative stricture ("webbing") is decreased if the ventral commissure of the vocal folds is left intact.

Permanent Tracheostomy

Permanent tracheostomy is indicated in animals with stage 3 collapse and patients that do not improve following partial arytenoidectomy and vocal fold resection. Permanent tracheostomy entails removing the ventral third of the tracheal cartilages over a 3- to 4-tracheal ring span and suturing the tracheal mucosa to the skin. During the initial postoperative period the tracheostoma should be checked every 1 to 3 hours for mucus accumulation and cleaned as needed. The amount of mucus produced gradually decreases so that long-term cleansing is necessary only one to three times daily. The hair of long-haired dogs should be kept trimmed to prevent matting with mucus, which could occlude the stoma. Some stenosis of the opening is expected. Dogs with permanent tracheostomy are predisposed to inhaled foreign bodies and obviously cannot be allowed to swim, but otherwise they seem to function well.

Suggested Reading

Ellison GW: Alapexy: an alternative technique for repair of stenotic nares in dogs, *J Am Anim Hosp Assoc* 40:484, 2004.

Hedlund CS: Surgery of the upper respiratory system. In Fossum TW, editor: *Small animal surgery*, ed 2, St Louis, 2002, Elsevier, p 716.

Monnet E: Brachycephalic airway syndrome In Slatter DH, editor: *Textbook of small animal surgery*, ed 3, Philadelphia, 2003, Saunders, p 808.

CHAPTER 142

Nasopharyngeal Disorders

GERALDINE B. HUNT, *Sydney, Australia*
SUSAN F. FOSTER, *Murdoch, Australia*

A variety of nasopharyngeal diseases are encountered in small animals. In cats nasopharyngeal disease is most commonly caused by cryptococcosis (dependent on location), nasopharyngeal polyps, neoplasia, and foreign bodies. In dogs nasopharyngeal disease may be caused by inflammation, neoplasia, foreign bodies, nasal mites (*Pneumonyssoides caninum*) or congenital abnormalities. Since clinical signs of disease resulting from different etiologies may be identical, a thorough and systematic approach to diagnosis is required to ensure that treatable diseases are not missed.

CLINICAL SIGNS OF NASOPHARYNGEAL DISEASE

Animals with disease limited to the nasopharynx present mainly with signs of upper airway obstruction (i.e., stertor/snoring). In dogs stertor is usually alleviated by open-mouth breathing. Cats are often unwilling or unable to breath through their mouths and thus may appear dyspneic. Some animals show signs of pharyngeal discomfort and make repeated attempts at swallowing; coughing and dysphagia may occur in cats. A cat with acute nasopharyngeal disease may paw at its nose and mouth. Dogs may also present with facial discomfort and pruritus. Reverse sneezing is a specific nasopharyngeal sign in dogs. Purulent nasal discharge and fetid breath may be identified in animals with foreign bodies.

Unless nasopharyngeal disease is accompanied by significant intranasal pathology, nasal discharge is usually mild or absent because secretions from the nasopharynx tend to be swallowed. Likewise, sneezing is not typical but may occur if the caudal nasal turbinates are irritated or if disease also affects the nasal cavity.

Enlargement of regional lymph nodes, in particular the mandibular and retropharyngeal nodes, may be the first detectable clinical sign in animals with nasopharyngeal neoplasia. Occasionally the main presenting signs are neurologic. Central nervous system signs may result from the spread of nasopharyngeal cryptococcosis or neoplasia. Signs of otitis media and vestibular disease may occur if there is extension of disease from the nasopharynx into the tympanic bulla (or vice versa) or if the opening to the eustachian tube is occluded. Horner's syndrome is encountered commonly in cats with involvement of the tympanic bullae. Animals with inflammatory or neoplastic disease extending beyond the tympanic bulla may also have signs of facial nerve dysfunction (facial asymmetry, absent palpebral reflex).

The duration of onset and severity of signs vary according to the underlying disease. Rapid onset of signs is suggestive of a nasopharyngeal foreign body, although some patients with foreign bodies have chronic signs. Gradual onset of stertor and attempted mouth breathing is more likely to indicate a slow-growing nasopharyngeal mass.

DIAGNOSIS OF NASOPHARYNGEAL DISEASE

Because of difficulties of access and the complex anatomy of surrounding structures, diagnosis of nasopharyngeal disease may be challenging. In the past investigation was often limited to digital palpation through the soft palate and visualization under anesthesia using dental mirrors and spay hooks. However, now many techniques of varying complexity are available to the veterinary practitioner.

Physical Examination

In quiet patients palpation through the soft palate may reveal masses in the nasopharynx. Regional lymph nodes should always be palpated and, if affected, may provide a convenient source of diagnostic material. Mucous membrane color should be evaluated for evidence of cyanosis, which may indicate serious respiratory compromise. Determination of oxygen saturation by means of pulse oximetry should be considered where available. Cardiopulmonary function should be evaluated carefully to rule out the possibility of intrathoracic disease in animals displaying signs of respiratory dysfunction. Likewise, an attempt should be made to differentiate stertor (a snoring-type noise arising from the nasopharynx or pharynx) from stridor (a high-pitched noise arising from disturbance of air flow through the larynx or trachea) before physical or chemical restraint. If possible, the effect of opening the mouth on stertor should be determined.

Direct Visualization of the Nasopharynx

If nasopharyngeal or caudal nasal disease is suspected, further evaluation under general anesthesia is required. Anesthesia is ideally induced using an intravenous technique enabling rapid airway control and maintained subsequently by inhalation agents in oxygen. The oropharynx, laryngopharynx, and larynx are inspected initially before placement of a cuffed endotracheal tube. When performing manipulations that may cause blood or other fluid to accumulate in the pharynx, it is critical that the cuff be inflated to ensure a leakproof seal and that the laryngopharynx be packed with gauze. The animal is best positioned in dorsal recumbency, with the maxilla held down firmly with tape applied over the upper canine teeth. Topical anesthesia of the nasopharynx is instituted with a small amount of local anesthetic (lidocaine, 1 mg/kg topically by means of a soaked surgical swab placed in the pharynx or trickled down from the external nares via the ventral nasal meatus). This avoids the necessity of deepening the plane of anesthesia excessively to abolish reflexes resulting from mechanical stimulation of sensitive nasopharyngeal structures. The nasopharynx is examined by palpation through the soft palate, followed by rostral retraction of the caudal edge of the soft palate using a spay hook. The caudal part of the nasopharynx is relatively well exposed in this fashion. The cranial nasopharynx and choanae can also be visualized in cats but not usually in dogs.

Nasopharyngeal Endoscopy

The mainstay of diagnosis of nasopharyngeal disease is retroflexed endoscopy. A flexible endoscope (appropriate to the size of the animal) is introduced into the pharynx and retroflexed above the soft palate. In some instances it may be simpler to retroflex the endoscope before insertion, introduce it into the pharynx and proximal esophagus, and then hook it above the soft palate. Rostral retraction, so that the retroflexed end advances towards the nose, enables visualization of the rostral nasopharynx, choanae, and caudal nasal cavities. Mass lesions may be apparent immediately; although in some cases lesions are obscured by mucus, blood, or pus. Vigorous flushing with saline (via the endoscope or through the nostrils) usually clears the field sufficiently to allow visualization of lesions. A technique of nasopharyngoscopy using an endoscope inserted via gastrotomy has been reported recently (Esterline, Radlinsky, and Schermerhorn, 2005) for use in situations in which a flexible endoscope of the size appropriate for a cat is not available. Since it involves a surgical approach to the stomach, this technique would only be recommended if no other means of visualizing the nasopharynx were practical.

Diagnostic Imaging

The normal nasopharynx is readily identified on plain lateral radiographs because of the presence of air dorsal to the soft palate. The hyoid apparatus and larynx define its caudal boundary. Space-occupying lesions of the nasopharynx may be delineated by surrounding air, and radiopaque objects may be apparent. However, because of the complex anatomy of the region, the presence of objects such as endotracheal tubes and esophageal stethoscopes, and secretions within the nasopharynx, radiographic details may be obscured. Positive-contrast studies of the nasal cavity and nasopharynx have been largely supplanted by endoscopy. In general, radiography provides little more information than thorough examination under anesthesia and palpation through the soft palate.

Ultrasonography can be useful in animals with soft tissue or fluid-filled masses in the nasopharynx and assist the acquisition of diagnostic samples using ultrasound-guided needle aspiration or biopsy. Large vascular structures may be present in some cases; thus Tru-Cut or incisional biopsies should be taken with care. Advanced imaging techniques such as computed tomography and magnetic resonance imaging are potentially useful for detecting nasopharyngeal lesions, determining precise anatomic information, and assessing involvement of nearby structures such as the middle ear and bones of the skull. These are also helpful in assessing tumor response to radiotherapy and/or surgery.

Obtaining Diagnostic Samples From the Nasopharynx

To make a definitive diagnosis, in many cases it is necessary to obtain representative specimens for cytology, histology, and microbial culture. Fine-needle aspiration may be performed readily through the soft palate. Blind Tru-cut biopsy of lesions through the soft palate is also technically feasible but carries a risk of inducing hemorrhage if large blood vessels lateral to the nasopharynx are perforated. Ideally tissue biopsies are obtained under direct visualization either by retracting or incising the soft palate or via endoscopic biopsy.

When a mass is present, vigorous massage of the lesion through the soft palate often dislodges or fragments the mass, and anterograde flushing via the nares may be successful in dislodging part or all of it. In dogs flushing is best achieved via soft catheters inserted into the ventral nasal meatus; however, in cats effective pressure can be generated by inserting the end of a 10-ml syringe directly into the nares and holding the nares closed with the fingers. Material dislodged from the nasal cavity or nasopharynx by flushing then bounces off the larynx or cuffed endotracheal tube to appear in the oropharynx or mouth. Anterograde passage of a catheter through the left and right ventral nasal meatus is helpful in dislodging foreign material and mucus.

Canine nasal mites may also be retrieved for diagnosis with nasal flushing, although endoscopic visualization is preferable. Flushing the nasal cavity with halothane has been reported to induce mites to migrate caudally in the nasopharynx, where they can be retrieved and identified easily (Marks, Moore, and Rishniw, 1997).

Adjunctive Tests for Diagnosis of Nasopharyngeal Disease

Cytologic examination and culture of nasal swabs may detect organisms such as *Cryptococcus* spp. Positive findings need to be interpreted carefully. Both cats and dogs can have asymptomatic carriage of *Cryptococcus* spp., and 30% to 40% of normal dogs with nasal neoplasia have *Aspergillus* or *Penicillium* spp. cultured from blind swabs (Sharp, 1998). Serology is useful to differentiate asymptomatic carriage of *Cryptococcus* spp. from infection because animals with cryptococcosis usually demonstrate a positive latex cryptococcal antigen agglutination test titer.

SURGICAL ACCESS TO THE NASOPHARYNX

When extraction of lesions such as inflammatory polyps, cryptococcal granulomas, or foreign bodies is not possible via palatine retraction or better access is required for obtaining diagnostic samples, the nasopharynx may be approached surgically via a longitudinal incision in the soft palate. In most cases adequate access is obtained by maximally opening the jaws, placing a mouth gag, and having an assistant hold the tube out of the way with a malleable retractor. Although placement of the endotracheal tube via a pharyngostomy incision improves the working area somewhat, it takes longer and results in more postoperative morbidity.

The soft palate is divided longitudinally from the caudal edge of the hard palate to within a centimeter of its caudal free edge. The caudal edge should be left intact to facilitate repair and support the incision during healing. Some bleeding from the rich vascular plexus within the soft palate should be anticipated but usually resolves spontaneously or with digital pressure. Surgical suction and good lighting should be available, as should a surgical assistant. When extensive dissection is likely to be undertaken in dogs, blood loss may be ameliorated somewhat by temporary occlusion of the carotid arteries using Rumel tourniquets placed through a ventral midline cervical incision. This technique is not recommended for cats because they often develop neurologic sequelae. In either species if major blood loss is anticipated, contingencies for replacement with whole blood or a blood replacement product should be made. The soft palate incision may be continued rostrally as a mucoperiosteal incision and ventral rhinotomy if indicated, providing excellent access to the ventral nasal cavity. Repair of the soft palate is performed in two or three layers. Polydioxanone in a continuous suture pattern in the nasal mucosal and muscularis layer and oral mucosa provides excellent closure. Postoperative management is usually uncomplicated. Animals display little evidence of pain associated with the incision and are usually willing to eat and drink within 24 hours of surgery unless systemic illness is present. Healing in this area is rapid and reliable, presumably because of its excellent blood supply. Soft food should be offered for 2 to 3 weeks after surgery, and the incision should be examined at weekly intervals to ensure that no areas of wound dehiscence are developing.

SPECIFIC NASOPHARYNGEAL DISEASES AND THEIR TREATMENT

Nasopharyngeal Foreign Bodies

Foreign bodies may include tablets, bones, fish heads, stones, plant material (blades of grass are especially common in cats), seaweed segments, and plastic. These materials are often coated with a layer of mucus or exudate. Nasopharyngeal foreign bodies may be dislodged by digital palpation or extracted under direct vision, endoscopically, or surgically. Visualization and removal are facilitated by laying the animal on its back and extending its head before retracting the soft palate. In many cases it is possible to dislodge foreign bodies caudally with a combination of anterograde flushing and passage of a urinary catheter. Alligator forceps may also be passed anterograde and used to push the foreign body caudally for retrieval in the pharynx. Small embolectomy or cardiovascular catheters, with an inflatable balloon passed via the nares and inflated at the choanae, can be useful to dislodge foreign bodies and push them into the pharynx. After removal of the foreign body, the nasopharynx should be flushed with saline. If local ulceration is severe, broad-spectrum antibiotics with efficacy against anaerobes may be administered for 3 to 5 days.

Nasopharyngeal Parasites

The canine nasal mite *P. caninum* is a parasite, reported from many countries (probably worldwide) that inhabits the nasal cavity, nasopharynx, and frontal sinus. Clinical signs described include sneezing, reverse sneezing, rhinitis, and impaired sense of smell. Diagnosis is established by direct observation of the mites in or around the external nares or endoscopically in the nasopharynx or nares. Nasal mites can be treated effectively with milbemycin, ivermectin, or topical selamectin. Milbemycin at 0.5 to 1 mg/kg once weekly orally for 3 consecutive weeks appears safe and efficacious; 0.5 mg/kg once monthly orally is the dose for heartworm prophylaxis (Gunnarsson et al., 1999). Selamectin at 6 to 24 mg/kg every 2 weeks topically for three treatments has also been demonstrated to be effective (Gunnarsson et al, 2004), but alopecia may develop at the higher doses; 6 to 12 mg/kg monthly topically is the dose used for heartworm prophylaxis. Ivermectin has been used at various doses (200 to 400 mcg/kg, subcutaneously [SC] or PO) and dosing frequencies (single dose or multiple doses at various intervals) and appears effective; but all doses have been higher than the licensed dose, and these doses may have serious adverse effects in ivermectin-sensitive breeds such as collies. One dog had nasal mites diagnosed while on ivermectin prophylaxis for heartworm (6 mcg/kg PO); thus lower doses may not be effective (Coleman, Walter, and Dickson, 2000). It is advisable to supply a single antiinflammatory dose of prednisolone (0.5 mg/kg PO) with the first treatment to be used either prophylactically or if signs worsen in severity after treatment. The transient increase in severity of signs that occurs in some dogs is presumed to be caused by a host reaction to the dead and dying mites. Although this reaction is only transient, it may be quite distressing to both the dogs and their owners.

Cuterebra larvae occasionally occur in the feline pharynx, most commonly in the retropharyngeal tissues but also on the soft palate. The parasite may be seen through the "breathing hole" in the mucosal surface or may be found within a resected mass lesion. *Cuterebra* larvae are removed by enlarging the breathing pore and grasping the parasite with forceps. Hypersensitivity reactions may occur if parasitic hemolymph escapes into the surrounding tissue; thus care must be taken not to damage the larva during extraction. Alternatively the entire granuloma may be excised (Levy and Ford, 1994).

Nasopharyngeal Cryptococcosis

In cats and dogs the nasal cavity is usually the primary site of infection with *Cryptococcus* spp. Rhinitis is the most common presentation, but caudal nasal cavity and nasopharyngeal involvement may occur, and nasopharyngeal signs may predominate. If nasopharyngeal cryptococcomas are present, debulking by vigorous nasal flushing or surgery is recommended to alleviate the upper airway obstruction and decrease residual infected tissue to be treated medically. The potential danger of complete upper airway obstruction in patients with nasopharyngeal cryptococcosis should not be underestimated, especially in cats, since they tend to be reluctant to resort to open-mouth breathing. In addition, since debulking has been found to hasten resolution in some cases that are responding slowly to medical management, debulking should be considered before medical therapy. Medical treatment for nasopharyngeal cryptococcosis requires oral itraconazole or fluconazole; ketoconazole is not very effective and likely to result in adverse side effects. Amphotericin is unnecessary unless there is central nervous system involvement. Fluconazole is a very effective agent for treating cryptococcosis and is well tolerated, even at high doses, in the majority of cases. The dose of fluconazole is 30 to 50 mg per cat every 12 hours orally, with dose based on cat size. Fluconazole penetrates the blood-brain barrier even in the absence of inflammation; thus it should be used in preference to itraconazole if there is concurrent nervous system involvement. Itraconazole is used more commonly because it is effective and considerably cheaper than fluconazole. It does not penetrate the blood-brain barrier and often causes a reversible hepatotoxicity at higher doses. Itraconazole is usually administered at 50 to 100 mg per cat once daily orally with food. Medium-size to large cats should receive 100 mg once daily, whereas cats weighing 3.5 kg or less should receive 50 mg daily or 100 mg on alternate days. Many cats eventually develop liver toxicity during therapy with itraconazole at these doses. This can take several weeks to months to develop and is manifest clinically as reduced appetite and sometimes vomiting. Invariably there is increased serum alanine aminotransferase activity. Itraconazole-induced hepatotoxicity is reversible on discontinuation of the drug, although appetite and demeanor may take up to 7 days to recover. Once the cat has recovered, it is generally possible to safely administer the drug again, albeit at a reduced dose, typically 50% of the original dose. In a minority of cases it is necessary to change therapy to fluconazole. Medical therapy with either drug should be continued until resolution of all clinical signs. Typically this takes 3 to 12 months, although some cases require longer periods of treatment. The serum cryptococcal antigen titer should be monitored, and a fourfold to fivefold reduction in titer suggests successful therapy. It is highly recommended that treatment be continued until the antigen titer declines to zero.

Nasopharyngeal Polyps

Nasopharyngeal polyps occur much more commonly in cats than dogs. Nasopharyngeal polyps in cats usually arise from the eustachian tube or the middle ear. They are composed of granulation tissue covered by a stratified squamous or ciliated columnar epithelial layer that is often ulcerated. The causes of inflammatory polyps in cats are unknown. It has been proposed that they result from either congenital defects or chronic inflammatory middle ear disease probably caused by viral upper respiratory tract infection. Clinical signs may be respiratory, otic, or both. Because of their caudal location in the nasopharynx, feline nasopharyngeal polyps are often amenable to removal by traction by an oral approach. Removal of nasopharyngeal polyps by traction is most likely to be successful if the polyp is well visualized. The animal is intubated, and the pharynx packed with gauze. A pair of grasping forceps with strong teeth is required. If they are not available, artery forceps are preferred to conventional alligator forceps. The cat is positioned in dorsal recumbency, and its head taped to the table or held by an assistant. The soft palate is drawn rostrally to visualize the polyp. The polyp is grasped firmly across as much of its body as possible, ensuring that pharyngeal mucosa is not included, and firm traction is applied. The polyp should be submitted for histopathology to confirm the diagnosis and eliminate the possibility of lymphosarcoma or cryptococcosis.

Owners should be warned of the likelihood of temporary Horner's syndrome after extraction. This usually resolves in 1 to 3 weeks. Recurrence of the polyp is possible, and some surgeons recommend ventral bulla osteotomy in all cats with this condition. However, a recent study suggested that traction/avulsion is a good first option in cats with no radiographic or computed tomography evidence of bullae involvement (Veir et al., 2002). The same study demonstrated that polyps do not always recur in cats with bulla involvement; therefore traction/avulsion is probably a reasonable first option in these cats also. Anderson, Robinson, and White (2000) showed that cats with nasopharyngeal polyps were nearly four times more likely to be cured by traction alone than cats with aural polyps and that treatment with antiinflammatory doses of prednisolone following traction reduced the recurrence rate.

In dogs polyps usually arise from the caudal nasal turbinates as a consequence of chronic rhinitis. They are usually situated rostrally in the nasopharynx, attached to the caudal nasal turbinates. This is also true of other forms of inflammatory granuloma. It may be possible to dislodge these with vigorous flushing or by grasping them endoscopically. In other cases a ventral surgical approach to the nasopharynx may be combined with a ventral rhinotomy to obtain diagnostic samples and debulk the lesions.

Nasopharyngeal Stenosis

Nasopharyngeal stenosis is most often seen in cats following chronic inflammation. Stricture formation may occur in both cats and dogs following infectious diseases, surgery, or other trauma or as a congenital abnormality (choanal atresia). Nasopharyngeal stenosis resulting from abnormally thickened palatopharyngeal muscles has also been reported in seven dachshunds (Kirkberger et al., 2006). Regardless of etiology, treatment aims are to establish patency of the choanae and nasopharynx and reduce the risk of restricture. Patency may be established by balloon dilation, bougienage, dilation using artery forceps, or surgical excision of the obstructing tissue. In some cases it may be possible to restore integrity of the nasopharyngeal mucosa by means of local flaps, but in most instances this is not feasible. Stents may be placed to maintain patency while epithelialization of the denuded area takes place, or intermittent redilation may be performed (similar to the approach for esophageal strictures). Underlying conditions leading to the inflammation and mucosal ulceration must also be addressed to achieve long-term resolution of the nasopharyngeal obstruction.

Nasopharyngeal Cysts

Nasopharyngeal cysts may arise as a result of caudal nasal turbinate disease (in dogs) or cystic malformation of structures adjacent to the nasopharynx, such as the thyroglossal duct or Rathke's cleft. In cases of cystic Rathke's cleft, embryonic pituitary development proceeds abnormally, resulting in a progressively expansile cystic lesion within the sphenoid bone. Signs are often progressive and may not prompt an owner to seek veterinary attention until the patient reaches adulthood. Cystic Rathke's cleft may or may not be associated with pituitary dwarfism. Other types of developmental cysts have been encountered in dogs. A cystic or multilobulated appearance may also occur with cartilaginous and bony neoplasms of the skull such as multilobular osteosarcoma. Therefore histopathology is a very important component of diagnosis and surgical decision making. Cystic Rathke's cleft or other developmental bony cysts require surgical débridement and debulking. Simple cysts of the nasal turbinates may be removed by traction or flushing or may require surgical débridement.

Nasopharyngeal Neoplasia

Cats with nasal lymphosarcoma may, but do not always, have very long remission times after radiation therapy, multiagent chemotherapy, or both. Radiation protocols vary but usually result in the delivery of 3 to 5 Gy per fraction for a total of 6 to 10 fractions (total dose of 30 to 50 Gy). Although long remission times have been reported with radiation therapy alone, multiagent chemotherapy is usually recommended in combination to treat any systemic lymphosarcoma. In particular, renal lymphosarcoma has been noted as a sequel to successful radiation treatment for nasal lymphosarcoma. Debulking by nasal flushing or surgery may be required with nasopharyngeal lymphosarcoma for both diagnosis and immediate relief of respiratory obstruction.

Nasopharyngeal lymphosarcoma in dogs is exceedingly rare, and little information is available on its treatment. Treatment usually involves multiagent chemotherapy protocols with prior surgical debulking only if respiratory signs are severe.

Nonlymphoid nasal tumors that may involve the nasopharynx in dogs and cats include osteosarcoma, chondrosarcoma, fibrosarcoma, and carcinomas. A variety of treatments have been reported, including surgery, cryosurgery, radiotherapy, chemotherapy, and combinations of these. Orthovoltage radiation (with cytoreductive surgery) and megavoltage radiation both increase survival times in dogs. Orthovoltage radiation with cytoreductive

surgery resulted in statistically longer survival times than megavoltage radiation in one study (LaDue et al., 1999). Chemotherapy alone has traditionally demonstrated little efficacy in the treatment of nonlymphoid nasal tumors in dogs or cats. However, 81% of canine nasal tumors have been shown to express cyclooxygenase-2 (COX-2) (Kleiter et al, 2004), and a recent small case series demonstrated that the treatment with oral piroxicam (a COX-2 inhibitor) in conjunction with alternating doses of doxorubicin and carboplatin was efficacious and well tolerated (Langova et al., 2004). It is not known whether this protocol will be useful in nonlymphoid feline tumors, but it may offer a feasible alternative when radiation is unavailable.

References and Suggested Reading

Anderson DM, Robinson RK, White RAS: Management of inflammatory polyps in 37 cats, *Vet Rec* 147: 684, 2000.

Coleman GT, Walter DE, Dickson CJ: *P. caninum* in a Queensland dog, *Aust Vet Pract* 30:83, 2000.

Esterline ML, Radlinsky MAG, Schermerhorn TS: Endoscopic removal of nasal polyps in a cat using a novel surgical approach, *J Feline Med Surg* 7:121, 2005.

Gunnarsson LK et al: Clinical efficacy of milbemycin oxime in the treatment of nasal mite infection in dogs, *J Am Animal Hosp Assoc* 35:81, 1999.

Gunnarsson L et al: Efficacy of selamectin in the treatment of nasal mite *(Pneumonyssoides caninum)* infection in dogs, *J Am Animal Hosp Assoc* 40:400, 2004.

Hunt GB et al: Nasopharyngeal disorders of dogs and cats: a review and retrospective study, *Compend Contin Educ Pract Vet* 24:184, 2002.

Kirkberger RM et al: Stenotic nasopharyngeal dysgenesis in the dachsund: seven cases (2002-2004) *J Am Anim Hosp Assoc* 42: 290, 2006.

Kleiter M et al: Expression of cyclo-oxygenase-2 in canine epithelial nasal tumours, *Vet Radiol Ultrasound* 45:255, 2004.

LaDue TA et al: Factors influencing survival after radiotherapy of nasal tumors in 130 dogs, *Vet Radiol Ultrasound* 40:312, 1999.

Langova V et al: Treatment of eight dogs with nasal tumours with alternating doses of doxorubicin and carboplatin in conjunction with oral piroxicam, *Aust Vet J* 82:676, 2004.

Levy JK, Ford RB: Diseases of the upper respiratory tract. In Shedrding RG, editor: *The cat: diseases and management*, ed 2, New York, 1994, Churchill Livingstone, p 947.

Little CJL: Nasopharyngeal polyps. In August JR, editor: *Consultations in feline internal medicine* 3, Philadelphia, 1997, Saunders, p 310.

Little L Patel R, Goldschmidt: Nasal and nasopharyngeal lymphoma in cats: 50 cases (1989-2005), *Vet Path* 44: 885, 2007.

Malik R et al: Nasopharyngeal cryptococcosis, *Aust Vet J* 75:483, 1997.

Marks SL, Moore, MP, Rishniw M: *Pneumonyssoides caninum*: the canine nasal mite, *Compend Contin Educ Small Anim Pract* 16:577, 1997.

Sharp NJH: Canine nasal aspergillosis-penicilliosis. In Greene CE, editor: *Infectious diseases of the dog and cat*, ed 2, Philadelphia, 1998, Saunders, p 404.

Veir JK: Feline inflammatory polyps: historical, clinical, and PCR findings for feline calici virus and feline herpes virus-1 in 28 cases, *J Feline Med Surg* 4:195, 2002.

CHAPTER 143

Laryngeal Diseases

CATRIONA M. MACPHAIL, *Fort Collins, Colorado*
ERIC MONNET, *Fort Collins, Colorado*

The larynx is a term used to describe the cartilages that surround the rima glottis and that are responsible for control of airflow during respiration. The four cartilages that make up the larynx are the paired arytenoids and the unpaired epiglottis, cricoid, and thyroid cartilages. The cricoarytenoideus dorsalis muscle is solely responsible for opening the glottis. The muscle originates on the dorsolateral surface of the cricoid and inserts on the muscular process of the arytenoids. The recurrent laryngeal nerve innervates all of the intrinsic muscles of the larynx except the cricothyroid muscle. The function of the larynx is to regulate airflow, protect the lower airway from aspiration during swallowing, and to control phonation. Diseases most commonly affecting the larynx include laryngeal paralysis, laryngeal collapse, and laryngeal masses. All of these conditions result in some degree of upper airway obstruction. Dogs and cats typically present for respiratory stridor, voice change, coughing, or gagging. Progression of clinical signs is highly variable.

LARYNGEAL PARALYSIS

Etiology

Laryngeal paralysis is a common unilateral or bilateral respiratory disorder that primarily affects older large-breed dogs. However, a congenital form does occur in certain breeds such as Bouvier des Flandres, Siberian huskies, and Alaskan malamutes. Laryngeal paralysis-polyneuropathy complexes have been described in dalmatians and rottweilers. Acquired laryngeal paralysis is caused by damage to the recurrent laryngeal nerve or intrinsic laryngeal muscles from polyneuropathy, polymyopathy, trauma, or intrathoracic or extrathoracic masses. In most dogs the cause remains undetermined, and these cases are classified as idiopathic. The Labrador retriever is by far the most common breed reported; but golden retrievers, Saint Bernards, Newfoundlands, and Irish setters are also overrepresented.

Clinical Signs

Laryngeal paralysis results in the arytenoid cartilages and consequently the vocal folds remaining in a paramedian position during inspiration, in effect causing an upper airway obstruction. Dogs typically present with noisy inspiratory respiration and exercise intolerance. Early clinical signs include voice change and mild coughing and gagging. Severe airway obstruction results in respiratory distress, cyanosis, and collapse. Dogs may also present with signs of dysphagia. Progression of clinical signs is highly variable, and dogs may have clinical signs for several months to years before significant respiratory distress ensues. However, clinical signs are easily exacerbated by heavy exercise or increasing environmental temperature. The majority of dogs present for surgical intervention in the late spring or early summer months (Snelling and Edwards, 2003). As respiratory rate increases, the arytenoids obstructing airflow may become inflamed and edematous, resulting in further airway obstruction. A vicious cycle ensues that if unaddressed may become life-threatening.

Diagnosis

Routine diagnostic evaluation for dogs thought to have laryngeal paralysis includes physical examination, complete blood count, biochemical profile, urinalysis, thyroid function screening, thoracic radiographs, and laryngeal examination. Dogs with bilateral laryngeal paralysis are at risk for aspiration pneumonia both before and after surgery. Therefore thoracic radiographs are a necessary part of the diagnostic workup in dogs suspected to have laryngeal dysfunction. For dogs that present with dysphagia or vomiting, an esophagram should be considered to rule out esophageal dysfunction or megaesophagus that may not be apparent on plain thoracic radiographs. Hypothyroidism is associated with laryngeal paralysis, although a direct link has yet to be established. Regardless, thyroid function screening is performed routinely in the workup for laryngeal paralysis. Thyroid supplementation should be instituted if indicated, although this does not typically improve clinical signs associated with laryngeal paralysis.

Definitive diagnosis of laryngeal paralysis requires visual examination of the larynx. However, laryngoscopy is a poorly specific diagnostic test since false-positives are common because of the influence of anesthetic agents on laryngeal function. Laryngeal paralysis should not be diagnosed solely on the lack of arytenoid movement. It can result in a fixed upper airway obstruction if there is secondary inflammation and swelling of the laryngeal cartilages. Diagnosis may also be confused by the presence of paradoxic movement of the arytenoids, resulting in a false-negative result. In this situation the arytenoid cartilages move inward during inspiration because of negative intraglottic pressure that is created by breathing against an obstruction. The cartilages then return to their original position during the expiratory phase, giving the impression of abduction. An assistant can state the stage of respiration during laryngoscopy to help distinguish normal from abnormal motion. Intravenous thiopental administered to effect is thought to be the best choice to allow for assessment of laryngeal function (Jackson et al., 2004). When a butorphanol-glycopyrrolate premedication is used, either thiopental or propofol allows excellent visualization of the larynx (Gross et al., 2002). Doxapram HCl (1mg/kg intravenously [IV]) has been advocated for routine use during laryngoscopy to increase respiratory effort and intrinsic laryngeal motion and should be administered if the diagnosis is in doubt (Miller et al., 2002; Tobias, Jackson, and Harvey, 2004). Transnasal laryngoscopy to diagnose laryngeal paralysis using intramuscular sedation alone has been reported in a small number of dogs (Radlinsky, Mason, and Hodgson, 2004).

Emergency Treatment

For dogs that present in acute respiratory distress, initial treatment is directed at improving ventilation, reducing laryngeal edema, and minimizing the animal's stress. A typical treatment regimen involves oxygen supplementation and administration of short-acting steroids (e.g., dexamethasone 0.2 to 1mg/kg IV) and sedatives (e.g., acepromazine 0.02mg/kg IV). Additional administration of buprenorphine (0.005mg/kg IV) or butorphanol (0.25mg/kg IV) may also be considered. These dogs are also often hyperthermic, and appropriate cooling procedures should also be instituted. If respiratory distress cannot be abated, intubation or a temporary tracheostomy should be considered.

Conservative Treatment

Often dogs are not severely affected clinically until they have bilateral laryngeal paresis or paralysis. Therefore dogs with unilateral laryngeal dysfunction are not surgical candidates. For dogs with bilateral laryngeal paralysis, the decision to recommend surgery is based on the quality of life of the dog, severity of clinical signs, and time of year. Conservative management of dogs with laryngeal paralysis involves environmental changes, owner education, weight loss, and consideration of antiinflammatory drugs to minimize laryngeal swelling. For dogs that are diagnosed with concurrent hypothyroidism, thyroid supplementation should be instituted, but this rarely improves the clinical signs of laryngeal paralysis.

Surgical Treatment

Numerous surgical techniques are available to treat laryngeal paralysis. Unilateral arytenoid lateralization is the current technique of choice for most surgeons. Bilateral lateralization has been shown to result in unacceptable morbidity. Other techniques include partial laryngectomy, castellated laryngofissure, and permanent tracheostomy.

Several variations of unilateral arytenoid lateralization have been described. The most common technique involves suturing the cricoid cartilage to the muscular process of the arytenoid cartilage. This mimics the directional pull of the cricoarytenoid dorsalis muscle and rotates the arytenoid cartilage laterally. An alternative technique involves suture placement from the muscular process of the arytenoid cartilage to the caudodorsal aspect of the thyroid cartilage. This pulls the arytenoid cartilage laterally rather than rotating it and increases the area of the rima glottis to a lesser degree than the cricoarytenoid suture (Griffiths, Sullivan, and Reid, 2001). However, differences in techniques do not appear to affect postoperative outcome.

Partial laryngectomy consists of various techniques for vocal cord excision and partial arytenoidectomy to increase the diameter of the glottis. Partial laryngectomy has been associated with various complications, including laryngeal webbing, laryngeal scarring, and aspiration pneumonia. Complication rates as high as 58% have been reported (Harvey and O'Brien, 1982). However, bilateral vocal fold resection alone resulted in fewer complications and better postoperative outcome than other partial laryngectomy techniques (Holt and Harvey, 1994). This is thought to be to the result of better laryngeal protection during swallowing and decreased laryngeal irritation by leaving the corniculate processes of the arytenoid cartilages intact.

Prognosis

Postoperative aspiration pneumonia has been reported in 8% to 19% of dogs (MacPhail and Monnet, 2001; Snelling and Edwards, 2003; Hamonel, Hottinger, and Novo, 2006). Although aspiration pneumonia occurs most likely in the first few weeks following surgery, it has been recognized that these dogs are at risk for aspiration pneumonia for the rest of their lives. Factors that have been significantly associated with a higher risk of developing complications include preoperative aspiration pneumonia, postoperative megaesophagus, temporary tracheostomy placement, and concurrent neoplastic disease. Without surgical complications, unilateral arytenoid lateralization results in less respiratory distress and stridor and improved exercise tolerance. Owner satisfaction with this procedure has been reported as excellent, with the majority of owners believing that the quality of their dog's life was dramatically improved.

Laryngeal Paralysis in Cats

Laryngeal paralysis is an uncommon condition in the cat. Clinical presentation is similar to that of the dog, and both unilateral and bilateral laryngeal paralysis have been reported. Cats with unilateral laryngeal paralysis can present with significant clinical signs, unlike dogs that are rarely symptomatic. There also appears to be a prevalence of left-sided unilateral laryngeal paralysis in cats, which is similar to that reported in humans and horses. The specific etiology of laryngeal paralysis in cats is unknown, but several cases have been associated with trauma, neoplastic invasion, and iatrogenic damage. Neoplastic infiltration can lead to fixed laryngeal obstruction with both inspiratory and expiratory dyspnea and noise. Successful surgical treatment primarily using unilateral arytenoid lateralization has been reported (Scharchter and Norris, 2000).

LARYNGEAL COLLAPSE

Etiology

Laryngeal collapse is a secondary component of brachycephalic airway syndrome (see Chapter 141). Brachycephalic airway syndrome refers to the condition of airway distress attributable to anatomic abnormalities of breeds such as English bulldog and Boston terrier. Chronic upper airway obstruction from the primary components of brachycephalic airway syndrome (stenotic nares, elongated soft palate) causes increased airway resistance and increased negative intraglottic luminal pressure. Over time this results in laryngeal collapse because of cartilage fatigue and degeneration. There are three stages of severity of laryngeal collapse. Stage 1 is the eversion of the laryngeal saccules into the glottis. The increased inspiratory effort creates a vacuum causing the mucosa of the laryngeal saccules to prolapse. In a retrospective study of dogs with brachycephalic airway syndrome, everted laryngeal saccules were present in almost 50% of affected dogs (Lorison, Bright, and White, 1997). The saccules are pulled from their crypts because of the high negative pressure within the glottis. Once the saccules are everted, the tissue is exposed to highly turbulent airflow, resulting in edema and inflammation, which further obstructs the airway. During stage 2 the cuneiform processes of the arytenoid cartilages lose rigidity and collapse into the laryngeal lumen. In addition, the aryepiglottic folds also collapse ventromedially. The most advanced phase of laryngeal collapse is stage 3 in which the corniculate process of each arytenoid cartilage fatigues and then collapses toward midline, resulting in complete laryngeal collapse.

Treatment

The early stage of laryngeal collapse is still amenable to surgical treatment. Resection of the everted laryngeal saccules is relatively simple. Each saccule is grasped with Allis tissue forceps and then sharply transected with Metzenbaum scissors. Suturing is not necessary. The difficulty of this technique lies is obtaining good visualization of the larynx and glottis. Often these dogs have redundant pharyngeal tissue that swells rapidly with minimal handling. The presence of an endotracheal tube can also make visualization difficult. It is for these reasons that some surgeons advocate using a temporary tracheostomy tube when performing this surgery. Stenotic nares and elongated soft palate should also be addressed if they have not been addressed previously.

Options for treatment of advance stages of laryngeal collapse are limited. First, all other underlying conditions (stenotic nares, elongated soft palate, everted laryngeal saccules) are addressed. Unilateral arytenoid lateralization techniques are rarely successful since the opposite cartilage continues to collapse medially. Bilateral arytenoid lateralization techniques are considered unacceptable because of the high risk for aspiration pneumonia. Partial arytenoidectomy procedures have also been associated with a high rate of complications and perioperative mortality. Permanent tracheostomy is the recommended treatment for stage 3 laryngeal collapse, although many owners consider this an unacceptable option.

The most common way to perform permanent tracheostomy is to create a window in the ventral trachea encompassing 3 to 5 tracheal rings longitudinally and one third of the diameter transversely. Tracheal collapse can occur if the created stoma is too large. Ideally only the tracheal rings are removed, leaving the mucosa intact. An I-shaped incision is then made in the mucosa, and the edges are sutured directly to the skin using small monofilament nonabsorbable sutures in a simple interrupted pattern. To minimize tension on the newly created stoma, some surgeons prefer to bring the trachea to a more superficial position by suturing the sternohyoideus muscles together dorsal to the trachea for the length of the proposed stoma.

The most significant complication associated with permanent tracheostomy comes from accumulation of mucus and secretions that may obstruct the trachea or stoma. Animals must be observed extremely closely in the first few days following surgery. Other complications include stricture of the stoma or occlusion of the stoma by excessive skinfolds. (See Chapter 141 for additional discussion of laryngeal collapse.)

LARYNGEAL MASSES

Neoplasia

Tumors of the larynx are uncommon in the dog and cat. Numerous types of tumor have been reported in the dog, including rhabdomyosarcoma, squamous cell carcinoma, adenocarcinoma, and mast cell tumor. Inflammatory nodules, especially involving the vocal folds, should be considered in the differential diagnosis. Squamous cell carcinoma and lymphoma are the most common tumors of the larynx in the cat.

Small lesions may be resected by partial laryngectomy. Aggressive surgical intervention involves complete laryngectomy with permanent tracheostomy but has only been reported in one dog. Radioresponsive tumors may be treated with radiation therapy. Otherwise most treatment is palliative, consisting of airflow bypass of the laryngeal area through permanent tracheostomy. Prognosis for laryngeal tumors is guarded because most cases are quite advanced at the time of diagnosis. There are only isolated reports of management of canine and feline laryngeal tumors (Jakubiak et al., 2005). Treatment of four cats with laryngeal squamous cell carcinoma with tube tracheostomy alone resulted in a median survival of only 3 days. Chemotherapeutic treatment of five cats with laryngeal masses resulted in a median survival of 141 days.

A recent study reported the placement of permanent tracheostomies in five cats with laryngeal carcinoma (Guenther-Yenke and Rozanski, 2007). Survival at home ranged from 2 to 281 days with two cats dying from tracheostomy site occlusion and three cats euthanized due to disease progression.

Benign Growths

Granulomatous laryngitis is an uncommon nonneoplastic proliferation of the arytenoid cartilages of the larynx that has been reported in both dogs and cats. Severe cases can result in laryngeal stenosis and significant upper airway obstruction. Mass biopsy is crucial to differentiate this disease from neoplasia. Treatment is palliative and consists of debulking of the mass, steroid therapy, or permanent tracheostomy.

Benign laryngeal cysts have also been described in isolated feline cases. Cysts are typically epithelial in origin and stem from the ventral aspect of the larynx. Surgical removal is usually curative. Some cysts are very large and can significantly obstruct airflow.

References and Suggested Reading

Griffiths LG, Sullivan M, Reid SW: A comparison of the effects of unilateral thyroarytenoid lateralization versus cricoarytenoid laryngoplasty on the area of the rima glottides and clinical outcome in dogs with laryngeal paralysis, *Vet Surg* 30:359, 2001.

Gross ME et al: A comparison of thiopental, propofol, and diazepam-ketamine anesthesia for evaluation of laryngeal function in dogs premedicated with butorphanol-glycopyrrolate, *J Am Anim Hosp Assoc* 38:503, 2002.

Guenther-Yenk CL, Rozanski EA: Tracheostomy in cats: 23 cases (1998-2006), *J Fel Med Surg* 9:451, 2007.

Hammel SP, Hottinger HA, Novo RE: Postoperative results of unilateral arytenoid lateralization for treatment of idiopathic laryngeal paralysis in dogs: 39 cases (1996-2002), *J Am Vet Med Assoc* 228:1215, 2006.

Harvey CE, O'Brien JA: Treatment of laryngeal paralysis in dogs by partial laryngectomy, *J Am Anim Hosp Assoc* 18:551, 1982.

Holt D, Harvey C: Idiopathic laryngeal paralysis: results of treatment by bilateral vocal fold resection in 40 dogs, *J Am Anim Hosp Assoc* 20:389, 1994.

Jackson AM et al: Effect of various anesthetic agents on laryngeal motion during laryngoscopy in normal dogs, *Vet Surg* 33:102, 2004.

Jakubiak MJ et al: Laryngeal, laryngotracheal, and tracheal masses in cats: 27 cats (1998-2003), *J Am Anim Hosp Assoc* 41:310, 2005.

Lorison D, Bright RM, White RAS: Brachycephalic airway obstruction syndrome—a review of 119 cases, *Canine Pract* 22:18, 1997.

MacPhail CM, Monnet E: Outcome of and postoperative complications in dogs undergoing surgical treatment of laryngeal paralysis: 140 cases (1985-1998), *J Am Vet Med Assoc* 218:1949, 2001.

Miller CJ et al: The effects of doxapram hydrochloride (Dopram-V) on laryngeal function in healthy dogs, *J Vet Intern Med* 16:524, 2002.

Radlinsky MG, Mason DE, Hodgson D: Transnasal laryngoscopy for the diagnosis of laryngeal paralysis in dogs, *J Am Anim Hosp Assoc* 40:211, 2004.

Scharchter S, Norris CR: Laryngeal paralysis in cats: 16 cases (1990-1999), *J Am Vet Med Assoc* 216:1100, 2000.

Snelling SR, Edwards GA: A retrospective study of unilateral arytenoids lateralization in the treatment of laryngeal paralysis in 100 dogs (1992-2000), *Aust Vet J* 81:464, 2003.

Tobias KM, Jackson AM, Harvey RC: Effect of doxapram HCl on laryngeal function of normal dogs and dogs with naturally occurring laryngeal paralysis, *Vet Anaesth Analg* 31:258, 2004.

CHAPTER 144

Medical Management of Tracheal Collapse*

MICHAEL E. HERRTAGE, *Cambridge, United Kingdom*

Tracheal collapse is a syndrome characterized by dorsoventral flattening of the tracheal rings with laxity of the dorsal tracheal membrane. The syndrome is associated with clinical signs of cough and varying degrees of dyspnea and is most frequently encountered in middle-aged to old toy or miniature dogs. Considerable controversy surrounds the precise cause of the syndrome; consequently there is still little agreement concerning the most effective approach to its management. Much attention has been focused on refining methods for surgical reconstruction of the collapsed trachea, but it is by no means clear that all cases require or benefit from surgery.

Recently tracheal stenting has been advocated as a therapeutic procedure for tracheal collapse (see Chapter 145). A clearer understanding of the cause of the syndrome and the role played by the secondary factors that initiate the symptomatic state are probably the most urgent goals for future research.

ETIOLOGY

The cause of tracheal collapse is complex; it is best regarded as a syndrome with multifactorial causes, many of which are incompletely understood. The development of the clinical condition appears to require the presence of both a primary cartilage abnormality, resulting in weakness of the tracheal rings, and secondary factors capable of initiating progression to the symptomatic state.

---

*This chapter was originally published in *Current Veterinary Therapy XIII* and has been updated for this edition. The original chapter was co-authored by Richard A.S. White, FRCVS.

A reduction in the glycoprotein and glycosaminoglycan content of the hyaline cartilage of the tracheal rings is considered the primary defect responsible for the intrinsic weakness of the tracheal rings. This, together with other pathologic changes in the matrix, is responsible for reducing the capacity of the cartilage to retain water, consequently diminishing its functional rigidity (Dallman, McClure, and Brown, 1985). The evidence to suggest that these underlying abnormalities of the matrix have a congenital origin is compelling. Both the onset of clinical signs during puppyhood in some dogs and the presence of clinical signs in most symptomatic dogs long before middle age, when the disease is classically recognized, support this concept. Therefore it seems likely that affected dogs begin life with an abnormal trachea; and, conversely, dogs with normal tracheas are rarely susceptible to the disease.

Many toy and miniature dogs with the anatomic tendency to tracheal collapse can remain asymptomatic throughout life unless secondary or inciting factors initiate the clinical syndrome. These potential factors may include obesity, recent endotracheal intubation, respiratory infection, cardiomegaly, cervical trauma, and inhalation of irritants or allergens (Fig. 144-1). The precise role of upper airway obstruction in the etiology of the syndrome remains unclear. The presence of laryngeal paralysis or collapse in some affected dogs has led to the view that these conditions can precipitate the tracheal changes. Conversely, chronic obstructive disease of the lower airway is capable of promoting dynamic upper airway collapse; thus the interrelation of both conditions remains controversial.

The dynamic changes of tracheal collapse may be confined to either the cervical or thoracic region of the trachea or may involve the entire length. Frequently the changes are most pronounced at the cervicothoracic junction. Collapse of the cervical tracheal segment occurs on inspiration because of the decreased pressure within the trachea, whereas the thoracic portion tends to collapse during the expiratory phase of respiration or during coughing as a consequence of increased intrathoracic pressure. In severely affected dogs these changes may also be detected more distally in the principal or proximal lobar bronchi. As a consequence of the flattened configuration of the tracheal rings, the dorsal membrane becomes widened, pendulous, and flaccid. The dorsal membrane contributes to the dynamic obstruction of the airway as it is drawn into the tracheal lumen during the respiratory cycle.

Once clinical signs are apparent, the syndrome is perpetuated by the cycle of chronic inflammation of the tracheal mucosa, which precipitates cough and in turn is exacerbated by the cough. Persistent inflammation of the tracheal mucosa leads to a loss of epithelium, fibrinous membrane formation, and squamous metaplasia with polypoid proliferation evident in advanced cases. The population of ciliated cells is reduced significantly by the metaplastic changes in the mucosa, and the hyperplastic subepithelial glands secrete increasingly viscid mucus. As a consequence, normal ciliary function is replaced progressively by cough as the major tracheobronchial clearing mechanism. Once the condition becomes symptomatic, the changes in the dorsal membrane and cartilage are believed to progress beyond those of the original anatomic abnormality; however, it has been difficult to document these worsening changes in individual cases.

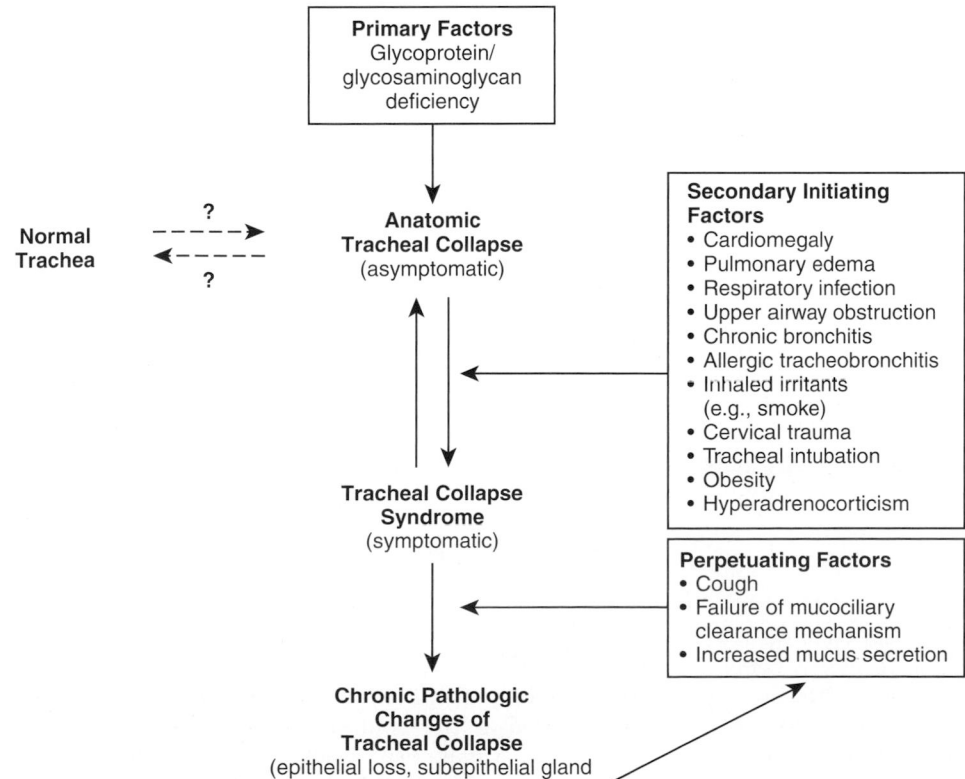

Fig. 144-1 Interrelation of probable factors involved in the etiology of tracheal collapse.

INCIDENCE

Tracheal collapse is confined almost exclusively to toy and miniature breeds and is only sporadically encountered in medium- to large-breed dogs. The Yorkshire terrier is the most commonly affected breed, but other commonly affected breeds include the miniature poodle, Chihuahua, and Pomeranian. Typically the patient is presented for evaluation at 6 to7 years of age, although careful investigation usually reveals that signs referable to the condition have been present for some years before presentation. Approximately 25% of affected dogs are symptomatic by the age of 6 months. The syndrome is equally distributed between the sexes.

CLINICAL SIGNS

Tracheal collapse syndrome is characterized by a chronic, paroxysmal cough precipitated by excitement, anxiety, or pulling on the leash. The cough is typically harsh, dry, and nonproductive and is easily elicited on tracheal palpation. A "goose honk" cough is a frequent but not consistent finding. Affected dogs may be otherwise asymptomatic and are often able to sustain prolonged periods of exercise without any clinical signs. However, more severely affected dogs may show varying degrees of tachypnea or even respiratory distress as a result of the severity of airway obstruction. Cyanosis or syncope from hypoxemia may be noted in advanced cases. The severity of clinical signs does not relate directly to the severity of the anatomic changes, and classification systems describing the degree of tracheal collapse are of limited help in this respect.

On physical examination turbulent air flow may be detected on auscultation directly over the cervical trachea, whereas referred musical or wheezing sounds may be heard on thoracic auscultation. The lung sounds in tracheal collapse may be normal or accentuated; however, in many cases bronchovesicular sounds are obliterated by referred sounds from the trachea. In dogs with tracheal collapse the heart rate is usually normal or slow at rest with pronounced sinus arrhythmia, whereas dogs with left ventricular heart failure often lose sinus arrhythmia because of increased sympathetic tone, and the heart rate is often increased. The cough in left ventricular heart failure is typically soft, moist, and mildly productive compared with the harsh, dry cough of tracheal collapse; however, left atrial enlargement can also cause left bronchial compression, which can mimic signs of tracheal collapse. Some dogs with tracheal collapse acquire pulmonary hypertension, which may result in a prominent or split second heart sound.

DIAGNOSIS

Confirmation of the diagnosis of tracheal collapse syndrome requires the combination of a persistent cough, a response to tracheal palpation, and demonstration of intratracheal changes, preferably by endoscopy. The dynamic dysfunction of the trachea can be demonstrated by a variety of diagnostic methods, including palpation, radiography, ultrasonography, or tracheoscopy.

Physical Examination

Collapse of the cervical portion of the trachea is usually readily appreciated on physical examination by careful palpation. The tendency of the dorsal membrane to invert into the tracheal lumen can be appreciated by gentle digital pressure once the trachea has been rolled laterally. More significantly, in affected dogs this maneuver usually initiates a cough.

Radiographic Examination

Radiography can be useful in demonstrating dynamic tracheal collapse during the different phases of the respiratory cycle. The most useful radiographic examinations include lateral projections of the thoracic inlet exposed during the inspiratory and expiratory phases, a tangential rostrocaudal (skyline) projection of the thoracic inlet, and fluoroscopic investigation to demonstrate movement of the dorsal membrane during the respiratory cycle. Luminal narrowing of the cervical trachea is seen on the lateral projection during inspiration, whereas ballooning of the same segment may be seen on expiration. These changes may be visible during expiration for the thoracic segment. These dynamic changes, including "fluttering" of the dorsal membrane during the respiratory cycle, are best viewed in real time using image-intensified fluoroscopy since radiographs tend to underestimate the frequency and degree of tracheal collapse (Macready et al., 2007). In the skyline projection the flattened trachea is seen as an oval, C, or crescent shape. In severe cases the cross section of the trachea at the thoracic inlet may be narrowed to a slitlike opening. Coughing in such cases may create the appearance of a highly redundant segment of trachea at the thoracic inlet. It should be emphasized that radiography may not highlight the dynamic changes of collapse in all cases.

Ultrasonography

Like fluoroscopy, ultrasonography provides real-time imaging that can be used to demonstrate dynamic changes in the tracheal profile. The technique has the distinct advantages of being noninvasive and safe and can be performed on minimally sedated or unsedated animals (Rudorf, Herrtage, and White, 1997). A high-frequency transducer with a standoff is required for imaging of the larynx and trachea. The transducer is positioned ventrally over the trachea just caudal to the cricoid cartilage; with the neck in a neutral position, a transverse scan is made of the air shadow between the cricoid and first tracheal ring. Beginning from this point, the transducer is moved caudally, imaging the profile of the tracheal air shadow during the phases of the respiratory cycle and during hyperextension of the neck. Interpretation requires some experience.

Endoscopy

Tracheoscopic examination of the tracheal lumen should be regarded as the gold standard for the purposes of completing a diagnosis. Tracheoscopy is useful to confirm not only the presence of the anatomic abnormality but also changes in the dorsal membrane along its entire length. The ventrodorsal movement of the dorsal membrane during the respiratory cycle can be appreciated in lightly anesthetized dogs. In some dogs with severe obstruction there may be an increased anesthesia risk, but this rarely proves to be a problem.

Microbiologic and Cytologic Studies

Tracheoscopy also permits the recovery of bacteriologic and cytologic samples from the lower respiratory system. Samples should be cultured for bacterial isolation and sensitivity, and cytologic studies should be performed to identify any cellular changes suggestive of an inhaled allergic or inflammatory airway response (see Chapter 146).

Other Tests

The identification of specific allergens or irritants often is not practical, although removal of the dog from cigarette smoke in the environment for a test period is often useful in investigating this as a common initiating cause.

Significant hepatic dysfunction is identified in many dogs with tracheal collapse (Bowes et al., 2006). Therefore liver function testing should be performed in cases of tracheal collapse, especially those with severe respiratory signs.

THERAPY

The clinician must be prepared to pursue several therapeutic avenues in the management of the individual dog to deal with the complex and multifactorial etiology of the syndrome (White and Williams, 1994). Since anatomic collapse alone does not guarantee a symptomatic state, every effort should be made to identify and correct any secondary causes. Successful long-term medical management is possible for the majority of patients provided the initiating factor or factors can be identified. This route should always be thoroughly investigated before a surgical solution is considered.

The Acute Case

The dog presenting in acute respiratory distress should be regarded as a medical emergency, and all diagnostic tests should be postponed until the dog has been stabilized. The dog should be sedated as required and subjected to as little stress as possible. Acepromazine (ProMACE, Fort Dodge) at a dose of 0.02 to 0.2 mg/kg intravenously, intramuscularly, or subcutaneously is generally effective. Oxygen therapy administered via a face mask may be the most practical means of improving the patient's oxygen status initially, but nasal intubation often causes the patient less anxiety for long-term management. We have used tracheostomy intubation as a temporary means of establishing an airway in hyperexcited dogs with severe obstruction with seemingly few long-term complications. In some dogs the tachypnea may promote hyperthermia, exacerbating the dyspnea. The dog should be kept in a cool environment or ice packs applied in severe cases to counter this problem. Short-acting glucocorticoids (e.g., dexamethasone sodium phosphate [Azium SP, Schering-Plough]) given once at a dose of 1 mg/kg intravenously

may be helpful for dogs with laryngeal edema or tracheal inflammation. Opioid agonist-antagonists such as butorphanol (Torbutrol, Fort Dodge) at a dosage of 0.05 to 0.11 mg/kg every 6 to 12 hours intravenously, intramuscularly, or subcutaneously or buprenorphine hydrochloride (Buprenex, Reckitt and Colman) at a dosage of 0.01 to 0.02 mg/kg every 12 hours intramuscularly are useful mild cough suppressants that cause little respiratory depression. When either of these drugs is combined with acepromazine, the resultant sedation can be significant.

Management of Secondary Initiating Causes

Weight Reduction
Many dogs with tracheal collapse are obese, and their intrathoracic adipose deposits may interfere with respiratory excursion, causing a reduction in thoracic wall compliance. Weight reduction should be pursued aggressively in all overweight patients to improve respiratory function; the clinical response can be dramatic in some cases. The daily caloric intake should be based on a high-fiber, low-calorie diet and restricted to 60% of the total daily requirement based on a lean body mass. Exercise restriction may limit the rate of weight loss. The veterinarian should monitor progress and encourage owner compliance with the regimen.

Congestive Heart Failure
Heart failure with pulmonary edema may initiate or exacerbate the clinical signs of tracheal collapse by increasing the volume of tracheobronchial secretions. In addition, the cough may be promoted by pressure of the enlarged left atrium on the left main-stem bronchus. Reduction of preload by diuresis and the use of angiotensin-converting enzyme inhibitors reduce pulmonary edema. Digitalization or administration of pimobendan may also be effective in suppressing the cough associated with congestive heart failure (see Chapter 171).

Inhaled Irritants
In some dogs the clinical syndrome of collapse may be precipitated by the inhalation of irritants or allergens. The removal of cigarette smoke from the dog's environment is an essential, although often difficult, part of the management regimen. The recognition and removal of other inhaled allergens is less straightforward but may prove beneficial in some dogs.

Respiratory Infections
Infections of the lower respiratory tract should be treated by appropriate antibacterial therapy optimally based on the results of bacterial culture from bronchoalveolar lavage. Treatment should be continued for a minimum of 14 days and in selected cases may need to be continued for prolonged periods for the control of deep-seated chronic infection. When antimicrobial therapy is initiated empirically, without microbiologic or cytologic confirmation of infection, doxycycline, cephalexin, or amoxicillin-clavulanate are common antibiotic choices.

Collars
The use of collars, particularly of a sliding chain design, should be discouraged because repeated external pressure

on the trachea may initiate mucosal irritation and promote coughing. Body harnesses are an alternative, although these may still pose some risk.

Management of the Coughing Animal

Antitussive Agents

Cough suppressants are recommended to reduce chronic irritation or damage to the tracheal epithelium caused by collapse of the dorsal membrane and to reduce shearing forces within the lung associated with chronic coughing. A variety of drugs are available, but we have had greatest success using co-phenotrope (Lomotil, Searle), which contains diphenoxylate hydrochloride and atropine.* The diphenoxylate acts as a narcotic antitussive agent, and the atropine reduces the volume of mucus secreted into the lower respiratory tract and also acts as an antimuscarinic bronchodilator. The recommended dosage of co-phenotrope is 0.2 to 0.5 mg of diphenoxylate per kilogram orally every 12 hours; this dosage can be maintained for extended periods until clinical signs subside. Constipation is an occasional problem but usually can be controlled by adding a stool softener to the diet. Other narcotic antitussive agents such as hydrocodone (Russigan, Daniels Pharmaceuticals; 0.22 mg/kg orally [PO] every 6 to 12 hours), codeine phosphate (Bronlex, Procter and Gamble Pharmaceuticals; 0.5 to 2.0 mg/kg PO every 12 hours) or butorphanol (Torbutrol, Fort Dodge; 0.5 to 1 mg/kg PO every 6 to 12 hours) may be used but are generally less effective than co-phenotrope.

Bronchodilators

The use of bronchodilators in the management of tracheal collapse is regarded as controversial by some authors. The rationale for their use is based on the dilation of pulmonary airways, which decreases intrathoracic pressure during expiration, thereby decreasing the tendency to tracheal narrowing during expiration. Use of bronchodilators is particularly important for patients with coexisting small airway disease with increased intrathoracic pressure on expiration and thus a greater tendency to tracheal collapse. Methylxanthine bronchodilators (theophylline) may be beneficial in achieving bronchodilation, improving mucociliary clearance, and reducing diaphragmatic fatigue in dogs with tracheal collapse. The preparations most commonly used include sustained-release theophylline (Theo-dur, Key Pharmaceuticals) at a dosage of 10 to 20 mg/kg orally every 12 hours and theophylline ethylenediamine (aminophylline, Roxane and Alpharma) at a dosage of 8 to 10 mg/kg orally every 8 hours. Older dogs often demonstrate apparent anxiety and restlessness when full doses of theophylline are administered, and clients should be warned to report any adverse drug effects.

β_2-Adrenergic agonists also can be used for bronchodilation. Terbutaline (Brethine, Ciba Geneva; 1.25 to 5 mg/

dog PO every 8 to 12 hours) and albuterol (Proventil, Schering; Ventolin, Glaxo-Wellcome; 50 mcg/kg PO every 8 hours) have been recommended for use in dogs. Signs of β-agonist toxicity include hypotension and tachycardia, and these could be reduced by inhalation administration. Care should be taken when using these drugs in dogs with congestive heart failure.

Glucocorticoids

Glucocorticoids should be used judiciously in the management of tracheal collapse. Drugs in this class may be beneficial in reducing laryngeal, tracheal, or bronchial inflammation but should be used for short periods only because their extended use may exacerbate bacterial infections, promote tachypnea, or cause iatrogenic hyperadrenocorticism. Glucocorticoids also promote weight gain and may make weight reduction difficult to achieve. Prednisolone (Prednistab, Vedco) may be used initially at a dosage of 0.5 mg/kg orally every 12 hours. Since the benefits of glucocorticoids are normally apparent within 7 to 10 days, the dosage should be tapered and withdrawn within this period. Inhaled corticosteroids may be used to reduce side effects of glucocorticoid administration (Bexfield et al., 2006).

Surgical Management

Surgical or device management of tracheal collapse is appropriate for dogs that remain persistently symptomatic despite vigorous medical management and attempts to eradicate all potential initiating factors. Candidates for reconstruction of the trachea should be selected carefully and should be free of other medical complications, including congestive heart failure and collapse of the lower airway, because these dogs rarely improve with surgical intervention.

A variety of surgical techniques have been described for the management of tracheal collapse. Most of these techniques, including tracheal ring chondrotomy, plication of the dorsal membrane, prosthetic mesh support, and intraluminal prosthetic supports, have little foundation in success and are no longer considered to be practical. Placement of external prosthetic supports currently is the preferred technique for surgical management of tracheal collapse, and both ring (Hobson, 1976) and spiral (Fingland, DeHoff, and Birchard, 1986) prostheses manufactured from polypropylene are used. Most authors suggest reconstruction of the cervical and, when affected, the thoracic segment. However, the results of surgical management of the thoracic portion of the trachea are frequently unrewarding because of the high morbidity associated with this procedure. A number of complications have been associated with implantation of prosthetic tracheal supports, including loosening or failure of the implant, infection, laryngeal paralysis, and tracheal necrosis. Isolation of the tracheal blood supply to accommodate the application of prostheses has been demonstrated to result in significant impairment of the tracheal blood flow, risking necrosis (Kirby et al., 1991). However, a modified dissection of the lateral pedicles permits preservation of the vascular supply to one side of the trachea and avoids serious ischemic complications (Coyne et al., 1993). Arytenoid lateralization at the time of surgical reconstruction of the trachea may improve

---

*Co-phenotrope (diphenoxylate hydrochloride with atropine) is not in widespread use as an antitussive agent in the United States, and no clinical trials demonstrating its efficacy and safety for this indication have been published. The potential adverse effects of atropine on the viscosity of airway secretions warrant further investigation.

the results of surgery (White, 1995). The prognosis for older dogs (>6 years of age at the time of surgery) is significantly worse than that for younger dogs, even though the degree of tracheal collapse, as assessed by tracheoscopy, may be less severe (Buback, Boothe, and Hobson, 1996). As emphasized previously, the severity of the grade of collapse does not appear to have any prognostic significance.

More recently intraluminal stent implantation has been used to treat dogs with severe tracheal collapse; this technique and its complications are discussed in Chapter 145.

References and Suggested Reading

Bauer NB et al: Liver disease in dogs with tracheal collapse, *J Vet Intern Med* 20:845, 2006.

Bexfield NH et al: Management of 13 cases of canine aspiratory disease using inhaled corticosteroids, *J Small Anim Pract* 47:377, 2006.

Buback JL, Boothe HW, Hobson P: Surgical treatment of tracheal collapse in dogs: 90 cases (1983-1993), *J Am Vet Med Assoc* 208:380, 1996.

Coyne BE et al: Clinical and pathologic effects of a modified technique for application of spiral prostheses to the cervical trachea of dogs, *Vet Surg* 22:269, 1993.

Dallman MJ, McClure RC, Brown EM: Normal and collapsed trachea in the dog: scanning electron microscopy study, *Am J Vet Res* 46:2110, 1985.

Fingland RB, DeHoff WD, Birchard SJ: Surgical management of cervical and thoracic tracheal collapse in dogs using extraluminal spiral prostheses: results in seven cases, *J Am Anim Hosp Assoc* 23:173, 1986.

Hobson HP: Total ring prosthesis for the surgical correction of collapsed trachea, *J Am Anim Hosp Assoc* 12:822, 1976.

Kirby BM et al: The effects of surgical isolation and application of polypropylene spiral prostheses on tracheal blood flow, *Vet Surg* 20:49, 1991.

Macready DM, Johnson LR, Pollard RE: Fluoroscopic and radiographic evaluation of tracheal collapse in dogs: 62 cases (2001-2006), *J Am Vet Med Assoc* 230:1870, 2007.

Rudorf H, Herrtage ME, White RAS: The use of ultrasonography in the diagnosis of tracheal collapse, *J Small Anim Pract* 38:513, 1997.

White RAS, Williams JM: Tracheal collapse in the dog—is there really a role for surgery? A retrospective study of 100 cases, *J Small Anim Pract* 35:191, 1994.

White RN: Unilateral arytenoid lateralization and extraluminal polypropylene ring prostheses for correction of tracheal collapse in the dog, *J Small Anim Pract* 36:151, 1995.

CHAPTER **145**

Intraluminal Stenting for Tracheal Collapse

CHICK W.C. WEISSE, *Philadelphia, Pennsylvania*

Tracheal collapse is a progressive degenerative disease of the cartilage rings in which hypocellularity and decreased glycosaminoglycan and calcium contents lead to dynamic airway collapse during respiration. This is a condition of predominantly small- and toy-breed dogs that can present with signs ranging from a mild, intermittent "honking" cough to severe respiratory distress from dynamic upper-airway obstruction. Although more commonly seen in older patients, dogs of all ages can be affected. Many of these patients are palliated first by conservative therapies, including general management strategies and medications (see Chapter 144). Weight loss, restricted exercise, and removal of second-hand smoke or inhaled allergens can reduce clinical signs. In addition, management of comorbidities such as cardiac disease or bronchopulmonary disease can help reduce the frequency of respiratory crisis episodes. These conditions, especially chronic bronchitis (see Chapter 146), should be sought and managed. Conservative treatment combinations used in dogs with tracheal collapse include antiinflammatory drugs, antitussives, sedatives/tranquilizers, or bronchodilators. These therapies, which are discussed in the previous chapter, may reduce the respiratory signs associated with tracheal collapse. The dog that has been evaluated comprehensively for other causes of cough and has failed aggressive conservative management for tracheal collapse is a candidate for surgical or interventional treatment.

The most commonly performed surgical treatment for patients with extrathoracic tracheal collapse is extraluminal polypropylene ring prostheses. This technique involves placing extraluminal support rings around the trachea during an open cervical approach and has a reported 75% to 85% overall success rate for reducing clinical signs in one report of 90 dogs (Buback, Boothe, and Hobson, 1996). However, this procedure is not without complications since 5% of animals died perioperatively, 11% developed laryngeal paralysis from the surgery, 19% required permanent tracheostomies (half within 24 hours), and ≈23% died of respiratory problems with a median survival of 25 months. In addition, only 11% of the dogs in this study had intrathoracic tracheal collapse (all dogs had extrathoracic tracheal collapse). The authors advised against this technique in patients with intrathoracic tracheal collapse because the resulting morbidity was unacceptably high.

The combination of surgical risk and the inability to adequately treat intrathoracic collapse led to the evaluation of human-intended, intraluminal tracheal stents for dogs with tracheal collapse. A number of stents have previously been evaluated in the canine trachea, including both balloon-expandable (Palmaz), and self-expanding (stainless steel, laser-cut nitinol, knitted nitinol) stents (Radlinsky et al., 1997; Norris et al., 2000; Moritz, Schneider, and Bauer, 2004). Clinical improvement rates in 75% to 90% of dogs treated with intraluminal, stainless steel, self-expanding metallic stents (SEMSs) have been reported (Norris et al., 2000; Moritz, Schneider, and Bauer, 2004). Immediate complications typically were minor, although there was a perioperative mortality rate of approximately 10%. Late complications included stent shortening, excessive granulation tissue formation, progressive tracheal collapse, and stent fracture. Some of these can be severe or life-threatening.

Neither surgery nor stenting is a cure for tracheal collapse. However, when used appropriately in the proper patient, both can improve the patient's quality of life significantly when medication alone is no longer adequate. My criteria for patient selection, method of stent selection, and technique for placing intraluminal tracheal stents follow.

PATIENT SELECTION AND EVALUATION

The diagnosis of tracheal collapse and other forms of respiratory dysfunction is beyond the scope of this chapter, but important rule-outs for chronic or recurrent coughing include chronic bronchitis, pneumonia, congestive heart failure, heartworm disease, and pulmonary neoplasia. Since comorbid disorders can complicate or even dominate the signs related to tracheal collapse, other primary or secondary respiratory disorders must be considered and managed before more invasive therapies for tracheal collapse. Animals with concurrent cardiac or bronchopulmonary disease can often benefit substantially from medical treatment such that invasive tracheal collapse treatments can be avoided or postponed.

Whether considering surgical rings or intraluminal stenting, it is important that aggressive medical management has been attempted and failed at providing a reasonable quality of life for the patient (see previous chapter). Although it is a subjective criterion, the veterinarian and owners must carefully evaluate the patient's status and agree when the time for more aggressive therapy is indicated. An exception to this rule is the emergent, intubated patient that has failed a number of attempts at extubation. It should be emphasized that an owner's inability to administer medication is not a valid reason to perform any invasive procedure for tracheal collapse since the majority of dogs will still require long-term medication.

RINGS OR STENT?

The decision to perform surgery versus stenting is complicated, and the best approach is still unresolved. Decisions must be made on an individual basis, but some guidelines can be advanced. In my opinion, if significant *intrathoracic* tracheal collapse is present, surgery is either unlikely to resolve the problem or will be associated with unacceptable morbidity; therefore an intraluminal stent should be considered in these cases. If only cervical tracheal collapse is present, surgical rings should be considered. An exception may be in a geriatric patient or one with cardiorespiratory or endocrine comorbidities that might make prolonged anesthesia or wound healing more of a concern.

The patient with extensive intrathoracic and extrathoracic tracheal collapse presents an even more complicated scenario. It can be argued that an intraluminal stent for the intrathoracic collapse and surgical rings for cervical collapse might avoid some of the complications associated with very long tracheal stents; however, the alternative view is that this approach would combine the potential complications associated with both procedures. In these cases I am currently placing a single long stent to span both the intrathoracic and extrathoracic trachea.

MAIN-STEM BRONCHIAL COLLAPSE

Much debate remains concerning the use of intraluminal stents in patients with main-stem bronchial collapse. Unfortunately no data are available to recommend or oppose the routine use of intraluminal stents in these patients; therefore one can only offer a personal opinion. The questions raised are twofold.

First, should stents be placed *within* collapsing main-stem bronchi? Currently I do not recommend stenting of collapsing main-stem bronchi routinely. Placing stents in main-stem bronchi will "cage-off" other bronchi and consequently prevent drainage from the associated lobes. In addition, secondary and tertiary bronchi will continue to collapse; therefore the benefit achieved from the bronchial stenting will likely be minimal and temporary when compared to the risks.

Second, should tracheal stents be placed in patients with main-stem bronchial collapse? Certain patients benefit from tracheal stenting, even with concurrent main-stem bronchial collapse. The patient should be carefully evaluated by fluoroscopy and endoscopy to determine the primary disorder. Tracheal collapse can lead to dyspnea, persistent cough, or both. If dyspnea is the major clinical sign and intrathoracic tracheal collapse is present, a tracheal stent can help relieve the dynamic obstruction. If the patient's primary problem is coughing, it becomes difficult to determine if the coughing is the result of the tracheal collapse, bronchial collapse, or another problem such as chronic bronchitis. In these patients I always warn the owner that continued coughing will likely be present after stenting because the main-stem bronchial collapse (as well as collapse of the smaller bronchi) will continue. In addition, in my experience continued, intractable coughing causes repeated cycling of the stent, increasing the risk of device fracture or formation of excessive granulation tissue. Persistent coughing must be treated aggressively to minimize the risk of these complications.

EXPECTATIONS/RISKS: DISCUSSION WITH OWNER

Once the decision has been made to consider tracheal stenting, an in-depth discussion with the owner reviewing all of the risks should take place. Neither surgery nor stenting has been demonstrated to slow the progression of disease, and both techniques are considered palliative. As indicated previously, clinical improvement rates of 75% to 90% were reported with intraluminal SEMSs (Norris et al., 2000; Moritz, Schneider, and Bauer, 2004). Most periprocedure complications were minor; however, in 10% of the dogs serious complications resulted in death. Late complications must be discussed with the owner, including stent shortening, excessive granulation tissue formation, progressive tracheal collapse, and stent fracture. Continued coughing should be expected in any dog with concurrent bronchial collapse, and these patients may carry a worse prognosis. In addition, the vast majority of dogs require continued medical therapy.

STENT PROPERTIES

A general review of stents is beyond the scope of this chapter; however, a brief discussion of certain stent characteristics will aid the reader in understanding the options available to the operator. The SEMS is used almost exclusively to treat tracheal collapse in dogs. (Balloon-expandable metallic stents are used rarely and are not discussed in this chapter). SEMSs are expanded to their stated measurements in the resting phase. Following manufacturing, the SEMSs are collapsed using a number of different techniques and loaded onto a delivery system covered by a sheath, which allows introduction through very small holes such as a vascular sheath or endotracheal (ET) tube. Following placement, the stent is deployed by retracting the surrounding sheath, allowing the stent to expand back to its original size and shape.

Stent Material

The majority of stents manufactured today are made of nitinol, which is classified as a shape-memory metal. The material is an alloy of nickel (Ni) and titanium (Ti) alloy developed by the Naval Ordinance Laboratory. Laser-cut nitinol stents are cut from hollow tubes of nitinol under extreme temperatures, altering the properties of

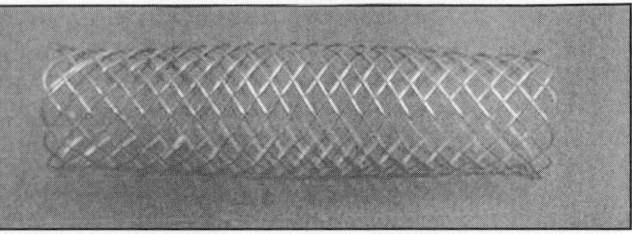

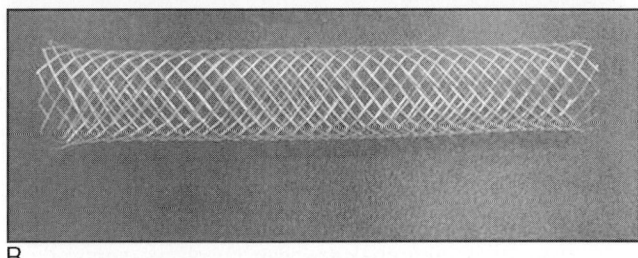

Fig. 145-1 **A,** Mesh nitinol stent (Vet Stent–Trachea, Infiniti Medical). Note the rounded edges of this stent chosen to reduce potential granulation tissue development. **B,** Mesh stainless steel stent (Courtesy Wallstent, Boston Scientific).

the metal and allowing compression of the stent onto a delivery system. On returning to ambient temperature, the stent favors its original design, which is achieved following release from the delivery system and sheath. Laser-cut nitinol SEMSs currently are not recommended for the treatment of tracheal collapse in veterinary patients because of an unacceptably high occurrence of stent fracture (personal experience). Woven, knitted, or mesh stents are designed to be compressed onto a delivery system at normal temperatures through design modifications. Examples of more commonly used nitinol stents in veterinary patients currently include mesh stents (Vet Stent–Trachea, Infiniti Medical)* or knitted stents (Ultraflex, Boston Scientific). Other commercially available stents used for tracheal collapse are made of stainless steel or similar alloys (Wallstent, Boston Scientific) (Fig. 145-1).

Foreshortening

The majority of stents currently placed for tracheal collapse in veterinary medicine are mesh or knitted SEMSs and undergo some degree of "foreshortening." This term refers to the shortening of the stent that is encountered as it is released from the delivery system. As indicated on the packaging, the stent size refers to the diameter and length at full expansion. If the stent does not achieve full expansion (i.e., the lumen in which it is placed prevents complete expansion to its original diameter), the stent will be *longer* than expected. In other words, the stents are significantly longer when viewed on the delivery system. As the stent expands it shortens, and as such the ultimate length of the stent is inversely proportional to the degree of expansion (the less the stent expands, the longer it will remain). This extremely important property of knitted and mesh stents

---

*The author is a consultant for Infiniti Medical, LLC and has been involved in the specifications chosen for the Vet Stent–Trachea and Delivery System.

must be recognized and accounted for during the stent selection process. For example, stent diameters of 10% to 15% greater than the diameter of the trachea are commonly chosen for tracheal stenting. The more oversized the stent, the longer the stent following initial deployment, and the greater the tendency for the stent to shorten over time (as it expands to its original diameter). This gradual shortening must be accounted for when choosing the appropriate stent length. An oversized stent may need to cover additional segments of normal trachea beyond the extremes of the collapse because future stent shortening should be anticipated. Typically the cranial end of the stent shortens in a caudal direction over time, most likely related to the larger diameter of the cervical trachea when compared to that of the intrathoracic trachea. When collapse extends to the larynx, the stent is placed to extend as far cranially as possible without contacting the cricoid cartilage. If the oversized stent gradually shortens over time, a single extraluminal ring can be placed surgically if clinical signs redevelop.

Stent Sizing

To choose an appropriately sized stent, it is important to determine the length of the collapse and the diameter of the trachea. The stent length and diameter are based on these metrics.

Stent Length

I prefer to identify the length of collapse in the awake animal using fluoroscopy. Although tracheoscopy historically has been regarded as the gold standard for identifying tracheal collapse, this procedure requires general anesthesia, which can add significant risk in these often debilitated patients. Simple radiography is not adequate for identifying the length of collapse because different areas of collapse are apparent during different phases of respiration (Fig. 145-2). I prefer to perform fluoroscopy in the fully awake dog. In addition, it is important to induce coughing if possible since these extreme airway pressures often reveal more extensive collapse than that identified during more relaxed breathing (Fig. 145-3). Anatomic landmarks are then identified to record the cranial-most and caudal-most extent of the collapse.

Occasionally a patient presents that is unable to be extubated following general anesthesia for an unrelated procedure. Under these circumstances the technique described previously is not possible. For these cases I use a homemade negative-pressure ventilation device (Fig. 145-4). Following preoxygenation with a series of positive-pressure ventilations, this apparatus is connected to the ET tube, and the dosing syringe plunger is withdrawn to −10 to −15 cm H_2O on the sphygmomanometer as a radiograph is taken to document the location of collapse (Fig. 145-5).

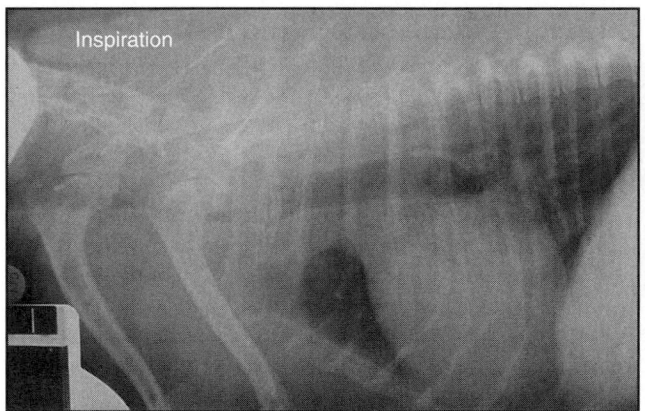
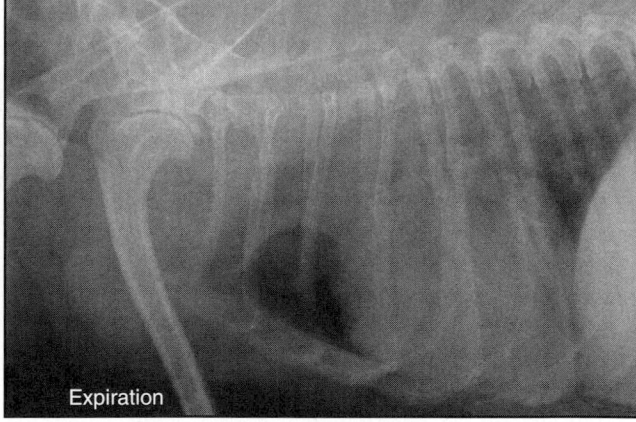

Fig. 145-2   Inspiratory and expiratory radiographs of the same dog demonstrating cervical tracheal collapse most apparent during inspiration *(top image)* and intrathoracic tracheal collapse most apparent during expiration *(bottom image)*.

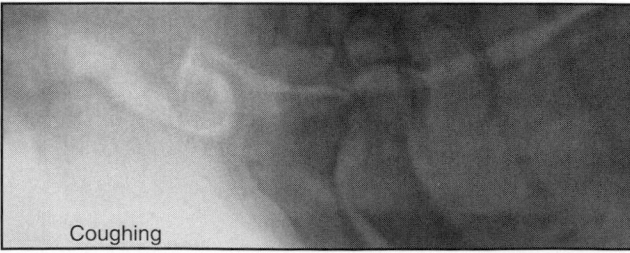

Fig. 145-3   Fluoroscopic images demonstrating dramatic difference in identification of length of tracheal collapse present during passive respiration *(top image with thoracic inlet tracheal collapse)* and a coughing episode *(bottom image)*. Note the extensive collapse and apparent folding of the caudal cervical trachea that occurs during coughing.

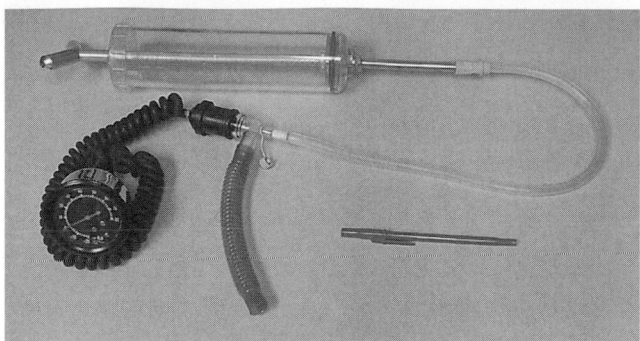

Fig. 145-4 Negative-pressure ventilation device attached to the endotracheal tube and used to identify the length of tracheal collapse in an anesthetized dog.

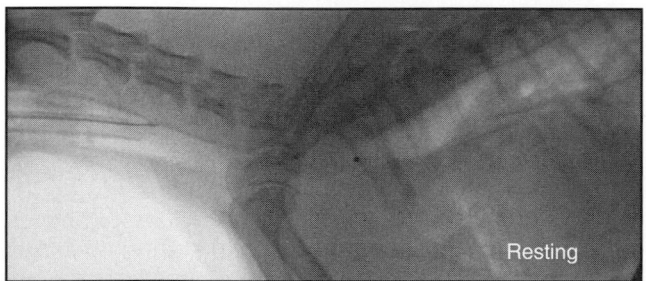

Resting

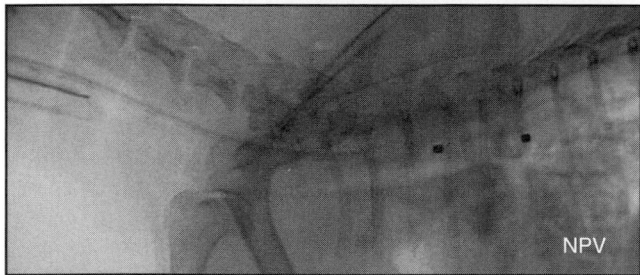

NPV

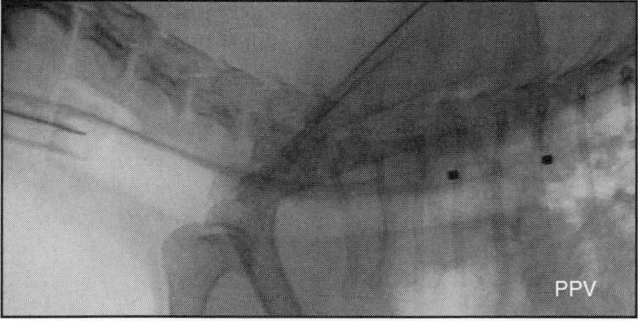

PPV

Fig. 145-5 Serial fluoroscopic images of the same dog under normal resting respiration, negative-pressure ventilation (NPV), and positive-pressure ventilation (PPV). Note the extensive tracheal collapse apparent under NPV; it is less clear under resting respiration. Under PPV dilation of the entire trachea is apparent.

Once the length of the collapse has been determined, the stent length is typically chosen to extend at *least 1 cm beyond the cranial and caudal extents of collapse*. If the entire length of the trachea is affected, the stent length is usually chosen to extend from approximately 1 cm cranial to the carina to 1 cm caudal to the cricoid cartilage of the

larynx. For shorter lengths of collapse, one must decide whether the animal will benefit from complete tracheal stenting versus covering a shorter segment. One study identified a potential increased risk of complications in animals receiving longer Wallstents; however, this finding was not corroborated in another study (Norris et al., 2000; Moritz, Schneider, and Bauer, 2004). A correlation between stent length and complication rate has not been apparent in my experience; and, if progression of tracheal disease is expected, the patient generally receives stenting across most of the tracheal length.

Stent Diameter

Typically the tracheal diameter is determined at the time of stent placement to prevent having to repeat general anesthesia. I place a measuring catheter within the esophagus to account for radiographic magnification (described later in the paragraph). Alternatively some other measuring device can be placed externally and included in the radiograph. The ET tube is withdrawn until the cuff is just caudal to the larynx. Positive-pressure ventilation of 20 cm H_2O is temporarily performed to achieve maximal tracheal expansion, and a radiograph is taken. The radiopaque marks on the marker catheter are 10 mm apart; this distance is measured on the radiograph and is also used to account for radiographic magnification. This extrapolation (known distance between markers plus magnification) is used to determine the actual maximal diameters of the intrathoracic and cervical tracheas (Fig. 145-6). The stent diameter chosen is usually ≈10% to 20% greater than the maximal tracheal diameter to minimize chances of stent migration. I generally inventory stents in 2-mm diameter increments (i.e., 8-mm, 10-mm, 12-mm, and 14-mm diameter). The cervical trachea is routinely larger in diameter than the intrathoracic trachea; however, the difference in these two measurements can vary dramatically. When the two diameters are similar (within 2 mm), the stent diameter chosen is equal to the maximal tracheal diameter or no more than 10% to 20% larger than the maximal diameter. For example, a dog with a maximal intrathoracic diameter of 8 mm and a maximal cervical tracheal diameter of 10 mm would likely receive a 12-mm diameter stent. When the tracheal diameter discrepancy is greater than 2 mm, stent sizing is more difficult. The risks of undersizing stent diameter are apparent (mucus trapping and stent migration); however, the risk of oversizing stent diameter is theoretical at this time (mucosal damage, excessive granulation, increased coughing). Therefore, one must consider the options: (1) Increase stent diameter by 10%-20% of largest tracheal diameter; (2) place two tracheal stents of different diameter; or (3) place cervical rings and intrathoracic tracheal stent. All of these options are reasonable and have been performed.

STENT PLACEMENT TECHNIQUE

The following description applies to placement of mesh SEMSs (Vet Stents–Trachea, Wallstents). Key issues include anesthesia and patient preparation, the specific procedural steps needed for successful stent deployment, and patient follow-up and aftercare.

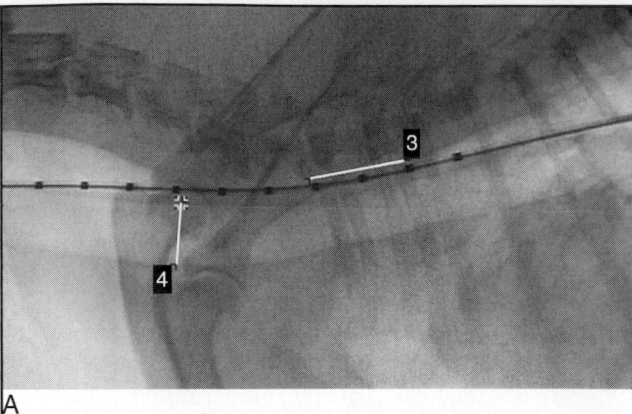

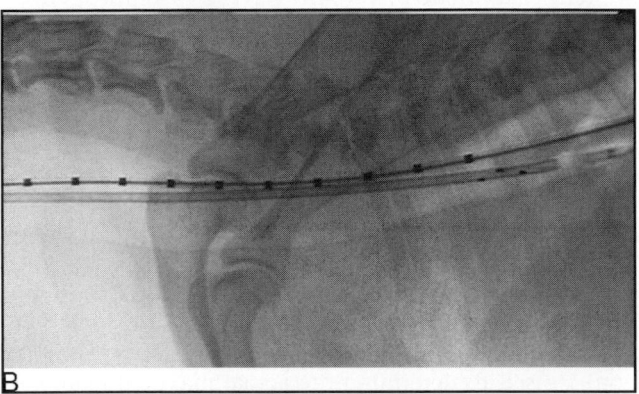

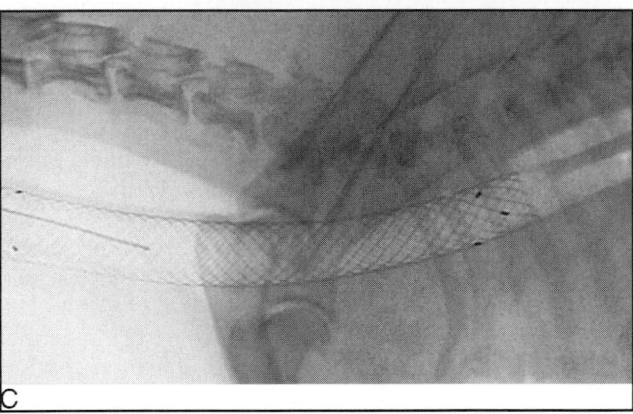

Fig. 145-6 Serial fluoroscopic images during tracheal sizing and stent placement. **A,** Using positive-pressure ventilation and an esophageal marker catheter, measurements are taken to determine the maximal tracheal diameter. **B,** The stent delivery system is advanced into the trachea. Note that the cervical and intrathoracic trachea are in line to facilitate passage of the stent. **C,** Restoration of a patent trachea immediately following placement of an intraluminal tracheal stent.

GENERAL ANESTHESIA AND PATIENT PREPARATION

Anesthesia protocols differ among institutions; however, I prefer a rapid induction and recovery. Premedication is routinely avoided unless intravenous catheterization creates excessive anxiety and respiratory distress. When necessary, an antitussive/tranquilization combination such as butorphanol (0.2 to 0.3 mg/kg intramuscularly [IM]) and acepromazine (0.05 to 0.01 mg/kg IM) can be an effective premedication. The patient is oxygenated before handling.

Unless contraindicated, a combination of intravenous propofol and diazepam is used with minimal inhalant anesthesia concentrations. Occasionally a propofol constant-rate infusion is used. The use of perioperative antibiotics is debatable, and they are chosen on an individual case basis. Unless contraindicated, these patients typically receive one perioperative dose of dexamethasone SP (0.1 to 0.25 mg/kg intravenously [IV]).

The largest ET tube possible should be selected (at least 4 mm inner diameter) to facilitate passage of the stent delivery system while permitting oxygen delivery and ventilation during the procedure. An ET tube with a radiopaque line or markers should be used when possible to avoid inadvertent deployment of the stent within the tube. The use of sterile ET tubes is debatable; I do not routinely require them. Following intubation the patient is placed in lateral recumbency.

A wet hydrophilic guidewire (Weasel Wire, Infiniti Medical) and flushed marker catheter (Marker Catheter, Infiniti Medical) combination is advanced into the mouth. Under fluoroscopic guidance the guidewire is gently advanced down the esophagus, and the marker catheter is advanced over the wire. The soft guidewire is always advanced first to avoid damage to the esophagus by the relatively stiffer marker catheter. The marker catheter is placed within the esophagus such that the radiopaque marks extend along the location of the tracheal collapse. The guidewire is then withdrawn.

Under fluoroscopic guidance the ET is withdrawn until the distal-most aspect is just beyond the larynx. The cuff is gently reinflated, and positive-pressure ventilation of 20 cm H_2O is held while a radiograph is taken. Subsequent measurements are used to determine the tracheal stent diameter as described previously. The radiographic landmarks previously obtained identifying the extent of the collapse are compared with those of the esophageal marker catheter to determine the length of stent necessary.

STENT PLACEMENT

Once the appropriately sized stent is chosen, it is removed from its packaging using sterile technique. The stent is prepared, and saline flushed according to manufacturer recommendations. A right-angle bronchoscope adapter (Fig. 145-7) is attached to the ET tube to facilitate passage of

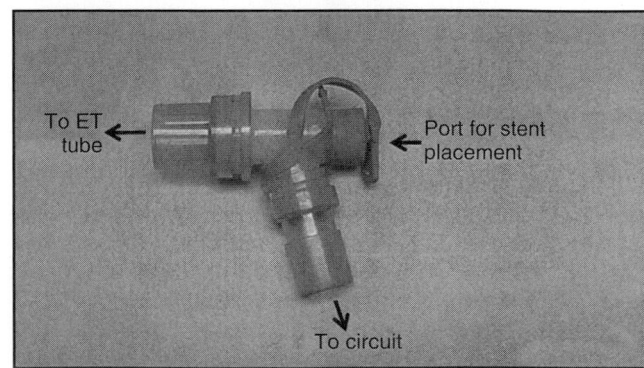

Fig. 145-7 Bronchoscope adapter used to maintain the anesthesia circuit while passing the stent delivery system through the endotracheal tube through the bronchoscope opening.

the stent delivery system while maintaining the anesthesia circuit system and patient oxygenation. Before passing the stent, the patient should be positioned such that the cervical and intrathoracic tracheas are in a straight line to facilitate placement of the relatively inflexible delivery system (see Fig. 145-6).

Because the stent is radiopaque, it is easily visualized under fluoroscopy, even when constrained within the delivery system. *All manipulations should be performed under direct fluoroscopic guidance.* The stent is directed to span the previously determined length of collapse. With one hand on the hub (or the cannula) and the other hand on the Y-piece (sheath), the sheath is gently withdrawn while *simultaneously* advancing the cannula (hub) in equal proportions. If done appropriately, as the stent is deployed, the distal end of the stent will remain in the same location throughout deployment. *Under no circumstances* should the cannula (hub) be advanced while the sheath remains stationary. This will force the stent caudally and traumatize the tracheal mucosa. These same circumstances apply to stent reconstrainment. If the operator is unhappy with the location of the partially deployed stent, reconstrainment should be performed via simultaneous withdrawal of the cannula and advancement of the sheath to avoid dragging the stent across the tracheal mucosa. The operator should practice these techniques outside of the patient before introducing the delivery system into the ET tube.

Following complete stent deployment, the delivery system is carefully removed. This should be performed under fluoroscopic guidance as well to ensure that the delivery system nose cone does not engage the distal end of the stent on removal. Radiographs are taken to document the final position of the stent (see Fig. 145-6). The patient is recovered immediately, typically in an intensive care unit setting and often within an oxygen cage. To facilitate smooth recovery from general anesthesia, the use of butorphanol (0.1 to 0.2 mk/kg IV) and/or acepromazine (0.005 to 0.01 mg/kg IV) can be useful.

POSTOPERATIVE CARE AND FOLLOW-UP

Patients routinely are discharged 1 or 2 days after stenting with a 3- to 4-week tapering dose of prednisone (initial dose of 1 to 2 mg/kg/day orally [PO]), continued antitussive therapy (hydrocodone 0.25 mg/kg PO q6–12h or higher doses if tolerated), and occasionally antibiotics if indicated. Patients with bronchial collapse or an observed "expiratory push" during exhalation may benefit from bronchodilator therapy as well.

Owners should be warned to anticipate an initial dry cough that should improve over the following 3 to 4 weeks. If the patient has documented bronchial collapse as well, the owners should expect continued coughing in the future. The majority of patients will require lifelong medication following tracheal stenting (see Chapter 144). The initial recheck examination is approximately 2 weeks after stenting or sooner if problems arise. Repeat examinations are then made according to the patient's clinical signs but should be performed regularly (every 3 to 6 months if possible).

References and Suggested Reading

Buback JL, Boothe HW, Hobson HP: Surgical treatment of tracheal collapse in dogs: 90 cases (1983-1993), *J Am Vet Med Assoc* 208(3):380, 1996.

Moritz A, Schneider M, Bauer N: Management of advanced tracheal collapse in dogs using intraluminal self-expanding biliary wall stents, *J Vet Intern Med* 18:31, 2004.

Norris JL: Intraluminal self-expanding stent placement for the treatment of tracheal collapse in dogs, Proceedings of the 10th Annual Meeting of the American College of Veterinary Surgeons (abstr), Arlington, VA 2000, p16.

Radlinsky MG: Evaluation of the palmaz stent in the trachea and main-stem bronchi of normal dogs, *Vet Surg* 26(2):99, 1997.

CHAPTER 146

Chronic Bronchitis in Dogs

LYNELLE R. JOHNSON, *Davis, California*

Chronic bronchitis is characterized by inflammation of the conducting airways and results in a chronic cough. The etiology of inflammation is unknown, although environmental pollutants, second-hand smoke, or inhaled irritants could be partly responsible for the induction of inflammatory airway disease in dogs. Chronic, low-grade aspiration injury might also play a role. In human medicine the role of bacterial infection in the generation or exacerbation of chronic bronchitis is widely debated, and in dogs no specific role has been established. Because chronic bronchitis is a disease of exclusion, treatment of the disease is based on all clinical information gathered from the individual animal.

Chronic airway inflammation is reflected by neutrophilic infiltration of the bronchial mucosa, which results in release of proteases, elastases, and oxidizing products. Mucosal injury is repaired by proliferation of the epithelium and hyperplasia of the surrounding tissue. Ongoing injury leads to a vicious cycle of airway injury and repair. These changes result in accumulation of mucus within the airway, which obstructs airflow and leads to clinical signs of cough and exercise intolerance. Airway collapse often accompanies chronic bronchitis, perhaps because of weakening of cartilage from inflammatory mediators or from affects on airway smooth muscle. Histologic examination of mucosal biopsy specimens from dogs with chronic bronchitis reveals hypertrophy and hyperplasia of mucous glands and goblet cells, smooth muscle hypertrophy, fibrosis of the lamina propria, and epithelial erosion with squamous metaplasia. The character of these lesions confirms the chronicity of disease. When a diagnosis of chronic bronchitis is made, it must be recognized that therapy is directed only at controlling clinical signs; once initiated, this disease is likely never cured.

CLINICAL FINDINGS

Chronic bronchitis is defined by the presence of a daily cough for at least 2 months of the year that lacks a specific cause. Usually the cough is described as a dry and hacking, but it can be moist or productive when copious amounts of respiratory secretions are produced. It may be overshadowed by a "goose honk" cough in small-breed dogs that have concurrent tracheal or airway collapse. Dogs are typically healthy and relatively active, although in the later stages of disease, exercise intolerance or heavy breathing may be reported. Severely affected animals may have intermittent cyanosis or collapse.

Chronic bronchitis occurs primarily in middle-aged to older dogs, and any breed (large or small) can be affected. On physical examination dogs are often overweight.

Some dogs are tachypneic, whereas dogs severely affected by bronchitis can have prolonged expiration or an expiratory push. Thoracic auscultation can be normal but often reveals coarse, diffuse crackles. Expiratory wheezes also may be noted and are considered the hallmark of chronic bronchitis. Tracheal sensitivity is usually present because of nonspecific airway inflammation. Airway collapse may be suspected on detection of a snapping sound over the thoracic cage as the intrathoracic airway collapses on expiration. In small-breed dogs a murmur of mitral insufficiency is a common coincident finding. When present, hepatomegaly is likely caused by obesity.

DIAGNOSIS

The diagnosis of chronic bronchitis is one of exclusion. The history of a long-term cough in a clinically well animal is highly suggestive of chronic bronchitis; however, airway infection (*Mycoplasma, Bordetella*, parasites), collapse, foreign body, or neoplasia can cause similar clinical signs. Therefore the diagnosis is based on the history, clinical findings, chest radiographs, and airway sampling for bacterial culture and cytologic examination.

Clinicopathologic abnormalities typically are absent in dogs with chronic bronchitis. Thoracic radiography is an important part of the diagnostic workup, both to confirm the likelihood of chronic bronchitis and to rule out other conditions. Classically a generalized increase in interstitial or peribronchial infiltrates is found in dogs with chronic bronchitis. End-on bronchi (doughnuts) and airways seen in longitudinal section (tram lines) represent airway walls thickened by inflammation. In the most advanced cases radiographic evidence of bronchiectasis may be identified. However, radiographs are relatively insensitive for chronic bronchitis, and in a case-controlled evaluation only increased thickness of airway walls and increased numbers of visible airway walls differed between normal dogs and dogs with bronchitis (Mantis, Lamb, and Boswood, 1998). In my opinion, normal chest radiographs are found relatively often in dogs with chronic bronchitis and do not rule out the diagnosis.

Collecting airway samples by tracheal wash or bronchoscopy is recommended to characterize the cellular infiltrate in the airway and to rule out infectious causes of cough. Bronchoscopy is particularly useful when typical radiographic findings of bronchitis are lacking. Dogs with chronic bronchitis have airway hyperemia, the airway mucosa has a cobblestone or irregular appearance, and many have increased mucus lining the airway. In animals with long-standing bronchitis fibrous nodules can be seen protruding into the bronchial lumen.

Cytologically chronic bronchitis is characterized by a preponderance of nondegenerate neutrophils. Some dogs have a predominance of eosinophils in airway washings or mixed inflammation. The importance of an eosinophilic infiltrate has not been investigated in dogs with chronic bronchitis. It may indicate systemic hypersensitivity (e.g., related to gastrointestinal parasites or ectoparasite infestation) or suggest an allergic basis for disease. Alternatively increased eosinophils in airway fluid may reflect the stage of disease. In humans airway eosinophilia is seen in patients with acute exacerbation of disease and indicates that noninfectious irritants, viruses, and *Mycoplasma* should be ruled out as causes of acute inflammation (Saetta et al., 1994). Increased mucus is present in many airway samples, and Curschmann's spirals (bronchial casts of airway mucus) are sometimes noted. Epithelial cells and squamous metaplasia may also be seen on cytologic examination.

Although suppurative inflammation is present on cytologic examination, bacterial infection is not a significant problem in the majority of dogs with chronic bronchitis. The trachea and large airway of dogs are not sterile; therefore various species of commensal bacteria and oral flora can be found in tracheal wash or bronchoalveolar lavage samples despite careful attention to technique. True bacterial infections of the lower respiratory tract are characterized by quantitative cultures of bronchoalveolar lavage fluid yielding more than 1.7×10^3 CFU/ml, lack of squamous cells on cytology, and a variably increased percentage of neutrophils (Peeters et al., 2000). Previously stable animals with bronchitis that have an acute exacerbation of disease may be experiencing true bacterial infection because dogs with chronic bronchitis might aspirate oral bacteria during episodes of coughing or panting. Aspirated bacteria become trapped in the mucus of the lower airway and may overwhelm host defenses because of the abnormal environment in the lower airway and cause infection. The airway is thus colonized and infected, and a septic suppurative inflammation would be seen on cytologic examination. Because *Mycoplasma* is part of the normal oral flora and can exacerbate lower airway injury, special culture techniques should be performed for these microorganisms in bronchitic animals.

Pulmonary function tests or advanced imaging can be performed to assess the severity of gas exchange or gas flow abnormalities. Arterial blood gas analysis generally shows only mild-to-moderate hypoxemia. Hypercarbia is not detected until late in the disease when respiratory failure ensues. Nuclear ventilation scans can be performed and may reveal patchy areas of deficient ventilation (Padrid et al., 1990). Flow volume loops are commonly performed in humans to assess maximal air flow. Tidal breathing flow volume loops have been performed in dogs with chronic bronchitis and have shown reductions in expiratory flow and loop shapes similar to those seen in humans with chronic bronchitis; however, these tests are not widely available.

THERAPY

Antiinflammatory Agents

Clinical signs of chronic bronchitis are caused by airway inflammation, and therapy with glucocorticoids is successful in resolving clinical signs in the majority of dogs. It is essential that infectious diseases be ruled out before the initiation of antiinflammatory treatment. In addition, it would seem wise to control coexisting diseases such as severe dental disease or congestive heart failure before using glucocorticoids.

Dosing of glucocorticoids should be tailored to the individual, with the severity of clinical signs, chronicity of disease, and general systemic health considered in decisions regarding treatment. Short-acting steroids such as prednisone or prednisolone are generally safe and effective in dogs with uncomplicated bronchitis. In the early stages of disease dogs often require dosages of glucocorticoids ranging from 0.5 to 1 mg/kg every 12 hours for 5 to 7 days to induce remission of clinical signs. As clinical signs abate, the dosage should be decreased by half every 5 to 7 days; and, when possible, drugs should be administered on an alternate-day basis to allow normalization of the pituitary-adrenal axis. Long-term therapy (2 to 3 months) can be anticipated in most cases, although discontinuation of medication may be possible. If disease worsens in the early stages of treatment, a return to the higher dose of glucocorticoid that controlled clinical signs is generally required. Alternatively treatment with inhaled steroids, bronchodilators, or antitussive agents can be added (see following paragraphs). Long-acting glucocorticoids such as dexamethasone, triamcinolone, and methylprednisolone acetate do not have a therapeutic advantage over prednisone and are associated with more severe derangements of the pituitary-adrenal axis. I have not used cytotoxic drugs or antihistamines in the treatment of chronic bronchitis.

To avoid systemic effects of glucocorticoids, inhaled medications can be considered in animals that tolerate administration via a face mask. Various types of steroids are available for inhalation in metered-dose inhaler canisters. I generally start with fluticasone propionate (Flovent, Glaxo Simith-Kline) using 110 mcg/puff– or 220 mcg/puff–strength administered at 1 puff BID to QID. To avoid the need for a voluntary respiratory maneuver to inhale the medication, the drug is dispensed using a spacing chamber and face mask. Spacing chambers are available through a variety of respiratory supply corporations or pharmacies; a tight-fitting face mask is critical for successful therapy. It is important that the dog have the nose and lips enclosed by the mask during actuation of the drug and that it breathes normally for 8 to 10 seconds (i.e., does not pant). Brachycephalic dogs are easily fit with face masks obtained from a local pharmacy or respiratory supply company because the shape of the face is more similar to that of humans. For dolichocephalic breeds, anesthetic or cone-shaped face masks are required, and an up-sizing adaptor may be required to fit properly on the spacer.

Bronchodilators

It is unlikely that bronchoconstriction plays a role in canine chronic bronchitis. Baseline pulmonary resistance increased in an experimental model of lung inflammation induced by *Bordetella bronchiseptica*; however, airway responsiveness as assessed by histamine challenge was unchanged (Cormier et al., 1993). The baseline increase in resistance was probably related to the presence of inflammatory products and mucosal edema rather than airway hyperreactivity. However, bronchodilators often are clinically helpful in reducing signs in dogs with bronchitis or in allowing a reduction in the dosage of glucocorticoid required to control signs. Both methylxanthine derivatives and β-agonists seem to act synergistically with glucocorticoids in the control of inflammatory lung disease. Bronchodilators may provide other beneficial effects by improving pulmonary perfusion, enhancing cardiac performance, reducing respiratory effort, and stimulating mucociliary clearance. In dogs that fail to respond adequately to glucocorticoids, a 2-week trial on a supplemental bronchodilator is a reasonable therapeutic option.

The two main classes of bronchodilators used in veterinary medicine are methylxanthine derivatives and β_2-agonists. Methylxanthine drugs were originally thought to act through phosphodiesterase inhibition, which causes smooth-muscle relaxation through accumulation of cyclic adenosine monophosphate. Current research suggests that the clinical effects of methylxanthines result from adenosine antagonism. Extended-release theophylline (Inwood Laboratories, 10 mg/kg orally [PO] q12h) has been shown to achieve plasma levels in dogs that approximate the human therapeutic range of 10 to 20 mcg/ml (Bach et al., 2004).

Adverse effects of methylxanthines are probably also related to adenosine antagonism and include gastrointestinal upset, tachycardia, and hyperexcitability. It is essential to individualize drug therapy because there is a wide variation in the dose that causes side effects. Theophylline metabolism is influenced by many factors, including fiber in the diet, smoke in the environment, congestive heart failure, and the use of other drugs. I recommend starting therapy with half the recommended dosage (5 mg/kg q12h) for the first week to reduce adverse side effects. If clinical signs improve and the dog tolerates the drug, the dosage may be increased as needed.

β_2-Agonists such as terbutaline and albuterol have also been used successfully in dogs with chronic bronchitis. Terbutaline is available through a wide number of pharmaceutical companies. Small dogs receive 0.625 to 1.25 mg orally every 12 hours, medium-sized dogs are given 1.25 to 2.5 mg orally every 12 hours, and larger dogs receive 2.5 to 5 mg orally every 12 hours. Albuterol at 50 mcg/kg orally every 8 hours was efficacious in reducing cough in almost half the dogs evaluated in a review of canine chronic bronchitis (Padrid et al., 1990). Interestingly, the bronchodilator also resulted in a reduction in the severity of the pulmonary infiltrate. As with methylxanthines, β-agonists may result in excitability or tremors during initial therapy, but animals usually become accustomed to the drug. β_2-Agonists are widely available for inhaled therapy and are inexpensive.

Antibiotics

When infection has been documented through appropriate culturing techniques and cytologic findings confirm infection, antibiotic treatment is warranted. Antibiotic choice should be based on culture and sensitivity results whenever possible and should have a broad spectrum of activity against bacteria commonly found in the lung such as *Pasteurella* spp., *Staphylococcus* spp., *Streptococcus* spp., and various gram-negative species. The antibiotic chosen should be lipophilic to facilitate penetration of the airway and should be relatively free of side effects. When possible, I prefer doxycycline (3 to 5 mg/kg PO q12h) because this drug has all of the desired attributes and is relatively devoid of side effects. Owners should be instructed to supply water after administering the drug to propel the pill fully into the stomach, thus avoiding the possibility of an esophageal stricture caused by delay in esophageal transit. Enrofloxacin (Baytril [Bayer], 2.5 to 5 mg/kg PO q24h) is generally reserved for severe infection. If needed, it is important to note that enrofloxacin inhibits metabolism of theophylline and the concurrent use of the two drugs results in toxic plasma levels of theophylline (Intorre et al., 1995). At least a 30% reduction in theophylline dosage is recommended when enrofloxacin is required to treat coincident infection. Length of antibiotic treatment depends on whether pneumonia is present or whether bronchial colonization and infection are suspected. True pneumonia generally requires 3 to 6 weeks of antibiotic therapy, whereas 5 to 10 days of treatment usually resolve signs related to bronchial colonization. If *Bordetella* is isolated from an airway wash, aerosolization with gentamicin (Gentocin, Schering Plough) would be recommended rather than oral antibiotics because of improved efficacy in reducing bacterial numbers in the airway (Bemis and Appel, 1977), although some dogs do seem to respond to long-term doxycycline. An ultrasonic nebulizer and face mask are used to administer 3 to 5 mg/kg of gentamicin once daily for 5 days.

Infection plays a predominant role in patients with concurrent bronchiectasis, and in these patients long-term antibiotic therapy is indicated. Bronchiectasis is defined as a dilation of the lower airways; suppuration is usually present. It may occur as a sequela to uncontrolled airway inflammation or infection. Mucus trapping and obstruction of the airway are severe, and recurrent pneumonia is commonly encountered. Chronic antibiotic therapy is often required in these patients, and broad-spectrum antibiotics or combinations of antibiotics should be chosen because infection may involve various gram-negative bacteria (especially *Pseudomonas*) and anaerobes. Chloramphenicol, trimethoprim-sulfa (15 mg/kg PO q12h), or clindamycin (Antirobe [Pharmacia & Upjohn], 11 mg/kg PO q12h) combined with enrofloxacin can be helpful in resolving long-standing pulmonary infection.

Antitussive Agents

The cough reflex is of major importance to the dog with bronchitis because it serves the essential function of clearing viscid secretions from the airway. Suppression of this reflex before resolution of inflammation can be deleterious because mucus can become trapped in small airways. Prolonged contact between inflammatory mediators in the mucus and epithelial cells perpetuates airway inflammation. When clinical signs suggest that inflammation is resolving yet the cough persists or in animals that have concurrent airway collapse with chronic bronchitis, cough suppression is desirable because chronic coughing can lead to repeated airway injury and syncopal events. Over-the-counter dextromethorphan-containing compounds seem to be useful in some animals. When more potent suppression of a dry cough is required, narcotic agents should be prescribed.

I prefer hydrocodone (Tussigon [Daniels Pharmaceuticals], 0.22 mg/kg PO q6–12h) or butorphanol (Torbutrol [Fort Dodge], 0.5 mg/kg PO q6–12h). These agents must be given at an interval that suppresses coughing without inducing excessive sedation or gastrointestinal effects. Long-term therapy may be required in some patients, particularly when tracheal collapse is also present.

ADDITIONAL THERAPY

Obesity worsens clinical signs in dogs with chronic bronchitis by decreasing thoracic wall compliance, increasing the work of breathing, and increasing abdominal pressure on the diaphragm. Improvements in exercise tolerance and arterial oxygenation can be seen with weight loss alone. Owners should be given reasonable goals for the dog's optimal weight and the time in which weight loss can be achieved. A 2% to 3% weight loss per week is desirable. This can be achieved through the use of a high-fiber, low-fat diet and by providing gradually increasing amounts of exercise. Close monitoring of owner compliance and accomplishments in the weight-loss program seems to enhance the overall success.

Animals with concurrent tracheal collapse or marked tracheal sensitivity benefit from having a harness instead of a collar. When stresses in the environment such as cigarette smoke, pollutants, heat, or humidity are encountered, the animal should be removed to a cool, clean area.

Some dogs benefit from intermittent airway humidification via steam inhalation or nebulization to improve clearance of airway secretions. An ultrasonic nebulizer is preferred for respiratory therapy because it produces sufficiently small particles of saline to penetrate deep into the airways. Coupage of the chest or gentle exercise after nebulization facilitates clearance of secretions.

PROGNOSIS

Owners should be aware that bronchitis is a chronic disease that can be controlled but never cured. The majority of animals have residual cough and exhibit clinical signs periodically throughout life. The presence of fibrosis and chronic inflammation on biopsy specimens confirms the irreversibility of airway disease. The goals of disease management are to control inflammation, thus limiting clinical signs; to diagnose and treat infection when it occurs; and to prevent the development of debilitating sequelae such as bronchiectasis and cor pulmonale.

References and Suggested Reading

Bach JE et al: Evaluation of the bioavailability and pharmacokinetics of two extended-release theophylline formulations in dogs, *J Am Vet Med Assoc* 224:1113, 2004.

Bemis DA, Appel MJG: Aerosol, parenteral, and oral antibiotic treatment for *Bordetella bronchiseptica* infections in dogs, *J Am Vet Med Assoc* 170:1082, 1977.

Cormier Y et al: Effect of inflammation on peripheral airway reactivity in dogs, *Clin Sci* 84:73, 1993.

Intorre L et al: Enrofloxacin-theophylline interaction: influence of enrofloxacin on theophylline steady-state pharmacokinetics in the beagle dog, *J Vet Pharmacol Ther* 19:352, 1995.

Mantis P, Lamb CR, Boswood A: Assessment of the accuracy of thoracic radiography in the diagnosis of canine chronic bronchitis, *J Small Anim Pract* 39:518, 1998.

Padrid PA et al: Canine chronic bronchitis: a pathophysiologic evaluation of 18 cases, *J Vet Intern Med* 4:172, 1990.

Peeters DE et al: Quantitative bacterial cultures and cytological examination of bronchoalveolar lavage specimens in dogs, *J Vet Intern Med* 14:534, 2000.

Saetta M et al: Airway eosinophilia in chronic bronchitis during exacerbations, *Am J Respir Crit Care Med* 153:1646, 1994.

CHAPTER 147

Bordetella bronchiseptica: Beyond Kennel Cough

RICHARD B. FORD, *Raleigh, North Carolina*

With the capacity to exist in the respiratory tract as a commensal organism and a pathogen, *Bordetella bronchiseptica* poses a unique and nearly ubiquitous threat to both dogs and cats of all ages. Most frequently implicated for its role in infectious tracheobronchitis (ITB) in dogs (also called *kennel cough*), clinical illness associated with colonization of *B. bronchiseptica* is ultimately defined by the ability of the bacterium to express various virulence factors, or determinants. Although the respiratory epithelium of the nasal cavity and trachea are principle targets of infection and a particularly common source of infectious cough and pneumonia, systemic infection associated with bacteremia and sepsis is reported.

THE BORDETELLAE

There are nine known *Bordetella* spp., four of which have been associated with respiratory infections in humans and other mammals: *Bordatella pertussis, Bordatella parapertussis, Bordatella holmesii,* and *B. bronchiseptica.* Associated with pertussis, or "whooping cough," *B. pertussis* and *B. parapertussis* are host-restricted human pathogens, most commonly associated with respiratory infection in children. On the other hand, *B. holmesii* has only been associated with respiratory illness in a limited number of humans since 1995. *B. bronchiseptica,* first isolated in the early 1900s, is somewhat unique in that it is able to infect the respiratory tract of several species of mammals, including humans (Mattoo and Cherry, 2005).

B. bronchiseptica is a gram-negative aerobic coccobacillus particularly well adapted to colonize the ciliated respiratory epithelium of dogs and cats. Today this organism is regarded as a principle bacterium associated with canine ITB (Ford, 2006). Dogs infected with canine parainfluenza virus (CPiV) or canine adenovirus-2 (CAV-2) may experience more severe respiratory disease when coinfected with *B. bronchiseptica. B. bronchiseptica* infection in the absence of either CPiV or CAV-2 (i.e., canine bordetellosis) is known to occur and can be associated with acute, fatal pneumonia, particularly in young dogs. Several commercial vaccines are available today and have been shown to induce high titers. However, *B. bronchiseptica* has been isolated from the nasal cavity of vaccinated animals, suggesting that vaccination does not necessarily prevent infection.

Virulence Factors and Pathogenesis

The complexity of *B. bronchiseptica* infection is characterized by its ability to become colonized persistently in the upper and lower respiratory tract yet cause no clinical signs or gross pathology. Histologic examination following experimental inoculation only rarely demonstrates inflammatory changes. When clinical signs associated with *B. bronchiseptica* do develop in dogs, the disease is characterized as tracheobronchitis. Congestion of tracheal and bronchial mucosa occurs with mucoid-to-mucopurulent exudates in airways. Lung parenchyma may also become infected since focal exudative pneumonia and petechiae are also reported. The most severe consequences of infection generally are seen in dogs and cats coinfected with other pathogens such as CPiV or feline calicivirus.

B. bronchiseptica exists both as a commensal organism in the respiratory tract of healthy dogs and cats and as a potentially life-threatening pathogen. The outcome of infection is highly variable and difficult to predict in the clinical setting. The complexity of this bacteria-host interaction is attributed to the fact that *B. bronchiseptica* possesses a virulence control system nearly identical to that found in *B. pertussis* and *B. parapertussis,* encoded by the *BvgAS* locus. *Bordetella* virulence genes A and S (BvgA and BvgS, respectively) are signaling proteins responsible for the expression of several virulence determinants (Table 147-1) and ultimately the pathologic consequences of infection.

The BvgAS locus controls at least three distinct phenotypic phases of *B. bronchiseptica:* Bvg$^+$, Bvg^i, and Bvg$^-$, which are believed to be involved with colonization, transmission, and survival (persistence), respectively. Interestingly, expression of a particular phase appears to be under the influence of various environmental conditions (such as coinfection or stress). The relevant signals that influence and regulate the BvgAS locus have yet to be determined.

Clinical Disease

In contrast to *B. pertussis* and *B. parapertussis,* which only infect humans, *B. bronchiseptica* is uniquely able to infect several species of mammals, including humans. Transmission of *B. bronchiseptica* occurs primarily through aerosolization of respiratory secretions. Bacteria can also be transmitted directly by contaminated dishware, human hands, and other fomites. Because *B. bronchiseptica* possesses several intrinsic mechanisms for evading host defenses, it is recognized for its role as a significant complicating factor in dogs with multiple-agent respiratory infections. The clinical consequences of infection range from subclinical

Table 147-1

Principle Virulence Determinants for *Bordetella bronchiseptica* and Summary of Actions

Virulence Determinant	Action
Filamentous hemagglutinin	Surface-associated and secreted protein; required for tracheal colonization; highly immunogenic
Fimbriae	Filamentous cell surface structure required for persistent tracheal colonization
Pertactin	Surface protein; enhances protective immunity
Vag8	Outer membrane protein
Adenylate cyclase	Calmodulin-activated toxin with dual adenylate cyclase/hemolysis activity; acts as an antiinflammatory and antiphagocytic factor during infection
Type III secretion	Allows *Bordetella* to translocate effector proteins into host cells; required for persistent tracheal colonization; inhibits host immune response; causes cell death
Dermonecrotic toxin	Heat-labile toxin; induces necrosis in vitro
Tracheal cytotoxin	Causes mitochondrial bloating, disruption of tight junctions, and damage to ciliated cells

From Mattoo and Cherry, *Clin Microbiol Rev* 18:326, 2005.

disease with shedding to suppurative pneumonia and death, especially in puppies.

B. bronchiseptica is frequently, although not exclusively, associated with canine ITB (i.e., kennel cough). The bacteria are commonly recovered from dogs with signs of upper and lower respiratory infection subsequent to having been housed in cluster environments such as boarding kennels, veterinary hospitals, and animal shelters. In addition, *B. bronchiseptica* recently has been reported as the most common cause of community-acquired infectious pneumonia in dogs less than 1 year of age (Radhakrishnan et al., 2007). Such findings support the fact that *B. bronchiseptica* is widely distributed throughout the canine population and poses a significant threat to susceptible dogs and to a lesser extent cats.

In practice the clinical signs vary considerably, depending on the extent of coinfection or the presence of another underlying respiratory disease. Typically dogs infected with *B. bronchiseptica* manifest clinical signs that range from purulent nasal discharge (without cough) to paroxysmal coughing episodes. In cats *B. bronchiseptica* infection is most commonly associated with lower respiratory signs characterized by cough, particularly in kittens. Clinical signs caused by *B. bronchiseptica* generally are described as self-limiting and in otherwise healthy animals are expected to last no more than about 2 weeks. Although clinical signs of *B. bronchiseptica* infection are reported to persist for only 1 to 2 weeks, bacteria can be shed from the respiratory tract for 2 to 3 months following recovery. Resistance to reinfection may last up

to 12 months. Dogs with signs persisting beyond 2 weeks should be evaluated for another underlying disease as the principle cause of cough.

Severe bronchopneumonia is described in dogs with no prior natural or vaccine exposure to the various agents that cause ITB or complicating bacterial infection. Affected dogs are likely to have a history of recent stays in a pet shop, boarding facility, kennel, or shelter. ITB may be associated with or without rhinitis and accompanying mucoid-to-mucopurulent nasal and ocular discharge. Complications associated with bronchopneumonia may become life threatening, particularly in puppies. On physical examination affected dogs are usually febrile and may be lethargic, anorexic, and dyspneic. Affected dogs are difficult to distinguish from those with canine distemper virus (CDV) infections or other pneumonias. Outbreaks of infectious pneumonia caused by *B. bronchiseptica* may affect more than 50% of dogs in a densely populated environment.

Several published reviews on bacterial endocarditis and sepsis in dogs and cats implicate *B. bronchiseptica* as common causative bacteria. Although the route of entry has not been characterized, *bordetella* is known for its ability to infect the cilia of respiratory epithelial cells. Ciliostasis subsequent to initial infection is followed by mucus production, damage to epithelium, and induction of an inflammatory response with the respiratory tract (Anderton, Maskell, and Preston, 2004). Injury to epithelial cells may represent a portal of entry into blood that in some patients culminates in bacteremia and sepsis with or without clinical evidence of respiratory tract infection.

Determining the actual prevalence of *B. bronchiseptica*–induced respiratory disease in dogs and cats is complicated by the facts that: (1) infectious respiratory disease is typically associated with other bacterial pathogens (e.g., *Mycoplasma* spp.) and viruses (e.g., parainfluenza virus, CDV, and calicivirus; and (2) *B. bronchiseptica* can be isolated from the respiratory tract of healthy dogs and cats (Moise et al., 1989).

Diagnosis

In the clinical setting diagnostic confirmation of *B. bronchiseptica* infection by culture is uncommon. Instead a clinical diagnosis of ITB is made on the basis of history and signs. Diagnostic confirmation entails collecting nasal swabs or fluid collected aseptically from a tracheal aspiration or bronchoscopic washing. These studies most commonly are done in patients with radiographic signs of bronchopneumonia or when coughing associated with kennel cough persists despite empiric antibiotic therapy. Airway samples are inoculated onto commercially available Bordet-Gengou agar supplemented with 0.004% cephalexin or 20 mcg of streptomycin and incubated for 48 hours at 37°C. Identity can be confirmed by use of a Gram stain.

Treatment

Therapy for any dog or cat with known or suspected respiratory infection caused by *B. bronchiseptica* varies with the severity of disease and the presence of an underlying disorder. Prompt antimicrobial intervention is important and may be lifesaving. Doxycycline is the preferred antimicrobial used in the treatment of infectious respiratory disease of dogs and cats. Tablets, capsules, or a liquid suspension may be administered at 5 mg/kg orally twice daily for 7 to 10 days. Alternatively doxycycline may be administered once daily at a dose of 10 mg/kg. The liquid suspension is preferred when treating cats and puppies. Although oral doxycycline can discolor the enamel of developing teeth in young animals, limiting the treatment to fewer than 10 days minimizes the risk. Shorter treatment durations (e.g., 5 to 7 days) have been effective in treating young puppies with severe bronchopneumonia caused by *B. bronchiseptica*. Azithromycin, amoxicillin-clavulanate, and cephalexin are alternative antimicrobials that could be used in lieu of doxycycline.

Although corticosteroids are recommended in the management of cough associated with viral tracheobronchitis in dogs, these drugs are contraindicated in any patient known to have pneumonia caused by *B. bronchiseptica*. Therefore empiric treatment should be limited to antibacterial therapy until a response to treatment can be evaluated.

Cough suppressants, including butorphanol and various forms of codeine, are often used in the treatment of kennel cough in dogs. When the infection is related only to a viral injury, judicious reduction of cough may be helpful to the patient (and client). However, in cases of bacterial infection caused by *B. bronchiseptica*, the response to antibiotics should be sufficient to reduce clinical signs of coughing, and antitussive therapy is not recommended. Furthermore, if bronchopneumonia is developing, suppression of cough can be dangerous by preventing clearance of bacteria, infected mucus, and other debris. Accordingly a chest radiograph should be considered before initiating any antitussive therapy, and the initial response to antibiotic therapy should be considered as a guide before attempting to suppress a kennel cough. This is especially true if there is fever or any constitutional signs of infection such as lethargy or anorexia.

Administration of fluids, either orally or parenterally, is indicated in any dog or cat with bacterial infection of the lower respiratory tract. Fluid therapy is particularly important in puppies and kittens with bacterial pneumonia. Within 24 hours significant insensible fluid loss through the respiratory tract can lead to increased viscosity of secretions, decreased clearance of lower airways, and greater risk of death.

Indications for nebulization, oxygen therapy, and coupage in patients with bacterial pneumonia are presented in detail in Chapter 149.

Vaccination

B. bronchiseptica vaccines are licensed in the United States for administration to both cats and dogs. The 2006 Report of the American Animal Hospital Canine Vaccine Task Force has classified all *B. bronchiseptica* vaccines as noncore. A parenteral, cellular antigen extract vaccine and an intranasal avirulent live vaccine are currently available for use in dogs. All *B. bronchiseptica* vaccines approved for intranasal administration in dogs contain modified-live parainfluenza vaccine. Some intranasal vaccines approved for use in

dogs also contain modified-live CAV-2 vaccine.* The only vaccine licensed for use in cats is an avirulent-live bacterial vaccine approved for intranasal administration only.

Canine Vaccination

The availability of both parenteral and intranasal *B. bronchiseptica* vaccine for dogs has led to questions concerning efficacy, onset of action, frequency of administration, and safety. Today most authors agree that both vaccine types are effective in reducing the severity of clinical illness (Edinboro et al., 2004; Gopinathan et al., 2007). No one vaccine type is known to be significantly better at reducing clinical illness than the other. However, *neither* parenteral nor intranasal vaccine appears to prevent infection subsequent to natural exposure.

Compared to parenteral *B. bronchiseptica* vaccine, intranasal vaccines provide a significantly faster onset of immunity at the time of initial vaccination. A single dose of intranasal vaccine has been shown to protect dogs against clinical illness as early as 72 hours, with most dogs responding by 4 to 14 days (Gore et al., 2005). Intranasal vaccines can be administered to puppies as young as 3 to 4 weeks of age.

On the other hand, initial vaccination with the parenteral vaccine *requires* that two doses be administered 3 to 4 weeks apart. Immunity cannot be expected for at least 1 to 2 weeks following administration of the second dose. The first of two doses should not be administered before 6 weeks of age. If the vaccination interval between the first and second parenteral doses exceeds 6 weeks, the entire two-dose series should be repeated. Two doses of parenteral vaccine result in higher antibody titers compared to titers derived from a single intranasal booster vaccination. However, antibody titers are less valid in assessing vaccine-induced immunity to *B. bronchiseptica* than are controlled challenge studies.

Challenge studies designed to assess the duration of immunity following vaccination are limited. However, there is reasonable evidence to support a sustained immune response lasting from between 10 and 14 months following intranasal vaccination. The duration of immunity following administration of the parenteral vaccine has not been published.

Current recommendations suggest that a single dose of either an intranasal or parenteral vaccine administered annually is sufficient to boost an individual patient's immunity. It is my opinion that annual booster with either vaccine type is sufficient for dogs having minimal risk of exposure. However, in the face of sustained exposure (e.g., regular boarding, dog day care), it is reasonable to recommend vaccination every 6 months as long as the risk of exposure exists. Although *B. bronchiseptica* is not the only pathogen associated with canine infectious respiratory disease, vaccination against *B. bronchiseptica* is justified because of its ability to seriously compromise the patient.

---

*The 2006 American Animal Hospital Association Canine Vaccine Guidelines recommend against the use of intranasal CAV-2 vaccine on the grounds that parenteral CAV-2 vaccine is considered to confer a superior immune response in preventing CAV-1 (canine infectious hepatitis virus) infection.

A recent study (Davis et al., 2007) has shown that intranasal vaccination prevents postchallenge shedding of bacteria, whereas the parenteral vaccine did not. Such studies support recommendations that either vaccine may be appropriate for use in households with one to two dogs. However, the intranasal vaccination is indicated to minimize transmission of *B. bronchiseptica* among dogs housed in a cluster environment (e.g., shelters, rescue groups).

Feline Vaccination

Currently only one feline vaccine is available for the prevention of *B. bronchiseptica* in cats. The vaccine consists of avirulent live bacteria and is administered to kittens as young as 4 to 6 weeks of age. Much less is known about the significance of *B. bronchiseptica* in the pathogenesis of feline infectious respiratory disease. As in dogs, the presence of *B. bronchiseptica* can cause pneumonia and seriously compromise respiratory function, particularly in kittens. It is possible that kittens coinfected with acute feline calicivirus or herpesvirus-1 may experience severe, even fatal, clinical illness in the presence of bacteria. Vaccination should be limited to kittens and young cats with a reasonable risk of exposure to other cats or dogs. The manufacturer recommends that annual boosters be administered to cats considered to be at risk of exposure. However, annual vaccination of healthy adult cats having little or no risk of exposure to cats or potentially infected dogs generally is not recommended.

Vaccine Complications

Clinical signs of respiratory disease, including purulent nasal discharge and cough, have been reported in both dogs and cats within a few days following intranasal vaccination. In most instances these signs resolve without treatment. However, some patients may become clinically ill and actually require short-term treatment with an antimicrobial. Postvaccinal nasal discharge and/or cough seem to occur more often in young animals than adults.

Inadvertent subcutaneous administration of the avirulent, live intranasal *B. bronchiseptica* vaccine is reported occasionally. Injection site abscess seems to be the most common physical manifestation. However, replication of the attenuated gram-negative bacteria in the subcutaneous space has been associated with death following liver failure. Endotoxemia rather that sepsis is speculated to be the cause. Anecdotal reports from practicing veterinarians suggest that some dogs do not manifest any adverse signs or illness. Treatment of a dog or cat that inadvertently receives the intranasal vaccine by the subcutaneous route includes administration of oral doxycycline, 5 mg/kg every 12 hours for 5 to 7 days.

It has been suggested that intranasal vaccine might have therapeutic benefit in dogs with active clinical signs consistent with ITB. However, in my experience in attempting to treat dogs involved in a shelter outbreak of infectious respiratory infection, intranasal vaccine neither lessened the severity of clinical signs nor did it shorten the course of infection. Intranasal vaccine should not be used in the attempt to treat preexisting respiratory infection.

Human Infection With Bordetella bronchiseptica

Of importance to veterinarians is the fact that *B. bronchiseptica* can be transmitted from animals (e.g., dogs, cats, rabbits) to other animal species and humans. Although generally considered to be rare and limited to individuals with immune compromise, unverified infections in humans have been reported (Woolfrey and Moody, 1991). The role of *B. bronchiseptica* as a zoonotic pathogen, particularly for those working directly with animals in high-density environments (e.g., shelters, rescue organizations) warrants additional study.

References and Suggested Reading

Anderton TL, Maskell DJ, Preston A: Ciliostasis is a key early event during colonization of canine tracheal tissue by *Bordetella bronchiseptica*, *Microbiology* 150:2843, 2004.

Davis R et al: Comparison of the mucosal immune response in dogs vaccinated with an intranasal avirulent live culture or a subcutaneous antigen extract vaccine of *Bordetella bronchiseptica*, *Vet Ther* 8:32, 2007.

Edinboro EH, Ward MP, Glickman LT: A placebo-controlled trial of two intranasal vaccines to prevent tracheobronchitis (kennel cough) in dogs entering a humane shelter, *Prev Vet Med* 62:89, 2004.

Ford RB: Canine infectious tracheobronchitis. In Greene CE, editor: *Infectious diseases of the dog and cat*, ed 3, St. Louis, 2006, Saunders, p 54.

Gopinathan L et al: Difference mechanisms of vaccine-induced and infection-induced immunity to *Bordetella bronchiseptica*, *Microbes Infect* 9:442, 2007.

Gore T et al: Intranasal kennel cough vaccine protecting dogs from experimental *Bordetella bronchiseptica* challenge within 72 hours, *Vet Rec* 156:482, 2005.

Mattoo S, Cherry JD: Molecular pathogenesis, epidemiology, and clinical manifestation of respiratory infections due to *Bordetella pertussis* and other *Bordetella* subspecies, *Clin Microbiol Rev* 18:326, 2005.

Moise NS et al: Clinical, radiographic, and bronchial cytologic features of cats with bronchial disease: 65 cases (1980-1986). *J Am Vet Med Assoc* 194:1467-1473, 1989.

Radhakrishnan A et al: Community-acquired infectious pneumonia in puppies: 65 cases (1993-2002), *J Am Vet Med Assoc* 230:1493, 2007.

Wassenaar TM, Gaastra W: Bacterial virulence: can we draw the line? *FEMS Microbiol Lett* 201:1, 2001.

Woolfrey BF, Moody JA: Human infections associated with *Bordetella bronchiseptica*, *Clin Microbiol Rev* 4:243, 1991.

CHAPTER 148

Chronic Bronchitis and Asthma in Cats

PHILIP PADRID, *Chicago, Illinois*

Chronic bronchial disease in cats occurs most commonly in two forms: chronic bronchitis and asthma. *Chronic bronchitis* is defined as an inflammatory disorder of the lower airways that causes a daily cough, for which other causes of cough (including heartworm disease, pneumonia, lungworms, and neoplasia) have been excluded. *Asthma* is more loosely defined as a disorder of the lower airways that causes airflow limitation, which may resolve spontaneously or in response to medical treatment. *Airflow limitation* is generally the result of some combination of airway inflammation, accumulated airway mucus, and airway smooth muscle contraction. The symptoms of asthma can be dramatic, including acute wheeze and respiratory distress. However, sometimes the only symptom of asthma-induced airflow limitation is a daily cough; in humans this is referred to as *cough-variant* asthma.

Definitive diagnosis of asthma is usually based on specific pulmonary function studies that require patient cooperation. Because both disorders, bronchitis and asthma, can cause a daily cough as the only clinical sign, there are many times when it is not possible to distinguish bronchitis from asthma in the feline patient. Nevertheless the diagnosis, prognosis, and treatment options for both diseases overlap with great frequency. The purposes of this article are to (1) review our current understanding of the pathophysiology of bronchial disease and asthma in cats, (2) review common clinical signs and diagnostic tests, (3) suggest rational and novel approaches for treating cats with these debilitating and frequently confusing airway disorders, and (4) discuss reasonable expectations for long-term care.

DIAGNOSIS

Reversible bronchoconstriction is one of the defining features of asthma and can be used to distinguish asthma from chronic bronchitis when the two diagnoses are not clearly separable by clinical means. However, demonstration of reversible bronchoconstriction via pulmonary function studies generally requires patient cooperation, and the equipment and expertise needed to perform these kinds of tests are not available in general veterinary practice. One maneuver can point the practitioner toward a diagnosis of asthma. If a patient is wheezing during the physical examination, I administer terbutaline by inhalation or parenterally (0.01mg/kg intramuscularly [IM]) and reevaluate the patient in 5 to 10 minutes. Resolution of the wheezing implies bronchoconstriction that was reversible and the result of the bronchodilating effects of the medication.

With the exception of this one maneuver, there are no specific tests practical for a general practice that can be used for definitive diagnosis of asthma or bronchitis in cats. Therefore I generally rely on clinical criteria, including:

- A history that includes one or more of these clinical signs: acute wheeze; tachypnea; or respiratory distress, including labored, open-mouth breathing. These signs are usually relieved quickly with some combination of oxygen, bronchodilators, and corticosteroids. The diagnosis of chronic bronchitis requires the presence of a daily cough. In some cases of asthma the only clinical problem may be daily or intermittent chronic cough.
- Radiographic evidence of bronchial wall thickening, usually described as *doughnuts* and *tramlines*. Air trapping may be evidenced by hyperinflated airways. This is seen most prominently on the lateral view and can be appreciated by recognizing the position of the diaphragmatic crus at approximately the level of L1-L2. Radiographs may also demonstrate atelectasis, most commonly of the right middle lung lobe. It is usually easier to see this pattern on a dorsoventral or ventrodorsal exposure because the right middle lung lobe silhouettes with the cardiac silhouette on the lateral view. Atelectasis most commonly occurs in the right middle lung lobe because of mucus accumulation within the bronchus; this airway is most commonly involved because it is the only airway that has a dorsoventral orientation within the bronchial tree and therefore is subject to the effects of gravity.
- Clinicopathologic evidence of airway inflammation, including the finding of large numbers of eosinophils recovered from tracheobronchial secretions in asthmatic airways and nonseptic neutrophils in bronchitic airways.

Response to Therapy As a Diagnostic Measure

Cats with asthma may stop coughing or wheezing within 10 minutes after administration of a bronchodilator. The great majority of cats with bronchitis or asthma respond to high-dose corticosteroid therapy within 5 to 7 days; a patient with a diagnosis of bronchitis or asthma that responds poorly should be reevaluated, and the diagnosis revisited.

These clinical findings, including reversible broncho-constriction and airway inflammation, are strikingly similar to the clinical findings in human asthma. Histologic similarities include hyperplasia and hypertrophy of the mucus-secreting apparatus and airway smooth muscle hyperplasia. Epithelial erosion also is frequently found in association with an eosinophilic infiltrate. Airway hyperreactivity, a defining feature of human asthma, has also been documented in cats with experimentally induced and naturally occurring asthma.

PATHOPHYSIOLOGY

The potential causes of bronchitis and asthma are numerous; however, the airways are capable of responding to noxious stimuli in a limited number of ways. Airway epithelium may hypertrophy, undergo metaplastic change, erode, or ulcerate. Airway goblet cells and submucosal glands may hypertrophy and produce excessive amounts of viscid mucus. Bronchial mucosa and submucosa are usually infiltrated with variable numbers and types of inflammatory cells and may become edematous. Bronchial smooth muscle may remain unaffected, become hypertrophied, or spasm. In almost all cases the unifying and underlying problem is chronic inflammation, but the exact cause remains unproven.

The resulting clinical signs of cough, wheeze, and lethargy are caused by limitation of airflow from excessive mucus secretions, airway edema, and airway narrowing from cellular infiltrates. In addition, cats with asthma may suffer acute airway narrowing from airway smooth muscle constriction. A 50% reduction in the luminal size of an airway results in a 16-fold reduction in the volume of air that flows across that airway. Clearly even small changes in airway diameter can result in dramatic changes in airflow. The clinical implications of this finding are twofold. First, relatively small amounts of mucus, edema, or bronchoconstriction can partially occlude airways and cause a dramatic fall in airflow. Conversely, therapy that results in relatively small increases in airway size may cause a dramatic improvement in clinical signs.

Cough may also result from stimulation of mechanoreceptors located in inflamed and contracted airway smooth muscle. Inappropriate airway smooth muscle contraction, in turn, seems fundamentally linked to inflammation. Although many inflammatory cell types are found within asthmatic airways of humans and cats, eosinophils appear to be primary effector cells in the development of asthmatic airway pathophysiology in both species. Highly charged cationic proteins within eosinophil granules are released into airways and cause epithelial disruption and sloughing. In addition, these granular proteins can make airway smooth muscle more "twitchy" and prone to contraction after exposure to low levels of stimulation (airway hyperreactivity).

Eosinophil–T Lymphocyte Interactions

The pathogenesis of asthmatic airway hyperreactivity is clearly multifactorial. Numerous investigations suggest that the interaction between T lymphocytes and eosinophils within airways may play an important role in the generation of airway inflammation and airway hyperreactivity in human asthma (Beasley et al., 1989; Bradley et al., 1991; NHLBI statement, 2006). Increased numbers of eosinophils and activated T lymphocytes are found in bronchoalveolar lavage (BAL) specimens and bronchial mucosa of patients with asthma. The presence of these cells is correlated with disease severity. Activated T cells are recruited into the airways of asthmatic individuals when they are exposed to aeroallergens. These CD4-positive lymphocytes (among other cells) secrete interleukin-5 (IL-5) to promote eosinophilopoiesis, survival, activation, and recruitment into airways. A Th2-driven cytokine profile has been demonstrated in antigen-induced asthma models in the feline species (Reinero et al., 2004).

Studies in Naturally Occurring Disease

Although coughing and wheezing cats have been identified by owners and veterinarians for almost a century, only in the last 15 years have veterinarians begun to study the disorder in earnest. Dye and associates (1996) identified pulmonary function abnormalities in cats with signs of chronic lower airway inflammation. Some of these cats had increased pulmonary resistance that resolved after treatment with terbutaline, a β_2-agonist, indicating the presence of reversible bronchoconstriction in these patients. In addition, some of these cats experience dramatic bronchoconstriction after exposure to low levels of methacholine, a drug with minimal effects on pulmonary function when used in equivalent doses in nonasthmatic cats. This was the first demonstration of *spontaneous*, naturally occurring airway hyperreactivity and reversible bronchoconstriction in a nonhuman species. In addition, histologic changes in airways from asthmatic cats include epithelial erosion, goblet cell and submucosal gland hyperplasia and hypertrophy, and an increased mass of smooth muscle, which are features of human asthmatic airways. Additional reviews have demonstrated the variation in clinical findings, radiographic patterns, and responses to therapy in cats with bronchitis and asthma (Adamama, 2004; Foster, 2004). This likely is a result of differences in staging these disorders and the fact that other disorders, including pulmonary fibrosis and occult heartworm infection, can mimic the symptoms of bronchial disease in cats (Cohn, 2004; Dillon, 2007).

Experimentally Induced Feline Asthma

Studies of cats with naturally occurring asthma are critical to the understanding and formulation of rational treatment strategies. However, diagnostic studies required for definitive diagnosis use specialized equipment and often require an anesthetized patient. This has limited evaluation of cats with spontaneous disease, and our understanding of the pathogenesis and natural course of asthma in cats has been hampered as a result. Recent technologic advances have allowed us to study pulmonary function in awake, unsedated cats and should yield new insights into the mechanisms of disease.

Experimental models of feline asthma have been developed to better understand the immunologic mechanisms operative in the pathogenesis and perturbation of asthma and as a means to objectively determine responses to therapy. The first model of feline asthma involved antigen sensitization and chronic aerosol challenge with *Ascaris suum* as an antigen. These cats developed persistent airway eosinophilia and hyperresponsiveness to nebulized acetylcholine along with typical morphologic changes observed in spontaneous bronchial disease of cats. These antigen-sensitized cats have elevated serum levels of soluble receptor for IL-2 found within 24 hours of antigen challenge and a decrease in the CD4:CD8 peripheral blood T cell ratio compared to control values. These findings suggest T cell activation in asthmatic cats similar to the findings in humans with asthma (Padrid et al., 1996, 1995b). In this experimental model we found that treatment with cyclosporine A (CsA) dramatically inhibited the pathologic changes in airway structure and function seen in cats not treated with CsA (Padrid, Cozzi, and Leff, 1996). (However, these findings should *not* be interpreted to mean that cyclosporine should be used to treat naturally occurring asthma in cats.) I have also shown that serotonin is a primary mediator in feline mast cells that contribute to airway smooth muscle contraction in vitro (Padrid et al., 1995a). This mediator is absent in human, equine, and canine airways. During an acute asthmatic attack, inhaled antigens within airways promote mast cell degranulation acutely with release of preformed serotonin. These mediators cause sudden contraction of airway smooth muscle. Interestingly, it has long been assumed that histamine released from feline mast cells caused acute bronchoconstriction. This assumption recently has been challenged by the finding that histamine nebulized into cat airways has an unpredictable effect from one cat to another. Specifically histamine may have no effect, it may cause bronchoconstriction, or it may actually dilate feline airways. These findings have potential therapeutic applications, as described later in the chapter.

Reinero and colleagues (2005) developed an experimental feline model in which cats were sensitized and chronically challenged with either Bermuda grass allergen (BGA) or house dust mites to mimic well-recognized antigenic triggers of human asthma. These cats produce allergen-specific immunoglobulin (Ig)E, allergen-specific serum and BAL fluid (BALF) IgG or IgA, airway hyperreactivity, airway eosinophilia, an acute Th2 cytokine profile in peripheral blood mononuclear cells and BALF cells, and histologic evidence of airway remodeling. This model has been particularly helpful in evaluating specific immunomodulating treatment strategies. For example, cats sensitized and challenged with BGA to develop the asthmatic phenotype were then treated with rush immunotherapy (parenteral high doses of BGA). These cats had significantly reduced eosinophil counts. More recently Norris and associates (2003) used CpG motifs (microbial oligodeoxynucleotide products that modulate activity in human and murine lymphocytes) in cats with BGA-induced airway inflammation and hyperreactivity. This approach dampened the eosinophilic response normally seen in these antigen sensitized and challenged cats; however, the hyperactivity within airways was not affected.

CLINICAL FINDINGS IN FELINE BRONCHITIS AND ASTHMA

Incidence and Prevalence

Currently there are no reliable data regarding the incidence and prevalence of asthma in cats. The prevalence of lower airway disease in the general adult cat population is estimated to be approximately 1%; prevalence in the Siamese breed may be 5% or greater. In 2000 a website (fritzthebrave.com) was developed to draw attention to the diagnosis and treatment of feline asthma. One result of this website was the generation of a "list-serve" with greater than 500 members, each of whom is the owner of one or more cats with asthma or bronchitis. A poll of these members revealed that more than 15% of the owners represented by this relatively random sample had Siamese cats (Kathryn Hopper, personal communication).

Clinical Signs

Clinical signs are variable. Cats with bronchitis have a daily cough and may be absolutely symptom free between episodes of cough. Alternatively they may be tachypneic at rest. Asthmatic cats may cough, wheeze, and struggle to breath on a daily basis. In mild cases symptoms may be limited to occasional and brief coughing. Some cats with asthma may be asymptomatic between occasional episodes of acute airway obstruction. Severely affected cats may have a persistent daily cough and experience many episodes of life-threatening acute bronchoconstriction.

As previously outlined, a common problem for the practitioner is to distinguish between chronic bronchitis and asthma as the cause of a chronic cough in cats. Although these two disorders are frequently lumped together under the title of chronic bronchial disease or lower airway disease, the two disorders may require different therapeutic approaches and often have different prognoses. By definition all cats with chronic bronchitis have daily cough. Some cats with asthma may be asymptomatic between occasional episodes of acute airway obstruction. Other asthmatic cats may cough occasionally and demonstrate frequent tachypnea. Importantly, asthmatic cats but not bronchitic cats may benefit from bronchodilator treatment.

Physical Examination

There are no consistent physical examination findings on which to base a diagnosis of asthma. In fact, cats with bronchitis or asthma may have a normal physical examination at rest. Conversely, respiratory distress primarily during expiration is the hallmark of these disorders in cats. Adventitious sounds, including crackles, often are heard. Wheezes are more characteristic of feline asthma.

DIAGNOSTIC TESTS

Thoracic Radiographs

Routine survey chest radiographs may be normal and should not cause the practitioner to abandon the diagnosis of asthma. However, frequently radiographs may demonstrate diffuse prominent bronchial markings consistent with inflammatory airways. Radiographic signs of increased lung lucency and flattening and caudal displacement of the diaphragm represent hyperinflation and suggest air trapping. In my experience approximately 10% of chest radiographs of cats with bronchial disease have increased density within the right middle lung lobe associated with a mediastinal shift to the right. This is evidence of atelectasis. In more extreme cases fluffy, ill-defined heavy interstitial infiltrates in multiple lung lobes may be appreciated. The cause of these changes in cats with lower airway disease may be multiple small areas of atelectasis in multiple lung lobes resulting from multiple diffuse small mucous plugs. This presents a diagnostic challenge because this radiographic change is consistent with a number of disorders, including neoplasia and diffuse interstitial pneumonitis.

Bronchoscopy

I emphasize that bronchoscopy is rarely required to make an accurate diagnosis of bronchitis or asthma in feline patients. Bronchoscopy in healthy cats is not a trivial undertaking. In cats with cough and respiratory compromise bronchoscopy may be a life-threatening procedure and should only be performed by persons adequately and formally trained in the technique (Johnson and Drazenovich, 2007). Instead the previously described historical and physical examination findings and results of chest radiography are sufficient to make a *tentative* diagnosis. *Definitive* diagnosis usually can be made in these patients by a strongly positive response to therapy. In fact, in my experience the primary indication for bronchoscopy in these patients occurs when there is not an otherwise predictable cessation or minimization of clinical signs after 6 to 7 days of aggressive corticosteroid treatment.

Tracheobronchial Culture

The presence of a mixed population of aerobic bacteria in airways has been reported previously in cats with bronchial disease. However, neither the lower airway nor the lung parenchyma of healthy cats is sterile. Organisms usually considered as pathogens such as *Klebsiella* and *Pseudomonas* spp. can be recovered from healthy feline airways. To my knowledge studies designed to correlate the clinical status of asthmatic or bronchitic cats with the presence or absence of bacteria within the airway have not been attempted or published. In fact, one well-designed study showed that cats with signs of bronchial disease had fewer positive airway cultures than a cohort population of healthy cats (Dye et al., 1996).

It is my experience that bacteria isolated from the asthmatic or bronchitic feline airway most commonly reflect colonization rather than true infection. The role of *Mycoplasma* may be an exception to this (Chandler and Lappin, 2002). *Mycoplasma* (and certain viruses) can degrade neutral endopeptidase, which is an enzyme that is responsible for biodegradation of substance P, a protein capable of causing bronchoconstriction and edema in the feline airway. *Mycoplasma* might then indirectly prolong the effects of substance P on airway smooth muscle. It is tempting to speculate that *Mycoplasma* or viruses such as herpes, which can remain dormant in feline airways, might be responsible for increasing the levels of substance P in cat airways and contribute to spontaneous bronchoconstriction.

Tracheobronchial Cytology

Until the 1980s it was generally assumed that eosinophils played only a beneficial role in the immune system by protecting against parasite infestation. However, within the last 20 years it has become clear that the presence of these cells in the wrong place at the wrong time can result in significant cellular and tissue damage. Therefore it is of great interest that eosinophils (often 20% to 25% of total count) can be recovered in large numbers from the tracheobronchial washings of many healthy cats (Padrid, 1991). These cells appear to cause no damage to the local tissue environment, and their presence should not be assumed to indicate allergy or parasitism. Similarly, alveolar macrophages are a normal cell within the lung parenchyma and are the most common cells recovered from BALF obtained from healthy cats. These cells do not reliably represent granulomatous or histiocytic inflammation when obtained in BAL from bronchitic or asthmatic cats.

Consistent with prior remarks regarding the role of bronchoscopy in the diagnosis of feline bronchial disease, I do not routinely collect tracheobronchial washings to make the diagnosis of asthma or bronchitis in felines. These diagnoses are made by careful history taking, physical examination findings, radiographic interpretation, and response to therapy. It is only when these criteria are not fulfilled, and especially if the patient does not respond to standard treatment protocols, that the diagnosis is revisited and bronchoscopy/tracheal washings are considered. Although some clinicians do prefer to obtain airway washings and culture before initiation of long-term respiratory therapy, the points made previously should be considered when interpreting the cytologic picture or culture results.

TREATMENT OF BRONCHITIS AND ASTHMA IN CATS

The primary signs of asthma include cough and wheeze, and these signs are frequently the result of some degree of airway smooth muscle contraction. In clinical practice it is usually difficult to distinguish between chronic bronchitis and asthma in feline patients. It is tempting to treat coughing cats with suspected bronchial disease by using only bronchodilators to relax the airway smooth muscle contraction. Although this is a central method of treatment when acute signs develop, it is critically important to understand that human (and perhaps feline) asthmatic and bronchitic airways show evidence of chronic ongoing inflammation whether the patient is symptomatic or not. Therefore treatment strategies are most successful if they are directed toward *decreasing the underlying inflammatory component* of the disease in addition to addressing the acute clinical signs of cough, wheeze, and increased respiratory effort.

Long-Term Corticosteroids

The most effective long-term treatment of chronic non-infectious bronchial disease is systemically administered corticosteroids. This class of drugs is most likely to suppress airway inflammation, a process orchestrated by a network of proteins (cytokines) that act on circulating and structural airway cells. An important effect of steroids is to inhibit the synthesis of genes for cytokines that are important in generating airway inflammation.

The side effects of these medications given for long periods are undesirable. Fortunately inhaled steroids have become available that do not cause systemic side effects, and this therapeutic approach has greatly enhanced our ability to treat patients with bronchial disease (see Aerosol Delivery of Steroids and Bronchodilators later in the chapter). I begin treatment of bronchitic or asthmatic cats with signs that occur more than once weekly (without medication) with prednisolone, 1 to 2 mg/kg orally every 12 hours for 5 to 7 days. At this point most newly diagnosed cats have greatly diminished signs. The dosage of steroids is then tapered slowly, over at least 2 to 3 months. This approach is much more effective than giving low doses of prednisone for short periods and in response to acute flare-ups.

Patients with symptoms that occur less than once weekly (without medication) are generally not considered to have chronic active inflammatory airways. These patients may be treated safely with bronchodilators when needed.

Some cats are managed effectively and safely by administration of low-dose, alternate-day corticosteroids. However, most cats with chronic bronchial disease continue to wheeze/cough when treated in this conservative manner. For patients with a positive response to higher doses of consistently administered systemic corticosteroids, inhaled corticosteroid therapy should be encouraged as an alternative to reduce adverse effects (see Aerosol Delivery of Steroids and Bronchodilators later in the chapter).

Injectable Steroids

Parenteral administration of long-acting corticosteroids is limited to patients for whom no other method of drug administration is feasible. In this setting injection of methylprednisolone (Depo Medrol, Phizer Animal Health, 10 to 20 mg IM total dose) once every 4 to 8 weeks may be effective. This therapy is very likely to result in significant/serious side effects, including weight gain, diabetes mellitus, and reduced immunity and represents the treatment of last resort.

Bronchodilators

The use of bronchodilators is based on the assumption that clinically significant bronchoconstriction is evident. Cats develop naturally occurring and clinically significant bronchoconstriction that in severe cases can be life threatening (Padrid, 2000). Bronchodilator drugs can be beneficial to these patients. These drugs are classified generally as β-receptor agonists, methylxanthine derivatives, or anticholinergics.

Most adrenergic agonists have variable α- and β-receptor affinity. Nonselective β-receptor agonists such as isoproterenol or mixed α- and β-receptor agonists such as epinephrine are more likely to produce cardiovascular side effects than similarly administered selective β-agonists. Consequently drugs with preferential affinity for β₂-receptors are likely to provide more effective bronchodilation with fewer side effects. The two principal β₂-agonists currently marketed in preparations that can be readily and regularly used in small animals are terbutaline sulfate and albuterol sulfate. A discussion of these drugs follows.

Terbutaline Sulfate

Terbutaline is a selective β₂-receptor agonist that produces relaxation of the smooth muscle found principally in bronchial, vascular, and uterine tissues. The exact mechanism by which activation of β₂-receptors results in smooth muscle relaxation is not totally understood, but it likely involves intracellular cyclic adenosine monophosphate–induced suppression of the kinase controlling myosin and actin interaction.

Terbutaline is available as a tablet, elixir, and injectable preparation suitable for subcutaneous or intramuscular use. The dosage rate has been reported to range from 0.01 mg/kg given subcutaneously or intramuscularly up to 0.1 to 0.2 mg/kg every 8 hours given by mouth. The *major clinical indication* for terbutaline is treatment of the patient with acute respiratory difficulty when inhaled albuterol therapy is not possible. Infrequently terbutaline is prescribed as a chronic oral treatment for bronchodilation.

Many veterinarians use terbutaline as an emergency drug to treat asthmatic cats that present in respiratory distress. The drug is similarly effective in humans. The home use of a rapid-acting bronchodilator such as inhaled albuterol or injected terbutaline can preclude the need for a stressful emergency room visit. I teach my clients to use an inhaler (see Aerosol Delivery of Steroids and Bronchodilators later in the chapter) or to administer terbutaline subcutaneously to their asthmatic cats at a dose of 0.01 mg/kg subcutaneously or intramuscularly. An obvious beneficial response generally occurs within 15 to 30 minutes. This may be repeated if a significant benefit is not observed after one dose. To determine if the drug has been absorbed and if a beneficial effect has occurred, heart rate and respiratory rate and effort are monitored before drug administration. A heart rate that approaches 240 beats/min suggests that the drug has been absorbed. A respiratory rate or effort (or both) that declines by 50% or more suggests a beneficial effect.

At usual doses terbutaline has little effect on β₁-receptors; thus direct cardiostimulatory effects are unlikely. However, terbutaline should always be used with care in patients that may have increased sensitivity to adrenergic agents—in particular cats with preexisting cardiac disease, diabetes mellitus, hyperthyroidism, hypertension, or seizure disorders. All β₂-agonists may lower plasma potassium; thus in at-risk patients receiving long-term terbutaline therapy, it may be prudent to monitor serum potassium levels. In clinical practice and experimentally it is rare to find β₂ agonist–associated hypokalemia in cats (Petruska et al., 1997). When terbutaline is used with other sympathomimetics or concurrently with digoxin, tricyclic antidepressants, and monoamine oxidase inhibitors, the risk of adverse cardiovascular effects increases. These potential effects are more likely in patients with preexisting cardiac disease, especially hypertrophic cardiomyopathy. Use with various inhalation anesthetics may predispose the patients to ventricular arrhythmias.

Albuterol Sulfate

Albuterol is a selective β_2-receptor agonist with pharmacologic properties similar to those of terbutaline. Albuterol is available as a tablet and syrup and is contained in various inhalants. I have only used the inhaled form of albuterol in feline patients. The inhaled form of albuterol comes as a single-strength 17g metered-dose inhaler (MDI) and delivers 90 mcg per actuation of the device.

The pharmacokinetic profile of albuterol in cats has not been reported. When administered by inhalation to humans, albuterol produces significant bronchodilation within 15 minutes that lasts for 3 to 4 hours. It is also well absorbed orally and may have bronchodilatory effects for up to 8 hours. Anecdotal experience with this drug in clinical practice suggests a similar pharmacokinetic profile in cats. Albuterol undergoes extensive hepatic metabolism. After oral administration approximately 58% to 78% of the dose is excreted in the urine over 24 hours, with 60% of the drug in an inactive form.

Rarely adverse effects include mild skeletal muscle tremors and restlessness, which generally subside after 2 to 3 days. As with terbutaline, care should be exercised when administering albuterol to patients with preexisting cardiac disease, diabetes mellitus, hyperthyroidism, hypertension, and seizure disorders. Potential drug interactions are similar to those of terbutaline.

Methylxanthines: Theophylline and Aminophylline

The methylxanthines relax smooth muscle, particularly bronchial smooth muscle, stimulate the central nervous system (CNS), and act as a weak cardiac stimulant and diuretic. Although I do not use this class of drugs to treat feline patients with asthma, methylxanthines are used frequently in the veterinary profession and thus are addressed briefly.

Theophylline is considered a less potent bronchodilator than the β-agonists (Bjermer, 2001). It has been shown in other species to produce centrally mediated increased respiratory effort for any given alveolar Pco_2; to improve diaphragmatic contractility with reduced diaphragmatic fatigue; to mildly increase myocardial contractility and heart rate; and to increase CNS activity, gastric acid secretion, and urine output. All of these effects have not been demonstrated in cats. Interestingly, at therapeutic concentrations of theophylline only adenosine receptor blockade has been reliably demonstrated. This has been suggested to explain the varied effects of theophylline.

Because of the relatively low therapeutic index and pharmacokinetic characteristics of theophylline, dosage rates should be based on lean body mass. The dosage depends on the preparation used. In standard preparations the recommended dosage for cats is 4 mg/kg every 8 to 12 hours. When using sustained-release preparations a dosage of 25 mg/kg every 24 hours should be considered.

The pharmacokinetics of theophylline have been studied extensively in a number of species (Boothe, 2006). After oral administration, peak plasma rates occur within 1.5 hours. The rate of absorption is limited principally by dissolution of the dosage form in the gut. Bioavailability in cats is generally greater than 90% when nonsustained-release preparations are used; however, sustained-release preparations may have a more variable bioavailability. In general the anhydrous theophylline tablet is preferred. A chronopharmacokinetic study in cats showed that evening administration is associated with better bioavailability and less fluctuation in plasma drug level (Dye et al., 1990).

Although theophylline can produce CNS stimulation and gastrointestinal disturbances, these effects are most often associated with excessive dosing and resolve with dosage adjustments. Seizures or cardiac arrhythmias may occur in severe toxicity. There are a number of known drug interactions with theophylline, including enrofloxacin (Baytril). The effects of theophylline may be diminished by phenytoin or phenobarbital and enhanced by cimetidine, allopurinol, clindamycin, and lincomycin. The effects of theophylline and β-adrenergic blockers may be antagonized if they are administered concurrently. Theophylline increases the likelihood of arrhythmias induced by adrenergic agonists and halothane and the likelihood of seizures with ketamine.

Antibiotics

There is no objective evidence that bacterial infection plays a significant role in the cause or continuation of feline chronic bronchitis or asthma. Similarly there is no objective evidence that antibiotic therapy has any effect on the duration or intensity of signs displayed by the cat with chronic bronchial disease. It is important to remember that the clinical signs of asthma in cats frequently wax and wane both in severity and in frequency of occurrence. Many anecdotal reports describe the therapeutic effect of antibiotics in controlling asthmatic symptoms, but these reports are consistent with the "waxing and waning" nature of the symptom in nontreated cases.

A positive culture result obtained from a tracheobronchial wash does not necessarily imply the presence of a clinically significant airway infection and should not automatically prompt the clinician to initiate antibiotic therapy. In my opinion antibiotics are rarely indicated for cats with chronic bronchitis or asthma and are appropriate only when there is strong evidence of superimposed airway infection. This may be inferred from the growth of a pure bacterial culture on a primary culture plate from material obtained from tracheobronchial secretions because the concentration of aerobic bacteria recovered from the airways of healthy cats rarely exceeds 5×10^3 organisms per milliliter. In contrast, growth of a single organism recovered without the use of enrichment broth implies more than 10^5 organisms per milliliter, and this is consistent with an infected airway in humans. Antibiotic therapy is then based on sensitivity data. Prophylactic or long-term therapy should be avoided unless there is documentation of a chronic airway infection, which is uncommon.

One possible exception to these statements involves *Mycoplasma* spp. *Mycoplasma* has been isolated from the airway of as many as 25% of cats with signs of lower airway disease, but it has not been cultured from the airway of healthy cats. For this reason and because it has the potential to cause significant structural damage to airway epithelium, it may be prudent to treat any cat with a *Mycoplasma*-positive airway culture with an appropriate antibiotic such as doxycycline or azithromycin.

Cyproheptadine

Cyproheptadine (Periactin, Merck Sharp and Dohme) is marketed as an antihistamine; however, it has been used for years as an appetite stimulant for depressed or anorectic cats because of its antiserotonin properties. As mentioned earlier, serotonin is a primary mediator released from activated mast cells into feline airways and causes acute smooth muscle contraction (bronchoconstriction) in cats but not in humans. I have shown that the ability of cyproheptadine to block serotonin receptors in muscle cells is effective in preventing antigen-induced airway smooth muscle constriction in vitro. Limited clinical observations in asthmatic cats have supported these in vitro findings. The primary indication for this drug is a trial in the symptomatic asthmatic cat already receiving maximal doses of terbutaline and corticosteroids. Cyproheptadine comes in both pill and liquid form and is dosed at 2 to 4 mg orally every 12 hours (Boothe, 2006). A beneficial therapeutic response may not be seen for 4 to 7 days; but depression, the primary side effect of this drug, may be observed 24 hours after administration. Depression is not life threatening but may cause the owner to discontinue cyproheptadine therapy.

Antileukotrienes: Zafirlukast, Montelukast, and Zileuton

Leukotrienes belong to a family of inflammatory mediators that are derived from arachidonic acid and are known collectively as eicosanoids. The leukotrienes LTC_4, LTD_4, and LTE_4 collectively are known as the cysteinyl leukotrienes and play an important role in airway inflammation. They produce mucus hypersecretion, increased vascular permeability, and mucosal edema; induce potent bronchoconstriction; and act as chemoattractants to inflammatory cells, particularly eosinophils and neutrophils.

The orally administered antileukotriene drugs are competitive, highly selective, and potent inhibitors of the production or the function of LTC_4, LTD_4 and LTE_4. Specifically, zileuton (Zyflo, Abbott Laboratories) blocks leukotriene biosynthesis by inhibiting production of the 5-lipoxygenase enzyme, whereas both montelukast and zafirlukast block adhesion of leukotrienes to their common leukotriene receptor (cys-LT1). In humans leukotrienes inhibit asthmatic responses to allergen, aspirin, exercise, and cold dry air. In addition, leukotriene blockade has been shown in many clinical trials to decrease the amount and frequency of administration of corticosteroids in steroid-dependent human asthmatics.

There have been few investigations regarding the role of leukotrienes in feline airway disease. Although LTE4 is found in increased concentrations in urine of asthmatic humans, no such increase in urinary LTE4 was found in 20 cats with signs of bronchial disease or in cats with experimentally induced asthma in unpublished studies that I conducted (1995) (Mellema, 1998). More recently in another experimental model of feline asthma, no increase in cysteinyl leukotrienes was found in either urine or BALF after challenge exposure to sensitizing antigen (Norris et al., 2003). In addition, zafirlukast did not inhibit airway inflammation or airway hyperreactivity in this feline asthma model (Reinero et al., 2005). Thus there is no current evidence that drugs that affect leukotriene synthesis or receptor ligation play a significant role in the treatment of feline or canine respiratory disease. However, there is at least one claim of efficacy using zafirlukast (1 to 2 mg/kg BID) or montelukast (0.5 to 1 mg/kg SID) for treatment of feline asthma (Mandelker and Padrid, 2000).

Aerosol Delivery of Steroids and Bronchodilators

Aerosol administration of the corticosteroid fluticasone and the bronchodilator albuterol rely on delivery of drug to the distal airways, which in turn depends on the size of the aerosol particles and various respiratory parameters such as tidal volume and inspiratory flow rate. Even in cooperative humans only approximately 10% to 30% of the inhaled dose enters the lungs. Recent studies in cats have demonstrated that passive inhalation through a spacer-mask combination (Aerokat, Aerokat Trudell Medical International, Inc.) is an effective method of delivering sufficient medication to be clinically effective (Reinero et al., 2005; Kirchvink et al., 2006).

Drugs for inhalation typically come in a rectangular MDI or a round "diskus" form. At the present time only the MDI form is practical for use in animals. Recently the propellants used for these medications have changed. The most effective means of using an MDI involves coordination between inhalation and actuation of the device, something that is not reliable in most infants, small children, or animals. For this reason an alternative involves the use of a spacer device and a mask specifically designed for cats (Fig. 148-1). A small, aerosol-holding chamber is attached to an MDI on one end and a face mask on the other. The spacer is approximately the size of the inner cardboard roll used with toilet paper. The MDI supplies precise doses of the aerosol drug, and the holding chamber contains the aerosol so it can be inhaled when the patients inspires. The mask is designed to cover the nose of the cat. The designers of the Aerokat spacer have shown that a holding chamber with a length of 11 cm and a diameter of 3.5 cm or larger delivered almost all of a therapeutically "ideal" aerosol (i.e., aerosol of equivalent aerodynamic diameter ≤2.8 μm) produced by an MDI; and in some cases delivery was enhanced because of evaporation of large, suspended particles (Foley, personal communication). The choice of spacer is relevant because cats have a tidal volume of between 5 to 10 ml of inspired air per pound of body weight. Currently only the Aerokat brand spacers have been designed specifically based on the tidal volume characteristics of the cat. Using these spacer devices, cats

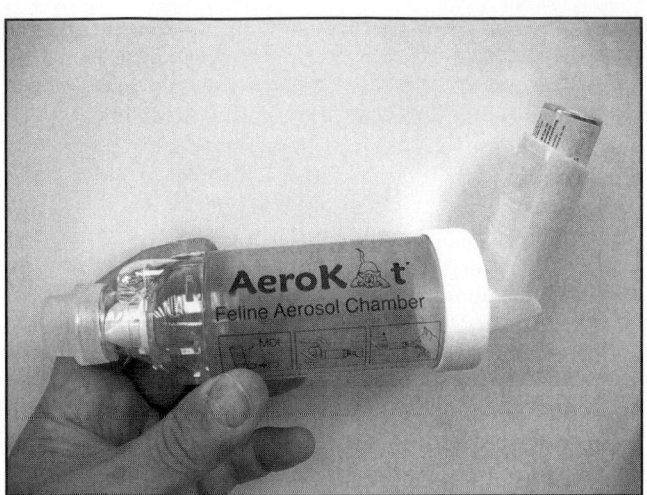

Fig. 148-1 The Aerokat spacer is specifically made for the feline species. The MDI fits snugly on one end, and the mask fits comfortably on the patient's nose. A float valve is built into the front of the spacer to let the owner know when the patient takes a breath.

inhale the majority of drug propelled into the spacer by breathing 7 to 10 times through the spacer-mask combination after actuation of the MDI. It is important to teach the owner to observe the pet actually breathing because cats initially may hold their breaths when introduced to this form of treatment.

The procedure is not time-consuming, but it can be helpful to acclimate the cat to the mask. When administering inhalation therapy, the MDI is first shaken to open an internal valve within the canister, and then it is attached to the spacer. The mask attached to the other end of the spacer is placed snuggly on the animal's nose or muzzle, and the MDI is pressed to release the medication into the spacer.

Fluticasone Propionate

The most commonly used inhaled corticosteroid is fluticasone propionate (Flovent, GlaxoSmithKline), a synthetic corticosteroid with an 18-fold higher affinity for the corticosteroid receptor when compared to dexamethasone. Binding of the steroid to this receptor results in a new molecular complex that leads to up- or down-regulation of the gene and its products. Like other corticosteroids, fluticasone acts to inhibit mast cells, eosinophils, lymphocytes, neutrophils, and macrophages involved in the generation and exacerbation of allergic airway inflammation by transcriptional regulation of these target genes. Preformed and newly secreted mediators, including histamine, eicosanoids, leukotrienes and multiple cytokines, are inhibited as well.

Fluticasone is a large molecule and acts topically within the airway mucosa. Because there is poor absorption across gut epithelium, there is minimal oral systemic bioavailability. Plasma levels do not predict therapeutic effects. This explains the lack of systemic side effects; however, it also suggests that clinically effective absorption into the airway mucosa is also delayed. Therefore optimal clinical effects may not occur for 1 to 2 weeks.

Fluticasone has been used to treat cats with bronchial asthma at least since 1993. Since then a number of manuscripts have demonstrated the clinical effectiveness of fluticasone for treatment of cats with allergic rhinitis, bronchitis, and asthma (both naturally occurring and experimentally induced). There have been no controlled published studies to determine the optimal dose or interval for use of fluticasone in cats; however, there are anecdotal reports that reference more than 500 small animal patients treated with fluticasone over a period covering 1995 through 2006. Dosage recommendations are based on these observations and recently published studies.

Fluticasone comes in three strengths: 44 mcg, 110 mcg, and 220 mcg per actuation. I have found that 44-mcg dosing twice daily does not consistently result in acceptable clinical responses. For cats with mild-to-moderate disease, 110 mcg given twice daily frequently results in clinical responses equivalent to that achieved by administration of 5-mg oral doses of prednisone given BID. Cats with more serious disease may require 220 mcg inhaled BID. In my experience administration of fluticasone more than twice daily has not resulted in clinical benefit.

Albuterol Sulfate

The pharmacology of albuterol, a selective β_2-adrenergic bronchodilator, has been described previously. This drug is available through different manufacturers and is commonly prescribed as Ventolin (GlaxoSmithKline) or Proventil (Schering Corp.). Albuterol only comes in a single uniform strength (90 mcg per inhalation). Albuterol usually results in relaxation of airway smooth muscles within 1 to 5 minutes; thus the effect is almost immediate. This drug should be used in animals with documented or assumed bronchoconstriction. Symptoms that may indicate bronchoconstriction are wheeze, noisy lower airway breathing, prolonged expiratory phase of ventilation, and coughing. Albuterol can be used once daily before administering fluticasone or as needed for acute coughing and wheezing. In emergency cases albuterol can be used every 30 minutes for up to 4 to 6 hours without serious side effects.

The use of inhaled medications to treat asthma and bronchitis is considered the standard of care in humans and is now widely recommended for cats with chronic bronchial disease. This approach avoids many of the side effects previously seen in patients treated with systemic medications.

References and Suggested Reading

Beasley R et al: Cellular events in the bronchi in mild asthma and after bronchial provocation, *Am Rev Respir Dis* 139:806, 1989.

Bjermer J: History and future perspectives of treating asthma as a systemic and small airways disease, *Respir Med* 95(9):703, 2001.

Boothe DM: Drugs affecting the respiratory system. In King LG: *Textbook of respiratory disease in dogs and cats*, St Louis, 2006, Elsevier, p 236.

Bradley BL et al: Eosinophils, T lymphocytes, mast cells, neutrophils, and macrophages in bronchial biopsies from atopic asthma: comparison with atopic non-asthma and normal controls and relationship to bronchial hyper-responsiveness, *J Allergy Clin Immunol* 88:661, 1991.

Chandler JC, Lappin MR: Mycoplasma respiratory infections in small animals: 17 cases (1988-1999), *J Am Anim Hosp Assoc* 38(2):111, 2002.

Dye JA et al: Chronopharmacokinetics of theophylline in the cat, *J Vet Pharmacol Ther* 13(3):278, 1990.

Dye JA et al: Bronchopulmonary disease in the cat: historical, physical, radiographic, clinicopathologic and pulmonary functional evaluation of 24 affected and 15 healthy cats, *J Vet Intern Med* 10:385, 1996.

Foley M: Trudell Medical International, Inc., London, Ontario, Canada, personal communication.

Johnson LR, Drazenovich TL: Flexible bronchoscopy and bronchoalveolar lavage in 68 cats (2001-2006), *J Vet Intern Med* 21(2):219, 2007.

Kirchvink N et al: Inhaled fluticasone reduces bronchial responsiveness and airway inflammation in cats with mild chronic bronchitis, *J Feline Med Surg* 8(1):45, 2006.

Mandelker L: Experimental drug therapy for respiratory disorders in dogs and cats, *Vet Clin North Am Small Anim Pract* 30(6):1357, 2000.

Norris CR et al: Concentrations of cysteinyl leukotrienes in urine and bronchoalveolar lavage fluid of cats with experimentally induced asthma, *Am J Vet Res* 64(11):1449, 2003.

Padrid PA: Feline asthma, *Vet Clin North Am Small Anim Pract* 30(6):1279, 2000.

Padrid PA, Cozzi P, Leff AR: Cyclosporine A attenuates the development of chronic airway hyper-responsiveness and histological alterations in immune-sensitized cats, *Am J Respir Crit Care Med* 154:1812, 1996.

Padrid PA et al: Cyproheptadine-induced attenuation of type-I immediate hypersensitivity reactions of airway smooth muscle from immune-sensitized cats, *Am J Vet Res* 56:109, 1995a.

Padrid PA et al: Persistent airway hyper-responsiveness and histological alterations after chronic antigen challenge in cats, *Am J Respir Crit Care Med* 151:184, 1995b.

Petruska JM et al: Cardiovascular effects after inhalation of large doses of albuterol dry powder in rats, monkeys, and dogs: a species comparison, *Fundam Appl Toxicol* 40(1):52, 1997.

Reinero CR et al: An experimental model of allergic asthma in cats sensitized to house dust mite or Bermuda grass allergen, *Arch Allergy Immunol* 135:177, 2004.

Reinero CR et al: Effects of drug treatment on inflammation and hyperreactivity of airways and on immune variables in cats with experimentally induced asthma, *Am J Vet Res* 66(7):1121, 2005.

CHAPTER 149

Bacterial Pneumonia

RICHARD B. FORD, *Raleigh, North Carolina*

Acquired inflammatory lung disease associated with bacterial colonization of tissues in the lower respiratory tract (lower airways and lung parenchyma) constitutes a clinical definition of bacterial pneumonia. Bacterial pneumonia occurs with moderate frequency in dogs but is considerably less common in cats. Ranking as one of the most complex life-threatening infections encountered in companion animal practice, bacterial pneumonia poses significant diagnostic and therapeutic challenges to the clinician.

INFECTION OF THE LOWER AIRWAYS AND LUNG

Complicating basic research into the pathogenesis of lung infection is the fact that experimentally induced bacterial pneumonia in healthy animals is difficult to achieve. In normal adult animals the oral cavity, the upper respiratory tract, and trachea are host to a variety of pathogenic bacteria, yet the ability of these pathogens to actually infect is limited by exceptionally effective host defenses unique to the lower respiratory tract. This suggests that other underlying mechanisms must work collectively to the point of causing airway or lung injury with subsequent bacterial colonization of airway epithelium or interstitial cells of the lung. The nature of bacterial infection and lower respiratory tract injury is complex.

The mere presence of bacteria in lower airways does not define bacterial pneumonia. In healthy dogs and cats resident bacteria from the oral-nasal cavity can be recovered from respiratory epithelium as far into the respiratory tract as the carina. For bacteria to actually infect the lung parenchyma, colonization must occur. This requires that organisms have access to a portal of entry. The larynx and trachea represent the most common portal for lower respiratory tract infections, but a second portal of entry to the respiratory tract is via hematogenous dissemination of bacteria from a point of distant infection. Bacterial pneumonia in dogs results predominantly from bacteria that enter via the larynx and trachea. Bacterial pneumonia in cats is poorly described in the literature. Most authors would agree that bacterial lung infections occur much less often in cats than in dogs; however, hematogenous dissemination of pathogenic bacteria leading to bacterial pneumonia actually may occur more often in cats than in dogs (Foster et al., 2004).

Subsequent to colonization, bacterial adherence must occur. This entails a complementary and specific interaction between receptors on the epithelial cell surface and macromolecules on the cell wall surface of bacteria called *adhesins. Bordetella bronchiseptica*, a common pathogen recovered from dogs and cats with bacterial pneumonia, expresses a common set of secreted and surface-associated adhesins such as filamentous hemagglutinin, fimbriae, and periactin that significantly influence colonization and virulence.

Extracellular proteins called *invasins* are produced by bacteria and act to break down host defenses and facilitate the spread of bacteria. Unique to the invading pathogen, these proteins serve as "spreading factors" (hyaluronidase, collagenase, and streptokinase). Other types of invasins, sometimes called exotoxins, cause direct injury to cell membranes, leading to cell lysis (hemolysins, leukocidins, streptolysin).

Pathogenic bacteria that are successful in their attempt to infect the patient possess structural or biochemical features that enable them to resist host defense mechanisms, specifically phagocytosis and adaptive immune responses (humoral and cell-mediated immunity). Specific to individual bacterial species are soluble proteins (toxins) secreted during periods of exponential growth. Bacterial toxins are highly specific in their action but are inherently unstable. Over time these proteins lose their toxic properties but retain antigen properties, as evidenced by their use in some vaccines. The activity of bacterial toxins has considerable influence on the virulence of the organism, the onset of clinical illness, the severity of infection, and even the prognosis.

RISK FACTORS

In addition to intrinsic virulence factors associated with individual bacterial pathogens, compromised host defenses play a critical role in an individual's risk of acquiring bacterial pneumonia. Increased age, underlying systemic illness, compromised immunity, and poor nutrition are often cited. However, these are largely intangible factors that are difficult to quantify and offer little predictive value in the clinical setting. In my experience young dogs and cats, in contrast to older animals, are at greatest risk of developing bacterial pneumonia. Critical factors contributing to morbidity include immunization status,

congenital disorders (megaesophagus, ciliary dyskinesia), environment (especially housing, sanitation, and ventilation), exposure to clusters of dogs, and coinfection (e.g., calicivirus infection in kittens or canine distemper virus in puppies). Aspiration pneumonia, commonly associated with acquired megaesophagus, myasthenia gravis, and laryngeal paralysis, is perhaps the single most common cause of bacterial pneumonia seen in adult dogs. Systemic or local bacterial infection (e.g., bacteremia, phlebitis, or periodontitis) is also a predisposing risk factor for bacterial pneumonia.

TYPES OF BACTERIA

Several studies have reported on the types of bacteria isolated from dogs and cats with bacterial pneumonia. These findings are summarized in Box 149-1. Gram-positive and gram-negative aerobes are commonly reported. Anaerobic infections, typically recovered in patients coinfected with either enteric or staphylococcal infections, do occur but are less frequently reported. Most *Mycoplasma* isolates recovered from the airways of animals have been found to coexist with other bacteria. Limited reports involving both dogs and cats with evidence of lower respiratory tract disease have identified *Mycoplasma* spp. as the sole bacterial isolate (Chandler and Lappin, 2002). Although the precise role of *Mycoplasma* spp. as a primary pathogen in bacterial pneumonia in dogs and cats requires further definition, some clinicians request culture for *mycoplasma* on separate media when attempting bacterial isolation from airway washings.

Bacterial pneumonia that develops subsequent to aspiration of gastric contents or opportunistic infections is more likely to be associated with gram-negative bacteria. However, from the available literature it is not possible to establish true prevalence of one bacterial pathogen over another as a causative agent in bacterial pneumonia. The most commonly reported gram-positive bacteria include *Staphylococcus, Streptococcus*, and *Enterococcus* spp. Among the gram-negative bacterial isolates, *B. bronchiseptica* and *Pasteurella* are the most frequently reported

---

Box 149-1

Pathogens Commonly Associated With Bacterial Pneumonia in Dogs and Cats

Canine
- *Bordetella bronchiseptica*
- *Staphylococcus* spp.
- *Streptococcus* spp.
- *Enterococcus* spp.
- *Escherichia coli*
- *Pseudomonas* spp.
- *Pasteurella* spp.
- *Klebsiella* spp.
- *Bacteroides*

Feline
- *Pasteurella* spp.
- *Bordetella bronchiseptica*
- *Streptococcus equi* spp. zooepidemicus
- *Pseudomonas* spp.
- *Mycoplasma* spp.

(Brady, 2004). A recent study into the cause of community-acquired infectious pneumonia among dogs under 1 year of age showed *B. bronchiseptica* to be the predominant bacterium recovered (at 49%) (Radhakrishnan et al., 2007). In several studies *B. bronchiseptica* has been cited as a predominant cause of bacterial pneumonia in dogs and cats. In dogs under 1 year of age, clinical disease caused by *B. bronchiseptica* pneumonia was determined to be more severe than pneumonia caused by other types of bacteria (Radhakrishnan et al., 2007).

DIAGNOSIS

The diagnosis of bacterial pneumonia generally is based on information derived from the history, physical examination findings, and thoracic radiography. However, in cats the clinical manifestation of bacterial pneumonia is quite different from that of the dog. Clinical findings characteristic of pneumonia in dogs can be completely absent in cats with active bacterial pneumonia.

Clinical History

The chief complaint associated with bacterial pneumonia does not routinely include cough, although this sign should prompt consideration of bronchopulmonary infection. Dogs and cats may be lethargic and have decreased exercise tolerance or interest in playing, inappetence, increased respiratory rate or effort, or persistent nasal discharge. Regurgitation related to esophageal disease, vomiting, and audible wheezing (as with laryngeal paralysis) are commonly reported findings in dogs with aspiration pneumonia. In contrast, owners of cats with pneumonia may not have observed any abnormal respiratory pattern or nasal discharge. Hospital-acquired pneumonia in both species has been associated with general anesthesia, administration of opiates, or lack of consciousness.

Physical Examination

Increased respiratory rate at rest and fever are anticipated but also inconsistent physical findings in patients with bacterial pneumonia. Cough, if present, may or may not be elicited on manipulation of the cervical trachea. Evidence of a purulent nasal and ocular discharge in a lethargic patient certainly warrants further assessment for lower respiratory disease.

Careful auscultation can be quite revealing. Evidence of fluid (mucus) in the airways during normal respiration and especially during cough supports a diagnosis of bacterial pneumonia. However, either the absence of normal breath sounds or a marked asymmetry in left- versus right-sided breath sounds is an additional clinical finding that supports a diagnosis of bacterial pneumonia with lobar consolidation.

Radiology

Historical signs, physical examination findings, and other signs of inflammation (fever, elevated white blood cell count) may be suggestive of bacterial pneumonia; but thoracic radiography is fundamental to establishing the diagnosis in both dogs and cats. Unless the patient is unable to be positioned, ventrodorsal and lateral projections are essential. In some patients obtaining both right and left lateral thoracic radiographs may be useful in assessing the extent of disease and ruling out other disorders (e.g., neoplasia). Although the ability to demonstrate lesions on thoracic radiography is important in establishing a diagnosis of bacterial pneumonia, the absence of abnormalities in a thoracic radiograph does not completely rule out a diagnosis of pneumonia.

Radiographic features of bronchopneumonia are variable and can vary from a diffuse, bronchointerstitial lung pattern to partial or complete alveolar density to consolidation. The cranioventral aspects of lung are most often affected in descending bacterial pneumonia. Although radiographs in cats with pneumonia can demonstrate classic lobar signs, the findings are more variable. Multifocal, patchy interstitial and alveolar changes may be evident; and even large nodules similar to those observed with metastatic lung disease may be identified. In cases of hematogenous pneumonia in either species the chest films may show diffuse interstitial-to-alveolar change, probably related in part to permeability (noncardiogenic) pulmonary edema. The presence of air in the esophagus may simply indicate aerophagia, but persistent esophageal dilation may indicate an underlying esophageal disorder such as megaesophagus or myasthenia gravis.

Bacterial Isolation

Although results of culture and sensitivity testing of transtracheal, endotracheal, or bronchoalveolar airway washes provide the optimal guidance for treatment of bacterial pneumonia, it is recognized that many patients are treated empirically in clinical practice. There are a number of reasons for this, including the inherent risks associated with collecting culture specimens from animals with respiratory distress. Empiric therapy is probably more justified in first-time cases of pneumonia or when radiographs or clinical signs do not suggest life-threatening bacterial pneumonia. Even when airway cultures are obtained, initial empiric antibiotic therapy is needed because it takes time for bacteria to grow in culture.

However, if initial treatment efforts appear to fail, the clinician is obligated to pursue the underlying etiology of suspected pneumonia. Cytology, Gram stain, and culture of fluid collected from the lower respiratory tract may be critical for therapeutic success in cases of hospital-acquired infection, when empiric treatment is failing, and in patients with pneumonia caused by unanticipated microorganisms (e.g., *Mycoplasma* spp. or in pulmonary blastomycosis). Recent treatment with antimicrobials does not necessarily predict negative culture results, and attempts to isolate the causative bacteria from patients receiving an antibiotic are still justified.

Collection of lower airway secretions may be accomplished by a number of methods. Transtracheal aspiration, a technique that does not require general anesthesia, is a particularly useful procedure in medium- to large-breed dogs with a productive cough. In small dogs and in cats endotracheal washing or bronchoalveolar lavage collected with or without a bronchoscope is preferable. However, since the latter procedures require short-term general or intravenous anesthesia, additional risks are incurred.

These techniques are described in detail elsewhere (Ford and Mazzaferro, 2006). When oropharyngeal contamination is a concern, the airways can be cultured using both an airway lavage sample and a guarded culture brush, which is passed through an endotracheal tube or optimally by bronchoscopic guidance. A positive brush culture may help distinguish contaminants when multiple organisms are isolated from the lavage.

Collected specimens should be handled appropriately for bacterial culturing. Some laboratories prefer to isolate *Mycoplasma* spp. using separate media, and sample handling should be discussed in advance with laboratory personnel.

In addition to culture, specimens collected from the lower respiratory tract should be examined cytologically. Leukocytes with intracellular bacteria confirm a diagnosis of bacterial pneumonia. However, the absence of bacteria does not exclude a diagnosis of bacterial pneumonia. The presence of the large bacterium *Simonsiella* (Cytophagales, Simonsiellaceae) in the airway cytology indicates that oropharyngeal contents have been aspirated into the airway or that samples have been contaminated during the collection. This finding may influence interpretation of culture results. When bacteria are evident, Gram staining of the specimen may provide some initial guidance for antibiotic therapy.

Transthoracic fine-needle lung aspiration using a 25- or 27-gauge, 1.5-inch needle is an alternative technique for obtaining diagnostic samples for cytology and culture. Patients with diffuse lung disease are better candidates for this procedure than cases of focal lung disease when the procedure is performed "blindly." Fine-needle aspiration of focal lung lesions is best accomplished under ultrasound or computed tomography guidance. However, neither technique ensures prevention of most common postaspiration complications, particularly pneumothorax.

TREATMENT

"The most important criterion for selection of an antibacterial is identification of the bacterial organism" (Greene and Reinero, 2006). However, antibiotic treatment generally is initiated in any patient suspected of having bacterial pneumonia, even in the absence of microbiologic diagnosis. The decision to initiate empiric antimicrobial therapy is justified when the risk associated with collecting adequate samples may further jeopardize the patient or when the time required to culture the offending organism represents a potentially life-threatening delay in managing the patient's infection.

Antibiotic therapy is the first treatment consideration in managing any patient suspected of having bacterial pneumonia. Initial selection of drug is usually based on the patient's overall health status. Oral antimicrobials such as trimethoprim/sulfonamide, doxycycline, cephalexin, or amoxicillin/clavulanate may be sufficient in the patient that has mild clinical disease, is still eating, and requires little to no supportive care. Oral antimicrobials, especially a liquid suspension, may be most practical when treating puppies or kittens, particularly when several animals from the same household are affected simultaneously. Adult patients with advanced disease benefit from intravenous administration of antibiotics and concurrent fluid therapy.

Simultaneous administration of two or more antibiotics to an individual patient is indicated in severely compromised patients, especially when bacterial susceptibility testing is not feasible. Table 149-1 summarizes recommendations for the empiric administration of antibiotics in cats and dogs suspected of having bacterial pneumonia.

There are no standard recommendations regarding treatment duration for patients with bacterial pneumonia. In puppies and kittens an effective antimicrobial may only need to be administered for 5 to 7 days. In mature patients with recurring signs of pneumonia associated with an underlying disorder such as megaesophagus, treatment periods may extend a month or longer. Generally the decision to discontinue antimicrobial therapy is based on the patient's activity, appetite, and evidence of resolution of the pneumonia based on follow-up thoracic radiographs. Generally treatment is continued for 1 to 2 weeks following resolution of radiographic lesions.

Supportive Treatment

Inflammation, fever, and insensible fluid loss (panting) dictate the need to maintain the hydration status of a patient with bacterial pneumonia. Patients that become dehydrated may experience decreased mucociliary clearance and alveolar emptying. Intravenous fluid therapy must be monitored carefully in the patient with bacterial pneumonia with the objective of avoiding overhydration.

Table **149-1**

Options for Empiric Treatment of Bacterial Pneumonia in Dogs and Cats

First-Choice Treatments (Uncomplicated Pneumonia)	Alternative Treatments (Severe Pneumonia With Complications)
Dogs	
Doxycycline: 5 mg/kg PO (suspension recommended for puppies) q12h	Enrofloxacin: 5 mg/kg PO q12h (use in puppies is restricted to life-threatening disease)
Trimethoprim/sulfonamide: 15 mg/kg PO or SQ q12h	Enrofloxacin: 5 mg/kg PO q12h *plus* Amoxicillin-clavulanate: 15 mg/kg PO q12h
Cephalexin: 22-44 mg/kg, PO q8h	Enrofloxacin: 5-10 mg/kg IV q12h *plus* Imipenem-cilastatin: 3-10 mg/kg IV q8h
	Chloramphenicol: 50 mg/kg PO or IV or SQ q6h
Cats	
Azithromycin: 5-10 mg/kg PO once daily	Clindamycin: 10-15 mg/kg, PO q12h
Amoxicillin-clavulanate: 15 mg/kg PO q12h	Chloramphenicol: 50 mg (total) PO or IV q12h
Cephalexin: 22-44 mg/kg PO q8h	Ticarcillin-clavulanate: 30-50 mg/kg IV q8h
Trimethoprim/sulfonamide: 15 mg/kg PO or SQ q12h	

IV, Intravenously; *PO*, orally; *SQ*, subcutaneously.

This is critical in patients with diffuse pulmonary infection in which increased pulmonary capillary permeability may be present. In most patients fluids should be administered at maintenance rates only. Higher than maintenance rates of administration may cause fluid overload and further compromise lung function.

Administration of a bronchodilator to a patient with bacterial pneumonia is controversial. Both methylxanthine (theophylline salts) and β-agonist bronchodilators (terbutaline, albuterol) have been administered as supplemental treatments in patients with bacterial pneumonia. The purported benefits of bronchodilator therapy include increased airflow, improved ciliary activity, increased serous component of bronchial secretions, inhibition of mast cell degranulation, and decreased microvascular "leak." Diaphragmatic muscle strength also may be enhanced by methylxanthines.

Use of a mucolytic drug such as N-acetylcysteine is rarely indicated in the treatment of bacterial pneumonia in dogs and cats. Despite the antioxidant effects and possible benefits in patients with pulmonary fibrosis, N-acetylcysteine administered by aerosol or direct inoculation into the trachea is an irritant and may cause reflex bronchoconstriction.

Nebulization of saline, 10 to 15 ml, administered over 15 to 20 minutes two to three times daily appears to provide relief to patients with bacterial pneumonia and may facilitate clearance of secretions accumulated in the lower airways. Some patients with pneumonia seem to respond to humidification of the air, particularly in arid climates. Although not a substitute for systemic antimicrobial therapy, antibiotics also can be administered by nebulization in cases in which such treatment might be beneficial (e.g., in resistant canine bordetellosis). Such treatment has been used in children for resistant respiratory infections with variable results. Drugs used in nebulization generally are those that are poorly absorbed from the respiratory mucosa and that generally would not be administered systemically because of risk of systemic toxicity. Examples include gentamicin (50 mg in 5 ml of saline twice daily), kanamycin (250 mg in 5 ml of saline nebulized twice daily), and polymyxin B (333,000 units in 5 ml of saline twice daily). Small particle size (0.5 to 3 μm) of nebulized fluids is critical for effective delivery of drugs or fluids into the lower respiratory tract. The use of a vaporizer or humidifier to deliver drugs is not effective. Pretreatment with inhaled albuterol may reduce irritation and attendant bronchial constriction.

Hypoxemia requiring administration of supplemental oxygen can develop in patients with severe pneumonia. Mechanisms for this functional disturbance include ventilation-perfusion inequality, arteriovenous shunting, and possibly diffusion impairment. Oxygen therapy is indicated in patients with a PaO_2 less than 85 mm Hg (or arterial oxygen saturation of less than 90%) while breathing room air. Oxygen can be administered through a nasal or nasopharyngeal catheter or an inexpensive hood or by housing the patient in a temperature-controlled oxygen cage (see Chapter 137). Patients receiving oxygen via a nasal catheter or a hood should receive humidified oxygen at rates of 50 to 100 ml/kg/minute. Higher flow rates are necessary for patients housed in an oxygen cage. In general, patients with PaO_2 of 60 mm Hg or less

while receiving supplemental oxygen are candidates for mechanical ventilation (see Chapter 138).

Physical therapy can be especially important in facilitating clearance of secretions from the lower airways, particularly in recumbent patients. Coupage, the administration of rapidly repeated, forceful chest compressions, is a means of stimulating cough and promoting clearance of airway secretions and should be performed several times daily. There is no role for the use of antitussive drugs in patients with bacterial pneumonia. Patients that are recumbent risk developing consolidating pneumonia and atelectasis. It is important that the recumbent patient be turned every 1 to 2 hours throughout the day. Upright positioning and encouraging the patient to take short walks can be important.

TREATMENT FAILURE

The clinician needs to follow the patient's response to therapy carefully, particularly in cases treated with empiric antibiotic therapy. Continued deterioration in the face of treatment, which can occur within 24 hours, may culminate in death if not managed appropriately and in a timely manner. Given the diverse causes of pneumonia, the clinician must be particularly aggressive in determining whether or not an underlying disorder, or principal primary cause, is contributing to the inability of an individual patient to respond. Pulmonary neoplasia, recurring regurgitation with aspiration, ciliary dyskinesia, laryngeal paralysis, and infection with an atypical microorganism are potential considerations.

Failure to respond may also be a consequence simply of having selected an antibiotic that is ineffective against the causative bacterium. For example, infections with B. bronchiseptica or Mycoplasma spp. may not respond to some broad-spectrum antibiotics but may demonstrate a positive response to doxycycline. In cases failing to respond, establishing the nature of the infection through isolation and susceptibility testing becomes imperative. Patients that clearly fail to respond to initial treatment and do not have an underlying disorder should receive aggressive antimicrobial therapy, preferably administered parenterally until such time that the causative organism can be confirmed.

References and Suggested Reading

Brady CA: Bacterial pneumonia in dogs and cats. In King LG, editor: *Textbook of respiratory disease in dogs and cats*, St Louis, 2004, Elsevier, p 412.

Chandler JC, Lappin MR: Mycoplasmal respiratory infections in small animals: 17 cases (1988-1999), *J Am Anim Hosp Assoc* 38:111, 2002.

Ford RB, Mazzaferro EM: *Kirk and Bistner's Handbook of veterinary procedures and emergency treatment*, ed 8, St Louis, 2006, Saunders-Elsevier.

Foster SF et al: Lower respiratory tract infections in cats: 21 cases (1995-2000), *J Feline Med Surg* 6:167, 2004.

Greene CE, Reinero CN: Bacterial respiratory infections. In Greene CE, editor: *Infectious diseases of the dog and cat*, ed 3, St Louis, 2006, Saunders-Elsevier, p 866.

Radhakrishnan A et al: Community-acquired infectious pneumonia in puppies: 65 cases (1993-2002), *J Am Vet Med Assoc* 230:1493, 2007.

CHAPTER 150

Noncardiogenic Pulmonary Edema

KENNETH J. DROBATZ, *Philadelphia, Pennsylvania*
H. MARK SAUNDERS, *Shelburne, Vermont*

Pulmonary edema is defined as an abnormal accumulation of fluid in the extravascular spaces of the lung. It is a dynamic clinical syndrome attributable to a variety of disease processes. Noncardiogenic pulmonary edema is caused by an increase in vascular endothelial permeability rather than from increased vascular hydrostatic pressure as seen in cardiogenic pulmonary edema.

Increased permeability in noncardiogenic pulmonary edema (NPE) originates from an injury to the pulmonary microvascular endothelium that separates the intravascular compartment from the pulmonary interstitium and alveoli. In contrast to hydrostatic or cardiogenic pulmonary edema, the increase in permeability results in extravascular fluid that is relatively high in protein and leads to an increase in extravascular lung water content at lower pulmonary hydrostatic pressures.

NPE can reflect the pulmonary response to a primary pulmonary injury only or to disease processes elsewhere in the patient. The common causes of primary pulmonary epithelial injury include aspiration of gastric contents, near drowning, inhalation of smoke or toxic gases, blunt trauma, or high inspired oxygen concentrations for prolonged periods. Extrapulmonary-mediated insults include systemic sepsis, neurogenic pulmonary edema, pancreatitis, uremia, systemic inflammatory response syndrome, and pulmonary embolism.

DIAGNOSIS

NPE is a reasonable differential diagnosis in any critical animal that is showing signs of respiratory distress. The clinical difficulty is to distinguish this form of pulmonary edema from that of cardiac origin; treatment varies depending on the etiology. The form of pulmonary edema is not always clear, and on rare occasions both cardiogenic and NPE may be present simultaneously. In the absence of direct measurement of pulmonary artery wedge pressures, clinical acumen and experience are essential to reaching a diagnosis, beginning with a thorough history and physical examination.

The history may provide information for a diagnosis, such as exposure to electrical cords, head or chest trauma, upper airway obstruction, exposure to toxins, or inhalation of smoke. A thorough physical examination should include all organ systems to detect the presence of systemic disease. Evaluation of the pulmonary and cardiovascular systems is essential for determining the presence and severity of pulmonary edema. There are no pathognomonic physical signs for NPE. Particular attention should be given to the presence of cardiac abnormalities such as a cardiac murmur, gallop, or arrhythmia; poor pulse quality; jugular pulses; and prolonged capillary refill time. Secondary cardiac signs may occur from NPE or mediators from systemic inflammation, confusing the physical determination of cardiogenic versus NPE. Unfortunately, when animals present with severe respiratory distress, restraint can be stressful and detrimental to the patient. Therefore a thorough physical examination may not be possible until the animal has been stabilized.

Thoracic radiographs should be obtained once the patient is stabilized. Review of the thoracic radiographs helps to differentiate cardiogenic from NPE, determine the extent and severity of pulmonary edema, reveal additional pulmonary or pleural space abnormalities, and serve as a reference point after instituting treatment. Interstitial or mixed interstitial-alveolar infiltrates in the more compliant perihilar region in dogs are more compatible with cardiogenic pulmonary edema and should be accompanied by left-sided cardiomegaly and pulmonary venous distention. Cardiogenic pulmonary edema in cats is rarely isolated to the perihilar region and is typically characterized by a diffuse distribution of multifocal interstitial or mixed interstitial-alveolar infiltrates. Early NPE typically appears radiographically as an interstitial pulmonary edema; although, by the time animals with acute edema are radiographed, the edema may have worsened, and the pulmonary pattern progressed to a mixed interstitial-alveolar or alveolar pattern. The location of NPE in the lung is variable, depending on the underlying etiology; caudodorsal and caudodorsal/diffuse involvement predominate. Symmetric or asymmetric distribution may depend on the inciting cause of the edema. For example, more systemic, extrapulmonary-mediated insults are more likely to cause symmetric involvement, whereas primary pulmonary epithelial injury such as inhalation of toxic fluids or near drowning may cause asymmetric pulmonary edema.

Arterial blood gases are not characteristic of NPE but often reflect pulmonary dysfunction, revealing hypoxemia caused by ventilation-perfusion mismatch. The partial pressure of alveolar carbon dioxide initially is low because of hyperventilation in response to the pulmonary parenchymal disease and, if severe, hypoxemia. In the later stages compromised pulmonary compliance can interfere with the animal's ability to ventilate, causing hypercapnia. Serum transferrin and total protein concentration have been suggested as diagnostic tests for differentiating permeability edema from cardiogenic pulmonary edema in humans (lower concentrations are more consistent with a permeability edema). This has not been evaluated in animals, but hypoproteinemia has been reported in dogs with acute respiratory distress syndrome. A complete blood count, serum chemistry profile, and urinalysis round out the initial diagnostic tests that should be performed in searching for an underlying cause of NPE. When available, echocardiography can be invaluable for identifying, or ruling out, evidence of left-sided heart disease. This study is especially helpful in cases of cardiomyopathy.

In summary, the diagnosis is not achieved by measuring one parameter. It involves assessing a combination of the history, physical abnormalities, thoracic radiographs, arterial blood gas measurements, and clinical laboratory test results. The measurement of pulmonary capillary wedge pressure (PCWP) is sometimes necessary for ruling out an increased hydrostatic cause of the pulmonary edema. However, such measurements are not yet routine in veterinary critical care.

INITIAL APPROACH AND MANAGEMENT

Ideally the identification and elimination of the inciting cause of NPE might result in dissipation of the pulmonary edema. Corticosteroids and blockers of the cyclooxygenase and leukotriene pathways have not been proven to definitely and consistently resolve the pulmonary inflammatory process occurring in most patients with NPE. A variety of other therapies have been attempted but also have not shown consistent promise; some are even detrimental. These frustrating results may be a reflection of how permeability edema varies over time within an animal, how it differs among animals, and how it sometimes varies even within the lungs of an affected animal. In lieu of specific therapies for the underlying disease process or resolution of the pulmonary endothelial inflammation, a nonspecific approach involving supporting the respiratory and cardiovascular systems is the current mainstay of treatment.

An animal that is presented in severe respiratory distress is a challenge; the restraint required for diagnosis and treatment could result in death. When possible, an intravenous catheter should be placed to allow rapid vascular access. Immediate oxygen therapy by oxygen cage, nasal oxygen, or intubation and ventilation can be lifesaving during the initial assessment and stabilization (see Chapter 137). The veterinarian may immediately be faced with the decision whether to sedate and/or anesthetize the patient for intubation and ventilation support (see Chapter 138). The acute, critical nature of some cases of NPE is such that ventilation may be required for obtaining initial stabilization.

Positive-pressure ventilation (PPV) opens collapsed alveoli and small airways to increase the number of ventilated alveoli, thereby decreasing intrapulmonary shunting. NPE decreases lung compliance so that greater than normal inspiratory pressures (20 cm H_2O) are usually necessary for generating adequate tidal volumes of 10 to 20 ml/kg.

Inspired oxygen concentrations of more than 50% for 12 hours or longer might cause oxygen toxicity. Maintaining the animal on the lowest oxygen concentration possible to correct hypoxemia minimizes the chances of toxicity. Positive end-expiratory pressure (PEEP) is often used as an adjunct to mechanical ventilation with the goal of providing an adequate partial pressure of oxygen in alveoli at a low mean airway pressure and low inspired oxygen concentration. It can also be used in spontaneously breathing patients. PEEP increases functional residual capacity, prevents alveolar and small airway collapse between breaths, and allows more alveoli to participate in gas exchange. The adverse effects of PEEP and PPV are similar. Both of these treatments can cause a decrease in venous return and cardiac output. In addition, barotrauma and pneumothorax are not unusual sequelae in patients with NPE receiving high PEEP and end-inspiratory pressures from PPV. More recently low lung-stretch ventilation techniques (permissive hypercapnia) have been shown to reduce ventilator-induced lung injury in people. It has also been postulated that the hypercapnia itself may attenuate lung and systemic organ injury.

Oxygen delivery to the tissues can be maintained despite hypoxemia if cardiac output is increased. Cardiac function in animals with NPE can be adversely affected by hypovolemia, depressed myocardial contractility, and vasoconstriction. Low blood volume results in poor venous return to the heart, poor cardiac output, and systemic hypotension. Fluid administration to increase blood volume, cardiac preload, and subsequent cardiac output helps improve tissue perfusion. However, the major concern with fluid infusion is the very real potential that *fluid therapy may increase pulmonary edema* in patients with NPE. The choice of crystalloids versus colloids is a continuing controversy. The decrease in intravascular oncotic pressure and the increase in hydrostatic pressure associated with crystalloid infusion promote pulmonary edema in patients with increased pulmonary capillary permeability. On the other hand, colloid solutions do not necessarily decrease the incidence of pulmonary edema and may be hazardous in the setting of altered pulmonary capillary permeability. The loss of colloid particles into the pulmonary interstitium would result in increased interstitial oncotic pressure and a subsequent increase in extravascular lung water. The relative permeability of the pulmonary microvasculature during disease states cannot be predicted clinically. A test infusion of a colloidal solution and monitoring the intravascular colloid osmotic pressure might provide insight into the ability of the vasculature to retain the infused colloids. No improvement, or a rapid decrease in colloid osmotic pressure, suggests that the colloid is rapidly lost from the vasculature, and its use in the patient should be restricted. Thus available data are contradictory on the comparative benefits of crystalloids and colloids with regard to pulmonary function in patients with NPE. Until more information is available, the choice of fluid therapy must be made on a patient-by-patient basis and according to the clinician's preference and experience.

Blood transfusions can optimize oxygen delivery. We recommend transfusion of whole blood or packed red blood cells to animals with NPE up to a packed cell volume of 30%. As the packed cell volume rises above 30%, the associated increase in blood viscosity and its deleterious effects on blood flow tend to negate any increases in oxygen delivery caused by the higher hemoglobin concentration.

High pulmonary microvascular hydrostatic pressure enhances fluid transudation across the vessel wall and worsens pulmonary edema. The goal is to achieve a normal pulmonary hydrostatic pressure (measured by PCWP) and to maintain tissue oxygen delivery. In the absence of PCWP measurement, measurement of central venous pressure (CVP) might be useful, keeping in mind that the CVP might not reflect PCWP in patients with pulmonary or cardiac disease. CVP and PCWP measure hydrostatic pressure and therefore may be poor criteria for predicting the development or monitoring the progression of pulmonary edema in animals with a capillary permeability defect.

Diuretics and vasodilators may be used to decrease pulmonary microvascular hydrostatic pressure. Our first choice for a diuretic is furosemide. In dogs the initial dose is a 2-mg/kg bolus intravenously or intramuscularly if intravenous access is not available. This dose is repeated every 6 to 8 hours. Continuous intravenous infusion of furosemide has been demonstrated to have an improved diuretic response in critically ill patients. We use a dosage of 0.1 mg/kg/hour of furosemide as a continuous infusion. If PCWP is very high, a systemic vasodilator such as nitroprusside (1 to 10 mcg/kg/minute constant-rate infusion) can rapidly lower PCWP. Systemic hypotension and decreased tissue oxygen delivery must be avoided if diuretics or vasodilators are being used as part of therapy. Monitoring blood pressure is warranted, particularly when one uses vasodilators. Systemic hypotension (mean arterial pressure <80 mm Hg) in an animal with adequate blood volume indicates the need for a positive inotrope. Both dopamine (5 to 10 mcg/kg/minute) and dobutamine (5 to 20 mcg/kg/minute) can be used to increase myocardial contractility and improve cardiac output and may prevent the volume overloading associated with excessive fluid therapy. More recently β-adrenergic stimulation has been shown to enhance alveolar edema clearance in some animal models of lung injury. More studies are necessary to determine if these drugs are useful in our clinical patients.

MONITORING THE EFFECTIVENESS OF THERAPY

Frequent assessment of mucous membrane color, capillary refill time, heart rate, pulse quality, thoracic auscultation, and respiratory rate and effort provides vital subjective information on the response to therapy. Serial pulse oximetry and arterial blood gas measurement provide more objective information about pulmonary function.

Total thoracic compliance can be measured in intubated patients. A decrease in this measure often precedes the clinical signs of pulmonary edema from fluid overload in humans. The resolution of NPE on thoracic radiographs is characterized by a shift from an alveolar to a mixed alveolar-interstitial and finally an interstitial pattern. Improvement of the radiographic pulmonary pattern lags behind the animal's clinical improvement.

Patients with NPE often have multiple organ problems and therefore warrant intensive monitoring of extrapulmonary organs such as the cardiovascular, central nervous, and renal systems. Measurement of blood pressure; cardiac rhythm; and more extensive cardiovascular parameters such as CVP, PCWP, cardiac output, systemic vascular resistance, oxygen delivery, and oxygen consumption provides more detailed information regarding the patient's cardiovascular status. Urine output, serial urinalyses, and serum creatinine and blood urea nitrogen provide assessment of renal function. In patients with systemic inflammation or sepsis, coagulation parameters should be serially evaluated for disseminated intravascular coagulation. The degree of monitoring should reflect the severity of the disease process, with the more severely affected patients requiring the most intensive monitoring.

Suggested Reading

Arif SK et al: Hypoproteinemia as a marker of acute respiratory distress syndrome in critically ill patients with pulmonary edema, *Intensive Care Med* 28:310, 2002.

Chonghaile MN, Higgins B, Laffey JG: Permissive hypercapnia: role in protective lung ventilatory strategies, *Curr Opin Crit Care* 11:56, 2005.

Demling RH, LaLonde C, Ikegami K: Pulmonary edema: pathophysiology, methods of measurement, and clinical importance in acute respiratory failure, *New Horiz* 1:371, 1993.

Drobatz KJ, Concannon K: Noncardiogenic pulmonary edema, *Compendium* 16:333, 1994.

Drobatz KJ et al: Non-cardiogenic pulmonary edema: 26 cases (1987-1993), *J Am Vet Med Assoc* 206:1732, 1995.

Marinelli WA, Ingbar DH: Diagnosis and management of acute lung injury, *Clin Chest Med* 15:517, 1994.

Marini JJ: Advances in the understanding of acute respiratory distress syndrome: summarizing a decade of progress, *Curr Opin Crit Care* 10:265, 2004.

Parent C et al: Clinical and clinicopathologic findings in dogs with acute respiratory distress syndrome: 19 cases (1985-1993), *J Am Vet Med Assoc* 208:1419a, 1996.

Parent C et al: Respiratory function and treatment in dogs with acute respiratory distress syndrome: 19 cases (1985-1993), *J Am Vet Med Assoc* 208:1428b, 1996.

Sibbald WJ, Cunningham MD, Chin DN: Non-cardiac or cardiac pulmonary edema? A practical approach to clinical differentiation in critically ill patients, *Chest* 84:453, 1983.

CHAPTER 151

Respiratory Parasites

ROBERT G. SHERDING, *Columbus, Ohio*

Various parasites, including nematodes, trematodes, protozoa, and arthropods, have a predilection for invading the nasal cavity, airways, lung parenchyma, or pulmonary arteries of dogs and cats. This chapter focuses on primary parasites of the respiratory system that live in the nasal cavity, airways, or lung tissue. Parasites that transiently migrate through the lung during development such as *Toxocara canis* and *Ancylostoma caninum* are not discussed here. Systemic parasitic infections that occasionally cause pulmonary involvement such as the protozoan *Toxoplasma gondii* also are not included. In addition, parasites that live primarily in the heart or pulmonary arteries (*Dirofilaria immitis*; *Angiostrongylus vasorum*) are beyond the scope of this chapter, although these are important causes of secondary cardiopulmonary disease.

NASAL PARASITES

Nasal parasites of clinical significance include worms, mites, and *Cuterebra* fly larvae. These cause nonspecific signs of chronic rhinitis that are difficult to distinguish from more common causes of nasal disease.

Eucoleus boehmi

Eucoleus boehmi is a small (1.5 to 4 cm in length) trichinelloid nematode that parasitizes the epithelial lining of the nasal mucosa, turbinates, and sinuses of dogs. Ova are passed into the environment with nasal discharges or with the feces when nasal secretions are swallowed. The life cycle is not well understood but may be direct or involve earthworms as transport hosts. Infection may spread among dogs kenneled together.

Clinical Signs and Diagnosis
Eucoleus infection may be clinically inapparent or it may cause signs of chronic rhinitis, including sneezing, mucopurulent or blood-tinged nasal discharge, nasal congestion, and reverse sneezing. The diagnosis is confirmed by the microscopic identification of characteristic double-operculated (bipolar) eggs in nasal flushes or on routine fecal flotation examination. Egg excretion may be cyclic and easily overlooked. *E. boehmi* ova are easily misidentified as ova of *Capillaria aerophila* (see section on *C. aerophila* later in the chapter) because of similarity in appearance; however, *E. boehmi* ova are slightly smaller and have distinctive, readily visible spaces between the egg shells and embryonated contents. The adult *E. boehmi* nematodes occasionally may be identified in nasal mucosal biopsies.

Treatment
Treatment is either an extended course of fenbendazole (Panacur, Intervet; 50 mg/kg q24h orally [PO]) for 14 days; or ivermectin (Ivomec, Merial Animal Health; 400 mcg/kg subcutaneously [SC] or PO) repeated at 2-week intervals for a total of two or three doses. Ivermectin should not be administered to collies, shelties, and other herding breeds without first determining safety with an MDR1 genotype test (available at www.vetmed.wsu.edu/vcpl). Relapses can occur after initial treatment, necessitating additional courses of therapy.

Mammomonogamus ierei

This small nematode, ranging in length from 6 to 20 mm, is widespread in cats in Puerto Rico and other islands of the Caribbean, where it is found attached to the mucosal lining of the nasal cavity and nasopharynx, causing mild chronic inflammation. Clinical signs generally are minimal. The life cycle is unknown. The diagnosis is confirmed by fecal flotation to identify the typical large embryonated ova, which appear very similar to hookworm eggs. Presumably ova may also be detected in rhinoscopic cytologies or nasal flushes. Treatment of *Mammomonogamus* in cats has not been well documented, but fenbendazole (dosed as for *Eucoleus*) is suggested.

Pneumonyssoides caninum

Pneumonyssoides caninum is a small mite (1 mm in length) found worldwide infecting the nasal cavity and sinuses of dogs. The parasite is endemic in Scandinavia with over 20% of dogs infected in some regions. Nasal mite transmission is probably through direct contact with infected animals, and infection can spread between dogs confined together in the same household or kennel.

Clinical Signs and Diagnosis
Nasal mites cause nonspecific clinical signs of rhinitis and nasal irritation such as sneezing, reverse sneezing, seromucoid nasal discharge, and impaired scenting ability (hyposmia). Facial pruritus also has been reported. The diagnosis is confirmed by direct visualization of yellow-white mites, 1 to 1.5 mm in length, at the external nares or in the nasal passages by rhinoscopy or by identification of mites in nasal discharge (swabs or flushes). In some cases the mites can evade detection by locating in the frontal sinuses and caudal choanae.

Treatment
Nasal mites can be treated effectively with selamectin (Revolution, Pfizer; 6 to 12 mg/kg, applied topically as a

"spot-on" to the skin over the shoulders) at 2-week intervals for a total of three doses or milbemycin oxime (Interceptor, Novartis; 0.5 to 1 mg/kg PO) at 1- to 2-week intervals for a total of three doses. Ivermectin, dosed as for *Eucoleus*, is an effective alternative, but it has a greater risk of adverse side effects. Clinical signs usually resolve rapidly with treatment. In dogs confined together effective control requires treating all animals in the household or kennel.

Cuterebra

Cuterebra spp. larvae are the larval forms (bots) of numerous species of arthropod flies that infect mostly rabbits and rodents. *Cuterebra* occasionally can infect outdoor dogs and cats in spring and summer, especially migrating in the subcutis of the face, head, and neck region. Rarely *Cuterebra* can cause respiratory disease when they migrate in the nasopharynx, causing sneezing and unilateral bloody nasal discharge, or in the wall of the cervical trachea, causing clinical signs of cough and dyspnea. The diagnosis is made by direct endoscopic visualization of the *Cuterebra* larvae embedded in the nasopharyngeal or upper airway mucosa. Airway *Cuterebra* can be treated by endoscopic extraction or by administering a single dose of ivermectin (200 to 400 mcg/kg SC; see precautions under the section on *Eucoleus*). The use of prednisone (1 mg/kg q12h PO) for 2 weeks may reduce the local inflammatory reaction to the parasite.

BRONCHOPULMONARY PARASITES

Most bronchopulmonary parasite infections are caused by metastrongyloid nematodes such as *Oslerus (Filaroides) osleri, Filaroides hirthi, Andersonstrongylus (Filaroides) milksi,* and *Crenosoma vulpis* in dogs and *Aelurostrongylus abstrusus* in cats. Both dogs and cats can also be infected with the trichurid lungworm, *C. aerophila* (also known as *Eucoleus aerophilus*), and the trematode lung fluke *Paragonimus kellicotti*.

Lungworm and lung fluke infections are relatively uncommon; young animals are most susceptible. Many infections are inapparent or subclinical; however, when clinical signs occur, chronic persistent cough is typical. Severe infections can cause dyspnea or be complicated by secondary bacterial bronchopneumonia. Abnormal bronchopulmonary infiltration patterns are often found on routine thoracic radiography in animals that manifest overt clinical signs. An increase in circulating eosinophils is sometimes seen on a complete blood count (CBC), but this is not consistent. Other routine laboratory evaluations are usually unremarkable. Definitive diagnosis requires identification of parasite ova or larvae in the feces or in respiratory cytology specimens.

Oslerus (Filaroides) osleri

O. osleri are metastrongyloid nematodes that live in granulomatous nodules located on the mucosal surface of the distal trachea, tracheal bifurcation, and first-division bronchi of dogs, especially puppies and young dogs less than 1 year of age. Wild canid species such as the North American coyote and Australian dingo have a high

prevalence of *O. osleri* infection and may serve as natural reservoirs of infection.

O. osleri has a direct life cycle that does not require an intermediate host; thus larvae that are coughed up, swallowed, and passed in the feces can be transmitted directly to another animal. In addition, larvae that are expelled from the trachea with respiratory secretions can be transmitted through saliva from dam to puppy during grooming behavior and regurgitative feeding. The prepatent period ranges from 10 to 18 weeks.

Clinical Signs

The primary clinical sign of *O. osleri* infection is chronic cough. A progressively enlarging granulomatous mucosal nodule or a series of confluent nodules may obstruct tracheobronchial airflow and cause exercise intolerance, dyspnea, or even death. Spontaneous pneumothorax has been reported.

Diagnosis

The distinctive tracheobronchial nodular lesions caused by *O. osleri* (Fig. 151-1) occasionally can be detected radiographically as large, space-occupying mucosal masses protruding into the lumen near the bifurcation (Fig. 151-2). These granulomatous mucosal nodules are most reliably identified by bronchoscopic visualization. The definitive diagnosis is based on finding mucosal nodules accompanied by thin-walled larvated ova (80 μm) and larvae (230 μm with kinked tail) in airway washings or bronchoscopic biopsies. Biopsies of parasitic nodules often reveal numerous *O. osleri* larvae embedded in granulomatous inflammatory tissue (Fig. 151-3).

Feces can also be examined for larvae, but this is less reliable than examination of airway specimens. For detection of *O. osleri* larvae in feces, zinc sulfate centrifugation-flotation is preferred over the Baermann technique; however,

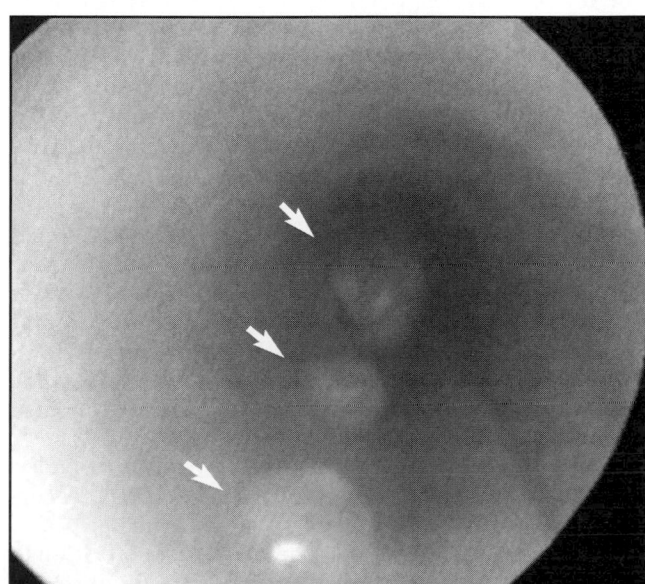

Fig. 151-1 Tracheoscopic image of the distal trachea from a dog with *O. osleri* infection. Three mucosal masses are evident. Mature parasites can be found within or adjacent to these nodules.

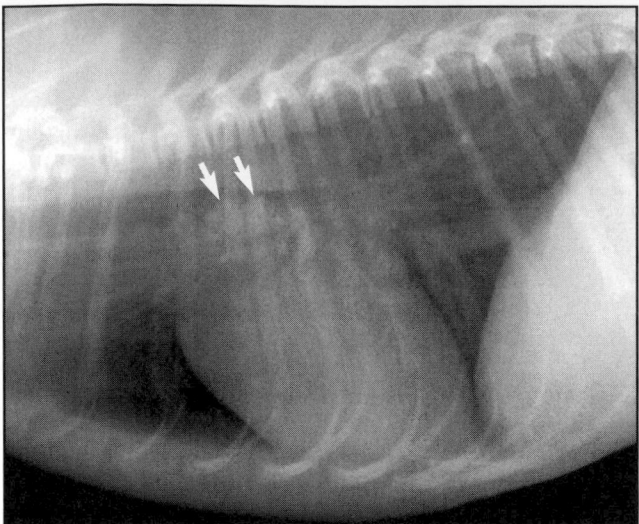

Fig. 151-2 Lateral radiograph from another dog with *O. osleri* infection. Notice that the mucosal nodules and inflammatory reaction have reduced the tracheal luminal diameter *(arrows).*

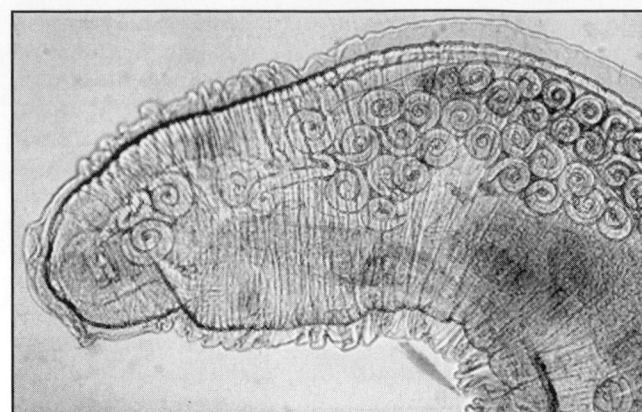

Fig. 151-3 Biopsy sample of a mucosal nodule demonstrating a portion of a female parasite carrying numerous larvae.

a negative fecal examination by either method is inconclusive, detecting less than one third of active infections. This may be attributable to the presence of few larvae and an intermittent pattern of larval shedding.

Treatment

The preferred treatment for *O. osleri* infection is either an extended course of fenbendazole (50 mg/kg q24h PO) for 14 to 21 days; or ivermectin (400 mcg/kg SC or PO) repeated at 2-week intervals for a total of three doses. Ivermectin should not be administered to collies, shelties, and other herding breeds without first determining safety with an MDR1 genotype test (available at www.vetmed.wsu.edu/vcpl). Additional doses of fenbendazole or ivermectin may be required to achieve remission in some dogs. Treatment has also been successful with albendazole, oxfendazole, thiabendazole, and levamisole. Albendazole has been associated with serious bone marrow toxicity and should be avoided or used cautiously. In rare cases severe airway obstruction may necessitate surgical or bronchoscopic removal or debulking of obstructing parasitic nodules.

Filaroides hirthi

F. hirthi are small metastrongyloid nematodes that live deep in the lung parenchyma (alveoli and terminal airways) of dogs, causing diffuse multifocal interstitial pneumonitis that may be eosinophilic, mononuclear, or granulomatous.

F. hirthi has a direct life cycle with a prepatent period of 32 to 35 days. First-stage larvae that are coughed up, swallowed, and passed in the feces are immediately infective and can cause direct feco-oral transmission through coprophagia. This mode of transmission has been shown to occur rapidly when infected and uninfected puppies are kenneled together. In endemically infected breeding colonies, dam-to-puppy transmission is common and can result in patent infections in puppies less than 3 months

of age. Because first-stage larvae are infective immediately, autoinfection can lead to massive overwhelming hyperinfections, with severe clinical disease and sometimes death in severely stressed or immunocompromised dogs.

Clinical Signs

F. hirthi usually causes subclinical interstitial pneumonia, but occasionally infected dogs are presented with acute or chronic progressive signs of cough and dyspnea. Fatalities have been reported in severe infections, especially in immunocompromised or corticosteroid-treated dogs and toy breed dogs.

F. hirthi has been found to be a prevalent endemic problem in breeding colonies of beagles and other research dogs, with infection rates approaching 100% in some colonies. Dogs from such colonies generally show minimal clinical signs; however, the parasite produces significant inflammatory lung lesions that can impair their usefulness in research.

Diagnosis

Routine thoracic radiography in infected dogs with clinical signs usually reveals diffuse bronchointerstitial infiltrates, with less frequent alveolar infiltrates. These changes may persist for several weeks. A peripheral eosinophilia may be seen in some dogs. The definitive diagnosis is based on finding larvated ova or first-stage larvae in airway or bronchoalveolar cytology specimens (e.g., aspirates or washings) or in the feces. The most reliable method for examining feces for *F. hirthi* larvae is with zinc sulfate (specific gravity 1.18) centrifugation-flotation, which is much more efficient for concentrating *F. hirthi* larvae than the Baermann procedure.

Treatment

F. hirthi can be treated with fenbendazole (50 mg/kg q24h PO) for 14 to 21 days or ivermectin (400 mcg/kg SC or PO) repeated at 2-week intervals for a total of three doses. Ivermectin should not be administered to collies, shelties, and other herding breeds without first determining safety with an MDR1 genotype test (available at www.vetmed.wsu.edu/vcpl). Albendazole (Valbazen; 25 to 50 mg/kg q12h PO) for 5 days and repeated in 2 weeks is also effective but has been associated with serious bone marrow toxicity and should be avoided or used cautiously. Dead and dying worms can elicit a multifocal granulomatous inflammatory response; thus clinical signs and radiographic changes may worsen initially after treatment. If severe, these changes can be controlled with prednisolone (1 to 2 mg/kg q12 to 24h PO) for 2 to 3 weeks and then tapered.

Control of *F. hirthi* infection in kennels and breeding colonies can be challenging because of high infection rates approaching 100% and direct transmission from dam to puppies. Isolation procedures and kennel sanitation measures are helpful adjuncts to medical management. Because they have longer residual activity than ivermectin, it has been suggested that selamectin and moxidectin should be investigated for efficacy in controlling *F. hirthi* reinfection in dog colonies.

Andersonstrongylus (Filaroides) milksi

A. milksi, also known as *F. milksi*, is a rare metastrongyloid nematode of dogs that has many similarities to *F. hirthi*. There is considerable confusion and some disagreement regarding the taxonomic classification of this parasite. Some of the early reports of this parasite in dogs are now considered to be misidentified *F. hirthi* infections. As in *F. hirthi*, this lungworm has a direct life cycle. Clinical findings, diagnosis, and treatment of *A. milksi* are thought to be similar to those of *F. hirthi* (see preceding section).

Aelurostrongylus abstrusus

A. abstrusus, the feline lungworm, is a metastrongyloid nematode that infects cats worldwide, especially feral, stray, and outdoor cats that eat prey. The adult *Aelurostrongylus* nematodes live in the terminal bronchioles and alveolar ducts, causing bronchiolitis, interstitial and alveolar pneumonia, and muscular thickening of the pulmonary arteries. The adult female worms are 9 to 10 mm in length, and the males are 4 to 6 mm. Eggs produced by the adult nematodes develop within the lung of the cat into first-stage larvae that are coughed up, swallowed, and passed in the feces. The indirect life cycle requires a molluscan intermediate host such as a terrestrial snail or slug. Cats can be infected either by ingesting infected snails and slugs or by eating transport and storage hosts such as rodents and birds that may harbor infectious larvae after feeding on infected snails and slugs. Infected cats begin excreting larvae 1 month after infection and continue for 6 to 9 months.

Bronchostrongylus subcrenatus and *Troglostrongylus subcrenatus* are metastrongyloid nematodes that are related to *A. abstrusus* and cause a similar lungworm disease in domestic cats and exotic felids in Africa.

Clinical Signs

Most *Aelurostrongylus* infections are clinically inapparent; however, severe infections can cause chronic cough, dyspnea, and debilitation. Pleural effusion, which may be eosinophilic, occurs rarely. Studies in experimentally infected kittens indicate that the severity of pulmonary disease and clinical signs are related to the infective dose of larvae, with heavy infections producing severe diffuse pulmonary inflammation and progressive clinical signs of cough, dyspnea, inappetence, debilitation, and sometimes death. In less severe infections the clinical signs and pulmonary lesions are self-limiting within 6 to 9 months. Thickening of the pulmonary arteries may persist for 2 years or more after recovery, but this does not appear to have adverse clinical consequences.

Diagnosis

A. abstrusus infection can mimic feline "asthma" and should be suspected in cats with bronchopulmonary disease that have a history of hunting birds and rodents. Radiographic findings of diffuse bronchointerstitial and patchy alveolar pulmonary infiltrates are typical and correspond to a dense inflammatory infiltration of lymphocytes, macrophages, and eosinophils around multifocal collections of eggs and larvae. An alveolar infiltrative radiographic pattern is most pronounced at 1 to 5 months after infection, followed by a bronchial or miliary interstitial nodular pattern that persists for up to 10 months after infection. Eosinophilia is found on CBC in some cats with aelurostrongylosis.

Confirmation of *Aelurostrongylus* infection is based on identification of first-stage larvae in airway or bronchoalveolar lavage cytology specimens or in the feces using either a Baermann fecal examination or zinc sulfate centrifugation-flotation. Larvae are 0.4 mm in length with a notched tail and configured in a coil or J shape. Although the Baermann fecal examination is considered a relatively sensitive clinical diagnostic test for *Aelurostrongylus* infection, larvae are shed intermittently in small numbers in feces; thus evaluation of respiratory cytology specimens for larvae can sometimes identify infections that are not detected by fecal examination.

Treatment

Mild *Aelurostrongylus* infections are generally self-limiting without treatment; however, cats with significant clinical pulmonary disease should be treated. The safest and most consistently effective treatment is fenbendazole (50 mg/kg q24h PO) for an extended duration of 14 to 21 days. Alternatives that are not as reliable include selamectin (6 to 12 mg/kg, as a topical "spot-on" application to the interscapular skin) at 2-week intervals for a total of three doses; or ivermectin (400 mcg/kg SC or PO) repeated at 1- to 2-week intervals for a total of two or three doses. Adjunctive therapy can include an antiinflammatory dosage of prednisolone (2 to 3 mg/kg q12 to 24h PO) for 2 weeks and then tapered; and a bronchodilator such as terbutaline (0.625 to 1.25 mg total dosage q8-12h PO) or inhaled albuterol (Ventolin; 90 mcg aerosol, 10 breaths by metered-dose inhaler q12h or as needed).

Crenosoma vulpis

C. vulpis is a metastrongyloid nematode that occasionally causes chronic bronchopulmonary disease and productive cough in dogs. Wild canids (wolves, foxes) and raccoons in North America and Europe serve as important natural reservoirs for this lungworm. In North America infection is widespread in the wild fox population and is endemic in red foxes in the northeastern United States and Atlantic provinces of Canada, with a prevalence of over 50% in red foxes of Nova Scotia, New Brunswick, and Prince Edward Island. In these regions *C. vulpis* can be an important cause of respiratory disease in dogs residing in rural or urbanized areas populated with foxes.

C. vulpis has an indirect life cycle that requires terrestrial snails and slugs as intermediate hosts, similar to *A. abstrusus* in cats. Dogs become infected by ingesting either infected snails and slugs or small prey that act as transport hosts after they feed on snails and slugs. The adult nematodes (females 12 to 16 mm in length and males 4 to 8 mm) live in the bronchi and bronchioles where they cause chronic bronchitis and bronchiolitis. After 17 to 21 days of infection the adult lungworms produce larvated eggs that develop into first-stage larvae that are coughed up, swallowed, and passed in the feces.

Clinical Signs

The predominant clinical sign of *C. vulpis* infection is chronic productive cough. Systemic signs such as fever, inappetence, or weight loss are usually absent.

Diagnosis

Thoracic radiography usually reveals a diffuse bronchial or bronchointerstitial pattern that may be indistinguishable from other causes of chronic bronchitis. Alveolar infiltrates are found less commonly. Hematologic findings can include eosinophilia, basophilia, or monocytosis.

Bronchoscopic findings vary from mild bronchial erythema to severe bronchitis with mucus accumulation and hyperplastic mucosal nodules. Bronchial hemorrhage is seen infrequently. Adult worms are visualized rarely. Tracheobronchial or bronchoalveolar lavage cytology specimens usually show increased mucus, high cellularity, and predominantly eosinophilic inflammation. First-stage larvae are identified cytologically in only 50% to 75% of cases.

Definitive diagnosis of *C. vulpis* infection depends on identification of first-stage larvae in airway cytology specimens or in feces, preferably using a Baermann procedure, which is reportedly a more reliable detection method for *C. vulpis* larvae than either zinc sulfate centrifugation-flotation of feces or bronchoalveolar lavage. *C. vulpis* larvae are approximately 300 µm in length with a blunt anterior end and a smooth tapering tail without notching or kinks.

Treatment

C. vulpis responds rapidly to treatment with fenbendazole (50 mg/kg q24h PO) for 3 to 7 days or a single dose of milbemycin oxime (0.5 mg/kg PO). Clinical signs and radiographic abnormalities generally improve within 1 week, and fecal larvae are absent within 2 to 4 weeks. Other successful treatments for *Crenosoma* have included febantel, levamisole, diethylcarbamazine, and ivermectin.

Capillaria aerophila

C. aerophila, also known as *E. aerophilus*, is a trichuroid nematode parasite found worldwide that infects the tracheobronchial mucosa of dogs, cats, and foxes. A prevalence rate of 1% to 5% is reported in various surveys of dogs and cats. The adult female worms are 20 to 38 mm in length, and the males are 12 to 25 mm. Adults begin producing ova 3 to 5 weeks after infection. These parasites embed deeply in the mucosa of the trachea and large bronchi, forming white, coiled masses surrounded by collections of ova. This results in chronic bronchitis. The direct life cycle involves ingestion of eggs from an infected host that are passed in the feces after being coughed up and swallowed. Earthworms may serve as transport hosts. Excreted eggs embryonate and become infective in about 40 days, remaining viable in the soil for extended periods of up to a year.

Clinical Signs

C. aerophila usually causes a clinically inapparent infection; however, occasionally it can cause chronic bronchitis with persistent cough. In severe cases dyspnea, loss of weight, poor body condition, or complicating bacterial bronchopneumonia may occur, especially in young animals.

Diagnosis

In animals with clinical signs thoracic radiographs may reveal a mixed pattern of diffuse peribronchial, interstitial, and alveolar infiltrates. Some dogs develop a marked peripheral eosinophilia. Airway cytology specimens may show increased mucus, eosinophilic inflammation, and the presence of *Capillaria* ova.

The diagnosis is based on identification of double-operculated yellow-brown ova in fecal flotation or airway cytology specimens. *Capillaria* ova must be differentiated from the similar-appearing ova of the intestinal whipworm (*Trichuris vulpis*) and the nasal nematode *E. boehmi* (see section on Nasal Parasites). *Capillaria* ova are smaller (<70 µm) than *Trichuris* ova, and they have asymmetric bipolar plugs that produce a distinctive lopsided appearance.

Treatment

The suggested treatment for *Capillaria* is fenbendazole (50 mg/kg q24h PO) for an extended duration of 14 to 21 days. It is not clear whether fenbendazole actually kills the adult nematodes or merely disrupts egg shedding by sterilizing the female worms. Ivermectin (200 to 400 mcg/kg SC or PO) repeated at 2-week intervals for a total of three doses can also be used to treat capillariasis; however, ivermectin should not be administered to collies, shelties, and other herding breeds without first determining safety with an MDR1 genotype test (available at www.vetmed.wsu.edu/vcpl). Levamisole has also been effective. A combination of febantel and praziquantel was not effective for treating *Capillaria* in cats.

Paragonimus kellicotti

P. kellicotti is a trematode lung fluke that infects wild carnivores and occasionally dogs and cats, especially in the Great Lakes and Gulf state regions of the United States. The lung fluke requires two intermediate hosts—the aquatic snail and the crayfish. Dogs and cats become infected by ingesting infected crayfish or by eating another animal that has recently ingested crayfish. Within 4 to 5 weeks after infection, the flukes are well established in radiographically visible pulmonary cysts, and they begin producing ova that appear in the feces. These cysts are most prevalent in the caudal lung lobes, especially on the right side. The adult flukes live in pairs within fibrous subpleural cysts that communicate directly with the bronchial system. This allows eggs to be readily expelled into the airway, where they are coughed up and then swallowed and passed in the feces to complete the life cycle.

Clinical Signs

The typical clinical signs of paragonimiasis are chronic cough, exercise intolerance, and weight loss. Hemoptysis is sometimes observed. In some cases sudden or recurrent episodes of dyspnea can be caused by spontaneous pneumothorax from cyst rupture. Clinically inapparent infections also occur.

Diagnosis

In dogs the diagnosis of *Paragonimus* infection should be suspected when radiographs reveal multiloculated thin-walled pulmonary cysts and large coalescing cavitations. Radiographic findings in cats are thick-walled cysts and large ill-defined nodular densities (granulomas). Some dogs and cats have radiographic evidence of spontaneous pneumothorax. Nonspecific peribronchial and linear interstitial infiltrates are common. Routine laboratory evaluations are unremarkable except for mild eosinophilia in some cases. Definitive diagnosis is based on identification of characteristic large yellow-brown, single-operculated ova in feces using fecal sedimentation technique or zinc sulfate centrifugation-flotation or in airway cytology specimens.

Treatment

P. kellicotti is treated effectively with either praziquantel (Droncit; 25 mg/kg q8h PO) for 3 days, or fenbendazole (50 mg/kg q24h PO) for an extended duration of 14 days. Albendazole (25 mg/kg q12h PO) for 10 days is also effective but should be avoided or used cautiously because of the potential for serious bone marrow toxicity. With successful elimination of the flukes, the radiographic lung lesions rapidly improve, and ova disappear from the feces.

References and Suggested Reading

Bihr T, Conboy GA: Lungworm (*Crenosoma vulpis*) infection in dogs on Prince Edward Island, *Can Vet J* 40:555, 1999.

Bowman DD et al: Evaluation of praziquantel for treatment of experimentally induced paragonimiasis in dogs and cats, *Am J Vet Res* 52:68, 1991.

Conboy G: Natural infections of *Crenosoma vulpis* and *Angiostrongylus vasorum* in dogs in Atlantic Canada and their treatment with milbemycin oxime, *Vet Rec* 155:16, 2004.

Dubey JP, Miller TB, Sharma SP: Fenbendazole for the treatment of *Paragonimus kellicotti* infection in dogs, *J Am Vet Med Assoc* 174:835, 1979.

Grande G et al: *Aelurostrongylus abstrusus* (cat lungworm) infection in five cats from Italy, *Vet Parasitol* 134:177, 2005.

Gunnarsson LK et al: Clinical efficacy of milbemycin oxime in the treatment of nasal mite infection in dogs, *J Am Anim Hosp Assoc* 35:81, 1999.

Gunnarsson L et al: Efficacy of selamectin in the treatment of nasal mite (*Pneumonyssoides caninum*) infection in dogs, *J Am Anim Hosp Assoc* 40:400, 2004.

Levitan DM et al: Treatment of *Oslerus osleri* infestation in a dog: case report and literature review, *J Am Anim Hosp Assoc* 32:435, 1996.

Marks SL, Moore MP, Rishniw M: *Pneumonyssoides caninum*: the canine nasal mite, *Compend Contin Educ Pract Vet* 16:577, 1994.

Outerbridge CA, Taylor SM: *Oslerus osleri* tracheobronchitis: treatment with ivermectin in 4 dogs, *Can Vet J* 39:238, 1998.

Schoning P, Dryden MW, Gabbert NH: Identification of a nasal nematode (*Eucoleus bohemi*) in greyhounds, *Vet Res Commun* 17:277, 1993.

CHAPTER 152

Interstitial Lung Diseases

BRENDAN M. CORCORAN, *Edinburgh, Scotland*

Strictly speaking, the lung interstitium is that part of the lung that does not include the airspaces, the capillary endothelial cells, and the alveolar lining epithelium. However, in disease it would be very unusual for only these structures to be affected, and inflammatory and infiltrative diseases of the true interstitium also affect the adjacent alveolar walls. With that consideration, it is often better to refer to the interstitial lung diseases (ILDs) as the diffuse parenchymal lung diseases. However, if infiltrative processes extend to include the alveolar spaces, the disease process is more properly categorized as pneumonia.

DISEASES OF THE LUNG INTERSTITIUM

Diseases of the lung interstitium are poorly defined in the dog and cat, and only recently are veterinarians beginning to properly understand the pathologic mechanisms involved in some of them. By inference these diseases involve pathologic processes that are restricted to the interstitial structures, but in reality they tend to also involve adjacent structures, giving a more complex pathologic profile. In addition, these diseases compromise respiratory function and can secondarily initiate other types of respiratory pathology. The most readily recognized disease entities are pulmonary infiltration with eosinophilia (PIE) (also known as eosinophilic bronchopneumopathy) and idiopathic pulmonary fibrosis (IPF). Parasitism in dogs and cats can be a contributory factor to the eosinophilic airway and lung diseases. The type of parasites involved depend on geographic location but can include *Filaroides* spp. (*Oslerus osleri*, *Filaroides hirhti*), *Crenosma vulpis*, *Aelurostrongylus abstrusus*, *Capillaria aerophilia*, and the heartworms *Angiostrongylus vasorum* and *Dirofilaria immitis* (see Chapter 151). In humans there is a large group of occupational and toxin- and drug-induced ILDs, but of these the only one that can be readily identified in the dog is paraquat poisoning (Box 152-1). Connective tissue and vasculitis disorders are also a significant problem in human medicine and can involve the lung; but identifying similar disease entities in the dog and cat is difficult, or it is difficult to show that such entities consistently affect the lung of dogs and cats. Several ILD conditions reported in humans are pathological descriptions, such as lymphocytic infiltrative disorders, and are unlikely to be identified in dogs and cats without more widespread availability of pathological data. Possibilities of infectious agents such as viruses and neoplastic processes (lymphoma) causing ILD exist. In addition groups of clinical conditions can involve the interstitium, such as pulmonary edema (cardiogenic and noncardiogenic) and lung parasitism, and syndrome entities such as acute respiratory distress syndrome; but

invariably these involve other parts of the lung and thus strictly speaking are not ILDs. Bacterial bronchopneumonia and the mycotic pneumonias (specific geographic locations worldwide) could also be included in this group. Interstitial lung changes detected radiographically can be the consequence of a disease process elsewhere such as metastatic mineralization with hyperadrenocorticalism or even a consequence of natural aging changes (Box 152-2). Many of the ILDs reported in human medicine are extremely rare, and it is possible that they exist in dogs and cats but that as yet they have not been identified. This chapter concentrates on IPF and PIE since they are the two best known examples of ILD.

DIAGNOSIS AND DIAGNOSTICS

Considering the possible disease entities included in the ILDs and the way many disease processes can involve the interstitium as part of their spectrum of pathologic changes, it can be difficult to definitively identify a "true" interstitial disease. In effect these diseases are suspected in dogs with tachypnea or lung crackles because of radiographic changes that are best described as "interstitial" and in which there is no (or minimal) radiographic evidence of bronchial or alveolar changes. The definition of the appearance of an interstitial lung pattern is itself problematic. Furthermore, the issue of radiographic quality is a major confounding factor in identifying interstitial lung patterns. An interstitial lung pattern can be best described as nodular or reticular linear densities where there is no evidence of increased bronchial markings or alveolar changes (i.e., air bronchograms). In a practical clinical situation the interstitial pattern is often determined by the exclusion of other obvious explanations for abnormal radiographic densities.

Radiography must be used with caution in the diagnosis of ILDs; and confounding factors such as exposure settings, body conformity, obesity, and stage of respiration need to be considered. In addition, subtle interstitial lung patterns are extremely difficult to identify with an acceptable degree of certainty. The use of high-resolution computed tomography (HRCT) can greatly improve the quality of thoracic imaging and the identification of genuine interstitial lung patterns, but its use is constrained by availability and cost. For IPF typical HRCT findings include ground glass opacity, subpleural bands, parenchymal bands, subpleural and peribronchovascular interstitial thickening, and traction bronchiectasis; and these changes appear to correlate well with the severity of disease (Johnson et al., 2005).

Routine hematology and biochemistry profiles are worth undertaking in suspect ILD cases, but they rarely give significant or specific changes. The presence of a

Box 152-1

Classification of Interstitial Lung Diseases in Humans

Examples (not exhaustive) of the types of diseases that might have similar analogous conditions in the dog and cat or may become recognized in the future

Drug or Toxin-Induced
Amiodarone
Paraquat
Radiation therapy
Chemotherapeutic drugs

Occupational
Farmer's lung disease

Primary Interstitial Lung Diseases
Eosinophilic pneumonia
Lymphoma
Lipoid pneumonia
Bronchoalveolar carcinoma
Adult respiratory distress syndrome
Metastatic calcification
Postinfection

Idiopathic Fibrotic Disorders
Idiopathic pulmonary fibrosis
Familial idiopathic pulmonary fibrosis
Lymphocytic interstitial pneumonitis
Bronchiolitis obliterans and organizing pneumonia
Autoimmune pulmonary fibrosis

Connective Tissue Disorders
Rheumatoid arthritis
System lupus erythematosus

Box 152-2

Diseases Involving the Pulmonary Interstitium

Pulmonary Fibrosis
Idiopathic pulmonary fibrosis
Fibrosis secondary to other disease processes (e.g., chronic bronchitis)
Normal aging change?

Eosinophilic Pneumonias
Pulmonary infiltration with eosinophilia
Eosinophilic bronchopneumopathy
Parasitic infections (pulmonary parasites, cardiac parasites)
Feline asthma (airways)

Pulmonary Mineralization
Hyperadrenocorticism
Pulmonary neoplasia
Idiopathic mineralization
Aging changes

Toxins
Paraquat

Miscellaneous
Pulmonary edema (cardiogenic, noncardiogenic)
Pulmonary neoplasia
Pneumonia (viral, bacterial, mycotic, protozoa)
(acute respiratory distress syndrome)

Note that the diseases listed here can present with radiographic evidence of interstitial lung involvement, but many are not classified as interstitial lung diseases.

circulation eosinophilia may be found in some cases of PIE, whereas the presence of basophilia would be very suspicious. A leukocytosis with a left shift should alert to the possibility of bacterial bronchopneumonia being present rather than an ILD.

Bronchoscopic evaluation of the respiratory system is invaluable in the investigation of the suspect ILD case, particularly in its ability to identify other disease entities that may be contributing to the respiratory problem or diseases that secondarily contribute to chronic interstitial lung changes. In PIE excess, often green-tinged secretions may be identified; whereas in IPF often little abnormality is detected apart from dynamic airway collapse. During bronchoscopy there is the opportunity to obtain airway samples and to carry out bronchoalveolar lavage. In PIE this should yield an eosinophil-rich sample (required for definitive diagnosis); but in IPF little abnormality is identified in samples, or there may be evidence of low-grade nonspecific inflammation.

Pulmonary function testing and blood gas analysis can be applied to the investigation of ILD, but the former is rarely used because it requires specialized equipment and training and there are limited normal reference values. Nevertheless the ILDs are likely to result in reduced lung compliance, and there is some unpublished evidence that this is the case with IPF. With respect to blood gas abnormalities, these diseases are most likely to result in ventilation-perfusion mismatch, and the degree of hypoxemia is determined by the severity of the disease. However, the contribution of true diffusion impairment to the blood gas picture is unknown. The degree of venous admixture can be derived from calculation of the alveolar-arterial PO_2 gradient, and in dogs with severe IPF it is abnormally high.

Definitive diagnosis of the ILDs can only be achieved by histopathologic assessment of lung tissue samples. Sufficient lung biopsy samples are rarely obtained. Transthoracic lung biopsy is usually ineffective in obtaining diagnostic material. This is in part because of the diffuse and patchy distribution typical of these diseases. Nevertheless, in some cases of PIE eosinophil-rich samples can be obtained in this manner, but it is usually only attempted if airway samples have been negative and there is a high index of suspicion that PIE is present. Open-chest and video-assisted thoracoscopic (VAT) lung biopsy are the only techniques that allow sampling of site-specific tissue. The techniques are rarely used because of the potential morbidity and mortality problems and the lack of skills or sophisticated thoracoscopic equipment. Nevertheless, greater use of VAT by specialized referral centers will make lung biopsy more common in veterinary practice. In IPF there is some information on the histopathologic appearance of diseased tissue, which includes patchy but extensive alveolar fibrosis, epithelial cell hyperplasia, squamous metaplasia, and varying degrees of inflammatory reaction; but the exact pathologic descriptors for IPF in the dog still need to be determined. VAT has allowed identification of cases of bronchiolitis obliterans with organizing pneumonia, lymphoplasmacytic ILD, and hypersensitivity pneumonitis in the dog and cat (Norris, Griffey, and Walsh, 2002). Pathological description of IPF in the cat is more complete, and both desquamative and usual interstitial pneumonitis (UIP) have been described (Rhind and Gunn-Moore, 2000; Williams et al., 2004). UIP is now recognized as the definitive pathological description of IPF in humans, but this pathological profile still has to be identified in the dog.

In practice ILDs are usually diagnosed on the basis of historical and clinical features supported by radiographic, bronchoscopic, and airway cytology results. For example, in IPF it is the clinical features of dyspnea with extensive pulmonary crackles in a predisposed middle- to old age–breed of (West Highland white terrier, cairn terrier) that gives the highest index of suspicion as to the diagnosis (Corcoran et al., 1999). In PIE it is the detection of large numbers of eosinophils in airway samples of a dog with respiratory signs or unexplained lung infiltrates that would support a diagnosis (Corcoran et al., 1991).

THERAPY

Therapy depends on identifying the underlying cause or the specific disease process. In some instances specific treatment modalities are used, but empiric or symptomatic therapy may be the only option. Depending on the degree of respiratory impairment and the chronicity of the clinical presentation, varying degrees of supportive care need to be considered. These can include periodic hospitalization, oxygen supplementation, nutritional care, obesity control, and planned exercise. PIE is treated with glucocorticosteroids (prednisone, 1 mg/kg q12h orally [PO], reducing to 0.25 mg/kg q48h over 2 to 3 weeks) and should result in a rapid and complete response. Subsequent recurrent or long-term maintenance therapy with oral prednisone may be required in some cases, but complete remission can occur in many cases. Concurrent treatment with a benzimidazole anthelmintic (fenbendazole, 50 mg/kg q24h PO for 7 days) is advisable in case there is parasitic involvement.

Effective medical treatment for IPF is not currently available. However, some affected dogs show a partial and transient favorable response to oral prednisolone at antiinflammatory doses (the suspicion is that such cases do not have IPF). The use of sildenafil in human patients and in dogs with IPF that also have concurrent pulmonary hypertension appears to be beneficial in some cases. The addition of bronchodilators can be beneficial in some cases but should be discontinued if there is no obvious response. The effectiveness of azathioprine and the antifibrotic agent colchicine in this disease are unknown in dogs and cats. Many other medications are being evaluated in human IPF, but the only agents that appear to have some promise are pirfenidone and hydroxyproline analogs. The possibility of these being effective in canine IPF is also unknown. The treatment of other conditions that can cause an interstitial lung pattern on radiographs such as pulmonary edema and the mycotic pneumonias is well described, and the reader should consult other chapters for exact treatment details.

References and Suggested Reading

Berry CR, Tyson AR: Thoracic mineralization. In King LG, editor: *Textbook of respiratory disease in dogs and cats*, ed 1, St Louis, 2004, Elsevier, p 569.

Clercx C et al: Eosinophilic bronchopneumopathy in dogs, *J Vet Intern Med* 14:282, 2000.

Corcoran BM: Idiopathic Pulmonary fibrosis. In King LG, editor: *Textbook of respiratory disease in dogs and cats*, ed 1, St Louis, 2004, Elsevier, p 581.

Corcoran BM et al: Pulmonary infiltration with eosinophilia in 14 dogs, *J Small Anim Pract* 32:494, 1991.

Corcoran BM et al: Chronic pulmonary disease in West Highland white terriers, *Vet Rec* 144:611, 1999.

Johnson VS et al: Thoracic high-resolution computed tomographic findings in dogs with canine idiopathic pulmonary fibrosis, *J Small Anim Pract* 46:381, 2005.

Norris CR, Griffey SM, Walsh P: Use of keyhole lung biopsy for diagnosis of interstitial lung diseases in dogs and cats: 13 cases, *J Am Vet Med Assoc* 221:1453, 2002.

Rhind SM, Gunn-Moore DA: Desquamative form of cryptogenic fibrosing alveolitis in a cat, *J Comp pathol* 123:226, 2000.

Williams K et al: Identification of spontaneous feline idiopathic pulmonary fibrosis, *Chest* 125:2278, 2004.

CHAPTER 153

Pleural Effusion

ELEANOR C. HAWKINS, *Raleigh, North Carolina*
THERESA W. FOSSUM, *College Station, Texas*

Pleural effusion is a common disorder of dogs and cats. This condition can represent a subtle sign of serious disease or a medical emergency. Causes of pleural effusion vary (Box 153-1), and determining the cause impacts both prognosis and therapy. Thoracic radiography, routine laboratory tests, thoracic/cardiac ultrasound, and cytologic and biochemical analyses of the pleural effusion are common diagnostic studies. Therapy can be medical, surgical, or both.

INITIAL MANAGEMENT OF PLEURAL EFFUSION

Respiratory distress from pleural effusion is caused by the inability of the lungs to expand; therefore immediate thoracocentesis is indicated to stabilize these animals. Thoracocentesis is also indicated for diagnostic purposes in animals with pleural effusion, and fluid for analysis should be collected *before* initiating antimicrobial therapy. The primary risk of thoracocentesis is laceration of underlying lung tissue (resulting in pneumothorax), hemothorax, or pulmonary hemorrhage in an already compromised animal. This risk is minimized by a well-restrained animal, careful technique, and appropriate catheter selection. Local anesthesia or manual restraint alone is often adequate when performing thoracocentesis, but mild sedation facilitates restraint in animals that are anxious or fractious.

Thoracocentesis is usually performed between the seventh and ninth intercostal spaces, above the costochondral junctions. Location of focal accumulation of fluid is identified radiographically or ultrasonographically. If available, ultrasonographic guidance facilitates insertion of the needle into localized pockets of fluid.

Butterfly catheters are commonly used because they are inexpensive, readily available, and convenient. Attached extension tubing prevents movement at the syringe from resulting in movement of the needle in the chest. A three-way stopcock facilitates retrieval of fluid and prevents the entrance of outside air into the thorax. The hand of the operator that holds the wings of the catheter should always rest gently on the body wall to minimize movement of the needle with respect to the body wall and to be prepared for immediate withdrawal if the surface of the lungs is felt through the needle or restraint of the animal is lost. Once the catheter has popped through the pleura, it should be laid against the body wall with the bevel facing toward the lungs. This avoids causing damage to the pulmonary parenchyma as the lungs expand with fluid removal. Specialized catheters for thoracocentesis are also available (Argyle Thoracocentesis System,

Sherwood Medical). Although more expensive, these catheter systems have safeguards to prevent damage to thoracic viscera. Alternatively over-the-needle catheters can be used (e.g., 3.25-inch or 5.25-inch 16- or 18-gauge Angiocath, Becton Dickinson); they have several advantages over butterfly catheters. Once over-the-needle catheters are in place, there is no needle in the thorax to lacerate the lung; it is even safe to reposition the animal to maximize retrieval of fluid. These catheters are also available in long lengths, which may be necessary to reach the pleural space in large-breed or obese dogs. Extension tubing and a three-way stopcock should be attached to the catheter to facilitate fluid removal. Side openings can be added to the catheter so that obstruction of a single opening is avoided. Gloves are worn, and a surgical blade is used to shave one or two side holes in the catheter while maintaining sterility. To prevent the catheter from breaking off in the pleural space on removal, holes should be no greater than one third the circumference of the catheter, spaced apart from each other, and have no rough edges. After thoracocentesis the modified catheter should be removed with care.

As much fluid is removed from the pleural space as is possible, except in animals with acute hemothorax. Respiratory distress in animals with hemothorax is often multifactorial (e.g., inadequate oxygen delivery, hypoventilation), and the blood within the pleural space can be resorbed. These animals benefit from restoration of oxygen-carrying capacity and blood volume, with thoracocentesis performed only as essential to allow lung expansion. Hemothorax may be diagnosed based on a history of acute trauma or rodenticide ingestion. Otherwise obtaining frank blood during thoracocentesis can also indicate a traumatic tap. Free blood in the pleural space is distinguished from a traumatic tap by the following: failure of the blood to clot, low packed cell volume relative to peripheral blood, and erythrophagocytosis identified by cytology.

Fluid retrieved from the pleural space should always be analyzed cytologically. Total cell count, protein quantitation, and examination of a concentrated slide preparation allow fluid to be classified as a transudate, modified transudate, septic or nonseptic exudate, or hemorrhagic effusion. Slides should be scrutinized for infectious agents or abnormal cell populations. Fluid is saved for further characterization as indicated by history, gross examination, or cytologic findings. If pyothorax is suspected, Gram staining is performed, and aerobic and anaerobic cultures are obtained. If chylothorax is among the differential diagnoses, fluid triglyceride concentrations are measured and

Causes of Pleural Effusion That Are Managed Directly

- Heart failure (modified transudate or chyle)
  - Heartworm disease
  - Cardiomyopathy
  - Tricuspid insufficiency
  - Congenital heart disease
- Obstruction or thrombosis of cranial vena cava
- Hypoproteinemia (pure transudate)
  - Protein-losing enteropathy
  - Protein-losing nephropathy
  - Liver failure
- Feline infectious peritonitis (nonseptic exudate)
- Coagulopathy (hemorrhagic effusion)
  - Rodenticide deficiency
  - Factor deficiency
- Trauma (hemorrhagic effusion or chyle)
- Lung lobe torsion (nonseptic exudate or hemorrhagic effusion)
- Diaphragmatic hernia (modified transudate, nonseptic exudate, or hemorrhagic effusion)
- Pulmonary thromboembolism (modified transudate, nonseptic exudate, or hemorrhagic effusion)

compared with triglyceride concentrations in a serum specimen obtained at the time of thoracocentesis (effusate triglycerides are higher in chylothorax).

In addition to managing respiratory compromise, the cardiovascular and systemic needs of the animal are met, including fluid therapy for dehydration or shock or antibiotics for sepsis syndrome. A complete diagnostic evaluation is undertaken after stabilization. Test selection is based on the history, physical examination, and cytologic characteristic of the effusion. When a primary cause is identified that can be managed directly (see Box 153-1), thoracocentesis is performed as needed to maintain the comfort of the animal until the underlying problem has resolved. The remainder of this article addresses the management of specific causes of pleural effusions: pyothorax, chylothorax, neoplastic effusion, lung lobe torsion (LLT), and idiopathic pleural effusion.

PYOTHORAX

The diagnosis of pyothorax is confirmed by the identification of a septic exudate through thoracocentesis. The diagnosis is generally straightforward when pleural fluid has been obtained before the initiation of antibiotic therapy, with organisms often visible cytologically. If antibiotics have already been given, the effusion may have the characteristics of a nonseptic exudate. Gram staining is helpful for characterizing organisms before culture results are available. A mixed infection, with anaerobes and aerobes, is generally present.

Often no source of infection is identified, especially in cats. In some of these cases pulmonary infection or a puncture wound may be the initiating event. A foreign body is another cause of pyothorax and can interfere with the

successful medical management of the disease. Although pyothorax is often idiopathic in dogs, the potential for the presence of foreign material is of greater concern in dogs than in cats.

It is necessary first to stabilize patients that are presented with severe dehydration, electrolyte imbalances, or sepsis. Thoracocentesis is performed for diagnostic and therapeutic purposes. Intravenous fluids and antibiotics are administered. Antibiotic recommendations are discussed in later paragraphs.

The two key components of successful treatment for pyothorax are drainage and antibiotics. Routine supportive care is also indicated. Aggressive treatment is begun immediately after the diagnosis of pyothorax to minimize the formation of adhesions, which interfere with drainage and decrease the likelihood of successful medical management. Drainage is achieved through indwelling chest tubes. Intermittent thoracocentesis is not nearly as effective as draining through chest tubes but can be considered in animals in which euthanasia is the only other option.

One chest tube is placed initially. The tube should be as large as can fit between the intercostal spaces to reduce the risk of obstruction of the tube with fibrin. Thoracic radiographs are evaluated after removal of as much fluid as possible through the tube. If remaining effusion is minimal, one tube is sufficient for treatment. However, if effusion persists on the opposite side, a second tube should be placed immediately. Inadequate positioning of a chest tube can result in persistent fluid on the ipsilateral side. Repositioning or replacing the tube is warranted. The continued presence of fluid despite multiple attempts to improve tube placement is suggestive of adhesions. Medical management with tube drainage can be attempted for 2 to 3 days, but the continued presence of localized fluid is an indication for thoracotomy and surgical débridement. The bandage securing the chest tube must not restrict the patient's ability to expand its chest during inspiration.

Continuous or intermittent suction of the chest tubes can remove the exudate from the pleural space. Continuous suction offers the advantage of maximal drainage, whereas intermittent suction is simpler logistically. Continuous suction is provided with a suction pump attached to a collection system that collects retrieved fluid, controls suction pressure, and maintains a one-way closed system. Convenient disposable collection systems are available commercially (e.g., Thora-Seal III, Sherwood Medical). Continuous suction does not greatly decrease the time required to manage pyothorax. Frequent monitoring is necessary to detect any problems with the system. Any leaks between the pleural cavity and the water seal can be rapidly and silently fatal. The system must also be evaluated periodically for obstructions caused by kinking of the tube or clogging with fibrin and debris.

Intermittent suction by syringe can be used successfully as long as the period between drainage attempts is short. Initially suction should be performed every 2 to 4 hours. As the volume of fluid produced decreases, often within the first few days, the interval can be lengthened. Ideally arrangements should be made for drainage to occur through the evening hours during the first 24 to 48 hours. If such arrangements are not feasible, the chest should be drained last thing in the evening and again first thing in the morning to minimize the time that fluid is allowed to accumulate.

Twice-daily lavage of the pleural space with sterile 0.9% saline helps maximize drainage. There is no obvious benefit from the addition of antibiotics, antiseptics, or enzymes. The addition of heparin (1500 units/100 ml) to the lavage fluid may decrease fibrin formation. The chest is drained as thoroughly as possible. A maximal volume saline (10 ml/kg of body weight) that has been warmed to body temperature is slowly infused into the chest. Less volume is used if discomfort is noted. The animal is rolled slowly from side to side for several minutes, and the fluid is then removed. The expected recovery is approximately 75% of the infused volume. Recovery of a greater volume of cloudy fluid may indicate that a pocket of exudate was reached. Recovery of much less volume suggests either pocketing of fluid in a region that is not getting adequate drainage through the existing tubes or severe dehydration. (Differentiation of these causes may be possible through ultrasonography.) It is important to maintain sterile technique whenever the system is opened to prevent the entrance of hospital-origin pathogens. Adapter ports are covered with sterile caps when not in use and wiped with alcohol or hydrogen peroxide before use.

Initial antibiotic selection is based on coverage for both gram-negative organisms and anaerobes. Culture and sensitivity data are used once they become available to make modifications in the treatment plan if a resistant organism is detected. Negative culture results can occur despite the presence of microorganisms and should not be used to exclude a diagnosis of pyothorax. Antibiotics are administered intravenously until the patient is alert and eating well; they are then given orally. Treatment with antibiotics is continued for 4 to 6 weeks after removal of the chest tube.

Amoxicillin with clavulanate (Clavamox, Pfizer Animal Health; 22 mg/kg q8h orally [PO]) is effective against nearly all anaerobes and gram-positive organisms and many (although not all) gram-negative organisms. Since amoxicillin with clavulanate is not available for intravenous administration, ampicillin with sulbactam is used initially (Unasyn, Pfizer Roering). The drug is dosed based on the ampicillin component (22 mg/kg q8h intravenously [IV]). Clindamycin (Antirobe, Pharmacia & Upjohn; 11 mg/kg q12h) also has good activity against anaerobes, including *Bacteroides fragilis*, but a second drug must always be added to treat gram-negative organisms. Fluoroquinolones or aminoglycosides can be used. Fluoroquinolones are preferred because they can be administered safely for prolonged periods. Initial antibiotic therapy may need to be modified, based on clinical response and results of culture and susceptibility testing.

Special antibiotic considerations must be made if "sulfur granules" are visible grossly in removed pleural fluid or if branching filamentous organisms are seen cytologically, indicative of *Actinomyces* or *Nocardia* spp. Acid-fast staining can help characterize the organisms. Acid-fast organisms are assumed to be *Nocardia*, although some *Nocardia* do not stain positively. Otherwise the more common *Actinomyces* is assumed, pending results of culture.

The final diagnosis is made through culture, and special techniques are required if these organisms are suspected. *Actinomyces* spp. are generally susceptible to penicillin derivatives. *Nocardia* are less predictable; but prolonged therapy with trimethoprim-sulfa drugs, tetracyclines, or aminoglycosides can be tried. A recent retrospective study supports early surgical intervention in dogs with infection caused by *Actinomyces*, presumably because of its association with plant foreign bodies (Rooney and Monnet, 2002).

It is extremely important to monitor patients regularly to ensure that days are not being wasted while the system is not providing adequate drainage, to determine the time to remove the chest tubes, and to determine whether surgical exploration is needed. Attempts to save money by foregoing regular monitoring often result in added expense in lengthened hospital stays or complications. Lateral and ventrodorsal or dorsoventral thoracic radiographs are evaluated at least every other day. Pockets of fluid that persist or increase in size indicate the need for replacement of chest tubes or surgical intervention if tube placement has been optimized. The volume of fluid recovered is measured, and a slide of the effusion is examined microscopically every day. The chest tube can be removed when the fluid has resolved radiographically, the volume of fluid recovered decreases to approximately 2 ml/kg of body weight per day, and signs of infection have resolved cytologically. Cytologic resolution is indicated by the absence of organisms. In addition, neutrophils decrease in numbers and lose their degenerative appearance, and macrophages appear. If these criteria for tube removal have not been met within 1 week of aggressive therapy, surgical exploration is considered.

Complete blood count and serum biochemical analysis are performed as indicated by the general condition of the animal. Electrolyte abnormalities are common until the patient is eating well.

Animals are discharged with oral antibiotics after removal of chest tubes. Reevaluation is indicated approximately 1 week after removal of the tubes and again approximately 1 week after discontinuation of antibiotics. Ideally an additional reevaluation occurs 1 month later. Thoracic radiographs are evaluated at these times. The purpose of these radiographs is to identify early recurrence of effusion. Early identification of recurrence greatly facilitates the ability of the surgeons to find a localized nidus of infection or foreign body. Thorough exploration of the chest cavity is extremely difficult, particularly in animals with a history of exudative disease. Localizing the disease provides a distinct advantage to the surgeon and increases the likelihood that a foreign body or nidus of disease can be found and removed.

Exploratory surgery is indicated for removal of a suspected foreign body or nidus of infection, for breakdown of adhesions when adequate drainage cannot be achieved, and for patients that do not show substantial improvement after 1 week of aggressive medical management. A sternotomy is performed so that both sides of the thorax can be accessed unless an obvious lesion is visible radiographically. Fibrin tags are broken down, grossly abnormal lung lobes are removed, and a search for foreign material is performed. As mentioned previously, most foreign material is extremely difficult to identify at surgery. A chest tube is placed for continued drainage after thoracotomy. The tube is pulled with medical management based on the criteria described, usually after 1 to 3 days.

The prognosis for pyothorax is fair to good. Animals that receive aggressive treatment early in the course of disease can recover with no further complications. Most patients that do not survive either die or are euthanized during the first few days when they are systemically ill or the owner declines treatment. When a foreign body is present, recurrence is likely unless surgical removal of the affected lung lobe or tissue is accomplished. Initial conservative treatment of pyothorax with oral antibiotics alone or with occasional thoracocentesis most often leads to adhesions, necessitating surgical débridement.

CHYLOTHORAX

Management of animals with chylothorax has been greatly refined since the initial report of its surgical treatment in three dogs and one cat in 1958. However, the ability to effectively treat affected animals has been hindered by a lack of understanding of the etiology of this devastating disease. Appropriate treatment of affected animals depends foremost on confirming the diagnosis and defining the cause. Once the diagnosis has been made and concurrent diseases ruled out, the value of medical versus surgical treatment must be considered.

Although the prevalence of chylothorax is unknown, a recent survey of 2000 veterinary clinics regarding the diagnosis and treatment outcomes of dogs and cats presenting with chylothorax suggested that cats were diagnosed with chylothorax approximately four times more often than dogs.* Of 795 veterinarians or veterinary hospitals returning the survey, nearly 40% had diagnosed at least one dog or cat with chylothorax in a 5-year period; information regarding 76 dogs and 297 cats with chylothorax was contributed.

Chylothorax was previously thought to be caused by thoracic duct (TD) rupture secondary to trauma; however, this is now known to be a relatively rare cause of chylothorax. Although traumatic rupture of the TD may occur, in most of these animals the TD spontaneously heals, and clinical signs associated with chylothorax are not recognized. More commonly recognized causes in dogs and cats include right heart failure, mediastinal masses, pericardial disease, paroxysmal atrioventricular block, fungal granulomas, and heartworm infection. Unfortunately, in a majority of animals despite extensive diagnostic workups, the underlying etiology is undetermined (idiopathic chylothorax). Because treatment of this disease varies considerably, depending on the underlying etiology, it is imperative that clinicians identify concurrent disease processes before instituting definitive therapy.

Because any disease that results in high systemic venous pressures (e.g., cardiomyopathy, pericardial effusion, congenital cardiac abnormalities, and heartworm

disease) may cause chylothorax, a complete cardiac workup is warranted in affected animals. Treatment of animals with cardiomyopathy or congenital heart disease and chylothorax should be based primarily on palliation when necessary with thoracentesis and improving cardiac output and decreasing venous pressures with appropriate drug therapy or interventions. If pericardial effusion is diagnosed, the underlying etiology should be determined, and pericardiectomy performed if indicated. Although heartworm infection is uncommon in felines, experimental infection with *Dirofilaria immitis* has been shown to result in chylothorax in a small number of cats. Naturally occurring heartworm disease has also been associated with chylothorax in cats. Therefore it is recommended that animals with chylothorax be screened for heartworm infection.

If an anterior mediastinal mass is identified, a fine-needle aspirate may be performed to determine the tumor or tissue type. Specific therapy (i.e., radiation therapy, chemotherapy, antifungal therapy, surgery) should then be instituted according to findings. In these animals the chylous effusion is probably secondary to compression of the cranial vena cava by the mass, and shrinkage of the mass may result in resolution of the pleural fluid. For prognostic purposes it is prudent to assess feline leukemia virus and feline immunodeficiency virus status in cats with mediastinal lymphosarcoma. In some animals with chylothorax the mediastinum and pericardium are thickened, associated with chronic irritation induced by chyle (Fossum et al., 2004). The pericardial thickening may lead to elevated right-sided venous pressures that may impede the drainage of chyle via lymphaticovenous communications after TD ligation.

When no obvious underlying disorder can be found, the term *idiopathic* chylothorax is used. Unfortunately management of animals with idiopathic chylothorax is difficult. Until the etiology of chylothorax in these animals is understood, therapy will remain palliative and less than optimal in many instances. One possibility is that in these animals increased volumes of lymph are being transported through the TD. These increased flows may occur secondary to abnormal right-sided venous pressures that cause much of the lymph that would normally be transported from the liver into the venous system to be shunted into the lymphatic system. It is possible that minimally elevated venous pressures, in association with other unknown factors, may be sufficient to substantially elevate lymphatic flows through the TD.

Clinical Signs/Signalment/History

Most animals with chylothorax present with a normal body temperature unless extremely excited or severely depressed. Additional findings in patients with chylothorax may include coughing, muffled heart sounds, depression, anorexia, weight loss, pale mucous membranes, arrhythmias, murmurs, and pericardial effusion.

Oriental breeds (i.e., Siamese and Himalayan) appear to have an increased prevalence of chylothorax. Although chylothorax may affect animals of any age, in one study older cats were more likely to develop chylothorax than young cats. This finding was believed to indicate an association

---

*Personal communication, Aguirre-Sanceledonio M, Fossum TW, 2005.

between chylothorax and neoplasia. Afghan hounds and Shiba Inu dogs are also thought to be predisposed to chylothorax.

Coughing is often the first (and occasionally the only) abnormality noted by owners until the animal becomes dyspneic. Many owners report that they first noticed coughing months before presenting the animal for veterinary care; therefore animals that cough and do not respond to standard treatment of nonspecific respiratory problems should be evaluated for chylothorax. Coughing may be a result of irritation caused by the effusion or related to the underlying disease process (i.e., cardiomyopathy, thoracic neoplasia).

Diagnosis

Animals that have collapsed lung lobes that do not appear to reexpand following removal of chyle or other pleural fluid should be suspected of having underlying pulmonary parenchymal or pleural disease such as fibrosing pleuritis. Diagnosis of fibrosing pleuritis is difficult. The atelectatic lobes may be confused with metastatic or primary pulmonary neoplasia, LLT, or hilar lymphadenopathy. Radiographic evidence of pulmonary parenchyma that fails to reexpand after removal of pleural fluid should be considered possible evidence of atelectasis with associated fibrosis. Fibrosing pleuritis should also be considered in animals with persistent dyspnea in the face of minimal pleural fluid.

Fluid recovered by thoracentesis should be placed in an ethylenediaminetetraacetic (EDTA) tube for cytologic examination. Placing the fluid in an EDTA tube rather than a "clot-tube" allows cell counts to be performed. Although chylous effusions are routinely classified as exudates, the physical characteristics of the fluid may be consistent with a modified transudate. The color varies, depending on dietary fat content and the presence of concurrent hemorrhage. The protein content is variable and often inaccurate because of interference of the refractive index by the high lipid content of the fluid. The total nucleated cell count is usually less than 10,000 and consists primarily of small lymphocytes or neutrophils, with lesser numbers of lipid-laden macrophages.

Chronic chylous effusions may contain low numbers of small lymphocytes because of the inability of the body to compensate for continued lymphocyte loss. Nondegenerative neutrophils may predominate with prolonged loss of lymphocytes or if multiple therapeutic thoracentesis have induced inflammation. Degenerative neutrophils and sepsis are uncommon findings because of the bacteriostatic effect of fatty acids, but they can occur iatrogenically because of repeated aspirations.

Pseudochylous effusion is a term that has been misused in the veterinary literature to describe effusions that look like chyle but in which a ruptured TD is not found. Given the known causes of chylothorax in dogs and cats, this term should be reserved for effusions in which the pleural fluid cholesterol is greater than the serum cholesterol concentration and the pleural fluid triglyceride is less than or equal to the serum triglyceride. Pseudochylous effusions are extremely rare in veterinary patients but may be associated with tuberculosis.

Chylothorax must be differentiated from other types of pleural effusion. Pyothorax may appear grossly similar to chylothorax, but the predominant cell type is a degenerative neutrophil in animals with infection of the pleural space. To help determine if a pleural effusion is truly chylous, several tests can be performed, including comparison of fluid and serum triglyceride levels, Sudan III stain for lipid droplets, and the ether clearance test. The most diagnostic test is comparison of serum and fluid triglyceride levels. If the effusion is truly chylous, it contains a higher concentration of triglycerides than simultaneously collected serum.

MEDICAL MANAGEMENT OF CHYLOTHORAX

If an underlying disease is diagnosed, it should be treated, and the chylous effusion managed by intermittent thoracentesis. If the underlying disease is treated effectively, the effusion often resolves; however, complete resolution may take several months. Surgical intervention should be considered in animals with idiopathic chylothorax or in those that do not respond to medical management. Chest tubes should only be placed in animals with suspected chylothorax secondary to trauma (very rare), when rapid fluid accumulation necessitates that thoracentesis be performed several times a week to prevent dyspnea, or after surgery. Electrolytes should be monitored since hyponatremia and hyperkalemia have been documented in dogs with chylothorax undergoing multiple thoracentesis (Willard et al., 1991). A low-fat diet may decrease the amount of fat in the effusion, which may improve the animal's ability to resorb fluid from the thoracic cavity.

Commercial low-fat diets are preferable to homemade diets; however, if commercial diets are refused, homemade diets are a reasonable alternative (Fossum, 2007). Medium-chain triglycerides (once thought to be absorbed directly into the portal system, bypassing the TD) are transported via the TD of dogs. Thus they may be less useful than previously believed. In addition, they are relatively unpalatable, and most cats and some dogs refuse to eat food to which they have been added. It is unlikely that dietary therapy will cure this disease, but it may help in the management of animals with chronic chylothorax. Clients should be informed that with the idiopathic form of this disease there is no effective treatment that stops the effusion in all animals. However, the condition may resolve spontaneously in some animals after several weeks or months.

Benzopyrene flavinoids such as rutin have been used for the treatment of lymphedema in humans for years and have been recommended for the treatment of chylothorax in cats. Although a small number of animals with chylothorax reportedly have resolved the effusion after treatment with this drug (Thompson, Cohn, and Jordan, 1999), the efficacy of rutin in the treatment of chylothorax is unproven. The recommended dosage is 50 to 100 mg/kg orally three times a day.

Somatostatin is a naturally occurring substance that has an extremely short half-live. It inhibits gastric, pancreatic, and biliary secretions (i.e., glucagon, insulin, gastric acid, amylase, lipase, and trypsin) and prolongs gastrointestinal transit time; decreases jejunal secretion; and stimulates gastrointestinal water absorption. In recent years analogs of somatostatin have been used to successfully treat chylothorax in humans with traumatic or postoperative chylothorax. In these patients reduced gastrointestinal secretions may aid healing of the TD by decreasing TD lymphatic flows (Markham, 2000). It has also been reported to result in early decreased drainage and early fistula closure in dogs with experimental transection of the TD. The mechanism by which nontraumatic chylothorax may benefit from this treatment is unclear; however, resolution of pleural fluid has been reported in cats with idiopathic chylothorax in whom octreotide (Sandostatin, Novartis Pharmaceutical Corp.), has been administered.* Octreotide (10 mcg/kg subcutaneously [SQ] three times a day for 2 to 3 weeks) is a synthetic analog of somatostatin that has a prolonged half-life and minimal side effects. Soft stools that resolve after withdrawal of the drug may occur. Prolonged treatment should be discouraged because in humans treatment for longer than 4 weeks has been associated with gallstone formation. I (TF) have used octreotide in two dogs; one with chylothorax and one with serosanguineous effusion after TD ligation. Although the latter dog resolved the effusion within a few days of treatment, the former case did not respond. The efficacy of octreotide in animals with chylothorax requires further investigation.

Fibrosing pleuritis is a life-threatening complication of chronic chylothorax, particularly in cats. In addition to chylothorax, pyothorax, feline infectious peritonitis, hemothorax, and tuberculosis have been associated with the development of fibrosing pleuritis. Although the cause of the fibrosis is unknown, apparently it can develop subsequent to any prolonged exudative or blood-stained effusion. Exudates are characterized by a high rate of fibrin formation and degradation. Fibrin formation probably increases because chronic inflammatory exudates such as chylothorax and pyothorax induce changes in mesothelial cell morphologic features, resulting in increased permeability, mesothelial cell desquamation, and triggering of both pathways of the coagulation cascade. These desquamated mesothelial cells have also been shown to produce type III collagen in cell culture, promoting fibrosis. In addition, the chronic presence of pleural fluid might lead to impairment in the mechanism of fibrin degradation. Fibrinolysis may decrease because direct injury to mesothelial cells may reduce inherent fibrinolytic activity of the cells and/or the increased fluid volume may dilute local plasminogen activator. Plasminogen activator converts the precursor plasminogen to its active form, plasmin. Fibrinolytic activity in mammals is attributable primarily to this serine protease. In animals with fibrosis the pleura is thickened by diffuse fibrous tissue that restricts normal pulmonary expansion. Pulmonary function testing in humans with fibrosing pleuritis have shown a decrease in vital capacity and static compliance, necessitating greater negative intrapleural pressures for any given change in lung volume when compared with healthy patients.

*Personal communication, Gretchen Sicard.

SURGICAL TREATMENT OF CHYLOTHORAX

Surgical intervention is warranted in animals that do not have underlying disease and in whom medical management becomes impractical, and the approaches I (TWF) advocate are summarized in the following paragraphs. Medical management becomes impractical when thoracentesis is required more frequently than once a week or when repeat thoracentesis fails to relieve the dyspnea. Surgical options include mesenteric lymphangiography and TD ligation, subtotal pericardiectomy, omentalization, passive pleuroperitoneal shunting, active pleuroperitoneal or pleurovenous shunting, and pleurodesis. Of these only the first two (TD ligation and pericardiectomy) are recommended as first-line therapies. Pericardectomy also may effectively treat or even prevent the serosanguineous effusions that occasionally occur after TD ligation in some animals.

In a recent study TD ligation with pericardectomy was performed in 17 animals, and pericardectomy alone was performed in 3 additional animals that presented over a 5.5 year period to one institution (Fossum et al., 2004). Nineteen animals presented for evaluation of idiopathic chylothorax (9 dogs, 10 cats), and 1 dog presented for serosanguineous pleural fluid after TD ligation that had been performed elsewhere. Clinical signs of pleural fluid resolved in 10 of 10 dogs and 8 of 10 cats after surgery. The overall success rate for surgical treatment of chylothorax (i.e., resolution of pleural fluid) in this study was 90% (100% in dogs and 80% in cats). These data suggest that TD ligation in conjunction with pericardectomy has a favorable outcome in animals with idiopathic chylothorax.

The only effective treatment for fibrosing pleuritis is decortication; however, the indications and value of decortication in animals are unknown. Decortication may give the best functional result when the pleuritis is of short duration and pulmonary parenchymal disease is minimal. In such cases the thickened pleura is not firmly adherent to the underlying parenchyma and can be removed without severely damaging the underlying lung; however, pneumothorax is a common sequelae and usually requires tube thoracentesis. Decortication in humans carries a good prognosis if only one or two lobes are involved; however, when the fibrosis is diffuse, as occurs in many animals with chylothorax, even with effective decortication a guarded prognosis is warranted. When more than one lung lobe is decorticated, reexpansion pulmonary edema may occur and is often fatal. If decortication is successful, lung expansion and pulmonary function may improve over a 2- to 3-month period. In a recent study several animals were reported to have severe fibrosing pleuritis despite the owners' claims that the clinical signs had been of recent onset (Fossum et al., 2004). In that study decortication was deemed necessary in two cats because the extent of the pleuritis was such that it was thought that respiratory distress might still be present after surgery, even if the pleural fluid resolved. Both of these cats developed severe pneumothorax and required prolonged intensive management of this condition. One cat was determined to have a tracheal rupture that healed spontaneously over a 2-week period. Neither cat developed reexpansion pulmonary edema after decortication; thus decortication may be of value in animals with severe fibrosing pleuritis in which increased lung expansion is deemed important. Owners must be cautioned about the increased morbidity and mortality associated with this condition, particularly with the development of reexpansion pulmonary edema. Duration of clinical signs appears to be a highly unreliable predictor of the success of surgery or the extent of fibrosing pleuritis in animals with chylothorax. Many owners simply do not recognize clinical signs of chylothorax until the disease is well advanced. In these animals fluid production may be offset by fluid resorption for months; thus clinical signs are mild until sufficient pleural thickening occurs that fluid resorption is diminished or eliminated completely. It is important to note that the degree of fibrosing pleuritis does not appear to warrant a poor prognosis. I have operated on cats with severe fibrosing pleuritis that later appear clinically normal once the effusion stops.

Thoracic Duct Ligation With Mesenteric Lymphangiography

Thoracic duct ligation is performed in cats from a left lateral intercostal thoracotomy or transdiaphragmatically. In dogs the ligation is performed from a right intercostal thoracotomy. The mechanism by which TD ligation is purported to work is that following TD ligation abdominal lymphaticovenous anastomoses form for the transport of chyle to the venous system. Therefore chyle bypasses the TD, and the effusion resolves. Advantages of TD ligation are that, if it is successful, it results in complete resolution of pleural fluid (as compared to palliative procedures described in the following paragraphs) and may prevent fibrosing pleuritis from developing. The disadvantages include that operative time is long, which is problematic in debilitated animals; there is a high incidence of continued or recurrent chylous or nonchylous (from pulmonary lymphatics) effusion; and mesenteric lymphangiography is often difficult to perform (particularly in cats). Without mesenteric lymphangiography, complete ligation of the TD cannot be ensured; however, lymphangiography in cats might not be uniformly successful in verifying complete ligation of the TD. In addition, some animals may form collateral lymphatics past the site of the ligature and thus reestablish TD flow. If chyle flow is directed into the diaphragmatic lymphatics, chylothorax may continue or recur.

For lymphangiography, food is withheld 12 hours before surgery. The left side of the thorax in cats (right side in dogs) and the abdomen, or just the abdomen if a midline celiotomy is being performed, is prepared for aseptic surgery. If a thoracic approach to the TD is used, a paracostal incision is made to exteriorize the cecum. Once the cecum has been exteriorized, a lymph node adjacent to the cecum is located. A small volume (0.1 to 1 ml) of methylene blue (USP 1%, American Quinine) diluted with saline to a light-to-medium blue color may be injected into the lymph node to increase visualization of lymphatics. Repeated doses of methylene blue should be

avoided because of the risk of inducing Heinz body anemia or renal failure. Careful dissection of the mesentery near this node allows large lymphatic vessels to be visualized and cannulated with a 20- or 22-gauge over-the-needle catheter. Cannulation of this lymphatic is more difficult in cats than in dogs because cats have more fat in their mesentery and their lymphatics are significantly smaller. Two sutures (4-0 silk) are placed in the mesentery and used to secure the catheter and an attached piece of extension tubing in place (the ends of the suture can be looped over the hub of the extension tubing). An additional suture may be placed around the extension tubing and through a segment of intestine to prevent dislodgement of the catheter. A three-way stopcock is attached to the end of the extension tubing, and a water-soluble contrast agent is injected at a dose of 1 ml/kg diluted with 0.5 ml/kg of saline. A lateral thoracic radiograph is taken while the last millimeter is being injected. This lymphangiogram can be used to help identify the number and location of branches of the TD, which need to be ligated, and it can be repeated following ligation to help determine the extent of lymphangiectasia present in the cranial thorax.

Typically the TD is approached via caudal intercostal thoracotomy (9th to 12th intercostal space) or via an incision in the diaphragm. Once the duct has been located, hemostatic clips can be used to ligate it. The advantage of using hemoclips (Edward Weck and Co. Inc.) is the reference point created for subsequent radiographs if further ligation is necessary. In addition, a nonabsorbable suture such as silk is also placed around the duct. Visualization of the TD can be aided by injecting methylene blue into the lymphatic catheter. If a catheter was not placed, the dye can be injected into a mesenteric lymph node, although this results in inferior visualization of the TD. Pericardiectomy may be performed from the same intercostal thoracotomy in most animals. If the pericardium cannot be reached, a second more cranial intercostal thoracotomy may be necessary.

Active Pleuroperitoneal or Pleurovenous Shunting

Active pleuroperitoneal or pleurovenous shunting (Denver double valve peritoneous shunt, Denver Biomaterials Inc.) has been recommended for the treatment of chylothorax in dogs and cats and may be a reasonable consideration in animals in which all other therapies have failed. Commercially made shunt catheters are available and can be used to pump fluid from the thorax to the abdomen. Under general anesthesia a vertical incision is made over the middle of the fifth, sixth, and seventh ribs. A purse-string suture is placed in the skin at this site; and, following the placement of fenestrations in the venous end of the shunt catheter; the catheter is bluntly inserted into the pleural space. A tunnel is created by blunt dissection under the external abdominal oblique muscle, and the pump chamber is pulled through the tunnel. The efferent end of the catheter is then placed into the abdominal cavity through a preplaced purse-string suture and incision located just caudal to the costal arch. The shunt must be placed with the pump chamber directly overlying a rib so that the chamber can be compressed effectively. Complications associated with pleuroperitoneal or pleurovenous shunts include: (1) the shunts are expensive; (2) they may easily occlude with fibrin; (3) some animals do not tolerate compression of the pump chamber; and (4) they require a high degree of owner compliance and dedication. In addition, thrombosis, venous occlusion, sepsis, and electrolyte abnormalities have been reported in humans.

Omentalization

Omentalization has been described as a technique to treat animals with chylothorax when other surgical treatments are not successful or deemed impossible. A fifth- or sixth-space intercostal thoracotomy is made to provide access to the cranial thorax. A paracostal incision is then made so that a dorsal omental pedicle flap can be raised. The omental flap is brought through an incision in the pars costalis of the diaphragm. Care should be taken to avoid rotation of or excessive tension on the omental pedicle. The omentum is spread out within the thorax to provide a large surface area. An omentopexy is performed by using synthetic absorbable suture to anchor the omentum to the mediastinum in the region of the lymphaticovenous anastomoses between the TD and the cranial vena cava. Sutures should be placed so that they do not interfere with the blood supply of the omentum. The success of this technique is unproven, and I (TWF) do not routinely recommend it.

Other Treatments

Passive pleuroperitoneal shunting has been recommended as treatment of chylothorax in cats, but this technique is no longer recommended. The goal of placing a fenestrated silastic sheet in the diaphragm was to allow drainage of the chylous fluid into the abdomen where the fluid could be resorbed by visceral and peritoneal lymphatics, thereby alleviating the respiratory distress and need for subsequent thoracentesis. This technique may be ineffective, and chronic irritation of the sheeting may be associated with neoplastic transformation of tissues.

Pleurodesis is the formation of generalized adhesions between the visceral and parietal pleura. Adhesions may occur spontaneously in association with pleural effusion, or in some species they can be induced following instillation of an irritating substance into the pleural cavity. This technique has been recommended for the treatment of chylothorax in dogs and cats, but I (TWF) do not recommend it. For pleurodesis to be successful the lungs must be able to contact the body wall; however, many animals with chronic chylothorax have some thickening of their visceral pleura, which prohibits normal lung expansion (see fibrosing pleuritis in previous paragraphs). Neither mechanical (surgical) pleurodesis or talc administration resulted in pleurodesis in experimental dogs; however, thickening of the pleura did occur in some animals. Chemical or surgical pleurodesis is unlikely to be successful in animals with chylothorax.

NEOPLASTIC EFFUSION

Any intrathoracic neoplasia potentially can result in pleural effusion through obstruction to lymphatic or venous drainage, inflammation, secondary infection, or hemorrhage. Effusion is most often associated with mediastinal lymphoma, pleural mesothelioma, and metastatic carcinoma.

Mediastinal lymphoma is a common tumor of cats and is treated with combination chemotherapeutic protocols as recommended for multicentric lymphoma. Response is often dramatic, with significant resolution of respiratory difficulties in 48 to 72 hours. Pending response, thoracocentesis is used to remove as much fluid from the thorax as possible. Stress is minimized, and an oxygen-enriched environment or nasal oxygen is provided as needed. Local radiation therapy can be administered when available and provides a similarly rapid response. Rates of remission as high as 92%, with durations as long as 29 months (median 6 months), have been reported for cats receiving combination chemotherapy (Cotter, 1983).

Remission is less likely in animals with mesothelioma and carcinoma involving the pleural surfaces. However, clinical signs in dogs sometimes can be relieved for prolonged periods through control of effusion with palliative therapy using intracavitary cisplatin (American Pharmaceutical Partners) with or without additional systemic treatment. Moore, Kirk, and Cardona (1991) reported resolution of pleural effusion in four dogs treated with intracavitary cisplatin. Effusion resolved in three dogs after one intracavitary treatment and in the fourth dog after two treatments. Recurrence of effusion ranged from 129 to longer than 306 days in a dog still alive and free of effusion at the time of the report. Two other dogs subsequently treated by the same author had decreased volumes, but not resolution, of effusion (Moore, 1992).

Cisplatin is able to reach high concentrations in tissues within a few millimeters of the contact surface. It is most likely to be effective in controlling effusion before actual nodules have formed. Systemic chemotherapy can be administered in addition to intracavitary treatment to reach the interior of larger, vascularized nodules. Cisplatin placed within the pleural cavity is absorbed systemically; if combined with systemic chemotherapy, dosages need to be adjusted to avoid significant toxicity.

The protocol for intracavitary delivery of cisplatin is not difficult. Dogs are administered 0.9% sodium chloride intravenously for 4 hours before treatment and for 2 to 4 hours after treatment at a rate of 10 ml/kg/hour. Cisplatin is given at a dose of 50 mg/m² diluted in 0.9% sodium chloride to a total volume of 250 ml/m². The solution is warmed to body temperature before administration. A 16-gauge over-the-needle catheter is placed into the pleural space using sterile technique, and as much fluid as possible is removed. Cisplatin is infused slowly into the pleural space through the same catheter, and the catheter is removed. Treatments were scheduled every 4 weeks in the study by Moore, Kirk, and Cardona (1991), and sometimes additional systemic treatment was given. The current protocol being used at our institution is to administer intracavitary carboplatin every 3 to 4 weeks as needed to control effusion. If the effusion resolves completely, intracavitary therapy is discontinued after the fourth treatment. Intracavitary therapy is reinstituted if effusion recurs.

Nonlymphomatous malignant effusions are rare in cats, and standard treatment has not been established. Cisplatin is not recommended for administration in cats because of acute pulmonary toxicity. Carboplatin has not been associated with pulmonary toxicity and has the potential to be effective as an intracavitary infusion.

Pleurodesis has been proposed to control malignant effusions in dogs and cats. Unfortunately a consistently effective technique has not been established (see section on Chylothorax earlier in the chapter).

The therapeutic response to any of these palliative measures is based primarily on clinical response, with the goal of therapy being a good quality of life with normal respiratory efforts. Thoracic radiographs can be taken for objective determination of progress. Animals with slowly forming effusion can be further managed with intermittent thoracocentesis. Placement of pleuroperitoneal shunts may provide symptomatic relief to patients requiring frequent thoracocentesis. By creating a path for pleural fluid to cross into the abdominal cavity, more space is available within the thoracic cavity for expansion of the lungs. Pleuroperitoneal shunts were discussed previously.

LUNG LOBE TORSION

LLT is a rotation of the lung lobe along its long axis, with twisting of the bronchus and pulmonary vessels at the hilus. Any mechanism that increases mobility of a lung lobe seems to favor development of torsion. Partial collapse of the lung (i.e., with pulmonary disease or trauma) frees it from its normal spatial relationships with the thoracic wall, mediastinum, and adjacent lung lobes and they may enhance mobility. Pleural effusion or pneumothorax, along with subsequent atelectasis of lung lobes, can allow increased movement of a lobe, predisposing to torsion. Although LLT has been reported to cause chylothorax in dogs, it is more likely that the chylothorax caused the LLT. LLT has been reported secondary to previous thoracic surgery, in which lung lobes are manipulated and may remain partially collapsed after thoracic closure.

Torsion of a lung lobe results in venous congestion of the affected lobe; however, the arteries remain at least partially patent, allowing blood to enter. As fluid and blood enter the alveoli, lung consolidation occurs, and the lobe becomes dark colored and firm, similar in shade to the liver. The shape of the affected lobe is often altered, and it may appear displaced from its normal location within the thorax radiographically. Pleural fluid usually accumulates because of continued venous congestion.

Clinical Signs/Signalment/History

Deep-chested large-breed dogs, especially Afghan hounds, are more commonly affected. LLT in Afghan hounds may be associated with chylothorax. In large breeds LLT has been reported to occur spontaneously, without previous history of disease or trauma. LLT has also been reported in small breeds, including pugs, but is usually secondary to primary pleural effusion, thoracic surgery,

or trauma. It is rare in cats. Middle-aged dogs are more commonly affected, but LLT may occur in animals of any age. Affected animals usually have moderate-to-severe respiratory distress. Pleural effusion is consistently present in animals with LLT; therefore findings often include muffled heart and lung sounds. Other findings may include depression, anorexia, coughing, fever, dyspnea, hemoptysis, hematemesis, and/or vomiting.

Diagnosis

Thoracic radiographic changes are variable, depending on the volume of pleural fluid, presence or absence of pre-existing disease, and duration of the torsion. The most consistent finding is the presence of pleural effusion accompanied by an opacified lung lobe. Initially air bronchograms are present in the torsed lobe and can be seen extending toward the abdomen. Air bronchograms eventually disappear as fluid and blood fill the bronchial lumen. The presence of a noninflated, radiopaque lung lobe that persists after removal of pleural fluid should increase suspicion for LLT. Positional radiographs using horizontal beam x-rays (lateral decubitus or upright ventrodorsal) are often helpful. Pleural fluid secondary to LLT may persist around the affected lobe rather than fall to the dependent side. Failure of the lobe to reinflate in the "up" or nondependent hemithorax is another indication of LLT. Ultrasonography or computed tomography may also allow confirmation of a LLT prior to surgery. The right middle lung lobe is the most commonly torsed lobe in dogs.

Laboratory findings with LLT are variable. Fluid analysis may reveal a sterile, inflammatory effusion or chyle; or the fluid may be bloody. However, pleural effusion of any etiology can initiate a secondary LLT, making results of pleural fluid analysis variable and confusing. The appearance of blood in a previously nonhemorrhagic pleural fluid may indicate occurrence of LLT. An inflammatory leukogram may be present; however, changes in the leukogram may reflect the initial disease process rather than the LLT.

MEDICAL MANAGEMENT

Initial therapy is aimed at stabilizing the animal and alleviating respiratory distress before surgery. Thoracentesis should be performed to remove pleural fluid. Persistent or massive pleural effusion may require placement of a chest tube. Oxygen therapy given by oxygen cage or nasal insufflation is beneficial to some animals. Underlying diseases such as pneumonia should be identified and treated with appropriate antibiotic therapy. Intravenous fluid therapy is beneficial before and during surgery to maintain hydration.

SURGICAL TREATMENT

Spontaneous correction of a torsed lung lobe is uncommon because of swelling of the lobe and rapid formation of adhesions. The treatment of choice for LLT is lobectomy of the affected lobe. Unless LLT is diagnosed very quickly (i.e., immediately after a surgical procedure), damage to the pulmonary parenchyma is generally severe enough that attempts to salvage the lobe are not warranted. Recurrence has been reported following surgical correction in which lobectomy was not performed. The prognosis is good for most animals with LLT if surgery is performed; however, animals have developed LLT in another lobe after surgery. Pleural effusion (unless it is chylous in nature) usually resolves within a few days of surgery.

IDIOPATHIC PLEURAL EFFUSION

A clinical diagnosis of idiopathic pleural effusion is made after complete diagnostic evaluation fails to identify a primary cause. The general diagnostic approach has been described earlier in the section on Initial Management of Pleural Effusion. Note that specific tests are required to identify the etiologies listed in Box 153-1. Although not strictly idiopathic, in our experience the most common cause of clinically diagnosed idiopathic effusion is occult neoplasia. Ultrasonography and computerized tomography are more sensitive than radiography in suggesting a diagnosis of neoplasia. Ultrasonography is best performed while effusion is present. In other cases or to confirm ultrasonographic findings, thoracoscopy or thoracotomy with gross examination and biopsy of pleura and lungs may be necessary to confirm a diagnosis of neoplasia. Another potential occult cause of apparently idiopathic effusion is infection with organisms that are not identified through routine cytologic or microbiologic methods, such as with occult mycobacteriosis. Thus a trial course of azithromycin can be considered (5 to 10 mg/kg q24h PO for 7 days and then q48h for 5 weeks).

Palliative treatment for patients with idiopathic pleural effusion begins with intermittent thoracocentesis. If it is difficult to remove the effusion adequately with routine thoracocentesis, ultrasound guidance may prove useful in identifying localized regions of fluid accumulation and directing needle or catheter placement. Corticosteroids and/or other immunosuppressive drugs have been successful in reducing the rate of fluid accumulation in some animals (but not all) with idiopathic pleural effusion. Pleuroperitoneal shunts are placed in patients that require frequent thoracocentesis to allow comfortable breathing (see section on Chylothorax earlier in the chapter).

References and Suggested Reading

Cotter SM: Treatment of lymphoma and leukemia with cyclophosphamide, vincristine, and prednisone. II. Treatment of cats, *J Am Anim Hosp Assoc* 19:166, 1983.

Fossum TW, Birchard SJ, Jacobs RM: Chylothorax in 34 dogs, *J Am Vet Med Assoc* 188:1315, 1986.

Fossum TW et al: Chylothorax in cats: 37 cases (1969-1989), *J Am Vet Med Assoc* 198:672, 1991.

Fossum TW et al: Severe bilateral fibrosing pleuritis associated with chronic chylothorax in 5 cats and 2 dogs, *J Am Vet Med Assoc* 201:317, 1992.

Fossum TW et al: Chylothorax associated with right-sided heart failure in 5 cats, *J Am Vet Med Assoc* 204:84, 1994.

Fossum TW et al: Thoracic duct ligation and pericardectomy for treatment of idiopathic chylothorax, *J Vet Intern Med* 18:307, 2004.

Fossum TW: *Small animal surgery*, ed 3, St Louis, 2007, Elsevier.

Kerpsack SJ et al: Evaluation of mesenteric lymphangiography and thoracic duct ligation in cats with chylothorax: 19 cases (1987-1992), *J Am Vet Med Assoc* 205:711, 1994.

Lee KA et al: Management of malignant pleural effusions with pleuroperitoneal shunting, *J Am Coll Surg* 178:586, 1994.

Markham KM et al: Octreotide in the treatment of thoracic duct injuries, *Am J Surg* 66:1165, 2000.

Moore AS: Chemotherapy for intrathoracic cancer in dogs and cats, *Probl Vet Med* 4:351, 1992.

Moore AS, Kirk C, Cardona A: Intracavitary cisplatin chemotherapy experience with six dogs, *J Vet Intern Med* 5:227, 1991.

Neath JN, Brockman JD, King LG: Lung lobe torsion in dogs: 22 cases (1981-1999), *J Am Vet Med Assoc* 217:1041; 2000.

Piek CJ, Robben JH: Pyothorax in nine dogs, *Vet Q* 22:107, 2000.

Pressler BM et al: Isolation and identification of Mycobacterium kansasii from pleural fluid of a dog with persistent pleural effusion, *J Am Vet Med Assoc* 220:1336, 2002.

Rooney MB, Monnet E: Medical and surgical treatment of pyothorax in dogs: 26 cases (1991-2001), *J Am Vet Med Assoc* 221:86, 2002.

Thompson MS, Cohn LS, Jordan RC: Use of ru tin for medical management of idiopathic chylothorax in four cats, *J Am Vet Med Assoc* 215:345, 1999.

Walker AL, Jang SS, Hirsh DC: Bacteria associated with pyothorax of dogs and cats: 98 cases (1989-1998), *J Am Vet Med Assoc* 216:359, 2000.

Willard MD et al: Hyponatremia and hyperkalemia associated with idiopathic or experimentally induced chylothorax in four dogs, *J Am Vet Med Assoc* 199:353, 1991.

CHAPTER 154

Pneumothorax

AMY K. VALENTINE, *Springfield, Oregon*
DANIEL D. SMEAK, *Columbus, Ohio*

Pneumothorax is the accumulation of air within the pleural space. The air source usually results from disruption of the thoracic wall, bronchial tree, pulmonary parenchyma, or esophagus, caused by injury or disease. Clinical signs of pneumothorax depend on the amount and rate of pleural air accumulation; but, when severe, signs may include tachypnea, dyspnea, abdominal breathing, or cyanosis. Affected animals compensate for reduced tidal volume by increasing frequency of ventilation, thus maintaining minute volume. Auscultation reveals diminished lung sounds, clear heart sounds, and increased resonance with percussion. Radiographic features of pneumothorax include air density within the pleural space, retraction of lung edges from the thoracic wall and diaphragm, and displacement of the cardiac silhouette away from the sternum on the lateral view. Pneumothorax causes decreased lung expansion with subsequent ventilation-perfusion mismatch, hypoxemia, and loss of intrapleural pressure gradients that impair the thoracic pump and venous return. These changes ultimately result in reduction of ventilatory capacity and cardiac output. Pneumothorax may be classified based on cause (traumatic or spontaneous) and pathophysiology (open or closed, simple or tension).

TRAUMATIC PNEUMOTHORAX

Traumatic pneumothorax, the most common type of pneumothorax in the dog, occurs in nearly half of all traumatic chest injuries (Kramek and Caywood, 1987). Traumatic pneumothorax is classified as open when it involves a penetrating injury to the chest wall as with a bite or stab wound, gunshot, or shearing injury. A closed traumatic pneumothorax usually is associated with blunt trauma resulting in laceration of the trachea, bronchial tree, or pulmonary parenchyma. Simple, closed pneumothorax is characterized by *nonprogressive* loss of intrapleural negative pressure. In contrast, tension pneumothorax develops when a disrupted airway, lung parenchyma, or chest wall functions as a one-way valve. This leads to *progressive* air leakage and elevation in intrapleural pressure, causing rapid deterioration of the patient.

Management

Management of traumatic pneumothorax is predicated on multiple factors, including the volume, source, and flow of air within the intrapleural space; the clinical condition of the patient; the severity of concurrent injury; and the availability of critical care resources. The most important means of stabilizing a patient in distress with pneumothorax, regardless of the cause, is evacuating free pleural air and reestablishing normal thoracic pressure gradients. This may be accomplished by various techniques, including closure of thoracic wall defect(s), thoracentesis (Fig. 154-1), tube thoracostomy (Fig. 154-2) with intermittent or continuous suction (Fig. 154-3), or a Heimlich flutter valve (Salci et al., 2005). Thoracentesis is usually performed as the initial treatment for pneumothorax since it is the simplest, least invasive means of pleural evacuation. Placement of a thoracostomy tube is indicated if the pneumothorax recurs rapidly, when persistent air leakage is anticipated, or if thoracentesis is unsuccessful in reestablishing negative intrapleural pressure. In cases in which air accumulation is so rapid that intermittent suction does not relieve respiratory distress,

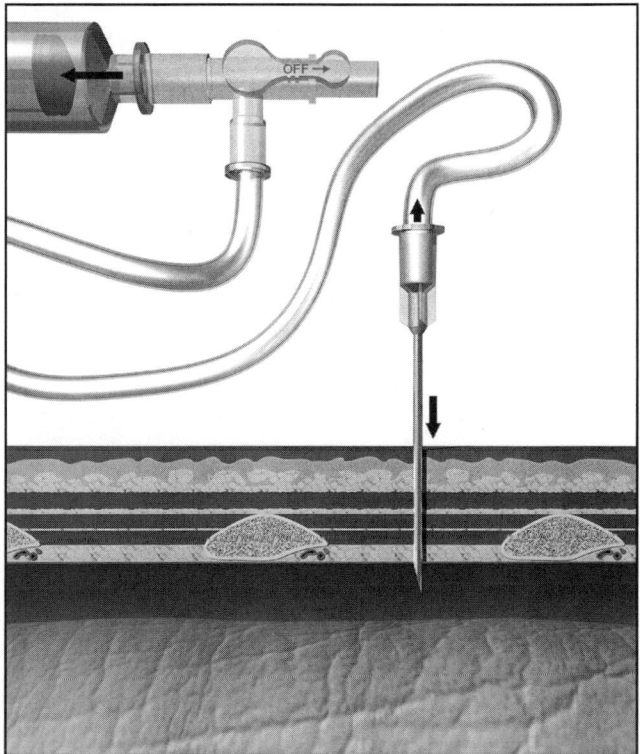

Fig. 154-1 Thoracentesis technique. A 20-gauge hypodermic needle or teat cannula is inserted into the eighth or ninth intercostal space in the upper half of the thoracic cage. Negative pressure is applied with a large syringe attached to an extension tube and a three-way stopcock. The collected air is expelled from the syringe by closing the stopcock to the patient and evacuating the syringe through the free open port on the stopcock (this process is repeated until no air remains in the pleural space).

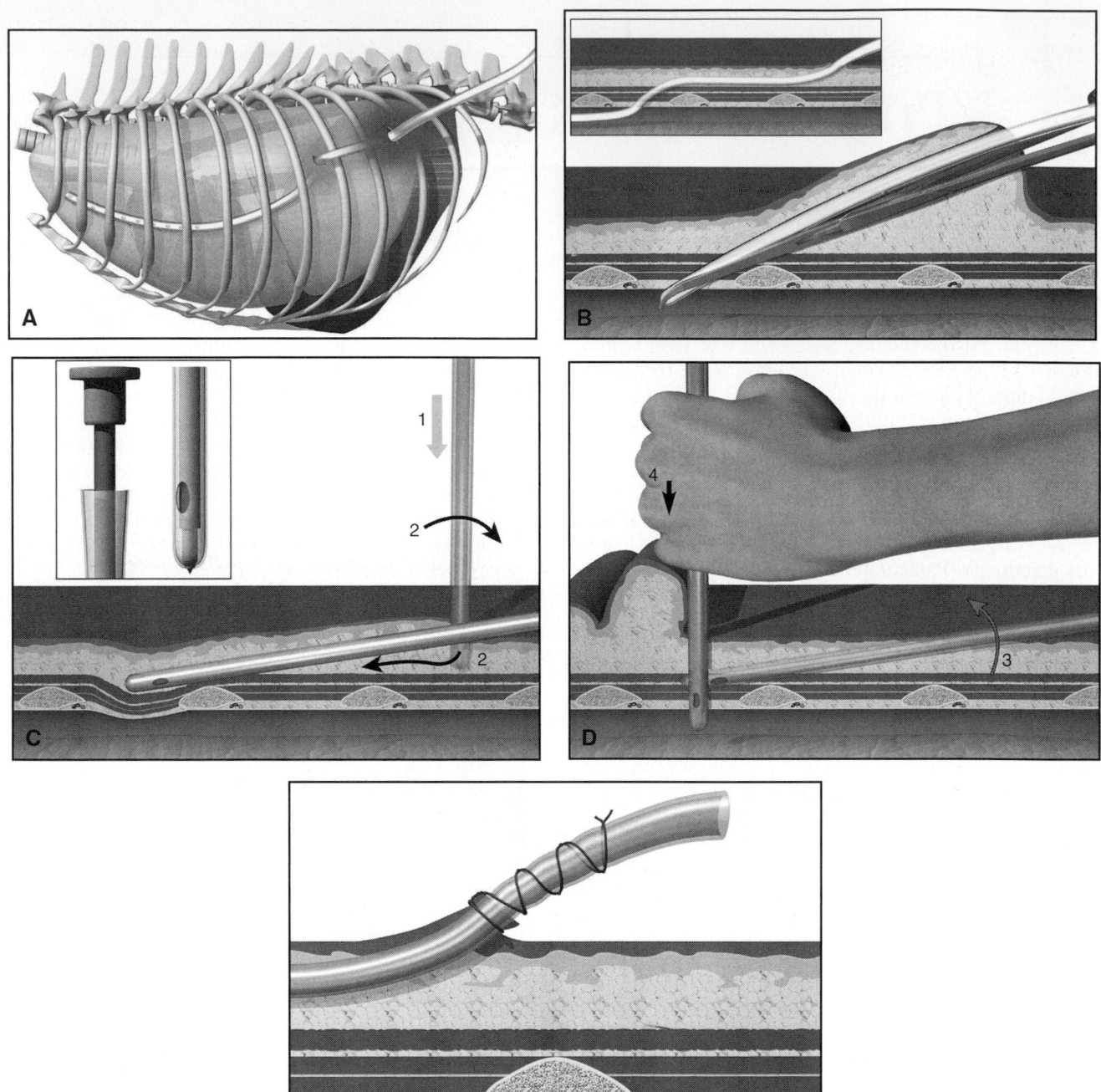

Fig. 154-2 Thoracostomy tube placement. **A,** A small skin incision is created in the dorsal one third of the 10th intercostal space. The tube is tunneled subcutaneously two intercostal spaces and inserted in the eighth intercostal space. It is then advanced cranioventrally to the level of the second rib. It is initially clamped to prevent further pleural air accumulation, connected to an adapter and stopcock for pleural aspiration, and finally fixed to the skin with suture. **B,** Placement of a thoracostomy tube with forceps. A small skin incision is made, and the forceps (with the tube grasped in the tips) is bluntly pushed through the subcutaneous, penetrating the eighth intercostal space. The forceps are spread open to release the tube and feed it into the cranial thorax. Alternately the loose skin can be pulled cranially several inches by an assistant, an incision is made directly over the eighth space, and the tube is inserted directly downward into the pleural space. Once the tube is advanced into the thorax, the skin is released, creating a tunnel and causing the tube to exit from the skin caudally. **C,** Placement of a trocar thoracostomy tube. The tube with stylet is inserted through a small skin incision, and the tube is advanced bluntly through the subcutaneous tissue to the middle of the eighth intercostal space. The flanged end is held with the dominant hand, with the thumb placed over the stylet to hold it firmly in place. **D,** The less dominant hand grasps the tube within an inch or two of the sharp tip. As progressive downward pressure is placed on the tube, it is "hinged" up to a perpendicular position. The hand at the flanged end drives the tube into the pleural space, and the hand holding the tube close to the tip functions as a guard against excessive trocar penetration. The stylet is removed as the tube is advanced to the cranioventral thorax. **E,** The tube is secured to the dog with a single purse-string suture placed within 5 mm of the skin incision. Either the free ends from the purse-string knot are used to hold the tube or a separate skin bite (shown) is taken adjacent to the knotted purse-string suture, and the suture is crisscrossed and knotted four to five times to produce a friction knot without occluding the tube lumen.

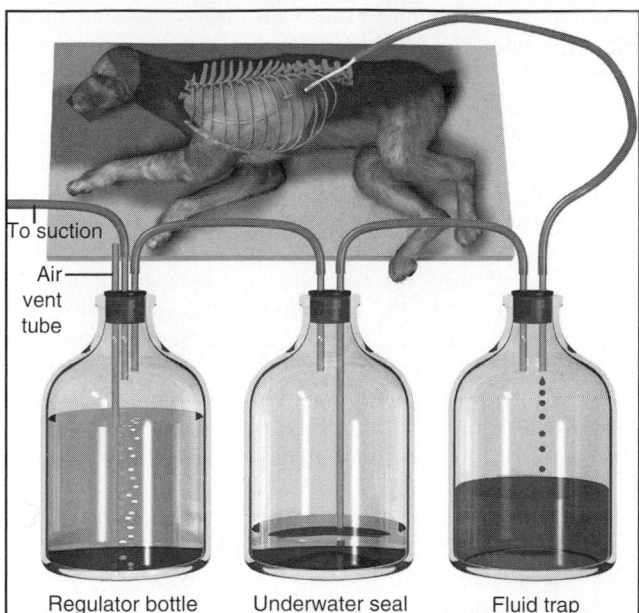

Fig. 154-3 Three-bottle continuous pleural evacuation system. The chest tube is securely attached to a long flexible tubing and connected to a bottle serving as a *fluid trap*. The fluid trap is attached to a bottle serving as an *air trap* with an air vent tube submerged in 1 to 2 cm of water (to prevent air from being drawn into the thorax if a leak were to occur within the last two bottles of the system). The air trap is connected to the *pressure regulator* bottle with an air vent tube submerged in water. The level of submersion of the air vent tube in the third bottle determines the amount of pleural suction (this should not exceed 15 to 20 cm of water). The third tube in the regulator bottle is connected to a suction system. Commercially available systems possess the same functions as the three-bottle system displayed, but they are contained within a small portable unit.

continuous suction should be instituted. Additional therapies may include supplemental oxygen, mild sedation, analgesics, intravenous fluids, and intravenous antibiotics, depending on the overall condition of the patient.

Open Pneumothorax
The thoracic wound is closed immediately with a clean cloth, bandage, or glove during initial patient evaluation and transportation to the treatment area. The wound is inspected briefly; the area surrounding it is clipped free of hair and debris; and a sterile, occlusive bandage with abundant amounts of antiseptic ointment is applied to seal the wound. Immediate thoracentesis is performed to evacuate air from the intrapleural space if the dog is dyspneic. Tube thoracostomy with intermittent or continuous suction should be considered if the pneumothorax progresses after initial thoracentesis. Thorough wound débridement and reconstruction can be performed once the patient has been stabilized and anesthetized under more controlled, sterile conditions.

Simple Pneumothorax
Simple pneumothorax, if not too severe, usually responds well to conservative management. Bilateral thoracentesis is performed if there is clinical indication based on tachypnea (especially if the respiratory rate exceeds 80 breaths/minute), dyspnea, or hypoventilation (cyanosis, abnormal

arterial blood gas measurements, or decreased oxygen saturation). Most pleural injuries seal within hours after thoracentesis and cage rest are instituted. Patients should be kept quiet, and ventilatory rate and pattern monitored closely for several days to detect recurrence or progression of pneumothorax.

Tension Pneumothorax
Tension pneumothorax, regardless of etiology, causes severe pathophysiologic consequences and can be rapidly fatal. Dogs with tension pneumothorax have severe and progressive dyspnea and distress, weakness, shallow respirations, abdominal breathing, and a barrel-shaped chest wall. Thoracic radiographs reveal a large amount of free air with flattening and displacement of the diaphragm caudally. Treatment should be rendered quickly and should include immediate thoracentesis followed by tube thoracostomy with intermittent or continuous suction. A flutter (Heimlich) valve may be used as an alternative to continuous suction; however, efficacy of the valve may be decreased by blood or effusion or in dogs weighing less than 15 kg (Orton, 1993). An exploratory thoracotomy for definitive treatment should be considered only after these measures have failed to stabilize the animal. It is often difficult at surgery to identify the site of traumatic injury causing the pneumothorax, and general anesthesia puts the dog at additional risk. If surgery is indicated, a median sternotomy is the preferred surgical approach for complete thoracic exploration since it allows visualization of both sides of the thorax (Bjorling, 1994).

Esophageal Perforation
Pneumothorax associated with esophageal perforation is usually caused by direct trauma or mucosal erosion from a sharp, intraluminal foreign body. Other etiologies may include gunshot injury, bite wound, or iatrogenic injury during endoscopic procedures. Pneumothorax from thoracic esophageal injury is often accompanied by pneumomediastinum and an inflammatory pleural effusion. Diagnosis of the perforation is confirmed using endoscopy or positive contrast radiography with an organic (iodinated) contrast agent. Medical treatment for esophageal perforation is discussed elsewhere (Johnson and Sherding, 1994; Kyles, 2003). Pneumothorax and pleural effusion are treated initially with chest tube drainage. Thoracotomy for esophageal surgery is reserved for significant esophageal injury or when esophageal healing is not progressing despite appropriate medical management. The severity of esophageal injury is usually based on subjective evaluation of the perforation, including the size of the defect, the health of the esophageal tissue around the defect, and evidence of focal versus generalized esophageal leakage of fluid or air (Johnson and Sherding, 1994).

SPONTANEOUS PNEUMOTHORAX

Spontaneous pneumothorax is defined as accumulation of air within the pleural space that is not associated with traumatic injury to the respiratory tract or chest wall. In contrast to traumatically induced pneumothorax, spontaneous pneumothorax is rare in dogs. Siberian huskies were overrepresented in one report (Puerto et al., 2002). Secondary spontaneous pneumothorax can stem from

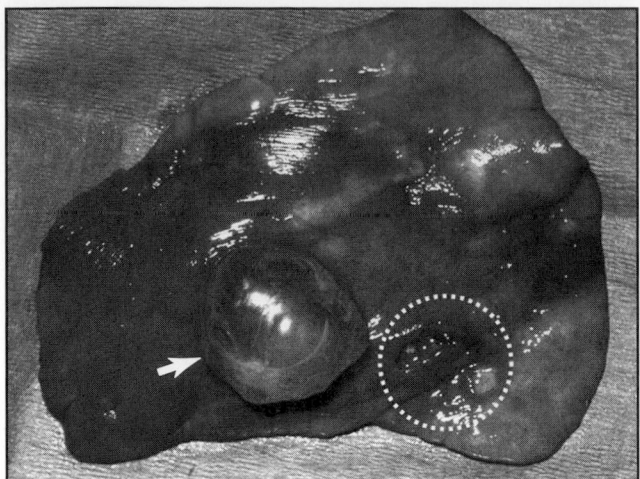

Fig. 154-4 Excised cranial lung lobe from a dog with primary spontaneous pneumothorax. The *white arrow* points to an intact pulmonary bleb. The *dashed circle* contains a ruptured (upper left) and an intact bullae (lower right).

respiratory tract rupture caused by an underlying lung disease such as parasitism (e.g., paragonimiasis), bacterial pneumonia, neoplasia, and pulmonary abscess. Primary spontaneous pneumothorax is caused by rupture of idiopathic pulmonary blebs or bullae (Fig. 154-4). Pulmonary blebs are defined as localized accumulation of air within the visceral pleura, whereas pulmonary bullae are confluent alveoli. Ruptured subpleural blebs in conjunction with bullous emphysema have been reported as the most common cause of spontaneous pneumothorax in dogs; however, 50% of the cases in one study had underlying (nonemphysematous) lung disease. Management and prognosis for spontaneous pneumothorax are determined in part by the underlying cause (Valentine et al., 1996). Approximately one third of dogs with spontaneous pneumothorax have tension pneumothorax (Holtsinger et al., 1993).

A general diagnostic protocol to identify underlying disease is recommended and should include a complete blood count, serum chemistry profile, examination for *Dirofilaria*, fecal flotation and sediment examination, and thoracic radiography. Serial evaluation of thoracic radiographs may be necessary after chest evacuation to help identify occult pulmonary disease. Computed tomography (CT), bronchoscopy, and thoroscopy represent advanced procedures for identification of pulmonary lesions responsible for pneumothorax (Lipscomb, Hardie, and Dubielzig, 2004; Au et al., 2006).

Initial management of spontaneous pneumothorax is similar to the previous discussion on management of traumatic pneumothorax. Thoracentesis is routinely performed and followed by tube thoracostomy if clinically significant pneumothorax recurs. If intermittent pleural evacuation is unsatisfactory, continuous suction should be administered to alleviate respiratory distress.

Secondary Spontaneous Pneumothorax (Underlying Parenchymal Disease)

Management of underlying pulmonary disease is important for appropriate treatment of dogs with secondary spontaneous pneumothorax. Parasitic disease such as

dirofilariasis or paragonimiasis should be treated medically; the pneumothorax usually responds well to conservative (chest drainage) therapy (Valentine et al., 1996). Underlying pneumonitis caused by foreign body (plant material) migration has a good prognosis for long-term resolution following lung lobectomy (Puerto et al., 2002). Underlying metabolic disease resulting in secondary pulmonary parenchymal or microvascular pathology may be refractory to treatment and therefore associated with a poorer prognosis for recovery and long-term survival (Valentine et al., 1996). Pulmonary masses documented with thoracic radiographs may be further defined with CT or magnetic resonance imaging, ultrasonography (difficult with the presence of free pleural air), bronchoscopy, fine-needle aspiration and cytologic studies, or exploratory thoracotomy. Prognosis and specific therapy are predicated on the diagnosis. The mortality rate for dogs with spontaneous pneumothorax from confirmed neoplasia has been reported to vary from 50% (Puerto et al., 2002) to 100% (Valentine et al., 1996). These high mortality rates include a 50% euthanasia rate following diagnosis of the primary or metastatic neoplasm. Spontaneous pneumothorax related to bacterial or fungal pneumonia or pulmonary abscess rupture has been associated with mortality rates as high as 80% (Valentine et al., 1996).

Primary Spontaneous Pneumothorax (Bullous Emphysema)

A presumptive diagnosis of bullous emphysema should be considered if no other pulmonary disease can be identified after the general diagnostic screen (listed earlier) is performed. Radiographic confirmation of pulmonary bullae in dogs is highly unreliable since most bullae that have ruptured and are actively leaking are not visible on plain radiographs. CT scanning may be useful for diagnosis and presurgical assessment of pulmonary bullae or blebs, but overall efficiency and predictive values for CT in dogs remain unknown (Lipscomb, Hardie, and Dubielzig, 2004; Au et al., 2006). Initial treatment for primary spontaneous pneumothorax may include thoracentesis followed by tube thoracostomy; however, the long-term recurrence rate with pleural evacuation alone may be as high as 70% (Valentine et al., 1996) to 87% (Holtsinger et al., 1993). A mortality rate of 59% caused by recurrent spontaneous pneumothorax following conservative treatment also has been reported (Puerto et al., 2002). In contrast, the long-term recurrence rate for dogs with ruptured pulmonary bullae or blebs following complete or partial lung lobectomy was 12.5% in one study (Valentine et al., 1996), and the mortality rate related to surgical complications was less than 5% (Holtsinger et al., 1993). Therefore early exploratory thoracotomy following CT or thoracoscopy is still recommended for diagnosis and treatment of primary spontaneous pneumothorax to optimize both survival and resolution (Puerto et al., 2002).

A median sternotomy is the standard surgical approach to adequately evaluate each hemithorax. Complete visual and tactile inspection of all lung lobes should be performed systematically. The thoracic cavity is subsequently filled with saline to identify the source(s) of air leakage from the affected lung during positive-pressure ventilation. Partial lung lobectomy may be considered if focal, peripheral pulmonary bullae are confirmed. Complete lung lobectomy should be performed if bullous disease is located toward the hilus or involving the majority of the lung lobe parenchyma. Histopathologic examination and bacterial or fungal culture or both should be considered if clinically indicated. Mechanical (gauze sponge) or chemical (tetracycline, sterile talc) pleurodesis may be performed if diffuse bullous emphysema is observed; however, the efficacy of this form of treatment for spontaneous pneumothorax in dogs is unknown (Orton, 1993). Mechanical abrasion and chemical sclerosis (talc slurry) were evaluated for efficacy of pleurodesis in normal dogs. Complete obliteration of the pleural space was not achieved after either treatment; however mechanical abrasion may be useful as an adjunctive treatment for bullous emphysema (Jerram et al., 1999). On rare occasion pneumothorax persists despite a negative thoracic exploratory. Chemical pleurodesis with tetracycline has met with some success in controlling air leakage.

Recently thoracoscopy has also been used to successfully locate and surgically excise the lung lobes affected with primary spontaneous pneumothorax in three dogs (Brissot et al., 2003). Visualization of bilateral hemithoraces was performed, and endoscopic excision of the affected areas documented bullous emphysema. All dogs recovered without recurrent pneumothorax through 18 to 29 months after surgery. Advantages of thoracoscopic evaluation and treatment may include easier identification of pulmonary bullae and decreased postoperative pain and morbidity.

References and Suggested Reading

Au JJ et al: Use of computed tomography for evaluation of lung lesions associated with spontaneous pneumothorax in dogs: 12 cases (1999–2002), *J Am Vet Med Assoc* 228(5):733, 2006.

Bjorling DE: Management of thoracic trauma. In Birchard SJ, Sherding RG, editors: *Saunders manual of small animal practice*, Philadelphia, 1994, Saunders, p 593.

Brissot HN et al: Thoracoscopic treatment of bullous emphysema in 3 dogs, *Vet Surg* 32(6):524, 2003.

Holtsinger RH et al: Spontaneous pneumothorax in the dog: a retrospective analysis of 21 cases, *J Am Anim Hosp Assoc* 29:195, 1993.

Jerram RM et al: The efficacy of mechanical abrasion and talc slurry as methods of pleurodesis in normal dogs, *Vet Surg* 28(5):322, 1999.

Johnson SE, Sherding RG: Disease of the esophagus and disorders of swallowing. In Birchard SJ, Sherding RG, editors: *Saunders manual of small animal practice*, Philadelphia, 1994, Saunders, p 637.

Kramek BA, Caywood DD: Pneumothorax, *Vet Clin North Am* 12:2, 1987.

Kyles AE: Esophagus. In Slatter D, editor: *Textbook of small animal surgery*, ed 3, Philadelphia, 2003, Saunders, p 582.

Lipscomb VJ, Hardie RJ, Dubielzig RR: CT scanning of dogs with spontaneous pneumothorax, *Vet Rec* 154(11):344, 2004.

Orton EC: Pleura and pleural space. In Slatter D, editor: *Textbook of small animal surgery*, ed 2, Philadelphia, 1993, Saunders, p 381.

Puerto DA et al: Surgical and nonsurgical management of and selected risk factors for spontaneous pneumothorax in dogs: 64 cases (1986-1999), *J Am Vet Med Assoc* 220(11):1670, 2002.

Salci H et al: Use of a Heimlich flutter valve in a dog with spontaneous pneumothorax, *Austr Vet Pract* 350:47, 2005.

Valentine AK et al: Spontaneous pneumothorax in dogs, *Compend Contin Educ* 18:1, 1996.

CHAPTER **155**

Pulmonary Thromboembolism

SUSAN G. HACKNER, *New York, New York*

Pulmonary thromboembolism (PTE) is the obstruction of a pulmonary vessel, or vessels, by a blood clot. Blood clots can develop locally or at a distant site and translocate to the pulmonary vasculature. Thromboemboli mechanically obstruct arterial blood flow, release humoral factors, and stimulate neurogenic reflexes. Subsequent alterations in respiratory and hemodynamic function are responsible for the clinical signs and diagnostic findings in patients with PTE. The condition ranges from incidental, clinically insignificant disease to massive embolism and death.

The actual incidence of PTE in small animals is uncertain. An incidence of 0.9% in the general canine necropsy population has been reported. However, necropsy studies underestimate the incidence of PTE because not all patients with PTE die and because thrombi lyse rapidly following death (50% dissolution within 3 hours). The incidence of PTE in critically ill animals and in patients with certain disease states is appreciable. Recognition of these conditions and their risk for thromboembolism (TE) is crucial to diagnosis and to decisions regarding prophylaxis.

PTE is extremely underdiagnosed in veterinary patients. Antemortem diagnosis is hindered by a lack of clinical awareness, clinical signs that resemble many other disease processes, and the relatively invasive or specialized tests required for definitive diagnosis. In retrospective studies PTE was suspected antemortem in less than 40% of affected dogs and 14% of affected cats.

Mortality rates of PTE in animals are unclear but are probably significant. Patient survival often depends on a prompt diagnosis and appropriate therapy instituted without delay.

ETIOLOGY

Thrombosis depends on three major risk factors: endothelial injury, blood stasis, and alterations in the blood constituents to favor thrombosis. This concept is known as Virchow's triad. Although all three factors are prothrombotic or thrombophilic, true hypercoagulability refers to a quantitative or qualitative defect in the coagulation system: platelet hyperaggregability, excessive activation or decreased removal of coagulation factors, deficiencies of natural anticoagulants (antithrombin, protein C), or defective fibrinolysis. The term *hypercoagulable states* in dogs and cats refers to acquired disorders in patients with underlying systemic disease known to be associated with an increased risk of thrombosis. In these patients the pathogenesis is generally multifactorial and complex. Inherited hypercoagulable states have not been reported in animals.

PTE has been shown to be associated with the following conditions in dogs: protein-losing nephropathy, neoplasia, cardiac disease (dirofilariasis, endocarditis, and cardiomyopathy), necrotizing pancreatitis, immune-mediated hemolytic anemia (IMHA), hypercortisolism (naturally occurring hyperadrenocorticism and corticosteroid therapy), diabetes mellitus, atherosclerosis, sepsis, trauma, and major surgical procedures. With the exception of cardiac disease, these conditions are all considered hypercoagulable states. In studies of necropsied dogs with PTE, the majority of dogs (59% and 64%) had more than one potentially hypercoagulable state. Many dogs had thrombosis in other organ systems.

PTE in cats is most commonly associated with cardiac disease (cardiomyopathy) and neoplasia. Other reported conditions include pancreatitis, IMHA, protein-losing nephropathy, protein-losing enteropathy, hypercortisolism, and sepsis. In one study 47% of cats had multiple disease processes that may have predisposed to TE.

PATHOPHYSIOLOGY

The pulmonary vascular bed filters venous blood. As a result, thromboemboli in the venous circulation become trapped in the pulmonary vasculature. In the healthy lung this vasculature has tremendous reserve capacity; minor occlusions are well tolerated. However, if occlusion is substantial or if it occurs in a patient with preexisting pulmonary or cardiac compromise, the consequences are clinically significant. Such sequelae may be pulmonary and/or hemodynamic.

Pulmonary consequences of PTE include ventilation-perfusion mismatch, bronchoconstriction, hypoxemia, and hyperventilation. Somewhat later (24 to 48 hours), two additional complications may occur (i.e., regional loss of surfactant and rarely pulmonary infarction). These result in atelectasis, edema, and effusion.

Hemodynamic consequences of PTE are related to the magnitude of the obstruction and the preexisting status of the cardiovascular and pulmonary systems. If reserve capacity is exceeded, pulmonary vascular resistance increases, resulting in increased right ventricular afterload and ventricular oxygen requirements. If these exceed supply, ischemia, arrhythmias, or right ventricular failure ensues. Obstruction to pulmonary blood flow and the resultant decrease in venous return may lead to decreased cardiac output.

The burden caused by massive PTE is largely the result of mechanical obstruction. This is exacerbated by hypoxia-induced vasoconstriction and the release of humoral substances from activated platelets on the surface of the thrombus. PTE is a dynamic event; thrombi can undergo lysis, fragmentation, or growth. Pathophysiologic consequences reflect such changes, and findings depend on the point in time at which they are examined.

CLINICAL PRESENTATION

The severity of clinical signs reflects the magnitude of respiratory and cardiac compromise and the ability of these systems to compensate for the insult. Signs range from mild to profound compromise and death. Symptoms are variable and inconsistent and can mimic a multitude of other diseases. The most common signs are dyspnea, tachypnea, and depression. Other signs include coughing, hemoptysis, cyanosis, and hypoperfusion. Collapse, shock, and sudden death can occur in patients with markedly decreased cardiac output.

Adventitious lung sounds may be auscultable in patients with pulmonary edema, hemorrhage, or bronchoconstriction. Pleural effusion may be detectable if present. Tachycardia occurs frequently. In patients with pulmonary hypertension a loud or split second heart sound may be auscultable. Signs of hypoperfusion occur in patients with marked hemodynamic compromise.

DIAGNOSIS

The diagnosis of PTE is often very difficult. It can resemble many other conditions such as pneumonia, pulmonary edema, intrapulmonary hemorrhage, neoplasia, and pleural effusion. Findings on routine tests are generally nonspecific, and specialized techniques are required for diagnostic confirmation. These techniques are either invasive or not widely available.

The first step in the diagnosis of PTE is an index of suspicion. PTE should be on the list of differentials in any patient with an acute onset of respiratory signs, particularly if the patient has no prior evidence of respiratory disease. The presence of predisposing diseases or potential hypercoagulable states increases the degree of suspicion.

Initial assessment of the patient involves thoracic radiography, arterial blood gas analysis, and routine hematologic and biochemical screening. If these are consistent with PTE or if they fail to identify another diagnosis, secondary assessment is indicated. Secondary assessment should include cardiac evaluation via echocardiography, determination of D-dimer concentrations, screening for possible underlying thrombophilic conditions, and testing for hypercoagulability (when possible). If results of these tests support a possible diagnosis of PTE, confirmatory tests should be considered. When confirmatory tests are not available or feasible, the diagnosis of PTE must be based on clinical likelihood determined from the aforementioned assessments and on elimination of other potential etiologies.

Initial Assessment

Thoracic Radiography

Most patients with PTE have abnormal thoracic radiographs, but findings are nonspecific. Two common radiographic patterns are described: regional oligemia (hypovascular lung regions) and pulmonary infiltration. Regional oligemia appears as areas of increased radiolucency and represents reduced vascular filling distal to the thrombotic occlusion. Oligemia is best identified on ventrodorsal and dorsoventral radiographic views. Pulmonary infiltrates represent areas of hemorrhage, atelectasis, or infarction. They are most commonly alveolar but may be interstitial or mixed alveolar-interstitial. They can be solitary or multiple and may involve more than one lung lobe. They are usually amorphous with indistinct borders. Less commonly radioopacity involves an entire lobe creating distinct lobar borders. Infiltrates are more common in the right and caudal lobes. Infrequently infiltrates appear as distinct, wedge-shaped densities with the apex toward the pulmonary hilus.

Pulmonary vessel changes may be evident, including enlargement of the main pulmonary artery segment and attenuation of a lobar artery or vein. Cardiomegaly may also occur. Pleural effusion is not common in dogs and is usually mild. It appears to be more common in cats.

Patients with PTE can have normal thoracic radiographs. In canine studies the percentage of dogs with normal radiographs ranged from 9% to 27%. In a feline study 7% had normal thoracic radiographs. Since these are necropsy studies and thus select for more severely affected patients, the occurrence of normal radiographs in animals with PTE is likely even higher. Thoracic radiographs that underestimate the degree of clinical respiratory compromise are an important clue to the presence of PTE.

Arterial Blood Gas Analysis

Arterial blood gas analysis can aid in the diagnosis of PTE and is relevant to the management thereof, but changes are not pathognomonic. The most common abnormalities are (in descending order): an increased alveolar-arterial oxygen tension gradient ($P_{(A-a)}O_2$), hypoxemia, hypocapnia, and decreased oxygen responsiveness. Hypercapnia is uncommon but can occur with severe compromise. When these changes are present, they are nonspecific indicators of inefficient gaseous exchange and do not confirm a diagnosis of PTE. Moreover, the presence of normal blood gas values does not exclude PTE.

Routine Hematologic and Biochemical Studies

These have limited value in the diagnosis of PTE. When abnormal results are present, they generally reflect inflammation, hypoxemia, or stress. However, results may be useful in identifying predisposing hypercoagulable states.

Secondary Assessment

Echocardiography

Echocardiography can be a valuable tool in the assessment of patients with suspected PTE. It may show changes consistent with PTE or evidence of compromise that impacts management decisions.

Rarely echocardiography demonstrates a right-sided thrombus ("thrombus in transit"), tricuspid valve thrombus, or organized thrombus in the main pulmonary artery. More commonly it demonstrates changes suggestive of PTE and pulmonary hypertension. These include dilation of the right ventricle, pulmonary artery, or inferior vena cava; right ventricular hypokinesis; tricuspid regurgitation; or abnormal septal wall motion. However, a normal echocardiogram does not exclude a diagnosis of PTE; a significant percentage of patients with PTE evidence no echocardiographic anomalies.

Right ventricular hypokinesis is associated with a doubling of the mortality rate in humans. Therefore its presence prompts a more aggressive approach to therapy. Arterial blood pressure is not a reliable indicator because hypokinesis can be present in normotensive patients.

D-Dimers

Of the laboratory markers, only D-dimers have proven clinical usefulness in the diagnosis of PTE in humans. D-dimer is a unique fibrin degradation product that is formed when cross-linked fibrin is proteolyzed by plasmin. Therefore it is specific for active coagulation and fibrinolysis and useful for detecting TE. However, the half-life of D-dimers is short (approximately 5 hours). As such they are only useful for detection of acute TE. D-dimers are not specific for TE. Elevated D-dimers have been demonstrated in dogs with neoplasia, hepatic disease, renal failure, cardiac failure, internal hemorrhage, disseminated intravascular coagulation, and following surgical procedures.

D-dimers in humans have a high negative predictive value for PTE and are used extensively as a screening test. Most workers recommend their use as part of a diagnostic algorithm to determine which patients require more definitive testing. They are considered most useful to rule out PTE in patients deemed to have a low clinical probability.

The use of D-dimers in small animal patients with suspected PTE is less clear but appears similar. Sensitivities of 89% to 100% have been reported in dogs, using the standard enzyme-linked immunosorbent assay test, a latex bead agglutination test (Accuclot D-dimer, Sigma), and a canine-specific point-of-care test (AGEN canine D-dimer test, Sigma). Reported specificity is approximately 70%. When semiquantitative methods have been used, specificity approaches 90%, with strong positive results (greater than 1000 ng/dl on latex agglutination) occurring only in patients with TE and with hemoabdomen.

Based on the available data in dogs, it appears that PTE can be considered extremely unlikely if the D-dimer test is negative and clinical suspicion is low. However, PTE is not excluded by a negative D-dimer, especially if the time period from event to presentation is prolonged. A positive test should always be interpreted in the light of other clinical findings. If these support PTE, further testing is indicated. A strong positive test in the absence of intracavitary hemorrhage is highly suggestive of TE.

Screening for Underlying Conditions

Since PTE occurs almost exclusively secondary to one or more underlying conditions, any suspicion of PTE should prompt a thorough investigation for these conditions. Although their presence does not confirm PTE, they provide further support when definitive diagnosis is not possible, and they are essential in clinical management.

Testing for Hypercoagulability

The presence of hypercoagulability neither confirms nor predicts TE. It merely indicates that TE is possible and, together with other compatible findings, enables the clinician to build a stronger case for a diagnosis. However, laboratory confirmation of hypercoagulability is difficult.

The use of thromboelastography (TEG) has been described in small animals for the assessment of overall hypercoagulability. Clinical experience is encouraging. However, few institutions offer TEG, and further studies are needed to fully elucidate clinical usefulness.

Significant hyperfibrinogenemia can indicate potential hypercoagulability but occurs in few of the hypercoagulable states (e.g., some cases of pancreatitis and sepsis). The majority of patients with PTE do not have hyperfibrinogenemia. Similarly, assay of antithrombin (AT-III) concentration or activity may be useful in some cases. A correlation with thrombotic risk has been shown when AT-III deficiency is the primary mechanism for thrombosis (e.g., protein-losing nephropathy). AT-III levels may also be decreased as a result of massive TE. Normal AT-III levels do not exclude hypercoagulability.

The routine coagulogram is not helpful in identifying hypercoagulation or TE. It is frequently normal. If abnormalities are present, they are nonspecific and generally reflect a consumptive process. There is no known correlation between thrombocytosis or shortened coagulation times and thrombosis.

Confirmation of Pulmonary Thromboembolism

Pulmonary scintigraphy has been shown to be sensitive and specific for experimental PTE and has been used successfully clinically in dogs and cats. The technique, however, is limited to few referral facilities with scanning equipment. The rationale of pulmonary scintigraphy is that occlusion of pulmonary vessels by a thrombus results in areas of the lung that continue to be ventilated despite the absence of perfusion. Radioactive labeling of the pulmonary blood (perfusion scan) followed by the inspired air (ventilation scan) allows demonstration of areas of the lungs with ventilation-perfusion mismatch. A normal perfusion scan virtually excludes a diagnosis of PTE, but an abnormal perfusion scan is not specific for PTE; perfusion defects can result from numerous nonthrombotic conditions, including pneumonia, edema, contusions, obstructive pulmonary disease, and atelectasis. However, these conditions are associated with decreased regional ventilation and an abnormal ventilation scan.

Spiral computed tomographic angiography (CTA) is used extensively for the diagnosis of PTE in humans. The technique allows precise visualization of the pulmonary vasculature and is rapid and noninvasive, making it an ideal modality in the unstable patient. Reported sensitivity in humans is as high as 95.5%, with a specificity of 97.6%. The technique has not yet been reported in small animals, but clinical experience at several institutions is encouraging.

Selective pulmonary angiography remains the gold standard for the diagnosis of PTE. It is indicated for the definitive diagnosis or exclusion of PTE when scintigraphy or spiral CT is unavailable or inconclusive. Iodinated contrast medium is rapidly injected via a large-bore catheter into the pulmonary arterial tree. The pulmonary arterial system can then be visualized via radiography. Intraluminal filling defects, abrupt termination of pulmonary arteries, and the complete absence of arterial branches are diagnostic for PTE. A regional loss of vascularity, asymmetric blood flow, tortuous pulmonary arteries, and abrupt tapering of peripheral vessels support a diagnosis of PTE but are nonspecific. A negative selective arteriogram essentially excludes clinically significant PTE. Because the procedure requires general anesthesia, which depresses cardiovascular function and is invasive, it constitutes a significant risk in the compromised patient. This limits the use of this technique in clinical veterinary practice.

Nonselective pulmonary angiography is easier and safer than selective techniques. General anesthesia and specialized equipment typically are not required. Contrast medium is injected via a large-bore catheter into the right side of the heart or the jugular vein. This study is less sensitive and more difficult to interpret than selective angiography because of dilution of the contrast medium by venous blood and the superimposition of vascular structures.

THERAPY

Therapy of PTE should begin as soon as possible. It should include support of the respiratory and cardiovascular systems, prevention of thrombus propagation and recurrence, and possibly thrombolysis. It appears that a relatively small percentage of PTE events are immediately fatal. In the normal dog thrombi begin to lyse spontaneously within hours. Even in patients with disturbed fibrinolysis, some degree of reorganization and lysis occurs in the days following the thromboembolic event. Therefore, if the patient can be supported through the respiratory and cardiovascular compromise and further exacerbations can be prevented, survival is possible. In some cases compromise may be so extreme that adequate support is not possible and survival unlikely. In such cases pharmacologic thrombolysis may be indicated.

Respiratory and Cardiovascular Support

Oxygen supplementation is indicated when dyspnea is evident and/or when partial pressure of arterial oxygen decreases below 70 mm Hg or arterial O_2 saturation to less than 92%. In addition to relieving hypoxemia, oxygen supplementation has been shown to dilate pulmonary vessels, improve hemodynamics, reduce pulmonary hypertension, and improve right ventricular function. Theoretically bronchodilators may be beneficial. Methylxanthine bronchodilators such as theophylline have small positive inotropic effects and produce sustained pulmonary vasodilation. Theophylline improves diaphragmatic contractility in dogs and reduces respiratory muscle fatigue. These effects may be beneficial in extremely dyspneic or tachypneic patients in which muscle fatigue can result in respiratory failure.

Perfusion should be optimized in any patient with hypoxemia. In these patients arterial oxygen content is deficient, and any decrease in perfusion further exacerbates the already reduced tissue oxygen delivery. In addition, optimizing perfusion reverses the prothrombotic effects of vascular stasis and hypoxia-induced endothelial injury.

Prevention of Propagation and Recurrence of Thrombi

Thrombi tend to propagate, especially in the thrombophilic and hypofibrinolytic patient, and this can result in further compromise. The patient with PTE has proved that it is thrombophilic and therefore at risk for additional thromboembolic episodes. When death occurs beyond the first few hours following PTE, it is likely caused by a recurrent embolic event. Therefore management should be focused on preventing such occurrences. Anticoagulants form the cornerstone of such management.

Anticoagulants
In general, anticoagulants do not lyse existing thrombi; they are indicated to inhibit propagation and prevent recurrent venous thrombosis. Since PTE is primarily a venous event, anticoagulants are indicated in all cases of PTE.

Unfractionated heparin. Heparin is the standard of care in humans with PTE. Until further data are available on alternate anticoagulants in small animal patients, unfractionated heparin remains the drug of choice for initial PTE therapy.

Unfractionated heparin is composed of mucopolysaccharides of varying molecular weights. The primary mechanism of action is the potentiation of AT-III activity, leading to the inactivation of thrombin (factor IIa), and factors Xa, IXa, XIa, and XIIa. Of these, thrombin and factor Xa are the most responsive to inhibition. The relative effect of heparin on these factors depends on its molecular size. Smaller heparin molecules (less than 18 saccharide units) are unable to catalyze thrombin inhibition. However, these molecules are effective in catalyzing the inhibition of factor Xa. Other effects of heparin include reduced blood viscosity, decreased platelet function, increased vascular permeability, and mildly enhanced fibrinolysis. These effects contribute to the hemorrhagic risk.

The anticoagulant effects of a standard dose of heparin vary widely among patients. Heparin may be poorly absorbed from subcutaneous sites. The plasma clearance of heparin depends on a rapid, dose-related, saturable cellular mechanism and a slower, nondose-related renal clearance. As such, the intensity and duration of effect increase disproportionately with increasing dose. Higher–molecular weight species are cleared more rapidly than lower–molecular-weight species, resulting in varied anticoagulant activity over time. Binding of heparin to plasma proteins, endothelial cells, and platelets contributes to the unpredictable response. In addition, some patients appear to have heparin resistance, requiring larger doses to achieve a therapeutic effect.

It has been shown in humans that, unless a prescriptive nomogram is used, many patients receive inadequate heparinization in the initial 24 to 48 hours of therapy, resulting in an increased incidence of recurrent TE. Successful heparin therapy necessitates monitoring the anticoagulant response and titrating the dose to the individual patient. Anticoagulant response can be monitored via the plasma heparin concentration or the partial thromboplastin time (PTT). The therapeutic range of heparin is a concentration of 0.3 to 0.7 units/ml by antifactor Xa assay, and 0.2 to 0.4 units/ml by protamine sulfate titration. However, the turnaround time for these assays makes them impractical for clinical monitoring of the PTE patient. In humans therapeutic heparin concentrations are achieved with a dose of heparin that prolongs the PTT to approximately 1.5 to 2.5 times that of controls. This range is also quoted in the veterinary literature. However, observations in canine studies suggest that this may be excessive (Mischke and Jacobs, 2001). When heparin doses were given to dogs to prolong the PTT to twice normal, plasma heparin concentrations were above therapeutic range. Until further data are available, the author uses a target PTT range of 1.5 to 2 × baseline. A limitation in the use of the PTT to guide heparin therapy is that it is not directly correlated with anticoagulant activity and clinical efficacy. This is largely because the PTT effect of heparin reflects primarily its antifactor IIa activity.

Heparinization guidelines for humans are established. However, it is impossible to give evidence-based recommendations in small animals. There are exceedingly few studies, and most quoted doses are anecdotal. Therefore it would appear prudent to use protocols established in humans and in animal models and to closely monitor PTT values and/or heparin concentrations. For humans the Consensus Conference on Antithrombotic Therapy recommends an intravenous bolus of heparin, followed by continuous-rate infusion (Hyers et al., 2001). Studies have demonstrated no increase in major bleeding compared to subcutaneous administration. The author uses an extrapolation of this protocol in dogs (Table 155-1). Because AT-III is required for heparin effect, plasma transfusion is recommended in patients with documented or suspected AT-III deficiency.

Subcutaneous administration of heparin is not recommended for acute PTE therapy. Although this protocol can reach target PTT ranges, they are rarely achieved rapidly. The use of subcutaneous heparin in patients with acute PTE should be reserved for patients in which intravenous heparin is not feasible. Published doses vary enormously. A small number of canine studies have shown marked individual variability in response, emphasizing the importance of monitoring. The author uses a dose of 200 units/kg every 6 hours, with adjustments based on regular PTT determinations. There is evidence that PTT results do not correlate reliably with plasma heparin concentrations in cats. For this reason heparin infusions are difficult in cats and alternative anticoagulation may be preferable.

Low–molecular weight heparin. Low–molecular weight heparins (LMWHs) are manufactured from unfractionated heparin to yield smaller molecules. These differ in several important respects: superior subcutaneous bioavailability; a prolonged half-life and predictable renal clearance, enabling once or twice daily dosing in humans; and predictable antithrombotic responses, permitting treatment

Table 155-1

Weight-Based Nomogram for the Intravenous Infusion of Heparin* in Dogs

PTT	Dose Change (units/kg/hour)	Additional Action	Next PTT
<1.2 × mean normal	+4	Rebolus with 80 units/kg	6 hours
1.2–1.5 × mean normal	+2	Rebolus with 40 units/kg	6 hours
1.5–2 × mean normal	0	0	6 hours for first 24 hours, then daily
2–3 × mean normal	−2	0	6 hours
>3 × mean normal	−3	Stop infusion 1 hour	6 hours

*An intravenous bolus administration of heparin of 80 to 100 units/kg is administered, followed by a continuous rate infusion of 18 units/kg/hour. A PTT is evaluated 6 hours after initiation of therapy. Adjustments are as indicated in the table.
PTT, Partial thromboplastin time.

based on body weight without laboratory monitoring. Other advantages are their ability to inhibit platelet-bound factor Xa and their decreased effect on platelet function and vascular permeability. These characteristics possibly account for fewer hemorrhagic effects at comparable antithrombotic dosages. Onset of action is rapid, with peak effects generally seen at 2 to 4 hours. Small–molecular weight fractions have little anti-IIa activity and cannot be monitored via PTT. Anticoagulant efficacy is monitored via an antifactor Xa assay. In humans favorable dose-response characteristics make monitoring unnecessary in most patients except those with renal failure.

In human clinical trials subcutaneous LMWH has shown similar or superior efficacy when compared with intravenous unfractionated heparin with regard to recurrent PTE and mortality. Although these drugs are considerably more expensive, the reduced risk and decreased need for monitoring contribute to cost-effectiveness.

Experience with LMWH in small animals is limited. Dalteparin (Fragmin, Pharmacia) at a dose of 150 units/kg every 8 hours subcutaneously was shown to achieve therapeutic ranges in five healthy dogs (Mischke et al., 2001). A study of pharmacokinetics of dalteparin in normal cats suggested that a dose of 100 units/kg every 24 hours subcutaneously was effective. However, clinical experience with this drug in cats indicates that every 6- to 8-hour dosing may be necessary for sustained therapeutic effects. Enoxaparin (Lovenox, Aventis) has also been used in small animals, but published reports are lacking. Until more information is available on effective dosing in small animals, it is hard to recommend LMWH as first choice in the initial therapy of PTE. However, it can be considered when intravenous heparin infusion is not feasible. In this role LMWH is likely preferable to intermittent subcutaneous unfractionated heparin.

Based on current knowledge and personal experience, the author recommends a starting dose of dalteparin of 150 units/kg every 8 to 12 hours in the dog and 100 units/kg every 8 hours in the cat. A reasonable starting dose of enoxaparin is 1 mg/kg every 12 hours. Regardless, it is imperative that anticoagulant efficacy be monitored via anti-Xa assay until an effective dose is established for that patient. Therapeutic range extrapolated from human subjects is an antifactor Xa of 0.3 to 0.7 units/ml. Samples should be collected 24 hours after initiation of therapy, just before injection, and 2 to 4 hours after injection to determine peak effect and duration. Dose and frequency are adjusted accordingly. Once an effective protocol is established for the patient, continued monitoring appears unnecessary, except for patients in renal failure.

Antiplatelet Drugs

Antiplatelet drugs should be considered together with but not in lieu of anticoagulant therapy. Antiplatelet drugs inhibit platelet aggregation, thereby preventing the formation of the primary platelet plug. Traditionally these drugs have been used for the prevention of arterial thrombosis (e.g., aortic, cerebrovascular) since arterial thrombi have a large platelet component compared to venous thrombi. However, there is compelling evidence to suggest a role for antiplatelet drugs as adjunctive therapy in PTE. Recent experimental studies of PTE in the presence of radiolabeled platelets have shown that platelets accumulate in venous thrombi in the early stages. As the thrombus ages, platelet acquisition slows, and the proportion of platelets decreases. Furthermore, venous thrombi activate platelets, causing release of serotonin, adenosine diphosphate (ADP), and thromboxane A_2 (TxA$_2$). Physiologic consequences include bronchoconstriction, vasoconstriction, and pulmonary hypertension. Antiplatelet drugs may ameliorate these effects. Finally, there is convincing clinical evidence in humans, with trials demonstrating a decrease in the incidence of PTE by over one third when antiplatelet therapy was included in the protocol.

Aspirin is the only antiplatelet drug that has been widely used in veterinary patients. It is a cyclooxygenase (COX) inhibitor, thus preventing the formation of various prostaglandins, including thromboxane A_2 (TXA$_2$) and prostacyclin (PGI$_2$). TXA$_2$ is produced by platelets, is largely a COX-1–derived product, and induces platelet aggregation. The antiplatelet effect of aspirin is irreversible, rapid, and saturable. Prostacyclin, produced by vascular endothelial cells is derived from both COX-1 and COX-2, and inhibits platelet aggregation. Aspirin is approximately fifty-fold more potent in inhibiting COX-1 than COX-2. Thus, intuitively, antiplatelet therapy with aspirin should require an ultra-low dose that inhibits TXA$_2$ production while sparing prostacyclin. Indeed, early veterinary studies in small numbers of dogs supported this hypothesis. More recent, large, human clinical trials demonstrate that aspirin is effective over a wide range of doses, including high doses, but that the adverse gastrointestinal effects of the drug are dose related.

The optimal antiplatelet dose of aspirin in dogs is not entirely established. Studies in healthy dogs, and in dogs with IMHA, indicate that a dose of 0.5 mg/kg q24hr may result in effective platelet inhibition. In cats, a dose of

81 mg/cat q3 days traditionally has been used. A retrospective study of aortic thromboembolism in cats revealed no statistical difference in outcome between traditional and low-dose (5 mg/cat q3 days) aspirin, but significantly fewer adverse effects with the low-dose protocol.

The thienopyridines (clopidogrel, ticlopidine) selectively inhibit ADP-induced platelet aggregation, and have no effect on cyclooxygenase (suggesting a synergistic effect with aspirin). Onset of action is not immediate; platelet inhibition occurs by 2 days, and reaches a steady state after 5 to 7 days. As with aspirin, the defect in platelet function persists for the life of the platelet.

Clopidogrel has largely superseded ticlopidine in human medicine due to superior potency, more rapid onset, and a lower incidence of adverse effects. Several large trials in human patients have demonstrated a marginal risk reduction of vascular events with clopidogrel compared with aspirin, with similar rates of gastrointestinal bleeding. Current recommendations are in most instances for aspirin therapy. Clopidogrel is reserved for patients who have an aspirin contraindication, have failed aspirin therapy, or who have a >20% risk of a vascular event.

Veterinary experience with these drugs is limited. Ticlopidine (62 mg/kg q24hr) has been shown to effectively inhibit ADP-induced platelet aggregation in healthy dogs. In heartworm-infected dogs, the dose required for this effect was greater and variable. A study in normal cats showed that, at ticlopidine doses sufficient to consistently inhibit platelet aggregability, cats became anorectic. A similar study of clopidogrel suggests that doses ranging from 18.75 to 75 mg q24hr are well-tolerated and result in significant inhibition of platelet aggregation. Dosages at 18.75 mg to 37.5 mg per day of clopidogrel are often used long-term in cats with cardiomyopathy and appear to be well tolerated.

Thrombolysis

Thrombolytic agents are plasminogen activators that result in the production of plasmin and subsequent dissolution of the fibrin thrombus. Advantages of thrombolytic therapy include rapid clot lysis, improved pulmonary perfusion, accelerated reversal of right heart failure, and improved hemodynamic stability. These must be weighed against the risk of massive hemorrhage, which is appreciable. The goal of thrombolytic therapy is to rapidly restore circulation so that the procedure is clinically beneficial and the risks of therapy justifiable.

Thrombolytic therapy is reserved for patients with life-threatening PTE that are unlikely to survive without rapid reperfusion. Contraindications include active internal bleeding, hypertension, recent (within 2 to 3 weeks) surgery or organ biopsy, and gastrointestinal ulceration.

To facilitate decisions regarding the use of thrombolytic therapy, humans with PTE are categorized according to hemodynamic stability and right ventricular function. Thrombolytic therapy reduces mortality in patients with massive PTE and shock. In hemodynamically stable patients pharmacologic thrombolysis has not been found to improve outcome, with the exception of patients with evidence of right ventricular dysfunction. This latter patient subset has a high mortality rate with anticoagulation alone, and

studies have shown that timely intervention with thrombolytic therapy increases survival. Anticoagulant therapy, with intravenous unfractionated heparin or subcutaneous LMWH, is recommended following thrombolysis.

Veterinary experience with thrombolytic agents is limited, making evidence-based recommendations for their use impossible. Risk-to-benefit ratios have not been investigated. As in humans, thrombolytic therapy may be indicated when PTE is accompanied by hemodynamic instability or right ventricular hypokinesis. However, we have yet to determine safe and effective protocols. Thrombolytic agents have been investigated in experimental canine PTE, but there are no published reports in clinical cases. There are a small number of reports involving the use of thrombolytics in animals with nonpulmonary TE.

The successful use of streptokinase (SK) has been described in four dogs with nonpulmonary TE. Protocols varied tremendously. Loading doses of 5,200 to 18,000 units/kg were administered over 30 minutes once or three times. Maintenance dosages ranged from 2083 to 9000 units/kg/hour, infused for 3 to 10 hours per day. The use of SK has been reported in cats with aortic TE, using a loading dose of 90,000 units over 20 to 30 minutes, followed by a maintenance dosage of 45,000 units/kg/hour for 3 or more hours. Most cats had evidence of thrombus dissolution, but bleeding complications were common, and mortality high.

Tissue plasminogen activator (t-PA) has a high affinity for fibrin, preferentially activating thrombus-associated plasminogen. Theoretically this decreases the risk of hemorrhage. In humans t-PA has shown higher success rates compared with SK and fewer adverse effects and is more effective in the lysis of aged thrombi. The successful use of t-PA has been described in a dog with aortic thrombosis. Bolus injections of 1 mg/kg every 60 minutes for a total of 10 doses resulted in resolution. Experience with t-PA in cats with aortic TE has not been encouraging. Treatment was successful in 43% of cats, but 50% died during therapy, most deaths resulting from reperfusion. The author has used t-PA (together with heparin) with some success in a small number of dogs with PTE. Bolus injections of 1 mg/kg are given over 15 to 20 minutes every 60 to 180 minutes until evidence of improvement and then repeated thereafter as needed. No major hemorrhage has been noted; minor hemorrhage has prompted only temporary discontinuation of the drug. Studies in humans indicate that a single infusion of t-PA over 2 hours may be superior to intermittent bolus injections. This remains to be evaluated in animals.

Ongoing Therapy

Initial therapy should be continued until the patient is stabilized and respiratory status is steadily improving. At that point the patient can be transitioned to ongoing therapy in preparation for hospital discharge. Ongoing therapy is aimed at preventing recurrent TE and is addressed in the section on Pharmacologic Prophylaxis later in the chapter. Therapy should be continued until the risk of TE is considered sufficiently decreased, but this is difficult to determine objectively. In patients with short-term reversible causes such as pancreatitis, I continue therapy for 1 to 2 weeks following clinical recovery. In patients with longer-term ongoing risk such as IMHA, anticoagulant therapy is continued until corticosteroids are weaned. Indefinite therapy is recommended in patients with recurrent TE, TE complicating malignancy, or cardiac disease.

PREVENTION

The mortality rate of PTE is substantial, with some deaths occurring rapidly before the diagnosis can be confirmed and effective treatment implemented. Moreover, diagnosis is difficult, and treatment of established PTE is not universally successful. This makes prevention imperative in the patient at risk for PTE. Prevention should address all aspects of Virchow's triad. This includes: (1) minimizing vascular stasis by maintaining adequate perfusion; (2) minimizing vascular injury by the appropriate handling of venous catheters; and (3) altering the hemostatic system via the appropriate use of drugs. Drugs are indicated when there is significant risk for PTE.

Objective determination of PTE risk in veterinary patients is difficult. The incidence of PTE in specific diseases is largely unknown, and few laboratory tools are available to confirm hypercoagulability. Assessment of risk remains largely subjective. Understanding the risk factors in patient groups and in individual patients forms the basis for such assessment.

Undoubtedly the single most convincing evidence of risk is a prior PTE episode. Prophylactic drugs are indicated until the cause is reversed. In many patients multiple risk factors are present, and the risks are cumulative (i.e., a thrombophilic patient may not develop PTE until precipitated by another hypercoagulable state or thrombophilic condition such as catheterization, surgery, hypoperfusion, or glucocorticoid therapy). Such a situation should prompt consideration of anticoagulant therapy. The author considers severe IMHA, severe acute pancreatitis, and sepsis to be indications for anticoagulant therapy. However, risk stratification is subjective and based on the severity of disease and concomitant risk factors. Nephrotic syndrome is a significant risk for PTE. Determination of AT-III level might asist in risk assessment. Risk may also be estimated by the severity of renal protein loss, the existence of potentially contributing factors, and any history of prior TE events.

Patients with hyperadrenocorticism or diabetes mellitus appear to have a low incidence of TE, and the need for prophylactic drugs in these patients is doubtful. Risk increases when another thrombophilic condition is applied. In humans with hyperadrenocorticism, TE risk is correlated with systemic hypertension. It is the author's opinion that this is true in dogs. Although anticoagulants are not generally indicated in the dog with uncomplicated Cushing's disease, the patient that is to undergo adrenalectomy, that has hypertension or protein-losing nephropathy, or that has had a prior TE episode is a candidate for anticoagulation.

Pharmacologic Prophylaxis

The choice of anticoagulant for PTE prophylaxis depends on the anticipated duration and the compliance and finances of the owner. Options include subcutaneous heparin, warfarin, and LMWH.

Prophylaxis is traditionally initiated with low-dose, subcutaneous, unfractionated heparin. Small fixed doses are used in humans. This protocol does not require laboratory monitoring and has been shown to reduce the rate of fatal PTE by two thirds. Recommended doses of heparin for prophylaxis in small animals range from 100 to 200 units/kg every 8 to 12 hours subcutaneously. These doses do not appear to result in major hemorrhage, but efficacy rates have yet to be assessed. Gradual weaning of heparin has been recommended in the veterinary literature, although there is little evidence to support this practice.

Warfarin is most commonly used for long-term outpatient TE prophylaxis. It is an oral vitamin K antagonist, thus inhibiting the activation of vitamin K–dependent factors. Because of the half-lives of these factors, the anticoagulant effect of warfarin is not immediate. During the first 24 to 48 hours of therapy, only factor VII and protein C are significantly affected. Inhibition of protein C is prothrombotic, thus potentially leading to thrombosis during initial therapy before other factors are inhibited. For these reasons heparin therapy should always overlap warfarin for at least the first 2 days and until therapeutic levels of warfarin are achieved. Warfarin is initiated at a dose of 0.05 to 0.1 mg/kg every 24 hours orally in the dog and the cat. A therapeutic range is generally achieved within 5 to 7 days. Therapy is monitored by use of the prothrombin time and the calculated International Normalization Ratio (INR) (Kirk and Bonagura, 1995). The therapeutic range for warfarin is an INR of 2.0 to 3.0. The INR should be assessed daily until a therapeutic range is achieved; heparin is then discontinued. Because of the risk of hemorrhage and the influence of diet, comorbidity, and various drugs, close continued monitoring of warfarin therapy on an outpatient basis is essential.

LMWHs are an attractive alternative to warfarin. They are less associated with hemorrhage and, after the initial establishment of an effective dose, do not require ongoing monitoring. Since onset of action is rapid, unfractionated heparin can be discontinued when LMWH is initiated. These benefits contribute to offsetting the costs of these drugs. However, until effective dosing protocols are established in small animals, initial dose adjustments based on anti-Xa assay are mandatory (see previous paragraphs).

Antiplatelet drugs are indicated as adjunctive therapy for TE prophylaxis. Together with the aforementioned rationales for the use of these drugs, most of the thrombophilic conditions in animals can result in both venous and arterial thrombosis. Therefore the addition of an antiplatelet drug has merit. In a recent study of dogs with IMHA, patients that received ultralow dose aspirin(with or without heparin) had improved outcomes without adverse gastrointestinal effects.

References and Suggested Reading

Donahue SM, Otto CM: Thromboelastography: a tool for measuring hypercoagulability, hypocoagulability, and fibrinolysis, *J Vet Emerg Crit Care* 15:9, 2005.
Hackner SG: Pulmonary thromboembolism. In King LG, editor: *Textbook of respiratory disease in dogs and cats*, St Louis, 2004, Saunders, p 526.

Hogan DF, Andrews DA, Talbott KK et al: Evaluation of antiplatelet effects of ticlopidine in cats, *J Am Vet Med Assoc* 65:327, 2004.

Hogan DF, Andrews DA, Green HW et al: Antiplatelet effects and pharmacodynamics of clopidogrel in cats, *J Am Vet Med Assoc* 225:1406, 2004.

Hyers TM et al: ACCP consensus conference on antithrombotic therapy: antithrombotic therapy for venous thromboembolic disease, *Chest* 119:176S, 2001.

Mischke R, Jacobs C: The monitoring of heparin administration by screening tests in experimental dogs, *Res Vet Sci* 70:101, 2001.

Mischke R et al: Amidolytic heparin activity and values for several hemostatic variables after repeated subcutaneous administration of high doses of a low molecular weight heparin in healthy dogs, *Am J Vet Res* 62:595, 2001.

Powell T, Muller NL: Imaging of acute pulmonary embolism: should spiral computed tomography replace the ventilation-perfusion scan? *Clin Chest Med* 24:29, 2003.

Smith AS et al: Arterial thromboembolism in cats: acute crisis in 127 cases (1992–2001) and long-term management with low-dose aspirin in 24 cats, *J Vet Intern Med* 17:73, 2003.

Stokol T: Plasma D-dimer for the diagnosis of thromboembolic disorders in dogs, *Vet Clin Small Anim* 33:1419, 2003.

Thompson MF, Scott-Montcrief JC, Hogan DF: Thrombolytic therapy in dogs and cats, *J Vet Emerg Crit Care* 11:111, 2001.

Weinkle TK et al: Evaluation of prognostic factors, survival rates, and treatment protocols for immune-mediated hemolytic anemia in dogs: 151 cases (1993–2002), *J Am Vet Med Assoc* 226:1869, 2005.

CHAPTER 156

Pulmonary Hypertension

ROSEMARY A. HENIK, *Madison, Wisconsin*

The recognition of pulmonary hypertension (PH) in dogs and cats has become more common with the widespread use of Doppler echocardiography in small animal practice. In addition, the development of drugs that both selectively lower pulmonary artery (PA) pressures and can be given orally lends an additional reason to identify and treat PH in cats and dogs. This chapter reviews the clinical classification of PH, its diagnosis, and treatment recommendations.

DEFINITION

Normal PA pressures in small animals, measured by cardiac catheterization under pentobarbital anesthesia, are 25 ± 5 mm Hg systolic, 10 ± 3 mm Hg diastolic, and mean of 15 ± 5 mm Hg. Similarly, mean PA pressure in 97 instrumented, nonsedated dogs was 14 ± 3.2 mm Hg, with a 95% confidence interval of 13.4 to 14.7 mm Hg (Haskins et al., 2005). PH is a sustained increase in the PA systolic, mean, or diastolic pressure. Based on these normal results, dogs and cats residing at sea level with a systolic PA pressure greater than 30 mm Hg, mean pressure greater than 20 mm Hg, or diastolic PA pressure greater than 15 mm Hg can be considered to have PH. Systolic PH is diagnosed most frequently in animals because of ease in estimating systolic PA pressure during Doppler echocardiography.

CLASSIFICATION AND ETIOLOGY

PH was previously classified into two categories: primary or secondary, depending on the absence or presence of identifiable causes. Primary PH, a diagnosis of exclusion,

has no known etiology and is rare, only recently documented in a dog (Glaus et al., 2004). Secondary PH develops as a result of impedance of pulmonary venous drainage (usually secondary to increased left atrial pressure), pulmonary overcirculation, or increased pulmonary vascular resistance.

PH in humans was reclassified by the World Health Organization in 1998 into five clinical categories based on shared pathophysiologic mechanisms, clinical presentation, and therapeutic options (Rich et al., 1998). The Evian Classification, named for the meeting site in France, was reviewed and modified in 2003 to ensure that it was accepted by experts in the field and was providing new information about disease mechanism and treatment efficacy. Minor modifications to the classification scheme were made based on recent published information (Simonneau et al., 2004). In addition, both the U.S. Food and Drug Administration and the European Agency for Drug Evaluation have used this clinical classification for labeling the newly approved drugs bosentan, treprostinil, and iloprost.

Although many of the diseases contributing to PH in companion animals differ from those in humans, it seems reasonable to adopt a clinical classification scheme (Box 156-1) to better define prognosis and therapeutic approach. This is especially important given that veterinarians are relatively new to identifying and addressing PH in companion animals and an organized approach to classification and treatment allows a more critical assessment of outcome.

The first category, termed *pulmonary arterial hypertension (PAH)*, includes a subgroup without identifiable cause, termed *idiopathic PAH (IPAH)*, the term *primary PH*

Box **156-1**

Clinical Classification of Pulmonary Hypertension in Veterinary Patients*

I. Pulmonary Arterial Hypertension (PAH)
Idiopathic pulmonary hypertension (IPAH)[†]
Familial pulmonary hypertension (FPAH)[†]
Associated with PAH:
    Heartworm disease
    Congenital systemic-to-pulmonary shunts
    Collagen vascular disease[†]
    Drugs/toxins[†]
    Persistent pulmonary hypertension of the newborn[†]

II. Pulmonary Hypertension With Left Heart Disease
Left-sided myocardial heart disease
Left-sided valvular heart disease

III. Pulmonary Hypertension Associated With Lung Diseases and/or Hypoxemia
Chronic obstructive pulmonary disease
Interstitial lung disease
Sleep-disordered breathing[†]
Alveolar hypoventilation disorders
Chronic exposure to high altitude
Developmental abnormalities[†]

IV. Pulmonary Hypertension Caused by Chronic Thrombotic or Embolic Disease
Thromboembolic obstruction of proximal or distal pulmonary arteries
Nonthrombotic pulmonary embolism
    Heartworm disease or other parasites
    Neoplasia
    Foreign material (i.e., catheter or coil)

V. Miscellaneous
Compression of the pulmonary vessels
Lymphadenopathy
    Neoplasia
    Fibrosing mediastinitis
Granulomatous disease
Other: sarcoidosis, histiocytosis X, lymphangiomatosis[†]

*Adapted for veterinary patients from Rich S et al., 1998 and Simonneau G, 2004.
[†]Questionable significance in veterinary patients at this time.

being discarded (Simonneau et al., 2004). PAH is both a vasoproliferative and a vasoconstrictive disorder. The pathogenesis of PAH involves an imbalance between endothelium-derived relaxing factors (e.g., nitric oxide and prostacyclin) and endothelium-derived constricting factors (e.g., endothelin-1, thromboxane, serotonin), which results in increased vasomotor tone, endothelial smooth muscle cell proliferation, vascular remodeling, and thrombosis (Sharma, 2003). Familial PAH (FPAH) is also included in this category but has not been documented in veterinary patients. Reports of related animals with lesions of PAH have all had underlying congenital heart disease.

A third subgroup includes a number of conditions or diseases associated with PAH that have in common the localization of lesions to the small pulmonary muscular arteries and arterioles (i.e., the precapillary segments of the pulmonary vasculature). The mechanisms responsible for the precapillary localization of the pulmonary vascular lesions are unknown, but the conditions share similar morphologic features and respond to pulmonary arterial vasodilators. Patients with PH caused by congenital systemic-to-pulmonary shunts, collagen vascular disease, or exposure to certain drugs or toxins are included in this category. Heartworm disease, besides fitting into the thromboembolic category, can also cause PH because of inflammatory changes in the pulmonary arterial endothelial lining.

Pulmonary vascular histopathologic changes that accompany congenital heart disease are usually indistinguishable from those of IPAH; the lesions include medial hypertrophy, intimal proliferation fibrosis, and in more severe PH plexiform lesions and necrotizing arteritis. The pulmonary vascular involvement from congenital heart disease in children usually follows a period in which pulmonary resistance is low and pulmonary blood flow is high. In these patients it is suspected that shear stress caused by high flow damages endothelial cells and produces PH (Simonneau et al., 2004). Large-diameter defects are also reported in many dogs with patent ductus arteriosus and PH; however, the retention of fetal pulmonary physiology cannot be ruled out as a cause of PH.

The second category, *PH with left heart disease*, is the most common condition leading to PH in veterinary patients (Johnson, Boon, and Orton, 1999). Left-sided valvular or myocardial diseases, resulting in high left atrial and pulmonary venous pressures, dictate that PH be addressed via unloading agents (i.e., systemic arterial vasodilators) or agents that improve myocardial performance. Blood must be able to leave the left side of the heart to reduce "back pressure" (high pulmonary venous and arterial pressures) caused by poor left-sided cardiac output or impaired ventricular filling. Once optimal arterial dilation and cardiac performance have been achieved, pulmonary arterial dilators may result in additional benefit to the patient.

The third category of PH results from *disorders of the lungs or hypoxemia*. Inadequate oxygenation of systemic arterial blood caused by intrinsic lung disease, impaired control of breathing, or residence at high altitude causes PH. Inspired oxygen results in a subsequent decrease in PA pressures. Veterinary patients in this category of PH include those with interstitial lung disease, chronic obstructive pulmonary disease, disorders leading to alveolar hypoventilation, chronic exposure to high altitude, or neonatal lung disease. In humans survival depends on the severity of the pulmonary disease rather than on pulmonary hemodynamics; and long-term oxygen therapy or relocation from high altitude may be needed in addition to treatment of the underlying lung disease (Simonneau et al., 2004).

The fourth clinical category of PH results from *thrombotic or embolic diseases* and includes heartworm disease in veterinary patients. Embolization of the pulmonary arteries may also occur as a result of thrombi, neoplasia, other parasites, or foreign material. In contrast to the previous categories, in which the pulmonary microcirculation is predominantly affected, thromboembolic disease usually involves the more proximal and larger segments of the pulmonary arterial tree. The therapeutic approach to thromboembolic PH is determined by the location of the emboli. Humans with large clots in major PAs require endarterectomy, a procedure not performed in veterinary patients. More peripheral emboli or thrombi can be treated with chronic pulmonary vasodilator therapy and lifelong anticoagulant therapy.

The fifth category is PH caused by *miscellaneous disorders*, which are rare in people and are of multiple etiologies, including sarcoidosis, histiocytosis X, lymphangiomatosis, or compression of the pulmonary vessels. Conditions causing central pulmonary vein compression do occur in veterinary patients; they include neoplasia, lymphadenopathy, fibrosing mediastinitis, or granulomatous disease. Granulomas from blastomycosis have resulted in PH in dogs.

CLINICAL EVALUATION

Presentation

PH is reported more commonly in dogs than in cats. Studies in dogs have shown that males and females are affected equally, with an age range from 2 months to 17 years (Johnson, Boon, and Orton, 1999; Pyle, Abbott, and MacLean 2004). Breed distribution mirrors breeds prone to chronic valvular disease or airway disease. Historical problems are related to underlying lung or cardiac disease such as cough, dyspnea, tachypnea, wheezing, exercise intolerance, or exertional weakness or collapse. A surprisingly high number (23%) of dogs with PH presented with syncope in one study, yet 13% of 53 dogs were asymptomatic (Johnson et al., 1999).

Physical Examination Findings

Systolic murmurs over the mitral valve are present in the majority of dogs with PH, which is expected given the high prevalence of left-sided cardiac disease in affected patients. Murmurs of tricuspid regurgitation (TR) may also be detected; however, diastolic murmurs of pulmonic insufficiency are not usually audible. With severe PH the intensity of the tricuspid regurgitant murmur tends to increase, and often there is a palpable precordial thrill associated with the murmur. Auscultation of a tympanic or a split S_2 may result from delayed pulmonic valve (PV) closure relative to aortic valvular closure. Signs of pulmonary dysfunction, including cyanosis, tachypnea, orthopnea, or wheezing, may be present. Right-sided congestive heart failure (CHF), although less common than left-sided CHF in dogs with PH, may result in jugular venous distention, muffled heart and breath sounds ventrally caused by pleural effusion, and ascites.

Diagnosis

Thoracic Radiography

Radiographic abnormalities reflect the severity of disease and vary with the etiology of PH. Animals with primary lung disease have parenchymal or bronchial abnormalities and secondary changes to the right heart. Right atrial (RA) and right ventricular (RV) enlargement, dilation of the PA segment, and pleural effusion may occur as PH worsens. Animals with valvular or myocardial disease of the left heart have radiographic changes typical of the underlying abnormality.

Electrocardiography

Electrocardiographic changes typical of right heart disease are not likely to occur until PH is moderate to severe. As the right ventricle becomes thicker than the left ventricle, a right axis deviation may develop in the frontal plane. P-pulmonale may occur with RA enlargement; and atrial arrhythmias, including atrial premature complexes or atrial fibrillation, may occur. Disease of the left heart, hypoxia, and ischemia may also contribute to a variety of other arrhythmias.

Doppler Echocardiography

Doppler echocardiography permits the estimation of right heart and PA pressures noninvasively, greatly lessening the need for cardiac catheterization. The ability to diagnose PH with Doppler echocardiography results from the tendency of the tricuspid and PVs to leak or become insufficient with high PA pressures. Since pressures across an open valve are equal if stenosis is not present, the RV systolic and PA systolic pressures are equal. If a RV-to-RA systolic regurgitant jet (i.e., TR) can be quantified, PA systolic pressure can be estimated (Fig. 156-1). Central venous pressure, usually unknown but estimated between 5 and 8 mm Hg in normal animals, may be added into the calculation; but this step is usually unnecessary in the determination of normal versus abnormal PA pressures.

A high-velocity TR jet is more likely to be present in PH than PV insufficiency (PI). However, in the absence of TR or if the regurgitant jet cannot be aligned with the Doppler cursor, a jet of PI may allow estimation of PA

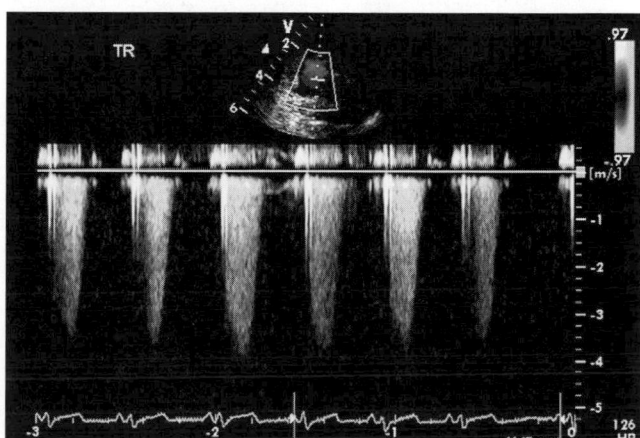

Fig. 156-1 Continuous wave spectral tracing of a tricuspid regurgitant jet in a dog with pulmonary hypertension and chronic valvular disease obtained from the left apical view. The maximum right ventricular to right atrial velocity is 3.9 M/sec, and the pressure is 61 mm Hg. If RA pressure is estimated to be 5 mm Hg, then PA systolic pressure is 66 mm Hg.

diastolic pressure, except when the RV diastolic pressure is increased. A TR jet of 2.8 M/sec or greater corresponds to an RV-to-RA gradient of 31 mm Hg or greater (i.e., PA systolic hypertension) using the modified Bernoulli equation:

$$4 \times V^2 = \text{pressure (mm Hg)}$$

where V is the maximum velocity in meters/second. A PI jet of 2 M/sec or greater corresponds to a diastolic PA-to-RV pressure of 16 mm Hg or greater, reflecting PA diastolic hypertension.

The degree of PH can be categorized as mild, moderate, or severe based on the absolute PA systolic pressure. Pyle, Abbott, and MacLean (2004) defined mild PH as a systolic PA pressure between 30 and 55 mm Hg , moderate between 56 and 79 mm Hg , and severe 80 mm Hg or greater. Quantification of PA pressure may better define prognosis or the need for treatment, although Johnson, Boon, and Orton (1999) found that disease course was not related to the RV-to-RA pressure gradient.

Changes in RV function and structure associated with PH can be recognized with M-mode and two-dimensional echocardiography, including hypertrophy and dilation of the right ventricle, flattening of the septum as RV pressures exceed LV pressures, and a decrease in the diameter of the LV (Fig. 156-2, *A* and *B*). PH alters the timing of PV opening and closure, the pattern of PV motion, and the shape of the pulmonary flow velocity profile (Weyman, 1994, Schober and Baade, 2006). As PA pressure increases, the effect of atrial contraction on PV motion decreases, and the PV opens later than normal. PH causes a rapid valve opening and rapid increase in velocity, a more rapid acceleration with an earlier peak velocity relative to total ejection time, an earlier decrease in velocity, and less flow or even flow reversal in late systole (Fig. 156-3). Despite changes in the pattern of flow, the peak outflow velocity usually does not differ from normal.

Other Diagnostic Tests

A stress or inflammatory leukogram may be present on a complete blood count, depending on the underlying etiology of the PH. Chronic hypoxemia may lead to an increased packed cell volume (PCV) and hemoglobin concentration, and nucleated red blood cells may be present. If right heart failure is present, alkaline phosphatase and increased alanine aminotransferase may occur secondary to passive congestion of the liver. If the etiology of PH is caused by chronic thromboembolic disease, D-dimer concentrations may support embolic disease if very high and rule out embolic disease if negative (Nelson, 2005).

THERAPEUTIC MANAGEMENT

The success of lowering PA pressure in veterinary patients depends on correctly identifying the underlying pathologic process and having medications that are orally effective. In humans the long list of drugs for PH has included nonselective vasodilators, inhaled oxygen, inhaled nitric oxide, diuretics, bronchodilators, prostacyclin analogs, endothelin receptor antagonists, and phosphodiesterase-5 (PDE5) inhibitors.

Vasodilators

The action of most vasodilators is not specific to the pulmonary circulation; therefore concomitant systemic vasodilation with hypotension has plagued this approach to PH treatment. In addition, systemic hypotension in the face of elevated RV chamber pressure may impair right

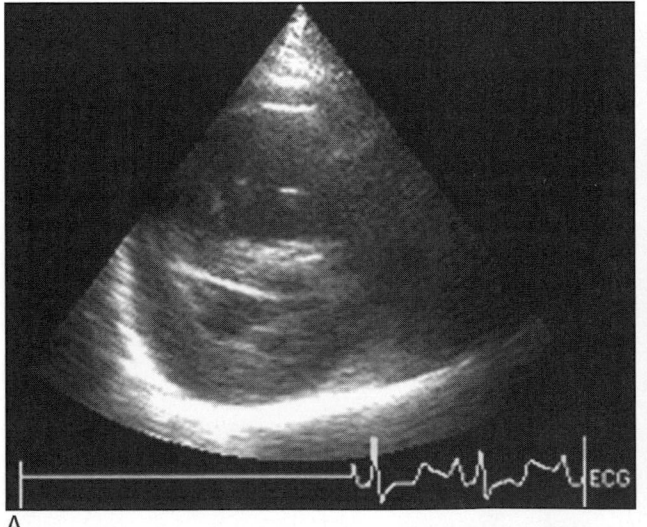 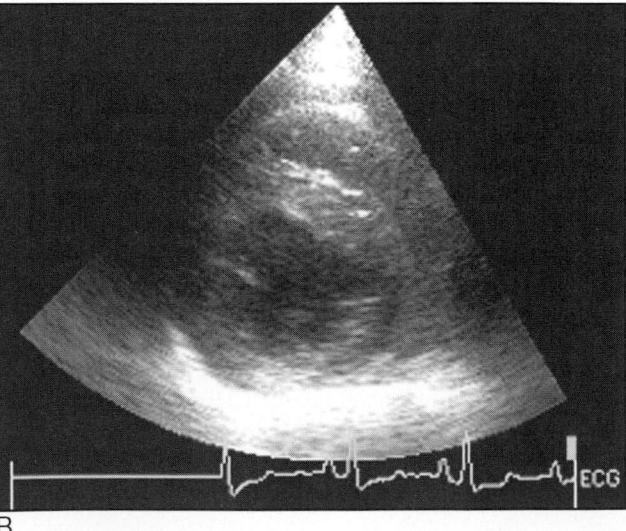

A B

Figs. 156-2 **A** and **B**, Right parasternal short axis views of the LV at end-diastole before (2a) and after (2b) treatment with sildenafil for right-sided congestive heart failure caused by pulmonary hypertension and chronic valvular disease. There is flattening of the septum and a decrease in the size of the LV **(A)**; PA systolic pressure was 72 mm Hg, and PA diastolic pressure was 55 mm Hg. Sildenafil treatment was added to enalapril and furosemide, and PA pressure decreased to 52/24 mm Hg within 12 hours. **B,** IVS flattening has disappeared, and the LV shape is normal. PA systolic pressure at this time was 40 mm Hg.

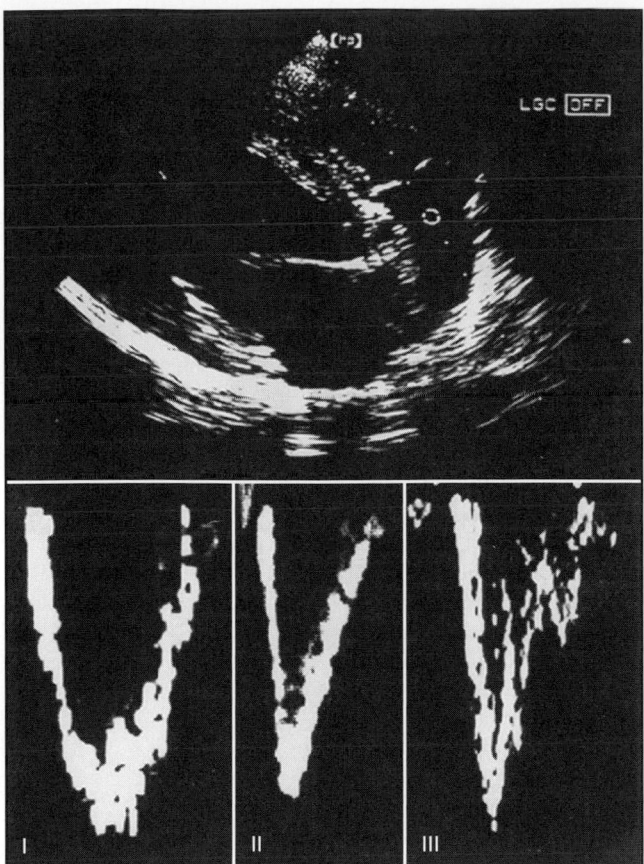

Fig. 156-3 Pulsed-wave pulmonary outflow velocity tracings in a normal dog (I), and dogs with PH (II and III). PH causes a rapid valve opening and rapid increase in velocity, an earlier peak velocity, an earlier decrease in velocity, and less flow or even flow reversal (III) in late systole. (Image courtesy Dr. Lynelle Johnson and Johnson L, Boon J, Orton EC: *J Vet Intern Med*, 1999.)

coronary artery perfusion and contribute to ischemic RV dysfunction (Mehta, 2003).

Prostanoids

Exogenous prostacyclin analogs (prostanoids) have been studied in humans with PAH. Prostacyclin is a potent vasodilator in both the pulmonary and systemic circulations and has antiplatelet activity. Chronic intravenous epoprostenol infusion, subcutaneous treprostinil infusion, inhaled iloprost, and oral beraprost all have been used with varying success in humans; but the method of delivery, short half-life, and expense make this drug class impractical for veterinary patients at this time.

Endothelin Receptor Antagonists

Bosentan (Tracleer, Actelion Inc.), a dual-receptor endothelin antagonist, is used singly or with other treatments in humans with PAH. Endothelin-1 is overexpressed in several forms of pulmonary vascular disease. Although endothelin mediates pulmonary vascular remodeling in a canine model of chronic embolic PH, bosentan is unlikely to be used in veterinary patients in the near future because of expense.

Phosphodiesterase-5 Inhibitors

The PDE5 inhibitor sildenafil (Viagra, Pfizer) has shown efficacy in reducing PA pressure. Phosphodiesterases are a superfamily of enzymes that inactivate cyclic adenosine monophosphate and cyclic guanosine monophosphate, the second messengers of prostacyclin and nitric oxide. The phosphodiesterases have different tissue distributions and substrate affinities, with abundant expression of PDE5 in lung tissues.

Currently there are three PDE5 inhibitors on the market for erectile dysfunction in men. In humans all three PDE5 inhibitors cause significant pulmonary vasorelaxation, with maximum effects being obtained after 40 to 45 minutes with vardenafil (Levitra, Bayer Pharmaceuticals), 60 min with sildenafil, and 75 to 90 min with tadalafil (Cialis, Lilly ICOS, LLC) (Ghofrani et al., 2004). Sildenafil and tadalafil, but not vardenafil, cause a significant reduction in the pulmonary-to-systemic vascular resistance ratio. Significant improvement in arterial oxygenation (equal to nitrous oxide inhalation) is only noted with sildenafil (Ghofrani et al., 2004). The effect of sildenafil on pulmonary vasculature is independent of the underlying cause of PH.

Sildenafil has been used successfully in dogs and cats with moderate-to-severe PH secondary to either left heart disease or primary lung disease. The currently recommended starting dosage is 1 mg/kg every 8 hours orally; dosages as high as 3 mg/kg orally every 8 hours have been tolerated but should be used only with careful monitoring of arterial blood pressure. Sildenafil is available in 25-, 50-, and 100-mg tablets, which are all approximately $10 in the United States, regardless of tablet size. Veterinary pharmacies can reformulate the 100-mg tablets into appropriately sized capsules. Information regarding adverse effects in dogs and cats, as well as dosage adjustment, is not currently available. Response to PDE5 inhibitors results in a decrease in measured TR or PI velocity, improvement in two-dimensional echocardiography abnormalities, increase in exercise tolerance, reduction in collapsing or syncopal episodes, and improved respiratory effort.

Treatment Recommendations Based on the Clinical Category of PH

Optimal treatment of PH depends on the underlying disease or condition. A major reason for the development of the clinical classification scheme was to tailor the approach to treatment based on the underlying disease process.

Pulmonary Arterial Hypertension

Pulmonary arterial vasodilators such as the PDE5 inhibitors are the treatment of choice for diseases characterized by lesions confined to the small arteries and arterioles. If left-to-right shunting lesions are present, correction should be performed if possible. If polycythemia is present because of right-to-left shunting disease, treatment with hydroxyurea in addition to PDE5 inhibitors is recommended to maintain PCV between 62% and 66%.

Heartworm disease and concomitant endarteritis should be treated with melarsamine HCl and low-dose aspirin, with care taken to protect the gastrointestinal track from aspirin-induced hemorrhage. In addition, the

PDE5 inhibitors provide a new therapeutic option in dogs with clinical signs caused by heartworm disease and PH.

Pulmonary Hypertension With Left Heart Disease

Diseases of the left heart, either valvular or myocardial, should be treated with cardiovascular drugs that reduce afterload, increase contractility, or both. Systemic arterial blood pressure measurements should be performed serially to produce optimal systemic vasodilation without signs of hypotension. Arterial vasodilators such as nitroprusside, angiotensin-converting enzyme inhibitors, and hydralazine can be used in combination to lower arterial blood pressure. Pimobendan, which is an "inodilator" with both systemic arterial and venous vasodilating and positive inotropic effects, also causes pulmonary arterial dilation. Once myocardial performance and arterial vasodilation are optimal, the addition of sildenafil or another PDE5 inhibitor may increase exercise tolerance and lessen syncope or other clinical signs in dogs with PH caused by left heart disease.

Pulmonary Hypertension Associated With Lung Diseases and/or Hypoxemia

Treatment of PH associated with lung disease or hypoxemia in humans is focused on the pulmonary problem rather than the vascular derangement and usually includes ambulatory oxygen administration. Dogs with chronic bronchitis should be managed with antimicrobials or antiinflammatory doses of prednisone, as dictated by cytology and culture of the airways. Administration of bronchodilators may lessen respiratory muscle fatigue and clinical signs. Pulmonary fibrosis or other interstitial lung disease, which is more likely to result in severe PH, should be treated aggressively with immunosuppressive, immunomodulatory, or antifibrotic treatment based on lung biopsy, culture, and histology. Ambulatory oxygen therapy is not a practical option in veterinary patients with lung disease and PH; therefore treatment of the underlying disease remains the cornerstone of treatment. Phosphodiesterase inhibitors should be considered in patients with PH and clinical signs refractory to specific pulmonary therapy.

Pulmonary Hypertension Caused by Chronic Thrombotic or Embolic Disease

The treatment approach to PH caused by thromboembolic disease varies with the location of the emboli and the underlying cause. Diseases (e.g., hyperadrenocorticism, heartworm disease) predisposing to pulmonary thromboembolism should be treated if possible. If the underlying disease process cannot be corrected, lifetime anticoagulant therapy should be administered (see Chapter 155) in addition to pulmonary arterial vasodilators (e.g., PDE5 inhibitors) for emboli in distal pulmonary arteries. Emboli in proximal pulmonary arteries are usually peracute and fatal in veterinary patients.

Miscellaneous Causes of Pulmonary Hypertension

PH caused by compression of the pulmonary vessels may occur in veterinary patients as a result of neoplasia, granulomatous disease, or lymphadenopathy. The etiology of the compressive lesion (e.g., blastomycosis, lymphosarcoma) must be identified to treat appropriately and cause regression of the mass; only then can PH be managed. Since the disorder is outside of the vessel, the use of antithrombotic drugs or PDE5 inhibitors would not be of benefit.

PROGNOSIS

The prognosis of animals with PH is variable and depends on the ability to treat or manage the underlying disease or condition. Animals with PH and CHF caused by left-sided valvular disease have a favorable prognosis and may live for over a year with careful attention to congestive signs, heart rate and rhythm, arterial blood pressure, serum electrolytes, and renal function. Dogs with right-to-left shunting congenital heart defects may live 4 to 5 years with management of polycythemia and PH. Animals with or severe lung disease or thromboembolic disease often have a poor prognosis because of disease progression. Finally, dogs with PH resulting from compressive lesions have a favorable prognosis if blastomycosis is the cause of the granuloma, whereas those with neoplastic compression of the pulmonary vessels have a guarded prognosis.

References and Suggested Reading

Ghofrani HA et al: Differences in hemodynamic and oxygenation responses to three different phosphodiesterase-5 inhibitors in patients with pulmonary arterial hypertension, *J Am Coll Cardiol* 44:1488, 2004.

Glaus TM et al: Clinical and pathological characterisation of primary pulmonary hypertension in a dog, *Vet Rec* 154:786, 2004.

Haskins S et al: Reference cardiopulmonary values in normal dogs, *Comp Med* 55:156, 2005.

Johnson L, Boon J, Orton EC: Clinical characteristics of 53 dogs with Doppler-derived evidence of pulmonary hypertension: 1992-1996, *J Vet Intern Med* 13:440, 1999.

Mehta S: Sildenafil for pulmonary hypertension, *Chest* 123:989, 2003.

Nelson OL: Use of the D-dimer assay for diagnosing thromboembolic disease in the dog, *J Am Anim Hosp Assoc* 41:145, 2005.

Pyle RL, Abbott J, MacLean H: Pulmonary hypertension and cardiovascular sequelae in 54 dogs, *Intern J Appl Res Vet Med* 2:99, 2004.

Rich S et al: Executive summary from the world symposium on primary pulmonary hypertension (Evian, France, September 6-10), 1998, A World Health Organization publication.

Schober KE, Baade H: Doppler echocardiographic prediction of pulmonary hypertension in West Highland white terriers with chronic pulmonary disease, *J Vet Intern Med* 20:912, 2006, PMID: 16955816 [PubMed – indexed for MEDLINE]

Sharma S: Treatment of pulmonary arterial hypertension, *Chest* 124:8, 2003.

Simonneau G et al: Clinical classification of pulmonary hypertension, *J Am Coll Cardiol* 43:5S, 2004.

Weyman AE: Right ventricular outflow tract. In Weyman AE: *Principles and practice of echocardiography*, ed 2, Baltimore, 1994, Lea & Febiger, p 863.

SECTION VIII

Cardiovascular Diseases

John D. Bonagura

VOLUME XIII CONTENT ON EVOLVE: http://evolve.elsevier.com/Bonagura/Kirks/

CHAPTER 157

Nutritional Management of Heart Disease

LISA M. FREEMAN, *North Grafton, Massachusetts*

GENERAL NUTRITIONAL ISSUES FOR ANIMALS WITH HEART DISEASE

For many years the role of nutrition in the management of heart disease consisted primarily of feeding a low-sodium diet. We now know that severe sodium restriction is not necessary in all animals with heart disease. It is also becoming apparent that supplementation of certain nutrients, either to correct a deficiency or to provide pharmacologic effects, may have profound benefits in animals with heart disease. Research is now beginning to show that nutrition can modulate heart disease by slowing the progression, minimizing the number of medications required, improving quality of life, or in rare cases actually curing the disease. Therefore attention to diet at all stages of heart disease is critical for optimal care of the cardiac patient.

A single diet does not work for all animals with heart disease, and dietary modifications need to be individualized. Patients with heart disease vary in their clinical signs, laboratory parameters, and food preferences, which all affect diet selection. For example, more severe sodium restriction would be required for a cat with congestive heart failure (CHF) than for a cat with asymptomatic heart disease. Animals with heart disease may be hyperkalemic, hypokalemic, or normokalemic, which influences the choice of diet. Concurrent diseases also alter diet choice and are present in many animals with heart disease (61% of dogs in one study; Freeman et al., 2003).

Based on these patient parameters, one or more diets can be selected for the individual patient. Currently a number of commercial veterinary cardiac diets are available, the specific characteristics of which vary, but they are all moderately to severely sodium restricted. Some cardiac diets also may include supplemental taurine, carnitine, arginine, antioxidants, or n-3 fatty acids. In some cases a veterinary diet designed for another disease or an over-the-counter diet may have the properties desired for an individual patient. I generally try to recommend multiple diets so the owner can determine which is most palatable to the pet. Having a number of choices is particularly beneficial for animals with severe CHF, a condition in which loss of appetite is common.

In addition to the pet food(s) selected, the owner must also receive careful instructions on treats and table food. In some cases animals may be eating an ideal pet food but are getting large amounts of sodium from treats. In one study over 90% of dogs with heart disease received treats, and these dogs were receiving up to 100% of their dietary sodium from them (Freeman et al., 2003). Examples of appropriate treats are shown in Table 157-1.

Therefore a diet must be selected that has the desired nutritional properties and palatability, but it also is important to devise an overall dietary plan that includes a satisfactory method for administering medications. Most people use food for this purpose, and the most commonly used foods are high in sodium (e.g., cheese, hot dogs, lunch meats). Therefore examples of appropriate methods of administering medications should be provided to the owner (Box 157-1). Including all sources of dietary sodium intake in the overall diet plan is important to achieve success with nutritional modifications.

All dietary changes should be made gradually over a period of 3 to 5 days. It may be difficult to make major dietary changes while the patient is sick or hospitalized. Often it is better to wait several days until the patient's condition has improved and then initiate the change. Food aversions develop in ill humans, and such aversions may prevent adequate intake of the food over the long term. It also is important to instruct the owner to notify the veterinarian if the patient does not eat adequate amounts of the new food so that other options can be devised.

NUTRITIONAL MODIFICATIONS BASED ON SEVERITY OF DISEASE

Asymptomatic Heart Disease

Nutritional therapy for dogs and cats with asymptomatic heart disease has been like a pendulum over the years. Initially very low–sodium diets were recommended to be fed when a heart murmur was first detected. Veterinarians then moved toward the approach that severe sodium restriction may not be ideal at this stage because of early activation of the renin-angiotensin-aldosterone (RAA) system, and this led to the idea that no nutritional modifications can or should be made for animals with asymptomatic heart disease. Veterinarians are now swinging back toward the middle because new research is supporting the idea that dietary modification in early heart disease might be beneficial and the nutritional management of animals with asymptomatic heart disease should not be ignored.

One of the earliest and major compensatory responses in heart disease is activation of the RAA system; and sodium restriction can further elevate renin, angiotensin, and aldosterone. Thus severe sodium restriction in animals with early heart disease theoretically could be

Examples of Low-Sodium Treats

Treat	Kilocalories per treat	Sodium (mg/treat)
Dogs		
Science Diet Adult Treats (medium)	20	13
Iams Original Formula Biscuits (small)	22	10
Hill's Prescription Diet Canine Treats	13	5
Stewart Fiber Formula Dog Biscuits (medium)	25	5
Baby carrots	4	4
Alpo Healthy Snacks Variety Snaps With Real Meat	13	1
Apple (raw, 1 slice) or orange (1 section)	10	0
Cats		
Purina Whisker Lickin's Brand Crunchy Cat Treats Tartar Control (all flavors)	3	3
Stewart Fiber Formula Cat Treats	1	1

detrimental by triggering early and excessive activation of the RAA system. I recommend only mild sodium restriction in asymptomatic heart disease (<100 mg/100 kcal for animals in International Small Animal Cardiac Health Council (ISACHC) Stage 1a and less than 80 mg/100 kcal for animals in ISACHC Stage 1b; see Chapter 171). However, this is an opportune time to begin talking to the owner about the animal's overall dietary patterns (i.e., the pet food, treats, table food, and how medications are administered) since it is generally much easier to institute dietary modifications when the animal is asymptomatic.

In addition to mild sodium restriction, the other main goal is to achieve or maintain optimal body condition. An estimated 25% to 40% of dogs and cats in the United States are overweight or obese. Therefore some animals with heart disease, particularly those in the asymptomatic stages,

Recommended Methods for Medication Administration

- Teach the owner to pill the animal without using foods.
- Use a Pet Piller or Pet Pill Gun (Jorgensen Laboratories).
- Switch from pills to a compounded, flavored liquid medication (NOTE: the pharmacokinetics may be altered).
- Use low-sodium foods to insert the pills before administration.
- Add to meat, home-cooked, without salt (not lunch meats).
- Fresh fruit (e.g., banana, orange, melon, berries).
- Add to low-sodium canned pet food.
- Add to peanut butter (labeled as "no salt added").

will be obese. Obesity can exacerbate heart disease, and weight loss in severely obese animals with heart disease usually results in a less dyspneic and a more active pet. Weight reduction programs can be challenging and run a high risk of failure without careful planning of a comprehensive program and regular monitoring and adjustment.

Finally, there is potential for benefit with nutritional modification in the asymptomatic animal. One recent study compared a moderately reduced sodium cardiac diet that was enriched with n-3 fatty acids, antioxidants, arginine, taurine, and carnitine to a placebo diet in dogs with asymptomatic chronic valvular disease (CVD) (Freeman et al., 2006). The cardiac diet increased circulating levels of key nutrients (e.g., antioxidants, n-3 fatty acids) and also moderately reduced cardiac size. This reduction in cardiac size did not appear to be an effect of sodium restriction. Future studies will help to build understanding of the role of nutritional modification in this early stage of disease.

Mild-to-Moderate Congestive Heart Failure

When CHF develops, additional nutritional concerns arise for the dog or cat with heart disease. Maintaining optimal body condition is of primary importance in the animal with CHF. Although obesity still can be present at this stage, animals with CHF more commonly begin to demonstrate weight loss. This weight loss, or cardiac cachexia, is unlike that seen in a healthy animal, which loses primarily fat. In an animal with CHF the primary tissue lost is lean body mass. The term *cachexia* does not necessarily equate with an emaciated, end-stage patient; and there is a spectrum of severity with cachexia. In the early stages it can be very subtle and may even occur in obese animals (i.e., an animal may have excess fat stores but still lose lean body mass). Loss of lean body mass usually is first noted in the epaxial, gluteal, scapular, or temporal muscles. Cardiac cachexia typically does not occur until CHF has developed but can occur with any underlying cause of CHF (e.g., dilated cardiomyopathy [DCM], CVD, congenital heart diseases). Cardiac cachexia is a common finding in animals with CHF and has deleterious effects on strength, immune function, and survival; thus it is important to recognize cachexia at an early stage for better opportunities to manage it effectively.

The loss of lean body mass in cardiac cachexia is a multifactorial process caused by anorexia, increased energy requirements, and an increased production of inflammatory cytokines such as tumor necrosis factor (TNF) and interleukin-1 (IL-1). These cytokines cause anorexia, increase energy requirements, and increase the catabolism of lean body mass. In addition, TNF and IL-1 also cause cardiac myocyte hypertrophy and fibrosis and have negative inotropic effects.

The nutritional management of animals with cardiac cachexia consists primarily of providing adequate calories and protein and modulating cytokine production. One of the most important issues for managing anorexia (which is defined here to include both a complete and partial loss of appetite) is to optimize medical therapy. An early sign of worsening CHF or the need for medication adjustment is a reduction in food intake in an animal that has previously been eating well. Medication side effects such as digoxin toxicity or azotemia secondary to angiotensin-converting enzyme (ACE) inhibitors or over-zealous diuretic use also can cause anorexia. Providing a more palatable diet can help to improve appetite (e.g., switching from a dry food to a canned food, changing to a different brand, having a balanced cooked homemade diet formulated by a veterinary nutritionist). It also may be useful to use flavor enhancers to increase food intake (e.g., yogurt, maple syrup, or applesauce in dogs; home-cooked meats or fish in cats). Modulation of cytokine production also can be beneficial for managing cardiac cachexia. Supplementation of fish oil, which is high in n-3 fatty acids, can decrease inflammatory cytokine production and improve cachexia (see following paragraphs).

Protein

As early as the 1960s protein restriction was recommended for animals with CHF to reduce the "metabolic load" on the kidneys and liver. Restricting protein is actually detri-mental to the animal with CHF because it can contribute to lean body mass loss and malnutrition. Animals with CHF should not be protein restricted unless they have concur-rent advanced renal disease. Some of the diets designed for dogs with cardiac disease are very low in protein (this is not a problem with feline cardiac diets). Similarly, protein-restricted renal diets are sometimes recommended for ani-mals with heart disease because these diets often (but not always) are moderately sodium restricted. Unless concurrent disease dictates otherwise, high-quality protein should be fed to meet canine (5.1 g/100 kcal) or feline (6.5 g/100 kcal) minimums. This should be a primary goal in animals with heart disease, particularly as CHF becomes more severe.

Another important issue with regard to protein is the still widespread misconception that dietary protein should be restricted in early renal disease. Some dogs receiving ACE inhibitors develop azotemia, although this is relatively uncommon. Azotemia occurs more frequently when ACE inhibitors are used in conjunction with diuretics, but in a small number of dogs azotemia can develop from ACE inhib-itors alone. When concurrent ACE inhibitor and diuretic use causes azotemia, reduction of the diuretic dose is indicated. A protein-restricted diet is not recommended in this situa-tion unless medication changes do not correct the problem and renal disease progresses.

Fat

In addition to being a source of calories and essential fatty acids, fat also can have significant effects on immune func-tion, inflammatory mediator production, and hemodynamics. Most canine and feline diets contain primarily n-6 fatty acids (e.g., linoleic acid, arachidonic acids). The n-3 fatty acids eicosapentaenoic acid (EPA) and docosahexaenoic acid (DHA) normally are found in very low concentrations in the cell membrane compared to the n-6 fatty acids, but they can be increased by a food or supplement enriched in n-3 fatty acids. The benefit of having a higher concentration of n-3 fatty acids in the membranes is that breakdown products of the n-3 fatty acids (eicosanoids) are less potent inflam-matory mediators than eicosanoids derived from n-6 fatty acids. This decreases the production of cytokines and other inflammatory mediators. Fish oil reduces the production of TNF and IL-1 and improves muscle mass. In some animals

fish oil supplementation also improves appetite. Another potential benefit is that n-3 fatty acids have antiarrhythmic effects.

Although an optimal dose of n-3 fatty acids has not been determined, I currently recommend a daily dos-age of 40 mg/kg of EPA and 25 mg/kg of DHA for animals with anorexia or cachexia. Unless the diet is one of a few specially designed therapeutic diets, supplementation is necessary to achieve this n-3 fatty acid dose. When rec-ommending a fish oil supplement, it is important to know the exact amount of EPA and DHA in a specific fish oil brand since supplements vary widely. However, the most common formulation of fish oil is 1-g capsules that con-tain approximately 180 mg of EPA and 120 mg of DHA. At this concentration fish oil can be administered at a dose of 1 capsule per 10 pounds of body weight to achieve my recommended EPA and DHA dosage. Fish oil supple-ments should always contain vitamin E as an antioxidant, but other nutrients should not be included to avoid tox-icities. Cod liver oil and flaxseed oil should not be used to provide n-3 fatty acids to dogs and cats.

Sodium

Sodium restriction is one method, along with the use of diuretics and venous vasodilators, to treat excessive increases in preload in patients with CHF. In the 1960s, when few medications were available for treating animals with CHF, dietary sodium restriction was one of the few methods of reducing fluid accumulation. In this situation severe sodium restriction clearly was beneficial in reduc-ing signs of congestion. However, with the current avail-ability of newer and more effective medications, the role of severe sodium restriction in early CHF (ISACHC stage 1 or 2) is no longer clear. I currently recommend moderate sodium restriction (i.e., 50 to 80 mg/100 kcal) for animals with ISACHC stage 2 heart disease.

Most owners are unaware of the sodium content of pet and human foods and need very specific instructions regard-ing appropriate pet foods, acceptable low-salt treats, and methods for administering medications. Owners also should be counseled on specific foods to avoid such as baby food; bread; canned vegetables (unless "no salt added"); cheeses, including "squirtable" cheeses (unless specifically labeled "low sodium"); condiments (e.g., ketchup, soy sauce); lunch meats and cold cuts (e.g., ham, corned beef, salami, sau-sages, bacon, hot dogs); most pet foods and treats; pickled foods; pizza; processed foods (e.g., potato mixes, rice mixes, macaroni and cheese); snack foods (e.g., potato chips, pack-aged popcorn, crackers); and soups (unless homemade with-out salt). Mildly to moderately reduced dietary sodium can be achieved with a veterinary diet designed for animals with early cardiac disease or with certain diets designed for use in senior pets. If using a diet designed for senior pets, it is impor-tant to look at the characteristics of the individual product. There is no legal definition for a senior diet; thus the levels of calories, protein, sodium, and other nutrients can vary dramatically between different companies' products.

Potassium and Magnesium

Potassium and magnesium are nutrients of concern in cardiac patients because depletions of these electrolytes can cause cardiac arrhythmias, decreased myocardial contractility, and muscle weakness and can potentiate the adverse effects of cardiac medications. Many of the medications used in animals with CHF such as loop diuretics (e.g., furosemide) and thiazide diuretics (e.g., hydrochlorathiazide) can predispose a patient to hypokalemia. Inadequate dietary intake of potassium, which occurred in nearly half of dogs with heart disease in one study, also can predispose an animal to hypokalemia (Freeman et al., 2003). However, it is also important to note that the increased use of ACE inhibitors, which results in renal potassium sparing, has made hyperkalemia just as likely as hypokalemia in animals with CHF. In addition, spironolactone, an aldosterone antagonist and potassium-sparing diuretic, is being used with greater frequency in dogs with heart disease and can cause hyperkalemia. Finally, some commercial cardiac diets are high in potassium, which can exacerbate hyperkalemia.

Magnesium plays a critical role in normal cardiovascular function; and many of the medications used to treat cardiac conditions, including digoxin and loop diuretics, are associated with magnesium depletion in people. Therefore animals with CHF have the potential to develop hypomagnesemia. Studies have reported variable prevalence rates of hypomagnesemia (from 2% to over 50%) in dogs with heart disease.

Serum potassium should be monitored routinely in CHF patients, particularly those receiving an ACE inhibitor or large doses of diuretics. Serum magnesium concentrations also should be measured, but clinicians should be aware that serum magnesium concentrations are a poor indicator of total body stores. Nonetheless, serial evaluations in an individual patient may be useful, especially in patients with arrhythmias or in those taking high doses of diuretics. Diets range greatly in their potassium content; thus if hypokalemia or hyperkalemia is present, a diet with a higher or lower potassium content, respectively, should be selected. Similarly, diets high in magnesium may be beneficial in a hypomagnesemic animal.

Severe or Refractory Congestive Heart Failure

In severe CHF greater restriction of dietary sodium (<50 mg/100 kcal) may allow lower dosages of diuretics to be used to control clinical signs. To achieve this level of sodium restriction it may be necessary to feed a commercial cardiac diet. Typically these diets are severely restricted in both sodium and chloride; levels of other nutrients vary with the individual product. There also is a higher risk for potassium and magnesium abnormalities in severe CHF; thus monitoring of electrolytes is important.

At this stage of disease cardiac cachexia becomes more common; thus it is critical to maintain adequate calorie and protein intake. This can be a challenge since appetite in severe CHF is often cyclical and owners should be warned that appetite can be highly variable. Another issue to consider is that anorexia in an animal that has been eating can be an early sign of worsening disease or the need for medication adjustment and should trigger a reevaluation. In addition to optimization of medical therapy, offering multiple choices of appropriate pet foods, a homemade diet, or even single food items that can increase calorie intake without exacerbating the underlying disease (e.g., home-cooked meat, low-sodium breakfast cereal, or Clif

Bars) can be very useful. Palatability enhancers also can be very helpful for pets with severe CHF (e.g., cooked fish, low-sodium tuna, or cooked meat for cats; cooked meat, yogurt, applesauce, or maple syrup for dogs). Encouraging the owner to try offering foods at different temperatures may increase food intake in some animals (e.g., warmed versus room temperature versus cold). n-3 fatty acid supplementation also can be beneficial in some animals in which appetite is poor. Other tips that may increase food intake include providing smaller, more frequent meals; feeding the recommended diet(s) from the owner's plate; or putting the recommended diet(s) into a treat jar.

SPECIAL SITUATIONS

Feline Dilated Cardiomyopathy

The role of taurine deficiency in feline DCM has been well described, and there has been a dramatic decline in the incidence of the disease since the late 1980s. Most current cases of feline DCM appear to be independent of taurine status. Still taurine deficiency should be suspected whenever the diagnosis of feline DCM is made. A complete diet history should be obtained because cats that are eating a vegetarian diet or other unconventional diet are at higher risk for taurine deficiency. Even commercial vegetarian diets, the ingredient lists of which include taurine, can be severely taurine deficient. Plasma and whole blood taurine should be analyzed, and treatment with taurine (125 to 250 mg orally [PO] q12h) should begin concurrent with medical therapy. If the cat is eating an unconventional diet, the owner also should be counseled to switch to a nutritionally balanced meat-based commercial cat food.

Canine Dilated Cardiomyopathy

Supplementation of certain nutrients, either in the diet or in the form of dietary supplements, is most often proposed for dogs with DCM. Although some studies have been conducted in these areas, making recommendations can be difficult because there are many unsubstantiated claims for dietary supplements that owners find when researching DCM. A discussion of the role for some of these nutrients in canine DCM follows:

Taurine
Unlike cats, dogs are thought to be able to synthesize adequate amounts of taurine endogenously, and taurine is not considered a requirement in canine diets. Although typical breeds with DCM (e.g., Doberman pinscher, boxer) do not appear to have reduced taurine concentrations, taurine deficiency has been documented in some dogs of certain breeds with DCM, such as the American cocker spaniel, Newfoundland, and golden retriever. Taurine deficiency may occur more commonly in certain breeds because of higher requirements or breed-specific metabolic abnormalities, but diet also may play a role. Lamb meal and rice and high-fiber or very low–protein/low-taurine diets have been associated with taurine deficiency, although the exact role of diet is not yet known.

The benefits of taurine supplementation are not as clear in canine DCM as in feline DCM. Although several small studies have shown some improvements in clinical or echocardiographic parameters in taurine-deficient dogs supplemented with taurine, the response is generally not as dramatic as is seen in cats with taurine deficiency–induced DCM (Kittleson et al., 1997). Although ongoing research in this area will help to better understand this disease and make better recommendations in the future, I currently recommend measuring plasma and whole blood taurine concentrations in dogs with DCM that are of high risk (e.g., cocker spaniel, Newfoundland, golden retriever) or atypical (e.g., corgi, bassett hound) breeds. In addition, taurine concentrations should be measured in dogs with DCM that are eating lamb meal and rice–based diets, high-fiber diets, or diets that are highly protein restricted. Although the extent of benefits of supplementation is not yet clear, I recommend taurine supplementation until plasma and whole blood taurine concentrations on the patient are available. The optimal dose of taurine for correcting a deficiency has not been determined, but the dosage currently recommended is 500 to 1000 mg every 8 to 12 hours.

L-Carnitine

L-Carnitine plays an important role in long-chain fatty acid metabolism and energy production. Carnitine is in high concentrations in the myocardium, and carnitine deficiency syndromes can be associated with primary myocardial disease in humans. Carnitine deficiency was reported in a family of boxers in 1991. Since that time L-carnitine has been supplemented in some dogs with DCM, but no blinded prospective studies have been done. However, one randomized, double-blind, placebo-controlled study in humans with DCM showed improved 3-year survival in patients receiving L-carnitine supplementation. One of the limitations on progress in the study of carnitine deficiency is that myocardial concentrations must be measured to document a deficiency since plasma concentrations are often normal even in the face of myocardial deficiency.

L-carnitine supplementation has few side effects, but it is an expensive supplement, and this may be a significant deterrent for some owners. I offer the option of L-carnitine supplementation to owners of dogs with DCM, especially boxers but do not consider it essential. The minimum or optimal dose of L-carnitine necessary to replete a dog with low myocardial carnitine concentrations is not known, but the dosage that has been recommended is 50 to 100 mg/kg orally every 8 hours.

Antioxidants

Although antioxidants have received a great deal of attention in the popular press in terms of preventing and treating cardiovascular diseases, most of the research in human cardiology has been on coronary artery disease. Antioxidants are produced endogenously but also can be supplied exogenously if there is an imbalance between the levels of oxidants produced and the antioxidant protection available. The major antioxidants include enzymatic antioxidants (e.g., superoxide dismutase, catalase, glutathione peroxidase) and oxidant quenchers (e.g., vitamin C, vitamin E, and β-carotene). Recent studies have shown that, in dogs with CHF from either DCM or CVD, there is an imbalance between oxidant production and antioxidant protection. Supplemental antioxidants are now included in many commercial veterinary diets, including at least one cardiac diet. The effect of antioxidant supplementation in dogs and cats with CHF is not yet known; however, this may hold promise for the future.

Coenzyme Q10

The roles of coenzyme Q10 in energy production and as an antioxidant have prompted some investigators to propose coenzyme Q10 deficiency as a possible cause for DCM. Coenzyme Q10 supplementation has anecdotally been reported to be beneficial; but most of the human studies of coenzyme Q10 supplementation have not been well controlled, and results are conflicting. The current recommended (but empiric) dosage in dogs is 30 mg orally BID, although up to 90 mg orally BID has been recommended for large dogs. The purported benefits of supplementation include correction of a deficiency, improved myocardial metabolic efficiency, and increased antioxidant protection. Controlled prospective studies are necessary to accurately judge the efficacy of this often expensive supplement.

Dietary Supplements: General Issues

In many cases the desired nutrient modifications can be achieved through diet alone. However, supplementation of certain nutrients may be desirable if they are not in a particular diet or not at high enough levels in the diet to achieve the desired effect. It is important to be aware that dietary supplements do not require proof of safety, efficacy, or quality control to be marketed. Therefore careful selection of type, dose, and brand is important to avoid toxicities or complete lack of efficacy. Much additional information is needed to define the role of dietary supplements in heart disease, when they should be used, when they should not be used, and optimal dosages.

Another important issue with the administration of dietary supplements is that they should not take the place of standard cardiac medications. Animals with severe CHF may already be receiving many pills each day, and it may not be clear to owners that it is more important to give the cardiac medications than the dietary supplements. In situations in which pill administration is becoming overwhelming for an owner, the veterinarian can assist the owner in determining which dietary supplements have the least potential benefits and can be discontinued.

References and Suggested Reading

Fascetti AJ et al: Taurine deficiency in dogs with dilated cardiomyopathy: 12 cases (1997-2001), *J Am Vet Med Assoc* 223:1137, 2003.

Freeman LM et al: Nutritional alterations and the effect of fish oil supplementation in dogs with heart failure, *J Vet Intern Med* 12:440, 1998.

Freeman LM et al: Dietary patterns in dogs with cardiac disease, *J Am Vet Med Assoc* 223:1301, 2003.

Freeman LM et al: Antioxidant status and biomarkers of oxidative stress in dogs with congestive heart failure, *J Vet Intern Med* 19:537, 2005.

Freeman LM et al: Effects of dietary modification in dogs with early chronic valvular disease, *J Vet Intern Med* 20:1116, 2006.

Kittleson MD et al: Results of the multicenter spaniel trial (MUST), *J Vet Intern Med* 11:204, 1997.

Pedersen H: Effects of mild mitral valve insufficiency, sodium intake, and place of blood sampling on the renin-angiotensin system in dogs, *Acta Vet Scand* 37:109, 1996.

CHAPTER 158

Syncope

MARC S. KRAUS, *Ithaca, New York*
CLAY A. CALVERT, *Athens, Georgia*

The evaluation of syncope in animals is often challenging. Difficulties arise from the very nature of syncope because these events are often unpredictably sporadic, infrequent, and characterized by intersyncopal periods that are often unremarkable. Syncope is defined as a sudden loss of consciousness associated with loss of postural tone from which recovery is spontaneous. Allowing for the occasional exception such as hypoglycemia, the common denominator leading to all forms of syncope is a decrease or brief cessation of cerebral blood flow. *Presyncope* is a term used to describe episodic rearlimb or generalized weakness, ataxia, or an altered level of consciousness. Presyncope is associated with a less severe or more transient cerebral insult. Severe heart rhythm disturbances are probably the most common causes of syncope in dogs and cats.

IS IT SYNCOPE?

Distinguishing syncope from seizure can be difficult. Situational triggers, prodromal symptoms, signs that occur during the episode, and the events that follow provide clues for differential diagnosis. Collapse episodes that are precipitated by exercise, stress, startle, cough, gag, deglutition, emesis, micturition, defecation, and pain are most likely syncope rather than seizure. Disorientation after the event with slow recovery of normal consciousness is more common with seizures. However, protracted cerebral hypoxia resulting from cardiac arrhythmia may also be followed by slow recovery. Differentiating seizure from syncope can be confounded by the possibility of "hypoxic convulsive syncope" caused by profound cardiac arrhythmia. Cats may demonstrate focal facial twitches that appear very much like a focal seizure. Syncope or presyncope without prodrome or violent tonic-clonic activity and with quick recovery suggests a heart rhythm disturbance. Although often associated with flaccid collapse, syncope caused by arrhythmia can be associated with extensor rigidity, opisthotonus, and spontaneous urination or defecation. Hypersalivation is rarely associated with syncope caused by heart rhythm disturbances.

NEUROCARDIOGENIC (VASODEPRESSOR) SYNCOPE

Neurocardiogenic syncope (also called the reflex-mediated syncope) is the result of an incompletely understood adrenergic-stimulated baroreceptor reflex mechanism. Sympathetic stimulation normally leads to vasoconstriction, increased heart rate, and increased cardiac contractility. However, in humans in the presence of dehydration, volume underloading of the left ventricle, and orthostasis, increased ventricular contractility (empty ventricle syndrome) stimulates afferent vagal traffic to the brainstem from ventricular mechanoreceptors. The next step in the reflex is sympathetic withdrawal, which results in vasodilation (vasodepressor syncope) along with increased vagal efferent traffic that results in bradycardia. This can be considered an abnormal and inappropriate activation of the baroreceptor reflex.

In dogs neurocardiogenic bradycardia and syncope are usually precipitated by fight, flight, fright, or startle situations. Furthermore, it is not evident that dehydration is a predisposing factor. In fact, in the most common scenario (i.e., the elderly small dog with advanced mitral valve disease), the patient is volume expanded and is often not being administered drugs. Nonetheless the hyperdynamic left ventricle of the patient with advanced mitral valve regurgitation may, under the influence of sympathetic surge, simulate the empty ventricle syndrome because of further increase in contractility and massive regurgitation. When vagal afferent receptors at the left atrium–pulmonary venous junctions are suddenly stretched by increased right ventricular output, they may also trigger the reflex. Reflex-mediated syncope also may develop in cases of ventricular outflow obstruction.

The common denominator of all neurally mediated syncopes is vagal input to the cardiovascular center of the brainstem with subsequent sympathetic withdrawal, usually accompanied by vagal outflow. In the clinical setting in dogs, the hallmark sign is bradycardia, including sinus bradycardia, sinus arrest, or transient atrioventricular (AV) block. Documentation of vasodilation caused by sympathetic withdrawal is problematic. For this reason the common assumption is that these syndromes are caused mainly by bradycardia. However, we have observed "apparent" neurocardiogenic syncope in the absence of bradycardia. Furthermore, weakness, pallor, and lethargy persist in some patients after bradycardia has resolved; these patients may well be hypotensive from protracted vasodilation, as is often observed in humans.

The "broad" diagnosis of neurally mediated syncope is usually presumptive and based on the triggering situation and underlying disorders such as bronchial lung disease, advanced mitral valve disease, dilated cardiomyopathy, or breed predilection. Cough, emesis, micturition, defecation, and exertional situations are common triggers to the "situational syncopes." Electrocardiogram (ECG) or auscultation is required for documentation of bradycardia; and an indwelling arterial catheter or reliable, noninvasive blood pressure device is required to document hypotension (of course this is rarely possible). The 24- to 48-hour ambulatory ECG and even a 5- to 7-day ECG event recording are somewhat insensitive tests since most episodes are infrequent. Usually the precipitating exertional situations are exertion with excitement, inactivity to sudden "normal" activity, startle, climbing stairs, physical restraint, bathing or grooming, or barking-jumping with excitement. In young adult golden retrievers most episodes occur during walking with the owner and are precipitated by an excitement event (e.g., seeing another animal or straining at the leash).

ETIOLOGY OF SYNCOPE

Many disorders can result in syncope (Box 158-1); they can be categorized into cardiac and noncardiac causes. Hypoglycemia, hypoxia, and anemia are the most common metabolic causes of syncope. Addison's disease rarely causes episodic signs but rather causes progressive and protracted signs.

By far the most common recognized cause of syncope is disturbance of the heart rhythm. Advanced heart block is the most common cause of syncope across all breeds and ages. On the other hand, sick sinus syndrome is the most common cause of bradycardia and syncope in middle-aged and older American cocker spaniels, West Highland white terriers, and miniature schnauzers. Situational bradycardia and syncope are common in small dogs of all ages but most common in older patients. With advanced mitral regurgitation and high preload, it is precipitated by a surge of adrenalin caused by fight, flight, and fright situations. Respiratory arrest, white mucous membranes, and cyanosis occur during severe and protracted bradycardia (and presumably vasodilation). Frequently the owner believes that death has occurred. Most episodes last for only seconds to minutes. However, when pulmonary edema is beginning, bradycardia can persist for as long as 30 minutes. As with most situational syncopes in elderly small dogs, neurocardiogenic bradycardia is seldom lethal. It is a warning of high preload, impending pulmonary edema, and a need to aggressively unload the heart. It can be lethal when precipitated in the hospital setting by physical restraint.

Neurocardiogenic bradycardia (syncope) can also occur in "normal" dogs, particularly in golden retrievers, boxers, and dogs undergoing attack training. In boxers it seems to have a bimodal age of first occurrence: 6 to 24 months of age and 7 to 10 years of age. It is usually triggered by exertion coupled either with excitement or startle and can occur without evidence of cardiomyopathy (based on the absence of ventricular arrhythmias, cardiac enlargement, and decreased contractility). However, since both syndromes are common, each can occur in the same dog. In such patients the differential diagnosis is confounding and requires Holter recording or event monitor recording. In our experience Holter recordings in boxers and Doberman pinschers performed within 48 hours following syncope caused by ventricular tachycardia usually contain thousands of ventricular premature contractions (PVCs) with couplets, triplets, and nonsustained ventricular tachycardia.

Neurocardiogenic bradycardia and syncope also occur in Doberman pinschers wherein it is a marker for cardiomyopathy; and the intermittent bradycardia usually coexists with ventricular tachyarrhythmias of variable severity. Cardiomyopathic patients may have a subtle autonomic dysfunction that predisposes to neurocardiogenic bradycardia.

Reflex-mediated syncopes may occur in specific circumstances. These situational syncopes are common in dogs of all ages but rare in cats. Situational syncope is most common in small, middle- to old-aged dogs; it is often associated with cough caused by tracheal or bronchial disease or advanced mitral valve disease with compression of a main-stem bronchus. In addition to tussive syncope, other situations include deglutition, gag-wretch, emesis, micturition, and defecation. Thus the situation defines the trigger (i.e., tussive syncope, deglutition syncope, emesis syncope, micturition syncope, and defecation syncope). We believe that advanced mitral valve disease in elderly small dogs predisposes to all situational syncopes, as does severe pulmonary hypertension. When the heart rate is documented during situational syncope, it is almost always slow. Far more difficult to document is the systemic blood pressure at the time of syncope; therefore the vasodepressor arm of the reflex is generally overlooked.

The presentation of neurally mediated syncope in affected dogs may not be consistently precipitated by any given situation. Patients can be variably affected so that cough, emesis, exertion-excitement, micturition, and defecation do not cause syncope each and every time.

DIAGNOSING THE CAUSE OF SYNCOPE

The diagnostic goal is to document the heart rhythm at the time of the event. The patient history, physical examination, situational activity, and symptoms that occur during and after the event are crucial to establishing the cause of syncope. Table 158-1 lists the cause and diagnostic associations.

Box 158-1

Common Causes of Syncope

Structural Cardiovascular Disease
- Outflow obstruction (pulmonic stenosis, aortic stenosis)
- Obstruction to right atrial filling (cardiac tamponade, constrictive pericarditis, tumor)
- Pulmonary hypertension
- Poor myocardial contractility

Electrical Disease (Extreme Bradycardia or Tachycardia)
- Sick sinus syndrome
- Advanced atrioventricular (heart) block
- Supraventricular tachyarrhythmias (most common are atrial fibrillation and reentrant tachyarrhythmias)
- Ventricular tachyarrhythmias

Metabolic Disorders
- Hypoglycemia
- Endocrine (Addison's)
- Hypoxia
- Anemia

Neurally Mediated Syncope
- Neurocardiogenic (reflex-mediated)
- Situational

General Diagnostic Tests

Routine laboratory tests generally do not identify the cause of syncope, but they should be performed when the history and physical examination are indications. A complete blood count is used to rule out anemia and infection. A serum chemistry profile is used to identify metabolic disorders (evaluate electrolyte abnormalities, blood urea nitrogen, creatinine, and glucose levels). An adrenocorticotropic hormone stimulation test is indicated in cases of suspected hypoadrenocorticism. Serum thyroxine is appropriate in cases of sinus bradycardia.

Imaging Studies

An echocardiogram with Doppler examination may be useful in patients with a heart murmur and to assess structure and function of the heart. It may also rule out occult pericardial disease, pulmonary hypertension, or intracardiac mass lesions. If a seizure is suspected, a computed tomography scan or magnetic resonance imaging may be indicated.

Testing for Arrhythmias

The only certain way to identify arrhythmias as the cause of syncope is to document the heart rate and rhythm during an episode. Real-time auscultation is useful because it documents the associated rate as fast, slow, or normal.

Table **158-1**

Signs Associated With Syncope

Type or Cause Of Syncope	Usual Associations
Classical situational syncope	Coughing, gagging, retching, swallowing, vomiting, micturition, or defecation
High preload in small breed dogs	Exertion-excitement precipitated Loud heart murmur Severe left atrial enlargement ECG: normal or chamber enlargements
Physical exertion in a dog with an aortic or pulmonic stenosis	Consider outflow obstruction May also involve ventricular arrhythmia or neurocardiogenic syncope
Pulmonary hypertension	Heartworm disease, mitral valve disease, severe lung disease, exertional signs, right-sided congestive heart failure
Sick sinus syndrome	Breed: miniature schnauzer, American cocker spaniel ECG: sinoatrial arrest, sinus bradycardia, junctional or ventricular escape beats and brief rhythm, atrial or junctional premature contractions, atrial or junctional tachycardia, and occasionally ventricular premature contractions
Atrial fibrillation	Advanced MR or dilated cardiomyopathy
Ventricular tachycardia	ECG: ventricular tachycardia, particularly cardiomyopathic boxers and Doberman pinschers
Heart block	ECG: bradycardia caused by advanced second- or third-degree AV block

AV, Atrioventricular; *ECG:* electrocardiogram; *MR,* mitral regurgitation.

Presumptive diagnosis of the cause of syncope is sometimes legitimate when specific arrhythmias are recorded on a standard ECG rhythm strip in breeds at high risk of syncope from that condition. For example, ventricular tachycardia should be presumed as the likely cause of syncope in Doberman pinschers and boxers when subsequent ECGs contain frequent PVCs (see Table 158-1). Specific clinical disorders or precipitating situations can be highly suggestive of a cause of syncope, but optimally the rhythm during an event should be known. In most cases rhythm disturbances are episodic, in which case a 24- to 48-hour Holter recording or a 5- to 7-day event recording is useful. For longer-term monitoring an implantable continuous-loop ECG recorder can be used. We sometimes issue a chest-press ECG (Veterinary Biolog) that enables the owner to document the heart rhythm associated with infrequent syncope. Humans with reflex-mediated syncope are evaluated by tilt-table, but this examination needs more development in dogs.

TREATMENT

Treatment of syncope varies with the cause and is aimed at managing the underlying disorder. If an arrhythmic etiology is discovered, antiarrhythmic medication or pacemaker therapy is indicated (Table 158-2).

Neurocardiogenic bradycardia and syncope caused by high preload often responds favorably to cardiac unloading therapy. Exertion-excitement–related syncope in elderly small dogs with loud mitral murmurs may be a warning of impending congestive heart failure. Treatment includes a furosemide, an angiotensin-converting enzyme inhibitor, and perhaps spironolactone. Furosemide should be considered even if pulmonary edema is not present on thoracic radiographs. After 1 to 2 weeks adjuvant afterload reduction using amlodipine can be added to the treatment regimen. The addition of digoxin may decrease the numbers of syncopal episodes. Although the exact mechanism is unknown, digoxin modulates baroreceptor function and inhibits sympathetic nerve discharge (the trigger for this type of neurally mediated syncope). Digoxin is not indicated in sinus bradycardia or in cases of AV block. The frequency of syncope can be further reduced by client education and the avoidance of instigating situations to whatever extent is practical. Treatment-resistant episodes sometimes respond favorably to sympathomimetic or anticholinergic therapy.

Fight or flight–stimulated neurocardiogenic syncope in boxers, Doberman pinschers, golden retrievers, and dogs undergoing attack training is best "treated" by avoiding the instigating situations. Preventive anticholinergic therapy is recommended only when episodes are predictable (i.e., scheduled exertion that might precipitate an event).

β-Blockade has been recommended for treatment of humans with neurocardiogenic syncope precipitated by sympathetic surge. β-Blockade is effective in some humans. However, this therapy is often ineffective and can be aggravating when bradycardia is the main component of the syndrome.

Syncope in cats is usually the result of a heart rhythm disturbance. Neurally mediated syncope and sick sinus syndrome are rare. In old cats intermittent or sustained heart blocks are the most common arrhythmic causes of

Table 158-2

Treatment of Syncope

Drug	Indication	Maintenance Dosage (mg/kg)	Frequency
Amiodarone (Cordarone)	Ventricular and supraventricular arrhythmias	10*	BID for 1 week (loading)
		5*	SID (maintenance)
Sotalol	Ventricular and supraventricular arrhythmias	0.5-2	BID
		Cat: 10 to 20	BID
Mexiletine	Ventricular arrhythmias	5-8	TID
Furosemide	Overt or impending CHF	1-2	BID-TID
ACE inhibitor	Overt or impending CHF		
Enalapril		0.5	SID
Benazepril		0.5	SID
Spironolactone	Overt or impending CHF Electrolyte control	1-2	BID
Digoxin	Atrial fibrillation (control ventricular response rate)	0.005-0.01[†]	BID
Diltiazem	Atrial fibrillation (control ventricular response rate)	Diltiazem XR (Dilacor)	TID
		Dog: 3-4 mg/kg	BID
		Cat: 30-60 mg total dose (start with 30 mg SID)	SID-BID
		Cardizem CD	
		Cat: 10 mg/kg	SID
		Cardizem	
		Dog: 0.5-1.5 mg/kg	TID (titrate dose to effect)
		Cat: 7.5 mg total dose	BID-TID (titrate dose to effect)
Amlodipine	Afterload reduction	0.3-0.4[‡]	BID
Pacemaker	Advanced heart block Sick sinus syndrome	Not applicable	
Hyoscyamine sulfate	Sick sinus syndrome	0.003-0.005[§]	TID
Propantheline bromide	Sick sinus syndrome	0.2-0.5	BID-TID

ACE, Angiotensin-converting enzyme; CHF, congestive heart failure.
*Recommended dosage range in veterinary medicine is testimonial and variable.
[†]In dogs weighing less than 20 kg.
[‡]Initiate at 0.1 mg/kg and up-titrate weekly while monitoring blood pressure. Target dosage is 0.4 mg/kg. Target systolic blood pressure is around 110 mm Hg. Initiate therapy once ACE inhibitor maintenance therapy has been established.
[§]Consider if positive response to intravenous atropine test (0.044 mg/kg). Pacemaker implantation is the treatment of choice.
Editor's note: Some patients with neurocardiogenic syncope respond (paradoxically) to sympathomimetic drugs such as terbutaline or theophylline.

syncope and episodic weakness. Some cats have a normal ECG during hospital examinations and are often misdiagnosed as having a seizure disorder. In young to middle-aged cats rapid ventricular tachycardia is a common cause of syncope. The majority of these cats have hypertrophic cardiomyopathy. Cats with hypertrophic cardiomyopathy and loud, apical systolic heart murmurs may also experience exertional syncope or presyncope as a result of left ventricular outflow tract obstruction. These patients usually respond favorably to β-blocker treatment. Metabolic causes of syncope are uncommon. Occasionally hypoglycemia can occur as a result of insulin treatment in diabetic cats. Profound anemia can result in exertional syncope or presyncope in cats and dogs.

Suggested Reading

Abboud FM: Neurocardiogenic syncope, N Engl J Med 15:1117, 1993.

Benditt DG, Brignole M, Raviele A, Wieling W, editors: Syncope and transient loss of consciousness, Malden, Mass, 2007, Blackwell Futura.

Benditt DG, Blanc JJ, Brignole M, Sutton R, editors: The evaluation and treatment of syncope, Malden, Mass, 2006, Blackwell.

Bright JM, Cali JV: Clinical usefulness of cardiac event recording in dogs and cats examined because of syncope, episodic collapse, or intermittent weakness: 60 cases (1997-1999), J Am Vet Med Assoc 216(7):1110, 2000.

Davidow EB, Jeffrey P, Woodfield JA: Syncope: pathophysiology and differential diagnosis, Compend Contin Educ Pract Vet 23:608, 2001.

Fogoros, RN: The evaluation of syncope. In Vlay SC: Electrophysiologic testing, ed 3, Oxford, England, 1999, Blackwell Science, p 241.

Kapoor WN: Syncope, N Engl J Med 343:1856, 2000.

Kittleson MD: Syncope. In Kittleson MD, Kienle RD, editors: Small animal cardiovascular medicine, St Louis, 1998, Mosby, p 495.

Oberg B, Thoren P: Increased activity in left ventricular receptors during hemorrhage or occlusion of caval veins in the cat: a possible cause of the vaso-vagal reaction, Acta Vet Scand 85:164, 1972.

Rush JE: Syncope and episodic weakness. in Fox PR, Sisson D, Moise NS, editors: Textbook of canine and feline cardiology, Philadelphia, 1999, Saunders, p 446.

CHAPTER 159

Systemic Hypertension

REBECCA L. STEPIEN, *Madison, Wisconsin*
ROSEMARY A. HENIK, *Madison, Wisconsin*

Systemic hypertension (pathologic elevation of systemic blood pressure [BP]) is increasingly recognized as a cause of morbidity in pet cats and dogs. Systemic hypertension (HT) usually represents a complication of other systemic diseases in dogs and cats and therefore is classified as *secondary* hypertension. However, in some cases a causative disease is not apparent after careful investigation, and the HT is deemed *primary* or *idiopathic*. Whether primary or secondary, persistent systemic HT indicates a failure of the body's physiologic adaptations to normalize BP in the setting of inappropriate elevation.

OVERVIEW OF SYSTEMIC HYPERTENSION IN THE POPULATION

Persistent elevation of systolic BP to values greater than 160 mm Hg is associated with progressive renal injury in dogs, and the severity of renal injury has been correlated to the degree of elevation (Finco, 2004). Potential renal pathologic changes induced by systemic HT include both glomerular and tubulointerstitial changes with resulting ischemia, necrosis, atrophy, and exacerbation of proteinuria. These gradual and additive changes may be difficult to quantify in living animals with preexisting renal disease, but systolic HT (>160 mm Hg) at the time of presentation increases the odds of uremic crisis and death in dogs with renal disease (Jacob et al., 2003). Systolic BP higher than 180 mm Hg has been associated with ocular injury, including retinal or intraocular hemorrhage; retinal vascular tortuosity; and retinal detachments and retinal degeneration that may cause acute blindness, especially in cats. Neurologic abnormalities, most often intracranial in nature, including seizures, mentation changes, and vestibular signs, have been noted in dogs and cats with HT and are more likely when systolic pressures exceed 180 mm Hg. Although variable cardiac hypertrophy has been documented in cats with naturally occurring HT (Henik, Stepien, and Bortnowski, 2004; Nelson et al., 2002; Chetboul et al., 2003) and has been shown to regress with successful antihypertensive therapy (Snyder, Sadek, and Jones, 2001), the degree of hypertrophy has not been shown to correlate with severity of HT. In dogs with experimentally induced HT, hypertrophy and diastolic dysfunction without fibrosis occurred within 12 weeks (Douglas and Tallant, 1991). Although congestive heart failure caused by systemic HT appears to be rare in either species, the onset, development, and clinical repercussions of cardiac changes resulting from sustained HT await further study in cats and dogs with naturally occurring systemic HT.

Systemic HT may be recognized when BP is measured as part of a diagnostic evaluation in animals known to have or suspected of having systemic diseases associated with the development of HT. Alternatively, elevated BP may be detected when clinical signs of HT (typically retinal detachment or intracranial neurologic signs) lead to BP measurement (Table 159-1). Although periodic BP evaluation in healthy patients has been advocated by some authors, the moderate sensitivity (53% to 71%) and specificity (85% to 88%) of oscillometric and Doppler methods to detect systolic BP greater than 160 mm Hg in conscious dogs increases the risk of false-positive and false-negative readings (Stepien et al., 2003). However, in cats these concerns may be modulated by the increased prevalence of diseases (chronic renal insufficiency and hyperthyroidism) associated with development of systemic HT in older cats. Because these diseases may have an insidious onset, annual BP screening of apparently healthy older cats may be warranted.

Detection of systemic HT as a complication of systemic disease requires an understanding of the diseases likely to produce systemic HT as a comorbid factor. Hypertension in the general canine population is thought to be approximately 1% to 10% (Bodey and Michell, 1996; Remillard, Ross, and Eddy 1991), and prevalence of HT in the healthy feline population is unknown. In both cases systemic HT is more common in subpopulations affected by particular diseases (Table 159-2). Published prevalence rates are highly variable for many diseases based on the criteria used for diagnosis (i.e., the number used as a "cut off" for normal values), advances in the early recognition of some diseases, and variability in BP measurement techniques.

In cats renal disease is the most likely cause of systemic HT. Renal disease is highly prevalent in the feline population, and HT occurs in approximately 20% to 30% of cats with this disease (Syme et al., 2002). In early studies as many as 86% of hyperthyroid cats had BP above the reference range; but more recent anecdotal evidence suggests that the prevalence rate of HT in hyperthyroid cats is much lower (≈10% to 30%), perhaps as a result of increased screening and earlier detection of hyperthyroidism (before hypertensive complications develop). Many elderly cats have both chronic renal insufficiency and hyperthyroidism, complicating analysis of the prevalence of HT in these diseases. The prevalence of HT in cats with diabetes mellitus is poorly documented, but BP screening in diabetic cats is warranted clinically, especially if proteinuria is present.

Numerous studies in dogs support chronic renal disease (especially glomerular disease), hyperadrenocorti-

Table 159-1

Indications for Measurement of Blood Pressure in Dogs and Cats*

Both Species	Dogs: Additional Indications	Cats: Additional Indications
• Intraocular hemorrhage • Retinal hemorrhage/detachment • Intracranial neurologic signs • Renal disease • Diabetes mellitus • Left ventricular hypertrophy not associated with outflow obstruction • Use of medications that can raise blood pressure • Sudden decompensation of left-sided cardiac disease	Both species list plus: • Hyperadrenocorticism • Acromegaly • Pheochromocytoma • Primary hyperaldosteronism	Both species plus: • Hyperthyroidism • Left ventricular hypertrophy • Heart murmur

*All cats should have systemic hypertension excluded as a cause of left ventricular hypertrophy before a diagnosis of idiopathic hypertrophic cardiomyopathy is made.

Table 159-2

Diseases Associated With Development of Systemic Hypertension in Dogs and Cats*

Disease	Estimated Prevalence of Systemic Hypertension (if known) (%)	Comment
Dogs		
Renal disease	60-90	Proteinuric animals may be at higher risk.
Hyperadrenocorticism	70-80	Proteinuric animals may be at higher risk.
Diabetes mellitus	25-50	Only small numbers of patients analyzed.
Pheochromocytoma	Unknown	Systemic hypertension may be periodic with catecholamine surges.
Primary hyperaldosteronism	Unknown	
Acromegaly	Unknown	
Use of hypertensive medications	Unknown	Phenylpropanolamine and corticosteroids most frequently implicated.
Cats		
Renal disease	20-65	Early studies documented higher prevalence.
Hyperthyroidism	10-86	Early studies documented higher prevalence.
Diabetes mellitus	Unknown	One study suggested a low prevalence.
Primary hyperaldosteronism	Unknown	
Use of hypertensive medications	Unknown	Corticosteroids are implicated most frequently.

*See text for references.

cism, and diabetes mellitus as the most common diseases associated with secondary systemic HT. Other uncommon endocrine diseases associated with HT in dogs include pheochromocytoma, primary hyperaldosteronism, and acromegaly. The use of hypertensive medications such as phenylpropanolamine or corticosteroids may elevate BP primarily or as an additive effect to a causative disease. Healthy sight hounds may have resting BP values up to 15 mm Hg higher than other breeds of similar size (Bodey and Michell, 1996) and should be assessed accordingly.

DIAGNOSIS OF SYSTEMIC HYPERTENSION

Studies of ease of use, accuracy, and precision of various noninvasive BP measurement systems have been performed in normal and hypertensive dogs and cats. In general, Doppler methods using a forelimb (radial) cuff are recommended for use in cats. In dogs oscillometric or Doppler methods with radial, metatarsal, or proximal tail cuffs are used. In all cases the patient should be calm and acclimated to the environment and position before measurement. Cuff width chosen should approximate 40% of the circumference of the limb at point of placement, and the limb or tail should be positioned such that the cuff site is at the level of the heart during measurement. Typically six consecutive BP measurements with simultaneous heart rates are recorded. The first measurement and any obviously spurious measurements are discarded, and the remaining values averaged for a representative reading. Careful training of specific personnel in the practice of measuring BP carefully and recording values consistently is highly recommended. Frequently cuff size is relatively too narrow to effectively occlude the artery, and measured pressure is higher than actual arterial pressure. The opposite occurs if the cuff is relatively too wide. When elevated ABP is identified, some clinicians recommend remeasuring pressure in the opposite limb or alternative site to exclude anatomic factors that may impact arterial occlusion.

Measurements obtained from an initial session should be interpreted in conjunction with the patient's clinical signs or concurrent disease and the observed level of patient agitation at the time of measurement. The recording of simultaneous heart rate is a helpful adjunct in assessing the patient's state of agitation. Either isolated systolic HT or combined systolic and diastolic HT is identified in the majority of hypertensive dogs. For this reason and because noninvasive measurement methods in current use most reliably deliver systolic BP measurements, decisions regarding diagnosis and therapy are usually based on systolic readings.

Studies of human hypertensive patients indicate a progressive increase in risk of end-organ damage as BP increases above normal values. Although antihypertensive therapy is indicated in an individual patient as soon as end-organ damage begins to occur, in veterinary patients the pressure at which an individual begins to sustain end-organ damage is usually unknown. Since recognizable injury to various organ systems has been documented when systolic BP exceeds 160 mm Hg chronically, antihypertensive medications currently are recommended for patients in this group (Brown et al., 2007). It is likely that this current cut-off value will change as more information becomes available.

If elevated BP is documented at a single session and no clinical signs of HT (ocular or neurologic) or obvious target organ injury are present, a repeated measurement should be scheduled, preferably within a week. If elevated BP is confirmed, a detailed diagnostic evaluation to search for a causative disease should be initiated (Box 159-1). If a known causative disease is present, therapy for HT can be started in conjunction with optimal management of the underlying disorder. If systolic BP is between 160 and 180 mm Hg and no clinical signs of HT are present, BP may be monitored until the diagnostic evaluation is complete. If BP remains elevated and causative disease is found, therapy of the underlying disease (e.g., hyperadrenocorticism) should be initiated, and BP monitored for response to treatment of the underlying disease. If thorough diagnostic evaluation fails to reveal a causative disease, animals with consistently elevated BP should be treated with antihypertensive medications and monitored for development of systemic disease or complications.

THERAPY OF SYSTEMIC HYPERTENSION

Multiple therapeutic options are available to treat the hypertensive veterinary patient. As is the case in humans, many animals need more than one medication to control HT adequately. This is predictable based on neurologic and endocrine control of the cardiovascular system. Mean arterial pressure is controlled by the interaction of systemic vascular resistance and cardiac output. In turn, cardiac output relies on the interaction of the heart rate and stroke volume, a value affected by preload (a reflection of blood volume), afterload, and contractile function. With intricate interplay of the sympathetic and parasympathetic nervous systems, endocrine control of blood volume, and vascular tone modulation through the renin-angiotensin-aldosterone and other systems, the cardiovascular system is capable of at least partially compensating for medication effects.

Thus it is reasonable to assume that better control of BP may be possible if direct vasodilating medications (e.g., amlodipine besylate) are combined with medications that limit the ability of the compensatory mechanisms to adjust to medication-induced changes (e.g., angiotensin-converting enzyme [ACE] inhibitors). For many clinicians the combination of amlodipine plus an ACE inhibitor represents typical therapy for feline HT. In addition, concern has been expressed regarding the possible detrimental effects of using calcium channel blockers as monotherapy. Calcium channel blockers cause preferential vasodilation of afferent renal arterioles and increase intraglomerular pressure in some circumstances. This afferent vasodilation, if combined with inadequate decreases in systemic BP, may actually promote glomerular damage (Brown et al., 1993; Jacob et al., 2003). In theory combining efferent arteriolar dilation associated with ACE inhibitors with the stronger antihypertensive effects of amlodipine or other dihydropyridine calcium channel blockers may provide optimal BP management while conferring some degree of renal protection against progressive injury. Finally, some conditions have recognized indications for specific medications (e.g., ACE inhibitors in proteinuric diseases, sympathetic nervous system blockade in symptomatic pheochromocytoma, aldosterone antagonists in hyperaldosteronism). In these cases indicated medications should form the basis for therapy, with additional medications with different mechanisms of action added as needed. In nonemergent cases (systolic BP less than 200 mm Hg, no evidence of ocular or neurologic signs), at least 7 days should elapse before adding new antihypertensive medications.

Systemic HT in cats (idiopathic or secondary to renal insufficiency or diabetes mellitus) responds well to therapy

---

Box **159-1**

Recommended Diagnostic Testing for Patients With Systemic Hypertension

Dogs	Cats
• Funduscopic examination	• Funduscopic examination
• Serum chemistries	• Serum chemistries
• Urinalysis	• Urinalysis
• Urine protein screening	• Urine protein screening
• Hyperadrenocorticism screening	• Thyroid screening if appropriate based on age
• Adrenocorticotropic hormone stimulation test	
• Dexamethasone suppression test	
• Abdominal ultrasound if indicated for additional renal and adrenal evaluation	

with amlodipine besylate (0.625 to 1.25 mg/cat q24h orally [PO]), and consistent administration typically results in long-term BP control (Elliott et al., 2001). In addition, early therapy with amlodipine in cats with blindness caused by retinal detachment may allow return of at least partial visual ability (Maggio et al., 2000). In cats with proteinuria addition of an ACE inhibitor to amlodipine therapy may reduce renal protein loss, but an ACE inhibitor alone is unlikely to control HT when used as a monotherapy. ACE inhibitors in common use for hypertensive cats are enalapril maleate (0.25 to 0.5 mg/kg q12-24h PO) and benazepril (0.25 to 0.5 mg/kg q24h PO). Benazepril may be preferred in cats with renal disease because of some hepatic elimination. Cats with controlled HT should be reevaluated at regular intervals to assess BP and renal function. Hypertensive cats with hyperthyroidism may benefit from amlodipine therapy with simultaneous β-blockade (e.g., atenolol, 6.25 to 12.5 mg/cat q12h PO) to help control tachycardia and other cardiovascular effects of thyrotoxicosis. If medical or surgical resolution of the hyperthyroidism occurs, antihypertensive medications can be tentatively reduced or eliminated, and the BP rechecked. Some cats remain hypertensive after resolution of thyrotoxicosis and require chronic antihypertensive therapy, often because of concurrent renal disease.

Canine HT typically is more challenging to control than feline HT. The reason for this disparity is unknown but makes dogs much more like humans, in whom the need for more than one antihypertensive medication to control BP is the norm. The BP effects of antihypertensive medications on BP are additive, but presumably so are the side effects. Ideal antihypertensive therapy would consist of optimal control of the causative disease paired with the minimal number of antihypertensive medications required to control BP to target systolic values of 145 to 160 mm Hg.

When specific abnormalities are identified (e.g., catecholamine excess in pheochromocytoma, excessive aldosterone secretion in primary hyperaldosteronism), targeted medical therapy such as α- and β-blockers or aldosterone antagonists (e.g., spironolactone, 1 to 2 mg/kg q12h PO) is indicated. If systemic HT persists, addition of an ACE inhibitor or amlodipine may be beneficial.

In dogs with renal disease, hyperadrenocorticism, or diabetes mellitus, a standard progressive protocol can be used and results in control of systemic HT in the majority of cases. ACE inhibitors such as enalapril (0.5 mg/kg q12-24h PO) or benazepril (0.5 mg/kg q12-24h PO) are indicated to limit renal protein loss in dogs with proteinuria, and administration usually results in an approximately 10% decrease in systolic BP in these and other patients with renal insufficiency. If systemic HT is mild, this 10% decrease may be sufficient to decrease BP to within an acceptable range. Although twice-daily dosing of an ACE inhibitor may result in more rapid onset of effect than once-daily dosing, it is unclear whether twice-daily dosing is more effective for BP control at steady state. Current recommendations for therapy for both proteinuria and HT are to begin at once-daily dosing and increase to twice-daily dosing if inadequate response is noted.

The calcium channel blocker amlodipine besylate (0.1 to 0.2 mg/kg q12-24h PO) is a direct vasodilator useful in the management of systemic HT of any cause. Amlodipine appears to cause minimal reflex tachycardia, a side effect of some other direct vasodilators. As is the case with an ACE inhibitor, once-daily dosing is used and increased to maximal doses as needed. Frequency may be increased to twice-daily dosing if response is inadequate. Some animals require higher doses of amlodipine than typically recommended; animals receiving doses above the recommended range should be monitored closely for hypotension, changes in renal function, and other side effects. The long elimination half-life of amlodipine in dogs may require a 1-week follow-up to more fully evaluate the antihypertensive effect.

Apparently refractory or difficult-to-manage systemic HT occurs occasionally in the canine population. In any case of apparently refractory HT, owner understanding and compliance with the dosing schedule should be checked. Ideally BP should be measured approximately 12 hours after steady state is attained; measurement of BP several hours after dosing may underestimate medication effects. Additional diagnostics may be required to identify additional causative factors in animals with more than one predisposing condition (e.g., discovery of hyperadrenocorticism in a patient with diabetes). In cases of truly refractory HT other medications (hydralazine, prazosin, spironolactone, diuretics) can be added to the patient's therapeutic plan. In general, addition of multiple medications based on theoretic benefit should be approached with caution, and all additional medications should be initiated at the low end of the dosing range with close BP and biochemical monitoring. There is a distinct shortage of clinical data supporting the safety and efficacy of multiple-drug regimens in the canine and feline hypertensive population. Additional medications may contribute to hypotension, dehydration with resultant renal dysfunction, and remote side effects such as inappetence or complicate the therapeutic plan for the caregiver without evidence of advantage over simpler routines.

Emergent hypertension with severe end-organ injury (active retinal detachment, intraocular bleeding, progressive central nervous system signs) should be treated in the hospital; amlodipine generally works very well in this setting. Rarely is sodium nitroprusside, hydralazine, or prazosin needed; and in such cases it is reasonable to contact a specialist to discuss therapy.

No clinical studies are available that address the prognosis for survival in cats and dogs affected with hypertension as a primary problem or a complication of systemic disease. Prognosis is likely varied based on the underlying disease, severity of hypertension, and presence and severity of clinical signs. Present therapeutic recommendations are aimed at ameliorating clinical signs and preventing progression of end-organ damage.

References and Suggested Reading

Bodey AR, Michell AR: Epidemiological study of blood pressure in domestic dogs, *J Small Anim Pract* 37:116, 1996.

Brown SA et al: Long-term effects of antihypertensive regimens on renal hemodynamics and proteinuria, *Kidney Int* 43:1210, 1993.

Brown S et al: Guidelines for the identification, evaluation, and management of systemic hypertension in dogs and cats, *J Vet Intern Med* 21:542, 2007.

Chetboul V et al: Spontaneous feline hypertension: clinical and echocardiographic abnormalities, and survival rate, *J Vet Intern Med* 17:89, 2003.

Douglas PS, Tallant B: Hypertrophy, fibrosis and diastolic dysfunction in early canine experimental hypertension, *J Am Coll Cardiol* 17:530, 1991.

Elliott J et al: Feline hypertension: clinical findings and response to antihypertensive treatment in 30 cases, *J Small Anim Pract* 42:122, 2001.

Finco DR: Association of systemic hypertension with renal injury in dogs with induced renal failure, *J Vet Intern Med* 18:289, 2004.

Henik RA, Stepien RL, Bortnowski HB: Spectrum of M-mode echocardiographic abnormalities in 75 cats with systemic hypertension, *J Am Anim Hosp Assoc* 40:359, 2004.

Jacob F et al: Association between initial systolic blood pressure and risk of developing a uremic crisis or of dying in dogs with chronic renal failure, *J Am Vet Med Assoc* 222:322, 2003.

Maggio F et al: Ocular lesions associated with systemic hypertension in cats: 69 cases (1985-1998), *J Am Vet Med Assoc* 217:695, 2000.

Nelson OL et al: Echocardiographic and radiographic changes associated with systemic hypertension in cats, *J Vet Intern Med* 16:418, 2002.

Remillard RL, Ross JN, Eddy JB: Variance of indirect blood pressure measurements and prevalence of hypertension in clinically normal dogs, *Am J Vet Res* 52:561, 1991.

Snyder PS, Sadek D, Jones GL: Effect of amlodipine on echocardiographic variables in cats with systemic hypertension, *J Vet Intern Med* 15:52, 2001.

Stepien RL et al: Comparative diagnostic test characteristics of oscillometric and Doppler ultrasonographic methods in the detection of systolic hypertension in dogs, *J Vet Intern Med* 17:65, 2003.

Syme HM et al: Prevalence of systolic hypertension in cats with chronic renal failure at initial evaluation, *J Am Vet Med Assoc* 220:1799, 2002.

CHAPTER 160

Permanent Cardiac Pacing in Dogs

MARK A. OYAMA, *Philadelphia, Pennsylvania*

D. DAVID SISSON, *Corvallis, Oregon*

Artificial pacing (AP) is extremely effective at resolving clinical signs of syncope, lethargy, and exercise intolerance secondary to bradyarrhythmias. The most common cardiac arrhythmias treated by pacing include sinus arrest (sick sinus syndrome), high-grade second- and third-degree (complete) atrioventricular block, and bradycardia associated with persistent atrial standstill. These rhythm disturbance disorders are discussed in more detail in Chapter 158 (also see Rishniw and Thomas, 1999). Temporary pacing is sometimes needed for patients with bradyarrhythmias and is reviewed in Chapter 8. This chapter emphasizes current developments in cardiac pacing in dogs.

In veterinary patients the most common method of permanent AP involves transvenous, single-lead, single-chamber ventricular pacing. This form of AP is performed routinely in academic and private referral hospitals and is associated with improved quality of life and high client satisfaction. Despite the relative ease of placement and satisfactory clinical results, optimal AP requires increasing attention to the growing list of pacemaker capabilities, programming parameters, and potential complications. Since the first veterinary

implantation in the early 1960s (Buchanan, 2003), AP has been the subject of much study. The reader is directed to several excellent reviews regarding the indications, equipment, technique, and practice of AP in veterinary medicine (Moise, 1999; Sisson, 1991; Rishniw and Thomas, 1999; Johnson, Martin, and Henley, 2007; Wess et al., 2006). After briefly reviewing the current method of AP, this update will highlight potential limitations of conventional AP and then introduce technologies that could advance the treatment of symptomatic bradyarrhythmias.

CONVENTIONAL ARTIFICIAL PACING

Conventional transvenous AP typically is accomplished by placing a pacing lead into the right ventricular apex via the jugular vein. The distal tip of the lead is secured into the ventricular endocardial surface, and the proximal end exits the jugular vein and is attached to a battery-powered generator. The vast majority of AP systems implanted in this manner are programmed to both detect and administer electrical impulses at the right ventricular apex. The usual mode of AP accomplished in this fashion is indicated by the three-letter code VVI, wherein the pacing system performs two functions. The first involves sensing of native cardiac depolarizations in the ventricle, during which time the AP system is quiescent (or inhibited). The second involves delivery of an electrical pacing discharge, following a prescribed time period of no detected native electrical activity. This so-called "demand" pacemaker function prevents periods of asystole and associated clinical signs.

The performance of modern AP systems can be fine-tuned using a wide array of programmable parameters, which, when properly set, allow safe, stable, and long-term treatment (Table 160-1). For example, the pulse duration and amplitude of the pacing discharge can be adjusted to maximize battery life while still ensuring functional depolarization of the ventricle. A number of pacing parameters can be adjusted after surgery via telemetric communication with a portable programming computer. To ensure safe and efficacious pacing, meticulous attention must be given to the proper programming of the pacemaker system parameters. Improper settings can lead to loss of pacing, inappropriate delivery of pacing stimuli, induction of ventricular arrhythmias, congestive heart failure, syncope, and sudden death. In a recent study, inappropriate asynchronous pacing was reported in 42% of dogs receiving AP systems, highlighting the need for follow-up examinations and proper programming (Moise and Estrada, 2002). In humans improper VVI pacing has been associated with sudden death (Zehender et al., 1992). The causative mechanism most likely involves sensing abnormalities, improper timing of pacing discharges, and induction of ventricular fibrillation. In canine AP patients a small but significant percentage of patients (13%)

experience sudden unexpected death, presumably from arrhythmia (Oyama, Sisson, and Lehmkuhl, 2001).

During the first several months following implant, routine electrocardiogram (ECG) examinations are advisable so that improper pacemaker function can be identified and corrected. Many modern pulse generators store their sensing and pacing activity in their resident memory, allowing the examiner to evaluate pacing system behaviors over a long period and thereby facilitate the identification of intermittent pacemaker dysfunction. In cases in which intermittent malfunction is suspected, 24-hour ambulatory ECG (Holter) monitoring can also be performed. Annual or biannual rechecks are advisable to ensure continuation of proper function and to monitor generator battery life.

Most commonly AP is performed in dogs with symptomatic advanced atrioventricular block or sick sinus syndrome. Although the clinical outcome of AP is very favorable, the incidence of complications, both major and minor, is relatively high. In a retrospective study of implantations performed in the early 1990s, 55% of dogs undergoing AP experienced some type of pacemaker-related complication (Oyama et al., 2001). The most commonly reported complication of AP implantation in dogs is dislodgement of the pacing lead from the right ventricle, occurring in 10% of one retrospectively studied canine population. Lead displacement typically results in a loss of sensing and/or pacing. Ventricular tachycardia is sometimes observed if the dislodged lead tip repeatedly impacts the right ventricular endocardium. Lead displacement typically requires a second operative procedure to reposition the lead properly and reestablish normal AP. Other reported AP complications include generator malfunction (6%), infection (5%), and right ventricular perforation by

---

Table 160-1

Common Programmable Parameters of Modern Artificial Pacing Systems

Parameter	Description
VVI Systems	
Pacing mode	Three-to-five letter code indicating chamber(s) paced, chamber(s) sensed, response, and programmability
Lower rate	Rate the pacemaker paces the heart in the absence of native electrical events; slowest rate the pacemaker allows
Pulse width	Duration of the pacemaker discharge in milliseconds
Amplitude	Intensity of the pacemaker discharge in volts
Sensitivity	Ability of the system to detect native electrical activity in the atria or ventricles
Refractory period	Duration of time following a sensed or paced event that all activity is ignored by the pacemaker
DDD Systems*	
Atrioventricular delay	Time duration between a sensed or paced atrial event and the delivery of a ventricular pacing discharge
Tracking rate	Fastest ventricular pacing rate that can be achieved in response to atrial-sensed events
Rate-Responsive Systems*	
Automatic mode switching	Ability of the pacemaker to automatically switch to a nonrate responsive mode if the atrial-sensed events exceed a programmed rate; helps prevent against excessive tachycardia
Upper rate	Fastest rate the ventricles may be paced in response to sensed atrial activity
Slope	The increase in pacing rate above baseline that occurs at different levels of patient activity
Threshold	Level of sensor activation that is needed to increase heart rate
Reaction time	Time allowed from threshold and the baseline heart rate to achievement of the programmed upper rate
Recovery time	Time allowed from the programmed upper rate to the baseline heart rate following cessation of patient activity

*Parameters found in the specific pacing mode in addition to those found in VVI.

the pacing lead (2%). The rate of complications decreases with increasing experience of the implanting veterinarian. It is our opinion that, as the profession has continued to gain experience, the overall rate of complications associated with transvenous pacemaker implantation has declined. Regardless of the propensity for complications, the remarkable improvement of clinical signs achieved by AP causes most owners (80%) to report a high level of satisfaction with the procedure. The long-term results of AP are encouraging, with nearly half of the patients surviving 3 years after implantation. The presence of severe preexisting heart disease and congestive heart failure negatively influences survival.

Although AP using the VVI mode is the most commonly performed procedure, this modality is accompanied by several important drawbacks. By virtue of its programming and placement within a single ventricular chamber, VVI pacing results in (1) a fixed heart rate, which leads to loss of native heart rate control during times of exercise and rest; (2) an abnormal sequence of cardiac depolarization, evidenced by the wide and bizarre morphology of the QRS complex seen on a surface ECG (Fig. 160-1); and (3) loss of coordinated atrial and ventricular contractions (AV synchrony), which reduces cardiac output and raises atrial pressure as the atria intermittently contract against a closed mitral and tricuspid valve (Fig. 160-2). In humans these deficiencies contribute to the development of "pacemaker syndrome" manifested as fatigue, dizziness, weakness, and on occasion congestive heart failure. Resolution of these signs is accomplished through more advanced and increasingly "physiologic" AP modes that use multiple pacing leads, alternate programming algorithms, or specialized single-lead systems.

ADVANCES IN ARTIFICIAL PACING

Rate-Responsive Ventricular Pacing

With conventional VVI pacing the patient's paced heart rate is fixed and does not change in response to the cardiovascular demands of the patient. Rate-responsive pacing (VVIR) uses an activity sensor that attempts to match the paced heart rate with the patient's activity. Most commonly the AP systems possess an accelerometer, minute-ventilation sensor, thermometer, gravitation sensor, and/or QT-interval sensor to detect increased patient activity. Once detected, the pacing rate increases to a programmed upper rate limit. In this way the AP system attempts to better mimic the normal heart rate response to activity and more closely resemble the normal physiologic response to exercise. In addition to the upper and lower rates, the operator can program the slope at which the heart rate increases and the activity threshold required to trigger the activity sensors (Fig. 160-3). In humans VVIR pacing improves exercise tolerance and alleviates signs of pacemaker syndrome as compared to VVI pacing. In veterinary medicine patients most likely to benefit from rate-responsive pacing are those with markedly disparate heart rates at rest and during activity. Dogs with a particularly active lifestyle and requirement for exercise are most likely to benefit from rate-responsive pacing systems.

Dual-Lead Dual-Chamber Pacing

Dual-lead dual-chamber pacing (DDD, DDDR) uses a second pacing lead positioned within the right auricular

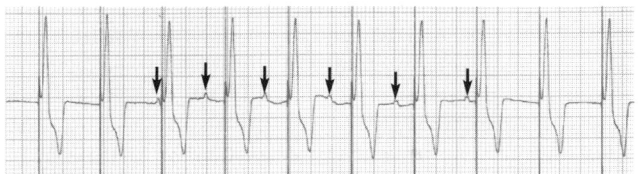

Fig. 160-2 Lead II ECG from a dog with a single-chamber pacemaker in VVI mode (50 mm/sec). Note that the patient's native P waves *(arrows)* and paced QRS complexes are independent of each other and not synchronized. Occasionally the P wave becomes superimposed on the QRS complex or T wave and is not visible. The resultant loss of atrial contribution to cardiac output and contraction of the atria against a closed atrioventricular valve can lead to weakness, dyspnea, and heart failure, which are components of the so-called *pacemaker syndrome.*

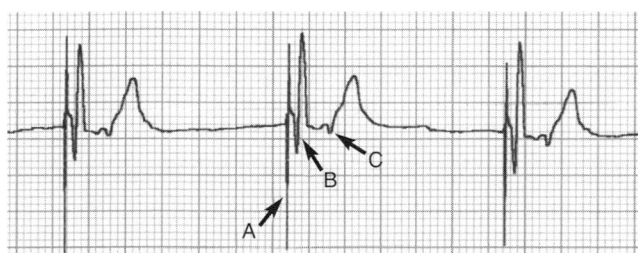

Fig. 160-1 Lead II electrocardiogram from a dog with a single-chamber pacemaker in VVI mode (50 mm/sec). The electrical discharge from the pacing lead **(A)** is immediately followed by a QRS complex representing ventricular depolarization **(B)**. Because of the location of the pacing lead within the right ventricular apex, the sequence of ventricular depolarization is altered and delayed, resulting in a QRS complex and T wave with abnormal morphology. Retrograde conduction of the ventricular impulse across the atrioventricular node and into the atrium is suggested by the biphasic P wave seen in the ST segment **(C)**.

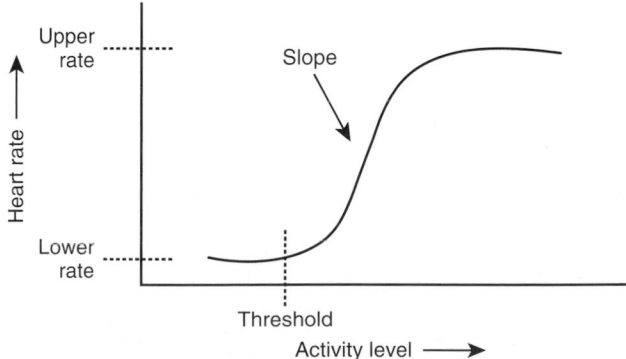

Fig. 160-3 Theoretic heart rate versus activity curve of a rate-responsive pacemaker. As patient activity increases, the pacing system increases heart rate to a maximum programmed upper rate. The rate at which the pacemaker increases the heart rate is represented by the slope of the line. The threshold represents the minimum level of activity that causes the pacing system to begin to increase the heart rate.

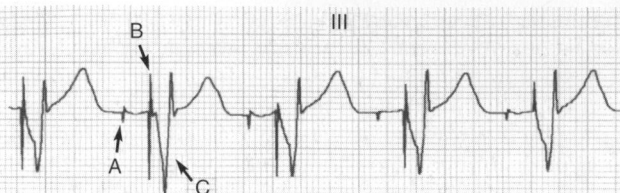

Fig. 160-4 Lead III electrocardiogram from a dog with a dual-chamber pacemaker (50 mm/sec). The atrial pacing lead delivers an electrical stimulus **(A)** followed by discharge of the ventricular pacing lead **(B)**. Dual-chamber pacing preserves synchrony between the atria and ventricles and therefore is more physiologic than single-chamber ventricular pacing.

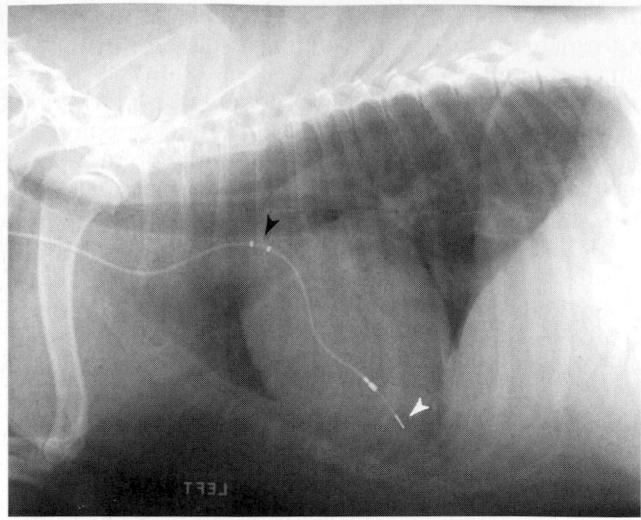

Fig. 160-5 Left lateral thoracic radiograph from a dog implanted with a single-lead VDD pacemaker. The pacing lead can be seen coursing from the cranial vena cava and into the right heart, with the distal tip of the lead positioned within the right ventricular apex *(white arrowhead)*. A set of atrial electrodes is seen positioned within the right atrium *(black arrowhead)*, where they are able to sense atrial electrical activity without having to use a separate atrial pacing lead. (Courtesy Dr. B. Bulmer.)

appendage to sense and pace the atrial chamber. Following atrial depolarization, the DDD system stimulates a timed ventricular depolarization via the lead positioned within the right ventricle (Fig. 160-4). In this way, DDD pacing maintains synchrony between the atrial and ventricular contractions and provides rate responsiveness via sensing the native electrical activity of the right atrium. For these reasons, DDD is the most widely used AP mode in humans. The ideal candidate for DDD pacing is one with advanced atrioventricular block but normal sinus node function. DDD pacing is not ideal in patients suffering from sinus node dysfunction (e.g., sick sinus syndrome) or atrial fibrillation because unregulated detection of rapid atrial depolarizations can lead to excessive ventricular pacing rates (pacemaker-mediated tachycardia). DDD pacing has been described in veterinary patients, but its practice is limited by expense, technical limitations in patients of small size, and complications associated with placement of the atrial lead.

Single-Lead Atrial Synchronous Pacing

Single lead synchronous pacing systems have been developed by including a proximal set of electrodes on the outer surface of the pacing lead that are able to detect atrial electrical activity as it conducts into the blood pool of the right atrial chamber (Fig. 160-5). The atrial electrodes are not in direct contact with the atrial tissue, and atrial depolarizations are "remotely" sensed by the "floating" atrial electrodes. With appropriate programming, detection of an atrial depolarization leads to ventricular pacing after an appropriate interval that is preselected to mimic the normal atrioventricular delay (roughly equivalent to the electrocardiographic PR interval) (Fig. 160-6). This cleverly designed single-lead synchronous VDD system accomplishes the goals of rate responsiveness and maintenance of atrioventricular synchrony without the need for the two pacing leads integral to DDD systems. Ideally this pacing modality is used in patients with advanced atrioventricular block but normal sinus node function. As compared to VVI, VDD pacing is associated with improved hemodynamics and less neurohormonal activation. VDD pacing increases stroke volume and cardiac output and decreases pulmonary capillary wedge pressure, left atrial size, and circulating atrial natriuretic peptide and norepinephrine concentrations in dogs with naturally occurring heart block (Bulmer et al., 2002; Bulmer, 2006).

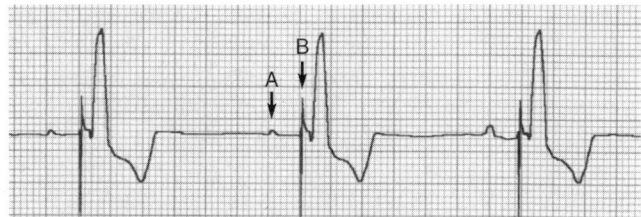

Fig. 160-6 Lead II electrocardiogram from a dog with a single-lead pacemaker in VDD mode. The atrial electrodes detect the patient's native P wave **(A)**; following a programmed delay, the pacemaker delivers a ventricular pacing stimulus **(B)**, resulting in ventricular depolarization. Note that, because the pacemaker senses native atrial depolarization, the VDD mode allows the patient to control its own heart rate and maintain synchrony between the atrial and ventricular contractions.

Temporary Transthoracic Artificial Pacing

Temporary AP is primarily used for emergency heart rate support in symptomatic patients and acts as a bridge to implantation of a permanent pacing system. Conventional temporary AP involves percutaneous placement of a transvenous pacing lead into the jugular vein and right ventricle (see Chapter 8). Because access to the jugular vein is achieved percutaneously, most cases of transvenous temporary pacing can be accomplished with local anesthesia and manual restraint or mild sedation. Although generally well-tolerated, placement of a transvenous temporary lead requires an experienced operator and can result in infection, hemorrhage, arrhythmias, and cardiac perforation. Temporary AP can also be accomplished in dogs via cutaneous electrodes placed on either side of the chest (DeFrancesco et al., 2003). Compared to temporary transvenous pacing, transthoracic pacing is noninvasive and can be instituted more quickly in an emergency. A major drawback of transthoracic pacing is pain associated with the delivery of the electrical impulse, necessitating the use of general anesthesia. For this reason we prefer transvenous temporary pacing in most circumstances.

ASSESSING ARTIFICIAL PACING NEEDS IN INDIVIDUAL PATIENTS

The advantages of rate-responsive pacing are self-evident, assuming that the systems function as intended. Simple exercise challenges can be used to assess the sensitivity and performance of rate-responsive AP systems during patient activity. A prospective study involving seven dogs with VVIR systems found a wide range of responses, depending on pacemaker manufacturer and programmed settings, suggesting that treadmill testing can be used to individualize the rate-response parameters of each patient (Ferasin et al., 2005). The value and need for more sophisticated synchronous AP systems are more difficult to determine in veterinary patients. Evidence of a pacemaker syndrome manifests as mild fatigue, dizziness, headaches, and loss of sense of well-being in humans; these symptoms are more difficult to detect in dogs. Without the ability to measure these correlates to these symptoms objectively, it is particularly challenging to identify the veterinary patients that would benefit from VVIR, DDD, or VDD pacing. Although recent attempts to objectively quantify the effects of AP through the use of exercise testing, neurohormone assay, and hemodynamic study show promise, these methods have not yet been refined for clinical use. Inasmuch as atrioventricular sequential pacing has certain hemodynamic advantages, the use of VDD or DDD AP systems should at least be considered for dogs with preexisting valvular or myocardial disease. Future studies are needed to further assess the physiologic responses to AP and to better identify patients that may benefit from synchronous AP modes.

References and Suggested Reading

Buchanan JW: First pacemaker in a dog: a historical note, *J Vet Intern Med* 17: 2003.

Bulmer BJ et al: Implantation of a single-lead atrioventricular (VDD) pacemaker in a dog with naturally occurring 3rd degree atrioventricular block, *J Vet Intern Med* 16:197, 2002.

Bulmer BJ et al: Physiologic VDD versus non-physiologic VVI pacing in canine third degree atrioventricular block, *J Vet Intern Med* 20:257, 2006.

DeFrancesco TC et al: Noninvasive transthoracic temporary cardiac pacing in dogs, *J Vet Intern Med* 17:663, 2003.

Ferasin L et al: Use of a multi-stage exercise test to assess the responsiveness of rate-adaptive pacemakers in dogs, *J Small Anim Pract* 46:115, 2005.

Johnson MS, Martin MW, Henley W: Results of pacemaker implantation in 104 dogs, *J Small Anim Pract* 48:4, 2007.

Oyama MA, Sisson DD, Lehmkuhl LB: Practices and outcome of artificial cardiac pacing in 154 dogs, *J Vet Intern Med* 15:229, 2001.

Sisson D et al: Permanent transvenous pacemaker implantation in forty dogs, *J Vet Intern Med* 5:322, 1991.

Moise NS: Pacemaker therapy. In Fox PR, Sisson DD, Moise NS, editors: *Textbook of canine and feline cardiology*, ed 2, Philadelphia, 1999, Saunders, p 400.

Moise NS, Estrada A: Noise reversion in paced dogs, *J Vet Cardiol* 4:13, 2002.

Rishniw M, Thomas WP: Bradyarrhythmias. In Bonagura JD, editor: *Current veterinary therapy: small animal practice XIII*, Philadelphia, 1999, Saunders, p 719.

Wess G et al: Applications, complications, and outcomes of transvenous pacemaker implantation in 105 dogs (1997-2002), *J Vet Intern Med* 20:877, 2006.

Zehender M et al: Prevalence, circumstances, mechanisms, and risk stratification of sudden cardiac death in unipolar single-chamber ventricular pacing, *Circulation* 85:596, 1992.

CHAPTER 161

Assessment and Treatment of Supraventricular Tachyarrhythmias

KATHY N. WRIGHT, *Cincinnati, Ohio*

Once considered relatively benign rhythm disturbances, supraventricular tachyarrhythmias (SVTs) are now known to be both a potential cause and a consequence of structural heart disease. SVTs can induce a variety of clinical signs, including weakness, syncope, and even congestive heart failure (CHF). Sustained or frequently recurrent SVTs may lead to tachycardia-induced cardiomyopathy, indistinguishable from idiopathic dilated cardiomyopathy (DCM) but potentially reversible with effective long-term control of the tachyarrhythmia. SVTs have rarely been known to precipitate sudden death if resultant myocardial ischemia leads to ventricular tachycardia, ventricular fibrillation, or electromechanical dissociation or should the antiarrhythmic drug used to treat an SVT exert a lethal proarrhythmic effect. Insights into SVT mechanisms provided by electrophysiologic studies during the past decade and the ability to cure certain SVTs have improved the diagnosis, treatment, and recognition of complications of these common arrhythmias.

DEFINITIONS

SVTs are rapid rhythms either originating in the atria or using the atria or atrioventricular (AV) junction above the bundle of His as a crucial component of the tachycardia circuit. The term *paroxysmal atrial tachycardia* was used generically by some cardiologists to mean SVT. This general term has become outdated as we learn the multiple mechanisms that are responsible for SVTs. One useful classification scheme with diagnostic and therapeutic applications broadly divides SVTs into atrial or junctional tachyarrhythmias (Wathen et al., 1993). Atrial tachyarrhythmias are SVTs using atrial tissue alone for initiation and maintenance of the arrhythmia. Examples include automatic atrial tachycardia, atrial flutter, and atrial fibrillation. Junctional tachyarrhythmias are SVTs that require the AV junction as an essential component of the initiation or maintenance of the tachycardia; the atrium may or may not be needed. Physiologic sinus tachycardia is in a unique class by itself, not included as a form of SVT.

ASSESSMENT OF SUPRAVENTRICULAR TACHYARRHYTHMIAS

Clues From the History and Physical Examination

History and signalment can provide useful initial information in determining the mechanism of SVTs. The physical examination should include careful evaluation for underlying structural heart disease and heart failure. A clinician should strongly suspect the presence of an accessory AV pathway and AV reciprocating tachycardia or automatic atrial tachycardia in young to middle-aged animals that present with rapid, narrow QRS complex tachycardia without apparent structural heart disease. Based on what is known about humans with similar clinical histories, AV nodal reentrant tachycardia and AV reciprocating tachycardia are the most common SVTs in this group. Animals with DCM and SVT may have SVT resulting from DCM, or, more commonly than previously recognized, DCM resulting from sustained SVT. Often reassessment of the structural heart disease after weeks to months of strict arrhythmia control is the only reasonable means of determining which disease process came first. If the structural heart disease involves primarily atrial dilation, intraatrial reentrant tachycardia, automatic atrial tachycardia, atrial flutter, and atrial fibrillation should be carefully considered.

Surface Electrocardiographic Features

A logical, mechanistic-based approach to the surface electrocardiogram is necessary when one evaluates SVTs. SVTs characteristically exhibit narrow QRS complexes. However, in rare cases a bundle branch block (preexistent or tachycardia-dependent) or conduction from atria to ventricles over an accessory AV pathway produces a wide QRS complex tachyarrhythmia that is supraventricular in origin. However, it is emphasized that the vast majority of tachyarrhythmias with wide QRS complexes are ventricular tachyarrhythmias, not aberrantly conducted SVTs.

Once narrow QRS complexes occurring at a rapid rate have been identified, one must decide whether the QRS complexes occur in a regular, regularly irregular, or irregularly irregular pattern. Atrial fibrillation is classically irregularly irregular. Other commonly encountered SVTs have regular patterns, although atrial tachycardias and atrial flutter may be conducted irregularly across the AV node, particularly after administration of a drug that blocks AV conduction. Variable degrees of AV block during an atrial tachyarrhythmia produce irregularity in the occurrence of QRS complexes, but the ventricular response may still have a pattern (i.e., it is regularly irregular). Electrical alternans is not uncommon in dogs with SVTs, and this may help the clinician distinguish the rhythm from a simple sinus tachycardia or a ventricular rhythm disturbance.

Identification of P' waves* or flutter (F) waves is the next important step in assessing the tachyarrhythmia; however, P' or F waves may be very hard to identify during a rapid SVT. This task is made more difficult when one examines only one or two limb leads. Instead, all possible leads should be run at both normal and maximal sensitivities. P' waves are often more easily identified in precordial (chest) leads than in standard limb leads. If an electrocardiograph is not equipped for precordial leads or if P waves remain obscure, the right and left arm (forelimb) electrodes of the standard electrocardiograph can be placed in various positions along the sternal borders of the chest wall (Lewis leads) while monitoring the "lead I" channel to better demonstrate atrial activity. Esophageal leads are also valuable, but lack of patient cooperation limits their use.

The presence or absence of visible P' waves, P' wave morphology, and the relationship of a P' wave to the preceding QRS complex all are helpful in SVT diagnosis (Fig. 161-1). The absence of visible P' waves during a regular SVT despite use of all of the tactics previously discussed is suggestive of typical AV nodal reentrant tachycardia, during which atrial and ventricular activation occur simultaneously. If the P' wave is closer to the preceding QRS complex than to the subsequent QRS complex so that the RP' interval is less than or equal to 50% of the RR interval, the SVT is classified as a short RP' SVT. On the other hand, if the P' wave is closer to the subsequent QRS complex with the RP' interval more than 50% of the RR interval, the SVT is known as a long RP' SVT. Fig. 161-1 and Table 161-1 review the electrocardiographic characteristics and mechanisms of the more common SVTs.

Initiation and termination of the tachyarrhythmia are very important diagnostic features. Sudden onset and offset of SVT without gradual rate acceleration and deceleration, respectively, are most characteristic of reentrant SVTs. Automatic SVTs (i.e., from discrete ectopic foci) typically exhibit a "warm-up" (rate acceleration on initiation) and "cool-down" (rate deceleration before termination) period. If a ventricular premature complex successfully terminates an SVT, it is almost certainly a junctional tachyarrhythmia. In cases of atrial flutter, sudden changes in conduction can lead to halving or doubling of the ventricular rate (e.g., a conduction sequence of flutter waves: QRS complexes changing from 1:1 to 2:1 or from 4:1 to 2:1).

---

*P' waves indicate atrial depolarization that does not originate in the sinoatrial node.

Electrophysiologic Testing

Within the past 20 years in human cardiology, electrophysiologic testing with the use of percutaneously placed multipolar catheters has become commonplace. This valuable tool is available at certain veterinary referral centers and has been an important addition in both the diagnosis and the treatment of particular SVTs. Catheters are advanced to strategic locations in the heart through accessed veins (and occasionally arteries) for pacing and recording. The response of a patient's SVT to programmed electrical stimulation, the sequence of atrial activation, and the location of the His bundle potential during the SVT are used to diagnose its mechanism and map its location.

THERAPY FOR SUPRAVENTRICULAR TACHYARRHYTHMIAS

Acute Management

Division of SVTs into atrial and junctional tachyarrhythmias has important implications for management (Wathen et al., 1993). Junctional tachyarrhythmias may be treated successfully with single-agent therapy directed at any essential component of the circuit. On the other hand, successful management of atrial tachyarrhythmias in terms of gaining both rate and rhythm control requires "dual therapy." One drug is used initially to slow AV nodal conduction; a second drug is used to terminate the atrial tachyarrhythmia itself. The site or sites of antiarrhythmic drug actions are shown in Fig. 161-2.

Vagal maneuvers lasting no more than 5 seconds (ocular pressure, gag reflex, single carotid sinus massage) may be helpful both diagnostically and therapeutically. These maneuvers may increase vagal tone, primarily slowing sinus nodal discharge and prolonging AV nodal conduction time and refractoriness. If an SVT abruptly terminates in response to a vagal maneuver, AV nodal reentrant tachycardia, orthodromic AV reciprocating tachycardia, or sinus nodal reentrant tachycardia is most probable. Unfortunately even SVTs using the sinus or AV nodes as essential circuit components typically fail to terminate with any vagal maneuver. Therefore the lack of response to a vagal maneuver should not be used to rule out an AV nodal–dependent SVT. Rare complications such as ventricular fibrillation may result, particularly from aggressive vagal maneuvers; thus careful electrocardiographic monitoring during the procedure is essential.

Intravenous antiarrhythmic drug therapy may be used to treat a rapid SVT causing hemodynamic compromise and often results in a "revealing" of the underlying mechanism. Hemodynamic (blood pressure) and electrocardiographic monitoring are important whenever one treats SVTs with intravenous agents. Diltiazem (Cardizem, Hoechst Marion Roussel; 0.125 to 0.35 mg/kg intravenously [IV]) comes in a parenteral formulation and is used widely in both human and small animal patients. Diltiazem rapidly slows AV nodal conduction and prolongs AV nodal refractoriness, making it ideal for slowing the ventricular response to rapid atrial tachyarrhythmias and for terminating junctional tachyarrhythmias (except for automatic junctional tachycardia). In cases of intraatrial tachycardia or atrial

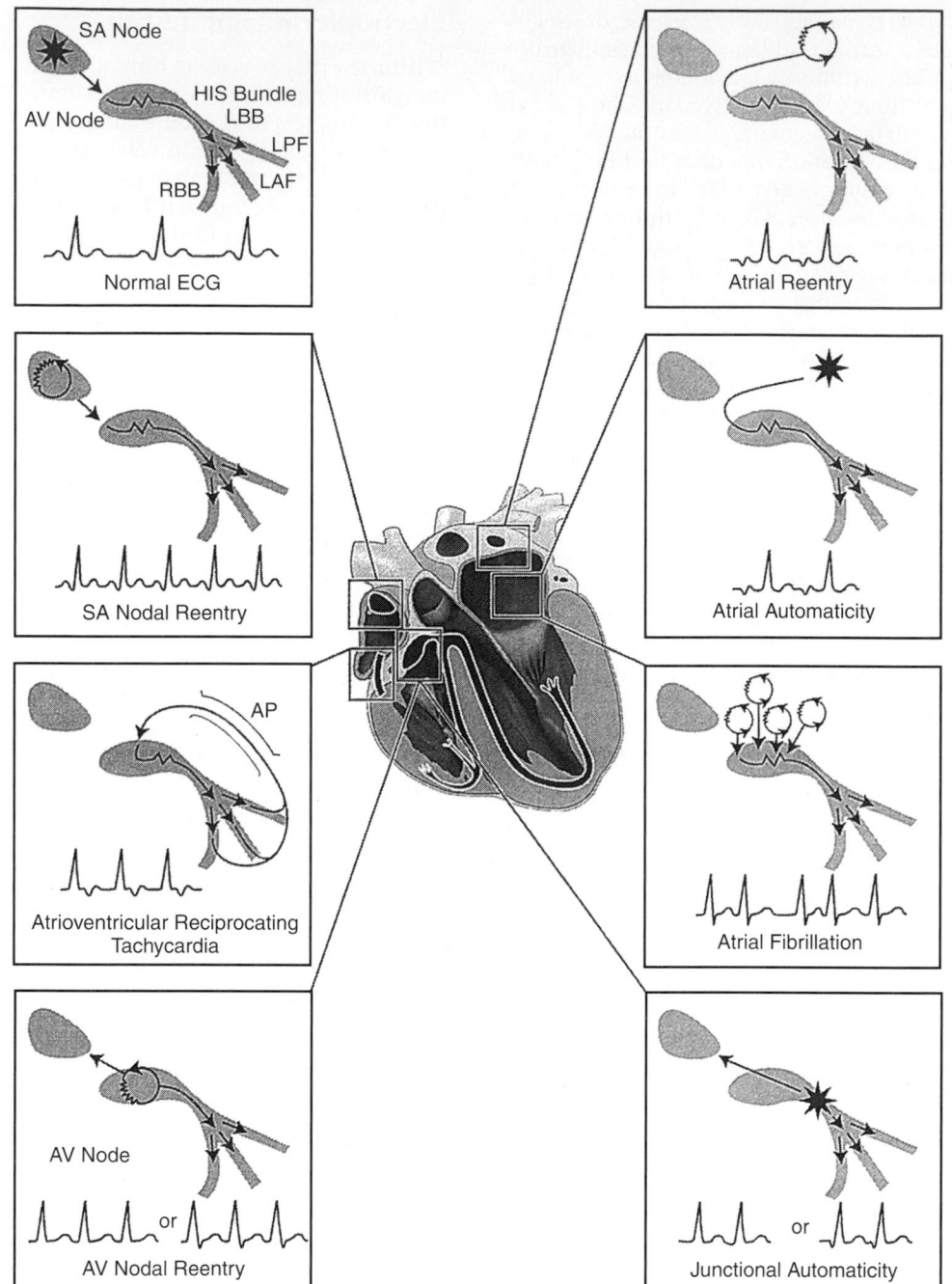

Fig. 161-1   Illustration of the mechanisms and characteristic electrocardiographic features of the most common supraventricular tachyarrhythmias. *AP,* Accessory pathway; *AV,* atrioventricular; *ECG,* electrocardiogram; *LAF,* left anterior fascicle; *LBB,* left bundle branch; *LPF,* left posterior fascicle; *RBB,* right bundle branch; *SA,* sinoatrial.

flutter, the consequences of diltiazem therapy are mainly on rate control, although occasionally there is conversion to sinus rhythm. The value of AV nodal block is not only therapeutic but also diagnostic since junctional reentrant tachyarrhythmias should not be associated with independent (blocked) P' or F-waves; conversely these are often observed following diltiazem in cases of intraatrial tachycardia or atrial flutter. Since diltiazem causes negative inotropic effects, cautious use is called for in the setting of left ventricular dysfunction. However, human clinical studies support its effective and safe use in patients with class III

and IV heart failure and rapid SVTs (Heywood et al., 1991; Goldenberg et al., 1994). I have used intravenous diltiazem in dogs with DCM and in dogs with severe tachycardia-induced cardiomyopathy secondary to an incessant SVT that present with rapid, hemodynamically compromising SVT (often atrial fibrillation) after initial treatment with parenteral furosemide if CHF is present. Diltiazem is as effective and appears to have far fewer adverse effects than parenteral verapamil.

Adenosine (Adenocard, Fujisawa USA) is another parenteral antiarrhythmic drug that slows AV nodal conduction

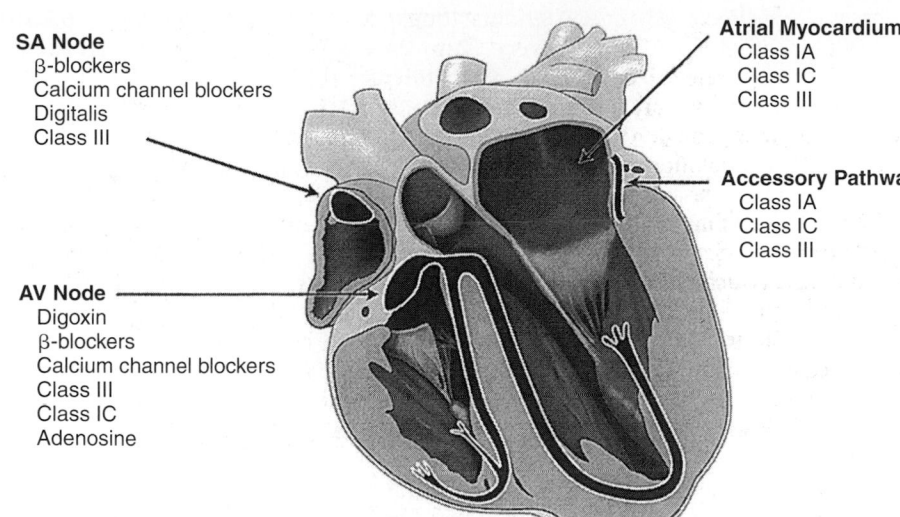

SA Node
β-blockers
Calcium channel blockers
Digitalis
Class III

AV Node
Digoxin
β-blockers
Calcium channel blockers
Class III
Class IC
Adenosine

Atrial Myocardium
Class IA
Class IC
Class III

Accessory Pathway
Class IA
Class IC
Class III

Fig. 161-2 Sites of action of anti-arrhythmic drugs, highlighting their use for specific supraventricular tachyarrhythmias. *SA,* Sinoatrial; *AV,* atrioventricular.

Table 161-1

Typical Electrocardiographic Characteristics of Supraventricular Tachyarrhythmias

SVT Mechanism	Visible P′ Waves	P′ Wave Morphology	RP′ Interval (vs. RR Interval)	Initiation/Termination	Response to AVB
Atrial					
SNRT	Yes	Same as sinus P	Long	Abrupt onset/offset at SVT rate	SVT continues
AAT	Yes	Variable, differs from sinus P	Often long, but varies with SVT rate	Gradual rate/acceleration	SVT continues
IART	Yes	Variable, differs from sinus P	Often long, but varies with SVT rate	Abrupt onset/offset at SVT rate	SVT continues
Atrial flutter	Flutter (F) waves	Identical saw-toothed F waves	Not applicable	Abrupt onset/offset at SVT rate	SVT continues
Atrial fibrillation	No; fibrillation (f) waves may be seen	Not seen	Not applicable	Abrupt onset/offset at SVT rate (often incessant)	SVT continues
Junctional					
Common AV nodal reentrant tachycardia	Generally no; may be seen as pseudo-S wave in II, III, aVF	Retrograde (if seen): (–) in II, III, aVF	Short	Abrupt onset/offset at SVT rate; critical PR prolongation to initiate	SVT terminates
OAVRT	Yes; within the ST-T segment	Retrograde: (–) in II, III, aVF	Typically short	Abrupt onset/offset	SVT terminates
AJT	Generally yes; AV dissociation common	Variable	Variable	Gradual rate acceleration/deceleration	SVT continues with AV dissociation

AAT, Automatic atrial tachycardia; *AJT,* automatic junctional tachycardia; *AV,* atrioventricular; *AVB,* atrioventricular block; *IART,* intraatrial reentrant tachycardia; *OAVRT,* orthodontic atrioventricular reciprocating tachycardia; *SNRT,* sinus nodal reentrant tachycardia; *SVT,* supraventricular tachyarrhythmia.

in humans. It must be administered as a rapid intravenous bolus, ideally through a central vein. Although adenosine is the drug of choice in humans for terminating a wide complex SVT and distinguishing this tachyarrhythmia from ventricular tachycardia, this agent has not been effective in dogs. Adenosine doses up to 2 mg/kg do not slow AV nodal conduction in dogs. In a small number of cases that I have treated, rapid doses of 0.5 mg/kg

intravenously have failed to terminate junctional SVTs, which would consistently terminate in a person at one third of that dosage.

An ultrashort-acting, selective β$_1$-blocker, esmolol (Brevibloc, Ohmeda), at 0.5 mg/kg intravenously over 1 minute has been used to slow AV nodal conduction and interrupt certain SVTs. Because its half-life is so brief compared to the longer-acting intravenous propranolol, esmolol is the preferred parenteral β-blocker because adverse effects such as negative inotropy are also short-lived. Nonetheless it should be used cautiously in animals with ventricular dysfunction. Esmolol appears less effective than parenteral diltiazem in terminating canine junctional SVTs and has become my second choice of intravenous AV nodal–blocking drugs. Both diltiazem and esmolol can be used in cats.

Procainamide is a class IA antiarrhythmic available in a parenteral formulation (Pronestyl, Elkins-Sinn) that prolongs the refractory periods of atrial and ventricular myocardium, retrograde AV nodal pathways, and accessory AV pathways. Dosages of 6 to 8 mg/kg intravenously over 3 minutes or 6 to 20 mg/kg intramuscularly have been successful in terminating or "converting" atrial tachyarrhythmias (after drugs to slow AV nodal conduction have been administered). When given immediately after induction of atrial fibrillation or flutter in dogs with "lone" atrial fibrillation, parenteral procainamide may be effective in converting the rhythm to sinus. This drug also has efficacy in acute and chronic management of AV reciprocating tachycardia in dogs. There is far less experience with parenteral procainamide in cats; however, I have used it cautiously and at a reduced dosage (1 to 3 mg/kg IV over 3 to 5 minutes). The adverse effects include hypotension with rapid intravenous administration and gastrointestinal upset. Myocardial contractility is minimally impaired except at higher doses (although the drug can cause vasodilation); therefore procainamide can be used in animals with left ventricular dysfunction.

Lidocaine generally is used for control of ventricular arrhythmias but has some efficacy in the treatment of atrial fibrillation of acute onset in dogs. The role of lidocaine generally is reserved for dogs in which the induction of the atrial arrhythmia is witnessed and the mechanism is related to elevated vagal tone.

Chronic Antiarrhythmic Drug Therapy

Chronic antiarrhythmic drug therapy for atrial tachyarrhythmias may involve dual therapy to control ventricular rate response and suppress the rhythm disturbance (see Acute Management Therapy for SVTs earlier in the chapter) or combination therapy to simply slow the ventricular response rate. This latter approach is often taken in dogs or cats with *persistent atrial fibrillation* and *severe structural heart disease*.

The canine patient with an atrial tachyarrhythmia and CHF is placed on digoxin (Lanoxin, Glaxo Wellcome; Cardoxin, Evsco Pharmaceuticals) at 0.005 to 0.01 mg/kg orally every 12 hours (dogs). In cats a lower dosage of 0.0312 mg orally every 24 to 48 hours is used. Digoxin represents the initial AV nodal–blocking drug in small animal patients with atrial fibrillation and CHF, except for the cat with hypertrophic cardiomyopathy and atrial tachyarrhythmias in which atenolol or diltiazem are considered the drugs of choice. Generally the ventricular response rate to atrial fibrillation is slowed insufficiently with digoxin monotherapy.

Adding a *second* AV nodal–blocking agent to digoxin generally produces the targeted ventricular response. The choice is between an oral calcium channel blocker and a β-blocker. There are theoretic reasons for supporting either choice. I prefer diltiazem at 0.5 to 1.5 mg/kg orally

every 8 hours (dogs) and atenolol typically at 6.25 mg orally every 12 to 24 hours (cats). Dogs in CHF subjectively appear to tolerate diltiazem better than the dose of β-blocker required to achieve ventricular rate control. The vasodilator properties of calcium channel blockers may partially offset their negative inotropic effects in the failing heart (Falk, 1996). Also, in a small percentage of cases diltiazem has converted an atrial tachyarrhythmia (presumed to be caused by triggered activity) to sinus rhythm. If inadequate heart rate control is achieved with digoxin and diltiazem, a small dose of atenolol or another β-blocker can be added to the antiarrhythmic regimen. Since many of the dogs are also in CHF, it is likely that a β-blocker (such as carvedilol) may later be prescribed for cardioprotection once CHF is stabilized. This type of triple therapy often results in good ventricular rate control.

Oral procainamide (Pronestyl, 10 to 20 mg/kg orally [PO] q4 to 6h [dogs] and 3 to 8 mg/kg PO every 6 to 8 hours [cats] has been used as one agent in dual-therapy regimens to suppress or convert atrial tachyarrhythmias and as single-agent therapy for treatment of junctional tachyarrhythmias. Higher dosages (up to 40 mg/kg PO q6h) have been required for controlling junctional SVTs in some dogs. Gastrointestinal side effects and proarrhythmic concerns (particularly in animals with structural heart disease) are the major factors limiting chronic procainamide use in small animals.

Sotalol (Betapace, Berlex Laboratories, 1 to 2 mg/kg PO q12h) is proving to be effective in both dogs and cats with certain SVTs. Sotalol combines both nonspecific β-blockade with class III antiarrhythmic activity (which prolongs repolarization). Because of this dual activity, sotalol can be used as a single agent in atrial or junctional tachyarrhythmias. Its negative inotropic effects are partially offset by the increased time for calcium entry (Antonaccio and Gomoll, 1990).

Other antiarrhythmic drugs currently under investigation for management of atrial and junctional SVTs in dogs include amiodarone (Cordarone, Wyeth-Ayerst) with the widest spectrum of antiarrhythmic actions and propafenone (Rhythmol, Reliant Pharmaceuticals). Clinicians should consult with a cardiac specialist before using these long-term for control of SVTs.

Nonpharmacologic Therapy

A few veterinary referral centers offer the possibility of curing rather than simply controlling certain SVTs. Transvenous catheter ablation with the use of radiofrequency energy has revolutionized the treatment of SVTs in humans. This procedure follows the mapping of an SVT circuit using multiple electrode catheters. A specialized catheter with a 4- to 5-mm distal-tip electrode is positioned at a critical site within the circuit; and radiofrequency energy is delivered through the distal electrode, causing thermal destruction of a small volume of tissue sufficient to cause interruption of the tachyarrhythmia. This technique has been used with great success in humans, and I have used it in over 40 canine cases.

Management of atrial fibrillation in dogs typically involves simple rate control. However, some centers use synchronized, biphasic cardioversion for rhythm control back to sinus rhythm. This approach is discussed more fully in Chapter 164.

References and Suggested Reading

Antonaccio MJ, Gomoll A: Pharmacology, pharmacodynamics, and pharmacokinetics of sotalol, *Am J Cardiol* 65:12A, 1990.

Chakko S, Kessler KM: Recognition and management of cardiac arrhythmias, *Curr Probl Cardiol* 6:59, 1995.

Falk RH: Pharmacologic control of heart rate in atrial fibrillation, *Cardiol Clin* 14:521, 1996.

Goldenberg IF et al: Intravenous diltiazem for the treatment of patients with atrial fibrillation or flutter and moderate-to-severe congestive heart failure, *Am J Cardiol* 74:884, 1994.

Heywood JT et al: Effects of intravenous diltiazem on rapid atrial fibrillation accompanied by congestive heart failure, *Am J Cardiol* 67:1150, 1991.

Santilli RA et al: Anatomic distribution and electrophysiologic properties of accessory atrioventricular pathways in dogs, *J Am Vet Med Assoc* 231:393, 2007.

Wathen MS et al: Classification and terminology of supraventricular tachycardia, *Cardiol Clin* 11:109, 1993.

Wright KN: Wolff-Parkinson-White syndrome. In Cote E, editor: *Vet Clin Adv,* Philadelphia, 2006, Elsevier, p 1166.

Wright KN: When, why, and how to perform cardiac radiofrequency catheter ablation, *J Vet Cardiol* 8: 95, 2006.

Wright KN: Interventional catheterization for tachyarrhythmias. In Abbott J, editor: *Veterinary clinics of North America: small animal practice,* Philadelphia, 2004, Elsevier, p 117.

Miller JM, Zipes DP: Therapy for cardiac arrhythmias. In Zipes DP et al,editors: *Heart disease: a textbook of cardiovascular medicine,* Philadelphia, 2005, Elsevier, p 713.

Olgin JE, Zipes DP: Specific arrhythmias: diagnosis and treatment. In Zipes DP et al, editors: *Heart disease: a textbook of cardiovascular medicine,* Philadelphia, 2005, Elsevier, p 803.

CHAPTER **162**

Ventricular Arrhythmias in Dogs

N. SYDNEY MOÏSE, *Ithaca, New York*
ANNA R.M. GELZER, *Ithaca, New York*
MARC S. KRAUS, *Ithaca, New York*

The treatment of ventricular arrhythmias (VAs) has dramatically changed over the last 30 years in human medicine. Reading this literature and more critically evaluating our standard of care in dogs also has altered our approach to the management of VAs. Decades ago recommendations for the treatment of VAs revolved around the number of premature complexes identified by routine electrocardiography, but today treatment is reserved for VAs that are judged to be truly dangerous. Furthermore, the success or failure of long-term treatment is more critically studied by 24-hour ambulatory electrocardiograph (ECG) monitoring (Holter monitoring). In this chapter the following topics are addressed in practical terms and in light of the medications most available to practitioners:

1. When should VAs be treated?
2. What are the most common diseases or circumstances that demand treatment?
3. What determines route of administration, and what medications should be selected?
4. How should the VA be monitored during therapy?

WHEN VENTRICULAR ARRHYTHMIAS SHOULD BE TREATED

VAs should be treated when they result in clinical signs or tachycardiomyopathy or harbor the risk of death. Hemodynamic consequences of VAs that cause clinical signs are related to hypotension. Sustained hypotension causes weakness, lethargy, exercise intolerance, and, if severe and prolonged, syncope. The development of low systemic blood pressure that persists long enough to result in clinical signs is primarily related to ventricular tachycardia (VT) that is rapid and prolonged (sustained) and not to single ventricular premature complexes. It is possible that the latter can lead to R-on-T phenomenon (i.e., when such beats fall within the vulnerable period of the T wave). Although such timing of a premature complex can induce ventricular fibrillation (VF), how frequently this occurs in the dog has not been ascertained. Thus the criterion to define the R-on-T interval that requires treatment in the dog is unknown. Polymorphic VAs also traditionally have been viewed as more ominous than monomorphic VAs; however, this is not necessarily true. Boxers with arrhythmogenic right ventricular cardiomyopathy (ARVC) have monomorphic VT 85% of the time, and their risk of sudden death is high. Older dogs with mitral regurgitation can have single ventricular premature complexes that are polymorphic and for which the frequency of sudden death is low. In contrast, Doberman pinschers with dilated cardiomyopathy (DCM) do have polymorphic VT and a high incidence of sudden death. Therefore the assessment of risk depends on the incorporation of multiple factors for each patient. It should be emphasized in this appraisal that underlying cardiac disease must be considered in addition to the type of VA present. Animals can tolerate sustained and rapid VT for more prolonged periods if they have adequate myocardial function and are capable of compensating (e.g., baroreceptor reflex) for the VT. Therefore, when there is underlying myocardial failure (e.g., DCM, ARVC, substantial AV valve regurgitation) or anesthetic depression of heart function, the need to suppress the VT is more important. However, because of additional physiologic issues such as renal perfusion and concurrent drug medication, treatment is also more challenging. It is important to note that, when a tachyarrhythmia persists, both structural and electrical remodeling can develop. These are detrimental electrically and can induce myocardial failure. This has been shown both experimentally and clinically in the dog (i.e., a dog that initially only has a tachyarrhythmia will develop myocardial failure if the rapid rate is not controlled). The myocardial failure can be permanent if the arrhythmia persists for a number of weeks or even days if the rate is very fast. Thus one of the major determinants of risk and need to treat rests in the rate of the arrhythmia. The faster and more sustained the VA, the more aggressive the treatment must be.

DISEASES AND CIRCUMSTANCES THAT DEMAND TREATMENT

By examining the natural history of a disease or the circumstances that are associated with VA, those that most often result in clinical signs or sudden death can be identified. Likely the two most common diseases that demand treatment for VT are ARVC in boxers and DCM in Doberman pinschers (and other afflicted breeds). Another breed with sudden death related to VT is the German shepherd. The other most common circumstances that cause VT are traumatic myocarditis, myocarditis, gastric torsion/volvulus, and splenic disease.

The VT identified in boxers is most frequently rapid (rates exceed 250 beats/min); monomorphic; and of a left bundle branch block pattern with an upright orientation in leads II and III and a VF. Holter recordings have documented that often the VT that causes clinical signs occurs when dogs are excited or exercising. The latter circum-

stances, which are associated with increases in sympathetic tone, are often the triggers for the VT. Controlling the triggers of arrhythmias can be as important in treatment as therapy to disrupt the substrate or mechanism of the arrhythmia. The mechanism of the VT in boxers is unknown. However, the origin of the VT, based on the morphology and the location of the pathology, is from the right ventricle. Recent studies raise the question of disruption of the intercalated disk proteins in affected boxers that could be an arrhythmogenic substrate (Oxford et al., 2007). Boxers with polymorphic VA often have heart failure, although it is common to observe rapid monomorphic VT in boxers with syncope alone (Kraus et al., 2002). In addition, Holter recordings of syncopal boxers have shown that, in addition to the VT, some dogs have sinus pauses of greater than 8 seconds that are responsible for the clinical signs. (This may represent a neurally mediated bradycardia as part of a neurocardiogenic reflex-mediated syncope). Thus treatment must be tailored to both arrhythmias. Studies are not available to prove that treatment of the VT in boxers actually decreases the risk of death, although some work does support the use of certain drugs for the antiarrhythmic effect. A drug may decrease the frequency of an arrhythmia, but this does not ensure that it will prevent sudden death.

Doberman pinschers with VA demanding treatment almost always have concurrent severe myocardial failure as a result of DCM. This is in contrast to the boxer, in which the echocardiogram often is normal. The polymorphic VT documented in Doberman pinschers may not be the cause of death since bradyarrhythmias have also been documented as another fatal rhythm. Because these dogs are usually on numerous medications and their hemodynamic status is more fragile, the negative inotropic effect of the antiarrhythmic drug must be considered. Most ventricular arrhythmias are affected markedly by elevations in sympathetic tone and circulating catecholamines; thus antiarrhythmics are often combined with β-adrenergic blockers (e.g., mexiletine plus atenolol) or adrenergic blockade as a component of the specific prescribed drug (sotalol, amiodarone). In the Doberman pinscher with DCM, titrating the dosage to have an appropriate antiarrhythmic effect with the least negative inotropic consequence is difficult. In general the comments here apply to other breeds afflicted with DCM.

In the German shepherd, an inherited (major gene is dominant) disease resulting in VA has been characterized by a rapid (>300 beats/min) polymorphic VT with occasional monomorphic VT. Myocardial structure and function appear normal as judged by echocardiography. Sudden death occurs in about 15% of affected dogs and in about 50% of dogs affected with more than 10 runs of rapid VT per 24 hours as determined by Holter monitoring. Death occurs usually between 15 and 52 weeks of age, although younger and older dogs have been reported to die. Most frequently, however, if a dog survives beyond 2 years of age, the risk of death is negligible. Triggered activity caused by early and delayed afterdepolarizations is hypothesized to initiate the VT, although the mechanism for sustained VT and deterioration to VF is unknown. The VT does degenerate into VF as the final, fatal rhythm. The autonomic nervous system plays an important role in the generation of the VA and the sudden death. Death is associated with sleep, exercise, and excitement shortly after sleep and with early morning excitement. In addition, VT is induced with certain anesthetics or analgesics (e.g., narcotics) that increased vagal tone, resulting in a slowing of the heart rate and exaggeration of sinus arrhythmia. Narcotics can be used in these dogs as long as the dogs also are given anticholinergics to avoid bradycardia. Although the component of the bradycardia is stressed in these dogs, many of the younger affected German shepherds have VA without a slow sinus rate.

Dogs with supposedly noninherited disorders do develop VAs. Some of the most severe VTs can occur in cases of myocarditis (see Chapter 177). Myocarditis does not mean an infectious process necessarily but inflammation. With the advent of markers of leakage proteins from myocytes such as troponin, the identification of myocarditis is more likely. Such patients can have VT that demands emergency care or rhythms in which oral treatment suffice. Controversy exists with regard to the management of dogs with traumatic myocarditis, gastric torsion and volvulus, and splenic disease. In these cases VAs are common, but rhythms that are potentially fatal develop uncommonly. However, because treatment risk usually is low and the treatment is short term and frequently effective, many clinicians prefer to treat the VT in these situations. However, most of the time treatment for traumatic myocarditis is not necessary unless the rate of the VT is greater than 160 to 180 beats/min or the impact on blood pressure is significant. With these diseases underlying insults are responsible for the arrhythmias, including the sympathetic nervous system, myocardial hypoxia or ischemia, decreased coronary perfusion, elevated circulating cytokines, and electrolyte shifts. Dogs with splenic masses often have VAs; these are most often benign and resolve with splenectomy. Of course the list of diseases and circumstances associated with VAs is extensive, but in general these principles are applicable.

DETERMINANTS OF ROUTE, MEDICATION, AND TREATMENT DOSAGE

At first it may seem obvious how one determines if intravenous medication is required; however, this is not always true because the wishes of the owner may not permit hospitalization. Dogs with VT and severe systemic hypotension leading them to a moribund, weak, or repeatedly collapsing state require intravenous treatment with the goal of conversion to sinus rhythm or slowing of the ectopic rate. Sometimes dogs in distress may be cardioverted if synchronization with the R wave is possible to avoid shocking on the T wave (see Chapter 164). Regardless of the type of VT or underlying disease or mechanism, lidocaine is the most common drug given intravenously for the treatment of VT in dogs today. The most common sequence of events is to administer one or several boluses of lidocaine at 1 to 2 mg/kg intravenously and follow this with a constant-rate infusion (CRI) of lidocaine at 40 to 80 mcg/kg/minute. Most frequently CRI dosages approximating 50 to 60 mcg/kg/minute are required to ensure effectiveness. Caution should be used if the total bolus

dosage approaches 6 mg/kg over a 15- to 30-minute period. Toxicity is recognized as twitching or seizures. Because the half-life of lidocaine is short, the side effects dissipate rapidly; but intravenous diazepam might be required. The most common reason for lidocaine toxicity is miscalculation of the dose in terms of decimal point location. Consequently clear written instructions with sample doses for the size of the animal are ideal for checking calculations in the emergency situation. Although lidocaine is the most commonly used drug, some prefer to use procainamide intravenously as a bolus (10 to 15 mg/kg slowly) followed by a CRI (25 to 50 mcg/kg/minute). This drug is uncommonly used orally but still remains as a possible drug for critical VT. Bolus treatment must be delivered with a slower push than lidocaine because more problems can develop with systemic hypotension (although lidocaine doses produce a momentary drop in systemic blood pressure, even in dogs with normal myocardial function).

Because lidocaine has multiple antiarrhythmic mechanisms, it can be effective regardless of disease or circumstance. However, when lidocaine is ineffective, understanding the reasons for failure is important, and alternate medications are needed. Sometimes the reason for a lack of response is that the dose used is too low; thus uptitration is important to eliminate this as an explanation for failure. The antiarrhythmic effects of lidocaine are hindered in the presence of hypokalemia or acid-base imbalance. After these examinations a trial with procainamide is logical. Other drugs can be tried as well, but availability is a major concern. When a drug is selected to treat VT, whether intravenously or orally, and the arrhythmia persists, the diagnosis of the rhythm may be incorrect. Although less frequent, wide QRS supra VT should be considered, as with atrial fibrillation with right bundle branch block. If additional antiarrhythmic drugs are not available for intravenous trial, oral medication and hemodynamic support can be given. Sotalol given orally in such situations has converted dangerous VT in several hours when usual intravenous medications failed. Some clinicians have had success with a slow bolus of amiodarone (5 mg/kg intravenously [IV] over 10 minutes). Finally some VT rhythms are *malignant* and will not terminate or slow. This happens with severe myocarditis, myocardial infarction, or myocardial neoplasia.

Oral medication is used when the VT is not immediately life threatening. The definition of life threatening is determined by both the type of VT and the hemodynamic response of the dog. Some dogs appear undisturbed by a rapid VT, particularly if they have preserved myocardial function and the VT is intermittent. To treat with oral medication usually suffices; however, there are management issues that are critical to knowing the effectiveness of the drug and the dosage selected (see following section). Other dogs may be presented with a history of syncope with the cause suspected to be intermittent VT based on ECG and Holter monitoring. The most commonly used oral drugs given for the treatment of VA are sotalol (2 to 2.5 mg/kg BID), mexiletine (4 to 8 mg/kg TID) combined with atenolol (0.5 to 1 mg/kg BID), or amiodarone. Amiodarone is commonly used in human medicine; however, thus far in the treatment of dogs with VT the published data have emphasized the problems (hepatotoxicity, thyroid dysfunction), with little evidence of effectiveness against the VT. It is vital to comment on the doses given. These are regarded as *usual* and not exact for a particular patient. Antiarrhythmic drugs and adrenergic blockers must be titrated to effect and with the intent to avoid side effects.

MONITORING TREATMENT OF VENTRICULAR ARRHYTHMIAS

When VT is treated in the intensive care situation with constant ECG monitoring, effective intravenous treatment is identified by conversion to a sinus rhythm. Still, critical evaluation is required if the VT occurs in intermittent runs because the "conversion" may occur simply by chance. With the advent of greater digital storage capacity on computers, electronic ECGs that continuously record the electrocardiogram of a critical patient can be evaluated effectively instead of the "by chance" paper recording. Selected electronic ECG systems currently available can store 1 or more hours of data at a time and then be reset. When dogs are treated by the intravenous route, a positive response to bolus therapy should be seen within minutes and maintained during CRI. If such treatment is given and no effect is documented, the medication plan should be reconsidered. After stabilization of the dog with intravenous treatment, transition to oral medication is initiated if deemed necessary. This transition is started with one to three oral medication doses before stopping the CRI. There is a crossover time when either excessive medication may cause side effects or too little permits the arrhythmia to return. It is important to note that, just because a drug is effective intravenously, it does not mean that it will be effective given orally or that a drug with a similar mechanism action will be effective. It is not uncommon to have a dog treated with lidocaine in the intensive care unit and then switched to sotalol orally with positive effect.

To know if a drug is having (1) no effect, (2) an antiarrhythmic effect, or (3) a proarrhythmic effect, Holter monitoring is required. To make this judgment a baseline recording is needed. Most often such a recording can be made for 24 hours, and treatment started immediately after removing the monitor. However, in some dogs the VT may be too dangerous to permit a full 24-hour baseline recording. For these dogs the longest baseline recording that is believed to be safe is performed, and the animal started on medication after this time. Because it is not known if medication will improve the VT, it can be argued that the baseline is as important as the treatment. This is true because some dogs do experience proarrhythmic effects from drugs used as antiarrhythmic medication. Therefore the standard of care for the treatment of VA is:

1. Obtain baseline 24-hour Holter monitor recording in the environment where the medication will be administered (home).
2. Treat with the selected medication and dosage.
3. Recheck 24-hour Holter recording in 7 to 10 days after questioning to ensure compliance.
4. Evaluate for change in frequency or severity of the VA and determine if treatment is successful or not.

If the VA counts and severity are not altered, the dosage of medication is usually increased if possible, and the Holter recording repeated 7 to 10 days later. If the VAs are not suppressed, an alternative or additional medication can be given. When combinations of antiarrhythmic drugs are used (e.g., sotalol plus mexiletine), caution and close monitoring are absolutely needed to avoid side effects.

In some dogs an oral medication that is effective cannot be found. In humans the use of the implantable cardioverter-defibrillator has supplanted many of the drugs in the treatment of VAs. This may be an option for some dogs afflicted with potentially fatal VT such as the boxer or the German shepherd; however, the use of these devices is limited to centers that have the ability to monitor and program them to ensure proper functioning.

In the evaluation of the Holter recordings an important consideration is the definition of an adequate antiarrhythmic response or a proarrhythmic response. Limited studies have been done in dogs, but it is likely that a marked reduction of VA by 75% and VT by 90% is required in an individual dog to state that a true antiarrhythmic effect has occurred. If such strict criteria are not met, the reduction actually may be the result of day-to-day variability. It is also possible for an antiarrhythmic effect to occur only with VT and not with single VAs. We have noted in the treatment of boxers that sotalol in some dogs suppresses the frequency of VT by more than 90%, but the number of single VAs does not change. Moreover, borrowing from human medicine, to say that a proarrhythmic effect has developed, a 10-fold increase in VT must be documented. Consequently, to try and monitor the drug effect on VA without Holter monitoring is ineffective.

Because most dogs undergoing treatment for VT have underlying structural or functional disease, monitoring requires attention to these aspects of cardiac function. Thus additional monitoring with thoracic radiography and echocardiography is common. Moreover, examination of blood chemistry profiles in such cases is warranted. It should be stressed that, if an owner reports any problems that are new after a medication has been started, it is wisest to blame the drug first. Assessment of side effects is important, and only if a critical approach is taken can serious problems be avoided. The most common problems reported are vague and relate to overall well-being in addition to complaints of anorexia. Other complaints reported include twitching, change in behavior, and disorders related to hepatotoxicity.

References and Suggested Reading

Basso C et al: Arrhythmogenic right ventricular cardiomyopathy causing sudden cardiac death in boxer dogs: a new animal model of human disease, *Circulation* 109(9):1180, 2004.

Brourman JD et al: Factors associated with perioperative mortality in dogs with surgically managed gastric dilatation-volvulus: 137 cases (1988-1993), *J Am Vet Med Assoc* 208(11):1855, 1996.

Calvert CA et al: Results of ambulatory electrocardiography in overtly healthy Doberman pinschers with echocardiographic abnormalities, *J Am Vet Med Assoc* 217(9):1328, 2000.

Kittleson MD, Kienle RD: Diagnosis and treatment of arrhythmias. In *Small animal cardiovascular medicine*, St Louis, 1998, Mosby, p 440.

Kraus MS et al: Morphology of ventricular arrhythmias in the boxer described by 12-lead electrocardiography with pace mapping comparison, *J Vet Int Med* 16:153, 2002.

Marino DJ et al: Ventricular arrhythmias in dogs undergoing splenectomy: a prospective study, *Vet Surg* 23(2):101, 1994.

Meurs KM et al: Comparison of the effects of four antiarrhythmic treatments for familial ventricular arrhythmias in boxers, *J Am Vet Med Assoc* 221(4):522, 2002.

Minors SL, O'Grady MR: Resting and dobutamine stress echocardiographic factors associated with the development of occult dilated cardiomyopathy in healthy Doberman pinscher dogs, *J Vet Intern Med* 12(5):369, 1998.

Moise NS: Diagnosis and management of canine arrhythmias. In Fox PR, Sisson D, Moise NS, editors: *Textbook of canine and feline cardiology,* ed 2, Philadelphia, 1999, Saunders, p 331.

Moise NS et al: Diagnosis of inherited ventricular tachycardia in German shepherd dogs, *J Am Vet Med Assoc* 210(3):403, 1997.

Muir WW: Gastric dilatation-volvulus in the dog, with emphasis on cardiac arrhythmias, *J Am Vet Med Assoc* 180(7):739, 1982.

Oxford EM et al: Molecular composition of the intercalated disc in a spontaneous canine animal model of arrhythmogenic right ventricular dysplasia/cardiomyopathy, *Heart Rhythm* 4:1196, 2007.

CHAPTER 163

Feline Cardiac Arrhythmias

ETIENNE CÔTÉ, *Prince Edward Island, Canada*
NEIL K. HARPSTER, *Boston, Massachusetts*

Normal cardiac impulse formation arises within specialized fibers of the sinoatrial (SA) node and when necessary in specialized atrial tissues and parts of the atrioventricular (AV) conduction pathways and His-Purkinje system. Alterations in normal cardiac rhythm, or cardiac arrhythmias, arise as a result of either focal or diffuse primary disorders affecting the heart. Examples include inflammation, infarction, ischemia, infiltration, degeneration, and primary cardiomyopathies. Arrhythmias also may develop secondary to generalized systemic disorders such as hypoxemia, systemic hypertension, hyperkalemia, sympathetic stimulation, hyperthyroidism, or severe anemia.

ETIOLOGY

The mechanisms responsible for cardiac arrhythmias are categorized generally as disorders of impulse formation, disorders of impulse conduction, or combinations of the two (Côté and Ettinger, 2005). Some arrhythmias may be initiated by one mechanism and perpetuated by another. The initiating factor in many arrhythmias involves a reduced resting cell membrane potential.

Because of the small size of domestic cats and their correspondingly small hearts, cats appear to be at reduced risk for the development of cardiac arrhythmias compared to other closely monitored species (dogs, horses, humans). Advanced heart disease may be present before the occurrence or recognition of arrhythmias, given the lifestyle of family pet cats that seem to pace themselves so well and minimize their clinical signs.

Primary cardiac disorders associated with cardiac arrhythmias include congenital cardiac disorders and acquired disorders. Cardiac arrhythmias are uncommon in cats with congenital cardiovascular disease (Harpster, 1987 and 1992) but have been recognized in severe conditions associated with marked cardiomegaly or heart failure. Exceptions include the tachyarrhythmias associated with ventricular preexcitation and conduction abnormalities associated with septal defects.

Most acquired cardiac disorders of cats, if sufficiently severe, can be associated with arrhythmias. The cardiomyopathies (hypertrophic, intermediate/ restrictive/ unclassified, and dilated) have commonly been associated with bradyarrhythmias and tachyarrhythmias. Generally tachyarrhythmias predominate when congestive heart failure (CHF) or aortic thromboembolism (ATE) occurs, whereas bradyarrhythmias are more common in association with episodes of syncope or in patients in cardiogenic or terminal shock (Fox and Harpster, 1999).

In cats hyperthyroidism is a well-documented cause of cardiac arrhythmias, including sinus tachycardia, supraventricular and ventricular premature complexes, or tachycardias; conduction abnormalities are also common, including first-degree AV block, left anterior fascicular block, and both right and left bundle branch block, although cause and effect are not proven and similar arrhythmias are seen in old cats.

Heartworm disease has been associated with cardiac arrhythmias in cats, mainly when cats are showing overt clinical signs caused by heartworm infection or following adulticidal therapy (Tilley, 1992; Harpster 1987; Harpster, 1992; Fox and Harpster, 1999). Ventricular premature complexes (VPCs) and other arrhythmias may occur.

Systemic diseases of noncardiac origin may be associated with cardiac arrhythmias, likely through altering circulatory blood volume, the presence of deleterious circulating levels of toxic substances or electrolytes, or high sympathetic tone (Tilley, 1992; Harpster 1992; Harpster 1987; Fox and Harpster, 1999). Specific recognized causes include reperfusion injury, acute shocklike states, thoracic or abdominal trauma, metabolic acidosis, disorders of the brain and spinal cord, hyperkalemia, hypokalemia, and hypomagnesemia.

Evaluation of the Arrhythmic Cat

Electrocardiographic recording in the cat with suspected cardiovascular disease or arrhythmia should include, minimally, leads I, II, III, aVR, aVL, and aVF, and a precordial lead (e.g., V4, also called CV6LU). Additional precordial leads may provide a clearer diagnosis, especially when motion artifact of the limbs is present or P waves are small.

Events reported by the owner, including episodic ataxia, collapse, vocalizing, syncope, or seizures, may lead the clinician to suspect intermittent arrhythmias. Clients and veterinarians can readily confuse syncope and seizures in cats. If arrhythmias are absent initially, diagnostic studies to differentiate between neurologic and cardiovascular events should be pursued. Ideally this should begin with a 24-hour period of observation in a veterinary critical care facility with continuous electrocardiographic monitoring. Beyond this, when primary neurologic episodes have tentatively been ruled out and/or the cost of additional hospitalization is prohibitive, additional options include Holter or event monitoring.

Electrocardiography is the diagnostic test of choice for cardiac arrhythmias in cats, but an ECG alone does not provide adequate information for identifying causes, selecting treatment, and establishing a prognosis that address the whole patient. Therefore every cat with an arrhythmia requires a complete clinical evaluation.

History

In cats, cardiac arrhythmias occur most commonly in conjunction with primary heart disease. Compared to dogs, cats less commonly have cardiac arrhythmias caused solely by extracardiac disturbances. Therefore the clinical history reflects manifestations of cats with heart disease in general, ranging from none (the arrhythmia is an incidental finding) to evidence of CHF or ATE.

Cardiac arrhythmias usually are found incidentally in cats; overt manifestations caused by arrhythmias are rare. For example, cardiac arrhythmias occur in 20% to 40% of cats with ATE, but syncope is rarely described in these cats (Laste and Harpster, 1995; Smith et al., 2003). Similarly, in 50 cats with atrial fibrillation the arrhythmia was found incidentally in 11 (22%), but no cat had a chief complaint convincingly attributable to arrhythmia

(Côté et al., 2004a). Therefore the presenting complaint of a cat with an arrhythmia generally appears to occur as a result of the underlying heart disorder and not the arrhythmia itself.

Physical Examination

The physical examination of a cat with an arrhythmia involves more than ausculting the heart and palpating the pulse. The examination begins with an initial, hands-off *observation* of respiratory effort, posture (e.g., flaccid neck ventroflexion as is seen with severe hypokalemia), mentation (e.g., extreme anxiety and concurrent dyspnea commonly noted with CHF or ATE), gait (e.g., deficits may be seen with ATE), and body condition (e.g., emaciation with hyperthyroidism). Assessment of *mucous membrane color* may reveal cyanosis with hypoxemia or pallor with hypoperfusion or anemia. Gentle *palpation of the ventral neck* evaluates the thyroid glands in older cats. *Palpation of the cardiac impulse and peripheral pulse* are essential; relevant abnormalities can include bilateral increase in the apex beat (cardiac enlargement), displacement of the apex beat to the right (right ventricular enlargement, apex shift, or mass lesion), a palpable thrill, or presence of a heartbeat without a corresponding pulse (intermittence suggests premature beats, but complete pulselessness suggests embolism or severe hypotension). *Cardiac auscultation*, including auscultation over the sternum in addition to both hemithoraces, reveals the heart rate; presence of a regular rhythm or arrhythmia; and presence or absence of murmurs, a gallop sound, or other abnormal sounds. Sudden pauses may indicate postextrasystolic pauses, AV block, or sinus pause or arrest. *Palpation* of the abdomen and limbs and assessment of the extremities for normal color and warmth are also essential.

Laboratory Testing

Routine laboratory tests consisting of a complete blood count (CBC), serum biochemistry profile, and urinalysis (and serum thyroxine level in cats >6 years old) are indicated as part of the minimum database in every cat with a cardiac arrhythmia. Broadly speaking, these tests seek to identify one of two classes of abnormalities: disturbances that are a clue toward finding the underlying cause of the arrhythmia (e.g., CBC evidence of leukemia in a cat with cardiac lymphoma) or disturbances that may directly alter the rhythm of the heart (e.g., hyperkalemia, hypokalemia, anemia, metabolic acidosis).

Serologic testing for feline leukemia virus (FeLV) and feline immunodeficiency virus (FIV) is warranted as part of the evaluation of any ill cat. However, FeLV- and FIV-associated disease is rarely associated with arrhythmias. Cardiac lymphoma, in association with FeLV or FIV, has been reported sporadically in a small number of cats.

Diagnostic Imaging

Thoracic radiographs are indicated in all cats with a cardiac arrhythmia. Possible abnormalities include findings consistent with heart disease (cardiomegaly; infiltrates suggesting pulmonary edema; pleural effusion) or systemic illness (pleural effusion, infiltrates suggesting pneumonia or metastases). The goals of obtaining radiographs are to guide treatment (e.g., thoracocentesis if large-volume pleural effusion; diuretics if pulmonary edema), to identify further points for testing (e.g., metastases warranting a tumor search), and to contribute to determining the prognosis.

Echocardiography remains the diagnostic test of choice for identifying structural heart disease in cats. An echocardiogram is indicated in every cat with a cardiac arrhythmia, even when there are no historical signs or other physical signs to suggest a cardiac disorder. This is because certain "silent" forms of heart disease such as restrictive/unclassified cardiomyopathy may produce no historical or physical signs other than the arrhythmia (Côté et al., 2004a).

Blood Pressure Measurement

Measurement of the arterial blood pressure, preferably by Doppler flow methodology, is indicated in all cats with cardiac arrhythmias. The normal range for systolic arterial pressure in a calm, unsedated cat is 100 to 170 mm Hg in the clinical setting.

Systemic hypertension may trigger cardiac arrhythmias via ventricular hypertrophy or through a comorbid condition such as hyperthyroidism. An arrhythmic hypertensive patient needs to be evaluated for causes (hyperthyroidism, chronic renal failure, white coat effect) and effects (retinopathy, neurologic deficits) of hypertension.

It is worth noting that arrhythmias other than inappropriate sinus tachycardia do not cause systemic hypertension; the more severe a bradycardia or a tachycardia becomes, the more likely it is to produce *hypo*tension. Systemic hypotension in cats with arrhythmias may be caused by a generalized disorder that predisposes to arrhythmia such as hypovolemia or cardiogenic shock. Alternatively, systemic hypotension may be caused by the arrhythmia itself, since both very high or very low heart rates can compromise cardiac output. An arrhythmic, hypotensive cat also needs to be evaluated for causes of hypotension other than the arrhythmia such as blood loss and profound dehydration.

Arterial blood pressure may be difficult to measure in a patient that is persistently arrhythmic. The solution is to wait until the arrhythmia has subsided (even briefly) to measure the blood pressure during sinus rhythm or at least during a period when the rhythm is fairly regular and at a rate that approaches normal. The gold standard is direct measurement using an intraarterial catheter and pressure transducer, which may be appropriate in critically ill cats but requires special skills and equipment.

CARDIAC ARRHYTHMIAS: DIAGNOSIS AND MANAGEMENT

Very little information has been published regarding the prevalence of cardiac arrhythmias in pet cats. Table 163-1 lists the results of an original retrospective study of abnormal ECGs from 170 consecutive cats with cardiovascular disease admitted to the cardiology service of the Angell Animal Medical Center over a 20-month period.

Table **163-1**

ECG Findings in 170 Consecutive Feline Patients With Recorded Abnormalities over a 20-Month Period

	Number	Percent
I. Cardiac bradyarrhythmias and conduction abnormalities		
A. AV conduction abnormalities (total)	(20)	(11.8)
1. First-degree AV block	10	5.9
2. Second-degree AV block	1	0.6
3. Third-degree AV block	10	5.9
B. IV conduction abnormalities	(82)	(48.2)
1. Left anterior fascicular block	32	18.8
2. Right bundle branch block	15	8.8
3. Left bundle branch block	5	2.9
4. Other IV conduction abnormalities	30	17.5
II. Cardiac tachyarrhythmias		
A. Supraventricular (SV)	(41)	(24.1)
1. Supraventricular premature complexes (SPCs)	26	15.3
2. Paroxysmal SV tachycardia	11	5.9
3. Atrial fibrillation	5	2.9
B. Ventricular (V)		
1. Ventricular premature complexes (VPCs)	(57)	(33.5)
a. Right ventricular origin[a]	19	11.2
b. Left ventricular origin[b]	29	17.1
c. Multiform[c]	9	5.3
2. Ventricular bigeminal rhythm	6	3.5
3. Ventricular triplets[d]	4	2.4
4. Paroxysmal ventricular tachycardia	3	1.8
5. Coupled ventricular premature complexes	7	4.1
C. Both SV and V arrhythmias[e]	17	10.0
III. Other ECG abnormalities		
A. Left ventricular hypertrophy pattern[f]	38	22.4
B. Gigantic P waves[g]	8	4.7

AV, Atrioventricular; *ECG,* electrocardiographic; *IV,* intraventricular.
[a]The characteristic feature of a right ventricle–origin premature complex is a dominant R wave deflection in leads II and CV6LU.
[b]The characteristic feature of left ventricle–origin premature complexes is a dominant S wave deflection in leads II and CV6LU.
[c]ECG recordings with multiform ventricular premature complexes have separate/individual premature complexes with the right ventricle–origin and the left ventricle–origin premature complex characteristics.
[d]A ventricular triplet consists of three consecutive ventricular premature complexes beats in a row.
[e]The 17 cats with both supraventricular and ventricular arrhythmias had an average left atrial:aortic ratio of 2.18 with a range of 1.21 to 3.32.
[f]Left ventricular hypertrophy pattern is characterized by the presence of R waves of 1 mV or greater in both leads II and CV6LU.
[g]Gigantic P waves are characterized by P waves in lead II that are 0.4 mV or greater in amplitude.

Normal sinus rhythm is the normal heart rhythm in resting cats. The heart rate is 110 to 180 beats/min. On ECG (Fig. 163-1) a P wave is followed by a QRS complex and a T wave; the R-R interval is constant, and the P waves; QRS complexes, and T waves maintain the same shape or morphology. In the home environment healthy cats on resting examination have a heart rate

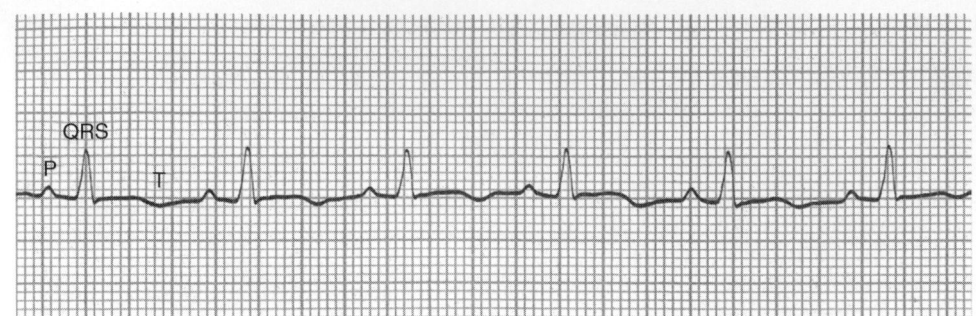

Fig. 163-1 Normal sinus rhythm in a cat. Heart rate = 160 beats/min, 50 mm/sec, 1 cm/mV.

of 118 ± 11 beats/min when examined by veterinary student-owners with a stethoscope (Hamlin, 1989) or a mean rate of 157 ± 3.7 beats/min on 24-hour Holter recordings (Ware, 1999).

Bradyarrhythmias (Bradycardias)

Sinus bradycardia has the same ECG features as normal sinus rhythm, but the heart rate is less than 110 beats/min. Because of the same ambient factors that cause sinus tachycardia, sinus bradycardia in cats in an examination room setting is extremely unusual. At home sinus bradycardia (rates as low as 68 beats/min) occurs routinely in the cat (Ware, 1999). However, in the clinical setting sinus rhythm at a rate less than 140 beats/min is unusual (Côté et al., 2004b) and can be considered to be a relative sinus bradycardia that warrants further diagnostic evaluation. Drugs (β-blockers) and anesthetics can create sinus bradycardia. Systemic disorders, including brain disease, hypothermia, and diseases causing high vagal tone should be a focus of diagnostic evaluation. The triad of shock, hypotension, and hypothermia is also commonly associated with sinus bradycardia in cats.

AV block (heart block) refers to hampered transmission of electrical activity through the AV conduction system. It may occur in one of three degrees of severity: all impulses successfully but slowly cross the AV system (first degree), some impulses cross but not others (second degree), or complete AV block (third degree). *First-degree AV block* is exclusively an ECG finding. It produces a PR interval greater than 0.09 seconds but no clinical or physical signs. Causes include digoxin toxicity, high vagal tone states, and structural heart disease.

Second-degree AV block, an intermittent failure of impulses to cross the AV node, produces P waves not followed by QRS complexes on ECG. Second-degree AV block traditionally is divided into two subtypes. With Mobitz type I or "Wenckebach" conduction through the AV node gradually slows over a few beats until ultimately block occurs. In Mobitz type II, conduction through the AV system has a fixed PR interval until, without forewarning, a P wave is blocked (Fig. 163-2). The occurrence of clinical signs depends on the number of blocked impulses and presence of escape activity. The greater the number of blocked impulses, the slower the resultant ventricular rate; therefore the more likely are overt signs such as syncope, especially if escape complexes do not develop. In the cat second-degree AV block is usually Mobitz type II and is most commonly associated with cardiomyopathy, conduction system degeneration, or the administration of such α-2 agonist drugs as medetomidine. Individual variation and digoxin toxicity are less common causes. Treatment is justified when AV block is causing overt signs such as hypotension or syncope. Except when caused by drugs, medications such as vagolytic drugs (e.g., propantheline) or β-agonists are not consistently beneficial for treating AV block, and treatment generally involves the implantation of a pacemaker.

With *third-degree AV block*, impulses are formed normally in the SA node, travel normally through the atria, and are all blocked in the AV conduction system. The ECG appearance is one of AV dissociation (Fig. 163-3). The atrial rate is faster than the ventricular (escape) rate. Ventricular activity is from an escape rhythm: QRS complexes that are different in shape from normal QRS complexes occur at a regular, slow (60 to 140/minute) rate. Notably the

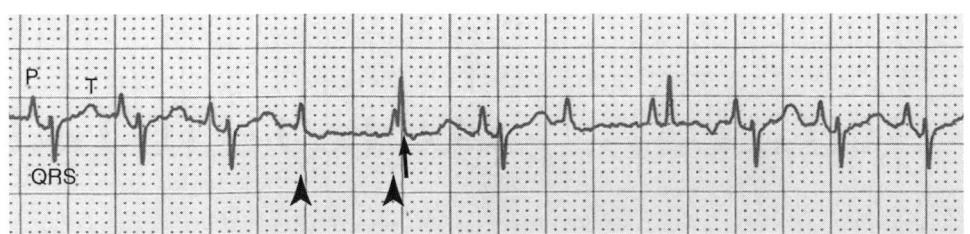

Fig. 163-2   Second-degree atrioventricular (AV) block in a cat—intermittent, Mobitz type II AV block. In this tracing the P waves are positive, and the normal sinus QRS complexes are negative. The fourth P wave is blocked *(first arrowhead)*, without a preceding lengthening of the PR interval. The fifth P wave is also blocked *(second arrowhead)*. Superimposed on the fifth P wave is a QRS complex that appears after a period of ventricular inactivity and is of a different shape than the normal QRS complexes; it is a ventricular escape beat *(arrow)*. The next P wave is conducted normally, but the seventh and eighth are not, and the same type of AV block is again apparent. The eighth P wave is followed by another ventricular escape. 25 mm/sec, 1 cm = 1mV.

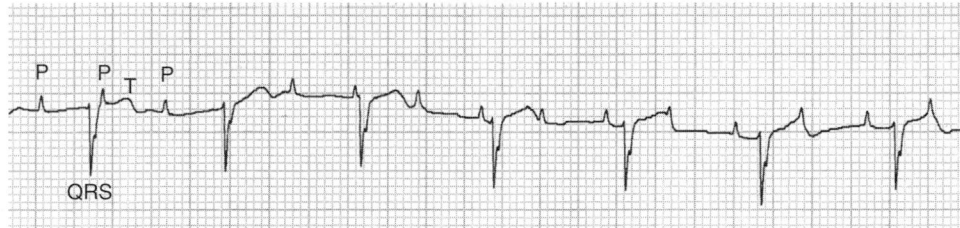

Fig. 163-3 Incidentally discovered third-degree arteriovenous block in a 17-year-old cat with hypertrophic cardiomyopathy. The fourth P wave is not seen because the second ventricular escape beat is superimposed over it. Artifactual undulation of the baseline is present and not clinically significant. Heart rate = 80 beats/min, 25 mm/sec, 1 cm = 1 mV.

escape rhythm is faster in cats than in dogs. Occasionally cats are observed with periods of profound ventricular asystole, which then recovers.

Third-degree AV block occurs almost exclusively in older cats (≥11 years old) and is caused by or associated with cardiomyopathies (Kaneshige et al., 2006). infiltrative heart disease (e.g., lymphoma), other structural heart diseases, or hyperthyroidism. It may occur idiopathically, probably from degeneration. It is generally permanent, although occasionally a cat may revert to second-degree AV block or to sinus rhythm (Kellum and Stepien, 2006). Chief complaints for cats with third-degree AV block include exertional dyspnea, respiratory distress, collapse, or none. Like second-degree AV block, the repercussions of third-degree AV block on a cat depend on stability of the escape activity and the ventricular rate. With low heart rates or erratic escapes, cats are more likely to show overt signs requiring treatment (pacemaker implantation). Such treatment is considered if the ventricular escape rate is constantly slow (<100 beats/min) and/or if the cat shows intermittent signs directly associated with bradycardia or asystole on ECG, Holter, or event monitor. The diagnosis of third-degree AV block in the cat does not in itself warrant treatment because, when the ventricular rate is adequate, there may be no signs, and the prognosis may not be affected. Some cats develop cardiomegaly and mild CHF that may be managed medically.

Atrial standstill (atrial paralysis, silent atria) involves complete absence of detectable atrial electrical activity. On ECG a regular R-R interval, generally with QRS complexes of the same shape and size, and no P waves are seen (Fig. 163-4). The two most common causes in cats are hyperkalemia and atrial myopathy (especially severe atrial stretching caused by primary heart disease). Two steps are essential when atrial standstill is suspected in a cat:

the evaluation of other ECG leads to seek out P waves (that may be isoelectric in one lead) and measurement of the serum potassium concentration to rule out hyperkalemia-induced atrial standstill. If serum potassium is less than 7 mEq/dl, an echocardiogram is warranted to evaluate the structure of the heart. Unlike dogs and humans, cats with severe hyperkalemia and atrial standstill do not necessarily have bradycardia, and heart rates as high as 240 beats/min are routinely present in cats despite severe hyperkalemia. Cats with hyperkalemia-induced atrial standstill require treatment of the underlying disorder as well as hyperkalemia. Although the optimal treatment is controversial, we use calcium gluconate (10% solution; 0.5 to 1.5 ml/kg infused slowly intravenously [IV] and discontinued if the heart rate decreases or the QRS complexes widen). Other possible treatments include sodium bicarbonate (1 to 2 mEq/kg very slow IV bolus) or the combination of regular insulin 0.25 to 0.5 units/kg IV with 2 g/kg of dextrose (= 4 ml/kg of 50% dextrose, preferably diluted before administration). Cats with normokalemia and atrial standstill require treatment specific to the form of underlying heart disease. Some cats in cardiogenic shock with apparent atrial standstill redevelop P waves with successful therapy.

Tachyarrhythmias (Tachycardias)

Tachyarrhythmias indicate a rapid heartbeat. In cats the suspicion of a pathologic tachyarrhythmia should be considered when the heart rate consistently approaches or exceeds 240 beats/min or when irregularities in the cardiac rhythm are noted. *Sinus tachycardia* (Fig. 163-5) has the same ECG features as normal sinus rhythm, but the heart rate is higher than 180 beats/min. The PR interval is normal (0.04 to 0.09 seconds) and is inversely proportional to heart rate. The significance of sinus tachycardia in the cat is highly variable. Most cats brought into a veterinary environment have sinus tachycardia even when healthy. The median heart rate on auscultation of 89 healthy cats in hospital was 180 beats/min (range: 140 to 260) (Côté et al., 2004b). The heart rate of 27 healthy cats undergoing an in-hospital ECG was 182 ±20 beats/min (Hamlin, 1989). Therefore sinus tachycardia is considered normal for a cat in a veterinary setting. However, sinus tachycardia also may occur in pathologic states. Anemia, hypotension, hyperthyroidism, sepsis, fever, pain, and other systemic disorders cause sinus tachycardia. Therefore the finding of sinus tachycardia must be placed in context. Sinus tachycardia does

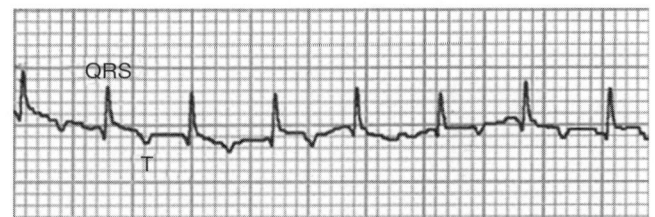

Fig. 163-4 Atrial standstill in a cat with hyperkalemia caused by urethral obstruction. Serum K^+ = 7.1 mEq/L. No P waves are seen, nor were they present in any other ECG lead. The heart rate is 205 beats/min. 25 mm/sec, 1 cm = 1 mV.

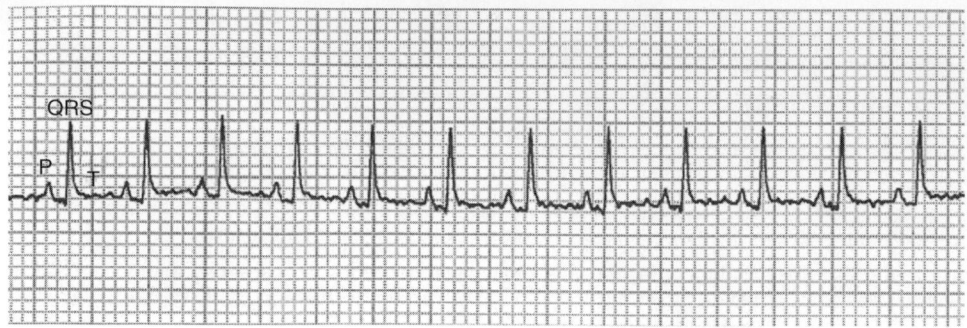

Fig. 163-5 Sinus tachycardia in a 15-year-old domestic shorthair cat with compensated hypertrophic cardiomyopathy and endocarditis of the aortic valve. The heart rate is 220 beats/min. The T wave is essentially isoelectric and poorly seen in this lead. A small amount of motion artifact is seen throughout the baseline. 25 mm/sec, 1 cm = 1 mV.

not cause clinical signs and rather is the result, not the cause, of physiologic or medical disturbances. It usually must not be suppressed because doing so would compromise the call for increased cardiac output or the need for reflex tachycardia. Some clinicians treat cats with severe sinus tachycardia (≈300/min) associated with hyperthyroidism with atenolol; however, this therapy typically is unnecessary once the thyrotoxicosis is controlled.

Supraventricular tachyarrhythmias are tachycardias in which the arrhythmia arises within the atria or the AV junction. Included are supraventricular (atrial) premature complexes, supraventricular (atrial, AV junctional) tachycardias, atrial flutter, and atrial fibrillation. Tachycardias mediated by an accessory pathway that bypasses the AV node such as Wolff-Parkinson-White syndrome can be considered supraventricular as well.

Supraventricular tachyarrhythmias usually develop secondary to enlargement, inflammation, or infarction of atrial myocardium. Common causes include AV valve regurgitation, diastolic dysfunction (hypertrophic or restrictive cardiomyopathies), atrial fibrosis or infarction, or less commonly in the cat primary valvular degeneration or infection (endocarditis). Other recognized causes include congenital cardiac disorders (i.e., atrial and ventricular septal defects, patent ductus arteriosus) and hyperthyroidism.

In most cases supraventricular tachyarrhythmias have the characteristic ECG features of normally conducted QRS-T complexes, except for the absence of a preceding P wave (Fig. 163-6). Atrial tachycardia is often an exception in that normal or abnormally conducted P waves are usually recorded. On occasion supraventricular tachyarrhythmias resemble ventricular arrhythmias when intraventricular conduction is abnormal (i.e., aberrant) in the former. Differentiation of an aberrantly conducted supraventricular tachycardia (SVT) from ventricular tachycardia (VT) might be accomplished during the recording of an ECG by the application of a vagal maneuver: for 10 to 15 seconds gentle pressure is applied to the region just dorsal and cranial to the larynx (unilateral carotid sinus massage), or moderate pressure is applied on the eyeballs bilaterally over closed eyelids, or the nasal planum is depressed gently for 10 to 15 seconds. If this fails, diltiazem (see following paragraphs) may create AV block, an alteration that should block abnormal P waves or flutter waves, terminate a reentrant SVT, or have no effect on a VT.

Supraventricular premature complexes (SPCs, including atrial premature complexes) are characterized by the premature occurrence of a normal QRS complex. Generally in cats there is no visible P wave for an SPC (Fig. 163-7), and only on occasion does a clear, premature P wave precede the premature QRS complex. Common associations with SPCs include structural heart disease, but on occasion they occur secondary to high stress or systemic disorders. Specific treatment of SPCs is not indicated unless they are frequent (i.e., accelerating the ventricular rate to >200/minute) or repetitive in nature. Under these circumstances they should be managed as for the patient with SVT (see next paragraphs).

SVT implies an accelerated cardiac rhythm that requires rapid activation above the ventricles (i.e., atria or AV tissues). The QRS complexes usually have the normal, expected configuration, but P waves generally are absent or buried in the prior QRS ST-T waves, and the heart rate commonly exceeds 240/min (see Fig. 163-6). As mentioned previously, on rare occasions the QRS complexes in SVT may resemble VT because of aberrant ventricular conduction, which is best demonstrated via a vagal maneuver.

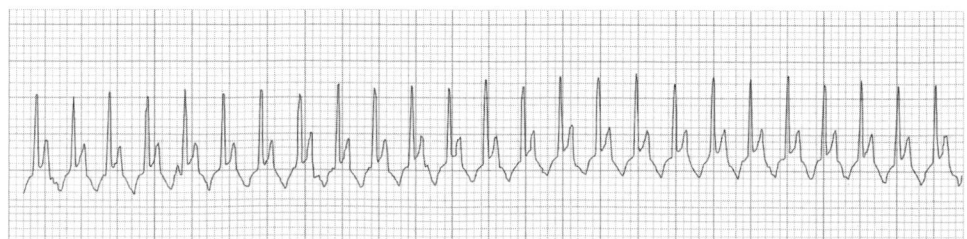

Fig. 163-6 Supraventricular atrial tachycardia. QRS complexes are narrow and positive in this lead II tracing, suggesting a supraventricular source for the initiating impulse. They are also tall, suggesting left ventricular enlargement. The rhythm is regular and rapid (heart rate = 290/min). Very large, abnormal P waves are seen clearly and repeatedly at the end of the QRS complex and are conducted with first-degree atrioventricular block. Ectopic P waves are often concealed within the preceding T wave or QRS complex. 25 mm/sec, 1 cm = 1 mV.

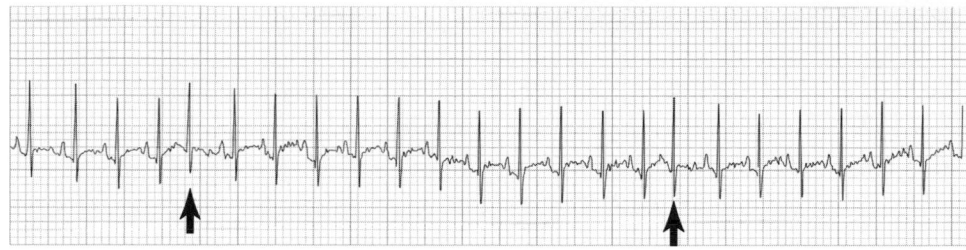

Fig. 163-7 Atrial premature complexes. The regularity of this sinus tachycardia (heart rate = 280/min) is interrupted by two supraventricular premature complexes, which are the fifth and seventeenth heartbeats *(arrows)*. The QRS complexes and T waves of these premature beats are the same as those of the sinus beats. 25 mm/sec, 1 cm = 1 mV.

Management of the cat with SVT usually requires combined management of both the arrhythmia and the heart failure that generally accompanies it. Therefore furosemide, oxygen therapy, and continuous ECG monitoring often are the cornerstones of initial care, frequently without antiarrhythmic drugs. In a cat with sustained SVT, specific management of the arrhythmia commonly is chosen in light of the underlying heart disease. For example, in addition to oxygen and diuretic therapies, sustained SVT in a cat with hypertrophic cardiomyopathy may be treated with either a calcium channel blocker or a β-blocker (see dosage under section on Ventricular Tachycardia later in the chapter), whereas SVT in a cat with dilated cardiomyopathy may be treated with digoxin with or without β- or calcium channel blockade.

Atrial fibrillation (AF) is characterized by a complete disorganization of atrial activity without effective atrial contraction. Characteristics on ECG are an isoelectric or irregularly undulating baseline, QRS complexes of a consistent though slightly varying shape, and an irregular ventricular rhythm that is generally rapid (mean: 223 ± 36 beats/min) (Fig. 163-8). In most cats the initiating factor appears to be advanced structural heart disease associated with marked left atrial enlargement. For example, the mean left atrial:aortic ratio in one study was 2.55 ± 0.80 (Côté, 2004a). Chief complaints commonly may be perceived as relating to heart disease (e.g., dyspnea, acute paralysis) but in 22% of cats AF is found incidentally. It occurs more often in males (Côté et al., 2004a).

In AF, ventricular rate control can be achieved by adequate control of CHF and use of medications that decrease conduction through the AV node. After control of fluid congestion, drugs chosen for ventricular rate control in AF are selected based in some cases on the underlying structural heart disorder (see previous paragraph on SVT). In general, diltiazem is most effective for blocking

AV nodal conduction and can be combined with digoxin or a β-blocker. The negative inotropic effects of diltiazem and atenolol must be appreciated. The prognosis with AF in cats is fair in our experience, with median survival of 165 days and 33% of cats with AF living 1 year or more.

Ventricular Tachyarrhythmias

A *ventricular tachyarrhythmia* occurs as a result of the early and unnecessary electrical activation of the ventricles. The resulting QRS-T complex precedes or obliterates the sinus P wave, and the QRS conformation is different from that of the normally conducted QRS complex (Figs. 163-9 and 163-10). In most instances the QRS complex in a ventricular tachyarrhythmia is producing a dominant R wave in leads II and V4 when the impulse originates in the right ventricle and a dominant Q wave, S wave, or QS complex when it arises in the left ventricle. In cats that also have an intraventricular conduction abnormality such as bundle branch block, the site of origin of the ventricular arrhythmia may be more difficult to accurately define. Four or more consecutive VPCs are a *ventricular run* or *VT*. Ventricular tachyarrhythmias are the second most common class of ECG abnormalities in cats (see Table 163-1).

In most cats with ventricular tachyarrhythmias, the arrhythmia is a marker of underlying myocardial disease. The presence of a ventricular tachyarrhythmia strongly identifies the need for a thorough patient workup as discussed initially in this chapter and ideally either a Holter monitor study or a 24- to 48-hour period of ECG monitoring in a veterinary critical care facility. Only by taking this approach can the significance of the arrhythmia be fully established and accurate decisions pertaining to therapeutic interventions made. Although the majority of cats with sporadic or infrequent ventricular tachyarrhythmias do not require antiarrhythmic therapy, frequent repetitive

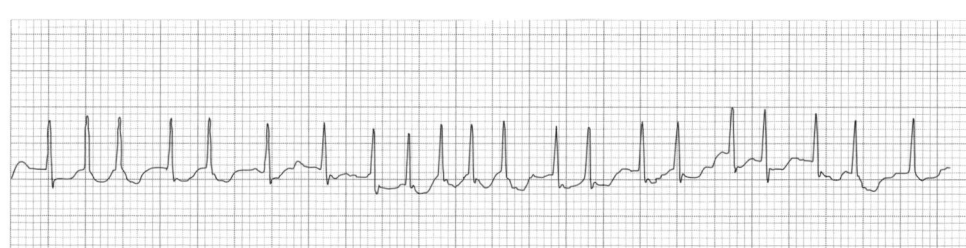

Fig. 163-8 Atrial fibrillation. The QRS complexes are supraventricular in appearance (narrow, upright in lead II), but the R-R interval is completely irregular, there are no visible P waves, and there is a finely undulating baseline. Heart rate = 260/minute, 25 mm/sec, 1 cm = 1 mV.

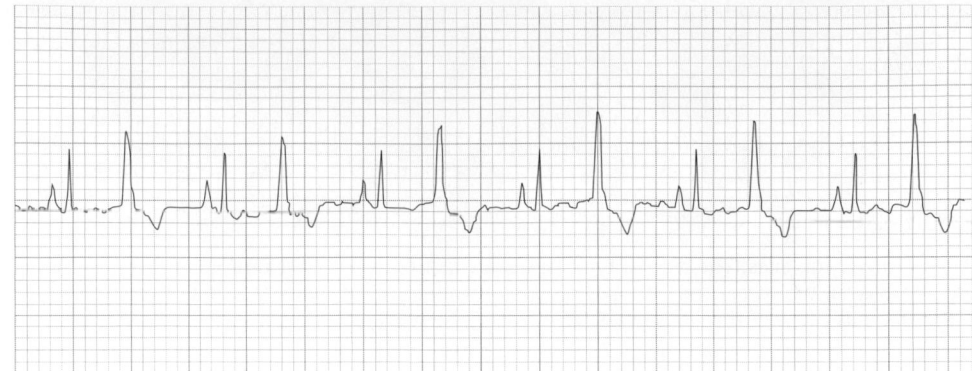

Fig. 163-9   Ventricular premature complexes (VPCs). The first QRS complex is a normal sinus complex, as evidenced by its preceding P wave and normal shape. The same is true for the other odd-numbered complexes on this tracing. The remaining complexes are wider, taller, and clearly different in shape compared to normal. They also occur prematurely. This alternating pattern between sinus beat and VPCs is termed *ventricular bigeminy*. The P waves also are tall, suggesting atrial enlargement. 25 mm/sec, 1 cm = 1 mV.

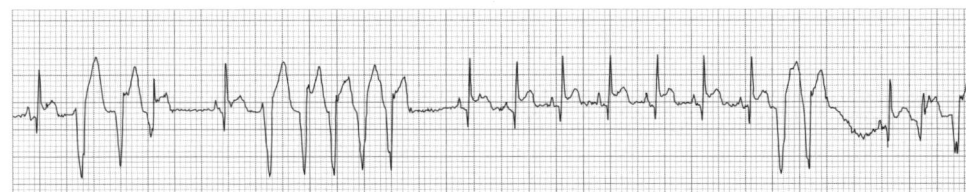

Fig. 163-10   Ventricular premature complexes (VPCs) and ventricular tachycardia (VT). The first is a normal sinus heartbeat, followed by two VPCs of varying morphology; the fourth beat appears to be a supraventricular premature beat occurring directly after the second VPC. The next beat is a normal sinus beat followed by five VPCs in a row—a run or "paroxysm" of VT that terminates spontaneously. During sinus rhythm there is substantial ST segment elevation (0.2 mV), suggesting myocardial hypoxia. 25 mm/sec, 1 cm = 1 mV.

VPCs or runs of VT that tend to promote cardiovascular instability (lethargy, low blood pressure, weakness or syncope, CHF) demand recognition and therapy.

Initial management must include identification and correction of precipitating factors such as hypokalemia, anemia, thyrotoxicosis, and hypoxemia. When aggressive (rapid, polymorphic) ventricular tachyarrhythmias are identified or when aggressive diuretic and oxygen therapy do not reduce the frequency of such arrhythmias in a cat with CHF, antiarrhythmic drug therapy should be introduced. Optimal therapy of ventricular arrhythmias in cats is poorly understood. Care must be used when giving negative inotropes such as β-blockers to cats with hypotension or uncontrolled CHF; with rare exceptions, these types of drugs are not initiated until such unstable conditions have improved or resolved.

A reasonable starting point is to evaluate the therapeutic response to an intravenous β-blocker (e.g., propranolol, 0.25 to 0.50 mg/*cat* IV slowly over 2 to 3 minutes; or esmolol, 0.05 to 0.5 mg/kg IV bolus over 1 to 2 minutes or administered as a constant rate infusion [CRI] at 50 to 200 mcg/kg/min). Alternatives include an intravenous lidocaine bolus (0.25 to 1.0 mg/kg over a 3- to 5-minute period; CAUTION: cats anecdotally are reported to be sensitive to the adverse effects of lidocaine) or procainamide (10 to 20 mcg/kg/min IV CRI); if this proves effective oral procainamide at 1/4 of a 250-mg tablet BID to TID is introduced as the IV infusion is gradually tapered down over 24 to 48 hours.

Following the acute control of life-threatening ventricular tachyarrhythmias or in the patient with less aggressive but worrisome ventricular tachyarrhythmias, oral antiarrhythmic agents should be considered. Options include procainamide (62.5 mg/*cat* PO BID to TID), propranolol (2.5 to 5 mg/*cat* PO BID to TID), or atenolol (6.25 to 12.5 mg/*cat* PO SID to BID). Others have used sotalol (2 mg/kg orally [PO] q12h). Beyond the initial patient evaluation and hospitalization, follow-up patient evaluation studies need to be pursued. These can range from periodic outpatient examinations with ECG recordings to the Holter monitor studies previously mentioned or even day-patient monitoring in a critical care facility when these facilities are available.

References and Suggested Reading

Côté E, Ettinger SJ: Electrocardiography and cardiac arrhythmias. In Ettinger SJ, Feldman EC, editors: *Textbook of veterinary internal medicine*, ed 6, St Louis, 2005, Elsevier, p 1040.

Côté E et al: Atrial fibrillation in cats: 50 cases (1979-2002), *J Am Vet Med Assoc* 225:256, 2004a.

Côté E et al: Assessment of the prevalence of heart murmurs in overtly healthy cats, *J Am Vet Med Assoc* 225:384, 2004b.

Fox PR, Harpster NK: Diagnosis and management of feline arrhythmias. In Fox PR, Sisson DD, Moïse NS, editors: *Textbook of canine and feline cardiology*, ed 2, Philadelphia, 1999, Saunders, p 386.

Hamlin RL: Heart rate of the cat, *J Am Anim Hosp Assoc* 25:284, 1989.

Harpster NK: The cardiovascular system. In Holzworth, J, editor: *Diseases of the cat*, Philadelphia, 1987, Saunders, p 820.

Harpster NK: Feline arrhythmias: diagnosis and management. In Kirk RW, Bonagura JD, editors: *Current veterinary therapy XI (small animal practice)*, Philadelphia, 1992, Saunders, p 732.

Kaneshige T et al: The anatomical basis of complete atrioventricular block in cats with hypertrophic cardiomyopathy, *J Comp Path* 135:25, 2006.

Kellum HB, Stepien RL: Feline third-degree atrioventricular block: clinical presentation, long-term outcome, and survival in 21 cats (1997-2004), *J Vet Intern Med* 20:97, 2006.

Laste NJ, Harpster NK: A retrospective study of 100 cases of feline distal aortic thromboembolism: 1977-1993, *J Am Anim Hosp Assoc* 31:492, 1995.

Smith SA et al: Arterial thromboembolism in cats: acute crisis in 127 cases (1992-2001) and long-term management with low-dose aspirin in 24 cases, *J Vet Intern Med* 17:73, 2003.

Tilley LP: *Essentials of canine and feline electrocardiography*, ed 3, Malvern, Penn, 1992, Lea & Febiger.

Ware WA: Twenty-four-hour ambulatory electrocardiography in normal cats, *J Vet Intern Med* 13:175, 1999.

CHAPTER 164

Cardioversion

JANICE M. BRIGHT, *Fort Collins, Colorado*
JULIE MARTIN, *Englewood, Colorado*

External electrical cardioversion refers to transthoracic delivery of a direct current (DC) shock for restoration of sinus rhythm in patients with ventricular or supraventricular tachyarrhythmias. The shock is synchronized to the R wave of the QRS complex to avoid induction of ventricular fibrillation. Synchronized energy delivery distinguishes cardioversion from defibrillation, which is unsynchronized. Until recently electrical cardioversion and defibrillation were done in humans and dogs using equipment that delivered a monophasic energy waveform (i.e., a high energy electrical shock sent a current across the chest in a single direction). However, newer cardioversion/defibrillation devices are available that deliver biphasic energy waveforms. These biphasic cardioverter/defibrillators use a lower-energy, self-reversing waveform that is safer and more effective than traditional monophasic shocks.

Biphasic electrical cardioversion has potential advantages over pharmacologic cardioversion in that a precisely regulated "dose" of electrical energy can restore sinus rhythm immediately and safely. Also, the distinction between supraventricular and ventricular tachycardia is less crucial with electrical cardioversion than with medical management. Finally, time-consuming titration of drugs with potential side effects is not an issue with DC cardioversion. However, a disadvantage of electrical cardioversion for emergency management of tachyarrhythmias is that the equipment and expertise may not be readily available. Moreover, when electrical cardioversion is done as an elective procedure, general anesthesia is required.

Electrical cardioversion appears to be most successful for termination of tachycardias resulting from impulse reentry such as atrial fibrillation, atrial flutter, atrioventricular node reentry, atrioventricular reciprocating tachycardias involving an accessory conduction pathway, and most forms of ventricular tachycardia. The electrical shock is believed to terminate the tachycardia by simultaneously depolarizing all excitable myocardium and possibly by prolonging refractoriness; in other words, the shock interrupts reentrant circuits and establishes electrical homogeneity, thereby terminating reentry.

INDICATIONS AND CONTRAINDICATIONS FOR DIRECT CURRENT CARDIOVERSION

Any tachycardia producing hypotension or congestive heart failure that does not respond promptly to medical management is a candidate for electrical cardioversion. The exception to this general rule would be a digitalis-induced tachyarrhythmia.

DC cardioversion done as an elective procedure is useful for restoring sinus rhythm in patients with sustained atrial fibrillation or atrial flutter. By improving hemodynamics (reducing ventricular filling pressures, augmenting cardiac output, decreasing ventricular rate, and providing atrioventricular synchrony), rhythm control is potentially beneficial for dogs with congestive heart failure and secondary atrial fibrillation (Dernellis, Stenfanadis, Toutouzas, 2000; Sisson, Brown, Riepe, 1995). Furthermore, restoring sinus rhythm circumvents the need for pharmacologic control of heart rate using drugs that often have a negative inotropic effect such as β-blockers and diltiazem (McNamara et al., 2003). In the absence of underlying heart disease, restoration of sinus rhythm in dogs with atrial fibrillation diminishes the risk of secondary thromboembolism and prevents tachycardia-induced cardiomyopathy. In athletic dogs there may also be an improvement in exercise tolerance. In dogs with atrial flutter, pharmacologic control of the ventricular rate is frequently difficult, and DC cardioversion is often our initial treatment of choice.

Electrical cardioversion is contraindicated in patients with cardiac glycoside toxicity, and there is an increased risk associated with electrical cardioversion in animals with sinus node dysfunction that do not have a pacemaker. Finally, DC cardioversion is contraindicated in patients with intraatrial thrombus because organized atrial contraction may dislodge the thrombus.

CARDIOVERSION PROCEDURE

Elective cardioversion is done under general anesthesia. Pretreatment with antiarrhythmic agents before electrical cardioversion of patients with atrial fibrillation is recommended to help prevent recurrence of atrial fibrillation after cardioversion. Unless the patient's condition is too critical to delay cardioversion, we treat for 2 weeks with amiodarone (12 to 15 mg/kg orally [PO] q24h) before the procedure. Although this antiarrhythmic agent causes pharmacologic restoration of sinus rhythm in some humans, we have not observed this in dogs. Amiodarone is continued after cardioversion at a maintenance dosage of 5 to 7 mg/kg orally every 24 hours. Preferably the cardioversion procedure should be scheduled for early afternoon so that serum levels of electrolytes may be obtained and electrolyte abnormalities corrected, if needed, before anesthesia. In addition the atria should be examined echocardiographically for thrombus in the morning on the day of the scheduled procedure. Successful cardioversion is more likely to be achieved if serum magnesium and potassium concentrations are in the mid to upper range of normal. We try to achieve a serum potassium concentration of 4.5 to 5.5 mEq/L and a serum magnesium concentration greater than 2 mEq/L immediately before cardioversion. Digoxin should be withheld on the day of the procedure; but, if digitalis toxicity is suspected, the cardioversion should be postponed until this problem has resolved.

Anesthetic premedication is recommended using an opioid (fentanyl 5 to 10 mcg/kg, hydromorphone 0.05 to 0.2 mg/kg, oxymorphone 0.05 to 0.1 mg/kg, or methadone 0.5 to 1 mg/kg) either alone or in combination with a benzodiazepine (midazolam 0.1 to 0.3 mg/kg) and administered subcutaneously or intramuscularly approximately 30 minutes before instrumentation and patient preparation. Before anesthetic induction the lateral thorax is clipped on each side from the axilla caudally and ventrally approximately 15 cm to facilitate placement and contact of the cardioversion paddles. Electrocardiographic electrodes are attached to the skin of the extremities and connected to the electrocardiographic (ECG) leads of the cardioversion device.

Anesthesia may be induced with fentanyl (5 to 20 mcg/kg), etomidate (0.5 to 2 mg/kg), or a combination of these two drugs combined with a benzodiazepine (diazepam 0.2 to 0.5 mg/kg or midazolam 0.1 to 0.3 mg/kg). An anticholinergic agent administered at a conservative dose is indicated if the heart rate decreases enough to adversely affect cardiac output and blood pressure. Short-term maintenance of anesthesia for cardioversion may require additional doses of the induction drugs or supplementation with low doses of propofol (0.25 to 1 mg/kg).

We recommend that patients be intubated and administered 100% oxygen using a standard small animal breathing circuit. Manual or mechanical ventilation of the patient may be necessary to avoid hypoventilation and respiratory acidosis during periods of deep sedation. Heart rate and rhythm, blood pressure, oxygen saturation, and end-tidal carbon dioxide should be monitored during and immediately after cardioversion. Inhalation agents are used by some clinicians but are generally not administered in our practices unless the patient needs an additional diagnostic or surgical procedure following the cardioversion.

Although cardioversion may be done by delivery of energy through either preplaced adhesive cardioversion pads or cardioversion paddles held against the thorax, we prefer paddles to achieve optimal positioning of electrodes and minimal transthoracic impedance. Immediately following induction of anesthesia, the patient is positioned in dorsal recumbency in a foam trough placed on a padded table. The forelimbs are secured cranially, and the rear limbs are secured caudally (Fig. 164-1). Care must be taken to ensure that neither the dog nor the operator is in contact with any metallic surface.

The synchronous mode (cardioversion mode) of the cardioverter/defibrillator is selected to prevent current delivery during the ventricular repolarization phase of the cardiac cycle. When the cardioverter/defibrillator device is used in its cardioversion mode, the device should recognize QRS complexes and identify them on the monitor. To prevent improper synchronization with accidental triggering of ventricular fibrillation, the operator should verify that the device is set to synchronous mode and that it is correctly identifying R waves before delivery of *each* shock. Some units require a resetting to synchronous mode following each shock. Erroneous identification of QRS complexes by the device is more likely to occur in patients with tall, peaked T waves or splintered QRS complexes. *Electrode paste* is applied to the cardioversion paddles, and the paddles are then held against the clipped areas of the thorax with the top of the paddles at approximately the level of the point of the shoulders (see Fig. 164-1). Pediatric paddles should be used for dogs less than 15 kg. Firm pressure on both paddles should be used to provide adequate electrical contact and reduce transthoracic impedance. The operator should give an "all clear" command and verify that no assistants are touching the animal or equipment before discharging the device.

It is recommended that the initial energy setting be low (10 to 20 J for atrial flutter and 35 to 50 J for atrial fibrillation) and additional shocks delivered, when necessary, using upward titration of energy until successful cardioversion is achieved or until the peak energy output of the device has been used. If a maximal energy biphasic shock fails to restore sinus rhythm, a low dose of quinidine gluconate may be administered (0.5 mg/kg

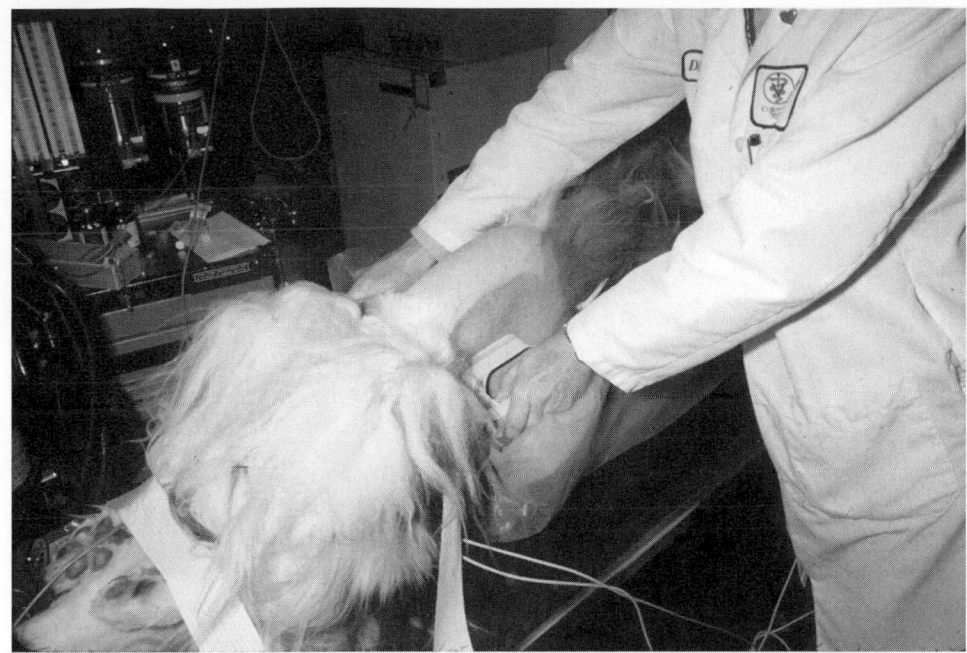

Fig. 164-1 Photo of a dog undergoing electrical cardioversion.

intravenously [IV]) in an attempt to facilitate cardioversion, and the maximal energy shock is then repeated. Reversing paddle polarity occasionally can be helpful. Ibutilide, a class 3 antiarrhythmic agent, has been used in humans as an alternative to quinidine to facilitate electrical cardioversion of atrial fibrillation. It is important to distinguish between inability to restore sinus rhythm, indicating inadequate energy delivery to the atria, and inability to maintain sinus rhythm after transient termination of atrial fibrillation. The latter situation (early reinitiation of atrial fibrillation) does not respond to higher energy shocks but may respond favorably to intravenous quinidine (0.5 to 1 mg/kg) or procainamide (6 to 8 mg/kg) given before delivery of an additional shock.

Following cardioversion the ECG should be monitored at least until full consciousness has been restored and preferably for several hours thereafter. If frequent premature atrial contractions are noted, suppression of supraventricular ectopy with a class 1A antiarrhythmic (procainamide 10 to 20 mg/kg intramuscularly [IM]) may possibly prevent early relapse into atrial fibrillation or atrial flutter. Dogs with structural heart disease should be maintained on medications for management of heart failure; however, drugs administered solely for heart rate control (e.g., digoxin, diltiazem) are discontinued.

EFFICACY OF BIPHASIC EXTERNAL CARDIOVERSION IN DOGS WITH ATRIAL FIBRILLATION

Retrospective evaluation of data from dogs with chronic atrial fibrillation has shown that transthoracic cardioversion with a biphasic waveform is a highly effective method of restoring sinus rhythm in canine patients (Bright, Martin, and Mama, 2005). In our experience successful cardioversion is achieved in more than 90% of dogs even in the presence of severe underlying heart disease. Restoration of sinus rhythm does not appear to be beneficially or adversely affected by pretreatment with amiodarone. In dogs undergoing biphasic cardioversion of atrial fibrillation at our hospital, the presence of underlying structural heart disease had no statistically significant effect on the current required to restore sinus rhythm. Similarly, the presence of structural heart disease did not significantly affect the total conversion energy or the conversion energy expressed as a function of body weight. The average current required to achieve cardioversion in our canine patients (mean 11.7 ± 4.5 A) was similar to the current required for biphasic transthoracic cardioversion of humans with atrial fibrillation (11 ± 1 A) (Mittal et al., 2000). This current is significantly less than that required for traditional cardioversion of humans using a monophasic energy waveform (41 ± 11 A) (Dorian et al., 2001). Fig. 164-2 shows a typical ECG strip recorded during biphasic electrical cardioversion of a dog with atrial fibrillation.

DURATION OF SINUS RHYTHM AFTER CARDIOVERSION OF ATRIAL FIBRILLATION

Antiarrhythmic agents generally are recommended to promote maintenance of sinus rhythm following cardioversion. In humans with chronic atrial fibrillation amiodarone is the most effective pharmacologic agent for maintenance of sinus rhythm (Kochiadakis et al., 2000). This drug is usually administered for 3 to 4 weeks before the cardioversion procedure. Other drugs that have proven useful for maintenance of sinus rhythm in humans include propafenone and sotalol. In dogs the importance of initiating antiarrhythmic agents before the cardioversion is debatable; however, data from our institution suggest a beneficial effect of pretreatment with amiodarone. We generally begin administration of amiodarone 2 weeks before the cardioversion procedure, but if it is not in the best interest of the patient or the owner to delay cardioversion, amiodarone

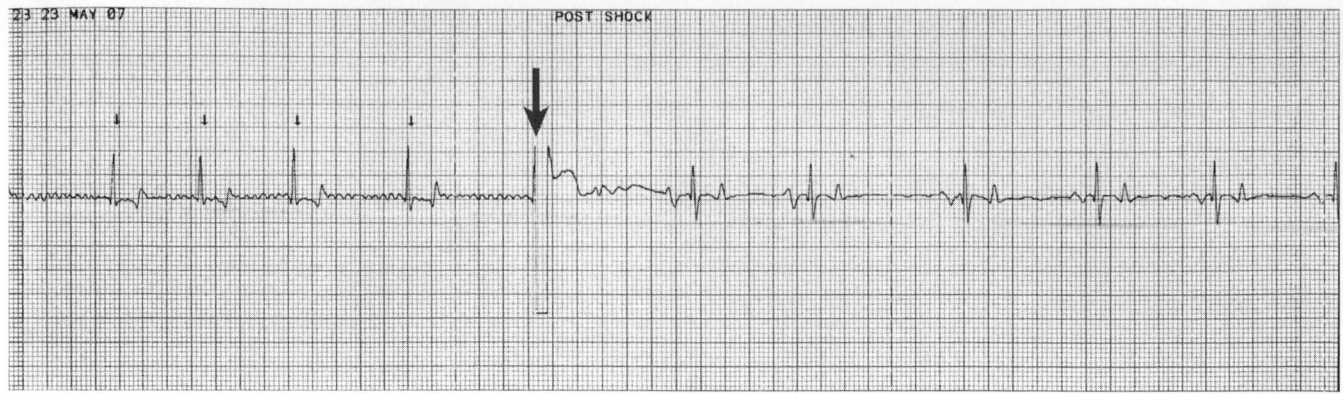

Fig. 164-2   A lead II ECG rhythm strip recorded during external electrical cardioversion of atrial fibrillation in a canine patient. The small arrows indicate QRS complexes appropriately identified by the device in its cardioversion (synchronized) mode. A biphasic shock of 100 J is delivered at the large arrow. After the shock there is normal sinus rhythm (paper speed 25 mm).

is begun as soon as possible after the dog awakens from anesthesia. Thyroid function and hepatic function should be monitored (every 3 to 6 months) in dogs receiving amiodarone. Because serum amiodarone concentration does not a correlate well to tissue concentration, serum drug levels are not routinely evaluated. Nonetheless, a serum amiodarone concentration below the therapeutic range may be helpful information to have when planning management of dogs with recurrence of atrial fibrillation after cardioversion. Amiodarone is continued indefinitely in dogs with underlying heart disease, particularly those with significant atrial enlargement. Because electrophysiologic remodeling of the atrial myocytes induced by atrial fibrillation is reversed after 2 to 4 weeks of sinus rhythm, consideration should be given to discontinuing amiodarone; however, the structural remodeling induced by atrial fibrillation is not completely reversible.

Although transthoracic biphasic cardioversion is a highly effective method of restoring sinus rhythm in dogs with naturally occurring chronic atrial fibrillation, the duration of sinus rhythm after cardioversion is quite variable. Unfortunately there is no consistently reliable way of determining which dogs will have an early recurrence of atrial fibrillation after electrical cardioversion. Recurrence of atrial fibrillation occurs earlier in dogs with underlying structural heart disease than in dogs with lone atrial fibrillation. Also, in a series of dogs undergoing cardioversion at our institution, those with atrial enlargement tended to have an earlier recurrence of the arrhythmia. Chronicity of atrial fibrillation before cardioversion is known to be inversely related to the duration of sinus rhythm following cardioversion in humans, and our data indicate that this relationship is valid in dogs as well. Atrial fibrillation is known to produce electrophysiologic and structural remodeling of the atrial myocardium, and this remodeling subsequently promotes both maintenance and recurrence of this arrhythmia ("atrial fibrillation begets atrial fibrillation") (Wijffels et al., 1995; Yu et al., 1999). Admittedly, the duration of atrial fibrillation before cardioversion is difficult to precisely determine in dogs, especially in dogs without underlying heart disease ("lone atrial fibrillation"). Therefore for many dogs the duration of the arrhythmia is only an estimate. Nonetheless our experience suggests that

the prognosis for long-term maintenance of sinus rhythm after cardioversion is less favorable when the arrhythmia has been present for more than 6 months.

POTENTIAL CLINICAL BENEFIT OF RESTORING SINUS RHYTHM

Treatment goals for patients with chronic atrial fibrillation are to reduce or eliminate clinical signs resulting from the arrhythmia and to prevent long-term complications. Although humans with atrial fibrillation often have impaired exercise tolerance and reduced quality of life, dogs without underlying heart disease may have no apparent clinical signs. Therefore in dogs with lone atrial fibrillation, restoration of sinus rhythm with DC cardioversion is done solely to prevent potential complications such as thromboembolism and tachycardia-induced myocardial failure. In dogs with underlying heart disease, initiation of atrial fibrillation frequently coincides with deterioration in clinical status, including the onset or the recurrence of congestive heart failure, weakness, anorexia, syncope, or collapse. Restoration of sinus rhythm, even if short term, is theoretically advantageous in these patients because of the salutary effects of sinus rhythm on ventricular filling pressures, cardiac output, heart rate, and coronary perfusion.

A controlled, prospective study is needed to confirm that rhythm control has a beneficial effect on the clinical status and survival of dogs with heart disease. However, in the meantime we have evaluated retrospectively the severity of heart failure in dogs successfully converted to sinus rhythm at our hospital. Using the International Small Animal Cardiac Health Council Heart Failure Classification to characterize the severity of clinical signs before and after cardioversion in 22 dogs, restoration of sinus rhythm was associated with reduction (9 of 22) or complete resolution (9 of 22) of clinical signs in 18 patients (81.8%). Before cardioversion 45.5% of the 22 dogs were in severe heart failure, and 54.5% were in mild- to-moderate failure. After cardioversion heart failure was severe in 0% and mild to moderate in 54.5%; 45.5% were asymptomatic. Thus preliminary data from our case series suggest that restoration of sinus rhythm

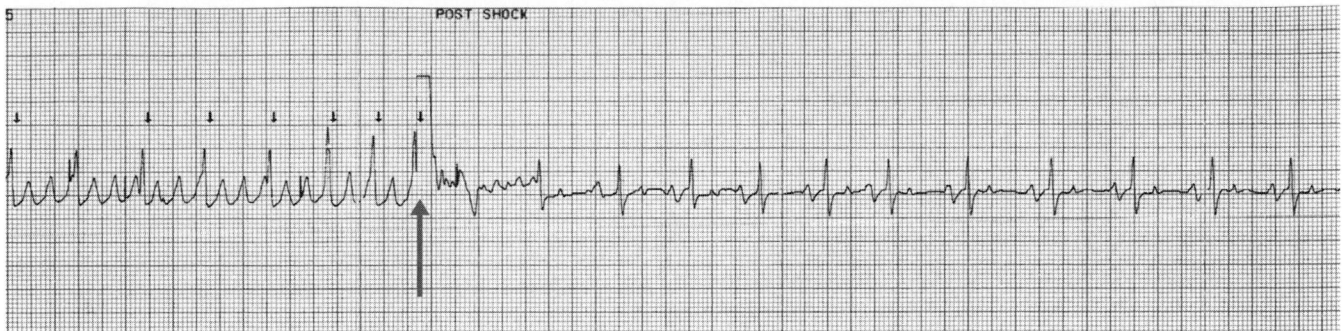

Fig. 164-3 A lead II ECG rhythm strip recorded during external electrical cardioversion of atrial flutter in a canine patient. The small arrows indicate QRS complexes appropriately identified by the device in its cardioversion (synchronized) mode. A biphasic shock of 20 J is delivered at the large arrow. After the shock there is normal sinus rhythm (paper speed 25 mm/second).

is helpful for stabilizing the clinical status of dogs with heart disease and that many dogs remain in sinus rhythm long enough to benefit from the procedure.

BIPHASIC EXTERNAL CARDIOVERSION IN DOGS WITH ATRIAL FLUTTER

Although sustained atrial flutter occurs far less frequently in dogs than sustained atrial fibrillation, pharmacologic rate control is often more difficult to achieve in patients with atrial flutter. Therefore biphasic transthoracic cardioversion provides an alternative method of managing this tachyarrhythmia. We have used biphasic transthoracic DC cardioversion in six dogs with atrial flutter; and restoration of sinus rhythm was achieved in all six, with conversion energies ranging from 15 to 30 J (0.4 to 1.2 J/kg) and conversion currents of 3 to 5 A. Atrial flutter recurred in two of these dogs after 42 and 124 days despite the use of amiodarone. Fig. 164-3 shows the ECG strip recorded during biphasic cardioversion of a dog with sustained atrial flutter.

BIPHASIC EXTERNAL CARDIOVERSION IN DOGS WITH VENTRICULAR TACHYCARDIA

Rapid and sustained ventricular tachycardia causes severe hemodynamic compromise. In most canine patients conversion to sinus rhythm and control of ventricular tachycardia can be accomplished with drugs. Occasionally pharmacologic conversion is not possible, or the side effects of the medications needed for conversion are intolerable. In these cases synchronized electrical cardioversion can be used to restore sinus rhythm. Pretreatment with an appropriate ventricular antiarrhythmic before cardioversion is recommended except in immediately life-threatening situations.

SAFETY OF EXTERNAL BIPHASIC CARDIOVERSION

To date we have observed no clinically significant adverse effects from biphasic DC cardioversion. Minor adverse effects noted have included brief asystole and nonsustained ventricular tachycardia immediately after shock delivery. Previous studies in dogs and other species have shown biphasic energy waveforms to be safe and minimally damaging to the myocardium. Although ventricular fibrillation has been described as a risk of traditional monophasic DC cardioversion in dogs, we have not observed this serious arrhythmia in any patient, including dogs with severe congestive heart failure and severe systolic dysfunction. We also have not observed significant adverse effects of amiodarone in our series of canine patients; however, others have reported serious adverse effects, particularly hepatotoxicity.

References and Suggested Reading

Bright JM, Martin JM, Mama K: A retrospective evaluation of transthoracic biphasic electrical cardioversion for atrial fibrillation in dogs, *J Vet Cardiol* 7:85, 2005.

Dernellis J, Stenfanadis C, Toutouzas P: From science to bedside: the clinical role of atrial function, *Eur Heart J* 2(suppl K):K48, 2000.

Dorian P et al: External cardioversion of atrial fibrillation with biphasic shocks requires less current and causes less patient discomfort, *Acad Emerg Med* 8:543, 2001.

Kochiadakis GE et al: Low-dose amiodarone and sotalol in the treatment of recurrent, symptomatic atrial fibrillation: a comparative, placebo controlled study, *Heart* 84:251, 2000.

McNamara RL et al: Management of atrial fibrillation: review of the evidence for the role of pharmacologic therapy, electrical cardioversion, and echocardiography, *Ann Intern Med* 139:1018, 2003.

Mittal S et al: Transthoracic cardioversion of atrial fibrillation: comparison of rectilinear biphasic versus damped sine wave monophasic shocks, *Circulation* 101:1282, 2000.

Sisson D, Brown R, Riepe R: Hemodynamic effects of atrial fibrillation in dogs with experimentally induced mitral regurgitation, *J Vet Intern Med* 9(abstr):200, 1995.

Wijffels MCEF et al: Atrial fibrillation begets atrial fibrillation: a study in awake, chronically instrumented goats, *Circulation* 92:1954, 1995.

Yu WC et al: Reversal of atrial electrical remodeling following cardioversion of long-standing atrial fibrillation in man, *Cardiovasc Res* 42:470, 1999.

CHAPTER 165

Patent Ductus Arteriosus

MATTHEW W. MILLER, *College Station, Texas*
SONYA G. GORDON, *College Station, Texas*

Patent ductus arteriosus (PDA) is a persistence of a fetal communication between the descending aorta and the main pulmonary artery. PDA is the second most common congenital cardiac malformation diagnosed in dogs. There is a higher incidence in females, with an odds ratio of approximately 3:1, although this is not evident in all breeds. Without correction, PDA has an estimated 1-year mortality that approaches 60%. Although subaortic stenosis (SAS) is reportedly the most commonly diagnosed congenital malformation, many diagnosed cases are of trivial hemodynamic significance, requiring no intervention and having little effect on an individual patient's life quality or duration. Therefore PDA is the most commonly diagnosed defect that routinely requires intervention.

DIAGNOSIS

The initial diagnosis of PDA still depends on careful physical examination and detection of the classic continuous murmur. In animals with very rapid hearts rates or elevations in pulmonary artery pressure, the diastolic component of the murmur may not be appreciated if careful auscultation is not performed. Ensuring that the stethoscope is placed high in the left axillary region increases the likelihood of an accurate initial diagnosis. Large volumetric left–to–right shunts frequently result in femoral pulses that are hyperdynamic or bounding.

Practicing veterinarians must be able to recognize the murmur of PDA so that appropriate diagnostic tests and treatments can be offered. In addition to concentrating on the dorsal left axillary region during auscultation, slowly moving the chest piece between the point of maximal murmur intensity and the left apex often allows the examiner to appreciate the continuous nature of the murmur at the base. In some puppies and kittens the continuous murmur may be equally loud or even more prominent immediately cranial to the left edge of the manubrium. In very young puppies or kittens and in cats with developing pulmonary hypertension the murmur may be very faint to absent at end diastole.

In a very small percentage of cases severe pulmonary vascular injury leads to shunt reversal (right-to-left PDA), a condition that is not amenable to closure in any manner. Dogs tend to develop pulmonary hypertension early in life and relatively quickly from a large PDA, but the development of pulmonary hypertension in cats typically is more gradual. This allows some cats to benefit from closure of the ductus, despite the presence of pulmonary vascular disease.

Diagnostic imaging allows for characterization of the type and severity of the defect. Classic radiographic findings include left ventricular and atrial dilation with pulmonary overcirculation, with venous prominence often evident. It is also common to appreciate dilation of both the main pulmonary artery and descending aorta. Pulmonary edema is present following the onset of congestive heart failure. A complete Doppler echocardiographic study is the test of choice for definitive diagnosis. Echocardiographic features of PDA include dilation of the left atrium, left ventricle, ascending aorta, and pulmonary artery. A portion of the PDA itself frequently can be visualized from several imaging planes, but the left cranial short axis view usually provides the optimal image. Saunders and colleagues (2007) at our institution recently described the transthoracic and transesophageal echocardiography (TEE) appearance of PDA as it relates to angiographic anatomy demonstrating the superiority of TEE for critical description of ductal anatomy in the dog. Doppler echocardiography confirms continuous flow in the main pulmonary artery with reversal of flow in diastole. Mild-to-moderate mitral regurgitation is a frequent finding, secondary to annular dilation. Depending on its severity, it usually resolves following ductal ligation or occlusion. Evidence of systolic dysfunction (elevated left ventricular internal diameter during systole, reduced percent fractional shortening) is common in dogs with large volumetric shunts and typically persists or appears worse following successful ligation or occlusion. Transaortic flow velocities commonly are accelerated and may be as high as 3.75 m/second with large shunts. This may lead to an erroneous diagnosis of concurrent SAS. Therefore caution should be used when interpreting transaortic flows in patients with large shunts.

Most patients are in sinus rhythm when the diagnosis is established. Although the electrocardiogram (ECG) often demonstrates criteria for left heart enlargement (widened P waves; increased QRS voltages), when the rhythm is normal an ECG contributes little to the overall diagnosis. An arrhythmia is the principal indication for recording an ECG in this disease. Atrial fibrillation may develop with long standing PDA, especially in larger-breed dogs, and is the most common arrhythmia seen with PDA.

Concurrent cardiac defects are relatively uncommon, but may be more likely in large-breed dogs. In our patient population approximately 9% of dogs with PDA have an additional congenital malformation, the most common of which is pulmonic stenosis.

THERAPY

Most canine patients and virtually all cats with PDA are referred for closure of the ductus. The best outcomes with PDA closure are likely to come from experienced operators, and this should be discussed with clients. Furthermore, closure of a ductus should never be delayed until a dog is "mature" or "develops symptoms" since irreversible myocardial damage, congestive heart failure, and death are likely outcomes. Currently there are two options: surgical ligation and catheter-based closure. The latter approach represents the most important advance in PDA management over the past decade. Surgical ligation of PDA has long been considered the standard of care for left-to-right shunting PDA and is a highly successful procedure with acceptable mortality (<5%) in experienced hands. However, in 1995 Snaps and colleagues published the first clinical report describing the use of vascular occlusion coils (Cook, Inc.) for treatment of PDA in a dog. Since that time, several devices have been evaluated for ductal occlusion in dogs.

Device Occlusion of Patent Ductus Arteriosus

Following the initial report by Snaps and colleagues, numerous reports detailed the use of either free-release or detachable occlusion coils. In addition, there have been two reports of the use of the human Amplatzer ductal occluder (AGA Medical Corp.) (Sisson, 2003). The high cost of this device and the requirement for transvenous delivery will most likely preclude its routine use in veterinary medicine. More recently the Amplatzer vascular plug (AGA Medical Corp.) and now the Amplatz canine ductal occluder (AGA Medical Corp.) have been available and evaluated in dogs (Hogan, 2006; Nguyenba, 2006). Generally these are deployed using a femoral artery catheter. Most canine patients can be treated successfully with one of these two devices (or with coils) provided the operator is experienced and the catheterization laboratory carries a sufficient inventory of devices.

All catheter-delivered devices are deployed under general anesthesia using fluoroscopic guidance following angiographic evaluation of ductal morphology. Fig. 165-1 shows a lateral radiograph with the three most commonly used occlusion devices deployed in clinical patients.

Device Selection
Selection of device type and size is substantially influenced by ductal morphology and minimal ductal diameter as determined by angiography or echocardiography. The vast majority of reports describe obtaining vascular access for angiography and device deployment via the femoral artery. Following routine anesthesia, arterial access is obtained by surgical cutdown to the right or left femoral artery. Following insertion of a vascular introducer, an angiographic catheter or transeptal sheath is positioned in the descending aorta or directly within the PDA. Angiograms are performed in the right lateral projection by injection of 0.5 to 2 ml/kg of radiographic contrast material either via power injector with 300 to 1050 PSI pressure or by vigorous hand injection.

Angiograms are recorded and reviewed with special emphasis on ductal morphology and minimal ductal diameter (Fig. 165-2). Although ductal morphology and minimal diameter substantially influence device selection, to date no consensus recommendations for device selection have been forthcoming. In our hospital TEE is used to screen patients before surgical or catheter-based intervention. If type III ductal morphology is diagnosed (tube with no taper), especially with a minimal ductal diameter in excess of 5 mm, catheter-based occlusion is not attempted, and the patient is sent directly to surgery for ligation.

Results of Device Occlusion in Dogs
Encouraging results with the various devices have been reported. The greatest number of cases and longest follow-up are available for patients in which vascular occlusion coils were used. The largest published study to date reported the results of 125 cases seen at a single institution (University of California, Davis) (Campbell et al., 2006). Coils were successfully deployed in 108 dogs (86%). Patients in which coil occlusion was not successful had significantly larger minimal ductal diameters than in those in which coil occlusion was successful, but specific ductal morphology was not described in this report. Complete ductal occlusion was documented in 61% of the dogs evaluated longer than 1 year following the procedure. Based on echocardiographic examination the residual ductal flow in the vast majority of the other 39% appeared to be hemodynamically inconsequential, such that repeat intervention was thought to be indicated in only four dogs (3.7%). The most common complication with the procedure was coil embolization of other vessels (n=27). There were three fatalities associated with the procedure.

Our group's experience is somewhat similar. From 1994 to 2005 we attempted coil embolization in 228 dogs. Ten procedures were aborted: seven because of an excessively large ductal diameter and three from inability to

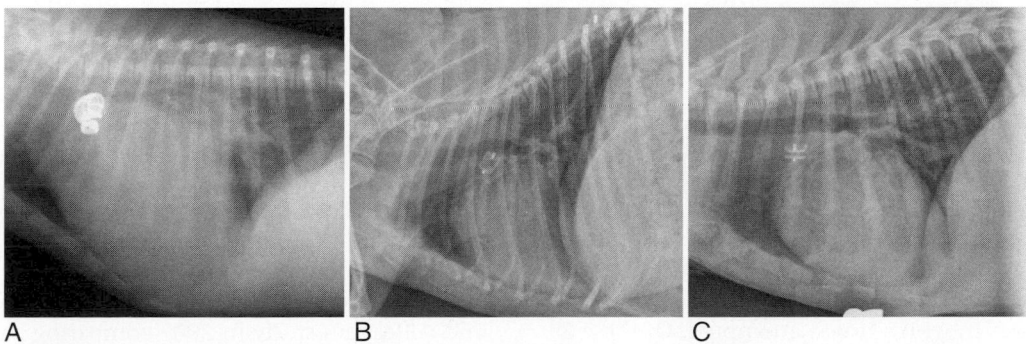

Fig. 165-1 Lateral radiographs from dogs with patent ductus arteriosus treated with (**A**) mutliple vascular occlusion coils, (**B**) Amplatzer vascular plug, and (**C**) Amplatzer canine ductal occluder.

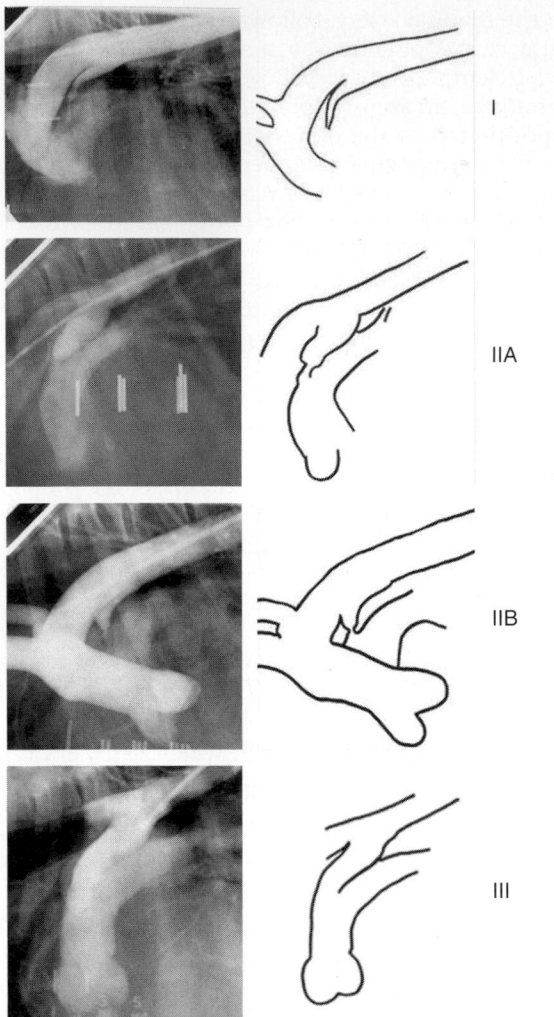

Fig. 165-2 Proposed angiographic classification scheme for canine patent ductus arteriosus.

obtain adequate arterial access because of small patient size. There were two fatalities, one caused by aortic rupture and one from aortic embolization and occlusion. Residual ductal flow was substantial enough to require a repeat procedure in three patients. Nonfatal complications included pulmonary coil embolization (nine), aortic embolization (four), and partial aortic deployment and femoral artery hematoma (four). All patients in which a femoral arterial hematoma developed underwent percutaneous arterial access. Follow-up longer than 6 months was available in 117 dogs. Of these dogs only 12% had residual flow. Based on this experience we do not attempt catheter-based occlusion in patients less than 2.5 kg despite that fact that success in this patient population has been reported. In addition, in patients with large, tubular (angiographic type III) ductal morphology we prefer surgical ligation for closure.

Achen and colleagues (2006) reported successful deployment of the Amplatzer vascular plug for closure of PDA in 29 of the 30 dogs in which it was attempted. Of these 29 dogs 22 had complete occlusion 24 hours after deployment, with complete occlusion documented in an additional two dogs within 4 months of deployment. Of the five dogs with residual flow, two had trivial-to-mild flow and no continuous murmur, and three were lost to follow-up. The plug embolized to the pulmonary vasculature in one dog (first dog), and that ductus was subsequently occluded with multiple vascular occlusion coils.

Hogan and colleagues (2006) reported successful deployment of the Amplatzer vascular plug in eight dogs without complication. Complete occlusion was achieved in seven dogs, and one dog had moderate residual flow. Smith and Martin reported (2007) complete occlusion in four of six dogs in which they deployed an Amplatzer vascular plug.

In 2006 Nguyenba and Tobias reported the initial clinical experience with the Amplatzer canine ductal occluder in 11 dogs. The device, specifically designed for dogs, was deployed successfully in 10 dogs. In one dog the device was undersized and embolized to the lung. The ductus was subsequently occluded using a larger device. Follow-up angiography in these dogs documented trivial residual flow in one case and complete occlusion in the remaining cases. No residual flow was detected by echocardiography 3 months after deployment in any of the six dogs evaluated at the time of presentation of this study.

Surgical Ligation of Patent Ductus Arteriosus

Despite the substantial advances in catheter-based interventions, surgical ligation of PDA should not be viewed as a less desirable option. In the hands of talented and experienced surgeons the success rates for ductal ligation approach 95%, with most institutions reporting mortality rates of less than 2% to 5%. Furthermore, surgical ligation can be performed with all ductal morphologies and in dogs of all sizes. For most cats surgery is probably the method of choice for closure because of the small feline size and unacceptably high embolization rates with coils. Currently catheter-based occlusion is not feasible in dogs less than 3 pounds and is difficult or not possible in all dogs less than 5 pounds or in dogs of any size with a type III ductal morphology (tube with no taper).

To our knowledge there is only one publication comparing the results of catheter-based versus surgical ligation at a single institution (Goodrich et al., 2007) In this study patient age, weight, gender distribution, and procedure times were similar for both groups. Initial success rate was higher for surgical ligation (94%) than with coil embolization (84%). There was no statistically significant difference in mortality between surgical ligation (5.6%) and catheter-based occlusion (2.6%), but this numeric difference requires more study in larger populations. It should also be emphasized that these techniques are not mutually exclusive. For example, Fujii and colleagues (2006) reported the successful use of vascular occlusion coils to occlude residual flow following surgical ligation.

Complications of Ductal Closure

The frequency of major complications in the Goodrich and colleagues study in 2007 comparing surgical ligation and catheter-based techniques showed a higher complication rate with surgery (12% versus 4.2 %). Major surgical complications included inadvertent damage to the left cranial lung lobe, necessitating partial or complete lung lobectomy; severe ductus hemorrhage; cardiac arrest; respiratory insufficiency requiring ventilatory, support, mesenteric torsion; and chylothorax. Major catheterization complications included hemorrhage associated with the femoral arteriotomy, hemorrhage secondary to inadvertent aortic perforation, and cardiac arrest at anesthetic induction.

Minor complications were more prevalent with catheter-based techniques (i.e., 26% in contrast to 12% for surgical ligation). Minor catheterization complications included inadvertent pulmonary or systemic coil embolization, partial aortic coil protrusion, ligation of both femoral arteries, femoral arteriotomy infection, and transient hemoglobinuria and thrombocytopenia. Minor complications associated with surgery included left thoracic limb lameness, suture reaction, postoperative hypoxia, incisional seroma, and minor hemorrhage.

FUTURE DEVELOPMENTS

PDA is arguably the most important congenital cardiac abnormality in dogs. Advances in catheter-based intervention make this therapeutic modality a practical alternative for all but a very small percentage of canine patients. Further technical improvements should ultimately provide the veterinary cardiologist with devices and techniques that will allow effective and safe occlusion of all ductal morphologies in any size patient. We can all look forward to ongoing advances in the growing field of interventional cardiology.

References and Suggested Reading

Achen SE et al: Transarterial ductal occlusion using the Amplatzer vascular plug in 30 cases, Proceedings of the 26th Annual Veterinary Forum, Seattle Wash, 2006, American College of Veterinary Internal Medicine.

Campbell FE et al: Immediate and late outcomes of transarterial coil occlusion of patent ductus arteriosus in dogs, *J Vet Intern Med* 20:83, 2006.

Fujii Y et al: Coil occlusion of residual shunts after surgical closure of patent ductus arteriosus, *Vet Surg* 35(8):781, 2006.

Goodrich KR et al: Retrospective comparison of surgical ligation and transarterial catheter occlusion for treatment of patent ductus arteriosus in two hundred and four dogs (1993-2003), *Vet Surg* 36(1):43, 2007.

Hogan DF et al: Use of a peripheral vascular occlusion device for correction of patent ductus arteriosus in dogs, Proceedings of the 25th Annual Veterinary Forum, Baltimore, Md, 2006, American College of Veterinary Internal Medicine.

Miller MW et al: Angiographic classification of patent ductus arteriosus morphology in the dog, *J Vet Cardiol* 8(2):109, 2006.

Nguyenba TP, Tobias AH: Patent ductus arteriosus occlusion with an investigational Amplatzer canine ductal occluder, American College of Veterinary Internal Medicine Forum, Seattle, 2006.

Saunders AB et al: Echocardiographic and angiographic comparison of ductal dimensions in dogs with patent ductus arteriosus, *J Vet Intern Med* 21(1):68, 2007.

Sisson D: Use of a self-expanding occluding stent for nonsurgical closure of patent ductus arteriosus in dogs, *J Am Vet Med Assoc* 223(7):999, 2003.

Smith PJ, Martin MWS: Transcatheter embolisation of patent ductus arteriosus using an Amplatzer vascular plug in six dogs, *J Small Anim Pract* 48:80, 2007.

Snaps FR et al: Treatment of patent ductus arteriosus by placement of intravascular coils in a pup, *J AmVet Med Assoc* 207(6):724, 1995.

CHAPTER 166

Ventricular Septal Defect

REBECCA E. GOMPF, *Knoxville, Tennessee*
JOHN D. BONAGURA, *Columbus, Ohio*

A ventricular septal defect (VSD) is a hole located in the (intra)ventricular septum that allows blood to communicate between the left and right sides of the heart. Essentially all VSDs in dogs and cats are present at birth. The prevalence of VSDs has been estimated to be 7% of dogs and 15% of cats with congenital heart defects. West Highland white terriers, Lakeland terriers, English bulldogs, and English springer spaniels are among the breeds considered at increased risk for VSDs. There are probably both national and regional differences in breed risk for VSDs. This malformation has been identified in isolation and in conjunction with other defects. In closely related English springer spaniels VSD was inherited, but the inheritance pattern was not determined. The finding of a VSD in many breeds is so sporadic that it is difficult to determine if the defect is genetic or simply a failure of normal embryogenesis. Generally no sex predilection has been noted for the development of VSD.

PATHOLOGY AND PATHOPHYSIOLOGY

Most VSDs are located dorsally in or around the membranous portion of the intraventricular septum. The typical defect is "high" and perimembranous, but there are certainly variations in location; appreciation of this point is relevant to auscultation, echocardiographic diagnosis, and catheterization or surgical intervention. The typical VSD is located just below the base of the right or noncoronary cusp of the aortic valve when viewed from the left surface of the ventricular septum. On the right side of the septum the defect is usually adjacent to the cranial edge of the septal tricuspid valve leaflet and just caudoventral to the supraventricular crest that separates the inflow from the outflow tracts. These defects are commonly classified as *perimembranous* or *paramembranous* and in older nomenclature were termed *subcristal* defects. A paramembranous defect can be very large, as with tetralogy of Fallot, encroaching on the supraventricular crest by extending toward the right ventricular outflow tract. Other subaortic defects communicate with the supracristal, subpulmonic portion of the ventricular septum. These holes are termed *supracristal*, *outlet*, *subarterial*, or *doubly-committed* defects, depending on the source. A defect located immediately ventral to the septal tricuspid leaflet is typical of an endocardial cushion defect, a malformation seen most often in cats in conjunction with an atrial septal defect and a common atrioventricular valve leaflet. Defects of the muscular or trabecular ventricular septum are encountered infrequently in dogs and cats, but can be single or multiple and apical or midventricular in location.

The clinical significance of the VSD depends on its size, location, and accompanying malformations. An uncomplicated, isolated VSD leads to left-to-right shunting. Blood flows at high velocity across the defect, moving from the higher-pressure left ventricle into the lower pressure right ventricle. The shunt flow usually enters adjacent to or just below the tricuspid valve. The velocity of shunting typically exceeds 4.5 to 5 m/second, as predicted by the transventricular pressure difference of approximately 100 mm Hg. This flow creates a prominent systolic murmur and the disturbed spectral and color-flow pattern in the right ventricle evident by Doppler echocardiographic studies. The shunt volume crosses the right ventricular outflow tract into the pulmonary artery, using the right ventricle largely as a conduit. From there the extra volume flows into the lungs and returns to the left heart, leading to left-sided volume overload. Small-to-moderate VSDs create cardiomegaly but clinically insignificant volume overload of the left heart. However, with larger defects the recirculated blood considerably increases left atrial and ventricular diastolic volumes and pressures, leading to left heart dilation and sometimes to left ventricular failure. As a result of the increased diastolic volume and associated increase in wall tension, compensatory hypertrophy of the left ventricle occurs over time.

When left-to-right shunts are large or complicated by other left heart defects, left-sided or biventricular congestive heart failure (CHF) may develop. This is especially likely when pulmonary artery flow is 2.5 to three times greater than aortic flow or when substantial aortic or mitral regurgitation is also present. In general, an isolated VSD in a dog or cat does not commonly cause CHF unless the VSD diameter is greater than 60% to 70% of the aortic diameter, and heart failure is more often diagnosed in cats than in dogs. Seemingly most puppies with an uncomplicated defect that survive to see a veterinarian for a first vaccine are "naturally selected" to live a relatively normal life span. This probably relates to the fact that a large VSD should cause CHF very early in life, at the time pulmonary vascular resistance drops. When CHF develops before 6 weeks of age, the consequences are those of a "fading puppy" or one that appears to have died of pneumonia. However, CHF can occur in older puppies or even later in life. This is especially likely when a large paramembranous or a subarterial VSD allows the aortic root to prolapse. The subsequent loss of valvular support can allow progressively severe aortic regurgitation. This additional volume overload to the left ventricle predisposes to CHF.

The effects of a VSD on the right heart and pulmonary circulation are variable and related to defect size and

748

location, pulmonary valve function, pulmonary vascular reactivity, and ventricular myocardial response. Generally speaking, the larger and less restrictive a VSD, the more likely the two ventricles will function as a common chamber with systolic and diastolic pressures beginning to equalize. This situation promotes significant right ventricular enlargement and hypertrophy. If right ventricular outflow is normal and pulmonary vascular resistance remains low, there is marked left-to-right shunting with pulmonary overcirculation. This increases the likelihood of left-sided or biventricular CHF. Pulmonary hypertension can occur in this setting, but it is mainly related to increased pulmonary blood flow along with left heart failure. Radiographs show a dilated main pulmonary artery and prominent pulmonary vascularity. In other animals with large shunts, the increased pulmonary blood flow damages the vasculature, increasing pulmonary vascular resistance markedly (Eisenmenger's physiology). This leads to high-resistance pulmonary hypertension, which increases the pressure load on the right ventricle and creates a thickened chamber. This reduces left-to-right shunting and promotes bidirectional or predominantly right-to-left shunting. In these cases the proximal pulmonary arteries may be dilated, but the peripheral vascular tree appears undercirculated radiographically. These patients develop clinical signs similar to those observed with tetralogy of Fallot described briefly in the following paragraph.

Although this chapter is focused on the isolated VSD, other cardiac lesions may be evident that alter the pathophysiology, clinical findings, and management approaches. In addition to severe aortic regurgitation and Eisenmenger's physiology described previously, two other obstructive conditions of the right ventricle can complicate a VSD. One of these is the tetralogy of Fallot, in which a large unrestricted VSD is complicated by right ventricular outflow tract obstruction and severe concentric hypertrophy of the ventricle. The second condition is the so-called double-chamber right ventricle, which is characterized by fibromuscular reaction and proliferation within the right ventricular cavity. This creates a midventricular obstruction just distal to the VSD in most cases, and the proliferation may actually close the defect, leaving only midventricular obstruction. Progressive tissue growth can cause severe obstruction, and high pressures in the proximal right ventricle lead to concentric hypertrophy in the proximal chamber. In both cases right-to-left or biventricular shunting may predominate. As a result of right-to-left shunting, both hypoxemia and secondary polycythemia can develop. A similar situation can occur in dogs or cats with VSD and severe pulmonic valvular stenosis or in the rare case in which the flow turbulence promotes progressive subpulmonic obstruction.

DIAGNOSIS

Signalment and Clinical Findings

Most cases of VSD are identified during the initial vaccination examination of puppies and kittens. Any breed may be affected; but English springer spaniels, West Highland white terriers, and Lakeland terriers seem predisposed.

In cats VSD is one of the more common congenital heart defects.

Most puppies and kittens with VSD are asymptomatic. However, puppies with large defects or with significant pulmonary hypertension are likely to have signs related to exercise intolerance. Respiratory problems such as coughing and dyspnea may indicate left heart failure. Cats with CHF are lethargic and dyspneic. Puppies with biventricular failure may develop ascites, whereas kittens are more likely to show pleural effusion.

The physical examination is remarkable for the presence of a murmur that is typically loud and often associated with a precordial thrill. Blood forced through a small VSD during systole causes turbulence in the right ventricular outflow tract and pulmonary artery, which is heard as a harsh, blowing systolic murmur over the right sternal border (just ventral to the tricuspid area). The murmur can radiate widely, including to the mitral area. In subpulmonic defects the murmur is louder at the left cranial sternal border and over the pulmonary artery. A VSD can close partially or fully because of adherence of the septal tricuspid leaflet or tissue proliferation; and during this process the shunt flow may be diverted caudally or cranially, leading to systolic murmurs in unexpected precordial locations. This finding is also the case when double-chamber right ventricle complicates a VSD. In larger defects there may also be a harsh, systolic murmur over the lower left base (pulmonic area) because of relative pulmonic stenosis caused by an increased volume of blood flowing through a normal-size valve. A diastolic murmur over the left heart base indicates aortic regurgitation caused by prolapse of the aortic valve.

Radiography

The size and shape of the heart on thoracic radiographs varies, depending on the size of the VSD. With small VSDs there is mild left atrial and left ventricular enlargement with some overcirculation of the lungs, which is seen as enlarged pulmonary veins and arteries and prominent small vessels (that may be misinterpreted as increased interstitial opacities). As the size of the VSD increases, so does the size of the left heart, and the right heart becomes more likely to enlarge as well. Pulmonary overcirculation should be commensurate with the magnitude of shunting but can be reduced by reactive pulmonary vascular change. The main pulmonary artery and lobar branches are dilated with high shunt volumes or in cases of pulmonary hypertension. With high-resistance pulmonary hypertension, the main pulmonary artery segment and proximal pulmonary arteries are dilated but the smaller vessels or veins are not.

Echocardiography and Doppler Studies

The changes found on the echocardiogram also depend on the location and size of the VSD, pulmonary vascular resistance, and accompanying lesions (see Pathology and Pathophysiology earlier in the chapter). The larger the VSD, the greater the volume overload of the left heart and the greater the dilation of the left ventricle and left atrium. With moderate-to-large VSDs, there is usually right heart enlargement as well. Right ventricular hypertrophy occurs when pulmonary vascular pressures increase and in cases of concurrent right ventricular outflow or midventricular obstruction.

The left heart responds to a chronic volume overload by dilating and then hypertrophying so that the thickness of the left ventricular wall and septum may be normal or slightly increased on echocardiography. The fractional shortening may increase initially in response to the left ventricular volume overload. However, a moderate-to-severe chronic volume overload of the left heart eventually results in decreased fractional shortening because of left ventricular dysfunction.

Imaging of an isolated VSD generally can be accomplished in the long axis view with the defect located just below the aortic valve on the left ventricular surface of the septum. On the right side the VSD is usually just ventral to the septal insertion of the tricuspid valve. The edges of the defect are sometimes quite bright. The short axis view at the base of the aorta should be used to decide where the defect enters the right ventricle. In cases of subarterial (subpulmonic) defects, the hole is not evident in long axis images but should appear readily in short or angled views.

To prevent misinterpretation of "echo drop-out," Doppler studies should be used to confirm the presence of the VSD, especially small lesions. Color is also best for finding muscular or apical defects. For a paramembranous defect, the long- or short-axis views from the right side show a jet of blood moving toward the transducer. On the short-axis view disturbed flow is also observed in the right ventricular outflow tract during systole.

Continuous-wave (CW) Doppler can measure the velocity of the blood flow through the VSD. The smaller the VSD, the higher the velocity of flow because of the greater differences in systolic pressures between the left ventricle ($\approx$120 mm Hg) and the right ventricle ($\approx$20 mm Hg). This usual 100 mm Hg pressure differential between the two ventricles produces a CW velocity of around 5 m/second, assuming good alignment to flow and no obstructive lesions on the right side that would increase right ventricular pressure. Small VSDs that maintain a normal pressure gradient and create little hemodynamic burden are generally called *restrictive* defects. Low-velocity diastolic shunting is also observed in most cases. The larger the VSDs, the smaller the pressure difference between the ventricles. The velocity of blood flow crossing a large VSD is much lower. Thus the peak shunting velocity of the blood flow through the VSD on CW Doppler is used to help define the size of the VSD.

The degree of pulmonary hypertension with a large VSD can be estimated by subtracting the pressure gradient across the VSD from the systemic blood pressure. The estimate of the right ventricular systolic pressure is equal to the pulmonary artery systolic pressure if pulmonic stenosis is not present. Pulmonary artery pressures less than 30 mm Hg are insignificant. Pressures of $\approx$50 to 80 mm Hg indicate moderate pulmonary hypertension, and pressures greater than 80 mm Hg indicate severe pulmonary hypertension.

Doppler studies should also interrogate any aortic regurgitation or right ventricular obstruction. These complicated cases are best referred to a cardiologist for assessment.

Cardiac Catheterization

Cardiac catheterization is rarely done to diagnose VSD today. However, if a dog is being considered as a surgical candidate, a catheterization may be done to document pulmonary vascular resistance and pulmonary-to-systemic flow ratio. Angiocardiography can further delineate the anatomic location of the VSD. Catheterization procedures are also needed for interventional device closure in which various clam shell or disc devices are used to close the defect without surgery.

TREATMENT

As stated previously, the vast majority of dogs and cats that survive to the first vaccine are unlikely to develop CHF or other complications such as pulmonary vascular disease. Double-chamber right ventricle can occur as a late complication. Patients are best evaluated at least once by a cardiologist, especially when there are complicated anatomic or physiologic issues. Medical therapy and surgical or catheter-based treatments are possible but rarely needed. Some VSDs close spontaneously, often associated with an adherence of the septal tricuspid leaflet or fibromuscular proliferation. Such closure can also create a ventricular septal aneurysm that generally causes no clinical consequence.

Medical Therapy of Ventricular Septal Defects

Small VSDs do not require therapy. Dogs and cats with moderate-to-large VSDs that are not in heart failure can be started on enalapril (0.25 to 0.5 mg/kg q12h) empirically as cardioprotection. However, there are no data to support benefits of such therapy. Patients with left heart failure or biventricular failure should be treated as any other volume-overloaded hearts with furosemide, enalapril, spironolactone, and pimobendan or digoxin (see Chapter 171). These patients are also candidates for pulmonary artery banding or more definitive repair.

Dogs with significant pulmonary hypertension due to high vascular resistance are very difficult to treat because the lung damage is not often reversible. Sildenafil (Viagra, 1 to 3 mg/kg orally [PO] q12h) may be helpful in some cases of pulmonary hypertension, but the benefit in dogs with pulmonary hypertension caused by large VSDs is unknown. If prescribed for clinical signs such as exercise intolerance, improvement should be noticed within 2 to 4 weeks.

Surgical Therapy of Ventricular Septal Defects

The two surgical options for VSDs are pulmonary artery banding, which reduces left-to-right shunting and the risk of CHF, and definitive closure of the defect. Pulmonary artery banding should be done only after consultation with a cardiologist. It is important to band for evidence of severe shunting or incipient CHF, not simply cardiomegaly, which occurs with even small-to-moderate left-to-right shunts. Definitive closure of a VSD requires open heart surgery using a right atrial or right ventricular approach, and this is limited to only a few referral centers. For more details see Section VIII on Evolve.

Transcatheter Closure of Ventricular Septal Defects

Several reports (Fujii et al., 2004; Shimizu et al., 2005) have detailed successful closure of small-to-moderate perimembranous VSDs with various transcatheter devices. Although detachable coils designed for closure of patent ductus arteriosus have been used, it is uncertain whether such defects even require closure. For larger, more significant holes, transcatheter devices with two discs are used. These can be delivered in larger dogs using traditional catheterization methods or through "hybrid" procedures in which a thoracotomy is used to deliver the system across the ventricle, but without need for cardiopulmonary bypass.

Management of Right-to-Left Shunting Ventricular Septal Defect

When VSD is complicated by right ventricular outflow obstruction or high pulmonary vascular resistance, CHF is rare; exercise intolerance, reversed shunting with hypoxemia, and polycythemia are more likely outcomes. Often animals with a sedentary lifestyle tolerate this disease for 5 or more years. Exercise creates vasodilation in skeletal muscle and increases tissue oxygen demands; accordingly, most affected animals have signs of tachypnea and exercise intolerance with exertion. Sudden death is common consequent to progressive hypoxemia, polycythemia, and cardiac arrhythmias. Any drug that causes systemic vasodilation should be avoided in these patients because right-to-left shunting can be exacerbated.

β-Blockage with the nonspecific β-blocker propranolol (starting at 0.25 mg/kg PO q8h and up-titrating over 4 weeks to 1 mg/kg PO q8h) may be beneficial by reducing exercise-induced right ventricle hypercontractility in tetralogy of Fallot since dynamic right ventricular outflow obstruction can be present. Theoretically the β_2-blocking effect should benefit by preventing some exercise-induced peripheral vasodilation.

Definitive surgical treatment for tetralogy of Fallot includes closure of the VSD and removal or bypass of the stenosis under cardiopulmonary bypass. Palliative surgery involves creation of an extracardiac shunt between the systemic and pulmonary circulations (e.g., Blalock-Tausig

shunt). Such shunts increase pulmonary flow, improve arterial saturation, and can produce significant clinical improvement. The major limitation is the extent to which these shunts will remain patent. Aspirin or another drug that inhibits platelet activation (such as clopidogrel) is indicated. Shunts are not an option when a reversed VSD is caused by pulmonary hypertension because the high pulmonary resistance obviates the value of the surgically created shunt. Partial balloon valvuloplasty of a stenotic pulmonary valve can reduce right ventricular pressures, but complete resolution of the pulmonic stenosis allows marked left-to-right shunting and will likely be fatal.

Medical management of polycythemia associated with right-to-left shunting may be necessary. Phlebotomy can be useful. A packed cell volume of 62% to 65% often is well tolerated, but values exceeding 68% to 70% are likely to cause exercise difficulties or predispose to thrombotic stroke or sudden death. When the need for phlebotomy becomes too frequent, bone marrow suppression can be attempted using hydroxyurea (10 to 20 mg/kg PO daily). This therapy may not work; and side effects, including anorexia, gastrointestinal disturbances, and skin rash can limit tolerability of the drug. A complete blood count and platelet count should be performed regularly when treating with this drug.

References and Suggested Reading

Bonagura JD, Lehmkuhl LB: Congenital heart disease. In Fox PR, Sisson D, Moise NS, editors: *Textbook of canine and feline cardiology*, ed 2, Philadelphia, 1999, Saunders, p. 471.

Boon JA: *Manual of veterinary echocardiography*. Baltimore, 1998, Williams & Wilkins, p 383.

Buchanan JW: Prevalence of cardiovascular disorders. In Fox PR, Sisson D, Moise NS, editors: *Textbook of canine and feline cardiology*, ed 2, Philadelphia, 1999, Saunders, p 457.

Fujii Y et al: Transcatheter closure of congenital ventricular septal defects in 3 dogs with a detachable coil, *J Vet Intern Med* 18:911, 2004.

Koffas H et al: Double-chambered right ventricle in 9 cats, *J Vet Intern Med* 21:76, 2007.

Shimizu M et al: Percutaneous transcatheter coil embolization of a ventricular septal defect in a dog, *J Am Vet Med Assoc* 226:69, 2005.

Thomas WP: Echocardiographic diagnosis of congenital membranous ventricular septal aneurysm in the dog and cat, *J Am Anim Hosp Assoc* 41:215, 2005.

CHAPTER 167

Pulmonic Stenosis

AMARA ESTRADA, *Gainesville, Florida*

Pulmonic stenosis (PS) is one of the most common congenital heart defects seen in dogs. Obstruction can occur anywhere along the right ventricular (RV) outflow tract into the main pulmonary artery. The lesion can be subvalvular, valvular, or supravalvular. Pulmonary valvular stenosis caused by commissural fusion of thin to moderately thickened valves that creates a dome-shaped valve is one type of PS. However, valvular stenosis caused by pulmonary valve dysplasia is different from the fused valve with a central orifice. Valvular dysplasia consists of markedly thickened valve leaflets with or without annular hypoplasia and fusion of the commissures. Most commonly, both types of stenosis are found to coexist whereby the valve is clearly dysplastic, but also exhibits degrees of commissural fusion. Pulmonary valvular stenosis can also occur in combination with a subvalvular fibrous or supravalvular ring. In English bulldogs and boxers, subvalvular stenosis may be caused by an anomalous origin of the left coronary artery. In these patients a single large coronary artery originates from the right aortic sinus (of Valsalva) and then divides into the left and right main branches. The left coronary artery then encircles the main pulmonary artery just below the valve, causing a subvalvular obstruction.

DIAGNOSIS

The diagnosis of PS can be made with reasonable certainty using knowledge of breed predilection, physical examination findings, and some simple diagnostic tools found in most veterinary hospitals. A presumptive diagnosis can easily be made following physical examination and electrocardiographic and radiographic evaluations. After this, echocardiography is used to make a definitive diagnosis, determine disease severity, identify any concurrent cardiac abnormalities, and guide treatment recommendations.

Breeds Affected

PS is most commonly encountered in terrier breeds, English bulldogs, Samoyeds, Chihuahuas, miniature schnauzers, Labrador retrievers, mastiffs, chow-chows, Newfoundlands, basset hounds, and cocker spaniels and is inherited in the beagle.

Clinical Signs

Most dogs with PS are asymptomatic as puppies. Most often auscultation of a cardiac murmur during a routine examination is the first clue that PS might be present. Clinical signs are more likely to occur in dogs older than 1 year of age. Symptoms may develop earlier in dogs with extremely severe stenosis or with the presence of other congenital cardiac abnormalities such as a patent foramen ovale (PFO), atrial septal defect (ASD), ventricular septal defect (VSD) or tricuspid valve dysplasia.

Initial clinical signs are related to low cardiac output, including exercise intolerance and shortness of breath. Dogs with extremely severe stenosis can have exertional dyspnea and syncope caused by the inability of the right ventricle to increase its output in response to exercise or excitement. Arrhythmias and reflex-mediated syncope are other causes for collapse; sudden death is a rare complication but has been reported. Signs of right-sided congestive heart failure (ascites, peripheral edema, pleural effusion) usually occur later in the course of the disease but can occur earlier in patients with concurrent tricuspid valve dysplasia or with development of atrial fibrillation. Right-to-left shunting of blood can occur in patients with an atrial or ventricular communication such as a PFO, an ASD, or a VSD. Cyanosis and polycythemia are usually minimal unless a large defect is present. Growth is usually normal in patients with PS, regardless of the severity of the obstruction.

Physical Examination Findings

Auscultation of a dog with PS allows detection of a left-sided systolic murmur heard best at the heart base. In general, the intensity of the murmur increases with the severity of obstruction. The murmur is described as a classic ejection-sounding, harsh murmur with a crescendo or crescendo-decrescendo quality. Rarely a diastolic murmur of pulmonic insufficiency can also be heard. Occasionally a pulmonary ejection click is heard. The click corresponds to the time when the doming pulmonary valve reaches its open position and snaps open. Jugular veins are usually normal in dogs with PS, but a prominent A wave is sometimes observed. However, with concurrent tricuspid valve dysplasia moderate-to-severe jugular distention or pulses can be identified. In cases with concurrent tricuspid dysplasia a murmur is also auscultated over the right apical region. The murmur associated with tricuspid valve insufficiency is more blowing in character than the PS murmur. Femoral pulse quality is usually normal in dogs with PS.

Electrocardiographic Findings

The electrocardiogram (ECG) may be normal in dogs with mild PS and therefore may be somewhat useful in assessing severity of obstruction. Dogs with more moderate-to-severe PS and RV hypertrophy usually have electrocardiographic evidence of right-sided enlargement (right axis deviation; deep S waves in leads I, II, III and aVF; prominent S waves in left-sided chest leads).

Radiographic Findings

Thoracic radiographs are very useful for supporting the clinical diagnosis of PS. However, it should be noted that, just as with the ECG, radiographs in mild cases of PS may be completely normal. Radiographs in dogs with moderate-to-severe PS usually demonstrate a prominent right ventricle and poststenotic dilation of the main pulmonary artery. Poststenotic dilation of the main pulmonary artery can be seen on a lateral view but is most impressive on a dorsoventral view. The pulmonary vasculature and parenchyma are usually normal, although sometimes they may appear undercirculated, especially in cases of right and left shunting.

Echocardiographic Findings

Obstruction in the RV outflow tract causes an increased resistance to flow and an increase in RV systolic pressure. The magnitude of increase in RV pressure depends on the severity of obstruction. The more severe the stenosis, the more pressure the right ventricle must generate to overcome the stenosed valve and maintain pulmonary perfusion. The response of the right ventricle to this pressure overload is concentric hypertrophy.

Two-Dimensional Echocardiography

Two-dimensional echocardiography allows for subjective evaluation of the severity of stenosis. Typical features of PS can be demonstrated clearly from both the right-sided long-axis and short-axis views (Fig. 167-1). In general, the thicker the right ventricle, the more severe the stenosis is likely to be. Concentric hypertrophy of the

right ventricle, narrowing in the region of the pulmonary valve, and poststenotic dilation of the pulmonary artery are hallmarks of PS. In severe cases septal flattening may occur as RV systolic pressure becomes higher than left ventricular systolic pressure (see Fig 167-1). Dogs with severe PS may also have hyperechoic regions visible within the right ventricle or septum related to areas of ischemia and fibrosis.

Three features of valvular stenosis that occur to varying degrees are: fusion of leaflets, valve thickening, and hypoplasia of the annular region. Valve leaflets may appear prominent because of thickening. Systolic motion of the valve leaflets is restricted, with inward curving of the tips of the leaflets known as *doming* apparent in stenosed but mobile valves. Dysplastic valves often appear very thickened and can be immobile, without the characteristic doming seen with the "typical" valvular stenosis of children. Poststenotic dilation of the pulmonary artery may be absent, and the pulmonary annulus may be hypoplastic in cases of valve dysplasia. The distinction between the two types of stenosis is often not clear, and pathologic features of both forms are usually present. For prognostic reasons dysplastic valves should be assessed for mobility, commissural fusion, and hypoplasia. Hypoplasia and immobile valves are likely to respond less favorably to interventional therapy.

Evidence of dynamic infundibular stenosis caused by hypertrophy may also be seen on two-dimensional evaluation. During systole, as the walls of the hypertrophied infundibulum come together, obstruction in this region can occur in addition to the valvular obstruction (Fig. 167-2). The severity of this dynamic stenosis may be impossible to estimate, but it is important to identify it before interventional procedures because this type of stenosis can become acutely more severe following balloon valvuloplasty and may require β-adrenergic blockade (see discussion of suicide right ventricle in the section on Therapy later in the chapter).

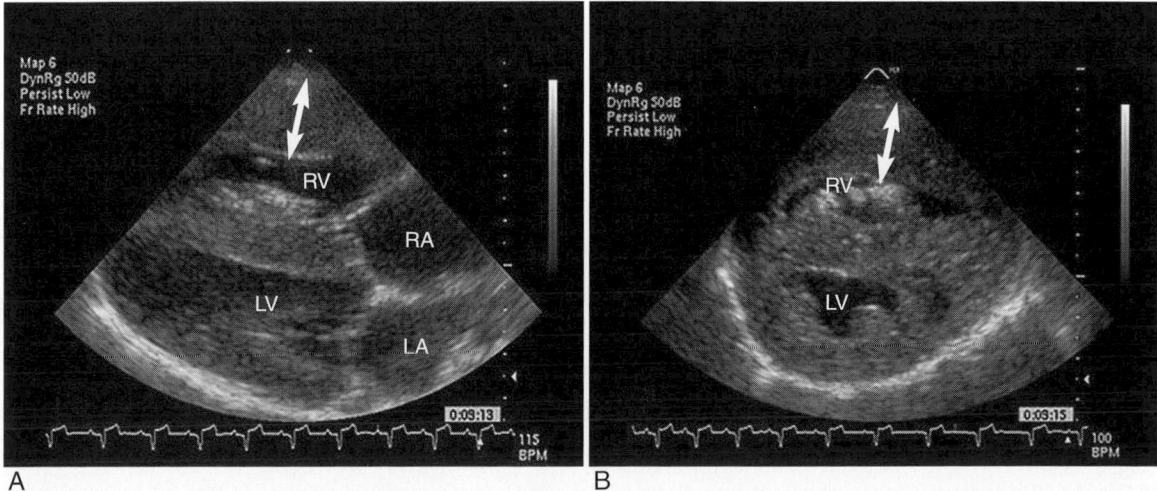

Fig. 167-1 Echocardiographic images from a dog with severe pulmonic stenosis. **A,** Right-sided four-chamber long-axis view, and **B,** right-sided short-axis view. Both echocardiographic images show dramatic right ventricular hypertrophy *(arrows)* and evidence of septal flattening, indicating higher right than left ventricular pressure. Notice also the increased echogenicity of the papillary muscles of the right ventricle, indicating probable ischemia of this portion of the myocardium. This degree of hypertrophy and septal flattening would be a typical appearance for a dog with severe pulmonic stenosis.

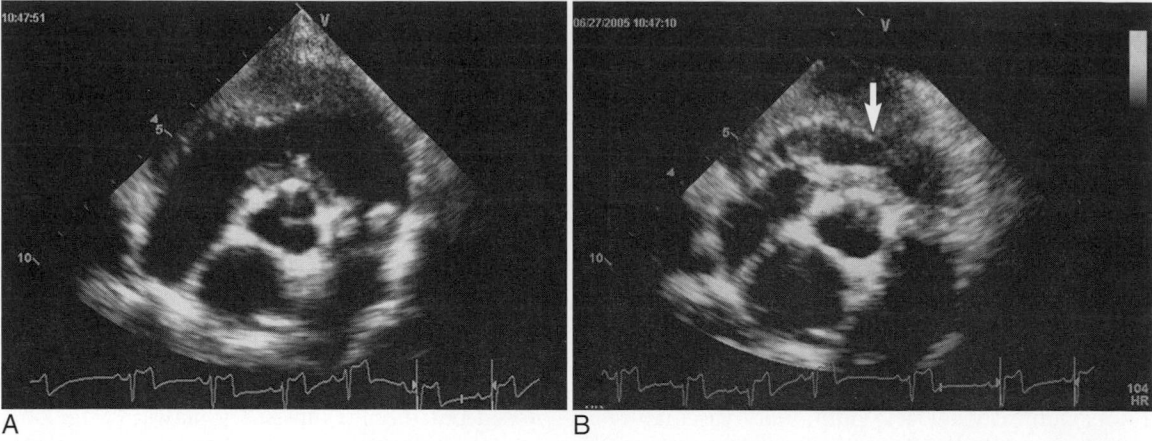

Fig. 167-2 Echocardiographic images from a dog with severe pulmonic stenosis; short axis images obtained at the level of the pulmonary valve. The pulmonary valve is severely thickened and dysplastic. There is no evidence of poststenotic dilation of the pulmonary artery beyond the dysplastic valve. The annulus is normal in size. During diastole **(A)** the infundibular or subvalvular region is open without evidence of subvalvular obstruction. However, during systole **(B)** the walls of the hypertrophied infundibulum come together and may create a dynamic subvalvular obstruction *(arrow)*. In some patients with significant infundibular hypertrophy, this subvalvular gradient can become acutely more severe following dilation of the stenosed pulmonary valve. This condition, termed *suicide right ventricle*, can occur immediately following balloon valvuloplasty. Right ventricular pressures dramatically increase as the hypertrophied infundibulum creates subvalvular obstruction that can sometimes become worse than the valvular obstruction.

Doppler Evaluation

Doppler echocardiography is useful in readily visualizing the turbulence that is created as blood flow encounters the stenosed valve. It can also help in recognizing dynamic obstruction, pinpointing exact locations of obstruction, and identifying any pulmonic insufficiency present. However, the major use of Doppler echocardiography is in determining the velocity of blood flow as it crosses the stenosed valve. Two-dimensional echocardiography allows for subjective and qualitative assessment of severity, whereas Doppler allows objective and quantitative assessment of the severity. Using the modified Bernoulli equation

$$\Delta \text{ pressure} = 4V^2$$

the measured velocity across the stenosed valve can be calculated into a pressure gradient across the valve. Gradients can be thought of as the difference in pressure between two chambers. In a normal dog without PS there is essentially no gradient across the pulmonary valve since systolic pressure in the right ventricle is equal to systolic pressure in the pulmonary artery. However, when the pulmonary valve is stenosed, the RV must generate enough pressure to overcome the obstruction and maintain pulmonary blood flow and systolic blood pressure.

For example, in a dog with PS, a velocity of 5.5 m/second is recorded (Fig. 167-3). This is calculated to equal a gradient of 121 mm Hg (Δ pressure = $4(5.5)^2$ = 121 mm Hg). Assuming that PA pressures are normal at about 25 mm Hg (121 mm Hg + 25 mm Hg), the right ventricle has a pressure burden of 146 mm Hg (versus a normal systolic pressure of 25 mm Hg).

For accurate measurement the echo beam must be aligned as parallel as possible with the main pulmonary artery trunk or in the direction of the flow seen on color Doppler. If the beam is not parallel, underestimation of

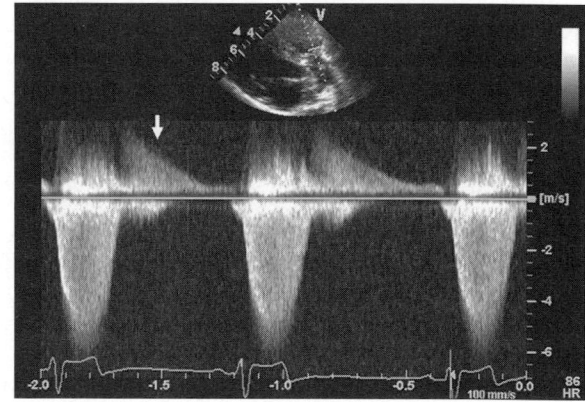

Fig. 167-3 Doppler interrogation in a dog with severe pulmonic stenosis. Pulmonic insufficiency *(arrow)* is also seen.

the severity of stenosis occurs. If tricuspid insufficiency is present, the same Doppler technique can be used to calculate the pressure difference between the right atrium and right ventricle by measuring the peak velocity of the tricuspid insufficiency jet. RV pressure then can be estimated by adding the pressure gradient to the estimated right atrial pressure. Echocardiographic-derived Doppler estimates of systolic pressure have shown very good correlation with invasive pressure measurements when done simultaneously.

Color Doppler imaging demonstrates an abnormal flow pattern originating at the stenotic valve. Normal flow is coded as red or blue, depending on whether it is directed toward or away from the transducer, respectively. High-velocity, turbulent flow through a stenotic valve appears as a mosaic of color or a turbulence encoding (often yellow or green). Visualization of the jet by color Doppler also facilitates optimal alignment of the Doppler beam, allowing for more accurate pressure gradient estimations. Color Doppler may also identify complicating factors, including atrial or ventricular shunts, tricuspid regurgitation, or dynamic obstruction in the *left* ventricular outlet related to altered ventricular geometry.

Classification of Disease Severity

In patients with relatively normal cardiac output, grading of lesion severity is based on RV pressure and valve gradient. The tighter the stenosis, the higher the RV pressure and valve gradient. Most cardiologists use the following Doppler-derived peak transvalvular pulmonary valve gradients to classify the severity of the stenosis:

- Mild: Doppler gradient up to 40 to 50 mm Hg
- Moderate: Doppler gradient between 40 and 80 (to 100) mm Hg
- Severe: Doppler gradient greater than 80 (to 100) mm Hg

TREATMENT

Firm guidelines for deciding which animals need to be treated have not been developed. In pediatric cardiology most interventionalists agree that treatment should be performed in any child with moderate stenosis or a gradient greater than 40 mm Hg. Most veterinary cardiologists would agree that animals with gradients in the severe range should be treated. The decision as to whether to treat dogs with moderate stenosis is not as clear. Many factors can be taken into consideration when making this decision such as degree of RV hypertrophy, presence of clinical signs, and severity of concurrent tricuspid insufficiency. However, it is my opinion that therapy should always be offered and recommended for any patient with a gradient over 60 mm Hg.

Medical Therapy

Medical therapy is of little benefit unless signs of right-sided congestive heart failure are present. In these cases standard therapy for heart failure is recommended in addition to, not in lieu of, interventional therapy. β-blockers such as atenolol (0.5 to 1 mg/1kg PO q12h) can be used in attempts to reduce arrhythmias, infundibular gradient, dynamic left ventricular outflow gradient, and syncopal events and to prevent sudden death. β-blockage is variable in terms of benefit and does not overcome the primary lesion.

Therapy

Pulmonary balloon valvuloplasty is the first line of treatment for PS. Valvuloplasty should be performed in any symptomatic patient as soon as PS is diagnosed. Even asymptomatic patients should be treated as soon as possible. Delay in treatment can lead to progression of RV and infundibular hypertrophy, not only making the procedure technically more difficult but also diminishing the immediate response to therapy. In fact, in some patients with significant infundibular hypertrophy, this subvalvular gradient can become acutely more severe following dilation of the stenosed pulmonary valve. This condition,

termed *suicide right ventricle*, occurs immediately following relief of severely stenosed valves. RV pressures dramatically increase as the hypertrophied infundibulum creates subvalvular obstruction that can sometimes become worse than the valvular obstruction. Therapy with intravenous β-blockers (esmolol 0.05 to 0.5 mg/kg slowly IV as a bolus) and volume loading of the right ventricle with intravenous fluid boluses can improve or alleviate this subvalvular obstruction.

As described previously, subvalvular PS in English bulldogs and boxers can be caused by an anomalous left coronary artery. Recognition of this abnormality on echocardiographic or angiographic studies is imperative because balloon dilation in these patients has been reported to cause rupture of the artery and sudden death of the patient. Balloon dilation in these patients is risky, and surgical conduit placement around the stenosis may be the only alternative. Less aggressive balloon dilation may also be performed in dogs with severe stenosis, right-sided congestive heart failure, or other clinical signs; but this procedure carries the same risks.

Interventional catheter-based procedures should only be performed by veterinarians with advanced training in these techniques. The technique for pulmonary balloon valvuloplasty involves placement of a dilation balloon across the stenosed valve. The entire procedure is performed under fluoroscopic guidance. A balloon that is 1.2 to 1.5 times the measured pulmonary annulus (from either echocardiographic or angiographic studies) is most often used. The balloon is placed from either a jugular or femoral vein using a vascular cutdown or percutaneous approach. Once the balloon is positioned across the stenosed valve, it is inflated with fluid under pressure to stretch or break open the valve. The balloon is kept inflated for only a few seconds. Multiple inflation-deflations are performed until a satisfactory degree of dilation is achieved. When the balloon is inflated initially, there is an indentation in the balloon at the region of the stenotic valve. This is called a *waist*. Successful dilation is achieved with visualization of a loss of this waist during inflation. On successful balloon dilation RV pressures and valve gradients decrease. This decrease following dilation can be detected immediately with intracardiac pressure monitoring. In pediatric cardiology a good outcome is defined as a residual Doppler gradient of 35 mm Hg or less. In veterinary cardiology reduction of the gradient to 50% of the original value is generally thought of as successful. Complete resolution of gradients across the valve in these patients is not possible because most valves are somewhat dysplastic and always cause at least some obstruction to flow. Accurate assessment of results requires evaluation of Doppler-derived gradients or gradients indexed to stroke volume in the ensuing weeks to months after catheterization.

Serious complications that can occur during this procedure are rare but include cardiac perforation causing pericardial effusion and tamponade, rupture of the pulmonary artery, suicide right ventricle, and fatal arrhythmias. Minor complications that occur with more frequency include damage to the tricuspid valve, creation of a right bundle branch block, temporary arrhythmias, and hemorrhage from vascular access sites. These latter complications are rarely clinically important, and most patients are discharged from the hospital the following day.

Follow Up

Short Term

Intracardiac pressure measurements are usually taken immediately before and after balloon dilation to guide therapeutic decisions. If the gradient or RV pressure has not decreased satisfactorily and there is not dynamic obstruction to explain the gradient, a larger balloon may be placed, and the procedure repeated.

Echocardiographic studies are performed the day following the procedure. Repeat of all measurements are made, with specific attention to valvular gradients and amount of pulmonary insufficiency and tricuspid insufficiency. Pulmonary insufficiency is virtually always increased following balloon valvuloplasty but is well tolerated by the right ventricle. However, tricuspid insufficiency is usually diminished because of the drop in the RV pressure created by the valvuloplasty procedure. Gradients measured the day after the procedure may not show as dramatic a drop as those measured immediately following the procedure. Pulmonary valve leaflets become swollen and edematous following balloon dilation and may temporarily increase the measured gradient until the swelling has subsided. Furthermore, stroke volume greatly influences gradients and is typically lower in dogs under general anesthesia.

Long Term

Long-term follow-up studies in pediatric cardiology show excellent results. Several recent veterinary studies have also shown that pulmonary balloon valvuloplasty significantly reduces valvular gradients and clinical signs in dogs with PS. Recheck evaluations are typically performed 3 and 6 months after the valvuloplasty procedure and then annually. Gradients can continue to decline in the first 3 to 6 months and possibly even longer as resolution of valve edema and regression of RV/infundibular hypertrophy occurs. Therefore determination of whether a valvuloplasty procedure has been successful should not be judged until several months following the procedure. Some cardiologists continue β-blockade in dogs with residual hypertrophy and dynamic RV outflow obstruction.

Suggested Reading

Brownlie SE et al: Percutaneous balloon valvuloplasty in four dogs with pulmonic stenosis, *J Small Anim Pract* 32:165, 1991.

Buchanan JW: Pulmonic stenosis caused by a single coronary artery in dogs: four cases (1965-1984), *J Am Vet Med Assoc* 196:115, 1990.

Bussadori C: Balloon valvuloplasty in 30 dogs with pulmonic stenosis: effect of valve morphology and annular size on initial and 1-year outcome, *J Vet Intern Med* 15:6, 2001.

Estrada AH, Moise NS, Renaud-Farrell S: When, how and why to perform a double ballooning technique for dogs with valvular pulmonic stenosis, *J Vet Cardiol* 7:1, 2005.

Estrada AH et al: Prospective evaluation of the balloon:anulus ratio for valvuloplasty in the treatment of pulmonic stenosis in the dog, *J Vet Intern Med* 20:4, 2006.

Johnson MS: Pulmonic stenosis in dogs: balloon dilation improves clinical outcome, *J Vet Intern Med* 18:5, 2004.

Johnson MS, Martin M: Results of balloon valvuloplasty in 40 dogs with pulmonic stenosis, *J Small Anim Pract* 45:3, 2004.

Martin MWS et al: Assessment of balloon pulmonary valvuloplasty in six dogs, *J Small Anim Pract* 33:443, 1992.

Sisson DD, MacCoy DM: Treatment of congenital pulmonic stenosis in two dogs by balloon valvuloplasty, *J Vet Intern Med* 2:92, 1988.

CHAPTER 168

Subaortic Stenosis

R. LEE PYLE, *Blacksburg, Virginia*
JONATHAN A. ABBOTT, *Blacksburg, Virginia*

Subaortic stenosis (SAS) resulting from a fibrous lesion that partially or completely encircles the subvalvular outflow tract is one of the most common cardiac malformations in the dog. Planned breeding experiments confirmed that SAS in Newfoundlands is heritable (Pyle, Patterson, and Chacko, 1976); and based on observed breed predispositions, it is likely that canine SAS generally has a genetic basis. The severity of the stenosis and associated clinical consequences vary widely. Dogs with severe SAS are at high risk of complications, including sudden death; but mild SAS seldom is responsible for morbidity or mortality.

The diagnosis of moderate or severe SAS generally is straightforward, although antemortem identification of mildly affected individuals can be difficult. SAS has been treated both medically with catheter-based methods and surgically, but evidence of efficacy for any specific management strategy currently is lacking.

ETIOLOGY

Studies performed during the 1970s confirmed that SAS in Newfoundlands has a genetic basis (Pyle, Patterson, and Chacko, 1976). The mode of inheritance was not completely defined, but the results of planned breeding experiments suggest that SAS is either a polygenic trait or an autosomal-dominant trait that is subject to modification by other genes or environmental factors. Because inheritance of SAS is not explained by simple Mendelian genetics, dogs with mild SAS may have severely affected offspring. As a result, detection of mild SAS is important despite the fact that mild outflow tract obstruction usually does not have clinical consequences.

SAS is observed most often in large- and giant-breed dogs. The German shepherd, boxer, golden retriever, Newfoundland, and rottweiler are all predisposed to the development of SAS. Mongrels are less likely to develop SAS than are purebred dogs, further suggesting that canine SAS is a genetic disorder. In recent years SAS has been identified in *many* other breeds.

PATHOLOGY

The subvalvular lesion is fibrous or fibrocartilaginous. In the mildest form of SAS the lesion consists of subvalvular nodules, and these cases may be clinically silent. More severe forms of SAS result in outflow tract obstruction caused by a ridge that partially or completely encircles the subvalvular left ventricular outflow tract (LVOT) (Fig. 168-1). The most severe forms consist of plaque or tunnel lesions that involve a large area of the LVOT (Fig. 168-2).

In pathologic studies of SAS in the Newfoundland, subvalvular lesions were detected only in pups that were older than 3 weeks. Based on this finding, SAS is not strictly congenital but rather develops early in life. This observation also has been made in humans. It has been speculated that the lesion arises because morphologic abnormalities in the LVOT increase shear stress and induce proliferation of cells in the LVOT (Freedom et al., 2005). In the dog the obstruction may progress for the first 12 months of life; this has important implications for diagnostic screening, genetic counseling, and patient prognosis.

PATHOPHYSIOLOGY

Outflow tract stenosis impedes ventricular ejection. To maintain normal perfusion pressure distal to the stenosis, the left ventricle must generate supraphysiologic systolic pressures. As a result there is a systolic pressure difference, or gradient, across the obstruction. This pressure gradient can be measured by selective catheterization but more often is estimated from Doppler echocardiographic studies. The pressure load that results from high resistance to ventricular ejection is a stimulus for the development of left ventricular concentric hypertrophy. Concentric hypertrophy is an increase in myocardial mass that is associated with a normal or reduced diastolic chamber dimension. As a result the ventricular walls are thick relative to lumen size. SAS is associated with arteriosclerotic lesions of the intramural coronary arteries. Abnormally narrow coronary vessels, large myocardial mass, and left ventricular systolic hypertension contribute to the development of myocardial ischemia, which is likely the predisposition for the ventricular arrhythmias that sometimes complicate SAS. Although a chronic left ventricular pressure load can result in the development of systolic myocardial dysfunction, this is relatively uncommon in dogs with SAS unless it is severe and chronic. Diastolic dysfunction can be shown by advanced Doppler studies.

In general dogs with mild or moderately severe obstructions are at low risk of premature death. However, a few patients in this category develop complications of longstanding SAS, including infective endocarditis and congestive heart failure. Dogs with severe obstruction are at much greater risk for serious sequelae. Sudden unexpected death, presumably the result of lethal ventricular tachyarrhythmia, occurs in the first 2 to 3 years of life in a substantive number of cases (Kienle, Thomas, and Pion, 1994).

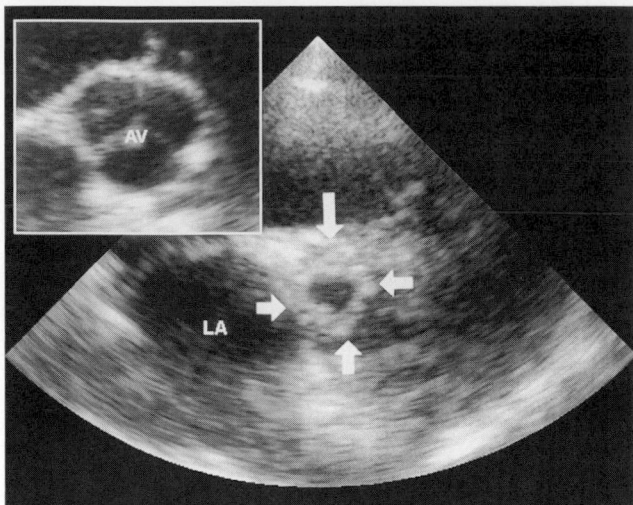

Fig. 168-1 Echocardiogram from an 11-month-old golden retriever with exercise intolerance and a grade IV/VI systolic murmur heard best in the left 4th to 5th intercostal spaces. The sector scan and the insert of the aortic valve (AV) were recorded from the right parasternal short-axis view. Note that the complete subaortic ring *(arrows),* which was immediately below the aortic valve (8 mm), encompasses considerably less area than the aortic valve. This stenosis resulted in a peak systolic pressure gradient of 150 mm Hg as measured by continuous wave Doppler. *LA,* Left atrium.

DIAGNOSTIC APPROACH

There are two distinct goals in the evaluation of patients suspected to have SAS: (1) identification and characterization of LVOT obstruction to provide prognostic information and guide therapy, and (2) elimination of affected dogs from the breeding population.

At the time of initial diagnosis most patients with SAS are asymptomatic; this is true regardless of the severity of obstruction. The history in mildly or moderately affected dogs is unremarkable and reflects normal behavior and activity. In severely affected dogs exercise intolerance, weakness, and syncope are noted occasionally. When left heart failure is present, signs can include coughing, dyspnea, and tachypnea.

In mildly or moderately affected dogs, a grade 1-4/6 systolic murmur can be heard best in the left fourth to fifth intercostal spaces at the costochondral junction. Severely affected dogs usually have a grade 4-6/6 systolic murmur often with a precordial thrill. Typically the murmur radiates widely and can be heard over the right lower hemithorax and in the thoracic inlet. In patients with severe SAS the arterial pulse is usually late rising and weak.

The diagnostic value of electrocardiography and radiography in the evaluation of SAS is low. Dogs with mild or moderate SAS usually have a normal electrocardiogram, but evidence of left ventricular hypertrophy may be detected in severely affected patients. Ventricular arrhythmias, including ventricular premature beats and ventricular tachycardia, are sometimes recorded. Depression of the ST segment suggests myocardial ischemia and is most evident on exercise or ambulatory electrocardiograms.

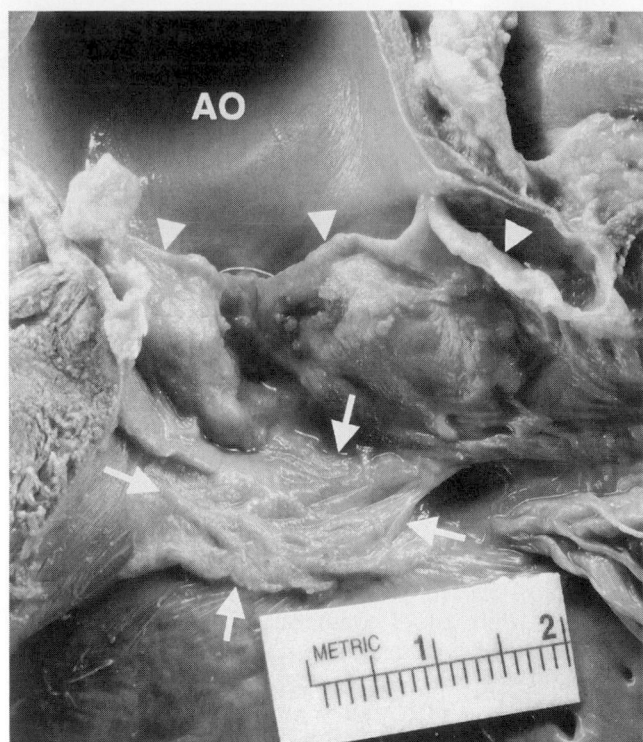

Fig. 168-2 Necropsy specimen from an Irish wolfhound with a plaque/tunnel–type subaortic stenosis (SAS) lesion. This dog developed bacterial endocarditis at 7 months from a urinary tract infection. The effects of the high-velocity SAS jet on the aortic valve leaflets predisposed to the infection. The arrows and the metric define the plaque SAS lesion in the left ventricular outflow tract. The three aortic valve leaflets *(arrowheads)* were thickened, nodular, and rigid. The center of each leaflet had a 2-mm perforation presumably caused by the erosive action of the bacteria. Echocardiographic studies revealed SAS, severe aortic regurgitation, a dilated left ventricle, mild mitral regurgitation, and extensive disease of the aortic valve caused by endocarditis and extension of the plaque material into the base of the aortic valve leaflets. The dog died suddenly at 27 months of age after long-term therapy for endocarditis. *AO,* Ascending aorta.

Thoracic radiographs are of limited value in identifying SAS. Left ventricular enlargement is usually not evident; however, poststenotic dilatation of the ascending aorta may be recognized in severely affected patients.

ECHOCARDIOGRAPY

SAS is an echocardiographic diagnosis. Except in cases for which balloon dilation is considered, echocardiography essentially has eliminated the need for cardiac catheterization for this disease. The subaortic lesion can often be visualized in severely affected dogs (see Fig. 168-1). Although the relationship between severity of obstruction and degree of hypertrophy is inconsistent, there is often echocardiographic evidence of concentric left ventricular hypertrophy in patients in which the lesion is visible. Left ventricular systolic performance evaluated by fractional shortening or ejection fraction is normal to hyperdynamic in most dogs. A few patients, typically those with long-standing SAS, develop ventricular dilation and evidence of systolic myocardial dysfunction.

Doppler echocardiography is required to confirm the presence of LVOT obstruction and provide an indirect assessment of stenosis severity. When a discrete obstruction is present, the resulting pressure gradient is associated with abrupt flow acceleration within the LVOT. The maximal instantaneous systolic pressure gradient (ΔP = mm Hg) across the stenosis is determined by the simplified Bernoulli equation

$$\Delta P = V^2 \times 4$$

where ΔP is the pressure gradient and V is the peak velocity (meters/second) across the LVOT. A gradient of 40 mm Hg or less reflects mild disease, and a gradient greater than 80 mm Hg is considered severe disease by most (Kienle, Thomas, and Pion, 1994). It is important to recognize that the pressure gradient across the LVOT is flow dependent, meaning that the gradient depends not only on the cross-sectional area of the stenotic orifice but also on stroke volume (Bonagura, 2001). Sympathetic activation associated with restraint and disorders such as aortic valve regurgitation or patent ductus arteriosus increase forward stroke volume and therefore peak aortic velocity. On the other hand, factors that decrease stroke volume and peak velocity include myocardial dysfunction, sedatives, anesthetics, and mitral regurgitation. The flow dependence of peak aortic velocity limits the usefulness of pressure gradient as a single index of stenosis severity.

The accuracy of the Doppler velocity estimate is critically dependent on the angle between the ultrasound beam and the direction of blood flow. Peak aortic velocities can be obtained using a caudal left parasternal or subxiphoid transducer site (Lehmkuhl and Bonagura, 1995) In most dogs the subxiphoid site provides superior alignment with the LVOT and is more accurate.

Other echocardiographic abnormalities occasionally are associated with SAS. The caudal border of the LVOT is bounded by the anterior mitral valve leaflet. Severe SAS involves the base of the anterior mitral leaflet, which probably explains the association of mitral dysplasia and SAS. In a few cases dynamic outflow tract obstruction caused by systolic anterior motion of the mitral valve complicates the fixed obstruction that results from the subaortic lesion. Occasionally mitral valve dysplasia creates marked LVOT obstruction and should be included in the differential diagnosis of left ventricular concentric hypertrophy.

IDENTIFYING MILD DISEASE

The diagnosis of moderate or severe SAS is not difficult. Typically imaging (2D) echocardiography reveals distinct abnormalities, and the diagnosis is confirmed and refined by Doppler studies. Identification of mildly affected dogs is a challenge and a source of considerable controversy. Auscultation is the initial method of screening for congenital heart disease. It is important to realize that a few dogs with mild disease are clinically normal in all respects, including auscultation (Pyle, Patterson, and Chacko, 1976). Consequently it is probable that dogs with mild disease occasionally are classified as free of congenital heart disease. In our practice dogs that do not have a murmur are not subject to further diagnostic

investigation. Because SAS may progress during the first 12 months of life, we frequently screen young pups of predisposed breeds but withhold a final determination until the animal is at least 1 year of age.

The prevalence of low-intensity ejection-type murmurs in dogs predisposed to SAS is high, and it seems unlikely that all of these murmurs are associated with LVOT pathology. Sometimes the murmur is intermittent and heard only after long diastolic intervals or alternatively when heart rate increases. Although we do not routinely do so, some examiners perform auscultation when the dog is at rest and again after exercise. The increase in stroke volume associated with exercise may provoke a murmur in patients with mild SAS and increase the sensitivity of auscultation as means to detect disease. However, this practice also amplifies many functional or innocent murmurs. Postexercise auscultation is made difficult by the increase in respiratory sounds. Furthermore, the prevalence of transient, exercise-induced functional murmurs in normal dogs is not known.

Thorough echocardiographic evaluation of dogs with congenital heart disease sometimes requires sedation. When necessary, we use buprenorphine (0.007 mg/kg intravenously [IV]) and acepromazine (0.03 mg/kg IV) because this sedative combination has minimal effects on Doppler variables. When mild SAS is suspected, we avoid sedation to eliminate the cardiodepressive effect of chemical restraint. There is more variability in the level of anxiety experienced by patients that are not sedated, and this needs to be considered when evaluating dogs for SAS.

In patients with mild SAS the outflow tract lesions are small and often impossible to detect using two-dimensional echocardiography. Detection of a velocity step-up during pulsed-wave Doppler interrogation of the LVOT is a characteristic feature of discrete obstruction. In cases in which mild SAS is suspected, this echocardiographic characteristic is seldom distinct, and it must be recognized that small pressure gradients and gradual flow acceleration are evident in normal individuals. Furthermore, the magnitude of acceleration in healthy dogs has not been defined. The detection of a systolic flow disturbance within the proximal aorta is another echocardiographic characteristic of subvalvular obstruction. Unfortunately it is difficult to define Doppler characteristics of disturbed (turbulent) flow objectively. Aortic valve incompetence (AI) is uncommon in normal dogs but is often associated with subaortic obstruction. The cause of AI in patients with SAS is likely multifactorial, but damage to the ventricular surface of the aortic valve leaflets from the high-velocity jet is probably important.

Because it is objective and easily quantified, peak aortic velocity generally is considered to be the primary diagnostic criterion for SAS. Although high velocities can be recorded in the absence of obstruction, the diagnosis of obstruction generally is not tenable when peak velocity is normal. Aortic velocities in most healthy dogs without systolic murmurs are less than 1.9 m/second, and the average velocity is close to 1.3 m/second. Nevertheless, there is an avid debate about the velocity that distinguishes normal dogs from dogs with mild SAS. Because peak velocity is determined by stroke volume and outflow tract geometry, there is a physical basis for high aortic velocities that occur in the absence of obstruction. For example, peak aortic velocities exceeding 2.25 m/second are commonly recorded when healthy dogs are subject to dobutamine infusion. However, the ventricle does not have a normal appearance when these high velocities are recorded. Instead the ventricle is hyperdynamic, and fractional shortening typically is greater than 45%. Similarly, when high aortic velocities are recorded from dogs with patent ductus arteriosus, the ventricle is dilated; and, provided fractional shortening is normal, this is indirect evidence of a large stroke volume. It seems unlikely that an echocardiographically normal ventricle that empties into an aorta of normal diameter will generate velocities that exceed 2.25 m/second. Although some breeds such as the boxer may have a relatively smaller aorta that might predispose to high flow rates, it is very unlikely that there is a *single* minimum velocity that identifies outflow tract obstruction in all cases. However, in our opinion under most circumstances a velocity greater than 2.25 m/second is suggestive of SAS. A velocity that is less than 2.25 m/second but greater than 1.9 m/second is difficult to interpret and represents an equivocal finding in our laboratory. Although Doppler studies do not overestimate velocity, sinus arrhythmia can cause marked variability in aortic velocities; therefore the use of an average of three to five consecutive velocities is recommended.

It should be recognized that studies of healthy dogs from which reference intervals have been derived excluded dogs with murmurs and have recruited dogs of different breeds. With respect to the possibility of a breed effect, boxers deserve mention. In a study of healthy boxers more than 50% had soft basilar ejection murmurs (Koplitz et al., 2003), and the boxers that had murmurs had higher aortic velocities than boxers that did not. The cause of these murmurs was not identified definitively, and it was speculated that an exaggerated response to sympathetic tone or an anatomic variant in the LVOT such as generalized aortic hypoplasia might explain the findings. Very possibly ejection murmurs heard in boxers result from two distinct causes: some are caused by SAS, and others are physiologic murmurs that relate to a breed-specific variation in outflow tract anatomy.

We believe that peak velocity is only a single variable in a dynamic system. Indeed some cases cannot be resolved as to cardiac status because objective, irrefutable evidence of SAS is lacking. Exclusion of a large proportion of the breeding population based on a single diagnosis may have a negative effect on the population genotype. Because of this, in equivocal cases the murmur and results of echocardiographic examination are documented, and the breeder is informed of the potential genetic implications of the findings. Breeding of animals in this equivocal category is not necessarily discouraged for dogs with otherwise strong characteristics, but careful evaluation of progeny is recommended. Only through breeding studies and/or necropsy evaluation does the real status of some dogs become known. Currently there is no available genetic test to identify affected dogs or carriers of SAS.

TREATMENT

Dogs with mild or moderate SAS typically are not treated in our practice. Generally these animals have few complications from their disease. Severely affected dogs do not fare as well and commonly die suddenly and unexpectedly presumably as a result of a lethal ventricular arrhythmia (Kienle, Thomas, and Pion, 1994). Unfortunately the treatment options are limited and of questionable value. A recent report (Meurs, Lehmkuhl, and Bonagura, 2005) summarized the results of transcatheter balloon dilation in dogs with severe SAS. Although short-term reduction of the peak systolic pressure gradient was found, there was no long-term benefit in survival times when compared to a group of dogs receiving atenolol; median survival in both groups was about 4 years. The weakness in this study was a lack of an untreated control group, although the median survival was longer than untreated dogs reported by Kienle, Thomas, and Pion (1994). Until a control group is studied, it is not possible to know with certainty whether balloon valvuloplasty or β-blocker therapy offers severely affected animals any benefit. The balloon dilation results are not surprising, considering the location of the SAS lesion and the nature of the stenotic lesion (see Figs. 168-1 and 168-2). In humans it has been stated that balloon dilation is rarely justified as a mode of therapy (Freedom et al., 2005).

When considering therapy with atenolol, we evaluate clinical signs, electrocardiographic findings, and echocardiographic results with particular emphasis on pressure gradient. Although we recognize the lack of data for the use of a beta blocker in this disease, we often recommend atenolol (0.5 to 1 mg/kg PO q12h) for severely affected animals. The presumed beneficial effect of β-blockade relates to the decrease in myocardial oxygen demand that is associated with the negative inotropic and chronotropic effects. Blunting of the chronotropic response to exercise may improve myocardial perfusion because coronary flow in patients with severe SAS occurs primarily during diastole (Pyle et al., 1973). In addition, a phenomenon of reflex-mediated bradycardia and hypotension has been described in people with aortic stenosis. It is possible that the same pathophysiologic mechanism explains syncopal episodes in dogs with SAS. Since adrenergic activation is believed to be the stimulus that initiates the reflex, atenolol or other β-blockers may be helpful.

It is possible that the effects of β-blockade reduce the frequency and potentially fatal outcome of arrhythmias in SAS; however, evidence to support this contention is lacking. In the absence of controlled studies or a precedent in pediatric medicine, it is also appropriate to consider the possibility that atenolol might harm patients with SAS. β-Blocker therapy could be detrimental because stroke volume in patients with severe SAS can be considered "fixed" by the structural impediment to ejection. The negative inotropic effect of β-blockers might limit the ability to generate the high ventricular pressures that are required to maintain stroke volume and coronary perfusion during exercise. Exercise restriction likely accomplishes many of the objectives of β-blockade; therefore exercise restriction is discussed with owners of dogs with severe SAS.

Other forms of medical therapy are seldom indicated. Medical management of congestive heart failure or atrial fibrillation is occasionally necessary for long-surviving patients with SAS. In these cases diuretic therapy is indicated, and digoxin is used to slow ventricular response rate when the presentation is complicated by atrial fibrillation. Historically vasodilators were believed to be contraindicated in patients with severe, fixed outflow tract obstruction. However, recent clinical data from humans with heart failure caused by aortic stenosis suggest that there may be a role for vasodilation when there is concurrent aortic stenosis and systolic myocardial dysfunction. Based on this, ACE inhibitors can be considered as adjunctive therapy for canine patients with SAS, heart failure, and echocardiographically confirmed myocardial dysfunction.

Infective endocarditis is a serious complication of SAS (see Fig. 168-2). Because many SAS dogs have abnormal aortic valve leaflets, antibiotics should be used before elective surgical or dental procedures that cause bacteremia.

Results of surgical correction have not been encouraging (Orton et al., 2000). Twenty-two dogs with severe SAS were treated with an open surgical approach; another 22 dogs were not treated with surgery. Intermediate-term outcome did not show a positive survival benefit; however, there was a decrease in systolic pressure gradient and a possible improvement in exercise tolerance. The reason this invasive procedure did not significantly improve the outcome is unknown, but the findings suggest the possibility that the substrate for sudden death, perhaps myocardial fibrosis, is established early in the course of the disease. As a result of this study, we do not recommend surgical correction.

References and Suggested Readings

Bonagura JD: Editorial: Problems in the canine left ventricular outflow tract, *J Vet Intern Med* 15:427, 2001.

Freedom RM et al: Thoughts about fixed subaortic stenosis in man and dog, *Cardiol Young* 15:186, 2005.

Kienle RD, Thomas WP, Pion PD: The natural history of canine congenital subaortic stenosis, *J Vet Intern Med* 8:423, 1994.

Koplitz SL et al: Aortic ejection velocity in healthy boxers with soft cardiac murmurs and boxers without cardiac murmurs: 201 cases (1997-2001), *J Am Vet Med Assoc* 222:770, 2003.

Lehmkuhl LB, Bonagura, JD: CVT Update: canine subvalvular aortic stenosis. In Bonagura JD, Kirk RW, editors: *Kirk's current veterinary therapy XII (small animal practice)*, Philadelphia, 1995, Saunders, p 822.

Meurs KM, Lehmkuhl, LB, Bonagura JD: Survival times in dogs with severe subvalvular aortic stenosis treated with balloon valvuloplasty or atenolol, *J Am Vet Med Assoc* 227:420, 2005.

Orton EC et al: Influence of open surgical correction on intermediate-term outcome in dogs with subvalvular aortic stenosis: 44 cases (1991-1998), *J Am Vet Med Assoc* 216:364, 2000.

Pyle RL, Patterson DF, Chacko S: The genetics and pathology of discrete subaortic stenosis in the Newfoundland dog, *Am Heart J* 92:324, 1976.

Pyle RL et al: Left circumflex artery hemodynamics in conscious dogs with congenital subaortic stenosis, *Circ Res* 33:34, 1973.

CHAPTER 169

Tricuspid Valve Dysplasia

DARCY B. ADIN, *Rochester, New York*

Tricuspid valve dysplasia is congenital malformation of the right atrioventricular valve apparatus and is thought to be caused by abnormal tissue undermining the right ventricle during embryogenesis (Garson et al., 1998). A variety of abnormalities are encountered, including thickened, shortened, or elongated leaflets; shortened or absent chordae tendineae; and abnormal papillary musculature. The major consequence of a malformed tricuspid valve is systolic regurgitation of blood into the right atrium, resulting in volume overload of the right heart. This tricuspid valve regurgitation can lead to right-sided congestive heart failure and atrial arrhythmias.

Tricuspid valve stenosis occasionally may be a feature of the disease and is characterized by impaired diastolic opening as a result of thickened and fused leaflets. Tricuspid valve stenosis induces atrial hypertrophy and enlargement and can also lead to congestive signs and arrhythmias. Cyanosis and polycythemia may occur in cases of concurrent atrial septal defect or patent foramen ovale.

Ebstein's anomaly is a related congenital defect whereby the origins of the tricuspid leaflets are apically displaced into the right ventricle. It may or may not be associated with leaflet dysplasia. Ebstein's anomaly has only rarely been documented in the veterinary literature (Chetboul et al., 2004, Takemura et al., 2003). Other congenital anomalies may be observed concurrently with tricuspid dysplasia, including mitral dysplasia, septal defects, pulmonic stenosis, and patent ductus arteriosus (Liu and Tilley, 1976). The foramen ovale may remain patent as a result of elevated right atrial pressure and dilation.

SIGNALMENT

Tricuspid dysplasia is a relatively uncommon defect, accounting for approximately 7% of canine congenital cardiac defects in retrospective studies (Baumgartner and Glaus, 2003; Tidholm, 1997). A variety of large-breed dogs have been reported, including Labrador retrievers, boxers, golden retrievers, Irish setters, Great Danes, and German shepherds (Andelfinger et al., 2003; Chetboul et al., 2004, Kornreich and Moïse, 1997; Liu and Tilley, 1976). The disease has been shown to be inherited in the Labrador retriever in an autosomal-dominant manner with incomplete penetrance and has been mapped to chromosome 9 in this breed (Andelfinger et al., 2003).

Tricuspid dysplasia is diagnosed less frequently in cats. It has been reported most commonly in the domestic shorthair cat but also in chartreux and Siamese cats (Chetboul et al., 2004; Kornreich and Moïse, 1997; Liu and Tilley, 1976).

DIAGNOSIS

Clinical Findings

Dogs and cats with tricuspid valve dysplasia may be clinically well with a heart murmur or presented for right-sided congestive heart failure. Although most animals are evaluated at a young age, it is not uncommon to make the diagnosis in an older animal at the time that clinical signs develop.

The hallmark physical examination feature for animals with tricuspid dysplasia is a right apical systolic murmur. The intensity of the murmur can vary from very soft to very loud with a precordial thrill and depends on the amount of regurgitation and the velocity of flow across the valve. Considering the latter factor, murmur intensity may not always reflect the severity of the disease. For example, a dog with a large tricuspid orifice resulting from severe malformation and volume overload of the right heart may have nearly laminar regurgitant flow because of pressure equilibration between the right atrium and right ventricle. Some of these dogs have a very soft murmur.

Dogs that are severely affected may be presented in right-sided congestive heart failure with jugular venous distention or pulsation, hepatomegaly, and ascites. Femoral arterial pulse quality is expected to be normal unless the disease is very severe. Mucous membrane color is normal unless a coexistent right-to-left shunt is present. Animals with right-sided congestive heart failure often have poor body condition.

Electrocardiography

The most common electrocardiographic finding in animals with tricuspid valve dysplasia is a splintered QRS complex, with as many as two thirds of dogs and cats showing this abnormality (Kornreich and Moïse, 1997). Splintering describes an Rr', RR', rR', or rr' morphology of the QRS complex (Fig. 169-1). The underlying mechanism for splintering is not known; however, several possibilities include ventricular fibrosis resulting in altered conduction, right bundle branch conduction disturbances, and accessory pathway conduction.

A right heart enlargement pattern may also be seen in approximately one third of dogs and one half of cats with tricuspid dysplasia (tall and sometimes wide P waves and deep S waves in leads I, II, and III and aVF with a right axis deviation) (Kornreich and Moïse, 1997). The use of precordial leads in dogs increases the sensitivity of the electrocardiogram to these changes.

Right atrial enlargement predisposes dogs and cats to atrial arrhythmias, including atrial premature complexes,

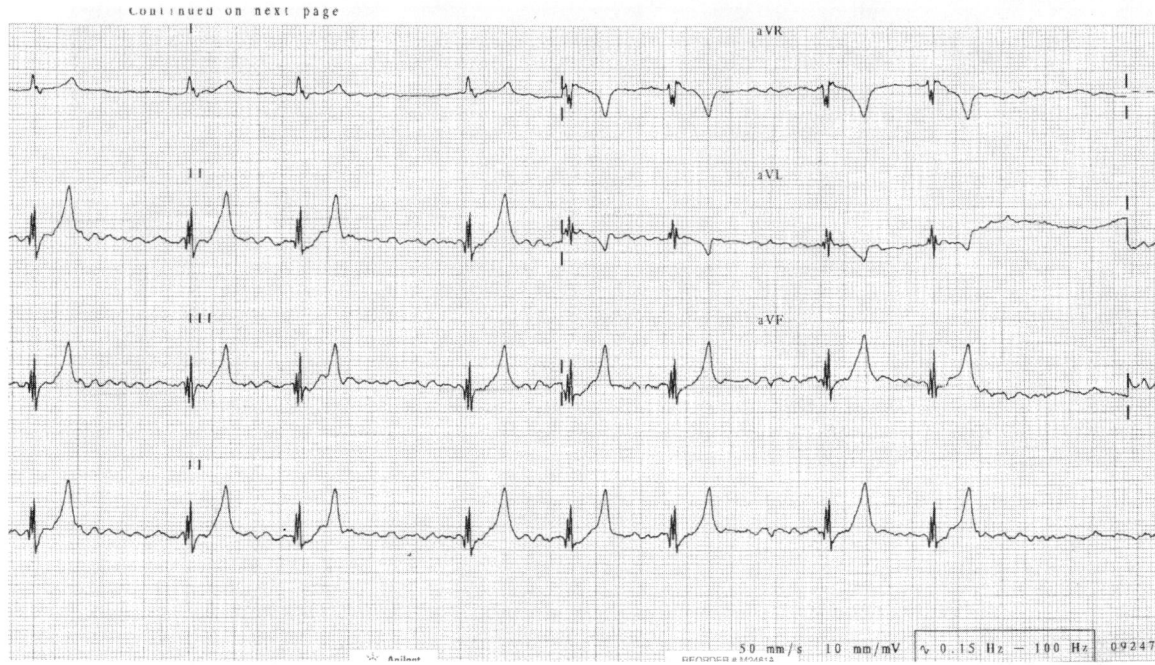

Fig. 169-1 Electrocardiogram from a dog with tricuspid dysplasia. Note the splintered QRS complex (rR'). The rhythm is atrial fibrillation.

atrial tachycardia, atrial flutter, and atrial fibrillation (see Fig. 169-1). The development of atrial tachyarrhythmias may decompensate a patient and initiate congestive symptoms because of the ensuing decrease in cardiac output and increase in atrial pressure.

Radiography

Right heart enlargement can be detected with thoracic radiography and can be profound in animals with severe tricuspid valve dysplasia (Fig. 169-2). The massive cardiomegaly in some cases may lead to differential diagnoses of dilated cardiomyopathy and pericardial effusion; however, physical examination and echocardiographic findings are definitive for tricuspid dysplasia. The right atrium is often the predominant chamber noted on thoracic radiographs, occupying the majority of the cardiac silhouette. The apex may be shifted dorsally on the lateral view and to the left and caudally on the ventrodorsal projection because of right heart enlargement. Notably the main pulmonary artery is normal, and the pulmonary vasculature may be normal or suggest decreased perfusion. Dogs that are in congestive failure with ascites have radiographic evidence of caudal vena caval enlargement (greater than the length of the fifth thoracic vertebrae).

Echocardiography

Echocardiography provides the definitive diagnosis for tricuspid valve dysplasia. The septal leaflet of the tricuspid valve often appears tethered to the interventricular septum. The leaflet tips are thickened and often curled. In severe cases it may be possible to identify a coaptation gap whereby the valve leaflets visibly do not meet in systole (Fig. 169-3). The papillary muscles are abnormally large with direct valve leaflet insertion. When chordae tendineae are present, they are thickened and short. Although both the right ventricle and right atrium are volume overloaded, right atrial enlargement predominates (see Fig. 169-3). The left ventricle is usually markedly volume underloaded. Doppler interrogation shows a large regurgitant jet across the tricuspid valve. The velocity of the tricuspid regurgitation is predictive of normal right ventricular pressure and generally less than 2.8 m/second. Ebstein's anomaly is identified by a marked apical displacement of the tricuspid valve insertions such that a portion of the right ventricle is "atrialized." The determination of apical displacement should be cautious, remembering that the normal insertion point of the tricuspid valve is slightly more apical than the normal insertion point of the mitral valve. In addition, care must be taken not to overinterpret any leaflet tethering that may be present. Ebstein's anomaly can be confirmed by invasively obtaining a ventricular electrogram and an atrial pressure pulse from this atrialized portion of the right ventricle.

When tricuspid stenosis is present, the right ventricle appears small, and the right atrium is enlarged. The resulting pressure overload induces right atrial hypertrophy and dilation. The thickened valve leaflets are usually observed to "dome" in diastole because their opening is restricted. Continuous-wave Doppler shows a delayed pressure gradient decay in early diastole as a result of the obstruction. In addition, the pressure gradient across the tricuspid valve is abnormally elevated and highest in late diastole after atrial contraction.

There is a growing interest among breeders to screen dogs for tricuspid dysplasia; however, there currently is no consensus among cardiologists regarding the optimal method of screening (auscultation only versus echocardiography) or regarding the precise echocardiographic

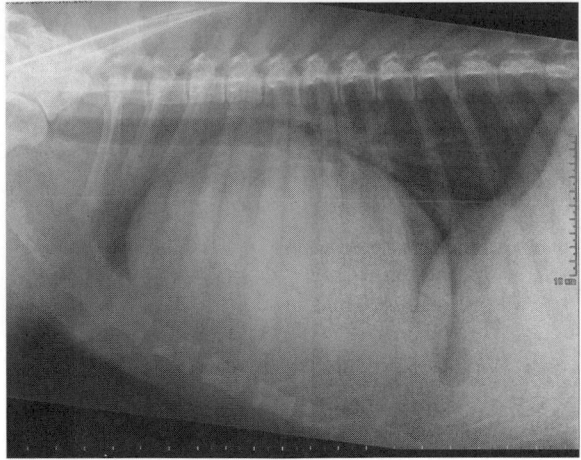

A

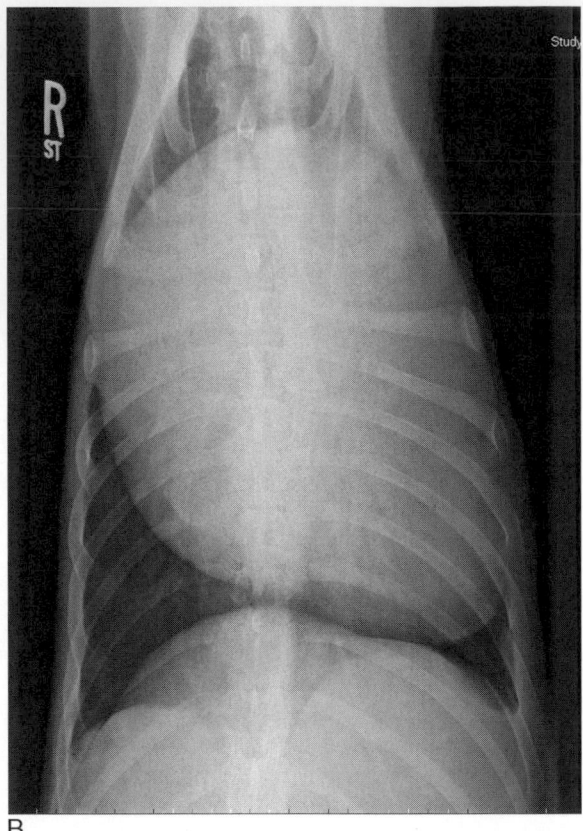

B

Fig. 169-2   Lateral **(A)** and ventrodorsal **(B)** radiographs from a dog with severe tricuspid dysplasia. Severe right-sided cardiomegaly is present. The apex is shifted dorsally on the lateral projection and to the left on the ventrodorsal radiograph.

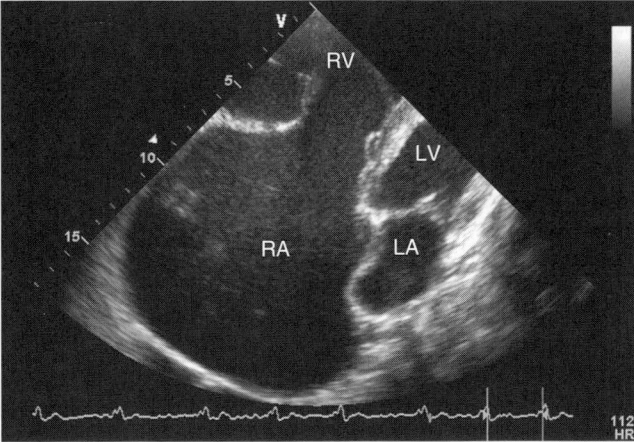

Fig. 169-3   Left apical parasternal echocardiographic image showing a severely enlarged right atrium and right ventricle. The tricuspid valve leaflets are thickened and attach directly to the papillary muscles. The septal leaflet is tethered to the interventricular septum. Based on the electrogram, the image is during systole when the valve leaflets should be closed; this valve has a very large coaptation gap.

criteria for the differentiation between normal and mildly affected dogs.

THERAPY

Medical therapy is instituted once ascites or, less commonly, pleural effusion develops. Diuretics (e.g., furosemide) and angiotensin-converting enzyme inhibitors (e.g., enalapril) are used to counteract fluid retention; however, it is uncommon for medications to eliminate third spacing of fluids entirely. Periodic manual removal of effusions (e.g., abdominocentesis) is often required despite concurrent diuresis. Because elevated hydrostatic pressure is the driving force for fluid accumulation, there should be no concern about complete evacuation of the peritoneal space as there would be for ascites caused by hypoproteinemia (aside from loss of protein). Excessive diuresis should be avoided, especially in cases in which low output signs are present (e.g., cool extremities, poor arterial pulses). A reduced sodium diet may help to control congestion; however, adequate nutritional intake is more important than a specific diet because many of these patients become cachectic with disease progression. The use of pimobendan can be considered, but it is not labeled for (or studied in) this disease.

Atrial tachyarrhythmias should be controlled since their development can further compromise a patient that is in or near congestive heart failure. Digoxin is used to slow the ventricular response rate in atrial fibrillation and provides some positive inotropic action; however, it often is inadequate as the sole agent. Diltiazem may be added to digoxin for heart rate control with atrial fibrillation and can be used for the treatment of atrial tachycardia.

Balloon valvuloplasty has been reported twice for the successful treatment of tricuspid stenosis (Brown and Thomas, 1995; Kunze et al., 2002). Surgical replacement of the tricuspid valve has been attempted in a limited number of cases with poor outcomes.

PROGNOSIS

The prognosis depends on the severity of the malformation and the resultant tricuspid regurgitation. Dogs with mild tricuspid valve dysplasia may have normal life spans. Most dogs with severe tricuspid valve dysplasia deteriorate within the first few years of life; however, occasionally congestive heart failure may not occur until later in life, and some dogs survive longer than 6 years even with severe disease.

References and Suggested Reading

Andelfinger G et al: Canine tricuspid valve malformation, a model of human Ebstein anomaly, maps to dog chromosome 9, *J Med Genet* 40:320, 2003.

Baumgartner C, Glaus TM: Congenital cardiac diseases in dogs: a retrospective analysis, *Schweiz Arch Tierheilkd* 145:527, 2003.

Brown WA, Thomas WP: Balloon valvuloplasty of tricuspid stenosis in a Labrador retriever, *J Vet Intern Med* 9:419, 1995.

Chetboul V et al: Les malformations congenitales de la valve tricuspide chez les carnivores domestiques: étude retrospective de 50 cas, *Schweiz Arch Tierheilkd* 146:265, 2004.

Garson A et al: The science and practice of pediatric cardiology, ed 2, Baltimore, 1998, Williams & Wilkins, p 1305.

Kornreich BG, Moïse NS: Right atrioventricular valve malformation in dogs and cats: an electrocardiographic survey with emphasis on splintered QRS complex, *J Vet Intern Med* 11:226, 1997.

Kunze CP et al: Balloon valvuloplasty for palliative treatment of tricuspid stenosis with right to left atrial-level shunting in a dog, *J Am Vet Med Assoc* 220:491, 2002.

Lui SK, Tilly LP: Dysplasia of the tricuspid valve in the dog and cat, *J Am Vet Med Assoc* 169:623, 1976.

Takemura N et al: Ebstein's anomaly in a beagle dog, *J Vet Med Sci* 65:531, 2003.

Tidholm A: Retrospective study of congenital heart defects in 151 dogs, *J Small Anim Pract* 38:94, 1997.

CHAPTER **170**

Mitral Valve Dysplasia

BARRET J. BULMER, *Corvallis, Oregon*

Appropriate opening and closing of the mitral valve allows unimpeded left ventricular filling and prevents valvular regurgitation. These functions depend on the integrated activity of all anatomic components of the mitral valve apparatus. Disruption or malformation of any of these components, including the mitral leaflets, the chordae tendineae, the mitral annulus, the left atrial wall, the papillary muscles, or the left ventricular wall may produce valvular dysfunction. Although acquired degenerative valve disease is the most common cause of mitral valve dysfunction in dogs, it should be recognized that mitral valve dysplasia (MVD) is a common form of congenital heart disease in both dogs and cats. Currently MVD may have surpassed ventricular septal defect as the most common congenital anomaly in cats. Alterations in cases of MVD include annular enlargement; short, thick leaflets with an occasional cleft; short and stout or long and thin chordae tendineae; upward malposition of atrophic or hypertrophic papillary muscles; and insertion of one papillary muscle directly into one or both leaflets (Liu and Tilley, 1975). Animals that appear to be overrepresented include cats of all breeds, Great Danes, German shepherds, bull terriers, golden retrievers, Newfoundlands, dalmatians, and mastiffs (Oyama et al., 2005).

PATHOPHYSIOLOGY

The pathophysiologic consequences of MVD relate to: (1) systolic regurgitation of blood from the left ventricle into the left atrium; (2) impaired left ventricular diastolic filling across a stenotic mitral valve; or (3) obstruction to left ventricular ejection via inappropriate, systolic displacement of the mitral valve into the left ventricular outflow tract. More than one functional disturbance can occur. Similar to acquired degenerative mitral valve disease, congenital insufficiency of the mitral valve produces volume overload of the left atrium and left ventricle. The two primary determinants of the volume of insufficiency are the regurgitant orifice area (ROA) and the left ventricular–to–left atrial pressure gradient. Therefore animals with a large ROA and those that must generate greater left ventricular pressures (e.g., MVD complicated by subaortic stenosis) suffer greater hemodynamic consequences compared to animals with small leaks and unimpeded left ventricular ejection. As the left atrial, pulmonary venous, and pulmonary capillary pressures rise secondary to the volume overload, left-sided heart failure develops with accumulation of fluid within the pulmonary interstitium and alveoli.

If the valvular dysfunction is manifested primarily as stenosis, it produces a different range of pathophysiologic consequences. Lesions that restrict pulmonary venous return and left atrial emptying, including mitral stenosis, supravalvular mitral stenosis, and cor triatriatum sinister, are accompanied by elevated left atrial and pulmonary venous pressures. The severity of this pressure increase depends on resistance of the stenotic valve and the volume of transmitral flow, which increases during exercise. In the initial stages of the disease the increased pressure maintains an adequate gradient for left ventricular filling. This elevated pressure gradient contributes to left atrial enlargement and hypertrophy, pulmonary venous congestion, and pulmonary edema because of increased pulmonary capillary hydrostatic pressure. The chronic hypoxia associated with lack of alveolar ventilation may produce reactive pulmonary arterial vasoconstriction in an attempt to diminish ventilation/perfusion mismatch. Ultimately right ventricular dysfunction and right-sided heart failure may develop from the pressure overload associated with long-standing pulmonary hypertension.

The third alteration that may accompany MVD is systolic displacement of the anterior mitral valve leaflet, a chordae tendineae, or papillary muscle into the left ventricular outflow tract. Although systolic anterior motion (SAM) or dynamic left ventricular outflow tract obstruction is most frequently associated with hypertrophic cardiomyopathy, it may also stem from mitral dysplasia independent of septal hypertrophy. Several mechanisms have been hypothesized for this association, including (1) a decrease in the ability of the papillary muscles to restrain the valve posteriorly; and (2) an interposition of the leaflets anteriorly into the outflow stream, which then propels them anteriorly into the outflow tract, and a geometry for mitral valve coaptation that favors SAM (Levine et al., 1995). Consequences of SAM include increases in systolic left ventricular pressure, wall tension, and myocardial work (promoting concentric hypertrophy); increased myocardial oxygen demand; reduced coronary perfusion pressure as aortic diastolic pressure falls and left ventricular diastolic pressure rises; and mitral regurgitation caused by incomplete valve closure (Sherrid, 1998).

DIAGNOSIS

History and Physical Examination

Similar to many forms of congenital heart disease, animals with MVD commonly are identified before the development of clinical signs related to abnormal cardiac auscultation during the initial veterinary examination. The absence of clinical signs often continues for a variable period of time until owners begin to recognize evidence of left-sided heart failure (i.e., coughing, tachypnea, restlessness, and exercise intolerance) predominantly. Uncommonly animals with mitral stenosis may also display evidence of right-sided heart failure (i.e., abdominal distention secondary to ascites formation and tachypnea resulting from pleural effusion). Severe mitral stenosis can be associated with recurrent bouts of flush pulmonary edema or hemoptysis. Less common historical complaints may include syncope, and on occasion animals may die suddenly without a previous history of clinical signs.

The wide range of phenotypic expressions and pathophysiologic consequences for MVD produce a variety of abnormal physical examination findings. No matter if the valve is primarily insufficient or stenotic or displays SAM, the most common auscultatory abnormality is a left apical systolic murmur of mitral valve regurgitation. Careful auscultation in animals with mitral stenosis may identify a left apical, diastolic, rumbling murmur of mitral valve stenosis; whereas patients with SAM often have a left-sided systolic murmur that varies in intensity directly with the heart rate (and sympathetic tone). Additional abnormal cardiac auscultatory findings may include S3 or S4 gallops, a variety of supraventricular or ventricular arrhythmias, and on very rare occasions an audible systolic click or opening snap. Animals with pulmonary edema may have increased bronchovesicular sounds or crackles, whereas those with pleural effusion may have muffled heart and lung sounds. Jugular venous distention or pulsation, a positive hepatojugular reflux, ascites, and/or hepatomegaly may signify the presence of right-sided heart failure.

Electrocardiography

Electrocardiographic alterations that may be identified in animals with MVD include chamber enlargement patterns, arrhythmias, and potentially ST segment alterations. An increased R wave amplitude and prolonged QRS duration may accompany left ventricular enlargement, whereas a prolonged or widened P wave is classically associated with left atrial enlargement (although tall P waves may also be encountered). If significant right ventricular enlargement is present as a result of mitral stenosis and pulmonary hypertension, deep S waves (in leads I, II, aVF, and V_{2-4}), and a right-axis shift in the mean electrical axis may be identified. Small amplitude QRS complexes (<1 mV) may be present in patients with pleural effusion. The most common arrhythmias in animals with MVD are supraventricular (i.e., atrial premature complexes and atrial fibrillation), although ventricular premature complexes also occur. Myocardial ischemia or hypoxia accompanying severe left ventricular concentric hypertrophy or pulmonary hypertension may produce ST segment elevation or depression.

Thoracic Radiography

Radiographic abnormalities in animals with MVD displaying primarily valvular insufficiency include left ventricular and left atrial enlargement. The most consistent radiographic finding in patients with mitral valve stenosis is left atrial enlargement (Lehmkuhl, Ware, and Bonagura, 1994). In cases in which pulmonary hypertension has developed, variable degrees of right ventricular and pulmonary arterial enlargement may be encountered. The concentric hypertrophy that accompanies animals with MVD and SAM may fail to produce significant chamber enlargement radiographically despite the presence of marked wall thickening. All three forms of MVD may contribute to the development of left-sided heart failure, with pulmonary venous congestion and perihilar interstitial edema ultimately giving way to an alveolar pattern. Hemoptysis creates a dense alveolar pattern. Because MVD is frequently accompanied by other forms of congenital heart disease, the predominant radiographic findings may not be representative of the mitral valve lesion.

Echocardiography

Two-dimensional, M-mode, spectral, and color flow Doppler echocardiography are invaluable in the assessment of animals with MVD. Ultrasonographers experienced with congenital heart disease can quickly ascertain the morphologic features of the dysplastic valve, the principal form (or forms) of valvular dysfunction, the myocardial response to the malfunctioning valve, and the presence or absence of concurrent cardiac anomalies (Fig. 170-1). Similar to electrocardiograms and radiographs, the echocardiographic findings depend on the primary manifestation and the severity of the valvular dysfunction. Two-dimensional echocardiography enables a detailed evaluation of the location, shape, motion, and attachments of the mitral valve leaflets to their respective chordae tendineae and papillary muscles. Animals with significant mitral insufficiency display eccentric left ventricular hypertrophy, left atrial dilation, and normal-to-hyperdynamic systolic function unless left ventricular dysfunction has developed. Virtually all patients with MVD have evidence of mitral regurgitation on color flow Doppler.

Common echocardiographic findings in patients with mitral stenosis include left atrial enlargement, thickened mitral valve leaflets, diastolic doming of the anterior mitral valve leaflet, and decreased excursion of the tips of the mitral valve. M-mode echocardiography may identify concordant motion of the anterior and posterior mitral valve leaflets, incomplete leaflet separation during

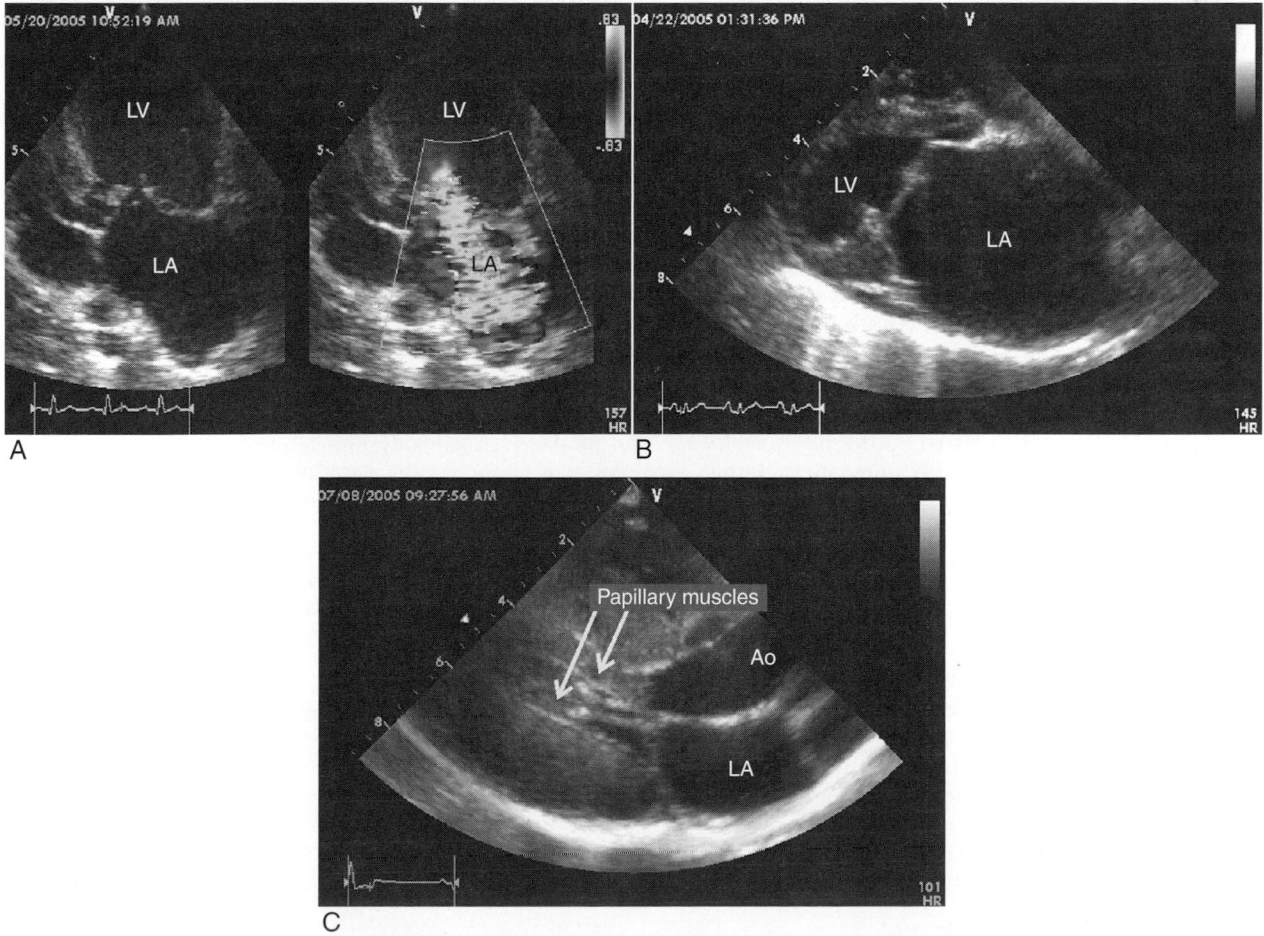

Fig. 170-1 **A,** Elongated and thickened mitral valve with abnormal chordal insertion on the anterior leaflet prevents appropriate closure of this valve. The result is a large volume of mitral insufficiency as evidenced by color Doppler with left atrial (LA) dilation and left ventricular (LV) eccentric hypertrophy in this 6-month-old dog. **B,** Marked left atrial dilation is present in this patient with severe mitral valve stenosis. The dysplastic mitral leaflets are tethered at their coaptation point, preventing the normal diastolic transit of blood from the left atrium into the left ventricle. **C,** This young rottweiler with mitral valve dysplasia displays asymmetrically elongated and displaced papillary muscles that inappropriately contact the chordae tendineae of the anterior mitral valve leaflet and interventricular septum during systole. Moderate-to-severe left ventricular concentric hypertrophy accompanies the dynamic left ventricular outflow tract obstruction because it impairs systolic ejection of blood into the aorta (Ao).

diastole, lack of leaflet closure during mid-diastole, a reduced EF slope, and an increased left atrium–to-aortic ratio (Lehmkuhl, Ware, and Bonagura, 1994). Increased transmitral flow velocities and prolonged pressure half-time are commonly recognized via spectral Doppler.

Animals with MVD and dynamic left ventricular outflow tract obstruction display systolic apposition of the anterior mitral valve leaflet, chordae tendineae, or papillary muscle with the interventricular septum as evidenced via two-dimensional and M-mode echocardiography. Additional echocardiographic findings include variable degrees of concentric left ventricular hypertrophy, partial premature closure of the aortic valve, and high-velocity turbulent flow within the left ventricular outflow tract accompanied by a posterolaterally directed jet of mitral insufficiency. Continuous-wave Doppler interrogation of the left ventricular outflow tract displays a characteristic concave and asymmetrically shaped pattern because the outflow tract obstruction occurs during mid-systole (versus cases of fixed subaortic stenosis). It should be noted that these findings are very similar, if not identical, to those recognized in hypertrophic obstructive cardiomyopathy; and in some cases it is extremely difficult to differentiate these two diseases.

THERAPY

Therapeutic decisions for the management of MVD are based on the form and severity of valvular dysfunction present, the presence or absence of clinical signs, and whether or not concurrent cardiac anomalies are present. Asymptomatic animals with primarily mitral valve insufficiency or mitral stenosis generally warrant client education and careful follow-up without specific medical management. In comparison, β-blockers are commonly administered to animals with systolic anterior motion of the mitral valve, even in the absence of clinical signs, if they have a significant resting or provoked left ventricular outflow tract gradient. Atenolol (0.5 to 1 mg/kg q24h orally [PO]) has been reported to successfully alleviate dynamic left ventricular outflow tract obstruction and left ventricular concentric hypertrophy in dogs with SAM (Connolly and Boswood, 2003). Animals with MVD and congestive heart failure are treated similarly to their counterparts with degenerative mitral valve disease via a regimen of diuretics and angiotensin-converting inhibitors, often with positive inotropic drugs (see Chapter 171). Care must be exercised to avoid overzealous diuretic administration in animals with mitral stenosis because their cardiac output is extremely preload dependent. Antiarrhythmics may be required to manage ventricular premature complexes or slow the ventricular response rate in cases with atrial fibrillation (see Chapter 161). Adequate rate control in animals with mitral stenosis complicated by atrial fibrillation should be a priority (Meisner et al., 1991). Surgical repair or replacement of the mitral valve using cardiopulmonary bypass has also been reported to palliate or resolve clinical signs in dogs with MVD (White et al., 1995; Griffiths, Orton, and Boone, 2004; Borenstein et al., 2004).

PROGNOSIS

The prognosis for animals with MVD depends on the type and severity of valvular dysfunction and, when required, response to medical therapy. Many animals with mild-to-moderate MVD live for prolonged periods of time free of clinical signs. Following the development of congestive heart failure, the natural history of congenital MVD appears similar to that of dogs with acquired degenerative valve disease. Overall a generally worse prognosis can be given for animals with mitral stenosis, and a generally better prognosis for those with outflow tract obstruction (assuming it and related ventricular hypertrophy are resolved with β-blocker administration) compared to those with valvular insufficiency predominantly. Depending on the morphology of the dysplastic valve and the manifestations of dysfunction, successful surgical repair or replacement of the valve may be curative in selected cases.

References and Suggested Reading

Borenstein N et al: Successful surgical treatment of mitral valve stenosis in a dog, *Vet Surg* 33(2):138, 2004.

Connolly DJ, Boswood A: Dynamic obstruction of the left ventricular outflow tract in four young dogs, *J Small Anim Pract* 44(7):319, 2003.

Griffiths LG, Orton EC, Boon JA: Evaluation of techniques and outcomes of mitral valve repair in dogs, *J Am Vet Med Assoc* 224(12):1941, 2004.

Lehmkuhl LB, Ware WA, Bonagura JD: Mitral stenosis in 15 dogs, *J Vet Intern Med* 8(1):2, 1994.

Levine RA et al: Papillary muscle displacement causes systolic anterior motion of the mitral valve: experimental validation and insights into the mechanism of subaortic obstruction, *Circulation* 91(4):1189, 1995.

Liu SK, Tilley LP: Malformation of the canine mitral valve complex, *J Am Vet Med Assoc* 67(6):465, 1975.

Meisner JS et al: Atrial contribution to ventricular filling in mitral stenosis, *Circulation* 84(4):1469, 1991.

Oyama MA et al: Congenital heart disease. In Ettinger SJ, Feldman EC, editors: *Textbook of veterinary internal medicine*, ed 6, St. Louis, 2005, Saunders, p 972.

Sherrid MV: Dynamic left ventricular outflow obstruction in hypertrophic cardiomyopathy revisited: significance, pathogenesis, and treatment, *Cardiol Rev* 6(3):135, 1998.

White RN et al: Mitral valve replacement for the treatment of congenital mitral dysplasia in a bull terrier, *J Small Anim Pract* 36(9):407, 1995.

CHAPTER 171

Management of Heart Failure in Dogs

BRUCE W. KEENE, *Raleigh, North Carolina*
JOHN D. BONAGURA, *Columbus, Ohio*

The heart is a deceptively complex organ that generates the force by which blood is continuously supplied to perfuse the metabolizing tissues. In all animals with closed circulatory systems (creatures above mollusks phylogenetically), control systems monitor the distention of selected arteries, veins, cardiac chambers, and respiratory organs, as well as some of the chemical properties of the arterial blood supply. These control systems coordinate an array of physiologic and neuroendocrine responses from the heart, blood vessels, kidney, lung, and central nervous system. Together these systems maintain blood volume, arterial pressure, venous pressure, heart rate, cardiac output, and ventilation. These critical variables are further adjusted to levels that support metabolic needs both at rest and during times of stress or exercise.

When the heart fails for any reason, the general outcome is activation of stereotypical responses that attempt to maintain blood pressure (BP) and vital organ perfusion. These compensations are both helpful and maladaptive. Understanding this pathophysiology is central to the therapy of heart failure (HF) and is the initial topic of this chapter.

HF is a syndrome, not a disease. The causes of HF in dogs differ, and the stages of heart disease and HF are often progressive. Appreciating these different causes and stages is helpful in constructing a general framework for managing dogs with heart disease and HF. This subject and the evidence for using specific drugs at various stages of HF is the second focus of this chapter.

Veterinarians have a number of powerful drugs for supporting a failing heart and managing the circulatory, renal, and neurohormonal consequences of HF. The clinical pharmacology of these drugs must be mastered for successful treatment of dogs with HF. Multidrug therapy provides the best outcome for dogs with advanced cardiac disease, and the experienced veterinarian learns to orchestrate these treatments. This chapter includes a brief review of the important clinical pharmacology of cardiac drugs. Finally, insofar as specific treatment recommendations can be advanced, we offer our own approaches to treating HF in dogs in the final portion of this chapter.

CLINICAL PATHOPHYSIOLOGY OF HEART FAILURE

The term *heart failure* describes a pathophysiologic situation in which the heart cannot maintain cardiac output sufficient to meet the perfusion needs of the metabolizing tissues while also maintaining normal venous pressures.

Invariably exercise capacity becomes limited in HF. Whether caused by systolic or diastolic heart dysfunction, decreased cardiac output and arterial BP are pivotal events in the syndrome of HF. In contrast, hemorrhagic or hypovolemic shock is also associated with reduced cardiac output and BP; but in these circumstances venous pressures are low, and the indicated therapy is quite different (see Chapter 1).

In both HF and hypovolemic shock the reduction in cardiac output and resultant decrease in arterial BP (arterial "under-filling") trigger a cascade of physiologic events coordinated by control systems focused primarily on restoring the arterial pressure toward normal. Activation of these control systems helps maintain basal (resting) BP and blood flow to selected organs within the normal range even in the face of initially reduced cardiac output. These mechanisms include sympathetic stimulation of the heart; vasoconstriction and redistribution of blood flow mediated by sympathetic, renin–angiotensin, vasopressin, and vascular endothelial systems; and sodium and water retention mediated by changes in renal blood flow, aldosterone, vasopressin, and inhibition of natriuretic hormones. These are powerful control systems for restoration of arterial BP. If the cause of decreased cardiac output and BP is reversible and transient, activation of these systems appears to cause no permanent harm, and they promptly return to their basal state once the crisis has passed. Conversely, when chronically activated, the physiologic balance shifts toward vasoconstriction, sodium retention, and mediators of inflammation and tissue growth. Furthermore, the heart itself is remodeled at the expense of structural and functional damage to cardiac muscle, including activation of fetal-gene programs, myocyte apoptosis, and interstitial and replacement fibrosis. These compensatory mechanisms may be so hemodynamically effective that clinical signs of cardiac failure may be absent or evident only with exercise until the time that pulmonary venous pressure increases sufficiently to cause edema or perfusion of skeletal muscles becomes severely limited. These effective but damaging compensations make heart diseases difficult to diagnose until they have caused extensive cardiac remodeling and damage.

Progression of heart disease and pump dysfunction triggers a spiral of increasing dependence on neurohormonal activity to maintain normal arterial BP and flow. Despite the hemodynamic benefits of these compensations (e.g., maintaining normal arterial BP at rest), their chronic activation is maladaptive—a concept central to the medical management of chronic HF. Clinical signs of congestive heart failure (CHF) are explained in part by chronically elevated venous pressures (causing pulmonary edema, pleural effusion, jugular venous distention, hepatomegaly, and ascites), inadequate tissue perfusion (exercise intolerance, lethargy, and azotemia), and metabolic disturbances (weight loss, insulin resistance, and azotemia). Although hemodynamic changes may explain the acutely life-threatening clinical signs of HF, morbidity and mortality in chronic HF patients appear to be related strongly to the tissue effects of the accentuated neurohormonal and cytokine-mediated compensations that develop in response to the reduced output of the failing heart.

The therapy of acute HF is directed primarily at identifying and "fixing" life-threatening hemodynamic derangements. The chronic therapy of HF is aimed at maintaining hemodynamic gains while modulating and blunting the maladaptive compensatory responses to protect tissues, prolong life, and minimize clinical signs.

CAUSES AND CLASSIFICATIONS OF HEART FAILURE

HF is not a specific disease but a clinical syndrome precipitated by a definable heart disease and characterized by the aforementioned cardiac, hemodynamic, renal, neurohormonal, and cytokine abnormalities. Causes of heart disease can be classified by etiology if known, but many heart diseases are genetic or idiopathic in origin. The classic pathophysiologic description of HF involves ventricular systolic dysfunction, diastolic dysfunction, or hemodynamic (volume or pressure) overload. However, most dogs in HF have elements of each of these categories. In the past HF has also been classified as forward or backward, which is instructive relative to the clinical signs observed in patients. Forward failure commonly refers to clinical signs resulting from low cardiac output and inadequate tissue perfusion, including weakness, lethargy, and prerenal azotemia. Insufficient BP or renal perfusion also triggers renal sodium retention. Backward failure refers to the failure of the heart to empty blood from the veins, leading to elevated venous and capillary pressures. The consequences of venous congestion include pulmonary edema, ascites, and pleural effusion, creating the well-recognized syndromes of left-sided, right-sided, or biventricular CHF. Cardiogenic shock is diagnosed when patients have severe signs of both forward and backward HF accompanied by systemic hypotension.

The anatomic location of the disease provides a useful framework for classification when considering the morphologic cardiac diagnosis. Heart diseases are commonly delimited as diseases of the pericardium, myocardium, endocardium and valves, impulse forming and conduction system, or vascular system. In dogs the most important diseases leading to HF are chronic degenerative valvular heart disease (DVD or valvular endocardiosis) causing mitral and tricuspid regurgitation, idiopathic or genetic dilated cardiomyopathy (DCM), pericardial effusion often caused by neoplasia, and pulmonary hypertension from heartworm disease. Taken as a group, congenital heart defects that include patent ductus arteriosus, subaortic stenosis, and various valve malformations can be considered important causes of HF in dogs. Cardiac rhythm disturbances often complicate structural heart disease, with atrial fibrillation (AF) and ventricular tachycardia representing the best examples. The diagnosis and management of these disorders are discussed in some detail in chapters throughout this section.

ESTABLISHING THE CARDIAC DIAGNOSIS IN HEART FAILURE

When a clinician suspects HF based on clinical signs, the first step in treatment is *establishing the underlying heart disease* responsible and determining the severity of the condition. This information allows the clinician to provide the most specific and appropriate therapy and a more accurate prognosis.

The reason for HF generally can be determined by appreciating the epidemiologic risk for heart disease (breed and age); the physical examination findings, emphasizing arterial and venous pulses, cardiac and thoracic auscultation, and abdominal palpation; the radiographic findings that support a diagnosis of HF and rule out bronchopulmonary or thoracic disease; and the results of 2D echocardiographic imaging for assessment of heart size, function, and overt lesions. Doppler echocardiographic studies are often important adjuncts to 2D and M-mode echocardiography in the assessment of some patients. Routine electrocardiography has a low specificity for heart disease in dogs but is pivotal when cardiac rhythm disturbances are suspected. Since BP may be elevated as a comorbid disease or low related to forward failure, noninvasive BP should be determined. Routine laboratory tests (complete blood count and serum chemistry) should also be obtained from suspected HF patients. In some patients a circulating biomarker such as N-terminal, pro-brain natriuretic peptide (N-pBNP) may assist in the differential diagnosis, assuming the laboratory has well-established cutoffs for HF (as opposed to simple heart disease).

In the vast majority of canine patients the underlying reason for HF is chronic atrioventricular valvular disease (see Chapter 172) or DCM (see Chapters 174 to 176). Pericardial disease (see Chapter 181) is an underrecognized cause of CHF and should be in the differential diagnosis of any dog with right-sided CHF or pleural effusion. In heartworm-endemic regions pulmonary hypertension caused by dirofilariasis should be a consideration for right-sided CHF. If the underlying reason for HF is not obvious from the workup described previously, the patient should be stabilized (e.g., diuresed) and referred to a cardiologist for a second opinion. If referral is not feasible, at a minimum thoracic radiographs taken before and after any therapy should be reviewed within the context of the history by a radiologist or cardiologist.

FUNCTIONAL CLASSIFICATION OF HEART DISEASE AND FAILURE

Because the clinical signs of HF are similar regardless of the underlying disease that causes the heart to fail, classification systems that grade the severity of HF or stage patients with HF have developed independently of anatomic or etiologic diagnoses. These *functional classifications of HF* include the four-stage New York Heart Association (NYHA) and the three-stage International Small Animal Cardiac Health Council (ISACHC) classifications along with some newer proposals described later in the chapter. Functional classification systems are designed to provide a framework for discussing and comparing the clinical signs of patients in HF and to some extent estimating the need for various therapies. These classification schemes vary in their details but serve to describe a semiquantitative method for judging the severity of a patient's clinical signs that can be generalized as follows:

- *Class I:* Heart disease is present, but no clinical signs are evident even with exercise.
- *Class II:* Heart disease is causing clinical signs only with strenuous exercise.
- *Class III:* Heart disease is causing clinical signs with routine daily activities or with mild exercise.
- *Class IV:* Heart disease is causing severe clinical signs even at rest.

Class I dogs are commonly identified in practice as the older but healthy dog with chronic mitral regurgitation (MR). Class II dogs are certainly underrecognized. Although exercise limitations are probably the most sensitive finding for a failing heart, most dogs do not engage in maximal exercise, and clients often disregard reduced exercise capacity as "just slowing down with age." Class III dogs have consistent clinical signs attributed to heart disease (classes II and III are combined in the ISACHC scheme). Dogs with class III left-sided HF pose a diagnostic dilemma in terms of distinguishing cough caused by primary tracheobronchial disease from that caused by left main-stem bronchial compression or pulmonary edema. Class IV dogs (class III in ISACHC scheme) are in obvious CHF and present more of a therapeutic than a diagnostic challenge.

Although some dogs with heart disease follow an orderly progression though a functional classification, these schemes allow the patient to move freely in both directions. For example, movement from class IV to class III or II might follow diuretic therapy. Progression from class I to class III or IV could occur following a large dietary salt load, the sudden structural deterioration of a mitral valve, or the onset of a hemodynamically significant arrhythmia such as AF.

The American College of Cardiology (ACC) and the American Heart Association (AHA) have developed a new approach to staging HF that emphasizes the progressive nature of most of the diseases that cause HF. This scheme (modified from *J Am Coll Cardiol* 38:2101, 2001) can be adapted for veterinary use as follows:

- *Stage A:* Patients are at high risk for the development of HF but without apparent structural abnormality at the present time. Examples would include cavalier King Charles spaniels; boxers; Doberman pinschers; and other dogs belonging to breeds, families, or demographic groups predisposed to heart disease.
- *Stage B:* Patients have a structural abnormality but have never had symptoms of HF. Examples include the asymptomatic miniature poodle with a murmur

of MR, an asymptomatic Doberman pinscher with systolic myocardial dysfunction and left ventricular dilatation, and an asymptomatic boxer with significant right ventricular ectopy on a Holter electrocardiogram (ECG).
- *Stage C:* Patients have a structural abnormality and current or previous clinical signs of HF. This stage includes all patients that have had an episode of clinical HF. They stay in this stage despite improvement of their clinical signs with standard medical therapy.
- *Stage D:* Patients have clinical signs of CHF that are refractory to standard treatment (defined in humans as standard doses of diuretics, angiotensin-converting enzyme [ACE] inhibitors, β-blockers, and digoxin).

The ACC/AHA staging system modified for dogs (and adopted by the European Society of Veterinary Cardiology and the American College of Veterinary Internal Medicine Study Groups) emphasizes that progressive structural abnormalities underlie the pathogenesis of HF. This system is meant to encourage a program of HF management and education that supports early detection and screening for heart disease and provides a loosely defined "stepped" plan of treatment intensification that may be applied appropriately as heart disease progresses. This program defines current *standard treatment* in humans as combination therapy of furosemide, an ACE inhibitor, digoxin (if no known contraindications exist), and a β-adrenergic blocking agent. What constitutes standard therapy for canine HF is still debated, but the principles of the classification still hold. This staging system departs from older functional classifications because a patient can still progress suddenly from stage B to stage C or even D, but that path cannot be traveled in reverse.

The modified ACC/AHA staging system provides a useful framework for thinking about heart disease and HF that is more analogous to the standard clinical approach to cancer. The parallels are obvious: screening and identification of patients that are known to be at risk for cancer (stage A); the identification and treatment of patients with in-situ disease (stage B); and the identification and treatment of patients with established (stage C) or widespread (stage D) disease.

FRAMEWORK FOR MANAGING HEART FAILURE IN DOGS

Considering what we know regarding the origin, pathogenesis, progression, and response to therapy of the common acquired heart diseases of dogs (valvular heart disease and DCM), a therapeutic framework for managing heart disease and HF in dogs should include specific diagnostic, treatment, and educational plans for each stage of heart disease. Management plans should consider the natural history of the disease and carefully weigh what is known regarding the potential benefits and risks of medications and their combinations when used in a specific clinical setting. This general scheme can be used to establish management plans for any type of heart disease. A brief example of a management strategy using these principles is described in the following paragraphs for DVD, with some additional comments inserted concerning the dog with DCM.

Stage A: Screening for Dogs At Risk But Without Clinical Signs

Cavalier King Charles spaniels, dachshunds, and other small breeds at increased risk for the development of chronic valvular heart disease should be screened by thorough cardiac auscultation. In otherwise healthy animals, the absence of a typical holosystolic murmur of mitral valve insufficiency over the left cardiac apex adequately rules out *significant* disease. This screening is repeated annually. If a screening examination is positive, the patient proceeds to stage B.

It should be emphasized that this stand-alone auscultation approach is inappropriate as the screening test for breeds at risk for cardiomyopathy. These disorders require echocardiography and possibly an ambulatory (Holter) ECG to obtain a reasonable sensitivity for diagnosis.

Stage B: Heart Disease Is Evident From Screening Examination

Now that heart disease (in this case a murmur of MR stemming from probable DVD) has been identified, the cardiac diagnosis is further refined by additional evaluations. The potential for early therapy is also considered.

Staging the severity of DVD includes imaging of the heart. In general one can recommend acquisition of high-quality thoracic radiographs exposed with a standard technique (e.g., right lateral and dorsoventral projections) if for no other reason than to have a comparison should the dog eventually develop respiratory signs. This approach improves differentiation of cardiac from primary respiratory causes of cough or dyspnea.

Depending on the circumstances, a two-dimensional echocardiogram might also be obtained to confirm the presence of anatomic valve lesions and provide additional quantitation of heart size and function. A Doppler echocardiographic study can confirm the auscultatory diagnosis and offers semiquantitative measures of severity. An echocardiogram is certainly indicated when the diagnosis is uncertain (e.g., is the MR murmur caused by endocardiosis or DCM in a cocker spaniel?). Furthermore, an echocardiogram is probably indicated in any dog younger than 6 years of age with a murmur to rule out the possibility of congenital heart disease. As with any system, common sense must also apply; and this last guideline would probably be inappropriate for a cavalier King Charles spaniel of 4 to 6 years of age, in which valvular endocardiosis may become evident in young adult dogs.

If thoracic radiographs are normal in the dog with a typical MR murmur of DVD, no further workup is indicated (although some clinicians measure arterial BP to screen for hypertension). Repeated imaging would be suggested in 1 year. However, if imaging demonstrates significant cardiomegaly or echocardiography shows hemodynamically important mitral valve regurgitation with left atrial enlargement, it would be prudent to consider the current evidence and treatment recommendations before the onset of clinical signs. Concurrently the client should be educated regarding the presence of significant heart disease; treatment options; and their potential impact of therapy on prognosis, cost, and quality of life.

Considering the current framework and example, how might one manage the dog with DVD and associated cardiomegaly? A number of therapeutic possibilities can be considered. Our personal recommendations and specific treatment guidelines are summarized later in this chapter.

Angiotensin-Converting Enzyme Inhibitors (Enalapril, Benazepril, Ramipril, Quinapril, and Lisinopril)

Early use of ACE inhibitors is still controversial. Evidence based on randomized, prospective, blinded clinical trials in dogs with chronic valve disease is mixed. One study (SVEP, Kvart et al., 2002) showed no benefit in delaying onset of CHF, whereas results from another trial (VETPROOF, Atkins et al., 2007) show a possible mild benefit. This was equivalent to approximately a 3-month extension of time before the onset of HF over a 3-year period. It should be emphasized that these points are pertinent only to the small-breed dog with DVD. Dogs with idiopathic DCM or large-breed dogs with significant MR might benefit from ACE inhibition based on some clinical reports. In an abstract from Guelph reporting results of an open-label trial, enalapril delayed onset of CHF for Doberman pinschers.

β-Blockers (Atenolol, Metoprolol, Carvedilol)

Therapy with β-blockers in stage B disease (or any other stage) is still debated because there are no data from sufficiently powered, controlled clinical trials in client-owned animals with DVD and only small studies in dogs with spontaneous DCM. Experimental evidence from relatively acute studies of induced mitral valve disease in larger dogs and from models of experimental canine myocardial disease, as well as extrapolation from human clinical trials, suggests a potential benefit of β-blockade. Overall these are relatively low grades of evidence on which to recommend a therapy. Proof of efficacy in asymptomatic DVD is difficult to obtain because the time course of chronic MR often exceeds 4 to 5 years before onset of CHF. In this ambiguous situation some cardiologists initiate a β-blocker therapy in asymptomatic dogs with moderate-to-advanced DVD; based on a recent survey of North American veterinary cardiologists, most do not. Again, dogs with DCM or large-breed dogs with advanced MR represent different patient groups, and it is more common for cardiologists to prescribe β-blockade in these groups aiming for myocardial protection. However, it is emphasized that no definitive studies have been published to support treatment with β-blockers in dogs with HF.

Digoxin

Cardiac glycosides are not recommended since there are no clinical trials and little experimental evidence supporting use of digoxin at this stage of disease in DVD (or in canine DCM).

Pimobendan (Vetmedin)

This inodilator is not recommended by most cardiologists at this stage of disease. Currently two clinical trials are investigating the efficacy and effects of pimobendan in asymptomatic dogs with DVD and with preclinical DCM.

Spironolactone

This aldosterone antagonist generally is not recommended based on absence of any convincing clinical evidence of efficacy at this stage of disease. Spironolactone demonstrates no significant diuretic effects in dogs with normal aldosterone levels (i.e., dogs not in CHF).

Neutraceuticals (Taurine, Carnitine, Coenzyme Q_{10}, ω-3 Fatty Acids, or Fish Oils)

These drugs generally are not recommended in dogs with DVD based on absence of any convincing clinical evidence at this stage of disease. Conversely, in particular canine breeds with primary myocardial diseases, there may be some indication for supplementation (see Chapter 159 for details).

Sodium (Salt)–Restricted Diet

Dietary modifications during stage B are controversial. Modest salt restriction, preferably without protein restriction (e.g., a "senior diet") may be of potential benefit in advanced DVD since experimental studies show abnormal sodium handling before the onset of HF. However, considering the long time course of chronic MR, this overall benefit is likely to be very small.

Stage C: Hemodynamically Significant Heart Disease With Signs of Heart Failure

Many dogs with DVD (and most with DCM) are first diagnosed and treated at this stage of disease. These patients usually are presented to the veterinarian because the owner has identified apparent dyspnea, often associated with orthopnea or a history of not wanting to lie down. Coughing is often present in the history along with days or weeks of exercise intolerance, lethargy, reduced appetite, and weight loss. The heart rate is often elevated for a resting dog (>140 beats/min), as is the respiratory rate (>40/min). Examination likely indicates cardiac abnormalities, including murmur(s) in dogs with DVD and possibly arrhythmias and gallop sounds. Lungs may crackle from pulmonary edema, but this is not always evident. In right-sided CHF jugular distention, hepatomegaly and possibly ascites may be evident.

If the animal is not too anxious or dyspneic, confirmation of the diagnosis with thoracic radiographs is always indicated as are other diagnostics as previously discussed. When life-threatening CHF is evident, aggressive management may be required as described for stage D and later in the treatment plans. For dogs that have been followed chronically through the various stages of heart disease, the likelihood of identifying early signs of HF is relatively high, and many of these dogs can be given a single dose of furosemide and sent home receiving oral medications for HF.

Unquestionably there are dogs with DVD in which the precise cause of coughing is not obvious. In these patients a more "restrained" HF treatment plan is indicated initially. This consists of a low daily dosage of furosemide plus an ACE inhibitor. This therapy generally improves signs when the problem is HF and thereby provides insight into the basis for coughing. Some dogs without overt CHF but affected by left main-stem bronchial compression also improve with this therapy and can be managed for some time with these two

drugs and occasional use of cough suppressants. However, in many canine patients there is no doubt about the diagnosis of CHF, and treatments that have been shown to reduce clinical signs and/or prolong life are recommended.

Most dogs with stage C failure are started on standard canine HF therapy. Based on the evidence and a recent survey of cardiologists, this includes preload reduction (furosemide), an ACE inhibitor, and pimobendan. There are clinical trials that show efficacy of these treatments in dogs with both advanced DVD and DCM. Some still prefer to prescribe an ACE inhibitor versus pimobendan, but a cogent argument can be made for starting both drugs simultaneously along with furosemide since these agents work differently. Spironolactone is often prescribed by cardiologists for advanced CHF, and this drug has recently been approved for treatment of CHF in dogs in Europe (although the specific trials are unpublished at this time). Digoxin has largely been supplanted by pimobendan, but cardiac glycosides may be useful in the setting of atrial arrhythmias or for potential benefits in sensitizing baroreceptors. As previously mentioned, the risk-benefits of a β-blocker in stable stage C (or D) failure is unresolved. If used, β-blockade should be delayed until the patient is free of any congestion and obviously is stable on a recheck examination. Drugs such as carvedilol should be started at low doses and gradually up-titrated.

Even with successful resolution of clinical signs, these patients remain on chronic drug therapy and never fall below a stage C classification. The diuretic dosage may be adjusted down to the lowest level needed. Chronic HF therapy is aimed at achieving two principal goals: (1) solidifying and maintaining hemodynamic improvements with a return to routine activities without clinical signs of HF; and (2) prolonging life by reducing the ongoing damage to the heart muscle inflicted by neurohormonal activation, as long as the therapy does not impair quality of life.

Stage D: Refractory Heart Failure

In the acute setting with previously untreated patients, it is impossible to tell which dogs will be refractory to treatment. For this reason stages C and D are considered together with respect to in-hospital management of HF. Chronic progression of stage C to stage D produces patients that are refractory to standard therapy with furosemide, spironolactone, ACE inhibition, pimobendan, and possibly β-blockers. Treatment of refractory HF from any cause is a challenging and potentially frustrating endeavor for both veterinarians and clients. A thorough search for factors commonly involved in the progression of HF is indicated, including anemia, hypertension, infection, and iatrogenic thyrotoxicosis.

Therapeutic principles for stage D failure include maintenance of whatever hemodynamic and cardioprotective regimens were well tolerated during stage C. It becomes important to evaluate critically client compliance, the current drug regimen, and the dosages. For example, it may be possible to "optimize" the dosages of the ACE inhibitor (to 0.5 mg/kg orally [PO] q12h for enalapril or benazepril), pimobendan (to 0.3 mg/kg PO q12h or 0.6 mg/kg daily divided TID), or spironolactone (2 mg/kg daily). If renal function is still normal, furosemide dosages can be increased, and digoxin can be added for its inotropic and baroreceptor activities. Regular subcutaneous dosing of furosemide may provide some additional benefit as described in the treatment plans. Others prefer to cautiously add hydrochlorothiazide (1 to 2 mg/kg QOD initially), although sequential nephron blockade of sodium resorption with three diuretics often predisposes to acute renal failure and marked electrolyte depletion. If a β-blocker is part of the regimen, the potential that the dose is too high should be considered. If a new arrhythmia has developed, especially AF, the addition of diltiazem to control ventricular rate may be pivotal (see Chapter 161 and following paragraphs). Some centers attempt direct current cardioversion to improve hemodynamics in dogs with CHF and AF. Although very effective in dogs with AF alone (see Chapter 164), in our experience some dogs with advanced heart disease do not cardiovert, and the majority revert. For dogs with documented severe pulmonary hypertension and exertional collapse, syncope, or advancing ascites or pleural effusion, a drug such as sildenafil (1 to 3 mg/kg PO q8–12h) or another phosphodiesterase V inhibitor may be useful for a trial course of therapy. When borderline or overt systemic hypertension complicates CHF, vigorous BP reduction should be undertaken (see Chapter 159). This generally involves a full dose of an ACE inhibitor and up-titrated doses of amlodipine (starting at 0.05 to 0.1 mg/kg PO q12h) to reduce systolic BP to the 90– to 120–mm Hg range.

The use of additional arterial or venous dilators, positive inotropes, or sophisticated electrical or mechanical circulatory aids may be of potential benefit for some clients and patients. Cardiologists may be helpful in discussing extralabel therapies or new drugs that may provide benefit. Cardiac pacemaker resynchronization therapy, valve repair, and other novel strategies may gain some foothold in advanced veterinary care. Consultation with or referral to an HF center or veterinary cardiologist is suggested if these resources are available.

For dogs with life-threatening pulmonary edema or cardiogenic shock, hemodynamic optimization and maintenance of BP and tissue oxygenation are the initial hospital treatment goals. Oxygen is administered. Thoracocentesis or abdominocentesis is indicated for large pleural effusions or tense ascites. Medical treatments may include intravenous boluses of furosemide supplemented by constant-rate infusions (CRIs); addition of nitroglycerin or sodium nitroprusside for acute load reduction; or infusion of dobutamine to manage cardiogenic shock. Details of these treatments follow.

DRUGS USED IN THE THERAPY OF CANINE HEART FAILURE

Cardiovascular therapy involves the use of a relatively large number of drugs. Some treatments for CHF elicit rapid hemodynamic effects (furosemide, dobutamine, sodium nitroprusside, and pimobendan). Others modulate neurohormonal or inflammatory mediators of CHF (ACE inhibitors, spironolactone, β–blockers, and fatty acids). Still others may be used for pure symptom relief (airway medications, sedatives, and oxygen). Understanding the clinical use of these drugs singly and in combination with others is critical.

Diuretics

Diuretics and dietary sodium restriction are critical for management of CHF. Furosemide (2 to 6 mg/kg intravenously [IV], intramuscularly [IM], subcutaneously [SQ], PO) is a potent loop diuretic used first for mobilization of edema and chronically to prevent fluid retention (on a BID-TID basis). Given initially by the intravenous or intramuscular route every 2 to 6 hours, furosemide also can be infused (after the initial bolus) for life-threatening pulmonary edema (6 to 8 mg/kg CRI over 24 hours). This approach appears to increase urine volume with less electrolyte disturbance. Spironolactone (2 mg/kg PO in one daily or two divided doses) is a very weak diuretic used mainly for cardioprotective and potassium-sparring actions and is given as cotherapy with furosemide in chronic management of CHF. Some clinicians use hydrochlorothiazide (starting at 1 to 2 mg/kg once daily or QOD) for refractory edema or ascites. Adverse effects of diuretics include polydipsia, polyuria, reduction in BP, azotemia, electrolyte depletion, and elevated blood potassium (with spironolactone). A thiazide can be dangerous when added to furosemide and spironolactone, and serum chemistries should be monitored carefully when three diuretics are prescribed. In the future nesiritide (genetically engineered, human-BNP) may be used as an adjunct to diuretic therapy of severe CHF.

Vasodilators and Angiotensin-Converting Enzyme Inhibitors

The ACE inhibitors and vasodilators are mainstays of CHF therapy. Venodilation pools blood in systemic veins and reduces venous pressure, whereas arterial dilation reduces BP and left ventricular afterload. MR is usually reduced considerably by arterial vasodilation and lowering of diastolic BP.

ACE inhibitors, including benazepril, enalapril, and ramipril, are typically dosed at 0.5 mg/kg PO once or twice daily). These drugs have modest vasodilator effects but importantly reduce angiotensin II and aldosterone levels and protect the cardiac muscle. The ACE inhibitors are the vasodilator drugs of choice for chronic CHF. In our practice we typically start at 0.25 mg/kg orally every 12 hours (or 0.5 mg/kg once daily) and increase the dosage to 0.5 mg/kg orally every 12 hours at the time of first follow-up if the drug is well tolerated. Major adverse effects include reduced BP, elevated blood urea nitrogen, and elevated serum potassium.

Direct vasodilator drugs (with usual dosages) include 2% nitroglycerin ointment (¼ to 1 inch topically q12h), sodium nitroprusside (0.5 to 5 mcg/kg/minute), and sildenafil (1.0 to 3 mg/kg PO q8-12h). Nitrates increase nitric oxide, and the phosphodiesterase V inhibitor sildenafil prevents degradation of the second messenger of this system (cyclic guanosine 5'-monophosphate). Nitrates are used for hospital therapy of CHF; sildenafil and related drugs are used for treatment of severe pulmonary hypertension (peak pressure >80 mm Hg).

L-arginine, the precursor of nitric oxide, is supplemented (empiric canine dose: 250 to 500 mg PO TID) when severe pulmonary hypertension is documented.

Amlodipine (0.05 to 0.1 mg/kg PO q12h in dogs with CHF; higher dosages for systemic hypertension) is a calcium channel blocker with vascular selectivity. It is used mainly in dogs with intercurrent systemic hypertension that do not respond sufficiently to an ACE inhibitor and diuretic therapy. Amlodipine can also provide additional vasodilation to unload the left ventricle in end-stage MR. The main adverse effect of all arterial vasodilator drugs is systemic hypotension. Some drugs, including amlodipine and hydralazine (1 to 3 mg/kg PO q12h), also may cause reflex neurohormonal activation.

Positive Inotropic Drugs

The positive inotropic drugs include catecholamines (dobutamine, dopamine), digoxin, and pimobendan. Dobutamine (2.5 to 10 mcg/kg/minute) is reserved for dogs with cardiogenic shock (BP <80 to 85 mm Hg; hypothermia; CHF) and is infused in 5% dextrose solution for 24 to 48 hours. Specifics on using dobutamine are outlined in Cardiogenic Shock later in the chapter.

Digoxin (0.005 to 0.0075 mg/kg PO q12h in dogs with normal renal function) is a modest positive inotropic drug that also slows heart rate. The main indication for digoxin is advanced CHF or CHF with AF, in which its vagal enhancement helps to slow atrioventricular nodal conduction and heart rate by improving baroreceptor sensitivity. Adverse effects of digoxin (i.e., anorexia, vomiting, diarrhea, depression, and cardiac arrhythmias) are best avoided by monitoring therapy with a serum digoxin level. A trough level of 0.8 to 1.2 ng/ml is the recommended target. Relative contraindications to digoxin use are complex ventricular ectopia, azotemia, sinus node dysfunction, and preexistent atrioventricular block.

Pimobendan (Vetmedin 0.2 to 0.3 mg/kg PO q12h; in end-stage CHF may administer off label) is a potent, orally administered inotropic drug with vasodilator properties. It is classified as a calcium sensitizer with phosphodiesterase III inhibition. Now widely available, pimobendan has largely replaced digoxin for management of moderate-to-severe CHF in dogs. No consistent adverse effects of pimobendan have been reported; however, clients may notice the heart "pounding" at higher dosages. Furthermore, it is likely that some dogs will experience an increase in ventricular ectopy following therapy with pimobendan (or any positive inotropic drug). The importance of any proarrhythmic effect awaits further study.

β-Adrenergic Blockers

β-Blockers, particularly carvedilol and metoprolol (long-acting) are used increasingly in HF to protect the heart muscle and with chronic use may improve left ventricular ejection fraction in cardiomyopathy. In model studies β-blockers are cardioprotective, but this was not evident in a preliminary clinical study in dogs with DCM. Carvedilol is now available in a very affordable generic form in some countries. It is a nonspecific β-blocker

with weaker α-adrenergic blocking effects. Also a potent antioxidant drug, carvedilol may protect myocardium from cytokine injury. Although β-blockers should never be used in uncontrolled CHF, gradual dose up-titration is possible in many dogs. For example, after an initial 2- to 4-week treatment to stabilize CHF, a starting dose of carvedilol (0.05 to 0.1 mg/kg PO once or twice daily) is usually well tolerated. The dosage may be increased slowly in DCM every 2 to 4 weeks, aiming for a target dosage of about 0.5 to 0.6 mg/kg orally every 12 hours. Higher doses are tolerated in asymptomatic dogs and in dogs with DVD in which myocardial dysfunction is usually less severe. Only very low doses tend to be tolerated in many dogs with severe DCM. Concurrent use of pimobendan seems to offset the negative inotropic effects of β-blockers. Major adverse effects are weakness, hypotension, bradycardia, and worsening of edema or effusions. Better known drugs such as atenolol are potentially beneficial in models of canine left ventricular dysfunction, but little is known clinically about their use for this purpose in canine HF.

Antiarrhythmic Drugs

Antiarrhythmic drugs are not used specifically for treatment of CHF. However, in AF heart rate control is usually gained by combination of digoxin plus diltiazem (starting dosage of diltiazem is 0.5 mg/kg PO q8h up-titrated to as high as 2 mg/kg PO q8h or 6 mg/kg daily of a long-acting preparation divided BID). Often the addition of carvedilol further slows the ventricular rate response to AF, allowing for a dosage reduction of diltiazem. Both drugs are negative inotropes and must be used carefully. Some clinicians prefer other β-blockers for control of heart rate in AF such as atenolol (starting dose of 0.1 mg/kg PO q12h in CHF with dosage up-titration to 0.25 to 0.5 mg/kg PO q12h).

Management of ventricular arrhythmias in the setting of CHF is difficult. Sotalol and many other antiarrhythmic drugs are negative inotropes and are best avoided if possible. Intravenous lidocaine (2 to 4 mg/kg intravenous boluses to 8 mg/kg; 50 mcg/kg/minute CRI) can be used in the hospital, and mexiletine (5 to 8 mg/kg PO q8h) may be effective if adverse effects (anorexia, vomiting, and tremors) are not severe. Reduced hepatic blood flow may lead to toxicity. Mexiletine and long-acting formulations of procainamide (12 to 20 mg/kg PO q8h) are ventricular antiarrhythmic drugs with minimal myocardial depression; however, other adverse effects, including anorexia and gastrointestinal signs, can be observed. Mexiletine can elevate liver enzymes in some dogs. Amiodarone is used increasingly for life-threatening arrhythmias at about 10 mg/kg orally once daily for 2 weeks and 4 to 6 mg/kg orally once daily thereafter. Liver enzymes/function tests and a complete blood count should be followed quarterly in dogs receiving amiodarone. Severe liver toxicity has been observed. The drug has a very long elimination half-life; therefore adverse effects may be persistent. Management of rhythm disturbances are discussed in more detail in Arrhythmias in CHF later in the chapter and in Chapters 161, 162, and 164).

SPECIFIC TREATMENT PLANS FOR CANINE HEART FAILURE

The management of HF in dogs involves consideration of the underlying cardiac diagnosis, the stage of heart disease, and the current clinical findings. Some dogs with stages C or D (or NYHA modified class IV) HF will likely succumb from tissue hypoxia, hypotension, or arrhythmia if not promptly treated in the hospital setting. Other patients with less severe signs are simpler to manage and often can be treated on an outpatient basis. There are few studies objectively assessing HF therapy in dogs; nevertheless, clinicians need to make decisions about patient management that are decisive and specific. In that vein the following are personal guidelines for hospital and home management of the dog with HR.

Asymptomatic Heart Disease

As noted previously, early introduction of cardiovascular drug therapy in preclinical or asymptomatic dogs with stage B heart disease is controversial. For dogs with DCM that is well-defined by echocardiography, we prescribe cardioprotective drugs in an attempt to delay onset of overt HF. We prescribe both an ACE inhibitor (enalapril 0.5 mg/kg PO q12h) and a β-blocker (usually carvedilol up-titrated every 2 weeks as described previously) to dogs with proven ventricular dysfunction caused by DCM. Large-breed dogs with chronic MR and demonstrable cardiomegaly or left ventricular dysfunction are treated as if they have occult DCM.

The SVEP and VETPROOF trials (Kvart et al., 2002; Atkins et al., 2007). together suggest a small benefit at best for small-breed dogs with preclinical DVD. We believe that, if an ACE inhibitor is started, it should be in a dog with well-advanced MR from DVD. We recommend regular chest radiographs or quantitative 2D echocardiograms to identify moderate-to-severe MR or a marked interval change in heart size compared to prior evaluations. In advanced or progressive cases we begin an ACE inhibitor empirically. We recommend a full dose of 0.5 mg/kg of enalapril/benazepril every 12 hours, considering that some dogs in these published trials were treated with relatively low doses. We also screen older dogs for hypertension, initiate ACE inhibitor therapy, and evaluate kidney and adrenal functions in dogs with hypertension and advanced MR.

We do not advocate the use of inotropic drugs such as digoxin or pimobendan in preclinical stage B unless radiographs indicate that pulmonary edema is imminent or left ventricular systolic dysfunction is markedly reduced and there is associated exercise intolerance. Breeds at risk for fulminant CHF such as the Doberman pinscher would be likely candidates for pimobendan in these situations. As stated earlier, clinical trials are under way to address the issue of early intervention with pimobendan in dogs with DCM and DVD.

Acute Pulmonary Edema

When CHF leads to life-threatening pulmonary dysfunction, the combination of parenteral furosemide, oxygen, topical nitroglycerin (or sodium nitroprusside), and sedation with butorphanol represents the initial treatment plan applicable to most dogs with CHF regardless of cause. In our experience butorphanol (0.25 mg/kg IM, repeated in 30 to 60 minutes if needed) is the safest sedative to use in this setting. With this protocol diuresis is initiated; hemoglobin oxygen saturation is increased, ventricular preload is reduced, the tendency toward pulmonary edema is decreased, and anxiety is relieved. If patients are heavily sedated, the torso is positioned in sternal recumbency, the chin supported with a towel or soft pad, the neck gently extended, and nasal oxygen inserted for better oxygenation.

A relatively high initial furosemide dose (4 to 5 mg/kg IV) is administered in cases of severe CHF because renal blood flow may be reduced. The dog should be checked every 30 minutes for evidence of diuretic effect (by observation for urination and palpation of the urinary bladder). Once diuresis ensues, the dose is reduced to 2 mg/kg every 8 to 12 hours intravenously or intramuscularly. In life-threatening pulmonary edema (i.e., severe dyspnea with poor response to initial therapy, expectoration of fluid, or "white-out" lung on chest radiograph), a CRI of furosemide and afterload reduction with nitroprusside (or oral hydralazine) should be considered.

Although topical nitroglycerin may function as a venodilator, reduction of systemic BP is one of the most effective methods for reducing the severity of MR. The addition of nitroprusside is indicated in cases of pulmonary edema characterized by severe dyspnea, hemoptysis, or expectoration of pink froth with marked alveolar infiltrates on the chest radiographs, especially those that don't improve clinically over the first 30 to 60 minutes of hospitalization (Fig. 171-1). The main contraindication to potent afterload reducers such as nitroprusside is preexistent hypotension (<90 mm Hg systolic BP). Frequent BP monitoring should be scheduled when administering nitroprusside, and the clinician should titrate the infusion dose to a systolic pressure of 85 to 100 mm Hg (as well as to clinical signs). Treatment duration is 24 hours (or less) in most cases. Less potent and less controllable alternatives to nitroprusside include an ACE inhibitor and oral hydralazine (0.5 to 2 mg/kg q8–12h). Initiation of pimobendan in the setting of acute pulmonary edema also can be considered since this drug reduces both afterload and preload.

Cardiogenic Shock

The finding of cardiogenic pulmonary edema or pleural effusion with severe hypotension (BP <80 mm Hg) and other indicators of low cardiac output (pallor, hypothermia, depression, and elevated blood lactate) is highly suggestive of cardiogenic shock. Dogs with DCM are most likely to be presented this way. Other potential causes include myocardial infarction, overdose of a β-blocker, and massive pulmonary embolus as might occur following treatment for adult heartworms or after a spontaneous pulmonary thromboembolism.

Initial treatment is the same as discussed previously, starting with furosemide-oxygen-nitroglycerin therapy. Since these patients are hypotensive and often very depressed, sedation is rarely needed. The need for

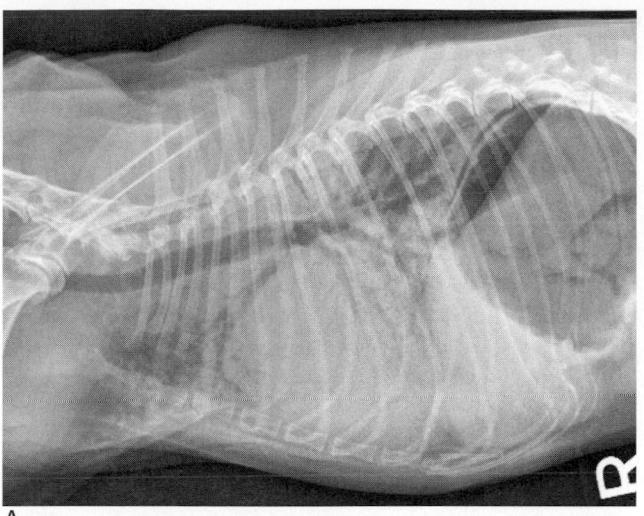
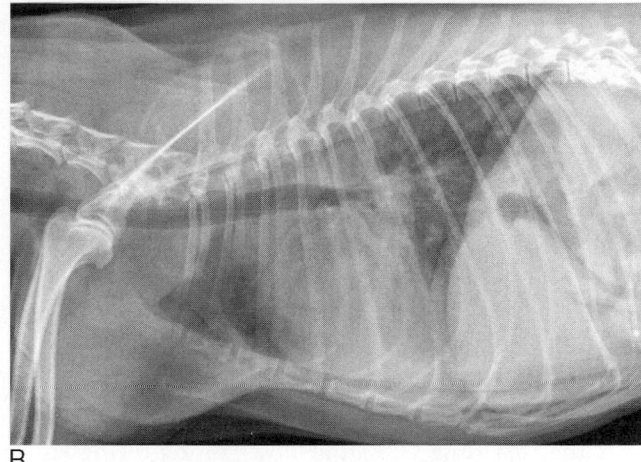

Fig. 171-1 **A,** Thoracic radiograph from a dog with severe pulmonary edema associated with DVD and ruptured chorda tendinea. **B,** Thoracic radiograph from the same dog 20 hours after aggressive diuresis and load-reducing therapy with sodium nitroprusside. The dog was released from the hospital.

thoracocentesis should be determined since dogs with cardiogenic shock may have both pulmonary edema and pleural effusion. Volume infusion is inappropriate to raise BP in this setting because it only worsens edema. In most cases the main goal is stimulation of myocardial contractility to improve pump function and facilitate diuresis.

In this situation the most important therapy to administer (along with diuretics) is a potent positive inotropic drug with a goal of increasing BP by augmenting cardiac output. No other drug seems as effective as dobutamine in this setting of cardiogenic shock. However, cotherapy with pimobendan may be very beneficial and can help dobutamine create a "bridge" to allow for long-term therapy with pimobendan, an ACE inhibitor, and diuretics. Digoxin is too weak to have much effect in cardiogenic shock and is only initiated in the setting of AF (for heart rate control).

Dobutamine (or dopamine if preferred) is administered as an intravenous CRI, starting at 2.5 mcg/kg/minute and increasing the infusion every 30 minutes until systolic BP is 90 mm Hg. The typical end point is 5 to 10 mcg/kg/minute. At higher infusion rates vasoconstriction and increased heart rate become increasingly important as factors that increase BP. However, neither vasoconstriction (which creates an afterload mismatch) nor sinus tachycardia (which increases oxygen demand) represents an advantage to a failing left ventricle. Therapeutic effects of dobutamine include increased cardiac output, elevated BP, increased tissue perfusion (better color and shorter refill time, stronger pulse), increasing body temperature, and improvement in attitude and strength. Adverse effects necessitating dose reduction include increasing heart rate, excessive vasoconstriction, and induction of extrasystoles. Seizure activity and vomiting are observed infrequently in dogs.

Once the BP is stable (systolic pressure in the 90- to 100-mm Hg range), other vasoactive drugs, either nitroprusside or an ACE inhibitor, can be initiated, and pimobendan started. After 24 to 48 hours of dobutamine therapy, the dobutamine rate is reduced by 50% every

2 to 4 hours, and after reaching 1 to 2 mcg/kg for 2 to 4 hours the infusion is discontinued.

Arrhythmias in Congestive Heart Failure

The most common rhythm considerations are atrial premature complexes, AF, ventricular ectopy (premature ventricular complexes and ventricular tachycardia), and sinus node disease in breeds at risk (e.g., miniature schnauzers, cocker spaniels, and West Highland white terriers), wherein digoxin and β-blockers should be avoided. Isolated atrial and ventricular premature complexes may respond to treatment of CHF and are not aggressively suppressed with drugs.

Digoxin is the initial drug chosen to control heart rate in dogs with AF and CHF; however, additional therapy is usually needed to prevent deleterious effects of persistent tachycardia. After confirming the rhythm diagnosis of AF with an ECG, digoxin can be started using a maintenance dosage (0.005 to 0.0075 mg/kg PO q12h) or a modified loading dose (0.01 mg/kg PO BID for two doses). To slow the heart rate further, after 24 to 48 hours of HF stabilization the calcium channel antagonist, diltiazem, is added to block the atrioventricular node (starting at 0.5 mg/kg PO q8h). Diltiazem added to digoxin better controls ventricular rate response. Provided systolic BP is higher than 90 mm Hg, one can rapidly up-titrate the dose of diltiazem at each subsequent dosing interval (i.e., increase the dose every 8 hours). Usual target doses of diltiazem are 1 to 2 mg/kg PO q8h (or an equivalent dose of long-acting diltiazem divided BID) to obtain a "resting" hospital heart rate of 120 to 160 beats/min. Some dogs require dosages as high as 6 mg/kg daily in divided doses. If follow-up examinations indicate stable CHF, a β-blocker also may be used to slow heart rate in AF. The clinician must beware of the negative inotropic effects of diltiazem and β-blockers.

Another option for treatment of AF is direct current cardioversion. Pros and cons of such therapy should be discussed with a cardiologist. Most dogs need to be kept on amiodarone to maintain sinus rhythm; and the time to relapse to AF may be short in some patients, related to severity of underlying disease, atrial remodeling, and duration of the rhythm (see Chapter 164).

When ventricular tachycardia complicates CHF, the optimal management is often uncertain. Treatment of isolated premature ventricular contractions with antiarrhythmic drugs is not recommended unless an ambulatory (Holter) ECG demonstrates "dangerous" rhythm disturbances at other times. Digoxin is *contraindicated* in the presence of complicated or repetitive ventricular arrhythmias. For management of ventricular tachycardia or dangerous ventricular ectopy, there are both intravenous hospital and long-term drugs. In the hospital lidocaine is the first drug chosen at doses of 2 to 4 mg/kg intravenous boluses up to 8 mg/kg over 10 minutes, followed by a 50- to 75-mcg/kg/minute CRI. Poor hepatic blood flow may lead to accumulation of drug and toxicity at relatively low doses. Procainamide (2 mg/kg boluses up to 10 to 20 mg/kg IV or 10 to 20 mg/kg IM, SQ, PO q6h) and amiodarone (2.5 to 5 mg/kg IV over 10 minutes) are alternatives for life-threatening ventricular tachycardia.

For chronic therapy of ventricular tachycardia, sotalol (1 to 2 mg/kg PO q12h) is best tolerated in dogs not yet in overt CHF, whereas mexiletine (5 to 8 mg/kg PO q8h) seems a better alternative in CHF if adverse effects (gastrointestinal or neurologic) are not severe. In some dogs the combination of mexiletine and low-dose sotalol is more effective. Amiodarone is used increasingly in patients with CHF (10 to 12 mg/kg PO once daily for 2 weeks; thereafter 4 to 6 mg/kg PO once daily). Appetite, history of gastrointestinal signs, liver enzymes/function tests, and complete blood and platelet counts should be followed every 1 to 3 months initially. Either mexiletine or amiodarone can be an effective antiarrhythmic if adverse effects do not supervene. Long-acting procainamide (12 to 20 mg/kg PO q8h) is another but infrequently used alternative.

Chronic (Home) Therapy of Congestive Heart Failure

The transition from hospital to home therapy of CHF may be nearly immediate in mild HF. However, when CHF is severe, a hospitalization period of 24 to 72 hours is typical. During this interval the initial diagnostic workup of thoracic radiographs, serum biochemical profile, ECG, and echocardiogram should be completed. Arterial BP should be measured frequently. Often a follow-up renal and electrolyte panel is obtained before release since vigorous diuretic therapy may alter serum biochemical values. Repeated thoracic radiographs may be obtained to ensure control of the CHF.

The typical transition to home therapy is as follows: (1) parenteral furosemide is replaced with oral furosemide; (2) oxygen is discontinued; (3) nitroglycerin is replaced with an ACE inhibitor (if not already on board); (4) pimobendan therapy is initiated; (5) digoxin is added if needed for rate control in AF; (6) spironolactone is initiated for cardioprotection; (7) the client is counseled regarding a sodium-restricted diet and the pros/cons of neutraceuticals; and (8) in dogs with echocardiographic evidence of left ventricular systolic dysfunction, carvedilol is prescribed; this therapy begins 2 to 4 weeks after initial CHF treatments and is up-titrated slowly as described previously; (9) in cases of severe pulmonary hypertension sildenafil therapy is discussed with the owner; (10) when AF complicates CHF, diltiazem is usually added to gain better heart rate control.

Most dogs respond well to multidrug treatment of CHF. The essential components of this therapy for confirmed dogs with CHF caused by DVD or DCM are dietary sodium restriction, furosemide, spironolactone, an ACE inhibitor, and pimobendan. These drugs are summarized in the previous section, and this strategy is detailed in Table 171-1. As HF progresses, fine tuning of this regimen is always necessary and should begin with drug dose optimization as discussed previously under management of stage D HF.

Follow-Up and Prognosis

Drug dosing and adverse drug effects are discussed with every client. Written instructions are optimal, including a summary of common adverse drug effects. Follow-up evaluations are rescheduled, emphasizing quality of life factors (eating, sleeping, mild exercise, family interaction, and clinical signs of disease or drug toxicity); home respiratory rate; physical examination findings; changes in body weight; current BP, renal function, and electrolyte values; heart rate and rhythm; and thoracic radiography. Renal function is particularly important to follow since HIF, sodium restriction, diuretic therapy, and ACE inhibitors can lead to an elevation of blood urea nitrogen and creatinine. Many dogs have primary renal disease, putting them at risk for development of azotemia or uremia. Common follow-up intervals are 7 to 14 days after initial diagnosis, 1 month later, and then every 3 months or immediately if problems develop.

COMPLICATING PROBLEMS IN CANINE HEART FAILURE

Severe pulmonary hypertension often occurs in dogs with chronic DVD, leading to exertional problems and ascites. This condition is likely related to elevated left atrial pressure, reactive pulmonary vascular change, and possibly concurrent lung disease. Ascites and pleural effusion are also common when AF develops later in the course of CHF, superimposed on pulmonary hypertension.

Some dogs with chronic left-sided CHF appear to develop pulmonary fibrosis and loud lung crackles at an accelerated rate; this should be recognized and not misdiagnosed as uncontrolled CHF. Dogs with chronic airway disease (tracheal or primary bronchial collapse or chronic bronchitis) may become symptomatic because of these diseases and require empiric courses of antibiotics (we use doxycycline initially) or even brief courses of prednisone at antiinflammatory doses.

Severe dental disease is often present as a comorbid condition in older small-breed dogs with DVD; this oral disease can reduce quality of life. This may require antibiotic therapy (amoxicillin with clavulanate or clindamycin) to reduce periodontal reaction or even a quick dental

Table **171-1**

Chronic (Home) Management of the Dog With Congestive Heart Failure

Treatment(s)	Treatment	Comments	Dosages | Guidelines
Dietary modifications	Reduce sodium intake; Consider OTC "senior diets" and prescription diets; optimal dosing of neutraceuticals in heart disease is generally not known	Discuss pros and cons of neutraceuticals (limited data; often expensive); consider taurine ± L-carnitine in cocker spaniels, L-carnitine in boxers, L-arginine for dogs receiving sildenafil for pulmonary hypertension; fish oils (EPA, DHA) in dogs with cardiac cachexia or poor appetite	Stringent restriction is <12 mg Na$^+$/kg of body weight daily; avoid high salt snacks, cheeses, and processed meats (hot dogs) Taurine: 250-500 mg PO q8-12h; L-carnitine: 40-50 mg/kg PO q8-12h; L-arginine: 250-500 mg PO q12h; ω-3 fatty acids: 40-50 mg/kg PO q12h
Furosemide	Prevent chronic sodium retention and edema	Dose to clinical/x-ray effect; follow BUN and BP	Furosemide: 2-6 mg/kg PO one to three times daily
Spironolactone	K$^+$ sparring, low-potency diuretic; cardioprotective	Mainly for heart protection; beware of ↑K$^+$	Spironolactone: ≈2 mg/kg PO once daily or divided BID
Inotropic drugs	Pimobendan (Vetmedin): potent oral inodilator Digoxin: modest inotrope that sensitizes baroreceptors increasing vagal tone	Pimobendan for CHF caused by DVD or DCM; also useful for other causes of canine CHF Digoxin for CHF with atrial fibrillation Digoxin contraindicated in renal failure, complex PVCs or bradycardia	Pimobendan: 0.2 to 0.3 mg/kg PO q12h Digoxin: 0.005 to 0.0075 mg/kg PO q12h
ACE-inhibitor	Enalapril, benazepril, and ramipril are most often used ACE-inhibitors in canine CHF	Maintain systolic BP above 85-90; follow BUN/Cr/K$^+$	Enalapril or Benazepril: 0.25-0.5 mg/kg PO q12h; the "full dose" is prescribed if BUN/Cr and BP are stable after 2 weeks of therapy
β-blocker	Carvedilol is the most often used β-blocker in canine CHF	Patient must be "dry" before beginning therapy Dosage is for dogs with DCM or left ventricular dysfunction; dogs without CHF can tolerate higher doses	Carvedilol: 0.05-0.5 mg/kg PO once or twice daily; start low and up-titrate every 2-4 weeks to target of ≈0.5 to 0.6 mg/kg PO q12h for the dog in CHF
Sildenafil	Phosphodiesterase V inhibitor that maintains the vasodilator effects of the nitric oxide messenger cyclic GMP	Sildenafil and related drugs are relatively specific pulmonary vasodilators used for treatment of severe PH with associated clinical signs	Initial dose is ≈0.5 to 1 mg/kg q8-12h Dosages up to 3 mg/kg q8h may be tolerated
Diltiazem	A calcium channel blocker used for control of heart rate in atrial fibrillation; not a drug treatment for CHF	Negative inotrope and vasodilator drug; can lower BP; initial dose is up-titrated rapidly (daily) to achieve rate control target of 120 to 160/minute at rest during hospital examination	Initial dose ≈0.5 mg/kg PO q8h of standard diltiazem (or 1.5 mg/kg *divided* BID for long-acting diltiazem); most dogs require *total daily dose* of 3 to 6 mg/kg

ACE, Angiotensin-converting enzyme; *BID,* twice a day; *BP,* blood pressure; *BUN,* blood urea nitrogen; *CHF,* congestive heart failure; *Cr,* creatinine; *EPA,* eicosapentaenoic acid; *DCM,* dilated cardiomyopathy; *DHA,* docosahexanoic acid; *DVD,* degenerative valvular heart disease; *GMP,* guanosine 5'-monophosphate; *K$^+$,* potassium ion; *NA$^+$,* sodium ion; *PH,* pulmonary hypertension; *PVC,* premature ventricular contraction; *OTC,* over the counter; *PO,* orally.

procedure to extract diseased teeth (with attendant risks of anesthesia).

Osteoarthritis is another common comorbid disease in older dogs with HF, especially in the larger breeds. The use of COX inhibitors can be beneficial, but initial doses should be one half of the regular dose, gastric protection (famotidine) should be prescribed daily, and renal function followed. A 4-week course of famotidine is also an empiric treatment for dogs with chronic CHF with recurrent anorexia.

The combination of primary renal failure and CHF is very difficult to manage because they require treatments directly opposed to one another (i.e., fluid repletion versus plasma volume control). When uremic signs develop, euthanasia may be prompted.

PROGNOSIS IN CANINE HEART FAILURE

The prognosis of canine CHF depends on the cause and severity of disease and the overall quality of management. Many dogs survive well beyond 1 year following the first signs of CHF with optimal veterinary and home care. It may take 2 to 4 weeks to obtain optimal stabilization of seriously ill dogs with CHF. Not every patient becomes well overnight, and clients should be so advised. As dogs become well managed, other problems may become evident.

The causes of death in chronic CHF vary but are most often related to one of the following: sudden electrical event (such as asystole or ventricular fibrillation); hypoxemia (pulmonary edema or pleural effusion); pulmonary embolism leading to fatal hypotension; multisystemic organ failure; or client desire for euthanasia. Client desire for euthanasia is a particularly common ending and depends on many factors that include effectiveness of therapy, severity of signs, client (and veterinarian) perceptions about quality of life, and issues of care (medication frequency, visits to the veterinary hospital, and costs) among other factors. It is important to ensure that clinical signs of disease are not caused by overmedication or drug toxicosis.

References and Suggested Reading

Atkins CE et al: Results of the veterinary enalapril trial to prove reduction in onset of heart failure in dogs chronically treated with enalapril alone for compensated, naturally occurring mitral valve insufficiency, *J Am Vet Med Assoc* 231(7):1061, 2007.

BENCH (BENazepril in Canine Heart disease) Study Group: The effect of benazepril on survival times and clinical signs of dogs with congestive heart failure: results of a multicenter, prospective, randomized, double-blinded, placebo-controlled, long-term clinical trial, *J Vet Cardiol* 1(1):7, 1999.

COVE STUDY GROUP: Controlled clinical evaluation of enalapril in dogs with heart failure: results of the Cooperative Veterinary Enalapril Study Group: the COVE Study Group, *J Vet Intern Med* 9(4):243, 1995.

Ericsson GF et al: Effects of enalapril maleate on survival of dogs with naturally acquired heart failure: the Long-Term Investigation of Veterinary Enalapril (LIVE) Study Group, *J Am Vet Med Assoc* 213(11):1573, 1998.

Fuentes VL: A double-blind, randomized, placebo-controlled study of pimobendan in dogs with dilated cardiomyopathy, *J Vet Intern Med* 16(3):255, 2002.

IMPROVE STUDY GROUP: Acute and short-term hemodynamic, echocardiographic, and clinical effects of enalapril maleate in dogs with naturally acquired heart failure: results of the Invasive Multicenter PROspective Veterinary Evaluation of Enalapril study: the IMPROVE Study Group, *J Vet Intern Med* 9(4):234, 1995.

Kvart C et al: Efficacy of enalapril for prevention of congestive heart failure in dogs with myxomatous valve disease and asymptomatic mitral regurgitation, *J Vet Intern Med* 16(1):80, 2002.

CHAPTER   172

Chronic Valvular Disease in Dogs

JOHN E. RUSH, *North Grafton, Massachusetts*

Chronic valvular disease (CVD) is the most common acquired heart disease in dogs, with an overall cumulative incidence of greater than 40%. CVD often results in congestive heart failure (CHF); and cardiac disease is responsible for approximately 10% of all canine deaths, with a higher incidence in some breeds of dogs such as the Cavalier King Charles spaniel. The mitral valve is most commonly affected, but concurrent tricuspid valve disease is often noted. Most veterinarians are very familiar with canine cardiac diseases, particularly CVD; thus the goal of this chapter is to discuss and highlight some important concepts, frequently discussed topics, and exciting diagnostic and therapeutic developments.

ETIOLOGY, PATHOLOGY, AND PATHOPHYSIOLOGY

The cause of CVD is currently unknown, although a genetic tendency to develop the disease has been proven in the Cavalier King Charles spaniel. As canine genomics develops it is likely that specific genes causing or contributing to the development of CVD will be identified. In addition, poorly defined environmental factors likely play a role in the rate of onset or severity of the disease.

Advanced valvular degeneration leads to grossly thickened and shortened valves with curled, nodular margins. Valvular hemorrhage and calcification may be seen. There is fibrosis of the valves, loss of collagen fibers, and an accumulation of acid-staining glycosaminoglycans within affected valves. Chordae tendineae are often affected and may become thickened, stretched, or ruptured. Electron microscopy has documented great variation in endothelial cell size and morphology of affected valves, with focal loss of the endothelial layer, collagen exposure, and activation of interstitial cells of the valve. It is not clear which of these findings is a result of the disease and which might be a cause or contributor to disease progression. CVD has historically been considered a noninflammatory, myxomatous degeneration of the atrioventricular valve, but there is growing interest in the role that serotonin or other inflammatory mediators may play in accelerating the pathology of the disease. There is one report of elevated C-reactive protein concentrations in the serum of affected dogs, suggesting a possible role of low-grade systemic inflammation in progression of the disease (Rush et al., 2006). Another study evaluating genomic expression patterns from the valves of dogs with CVD confirmed activation of several pathways involved in cell signaling, inflammation, and extracellular matrix activation, with several inflammatory cytokines and serotonin-transforming growth factor β pathways identified as contributory to the development of the degenerative process in the valve (Oyama and Chittur, 2006). Separate from the valve, many dogs with CVD have histopathologic lesions in the myocardium, including small foci of myocardial fibrosis and necrosis, as well as more widespread intramural coronary arteriosclerosis (Falk et al., 2006). The role that arteriosclerosis, myocardial fibrosis, and microinfarction resulting from occlusion of these arteriosclerotic lesions might play in the progression toward ventricular dilation and CHF is not well understood at this time, but these lesions seem to offer possible alternative avenues for investigation as treatment or interventional opportunities.

Progressive valvular thickening leads to valvular regurgitation and progressive dilation and hypertrophy of the atria and ventricles. Classic compensatory mechanisms (sympathetic nervous system activation, enhanced renin-angiotensin system activity) are activated in an attempt to restore blood pressure and tissue perfusion. As long as the dilated left atrium remains sufficiently compliant to accept the regurgitant blood volume, CHF does not develop, although coughing may develop from left bronchial compression. Eventually, as the volume of regurgitated blood becomes overwhelming, chordal rupture suddenly increases the regurgitant fraction, or the left ventricular myocardium starts to fail, CHF develops. This is typically in the form of pulmonary edema for mitral valve disease. Chronic left heart failure often leads to pulmonary hypertension (PHTN), posing added strain to the right heart and leading to signs of right-sided CHF with accumulation ascites and possibly pleural effusion. Atrial rhythm disturbances, including atrial fibrillation, can contribute to cardiac dysfunction.

Clinical Evaluation of the Dog With Chronic Vascular Disease

CVD is identified most commonly in middle-aged or older, small- to medium-sized breeds of dogs. Although CVD also occurs in large-breed dogs, dilated cardiomyopathy is a more common cause of CHF in these breeds than CVD. When large-breed dogs develop CVD, concurrent myocardial failure is often noted early in the disease. The incidence of CVD is increased in male dogs relative to females (1.5 to 1).

Clinical Presentations in Chronic Vascular Disease

Most dogs are first diagnosed with CVD based on the finding of a cardiac murmur in the absence of any signs of cardiac decompensation. The period between first identification of a murmur and onset of clinical signs is generally years. As the disease advances, many dogs develop a cough as the first sign of CVD, caused by either early CHF or atrial enlargement causing compression of the airways. Panting, dyspnea, exercise intolerance, weight loss, weakness, and syncope can also be causes for presentation to a veterinarian. Specific triggers that acutely increase fluid volume retention or decrease cardiac performance may precipitate CHF. These include dietary intake of salty foods, vigorous exercise or exertion in the prior 48 hours, recent onset of a rapid tachyarrhythmia, glucocorticoid administration, overzealous fluid therapy, or general anesthesia.

EVALUATION OF THE ASYMPTOMATIC DOG WITH A HEART MURMUR

Many dogs with CVD have an audible murmur for years before the onset of cardiac decompensation and CHF. An extra systolic sound known as a midsystolic "click" is often detected before the onset of this murmur and has been associated with mitral or tricuspid valve prolapse; this is a sign of early CVD. With rare exception, clinically significant CVD is accompanied by a cardiac murmur of medium intensity to loud murmur. Point of maximal murmur intensity is over the left apex with radiation dorsally and to the right in most cases. In most dogs the intensity of the murmur is roughly correlated with the severity of mitral regurgitation (MR) as long as arterial blood pressure is normal.

When a murmur is auscultated in a dog without clinical signs, baseline testing can be offered to the owner and is often helpful for comparison at subsequent examinations. At a minimum the client should be clearly informed of the presence of the murmur and the fact that the disease may ultimately progress to CHF. Baseline testing might include thoracic radiographs to assess for cardiomegaly and/or echocardiography to confirm the diagnosis and help assess cardiac size and function. A blood pressure measurement is indicated to exclude systemic hypertension, which might accelerate progression of MR. If hypertension is identified, an underlying cause such as renal or adrenal disease should be sought.

EVALUATION OF THE DOG WITH SIGNS OF CARDIAC DYSFUNCTION

Once heart failure develops, a range of clinical presentations are possible, related to the degree and duration of valvular dysfunction. In an acute setting clinical signs are usually pulmonary or behavioral in origin and include cough, tachypnea, retching/gagging, nocturnal dyspnea, orthopnea or "reluctance to settle," and sometimes either excessive "clinginess" or social isolation. Less commonly abdominal distention from ascites may be present, or the client may detect a "racing heart." Syncope may be the initial sign of heart disease and can occur as a result of significant arrhythmias, secondary to low cardiac output, in association with a vasovagal (reflex-mediated) response, or following a coughing spell (tussive syncope). In my experience syncope is common at the time of the initial presentation of heart failure, and syncope in this setting likely has a reflex-mediated or vasovagal component. Some dogs exhibit decreased exercise tolerance and weight loss for weeks to months before the onset of CHF, but these are often overlooked and are rarely the causes for presentation to a veterinarian.

Physical Examination

Pulmonary auscultation may reveal loud bronchial sounds that can progress to pulmonary crackles with the onset of alveolar edema. The latter may be particularly prominent over the hilar or caudal lung fields on inspiration. Hepatomegaly and ascites may be evident in dogs with right-sided CHF from advanced mitral disease with PHTN. Jugular venous distention is commonly appreciated in dogs with ascites. Often the femoral pulses are easily palpated and prominent, even at the time of onset of CHF. Irregularities in pulse rate and strength may be noted in association with an arrhythmia. In animals with CHF the heart rate is usually elevated or in the upper normal range, and sinus arrhythmia is typically absent, although this is variable. The ventricular apex beat is hyperdynamic and is progressively shifted caudally from the fifth intercostal space with increasing disease severity. If present, a precordial thrill is also palpable over the apex. There may be a left ventricular heave or apical thrust. There may be other abnormalities since most CVD patients are geriatric; therefore a complete physical examination is warranted.

Thoracic Radiography

Thoracic radiographs are *essential* to the management of CVD. The earliest characteristic findings on thoracic radiographs are mild left ventricular enlargement and left atrial enlargement, which may be best noted as auricular prominence on the dorsoventral (DV) view at the 2 to 3 o'clock location. Left atrial and left ventricular enlargement elevate the trachea and carina on the lateral radiographic projection, with a decrease in the angle between the trachea and the thoracic spine. The left mainstem bronchus may become elevated and compressed in cases of moderate-to-severe left atrial enlargement. There is straightening of the caudal cardiac border and loss of the caudal cardiac waist. Pulmonary venous dilation occurs; this finding may be best appreciated in the cranial lung fields in the lateral view. Distended pulmonary veins (and arteries in severe cases) can also be identified in the caudal lung fields on the dorsoventral or ventrodorsal projections. Early pulmonary edema is seen as a diffuse increase in interstitial density in the hilar or caudal lung fields, progressing to perihilar fluffy densities and air bronchograms with the onset of alveolar edema. Cardiogenic pulmonary edema appears to have a propensity for the right caudal lung fields, and this finding is noted on the DV view. With tricuspid regurgitation (TR) and right-sided or biventricular CHF, the cranial aspect of the trachea may be elevated, and the caudal vena cava increases in size.

Radiograph evaluation is not only useful for monitoring cardiac chamber size and documenting CHF, but it also serves to guide therapy and exclude other disorders.

Pneumonia can develop in an older dog with CVD and CHF; thus in a patient with new signs or a poor response to therapy, infection or other problem such as lung cancer should be considered. Chronic bronchitis is also common in many dogs with CVD and occasionally can be recognized by the presence of severe bronchial patterns or bronchiectasis.

Electrocardiography

Electrocardiographic findings can include evidence of left ventricular hypertrophy, widened P waves of left atrial enlargement (P mitrale), and infrequently P pulmonale (P >0.4 mV). P pulmonale is seen more frequently in dogs with concurrent respiratory disease. ST segment slurring or depression, which may result from myocardial disease, ischemia, or hypoxia, is evident in some dogs with left ventricular hypertrophy. Sinus rhythm or sinus tachycardia is typical of dogs with CVD and CHF. Atrial arrhythmias, especially atrial premature depolarizations, are common. Atrial fibrillation develops in some dogs with marked atrial enlargement. Conversely, ventricular arrhythmias are relatively uncommon in animals with compensated disease, and even in dogs with CHF ventricular ectopy is far less common than with dilated cardiomyopathy.

Echocardiography

Echocardiography is valuable in assessing cardiac changes, although thoracic radiographs are more useful in identifying CHF. Valvular thickening and valvular prolapse into the atria can be appreciated early in the course of disease. With advancing disease the valve becomes progressively thickened, and left atrial and ventricular enlargement is noted. With severe MR the left atrium enlarges disproportionately to the left ventricle. Rupture of a chordae tendineae leads to a flail mitral leaflet with chaotic valve motion and a tip of the leaflet pointing dorsally into the left atrium in systole. Fractional shortening is normal or increased in the early stages of the disease and increases with increasing regurgitant fraction. Fractional shortening returns toward "normal" or becomes diminished with disease progression and the onset of myocardial failure; this finding is often noted early in large-breed dogs. The left ventricular free wall often develops a relatively reduced excursion when compared to the septum (the opposite of normal dogs). Although left atrial size is a better objective measure of severity of chronic MR, Doppler methods also can be used. The location and extent of the regurgitant jet can be mapped using color flow Doppler echocardiography as a crude indicator of disease severity. Additional Doppler methods such as measurement of jet diameter or analysis of the proximal isovelocity area may permit more accurate estimation of the regurgitant flow fraction using color Doppler methods.

Frequently there is evidence of tricuspid valve disease. This can include tricuspid prolapse, valvular thickening, and Doppler evidence of TR. High-velocity TR is a marker for PHTN, which can become very severe in some dogs with CVD. Pericardial effusion is observed occasionally on echocardiography related to right-sided CHF or left atrial tear (see Left Atrial Tear or Splitting later in the chapter).

Biomarkers

Natriuretic peptides, including B-type natriuretic peptide (BNP) and atrial natriuretic peptide, are released in response to ventricular and atrial stretch, and the levels of these peptides increase progressively with the onset of CHF. Studies have documented that these peptides are elevated in dogs with CVD and CHF, with progressive increases as the heart enlarges. Natriuretic peptides hold great promise for early identification of patients at risk of developing CHF and for confirming the diagnosis in those dogs with signs that would be consistent with CHF such as shortness of breath or cough. Natriuretic peptides also may offer some prognostic information, and it remains to be seen whether they can be used to assist in treatment decisions or response to therapy. A commercial assay for canine NT-proBNP has recently become available, and in-house natriuretic peptide testing may be available soon. One issue that requires better definition are the "cutoffs" that prove reliable (both sensitive and specific) for the diagnosis of CHF.

TREATMENT OF CHRONIC VALVULAR HEART DISEASE

The therapy for dogs with CVD includes consideration of the patient with preclinical disease and the dog coughing from bronchial compression, the need for both hospital and home treatment plans for the dog with overt CHF, and the management of additional complications of this disorder.

Management of Asymptomatic Dogs

Treatment of asymptomatic CVD in the dog is controversial. Although angiotensin-converting enzyme (ACE) inhibitors are useful in the treatment of overt CHF, the SVEP trial evaluating the ACE-inhibitor enalapril in asymptomatic cavalier King Charles spaniels failed to show a significant prevention benefit in terms of delaying onset of CHF (Kvart et al., 2002). However, the recently published VETPROOF enalapril trial suggested a possible long-term survival benefit of enalapril in dogs with advanced mitral disease treated before the onset of CHF (Atkins et al, 2007). Clearly more studies are needed before definitive recommendations can be made. In view of these studies most cardiologists do not initiate therapy in small-breed dogs with chronic MR in the absence of significant cardiomegaly. Some clinicians initiate ACE inhibitor therapy in preclinical disease when there is moderate-to-severe heart enlargement or when marked change is observed on serial examinations. However, this therapy is still considered empiric, and there is no unanimity about such treatment.

Aside from the controversy noted previously, there may be some other reasons to consider ACE-inhibition in CVD. For example, in larger-breed dogs with MR, cardioprotective therapy with an ACE-inhibitor and/or β-blocker may be reasonable, especially when there is evidence of volume overload, because progressive left ventricular dysfunction seems more common in this patient group. The dog with left atrial enlargement that is coughing from presumed bronchial compression may benefit from ACE inhibitor therapy (or ACE-inhibitor and low-dose diuretic or cough suppressant).

Dogs with CVD and concurrent systemic hypertension should have their hypertension managed, and ACE inhibitors generally are selected first in this particular setting.

β-Blockers are dangerous in uncontrolled CHF, but there may be a role for these drugs in treated heart failure or asymptomatic disease. There is certainly some enthusiasm for implementation of β-blockers in the preclinical phase of CVD based on extrapolation from research studies. However, clinical studies documenting a clear clinical benefit in dogs with spontaneous CVD are still ongoing, and evidence of benefit is completely lacking in this disease. When prescribed, most cardiologists use carvedilol or metoprolol (see Chapter 171). Again, large-breed dogs with significant CVD may be the best candidates for such myocardial protective strategies.

Severe dietary sodium restriction is not recommended in the asymptomatic stage because of early activation of the renin-angiotensin-aldosterone system. However, client education on avoiding high-sodium diets, treats, and table foods is important. One study evaluating the use of a novel diet for management of dogs with asymptomatic CVD identified a reduction in cardiac size during the 4-week dietary trial, demonstrating the impact of dietary sodium on plasma volume and cardiac size (Freeman, Rush, and Markwell, 2006). Studies that document a clear clinical benefit such as a delay in the onset of CHF or improved survival are lacking; thus firm treatment recommendations cannot be made at this time.

Management of Dogs With Congestive Heart Failure

Once CHF develops, many options are available for patient management (see Chapter 171). The patient with severe pulmonary edema requires diuresis. Oxygen administration and sedation (e.g., butorphanol at 0.1 to 0.2 mg/kg intramuscularly [IM] as needed) are helpful supplements to treating hospitalized patients. Some clinicians use topical 2% nitroglycerin as a venodilator for dogs in the hospital setting, but efficacy data for this approach are lacking. Sodium nitroprusside is useful in life-threatening lung edema caused by ruptured chordae tendineae (see Rupture of the Chordae Tendineae later in the chapter). Once stabilized, most dogs are treated with a combination of oral drugs in the home setting to prevent recurrence of CHF, minimize clinical signs, and prolong life.

Furosemide is the most commonly used diuretic, and the dose is titrated to effect (i.e., to limit clinical signs resulting from fluid accumulation). In patients with severe pulmonary edema intravenous boluses of furosemide are indicated, and some clinicians supplement these with a constant-rate infusion of furosemide. The dose of furosemide required to clear significant edema accumulations and cause the animal to be minimally symptomatic (the desired dose) is often close to that resulting in electrolyte disturbance, dehydration, and the development of prerenal azotemia. Doses of furosemide can vary from 2 mg/kg/day in mild CHF up to 4 to 6 mg/kg every 8 hours in advanced disease. Azotemia and electrolyte imbalance can result from the combined use of ACE inhibitors and diuretics; thus serial monitoring of these parameters is indicated. A baseline evaluation of blood urea nitrogen

(BUN), creatinine, and serum electrolytes should be obtained, with serum chemistry recheck done 5 to 10 days after starting these drugs and 5 to 10 days after any significant dosage adjustment, followed by routine evaluation every 3 to 6 months. ACE inhibitors combined with diuretics may not be well tolerated in some dogs with preexisting renal disease; careful monitoring of clinical signs (appetite and activity) and more frequent assessment of electrolytes and BUN/creatinine are advisable.

Several clinical trials in dogs with CVD and CHF have demonstrated the clinical benefits of ACE inhibitors in reducing clinical signs or delaying the time until clinical deterioration or death. Drugs such as enalapril or benazepril can be initiated in the hospital or home setting. A full dosage of these drugs is generally considered 0.5 mg/kg orally every 12 hours, but many clinicians initiate therapy at one half that dosage and later increase it at the time of first or subsequent follow-up. Blood pressure and renal function are often used to monitor treatment.

The recent approval of pimobendan (Vetmedin), a calcium sensitizer and phosphodiesterase inhibitor, provides an additional effective drug for management of CHF. The positive inotropic and mixed vasodilator properties of pimobendan result in improved control of CHF and clinical signs of heart failure. Several small clinical trials have documented that pimobendan combined with diuretic therapy is at least as effective as furosemide and ACE inhibitors and may have fewer side effects than many of the commonly used cardiovascular medications (Smith et al., 2005). Pimobendan does not appear to have proarrhythmic properties at commonly used clinical doses, but this requires more study. Cardiologists hold some differing opinions on the role that pimobendan plays in the management of CHF in dogs with CVD. Some believe that initial management of CHF should revolve around furosemide and pimobendan, whereas others opt for furosemide with an ACE-inhibitor. I believe that the initial treatment strategy for dogs with CVD and well-defined CHF should include the "triple therapy" of furosemide, pimobendan, and an ACE inhibitor.

As cardiac disease progresses, additional medications will be required to control advancing CHF. This therapy may include a dose escalation of furosemide, the addition of other diuretics to combat diuretic resistance, treatment with digoxin or antiarrhythmics as necessary, and various dietary manipulations. I usually consider that diuretic resistance has developed when doses of furosemide in excess of 2.2 mg/kg twice a day are required to control congestive signs during chronic CHF therapy. In this situation the addition of spironolactone (1 to 2 mg/kg orally [PO] once or twice daily) or a combination of hydrochlorothiazide with spironolactone is recommended. If hydrochlorothiazide is prescribed, initial dosages should be conservative, and renal function and electrolytes should be evaluated within 5 to 7 days. In addition, careful scrutiny of other causes of fluid retention such as high-sodium diets, salty treats, or glucocorticoid therapy is indicated.

Digoxin still has some role in the management of CVD, although it has largely been supplanted by newer drugs with fewer side effects. Digoxin is indicated in CVD dogs in the setting of CHF with atrial fibrillation and in cases with frequent or sustained supraventricular arrhythmias. In addition, digoxin may be useful in management of syncope in dogs with CVD when no clear cause for collapse (such as arrhythmia) can be established. Toxicity in veterinary patients has the very real potential to contribute to a decision for euthanasia, and the narrow therapeutic window for digitalis glycosides predisposes to the development of toxicity. Serial monitoring of serum digoxin levels is advisable, with target 8-hour postpill serum concentrations in the 0.8- to 1.2-mg/ml range. For dogs with rapid ventricular rate response to atrial fibrillation, either diltiazem or a β-blocker may be required in addition to digoxin to reduce the heart rate to less than 160 beats/min.

β-Blockade has gained favor recently as a therapeutic modality for treatment of CHF. Several studies on the use of β-blockers have documented benefits that accrue from chronic treatment in people with CHF, although these effects often are not seen for several months. Reported benefits include up-regulation of previously down-regulated β-receptors, improved cardiac performance (improved stroke volume), and improved survival. These clinical benefits appear to have sound theoretic basis, but there is not consensus among cardiologists about the use of β-blockers in dogs with CVD. Currently carvedilol is under evaluation in veterinary patients with naturally occurring CHF caused by both cardiomyopathy and CVD. Since β-blockers are negative inotropes, the most demonstrable effect when used in dogs with active CHF is likely to be a worsening of CHF. The negative inotropic and chronotropic effects of β-blockers can be harmful to dogs with active failure or those at the edge of compensation. β-Blockers are best used in patients that are minimally symptomatic with early/mild heart failure or in later stages of CHF that are already well controlled on a stable cardiac drug regimen (see Chapter 171 for more details). Carvedilol, metoprolol, and atenolol all have been used for cardioprotection in dogs with CVD, but carvedilol may have some advantages in terms of concurrent α-blockade (lowing vascular resistance), potent antioxidant effects, and more convenient dosing formulations.

Dietary sodium restriction is also important for the management of dogs with CVD. The owners of an asymptomatic dog with CVD should be counseled to avoid diets high in sodium and to avoid treats or table food (and any foods used to administer medications) that are high in sodium. Initially the selected diet should have a sodium content of less than 100 mg/100 kcal of energy. Once CHF develops, additional sodium restriction is recommended (<80 mg/100 kcal). This does not necessarily require a commercial cardiac diet, and care should be taken to avoid diets designed for dogs with renal disease or cardiac diets that are low in protein since these can contribute to loss of muscle mass and cardiac cachexia. As CHF progresses, stricter dietary sodium restriction may allow for use of lower dosages of diuretics to control clinical signs. A variety of other dietary considerations may be important in individual cases. Some diets are designed or supplemented with various levels of certain nutrients such as potassium, magnesium, taurine, L-carnitine, arginine, antioxidants, or ω-3 fatty acids (see Chapter 157).

Exercise restriction with severe CHF is essential; however, limited exercise in dogs with stable chronic heart failure is often well tolerated and improves quality of life scores. Repetitive or strenuous activities such as ball chasing and running should be restricted once advanced heart disease or serious arrhythmias develop.

CLINICAL COMPLICATIONS AND CHALLENGES

Cough in the Dog With Concurrent Chronic Valvular Disease and Respiratory Disease

The cause of the cough can be difficult to determine in dogs with concurrent cardiac and respiratory disease. Dogs coughing from primary pulmonary disease often are overweight or have no history of weight loss, and auscultation may indicate only a soft murmur or no murmur at all. Many dogs with tracheobronchial disease demonstrate tracheal sensitivity, a very productive cough, or a cough of long-standing duration (often longer than 2 to 4 months). In contrast, most dogs with a cardiac cough have a loud murmur, some weight loss, and a cough of more recent onset. Sinus arrhythmia is more common in the dog with respiratory disease; whereas the dog with CHF often has normal sinus rhythm, sinus tachycardia, or atrial arrhythmias. Both CHF and respiratory diseases such as chronic bronchitis and pulmonary fibrosis can cause crackles and wheezes on auscultation; thus this is rarely a helpful discriminating factor. The radiographic finding of pulmonary edema with interstitial-to-alveolar infiltrates in the perihilar regions, pulmonary venous prominence, and an enlarged left atrium supports a diagnosis of CHF. Marked left atrial enlargement may compress the main-stem bronchi and lead to cough; this cough often improves with therapy for heart failure, which results in a decrease in the size of the left atrium. Dogs with more respiratory findings often have right heart enlargement and a lack of left atrial enlargement on thoracic radiographs.

Rupture of the Chordae Tendineae

Acute rupture of a chordae tendineae may lead to catastrophic heart failure and may be clinically appreciated by a marked change in the murmur intensity and sudden-onset pulmonary edema. Acute CHF develops as the left atrium is unable to compensate for an acute increase in regurgitant volume. Historically chordal rupture has been associated with a grave prognosis. However, a recent review (Serres et al., 2007) concluded that survival time of affected dogs was longer than previously described, with 58% of affected and aggressively treated dogs surviving more than 1 year after diagnosis. Although cardiologists do not always agree on the echocardiographic criteria used in this study for diagnosis of ruptured chordae tendineae, these data suggest that not all chordal ruptures are lethal and that it is reasonable to undertake therapy. In addition to aggressive diuresis, oxygen therapy, and sedation as required, the use of sodium nitroprusside infusion at a rate of 1 to 5 mcg/kg/minute for 24 to 48 hours can be successful in acute load reduction and management of catastrophic heart failure and severe pulmonary edema in dogs with CVD. The dose of nitroprusside is generally titrated to a systolic blood pressure of ≈90 mm Hg.

Left Atrial Tear or Splitting

Left atrial tear can result from atrial stretch from MR or from endocardial damage caused by the jet of blood chronically impinging on the endocardial aspect of the left atrium. The weakened endocardium can split; and at times the entire left atrial wall ruptures, allowing blood to escape into the pericardial sac. The resultant cardiac tamponade may be fatal. The tear may more accurately be characterized as endocardial splitting since this process may occur without rupture of the atrial wall, or rupture may occur without pericardial bleeding (e.g., rupture in the atrial septum leads to an acquired atrial septal defect). Treatment of left atrial tear is directed at aggressively lowering left atrial pressure through treatment of volume overload. Pericardiocentesis is rarely indicated unless tamponade is life-threatening. The volume of blood identified by echocardiography may be relatively small; and great care should be used when tapping the pericardium, especially from the left side, because the dilated left auricle is easily punctured.

Pulmonary Hypertension

PHTN is defined as a resting mean pulmonary arterial pressure of greater than 25 mm Hg. Pulmonary hypertension may occur as an isolated entity, secondary to pulmonary thromboembolism or chronic respiratory disease, or as a result of long-standing left-sided CHF. PHTN often leads to syncope and signs of right-sided CHF such as ascites or even pleural effusion. PHTN is most often diagnosed by noninvasive continuous-wave Doppler echocardiography with application of the Bernoulli equation to the tricuspid regurgitant jet velocity:

$$\text{PA pressure} = \text{peak velocity}^2 \times 4 + \text{estimated right atrial pressure}$$

where velocity units are in meters per second. Moderate PHTN is common in advanced CVD and can be well tolerated, but severe PHTN is generally associated with a poor prognosis. Pimobendan may reduce pulmonary artery pressures in selected cases. Recently sildenafil (Viagra, Revatio) and tadalafel (Cialis) have been described as a therapeutic option in both humans and dogs with PHTN. I currently add sildenafil or tadalafel to the treatment regimen of dogs with CVD and severe PHTN (estimated systolic pulmonary artery pressures >80 mm Hg) and to those with moderate PHTN (estimated systolic pulmonary artery pressures between 50 and 80 mm Hg) and unresolved syncope or tachypnea following resolution of radiographic evidence of pulmonary edema. It is important to recall that concurrent sildenafil and nitrate therapy is contraindicated because of the potential for severe hypotension. Currently the extralabel prescription of these drugs in most countries is quite expensive.

Surgical Intervention in Chronic Valvular Disease

Surgical procedures have been developed to repair or replace the mitral valve in dogs with CVD. Cardiopulmonary bypass is required for these procedures; successful cardiopulmonary bypass requires a dedicated team of surgeons, perfusionists, anesthesiologists, cardiologists, intensive care specialists, and strong veterinary technician support. The cost associated with surgery can be prohibitive ($8,000 to $12,000). Once these techniques are mastered and refined for veterinary medicine, it seems probable that surgery or developing catheter-based interventions (or hybrid procedures) to limit MR will become the preferred treatment for those that can afford the procedure.

References and Suggested Reading

Atkins CE et al: Results of the veterinary enalapril trial to prove reduction in onset of heart failure in dogs chronically treated with enalapril alone for compensated, naturally occurring mitral valve insufficiency, *J Am Vet Med Assoc* 231:1061, 2007.

Falk T et al: Arteriosclerotic changes in the myocardium, lung and kidney of dogs with chronic congestive heart failure and myxomatous mitral valve disease, *Cardiovasc Pathol* 15:185, 2006.

Freeman LM, Rush JE, Markwell PJ: Effects of dietary modification in dogs with early chronic valvular disease, *J Vet Intern Med* 20: 1116, 2006.

Gordon SG, Miller MW, Saunders AB: Pimobendan in heart failure therapy—a silver bullet? *J Am Anim Hosp Assoc* 42:90, 2006.

Griffins LG, Orton EC, Boon JA: Evaluation of techniques and outcomes of mitral valve repair in dogs, *J Am Vet Med Assoc* 224:1941, 2004.

Kvart C et al: Efficacy of enalapril for prevention of congestive heart failure in dogs with myxomatous valve disease and symptomatic mitral regurgitation, *J Vet Intern Med* 16:80, 2002.

Oyama MA, Chittur SV: Genomic expression patterns of mitral valve tissues from dogs with degenerative mitral valve disease, *Am J Vet Res* 67:1307, 2006.

Rush JE et al: C-reactive protein concentration in dogs with chronic valvular disease, *J Vet Intern Med* 20:635, 2006.

Serres R et al: Chordae tendineae rupture in dogs with degenerative mitral valve disease: prevalence, survival and prognostic factors (114 cases, 2001-2006), *J Vet Intern Med* 21:258, 2007.

Smith PJ et al: Efficacy and safety of pimobendan in canine heart failure caused by myxomatous mitral valve disease, *J Small Anim Pract* 46:121, 2005.

CHAPTER 173

Infective Endocarditis

KRISTIN A. MACDONALD, *Davis, California*

Infective endocarditis (IE) is an uncommon, often deadly, and sometimes difficult to diagnose disease in veterinary medicine. IE is caused by invasion of a microbe into the endothelium of the valves of the heart, resulting in proliferative or erosive lesions and consequently valvular insufficiency. The incidence of IE in dogs referred to a veterinary teaching hospital is low (0.09% to 6.6%) (MacDonald et al., 2004; Calvert, 1982). Given the difficulty in diagnosis, the nebulous clinical signs, and lack of necropsy examinations, the true incidence of IE in the canine population is likely much higher. IE in cats is extremely rare. In small animals the mitral and aortic valves are almost exclusively affected with nearly equal distribution. Patients often succumb to congestive heart failure (CHF), sudden death, or thromboembolic disease. Immune-mediated diseases, including polyarthritis or glomerulonephritis, are also common secondary sequelae. Identification of the offending organism is paramount for effective treatment with long-term antibiotics. Blood culture is especially helpful to identify the offending organism and determine the spectrum of antibiotic sensitivity. However, the incidence of culture-negative IE in dogs is high at 60% to 70% (MacDonald et al., 2004; Sisson and Thomas, 1984). This update considers IE in the dog and discusses the emergence of *Bartonella* as a cause of IE in dogs with blood culture negative for traditional bacteria. Recent advances in diagnosis, treatment, and prognosis of IE in dogs are also reviewed.

PREDISPOSING FACTORS

Bacteremia of any cause may predispose a patient to develop IE. Common sources of bacteremia include discospondylitis, prostatitis, pneumonia, urinary tract infection, pyoderma, periodontal disease, and long-term indwelling central venous catheters. Subaortic stenosis is the only structural heart disease that significantly predisposes dogs to development of aortic valve IE (Sisson and Thomas, 1984). Dogs with myxomatous valvular degeneration rarely develop IE despite dental prophylaxis procedures and other causes of bacteremia and therefore are not likely to have a substantially increased risk for development of IE. The role of immunosuppressive therapy (i.e., corticosteroids) as a predisposing factor for development of IE is controversial. In a recent study of IE in dogs only 1 of 18 dogs (5%) had been recently administered immunosuppressive therapy for treatment of pemphigus foliaceus. However, an earlier study found that 17 of 45 dogs (38%) with IE received corticosteroids at some time during the course of disease (Calvert, 1982).

PATHOPHYSIOLOGY

Vegetative Lesions

The inciting event in formation of IE is bacterial adherence to the disrupted endothelial surface of a cardiac valve. Mechanical lesions (i.e., subaortic stenosis or cardiac catheterization procedure) or inflammatory disease can promote bacterial seeding within the endothelium. During disruption of the endothelium, extracellular matrix proteins, thromboplastin, and tissue factor all trigger coagulation; and a coagulum forms on the damaged endothelium. This coagulum contains fibrinogen, fibrin, and platelet proteins and avidly binds bacteria. Inflammation induces endothelial cell expression of integrins that bind bacteria and fibronectin to the extracellular matrix. Some bacteria (i.e., *Staphylococcus aureus*) carry fibronectin-binding proteins and also can trigger active internalization by host cells. Organisms that commonly cause IE are those that have the greatest ability to adhere to damaged valves and include *Staphylococcus* spp. and *Streptococcus* spp. These bacteria can trigger tissue factor production and induce platelet aggregation. Platelets release bactericidal proteins, but many of the bacteria that cause IE are resistant to these proteins. Bacteria such as *S. aureus* and *Bartonella* may become internalized within the endothelial cells and escape detection by the immune system. *Bartonella* also evade the immune system by colonizing red blood cells without causing hemolysis. Bacteria also can excrete enzymes that lead to destruction of valve tissue and proliferation of the vegetative lesion. The fibrinous vegetative lesion shields bacteria from the bloodstream and inflammatory cells and provides a formidable obstacle for antibiotic penetration.

Congestive Heart Failure

CHF generally develops subsequent to severe aortic or mitral insufficiency in dogs with IE of those valves. Rarely vegetation also creates stenosis of the valve. Increased left ventricular end-diastolic pressure occurs secondary to severe valvular insufficiency and leads to elevated left atrial and pulmonary capillary wedge pressures with development of cardiogenic pulmonary edema.

Immune-Mediated Disease

Patients with IE tend to develop high titers of antibodies against causative microorganisms, and there is continuous formation of circulating immune complexes. Subacute IE in humans is more likely to result in immunologic disease (Baddour et al., 2005). Immune complexes consist of immunoglobulin (Ig)M and IgG, as well as C3 (complement). Factors such as rheumatoid factor may impair the ability of complement to solubilize immune complexes and may lead to formation of large immune complexes. Extracardiac disease manifestations are caused by immune complex deposition and further complement activation and tissue destruction in the glomerular basement membrane, joint capsule, or dermis. Circulating immune complexes are greatly reduced shortly after antibiotic therapy in humans with IE.

CLINICAL PRESENTATION

Medium- to large-breed, middle age–to-older male dogs are most commonly affected with IE. German shepherds were predisposed to develop IE in a postmortem study. In a recent study the most frequent presenting complaint of dogs with IE was lameness (44% of dogs), followed by nonspecific signs such as lethargy, anorexia, respiratory abnormalities, weakness, and collapse (MacDonald et al., 2004). Some dogs exhibit signs that suggest fever such as shaking or shivering.

Cardiopulmonary Abnormalities

A murmur is ausculted in a majority of dogs with IE (89% to 96%) (MacDonald et al., 2004; Sisson and Thomas, 1984). Clinical findings of a diastolic murmur and bounding femoral pulses should trigger a high level of suspicion of aortic valve IE, and further diagnostics should be pursued immediately as outlined in the following paragraphs. Fever is often present (50% to 74%). Arrhythmias are present in 40% to 70% of dogs and include in order of incidence ventricular arrhythmias, supraventricular tachycardia, third-degree atrioventricular block, and atrial fibrillation. The highest reported frequency of arrhythmias was seen in dogs with aortic IE, with 62% of dogs having ventricular arrhythmias (Sisson and Thomas, 1984). Third-degree atrioventricular block may occur with periannular abscess formation secondary to aortic valve IE. CHF is present in almost half of patients and is diagnosed by identification of perihilar to caudodorsal pulmonary infiltrates. Acute CHF occurs in the absence of significant left atrial enlargement in a majority of cases of IE (75%) (MacDonald et al., 2004). There is no difference in the occurrence of CHF between IE of the mitral or aortic valves.

Other Systemic Sequelae

Thromboembolism (septic and aseptic) commonly occurs in 70% to 80% of dogs with IE examined in the pathology table (MacDonald et al., 2004). Risk of thromboembolic disease is greatest with vegetative lesions larger than 1 cm in size or with increasing lesion size during antibiotic therapy in people. Infarction of the kidneys and spleen is most common in dogs, followed by myocardium, brain, and systemic arteries.

Immune-mediated disease, including polyarthritis and glomerulonephritis, is commonly seen in dogs with IE (6 of 8 or 75% and 4 of 11 or 36%, respectively, in our study). Joint fluid analysis and culture should be performed in any dog with lameness. Urine protein:creatinine ratio should be evaluated in any dog with proteinuria to support the diagnosis of glomerulonephritis.

Clinicopathologic Abnormalities

Complete blood count commonly reveals leukocytosis (78%) with a mature neutrophilia and monocytosis. Mild-to-severe thrombocytopenia is commonly seen in over half of all cases. Mild nonregenerative anemia is also commonly seen. Serum chemistry may show hypoalbuminemia, elevated hepatic enzyme activity, and acidosis.

Azotemia may be prerenal or renal. Renal infarction may be seen secondary to thromboembolic disease in IE and may cause severe azotemia. Urinalysis commonly reveals hemoglobinuria, hematuria, proteinuria, and cystitis. Urine culture should be obtained in all cases in an effort to identify possible offending microbes.

DIAGNOSIS

Blood Culture

Blood culture before treatment with antibiotics is an essential tool to support the diagnosis of IE and to aid in proper selection of antimicrobial treatment. Unfortunately many patients (78% in one study) have been treated with antibiotics before blood culture, thus reducing the likelihood of a positive blood culture. Three or four blood samples (5 to 10 ml) should be collected aseptically from different venous sites at least 30 minutes to 1 hour apart and submitted for aerobic and anaerobic culture. Lysis centrifugation tubes (Isolator, Isostat microbial system, Wampole

Laboratories) may increase diagnostic yield. For culture of *Bartonella*, a fastidious gram-negative intracellular bacterium, 2 ml of aseptically collected blood is placed in a plastic tube containing ethylenediaminetetraacetic acid (EDTA) (K_2EDTA blood tubes, Becton Dickinson VACUTAINER Systems) and frozen at $-70°$ C until plated. Samples are plated on specialized culture medium of heart infusion agar and incubated in 5% CO_2 for up to 4 weeks.

Bacterial Isolates

There is a high incidence of negative blood cultures in dogs with IE ranging from 60% to 70% (MacDonald et al., 2004; Sisson and Thomas, 1984) The most common bacterial isolates are *Staphylococcal* spp. (*S. aureus*, *S. intermedius*, coagulase-positive, and coagulase-negative), *Streptococcus* spp. (*S. canis*, *S. bovis*, and β-hemolytic), and *Escherichia coli* (Table 173-1). Other isolates cultured in our teaching hospital and reported in other case series include

Table 173-1

Common Etiologic Agents, Typical Antimicrobial Sensitivity Profiles, and Treatment Recommendations for Dogs With Infective Endocarditis

Etiologic Agent	Typical Sensitivity Profile	Recommended Antibiotic
Staphylococcus Intermedius	Usually sensitive	**Acute:** Timentin 50 mg/kg IV QID, or enrofloxacin 10 mg/kg IV BID, or amikacin 20 mg/kg IV q24h, with fluid support **Chronic:** Clavamox 20 mg/kg PO TID, or enrofloxacin 5-10 mg/kg PO BID × 6-8 weeks Individually dependent, evaluate MIC
Staphylococcus aureaus	Often resistant If methicillin resistance, avoidance of β-lactams	**Acute:** May require amikacin or vancomycin, and oxacillin, nafcillin, or cefazolin IV × 2 weeks **Chronic:** If not methicillin resistant, high-dose first-generation cephalosporin PO 6-8 weeks
Streptococcus canis	Usually sensitive If resistant, amikacin and high-dose penicillin	**Acute:** Ampicillin 20-40 mg/kg IV TID-QID, or ceftriaxone 20 mg/kg IV BID × 2 weeks **Chronic:** Amoxicillin or Clavamox PO 6-8 weeks Individually dependent, evaluate MIC
Escherichia coli	Often resistant because of β-lactamase, need extended MIC	**Acute:** Amikacin and/or imipenem 10 mg/kg IV TID **Chronic:** Imipenem 10 mg/kg SQ TID 6-8 weeks Individually dependent, evaluate MIC
Pseudomonas	Resistant, need extended MIC	**Acute:** Amikacin, Timentin, or imipenem IV **Chronic:** Imipenem SQ or possibly Clavamox PO
Bartonella	MIC not predictive of MBC	**Acute:** Amikacin 20 mg/kg IV × 1-2 weeks, and β-lactam (i.e., Timentin 50 mg/kg IV QID × 1-2 weeks) **Chronic:** β-lactam PO × 6-8 weeks Doxycycline 5 mg/kg PO q24h × 6-8 weeks Azithromycin 5 mg/kg PO q24h × 7 days and then EOD
Unknown etiologic agent	Culture negative	**Acute:** Amikacin and Timentin IV × 1-2 weeks **Chronic:** Clavamox 20 mg/kg TID × 6-8 weeks and Enrofloxacin 5-10 mg/kg PO BID × 6-8 weeks

Typical MIC profiles derived from University of California Davis Veterinary Medical Teaching Hospital's microbial service database of antimicrobial sensitivity of cultured microorganisms. Recommended antibiotics for particular bacteria were chosen based on >90% of the cultured isolates sensitive to the particular antibiotic.
BID, Twice a day; *EOD,* every other day; *IV,* intravenously; *MBC,* minimum bactericidal concentration; *MIC,* minimum inhibitory concentration; *PO,* orally; *QID,* four times a day; *SQ,* subcutaneously; *TID,* three times a day.

Pseudomonas spp., *Erysipelothrix rhusiopathiae*, *Enterobacter* spp., *Pasteurella* spp., *Corynebacterium* spp., and *Proteus* spp. Rare bacterial isolates include *Bordetella avium*–like organism, *Erysipelothrix tonsillarum*, and *Actinomyces turicensis*.

Bartonella Infective Endocarditis

Bartonella has emerged as an important cause of culture-negative IE in humans and dogs (Houpikian and Raoult, 2005; MacDonald et al., 2004). *Bartonella* was the cause of 28% of IE in dogs in a recent study and of IE in 45% of dogs with negative blood cultures. *Bartonella vinsonii berkhoffii* is the most common species to cause IE in dogs, followed by *B. henselae*, *B. clarridgeiae*, *B."clarridgeiae–like"*, and *B. washoensis*. *Bartonella* primarily affects the aortic valve and less commonly affects the mitral valve in dogs. *Bartonella* causes unique valvular lesions characterized by fibrosis, mineralization, endothelial proliferation, and neovascularization (Pesavento et al., 2005). *Bartonella* evades the immune system by colonizing red blood cells and endothelial cells and also impairs the immune system by reducing the number of CD8+ lymphocytes and their cell adhesion molecule expression, inhibiting monocyte phagocytosis, and impairing B cell antigen presentation within lymph nodes (Pappalardo et al., 2001). The clinical characteristics of dogs with IE caused by *Bartonella* are not different from those of dogs with IE caused by traditional bacteria. Despite the use of specialized culture medium and long incubation periods, *Bartonella* is rarely cultured from the blood of dogs with IE. Dogs with polymerase chain reaction (PCR)–confirmed IE caused by *Bartonella* were highly seroreactive to *Bartonella* spp., and titers were higher than 1:1024 in one study (MacDonald et al., 2004). There is cross-reactivity to different *Bartonella* spp., as well as to *Chlamydia* spp. and *Coxiella burnetii*. PCR of the infected valve or possibly blood may be useful to confirm a diagnosis of *Bartonella*. In my experience dogs with IE caused by traditional bacteria do not have coinfections with *Bartonella* (MacDonald et al., 2004; Pesavento, 2005). Several epidemiologic studies have suggested that ticks and fleas may be vectors for *Bartonella*. Concurrent seroreactivity to *Anaplasma phagocytophilum*, *Ehrlichia canis*, or *Rickettsia rickettsii* is common in dogs with IE caused by *Bartonella*, and titers should be submitted for tick-borne diseases in any dog that is seroreactive to *Bartonella* antigen (MacDonald et al., 2004; Breitschwerdt et al., 1998).

Echocardiography

Diagnosis of IE in dogs relies primarily on visualization of a characteristic vegetative lesion of the valve by echocardiography (ECHO). Vegetative lesions appear hyperechoic and oscillating and move independently from the valve. Smaller lesions may be most obvious on the valvular surface facing blood flow. Chronic lesions may appear hyperechoic or rarely calcified. The mitral and aortic valves are almost exclusively affected in small animals. Severe proliferative myxomatous valve degeneration must be differentiated from vegetative lesions. Patient signalment is often helpful since dogs with marked myxomatous mitral valve degeneration are small breeds that rarely develop IE and dogs with IE are medium to large breeds that do not commonly develop marked valvular thickening as a result of myxomatous valve degeneration. In humans transthoracic ECHO has a low sensitivity of 55% for detection of vegetative valvular lesions compared to transesophageal ECHO (Reynolds et al., 2003). Although no veterinary study has compared the sensitivity of transthoracic ECHO versus transesophageal ECHO, the sensitivity of transthoracic ECHO is likely higher given the smaller size of our veterinary patients and the adequate visualization of the mitral and aortic valves in most dogs. Erosive lesions may be more difficult to identify. Presence of moderate or severe aortic insufficiency on color flow Doppler should greatly raise the suspicion of aortic IE, and careful interrogation of the aortic cusps in several views may be necessary to identify the vegetation. Subaortic stenosis may be present and can be diagnosed by two-dimensional evidence of fibrotic narrowing of the left ventricular outflow tract, and severity can be determined by measurement of aortic blood flow velocity by continuous-wave Doppler using the left apical five-chamber view. Severity of aortic insufficiency may be estimated by the width of the jet origin, possibly by the length of the insufficiency jet on color flow Doppler, and by the slope of the aortic insufficiency on continuous-wave Doppler (i.e., steep slope, severe aortic insufficiency). Mitral regurgitation may occur secondary to vegetative or erosive mitral lesions. Left atrial enlargement or eccentric hypertrophy of the left ventricle may not be present if the IE is acute in nature. If there is a high clinical suspicion of IE (new valvular insufficiency, fever, polyarthritis, leukocytosis, bacteremia) and no vegetative lesions are seen by transthoracic ECHO, transesophageal ECHO is recommended to better evaluate the mitral and aortic valves.

Suggested Criteria for Diagnosis of Infective Endocarditis

Definitive diagnosis of IE depends on identification of a vegetative or erosive lesion by ECHO or pathology. The modified Duke criteria have been developed to identify humans at high risk for IE and have been further modified for use in dogs evaluated for possible IE (Box 173-2). Since transthoracic ECHO is relatively insensitive in humans for detection of IE, other major and minor criteria are used to determine a possible diagnosis (Baddour et al., 2005). Cases of possible IE with high clinical suspicion should undergo transesophageal ECHO to better evaluate the valve morphology, or transthoracic ECHO should be repeated in a few days. Specific serologic data (*Coxiella burnetii* IgG titer >1:800) have recently been added to the Duke criteria to identify an etiologic agent in culture-negative cases in humans. Based on the veterinary literature, high seroreactivity to *Bartonella* (>1:1024) may be an additional minor criterion for diagnosis of IE caused by *Bartonella* in dogs. A titer of greater than 1:800 for IgG antibodies to *B. henselae* or *B. quintana* had a positive predictive value of 0.96 for detection of *Bartonella* infection in humans with IE and confirmed the diagnosis in 45 of 145 humans (31%) with-culture negative IE with 100% sensitivity (Fournier et al., 2002). PCR on serum from humans with confirmed

Box 173-1

Suggested Criteria for Diagnosis of Infective Endocarditis in Dogs

Major Criteria
- Positive echocardiogram
- Vegetative, oscillating lesion
- Erosive lesion
- Abscess
- New valvular insufficiency
- >Mild AI in absence of subaortic stenosis or annuloaortic ectasia
- Positive blood culture
- >2 positive blood cultures
- >3 with common skin contaminant

Minor Criteria
- Fever
- Medium to large dog (>15 kg)
- Subaortic stenosis
- Thromboembolic disease
- Immune mediated disease
- Polyarthritis
- Glomerulonephritis
- Positive blood culture not meeting major criteria
- *Bartonella serology >1:1024
- No pathologic evidence

Diagnosis
Definite
- Pathology of valve
- Two major criteria
- 1 major and 2 minor

Possible
- 1 major and 1 minor
- 3 minor

Rejected
- Firm alternative Dx
- Resolution <4 days of Rx

AI, Aortic insufficiency; *Dx,* diagnosis; *Rx,* treatment.
*Proposed minor criterion in dogs; not officially accepted as criterion.
Veterinary criteria are modified from the modified Duke criteria used in human medicine for diagnosis of infective endocarditis.

IE caused by *Bartonella* is relatively insensitive (58%) but specific (100%) (Zeaiter et al., 2003).

TREATMENT

Long-term bactericidal antibiotics are the cornerstone of therapy for IE. Common etiologic agents, their typical sensitivity profile, and therapeutic regimens are included in Table 173-1. Therapeutic recommendations were derived from the University of California Davis Veterinary Medical Teaching Hospital's microbial service database of antimicrobial sensitivity of microorganisms. Recommended antibiotics for particular bacteria were chosen based on greater than 90% of the cultured isolates sensitive to the particular antibiotic. However, general antibiotic sensitivities and resistance profiles may vary, depending on the hospital. Hospital-acquired infections may be much more resistant than infections acquired within the community. High serum concentration of antibiotics with good tissue and intracellular penetrating properties is needed to enter the vegetative lesion and kill the bacteria. The optimal antibiotic treatment depends on culture of the microorganism and minimum inhibitory concentration (MIC) of the antibiotics. While the culture results are pending or if there is no known microbial etiology, empiric treatment with broad-spectrum antibiotics is recommended, including aminoglycosides and β-lactam antibiotics. There is significant resistance of many bacteria isolated from our hospital to enrofloxacin; therefore it cannot be recommended as an empiric, acute first line of defense when an MIC is unavailable. Patients should be supported with fluid therapy while being treated with aminoglycosides, and concurrent administration of furosemide is contraindicated because it worsens nephrotoxicity. This limits the use of aminoglycosides to patients that are not in CHF. Initial intravenous antibiotic therapy for 1 to 2 weeks is recommended for aggressive therapy, followed by long-term oral antibiotic therapy for 6 to 8 weeks or longer. Subcutaneous administration of antibiotics on an outpatient basis rather than oral antibiotics has been suggested by some clinicians, but there is no clear advantage over chronic oral treatment. One exception is in the chronic treatment of resistant infections using imipenem administered subcutaneously after an initial 1- to 2-week course administered intravenously (Barker et al., 2003). Subcutaneous administration of antibiotics often requires frequent daily injections, and client compliance may be suboptimal. In addition, bioavailability of oral antibiotics such as the β-lactams (i.e., amoxicillin and Clavamox) and fluoroquinolones is very high (>75%, >90%, >90%, respectively). According to the resistance profiles of bacteria cultured from patients within our hospital, many bacteria are resistant to ampicillin, and empiric use of ampicillin cannot be recommended without an MIC.

The treatment of choice for *Bartonella* infections has not been defined in human or veterinary medicine. MICs are not indicative of therapeutic efficacy of antibiotics against intracellular bacteria, including *Bartonella,* and minimum bactericidal concentration may be more appropriate. In an in vitro study only gentamicin and not ciprofloxacin, streptomycin, erythromycin, ampicillin, or doxycycline exerted bactericidal activity against *Bartonella* (Rolain et al., 2000). Treatment with at least 2 weeks of aminoglycosides has been shown to improve survival in humans with *Bartonella* IE (Raoult et al., 2003). Current treatment recommendations in humans include aminoglycosides and β-lactam antibiotics for 4 to 6 weeks (Baddour et al., 2005). In 24 dogs with various systemic manifestations secondary to bartonellosis, treatment with the following antibiotics resulted in clinical recovery and negative post-treatment titers: doxycycline, azithromycin, enrofloxacin, and amoxicillin/clavulanate (Breitschwerdt et al., 2004). In dogs with severe life-threatening IE caused by *Bartonella,* aggressive treatment with aminoglycosides may be necessary, with careful monitoring of renal enzymes and supportive intravenous fluid administration. Azithromycin achieves high intracellular concentrations and may be given with careful monitoring of the hepatic enzymes since it may cause hepatotoxicity with chronic therapy.

Anticoagulant therapy is not currently recommended since there has been a trend of increased bleeding episodes and no benefit in vegetation resolution or reduced embolic events in humans with IE treated with aspirin (Baddour et al., 2005).

Treatment of CHF

Dogs with CHF should be treated with furosemide at the appropriate dose, depending on severity of pulmonary edema (stable mild-to-moderate CHF, 1 to 4 mg/kg orally [PO] BID-TID; acute fulminant CHF, 5 to 8 mg/kg intravenously [IV] q 2–4h initially and then reduced according to patient's response). In dogs with significant aortic insufficiency secondary to aortic IE or massive mitral regurgitation, afterload reduction using amlodipine, hydralazine, or nitroprusside should be instituted providing the dog is not hypotensive at baseline. Aggressive afterload reduction in hypertensive patients is warranted. In normotensive animals the target reduction of blood pressure from baseline is 10 to 15 mm Hg. Adjunctive therapy for chronic CHF includes an angiotensin-converting enzyme inhibitor and possibly digoxin if there is myocardial failure (see Chapter 171). Antiarrhythmic treatment may be necessary, especially if there are high-grade ventricular arrhythmias (see Chapter 162).

Follow-up

In patients with initially positive cultures (blood or urine), repeat culture is recommended 1 to 2 weeks after starting antibiotic therapy and 2 weeks following termination of antibiotic therapy. An echocardiogram should be performed after 2 weeks of antibiotic treatment, in 4 to 6 weeks, and 2 weeks following termination of antibiotic therapy to assess size of vegetative lesion and severity of valvular insufficiency. In patients affected with *Bartonella*, repeat serology should be performed a month after initiation of treatment, and titers should be reduced. If titers are elevated persistently, a different antibiotic may be needed.

Prophylaxis

In dogs with congenital heart disease, in particular subaortic stenosis, perioperative parenteral antibiotics such as a β-lactam or a cephalosporin should be given 1 hour before surgery or dentistry and 6 hours after the procedure. Clindamycin may be useful as a prophylactic antibiotic for dental procedures. Prophylactic antibiotics for dogs with myxomatous valve degeneration undergoing a dental procedure is controversial since these dogs are not at an increased risk for development of IE; however, bacteremia does occur, and other tissues may be at risk.

Prognosis

Dogs with aortic IE have a grave prognosis, and median survival in one study was only 3 days compared to a median survival of 476 days for dogs with mitral IE (MacDonald et al., 2004). Dogs with *Bartonella* IE have short survival times since the aortic valve is almost exclusively affected. Similarly, in another case series 33% of dogs with aortic IE died within the first week, and 92% died within 5 months of diagnosis (Sisson, 1984). Glucocorticoid administration before treatment of IE is associated with higher mortality in dogs with IE (Calvert, 1982). Short-term death is most often caused by CHF or sudden death. Likewise, in humans with IE the presence of CHF has the greatest impact on poor prognosis. Other causes of death in dogs with IE within the first week of treatment include renal failure, pulmonary hemorrhage, and severe neurologic disease. (Acknowledgement: Dr. Valerie Wiebe, PharmD [Pharmacy], for assistance with antibiotic recommendations and Dr. Barbara Byrne, DVM [Microbiology], for MIC data, University of California Davis, Veterinary Medical Teaching Hospital.)

References and Suggested Reading

Baddour LM et al: Infective endocarditis: diagnosis, antimicrobial therapy, and management of complications, AHA scientific statement, *Circulation* 111:e394, 2005.

Barker CW et al: Pharmacokinetics of imipenem in dogs, *Am J Vet Res* 64:694, 2003.

Breitschwerdt EB et al: Sequential evaluation of dogs naturally infected with *Ehrlichia canis, Ehrlichia chaffensis, Ehrlichia equi, Ehrlichia ewingii,* or *Bartonella vinsoniii, J Clin Microbiol* 36:2645, 1998.

Breitschwerdt EP et al: Clinicopathological abnormalities and treatment response in 24 dogs seroreactive to *Bartonella vinsonii (berkhoffii)* antigens, *J Am Anim Hosp Assoc* 40:92, 2004.

Calvert CA: Valvular bacterial endocarditis in the dog, *J Am Vet Med Assoc* 180:1080, 1982.

Fournier PE et al: Value of microimmunofluorescence for diagnosis and follow-up of *Bartonella* endocarditis, *Clin Diagn Lab Immunol* 9:795, 2002.

Houpikian P, Raoult D: Blood culture-negative endocarditis in a reference center, etiologic diagnosis of 348 cases. *Medicine* 84:162, 2005.

MacDonald KA et al: A prospective study of canine infective endocarditis in northern California (1999-2001): emergence of *Bartonella* as a prevalent etiologic agent, *J Vet Intern Med* 18:56, 2004.

Pappalardo BL et al: Immunopathology of *Bartonella vinsonii (berkhoffii)* in experimentally infected dogs, *Vet Immunol Immunopathol* 83:125, 2001.

Pesavento PA et al: Pathology of *Bartonella* endocarditis in six dogs, *Vet Pathol* 42:370, 2005.

Raoult D et al: Outcome and treatment of *Bartonella* endocarditis, *Arch Intern Med* 163:226, 2003.

Reynolds HR et al: Sensitivity of transthoracic versus transesophageal echocardiography for the detection of native valve vegetations in the modern era, *J Am Soc Echocardiogr* 16:67, 2003.

Rolain JM et al: Bactericidal effect of antibiotics on *Bartonella* and Brucella spp.: clinical implications, *J Anti Chemother* 46:811, 2000.

Sisson D, Thomas WP: Endocarditis of the aortic valve in the dog, *J Am Vet Med Assoc* 184:577, 1984.

Zeaiter Z et al: Diagnosis of *Bartonella* endocarditis by a real-time nested PCR assay using serum, *J Clin Microbiol* 41:919, 2003.

CHAPTER 174

Dilated Cardiomyopathy in Dogs

DANIEL F. HOGAN, *West Lafayette, Indiana*
HENRY W. GREEN, III, *West Lafayette, Indiana*

Dilated cardiomyopathy (DCM) is an idiopathic myocardial disease characterized by systolic and diastolic dysfunction with chamber dilation primarily involving the left ventricle and variable right ventricular changes. This disorder represents one of the most common acquired cardiac diseases in dogs (13.6%), with only degenerative valve disease (47.8%) and in some regions heartworm disease more prevalent. Typically DCM results in clinically important morbidity and mortality, including congestive heart failure (CHF) and sudden death, which is often secondary to ventricular arrhythmias. The latter appears to be breed related with the highest incidence within the Doberman pinscher and boxer breeds (Sisson, O'Grady, and Calvert, 1999) (see Chapters 175 and 176). This chapter considers the etiology, diagnosis, and chronic therapy of dogs with DCM. Chapter 171 provides additional recommendations for treatment of CHF, including hospital therapy.

ETIOLOGY

Systolic dysfunction with resultant cardiac dilation is thought to be the final common outcome of a variety of myocardial insults, including cytosolic, metabolic, immunologic, genetic, and infective mechanisms. In canine DCM most of these potential insults remain to be studied; thus the term *idiopathic* is most appropriate. Sporadically recognized causes of canine DCM include viral myocarditis, incessant tachycardia, taurine depletion, and possibly carnitine deficiency. In cases in which specific causes can be identified, an appropriate modifier should be used to describe the etiology of the disorder (i.e., taurine-deficiency cardiomyopathy). In humans familial inheritance of numerous genetic mutations, often those encoding cytoskeletal proteins, appear to be the most common basis for DCM and represent 20% to 50% of DCM patients (Wynne and Braunwald, 2001). The overrepresentation of certain breeds and familial inheritance patterns suggest a genetic cause for canine DCM as well. Recently the giant myofilament protein titin has gained considerable interest in Doberman pinchers (Meurs, 2005).

CLINICAL DIAGNOSIS

Although DCM generally is described as one disease, clinical signs and progression of the disease demonstrate some breed variation. Because of these differences, the specific breed should be considered when assessing an individual animal with respect to etiology, therapeutic protocol, and prognosis.

Signalment and History

Dilated cardiomyopathy is usually considered a disease of large- and giant-breed dogs, with males generally having a higher incidence. Certain breeds are overrepresented, and there is some geographic variation. North American surveys suggest increased prevalence in the Doberman pinscher, Irish wolfhound, Great Dane, boxer and American cocker spaniel; whereas European surveys identified an increased risk for the Airedale terrier, Newfoundland, Doberman pinscher, and English cocker spaniel (O'Grady and Sullivan, 2004). Other breeds that we commonly observe include Dalmatians, German shepherds, and standard poodles. With the exception of the Portuguese water dog, in which clinical signs are often manifested before 12 weeks of age, DCM is commonly regarded as an adult-onset genetic disorder. Because of the potential benefit from early intervention, evaluation for occult (asymptomatic) disease can be considered in the breeds listed here. Clinical signs in dogs with DCM may be absent (preclinical or occult disease) or so subtle that they are overlooked. Some historical signs that should raise suspicion include mild exercise intolerance and weight loss. However, most often DCM is not diagnosed until clinical signs of overt CHF (coughing, tachypnea, dyspnea, and ascites) are present. As mentioned previously, sudden death is sometimes the first clinical sign of DCM in previously asymptomatic dogs.

Physical Examination

Although not present in every case, it is common for a soft (grade 1-3/6) systolic murmur to be heard over the mitral or tricuspid valve regions as a result of mitral or tricuspid valve insufficiency. Louder murmurs can be heard if there is concurrent degenerative valvular disease. A low-frequency early diastolic sound (S3 gallop) may be noted over the left apex, indicating ventricular dilation and elevated atrial pressure. Femoral arterial pulses are usually weak as a result of reduced stroke volume from decreased systolic function. Pulse deficits are the hallmark of an arrhythmia such as atrial fibrillation. Pulmonary auscultation may reveal crackles and increased bronchovesicular lung sounds secondary to pulmonary edema or muffled sounds if pleural effusion is present. Jugular venous distention, hepatomegaly, and ascites may be noted in dogs with biventricular CHF.

Electrocardiography

Most dogs with systematic DCM exhibit changes consistent with left ventricular enlargement and possibly left atrial enlargement. Cardiac arrhythmias, including sinus tachycardia, atrial fibrillation, and ventricular arrhythmias, are commonly identified. Conduction disturbances, including partial or complete left bundle branch blocks, are seen occasionally.

Ventricular premature complexes (VPCs) are common in Doberman pinschers and boxers with DCM and may require 24-hour ambulatory electrocardiographic (AECG) monitoring to fully characterize the rhythm disturbances. However, frequent VPCs may also be seen in boxers with what has been called *arrhythmogenic right ventricular cardiomyopathy* (previously described as boxer cardiomyopathy) (see Chapter 175) or similar clinical variant without concurrent DCM. The presence of VPCs may be a marker for occult DCM. Several studies in Doberman pinschers have found a clinical association between the number and complexity of ventricular arrhythmias and the development of DCM. One study demonstrated that nearly all dogs with frequent VPCs on AECG (>50 to 100/24 hour) went on to develop overt DCM (Sisson, O'Grady, and Calvert, 1999).

Atrial fibrillation appears to be more prominent in but not limited to giant-breed dogs such as Irish wolfhounds, Great Danes, and Newfoundlands. Two studies of giant-breed dogs revealed a 75% to 97% incidence of atrial fibrillation on initial presentation (O'Grady and Sullivan, 2004).

Thoracic Radiography

Dogs with DCM usually exhibit moderate-to-severe generalized cardiomegaly. Because of conformational differences (deep thorax and upright heart), Doberman pinschers and boxers often have less impressive radiographic changes. Pulmonary venous distention and pulmonary edema are the hallmarks of left-sided CHF, whereas pleural effusion is often a sign of biventricular CHF.

Echocardiography

Although a presumptive diagnosis of DCM can be made based on historical, physical examination, and ECG data, transthoracic echocardiography (TTE) allows a definitive diagnosis. Semiquantitative assessment of disease severity can also be determined. The hallmark of DCM from TTE is evidence of systolic dysfunction through alterations in multiple systolic indices, including reductions in percent fractional shortening, ejection fraction, and left ventricular area shortening along with increases in the E-point-to-septal separation and end-systolic diameter indexed to weight (Sisson, O'Grady, and Calvert, 1999). There is dilation of the left ventricle and left atrium (increased diameter indexed to weight). The thickness of the interventricular septum and left ventricular free wall are normal to decreased. The right ventricle and right atrium are variably affected and may appear normal to severely dilated. Mitral valve leaflet excursions typically are diminished because of low cardiac output and decreased venous return. Color Doppler often documents a central jet of mitral regurgitation derived from mitral annular and papillary muscle distortion, although this may be prominent if there is concurrent degenerative mitral valve disease.

Diagnosis of affected dogs in the occult stage is far more difficult and controversial. In Doberman pinschers, in which occult disease has been studied most extensively, dilation of the left ventricle tends to precede systolic dysfunction; this may not be true for other breeds. Newer echocardiographic modalities may prove useful in the future to allow earlier detection of disease and potentially affirm equivocal results from TTE. One such modality is tissue Doppler imaging with determination of myocardial velocity gradient and mitral annular systolic motion velocity (S_m). Others include myocardial strain and left ventricular torsion. With further experience these novel techniques may be considered useful inclusions in any screening program for detection of occult DCM. Additional echocardiographic data that may differentiate equivocal cases include systolic time intervals, diastolic performance indices, and stress echocardiography.

PROGNOSIS

Generally DCM carries a guarded-to-poor prognosis, although this is influenced by factors such as etiology and stage of disease at the time of diagnosis. For example, DCM in some American cocker spaniels has been associated with taurine deficiency, in which supplementation (see section on Therapeutic Considerations) can result in improved function and prognosis. The prognosis for English cocker spaniels treated with conventional drugs only can be surprisingly long, often more than 2 years. Occult disease in Doberman pinschers can last from 2 to 4 years before overt disease develops, but it is not known if this holds true for other breeds. Once overt CHF is present, the prognosis is highly variable. In our experience most naive dogs (no treatment) with DCM that present in CHF and respond to initial therapy survive for at least 6 to 12 months, with some surviving 12 to 24 months and only a minority longer than 24 months. However, age at onset of CHF (younger is worse), breed, concurrent presence of dyspnea and ascites, and the presence of atrial fibrillation all appear to be negative prognostic indicators, as would be logical by the severity of the clinical signs (O'Grady and Sullivan, 2004).

THERAPEUTIC CONSIDERATIONS

There are many different views regarding the best therapeutic protocol for DCM and very few studies of high-grade evidence. It would seem reasonable, at least as a starting point, to parallel the commonly used triple-therapy protocol (diuretic, angiotensin-converting enzyme (ACE) inhibitor, and positive inotrope) from the human literature; and there are published data to support the use of furosemide, ACE inhibitors, and pimobendan in dogs.

Diuretics

Most dogs with DCM present in CHF; thus diuretics play a large role in initial treatment and long-term control of fluid retention. However, if CHF is absent at the time of presentation, diuretics are not used because they result in further activation of detrimental neurohormonal responses. In addition, because of the unregulated activation of these responses, diuretics should never be used as sole therapy.

Furosemide

Furosemide is the most commonly used diuretic and has a rather large dosage range (2 to 4 mg/kg q24-8h orally [PO]). It is prudent to use the lowest possible dose to avoid adverse effects such as dehydration and hypokalemia. The concurrent use of ACE inhibitors and positive inotropes allows less dependence on diuretics. Therefore a lower required dosage of furosemide, often in the range of 0.5 to 2 mg/kg/day divided BID or TID, can be effective in some dogs. Another reason for using the lowest possible dose of furosemide is that, if excessive diuresis occurs while receiving ACE inhibitors, an acute reduction in glomerular filtration rate (GFR) can lead to acute renal failure.

Thiazides

With chronic refractory CHF the dosage of furosemide can be increased progressively, or another diuretic may be added. The thiazides (hydrochlorothiazide, 2.2 to 4.4 mg/kg q12h PO; chlorothiazide, 20 to 40 mg/kg q12h PO) are commonly chosen in this setting. The enhanced diuresis from their addition can be quite dramatic and, in fact, may be too great and result in dehydration, acute renal failure, and severe electrolyte derangements. We have found that the addition of these agents in a modified pulse therapy protocol (q12h given every third day) allows enhanced diuresis without inducing dehydration or hypokalemia. As the cardiac disease progresses, administration can be increased to every other day and then every day.

Spironolactone

Spironolactone, an aldosterone antagonist that has been classified as a potassium-sparing diuretic, can also be added to furosemide. Recent experimental data in dogs suggest that standard doses (2.2 to 4.4 mg/kg q12h PO) do not result in an appreciable diuresis in healthy dogs. The situation in CHF is less certain. Historically spironolactone has been used to help prevent hypokalemia induced by chronic diuretic therapy in the pre-ACE inhibitor era. With the advent of ACE inhibitor therapy, there was concern that concurrent use of spironolactone with ACE inhibitors might result in hyperkalemia from excessive depression of aldosterone action and levels, respectively. However, clinically this is not commonly recognized and might be the result of the well-recognized phenomenon of aldosterone escape with ACE inhibitor therapy. Routine monitoring of potassium levels in dogs receiving concurrent spironolactone and ACE inhibitors is prudent, and excessive potassium intake should be avoided.

Angiotensin-Converting Enzyme Inhibitors

The development of ACE inhibitors has made perhaps the greatest impact on medical management of DCM over the past 50 years. These agents prevent the formation of angiotensin II, which induces vasoconstriction, fluid retention, myocardial and vascular smooth muscle hypertrophy/fibrosis, aldosterone release, and enhancement of sympathetic nervous system activity. There are numerous drugs within the ACE inhibitor class; and, although there are some unique differences among the individual drugs, beneficial effects are seen across the class when used in dogs with DCM. These benefits include reduced signs of CHF and improved survival. Enalapril and benazepril are probably the best studied in dogs, but this is changing rapidly as additional drugs within this class become approved for use in dogs in Europe (Table 174-1).

Unlike in mitral insufficiency, there appears to be a therapeutic role for ACE inhibitors in dogs with DCM of all stages because the renin-angiotensin-aldosterone system is activated early in the course of DCM, even before development of CHF. Many of these agents are labeled for use once or twice a day, but we generally use enalapril at a dosage of 0.5 mg/kg every 12 hours orally, especially with CHF. Some clinicians initiate therapy at 0.25 mg/kg every 12 hours orally and increase the dosage after follow-up renal function tests. Potential adverse effects for drugs of this class include gastrointestinal (inappetence, vomiting), renal (acute renal insufficiency), and hypotension. However, in our experience it is very uncommon for dogs to experience clinically evident hypotension. This may be because of a species difference in sensitivity to these drugs. The greatest risk appears to be a reduction in GFR usually associated with volume depletion, possibly from aggressive diuretic use. Therefore routine monitoring of renal parameters is recommended in dogs receiving ACE inhibitors. This is commonly done in practice by measuring renal values before drug therapy, 3 to 5 days after starting therapy or increasing dose or dosing frequency

Table 174-1

List of Commonly Used Angiotensin-Converting Enzyme Inhibitors in Dogs and Cats

Generic Name	Trade Name	Dose (Dog)	Dose (Cat)
Benazepril	Fortekor, Lotensin	0.25-0.5 mg/kg q24-12h	0.25-0.5 mg/kg q24-12h
Enalapril	Enacard, Vasotec	0.25-0.5 mg/kg q24-12h	0.25-0.5 mg/kg q24-12h
Imidapril	Prilium	0.25 mg/kg q24h	
Lisinopril	Prinivil, Zestril	0.25-0.5 mg/kg q24-12h	0.25-0.5 mg/kg q24h
Ramipril	Altace	0.5 mg/kg q24-12h	0.5 mg/kg q24h

of the ACE inhibitor or diuretic, and every 3 to 6 months while on chronic stable therapy. Renal values should also be measured any time a dog exhibits clinical signs such as vomiting, inappetence, or reduced urination. The concurrent use of nonsteroidal antiinflammatory drugs may increase the risk of renal insufficiency and reduce the clinical efficacy of these drugs. Two drugs within this class that should be highlighted because of their unique pharmacokinetic properties are lisinopril and benazepril. Lisinopril, unlike the remainder of the ACE inhibitors, is not a prodrug. Therefore it does not require metabolism to the active metabolite and can be used in dogs with concurrent hepatic insufficiency. Benazepril is excreted through both renal and hepatic routes and therefore does not appear to require altered dosing in dogs with mild-to-moderate concurrent renal insufficiency. The therapeutic advantage of these characteristics requires further study.

Positive Inotropes

Increasing the strength of ventricular contractions in dogs with ventricular systolic dysfunction is naturally intuitive. However, only a few oral drugs confer a positive inotropic effect. These drugs as a class are associated with increased frequency of ventricular arrhythmias, especially in humans. The arrhythmogenic potential of inotropic drugs in dogs requires more study.

Digitalis Glycosides

Until recently digoxin was the only positive inotrope available orally in many countries, including the United States. Digoxin not only exhibits a weak inotropic effect but has the additional benefit of neurohormonal modulation. This results from a normalization of baroreceptor function, which leads to reduction in sympathetic and enhancement of parasympathetic nervous system activity. Although there has been no prospective study in veterinary medicine to evaluate the clinical efficacy of digoxin in DCM, there are anecdotal reports of increased quality of life. A large clinical trial in humans demonstrated reduced cardiovascular mortality, an overall significant reduction in hospital visits, and an improvement of quality of life. In addition, lower blood levels of digoxin have been shown to confer measurable benefits while reducing the risk for toxicity. There is a trend among veterinary cardiologists to achieve digoxin levels that are lower than those previously accepted as therapeutic in dogs (approximately 1 to 2 ng/ml). We prefer to use a dosing protocol of 0.003 to 0.005 mg/kg every 12 hours orally; the lower end is used for medium and large dogs or in dogs with concurrent renal insufficiency since digoxin is cleared primarily by the kidney. In very large dogs we often use 0.22 mg/m² every 12 hours orally, but the initial dose should never exceed 0.25 mg every 12 hours. Digoxin levels are required to monitor therapy so appropriate up-or-down dose titrations can be made. In our practice digoxin levels are usually measured 6 to 8 hours after dosing, 7 to 10 days after initiating or changing the dose, whenever renal insufficiency is recognized or clinical signs of toxicity are present (inappetence, vomiting, diarrhea, arrhythmias), or every 6 months with stable chronic therapy. Some cardi-

ologists prefer to sample a trough 10 to 12 hours after the previous dose; however, this timing can be more difficult to achieve in the outpatient clinic. If toxicity is suspected, therapy should be discontinued until the digoxin level is known. For uncomplicated cases we consider levels from 0.7 to 1.5 ng/ml to be therapeutic. If toxicity is suspected within this range, we consider cutting the dose in half to see if signs abate. If clinical signs persist, we consider concurrent medication, or clinical disease. Higher serum levels (1.5 to 2.5 ng/ml) may be required to help manage atrial fibrillation with attendant risk of adverse effects. When atrial fibrillation with rapid ventricular response rate (>200 beats/min) is present, an oral loading protocol of 0.003 to 0.005 mg/kg every 8 hours orally for 48 hours can be used. This hastens the development of a therapeutic level.

Pimobendan

Pimobendan (Vetmedin) is a positive inotropic drug recently approved for use in dogs. The positive inotropic effect is caused by an increased sensitivity of troponin C for calcium and also by phosphodiesterase III inhibition. The latter mechanism also results in venous and arterial vasodilation, which is the reason this drug is referred to as an "inodilator." Pimobendan also exhibits beneficial neurohormonal effects, which include a reduction in plasma norepinephrine levels and inflammatory cytokines such as tumor necrosis factor (TNF)-α and interleukin (IL)-1β. Adverse effects could include an increase in sinus rate and enhanced arteriovenous nodal conduction. Whether or not pimobendan is proarrhythmic requires more study. Clinical studies in dogs have revealed improved survival and improved quality of life and functional class of heart failure (Luis Fuentes, 2004). The standard dosing protocol is 025 to 0.3 mg/kg every 12 hours orally.

Antiarrhythmic Therapy

Supraventricular Arrhythmias

Cardiac arrhythmias are commonly encountered with DCM, with atrial fibrillation most frequently requiring clinical management. The focus of atrial fibrillation treatment is management of the ventricular response rate in most cases. However, pharmacologic and electrocardioversion techniques have been used successfully in some dogs (see Chapter 164). Pharmacologic management of atrial fibrillation is centered on slowing atrioventricular (AV) nodal conduction velocity through the use of digoxin, calcium channel blockers, and β-blockers. Digoxin is usually the first-line drug but is often ineffective by itself. For this reason diltiazem (0.5 to 1.5 mg/kg q8h PO) or atenolol (0.5 to 1 mg/kg q24–12h PO) is commonly added to the protocol. The β-blockers are hampered by the risk of decompensation at the doses commonly required to effectively control the ventricular response rate. For this reason we most commonly add diltiazem to digoxin and find this combination very effective. The use of cardioprotective β-blocker therapy for CHF will be discussed separately.

Ventricular Arrhythmias

Certain breeds have a higher incidence of ventricular arrhythmias, including boxers and Doberman pinschers (see Chapters 175 and 176). The class III agents (sotalol, amiodarone) appear particularly effective at abolishing these arrhythmias. However, sotalol (1 to 2 mg/kg q12h PO) does have β-blocking properties and should be used very cautiously in these patients to avoid cardiac decompensation, although this is not a complete contraindication. Amiodarone (10 mg/kg q24–12h PO for 7 to 10 days and then 5 to 10 mg/kg q24h PO) can be a very effective antiarrhythmic drug with less negative inotropy then sotalol. However, amiodarone can be associated with adverse effects, including hepatotoxicity and altered thyroid function. The class Ib drug, mexiletine (4 to 10 mg/kg q8h orally) also appears to be quite effective. Efficacy may be enhanced with concurrent use of atenolol, sotalol, or another β-blocker.

Ancillary Treatments

Nutritional Therapy

Amino acid supplementation. There is growing evidence that amino acid deficiencies may be more common in dogs with DCM than previously suspected, but these cases still comprise a small minority of the DCM population (Bonagura, 2000). The prevalence of carnitine deficiency with DCM does not appear large, and many dogs do not demonstrate a clinical response to supplementation alone. An accurate diagnosis usually requires an endomyocardial biopsy because serum levels are often normal or even elevated with myocardial deficiency. Carnitine supplementation (50 to 100 mg/kg q12–8h PO) is relatively expensive but may be helpful in some dogs. Taurine deficiency has also been recognized, especially in some specific breeds such as the American cocker spaniel, golden retrievers, and Newfoundlands and in dogs eating custom and lamb-rice diets. Unlike carnitine, an accurate assessment of taurine status can be determined by measuring serum or whole blood levels, and supplementation has been associated with a positive clinical response. Taurine levels should be measured when DCM is recognized in a dog from one of the previously mentioned breeds, in a breed uncommonly diagnosed with DCM, or in a dog receiving an unusual or unbalanced diet. Taurine supplementation (500 mg q12h PO) should be given to dogs with a documented deficiency or while levels are pending in dogs suspected as being deficient. Taurine supplementation is not expensive; thus a 3- to 6-month therapeutic trial in lieu of a documented deficiency could be considered.

Reduced sodium intake. Reduced dietary intake of sodium helps prevent excessive fluid retention and less dependence on diuretics. Modest-to-moderate sodium restriction is prudent, but excessive restriction results in reduced diet palatability and possibly activation of neurohormonal systems. We have found the following diets helpful: Purina (CV, NF) and Hill's (k/d, g/d, and h/d). However, this list should not be considered exhaustive. See Chapter 157 for more details about diet and supplementation.

Antioxidants

There is some evidence that antioxidants may play a beneficial role in cardiovascular disease through reduction in inflammatory cytokines (i.e., TNF-α and IL-1β). Supplementation with omega-3 fatty acid products (780 mg of eicosapentaenoic acid [EPA] and 497 mg of docosahexaenoic acid [DAA] per day) is safe, inexpensive, and has been shown to exhibit beneficial effects (Smith, 2007).

β-Blockers. Chronic activation of the sympathetic nervous system can result in myocardial remodeling, fibrosis, and reduced function. Clinical data from humans suggest that chronic β-blocker therapy results in improved cardiac function and survival. Although data are absent in veterinary medicine, it is possible that dogs with DCM may also benefit from these agents. However, these agents can cause decompensation if the dose is too high or the animal particularly sensitive to sympathetic withdrawal. For these reasons these drugs should only be used in dogs with occult or compensated disease, or treated DCM and at very low initiating doses. The two drugs that have received the most attention in veterinary medicine are metoprolol and carvedilol. Both of these drugs provide nonspecific β-blockade; but carvedilol also exhibits potent antioxidant properties and α–blockade, although this last effect seems to be weak and may not exert a clinical impact. Both of these agents appear to be relatively safe in dogs when used in a slow up-titration dosing regimen (metoprolol, 0.1 mg/kg q12–8h PO; carvedilol, 0.04 to 0.1 mg/kg q12h PO) when the dose is increased every 7 to 14 days to a maximum tolerated dose or 1 mg/kg for either drug (Abbott, 2004).

Spironolactone. Spironolactone may exhibit a weak diuretic effect at best in the dog, but it may hold greater promise as an antimitogenic agent by interfering with the remodeling and fibrotic effects of aldosterone. In a large human clinical trial it was found that the addition of a once-a-day, subdiuretic dose of spironolactone to standard cardiac therapy resulted in a reduction in overall mortality by more than 30%. Although there are no clinical data in veterinary medicine to support a similar effect in dogs with DCM, it is now common to use spironolactone in this manner. There is no established once-a-day low dose for dogs, but we use an empiric regimen of 6.25 mg q24h orally for dogs less than 10 kg, 12.5 mg q24h orally for dogs 10 to 25 kg, and 25 mg q24h orally for dogs more than 25 kg.

Intermittent dobutamine infusion. Dobutamine is a very effective drug for treatment of cardiogenic shock in dogs with DCM (see Chapter 171). It has been documented in the human literature that some chronic refractory heart failure patients demonstrate a positive clinical response to intermittent dobutamine therapy. These beneficial effects are sometimes seen for a period of time longer than the infusion period. We have used this protocol occasionally; dobutamine is infused at 5 to 10 mcg/kg/min intravenously for a 12- to 24-hour period. It is difficult to say whether this therapy is effective, but some dogs seem to have had a positive clinical response.

References and Suggested Reading

Abbott JA: Beta-blockade in the management of systolic dysfunction, *Vet Clin Small Anim* 34:1157, 2004.

Bonagura JD, editor: *Kirk's current veterinary therapy XIII (small animal practice)*, Philadelphia, 2000, Saunders, p 761.

Fuentes VL: Use of pimobendan in the management of heart failure, *Vet Clin North AM (small Anim Pract)* 34:1145, 2004.

Meurs KM: Primary myocardial diseases in the dog. In Ettinger SJ, Feldman EC, editors: *Textbook of veterinary internal medicine*, ed 6, St Louis, 2005, Elsevier, p 1077.

O'Grady MR, O'Sullivan ML: Dilated cardiomyopathy: an update, *Vet Clin Small Anim* 34:1187, 2004.

Sisson DD, Kittleson MD: Management of heart failure: principles of treatment, therapeutic strategies, and pharmacology. In Fox PR, Sisson DD, Moïse NS, editors: *Textbook of canine and feline cardiology: principles and clinical practice*, ed 2, Philadelphia, 1999, Saunders, p 216.

Sisson DD, O'Grady MR, Calvert CA: Myocardial diseases of dogs. In Fox PR, Sisson DD, Moïse NS, editors: *Textbook of*

canine and feline cardiology: principles and clinical practice, ed 2, Philadelphia, 1999, Saunders, p 581.

Smith CE et al: Omega-3 fatty acids in boxer dogs with arrhythmogenic right ventricular cardiomyopathy, *J Vet Intern Med* 21:265, 2007.

Wynne J, Braunwald E: The cardiomyopathies and myocarditides. In: Braunwald E, Zipes DP, Libby P, editors: *Heart disease: a textbook of cardiovascular medicine*, ed 6, Philadelphia, 2001, Saunders, p 1751.

CHAPTER 175

Cardiomyopathy in Boxer Dogs

KATHRYN M. MEURS, *Pullman, Washington*
ALAN W. SPIER, *Tampa, Florida*

Boxer cardiomyopathy is a primary myocardial disease that typically presents in one of three forms: an asymptomatic form with ventricular premature complexes (VPCs); a symptomatic form with VPCs; and a form with ventricular dilation, myocardial dysfunction, and ventricular and supraventricular tachyarrhythmias. Affected dogs may live for years with the disease and remain asymptomatic, may die of sudden death, or may gradually progress to congestive heart failure. This disease is most commonly referred to as *arrhythmogenic right ventricular cardiomyopathy (ARVC)*. ARVC is an adult-onset familial disease that appears to be inherited in an autosomal-dominant fashion. The frequency of disease, as well as disease severity, increases with age.

A small percentage of boxers with myocardial disease present for the first time with ventricular dilation and myocardial dysfunction without a history of ARVC. It is possible that these boxers have a separate myocardial disease with an etiology that might include an inherited carnitine deficiency, viral myocarditis, or some other myocardial insult that results in the development of a cardiomyopathic state.

DIAGNOSIS

Arrhythmogenic Right Ventricular Cardiomyopathy

A single diagnostic test for boxer ARVC is unavailable, and the diagnosis is best based on the presence of a combination of findings that may include a family history of disease, the presence of a ventricular tachyarrhythmia, a history of syncope or exercise intolerance, and the exclusion of other systemic and cardiovascular diseases that could be responsible for the clinical presentation. Generally a thorough physical examination, electrocardiogram, blood pressure measurement, and echocardiogram should be performed when a diagnosis is suspected. In addition, a Holter monitor provides important information for both the initial treatment and long-term management of the case and should be performed whenever possible.

Physical examination findings may include the auscultation of a tachyarrhythmia, although it should be emphasized that many affected dogs have very intermittent bouts of the arrhythmia and the absence of a tachyarrhythmia during examination does not rule out the diagnosis. In addition, since this is primarily an electrical disease, the majority of affected boxers do not have a heart murmur, although a left apical systolic murmur of mitral regurgitation may be identified in the cases that also have myocardial dysfunction and many boxers have a left basilar ejection murmur of uncertain etiology.

The classic electrocardiographic findings of ARVC include the presence of an upright VPC (left bundle branch block morphology) on a lead II electrocardiogram (Harpster, 1991). However, some affected dogs have a different morphology to their VPCs; or, since the arrhythmia is so intermittent, the electrocardiogram may not demonstrate any VPCs at all. It is important to note that a normal electrocardiogram does not exclude a diagnosis of ARVC; if suspicion exists because of clinical signs (syncope, exercise intolerance), auscultation of an arrhythmia, or a family history of disease, a 24-hour Holter monitor is strongly suggested. Even if occasional VPCs are identified on an in-house electrocardiogram, we generally recommend a Holter monitor to help provide the best assessment of overall frequency and complexity of the arrhythmia. In addition, a pretreatment Holter provides useful information when attempting to determine the efficacy and the potential proarrhythmia of treatment once it has started.

The results of the Holter monitor can be very useful in establishing a diagnosis of ARVC, particularly if the electrocardiogram is within normal limits. It is unusual for mature adult dogs to have ventricular ectopy. The median number of VPCs detected on the Holter reading from 600 mature asymptomatic boxers was 10 VPCs in 24 hours. Therefore the identification of frequent ventricular ectopy (>100 VPCs/24 hours) in an adult boxer is strongly suggestive of a diagnosis of ARVC, particularly if there is significant complexity (couplets, triplets, bigeminy, or ventricular tachycardia) to the arrhythmia. However, in some cases a diagnosis of ARVC in the boxer is greatly suspected based on the breed and presence of syncope, but the Holter monitor reading is not clearly abnormal. This may be because of the significant day-to-day variability of VPC number (up to 83%) in affected dogs. In highly suspect cases it may be worth performing a second Holter monitor or an event monitor if the dog is syncopal.

A blood pressure measurement and echocardiogram are recommended in cases of suspect ARVC. Although in the majority of cases the blood pressure, cardiac chamber sizes, and systolic function are within normal limits, an echocardiogram can rule out other less common causes of ventricular ectopy (e.g., neoplasia). Blood pressure measurement may give insights into additional systemic diseases that are capable of causing syncope. In addition, the echocardiogram is necessary to identify the small percentage of dogs with ARVC that develop right and left ventricular enlargement and myocardial dysfunction.

Dilated Cardiomyopathy

A small percentage of boxers have a clinical presentation consistent with dilated cardiomyopathy. Affected dogs may present with syncope or signs of left heart failure, including coughing; tachypnea; or biventricular failure, including coughing, tachypnea, and ascites. Thoracic radiographs may demonstrate left or biventricular enlargement, pulmonary edema, and pulmonary venous congestion. The echocardiogram may demonstrate left or biventricular enlargement with systolic dysfunction. The etiology of these cases is unknown. A small percentage of the cases may have progressed gradually from ARVC; however, other etiologies for myocardial dysfunction, including L-carnitine deficiency or myocarditis, should be considered.

SCREENING

Given the inheritable nature of ARVC, there is significant interest by breeders and enthusiasts of the boxer breed for the development of a screening program. However, at this time there is no single ideal screening test, and consideration should be given to multiple factors, including a family history of ARVC and repeated abnormal Holter monitor readings. Given the adult-onset nature, many perform the first Holter monitor at the age of 3 years and continue on an annual basis. Holter monitor results should be evaluated for both the number of VPCs and the complexity of arrhythmia (e.g., singles, couplets, triplets, ventricular tachycardia). However, there are still many unanswered questions about ARVC and the relationship of the ventricular arrhythmia to the development of clinical signs. Some affected dogs can have thousands of VPCs and never develop clinical signs; others demonstrate severe clinical signs with a fairly low number of VPCs. We have not found the number of VPCs or the complexity of the arrhythmia to be statistically different in symptomatic (syncopal) dogs compared to asymptomatic affected dogs. Therefore the factors that determine which dogs will eventually become clinical for the disease are not known, which leads to additional frustration in screening for this disease. Breeders should be strongly encouraged to screen for the disease but should be advised about the significant complexities of screening and counseled not to remove dogs completely from a breeding program because of a single abnormal Holter reading. Annual Holter monitoring is strongly recommended, and an emphasis should be placed on the results of multiple annual Holters in an asymptomatic animal.

The results of 24-hour Holter monitoring from over 600 asymptomatic adult boxers identified a median number of VPCs of 10, with 25% and 75% confidence intervals of 2 and 110 VPCs per 24 hours, respectively. Based on this information we have developed the following initial system for screening asymptomatic dogs.

1. 0 to 50 single VPCs/24 hour: interpreted as within normal limits
2. 51 to 100 VPCs/24 hours: interpreted as indeterminate; suggest repeating in 6 to 12 months
3. 100 to 300 single VPCs/24 hours: interpreted as suspicious; consider keeping out of the breeding program for 1 year and repeating the Holter study
4. 100 to 300 VPCs/24 hours with increased complexity (frequent couplets, triplets, ventricular tachycardia) or 300 to 1000 single VPCs/24 hours: interpreted as likely affected
5. More than 1000 VPCs/24 hours: interpreted as affected, may consider treatment as discussed in the following paragraphs

These criteria are based on the evaluation of single Holter monitors in mature boxers with no history of syncope. Additional studies to evaluate the long-term outcome of boxers with arrhythmias are currently being performed. This information has been provided as a possible starting point for making screening recommendations. Multiple criteria should be considered for each dog before making any strict recommendations, including family history, evidence of any ongoing systemic disease that could be associated with the development of the ventricular arrhythmia, and repeated Holter studies.

TREATMENT

In affected boxers antiarrhythmic therapy has been shown to decrease the number of VPCs, the complexity (grade) of the arrhythmia, and the presence of syncope (Meurs et al., 2002). However, the ability of antiarrhythmic therapy to decrease the risk of sudden death in affected dogs has never been proved or disproved. In addition, ventricular antiarrhythmics can demonstrate important proarrhythmic effects. Therefore the risks and benefits should always be assessed when considering treatment. In the asymptomatic dog we generally recommend therapy to decrease the number and complexity of the arrhythmias if there are at least 1000 VPCs/24 hours or if runs of ventricular tachycardia or evidence of the R-on-T phenomenon exist. It should be remembered that some ARVC dogs die of sudden death without ever having any documented episodes of syncope; thus the absence of a syncopal history does not imply a lack of risk. Ideally boxers with syncope and ventricular arrhythmias should be treated after a 24-hour Holter monitor is performed to quantify the pretreatment arrhythmia. If the syncope is frequent or ventricular tachycardia is observed, a Holter monitor evaluation may not be performed so that therapy can be started as soon as possible. However, in these cases the absence of a pretreatment monitor may make it difficult to fully assess the response to therapy. Therefore, whenever possible, a Holter monitor evaluation is performed first, and the owner is then advised to start therapy immediately after removing the Holter (before the results are available) if great concern exists.

Two therapeutic protocols appear to be most effective at reducing the number of VPCs and the degree of complexity of the arrhythmia. The first is sotalol (1.5 to 2.5 mg/kg q12h orally [PO]); the second is a combination of mexiletine (5 to 6 mg/kg q8h PO) with a β-blocker (atenolol (0.5 mg/kg q12h PO) or sotalol (1.5 to 2 mg/kg q12h PO)). Sotalol as a monotherapy is generally chosen first because of the low level of side effects and ease of dosing twice a day. However, in some dogs sotalol is less effective. In these cases adding mexiletine or switching to mexiletine and atenolol may be useful. Mexiletine can cause a loss of appetite or mild gastrointestinal upset, but the addition of a β-blocker allows a lower dose of mexiletine to be used to help reduce this side effect. In addition, mexiletine should always be given with a meal.

Despite their potential for beneficial antiarrhythmic effects, the medications listed here can have a proarrhythmic effect or may be less effective in some individual boxers with ARVC. Therefore, if possible, patients should be managed by assessing both a pretreatment and posttreatment (2 to 3 weeks after starting treatment) Holter monitor evaluation. This can help determine the effect of treatment and confirm that the arrhythmia has not gotten worse. Significant day-to-day variability (up to an 83% change in daily VPC number) has been observed in affected boxers (Spier and Meurs, 2004). Therefore a therapeutic response is considered when at least an 80% reduction in VPC number and a reduction in the complexity of the arrhythmia are observed on the posttreatment Holter reading. In addition, an increase in symptoms after starting treatment or a greater than 80% increase in the number of daily VPCs may suggest a proarrhythmic effect.

New Advances in Therapy

The use of implantable cardioverters-fibrillators has gained popularity in humans with ventricular tachyarrhythmias. A defibrillator was successfully placed in one boxer with ARVC, although some complications were observed that were associated with programming limitations of the device. The long-term benefits of this type of therapy in dogs with this myocardial disease have yet to be studied.

References and Suggested Reading

Basso C et al: Arrhythmogenic right ventricular cardiomyopathy causing sudden death in boxer dogs: a new animal model of human disease, *Circulation* 109:1180, 2004.

Harpster N: Boxer cardiomyopathy, *Vet Clin North Am Small Anim Pract* 21:989, 1991.

Keene B: l-carnitine supplementation in the therapy of dilated cardiomyopathy, *Vet Clin North Am Small Anim Pract* 21:1005, 1991.

Meurs KM et al: Familial ventricular arrhythmias in boxers, *J Vet Intern Med* 13:437, 1999.

Meurs KM et al: Comparison of in-hospital versus 24-hour ambulatory electrocardiography for detection of ventricular premature complexes in mature boxers, *J Am Vet Med Assoc* 218:222, 2001.

Meurs KM et al: Comparison of the effects of four antiarrhythmic treatments for familial ventricular arrhythmias in boxers, *J Am Vet Med Assoc* 221:522, 2002.

Spier AW, Meurs KM: Spontaneous variability in the frequency of ventricular arrhythmias in boxers with arrhythmogenic cardiomyopathy, *J Am Vet Med Assoc* 224:538, 2004.

CHAPTER 176

Cardiomyopathy in Doberman Pinschers

CLAY A. CALVERT, *Athens, Georgia*
KATHRYN M. MEURS, *Pullman, Washington*

Cardiomyopathy (CM) in Doberman pinschers (DPs) is a common, inherited, slowly progressive primary myocardial disease. Based on anecdotal reports, we believe that CM in this breed was present in the United States and Canada as far back as the mid-1940s and the incidence of CM in DPs has reflected the breed population since that time. The hallmarks of CM in DPs are heart rhythm disturbances (mostly ventricular tachyarrhythmia, sudden death [SD], or end-stage congestive heart failure [CHF]).

Affected DPs appear to progress through a long asymptomatic preclinical or occult phase (Fig. 176-1). Ventricular premature complexes (VPCs) are often the first markers for CM in this stage and are initially infrequent. Some DPs have slightly increased left ventricular internal dimensions for several years, even from early adulthood, before VPCs appear. Holter recording evaluation is usually needed for earliest detection of VPCs, and the echocardiogram parameters are usually within the "normal" ranges at that time. Typically within 1 year after ventricular ectopy is identified the echocardiogram findings become equivocally abnormal. Within 2 years the echocardiogram findings become unequivocally abnormal. As left ventricular dilation and contractility worsen, VPCs tend to worsen, and potentially lethal ventricular tachycardia (VT) develops in at least 50% of affected DPs. SD is often the first sign of CM and is the outcome in 30% to 50% of patients. It typically occurs between 6 and 8 years of age, is associated with at least moderate dilation and decreased contractility of the left ventricle, and often occurs about 1 year before overt CHF would be anticipated. Over 50% of all overtly healthy DPs over 10 years of age have numerous VPC and/or echocardiographic abnormalities. Many of these DPs die of comorbid disease, and CM is often not identified because cardiac workups have not been performed.

ETIOLOGY AND GENETICS

The breeding history of the DP in North America is one of extreme inbreeding. Until recently virtually all DPs born in the United States and Canada could be traced to one of seven sires. "The seven sires" came from champion German stock imported into the northeastern United States and Canada during the late 1930s and early 1940s and were all closely related; the older three sired the younger four. Three of the seven died suddenly and unexpectedly in middle age. Many related DPs have been exported throughout Europe since 1945, and many have been exported throughout the world in the past 30 years. In many cases the sires and/or dams of these dogs have subsequently died of CM. There is a distinct American flavor to the Dutch, English, and Australian DP. In addition, we have identified CM in numerous DPs imported to the United States from Europe. However, in general we believe that the incidence of CM in Europe is lower than in the United States and Canada.

Although CM is known to be a familial disease, the genetics in DPs are not well understood. In humans approximately 25% to 30% of all cases are familial and can be autosomal dominant (about 50%), autosomal recessive, or X-linked. The mode of inheritance in DP was suggested to be autosomal dominant in one retrospective study. Mutations, usually single, each causing CM in humans, have been identified in most of the proteins of the sarcomere, cytoskeleton, and sarcolemma. If CM in DPs is an autosomal-dominant trait, it should appear with almost equal prevalence in both genders, and there should not be any silent carriers. All affected dogs should have at least one affected parent. However, in some cases it may appear as if neither parent was affected if the dogs died of noncardiac disease before the CM has developed. Although several studies have been performed to try to determine the molecular basis for the disease, and two genes (actin, desmin) have been eluded, the genetic etiology remains undefined.

SCREENING AND EARLY DIAGNOSIS

We strongly recommend annual screening of adult DPs for preclinical CM. Without careful screening SD is often the first sign of CM, or CM is unrecognized until the end-stage of CHF is reached. CHF carries a short and subsequent survival time of less than 1 to 6 months (mean 3 to 4 months) in most DPs treated with conventional drugs. Screening should include both echocardiography and Holter monitor evaluation beginning at 2 to 3 years of age. The likelihood of finding VPCs and echocardiographic markers for CM increases with age.

The most important Holter recording markers for CM are VPCs that usually arise from the left ventricle. Twenty-four–hour Holter recordings containing more than 50 VPCs, any couplets or triplets of VPCs, or runs of VT indicate in our experience that the echocardiogram will be abnormal or equivocally progress to this stage within 1 year. Statistical analyses of large numbers of DPs

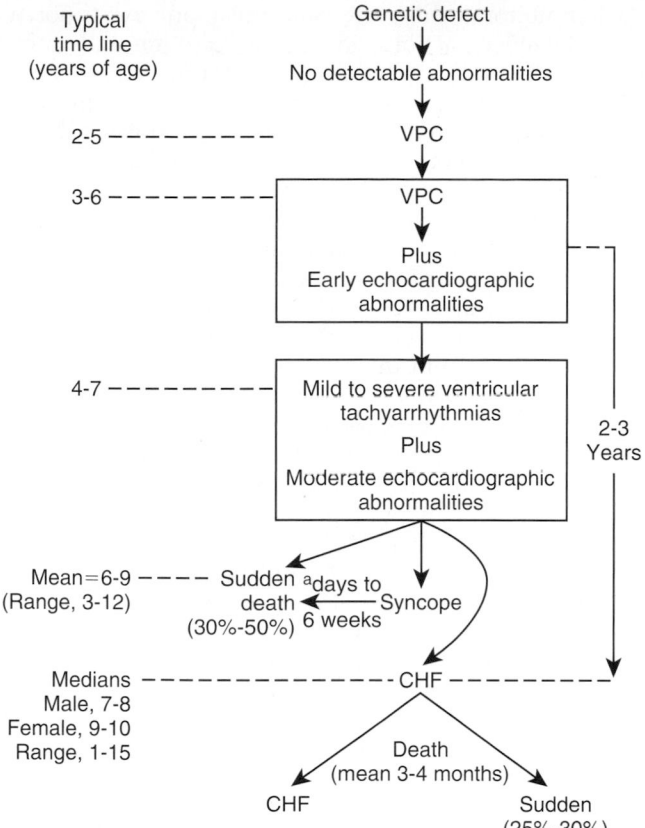

Typical
time line
(years of age)

Genetic defect
↓
No detectable abnormalities
↓
2-5 — — — — — — —   VPC
↓
3-6 — — — — — — —   VPC
↓
Plus
Early echocardiographic
abnormalities

4-7 — — — — — — —   Mild to severe ventricular
tachyarrhythmias
Plus
Moderate echocardiographic
abnormalities

2-3
Years

Mean=6-9 — — — — Sudden ᵃdays to
(Range, 3-12)   death ← 6 weeks → Syncope
(30%-50%)

Medians — — — — — — — — — — CHF — — — — — —
Male, 7-8
Female, 9-10
Range, 1-15
                                Death
                        (mean 3-4 months)
        CHF   Sudden
                                        (25%-30%)

Fig. 176-1 Typical evolution of cardiomyopathy in Doberman pinschers. Arrhythmia and echocardiographic abnormalities can begin as early as 1 year of age or as late as at least 11 years of age. Disease evolution is accelerated when markers appear at a young age and is slower when markers first appear at old age. Syncopeᵃ due to ventricular tachycardia is a marker that survival to the end-stage of congestive heart failure is unlikely; rather sudden death intervenes in spite of therapy.

indicate that even one VPC correlates with increased risk of CM. However, for any one DP, on rare occasions fewer than 50 isolated VPCs may be considered "normal." Any VPC detected during static electrocardiogram (ECG) in DPs is probably the result of CM unless another etiology can be identified. Arrhythmias can begin as young as 9 to 12 months of age and often begin around 2 to 4 years of age; by 6 years of age about 50% of all overtly healthy DPs have VPCs. In DPs with normal to equivocally abnormal echocardiograms the severity of arrhythmia is generally mild, total VPCs/24 hours vary from less than 100 to a few thousand, and life-threatening VT is generally absent. Rapid VT is common after the left ventricular end-systolic dimension exceeds 40 mm, end-systolic dimension exceeds 50 mm, and the fractional shortening declines to less than 23%. Although arrhythmias very often begin when echocardiographic parameters are within the normal ranges, retrospective analyses of serial echocardiograms in these DPs indicate that these parameters progressively change from normal to abnormal. By 1 to 2 years after the onset of VPCs, echo parameters become unequivocally abnormal. Thus, unless screening is begun at 2 to 3 years of age, the odds are that, when the arrhythmias are first

detected, even by Holter recordings, the echocardiogram will be abnormal.

The standard ECG is useful if VPCs are detected, and in most cases at least moderate dilation and systolic dysfunction of the left ventricle are present. Prolongation of the P wave and/or QRS complex duration often correlates with severe myocardial failure. Without treatment, SD or CHF is likely within 9 months. Low-voltage, wide R waves with a "sloppy" or slurred down-stroke of the R wave also suggest advanced myocardial failure and impending CHF.

Compared to age, gender, and size, matched breeds of dogs that have a low incidence of CM, it is our experience that the heart of most normal DPs is not as muscular. Thus the normal echocardiographic parameters that we use are specific for the DP. The most useful M-mode echocardiographic markers of occult CM in order of importance are left ventricular end-systolic dimension, end-diastolic dimension, and fractional shortening. The distinction between a normal and equivocally abnormal echocardiogram is confounded by the limited accuracy of the test, interexaminer variability, and stress level (adrenaline) during the test. Generally overt signs of depressed left ventricular function in sedentary dogs are not evident until the left ventricular end-diastolic dimension and fractional shortening are greater than 55 mm and less than 20%, respectively. In active dogs the owners may recognize exercise intolerance in dogs with mild ventricular dysfunction but often attribute it to age.

Mitral regurgitation (MR) is found by Doppler when the left ventricular end-systolic dimension is moderately increased. MR is often the result of dilation and decreased systolic contraction of the annulus or papillary muscles, but myxomatous mitral and tricuspid valve degeneration are also common in middle-aged and older DPs. MR is relatively severe in some DPs and confounds the differential diagnosis of "large-dog MR" versus CM. Moderate-to-severe MR facilitates fractional shortening and worsens left atrial dilation. In these DPs left atrial dilation is disproportionately severe relative to reduced fractional shortening compared to DPs with mild CM and mild MR. However, standard ECG and Holter recordings from these DPs consistently demonstrate ventricular ectopy, and SD is sometimes the outcome.

SYNCOPE

Syncope in DP is usually caused by rapid, sustained VT. The likelihood of surviving an episode of rapid, sustained VT is probably related to the left ventricular ejection fraction. The lower the ejection fraction, the more likely VT will degenerate to fibrillation and cause SD. Aggressive antiarrhythmic treatment is indicated and usually retards SD, but our experience is that "syncopal" dogs nonetheless will die suddenly usually within 1 year. A less common cause of collapse in this breed is reflex-mediated (neurocardiogenic) syncope. This is an adrenergic-stimulated vagal reflex of bradycardia and vasodilation triggered by fight, flight, fright, or startle scenarios. In this breed neurocardiogenic bradycardia can be benign but is still a marker for CM and must be distinguished from VT-induced episodic weakness or syncope. The presence of numerous VPCs or VT contained in routine ECG or Holter recording indicates VT as the likely cause of syncope. The onset of atrial fibrillation can also precipitate episodic weakness and syncope.

SUDDEN DEATH

Sudden death is the outcome in at least 30% of affected DPs, is as high as 50% in some lines, and exceeds 50% in some families. Syncope, presyncope, and SD are the result of sustained (greater than 30 seconds), rapid VT. If VT stops spontaneously, the patient quickly recovers; but SD is the outcome if the VT degenerates into ventricular fibrillation. Premonitory events of syncope may not precede SD; in other words, the first faint is the last one. Should spontaneous recovery occur and antiarrhythmic treatment not be initiated, another episode is likely within hours to weeks. Rarely does a DP survive three separate episodes. Left untreated, syncope or presyncope caused by VT usually is followed by SD within 1 or 2 weeks, and survival beyond 6 weeks is rare. Sudden death occurs more often in the morning and during or immediately following exertion-excitement, but it can occur during sleep.

In our experience life-threatening ectopy does not occur until left ventricular systolic function is at least moderately depressed. Lethal VT is often associated with end-diastolic dimension greater than 50 mm, end-systolic dimension greater than 45 mm, and fractional shortening between 18% and 23%. Among the surviving subset, progression of left ventricular dysfunction is associated with a lower incidence of SD until the onset of CHF.

TREATMENT GUIDELINES

There is no general agreement regarding treatment guidelines for occult CM. We recommend treatment for myocardial failure when the echocardiogram is unequivocally abnormal (i.e., when the left ventricular end-systolic dimension is greater than 40 mm, the end-diastolic dimension is greater than 50 mm, and the fractional shortening is less than 25%). Ideally treatment is based on all three parameters, but in selected DP it may be based on one or two measures because early myocardial failure is not always "textbook". In addition, we usually do not initiate treatment until the E-point-to–septal separation is greater than 10 mm, a finding typical of ventricular dilation and myocardial failure.

Based on studies in humans, three available classes of drugs may exert a favorable influence on progression of myocardial degeneration and systolic dysfunction: angiotensin-converting enzyme (ACE) inhibitors, aldosterone receptor antagonists, and β-adrenergic receptor blockers. There is little documentation on the influence of these drugs on disease progression in DPs with occult CM. We believe that therapy with an ACE inhibitor initiated before onset of CHF can significantly retard the progression of myocardial failure or CHF. Suggested dosage schedules include enalapril (Enacard, Merial; 0.25 mg/kg q12h orally [PO] for 1 week and then 0.5 mg/kg q12h orally) or benazepril (Lotensin, Novartis; 0.25 mg/kg q24h PO or q12h for 1 week and then 0.5 mg/kg q 24h PO or q12h PO). Also consider spironolactone (Aldactone, Searle; 1 to 2 mg/kg q 12 PO) in combination with the

ACE inhibitor at this stage. Spironolactone exerts potentially beneficial actions on the myocardium and vasculature. The ACE inhibitor–spironolactone combination increases potassium and magnesium serum concentrations, which may reduce arrhythmia. Spironolactone may exert an antifibrotic action (blocking cardiac fibroblast receptors) and may slow progressive myocardial fibrosis. β-Blockade has been shown in numerous human studies to exert a favorable influence on both SD risk and progression of myocardial degeneration. Clinical studies in DPs have not been reported. The addition of carvedilol to the treatment regimen 2 weeks after initiating ACE inhibitor treatment can be considered in DPs with occult CM. We use carvedilol (Coreg, SmithKline Beecham) at 12.5 mg every 12 hours orally for 1 week and then 25 mg every 12 hours orally because it may be the most effective β-blocker in humans with CM. Carvedilol is also a vasodilator (α-blockade) and a potent antioxidant, and it has anti-endothelin activity. The drug is expensive currently. A dosage of 25 mg every 12 hours produces blood levels that are associated with mild-to-moderate β-blockade in DPs, depending on patient size. After 2 additional weeks an increase to 37.5 mg every 12 hours is recommended in patients greater than 35 kg. In spite of its α-blocking (afterload reducing) activity, carvedilol embarrasses contractility if myocardial failure is severe. It is critical that high doses of carvedilol *not* be initiated in DPs with overt or impending CHF. For example, DPs with overt CHF and sinus rhythm sometimes cannot tolerate a starting dosage of 3.125 mg every 12 hours, and those with CHF and atrial fibrillation may not tolerate even 1.56 mg every 12 hours. However, overt adverse affects are uncommon if the fractional shortening is greater than 18%. The dosage of carvedilol may need to be adjusted downward should severe CHF occur.

These regimens are based on the pathophysiology of CM and the success of these medications in humans. Extrapolating data from human studies and applying it to dogs are often inappropriate. We have not observed an obviously favorable influence of carvedilol or spironolactone on disease progression. A large randomized prospective study is needed.

At least 30% of DPs with CM eventually experience life-threatening ventricular ectopy. Such an incidence would seem to dictate aggressive therapy. However, most antiarrhythmic drugs have proarrhythmia activity, some are negative inotropes, and sustained efficacy has not been proven. In addition, adverse effects, mostly gastrointestinal disturbances, are common. Although SD in DPs with occult CM can be retarded, it probably cannot be prevented. Criteria for initiating antiarrhythmic treatment are controversial. We initiate treatment for:

1. Rapid (>200 beats/min) VT (Lown class 4)
2. Syncope with subsequent documentation of many VPCs (presumed Lown class 4)
3. Couplets or triplets of VPCs (Lown class 3) with greater than approximately 6000 to 8000 VPCs/24 hours.

A standard ECG and even a 24h Holter ECG are short samples-in-time. Frequent (at least every 3 months) Holter recordings should be performed in affected dogs when possible because of the dynamic and progressive nature of arrhythmias in many DPs. In the face of refractory rhythm disturbances, Holter recordings may need to be repeated at 1- to 4-week intervals until the rhythm is stabilized. Because of the high risk of SD, some veterinarians prefer to treat all affected DPs presenting with VPCs or VT.

In therapy of ventricular ectopy we recommend mexiletine (Mexitil, Boehringer Ingelheim) at 5 to 6 mg/kg every 8 hours orally for maintenance treatment. Mexiletine frequently causes gastrointestinal upset, but this may be significantly reduced if each dose is given with a small amount of food. If the patient is not already being administered carvedilol, initiate it at this time (if CHF is neither present nor imminent) since the combination of a β-blocker and mexiletine is more effective (in the short-term) than either alone. Rapid and remarkable improvement in VT severity is usual following the initiation of mexiletine. However, in spite of treatment at least 50% of the ventricular arrhythmias in DPs with occult CM become refractory within 3 to 9 months. Under these circumstances consider the addition of amiodarone (10 mg/kg q12h PO for 5 days and then 5 mg/kg q24h PO). Initial follow-up Holter recordings in DPs administered amiodarone sometimes document improvement in the severity of VT, but long-term efficacy has not been proven, and all of the DPs that we have treated with amiodarone have died suddenly. Whether amiodarone exerts a favorable, unfavorable, or neutral effect on time to SD has not been determined. Amiodarone is associated with numerous adverse effects in humans. Even in large DPs we have consistently encountered gastrointestinal disturbances and reversible hepatotoxicity at a maintenance dosage of 400 mg once daily. A maintenance dosage of 200 mg once daily sometimes causes hepatotoxicity. Baseline, 1 week, and then monthly serum chemistry profiles are required.

As myocardial failure worsens, a positive inotrope should be considered. Pimobendan (Vetmedin, Boehringer Ingelheim) administered at 0.3 mg/kg every 12 hours orally is a potent inodilator that exerts a significant positive inotropic action in DPs with advanced CM. We do not recommend pimobendan in dogs with fractional shortening values of 20% or greater. Of major concern is the protracted administration of a powerful positive inotrope in patients with myocardial disease. Past experiences with such drugs have been unfavorable in dogs and humans because of increased SD risk. We have encountered worsening of VT and SD in some DPs treated long term with pimobendan. However, to be determined is whether SD risk in DPs administered pimobendan is greater than in those not administered pimobendan. In one study of overt CHF, pimobendan was associated with prolonged survival in DPs with CM (Luis Fuentes et al., 2002).

We do not recommend digoxin for the treatment of CM in DPs except in the face of atrial fibrillation or sustained or frequent paroxysmal atrial tachycardia. In addition, we do not recommend furosemide treatment until CHF is imminent. Furosemide is used when patients develop nocturnal dyspnea, a gallop heart rhythm, or distended pulmonary veins or based on echocardiographic measurements of high preload.

References and Suggested Reading

Luis Fuentes V et al: A double-blind, randomized, placebo-controlled study of pimobendan in dogs with dilated cardiomyopathy, *J Vet Intern Med* 16:255, 2002.

Meurs KM: Primary myocardial disease in the dog. In Ettinger SJ, Feldman EC, editors: *Textbook of veterinary internal medicine*, Philadelphia, 2005, Saunders, p 1077.

CHAPTER 177

Myocarditis

KARSTEN E. SCHOBER, *Columbus, Ohio*

Myocarditis is one of the most challenging diagnoses in small animal cardiology and may be even more difficult to manage. The entity is rarely recognized clinically, the prevalence unknown and probably underestimated, the pathophysiology poorly understood, and the clinical presentation and course variable. Furthermore there is no commonly accepted diagnostic gold standard, and all current specific treatments are controversial.

Myocarditis is defined as an insidious inflammatory disorder of the myocardium characterized by leukocytic infiltration and nonischemic myocyte degeneration and necrosis (Feldman and McNamara, 2000). Because there is no consistently recognizable clinical syndrome or specific noninvasive diagnostic test, the clinical diagnosis of both acute and chronic myocarditis remains problematic and is often only presumptive. There are a variety of causes; infectious agents seem most relevant. Primary myocarditis is presumed to be caused by an acute viral infection or a postviral autoimmune response, neither of which are well studied in dogs or cats. Secondary myocarditis is inflammation caused by a specific pathogen, including bacteria, protozoa, fungi, drugs, chemicals, physical agents, and systemic inflammatory diseases. The causal link between active, viral myocarditis and the subsequent development of dilated cardiomyopathy (DCM) is documented in humans but much less appreciated and explored in small animals. This chapter briefly considers some of the current ideas regarding the manifestations, potential importance, and management of myocarditis in dogs and cats.

PATHOPHYSIOLOGY

Myocarditis has both infectious and noninfectious causes (Table 177-1). Cardiotropic viruses, including those with ribonucleic acid (RNA) and deoxyribonucleic acid cores, are the predominant pathogens that lead to myocardial inflammation in humans (Feldman and McNamara, 2000). Current speculation is that 10% to 30% of human myocarditis is virus associated. However, with the exception of canine parvovirus, the importance of viruses in the development of myocarditis is largely undetermined in dogs and cats.

Current knowledge of the pathogenesis of viral myocarditis stems mostly from laboratory animal studies. A viral infection of the heart follows a standard progression. Most viral pathogens enter the body through the upper respiratory or gastrointestinal tracts. Genetic susceptibilities that alter the autoimmune response to viral infections may be important at this stage. The *acute phase* (days 0 through 3; viremic phase; fulminant myocarditis) is characterized by systemic viremia, virus binding to myocyte coreceptors, virus invasion into cardiomyocytes, and virus replication causing myocytolysis. Macrophage activation leads to the production and release of proinflammatory cytokines, including tumor necrosis factor (TNF), interferon-γ, various interleukins, and inducible nitric oxide (iNO). The *subacute phase* (days 4 through 14; inflammatory phase; postviral or lymphocytic myocarditis) is characterized by clearance of the viruses by natural killer cells, cytokines, perforin, and neutralizing antibodies. Attracted by cytokine release, mononuclear cells such as cytotoxic T and B lymphocytes enter the myocardium and may cause extensive cellular damage. By the end of this stage the virus has already been cleared from the body, but the ongoing immune response mediates the myocardial damage and cell death. In the final or *chronic phase* (days 15 and beyond; healing phase; chronic myocarditis) there is evidence of myofiber dropout and replacement fibrosis. Most patients recover completely. However, in others viral persistence and host-pathogen interactions lead to chronic inflammation, repetitive cycles of myocardial injury and repair, apoptosis, coronary microvascular spasm, and autoimmune effects. These responses can result in continued myocardial injury and slow evolution to DCM and heart failure. This may occur even after many years, and some cases of idiopathic DCM in dogs and cats may represent unrecognized viral myocarditis.

Slow-growing nonviral agents such as *Trypanosoma cruzi* may also cause chronic myocarditis with progressive DCM-like pathology after a prolonged latent period (Bonagura, 1995, p 850). Cardiotoxic drugs and drug hypersensitivity reactions have been associated with myocarditis. The severity of histopathologic lesions resulting from any of these agents varies with the severity of the insult and the nature and magnitude of the host-toxin interaction. Cardiac injury and myocarditis in critically ill patients is often severe but remains most commonly unrecognized. Potential mechanisms for myocarditis in such patients include excess NO and proinflammatory cytokine production, endotoxins, direct bacterial damage, and ischemia and reperfusion. Traumatic injury of the heart caused by nonpenetrating chest trauma (referred to as *traumatic myocarditis*) may be associated with myocardial contusion, intramyocardial bleeding, inflammation, and myocardial degeneration and necrosis. Myocardial dysfunction is a rare consequence and almost always reversible, and arrhythmias are usually benign. There is no evidence of long-term myocardial damage and dysfunction after traumatic myocarditis in dogs and cats (Bonagura, 1995, p. 846).

Table 177-1

Causes of Myocarditis in Dogs and Cats

Infectious	Viral (parvovirus,* distemper virus,* herpesvirus, coronavirus, others)
	Bacterial* (various)
	Rickettsial (Rickettsia, Ehrlichia, Bartonella*)
	Spirochetal (Borrelia,* Leptospira*)
	Fungal (various)
	Algaelike (Prototheca)
	Protozoal (Trypanosoma,* Toxoplasma,* Neospora, Hepatozoon)
	Parasitic (Toxocara, Trichinella)
Physical	Traumatic chest or body impact
	Hyperthermia
Immune-mediated	Postinfectious
	Systemic disorders
	Drug hypersensitivity
Toxic	Drugs
	Toxins
Other	Idiopathic

*Most commonly described.

PATHOLOGY

Inflammation may cause the myocardial pallor with occasional areas of minute hemorrhage. Microscopically there is distortion of muscle fibers caused by interstitial edema and fiber necrosis. The inflammatory infiltrate is usually lymphocytic. Morphometric quantification of the lesions is essential, with 14 leukocytes/mm^2 being the cutoff to distinguish between the presence and absence of myocarditis in humans. Immunohistochemical staining for T lymphocytes may be needed to establish the diagnosis. Depending on the causative agent, there may be more specific histologic features. Healing is often associated with interstitial fibrosis. A viral origin of myocarditis can only be proved if viral particles such as inclusion bodies or the virus itself are detected within an altered myocardium. This has become possible through molecular analysis of necropsy and endomyocardial biopsy specimens using new techniques of viral gene amplification, including polymerase chain reaction (PCR) and in situ hybridization. The *histologic* diagnosis of myocarditis was clarified by the Dallas criteria (see the following section on Clinical Manifestations and Diagnosis), but these unfortunately did not include immunohistochemistry to demonstrate a T cell–mediated immune response. The *clinicopathologic* classification of primary myocarditis originally proposed by Braunwald and associates is based on the onset of illness, left ventricular function, endomyocardial biopsy (EMB) findings, and clinical and histologic outcomes and led to four classes of myocarditis: fulminant, subacute, chronic active, and chronic persistent. This classification has not yet gained wide acceptance in veterinary medicine.

CLINICAL MANIFESTATIONS AND DIAGNOSIS

Myocarditis can create diverse clinical features. The diagnosis of acute myocarditis is made largely by clinical history and a high index of suspicion rather than a definitive diagnostic test. It may follow upper respiratory or gastrointestinal infection, surgery, or recent drug exposure. General constitutional symptoms, particularly fever, anorexia, soft cough, muscle pain, exercise intolerance, and diarrhea, are often reported. There is no specific *clinical sign* on which to base the diagnosis. Classically the combination of an acute infective illness and myocardial abnormalities such as a sudden onset of unexplained ventricular arrhythmia, syncope, episodic weakness, acute congestive heart failure (CHF), anesthetic death, or sudden death may suggest the diagnosis. Thoracic auscultation may disclose evidence of an arrhythmia, a cardiac murmur, or abnormal lung sounds such as crackles.

Electrocardiography may reveal a variety of findings, including persistent sinus tachycardia, ST segment, QT and T wave abnormalities, ventricular or supraventricular ectopy, and atrioventricular (AV) conduction disturbances, including complete AV block (Kaneshige et al., 2007). Although such electrocardiogram (ECG) findings are nonspecific, the ECG has the virtue of drawing attention to the heart and leading to echocardiographic and other investigations.

Radiography may be unremarkable or reflect cardiomegaly, venous congestion, and pulmonary interstitial and alveolar densities suggestive of CHF or pulmonary infection. As with other noninvasive techniques, *echocardiography* may be unremarkable or display nonspecific findings. Diffuse or focal nodular thickening and heterogeneous granular texture of the myocardium caused by cellular infiltrates and pericardial effusion have been observed in association with acute (or fulminant) myocarditis. Segmental or generalized ventricular wall motion abnormalities and hypokinesis have been reported in humans and cats with histologically proven myocarditis. However, such changes may be confused with abnormalities caused by myocardial ischemia or infarction. The most important aspect of echocardiography may be its ability to exclude other types of myocardial and valvular heart diseases.

Laboratory tests, including the analysis of serum cardiac troponin (cTn) concentration, is a promising approach to specifically diagnose acute myocardial injury. Unfortunately blood cTn is not altered consistently in myocarditis, nor is it specific of myocardial inflammation. In addition, the window for diagnosis may be relatively brief. Nevertheless, elevation of serum cTn in association with a strong clinical suspicion may aid in the early presumptive diagnosis of acute myocarditis in which significant myocytolysis and myocardial necrosis may occur (Fig. 177-1). Experimental studies in mice (Smith et al., 1997) and clinical studies in humans (Lauer et al., 1997) with histology-proven myocarditis reported on the high sensitivity of cTn in the diagnosis of acute myocarditis and the close relationship between serum concentrations of cTn and the severity of myocardial inflammation. The value of cTn in the diagnosis of chronic myocarditis is limited. *Serologic testing* for known infectious causes (including toxoplasmosis, borreliosis, rickettsial diseases, bartonellosis, and Chagas' disease) may identify the causative antigen and assist in further treatment plans.

EMB continues to be the most definitive test and gold standard to confirm myocarditis in vivo in humans; but it

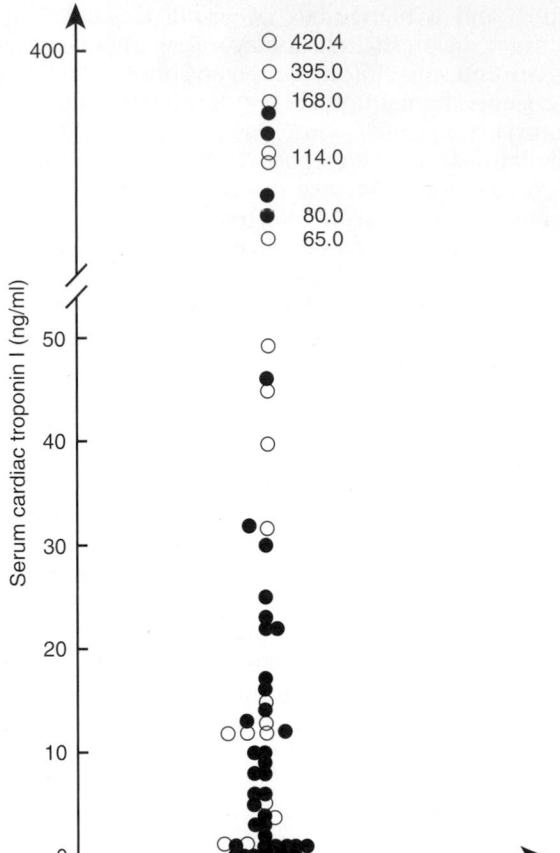

Fig. 177-1 Serum cardiac troponin I (cTnI) concentration in 60 dogs with the clinical diagnosis of acute myocarditis. Diagnostic criteria were the sudden onset of unexplained ventricular or supraventricular ectopy, abnormal diffuse or focal thickening of the left ventricle with granular texture of the myocardium on two-dimensional echocardiography, left ventricular systolic dysfunction with no or only minor chamber dilation, or vegetative endocarditis associated with ventricular tachyarrhythmias. Dogs with known structural heart disease (congenital and acquired), recent trauma, a splenic mass, and gastric dilation-volvulus syndrome were excluded. Open circles represent dogs with acute myocarditis confirmed by histopathology. Zero cTnI refers to the lower limit of detection of the immunoassay used (0.1 ng/ml; OPUS Troponin I, Dade-Behring Diagnostics Inc.). (From the veterinary medical data base of the Department of Small Animal Medicine, University of Leipzig, Germany (unpublished data).)

is used infrequently in small animals because of its invasive nature, limited sampling access, small sample size, relevant interobserver variability in the histologic assessment of the sample, and relatively low diagnostic yield. The diagnosis depends on the presence of inflammatory infiltrates and myocyte degeneration or necrosis. To standardize the histologic diagnosis of myocarditis in human- (and animal)-model EMB specimens, the Dallas criteria were introduced by Aretz and colleagues in 1987. Such criteria distinguish between *active* myocarditis (presence of lymphocytes and myocytolysis), *borderline* or ongoing myocarditis (lymphocytic infiltration and absence of myocytolysis), and *negative* findings (absent lymphocytic infiltrates and myocytolysis). Since EMB does not appear to be a reliable method for making the diagnosis of myocarditis, biopsy is usually reserved

for refractory cases. Interestingly, PCR of tracheal aspirate samples looking for viral RNA has correlated highly with EMB results in humans and seems to be an alternative to EMB in situations in which acute viral myocarditis is suspected.

MANAGEMENT PRINCIPLES

The treatment of myocarditis is controversial, and no generally applicable therapeutic regimen has been established. Supportive care directed toward alleviating clinical signs is the first line of therapy. Specific aims of management are to stabilize cardiac pump function and reduce the risk of progression to heart failure, manage arrhythmias, and identify and remove infectious or toxic agents. There is good evidence from animal work that exercise in the setting of acute myocarditis is detrimental and therefore should be restricted. If an infectious cause can be identified or is suspected, it should be treated aggressively with effective antimicrobials. In patients with symptoms of heart failure, medical therapy should focus on reduction of cardiac load, improvement of ventricular pump function, suppression of exaggerated neuroendocrine activation and arrhythmias, and long-term cardiac protection. Treatment options include diuretics, angiotensin-converting enzyme (ACE) inhibitors, positive inotropes, spironolactone, and β-adrenergic blocking agents once clinical stability has been achieved.

There is evidence from murine models that commonly used drugs for the treatment of CHF may have additional beneficial and more specific effects in acute myocarditis. The following treatments might be useful based on extrapolation from models. ACE inhibitors have been shown to directly decrease the amount of myocardial inflammation. Cytokine activation secondary to the inflammatory process results in the stimulation of nitric oxide synthase and the production of excessive amounts of NO from injured myocytes. This effect may be blunted with the positive inotrope pimobendan (Vetmedin, Boehringer Ingelheim) (0.2 to 0.3 mg/kg orally [PO] q12h) and the calcium channel antagonist amlodipine (Norvasc, Pfizer). In contrast, digitalis may increase the myocardial production of proinflammatory cytokines, induce vascular spasm, worsen myocardial injury, induce arrhythmias, and increase mortality in viral myocarditis. Therefore digoxin should be avoided or only used with extreme caution. β-Blockade may decrease the extent of myocardial damage and improve survival, presumably by relief of coronary vasospasm. Propranolol, sotalol, and carvedilol are preferred because of their nonselectivity. Hemodynamically relevant arrhythmias occur frequently and necessitate antiarrhythmic treatment (see section on Arrhythmogenic Right Ventricular Cardiomyopathy later in the chapter). Arrhythmias are commonly labile in acute myocarditis; and both the type of arrhythmia and the underlying electrophysiologic mechanism may change quickly. In addition, effective doses of antiarrhythmics are difficult to predict in dogs and cats with acute myocarditis and are often substantially different from commonly recommended doses. Occasionally dogs and cats with myocarditis need temporary or permanent cardiac pacing for AV block to achieve hemodynamic stabilization and relief of clinical signs.

A variety of new therapies for myocarditis are available in humans, including antiviral agents and vaccines, immunosuppression, and modulation of the biologic response to inflammation. The specific question for patients with myocarditis is whether regimens designed to reduce or eliminate inflammation can provide clinical benefits compared to conventional heart failure therapy. A number of agents, including nonsteroidal antiinflammatory drugs, intravenous immunoglobulin, methylprednisolone, cyclosporine, azathioprine, antiviral drugs, and anti-TNF, have been used to treat acute myocarditis in humans and experimental animals. However, results of recent randomized, placebo-controlled human trials have failed to demonstrate beneficial effects of immunosuppression. Moreover, nonsteroidal antiinflammatory drugs may be detrimental because they may reduce viral clearance, attribute to an exaggerated cytotoxic response, induce coronary vascular spasm, and delay myocardial repair (and many are toxic to dogs and to cats) (Meune et al., 2003). The future development of effective treatment will depend on early diagnosis and detailed knowledge of the pathogenesis of myocarditis and subsequent immune response.

FELINE MYOCARDITIS AND CARDIOMYOPATHY

The incidence of myocarditis in cats is largely unknown. However, there is some evidence that acute endomyocarditis (EMC) may be of particular importance in the cat. In a series of 461 cats with cardiomyopathy first published by Liu in 1977 and later summarized in his review of cardiomyopathy (Liu, 1985). about 6% were diagnosed with EMC. Affected cats were young, with a mean age of 2.6 years (range 2.5 months to 8 years). Most cats (85%) with acute myocarditis died suddenly. Some cats were dyspneic and depressed and had leukocytosis for 1 to 2 days before death. In another retrospective study considering 1472 feline necropsies performed over a 7-year period, Stalis, Bossbaly, and Van Winkle (1995) reported on 37 (2.5%) cases of EMC and 25 (1.7%) cases of left ventricular endocardial fibrosis. Four (0.3%) cats had histologic evidence of both diseases. Similar to Liu's study, cats with EMC were young (mean age at death 3.4 years, range 6 months to 14 years). Interstitial pneumonia was found in 71% of cats with EMC. Based on such studies it seems that antecedent respiratory infections and stress are potential precursors of EMC in cats and that restrictive cardiomyopathy and left ventricular endocardial fibrosis represent one late sequel to EMC (Stalis et al., 1995). Therapy of EMC in cats is symptomatic, mainly for CHF.

Arrhythmogenic Right Ventricular Cardiomyopathy

Arrhythmogenic right ventricular cardiomyopathy (ARVC), a newly described myocardial disease in cats (Fox et al., 2000), is also characterized by a high incidence of myocarditis reaching 83% of affected cats in a small case series. Of note, the histopathologic changes of ARVC were not confined to the right ventricle. Similar but generally less marked lesions of myocardial injury and repair were also observed in the ventricular septum or the left ventricular free wall of most animals. However, the possible pathogenic role of myocardial inflammation as a potential injury mediator in ARVC is still undetermined. Conventional heart failure therapy with furosemide, enalapril, and nitroglycerin and antiarrhythmic treatment with atenolol, sotalol, or procainamide are recommended. In the near future the use of pimobendan for inotropic support of the failing heart may be an additional treatment option in cats with ARVC and heart failure.

Toxoplasmosis

Toxoplasmosis is a common but largely underappreciated cause of myocarditis in cats. Two case series of *Toxoplasma gondii*–infected cats (Dubey et al., 1993, 1996) revealed myocarditis in 62.7% and 100% of the animals by histopathology. However, there is only one single published report on the antemortem diagnosis of toxoplasmosis in a cat (Simpson et al., 2004). Oral clindamycin (8 mg/kg q8h or 12 mg/kg q12h PO) is the treatment of choice to clear the infection.

Transmissible myocarditis and diaphragmitis (TMD) has been described in cats in northern California. Clinical signs included transient fever, depression, lethargy, and lymphadenopathy (Pedersen et al., 1993). All cats had histology-proven acute myocarditis and diaphragmitis characterized by small pale foci within the myocardium, intramyocardial hemorrhage, myonecrosis, and mononuclear cell infiltrates. A causative organism could not be identified.

MYOCARDITIS IN THE DOG

As with cats, the incidence of myocarditis in the general canine population is unknown. However, very similar to cats, a retrospective necropsy study, including 4638 consecutive dogs seen in the pathology department over a 9-year period at a European Veterinary Teaching Hospital, reported on 70 (1.5%) dogs with the histopathologic diagnosis of myocarditis (Venzin et al., 1990). Dyspnea was the most often encountered clinical sign, and arrhythmias occurred frequently, but sudden cardiac death was rare (4.2%). Inflammatory lesions were found equally distributed between both ventricles. Myocarditis was judged as primary in 33% and secondary in 67% of dogs and was suppurative in 67% of cases. Canine distemper, toxoplasmosis, leptospirosis, and leishmaniosis were the most often determined causes of secondary myocarditis.

Parvovirosis. Parvovirus myocarditis was an extensive problem in young puppies in the late 1970s and early 1980s, when the virus first appeared. Sudden cardiac death or acute death secondary to pulmonary edema was common. Apparently some dogs survived the neonatal infection and developed a disease clinically indistinguishable from DCM. Histopathologic characteristics were myofiber loss, myocytolysis, and lymphocytic and plasmacytic infiltrates (Liu, 1985). Large, basophilic intranuclear inclusion bodies found in the myocardium of acutely infected puppies were pathognomonic findings. No cases of parvovirus-induced myocarditis have been identified in the canine literature since the early 1980s.

Chagas' disease. Chagas' disease is a leading cause of myocarditis and myocardial failure in humans and dogs in Latin America. It is a rare disease in North America and is caused by *T. cruzi*, a hemoflagellate protozoon parasite (see Bonagura, 1995, p 850).

Lyme disease. Lyme carditis is a rare cause of myocardial disease in dogs. It is caused by infection with the spirochete *Borrelia burgdorferi*. Classically AV block, including complete heart block, is seen; but ventricular arrhythmias and myocardial failure occasionally occur. If Lyme carditis is suspected, diagnosis can be confirmed by antibody titers. The efficacy of antibiotic therapy (intravenous penicillin G and tetracycline) in Lyme carditis associated with AV block is not established. Symptomatic dogs with AV block may require temporary or permanent cardiac pacing.

Bartonellosis. Severe multifocal myocarditis and valvular endocarditis secondary to *Bartonella vinsonii* ssp. *berkhoffi* infection has recently been described in dogs. Diagnosis was based on seroreactivity to *B. vinsonii* antigens as determined by immunofluorescent assay testing. Conventional blood cultures generally failed to result in bacterial growth. Treatment with enrofloxacin, doxycycline, and azithromycin should be attempted; however, complete elimination of the infection may be difficult to attain.

Atrial myocarditis. A particular form of cardiomyopathy that preferentially destroys the atrial myocardium has been observed in dogs, most commonly in English springer spaniels. Myocardial destruction is most likely the result of a myocarditis of unknown etiology. Atrial standstill, a nodal escape rhythm, and complete AV block are observed frequently. The atrial cardiomyopathy may be followed by ventricular myocardial failure. Treatment includes permanent cardiac pacing and symptomatic medical therapy, including furosemide, spironolactone, an ACE inhibitor, and pimobendan. Long-term prognosis is poor because CHF or sudden death occurs early.

Arrhythmogenic right ventricular cardiomyopathy. As in cats, ARVC is associated with myocarditis in almost two thirds of cases, frequently affecting both the right and left ventricles. Because myocarditis was conspicuously present in all ARVC dogs with sudden cardiac death in one study (Basso et al., 2004), it is assumed that myocardial inflammation may also play a role in arrhythmogenesis. Therapy with class III antiarrhythmics, preferentially sotalol at 1.5 to 3.5 mg/kg every 12 hours orally, is the preferred treatment option. Alternatively the combination of mexiletine (4-6 mg/kg q8h PO) and sotalol or atenolol (12.5 mg/dog q12h PO) has been used (see Chapter 175). However, evidence is lacking that antiarrhythmic therapy prevents sudden cardiac death in dogs with ARVC. The minority of dogs with ARVC that develop CHF should be treated symptomatically.

References and Suggested Reading

Aretz HT et al. Myocarditis: a histopathological classification, *Am J Cardiovasc Pathol* 1:3, 1987.

Bonagura JD, editor: *Kirk's current veterinary therapy XII (small animal practice)*, Philadelphia, 1995, Saunders.

Dubey JP, Carpenter JL: Histologically confirmed clinical toxoplasmosis in cats: 100 cases (1952-1990), *JAVMA* 1556:2003, 1993.

Dubey JP, Mattix ME, Lipscomb TP: Lesions of neonatally induced toxoplasmosis in cats, *Vet Path* 33:290, 1996.

Feldman AM, McNamara D: Myocarditis, *N Engl J Med* 343:1388, 2000.

Kaneshige T et al: Complete atrioventricular block associated with lymphocytic myocarditis of the atrioventricular node in two young dogs, *J Comp Pathol* 137:146, 2007.

Lauer B et al: Cardiac troponin T in patients with clinically suspected myocarditis, *J Am Coll Cardiol* 30:1354, 1997.

Liu SK: Myocarditis and cardiomyopathy in the dog and cat, *Heart Vessels* 1(suppl):122, 1985.

Meune C et al: Risks versus benefits of NSAIDs, including aspirin in myocarditis: a review of the evidence from animal studies, *Drug Safety* 26:975, 2003.

Smith SC et al: Elevations of cardiac troponin I associated with myocarditis: experimental and clinical correlates, *Circulation* 95:163, 1997.

Stalis H, Bossbaly MJ, Van Winkle TJ: Feline endomyocarditis and left ventricular endocardial fibrosis, *Vet Pathol* 32:122, 1995.

Venzin I, Ossent P, Glardon O: Myocarditis in the dog: Retrospective study on clinical and pathologic findings in 70 cases, *Kleintierpraxis* 35:161, 1990.

CHAPTER 178

Management of Feline Myocardial Disease

VIRGINIA LUIS FUENTES, *Hatfield, Hertfordshire, United Kingdom*

CLASSIFICATION OF MYOCARDIAL DISEASE

Ever since the descriptions of cardiomyopathy in cats in the early 1970s, the management of feline myocardial disease has been complicated by problems in distinguishing the different forms of myocardial disease. Although echocardiography has become the standard for recognition and staging of cardiomyopathy (Table 178-1), often the situation is not straightforward. Using the WHO classification of human cardiomyopathies as a basis for feline myocardial disease, feline cardiomyopathies were originally categorized as hypertrophic, dilated, restrictive, or unclassified, with the subsequent addition of arrhythmogenic right ventricular cardiomyopathy. However, the exact classification of the disease in individual cats has continued to be challenging, particularly since end-stage disease can result in a phenotype that does not fit comfortably in any category except "unclassified."

The problems of a classification with anatomic, functional, and etiologic roots have recently been addressed in a scientific statement by the American Heart Association (Maron et al., 2006). Human cardiomyopathies are now divided into primary (in which the myocardial changes are the major abnormality such as hypertrophic cardiomyopathy) and secondary (in which a multiorgan systemic disease such as hyperthyroidism also affects the myocardium). Primary cardiomyopathies are divided into those with a genetic basis, those with an acquired etiology, or those with a combination of genetic and acquired factors (mixed). Hypertrophic cardiomyopathy (HCM) and arrhythmogenic cardiomyopathy are considered genetic in humans, whereas dilated cardiomyopathy (DCM) and restrictive cardiomyopathy (RCM) are classed as mixed. There is now firm evidence that HCM can be genetic in cats: two separate mutations in myosin-binding protein C have been documented in Maine coons and rag dolls with HCM. There is also evidence that DCM can be acquired in cats with taurine-deficient diets. Nevertheless, in the majority of feline cardiomyopathy cases, we can only guess at the etiology. Cats are also affected with secondary cardiomyopathies such as hyperthyroidism and systemic hypertension, which commonly affect myocardial function.

To add to these difficulties in classification, cats may progress from one phenotype to another. Myocardial infarction can complicate HCM, RCM, or DCM, resulting in regional wall thinning and hypokinesis irrespective of the original left ventricular (LV) morphology.

An end-stage form of HCM has also been described in human and feline patients, characterized by LV hypertrophy with dilation and reduced systolic function. Even on a genetic level, some mutations can be characterized by a DCM or HCM phenotype; thus it is no surprise that some feline patients are difficult to classify.

For those who manage cats with myocardial disease in practical settings, it may be more important to stage the disease in individual cats rather than agonize over the correct classification of the type of cardiomyopathy. Asymptomatic cats with myocardial disease require different management from those with congestive heart failure (CHF). Table 178-2 outlines the use of different therapies according to the stage and type of cardiomyopathy. Specific clinical problems include distinguishing asymptomatic cats with HCM from cats with functional murmurs and distinguishing cats with CHF caused by myocardial disease from those with other causes of respiratory distress.

APPROACH TO THE ASYMPTOMATIC CAT WITH A MURMUR

The prevalence of murmurs in the healthy cat population is high, and many of these murmurs are probably associated with HCM (Côté et al., 2004). However, the finding of a murmur is never an indication for empiric therapy for heart disease. Some cats have low-to-moderate intensity systolic murmurs associated with high cardiac output and adrenergic states associated with anemia, hyperthyroidism, or fever. Other causes of sympathetic activation (stress, drugs) can be associated with a systolic murmur in healthy cats, and the murmur sometimes seems related to a hyperdynamic contraction of the right or left ventricle. Other disorders that may be associated with heart murmurs include systemic hypertension, congenital heart defects, and idiopathic aortic dilation. A significant number of cats have no obvious anatomic or physiologic cause of a heart murmur (functional murmurs).

A good clinical workup considers each of these diagnoses; but once hyperthyroidism and anemia (high cardiac output states) have been ruled out, further diagnostics are usually necessary. A normal cardiac silhouette on radiographs does not rule out cardiomyopathy, but it is a good indication that minimal structural changes are present (i.e., the murmur is functional, or LV hypertrophy is mild). The six-lead electrocardiogram (ECG) probably has relatively good specificity for heart disease, but the sensitivity seems too low since many cats with structural heart

Table 178-1

Two-Dimensional and M-Mode Echocardiographic Characteristics of the Main Feline Cardiomyopathies

	Normal	Hypertrophic Cardiomyopathy	Restrictive Cardiomyopathy	Dilated Cardiomyopathy	Arrhythmogenic Right Ventricular Cardiomyopathy
Left atrial diameter	LA:Ao > 1.6 LAx <16 mm	Normal, ↑, ↑↑	↑↑	↑, ↑↑	Normal
Left ventricular wall thickness	IVSd, LVFWd <6 mm	↑, ↑↑	Normal, ↑, ↓	Normal, ↓	Normal
Left ventricular diameter	LVDd 10-20 mm LVDs 4-12 mm	↓, normal, ↑	Normal	↑, ↑↑	Normal
Right atrial diameter	Similar to LA diameter in right parasternal LAx and left apical views	Normal, ↑	↑, ↑↑	↑, ↑↑	↑, ↑↑, ↑↑↑
Right ventricular diameter	Less than LV diameter in right parasternal LAx and left apical views	Normal	Normal	Normal, ↑	↑↑, ↑↑↑
Systolic Function	FS% 30%-60%	↓, normal, ↑	Normal, ↓	↓↓	Normal
Dynamic LVOT obstruction	No systolic anterior motion, LVOT velocities <2.0m/s	+/−	−	−	−

FS%, LV fractional shortening; *IVSd,* interventricular septal thickness in diastole; *LA,* left atrial; *LA:Ao,* left atrial:aortic diameter in two-dimensional echocardiographic short-axis view; *LAx,* right parasternal long-axis view; *LV,* left ventricular; *LVDd,* LV diameter in diastole; *LVDs,* LV diameter in systole; *LVFWd,* left ventricular free wall thickness in diastole; *LVOT,* LV outflow tract; *RA,* right atrial; *RV,* right ventricular.

disease have a normal ECG. Echocardiography certainly should be recommended if cardiomegaly is identified on radiographs or by analysis of the ECG. The NT-proBNP and NT-proANP assays also offer some promise as initial screening tests for cardiomyopathy (Feline Cardiocare, Veterinary Diagnostics Institute; Vetsign CardioSCREEN, Guildhay) since natriuretic peptide concentrations may be increased in asymptomatic cats with myocardial disease (Connolly et al., 2008), but echocardiography remains the gold standard for diagnosis of cardiomyopathy or exclusion of serious heart disease. The use of a cardiac troponin (cTnI) as a marker of myocardial injury has been suggested in a number of reports; but. as with natriuretic peptides, specific cutoffs for sensitivity and specificity require further study. Some standardization among laboratories and kits is also required if biomarkers are to be used effectively for diagnosis.

Table 178-1 lists a summary of echocardiographic features characteristic of the different types of cardiomyopathies. Echocardiography is useful to document dynamic outflow tract obstruction (LV or right ventricular) and the presence of LV hypertrophy. Echocardiography also can be used to assess risk of CHF, with left atrial (LA) dilation being a useful simple indicator of increased risk for CHF

and thromboembolism and transmitral flow and tissue Doppler imaging contributing to more sophisticated assessments. Although cats with mild asymptomatic disease are unlikely to require treatment, they are still at risk of developing CHF with interventions such as intravenous fluid therapy or anesthesia. It is unusual to diagnose RCM or DCM in asymptomatic cats; they more commonly present with CHF or arterial (aortic) thromboembolism (ATE).

MANAGEMENT OF ASYMPTOMATIC HYPERTROPHIC CARDIOMYOPATHY

Goals of therapy include prevention of CHF, ATE, and sudden cardiac death and the prevention or reversal of myocardial abnormalities, although it is far from clear how to achieve these goals. It may not even be necessary to aspire to these goals in all cats, since the prognosis for life appears very favorable in most cats without any therapy. Other asymptomatic cats clearly are at risk for CHF and ATE. LA enlargement and massive global or segmental LV hypertrophy (as opposed to focal thickening) are sometimes taken as predictors for these risks. However, objective risk factors for development of CHF, ATE, or fatal arrhythmia have not been well defined in prospective studies.

Table **178-2**

Drugs Used for Feline Myocardial Disease

	ASYMPTOMATIC				ACUTE CHF	LOW OUTPUT FAILURE	MILD-MODERATE CHF				REFRACTORY CHF
	HCM*	HOCM*	RCM	DCM	(Any)	(Any)	HCM	RCM	DCM	ARVC	(Any)
Furosemide	–	–	–	–	+	+	+	+	+	+	+
2% Nitroglycerin	–	–	–	–	+	+	–	–	–	–	
ACE inhibitor	±	±	+	+	+	± Care with hypotension	+	+	+	+	+
Atenolol	±	±	–	–	–	–	± Not if CHF still present,* not with diltiazem	–	–	–	–
Diltiazem	±	–	–	–	–	–	± Care with CHF, not with β-blocker	–	–	–	–
Spironolactone	±	±	±	±	–	–	±	±	±	+	+
Thiazide	–	–	–	–	–	–	–	–	–	–	±
Digoxin	–	–	–	±	–	–	–	–	±	–	± Not with HOCM
Pimobendan	–	–	–	±	–	±	–	±-	+	–	± Not with HOCM
Antithrombotic therapy	±	±	±	±	±	±	+	+	+	+	+

*See text for details.

–, Not indicated; ±, no clear indication or indicated in selected cases; +, indicated; *ACE*, angiotensin-converting enzyme; *ARVC*, arrhythmogenic right ventricular cardiomyopathy; *CHF*, congestive heart failure; *DCM*, dilated cardiomyopathy; *HCM*, hypertrophic cardiomyopathy; *HOCM*, hypertrophic obstructive cardiomyopathy; *RCM*, restrictive cardiomyopathy.

Although regression of LV hypertrophy may be a desirable goal, the mechanisms of hypertrophy may be so diverse in different forms of HCM that one common therapeutic strategy may not be capable of achieving this result. Angiotensin-converting enzyme (ACE) inhibitors or angiotensin II antagonists, spironolactone, and statins have all been used successfully in experimental HCM models. However, in one prospective 12-month study of Maine coons with HCM, treatment with the ACE-inhibitor ramipril (0.5 mg/kg q24h orally [PO]) *failed to show any effect* on either LV hypertrophy or diastolic function (MacDonald et al., 2006).

The specific risk of ATE in asymptomatic cats with HCM has not been published. Most clinicians view LA enlargement as a likely risk factor for this complication, and many consider antithrombotic therapy appropriate in HCM cats with this echocardiographic finding. This treatment is discussed in the following paragraphs and in Chapter 180.

DRUG THERAPY CONSIDERATIONS IN ASYMPTOMATIC CATS

Although there might be value in treating asymptomatic HCM cats considered to be at high risk, there is no consensus about which therapy should be used, and there are no published prospective studies demonstrating major end-point benefits of treatment. In situations in which either the owner or cat is reluctant to undertake lifelong medication, treatment remains difficult to justify (particularly if this is a source of daily stress for the patient). β-Adrenergic antagonists (atenolol), calcium channel antagonists (diltiazem), and ACE inhibitors each have their advocates. The use of these drugs in asymptomatic disease is based mostly on theoretic benefit or studies with relatively low-grade clinical evidence.

β-Blockers reduce myocardial oxygen consumption, an effect that should reduce demand ischemia. This benefit, along with slowing heart rate and prolonging diastolic filling, may have some overall benefit on diastolic function in HCM. Atenolol also reduces stress-related dynamic outflow obstruction (see following paragraph). The total daily dose of atenolol is generally 1 to 4 mg/kg daily, with some clinicians using a single dose and others preferring twice-a-day dosing. When twice-daily dosing is prescribed, the two doses may be unequal (e.g., ½ of a 25-mg tablet in the AM and ¼ of a 25-mg tablet in the PM). Liquid atenolol can be easier to dose than tablets. Many clinicians seem to dose atenolol to a heart rate effect (e.g., to achieve a rate of 120 to 160/min during physical examination). Doppler echocardiography can be used to confirm that the dose of atenolol is sufficient to control outflow tract obstruction. Adverse effects of atenolol can include excessive bradycardia and cardiac dilation.

The calcium channel antagonist diltiazem may improve LV relaxation, although definitive evidence of this effect in cats is lacking. Diltiazem also slows heart rate and reduces dynamic outflow obstruction, although less consistently than atenolol. Standard diltiazem is dosed at 7.5 mg every 8 hours orally, which is impractical for most cat owners. Extended-release preparations of diltiazem permit once– or twice–daily dosing using preparations such as Dilacor XR (Watson Pharma, Inc.) at 15 to 30 mg every 12 to 24 hours orally. These long-acting diltiazem compounds can achieve therapeutic plasma levels; however, precise dosing guidelines are still needed for these drugs. Adverse effects of diltiazem include anorexia, weight loss, and skin lesions, with an overall incidence of side effects seemingly higher than with atenolol or ACE inhibitors.

Although ACE inhibitors have theoretic benefits in cardiomyopathy, there are no data supporting their use in asymptomatic cats. As cited previously, well-controlled studies in asymptomatic Maine coon cats have failed to show benefit of the ACE inhibition. However, I do consider an ACE-inhibitor for treatment of asymptomatic cats demonstrating LA enlargement. In theory vasodilation might worsen dynamic LV outflow tract (LVOT) obstruction unless a β-blocker or calcium channel blocker is also prescribed; however, the practical importance of this in cats is undetermined.

HYPERTROPHIC CARDIOMYOPATHY WITH DYNAMIC LEFT VENTRICULAR OUTFLOW TRACT OBSTRUCTION

In human HCM patients LVOT obstruction is associated with increased risk of heart failure and death (Maron et al., 2003). Control of LVOT obstruction is usually instigated when patients become symptomatic. In cats there is some controversy over the clinical significance of dynamic LVOT obstruction. One retrospective feline study suggested that systolic anterior motion of the mitral valve was associated with longer survival times (Rush et al., 2002). It is often possible to control dynamic LVOT obstruction with β-blockers in cats, and anecdotal evidence suggests that some apparently asymptomatic cats show an improvement in exercise tolerance or energy levels following administration of β-blockers. It is possible that symptomatic cats are more difficult to identify than symptomatic humans, particularly since human symptoms include signs such as chest pain. Cats with severe dynamic LVOT obstruction may be treated with atenolol and reexamined within the first month of treatment to confirm that LVOT obstruction has been controlled and no adverse effects have developed (such as bradycardia or an increase in LA size). The dose of atenolol can be titrated to a point at which the LVOT gradient has resolved (and the murmur has diminished or disappeared) without causing severe bradycardia.

SYMPTOMATIC CATS WITH CONGESTIVE HEART FAILURE: CLINICAL APPROACH

Physical examination findings that might arouse suspicion of myocardial disease with CHF include combinations of a systolic murmur, gallop sounds or arrhythmias with tachypnea, pulmonary crackles, and jugular distention. Sometimes no auscultatory abnormalities are present, although respiration is generally labored in inspiration and often in expiration. A prolonged inspiratory phase with noise should prompt consideration of upper airway obstruction. Prolonged expiratory efforts, especially with wheezing, are more suggestive of asthma or a fixed major airway obstruction. Crackles are a helpful finding for parenchymal disease but are not always evident. Muffled sounds ventrally may suggest pleural effusion or lung consolidation.

Imaging is critical to diagnosis. Radiography can be helpful for documenting pulmonary infiltrates or pleural effusion associated with CHF and excluding other causes of respiratory distress, although great care should always be taken when handling dyspneic cats. Sedation (butorphanololbutorphanolol 0.1 mg/kg intramuscularly [IM], repeated to 0.3 mg/kg cumulative dose) may allow safer handling in stressed feline patients. These cats are very fragile, and thoracic ultrasound may offer a safer option for identifying pleural effusions in particular and perhaps the "comet tail artifacts" often related to pulmonary infiltration or edema.

Echocardiography is the only practical way of identifying the underlying structural and functional abnormality of the heart, and demonstration of LA enlargement can be extremely useful as a means of supporting a clinical suspicion of CHF. A full echocardiographic examination can always be delayed until the cat is more stable because characterization of the underlying myocardial disease is not crucial for initial management.

Additional diagnostic study should be accomplished as permitted by the clinical situation. Blood pressure should be measured. Routine laboratory tests (complete blood count, serum biochemistries), cytologic examination of effusions, and biomarker studies (troponin, natriuretic peptides) generally are indicated but may need to be delayed pending initial stabilization.

The differential diagnosis of CHF in cats includes other causes of respiratory distress, pulmonary infiltration, pleural effusion, or airway obstruction. Acute pulmonary infiltration with tachypnea can be associated with thoracic trauma, overinfusion of crystalloid, noncardiogenic pulmonary edema (see Chapter 150); severe pulmonary infections; lung parasitism (see Chapter 151); or spontaneous heartworm death (see Chapter 182). The two most common types of pleural effusions identified in cats with CHF are the modified transudate (with small lymphocytes in the cytology) and true chylothorax related to obstruction of systemic venous and lymphatic return. The differential diagnosis of pleural effusion is extensive and is considered in Chapter 153. Bronchial asthma in cats can be associated with acute dyspnea but is readily distinguished from CHF by examination and radiography (see Chapter 148). Uncommonly cats with dyspnea are found to have major airway obstruction related to nasopharyngeal polyps (see Chapter 142 and Section VII on Evolve), laryngeal paresis (see Chapter 143), or tracheal obstruction.

MANAGEMENT OF THE SYMPTOMATIC CAT WITH CONGESTIVE HEART FAILURE

Short-term goals of therapy in cats with CHF include relieving life-threatening hypoxemia, lowering LA pressures, and improving hemodynamic function; improving hemodynamic function is particularly difficult in cats with diastolic dysfunction.

ACUTE CONGESTIVE HEART FAILURE

Fortunately the type of myocardial disease has less bearing on management than the stage of presentation. Oxygen, diuresis, and venodilation are all appropriate treatments for any cat with left heart failure. Pleural effusions must be drained if they cause respiratory distress, and this can be achieved with a 23-G butterfly cannula. Furosemide is the mainstay of treatment for cats presenting with acute pulmonary edema. Doses should be lower than those used in dogs, but some cats still require aggressive diuresis. For unresponsive cases intravenous furosemide at doses of 1 to 2 mg/kg can be repeated every 1 to 2 hours initially; but renal function, electrolytes, and blood pressure must be monitored. A constant-rate infusion of furosemide also can be considered (see Chapter 171). Topical 2% nitroglycerin cream (1/4 to 1/2 inch q8h) can be added for its potential venodilatory effect. Severely dyspneic cats must be handled with care, and stress should be avoided at all costs. Some cats benefit from low doses of butorphanol (0.1 mg/kg, repeated as needed) as sedation. Although ACE inhibitors may have some favorable venodilating effects, great caution should be used in cats with hypotension; and these agents are best avoided until systemic arterial pressures are at least 90 mm Hg.

LOW-OUTPUT HEART FAILURE

Some cats develop low output signs in addition to CHF. These cats typically present with hypothermia, bradycardia, and severe hypotension (systolic blood pressure <70 mm Hg). Although this is more common in RCM and DCM, some HCM cats may also present in this way, possibly related to acute ischemic events or myocardial infarctions. Traditionally positive inotropes are considered to be contraindicated in HCM because of the likelihood of increasing myocardial oxygen consumption. However, despite this admonition, dobutamine appears to be very effective in improving cardiac output and clinical signs in low-output cats irrespective of the type of underlying cardiomyopathy. Doses should be started at lower ranges than those used for dogs, with initial infusion rates of 1 to 2 mcg/kg/minute cautiously titrated upwards (to a maximum of 5 mcg/kg/min) over several hours. The therapeutic targets are improvements in systolic blood pressure to higher than 100 mm Hg, increase in heart rate, and normal body temperature, at which point the infusion can be maintained for 12 to 24 hours. Some cats show signs of nausea or restlessness with relatively low doses, and infusions exceeding 24 hours are rarely needed; the risk of seizures become higher after 24 hours. Although dynamic LVOT obstruction is a definite contraindication to dobutamine, it is rarely evident during these low-output episodes, even in cats with HCM. Absence of a murmur makes LVOT obstruction especially unlikely. Warmth and supportive care are important; and, in the rare cases in which low output signs are present in the absence of CHF, it may even be necessary to consider cautious intravenous fluid therapy with low–sodium containing fluids.

HOME MANAGEMENT OF CONGESTIVE HEART FAILURE

Long-term goals of therapy include prevention of abnormal sodium and water retention, modulation of adverse neurohormonal activation, delay or reversal of myocardial changes, and prevention of thromboembolism. The first two goals may be achievable with oral furosemide and an ACE inhibitor alone in many cats. Furosemide should be titrated to effect (usually 1 to 3 mg/kg q8 to 24h PO), to achieve resolution of pulmonary edema and pleural effusions. Once congestive signs have resolved, the furosemide dose should be reduced as far as possible. Some cats suffer an acute episode of pulmonary edema but, once stable, remain well compensated for long periods with minimal doses of furosemide (and furosemide may even be withdrawn in a few cats). In hypotensive cats ACE inhibitors should be introduced cautiously, at quarter or half dose. Such cats often tolerate the full dose of ACE inhibitor in the long term but are vulnerable to worsening hypotension and azotemia following acute administration. ACE inhibitors do not appear to have an adverse effect on dynamic LVOT obstruction (Oyama, 2003) and should counteract adverse renin-angiotensin system (RAS) activation triggered by concurrent furosemide administration. There is no clear advantage of one ACE inhibitor over another; enalapril (0.25 to 0.5 mg/kg q24h PO), benazepril (0.25 to 0.5 mg/kg q24h PO), and ramipril (0.5 mg/kg q24h PO) all have been used. The individual types of cardiomyopathies may benefit from tailored therapy specific to the underlying functional disturbance.

Hypertrophic Cardiomyopathy

Asymptomatic cats *already receiving* diltiazem or atenolol can be treated with furosemide and an ACE inhibitor as listed previously in addition to the therapy they are already receiving. In some cases congestive signs may be easier to control if the β-blocker is withdrawn or at least reduced by 50%. Therapy with β-blockers should *never be started* while cats have any signs of CHF and are probably only indicated in cats with well-compensated HCM with obstruction. Spironolactone might have several theoretic benefits in cats with HCM and CHF since it has resulted in regression of LV hypertrophy in other HCM models and also helps to counteract RAS activation. However, spironolactone did not reduce fibrosis in a model of spontaneous feline cardiomyopathy, and a significant percentage of cats developed skin lesions with chronic administration (MacDonald et al., 2007). Overall spironolactone appears to be well tolerated and can be given as 1/4 of a 25-mg tablet per cat every 24 hours.

Dilated Cardiomyopathy

Oral taurine (250 mg q12h) should be given to cats with global systolic dysfunction until plasma taurine concentration results are available. Genuinely taurine-deficient cats are now rare, but they have a good prognosis with taurine supplementation. Cats with idiopathic DCM are unlikely to show any response to taurine supplementation and have a much poorer prognosis. Digoxin traditionally has been give to cats with systolic dysfunction, but dosing can be problematic. Generally 1/4 of a 0.125-mg tablet is given every 48 hours for cats weighing less than 3 kg; every 24 to 48 hours for cats weighing 3 to 6 kg; and every 24 hours for cats over 6 kg. Toxicity is common, and the hemodynamic benefits are not dramatic. The effects of pimobendan have not been studied in cats, but there are anecdotal reports of benefit in cats with systolic dysfunction using extralabel pimobendan (Vetmedin) at oral doses of 0.625 mg to 1.25 mg per cat every 12 hours orally.

Restrictive Cardiomyopathy

There is little in the way of specific therapy for either the myocardial or endomyocardial forms of RCM. Furosemide and an ACE inhibitor are standard therapy, but these cats are quite likely to become refractory to treatment and require additional diuretics (see following paragraph).

MANAGEMENT OF RECURRENT OR REFRACTORY CONGESTIVE HEART FAILURE

Furosemide can be titrated up or down to effect, but some cats have recurrent or persistent congestive signs. In the cat with progressive fluid accumulation it is reasonable to introduce spironolactone as an additional diuretic and neurohormonal modulator. Cats that become truly refractory to furosemide tend to lack both the beneficial and the adverse effects of furosemide such as azotemia. In these cases the dosage of furosemide and ACE inhibitors can be increased, or clients (if accepting) can be given preloaded syringes with furosemide (1 mg/kg) that can be administered subcutaneously two or three times weekly. An alternative is addition of a thiazide diuretic such as hydrochlorothiazide (1 to 2 mg/kg q12 to 24h PO). This should be started without subtracting any of the prior therapy. Thiazides should be added at the lowest end of the dosage range and titrated up to effect with careful monitoring of renal function and serum electrolytes. Extralabel use of pimobendan (0.625 to 1.25 mg twice daily) is also potentially beneficial for these cats. Many cats with CHF can tolerate between 0.25 and 0.5 mg/kg of enalapril or benazepril twice daily, and this may be another consideration. Periodic thoracocentesis or a brief hospitalization and parenteral diuresis may be needed for decompensation associated with marked dyspnea.

PROGNOSIS

There have been no prospective, multicenter, randomized trials of drug therapy of cats with CHF; and published data, although instructive, do not compare specific treatment approaches or correct for client perceptions that may prompt euthanasia. Perhaps surprisingly to some, a 1-year or longer survival is not uncommon for a cat following the first bout of CHF provided there is good initial therapy, excellent home therapy, continuing veterinary support, and a willing owner. Many cats can tolerate small-to-moderate amounts of pleural fluid as long as they are not stressed; and clients can be taught to monitor respiratory rate and depth, activity, appetite, and attitude as markers of quality of life and control of CHF. Ultimately the combination of progressive CHF and advanced kidney failure tends to limit the success of these therapies. Other cases are complicated by ATE or sudden death.

ARTERIAL (AORTIC) THROMBOEMBOLISM

Cats with all forms of cardiomyopathy are at risk of ATE and this is particularly true of the more advanced stages of myocardial disease. Some cats present with an episode of ATE as their first sign of myocardial disease. Typically these cats have sudden onset signs of pain, vocalizing, and paresis when the aortic trifurcation is affected. Forelimbs can also be affected, sometimes with quick spontaneous recovery. Clinical signs may be more confusing with cerebral, mesenteric, or coronary embolism.

MANAGEMENT OF ACUTE THROMBOEMBOLISM

Affected cats are acutely distressed, and pain management is paramount. Epidural anesthesia is an ideal solution; otherwise opiates are necessary. Hypothermia is a poor prognostic sign and may be helpful in triaging which patients to treat. It can be difficult to distinguish tachypnea from pain versus CHF without radiography, and some cats die acutely in the first 24 hours from sudden hyperkalemia associated with reperfusion. There is still controversy over the risk-benefit ratio of thrombolytic therapy, and most clinicians opt for prevention of thrombus extension. Aspirin, unfractionated heparin (100 to 500 units/kg as an initial dose intravenously [IV]), and low–molecular weight heparin are all used. Supportive care is important, and confirmed concurrent congestive signs should be treated as described earlier. Management and prevention of ATE are discussed in Chapter 180.

PREVENTION OF THROMBOEMBOLISM

There is no consensus on the optimal therapy for prevention of aortic thromboembolism. Aspirin has been used for many years with a relatively low rate of side effects. Its efficacy has not been established, and a low-dose compounded dose (5 mg/cat q3d) does not appear any less effective than a higher dose (81 mg/cat q3d) based on retrospective analysis. Lower dosages do appear to have a lower rate of side effects (often related to gastrointestinal ulceration). Warfarin is associated with an unacceptable rate of side effects and an impractically high level of monitoring requirements. Pimobendan is also said to have antithrombotic effects, which may be pertinent to cats receiving this drug for CHF therapy.

Clopidogrel (Plavix, 18.75 mg/cat q24h orally) offers some hope as a new antithrombotic treatment and is currently under evaluation (FATCAT trial). Clopidogrel shows in vitro inhibition of feline platelets and seems to be well tolerated, although ulceration is still a potential concern. Clopidogrel can be combined with aspirin, although it is probably safest to use the lowest aspirin dose (5 mg q3d) and to have clients monitor appetite as a marker of gastrointestinal side effects.

References and Suggested Reading

Connolly DJ et al: Circulating natriuretic peptides in cats with heart disease, *J Vet Intern Med* 22:946, 2008.

Côté E et al: Assessment of the prevalence of heart murmurs in overtly healthy cats, *J Am Vet Med Assoc* 225:384, 2004.

Fox PR: Feline cardiomyopathies. In Fox PR, Sisson D, Moise NS, editors: *Textbook of canine and feline cardiology, principles and clinical practice*, ed 2, Philadelphia, 1999, Saunders, p 621.

Fox PR: Endomyocardial fibrosis and restrictive cardiomyopathy: pathologic and clinical features, *J Vet Cardiol* 6:25, 2004.

MacDonald KA et al: The effect of ramipril on left ventricular mass, myocardial fibrosis, diastolic function, and plasma neurohormones in Maine coon cats with familial hypertrophic cardiomyopathy without heart failure, *J Vet Intern Med* 20:1093, 2006.

MacDonald KA et al: Effect of spironolactone on diastolic function and left ventricular mass in Maine coon cats with familial hypertrophic cardiomyopathy, *J Vet Intern Med* 21:611, 2007.

Maron BJ et al: American College of Cardiology/European Society of Cardiology clinical expert consensus document on hypertrophic cardiomyopathy, *J Am Coll Cardiol* 42:1687, 2003.

Maron BJ et al: Contemporary definitions and classification of the cardiomyopathies: an American Heart Association scientific statement, *Circulation* 113:1807, 2006.

Oyama MA et al: Effect of ACE-inhibition on dynamic left-ventricular obstruction in cats with hypertrophic obstructive cardiomyopathy, *J Vet Intern Med* 17:2003.

Rush JE et al: Population and survival characteristics of cats with hypertrophic cardiomyopathy: 260 cases (1990-1999), *J Am Vet Med Assoc* 220:202, 2002.

CHAPTER **179**

Right Ventricular Cardiomyopathy in Cats

PHILIP R. FOX, *New York, New York*

OVERVIEW OF MYOCARDIAL DISEASE

Heart disease in the cat is caused principally by conditions that affect the myocardium. Cardiomyopathy describes a heterogeneous class of disorders, the dominant features of which are structural abnormality and functional impairment of the heart muscle (Fox, 1999). This excludes conditions resulting from valvular, hypertensive, vascular, pericardial, pulmonary, or congenital derangements. A variety of schemes have been proposed to define the cardiomyopathies. The term *idiopathic* (primary) cardiomyopathy has been applied classically to describe the myocardium as the sole source of heart disease when etiology cannot be identified; whereas *secondary* cardiomyopathy denotes heart muscle disease resulting from an identifiable systemic, metabolic, or nutritional disorder. This original classification has been expanded by The World Health Organization/International Society and Federation of Cardiology Task Force to include four types of idiopathic heart muscle disease (Richardson et al., 1996): hypertrophic, dilated, restrictive, and arrhythmogenic right ventricular cardiomyopathy (ARVC). Advancements in echocardiography and the increasing affordability of this technology have increased clinical diagnostic reliability and awareness of these conditions.

INCIDENCE

Of the four types of idiopathic heart muscle disease in the cat, ARVC is the least common (Fox, 1999). In my cardiovascular clinic the prevalence of ARVC in cats examined by echocardiography is approximately 2% to 4%. Although still underrecognized, diagnosis of this disorder can be improved by rigorous application of diagnostic testing and appropriate clinical awareness.

ETIOLOGY AND PATHOGENESIS

ARVC has been described in dogs (Basso et al., 2004), humans (Nava, Rossi, and Thiene, 1997; Basso et al., 1996), and cats (Fox et al., 2000). Etiology and pathogenesis remain unresolved. Ventricular arrhythmias and ARVC are inherited as an autosomal-dominant trait in boxer dogs (Meurs et al., 1999). In humans autosomal-dominant familial transmission has been reported, with a mutation identified at the cardiac ryanodine receptor 2 gene (Ryr2) in ARVC type 2 (Tisso et al., 2001; Rampazzo et al., 1994). In addition, autosomal-dominant and autosomal-recessive forms of human ARVC have been related to mutations in desmoplakin. Abnormalities in genes encoding for cell junctional proteins, including plakoglobin, desmoplakin, and plakophilin, are the focus of increasing attention (Sen-Chowdhry, Syrris, and McKenna, 2005; Gerull et al., 2004). Because desmosomes (organized intercellular junctions) lend cells mechanical integrity and stability, impaired function of cell adhesion junctions during shear stress may promote inflammation, myocyte detachment, myocyte death, and fibrolipomatous repair (Thiene et al., 2005). Therefore ARVC increasingly has been considered to be a disease of the desmosome. Although I have noted familial tendencies of ARVC in cats, pedigree analysis is currently lacking. Neither the specific gene defects nor the defective coded proteins have been identified to date.

PATHOPHYSIOLOGY

Progressive atrophy of the right ventricular (RV) myocardium with fibrous and/or fatty replacement are common sequelae of ARVC in cats (Fox et al., 2000), dogs (Basso et al., 2004), and humans (Basso and Thiene, 2005). Gap junction remodeling secondary to altered mechanical coupling may promote arrhythmogenicity (Thienne et al., 2005). Abnormal myocardial structure and function are accelerated by myocarditis, programmed cell death, and fibrous and fatty infiltrates. Apoptosis is present in a high percentage of felines with ARVC (Fox et al., 2004), similar to that reported in humans (Valente M et al., 1998) and dogs (Basso et al., 2004). Both apoptosis and myocarditis in affected cats may contribute to myocyte injury and repair in susceptible felines. Atrophy of RV myocardium with fibrofatty replacement reduces cardiac reserve and provokes right-sided congestive heart failure (CHF). RV dilation and remodeling alter the geometry and function of the tricuspid valve apparatus and result in tricuspid valve insufficiency. The histopathologic changes of ARVC are not confined to the right ventricle, and similar but less marked lesions of myocardial injury and repair may be present in the ventricular septum or left ventricular (LV) free wall. This suggests that the ARVC disease process may progress over time to involve the left ventricle (Basso et al., 1996; Corrado et al., 1997).

SIGNALMENT

Right-sided heart failure is most frequently detected in middle-aged cats, although affected cats range in age from 1 to 20 years old. Currently there has been no documented gender predisposition. ARVC has been documented in many breeds; I have identified this condition most commonly in domestic shorthair and Birman cats.

CLINICAL PRESENTATION

Frequently the first clinical presentation is for CHF. Affected cats may show tachypnea, jugular venous distention, effusion (pericardial, thoracic, abdominal), or hepatosplenomegaly. Right-sided heart failure is usually severe. Syncope has been documented with sustained ventricular tachycardia, but this finding is uncommon. Many cats are asymptomatic, and diagnosis is made during echocardiographic examination performed to assess a heart murmur or arrhythmia.

PHYSICAL EXAMINATION

Thoracic auscultation usually reveals a pansystolic heart murmur consistent with tricuspid regurgitation. This is often loudest along the right sternal or right costochondral border. Arrhythmias and associated femoral arterial pulse deficits may be detected. With right-sided heart failure affected cats may be tachypneic or dyspneic. Many of these animals have distended jugular veins, and some also have ascites and hepatosplenomegaly. The presence of pleural and pericardial effusion may cause heart and lung sounds to be muffled.

RADIOGRAPHY

Classic findings include enlargement of the right atrium and right ventricle. Often these changes are dramatic. Left atrial enlargement may be present in some cats. In cases with right-sided heart failure pleural effusion, ascites, hepatosplenomegaly, and cardiomegaly (often augmented by the associated pericardial effusion) may be present.

ELECTROCARDIOGRAPHY

A variety of arrhythmias have been documented, including supraventricular tachyarrhythmias (particularly atrial fibrillation); complex ventricular ectopy, including ventricular tachycardia (of RV and LV origin); and major conduction abnormalities. Ventricular tachycardia can be sustained in some cases. The frequency of atrial fibrillation is consistent with severe right atrial (RA) enlargement.

ECHOCARDIOGRAPHY

The most obvious echocardiographic finding is marked RV enlargement (Fig. 179-1). Abnormal RV muscular trabecular patterns (particularly in the apical cavity) are often a characteristic finding when coupled with RV dilation. Additional right heart changes include RA enlargement, paradoxic ventricular septal motion, and localized RV aneurysm formation (i.e., akinetic or dyskinetic areas with diastolic outward bulging) in the apical or subtricuspid region. Ventricular septal and LV wall thickness at end-diastole, LV end-diastolic and end-systolic cavity dimensions, and percent fractional shortening (in the absence of paradoxic septal motion) are generally within normal ranges. In some cats left atrial enlargement may be present. Doppler color flow imaging invariably demonstrates tricuspid regurgitation.

MAGNETIC RESONANCE IMAGING

Magnetic resonance imaging using T1 weighted images has demonstrated morphologic evidence of RV fatty infiltration in formalin-fixed ARVC hearts. When available, this technique may facilitate antemortem diagnosis.

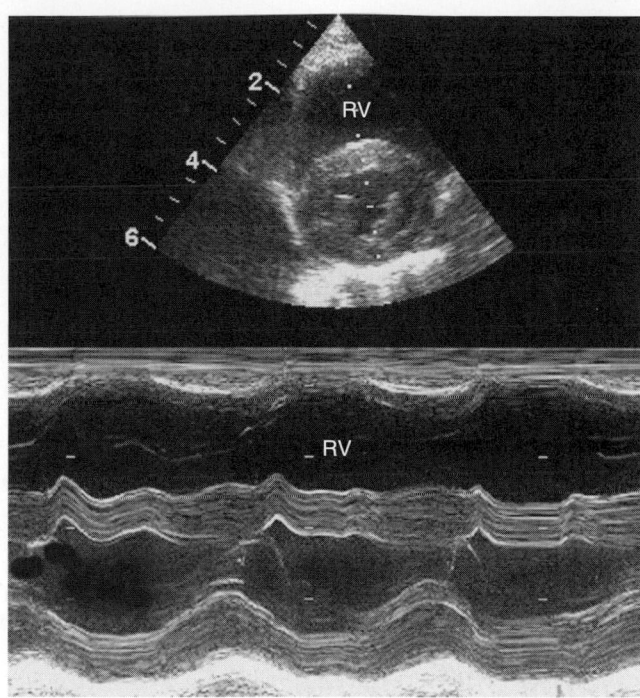

Fig. 179-1 Echocardiograms from a cat with arrhythmogenic right ventricular cardiomyopathy. The right ventricle is severely dilated. *RV,* Right ventricle.

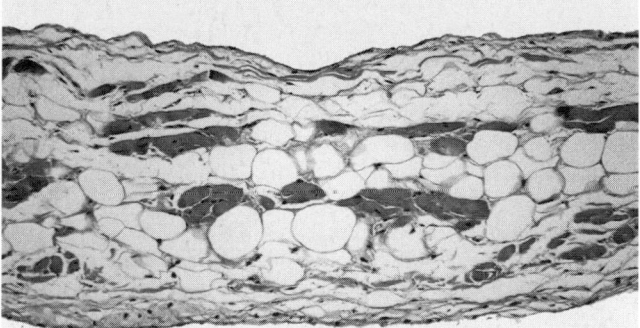

Fig. 179-2 Histologic section taken from a region of thinned, right ventricular wall in a cat with arrhythmogenic right ventricular cardiomyopathy. Myocardium is replaced by fatty tissue. Islands of residual myocytes are surrounded by adipocytes. (H&E stain, × 200.)

GROSS PATHOLOGY

Morphologic abnormalities are striking in feline ARVC (Fox et al., 2000). Typical findings include moderate-to-severe RV dilation; RV wall thinning (diffuse or segmental); flattened appearance of RV wall trabeculae; and prominent RV septo-parietal bands in the RV apex. Aneurysms in apical, subtricuspid, and infundibular regions of the RV wall may be small or extensive and appear translucent. Right atrial cavity dilation generally is present and severe, and segments of RA walls are markedly thinned. Mural thrombosis is observed occasionally in the right ventricle or left artery.

HISTOPATHOLOGY

The hallmark histopathologic feature of ARVC is partial or almost entire replacement of the RV free wall by fatty (25% of cases) or fibrofatty (75% of cases) tissue (Fox et al., 2000). These lesions closely resemble those characteristic of ARVC in humans and dogs. The fibrofatty pattern consists of focal or diffuse RV myocardial atrophy associated with adipose tissue and replacement-type fibrosis. The fatty pattern within the RV wall and trabeculae is characterized by multifocal or diffuse areas of adipose cell infiltration with only scant interstitial fibrosis (Fig. 179-2). Islands of myocytes are often surrounded by fat or fibrofatty tissue. In both forms residual surviving myocytes are usually scattered within the areas of fibrosis or fat, and fibro-fatty replacement usually extends from the epicardium toward the endocardium. Focal or multifocal RV myocarditis is most prevalent in ARVC cats with the fibrofatty pattern. It consists mostly of T lymphocytes associated with myocyte cell death and mild-to-severe fibrous tissue deposition. Similar findings may also be present in left and RA walls, the LV free wall, and the ventricular septum. Fatty infiltration is present occasionally in the LV free wall but not in the ventricular septum. Abnormal intramural small vessels with thickened walls (caused primarily by medial hypertrophy) are uncommon. Apoptotic myocytes have been identified by terminal dUTP nick-end labeling (TUNEL) histochemical investigation in 75% of affected cats.

DIFFERENTIAL DIAGNOSIS

Radiographic and echo-Doppler examinations provide a reliable assessment of cardiac structure and function and help differentiate other forms of heart disease, such as atrial septal defect. Feline ARVC is characterized by severe RV and RA dilation, and tricuspid valvular regurgitation is usually present. Consequently ARVC is invariably misdiagnosed as tricuspid valvular dysplasia. Congenital tricuspid valvular dysplasia, when severe, is usually apparent in the very young cat but rarely results in profound RV enlargement as occurs in ARVC. Also, tricuspid valve dysplasia is characterized by marked dysplasia of the tricuspid valve apparatus, including direct attachment of valve leaflets to papillary muscles and papillary muscle or valve leaflet fusion. These lesions are generally discernible by two-dimensional echocardiography. Other causes of RV dilation in the cat can be differentiated by careful echo-Doppler examination. RV enlargement can be present with pulmonic stenosis, tetralogy of Fallot or other causes of cyanotic heart disease, or pulmonary hypertension. However, such cases also have RV hypertrophy with other specific lesions. Because the left ventricle is generally unremarkable in ARVC cats, this condition cannot be confused with hypertrophic cardiomyopathy or endomyocardial fibrosis, two diseases characterized by distinctive LV alteration. Moreover, most cases of restrictive cardiomyopathy do not have the severe right heart dilation and RV wall thinning that typifies ARVC.

THERAPY

With right-sided CHF dyspnea may result from effusions, and prompt mechanical fluid removal (centesis) is indicated in such circumstances. Standard pharmacologic therapy for CHF includes diuretics, angiotensin-converting enzyme (ACE) inhibitors, and digoxin. Furosemide (2 to 6 mg/kg/day) and spironolactone (¼ to ½ of a 25-mg tablet daily), are administered. Hydrochlorothiazide (1/4 of a 25-mg tablet daily) may be added in refractory cases. When multiple diuretics are administered, close monitoring of serum blood urea nitrogen (BUN) creatinine, and electrolytes is advocated. An ACE inhibitor (enalapril, 0.5 mg/kg daily) is also given. Digoxin (¼ of a 0.125-mg tablet daily or every other day) may be added when the animal appears stable. Because of renal clearance of digoxin, BUN/creatinine should be monitored. Unresponsive CHF may improve with extralabel administration of pimobendan (0.25 mg/kg orally [PO] q12h). Symptomatic ventricular tachycardia is treated with lidocaine HCl (0.25 to 1 mg/kg intravenously [IV] given over 2 minutes or in 1-mg boluses [up to a total of 4 mg for an average-sized cat]). Esmolol (150 to 500 mcg/kg IV bolus or 100 to 300 mcg/kg/min constant-rate infusion) may be added in refractory circumstances with careful blood pressure monitoring. For long-term management of ventricular tachycardia, sotalol (10 to 20 mg q12-24h PO) has been used safely, although efficacy has not been demonstrated. Sequential echocardiograms, thoracic radiographs, and electrocardiograms may assist long-term monitoring.

PROGNOSIS

Generally the treatment of cats with right-sided heart failure has been unrewarding. Heart failure is generally progressive and becomes unresponsive in most cases. Conversely, some affected cats may never become clinically affected. This condition appears to be familial in some breeds. Therefore screening echocardiograms are recommended for siblings of affected animals.

References and Suggested Reading

Basso C, Thiene G: Adipositas cordis, fatty infiltration of the right ventricle, and arrhythmogenic right ventricular cardiomyopathy: just a matter of fat? *Cardiovasc Pathol* 14:37, 2005.

Basso C et al: Arrhythmogenic right ventricular cardiomyopathy: dysplasia, dystrophy, or myocarditis? *Circulation* 94:983, 1996.

Basso C et al: Arrhythmogenic right ventricular cardiomyopathy causing sudden cardiac death in boxer dogs: a new animal model of human disease, *Circulation* 109:1180, 2004.

Corrado D et al: Spectrum of clinicopathologic manifestations of arrhythmogenic right ventricular cardiomyopathy/dysplasia: a multicenter study, *J Am Coll Cardiol* 30:1512, 1997.

Fox PR: Feline cardiomyopathies. In Fox PR, Sisson DD, Moise NS, editors: *Textbook of canine and feline cardiomyopathy principles and clinical practice*, ed 2, Philadelphia, 1999, Saunders, p 621.

Fox PR et al: Spontaneous occurrence of arrhythmogenic right ventricular cardiomyopathy in the domestic cat: a new animal model of human disease, *Circulation* 102:1863, 2000.

Gerull B et al: Mutations in the desmosomal protein plakophilin-2 are common in arrhythmogenic right ventricular cardiomyopathy, *Nat Genet* 36:1162, 2004.

Meurs KM et al: Familial ventricular arrhythmias in boxers, *J Vet Intern Med* 13:437, 1999.

Nava A, Rossi L, Thiene G, editors: *Arrhythmogenic right ventricular cardiomyopathy/dysplasia*, Amsterdam, 1997, Elsevier.

Richardson P et al: Report of the 1995 World Health Organization/International Society and Federation of Cardiology Task Force on the Definition and Classification of cardiomyopathies, *Circulation* 93:841, 1996.

Rampazzo A et al: The gene for arrhythmogenic right ventricular cardiomyopathy maps to chromosome 14q23, *Hum Mol Genet* 3:959, 1994.

Sen-Chowdhry S, Syrris P, McKenna WJ: Genetics of right ventricular cardiomyopathy, *J Cardiovasc Electrophysiol* 16:927, 2005.

Thiene G et al: Twenty years of progress and beckoning frontiers in cardiovascular pathology cardiomyopathies, *Cardiovasc Pathol* 14:165, 2005.

Tisso N et al: Identification of mutations in the cardiac ryanodine receptor gene in families affected with arrhythmogenic right ventricular cardiomyopathy type 2 (ARVD2), *Hum Mol Genet* 10:189, 2001.

Valente M et al: In vivo evidence of apoptosis in arrhythmogenic right ventricular cardiomyopathy, *Am J Pathol* 152:479, 1998.

CHAPTER 180

Arterial Thromboembolism in Cats

ANTHONY H. TOBIAS, *St. Paul, Minnesota*
DEBORAH M. FINE, *Columbia, Missouri*

Arterial thromboembolism (ATE) in cats most frequently occurs when a thrombus that develops within the left atrium embolizes a remote site. The most commonly affected site of embolization is the aortic trifurcation, resulting in abrupt occlusion of blood supply to the hind limbs and ischemia of an extremely large muscle mass. Pathologic conditions within the left atrium such as endocardial damage and blood stasis form the substrate for thrombus formation (Smith and Tobias, 2004). In most cases ATE is a devastating complication of serious underlying heart disease.

A recent retrospective study of 127 cats with ATE conducted at the University of Minnesota Veterinary Medical Center (UMVMC) (Smith et al., 2003) demonstrated that ATE is fairly common in referral hospitals, with an incidence rate of 0.57% or 1 in every 175 new feline admissions. Male cats were affected more frequently (67%) than females and were overrepresented when compared to the general feline hospital population (odds ratio = 1.75; P=0.003). This likely reflects the higher incidence of hypertrophic cardiomyopathy among males. Middle-aged cats were affected most commonly, but the age range was wide (8.6 ± 4.2 years). Most cases of ATE (81%) occurred in mixed-breed cats, although some purebreds (i.e., Abyssinian, Birman, and Ragdoll) were overrepresented.

A remarkable and striking feature of ATE is the occult nature of predisposing or underlying disease in the great majority of cases. Some cats have a history of cardiac or other predisposing diseases, but ATE was the first indication of any abnormality in 97 (76%) of the 127 cats studied. The only fairly common prodromal feature reported in 16% of cases was vomiting, which occurred minutes to hours before the onset of acute limb signs.

DIAGNOSIS

The diagnosis of ATE is seldom challenging. Most affected cats present because of acute-onset limb lameness, weakness, or paralysis. Affected limbs are virtually always painful (often severely), especially when manipulated, although occasional cats may not manifest overt pain possibly because of a combination of shock and stoicism. Long-standing ischemia eventually reduces pain as a result of peripheral ischemic neuropathy. Musculature frequently is firm, and pulses in the affected limbs are weak or nonpalpable. Nail beds and pads may appear pale to cyanotic. Evaluation of arterial blood flow to the affected limb by Doppler is a useful adjunct to physical examination. Absence of arterial blood flow lends strong support to a diagnosis of ATE.

The distribution of sites affected by ATE in cats from the aforementioned (UMVMC) study population is presented in Fig. 180-1. Signalment, clinical and vital signs, and results of initial diagnostic procedures are provided in Table 180-1. Important features include the following:

1. In most cats with ATE (72% in the UMVMC study), both hind limbs are affected.
2. Some residual motor function is present in approximately one third of cases, usually among cats in which either a forelimb or single hind limb is affected.
3. Rectal hypothermia is common in cats with both forelimb and hind limb signs, reflecting the profound shock that frequently accompanies ATE.
4. Respiratory rate is markedly elevated in the great majority of cats with ATE, and some show panting or open-mouth breathing. Further, respiratory rate and pattern alone do not provide sufficient clinical information to discriminate between cats with and without concurrent congestive heart failure (CHF). Other diagnostic procedures, especially thoracic radiographs, are required to make this important distinction. Among the UMVMC study cats tachypnea was present in more than 90% of cases, but radiologic or postmortem examination evidence of CHF was present in only 44%. In many cats increased respiratory rate and abnormal breathing patterns are ascribable to pain and metabolic disorders such as acid-base disturbances.
5. Heart murmurs, gallops, and arrhythmias were detected in 57% of the cats in the UMVMC study population, emphasizing the frequently occult nature of underlying disease.
6. Serum concentrations of glucose, alanine transaminase, aspartate aminotransferase, and creatine phosphokinase are frequently elevated, occurring in more than 70% of the UMVMC study cats in which these variables were measured. Other serum biochemistry and electrolyte abnormalities are common but less consistent.

Antemortem diagnostic procedures that included echocardiography or postmortem examinations were performed in 105 of the 127 UMVMC study cats. Underlying disorders among these cats mainly demonstrated

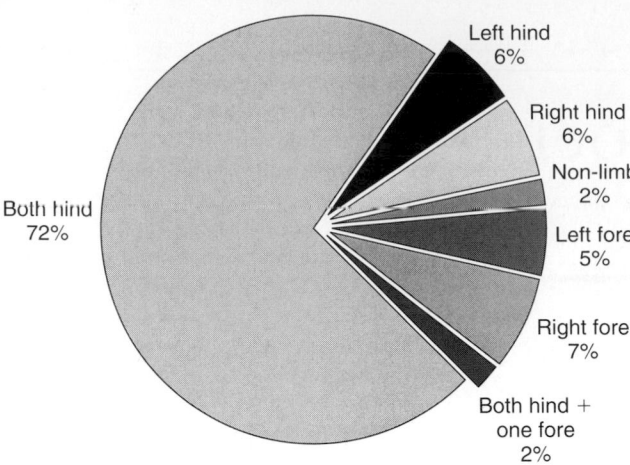

Fig. 180-1 Body areas affected by arterial thromboembolism in 127 cats. The nonlimb sites were cerebral and renal. (Modified from Smith SA et al: *J Vet Intern Med* 17:73, 2003.)

underlying heart disease as presented in Fig. 180-2. Primary or secondary cardiac disorders were identified in 94 (89%) of the 105 cases. Clearly a thorough cardiac evaluation that includes echocardiography should form part of the evaluation for any cat with ATE. Hypertrophic and unclassified cardiomyopathies were the most common diagnoses, but all forms of cardiomyopathy were represented.

Seven cats had a prior diagnosis of hyperthyroidism but were euthyroid with therapy at the time of their ATE episode. It remains to be established whether hyperthyroidism per se is a risk factor for ATE or whether cardiac pathology caused by hyperthyroidism predisposes cats to ATE. The UMVMC data do not provide a definite answer to this question, but most of the study cats with current or treated hyperthyroidism had evidence of cardiac abnormalities at the time of their ATE episode. In our opinion hyperthyroidism is likely to predispose cats to ATE by causing cardiac disease.

Table 180-1

Signalment, Clinical and Vital Signs, and Results of Initial Diagnostic Procedures From 127 Cats With Arterial Thromboembolism

	Reference Range	Data*	n[†]	%[‡] Cases Increased	%[‡] Cases Decreased
Signalment					
Gender (male: female)		85:42 (67%:33%)	127		
Age (years)		8.6 ± 4.2	127		
Clinical and Vital Signs					
Limbs affected (1:2 or more)		31:94 (25%:75%)	125		
Motor function (present:absent)		39:77	116		
Rectal temperature (°F)	100.0-102.5	98.7 (90.0-103.4)	110	5	66
Heart rate (beats per minute)	150-240	191 ± 46	112	11	16
Respiratory rate (breaths per minute)	12-38	60 (20-200)	109	91	0
Cardiac					
Left atrial dimension in systole (mm)	10.0-14.0	19.7 ± 4.2	78	91	0
Congestive heart failure (present:absent)		55:70 (44%:56%)	125		
Serum Biochemistry					
Albumin (g/dL)	2.2-3.0	2.7 ± 0.4	71	14	7
Glucose (mg/dL)	64-145	179 (17-500)	86	72	3
Blood urea nitrogen (mg/dl)	13-35	34 (15-151)	87	41	0
Creatinine (mg/dl)	0.1-2.1	1.8 (0.6-6.6)	87	26	0
Sodium (mmol/l)	147-155	150 (133-170)	84	11	7
Potassium (mmol/L)	3.7-5.3	4.4 (2.7-9.6)	84	12	14
Phosphorous (mg/dL)	1.2-7.6	5.6 (1.8-20.9)	77	16	0
Calcium (mg/dl)	8.7-11.1	9.5 (6.0-12.1)	81	6	16
Alanine aminotransferase (Units/L)	8-98	199 (15-7650)	81	73	1
Aspartate aminotransferase (Units/L)	9-37	279 (29-7560)	77	99	0
Creatine phosphokinase (Units/L)	5-400	287,434 ± 276,832	10	100	0

Modified from Smith SA et al: *J Vet Intern Med* 17:73, 2003.

*A ratio is reported for categorical data; median (range) is reported for nonnormally distributed continuous date; all other data are reported as mean ± standard deviation.

[†]Number of cases for which data were reported.

[‡]Percentage of cases for which data were reported.

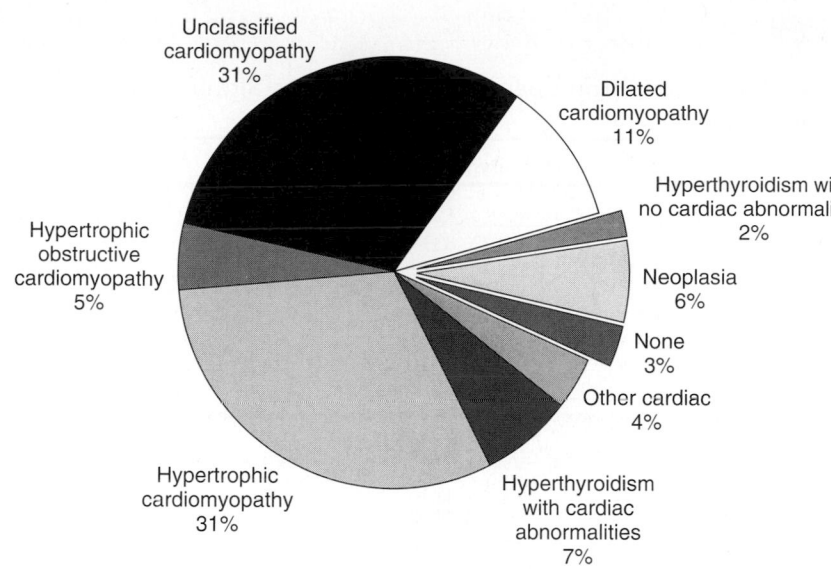

Fig. 180-2 Underlying disorders in 105 cats with arterial thromboembolism in which antemortem diagnostic procedures that included echocardiography or postmortem examinations were performed. (Modified from Smith SA et al: *J Vet Intern Med* 17:73, 2003.)

Neoplasia was second to cardiac disease as the underlying disorder in cats with ATE, occurring in 6% of the UMVMC study cases. No antemortem or postmortem evidence of cardiac disease was present in these six cats. Pulmonary carcinoma is one of the more common tumors associated with ATE, and neoplastic cells may be found within the emboli, suggesting that these may be tumor emboli that originate from the lungs rather than thromboemboli that originate in the left heart (Ibarrola et al., 2004; Smith et al., 2003). In the UMVMC study population tumor types other than pulmonary carcinoma (including hepatocellular carcinoma, vaccine-associated sarcoma, and squamous cell carcinoma) were also associated with ATE. The pathophysiology by which these tumors predispose cats to ATE remains to be established but probably involves paraneoplastic hypercoagulability.

Underlying disorders other than primary or secondary heart disease and neoplasia are uncommon among cats with ATE. Occasionally no cause for ATE is found, and no underlying diseases were identified in 3% of the 105 UMVMC study cases.

PROGNOSIS

Optimal treatment for cats with ATE has yet to be established. Many owners elect euthanasia when confronted with the reality that their cat with ATE has a life-threatening complication superimposed on serious underlying disease. In the UMVMC study population, euthanasia was elected in 25% of cases soon after ATE, and the underlying disease in some cases was diagnosed. Data from this study provide additional prognostic information that should allow both owners and clinicians to make more informed decisions.

A total of 87 of the 127 UMVMC study cats with acute-onset ATE (having occurred within 2 days of presentation) leading to limb signs were treated. Treatments were provided according to the preferences of the attending clinicians. Thrombolysis with streptokinase was attempted in four cases. The remaining cats received unfractionated heparin, aspirin, or both, using a variety

of dosage regimens. Various analgesics were administered (butorphanol, oxymorphone, fentanyl dermal patches, and morphine); and supportive care was provided, as well as treatment for CHF when appropriate. The results of this retrospective study provide the following clinically relevant data:

1. Among the 87 cats with acute ATE in which treatment was provided, 39 (45%) survived to discharge, reflecting the poor prognosis that accompanies this condition. These data are similar to previous retrospective reports.
2. Among the cats that survived to discharge, the period of hospitalization was fairly short (median = 2 days; range = 0 to 10 days). The clinical status of cats with ATE often improves or deteriorates rapidly.
3. Table 180-2 lists the variables that on initial evaluation were significantly different between cats that survived to discharge and those that did not survive. These data show:
   a. In survivors frequently only one limb was affected, and they demonstrated some motor function.
   b. Rectal temperature and heart rate both were higher among survivors.
   c. Serum phosphorous was lower among survivors.
4. Variables that on initial evaluation were not significantly different between survivors to discharge and nonsurvivors were: gender; age; respiratory rate; left atrial dimension; presence or absence of CHF; and serum concentrations of albumin, glucose, blood urea nitrogen, creatinine, sodium, potassium, calcium, alanine aminotransferase, aspartate aminotransferase, and creatine phosphokinase.
5. A logistic regression model for predicting survival to discharge was developed using the variables that were significantly different between survivors and nonsurvivors. Once rectal temperature at presentation was included in the model, accuracy of prediction was not significantly improved by adding any other variables. The model is presented in Fig. 180-3, and it predicts a 50% probability of survival in cases with a

Table **180-2**

Clinical And Biochemical Variables From Cats With Acute Thromboembolism That Were Significantly Different Between Survivors to Discharge and Nonsurvivors

	Survivors* (n = 39)	n†	Nonsurvivors* (n = 48)	n†	P value
Clinical and Vital Signs					
Limbs affected (1:2 or more)	17:22 (44%:56%)	39	8:40 (17%:83%)	48	0.008
Motor function (present:absent)	20:13 (61%:39%)	33	11:35 (24%:76%)	46	0.001
Rectal temperature (°F)	99.9 ± 2.0	37	96.5 ± 3.4	45	<0.001
Heart Rate (beats per minute)	210 (100–300)	37	188 (80-350)	43	0.038
Serum Biochemistry					
Phosphorous (mg/dl)	5.4 (3.3-9.7)	29	6.4 (1.8-20.9)	37	0.024

Modified from Smith SA et al: *J Vet Intern Med* 17:73, 2003.
*The data are from 87 cases with acute limb signs in which treatment was provided.
†A ratio is reported for categorical data; median (range) is reported for nonnormally distributed continuous data; all other data are reported as mean ± standard deviation.
‡Number of cases for which data were reported.

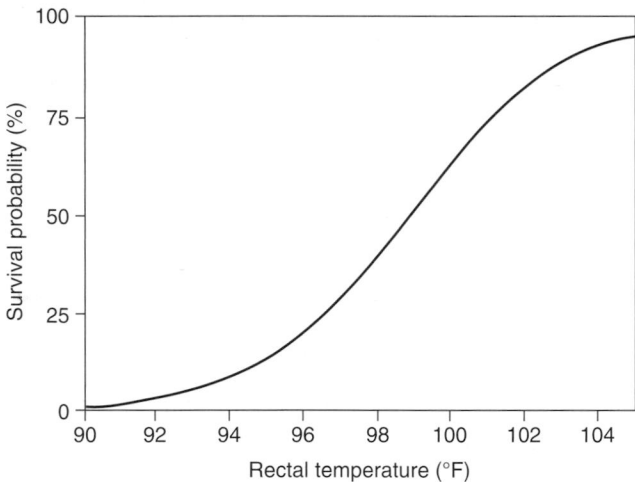

Fig. 180-3 Logistic regression model predicting survival probability to discharge (P) based on rectal temperature (T) at presentation. The equation for the model is: $P=1/(1+e^{-47.59+0.48T})$. (Modified from Smith SA et al: *J Vet Intern Med* 17:73, 2003.)

rectal temperature of 98.9° F. The predictive value of rectal temperature probably stems from the fact that it reflects overall hemodynamic status and that cats with profound hypotension are often hypothermic and bradycardiac.

A predictive model based on a simple and rapidly measured physical examination variable such as rectal temperature is extremely useful. However, it is also important to recognize its limitations and to interpret the results with care. First, although the model correctly classified 67% of survivors and 79% of nonsurvivors in our study, some cats with ATE are incorrectly classified. Second, the predictive model is based on cats that received a variety of anticoagulant protocols. It remains to be determined how (and whether) more standardized anticoagulant protocols can affect survival to discharge. These approaches are described in the following paragraphs.

Forty-four study cats were discharged from the UMVMC following their acute ATE episodes. This number includes the 39 cases discussed previously, as well as five cats that survived to discharge after referral for further management following ATE of greater than 2 days' duration. Eighteen cats (41%) were discharged on high-dose aspirin (≥40 mg total dose/cat orally [PO] q72h), 24 (55%) received low-dose aspirin (5 mg total dose PO q72h), and 2 (4%) received no anticoagulant therapy. Treatment for CHF was prescribed when appropriate (34% of the 44 survivors).

Follow-up of these study cats demonstrated:

1. Eleven of the 44 cats (25%) experienced a total of 16 additional ATE episodes. The episodes were fatal in nine (20.5%) of the cases (three died, six were euthanized). Based on these data, recurrent ATE should be anticipated in about 25% of the cases when aspirin is used for long-term thromboprophylaxis.
2. Among the cats that had additional ATE episodes, average time to first recurrence was 191 ± 152 days (approximately 6 months), but the range was extremely wide.
3. Permanent limb damage is the exception rather than the rule, although time to complete recovery of limb function may be days, weeks, or even months. Complications ascribable to limb ischemia occurred in five (11%) of the 44 discharged cats and ranged from minor tissue necrosis requiring wound management (n=2) to limb contracture (n=1) and limb necrosis requiring amputation (n=2). These results are compatible with previously published reports and textbook descriptions.
4. Nine (20.5%) of the 44 discharged cats were alive at the end of the study period, 9 (20.5%) died or were euthanized because of recurrent ATE, and 26 (59%) died or were euthanized because of progression of their underlying cardiac disease. Recurrent ATE in cats following an acute episode is a significant cause of morbidity and mortality. However, progression of underlying cardiac disease is the single most important cause of morbidity and mortality among cats that

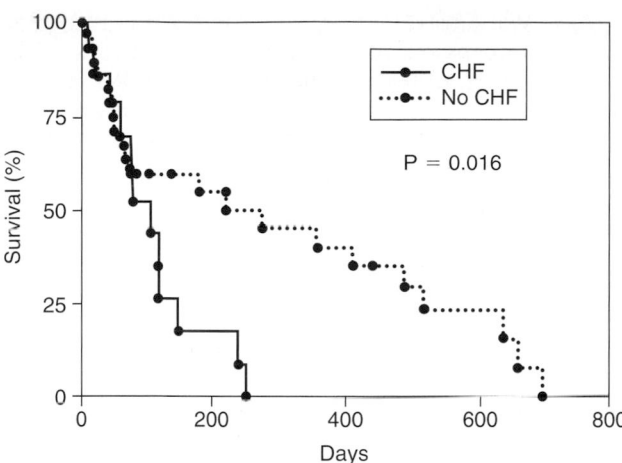

Fig. 180-4 Kaplan-Meier curves for cats that survived to discharge following acute arterial thromboembolism. (Modified from Smith SA et al: *J Vet Intern Med* 17:73, 2003.)

recover from an acute episode of ATE. Mortality from progressive heart disease was almost three times more common than mortality from recurrent ATE.

5. Kaplan-Meier curves for cats that were discharged following an acute ATE episode are presented in Fig. 180-4. The curves are plotted by the presence or absence of CHF at the time of their initial episode. Survival time for cats diagnosed with CHF (n=15) was significantly shorter than for cats without CHF (n=29) (median survival times = 77 versus 223 days, P=0.016). Thus, although the presence or absence of CHF does not affect survival to discharge among cats with acute ATE, it does have a statistically significant and clinically important effect on mortality following discharge.

6. No significant difference in survival was detected between cats that received high- or low-dose aspirin (median survival times = 149 and 105 days, respectively; P=0.882), although the numbers treated were relatively low. Further, the proportion of cats that experienced ATE recurrences was similar in the two groups (28% and 25%, respectively). However, 22% of the cats in the high-dose aspirin group showed gastrointestinal side effects versus 4% in the low-dose aspirin group. Thus in this retrospective study efficacy of the two aspirin dosage regimens was not statistically different in terms of survival and ATE recurrence, but adverse gastrointestinal effects were less common among cats receiving low-dose aspirin. Consequently low-dose aspirin is our current recommendation for long-term thromboprophylaxis in cats.

THERAPY

The therapeutic approach that we describe here for the short- and long-term management of cats with ATE involves unfractionated heparin, low-dose aspirin, analgesia, supportive care, and treatment for CHF when appropriate. This therapy is both conventional and conservative. However, we are frequently disappointed and frustrated by the indifferent results obtained in some cats treated in this manner. Given the magnitude of the perturbation to the system caused by acute ATE, the massive amount of tissue damage, and the seriousness of the underlying disorders in most cases, such responses are not surprising. Nevertheless, many of us continue to search for other therapeutic approaches for both the management of cats with acute ATE and long-term thromboprophylaxis. Some of the alternate strategies that have been proposed and attempted for the management of acute ATE include thrombolytic agents such as tissue type plasminogen activator and streptokinase and surgical and catheter-based removal of thromboemboli from obstructed sites. Currently available information indicates that these strategies are: (1) associated with outcomes that are either worse or no better than those obtained with a more conventional and conservative approach, and (2) based on studies of very few cases with little outcome- or evidence-based comparative data.

Initial management of ATE should include pain control. Butorphanol is too weak and short-acting for this purpose, and for the first 24 to 48 hours opioids are recommended (see Chapter 2). Fentanyl (1 to 3 mcg/kg/hr), hydromorphone, or morphine generally reduces the magnitude of pain. Rectal temperature should be monitored. CHF should be documented by radiography since pain and opioids can affect ventilatory pattern. Furosemide (2 mg/kg intravenously [IV]) and oxygen are appropriate treatments for CHF (also see Chapter 178).

In addition to analgesia, other supportive measures, and treatment for CHF when appropriate, our current anticoagulant recommendations for cats with ATE are:

1. Unfractionated heparin 250 to 300 units/kg subcutaneously every 8 hours, with the first dose administered intravenously for cases in shock.*
2. Low-dose aspirin (5 mg total dose/cat PO q72h) initiated as soon as the patient is eating.†
3. Discontinue heparin gradually over 2 to 3 days once the patient is hemodynamically stable and receiving low-dose aspirin.‡

---

*In humans a plasma heparin concentration of 0.35 to 0.70 units/ml measured by the chromogenic factor Xa assay is associated with the greatest clinical efficacy and fewest hemorrhagic complications. In normal cats an unfractionated heparin dose of 300 units/kg subcutaneously every 8 hours most consistently provides this concentration. The chromogenic factor Xa assay is the test of choice for heparin monitoring and dose titration, but the assay is not widely available at present. We do not recommend titrating the heparin dose based on activated partial thromboplastin time or activated clotting time. In cats both of these variables correspond very poorly with plasma heparin concentrations measured by the chromogenic factor Xa assay (Smith and Tobias, 2004).

†The rationale for the use of aspirin in general and the low dose of 5 mg/cat orally every 72 hours in particular is provided in Smith and colleagues, 2003.

‡This recommendation is based on the fact that abrupt cessation of heparin in humans may lead to thrombotic complications.

PREVENTION

A variety of drugs for long-term thromboprophylaxis in cats have been investigated either as an alternative or adjunct to aspirin. These include warfarin, low–molecular weight heparin (dalteparin, enoxaparin), ticlopidine, clopidogrel, eptifibatide, and abciximab. Some of these drugs show potential for thromboprophylaxis in cats, and research is ongoing (Smith and Tobias, 2004). In a recent clinical study involving cats with cardiomyopathy, the low–molecular weight heparin dalteparin at a median dose of 99 units/kg subcutaneously every 12 or 24 hours was administered easily by owners and was well tolerated by cats with few side effects (Smith et al., 2004). In another recent study involving five experimental cats, clopidogrel (Plavix), Bristol-Myers Squibb/Sanofi Pharmaceuticals, at total doses ranging from 18.75 to 75 mg/cat q24h PO demonstrated significant antiplatelet activity (Hogan et al., 2004). Many cardiologists empirically use clopidogrel (typically at 18.5 mg PO q24h) as antithrombotic therapy in cats. Currently a multicenter trial of clopidogrel is ongoing. However, it remains to be established whether these drugs can reduce the frequency and severity of ATE in predisposed cats.[4]

We do not recommend warfarin long-term thromboprophylaxis in cats that survive acute ATE episodes. In a study reported by Moore and colleagues (2000) median survival of warfarin-treated cats was only 51 days. Further, the frequency of fatal hemorrhage among the warfarin-treated cats was 17%. Warfarin provides no demonstrable survival benefit over aspirin, is associated with a higher risk of fatal hemorrhage, and requires frequent monitoring of coagulation variables.

A significant subset of cats that survive the acute episode have recurrent ATE, as confirmed by UMVMC study data. Long-term thromboprophylaxis is appropriate for such cases. However, the situation among cats with disorders such as primary or secondary heart disease with or without CHF and no prior history of ATE is more controversial. We are not aware of any studies that have established the frequency of ATE among such cases. Historically large atrial size and the presence of spontaneous contrast or "smoke" on echocardiography have been considered risk factors

for ATE. We subscribe to these notions but recognize that they are based on clinical impression, anecdote, and extrapolation from human medicine. We usually recommend long-term thromboprophylaxis in cats with more severe cardiac disease, prominent atrial enlargement, and spontaneous contrast on echocardiography. Currently low-dose aspirin (5 mg total dose PO q72h) is our drug of choice for long-term thromboprophylaxis in these situations, as it is for cats that survive an acute ATE episode. Low-dose aspirin must be compounded, but it is otherwise easy to administer and requires no specific monitoring. Further, the available data, albeit limited, indicate that the use of low-dose aspirin in cats is associated with minimal adverse effects. Other clinicians use clopidogrel, combinations of low-dose aspirin and clopidogrel, or low–molecular weight heparin as described previously. All of these treatments are empiric at this point, and there have been no blinded, prospective studies comparing treatments or therapy to placebo. It is incumbent on us to search for and embrace new therapies for long-term thromboprophylaxis as soon as their safety and superior efficacy have been established in clinical trials. However, to date no drug or drug combination has been shown to be safer or more effective than low-dose aspirin for long-term thromboprophylaxis in cats that are predisposed to ATE.

References and Suggested Reading

Hogan DE et al: Antiplatelet effects and pharmacodynamics of clopidogrel in cats, *J Am Vet Med Assoc* 225:1406, 2004.

Ibarrola P et al: Appendicular arterial tumor embolization in two cats with pulmonary carcinoma, *J Am Vet Med Assoc* 225:1065, 2004.

Moore KE et al: Retrospective study of streptokinase administration in 46 cats with arterial thromboembolism, *Vet Emerg Crit Care* 10:245, 2000.

Smith CE et al: Use of low molecular weight heparin in cats: 57 cases (1999–2003), *J Am Vet Med Assoc* 225:1237, 2004.

Smith SA, Tobias AH: Feline arterial thromboembolism: an update. In Abbott JA, editor: *Veterinary Clinics of North America small animal practice*, Philadelphia, 2004, Elsevier Saunders, p 1245.

Smith SA, Tobias AH, Jacob KA, et al: Arterial thromboembolism in cats: acute crisis in 127 cases (1992-2001) and long-term management with low-dose aspirin in 24 cases, *J Vet Intern Med* 17:73, 2003.

---

[4]This statement is true for aspirin as well. There have been no clinical studies to show that aspirin reduces the frequency or severity of ATE or that it provides a significant morbidity and mortality benefit over no therapy in cats at risk for ATE.

CHAPTER 181

Pericardial Effusion

O. LYNNE NELSON, *Pullman, Washington*
WENDY A. WARE, *Ames, Iowa*

The double-layered pericardial sac surrounding the heart normally contains a small volume (≈0.25 ml/kg) of serous fluid between its outer fibrous layer (parietal pericardium) and inner serous membrane (visceral pericardium or epicardium). Excessive fluid accumulation (pericardial effusion) is the most common pericardial disorder in small animals. This occurs much more frequently in dogs than in cats.

PATHOPHYSIOLOGY

Pericardial effusion disturbs cardiac function by impeding filling. Because the pericardium is relatively noncompliant, increases in pericardial fluid volume can sharply increase intrapericardial pressure. When intrapericardial pressure equals or exceeds normal cardiac filling pressure and impairs filling, the condition of cardiac tamponade exists. The fluid accumulation rate and the distensibility of the pericardial sac determine whether and how quickly cardiac tamponade develops. Rapid accumulation of a small volume (e.g., 50 to 100 ml) can raise intrapericardial pressure markedly because the pericardium can stretch only slowly. Fibrosis and pericardial thickening further limit the compliance of this tissue. Pericardial fibrosis and inflammatory cell infiltrates are seen with idiopathic and neoplastic causes of effusion. Conversely, if effusion accumulates slowly, the pericardium may enlarge sufficiently to accommodate the increased volume at low pressure. As long as intrapericardial pressure is lower than venous pressures, cardiac filling and output remain relatively normal, and signs of tamponade are absent. Therefore large-volume pericardial effusion implies a gradual process.

The external cardiac compression that occurs with tamponade progressively limits filling, initially of the right heart but subsequently the left as well. Systemic venous pressure increases while cardiac output falls. Diastolic pressures in all cardiac chambers and great veins eventually equilibrate. Neurohumoral compensatory mechanisms of heart failure become activated as cardiac output falls. External signs of systemic venous congestion and right-sided congestive heart failure become especially prominent with time.

Cardiac tamponade exaggerates the variation in arterial blood pressure that occurs normally during the respiratory cycle. The inspiratory reduction in left heart output can cause a 10–mm Hg or greater fall in arterial pressure during inspiration; this is known as *pulsus paradoxus*. Although myocardial contractility is not affected directly by pericardial effusion, reduced coronary perfusion during tamponade can lead to systolic and diastolic impairment. Low cardiac output, arterial hypotension, right-sided congestive heart failure, and poor perfusion of other organs, as well as the heart, can ultimately lead to cardiogenic shock and death.

PRESENTATION

Cardiac tamponade is relatively common in dogs but rare in cats. Clinical signs reflect the consequences of systemic venous congestion and poor cardiac output. Right-sided congestive signs usually predominate, especially abdominal enlargement (ascites). Tachypnea and weakness or syncope with exertion is common in the history. Lethargy, poor exercise tolerance, inappetence, cough, and other nonspecific signs can occur before obvious ascites develops. Loss of lean body mass (cachexia) is apparent in some chronic cases. Rapid pericardial fluid accumulation can cause acute tamponade, shock, and death. In such cases pulmonary edema, jugular venous distention, and hypotension may be evident without signs of pleural effusion, ascites, or radiographic cardiomegaly.

Physical examination findings typically include jugular vein distention and/or positive hepatojugular reflux, hepatomegaly, ascites, labored respiration, and weakened femoral pulses. Femoral pulse attenuation during inspiration may be discernible in occasional patients with pulsus paradoxus because of the phasic reductions in pulse (as well as mean arterial) pressure. High sympathetic tone associated with reduced cardiac output causes sinus tachycardia, mucous membrane pallor, and prolonged capillary refill time. The precordial impulse is palpably weak when pericardial fluid volume is large. Subcutaneous edema occasionally is evident. Heart sounds are muffled by moderate-to-large pericardial effusions. Lung sounds are muffled ventrally with pleural effusion. Although pericardial effusion does not cause a murmur, concurrent cardiac disease may do so. Large-volume pericardial effusions sometimes cause clinical signs by virtue of their size, even in the absence of overt tamponade. Lung or airway compression can provoke dyspnea or cough; esophageal compression can cause dysphagia or regurgitation. Fever may accompany infectious pericarditis, and affected patients may appear very ill.

ETIOLOGY

Most pericardial effusions in dogs are serosanguineous or sanguineous and are either neoplastic or idiopathic ("benign") in origin. Transudates, modified transudates, and exudates are found occasionally in both dogs and cats. Pericardial effusions secondary to feline infectious peritonitis and congestive heart failure (especially hypertrophic cardiomyopathy) are identified most often in cats. Pericardial effusion from lymphoma, systemic infections, and rarely renal failure also are reported in cats. Cardiac tumors are relatively infrequent in dogs; they are rare in cats. Peritoneopericardial diaphragmatic hernia or (rarely) other congenital pericardial malformations may be associated with effusion in both species.

Hemorrhagic effusions tend to be dark red, with a packed cell volume greater than 7%, specific gravity greater than 1.015, and protein greater than 3 g/dl. Besides red blood cells, reactive mesothelial, neoplastic, or other cells may be seen on cytology. The fluid does not clot unless hemorrhage was very recent. Neoplastic hemorrhagic effusions are more common in older dogs, although middle-aged and even younger dogs are sometimes affected. Hemangiosarcoma (HSA) is by far the most common cause, followed by heart base tumors and pericardial mesothelioma. HSA usually arises within the right heart, especially the right auricular appendage. HSA appears to have an increased prevalence in certain breeds such as the German shepherd, golden retriever, Afghan hound, English setter, American cocker spaniel, Doberman pinscher, Labrador retriever, and miniature poodle.

Chemodectoma or aortic body tumor (arising from chemoreceptor cells at the base of the aorta) is the most common heart base tumor. Breed predilections include boxers, Boston terriers, and bulldogs; but not all dogs with chemodectomas are of brachycephalic breeds. Other heart base tumors include thyroid, parathyroid, lymphoid, or connective tissue neoplasms. Pericardial mesothelioma is confirmed occasionally in the dog and cat. Pericardial effusion secondary to metastatic tumors appears to be rare. Neoplastic pericardial effusion in cats is most often associated with lymphoma; various other cardiac tumors are rarely involved.

Idiopathic pericardial effusion is most common in medium-to-large dog breeds. Although dogs of any age can be affected, the median age appears to be about 6 to 7 years. Mild inflammation with areas of hemorrhage and diffuse pericardial fibrosis have been described histologically. Less common causes of intrapericardial hemorrhage include left atrial rupture from severe chronic mitral regurgitation, coagulopathy, and penetrating trauma.

Transudative effusions are usually modified rather than pure transudates. Transudative effusions can occur with congestive heart failure, peritoneopericardial diaphragmatic hernia, hypoalbuminemia, pericardial cysts, or toxemias that increase vascular permeability (including uremia). Usually these conditions are associated with a small volume of pericardial effusion, and cardiac tamponade rarely develops. Effusions caused by cardiac lymphoma and rarely by heart base masses can appear transudative rather than hemorrhagic.

Exudative pericardial effusions are rare in small animals. Exudates appear cloudy to opaque or serofibrinous to serosanguineous. They are characterized by high nucleated cell count (well over 3000 cells/μl), protein concentration (usually much higher than 3 g/dl), and specific gravity (>1.015). Cytologic findings are related to the etiology. Infectious causes usually stem from plant awn migration, bite wounds, or extension of infection in nearby structures. Various aerobic and anaerobic bacteria, actinomycosis, coccidioidomycosis, disseminated tuberculosis, and rarely systemic protozoal infections have been identified. Sterile exudative effusions have occurred with leptospirosis, canine distemper, uremia, and idiopathic pericardial effusion in dogs and with feline infectious peritonitis and toxoplasmosis in cats.

DIAGNOSTIC EVALUATION OF PERICARDIAL EFFUSION

Blood Pressure

Arterial blood pressure should be measured in all cases of suspected pericardial disease. Hypotension (arterial blood pressure <90) is generally an indication of critical tamponade. Doppler flow detectors may document respiratory variation in audible signal strength compatible with pulsus paradoxus.

Radiography

Thoracic radiography classically reveals a very round cardiac silhouette with large-volume pericardial effusion. The globoid cardiac shadow is especially apparent on the ventrodorsal or dorsoventral projection. However, smaller volumes of pericardial fluid often result in mild-to-moderate generalized cardiomegaly with normal chamber contours, making radiographic diagnosis of pericardial effusion less certain. Sometimes pleural effusion is present. Other radiographic findings commonly associated with pericardial effusion and tamponade include caudal vena cava distention, hepatomegaly, and ascites. Pulmonary vascular underperfusion and interstitial pulmonary edema may be noted. A soft-tissue mass effect may be evident in cases of heart base tumor. The trachea may be deviated or appear displaced dorsally and to the right, distinctly separate from the heart base. Thoracic radiographs are also helpful to screen for other potentially associated lesions such as metastatic lung disease and lymphadenopathy.

Electrocardiography

Electrocardiography is fairly insensitive for detecting pericardial effusion; in many cases the electrocardiogram (ECG) appears normal. However, ECG findings that can suggest pericardial effusion include diminished complex size (<1 mV in all leads), electrical alternans, and ST segment elevation (epicardial injury). Electrical alternans or altering QRS complex height results from physical swinging of the heart within the pericardium. It is best appreciated in large-volume pericardial effusion with the ECG obtained from a standing position. Sinus tachycardia is the most common cardiac rhythm associated with pericardial effusion, but atrial or ventricular tachyarrhythmias may also be noted. Atrial fibrillation can complicate chronic pericardial disease in large-breed dogs.

Echocardiography

Echocardiography is a very sensitive test to detect even small volumes of pericardial effusion. In most cases the

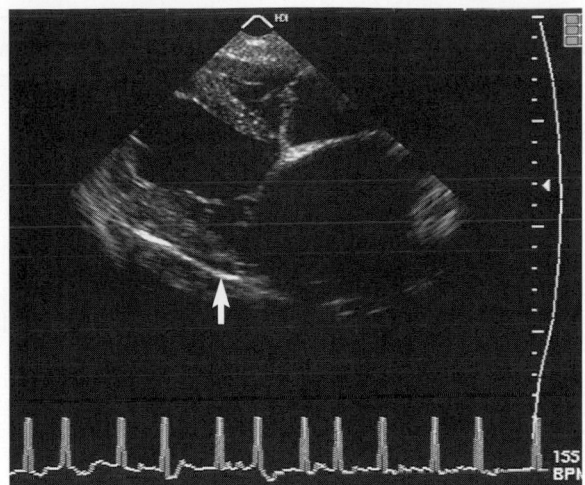

Fig. 181-1 Echocardiogram from a dog with a very tiny of amount of pericardial fluid. In this case the fluid is best noted along the caudal left atrial wall at the atrioventricular junction *(arrow)*.

pericardial fluid is hypoechoic; thus pericardial effusion appears as an echo-free space between the epicardium and the intensely hyperechoic parietal pericardium. Because the pericardium is more tightly adhered to the heart base and fluid initially collects ventrally, the apical and caudal left atrial regions are good places to screen for small amounts of pericardial effusion (Fig. 181-1). Occasionally pleural effusion, a markedly enlarged left atrium, or a persistent left cranial vena cava can be confused with pericardial effusion. A thorough scan from numerous positions differentiates these conditions. Particularly when scanning from the right parasternal window, the right ventricular free wall commonly appears hyperechoic because of the dramatic difference in density between the pericardial effusion and epicardium. This should not be interpreted as a right ventricular abnormality or thickened epicardium.

Echocardiography is especially useful in determining the severity of tamponade, which correlates to clinical severity. Tamponade is seen as diastolic collapse of the right atrium and sometimes the right ventricle and is a direct reflection of intrapericardial pressures (Fig. 181-2, *A* and *B*). Echocardiography can establish an etiology of pericardial effusion if cardiac or heart base masses are identified and can screen for concurrent disease such as valvular disease, cardiomyopathy, or congenital abnormalities. Whenever possible it is best to perform echocardiographic evaluation before the removal of pericardial fluid. The presence of fluid generally improves visualization of the heart base and location or point of adherence of any mass lesions. Thorough examination of the right atrium and auricle (especially from the left cranial long axis position), ascending aorta, and parietal pericardium are important to screen for neoplasia. In some cases the localization of a lesion may narrow the list of differentials for the effusion (e.g., masses of the right atrium or auricular appendage are consistent with a diagnosis of HSA). Transesophageal echocardiography can be especially useful in examination of the heart base regions for suspected mass lesions and enlarged lymph nodes. Positive and negative predictive values of echocardiography for recognizing cardiac mass lesions have not been reported.

Pericardiocentesis

Pericardiocentesis is the treatment of choice for initial stabilization of animals with pericardial effusion and cardiac tamponade. Pericardial fluid analysis is also a part of the diagnostic process. Aspiration of even a small amount of fluid can markedly reduce intrapericardial pressure and improve clinical status. Diuretic therapy without pericardiocentesis is usually not helpful for cardiac tamponade (except for effusion caused by congestive heart failure). Diuretics can worsen hypotension or precipitate cardiogenic shock.

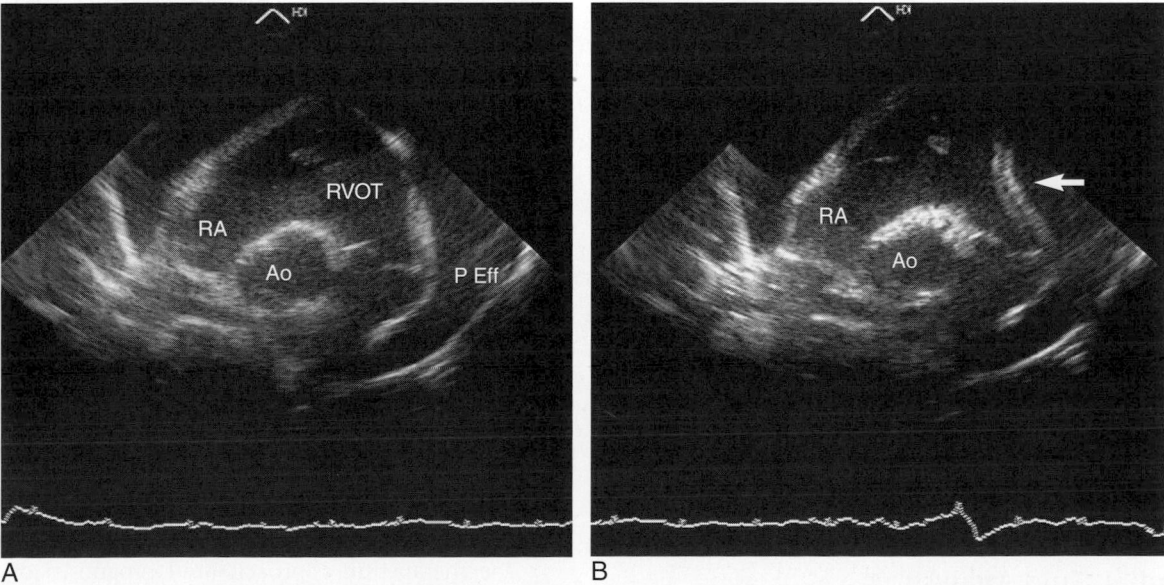

A   B

Fig. 181-2 **A,** Echocardiogram from right parasternal short-axis view of the heart base in a dog with pericardial effusion (end-systolic frame). **B,** The same view in diastole revealing tamponade, with collapse of the right ventricular wall *(arrow)*. *Ao,* Aorta; *P Eff,* pericardial effusion; *RA,* right atrium; *RVOT,* right ventricular outflow tract.

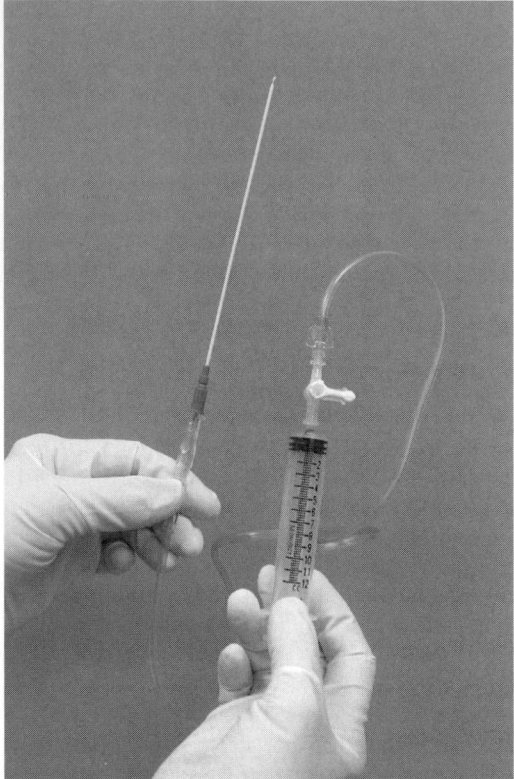

Fig. 181-3 Common apparatus for pericardiocentesis procedure; a 16-gauge, 6-inch over-the-needle catheter connected to extension tubing and a three-way stopcock.

Pericardiocentesis is performed most routinely from the right side because the cardiac notch reduces the potential for lung injury and the major coronary vessels are located on the left. On a standard examination table the animal is more securely restrained in sternal or left lateral recumbency. A radiographic wedge can be used to elevate the spine slightly. Some clinicians do perform pericardiocentesis in the standing dog. If an echocardiography table or other elevated table with an appropriately sized cutout is available, the animal can be placed in right lateral recumbency and tapped from underneath. Sedation is seldom required for dogs. Echo-guidance may be used but is not often necessary. The ECG should be carefully monitored during the procedure. Needle/catheter contact with the epicardium often induces ventricular arrhythmias (usually with an upright configuration in lead II) and should prompt retraction of the device.

An over-the-needle type catheter is used most commonly for pericardiocentesis (Fig. 181-3). Depending on the size of the animal, a 12- to 20-gauge, 2- to 6-inch-long catheter is selected. Extra side holes may be cut near the catheter tip to facilitate drainage of large-volume or flocculent fluid. Extension tubing is attached to the needle stylet, and a three-way stopcock is placed between the tubing and collection syringe (see Fig. 181-3). Box 181-1 summarizes the pericardiocentesis procedure.

Pericardial Fluid Analysis

Pericardial fluid is submitted routinely for cytology and culture. If obvious masses are not identified by echocar-

Box 181-1

Step-by-Step Approach to Pericardiocentesis

1. Shave the hair over the right precordium (third to seventh rib spaces, sternum to costochondral junction). Prepare the area with aseptic surgical scrub technique.
2. Attach ECG monitor and noninvasive blood pressure if available.
3. Identify the catheter insertion site by palpating the strongest precordial impulse and considering radiographic evaluation and echo-guidance.
4. Local anesthesia should be used, especially with large catheters.
   a. Infiltrate lidocaine (2%) from the insertion site into the underlying intercostal muscles and pleura.
   b. Make a small stab incision in the skin (No. 11 blade) if using a large catheter.
5. Insert the catheter with care to avoid the intercostal vessels just caudal to the ribs.
6. Once the needle penetrates the skin and after every increment of advancement, apply gentle negative pressure to the syringe and observe for fluid.
   a. Pleural fluid is typically straw colored.
   b. Pericardial fluid is typically dark and bloody; typically this fluid is under a positive pressure.
7. Subtle scratching of the needle tip on the pericardial surface may be noted, or a loss of resistance may be felt as the needle enters the pericardial space. This is not usually associated with ventricular arrhythmias.
8. If the needle contacts the epicardium, marked scratching or pulsing sensation is usually felt. This is usually associated with ventricular arrhythmias. Retract the needle.
9. When a catheter system is used and especially in smaller-volume pericardial effusion, remove the needle and attach extension tubing to the catheter.
10. After a small bit of fluid is obtained, take steps to differentiate the bloody pericardial fluid from hemorrhage.
    a. Place a drop of fluid onto the table or in a clot tube and observe for clotting (pericardial effusion should not clot).
    b. Obtain a packed cell volume (PCV) on the fluid and compare it to the peripheral PCV.
11. Aspirate as much fluid as possible from the pericardial space. Submit samples for cytology (and culture if indicated).
12. Verify reduction of effusion and tamponade by echocardiography.

diography, fluid analysis may take on a more important role in determining the next diagnostic and therapeutic steps. Standard laboratory and cytologic evaluation may identify suppurative, mycotic, or chylous effusions but is rarely helpful in distinguishing neoplastic from benign hemorrhagic pericardial effusion. In addition, mesothelial cells lining the pericardium can become reactive and may exfoliate into the effusion. These cells can be difficult to differentiate from neoplastic cells, particularly mesothelioma. Other cardiac-related tumors rarely exfoliate cells into the effusion, with the possible exception of lymphoma.

The therapeutic approach (and prognosis) of animals with pericardial effusion directly depends on the underlying cause of the effusion. Neoplasia and idiopathic pericardial effusion are the most common causes of pericardial effusion in the dog, but unfortunately fluid cytology does not reliably sort these causes. In addition, certain neoplastic disorders have notoriously short survival times (e.g., HSA). Reports in humans and dogs have examined the use of fluid pH measurement to distinguish between inflammatory and noninflammatory causes of pericardial effusion. Studies in dogs have been conflicting. Theoretically effusions with high pH values are likely from noninflammatory causes (neoplasia), and effusions with low pH values are most likely associated with inflammatory causes (idiopathic or infectious pericarditis). A recent prospective report of 37 dogs with pericardial effusion (Fine, Tobias, and Jacob, 2003) found no correlation between pH and etiology of effusion. Data from this report overlapped 89% of the time between neoplastic and idiopathic effusion groups. At this time there is likely little justification to use pH measurement as a diagnostic test in cases of pericardial effusion.

Advanced Imaging Techniques

The major advantage of computed tomography (CT) and magnetic resonance imaging (MRI) techniques is the ability to noninvasively view internal structures such as the heart. With CT, information is collected from the penetration of x-ray beams projected in a circumferential manner around the chest cavity, and the resulting information is arranged digitally into a two-dimensional image. The images can be reformatted into differing imaging planes corresponding to major anatomic planes (i.e., long axis, short axis planes). On a CT image, black is associated with fluid or air, soft tissues appear as various shades of grey, and bone is white. The relative grayness of the image depends on the relative density of the tissues imaged. Tissue characterization (other than calcium) is limited compared to MRI. Thus the major limitations of CT include the use of ionizing radiation and the frequent need for iodinated contrast to enhance differing tissue densities such as tumors.

Since MRI relies on the magnetic environment of the cellular nuclei, ionizing radiation is avoided. The resulting information is also computer processed to form a two-dimensional image. Cine sequences that loop through the cardiac cycle phases may also be obtained. With advances in software, many pulse sequences can be used for cardiac imaging. They are generally divided into dark (black)-blood and bright (white)-blood techniques. Vessels, cardiac chambers, and soft tissues of varying densities are more easily distinguished; and contrast enhancement is needed less often. In most cases image acquisition must be gated to a point in the cardiac cycle to avoid image blur. MRI may become a valuable tool to detect mass lesions not identified by echocardiography in veterinary patients (Fig. 181-4).

Diagnosis Problems

The most difficult diagnosis involves the mature dog with a hemorrhagic effusion but no overt mass lesion or metastatic disease on cardiac, abdominal, and thoracic imaging. In most cases serial imaging over 2 to 3 months identifies HSA or chemodectoma. Breeds at risk for HSA should undergo careful examination of the spleen and liver.

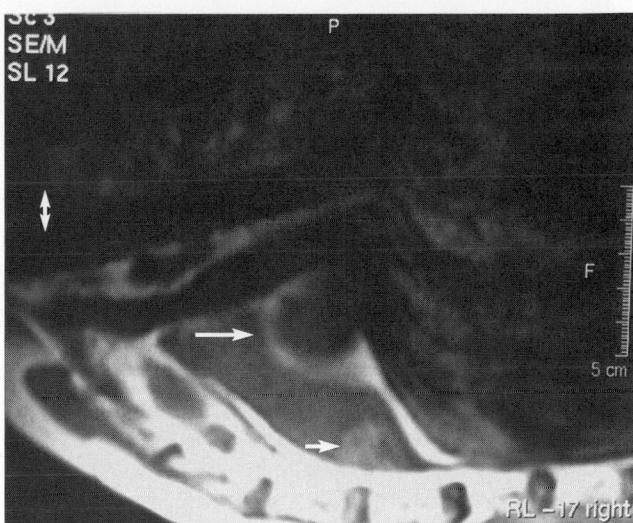

Fig. 181-4 T1-weighted (black blood) magnetic resonance image of a dog with pericardial effusion. This cystic lesion cranial to the heart *(long arrow)* was not appreciated on transthoracic echocardiography. Histopathologic evaluation revealed the structure to be a rare thyroglossal cyst. An enlarged sternal lymph node is also noted *(short arrow)*.

The most common diagnostic challenge is differentiating idiopathic versus mesothelioma-related pericardial effusion. Multiple studies have compared presenting clinical signs and diagnostic and histopathologic findings in cases ultimately diagnosed with pericardial mesothelioma versus idiopathic pericardial effusion. Unfortunately clinical signs and results of noninvasive diagnostic tests are insufficient to differentiate idiopathic effusion from mesothelioma unless a discrete pericardial/intrapericardial mass is observed. Surgical pericardial biopsy can be misleading since both conditions lead to extensive pericardial fibrosis with a mixed inflammatory response incorporating large numbers of reactive mesothelial cells. One retrospective evaluation suggested that recurrence of pleural effusion within 120 days of pericardiectomy increases the likelihood of a diagnosis of mesothelioma (Stepien, Whitley, and Dubielzig, 2000). Survival longer than 120 days after pericardiectomy without chemotherapeutic intervention was unusual in dogs ultimately diagnosed with mesothelioma.

Immunohistochemical staining of biopsy material may be useful to determine etiology of pericardial effusion in questionable cases. Preliminary investigations have evaluated the staining patterns of cardiac HSA, chemodectoma, mesothelioma, and idiopathic pericardial effusion using antibodies specific for CD31, desmin, cytokeratin, vimentin, synaptophysin, chromogranin, and endothelin. In this study the antibody for CD31 was specific for HSA. Synaptophysin and chromogranin demonstrated high specificity but only moderate sensitivity for chemodectoma. Cytokeratin was specific for mesothelial tissue, and desmin occasionally differentiated mesothelioma from reactive mesothelial tissue. If staining characteristics performed on pericardial fluid yield similar results, immunocytochemical stains could potentially improve the diagnostic capability of pericardial fluid analysis. Flow cytometry methods also have shown preliminary value for isolation of neoplastic cells in fluid or blood.

MANAGEMENT OF PERICARDIAL EFFUSION

Initial Management

In most cases systolic function is normal, and positive inotropic drugs are not warranted. Likewise vasodilators and diuretics have a negligible effect on intrapericardial fluid (and pressures) and may only serve to lower systemic arterial pressures. Initial therapy of patients with pericardial effusion is directed at acutely reducing the intrapericardial pressures and enhancing cardiac filling. Thus pericardiocentesis is the treatment of choice and potentially provides some diagnostic information. If a significant volume of fluid is removed, the signs of right heart failure should resolve within days.

After initial pericardiocentesis the next therapeutic step depends on the underlying cause of the effusion. In animals with infectious pericarditis, treatment depends on the organism identified by cytology, culture, or possibly serologic results. Most cases of infectious pericarditis benefit from surgical pericardiectomy; this provides more effective drainage and helps avoid subsequent constrictive pericardial disease. Dogs with idiopathic pericarditis (culture-negative) are often treated conservatively with one or more centesis procedures followed by a course of broad-spectrum antibiotic and antiinflammatory doses of prednisone (1 mg/kg/day) tapering over 2 to 4 weeks. Recovery appears to occur with this approach in about 50% of cases. In cases with recurrent effusion, surgical subtotal pericardiectomy and pericardial biopsy are indicated and associated with very long median survival times. Pericardial removal allows the fluid to drain onto the larger absorptive surface of the pleura.

Neoplastic pericardial effusion with tamponade is also initially treated by pericardiocentesis. Chemotherapy may be palliative in some cases of lymphosarcoma or more rarely HSA and mesothelioma. Periodic pericardiocentesis can be done in some animals with neoplastic disease until the effusion becomes unmanageable. In some cases surgical approaches offer the best management options for neoplastic effusions.

Surgical Management

Pericardiectomy is indicated when multiple pericardiocentesis procedures fail to resolve the effusion, when pericardial constrictive disease is suspected, and when exploration and biopsy are needed to rule out suspected neoplastic or infectious disease. Subtotal pericardiectomy has been done most commonly, with removal of the pericardium below the phrenic nerves; but thoracoscopic partial pericardectomy has also been described with good results. The pericardium and biopsies of any masses are submitted for histopathologic evaluation. It is unusual to find a discrete mass that can be excised completely since most neoplastic conditions are too extensive at the time of diagnosis.

Animals with idiopathic pericardial effusion typically have a good prognosis after pericardiectomy because the pleural space can readily absorb the relatively small amount of fluid. Animals with neoplastic disease have a more variable prognosis. Cardiac HSA often has a rapidly progressive course, and metastases are commonly present at the time of diagnosis. Pericardiectomy should be performed cautiously in animals with cardiac HSA because tumor rupture and bleeding into the chest cavity could have dire consequences. Chemotherapy may be palliative in a select group, although there is no compelling evidence that survival times are prolonged significantly. Mean survival times of dogs with cardiac HSA are short, usually 2 to 4 weeks.

Pericardiectomy typically is helpful to alleviate cardiac tamponade in animals with pericardial mesothelioma; however, the procedure is thought to facilitate metastatic dissemination throughout the thoracic cavity. Even so, animals may survive longer with pleural effusion versus pericardial effusion; and in general periodic thoracocentesis is easier to perform. Intracavitary chemotherapy has been attempted in thoracic mesothelioma with limited success. Survival times after identification of pericardial effusion range from 3 to 10 months.

Chemodectoma tends to be slow growing and locally invasive but has a low rate of metastasis. Pericardiectomy in animals with chemodectoma can prolong quality of life for many months to sometimes years and is a good option in many cases.

A newer procedure, percutaneous balloon pericardiotomy, is gaining in popularity in humans for the management of chronic pericardial effusions. This technique also has been shown to be useful in dogs with chemodectoma and idiopathic pericardial effusion. Using general anesthesia and fluoroscopic guidance, a balloon-dilating catheter (14 to 20 mm diameter) may be placed percutaneously (fifth intercostal space) through a catheter-introducer sheath and positioned across the parietal pericardium. Multiple dilations are used to create a small window into the pericardium to allow for drainage. The advantages of this technique include low morbidity and mortality compared to thoracotomy, minimal recovery time, and decreased cost. Disadvantages include the need for special imaging equipment and possible premature closure of the stoma with recurrence of pericardial effusion. An alternative approach is to use a "mini-thoracotomy" and long surgical or laparoscopic instruments to remove a segment of pericardium via the small incisions.

References and Suggested Reading

Aronsohn MG, Carpenter JL: Surgical treatment of idiopathic pericardial effusion in the dog: 25 cases (1978-1993), *J Am Anim Hosp Assoc* 35:521, 1999.

Church WM et al: Characterization of immunohistochemical staining patterns for cardiac hemangiosarcoma, idiopathic pericarditis, heart base chemodectomas, and pericardial mesothelioma, *J Vet Intern Med* 19:416, 2005.

Day MJ, Martin MWS: Immunohistochemical characterization of the lesions of canine idiopathic pericarditis, *J Small Anim Pract* 43:382, 2002.

Ehrhart N et al: Analysis of factors affecting survival in dogs with aortic body tumor, *Vet Surg* 31(1):44, 2002.

Fine DM, Tobias AH, Jacob KA: Use of pericardial fluid pH to distinguish between idiopathic and neoplastic effusions, *J Vet Intern Med* 17:525, 2003.

Jackson J, Richter KP, Launer DP: Thoracoscopic partial pericardiectomy in 13 dogs, *J Vet Intern Med* 13:529, 1999.

Savitt MA et al: Physiology of cardiac tamponade and paradoxical pulse in conscious dogs, *Am J Physiol* 265:H1996, 1993.

Sidley JA et al: Percutaneous balloon pericardiotomy as a treatment for recurrent pericardial effusion in 6 dogs, *J Vet Intern Med* 16:541, 2002.

Stepien RL, Whitley NT, Dubielzig RR: Idiopathic or mesothelioma-related pericardial effusion: clinical findings and survival in 17 dogs studied retrospectively, *J Small Anim Pract* 41(8):342, 2000.

Tobias AH: Pericardial disorders. In Ettinger SJ, Feldman EC, editors: *Textbook of veterinary internal medicine*, St Louis, 2005, Elsevier, p 1104.

Ware WA, Hopper DL: Cardiac tumors in dogs: 1982-1995, *J Vet Intern Med* 13:95, 1999.

CHAPTER 182

Feline Heartworm Disease

CLARKE E. ATKINS, *Raleigh, North Carolina*

PREVALENCE IN THE UNITED STATES

Heartworm infection is less common in cats than in dogs, approximating 5% to 20% of the canine prevalence in a given geographic area (Ryan, Gross, and Soll, 1996). This has led to a low index of suspicion for feline heartworm disease (FHWD), with resultant underdiagnosis. In addition, the diagnosis of FHWD is often obscured because (1) cats are frequently amicrofilaremic; (2) serologic tests (specifically the enzyme-linked immunosorbent assay [ELISA] antigen and antibody tests) have lacked sensitivity or specificity in cats; (3) worm burdens are small; (4) aberrant sites are more common than in dogs; (5) clinical signs are often nonspecific and different from those seen in dogs; and (6) FHWD can easily be mistaken for feline bronchial disease (asthma) and responds to similar therapies. For these reasons, despite recent efforts at defining the scope of this problem in cats, the exact prevalence of FHWD is unknown and likely underestimated.

The greatest numbers of cases of feline heartworm infection (FHWI) have been reported from the southeastern United States, the Eastern Seaboard, the Gulf Coast, and within the Mississippi River valley (Ryan and Newcomb, 1996). Prevalence studies have focused mainly on cats from shelters (Fig. 182-1). Although this population choice has allowed the use of the relatively sensitive and very specific postmortem diagnosis, these studies are not necessarily applicable to pet cats, even in the same geographic region. These studies have revealed a prevalence of FHWI ranging from 0% to 14% (see Fig. 182-1). There are limited data in pet cats, but a joint study performed on such cats presented to the teaching hospitals of North Carolina State University (NCSU) and Texas A&M University for evaluation of cardio-respiratory signs demonstrated an infection prevalence of 9% and an exposure rate of 26%; the latter figure was based on antibody titers (Atkins et al., 1998). A number of serologic surveys, largely in asymptomatic cats, have demonstrated exposure rates (antibody seropositivity) of 5% to 36%, even in areas not considered heavily heartworm endemic and as high as 44% in symptomatic cats (Robertson-Plough, 1998). The largest survey to date evaluated over 2000 largely asymptomatic cats in areas by and large not thought to be regions of heavy exposure (Miller et al., 1998). The exposure rate was nearly 12% nationwide (Fig. 182-2). In my opinion heartworm infection should be considered a risk for cats in any locale in which dogs are considered at risk.

DIAGNOSIS

The diagnosis of FHWI or FHWD poses a unique and problematic set of issues. First, the clinical signs in cats are often different from those in dogs, and the index of suspicion is still generally low. Furthermore, the diagnosis is often elusive because eosinophilia is transient or absent and most cats are amicrofilaremic. Radiography, although helpful, is neither adequately sensitive nor specific, requires expertise in interpretation, and is excessively expensive as a screening tool. Echocardiography shows promise in terms of specificity but is costly, only moderately sensitive, and requires special equipment and expertise. Currently the most useful tests are the ELISA serologic tests, but these too are imperfect. The antigen test is very specific but is inadequately sensitive, missing over 50% of natural infections (McCall et al., 1995). On the other hand, the laboratory feline antibody test is very sensitive for exposure (and at least partial larval

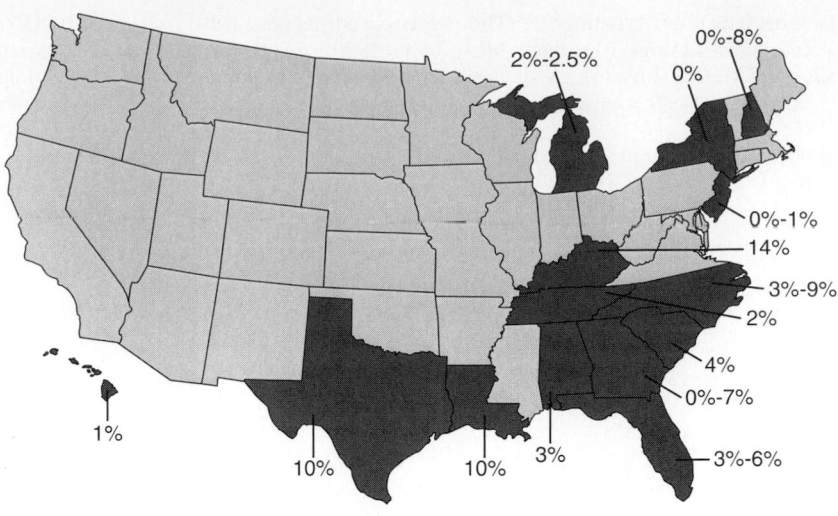

Fig. 182-1 Necropsy-proven prevalence of heartworm infection in shelter cats. The shaded states are those in which such studies have been completed. One Michigan study, which showed a prevalence of 2%, was an antigen study.

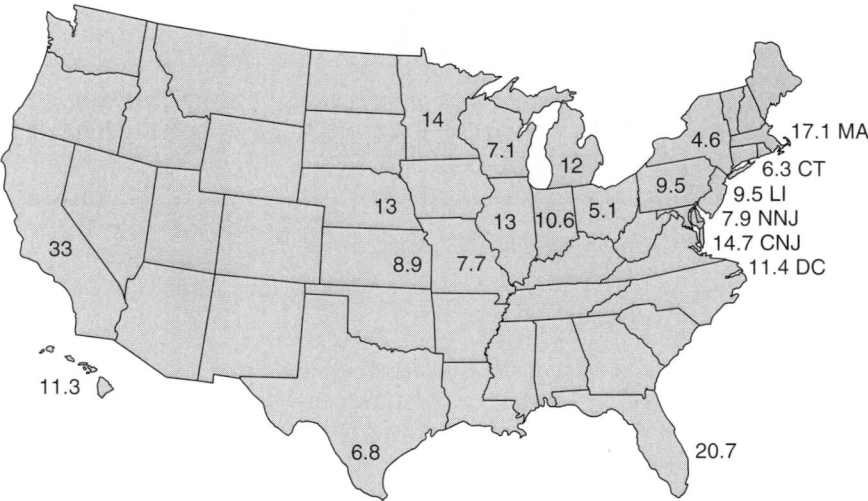

Fig. 182-2 Prevalence (percent antibody-positive) of heartworm exposure in over 2000 largely asymptomatic cats in 19 states (21 regions). *NNJ*, north New Jersey; *CNJ*, central New Jersey; *LI*, Long Island, NY (Miller et al., 2000).

development), but its specificity is low for mature infection, meaning that a positive test indicates exposure but not necessarily adult infection (McCall et al., 1995 and 1998). These two tests are often used in combination or in sequence. If used in sequence, the antibody test is performed first; if positive, the antigen test is then run.

Signalment, History, and Clinical Signs

Although no breeds of cat have been shown to be at increased risk for FHWI, most authors do suspect a male predisposition. This suspicion is based on the overall preponderance of male cats diagnosed with FHWI (71%; Ryan, Gross, and Soll, 1996) and the greater experimental infection rate in males than in females (McTier et al., 1993). However, the experience at NCSU suggests that, although more males (61%) than females are diagnosed with FHWI, the male-to-female ratio is not significantly different from that of the general population of cats seen at a teaching hospital (53% male; Atkins et al., 2000) or the population of cats presented with cardiorespiratory signs (60% male; Atkins et al., 1997). The typical cat with FHWI is 4 to 6 years of age, but the age range varies widely (range <1 to 19 years). The history of outdoor exposure

predicts a heightened risk of heartworm exposure (Miller et al., 1998). Nevertheless, over one fourth of heartworm-infected cats are reported by their owners to be housed totally indoors (Atkins et al., 2000). This may mean that indoor cats can be infected, that owners misinterpret the question when asked, or both. Although a seasonal incidence (August to December) has been suggested for FHWD (Guerrero et al., 1992), other studies do not support this contention (Atkins et al., 2000).

Heartworm-infected cats are often asymptomatic; and clinical manifestations, when present, may take either an acute (often cataclysmic) or a chronic (often waxing and waning) course. Acute or peracute presentation is usually caused by dead worm embolization, anaphylaxis, or migration of worms to the central nervous system. Signs variably include salivation, tachycardia, shock, dyspnea, cough, hemoptysis, vomiting and diarrhea, syncope, dementia, ataxia, circling, head tilt, blindness, seizures, and death. Sudden death, with little or no premonitory signs, has been observed in approximately 10% to 23% of cases (Atkins et al., 2000, Ryan, Gross, and Soll, 1996). Postmortem examination typically reveals pulmonary congestion and edema. Caval syndrome has also been recognized in cats.

Findings in chronic FHWD may include cough, dyspnea, anorexia, weight loss, lethargy, exercise intolerance, vomiting, and signs of right heart failure. Cough is a relatively consistent finding (>50% of cases, compared with 15% in cats with cardiorespiratory signs but not FHWI). When noted in cats in endemic areas, the suspicion of FHWD should increase. Likewise dyspnea, although less specific than cough, is present in 40% to 60% of cases. The pulmonary response to in situ heartworms in cats includes type II cell hyperplasia and activation of pulmonary intravascular macrophages. The latter response, not recognized in dogs, may explain the asthmalike syndrome recognized in some cats, even after they have been cleared of *Dirofilaria immitis* (Dillon, Warner, and Molina, 1996).

Physical examination is often unrewarding, although a murmur, a gallop, and/or diminished or adventitial lung sounds may be noted. In addition, cats may be thin and/or dyspneic. If heart failure is present, elevated heart rate, jugular venous distention, pleural effusion (often chylous), and rarely ascites are detected.

Hematology and Microfilarial Tests and Serology

Hematology

Although the presence of eosinophilia or basophilia may increase the index of suspicion for FHWI, tests for these conditions are of limited value. This is true because these hematologic changes are transient (present at 4 to 7 months after infection) and present in only 33% of cases (Dillon, 1984). In a prospective study of cats with cardiorespiratory signs, those with FHWD were not significantly more apt to have eosinophilia or basophilia than those not shown to be infected (Atkins et al., 1997).

Microfilarial Tests

A definitive diagnosis of FHWI can be made by the detection of circulating microfilariae using the modified Knott test, Millipore filter, direct smear, or microhematocrit techniques. One literature review indicated that 36% of 45 cats with FHWD were microfilaremic (Ryan, Gross, and Soll, 1996), whereas other reports have indicated that no more than 20% of infected cats are microfilaremic (Dillon, 1984; Atkins et al., 1997). This discrepancy probably reflects the fact that at the time of early reports diagnostic methods were limited to microfilarial tests and postmortem examination. Although increasing the volume of blood samples, multiple testing, and drawing evening samples may increase the diagnostic efficiency of the microfilaria-dependent tests, the low percentage of cats that become microfilaremic, the transient nature of microfilaremia, and the low microfilarial numbers seriously limit their usefulness.

Antigen Tests

All heartworm antigen tests currently marketed for dogs can be used in cats. There is now one antigen test kit designed specifically for the cat (SNAP Feline Heartworm Antigen Test, IDEXX Laboratories). Although virtually 100% specific, ELISA antigen tests have been of somewhat limited use in cats because of their inability to detect low worm burdens (one to two or fewer mature female worms); in general, naturally infected cats have one to three (most often one, almost always less than five) worms. In addition, since current tests detect antigens presumably produced in the reproductive tracts of mature female worms, they do not detect immature (<7 months) or all-male infections. These factors may result in false-negative results, and their importance is underscored by a review of 108 reported naturally occurring cases of feline HWD that revealed that 53% harbored single-worm infections and 18% had all-male infections (Ryan, Gross, and Soll, 1996). Furthermore, it is now clear that pulmonary pathology and presumably clinical signs may exist before worm maturation, at a time when cats are antigen negative (Selcer et al., 1996; Browne et al., 2005). These limitations are demonstrated in two studies. First, in a study of six commercial ELISA antigen tests, positive test results were obtained 36% to 93% of the time from the sera of 31 known positive cats harboring one to seven female worms (McTier et al., 1993). Although sensitivity increased with greater female worm burdens, no all-male heartworm infections were detected. Second, a commercial antigen test allowed detection of fewer than 40% of necropsy-proven, natural infections (McCall et al., 1995). False-negative antigen test results occur frequently, depending on the test used, the maturity and gender of the worms, and the worm burden. Advances in the sensitivity of ELISA antigen tests will probably improve their efficiency in the diagnosis of infections containing at least one female worm. Although the specificity of antigen tests is well accepted, the risk of false-positive results does increase with low prevalence areas. Therefore positive test results should be confirmed by a second test or supported by the presence of appropriate clinical findings (e.g., cough, radiographic lesions, echocardiography).

Antibody Tests

Three "send-off" ELISA antibody tests designed specifically for the diagnosis of FHWI (Animal Diagnostics, Inc., HESKA Corporation, and Antech Diagnostics) and one ELISA antibody test (Solo Step FH, HESKA Corp) designed for in-house use are available commercially. Published data on the "send-off" tests suggests higher specificity than has been found with previous antibody tests (McCall et al., 1998). Although less specific for mature infections than the antigen tests, the commercial ELISA antibody test is capable of detecting male-only and immature infections and has been shown to be useful in the detection of FHWI, even when antigen test results are negative (McCall et al., 1995). The antibody tests were shown to be 100% specific in determining cats to be heartworm negative before infection and detected 80% of experimental infections by 2 months, 97 to 100% by 3 months, and 100% by 4 months after infection (McCall et al., 1998). The antibody test was used to screen 215 random-source cats and detected 7 of 8 necropsy-proven cases (sensitivity = 88%) but at the same time gave false-positive results for 21 cats (90% specificity). The strength of this test is in *ruling out infection* (>99% negative predictive value), but a positive test clearly does not always indicate mature or current infection (positive predictive value <25%). A negative antibody test indicates either no infection or an early (<60- to 90-day) infection. A positive test result is thought to mean that (1) adults are present in the heart and/or pulmonary arteries, (2) past resolved infection with anti-bodies is still present, (3) precardiac late larva 4 (L4) or immature L5 infection exists, or (4) ectopic infection is present. Ideally a positive test result should be confirmed with an antigen test, echocardiography, or angiography and supported by the presence of appropriate clinical findings (e.g., cough, radiographic lesions). In addition to aiding in making a diagnosis of FHWI, the antibody test may be useful as a marker for exposure to heartworms, even in cats that never develop mature infection. Finally, the antibody test is currently the most logical single screening test for asymptomatic (and symptomatic) cats.

Imaging: Radiography and Echocardiography

Radiography
Radiographic findings of FHWD (Fig. 182-3) include enlarged caudal pulmonary arteries, often with ill-defined margins; pulmonary parenchymal changes, including focal or diffuse infiltrates (interstitial, bronchointerstitial, or even alveolar); perivascular density; and occasionally atelectasis or pleural effusion. Pulmonary hyperinflation and right heart enlargement may also be evident. Thoracic

radiography has been suggested as an excellent screening test for FHWD. However, although often helpful, thoracic radiography is neither sensitive nor specific in making the diagnosis of FHWD. The single most sensitive radiographic criterion (left caudal pulmonary artery diameter greater than 1.6 times that of the ninth rib at the ninth intercostal space) can be identified in only 53% of cases (Schafer and Berry, 1995) and may also be noted in heartworm-free cats with heart failure. Likewise, pulmonary parenchymal changes are only detectable radiographically in approximately 50% of natural cases (Schafer and Berry, 1995). Even though most cats with clinical signs have some radiographic abnormality, the findings are not specific for FHWD, are variable, and are often transient (Selcer et al., 1996). Finally, radiographic abnormalities have been detected in experimentally exposed cats that ultimately resisted heartworm maturation and were negative on postmortem examination (i.e., false-positive; Selcer et al., 1996). On the other hand, pulmonary angiography can be used to make a definitive diagnosis by the demonstration of radiolucent intravascular "foreign bodies" and enlarged, tortuous, and blunted pulmonary arteries.

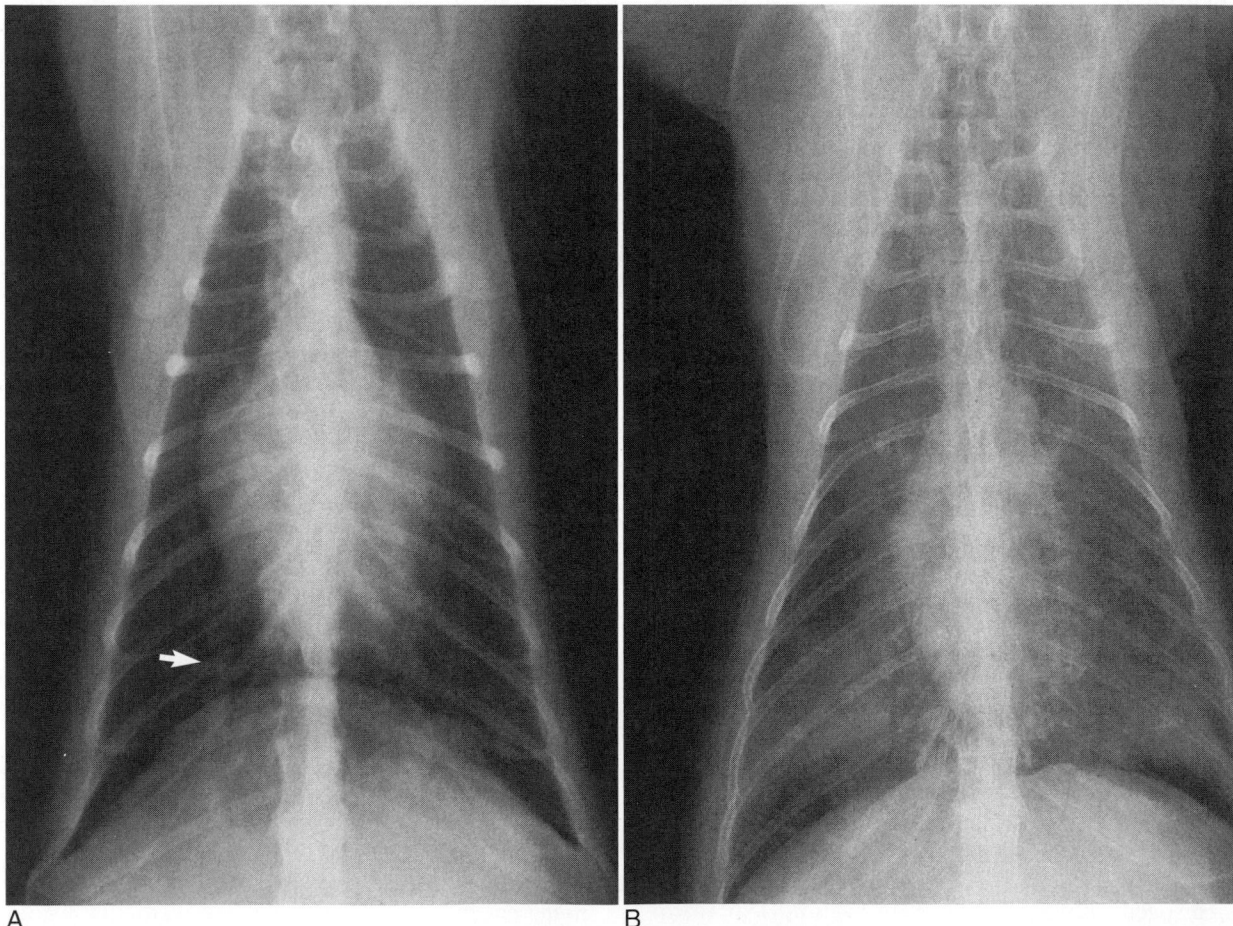

A   B

Fig. 182-3   A, Thoracic radiograph of a cat with mild radiographic signs of heartworm disease. Note the right caudal pulmonary artery *(arrow)*. The arrow is located at the ninth intercostal space, the site for comparison of the ninth rib with the caudal lobar pulmonary artery (either right or left). The finding of a pulmonary artery ≥1.6 times the radiographically-measured diameter of the ninth rib is suggestive of heartworm disease in the cat. **B,** Thoracic radiograph obtained from a more severely affected cat. Note the alveolar infiltrate in caudal lung lobes. (From Schafer M, Berry CR: *Vet Radiol Ultrasound* 36:499, 1995, with permission).

Echocardiography

Echocardiography is more sensitive in cats than in dogs for the detection of heartworm infection. Typically a "double-lined echodensity" (Fig. 182-4) is evident in the main pulmonary artery, one of its branches, the right ventricle, or occasionally the heart at the right atrioventricular junction. FHWI was detected echocardiographically in seven of nine natural cases and 12 of 16 experimental infections (Atkins et al., 1997; Selcer et al., 1996). A thorough examination that allows visualization of the bifurcation of the pulmonary artery is essential. A retrospective review of a larger case series (DeFrancesco et al., 1998) revealed a lower sensitivity when worms were not specifically sought and particularly when studies were performed by noncardiologists. This observation underscores the need for a high index of suspicion and expertise if this technique is to be of value in the diagnosis of FHWI. Although echocardiography can be a useful diagnostic tool, it cannot reliably determine worm numbers because of the coiling "posture" of heartworms that produces redundant shadows.

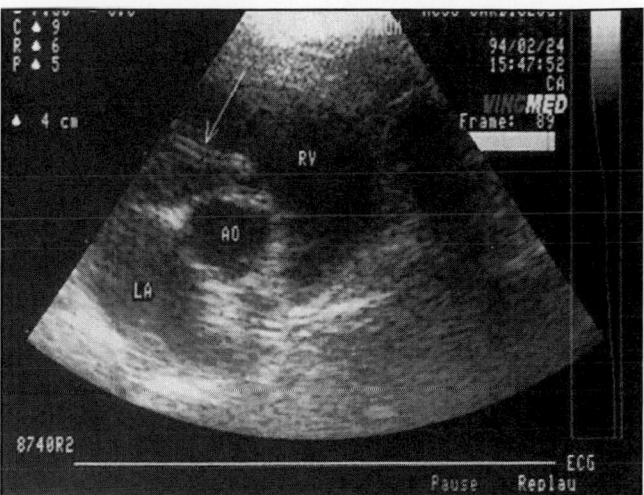

Fig. 182-4 A two-dimensional echocardiogram obtained from a cat with heartworm disease. A double-lined density (adult heartworm, indicated by arrow) is evident and is diagnostic for heartworm infection. *Ao,* Aorta; *RV,* right ventricle; *LA,* left atrium.

PREVENTION

The question arises as to whether heartworm prophylaxis is warranted for cats because they are not the natural host to *D. immitis* and because the incidence in cats is low. When deciding whether to institute prophylaxis, it is worth considering that the prevalence of FHWI in the southeastern United States and the Mississippi River valley approximates or even exceeds that of feline leukemia virus and feline immunodeficiency virus infections in the United States (Levy, 2006). Furthermore, a 1998 nationwide antibody survey of over 2000 largely asymptomatic cats revealed an exposure prevalence of nearly 12% (see Fig. 182-2; Miller et al., 1998). Finally, the consequences of FHWD are potentially dire, with no clear therapeutic solutions. Therefore I advocate preventive therapy in cats in endemic areas.

Four heartworm preventives with Food and Drug Administration approval are marketed for use in cats in the United States (Table 182-1). Ivermectin (Heartgard, Merial, Ltd.) is provided in a chewable formulation; milbemycin (INTERCEPTOR, Novartis Animal Health) as a flavored tablet; selamectin (Revolution, Pfizer Animal Health), a broad-spectrum parasiticide, comes in a topical formulation; and 10% imidacloprid/1% moxidectin (Advantage Multi, Bayer Animal Health), a broad-spectrum parasiticide is supplied in a topical formulation. It is important to emphasize that four feline heartworm preventives are available, all highly effective with monthly administration and with varied spectra and methods of administration to meet the needs of most clients.

Because cats are rarely microfilaremic, when present, microfilariae occur in low numbers; and, because rapid microfilarial elimination is not seen with most monthly preventives, screening for FHWI before initiation of a preventive is not absolutely necessary. Even though there is no reason to expect adverse reactions to prophylaxis in cats with existing FHWI, it may still be useful to know the heartworm status of cats before institution of a preventive as a gauge of heartworm risk (both for the individual and for other animals in the practice area). The current ELISA antigen tests are not adequately sensitive for this purpose and are not recommended unless the client is properly educated about the limitations of the test. The ELISA antibody test (alone or with an antigen test) is currently more appropriate because of its higher sensitivity and ability to identify cats at risk (infected or exposed).

Based on the severity of FHWD, the lack of an effective and safe adulticidal therapy, and the difficulty in making a definitive diagnosis, I believe that cat owners in endemic areas should be offered heartworm preventive for their feline pets. In addition, cats already infected with heartworms and their housemates should be placed on a preventive.

Table **182-1**

Comparisons of Macrolides Currently in Use in Cats for Heartworm Prevention

Drug	HW	Hook	Whip	Round	Tape	Flea/Eggs	Tick	Sarcoptes	Ear Mites
Ivermectin	+	+							
Milbemycin	+	+		+					
Selamectin	+	+		+		+/+			+
Imidacloprid/ moxidectin	+	+		+		+/−			+

THERAPY

Since the vast majority of cats are amicrofilaremic, microfilaricidal therapy is unnecessary in this species. The use of arsencial-adulticides is problematic. Thiacetarsemide is no longer available, and the data on melarsomine in experimental (transplanted) FHWI are limited and contradictory. Although there is an abstract report in which one injection (2.5 mg/kg; one half the recommended canine dose) of melarsomine was administered to experimentally infected cats without treatment-related mortality, the worm burdens after treatment were not significantly different from those found in untreated control cats (Goodman et al., 1996). Diarrhea and heart murmurs were noted frequently in treated cats. A second abstract report, using either the standard canine protocol (2.5 mg/kg twice over 24 hours) or the "split-dosage" (one injection followed by two injections 24 hours apart in 1 month), gave more favorable results (McLeroy et al., 1998). The standard treatment and split-dosage regimens resulted in 79% and 86% reduction in worm burdens, respectively, and there were no adverse reactions. Although promising, these unpublished data need to be interpreted with caution since the transplanted worms were young (<8 months old) and more susceptible and the control cats experienced a 53% worm mortality (average worm burden was reduced by 53% simply by the act of transplantation). In addition, the clinical experience in naturally infected cats has been generally unfavorable, with an unacceptable mortality. Because of the inherent risk, lack of clear benefit, and short life expectancy of heartworms in this species, I do not advocate adulticidal therapy in cats. Surgical or catheter-based removal of heartworms has been successful and is attractive because it minimizes the risk of thromboemboli. Unfortunately the mortality seen in the only published case series was unacceptable (two of five cats; Venco et al., 1999). However, this procedure may hold promise for the future using a less traumatic loop snare, thereby presumably reducing anaphylaxis resulting from worm trauma.

Cats with HWI should be placed on a monthly preventive, and short-term corticosteroid therapy (prednisone, 1 to 2 mg/kg q48h TID) used to manage respiratory signs. If signs recur, alternate-day steroid therapy (at the lowest dosage that controls signs) can be continued indefinitely. For embolic/anaphylactic emergencies, oxygen, corticosteroids (dexamethasone, 1 mg/kg intravenously [IV] or intramuscularly [IM]; or prednisolone sodium succinate, 50 to 100 mg IV/cat), and bronchodilators (aminophylline at 6.6 mg/kg IM q12h; theophylline, sustained release 5 to 7 mg/kg orally [PO] BID; or terbutaline, 0.01 mg/kg subcutaneously [SC]) may be used. Bronchodilators based on the ability of agents such as the xanthines (aminophylline and theophylline), to improve function of fatigued respiratory muscles. In addition, the finding of hyperinflation of lung fields may indicate bronchoconstriction, a condition for which bronchodilation would be indicated. Nevertheless I do not use bronchodilators routinely in FHWD.

The use of aspirin has been questioned because vascular changes associated with FHWI consume platelets, increasing their turnover rate and effectually diminishing the antithrombotic effects of the drug. Conventional doses of aspirin did not prevent angiographically detected vascular lesions (Rawlings, 1990). Dosages of aspirin necessary to produce even limited histologic benefit approached the toxic range. Despite this, because therapeutic options are limited, aspirin at conventional doses (80 mg PO q72h) is well tolerated, generally harmless, inexpensive, and convenient; and, because the quoted studies were based on relatively insensitive estimates of platelet function and pulmonary arterial disease (thereby possibly missing subtle benefits), I continue to advocate aspirin for *asymptomatic* cats with HWI. Aspirin is *not* prescribed concurrently with corticosteroid therapy. Management of other signs of HWD in cats is largely symptomatic.

PROGNOSIS

In the aforementioned study of 50 cats with natural heartworm infection, at least 12 cats died of causes other than heartworm disease. Seven of these and two living cats were considered to have survived heartworm disease (lived ≥1000 days; Atkins et al., 2000). The median survival for all heartworm-infected cats living beyond the day of diagnosis was 1460 days (4 years; range 2 to 4015 days), whereas the median survival of all cats (n=48 with adequate follow-up) was 540 days (1.5 years; range 0 to 4015 days). Survival of 11 cats treated with sodium thiacetarsemide (mean 1669 days) was not significantly different from that of the 30 managed without adulticide (mean 1107 days). Likewise youth (≤3 years of age), presence of dyspnea, cough, ELISA-positivity for heartworm antigen, presence of echocardiographically identifiable worms, or gender of the cat did not appear to affect survival. Comparison of other cardiovascular disease prognoses to FHWI reveals that survival is roughly equivalent to that of hypertrophic cardiomyopathy (Atkins et al., 2003).

References and Suggested Reading

Atkins CE: Veterinary CE Advisor: Heartworm disease: an update, *Vet Med* 93(suppl):12:2, 1998.

Atkins CE et al: Prevalence of heartworm infection in cats with signs of cardiorespiratory abnormalities, *J Vet Med Assoc* 212:517, 1997.

Atkins CE et al: Heartworm infection in cats: 50 cases (1985-1997), *J Vet Med Assoc* 217:355, 2000.

Atkins et al: Prognosis in feline heartworm infection: comparison to other cardiovascular disease. In Seward LR, Knight DH, editors: *Proceedings of the heartworm symposium '01*, Batavia, Ill, 2003, American Heartworm Society, p 41.

Browne LE et al: Pulmonary arterial disease in cats seropositive for *Dirofilaria immitis* but lacking adult heartworms in the heart and lungs, *Am J Vet Res* 66:1544, 2005.

DeFrancesco TC et al: Diagnostic utility of echocardiography in feline heartworm disease. In Soll MD, Knight DH, editors: *Proceedings of the American heartworm symposium '98*, Batavia, Ill, 1998, American Heartworm Society.

Dillon AR: Feline dirofilariasis, *Vet Clin North Am* 114:1184, 1984.

Dillon AR, Warner AE, Molina RM: Pulmonary parenchymal changes in dogs and cats after experimental transplantation of dead *Dirofilaria immitis*. In Soll MD, Knight DH, editors: *Proceedings of the heartworm symposium '95*, Batavia, Ill, 1996, American Heartworm Society, p 97.

Goodman DA et al: Evaluation of a single dose of melarsomine dihydrochloride for adulticidal activity against *Dirofilaria Immitis* in cats, *Proc Am Assoc Vet Parasitol* 41(abstr):64; 1996.

Guerrero J et al: Prevalence of *Dirofilaria immitis* infection in cats from the southeastern United States, In Soll MD, editor: *Proceedings of the heartworm symposium '92*, Batavia, Ill, 1992, American Heartworm Society, p 91.

Levy JK et al: Seroprevalence of feline leukemia virus and immunodeficiency virus infection among cats in North America and risk factors for Seropositivity, *J Vet Med Assoc* 228: 371, 2006.

McCall JW et al: Utility of ELISA-based antibody test for detection of heartworm infection in cats. In Soll MD, Knight DH, editors: *Proceedings of the American heartworm symposium '95*, Batavia, Ill, 1995, American Heartworm Society, p 127.

McCall JW et al: Evaluation of antigen and antibody tests for detection of heartworm infection in cats. In Soll MD, Knight DH, editors: *Proceedings of the American heartworm symposium '98*, Batavia, Ill, 1998, American Heartworm Society, p 127.

McLeroy LW et al: Evaluation of melarsomine dihydrochloride (Immiticide) for adulticidal activity against *Dirofilaria immitis* in cats, *Proc Am Assoc Vet Parasitol* 43(abstr):67; 1998.

McTier TL et al: Evaluation of ELISA-based adult heartworm antigen test kits using well-defined sera from experimentally and naturally infected cats. In Proceedings of the 38th Annual Meeting of the American Association of Veterinary Parasitologists (abstract), Minneapolis, 1993, p 37.

Miller MW et al: Prevalence of exposure to *Dirofilaria immitis* in cats from multiple areas of the United States. In Soll MD, Knight DH, editors: *Proceedings of the heartworm symposium '98*, American Heartworm Society, 1998, Batavia, Ill, p 161.

Rawlings CA: Pulmonary arteriography and hemodynamics during feline heartworm disease, *J Vet Intern Med* 4:285, 1990.

Robertson-Plough CK et al: Prevalence of feline heartworm infection among cats with respiratory and gastrointestinal signs: results of a multicenter study. In Soll MD, Knight DH, editors: *Proceedings of the heartworm symposium '98*, Batavia, IL, 1998, American Heartworm Society, p 127.

Ryan WG, Newcomb KM: Prevalence of feline heartworm disease: a global review. In Soll MD, Knight DH, editors: *Proceedings of the heartworm symposium '95*, Batavia, Ill, 1996, American Heartworm Society, p 79.

Ryan WG, Gross SJ, Soll MD: Diagnosis of feline heartworm infection. In Soll MD, Knight DH, editors: *Proceedings of the heartworm symposium '95*, Batavia, Ill, 1996, American Heartworm Society, p 121.

Schafer M, Berry CR: Cardiac and pulmonary artery mensuration in feline heartworm disease, *Vet Radiol Ultrasound* 36:499, 1995.

Selcer BA et al: Radiographic and 2-D echocardiographic findings in eighteen cats experimentally exposed to *D. immitis* via mosquito bites, *Vet Radiol Ultrasound* 37:37, 1996.

Venco L et al: Surgical Removal of heartworms in naturally infected cats. In Seward RL, Knight DH, editors: *Proceedings of the heartworm symposium '98*, Batavia, Ill, 1999, American Heartworm Society, p 241.

CHAPTER 183

Canine Heartworm Disease

MATTHEW W. MILLER, *College Station, Texas*
SONYA G. GORDON, *College Station, Texas*

Despite the availability of several very effective and safe preventive medications, heartworm disease continues to be an important disease of both dogs and cats. This chapter briefly reviews the life cycle of this parasite, diagnostic studies, and staging of disease. Treatment and prevention of canine dirofilariasis is the focus of this chapter. Feline heartworm disease is described in the preceding chapter.

DIAGNOSIS AND STAGING OF CANINE HEARTWORM DISEASE

Life cycle of *Dirofilaria immitis*

A basic knowledge of the life cycle of the heartworm parasite is important for understanding strategies for prevention, diagnosis, and therapy. The mosquito is a requisite intermediate host for transmission of this disease. The first-stage larvae (L_1) or microfilaria are ingested by the mosquito following a blood meal from an infected animal. The parasite molts twice within the mosquito, and these molts are required for the parasite to develop into the infective third stage (L_3). The parasite maturation within the mosquito from L_1 to L_3 requires approximately 2 to 3 weeks. In addition, appropriate environmental conditions are necessary for development. One of the most important of these is an average daily temperature in excess of 64° F for longer than 30 consecutive days.

The L_3 larvae are the infective stage of the parasite and are transmitted to a susceptible host following a bite from an infected mosquito. The third larval stage travels within the subcutaneous tissues of the new host, molting to the fourth larval stage (L_4) in approximately 1 to 2 weeks and becomes a young adult (L_5) in 30 to 60 days. These young adults enter the systemic venous system and are carried to the lungs approximately 100 days after infection. Under ideal conditions the infection can become patent (adult worms producing microfilaria) in 5 months, but more often this complete cycle requires in excess of 6 months.

Establishing a Diagnosis

The American Heartworm Society (AHWS) (www.heartwormsociety.org) recommends that an adult heartworm antigen (Ag) be used as the primary screening test for the disease in dogs. There are numerous suppliers of the heartworm Ag test, and readers are referred to excellent comparative articles (Atkins, 2003; Courtney, 2001) for relative sensitivity and specificity of these tests. Ag testing is substantially more sensitive than microfilarial concentration tests. In addition, the widespread use of monthly preventive medication has decreased the sensitivity of the microfilarial tests by rendering the vast majority of infections amicrofilaremic (occult) while having no effect on the sensitivity of the Ag tests. Circulating Ag is generally undetectable until 6 to 7 months following infection.

As a general rule, weakly positive test results should be rechecked by either repeating the original test or submitting a sample for evaluation using a different Ag test, preferably at a reference laboratory. False-positives occur infrequently but are almost always associated with technical errors. False-negative tests are usually the result of immature infections, infection with low female worm numbers, or all male infections. Another potential but less likely cause for a false-negative test is complexing of circulating Ag with antibody, leaving insufficient free Ag available for detection.

The use of concentration tests for detection of circulating microfilaria is no longer recommended for routine screening of patients with suspected infection. The simultaneous use of both an Ag and a concentration test has been advocated by some since it may increase the likelihood of establishing a definitive diagnosis on the small percentage of cases in which a very low number of gravid females is present or on the patient in which all Ag is complexed. However, once a positive Ag test is obtained, performing a concentration test to determine the concentration of circulating microfilaria is important. This information may

dictate the preventive medication used. Some preventive medications (milbemycin) are potent microfilaricides at the suggested preventive dose and may be associated with substantial risk of a shocklike reaction when administered to heavily microfilaremic dogs. It is prudent to recommend that the client observe a microfilaremic patient for the entire day following administration of the first dose of preventive, no matter what preventive is used.

Classification and Staging

Before heartworm therapy the dog with heartworm infection should be classified, optimally based on radiographic findings and laboratory studies. When heartworm disease causes clinical signs, these are generally attributable to pulmonary parenchymal injury, pulmonary arterial injury, or cardiac dysfunction. Additional infrequently encountered clinical syndromes include severe glomerular disease, caval syndrome, and disseminated intravascular coagulopathy.

There are a number of ways to classify patients with positive heartworm tests. One approach is related to the use of the Immiticide brand of melarsomine and is based on the Food and Drug Administration (FDA)–approved label (Table 183-1). The drug package insert for Immiticide provides very detailed and specific information about this classification system. Another way is to consider heartworm patients in terms of clinical syndromes or presentations, an approach that overlaps the aforementioned classification system but also provides additional perspective regarding treatment approaches. Dogs can be characterized clinically as follows:

- *Asymptomatic* or equivocal signs: Heartworm infection is evident, but there is no clear evidence of disease.
- *Respiratory signs* of heartworm disease, including cough and tachypnea with exercise: These problems are often related to heartworm-induced pneumonitis or lung fibrosis; some but not all dogs also have evidence of pulmonary vascular disease.
- *Cor pulmonale*—Radiographic evidence of significant pulmonary vascular disease: Typical clinical findings include limited exercise capacity and possibly

Table **183-1**

Classification of Heartworm Disease Severity in Dogs

Class	Clinical Signs	Radiographic Signs	Clinicopathologic Abnormalities
1: Mild	None or occasional cough; fatigue with exercise or mild loss of condition	None	None
2: Moderate	None or occasional cough; fatigue with exercise; mild or moderate loss of condition	Right ventricular enlargement and/or some pulmonary enlargement ± perivascular and mixed alveolar-interstitial opacities	± Mild anemia (PVC 20%-30%); ± proteinuria
3: Severe	General loss of condition or cachexia; fatigue on exercise or mild activity; occasional or persistent cough ± dyspnea or right sided heart failure	Right ventricular ± right atrial enlargement; moderate-to-severe pulmonary artery enlargement; perivascular and mixed alveolar-interstitial opacities	± Anemia (PVC <30%); ± proteinuria
4: Very severe	Caval syndrome		

PVC, Premature ventricular contraction.

exertional collapse or syncope; some but not all dogs have significant pulmonary parenchymal changes.

- *Congestive heart failure* (CHF): Right-sided heart failure is a complication of severe pulmonary vascular disease and pulmonary hypertension and cor pulmonale that follow.
- *Caval syndrome*—an acute syndrome related to a large worm burden, severe pulmonary hypertension, and right ventricular dysfunction with tricuspid regurgitation: Hepatic congestion and intravascular hemolysis with hemoglobinuria are classic clinical signs
- Heartworm infection or disease in a dog with *serious comorbid conditions*: Examples include malignant neoplasia, diabetes mellitus, and chronic renal failure.

ADULTICIDE THERAPY FOR CANINE HEARTWORM DISEASE

If necessary, dogs with heartworm disease should be classified and stabilized before adulticidal therapy. Dogs with *significant respiratory signs* and pulmonary infiltration generally are treated with glucocorticoids, typically prednisone at 0.5 mg/kg once or twice daily for 7 to 14 days. Patients with eosinophilic pneumonitis often show a marked improvement in clinical signs. Dogs with *severe cor pulmonale* based on radiographic signs (or evidence of heart failure) should be given strict rest before and after adulticidal treatment. Other therapies, including aspirin and heparin, have been used empirically in dogs with severe cor pulmonale, but there is no consensus for their use, and we do not recommend these drugs. There is a clear risk of gastrointestinal bleeding with aspirin therapy, and the risk is extremely high if nonsteroidal antiinflammatory drugs are combined with corticosteroids. When *right-sided CHF* is evident, adulticide therapy is delayed for a number of weeks until CHF has been stabilized and resolved medically (see Chapter 171). In general, the management of CHF in heartworm disease involves strict rest, furosemide to effect, an angiotensin-converting enzyme inhibitor, and possibly pimobendan. Dogs with caval syndrome should be referred immediately to a hospital experienced in removing filarial parasites. Melarsomine should not be given to dogs with caval syndrome. Patients with heartworm infection suffering from other serious systemic disorders are generally handled on a case-by-case basis.

Melarsomine Dihydrochloride (Immiticide)

The only currently approved drug for adulticide therapy is melarsomine dihydrochloride (Immiticide) (Merial). It is safer and more efficacious than its predecessor (sodium caparsolate). Most often the drug is administered at 2.5 mg/kg intramuscularly twice, 24 hours apart. In more severe cases, especially in dogs with marked cor pulmonale (heartworm class 3; see Table 183-1), melarsomine should be administered in a "split dose," which consists of an initial injection followed in approximately 1 month by a series of two injections over a 24-hour period. This lowers the initial kill rate, thereby diminishing the impact of dying worms on the pulmonary vasculature.

Despite the enhanced safety of this product, adverse reactions are still noted. In fact, by definition successful pharmacologic adulticidal therapy dictates thromboembolic events. The severity of this complication can be diminished by restricting exercise after melarsomine administration and by using the split-dose regimen recommended for class 3 heartworm disease. A 4- to 6-week period of severe exercise restriction after adulticidal therapy is recommended. The method and degree of exercise restriction varies with the client needs and the pet's inherent activity level but might include hospitalization, cage rest, sedation, housing in a restricted room of the house or garage, and only gentle leash walks.

Nevertheless, some owners do not or cannot restrict exercise, resulting in or worsening thromboembolic complications. In addition, severe adverse reactions may be noted when dogs are incorrectly (or even correctly) categorized as class 1 or class 2 heartworm disease severity and subsequently treated with the traditional two-injection regimen. To minimize the chance of thromboembolic complication it would be reasonable to adapt an alternative approach, using the three-injection (split-dose) method in all class 1, 2, or 3 heartworm infections.

Split versus Standard Dosing of Melarsomine

Studies have shown that patients treated with the split-dose regimen (three total doses) have a higher seroconversion to a negative Ag status (89.7%) rate than patients treated with either caparsolate (65.9%) or the standard melarsomine dosing regimen of a total of two doses 24 hours apart (76.2%). In addition, in a study using experimental heartworm infection in dogs, more effective adulticide activity did not appear to increase the severity of clinically apparent pulmonary hypertension or thromboembolism. Perhaps more important, killing worms in two increments of approximately 50% each diminishes the insult to the lung and pulmonary vasculature. This approach is critical in dogs with advanced cor pulmonale. After approximately 50% of the worms are destroyed, there is a 1-month interval for the lungs to heal before the second insult of dying worms starts. Furthermore, if there is a significant adverse reaction to the initial adulticidal injection, the second and third injections can be delayed (or even cancelled) until clinical signs have resolved and damaged tissue can heal (i.e., typically in 2 to 3 months).

Disadvantages to this split or two-step approach include the added cost of the third injection. This may be counteracted by reduction in adverse reactions, which often require hospitalization and intensive therapy. Second, the total arsenic dosage is increased, which may be an issue in the dog with significant renal disease. Despite these concerns, we have found the approach to be well tolerated generally, and we advocate a two-dose regimen with supportive fluid therapy for dogs with significant renal disease requiring heartworm adulticidal therapy. Finally, exercise restriction is often a problem for owners, and the "split dose" regimen requires approximately 2 months' exercise restriction (Fig. 183-1). This may prove difficult for some owners.

We believe that the split, three-injection approach of melarsomine administration provides the best management strategy for virtually all heartworm infections.

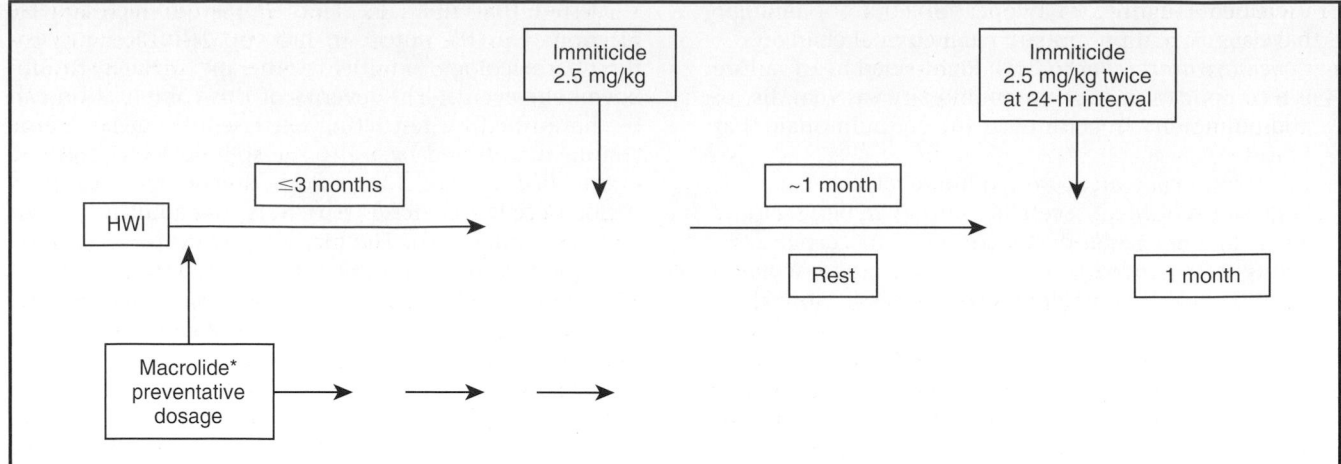

Fig. 183-1 Our preferred approach to adulticidal therapy in all dogs infected with heartworms includes three doses of melarsomine. Macrolide prophylaxis is begun at the time of diagnosis, if not already in use. *If microfilaremic, care should be given to prevent or observe and treat adverse reactions, based on microfilarial numbers and macrolide used. See text for complete description.

This treatment regimen is safer and probably more effective than the two-dose regimen, justifying the increased cost. The AHWS now advocates this approach as well. Even if owners cannot afford the minimum database for evaluation of general health and the presence and severity of heartworm disease, they may still benefit financially by use of the three-dose regimen. In such instances, even though the attending clinician has more difficulty predicting an adverse reaction without thoracic radiographs, the likelihood of adverse reaction (and attendant costs) can be reduced by this approach.

Administration and Clinical Use of Melarsomine

At the time of heartworm diagnosis by a positive Ag test, we recommend completing a database that includes a patient history, complete physical examination, microfilaria test, serum chemistry panel, complete blood count, urinalysis, and thoracic radiographic evaluation. At this time a monthly macrolide preventive is prescribed (see Figure 183-1). This approach is used to prevent further infection; to eliminate microfilariae (since this renders the dog risk free as a reservoir of infection); and to destroy developing L_4 larvae, a stage not susceptible to adulticidal therapy. The risk of an adverse reaction in microfilaria-negative dogs (occult infection) is very low with any preventive. In microfilaremic dogs the first macrolide dosage is administered in the hospital or at home with observation so that an adverse reaction might be recognized and treated promptly. Corticosteroids with or without antihistamines (either dexamethasone at 0.25 mg/kg intravenously [IV] and Benadryl at 2 mg/kg intramuscularly [IM] *or* 1 mg/kg of prednisolone orally [PO] 1 hour before and possibly 6 hours after administration of the first dose of preventive) are administered in our practice to reduce the potential for adverse reaction in patients with high microfilaria counts. It is important to emphasize that adverse reactions are unusual with macrolides at preventive doses; however, the risk is probably greater with milbemycin than with the doses of ivermectin, selamectin, or moxidectin used for prevention of heartworm infection.

Depending on the time of year, as long as 2 to 3 months might be allowed to lapse before adulticidal therapy is administered. Monthly macrolide administration ensures that the dog is at no risk of additional infection and prevents maturation of infections of 3 months' duration or less. Theoretically infections of 4 months but less than 6 months are too old to be prevented with monthly preventives, but the immaturity of the worms would make them relatively resistant to therapy with melarsomine. Administering preventives for 2 to 3 months before administration of the first dose of melarsomine would not only prevent young infections from maturing, but the delay also would allow larval maturation to adulthood, ensuring that the only stage of the life cycle present is the mature L_5, which is vulnerable to melarsomine therapy. This delay is particularly important if the diagnosis is made during or at the end of a mosquito exposure season. If the diagnosis is made in the spring or late winter when infective larvae are most likely mature, adulticidal therapy may be initiated immediately (see Fig. 183-1).

The first injection of melarsomine is administered by deep intramuscular injection (2.5 mg/kg) in the lumbar musculature as described fully in the package insert. The injection needle is changed before injection, and care is taken to inject deep into the muscle. The injection site is recorded. It is important to place the injection in the center of the epaxial muscle. Typically patients are hospitalized for the day of the injections. Some dogs seem to experience discomfort, depression, or nausea following injection; for this reason some clinicians administer butorphanol (0.3 to 0.4 mg/kg IM) before injection. Sedation also helps to ensure excellent injection technique. The need for exercise restriction for at least 1 month is emphasized, and sedation is provided if necessary. Owners are also advised regarding potential adverse reactions (fever, lethargy, inappetence, cough, dyspnea, and collapse) and to call if they have concerns. Since these signs are often related to the predictable pulmonary reaction to dead worms, some clinicians routinely dispense prednisolone (0.5 mg/kg daily) to be used specifically for signs of increased coughing, tachypnea, or lethargy. Generally 5 to 7 days of therapy are sufficient to overcome pulmonary reactions to dead worms. The owners are advised that they must return for a second series of two injections in approximately 1 month.

If serious systemic reaction results, the second stage of the adulticidal treatment may be delayed or even cancelled. However, even with severe postadulticide reactions, the entire treatment protocol generally is completed within 2 to 5 months (see Fig. 183-1). After a minimum of 1 month the melarsomine injection procedure is repeated; the injection site is recorded again. If significant local reaction was noted after the first injection, dexamethasone or oral nonsteroidal antiinflammatory drugs are used to minimize pain at the injection site that accompanies subsequent injections. Butorphanol can also be used as described previously. The following day (approximately 24 hours after the first injection) the process is repeated with injection into the *opposite* lumbar area. Client instructions are similar to those previously given, with reemphasis of the need for strict exercise restriction.

Ag testing is repeated 6 months following the second series of injections; a positive test result indicates incomplete adulticidal efficacy. It is emphasized that, despite the proven efficacy of melarsomine, not all worms are killed in every patient. Typically worm burden is markedly reduced; but if as few as one to three adult female worms remain, positive Ag tests are likely. Whether or not repeat adulticidal therapy is warranted under these circumstances is decided on a case-by-case basis, with input from the owners and perhaps a specialist.

The Role of Wolbachia

Like most filarial nematodes, *D. immitis* harbors obligate, intracellular, gram-negative bacteria belonging to the genus *Wolbachia* (*Rickettsiales*). Studies in non-*D. immitis* filariae demonstrated that treatment with tetracyclines during the first month of infection was lethal to some *Wolbachia*-harboring filariae but not to a filaria that did not harbor *Wolbachia*. In addition, treatment of *Wolbachia*-harboring filariae suppressed microfilaremia. Although similar studies with *D. immitis* have not yet been reported, in one study tetracycline treatment of heartworm-infected dogs resulted in infertility in the female worms. It has been suggested that *Wolbachia* contributes to pulmonary and renal inflammation through its surface protein WSP, independently from its endotoxin component. Studies to determine the role of *Wolbachia* in the pathogenesis of heartworm disease and the clinical use of suppressing these populations with doxycycline before adulticide therapy may provide an additional means by which to reduce the severity of postadulticide therapy. Some clinicians are already suggesting pretreatment of animals with doxycycline for 30 days before adulticide therapy; however, there are no published data to demonstrate better outcomes with this approach.

Monthly Preventives as Adulticides

Much has been written about the adulticidal properties of the monthly preventives. Some individuals have suggested that the adulticidal properties represent an alternative to melarsamine. The variable efficacy of the preventives is correlated with what is frequently called *reach-back*. This term is misleading in that the property that is being described is simply a reflection of efficacy against older infections. Based on data published thus far, ivermectin has the highest efficacy against mature infections. McCall and colleagues (2001) reported that, when given monthly for longer than 24 months at the standard preventive dose, ivermectin is 98% effective against 5-month-old worms and 95% effective against 7-month-old worms. The same efficacy data have not been published in older infections. Despite these intriguing results Rawlings and colleagues (2001) showed that dogs with 5.5- to 6.5-month-old infections started on the label doses of either ivermectin or milbemycin developed radiographic changes and necropsy findings similar to dogs with the same age infections that were untreated. These results reinforced the recommendations of the AHWS that dogs be tested with an Ag test *before* being started on preventive medication and that *dogs found to be AG positive receive treatment with an adulticide* before starting on a preventive medication.

Elimination of Circulating Microfilaria

Historically, elimination of circulating microfilaria has been attempted several months following adulticide therapy as the second step in the treatment of a patent infection. The general recommendation now is that elimination of circulating microfilaria be accomplished as a secondary benefit of chemoprophylaxis, although some argue that rapid elimination of circulating microfilaria will more quickly eliminate a potential disease reservoir. Despite this concern, the monthly preventives will eliminate microfilaria and also that reservoir of infection.

It is sometimes difficult to eliminate circulating microfilaria before completion of adulticide therapy. However, even without adulticide therapy, circulating microfilaria can be eliminated with several sequential months of therapy with a macrocyclic lactone, including ivermectin, milbemycin oxime, moxidectin, and selamectin. As previously mentioned, administration of a macrocyclic lactone should begin as soon as a definitive diagnosis is established.

The macrocyclic lactones are the safest and most effective microfilaricidal drugs to date. However, none of these drugs is approved currently as a microfilaricide by the United States FDA. Use of the monthly preventives for this purpose is covered by the Animal Medicinal Drug Use Clarification Act of 1994, which allows licensed veterinarians extralabel use of certain drugs that have an established clinical application, provided a valid veterinarian-client-patient relationship exists. Ensuring proper dose administration and providing appropriate aftercare when products are used in an extralabel application are the personal responsibilities of the dispensing veterinarian. The AHWS has taken a firm stance on the use of high-dose ivermectin for rapid elimination of microfilaria. The following is from the current treatment guidelines: "It is both unnecessary and dangerous to use livestock preparations of these drugs (ivermectin) to achieve higher doses for the purpose of achieving more rapid results." They go on to suggest that, if rapid elimination of circulating microfilaria is deemed important, milbemycin oxime should be used since it is the most potent microfilaricide producing the most rapid rate of microfilaria clearance. Clearance of circulating microfilaria can also be accelerated by administering the monthly preventive dose of any of the currently available macrolides every 2 weeks. Once the microfilaria are cleared, the standard dose should be administered monthly.

Again, the need for rapid clearance of microfilaria is controversial and not without potential complications. Although most reactions are mild and transient (lethargy, inappetence, salivation, and retching), important clinical manifestations of rapid microfilaria death can occur and include hypotension, pale mucous membranes, tachycardia, and collapse. High-risk dogs should be observed for the first 8 to 12 hours following administration of potentially microfilaricidal drugs. We pretreat these dogs with prednisolone, 1 mg/kg orally, or dexamethasone, 0.25 g/kg intravenously, 1 hour before administration of the first dose of monthly preventive to a microfilaria-positive dog Although severe reactions are seen most commonly in dogs with high microfilaria counts, occasionally dogs with microfilaremia as low as 5000 microfilaria per milliliter develop acute circulatory collapse.

HEARTWORM PREVENTION IN DOGS

Canine heartworm disease is an almost completely preventable disease despite the fact that the dog is an exceptionally susceptible host. Administration of heartworm prophylaxis is suggested for all dogs living in endemic areas. Although year-round chemoprophylaxis may not be necessary throughout the northern half of the country, it is important to remember that successful seasonal prophylaxis depends on proper timing of heartworm *preventive* administration. When heartworm transmission can potentially occur over more than 6 months, seasonal chemoprophylaxis may not be the most effective method of prevention. Year-round treatment should be considered to enhance compliance and control other parasitic infections.

The currently available macrolides (ivermectin, milbemycin, moxidectin, and selamectin) have all been shown to have exceptional efficacy when administered appropriately at recommended doses and dosing intervals. The ideal *preventive* medication is the product that best promotes client compliance.

Product Switching

Occasionally the type of preventive medication used needs to be switched. Rarely does this result from intolerance to the product. More often it is related to perceived superiority or preference of administration route (topical versus oral) by the client, the prescribing veterinarian, or both. When product switching occurs, it is important to establish a temporal line of evidence regarding the Ag status of that animal so that, in the unlikely event of a prevention failure, the circumstances of the break can be ascertained.

Although this may seem superfluous, there have been so-called prevention failures with heartworm preventives, and this approach establishes the most likely cause. We recommend obtaining a contemporary Ag test at the time of product switch. Any infection that is 6 months old or older would be expected to result in an Ag-positive status and therefore implicate the first product as responsible for prevention failure. If the Ag test is negative, the new product is begun at the appropriate dosage, and a retesting schedule established. Any infection that is 3 months old or younger will almost certainly be prevented by monthly administration of all the currently available preventives. Conversely, a 4-month-old infection, although not identified by the initial Ag test, will, depending on the product used, probably go on to become a mature infection. Seroconversion will most likely occur 6 to 7 months after infection or 2 to 4 months after the Ag tests performed at the time of product switching. Any new infection associated with exposure during that time would be too young to be detected by an Ag test. Therefore repeating the Ag test 4 months after the product was switched allows the veterinarian to determine if a prevention break occurred while the patient was receiving the initial product. If the Ag test at 4 months is negative, it is very strong evidence that the initial product was effective. Seroconversion to a positive status 4 months or more after product switching implicates the replacement product as the cause for the prevention break.

References and Suggested Reading

Atkins CE: Comparison of results of three commercial heartworm antigen test kits in dogs with low heartworm burdens, *J Am Vet Med Assoc* 222(9):1221, 2003.

Case JL et al: A clinical field trial of melarsomine dihydrochloride (RM340) in dogs with severe (class 3) heartworm disease. In Soll MD, Knight DH, editors: *Proceedings of the American Heartworm Symposium, 1995*, Batavia, Ill, 1995, American Heartworm Society, p 243.

Courtney CH, Zeng Q: Comparison of heartworm antigen test kit performance in dogs having low heartworm burdens, *Vet Parasitol* 96(4):317, 2001.

Kramer L et al: Is Wolbachia complicating the pathological effects of *Dirofilaria immitis* infections? *Vet Parasitol* 133(2-3):133, 2005.

McCall JW et al: Further evidence of clinical prophylactic, retroactive (reach-back) and adulticide activity of monthly administrations of ivermectin (HeartGard Plus) in dogs experimentally infected with heartworms. In Seward RL, Knight DH, editors: *Proceedings of the American Heartworm Symposium, 2001*, Batavia, Ill, 2001, American Heartworm Society, p189.

Miller MW et al: Clinical efficacy of melarsomine dihydrochloride (RM340) and thiacetarsemide in dogs with moderate (class 2) heartworm disease. In Soll MD, Knight DH, editors: *Proceedings of the American Heartworm Symposium 1995*, Batavia, Ill, 1995, American Heartworm Society, p 233.

Rawlings CA et al: Disease response to trickle kill when ivermectin or milbemycin is started during *Dirofilaria immitis* infection in dogs. In Seward RL, Knight DH, editors: *Proceedings of the American Heartworm Symposium 2001*, Batavia, Ill, 2001, American Heartworm Society, p 179.

Simón F et al: Immunopathology of *Dirofilaria immitis* infection, *Vet Res Commun* 1(2):161, 2007, Epub Dec 23, 2006.

SECTION IX

Urinary Diseases

India F. Lane

VOLUME XIII CONTENT ON EVOLVE: http://evolve.elsevier.com/Bonagura/Kirks/

CHAPTER 184

Managing the Patient With Polyuria and Polydipsia

KATHARINE F. LUNN, *Fort Collins, Colorado*

Polyuria and polydipsia are common problems in small animal medicine. Although a client may report only polyuria or polydipsia, these two disorders generally are considered as one problem, typically termed *polyuria/polydipsia (PU/PD)*, as neither polyuria nor polydipsia can persist in isolation. The textbook definitions of polyuria and polydipsia include urine output in excess of 50 ml/kg/day and water intake greater than 100 ml/kg/day, respectively. In practice, these definitions are rarely used to determine if a patient exhibits PU/PD. Measurement of water intake can be difficult or inconvenient for many clients, and measurement of urine output is rarely if ever performed in patients in their home environment. Although measurement of these parameters is more feasible in a hospital setting, they may not provide a true reflection of the patient's usual behavior. It should also be recognized that an individual patient can be polyuric and polydipsic without exceeding the limits described here. For example, a 5-kg cat would have to consume more than 500 ml of water per day to meet the classical definition of polydipsia; most cat owners would recognize increased water intake at a considerably lower volume than this. *Therefore it is more clinically useful to place PU/PD on the problem list if the owner has observed that water intake and/or urine output are increased compared to their usual observations and the urine specific gravity (USG) is found to be persistently low.* Measurement of the pet's water intake at home is perhaps most useful in cases in which there is discordance between the owner's observations and the USG. In some patients PU/PD may be placed on the problem list regardless of owner observations if the clinician notes a persistently low USG on urinalysis.

NORMAL PHYSIOLOGY

Water intake and urine production are controlled by the hypothalamus, pituitary gland, and kidney. Thirst is stimulated primarily by small changes in plasma osmolality. Thus a water deficit leads to hyperosmolality, which stimulates osmoreceptors, resulting in thirst. Arterial hypotension, fever, pain, and certain drugs also can stimulate thirst. Antidiuretic hormone (ADH; vasopressin; arginine vasopressin [AVP]) is synthesized in the supraoptic and paraventricular nuclei of the hypothalamus and stored in the pituitary. Release of ADH is stimulated by the same factors that stimulate thirst. ADH secretion can also be stimulated by nausea, hypoglycemia, stress, pain, fever, exercise, and some drugs. In the healthy kidney fluid leaving the ascending loop of Henle and early distal convoluted tubule is always dilute, regardless of the level of ADH. In the late distal convoluted tubule and the collecting duct, ADH promotes the passive resorption of solute-free water. In the absence of ADH the membranes in this part of the nephron are impermeable to water. ADH exerts its effects by binding to vasopressin (V2) receptors in the distal renal tubule, ultimately leading to the insertion of water channels (aquaporin-2) into the apical membrane of the epithelial cells. These channels allow water to flow along the osmotic gradient between the distal convoluted tubule/collecting duct and the hypertonic renal medulla. The countercurrent multiplier system of the renal tubules establishes hypertonicity in the renal medullary interstitium, and this is maintained by the vasa recta. Slow blood flow in the vasa recta prevents "wash-out" of medullary solutes such as sodium, chloride, and urea.

CAUSES OF POLYURIA AND POLYDIPSIA

PU/PD are the clinical manifestations of failure to produce concentrated urine. As described previously, the physiologic processes that allow for concentration of the urine include the presence of ADH, the ability of the renal tubules to respond to ADH, and the presence of an osmotic gradient between the hypertonic renal medulla and the fluid in the distal convoluted tubule and collecting duct. Thus PU/PD can result from reduced or absent ADH synthesis or release, failure of the renal tubule to respond to ADH, or reduction in the osmotic gradient between the filtrate in the distal convoluted tubule and the renal medullary interstitium. Reduction in the osmotic gradient can be caused by the presence of osmotically active particles in the filtrate or decreased medullary hypertonicity. In all of these situations polyuria is the primary problem, resulting from an inability to produce concentrated urine, and the animal manifests a compensatory polydipsia. In contrast, primary polydipsia is a disorder of thirst and may result from a psychogenic (behavioral) abnormality in which hypothalamic, pituitary, and renal function are normal. Fever, pain, and hyperthyroidism can also cause polydipsia. In addition, polydipsia can be a normal physiologic response to environment changes such as elevated ambient temperature or the feeding of a dry diet.

It is rarely possible to distinguish clinically between primary polydipsia and primary polyuria; although the evaluation of serum sodium concentration [Na⁺] or measured osmolality, when available, may be helpful in some cases. Serum [Na⁺] at or below the lower limit of the reference range is suggestive of a primary polydipsia. In contrast, high-normal or elevated serum [Na⁺] supports the presence of primary polyuria. This distinction is not helpful in all patients with PU/PD since many have a normal serum [Na⁺]. In addition, low serum [Na⁺] may be associated with hypovolemia. It is also important to recognize that some conditions that cause PU/PD may do so by more than one mechanism. For example, patients with hyperadrenocorticism may demonstrate PU/PD because of impaired central release of ADH, reduced renal responsiveness to ADH, or psychogenic polydipsia. Patients with liver failure may manifest both psychogenic polydipsia and decreased renal concentrating ability as a result of decreased blood urea nitrogen (BUN) production and reduced renal medullary hypertonicity.

Primary Polydipsia

Primary polydipsia may be a behavioral problem, sometimes attributed to insufficient exercise or a stressful environment or associated with particular personality types or breeds of dogs. This condition is uncommon in dogs and rare in cats. Primary polydipsia may explain the PU/PD seen in cats with hyperthyroidism, and it has been suggested to accompany primary gastrointestinal disease in dogs. Primary polydipsia can also be a manifestation of hepatic encephalopathy, and it may at least partly explain the PU/PD that accompanies canine hyperadrenocorticism. Patients with primary polydipsia are able to concentrate their urine in response to water deprivation.

Primary Polyuria

Primary polyuria may result from absent or reduced ADH synthesis or release or from failure of the renal tubules to respond to ADH. The former condition is termed *central diabetes insipidus (CDI)*. Failure of the renal tubules to respond to ADH is called *nephrogenic diabetes insipidus (NDI)*. This may be a primary disorder, or it may be secondary to many other conditions.

Central Diabetes Insipidus
In CDI the deficiency of ADH may be partial or complete and the result of trauma, neoplasia, congenital defects, or idiopathic causes. The diagnosis is made by demonstrating that the patient is unable to produce concentrated urine in response to water deprivation but responds to the administration of exogenous ADH.

Primary Nephrogenic Diabetes Insipidus
This is a rare congenital disorder in which the renal tubules are unable to respond to ADH. Affected animals have an obligate polyuria and do not concentrate their urine in response to water deprivation or administration of exogenous ADH.

Secondary Nephrogenic Diabetes Insipidus
Table 184-1 lists the many causes of secondary NDI. This category encompasses the vast majority of causes of PU/PD in the dog and cat and includes the most common causes of PU/PD, as well as many uncommon disorders. Polyuria is the primary problem in these disorders and is the result of an acquired inability of the renal tubules to respond to ADH. This may be because of a loss of the normal osmotic gradient between the renal medullary interstitium and the fluid in the distal renal tubule, or it may result from interference with the actions of ADH on the renal tubular cells. A water deprivation test is of no value in the investigation of secondary NDI; each disorder must be ruled out by specific diagnostic tests.

Renal Medullary Solute Washout
Fluid therapy, diuretic therapy, and chronic PU/PD may result in the loss of renal medullary solutes, leading to an impaired renal response to ADH. This can interfere with renal concentrating ability in response to water deprivation or a 1-desamino-8-D-AVP (desmopressin) (DDAVP) trial; therefore a gradual period of water restriction to restore a normal concentration gradient may be recommended before these tests are performed.

Miscellaneous Causes of PU/PD

Diet, drugs, and toxins can lead to PU/PD through a variety of mechanisms. Therefore a thorough diet and drug history is an essential part of the evaluation of the patient with PU/PD. Many clinicians have noted that dogs with splenomegaly, splenic masses, or bladder tumors may have a history of PU/PD; however, the mechanism is not known. Similarly dogs with gastrointestinal disease may be polyuric and polydipsic; this is suggested to be a psychogenic problem, perhaps in response to gastrointestinal pain or discomfort.

DIAGNOSTIC APPROACH TO POLYURIA AND POLYDIPSIA

Table 184-1 includes the primary diagnostic tests that are used to investigate specific causes of secondary NDI. The diagnosis of CDI and primary polydipsia is discussed in the Stages of Testing in PU/PD later in the chapter. The following guidelines should be kept in mind when formulating a diagnostic plan for a polyuric and polydipsic dog or cat:

1. Investigate the common disorders first. The most common causes of PU/PD in the dog are chronic renal failure, hyperadrenocorticism, and diabetes mellitus. In the cat the most common causes are chronic renal failure, diabetes mellitus, and hyperthyroidism.
2. CDI is rare, primary NDI is very rare, and primary polydipsia is uncommon. Therefore do not pursue diagnostic tests for these disorders until more common differential diagnoses have been thoroughly ruled out.
3. Always begin the diagnostic plan with tests that are simple to perform and interpret, safe for the patient,

Table **184-1**

Causes of Secondary Nephrogenic Diabetes Insipidus, Underlying Mechanisms, and Recommended Diagnostic Tests

Cause	Mechanism(s)	Recommended Diagnostic Tests	Comments
Diabetes mellitus	Osmotic diuresis	Urinalysis Blood glucose Serum fructosamine	
Primary renal glycosuria	Osmotic diuresis	Urinalysis	
Fanconi syndrome and other tubulopathies	Osmotic diuresis	Urinalysis Urine electrolyte and amino acid levels	
Chronic renal failure	Osmotic diuresis	Serum chemistry Urinalysis GFR measurement	Absence of azotemia does not rule out chronic renal failure Patients with mild to moderate renal failure retain urine diluting ability
Polyuric acute renal failure	Osmotic diuresis	Serum chemistry Urinalysis	
Postobstructive diuresis	Osmotic diuresis Down regulation of aquaporin-2	History Physical examination	
Chronic partial ureteral obstruction	Down regulation of aquaporin-2	Abdominal radiography Abdominal ultrasonography Excretory urography	
Renal medullary solute washout	Decreased renal medullary tonicity with loss of osmotic gradient	Find underlying cause	
Pyelonephritis	Bacterial endotoxin reduces tubular sensitivity to ADH Damaged countercurrent mechanism	Urinalysis and urine culture Abdominal ultrasonography Ultrasound-guided pyelocentesis Excretory urography	A single negative urine culture does not rule out pyelonephritis
Pyometra	Bacterial endotoxin reduces tubular sensitivity to ADH	History and physical examination Abdominal imaging	"Stump" pyometra is possible in a spayed female
Liver failure	Loss of medullary hypertonicity Impaired hormone metabolism	Fasting and postprandial bile acids	PU/PD may also have a psychogenic component
Portosystemic shunt	Loss of medullary hypertonicity Increased GFR	Fasting and postprandial bile acids Abdominal ultrasonography Portography Rectal scintigraphy	PU/PD may also have a psychogenic component

Condition	Mechanism	Diagnostic tests	Comments
Hyperadrenocorticism	Impaired tubule response to ADH	ACTH stimulation test Low-dose dexamethasone suppression test	Impaired release of ADH and psychogenic polydipsia may also contribute to PU/PD in patients with hyperadrenocorticism
Hypoadrenocorticism	Loss of medullary hypertonicity	ACTH stimulation test	
Hyperthyroidism	Loss of medullary hypertonicity	Total T$_4$ Free T$_4$ by equilibrium dialysis Thyroid scintigraphy	PU/PD may also have a psychogenic component
Acromegaly	Osmotic diuresis due to diabetes mellitus Interference with action of ADH?	History and physical examination GH levels (not readily available) IGF-I levels Brain imaging	Partial CDI may contribute to PU/PD in some patients
Pheochromocytoma	Excessive catecholamines	History and physical examination Abdominal imaging Hormonal assays	Hormonal assays not commonly performed in veterinary medicine
Primary hyperaldosteronism	Impaired tubule response to ADH	Aldosterone levels Renin activity	Impaired release of ADH may also lead to CDI
Hypercalcemia	Interferes with action of ADH on renal tubule	Serum chemistry Ionized calcium	Many possible causes of hypercalcemia
Hypokalemia	Down regulation of aquaporin-2 Loss of medullary hypertonicity	Serum chemistry	
Hyponatremia	Loss of medullary hypertonicity	Serum chemistry	
Leiomyosarcoma	Impaired tubule response to ADH	Abdominal imaging	
Polycythemia	Action of atrial natriuretic peptide	Complete blood count	Impaired release of ADH may also lead to CDI
Leptospirosis	Mechanism(s) unknown	Serology Polymerase chain reaction	Renal failure is not the cause of PU/PD in all cases

ACTH, Adrenocorticotropic hormone; *ADH,* antidiuretic hormone; *CDI,* central diabetes insipidus; *GFR,* glomerular filtration rate; *GH,* growth hormone; *IGF-I,* insulin-like growth factor I.

and inexpensive for the client. The water deprivation test does not meet these criteria.

4. Take advantage of a written reference list of differential diagnoses for PU/PD so that disorders can be removed from the list as they are ruled out.
5. Do not completely rule out differential diagnoses for PU/PD without definitive evidence. For example, not all dogs with hyperadrenocorticism "look cushingoid," and not all patients with pyelonephritis have an active urine sediment. Use specific diagnostic tests to investigate these differential diagnoses.

The following sections review a logical, stepwise approach to PU/PD. In some cases diagnostic tests are chosen from more than one stage concurrently, based on the overall clinical picture and the most likely diagnoses.

Stage One Testing in Polyuria and Polydipsia: the "Minimum Database"

A careful history, complete physical examination, urinalysis, complete blood count (CBC), serum chemistry profile, and urine culture are mandatory in the initial evaluation of all patients with PU/PD. Consideration of the species, breed, age, sex, and history of the patient allows the differential diagnoses for PU/PD to be placed in order of likelihood. For example, chronic renal failure, hyperadrenocorticism, and diabetes mellitus are more likely in middle-aged dogs than in puppies. A careful history of the reported PU/PD also helps to rule out other disorders of urination such as pollakiuria or urinary incontinence. As indicated previously, a complete diet and medication history is essential to rule out iatrogenic causes of PU/PD such as glucocorticoid administration or the feeding of a highly protein–restricted diet. The physical examination may be normal in many patients with PU/PD, but it may also reveal signs of disorders such as hyperadrenocorticism or neoplasia. A complete urinalysis, serum chemistry profile, and CBC allow many of the disorders listed in Table 184-1 to be ruled out. Subtle changes in the chemistry profile and CBC may also provide diagnostic clues. For example, minor changes in serum [Na⁺] may help to distinguish between primary polyuria and primary polydipsia. Decreases in cholesterol, albumin, and BUN may suggest liver failure, and thrombocytosis and a stress leukogram may prompt further evaluation for hyperadrenocorticism.

Urine culture should be performed in all patients with PU/PD to investigate pyelonephritis and because many causes of PU/PD predispose the patient to the development of urinary tract infections (e.g., diabetes mellitus, hyperadrenocorticism, and chronic renal failure). Although sediment evaluation is important, it cannot be used to rule out infection because it is difficult to visually detect bacteria in the sediment prepared from a urine sample with a low USG and because several disorders that cause PU/PD also inhibit the development of an active urine sediment. If pyelonephritis is suspected, a single negative urine culture cannot rule this out; additional cultures, as well as further diagnostic tests outlined in Stage Three Testing in PU/PD, should be performed.

Serum total thyroxine (T₄) measurement in cats and leptospirosis titers in dogs are also considered part of the minimum database for PU/PD. Leptospirosis is recognized increasingly as a cause of PU/PD in dogs, and serologic testing is recommended in all geographic locations with the exception of desert environments.

Interpretation of Urine Specific Gravity

The terms *isosthenuria, hyposthenuria, and hypersthenuria* refer to urine that is isoosmolar, hypoosmolar, or hyperosmolar, respectively, compared to plasma. Thus an accurate assessment of urine concentration requires measurement of urine and plasma osmolality. In practice osmolality is not measured routinely; therefore ranges of USG are used to define isosthenuria (USG of 1.008 to 1.012), hyposthenuria (USG <1.008), and hypersthenuria (USG >1.012). By convention the term *hypersthenuria* is often used to refer to highly concentrated urine (USG >1.035 in the dog; USG >1.045 in the cat); and the term *minimally concentrated urine* describes USG in the range of 1.013 to 1.030 (dog) and 1.013 to 1.040 (cat). Measurement of several random USGs can be useful in the evaluation of the patient with PU/PD. Detection of a random USG greater than 1.030 indicates that the patient does not have an obligate polyuria and suggests that the problem is one of primary polydipsia. In most cases a definitive diagnosis cannot be obtained by evaluation of USG alone; however, certain differential diagnoses can be rendered more or less likely by the evaluation of several USGs. For example, marked hyposthenuria is most likely with CDI or primary polydipsia, and hyposthenuria can occur with many diseases causing secondary NDI (e.g., hypercalcemia, hyperadrenocorticism, and pyelonephritis). Although it is true that patients with chronic renal failure normally produce isosthenuric or minimally concentrated urine, if renal failure is mild to moderate, the patient is still *capable* of diluting the urine if another disorder is present. For example, an animal with both chronic renal failure and psychogenic polydipsia would be able to produce hyposthenuric urine unless the renal failure was advanced. Conversely it is important to note that several renal disorders other than chronic renal failure interfere with concentrating ability. These disorders may lead to production of hyposthenuric urine, and this finding should not lead the clinician to eliminate the possibility of renal *disease* as a cause of PU/PD. Important examples include pyelonephritis and hypercalcemia, which can lead to irreversible renal failure if not suspected, diagnosed, and managed.

Stage Two Testing in PU/PD: Ruling Out Specific Differential Diagnoses

If the minimum database has failed to diagnose the cause of PU/PD, further tests are recommended to continue to rule out the many causes of secondary NDI. Although the index of suspicion may be low for many of these disorders, it is important to rule them out before proceeding to a potentially harmful test such as water deprivation. The adrenocorticotropic hormone (ACTH) stimulation test is a valuable test in the investigation of PU/PD in the dog. This test is sensitive and specific for the diagnosis of hypoadrenocorticism, and the results may also identify iatrogenic hyperadrenocorticism. The ACTH stimulation test has a moderate sensitivity for the diagnosis of pituitary-dependent hyperadrenocorticism and lower sensitivity for the diagnosis of adrenal-dependent hyperadrenocorticism; therefore a normal ACTH stimulation test result should prompt follow-up with a low-dose dexamethasone suppression test if there is any clinical suspicion of hyperadrenocorticism. Fasting and postprandial bile acids are recommended in the evaluation of the patient with PU/PD to rule out either acquired liver failure or a congenital portosystemic shunt. Not all patients with these disorders have elevated liver enzymes or decreased liver products (BUN, cholesterol, albumin, and glucose) on a chemistry panel; therefore a more specific and sensitive test of liver function is recommended. Serum T_4 levels should be part of the minimum database in the feline patient with PU/PD. In dogs, although hyperthyroidism is rare, this differential diagnosis is simply ruled out with a serum total T_4 assay. If hyperthyroidism is suspected in a cat but not confirmed by the total T_4, repeated T_4 measurements, free T_4 by equilibrium dialysis, or thyroid nuclear scintigraphy should be considered.

Stage Three Testing in PU/PD: Imaging Studies

Imaging studies in the patient with PU/PD may be used to screen for a range of disorders that were not detected on initial testing. For example, thoracic and abdominal radiographs may reveal evidence of neoplasia, and abdominal ultrasound may demonstrate splenic or adrenal masses. Imaging studies may also be indicated in the pursuit of specific diagnoses. Examples include abdominal ultrasound to look for "stump" pyometra or partial urinary tract obstruction, excretory urography or ultrasound-guided pyelocentesis to investigate suspected pyelonephritis, and imaging of the brain in suspected acromegaly or CDI.

Stage Four Testing in PU/PD: Uncommon Disorders

Assessment of Glomerular Filtration Rate

Glomerular filtration rate (GFR) studies are indicated in the evaluation of patients with PU/PD that demonstrate persistent unexplained isosthenuria or minimally concentrated urine with normal BUN and creatinine (see Chapter 189). Loss of approximately 66% of functional renal mass results in loss of concentrating ability, but azotemia does not develop until more than 75% of functional renal mass is lost. Therefore normal BUN and creatinine cannot be used to rule out chronic renal failure in a patient that has lost more than 66% but less than 75% of functional renal mass. Commonly used methods of GFR assessment include iohexol clearance, exogenous creatinine clearance, and nuclear scintigraphy. Water deprivation could potentially lead to decompensation in a patient with undetected chronic renal failure; therefore assessment of GFR is recommended before considering this step.

Response to DDAVP

DDAVP, or desmopressin, is a synthetic analog of ADH. Desmopressin is used to treat CDI and is also used in the final stages of a water deprivation test to determine if the patient is able to respond to exogenously administered ADH (as would be expected in CDI but not in NDI). A therapeutic trial with DDAVP has been described (Nichols, 2000); this approach is a recommended alternative to the water deprivation test. Desmopressin is available as tablets (0.1 and 0.2 mg), nasal solution (0.1 mg/ml or 1.5 mg/ml) and parenteral injection (4 mcg/ml). For the DDAVP trial the 0.1-mg/ml nasal solution is preferred and is administered into the conjunctival sac (1 to 4 drops q12h for 5 to 7 days). Before starting the DDAVP trial the patient's water intake is measured over 2 to 3 days to provide a baseline value. A positive response to the DDAVP trial is indicated by a reduction in water intake or an increase in USG. These findings support a diagnosis of CDI but may also be seen in patients with hyperadrenocorticism. A DDAVP trial should only be considered under the following circumstances:

1. Stages 1, 2, and 3 of the diagnostic plan have been completed, and all testable causes of secondary NDI have been ruled out.
2. Patient signalment, history, and serum [Na+] are more consistent with CDI than primary polydipsia.
3. The patient will be closely observed and given free access to water.

Success of a DDAVP trial depends on appropriate owner compliance and objective monitoring of water intake and USG during the trial. Although rare, hyponatremia or volume overload could result from excess DDAVP activity in an animal without CDI.

Gradual At-Home Water Deprivation

If patient signalment, history, and serum [Na+] are more consistent with primary polydipsia than CDI, gradual water deprivation may be considered in selected cases. This approach is not recommended unless the following conditions are satisfied:

1. All causes of primary polyuria have been considered and ruled out.
2. The patient has a normal or low-normal serum [Na+].
3. The patient has a normal BUN and creatinine.
4. The patient is not clinically sick or dehydrated.
5. The client and veterinarian are committed to frequent evaluation of patient body weight and USG, as well as daily measurement of BUN and serum [Na+].
6. The client is motivated, well informed, observant, and compliant.

Before starting water deprivation, the patient's normal water intake should be established over 3 to 5 days. This amount can then be decreased by no more than 5% per day while normal food intake and activity level are continued. The test is discontinued if the patient loses 5% or more of body weight, serum [Na+] or BUN become elevated, clinical signs of illness develop, or USG increases to 1.030 or greater. If USG is 1.030 or higher at any point, the diagnosis of primary polydipsia has been confirmed. Again, because of the significant risks associated with water deprivation in a patient with an obligate polyuria, this test is not recommended unless the conditions listed previously have been satisfied. Animals may be referred for more intensive in-hospital water deprivation assessment in unusual cases.

References and Suggested Reading

Cohen M, Post GS: Nephrogenic diabetes insipidus in a dog with intestinal leiomyosarcoma, *J Am Vet Med Assoc* 215 (12):1818, 1999.

Cohen M, Post GS: Water transport in the kidney and nephrogenic diabetes insipidus, *J Vet Intern Med* 16 (5):510, 2002.

Feldman EC, Nelson RW: *Canine and feline endocrinology and reproduction*, ed 3, St Louis, 2004, Saunders, p 2.

Finco DR, Braselton WE, Cooper TA: Relationship between plasma iohexol clearance and urinary exogenous creatinine clearance in dogs, *J Vet Intern Med* 15 (4):386, 2001.

Henderson SM, Elwood CM: A potential causal association between gastrointestinal disease and primary polydipsia in three dogs, *J Small Anim Pract* 44 (6):280, 2003.

Nichols R: Clinical use of the vasopressin analogue DDAVP for the diagnosis and treatment of diabetes insipidus. In Bonagura JD, editor: *Kirk's current veterinary therapy XIII*, Philadelphia, 2000, Saunders, p 325.

Rijnberk A et al: Aldosteronoma in a dog with polyuria as the leading symptom, *Domest Anim Endocrinol* 20:227, 2001.

van Vonderen IK et al: Polyuria and polydipsia and disturbed vasopressin release in 2 dogs with secondary polycythemia, *J Vet Intern Med* 15 (5):300, 1997.

van Vonderen IK et al: Vasopressin response to osmotic stimulation in 18 young dogs with polyuria and polydipsia, *J Vet Intern Med* 18 (6):800, 2004.

CHAPTER 185

Interpreting and Managing Crystalluria

JOSEPH W. BARTGES, *Knoxville, Tennessee*
CLAUDIA A. KIRK, *Knoxville, Tennessee*

Crystalluria is defined as the observation of crystals during microscopic examination of a centrifuged urine sample. Occasionally crystalluria may be heavy enough to be observed macroscopically. Crystalluria represents elimination of a solid (minerals and electrolytes) in a liquid medium (urine).

The most common crystals observed in dog and cat urine are struvite (magnesium ammonium phosphate hexahydrate), calcium oxalate dihydrate, ammonium urate, and cystine. In addition, other ions and certain drugs are capable of forming crystals in urine. Amorphous crystals, which lack a classic symmetric structure, are commonly observed in dog urine and sometimes in cat urine. Typically amorphous crystals are variant forms of struvite; however, other ions such as ammonium urate may appear amorphous.

CRYSTAL FORMATION

Crystals form when the urine is or has recently been oversaturated with the ions that make up the crystals. With oversaturation the minerals cannot remain dissociated (dissolved), and they combine to form an organized structure (a crystal). The microscopic appearance of the crystals depends on their composition. The concentrations of minerals, urine volume, urine pH, temperature, and the presence of promoters and absence of inhibitors of crystal formation all influence crystal formation. The

concentration of crystallogenic compounds depends on the ion excretion rate and the volume of urine produced. The less urine excreted, the higher the concentrations of solids in the urine. In addition, urinary pH and the presence of other ions affect the relative concentration and the solubility of certain compounds in urine (Table 185-1); and the presence of cellular debris, foreign bodies, mucosal erosions, or even other crystals can serve as a surface or scaffolding to enhance crystal formation.

Temperature influences crystal formation as well. Temperature variation is not likely in the urinary bladder, but it does influence precipitation of crystals after collection. If the urine is allowed to cool below body temperature, crystals are likely to precipitate. Most crystals form in an acidic urine (pH <7.0), whereas a few (particularly struvite) form when the urine pH is greater than 7.0 (see Table 185-1). The presence of a surface such as denuded mucosa, a piece of suture, or another mineral promotes crystal formation. Finally, certain compounds inhibit crystal and stone formation. For example, Tamm-Horsfall mucoprotein and nephrocalcin are protein inhibitors of crystal formation (Carvalho et al., 2003). Although the role of these proteins in canine and feline crystal formation is not well defined, the inhibitory activity can be influenced by urine pH.

Crystalluria is influenced by both diet and water intake. Dietary influence on crystal formation may

Table 185-1

Common Characteristics of Canine and Feline Urinary Crystals

		pH WHERE COMMONLY FOUND		
Type	Appearance	Acid	Neutral	Alkaline
Ammonium urate	Yellow-brown spherulites, thorn apples	+	+	±
Amorphous urates	Amorphous or spheroid, yellow-brown structures	+	±	−
Ampicillin	Long, thin needles that are colorless	+	?	?
Bilirubin	Reddish-brown needles or granules	+	−	−
Calcium carbonate	Large yellow-brown spheroids with radial striations or small crystals with spheric ovoid or dumbbell shapes	−	±	+
Calcium oxalate dihydrate	Small colorless envelopes (octahedral form)	+	+	±
Calcium oxalate monohydrate	Small spindles, "hemp seeds" or dumbbells	+	+	±
Calcium phosphate	Amorphous, or long, thin prisms	±	+	+
Cholesterol	Flat, colorless plates with corner notch	+	+	−
Cystine	Flat, colorless hexagonal plates	+	+	±
Hippuric acid	4- to 6-sided colorless elongated plates or prisms	+	+	±
Leucine	Yellow-brown spheroids with radial and concentric laminations	+	+	−
Sodium urate	Colorless or yellow-brown needles or slender prisms, sometimes in clusters or sheaves	+	±	−
Struvite	3- to 6-sided colorless prisms	−	±	+
Sulfa metabolites	Sheaves of needles with central or eccentric binding; shucks of wheat comprised of slender sheaves that grow in such a way as to form two half circles with central budding; sometimes fan-shaped clusters; sometimes globules with striations	+	±	−
Tyrosine	Fine, colorless or yellow needles arranged in sheaves or rosettes	+	−	−
Uric acid	Diamond or rhombic rosettes, or oval plates, structures with pointed ends. Occasionally six-sided plates	+	−	−
Xanthine	Amorphous, spheroid, or ovoid structures with a yellow-brown color	+	±	−

±, Crystals may occur at this pH but are more common at the other pH.

include (1) altered excretion of dietary constituents or metabolites; (2) dietary-induced alteration of urinary pH; or (3) changes in urine volume. Alterations in urinary pH, ion excretion, and urine concentration can be observed following the initial consumption of a new food and may not reflect a pathologic process (e.g., a hospitalized patient consuming a novel diet). However, in most cases of dietary change, urine composition stabilizes in 4 to 7 days. Time of feeding with respect to urine collection and feeding method can have a significant influence on the urine pH and possibly crystalluria. A postprandial alkaline tide (urine alkalinization) is common 3 to 6 hours after eating, particularly in meal-fed animals. Some pharmacologic agents result in crystalluria. Identification of unusual crystals in urine should prompt review of medications that the animal may be receiving. Drugs associated with crystalluria include sulfadiazine and its metabolites, ampicillin, and radiopaque contrast agents (see Table 185-1) (Osborne et al., 1999). In humans ciprofloxacin, primidone, 5-fluorocytosine, 6-mercaptopurine, and acyclovir also have been associated with crystalluria.

Occasionally foreign material may be mistaken for crystalluria, depending on method of urine collection. Pollen and other environmental contaminants (e.g., clay litter) may be collected with voided urine samples. Talc powder crystals from surgical gloves may be introduced into urine samples during collection of a midstream voided sample or during insertion of a urinary catheter.

SIGNIFICANCE OF CRYSTALLURIA

Crystalluria is not synonymous with urolithiasis. Crystalluria occurs when urine is or has recently been oversaturated with crystallogenic compounds; however, crystalluria by itself is not pathologic. For example, many adult dogs have struvite crystalluria; however, struvite uroliths do not form in adult dogs unless there is a urinary tract infection with a urease-producing microbial organism (typically *Staphylococcus* spp. or *Proteus* spp.). Therefore struvite crystalluria in adult dogs is rarely a concern unless an infection is present. Likewise, many animals with cystinuria have crystalluria, but the incidence of cystine urolith formation is low (Tsan et al., 1972). Urolith formation in immature Dalmatians occurs uncommonly despite the presence of urinary urate crystals; and in immature Dalmatians urate crystalluria is not predictive of future urolith formation in adulthood (Bartges et al., 1999a). Nonetheless, crystalluria does represent a potential risk factor for urolith formation.

In contrast to the observation that crystalluria does not predict urolithiasis, uroliths can occur without observable crystalluria. Patients may have active urolith disease but not have crystalluria. Two potential explanations for this phenomenon are (1) oversaturation is intermittent, and the urine sample was collected during a period of relatively low saturation; or (2) precipitating crystals are rapidly incorporated into a preexisting urolith (Bartges et al., 1999b). In practice most dogs and cats with struvite and ammonium urate uroliths do have crystalluria; however, more than 50% of dogs and cats with active calcium oxalate uroliths do not have crystalluria (Lulich et al., 1999).

Interpretation of crystalluria depends highly on how the sample was collected and how it was analyzed. Most important, crystals may form in urine after it is collected (in vitro crystallization). Crystals may not be present in urine while at body temperature in the urinary bladder; however, if it is cooled after collection (e.g., by refrigerating the sample), crystals may form. Crystals may also form if the urine sample undergoes evaporation. To correctly assess crystalluria, a urine sample should be collected fresh and examined within 15 to 20 minutes (unrefrigerated) and immediately if refrigeration of the sample is anticipated. It may be beneficial to keep the urine at body temperature. Refrigerated samples should be allowed to return to room temperature before urinalysis and urine sediment examination are completed.

Crystal aggregates occur when crystals stick together in clumps. This implies a propensity for the microscopic crystals to adhere together and organize over time, which is a prerequisite for macroscopic urolith formation. However, presence of crystal aggregates must be interpreted in light of how the sample was collected and processed and taking into account factors such as animal species and gender (Osborne et al., 1986).

In addition to these factors, the significance of crystalluria is determined by the type of crystal, the medical history of the animal, and the persistence of crystalluria in serial urinalyses. As implied previously, the presence of crystalluria does not necessarily warrant a change in diet or the administration of medication. Based on review of all available information, the clinician must determine the likelihood of stone formation in an individual animal. In male dogs or cats the clinician must also consider the risk of urethral obstruction. Crystalluria is more likely to be significant in animals with (1) known urolithiasis; (2) a prior history of urolithiasis or urinary obstruction; (3) clinical signs of lower urinary tract disease, or (4) persistent or particularly heavy crystalluria.

MANAGING CRYSTALLURIA

Bilirubin

Bilirubin crystals appear as yellow-red or red-brown needles or granules (Fig. 185-1). Bilirubin crystalluria can be normal in dogs (Reilly et al., 2001), especially in concentrated urine; however, these crystals are always abnormal in cats. Bilirubin crystalluria may occur with diseases associated with hyperbilirubinemia and bilirubinuria, including prehepatic, hepatic, and posthepatic causes.

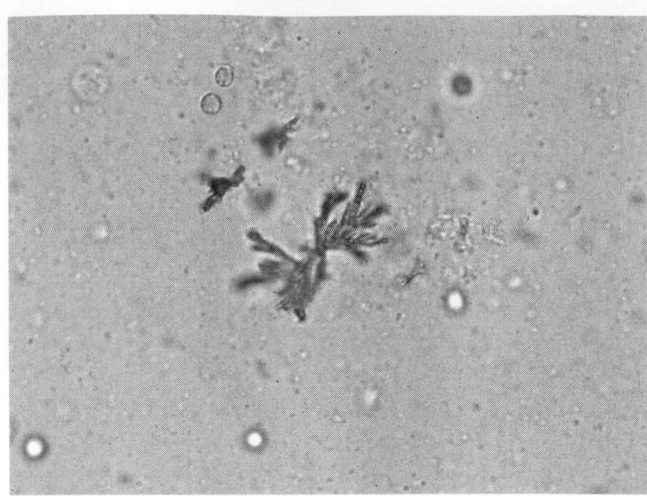

Fig. 185-1 Bilirubin crystals. (Photomicrograph courtesy Dr. India Lane, The University of Tennessee.)

Calcium oxalate

Calcium oxalate crystals (Fig. 185-2) may occur with urolith formation but also with diseases associated with hypercalcemia (e.g., hyperparathyroidism or neoplasia) or with ethylene glycol toxicity (usually these crystals are calcium oxalate monohydrate). Presence of calcium oxalate crystalluria should prompt evaluation of the patient for a predisposing disease, especially if hypercalcemia is present. As with other crystals, the presence of calcium oxalate crystalluria is not synonymous with urolith formation, nor does the absence of calcium oxalate crystalluria rule out urolithiasis. Over 50% of dogs and cats with active calcium oxalate urocystolithiasis do not have crystalluria (Osborne et al., 1996). If calcium oxalate crystalluria is persistent and other diseases have been ruled out, preventive strategies should be considered. Several diets are available for managing calcium oxalate urolithiasis in dogs and cats. In addition, potassium citrate administration may be beneficial as an alkalinizing agent; citrate is a calcium oxalate inhibitor. Thiazide diuretics decrease urinary calcium excretion in dogs and are used in humans with idiopathic hypercalciuria and calcium oxalate urolithiasis; however, there are no long-term studies in dogs and cats evaluating their efficacy or safety.

Cystine

Cystine crystals typically occur in urine with a pH less than 7.0 (Fig. 185-3). Cystine urolithiasis occurs uncommonly—in fewer than 2% of dogs and fewer than 0.2% of cats. Cystine is a disulfide-containing amino acid and is normally filtered at the glomerulus and resorbed in the proximal tubule. Therefore cystinuria and cystine crystalluria occur because of a defect in resorption in the proximal renal tubule. Management of cystine crystalluria and urolithiasis involves feeding a low-protein diet (since cystine is an amino acid), increasing urine volume (decreasing urine specific gravity), and increasing urine pH. Because cystine solubility increases exponentially when the urine pH is greater than 7.2, urine alkalinization to 7.5 is recommended.

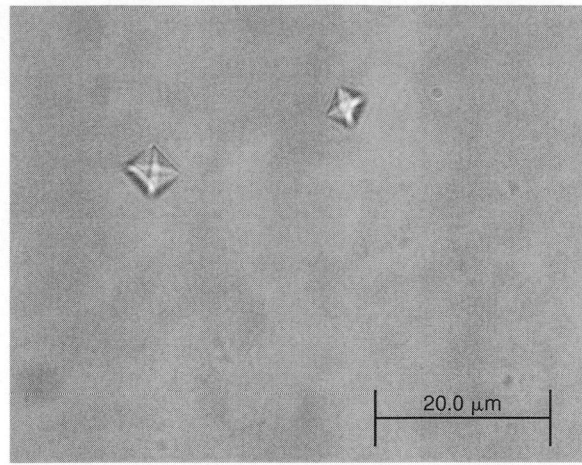

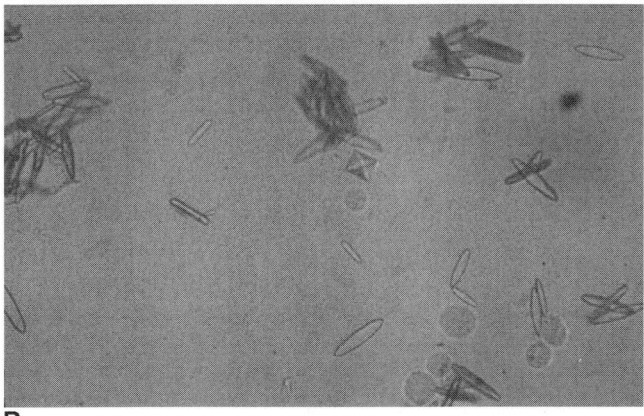

Fig. 185-2 **A,** Calcium oxalate dihydrate crystals (photomicrograph courtesy of Dr. Michael Fry, The University of Tennessee). **B,** Calcium oxalate monohydrate crystals. (Photomicrograph courtesy Dr. India Lane, The University of Tennesse.)

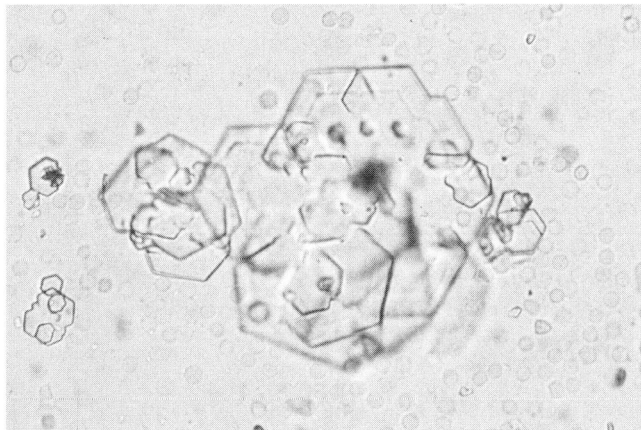

Fig. 185-3 Cystine crystals.

Pharmacologically cystine crystalluria can be decreased by administering a drug that cleaves the disulfide bond, resulting in a more soluble compound. These drugs include D-penicillamine and 2-mercaptopropionylglycine (2-MPG). 2-MPG is associated with fewer side effects.

Struvite

Struvite crystals occur commonly in dogs and cats, and struvite is the most common mineral occurring in uroliths from dogs and cats. Struvite crystals typically form in concentrated urine that has a pH greater than 7.0 in the dog and greater than 6.5 in the cat (Fig. 185-4). Two types of struvite uroliths occur: infection-induced and sterile. Infection-induced struvite uroliths occur most commonly in dogs, in pediatric dogs and cats, and in animals that are immunocompromised. For infection-induced struvite stones to form, the microbe must produce urease, which is an enzyme that metabolizes urea, resulting in oversaturation of urine. Therefore struvite crystalluria in dogs that do not have a urinary tract infection is rarely a concern and requires no treatment. Adult cats typically form struvite uroliths without a urinary tract infection (sterile struvite uroliths); therefore struvite crystalluria is more of a clinical concern in an adult cat. This is particularly true in male cats because greater than 80% of urethral matrix-crystalline plugs contain struvite as the predominant mineral (Lekcharoensuk et al., 2002). Management of struvite crystalluria in cats involves increasing urine volume (decreasing urine specific gravity) and feeding a diet that is formulated to contain lower quantities of magnesium, protein (source of ammonium), and phosphate and that induces an acidic pH. Therapeutic foods are available for both struvite dissolution and struvite prevention.

Uric Acid

Uric acid or urate salts (ammonium or sodium) usually occur in acid urine. They are often yellow or yellow-brown and may occur in a variety of shapes (Fig. 185-5). Uric acid crystalluria occurs uncommonly except in Dalmatians and English bulldogs that have a breed-associated crystalluria and urolithiasis. Uric acid crystalluria may occur in animals with hepatic disease, especially portosystemic shunts. For this reason, liver function should be evaluated in dogs and cats with uric acid crystalluria. If uric

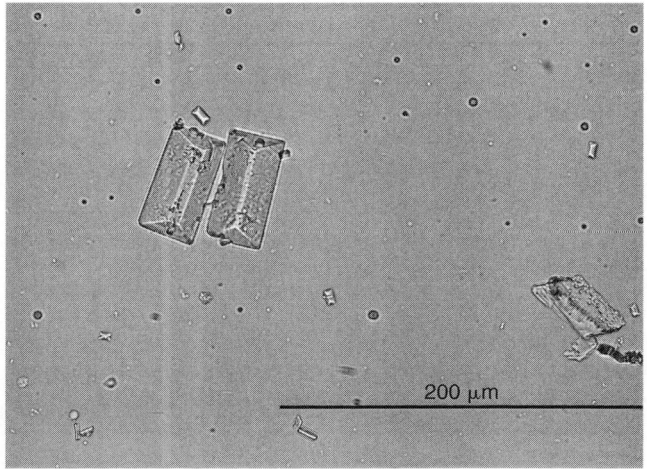

Fig. 185-4 Struvite crystals. (Photomicrograph courtesy Dr. Michael Fry, The University of Tennessee.)

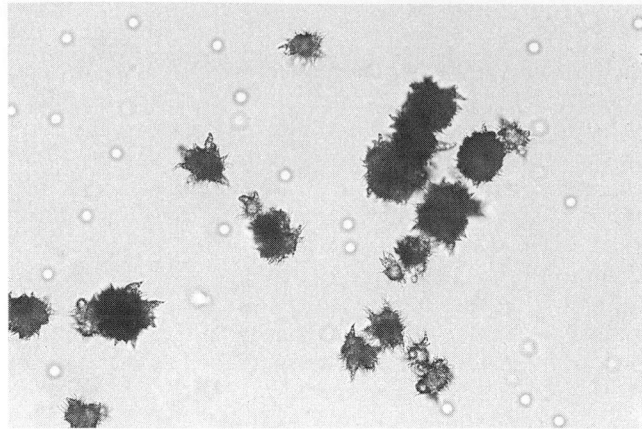

Fig. 185-5   Ammonium urate crystals.

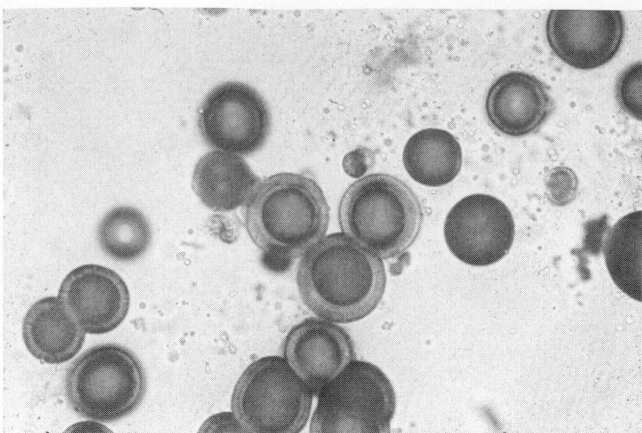

Fig. 185-6   Xanthine crystals.

acid crystalluria is associated with liver disease, managing the underlying liver disease may help prevent urolith formation.

In dogs and cats with no underlying hepatic dysfunction (e.g., Dalmatians), crystalluria may or may not lead to urolith formation. Persistent crystalluria, especially with concentrated urine, increases the risk for urolith formation. Dietary manipulation to reduce protein consumption and induce alkaline urine is often sufficient to minimize uric acid crystallization. Allopurinol, a xanthine oxidase inhibitor that competitively inhibits the conversion of xanthine to uric acid, may be required in dogs in which dietary therapy is not completely effective. Allopurinol therapy has not been evaluated in cats, although it has been used.

Xanthine

Xanthine crystals (Fig. 185-6) occur rarely in dogs and cats unless they are receiving allopurinol, a xanthine oxidase inhibitor that inhibits the metabolic conversion of xanthine to uric acid. Concurrent consumption of a nonprotein-restricted diet increases the risk of xanthine crystalluria and urolithiasis in dogs and cats receiving allopurinol. Higher-protein foods increase the dietary intake of urate precursors and thereby increase xanthine levels. Naturally occurring xanthinuria and xanthine crystalluria have been described in cavalier King Charles spaniels (van Zuilen et al., 1997) and cats (Osborne et al., 2004). Xanthine crystalluria represents an increased risk for xanthine urolith formation. Treatment involves feeding a restricted protein diet, inducing production of more dilute urine, and urinary alkalinization.

Crystalluria occurs commonly in dogs and cats and represents renal excretion of ions in a given urine sample. It may occur normally in healthy animals and does not necessarily imply that a pathologic condition is present or that uroliths will form. The significance of crystalluria should be interpreted in association with other historical, physical examination, laboratory, and imaging information. Understanding factors associated with crystal type and when and how crystals form helps to determine the significance of the crystalluria and the need, if any, for medical therapy.

References and Suggested Reading

Bartges JW, Osborne CA: Influence of diet on laboratory tests. In Kirk RW, Bonagura JD: *Current veterinary therapy XII*, Philadelphia, 1995, Saunders, p 20.

Bartges JW et al: Canine urate urolithiasis: etiopathogenesis, diagnosis, and management, *Vet Clin North Am Small Anim Pract* 29(1):161, 1999a.

Bartges JW et al: Methods for evaluating treatment of uroliths, *Vet Clin North Am Small Anim Pract* 29(1):45, 1999b.

Carvalho M et al: Role of urinary inhibitors of crystallization in uric acid nephrolithiasis: dalmatian dog model, *Urology* 62(3):566, 2003.

Daudon MP et al: Clinical value of crystalluria study, *Ann Biol Clin (Paris)* 62(4):379, 2004.

Lekcharoensuk C et al: Evaluation of trends in frequency of urethrostomy for treatment of urethral obstruction in cats, *J Am Vet Med Assoc* 221(4):502, 2002.

Lulich JP et al: (1999). Canine lower urinary tract disorders. In Ettinger SJ, Feldman EC: *Textbook of veterinary internal medicine*, Philadelphia, 1999, Saunders, 1747.

Osborne CA et al: Crystalluria: observations, interpretations, and misinterpretations, *Vet Clin North Am Small Anim Pract* 16(1):45, 1986.

Osborne CA et al: Feline crystalluria: detection and interpretation, *Vet Clin North Am Small Anim Pract* 26(2):369, 1996.

Osborne CA et al: Drug-induced urolithiasis, *Vet Clin North Am Small Anim Pract* 29:251, 1999.

Osborne CA et al: Feline xanthine urolithiasis: a newly recognized cause of urinary tract disease, *Urol Res* 32(2)(abstr):171, 2004.

Reilly HJ et al: Influence of diet on urine pH and serum biochemical values in healthy dogs, *Vet Ther* 2(1):61, 2001.

Tsan MF et al: Canine cystinuria: its urinary amino acid patterns and genetic analysis, *Am J Vet Res* 33:2455, 1972.

van Zuilen CD et al: Xanthinuria in a family of cavalier King Charles spaniels, *Vet Q* 19(4):172, 1997.

CHAPTER 186

Diagnostic Approach to Acute Azotemia

JENNIFER E. STOKES, *Knoxville, Tennessee*

GENERAL INFORMATION

Acute azotemia occurs as a result of rapid hemodynamic, filtration, tubulointerstitial, or excretory damage to the upper and/or lower urinary tract. The abrupt decrease in glomerular filtration rate (GFR) results in accumulation of uremic toxins and metabolic byproducts; metabolic dysfunction; and dysregulation of fluid, electrolyte, and acid-base balance. Because kidneys receive 20% of cardiac output, these organs are particularly susceptible to ischemic and toxicant-induced damage. Acute azotemia can develop as a result of prerenal, intrinsic renal, or postrenal disease.

Prerenal disease develops when GFR declines because of decreased renal blood flow or increased renal vascular resistance. Prerenal azotemia is a functional abnormality that is potentially reversible. Prerenal disease can coincide with intrinsic renal failure; and prolonged prerenal azotemia can progress to structural damage and intrinsic, irreversible renal failure. Patients with prerenal azotemia generally have concentrated urine (specific gravity >1.025), unless an underlying condition (Addison's disease) or concurrent medications (prednisone, furosemide) prevent maximal concentrating ability. Intrinsic causes of acute azotemia result from renal parenchymal damage caused by ischemic, glomerular, or tubular disease. In dogs and cats toxic, infectious, and ischemic causes occur most commonly. Postrenal azotemia is caused by obstruction or rupture of the urinary tract. If postrenal acute renal failure is recognized and treated early, most cases are reversible (see Chapter 191).

Establishing the cause of acute azotemia can help predict prognosis and determine if specific therapy is indicated in addition to standard supportive care. Specific medical treatments for some causes of acute azotemia include antimicrobials for leptospirosis and bacterial pyelonephritis and 4-methylpyrazole or ethanol for ethylene glycol (EG) toxicity (see Chapter 29). Prognosis for acute azotemia is variable and associated with the underlying cause. Animals with EG nephrotoxicity have a survival of 20% or less compared to the overall survival rate of acute renal disease of approximately 60% (Cowgill and Francey, 2005). Differential diagnoses for acute azotemia, including potential nephrotoxins and potential predisposing factors, are listed in Boxes 186-1 and 186-2.

DIAGNOSTIC PLAN FOR ACUTE RENAL AZOTEMIA

Signalment

During initial assessment the signalment may provide insight to the possible cause of acute azotemia. In general, young animals are more prone to dietary indiscretion; owners should be asked if their pet had access to zinc (pennies, bolts), lilies, raisins, grapes, or any medications. Congenital renal disease typically manifests as a chronic condition rather than as acute azotemia and is not discussed further. Neoplasia should be considered in geriatric patients, although lymphoma and nephroblastoma are encountered in the middle-aged and young pet. Urolithiasis is more common in certain breeds (Table 186-1) (see Chapter 203).

History

A thorough patient history assists in determining the cause of acute azotemia. The pet's current and past medical history should be reviewed for concurrent medical diseases, episodes of urolithiasis, urinary tract infection, recent sedation, or anesthesia. The pet's usual environment, travel history, and exposure to wild or domestic animals and ticks influences decisions concerning testing for infectious diseases. If leptospirosis is suspected, an accurate vaccine history must be collected since multivalent leptospiral vaccines are available.

The owner should be asked about the pet's exposure to *specific* nephrotoxins, as well as specific medications (see Box 186-1). Nonsteroidal antiinflammatory agents and angiotensin-converting enzyme inhibitors are the most commonly prescribed of the potentially nephrotoxic agents. In addition to medications prescribed for the pet, it is useful to determine if the pet has access to an owner's medications, such as oral medications with potential nephrotoxicity like topical zinc oxide or calcipotriol (a topical synthetic cholecalciferol antipsoriasis medication) (Welch, 2002). The possibility of recent exposure to antifreeze, cholecalciferol rodenticides, or toxic plants should be established. For many potential nephrotoxins, including raisins/grapes and lilies, determining their role in causing acute azotemia is usually made based on history.

Box 186-1

Potential Nephrotoxins Encountered in Small Animal Practice

Medications
- Antimicrobial agents
  - Aminoglycosides
  - Amphotericin B
  - Carbapenems
  - Cephalosporins
  - Fluoroquinolones
  - Penicillins
  - Rifampin
  - Sulfonamides
  - Tetracyclines
  - Vancomycin
- Immunosuppressants
  - Azathioprine
  - Cyclosporine
  - Cancer chemotherapy
  - Bisphosphonates
  - Carboplatin
  - Cisplatin
  - Doxorubicin
  - Methotrexate
- Miscellaneous medications
  - Acyclovir
  - Angiotensin-converting enzyme inhibitors
  - Allopurinol
  - Apomorphine
  - Calcium
  - Cimetidine
  - Dextran 40
  - Mannitol
  - Nonsteroidal antiinflammatory drugs
  - Penicillamine
  - Streptokinase
  - Thiacetarsemide
  - Vitamin D (cholecalciferol)

Additional Substances
- Ethylenediaminetetraacetic acid
- Ethylene glycol
- Radiocontrast media
- Grapes, raisins
- *Lilium* spp.
  - Easter lily, tiger lily, stargazer lily, Asiatic hybrid lily
- *Hemerocallis* spp.
  - Common day lily, early day lily
- Heavy metals
  - Mercury, gold, nickel, thallium, lead, zinc
- Carbon tetrachloride
- Snake and bee venom
- Hemoglobin, myoglobin
- *Amanita phalloides* (mushroom)

Box 186-2

Potential Causes and Risk Factors for Acute Azotemia in Dogs and Cats

Vascular or Ischemic
- Anesthesia
- Cutaneous and renal glomerular vasculopathy ("Alabama rot")
- Decreased cardiac output
- Dehydration
- Disseminated intravascular coagulation
- Hyperviscosity syndrome
  - Hyperglobulinemia
  - Multiple myeloma
  - Polycythemia
- Hypotension
- Surgery
- Systemic arterial hypertension
- Thrombosis/infarction
- Vasculitis

Concurrent administration of potential nephrotoxins (see Box 186-1)

Infectious
- Bacterial and fungal pyelonephritis
- Leptospirosis
- Babesiosis
- Borreliosis
- Leishmaniasis

Metabolic/Systemic Disease
- Acidosis
- Diabetes mellitus
- Hepatic insufficiency
- Hyperadrenocorticism
- Hypercalcemia
- Hypoadrenocorticism
- Hypoalbuminemia
- Hypocalcemia
- Hypokalemia
- Hypomagnesemia
- Hyponatremia
- Pancreatitis
- Pre-existing renal disease
- Sepsis

Other
- Advanced age
- Immune-mediated disease
  - Acute glomerulonephritis
  - Renal transplant rejection
  - Systemic lupus erythematosus
- Urolithiasis
- Urinary tract rupture
- Envenomation
- Hyperthermia
- Neoplasia, infiltrative
- Tumor lysis syndrome (some causes can be placed under multiple categories)

Evidence of a specific toxin may be observed in the vomitus. Although a nephrotoxic substance has been extracted from Easter lilies, there is no commercial diagnostic test for this toxin; and the toxic agent of other lilies, raisins, and grapes is unknown (Rumbeiha et al., 2004).

Table 186-1

Breeds at Increased Risk of Urolithiasis (Canine Unless Otherwise Indicated)

Stone type	Breed
Calcium oxalate	Miniature schnauzers, Lhasa apso, Yorkshire terrier, bichon frise, Pomeranian, Shih Tzu, cairn terrier, Maltese, miniature poodle, Chihuahua
Calcium oxalate (feline)	Domestic shorthair, Himalayan, Persian, rag doll, British shorthair, exotic shorthair, Havana brown, Scottish fold
Struvite (magnesium ammonium phosphate)	Miniature schnauzers, Lhasa apso, Yorkshire terrier, Shih Tzu, bichon frise, miniature poodle, cocker spaniel
Urate/xanthane	Dalmatian, English bulldog, miniature schnauzer, Shih Tzu, Yorkshire terriers
Cystine	Mastiff, Australian cattle dog, English bulldog, dachshund, Staffordshire bull terrier, Newfoundland
Calcium phosphate	Yorkshire terrier, miniature schnauzer, bichon frise, Shih Tzu, springer spaniel, Pomeranian, miniature poodle, cocker spaniel
Silica	German shepherd, Old English sheepdog, cocker spaniel, bichon frise, Labrador retriever, golden retriever, miniature schnauzer, Shih Tzu

An accurate description of the current illness is important as well, including the duration of clinical signs and the specific nature of the clinical syndrome. A pet with signs of illness for several months' duration may have an acute exacerbation of chronic kidney disease. Dysuria, stranguria, and pollakiuria suggest lower urinary tract disease. Pets with a history of recent trauma may have uroabdomen or other renal or postrenal injury.

Physical Examination

A thorough physical examination should include routine evaluation, assessment of hydration status, and general body condition; a digital rectal examination; and an ophthalmic examination. Anterior uveitis is common with leptospirosis but may be present in animals with other infectious diseases or lymphoma. Leptospirosis should also be suspected in any icteric dog with acute azotemia (see Chapter 269). If pallor and red urine are present, intravascular hemolytic anemia from zinc intoxication or babesiosis should be considered. Infectious diseases should be ruled out in a febrile patient. Bradycardia should prompt investigation for hypoadrenocorticism, although bradycardia can be caused by hyperkalemia or excessive vagal tone from other causes. If dysphoria is present, further questioning of the owner and testing for EG toxicity are indicated. Cranial abdominal pain is a nonspecific finding but should increase one's index of suspicion of pancreatitis, particularly in dogs. If abdominal fluid is detected, diagnostic procedures should be done to rule uroabdomen in or out.

The kidneys should be palpated to determine renal size, symmetry, and pain. Finding small kidneys would suggest chronic renal disease with an acute exacerbation. Bilaterally large kidneys are palpated in animals with acute renal disease because of toxicity, infection, or lymphoma. The finding of frequently asymmetric kidneys (one large and one small) in a cat should prompt the clinician to assess the cat more closely for ureteral obstruction.

Local cellulitis may be consistent with envenomation from snake or bull ant bites. Generalized lymphadenomegaly should prompt a clinician to assess the pet more closely for lymphosarcoma or infectious diseases. If the pet has a poor body condition suggesting a chronic disease process, it is important to determine if chronic renal disease or hypoadrenocorticism is present. In animals with lower urinary tract signs, the lower urogenital area should be examined closely to assess for obstructive lesions. Urolithiasis or neoplasia may be suspected if urethral or anal gland masses, urethral thickening, or enlarged intrapelvic lymph nodes are palpated on digital rectal examination.

Initial Diagnostic Testing

If there are no definitive historical or physical examination findings to guide initial diagnostic testing, a complete blood count, serum biochemistry profile, electrolytes, urinalysis, urine culture, abdominal radiographs, and abdominal ultrasound should be performed. Leptospirosis testing is recommended in any dog with acute azotemia. Testing cats for feline leukemia and feline immunodeficiency virus may be indicated. Neither disease directly causes acute azotemia, but each may predispose to neoplasms or infections that adversely affect renal function. If available, measuring systemic blood pressure, blood gas values, and coagulation status can provide useful information, particularly for acute and long-term management.

Evaluation of Complete Blood Count

A clinician should be suspicious of leptospirosis, pyelonephritis, or other infectious disease if a leukocytosis and left shift are diagnosed. Testing for babesiosis and zinc intoxication are indicated if a strongly regenerative anemia is observed since both conditions cause intravascular hemolysis. Thrombocytopenia may be seen with leptospirosis, babesiosis, and rickettsial diseases. Hyperviscosity syndrome would be suspected in a patient with polycythemia or hyperglobulinemia. Relative polycythemia (hemoconcentration) may be evident in a pet with prerenal azotemia. Absolute polycythemia may be present as a result of polycythemia vera or secondary polycythemia caused by chronic hypoxemia or a paraneoplastic syndrome (e.g., renal neoplasia).

A sick azotemic animal with a lack of a stress leukogram or relative eosinophilia should be tested for hypoadrenocorticism (adrenocorticotropic hormone stimulation test). *Babesia* organisms may be seen on peripheral blood smears, but an absence of hemoparasites does not rule out such an infection, and serologic testing is indicated in suspect cases.

Evaluation of Serum Biochemical Results

Further diagnostic tests are indicated in hypercalcemic animals (also see Chapter 54). Hypercalcemia is most commonly caused by neoplasia, chronic renal failure, hypoadrenocorticism, hyperparathyroidism, and vitamin D toxicosis in dogs. In cats neoplasia, renal disease, and idiopathic hypercalcemia are the most common causes of elevated serum total calcium. Hypercalcemic animals should have ionized calcium and ideally blood pH measurements performed. Hypercalcemia-induced acute azotemia is most commonly associated with neoplasia, vitamin D toxicosis, and primary hyperparathyroidism. Hypoglycemia may suggest sepsis or hypoadrenocorticism in an azotemic patient. Hyperkalemia with concurrent hyponatremia may be caused by hypoadrenocorticism, acute renal failure (of any cause), and uroabdomen. Elevations in liver enzyme activity, bilirubin concentration, or creatinine kinase activity should increase the clinician's index of suspicion for leptospirosis. In dogs elevated amylase and lipase suggest pancreatitis but are not specific markers for the disease. Currently the most sensitive laboratory test for pancreatitis in cats is a species-specific pancreatic lipase immunoreactivity test (see Chapter 124).

Hypocalcemia occurs in 50%, and hyperglycemia occurs in more than 70% of cats and dogs with EG intoxication. Marked acidosis and elevated anion gap (Gaynor and Dhupa, 1999) also should increase suspicion for EG intoxication. Acidosis can be estimated by assessing serum total carbon dioxide levels, although measuring blood pH is preferable. Hyperphosphatemia can also occur because of the presence of phosphate-containing rust inhibitors in EG.

Urinalysis

A urinalysis should be performed in all azotemic patients. Leptospirosis has been associated with glucosuria, proteinuria, bilirubinuria, increased granular casts, leukocytes, and erythrocytes. Leptospires are not observed in urine without special staining or dark-field microscopy. Crystalluria occurs in healthy animals but may be associated with urolithiasis (see Chapter 185). Both dihydrate and monohydrate calcium oxalate crystals (especially the latter) may be observed in EG cases, although both can be seen in normal animals. Pyelonephritis should be suspected when pyuria, hematuria, and increased granular casts are present; however, absence of bacteriuria does not rule out upper urinary tract infection. Yeast or fungi may be seen cytologically. Urine culture is indicated in all patients with acute azotemia.

Imaging Studies

Routine abdominal imaging is also indicated in dogs and cats with acute azotemia. Survey abdominal radiography is useful in determining renal size and detecting uroliths, abdominal fluid, metallic gastrointestinal foreign bodies, mass lesions, and bony trauma. Severe vitamin D toxicosis may be suspected if generalized soft-tissue mineralization is seen radiographically. Contrast studies (excretory urography or cystourethrography) are the most sensitive methods for detecting urinary tract rupture.

Abdominal ultrasound is extremely useful for assessing the structure of the urinary tract and surrounding tissues. Sonography may detect renal cysts or masses, abdominal fluid, uroliths, hydronephrosis, outflow obstruction, pancreatitis, lymphadenomegaly, bilaterally small adrenal glands, and abdominal masses. Doppler techniques can be used to assess for renal vascular changes such as thromboemboli and occlusive mass lesions. Specific sonographic renal abnormalities detected in dogs with leptospirosis include renomegaly, pyelectasia, hyperechoic cortices, perirenal fluid accumulation, and a hyperechoic medullary band, which corresponds to necrosis and hemorrhage (Greene et al., 2006). Sonographic abnormalities reported in dogs and cats with known or probable EG toxicity include hyperechoic renal cortices and medulla, which can progress to severe intensity, and a "halo" sign, which is a band of relative hypoechogenicity at the corticomedullary junction and central medulla surrounded by hyperechoic cortex and medulla. The changes vary, depending on the stage of toxicity (Adams, Toal, and Breider, 1991).

Imaging studies also are critical for the detection of ureteral obstruction. Radiographic abnormalities documented in cases of ureteral obstruction in cats include bilateral renomegaly, renal asymmetry, expansion of the retroperitoneal space, or ureteroliths. Radiography or ultrasonography may diagnose ureteral obstruction, but in 20% to 30% of cats no discrete mineralized material is identified with routine abdominal imaging. The sensitivity for detecting ureteroliths increases when radiographs and serial ultrasound examinations are used in tandem (see Chapter 202). Antegrade pyelography using ultrasound guidance to inject contrast media into the renal pelvis can be performed to detect and characterize ureteral obstructions that are not apparent with routine radiographic techniques (Kyles et al., 2005). Advanced imaging techniques (such as computed tomography or urethrocystoscopy) are sometimes required in challenging cases of ureteral obstruction or other unusual types of acute azotemia.

When To Consider a Renal Biopsy

Renal biopsy occasionally is indicated for determining the underlying cause of disease and prognosis in a patient with acute azotemia. It should be considered if the definitive cause, extent of injury, chronicity, or prognosis cannot be established by less invasive means. It is also recommended in patients for which peritoneal dialysis or hemodialysis is considered. Histologic evidence of intact renal tubular epithelial basement membranes and regenerating epithelial cells are favorable indicators for recovery. Renal tissue samples also can be analyzed for EG content. Calcium oxalate crystals may be seen histologically, although crystals are not pathognomonic for EG toxicity. Leptospirosis may also be diagnosed histologically using Giemsa or silver stain in biopsy or postmortem tissue samples. Renal biopsy to diagnose leptospirosis usually is indicated in determining zoonotic potential for exposed people and pets rather than as a means of determining an antemortem clinical diagnosis.

Additional Diagnostic Tests

Infectious Disease Testing

As mentioned previously, leptospirosis is a key differential diagnosis for acute renal azotemia. The standard serologic test for leptospirosis is the microscopic agglutination test (MAT). It is serogroup specific but not serovar specific. Testing for multiple serovars, including canicola, icterohaemorrhagiae, bratislava, hardjo, pomona, grippotyphosa, and autumnalis is recommended. Ideally serologic diagnosis of leptospirosis is based on a fourfold increase in paired titers completed at a 2- to 4-week interval. Dogs can be seronegative the first seven to ten days of clinical illness. A single titer of 1:800 can be used to support a presumptive diagnosis of leptospirosis when compatible clinical disease is present and there is no history of leptospiral vaccination within the previous 3 months. Vaccine titers usually are less than 1:400 for the first 3 months after vaccination, but titers as high as 1:800 have been observed to persist for 9 months after vaccination. An immunoglobulin M enzyme-linked immunosorbent assay (ELISA) is more sensitive in detecting early infection than the MAT but is not yet widely available for clinical use.

In addition to serologic testing, it is also useful to submit urine for polymerase chain reaction (PCR) tests for leptospiral organisms. Although organisms may not be shed in urine for 4 to 10 days after onset of illness and antimicrobial therapy may decrease renal shedding, urinary PCR is highly sensitive (perhaps oversensitive) for leptospirosis. The presence of leptospiral organisms in the urine (based on PCR results), and clinical findings compatible with leptospirosis, the dog should be considered a potential zoonotic source of disease for humans (Greene et al., 2006).

Babesiosis is a rare cause of acute azotemia in dogs, but it should be considered in a dog with acute azotemia and regenerative anemia and/or thrombocytopenia. Indirect fluorescent antibody testing is probably the most specific and commonly used test to detect *Babesia* antibodies. Usually a titer of ≥1:80 to *B. canis* or ≥1:320 to *B. gibsoni* is sufficient for diagnosis (Taboada and Lobetti, 2006). Dogs may be seronegative early in the disease; thus measuring convalescent titers is necessary in some cases to make a diagnosis. PCR testing is also available and is the most sensitive and specific means of diagnosis.

Although acute azotemia has not been proven to be a result of infection with *Borrelia burgdorferi* in dogs, there is an association between Lyme disease and acute azotemia. In dogs in Lyme-endemic areas that develop a progressive, proteinuric form of acute azotemia, testing for borreliosis is recommended. The most common screening procedures include ELISA and indirect fluorescent antibody techniques, but false-positives caused by cross-reactivity with other organisms or to vaccination occur. Any such positive result should be followed by a confirmation test such as Western blot or an ELISA test for antibodies against specific proteins (recombinant Osp C or C6). A commercial test, SNAP 3DX (IDEXX Laboratories) is available for testing for antibody to the C6 peptide and

is likely the most sensitive and specific test to diagnose active infection (as opposed to recovered infection or vaccine or cross-reactivity). Dogs can be seropositive and not be ill from infection; thus diagnosis should not be made on serologic testing alone (Greene and Straubinger, 2006).

Evaluation of Abdominal Fluid

If present, abdominal fluid should be collected for fluid analysis and cytologic examination. A sample should be saved for future culture. Fluid protein should be measured. Fluid potassium, creatinine, and urea nitrogen should be measured and compared to serum values to diagnose or rule out uroabdomen.

Ethylene Glycol Assays

Measuring serum or urine EG levels by gas chromatography is the most specific diagnostic test for EG toxicity, but such testing is not readily available. A commercially available test kit (Allelic Biosystems Ethylene Glycol Test Kit, PRN Pharmacal, Inc.) measures blood EG concentrations of 50 mg/dl or above. Levels are highest 3 hours after ingestion and are nondetectable within 48 hours of ingestion. This test is most useful 1 to 12 hours after ingestion but may detect EG for up to 24 hours or longer after exposure since EG is excreted slowly in acute renal failure. The test may be falsely negative in cats, which can develop acute azotemia at lower serum EG levels. False-positive results occur in animals exposed to glycerol, metaldehyde, and propylene glycol (e.g., anticonvulsants, activated charcoal) (Gaynor and Dhupa, 1999).

Zinc Assays

A presumptive diagnosis of zinc toxicity is made in an azotemic, anemic patient with evidence of a metallic gastrointestinal foreign body. Zinc is a common element in United States pennies (minted after 1982), cage nuts, cage wire, brass buttons, and zinc oxide ointment. Diagnosis is confirmed by measuring plasma zinc levels. Correct sample collection is imperative; many ethylenediaminetetraacetic acid and heparin collection tubes contain zinc in their rubber stoppers, which may contaminate the sample. Royal blue-top tubes are zinc free. Assessment of tissue levels in the liver or kidney may also be diagnostic.

References and Suggested Reading

Adams WH, Toal RL, Breider MA: Ultrasonographic findings in dogs and cats with oxalate nephrosis attributed to ethylene glycol intoxication: 15 cases (1984-1988), *J Am Vet Med Assoc* 199:492, 1991.

Cowgill LD, Francey T: Acute Uremia. In Ettinger SJ, Feldman EC, editors: *Textbook of veterinary internal medicine*, Philadelphia, 2005, Saunders Elsevier, p 1731.

Gaynor AR, Dhupa N: Acute ethylene glycol intoxication, *Compend Contin Educ Pract Vet* 21:1014, 1999.

Greene CE, Straubinger RK: Borreliosis. In Greene CE, editor: *Infectious diseases of the dog and cat*, 2006, p 417.

Greene CE et al: Leptospirosis. In Greene CE, editor: *Infectious diseases of the dog and cat*, St. Louis, 2006, Saunders, p 402.

Khan KN et al: Interspecies differences in renal localization of cyclooxygenase isoforms: implications in nonsteroidal antiinflammatory drug-related nephrotoxicity, *Toxicol Pathol* 26:612, 1998.

Kyles AE et al: Clinical, clinicopathologic, radiographic, and ultrasonographic abnormalities in cats with ureteral calculi: 163 cases (1984-2002), *J Am Vet Med Assoc* 226:932, 2005.

Mazzaferro EM et al: Acute renal failure associated with raisin or grape ingestion in 4 dogs, *J Vet Emerg Crit Care* 14:203, 2004.

Rumbeiha WK et al: A comprehensive study of Easter lily poisoning in cats, *J Vet Diagn Invest* 16:527, 2004.

Taboada J, Lobetti R: Babesisosis. In Greene CE, editor: *Infectious diseases of the dog and cat,* St. Louis, 2006, Saunders, p 722.

Tefend M: *Acute renal failure: diagnosis and treatment, Proceedings of the ACVIM Forum,* Baltimore, Md, 2005.

Welch SL: Oral toxicity of topical preparations, *Vet Clin North Am Small Anim Pract* 32:443, 2002.

CHAPTER 187

Proteinuria: Implications for Management

GREGORY F. GRAUER, *Manhattan, Kansas*

Persistent proteinuria of renal origin is an important marker of chronic kidney disease (CKD) in both dogs and cats. Albumin is usually the primary component of proteinuria in CKD. Not only is proteinuria a diagnostic marker for CKD, but the potential for proteinuria/albuminuria to mediate CKD progression has also been recognized. The recent development of species-specific albumin enzyme-linked immunosorbent assay technology has enabled detection of low concentrations of canine and feline albuminuria. This advance has stimulated discussion of what levels of proteinuria/albuminuria are normal and what values may be associated with renal disease progression. For these reasons detection, monitoring, and treatment of dogs and cats with renal proteinuria have received renewed interest. Just as our definition and treatment guidelines for systemic hypertension are changing, so perhaps is our approach to recognizing, monitoring, and treating proteinuria.

DETECTION OF PROTEINURIA

Proteinuria is routinely detected by semiquantitative screening methods such as the conventional dipstick colorimetric test (very common) and the sulfosalicylic acid (SSA) turbidimetric test (less common). The dipstick test is inexpensive, easy to use, and primarily measures albumin; however, both the sensitivity and specificity for albumin are relatively low with this methodology. False-positive results (decreased specificity) may be obtained if the urine is alkaline, if the urine sediment is active (pyuria, hematuria, and/or bacteriuria; often termed *postrenal* proteinuria), or if the dipstick is left in contact with the urine

long enough to leach out the citrate buffer that is incorporated in the filter paper pad. False-positive results with the dipstick occur more frequently in cats than in dogs but occur in both. False-negative results (decreased sensitivity) may occur in the setting of Bence Jones proteinuria, low concentrations of albuminuria, and/or dilute or acidic urine. The conventional dipstick test has a detection level of greater than 30 mg/dl.

The SSA test is performed by mixing equal quantities of urine supernatant and 5% SSA in a glass test tube and grading the turbidity that results from precipitation of protein on a 0 to 4+ scale. In addition to albumin, the SSA test can detect globulins and Bence Jones proteins. False-positive results may occur if the urine contains radiographic contrast agents, penicillin, cephalosporins, sulfisoxazole, or the urine preservative thymol. The protein content may also be overestimated with the SSA test if uncentrifuged, turbid urine is analyzed. False-negative results are less common than with the conventional dipstick test because of the increased sensitivity of the SSA test (>5 mg/dl). Because of the relatively poor specificity of the conventional dipstick analysis, many reference laboratories confirm a positive dipstick test result for proteinuria with the SSA test. Still, grading of both the color change on the dipstick test and the turbidity on the SSA test is subjective; results can vary among individuals and laboratories.

Proteinuria detected by these semiquantitative screening methods has historically been interpreted in light of the urine specific gravity and urine sediment. For example, a positive dipstick reading of trace or 1+ proteinuria in hypersthenuric urine has often been attributed to urine concentration rather than abnormal proteinuria. In addition, a positive dipstick reading for protein in the presence of hematuria or pyuria was often attributed to urinary tract hemorrhage or inflammation. In both examples the interpretation may not be correct. Given the limits of the conventional dipstick test sensitivity, any positive result for protein regardless of urine concentration may be abnormal (except in the case of false-positive results). Likewise, hematuria and pyuria have an inconsistent effect on urine albumin concentrations; not all dogs with hematuria and pyuria have albuminuria.

DETECTION OF ALBUMINURIA

Albuminuria can be measured by point-of-care, semiquantitative tests (e.g., E.R.D.-HealthScreen Urine Test, Heska Corporation) and with quantitative immunoassays at reference laboratories. Microalbuminuria (MA) is defined as concentrations of albumin in the urine that are greater than normal but below the limit of detection using conventional dipstick urine protein screening methodology. Because of the sensitivity of the conventional dipstick test, the upper end of urine albumin concentration that is considered to represent MA is 30 mg/dl. Urine albumin concentrations above 30 mg/dl are referred to as overt albuminuria and can often be detected using the urine protein/creatinine (UP/C) ratio (see Quantitation of Proteinuria later in the chapter). The lower end of the MA range has been less easily defined because of the requirement that this concentration be greater than "normal" and the necessity that this concentration be reliably detected. In the dog and cat the lower limit was defined based on the log mean + 2 standard deviations of populations of apparently healthy dogs and cats as greater than 1 mg/dl. Urine albumin concentrations can be adjusted for differences in urine concentration by dividing by urine creatinine concentrations. For example, a urine albumin/creatinine ratio greater than 0.03 is considered abnormal in humans. Alternatively urine can be diluted to a standard concentration such as 1.010 before assay. In one study of dogs normalizing urine albumin concentrations to a 1.010 specific gravity yielded similar results to the ratio of urine albumin/creatinine (Lees et al., 2002).

Indications for the use of MA tests include: (1) when conventional screening tests for proteinuria produce equivocal or conflicting results or false-positive results are suspected; (2) when conventional screening tests for proteinuria are negative in apparently healthy older dogs and cats and a more sensitive screening test is desired; (3) when conventional screening tests for proteinuria are negative in apparently healthy young dogs and cats with a familial risk for developing proteinuric renal disease and a more sensitive screening test is desired; or (4) when conventional screening tests for proteinuria are negative in dogs and cats with chronic illnesses associated with a high risk for proteinuric renal disease and a more sensitive screening test is desired.

LOCALIZATION OF PROTEINURIA

When proteinuria is detected by screening tests, it is important to try to identify its source. Proteinuria may be caused by physiologic or pathologic conditions. Physiologic or benign proteinuria is often transient and abates when the underlying cause is corrected. Strenuous exercise, seizures, fever, exposure to extreme heat or cold, and stress are examples of conditions that may cause physiologic proteinuria. The mechanism of physiologic proteinuria is not completely understood; however, transient renal vasoconstriction, ischemia, and congestion may be involved. Decreased physical activity may also affect urine protein excretion in dogs; one study showed that urinary protein loss was higher in dogs confined to cages than in dogs with normal activity levels (McCaw, Knapp, and Hewet, 1985).

Pathologic proteinuria may be caused by urinary or nonurinary abnormalities. Nonurinary disorders associated with proteinuria often involve the production of small–molecular weight proteins (dysproteinemias) that are filtered by the glomeruli and subsequently overwhelm the resorptive capacity of the proximal tubule. An example of this "prerenal" proteinuria is the production of immunoglobulin light chains (Bence Jones proteins) by neoplastic plasma cells. Genital tract inflammation (e.g., prostatitis or metritis) can also result in pathologic nonurinary proteinuria. Obtaining urine samples via cystocentesis reduces the potential for urine contamination with protein from the lower urinary tract.

Pathologic urinary proteinuria may be renal or nonrenal in origin. Nonrenal proteinuria most frequently occurs in association with lower urinary tract inflammation or hemorrhage (also referred to as postrenal proteinuria). Changes observed in the urine sediment are usually compatible with the underlying inflammation (e.g., pyuria, hematuria, bacteriuria, and increased numbers of transitional epithelial cells). On the other hand, renal proteinuria is most often caused by increased glomerular filtration of plasma proteins associated with intraglomerular hypertension, glomerular capillary wall structural abnormalities, or the presence of immune complexes or vascular inflammation in the glomerular capillaries. Renal proteinuria may also be caused by decreased resorption of filtered plasma proteins caused by tubulointerstitial disease. In some cases tubulointerstitial proteinuria may be accompanied by normoglycemic glucosuria and increased excretion of electrolytes (e.g., Fanconi syndrome and acute tubular damage). Glomerular lesions usually result in higher-magnitude proteinuria compared with proteinuria associated with tubulointerstitial lesions. In addition to glomerular and tubulointerstitial disease, renal proteinuria may be caused by inflammatory or infiltrative disorders of the kidney (e.g., neoplasia, pyelonephritis, and leptospirosis), which are often accompanied by an active urine sediment.

MONITORING RENAL PROTEINURIA

Transient renal proteinuria/albuminuria is likely of little consequence and does not warrant treatment. On the other hand, persistent renal proteinuria/albuminuria indicates the presence of CKD. Persistent proteinuria/albuminuria can be defined as positive test results on three or more occasions 2 weeks or more apart. Because persistent proteinuria/albuminuria can be constant or increase or decrease in magnitude over time, monitoring should use quantitative methods to determine disease trends and/or response to treatment. Changes in the magnitude of proteinuria should always be interpreted in light of the patient's serum creatinine concentration since proteinuria may decrease in progressive renal disease as the number of functional nephrons decrease. Decreasing proteinuria in the face of a stable serum creatinine suggests improving renal function, whereas decreasing proteinuria in the face of an increasing serum creatinine suggests disease progression.

QUANTITATION OF PROTEINURIA

If persistent proteinuria is detected by screening tests, urine protein excretion should be quantified. This helps to evaluate the severity of renal lesions and to assess the response to treatment or the progression of disease. Methods used to quantitate proteinuria include the UP/C ratio and immunoassays for albuminuria that are expressed as either urine albumin/creatinine ratio or in milligrams per deciliter in urine samples that have been diluted to a standard urine specific gravity (e.g., 1.010). Albumin concentration of 30 mg/dl or greater in urine standardized in this fashion usually results in UP/C ratios of 0.4 and 0.5 or greater in cats and dogs, respectively. The UP/C and urine albumin/creatinine ratios from spot urine samples have been shown to accurately reflect the quantity of protein/albumin excreted in the urine over a 24-hour period. Because of the difficulty of 24-hour urine collection, this methodology has greatly facilitated the diagnosis of proteinuric renal disease in veterinary medicine. Most studies have shown that normal urine protein excretion in dogs and cats is 10 mg/kg/24 hours or less and that normal UP/C ratios are 0.2 to 0.3 or less. Initially recommended normal values for canine UP/C ratios of less than 1.0 were likely too liberal and have recently been lowered. Today UP/C ratios less than 0.5 and 0.4 are considered as normal for dogs and cats, respectively. Persistent proteinuria that results in UP/C ratios greater than 0.4 and 0.5 in cats and dogs, respectively, when prerenal and postrenal proteinuria have been ruled out, is consistent with either glomerular or tubulointerstitial CKD. Urine protein/creatinine ratios greater than 2.0 are strongly suggestive of glomerular disease. It is possible that the definition of normal will continue to change with additional research. For example, even the ultralow-level, single-nephron proteinuria that occurs secondary to intraglomerular hypertension in hypertrophied nephrons in CKD is abnormal in the face of what may be considered normal whole-body or whole-kidney proteinuria.

TREATMENT OF RENAL PROTEINURIA

Once persistent proteinuria has been documented by monitoring, the appropriate response depends on the magnitude of the proteinuria and the health status of the patient (e.g., the presence or absence of azotemia and/or hypertension). In nonazotemic, persistently proteinuric patients, further investigation (and appropriate treatment) of potential concurrent infectious, inflammatory, or neoplastic diseases is warranted. For example, proteinuria associated with dirofilariasis in dogs often improves or resolves after successful treatment of the infection. Neoplasia, infection, polyarthritis, hepatitis, hyperadrenocorticism, immune-mediated hemolytic anemia, and systemic hypertension are commonly identified concurrent medical problems in dogs with renal proteinuria. In cats viral diseases, neoplasia, immune-mediated disease, polyarthritis, and systemic hypertension are some of the more common conditions associated with renal proteinuria. Unfortunately in many cases an underlying disease may not be identified or may be impossible to eliminate (e.g., neoplasia). In a retrospective study of over 100 dogs with glomerulonephritis, 43% had no identifiable concurrent disease. (Cook and Cowgill, 1996).

When an underlying disorder cannot be identified or treated, treatment strategies for persistent proteinuria depend on its magnitude. Proteinuria resulting in UP/C ratios greater than 1.0 to 3.0 should be treated, whereas continued monitoring and patient investigation should be the primary focus in cases with lesser-magnitude proteinuria. Treatment recommendations usually include reduced dietary protein (early renal failure diets), n-3 fatty acid supplementation (early renal failure diets), low-dose aspirin (0.5 mg/kg q24h orally [PO]), and angiotensin-converting enzyme (ACE) inhibitors (e.g., enalapril, benazepril, 0.5 to 1 mg/kg q24h PO), although it is difficult to separate the effects of individual treatments when they are used in combination. The recommendation to treat proteinuria of this magnitude comes primarily from the results of a blinded, multicenter clinical trial in dogs with spontaneous glomerulonephritis. All dogs in this study had UP/C ratios 3.0 or higher, and all dogs were fed a renal failure diet and treated with low-dose aspirin in addition to either enalapril or placebo (Grauer et al., 2000). Therefore it is possible that the beneficial effects of ACE inhibitors observed in this study (1) would not be observed in dogs with lesser-magnitude proteinuria, and (2) were dependent on the concurrent dietary and aspirin treatment. In another study enalapril treatment, initiated before the onset of proteinuria and azotemia in male Samoyed dogs with X-linked hereditary nephritis, attenuated the eventual proteinuria and azotemia, decreased glomerular basement membrane splitting, and prolonged survival (Grodecki et al., 1997).

Treatment for persistent proteinuria in azotemic dogs and cats should be initiated when the UP/C is 0.5 and 0.4 or greater, respectively. Treatment recommendations in this case usually include ACE inhibition and renal failure diets. These recommendations come from (1) studies in dogs and cats with naturally occurring chronic renal failure (CRF) that document reduced survival associated with proteinuria (Jacob et al., 2005; Syme et al., 2006); and (2) studies in dogs with the remnant kidney model of CRF in which ACE inhibition and n-3 fatty acid supplementation reduced proteinuria and slowed renal disease progression (Brown et al., 1998, 2003). Additional management considerations for CKD are given in several chapters in this section, including Chapters 190 and 192.

SUPPORTIVE CARE

In addition to the previous considerations, supportive therapy is also important in the management of proteinuric renal disease. This supportive care should be aimed at decreasing hypertension, edema, and the tendency for thromboembolism to occur. Reduction of systemic hypertension may reduce intraglomerular hypertension, especially in dogs and cats with renal disease, that has resulted in loss of autoregulation of renal blood flow. Measurement of antithrombin III and fibrinogen concentrations may be helpful in determining which patients should be treated with anticoagulant therapy. Dogs with antithrombin III concentrations less than 70% of normal and fibrinogen concentrations greater than 300 mg/dl are candidates for therapy. Low-dose aspirin is easily administered on an outpatient basis and does not require extensive monitoring. Since fibrin accumulation within the glomerulus is a frequent consequence of proteinuric renal disease, aspirin treatment may serve a dual purpose. Finally, reduced-quantity, high-quality protein diets with n-3 fatty acid supplementation should also be recommended in an attempt to decrease glomerular hyperfiltration and proteinuria. For additional, specific treatment strategies for glomerular disorders, see Chapter 188.

References and Suggested Reading

Brown SA et al: Beneficial effects of chronic administration of dietary w-3 polyunsaturated fatty acids in dogs with renal insufficiency, *J Lab Clin Med* 131:447, 1998.

Brown SA et al: Evaluation of the effects of inhibition of angiotensin-converting enzyme with enalapril in dogs with induced chronic renal insufficiency, *Am J Vet Res* 64:321, 2003.

Burkholder WJ et al: Diet modulates proteinuria in heterozygous female dogs with x-linked hereditary nephropathy, *J Vet Intern Med* 18:165, 2004.

Cook AK, Cowgill LD: Clinical and pathological features of protein-losing glomerular disease in the dog: a review of 137 cases (1985-1992), *J Am Anim Hosp Assoc* 32:313, 1996.

Grauer GF et al: Effects of enalapril vs. placebo as a treatment for canine idiopathic glomerulonephritis, *J Vet Intern Med* 14:526, 2000.

Grauer GF et al: Comparison of conventional urine protein test strips and a quantitative ELISA for the detection of canine and feline albuminuria, *J Vet Intern Med* 18 (Abstract):418, 2004.

Grodecki KM et al: Treatment of X-linked hereditary nephritis in Samoyed dogs with angiotensin-converting enzyme (ACE) inhibitor, *J Comp Pathol* 17:209, 1997.

Jacob F et al: Evaluation of the association between initial proteinuria and morbidity or death in dogs with naturally occurring chronic renal failure, *J Am Vet Med Assoc* 226:393, 2005.

Lees GE et al: Persistent albuminuria preceded onset of overt proteinuria in male dogs with X-linked hereditary nephropathy, *J Vet Intern Med* 16 (Abstract):353, 2002.

Lees GE et al: Assessment and management of proteinuria in dogs and cats: 2004 ACVIM Forum Consensus Statement (Small Animal), *J Vet Intern Med* 19:377, 2005.

McCaw DL, Knapp DW, Hewet JE: Effect of collection and exercise restriction on the prediction of urine protein excretion using urine protein/creatinine ratio in dogs, *Am J Vet Res* 46:1665, 1985.

Syme HM et al: Survival in cats with naturally occurring chronic renal failure is related to severity of proteinuria, *J Vet Intern Med* 20:528, 2006.

CHAPTER **188**

Glomerular Disease

SHELLY L. VADEN, *Raleigh, North Carolina*
CATHY A. BROWN, *Athens, Georgia*

Glomerular diseases are a leading cause of renal disease in dogs, but they occur less commonly in cats. The standard of care for management of dogs and cats with glomerular disease is nonspecific, but the standard of care in humans often includes additional therapy based on the histologic diagnosis of the glomerular disease. The recent movement to improve the evaluation of renal biopsy specimens from dogs and cats should eventually lead to implementation of disease-specific protocols for the treatment of dogs and cats with glomerular disease. The purpose of this chapter is to discuss the glomerular diseases that occur in dogs and cats, including specific management suggestions.

NONSPECIFIC MANAGEMENT OF GLOMERULAR DISEASE

Nonspecific management is indicated in all dogs and cats with glomerular disease, regardless of the histologic diagnosis. Nonspecific management can be divided into four major categories, based primarily on the stage of progression of chronic kidney disease (CKD) in an individual patient (see Chapter 192). The management categories are (1) treatment of potentially underlying diseases processes (CKD stages 1 to 4); (2) reduction of proteinuria (CKD stages 1 to 4); (3) modification of factors known to contribute to progression of renal disease (CKD stages 3 to 4); and (4) management of uremia and other complications of generalized renal failure (CKD stages 3 to 4). Detailed discussions of each of these categories can be found in other chapters in this section. However, the need to evaluate an animal with persistent glomerular proteinuria for systemic diseases cannot be overemphasized. Many of the glomerular diseases that occur in dogs and cats are believed to develop secondary to a systemic neoplastic, infectious, or noninfectious inflammatory disease process (NIN). However, a NIN may not be obvious at first presentation because it is either resolved or occult. Because occult diseases may become overt months after initial presentation, continued observation and scrutiny are necessary. Identification and treatment of a NIN is the initial and perhaps most important step in the management of a persistently proteinuric dog or cat. The animal should be evaluated subsequently for resolving proteinuria, which may occur slowly over a period of months (see Chapter 187).

PROCUREMENT AND EVALUATION OF THE RENAL BIOPSY

Specimen Preparation

If proteinuria does not resolve or worsens over time or following treatment of a potentially underlying NIN, a renal biopsy to determine the specific glomerular disease present may be warranted. More study is needed to determine which dogs and cats with glomerular disease benefit the most from the results of a renal biopsy. However, it is likely that the animals with CKD stages 1 or 2 (possibly 3) and with magnitude of proteinuria that is either in or nearing nephrotic range are the ones that will benefit the most. Once collected, renal biopsy specimens should be divided into three pieces, each of which contains glomeruli. The largest piece should be placed in formalin, a smaller piece should go into a fixative suitable for electron microscopy (EM; e.g., 4% formalin plus 1% glutaraldehyde in sodium phosphate buffer), and another small piece should either be frozen or placed in a fixative suitable for immunofluorescent microscopy (IFM); (i.e., ammonium sulfate-N-ethylmaleimide fixative, also known as Michel's solution). Although light microscopy may be highly suggestive of a particular glomerular disease, particularly with more advanced disease, EM is required to verify the presence of immune deposits, to detect small deposits not evident by light microscopy, to identify the location of the deposits in the glomerulus (subendothelial, subepithelial, intramembranous, mesangial), and to detect basement membrane or podocyte abnormalities. IFM is used to determine the specific nature of the immune deposits (immunoglobulin [Ig]G, IgA, IgM, complement) and further defines the disease process.

Evaluation of Biopsy Specimens

The normal renal cortex contains scattered glomeruli and numerous tubules within a scant interstitium. These renal components are evaluated initially in slides stained with hematoxylin and eosin (H&E) to determine lesion distribution, severity, and the primary site of renal disease (interstitial or glomerular). The evaluation of the glomeruli is the focus of this discussion; a description of the evaluation of the entire biopsy sample can be found elsewhere. The glomerulus is a tuft of highly branched capillaries that invaginate into an extension of the proximal tubule. The afferent arteriole enters and arborizes to form the glomerular capillary tuft and exits as the efferent arteriole; these arterioles enter and exit at the vascular pole. The capillary loops are supported by scaffolding that is made up of mesangial cells and their surrounding extracellular mesangial matrix. The capillary tuft is draped by glomerular basement membrane (GBM) and is covered by a layer of interdigitating visceral epithelial cells (podocytes). The glomerular filtration barrier consists of endothelium, GBM, and podocytes.

Proteinuria results when there is disruption of the filtration barrier, which may be caused by the deposition of immune complexes, complement, or amyloid; by a change (either acquired or congenital) in the composition of the GBM; or by injury to the endothelial cells or podocytes. Glomerular injury may also affect mesangial cells, resulting in mesangial cell proliferation and/or increased production of mesangial matrix. Since injury primarily affecting mesangial cells does not directly disrupt the filtration barrier, proteinuria is not typically a prominent feature of diseases involving mesangial cells. Glomerular involvement observed by light microscopy may be *focal* (less than 50% of glomeruli involved) or *generalized* (all or almost all glomeruli involved). Within an affected glomerulus, the lesion may be *segmental* (only part of the capillary tuft affected) or *global* (the entire tuft involved). Although most glomerular diseases in dogs and cats are generalized and global, focal segmental disease may also occur. Glomeruli should be evaluated for cellularity, matrix increase, amyloid deposition, hyalinization, necrosis, fibrin thrombosis, crescents, protein deposits, adhesions, and GBM changes. Because thicker sections appear more cellular, have more mesangial matrix, and have thicker capillary loops, renal biopsies should be routinely sectioned and evaluated at 3 to 4 μm. Biopsies with glomerular deposits suggestive of amyloid should be cut at 6 to 8 μm, stained with Congo red or standard toluidine blue, and viewed with polarized light to confirm this diagnosis. Periodic acid–Schiff hematoxylin (PASH) and Masson's trichrome stains, in addition to H&E, should be used when evaluating glomerular morphology in diseases other than amyloidosis. Basement membrane, mesangial matrix, and cell cytoplasm (including podocytes and endothelium) stain pink with PASH; trichrome stains basement membrane and mesangial matrix blue to blue-grey and immune deposits within the capillary walls magenta. In the normal glomerulus stained with PASH, the thickness of the capillary walls should be assessed in peripheral capillary loops; and, when cut at a right angle, the normal loops are thin, uniform, and crisp. The mesangial matrix can be seen as disconnected branches containing mesangial cells. Matrix typically surrounds one or two mesangial cell nuclei; mesangial matrix expansion is present if matrix extends to encircle more cells. More than three mesangial cell nuclei in close proximity are indicative of mesangial hypercellularity.

MEMBRANOPROLIFERATIVE GLOMERULONEPHRITIS

Glomerulonephritis is an immune-mediated disease most often associated with deposition of immune complexes within the glomerulus. The site of complex deposition may be subendothelial, subepithelial, and/or mesangial, with the associated immunologic and glomerular responses resulting in different forms of glomerulonephritis. These immune complexes may be circulating and passively trapped in mesangial or subendothelial sites; or they may form "in situ" when antibody binds to normal glomerular antigens or to soluble antigens localized within subendothelial, subepithelial, or mesangial areas. Membranoproliferative glomerulonephritis (MPGN) is probably the most common form of glomerulonephritis in dogs, accounting for 20% to 60% of cases in various studies, and is rare in cats. The term MPGN refers to the light microscopic findings of increased "membranelike" thickening of the capillary wall with increased glomerular cellularity and is caused by the presence of immune complexes on the subendothelial aspect of the GBM (type I MPGN), with additional deposits within the mesangium or on the subepithelial aspect of the GBM (type III MPGN). Dense deposit disease (type II MPGN) is characterized by intramembranous dense deposits, is not associated with infectious diseases, and is probably uncommon in dogs. On light microscopy larger immune deposits may stain magenta with trichrome stain, making a diagnosis of MPGN more likely. However, confirmation of this diagnosis depends on demonstration of subendothelial deposits (immune complexes) via EM. In this location the immune deposits, which contain primarily IgG, are associated with proliferation of resident glomerular cells and activation of complement. Subendothelial deposits are readily accessible to circulating inflammatory cells and platelets and thus may be associated with more severe capillary wall injury. Crescents may be observed in some cases of MPGN because breaks or gaps in the damaged GBM allow the passage of fibrinogen, and later macrophages, into the urinary space. Fibrin and macrophages induce parietal epithelial cell and fibroblast proliferation, and glomerular crescents form. Glomerular diseases with significant crescent formation typically are more severe and have a rapidly progressive clinical course.

MPGN may be of unknown cause or secondary to a variety of underlying systemic and infectious diseases. In some cases of MPGN, glomeruli may be infiltrated with monocytes or neutrophils; this inflammatory infiltrate is characteristic of exudative or postinfectious glomerulonephritis. Postinfectious glomerulonephritis of humans most commonly occurs following a streptococcal infection but has also been identified with other infections (e.g., staphylococcal infection). Interestingly, this pattern of disease is usually caused by transient infections, often resolved before clinical signs of glomerular disease.

Effective treatment of the underlying infectious, inflammatory, or neoplastic disease is the cornerstone of management of patients with MPGN. Because activation of platelets appears to be involved in the pathogenesis of this disease, antiplatelet drugs also should be used. Specific data regarding the prognosis of MPGN in dogs are lacking. In humans azotemia, severe proteinuria, systemic hypertension, and marked tubulointerstitial lesions at presentation are the most significant predictors of an unfavorable outcome.

MEMBRANOUS GLOMERULONEPHRITIS OR MEMBRANOUS NEPHROPATHY

Membranous glomerulonephritis (MGN) results from the deposition of immune complexes, most often containing IgG, on the subepithelial aspect of the GBM. Although the glomerular tufts are of normal cellularity, the capillary loops are thickened, and spikes may be evident with PASH as the basement membrane extends between the unstained immune deposits. Advanced cases may have irregular thickening and distortion of the capillary walls with occasional widening of the mesangium. The morphologic changes that occur in the glomerulus in response to immune complexes on the urinary side of the GBM are restricted because the immune complexes are separated from the vascular space and circulating inflammatory mediators. Instead the subepithelial immune deposits primarily induce complement-mediated podocyte injury with diffuse foot process effacement ultrastructurally. The podocytes also produce more basement membrane between and eventually around the immune deposits, resulting in the spikes that may be visualized with PASH staining. Confirmation of a diagnosis of MGN depends on ultrastructural demonstration of the subepithelial deposits. In animals with secondary MGN, deposits may be found elsewhere in the glomeruli.

MGN occurs in 10% to 45% of reported cases of glomerulonephritis in dogs and is the most common type of glomerulonephritis in cats. MGN appears to be more common in male dogs and cats than in females. The mean age of affected dogs is 8 years; the mean age of affected cats is only 3.6 years. Because proteinuria in affected animals may be severe, many of them present with complete or partial nephrotic syndrome.

In humans MGN is considered to be either primary (i.e., idiopathic) or secondary to another disease process; primary disease is most common. EM is used to confirm the location of the immune deposits and to characterize the stage of disease progression. Deposition of immune complexes (stage I), progressive engulfment of the complexes by the surrounding GBM (stages II and III), and eventual resolution of the deposits (stage IV) characterize the stages of MGN. These stages correlate with temporal evolution of the disease and clinical presentation in dogs, cats, and humans. In early stages proteinuria and nephritic syndrome are likely; progressive azotemia is likely during more advanced stages in cats and dogs. However, accurate staging of MGN is difficult in some animals; multiple disease stages may be present simultaneously.

In addition to identification of potentially inciting disease processes and nonspecific management, immunosuppressive therapy may be warranted in dogs or cats with persistent proteinuria caused by MGN, particularly if they appear to have idiopathic disease and are not azotemic. The clinical course of idiopathic MGN in humans varies from spontaneous complete remission in 33% to 65% of patients to rapid progression to end-stage renal disease. The risk of progression in humans appears to correlate with the magnitude of proteinuria and renal functional impairment; patients with the highest degree of proteinuria and azotemia are more likely to have more rapid progression when compared with other patients. Although treatment of MGN in humans is controversial, some patients may respond to immunosuppressive therapy of corticosteroids combined with an alkylating agent. The approach that has proven to be most beneficial is alternating methylprednisolone and chlorambucil every other day for 6 months. Cyclosporine may be a valid option for patients not responding to corticosteroids and alkylating agents. There is evidence to suggest that humans with MGN stage I or II may be more likely to respond to immunosuppressive therapy than patients with MGN stage III or IV. Although MGN appears to be progressive in some dogs and cats, progression may be slow enough that many animals can lead relatively normal lives. In cats stages III and IV MGN may be associated with a poorer prognosis.

MESANGIOPROLIFERATIVE GLOMERULONEPHRITIS

Mesangioproliferative glomerulonephritis accounted for only 2% to 16% of glomerular lesions in dogs of two studies (MacDougall et al., 1986; Koeman et al., 1987). The mean age of affected dogs was between 7 and 9 years. Proteinuria and renal failure (mild-to-moderate, acute, or chronic) are the expected presenting signs in affected dogs. Like MPGN and MN, mesangioproliferative glomerulonephritis is an immune complex–mediated disease.

Mesangioproliferative glomerulonephritis is characterized by mesangial cell hyperplasia, defined as more than three cells per mesangial area, which is often accompanied by an increase in mesangial matrix. On EM immune complexes are present primarily within the mesangium and are mainly of the IgA class (IgA nephropathy). The diagnosis of IgA nephropathy requires a predominance of IgA positivity when examined by IFM.

IgA nephropathy is the most common type of chronic, progressive glomerulonephritis in humans and is an important cause of end-stage renal disease. As with many glomerular diseases, the severity of the tubulointerstitial lesions is a better predicator of progression than the severity of the glomerular changes. There have been several studies of canine glomerular disease that demonstrated mild-to-moderate frequency of IgA positivity via IFM, suggestive of IgA nephropathy. In one study dogs with enteric or hepatic diseases had the highest incidence of IgA deposition (Miyauchi, 1992). Excessive IgA immune complex formation caused by enteric disease or decreased clearance of IgA complexes in association with liver disease have been proposed in the pathogenesis of secondary IgA nephropathy in humans. Treatment of humans with secondary IgA nephropathy is directed toward treatment of the associated systemic disease. Control of systemic hypertension is also a cornerstone of therapy. Administration of fish oil rich in ω-3 fatty acids slowed progression of renal disease in humans but did not lead to a reduction in proteinuria.

AMYLOIDOSIS

Amyloidosis is one of the most common glomerular diseases in dogs, accounting for approximately one fourth of dogs with glomerular disease; cats rarely develop glomerular amyloidosis. With the exception of the Chinese sharpei, amyloid is deposited primarily in the glomeruli of affected dogs. Reactive amyloidosis is the most common form of amyloidosis in dogs and cats, and older animals are more commonly affected. Females appear to be affected more often than males. Beagles, English foxhounds, collies, and walker hounds may be at increased risk for amyloidosis; it may be familial in the former two breeds. Amyloid is first deposited in mesangial areas, with eventual subendothelial deposition. Because proteinuria associated with glomerular amyloidosis may be massive, many dogs present with nephrotic syndrome or pulmonary thromboembolism (caused by loss of antithrombin III). Chinese shar-pei dogs and Abyssinian cats have a familial form of reactive amyloidosis that is characterized by glomerular and medullary amyloid deposition, with medullary deposits typically predominating. In a study of shar-pei dogs only 64% had glomerular involvement, and as few as 25% to 43% of affected dogs were reported to have proteinuria (Dibartola et al., 1990). Affected shar-pei dogs and Abyssinian cats are more likely to present with azotemia rather than proteinuria since medullary interstitial amyloid deposition leads to ischemia, chronic interstitial fibrosis, papillary necrosis, and nephron loss.

In H&E stained slides glomerular amyloid appears as eosinophilic nodular deposits that expand the mesangium and glomerular capillary walls. Interstitial amyloid may be present as perivascular and peritubular deposits throughout the medulla. When stained with Congo red and evaluated by conventional light microscopy, amyloid deposits take on various shades of red, depending on the amount of amyloid and the thickness of the section. Deposits stained with Congo red and evaluated by polarizing microscopy are birefringent and have an apple-green color.

The β-pleated sheet configuration of amyloid fibrils leads to their insolubility and resistance to proteolysis, making specific treatment relatively ineffectual. Familial renal amyloidosis in shar-pei dogs and Abyssinian cats has been compared to familial Mediterranean fever in humans, which is characterized by fever of unknown origin, renal amyloidosis, and pleuritis, peritonitis, and/or synovitis. In affected humans the development of renal amyloidosis may be prevented by colchicine therapy, even in patients who continue to have recurrent febrile episodes. This has led to the recommendation that colchicine be given to shar-pei dogs with renal amyloidosis during the predeposition phase of disease, which is presumably characterized by recurrent fevers and swollen hocks. However, colchicine administration may lead to remission of proteinuria even after the appearance of amyloid deposits. There is no evidence to support that colchicine is effective once amyloidosis has resulted in renal failure. The dose of colchicine is 0.01 to 0.03 mg/kg given orally every 24 hours. Gastrointestinal upset is the primary side effect.

Dimethylsulfoxide (DMSO) has been shown to be beneficial in a limited number of dogs with renal amyloidosis, although the true benefit remains controversial (Dibartola, 1989). DMSO does not solubilize amyloid fibrils; the amount of amyloid deposited will likely remain unchanged. The antiinflammatory effects of DMSO may account for some of its beneficial effects. Reduction of interstitial fibrosis and inflammation may lead to improved renal function and reduced proteinuria. DMSO has an unpleasant odor that may lead to poor owner compliance. The recommended dosage is 90 mg/kg given orally or subcutaneously three times weekly. To reduce injection site pain DMSO should be diluted 1:4 with sterile water before administration. Nausea and anorexia are side effects in some dogs. Neither DMSO nor colchicine is effective once the plateau phase of deposition has been reached. The prognosis for dogs and cats with renal amyloidosis is generally poor.

GLOMERULOSCLEROSIS

Nonspecific glomerulosclerosis develops as an end-stage lesion in response to glomerular injury or decreased functioning renal mass. When nephron numbers are decreased, the normal response of the remaining nephrons is hypertrophy and hyperfunction. Although these adaptations have beneficial effects in increasing glomerular filtration rate, they also may cause glomerular injury, glomerulosclerosis, and in some animals a progressive decline in renal function. On light microscopy glomerulosclerosis is characterized by mesangial cell hyperplasia and mesangial expansion of portions of the glomerulus. Secondary changes such as hyalinosis and adhesions of the sclerotic portion of the tuft to Bowman's capsule are common. Animals with glomerulosclerosis secondary to chronic renal disease may be proteinuric, but their proteinuria is mild. In contrast, focal segmental glomerulosclerosis (FSGS) is a specific glomerular disease that is associated with severe proteinuria in humans. FSGS is the most common cause of the nephrotic syndrome in adult humans, but this lesion has seldom been described in nephrotic dogs and cats.

MINIMAL CHANGE DISEASE

Minimal change disease is a common cause of nephrotic syndrome in humans, but it is described uncommonly in the dog. The low prevalence in dogs may be a true finding or may be to the result of failure of detection when only light microscopy is used. Affected patients would be expected to have heavy proteinuria and a high incidence of nephrotic syndrome. In minimal change disease glomeruli are essentially normal on light microscopy, but characteristic ultrastructural lesions of diffuse foot process effacement are observed on EM. Humans with minimal change diseases tend to be highly responsive in corticosteroids, with an expected response rate of 80% to 90%.

HEREDITARY NEPHRITIS

Inherited defects in the structure of the GBM involving mutations in type IV (basement membrane) collagen have been described in several breeds of dogs. Although the light microscopic lesions are variable and nonspecific, the ultrastructural lesions of irregular GBM splitting are unique to this disease. Therefore diagnosis of this disease depends on electron microscopic evaluation of renal tissue. There is no specific treatment for this disease, but nonspecific management by feeding a renal diet and administering angiotensin-converting enzyme inhibitors has proven beneficial.

FOLLOW-UP EVALUATION

Successful management of the dog or cat with glomerular disease requires adequate patient follow-up. The urine protein/creatinine (UP/C) ratio, urinalysis, body weight, body condition score, systemic blood pressure, and serum albumin and creatinine concentrations should be evaluated monthly when modifications in the therapeutic plan are being made. However, the patient may only need to be evaluated every 3 to 6 months if the clinical signs are stable and therapeutic changes are unlikely. Day-to-day variations in the UP/C ratios of up to 50% in dogs and 90% in cats have been described. Ideally, averaging the results of 2 to 4 UP/C ratios measured over a 3- to 5-day period provides the best estimate of proteinuria for an individual patient. Serial ratios that increase or decrease by greater than 50% in dogs and 90% in cats support a meaningful change in the magnitude of proteinuria. In dogs or cats with isosthenuric or dilute urine, a urine sample should also be submitted for bacterial culture and susceptibility testing every 6 months. Because histologic lesions do not necessarily resolve even though renal function may improve, repeat biopsies generally are not recommended.

References and Suggested Reading

Arthur JE et al: The long-term prognosis of feline idiopathic membranous glomerulonephropathy, *J Am Anim Hosp Assoc* 22:731, 1986.

Cattran D: Management of membranous nephropathy: when and why for treatment, *J Am Soc Nephrol* 16:1188, 2005.

DiBartola SP et al: Clinicopathologic findings in dogs with renal amyloidosis: 59 cases (1976-1986), *J Am Vet Med Assoc* 195:358, 1989.

DiBartola SP: The pathogenesis of reactive systemic amyloidosis, *J Vet Intern Med* 3:31, 1989.

DiBartola SP et al: Familial renal amyloidosis in Chinese shar-pei dogs, *J Am Vet Med Assoc* 197:483, 1990.

Harris CH et al: Canine IgA glomerulonephropathy, *Vet Immunol Immunopathol* 36:1, 1993.

Jennette JC et al: *Heptinstall's pathology of the kidney*, ed 5, Philadelphia, 1998, Lippincott-Raven.

Koeman JP et al: Proteinuria in the dog: a pathomorphological study of 51 proteinuric dogs, *Res Vet Sci* 43:367, 1987.

MacDougall DF et al: Canine chronic renal disease: prevalence and types of glomerulonephritis in the dog, *Kidney Int* 29:1144, 1986.

Miyauchi Y et al: Glomerulopathy with IgA deposition in the dog, *J Vet Med Sci* 54:969, 1992.

Nangaku M, Couser WG: Mechanisms of immune-deposit formation and the medication of immune renal injury, *Clin Exp Nephrol* 9:183, 2005.

Vaden SL et al: Renal biopsy: a retrospective study of 283 dogs and 65 cats, *J Vet Intern Med* 19:794, 2005.

Vilafranca M et al: A canine nephropathy resembling minimal change nephrotic syndrome in man, *J Comp Pathol* 109:271, 1993.

Vilafranca M et al: Histological and immunohistological classification of canine glomerular disease, *J Vet Med* 41:599, 1994.

Wright NG et al: Membranous nephropathy in the cat and dog: a renal biopsy and follow-up study of sixteen cases, *Lab Invest* 45:269, 1981.

CHAPTER **189**

Measuring Glomerular Filtration Rate: Practical Use of Clearance Tests

SHERRY LYNN SANDERSON, *Athens, Georgia*

With declining renal function, urine concentrating ability is impaired when 66% of nephrons are no longer functioning, and azotemia develops when 75% of nephrons are no longer functioning. Although urine specific gravity, blood urea nitrogen (BUN), and serum creatinine are commonly used to assess renal function, these tests are affected by many variables not necessarily related to renal function.

FLAWS IN TRADITIONAL TESTS FOR RENAL FUNCTION

Nonrenal Variables Affecting Urine Concentration (Urine Specific Gravity)

Urine concentrating ability is commonly used to detect renal dysfunction; however, many variables can affect urine concentration. These include drugs, diet, concurrent disease, and even temperament.

Drugs

It is well known that certain medications can result in the production of dilute urine in dogs and cats with normal renal function. For example, corticosteroids inhibit antidiuretic hormone in dogs and produce dilute urine. Similarly, phenobarbital can also produce a low urine specific gravity in dogs with normal renal function. Furosemide, hydrochlorothiazide, and mannitol can affect urine concentration in both dogs and cats with normal renal function by producing diuresis.

Diet

Diet can influence urine concentration without impairing renal function. In particular, feeding a dog a protein-restricted diet may result in medullary washout and production of dilute urine. Many diets prepared for renal or hepatic insufficiency, geriatric patients, and dissolution or prevention of urolithiasis are formulated to reduce protein intake. In fact, evaluating urine specific gravity and BUN levels are two methods for assessing owner compliance with the feeding of a protein-restricted diet.

Diseases

Nonrenal diseases such as diabetes mellitus, neurogenic (central) diabetes insipidus, hyperadrenocorticism, and liver failure can produce a low urine specific gravity in animals with normal renal function. The mechanism of polyuria varies, depending on the disease.

Temperament

The activities of a dog and its temperament can also influence water intake and urine concentration. These behaviors may not be considered necessarily inappropriate or suggestive of renal dysfunction.

Although it is true that urine concentrating ability is impaired when 66% of nephrons are no longer functioning, finding dilute urine does not always equate with renal disease (see chapter 184 for more information about polyuric disorders).

Nonrenal Variables Affecting BUN and Serum Creatinine

Blood Urea Nitrogen

BUN values are influenced by several factors other than glomerular filtration rate (GFR). For example, consuming a high-protein diet can increase BUN levels. Similarly, bleeding into the gastrointestinal tract can create the same effect as consuming a high-protein diet. BUN is also highly influenced by tubular resorption and is inferior to serum creatinine for estimating GFR. Therefore the main clinical use of BUN in patients with renal disease is as an indicator of retention of harmful nitrogenous wastes in the body rather than for its value for determining renal function.

Serum Creatinine

Although serum creatinine is a better indicator of GFR than BUN, it gives only a crude estimate of GFR. Differences in the rate of creatinine production relative to diet and muscle mass may affect this value. For example, serum creatinine concentrations may decrease in dogs and cats with advanced chronic kidney disease (CKD) because of muscle wasting rather than improvement in GFR.

The analytic method used to measure serum creatinine can also influence the results. The most common method used for measuring serum creatinine is the Jaffe method. This method is not specific for creatinine, and in other species over 50 compounds found in blood can react positively by the Jaffe reaction. Nonrenal compounds contribute to as much as 50% of the value reported for serum creatinine in dogs. Most of these compounds are not excreted by the kidneys; therefore their presence in blood has nothing to do with renal function; however, these factors can falsely increase serum creatinine concentrations. In addition, great variations in serum creatinine measurements have been found among different laboratories and among different breeds of healthy dogs.

Nonlinear relationship between serum creatinine concentration and glomerular filtration rate. Although serum creatinine increases as GFR declines, this relationship is not linear. Early in CKD large decreases in GFR cause only small increases in serum creatinine; whereas in advanced stages of CKD small decreases in GFR result in large changes in serum creatinine. This occurs because the insidious loss of nephrons occurring with CKD is accompanied initially by compensatory hypertrophy of residual functional nephrons so that their single-nephron GFR may more than double. This results in enhanced excretion of nitrogenous wastes and delays onset of azotemia until more nephrons are lost. Studies with the remnant kidney model of renal failure also indicate that renal mass and nephron numbers are reduced to 10% to 15% of normal when GFR is still 25% of normal because of compensatory hypertrophy of the remaining nephrons. These findings indicate that patients are often worse off in terms of number of functional nephrons than surmised by considering GFR values. This interpretation, as well as the abundance of nonrenal influences on urine concentration, BUN, and serum creatinine levels, provides a strong argument for pursuing more sensitive methods for evaluating renal function than tests of urine concentration and azotemia currently offer.

Reciprocal of serum creatinine versus time as an indicator of glomerular filtration rate. Some investigators have suggested that plotting the reciprocal of the serum creatinine (1/SCr) versus time shows a linear decrease in renal function with time, providing a method for estimating GFR to follow the progression of renal disease. Others have suggested that this method often gives erroneous estimates of rates of progression because a perfect linear correlation between 1/SCr and GFR does not always occur.

In a recent study (Sanderson et al., 2005) the reciprocal of serum creatinine as an estimate of GFR was compared to a plasma clearance test (iohexol clearance test) in dogs in various stages of naturally occurring CKD. Results showed that in early stages of CKD, defined as a serum creatinine less than 4 mg/dl, the reciprocal of serum creatinine was a modest indicator of GFR. However, in moderate-to-severe stages of CKD, defined as a serum creatinine of 4 mg/dl or higher, the reciprocal of serum creatinine was a poor indicator of GFR.

MORE SENSITIVE METHODS OF ASSESSING GLOMERULAR FILTRATION RATE

GFR is defined as the milliliters of plasma that are cleared of a substance over time and is expressed as milliliters per minute per kilogram of body weight. Therefore renal clearance assays are used to define GFR by determining the clearance of a plasma-borne solute from urine. The measured solute optimally should not be protein bound, should be freely filtered across the glomeruli, and should be neither secreted nor resorbed by the renal tubules. The clearance of this solute is proportional to GFR. Inulin and creatinine are well suited for this purpose.

Plasma Clearance Tests

Inulin Clearance Test

Inulin clearance is considered the gold standard for estimating GFR. However, performing an inulin clearance is labor intensive and requires continuous infusion of inulin and arduous laboratory measurements, making this technique impractical for routine use in clinical practice.

Nuclear Imaging Techniques

Nuclear imaging techniques may be an alternative method for calculating GFR. However, because of the need for specialized equipment and handling of radioactive materials, the use of this test is limited primarily to veterinary teaching hospitals and larger referral centers. Therefore this approach is largely impractical for routine use in clinical practice.

Endogenous and Exogenous Creatinine Clearance Tests

Less precise alternatives for estimating GFR include endogenous or exogenous creatinine clearance. Both endogenous and exogenous creatinine clearance tests require that urine be collected during precisely defined time intervals. Accurate urine collections require intermittent catheterization of the urinary bladder, procedures that are labor intensive and stressful for the patient.

Endogenous creatinine clearance test. The endogenous creatinine clearance test is not suitable for detecting slight changes in renal function because noncreatinine chromagens constitute a large percentage of plasma chromagens and lead to underestimation of renal function. Another criticism of the endogenous creatinine clearance test is the considerable variability inherent in this measurement.

Exogenous creatinine clearance test. In the exogenous creatinine clearance test a larger dose of creatinine is administered to minimize the effects of noncreatinine chromagens. However, creatinine clearance may not accurately estimate GFR in heavily proteinuric patients because, as glomerular disease worsens, there is progressive hypersecretion of creatinine by remnant renal tubules (Shemesh, 1985).

Iohexol Clearance as an Alternative Test of Glomerular Filtration Rate

Until recently diagnosing early (preazotemic) renal disease in dogs and cats was limited primarily to renal clearance tests such as inulin or creatinine clearance. The inability to readily assess renal function in a practical way often posed a dilemma for clinicians with patients in which the only finding was a low urine specific gravity. As a result, detection of early (preazotemic) renal disease was often missed. In addition, assessing renal function in patients with azotemic renal failure also has inherent limitations, as outlined previously.

Iohexol Clearance Test
The iohexol clearance test can be used in clinical practice to estimate GFR in dogs or cats. It is easy to perform and does not require specialized equipment or collection of urine. The relative ease in performing plasma or serum clearance procedures compared to urinary clearance procedure makes this test especially attractive.

Iohexol (Omnipaque) is a low-osmolar, nonionic, iodinated radiographic contrast medium used for radiographic procedures in both human and veterinary medicine. By measuring the plasma or serum disappearance of iodine following a single intravenous dose of iohexol, GFR can be estimated (see Table within Box 189-1 for complete protocol for performing iohexol clearance).

Iohexol clearance was compared to urinary clearance of exogenous creatinine in 10 dogs with normal renal function and in 12 dogs with surgically reduced renal mass (Finco, Braselton, and Cooper, 2001). Plasma was analyzed for iohexol by three assay methods: chemical, high-performance liquid chromatography (HPLC), and inductively coupled plasma emission spectroscopy (ICP). Results showed significant correlation between iohexol clearance and urinary clearance of exogenous creatinine using all three of the assay methods (chemical: $R^2 = 0.90$; HPLC: $R^2 = 0.96$; and ICP: $R^2 = 0.96$). The investigators concluded that iohexol clearance is a reliable marker of GFR in dogs.

Iohexol clearance has also been evaluated in cats. In one study (Miyamoto, 2001a) four renal-intact and six partially nephrectomized adult cats were evaluated. Iohexol clearance results were compared to (exogenous) urinary clearance of creatinine. Correlation between iohexol clearance and (exogenous) urinary clearance of creatinine for all cats was high ($R = 0.951$). In a second study by the same author (Miyamoto, 2001b) 52 cats presenting for a variety of problems were studied. Results indicated that the iohexol clearance test was a much more sensitive indicator of renal dysfunction than BUN and plasma creatinine. Therefore, as in dogs, iohexol clearance in cats provides a reliable and sensitive estimate of GFR.

Indications for Iohexol Clearance Tests
The following is a list of potential indications for performing an iohexol clearance test:

1. Assessing renal function in nonazotemic patients in which the only clinical signs are polyuria and polydipsia. Although administering iohexol to dogs and cats has the potential to be associated with adverse reactions, the risks of performing this test are far fewer than the risks of performing an inappropriately conducted water deprivation test (see Chapter 184). The iohexol clearance test often yields more useful results than the water deprivation test. The author recommends that an iohexol clearance test be performed in all patients before considering a water deprivation test.
2. Identifying occult renal dysfunction before procedures or therapy that may be detrimental to renal function.
3. Optimizing dosing schedules for drugs eliminated by glomerular filtration in patients with renal dysfunction, especially in patients receiving nephrotoxic drugs.
4. Screening nonazotemic patients with a familial history of renal dysfunction with the goal of identifying affected individuals and initiating appropriate therapy before the onset of azotemia.
5. Assessing discrepancies between serum creatinine and BUN. Since nonrenal parameters can affect both of these tests, it is often difficult to determine which one of the tests is responsible when a disparity exists.
6. Accurately assessing severity of renal dysfunction in patients with CKD and monitoring changes in renal function after initiating therapy.

Potential Complications and Adverse Effects of the Iohexol Clearance Test
Although uncommon, adverse reactions to iohexol can occur. Similar to other radiographic contrast media, potential adverse effects include anaphylaxis, cardiac arrhythmias and hypotension, gastrointestinal symptoms (nausea and vomiting), and acute renal failure.

Anaphylaxis. If the clinician is concerned that a patient may be at risk for developing an anaphylactic reaction to intravenous iohexol, the patient can be premedicated with diphenhydramine (0.5 mg/kg intramuscularly). In an ongoing study of CKD, one dog (a 10-year-old, male castrated Shetland sheepdog) had a history of having a mild adverse reaction (vomited) to a radiographic contrast agent administered for an excretory urogram. Multiple iohexol clearance tests were performed safely in this dog after pretreatment with diphenhydramine. Although the potential for anaphylactic reactions exists and clients need to be counseled accordingly, the incidence appears infrequent.

Cardiac arrhythmias and hypotension. In humans cardiac arrhythmias and hypotension are rare (0.7% to 2%) complications associated with intravenous administration of iohexol. It is unknown how often this occurs in dogs and cats. Nonetheless it would be prudent to keep this in mind in patients with preexisting heart disease.

Gastrointestinal complications. Nausea and vomiting are also infrequent complications (0.7% to 2%)

Box **189-1**

Protocol for Estimation of Glomerular Filtration Rate In Dogs and Cats by Serum Iohexol Clearance

1. Patient should be well hydrated and fasted for 12 hours before the iohexol clearance study (do not restrict water intake).
2. Record an accurate body weight in kilograms.
3. Place an intravenous catheter and flush with sterile saline to ensure catheter patency before the administration of iohexol.
4. If concerned about an adverse reaction to iohexol, pretreat the patient with diphenhydramine.
5. Administer a single dose of iohexol (150 to 300 mg/kg) as a rapid intravenous bolus and record time administered to the nearest minute. Iohexol is relatively expensive, especially when used in a large dog. Severity of azotemia may impact the dose of iohexol used:
   A. With mild azotemia it is best to choose a 300-mg/kg intravenous dose of iohexol to ensure that sufficient iohexol will remain in the blood to be detected by the assays used to measure it.
   B. With moderate-to-severe azotemia, it is acceptable to use a 300-mg/kg intravenous dose of iohexol. However, because renal clearance of iohexol is impaired, a lower dose (150 mg/kg intravenously) of iohexol often can be used.
6. After administering the intravenous dose of iohexol, blood is collected in a clot tube at 2, 3, and 4 hours after iohexol injection. *It is VERY important to record the times samples were collected to the nearest minute.* See following table.
7. Allow the blood sample to clot before centrifuging, and transfer serum (0.4 ml or more) into a plastic appropriately labeled vial. Serum samples may be refrigerated or frozen.
8. Ship chilled or frozen serum samples to the analytical laboratory in an insulated container. Be certain to include the exact dose of iohexol administered (milligrams of iodine per kilogram of body weight), the exact time of iohexol administration, and the exact time samples were collected (see following table).
9. One laboratory that is equipped for analysis of iohexol clearance is the University Animal Diagnostic Laboratory, at Michigan State University (B629 West Fee Hall, East Lansing, MI 48824; phone: 517-355-0281).
10. GFR will be reported in ml/min/kg body weight.

Example of a Table Used For Iohexol Clearance

Animal Name and ID	Body Wt (kg)	Test Date	Iohexol Dose	Time of Administration	Sample Times (AM or PM)		
					2 hr	3 hr	4 hr

From Kruger et al., 1998.

associated with iohexol administration in humans. Although the potential for similar complications exists in dogs and cats, gastrointestinal effects appear to be very rare.

Acute renal failure. Radiographic contrast agents markedly aggravate outer medullary hypoxia and generate cytotoxic reactive oxygen species (Heyman, Reichman, and Brezis, 1999). The pathophysiology of contrast-induced nephropathy results from enhanced medullary metabolic activity and oxygen consumption as a result of osmotic diuresis and increased salt delivery to the distal nephron. The major risk factors for radiocontrast nephropathy in humans are (1) administering high doses of contrast media; (2) dehydration; (3) decreased effective arterial volume secondary to congestive heart failure, cirrhosis, or nephrotic syndrome; (4) factors favoring prerenal failure problems such as administration of nonsteroidal antiinflammatory drugs or angiotensin-converting enzyme inhibitors; and (5) preexisting renal failure (Esnault, 2002).

The majority of complications associated with administering radiographic contrast material occur when *high-osmolality, nonionic radiocontrast media* is used. Since the introduction of *low-osmolality, nonionic radiocontrast media (including iohexol),* acute adverse reactions to radiographic contrast media are uncommon. I have performed more than 50 iohexol clearance tests in dogs with various stages

of naturally occurring CKD and have not encountered any known adverse reactions to iohexol in these patients.

References and Suggested Reading

Esnault VLM: Radiocontrast media-induced nephrotoxicity in patients with renal failure: rationale for a new double-blind, prospective, randomized trial testing calcium channel antagonists, *Nephrol Dial Transplant* 17:1362, 2002.

Finco DR, Braselton E, Cooper TA: Relationship between plasma iohexol clearance and urinary exogenous creatinine clearance in dogs, *J Vet Intern Med* 15:368, 2001.

Heyman SN, Reichman J, Brezis M: Pathophysiology of radiocontrast nephropathy: a role for medullary hypoxia, *Invest Radiol* 34:685, 1999.

Kruger JM et al: Putting GRF into practice: clinical applications of iohexol clearance, Proceedings of the 16th ACVIM Forum Proceedings, San Diego, 1998, p 657.

Miyamoto K: Use of plasma clearance of iohexol for estimating glomerular filtration rate in cats, *Am J Vet Res* 62:572, 2001a.

Miyamoto K: Clinical application of plasma clearance of iohexol on feline patients, *J Feline Med Surg* 3:143, 2001b.

Sanderson SL et al: Relationship between serum iohexol clearance and reciprocal of serum creatinine in dogs with naturally occurring chronic renal failure, *J Vet Intern Med* 19(abstr):433, 2005.

Shemesh O et al: Limitations of creatinine as a filtration marker in glomerulopathic patients, *Kidney Int* 28:830, 1985.

CHAPTER 190

Evidence-Based Management of Chronic Kidney Disease

DAVID J. POLZIN, *St. Paul, Minnesota*
CARL A. OSBORNE, *St. Paul, Minnesota*
SHERI ROSS, *St. Paul, Minnesota*

OVERVIEW OF EVIDENCE-BASED MEDICINE

The purpose of evidence-based medicine is to facilitate application of current standards of medical care based on best available evidence of the benefits, limits, and risks of treatment recommendations. Several factors should be considered when making a recommendation for treatment, including: (1) the established goal of the treatment, (2) whether there is reasonable assurance of safety and effectiveness for the treatment, (3) the magnitude of benefit expected to accrue from the proposed therapy, and (4) the likely impact of owner compliance and satisfaction with the treatment. Ideally therapy should both prolong and enhance the pet's quality of life, be free of significant adverse effects or risks, place manageable demands on the owner's time and financial resources, and not disrupt the relationship between the owner and pet. When the therapeutic plan fails to achieve these goals, poor compliance, treatment failure, or euthanasia may result because the needs of the pet and owner have not been met. Therapeutic success may be facilitated by using best available evidence to prioritize treatment recommendations and educate pet owners as to what they can reasonably expect from treatment.

Whenever possible, treatment recommendations should be based on results of rigorous, controlled scientific studies. Of course, not all recommendations can be based on such studies. Nonetheless, it is important to recognize the inherent limitations of recommendations based on less secure forms of evidence. Unfortunately many therapies recommended for dogs and cats with chronic kidney disease (CKD) have never been examined in an appropriate and systematic fashion in clinical patients. Often treatments are recommended on the basis of less convincing forms of evidence such as clinical experience, expert opinion, pathophysiologic rationale, studies performed in other species, or studies in dogs or cats with induced disease. Evidence from the recalled experiences of clinicians and other experts tends to overestimate the efficacy of a therapy or other interventions.

One suggested method of accommodating concerns regarding these limitations in evidence is to assign a score defining the strength and quality of the recommendation. We have chosen to use a four-point system of grading for this purpose. Grade 1 evidence, the highest-quality evidence, is that obtained from at least one properly randomized controlled clinical trial (RCCT) or a meta-analysis of multiple RCCTs. Such studies yield an estimate of effectiveness that reflects the likely effect of the treatment when applied to patients in a clinical setting. Grade 1 evidence provides strong support for a recommendation. Grade 2 evidence is data collected from studies performed using acceptable laboratory models or simulations in the target species. These studies yield an estimate of efficacy (rather than effectiveness) that reflects the effect of the treatment in an idealized setting that may or may not represent the true conditions under which the treatment is typically applied clinically. Grade 3 evidence is data obtained from at least one well-designed clinical trial without randomization, from cohort or case-controlled analytic studies, or from uncontrolled studies in which dramatic results are obtained. Grades 2 and 3 evidence provides intermediate or moderate support for a recommendation. Grade 4 evidence includes recommendations based on the opinions of respected authorities derived from clinical experience, descriptive studies, studies in other species (e.g., humans and rodent models), pathophysiologic justification, and reports of expert committees. Grade 4 evidence provides weak support for a recommendation.

An additional element to consider when examining evidence supporting or refuting a therapeutic claim is whether the evidence is clinically relevant. Treatments are indicated when they provide important clinical benefits. Unfortunately studies often focus on outcomes that may or may not have any clinical relevance to pets and their owners. For example, a study linking calcitriol therapy to correcting hyperparathyroidism does not necessarily provide sufficient reason for recommending such therapy in terms of major clinical outcomes of survival and quality of life. Parathyroid hormone activities or other physiologic or laboratory measurements are often used as "substitute" or "surrogate" end points in studies because typically they are obtained more easily than more important clinical outcomes. Such results only provide a pathophysiologic rationale for applying the treatment to patients (i.e., grade 4 evidence). It is of primary importance to provide evidence that the treatment influences major outcomes that are important to pets and their owner. These include increased activity or appetite, decreased vomiting, decreased incidence of uremic crises requiring urgent hospitalization, and prolonged good-quality life span.

In this chapter we provide guidelines for managing dogs and cats with CKD and the strength of evidence supporting the recommended guidelines. The strength of evidence supporting the guidelines can be used to assess the relative priorities of various therapies. It is appropriate that the owner and veterinarian commit substantial effort toward treatment recommendations supported by strong evidence as compared to efforts expended on carrying out treatments supported only by weak evidence.

LINKAGE BETWEEN STAGE OF CHRONIC KIDNEY DISEASE AND TREATMENT RECOMMENDATIONS

Classification of CKD according to guidelines developed by the International Renal Interest Society is an important advance in our approach to managing CKD in dogs and cats (see Chapter 192). According to this classification system, treatment recommendations can be rationally

linked to the magnitude of reduction in kidney function and the presence or absence of proteinuria and hypertension. These three core characteristics of CKD patients (the magnitude of renal dysfunction, proteinuria, and hypertension) are related to the risk for development of clinical complications and additional loss of kidney function and therefore serve as a logical basis for evaluating and justifying therapeutic intervention. Indications for treatment recommendations are provided using this staging system (Table 190-1).

CONSERVATIVE MANAGEMENT OF CHRONIC KIDNEY DISEASE: THERAPEUTIC OPTIONS

Conservative medical management of CKD can be synthesized into the following four general treatment goals:

Table **190-1**

Evidence-based Management of Chronic Kidney Disease in Dogs and Cats

Recommendation	Indication	Treatment Options	Goal of Treatment	Evidence Supporting Recommendation
Feed a renal diet	D: CKD stages III,IV C: CKD stages II*,III,IV	Manufactured diets Homemade diets	Ameliorate risk of developing uremia or premature death Slow progression of CKD Maintain or improve nutrition Control phosphorus intake	**Grade 1** D & C: RCCT
Ameliorate GI signs[†]	CKD stages III, IV with GI signs attributable to CKD present	H_2 blockers[‡] Sucralfate Antiemetics	Ameliorate and/or prevent GI signs associated with uremia, including anorexia, nausea, vomiting, GI ulceration, and blood loss	**Grade 4** Opinion and pathophysiologic justification
Optimize nutrition	CKD stages III,IV with inadequate oral calorie intake	Esophagostomy tube Gastrostomy tube	Provide adequate calorie intake Achieve and maintain a body condition score of 5/9	**Grade 4** Opinion and descriptive studies
Supplement ω-3 PUFAs	CKD stages II-IV	Supplements containing ω-3 PUFAs	To slow progression of CKD	**D: Grade 2** Induced model of CKD **C: Grade 4** Pathophysiologic justification; extrapolation from other species; retrospective study in cats
Correct hyperphosphatemia	CKD stages II, III,IV	Reduced phosphorus diet Intestinal phosphorus binders	Slow progression of CKD CKD Stages 2 and 3: Serum phosphorus of ≤4.5 or ≤5 mg/dl or lower, respectively CKD Stage 4: Serum phosphorus of 6 mg/dl or lower	**D: Grade 2** Induced model of CKD **C: Grade 4** Pathophysiologic justification; extrapolation from other species; inference from clinical trials in cats
Correct hypokalemia	CKD stages III,IV with serum potassium concentration <3.5 mEq/L	Potassium supplementation (e.g., potassium gluconate or citrate)	Maintain serum potassium concentration 4.0 to 5.4 mEq/L Stabilize kidney function (?) Correct hypokalemic polymyopathy	**Grade 4** Opinion and pathophysiologic justification
Correct metabolic acidosis	CKD stages I-IV	Sodium bicarbonate Potassium citrate Renal diet	Maintain serum bicarbonate concentration 18 to 24 mEq/L Minimize protein catabolism	**Grade 4** Opinion and pathophysiologic justification

(Continued)

Table 190-1—Cont'd

Evidence-based Management of Chronic Kidney Disease in Dogs and Cats

Recommendation	Indication	Treatment Options	Goal of Treatment	Evidence Supporting Recommendation
Maintain hydration	CKD stages III,IV with evidence of chronic or recurrent dehydration	Long-term subcutaneous fluid therapy Provide water through feeding tube	Correct clinical signs associated with dehydration Reduce magnitude of azotemia Stabilize or improve kidney function	**Grade 4** Opinion and pathophysiologic justification
Ameliorate proteinuria	CKD stages I-IV Stage I UP/C ≥2.0 D: Stages II-IV UP/C >0.5 C: Stages II-V UP/C >0.4	Angiotensin-converting enzyme inhibitors Angiotensin receptor bockers	Reduce proteinuria (by at least one half, or, ideally, to UPC <1.0) Slow progression of CKD Reduce risk of premature death	**Grade 1** D and C: For reducing proteinuria (RCCT) **Grade 4** For slowing progression of CKD in dogs and in cats (pathophysiologic justification; findings in humans)
Ameliorate hypertension	CKD stages II-IV with blood pressures above 160/100	Angiotensin-converting enzyme inhibitors Amlodipine Other antihypertensives Limit sodium intake (?)	Reduce blood pressure below 160/100 Reduce risk of hypertension-induced injury to eyes, kidneys, CNS, and cardiovascular system	**C: Grade 2** Evidence of lowered risk of hypertensive retinopathy (RCCT using amlodipine) **D: Grade 4** Opinion and pathophysiologic justification
Correct anemia	CKD stages III,IV	Minimize blood loss rHuEPO or darbepoetin	D: Maintain hematocrit between 38 and 48 C: Maintain packed cell volume between 30 and 40	**Grade 3** rHuEPO: Nonrandomized trial in dogs and cats **Grade 4** Darbepoetin: Opinion and pathophysiologic justification
Administer calcitriol	CKD stages III,IV	Oral calcitriol	Slow progression of CKD Reduce risk of premature death Minimize renal secondary hyperparathyroidism	**D: Grade 1** RCCT **C: Grade 4** RCCT does not support; pathophysiologic justification; extrapolation from other species

C, Cats; CKD, chronic kidney disease; CNS, central nervous system; D, dogs; GI, gastrointestinal; PUFA, polyunsaturated fatty acid; rHuEPO, recombinant human erythropoietin; RCCT, randomized controlled clinical trial; UPC, urine protein/creatinine.
*Evidence in cats supports intervention for cats with serum creatinine 2 mg/dl (mid-stage 2).
†GI signs: gastrointestinal signs such as anorexia, nausea, vomiting, and GI bleeding.
‡Ranitidine, famotidine.

(1) to provide adequate and appropriate nutritional support; (2) to correct deficits and excesses in fluids, acid-base, and electrolytes (i.e., sustain a normal internal milieu); (3) to ameliorate clinical signs of CKD; and (4) to provide renoprotective therapy to slow progression of CKD. The guidelines provided in this chapter provide a framework for achieving these treatment goals.

Provide Adequate and Appropriate Nutritional Support

Guideline 1: Recommend Feeding a Renal Diet

There is strong evidence (grade 1) supporting a recommendation to feed a renal diet to dogs and cats with serum creatinine concentrations in excess of 2 mg/dl (CKD stages III and IV in dogs and mid-II through IV in cats). Benefits shown to accrue from dietary therapy in dogs and cats include preventing or delaying the onset of uremia and premature death from complications of CKD. At least in dogs, these benefits have been shown to accrue from slowing progression of CKD. In addition, these diets have been shown to maintain or improve nutrition. Evidence supporting the recommendation to feed renal diets includes findings of randomized controlled clinical trials in dogs and cats with spontaneous CKD (Jacob, Polzin, and Osborne, 2002; Polzin, Osborne, and Ross, 2005; Ross et al., 2006). The canine RCCT indicated that diet therapy reduced the risks of uremic crisis and renal death by 72% and 69%, respectively, over the 2 years of study, with a median survival time of 594 days in dogs fed the renal diet compared to 188 days in dogs fed a maintenance-type diet. In the feline RCCT there was sufficient survival in both diet groups after 2 years of study that median survival times could not be compared (Ross et al., 2006). However, in a nonrandomized clinical trial performed in cats with naturally occurring CKD, the median survival time for cats consuming the renal diet was 633 days compared to 264 days for cats that did not switch to a renal product (Elliot et al., 2000). Patient and owner acceptance of the diets used in these studies was excellent, perhaps in large part because of gradual introduction of the diets over several weeks.

Guideline 2: Ensure Adequate Nutrition
Owners often consider food consumption to be a premier indicator of their pet's quality of life, and they are happy when their pet shows any interest in food. However, it is inappropriate to accept the pet's consumption of "some" food as a goal of therapy. Malnutrition is a major cause of morbidity and mortality in dogs and cats with CKD stages 3 and 4. Ideally patients should consume enough calories from an appropriate diet to maintain a body condition score of 4 to 5/9. Increased efforts are indicated to ensure sufficient calorie intake for patients with body condition scores of 3/9 or lower or when patients fail to consume adequate calories to maintain a stable, appropriate body weight. In addition to inattention to adequate nutrition, some factors that may contribute to malnutrition in dogs and cats with CKD include consumption of inappropriate diets and metabolic factors related to uremia (especially uremic gastrointestinal signs and metabolic acidosis). Since inappropriate diets can exacerbate clinical signs of uremia and/or promote progression of CKD, cats and dogs with CKD should be fed a renal diet. Failure to adequately address uremic gastritis, uremic stomatitis, and dental health can promote anorexia. Metabolic acidosis can promote protein catabolism and malnutrition.

It is appropriate to consider placing a feeding tube when patients fail to spontaneously consume adequate food. Feeding via gastrostomy or esophagostomy tube is a simple and effective way to provide an adequate intake of calories and water. In addition, feeding tubes simplify drug administration (see also Chapter 196). Based on this line of reasoning, use of feeding tubes has been recommended for CKD patients. However, there is only weak evidence to support use of feeding tubes to meet caloric needs of dogs and cats with CKD (grade 4).

Guideline 3: Provide Omega-3 Polyunsaturated Fatty Acids
Omega-3 (ω-3) Polyunsaturated fatty acid (PUFA) supplementation should be considered for dogs and cats with CKD stages II through IV and stage I patients with proteinuria. However, the ideal quantity of ω-3 PUFA supplementation is not known, nor is it clear whether it is the quantity of ω-3 PUFAs or the ratio of ω-6: ω-3 PUFAs that is of primary importance. Most renal diets are supplemented with ω-3 PUFAs or have an enhanced ω-6: ω-3 PUFA ratio.

Potential benefits of ω-3 PUFAs include stabilization or improvement in renal function; preservation of renal structure; and reductions in proteinuria, intraglomerular hypertension, systemic hypertension, and hyperlip-

idemia. These benefits are thought to accrue, at least in part, as a result of antiinflammatory, antithrombotic, and antioxidant effects associated with modification of prostanoid, thromboxane, and leukotriene production.

There is moderate evidence (grade 2) to support the recommendation to provide ω-3 PUFAs in dogs with CKD but only weak evidence (grade 4) to support providing it in cats with CKD. Evidence of therapeutic efficacy of ω-3 PUFA supplementation has been demonstrated in induced CKD in dogs, in which it was associated with improved renal function, renal structure, and survival (Brown, 1998). In cats evidence is limited to results of a retrospective study of cats with spontaneous CKD in which those surviving the longest were receiving the diet with the highest ω-3 PUFA content (Plantinga et al., 2005).

Correct Deficits and Excesses in Fluids, Acid Base, and Electrolytes

Guideline 4: Maintain Serum Phosphorus Concentration Below Target
Intervention to manage serum phosphorus concentration is indicated for dogs and cats with CKD stages II to IV when serum phosphorus concentration rises above the therapeutic target concentration. Ideally serum phosphorus concentration should be maintained below 4.5 mg/dl in stage II, below 5 mg/dl in stage III, and below 6 mg/dl in stage IV. When serum phosphorus concentration exceeds the target concentration, dietary phosphorus restriction should be initiated using a renal diet. In most dogs and cats with CKD stages II and III, dietary phosphorus restriction alone maintains the desired serum phosphorus concentration. However, in some CKD stage III patients and most CKD stage IV patients, addition of an intestinal phosphate binding agent is necessary to reduce serum phosphorus concentration below the target concentration. The most commonly used intestinal phosphate binding agents in dogs and cats contain aluminum as hydroxide, oxide, or carbonate salts. Because of concern about aluminum toxicity in humans, aluminum-containing binding agents are becoming more difficult to obtain. Although there have been isolated reports of hematologic, skeletal, and neurologic complications of aluminum toxicity in CKD dogs, aluminum-containing binding agents usually appear to be well tolerated and safe in dogs and cats. Alternative drugs that do not contain aluminum include calcium carbonate, calcium acetate, sevelamer hydrochloride, or lanthanum carbonate. Experience with these drugs in dogs and cats is limited, but hypercalcemia may be a problem with the calcium-based products, particularly when administered with calcitriol.

There is moderate (grade 2) evidence to support recommending a phosphorous-restricted diet for dogs with CKD (Brown et al., 1991); however, the evidence in cats with CKD is weak (grade 4). Although strong evidence supports feeding a renal diet in CKD in both species, the specific effect of phosphorus intake on clinical outcome has only been documented in dogs with induced CKD in which dietary phosphorus restriction was shown to slow progression of CKD and improve survival. Similar studies have not been reported in cats, although phosphorus restriction has been shown to reduce renal mineralization in cats with induced CKD. There is only weak (grade 4) evidence supporting the specific targets for serum phosphorus concentration given in this chapter.

There is only weak evidence (grade 4) supporting a recommendation to use intestinal phosphate binding agents to achieve target blood phosphorus concentrations in dogs with CKD. To date there have been no studies reporting the effect of phosphate binders on clinical outcomes in dogs and cats with CKD, although there are descriptive studies suggesting that intestinal phosphate binders are effective in reducing serum phosphorus concentrations.

Guideline 5: Maintain Serum Potassium Concentration Within the Target Range

Intervention to manage serum potassium concentration is indicated for dogs and cats with CKD stages I through IV when serum potassium concentration decreases below or rises above the target range of 3.5 to 5.5 mEq/L. The goal of therapy is to bring serum potassium concentration above 4 mg/dl. Hypokalemia is primarily of concern in cats with CKD or cats and dogs with renal tubular disorders such as Fanconi syndrome. Hypokalemia in cats with CKD is presumed to result from inadequate intake and enhanced urinary losses. It has been suggested that increased urinary losses may result in part from enhanced activation of the renin-angiotensin-aldosterone system in response to low-sodium diets. Clinical effects of hypokalemia may include varying degrees of skeletal, smooth, and cardiac muscle weakness and impairment in kidney function. Treatment of hypokalemia usually involves oral or parenteral administration of potassium salts and enhancing food intake. Potassium gluconate and potassium citrate are the preferred salts for oral administration; potassium chloride is used parenterally.

Hyperkalemia is primarily of concern in CKD stage IV when the renal excretory capacity for potassium excretion is no longer able to excrete the daily potassium load provided by the diet. However, it may also occur in association with therapeutic blockade of the renin-angiotensin system and with hyporeninemic hypoaldosteronism. The primary clinical consequence of hyperkalemia is cardiotoxicity. Treatment usually involves reducing the potassium content of the diet. Hyperkalemia resulting from blockade of the renin-angiotensin system may require reduction in drug dosage should the risk of significant cardiotoxicity develop.

There is only weak evidence (grade 4) supporting a recommendation to provide potassium supplementation to stabilize or improve renal function in cats with CKD. A randomized controlled clinical trial examining the effect of oral potassium supplementation on total body potassium and kidney function failed to yield conclusive findings (Theisen et al., 1997). Recommendations for managing hyperkalemia are based on descriptive studies and pathophysiologic justification (evidence grade 4).

Guideline 6: Correct Metabolic Acidosis

Intervention to correct metabolic acidosis is indicated for dogs and cats with CKD stages I to IV when blood bicarbonate concentration drops below the therapeutic target concentration of 18 mEq/L (19 mEq/L for total carbon dioxide concentration). Metabolic acidosis in CKD results primarily from impaired renal ammoniagenesis, although impaired excretion of titratable acid and impaired resorption of bicarbonate may contribute as well. Metabolic acidosis also occurs in patients with renal tubular acidosis (RTA) because of either impaired bicarbonate resorption (proximal RTA) or impaired urine acidification (distal RTA). Clinical effects of metabolic acidosis may include progressive renal injury and increased protein catabolism with loss of lean tissue. Treatment of metabolic acidosis involves administration of an alkalinizing salt, usually sodium bicarbonate or potassium citrate, in a sufficient amount to increase blood bicarbonate concentration into the normal range. However, there is only weak evidence (grade 4) to support the recommendation to maintain blood bicarbonate concentration above the target concentration. The recommendation is based on extrapolation from studies in other species and pathophysiologic justification.

Guideline 7: Maintain Hydration

Intervention to correct and prevent dehydration is indicated for dogs and cats with CKD stages II through IV with clinical evidence of dehydration. Maintenance of hydration in CKD depends on adequate compensatory polydipsia. Cats with CKD appear to be particularly susceptible to chronic dehydration, perhaps because the magnitude of compensatory polydipsia is inadequate. However, lack of adequate access to good-quality drinking water, certain environmental conditions, and intercurrent illnesses that limit fluid intake or promote fluid losses (e.g., pyrexia, vomiting, or diarrhea) may lead to dehydration. The clinical consequences of chronic dehydration include decreased appetite, lethargy, weakness, constipation, prerenal azotemia, and predisposition to acute kidney injury. Additional loss of kidney function from acute kidney injury is a potentially important cause for progression of CKD. The goal of therapy is to correct and prevent dehydration and its clinical effects.

Acute dehydration should be corrected quickly to minimize the risk of additional renal injury. Ideally fluid restoration should be provided promptly via intravenous administration of a balanced electrolyte solution. However, in mild dehydration and when economic considerations prohibit an intravenous approach, oral or subcutaneous therapy may be considered. The key goal of therapy with acute dehydration is rapid restoration of adequate renal perfusion to limit the risk of additional renal injury.

In patients with chronic or recurrent evidence of dehydration and in which conditions responsible for dehydration cannot be identified and corrected, long-term subcutaneous fluid therapy may be considered. Typically a balanced electrolyte solution (e.g., lactated Ringer's solution) is administered subcutaneously every 1, 2, or 3 days as needed. The volume administered depends on the size of the patient, with a typical cat receiving about 75 to 100 ml per dose. If the clinical response of the patient is less then desired, the dose can be increased cautiously. However, it is important to recognize that, although the patient is polyuric, it is possible to induce fluid overload with excessive administration of subcutaneous fluids. In addition, sodium-containing fluids used for subcutaneous therapy do not provide electrolyte-free water and may promote systemic hypertension, hypernatremia, or circulatory overload in patients with compromised cardiac function. A more physiologically appropriate approach to maintaining hydration is to place a feeding tube and provide water via the feeding tube. This approach may also be easier for clients that find it difficult to administer fluids subcutaneously.

There is only weak evidence (grade 4) supporting a recommendation to provide long-term subcutaneous fluid therapy to patients with CKD. The recommendation is based on descriptive studies and pathophysiologic justification.

Ameliorate Clinical Effects of Chronic Kidney Disease

Guideline 8: Correct Clinically Apparent Anemia
Treatment of anemia of CKD is indicated in dogs and cats with CKD stages III and IV when the hematocrit declines below acceptable levels and the patient has clinical signs attributable to anemia. Clinical signs that may be attributable to anemia in patients with CKD include impaired appetite, lethargy, weakness, and decreased social interaction. The primary cause for anemia of CKD is impaired erythropoietin (EPO) production caused by loss of functioning kidney tissue. Other factors that may exacerbate anemia include blood loss, iron deficiency, poor nutrition, hyperparathyroidism, and infections.

The most effective means of correcting anemia of CKD is administration of EPO, either as recombinant human EPO (rHuEPO; Epogen, Procrit) or darbepoetin (Aranesp). There is moderate evidence (grade 3) to support a recommendation to use rHuEPO to correct the anemia of CKD. An uncontrolled clinical trial confirmed that rHuEPO was effective in increasing hematocrit values in dogs and cats with CKD (Cowgill et al., 1998). The increase in hematocrit appeared to be associated with improved appetites and other clinical signs attributable to anemia in cats. However, anti-EPO antibodies developed in some dogs and cats, leading to progressive nonregenerative anemia unresponsive to further rHuEPO administration. Patients treated with rHuEPO should be monitored closely for recurrence of anemia, which may herald the onset of anti-EPO antibodies. Treatment should be terminated if antibody-associated anemia is suspected to minimize antibody production. Darbepoetin may be less likely to induce anti-EPO antibodies. However, experience with darbepoetin is limited, and there is only weak evidence (grade 4) to support its use in dogs and cats with anemia of CKD. See Chapter 198 for an extensive discussion of this topic.

Guideline 9: Ameliorate Gastrointestinal Signs of Chronic Kidney Disease
Dogs and cats in CKD stages III and IV may have gastrointestinal complications of CKD, including reduced food intake, nausea, vomiting, uremic stomatitis and halitosis, gastrointestinal hemorrhage, diarrhea, and hemorrhagic colitis. In addition, gastrointestinal hemorrhage may lead to iron deficiency anemia. Treatment for these gastrointestinal signs largely focuses on ameliorating uremic gastritis by: (1) limiting gastric acidity using H_2 blockers (ranitidine, famotidine); (2) suppressing nausea and vomiting using antiemetics (metoclopramide, 5-HT_3 receptor antagonists such as ondansetron HCl or dolasetron mesylate, the newer NK_1 antagonist maropitant, or low doses of the phenothiazine tranquilizer prochlorperazine); and (3) providing mucosal protection using sucralfate. Of these treatments, H_2 blockers are by far the most commonly used, and few adverse effects have been attributed to their use in CKD patients. Antiemetics typically are added when anorexia, nausea, or vomiting persists despite the use of an H_2 blocker. Sucralfate is added when gastrointestinal ulcerations and hemorrhage are suspected. Unfortunately there is only weak evidence to support a recommendation for any of the drugs described here in dogs and cats with CKD. Evidence of therapeutic effectiveness is limited to pathophysiologic justification and clinical experience (grade 4).

Provide Renoprotective Therapy to Slow Progression of Chronic Kidney Disease

Guideline 10: Reduce the Magnitude of Proteinuria
It is appropriate to initiate efforts toward reducing glomerular proteinuria in dogs and cats with CKD stages I through IV. Therapeutic intervention is indicated when the urine protein/creatinine (UP/C) ratio exceeds 2.0 in dogs and cats with CKD stage I and the UP/C ratio exceeds 0.5 in dogs and 0.4 in cats with CKD stages II through IV. Proteinuria has been shown to adversely affect outcomes in humans, dogs, and cats with CKD (grade 3 evidence). In dogs the risk of an adverse event (uremic crisis or death) was found to increase by 1.5-fold for every 1-unit increase increment in the UP/C ratio above 1.0. These adverse effects associated with proteinuria likely occur because proteinuria itself appears to injure the renal tubules, thereby promoting progression of CKD. It is now well established in humans that therapeutically reducing proteinuria by suppressing the renin-angiotensin-aldosterone system ameliorates proteinuria and slows progression of renal injury. (An alternative explanation is that proteinuria is a marker for or a part of another injurious process.) The evidence in dogs and cats is similar although somewhat less compelling. In an RCCT in dogs with glomerulopathies, treatment with the angiotensin-converting enzyme (ACE)-inhibitor enalapril significantly reduced proteinuria, but the duration of the study was too brief to adequately assess renoprotective value of the therapy. However, in a study examining the effects of enalapril in Samoyed dogs with hereditary nephritis, treated dogs survived 1.36-fold longer than untreated dogs. In cats with UP/C ratio values greater than 1.0, treatment with benazepril was associated with longer survival times. However, in cats with UP/C ratio values less than 1.0, the data were equivocal. This latter finding is consistent with observations in humans suggesting that the magnitude of benefit accruing from ACE inhibitors is proportional to the magnitude of reduction in proteinuria.

There is weak evidence (grade 4) that ACE inhibitor therapy slows progression of kidney disease or prolongs survival in dogs and cats (Grauer et al., 2000; Lees et al., 2005).

Guideline 11: Minimize Systemic Hypertension

Drug therapy to lower blood pressure is indicated in dogs and cats with CKD stages II through IV when blood pressure exceeds 160/100 mm Hg and in dogs and cats with CKD stage I when blood pressure exceeds 180/120. Unless evidence of hypertensive retinal lesions or central nervous system lesions are present, blood pressure values should be determined on at least three separate episodes before establishing the need for therapeutic intervention. The goal of therapy is to reduce blood pressure to at least below 160/100 mm Hg. Untreated, persistently elevated blood pressure may promote progressive renal injury, retinopathy, central nervous system injury, and cardiovascular complications. Elevated blood pressure has been linked to increased mortality in dogs with CKD stages III and IV. In addition, in an induced model of hypertensive CKD, elevated blood pressure was shown to result in reduced renal function, increased proteinuria, and more severe renal lesions.

There is moderate evidence (grade 2) to support a recommendation for amlodipine in managing elevated blood pressure in cats with CKD (Mathur et al., 2002). In cats with induced hypertensive CKD, amlodipine was shown to significantly reduce development of retinal lesions. Amlodipine, the first-choice antihypertensive drug in cats, typically is highly effective in reducing blood pressure in cats, often by as much as 30 to 50 mm Hg. In contrast, there is only weak evidence (grade 4) to support a recommendation to treat elevated blood pressure in dogs with CKD. There are no comparative studies documenting a clinical benefit to treatment of elevated blood pressure in dogs with CKD. Antihypertensive therapy in dogs is recommended based on pathophysiologic justification and extrapolation from observations in humans and rodents. Hypertension in dogs is more resistant to drug therapy than in cats. Because ACE inhibitors such as benazepril and enalapril reduce intraglomerular pressure even when systemic blood pressure is not effectively ameliorated, these drugs are currently considered first-line drugs in dogs with CKD in mitigating the renal effects of hypertension. However, since ACE inhibitors are often ineffective as antihypertensive drugs in dogs, amlodipine is commonly added to ACE inhibitor therapy in an attempt to achieve the therapeutic goal. This combined therapy is particularly important when target organ injury to the eyes or brain is evident. Additional information about hypertensive renal disease can be found in Chapters 159 and 197.

Guideline 12: Provide Calcitriol

Calcitriol is indicated for dogs with CKD stages III and IV to slow progression of CKD and extend survival. However, calcitriol therapy should not begin until the patient's serum phosphorus concentration has been reduced to 6 mg/dl or less. Calcitriol (1,25-dihydroxycholecalciferol), the most active form of vitamin D, is formed in the kidneys by hydroxylation of 25-hydroxycholecal-

ciferol. Calcitriol deficiency occurs in CKD as a result of the combined effects of phosphorus retention and reduction in renal mass. Renal secondary hyperparathyroidism occurs in large part as a consequence of this deficiency of calcitriol. Calcitriol therapy may induce its clinical effects either indirectly by suppressing hyperparathyroidism or directly by an effect on systemic calcitriol receptors. There is strong evidence (grade 1) to support a recommendation for carefully monitored calcitriol therapy in dogs with CKD (calcitriol was shown to reduce mortality in dogs with CKD in an RCCT comparing calcitriol treatment to placebo). The survival benefit appeared to result from reduced progression of CKD. Studies in human patients with CKD have confirmed a similar survival benefit of calcitriol therapy. There is only weak evidence (grade 4) supporting a recommendation for or against calcitriol therapy in cats with CKD. An RCCT performed in cats with CKD failed to detect a survival benefit of calcitriol therapy. However, this study was a 1-year study, and the possibility that a clinical benefit could have been missed because of the short duration of study compared to the long survival time typical of feline CKD cannot be excluded. There is only weak evidence (grade 4) to support a recommendation for or against using calcitriol to manage clinical signs associated with CKD in dogs or cats. In both the dog and cat RCCT, a benefit of calcitriol in improving appetite, increasing activity, or enhancing quality of life was not detected. See Chapter 193 for more details on these references and appropriate use of this agent.

References and Suggested Reading

Brown SA et al: Beneficial effect of dietary mineral restriction in dogs with marked reduction of functional renal mass, *J Am Soc Nephrol* 1:1169, 1991.

Brown S et al: Beneficial effects of chronic administration of dietary omega-3 polyunsaturated fatty acids in dogs with renal insufficiency, *J Lab Clin Med* 131:447, 1998.

Cowgill L et al: Use of recombinant humans erythropoietin for management of anemia in dogs and cats with renal failure, *J Am Vet Med Assoc* 212:521, 1998.

Elliot J et al: Survival of cats with naturally occurring chronic renal failure: effect of dietary management, *J Small Anim Pract* 41:235, 2000.

Grauer G et al: Effects of enalapril versus placebo as a treatment for canine idiopathic glomerulonephritis, *J Vet Intern Med* 14:526, 2000.

Jacob F et al: Clinical evaluation of dietary modification for treatment of spontaneous chronic renal failure in dogs, *J Am Vet Med Assoc* 220:1163, 2002.

Lees G et al: Assessment and management of proteinuria in dogs and cats: 2004 ACVIM Forum consensus statement (small animal), J Vet Intern Med 19:377, 2005.

Mathur S et al: Effects of the calcium channel antagonist amlodipine in cats with surgically induced hypertensive renal insufficiency, *Am J Vet Res* 63:833, 2002.

Plantinga EA et al: Retrospective study of the survival of cats with acquired chronic renal insufficiency offered different commercial diets, *Vet Rec* 157:185, 2005.

Polzin DJ, Osborne CA, Ross S: Chronic kidney disease. In Ettinger S, Feldman E, editors: *Textbook of veterinary internal medicine*, ed 6 Philadelphia, 2005, Saunders, p 1756.

Ross SJ et al: Clinical evaluation of dietary modification for treatment of spontaneous chronic kidney disease in cats, *J Am Vet Med Assoc* 229(6):949, 2006.

Theisen S et al: Muscle potassium content and potassium gluconate supplementation in normokalemic cats with naturally occurring chronic renal failure, *J Vet Intern Med* 11:212, 1997.

CHAPTER **191**

Acute Renal Failure

LINDA ROSS, *North Grafton, Massachusetts*

Acute renal failure (ARF) is defined as the rapid loss of nephron function (over hours to several days) resulting in azotemia; fluid, electrolyte and acid-base abnormalities; and uremia. Many causes of ARF have been identified in dogs and cats (also see chapter 186). Although supportive therapy is similar regardless of etiology, the prognosis and clinical outcome have been shown to vary, depending on the cause (Vaden, Levine, and Breitschwerdt, 1997).

Classically ARF is divided into three stages. The first (initiation) occurs during and immediately following the renal insult, when pathologic damage to the kidneys is occurring. The latter part of the initiation phase has recently been termed the *extension phase*. During this time ischemia, hypoxia, inflammation, and cellular injury continue, leading to cellular apoptosis and/or necrosis. The initiation phase usually lasts less than 48 hours, during which time clinical and laboratory abnormalities may not be apparent. The second stage (maintenance) is characterized by azotemia and/or uremia and may last for days to weeks. Oliguria (<1 ml of urine per kilogram of body weight per hour) or anuria (no urine production) may occur during the maintenance stage. Urine production can be highly variable. The third stage is recovery, during which time azotemia improves and renal tubules undergo repair. Marked polyuria may occur during this stage as a result of partial restoration of renal tubular function and of osmotic diuresis of accumulated solutes. Renal function may return to normal, or the animal may be left with residual renal dysfunction. It is possible for animals to have ARF with sufficient tubular damage to cause polydipsia and polyuria but not enough nephron loss to cause azotemia.

Treatment of ARF consists of therapy specific for the cause, and supportive therapy based on the stage of ARF and the animal's fluid, electrolyte, and acid-base status. It is important to remember that the doses of drugs excreted primarily by the kidneys should be reduced or the dosage interval extended in proportion to the degree of azotemia.

SPECIFIC THERAPY

Specific therapy to correct or eliminate the cause of ARF should be instituted if the cause is known or suspected. For example, animals with known ethylene glycol ingestion should have vomiting induced if the ingestion occurred within 3 hours and/or should receive drugs such as 4-methylpyrazole or ethanol to prevent the metabolism of ethylene glycol to its toxic components (Chapter 29). In geographic areas where leptospirosis occurs, all dogs with presumed ARF should receive antibiotics effective against leptospires (penicillin, amoxicillin, or doxycycline). Empiric antibiotic therapy is indicated until pyelonephritis is ruled out by urine or renal tissue culture.

SUPPORTIVE THERAPY

Fluid Therapy

Intravenous fluid therapy remains the mainstay of treatment for ARF. Frequent monitoring of the animal's hydration status, renal function, acid-base status, and electrolytes are necessary to determine appropriate intravenous fluid types and amounts. The increasing availability of in-house or bedside blood chemistry analyzers facilitates such monitoring. Placement of a catheter in the jugular vein allows monitoring of central venous pressure and more precise assessment of intravascular volume status. However, if hemodialysis is a treatment option, the jugular veins should not be used for intravenous catheters or even venipuncture for blood samples; rather they should be preserved for placement of the hemodialysis catheter (see Chapter 194).

The initial volume of fluid to be administered should be calculated based on the animal's body weight and degree of hydration. Water deficits should be replaced within 4 to 6 hours to restore renal blood flow (RBF) to normal as soon as possible. Maintenance fluid requirements (44 to 66 ml/kg/day) and estimated fluid losses from vomiting or diarrhea must be met. Urine production should be monitored during the first few hours of fluid therapy. Placement of an indwelling urinary catheter is the most accurate method for this determination. However, the benefits of an indwelling catheter must be weighed against the risks of ascending infection and (in cats) sedation or anesthesia to place the catheter.

An isotonic, polyionic fluid such as lactated Ringer's solution (LRS) or Plasma-Lyte A (Baxter) may be administered initially. If hyperkalemia is present or suspected because of oliguria or anuria, a potassium-free fluid such as 0.9% sodium chloride is indicated. Following rehydration, the type of fluid should be adjusted based on the animal's fluid and electrolyte status. Polyionic fluids may contain too much sodium for maintenance; and half-strength LRS or 0.45% sodium chloride in 2.5% dextrose may be used for long-term therapy.

Management of Oliguria or Anuria

Once the animal has been hydrated, urine flow should increase rapidly to 2 to 5 ml/kg/hour, depending on the rate of intravenous fluid administration. If urine production is not sufficient, the clinician should first reassess the animal's circulating blood volume. This assessment can include physical examination of hydration status, visual estimation of jugular venous pressure, measurement of PCV and total solids, thoracic radiographs to evaluate cardiac size and pulmonary vascular markings, or ultrasound imaging of the cardiac chambers and hepatic veins. Failure to restore circulating volume to normal is a common reason for decreased urine volume. If the animal is normovolemic, the rate of fluid administration should be slowed to prevent fluid overload and associated adverse effects, particularly respiratory complications related to pulmonary edema. An indwelling urinary catheter should be placed if not already present. Calculation of "ins and outs" can then be used to provide appropriate quantities of intravenous fluids to match urine output. The maintenance fluid requirement (estimated at 20 ml/kg/day for insensible losses) is calculated for a short interval of time, typically 4 hours. The volume of urine produced during the previous time interval is added to the maintenance amount, giving the volume of intravenous fluids to be administered over the subsequent 4-hour period. This regimen helps maintain hydration while minimizing the risk of fluid overload.

Specific therapy to increase urine flow, consisting of administration of one or more diuretics, should next be instituted (Table 191-1). Furosemide is the first diuretic to be administered. Traditionally it has been administered as a bolus at an initial dose of 2 mg/kg intravenously (IV), with escalating doses to 4 to 6 mg/kg at hourly intervals if the initial dose fails to increase urine production. However, a loading dose of 0.66 mg/kg followed by

Table 191-1

Drugs To Promote Urine Production in Animals With Oliguria or Anuria

Drug	Dosage
Furosemide	0.66 mg/kg IV bolus, followed by 0.66 mg/kg/hr CRI *or* 0.5-1 mg/kg/hr CRI *or* 2 mg/kg IV bolus If effective, diuresis begins within 15-30 minutes Increase dose to 4-6 mg/kg intravenously at hourly intervals if initial dose does not induce diuresis
Osmotic diuretics	Contraindicated if animal has fluid overload, pulmonary edema, or congestive heart failure
Mannitol 20% Dextrose 20%	0.5-1 g/kg IV bolus slowly, then 1-2 mg/kg/minute IV infusion or repeat bolus every 4-6 hours at a dose of 0.25-0.5 g/kg intravenously *or* 2 to 10 ml/min for the first 10 to 15 minutes intravenously, then 1 to 5 ml/minute intravenously for a total daily dose of 22 to 66 ml/kg; alternate administration with a polyionic solution
Dopamine	Dogs: 0.5-3 mcg/kg/min CRI intravenously; do not dilute in alkaline solution

CRI, Continuous-rate infusion; *IV,* intravenous.

continuous rate infusion (CRI) at 0.66 mg/kg/hour has been shown to be more effective in producing diuresis in normal dogs (Adin et al., 2003), and is the protocol I currently use. Others have suggested a CRI of 0.5 to 1 mg/kg/hour.

If furosemide fails to increase urine flow, osmotic diuresis can be attempted. A 20% dextrose solution can be given at 2 to 10 ml/min for the first 10 to 15 minutes, followed by a rate of 1 to 5 ml/min for a total daily dosage of 22 to 66 ml/kg. Administration of hypertonic dextrose should be alternated with a polyionic solution to prevent dehydration from osmotic diuresis. Urine should be monitored for glucose to determine the effectiveness of this therapy. Alternatively, 20% mannitol can be given as a bolus dose of 0.5 to 1 g/kg of body weight over 15 to 20 minutes. If effective, urine flow will increase within 1 hour. Repeat bolus doses can then be administered every 4 to 6 hours, or it can be administered as a CRI at a dose of 1 to 2 mg/kg/min. Mannitol may have additional beneficial effects in addition to its action as a diuretic. It inhibits renin release because of its hyperosmolar effect on tubular luminal filtrate. In addition, it acts as a free-radical scavenger, blunts damaging increases in intramitochondrial calcium, and may result in a beneficial release of atrial natriuretic peptide. Because mannitol is not metabolized, its effects remain in the intravascular space longer than those of dextrose. Administration of hypertonic solutions is contraindicated in oliguric animals that are overhydrated because it results in increased serum osmolality, circulating blood volume, and blood pressure.

Dopamine infusion has traditionally been recommended for oliguric or anuric animals. Dopamine stimulates two types of dopamine receptors (DA-1 and DA-2) as well as α- and β-adrenergic receptors. In dogs it causes an increase in RBF and urine volume; glomerular filtration rate (GFR) either increases or is unchanged. In cats increased urine production occurs in the absence of increases in RBF or GFR. This is most likely caused by α-adrenergic stimulation, which increases cardiac output and blood pressure and induces natriuresis. The benefit of dopamine infusion in humans with or at risk of ARF has come under increasing scrutiny. Dopamine has been used in humans because it was thought to increase RBF and therefore reduce ischemic damage to renal tubules. However, the etiology of ARF in humans with critical illnesses is now believed to be multifactorial. A recent meta-analysis found that dopamine infusion did not prevent mortality or need for dialysis and concluded that the use of dopamine for the treatment (or prevention) of ARF could not be justified and should be eliminated from routine clinical use (Kellum and Decker, 2001). There is little or no documentation of the efficacy of dopamine in dogs and cats with ARF. It may have some benefit in dogs with oliguria or anuria because increasing urine production is beneficial in managing fluid therapy. Its use in cats is less clear because the higher doses necessary to promote urine production may result in adverse physiologic consequences (see following paragraphs) that may negate its benefit.

For dogs dopamine is diluted in an isotonic fluid and administered as an intravenous infusion at the rate of 0.5 to 3 mcg/kg/min. High rates of infusion (greater than 10 mcg/kg/min) are to be avoided because they may cause arrhythmias, increased blood pressure, and vasoconstriction. The last may reduce RBF as well as that to other organs. Sodium bicarbonate should not be added to the fluids since dopamine is inactivated in alkaline solutions. Electrocardiographic monitoring is recommended during dopamine infusion because of its arrhythmogenic properties. If arrhythmias occur, discontinuation of the drug for 30 to 60 minutes and reinfusion at a lower rate usually alleviate the problem. Furosemide may be administered concurrently with dopamine. The combination has been shown to be synergistic in maintaining GFR, RBF, and urine flow in dogs with experimental ARF and to reduce the severity of some forms of experimental ARF when administered before the renal insult. If oliguria persists despite these measures, dialysis would be the next therapeutic step.

Recently a selective DA-1 agonist (fenoldopam) has become available. Preliminary studies of its renoprotective effects in people have been promising. One experimental study in healthy cats found that an infusion of 0.5 mcg/kg/min produced more diuresis than dopamine (Simmons et al., 2006). However, a study in experimental dogs undergoing nephrotomy showed no difference in GFR or urine volume between dogs receiving fenoldopam or saline (Zimmerman-Pope et al., 2003). No clinical studies have been reported in dogs or cats with ARF,

and its role in management of oliguric ARF is not yet known.

Corrections of Acid-base and Electrolyte Abnormalities

Metabolic acidosis occurs in ARF. Alkalinizing therapy is not recommended unless the blood pH is less than 7.2 or the serum bicarbonate is less than 14 mEq/L after correcting fluid deficits because it can result in significant complications, including paradoxic cerebrospinal fluid acidosis, decreased ionized serum calcium, and hypernatremia. If necessary, the bicarbonate deficit is calculated as:

$$\text{Body weight (kg)} \times 0.3 \times (24 - \text{measured bicarbonate})$$
$$= \text{mEq bicarbonate deficit.}$$

One-quarter of the deficit is added as sodium bicarbonate to the intravenous fluids over 12 hours, and acid-base status reassessed before further administration.

Moderate-to-severe life-threatening hyperkalemia may occur if the animal is oliguric or anuric. The first and most important step in therapy for hyperkalemia is to ensure urine production and excretion. Animals with severe hyperkalemia or those in which oliguria persists may benefit from additional specific therapy such as sodium bicarbonate, regular insulin, and glucose, or in life-threatening situations calcium gluconate. Hypokalemia may occur during the diuretic phase of ARF. Therapy consisting of intravenous or oral potassium chloride is indicated if the serum potassium concentration is below the normal range, although clinical signs are not usually apparent until it falls below 2.5 mEq/L.

Treatment of Other Uremic Signs

Vomiting can be a significant problem in animals with ARF. Drugs that inhibit gastric acid production are indicated because uremia results in hypergastrinemia. Such drugs include histamine receptor antagonists such as famotidine (0.5 to 1 mg/kg q24h orally [PO]) and proton pump inhibitors such as omeprazole (Prilosec OTC, Proctor & Gamble) (0.7 mg/kg q24h PO or lansoprazole (Prevacid, TAP Pharmaceutical Products Inc.) (0.6 to 1 mg/kg q24h IV). Centrally acting antiemetics may also be necessary. Metoclopramide, a dopamine antagonist, may be given as intermittent therapy at a dosage of 0.2 to 0.5 mg/kg q8h IV or as a CRI at 1 to 2 mg/kg/day IV. Other centrally acting drugs include dolasetron (Anzemet, Aventis Pharmaceuticals) (0.6 mg/kg q24h PO or subcutaneously [SQ] or diluted in compatible intravenous fluid and administered over 15 min IV) and ondansetron (Zofran, GlaxoSmithKline) (0.1 to 0.2 mg/kg q8h SQ or 0.5 mg/kg intravenous loading dose and then 0.5 mg/kg/hr CRI). Phenothiazine derivative antiemetics such as chlorpromazine (0.2 to 0.5 mg/kg q6-8h, SQ, intramuscularly, or IV) can be tried if vomiting persists despite other therapy. Side effects of phenothiazines include sedation and decreased blood pressure. A newer NK1 antagonist, maropitant (Cerenia, Pfizer) (1 mg/kg q 24h, SQ for up to 5 days), is effective as a central and peripheral acting antiemetic in treating nausea and vomiting from renal failure.

Hypertension

Arterial hypertension is common in animals with ARF and is often the result of fluid overload. Treatment includes reducing the rate of intravenous fluid administration, administration of diuretics, and dialysis to remove excess fluid if the animal is oliguric or anuric. Pharmacologic treatment is limited because most antihypertensive drugs are available only in oral formulations and the vomiting associated with ARF often precludes oral medication. If hypertension is severe, parenteral antihypertensives include nitroprusside (initial dose 1 to 2 mcg/kg/min CRI IV; titrate up q5min to achieve desired blood pressure) and hydralazine (0.5 to 3 mg/kg q12h IV or 0.1 mg/kg loading dose IV and then 1.5 to 5 mcg/kg/min CRI IV). Administration of both drugs requires close monitoring. Oral antihypertensives include amlodipine (Norvasc, Pfizer) (0.1 to 0.25 mg/kg q12–24h PO in dogs; 0.625 to 1.25 mg/cat q24h PO in cats) and angiotensin-converting enzyme (ACE) inhibitors such as enalapril (0.25 to 0.5 mg/kg q12–24h PO) and benazepril (Lotensin, Novartis) (0.25 to 0.5 mg/kg q24h PO). ACE inhibitors have been associated with worsening of renal function in humans.

Nutritional Management

Nutritional support has been shown to be important for recovery from ARF. These animals are in a state of negative nutritional balance at a time when protein and energy are needed to support regeneration of damaged renal tissue. Enteral nutrition via an esophagostomy or gastrostomy tube can be used if the animal is not vomiting (see Chapter 196); otherwise parenteral nutrition is indicated.

Prognosis and Duration of Treatment

The prognosis for dogs and cats with ARF depends on the cause and the response to therapy. Those in which the cause is identified and treated early in the course of the disease (e.g., pyelonephritis and leptospirosis) have a relatively good prognosis. Animals with ethylene glycol toxicity that are already azotemic when diagnosed have been shown to have a poor-to-grave prognosis, even with

therapy. Other criteria that have been shown to confer a poor prognosis include severe azotemia (serum creatinine >10 mg/dl), lack of improvement or worsening of azotemia with appropriate fluid and supportive therapy, and concurrent systemic disease such as pancreatitis or sepsis.

Supportive and specific treatment should be continued until one of the following occurs: (1) renal function returns to normal; (2) renal function improves and stabilizes, although not to normal levels, and the animal is doing well clinically; (3) renal function worsens, fails to improve, or does not improve sufficiently for the animal to be managed medically at home for the resulting renal insufficiency. In the first two scenarios fluid therapy can be tapered, and other supportive medications adjusted in response to the animal's clinical signs. In the third scenario dialysis may be considered to support the animal for a longer period of time to see if renal function will improve. If dialysis is not an option, euthanasia may be indicated at this point.

References and Suggested Reading

Adin DB et al: Intermittent bolus injection versus continuous infusion of furosemide in normal adult greyhound dogs, *J Vet Intern Med* 17:632, 2003.

Chew DJ, Gieg JA: Fluid therapy during intrinsic renal failure. In DiBartola SP, editor: *Fluid, electrolyte, and acid-base disorders in small animal practice*, ed 3, Philadelphia, 2006, Saunders Elsevier, p 518.

Cowgill LD, Francey T: Acute uremia. In Ettinger SF, Feldman EC, editors: *Textbook of veterinary internal medicine*, ed 6, Philadelphia, 2005, Saunders Elsevier, p 1731.

Kellum JA, Decker JM: Use of dopamine in acute renal failure: a meta-analysis, *Crit Care Med* 29:1526, 2001.

Ross LA: Acute renal failure, *Standards of Care, Emerg Crit Care Med* 2006, 16:96, 2006.

Simmons JP et al: Diuretic effects of fenoldopam in healthy cats, *J Vet Emerg Crit Care*, in press.

Vaden SL, Levine J, Breitschwerdt EB: A retrospective case-control of acute renal failure in 99 dogs, *J Vet Intern Med* 11:58, 1997.

Whittemore JC, Webb CB: Beyond fluid therapy: treating acute renal failure, *Compend Contin Educ Pract Vet* 27:288, 2005.

Zimmerman-Pope N et al: Effect of fenoldopam on renal function after nephrotomy in normal dogs, *Vet Surg* 32:566, 2003.

CHAPTER 192

Chronic Kidney Disease: Staging and Management

JONATHAN ELLIOTT, *London, United Kingdom*
A.D.J. WATSON, *Glebe, New South Wales, Australia*

The International Renal Interest Society (IRIS) was formed to undertake the task of producing tools to help practitioners better diagnose, stage, and treat chronic kidney disease (CKD) in dogs and cats.* The group has formulated consensus positions based on their own clinical experience and recommendations made by expert panels that have reported recently on hypertension and proteinuria.† The results of these deliberations are described here.

DIAGNOSIS OF KIDNEY DISEASE

Kidney disease is identified in patients examined because of illness or screened because of their age. Fig. 192-1 presents a decisional algorithm for the diagnosis of kidney disease. The classic findings suggestive of kidney disease recognized by members of the IRIS group are presented in Box 192-1. Many but not all of these abnormalities may have been noted by the owner over a relatively long period (weeks to months), perhaps gradually becoming more noticeable if the disease is truly chronic; but not all animals show classic signs of CKD.

When faced with an animal suspected of having CKD, practitioners should adopt a logical approach to diagnosis. The recommended minimum database to be collected from such patients is shown in Fig. 192-2. During this process it is helpful to review the historical and physical abnormalities that led to this suspicion since these and other available evidence may highlight specific problems that warrant further investigation to determine the type of kidney disease present. This review may also indicate whether an underlying cause is likely to be identified by further investigations and whether concomitant diseases should be suspected.

The laboratory database obtained should include appropriate blood biochemistry tests, hematologic examination, and complete urinalysis. These should serve to confirm the clinical diagnosis but may also give indications of the etiology and possible presence of underlying diseases. The results also enable classification of the kidney disease, with the aim of facilitating treatment decisions and providing a prognosis for the owners. Because kidney disease increases in prevalence as dogs and cats age, the practice of running geriatric screens to detect kidney dysfunction has become more widespread in veterinary practice. The IRIS minimum recommended geriatric screen for this purpose is presented in Box 192-2, together with a more ideal complete version.

The key factor in the proposed staging system is the blood creatinine concentration, determined in plasma or serum when the patient is fasted and well hydrated. Because the staging applies only to CKD, it is imperative for other possible causes of increased creatinine concentrations (acute renal failure, prerenal and postrenal azotemia) to be excluded (Fig. 192-3). Furthermore, the creatinine concentration should be stable, ideally over several days or weeks, because staging is inaccurate if azotemia is changing in severity. CKD is generally accompanied by relatively long-standing clinical signs of kidney disease (see Box 192-1). If these signs have been present in an animal that is acutely sick and has an unstable plasma creatinine concentration, it may be suffering an acute uremic crisis. One should manage this crisis and wait until blood creatinine concentration is stable before attempting to stage the disease. Acutely ill dogs and cats with renal azotemia (acute renal failure) but no clinical history compatible with CKD may stabilize after treatment with persistent abnormalities in kidney function. These cases should be staged once the plasma creatinine concentration is stable over a 2- to 4-week period.

Although blood creatinine concentration is considered a relatively crude index of glomerular filtration rate (GFR), it is currently the best GFR indicator available in routine practice. In future iterations of the staging system, the basal creatinine concentration might be replaced by a more precise indicator. Another potential future modification concerns the patient's muscle mass. This governs the production rate of creatinine and thereby influences its blood concentration. Thus cachexia with marked loss of lean body mass leads to lowered creatinine production and may cause underestimation of the severity of kidney dysfunction, particularly in cats. The opposite may occur in well-muscled individuals. The importance of these changes has yet to be assessed, but it is something to consider when staging borderline cases. Staging on blood creatinine concentration should be followed, if possible, by further substaging on the basis of proteinuria and blood pressure since both of these factors may influence treatment selection and prognosis.

STAGES OF CHRONIC KIDNEY DISEASE

The staging system for CKD developed as an IRIS consensus document and was modified following use by

---

*The IRIS group recommend the use of the term *chronic kidney disease* in place of *chronic renal failure* to bring the veterinary profession in line with current terminology used in human medicine.
†Members of the IRIS Board are listed at www.IRIS-Kidney.com.

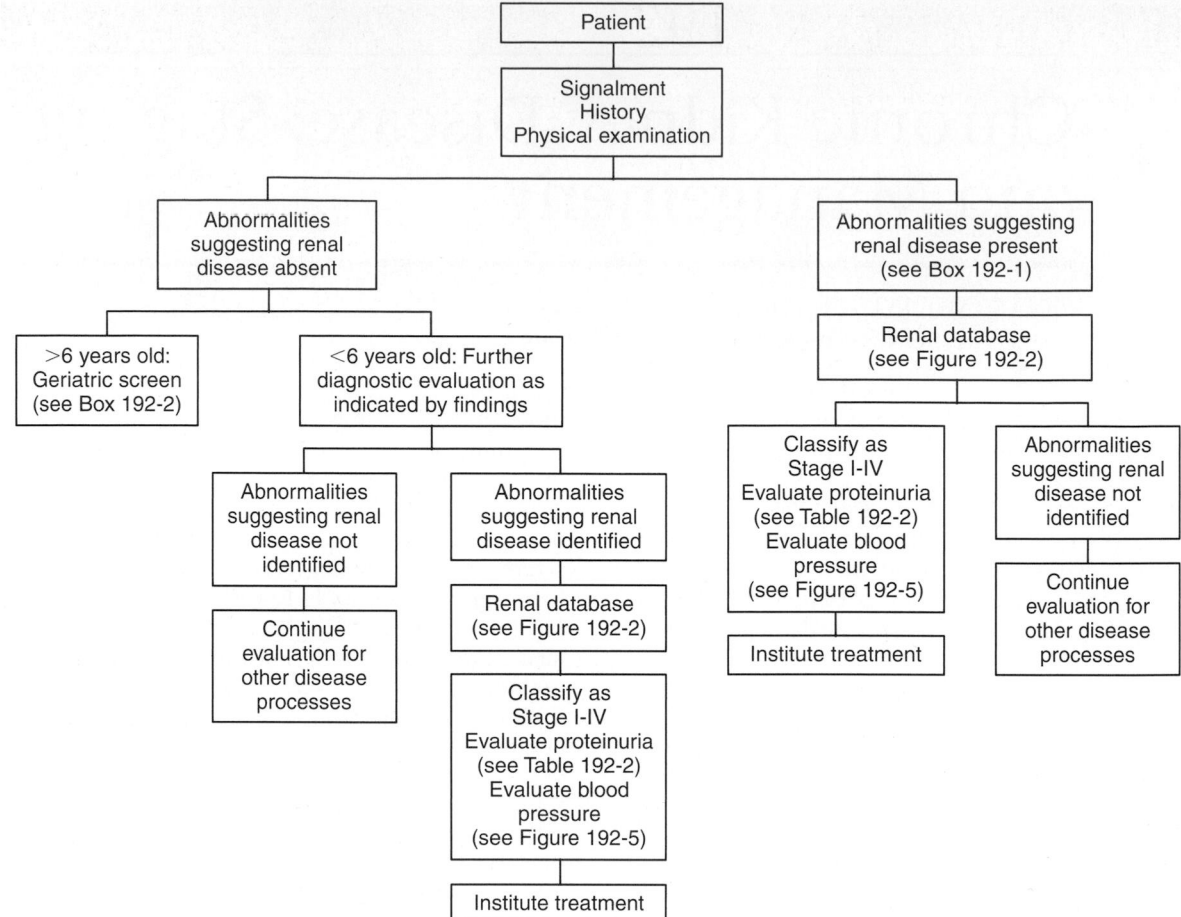

Fig. 192-1   Decisional algorithm for diagnosis of chronic kidney disease.

IRIS Board members in clinical practice and discussion with members of the American and European Societies of Veterinary Nephrology and Urology. This has resulted in separate but similar algorithms for staging CKD in cats and dogs (Fig. 192-3 and Table 192-1) categorizing the severity of disease as is done with congestive heart failure. This system and the associated treatment recommendations should help veterinary practitioners diagnose, understand, and treat CKD. In the longer term, consistent and widespread application of staging should facilitate collection and analysis of clinical data from various sources, thereby improving knowledge of causes, consequences, and treatments of CKD in cats and dogs.

SUBSTAGES OF CHRONIC KIDNEY DISEASE

Proteinuria

The goal is to identify renal proteinuria, having first ruled out potential prerenal and postrenal causes. Ideally the urine protein/creatinine (UP/C) ratio should be measured in all cases, provided there is no evidence of urinary tract inflammation or hemorrhage and plasma protein evaluation has ruled out dysproteinemias. Renal proteinuria can be of glomerular or tubular origin. Patients are classified as proteinuric (P), nonproteinuric (NP) or borderline (BP), as shown in Table 192-2.

The IRIS algorithm for substaging on proteinuria reflects the recent ACVIM Consensus Statement on renal proteinuria (Lees et al., 2005) and is presented in Fig. 192-4. Ideally decisions should be made on the basis of at least three urine samples collected over a period of at least 2 weeks. This will determine whether proteinuria is transient (and therefore likely to be functional/physiologic) or persistent (and therefore likely to be pathologic and of tubular or glomerular origin). The higher the UP/C ratio, the more likely the animal is to have primary glomerular disease. Patients with persistent proteinuria in the BP substage should be reevaluated within 2 months and reclassified as appropriate. Proteinuria may decline as renal dysfunction worsens and thus may be less frequent in CKD stages III and IV. Response to any treatment given to reduce glomerular filtration pressure and proteinuria should be monitored at intervals using the UP/C ratio.

A finding of persistent proteinuria probably has important implications for the potential benefits of both dietary and pharmacologic management of CKD in the dog and cat. Recent evidence suggests that the severity of proteinuria is inversely related to the occurrence of uremic crises and renal mortality in dogs

---

Box **192-1**

Abnormalities Suggestive of Kidney Disease*

History
- Signalment (breed, age, gender)
- Polydipsia/polyuria
- Loss of body weight
- Reduced or irregular appetite
- Hair coat changes
- Vomiting
- Lethargy
- Exercise intolerance
- Decline in sociability or other behavioral changes
- Recent travel to region endemic for infectious renal disease
- Current or previous therapy with effects on renal function
- Blindness (especially if sudden onset)

Physical Examination
- Pale mucous membranes, dehydration
- Abnormal hair coat
- Dental calculus, gingivitis, periodontitis
- Oral ulceration, stomatitis, halitosis, uremic breath
- Abnormal renal palpation (small, firm and irregular, or enlarged)
- Abnormal rectal palpation (prostate or urethra)
- High systemic arterial blood pressure
- Ocular changes consistent with hypertension
- Decline in body weight or low body condition score
- Evidence of osteodystrophy (e.g., pliable mandible, fractures with little or no trauma, bone pain)
- Edema

*There is considerable interanimal variability and not all these findings may be present in an individual with kidney disease.

Box **192-2**

Geriatric Screen (for All Dogs and Cats More Than 6 Years Old)

- Minimum
  - Hematocrit
  - Total solids
  - Urinalysis
  - Creatinine
  - Urea
- More complete
  - Complete hematology
  - Full biochemical panel
  - Complete urinalysis

(Jacob et al., 2005) and all-cause mortality in cats (Syme et al., 2006). Experimental evidence supports the beneficial effects of dietary therapy (particularly n-3 polyunsaturated fatty acid [PUFA] supplementation; Brown et al., 1998) and angiotensin-converting enzyme inhibitor (ACEI) therapy in dogs and ACEI therapy in cats in lowering UP/C ratio and glomerular filtration pressures, limiting structural changes in remnant kidneys, and/or slowing the decline in GFR. Clinical studies also suggest beneficial effects of dietary intervention (n-3 PUFA supplementation and restriction of protein, phosphate, and sodium intake) in dogs (Jacob et al., 2002) and cats (Elliott et al., 2000; Plantinga et al., 2005). However, all of these studies involved clinical kidney diets rather than manipulation of single dietary components; thus the precise factor(s) responsible for the outcomes cannot be determined. Similarly, clinical studies in dogs and cats confirm the beneficial effects of ACEI therapy (Grauer et al., 2000; King et al., 2006). The IRIS recommendations on substaging result from this accumulating evidence and are linked to the treatment recommendations specifically addressing proteinuria in the following paragraphs.

Blood Pressure

Measurement of blood pressure is important in substaging CKD in dogs and cats. The kidney is at risk of damage from hypertension. Although systemic arterial blood pressure is labile and varies according to physiologic state, hypertension is defined as a blood pressure that causes harm. The 2003 ACVIM Consensus Statement on blood pressure defined pressures that, in the experience of the cardiologists, nephrologists, neurologists and ophthalmologists involved, were associated with end-organ damage (Brown et al., 2007). The four organs most prone to damage from systemic hypertension are the heart, kidneys, brain, and eyes. Table 192-3 defines blood pressure ranges associated with minimal, low, moderate, and severe risk of end-organ damage. The algorithm in Fig. 192-5 shows the IRIS group's recommendations for using these data, together with relevant clinical findings in substaging cases of canine and feline CKD.

History	Laboratory
Water intake Body weight Food intake Vomiting	Obtain samples prior to therapy *Hematology* (at least): • Hematocrit • Reticulocyte count • Total solids by refractometry
Physical examination Body temperature Hydration status Body weight and body condition score Mucous membrane color Kidney palpation Coat condition Oral examination Rectal palpation Fundic examination Thyroid palpation (cat) Blood pressure (if available)	*Blood biochemical tests* (at least): • Creatinine • Urea (blood urea nitrogen) • Phosphate • Calcium and albumin • Bicarbonate (or total carbon dioxide) • Potassium *In cats >10 years old:* check ALT and screen for hyperthyroidism *Urinalysis* (at least): • Cystocentesis preferred (record method) • Dipstick of supernatant to determine pH, glucose, hemoglobin, protein • Specific gravity by refractometry • Sediment examination (centrifuge at least 3 ml of urine)

Fig. 192-2 Minimal database for patients with signs of kidney disease.

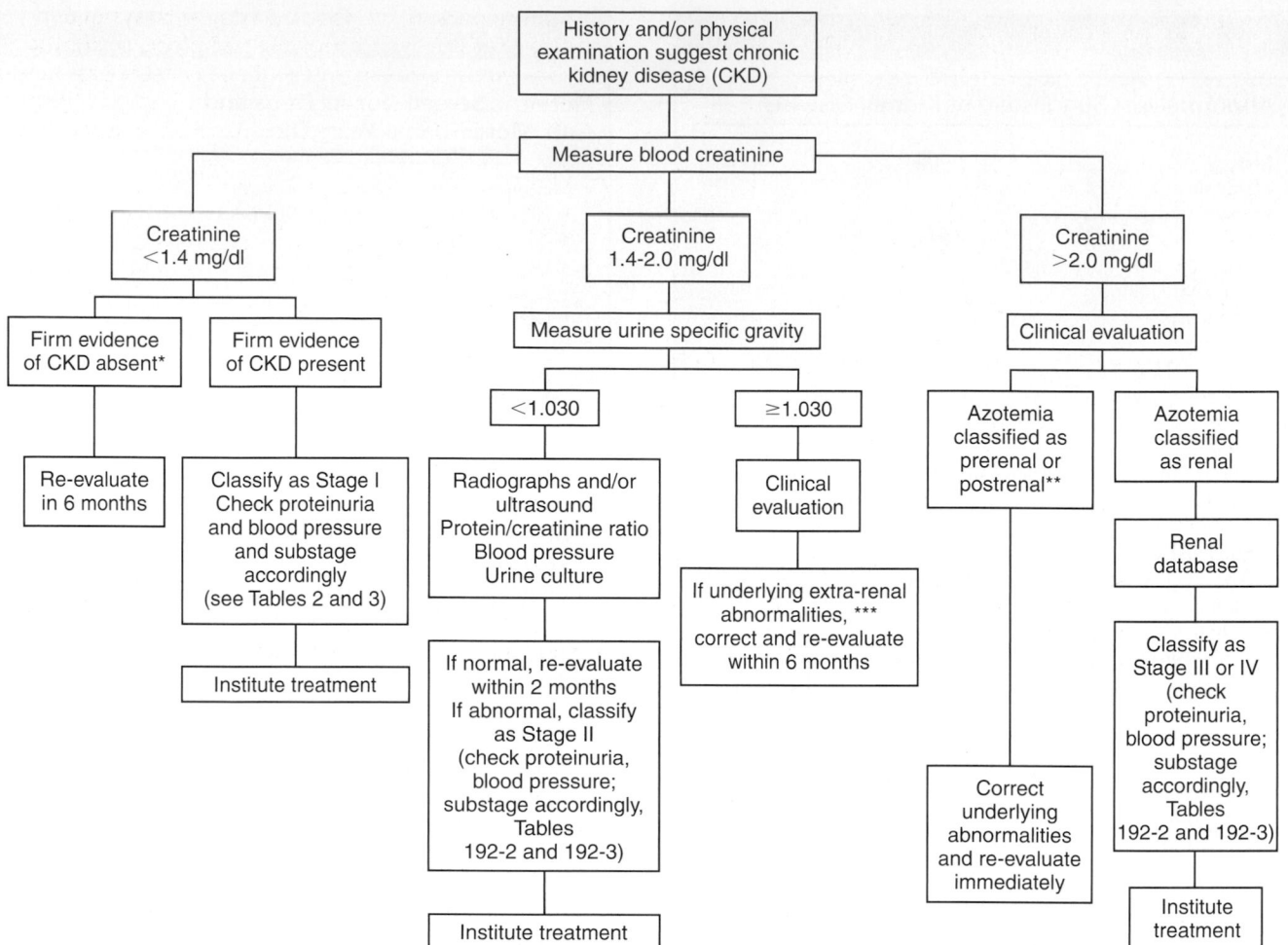

Fig. 192-3 Staging for chronic kidney disease. The algorithm for dogs is shown; the algorithm for cats is similar but uses the creatinine concentrations shown in Table 192-1 and a urine specific gravity of ≥1.035 as an indicator of concentrating ability.

Table 192-1

Staging on Blood Creatinine Concentration

Stage	Creatinine (mg/dl) (µmol/l)	Comments
I	<1.4 (125) dogs <1.6 (140) cats	Nonazotemic Some other renal abnormality present (e.g., inadequate urinary concentrating ability without identifiable nonrenal cause; abnormal renal palpation and/or abnormal renal imaging findings; proteinuria of renal origin; abnormal renal biopsy results; increasing blood creatinine concentrations in samples collected serially)
II	1.4-2 (125-180) dogs 1.6-2.8 (140-250) cats	Mild renal azotemia (lower end of the range lies within reference ranges for many laboratories, but the insensitivity of creatinine as a screening test means that animals with creatinine values close to the upper reference limit often have excretory failure) Clinical signs usually mild or absent
III	2.1-5 (181-440) dogs 2.9-5 (251-440) cats	Moderate renal azotemia Many extrarenal clinical signs may be present
IV	>5 (>440) dogs and cats	Severe renal azotemia Many extrarenal clinical signs are usually present

The IRIS group does not specify the method to be used for blood pressure measurement. The type of equipment used, the protocol followed (probably more important), and the conditions in the practice when measurements are done undoubtedly affect the values obtained and the reproducibility of results between sessions. However, blood pressures persisting in the moderate- or high-risk range on three occasions over at least 2 weeks suggest that therapeutic intervention may be warranted, even if end-organ damage is not apparent.

Table 192-2

Substaging on Urine Protein/Creatinine (UP/C) Ratio

UP/C Value*	Interpretation
<0.2 dogs and cats	Nonproteinuric (NP)
0.2-0.4 cats 0.2-0.5 dogs	Borderline proteinuric (BP)
>0.4 cats >0.5 dogs	Proteinuric (P)

*Calculated using mass units.

COMBINING CHRONIC KIDNEY DISEASE STAGES AND SUBSTAGES

The IRIS scheme allows CKD in dogs and cats to be staged on the basis of the fasting blood creatinine concentration and further characterized according to urine protein content and systemic blood pressure, as shown in the following examples:

1. A proteinuric (UP/C ratio 0.7) dog with systolic blood pressure of 120 mm Hg and blood creatinine concentration 3.4 mg/dl would be classified as stage III-P-N (where P denotes proteinuric and N denotes blood pressure status with minimal or no associated risk of end-organ damage).

2. A dog with borderline proteinuria (UP/C ratio 0.35) and blood creatinine concentration of 5.4 mg/dl that did not have blood pressure assessment would be classified as stage IV-BP-RND (where BP denotes borderline proteinuria and RND denotes that the risk of end-organ damage associated with blood pressure has not been determined).

3. A nonproteinuric (UP/C ratio 0.12) cat with systolic blood pressure of 210 mm Hg having bilateral retinal detachments and blood creatinine concentration of 2 mg/dl would be classified as stage II-NP-Hc (where NP denotes nonproteinuric and Hc denotes blood pressure associated with a high risk of end-organ damage and existing complications of end-organ damage).

It should then be possible to make empiric recommendations about treatments that can logically be considered for the patient and to prognosticate on the likely response to such therapy based on accumulated clinical experience.

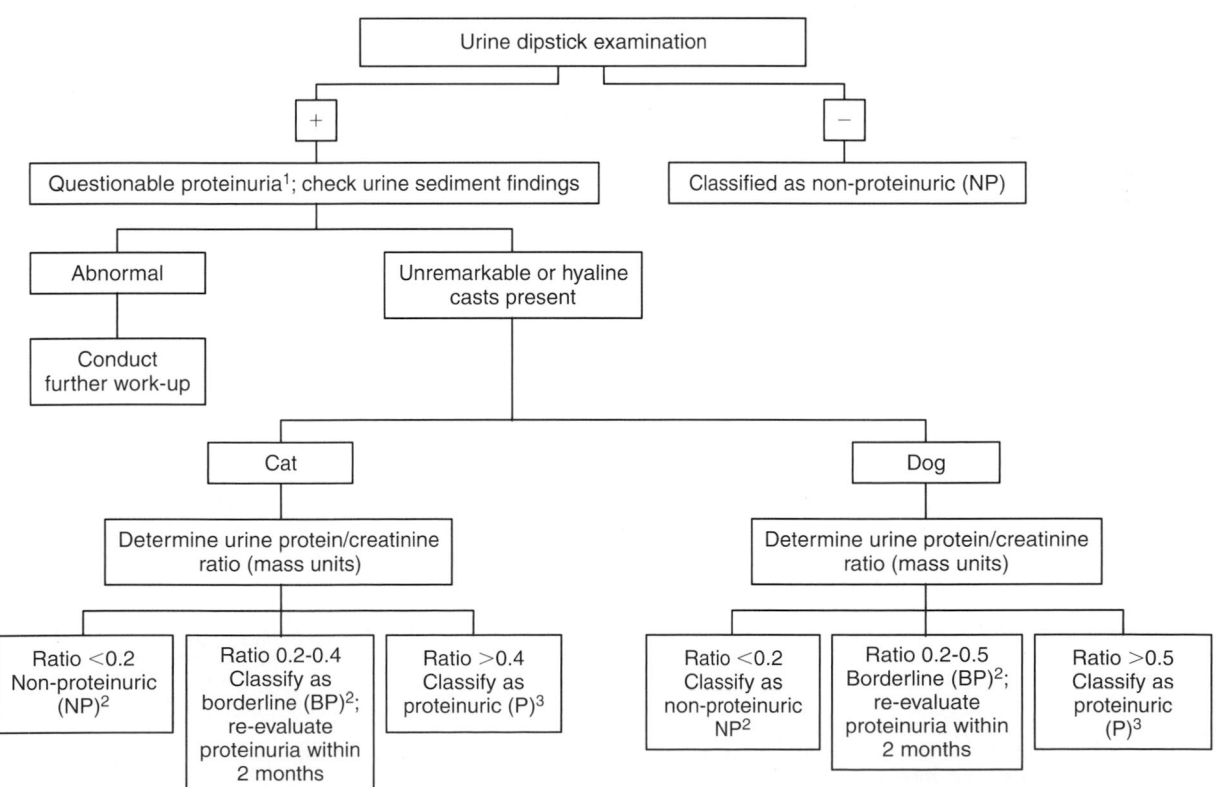

1. Standard urine dipstick tests can give false positive results (particularly 1+); practitioners should consider using a more specific screening test (e.g., sulphosalicyclic acid turbidometric test or the ERD test (Heska Ltd.).
2. UP/Cs in the NP or BP range may be categorized as "microalbuminuric" on the ERD test; the significance of microalbuminuria in predicting future renal health is not understood at present; the IRIS recommendation is to continue to monitor this level of proteinuria.
3. Proteinuria of this magnitude requires therapeutic intervention in CKD Stages II to IV.

Fig. 192-4 Urine dipstick examination.

Table 192-3

Substaging on Blood Pressure

Risk*	Systolic (mm Hg)	Diastolic (mm Hg)
Minimal	<150	<95
Low	150-159	95-99
Moderate	160-179	100-119
High	≥180	≥120

*Risk = likelihood that high pressure will further damage the kidney and other end-organs (i.e., heart and blood vessels, brain, and chorioretina).

RECOMMENDATIONS FOR TREATING CHRONIC KIDNEY DISEASE IN DOGS AND CATS

Empirical recommendations developed, through consensus of the IRIS group, for management of CKD in dogs and cats according to stage are presented in Table 192-4. They represent suggested starting points and should always be tailored to the individual patient. Frequent monitoring and readjustment of therapy according to response are the keys to success. As many of the complications of CKD increase in prevalence with the stage, so the intensity of treatment required also increases.

General Management for Patients Diagnosed With CKD

- Discontinue all potentially nephrotoxic drugs
- Identify and treat any prerenal and postrenal abnormalities
- Rule out any treatable conditions within the urinary tract (e.g., renal urolithiasis and pyelonephritis)
- Rule out any treatable underlying disease outside the urinary system that can perpetuate renal damage (e.g., hyperthyroidism, hyperadrenocroticism, pyometra)

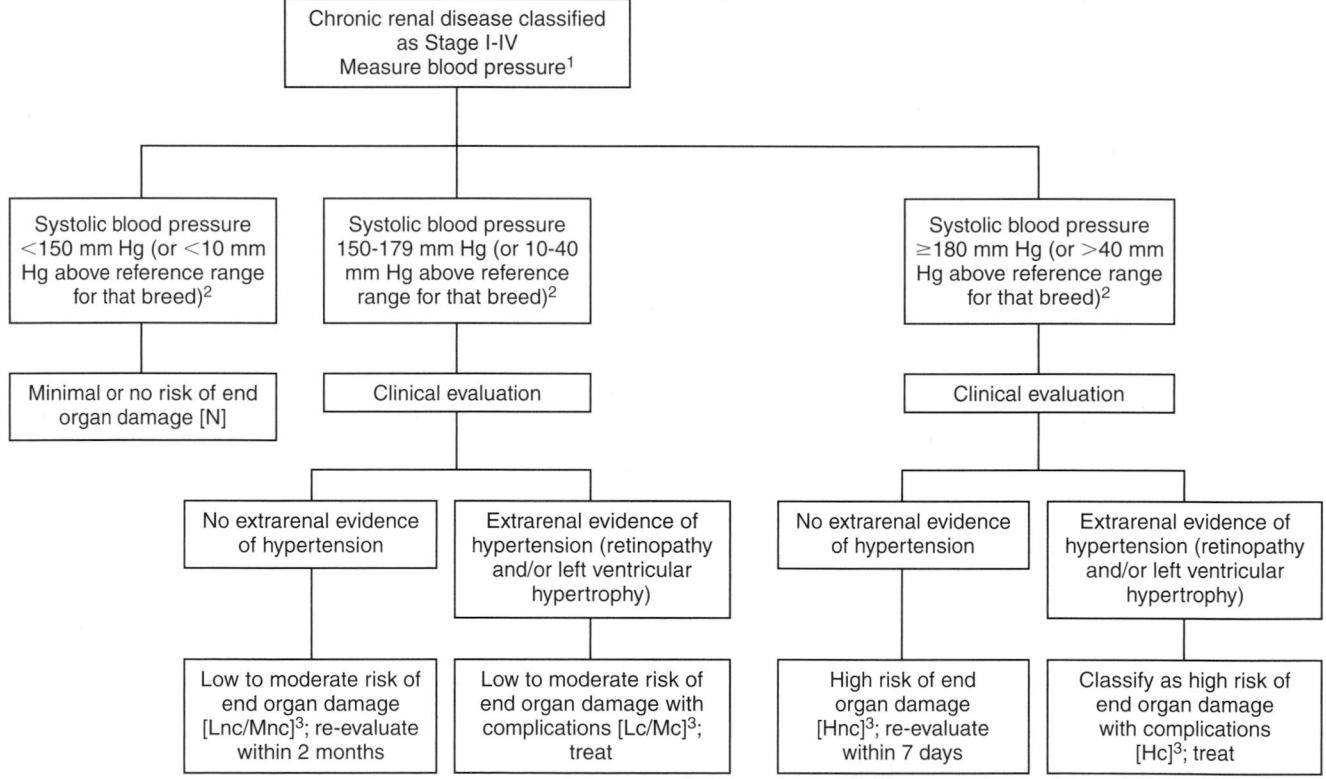

1. Blood pressure should be evaluated using a standard protocol that accounts for difficulties associated with indirect measurement of blood pressure. This should include patient acclimation to measurement conditions and multiple measurements during each measurement session. Because prognosis and therapy depend on this assessment, the final classification should rely on multiple pressure determinations (preferably involving repeat visits to the clinic on separate days, but "acceptable" if done during the same visit with at least 2 hours between determinations). This algorithm only classifies on the basis of systolic blood pressure, but Table 192-3 provides definitions based on systolic and diastolic pressures. In many cases both values will fall in the same category. When they do not, classification should be that of the higher category.
2. Comparison should be made with the upper limit of the breed-specific reference ranges, where available. Sight hounds, in particular, have higher reference ranges than most other dog breeds.
3. Patients are classified according to risk of end organ damage (see Table 192-3) and actual presence of extrarenal end organ damage or complications (e.g., hypertensive ocular lesions and/or left ventricular hypertrophy). Patients are then categorized according to the level of risk (N, minimal or none; L, low; M, moderate; H, high) and whether there is evidence of end organ damage/complications (nc, no complications; c, complications). Thus a patient with systolic blood pressure of 165 mm Hg and hyphema would be substaged as Mc (moderate risk with end organ complications). If blood pressure is not determined, the patient is classified as "blood pressure risk not determined" (RND).

Fig. 192-5   Algorithm for substaging on systemic blood pressure.

Table 192-4

Treatment Recommendations According to Stage of Chronic Kidney Disease

Stage	Complications to Address	Recommended Approach in the Dog	Differences in the Cat	Monitoring Required to Detect Adverse Events
I	Dehydration	See general comments in text	As for dog	See comments in text
	Systemic hypertension	See general comments in text	Treatment approach differs (see text for details)	See comments in text
	Proteinuria	If UP/C >2.0, investigate for disease processes leading to proteinuria*† and start antiproteinuric therapy‡§	As for dog	ACEI use is contraindicated in any animal that is clinically dehydrated and/or showing signs of hypovolemia
		UP/C >1.0 but <2.0 requires thorough investigation,*† and close monitoring¶	As for dog	Correct dehydration before using these drugs otherwise GFR may drop precipitously
		UP/C >0.5 but <1.0 requires close monitoring¶	Close monitoring should start at UP/C >0.4	
II	Dehydration	See general comments in text	As for dog	See comments in text
	Systemic hypertension	See general comments in text	Treatment approach differs (see text for details)	See comments in text
	Proteinuria	Recommendations as for stage I except intervention point for antiproteinuric therapy‡§ is UP/C >0.5	As for dog except treatment should commence if UP/C is >0.4	See comment about ACEI use for stage I
		UP/C >0.2 but <0.5 requires close monitoring¶	UP/C <0.2 but <0.4 requires close monitoring	
	Metabolic acidosis	If blood HCO_3/TCO_2 is <18 mEq/L) once patient is stabilized on diet of choice, give oral sodium bicarbonate or potassium citrate to maintain blood HCO_3/TCO_2 at 18-24 mEq/L	Intervention point for treatment of metabolic acidosis is blood HCO_3/TCO_2 of 16 mEq/L	Treatment with phosphate binders should be to effect, with signs of toxicity limiting the upper possible dose rate in each patient
	Hypokalemia	Not a problem in dogs with CKD	If the patient is hypokalemic, give potassium gluconate orally to correct this (typically 1-2 mEq/kg/day)	Monitor blood calcium and phosphate concentrations every 4-6 weeks until stable and then every 12 weeks
	Hyperphosphatemia/ hyperparathyroidism	Chronic reduction of phosphate intake to maintain plasma phosphate concentration at 2.7-4.5 mg/dl (0.9 to 1.45 mmol/L) is beneficial to patients with CKD—by first restricting dietary phosphate intake and then by adding intestinal phosphate binders¶ if required	Cats in stage 2 have normal plasma phosphate concentrations but often have increased plasma PTH concentration	Microcytosis and/or generalized muscle weakness suggests aluminium toxicity if using an aluminium containing binder; switch to another form of phosphate binder should this occur. Hypercalcemia should be avoided; combinations of aluminium and calcium containing phosphate binders may be necessary in some cases
III	Systemic hypertension Proteinuria Metabolic acidosis Hypokalemia	As for stage II	As for stage II	See stage II
	Dehydration	As for stage II— routine, regular administration of parenteral fluids could be considered to prevent dehydration	As for dog	Calculate daily fluid requirements carefully and avoid overhydration or sodium overload

(Continued)

Table 192-4—Cont'd

Treatment Recommendations According to Stage of Chronic Kidney Disease

Stage	Complications to Address	Recommended Approach in the Dog	Differences in the Cat	Monitoring Required to Detect Adverse Events
	Hyperphosphatemia/ hyperparathyroidism	If plasma phosphate exceeds 4.5 mg/dl (1.45 mmol/L) after maximum palatable phosphate binder dose has been achieved and hyperparathyroidism (increased blood PTH concentration) is documented, consider using ultralow dose calcitriol (1.5 to 3.5 ng/kg/day); evidence suggests judicious use prolongs survival in dogs at stages III and IV when phosphate is controlled and ionized calcium and PTH are monitored	Beneficial effects of ultra-low dose calcitriol have not been established in cats	Monitor blood ionized calcium and phosphate and avoid hypercalcemia
	Raised plasma urea concentration	Restrict dietary protein if blood urea is >30 mmol/L to decrease urea concentration	As for dog, but level of protein to be fed will be higher	Avoid protein malnutrition; monitor body condition score
	Anemia	Consider treatment for anemia if affecting patient's quality of life (typically with PCV ≤ 20% [0.20 l/l]). Human recombinant erythropoietin is the most effective treatment but is not approved for veterinary use. Anabolic steroids are of no proven benefit and may be detrimental	As for dog	Monitor PCV to avoid erythrocytosis and to detect when patient is becoming refractory to treatment
	Nausea and vomiting	Treat with H$_2$ receptor blocker (e.g., ranitidine) and antiemetic (e.g., metoclopramide)	As for dog, although vomiting is less common	
	Drug therapy	Drugs that rely predominantly on renal function for elimination should be used with caution in CKD stages III and IV; it may be necessary to adjust dose of these drugs (depending on their therapeutic indices) to avoid accumulation	As for dog	
IV	All complications listed under Stage III apply	All recommendations made for stage III apply to stage IV, but as azotemia worsens, need to: (a) Intensify efforts to prevent protein/calorie malnutrition. (could consider placing feeding tube—e.g., percutaneous gastrostomy tube) (b) Intensify efforts to prevent dehydration (can administer fluids as well as food through tube) (c) Consider dialysis, renal transplantation, or euthanasia	As for dog; recommendations for stage III in cat also apply	As for stage III Do not introduce ACEI to unstable, dehydrated animal; GFR may drop precipitously if used before patient is adequately hydrated

ACEI, Angiotensin-converting enzyme inhibitor; *CKD*, chronic kidney disease; *GFR*, glomerular filtration rate; *HCO$_3$*, bicarbonate; *PCV*, packed cell volume; *PTH*, parathyroid hormone; *TCO$_2$*, total carbon dioxide; *UP/C*, urine protein/creatinine ratio.

*Look for any concurrent associated disease or process that can be treated or corrected.

†Consider kidney biopsy to help identify underlying disease (consult expert if unsure of indications for biopsy).

‡ACEI with dietary n-3 PUFA supplementation and dietary protein restriction.

§ACEI Low-dose aspirin (0.05-0.5 mg/kg/day) if serum albumin is < 2 g/dl (20 g/L).

¶Monitor response to treatment/progression of disease: stable plasma creatinine concentration and decreasing UP/C: good response; serially increasing plasma creatinine concentration and/or increasing UP/C: disease progressing.

¶Aluminium hydroxide, aluminium carbonate, calcium carbonate, calcium acetate dosed to effect (starting at 30-60 mg/kg with each feeding mixed with the food if possible). The dose required varies according to the amount of phosphate being fed and the stage of CKD.

Management of Dehydration

At all stages of CKD patients have decreased urine concentrating ability and therefore one should correct clinical dehydration with isotonic, polyionic replacement fluids **and** have fresh water available at all times.

Management of Hypertension*

Hypertension can occur at any stage of CKD. Recommended treatments and monitoring are the same regardless of stage (Table 192-5). The goal is to reduce systolic blood pressure (SBP) to <160 mm Hg, minimizing risk of extrarenal end organ damage (e.g., CNS, retinal, cardiac)[†]. If evidence of such damage is lacking but SBP persistently exceeds 160 mm Hg, treatment should be instituted. *Persistence* should be judged on multiple SBP measurements made over 2 months (if at low to moderate risk [i.e., 150 to 179 mm Hg SBP]) or over 1 to 2 weeks (if at severe risk [i.e., ≥180 mm Hg]). Animals with end organ damage should be treated without the need to demonstrate persistence. Reducing blood pressure is a long-term treatment aim; gradual and sustained reduction should be the goal, avoiding sudden/severe decreases leading to hypotension. The recommended approach differs slightly in the dog and cat. In both species there is limited evidence that lowering dietary sodium alone is beneficial, but if attempted as part of a treatment protocol it should be done gradually (Table 192-4).

Lifelong antihypertensive therapy is usually required, and serial SBP monitoring is essential. After stabilization, monitoring every 3 months is the minimum. SBP <120 mm Hg and/or weakness/tachycardia indicate hypotension, which is to be avoided. Reducing blood pressure may lead to small and persistent increases in creatinine (<0.5 mg/dl), usually within 5 to 7 days of adjusting treatment. Marked acute increases in creatinine suggest an adverse drug effect, whereas gradual increases indicate deteriorating kidney function.

Other Management Procedures

Other aspects of management are summarized in Table 192-4. Specific dose rates are not stipulated. Standard dose rates apply for starting therapy with most agents, although caution is advisable with drugs eliminated mainly by renal mechanisms. Most complications of CKD, at which therapy is directed, become more prevalent with severity of CKD. In contrast, proteinuria and systemic hypertension can occur at any stage. They are integral to substaging because they are targets for therapy at all stages and are considered risk factors for CKD progression.

Diet can be manipulated to achieve multiple management goals in CKD. Each is dealt with in Table 192-4.

Table 192-5

A Logical Stepwise Approach to Managing Canine and Feline Hypertension

Step	Canine	Feline
1	ACEI therapy at the standard dose	Administer a CCB (generally amlodipine besylate)
2	Double dose of ACEI (improves antihypertensive effect in some patients)	Increase the dose of amlodipine up to 0.5 mg/kg/day
3	Combined treatment with an ACEI and a long-acting calcium channel blocker (CCB, generally amlodipine besylate)	Combined treatment with CCB and an ACEI
4	Combined treatment with ACEI, CCB and hydralazine	

Thus, dietary management often addresses several therapeutic targets including the following:

- Hyperphosphatemia and hyperparathyroidism: Limiting the dietary phosphate is beneficial in dogs and cats with CKD
- Proteinuria: Supplementing n-3 PUFAs and restricting protein intake address this problem
- Hypertension: Many commercial diets formulated for CKD patients have restricted sodium content (see above)
- Hypokalemia: Commercial diets formulated for feline CKD patients often have increased potassium content, but additional potassium may be required
- Azotemia: In the later stages of CKD, restriction of protein intake can reduce nitrogenous waste products within the blood.

The stage at which each therapeutic strategy is appropriate varies (see Table 192-4). The need for frequent monitoring and adjustment of therapy is an important principle here.

SUMMARY

The IRIS staging system reflects current knowledge and opinion about CKD in dogs and cats and will continue to evolve. Consistent, widespread use of such staging should help practitioners with diagnosis and prognosis in CKD, provide a framework for formulating treatment plans, and facilitate communication within the veterinary community.

ACKNOWLEDGMENT

The work of the IRIS Group is facilitated by generous funding from Novartis Animal Health. Updates can be accessed at http://www.iris-kidney.com.

---

* These recommendations are based on systolic blood pressures. Corresponding diastolic pressures presented in Table 192-3 can also be used to aid treatment decisions.
† The target posttreatment blood pressure necessary to prevent hypertensive renal damage is currently unknown.

References and Suggested Reading

Brown SA et al: Beneficial effects of chronic administration of dietary omega-3 polyunsaturated fatty acids in dogs with renal insufficiency, *J Lab Clin Med* 131:447, 1998.

Brown S et al: Guidelines for the identification, evaluation and management of systemic hypertension in dogs and cats, *J Vet Intern Med* 21:542, 2007.

Elliott J et al: Survival of cats with naturally occurring chronic renal failure: effect of dietary management, *J Small Anim Pract* 41:235, 2000.

Grauer GF et al: Effects of enalapril versus placebo as a treatment for canine idiopathic glomerulonephritis, *J Vet Intern Med* 14:526, 2000.

Jacob F et al: Clinical evaluation of dietary modification for treatment of spontaneous chronic renal failure in dogs, *J Am Vet Med Assoc* 220:1163, 2002.

Jacob F et al: Evaluation of the association between initial proteinuria and morbidity rate or death in dogs with naturally occurring chronic renal failure, *J Am Vet Med Assoc* 226:393, 2005.

King JN et al: Benazepril in renal insufficiency in cats study group: tolerability and efficacy of benazepril in cats with chronic kidney disease, *J Vet Intern Med* 20:1054, 2006.

Lees GE et al: Assessment and management of proteinuria in dogs and cats: 2004 ACVIM Forum Consensus Statement (Small Animal), *J Vet Intern Med* 19:377, 2005.

Plantinga EA et al: Retrospective study of the survival of cats with acquired chronic renal insufficiency offered different commercial diets, *Vet Rec* 157:185, 2005.

Syme HM et al: Survival of cats with naturally occurring chronic renal failure is related to proteinuria, *J Vet Intern Med* 20(3):528, 2006.

CHAPTER 193

Calcitriol

DAVID J. POLZIN, *St. Paul, Minnesota*
SHERI ROSS, *San Diego, California*
CARL A. OSBORNE, *St. Paul, Minnesota*

OVERVIEW OF CALCIUM AND PHOSPHORUS METABOLISM

Precise control of both phosphate and calcium homeostasis is essential to the normal functioning of virtually all life-sustaining physiologic processes. Disturbances in metabolism of the divalent ions calcium and phosphorus are common in patients with chronic kidney disease (CKD). Typical abnormalities seen in patients with CKD include hyperphosphatemia, hypocalcemia, hypercalcemia, renal secondary hyperparathyroidism, and calcitriol deficiency. Because these disturbances have been linked to increased morbidity and mortality in CKD, therapeutic intervention directed at minimizing these abnormalities and their systemic effects is an important component of conservative medical management of CKD.

The principal components involved in divalent ion metabolism that are relevant to patients with CKD include calcium, phosphorus, parathyroid hormone (PTH), and calcitriol. The primary goal of this system seemingly is to maintain normal blood calcium concentrations. Although calcium occurs in ionized, complexed, and protein-bound forms in blood, ionized calcium concentration is the primary component monitored and regulated. A reduction in blood ionized calcium concentration stimulates secretion of PTH. The amount of pre-formed PTH present in parathyroid cells is limited, and PTH degrades rapidly. Hypocalcemia increases PTH secretion by a posttranscriptional mechanism acting through the parathyroid gland membrane calcium-sensing receptor to stabilize PTH messenger ribonucleic acid. Increased PTH secretion acts to restore ionized calcium levels by three mechanisms: (1) increasing renal calcium resorption from the ascending loop of Henle, distal tubule, and collecting tubule; (2) increasing calcium resorption from bone; and (3) enhancing formation of calcitriol (1,25-dihydroxycholecalciferol) from 25-hydroxycholecalciferol by the kidneys. Calcitriol promotes elevation of serum calcium levels by enhancing absorption of calcium from the intestines and facilitating the effect of PTH on bone. The resulting increase in serum calcium levels reduces secretion of PTH. In addition, through a mechanism independent of blood calcium concentration, increased calcitriol levels inhibit synthesis and storage of PTH by activating vitamin D receptors (VDR), resulting in decreased PTH gene transcription.

Serum phosphate levels reflect the balance between intestinal absorption and renal excretion of phosphate. Intestinal absorption of phosphate is a function of: (1) dietary phosphorus content, (2) the amount of phosphate rendered insoluble by formation of nonabsorbable phosphate complexes within the intestinal lumen (e.g., calcium phosphate), and (3) the action of calcitriol to enhance intestinal phosphate absorption. Serum phosphate levels influence intestinal calcium and phosphorus absorption through an effect on renal calcitriol production. Phosphate retention and hyperphosphatemia inhibit renal 1-α hydroxylase activity, the enzyme responsible for renal conversion of 25-hydroxycholecalciferol to calcitriol, the most active form of vitamin D. By decreasing calcitriol levels, phosphate retention and hyperphosphatemia reduce intestinal phosphate absorption. In contrast, hypophosphatemia may be associated with elevated calcitriol levels, leading to increased intestinal absorption of phosphate. Renal phosphate excretion results from a combination of glomerular filtration and proximal tubular resorption. If phosphate intake remains unchanged, reduced glomerular filtration rate consistently increases retention of phosphate and promotes hyperphosphatemia. As described previously, hyperphosphatemia promotes elevated PTH activity. This increase in PTH activity is appropriate because PTH blocks proximal renal tubular resorption of phosphate, thus promoting phosphaturia, which facilitates restoration of normal serum phosphate concentrations.

PATHOPHYSIOLOGY OF RENAL SECONDARY HYPERPARATHYROIDISM

The inciting event in development of renal secondary hyperparathyroidism is retention of phosphate caused by reduced renal excretion (Fig. 193-1). Phosphate retention stimulates increased PTH production and secretion both by a direct effect of phosphate on the parathyroid gland and by reducing renal production of calcitriol by inhibiting renal 1-α hydroxylase activity. Hyperphosphatemia

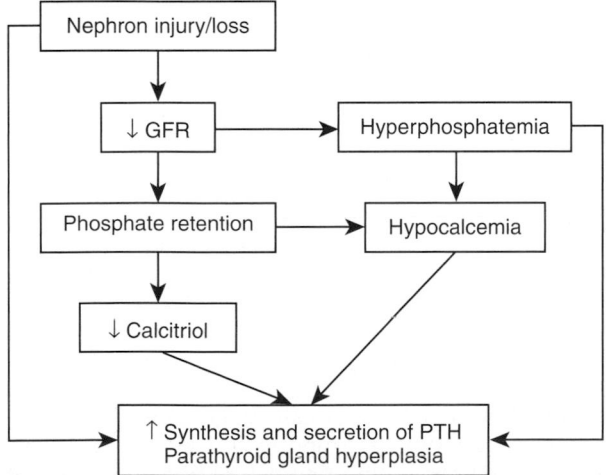

Fig. 193-1 Mechanism of development of renal secondary hyperparathyroidism. Reduced glomerular filtration rate initiates development of hyperparathyroidism by promoting phosphate retention and hyperphosphatemia. Phosphate retention suppresses the renal enzyme 1-α hydroxylase, which catalyzes the conversion of 25-hydroxycholecalciferol to 1,25-dihydroxycholecalciferol or calcitriol, the most active form of vitamin D. Calcitriol deficiency, hypocalcemia, and hyperphosphatemia all potentially contribute to development of hyperparathyroidism and parathyroid gland hyperplasia.

may also promote PTH secretion by complexing with ionized calcium, thereby lowering ionized calcium concentration. Elevated PTH levels increase phosphaturia, thereby maintaining serum phosphate within normal limits. Thus, at least initially, secondary hyperparathyroidism and its consequences are the long-term "trade-off" for the short-term benefit of maintaining normal serum phosphate concentrations. However, as renal disease progresses, the capacity to increase phosphaturia becomes insufficient to prevent hyperphosphatemia. In addition, loss of nephrons progresses to the point at which insufficient renal mass remains to sustain adequate production of calcitriol.

Persistent calcitriol deficiency may lead to parathyroid gland hyperplasia and hypertrophy with sustained autonomous secretion of PTH, a condition often referred to as *tertiary hyperparathyroidism*. Tertiary hyperparathyroidism typically is resistant to conventional medical interventions, and surgical reduction in the renal mass may be required to normalize PTH levels. Maintaining adequate levels of calcitriol throughout the course of CKD is important in preventing development of tertiary hyperparathyroidism because calcitriol has antiproliferative properties, decreases PTH gene transcription, and represses parathyroid cell proliferation.

RECOMMENDATIONS FOR USE OF CALCITRIOL IN CHRONIC KIDNEY DISEASE

Managing Divalent Ion Disorders in Chronic Kidney Disease

Minimizing development of calcium and phosphate disturbances and their consequences is a critical component of therapy for patients with CKD. The goals of management of divalent ion disturbances and renal secondary hyperparathyroidism in CKD are to: (1) reduce hyperphosphatemia and the mechanisms underlying phosphate retention; (2) restore adequate levels of active vitamin D (calcitriol), and (3) normalize serum calcium concentrations.

Therapy should begin by introducing a reduced phosphorus diet. The goal is to reduce serum phosphate concentration below 6 mg/dl (ideally, serum phosphate concentration should probably be in the range of 4.5 to 5.5 mg/dl). Diets designed for patients with CKD are appropriate for this purpose in that phosphorus content is typically reduced by 75% or more compared to typical maintenance-type diets. This dietary modification normalizes serum phosphate concentrations and reduces or normalizes PTH levels in most patients with CKD stage II and many patients with CKD stage III. Diet alone is unlikely to be sufficient therapy for patients with CKD stage IV (see Chapter 192).

When diet therapy alone fails to normalize serum phosphate concentrations and/or PTH levels, uptake of phosphorus can be further reduced by addition of an intestinal phosphate binding agent. Intestinal phosphate binding agents typically release cations (e.g., aluminum, calcium, or lanthanum), which bind irreversibly to phosphate in the intestinal lumen, thus rendering bound phosphate nonabsorbable. However, a potential disadvantage of intestinal phosphate binders is that some of the cations released may be absorbed and produce adverse effects. For example, aluminum retention has been associated with adverse hematologic, skeletal, and nervous system effects; and calcium-based binders may promote hypercalcemia. One product, sevelamer hydrochloride (Renagel, Genzyme Corp.) is a polyhydrochloride polymer that does not release cationic metals; however, it is very expensive and appears to be no more effective than less expensive binding agents.

The initial dosage of aluminum or calcium-based phosphate binders is 30 to 90 mg/kg/day given orally with food. It is important to administer the phosphate binder with food because the goal of this therapy is to bind the phosphorus contained in food so that it is not absorbed. Administering phosphate binders between meals is likely to markedly reduce the effectiveness of phosphate binding while promoting absorption of the cation contained in the binder. The dose of phosphate binding agent should be adjusted to achieve the goal of reducing serum phosphate concentration to below 6 mg/dl. In general, use of calcium-based phosphate binding agents is not recommended for patients receiving calcitriol. The exception to this rule may be in patients with overt hypocalcemia.

Once serum phosphorus has been reduced to below 6 mg/dl, calcitriol therapy may be initiated. Because calcitriol promotes intestinal absorption of both calcium and phosphorus, failure to adequately control serum phosphate concentration before initiating calcitriol may result in hyperphosphatemia, elevation in the serum calcium x phosphate product, and soft-tissue mineralization.

Benefits of Calcitriol Therapy

A host of clinical benefits have been hypothesized to accrue from calcitriol therapy in dogs and cats with CKD, including enhanced survival, appetite, activity, alertness, and interactivity with owners. It is common to use calcitriol in management of renal osteodystrophy in humans, but clinical signs of this condition are less prominent in most dogs and cats with CKD. The most important proposed benefit of calcitriol therapy, prolonged survival, has been confirmed in dogs with stages III and IV CKD (Polzin et al., 2005b) but remains unproven in cats with CKD. Evidence supporting the other clinical benefits of calcitriol is limited to pathophysiologic justification and clinical observations. Randomized clinical trials have failed to confirm that calcitriol ameliorates clinical signs in dogs and cats with CKD, but these studies were performed in stable CKD patients that were not exhibiting overt signs or anorexia, lethargy, or depression. Serum phosphate concentrations were aggressively managed in these studies; thus the magnitude of hyperparathyroidism was limited in both control and calcitriol groups. As a consequence, the hypothesized benefits of calcitriol on appetite, activity, and alertness may not have been observed. The fact that calcitriol forestalled onset of clinical signs of uremia in dogs may be interpreted as evidence of limiting development of the adverse clinical signs associated with uremia. Further clinical trials will be necessary to validate whether calcitriol ameliorates clinical signs associated with CKD.

Although the beneficial effects of calcitriol have traditionally been ascribed to suppression of PTH, this may not be the only mechanism of action of calcitriol. Recent epidemiologic studies in humans have suggested an important systemic role for direct activation of the VDR. Emerging data suggest that vitamin D therapy may prolong survival by mechanisms independent of calcium, phosphorus, and PTH. In canine studies demonstrating a beneficial effect of calcitriol on survival, differences in serum phosphorus, calcium, and PTH levels between the calcitriol group and placebo group were small. Further, studies in humans have shown that paricalcitol, a selective activator of the VDR, is associated with a more favorable efficacy to side-effect profile than calcitriol, with less morbidity and better survival.

Indications for Calcitriol

Dogs With Chronic Kidney Disease
In a randomized controlled clinical trial, calcitriol was shown to prolong survival and forestall development of uremic crises in dogs with stage III and early stage IV CKD. Because the rate of progression of CKD was slower in dogs receiving calcitriol in this study, it was concluded that calcitriol favorably influenced clinical outcome as a consequence of providing a renoprotective effect. These findings are consistent with observations in humans with CKD. On the basis of these findings, calcitriol therapy is indicated for dogs with stage III and early stage IV CKD. Calcitriol therapy is indicated in these patients even if PTH levels are not elevated. Because advanced hyperparathyroidism may be difficult or impossible to manage medically, early intervention or prophylaxis is recommended. However, the value of calcitriol therapy in dogs with stages I and II CKD has not been established.

Cats With Chronic Kidney Disease
There are insufficient data on which to base a recommendation for or against calcitriol administration to cats with any stage CKD. A 1-year–duration randomized, controlled clinical trial in our hospital failed to confirm any clinical benefits for cats in stages II, III, and IV CKD; but the possibility that calcitriol is of benefit was not excluded by this study.

Dosing Calcitriol

Baseline values for serum calcium (ideally ionized calcium) concentration, phosphorus concentration, and PTH activity should be established before beginning calcitriol therapy and then repeated after 2 to 4 weeks of therapy. We recommend starting calcitriol at a dosage of 2.5 ng/kg orally once daily. Calcitriol dosage should be adjusted so that PTH levels are reduced into the normal range without inducing hypercalcemia. If PTH remains elevated after 2 to 4 weeks of therapy, calcitriol dose may be increased to 3.5 ng/kg. Calcium and PTH levels should be reassessed after an additional 2 to 4 weeks; and if PTH remains elevated, calcitriol dose may be increased cautiously to 4.5

to 5 ng/kg. At this level monitoring serum calcium concentration becomes even more essential. We do not recommend increasing daily calcitriol dosage above 5 ng/kg/day. We have found that, in most dogs and cats in stages II and III CKD, doses between 1.5 and 5 ng/kg are effective in normalizing PTH activities. Effectiveness of calcitriol therapy at relatively low doses is not surprising given that a near maximal effect of calcitriol on PTH gene transcription occurs at or near physiologic levels. However, the effectiveness of calcitriol in lowering PTH levels may be impaired by overt hypocalcemia. In such instances it may be necessary to cautiously provide oral calcium supplementation. Long-standing hyperparathyroidism with parathyroid hyperplasia may be associated with a deficiency of VDR on the hyperplasic parathyroid cells, resulting in hyperparathyroidism that is refractory to calcitriol therapy. Since calcitriol induces formation of the VDR on parathyroid cells, long-standing deficiency of calcitriol may contribute to the deficiency of VDR in this setting. In such instances a more prolonged course of calcitriol therapy or "pulse" therapy (see following paragraphs) may be attempted to determine if PTH levels can be reduced.

Should calcitriol therapy induce an increase in ionized calcium concentration, it may be necessary to reduce calcitriol dosage. Calcitriol-induced hypercalcemia may also be ameliorated by administering calcitriol in the evening on an empty stomach when calcitriol is less likely to promote enhanced intestinal calcium absorption. If hypercalcemia persists, pulse dosing may be considered.

Pulse therapy involves administration of larger doses of calcitriol at less frequent intervals. Pulse therapy may induce formation of greater numbers of VDR on parathyroid cells, rendering the gland more responsive to the action of calcitriol. In addition, pulse therapy may minimize the tendency for calcitriol therapy to induce hypercalcemia since it induces hypercalcemia by promoting intestinal absorption of calcium. Calcitriol promotes intestinal absorption of calcium through its effect on newly formed intestinal cells leaving the crypts of Lieberkühn. The tendency of these cells to absorb calcium is determined largely by their exposure to calcitriol only during this early developmental phase. Since calcitriol has a relatively short half-life (about 4 to 6 hours), less frequent administration limits the number of intestinal cells primed to enhanced calcium absorption, thereby moderating the predisposition of calcitriol to induce hyperabsorptive hypercalcemia. Pulse therapy is usually provided at twice the usual daily dose (for a total dose of 5 to 10 ng/kg) administered orally every other day. Once hyperparathyroidism is controlled using pulse therapy, an attempt should be made to revert to daily low-dose administration of calcitriol.

Calcitriol must be compounded into a dose size appropriate for dogs and cats. It is important to remember that the quantity of calcitriol contained in capsules designed for use in humans contains a considerable overdose when administered to dogs and cats; this quantity should never be used in these species.

Potential Complications of Calcitriol Therapy

In our studies we found low-dose calcitriol therapy to be quite safe. No obvious adverse effects were noted, although calcitriol doses occasionally had to be reduced because of development of hypercalcemia. Hyperphosphatemia, hypercalcemia, and elevated calcium x phosphate product are relative contraindications to calcitriol therapy. Development of hypercalcemia and soft-tissue mineralization, particularly of the vascular system, is of great concern in humans with CKD. Because of the tendency for calcitriol to promote hypercalcemia, selective VDR activators such as paricalcitol (Zemplar) and doxercalciferol have been developed. In humans with CKD these compounds appear to provide adequate control of hyperparathyroidism with minimal changes in serum calcium and phosphate concentrations, even when calcium-based intestinal phosphate binding agents are used. As mentioned previously, these compounds appear to have less morbidity and mortality associated with their use compared to calcitriol. However, the long-term benefits of these compounds remain to be established. There are no reports on the use of paricalcitol in dogs or cats with spontaneous CKD.

Monitoring Patients With Calcitriol

Although low-dose calcitriol appears to generally be safe, monitoring is advocated to optimize therapy and avoid iatrogenic complications. Ideally serum calcium, ionized calcium, phosphate, and PTH levels should be evaluated every 2 to 4 weeks until the desired dosage is established. Thereafter these parameters and serum creatinine concentration should be monitored every 3 to 6 months; however, the frequency of monitoring should be individualized to each patient based on response to therapy and stability of the monitored values. The goal of therapy is to maintain serum phosphate, calcium, and PTH levels within normal limits.

References and Suggested Reading

Andress DL: Vitamin D in chronic kidney disease: a systemic role for selective vitamin D receptor activation, *Kidney Int* 69:33, 2006.

Brown SA et al: Beneficial effect of dietary mineral restriction in dogs with marked reduction of functional renal mass, *J Am Soc Nephrol* 1:1169, 1991.

Gerber B, Hassig M, Reusch CE: Serum concentrations of 1, 25-dihydroxycholecalciferol and 25-hydroxycholecalciferol in clinically normal dogs and dogs with acute and chronic renal failure, *Am J Vet Res* 64(9):1161, 2003.

Nagode LA, Chew DJ, and Podell M: Benefits of calcitriol therapy and serum phosphorus control in dogs and cats with chronic renal failure. Both are essential to prevent of suppress toxic hyperparathyroidism, *Vet Clin North Am Small Anim Pract* 26:1293, 1996.

Polzin DJ, Osborne CA, Ross S: Chronic kidney disease. In Ettinger S, Feldman E, editors: *Textbook of veterinary internal medicine*, ed 6, Philadelphia, 2005b, Saunders, p 1756.

Polzin D et al: Clinical benefit of calcitriol in canine chronic kidney disease, *J Vet Intern Med* 19:433A, 2005.

CHAPTER 194

Hemodialysis

CATHERINE E. LANGSTON, *New York, New York*

The most common application of hemodialysis is therapy of renal failure that is not responsive to medical management. Hemodialysis also can be used for the removal of ingested toxins (e.g., ethylene glycol), selected drug overdoses, and volume overload. Dialysis modalities, including intermittent hemodialysis (IHD) and continuous renal replacement therapy (CRRT), are becoming more readily available, and Internet-savvy clients are requesting referral for these therapies for their pets. This chapter covers the information of importance to practicing veterinarians regarding hemodialysis and highlights some of the exciting developments in this field.

PRINCIPLES OF DIALYSIS

Hemodialysis removes uremic toxins from the bloodstream by diffusion. During the treatment a continuous flow of blood from the patient is carried to the dialyzer through disposable tubing (extracorporeal circuit, Fig. 194-1). The dialyzer, or artificial kidney, contains a porous membrane. As with the kidney, size and charge are major determinants determining which particles are filtered by the dialyzer. Small to middle-sized molecules in high concentration in the bloodstream, such as urea and creatinine, diffuse through the pores into a dialysate solution on the opposite side of the membrane. Large molecules such as albumin and cells are too large to pass through the pores and remain in the bloodstream. Because necessary electrolytes such as sodium can pass through the membrane easily, the dialysate solution has physiologic concentrations of these electrolytes, preventing significant loss from the patient. After passing through the dialyzer, the blood is returned to the patient. In a standard 4- to 5-hour intermittent dialysis treatment, a patient's blood volume may be circulated through the machine the equivalent of 20 to 30 times. Ultrafiltration removes fluid from the patient by creating a hydrostatic pressure gradient between the blood compartment and the dialysate compartment.

DIALYSIS EQUIPMENT

Dialysis Machines

There are a variety of models and manufacturers of dialysis machines, but all must circulate blood in the extracorporeal circuit, circulate dialysate, and precisely control ultrafiltration. Most machines also have an integrated syringe pump to deliver a constant infusion of heparin or other anticoagulant during the treatment.

Intermittent hemodialysis generally involves rapid blood and dialysate flow for efficient removal of uremic toxins and fluid, allowing treatments to occur at intervals. A typical regimen would include several hours per treatment, three to four times per week. Machines designed for IHD are capable of supplying the large volume of dialysate necessary by mixing purified water with concentrated electrolyte solutions. Sodium and bicarbonate concentrations can be adjusted independently and tailored to the patient's needs. The resulting dialysate is purified but not sterile; thus low levels of endotoxins may contribute to chronic inflammation in IHD patients. Newer IHD machines include an additional filtration step in dialysate delivery, creating what is termed *ultrapure* dialysate. IHD machines require a water treatment system, which may be a large-capacity system that pipes water to the dialysis unit or a contained water treatment system that can supply purified water for a single machine. These machines can be programmed to perform at a wide variety of blood flow rates to allow for variability of patient size and can provide a high or low efficiency treatment. Because of the complexity of equipment and the possibility of acute changes in patient status during treatment, IHD is usually performed by specially trained dialysis personnel.

CRRT uses the same general principles as IHD, with the exception of timing. CRRT is intended to be a continuous dialysis treatment, which is sustained until renal recovery occurs or until the patient is stable and can be transitioned to IHD. CRRT machines do not create dialysate, and prepackaged sterile dialysate is used with these machines. Dialysate flow rates are much slower with CRRT (up to 6 L/hour) compared to IHD (20 to 50 L/hour). In many human facilities, CRRT is instituted by the dialysis personnel, who are available for machine preparation and scheduled dialyzer and tubing changes (manufacturer's recommendation is to change materials every 3 days). The patient and machine are then monitored around the clock by CRRT-trained intensive care unit nursing staff. A dialysis team member is usually available (either by phone or on call) for troubleshooting. Common problems with CRRT include poor blood flow (usually caused by catheter size or malposition) and excessive clotting in the dialyzer, necessitating unscheduled changes of the extracorporeal circuit. "Hybrid" machines that can perform either modality recently have become available, allowing low-efficiency continual therapy initially until the patient is more hemodynamically stable and then more aggressive intermittent treatments as needed.

Monitoring Devices

Careful monitoring of the dialysis patient is necessary. Some of the parameters that require close monitoring during treatment include blood pressure, coagulation status,

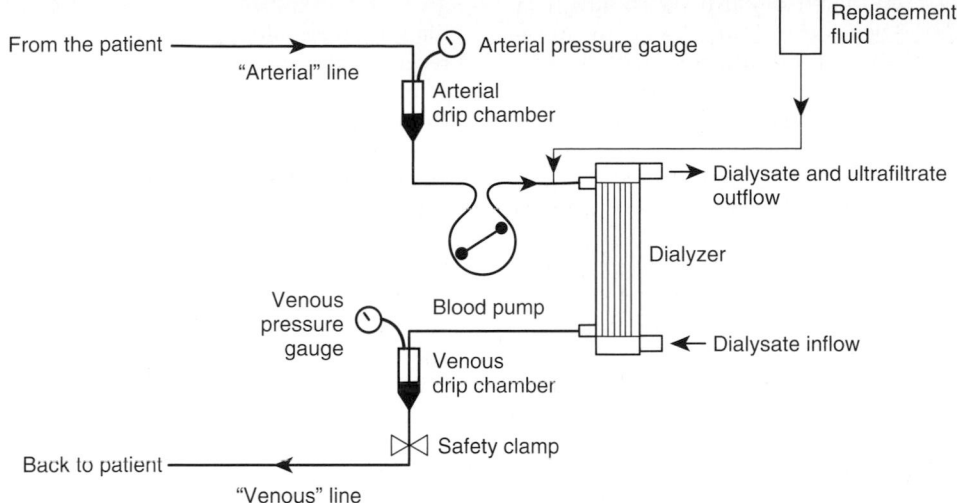

Fig. 194-1 Pathway of blood from the vascular access in the patient through the extracorporeal circuit and back to the patient.

and blood volume. Indirect blood pressure measurement can be accomplished with a variety of devices. Typically during treatment blood pressure is monitored every 15 to 30 minutes for IHD, and slightly less frequently in a stable patient on CRRT. Rapid assessment of coagulation parameters is necessary to adjust anticoagulant dosing during treatment (see section on Anticoagulation later in the chapter). Multiple devices are available specifically for monitoring dialysis patients, and newer dialysis machines incorporate these technologies into the system design. A hemoglobin sensor placed on the blood tubing can continuously determine the hematocrit and is used to determine relative blood volume changes, working under the presumption that red blood cells are neither being added nor removed from the patient during the treatment. Hematocrit will change related to plasma volume expansion (decreased hematocrit) or contraction (increased hematocrit). Rapid ultrafiltration can remove volume from the intravascular compartment faster than it can refill from the interstitium, and this situation can lead to symptomatic hypotensive episodes during dialysis. Close monitoring of the relative blood volume should minimize the likelihood of a hypotensive event.

Vascular Access

Both IHD and CRRT require vascular access. Depending on the predicted duration of dialysis treatments, the dialysis nephrologist may choose to select a catheter for short-term (temporary) or long-term (permanent) use. For short-term treatment double-lumen catheters placed percutaneously with a guidewire (Seldinger technique) or via minor surgical exposure of the vessel are the most commonly used type of vascular access. These catheters can be placed with a local anesthetic and mild sedation. Regardless of the anticipated treatment duration, generally the largest feasible catheter size is selected to ensure sufficient blood flow (up to 20ml/kg/minute for IHD) for an efficient dialysis treatment. An 11.5-Fr dual-lumen hemodialysis catheter (MedComp) can be placed in most medium-to-large dogs and provides up to 350ml/minute

blood flow; these catheters can be maintained for 4 weeks or longer. In cats a 7-Fr dual-lumen central catheter (Arrow International) can be placed percutaneously. The 7-Fr catheter accommodates up to 100ml/min blood flow in in vitro experiments; however, in clinical use these catheters frequently do not provide sufficient blood flow for medium- to high-efficiency treatments. Smaller catheters such as a 5.5-Fr double- or triple-lumen catheter can be placed in smaller cats and provide 5- to 10-ml/minute blood flow, which would be appropriate for early IHD (low efficiency regimens) and potentially for CRRT.

Long-term dialysis catheters are placed surgically, leaving the proximal portion of the catheter in a subcutaneous tunnel. The tunnel separates the skin exit site from the venotomy site, decreasing infectious complications, and a Dacron cuff helps anchor the catheter in place. These catheters have remained functional for 6 to 9 months in dogs. New catheter designs, including separation of the two catheter lumens in the same vessel, have helped decrease catheter malfunction from thrombus formation in and around the catheter.

For chronic dialysis a subcutaneous graft or fistula is the most common method of access in humans but must be surgically created at least a month before use. A model of surgically created grafts has been developed in dogs but is not in widespread use.

ANTICOAGULATION

Some form of anticoagulation is needed during dialysis to prevent thrombosis in the extracorporeal circuit. Unfractionated heparin is the most commonly used anticoagulant. Activated clotting time (ACT) has traditionally been monitored during treatment, and the results have been used to adjust the heparin dose, with a goal of maintaining the ACT at 1.6 to 2 times normal. Excessive clotting and bleeding are potential complications of heparin anticoagulation. Low–molecular weight heparin is not commonly used in veterinary hemodialysis, and its use in human hemodialysis generally is limited to high-risk patients because of the high cost compared with unfractionated heparin. With advances in technology, use of bedside monitors that can accurately measure partial thromboplastin time with a small volume of blood may replace ACT monitoring in the future of veterinary hemodialysis.

Regional citrate anticoagulation is used in some human and veterinary CRRT units. Citrate, administered as a constant-rate infusion into the extracorporeal circuit, binds calcium, preventing coagulation in the circuit. Since the anticoagulation occurs outside of the patient, bleeding complications associated with anticoagulation are minimized. Calcium chloride is administered through a centrally placed intravenous catheter or via the extracorporeal circuit just at the point where the blood is reentering the body to avoid hypocalcemia in the patient. This procedure is complex and requires frequent blood calcium monitoring and dose adjustments of both citrate and calcium infusions, but it diminishes the risk of hemorrhage associated with long-term heparinization. Citrate is relatively contraindicated in the face of hepatic dysfunction.

INDICATIONS FOR DIALYSIS

IHD and CRRT are most commonly used to treat acute renal failure (ARF). The goal of acute dialysis is to resolve life-threatening disorders (i.e., hyperkalemia, pulmonary edema) and control uremia, thus decreasing subsequent uremic complications, allowing time for renal repair to occur. In contrast, chronic dialysis is used to control signs associated with end-stage renal failure for the remainder of the patient's life.

Dialysis is appropriate for any disease causing ARF. Common reasons for acute dialysis include leptospirosis, bacterial pyelonephritis, toxic nephropathy (e.g., ethylene glycol, lily ingestion, grapes/raisins, aminoglycosides), and renal ischemia. Dialysis can also be used in patients with acute uremia syndrome associated with ureteral obstruction. Dialysis is being used to manage these patients before surgery, allowing control of hyperkalemia and other life-threatening uremic complications, allowing time for diagnostic evaluation, and improving patient stability in preparation for anesthesia. Generally one to three treatments before surgery are adequate. Two to four dialysis treatments before renal transplantation surgery have also been used in some institutions to stabilize patients with acute uremic crisis or severe uremia (Cowgill and Francey, 2006).

Client demand for chronic hemodialysis for chronic kidney disease (CKD) is increasing. Because of the irreversible nature of CKD, dialytic treatment is ongoing, typically three treatments a week; treated patients can maintain an excellent quality of life for extended periods of time (6 to 12 months or more).

Certain drugs and toxins can be removed with dialysis. Substances with low–molecular weight and minimal protein binding are more readily removed. Rapid removal of the offending substance is generally desired. With IHD a charcoal perfusion cartridge can be placed in series with the dialyzer, expanding the possible toxicities that can be treated. In contrast to dialytic removal, charcoal perfusion involves filtering the blood across microencapsulated charcoal beads, which adsorb the toxic compound, removing it from the circulation. Because medications given for therapeutic purposes also can be removed by dialysis, dose alterations may be necessary in patients receiving dialysis.

Slow continuous ultrafiltration (removal of fluid from the patient) without concurrent dialysis can be used to treat volume overload situations that are not associated with renal failure (i.e., diuretic-resistant congestive heart failure). Therapeutic plasmapheresis can also be performed, using a plasmapheresis cartridge instead of a dialyzer, although appropriate indications for plasmapheresis are not well established. Plasmapheresis differs from dialysis in that large pores in the cartridge allow removal of albumin and globulins, separating the plasma from the cellular components. There is little veterinary experience with either of these techniques.

INITIATING DIALYSIS

Anuria or oliguria that does not respond to volume expansion and diuretics is a clear indication for starting dialysis. Volume overload, which may manifest as life-threatening pulmonary edema or pleural effusion, can occur with oliguria or anuria or in patients with an inappropriate urine output relative to the volume of administered fluid; they are both indications for dialysis. Hyperkalemia is an immediately life-threatening complication. Medical strategies for hyperkalemia (i.e., insulin, dextrose, bicarbonate, or calcium) can be used as temporary measures but do not remove the excess potassium from the body (see Chapter 191). IHD can remove potassium rapidly and minimize cardiac toxicity, normalizing the electrocardiogram. Severe uremia (blood urea nitrogen >100 mg/dl, creatinine >10 mg/dl) and uremia that does not respond to the first 24 hours of medical management are other indications for dialysis (Box 194-1). In humans instituting dialysis earlier in the course of renal failure improves outcome and the likelihood of return of renal function; early referral for dialysis, before the onset of severe extrarenal manifestations of uremia, is prudent in the veterinary field also (Box 194-2).

The decision to start dialysis for CKD generally is based on failure of medical management to control signs of uremia such as anorexia, lethargy, or vomiting. Frequently a feeding tube is placed at the time of dialysis catheter placement in these patients to provide nutritional support

---

Box 194-1

Indications for Hemodialysis

- Oliguria or anuria unresponsive to therapy
- Volume overload
- Hyperkalemia
- Severe uremia (blood urea nitrogen >100 mg/dl, creatinine >10 mg/dl)
- Uremia unresponsive to medical management for 24 hours
- Poisoning or drug overdose (ethylene glycol, aspirin, acetaminophen, phenylbutazone, digoxin, amikacin, azathioprine, cyclophosphamide, enalapril, procainamide, phenobarbital, theophylline, many others)

during the initial few weeks of dialysis and during periods of stress. Dialysis for toxin removal should be instituted as rapidly as possible. Patients with antifreeze ingestion should receive a dose of 4-methylpyrazole (dogs) or ethanol (cats) to slow metabolism of ethylene glycol while arrangements for dialysis are being made.

TREATMENT PROTOCOLS

IHD is an efficient method of solute removal and an appropriate treatment modality for ARF, CKD, acute toxicities, and fluid removal. With severe azotemia rapid reduction of urea can lead to untoward effects; thus the first few IHD treatments are abbreviated. Several (usually three to seven) short daily treatments are applied to gradually control metabolic derangements associated with severe uremia. Ongoing treatments, typically of 4- to 5-hour duration three times a week, are performed until the patient has regained renal function. Some patients can be discharged from the hospital after the first 2 weeks of treatment and return for outpatient dialysis treatments over the next several weeks. With severe uremia in an unstable patient, the first treatment may be long (6 to >24 hours) with slow blood flow to gradually control the uremic manifestations while diminishing risk of complications, a prescription referred to as slow low-efficiency dialysis.

CRRT is an appropriate treatment modality for ARF and fluid removal and is usually applied for a short-term duration. CRRT treatments in human pediatric patients have a mean duration of about 4 days (range 0.5 to 30 days). CRRT typically is started with a modest blood flow rate (2 to 3 ml/kg/minute compared to 5 to 20 ml/kg/minute with IHD) and slow dialysate flow rate (8 to 34 ml/minute compared to 500 ml/minute with IHD). The clinician determines the desired net fluid removal rate based on patient hydration status. Additional ultrafiltration with fluid replacement to enhance convective solute clearance (removal of solutes dissolved in the fluid that is removed from the patient) ranges from 0 to 35 ml/kg/hour. Once treatment is started, these parameters may be adjusted to achieve the desired clearance. Clinical indicators of recovery (e.g., increase in urine output) may prompt the clinician to decrease the blood or dialysate flow rate in attempt to wean the patient off CRRT.

COMPLICATIONS

Complications encountered during dialytic management may be a result of the dialysis procedure or of the underlying renal failure.

Procedural Complications

Dialysis disequilibrium syndrome is a condition characterized by a rapid decline in blood osmolality caused by removal of osmoles (especially urea) by dialysis. Because the osmoles can be removed from the blood faster than they can diffuse from the intracellular compartment, a state of relative intracellular hyperosmolality ensues. Subsequent cellular swelling leads to central nervous system signs (i.e., seizures, mentation changes). Patients at increased risk for dialysis disequilibrium syndrome include those with severe azotemia, smaller blood volumes, or preexisting neurologic signs. Slow, low-efficiency dialysis or CRRT can be used to reduce the likelihood of this complication, as can prophylactic administration of the osmotic agent mannitol.

In small patients removal of the blood volume necessary to fill the dialysis circuit can result in hypotension. In an effort to minimize this complication, colloidal substances (e.g., dextran) may be used to prime the circuit. Administration of colloids or blood products may be required to maintain blood pressure throughout treatment. Ultrafiltration can also cause significant hypovolemia. Temporarily stopping ultrafiltration may be sufficient to manage a hypotensive event.

Hemorrhage related to heparin anticoagulation is most likely during the first few dialysis treatments, while the individual response to heparin is being determined, and with prolonged sessions (>6 hours). Thrombosis at the tip of the dialysis catheter in the right atrium is common with catheters in place for over 3 weeks and impairs adequate blood flow. Clinically significant pulmonary thromboembolism is uncommon, but vena caval thrombosis or stenosis (with intermandibular edema) is a well-recognized complication in dogs. Early treatment of complete or partial catheter occlusion with human recombinant tissue plasminogen activator (alteplase, Cathflo Activase, Genetech) may salvage a malfunctioning catheter.

The tips of a dual-lumen hemodialysis catheter are staggered. The more proximal tip removes blood from the patient to carry it to the dialyzer. Blood coming from the dialyzer, which has been cleared of uremic toxins, is returned through the distal tip and swept forward in the bloodstream. A poorly functioning catheter may create turbulence and pressure gradients that allow uptake of the returning dialyzed blood, decreasing the efficiency of solute clearance. The amount of recirculation can be measured by a variety of methods to determine if intervention is indicated.

Uremic Complications

Manifestations of uremia (e.g., oral, gastrointestinal) are common in ARF patients. With dialytic management survival can be enhanced such that a variety of less common uremic complications are also observed. Respiratory dysfunction, presumptively from pulmonary edema or uremic pneumonitis, is encountered frequently. Pulmonary hemorrhage associated with leptospirosis is another cause of respiratory compromise. Interestingly, a frequent uremic complication in patients on dialysis for ARF is moderate-to-severe fulminant pancreatitis, although it may not be detected antemortem. Common clinical signs of pancreatitis (anorexia, vomiting, abdominal pain) overlap with signs of ARF; when these signs persist despite adequate control of uremia by dialysis, careful evaluation for pancreatitis is warranted.

OUTCOME

Overall 40% to 60% of patients with ARF treated with dialysis survive, a notable achievement given that the patient

Box 194-2

Dialysis Facilities Offering Intermittent Hemodialysis or Continuous Renal Replacement Therapy in United States

Animal Medical Center (IHD)
New York, NY
(212)838-8100
hemodialysis@amcny.org
Dr. Cathy Langston

Tufts Foster Hospital for Small Animals (IHD)
North Grafton, MA
(508)839-5395
Dr. Mary Labato
Dr. Linda Ross

University of California (IHD)
Veterinary Medical Teaching Hospital
Companion Animal Hemodialysis Unit
Davis, CA
(530)752-1393
Dr. Larry Cowgill

University of California (IHD)
Veterinary Medical Center at San Diego
Renal Medicine/Hemodialysis Service
San Diego, CA
(858)875-7505
Dr. Julie Fischer
Dr. Larry Cowgill

Advanced Critical Care and Internal Medicine (CRRT)
Tustin, CA
(949)654-8950
Dr. Ravi Seshadri

Advanced Critical Care (CRRT)
City of Angels Veterinary Specialty Center
Culver City, CA 90232
(310)558-6100
Dr. Richard Mills
Dr. Jon Perlis

California Animal Referral and Emergency Hospital (CRRT)
Santa Barbara, CA
(805)899-2273
Dr. Andrea Wells

Center for Specialized Veterinary Care (CRRT)
Westbury, NY
(516)420-0000
Dr. Diane Levitan

Chicago Veterinary Kidney Center (CRRT)
Buffalo Grove, IL
(847)459-7535
Dr. Jerry Thornhill

Veterinary Specialist of South Florida (CRRT)
Cooper City, FL
(954)432-5611
Dr. Brian Roberts

Louisiana State University (CRRT)
Veterinary Medical Teaching Hospital
Baton Rouge, LA
(225)578-9600
Dr. Mark Acierno

CRRT, Continuous renal replacement therapy; *IHD,* intermittent hemodialysis. Facilities listed are those available at the time of writing, and this table may not include all available centers.

population is comprised of animals unresponsive to conventional medical management (Langston, 2003). However, there are marked differences in survival for different etiologies of ARF. The survival rate for ARF from infectious causes was about 60% to 70% (Francey and Cowgill, 2002; Francey, 2004). Hemodynamic and metabolic causes had a 40% to 56% survival rate. Only 20% to 30% of patients with ARF from toxic causes (e.g., ethylene glycol) survived. In addition to providing lifesaving benefits for acute scenarios, dialytic support may be extended to provide additional time for renal repair and recovery. Although the majority of renal recovery has traditionally been thought to occur within 4 weeks of renal injury, I have seen patients with continued recovery over 3 to 6 months.

References and Suggested Reading

Cowgill LD, Francey: Hemodialysis. In Dibartola SP, editor: *Fluid therapy in small animal practice,* ed 3, Philadelphia, 2006, Saunders, p 650.

Fischer JR: Veterinary hemodialysis: advances in management and technology, *Vet Clin North Am* 34:936, 2004.

Francey T: Outcome of dogs and cats treated with hemodialysis, Proceedings of the Advanced Renal Therapies Symposium 1, New York, 2004.

Francey T, Cowgill LD: Use of hemodialysis for the management of acute renal failure in the dog: 124 cases (1990-2001), *J Vet Intern Med* 16(abstr):352, 2002.

Langston CE: Advanced renal therapies: options when standard treatments are not enough, *Vet Med* 98:999, 2003.

CHAPTER 195

Renal Transplantation

CHRISTOPHER A. ADIN, *Rochester, New York*

Renal transplantation is widely accepted as the most successful and cost-effective method for the treatment of end-stage renal disease in humans; application of this technique is limited primarily by the availability of suitable organ donors. Pioneering work by Drs. Clare Gregory and Gary Gourley in the late 1980s made clinical application of renal transplantation a reality for dogs and cats with naturally occurring renal disease (Bonagura and Kirk, 1992). However, organ transplantation presents a number of unique surgical, immunosuppressive, ethical, and financial challenges in veterinary patients, slowing widespread application of this technique in veterinary medicine. Fortunately a number of recent advances in each of these areas have improved the success rate and availability of organ transplantation for dogs and cats. These events, coupled with an increasing demand for advanced medical and surgical therapies in veterinary patients with end-stage renal disease, have fueled a strong interest among pet owners seeking the highest level of care for their animals. This chapter summarizes recent advances in veterinary renal transplantation and provides up-to-date information for the veterinary practitioner for identification and referral of appropriate candidates.

PREPARATION FOR RENAL TRANSPLANTATION

Indications for Renal Transplantation

Renal transplantation is offered as one of several methods to manage cats and dogs with moderate-to-severe end-stage renal disease. Evidence from large retrospective studies performed in humans would indicate that early and aggressive management of renal disease with hemodialysis or renal transplantation leads to improved outcome in affected patients. In fact, the 1993 National Institute of Health Consensus Statement on the Morbidity and Mortality of Dialysis recommended that men with a serum creatinine concentration of 2 mg/dl should be referred to a nephrologist for predialysis and transplant evaluation. Similarly, early referral is recommended by veterinary transplant centers to allow development of a relationship with the client, to allow time for adequate screening of recipients, and to facilitate a well-informed client decision when the time for intervention arises. Renal transplantation is most successful when performed as an elective procedure in stable cats and dogs with serum creatinine between 3 g/dl and 10 mg/dl. In animals with more severe degrees of azotemia, preoperative hemodialysis may be required.

Screening of Transplant Candidates

Original screening criteria for veterinary transplant candidates were based on exclusion criteria used in human medicine. A broad array of preoperative tests was recommended; and identification of any serious organ dysfunction, endocrine disease, or infectious process not related to the primary renal disease was considered a contraindication for kidney transplantation. As experience in veterinary renal transplantation accumulates, retrospective analysis has allowed us to revise these screening criteria and in general has led to a less restrictive policy at most institutions (Fig. 195-1). For example, original guidelines suggested that any cat with abnormal findings on echocardiogram should be declined for renal transplantation. However, a recent retrospective analysis indicated that mild, focal changes in ventricular septal wall thickness were present in the majority of cats with chronic renal failure and may represent changes secondary to hypertension or uremia rather than primary cardiac disease (Adin et al., 2000). Minor echocardiographic changes were not predictive of postoperative complications and should not serve as an absolute contraindication to renal transplantation (Adin et al., 2000). Instead more severe changes representative of primary hypertrophic cardiomyopathy (diffuse or severe hypertrophic changes) or evidence of preexisting heart failure is now considered to be of more significance in screening of feline transplant candidates. A variety of other factors such as severe preoperative azotemia or unmanaged hypertension have now been shown to contribute to the occurrence of postoperative neurologic abnormalities (Adin et al., 2001; Kyles et al., 1999). Although these factors are not absolute contraindications to renal transplantation, correction of preoperative azotemia and hypertension through medical therapy or hemodialysis is recommended in cats with more severe stages of renal dysfunction. Other preoperative findings such as severe cachexia or urinary tract infection may be addressed with aggressive medical therapy and reevaluated by the transplant center, as indicated in Fig. 195-1.

Animals with preexisting infectious diseases are at particularly high risk of experiencing complications after immunosuppressive therapy is initiated; renal transplantation may not be the most advisable method of treatment in these animals. For this reason, renal transplantation is not recommended in cats with feline leukemia virus infection or active feline immunodeficiency virus infection. Caution in also advised in cats housed in multicat households that include cats with known infectious diseases. Positive immunoglobulin (Ig)G titers to *Toxoplasma gondii* are not an absolute contraindication to renal transplantation, and veterinarians should consult with the

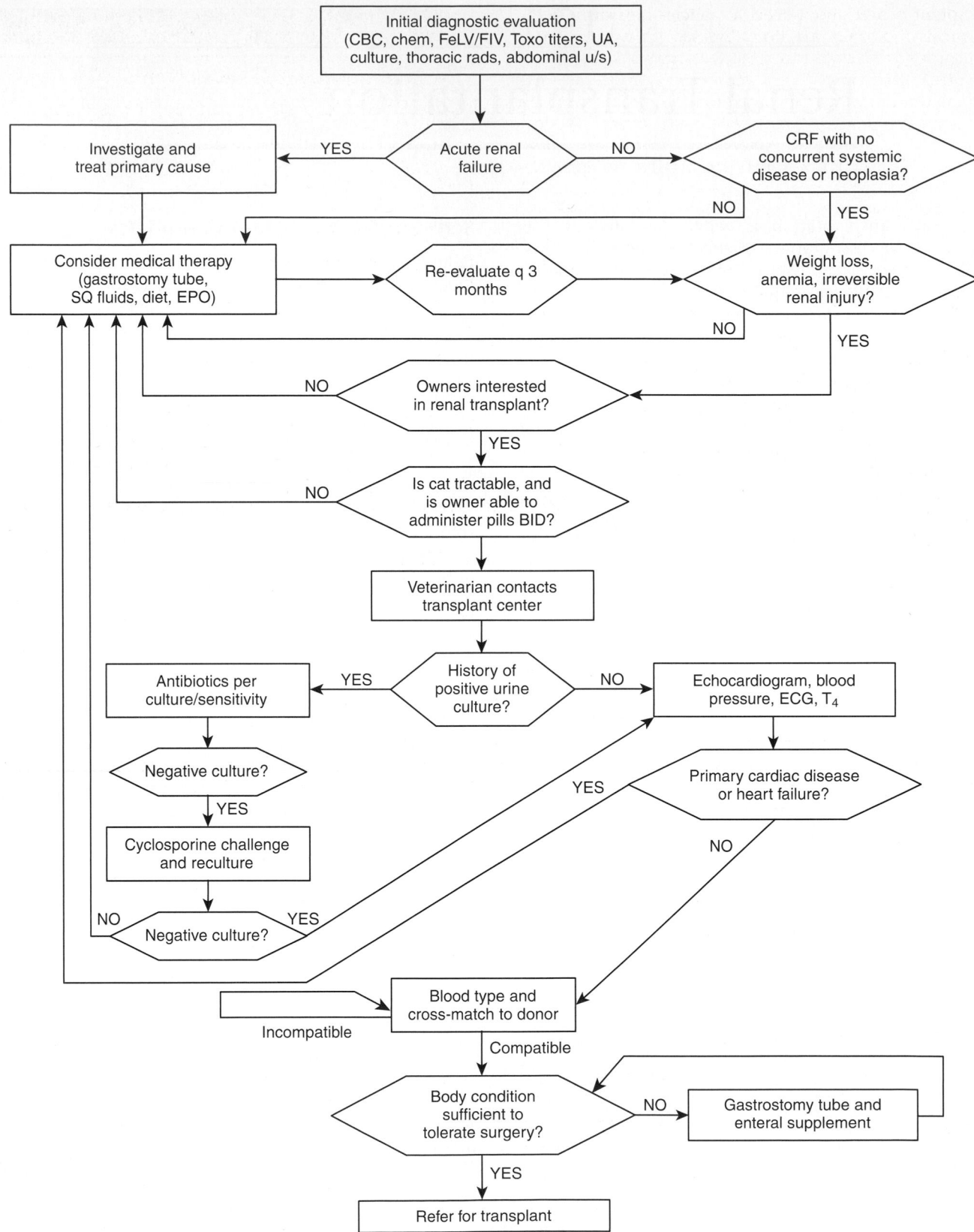

Fig. 195-1 Screening criteria for transplants.

transplant center about specific policies regarding toxoplasmosis and other infectious diseases. Transplant center clinicians are often able to provide assistance in maximizing medical therapy for end-stage renal disease, even if transplantation is not recommended. In some animals with more moderate degrees of azotemia (creatinine less than 6 mg/dl), aggressive therapy with gastrostomy tube placement, fluid therapy, dietary modification, and erythropoietin may provide survival times that parallel those following renal transplantation (see Chapter 190 and other chapters in this section).

Identification and Screening of Renal Transplant Donors

Using modern immunosuppressive protocols, feline kidney transplantation may be performed using unrelated donors with low risk of organ rejection. As a result, feline kidney donors may be obtained from a source of healthy cats that are in need of adoption such as a research colony or animal shelter. Screening of the donor involves standard hematologic analysis, serum biochemistry panel, urinalysis, and infectious disease screening (feline leukemia virus, feline immunodeficiency virus, and IgG/IgM titers for *Toxoplasma*). Imaging of the urinary tract is performed by intravenous pyelography or abdominal ultrasound to confirm the presence of two structurally normal kidneys. Prospective recipients are blood typed and then crossmatched to three or more donors. Tissue typing is not typically performed.

Allograft rejection is more difficult to prevent in dogs than in cats; the best successes are achieved when using related or tissue-matched donors. Aside from screening for general health and blood crossmatching as described previously, additional dog lymphocyte antigen (DLA) typing is recommended before selecting a canine kidney donor. Coordination of DLA typing can be completed by the transplant center before referral of canine transplant candidates.

Use of animal organ donors has stimulated an ethical debate in veterinary medicine that is similar to the one that surrounds live organ donation in humans. In retrospective studies of both veterinary and human transplant donors, the risks of perioperative complications or long-term morbidity associated with kidney donation are extremely small. Currently all veterinary transplant centers require that the owner of the organ recipient, regardless of outcome, adopt the kidney donor and provide lifelong care—a process that has provided excellent homes to over 400 cats in the United States over the last 20 years. Alternative sources of organs are extremely limited in veterinary medicine, and the resources required to form an organ-sharing network modeled on the human transplant system are not available. However, with improvements in cold organ preservation in dogs and cats, cadaveric organ donation may become available in the future.

Availability of Renal Transplantation

A number of veterinary transplant programs have been established across the country since the inception of clinical renal transplantation in the late 1980s, providing

---

Box **195-1**

Regional Transplant Centers and Informational Websites

North Carolina State University, College of Veterinary Medicine, Raleigh, NC.
http://www.cvm.ncsu.edu/docs/surgery_felinerenaltransplant unit.html
University of California, Davis, College of Veterinary Medicine, Davis, CA
http://www.vmth.ucdavis.edu/vmth/clientinfo/info/sasurg/ felrenaltransplant.html
University of Florida, College of Veterinary Medicine, Gainesville, FL
http://sacs.vetmed.ufl.edu/Sas/SurgeryWebpage/Renal.htm
University of Pennsylvania, College of Veterinary Medicine, Philadelphia, PA
http://www.vet.upenn.edu/departments/csp/surgery/programs/
University of Wisconsin, College of Veterinary Medicine, Madison, WI
http://www.vetmed.wisc.edu/dss/mcanulty/felinekidneytransplant/
The Animal Medical Center, New York, NY
http://www.amcny.org/department/kidneytransplantdefault. htm
Vet Surgery Central, Inc., Southfield, MI
http://www.vetsurgerycentral.com/transplant_vet.htm

---

services to clients in each major region of the United States (Box 195-1). Most centers maintain informative websites, with general information about renal transplantation, specific guidelines, and contact information for each institution. For most efficient communication of medical information, it is recommended that the referring veterinarian (not the client) make the initial contact with the referral center.

THE TRANSPLANT PROCEDURE

Surgical Procedure

In principle the current surgical technique for implantation of a renal allograft in the dog and cat is similar to that established by Gregory and Gourley in their original description of clinical renal transplantation (Gregory et al., 1987). Renal allograft transplantation involves implantation of the donor kidney into the caudal abdomen of the recipient. Blood supply to the kidney is established through surgical anastomoses of the donor artery and vein to the recipient vasculature; urine drainage is established by implantation of the ureter into the urinary bladder. With few exceptions the native kidneys are retained to provide a baseline level of renal function and fluid removal during periods of allograft dysfunction (a fact that is often surprising to pet owners). As with any complex procedure, technical experience obtained over the past 20 years has led to discovery of a number of species-specific surgical complications. Subsequently procedures have been modified in an attempt to minimize surgical morbidity and mortality.

Ureteral implantation is perhaps the most technically challenging aspect of renal transplantation in the cat, and the high incidence of ureteral obstruction in the immediate postoperative period is a major cause of delayed graft function. Originally intravesicular techniques were used, progressing from a simple "drop in" technique in which the ureter was pulled through a defect in the bladder wall and tacked to the interior of the bladder with a single transmural suture (Kochin et al., 1993) to direct apposition of the ureteral and bladder mucosal using interrupted sutures (Gregory et al., 1996). Unfortunately intravesicular techniques were associated with a high rate of granuloma formation and ureteral obstruction. More recently experimental studies have demonstrated that extravesicular implantation of the ureter into the bladder may decrease the incidence and severity of postoperative ureteral obstruction, as well as the duration and technical difficulty of the procedure (Mehl et al., 2005). Excision of the entire ureteral papilla from the donor cat also decreases the risk of ureteral obstruction during implantation (Hardie et al., 2005). Improvements in ureteral implantation techniques not only have benefited cats receiving renal transplants but are frequently applied in cats with upper urinary tract obstructions secondary to ureteral calculi or ureteral trauma.

Despite a number of innovations in methods for vascular anastomoses, most transplants are still performed by hand suturing of the vessels using microsurgical techniques. Surprisingly, vascular obstruction or primary failure of vascular anastomoses is not encountered frequently in veterinary transplantation, despite the small size of the patients and the technically demanding nature of vascular surgery. However, other complications have led to important modifications of the originally described surgical techniques over the past decade. For example, transplanted kidneys are quite mobile after implantation into the abdomen; and initial attempts to stabilize the kidney with interrupted sutures placed between the renal capsule and body wall were found to be inadequate, resulting in the tragic occurrence of postoperative renal pedicle torsion in a small number of animals. In both dogs and cats the implanted kidney is now stabilized using a *transversus abdominis* muscle flap, which is raised from the lateral aspect of the abdominal wall and sutured to the renal capsule, cradling the kidney in a sling of muscle. Unilateral hind limb ischemia is a similarly devastating but infrequent complication in feline renal transplant recipients secondary to use of the external iliac artery and common iliac vein as recipient vascular pedicles. Vascular anastomoses are now performed to the caudal abdominal aorta and vena cava in an end-to-side fashion, eliminating problems with hind limb ischemia (Bernsteen et al., 1999). As an added benefit, end-to-side anastomotic techniques circumvent problems associated with differences in size of donor and recipient vessels that cause difficulty when performing end-to-end anastomoses.

A final area of surgical technique modification has been the application of enteroplication in dogs receiving renal allograft transplantation. Interestingly, experimental and clinical experiences have shown that dogs have a high incidence of intussusception following renal allograft implantation. Accordingly, surgeons now recommend enteroplication as part of the transplant procedure (Kyles et al., 2003). Preoperative and intraoperative opioid administration is also believed to decrease the incidence of this complication in dogs and has been incorporated into the standard anesthetic regimen for canine renal transplantation. Postsurgical intussusception appears to be a species-specific problem, and enteroplication is not currently recommended in cats undergoing renal transplantation.

Organ Preservation

Recent experimental evidence and clinical data from human renal transplantation have indicated that early ischemic injury to the transplanted organ leads not only to delayed function of the graft but also causes an antigen-independent stimulation of the immune system and can lead to chronic rejection of the organ. This new recognition of the significance of ischemic injury has bolstered research into methods of graft preservation, even with the brief periods of organ storage that are encountered when using live donors in veterinary transplantation. Several preservation solutions are available for use in humans receiving organ transplants, but the cost and inconvenience of storing and using these solutions has limited their use in veterinary transplant centers. Fortunately a simple and inexpensive preservation solution has been introduced for use in feline renal transplantation, replacing the cold heparinized saline flush that was used for the past two decades in many transplant centers (McAnulty, 1998).

POSTTRANSPLANTATION ISSUES

Immunosuppression

The discovery of cyclosporine, a calcineurin inhibitor with specific anti–T cell activity, was arguably the crucial development that transformed renal transplantation from an interesting idea into the treatment of choice for humans with end-stage renal disease. The simple combination of cyclosporine with a corticosteroid, one of the original immunosuppressive protocols, has proven to provide long-term success in feline renal transplant recipients with few side effects. As a result, this protocol is still used as the primary method of therapy for cats receiving renal allografts. Pharmacokinetics of cyclosporine varies greatly in cats; therapeutic drug monitoring is required at frequent intervals for the remainder of the recipient cat's lifetime. Transplant recipients initially receive cyclosporine at a dosage of 4 to 5 mg/kg every 12 hours; subsequent doses are titrated to maintain 12-hour trough blood levels between 250 and 300 ng/ml. Various formulations of cyclosporine are available, and each form has different bioavailability. The microemulsified form of oral cyclosporine (Neoral, 100 mg/ml, Novartis) is currently recommended. To ensure complete dosing of this liquid and to avoid a negative association with the bad taste of oral cyclosporine, the drug is drawn up in a tuberculin syringe and injected into an empty gelatin capsule (size 000 or 0000). Prednisolone tablets may also be added to the capsule before administration to decrease the number of tablets or capsules administered. In patients that are resistant to oral medication, long-term maintenance of a low-profile gastrostomy tube can allow direct administration of liquid cyclosporine followed by 5 to 10 ml of water flush. High-profile lipid chromatography analysis continues to be the most accurate cyclosporine assay; clients must mail blood samples to specific centers that offer this method of analysis. Drug level monitoring is performed weekly in the initial postoperative period and is then continued at a minimum interval of 2 to 3 months in stable patients. At this time immunosuppressive drugs are continued for the life of the animal.

Recent studies in the area of transplant immunosuppression have not only led to novel agents for immunosuppression but have described novel combinations of existing immunosuppressive drugs. One important contribution has been the discovery that ketoconazole, an antifungal agent, may be used at subtherapeutic doses to decrease the amount of cyclosporine required in both dogs and cats (Dahlinger, Gregory, and Bea, 1998; McAnulty and Lensmeyer, 1999). Ketoconazole acts by inhibiting hepatic cytochrome P-450 enzymes involved in metabolism of cyclosporine and when given concurrently with cyclosporine the dose of cyclosporine can be reduced. When ketoconazole was given to dogs (5 to 14 mg/kg once a day), the total dose of cyclosporine could be decreased by 38% to 75%. Cats given ketoconazole (10 mg/kg/day) administration allowed conversion to a once-a-day regimen for cyclosporine (usually 4-5 mg/kg). The benefits of ketoconazole administration are numerous, with potential for increased compliance (once-a-day dosing of cyclosporine is possible), up to 58% decrease in cost of medications, decreased incidence of opportunistic fungal infections, and potential for decreased rejection rate in patients receiving combination therapy. Because of cytochrome P-450 inhibition, ketoconazole may cause hypoalbuminemia, weight loss, and hepatotoxicity in some animals; periodic monitoring of liver enzymes is indicated in patients receiving chronic combined cyclosporine and ketoconazole therapy.

In contrast to the situation in cats, it has proven extremely difficult to achieve a balanced, affordable immunosuppressive protocol that consistently results in long-term survival following renal transplantation in unrelated dogs. However, recent successes in both clinical and experimental canine transplantation would suggest that improvements might be on the horizon for dogs with end-stage renal disease. A group at the University of California, Davis, have reported their clinical experience in 15 dogs using three well-known immunosuppressive drugs (prednisolone, azathioprine, and cyclosporine) in a novel combined protocol (Gregory et al., 2006). Allograft rejection was prevented with this three-drug protocol, but the frequent occurrence of opportunistic infections in many recipients suggested an excessive level of immunosuppression. Perioperative thromboembolic events also led to several deaths early in the study, although addition of enoxaparin (a low–molecular weight heparin compound) prevented this complication in the last six dogs treated. Meanwhile, an experimental study performed at the University of Wisconsin, Madison, evaluated the efficacy of an exciting new pyrimidine antimetabolite

capecitabine (Xeloda, F. Hoffman, La Roche Ltd.), in dog lymphocyte antigen (DLA)–matched beagles (Schmiedt et al., 2006). Capecitabine used in combination with prednisolone and cyclosporine was highly effective in preventing allograft rejection. Another group at Auburn University has begun an aggressive attempt to induce immunologic tolerance (long-term allograft function without a requirement for immunosuppressive drugs) in the dog (Broaddus et al., 2006). In this protocol dogs are exposed to myeloablative (whole body) irradiation followed by concurrent donor bone marrow and renal allograft transplantation. Dogs were administered cyclosporine and mycophenolate-mofetil for 60 days after surgery; immunosuppressive drugs were then tapered and discontinued. DLA-mismatched dogs had long-term survival and allograft function even after drug withdrawal, although there was histologic evidence of allograft rejection in all samples at 228 to 580 days. Although success in canine renal transplantation continues to lag behind that achieved in cats, a number of novel approaches to manipulate the immune response to allograft tissues may provide a solution to this difficult problem in the near future.

Cost

The cost of renal transplantation varies at each institution, ranging from $5000 to $8000 for cats and from $7,000 to $12,000 for dogs. Extended postoperative care can double the overall cost in some animals that experience postoperative complications. In addition, clients should be warned of the recurring cost of lifelong immunosuppressive drugs and laboratory testing, with costs ranging from $100 to $200/month in cats and from $400 to $600/month or more in dogs.

Outcome

Reliable statistics on outcome of veterinary transplantation in cats are now becoming available as transplant centers report the results of renal transplantation in large numbers of animals. Published data suggest that approximately 80% of cats survive the perioperative period and are discharged from the hospital and approximately 60% survive the first 6 months after kidney transplantation (Adin et al., 2001). Interestingly, the majority of cats that survive the first 6 months go on to enjoy long-term survival, with 42% of cats remaining alive 3 years after surgery. Overall median survival in the largest reported case series was 22 months (Matthews and Gregory, 1997). At the time of renal transplantation, mean serum creatinine values were approximately 8 mg/dl, and medical options typically had been exhausted. These figures reflect an important message for clients of prospective transplant recipients—renal transplantation has the potential to markedly increase the quality and duration of life in cats with advanced renal failure, but recipients are not expected to have life spans comparable to that of a normal cat.

Prognosis for dogs after renal transplantation is much more difficult to gauge because of the small number of canine transplants that are performed and the variation in immunosuppressive regimens that are used at different institutions. In addition, survival of dogs in experimental studies of renal transplantation often exceeds that of dogs with naturally occurring renal disease that are treated with the same protocol. Current clinical reports suggest that only about 50% of dogs survive the first 2 months after kidney transplantation and that a high rate of opportunistic infections may occur in patients that survive long term (Gregory et al., 2006). As clinical experience increases and novel immunosuppressive protocols are developed, it is expected that survival and quality of life will improve for dogs much as it did for cats receiving renal transplants over the last 20 years.

References and Suggested Reading

Adin DB et al: Echocardiographic evaluation of cats with chronic renal failure (Abstract), *J Vet Intern Med* 14:337, 2000.

Adin CA et al: Diagnostic predictors of complications and survival after renal transplantation in cats, *Vet Surg* 30:5151, 2001.

Bernsteen L et al: Comparison of two surgical techniques for renal transplantation in cats, *Vet Surg* 28:417, 1999.

Broaddus KD et al: Renal allograft histopathology in dog leukocyte antigen mismatched dogs after renal transplantation, *Vet Surg* 35:125, 2006.

Dahlinger J, Gregory C, Bea J: Effect of ketoconazole on cyclosporine dose in healthy dogs, *Vet Surg* 27:64, 1998.

Gregory CR et al: Preliminary results of clinical renal allograft transplantation in the dog and cat, *J Vet Intern Med* 1:53, 1987.

Gregory CR et al: A mucosal apposition technique for ureteroneocystostomy after renal transplantation in cats, *Vet Surg* 25:13, 1996.

Gregory CR et al: Results of clinical renal transplantation in 15 dogs using triple drug immunosuppressive therapy, *Vet Surg* 35:105, 2006.

Hardie RJ et al: Ureteral papilla implantation as a technique for neoureterocystostomy in cats, *Vet Surg* 34:393, 2005.

Kochin EJ et al: Evaluation of a method of ureteroneocystostomy in cats, *J Am Vet Med Assoc* 202:257, 1993.

Kyles AE et al: Modified noble plication for the prevention of intestinal intussusception after renal transplantation in dogs, *J Invest Surg* 16:161, 2003.

McAnulty JF: Hypothermic storage of feline kidneys for transplantation: successful ex vivo storage up to 7 hours, *Vet Surg* 27:312, 1998.

McAnulty JF, Lensmeyer GL: The effects of ketoconazole on the pharmacokinetics of cyclosporine A in cats, *Vet Surg* 28:448, 1999.

Mehl ML et al: Comparison of 3 techniques for ureteroneocystostomy in cats, *Vet Surg* 34:114, 2005.

Schmiedt C et al: Use of capecitabine after renal allograft transplantation in dog erythrocyte antigen-matched dogs, *Vet Surg* 35:113, 2006.

CHAPTER **196**

Gastrostomy Tube Feeding in Kidney Disease

DENISE A. ELLIOTT, *St. Charles, Missouri*

Dietary therapy has remained the cornerstone of management of chronic kidney disease for decades. The goals of dietary modification are to meet the patient's nutrient and energy requirements; alleviate clinical signs and consequences of the uremic intoxication; minimize disturbances in fluid, electrolyte, vitamin, mineral, and acid-base balance; and slow progression of the renal failure. Recent clinical studies have clearly demonstrated the beneficial effects of dietary therapy in reducing uremic symptoms and slowing disease progression (Elliott et al., 2000; Jacob et al., 2002) (see Chapter 190). However, for the nutritional modifications to be effective at amelio-

rating the clinical signs of uremia, the pet must be prescribed and consume the appropriate diet. This task can clearly be challenging in the patient with renal disease.

Patients with chronic kidney disease are often anorectic and have reduced appetites. Adequate daily dietary intake is further hampered by uremic manifestations such as nausea, vomiting, and gastric ulcerations. In addition, an altered sense of taste and smell, reported in uremic people, may also affect dogs and cats. These factors combine to reduce caloric intake and refusal of the diet, a common problem reported by many owners. The subsequent protein-calorie malnutrition and wasting contribute to many aspects of uremia, including impaired immune function, increased susceptibility to infection, delayed wound healing, decreased strength and vigor, and increased morbidity and mortality. Indeed, protein-calorie malnutrition has been implicated as a key factor influencing outcome in humans with renal failure. Therefore prevention of malnutrition by ensuring adequate nutrient intake is considered crucial in the management of renal failure.

NUTRITIONAL ASSESSMENT IN CHRONIC KIDNEY DISEASE

Optimal initiation of nutritional support requires early assessment of patients to identify those either at risk of malnutrition or that already require nutritional support. Nutritional assessment includes evaluation of the history, physical examination, body weight (BW), body condition score (BCS), and laboratory data. The type, amount, and frequency of food intake and the incidence of vomiting should be noted. A food diary can be used to record daily intake. The daily caloric intake should be compared with the calculated daily caloric requirements. Manifestations of inadequate nutrient intake include loss of BW or BCS, hypoalbuminemia, and anemia. However, alterations of common laboratory indicators of malnutrition (albumin, blood urea nitrogen, cholesterol, erythrocyte mass, and lymphocyte counts) are often indistinguishable from those that can occur with chronic kidney disease and other concurrent disease processes. Other markers of nutritional status, including prealbumin, transferrin, and ceruloplasmin, have not been fully evaluated in feline and canine patients. Objective determination of alterations in fat mass or lean body mass using total body water, dual energy x-ray absorptiometry, and bioelectrical impedance analysis are more precise measures of body condition but are not widely available.

RATIONALE FOR GASTROSTOMY TUBE FEEDING

Practical measures to improve food intake include the use of highly odorous foods, warming food before feeding, and stimulating eating by positive reinforcement (such as petting and stroking behavior). Appetite stimulants such as benzodiazepines or serotonin antagonists may be administered judiciously; however, these methods are often ineffective in the uremic patient. Effective dietary management for patients in which daily caloric intake cannot be sustained with oral feeding can be accomplished with the aid of a gastrostomy tube. Gastrostomy tubes are ideal for long-term enteral access because they are associated with fewer upper airway complications and have a larger diameter than nasogastric and most esophagostomy tubes. Esophagostomy tubes are useful for short-term (days to weeks) dietary management in animals expected to recover from a transient insult or crisis (also see Chapter 136).

Gastrostomy tubes should be instituted for nutritional support on documentation of a 10% to 15% loss of BW in conjunction with a declining BCS and a history of poor dietary intake. Enteral feeding such as with a gastrostomy tube is indicated for patients with an intact, functional gastrointestinal system. Gastrostomy tubes are advantageous not only for supplying nutrients but also for easing the administration of fluid and medications, all of which can be delivered via the tube.

At first some owners are concerned not only about the appearance of the gastrostomy tube on their pet but about the time commitment and technical ability required for at home care of gastrostomy tubes. Therefore part of patient selection process necessitates detailed discussions and reassurance that the client can provide the appropriate resources to optimize the care of the patient.

GASTROSTOMY TUBE PLACEMENT

Equipment Requirements

Gastrostomy tubes are available in several sizes; 18 to 20 Fr are appropriate for cats or small dogs, and 24 Fr are adequate for larger dogs. Gastrostomy tubes generally are composed of latex or silicone. The selection of tube composition depends on the expected duration of use, biocompatibility, and cost. Latex tubes are less expensive but generally require replacement within 8 to 12 weeks because of tube wear and tear. Silicone tubes are softer and flexible and have a long life; however, they are generally more expensive than the other tubes. Silicone tubes typically survive 6 to 12 months and appear to be less irritating at the stoma site.

Various designs are available. The most common choice for initial placement is a latex Pezzer catheter (with a mushroom tip). Cost-effective preassembled kits are available commercially. Replacement tubes typically are Foley catheters (with a balloon at the tip). An array of feeding adapters can be attached to the gastrostomy tube; I prefer a Y-port device that has both catheter and Luer tip syringe ports (Bard Dual Port Feeding Adapter, Bard Access Systems, Inc.). Blended food can be delivered easily using the catheter port, and oral medications can be administered via the Luer port.

Low-profile gastrostomy tube devices (LPGDs) have been developed for use as both initial and replacement tubes. These devices are positioned flush with the body wall. Client and patient acceptance is much higher than with traditional tubes because the patient still appears "normal," without a long tube attached to the body or an obtrusive stockinette cover. Indeed, in one study LPGDs were the preferred replacement devices in 62% of dogs (Elliott, Riel, and Rogers, 2000). LPGDs are constructed of silicone, which improves tissue biocompatibility and appears to cause less stoma site inflammation. In addition, the mushroom tip has an antireflux valve design to prevent reflux of gastric contents. A feeding adapter is attached to the end of the device during the feeding procedure. LPGDs are expensive but have been documented to last at least 12 months. Thus the additional cost of the LPGD may be offset by the decreased frequency of replacement.

Tube Placement Procedure

Gastrostomy tubes can be placed using a surgical or percutaneous approach. Percutaneous placement is preferred since it requires a shorter period and lighter plane of anesthesia compared to surgical placement. There are two percutaneous techniques, one using an endoscope (percutaneous endoscopic gastrostomy (PEG) tubes) and one performed as a blind technique.

Gastrostomy tube placement is a 10- to 20-minute procedure requiring general anesthesia. Selection of anesthetic agent depends on the patient; however, special considerations are relevant in renal failure patients. Agents should be selected for their minimal effect on the cardiovascular and renal systems, lack of nephrotoxicity, and minimal requirement for renal excretion. A preanesthetic antimuscarinic (atropine) and sedative (oxymorphone or butorphanol), followed by an intravenous anesthetic induction agent (propofol-diazepam combination) and inhalation anesthesia (isoflurane) are appropriate choices. Intraanesthetic preservation of renal function may be supported by maintaining adequate intravascular volume with crystalloid fluids (e.g., lactated Ringer's solution) and supporting intravascular pressure. Low-dose dopamine (dogs) or mannitol (dogs and cats) infusion may be required to increase renal blood flow, glomerular filtration rate, and diuresis in individual cases.

The patient is placed in right lateral recumbency to allow the gastrostomy tube to be positioned on the left side along the greater curvature of the stomach. An area on the left of the patient, 1 to 2 cm caudal to the last rib and midway between the dorsal and ventral midline, is clipped and prepared with an antiseptic regimen. A mouth gag is placed to protect the endoscope from accidental damage. The endoscope is passed into the stomach, and the stomach is insufflated with air until it is distended. Gastric distention facilitates the positioning of the gastrostomy tube by pushing the stomach against the abdominal wall, displacing the spleen caudally and ventrally and moving the colon caudally. Monitoring oxygen saturation with a pulse oximeter or mechanical ventilatory assistance is important because gastric distention can cause ventilatory and circulatory compromise. An assistant wearing sterile gloves gently probes the area behind the last rib (about one third of the distance from the epaxial musculature to the ventral midline) with a finger while the endoscopist selects the appropriate location on the greater curvature of the stomach. Transillumination and palpation should ensure that the spleen is not present between the stomach and the abdominal wall. An 18-gauge, 1½-inch needle is inserted transabdominally into the gastric lumen. Sterile nylon suture (0–0) is passed through the hub of the needle and advanced into the gastric lumen. The suture is grasped using endoscopic retrieval forceps, and the endoscope and forceps with attached suture are slowly withdrawn out the mouth. A pair of hemostats placed on the other end of the suture material ensures that the abdominal end of the suture is not inadvertently pulled though the abdominal wall. The oral end of the suture is secured to the catheter tip of the gastrostomy tube, and the gastrostomy tube is lubricated to facilitate passage through the oral pharyngeal region. The needle is then removed from the abdominal wall, and the assistant pulls the suture with attached gastrostomy tube through the mouth and into the stomach using gentle traction. A small skin incision is necessary to aid the passage of the gastrostomy tube through the abdominal wall. The endoscope is replaced into the stomach, and the gastrostomy tube site is examined. The mushroom tip should sit comfortably on the gastric wall without "blanching" the gastric mucosa; however, close apposition of the gastric and abdominal walls should be maintained. If the tube is pulled too tight, it may cause pressure necrosis of the gastric wall with subsequent complications (intraperitoneal leakage of gastric contents, tube migration). The stomach should be deflated, and the position of the tube rechecked before exit of the endoscope. The position of the tube on the exterior abdominal wall is marked with a permanent marker to facilitate identification of tube migration. A phalange is placed on the exterior portion of the tube to aid immobilization, and the tube is sutured to the external body wall using butterfly wings. The external clamps and feed adaptor devices are attached to the tube. Antibiotic ointment is applied to the stoma site, and a stockinette and Elizabethan collar are placed on the patient to prevent tube dislodgement.

Dietary Selection and Gastrostomy Tube Management

Water is introduced through the tube 12 to 18 hours following initial placement, and feeding is scheduled to begin within 24 to 36 hours. Several commercial diets specifically formulated for the management of the renal patient are available. Human enteral products are inappropriate because of expense and nutritional inadequacy for dogs and cats (e.g., insufficient protein, taurine, arachidonic acid, arginine). On selection of the diet the daily energy and requirements should be calculated. Dogs should be fed $132 \times BW(kg)^{0.75}$, and cats require 60 kcal/kg/day. Caloric requirements can vary by 25%; thus actual caloric intake needs to be individualized based on serial BW and BCS. An estimation of daily caloric intake can be determined by reviewing the caloric intake that sustained ideal BW when the pet was healthy. The diet is blended with the least amount of water required to achieve syringability. The total volume of food is divided into four to six equal-sized meals, which should not exceed the gastric capacity of the patient (45 to 90 ml/kg). Generally one fourth to one third of the daily caloric intake is administered on the first day. If no complications occur, the amount fed is successively increased to reach total caloric requirements by the third or fourth day. With time and adaptation to the feeding procedure, the meal frequency may be reduced to a convenient BID-to-TID daily schedule. The patient's appetite may wax and wane; thus a meal can be offered orally and, if not consumed, can be blended and administered via the tube.

Before every meal, the gastric contents should be aspirated with a syringe. If more than 50% of the prior feeding is present, the contents should be returned to the stomach, and the feeding skipped until the next scheduled time. Frequent aspiration of the previous meal may suggest delayed gastric emptying and warrant medical management (e.g., metoclopramide 20 to 30 minutes before feeding).

Oral medications should be administered before feeding, with the exception of phosphate binders, which must be mixed directly with the food. The food should be warmed to room temperature and administered slowly over 5 to 15 minutes. Salivation and patient discomfort suggest nausea, which may be handled by slowing the rate of feeding. On completion the tube should be flushed with 5 to 10 ml of water.

The position of the tube on the body wall should be examined daily for migration; and the stoma site inspected for pain, redness, odor, and discharge. The site should be cleaned daily with an antiseptic solution, and antimicrobial ointment applied. Food residue should not be left near the stoma.

COMPLICATIONS OF GASTROSTOMY TUBE FEEDING

Complications of Tube Placement

Splenic laceration, gastric hemorrhage, pneumoperitoneum, displacement into the peritoneal cavity, and peritonitis have been reported as infrequent gastrostomy tube placement complications. The risk of splenic laceration can be reduced by adequate insufflation of the stomach and palpation to ensure that the spleen is not located between the stomach and the body wall. Postplacement intragastric bleeding, likely a complication of severe uremia and gastroenteritis, was the most frequent complication noted in one study of dogs with chronic kidney disease (Elliott, Riel, and Rogers, 2000). However, the bleeding did not cause any apparent clinical morbidity. Gastrostomy tube displacement into the abdominal cavity may be recognized by the development of fever and abdominal pain. Tube displacement is more likely if (1) the gastrostomy tube is secured too tightly, leading to pressure necrosis of the abdominal wall; (2) an internal flange is absent; (3) and the external flange is adjusted inappropriately.

Stoma Site Complications

Abnormalities at the stoma site may include discharge, pain, tissue swelling, erythema, abscess formation, and ulceration. Stoma site complications have been reported in 46% of dogs with chronic kidney disease (Elliott, Riel, and Rogers, 2000). This seemingly high incidence may be a consequence of impaired immune function, increased susceptibility to infection, and delayed wound healing associated with malnutrition and/or uremia. The high incidence of peristomal complications highlights the necessity of meticulous stoma site care. Abnormalities at the stoma site can be minimized by strict attention to cleaning of the stoma site with an antiseptic solution and application of an antibiotic ointment around the stoma site. In addition, the patient should be prohibited from licking the site through the permanent placement of a stockinette. Warm packs containing antiseptic solution placed on the stoma site may minimize problems or hasten recovery.

Patient Removal of the Tube

Inappropriate patient removal of the tube is undoubtedly the most problematic complication. In one study approximately 20% of dogs removed their gastrostomy tubes,

which emphasizes the importance of restraining the gastrostomy tube in a stockinette and using Elizabethan collars (Elliott et al., 2000). Patient removal of the gastrostomy tube is considered an emergency situation and indeed may lead to life-threatening intraperitoneal leakage of gastric contents if the stomach has not yet adhered to the body wall. In most situations a new tube can be placed through the existing stoma site using a guide catheter. On the other hand, if the tube has been in place for less than 7 days or there is evidence of peritonitis or radiographic contrast agent leakage, an exploratory laparotomy is required to correct the situation. Because of their short length and inaccessibility, the use of LPGDs may reduce the incidence of inadvertent gastrostomy tube removal.

Complications during the feeding process, including salivation, gulping, retching, and vomiting, can be minimized by reducing either the total volume at each feeding (increasing the frequency of feeding to maintain caloric intake) or the rate of administration. Simultaneous management of fluid, electrolyte, and acid-base disturbances contributing to uremic gastritis may reduce the incidence of vomiting.

Periodically gastroscopy tubes become blocked with food. Techniques to facilitate removal of the obstruction include massaging the outside of the tube while simultaneously flushing and aspirating with water; instilling carbonated drinks, meat tenderizers, or pancreatic enzyme solutions (allow to soak within tube for 15 to 20 minutes); or gently using a polyurethane catheter to dislodge the obstruction. The final resort for a blocked tube is tube removal and replacement.

REPLACEMENT OF GASTROSTOMY TUBES

Reasons to replace the initial gastrostomy tube include inappropriate patient removal, the convenience of the LPGD, tube malfunction, blockage, or tube wear and tear. If the original gastrostomy tube has been in place for more than 7 to 10 days, adhesion of the stomach to the body wall should have occurred. In this situation the original gastrostomy tube can be removed by placing firm traction on the outside of the tube. The method of replacement depends on the type of replacement tube. For LPGD devices an obturator is inserted down the center of the LPGD and used to stretch the end of the device to form a transient linear structure, which then is inserted into the stoma. Once placed in the stomach, the obturator is removed.

For replacement with a traditional balloon-type gastrostomy tube, a polyurethane catheter is inserted through the stoma. The polyurethane catheter is used as a guide, and the replacement gastrostomy tube is threaded over this guide into the stomach. Once in place, the balloon is insufflated, and the polyurethane catheter removed. Regardless of the replacement technique used, appropriate replacement of the tube within the gastric lumen should be verified radiographically using survey radiographs or after iodinated contrast media is injected through the new tube.

Exploratory laparotomy is necessary for replacement if the gastrostomy tube has been removed before gastric-abdominal adhesion formation, if the tube tip is displaced into the abdominal cavity, or if the sealed stoma is perforated inadvertently during percutaneous replacement.

MONITORING AND OUTCOME

Gastrostomy tubes have been used to provide nutritional support in dogs with chronic kidney disease for as long as 438 days. Elliott, Riel, and Rogers (2000) reported that BW increased in 22% of dogs with chronic kidney disease following gastrostomy tube placement. Declining BW was stabilized in a further 31% of dogs. However, 30% of dogs continued to lose BW despite gastrostomy tube placement. These results highlight the necessity for repeated nutritional assessment and aggressive alterations in dietary intake to ensure stabilization or gain of BW rather than continued loss of BW. In addition to low caloric intake, BW changes in uremic patients may be influenced by metabolic acidosis and chronic inflammation; both stimulate protein catabolism and loss of lean body mass. Thus every effort must be made be control metabolic acidosis and aggressively manage coexisting catabolic illnesses.

References and Suggested Reading

Armstrong PJ, Hardie EM: Percutaneous endoscopic gastrostomy: a retrospective study of 54 clinical cases in dogs and cats, *J Vet Intern Med* 4:202, 1990.

Bright RM, Burrows CF: Percutaneous endoscopic tube gastrostomy in dogs, *Am J Vet Res* 49:629, 1988.

Bright RM, DeNovo RC, Jones JB: Use of a low-profile gastrostomy device for administering nutrients in two dogs, *J Am Vet Med Assoc* 207:1184, 1995.

DeBowes LJ, Coyne B, Layton CE: Comparison of French-pezzer and Malecot catheters for percutaneously placed gastrostomy tubes in cats, *J Am Vet Med Assoc* 202:1963, 1993.

Elliott DA, Riel DL, Rogers QR: Complications and outcomes of gastrostomy tubes used for the nutritional management of renal failure in dogs: 56 cases (1994-1999), *J Am Vet Med Assoc* 217(9):1337, 2000.

Elliott J et al: Survival of cats with naturally occurring chronic renal failure: effect of dietary management, *J Small Anim Pract* 41:235, 2000.

Fulton RB, Dennis JB: Blind percutaneous placement of a gastrostomy tube for nutritional support in dogs and cats, *J Am Vet Med Assoc* 201:697, 1992.

Jacob F et al. Clinical evaluation of dietary modification for treatment of spontaneous chronic renal failure in dogs, *J Am Vet Med Assoc* 220:1163, 2002.

Ireland LM et al: A comparison of owner management and complications in 67 cats with esophagostomy and percutaneous endoscopic gastrostomy feeding tubes, *J Am Anim Hosp Assoc* 39(3):241, 2003.

Marks SL: The principles and practical application of enteral nutrition, *Vet Clin North Am* 28:677, 1998.

CHAPTER **197**

Systemic Hypertension in Renal Disease

MARK J. ACIERNO, *Baton Rouge, Louisiana*

Hypertension is a common sequela to kidney disease and is thought to affect as many as 19.4% of feline and 61% of canine renal failure patients. Normal blood pressure is the result of complex interactions among the heart, kidney, endothelial signaling mechanisms, and the autonomic nervous system (Fig. 197-1). These factors establish systemic vascular resistance and cardiac output, which are the final determinants of blood pressure. Although the association between renal failure and hypertension has been studied extensively in humans and in animal models, the exact cause of the blood pressure elevation is not known.

DEFINITION AND SIGNIFICANCE OF HYPERTENSION

In recent years clinicians and investigators have achieved a better understanding of blood pressure measurements expected in healthy dogs and cats. As a result, the definition of hypertension has been refined. It is now believed that blood pressure measurements greater than 150/95 mm Hg on three separate visits in a patient that demonstrates no clinical signs directly attributable to the blood pressure elevation is compatible with systemic hypertension, as is a single reading of greater than 150/95 mm Hg in a symptomatic patient (see also Chapter 159).

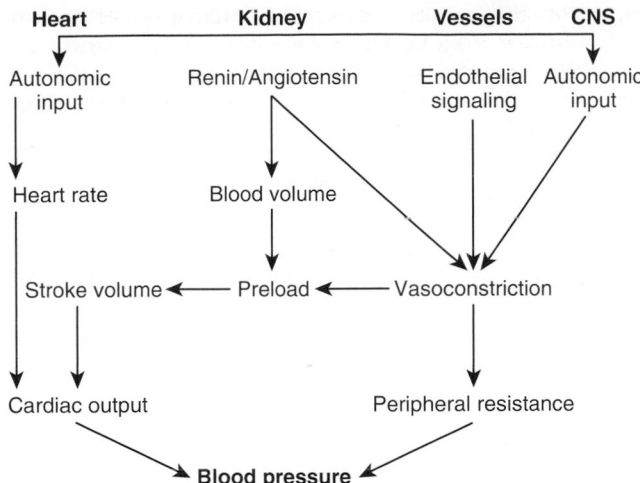

Fig. 197-1 The complex relationship between the heart, kidneys, endothelial signaling, and autonomic nervous system and how they establish blood pressure.

Although patients with mild increases in blood pressure fail to demonstrate clinical signs directly attributable to their hypertension, more dramatic pressure increases can lead to significant renal, ocular, cardiac, or central nervous system injuries. Renal disease is a recognized cause of hypertension, however, persistent blood pressure elevations from any cause can contribute to glomerular and tubular damage. Hypertensive retinopathy and choroidopathy, manifested as retinal edema, tortuous vessels, hemorrhage, and retinal detachment, are common manifestations of hypertension. Cats with chronic kidney disease are often brought to the veterinarian for blindness rather than clinical signs directly attributable to kidney disease. In some cases hypertension may precede overt azotemia in cats with early chronic kidney disease. A cardiac murmur, arrhythmia, and gallop rhythm can develop as increased systemic blood pressure leads to cardiac muscle hypertrophy. Hypertensive encephalopathy manifested as head tilt, ataxia, depression, or seizures may develop as blood pressure overwhelms the cerebral vasculature autoregulatory mechanisms.

PRESSURE MEASUREMENT TECHNIQUES

Hypertension secondary to renal disease is common and is associated with significant morbidity and mortality; therefore blood pressure should be measured periodically in affected animals. Direct measurement of patient blood pressure requires the catheterization of a suitable artery and the determination of systolic and diastolic pressure by an electronic transducer. Although this is considered to be the gold standard of blood pressure measurement, it is neither convenient nor practical in the clinical setting. Rather veterinarians rely on Doppler and oscillometric techniques as noninvasive, indirect measures of patient blood pressure.

Because of its low cost, ease of use, and suitability for use in all companion animals, the Doppler flow detector is a common method for measuring blood pressure.

The only equipment needed other than the detector is a sphygmomanometer and a selection of cuffs in different sizes. Doppler flow detectors work by emitting ultrasound waves and then "listening" for the waves to be reflected back. If there is movement such as blood cells racing through an artery, the frequency of the returned wave is shifted (the Doppler effect). This change in frequency is amplified by the detector and heard by the user as a characteristic "swoosh" sound.

When using the Doppler flow detector, blood pressure is measured by snugly placing a cuff on the proximal portion of any extremity. Ultrasound gel is placed on the Doppler probe, and the probe is then gently placed over any artery distal to the cuff. To improve conduction, the hair over the artery is usually clipped. The cuff is then inflated 20 to 30 mm Hg past the pressure at which blood flow can no longer be heard. Then the cuff is gradually deflated while the operator observes the pressure displayed by the sphygmomanometer. The point at which blood flow can be first heard is the systolic pressure. Often a second sound, which represents the diastolic pressure, can be heard as deflation of the cuff continues. The Doppler flow detector has been validated for use on all cats and dogs, although the limits of agreement between direct and indirect measurements may be somewhat wide. Systolic blood pressure measurement is easily obtained, but determining diastolic pressure is technically challenging.

Oscillometric units are also quite popular because they are automated and can determine systolic pressure, diastolic pressure, mean arterial pressure, and heart rate. These devices work by inflating a cuff around an extremity until arterial blood flow is stopped and then, while slowly decreasing the pressure of the cuff, they monitor for the return of arterial pulsations and arterial vibrations. Despite their convenience, these units can underestimate blood pressure significantly when used on cats and small dogs and is not recommended in these patients.

Regardless of which pressure-measuring technique is used, there are four principles that help to ensure accurate blood pressure measurement: proper cuff size, consistency of personnel and technique, reproducibility of results, and acclamation of the patient. Perhaps the most important factor in attaining accurate blood pressure measurement is the selection of a proper cuff. The width of the cuff should be 30% to 40% of the circumference of the extremity. A cuff that is too wide underestimates blood pressure, whereas an undersized cuff leads to artificially elevated values. A tape measure can be helpful in measuring the circumference of the limb and selecting an appropriate cuff width.

Consistency of technique and personnel is essential to ensure accurate blood pressure measurement. Whenever possible, the same team should be involved in the blood pressure measurement process, and they should use the same technique each time blood pressure is measured. This allows for mastery of blood pressure–taking techniques and development of a consistent methodology.

Blood pressure measurements should be repeated at least three and preferably five times. If there is significant variation between measurements (10%), the entire series should be disregarded and repeated until reproducible results are obtained. A diagnosis of hypertension in an asymptomatic patient should be confirmed by repeating the blood pressure measurements on two additional office visits.

The stress created by a visit to a veterinary office, known as the *white coat effect*, can cause a profound increase in patient blood pressure. To minimize its impact, blood pressure should always be measured in a quiet area away from other animals and before other procedures are performed. The patient should be allowed to acclimate to its surroundings, and whenever possible the owner should be present. Restraint should be kept to a minimum. Blood pressure measurement should not be attempted in obviously agitated animals.

TREATMENT OF HYPERTENSION

Angiotensin-converting enzyme (ACE) inhibitors are generally considered to be the initial drug of choice in treating canine hypertension (Table 197-1). ACE inhibitors exert their effect by blocking the conversion of angiotensin I to angiotensin II and can lower blood pressure in three ways. First, angiotensin II is a powerful vasoconstrictor; systemic vasodilation occurs when its synthesis is inhibited. Second, angiotensin II directly promotes sodium absorption in the proximal tubule of the kidney leading to intravascular volume expansion. Last, angiotensin II stimulates the release of aldosterone, which also promotes renal sodium and water resorption. Renal insufficiency patients should have their serum chemistry values checked after starting treatment since ACE inhibitors may have the potential to worsen azotemia. As with all antihypertensive medication, ACE inhibitors should be started at the lowest possible dose and increased as needed.

Enalapril is eliminated entirely through renal excretion, whereas both the renal and hepatic mechanisms are involved in the clearance of benazepril. The half-life of enalapril is prolonged in renal failure patients, but the clearance of benazepril appears to be unchanged. This may be because of up-regulated hepatic excretion of benazepril into the bile when renal clearance is compromised. For this reason benazepril may be preferable to enalapril in the treatment of hypertension in renal failure patients. In my experience benazepril is also less likely to cause gastrointestinal upset; however, there are no well controlled studies in clinical patients comparing efficacy or adverse effects in dogs or cats with spontaneous hypertension. Furthermore, in dogs with severe hypertension and critical target organ injury to the retina or brain, monotherapy with an ACE inhibitor is unlikely to reduce blood pressure sufficiently. In those patients, other treatments are generally required (see below).

ACE inhibitors are less effective in treating hypertension in cats. Studies have shown that as many as 50% of hypertensive cats fail to respond to enalapril. Another study using benazepril demonstrated that, although cats did have a statistically significant decrease in blood pressure, the actual response may be too small to make benazepril useful as a monotherapy agent (Brown, 2001). Therefore dihydropyridine calcium channel blockers are generally considered to be the drug of choice in controlling feline hypertension. Calcium channel blockers exert their effects by blocking the influx of calcium needed to cause smooth muscle contraction and thereby act to decrease systemic vascular resistance. Amlodipine besylate (see Table 197-1) is perhaps the most widely used drug for controlling hypertension in cats. Amlodipine is long acting, gradual in effect, and allows for once-a-day dosing. In humans and dogs calcium channel blocker administration can worsen renal disease despite a significant blood pressure decrease. One possible explanation for this paradoxic effect is that calcium channel blockers preferentially dilate the afferent arteriole of the glomerulus, resulting in glomerular hypertension. Therefore these drugs should not be used as a monotherapy antihypertensive agent in dogs with renal disease. For reasons that are not clear, calcium channel blockers do not appear to have the same effect in cats. Studies have shown that feline patients treated with amlodipine live longer and have fewer hypertensive compilations. Therefore calcium channel blockers are considered safe for monotherapy use in cats.

β-Blockers are useful adjunctive therapy in dogs or cats when the initial antihypertensive agent has failed to achieve the desired pressure reduction. β-Adrenergic receptors are found in both the heart (β-1) and lungs (β-2). Blockade of the β-1 receptors slows the heart and lowers blood pressure, but blockade of the β-2 receptors can trigger bronchial constriction and respiratory distress. Therefore a β-1 selective antagonist such as atenolol (see Table 197-1) is preferred for the management of

Table 197-1

Commonly Used Antihypertensive Medications and their Dosages

Drug	Class	Canine Dose	Feline Dose
Enalapril (Enacard, Merck)	ACE inhibitor	0.5-1 mg/kg q12-24h PO	0.25-0.5 mg/kg q12-24h PO
Benazepril (Lotensin, Novartis)	ACE inhibitor	0.25-0.5 mg/kg q12-24h PO	0.25-0.5 mg/kg q12-24h PO
Amlodipine (Norvasc, Pfizer)	Ca^{++} channel blocker	0.05-0.2 mg/kg q24h PO*	0.625-1.25 mg/cat q24h PO
Atenolol (Tenormin, AstraZeneca)	β-Blocker	0.25-1 mg/kg q12-24h PO	6.25-12.5 mg/cat q12-24h PO
Metoprolol (Lopressor, Novartis)	β-Blocker	0.5-1.0 mg/kg q 8-12h PO	2-15 mg/cat q8h PO
Prazosin (Minipress, Pfizer)	α-Blocker	0.5-2 mg/dog q12h	Not recommended
Spironolactone (Aldactone, Searle Pharmaceuticals)	Aldosterone inhibitors	1-2 mg/kg q12h, PO	1 mg/kg q12h PO

*Higher dosages up to 0.4 to 0.5 mg/kg have been required in refractory patients

hypertension. Atenolol is water soluble and is eliminated by the kidney. The impact of this elimination in patients with azotemia has not assessed clinically. Atenolol also can be used as cotherapy with amlodipine in the treatment of hypertension associated with hyperthyroidism. However, monotherapy with atenolol is generally ineffective in management of significant hypertension in these cats.

α-Blockers selectively antagonize vascular α-receptors, resulting in vasodilation and decreased blood pressure. Prazosin, a potent α-adrenergic inhibitor, has been used successfully as a primary and adjunctive treatment for hypertension in the dog. Its effectiveness as an antihypertensive agent in cats has not been investigated fully; therefore its use is not recommended except in the most refractory cases.

Recent studies have shown that drugs that antagonize aldosterone may protect the heart, brain, and kidneys from the deleterious effects of hypertension. Although inhibition of aldosterone results in small decreases in blood pressure, the real benefit may be a decrease in hypertension-induced fibrosis of target organs. Therefore hypertensive patients may benefit from the use of spironolactone as an adjunctive treatment (see Table 197-1). Since spironolactone decreases sodium resorption and potassium excretion, it is possible that electrolyte abnormalities could occur when using this drug. Although these abnormalities are unlikely at the dosage recommended, special attention should be paid to electrolytes when rechecking serum chemistries. Additionally, some cats develop skin lesions while receiving spironolactone, and clients should be so-warned.

THERAPEUTIC GOALS AND MONITORING

The goal of treating hypertensive patients is to gradually lower systolic pressure to less than 170 mm Hg; blood pressure may not completely normalize. In the initial stages of treatment it is important to monitor the patient regularly and avoid making rapid adjustments in medication. Therapeutic changes can be made at 1- to 2-week intervals unless the patient's condition deteriorates and more immediate modifications are needed. When increasing the dose of the primary antihypertensive medication fails to produce the desired decrease in blood pressure, a secondary antihypertensive in a different drug class should be started. Once systolic pressure has stabilized at acceptable measurements, the patient should be rechecked every 3 months, with complete blood count and serum chemistry results reevaluated at least twice a year (see Chapter 192).

References and Suggested Reading

Acierno MJ, Labato MA: Hypertension in renal disease: diagnosis and treatment, *Clin Tech Small Anim Pract* 20:23, 2005.

Belew AM, Barlett T, Brown SA: Evaluation of the white-coat effect in cats, *J Vet Intern Med* 13:134, 1999.

Binns SH et al: Doppler ultrasongraphic, oscillometric sphygmomanometric, and photoplethysmographic techniques for noninvasive blood pressure measurement in anesthetized cats, *J Vet Intern Med* 9:405, 1995.

Brown SA et al: Effects of the angiotensin converting enzyme inhibitor benazepril in cats with induced renal insufficiency, *Am J Vet Res* 62:375, 2001.

Epstein M: Aldosterone as a mediator of progressive renal disease: pathology and clinical implications, *Am J Kidney Dis* 37:677, 2001.

Hostetter TH, Ibrahim HN: Aldosterone in chronic kidney and cardiac disease, *J Am Soc Nephrol* 14:2395, 2003.

Stepien RL et al: Comparative diagnostic test characteristics of oscillometric and doppler ultrasound methods in the detection of systolic hypertension in dogs, *J Vet Intern Med* 17:65, 2003.

Syme HM et al: Prevalence of systolic hypertension in cats with chronic renal failure at initial evaluation, *J Am Vet Assoc* 220:1799, 2002.

Mathur S et al: Effects of the calcium channel antagonist amlodipine in cats with surgically induced hypertensive renal insufficiency, *Am J Vet Res* 63:833, 2002.

CHAPTER 198

Treatment of Anemia in Renal Failure

MARIE E. KERL, *Columbia, Missouri*
CATHERINE E. LANGSTON, *New York, New York*

Renal failure is a common disease presentation for both dogs and cats. Although patients with either acute renal failure or chronic kidney disease can become anemic, anemia occurs more commonly in patients with chronic kidney disease. Moderate-to-severe anemia is a serious complication of chronic kidney disease. Formulating the differential diagnosis for anemia and accurately identifying the cause or causes provides the clinician with the best means to administer appropriate and timely treatment. This article reviews the common causes of anemia associated with renal failure, suggests diagnostic plans, and outlines currently available treatment options.

ETIOLOGY OF ANEMIA

The basic mechanisms of anemia include blood loss, red blood cell (RBC) destructive processes, and failure of bone marrow production. In some animals with renal failure, more than one etiology contributes to anemia. All possible mechanisms should be considered in each anemic patient regardless of renal disease status to avoid "tunnel vision." The basis for anemia of renal failure in the majority of dogs and cats is blood loss or lack of RBC production.

Blood-Loss Anemia

Blood loss can occur for a variety of reasons in the animal with renal failure. Iatrogenic blood-loss anemia from frequent blood sampling for diagnostic testing is the first consideration for hospitalized animals. The blood volume for diagnostic testing of cats or small-breed dogs should be minimized to limit iatrogenic loss. Other possible sources of blood loss include gastrointestinal bleeding, ectoparasitism or endoparasitism, and uremia-induced defects in platelet function. Animals receiving hemodialysis have mild ongoing RBC loss in the dialysis circuit. Typically blood loss should initiate a regenerative response from the bone marrow; however, animals with chronic kidney disease cannot mount an appropriate regenerative response because of relative erythropoietin (EPO) deficiency. In addition, iron deficiency occurs with prolonged blood loss, which attenuates a regenerative response.

Uremic Gastropathy

Gastric ulceration and necrosis are common findings in humans with chronic kidney disease. Gastric histopathology findings in dogs with renal failure include gastric edema, vasculopathy, glandular atrophy, mineralization, and submucosal arteritis, with ulceration or necrosis being relatively uncommon findings (Peters et al., 2005). However, clinical experience with animals in renal failure indicates that significant gastrointestinal bleeding occurs in certain patients. Gastrin, a polypeptide hormone produced in the G cells in the stomach, is renally excreted; and cats with chronic kidney disease have increased gastrin levels, although the relationship between creatinine and serum gastrin levels is not linear (Goldstein et al., 1998). Persistent increases in serum gastrin can result in gastric hyperacidity and mucosal erosions. Additional factors that can contribute to gastrointestinal bleeding include concurrent use of nonsteroidal antiinflammatory medications or corticosteroids. Although ongoing blood loss from uremic enterocolitis might contribute to anemia, it would be unlikely for this disorder to represent the sole cause of anemia. Animals with acute renal failure can experience gastrointestinal signs similar to patients affected by chronic kidney disease; however, the relatively short duration of pathologic changes with acute renal failure make blood-loss anemia from gastrointestinal sources a less frequent occurrence.

Clinical signs of upper gastrointestinal bleeding include hematemesis, melena, or hematochezia. Melena is not always seen in animals with chronic gastrointestinal blood loss since loss can occur in relatively small quantities over time. Uremic enterocolitis causes marked large bowel diarrhea with frank blood. Other indicators of blood loss include an elevated blood urea nitrogen (BUN)/creatinine ratio and microcytic, hypochromic anemia when chronic loss has been sufficient to result in iron deficiency.

Increased Bleeding Tendency

The chief hemostatic change that occurs with uremia is impaired platelet function. Total platelet count in animals with renal failure is usually within or slightly below reference range unless the underlying etiology of the renal failure also results in thrombocytopenia (e.g., leptospirosis). Platelet counts typically have to be severely reduced ($< 30,000$ to $40,000/\mu l$) for clinical bleeding to result from thrombocytopenia alone. Prolonged skin bleeding times have been described in humans with renal failure, and prolonged buccal mucosal bleeding time has been reported in dogs with renal failure. Proposed mechanisms for platelet dysfunction in dogs include defective platelet cyclooxygenase causing reduced thromboxane

A2 production, abnormal concentration of large multimers of von Willebrand factor, abnormal intracellular cyclic adenosine monophosphate concentration, and abnormal intracellular calcium mobilization. These changes cause impaired subendothelial adhesion of platelets and abnormal platelet aggregation. Total von Willebrand factor has been found to be normal in dogs with renal failure.

Red Cell Destruction

The uremic environment decreases RBC survival in some humans, but dogs with renal failure had no evidence of increased RBC fragility. Parathyroid hormone has been proposed as a cause of hemolysis, but the evidence is inconclusive.

Decreased Erythropoiesis

Erythropoietin deficiency. EPO is the hematopoietic growth factor that stimulates erythrogenesis in anemia, and deficiency is the most commonly recognized contributor to anemia of chronic kidney disease. Most EPO is produced in the peritubular interstitial cells of the outer medulla and inner cortex of the kidney; however, between 10% and 15% of total EPO is produced by the liver. Renal hypoxemia caused either by anemia or hypoxia is the main trigger for EPO production, and the main effect of EPO is to stimulate RBC growth and differentiation is on the colony-forming unit–erythroid cells of the bone marrow. Following an increase of EPO production, a time period of approximately 5 days is required for the release of erythrocytes into the circulation. Additional effects of EPO to benefit the anemic patient includes induction of hemoglobin and RBC membrane protein synthesis and facilitation of RBC release from the bone marrow to the bloodstream. With chronic kidney disease and reduced renal mass, renal EPO production is attenuated, which causes relative EPO deficiency. In anemic dogs with chronic kidney disease, measured EPO can be above normal but not as elevated as in dogs with similarly severe anemia that are not uremic. Cats with chronic kidney disease have EPO levels that are similar to those of normal cats.

Other factors contributing to decreased erythropoiesis. Humans with chronic kidney disease and poor nutritional status can develop deficiencies of certain vitamins, especially B vitamins. These vitamins, particularly B_{12} (cobalamin), folic acid, niacin, B_2 (riboflavin), and B_6 (pyridoxine), are all important in erythropoiesis. Although deficiencies have been documented in humans with chronic kidney disease, evaluation of B-vitamin concentrations has not been reported in dogs or cats with chronic kidney disease. Protein-calorie malnutrition can contribute to nonregenerative anemia.

A variety of possible uremic toxins have been identified in humans, and some of these toxins may contribute to poor regenerative response of the bone marrow. The hematologic effects of these substances have not been investigated in dogs and cats.

Iron deficiency can be caused by chronic blood loss and poor iron intake in renal failure. Iron deficiency anemia must be differentiated from anemia of chronic inflammatory disease, which also causes a nonregenerative anemia.

The distinction between these etiologies is important relative to therapy; iron deficiency anemia would be expected to respond to supplemental iron therapy, but anemia of chronic inflammatory disease persists with iron therapy, and iron overdose can result.

DIAGNOSIS

When determining a cause for anemia in the animal with renal failure, specific historical questions to consider include evidence of listlessness, exercise intolerance, hematemesis, melena, hematochezia, and/or recent hospitalization with frequent blood sampling. In addition, reports of a sudden decline in attitude or activity might increase suspicion of acute blood loss either externally or internally. Physical examination can reveal pallor consistent with either anemia or hypovolemia. Examination findings that occur with clinically significant anemia include lethargy, poor responsiveness, tachypnea, tachycardia, weakness, and deviations from normal pulse quality (e.g., bounding or weakly palpable pulses). If a rapid clinical decline was noted historically, hemorrhage into a body cavity may be considered, or melena may be identified by digital rectal examination. Identification of mucosal blood loss, most commonly seen as gingival bleeding, would be consistent with uremic platelet function defect. Profound anemia can result in retinal hemorrhages, although this is seen uncommonly with the anemia of chronic kidney disease.

Complete blood count in the anemic renal failure patient should reveal normocytic, normochromic, nonregenerative anemia. This finding is consistent with the relative EPO deficiency of chronic kidney disease; however, it is also consistent with anemia of chronic inflammatory disease and iron sequestration. White blood cell count, differential, and platelet count are not affected. Any abnormalities in these cell lines should be evaluated as separate problems. A regenerative response (i.e., reticulocytosis, polychromasia, macrocytosis) is not a feature of anemia of chronic kidney disease caused by relative EPO deficiency. These findings are strongly suggestive of blood loss or hemolysis of longer than 5 days' duration. Microcytosis and hypochromasia should be seen in animals with chronic iron deficiency. RBC deformities (echinocytes, burr cells) can occur in uremic patients.

Additional tests may be needed to determine the cause of anemia. If clinical evidence of mucosal bleeding was evident on examination and platelet count was within reference ranges, buccal mucosal bleeding time should be considered to diagnose underlying platelet function defect. Specific testing can be performed to distinguish iron deficiency anemia from anemia of chronic inflammatory disease; however, results are not always straightforward. An iron panel consisting of serum iron (a mobile form of iron), total iron-binding capacity (an indirect measurement of transferrin, the serum carrier molecule for iron), and ferritin (a storage form of iron) can be performed. With iron deficiency anemia, all results would be expected to be low. With anemia of chronic inflammatory disease, serum iron is low, and transferrin is normal to low because of sequestration of iron; however, ferritin levels should be normal or increased. Bone marrow core biopsy samples can also be evaluated for presence of iron stores in the form of hemosiderin. Evidence of decreased iron stores in the bone marrow would be consistent with true iron deficiency; however, this is a more invasive testing modality, and the core biopsy instrument may not be readily available in general practice. If anemia of chronic inflammatory disease is suspected, appropriate testing to identify the inflammatory disease (e.g., imaging studies, serologic testing) should be performed. Thoracocentesis or abdominocentesis are indicated with historical evidence of acute blood loss and suggestive physical examination findings.

Although EPO deficiency is the most likely explanation for nonregenerative anemia with chronic kidney disease, EPO levels are not typically measured in the clinical setting because of expense and delay in receiving results, and a normal EPO level does not rule out relative EPO deficiency. When all other causes of anemia are ruled out, therapeutic response to EPO is the usual means to identify EPO deficiency.

TREATMENT

Minimize Blood Loss

The mainstays of treatment of anemia associated with chronic kidney disease include minimizing ongoing blood loss and increasing RBC number and production. Hospitalized patients should have blood sampling frequency and volume minimized to what is clinically necessary. For patients less than 4.5 kg (10 lbs), pediatric blood sampling tubes containing anticoagulant appropriate for less than 1 ml of blood can be used to perform most biochemical tests. The clinician should determine if daily monitoring of biochemical values is necessary for treatment decisions; in many cases every-other-day testing of BUN and creatinine is sufficient.

Treatment for endoparasitism or ectoparasitism should be performed if indicated. Gastrointestinal blood loss secondary to uremic gastropathy can be minimized by resolving the uremic crisis and providing gastroprotective drugs. Gastroprotective treatments to consider include histamine-2 receptor antagonists such as famotidine (0.5 mg/kg orally [PO], intramuscularly [IM], intravenously [IV] SID) or ranitidine (1 mg/kg PO, IM, IV, BID), locally acting gastric protectants such as sucralfate (0.25 to 1 g PO TID), or proton pump inhibitors such as omeprazole (0.5 to 1 mg/kg PO SID). These doses reflect a dose reduction for renally excreted drugs such as histamine-2 receptor antagonists. Resolution of anemia and improvement of the BUN:creatinine ratio would be evidence of response to treatment.

Maximize Regenerative Capability

Iron Deficiency

Iron deficiency anemia should be treated with iron supplementation; however, treatment with iron alone does not resolve anemia from EPO deficiency, and treatment of anemia of chronic inflammatory disease with iron does not resolve anemia and can result in iron overdose. If a chronic inflammatory disease has been diagnosed in addition to chronic kidney disease, specific treatment for the inflammatory disease can be initiated. With true iron deficiency and when recombinant EPO therapy is initiated, oral supplementation with ferrous sulfate (dogs: 100 to 300 mg total daily dosage PO; cats: 50 to 100 total daily dosage PO) is the traditional treatment method. Oral iron therapy can result in gastrointestinal upset in certain individuals. Dividing the daily dosage and administering with food may help to prevent this side effect. Oral iron supplementation is generally insufficient to meet the demands of erythropoiesis in humans receiving EPO therapy; parenteral iron administration is recommended. Serum iron and ferritin decreased and evidence of iron deficiency developed in dogs treated with oral iron supplementation during EPO therapy (Randolph et al., 2004a). Iron dextran (50 mg/cat or 10 to 20 mg/kg/dog IM q3-4 weeks) can be administered by intramuscular injection. A risk of anaphylaxis exists with this treatment when administered intravenously, and iron overdose can result.

Nutritional Status

If malnutrition is considered to be contributing to anemia, calorie and nutrient intake should be optimized. Resolving a uremic crisis can improve voluntary food intake in some animals. Providing a balanced diet for animals with renal impairment can prevent protein-calorie malnutrition and optimize vitamin intake. In humans with renal failure B vitamin supplementation can improve anemia of chronic kidney disease modestly; however, no studies exist on providing supplemental B vitamins to animals in renal failure. If voluntary food intake is inappropriately low, enteral nutrition can be provided by way of a nasoesophageal, esophagostomy, or gastrostomy feeding device (Chapter 196).

Erythropoietin Therapy

Erythropoietin can be used for treatment of anemia in dogs and cats with chronic kidney disease. The only commercially available EPO is recombinant human EPO (r-HuEPO), which has approximately 80% amino acid sequence identity to canine and feline EPO. This degree of variation in sequence homology allows r-HuEPO to be effective in increasing RBC production in dogs and cats, but it also causes the major complication of EPO therapy: anti-EPO antibody formation. Both recombinant canine and feline EPO have been studied in a research setting, but neither product is available commercially (Randolph et al., 2004a; Randolph et al., 2004b.) r-HuEPO is not approved for use in animals by the Food and Drug Administration; therefore clients should sign an informed consent before veterinary use. Although a number of products are currently available for humans, Epogen (Amgen) and ProCrit (Ortho Biotech Products) have been the most commonly used for veterinary applications. Therapy should be reserved until anemia is clinically significant because of the potentially life-threatening nature of anti-EPO antibody formation. The recommended starting dose of EPO is 100 units/kg subcutaneously three times weekly until the packed cell volume (PCV) is at the low end of the reference range (dogs 30% to 35% PCV; cats 25% to 30% PCV). Iron supplementation is imperative with initiation of EPO therapy at doses previously described.

The desired PCV typically takes 4 to 12 weeks to achieve. At this point, dosing interval is reduced to twice weekly until PCV is in the middle of the desired range. Maintenance dosage is typically 50 to 100 units/kg once to twice weekly. The PCV and reticulocyte count should be checked weekly during treatment until four consecutive readings are stable at a specific dose and then monthly thereafter. Overproduction of RBCs can cause polycythemia, hyperviscosity, and hypertension and should be avoided.

Laboratory evidence of anti-EPO antibodies has been reported to occur in 60% to 100% of dogs receiving r-HuEPO; whereas clinically significant anemia has been reported to occur in 20% to 70% of dogs and cats receiving EPO, presumptively as a result of anti-r-HuEPO antibody formation (Cowgill et al., 1998; Langston et al., 2003). Antibodies typically develop within the first few months of therapy but could have a later onset. If anti-EPO antibody formation occurs, the antibodies suppress native EPO action on bone marrow precursor cells, resulting in profound anemia. The primary sign of immunologic reaction is a precipitous decline in PCV following a prior response to therapy. Reticulocyte counts decrease to zero before a decline of PCV. If clinical evidence supports this drug complication in dogs or cats, EPO therapy should be discontinued, and transfusion therapy initiated. Antibody levels can decline and resolve over 2 to 12 months, and PCV can return to the pretreatment level. Although the anemia associated with antibody formation can be reversed, the patient can remain transfusion dependent for weeks to months. The need for multiple transfusions over time causes crossmatch incompatibility even when blood-type compatibility is addressed before transfusion, and incompatibility adds to the cost and complexity of the management of anemia. In addition, the anemia that required EPO therapy initially would still be present following resolution of antibodies. Therefore development of this complication frequently results in death or euthanasia of the animal.

Hypertension is a complication of EPO administration in humans, and blood pressure increases in almost 60% of cats treated with EPO. Blood pressure should be monitored weekly during the initial administration of EPO (Chapter 197). Other reported complications of EPO administration include seizures, vomiting, injection discomfort, skin reactions, cellulitis, cutaneous or mucocutaneous reactions, fever, and arthralgia; but these complications are rare.

Darbepoetin (Aranesp, Amgen) is a derivative of r-HuEPO that has more attached carbohydrate groups to slow clearance and decrease the frequency of administration. The initial regimen calls for weekly injections, which decreases to once every 3 weeks for maintenance therapy in humans. Experimental evidence suggests that it is less likely to cause an immunologic reaction in nonhuman subjects. All antibodies to r-HuEPO described to date are directed against the protein component, and the additional carbohydrate moieties of darbepoetin may shield the protein backbone from immunologic exposure. Experience with this drug is limited in veterinary medicine but promising. It appears to be effective, although apparently at least one dog has developed neutralizing antibodies (personal observation).

Over the last 5 years anti-r-HuEPO antibody formation in humans has been reported with increasing frequency, a condition that had been reported in only three humans before 1998. Extensive evaluations have led many to suspect that the risk of antibody formation is higher with subcutaneous administration compared to the intravenous route, perhaps because of slower clearance with subcutaneous administration. Optimal treatment for this condition in humans is unclear, but immunosuppressive therapy appears helpful.

Future Directions
Virus-vectored feline EPO gene therapy has been investigated and holds some promise, although control of gene expression and distribution is a problem that still must be overcome. Continuous EPO receptor activator has a significantly longer half-life than EPO or darbepoetin and is being investigated in humans. A drug that inhibits enzymatic degradation of hypoxia-inducible factor, a molecule that stimulates EPO production, is being investigated and would not be expected to induce antibody formation.

When to Transfuse?

Transfusion should be considered when RBC mass has declined sufficiently to limit oxygen-carrying capacity and cause clinical signs of anemia and when rapid increase of oxygen-carrying capacity is needed (e.g., before general anesthesia, following development of anti-EPO antibodies). There is no set PCV at which transfusion is always indicated. The decision to transfuse is based on clinical signs (i.e., fatigue, pallor, tachypnea, tachycardia, and weakness) and duration and degree of anemia. Mild-to-moderate reductions in PCV are often tolerated reasonably well in animals with renal failure because of gradual onset, increased levels of 2,3-diphosphoglycerate, and increased cardiac output to facilitate tissue oxygen delivery. In addition, cats in particular are talented at limiting physical activity to tolerate anemia.

Oxygen-carrying capacity can be increased with administration of whole blood or packed RBCs. Risks of blood transfusion include volume overload with rapid administration, acute hypersensitivity reaction, and transmission of infectious disease. Incompatibility reactions can be minimized by accurate blood-typing of donor and recipient in cats, using canine universal donors, and crossmatching for dogs and cats if the recipient has received a prior transfusion (Chapter 56). In addition, the life span of transfused RBCs in a uremic recipient is shortened. The goal for transfusion is to restore the patient PCV to the low end of the normal range to avoid a rapid increase in blood viscosity. If blood products are not available, oxygen-carrying capacity can be increased with administration of a hemoglobin-based oxygen carrier (HBOC) (Oxyglobin, Biopure). This product does not result in increased PCV; patient hemoglobin can be monitored to evaluate response to treatment. HBOCs are strong colloids and must be administered judiciously to prevent volume overload with resultant pulmonary edema or pleural effusion. Cats are more likely than dogs to experience volume overload with this product. The color of the HBOC imparts a red color to the recipient's serum that interferes with colorimetric tests. This change causes creatinine to be underestimated; however urea nitrogen and electrolytes are measured accurately.

References and Suggested Reading

Cowgill LD et al: Use of recombinant human erythropoietin for management of anemia in dogs and cats with renal failure, *J Am Vet Med Assoc* 212:521, 1998.

Goldstein RE et al: Gastrin concentrations in cats with chronic renal failure, *J Am Vet Med Assoc* 213:826, 1998.

Langston CE, Reine NJ, Kittrell D: The use of erythropoietin, *Vet Clin Small Anim Pract* 33:1245, 2003.

Peters RM et al: Histopathologic features of canine uremic gastropathy: a retrospective study, *J Vet Intern Med* 19:315, 2005.

Randolph JF et al: Clinical efficacy and safety of recombinant canine erythropoietin in dogs with anemia of chronic renal failure and dogs with recombinant human erythropoietin-induced red cell aplasia, *J Vet Intern Med* 18:81, 2004a.

Randolph JF et al: Expression, bioactivity, and clinical assessment of recombinant feline erythropoietin, *Am J Vet Res* 65:1355, 2004b.

CHAPTER **199**

Uncomplicated Urinary Tract Infection

MARY ANNA LABATO, *North Grafton, Massachusetts*

DEFINITIONS

Urinary tract infection (UTI) is defined as the adherence, multiplication, and persistence of an infectious agent in the urinary system. Infection occurs when there is a break in the host defense mechanisms and sufficient numbers of a virulent microbe are allowed entrance. UTIs usually are caused by bacterial organisms; infections often involve bacteria that are normally present in the distal urogenital tract. However, fungi and viruses occasionally are the causative agent.

Uncomplicated UTIs are uniformly caused by bacterial organisms. An *uncomplicated (or "simple") infection* is one in which no underlying structural, neurologic, or functional abnormalities of the host are known or suspected.

Pyuria refers to the presence of white blood cells (WBCs) in urine. Significant pyuria is defined as finding greater than three to five WBCs per high-power field during examination of urine sediment from a sample collected by cystocentesis. If the urine is collected by urethral catheterization or voiding and has greater than five to 10 WBCs per high-power field, it should be considered significant. Pyuria indicates urinary tract inflammation and is not synonymous with UTI. A number of disease processes result in inflammation of the urinary system without the presence of an infectious agent.

Bacteriuria refers to the presence of bacteria in urine. The presence of bacteria in urine is not synonymous with UTI as it may represent contamination of the urine sample. High bacterial numbers in a properly collected and cultured urine sample indicate a bacterial urinary tract infection (Table 199-1).

PATHOGENESIS OF URINARY TRACT INFECTION

UTIs are considered common; however, it has been reported that the incidence of a bacterial UTI is 2% to 3% in dogs and less than 1% in cats. Another report indicated that 14% of all dogs will have a bacterial UTI during their lifetime, and that UTI it is more common in female dogs (Chew and Kowalski, 2001). In cats bacterial UTIs occur more often in older animals (>10 yrs old). By comparison, during any given year, 11% of women report having a UTI.

Most UTIs are caused by ascending migration of pathogenic organisms from the distal urogenital tract. Normally a population of bacteria residing in the lower urogenital tract serves as a defense mechanism to prevent colonization of a pathogenic organism; these resident bacteria may emerge as uropathogens if other host defenses are altered. There are a number of other natural and acquired host defenses of the urinary tract. For example, the act of normal micturition is a host defense; it entails frequent and complete voiding of adequate urine volume. A number of anatomic structures serve as defense mechanisms, including a high-pressure zone within the urethra, surface characteristics of the urothelium, and urethral peristalsis. In addition, the length of the urethra may provide protection against ascending

Table **199-1**						
Interpretation of Quantitative Urine Cultures in Dogs and Cats						
	SIGNIFICANT (cfu/ml)		**SUSPICIOUS**		**CONTAMINATION**	
Source	Dogs	Cats	Dogs	Cats	Dogs	Cats
Cystocentesis	>1000	>1000	100-1000	100-1000	<100	<100
Catheterization	>10,000	>1000	1000-10,000	100-1000	<1000	<100
Voiding	>100,000	>10,000	10,000-99,000	1000-10,000	<10,000	<1000

Modified from Bartges JW: Urinary tract infections. In Ettinger SJ, Feldman EC, editors: *Textbook of Veterinary Internal Medicine,* ed 6, Philadelphia, 2005, Elsevier, p 1805.
cfu/ml, Colony-forming units per milliliter of urine.

infection. In male dogs prostatic secretions contain immunoglobulins and antibacterial components. Upper urinary tract host defense mechanisms include an extensive renal blood supply and flow, ureterovesical flap valves, and ureteral peristalsis. There are a number of mucosal defense barriers within the urogenital tract. These are comprised of antibody production, the surface layer of glycosaminoglycans, and intrinsic mucosal antimicrobial properties. Equally important are the rapid turnover and exfoliation of urothelial cells. Normal urine also has antimicrobial properties. Urine pH (high and low ranges), hyperosmolality, Tamm-Horsfall mucoproteins, and high concentrations of urea and organic acids impede bacterial growth.

The organisms that commonly cause UTI in dogs and cats are similar. Infections caused by *E. coli* are most common. Gram-positive cocci are the second most common isolates (enterococci, staphylococci, and streptococci). *Proteus, Klebsiella, Pasteurella,* and *Pseudomonas* are also frequent isolates. Most UTIs are the result of ascending infections from the distal urogenital tract. The bacteria must gain access to the urinary tract and adhere to and colonize the urothelial surface. Infection depends on the number and virulence of the organism and the interaction with the host defenses. Fortunately most acute lower UTIs are uncomplicated and are not associated with signs or symptoms of upper UTIs. UTI or prostatitis is uncommon in male dogs. Acute or chronic prostatitis should be considered a complicated infection and treated accordingly. It is equally important to rule out underlying causes for the infection (e.g., hyperadrenocorticism, prostatic neoplasia, benign prostatic hypertrophy).

CLINICAL FINDINGS

Dogs and cats with UTI may or may not demonstrate signs of urinary tract disease. The development of clinical signs depends on the site and duration of infection, the presence or absence of predisposing causes, the body's compensatory response, and the virulence and numbers of the uropathogen. Lower tract UTIs may present with pollakiuria, stranguria, dysuria, hematuria, and inappropriate urinations. The bladder and proximal urethra are so closely associated that inflammation in one is thought to affect the other. Female dogs with abnormalities of the vulva, perivulvar dermatitis, or vaginal stenosis may have an increased risk of UTI. Gross hematuria at the beginning of urination or a urethral discharge may be associated with urethral or prostatic disease. Prostatic disease is a more common cause of urethral discharge independent of urination than is urethral disease. Differential diagnoses for dysuria, pollakiuria, and hematuria consist not only of bacterial cystitis but include cystic calculi, neoplasia, detrusor overactivity ("urge incontinence"), prostatitis, idiopathic or interstitial cystitis in cats, and urethritis. Clinical signs associated with upper urinary tract involvement may include fever, pain, hematuria, septicemia, polyuria or renal failure.

Historical or clinical findings that would lead a UTI to be classified as *complicated* include recurrence, persistence in the face of appropriate treatment, or the presence of host abnormalities (e.g., hyperadrenocorticism or corticosteroid administration, diabetes mellitus, renal failure, neurogenic bladder dysfunction).

DIAGNOSIS

Diagnosis should be based on urinalysis, urine culture, and antimicrobial susceptibility testing. The urine sample should be obtained in a sterile manner, preferably by cystocentesis. Urine culture with sensitivity is a valuable diagnostic tool even in the first-time, uncomplicated infection. Quantification of bacterial numbers helps to identify contamination (collection via free-catch or manual expression) versus true infection. Once bacterial identification is determined, selection of the appropriate antibiotic makes treatment efficient and economical. If infection recurs, prior urine cultures also help determine whether the "new" infection is a relapse of the initial infection or reinfection with a different organism. Additional testing ideally should include a complete blood count, chemistry profile, and some form of diagnostic imaging (survey radiographs, abdominal ultrasound, or contrast radiography). Quite frequently, especially in cats or immature dogs, it is difficult to obtain a sterile urine sample. The bladder may be too small to safely obtain a sample as a result of the pollakiuria, or the animal may be too uncooperative to safely restrain without sedation. In these cases the presumptive diagnosis of UTI is made based on history, clinical signs, physical examination, and response to treatment.

The Minimum Inhibitory Concentration

It is important to understand the meaning of culture and susceptibility results to select the ideal antimicrobial agent. The minimum inhibitory concentration (MIC) is the lowest drug concentration that inhibits microbial growth (this does not necessarily mean all bacteria are killed outright). In vitro MIC cannot be interpreted as absolute values since they are based on the ability of the drug to reach a given concentration in plasma. Plasma and urine concentration may vary in an individual patient for many reasons. The criteria for categorizing bacteria as *susceptible, intermediate,* or *resistant* to a given antimicrobial plasma concentration are based on knowledge of the predictable susceptibility of the organism and on another dilution, the *breakpoint value.* The breakpoint is an arbitrary criterion, generally set at the point at which the majority of all isolates for that microbe are inhibited, and should be provided by the veterinarian's microbiology laboratory. These data are obtained from thousands of cultures and sensitivities and are determined by a regulatory agency, the National Committee for Clinical Laboratory Standards (NCCLS). Knowing the breakpoint is a key step in choosing the appropriate antibiotic. The farther the MIC of an individual organism is from the breakpoint, the more likely a drug is to be effective. For example, *E. coli* is cultured from a urine sample. The organism is sensitive to cephalexin with an MIC of 2 mcg/ml. This is four dilutions away from the breakpoint of 32 mcg/ml. It is also sensitive to trimethoprim-sulfa with an MIC of 40 mcg/ml, only one dilution away from the breakpoint of 80 mcg/ml. Assuming that all other factors are equal, the chance of successful treatment is greater with cephalexin than trimethoprim-sulfa.

As a general rule, one should avoid choosing a drug when the MIC is approaching the breakpoint (often reported as "intermediate" susceptibility). If the only antimicrobial choice is a drug with an MIC near the breakpoint, the antimicrobial dose selected should be in the high end of the dosing range. If an antimicrobial is cleared through the kidney and reaches a high concentration in urine, even a drug with an intermediate sensitivity may be effective in treating the infection. Antimicrobials categorized as "resistant" for an organism do not inhibit the organism at the usual blood or tissue concentrations and are unlikely to be effective.

TREATMENT

Treatment of an uncomplicated lower UTI should resolve during a 7- to 10-day course of antibiotics. If an upper tract infection is suspected or definitively diagnosed, treatment should continue for a minimum of 4 weeks. In human medicine it is recommended that a simple, uncomplicated infection be treated for 3 days and acute uncomplicated pyelonephritis for 14 days. More studies are needed in veterinary medicine to establish optimum length of therapy for dogs and cats. Clinical signs should resolve within 48 hours of starting treatment.

If culture results are available, antimicrobial choice should be based on the susceptibility as described previously. Treatment of an uncomplicated infection may be undertaken without culture results if this is an initial infection and the patient has not received antibiotics within the last 4 to 6 weeks. In these cases the choice of antibiotics should be based on the knowledge of the bacteria most commonly causing UTI (Table 199-2). Gram stain of urine sediment may provide an indication regarding the type of organism causing the infection and guidance about which antibiotic to use. As stated previously, the most common isolate is *E. coli,* which is a gram-negative rod associated with an acidic urine. Staphylococci are gram positive and associated with alkaline urine because they produce urease.

When instituting empiric therapy, a broad-spectrum antibiotic should be the first choice (Table 199-3). Cephalosporins usually have activity against both *E. coli* and *Staphylococcus* spp. Another alternative is trimethoprim-sulfa. Drugs related to penicillin should also be considered. The use of fluoroquinolones for the empiric treatment of UTIs is contraindicated because of the inherent resistance of many gram-positive bacteria

Table 199-2

Antimicrobial Selections for Common Urinary Tract Pathogens

Organism	Drug	Alternative
Gram-Negative Organisms		
Escherichia coli	Cephalexin Trimethoprim-sulfonamide	Fluoroquinolone
Proteus spp.	Ampicillin Amoxicillin-clavulanate	Cephalexin
Klebsiella spp.	Cephalexin	Trimethoprim-sulfonamide
Pseudomonas aeruginosa	Fluoroquinolone	Tetracyclines
Gram-Positive Organisms		
Staphylococcus spp.	Ampicillin Amoxicillin-clavulanate	Cephalexin
Streptococcus spp.	Ampicillin Amoxicillin-clavulanate	Cephalexin
Enterococcus spp.	Trimethoprim-sulfonamide	Fluoroquinolone

Table 199-3

Guidelines for Antibiotic Usage for Urinary Tract Infections

Drug	Recommended Dosage
Ampicillin	25 mg/kg q8h PO
Amoxicillin-clavulanate	15 mg/kg q12h PO
Cephalexin	22 mg/kg q8h PO
Doxycycline	5 mg/kg q12h PO
Enrofloxacin	5 mg/kg q12h PO
Trimethoprim-sulfa	15 mg/kg q12h PO

and the development of resistance patterns in many gram-negative organisms, especially *E. coli*, to this class of antibiotics. After the completion of the course of antibiotics, it is preferable to perform a urine culture to ensure that the infection has been resolved. The culture should be obtained at least 4 to 5 days after completion of the course of therapy. If antimicrobial treatment does not result in sustained clinical response and negative urine culture, further investigation of owner compliance and host defenses is indicated.

References and Suggested Reading

Bartges JW: Urinary tract infections. In Ettinger SJ, Feldman EC, editors: *Textbook of veterinary internal medicine*, ed 6, Philadelphia, 2005, Elsevier, p 1800.

Chew DJ, Kowalski J: Diagnosing initial and recurrent urinary tract infections in dogs, *Bayer Selected Proceedings*, TNAVC, Orlando, Fla, Jan. 2001.

Cooke CL et al: Enrofloxacin resistance in *Escherichia coli* isolated from dogs with urinary tract infections, *J Am Vet Med Assoc* 220:190, 2002.

Fihn SD: Acute uncomplicated urinary tract infection in women, *N Engl J Med* 349:259, 2003.

Forrester SD, Troy GC: Urinary tract infections associated with endocrine disorders in dogs. In Bonagura JD, editor: *Kirk's current veterinary therapy XIII*, Philadelphia, 2000, Saunders, p 878.

Ling GV et al: Interrelations of organism prevalence, specimen collection method, and host age, sex and breed among 8,354 canine urinary tract infections (1969-1995), *J Vet Intern Med* 15:341, 2001.

Mehnert-Kay SA: Diagnosis and management of uncomplicated urinary tract infections, *Am Fam Physician* 72:451, 2005.

Nicolle LE et al: Infectious disease society of America guidelines for the diagnosis and treatment of asymptomatic bacteriuria in adults, *Clin Infect Dis* 40:643, 2005.

Sannes MR, Kuskowski MA, Johnson JR: Antimicrobial resistance to *Escherichia coli* strains isolated from urine of women with cystitis or pyelonephritis and feces of dogs and healthy humans, *J Am Vet Med Assoc* 225:368, 2004.

CHAPTER 200

Multidrug-Resistant Urinary Tract Infection

JEANNE A. BARSANTI, *Athens, Georgia*

Urinary tract infections (UTIs) are common in dogs and in geriatric cats. Most are caused by common bacterial organisms and easily treated successfully with short (7 to 10 days) courses of commonly available antibiotics. However, some UTIs are difficult because infection recurs frequently. Multidrug-resistant organisms cause approximately 30% of such difficult UTIs (Sequin et al., 2003). A case from a private practice is presented to illustrate the important concepts in dealing with difficult UTIs.

CASE EXAMPLE

A 12-year-old, female, spayed, mixed-breed dog weighing 9 kg was presented for hematuria, dysuria, and licking the vulva. The client owned this dog for 1 year. The previous owner told the client that the dog had been licking its vulva on occasion for the past 2 years. Hematuria and dysuria were new problems. The dog appeared to be normal on physical examination, so the veterinarian prescribed a quinolone antibiotic without doing a urinalysis or culture. The dog did not improve. On the second presentation a cystocentesis urine sample was submitted for culture. The result was a hemolyzing *E. coli* (>100,000 colony-forming units [CFU]/ml). The organism was reported to be sensitive only to nitrofurantoin and imipenem. Nitrofurantoin was prescribed at 4 mg/kg every 8 hours for 4 weeks. The dog's clinical signs resolved, and a complete urinalysis performed during therapy was normal.

Within 3 days of discontinuing therapy, the dog's clinical signs returned. A culture of urine collected by cystocentesis again revealed hemolyzing *E. coli* (>100,000 CFU/ml) with the same sensitivity pattern. A third-generation cephalosporin that was not on the sensitivity panel was administered subcutaneously once a day for 4 weeks. Again clinical signs resolved, and a complete urinalysis performed during therapy was normal with no bacteria seen. Within 1 week of discontinuing therapy, clinical signs returned, and culture revealed hemolyzing *E. coli* with the same sensitivity pattern. Imipenem was used intravenously three times a day for 2 weeks.

Ten days after stopping therapy clinical signs returned, and urine culture results were the same as on previous occasions. A complete blood count (CBC) and serum biochemical profile were normal. An adrenocorticotropic hormone response test suggested hyperadrenocorticism, which was controlled with trilostane. After controlling the hyperadrenocorticism, the third-generation cephalosporin was used subcutaneously for 6 weeks, and again the dog's UTI returned within 1 week of discontinuing therapy. Radiology and ultrasound of the urinary tract were normal except for an equivocal increase in renal echogenicity. Cystoscopy was performed, and the only abnormality was inflammation around the openings of both ureters, which was confirmed by histopathology. The vagina, urethra, and rest of the bladder mucosa appeared to be normal. This is a frustrating, difficult UTI for the dog, the owner, and the veterinarian.

DIAGNOSTIC APPROACH

This case is an example of recurrent UTI. The first diagnostic step in such a case is to differentiate *relapse* from *reinfection*. A relapse is a UTI caused by the same organism that recurs after therapy is discontinued. Although most relapsing UTIs recur quickly, some do not relapse for months (Freitag et al., 2006). When recurrence of a UTI with the same organism does not occur for months, it is difficult to distinguish a relapsing infection from a reinfection caused by the same organism, perhaps derived from the gastrointestinal tract. A reinfection is generally defined as a UTI caused by a different organism that recurs at variable intervals after therapy is discontinued. Less common types of difficult UTIs are persistent infections and superinfections. Distinguishing between these types of UTIs requires performing urine cultures before, during, and after therapy.

Relapsing Infections

Distinguishing relapses from reinfections is difficult because one must determine whether the organism is the same or different. If the species type changes (e.g., from *Proteus* to *E. coli*), the decision is simple. However, *E. coli* is the most common cause of UTIs and there are many varieties of *E. coli*. Clinicians have relied mainly on the sensitivity pattern of the organism to help determine whether the current infection is caused by a new or the same *E. coli*. However, the same *E. coli* can shift in regard to antibiotic sensitivity; thus this method is not very accurate (Drazenovich, Ling, and Foley, 2004; Freitag et al., 2006). Unfortunately more accurate methods such as pulsed-field gel electrophoresis are not readily available. The UTI in the example case fits a relapsing infection best: the infection recurs rapidly with discontinuation of treatment, and the organism is the same type with the same antibiotic sensitivity pattern. This is an important determination since the pathophysiology of relapsing infections differs from that of reinfections.

In relapsing infections the problem is usually that the organism has found a deep-seated niche in the urinary tract, protected from antimicrobial action. The antimicrobial kills the bacteria that are in the urine but cannot reach those deep in tissue sites. The likely tissue sites are the kidney (chronic pyelonephritis) and the prostate gland in intact males. Struvite uroliths are another potential site of infection. Other sites are the submucosa of the bladder and any location associated with a partially obstructive process such as a ureterolith. Experimentally it has been found that uropathogenic *E. coli* can enter host bladder epithelial cells and remain quiescent for a period of time before leaving the cell and replicating again (Mulvey, 2002; Schilling, Mulvey, and Hultgren, 2001).

The appropriate diagnostic approach in a relapsing UTI is finding the site where the bacteria are hiding. This involves imaging the entire urinary tract, as well as evaluating prostatic fluid in intact male dogs. The example case is typical of relapsing infections: the infection appears to respond to antibiotics because the clinical signs are secondary to bacteria from elsewhere in the urinary tract entering the bladder and resulting in signs of cystitis. When antibiotics effective against the organism are administered, the bacteria in the urine are killed, and the cystitis abates. Not all relapsing UTIs are associated with clinical signs. Some recur and remain silent, detected only by repeated urine cultures. The veterinarians in the example case tried to determine the site of infection. They found that the most likely site was the ureters/kidneys because the cystoscopy found chronic inflammation around the ureteral orifices and the ultrasound suggested increased renal echogenicity. An excretory urogram would also be indicated to evaluate the kidneys and ureters more fully.

Reinfections

With reinfections, the problem is not curing the infection. In this instance each infection is cured. However, the pet becomes reinfected with a different organism at a variable interval. The causes are multiple and include poor systemic immune function (such as hyperadrenocorticism or immunosuppressive drug therapy), loss of one of the antimicrobial properties of urine (such as glucosuria associated with diabetes mellitus or poor urine-concentrating ability from any one of many causes), an anatomic predisposition to infection (such as a stricture, a urolith, a prior urethrostomy, or a neoplasm), or a physiologic predisposition to infection (such as urine retention from a neurologic problem or decreased urethral sphincter tone). Diagnostic tests should include physical examination of the vulva or prepuce, palpation of the urinary tract and prostate gland, CBC, serum biochemical profile, complete urinalysis, urinary tract imaging, and determination as to whether the pet can empty the bladder normally. In some cases, especially female dogs, all of the above are normal. For example, almost 30% of 100 dogs in one retrospective study had no identifiable underlying reason for reinfections (Sequin et al., 2003). I have assumed that such dogs have a defect in local immunity, allowing bacteria to adhere to the reproductive and urinary tract mucosa and make their way to the bladder.

Persistent Infections

A persistent infection is one in which the original causative bacteria continue to be present during therapy that should be effective based on culture and sensitivity. Such infections can be diagnosed only by performing a urine culture during therapy to document that bacteriuria continues. A common misconception is that urine cultures of animals given antimicrobials will always be negative. This is correct only if the drug is effective, as is true in most UTIs because of high concentrations of antibiotics in urine. However, if the organism is resistant to the drug chosen for therapy, bacteria grow despite the presence of the drug. Persistent UTI is a very difficult situation and fortunately rare. Usually a persistent infection indicates that there is a failure of host defense mechanisms. There may be a structural abnormality in the urinary tract that must be corrected to resolve the infection. The causative organism is often highly antibiotic resistant or unusual. It is also possible that the drug administered is not getting into the urine at antibacterial concentrations. How the prescribed drug is metabolized and excreted should be reviewed. The possibility that the drug is not being administered by the client should also be considered by asking the client how he or she is giving the medication and how he or she knows that the pet ingests it. If client and patient compliance are not issues, the diagnostic approach must include a serum biochemical profile to evaluate liver and kidney function. Urinary tract imaging should be performed to find any underlying structural problem.

The veterinarians in the example case performed a complete urinalysis during therapy to confirm drug efficacy and rule out persistent infection. A urine culture would have been useful to confirm the urine cytology since bacteria can be present in urine and difficult to detect by cytology unless Wright's stained smears are used (Swenson et al., 2004). Although a urine culture was not performed in the example case to completely exclude a persistent infection, the facts that urinalyses performed during therapy were normal and that clinical signs resolved with therapy support the conclusion that the infection was not persisting during therapy.

Superinfections

A superinfection is an infection with a different organism that arises during the course of treatment for the original organism. A superinfection can be diagnosed only by doing a urine culture during therapy. Superinfections usually are associated with indwelling urinary tubes.

THERAPEUTIC APPROACH TO RECURRENT INFECTIONS

Even difficult UTIs usually are caused by aerobic, common bacterial organisms. Unfortunately the most common organism, *E. coli*, is highly diverse with the ability to develop multidrug resistance (MDR). One recent pilot study in dogs showed that MDR developed within 3 days of treatment with amoxicillin or enrofloxacin (Debavalya et al., 2007). Although MDR resolved within 3 weeks after treatment with amoxicillin, MDR did not resolve after treatment with enrofloxacin. In the example case a quinolone was used without doing a urine culture. On the first culture the *E. coli* was resistant to multiple drugs. Without an initial urine culture, it is impossible to know whether quinolone therapy induced MDR or whether the organism was originally resistant. This emphasizes the importance of doing urine cultures before therapy, especially when using a quinolone, which generally should not be used as first-line therapy. If the bacteria identified exhibit MDR, many laboratories will do extended antimicrobial testing on request.

Relapsing Infections

The goal with relapsing infections is to find the site and determine if any predisposing factors at that site can be corrected. For example, if a chronic prostatic infection is found, neutering assists in elimination of infection. In the example case hyperadrenocorticism was present, but controlling the hyperadrenocorticism did not help with treatment of the UTI. It is possible that the infection occurred independently of that condition or was firmly established before the hyperadrenocorticism was controlled. It is not recommended to remove kidneys affected by pyelonephritis since nephrectomy rarely results in control of UTI (both kidneys are often affected). Because the site of infection should not be removed and since it is very difficult for antimicrobial agents to penetrate and act effectively in the renal medulla, prognosis for cure of chronic pyelonephritis is always guarded. A similar prognosis appears warranted for dogs with nephroliths and recurrent upper-tract UTIs because complete elimination of the nephroliths and clearance of accompanying deep-tissue infection is difficult in many cases. The example case illustrates these frustrating facts well. The drugs were not failing to kill the organism; they were failing to reach the primary site of infection. Few antibiotics are thought to penetrate renal tissue: trimethoprim, chloramphenicol, nitrofurantoin, some of the quinolones, and the aminoglycosides. Aminoglycosides are not recommended in chronic pyelonephritis because of nephrotoxicity with long-term use. Optimal duration of therapy is unknown, but generally 4 to 6 weeks is recommended. In the example case it may have been better to extend the duration of treatment with nitrofurantoin to 2 to 3 months since it seemed to control the UTI without adverse effects. One must consider potential drug toxicity when using an antibiotic for longer than normal periods of time. When a case with a relapsing infection appears to have responded to therapy (negative urine culture after therapy completed), it is important to reculture the urine at 1 month and then every 3 months for at least a year to detect another recurrence.

When up to 3 to 6 months of full-dose therapy fails to prevent relapse, one can use suppressive therapy. There is some evidence that in difficult cases in dogs in which no underlying abnormality can be corrected, low-dose, long-term antimicrobial regimens can assist in UTI control (Sequin et al., 2003). This involves administration of a single dose of the effective antimicrobial once a day. The dose is the usual single dose of the drug chosen. If the animal is confined at night, administration after the last urination of the day is recommended so that the urine contains the antimicrobial for the night. This should be started when the infection is under control (negative urine culture). Drugs typically considered for suppressive therapy are trimethoprim, nitrofurantoin, cephalexin, and enrofloxacin. All of these drugs can be potentially toxic. In the example case nitrofurantoin would be a reasonable choice since it was effective at full-dose therapy. Neurologic and hepatic toxicity are possible with nitrofurantoin. Risks of suppressive therapy are induction of antibiotic resistance and/or drug toxicity. The alternative is not treating the infection unless clinical signs are apparent. The risk is that the infection will become systemic. Urine should be cultured monthly during suppressive therapy to ensure that the drug continues to be effective.

Reinfections

An effort should be made to eliminate the underlying predisposing factor. Each infection should be treated for 7 to 10 days in spayed female and neutered male dogs and in cats. Intact male dogs should be treated for 3 to 4 weeks and neutered because of the risk of prostatic infection. Drug choice should be based on urine culture and sensitivity. In intact male dogs an antimicrobial with prostatic penetrance such as trimethoprim, chloramphenicol, or a quinolone should be considered if the organism is reported sensitive. Unless clinical signs are severe, one can wait for these results before prescribing therapy.

If infections recur frequently (more than 4 to 6 times a year), prophylactic (preventive) therapy can be considered. Prophylactic therapy is defined as the administration of an antimicrobial drug to prevent establishment of infection in uninfected sites. Before beginning prophylactic therapy, the current infection should be eliminated with standard full-dose therapy, and then once-a-day therapy begun with a drug to which the organism was sensitive. A urine culture should be performed at the end of full-dose therapy to ensure that the infection was controlled. The chosen drug is given once a day just before a 6- to 12-hour period when urine will be retained in the bladder such as at night in house dogs. The dose is the usual single dose of the drug chosen administered for 6 months in an effort to break the cycle of infections. Urine should be cultured once a month during prophylactic therapy to ensure that UTI is prevented. If the urine remains sterile for 6 months, the drug is discontinued, and the animal monitored for recurrence. The risks of preventive therapy are the development of antibiotic resistance and drug toxicity. Therefore this approach should be used only if the underlying cause of reinfections cannot be determined or eliminated and if the frequency of reinfections is every few months. It should be noted that there is only anecdotal evidence and one study with a small number of cases to support the effectiveness of this approach in dogs (Sequin, 2003). A recent study of a large number of children indicated that prophylactic therapy did not reduce risk of reinfection but did increase the chance that a second infection would be antibiotic resistant (Conway et al., 2007). Therefore further evaluation of this approach in pets is warranted.

There is some evidence that cranberry juice is helpful in women with frequent reinfections but no such evidence in dogs. The mechanism of action is prevention of bacterial adherence to reproductive and urinary lower tract mucosa. One can use cranberry juice in conjunction with prophylactic antimicrobial therapy, although efficacy is questionable.

Persistent Infections

The first goals with persistent infections are to find and correct any underlying predisposing factors and to question the owner to insure the drug is actually administered. If no cause for treatment failure can be found or corrected, the goal is to find a drug that will work by using measurement of the minimum inhibitory concentration (MIC) of each antimicrobial for that organism and comparing that concentration to concentrations of the antimicrobial in urine (see also Chapter 199). The potential efficacy of each drug is estimated by multiplying the MIC by 4. If the product is less than the mean urine concentration for that drug, it is likely the drug will be effective in killing the bacteria in the urine (though not necessarily in tissue sites) (Bartges, 2005; Polzin, 2006). This assumes that the pet has normal urine concentrating ability. If it does not, the MIC should be compared to serum concentrations of that drug. Once a potentially effective drug is identified, that drug should be started, and urine recultured in approximately 1 week. If the urine culture is negative, the duration of time to use the drug should be based on its safety and the reversibility of the underlying condition.

Superinfections

If possible, the urinary tube should be removed. If this is not possible and the animal is asymptomatic, antimicrobial therapy should be stopped. Antiseptics can be used systemically (e.g., methenamine mandelate) or locally (e.g., Tris-ethylenediaminetetraacetic acid) until the tube can be removed. If the animal has localized symptoms, urinary antiseptics should be tried first. Antimicrobial therapy should be dictated by culture and sensitivity and used if systemic signs of infection develop.

SUMMARY

Urine cultures are an essential component of diagnosing and effectively treating recurrent UTIs. One must differentiate relapsing infections, persistent infections, reinfections, and superinfections to determine appropriate therapy. It is important to look for underlying factors that predispose to recurrent infections and eliminate these for therapy to be effective (Sequin, 2003). The search for such underlying factors involves history; physical examination of the urinary and reproductive tracts; hematology and biochemical laboratory testing; urinalyses; and urinary tract imaging via radiography, ultrasonography, and endoscopy. Antibiotic therapy should be carefully chosen based on antibiotic sensitivity testing and knowledge of antimicrobial metabolism and excretion, toxicity, and ability to reach tissue sites of infection. It is also very important to discuss the need for diagnostic testing and the requirements of potential therapy with the client to be sure the client is able to comply with recommendations.

References and Suggested Reading

Barsanti JA: Genitourinary Infections. In Greene CE, editor: *Infectious diseases of the dog and cat*, ed 3, St. Louis, 2006, Elsevier, p 935.

Bartges JW: Urinary tract infections. In Ettinger SJ, Feldman EC, editors: *Textbook of veterinary internal medicine*, ed 6, St, Louis, 2005, Saunders, p 1800.

Conway PH et al: Recurrent urinary tract infections in children, *JAMA* 298:179, 2007.

Debavalya N et al: Impact of routine antimicrobial therapy on canine fecal *Escherichia coli* antimicrobial resistance: a pilot study, *J Vet Intern Med* 21:660, 2007.

Drazenovich N, Ling GV, Foley J: Molecular investigation of *Escherichia coli* strains associated with apparently persistent urinary tract infections in dogs, *J Vet Intern Med* 18:301, 2004.

Freitag T et al: Antibiotic sensitivity profiles do not reliably distinguish relapsing or persisting infections from reinfections in cats with chronic renal failure and multiple diagnoses of *Escherichia coli* urinary tract infection, *J Vet Intern Med* 20:245, 2006.

Mulvey MA: Adhesion and entry of uropathogenic *Escherichia coli*, *Cell Microbiol* 4:257, 2002.

Polzin DJ: Difficult urinary tract infections, *Compend Contin Educ Pract Vet* 28(suppl):7, 2006.

Schilling JD, Mulvey MA, Hultgren SJ: Structure and function of *Escherichia coli* type 1 pili: new insight into the pathogenesis of urinary tract infections, *Infect Dis* 183(suppl 1):S36, 2001.

Sequin MA et al: Persistent urinary tract infections and reinfections in 100 dogs (1989-1999), *J Vet Intern Med* 17:622, 2003.

Swenson CL et al: Evaluation of modified Wright-staining of urine sediment as a method for accurate detection of bacteriuria in dogs, *J Am Vet Med Assoc* 224:1282, 2004.

CHAPTER **201**

Cancer and the Kidney

BARRAK M. PRESSLER, *West Lafayette, Indiana*

Primary renal neoplasia is extremely uncommon in dogs and cats. Excluding lymphoma, published case series and reviews suggest that primary renal tumors account for 0.6% to 1.7% of all neoplasms in dogs and 1.6% to 2.5% in cats. Retrospective review of cases evaluated by the Oncology Service at North Carolina State University (NCSU) over an 18-year period revealed an incidence of 1.5 cases referred for treatment of renal neoplasms (including renal lymphoma) per year, comprising 0.4% of all patients presenting to this service (unpublished data). This chapter reviews the differential diagnoses for renomegaly and provides an overview of the various subtypes of primary renal neoplasia. Paraneoplastic syndromes associated with renal cancer, the effects of extrarenal tumors on the kidney, and the effects of chemotherapy on the kidney are also reviewed.

RENOMEGALY

Normal Renal Size

In dogs and cats kidney length and volume are linearly correlated to body weight. The right kidney is usually slightly larger than the left, and males have larger kidneys than females; however, these differences are small enough to be clinically irrelevant. Palpation of the kidneys in dogs is difficult; thus renomegaly typically is detected on physical examination only when severe. On the contrary, subtle increases in kidney size may be detected earlier in cats because of the ease of palpation of the kidneys. Normal kidney length in dogs can be approximated by the formula:

$$\text{Kidney length in centimeters} = (0.07 \times \text{body weight in kilograms}) + 4.75$$

but the standard deviation from this result is relatively large, particularly in small- and giant-breed dogs (Barr, Holt, and Gibbs, 1990). On survey radiographs the kidney length is usually between 2.5 and 3.5 times the length of the L_2 vertebra in dogs, and in cats it is between 2.4 and 3 times the same measurement. Although results obtained using this technique correlate well with actual kidney length in most dogs, the large degree of dog-to-dog variations in kidney size makes this comparison only suitable for approximations; thus it should not be used as an inflexible reference range for kidney size. Contrast studies may improve visualization of the kidneys and thus facilitate more exact measurement of length; measurements after contrast administration are slightly longer than those made using plain survey radiographs. Ultrasonography is necessary for measurement of kidney volume and can also be used to measure kidney length.

Differential Diagnosis

Renomegaly may be unilateral or bilateral, symmetric or asymmetric. The most common causes of renomegaly are listed in Box 201-1, as well as the relative expected change in renal size (mild to moderate or severe) and species affected. Primary renal neoplasia is the most common cause of renomegaly in dogs. Common causes of renomegaly in cats include renal neoplasia (particularly lymphoma), granulomatous infiltration (caused by feline infectious peritonitis), perinephric pseudocysts, hydronephrosis, and polycystic kidney disease. Focal renal lesions (such as tumors, intraparenchymal cysts, or abscesses) do occur but rarely cause clinical signs unless they have resulted in distortion of the entire organ. Most focal lesions are incidental findings discovered during diagnostic imaging of the abdomen for another purpose.

Box 201-1

Causes of Renomegaly in Dogs and Cats*

UNILATERAL RENOMEGALY

Moderate-to-severe
- **Primary renal neoplasia (C, D)**
- **Hydronephrosis (C, D)**
- **Lymphoma (C, D)**
- **Perinephric pseudocyst (C)**

Mild
- Compensatory hypertrophy (D)
- Solitary cysts (D)
- Glomerulonephritis (C, D)

Variable
- Renal abscess (C, D)

BILATERAL RENOMEGALY

Moderate-to-severe
- Primary renal neoplasia (C, D)
- Hydronephrosis (C, D)
- **Feline infectious peritonitis (C)**
- **Lymphoma (C, D)**
- **Perinephric pseudocysts (C)**
- Perirenal abscesses (C, D)
- **Polycystic kidney disease (C)**

Mild
- Acute pyelonephritis (C, D)
- Amyloidosis (D)

Variable
- Acromegaly (C)
- Acute renal failure (C, D)
- Portosystemic shunts (D)

*The most common causes of renomegaly are in bold type.
C, Cat; D, dog.

Determining whether renomegaly is unilateral or bilateral is usually the first step in narrowing the differential diagnosis list and prioritizing diagnostic tests. Diagnostic imaging, particularly ultrasonography, is usually sufficient to diagnose polycystic kidney disease, hydronephrosis, and perinephric pseudocysts. Diseases that cause distortion of the renal parenchyma such as primary renal neoplasia, lymphoma, or feline infectious peritonitis may require cytologic or histopathologic examination for definitive diagnosis. Other causes of diffuse, mild, bilateral renomegaly, including acute pyelonephritis, amyloidosis, acute renal failure, or portosystemic shunting (in dogs), should be suspected based on concurrent clinical and clinicopathologic findings.

RENAL NEOPLASIA

Detection of a hyperechoic or isoechoic mass effacing normal renal architecture is highly suggestive of renal neoplasia. Histologic determination of the tumor type is required for accurate prognosis and to guide treatment. Although ultrasound-guided percutaneous biopsy can be considered, in the absence of metastatic disease nephrectomy is usually preferred since this may be curative and decreases the risk of iatrogenic seeding of tumor cells. Clinicians should perform careful assessment of renal function before complete nephrectomy. Serum creatinine is an insensitive indicator of kidney disease; determination of glomerular filtration rate should be considered in some cases (Chapter 189).

Renal Cell Carcinomas

Renal cell carcinomas (RCCs) are the most common primary renal neoplasms in dogs, and in cats they are second in frequency only to primary renal lymphoma (Henry et al., 1999; Klein et al., 1988). In published reports RCCs account for 74% to 85% of nonlymphoma primary renal tumors in dogs and cats and have accounted for 59% of all renal tumors in dogs (including lymphoma) presenting to the NCSU Oncology Service; no cats with primary renal carcinoma were evaluated at NCSU during the same time period. Median age of affected animals is 9 to 11 years. In humans there is a moderate increase in risk of RCC for males, a predilection that may exist in dogs as well (Klein et al., 1988). RCCs usually are clinically occult until they have (1) become large space-occupying masses, (2) metastasized and caused other organ dysfunction, or (3) elaborated sufficient cytokines to cause systemic (paraneoplastic) illness or cachexia (Fig. 201-1). In both dogs and cats owners typically seek veterinary care for nonspecific signs such as lethargy, anorexia, and weight loss (Henry et al., 1999; Klein et al., 1988). Less common clinical findings include hematuria, abdominal pain, palpable abdominal mass, or signs associated with renal failure. Azotemia and uremia typically only occur when both kidneys are affected or when neoplasia develops in a patient with preexisting renal disease. Clinicopathologic abnormalities are absent in most dogs with RCCs; but anemia, polycythemia, hypoalbuminemia, leukocytosis, or abnormalities secondary to renal failure may be present (Klein et al., 1988).

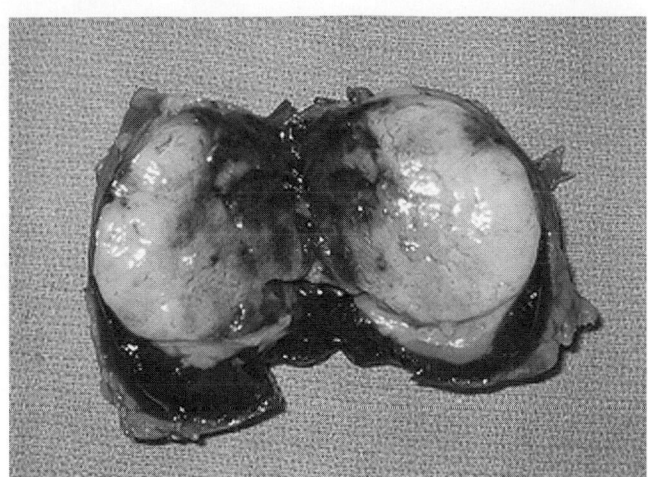

Fig. 201-1 Unilateral renal cell carcinoma (longitudinally sectioned) from an 11-year-old Siamese cat. The mass has displaced most of the normal renal parenchyma and caused a moderate amount of subcapsular hemorrhage. As is typical for renal tumors, despite the advanced nature of this neoplasm the cat presented with only vague clinical signs of anorexia and lethargy, and moderate renomegaly was detected on physical examination. No clinical signs referable to disease of the urinary tract disease were reported by the owner; and complete blood count, serum chemistry panel, and urinalysis were unremarkable.

Clinical experience suggests that ultrasonography has high sensitivity and reasonable specificity for diagnosis of primary renal neoplasms. Plain film radiography is less accurate for identification of masses and for confirming that masses are renal in origin, although contrast studies may improve detection. Computed tomography and magnetic resonance imaging have not been evaluated systematically in veterinary patients but are considered superior to ultrasonography in humans. In dogs and cats with renal tumors metastasis usually has occurred at the time of initial diagnosis, most often from delayed diagnosis rather than tumor aggressiveness. The most common sites of metastasis are the regional lymph node, liver, and contralateral kidney; the central nervous system (including the spine, spinal cord, and brain); and lungs (Klein et al., 1988). Local extension may involve the ipsilateral adrenal gland and abdominal serosal surfaces.

Histologic subclassification of RCCs has not been evaluated extensively in dogs and cats. In humans RCCs are subdivided into four main categories, which differ in etiology and prognosis (Moch et al., 2000; Renshaw 2002). Clear cell carcinomas (CCCs, more recently referred to as conventional carcinomas) comprise 75% of cases of renal carcinomas in humans and are so named because many tumor cells have clear cytoplasm. CCCs are thought to arise from renal proximal tubular epithelial cells. There is a strong association between CCCs and deletion or inactivation of the von Hippel-Lindau gene, a tumor suppressor gene that regulates hypoxia-inducible factors and the absence of which results in dysregulated vascular endothelial growth factor expression (Rathmell, Godley, and Rini, 2005). Other subtypes of RCC are papillary RCC, chromophobe RCC, and collecting duct RCC; differentiation and subtype classification of RCCs in humans may

require immunohistochemistry, most commonly using antivimentin, anticytokeratin 7, and anti-RCC marker antibodies (Renshaw, 2002). Likewise there is variation in histologic types of RCC in dogs and cats—tubular, papillary, tubulopapillary, and solid/undifferentiated forms have been reported, with the tubular subtype predominating (Henry et al., 1999).

Nephrectomy is the treatment of choice for solitary renal tumors without azotemia or evidence of metastasis. Partial nephrectomy is often performed in humans and can be considered in dogs and cats if complete excision appears feasible. However, the majority of tumors in veterinary patients are locally extensive by the time of diagnosis, and total nephrectomy usually is required. Unfortunately there are no standardized adjuvant chemotherapy protocols for RCC, and these tumors appear to respond poorly to most agents. Doxorubicin and cisplatin are often administered, but reports of efficacy are lacking. Immunotherapy with interferon-α and interleukin-2 is the treatment of choice for nonresectable or metastatic RCCs in humans, with up to 50% of patients exhibiting a measurable response (Rathmell, Godley, and Rini, 2005). Anecdotally interferon-α (1.5 to 2 million units/m^2 subcutaneously three times per week) may have therapeutic effect in some dogs with RCC.

Sarcomas

Primary renal sarcomas are the rarest primary renal tumors in dogs and cats in published case series, accounting for 4% to 11% of all nonlymphoma primary renal tumors (Henry et al., 1999; Klein et al., 1988). However, in the NCSU Oncology Service referral population 24% of primary renal tumors in dogs were hemangiosarcomas. Other reported renal sarcomas include fibrosarcoma, osteosarcoma, and anaplastic sarcoma. Clinical signs of renal sarcomas other than hemangiosarcoma are usually identical to those seen with RCC, and treatment and typical disease progression appear to be similar. Primary renal hemangiosarcoma may be less aggressive than visceral hemangiosarcoma arising from other sites, including slower rate of progression and decreased frequency of macroscopic metastasis at the time of diagnosis (Locke and Barber, 2006). Mean survival of 14 dogs was 278 days, with the worst outcome associated with hemoperitoneum at the time of diagnosis. Chemotherapy protocols for renal hemangiosarcoma have not been evaluated thoroughly, although a doxorubicin-based protocol likely is appropriate (see Chapters 65 and 66). Insufficient cases exist to reliably predict behavior or prognosis of other renal sarcomas, although a combination of surgery and adjuvant chemotherapy is recommended.

Nephroblastomas

Nephroblastomas are renal tumors that are thought to arise from undifferentiated embryonic elements (blastema). Diagnosis requires the presence of epithelial, stromal, and blastema elements within the tumor (Khoury, 2005). These tumors are histologically diverse and often may be confused with RCCs or sarcomas because of the predominance of one cell type. In humans nephroblastomas are also called Wilms' tumor and occur at much higher frequency in children (Khoury, 2005). Specific chromosomal mutations have been noted in many humans, but nephroblastomas in dogs and cats have not been examined yet for similar genetic alterations. Veterinary patients with nephroblastoma are often younger than patients with other primary renal tumors. Although dogs and cats as young as 1 year of age have been reported, clinical experience and published cases suggest that a second peak of occurrence exists at approximately the same age as other primary renal tumors. Hematuria is reported more frequently in patients with nephroblastoma than with other primary renal tumors. It appears that nephroblastomas are less likely to metastasize than other primary renal tumors and have a much better long-term prognosis; nephrectomy may be curative, although adjunctive chemotherapy should be given in cases in which histology suggests a less differentiated, more aggressive tumor. When metastasis does occur, the spinal cord is a common site.

Multifocal Renal Cystadenocarcinoma and Nodular Dermatofibrosis

Several related families of German shepherd dogs and German shepherd crossbreeds develop a syndrome of bilateral multifocal renal cystadenocarcinomas, nodular dermatofibrosis, and uterine leiomyomas; this disease also occurs sporadically in non-German shepherd dogs. Evidence suggests that affected dogs may have mutation in one allele of folliculin, a protein of unknown function; homozygous mutants are thought to die in utero. Histopathologic changes are similar to those noted in vitro with transforming growth factor–β dysregulation. Multiple renal cysts can be detected by imaging studies as early as 4 to 5 years of age, although diagnosis usually does not occur until later. Owners most commonly present their dogs for evaluation of diffuse skin nodules between 3 and 12 years of age (mean 8 years) (Moe and Lium, 1997). Renomegaly can be palpated in most dogs at the time of presentation. Long-term prognosis is poor since metastasis and renal failure are common; mean age at death is 9 years (Moe and Lium, 1997). Nephrectomy is contraindicated because both kidneys invariably are affected. Chemotherapy may be attempted, but successful therapy has not been reported; drugs that theoretically may be useful include paclitaxel and pirfenidone, although neither has been evaluated in clinical cases.

Lymphoma

Renal lymphoma is the most common kidney tumor in cats. At the NCSU Oncology Service 91% of renal tumors in this species were diagnosed as isolated or primary renal lymphoma. Unlike patients with other primary renal tumors, cats with renal lymphoma do present with signs and clinicopathologic changes of acute renal failure; up to 80% of cats have increased serum creatinine concentrations at the time of diagnosis (Mooney et al.,

1987). On physical examination the kidneys are usually bilaterally enlarged and irregular and may be painful when palpated. Renal shape and size are very similar to those in cats with severe polycystic kidney disease; abdominal ultrasound can be used for differentiation of the two diseases. The urinalysis is usually unremarkable with the exception of decreased urine concentration. Feline leukemia virus (FeLV) is strongly associated with development of renal lymphoma—approximately 50% of affected cats are FeLV positive (Mooney et al., 1987). Central nervous system involvement occurs at an increased frequency in cats with renal lymphoma, with approximately one third of cats developing neurologic abnormalities; most cats first exhibit signs of central nervous system involvement after disease recurrence rather than at the time of initial diagnosis (Mooney et al., 1987). Renal lymphoma is considered as advanced disease in most staging schemes; some oncologists classify affected cats as having stage III lymphoma, whereas others describe lymphoma in cats solely based on anatomic site.

Chemotherapy protocols for cats with renal lymphoma typically are the same as those for lymphoma affecting other parenchymal organs, usually incorporating L-asparaginase, vincristine, doxorubicin, cyclophosphamide, and prednisone (see Chapters 65 and 73). Approximately 60% of cats achieve complete remission, with a mean duration of remission of 372 days (median 127 days) and mean survival of 408 days (median 169 days) (Mooney et al., 1987). Nephrectomy is not recommended because, even though disease may not be overtly bilateral, both kidneys invariably are affected. Negative prognostic indicators include involvement of other organ systems (particularly the central nervous system), FeLV infection, and severity of renal failure, although larger studies are still needed to determine the relative weight of these factors (Mooney et al., 1987). Azotemia often improves dramatically with treatment of lymphoma so that renal failure is the eventual cause of death in a minority of cases. However, residual renal damage does persist in most cases and may affect ongoing decisions regarding treatment.

Dogs with stage V lymphoma may have neoplastic infiltration of the kidneys, particularly once disease has progressed to the terminal stages. As with cats, primary renal lymphoma cases do occur, although less frequently than carcinomas, sarcomas, or nephroblastomas. Dogs with renal lymphoma are less likely than cats to present with signs of uremia. Affected patients are more likely to show nonspecific signs of illness, with renal masses diagnosed on subsequent physical examination or diagnostic imaging studies. Both unilateral and bilateral renal involvement may occur; affected kidneys may be diffusely infiltrated or have masslike lesions. Dogs with primary renal lymphoma typically have limited involvement of other organs. As with cats, chemotherapy is the primary treatment for primary renal lymphoma in dogs. Protocols are the same as for dogs with nonrenal lymphoma (see Chapters 65 and 72), although dose modifications or alternate drug choices should be considered for renally excreted or nephrotoxic drugs. Unlike in cats, nephrectomy is a potential treatment option for dogs with unilateral renal lymphoma. However, nephrectomy should be considered only if azotemia and decreased urine concentrating ability are absent, if abdominal ultrasound or contrast radiography suggests only unilateral disease, and if no other sites of disease are identified. Adjunctive chemotherapy is recommended following nephrectomy.

Transitional Cell Carcinomas

Transitional cell carcinomas (TCCs) arise from the renal pelvis and make up approximately 20% to 30% of primary renal neoplasms in dogs and cats (Henry et al., 1999; Klein et al., 1988). Although not considered to be of renal origin, these tumors usually invade the renal parenchyma and have the same clinical course and treatment options as RCC and primary renal sarcomas. Compared to those tumors, TCCs are more likely to cause urinary obstruction, hydronephrosis, and hematuria. Differentiation of TCCs from high-grade/undifferentiated RCCs may be difficult; on careful review tumors in both groups are often reclassified (Henry et al., 1999).

Metastasis of Extrarenal Neoplasms

Because renal blood flow makes up approximately 15% of total cardiovascular output, metastasis of neoplastic cells to the kidney often occurs. Microscopic or gross infiltration by tumor cells is a common postmortem finding in animals that have died of metastatic neoplasia. Of the three tumor subtypes (carcinoma, sarcoma, and round cell tumors), carcinomas are most often implicated in metastatic spread of cancer to the kidneys. Interestingly, azotemia or clinical signs of renal failure are rare even when a large proportion of renal parenchyma has been infiltrated. Nonspecific treatment of renal failure (e.g., change to a renal-formulated diet, phosphate binders) should be instituted when necessary. Standard chemotherapy protocols should be altered to minimize administration of nephrotoxic agents if concurrent renal disease is suspected or confirmed.

Benign Tumors

Benign tumors account for 5% to 17% of primary renal tumors in dogs and cats (Henry et al., 1999; Klein et al., 1988). Adenomas, transitional cell papillomas, fibromas, mesoblastic nephromas, and hemangiomas have been reported. These tumors are most commonly incidental postmortem findings, although occasionally they may cause microscopic or gross hematuria or urinary obstruction. If diagnosed antemortem, vigilant monitoring or partial nephrectomy should be considered since insufficient cases have been described to exclude the possibility of malignant transformation.

Other Considerations

Paraneoplastic Syndromes
Primary renal tumors are rarely associated with paraneoplastic syndromes. Published case series of renal tumors in dogs and cats report an apparent incidence of less than 5% (Henry et al., 1999; Klein et al., 1988). Polycythemia

secondary to excess production of erythropoietin is the most common paraneoplastic syndrome caused by renal neoplasia. Although not a true paraneoplastic syndrome, polycythemia may also occur when renal tumors decrease local oxygen concentration, resulting in excess erythropoietin production by nonneoplastic renal epithelial cells. Polycythemia may be an incidental finding noted on complete blood count, or animals may present with epistaxis or central neurologic abnormalities such as disorientation or seizures. Measurement of serum erythropoietin concentration is of questionable value; erythrocytosis and presence of a renal mass usually are sufficient for diagnosis. Renal tumors reported to cause polycythemia in dogs include renal carcinomas, fibrosarcoma, and lymphoma; renal carcinoma has been associated with polycythemia in a cat. Nephrectomy typically results in resolution of the polycythemia, although metastasis of functional neoplastic cells may prevent resolution.

Other paraneoplastic syndromes reported in dogs with renal tumors include extreme leukocytosis, hypertrophic osteopathy, and hepatopathy. Paraneoplastic leukocytosis is caused by excess production of granulocyte-macrophage colony-stimulating factor. The profound leukocytosis is the result of a mature neutrophilia (although low numbers of immature cells are occasionally seen), with as many as 200,000 neutrophils/µl blood reported. This extreme neutrophilia usually does not result in any clinical signs, although mild hypoglycemia may occur. Hypertrophic osteopathy usually is palpable as firm swelling of the distal long bones, most prominent in the metaphyseal regions, and can be very painful. These two syndromes may occur concurrently, and both may resolve following successful tumor resection. Mild hepatopathy, characterized by elevations in alkaline phosphatase and γ-glutamyltransferase without concurrent hyperbilirubinemia, is common in humans with renal tumors; this syndrome has been reported in a dog with a sarcomatoid RCC.

Complications of Extra-Renal Cancer on the Kidney
Azotemia is common in dogs and cats with paraneoplastic hypercalcemia. A variety of tumor types may secrete parathyroid hormone–related protein (PTHrp) or other humoral factors that increase calcium release from bones and promote calcium absorption from the gastrointestinal tract (see Chapter 54). Although PTHrp is thought to exert its function by the same mechanisms as PTH, dogs and cats with hypercalcemia of malignancy usually have higher serum calcium and phosphorus concentrations and are more likely to develop kidney disease than those with hyperparathyroidism. Kidney damage may occur through a combination of mineralization of tubular basement membranes, dysregulated renal tubular cell mitochondrial function, dehydration secondary to hypercalcemia-induced polyuria, and alterations to glomerular filtration rate. Therapy for patients with hypercalcemia and kidney disease should include diuresis with 0.9% sodium chloride. Loop diuretics (e.g., furosemide) may be used to increase renal calcium excretion but should not be used before rehydration, and patients should be maintained on intravenous fluid therapy during administration. Bisphosphonate drugs inhibit osteoclast function and reduce mobilization of calcium stores

from bones. Pamidronate is highly effective when given at a dose of 1 to 2 mg/kg intravenously diluted in 0.9% NaCl and administered over 4 hours; faster infusions may cause nephrotoxicity. Prednisone may also be used to promote calciuresis but should only be considered once lymphoma has been excluded definitively as the cause of hypercalcemia; glucocorticoids can mask disease, making diagnosis more difficult, and also may worsen long term prognosis.

Kidney disease is found in a high proportion of humans with monoclonal gammopathies secondary to multiple myeloma or B-cell lymphoma. Contributing factors may include obstruction of renal tubules by light chains, toxicity to renal tubular epithelial cells via large-scale resorption and degradation of proteins, deposition of immunoglobulin light chains within the renal parenchyma, decreased renal perfusion caused by serum hyperviscosity, and tumor infiltration of the kidney. Obstruction of renal tubules and tubular cell toxicity (so-called *cast nephropathy*) has not been described definitively in dogs or cats. Immunoglobulin light chains also may cause amyloidosis or fibrillary nephropathy in humans, although only sporadic cases of light-chain–associated renal amyloidosis have been reported in dogs and cats. Syndromes of tubular cell dysfunction such as Fanconi syndrome or renal tubular acidosis have been reported in humans with multiple myeloma but have not been described in dogs or cats.

Glomerulonephritis in dogs and cats presumptively may occur secondary to any extrarenal inflammatory disease, including neoplasia. Membranous glomerulopathy is associated with carcinomas in humans in whom protein-losing nephropathies may develop while neoplasia remains occult. In dogs, although only approximately 30% of patients with glomerulonephritis are reported to have an identifiable concurrent extrarenal disease, the true incidence is likely much higher. Neoplasms reported to cause protein-losing nephropathies in dogs and cats include leiomyosarcoma, adrenal adenocarcinoma, and parathyroid adenoma (membranoproliferative glomerulonephritis); hemangiosarcoma, osteosarcoma, and mast cell tumor (membranous glomerulopathy); and mammary tumors and Sertoli cell tumor (reactive amyloidosis). TCC, bronchogenic adenocarcinoma, and lymphoma have also been reported to cause glomerulonephritis, although the histologic subtype was not described. Dogs with lymphoma or osteosarcoma may have microalbuminuria despite the absence of overt (positive standard urine dipstick) proteinuria.

Urinary obstruction secondary to neoplasms of the ureters, bladder, or urethra is a rare cause of postrenal azotemia and progressive renal injury. Surgical relief of obstruction is indicated, although azotemia in the presence of unilateral renal obstruction implies significant dysfunction of the contralateral kidney.

Tumor lysis syndrome, which occurs secondary to massive release of intracellular contents (particularly phosphorus, uric acid, and potassium) after chemotherapy in some dogs or cats with lymphoma, is another rare cause of renal failure. Precipitation of uric acid, calcium phosphate, or hypoxanthine in renal tubules, as well as cytokine-induced perturbations in renal blood flow, leads to rapid renal failure and often death in humans. Treatment should include rehydration and maintenance of renal perfusion via isotonic crystalloids, alkalinization of urine to inhibit uric acid precipitation, and appropriate treatment of life-threatening hyperkalemia and hypocalcemia.

Effects of Chemotherapy on the Kidney

Several chemotherapy agents are either regularly associated with nephrotoxicity or have been reported to cause renal disease as idiosyncratic reactions (also see chapters 65 and 66). The platinum compounds (primarily cisplatin) cause acute tubular necrosis by accumulation of platinum within proximal convoluted tubular cells. Diuresis with 0.9% saline is recommended both before and following treatment with cisplatin. Recommended protocols vary, but the NCSU Oncology Service administers 0.9% saline at 18.3 ml/kg/hour intravenously for 4 hours, and then administers cisplatin at the same diuresis rate over 20 minutes, followed by 2 more hours of diuresis at the same rate. Pretreatment with mannitol has also been suggested but is no longer routinely used. Streptozotocin also causes tubular necrosis, and a similar diuresis protocol is recommended.

Doxorubicin causes renal disease in cats by unknown mechanisms. Clinicians should consider alternative agents or more aggressive diuresis in cats with preexisting renal disease, and doxorubicin should be stopped in cats that develop proteinuria or azotemia during therapy. Methotrexate has been reported to cause tubular necrosis in dogs, although this is uncommon. Lomustine (CCNU) may cause idiosyncratic acute renal failure, although this is also very rare.

References and Suggested Reading

Barr FJ, Holt PE, Gibbs C: Ultrasonographic measurement of normal renal parameters, *J Small Anim Pract* 31:180, 1990.

Henry CJ et al: Primary renal tumours in cats: 19 cases (1992-1998), *J Feline Med Surg* 1:165, 1999.

Khoury JD: Nephroblastic neoplasms, *Clin Lab Med* 25:241, 2005.

Klein MK et al: Canine primary renal neoplasms: a retrospective review of 54 cases, *J Am Anim Hosp Assoc* 24:443, 1988.

Locke JE, Barber LG: Comparative aspects and clinical outcomes of canine renal hemangiosarcoma, *J Vet Intern Med* 20:962, 2006.

Moch H et al: Prognostic utility of the recently recommended histologic classification and revised TNM staging system of renal cell carcinoma: a Swiss experience with 588 tumors, *Cancer* 89:604, 2000.

Moe L, Lium B: Hereditary multifocal renal cystadenocarcinomas and nodular dermatofibrosis in 51 German shepherd dogs, *J Small Anim Pract* 38:498, 1997.

Mooney SC et al: Renal lymphoma in cats: 28 cases (1977-1984), *J Am Vet Med Assoc* 191:1473, 1987.

Rathmell WK, Godley PA, Rini BI: Renal cell carcinoma, *Curr Opin Oncol* 17:261, 2005.

Renshaw AA: Subclassification of renal cell neoplasms: an update for the practicing pathologist, *Histopathology* 41:283, 2002.

CHAPTER 202

Management of Feline Ureteroliths

ANDREW E. KYLES, *Davis, California*
JODI L. WESTROPP, *Davis, California*

URETEROLITHIASIS

Ureterolithiasis has emerged as an important cause of acute and chronic renal disease in cats over the last 15 years (Fig. 202-1). The emergence of ureterolithiasis has coincided with a dramatic change in the relative frequency of struvite and calcium oxalate (CaOx) uroliths in cats. In the 1970s and 1980s struvite urolithiasis predominated, but in 1993 CaOx superseded struvite as the most common urolith type and continues to be the most common mineral analyzed from cats at the Gerald V. Ling Urinary Stone Analysis Laboratory (Fig. 202-2). This change in urolith composition presumably is at least partially associated with dietary modification, such as urine acidification of proprietary cat food, to reduce the prevalence of struvite urolithiasis. Formation of CaOx uroliths does not depend on urine pH; however, highly acidifying diets can cause mobilization of calcium and phosphorus from the bone and therefore increase the concentration of these minerals in the urine. In a recent study we reported that 98% of feline ureteroliths contained CaOx (Kyles et al., 2005a). Therefore the emergence of ureterolithiasis may be associated with an increased prevalence of CaOx urolithiasis in cats, an increased awareness of ureterolithiasis, and/or an increased use of diagnostic imaging in cats with renal dysfunction.

The pathogenesis of CaOx urolithiasis in cats is poorly understood. Certain breeds such as Himalayan and Persian have an increased risk ratio for CaOx urolithiasis (OR = 4.39 and 2.82, respectively). In humans approximately 75% of kidney stones are composed predominantly of CaOx, and oxalate metabolism is thought to play a crucial role in stone development. Hyperoxaluria can occur from increased dietary intake, as well as from a loss or diminished activity of oxalate-degrading bacteria in the colon (*Oxalobacater formigenes*). Humans are also much more prone to developing nephrolithiasis, particularly in industrialized nations. Although urinary supersaturation with crystals is implicated in stone formation in humans, several studies have investigated the possibility that the urine is not the initial site of stone development. A vascular etiology for nephrolithiasis in humans has been proposed, suggesting that vascular abnormalities (e.g., hypertensive vascular injury, atherosclerosis) can lead to Randall's plaques (papillary lesions that are usually associated with calcium and phosphate or CaOx deposition) (Stoller et al., 2004). It has been hypothesized that the initiating event in CaOx nephrolithiasis in humans may occur in the vascular bed at the tip of the renal papilla, a deviation from traditional concepts regarding urolith initiation (e.g., urinary stasis, infection). No studies investigating this hypothesis have been published in cats or dogs.

Other intraluminal causes of ureteral obstruction include soft-tissue plugs (which sometimes contain flakes of mineralized material), pyelonephritis debris, and calculi that appear to be composed of dried solidified blood

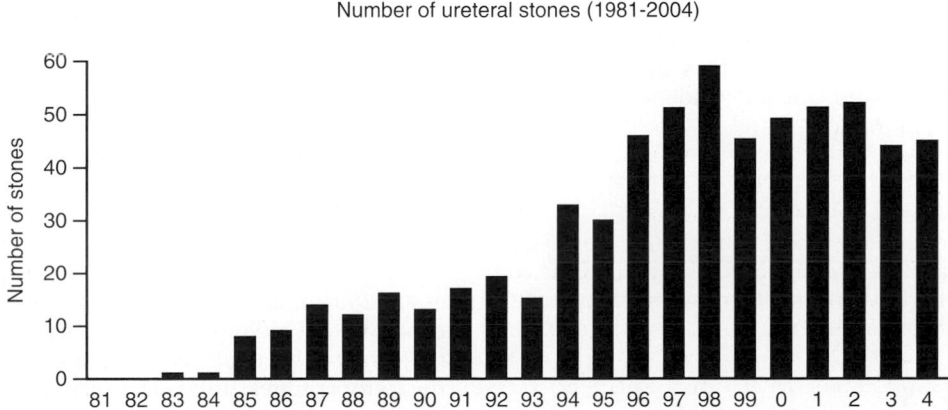

Number of ureteral stones (1981-2004)

Fig. 202-1 Number of calcium oxalate calculi from the upper urinary tract of cats submitted to the Gerald V. Ling Urinary Stone Analysis Laboratory, University of California, Davis. (Courtesy Dr. A. Cannon, University of California, Davis.)

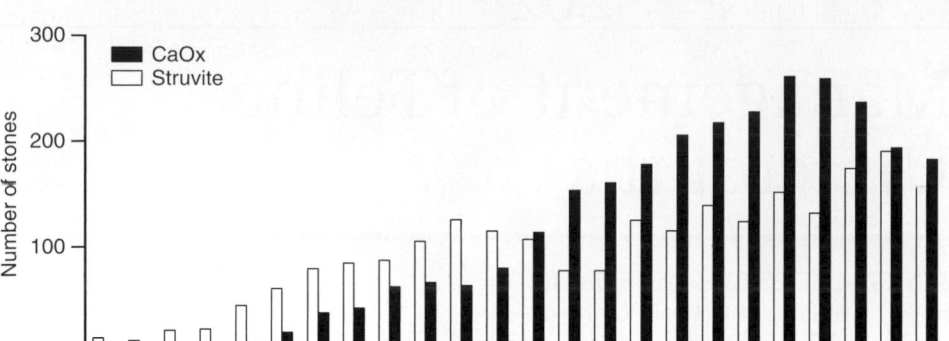

Fig. 202-2   Total number of calcium oxalate and struvite containing uroliths in cats submitted to the Gerald V. Ling Urinary Stone Analysis Laboratory, University of California, Davis. (Courtesy Dr. A. Cannon, University of California, Davis.)

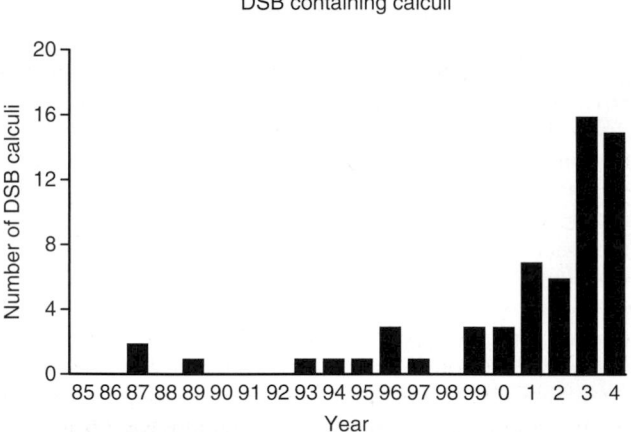

Fig. 202-3   Total number of calculi containing dried solidified blood from cats submitted to the Gerald V. Ling Urinary Stone Analysis Laboratory, University of California, Davis. (Courtesy Dr. A. Cannon, University of California, Davis.)

(DSB). These DSB calculi are very firm and "stonelike" but usually do not contain crystalline material (Westropp et al., 2006). The incidence of DSB calculi in cats also seems to be increasing (Fig. 202-3). These calculi are a particular diagnostic challenge because they are not visible on survey radiographs and are rarely identified during ultrasonographic examination.

SIGNALMENT

Ureterolithiasis tends to develop in middle-aged or older cats, with a median age at diagnosis of 7 years. Cats as young as 8 months have been diagnosed with ureteral calculi. There is no sex predilection.

CLINICAL SIGNS

Clinical signs are commonly nonspecific, including reduced appetite, weight loss, lethargy, and hiding. Cats also may present with hematuria without concurrent lower urinary tract signs such as stranguria, pollakiuria, and dysuria. Often cats may present with variable signs of renal failure, including vomiting, polyuria and polydipsia, and anuria. Some obstructed cats with severe azotemia experience surprisingly few clinical signs, whereas a few present in a moribund, hypothermic state. Kidney size can be normal, increased, or decreased and is frequently asymmetric. Abdominal pain, which is commonly reported in humans with ureteral calculi, is rarely recognized in cats.

CLINICOPATHOLOGIC FINDINGS

There is marked variation in serum creatinine and blood urea nitrogen concentrations in cats with ureteroliths. Factors that affect the degree of azotemia include whether the ureteral calculi are unilateral or bilateral, the degree of ureteral obstruction, the degree of impairment of renal function in each kidney, and the severity of prerenal azotemia. Although cats with bilateral ureterolithiasis tend to have higher serum creatinine and blood urea nitrogen concentrations, 76% of cats with unilateral ureteral calculi are azotemic, indicating impairment of renal function in the contralateral kidney, obstruction of the contralateral ureter, or prerenal azotemia (Kyles et al., 2005a).

DIAGNOSTIC IMAGING

Diagnostic imaging of the abdomen should be performed in all cats with acute or chronic renal failure. With the exception of most DSB calculi, all the ureteral calculi we have analyzed contain CaOx or calcium phosphate and therefore are radiopaque. The sensitivity of survey abdominal radiography for the diagnosis of ureterolithiasis is 81% (Kyles et al., 2005a). Small calculi, calculi overlying the colonic contents, and radiolucent calculi may be missed on survey radiographs. Ureteral calculi are most readily identified in the retroperitoneal area on the lateral radiographic projection; however, visibility on lateral radiographs alone can lead to difficulty in determining which ureter is involved or whether one or both ureters are affected.

The sensitivity of abdominal ultrasonography for the diagnosis of ureteral calculi is 77% (Kyles et al., 2005a). Partial or complete ureteral obstruction, indicated by dilation of the renal pelvis, ureter, or both, is observed in 92% of cats. Ureteral dilation tends to begin proximally and, as the degree of hydroureter increases, extend distally. The hydroureter often does not extend to the level of the ureteral calculus; this may explain why the calculus is not identified in 23% of cases. A combination of survey radiography and ultrasonography is recommended and has a sensitivity of 90% for the diagnosis of ureterolithiasis.

Additional imaging modalities such as antegrade pyelography or computed tomography (CT) may be necessary to identify calculi that are not apparent on survey radiographs or ultrasonography. Percutaneous antegrade pyelography can be used to determine if ureteral obstruction is present. A 2.5-inch, 25-gauge spinal needle is placed through the parenchyma of the kidney into the renal pelvis under ultrasound guidance. Urine is withdrawn, which can be submitted for cytologic examination and bacteriologic culture. A volume of aqueous, iodinated contrast media equal to half the volume of urine removed is infused into the pelvis. Care should be taken not to inadvertently advance the needle through the renal pelvis into the abdomen because this can result in uroabdomen. Contrast-enhanced CT is superior to other imaging modalities for determining the presence of ureteroliths, their number, and position. In our practice CT has largely replaced antegrade pyelography for imaging cats with apparent ureteral obstruction if ureteral calculi cannot be identified by survey radiographs and ultrasound.

Intravenous urography and nuclear scintigraphy are of limited use because ureteral obstruction reduces the filtration of contrast media or isotope. This results in poor opacification of the upper portion of the urinary tract during intravenous urographic studies and an artificial decrease in the calculated glomerular filtration rate (GFR) with nuclear scintigraphy. Scintigraphic measurement of individual kidney GFR may aid in prognosis and management decisions, particularly if nephrectomy of the obstructed kidney is considered.

MEDICAL MANAGEMENT

All cats with ureteral calculi receive medical management until it is determined whether the ureteral calculi will pass into the bladder. Conservative medical management for stable cats generally consists of supportive therapy for renal failure (Chapters 190 and 191) and treatments designed to increase the likelihood of relief of ureteral obstruction. Fluid diuresis alone or in combination with diuretic drug therapy (furosemide, mannitol) may improve the likelihood of passage of ureteral calculi. In humans intravenously administered glucagon causes relaxation of the ureteral smooth muscle and promotes passage of calculi. In cats we did not observe any beneficial effects of glucagon (0.1 mg per cat intravenously). Other drugs such as α-adrenergic antagonists (prazosin, tamsulosin), amitriptyline (a tricyclic antidepressant), and calcium channel blockers have also been used to facilitate ureterolith passage in humans; but there are no reported studies of the use of these drugs in cats with ureterolithiasis.

Cats with markedly high serum creatinine concentrations at the time of initial examination benefit from aggressive medical management such as hemodialysis or emergency nephrostomy catheter placement, although the mortality rate in cats undergoing these treatments is significantly higher than in cats that do not undergo them (Kyles et al. 2005b). The aim of dialysis or emergency nephrostomy catheter placement is to reduce the degree of azotemia, allow time to determine whether the calculus will pass on its own, and improve the clinical condition of the cat in preparation for surgery. Seventy-two percent (13 of 18) of cats treated with dialysis survived to surgery, three cats died, and two experienced a marked reduction in the degree of azotemia without surgery, presumably because of passage of the ureterolith (Kyles et al., 2005b). Nephrostomy catheters can be placed either via an emergency laparotomy or by an ultrasound-guided, percutaneous technique. By alleviating the postrenal component of azotemia, preoperative nephrostomy catheter placement has the added advantage of allowing a preoperative assessment of the remaining renal function in the obstructed kidney.

During conservative management cats are monitored by serial measurement of serum creatinine and blood urea nitrogen concentrations and serial ultrasonography or abdominal radiography. Repeated imaging studies should be performed in cats undergoing medical therapy to document passage of calculi. The degree of improvement in renal function after passage of the ureteral calculus is variable, with some cats experiencing a marked decrease in azotemia and others showing little or no change in the serum creatinine concentration, presumably reflecting the underlying degree of irreversible renal dysfunction. In cats treated medically that survived longer than 1 month after diagnosis, the 12-month survival rate was 66%, with a number of cats dying of causes related to chronic renal insufficiency or recurrent ureterolithiasis (Kyles et al., 2005b). Fifty percent of cats (6 of 12) had a serum creatinine concentration greater than the upper reference limit at 6 to 12 months after diagnosis (Kyles et al. 2005b).

SURGICAL MANAGEMENT

Surgical removal of ureteral calculi is warranted when there is evidence of partial or complete ureteral obstruction, as indicated by hydronephrosis and dilation of the ureter proximal to the obstruction, and when the calculus is immobile on repeated imaging examinations. Major factors determining the recovery of renal function after reestablishing ureteral patency include the duration and extent of the obstruction. In research dogs GFR is almost completely recovered after relief of complete ureteral obstruction within 4 days, 46% of GFR returned after 14 days of obstruction, and almost no GFR returned after 40 days of obstruction. In cats the optimal time for medical management before making a decision to pursue surgery has not been determined. The reported median interval between diagnosis and surgery was 3 days (Kyles et al., 2005b).

The surgical technique used depends on the location of the calculus and the preference of the surgeon. The two most common techniques for removing ureteral calculi are *ureterotomy* and *partial ureterectomy combined with ureteroneocystostomy*. For both techniques surgical magnification is required, and use of an operating microscope preferred.

Ureterotomy

Ureterotomy is indicated in cats for the removal of intraluminal ureteral obstructions and can be performed at any level of the ureter. If the ureteral calculus cannot be readily identified, a piece of suture material can be advanced up the ureter from the bladder to identify the level of the obstruction. The ureter should be handled with care, and the blood supply preserved. The ureter is surrounded by fat, which should be dissected away from the ureter. A longitudinal incision is made with a scalpel blade and extended with scissors. Normally the calculus is readily removed, although occasionally it becomes embedded in the ureteral wall. Care should be taken to prevent a ureteral calculus from inadvertently being pushed back into the renal pelvis. After calculus removal the ureter is flushed with sterile saline, and a catheter or length of suture material is passed proximally into the renal pelvis and distally to the level of the bladder to ensure that the ureter is patent. The ureterotomy is closed with 8-0 monofilament suture material. A simple continuous suture pattern is preferred. The most common complication in cats is urine leakage and uroabdomen, which is reported in 16% of cats after ureterotomy (Kyles et al., 2005b).

Partial Ureterectomy and Ureteroneocystostomy

Ureteroneocystostomy involves reimplantation of the distal ureter into the bladder and is used to reestablish urine flow after resection of the distal ureter. The technique is most often performed to remove distal ureteral calculi, although up to 80% of the feline ureter can be resected, and ureteroneocystostomy successfully achieved if appropriate tension-relieving techniques are applied. Techniques for ureteroneocystostomy can be divided into intravesicular (e.g., the mucosal apposition technique), which are performed from within the bladder and require a cystotomy for access, and intravesicular (e.g., the modified Lich-Gregoir technique). The modified Lich-Gregoir technique is preferred in cats, particularly cats with minimum preexisting ureteral dilation, because it is associated with a reduced degree of postoperative swelling and ureteral obstruction (Mehl et al., 2005).

For the modified Lich-Gregoir technique, a 1-cm seromuscular incision is made at the apex of the bladder, and a 0.5-cm incision is made in the mucosa at the caudal aspect of the seromuscular incision. The distal 0.5- to 1-cm of the ureter is dissected free from the periureteral fat and spatulated. The mucosa of the ureter is sutured to the bladder mucosa using a simple interrupted pattern and 8-0 monofilament suture material. The first suture is placed at the apex of the spatulation, and the second at the distal end of the spatulation. A length of 5-0 suture material is placed into the ureter to ensure patency. A minimum number of mucosal sutures, usually six, is required because an excessive number of sutures increase the risk of postoperative ureteral obstruction. The seromuscular layer is closed using a simple interrupted pattern

and 5-0 monofilament suture material. The mucosal layer should provide accurate mucosal apposition, whereas the seromuscular layer provides the watertight seal. Uroabdomen is the most common complication of ureteroneocystostomy and occurs with a similar frequency to that observed after ureterotomy in cats with ureteral calculi (15%)(Kyles et al., 2005b). Cats should be evaluated carefully for postoperative ureteral obstruction at the level of the stoma after ureteroneocystostomy. Routine monitoring of serum creatinine concentrations with serial ultrasound examinations is indicated in the postoperative period.

Ureteroureterostomy

Ureteroureterostomy is performed rarely in cats with intraluminal obstructions. The technique is technically more difficult than ureteroneocystostomy and can be recommended only when a portion of the proximal ureter is resected and the ureter cannot be reimplanted into the bladder. The chances of ureteral stricture are reduced by increasing the circumference of the anastomosis by spatulation. It is also possible to attach the ureter to the contralateral ureter (transureteroureterostomy).

Techniques for Tension Reduction

Tension on the ureteroneocystostomy or ureteroureterostomy anastomosis increases the risk of dehiscence or stricture formation and should be avoided. Tension can be reduced by *renal descensus* and *psoas cystopexy*. Renal descensus involves dissecting the kidney from its retroperitoneal attachments and performing a nephropexy to attach the kidney to the body wall in a more caudal location. Psoas cystopexy involves pulling the apex of the bladder craniolaterally toward the kidney and suturing the bladder to the psoas muscle dorsally. It is also possible to dissect the kidney from its retroperitoneal attachments and suture the kidney directly to the bladder (nephrocystopexy) if necessary.

Nephrostomy Catheters

The feline ureter is too small to allow placement of a ureteral stent. Nephrostomy tubes have been recommended for urine diversion following ureterotomy in cats. However, complications related to nephrostomy catheter placement are common and include uroabdomen, poor drainage, and catheter dislodgment. In cats with ureteral calculi a ureterotomy can be performed without placement of a nephrostomy catheter (Kyles et al., 2005b).

Nephrotomy

Nephroliths are common in cats with ureteral calculi. One study reported radiographic or ultrasonographic evidence of nephroliths in 62% of cats with ureterolithiasis (Kyles et al., 2005a), although this is probably an overestimation since it can be difficult to differentiate renal calculi from renal pelvic calcification. In most of these cats a nephrotomy is not indicated based on traditional criteria such as obstruction of urine flow, pain, or chronic pyelonephritis. However, there is justifiable concern that a nephrolith may move into the ureter and cause another episode of ureteral obstruction. The counter argument is that a cat with a degree of ureteral obstruction may be more likely to leak urine through a concurrent nephrotomy incision. We have not routinely performed a nephrotomy in cats with concurrent ureteral and renal calculi. One interesting approach is to perform a mini-nephrotomy approach to allow insertion of an endoscope and endoscopic retrieval of calculi in the renal pelvis or proximal ureter (Kuntz, 2005). Unfortunately recurrence of urolithiasis and ureteral obstruction is possible regardless of whether or not nephroliths are removed.

Nephrectomy

Nephrectomy can be considered in cats with unilateral ureteral obstruction and adequate function in the contralateral kidney. However, ureteral obstruction may be bilateral, and renal function is often already compromised in both kidneys in affected cats, precluding sacrifice of one kidney. Furthermore, there is a risk of recurrence of obstruction in the contralateral kidney. For these reasons definitive surgery rather than nephrectomy is usually indicated.

Renal Transplantation

Renal transplantation is a viable treatment for chronic kidney disease in cats after relief of the ureteral obstruction. There is a risk of formation of calculi in the allograft. In transplant patients with a history of urolithiasis, it is recommended to use absorbable suture material in the urinary tract, to carefully monitor for urinary tract infection, and to feed a diet designed to prevent the recurrence of CaOx calculi. In one group of cats there was no difference in the long-term outcome for allograft recipients when stone formers were compared to cats with an underlying cause of renal failure that was not related to urolithiasis (Aronson et al., 2006).

Prognosis for Surgical Treatment

The overall morbidity and mortality rates for the postoperative period, defined as the first month after surgery, are 31% and 18%, respectively (Kyles et al., 2005b). In cats that survived longer than 1 month after surgery, the 12-month survival rate was 91%, with a number of cats dying of causes related to chronic renal insufficiency, recurrent ureterolithiasis, or nonregenerative anemia (Kyles et al. 2005b). Fifty-two percent of cats (23 of 44) had a serum creatinine concentration greater than the upper reference limit at 6 to 12 months after diagnosis (Kyles et al. 2005b).

RECURRENCE

Because of the possibility of recurrence of CaOx uroliths, several proposed management strategies should be implemented. If serum calcium concentration is elevated, a search should be initiated for underlying causes such as primary hyperparathyroidism, neoplastic processes, renal secondary hyperparathyroidism, and idiopathic hypercalcemia in cats (Chapter 52). Appropriate medical and dietary management should be instigated in cats with renal failure. Hypocitraturia is a risk factor for CaOx

---

Box **202-1**

Commercial Diets Marketed To Assist With Prevention of the Formation of CaOx Calculi in Cats

- Eukanuba Veterinary Diets Nutritional Urinary Formula Moderate pH/O/Feline canned and dry
- Hill's Prescription Diet Feline x/d canned and dry
- IVD Feline Mature Formula canned and dry
- IVD Feline Modified Formula canned and dry
- Purina Veterinary Diets NF Kidney Function Feline Formula canned and dry
- Royal Canin Veterinary Diet Feline Urinary SO canned and dry

---

stone formation in humans because citrate is chelated to calcium, forming a more soluble salt. Citrate supplementation appears beneficial in humans, but no studies are available in cats that evaluate the effect of citrate supplementation on CaOx calculus formation. If supplementing potassium citrate (75 mg/kg orally BID), the serum potassium concentration should be evaluated periodically, particularly if renal function is compromised, to be certain the cat does not become hyperkalemic. Potassium citrate is also reported to interact with aluminum-containing phosphate binders. Hydrochlorothiazide is a diuretic that decreases urine calcium excretion in humans and has been recommended to prevent recurrence of CaOx formation in dogs. Again, studies in affected cats are lacking.

Many diets are marketed to prevent the recurrence of CaOx uroliths in cats with normal renal function (Box 202-1). The cat should never be offered the new diet while hospitalized, and the new diet should be placed next to the old one so the cat can transition to the preferred diet slowly. Periodic urine samples should be evaluated. The urine should be relatively dilute (<1.025), and the sediment should be free of pronounced crystalluria. Serial abdominal imaging studies should be performed to detect recurrence of CaOx urolithiasis. Further information on CaOx urolith prevention can be found at: http://www.vetmed.ucdavis.edu/vme/stonelab.

References and Suggested Reading

Aronson LR et al: Renal transplantation in cats diagnosed with calcium oxalate urolithiasis: 19 cases (1997-2004), *J Am Vet Med Assoc* 225(5):743, 2006.

Kuntz CA: Retrieval of ureteral calculus using a new method of endoscopic assistance in a cat, *Aust Vet J* 83:480, 2005.

Kyles AE et al: Clinical, clinicopathologic, radiographic and ultrasonographic abnormalities in cats with ureteral calculi; 163 cases (1984-2002), *J Am Vet Med Assoc* 226:932, 2005a.

Kyles AE et al: Management and outcome of cats with ureteral calculi; 153 cases (1984-2002), *J Am Vet Med Assoc* 226:937, 2005b.

Mehl ML et al: Comparison of 3 techniques for ureteroneocystostomy in cats, *Vet Surg* 34:114, 2005.

Stoller ML et al: The primary stone event: a new hypothesis involving a vascular etiology, *J Urol* 171:1920, 2004.

Westropp JL et al: Dried solidified blood calculi in the urinary tract of cats, *J Vet Intern Med* 20(4):828, 2006.

CHAPTER 203

Incomplete Urolith Removal: Prevention, Detection, and Correction

JODY P. LULICH, *St. Paul, Minnesota*
CARL A. OSBORNE, *St. Paul, Minnesota*

Recurrence of uroliths following surgery is commonly attributed to failure of medical therapy to adequately reduce factors promoting urolith formation. However, this hypothesis is based on the premise that all stones were completely removed from the urinary tract before therapeutic intervention. We performed a retrospective study of cystotomies performed to remove urocystoliths from 37 dogs and 29 cats in our veterinary teaching hospital. Incomplete removal of uroliths was documented in eight dogs and four cats. The observation that uroliths were detected in the lower urinary tract following cystotomy in 20% of cats and 14% of dogs in a teaching hospital with board-certified surgeons on the staff emphasizes an inherent risk associated with this procedure. Based on our experience and consultations with our colleagues in private practice, incomplete removal of uroliths occurs more frequently than is recognized. Remaining uroliths are commonly discovered several weeks or months following surgery when patients are reevaluated because of persistent or recurrent signs of lower urinary tract disease. In this situation delayed detection of uroliths often is erroneously attributed to recurrence (or rather pseudorecurrence). This in turn may result in inaccurate and inappropriate prognostic and therapeutic recommendations to prevent future recurrence. The most common cause of rapid recurrence of uroliths is incomplete surgical removal.

Pseudorecurrence can also occur when uroliths are eradicated by other modalities (e.g., medical dissolution, voiding urohydropropulsion, laparoscopic-assisted cystotomy, lithotripsy). The following discussion describes techniques to prevent, detect, and correct pseudorecurrence following surgical removal of uroliths. In most instances these principles and procedures can be applied to other methods of urolith eradication as well.

PREVENTING PSEUDORECURRENCE

Avoiding incomplete urolith removal requires a high degree of suspicion that, even when using best surgical techniques, considers that uroliths can evade detection and removal. To minimize this complication, the following procedures should be considered.

Inform the Client

When discussing the option of surgery to remove uroliths from the lower urinary tract, clients should be informed that even in the hands of experienced surgeons there is a risk that not all of the uroliths will be removed. To minimize this complication, appropriate procedures to assess success will be performed following surgery. Clients should also be informed of the consequences of incomplete removal of uroliths and the benefits and risks of therapeutic strategies available to manage this complication.

Confirm Urolith Location and Number Before Removal

Uroliths often migrate to lower portions of the urinary tract. Therefore, if several days have elapsed between the date of diagnostic imaging and the date of surgery scheduled to remove uroliths, the number and location of stones should be reevaluated by appropriate imaging methods just before surgery. This number can be compared with the number of stones removed. Disparities should arouse sufficient concern to pursue diagnostic procedures to rule out pseudorecurrence.

Reposition Urethroliths to the Urinary Bladder

To avoid performing two surgical incisions, urethroliths should be flushed into the urinary bladder before surgery. Retrograde urohydropropulsion is a simple and effective method of dislodging and propelling urethral stones into the urinary bladder. Following general anesthesia and just before surgery, approximately 30 ml of sterile lactated Ringer's solution or normal saline should be rapidly and forcefully flushed through the urethra using a flexible wide-bore catheter. It is important to remember to remove most of the urine from the urinary bladder (by decompressive cystocentesis or manual expression) before hydropropulsion to permit maximal retrograde hydrostatic pressure and to avoid iatrogenic bladder rupture caused by overfilling.

Consider Presurgical Urethral Catheterization

Placement of large-diameter catheters following retrograde urohydropropulsion has both benefits and risks.

Urethral catheterization can minimize the migration of urocystoliths back into the urethra. Placement of a cuffed (Foley) catheter such that the inflated balloon obstructs the trigone may more effectively prevent urolith migration than catheters without dilation capabilities. However, urethral catheterization increases the risk of iatrogenic infection. In addition, stones that enter the urethra with the catheter in place may become more securely wedged in the urethra as the catheter is withdrawn.

Strive for Complete Urolith Removal

Appropriate care should be taken to remove all uroliths from the bladder lumen, bladder neck, and urethra. Uroliths may be removed with the aid of spoons, forceps, gauze sponges, or suction devices. The lumen of the bladder and bladder neck should be explored with a finger to detect remaining uroliths. In addition, the bladder lumen should be flushed with an isotonic solution to remove subvisual uroliths.

Flush the Urethra Before Closing the Urinary Bladder

Uroliths that have passed into the urethral lumen during cystotomy are easily flushed back into the bladder lumen by injecting appropriate quantities of physiologic saline through a catheter placed in the external urethral orifice. It is important that the catheter tip reside only in the most distal portion of the urethra. The external urethral orifice should be occluded around the catheter to facilitate flushing of the urethroliths back into the bladder lumen. If the distal urethra is not occluded, fluid may flow around small urethroliths without moving them into the bladder. Appropriate caution must be used to minimize retrograde flushing of bacteria that normally colonize the mucosa of the distal urethra and genital tract into the urinary bladder and surgical site.

Normograde urethral flushing (i.e., inserting a flexible catheter in the urethral lumen via the urinary bladder) may also enhance patency of the urethra by forcing small uroliths out the distal urethral orifice. However, caution must be considered when flushing larger stones unable to exit the external urethral orifice. If attempted, some uroliths may become securely lodged in the urethra lumen such that their placement is not easily reversed by retrograde urohydropropulsion.

DETECTING PSEUDORECURRENCE

Procedures that facilitate immediate detection of uroliths inadvertently left in the urinary tract following surgery have become a standard of practice. If uroliths obstruct the urethra before the cystotomy incision heals, life-threatening complications may develop. Also, if uroliths remaining in the lower urinary tract following surgery are first detected by radiography or ultrasonography several weeks after surgery, it may be assumed erroneously that the patient is highly predisposed to recurrent urolithiasis. The following options should be considered to accurately detect pseudorecurrence.

Urolith Number

When possible, the number of uroliths removed from the lower urinary tract should be compared with the number of uroliths detected by radiography, ultrasonography, or via cystoscopy. Incongruities in the count should raise suspicion that uroliths remain in the lower urinary tract, are deposited in the abdomen, or have been evacuated by suction.

Transurethral Catheterization

Normograde and retrograde passage of urinary catheters is a common method of assessing complete urolith removal. However, it is our opinion that it is an insensitive tool. This is especially true for uroliths with an irregular contour (e.g., calcium oxalate and silica) that allow catheters and flushing solutions to slide past when lodged in the urethral lumen.

Therefore large-bore catheters should be selected. Any resistance to advancement of the catheter through the urethral lumen should prompt appropriate evaluation of the urethra for persistent uroliths. Under these conditions forceful attempts to advance the catheter through the urethral lumen may inadvertently tear the wall of the urethra or cause the uroliths to become so firmly lodged in the urethral lumen that retrograde urohydropropulsion is ineffective.

Radiography

Radiography is a valuable technique in the diagnosis of pseudorecurrence and has become the standard of care. In a recent case review by the Professional Liability Insurance Trust (PLIT) for the American Veterinary Medical Association, a veterinarian who does not perform radiography to verify complete removal of uroliths following cystotomy is practicing substandard care (PLIT, 2005). Therefore we recommend that appropriate medical imaging be performed following cystotomy to verify complete urolith removal.

Radiographic detection of residual uroliths depends on their size, location, and mineral composition. Although survey radiography is suitable for identification of radiopaque uroliths greater than approximately 2 to 3 mm in diameter, contrast-enhanced procedures are needed to identify uroliths composed of compounds similar to the radiographic density of soft tissue (e.g., ammonium urate, cystine, xanthine). Double-contrast cystography is the preferred technique because it has been associated with the highest sensitivity and lowest false-negative detection rates (Fig. 203-1). Although we commonly inject room air as the negative contrast agent, carbon dioxide (CO_2 refills and dispenser, Genuine Innovation) or nitrous oxide is preferred to minimize the risk of air embolization. Following instillation of negative contrast agent, we inject 1 to 4 ml of iodinated contrast, depending on bladder size. A minimum of three orthogonal views are recommended by some to completely evaluate the urinary bladder: left lateral, right lateral, and a ventrodorsal view. We routinely evaluate the urinary bladder with two lateral views, one before and one following bladder instillation of contrast

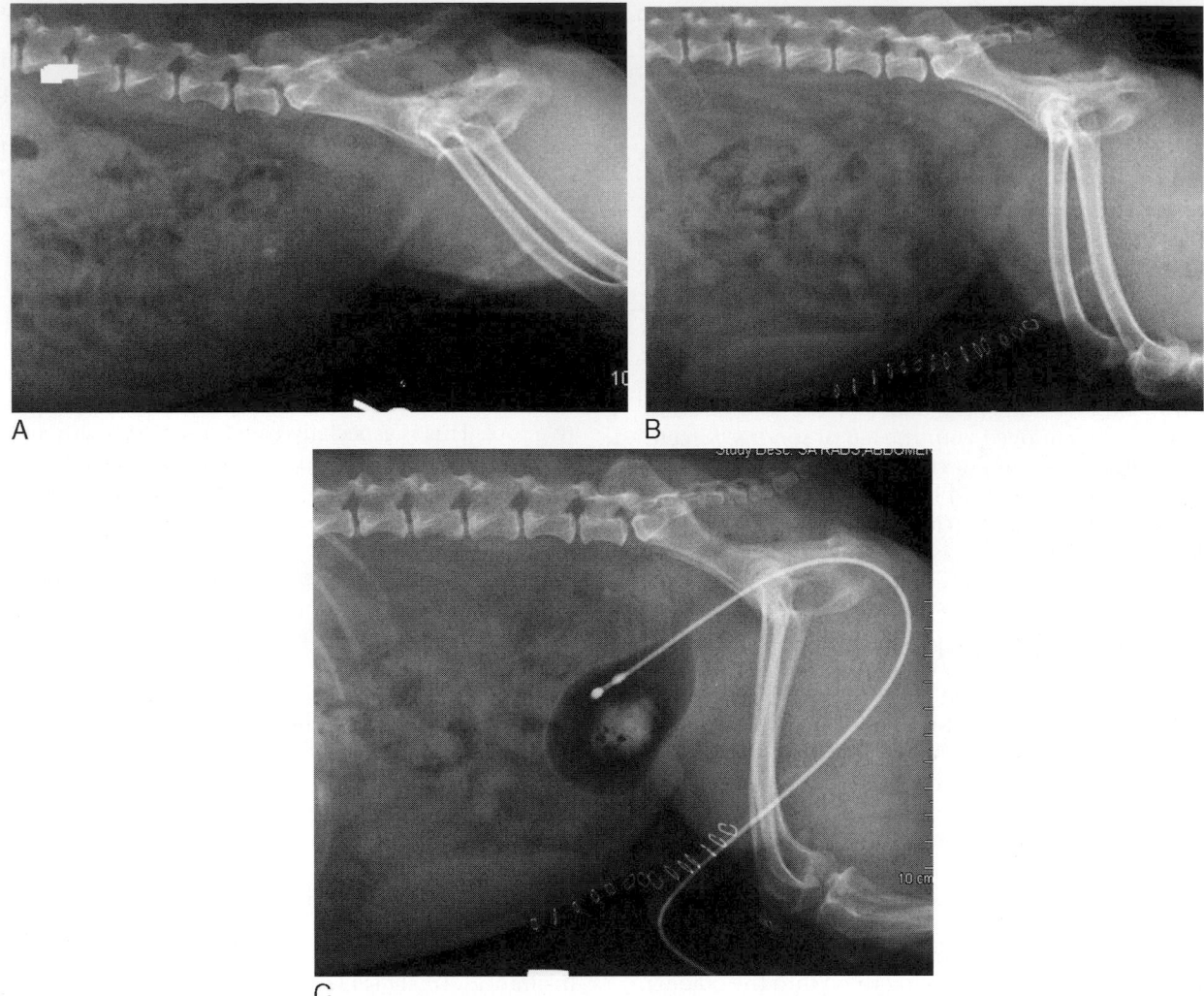

Fig. 203-1 Presurgical **(A)** and postsurgical **(B)** lateral survey radiographs of a 5-year-old male miniature Schnauzer illustrating multiple calcium oxalate uroliths in the bladder and urethra. Double contrast cystography **(C)** confirmed the number and location of pseudorecurrent uroliths.

agents. In some cases stones lodged in the pelvic urethra escape radiographic detection because they become obscured by the bones of the pelvis. If this is likely, rectal palpation of the pelvic urethra should be sufficient to detect their presence. Ultrasonographic examination is rarely useful immediately following surgery because additional air in the abdomen limits visualization. In addition, ultrasound examination does not detect residual stones located in the urethra.

Postsurgical Endouroscopy

For clinics with endoscopic capabilities, visually evaluating the lumen of the urinary tract is one of the most sensitive methods of detecting pseudorecurrence of urethroliths. Small-diameter flexible endoscopes are used in male dogs. Endouroscopy is of limited benefit in male cats because the narrow urethral lumen limits the availability of suitable equipment that can pass through the urethral lumen. Larger, rigid endoscopes are suitable for female dogs and cats. Endouroscopy not only has the advantage of identifying uroliths, but small stones capable of passing

through the urethra can be retrieved and removed (see sections on Basket Retrieval and Intracorporeal Lithotripsy later in the chapter).

CORRECTING PSEUDORECURRENCE

Depending on urolith size and shape, stones remaining after surgery may obstruct the urethra, contribute to hematuria, perpetuate urinary discomfort, and/or increase the risk of urinary tract infection. Therefore, to avoid these complications, uroliths should be removed promptly. Below are several therapeutic options for managing pseudorecurrent uroliths.

Spontaneous Voiding

Small uroliths capable of passing through the urethra may pass spontaneously, obviating the need for additional therapy. Following surgery normal bladder healing is associated with increased dysuria and pollakiuria, favoring increased bladder evacuation and subsequent urolith expulsion. It has been our experience that, if uroliths have not voided spontaneously after 1 to 3 months, their spontaneous evacuation is unlikely to occur. After this time other methods of urolith removal should be considered.

Medical Dissolution

Pseudorecurrent uroliths composed of magnesium ammonium phosphate, cystine, or salts of urate can be dissolved medically. It is important to recognize that uroliths located in the urethra are not likely to dissolve because they are not surrounded by urine that is undersaturated for that particular mineral. Therefore urethroliths need to be flushed back into the urinary bladder, and their position periodically monitored to improve success of dissolution therapy.

Surgical Removal

Ideally patients should be evaluated for complete urolith removal immediately after completion of surgery and before recovery from anesthesia. This facilitates the surgeon's ability to reexplore the lower urinary tract without reanesthetizing the patient. If the patient's cardiovascular system is unstable, anesthesia should be discontinued, and the surgery postponed until potentially life-threatening complications can be controlled.

For some patients retrograde urohydropropulsion needs to be performed to flush urethroliths back into the urinary bladder. This should be performed before entering the surgical area. By doing so, the surgeon can better anticipate the approach to remove retained uroliths.

Basket Retrieval

Retrieving stones cystoscopically with a stone basket is ideal for removing small stones that can easily be pulled through the urethra. A variety of stone baskets are available to facilitate this technique (Stone Retrieval Grasping Forceps, Boston Scientific; N-Circle Nitinol Tipless Stone Extractor, Cook Urologic, Inc.).

It is logical to ask, "Why can't they be removed by voiding urohydropropulsion?" Voiding urohydropropulsion is a simple and effective technique for urolith removal. However, excessive distention of the urinary bladder with saline and/or manual expression of the urinary bladder following surgery increases the chance of bladder rupture. Therefore voiding urohydropropulsion should be avoided.

Intracorporeal Lithotripsy

Intracorporeal lithotripsy is ideal for uroliths that become lodged in the urethra following surgery. In this situation the urethra often holds the urolith stationary, facilitating accurate and consistent delivery of laser energy. Under these conditions urethroliths are quickly fragmented into smaller pieces that can be retrieved or flushed out of the urinary tract. Lithotripsy can also be used to manage uroliths left in the bladder (see Chapter 204). Combined with basket retrieval techniques, lithotripsy is a safe and effective method of correcting pseudorecurrent uroliths.

References and Suggested Reading

Feeney DA et al: Imaging canine urocystoliths: detection and prediction of mineral composition, *Vet Clin North Am Sml Anim Pract* 29:59, 1999.

Lulich J et al: Incomplete removal of canine and feline urocystoliths by cystotomy, *J Vet Intern Med* 7:124, 1993.

Lulich JP et al: Voiding urohydropropulsion: lessons learned from 5 years of experience, *Vet Clin North Am Small Anim Pract.*29:283, 1999.

Osborne CA et al: Canine retrograde urohydropropulsion: lessons from 25 years of experience. *Vet Clin North Am Small Anim Pract* 267, 1999.

Professional Liability Insurance Trust (PLIT): Omission of radiograph falls below standard of care, *Summer newsletter* 24(3):1, 2005.

CHAPTER 204
Laser Lithotripsy for Uroliths

LARRY G. ADAMS, *West Lafayette, Indiana*
JODY P. LULICH, *St. Paul, Minnesota*

Lithotripsy is crushing or fragmenting uroliths by shock waves or laser energy. Types of lithotripsy include extracorporeal shock wave lithotripsy (SWL), electrohydraulic lithotripsy, and laser lithotripsy. SWL is mainly used for treatment of nephroliths and ureteroliths (Adams and Senior, 1999). Although electrohydraulic lithotripsy can be performed to fragment urocystoliths in larger female dogs (Adams and Senior, 1999), this technique has been replaced by the safer and more efficient laser lithotripsy method. Laser lithotripsy is a relatively new option for fragmentation and removal of lower tract uroliths visualized using rigid or flexible endoscopes (Adams and Lulich, 2006).

In humans laser lithotripsy using the holmium: YAG (Ho:YAG) laser has become the standard of care for intracorporeal fragmentation of uroliths. In humans laser lithotripsy is principally used for fragmentation of ureteroliths and small nephroliths (Lingeman, Lifshitz, and Evan, 2003). Although the Ho:YAG laser can be used to fragment and remove large staghorn nephroliths in humans, this approach is often not practical because the large stone burden requires prolonged or multiple procedures. Likewise, SWL has a lower success rate than percutaneous nephrolithotomy for removal of staghorn nephroliths (Lam et al., 1992). Therefore percutaneous nephrolithotomy is considered the procedure of choice for most large staghorn nephroliths (Lingeman, Lifshitz, and Evan, 2003).

Urolith size, number, and location are important considerations for selecting minimally invasive procedures (e.g., voiding urohydropropulsion, laparoscopic-assisted cystotomy, and laser lithotripsy) for urolith management in dogs and cats (see also Chapter 203). Voiding urohydropropulsion may be used to remove uroliths that are smaller than the diameter of the dilated urethra. Laser lithotripsy effectively extends the use of voiding urohydropropulsion to larger uroliths by fragmenting uroliths into smaller pieces before transurethral evacuation (Figs. 204-1 and 204-2).

Prior in vitro studies confirmed that the Ho:YAG laser can efficiently fragment uroliths from dogs regardless of chemical composition (Wynn et al., 2003). Likewise, experimentally implanted urethroliths in male dogs were safely fragmented by laser lithotripsy using the Ho:YAG laser (Davidson et al., 2004). We recently reported successful laser lithotripsy fragmentation and removal of bladder and urethral calculi from dogs with spontaneously occurring uroliths (Adams and Lulich, 2006).

EQUIPMENT NEEDED FOR LASER LITHOTRIPSY

The Ho:YAG laser is the preferred laser for lithotripsy. The active medium of this laser is a crystal of yttrium, aluminum, and garnet (YAG) doped with holmium, with a wavelength of 2100 nm, which is in the near infrared portion of the electromagnetic spectrum. Because the 2100-nm wavelength of the Ho:YAG laser is absorbed in 0.5 mm of fluid, it can be used to safely fragment uroliths within the urethra or urinary bladder with minimal or no damage to the urothelium. The Ho:YAG laser energy is delivered in 350-microsecond pulses and is quickly dispersed in water surrounding the tip of the laser fiber. Ho:YAG lasers are available with total power ranging from 20 to 100 watts, but the lower-power lasers (20 to 30 watts) are adequate for laser lithotripsy.

Laser lithotripsy can be performed through small-diameter flexible ureteroscopes (e.g., 7.5 to 8.5 Fr), which are used for urethrocystoscopy in male dogs, and rigid cystoscopes (e.g., 9 to 19 Fr), which are used in female dogs and cats. The size of the cystoscope is based on the size of the dog or cat. The laser energy of the Ho:YAG laser is transferred from the laser unit to the surface of the stone through small-diameter (200- to 550-micron) flexible quartz laser fibers. These special fibers are passed through the working channel of the cystoscope. When working through the biopsy channel of rigid cystoscope, we use a 365- or 550-micron quartz laser. Both 200- and 365-micron fibers pass through the 3-Fr working channel of a flexible endoscope, although care must be used to avoid damaging the working channel with the rigid tip of the fiber. To protect the working channel from damage, a laser catheter can be passed through it before passage of the laser fiber. In the event of accidental discharge of the laser while the fiber tip is within the working channel of the scope, the laser catheter provides minimal protection to the scope. The smaller-diameter fibers have minimal impact on the ability to deflect the tip of flexible ureteroscopes and allow for efficient targeting of urethral calculi.

Additional equipment required for laser lithotripsy includes stone baskets used for extraction of urolith fragments. A variety of stone baskets are available from various manufacturers. We prefer tipless baskets that facilitate capture of small stone fragments within the urethra or bladder lumen. Although not essential, C-arm fluoroscopy is helpful to document urolith size and location during laser lithotripsy. This is most helpful in male dogs because

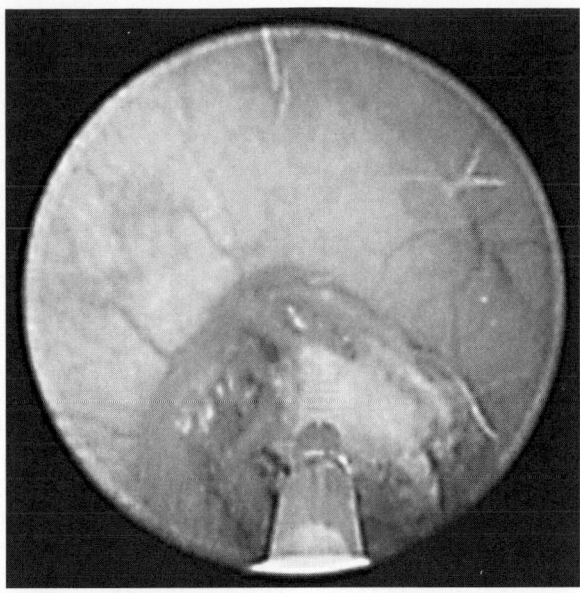

Fig. 204-1 Cystoscopic view of laser lithotripsy of a calcium oxalate urolith within the bladder lumen of a female dog. Note that the quartz laser fiber tip is in direct contact with the urolith surface. Small urolith debris can be seen as streaks within the saline used to distend the urinary bladder.

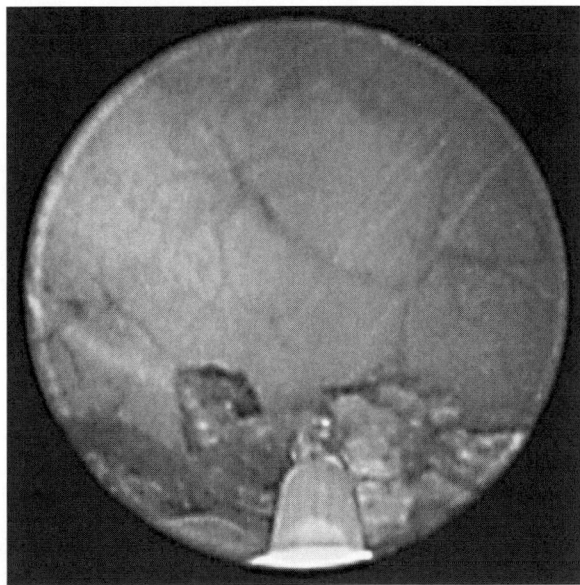

Fig. 204-2 Multiple urolith fragments in bladder lumen after laser lithotripsy fragmentation of the calcium oxalate urolith. The remaining urolith fragments are small enough to pass through the urethra.

of the limited visualization provided through flexible ureteroscopes. Fluoroscopy-aided retrograde contrast studies can also be performed to detect anatomic abnormalities associated with the uroliths and to document complete urolith removal. In female dogs and cats the entire bladder lumen can be readily visualized through the rigid cystoscope, making concurrent fluoroscopy less essential.

LASER LITHOTRIPSY TECHNIQUE

Laser lithotripsy is performed with urolith visualization by urethrocystoscopy. Detailed description of urethrocystoscopy is beyond the scope of this chapter and has been described elsewhere (Adams, 2006; Chew et al., 1996). We prefer to position female dogs and cats in dorsal recumbency and male dogs in lateral recumbency for laser lithotripsy. The area around the vulva or prepuce is clipped to remove surrounding hair and prepped for aseptic introduction of the cystoscope into the urethra and bladder. During cystoscopy irrigation of sterile warmed normal saline is used to distend the urinary tract and facilitate cystoscope passage. Once the uroliths are visualized in the urethra or bladder, a flexible quartz laser fiber is advanced through the working channel of the scope and connected to the laser unit.

To achieve optimum fragmentation of the urolith, the quartz fiber tip must be guided with the aid of a cystoscope so that it is in direct contact with the surface of the urolith before laser activation. During laser lithotripsy continuous irrigation of warmed sterile normal saline serves to absorb stray laser energy and flush urolith debris and fragments out of the visual field to maintain visibility. We use initial power and frequency settings of 0.5 to 0.7 joules per pulse and 6 to 10 Hz for laser lithotripsy. Increasing the frequency of laser pulses (Hz) increases the efficiency of urolith fragmentation but decreases the operator's potential reaction time in the event that the laser fiber tip inadvertently contacts the urothelium. Therefore the lowest laser settings that result in effective urolith fragmentation should be used during laser lithotripsy.

During laser activation the energy is limited to an area directly in front of the quartz laser fiber tip. An aiming beam within the visible spectrum is used to facilitate targeting the laser energy. The laser fiber should not be aimed directly at the mucosal surface and should be kept 0.5 mm or more away from the mucosal surface during laser activation. Therefore it is preferable to apply laser energy to the urolith surface while working parallel rather than perpendicular to the mucosa (see Figs. 204-1 and 204-2). In the event of brief laser application directly to the mucosal surface, mucosal injury is usually limited to superficial damage and associated bleeding. When in contact with the mucosal surface, the Ho:YAG laser is capable of making incisions into the bladder or urethral wall; perforation is possible during laser lithotripsy. The Ho:YAG laser can be used effectively in contact mode to remove small pedunculated polyps or tumors within the urinary tract without creating full-thickness incisions. With proper technique the risk of bladder or urethral perforation is minimal during laser lithotripsy.

Once uroliths are fragmented so that the fragments are small enough to pass through the urethra, larger fragments are removed initially with a stone basket to verify that the fragments are small enough to allow removal by antegrade voiding. Urolith fragments retrieved with stone baskets using aseptic technique should be submitted for bacterial culture and quantitative urolith analysis. If the larger fragments were safely retrieved through the urethra, voiding urohydropropulsion is performed to evacuate remaining fragments.

Because of their larger urethral diameter, laser lithotripsy is successful in most female dogs and cats, and all stone fragments can be removed from the lower urinary tract. When all urolith fragments are documented to have been removed, the patient is considered stone free. Transurethral cystoscopy and laser lithotripsy results in stone-free status in approximately 80% of male dogs and 100% of female dogs (Adams and Lulich, 2006). In some male dogs laser lithotripsy of urethroliths may be followed by cystotomy to remove larger urocystoliths.

INDICATIONS FOR LASER LITHOTRIPSY

Minimally invasive removal of urethrocystoliths via laser lithotripsy is possible for female dogs and cats and for most male dogs larger than approximately 6 kg of body weight. With additional training and experience, laser fragmentation of ureteroliths and nephroliths in larger dogs is also feasible.

In male dogs the narrow urethral diameter along with curved course of the urethra around the ischial arch effectively limits the size of dog in which a transurethral approach is possible. The dog's size along with the size and number of uroliths that must be fragmented and removed transurethrally are considered to determine if male dogs are suitable candidates for laser lithotripsy. Alternative minimally invasive approaches for removal of urocystoliths in small male dogs include percutaneous cystoscopy, laparoscopic-assisted cystoscopy, and SWL fragmentation of bladder stones followed by voiding urohydropropulsion. Laser lithotripsy via transurethral approach may not be the best option for removal of very large stone burdens in male or female dogs because of the volume of fragments that must be flushed through the urethra following laser fragmentation.

ADVANTAGES OF LASER LITHOTRIPSY

Laser lithotripsy offers many advantages for urolith removal when compared to surgical approaches. One significant advantage of minimally invasive stone removal is reduced postprocedural dysuria and hematuria. Therefore owner preference plays a significant role when choosing whether to remove urocystoliths by open cystotomy or minimally invasive techniques such as laser lithotripsy. Laser lithotripsy can rapidly correct life-threatening urethral obstruction caused by uroliths. In fact, the procedural time is often shorter than surgery. Because cystoscopy can be performed safely immediately following cystotomy, uroliths not completely removed surgically can be fragmented and basketed without an additional incision (see Chapter 203). Dogs with recurrent uroliths may be managed repeatedly with laser lithotripsy via a transurethral approach to avoid repeated cystotomy. We have performed laser lithotripsy three times over a 23-month period in one male dog with recurrent calcium oxalate urolithiasis.

CONTRAINDICATIONS TO LASER LITHOTRIPSY

One relative contraindication to transurethral laser lithotripsy is the presence of an active urinary tract infection.

Because increases in intravesicular pressure during voiding urohydropropulsion may induce vesicoureteral reflux (and contribute to ascending pyelonephritis), urinary tract infections should be controlled with antimicrobics before lithotripsy. With an active urinary tract infection, small perforations of the bladder wall also could spread microorganisms into the abdominal cavity. Perioperative antimicrobics should be administered to dogs or cats with any history of current or prior urinary tract infection, because fragmentation of infected uroliths may liberate viable bacteria from the inner layers of the urolith.

Other contraindications to transurethral laser lithotripsy include coagulopathy and obstruction of the urinary outflow distal to the urolith (e.g., urethral stricture). With coagulopathies transurethral passage of the cystoscope and laser lithotripsy may result in intraluminal or periurethral hemorrhage. Therefore coagulopathies should be resolved if possible before attempting laser lithotripsy. Urethral strictures may preclude the passage of the cystoscope and make removal of urolith fragments more difficult because of the narrow urethral lumen through the strictured region.

POTENTIAL COMPLICATIONS OF TRANSURETHRAL LASER LITHOTRIPSY

Complications resulting from laser lithotripsy have been uncommon. The most common complication seen during prolonged transurethral cystoscopy is swelling of the urethral mucosa, which becomes particularly important in male dogs because of the narrow diameter of the urethral lumen. Acute mucosal swelling may preclude transurethral passage of the flexible ureteroscope in and out of the urinary bladder and prevent complete urolith fragmentation and removal. If this occurs, allowing 1 to 3 days for the urethral swelling to resolve may permit complete urolith removal. Urethral swelling may also result in transient outflow obstruction in some dogs after prolonged transurethral laser lithotripsy procedures.

Mucosal bleeding during laser lithotripsy may result in extravasation of blood and formation of blood clots within the bladder lumen. Blood clots tend to trap smaller urolith fragments against the mucosal surface, which may preclude complete removal of all fragments by voiding urohydropropulsion. In humans "second-look" procedures (such as percutaneous nephroscopy) are often used to remove any residual urolith fragments 1 to 2 days after the initial minimally invasive urolith removal technique. Similarly, second-look cystoscopy and voiding urohydropropulsion are required in some dogs and cats after laser lithotripsy.

Because Ho:YAG laser energy can be used to incise tissues, laser perforation of the urethra or bladder is possible. Given the small diameter of the quartz laser fibers, small-diameter holes caused by laser perforation of the bladder or urethra most likely can be resolved by placing an indwelling transurethral catheter and keeping the urinary tract decompressed for 3 to 5 days. If laser perforation is suspected, retrograde contrast studies should be used to document any leakage from the urinary tract and to confirm that the perforation has healed before removal of the indwelling urinary catheter.

Another potential source of complications from trans-urethral laser lithotripsy and removal of the fragments is trauma to the bladder or urethra during voiding urohy-dropropulsion to remove the urolith fragments. Transient urethral obstruction may occur when large numbers of urocystolith fragments are voided simultaneously through the urethra. If this occurs, repeat laser fragmenta-tion of fragments within the urethral lumen can be used to resolve the obstruction. In addition, excessive intrave-sicular pressure applied to the bladder during transient urethral obstruction (in an attempt to flush out urolith fragments) could lead to bladder perforation. Proper void-ing urohydropropulsion technique is required to prevent this complication.

SWL fragments stones mechanically, whereas laser fragmentation relies on a photothermal mechanism, pos-sibly inducing chemical alterations in stone composi-tion (Chan et al., 1999). This difference is not clinically relevant for most stone types; however, laser lithotripsy converts uric acid uroliths to small quantities of cyanide. Although cyanide can by absorbed into systemic circula-tion, the risk of clinical toxicity is very low (Teichman et al., 1998). We have safely removed uric acid uroliths from several dogs and one cat without complications related to cyanide toxicity. Our attempts to detect cya-nide production in the effluence during cystoscopy and lithotripsy have been unsuccessful. Nonetheless, constant irrigation of saline and frequent evacuation of the urinary bladder during the procedure are recommended to pre-vent cyanide from potentially accumulating in higher concentrations.

References and Suggested Reading

Adams LG: Cystoscopy. In Elliot J, Grauer GF, editors: *Manual of small animal nephrology and urology*, ed 2, London, 2006, British Small Animal Veterinary Association, p 192.

Adams LG, Lulich JP: Laser lithotripsy for removal of uroliths in dogs. In Kollias N et al, editors: Proceedings of SPIE, ed 6078, Bellingham, Wash, 6078:36, 2006.

Adams LG, Senior DF: Electrohydraulic and extracorporeal shock-wave lithotripsy, *Vet Clin North Am Small Anim Pract* 29:293, 1999.

Chan KF et al: Holmium:YAG laser lithotripsy: a dominant pho-tothermal ablative mechanism with chemical decomposition of urinary calculi, *Lasers Surg Med* 25:22, 1999.

Chew DJ et al: Urethroscopy, cystoscopy, and biopsy of the feline lower urinary tract, *Vet Clin North Am Small Anim Pract* 26:441, 1996.

Davidson EB et al: Laser lithotripsy for treatment of canine uro-liths, *Vet Surg* 33:56, 2004.

Lam HS et al: Staghorn calculi: analysis of treatment results between initial percutaneous nephrostolithotomy and extra-corporeal shock wave lithotripsy monotherapy with reference to surface area, *J Urol* 147:1219, 1992.

Lingeman JE, Lifshitz DA, Evan AP: Surgical management of uri-nary lithiasis. In Retik AB et al, editors: *Campbell's urology*, ed 8, Philadelphia, 2003, Saunders, p 3361.

Teichman JM et al: Holmium:YAG lithotripsy: photothermal mechanism converts uric acid calculi to cyanide, *J Urol* 160:320, 1998.

Wynn VM et al: In vitro effects of pulsed holmium laser energy on canine uroliths and porcine cadaveric urethra, *Lasers Surg Med* 33:243, 2003.

CHAPTER 205

Management of Feline Nonobstructive Idiopathic Cystitis

JOHN M. KRUGER, *East Lansing, Michigan*
CARL A. OSBORNE, *St. Paul, Minnesota*

In approximately 65% of nonobstructed male and female cats with naturally occurring lower urinary tract disease, the exact cause(s) of hematuria, dysuria, pollakiuria, stranguria, and periuria (urinating outside the litter box) are still unknown. After appropriate diagnostic evaluations, these cats are classified as having idiopathic feline lower urinary tract disease, idiopathic cystitis, or interstitial cystitis. In the past four decades over 70 agents or procedures have been recommended for management of nonobstructive idiopathic cystitis in cats; yet fewer than 10% of these proposed treatments have been evaluated in controlled clinical trials (Box 205-1). Debate surrounding the efficacy of various treatments is complicated by the self-limiting nature of clinical signs associated with the majority of cases of idiopathic cystitis. In this setting any form of therapy might appear to be beneficial as long as it is not harmful. The self-limiting nature of clinical signs in many cats with idiopathic cystitis underscores the need for controlled prospective double-blind clinical studies to prove the efficacy and safety of various forms of therapy.

BIOLOGIC BEHAVIOR

Periuria, pollakiuria, stranguria, and gross hematuria are the most common clinical signs observed in cats with nonobstructive idiopathic cystitis. Remarkably these clinical signs subside within 5 to 7 days (without therapy) in up to 92% of cats with acute nonobstructive idiopathic cystitis (Barsanti et al., 1982, Kruger et al., 2003; Osborne et al., 1996). Signs may recur after variable periods of time and again subside without treatment. Approximately 40% to 50% of cats with acute idiopathic cystitis experience recurrence of signs within 1 to 2 years (Barsanti et al., 1982; Kruger et al., 2003). Our impression is that recurrent episodes of acute idiopathic cystitis tend to decrease in frequency and severity as the cats become older (Kruger et al., 2003). Although recurrent clinical signs in patients with idiopathic cystitis are often assumed to be recurrence of the original disease, they may also be the result of a delayed manifestation of the original disease (e.g., spontaneous or iatrogenic urethral stricture) or onset of a different lower urinary tract disease associated with similar clinical signs (e.g., urolithiasis).

We have also encountered a small subset of cats with idiopathic cystitis in which clinical signs persist for weeks to months or recur frequently. These cats are classified as having chronic idiopathic cystitis. In our experience fewer than 15% of cats evaluated because of acute idiopathic cystitis will develop chronic forms of the disease. Whether chronic idiopathic cystitis represents one extreme in the spectrum of clinical manifestations associated with similar etiologic factors or whether it represents an entirely different mechanism of disease than that associated with acute self-limiting idiopathic disease is unknown.

TREATMENT OF IDIOPATHIC CYSTITIS

Overview

Specific recommendations for management of cats with acute and chronic idiopathic cystitis ideally should be based on results of controlled clinical trials that document the efficacy and safety of therapeutic agents. We emphasize that all of the following general recommendations for treatment of nonobstructive idiopathic cystitis have not been substantiated by experimental and/or clinical investigations. Some of our recommendations are based on our uncontrolled clinical observations and personal opinions and should be considered within this framework.

Management of cats with nonobstructive idiopathic cystitis should encompass (1) thorough diagnostic evaluation to exclude other causes of lower urinary tract disease (Table 205-1); (2) client education emphasizing the biologic behavior of the disease and lack of controlled studies demonstrating efficacy of proposed therapies; (3) strategies to minimize urethral obstruction; (4) consideration of use of pharmacologic agents to reduce the severity and duration of clinical signs; (5) strategies to minimize risk of recurrence; and (6) prevention of iatrogenic disease. We approach treatment of cats with acute idiopathic cystitis by (1) emphasizing client understanding of the disease, and (2) minimizing the risk of recurrence through use of long-term dietary and environmental management strategies. Short-term use of pharmacologic agents is considered for any patient with severe clinical signs. Long-term pharmacologic inventions usually are reserved for cats with more severe chronic forms of the disease in which dietary and environmental management strategies have failed to adequately control clinical signs or frequency of recurrences.

944

Box 205-1

Therapeutic Agents or Procedures Advocated by Veterinarians for Management of Nonobstructive Feline Idiopathic Cystitis Over a 3-Year Period From 2003 To 2005

Antiinflammatories/Analgesics
- Prednisolone*
- Methylprednisolone
- Dexamethasone
- Piroxicam
- Meloxicam
- Ketoprofen
- Carprofen
- Tolfenamic acid
- Tepoxalin
- DMSO
- Zafirlukast
- Montelukast
- Butorphanol
- Buprenorphine
- Oxymorphone
- Fentanyl
- Tramadol

Environmental Management
- Environmental enrichment
- Litter box management
- Facial pheromone*

Antidepressants/Anxiolytics
- Amitriptyline*
- Nortriptyline
- Imipramine
- Clomipramine
- Fluoxetine
- Paroxetine
- Diazepam
- Oxazepam
- Alprazolam
- Buspirone

Antispasmodics
- Propantheline*
- Oxybutynin
- Aminopentamide
- Atropine
- Acepromazine
- Prazosin
- Phenoxybenzamine
- Dantrolene
- Flavoxate

Antimicrobics
- Doxycycline
- Enrofloxacin
- Amoxicillin
- Amoxicillin/clavulanate

Dietary Management
- Canned diets*
- Acidifying diets
- Hypoallergenic diets
- Omega 3 fatty acids
- Supplemental water

Glycosaminoglycans
- Pentosan polysulfate
- Glucosamine*
- Chondroitin sulfate
- Polysulfated glycosaminoglycans
- Hyaluronate

Miscellaneous
- Parenteral fluids*
- Furosemide
- Megestrol acetate
- Hydroxyzine
- Cyproheptadine
- Trimeprazine
- Cromolyn
- Arginine
- Hydrodistention

Alternative Medicine
- Acupuncture
- Colloidal silver
- Cantharis
- Terebinthina
- Marshmallow root
- Parsley root
- Uva ursi leaf
- Corn silk
- Dandelion
- Polyporus mushroom
- Others

Compiled from the Veterinary Information Network http://www.vin.com.
*Indicates therapies that have been evaluated by controlled clinical trials.

Antimicrobial Agents

Antimicrobial agents commonly have been used for decades as empiric therapy for hematuria, dysuria, and pollakiuria in cats. However, the infrequency (1% to 3%) with which bacteria have been identified at the onset of clinical signs of lower urinary tract disorders in young to middle-aged cats has been well established. The uselessness of antimicrobial agents in the treatment of abacteriuric cats with lower urinary tract disease also has been documented (Barsanti et al., 1982). Widespread empiric use of antimicrobial agents for treatment of cats with lower urinary tract signs may have been perpetuated at least in part by misinterpretation of "pseudobacteria" observed in unstained urine sediment and failure to perform diagnostic quantitative urine cultures to confirm bacterial urinary tract infection. In a recent study in our laboratory, up to 89% of unstained feline urine sediments reported as positive for bacteriuria by light microscopy were found to be sterile when compared to results of quantitative

Table 205-1

Diagnostic Plan for Feline Dysuric Hematuria Without Urethral Obstruction

Factor	CLINICAL PRESENTATION	
	First or Infrequent Episodes	Frequent or Persistent Episodes
Defined history	+++++†	+++++
Defined physical examination	+++++	+++++
Urinalysis (with sediment)*	+++++	+++++
Screening, quantitative urine culture*	+++	++++
Serum chemistry profile (esp. serum urea nitrogen, creatinine, potassium ion, and bicarbonate)	+	++
Assess lesion(s), site(s), and cause(s)		
Palpation	+++++	+++++
Survey radiography	+++	+++++
Ultrasonography	+++	+++++
Contrast radiography (retrograde urethrocystography or antegrade cystourethrography)	+	++++
Urethrocystoscopy	+	++++
Complete blood count	+	+++
Cystotomy and biopsy‡	Infrequent	±

*Urine sample preferably collected by cystocentesis. CAUTION: cystocentesis commonly causes hematuria.
†The number of +'s indicates relative importance.
‡Exploratory cystotomy is only indicated when there is reason to believe that the results will justify the risks to the patient and associated costs to the client.

urine culture. Staining of urine sediment with a modified Wright-stain procedure (Diff Quik) significantly reduces the frequency of false-positive bacteriuria.

Amitriptyline and Other Antidepressants

Amitriptyline hydrochloride (Elavil, Astra-Zeneca Pharmaceuticals) has been advocated for the treatment of severe recurrent idiopathic cystitis in cats. Amitriptyline is a tricyclic antidepressant drug with anticholinergic, antihistaminic, sympatholytic, analgesic, and antiinflammatory properties. In humans several weeks to months of treatment are often necessary before the antidepressant actions of amitriptyline are clinically evident. In contrast, the anticholinergic, antihistaminic, sympatholytic, analgesic, and antiinflammatory effects of amitriptyline and other tricyclic antidepressants are more rapid in onset (often within several days). Consequently amitriptyline and other tricyclic antidepressants have been used in humans for treatment of various nonpsychiatric conditions. Amitriptyline has been used extensively for treatment of humans with interstitial cystitis. In a recent randomized placebo-controlled, double-masked study of amitriptyline for treatment of interstitial cystitis in humans, 63% of patients receiving amitriptyline for 4 months rated satisfaction with the therapeutic outcome as good or excellent compared to only 4% of patients receiving a placebo. In an uncontrolled study of cats with severe recurrent idiopathic cystitis, clinical signs decreased in 9 of 15 (60%) cats treated with amitriptyline for 6 months (Chew et al., 1998). However, in a randomized double-masked, placebo-controlled clinical trial to evaluate the efficacy of short-term (7-day) amitriptyline therapy in ameliorating clinical signs in 31 cats with acute nonobstructive idiopathic cystitis, amitriptyline did not appear to reduce the duration of pollakiuria

and hematuria (Kruger et al., 2003). In addition, clinical signs recurred sooner and with higher frequency in amitriptyline-treated cats than in cats receiving a placebo. Adverse events associated with amitriptyline treatment included urinary tract infection, sedation, hyperbilirubinemia, and increased serum alanine aminotransferase (ALT) activity. In another placebo-controlled study of cats with idiopathic cystitis performed by other investigators, differences were not observed in the magnitude of change in severity of clinical signs after short-term (7-day) treatment with amitriptyline and amoxicillin compared to a placebo and amoxicillin (Kraijer, Fink-Gremmels, and Nickel, 2003).

These results suggest that short-term (7-day) amitriptyline treatment is of little benefit in resolving pollakiuria and hematuria in cats with acute idiopathic cystitis. However, the apparent lack of beneficial effects of short-term administration does not preclude the possibility that long-term amitriptyline administration may be of value for cats with more severe or persistent forms of idiopathic cystitis. Pending results of controlled clinical trials, we reserve amitriptyline for cats with severe chronic idiopathic cystitis who have not responded to other forms of pharmacologic, dietary, and environmental management (Table 205-2). If improvement in clinical signs is not observed after 2 to 4 months of therapy, the dosage of the drug should be tapered gradually over several weeks and then stopped. In humans abrupt discontinuation of tricyclic antidepressants may result in a withdrawal syndrome characterized by gastrointestinal, somatic, neurologic, and psychiatric disturbances. The efficacy and safety of other tricyclic antidepressants, selective serotonin reuptake inhibitors, and anxiolytics advocated for management of chronic or frequently recurrent forms of idiopathic cystitis have not been evaluated by controlled clinical trials (see Table 205-2).

Table 205-2

Therapeutic Options for Pharmacologic Management of Feline Idiopathic Cystitis

Agent	Properties	Dose*	Controlled Trial?	INDICATIONS AND OUR FORECAST[†]		Adverse Effects/Special Considerations
				Acute FIC	Chronic FIC	
Butorphanol (Torbugesic)	Analgesic	0.2-0.4 mg/kg q8h PO for 1-3 days	NR	++		Sedation, ataxia, anorexia, diarrhea
Buprenorphine (Buprenex)	Analgesic	0.01-0.02 mg/kg q6-12h IM, SQ, buccally for 1 to 3 days	NR	++		Sedation, respiratory depression
Fentanyl (Duragesic)	Analgesic	1.25-2.5 mg q72h transdermally	NR	+		Respiratory depression, bradycardia, urine retention, constipation, dysphoria, agitation
Tramadol (Ultram)	Analgesic	ND (4 mg/kg q12h PO for 1-3 days)	NR	+		Respiratory depression, anorexia, constipation, diarrhea, behavior changes; avoid concurrent administration of antidepressants; combination product containing acetaminophen (Ultracet, Ortho-McNeil Pharmaceutical) is contraindicated in cats
Tolteridine (Detrol)	Anticholinergic, antispasmodic	ND (0.05 mg/kg q12h PO)	NR	+	+	Vomiting, diarrhea, constipation, urine retention, sedation; amitriptyline may potentiate adverse effects
Pentosan polysulfate (Elmiron)	GAG analog	50 mg q12h PO	NR		+	Diarrhea, vomiting (rare)
Chondroitin sulfate/ Glucosamine hydrochloride	GAG/ GAG precursor	Chondroitin sulfate 8.8 mg/kg 22/Glucosamine HCl 22 mg/kg q24h PO	NR		+	Gastrointestinal upset (rare)
Amitriptyline (Elavil)	Antidepressant, sympatholytic, Anticholinergic, antihistamine, analgesic	5-12.5 mg q12-24h PO	Yes (acute) NR (chronic)		++	Sedation, weight gain, urine retention, urolith formation, UTI, increased liver enzymes; avoid short-term use or rapid discontinuation
Clomipramine (Clomicalm)	Antidepressant, sympatholytic, anticholinergic, antihistamine, analgesic	0.5 mg/kg q24h PO	NR		+	Sedation, vomiting, diarrhea, anticholinergic effects; avoid short-term use or rapid discontinuation
Buspirone (BuSpar)	Anxiolytic	2.5-5 mg q12h PO	NR		+	Sedation (rare), behavior changes
Fluoxetine (Prozac)	Antidepressant	0.5-1 mg/kg q24h PO	NR		+	Diminished appetite, vomiting, lethargy, anxiety, irritability, sleep disturbances

GAG, Glycosaminoglycan; IM, intramuscularly; ND, not determined; NR, not reported; PO, orally; SQ, subcutaneously; UTI, urinary tract infection.
*Values in parentheses indicate an approximate dose extrapolated from human dosages.
[†]Our predictions of efficacy if agent was evaluated by a controlled clinical trial: +++ highly effective; ++ moderately effective; + occasionally effective.

Antiinflammatory Agents and Analgesics

Mucosal ulceration and submucosal edema, hemorrhage, fibrosis, neovascularization, mastocytosis, and mononuclear inflammatory cell infiltration are common light microscopic lesions observed in the urinary bladders of cats with chronic idiopathic cystitis. These abnormalities are consistent with inflammation. However, the specific cause(s) of inflammation in many cats with idiopathic cystitis is (are) unknown. The lack of specific therapy for cats with idiopathic cystitis has resulted in widespread use of antiinflammatory agents in an attempt to reduce the severity of inflammation-associated clinical signs. Unfortunately there have been few controlled clinical trials to study the short- and long-term effectiveness of antiinflammatory agents in the symptomatic treatment of pollakiuria and hematuria in cats.

Glucocorticoids

By virtue of their potent antiinflammatory properties, glucocorticoids are a logical therapeutic choice to minimize pollakiuria and hematuria in cats with idiopathic cystitis. However, results of a small, double-blind, placebo-controlled study of untreated male and female cats with idiopathic cystitis indicated that antiinflammatory doses of prednisolone (1 mg/kg orally q12h for 10 days) was of no benefit in reducing the severity or duration of clinical signs in affected cats (Osborne et al., 1996). Clinical signs subsided within 1 to 2 days in both prednisolone (n=6)– and placebo (n=6)– treated cats; urinalysis abnormalities of hematuria and pyuria subsided in approximately 2 to 5 days in both groups.

Nonsteroidal Antiinflammatory Drugs

Nonsteroidal antiinflammatory drugs (NSAIDs) are widely used for their antiinflammatory and analgesic properties in veterinary and human medicine. Although generally considered mild analgesics, NSAIDs may be more effective in settings in which inflammation has caused sensitization of pain receptors to normally painless mechanical and chemical stimuli. NSAIDs have been used for management of mild discomfort in humans with interstitial cystitis. Similarly the NSAIDs meloxicam, ketoprofen, tolfenamic acid, and piroxicam have been recommended for treatment of dysuria and inflammation in cats with idiopathic cystitis. However, the safety and efficacy of NSAIDs in the treatment of either humans with interstitial cystitis or cats with idiopathic cystitis have not been evaluated by controlled clinical trials. It is noteworthy that certain NSAIDs have been associated with sterile hemorrhagic cystitis in humans and have been shown to induce histopathologic lesions typical of interstitial cystitis in rodents. Pending further safety and efficacy studies, one must use appropriate caution when considering use of NSAIDs to treat feline idiopathic cystitis.

Opioid Analgesics

Narcotic analgesics are often used for initial management of severe visceral pain in humans with interstitial cystitis. Similarly the opiate agonists butorphanol, buprenorphine, fentanyl, and tramadol have been advocated for short-term analgesia in cats with idiopathic cystitis (see Table 205-2). Our anecdotal observations and those of others suggest that short-term opioid analgesic therapy for 24 to 72 hours may be of benefit in alleviating acute "flare-ups" of severe pollakiuria, dysuria, stranguria, and periuria in cats with idiopathic cystitis. In addition, combination of an opioid analgesic and a short-term tranquilizer (e.g., acepromazine) may facilitate collection of urine specimens for urinalysis and culture from acutely symptomatic cats. However, we emphasize that there have been no reports of controlled studies evaluating the efficacy and safety of short-term opioid analgesics for management of cats with idiopathic cystitis.

Anticholinergics and Antispasmodics

Pollakiuria is a common feature of feline idiopathic cystitis. Inappropriate voiding of urine occurs at low volumes of bladder filling and may be associated with sensations of pain, bladder fullness, and urgency. Presumably, pollakiuria is the result of inflammation-induced stimulation of urinary bladder sacral sensory afferent nerves. Sensations of pain and perception of fullness and urgency induce a premature micturition reflex and subsequent inappropriate or involuntary voiding of small quantities of urine. Because cholinergic parasympathetic efferents are normally responsible for detrusor contraction, anticholinergics agents may logically be considered as symptomatic treatment of pollakiuria and urge incontinence.

The quaternary ammonium anticholinergic agent propantheline (Pro-Banthine, Schiapparelli Searle) is a potent nonselective muscarinic antagonist that minimizes the force and frequency of uncontrolled detrusor contractions. However, the clinical use of propantheline has been limited by lack of selectivity for urinary bladder compared to other smooth-muscle organs. In a controlled clinical study of the efficacy of propantheline (7.5 mg given orally on one occasion) for treatment of acute nonobstructive idiopathic cystitis, no difference in rate of recovery was observed between cats treated with propantheline and control groups (Barsanti et al., 1982). Potential adverse effects include urinary retention, tachycardia, vomiting, and constipation. Unfortunately the optimal dose and maintenance intervals for cats have not been determined. Further studies using appropriate doses are required to substantiate a beneficial symptomatic effect of propantheline in cats with idiopathic cystitis.

Oxybutynin chloride (Ditropan, Alza Corp.) and tolterodine (Detrol, Pfizer US Pharmaceuticals) are synthetic tertiary amine muscarinic receptor antagonists used for management of overactive bladder and urge incontinence in humans, dogs, and cats (see Table 205-2). Oxybutynin is a moderately potent anticholinergic agent with additional independent musculotropic relaxant and local anesthetic effects. As a result, intravesicular oxybutynin has been used for symptomatic management of human interstitial cystitis. Although tolterodine is a pure muscarinic antagonist, pharmacologic studies in healthy anesthetized cats indicate that it has a significantly more pronounced in vivo effect on urinary bladder than on salivary gland, whereas oxybutynin has greater selectivity for salivary gland (Nilvebrant et al., 1997). It is tempting to speculate that tolterodine may be of value in reducing pollakiuria associated with feline idiopathic cystitis. However, controlled studies evaluating the efficacy of oxybutynin or tolterodine in reducing the magnitude of pollakiuria in cats with idiopathic cystitis have not been reported. Potential adverse effects associated with tolterodine or oxybutynin administration include vomiting, diarrhea, constipation, urine retention, and sedation. Coadministration of oxybutynin or tolterodine with other anticholinergic agents (e.g., amitriptyline) may intensify adverse effects and should be avoided.

Glycosaminoglycans

Transitional epithelium of the urinary bladder is covered by a glycocalyx composed of hydrated glycoconjugates, including glycoproteins and glycosaminoglycans (GAGs). Urothelial GAGs minimize adherence of microorganisms and crystals to the bladder urothelium and limit movement of urine proteins and other ionic and nonionic solutes from the bladder lumen into surrounding tissues. Quantitative or qualitative defects in surface GAGs and subsequent increased urothelial permeability have been hypothesized to be causative factors in the pathogenesis of feline idiopathic cystitis and human interstitial cystitis.

Pentosan Polysulfate

Oral or intravesicular administration of GAGs is commonly used to manage interstitial cystitis in humans. Pentosan polysulfate sodium (Elmiron, Ortho-McNeil Pharmaceutical) is a semi-synthetic low–molecular weight heparin analog that reinforces urothelial GAGs and reduces transitional cell injury. Pentosan polysulfate is the only oral medication approved by the Food and Drug Administration for treating interstitial cystitis in humans in the United States. Symptomatic remission was observed in 28% to 40% of humans with interstitial cystitis treated with oral or intravesicular pentosan polysulfate sodium compared to 13% to 20% remission in patients treated with a placebo. Maximum benefit in overall improvement in pain and urgency in humans with interstitial cystitis was noted after 6 to 11 months of therapy. Prolongation of prothrombin time, epistaxis, gingival bleeding, alopecia, abdominal pain, diarrhea, and nausea have been observed uncommonly in humans treated with pentosan polysulfate. Our empiric clinical impression and the impression of others is that oral or parenteral pentosan polysulfate may benefit some cats with chronic idiopathic cystitis (see Table 205-2). Results of controlled clinical studies evaluating the safety and efficacy of pentosan polysulfate for treatment of feline idiopathic are warranted.

Glucosamine and Chondroitin Sulfate

Glucosamine, an amino sugar naturally produced in the body, is an important intermediate for the formation of GAGs. Chondroitin sulfate is one of the most abundant GAGs in the bladder surface GAG layer. Oral glucosamine and intravesicular chondroitin sulfate have been reported to have moderate beneficial effects in uncontrolled studies of humans with interstitial cystitis. Anecdotally oral glucosamine alone or in combination with oral chondroitin sulfate has been of apparent benefit to some cats with chronic forms of idiopathic cystitis (see Table 205-2). However, a recent 6-month randomized placebo-controlled clinical trial of oral glucosamine in cats with idiopathic cystitis did not reveal any significant difference between the severity of clinical signs in cats treated with glucosamine and those treated with a placebo (Gunn-Moore and Shenoy, 2004). The efficacy of oral glucosamine combined with chondroitin sulfate for management of cats with idiopathic cystitis has not been evaluated. Because of potential synergy between glucosamine and chondroitin sulfate, a randomized controlled, double-masked clinical trial is clearly warranted.

Dietary Management

Unless complicated by other illness, cats with idiopathic cystitis typically have concentrated and acidic urine. The prevalence and magnitude of crystalluria are variable. However, the prevalence of crystalluria in cats with idiopathic cystitis does not differ significantly from that of unaffected cats. Although crystalluria per se does not appear to be a risk factor for nonobstructive idiopathic cystitis, it has been hypothesized that high concentrations of normal and/or abnormal components in urine may be toxic to urinary bladder tissues in affected cats. The comparative effects of wet and dry forms of a diet designed to lower urine pH on the frequency of recurrence signs in cats with idiopathic cystitis was evaluated in a nonrandomized, open, prospective study (Markwell et al., 1999). Signs of lower urinary tract disease recurred in 11 of 28 (39%) cats fed the dry diet and in 2 of 18 (11%) cats fed the canned diet. Although the basis for the beneficial response associated with the canned diet was not determined, cats consuming the canned diet had a significantly lower urine specific gravity than those consuming the dry diet. Based on these results and until other randomized controlled studies are available, we routinely recommend increasing dietary water intake by feeding canned food or by use of other strategies designed to increase water consumption (Westropp, Buffington, and Chew, 2005).

Urethral obstruction is a potentially life-threatening sequela in cats with idiopathic cystitis that may result from formation of matrix-crystalline urethral plugs. Because insoluble microscopic crystals appear to be an integral part of many matrix-crystalline urethral plugs encountered in male cats, using medical protocols to prevent crystal formation in patients at risk for urethral obstruction is logical. Struvite is the primary mineral component of most urethral plugs, although other mineral types may be encountered. Successful prevention of recurrent urethral obstruction caused by struvite-containing urethral plugs using diets to reduce urine pH and urine magnesium and phosphorous concentrations has been reported.

Stress Management

Clinical observations suggest that stress may play a role in precipitating or exacerbating signs associated with idiopathic cystitis. Neuroendocrine abnormalities identified in cats with chronic idiopathic cystitis are indicative of increased activity of the sympathetic nervous system and diminished adrenocortical responsiveness (Westropp, Buffington, and Chew, 2005). Based on these observations, therapeutic strategies designed to normalize reactivity of the stress response system have been advocated as primary therapy for prevention and recurrence of feline idiopathic cystitis.

Environmental Enrichment

Environmental enrichment for indoor-housed cats entails providing necessary resources (food, water, litter boxes, space, play), refining cat-owner interactions, managing conflict, and minimizing the impact of change (Westropp, Buffington, and Chew, 2005). Although the ease, safety, and economy of these activities are appealing, controlled studies evaluating the efficacy of environmental enrichment strategies for management of idiopathic cystitis have not been reported.

Facial Pheromone

Feline facial pheromone fraction F3 (Feliway, Veterinary Products Laboratories) is a synthetic pheromone that was developed for management of anxiety-related behaviors in cats. Application of pheromones to the living environment has been recommended as adjunctive therapy to environmental enrichment for management of cats with idiopathic cystitis. However, a recent randomized double-blind, placebo-controlled, crossover study of nine cats with idiopathic cystitis treated for 2 months with feline facial pheromone or a placebo did not reveal significant differences in severity of clinical signs, behavior, or overall health between treatment groups (Gunn-Moore and Cameron, 2004).

References and Suggested Reading

Barsanti JA: Feline urologic syndrome: further investigations into therapy, *J Am Anim Hosp Assoc* 18: 387, 1982.

Chew DJ et al: Amitriptyline treatment for severe recurrent idiopathic cystitis in cats, *J Am Vet Med Assoc* 213:1282, 1998.

Gunn-Moore DA, Cameron ME: A pilot study using synthetic feline facial pheromone for the management of feline idiopathic cystitis, *J Feline Med Surg* 6:133, 2004.

Gunn-Moore DA, Shenoy CM: Oral glucosamine and the management of feline idiopathic cystitis, *J Feline Med Surg* 6:219, 2004.

Kraijer M, Fink-Gremmels J, Nickel RF: The short-term clinical efficacy of amitriptyline in the management of idiopathic feline lower urinary tract disease: a controlled clinical study, *J Feline Med Surg* 5:191, 2003.

Kruger JM et al: Randomized controlled trial of the efficacy of short-term amitriptyline administration for treatment of acute, nonobstructive idiopathic lower urinary tract disease in cats, *J Am Vet Med Assoc* 222:749, 2003.

Markwell PJ et al: Clinical evaluation of commercially available acidification diets in the management of idiopathic cystitis in cats, *J Am Vet Med Assoc* 214:361, 1999.

Nilvebrant L et al: Tolteridine—a new bladder selective antimuscarinic agent, *Eur J Pharm* 327:195, 1997.

Osborne CA et al: Prednisolone therapy of idiopathic feline lower urinary tract disease: a double-blind study, *Vet Clin North Am Small Anim Pract* 26: 563, 1996.

Westropp JL, Buffington CAT, Chew D: Feline lower urinary tract diseases. In Ettinger SJ, Feldman EC, editors: *Textbook of veterinary internal medicine*, ed 6, St Louis, 2005, Elsevier Saunders, p 1828.

CHAPTER 206

Urethral Obstruction in Cats

KENNETH J. DROBATZ, *Philadelphia, Pennsylvania*

Feline urethral obstruction is a relatively common complaint compromising approximately 10% of cats presenting to a large urban veterinary emergency service in a recent report (Lee and Drobatz, 2003). The most common cause of obstruction is a mucous or mucocrystalline plug secondary to feline lower urinary tract disease, although obstruction by calcium oxalate stones is becoming more frequent. The majority of cats presented with urethral obstruction are relatively stable, but approximately 12% have severe physiologic compromise with significant electrolyte and acid-base changes. In this latter group of patients the initial approach can make the difference between life and death in this relatively reversible condition. This chapter focuses on the initial evaluation, treatment, and monitoring of these physiologically dynamic and fragile patients.

CLINICAL SIGNS AND DIAGNOSIS OF URETHRAL OBSTRUCTION

The most common clinical sign specific to urethral obstruction is straining to urinate without passing any urine. This is often preceded by complaints such as excessive licking at the perineal area, vocalizing, pollakiuria, dysuria, hematuria, and urinating small amounts outside the litter box. The median duration of clinical signs is about 3 days, with the owner becoming concerned when the cat cannot pass urine despite prolonged attempts in the litter box. Many owners confuse the prolonged urinating posture as straining to defecate and complain that their cats are constipated or reluctant to walk. More severely affected cats become lethargic, stop eating, vomit, and become extremely weak. Some cats are found lying in their litter boxes, extremely weak and minimally responsive when the inability to pass urine is prolonged.

The diagnosis of urethral obstruction is relatively straightforward when the cat is presented with a history of straining to urinate and a large, firm urinary bladder is palpated. Care should be taken not to apply too much pressure to a severely distended urinary bladder because the bladder wall may be compromised as a result of prolonged ischemia. A more challenging diagnosis is when astute owners bring their cat in for straining to urinate early on before bladder distention has become excessive. In these instances the urinary bladder may be mildly-to-moderately distended but cannot be expressed.

FLUID BALANCE, TISSUE PERFUSION, AND INITIAL DATABASE

Because of the severe fluid deficits and dramatic electrolyte changes that develop, cardiovascular compromise is the most common and immediate life-threatening sequela to urethral obstruction. The initial physical evaluation should focus on assessment of mucous membrane color, capillary refill time, pulse quality and rate, and cardiac auscultation. An inappropriate slow heart rate indicates clinically significant hyperkalemia and should prompt immediate electrocardiogram (ECG) evaluation and measurement of serum potassium. However, it also should be noted that in cats life-threatening hyperkalemia also can be associated with a normal to rapid heart rate.

To optimize tissue oxygen delivery, supplemental oxygen via mask or flow-by should be administered; and intravenous access should be obtained to facilitate emergency drug therapy, fluid administration, and collection of blood. An emergency database ideally includes packed cell volume (PCV), total solids (TS), blood glucose, dipstick blood urea nitrogen (BUN), sodium, potassium, ionized calcium, and a venous blood gas. Both serum BUN and creatinine can be severely elevated in cats with obstructive uropathy; however, these values are not prognostic per se and often return to normal levels within a few days. A lead II ECG should be reviewed for hyperkalemia-induced cardiac conduction abnormalities. ECG abnormalities consistent with hyperkalemia include tall positive or large negative T-waves, diminished or absent P-waves, prolonged P-R intervals, widened QRS complexes, and sine waves. The sine wave is an end-stage ECG finding that develops when the QRS and T waves merge. Rarely ventricular tachycardia can be seen in cats with hyperkalemia; however, sinoventricular rhythm with intraventricular conduction delay may be misinterpreted as ventricular tachycardia. Although textbooks describe characteristic ECG findings developing with specific, progressively increased blood potassium concentrations, the association is inconsistent clinically. Some cats are hyperkalemic without exhibiting major ECG changes. Conversely, when ECG changes are observed, clinically significant hyperkalemia is present.

Physical assessment, oxygen administration, ECG evaluation, and intravenous access should occur within minutes of presentation; fluid administration can then be initiated quickly. Although potassium-free solutions such as 0.9% saline are recommended in cats with urethral obstruction, any balanced electrolyte solution suffices to provide vascular volume support and does not contribute substantially to the potassium concentration on an acute basis. Theoretically administration of 0.9% saline contributes to the metabolic acidosis in obstructed, dehydrated cats. In a recent randomized clinical trial at our hospital, 0.9% saline was slower to correct metabolic acidosis in critically ill cats with urethral obstruction when compared to Normsol-R (Abbott Laboratories), but the outcome was similar between the two treatments. The dilution provided by 0.9% saline or a balanced electrolyte solution helps to lower the potassium concentration but does not lower it rapidly enough in patients that are affected by the hyperkalemia. I recommend administering 20 to 30 ml/kg of body weight as an intravenous bolus and monitoring tissue perfusion status (mucous membrane color, capillary refill time, pulse quality) as fluid is being administered. I adjust the dose and administration rate, depending on the response to this fluid challenge, as well as the response to treatment of the electrolyte and acid-base abnormalities.

Rapid assessment of the emergency database results provides information for further therapy. A variety of electrolyte and acid-base derangements occur in critically ill cats with urethral obstruction, leading to significant physiologic consequences. The most important abnormalities are hyperkalemia, metabolic acidosis, and ionized hypocalcemia, often developing concurrently.

Hyperkalemia

Potassium concentration can be extremely high (>10 mEq/L) in cats with urethral obstruction. The primary clinical concern is the effect of potassium on cardiac conduction. When ECG changes are recognized as described earlier, the potassium concentration is usually quite high; the clinician can also assume other electrolyte and acid-base changes to be severe as well. Since the severity of ECG signs does not always correlate with the magnitude of hyperkalemia, treatment should be guided by its functional consequences by monitoring the ECG. A cat with a high potassium concentration but no functional consequence does not require specific therapy for hyperkalemia and responds well to intravenous fluid therapy and relief of the urethral obstruction. A cat with cardiac conduction disturbances requires specific therapy directed at the hyperkalemia or its functional effects. Reversing the effects of hyperkalemia can be achieved by direct antagonism of the actions of the high potassium on the membrane potentials and by lowering the plasma potassium concentration. Plasma potassium concentration may be lowered by driving potassium intracellularly or by removal of potassium from the body.

Calcium gluconate directly antagonizes the cardiac effects of hyperkalemia. Administration of 50 to 100 mg/kg of calcium gluconate intravenously over 2 to 3 minutes is recommended for the average cat, with continuous ECG evaluation (to observe for calcium-induced cardiac arrhythmias). The effects of calcium gluconate administration are immediate; thus it is the first drug of choice in cats that have significant cardiac rhythm disturbances caused by hyperkalemia. The effects last approximately 20 to 30 minutes.

Regular insulin at 0.1 to 0.25 unit/kg intravenous bolus promotes the intracellular movement of potassium. Insulin administration should be followed by a slow bolus of 1 to 2 g of 25% glucose per unit of insulin given to prevent hypoglycemia. Plasma potassium concentration should begin to decrease within several minutes to 1 hour. Blood glucose monitoring should be maintained for several hours after the administration of the insulin, and the intravenous fluids should be supplemented with glucose as needed to maintain normoglycemia.

Sodium bicarbonate administration can lower plasma potassium concentration by raising the pH and driving potassium into the cells (see the section that follows on Metabolic Acidosis). The effect on the plasma potassium concentration begins within 30 to 60 minutes and may persist for hours.

The effects of calcium, insulin and dextrose, and sodium bicarbonate are transient. The administration of these drugs buys the clinician time to remove the urethral obstruction and induce fluid diuresis to correct the underlying problem.

Metabolic Acidosis

Metabolic acidosis can be severe in critically ill cats with urethral obstruction. Blood pH drops below 7.0 in some cats. Severe acidosis (<7.0) can predispose the heart to ventricular arrhythmias, decrease cardiac contractility, decrease the inotropic response to catecholamines, and cause peripheral vasodilation, all of which may contribute to poor tissue perfusion.

The main treatments for metabolic acidosis include relief of obstruction, fluid diuresis, and bicarbonate therapy. The first two are usually adequate in the majority of cats. In the unstable cat with severe metabolic acidosis, administration of sodium bicarbonate should be considered. The formula recommended to approximate the total body deficit is $0.3 \times$ body weight (kilograms) $\times$ the base deficit. One third of this deficit should be given slowly intravenously (over approximately 15 minutes), and the rest placed in the intravenous fluids to be administered over several hours. (If blood gas analysis is not available, 1 to 2 mEq/kg of sodium bicarbonate can be administered slowly to critically ill cats.) Rapid intravenous boluses of sodium bicarbonate should be avoided because of the production of CO_2 and its diffusion into the central nervous system, making cerebrospinal fluid acidosis even worse. In addition, because bicarbonate administration raises blood pH, sodium bicarbonate might lower the ionized calcium concentration (see following paragraphs). Bicarbonate should be administered after calcium supplementation in cats with very low blood-ionized calcium.

Ionized Hypocalcemia

Severe ionized hypocalcemia may occur in the more critically ill cats. Hypocalcemia exacerbates the effects of hyperkalemia on membrane excitability. Treatment of severe ionized hypocalcemia is reserved for cats that have clinical signs such as muscle stiffness, tetany, and cardiovascular disturbances. Treatment is similar to calcium gluconate therapy for hyperkalemia mentioned previously (50 to 100 mg/kg of calcium gluconate intravenously over 2 to 3 minutes). Continuous ECG monitoring is recommended when administering calcium.

SEDATION FOR URETHRAL CATHETERIZATION

Ongoing resolution of metabolic derangements depends on catheterization and relief of urethral obstruction. The most severely affected (i.e., moribund) cats may not require sedation for urethral catheterization and are so compromised that administration of a sedative may result in death. In other cats mentation and responsiveness are improved after emergency stabilization; sedation may be required to provide a relatively stress-free urethral catheterization. Ketamine (5 to 10 mg/kg intravenously [IV]) with diazepam (0.2 to 0.5 mg/kg IV) or midazolam (0.2 to 0.5 mg/kg IV) can be used. Alternatively butorphanol (0.2 mg/kg) combined with diazepam (0.2 to 0.5 mg/kg IV) or midazolam (0.2 to 0.5 mg/kg IV) along with ketamine (2 mg/kg IV) is preferred by some clinicians. The butorphanol or benzodiazepine doses may be repeated if passage of a urinary catheter is prolonged. Alternatively ongoing sedation can be maintained with propofol (small slow boluses of 2 to 4 mg/kg IV titrated to effect). Respiratory rate should be monitored carefully when propofol is used since apnea can sometimes be a side effect when it is given too quickly. Ketamine should be avoided if cardiac abnormalities are detected on physical examination or if cardiac disease is suspected.

INSTRUCTIONS FOR URETHRAL CATHETERIZATION

Supplies needed for urethral catheterization include a sterile open-end 3.5-Fr tomcat catheter (Sovereign, Covidien), 3.5- or 5-Fr red rubber feeding tube (Sovereign, Tyco Health Care Group LP), sterile lubricating gel, sterile gloves, intravenous extension set, sterile 0.9% saline flush, several 10-ml syringes for flushing the urinary catheter, sterile urine collection bag, and sterile intravenous line for connection of indwelling urinary catheter to sterile urine collection bag (catheter adaptor, Becton Dickinson Co.).

The following are the usual steps taken to relieve the urethral obstruction. Position the cat in lateral or dorsal recumbency (based on the preference of the operator). Clip the hair on and around the prepuce and gently scrub the area as for a sterile procedure. Extrude the penis and pinch the prepuce to maintain extrusion. Clear any plugs from the tip of the penis (rarely this is the only source of obstruction). Using sterile technique, place the tip of the tomcat catheter into the tip of the penis. While maintaining the catheter in the tip of the penis, allow the penis to slip back into the prepuce. Pull the prepuce caudally and dorsally to "straighten out" the urethra and then gently advance the urinary catheter until resistance is encountered. Place the male end of the intravenous extension line onto the dilated end of the tomcat catheter. Place the 10-ml syringe filled with sterile saline flush onto the female end of the extension set and flush sterile saline into the urinary catheter. If resistance to flushing is encountered, slightly back the urinary catheter out until flushing can be continued. Slowly advance the urinary catheter again while flushing. If resistance to flushing is encountered again, slightly back the urinary catheter out

again until flushing can be continued. Repeat as needed multiple times. This gentle flushing eventually results in dislodgement of the urethral obstruction and successful passage of the urinary catheter into the urinary bladder. Be patient and remember to maintain adequate sedation during flushing.

Rarely a urinary catheter cannot be passed using the previous method. In this instance perform a cystocentesis, placing a 22-gauge needle in the ventral body of the bladder angled caudally. Drain the urinary bladder completely and then repeat the urethral flushing and catheterization procedure described. Relief of back pressure from the distended urinary bladder may now allow retrograde flushing of the urethral plug and passage of the urinary catheter. Be aware that cystocentesis is considered a back-up alternative for facilitating urinary catheterization because passing a needle into a urinary bladder with compromised blood flow and damaged tissue may contribute to urinary bladder rupture. Should the above methods fail, emergency perineal urethrostomy or temporary prepubic cystostomy has to be performed to allow for urine flow.

Once the urinary catheter tip is passed into the urinary bladder neck, drain the urine and flush the bladder multiple times with sterile saline. Slowly remove the tomcat catheter while continuing to flush saline through the catheter to maintain urethral patency. Then sterilely place the 5-Fr red rubber feeding tube into the urethra (a 3.5-Fr catheter is the second choice if the 5-Fr cannot be passed). Take care that the red rubber catheter is not placed too far into the urinary bladder since a knot in the catheter can develop as it follows the contour of the bladder wall. Suture (3-0 nylon) the catheter to the prepuce using a white tape butterfly around the urinary catheter where it exits the tip of the penis. Connect the red rubber catheter to the sterile intravenous line and connect the other end of the line to the sterile urine collection bag.

CONTINUED INPATIENT CARE

After initial stabilization continued monitoring of physical perfusion parameters, body temperature, mentation, continuous ECG, PCV, TS, dipstick glucose, dipstick BUN, serum sodium, serum potassium, ionized calcium concentration, acid-base status, and urine output should be done. Most cats do well if they remain stable after the first two hours. Post-obstructive diuresis can be profound, especially in the 24 to 48 hours following relief of the obstruction. Urine output may exceed 120 ml/hour in some cats. Fluid therapy should be adjusted according to measured urine output, perfusion parameters, PCV, and TS. Once renal function has returned to near normal levels, it may be necessary to reduce the rate of fluid administration to insure continued diuresis is not iatrogenic. The most common electrolyte problem encountered after the initial stabilization period is hypokalemia. Many cats require potassium supplementation within several hours. Another (rare) complication of urethral obstruction is severe hematuria resulting in anemia. If the urine appears unusually bloody, a PCV should be performed on the urine, and the cat's peripheral blood PCV should be monitored closely. A transfusion is rarely required to maintain the PCV and tissue perfusion at reasonable levels. Pain management is also important in the postobstructive period. Anecdotally butorphanol (0.1 mg to 0.2 mg/kg IV q6-8h) or buprenorphine (0.01 mg/kg IV q6-12h) appears to work well. An Elizabethan collar should be placed to prevent the cat from dislodging the urinary catheter.

The urinary catheter is usually kept in place for 1 to 2 days. It can be removed when urine appears relatively free of crystalline material (grit) and is not grossly cloudy or bloody. It should be removed in the morning on the day of discharge, and the cat monitored to make sure it can urinate before going home. If the cat cannot urinate, a urethral plug may still be present, or there may be a functional voiding problem because of urethral spasm or bladder atony. Sedation and urinary catheterization are required to determine the cause. A physical obstruction should be detected during passage of the urinary catheter; however, the urinary catheter passes relatively easily if urethral spasm is the cause.

Urethral spasm may be treated with phenoxybenzamine (2.5 to 7.5 mg/cat orally q12-24h). The onset of action is relatively slow (hours), and effectiveness increases over several days. For this reason some clinicians advocate starting phenoxybenzamine soon after initial urinary catheterization when the cat is stable and can tolerate oral drugs.

LONG-TERM MANAGEMENT

Recurrent bouts of obstructive or nonobstructive feline lower urinary tract disease are common. Long-term management has been extensively reviewed (Kruger, Osborne, and Lulich, 2000; also see Chapter 205). Most authors agree that increasing water intake is important. Water intake can be maximized by changing the diet to wet food, ensuring availability of adequate fresh water, and encouraging the cat to take in as much water as possible. Flare-ups of idiopathic cystitis may be precipitated by stress; therefore creating a stress-free environment for the cat is also beneficial. Recommendations for pharmacologic treatments as home management of affected cats are often supported by anecdote and little objective evidence of efficacy.

The owner should be warned about the possibility of reobstruction and advised to monitor the cat's urination carefully. The most common time for reobstruction appears to be within the first few days or week after discharge from the hospital. In my experience reobstruction is not common when cats are hospitalized and treated as described here.

If a cat has multiple obstructive episodes despite appropriate preventive medical therapy, a perineal urethrostomy can be performed to minimize obstructive complications of feline lower urinary tract disease. The owner should be warned of the potential adverse effects of perineal urethrostomy, including stricture formation or recurrent urinary tract infections. In addition, the owner should clearly understand that the procedure does not eliminate the underlying causes of lower urinary tract inflammation.

References and Suggested Reading

Cole SG, Hilton A, Drobatz KJ: The influence of crystalloid type on acid-base and electrolyte status of cats with urethral obstruction, *J Vet Emerg Crit Care,* in press.

Drobatz KJ, Hughes D: Concentration of ionized calcium in plasma from cats with urethral obstruction, *J Am Vet Med Assoc* 211(11):1392, 1997.

Kruger JM, Osborne CA, Lulich JP: Nonobstructive idiopathic feline lower urinary tract disease: therapeutic rights and wrongs. In Bonagura JD, editor: *Kirk's current veterinary therapy XIII,* Philadelphia, 2000, Saunders, p 888.

Lee JA, Drobatz KJ: Characterization of the clinical characteristics, electrolytes, acid-base, and renal parameters in male cats with urethral obstruction, *J Vet Emerg Crit Care* 13(4): 227, 2003.

Lee JA, Drobatz KJ: Historical and physical parameters as predictors of severe hyperkalemia in male cats with urethral obstruction, J Vet Emerg Crit Care, 16(2):104, 2006.

Gunn-Moore DA: Feline lower urinary tract disease, *J Feline Med Surg* 5:133, 2003.

CHAPTER 207

Urinary Incontinence and Micturition Disorders: Pharmacologic Management

INDIA F. LANE, *Knoxville, Tennessee*
JODI L. WESTROPP, *Davis, California*

Although the primary pharmacologic agents useful in the management of micturition disorders have not changed in the past decade, the availability of many compounds has varied. Alternative products often are sought during times of reduced availability and when first-line treatment choices fail. In this chapter we present a brief review of the rationale for pharmacologic manipulation of micturition and updates on available agents and new approaches. Drug information and dosing recommendations can be found in Tables 207-1 and 207-2.

PHARMACOLOGIC MANAGEMENT OF URINARY RETENTION

To enhance urine voiding, pharmacologic agents are chosen to improve urinary bladder contractile function, relax urethral outlet resistance, or both. In most instances the urethral outlet resistance is manipulated first, with bladder function assessed and treated after urethral resistance declines.

Urethral outlet resistance is maintained by smooth and striated muscle components of the urethra, as well as physical features of the urethra that aid closure (urethral folds, moist epithelial seal, urethral length and position). Manipulation of urethral resistance has relied on manipulation of the muscular components, primarily smooth muscle. In general, smooth muscle relaxation is effective in many dogs with functional urinary obstruction, in some dogs and cats with neurogenic disorders of micturition (e.g., postintravertebral disk disease [IVDD]), and for relaxing the urethral outlet during bethanechol administration. Agents directed at smooth muscle are only partially effective for cats with urethrospasm when striated muscle contraction predominates. Similarly they are less effective for detrusor-striated urethral muscle dyssynergia associated with neurogenic disorders and for some cases of idiopathic dyssynergia. Because it is clinically difficult to discern the relative influence of smooth or striated muscle in voiding dysfunction, smooth muscle relaxants are often administered first, with striated muscle relaxants added if necessary.

Activation of terminal α-adrenergic receptors elicits contraction of smooth muscle in the urinary bladder neck and urethra; selective or nonselective antagonism of these receptors can be achieved pharmacologically. The nonselective agent phenoxybenzamine is reasonably effective in dogs. The agent may not be available in some countries, and pricing has been variable. Prazosin has been a useful, potent, and inexpensive alternative in dogs and cats, although the drug must be compounded for accurate administration in small dogs and cats. Prazosin is usually effective when given once or twice daily; some earlier texts recommended more frequent administration. Hypotension and sedation are the most common and worrisome adverse effects of α-antagonists. Uroselective α₁-antagonists (terazosin, doxazosin, tamsulosin) are readily available for human use and are most commonly used to modulate prostatic and urethral smooth muscle in men with prostatic hypertrophy. No studies evaluating these drugs in dogs are available. Phenothiazine derivatives (e.g., acepromazine) antagonize α-receptors and can be highly effective urethral relaxants in stable, normotensive patients. Sedation may be an unwanted adverse effect.

Striated muscle relaxation is most commonly obtained using benzodiazepines such as diazepam or alprazolam. Sedative effects limit the long-term use of these agents for urologic disorders. Oral diazepam has a very short half-life; and, if this drug is administered for urethral relaxation, it should be given 15 to 30 minutes before taking the pet outdoors to void. Dantrolene, baclofen, and cyclobenzaprine have also been recommended as striated muscle relaxants for small animals, but their use has been limited by side effects.

The effect of α-antagonists on voiding is appreciated relatively quickly, but full effect may take several days. If urinary bladder function is weak, other agents can be administered to improve bladder contraction. Urinary bladder contraction is enhanced by activating the terminal receptors for parasympathetic input or antagonizing the (sympathetic) adrenergic input on β-receptors in detrusor muscle. Bethanechol, a parasympathomimetic agent, remains the primary treatment for detrusor atony or dysfunction, although the efficacy of orally administered bethanechol is questionable. Cholinesterase inhibitors (neostigmine, pyridostigmine) have been used to increase parasympathetic activity when bethanechol is unavailable. Other drugs that stimulate urinary bladder contraction include the prokinetic agent cisapride and β-blocking agents such as propranolol. When pharmacologic intervention for bladder evacuation is unsuccessful,

Table 207-1

Pharmacologic Agents Useful in the Management of Urine Retention

Category/Agent	Mechanism	Recommended Dosage	Possible Adverse Effects	Contraindications or Comments
Agents That Facilitate Urethral Relaxation				
Acepromazine	Skeletal muscle relaxation via neuroleptic effect; smooth muscle relaxation via α-antagonism	Up to 0.1 mg/kg IV q12-24h (doses as low as 0.02 mg/kg IV may be effective) 1.1-2.2 mg/kg PO q12-24h	Hypotension Sedation Disinhibition	Hypovolemia Cardiac disease Seizure disorder
Alprazolam	Centrally acting anxiolytic benzodiazepine	Cat: 0.125-0.25 mg/cat PO q12h	As for diazepam, except that idiopathic hepatic necrosis has not been documented.	May be a good alternative to diazepam if oral therapy is needed
Baclofen	Skeletal muscle relaxation	Dog: 1-2 mg/kg PO q8h Cat: not recommended	Weakness GI upset Pruritus	
Dantrolene	Skeletal muscle relaxation via direct effects	Dog: 1-5 mg/kg PO q8-12h Cat: 0.5-2 mg/kg PO q8h 1 mg/kg IV	Weakness Sedation GI upset Hepatotoxicity	Cardiac disease
Diazepam	Skeletal muscle relaxation via central effects (benzodiazepine)	Dog: 2-10 mg/dog PO q8h Cat: 1-2.5 mg/cat PO q8h or prn	Sedation Paradoxic excitation Idiopathic hepatic necrosis (with PO use in cats only) Polyphagia	Pregnancy Hepatic disease
Phenoxybenzamine	Smooth muscle relaxation via nonspecific α-antagonism	Dog: 0.25 mg/kg PO q8-12h or 2.5-20 mg/dog PO q8-12h Cat:1.25-7.5 mg/cat PO q8-12h	Hypotension Tachycardia GI upset	Cardiac disease Hypovolemia Glaucoma Renal failure Diabetes mellitus (type II)
Prazosin	Smooth muscle relaxation via α-1 antagonism	Dog: 1 mg/15 kg PO q8-12h Cat: 0.25-0.5 mg/cat PO q12-24h	Hypotension Mild sedation Ptyalism	Cardiac disease Renal failure
Terazosin	Smooth muscle relaxation via α-1 antagonism	Dog: 0.5-5 mg/dog q12-24h Cat: not determined	Hypotension Mild sedation Ptyalism	Cardiac disease Renal failure
Tamsulosin*	Uroselective relaxation via α-1 antagonism	Dog: 0.1 mg/10 kg q24h	Hypotension	Empiric dosage
Agents that Facilitate Urinary Bladder Contractility				
Bethanechol	Parasympathomimetic	Dogs: 5-25 mg PO q8h Cats: 1.25-5 mg PO q8h	Ptyalism Vomiting Diarrhea	Outlet obstruction or high outlet resistance GI obstruction Atropine is antidotal
Cisapride	Prokinetic; may enhance acetylcholine release	Dogs 0.5 mg/kg PO q8h Cats: 1.25-5 mg/cat PO q8-12h	Diarrhea Possible abdominal pain	GI obstruction Reduce dose with hepatic insufficiency

Modified from Fischer JR, Lane IF: Incontinence and urine retention, BSAVA Manual of canine and feline urology, ed 2, Gloucester, England, 2007, pp 26-40.
GI, Gastrointestinal; *IV*, intravenously; *PO*, orally; *prn*, as needed.
*Dosage and safety of this drug are not determined. Contraindicated in cats.

urine removal via multiple catheterizations or placement of a tube cystotomy is warranted.

PHARMACOLOGIC MANAGEMENT OF URINARY INCONTINENCE

Manipulations to improve urine storage include those aimed at increasing urethral outlet resistance or increasing urinary bladder accommodation and storage function. Because urethral incompetence (urethral or primary sphincter mechanism incompetence) is the most common micturition disorder in dogs, the most common treatments include reproductive hormones and α-agonists. Other agents have indirect effects on urethral function or combined effects on the urinary bladder and urethra.

Reproductive hormones are reasonably effective in improving continence in dogs with urinary incontinence. Estrogens such as diethylstilbestrol (DES), stilbestrol,

Table 207-2

Pharmacologic Agents Useful in the Management of Urinary Incontinence

Agent	Classification	Recommended Dosage	Possible Adverse Effects	Contraindications or Comments
Diethylstilbestrol (DES) Stilbestrol	Reproductive hormone	Dogs: 0.1-1 mg/dog PO q24h for 5-7 days, then weekly or as needed	Estrus Behavior change Myelosuppression Pyometra in intact female	Males Cats Pregnancy
Stilbestrol (alternate regimen)	Reproductive hormone	Dogs: 0.04-0.06 mg/dog PO q24h for 7 days, reduced weekly to 0.01-0.02 mg/dog/day	As with DES	As with DES
Premarin	Conjugated estrogen	Dogs: 0.02 mg/kg PO q24h for 5-7 days, then q2-4days or as needed	As with DES	As with DES
Estriol	Reproductive hormone	Dogs: 0.5-1 mg/dog PO q24h for 5-7 days, then q2-3days as needed	As with DES	As with DES
Estriol (alternate regimen)	Reproductive hormone	Dogs: 2 mg/dog PO q24h for 7 days; then reduce daily dose by 0.5 mg each week to establish minimal effective daily dose; then try every other day administration	As with DES Adverse effects more common at higher doses	As with DES
Testosterone cypionate	Reproductive hormone	Dogs: 2.2 mg/kg IM q4-8weeks	Behavior change Perianal adenoma perineal hernias, prostatic disorders Aggression	Cardiac, renal or hepatic disease
Testosterone propionate	Reproductive hormone	Dogs: 2.2 mg/kg IM q2-3days	As for testosterone cypionate	As for testosterone cypionate
Phenylpropanolamine (PPA)	Indirect α-agonist	Dogs: 1.5 mg/kg PO q8-12h or 12.5-75 mg PO q8-12h	Anxiety Aggression Anorexia Hypertension Tachycardia	Some cardiac disease Hypertension ± anxiety disorders
Ephedrine	α-Agonist	Dogs: 1.2 mg/kg PO q8h	As with PPA	As with PPA
Pseudoephedrine	α-Agonist	Dogs: 0.2-0.4 mg/kg (practically, 15-60 mg total dose per dog) PO q8-12h	As with PPA	As with PPA
Imipramine	Antimuscarinic, α/β-agonist	Dogs: 5-15 mg PO q12h	Sedation Dry mouth Urinary retention GI upset	Seizure disorders Use of other anticholinergic or CNS depressants, glaucoma, GI obstruction, renal or hepatic disease, cardiac arrhythmias
Oxybutynin	Antimuscarinic	Cats and small dogs: 0.5-1.25 mg total per dose Larger dogs: 2.5-3.75 mg total per dose	As for imipramine	Glaucoma, GI obstruction, renal or hepatic disease, cardiac arrhythmias, hypertension
Dicyclomine	Antimuscarinic	Dogs: 5-10 mg/dog PO q8h	As for imipramine	As for oxybutynin
Depot leuprolide	GnRH analog	Dogs: 11.25 mg/dog		May be redosed as needed May be used in combination with α-agonists
Depot deslorelin	GnRH analog	Dogs: 5-10 mg/dog		May be redosed as needed As for leuprolide

Modified from Fischer JR, Lane IF: Incontinence and urine retention, BSAVA Manual of canine and feline urology, ed 2, Gloucester, England, 2007, pp 26-40.
CNS, Central nervous system; *GI,* gastrointestinal; *GnRH,* gonadotropin-releasing hormone; *IM,* intramuscularly; *IV,* intravenously; *PO,* orally; *prn,* as needed.

estriol, and conjugated estrogens (Premarin) improve urethral resistance by increasing α-adrenergic receptor responsiveness and improving urethral vascularity and other mucosal epithelial characteristics. Estrogen compounds are particularly useful in spayed females. Although many estrogen products are readily available as hormone replacement treatment for women, the most reliable veterinary product, DES, is no longer commercially available because of human health risks associated with the drug. DES is available from many veterinary compounding agencies; reliability depends on the source. The effectiveness of most estrogen treatments is improved by using a "loading" dose regimen followed by a frequency of administration tailored to the individual patient and drug (see Table 207-1). Estrogens can also be used concurrently with phenylpropanolamine (PPA) and are theorized to be synergistic when combined therapy is used. Estrogens are often chosen for dogs that do not tolerate α-agonists, those that are not completely continent on α-agonists alone, and for clients who prefer the intermittent treatment regimen. Some dogs treated with commercially available estrogen products require more frequent administration than with DES.

Estrogen treatment improves continence in 60% to 80% of treated dogs; in a recent open-label trial of estriol, veterinarians reported continence in 61% of 129 dogs and improvement in an additional 22%; owner-reported responses were slightly less favorable (Mandigers and Nell, 2001). A prolonged residual effect of estrogen administration can be seen in some dogs after a period of successful treatment. Administration can be stopped on a trial basis and restarted when incontinence returns (usually weeks to months).

Possible adverse effects of estrogens include signs of estrus, hair loss, behavioral changes, and bone marrow suppression. Estrogenic side effects are most common during the loading dose of estriol and with higher doses of DES. Bone marrow suppression is unlikely in dogs treated with appropriate doses of the drugs listed here, but owners should be advised of this potentially fatal adverse effect. Estradiol cypionate (ECP), a repository preparation, should never be used for urinary incontinence in dogs because of the higher risk of bone marrow suppression. Estrogen administration should be avoided in male dogs and in dogs with a history or breed predilection for immune-mediated disease, since estrogens are immunostimulatory. Estrogens are not very effective and poorly tolerated in cats.

Another reproductive hormone treatment using gonadotropin-releasing hormone (GnRH) analogs has recently been applied to the treatment of urinary incontinence. Reichler and associates (2003) reported their experience with leuprolide, buserelin, and deslorelin, GNRH analogs that suppress sex hormone release. In theory, chronically unsuppressed follicle-stimulating hormone (FSH) and luteinizing hormone (LH) release (because of lack of negative feedback) in ovariectomized dogs may contribute to urinary incontinence. Administration of GnRH analogs paradoxically results in reduced FSH and LH over time. In Reichler's series the drugs appeared useful in 12 of 13 dogs with refractory incontinence, either alone or in combination with α-agonists. In a more recent trial 9 of 23 incontinent dogs treated with long-acting leuprolide were continent for prolonged periods (70 to 575 days); another 10 of the dogs had partial response. However, these 23 dogs also responded to phenylpropanolamine, with 92% overall reduction in urine leakage. There were no apparent adverse effects of GnRH treatment reported in this study, but long-term use of these drugs in dogs has not been evaluated. GnRH analog administration may prove to be a valuable long-acting treatment that would alleviate the need for daily or weekly medication; however, availability of GnRH analogs is limited in the United States.

Sympathomimetic drugs with α-agonist effects, including phenylpropanolamine, phenylephrine, and pseudoephedrine, have been extremely effective in improving or controlling urinary incontinence. Like DES, phenylpropanolamine has been removed from commercial production for humans but is produced under a Food and Drug Administration–compassionate use provision by veterinary compounding pharmacies. Over-the-counter (OTC) pseudoephedrine products are now semicontrolled by pharmacies to limit availability of the compound for methamphetamine production. In many states products containing pseudoephedrine in tabular form must be requested from the pharmacist and signed for by the consumer. Many products have been replaced with phenylephrine at this time. Although phenylpropanolamine has been studied most often, all α-agonists have the same mechanism of action and approximate dose range for the treatment of urethral incompetence. OTC products containing antihistamines or acetaminophen should be avoided. Tolerability and severity of side effects, including restlessness, tachycardia, systemic hypertension, anorexia, gastrointestinal side effects, and aggression and other behavioral changes, may vary among products. For an individual dog the treatment response also may vary among drugs and among formulations of the same drug (e.g., regular versus time-released products).

Although most dogs usually will become continent or improve dramatically with either estrogen or α-agonist administration, the two drugs can also be combined for synergistic effect in the same patient. Combination treatment allows estrogen to "prime" the urethral receptors for α-agonist treatment. Starting doses are the same as for each drug when used individually, but the dose of both products often can be reduced slightly over time if the combination is effective.

Other pharmacologic agents that may be useful in unusual or refractory cases include anticholinergic (antimuscarinic) agents that enhance bladder storage or agents that act on both urinary bladder and urethral smooth muscle to improve storage (imipramine, duloxetine), but these drugs have not been evaluated in clinically affected dogs. Anticholinergic agents are quite effective for detrusor instability (overactive bladder or urge incontinence) in which involuntary detrusor contractions occur and cause inappropriate leakage of urine. True detrusor instability is rare in animals, but these agents can be helpful in improving urine storage in select animals, either alone or in combination with α-agonists or reproductive hormones. Without urodynamic documentation of poor bladder storage function or detrusor instability, trial treatment can be considered in animals in which urge incontinence appears likely. These dogs or cats usually leak urine when active (i.e., when walking, jumping, or moving); urine dribbling may appear behavioral. Oxybutynin is the most commonly recommended anticholinergic agent. The authors have limited experience using the new anticholinergic tolterodine (Detrol, Pharmacia and Upjohn). Other agents, including amitriptyline, imipramine, flavoxate, and dicyclomine, also have anticholinergic effects. Imipramine and amitriptyline, tricyclic antidepressants, may improve urine storage by several mechanisms, including anticholinergic, α-adrenergic and β-adrenergic effects. However, imipramine has not proven very effective in clinical application. Side effects of antimuscarinic agents include dry mouth, blurred vision, urine retention, and gastrointestinal upset; they significantly limit tolerance of the drugs in humans but appear well tolerated by dogs. Ptyalism and gastrointestinal symptoms are possible in dogs and usually are remedied by reducing the dose. Clients may be familiar with the heavily marketed product tolterodine for overactive bladder in humans. This antimuscarinic agent is touted for once-daily administration and reduced side effects when compared to other available agents. There are no published reports of the use of the drug in small animals at this time.

Duloxetine, a serotonin and norepinephrine reuptake inhibitor, may improve urethral striated muscle resistance and bladder capacity and has proven useful in women with stress incontinence. The most common adverse effect in women was nausea, which can be minimized by slow dose escalation (Norton et al., 2002; Oelke, Roovers, and Michel, 2006). Experience is limited in small animals at this time.

Other diagnostic considerations and management recommendations for patients with refractory micturition disorders can be found in the references (Lane, 2003; Fisher and Lane, 2003). Endosurgical approaches to urinary obstruction and urinary incontinence are described in other chapters in this volume (see Chapters 208 and 209).

References and Suggested Reading

Fischer JR et al: Urethral pressure profile and hemodynamic effects of phenoxybenzamine and prazosin in non-sedated male beagle dogs, *Can J Vet Res* 67:30, 2003.

Lane IF: Treating urinary incontinence, *Vet Med* 98:58, 2003.

Fischer JR, Lane IF: Treating functional urinary obstruction, *Vet Med* 98:67, 2003.

Mandigers PJJ, Nell T: Treatment of bitches with acquired urinary incontinence with oestriol, *Vet Rec* 149:765, 2001.

Norton PA et al: Duloxetine versus placebo in the treatment of stress urinary incontinence, *Am J Obstet Gynecol* 187:40, 2002.

Oelke M, Roovers JP, Michel MC: Safety and tolerability of duloxetine in women with stress urinary incontinence, *Br J Obstet Gynecol* 113(suppl 1):22, 2006.

Reichler IM et al: The effect of GnRH analogs on urinary incontinence after ablation of the ovaries in dogs, *Theriogenology* 60:1207, 2003.

Reichler IM et al: Effect of a long-acting GnRH analogue or placebo on plasma LH/FSH, urethral pressure profiles and clinical signs of urinary incontinence due to sphincter mechanism incompetence in bitches, *Theriogenology* 66:1227, 2006.

Scott L et al: Evaluation of phenylpropanolamine in the treatment of urethral sphincter mechanism incompetence in the bitch, *J Small Anim Pract* 43:493, 2002.

CHAPTER 208

Urinary Incontinence: Treatment With Injectable Bulking Agents

JULIE K. BYRON, *Urbana, Illinois*
DENNIS J. CHEW, *Columbus, Ohio*
MARY A. McLOUGHLIN, *Columbus, Ohio*

Few problems in small animal practice are as frustrating to the owner and veterinarian as urinary incontinence. Although not life threatening, urinary incontinence is unacceptable to most pet owners. Affected dogs that cannot be managed successfully often are euthanized, surrendered to a humane shelter, or kept permanently outdoors. A search of records submitted to the Veterinary Medical Database revealed that 0.5% of dogs seen at veterinary teaching hospitals from 1994 to 2003 were diagnosed with urinary incontinence (VMDB, 2005).

The causes and manifestations of urinary incontinence vary; thus accurate diagnosis and elucidation of the underlying etiology is essential for therapeutic success. However, even for patients in which the disease is localized to urethral sphincter mechanism incompetence (USMI), complete continence with medical treatment is not guaranteed (see Chapter 207). Recently use of injectable bulking agents has been increasing in treating dogs that fail medical therapy. This approach, adopted from human therapeutics, shows promise in both reducing the need for medical therapy and improving response to it.

ETIOLOGY

Maintenance of urinary continence relies on many factors. Normally the major component of urethral tone is comprised of smooth muscle. Mucosal integrity, vasculature, and connective tissue surrounding the urethra also play important roles in preserving continence. In addition, healthy urothelium, surface tension from glandular secretions, and the pliability of the mucosa contribute significantly to coaptation of the urethral walls.

Bladder position and the exposure of the vesicourethral junction and proximal urethra to intraabdominal pressure also are important in preserving continence. When sudden increases in abdominal pressure occur, an increase in pressure occurs both within the bladder and in the proximal and midurethra, termed *pressure transmission* (Gregory and Holt, 1994). Several studies have evaluated the relationship of urethral position and length, as well as the vesicourethral angle to incontinence (Gregory, 1994; Gregory et al., 1996). However there is a large amount of overlap in these measurements between normal and affected dogs; many incontinent dogs have been found to have short urethras and intrapelvic bladders. Despite lack of definitive evidence for a direct cause-and-effect relationship, bladder and urethral position appear to be an important risk factor for incontinence.

The relationship of hormone status to incontinence has long been recognized. As many as 20% of neutered female dogs are expected to develop some degree of urinary incontinence during their lives, and 75% of these dogs will do so within 3 years of neutering. Decreased estrogen concentrations in women are associated with loss of urethral muscle tone, urethral vascular atrophy, and decreased glandular secretions, affecting major components of the continence mechanism. Decreased estrogen concentrations are likely a factor in the development of incontinence in dogs, but the lack of clinically recognized incontinence in anestrus-intact females (and the many ovariectomized dogs without incontinence) supports a more complex mechanism than a simple lack of trophic effect (Richter and Ling, 1985). Recent evidence suggests that increases in luteinizing hormone and follicle-stimulating hormone associated with estrogen decrease also may play a role in the development of incontinence in dogs, but the mechanism has yet to be determined (Reichler et al., 2005).

Other risk factors for incontinence are breed, body weight, and tail docking. Among the breeds found to be at increased risk for urinary incontinence are Old English sheepdogs, Doberman pinschers, German shepherd dogs, boxers, weimeraners, rottweilers, and Irish setters. Interestingly, of the breeds evaluated, Labrador retrievers appeared to have a decreased risk of incontinence, particularly among large-breed dogs (Holt and Thrusfield, 1993). Large- and giant-breed dogs and dogs weighing over 20 kg have been found to have a significantly increased risk of developing incontinence, whereas small-breed dogs have decreased risk. Tail docking has been suspected to be a contributor to the onset of incontinence in dogs because damage to the muscles of the pelvic floor is considered to be a contributing factor in the development of stress incontinence in women, but no studies have directly related tail docking to incontinence. However, tail docking is common; and among the breeds with increased risk of incontinence many females are docked as neonates but develop the disorder only after they are neutered, sometimes as older adults.

Although the risk factors remain unclear, the most common type of urinary incontinence recognized in female dogs is USMI. Incontinent female dogs have been found to have lower urethral closure pressures than continent dogs, and closure pressure increases in patients successfully managed with medical therapy. As noted previously, the closure pressure of the urethra depends on multiple factors; however, α-adrenergic receptor number and stimulation have been identified as primary therapeutic targets.

DIAGNOSIS

History and Minimum Database

The International Continence Society defines incontinence as "the complaint of any involuntary leakage of urine." There are several underlying reasons for the client complaint of "leaking urine," including behavioral, endocrine, and infectious causes, as well as USMI. The most important point to establish with owners is the involuntary nature of the problem. Many owners perceive submissive urination, pollakiuria, or polyuria as incontinence. For this reason the owner needs to be questioned extensively to establish the diagnosis. Water and food intake; general health; medical treatments; and appearance, frequency, and volume of urine voiding are all factors that should be discussed. It is essential to the diagnosis that the dog seem unaware of the leakage at the time it occurs, although it may "clean up" afterwards or lick the vulvar area frequently. Irritation of the vulva can occur because of a constantly wet environment or secondary bacterial infection. In addition, although difficult to definitively diagnose without urodynamic studies, detrusor instability (overactive bladder) may play a role in some incontinent patients.

Many incontinent dogs, especially those older than 7 years of age, develop incontinence after becoming polyuric from an unrelated disease process or following diuretic therapy of heart failure. Development of incontinence can therefore signal another, more serious problem that has otherwise escaped the owner's observation. We recommend that all incontinent dogs receive a general health screen, including complete blood count, serum electrolyte and chemistry evaluation, urinalysis (collected by cystocentesis), and systolic blood pressure measurement. In addition, because pollakiuria may be misinterpreted as incontinence by some owners and because of the increased risk of urinary tract infection in incontinent dogs, a quantitative urine culture should be performed.

Urodynamic Evaluation

The term *urodynamics* refers to several tests evaluating lower urinary tract function. The rationale behind the development of this technique is the theory that to maintain continence urethral pressure must be higher than intravesical pressure during the filling and storage phases of micturition. The three most commonly performed tests are the cystometrogram (CMG, an evaluation of bladder storage and contractile function), the Valsalva leak point pressure (VLPP), and the urethral pressure profile (UPP). These tests can be used to differentiate between detrusor instability and USMI, and they can assist in establishing severity of disease. The predictive value of urodynamic results is still debated, and improved

standardization of techniques will increase its reliability and diagnostic worth. At this time no studies have been published evaluating the predictive value of the UPP or VLPP on response to periurethral bulking agents in dogs. Studies in women have had mixed results, with the complicating factor that the VLPP does not always increase in patients with real improvement in continence. Based on our experience, there does not appear to be a strong correlation between the UPP and the success of periurethral bulking agent therapy. However, this does not mean that there is no role for urodynamics in the assessment of patients for bulking agent treatment. It is important to verify the presence of USMI and any component of overactive bladder before placing bulking agents because the relative contribution of each of these disorders will guide therapeutic decisions. Many dogs may have a significant component of overactive bladder and require anticholinergic therapy in addition to bulking agents to attain continence.

TREATMENT

Treatment of urinary incontinence has taken several avenues. Pelvic floor muscle training and pharmacologic treatments are considered primary therapy in humans, but surgical procedures for stress incontinence in women have been described for over 100 years and are still applied extensively. Both medical and surgical treatments have been adapted for small animals, including sympathomimetic drugs, estrogens, periurethral injections, and colposuspension. The use of injectable bulking agents is becoming more widespread and, with the advent of newer materials, shows significant promise in treating incontinence in dogs.

Injectable Bulking Agents

Injection of bulking agents to prevent urine leakage has been reported as early as 1938, with a description of cod liver oil injection in women. Although many materials have been investigated, the theory behind all injectable bulking agents is to narrow the diameter of the urethral lumen, thus creating outflow obstruction and allowing the urethral sphincter to close more easily. In veterinary medicine injection of bulking agents has been performed in selected centers for many years but is now seeing more widespread application following the introduction of safer and more effective bulking materials.

Patient Selection

Because of cost and concerns about duration of postprocedure continence, patient selection for urethral injection is important. The ideal patient has USMI without additional active lower urinary tract disease, including urinary tract infection. Patients should be screened via the CMG and any significant degree of detrusor instability managed medically before the injection procedure. As discussed in the following paragraphs, patients with ectopic ureters may benefit from the procedure; however, the location of the ureteral stomata is important. The majority of our periurethral injection patients have previously tried and failed medical therapy. In spite of this, many of these patients have an improved response to α-agonists after injection. Based on anecdotal data, previous response to medical therapy does not appear to predict outcome of injection therapy. Currently injection therapy is recommended most frequently to those patients with USMI and failure or declining efficacy of α-agonist or estrogen therapy.

Procedure

The bulking material is injected into the submucosa of the proximal urethra through a transurethral cystoscope or via a periurethral approach (Fig. 208-1). The periurethral approach has been found to have a slightly higher risk of early postoperative complications in women and has not been used in dogs. Using the transurethral approach, three blebs are created in the urethral wall at the 2, 6, and 10 o'clock positions, approximately 1 cm distal to the bladder neck, effectively narrowing the urethra (Figs. 208-2 and 208-3).

Following standard protocols, a cystoscope is passed into the external urethral meatus and advanced to the level of the trigone. The scope is then withdrawn to a point just caudal to the bladder neck. When the urethra and bladder are moderately infused with fluid, the demarcation between urethra and bladder at this level is relatively clear. The injection needle is passed into the instrument port and advanced submucosally with the bevel pointing toward the mucosa. The bevel of the needle is then rotated 180 degrees, and the injection is begun. The material must be injected slowly with the scope held very still because the urethral mucosa tears easily, leading to loss of the injected material and the need for reseating of the needle. Each bleb is filled with approximately 0.5 to 1 ml of material initially; however, the exact amount needed varies, depending on patient size and conformation, as well as the material injected. Some blebs may be larger than others because the more lateral portions of the wall are easier to fill. The goal is visual occlusion of the urethra; however, there is little risk of functional obstruction to voiding. If a concern about obstruction exists, a red rubber catheter gently passed into the urethra flattens the injected material and opens the urethra. Each bleb of

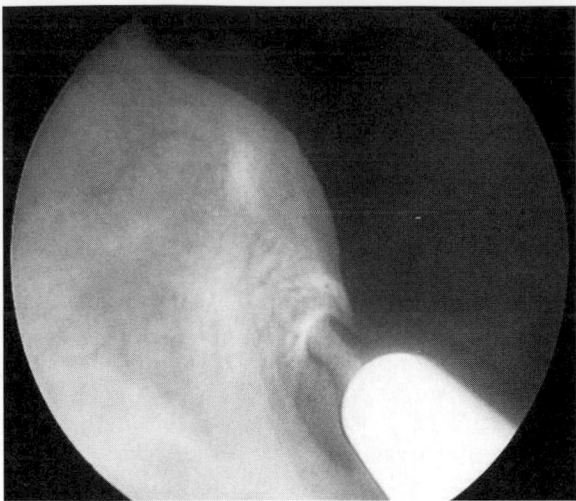

Fig. 208-2   Cystoscopic view of the urethra of a female dog. The injection needle is placed through the mucosa, and glutaraldehyde cross-linked bovine (GAX) collagen is being injected under the mucosa.

material should be placed in the same plane of the urethra to improve coaptation of the urethra.

Bulking agents

The ideal injectable bulking agent is easily delivered, biocompatible, nonantigenic, noncarcinogenic, stable within tissue, and reasonably cost-effective. Over the past 70 years several different agents have been used as the injected material; however, improvement in continence was rarely achieved without significant scarring or sloughing of the urethra. Recent application of safer injectable agents, particularly collagen preparations, has improved the outcome of the procedure. Veterinary experience with collagen compounds, as well as their precursor Teflon, are summarized here.

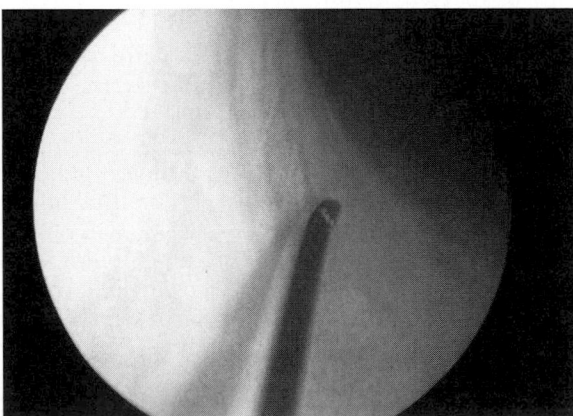

Fig. 208-1   Cystoscopic view of the urethra of a female dog. The needle in the foreground is the transurethral injection needle extending from the instrument channel of the scope.

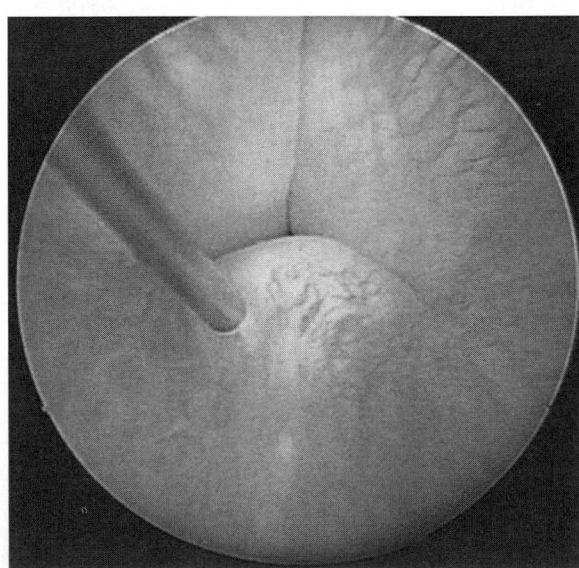

Fig. 208-3   Cystoscopic view of the urethra of a female dog after proper placement of submucosal glutaraldehyde cross-linked bovine (GAX) collagen.

Polytetrafluoroethylene paste. Polytetrafluoroethylene (PTFE; Teflon Polytef Paste, Dupont) was the first widely used urethral bulking agent in both humans and dogs. The procedure was reported in one study to improve continence in 57% of 298 women treated with just one set of injections (Lampante, Sparwasser, and Charvalakis, 1984). Its use in women decreased after it was found that the PTFE particles migrated after just a few months from the injection site to other parts of the body, including the brain, lungs, and lymph nodes. In addition, the PTFE caused a severe inflammatory reaction at the site of injection and often was extruded, leaving ulcers in the urethral mucosa. The results of PTFE injection have been reported for 22 dogs that either had failed α-agonist treatment or for which such treatment was unsuitable (Arnold et al., 1989). In this group of dogs 36% were continent after one PTFE injection, and an additional 41% were continent after a second injection. The majority of these dogs required adjunct treatment with phenylpropanolamine (PPA) to maintain continence. Fourteen (64%) dogs relapsed after 4 to 17 months. Necropsy was performed in 3 dogs 2 to 11 months after injection; PTFE was not found at sites other than the periurethral tissues. Due to granulomatous reactions at the injection site and the development of improved injection materials, PTFE has been abandoned as a periurethral injection material in women and is currently unavailable in North America. However, PTFE is still used by some European veterinarians as a more economical alternative to cross-linked collagen, particularly in large breed dogs.

Bovine cross-linked collagen. Glutaraldehyde cross-linked bovine (GAX) collagen (Contigen Bard Collagen Implant, Bard Urological Division) today is the most widely used periurethral bulking agent in humans. Before its use in urology, collagen had been used safely by plastic surgeons and dermatologists in a variety of tissues; migration of injected collagen was not observed (Kershen, Dmochowski, and Appell, 2002). The collagen is supplied in 2.5-ml syringes and is injected using a 5-Fr transurethral injection needle (Contigen Transurethral Injection System, Bard Urological Division) placed through the instrument port of a rigid cystoscope (Figs. 208-4 and 208-5). Rather than causing an inflammatory reaction, the GAX implant is vascularized and invaded by fibroblasts. Fibroblasts lay down new endogenous collagen, stabilizing the implant. In humans no evidence of migration within the body has been found during 15 years of GAX use. The postoperative cure rates have been very good; but, as with any injectable treatment, long-term outcome is poor compared to that of other surgical procedures in women. Reported cure rates in women range from 60% to 80%, but this success decreases to 40% after 2 years (Winters et al., 2000; Kershen, Dmochowski, and Appell, 2002). In one metaanalysis of studies performed before February 2003, it was found that there were no subjective or objective benefits in the outcome when compared to surgery, but few studies were available for analysis (Pickard et al., 2003). The biggest advantage of collagen injection in humans is the low morbidity associated with this outpatient procedure. The procedure is especially useful in elderly or frail patients who cannot undergo general anesthesia and surgery. The low morbidity and minimally

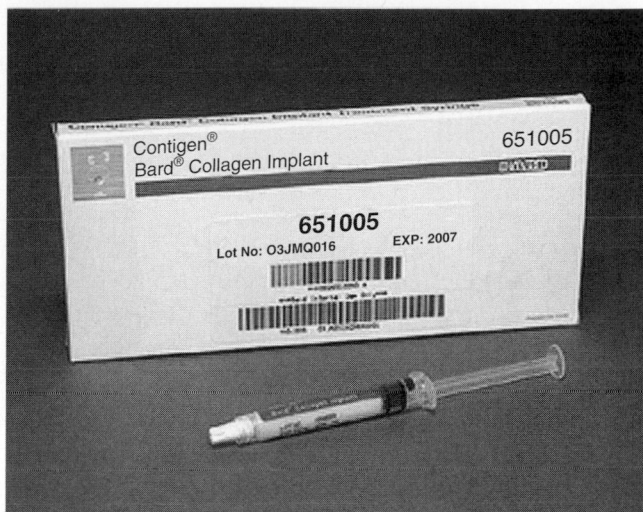

Fig. 208-4   Packaging of the glutaraldehyde cross-linked bovine (GAX) collagen. (Courtesy Contigen, Bard Urological Division.)

invasive nature of collagen injection also makes this procedure attractive for the treatment of refractory incontinence in dogs. In this species surgical procedures for incontinence have not proved advantageous for either short- or long-term outcomes.

Response to Collagen Injection in Dogs

Three reports have described the outcomes of collagen injection in the incontinent female dog. The first report included 32 spayed female dogs refractory to PPA treatment and subsequently treated with periurethral collagen injection (Arnold et al., 1996). Of these dogs, 53% were continent after one or two injections without the addition of PPA. With PPA the success rate increased to 75%. No postoperative complications were observed, and six of these dogs (19%) were observed to be continent longer than 30 months after the first injection. A longer-term follow-up study was performed by the same group of investigators involving 40 dogs over 7 years (Barth et al., 2005).

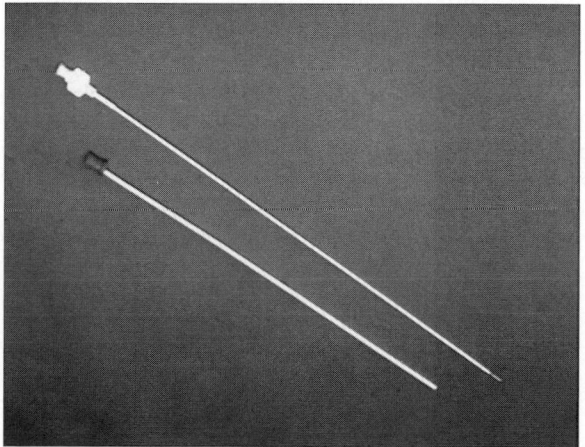

Fig. 208-5   5-Fr transurethral injection needle system. (Courtesy Contigen, Bard Urological Division.)

In the larger study 68% of the dogs were continent for a mean of 17 months (range 1 to 64 months) after collagen injection. Improvement was also observed in an additional 25%, and of these 60% became continent after the addition of α-agonist therapy. Mild and transient side effects were noted in 15% of treated dogs, including stranguria, hematuria, and vaginitis. A recent retrospective study evaluated the outcome of 34 collagen injections in 29 female dogs (Byron et al., 2005). Seven of these dogs had been diagnosed with ureteral ectopia; six had received corrective surgery but had persistent postoperative incontinence Of the treated dogs, 66% achieved complete continence immediately after the procedure, and an additional 32% were improved. Of the dogs with improved continence, 55% achieved full continence after the addition of medical therapy. The mean duration of complete continence after the procedure was 12.1 months without additional medical therapy. The majority of dogs had an improved response to medical therapy if added after continence declined. Overall client satisfaction with the procedure was 88%, with 76% of the clients being 100% satisfied with the procedure. Although little data are available, addressing the success of reinjection following decline in continence after collagen injection in dogs, studies in women have been encouraging. In our experience repeated injection of collagen, either by "enhancing" the previously placed blebs or by addition of new ones, has led to improved response and reinduction of continence. Currently we recommend reinjection in patients who do not improve after initial collagen injection or who experience a decline in continence after a period of time.

A newer use of injectable collagen is in some patients with ectopic ureters. Approximately 50% of these patients continue to have some degree of incontinence after neoureterostomy. Although technically more challenging to implant because of scarring of the urethral mucosa, periurethral injection of collagen appears to improve continence. In addition, injection of collagen distal to the ectopic stoma in patients with proximally placed ureteral ectopia may reduce incontinence without more invasive surgical intervention.

Newer agents. As mentioned previously, the ideal injectable bulking agent should be easily delivered, anatomically stable, safe, biocompatible, nonantigenic, noncarcinogenic, and inexpensive. Several agents on the horizon are nearly ideal in these respects. These include but are not limited to carbon-coated zirconium beads, autologous cartilage and fat grafts, silicone microimplants, microballoons, and acellular extracellular matrix substances (Kershen, Dmochowski, and Appell, 2002; van Kerrebroeck et al., 2003). As tissue engineering advances, more potential materials will be tested. The current limitation of injection therapy is the poor long-term outcome, and this obstacle must be overcome by those working to design new injectable agents.

References and Suggested Reading

Arnold S et al: Treatment of urinary incontinence in dogs by endoscopic injection of Teflon, *J Am Vet Med Assoc* 195:1369, 1989.

Arnold S et al: Treatment of urinary incontinence in bitches by endoscopic injection of glutaraldehyde cross-linked collagen, *J Small Anim Pract* 37:163, 1996.

Barth A et al: Evaluation of long-term effects of endoscopic injection of collagen into the urethral submucosa for treatment of urethral sphincter incompetence in female dogs: 40 cases (1993-2000), *J Am Vet Med Assoc* 226:73, 2005.

Byron JB et al: Transurethral collagen implantation for treatment of canine urinary incontinence, ACVIM Forum, Baltimore, Md, Abstract 120, 2005.

Gregory SP: Developments in the understanding of the pathophysiology of urethral sphincter mechanism in competence in the bitch, *Br Vet J* 150:135, 1994.

Gregory SP, Holt PE: The immediate effect of colposuspension on resting and stressed urethral pressure profiles in anaesthetized incontinent bitches, *Vet Surg* 23:330, 1994.

Gregory SP, Cripps PJ, Holt PE: Comparison of urethral pressure profilometry and contrast radiography in the diagnosis of incompetence of the urethral sphincter mechanism in bitches, *Vet Rec* 138:58, 1996.

Holt PE, Thrusfield MV: Association in bitches between breed, size, neutering and docking, and acquired urinary incontinence due to incompetence of the urethral sphincter mechanism, *Vet Rec* 133:177, 1993.

Kershen, RT, Dmochowski RR, Appell RA: Beyond collagen: injectable therapies for the treatment of female stress urinary incontinence in the new millennium, *Urol Clin North Am* 29:559, 2002.

Lampante L, Sparwasser H, Charvalakis C: Behandlungsergebnisse der harninkontinenz durch endourethrale submukose tefloninjektion, *Urologe [B]* 24:83, 1984.

Pickard R et al: Periurethral injection therapy for urinary incontinence in women, *Cochrane Database Syst Rev 2*, 2003.

Reichler IM et al: FSH and LH plasma levels in bitches with differences in risk for urinary incontinence, *Theriogenology* 63:2164, 2005.

Richter KP, Ling GV: Clinical response and urethral pressure profile changes after phenylpropanolamine in dogs with primary sphincter incompetence, *J Am Vet Med Assoc* 187:605, 1985.

van Kerrebroeck P et al: Treatment of stress urinary incontinence: recent developments in the role of urethral injection, *Urol Res* 30:356, 2003.

Veterinary Medical Databases Search Request #05–139: December 1, 2005, the Veterinary Medical Database, http://www.vmdb.org. *VMDB does not make any implicit or implied opinion on the subject of the paper or study.*

Winters JC et al: Collagen injection therapy in elderly women: long-term results and patient satisfaction, *Urology* 55:856, 2000.

CHAPTER 209

Interventional Radiology in Urinary Diseases

CHICK W.C. WEISSE, *Philadelphia, Pennsylvania*
ALLYSON C. BERENT, *Philadelphia, Pennsylvania*

With *interventional radiology (IR)*, contemporary imaging techniques are used to selectively access vessels and other structures to deliver materials for therapeutic purposes. These techniques are most commonly performed in veterinary medicine for occlusion of patent ductus arteriosus (Chapter 165), embolization of portosystemic shunts (Chapter 134), and placement of tracheal stents (Chapter 145). *Endosurgery* involves the use of endoscopic equipment, with or without concurrent fluoroscopy, to perform minimally invasive interventions in virtually any part of the body.

Currently the investigation and application of these techniques is expanding in veterinary medicine, particularly in applications pertaining to the urinary tract. The relatively common incidence of urinary tract obstruction neoplasia and trauma, combined with the morbidity associated with traditional surgical techniques, makes the use of less invasive procedures such as laparoscopy, endoscopy, and IR highly appealing. Such interventional procedures are already considered the standard of care in human medicine. This chapter contains a brief review of some of the interventional procedures currently performed in veterinary patients, as well as some promising future urologic applications.

ADVANTAGES

The use of IR and endosurgical techniques in veterinary patients offers a number of advantages compared to more traditional therapies. These procedures are minimally invasive and lead to reduced perioperative morbidity and mortality, shorter anesthesia times, and shorter hospital stays. The less equipment-intensive procedures can result in reduced cost as well. In addition, some techniques such as palliative stenting for malignant obstructions offer alternative treatment options for conditions that may not be amenable to standard surgical or medical approaches.

EQUIPMENT

Most of these minimally invasive procedures (performed through catheters, orifices, or small percutaneous holes) are performed in clean angiography suites; traditional sterile operating rooms are not required. Entry sites receive a standard sterile scrub; operators wear full lead gowns, lead thyroid shields, caps, gowns, and masks. The radiation exposure during conventional or C-arm fluoroscopy can be substantial; thus the operator should review radiation safety guidelines, minimize exposure time and beam size, and maximize shielding and distance from the beam whenever possible.

For many of the more commonly performed IR procedures, a traditional fluoroscopy unit is sufficient. A C-arm fluoroscopy unit has the advantage of mobility of the image intensifier, permitting multiple tangential views without moving the patient. Occasionally ultrasonography is useful for percutaneous needle access into vessels or other structures (e.g., urinary bladder, renal pelvis).

Various flexible and rigid endoscopes are used for traditional interventional endosurgical procedures. Rigid cystoscopy is performed commonly in female animals for urethral, urinary bladder, and ureteral access. Recommended diameters range from 1.9 to 6.5 mm, depending on the size of the patient. Flexible ureteroscopes (2.5- to 2.8-mm diameter) are used for lower urinary tract access in male dogs and for ureteral access in larger animals. Rigid nephroscopes (5.3- to 7.3-mm diameter) are commonly used for percutaneous nephrolithotomy. Different types of intracorporeal lithotripters and lasers are available for these procedures such as ultrasonic lithotripters, Holmium:YAG lasers, and diode-type lasers (also see Chapter 204).

TECHNIQUES

Kidney and Ureter

Percutaneous Nephrostomy

Ureteral obstruction secondary to ureteroliths or malignancy can result in severe hydronephrosis and/or life-threatening azotemia when present bilaterally or in animals with concurrent renal insufficiency. Although some patients can be managed with supportive care until a ureterolith passes, others may require surgery (see Chapter 202). Ureterotomy or other surgical approaches can require prolonged operating time and complex microsurgical technique in these often debilitated patients. An alternative strategy is to place a nephrostomy tube to relieve obstruction and thoroughly assess the patient before prolonged ureteral surgery. Nephrostomy drainage also allows aggressive fluid support and medical management of metabolic derangements to proceed in the interim. Although nephrostomy tubes are often placed surgically, *percutaneous nephrostomies* can be performed safely and efficiently in select patients to accomplish the same goals.

Under general anesthesia the skin over the paracostal area is clipped and prepared. Percutaneous needle access to the renal pelvis is obtained, and a contrast pyelogram is performed under fluoroscopic visualization (Fig. 209-1, *A*). A guidewire is placed, tract dilation is performed, a locking-loop drainage catheter is advanced over-the-wire, and the loop is formed within the renal pelvis (Figs. 209-1, *B* and 209-1, *C*). The catheter is attached to a urine collection system and secured in place with a finger-trap suture and multiple tacking sutures to the body wall (Fig. 209-1, *D*). The patient is recovered from anesthesia, and urine output is carefully monitored. The presence of the nephrostomy tube allows drainage of urine produced by this kidney and renal pelvic access for subsequent contrast ureterography. Serial radiographic studies can be performed to determine if the obstruction resolves sufficiently without ureteral surgery.

Ureteral Stenting

Ureteral stents are placed to divert urine from the renal pelvis into the urinary bladder. This technique can be useful in patients with ureteral obstruction and has been performed in animals to circumvent inflammation following ureteroscopy or ureteral stone retrieval (basket retrieval or laser lithotripsy), to prevent nephrolith stone fragments from causing a ureteral obstruction following lithotripsy, and to alleviate obstructions secondary to ureteral neoplasia. In addition, the presence of the ureteral stent may create sufficient ureteral dilation to permit passage of previously obstructive ureteroliths. This technique is currently under investigation for use in veterinary patients with ureterolith-induced obstructions.

Under general anesthesia concurrent cystoscopy and fluoroscopy are used to introduce a guidewire into the ureteral opening and advance the guidewire proximally (retrograde approach). A hydrophilic catheter is advanced over-the-wire under fluoroscopic guidance, the guidewire is removed, and a retrograde contrast ureteropyelogram is performed to help identify any lesions, stones, or filling defects in the renal pelvis or ureter. A stiffened guidewire is then advanced retrograde through the catheter, which

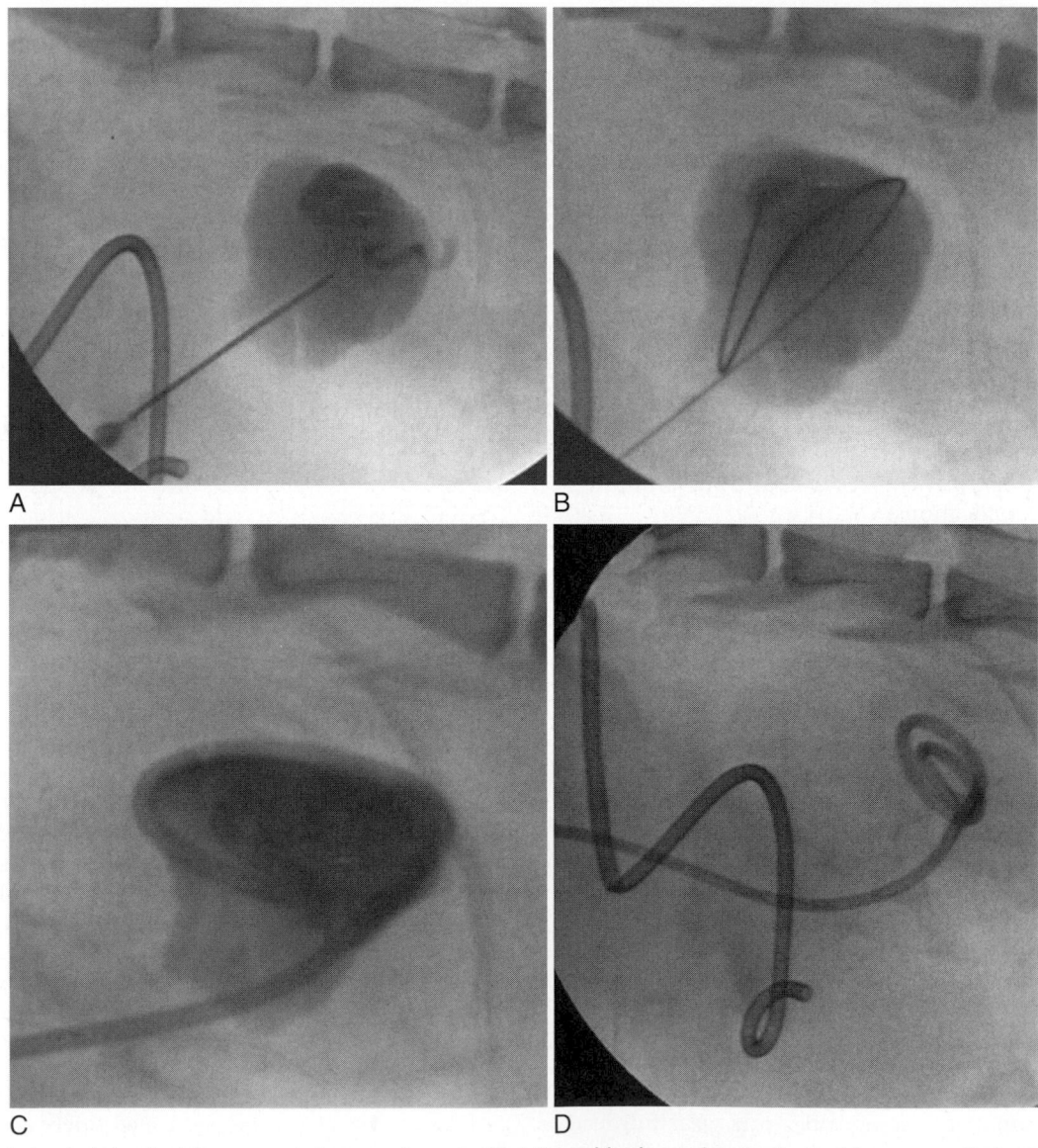

Fig. 209-1   Lateral abdominal fluoroscopic image of a cat with bilateral hydronephrosis. **A,** An 18-gauge catheter is percutaneously placed in the renal pelvis, and a contrast pyelogram is performed. **B,** Stiffened 0.035-inch guidewire advanced into the renal pelvis. **C,** Pigtail drainage catheter within renal pelvis following removal of the guidewire. **D,** Bilateral percutaneous nephrostomy tubes.

is replaced with either an indwelling double pigtail ureteral stent (Fig. 209-2) or an exteriorized pigtail catheter (see Fig. 209-6, *F*). In an antegrade technique, percutaneous nephrostomy access is achieved as described in the previous section; and the guidewire is passed down the ureter, into the bladder, and out the urethra. A ureteral dilator is passed over-the-wire and exchanged for an indwelling ureteral stent or a nephroureteral stent.

Percutaneous Nephrolithotomy

Urinary obstruction by nephroliths or proximal ureteroliths can result in progressive renal insufficiency, intractable pyelonephritis, and hydronephrosis. Small stones may pass spontaneously into the lower urinary tract; however, other uroliths require surgery to relieve the obstruction and avoid permanent renal damage. Nephrotomies, pyelotomies, or ureterotomies can be prolonged, invasive, and complicated surgeries with significant morbidity. In human patients percutaneous nephrolithotomy is considered the standard of care for large nephroliths and proximal ureteroliths (those not amenable to extracorporeal shock-wave lithotripsy or endosurgical techniques). This minimally invasive procedure aims to minimize morbidity and preserve as much renal function as possible.

Under general anesthesia the skin over the paracostal area is clipped and prepared. A retrograde ureteropyelogram is performed using the technique described previously for ureteral stenting. Ureteral catheter access is maintained to protect the ureter from stone fragment escape down the ureter and to allow for repeat ureteropyelography if necessary. The retrograde approach may not be possible in male cats or small male dogs, in which case antegrade access is obtained via a percutaneous nephrostomy. Following percutaneous needle and wire access into the renal pelvis, serially larger dilators are advanced over-the-wire to dilate the tract sufficiently for the placement of a large nephroscope sheath (Fig. 209-3). Alternatively a balloon dilation set can be used for this purpose. The nephroscope is then placed through the access sheath, and the nephrolith or proximal ureterolith is identified and fragmented using ultrasonic or laser lithotripsy. The fragments are removed via suction, grasping-forceps, or basket-retrieval methods, with instruments directed through the instrument channel. Following urolith removal a percutaneous nephrostomy tube is left in place for approximately 2 to 3 weeks to allow for progressive closure of the access tract. If there is ureteral trauma or inflammation, a percutaneous nephroureteral stent can be placed, maintaining patency from the skin tract, into the renal pelvis, and down the ureter into the bladder.

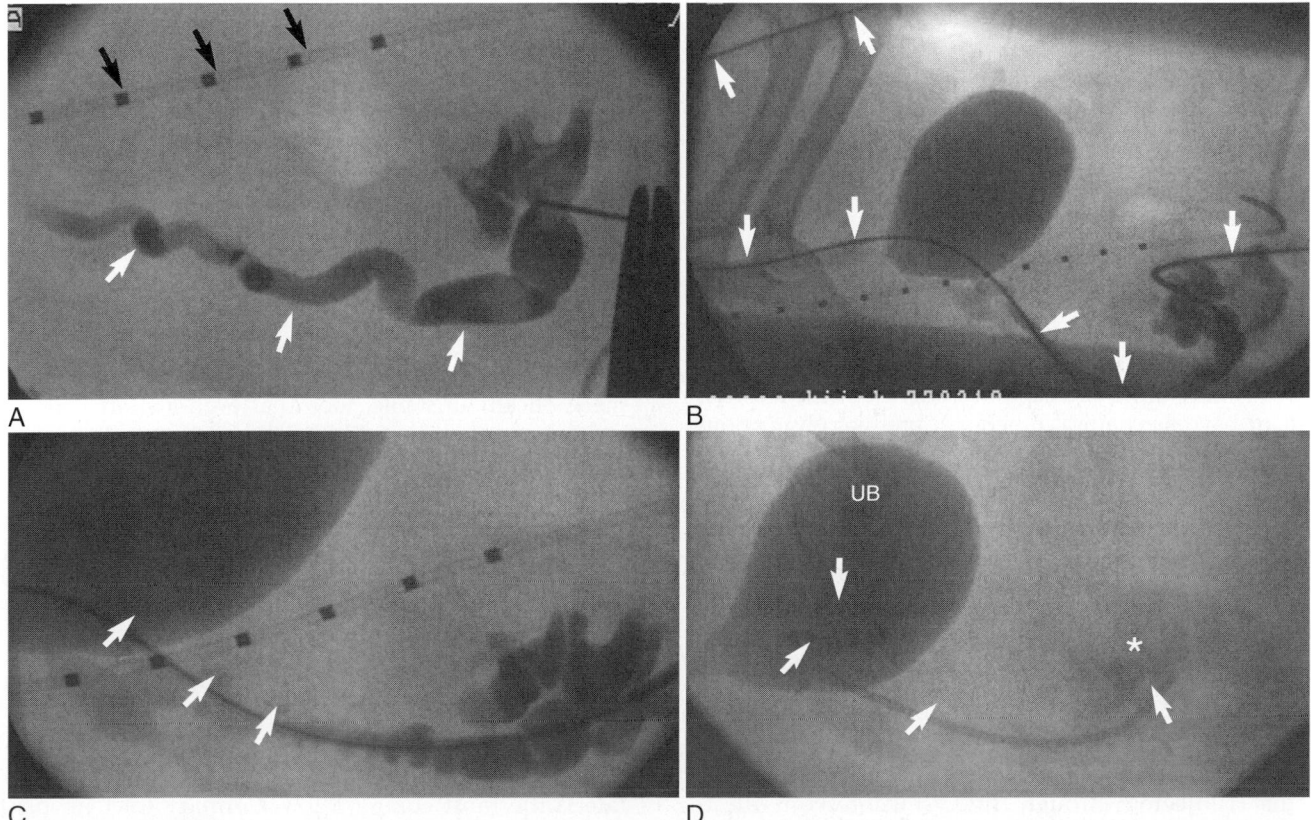

Fig. 209-2 Lateral abdominal fluoroscopic image of a 6.5-kg dog (dorsal recumbency) with transitional cell carcinoma–induced obstruction of the left ureteral stoma. **A,** Percutaneous pyelocentesis with an 18-gauge catheter and subsequent contrast ureteropyelogram demonstrating hydronephrosis and hydroureter *(white arrows)*. A colonic marker catheter *(black arrows)* has been placed for measurement purposes. **B,** Antegrade placement of a 0.035-inch angled hydrophilic guidewire and catheters *(white arrows)* through the percutaneous nephrostomy, across the malignant obstruction and out the penis for through-and-through access. **C,** Retrograde ureteral dilation with a 6-Fr ureteral dilator placed over-the-wire and across the malignant obstruction. **D,** Indwelling 4.7-Fr ureteral stent *(white arrows)* placed over-the-wire from the renal pelvis *(white asterisk)* to the urinary bladder *(UB)*.

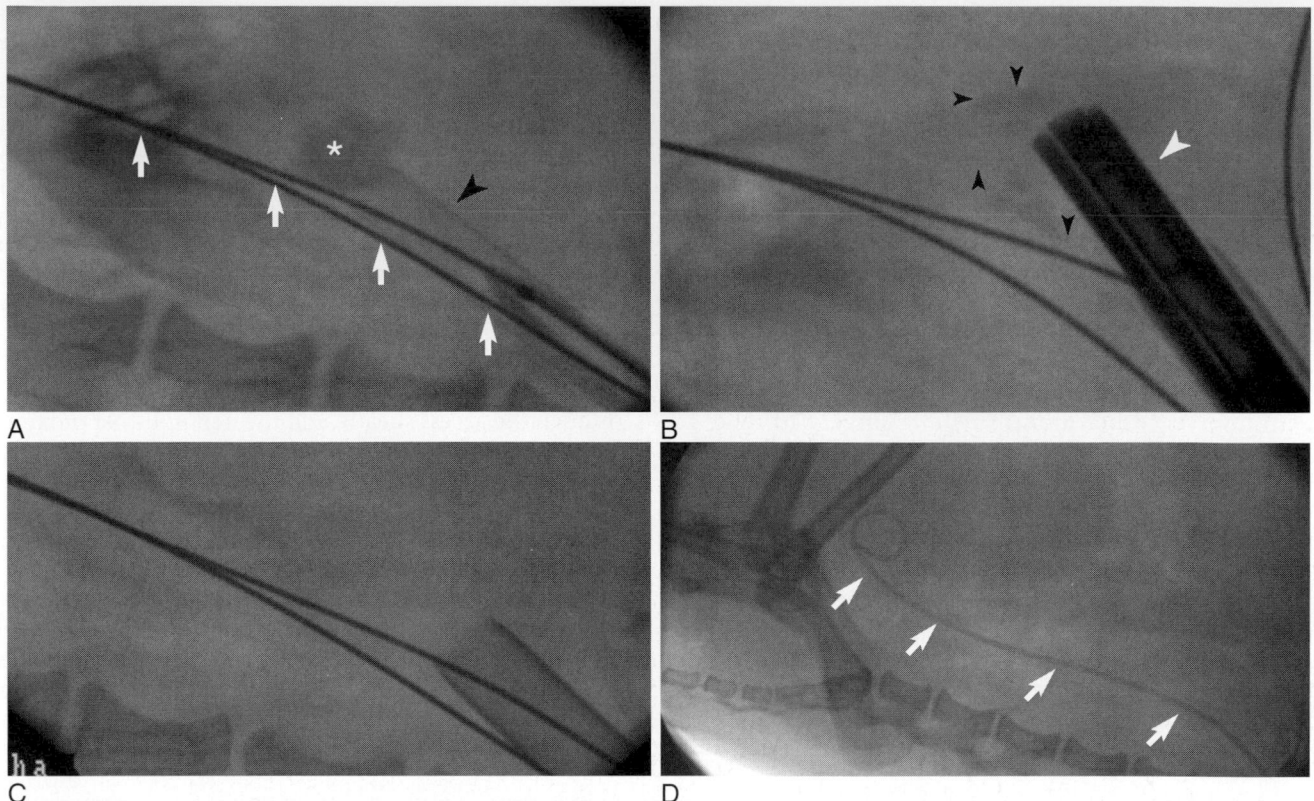

Fig. 209-3 Lateral fluoroscopic image of a dog (dorsal recumbency) with bilateral nephroliths undergoing a percutaneous nephrolithotomy. **A,** Following percutaneous nephrostomy and through-and-through guidewire and safety guidewire access *(white arrows)*, an access sheath *(black arrow)* is placed up to the nephrolith *(white asterisk)*. **B,** A nephroscope and lithotripter *(white arrow)* are placed within the sheath, and the nephrolith is fragmented *(black arrowheads)*. **C,** Fluoroscopic image following nephrolith fragmentation and removal. **D,** Nephroureteral stent *(white arrows)* placement following lithotripsy to maintain ureteral patency and allow nephrostomy tract to heal.

Urinary Bladder and Urethra

Antegrade Urethral Catheterization

Urethral catheterization is typically a simple and routine procedure in veterinary patients to monitor urine output, establish urine drainage in patients that are recumbent or have mechanical/functional urethral obstructions, or ensure urethral patency following surgical procedures. Occasionally retrograde catheterization can be difficult in very small (female) patients or in feline patients with significant urethral trauma (e.g., following manipulations to relieve urethral obstruction). Antegrade urethral catheterization performed under direct fluoroscopic visualization can be performed rapidly, easily, and safely in patients in which attempts at routine retrograde catheterization have failed.

Under general anesthesia (recommended) or heavy sedation, the patient is placed in lateral recumbency, and the flank and caudal ventral abdomen are clipped and scrubbed. Cystocentesis is performed, and contrast media is injected through the cystocentesis needle to define the urinary bladder and urethra (Fig. 209-4). Under fluoroscopic guidance a guidewire is advanced antegrade into the bladder and through the urethra until exiting the penis or vulva. A urinary catheter is then advanced over-the-wire in a retrograde fashion into the urinary bladder, and the guidewire is removed. The urinary catheter is secured in place in a routine fashion.

Percutaneous Cystostomy Tubes

Cystostomy tubes are placed regularly during surgery to manage veterinary patients with urinary obstructions or to divert urine away from a traumatized urethra. Occasionally these patients are severely debilitated and metabolically unstable, such that even a short period of general anesthesia would be dangerous. A variety of cystostomy tubes and techniques are available for percutaneous placement to quickly and safely establish urine drainage and/or diversion. Locking-loop drainage catheters have been used for such purposes in veterinary patients. These tubes can be placed directly into the urinary bladder via palpation alone or with fluoroscopic or ultrasound guidance.

Urethral Stenting for Malignant Obstructions

Malignant obstruction of the urethra can cause severe dysuria and life-threatening azotemia in some patients. Transitional cell carcinoma of the urethra and/or prostate is the most common lower urinary tract neoplasia encountered in small animal patients, with greater then 80% of dogs experiencing dysuria and approximately 10% developing complete urinary tract obstruction (Norris et al., 1992; Knapp et al., 2000). Chemotherapy has been successful in slowing tumor growth, but complete cures are uncommon. When signs of obstruction occur, more aggressive therapy is indicated. Cystostomy tube place-

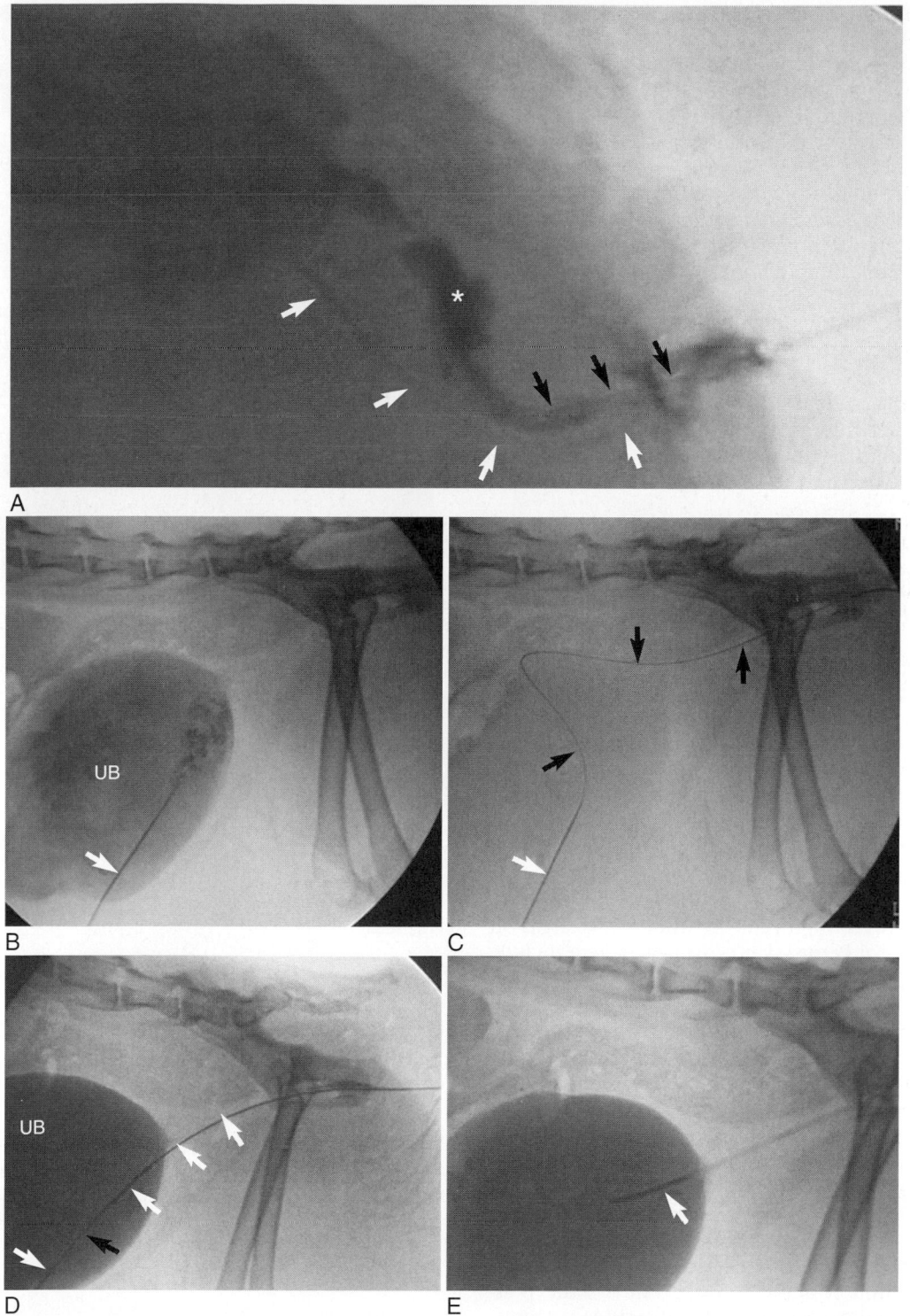

Fig. 209-4 Lateral abdominal fluoroscopic image of cat with an iatrogenic urethral tear secondary to traumatic catheterization. **A,** Retrograde contrast urethrogram demonstrating misplaced tomcat catheter *(black arrows)* and periurethral contrast extravasation *(white asterisk)*. Contrast within the normal urethra can be identified as well *(white arrows)*. **B,** Percutaneous cystocentesis with 18-gauge over-the-needle catheter *(white arrow)* and contrast cystourethrogram demonstrating extremely distended urinary bladder (UB). **C,** Angled hydrophilic 0.035-inch guidewire *(black arrows)* advanced through catheter *(white arrow)* and down urethra. **D,** Urinary catheter *(white arrows)* advanced retrograde over guidewire *(black arrow)* and into urinary bladder *(UB)*. **E,** Urinary catheter *(white arrow)* placement following removal of guidewire and cystocentesis catheter. Urinary bladder drainage can now be performed.

ment, transurethral resection, and surgical diversion have been described but are either invasive or associated with significant morbidity (complications of manual urine drainage, frequent urination, urinary tract infection)

(Stiffler et al., 2003; Liptak et al., 2004; Fries et al., 1991; Stone et al., 1988). Placement of self-expanding metallic stents using fluoroscopic guidance through a transurethral approach can provide a fast, reliable, and safe alternative to establish urethral patency in both males and females. We have experienced good-to-excellent palliative outcomes in greater than 75% of cases (Weisse et al., 2006). Urethral stenting may also be useful in patients with benign urethral strictures when traditional therapies have failed or when surgery is refused or not indicated.

A contrast cystourethrogram is performed, and transurethral retrograde or antegrade guidewire access across the malignant narrowing is obtained. Measurements of the normal urethral diameter and the length of obstruction are obtained (Fig. 209-5), and an appropriately sized self-expanding metallic urethral stent is chosen (approximately 10% to 15% greater than the normal urethral diameter and 1 cm longer than the obstruction on both the cranial and caudal ends). The stent is deployed under fluoroscopic guidance, and a repeat contrast cystourethrogram is performed to document restored urethral patency.

Additional Procedures

Additional IR techniques include novel approaches to control hemorrhage, occlude vascular malformations, or reduce tumor growth. Arterial embolization involves selective, catheter-directed delivery of particulate material (typically polyvinyl alcohol) performed under fluoroscopic guidance. Chemoembolization involves the addition of chemotherapy to the particle and contrast mixture to achieve extremely high regional concentrations of chemotherapy to enhance effectiveness and minimize systemic toxicity (Weisse et al., 2002). These therapies have been performed in veterinary medicine for urogenital neoplasia and associated hemorrhage (Weisse, 2002).

Other endosurgical procedures under investigation at the University of Pennsylvania and elsewhere include ureteral cauterization for idiopathic renal hematuria, urinary polyp removal, endosurgical repair of ectopic ureters, and endoscopic-guided collagen injection for urethral sphincter mechanism incompetence. Idiopathic renal hematuria is a rare condition in which a focal area of bleeding in the upper urinary tract results in long-term hematuria, iron deficient anemia (chronically), and the potential for clot formation resulting in ureteral colic or signs of lower urinary tract disease. Surgical nephrectomy or partial renal artery occlusion of the affected side has been considered the standard treatment, although this can result in loss of a functional kidney and significant morbidity (Mishina et al., 1997). In humans the presence of a hemangioma has been visualized via ureteroscopy, which is cauterized through the instrument port of a ureteroscope (Tawfiek and Bagley, 1998). This has also been performed in a small number of dogs (Fig. 209-6) (personal communication, Larry Adams). Bladder polyps are common findings in dogs and can be associated with chronic, recurrent urinary tract infections and cystolith formation and are often misinterpreted for cystic neoplasia. Using cystoscopy and laser lithotripsy (Holmium: YAG), the polyps can be removed without surgical intervention by cauterizing the stalk. Alternatively a basket can be used trap the polypoid tissue and break the stalk

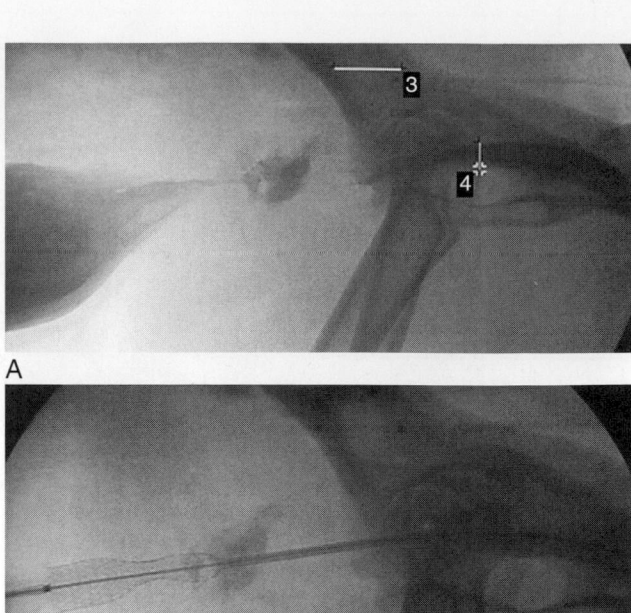

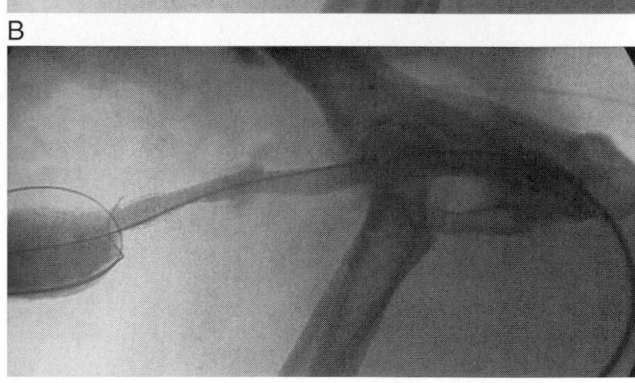

Fig. 209-5 Lateral abdominal fluoroscopic image of a dog with prostatic and urethral transitional cell carcinoma. **A,** Contrast cystourethrogram demonstrating extravasation of contrast into prostatic tissue and contrast attenuation caused by urethral narrowing at the level of the prostate. (3) 2-cm marker catheter placed within the rectum for measuring purposes. (4) Urethral diameter measurement taken caudal to the diseased urethra to choose appropriately sized stent. **B,** Partial self-expanding metallic stent deployment placed during fluoroscopic visualization. **C,** Contrast cystourethrogram immediately following complete stent deployment demonstrating restored urethral patency.

with mild tension. Ectopic ureters are a common congenital anatomic deformity in dogs. Endoscopic repair of ectopic ureters is a common procedure in humans with similar conditions and has been performed in a few dogs successfully with the use of fluoroscopy, cystoscopy, and diode laser ablation. Collagen injection via urethroscopic guidance has been performed for USMI at many institutions. This procedure is indicated if medical management has failed, is contraindicated, or not tolerated (see Chapter 208).

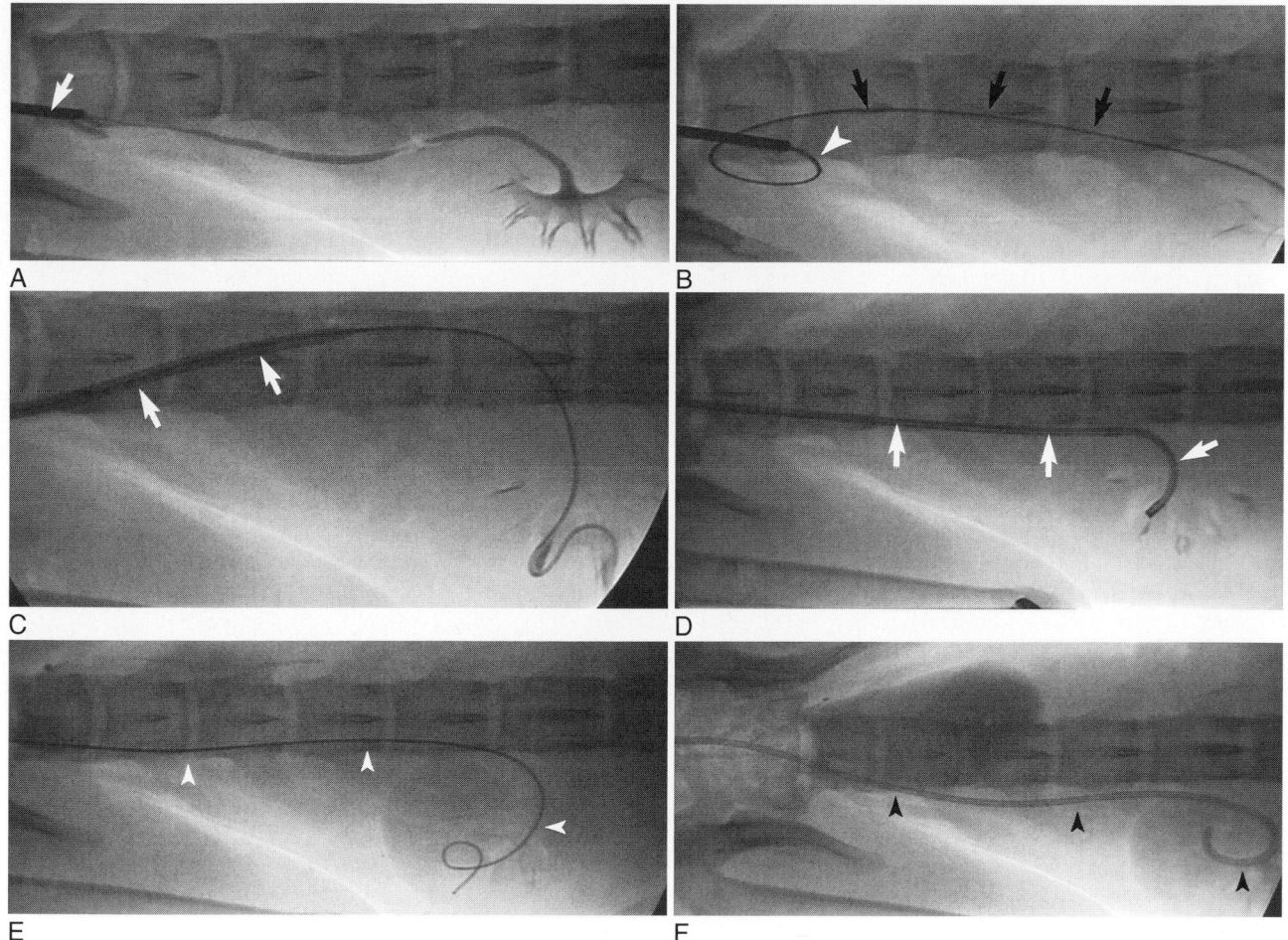

Fig. 209-6   Dorsoventral abdominal fluoroscopic image of a dog with unilateral idiopathic renal hematuria. **A,** A cystoscope *(white arrow)* is used to place a cone-tipped catheter in the most distal aspect of the ureter to perform a retrograde contrast ureteropyelogram. **B,** An angled-tipped hydrophilic 0.035-inch guidewire *(black arrows)* is advanced through the scope, up the ureter, and into the renal pelvis. The J-hooked distal ureter is apparent *(white arrowhead).* **C,** The cystoscope is removed over-the-wire, and a ureteral dilator *(white arrows)* is advanced over-the-wire under fluoroscopic guidance. **D,** The ureteral dilator is removed, and the ureteroscope *(white arrows)* is advanced over-the-wire. **E,** Once evaluation for cautery or stone retrieval is complete, the guidewire *(white arrowheads)* is replaced through the working channel. **F,** A single pigtailed locking-loop ureteral stent is placed over the guidewire *(black arrowheads).* The loop is locked in place in the renal pelvis, with the distal end exiting the urethra to provide temporary patency.

References and Suggested Reading

Fries CL et al: Enterocystoplasty with cystectomy and subtotal intracapsular prostatectomy in the male dogs, *Vet Surg* 20(2):104, 1991.

Knapp DW et al: Naturally occurring canine transitional cell carcinoma of the urinary bladder: a relevant model of human invasive bladder cancer, *Urol Oncol* 5:47, 2000.

Liptak JM et al: Transurethral resection in the management of urethral and prostatic neoplasia in 6 dogs, *Vet Surg* 33:505, 2004.

Mishina M et al: Idiopathic renal hematuria in a dog ; the usefulness of a method of partial occlusion of the renal artery, *J Vet Med Sci* 59(4):293, 1997.

Norris AM et al: Canine bladder and urethral tumors: a retrospective study of 115 cases (1980-1985), *J Vet Intern Med* 16:145, 1992.

Stiffler KS et al: Clinical use of low-profile cystostomy tubes in four dogs and a cat, *J Am Vet Med Assoc* 223(3):325, 2003.

Stone EA et al: Ureterocolonic anastomosis in ten dogs with transitional cell carcinoma, *Vet Surg* 17:147, 1988.

Tawfiek ER, Bagley DH: Ureteroscopic evaluation and treatment of chronic unilateral hematuria, *J Urol* 160:700, 1998.

Weisse C et al: Percutaneous bland arterial embolization and chemoembolization for the treatment of benign and malignant diseases, *J Am Vet Med Assoc* 221:1430, 2002.

Weisse C et al: Evaluation of palliative stenting for management of malignant urethral obstructions in dogs, *J Am Vet Med Assoc* 229:226, 2006.

SECTION X

Reproductive Diseases

Margaret V. Root Kustritz

CHAPTER 210

Breeding Management of the Bitch

GARY C.W. ENGLAND, *Nottingham, England*
MARCO RUSSO, *Naples, Italy*

In the bitch the most significant problem with the management of breeding is the large variation that occurs in the time between the onset of proestrus behavior and the timing of ovulation. In addition, there is poor correlation of the behavior of the bitch with the underlying endocrine events. It is usually a misunderstanding of these two components of the normal physiology that results in mating at a time remote from the fertilization period and a failure to achieve a pregnancy.

The aim of this chapter is to review the methods that are available for the identification of the optimal time for breeding, which include observational assessments, measurement of plasma hormone concentrations, examination of exfoliated vaginal cells, vaginal endoscopy, and ovarian ultrasonography.

Unlike other domestic species, which are polyestrus, a nonpregnant bitch undergoes a 65-day luteal phase followed by a 5- to 6- month period of anestrus. The monoestrus nature of the bitch and the extended time until the return of estrus highlights for the breeder the importance of determining the timing of the period of greatest fertility.

REPRODUCTIVE PHYSIOLOGY

The basic endocrinologic events in the bitch are not unlike those of other species in that there is a preovulatory surge of luteinizing hormone (LH) that occurs approximately 2 days before ovulation. However, at the time of ovulation oocytes are immature and cannot immediately be fertilized. Fertilization can occur only after extrusion of the first polar body and completion of the first meiotic division to form the secondary oocyte. Interestingly, oocytes remain viable within the reproductive tract for 4 to 5 days after they have become fertilizable (i.e., they do not begin to undergo degeneration until 6 to 7 days after ovulation).

When compared with other species, this relative delay in the availability of oocytes for fertilization combined with their lengthened survival time has a significant impact on the onset and duration of the fertilization period of this species.

The Fertilization Period

For all species the fertilization period is the time when oocytes are available to be fertilized. In the bitch this period commences 2 days after ovulation and extends until approximately 5 days after ovulation (Fig. 210-1). The fertilization period is likely to be the approximate time of maximal fertility, which subsequently declines rapidly over the next few days because of degeneration of the oocytes and closure of the cervix, which prevents sperm from entering the reproductive tract.

Although the fertilization period is extremely important in the bitch, it is not the only period of time during which a breeding can result in pregnancy. Intrauterine insemination after the end of the classically defined fertilization period has resulted in pregnancies of a small litter size (presumably by fertilization of aging oocytes), whereas breeding before the fertilization period commonly results in pregnancy (by virtue of sperm survival in the female reproductive tract).

The Fertile Period

The fertile period is the time during which a breeding could result in a conception. Therefore it includes the fertilization period, but it also precedes the fertilization period by several days because sperm can survive within the female reproductive tract (see Fig. 210-1). Sperm survival within the bitch means that a breeding before the fertilization period can result in a pregnancy. Interestingly, in fertile stud dogs sperm survival for up to 7 days does not appear to be uncommon, thus enabling the fertile period to commence 5 days before ovulation (i.e., sperm surviving for 7 days fertilize oocytes 2 days after ovulation).

Clearly not every stud dog produces sperm able to survive such a protracted period of time within the female reproductive tract. Dogs with poor semen quality generally have reduced sperm survival, and this accounts largely for the poor fertility seen in these individuals. Sperm that have been preserved also have a short survival time within the female reproductive tract. Therefore the potential fertile period is a feature of male fertility combined with female physiology.

THE OPTIMAL TIME FOR BREEDING

The period of peak fertility for natural breedings with fertile animals ranges from the day of until 4 days after ovulation (Table 210-1). There does not appear to be a difference in litter size when bitches are mated on any one of these days. Breedings earlier or later commonly result in lower pregnancy rates and smaller litters. In general it is thought that peak fertility commences before the true

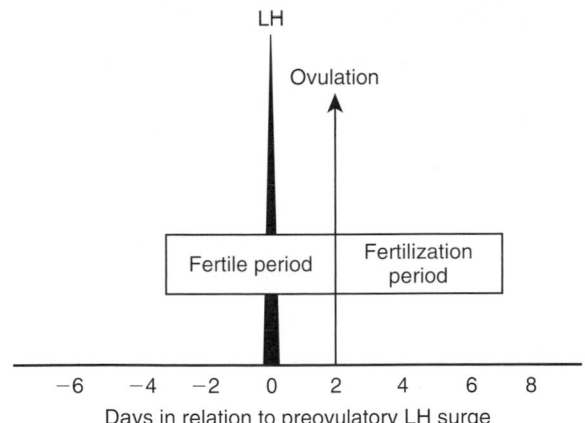

Fig. 210-1 Schematic relationship among the fertilization period, fertile period, ovulation, and the luteinizing hormone surge.

fertilization period since sperm are required to mature within the female reproductive tract and this process of capacitation may take approximately 6 hours or more.

For the accurate prediction of the optimal time to breed, the most sensible option clearly is detection either of the LH surge or of ovulation itself. However, documentation of these events can be difficult.

Observational Assessments

Although in other species there are reasonable relationships between the time of ovulation and several aspects of the reproductive cycle, in the bitch this may not be the case. Both the time of ovulation in relation to the onset of proestrus and the behavioral characteristics typical of estrus have a poor relation with the fertilization period.

The Number of Days From the Onset of Proestrus
Many breeders rely on counting the number of days from the onset of proestrus and believe that bitches always

ovulate a defined number of days from the onset of this event. This is not the case for any breed (Fig. 210-2). The duration of proestrus is variable among bitches; and, although the "average bitch" may ovulate 12 days after the onset of proestrus, some bitches ovulate as early as day 5, and others as late as day 30 after the onset of proestrus.

The large variation in the time of ovulation (and therefore the fertilization period) explains most of the infertility that arises when bitches are bred on the 12th and 14th day, which is common breeding practice. Furthermore, it is clear that the events of one estrus are not necessarily the same at the subsequent cycle; some bitches may vary in the day of ovulation by as much as 12 days from one cycle to the next (e.g., they ovulate on day 12 of one cycle and on day 24 of the next cycle).

The Onset of Estrus Behavior
In some species the onset of the behavioral signs of estrus (acceptance of mating) can be used to determine the optimal time for breeding. However, in the bitch there is often a poor correlation between endocrine events and behavioral events. Studies on laboratory-kept bitches suggested that the onset of standing estrus occurred on average at approximately the same time as the LH surge. Using these data, 3 or 4 days after the onset of standing estrus would be a suitable time for mating. However, in many other bitches the behavioral responses correlate poorly with the underlying hormonal events. This may be because bitches are housed away from the male and introduced only when the breeder considers that the time is correct, thus inhibiting natural courtship responses; or it may simply represent greater variation than was originally thought. A further complication is that in some bitches the behavioral changes may be displayed poorly and therefore the onset of estrus may be indistinct.

It may be that, with regular examination using a standard stimulation (e.g., possibly with the use of a teaser male), the value of assessing estrous behavior could be improved. However, male dogs have been shown to

---

Table **210-1**

Timing of Events in Relation to the Luteinizing Hormone Surge and Ovulation in the Bitch

Event	Days From Luteinizing Hormone Surge	Days From Ovulation
Period of potential fertility: the fertile period	3 days before LH surge until 7 days after LH surge	5 days before ovulation until 5 days after ovulation
Approximate time of oocyte maturation	4 or 5 days after LH surge	2 or 3 days after ovulation
Period of actual fertility: the fertilization period	4 days after LH surge until 7 days after LH surge	2 days after ovulation until 5 days after ovulation
Period of peak fertility	2 days after LH surge until 6 days after LH surge	The day of ovulation until 4 days after ovulation
Preferred breeding time using natural service or fresh semen insemination	2 days after LH surge until 6 days after LH surge	The day of ovulation until 4 days after ovulation
Preferred breeding time for males with poor quality semen or frozen-thawed semen insemination	4 days after LH surge until 6 days after LH surge	2 days after ovulation until 4 days after ovulation

Modified from England and Concannon, 2002.
LH, Luteinizing hormone.

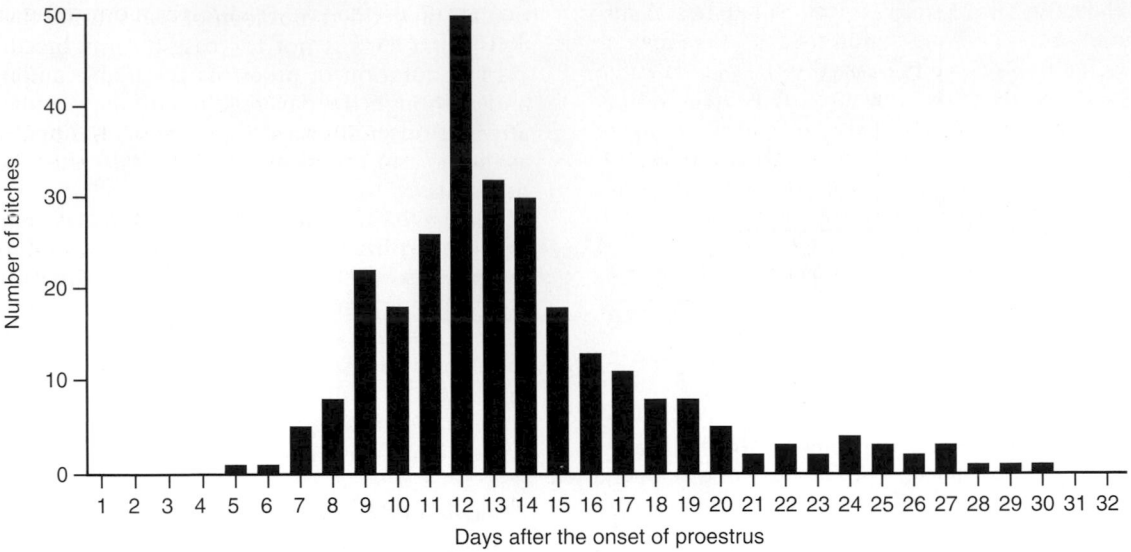

Fig. 210-2 The relationship between day of ovulation and the onset of proestrus for normal fertile bitches.

demonstrate clear preferences for some females over others, thus making the interpretation of this criterion very difficult to assess.

When relying solely on the receptivity of the bitch, breeding should be planned shortly after the onset of estrus and should continue throughout the period of female receptivity.

The Onset of Vulval Softening

One observational assessment that may be useful in establishing the optimal time for breeding is the change in the tone of the vulva. During proestrus the reproductive tract becomes edematous, and the vulva and perineal tissues become enlarged. In proestrus there is increasing turgidity of the vulva in response to increasing concentrations of estrogen. At the time of the LH surge there is a decline in estrogen concentration combined with a concomitant rise in progesterone. This results in a reduction in edema with a consequent distinct softening of the vulva. Subjective examination of the vulva once or twice daily by gentle palpation easily demonstrates when this event has occurred. Ovulation generally occurs 2 days later; therefore breeding should commence 3 days after this event has been observed.

In cases in which only observational assessments are available for the determination of the optimum time for breeding, a combination of the onset of standing estrus and the timing of vulval softening may be used. Each of these events occurs on average 1 or 2 days before ovulation. Therefore breeding should be planned commencing 2 or 3 days later for natural mating or fresh semen insemination. These assessments are not accurate enough for use with insemination of preserved semen, which frequently has a short longevity within the female reproductive tract.

Measurement of Plasma or Serum Hormone Concentration

There is a significant surge in LH concentration approximately 2 days before ovulation in the bitch; therefore detection of this event could be used to predict ovulation. However, there is a further preovulatory event: the luteinization of the follicle wall before ovulation (Fig. 210-3). This preovulatory luteinization results in a significant increase in plasma (serum) concentrations of progesterone before ovulation, which can be detected by conventional assay methods.

Measurement of Plasma or Serum Luteinizing Hormone Concentration

The detection of a significant increase in plasma LH concentration is a reliable and accurate method for determining the time of ovulation and therefore the optimal time to breed. In most countries there is no readily available commercial assay for canine LH, and measurement relies on radioimmunoassay techniques. As a result, this method is not used frequently since radioimmunoassays are commonly expensive and result in a delay in obtaining

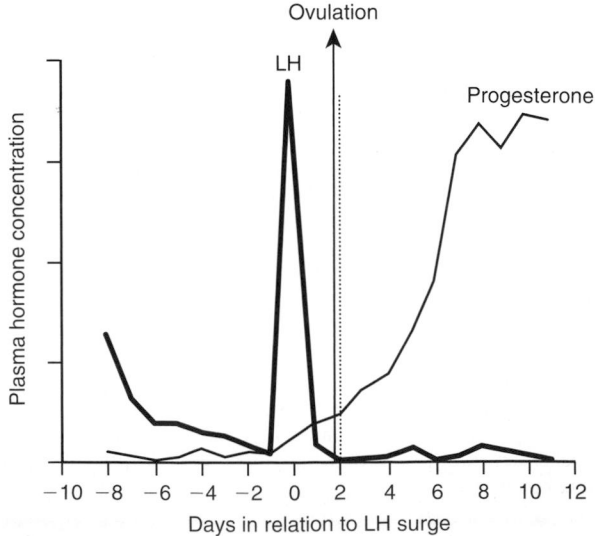

Fig. 210-3 Schematic relationship among ovulation, the luteinizing hormone surge, and plasma progesterone concentration.

the results because samples are assayed in batches. A further potential problem is the requirement to take regular (daily) blood samples since the duration of the LH surge is relatively short. Recently however, an enzyme-linked immunosorbent assay (ELISA) has been marketed for the measurement of canine LH in the practice laboratory. The method is simple and rapid and has been used successfully, although it has not yet been subjected to wide investigation.

When using these methods to detect the LH surge, breeding should commence 3 or 4 days after the surge has been identified since this coincides with the onset of the fertilization period.

Measurement of Plasma or Serum Progesterone Concentration

Luteinization of the follicle wall before ovulation results in plasma progesterone concentrations beginning to increase rapidly from baseline approximately 2 days before ovulation during the LH surge. This distinct increase can be detected by serial monitoring, which allows for the anticipation of ovulation. A further increase in progesterone concentration allows confirmation of ovulation and detection of the onset of the fertilization period. Since the initial rise in progesterone is progressive, it is only necessary to collect blood samples every second or third day, unlike the daily requirement for sampling to detect the LH surge. However, when the sampling interval is increased, the accuracy of detecting ovulation is decreased. Therefore, when there is poor-quality semen, it is often prudent to perform daily estimations close to the anticipated time of ovulation.

Progesterone concentrations may be measured by radioimmunoassay, quantitative or qualitative ELISA, or immunochemilluminesce assay. Many veterinary diagnostic laboratories offer measurement of progesterone with reporting of results the same day. Several qualitative or semiquantitative progesterone ELISA test kits have become available commercially for use in the veterinary practice. Results are usually obtainable within 45 to 60 minutes of sample collection.

In general it is considered that progesterone concentrations exceed 2 ng/ml (6.5 nmol/L) on the day after the LH surge; therefore breeding can be planned in relation to this event (i.e., 4 to 6 days later). Some reports suggest that breeding should commence 1 day after progesterone concentrations exceed 8 to 10 ng/ml (25 to 32 nmol/L), which are typically seen at the beginning of the fertilization period. There are little data to link absolute progesterone concentrations with the timing of the end of the fertilization period, and this is best detected using vaginal cytology (see later paragraphs).

Examination of the Caudal Reproductive Tract

Both estrogen and progesterone have significant effects on the female reproductive tract. Although evaluation of changes within the uterine tubes and uterus is not possible, it is relatively simple to monitor changes of the vaginal wall that are induced by fluctuations in hormonal concentration, thereby indirectly monitoring changes in these hormones.

Exfoliative Vaginal Cytology

Collection, staining, and microscopic examination of exfoliated vaginal cells is a simple method for monitoring the stage of the estrous cycle, especially when examination is performed serially. The increase in plasma estrogen during proestrus and estrus causes thickening of the vaginal wall predominantly via an increase in the number of cell layers, probably as a mechanism to protect the otherwise delicate mucosa at the time of mating. The mucosa changes from a cuboidal epithelium (in anestrus) through a transitional phase (during procstrus) into a stratified, keratinized squamous epithelium (during the fertile period). After the end of the fertilization period, as progesterone concentrations increase there is rapid sloughing of the newly developed epithelium and an uncovering of a simple cuboidal epithelium similar to that observed during anestrus.

Vaginal cells may be collected by aspiration of the vaginal cavity using a plastic catheter or by using a saline-moistened cotton swab gently rolled over the surface of the vaginal mucosa. When using the latter method, it is important not to allow contact of the swab with the vestibule or skin since collection of these cells can give erroneous results. Swabs should be introduced and removed using a small speculum or guard.

Once collected, cells should be placed onto a glass microscope slide by lightly rolling the cotton swab or by application of the aspirated fluid, which is then spread into a thin film. Smears can be stained using either a simple Wright-Giemsa stain or a modified trichrome stain. The former is readily available and has the advantage that sample preparation may take only minutes; the latter has the advantage of identification of keratinized cells, but the staining technique is laborious.

During proestrus, as plasma estrogen concentrations increase, the surface epithelial cells alter in their shape, size, and staining character. They change from small, circular cells with little cytoplasm (parabasal cells) to larger, irregularly shaped, flat (squamous) nucleated cells (intermediate cells). Ultimately they become anuclear cornified squamous cells (superficial cells) and are characterized as having no nucleus or a faint and/or small pycnotic nuclear remnant. After the end of the fertilization period during sloughing of the epithelium, the superficial cells disappear, and small parabasal cells reappear in the vaginal smear.

Polymorphonuclear leukocytes generally are present in small numbers in the anestrus vaginal smear but disappear from the smear during the fertile period because the thickened mucosa is a barrier to their migration to the surface. These polymorphonuclear leukocyte cells reappear, often in large numbers, at the end of the fertilization period as epithelial sloughing results in a thinner mucosa at the same time as there is a significant chemotractant effect within the vaginal lumen.

The relative proportions of different types of epithelial cells can be used as broad markers of the endocrine environment. Several indices of cornification and keratinization have been used; in general the fertile period can be crudely predicted by calculating the percentage of epithelial cells that appear anuclear when using a modified Wright-Giemsa stain (Fig. 210-4). Breeding should be attempted throughout the period when more than 75% of epithelial cells are anuclear because in most bitches this coincides with the fertile period.

However, there is great variation among bitches, and in some cases the percentage of cornified cells reach nearly 100% as early as 9 days before or as late as 2 days before ovulation. Conversely, in some cases peak values of anuclear cells may reach only 60%. Therefore changes in the vaginal cytology cannot be used to accurately time ovulation prospectively. Nevertheless, vaginal cytology permits monitoring of the normal progress of proestrus, and waiting for significant cornification allows unnecessary testing, transportation, or breeding to be avoided until the proestrus rise in estrogen is nearly complete.

As previously discussed, at the end of the fertilization period the vaginal smear rapidly becomes dominated by small- and intermediate-sized epithelial cells, cellular debris, bacteria, and polymorphonuclear leukocytes; the anuclear cell index declines dramatically. This time has been referred to as the onset of vaginal metestrus, and it is important to note that natural mating or vaginal insemination is rarely fertile when performed after this stage. In view of this, vaginal cytology is extremely valuable for demonstrating the end of the fertilization period, an event that is often not clear when using qualitative progesterone ELISA tests.

Changes in Vaginal Fluid

Measurement of the electrical resistance of the vaginal fluid (vaginal wall) has been purported as being useful for detecting the optimal time for breeding. This method is used to detect the optimal time of insemination in fox vixen. However, we recently used a commercial probe to measure electrical resistance daily in 48 bitches and found that only in two bitches were any useful trends apparent.

Similarly, the measurement of vaginal glucose concentration has failed to stand up to scientific scrutiny for the prediction of the optimal time to breed.

However, in a small number of bitches crystallization of mucus collected from the anterior vagina has been found to develop after the peak in plasma estrogen concentration. Assessment of the mucus, which originates from cervical glandular tissue, may be useful in combination with vaginal cytology for determining the optimal mating time.

Vaginal Endoscopy

Vaginal endoscopy (vaginoscopy) is the examination of the luminal surface of the vaginal mucosa using a rigid endoscope. The principle underlying the technique is that endocrinologic changes influence the nature of the epithelium (as discussed previously) and therefore the appearance of the vaginal wall.

Vaginoscopic examination is well tolerated in most nonsedated bitches that are in proestrus or estrus. Examination is normally performed with the bitch standing. In most cases it can take as little as 2 minutes to make an evaluation of the stage of the cycle. The evaluation is based on assessment of the appearance of the vaginal wall (i.e., the mucosal fold contours and profiles and the color of the mucosa and of any fluid present) and the changes in this appearance at specific times of the estrous cycle.

During anestrus the vaginal mucosa is relatively thin; therefore, when examined endoscopically it is flat and dry in appearance. Furthermore it has a red coloration because the submucosal vasculature is visible. At the onset of proestrus the mucosa becomes thickened and edematous as a result of the increase in plasma concentrations of oestrogen. Therefore the mucosal folds appear greatly enlarged, thickened, and edematous and have a pink or pink/white color. Serosanguinous fluid can be observed within the lumen and may be seen to exit from the cervix.

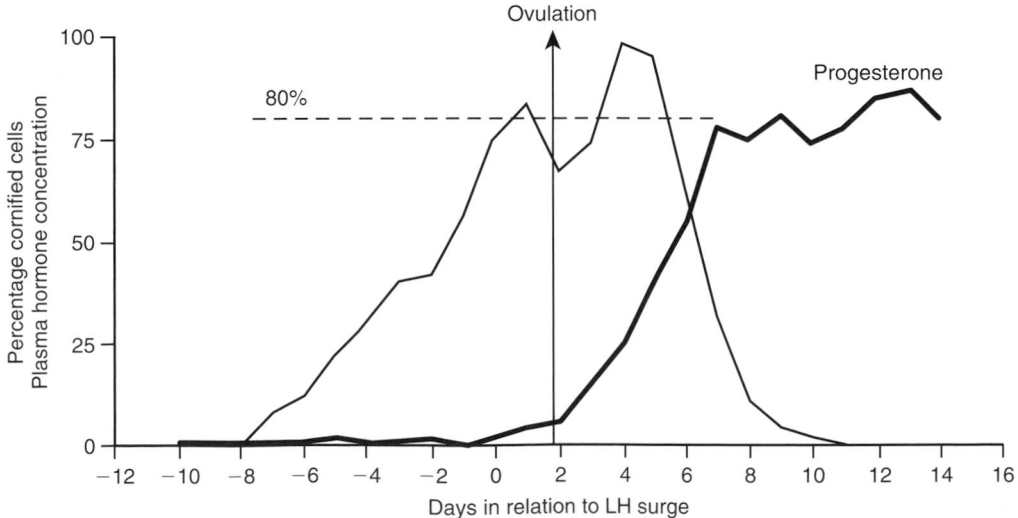

Fig. 210-4 Schematic relationship among ovulation, plasma progesterone concentration, and the percentage of cornified epithelial cells.

As proestrus progresses, the mucosal surface becomes progressively less pink and typically appears white in color because the thickened mucosa prevents the underlying capillaries that were visible during anestrus from being seen. In very late proestrus or early estrus at approximately the same time as the LH surge, there is a progressive shrinking of the folds that is accompanied by further pallor. These effects are the result of an abrupt withdrawal of estrogen. Estrogen concentrations decline rapidly during and after the LH surge. Subsequently over the next several days mucosal shrinkage is accompanied by gross wrinkling of the mucosal folds that now become distinctly angulated and retain a dense cream to white color.

The onset of the fertile period can be detected by observing the onset of mucosal shrinkage without excessive angulations, whereas gross shrinkage of entire mucosal folds with obvious angulation is characteristic of the fertilization period.

Breeding is best planned approximately 4 days after the first detected mucosal shrinkage or at the onset of the period of obvious angulation of mucosal folds. The end of the fertilization period can be detected by observing sloughing of the vaginal epithelium (see section on Exfoliative Vaginal Cytology earlier in the chapter) and development of a variegated appearance to the color of the mucosal surface.

Observation of Follicular Dynamics Using Ultrasound

It has been clearly demonstrated that the ovaries of a bitch can be identified using real-time diagnostic B-mode ultrasound. In some bitches there is significant amount of fat within the ovarian bursa, which makes imaging difficult. However, with careful and repeated examination it is possible to monitor follicular growth and detect the time of ovulation. In general, ovulation is difficult to identify because follicles do not collapse, changes in echogenicity are not always consistent, and new corpora lutea also have central fluid-filled cavities similar to those of the follicles.

Follicles appear as anechoic (black) structures that increase in size throughout proestrus and estrus to reach approximately 8 mm in diameter just before ovulation. Although difficult, it is possible to determine the time of ovulation using ultrasound. Usually there is an apparent decrease in the number of large anechoic follicles or their complete disappearance because of an increase in echogenicity and/or a related apparent decrease in follicle size. The absence of anechoic structures may be best detected by repeated examination, during which it can be seen to persist for 1 to 2 days commencing approximately at the time of ovulation. It is often followed by the reappearance of anechoic structures in the ovaries, representing the early developing corpora lutea. Corpora lutea generally have thicker walls than preovulatory follicles and also

contain central fluid. Cavitated corpora lutea are visible for several days to 2 weeks after ovulation. In clinical practice using ovarian ultrasound to determine the fertilization period has little clinical application at the present time because of the difficulties in imaging the ovaries and the requirement for frequent examination.

CONCLUSION

When considering the optimum time to breed, an important consideration is the unique reproductive physiology of the bitch. Although there is a protracted fertilization period compared with other species, it is important to remember that the most common causes for apparent infertility are misunderstanding of the normal physiology and thus breeding at the incorrect time.

In general, the optimal time to breed is during the fertile period. However, this period is influenced by the male, and in animals with poor-quality semen or in which semen has been preserved there may be shortened survival of sperm within the female reproductive tract. Therefore understanding the normal physiology and detecting the fertilization period are among the most important aspects of investigating infertility in canine reproduction.

Suggested Reading

England GCW: Vaginal cytology and cervicovaginal mucus arborisation in the breeding management of bitches, *J Small Anim Pract* 33:577, 1992.

England GCW, Allen WE: Crystallization patterns in anterior vaginal fluid from bitches in oestrus, *J Reprod Fertil* 86:335, 1989.

England GCW, Concannon PW: Determination of the optimal breeding time in the bitch: basic considerations, accessed 2002 from www.ivis.org.

England GCW, Yeager AE: Ultrasonographic appearance of the ovary and uterus of the bitch during oestrus, ovulation and early pregnancy, *J Reprod Fertil* 47(suppl):107, 1993.

Goodman M: Ovulation timing: concepts and controversies, *Vet Clin North Am Small Anim Pract* 31:219, 2001.

Hiemstra M et al: The reliability of vaginal cytology in determining the optimal mating time in the bitch, *Tijdschr Diergeneeskd* 126:685, 2001.

Jeffcoate IA, England GCW: Urinary LH, plasma LH and progesterone and their clinical correlates in the periovulatory period of domestic bitches, *J Reprod Fertil* 51(suppl):267, 1997.

Jeffcoate IA, Lindsay FEF: Ovulation detection and timing of insemination based on hormone concentrations, vaginal cytology and the endoscopic appearance of the vagina of domestic bitches, *J Reprod Fertil* 39(suppl):277, 1989.

Lindsay FEF, Concannon PW: Normal canine vaginoscopy. In Burk T, editor: *Small animal reproduction and infertility*, Philadelphia, 1986, Lea & Febiger p 112.

van Klaveren NJ et al: The optimal mating time in the bitch based on the progesterone concentration in peripheral blood: a comparison of reliability between three ELISA test kits and a 125-iodine radioimmunoassay, *Tijdschr Diergeneeskd* 126:680, 2001.

CHAPTER 211

Use of Vaginal Cytology and Vaginal Cultures for Breeding Management and Diagnosis of Reproductive Tract Disease

BEVERLY J. PURSWELL, *Blacksburg, Virginia*

Breeding management in the dog has evolved over the last few years to a fairly sophisticated level compared to previous times. With the advent and routine use of progesterone testing in breeding management, the use of cooled shipped semen and frozen semen has allowed clinical canine reproduction to approach the level of technology commonplace in other species. Yet there remains much hearsay and lay opinion influencing the breeder and their requests for veterinary care. Vaginal cytology is a traditional technique used in breeding management. The limitations of the information gained from vaginal cytology must be appreciated by the veterinarian and the breeder. Vaginal cultures are another area in which misinformation abounds. For vaginal cultures to result in any meaningful information, the culture must be obtained correctly, and knowledge of the normal flora of the vagina must be applied to culture results. Both techniques, vaginal cytology and vaginal cultures, can be extremely informative in breeding management situations and in diagnosis of reproductive tract disease when placed in context with the total clinical picture.

VAGINAL CYTOLOGY

Vaginal cytology can be used in breeding management because of the changes that occur to the vaginal epithelium when under the influence of estrogen (also see Chapter 210). Normally the vaginal epithelium is only a few cell layers in thickness. Under the influence of estrogen, the vaginal epithelium thickens to 20 to 30 cell layers in thickness. This cornification process of the vaginal epithelium protects the vagina from the physical trauma experienced at breeding. The exfoliative cytology of the vagina reflects the cornification process by the cell types that predominate. The basal cells closest to the basement membrane are small and round and have prominent nuclei. This cell type predominates the cytology taken when the bitch is not under the influence of estrogen. As the vaginal epithelium thickens because of the influence of estrogen, the cells that are further from their basement membrane undergo cornification. These cells are large and have angular cell borders and small pyknotic

nuclei or no nuclei at all. When the bitch is in proestrus or estrus and under the influence of estrogen, the cornified cell type predominates the vaginal cytology.

Vaginal cytology is extremely helpful to the clinician in diagnosing *inflammation in the reproductive tract*. Normally only the occasional neutrophil is present in vaginal cytology. As the bitch progresses through proestrus into estrus, the neutrophils disappear altogether. This is most likely a result of the increase in thickness of the vaginal epithelium impeding the migration of neutrophils into the vaginal lumen. In cases of uterine or vaginal inflammation, the numbers of neutrophils in the vaginal cytology increase dramatically. During early diestrus there is an influx of nondegenerate neutrophils, which is considered normal for that stage of the estrous cycle. At all other times large numbers of neutrophils indicate an inflammatory process. In inflammatory processes the majority of the cells present are degenerate neutrophils.

Vaginal cytology is useful in breeding management and in detecting disease processes within the reproductive tract. Vaginal cytology indicates the influence of estrogen on the reproductive tract and the presence of inflammation. Beyond these two helpful pieces of information, it is limited in relaying other information concerning the hormonal status of the bitch. Vaginal cytology cannot accurately determine ovulation or the ideal time to breed. However, it does indicate accurately the onset of diestrus. There is a dramatic and sudden change from cornified to noncornified epithelial cells at the onset of diestrus. This determination can be useful in predicting gestation length. Most bitches whelp 56 to 57 days after the onset of cytologic diestrus.

VAGINAL CULTURE

Vaginal cultures are often requested by a stud dog owner before breeding a bitch outside of its kennel. This practice of requesting vaginal cultures is an attempt to protect the male dog from contracting disease organisms from the bitch. Without evidence of an ongoing disease process, positive vaginal cultures only reflect the normal flora that are present in a majority of bitches. A variety of bacteria are commonly isolated from the vagina of

980

normal breeding bitches. This clinical picture becomes further confounded when the vaginal culture is taken during proestrus and estrus. At this time it is not unusual to obtain bacterial cultures that reflect heavy growth of a single organism. It is thought that the serosanguineous discharge present during proestrus and estrus promotes the proliferation of bacteria within the vagina. Therefore results of vaginal cultures must be interpreted with this information in mind and correlated with the entire reproductive picture presented by each clinical case.

When culturing the vagina, a guarded swab culture instrument (Kalayjian Industries) is necessary to sample the anterior vagina while preventing contamination from the distal tract. The distal vagina and vestibule normally harbor large numbers of bacteria. To accurately diagnose and assess bacteria that may be present in the uterus and causing reproductive dysfunction, anterior vaginal cultures are needed because these are most reflective of the disease process.

Canine vaginal flora have been well documented in a number of studies over the last 30 years (Table 211-1). It has been observed by investigators that the normal flora of the canine vagina contain bacteria that may cause reproductive tract disease (e.g., *E. coli* and *Mycoplasma* spp.). These bacteria are opportunistic pathogens in addition to being normal flora. Their presence in the vagina does not necessarily indicate disease or infection. It is interesting to note that the same organisms found as normal flora in the canine vagina can also been found as normal flora on the penis and prepuce of the dog (Table 211-2).

There is one microorganism that, when present, always indicates an infection: *Brucella canis*. The pre-ferred screening test for *Brucella canis* infection is serology, either by a rapid slide agglutination assay, tube agglutination test, or agar gel immunodiffusion test. Serology for *B. canis* should be a part of any prebreeding management strategy.

When interpreting the results of a vaginal culture, the clinician must consider a number of other factors. The medical and reproductive histories are helpful in identifying previous problems with infections or infertility. Vaginal cytology should always be collected and evaluated in concert with vaginal cultures. When there is no evidence of inflammation in the vaginal cytology, the results of the culture most likely reflect normal flora. If there is an abnormal vulvar discharge, inflammation is documented by vaginal cytology, or the bitch is exhibiting systemic signs of disease, the vaginal culture is essential for identifying the causative organism and determining the appropriate antimicrobial therapy.

Other Diagnostic Tests

Other diagnostic tests that may be indicated include vaginoscopy and ultrasonography. These studies assist in adequately and appropriately diagnosing the location and cause of reproductive disease. Vaginoscopy is essential in determining the physical source of a vulvar discharge and can be useful for determining the stage of the reproductive cycle (also see Chapter 210). Ultrasonography often demonstrates the presence of uterine pathology by allowing visualization of fluid within the uterine lumen or demonstrating cystic endometrial hyperplasia.

Table **211-1**

Aerobic Bacteria Isolated From the Vagina of 59 Bitches (826 Vaginal Swab Specimens)

Organism	ISOLATES		BITCHES FROM WHICH ORGANISMS WERE ISOLATED	
	Number	Percent	Number	Percent
Pasteurella multocida	492	59.6	58	98.3
β-Hemolytic streptococci	392	47.5	53	89.8
Escherichia coli	263	31.8	50	84.7
Gram-positive rods (unclassified)	141	17.1	53	89.8
Gram-negative rods (unclassified)	134	16.2	51	86.4
Mycoplasma spp.	73	8.8	35	59.3
Streptococcus spp. (α-hemolytic, nonhemolytic)	72	8.7	33	55.9
Pasturella spp.	60	7.2	40	67.8
Enterococci	51	6.2	26	44.1
Proteus mirabilis	40	4.8	15	25.4
Staphylococcus intermedius	34	4.1	20	33.9
Coryneforms	25	3.0	24	40.7
Coagulase-negative staphylococci	17	2.1	13	22.0
Pseudomonas spp.	6	0.7	6	10.2
Total	1800	(2.3 isolates/bitch)		
No bacterial growth	43	5.2		

With permission from Bjurstrom L, Linde-Forsberg C: *Am J Vet Res* 53(5):665, 1992a.

Table 211-2

Aerobic Bacteria Isolated From the Prepuce of 15 Stud Dogs (232 Samples)

Organism	ISOLATES		DOGS FROM WHICH ORGANISMS WERE ISOLATED	
	Number	Percent	Number	Percent
Pasteurella multocida	123	54.7	15	100.0
β-Hemolytic streptococci	76	32.8	11	73.3
Escherichia coli	42	18.1	8	53.3
Coagulase-negative staphylococci	39	16.8	10	66.7
Mycoplasma spp.	25	10.8	12	80.0
Staphylococcus intermedius	22	9.5	9	60.0
Gram-negative rods (unclassified)	19	8.2	9	6.0
Gram-positive rods (unclassified)	11	4.7	6	40.0
Streptococcus spp. (α-hemolytic, nonhemolytic)	7	3.0	4	26.7
Pasturella spp.	7	3.0	6	40.0
Coryneforms	4	1.7	3	20.0
Enterococci	4	1.7	4	26.7
Pseudomonas spp.	1	0.4	1	6.7
Proteus mirabilis	1	0.4	1	6.7
Total	381	(1.9 isolates/dog)		
No bacterial growth	33	14.2		

With permission from Bjurstrom L, Linde-Forsberg C: *Am J Vet Res* 53(5):670, 1992b.

Antimicrobial Therapy

Hard-and-fast rules for management based on culture results are untenable when culturing sites that are not normally sterile. Vaginal culture and cytology are invaluable when diagnosing reproductive tract disease, but routine cultures in normal animals must be interpreted with great care. Prophylactic antibiotics before and during breeding have been shown to be *detrimental* in the normal animal. Inappropriate antimicrobial therapy can alter the vaginal flora, causing overgrowth of opportunistic pathogens and creating abnormal vulvar discharges. Thus such use of antibiotics must be avoided.

Suggested Reading

Bjurstrom L, Linde-Forsberg C: Long-term study of aerobic bacteria of the genital tract in breeding bitches, *Am J Vet Res* 53(5):665, 1992a.

Bjurstrom L, Linde-Forsberg C: Long-term study of aerobic bacteria of the genital tract in stud dogs, *Am J Vet Res* 53(5):670, 1992b.

Johnston SD, Root Kustritz MV, Olson PNS: *Canine and feline theriogenology*, Philadelphia, 2001, Saunders, p 32.

Olson PN, Jones RL, Mather EC: The use and misuse of vaginal cultures in diagnosing reproductive diseases in the bitch. In Morrow DA, editor: *Current therapy in theriogenology 2*, Philadelphia, 1986, Saunders, p 469.

Strom B, Linde-Forsberg C: Effects of ampicillin and trimethoprim-sulfamethoxazole on the vaginal bacterial flora of bitches, *Am J Vet Res* 54(6):891, 1993.

CHAPTER 212

Endoscopic Transcervical Insemination

MARION S. WILSON, *Te Kuiti, New Zealand*

It is widely recognized in many species that thawed frozen semen must be deposited into the uterus rather than vaginally to achieve good conception rates. The options available to achieve intrauterine semen deposition are surgical or transcervical insemination (TCI). In many parts of the world the surgical option is the method of choice in the bitch because it is easy to perform, without any major learning period. However, surgery has some drawbacks, including the risks associated with general anesthesia and surgery and the restriction to a single insemination. Accordingly many owners and veterinarians prefer a nonsurgical option.

I developed the TCI technique using a rigid endoscope specifically to deposit frozen semen into the uterus of the bitch. In researching the technique several features relating to the anatomy of the canine reproductive tract were identified. These points are relevant to endoscopic TCI and are considered first, followed by a description of relevant procedures for TCI.

ANATOMY

The cranial vagina (paracervix) is dominated by the dorsal median fold (DMF), which significantly reduces the vaginal lumen in the approach to the cervix. The restricted vaginal lumen limits the diameter of equipment that can be passed through the area. This feature, together with a particularly long vagina in the bitch, limits the number of endoscopes suitable for the technique. The DMF ends cranially at the vaginal portion of the cervix, which exists as a distinct tubercle (cervical tubercle). The paracervix is limited cranially by the fornix, which is a slitlike space cranioventral to the cervical tubercle. It appears as a blind end when viewed through the endoscope and is another important landmark. The cervix lies diagonally across the uterovaginal junction with the canal of the cervix directed craniodorsally from the vagina to the uterus. Consequently the external os is located ventrally in the cervical tubercle.

EQUIPMENT

The endoscope identified as meeting the criteria with regard to length and diameter is a rigid extended length cystourethroscope.* An 8-Fr-gauge urinary catheter is used for insemination in the majority of bitches, although a 6-Fr-gauge is sometimes required in small or maiden

bitches. A specially designed platform is used to restrain the bitch in the standing position; the platform provides a tie point to the dog's collar and a canvas band around the abdomen to restrict sideways movement and discourage any attempt to sit. A hydraulic chair together with a hydraulic table for the platform ensures the optimum position of the bitch relative to the operator during the procedure; this is particularly important when the endoscope is being used without a camera. Bitches in oestrus exhibiting standing behavior show excellent tolerance to the technique; sedation has never been necessary.

TECHNIQUE

The endoscope is introduced into the vagina, taking care to avoid the clitoris and urethral orifice. It is advanced through the vaginal folds by observing the direction of the vaginal lumen. In proestrus and early oestrus the rounded vaginal folds can make advancing the endoscope more difficult as they tend to fill the lumen; as oestrus progresses, dehydration of the folds results in a more obvious route forward. The DMF and crescentic lumen represent an important landmark in locating the cervical os. At this point the lumen can be quite narrow in some bitches, requiring manipulation of the endoscope to the widest space. This may result in the endoscope being pushed to one side of the DMF rather than continuing ventrally under the DMF. The ventral location of the os means that it is not immediately obvious and the scope has to be directed under the cervical tubercle until the os, located in the center of a rosette of furrows, can be identified. The catheter is advanced into the cervical os by manipulation of the endoscope and catheter. The rigidity of the endoscope is used to move the cervical tubercle, line up the os, and change the angle of the canal.

Once the tip of the catheter is introduced into the os, it is advanced steadily using a twisting movement to aid its passage through the cervical canal; it is passed in as far as it will go without force. The semen is inseminated slowly under continual observation to ensure that there is no significant backflow of semen into the vagina. If this happens the catheter should be relocated, either further in or back slightly, and insemination begun again.

PRACTICAL CONSIDERATIONS

The cost of the equipment makes it a major decision to take on board endoscopic TCI in a practice. Veterinarians must understand what they can expect from the technology,

---

*Storz Extended Length Cystourethroscope: telescope 30° 325 B, 3.5-mm sheath, 027KL, Bridge 027NL.

how easy the techniques are to learn, and what problems and results they can expect.

Theoretically the technique is very simple but takes time, patience, and practice to perfect. The attachment of a video camera to the endoscope allows for direct training by an experienced operator and is extremely helpful in training. However, many people have taught themselves to perform TCI. Most find the prospect of getting the catheter into the os to be a challenge they can confidently overcome in a relatively short time. However, mastering the peculiarities of all breeds and sizes takes much longer.

The Limiting Factors/Problems

For the technique to be widely adopted, it is essential that it can successfully be applied to all, or at least, most bitches. It is also important that the majority of bitches can be inseminated using the same endoscope. Looking at the vast array of breeds presented with regard to size and shape, this would seem unlikely, but for the most part it is possible.

Length of the Vagina
So far no bitch has been examined when the cervix is beyond the reach of the equipment described; thus vaginal length is not a limiting factor, provided the correct endoscope is purchased.

Diameter of the Paracervix
The one limiting factor identified thus far is the amount of space available in the paracervix. In a small percentage of bitches it is impossible to advance the endoscope through this area. This occurs in some maiden bitches of small or medium-sized breeds and in some toy breeds such as the Chihuahua. Endoscopes of smaller diameter are available, but they are also considerably shorter and only solve the problem for toy breeds when the vaginal length is short. The standard endoscope described here has been used successfully on many small/toy breeds, including pugs, Pekingese, griffon Bruxellois, cavalier King Charles spaniels, and miniature dachshunds; thus it is suitable for the majority of bitches. More recently a smaller-diameter sheath has been developed for use with the standard telescope, solving the space problem in some bitches; however, a 6-Fr-gauge catheter is required for insemination with this sheath. With the very small toy breeds restraint of the bitch while trying to manipulate a relatively long scope is a large part of the problem. In these cases sedation may improve success.

Identification of the Cervical Os
Theoretically once the endoscope has passed through the paracervix it should be possible to catheterize all bitches. The ability to identify the os comes from experience (i.e., appreciating what it looks like, where it is usually located, and how to search for it when it is not obvious). Some bitches have folds that can be mistaken for the os, but obviously there is no opening for the catheter. Fluid issuing from the os identifies the correct location.

Cannulation of the Cervix
Ensuring that the catheter advances once the tip is with the os depends on application of appropriate pressure and at the correct angle to account for the angle of the cervical canal. Sometimes progress is limited by the diameter of the canal, and a smaller-gauge catheter is necessary.

Visibility
Vaginal discharges resulting in poor visibility can cause significant problems, particularly in the learning phase of TCI.

Most of the problems encountered result from not appreciating the anatomy of the female reproductive tract or not having developed the knack of manipulating the endoscope and catheter together. However, not all bitches are easy to catheterize. Difficult entry angles, ongoing poor visibility, and fidgeting patients occasionally defy all attempts from even the most skilled operator.

Confidence in the Technique

Intrauterine Deposition
With visualization of the cervix there can be no doubt that the catheter is intrauterine. Continued viewing of the insemination process ensures that the semen is deposited in the uterus. A video camera allows the client and the operator to observe the intrauterine deposition of the semen. This is a particularly positive aspect of videoendoscope technology.

Safety
The risk of trauma or infection resulting from the procedure is an important consideration. It is difficult to imagine that the plastic urinary catheter could ever perforate the vaginal or uterine wall during estrus unless a pathologic condition preexisted. However, the paracervical area can be traumatized by the use of inappropriate force with the endoscope. If advancing the endoscope causes obvious discomfort to the bitch, the procedure should be stopped. It has been suggested that TCI could introduce infection to the uterine environment. During proestrus and oestrus bacteria are routinely isolated from the uterus and vagina apparently without causing any problems, perhaps because of a greater resistance to infection at this time. Therefore it is reasonable to assume that advancing a catheter from the vagina to the uterus at this time will not cause any problems. However, care must be taken to prevent introduction of new infections as a result of inadequately cleaned equipment or from environmental contamination caused by poor technique.

The equipment can be readily cleaned and disinfected, and standard techniques and procedures should be established.

Frozen Semen
This technique provides for the intrauterine deposition of semen, a vital part of frozen semen technology. Equally important to the successful use of frozen semen are the timing of insemination, semen quality, and bitch fertility. Endoscopic TCI, like any other intrauterine insemination method, will be successful only if all of these factors are taken into account.

TCI also can be performed using the so-called *Norwegian method*. This method uses a nylon sheath and metal catheter, which are produced in three sizes to suit different-size bitches. The technique requires palpation and fixation of the cervix through the abdominal wall; manipulation of the cervix enables catheterization with the metal catheter. The Norwegian method has been described in several previous reports.

Results from a trial comparing Norwegian and endoscopic TCI demonstrated that conception rates of 83.3% and average litter size of 7.5 were possible using TCI in bitches of unknown breeding history. These results compare favorably with results from other trials using frozen semen, indicating there are no undesirable effects from TCI. There are no trials making a direct comparison between surgical and endoscopic TCI; thus it is impossible to know if the results are better using TCI.

The ability of repeat inseminations has been reported to increase conception rates or litter size. TCI allows for this approach, whereas surgery does not. When the semen is of lower quality, repeat inseminations allow more semen to be inseminated over an extended period. Repeat inseminations are also useful when the bitch is difficult to time relative to phase of the estrus cycle.

Fresh or Chilled Semen

In any insemination, if the semen can be deposited intra-uterine, it is reasonable to expect that the results may be better than vaginal deposition; this applies to both chilled and fresh semen, particularly when semen quality is poor. Using TCI for fresh and chilled inseminations not only results in excellent conception rates and litter sizes but provides the opportunity to develop experience and expertise for many more situations.

Other Uses

The endoscope also can be used for routine vaginoscopy to determine the progression through the reproductive cycle, as well as for diagnostic vaginoscopy, cystoscopy, and hysterography. TCI has been used to study the intra-uterine environment with respect to microbiology and cytology throughout the reproductive cycle of the bitch, providing valuable research data (Watts and Wright, 1995). When examinations are performed during anestrus and diestrus, the vaginal walls are thinner and more susceptible to trauma; extreme care must be taken in these situations. Bitches not in standing heat do not tolerate the endoscope very well; thus sedation is usually required in these cases. Sedation diminishes the dog's reaction to inappropriate manipulation of the endoscope, emphasizing the need for extreme care. Air insufflation is also helpful for examination during anestrus and diestrus. The uterus is likely to be more susceptible to infection during diestrus when under the influence of high progesterone levels. Special care and aseptic examination technique are crucial at this stage of the cycle.

Presumably the routine ability to catheterize the cervix will lead to the development of new diagnostic procedures and treatments.

References and Suggested Reading

Andersen K: Insemination with frozen dog semen based on a new insemination technique, *Zuchthygiene* 10:1, 1975.

Linde-Forsberg C: Achieving canine pregnancy by using frozen or chilled extended semen, *Vet Clin North Am Small Anim Pract* 21:467, 1991.

Lindsay FEF: The normal endoscopic appearance of the caudal reproductive tract of the cyclic and non-cyclic bitch: post uterine endoscopy, *J Small Anim Pract* 24:1, 1983.

Watts JR, Wright PJ: Investigating uterine disease in the bitch: uterine cannulation for cytology, microbiology and hysteroscopy, *J Small Anim Pract* 36: 201, 1995.

Wilson MS: Transcervical insemination techniques in the bitch, *Vet Clin North Am: Small Anim Pract* 31: 291, 2001.

CHAPTER 213

Pregnancy Loss in the Bitch

JONI L. FRESHMAN, *Colorado Springs, Colorado*

Pregnancy loss in the bitch can occur for a multitude of reasons. Pregnancy loss earlier than 21 days is difficult to diagnose because of the unavailability of a definitive pregnancy test for this time period. Pregnancy can be diagnosed by abdominal ultrasound as early as 16 to 18 days after ovulation but more reliably from days 20 to 26. Relaxin assay (Witness Relaxin, Synbiotics) can diagnose pregnancy later than 21 days from the luteinizing hormone (LH) surge, and radiographs are useful for pregnancy diagnosis after 42 to 45 days of gestation. Abdominal palpation is not sensitive enough to document pregnancy for the purposes of confirming pregnancy loss.

Fetal death in the first half of pregnancy typically results in resorption of the fetuses or unobserved abortion. Fetal death in the second half of gestation typically results in abortion or stillbirth, although resorption may still occur. Abortion may not be recognized because the bitch may ingest the aborted material. Fetal death in late gestation in the presence of continuing luteal influence may also result in mummification when fetal and placental fluids are resorbed, leaving dried structures in the uterus.

DIAGNOSTICS

The most useful step in diagnosis and prevention of future pregnancy loss is submission of the aborted fetus and placenta, in total, to a diagnostic laboratory experienced in reproductive histopathology. The materials should be submitted immediately, refrigerated but not frozen. Vaginal swabs from the bitch for culture and serum from the bitch for titers may also be useful. Aborting/resorbing bitches should have a diagnostic panel to include a complete blood count, serum biochemistry panel, urinalysis, *Brucella canis* test, serum progesterone test, and vaginal cytology, with culture and sensitivity if inflammation is evident.

Pregnancies of bitches with a history of pregnancy loss should be monitored by ultrasound, ideally at least weekly. Fetal heart rates are good indicators of fetal health and should be in the 170 to 220 beats/min range. Rates should vary with the fetus's activity and sleep status.

There are many potential causes of pregnancy loss in the bitch. These can be separated into two main categories, infectious and noninfectious. Even with use of all available diagnostics, some cases of pregnancy loss remain idiopathic.

INFECTIOUS CAUSES OF PREGNANCY LOSS

Infectious causes of pregnancy loss are those most commonly diagnosed. Aborted fetuses, placentas, and vaginal swabs from the bitch should be submitted for testing. In addition, analysis of serum submitted from the bitch may be helpful in diagnosis.

Brucella canis

Brucella canis is a gram-negative, aerobic reproductive pathogen in the dog, most commonly spread by contact with infected aborted fetuses, placentas, infected vulvar discharge, and urine (Greene and Carmichael, 2006). Although brucellosis can cause early embryonic death (10 to 20 days), it most commonly causes abortion at 45 to 59 days of gestation (Greene and Carmichael, 2006). Initial screening for brucellosis is made with the rapid card agglutination test (RCAT, Synbiotics). This test is very sensitive, and a negative initial test can be relied on unless the bitch has been receiving antibiotics. Early infection may also be negative, and testing 4 to 8 weeks after exposure is recommended. A test that is initially positive but clears with the addition of the included chemical 2-mercaptoethanol can result from cross-reacting antibodies or from immunoglobulin (Ig)M antibodies, denoting an early *Brucella* infection. These dogs should have tests repeated in 30 days or have other diagnostic tests performed. The cytoplasmic antigen agar gel immunodiffusion (AGIDcpa) test is a specific confirmatory test, but it may not become positive until 4 weeks after the RCAT (Hollet, 2006). Blood cultures typically are positive at 2 to 4 weeks after infection (Greene and Carmichael, 2006). Because of labor and expense, blood cultures typically are not used as a first test for *Brucella*. Brucellosis can be a difficult organism to grow; thus multiple negative cultures (three) are required to rule out infection.

Antibiotic therapy for canine brucellosis is controversial. Antibiotics are not proven to cure the disease since dogs may relapse after apparent remission. *Brucella canis* does pose a risk to immunosuppressed humans. If treatment is attempted, the bitch should be ovariohysterectomized and isolated from other dogs. Antibiotics used are a combination of streptomycin 20 mg/kg every 24 hours for 14 days and tetracycline 30 mg/kg every 12 hours for 28 days (Greene and Carmichael, 2006). Recently the use of long-term enrofloxacin has resulted in regression of the disease and production of puppies by infected dogs and bitches (Wanke, Delpino, and Baldi, 2006). The clinician should understand the adverse effects of these antibiotics. Canine brucellosis is a reportable disease in many states. Procedures for management of infected kennels have been published (Hollet, 2006).

Other Bacteria

The bitch's reproductive tract contains normal flora (Box 213-1) (Bjurstrom, Linde-Forsberg, 1992), thus positive vaginal cultures are not diagnostic for infection. Any bacterial species is capable of overgrowth and can cause infection and pregnancy loss. Diagnosis requires cultures from aborted material and inflammatory cytology from vagina or uterus. Submission of fetal stomach contents is particularly valuable.

Normal bitches given prophylactic antibiotics developed increased numbers of *Escherichia coli* and *mycoplasma*, and two out of five developed vaginal discharge (Ström and Linde-Forsberg, 1993). For this reason empiric antibiotic use in the bitch is strongly discouraged. Although most sources consider the canine uterus to be a sterile environment, one study found uterine flora in 68% of bitches studied (Baba et al., 1983). In this study, these organisms were most commonly *staphylococcus* spp. and *mycoplasma* spp. No histopathologic abnormalities were seen in the uteri of these bitches.

Salmonella

Salmonella spp. are not found as normal flora in the bitch's reproductive tract. *Salmonella panama* has been identified as the cause of canine abortions. Infection can occur by contact with infected food, water, or fomites. Diagnosis is by culture of aborted materials or vaginal discharge. Cure of *Salmonella* infection has been reported with trimethoprim sulfa antibiotics; however, treatment may simply prolong the carrier state (Johnston et al., 2001). Prophylactic antibiotics increase the risk of infection by decreasing the number of organisms needed to cause infection because of suppression of normal flora. The infected bitch should be isolated, and excellent sanitation should be provided. Removing her from the breeding population may be necessary. Owners should be cautioned about zoonotic potential.

Campylobacter

Campylobacter has also been documented as a cause of abortion and fetal resorption in the bitch. The bitch may be otherwise asymptomatic. Aborted materials and vaginal cultures need to be submitted in special media. Owners should be cautioned about the zoonotic potential of *campylobacter*. Treatment is with erythromycin 10 to 15 mg/kg every 8 hours orally for 10 to 14 days.

Box 213-1

Selected Common Normal Vaginal Flora in the Bitch

- Pasteurella
- Group B streptococcus
- *E. Coli*
- Enterococci
- Bacteroides
- *Staphylococcus intermedius*
- *Mycoplasma*

Mycoplasma/Ureaplasma

These organisms have been documented as normal flora in the bitch. *Ureaplasma* has alternatively been considered an obligate reproductive pathogen. These organisms are most likely to cause reproductive dysfunction in overcrowded kennel situations. Dispersal of dogs decreases the number of organisms. Treatment with antibiotics reduces the number of organisms present, but the numbers rise once antibiotics are stopped unless husbandry is addressed.

Canine Herpesvirus

Canine herpesvirus (CHV) is a common, mild, upper respiratory infection in dogs, and as such is a ubiquitous organism. Bitches infected during their last 3 weeks of gestation develop a systemic infection and placentitis, which results in abortion. Mummification of fetuses can also occur. The bitch is otherwise typically asymptomatic. Puppies exposed during their first 3 weeks of life are also at high risk of death. Recurrence in the same bitch is uncommon but can occur. Diagnosis of CHV is by examination and virus isolation of the aborted fetus and/or placenta. The infected placenta is underdeveloped and congested with gray-to-white foci. No treatment is available for CHV abortion. However, isolation of the pregnant bitch from other dogs for the danger period (3 weeks' prepartum through 3 weeks' postpartum) can prevent infection. Vaccination is available in Europe (Merial).

Canine Parvovirus 1 (Minute Virus of Canines)

Minute virus of canines (canine parvovirus 1) has been documented as a cause of fetal death and resorption in early pregnancy, most notably the first trimester (Carmichael et al., 1991). No clinical illness is seen. The viral infection is short, with a 2-week incubation and disappearance of the virus about 2 weeks after fetal death (Carmichael, Schlafer, and Hashimoto, 1981). Bitches infected in the last trimester usually deliver normal puppies. Diagnosis is difficult since there is only one cell line that currently supports viral isolation. There is no known treatment.

Other Viruses

Other viruses have been implicated in canine pregnancy loss. A calicivirus has been isolated from the canine vaginal tract in cases of vesicular vaginitis. Calicivirus does cause abortion in other species and may do so in the canine. Virus isolation from aborted material is recommended for diagnosis.

Canine distemper virus (CDV) can cause placental separation and subsequent pregnancy loss. Other clinical signs consistent with CDV should be present.

A canine vaccine contaminated with bluetongue virus was documented to cause canine abortion (Wilbur et al., 1994). Natural exposure to bluetongue virus and abortion have not been identified.

Protozoa

Toxoplasmosis is an uncommon cause of canine abortion. Ingestion of cat feces or infected raw meat can produce infection. In experimental conditions injection with *Toxoplasma* caused abortion 4 to 6 days after inoculation, with systemic illness appearing 3 to 5 days after inoculation. Diagnosis is made with paired serum samples from the bitch. Avoiding exposure to feline feces and raw meat should prevent infection.

Neospora caninum has been transmitted transplacentally in experimental conditions. Although it is unknown if this occurs naturally, *Neospora* may be responsible for cases of abortion previously attributed to *Toxoplasma*.

NONINFECTIOUS CAUSES OF PREGNANCY LOSS

Maternal Health

Maternal disease can cause pregnancy loss. Bitches should be evaluated for endocrine diseases such as hypothyroidism, diabetes mellitus, hypoadrenocorticism, and hyperadrenocorticism, which are all documented as causes for pregnancy loss in women. In borzoi hypothyroidism was identified as the cause of abortion and mummified fetuses (Johnson, 1987).

Uterine health can also play a role in pregnancy loss. Cystic endometrial hyperplasia (CEH) can create a uterine environment that will not support fetal growth to term. Diagnosis of this disease is made only by histopathologic examination of uterine biopsies. No known treatment is available.

Bitches decrease production of puppies between 4 and 8 years of age, with increasing effect after 8 years (Fox, 1963). This may be to the result of a combination of CEH and aging of ova.

Dietary deficiencies in the bitch may affect fetal survival. Deficiency of vitamin A, manganese, or iodine may cause fetal loss. However, these are unlikely in dogs fed a good commercial diet.

Abdominal trauma is an uncommon cause of pregnancy loss. However, significant abdominal trauma can result in abortion or resorption. History and physical examination should reveal this cause. Risky exercise should not be continued during pregnancy. Dogs should be walked and exercised on the flat as they are willing; however, strenuous exercise such as field training or exercise that carries risk of trauma such as agility, herding, or fly ball should be suspended during pregnancy.

Maternal exposure to chemicals may also affect fetal health. Heavy metals, solvents, and plastics may all have adverse effects. A careful history of exposure before and during pregnancy is important. In addition, an increased abortion rate in wives of men exposed to these chemicals has been documented; thus exposure of the sire should also be considered.

Finally, dystocia contributes to late pregnancy loss. The average term stillbirth rate is 2.2% to 4.5%. The incidence of fetal mortality increases to 22.3% with dystocia (Johnston et al., 2001). Late pregnancy can be monitored with a uterine monitoring system (Whelpwise). This alerts the owner and veterinarian to a problem earlier than may otherwise occur, enabling intervention with problem deliveries.

Gamete Aging

In bitches that are bred too early in their cycle, sperm may be aged by the time fertilization occurs. Conversely, bitches bred late in their cycle may have ova that are at the end of their functional lives. In humans this increases the risk of abortion. It is unknown if this is also true in the dog.

Genetic and Chromosomal Causes

The fetal mortality rate is higher in purebred than hybrid dogs (Fox, 1963). In a study of outbred and inbred studs bred to outbred and inbred bitches, the inbred producers had a decreased conception rate and fewer live births (Wildt et al., 1982). Evaluation of pedigrees of the dam and sire is useful when there is pregnancy loss. Programs are available to calculate the coefficient of inbreeding (COI). Breeding the bitch to an unrelated proven male may be helpful.

In women 50% of human fetuses that implant are lost in the first or second trimester (Jacobs, 1982). Genetic causes, especially chromosome loss, are responsible for many. Lethal defects cause early embryonic death and resorption. The incidence of such losses is unknown in the canine. Karyotyping of aborted fetuses shows gross chromosomal defects such as triploidy or x-monosomy, but does not diagnose single gene defects (Post, 1995). The canine genome project may help advance knowledge in this area.

Drug Administration

The critical period for embryotoxicity in the bitch is 6 to 20 days after LH surge. Drug administration should be avoided during this time period. Certain drugs are known to be a risk for pregnancy loss (Box 213-2).

Hypoluteodism

The lack of sufficient progesterone to maintain pregnancy is an extremely uncommon cause of pregnancy loss in the bitch. Because progesterone decrease rapidly follows abortion from any cause, this decline may be mistaken as the cause itself. Thorough diagnostics should be performed to rule out other causes, especially infectious ones, before any progesterone supplementation.

In the bitch serum progesterone higher than 2 ng/ml is required to maintain pregnancy. Serial monitoring of progesterone can be performed. Values higher than 20 ng/ml are common. Levels of 5 to 10 ng/ml may necessitate

---

Box **213-2**

Drugs That May Cause Pregnancy Loss

- Dexamethasone
- Misoprostol
- Verapamil
- Diltiazem
- Xylazine
- Pentobarbital
- Chemotherapeutics
- Organophosphates

Table **213-1**	

Pharmacologic Progesterone Supplementation in the Bitch

Drug	Dose
Progesterone in oil	2-3 mg/kg q24-48h IM
Ally-trenbolone*	0.088 mg/kg q24h PO

*Regumate, Hoechst-Roussel, Summerville, NJ.
IM, Intramuscularly; *PO*, orally.

weekly or every-other-day monitoring. Supplementation is provided if the progesterone level reaches 5 ng/ml with a week or more left in gestation. Two options for progesterone supplementation exist (Table 213-1). When using progesterone in oil, monitor to maintain a serum progesterone level of 10 ng/ml. Ally-trenbolone (Regumate) has an advantage in that it does not cross-react in progesterone assay; thus the endogenous progesterone level can continue to be monitored. The pregnancy should be monitored with ultrasound because of the increased risk of pyometra.

Progesterone supplementation should be avoided during the first trimester because of the risk of masculinizing female fetuses. In addition, ovulation timing is necessary to document the correct due date. Progesterone supplementation should be stopped 2 to 3 days before expected parturition so that fetuses are not retained too long. Finally, milk production is often inadequate, possibly because of prolactin suppression; thus milk supplementation of pups often is needed.

References and Suggested Reading

Baba E et al: Vaginal and uterine microflora of adult dogs, *Am J Vet Res* 44: 606, 1983.

Bjurstrom L, Linde-Forsberg C: Long-term study of aerobic bacteria of the genital tract in breeding bitches, *Am J Vet Res* 53, 1992.

Carmichael LE, Schlafer DH, Hashimoto A: Pathogenicity of minute virus of canines (MCV) for the canine fetus, *Cornell Vet* 81:151, 1991.

Eilts BE: Pregnancy maintenance in the bitch using regumate, Proceedings of the Society of Theriogenology Annual Meeting, San Antonio, 1992, p 144.

Fox MW: Neonatal mortality in the dog, *J Am Vet Med Assoc* 143:1219, 1963.

Greene CE, Carmichael LE: Canine brucellosis. I: *Infectious diseases of the dog and cat*, ed 3, St Louis, 2006, Saunders Elsevier, p 369.

Hollet RB: Canine brucellosis: outbreaks and compliance, *Theriogenology* 66:575, 2006.

Jacobs PA: Pregnancy losses and birth defects. In Austin CR, Short RV, editors: *Reproduction in mammals. 2. Embryonic and fetal development*, Cambridge, 1982, Cambridge University Press, p 142.

Johnson CA, Grace JA, Probst MR: The effect of maternal illness on perinatal health, *Vet Clin North Am Small Anim Pract* 17:555, 1987.

Johnston SD, Root Kustritz MV, Olson PNS: Canine and feline theriogenology, Philadelphia, Saunders, 2001.

Post K: Embryo and fetal loss in the canine: a review, Hastings, Nebraska, 1995, Theriogenology Handbook, Society for Theriogenology.

Ström B, Linde-Forsberg C: Effects of Ampicillin and trimethoprim-sulfamethoxazole on the vaginal bacterial flora of bitches, *Am J Vet Res* 54:891, 1993.

Wanke MM, Delpino MV, Baldi PC: Use of enrofloxacin in the treatment of canine brucellosis in a dog kennel (clinical trial), *Theriogenology* 66(6-7):1573, 2006.

Wilbur LA et al: Abortion and death in pregnant bitches associated with a canine vaccine contaminated with bluetongue virus, *J Am Vet Med Assoc* 204:1762, 1994.

Wildt DE et al: Influence of inbreeding on reproductive performance, ejaculate quality, and testicular volume in the dog, *Theriogenoloy* 17:445, 1982.

CHAPTER 214

False Pregnancy in the Bitch

DANA R. BLEIFER, *Woodland Hills, California*

False pregnancy, also called *pseudopregnancy* or *pseudocyesis*, is a common condition in intact bitches. The exact incidence may not be known, but one report found 87% of intact females to exhibit signs of false pregnancy two or more times in their lifetime (Janssens, 1986). On rare occasions it is also seen in spayed females. Usually clinical signs are mild and often ignored or unnoticed; but when disorders are manifest or if behavioral clinical signs are present, treatment may be warranted.

CLINICAL SIGNS

Clinical signs of pseudopregnancy are not associated with an endocrine abnormality; they are related to normal elevated plasma concentration of prolactin (England and Harvey, 1998). As progesterone concentration decreases in the second half of diestrus, prolactin concentration increases. A rise in the prolactin also can be seen if plasma progesterone drops for other reasons such as ovariohysterectomy during the luteal phase. Progesterone may also decrease suddenly consequent to spontaneous or pharmacologic abortion. Because all intact bitches experience this drop in progesterone and rise in prolactin in diestrus, one could say all bitches experience a physiologic pseudopregnancy. What makes some bitches experience clinical or overt pseudopregnancy is unclear. Perhaps it is excessively elevated prolactin concentration (Gobello, de la Sota, and Goya, 2001) or maybe an increase in sensitivity to the hormone in those bitches (Gobello et al., 2001). There are no differences in progesterone concentrations between pregnant and nonpregnant bitches, nor is there a difference in progesterone concentrations in bitches with overt and covert false pregnancy. Thus any bitch with a history of false pregnancy should be spayed in late anestrus, early proestrus, or anytime that progesterone levels are low.

Clinical signs of overt pseudopregnancy vary. The most common sign is mammary gland enlargement, with or without milk production. In some cases lactation may result in mastitis. Other signs associated with whelping may be observed such as nesting, nursing a "litter" of toys, nervousness, aggression, dullness, or a milky vulvar discharge. Signs of pseudopregnancy usually manifest 6 to 12 weeks after estrus and may last from weeks to months. Cases manifesting behavioral changes only may be difficult to diagnose; but when there is a recurrent cyclic pattern, pseudopregnancy should be considered. The severity of clinical signs also can vary dramatically. Often it is the severity of clinical signs or the necessity of participating in a show, performance trial, or work that dictates the need for treatment.

DIAGNOSIS OF THE AFOREMENTIONED CLINICAL SIGNS

Differential diagnosis of the aforementioned clinical signs includes pregnancy, pyometra, and ovarian remnant syndrome in spayed bitches. Generally the medical history, physical examination, ultrasound to rule out pregnancy or pyometra, vaginal cytology to identify cornification, and hormone testing for progesterone and/or estrogen can differentiate the conditions. Mammary gland development has also been reported in hypothyroidism, but it is unclear if the hypothyroidism was a cause or a coincidence with a normal false pregnancy (Chastain and Schmidt, 1980). The first condition to rule out is true pregnancy. Depending on the number of weeks following estrus, the fetus should be evident by ultrasound if longer than 25 to 28 days or by radiograph if longer than 50 days. Even if the time period exceeds gestational length, it is wise to rule out a mummified fetus.

If the clinical signs include lethargy, poor appetite, or vulvar discharge, pyometra, hydrometra, or mucometra should be ruled out. Ultrasound can identify the presence of fluid in the uterus. If there is a vulvar discharge, a vaginal cytology demonstrating excessive white blood cells also may increase the suspicion of pyometra. In the case of a closed cervix pyometra, there may be an elevated systemic white blood cell count with an immature neutrophilia (see Chapter 218).

In spayed bitches an ovarian remnant should be ruled out if there is a cyclic pattern to the pseudopregnancy signs. Vaginal cytology performed at the time of suspected estrus should show cornification of the vaginal epithelial cells if there is active ovarian tissue. Progesterone levels higher than 2 ng/ml in the weeks following a suspected "heat cycle" would also confirm the presence of ovarian tissue. Removal of the ovarian remnant is the treatment of choice. It is my experience that the ovarian remnant is easier to find during a heat cycle.

THERAPY

The majority of cases of pseudopregnancy require no treatment. False pregnancy does not predispose the bitch to reproductive disease. Spontaneous resolution usually occurs. After the luteal phase, serum prolactin is highest and then gradually declines. After a few weeks clinical signs should start to regress (typically about 12 weeks after estrus). Restricting food and water intake and increasing exercise have been suggested to shorten this period (Lawler et al., 1999). Sedatives can be used to minimize certain behaviors, but phenothiazines such as acepromazine maleate (Promace, Fort Dodge) should be avoided. Phenothiazides are dopamine antagonists and may increase prolactin levels. Although diuretic therapy may decrease mammary gland secretions, such treatment should only be used with great care.

Occasionally pseudopregnancy persists for many months or years. The reason for this is unknown but may relate to lack of hormonal interaction between the pituitary/hypothalamus and the ovary. The recurrence of false pregnancy in spayed females is perplexing but may be related to the point in their cycle at which they were spayed, as well as other hormonal interactions.

Reproductive hormones have been used successfully to treat pseudopregnancy. Progestogens work well by suppressing the release of prolactin, but signs may recur if the progestogen is discontinued quickly. The dosage should be decreased gradually. Megestrol acetate (Ovaban, Schering-Plough) dosed at 2.5 mg/kg every 24 hours orally for 8 days is the only approved product available in the United States. Estrogen and androgen treatments have also been successful and are thought to work in the same way as progesterone. Both estrogens and androgens may be associated with adverse side effects; thus they should be used carefully if at all for this purpose. Until recently mibolerone (Cheque Drops, Upjohn) was available in the United States and was a very effective treatment. There are a variety of suggested dosages, but typically mibolerone 16 mcg/kg every 24 hours orally for 5 days diminishes clinical signs.

The treatment of choice for false pregnancy in the bitch now appears to be the antiprolactin drug cabergoline (Dostinex, Pharmacia & Upjohn). Cabergoline is a long-acting serotonin antagonist. A dosage of 5 mcg/kg every 24 hours orally for 5 days seems to be optimal (Jochle et al., 1989). The drug typically is well tolerated and very effective, but it is also expensive. The dopamine agonist bromocriptine mesylate (Parlodel, Sandoz) is also effective but associated with a high incidence of gastrointestinal side effects. Compounding bromocriptine into a suspension and gradually increasing the dosage up to 10 mcg/kg daily for 19 days may decrease some side effects. Concurrent treatment with metoclopramide HCl (Reglan, Robbins) may be used to reduce vomiting; this drug can oppose dopaminergic action. Other dopaminergic agonists have been used successfully but are not readily available in the United States.

References and Suggested Reading

Buckrell BC, Johnson WH: Anestrus and spontaneous galactorrhea in a hypothyroid bitch, *Can Vet J* 27:204, 1986.

Chastain CB, Schmidt B: Galactorrhea associated with hypothyroidism in intact bitches, *J Am Anim Hosp Assoc* 16:851, 1980.

England Gary, Harvey Mike: *Manual of small animal reproduction and neonatology*, Shurdlington, Cheltenham UK, 1998, British Small Animal Veterinary Association, p 39.

Gobello C, de la Sota RL, Goya RG: Study of the change of prolactin and progesterone during dopaminergic agonist treatments in pseudopregnant bitches, *Anim Reprod Sci J* 66(3-4):257, 2001.

Gobello C et al: *Advances in reproduction in dogs, cats and exotic carnivores*, Cambridge UK, 2001, Journals of Reproduction and Fertility Ltd, p 55.

Janssens LAA: Treatment of pseudopregnancy with bromocriptine, an ergot alkaloid, *Vet Rec* 119:172, 1986.

Jochle W et al: *Dog and cat reproduction, contraception and artificial insemination*, Cambridge, UK, 1989, Journals of Reproduction and Fertility Ltd, p 199.

Johnston SD, Kustriz, MR, Olson PNS: Canine and feline theriogenology, Philadelphia, 2001, Saunders.

Lawler DF et al: *Journals Abstract, Am J Vet Res* 60{7}:820, 1999.

Okens AC et al: Plasma prolactin concentration and the effect of metergoline in pseudopregnant Afghan hounds: Journals Abstract, *Tijdschr Diergeneeskd* 125(3):81 2000 Infertility and Hormone Treatment in the Female. pp 66-67.

CHAPTER 215

Dystocia Management

AUTUMN P. DAVIDSON, *Davis, California*

Although many bitches whelp in the home or kennel setting without difficulty, requests for veterinary participation in the field of canine obstetrics have become more common. The increased financial and emotional value of stud dogs, brood bitches, and their offspring to the dog fancier makes the preventable loss of even one neonate undesirable. Breeding colonies in academic, scientific, and industrial facilities need to maximize neonatal survival for financial and ethical reasons. Veterinary involvement in canine obstetrics has several goals: to increase neonatal viability (minimizing puppies born dead from the difficulties in the birth process), to minimize morbidity and mortality in the brood bitch, and to contribute to better survival rates of neonates during the first week of life. Neonatal survival is directly related to the quality of labor (Johnson, Smith, and Baile, 1983; Neutra, 1978; Tutera and Newman, 1975). Optimal management of whelping requires an understanding of normal labor and delivery in the bitch, as well as the clinical ability to detect and treat abnormalities in the whelping process.

Dystocia is defined as difficulty in the normal vaginal delivery of a neonate from the uterus. Dystocia must be detected in a timely fashion for medical or surgical intervention to improve outcome. In addition, the etiology of dystocia must be identified for the most appropriate therapeutic decisions to be made.

NORMAL GESTATION IN THE BITCH

Clinicians commonly are asked to ascertain if a bitch is at term pregnancy and ready chronologically to deliver a litter and to intervene if labor has not begun on time. Prolonged gestation is a form of dystocia. Normal gestation in the bitch is 56 to 58 days from the first day of diestrus (detected by serial vaginal cytologies, defined as the first day that cytology returns to 50% or fewer cornified/superficial cells) or 64 to 66 days from the initial rise in progesterone from baseline (generally >2ng/ml), which equates to the day of the luteinizing hormone (LH) surge or 58 to 72 days from the first instance that the bitch permitted breeding (Concannon, Whaley, and Lein, 1983). Predicting gestational length without prior ovulation timing is difficult because of the disparity between estrual behavior and the actual time of conception in the bitch and the length of time semen can remain viable in the bitch reproductive tract, often up to more than 7 days (Feldman and Nelson, 1996). Breeding and conception dates do not correlate closely enough to permit highly accurate prediction of whelping dates. In addition, clinical signs of term pregnancy are not specific: the radiographic appearance of fetal skeletal mineralization varies at term, fetal size varies with breed and litter size, and the characteristic drop in body temperature (typically less than 100° F) may not be detected in all bitches and varies in others.

Breed, parity, and litter size also can influence gestational length (Eilts et al., 2002). Astute dog owners and clinicians may be able to detect subtle signs of impending delivery such as relaxation of the perineum, mammary engorgement, or a change in the appearance of the gravid abdomen, but these are not sensitive or specific. The inability to clinically manage prematurity in the canine effectively makes hastened intervention in the whelping process undesirable. Unfortunately an excessively conservative approach resulting in intrauterine fetal death is undesirable as well (Wallace, 1994).

Bitches typically enter stage I labor within 24 hours of a decline in serum progesterone to below 2 to 5 ng/ml (Concannon, McCann, and Temple, 1989), which occurs in conjunction with elevated circulating prostaglandins and is commonly associated with a transient drop in body temperature usually to less than 100° F. Monitoring serial progesterone levels for impending labor is problematic because in-house kits enabling rapid results are inherently inaccurate between 2 and 5 ng/ml. Commercial laboratories offering quantitative progesterone by chemiluminescence typically have a 12- to 24-hour turnaround time, which is not rapid enough to enable decisions about an immediate indication for obstetric intervention. Clearly it is beneficial to obtain information about ovulation timing, minimally by determining the onset of cytologic diestrus, for evaluating gestational length at term. If only breeding dates are available, the clinician should avoid electively delivering puppies younger than 62 gestational days, unless an indication of impending fetal demise is present. Fetal heart rate monitoring may be helpful; if fetal heart rates are consistently less than 150 beats/min, fetal stress may be present.

NORMAL LABOR AND DELIVERY

Stage I labor in the bitch normally lasts from 12 to 24 hours, during which time the uterus has myometrial contractions of increasing frequency and strength associated with cervical dilation. No abdominal effort (visible contractions) is evident during stage I labor. Bitches may exhibit changes in disposition and behavior, becoming reclusive and restless and nesting intermittently, often refusing to eat, and sometimes vomiting. Panting and trembling may occur. Vaginal discharge typically is clear and watery.

Normal stage II labor is defined to begin when external abdominal efforts can be seen accompanying myometrial contractions to culminate in the delivery of a neonate. Presentation of the fetus at the cervix triggers the Ferguson reflex, promoting the release of endogenous oxytocin from the hypothalamus. Typically these efforts should not last longer than 1 to 2 hours between puppies, although great normal variation exists. The entire delivery can take between 1 to longer than 24 hours; however, normal labor outcome is associated with shorter total delivery time and intervals between neonates (Darvelid, 1985; Gaudet, 1985; Gaudet and Kitchell, 1985). Vaginal discharge can be clear, serous to hemorrhagic, or green (uteroverdin). Typically bitches continue to nest between deliveries and may nurse and groom neonates intermittently. Anorexia, panting, and trembling are common.

Stage III labor is defined as the delivery of the placenta. Bitches typically vacillate between labor stages II and III until the delivery is complete. During normal labor all fetuses and placentae are delivered vaginally, although they may not be delivered together in every instance. Occasionally placentae are delivered hours after delivery of puppies is complete. Bitches typically consume placentae, making client counts potentially inaccurate.

DETECTING ABNORMALITIES IN CANINE LABOR

The standard approach to labor management in the bitch has involved subjective monitoring of the bitch's behavior, rectal temperature, progression of whelping, and the physical condition of the neonates. Little accurate, timely, and evidence-based information is made available to the clinician concerning actual uterine activity or prepartum fetal viability with this methodology. Telephone consultations between the veterinarian and breeder or kennel manager usually entail interpretation of indirect information such as time between deliveries, color of vaginal discharge, presence and nature of externally visible abdominal contractions, and occurrence of stillborn puppies. Although generally acceptable (associated with a favorable outcome) for the uneventful delivery in a young, healthy bitch, whelping associated with fetal and maternal morbidity and mortality is familiar to most clinicians in reproductive practice. For these cases, improved diagnostic tools are desirable, such as those used in human obstetrics. Clinical information about the onset, duration, and progression of the stages of labor, frequency and strength of myometrial contractions, progression of delivery of fetuses into the uterine body and vagina for birth, and physical status of the fetuses is helpful for obstetric decision making (Friedman, 1968). Evaluating the metabolic status of bitches presented for dystocia is important if hypocalcemia or hypoglycemia is suspected but neither is commonly detected.

Recently a system for monitoring labor and fetal viability in the bitch has become available commercially (Veterinary Perinatal Services, Inc.). This system is intended for use by veterinarians in the clinical setting when evaluating a bitch in labor or by dog fanciers or kennel managers with veterinary supervision in the home or kennel setting. The Veterinary Perinatal Service (VPS) design is based on labor monitoring systems used routinely in human obstetrics. The uterine monitoring system consists of a tocodynamometer (sensor), a recorder, and a modem (Healthdyne Inc.; Sonicaid, Oxford Instruments) (Fig. 215-1). The uterine sensor detects changes in intrauterine and intraamniotic pressures. The sensor is strapped over a lightly clipped area of the bitch's caudolateral abdomen using an elasticized strap. The sensor's recorder is worn in a small backpack placed over the caudal shoulder area (Fig. 215-2). Bitches should be at rest in the whelping box, cage, or a crate during the monitoring sessions. The monitoring equipment is well tolerated. Subsequent to each recording session, data are transferred from the recorder to the service center using a modem with the telephone.

Fetal heart rate assessments can be performed easily by using either real-time ultrasound or a handheld Doppler unit. Normal fetal heart rates generally range above 220 beats/min. Normal beagles at term have heart rates at least twice the maternal rate. Fetal distress is evident by persistent fetal bradycardia of 120 to 150 beats/min. In a model of impaired oxygen delivery, heart rates in fetal dogs were recorded during hypoxic episodes; they showed that decelerations were an early sign of fetal hypoxia (Monheit, Stone, and Abitobol, 1988).

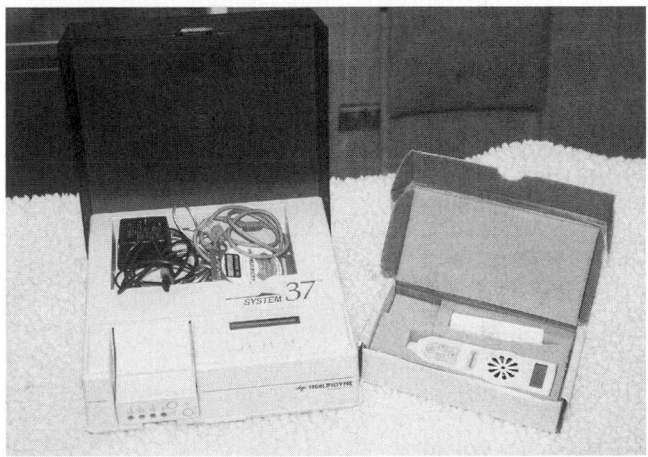

Fig. 215-1 Veterinary obstetrical monitoring equipment consists of a tocodynamometer (sensor, recorder, and modem, *left*) and hand-held Doppler unit (*right*).

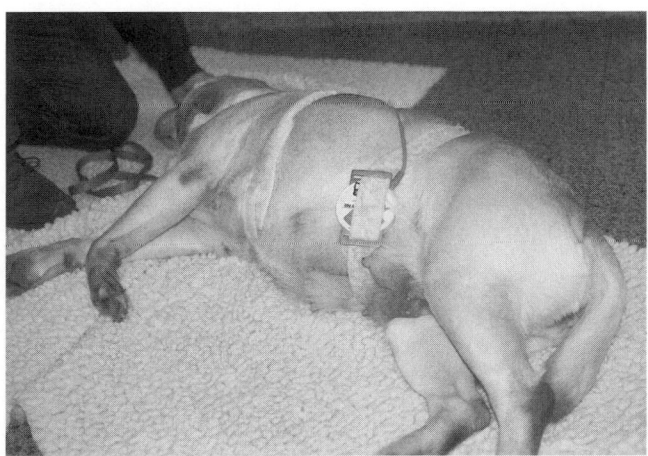

Fig. 215-2 A monitoring session showing a pregnant Labrador retriever bitch with tocodynamometer sensor in place. The sensor is placed over a lightly clipped area of the gravid lateral abdomen.

Fetal heart rate monitoring, performed with either a real-time ultrasound probe (5 to 7.5 MHz) or a handheld Doppler unit, is best used with bitches in lateral recumbency, using acoustic coupling gel (Fig. 215-3). Visualization of the fetal cardiac valve motion enables estimation of the heart rate with real-time ultrasound. Directing the handheld Doppler perpendicularly over a fetus results in a characteristic amplification of the fetal heart sounds, distinct from maternal arterial, digestive, or cardiac sounds, enabling audible determination of fetal heart rates. The presence of fetal distress is reflected by sustained deceleration of the heart rates. Decelerations associated with uterine contractions suggest mismatch between the size of the fetus and the birth canal or fetal malposition or malposture. Malpresentation is generally not a problem in canine deliveries. Transient accelerations occur with normal fetal movement (England and Gary, 1998; Verstegen et al., 1993; Shenker, Post, and Seiler, 1975).

THE PREPARTUM VISIT

Dog fanciers or kennel personnel can perform labor and fetal monitoring with veterinary guidance by telephone after previous demonstration of equipment in the clinic or on site. Ideally such demonstration should take place during a prepartum office visit or kennel call. After performing a physical examination of the gravid bitch, the clinician reviews labor management with the client or kennel personnel, including the use of monitoring equipment and administration of any medications, as well as whelping equipment and neonatal resuscitation. Light clipping of the hair coat over the gravid area of the lateral flanks allows proper contact later of the uterine sensor and fetal Doppler. In addition, proper technique for the subcutaneous administration of injectable drugs is taught during the prepartum consult. Calcium gluconate, 10% solution with 0.465 mEq Ca++ (Fujisawa Inc.), and oxytocin, 10 USP units/ml (American Pharmaceutical Partners, Inc.) can be dispensed in predrawn syringes for later use on veterinary prescription.

Specific orders (Fig. 215-4) are written for each bitch by the attending veterinarian concerning the indica-

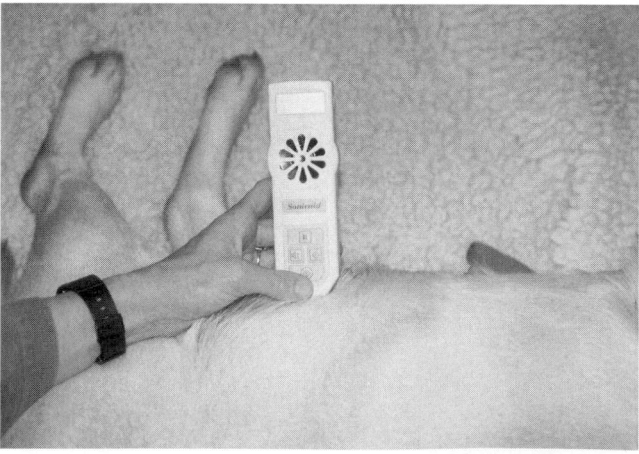

Fig. 215-3 Evaluating fetal heart rate with a hand-held Doppler. Fetal heart rates can be detected audibly or read from the unit.

tion, frequency of administration, and dosage of medications (calcium and oxytocin) and faxed to VPS. A copy is retained for the medical record. An abdominal radiograph may be obtained at the prepartum visit to best estimate litter and relative fetal size (Eneroth et al., 1999).

CLINICAL LABOR MONITORING

Use of this monitoring equipment in a veterinary clinical setting is dictated by the presentation or referral of bitches for labor evaluation and is very helpful in making immediate assessment of the quality of labor and fetal viability. Minimal monitoring of uterine activity for 30 minutes is advised. Fetal heart rate monitoring can be performed immediately after uterine monitoring while uterine data are being sent via modem and generally takes 5 to 10 minutes, depending on the number of fetuses and skill of the operator.

For labor evaluation during whelping in the home or kennel setting, uterine and fetal monitoring should be initiated at least 1 week before the first predicted whelping date and are generally performed twice daily for 1 hour at each episode approximately 12 hours apart. This permits prospective identification of normal prelabor myometrial activity and the onset and duration of stages I and II of labor (Figs. 215-5 and 215-6). Owners should attempt to identify a heartbeat for each fetus with the Doppler unit at each monitoring session. Obstetric personnel (licensed human obstetric nurses) are available 24 hours a day at the VPS central office to receive and interpret uterine contractile recordings and subsequently communicate such findings by telephone to the attending veterinary clinician. Once a bitch enters stage I labor, the subsequent frequency of uterine and fetal monitoring is based on the recommendation of such obstetric personnel and the attending veterinarian evaluating the progression of labor and neonatal condition. Obstetric personnel generally consult by telephone with the veterinary clinician continuously during actual labor monitoring.

THERAPEUTIC INTERVENTION IN DYSTOCIA

The diagnosis of dystocia can be made objectively if uterine contractility is determined to be inappropriate (generally infrequent, weak myometrial contractions) for the stage of labor (Fig. 215-7) or if excessive fetal stress as determined by fetal heart rate monitoring is resulting from labor. Subjectively the diagnosis of dystocia can be made if stage I labor is not initiated at term, if stage I labor is longer than 24 hours without progression to stage II, if stage II labor does not produce a vaginal delivery within 1 to 4 hours, if fetal or maternal stress is excessive, if moribund or stillborn neonates are resulting, or if stage II labor does not result in the completion of deliveries in a timely manner (within 12 to 24 hours).

Dystocia results from maternal factors, fetal factors, or a combination of both. Maternal factors include uterine inertia, fluid abnormalities, and pelvic canal anomalies. Uterine inertia (i.e., failure of the uterine muscle to contract in an effective manner) can be primary or secondary. Primary

WhelpWise™ Veterinary Orders
Please circle all that apply

Client _____ Client phone _____ Date _____

Animal name _____ Breed _____ Wt. _____

1. Initiate the WhelpWise™ service. Instruct client in use of equipment. Encourage client to monitor uterine contractions twice daily, preferably 10 to 12 hours apart. At the onset of an active labor pattern, client and WhelpWise staff will determine the frequency and duration of subsequent monitor sessions.
   Notify me of onset of labor: **YES NO**   After hours: **YES NO**

2. In the presence of inertia as documented by the external uterine contraction monitor, begin labor augmentation per protocol. **YES NO**
   Notify me before beginning medications: YES NO

3. All medication doses are based on the uterine contraction pattern, and used to treat inertia only.
   Medication will not be given in the presence of a strong, regular contraction pattern

   Oxytocin: _____ to _____ **UNITS** administered **Sub Q or IM** every _____ minutes (Usual dose **.25** to 4 units every 30-90 minutes)
   Calcium solution (10%) _____ cc, **subcutaneously** every _____ hrs. (Usual dose: 1 ml/10 lbs BW or 4.5 kg BW min.
   to maintain an adequate uterine contraction pattern every 4-6 hours.)
   Cleanout shot of: _____ , after deliveries are complete.

Suggested breakdown:
Oxytocin: 2 syringes with .5 units (one half unit), 3 syringes with 1 unit, 3 syringes with 2 units, 2 syringes with 3 units. In breeds over 70 lbs: add 2 syringes with 4 units, breeds over 100 lbs: add 1 additional syringe of 5 units.
Calcium: 1/2 cc/10 pounds drawn into 3 syringes. Example: Dog's weight 30 pounds: 3 syringes of 1.5 cc.

4. Encourage client to monitor the fetal heart rates a minimum of once a day prior to labor, and every 1-2 hours or more frequently during active labor. Notify me if decelerations or absence of fetal heart rates are noted. Recommend that the client assess the fetal heart rates prior to administration of any medication.

5. If the case being monitored is a planned cesarean section, notify me at the onset of labor.

6. Notify me of the outcomes at the conclusion of service by _____ phone _____ fax

Other instructions:

_____

_____

_____

Signature _____ Veterinarian _____

Clinic name _____ Address _____

Clinic phone _____ Fax _____ After hours _____

Veterinary Perinatal Specialties Inc.   9111 W. 38th Ave. Wheat Ridge, CO 80033
1-888-281-4867   (303) 423-3429   Fax: (303) 423-8242

Fig. 215-4 Veterinary orders form. The supervising veterinarian determines whether medications (calcium gluconate and oxytocin) may be given by an owner and if so, under which circumstances and at what dosage. This form is faxed to Veterinary Perinatal Services when home monitoring is initiated.

uterine inertia is multifactorial, with genetic, mechanical, hormonal, and physical components. Bitches exhibiting primary inertia fail to proceed into an effective labor pattern, and cesarean section is indicated. Bitches exhibiting secondary inertia fail to complete expulsion of all fetuses because of exhaustion of the uterine muscle. Medical man-agement may be successful. Clinically secondary uterine inertia is the most common maternal cause of dystocia. Abnormalities of fetal/placental fluids include hydrops, an excessive accumulation of allantoic fluid associated with each fetus, causing the fetal unit to be markedly oversized. Rarely underproduction of fetal fluids occurs, resulting in

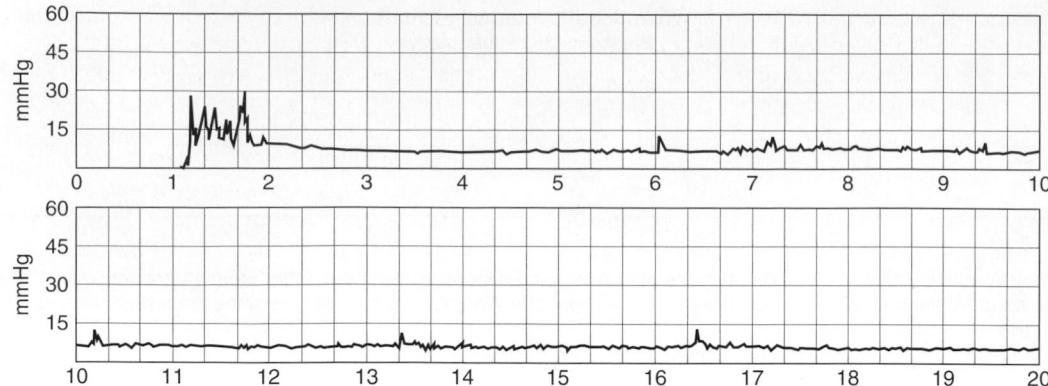

Fig. 215-5 Normal uterine baseline recording (prelabor), no contractions evident. X-axis represents time in minutes; Y-axis strength of contraction in millimeters of Mercury.

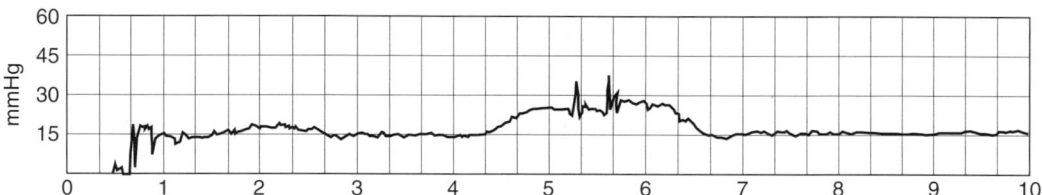

Fig. 215-6 Normal myometrial contraction, prelabor. Note excursion off baseline during contraction with return to baseline.

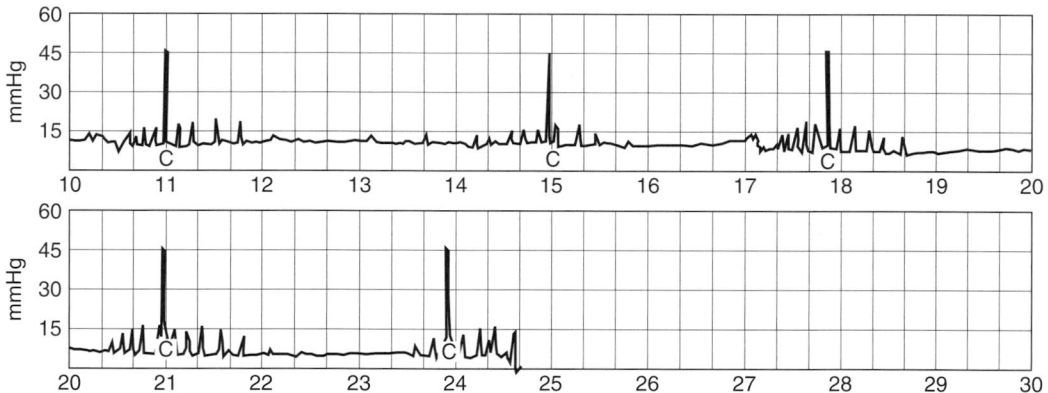

Fig. 215-7 Uterine inertia: abdominal efforts (seen as vertical spikes) with no myometrial contractions evident.

dystocia caused by a lack of lubricating fluids. Disorders of the birth canal contributing to dystocia include pelvic abnormalities such as narrowing from a healed fracture or congenital disorders and vaginovulvar abnormalities such as strictures. Successful natural breedings can occur despite the presence of septate (vertical) bands in the vaginal vault. Unfortunately subsequent vaginal delivery of fetuses is usually impaired. Septate bands and strictures should be detected by the veterinarian at the time of the soundness examination before breeding and resolved if possible. Annular (circular) strictures are often detected at the time of breeding since they can interfere with the ability to attain a natural tie. These may be repaired before breeding; however, recurrence is common, and elective cesarean delivery may be less problematic. Bitches with unusually small vulvar openings may require a partial episiotomy to deliver puppies vaginally.

Fetal causes of dystocia include fetal oversize; fetal anomalies; and abnormal fetal position, presentation, or posture. Fetal oversize can occur with prolonged gestation in abnormally small litters and is the most common fetal cause of dystocia. Fetal anomalies such as anasarca and hydrocephalus (abnormalities of body fluid distribution) can cause a mismatch between the size of the birth canal and the fetus. Because both an anterior (head first) and posterior (breech) presentation are normal in the bitch, only a transverse (sideways) presentation is associated with dystocia and is rare. Puppies normally are positioned with the fetal backbone adjacent to the top surface of the uterus. Malpositioning (fetal backbone adjacent to ventral surface of uterus) can cause mild dystocia. Abnormalities of posture, normal being fully extended forlimbs (as if diving), are the second most frequent fetal cause of dystocia. Malpositioning of the head, forelimbs, or hind limbs of the canine fetus is not readily corrected with the use of forceps, traction, or digital manipulation because of the limitations of the size of the birth canal of the bitch.

The use of uterine and fetal monitors allows the veterinary clinician to detect and monitor labor and manage dystocia medically or surgically with insight. Clinical use of the monitoring equipment should dictate subsequent medical or surgical intervention. In the home or kennel setting, the administration of medications is initiated as indicated by monitoring information and only with authorization from the attending veterinary clinician. Continued monitoring permits evaluation of the response to therapy (Fig. 215-8). Unresponsive uterine inertia, obstructive dystocia, aberrant uterine contractile patterns, or progressive fetal distress without response to medical management are indications for return to the veterinary facility for cesarean section (Davidson, 2001).

Medical management revolves around the administration of calcium gluconate and oxytocin, based on the results of monitoring. Drugs are given only after 8 to 12 hours of an established contraction pattern (stage I labor) as detected by the uterine monitor and only if inertia is detected when stage II labor is anticipated. Premature administration of drugs results in suboptimal response; for this reason prelabor monitoring permitting recognition of the onset of labor is ideal.

Generally the administration of calcium increases the strength of myometrial activity, and oxytocin increases the frequency of myometrial contractions. Interestingly, despite normocalcemia, the administration of calcium gluconate usually results in improved myometrial tone. Calcium gluconate, 10%, is given when ineffective, weak uterine contractions are detected. A 10% solution of calcium gluconate can be given subcutaneously, avoiding the potential for cardiac irritability associated with intravenous administration. Calcium gluconate 10% (0.465 mEq/ml) is dosed at 1 ml/4.5 kg of body weight, generally every 4 to 6 hours.

Oxytocin is administered when uterine contractions are less frequent than expected for the stage of labor. Oxytocin given too early or too late during whelping has a minimal effect on the contractile pattern. The most effective time for dosing is when uterine inertia begins to develop, before the complete cessation of uterine contractility occurs. High doses of oxytocin saturate the receptor sites and make it ineffective as a uterotonic. Substantially lower than traditional doses of oxytocin are now known to be effective in improving the quality of myometrial contractions. Oxytocin is available at a concentration of 10 units/ml, permitting accurate small dosing. Refrigeration is not required. An initial dose of 0.25 to 0.5 units per dog administered subcutaneously is advised. Subsequent doses range from 0.50 to 2 units per dog. Higher doses of oxytocin or intravenous boluses can cause tetanic, ineffective uterine contractions that compromise fetal oxygen supply during placental compression. If fetal stress is evident (persistent bradycardia) and response to medications poor, surgical intervention is indicated. Uterine hyperstimulation with elevated baseline levels of contractility compromising placental blood supply (Fig. 215-9) or a uterine obstructive pattern also negates

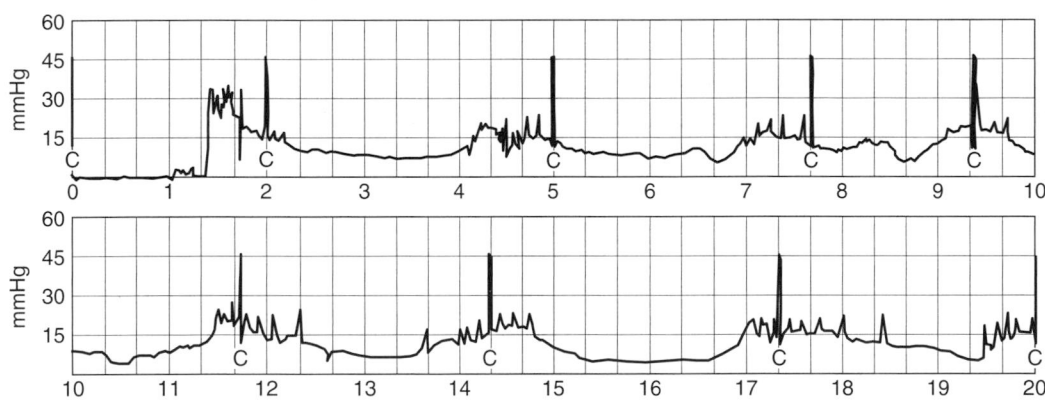

Fig. 215-8   Inertia as seen in Fig. 215-7 treated with 1 unit of oxytocin subcutaneously; normal contraction pattern evident.

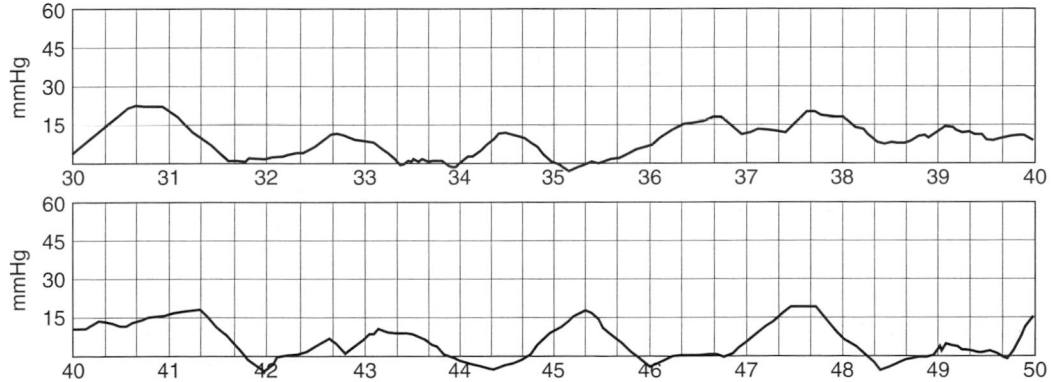

Fig. 215-9   Uterine hypercontractility; note minimal return to baseline.

further use of calcium gluconate or oxytocin (Lopez-Zeno et al., 1992). Use of intrapartum monitoring has been demonstrated to lead practitioners to perform cesarean section earlier in some cases of dystocia, decreasing puppy mortality in these cases.

A written summary concerning the labor pattern and response to medical intervention can ultimately be incorporated into the dog's medical record for reference in future breedings. The monitoring equipment can be leased for constant use in a busy reproductive practice for a monthly fee. Alternatively, the equipment may be leased and shipped directly to the veterinary client for use during with an individual dog during labor. Practitioner and client acceptance of the equipment once familiarity is established is generally very good.

References and Suggested Reading

Bennett D: Canine dystocia—a review of the literature, *J Small Anim Pract* 15:101, 1974.

Concannon P, McCann J, Temple M: Biology and endocrinology of ovulation, pregnancy and parturition in the dog, *J Reprod Fertil* 39(suppl):3, 1989.

Concannon P, Whaley S, Lein D: Canine gestation length: variation related to time of mating and fertile life of sperm, *Am J Vet Res* 44:1819, 1983.

Darvelid A, Linde-Forsberg C: Dystocia in the bitch: a retrospective study of 182 cases, *J Small Anim Pract* 35:402, 1985.

Davidson AP: Uterine and fetal monitoring on the bitch, *Vet Clin North Am: Small Anim Pract* 31(2):305, 2001.

Eilts B et al: Factors influencing gestation length in the bitch. Proceedings of the Third European Veterinary Society for Small Animal Reproduction; European Congress on Companion, Exotic and Laboratory Animals, Liege, Belgium, 2002, p128.

England GC: Ultrasound assessment of abnormal pregnancy, *Vet Clin North Am: Small Anim Pract* 28(4):281, 1998.

Eneroth A et al: Radiographic pelvimetry for assessment of dystocia in bitches: a clinical study in two terrier breeds, *J Small Anim Pract* 40:257, 1999.

Feldman EC, Nelson RW: Canine reproduction. In *Veterinary reproduction and endocrinology*, Philadelphia, 1996, Saunders.

Friedman EA: Use of labor pattern as a management guide, *J Reprod Med* 8:57, 1968.

Gaudet DA: Retrospective study of 128 cases of canine dystocia, *J Am Anim Hosp Assoc* 21:813, 1985.

Gaudet DA, Kitchell BE: Canine dystocia, *Compend Contin Educ Small Anim Pract Vet* 7(5):1406, 1985.

Johnson S, Smith F, Baile N: Prenatal indicators of puppy viability at term, *Compend Contin Educ Small Anim Pract Vet* 5:1013, 1983.

Lopez-Zeno JA et al: A controlled trial of a program for the active management of labor, *N Engl J Med* 326(7):450, 1992.

Monheit AG, Stone ML, Abitbol MM: Fetal heart rate and transcutaneous monitoring during experimentally induced hypoxia in the fetal dog, *Pediatr Res* 6:548, 1988.

Neutra RR: Effect of fetal monitoring on neonatal death rates, *N Engl J Med* 229(7):324, 1978.

Shenker L, Post R, Seiler J: Routine electronic monitoring of fetal heart rate and uterine activity during labor, *Obstet Gynecol* 46:185, 1975.

Tutera G, Newman R: Fetal monitoring: its effect on perinatal mortality and cesarean section rates and its complications, *Am J Obstet Gynecol* 122:750, 1975.

Verstegen J et al: Echocardiographic study of heart rate in dog and cat fetuses in utero, *J Reprod Fertil* 47(suppl):175, 1993.

Wallace M: Management of parturition and problems of the periparturient period of dogs and cats, *Semin Vet Med Surg (Small Anim)* 9:28, 1994.

CHAPTER 216

Canine Postpartum Disorders

MICHELLE ANNE KUTZLER, *Corvallis, Oregon*

The interval from parturition to weaning, the postpartum period, is typically 6 to 8 weeks in the dog. During the postpartum period uterine remodeling of the placental sites occurs, which is histologically complete by 12 weeks after delivery. Postpartum vaginal discharge, initially dark green in color, may persist for 3 to 6 weeks, over which time fibrin and blood are voided, and the discharge changes to reddish-brown. Abnormal events arising during the postpartum period are described in the following paragraphs with a summary of recommended therapies appearing at the end of this chapter (Table 216-1).

HEMORRHAGE

Scant bleeding after parturition is normal; however, excessive bleeding may indicate uterine or vaginal parturient trauma or be evidence of an underlying coagulopathy. Vaginoscopy may be useful to identify the source of bleeding. Intravenous fluid support and blood transfusions may be needed to stabilize the patient, depending on the overall condition of the animal and the total amount of blood lost. It is important to consider when correcting blood volume deficits that the normal hematocrit in most bitches at term is 30%. Although oxytocin (0.5 to 1 unit/kg, not to exceed 20 units intramuscularly [IM]) or ergonovine maleate (15.4 mcg/kg IM) is reported to reduce the size of the uterine lumen, their efficacy for the treatment of acute postpartum hemorrhage has not been evaluated critically, and ovariohysterectomy is often indicated.

SUBINVOLUTION OF PLACENTAL SITES

Subinvolution of the placental sites (SIPS) involves the delay in the normal process of placental degeneration and endometrial reconstruction with an unclear etiopathogenesis. Instead of degenerating after parturition, trophoblast cells persist within the endometrium, preventing endometrial blood vessels from developing thromboses, resulting in persistent bleeding. In addition, trophoblast cells invade the myometrium and on rare occasions may erode through the serosa, resulting in peritonitis (Beck and McEntee, 1966).

The incidence of SIPS in postpartum bitches is 10% to 20%; generally it occurs in primiparous bitches younger than 2½ years old. The only clinical sign of SIPS is persistent serosanguineous discharge for longer than 6 weeks after delivery. However, SIPS may occur in the absence of any vaginal discharge (Al-Bassam, Thomson, and O'Donnell, 1981). A presumptive diagnosis of SIPS is made based on the clinical history. Bitches with SIPS are afebrile and otherwise healthy, which differentiates SIPS from metritis; however, abnormalities within the bladder or vagina should also be ruled out. Abdominal palpation, contrast radiography, or ultrasonography may identify discrete, firm spheroid enlargements within the uterine horns (≈2.5 cm in diameter). Identification of multinucleated, basophilic staining trophoblast cells with highly vacuolated cytoplasm on cytologic examination of the discharge or histologic examination of a uterine biopsy provides a definitive diagnosis. A cystocentesis with urinanalysis and vaginoscopic examination should rule out the urinary tract and vagina as the source of the discharge.

The clinical management of SIPS must be based on the individual patient and client. Most cases of SIPS are self-limiting, which is fortunate, since medical treatment has not proven to be effective. Administration of antibiotics, progestins, or oxytocin does not decrease the duration, amount, or character of the vaginal discharge (Dickie and Arbeiter, 1993; Smith, 1986; Schall et al., 1971). Bitches intended for future breeding should be monitored cautiously until the discharge resolves spontaneously. Monitoring includes deliberate daily observation of the bitch's general appearance by the owner and weekly vaginal cytologic examinations and complete blood cell counts to confirm the absence of metritis or anemia. However, in cases of uterine rupture or severe hemorrhage or if the patient is no longer a valuable breeding animal, ovariohysterectomy is recommended. Normal fertility has been reported in bitches following recovery from SIPS.

UTERINE PROLAPSE

Uterine prolapse is relatively uncommon in the bitch and can occur during or within a few hours after parturition, involving either one or both uterine horns. Dystocia, delivery of large litters, incomplete placental separation, advanced maternal age, and excessive relaxation of the pelvic and perineal region are considered predisposing factors. Examination reveals a firm soft-tissue mass protruding from the vagina, which should be differentiated from a vaginal prolapse or neoplasia by palpation of the cervix and clinical appearance. Patients with a uterine prolapse can quickly develop hypotensive or hemorrhagic shock, especially if the ovarian or uterine vessels have been ruptured. While stabilizing the patient, the prolapsed tissues should be covered with warm, saline-moistened towels. After gentle cleaning and copiously lubricating the tissue, manual reduction,

Table 216-1

Recommended Therapies for Canine Postpartum Disorders

Drug	Dosage	Indications	Side Effects	Additional Information
Acepromazine	0.5-2 mg/kg SQ	Agalactia	Bradycardia, hypotension	
Cabergoline	5 mcg/kg q24h PO for 5 days	Adjunctive therapy for treating mastitis or puerperal tetany to suppress lactation	None observed at this dosage	
Calcium carbonate	100 mg/kg q24h PO	To prevent recurrence of puerperal tetany	May cause gastrointestinal irritation and constipation	
Calcium gluconate (10%)	0.22-0.44 ml/kg IV (slowly)	Puerperal tetany	Bradycardia and other arrhythmias	Should be administered in conjunction with careful cardiac monitoring
Cefadroxil	22 mg/kg q12h PO	Susceptible bacterial infections in lactating bitches	May cause gastrointestinal effects in susceptible animals	Has not been observed to affect nursing pups
Ergonovine maleate	15.4 mcg/kg IM	Postpartum hemorrhage	Uterine rupture has been reported	
Oxytocin	0.5-1 unit/kg, not to exceed 20 units q4-6h IM	Postpartum hemorrhage, secondary agalactia	Uterine cramping and abdominal discomfort	Milk will let down within 2 minutes of injection
PGF-2α (Lutalyse, UpJohn)	250 mcg/kg q24h SQ	Metritis	Hypersalivation, vomiting, diarrhea, abdominal discomfort	This dose minimizes the severity of side effects while using the least number of treatments

IM, Intramuscularly, *IV,* intravenously; *PGF,* prostaglandin F; *PO,* orally; *SQ,* subcutaneously.

with or without an episiotomy, under epidural or general anesthesia should be attempted. Manual reduction may be accomplished with a gloved finger, test tube, or syringe case. Systemic antibiotics are warranted because the risk of metritis following a uterine prolapse is high. Cefadroxil (22 mg/kg q12h orally [PO]) is recommended because it has broad-spectrum antibacterial activity and has not been observed to affect nursing pups (Bonagura, 2000, p 933). If the uterine tissue is not viable or the bitch is no longer intended for breeding, manual reduction should be followed by an ovariohysterectomy. If the uterus cannot be reduced manually, the urethra should be catheterized, and the uterus may be externally amputated. The amputation procedure involves individual ligation of the uterine arteries, transection, and oversewing of the base of the uterine body. A laparotomy should follow amputation to complete the ovariohysterectomy.

SEPTIC METRITIS

Septic metritis is an acute ascending bacterial (usually *Escherichia coli*) infection of the uterus, typically at the sites of placental attachment, occurring in the immediate postpartum period. Obstetric manipulations during a dystocia, abortion, retained fetal or placental tissue, and uterine prolapse are considered predisposing factors. Clinical signs include rectal temperature higher than 39.5° C (>103° F), dehydration and anorexia, depression, disinterest in pups and agalactia, and malodorous sanguineous vaginal discharge. Abdominal palpation may reveal a doughy, enlarged, and painful uterus. Vaginal cytology reveals large numbers of degenerative neutrophils, bacteria, and debris. Clinical pathology often shows elevated total solids (secondary to dehydration) with immature leukocytosis; however, leukopenia can occur in severely ill bitches. Abdominal radiography with or without contrast studies, ultrasonography, or hysteroscopy may aid in identifying an underlying cause. Although not diagnostic for metritis, cranial vaginal cultures with sensitivity may be helpful in determining appropriate antibiotic therapy.

Removal of pups from the bitch and administration of intravenous fluids and broad-spectrum antibiotics are necessary for treatment of accompanying septicemia. Amikacin (5 to 10 mg/kg q12h intravenously [IV]) with cephalothin (22 mg/kg q8h IV) is recommended; however, antibiotics alone may be ineffective in treating postpartum metritis (Durfee, 1968). Uterine evacuation using prostaglandin F$_2\alpha$ tromethamine (Lutalyse, UpJohn) at a dosage of 250 mcg/kg q24h subcutaneously has been determined to minimize the occurrence of side effects while obtaining a clinical cure with the least number of treatments (Feldman and Nelson, 1996). If the patient is no longer needed for breeding, ovariohysterectomy is recommended when the patient is stable for general anesthesia. Bitches recovering from acute postpartum metritis have retained their fertility, demonstrated by normal subsequent whelpings without future postpartum complications (Durfee, 1968).

AGALACTIA

Agalactia can present as either complete failure of mammary gland development (primary) or failure of milk to letdown (secondary). Debilitating maternal illness, malnutrition, and endocrine imbalances are predisposing factors. In addition, extremely stressed bitches may have elevated adrenaline concentrations, leading to decreased pituitary release of oxytocin or entry of oxytocin into the mammary gland. Acepromazine (0.5 to 2 mg/kg subcutaneously [SQ]) promotes prolactin secretion and may improve endogenous oxytocin release. Oxytocin administered either parenterally (0.5 to 1 unit/kg, not to exceed 20 units q4-6h [SQ]) or intranasally using a nebulizing spray (Syntocinon, Sandoz) into one nostril (q6-8h) results in milk letdown within 2 minutes. In addition, efforts should be made to correct the underlying maternal condition. Pups should be offered supplemental feedings or reared as orphans if the condition persists.

SEPTIC MASTITIS

Acute septic mastitis, an ascending bacterial infection involving one or more of the mammary glands, can occur secondary to galactostasis and in the presence of unsanitary housing. Clinical signs include rectal temperature higher than 39.5° C (>103° F); dehydration and anorexia; depression; disinterest in pups and agalactia; and painful, firm, and reddened mammary glands. Expressed mammary secretions tend to be sticky and discolored (either purulent or blood tinged). Clinical pathology reveals a leukocytosis with marked immature neutrophilia. Cytologic examination of the mammary secretions may reveal bacteria, white blood cells, and erythrocytes; whereas a Gram stain may improve antibiotic selection. Bacterial culture of mammary secretions typically yields *Staphylococcus* spp., *Streptococcus* spp., and *E. coli* as causal organisms. Milk white blood cell counts have been recommended in the past for diagnosing mastitis, but this test has not been reliable because cell counts tend to differ from bitch to bitch and within glands from the same bitch (Olson and Olson, 1984).

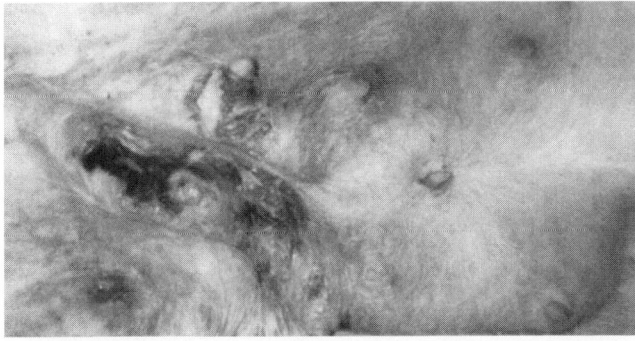

Fig. 216-1 This 5-year-old yellow Labrador retriever bitch was 2 weeks postpartum when the owner first noticed swelling in her left hind leg (note presence of dermatitis in the medial thigh). When examined in left lateral recumbency, both pairs of mammary glands (caudal abdominal and inguinal) are swollen and erythematous. In addition, the overlying skin is necrotic in multiple areas of necrosis with evidence of abscessation.

Until culture and sensitivity results are obtained, cefadroxil (22 mg/kg q12h PO) is recommended because it has broad-spectrum antibacterial activity and has not been observed to affect nursing pups (Bonagura, 2000). Pups should be allowed to nurse because nursing may speed resolution of the disease. However, if many glands are affected or the mother is severely ill, the pups should be hand raised. If the pups are weaned, cabergoline (Dostinex, Pharmacia & Upjohn) (5 mcg/kg SID PO for 5 days) may be useful to reduce lactation and prevent further bacterial extension. Warm compresses can be applied two to three times a day along with milking out the affected glands. In cases of abscessation or gangrenous mastitis (Fig. 216-1), surgical drainage and removal of the affected mammary gland may be necessary. In these cases there is a clear line of demarcation separating the healthy tissue from the gangrenous tissue.

PUERPERAL TETANY

Puerperal tetany, also known as postpartum hypocalcemia or eclampsia, generally develops less than 28 days after delivery but can occur during late pregnancy or during parturition. In the dog puerperal tetany occurs most commonly in small-breed bitches, less frequently in medium-sized bitches, and very rarely in large-breed bitches. Other than breed, predisposing factors include young age, large litter size in relation to body weight, and diet during pregnancy. Diets high in animal protein (egg or meat) or containing cereals with phytates, a compound that binds ionized calcium, making it biologically unavailable, have also been suggested to predispose to puerperal tetany.

Puerperal tetany occurs when there is an acute decrease in ionized calcium concentration. A reduction in calcium levels increases membrane permeability in nerve cells to sodium ions, causing increased frequency of spontaneous nervous activity noticeable as muscle fasciculations. Clinical signs are related not only to the absolute decrease in ionized calcium concentrations but also to the rate and progression of its decline. The onset of clinical signs is usually rapid, and the progression of signs is predictable. Early clinical signs in dogs and cats include restlessness, whining, panting, salivation, anorexia, vomiting, and behavioral changes. As the signs progress, muscle fasciculations, stiffness, ataxia, tonic-clonic muscle spasms, hyperthermia, tachycardia, seizures, and death may ensue. Ionized serum calcium concentrations less than 0.6 to 0.8 mmol/L are definitive for diagnosing puerperal tetany (Drobatz and Casey, 2000). If ionized calcium quantification is not available, total serum calcium measurements can be used, with concentrations less than 1.625 mmol/L highly indicative of puerperal tetany. Ionized calcium concentrations are typically 30% to 50% of total calcium concentrations; however, alkalosis resulting from hypersalivation may increase the protein-bound calcium fraction, resulting in a lower net decrease in ionized calcium levels (Biddle and Macintire, 2000). In addition to measuring calcium levels, a full serum chemistry evaluation is necessary because hypoglycemia and other electrolyte disturbances may develop concurrently with puerperal tetany.

Treatment for puerperal tetany is aimed at returning ionized calcium concentrations to normal values.

This is achieved by slow intravenous administration of 10% calcium gluconate (0.22 to 0.44 ml/kg) in combination with careful cardiac auscultation or electrocardiography. The development of bradycardia and other arrhythmias during intravenous calcium administration is indicative of too-rapid replacement. Full recovery or clinical cure occurs within minutes of the intravenous treatment. Judicious administration of intravenous fluids and anticonvulsants (diazepam 1 to 5 mg IV once) is indicated for treatment of hyperthermia and seizures. The pups should be removed from the dam and hand fed a milk supplement for 12 to 24 hours to prevent a relapse. If the litter is older than 4 weeks old, they should be weaned. Lactation may be suppressed using cabergoline (Dostinex, Pharmacia & Upjohn) (5 mcg/kg SID PO for 5 days). Oral supplementation with calcium carbonate (100 mg/kg q24h) and vitamin D (10,000 to 25,000 units q24h) is also recommended to prevent a relapse. Bitches may suffer from a puerperal tetany at the next whelping. However, bitches should not be supplemented with calcium during pregnancy since this increases the likelihood of developing puerperal tetany rather than preventing its recurrence.

References and Suggested Reading

Al-Bassam MA, Thomson RG, O'Donnell L: Involution abnormalities in the postpartum uterus of the bitch, *Vet Pathol* 18:208, 1981.

Beck AM, McEntee K: Subinvolution of placental sites in a postpartum bitch: a case report, *Cornell Vet* 56:269, 1966.

Biddle D, Macintire DK: Obstetrical emergencies, *Clin Tech Small Anim Pract* 15(2):88, 2000.

Bonagura JD, editor: *Kirk's current veterinary therapy XIII (small animal practice)*, Philadelphia, 2000, Saunders, p 933.

Dickie MB, Arbeiter K: Diagnosis and therapy of the subinvolution of placental sites in the bitch, *J Reprod Fertil* 47(suppl):471, 1993.

Drobatz KJ, Casey KK: Eclampsia in dogs: 31 cases (1995-1998), *J Am Vet Med Assoc* 217(2):216, 2000.

Durfee PT: Surgical treatment of postparturient metritis in the bitch, *J AmVet Med Assoc* 153(1):40, 1968.

Feldman EC, Nelson RW: Periparturient diseases. In Feldman EC, Nelson RW, editors: *Canine and feline endocrinology and reproduction*, ed 2, Philadelphia, 1996, Saunders, p 572.

Olson PN, Olson AL: Cytologic evaluation of canine milk, *Vet Med Small Anim Clin* 79:641, 1984.

Schall WD et al: Spontaneous recovery after subinvolution of placental sites in a bitch, *J Am Vet Med Assoc* 159(12):1780, 1971.

Smith FO: Postpartum diseases, *Vet Clin North Am Small Anim Pract* 16(3):521, 1986.

CHAPTER 217

Nutrition in the Bitch During Pregnancy and Lactation

DAVID A. DZANIS, *Santa Clarita, California*

Gestation and lactation place some of the most rigorous nutritional demands on the bitch, especially when compared to the adult, nonreproducing animal. This should not be surprising, since she is "eating for two" (or more). A dietary deficiency or excess in one or more nutrients during this life stage can have profound effects on the ability of the bitch to conceive, whelp, and raise a healthy litter.

Successful nutritional management of the bitch during pregnancy and lactation takes more than just recommending a particular brand of dog food. Rather, considering the nutrient needs of the individual animal, assessing the qualities of the ration in meeting those needs, and feeding the ration in an appropriate manner are all critical elements. The American College of Veterinary Nutrition has developed a graphic representation to help demonstrate these basic principles (Fig. 217-1).

DETERMINING NUTRIENT REQUIREMENTS

The nutrient of greatest increased demand during pregnancy and especially lactation is energy. Since daily caloric need of a given individual is also greatly influenced by body size, breed, age, activity, and environmental conditions, perhaps the best means of expressing energy needs for pregnancy and lactation is as a proportion of the normal energy requirements of the same animal at maintenance. However, to do that one must first know what the bitch's energy needs are at maintenance.

A number of equations are used to determine maintenance energy requirements of the dog, but perhaps the most widely accepted equation is:

$$\text{Metabolizable energy (ME) (kilocalories per day)}$$
$$= 132 \times (\text{body weight in kilograms})^{0.75}$$
$$(\textit{National Research Council [NRC], 1985})$$

Although equations are available that do not rely on an exponent and thus are easier to calculate, determination of metabolic body weight by this method better accounts for the great diversity in adult body size in dogs. The constant (132) in the formula was determined in dogs under laboratory conditions; thus it assumes the dog to be at a moderate activity level and in environmentally favorable conditions during most of the day. Actual maintenance requirements of a given individual may vary up to 30% either way. A mostly indoor, sedentary house pet requires less to maintain body weight, whereas an outdoor kenneled dog needs more. Breed and body size are also factors. For example, the equation coefficient may vary from 94 for a large-sized pet dog to 175 for a highly active pet Border collie (NRC, 2006).

Because of the potentially large variation in caloric requirements, perhaps a more practical means of determining needs of an individual is simply to monitor the amount of a given food (and number of calories that amount of food delivers) needed to keep the animal in optimum body condition during prebreeding. During gestation and lactation the amount of the same food can then be adjusted by the appropriate proportion. If a more calorie-dense food is fed during these periods, the proportional increase would be modified relative to the calorie content of the old and new diets.

Regardless of the actual maintenance needs, the energy requirements for early and midgestation are approximately the same as those for maintenance (Fig. 217-2). This is because, although the fetuses are developing rapidly, they remain relatively small. Only in the last few weeks of gestation are additional calories needed for growth of the puppies and maternal tissues. Depending on the number of fetuses, total weight gain by the time of parturition should be around 15% to 25% (Case et al., 2000; Debraekeleer, Gross, and Zicker, 2000). At this time the bitch likely is consuming approximately 150% of her normal maintenance needs. Expressed differently, the increase in energy requirements above maintenance from the fourth week after mating until whelping is approximately 26 kcal of ME per kilogram of body weight per day (NRC, 2006).

Dramatic increases in energy needs are seen after the first week of lactation, even though the bitch may be approaching or even falling below her prebreeding body weight after whelping. Increased energy is needed to meet the monumental nutritional demands of milk production for the ever-growing offspring. The calorie requirement of a given individual depends on the amount of milk production, which in turn is correlated with the number of puppies. For litters of one to four puppies, milk production can be estimated at 1% of the bitch's body weight per pup, which increases the bitch's energy requirement by 24 kcal of ME per kilogram of body weight per day for each puppy in the litter (NRC, 2006). For litters larger than four, milk production and caloric needs per additional pup are approximately half of these values, and the increase in milk yield as litters exceed eight pups is negligible. Put more simply, in a bitch in peak lactation (4 weeks after whelping) with a moderate-to-large litter, energy needs three times the normal maintenance requirements

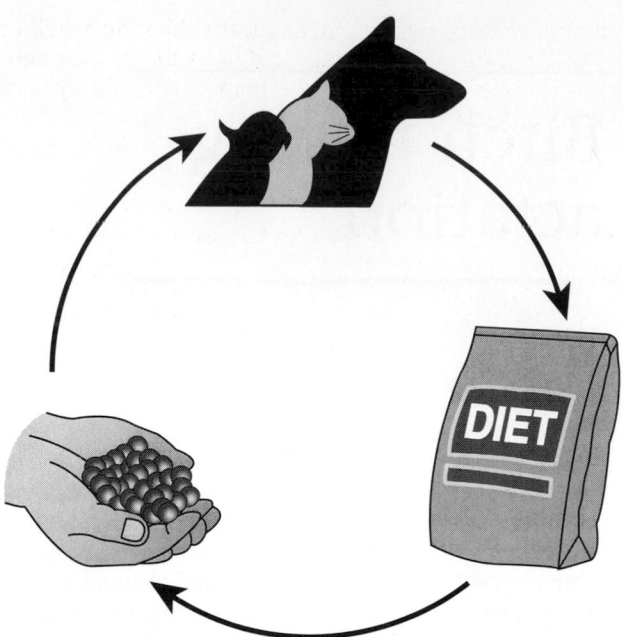

Fig. 217-1 The American College of Veterinary Nutrition Iterative Process of Nutritional Assessment requires consideration of the animal, the ration, and the feeding management (Courtesy American College of Veterinary Nutrition.)

would not be surprising. As the puppies are weaned and milk production declines, the calorie needs for lactation drop, and more energy can be directed toward reestablishing normal body weight.

In addition to calories, the needs for most other essential nutrients increase during this life stage. For example, more protein, calcium, and phosphorus are needed for proper growth and bone development of the puppies. Added intake of dietary salt also is required for normal milk production. The Association of American Feed Control Officials (AAFCO) Dog Food Nutrient Profiles indicate for which nutrients there are increased dietary needs above maintenance of the reproducing bitch (see Appendix III). Absence of an established difference in the profiles between growth/reproduction and maintenance reflects the lack of data showing a decreased need in the adult at maintenance. Also, although the amount in the diet may appear to remain the same, the actual daily intake of a given nutrient is higher because of increased food intake.

One recent recommendation by the NRC that has not been incorporated into the AAFCO Dog Food Nutrient Profiles to date is for dietary ω-3 fatty acids, specifically of α-linolenic acid (ALA) and eicosapentaenoic acid (EPA) and docosahexaenoic acid (DHA) in combination. Although dietary essentiality of these fatty acids has not been established definitively, small amounts in the diet of the bitch may be helpful in normal brain and retinal development of pups, perhaps in utero but more likely via the milk during the early neonatal period. The NRC-recommended allowance for ALA and for EPA and DHA in combination in foods for dogs in gestation and lactation is 0.08% and 0.05% dry matter, or 0.2 and 0.13 g/1000 kcal ME, respectively (NRC, 2006). Notwithstanding the lack of similar recommendations in the AAFCO Profiles, no apparent developmental abnormalities caused by ω-3 fatty acid deficiencies have been reported to date for any commercial dog food.

Eclampsia, a condition characterized by periparturient hypocalcemia in the bitch (especially during early lactation), would at first thought imply that dietary calcium requirements of late gestation have not been met, such that further supplementation is indicated. Although definitive studies on the prevention of this condition in dogs are lacking, a lesson may be drawn from what is known about milk fever, a similar condition in dairy cows. Contrary to intuition, the calcium needs of the growing fetus are relatively low, and a high dietary

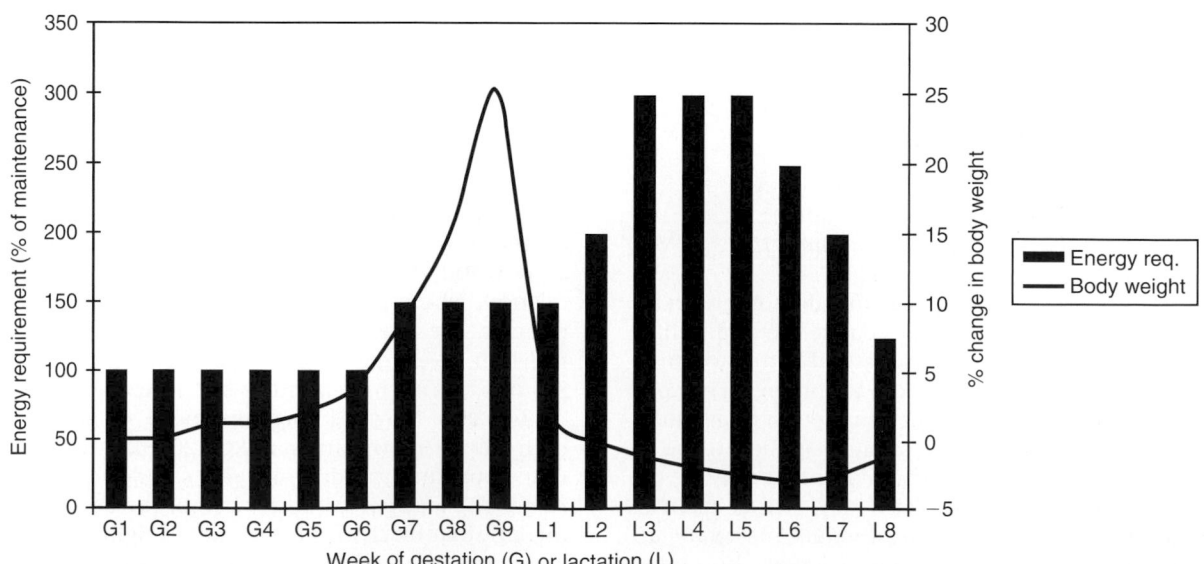

Fig. 217-2 Energy needs and expected body weight changes of the bitch during gestation and lactation. (Modified from Case et al., 2000; Debraekeleer, Gross, and Zicker, 2000.)

calcium intake during gestation initiates responses to suppress calcium intestinal absorption and bone and kidney resorption in the mother. Then, when lactation ensues, the dramatic loss of calcium into the milk cannot be countered by normal metabolic responses, and the animal cannot maintain normocalcemia regardless of dietary intake of calcium at that stage. On the other hand, a low calcium intake in cattle helps ensure that bone calcium remains relatively mobile and responsive to the sudden demands of lactation. However, the syndromes in dogs and cows are different, and data are lacking to indicate that a low-calcium diet in late gestation is an effective preventive in dogs. However, it does suggest that calcium supplementation beyond that already provided in a balanced diet is imprudent at best (Case et al., 2000; Debraekeleer, Gross, and Zicker, 2000).

Although carbohydrates are not recognized as essential nutrients in the dog, some authors recommend that the diet contain a carbohydrate source (Debraekeleer, Gross, and Zicker, 2000) to mitigate the slight risk of periparturient hypoglycemia in the bitch, ensure ample glucose for the developing fetuses, and help maintain lactose levels in the milk. Except for some exclusive canned and frozen pet food products (e.g., "all beef"), most dog foods (and all dry or semi-moist foods) should contain an ample source of carbohydrates.

CHOOSING THE APPROPRIATE FOOD

An abundance of high-quality, nutritionally "complete, and balanced" commercial foods are available for feeding bitches in gestation and lactation. The flavor, form (dry versus canned), and presence or absence of a particular ingredient are not as important as the product's substantiation of nutritional adequacy. To ensure that the product is suitable to be fed as the sole source of nutrition, the information panel on the label should bear either of the following: "(Product Name) is formulated to meet the nutritional levels established by the AAFCO Dog Food Nutrient Profiles," or "Animal feeding tests following AAFCO procedures substantiate that (Product Name) provides complete and balanced nutrition." If it bears the statement that it is intended "for intermittent or supplemental feeding only," bears reference to AAFCO in a manner other than either of the previous statements, refers to an organization other than AAFCO, or bears no nutritional adequacy statement, the product should not be presumed to be nutritionally sufficient.

The first AAFCO nutritional substantiation method requires that the product contain adequate but not excessive quantities of all recognized essential nutrients compared to the AAFCO Profiles, such as amino acids, calcium, and vitamin A. These levels were established using the results of scientific studies demonstrating adequacy of a given nutrient and then adding adjustment factors to allow for differences in bioavailability of nutrients in commonly used ingredients. For the feeding trial method, a specified number of bitches must be fed the product as the sole source of nutrition (except water) from breeding through peak lactation (4 weeks after whelping). Performance is judged on acceptable maintenance of body weight compared to prebreeding, normal

hematologic and serum biochemical values, and lack of any other clinical or pathologic sign of nutritional deficiency or excess. In addition, litter size, survivability, and weight of the puppies at the end of the trial must compare favorably to animals fed a ration previously shown to be nutritionally complete and balanced.

Both the profile method and the feeding trial method have their advantages and disadvantages, and neither is perfect (Dzanis, 2003). Overall the feeding trial method is the preferred choice of substantiation. However, under current AAFCO Model Pet Food Regulations for a "product family," a pet food deemed to be "nutritionally similar" to a tested product can bear a statement suggesting completion of animal feeding tests, even though the food actually never underwent the feeding trial. This may be particularly troublesome in light of the fact that products substantiated under the product family criteria share the disadvantages of both the profile and the feeding trial methods and hence offer the least assurance of nutritional adequacy. Some product family member labels may bear a statement that accurately reflects the fact that the product is "nutritionally similar" to a tested product; but, because of a provision in the regulations, most circumvent this statement. Rather most product family members bear the same statement allowed on the tested "lead member" products. Thus it may be impossible for the veterinarian or pet owner to know whether the particular food was tested or not solely on the basis of labeling.

The good news is that the majority of products bearing the "animal feeding tests" label statements also are formulated to meet the AAFCO Profiles but simply do not allude to that fact on the label. On the other hand, a product bearing the AAFCO Profile statement most probably has not been subject to a feeding trial. Because each method has its pros and cons, the best assurance of nutritional adequacy is if the product meets *both* criteria. If there is a question about a specific product, the manufacturer's representative should be able to attest to and document its product family status and whether the feeding-tested product also meets the AAFCO Profiles.

Another component of the nutritional adequacy statement is that it be suitable for the intended life stage. Few if any labels bear reference to nutritional adequacy for female reproduction. Rather most cite suitability for "all life stages," which includes the rigorous demands of gestation and lactation. It must also be noted that not all intended uses of the product may be evident from the front panel designation. Many of the higher-end "adult" foods may in fact be suitable for all life stages, as would be indicated on the information panel. This is often done to distinguish the product from the manufacturer's "puppy" product, which is generally a bit higher in nutrient density than the adult formula. Regardless, both have been held up to the same nutritional criteria; and, although relatively more of the adult formula may need to be fed compared to the growth formula, both should perform as expected. In some cases the all–life stage "adult" formula may be more appropriate for the bitch with a propensity for excessive weight gain.

For clients who prefer to offer a raw or other home-formulated food rather than a commercial food, it must be noted that there are no regulatory requirements that a given recipe from books, Internet websites, or elsewhere be "complete and balanced." Although testimonials or other assurances of the suitability of a given home formulation may abound, it is highly prudent to seek the advice of a board-certified veterinary nutritionist or other professional sufficiently trained to scientifically evaluate the nutritional content of the proposed diet. Also, recipes in which ingredients are not cooked may present an increased risk of harboring potentially pathogenic organisms. To mitigate the possible risk to both animal and human health, appropriate handling and sanitary measures need to be followed.

FEEDING MANAGEMENT

Feeding management of the reproducing bitch should begin well before breeding. Difficulties in conception, parturition, and successful rearing of healthy pups may occur in a bitch that is either underconditioned or overweight. Strategies to bring the bitch to optimum weight should begin many months before expected breeding. By the time of mating, the bitch should be at a stable, if not ascending, plane of nutrition. By no means should success be assumed if the animal is on a weight loss diet at the time of breeding.

Under AAFCO Model Pet Food Regulations, feeding directions are required on all "complete and balanced" product labels, although the ranges of recommended feeding amounts are often too broad to be useful. Also, foods designated just for adult use may not have directions for the pregnant or lactating bitch. A preferred method to determine amounts to be fed is by calculating the energy needs of the animal as described previously and then comparing them to the calorie content of the diet. Voluntary calorie content label statements are allowed; but, except as required for "lite" or "less calories" products intended for weight loss, these statements rarely appear on the label. If stated, the energy content must be expressed in terms of kilocalories per kilogram of food as fed. More consumer-friendly units (e.g., kilocalories per cup or can) also may be given. If the latter information is not provided, measuring the number of cups in a known weight of food such as a 20-pound bag usually gives a more accurate estimate than trying to precisely weigh a single cup of product.

In 2005 the American College of Veterinary Nutrition proposed an amendment to the AAFCO regulations to require calorie content statements on all dog and cat food labels and to require these statements both in terms of kilocalories of ME per kilogram and kilocalories of ME per cup or can. This proposal has not been adopted by AAFCO to date. Until and unless this proposal is passed, alternative methods of determining calorie content may be necessary. If the label calorie content information is absent or incomplete, the manufacturer's representative may be able to provide that information. Alternatively calorie content can be estimated from the guaranteed analysis values using the following formula:

$$ME \text{ (kcal/kg as fed)} = ((3.5 \times CP) + (8.5 \times CF) + (3.5 \times NFE)) \times 10$$

where CP = percentage of crude protein, CF = percentage of crude fat, and NFE = percentage of nitrogen-free extract (carbohydrate), which is 100 minus the sum of percentages for crude protein, crude fat, crude fiber, moisture, and ash (AAFCO, 2007). This formula tends to overestimate the true calorie content of high-fiber or poor-quality foods and underestimate that of very digestible products (NRC, 2006). A reportedly more accurate, albeit more complicated, calculation of ME has been suggested:

$$\text{Gross Energy (GE)} = (5.7 \times CP) + (9.4 \times CF) + (4.1 \times (NFE + \% \text{ crude fiber}))$$

$$\text{Percentage energy digestibility (PED)} = 91.2 - (1.43 \times (\% \text{ crude fiber/proportion dry matter}))$$

$$\text{Digestible energy (DE)} = GE \times PED/100$$

$$ME = (DE - (1.04 \times CP)) \times 10 \text{ (NRC, 2006)}$$

An example of estimation of ME using both methods on the same guaranteed analysis values is found in Fig. 217-3. The NRC method does yield a higher estimate for this relatively higher-fat, lower-fiber example. As an alternative to using the NRC method, substitution of the coefficients for CP, CF, and NFE with the values 4, 9 and 4, respectively, in the previous AAFCO formula may yield more accurate results when estimating the calorie content of a higher-quality diet. Regardless, the AAFCO formula is still a good means of comparing energy content among products. Since this formula calculates energy on an as-fed basis, further conversion to dry matter (i.e., the derived value divided by the proportion of the non-moisture component of the diet) is necessary to compare among products of very different moisture contents such as a dry versus a canned or semi-moist product.

Regardless of feeding directions or previous estimates of energy needs, an individual animal may vary greatly in its true requirements. Thus careful monitoring of both body weight and body condition score, with adjustment in intake as needed to maintain optimum condition, is warranted.

No change in food, feeding amount, or frequency is usually indicated the first two thirds of gestation. A temporary drop in voluntary food consumption may be observed during estrus and in midgestation, but this is normal and does not indicate a need for adjusting the feeding management as long as body weight and condition are acceptable. Beginning about 3 weeks before expected whelping, a gradual increase in nutrient intake should be initiated. This can be done simply by increasing the amount of food offered or by switching to a more calorie-dense food. The frequency of feeding may need to be increased to accommodate the increased intake. By time of parturition, a calorie intake approximately 50% above prebreeding needs should be anticipated.

As the bitch enters peak lactation, caloric requirements may triple. If not already switched during gestation, switching the diet to a more energy-dense product generally is indicated. Offering food free choice may be necessary for the bitch to be able to consume adequate quantities throughout the day. Some degree of weight loss

Guaranteed analysis:

Crude protein	28%
Crude fat	16%
Crude fiber	3%
Moisture	10%
Ash	5%

62% Nitrogen-free extract (NFE) = 100% − 62% = 38%

Proportion dry matter = (100% − 10%)/100% = 0.9

AAFCO Method

$28 \times 3.5 = 98$
$16 \times 8.5 = 136$
$38 \times 3.5 = \underline{133}$
Total   367

Calorie content = 367 × 10 = 3670 kcal ME/kg as fed
           = 3670/0.9 = 4078 kcal ME/kg dry matter

NRC Method

$28 \times 5.7 = 159.6$
$16 \times 9.4 = 150.4$
$41 \times 4.1 = \underline{168.1}$
Total   478.1

$91.2 - (1.43 \times 3/0.9) = 86.4$
$478.1 \times 86.4/100 = 413$
$413 - (1.04 \times 28) = 384$

Calorie content = 384 × 10 = 3840 kcal ME/kg as fed
           = 3840/0.9 = 4267 kcal ME/kg dry matter

Fig. 217-3 Example of estimating calorie content from label guaranteed analysis values using Association of American Feed Control Officials and National Research Council formulas.

compared to prebreeding may be anticipated; but, if body weight drops more than a few percent below weight at maintenance, a more calorie-dense food should be offered. As the puppies are weaned and the bitch regains any lost weight, the amounts offered can be cut back slowly so that she is near normal food intake and body weight by the time milk production has ceased.

Assuming that the appropriate food is selected as discussed previously, no dietary supplementation should be necessary. At best supplements may do no harm, but injudicious use may create nutrient excesses. The example of calcium is given earlier. However, even something as simple as added fat to increase total caloric intake may be detrimental if it suppresses intake of the mainstay diet since it decreases intake of all other essential nutrients.

References and Suggested Reading

Association of American Feed Control Officials: *Official publication*, Oxford, Ind, 2007, AAFCO.

Case LP et al: *Canine and feline nutrition*, ed 2, St Louis, 2000, Mosby.

Debraekeleer J, Gross KL, Zicker SC: Normal dogs. In Hand MS et al, editors: *Small animal clinical nutrition*, ed 4, Topeka, Kan, 2000, Mark Morris Institute, p 214.

Dzanis DA: Ensuring nutritional adequacy. In Kvamme JL, Phillips TD, editors: *Pet food technology*, Mt. Morris, ILL, 2003, Watt Publishing, p 62.

National Research Council: *Nutrient requirements of dog.* Washington, DC, 1985, National Academy Press.

National Research Council: *Nutrient requirements of dogs and cats*, Washington, DC, 2006, National Academies Press.

CHAPTER 218

Pyometra

FRANCES O. SMITH, *Burnsville, Minnesota*

Pyometra is a disease of the uterus, literally meaning *pus in the uterus*. Similar clinical entities include mucometra and hydrometra. Pyometra typically occurs in the estrogen-primed uterus during the period of progesterone dominance (diestrus) or thereafter (anestrus). It is most commonly diagnosed in an intact bitch from 4 weeks to 4 months following an estrous cycle. Many studies highlight an increased incidence of pyometra in nulliparous bitches and in bitches over 4 years of age. Pregnancy has a sparing effect on the uterus. There is no correlation between clinical signs of false pregnancy and pyometra in the bitch.

PATHOGENESIS

In one colony of beagles the incidence of pyometra was 15.2% of bitches older than 4 years of age, with the average age of onset 9.36 ± 0.35 years (Fakuda, 2001). In a population of insured dogs in Sweden in which routine ovariohysterectomy is disallowed, the crude 12-month incidence of pyometra over the 2-year period from 1995 through 1996 was approximately 2% in bitches under 10 years of age (Egenvall et al., 2001).

The pathogenesis of pyometra in the bitch involves estrogen stimulation followed by prolonged periods of progesterone dominance. Progesterone results in endometrial proliferation, glandular secretions, and decreased myometrial contractions. Leukocyte inhibition in the progesterone-primed uterus tends to support bacterial growth. These effects are cumulative with each estrous cycle, exacerbating the uterine pathology. Dow (1957) described four stages of cystic endometrial hyperplasia (CEH) pyometra. Type one is uncomplicated CEH; type two is CEH with infiltration of plasma cells. Type three is CEH with acute endometritis. Finally, type four is CEH with chronic endometritis.

Estrogen therapy is associated with an increased risk of pyometra in bitches from 1 to 4 years of age (Chastain, Panciera, and Waters, 1999). Use of estrogens (estradiol cypionate) for mismating in diestrous bitches is particularly dangerous and has resulted in approximately a 25% occurrence rate of pyometra (Bowen et al., 1985). Furthermore, use of estrogens in the bitch has a potential for idiosyncratic, nondose-related bone marrow suppression. The one (and only) time I used estradiol cypionate for mismating in an 18-month old golden retriever resulted in an open-cervix pyometra.

There is an increased risk for pyometra in several breeds, including the golden retriever, miniature schnauzer, Irish terrier, Saint Bernard, Airedale terrier, cavalier King Charles spaniel, rough collie, rottweiler, and Bernese mountain dog (Chastain, Panciera, and Waters, 1999; Egenvall et al., 2001).

CLINICAL FINDINGS

The medical history of a female dog with pyometra can be nonspecific. In older bitches the client may not recognize an estrous cycle and assume that the bitch has experienced "menopause." The client may also mistake a serosanguineous vaginal discharge associated with pyometra with that of a normal estrus. Vaginal cytology assists in differentiating the prevailing hormonal events at the time of initial examination. Clinical history of bitches with pyometra often includes depression, inappetence, polydipsia, polyuria, lethargy, and abdominal enlargement—with or without vaginal discharge. Pyometra should always be in the differential diagnosis of a sick, intact bitch.

Bitches with pyometra typically are afebrile. An elevated white blood count is typical, and hyperproteinemia and hyperglobulinemia also are common. Prerenal azotemia accompanies dehydration, but urine-concentrating ability may be impaired. Cystocentesis is associated with the risk of perforation of the fluid-filled uterus and possible spillage of uterine contents into the abdomen. The most common organism isolated from the uterus or vaginal discharge of a bitch with pyometra is *Escherichia coli*. Culture and sensitivity of the vaginal discharge or of intrauterine fluid at the time of ovariohysterectomy should be performed to guide antibiotic therapy.

The vaginal discharge in the CEH/pyometra complex may be purulent, sanguinopurulent (tomato soup), mucoid, or frankly hemorrhagic (Troxel et al., 2002). Vaginal discharge of any description should alert the clinician to include pyometra in the differential diagnosis. Other causes of vaginal discharge include vaginitis, estrus, immune-mediated thrombocytopenia (bloody discharge), anticoagulant toxicity, metritis, and subinvolution of placental sites.

Diagnosis is best accomplished with ultrasonography and/or radiography. The classic radiographic finding is a fluid-filled, tubular organ between the descending colon, which presents a sausagelike appearance. The uterus is best visualized with a lateral abdominal radiograph. Ultrasonographically a fluid-filled organ can again be identified, and uterine wall thickness and proliferative changes noted as well.

THERAPY

The treatment of choice for any aged or ill bitch or for a bitch with closed-cervix pyometra is complete ovariohysterectomy. Medical treatment of bitches with closed-cervix pyometra may result in uterine rupture or in seepage of uterine contents into the abdomen. I do not advocate the use of medical management for any bitch with a closed-cervix pyometra. Bitches that are seriously ill should be stabilized medically with appropriate intravenous fluid therapy and broad-spectrum antibiotics before surgery. The clinician should be prepared to deal with bacteremia and endotoxemia. Disseminated intravascular coagulation is an infrequent but possible complication of pyometra.

Young bitches with breeding value and an open cervix, normal organ function, together with a compliant and reasonable owner, may be treated with prostaglandins. Prostaglandins increase myometrial contractility, encourage cervical relaxation, allow expulsion of the uterine contents, and with repeated doses result in lysis of the corpus luteum. Serum progesterone should be measured before treatment with prostaglandins.

The most frequently administered drug is prostaglandin $F_2\alpha$ ($PGF_2\alpha$) at a dose of 250 mcg/kg every 12 hours subcutaneously until the uterus reduces to near normal in size, which typically takes 3 to 5 days. Therapy that requires a longer treatment period or a recurrence of fluid in the uterus signals a negative prognosis for prostaglandin treatment success. A vaginal culture should be obtained before treatment, and appropriate antibiotics administered for 3 to 4 weeks following therapy. Prostaglandins are not approved for small animal usage in the United States; thus an informed-consent form, including risks of treatment, should be obtained before therapy. Many other protocols have been published, starting with doses of $PGF_2\alpha$ as low as 50 mcg/kg and gradually increasing to 250 mcg/kg over the treatment period to decrease the side effects of panting, nausea, salivation, vomiting, and diarrhea—all of which are commonly seen 15 to 45 minutes after each injection. One study described the use of $PGF_2\alpha$ (150 mcg/kg) in 17 bitches with pyometra administered by infusing 0.3 ml/10 kg of body weight into the vaginal canal one or two times daily for 4 to 12 days. Bitches received intramuscular antibiotics as well as the intravaginal infusion. Treatment was effective in 86.6% of these bitches (Gabor, Siver, and Szenci, 1999). It has been noted that cloprostenol, a prostaglandin analog, has been used successfully for treatment of open-cervix pyometra (Johnston, Kustritz, and Olson, 2001). However, I do not use cloprostenol because it is far more potent and

has great potential for accidental overdosage. Also of note are the antiprogestins RU46534 and aglipristone, which have been used to treat open-cervix pyometra in Europe (Johnston, Kustritz, and Olson, 2001). These antiprogestins are not available in the United States. In my opinion, prostaglandins should *never* be dispensed for client administration because of the narrow safety index and the potential for triggering asthmatic events and pregnancy loss in humans.

Bitches treated with prostaglandins may have their interestral interval shortened slightly. The bitch should have a vaginal culture, be treated with appropriate antibiotics, and be bred to a fertile male at her next estrous cycle. Success results in conception rates of 50% to 65%. Fertility in bitches after pyometra therapy is decreased when compared to normal bitches. Failure to conceive or failure to be bred results in a high incidence of recurrence of pyometra, with recurrence rates as high as 77%. I have observed pyometra in subsequent generations of both chow-chows and English setters of young age, suggesting that there may be a familial tendency toward early development of CEH in these animals.

References and Suggested Reading

Bowen RA et al: Efficacy and toxicity of estrogens commonly used to terminate canine pregnancy, *J Am Vet Med Assoc* 186:783, 1985.

Chastain CB, Panciera D, Waters C: Associations between age, parity, hormonal therapy and breed, and pyometra in Finnish dogs, *Small Anim Clin Endocrinol* 9(2):18, 1999.

Dow C: The cystic hyperplasia-pyometra complex in the bitch, *Vet Rec* 69:1409, 1957.

Egenvall A, Hagman R, Bonnett B et al: Breed risk of pyometra in insured dogs in Sweden, *J Vet Intern Med* 15[6]:530, 2001.

Fakuda S: Incidence of pyometra in colony-raised beagle dogs, *Exp Anim* 50(4):325, 2001.

Gabor G, Siver L, Szenci O: Intravaginal prostaglandin F2 alpha for the treatment of metritis and pyometra in the bitch, *Acta Vet Hung* 47(1):103, 1999.

Johnston SD, Kustritz MVR, Olson PNS: Disorders of the canine uterus and uterine tubes (oviducts). In Johnston SD, Kustritz MVR, Olson PNS: *Canine and feline theriogenology*, Philadelphia, 2001, Saunders, p 219.

Troxel M et al: Severe hematometra in a dog with cystic endometrial hyperplasia/pyometra complex, *J Am Anim Hosp Assoc* 38:85, 2002.

CHAPTER 219

Vaginitis

MARGARET V. ROOT KUSTRITZ, *St. Paul, Minnesota*

Vaginitis is inflammation of the vaginal epithelium. This term is clinically inclusive of inflammation within the vaginal vault, around the urethral papilla, or in the clitoral fossa. Reported incidence of canine vaginitis is 0.7%. Vaginitis is not a clinical entity in cats.

Inflammation of the vaginal mucosa is not caused by primary bacterial infection. A primary cause of vaginal inflammation allows colonization of normal vaginal flora. The most common conditions reported to cause primary vaginal inflammation are chronic urinary tract infection and presence of vaginal anatomic anomalies. The mechanisms responsible for vaginitis secondary to vaginal anomalies include pooling of urine in the vagina and urine scald of the vaginal mucosa.

Two clinical forms of vaginitis occur. Juvenile or "puppy" vaginitis occurs in bitches before their first estrus. These young dogs present with a small amount of clear, sticky, odorless vulvar discharge that often is found incidentally at the time of physical examination before vaccination. Most bitches exhibit no clinical signs; the occasional bitch has excessive vulvar discharge and behaviors indicative of vaginal irritation such as licking of the vulva, scooting the hindquarters on the ground, or pollakiuria.

Adult-onset vaginitis may occur in spayed or intact adult female dogs but most commonly is seen in spayed bitches, perhaps because there are more spayed bitches in the North American population. These dogs present with a history of vulvar discharge varying in amount and character from scant and mucoid to copious and purulent. The vaginal discharge of vaginitis rarely is blood tinged or frankly hemorrhagic. Often these dogs exhibit other signs of disease such as licking of the vulva and positional urinary incontinence. Vaginitis and vulvar licking can occur with related conditions such as perivulvar dermatitis and atopy; clinical signs of these disorders also may be present.

On physical examination vulvar discharge may be evident in the vulvar cleft or dried and adhered to the perivulvar hair. The vulva may be swollen, and the clitoris hypertrophied if the dog has been licking at the area excessively. Some prepuberal or spayed dogs have an infantile vulva that is tucked up well within the perivulvar folds; these dogs also may have urinary incontinence, especially if they are overweight. Physical examination may reveal evidence of concurrent disease such as atopy.

To diagnose vaginitis, inflammation of the vaginal mucosa must be identified. The source of any vulvar discharge should be localized to the urinary tract, vagina, uterus (intact dogs), or uterine stump (spayed dogs). Digital vaginal examination and vaginoscopy can be used to identify the presence of vaginal anatomic anomalies and to investigate for unusual underlying causes of inflammation such as foreign objects or vaginal masses. A vaginal cytology specimen should be collected and evaluated for cornification. Presence of cornified cells in a spayed bitch indicates that estrogen-secreting tissue is present; this dog should be evaluated further for ovarian remnant syndrome (Box 219-1).

Treatment of canine vaginitis requires identification and correction of any underlying causes of inflammation and symptomatic therapy if an underlying cause cannot be identified. Key questions that should be addressed in all cases include:

- Is the dog prepuberal?
- Is the dog postpuberal or spayed?
- Is the dog symptomatic?
- Is the dog asymptomatic?

No treatment is required for the dog with juvenile vaginitis with manifestations of disease beyond the presence of slight vulvar discharge. Empiric short-term therapy with a broad-spectrum antibiotic may be beneficial in some cases. A common antibiotic choice is amoxicillin-clavulanate (Clavamox [Pfizer Animal Health], 14 mg/kg twice daily orally [PO] for 14 days). Prepuberal bitches may benefit from estrous cycling as well since exposure to endogenous estrogen thickens the vaginal epithelium and allows enhanced movement of white blood cells into the vagina. The bitch's immune system may mature in that time as well. Anecdotal reports suggest that topical therapy of the perivulvar area and vulvar mucosa with antibiotic ointment may decrease vulvar licking and self-trauma. The majority of dogs with juvenile vaginitis undergo spontaneous resolution of the condition within months of diagnosis.

No treatment is required for the dog with adult-onset vaginitis showing no signs beyond the presence of slight vulvar discharge. A complete diagnostic workup should be performed before instituting antibiotic therapy. If urinary tract infection is present, the urine should be cultured and treated with an appropriate antibiotic. If a vaginal anomaly, secondary urine pooling, or a vaginal mass is present, surgical repair should be considered. Episioplasty (vulvoplasty) is appropriate treatment for dogs with concurrent vaginitis and perivulvar dermatitis and also may be beneficial for treatment of idiopathic adult-onset vaginitis. Medical therapy for idiopathic adult-onset vaginitis is symptomatic. It should be treated with an appropriate antibiotic based on culture and sensitivity testing for 1 month. If quantitative aerobic vaginal culture is not significant, empiric short-term therapy with a broad-spectrum antibiotic may be beneficial. A common

Box 219-1

Scheme for Diagnosis of Canine Vaginitis

I. Verify inflammation of the vagina, vestibule, or clitoral fossa by vaginoscopy. An otoscope makes an adequate vaginoscope in practice. Also assess for presence of a vaginal anatomic anomaly, foreign object, or mass.

II. Localize the site of vulvar discharge.

A. Urinary tract
1. Urinalysis and urine culture on sample collected by cystocentesis

B. Uterus or uterine stump
1. Abdominal palpation
2. Abdominal radiographs and/or ultrasound

C. Vagina
1. Vaginal cytology
   a. Cornified: normal estrus? ovarian remnant?
   b. Noncornified: normal for bitch not in estrus and for spayed bitch
2. Quantitative aerobic vaginal culture; moderate-to-heavy growth of any single organism is significant; organisms most commonly identified are those of the normal vaginal flora (*Escherichia coli, Staphylococcus* spp., *Streptococcus* spp., *Proteus mirabilis*); sensitivity testing should be used to guide antibiotic therapy
3. Vaginoscopy

antibiotic choice is amoxicillin-clavulanate (14 mg/kg twice daily PO for 14 days). Some dogs require long-term, low-dose antibiotic therapy, as might be used for dogs with chronic cystitis. Concurrent therapy with diethylstilbestrol (1 mg once daily PO for 5 days and then 1 mg every 3 to 4 days PO for 1 month), phenylpropanolamine (1.5 to 2 mg/kg PO twice daily), or prednisone (decreasing dose over 2 to 3 weeks) may be of benefit to some dogs. Prednisone should not be administered to bitches with urinary incontinence. Treatment with testosterone also may hasten resolution of clinical signs. Vaginal douches never have been demonstrated to be of benefit because of the unusual angulation and extreme length of the canine vagina. Anecdotal reports suggest that topical therapy of the perivulvar area and vulvar mucosa with antibiotic ointment may decrease vulvar licking and self-trauma.

References and Suggested Reading

Hammel SP, Bjorling DE: Results of vulvoplasty for treatment of recessed vulva in dogs, *J Am Anim Hosp Assoc* 38:79, 2002.

Hirsh DC, Wiger N: The bacterial flora of the normal canine vagina compared with that of vaginal exudates, *J Small Anim Pract* 18:25, 1977.

Johnson CA: Diagnosis and treatment of chronic vaginitis in the bitch, *Vet Clin North Am: Small Anim Pract* 21:523, 1991.

Kyles AE et al: Vestibulovaginal stenosis in dogs: 18 cases (1987-1995), *J Am Vet Med Assoc* 209:1889, 1996.

Parker NA: Clinical approach to canine vaginitis: a review. Proceedings of the Annual Meeting of the Society for Theriogenology, Baltimore, Md, 1998, p 112.

Root MV, Johnston SD, Johnston GR: Vaginal septa in dogs: 15 cases (1983-1992), *J Am Vet Med Assoc* 206:56, 1995.

CHAPTER 220

Surgical Repair of Vaginal Anomalies in the Bitch

ROBERTO E. NOVO, *St. Paul, Minnesota*

A number of developmental and acquired conditions affect the canine vagina and vulva. Congenital conditions, which primarily affect younger dogs, include rectovaginal fistula; vulvar/vaginal hypoplasia; anovulvar cleft; clitoral enlargement; and vaginal septa, bands, or strictures. Acquired conditions generally affect older dogs and include vaginal neoplasia and vaginal prolapse. Some acquired conditions such as vaginal hyperplasia and perivulvar dermatitis can affect younger dogs. Invariably there is some overlap between congenital and acquired abnormalities because some acquired problems may develop secondary to abnormal anatomy of the reproductive tract. Surgery to correct these abnormalities often corrects the presenting clinical signs. These procedures may be as simple as digital breakdown of a thin vaginal band or more complex (e.g., complete vaginal ablation).

SURGICAL APPROACHES TO THE CANINE VAGINA

Most surgical procedures of the vagina (and vestibule) can be approached via a caudal episiotomy. More involved procedures may require a ventral approach, which necessitates a pubic osteotomy. With either surgical approach, strong consideration should be given to management of postoperative pain. The use of a fentanyl patch or epidural analgesia should be considered before surgery. An appropriately sized fentanyl patch (4 mcg/kg/hour in dogs) should be applied the day before surgery. Alternatively, an epidural with the use of morphine (0.1 mg/kg), bupivacaine (1 mg/kg), or a combination of both can be administered before or immediately after surgery. If epidural analgesia is elected, the surgeon should review the various techniques and dosing guidelines described in the veterinary literature.

Caudal Approach (Episiotomy)

When performing an episiotomy, the animal is placed in sternal recumbency with the pelvic limbs hanging over the end of the table. The edges of the table should be well padded to avoid trauma to the limbs. The table is tilted so the animal's head is down about 30 degrees and the vulva is at a comfortable working height. This head-down position may make ventilation of the patient more difficult, requiring assisted manual or mechanical ventilation to maintain adequate oxygenation and anesthetic plane. These patients are also at increased risk of gastric reflux/

regurgitation and subsequent aspiration. It is imperative that these animals be fasted at least 12 hours before surgery and receive H_2 blockers to decrease gastric acidity. In addition, a cuffed endotracheal tube should be used, and the pharynx should be evaluated and suctioned at the end of the procedure. A purse-string suture is placed around the anus to prevent fecal contamination of the surgical field. A piece of surgical tape marked *purse string* should be placed on the patient's head to remind the surgeon and anesthetist to remove the sutures once the procedure is finished. The vestibule and caudal vagina should be flushed with dilute Betadine solution as part of the surgical scrub. Three to four flushes of a 1:10 dilution of Betadine (Vedco Inc.) with sterile water should be used to minimize vaginal mucosal irritation.

An incision along the median raphe is made from the level of the caudodorsal aspect of the horizontal vaginal canal, descending to the dorsal commissure of the vulvar cleft. The incision is continued along the same plane of the skin incision through the vaginal musculature and mucosal layers. Placement of a flat instrument (i.e., scalpel handle) in the vestibule can be used to stabilize the tissues while the incision is made through the dorsal vestibular mucosa. Alternatively Metzenbaum scissors can be used to cut the mucosal layer. Cautery and ligation should be used for hemostasis. Hemorrhage is often associated with surgery to this region because of the increased vascularity to the vaginal tissues. Exposure is maintained with the use of self-retaining retractors (i.e., Gelpi or Weitlander retractors) or stay sutures (Fig. 220-1). A urinary catheter should be placed if there is potential for tissue manipulation around the urethra and urethral tubercle.

Closure of the episiotomy is performed in four layers: mucosa, muscular and subcutaneous tissues, and skin. A simple interrupted or continuous pattern of 3-0 monofilament absorbable suture is used for the mucosa. The muscular and subcutaneous tissues can be closed together or separately, depending on the size of the animal, using a simple continuous pattern of 3-0 or 4-0 absorbable suture. The skin edges can be closed with sutures (simple interrupted or cruciates) or surgical staples.

Ventral Approach

Fortunately the ventral approach to the canine vagina is not used often since it requires a pelvic osteotomy. This approach is often used for vaginal ablations or segmental resections of vaginal strictures. The urethra should be

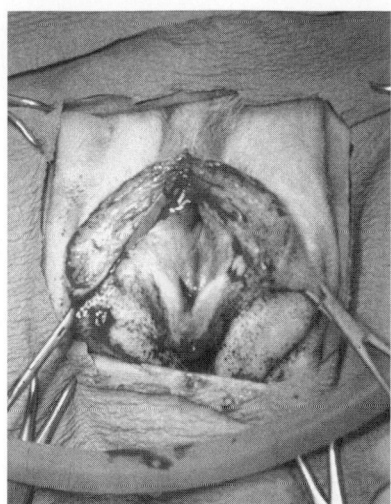

Fig. 220-1 An episiotomy over the dorsal aspect of the vulva allows access to the lumen of the vestibule/vagina. Doyens placed on the edges of the incision allow for control of hemorrhage and visualization.

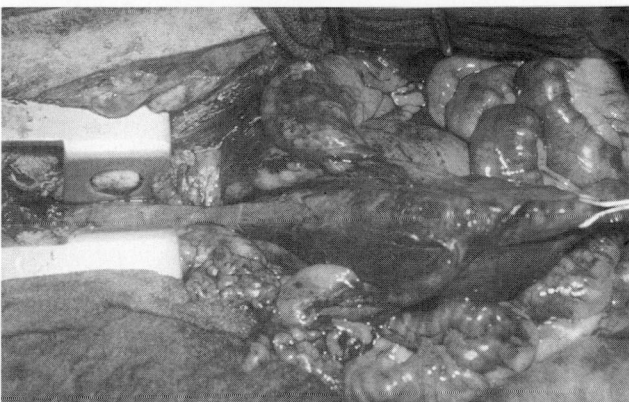

Fig. 220-2 A ventral approach to the female urogenital system via a pubic symphysis osteotomy. Finochietto retractors increase exposure and allow for visualization of the structures within the pelvic canal.

catheterized to aid in identification and prevent iatrogenic trauma.

A standard ventral midline approach is performed in the caudal abdomen up to the cranial pelvic rim. The urinary bladder can be manipulated aside to provide access to the vagina. The pelvic osteotomy is performed to increase the exposure to the vagina and urethra. The incision is extended caudally over the midline of the pubic symphysis. The adductor muscles are elevated laterally with periosteal elevators to expose the pubic and ischial rami. A partial or complete pelvic osteotomy can be performed, depending on the location and amount of exposure needed. A partial pelvic osteotomy involves osteotomies both through pubic rami and across the pubic symphysis at the level of the obturator foramen. A complete pelvic osteotomy through both pubic rami and ischial rami gives the greatest exposure. Once the surgeon has determined the location of the osteotomy, holes are predrilled on either side of the osteotomy site. It is much easier to drill these holes before performing the osteotomy, especially if using a hand chuck and pin. The osteotomy is performed with Gigli wire, rotating burr, sagittal saw, or bone cutters. The internal obturator muscle is elevated off the pubic symphysis on one side of the pelvis and hinged on the contralateral internal obturator muscle to expose the pelvic canal.

Alternatively an osteotomy through the pubic symphysis, separating the hemipelvis, can be performed. The flexibility of the pelvis allows the placement of retractors to separate the hemipelvis, giving exposure to the pelvic canal. Holes can be predrilled on either side of the pubic symphysis. Self-retaining retractors (i.e., Finochietto retractors) facilitate exposure (Fig. 220-2). Care must be taken not to put excessive stress on the hemipelvis, which can create a fracture or sacroiliac luxation (especially in young dogs or cats).

Closure of this approach begins with reduction of the pelvic floor, using 18- to 20-gauge cerclage wire. The predrilled holes allow for rapid and accurate alignment of

the pubic and ischial rami. The obturator and adductor muscle fascia from either side is sutured to its contralateral partner along the midline. Closure of the linea, subcutaneous, and skin is performed routinely. Because of the osteotomy, restricted activity should continue for 4 months following surgery. In small patients the pubic symphysis does not have to be replaced. Closure of the obturator and adductor muscles along the midline provides adequate support of the pelvic floor.

CONGENITAL ABNORMALITIES

Anovulvar Cleft

A cleft or trough is located between the ventral anus and dorsal vulva. This rare defect occurs as a result of inappropriate fusion of the urogenital folds and can be observed in sexually normal female dogs or with intersex disorders. The vestibular floor and clitoris are exposed, resulting in fecal contamination and hyperemia. Correction of this defect with a perineoplasty reduces infection and abrasion of the exposed mucous membranes and provides a more cosmetic appearance.

An H-shaped or inverted V-shaped incision is made along the mucocutaneous junction of the anovulvar cleft. The vestibular mucosal margin and skin edge must be separated. Interrupted sutures of an absorbable suture are used to close the vestibular mucosa and submucosa. This is followed by subcutaneous and skin sutures. Because of the proximity of the incision to the anus, the incision may become infected. The area must be kept clean until sutures are removed. Prophylactic antibiotics may be used, but they are not necessary. An Elizabethan collar is recommended to prevent self-mutilation to the incision.

Vulvar Hypoplasia

Vulvar hypoplasia occurs frequently in spayed female dogs. The vulva is small and recessed into the perineal skin folds. This condition is also referred to as a *juvenile/infantile vulva*. Dogs with juvenile vulva often present for perivulvar moist dermatitis (Fig. 220-3), which is

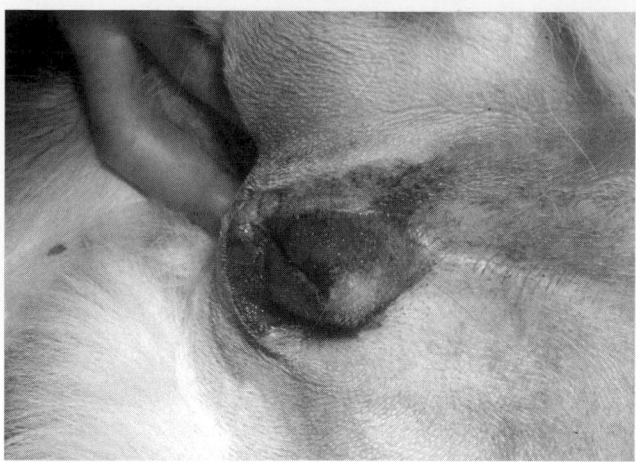

Fig. 220-3 Dog with vulvar excoriations secondary to self-mutilation associated with perivulvar fold dermatitis.

aggravated by retention of urine and/or feces within the folds of skin. A similar condition occurs in obese dogs when the redundant perineal skin covers the vulvar cleft. Recurrent vaginitis and urinary tract infections are common in these patients. Surgical removal of the perivulvar folds and antibiotic management help to alleviate clinical signs. In obese patients weight reduction may help alleviate the perivulvar dermatitis. However, before surgery is recommended, medical management should be instituted to decrease the inflammatory and infectious process around the vulva. Gentle cleansing of the affected area with a benzoyl peroxide shampoo and a mild topical astringent is started. The use of oral antibiotics and topical antibiotic-steroid cream can also be recommended. Once the inflammatory reaction has subsided, an episioplasty can be performed.

An episioplasty is performed to remove the excess perivulvar skinfolds and the underlying subcutaneous fat. Before surgery the perivulvar skin is plicated to determine how much skin should be removed. The goal is to remove enough skin so that the vulva is no longer recessed without creating excessive tension on the incision site. A crescent-shaped skin incision is made around the vulva, starting lateral to the ventral vulvar commissure, extending laterally and dorsally to a point about 1 cm dorsal to the dorsal vulvar commissure, and then extending ventrolaterally to the contralateral side. A second crescent-shaped incision begins and ends at the same points as the first incision; however, this incision extends wider than the first (Fig. 220-4). The perivulvar skin between the incisions is excised with Metzenbaum scissors. If uncertainty exists about how much skin to remove, the surgeon should consider starting the second incision with a narrow arch and, if the vulva is still recessed, creating a wider incision to remove more skin. This prevents unnecessary tension on the incision line.

Excessive subcutaneous fat dorsal to the vulva is removed. This is critical in obese animals. Hemorrhage is controlled with cautery and ligation. The subcutaneous tissues are closed using absorbable suture in a simple interrupted pattern. The first subcutaneous suture should be placed at the dorsal midpoint, followed by additional sutures at the midpoints of the remaining defect. The skin is closed with simple interrupted nonabsorbable sutures. Again skin sutures are placed at 12, 9, and 3 o'clock positions to ensure a cosmetic closure.

Rectovaginal/Vestibular Fistula

This fistula is an abnormal communication between the rectum and the dorsal aspect of the vagina or vestibule. Affected dogs often have atresia ani or an imperforate anus. The dogs present because of passage of soft feces through the vulva. Severity of clinical signs varies with size of the fistula, type of diet, and presence of atresia ani. Dogs with atresia ani may have megacolon as a complicating factor. Vaginography or a barium sulfate enema can be used to demonstrate the location and size of the fistula.

Repair of this defect is twofold, involving restoration of the vaginal/vestibular lumen followed by restoration of the rectal lumen and anal orifice. Surgery is performed via a perineal approach. An incision is made between the anus (or region of the anus) and the dorsal vulvar cleft, along the median raphe. The subcutaneous tissues are bluntly dissected until the fistula is identified. A red rubber catheter placed within the fistula may aid in identification. The communications with the rectum and vagina/vestibule are ligated and resected. The rectal mucosa should be oversewn to ensure a tight seal. If the fistula is short and wide, ligation may not be possible. The stoma should be resected and then closed primarily with absorbable simple interrupted sutures. Again the defects should be oversewn. The subcutaneous tissues and skin should be closed routinely.

In the event of anal atresia, surgery must be performed to recreate a stoma between the rectum and anus (if present). The degree of anal abnormalities may vary from an imperforate anus in which a membrane remains at the level of the anus to complete anal atresia in which the anus and associated anal muscles are absent. Patients with an imperforate anus require opening of the anal canal. This can be performed by breaking down the membrane digitally, by blunt dissection, or by surgical resection of the membrane. Dogs with an imperforate anus must be evaluated carefully with a barium contrast study to differentiate the disorder from anal atresia, which may clinically appear the same. Dogs with an imperforate anus generally have normal anal function and tone. If anal atresia is present, there is minimal-to-no evidence of an anus, and on contrast radiography of the colon there is an absent section of rectum caudal to the fistula. A rectal pull-through procedure is performed, creating a new anal orifice. Because the anal musculature and innervation are absent, these animals have fecal incontinence. Muscle flaps can be attempted to increase tone to the new opening; however, results have been inconsistent.

Clitoral Hypertrophy/Os Clitidoris

Clitoral hypertrophy may occur in dogs with intersex disorders, dogs receiving anabolic steroids, or dogs with hyperadrenocorticism; however, this condition also may

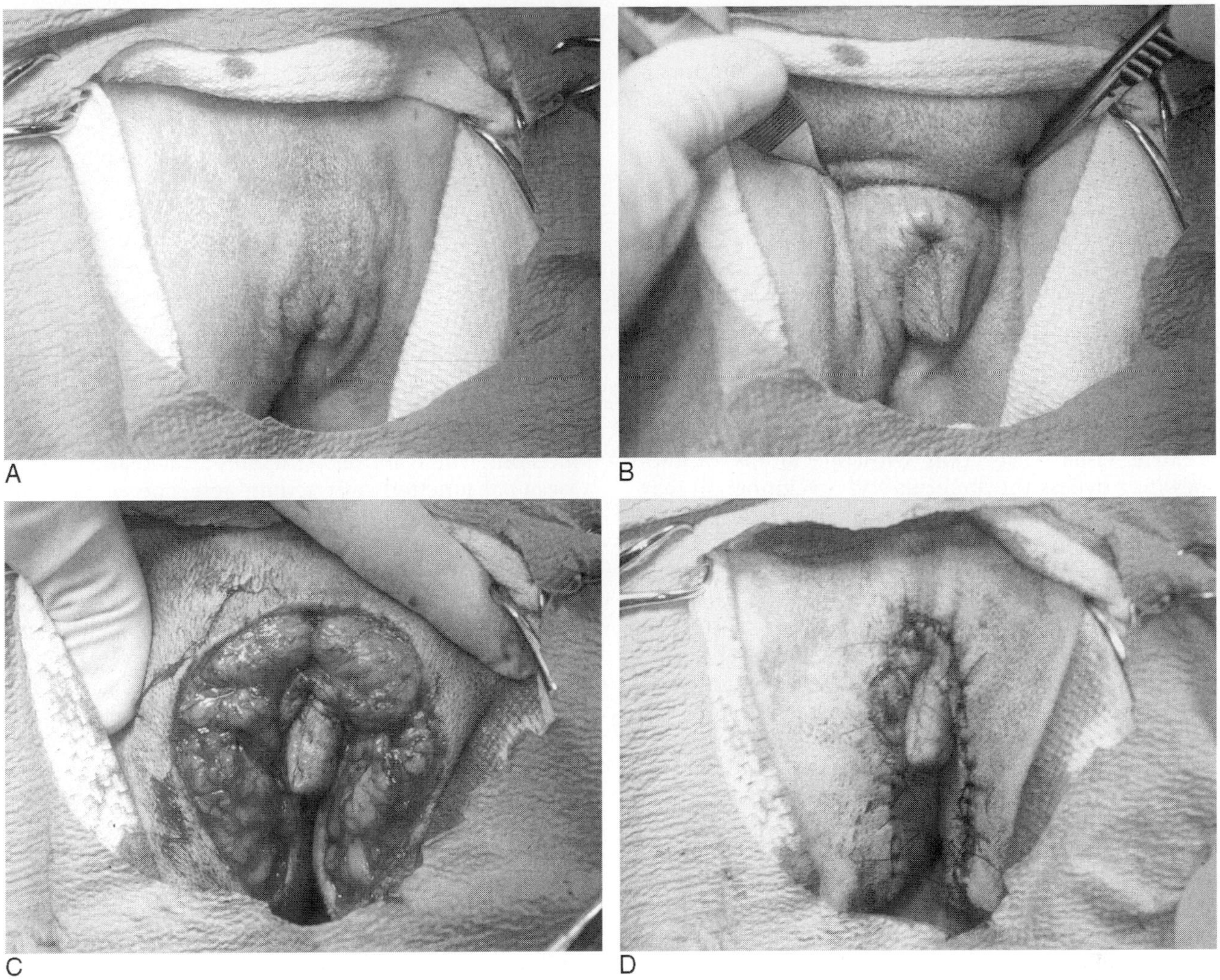

Fig. 220-4 Episioplasty for correction of a recessed juvenile vulva or for redundant perivulvar skin. **A,** Appearance of a dog with a recessed vulva. Note that the vulva is not visible under the redundant skinfolds. **B,** The redundant skin is retracted to visualize the vulva. The excess skin is plicated to determine the amount of skin that will need to be excised. **C,** Two crescent-shaped skin incisions are made around the vulva. **D,** The subcutaneous tissue and skin are closed with multiple simple interrupted sutures.

be found in normal females. Some dogs with chronic vaginitis may present with clitoral hypertrophy caused by excessive vulvar licking. The clitoris often protrudes through the vulvar cleft and may contain an os clitidoris (Fig. 220-5). These dogs generally are presented by an owner for cosmetic reasons, clitoral irritation and vestibular inflammation, or mutilation of the protruded clitoris. Treatment of hyperadrenocorticism or termination of steroid administration may cause resolution of clitoral hypertrophy. If an os clitoris is present, clitoral enlargement may persist after gonadectomy. In cases in which the clitoris is protruding through the vulvar cleft, amputation of the clitoris is recommended. Clitoral amputation is performed by simple submucosal dissection. Dogs with intersex disorders may have significant bleeding during the dissection because of the presence of erectile tissue. Performing an episiotomy may improve visualization and assist with hemostasis.

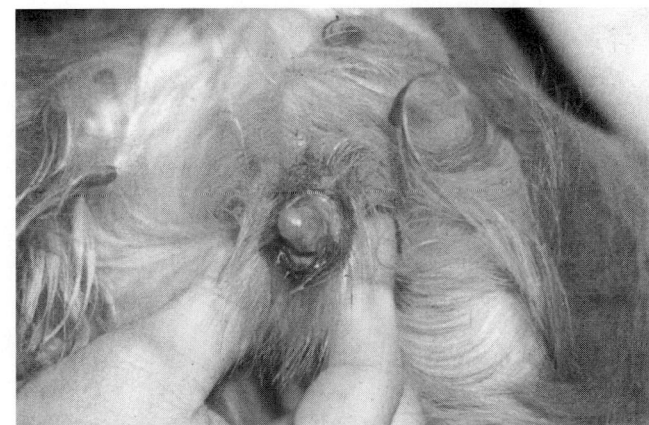

Fig. 220-5 Dog with an os clitoris. The end of the enlarged clitoris is extruded between the vulvar cleft.

Vaginal Band, Septa, and Stenosis

A number of vaginal and vestibular congenital abnormalities occur as a result of imperfect joining of the genital folds, genital swellings, or Müllerian ducts. These conditions may be incidental findings on a physical examination, or occasionally they cause a variety of clinical presentations. Bitches with stenosis or bands may present with clinical signs of chronic vaginitis, which may be associated with urine pooling in the anterior portion of the vagina. Other bitches may present for artificial insemination after unsuccessful attempts at natural breeding. The female and/or male may demonstrate pain when attempting to breed. Vaginal bands are also frequently associated with dogs having ectopic ureters. A digital vaginal examination may be most informative since visual inspection with speculums or otoscopes may bypass the abnormality. A vaginogram may be necessary to determine the extent and severity of the abnormality.

A persistent or imperforate hymen can be corrected with digital breakdown of the membrane. Vaginal bands or septa that cannot be corrected digitally may require an episiotomy and surgical resection (Fig. 220-6). Depending on the extent of the mucosal defect remaining after surgical removal of the band or septa, the defect can be left to heal by second intention or surgically closed using an absorbable suture in a simple continuous manner.

Vestibulovaginal stenosis is diagnosed as a palpable submucosal fibrous ring at the level of a persistent hymen. Vaginal stenosis is a region of vaginal hypoplasia, in which the lumen over a given area is narrower than the rest of the vagina or vestibule. Bitches with stenosis of the vestibulovaginal junction that exhibit clinical signs tend to respond poorly to digital and surgical attempts at dilation. If surgery is indicated, a vaginogram should be performed to determine the extent of the affected region. Three surgical techniques have been recommended for correction of these defects: T-vaginoplasty, stenosis resection, and partial/complete vaginectomy. Resection of

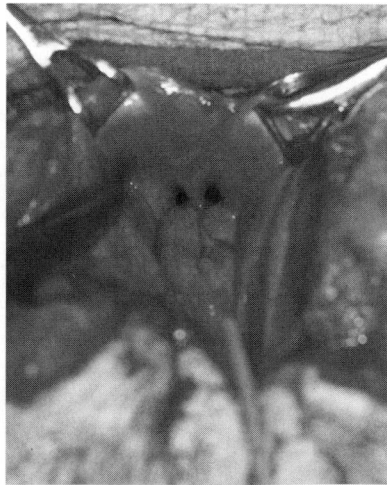

Fig. 220-6 Episiotomy performed for visualization of a vaginal band. A urinary catheter identifies the urethral opening at the base of the vestibulovaginal junction.

the stricture/stenosis has a better outcome than the T-vaginoplasty for complete resolution of clinical signs; however, the procedure is more difficult technically and therefore can have higher surgical complications. The T-vaginoplasty has been shown to resolve clinical signs in some dogs. Surgical recommendations vary with severity of the stenosis. Severe stenosis would most likely respond to resection and anastomosis, whereas the milder stenosis would probably respond to a less invasive T-vaginoplasty.

The T-vaginoplasty is performed via a standard episiotomy approach. A longitudinal incision is made on the dorsal aspect of the vaginal stricture, followed by a T-shaped closure to increase the vaginal diameter. However, this procedure has met with variable results. Bitches with submucosal fibrous rings may not require full-thickness incisions. These annular strictures located at the vestibulovaginal junction only require resection of the fibrous tissue through a mucosal incision. The fibrous ring is resected, and the remaining mucosal defect is closed so that none of the deeper vaginal tissues are exposed. In spayed bitches only the ventral 180 degrees of the stricture is removed in mild cases to allow adequate drainage of vaginal fluids. Positive postoperative results have been reported on the few cases in which complete resection and anastomosis of the defect were performed. This technique is technically more difficult since it requires a 360-degree dissection of the stenosis. A standard episiotomy may give the surgeon adequate visualization of the defect in the event of a small stricture or stenosis; however, if the defect is more extensive, as often occurs with vaginal stenosis, a ventral approach may be necessary. Full-thickness excisions of vaginal stenosis are always required. Two circumferential incisions are made cranial and caudal to the defect. Catheterization and protection of the urethra are critical when performing a vaginal resection and anastomosis. Ligation and cautery of superficial and muscular vessels are mandatory. Closure of the remaining defect can be performed once the stenosis is resected using absorbable suture in a simple interrupted pattern.

A complete vaginectomy is the final option for correction of vaginal stenosis in bitches that are not intended for breeding. Results with this technique seem to be very favorable. A standard episiotomy may be used in spayed bitches, whereas a ventral approach combined with a midline laparotomy may be used in intact bitches. The vagina is resected anterior to the urethral tubercle, making sure that the entire stenotic vagina is removed. A Parker-Kerr oversew or other inverting suture patterns are used to close the vagina.

ACQUIRED ABNORMALITIES

Vaginal Prolapse

Vaginal prolapse includes two very different disease processes. One process involves prolapse of edematous mucosa on the floor of the vaginal vault. This disease is also referred to as *vaginal edema* and was previously also referred to as *vaginal hyperplasia*. The second process involves a true prolapse of the vagina, in which the prolapse is circumferential and often includes the cervix. These dogs have *true vaginal prolapse*. For ease of discussion, the terms *vaginal edema* and *true vaginal prolapse* are used when discussing the two disease processes.

Vaginal Edema/Hyperplasia

Young intact bitches in proestrus or estrus are frequently reported with this condition. Large and brachycephalic breeds are overrepresented. Normally during the follicular phase of the estrous cycle the vaginal and vestibular mucosa becomes thickened and edematous. Occasionally an exaggerated response occurs, resulting in excessive edema. The submucosal tissue edema and redundant mucosa at the floor of the vagina just cranial to the urethral tubercle can protrude through the vulvar labia as a fleshy red mass (Fig. 220-7). The exposed tissue is prone to trauma, desiccation, and self-mutilation. The urethra is not exteriorized and can be catheterized at the base of the edematous tissue. The location of the urethral tubercle helps distinguish vaginal edema from vaginal prolapse, in which the urethral opening may be exteriorized with the prolapsed vagina.

Conservative management consists of protection of the exteriorized portion of the mass with lubricants and prevention of self-mutilation with an Elizabethan collar. Vaginal edema is most commonly seen during the first estrous period and regresses spontaneously during the luteal phase. However, recurrence is common during following estrous cycles. Owners should be cautioned that the edematous tissue may also recur at parturition,

resulting in dystocia. Hormonal therapy with megestrol acetate (2 mg/kg orally daily for 7 days) or gonadotropin-releasing hormone (50 mcg intramuscularly once) may also be attempted. Owners should be advised of specific side effects of hormonal therapy.

Ovariohysterectomy is curative and should be considered to prevent recurrence. Surgical resection of the mass should be considered if the bitch is intended for breeding or if the tissues are traumatized. A standard episiotomy is performed to expose the base of the edematous tissue. The mass is lifted off of the vestibular floor, and the urethra catheterized to prevent iatrogenic trauma. A transverse elliptical incision is made around the base, and the redundant vaginal tissue is amputated. The vaginal mucosal defect is closed with absorbable suture in a simple continuous pattern, carefully avoiding the urethral orifice.

True Vaginal Prolapse

True vaginal prolapse occurs less frequently than vaginal edema and can be either partial or complete. In a complete true vaginal prolapse the cervix is exteriorized. In both cases there is a doughnut-shaped eversion of the vaginal tissues. This is differentiated from vaginal edema in that there is circumferential involvement of the vaginal mucosa and the urethral tubercle. Brachycephalic breeds in normal estrus are predisposed to vaginal prolapse.

No treatment may be necessary in cases with mild prolapse since spontaneous regression occurs during

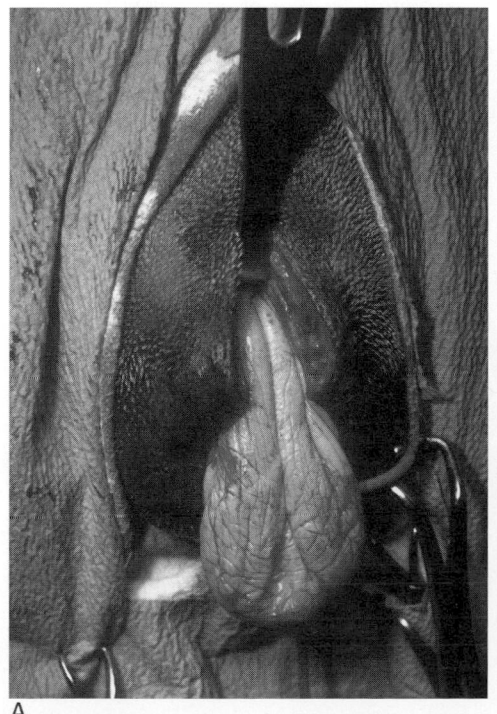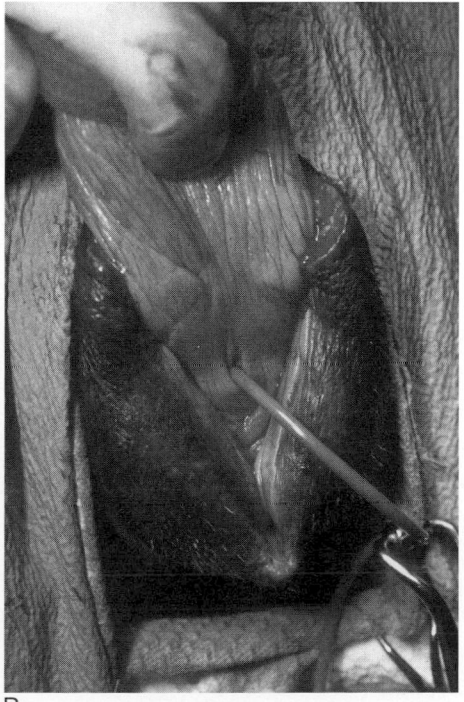

Fig. 220-7 Hyperplasia of the vaginal floor. **A,** An episiotomy is performed to expose the base of the hyperplastic tissue. **B,** The pedunculated hyperplastic tissue is elevated, exposing the urethral opening. A urinary catheter is inserted to maintain visual recognition and protection of the urethra during resection of the hyperplastic tissue.

diestrus. More severe prolapses may require protection of exposed tissues. General anesthesia is required if attempting to replace the prolapsed mucosa. The everted tissue is cleaned with a dilute antiseptic solution or saline. If the edema is severe, manual compression or application of 50% dextrose solution to the mucosal surface may decrease its size, therefore facilitating reduction. A lubricated plastic syringe can be used to reduce the tissues. An episiotomy may be necessary to provide better exposure for reduction. Reduction can also be assisted by traction on the uterus via a ventral abdominal approach. Once the vagina is reduced, reprolapse can be minimized by suturing the uterine body or the broad ligament to the abdominal wall. A urinary catheter should be maintained until the vaginal swelling resolves.

Dogs with long-standing prolapses may have secondary necrosis, infection, or hemorrhage of the prolapsed tissues. These dogs should be evaluated and treated as necessary for hypotension and/or sepsis. Surgical resection of the devitalized tissues is indicated in these patients to prevent further sepsis and self-mutilation. An episiotomy helps with exposure and placement of a urinary catheter. A stepwise full-thickness circumferential incision is made in the vaginal wall. A section of 1 to 2 cm of the outer mucosal layer is incised, followed by resection of the inner noninverted mucosal layer. Horizontal mattress sutures are used to close the incision edges. Hemorrhage can be significant and should be controlled with cautery and ligation. This is continued circumferentially in small sections until the entire prolapsed tissue is resected.

Suggested Reading

Crawford JT, Adams WM: Influence of vestibulovaginal stenosis, pelvic bladder, and recessed vulva on response to treatment for clinical signs of lower urinary tract disease in dogs: 38 cases (1990-1999), *J Am Vet Med Assoc* 221:995, 2002.

Hedlund CS : Surgery of the reproductive and genital systems. In Fossum TW, editor:, *Small animal surgery* St. Louis, 2002, Mosby, p 610.

Johnston SD: Vaginal prolapse. In Kirk RW, editor: *Current veterinary therapy X*, Philadelphia, 1989, Saunders, p 1302.

Kyles AE et al: Vestibulovaginal stenosis in dogs: 18 cases (1987-1995), *J Am Vet Med Assoc* 209:1889, 1996.

Marretta SM: Vagina and vulva: episioplasty. In Bojrab MJ, editor: *Current techniques in small animal surgery*, Baltimore, 1998a, Williams & Wilkins, p 506.

Marretta SM: Vagina and vulva: episiotomy. In Bojrab MJ, editor: *Current techniques in small animal surgery*, Baltimore, 1998b, Williams & Wilkins, p 508.

Mathews KG: Surgery of the canine vagina and vulva, *Vet Clin North Am: Small Anim Pract* 31: 271, 2001.

Pettit GD: Vagina and vulva: surgical treatment of vaginal and vulvar masses. In Bojrab MJ, editor: *Current techniques in small animal surgery*, Baltimore, 1998, Williams & Wilkins, p 503.

Rahal SC et al: Rectovaginal fistula with anal atresia in 5 dogs, *Can Vet J* 48:827, 2007.

Root MV, Johnston SD, Johnston GR: Vaginal septa in dogs: 15 cases (1983-1992), *J Am Vet Med Assoc* 206:56, 1995.

Soderberg SF: Vaginal disorders, *Vet Clin North Am: Small Anim Pract* 16:543, 1986.

Soderberg SF: Surgical diseases of the canine vulva and vagina. In Bojrab MJ, editor: *Disease mechanisms in small animal surgery*, Philadelphia, 1993, Lea & Febiger, p 574.

Wang KY et al: Vestibular, vaginal and urethral relations in spayed dogs with and without lower urinary tract signs, *J Vet Intern Med* 20:1065, 2006.

Wykes PM, Olson PN: Vagina, vestibule, and vulva. In Slatter D, editor: *Textbook of small animal surgery*, Philadelphia, 2002, Saunders, p 1502.

CHAPTER 221

Early-Age Neutering in the Dog and Cat

LISA M. HOWE, *College Station, Texas*

Veterinarians in the United States have typically recommended that female dogs and cats undergo ovariohysterectomy before the first estrus (prepubertal) to decrease the risk of mammary neoplasia and prevent unwanted pregnancy. Traditionally female dogs and cats not intended for breeding purposes have been neutered at approximately 6 months of age, and male dogs and cats have been neutered at approximately 6 to 9 months of age. In an attempt to address the dog and cat overpopulation problem in the United States, veterinarians have been advocating early-age neutering in which the animal is neutered as early as 6 weeks of age.

Although animal shelters often request that neuter contracts be signed at the time of pet adoption, many new owners fail to comply with the contract, even when financial reimbursement is available for the neuter surgery. One survey by the Massachusetts Society for the Prevention of Cruelty to animals reported that in 500 households with dogs and cats, 73% of dogs and 87% of cats were neutered, but nearly 20% of the neutered animals had produced at least one litter of offspring before neutering. In Texas a study examining over 43,000 dogs and cats 6 months and older reported that only 27% of dogs and 33% of cats were sterilized (Mahlow, 1999). It was estimated that if 80% of the estimated 10 million dogs and cats in Texas are sexually mature (believed to be a conservative estimate) and 71% of those are sexually intact, approximately 5.7 million dogs and cats would be capable of reproducing. Prepubertal gonadectomy performed before adoption on puppies and kittens can result in compliance rates of 100% for neutering and improved staff morale.

Scientific data regarding the ideal age at which dogs and cats should be sterilized are lacking. Thus, despite approval of the concept of early-age neutering by the American Veterinary Medical Association, American Animal Hospital Association, American College of Theriogenologists, Humane Society of the United States, American Humane Association, Association of Veterinarians for Animal Rights, Cat Fanciers Association, and numerous state veterinary associations, the concept remains controversial to many veterinarians. Studies conducted in the early to mid 1990s suggest that prepubertal gonadectomy surgery is safe in dogs and cats as young as 6 weeks of age (Aronsohn and Faggella, 1993; Faggella and Aronsohn, 1993; Faggella and Aronsohn, 1994). Studies demonstrated that the effects of early neutering on skeletal and physical development and behavior are similar to those of traditionally timed gonadectomy (Salmeri et al., 1991; Stubbs et al., 1996). More recent scientific studies examining both short- and long-term outcomes of early-age neutering further support the safety of the procedure and have addressed concerns, including morbidity/mortality during and after surgery and urinary obstruction in male cats in greater depth.

SCIENTIFIC STUDIES

Although the anesthetic and surgical techniques of early-age neutering have been reported to be safe, veterinarians have persistently expressed concerns about the short- and long-term health risks. Concerns include increased susceptibility to infectious diseases, safety of anesthesia and surgery in young patients, bone growth abnormalities, urinary tract obstruction in male cats, penile and preputial development problems in male cats, perivulvar dermatitis in female dogs, urinary incontinence in female dogs, obesity, and adrenal tumors. Since the late 1990s numerous studies have been conducted that address many of these concerns and have demonstrated most of the concerns to be unfounded.

Infectious Diseases and Short-Term Morbidity/Mortality

In studies conducted in association with animal shelters, puppies and kittens undergoing early-age neutering were at no greater risk of infectious diseases or anesthetic or surgical complications than older animals. In one study of 1988 shelter animals undergoing neutering in association with the fourth-year student surgical teaching program of a veterinary college, 12 animals (0.6%) died or were euthanized because of severe infections of the respiratory tract or as a result of parvoviral enteritis during the 7-day postoperative period (Howe, 1997). All of the deaths were seen in the shelter with the shortest animal holding period; however, the incidence of infectious diseases did not differ among age-groups (<12, 12 to 23, and ≧24 weeks of age). When anesthetic and surgical complication rates were examined in that 7-day study, animals neutered at 24 weeks of age or older had a significantly higher minor complication rate than animals neutered at younger than 12 weeks of age, but the complication rate did not differ from animals neutered at 12 to 23 weeks of age. Minor complications included such problems as incisional swelling or suture reactions, scrotal swelling, mild gastrointestinal upsets, and cardiac rate and rhythm abnormalities during anesthesia. Differences in major complications were not detected among groups. In that study younger patients did relatively better than older animals, even when immunity to infectious diseases may not have been strong or when veterinary students were performing anesthesia and delicate pediatric surgeries.

In a long-term study (48-month median follow-up) of these same animals (269 dogs) after adoption, there was an increased incidence of parvoviral enteritis in the puppies neutered at an early age (median age = 10 weeks) compared to the traditional age (median age = 52 weeks) (Howe et al., 2001). Parvoviral enteritis is common in puppies from shelter environments but uncommon in older dogs. The potential influence of anesthesia and surgery on the incidence of parvoviral enteritis in puppies that underwent gonadectomy could not be determined because comparisons with puppies that did not undergo gonadectomy were not performed. A similar long-term study (36-month median follow-up) of 263 cats showed that prepubertal gonadectomy did not result in an increased incidence of infectious diseases after adoption compared with traditional-age gonadectomy (Howe et al., 2000).

Long Bone Growth

Historically veterinarians believed that puppies and kittens neutered at young ages might have stunted growth. Several research studies have shown this concern to be unfounded and have demonstrated that neutering at both 7 weeks and 7 months of age results in delayed closure of the distal radial physis compared with intact animals. In the first it was shown in dogs that growth rates were unaffected by gonadectomy, but the growth period and final radial/ulnar length was extended in all neutered male dogs (neutered at 7 weeks and 7 months of age) and in females neutered at 7 weeks of age (Salmeri et al., 1991). Thus the dogs were not stunted in growth but actually were slightly taller as determined by radiographs. Another study in cats showed that males gonadectomized at 7 weeks or 7 months of age reached the growth plateau (the time when bone length no longer increases) on average 35% later and achieved radial length of 13% greater than intact males (Root, Johnston, and Olson, 1997). Female cats gonadectomized at 7 weeks or 7 months of age reached the growth plateau on average 18% later and achieved a 9% longer radial length compared to intact females. An earlier study in cats found that gonadectomy at both 7 weeks and 7 months of age in male and female cats delayed distal radial physeal closure by approximately 8 weeks compared to intact cats (Stubbs et al., 1996). The clinical significance of delayed closure of growth plates is not clear, and it is unknown whether it might make the growth plates more susceptible to injury. In long-term studies of 263 cats and 269 dogs examining outcome of gonadectomy performed at an early age or traditional age, no differences in the incidence of musculoskeletal problems (including fractures or hip dysplasia in dogs) was seen between groups in either species (Howe et al, 2000; Howe et al., 2001).

Urethral, Penile, and Preputial Development in Male Cats

One of the major concerns of veterinarians about performing early age neutering is that of lower urinary

tract disease (LUTD) and urethral obstruction in male cats. Numerous studies dating to the 1960s have examined this issue, and more currently both experimental and clinical studies have been conducted. Two experimental studies examining cats castrated at 7 weeks and 7 months of age compared to sexually intact cats have addressed this concern. The first study examined urethral development when cats were 1 year of age and found that urethral diameters as determined by contrast retrograde urethrography were similar between both groups of neutered cats compared to intact cats (Stubbs et al., 1993). Further, no difference in urethral dynamic function as determined by urethral pressure profiles was seen between groups. In the second study the diameter of the preprostatic and penile urethra as measured on voiding cystourethrograms when cats were 22 months of age was examined (Root et al., 1996). As with the previous study, no differences were seen in urethral diameter of male cats neutered at 7 weeks or 7 months of age compared to intact cats. Findings of these studies are consistent with findings of an older study examining the urethral diameter at three penile locations (just distal to the os penis, just proximal to the os penis, and 2 mm further proximal to the os penis) in cats castrated at 5 months of age compared to intact cats (Herron, 1972). At maturity (10 months of age) the urethral circumference of both groups of cats was the same in all locations.

In addition to experimental studies, a recent clinical study examined the effect of castration on the incidence of urinary system problems in a long-term follow-up of 263 cats neutered at an early age compared to the traditional age (Howe et al., 2000). The median follow-up was 37 months and included 108 male cats divided into two groups based on age at the time of castration: early age (median age at castration = 9 weeks; n = 70) and traditional age (median age at castration = 51 weeks; n = 38). In that study *traditional-age* cats had significantly more overall urinary tract problems (17%) compared to early-age cats (3%). Cystitis was the most common problem seen, and the incidence was significantly greater in traditional-age cats. There was no significant difference in the rate of urethral obstruction between groups, although 2/38 (5%) traditional-age cats suffered urinary obstruction, whereas 0/70 (0%) early-age cats became obstructed. The findings of this study support findings of a much older study that examined cats castrated from 3 months to 3 years compared to sexually intact cats, in which cats were fed a calculi-inducing diet for 16 months (Duch et al., 1978). No difference was noted in the obstruction rate between the castrated and intact groups; however, a trend toward a protective effect in the castrated group was noted in that there was a longer time before occurrence of obstruction in that group.

All of these studies examined together indicate that *urethral* development and diameter in male cats is not an androgen-dependent process, even though *penile* size and development is androgen dependent. Therefore it would appear that veterinarians should not be any more concerned about obstructive or nonobstructive LUTD in male cats castrated at an early age than those castrated at a traditional age.

Concerns have also been expressed about penile and preputial development in male cats castrated early. The balanopreputial fold is a fold of tissue (a continuous layer of epithelium) that connects the penis to the prepuce at birth. The separation process of the balanopreputial fold is androgen dependent and is complete at birth in some species but not until after puberty in other species. It has been suggested that prepubertal castration in cats might delay or prevent dissolution of the membrane, which may predispose to ascending urinary tract disease since these cats may not be able to fully extrude the penis for cleaning (Herron, 1971). Studies examining separation of the balanopreputial fold have reported mixed findings. In one study it was reported that at 1 year of age the penis could be fully extruded in all males, including those castrated at 7 weeks of age (Stubbs et al., 1996). Penile spines were absent in those castrated at 7 weeks of age and were atrophied in those castrated at 7 months. However, another study reported different findings on penile extrusion in cats at 22 months of age (Root et al., 1996). Of the cats neutered at 7 weeks of age, the penis could be fully extruded in 0% of cats; whereas in intact cats the penis could be fully extruded in 100% of the cats. Of the cats neutered at 7 months of age, the penis could be fully extruded in 60%. In males incapable of complete penile extrusion, only one third to two thirds of the length of the penis could be visualized. On the basis of the long-term clinical cat study, it would appear that failure of separation of the balanopreputial fold (when present) does not cause a clinical problem in cats neutered early (Howe et al., 2000). However, should cats become obstructed, penile manipulations for catheterization may be more challenging because of small penile size and potential inability to fully extrude the penis.

Genitalia Development in Dogs

The penis, os penis, and prepuce of puppies neutered at 7 weeks of age are infantile in appearance compared to those neutered at 7 months or left intact (Salmeri et al., 1991). To date there have been no published reports of an increased incidence of balanoposthitis as a result of infantile genitalia. In females vulvas of puppies neutered before puberty are small when compared to those of intact dogs (Salmeri et al., 1991). However, vulvas may also appear small in some female dogs spayed later in life or in intact females during anestrus. Perivulvar dermatitis can occur in female dogs with small or recessed vulvas, especially if the dog is fat or has excessive skin covering the vulva. To date there is no information to suggest that the incidence of perivulvar dermatitis is higher in female dogs spayed at an early age compared with those spayed at the traditional age. Regardless of the age at gonadectomy, the vulva, vestibule, and vagina undergo atrophy.

Urinary Incontinence in Female Dogs

In the female dog an increased incidence of urinary incontinence has been associated with ovariohysterectomy. Although there are many causes of urinary incontinence, hormone responsive incontinence is most frequently associated with ovariohysterectomy. Since the onset of urinary incontinence in neutered dogs is variable and may occur in sexually intact animals, the cause of incontinence is most likely multifactorial in etiology. Currently there is no evidence to suggest that prepubertal gonadectomy potentiates the problem. In the long term (median follow-up time = 48 months) study in 269 dogs from animal shelters, urinary incontinence developed in three dogs (Howe et al., 2001). Two of these dogs were in the traditional age-group (median age at gonadectomy = 52 weeks), and one was in the early age-group (median age at gonadectomy = 10 weeks). Of these three dogs only one (traditional age-group) had a history consistent with hormone-responsive urinary incontinence. A difference was not detected between age-groups for incidence of incontinence.

Behavior

Concerns regarding potential negative behavioral consequences of prepubertal gonadectomy have been cited as a reason to avoid early neutering. One study demonstrated that of seven behavioral characteristics assessed in dogs neutered at 7 weeks or 7 months of age compared with intact dogs, only general activity and excitability differed among groups (Salmeri et al., 1991). All neutered dogs were judged to be more active than intact dogs, and dogs neutered at 7 weeks of age were judged to be more excitable than sexually intact dogs. The most common problems reported in the long-term follow-up of dogs neutered early or at a traditional age were behavioral in nature (Howe et al., 2001). Overall 32% of dogs neutered early and 34% of dogs neutered at a traditional age had at least one behavioral problem; aggressive and destructive behaviors were most common. A difference between age-groups was not detected in incidence of overall or specific behavioral problems.

In cats the effects of neutering on behavior were examined, and it was found that cats gonadectomized at 7 weeks and 7 months were more affectionate and demonstrated less intraspecies aggression than sexually intact cats (Stubbs et al., 1996). In the 3-year follow-up study of 263 cats, no difference in the incidence of behavioral problems in cats gonadectomized at an early age (median age = 9 weeks; 26% incidence) compared to those neutered at a more traditional age (median age = 51 weeks; 35% incidence) was found. The most commonly encountered behavior problems in both groups of cats included destructive behavior and inappropriate elimination.

Obesity

Both male and female cats may become obese after gonadectomy; however, no difference between cats neutered at 7 weeks and 7 months of age was identified (Stubbs et al., 1996). In both of these groups there was increased body weight and increased depth of falciform ligament compared to intact cats. A second study demonstrated lower resting metabolic rates and lower maintenance energy requirement as measured by indirect calorimetry in cats neutered at 7 weeks and 7 months compared to sexually intact cats (Root et al., 1996). The study showed that both male and female gonadectomized cats (regardless of the age at which they are neutered) need approximately 30% fewer calories than intact cats. Another study confirmed these findings and demonstrated that the maintenance energy requirement is substantially lower for spayed female cats than for sexually intact female cats (Flynn, Hardie, and Armstrong, 1996). It was noted that sexually intact cats appeared to self-regulate food intake, whereas spayed cats tended to eat all food available.

In dogs information regarding the propensity of animals to gain weight following neutering is less clear. One study found no difference in food intake, weight gains, or back-fat depth among puppies neutered at 7 weeks or 7 months of age or left intact (Salmeri et al., 1991). However, an older retrospective study from the United Kingdom examining 8000 dogs showed that spayed female dogs were almost twice as likely to be obese as intact female dogs (Edney and Smith, 1986).

Miscellaneous

Retention in the original adoptive household and the physical status of all body systems, including integumentary, gastrointestinal, musculoskeletal, and cardiopulmonary, were examined as part of the long-term dog and cat follow-up studies (Howe et al., 2000; Howe et al., 2001). In both cats and dogs age at neutering had no effect on the rate of retention in the original adoptive household or on problems associated with any body system except the gastrointestinal tract in dogs. Dogs neutered at a traditional age had more gastrointestinal tract problems than did dogs neutered at an early age. Most of these problems were minor, and the cause of this increased incidence was undetermined.

Concerns have been expressed that puppies and kittens neutered at early ages could be at risk for developing adrenal tumors. Although these concerns have arisen from reports that adrenal tumors in ferrets were found more often in neutered animals, there is no documentation of adrenal tumors associated with prepubertal gonadectomy in cats or dogs.

ANESTHETIC AND SURGICAL TECHNIQUES AND CONSIDERATIONS

Preoperative and Operative Considerations

Anesthetic and surgical considerations for the pediatric puppy or kitten include the potential for hypothermia and hypoglycemia, the delicate nature of pediatric tissues, and a relatively small blood volume compared to that of the adult dog or cat. Hypothermia can be minimized by using circulating warm water or air blankets and by the use of warmed intravenous fluids (if used). Excessive wetting of the pediatric patient during surgical site preparation should be avoided; and the use of warmed scrub agent (chlorhexidine) and avoidance of alcohol help preserve body heat. Minimizing operative time also helps to decrease the severity of hypothermia.

Prolonged fasting of the pediatric puppy or kitten may result in hypoglycemia since hepatic glycogen stores are minimal in neonates. Food should be withheld no longer than 8 hours, with 3 to 4 hours recommended for the youngest patients (6 to 8 weeks old). Animals should be fed a small meal within 1 to 2 hours after recovery from anesthesia.

Pediatric tissues are very friable and should be handled with care. The relatively small blood volume of pediatric puppies and kittens makes meticulous hemostasis imperative. Fortunately the small size of blood vessels and the presence of minimal abdominal and ovarian bursal fat permit excellent visualization of the vasculature and precise hemostasis.

Numerous protocols for anesthetic management of the pediatric puppy or kitten undergoing early-age neutering have been reported and typically involve balanced anesthesia techniques. Efficacious protocols include:

1. Puppies
   a. For females: atropine (0.04 mg/kg intramuscularly [IM]) and oxymorphone (0.11 mg/kg IM), followed by propofol (3.4 mg/kg IV) 15 minutes later with isoflurane for maintenance
   b. For males: atropine (0.04 mg/kg IM) and oxymorphone (0.22 mg/kg IM), followed by propofol (6.5 mg/kg intravenously [IV]) 15 minutes later with isoflurane if additional analgesia is needed
   c. For males or females: glycopyrrolate (0.011 mg/kg IM) and butorphanol (0.22 mg/kg IM), followed by pentothal (22 mg/kg IV) to effect 15 minutes later with halothane or isoflurane for maintenance
2. Kittens
   a. For females: midazolam (0.22 mg/kg IM) and ketamine (11 mg/kg IM) with isoflurane for maintenance
   b. For males: tiletamine-zolazepam (11 mg/kg IM) followed by isoflurane if additional analgesia is needed
   c. For males or females: glycopyrrolate (0.011 mg/kg IM), butorphanol (0.22 mg/kg IM), acepromazine (0.055 mg/kg IM), and ketamine (11 mg/kg IM) with halothane or isoflurane for maintenance

When performing early-age neutering, perioperative antimicrobial therapy is not indicated unless a preexisting bacterial skin condition is present at or near the surgical site, another medical condition necessitates antibiotic therapy, or a break in aseptic technique occurs. If necessary, intravenous cefazolin may be administered (22 mg/kg) during anesthetic induction or if a break in surgical asepsis occurs.

To prevent unnecessary abdominal exploratory surgery in the future, all puppies and kittens undergoing early-age neutering should be tattooed to identify their neutered status. The recommended tattoo site is the prepubic area in females and the inguinal area in males. The appropriate female or male gender symbol along with an encircled "X" is used to denote the neutered status. Tattooing may be performed after the surgical site has been clipped but before surgical preparation of the area.

Ovariohysterectomy

Pediatric ovariohysterectomy may be performed similarly to adult ovariohysterectomy with slight modifications. Puppy incisions are started relatively more caudal to the umbilicus than in adult dogs. Typically the uterus is more easily exposed in puppies if the incision is started at least 2 to 3 cm caudal to the umbilicus. This placement results in the incision being nearer the middle third of the distance from the umbilicus to the cranial brim of the pelvis, similar to a cat incision. In kittens the incision is placed in a location similar to that of adult cat incisions. Substantial amounts of serous fluid may be an incidental finding in the abdominal cavity of both puppies and kittens. To improve visualization of the abdominal contents, it may be necessary to use gauze sponges to remove some of the fluid. Because of incision location in both puppies and kittens, the uterus may be located easily by looking between the urinary bladder and colon. In contrast to adult dogs and cats, it is recommended that the use of a Snook ovariohysterectomy hook be avoided in pediatric puppies and kittens because of the delicate nature of the tissues.

Uterine tissue is extremely fragile and friable in both puppies and kittens; therefore care must be used to avoid excess traction. After the uterus has been located, the suspensory ligament may be broken down carefully to improve visualization. The ovarian vessels are double ligated using 3-0 to 4-0 absorbable suture material or appropriately sized stainless steel hemostatic clips. In very small pedicles a single ligature may be sufficient to prevent hemorrhage.

After the ovarian pedicles have been ligated on both sizes, the remaining broad ligaments are broken down, and the uterus ligated at the junction of the uterine body and cervix using absorbable suture material or hemostatic clips. Once the reproductive tract has been removed, it should be examined for complete removal (of ovaries and uterine body), and the abdomen should be examined for evidence of hemorrhage. The ventral fascia (external rectus sheath) can be closed with either a simple interrupted or continuous pattern using 3-0 (or possibly 2-0 on large puppies) absorbable (polydioxanone, polyglyconate, or polyglactin 910) or monofilament nonabsorbable (polypropylene, polybutester, or nylon) suture material. It is important to differentiate the ventral fascia from overlying subcutaneous tissue, which requires careful attention, particularly in young puppies. The subcutaneous layer may be closed with an absorbable suture material (3-0 or 4-0, poliglecaprone 25 is preferred) in a continuous intradermal pattern to avoid the use of skin sutures. Some veterinarians avoid using skin sutures in pediatric puppies and kittens to prevent premature suture removal by the patient; however, I routinely use *loosely* placed skin sutures without complication.

Castration

Pediatric puppy castration is also performed with modifications to the techniques used in adult dogs. Because puppy testes are mobile and can be difficult to identify, careful palpation must be used to determine whether both testicles have descended before beginning surgery. If one or both testes have not descended, standard cryptorchidectomy techniques may be used for castration, or surgery postponed pending descent of the testicle(s) or increased patient size. The entire scrotal region is clipped and surgically prepared to permit the scrotum to be included in the surgical sterile field. Because of the small size and mobility of the puppy testicles, including the scrotum in the surgical field can facilitate locating and manipulating the testicles. Clipping and surgical preparation of the scrotum does not cause scrotal irritation in puppies as it does in adult dogs because the scrotal sac of puppies is not well developed compared to that of adult male dogs. Puppies may be castrated through a single midline prescrotal or scrotal incision or through two scrotal incisions similar to a feline castration. When a midline incision is used, the testicles must be held securely underneath the incision site to prevent iatrogenic penile trauma. Following exposure of the testicle and spermatic cords in closed fashion (testes remain enclosed in the parietal vaginal tunic during castration), the spermatic cords are ligated (double ligations preferred) with 3-0 absorbable suture material or stainless steel hemostatic clips. Adequate hemostasis should be verified before return of the pedicle to the inguinal region. Incisions may be closed using one or two buried interrupted sutures in the subcuticular layer, or incisions may be left open to heal by second-intention healing. Closure of the incision prevents postoperative contamination with urine or feces and extrusion of fat from the incision.

Kitten castration is performed using identical techniques (closed or open techniques using spermatic cord tissues for knot tying or sutures or hemostatic clips for hemostasis) as in the adult cat. Care should be used when exteriorizing and manipulating tissues to prevent rupture or tearing of the small and fragile spermatic cord. As with adult cat castrations, scrotal incisions are left open to heal by second-intention healing.

Postoperative Considerations

During the postoperative period puppies and kittens should by monitored closely for hypoglycemia, hypothermia, pain, or dysphoria. Supplemental heat, corn syrup (if dextrose-containing intravenous fluids are not used during surgery), or additional analgesics or sedatives may be used to ensure smooth recovery from anesthesia.

Pediatric patients recover much more quickly from anesthesia than older dogs and cats and may be fed a small meal 1 to 2 hours after recovery. Puppies and kittens typically are hungry at this time and are often ready to eat and play, unlike traditional-age patients undergoing gonadectomy.

Prepubertal gonadectomy of puppies and kittens (as early as 6 weeks of age) is slowly increasing in popularity in the United States as a result of mounting evidence of the safety of the procedure on both a short- and long-term basis. Puppies and kittens undergoing prepubertal gonadectomy have shorter recovery rates, lower morbidity, and similar mortality rates compared to those neutered at a more traditional age (≥6 months of age). Long-term outcome in cats and dogs undergoing early neutering is similar to the outcome in those undergoing traditional-age neutering. As with any surgical procedure, early-age neutering is a safe procedure when appropriate attention is paid to anesthetic and surgical techniques.

References and Suggested Reading

Aronsohn MG, Faggella AM: Surgical techniques for neutering 6-to 14-week-old kittens, *J Am Vet Med Assoc* 202:53, 1993.

Duch DS et al: The effect of castration and body weight on the occurrence of the feline urological syndrome, *Feline Pract* 8:35, 1978.

Edney ATB, Smith PM: Study of obesity in dogs visiting veterinary practices in the United Kingdom, *Vet Rec* 118:391, 1986.

Faggella AM, Aronsohn MG: Anesthetic techniques for neutering 6- to 14-week-old kittens, *J Am Vet Med Assoc* 202:56, 1993.

Faggella AM, Aronsohn MG: Evaluation of anesthetic protocols for neutering 6- to 14-week-old pups, *J Am Vet Med Assoc* 205:308, 1994.

Flynn MF, Hardie EM, Armstrong J: Effect of ovariohysterectomy on maintenance energy requirements in cats, *J Am Vet Med Assoc* 209:1572, 1996.

Herron MA: A potential consequence of prepubertal feline castration, *Feline Pract* 1:17, 1971.

Herron MA: The effect of prepubertal castration on the penile urethra of the cat, *J Am Vet Med Assoc* 160:208, 1972.

Howe LM: Short-term results and complications of prepubertal gonadectomy in cats and dogs, *J Am Vet Med Assoc* 211:57, 1997.

Howe LM et al: Long-term outcome of gonadectomy performed at an early age or traditional age in cats, *J Am Vet Med Assoc* 217:1661, 2000.

Howe LM et al: Long-term outcome of gonadectomy performed at an early age or traditional age in dogs, *J Am Vet Med Assoc* 218:217, 2001.

Mahlow JC: Estimation of the proportions of dogs and cats that are surgically sterilized, *J Am Vet Med Assoc* 215:640, 1999.

Root MV, Johnstron SD, Olson PN: Effect of prepubertal and postpubertal gonadectomy on heat production measured by indirect calorimetry in male and female domestic cats, *Am J Vet Res* 57:371, 1996.

Root MV, Johnston SD, Olson PN: The effect of prepubertal and postpubertal gonadectomy on radial physeal closure in male and female domestic cats, *Vet Radiol Ultrasound* 38:42, 1997.

Root MV et al: The effects of prepubertal and postpubertal gonadectomy on penile extension and urethral diameter in the domestic cat, *Vet Radiol Ultrasound* 37:363, 1996.

Salmeri KR et al: Gonadectomy in immature dogs: effects on skeletal, physical, and behavioral development, *J Am Vet Med Assoc* 198:1193, 1991.

Stubbs WP et al: Prepubertal gonadectomy in the domestic feline: effects on skeletal, physical, and behavioral development, *Vet Surg* 22:401, 1993.

Stubbs WP et al: Effects of prepubertal gonadectomy on physical and behavioral development in cats. *J Am Vet Med Assoc* 209:1864, 1996.

CHAPTER 222

Estrus Suppression in the Bitch

PATRICK CONCANNON, *Ithaca, New York*

During the last two decades no new methods or products for estrus prevention or suppression in small animals have been introduced in North America (Concannon, 1995a; Concannon, 1995b; Concannon and Meyers-Wallen, 1991; Concannon, 1983; Burke, 1982). This is the case despite the need for more choices in contraception to address the dog and cat overpopulation problem and despite research reports on several promising new methods. In fact, contraceptive options have decreased with the recent cessation in the manufacture and sale of the commercial liquid formulation of the androgen mibolerone (Cheque Drops, Pharmacia-Upjohn) as an estrus preventive. In North America the oral progestin megestrol acetate remains the only drug marketed for suppression of ovarian cycles, and it is only approved for use in dogs; there is no contraceptive product approved for use in cats. Options available to veterinarians in Europe and some Latin American countries are less limited in terms of contraceptive progestins marketed with an indication for use in small animals. These often include proligestone and medroxyprogesterone acetate (MPA) in addition to megestrol acetate (England, 1998; Concannon, 1995a; Concannon, 1995b). Furthermore, in some countries one or more progestins is marketed with an indication for use in cats, prepubertal dogs, and adult dogs, whereas in the United States megestrol acetate is sold with an indication for use in adults dogs only.

Steroid drugs marketed for human use are sometimes discovered to have been administered as contraceptive treatments in small animals by or at the request of owners; practitioners should be aware of these and their possible application and side effects. In North America these include depot MPA and various anabolic androgens, including testosterone. Annual or semiannual administration of gonadotropin-releasing hormone (GnRH)-agonist implants can be used to suppress ovarian cycles in bitches; and the marketing of such implants with that indication in Australia, New Zealand, and Europe is expected within a few years.

The best cycle preventive measures for bitches and queens not intended for future breeding remain ovariectomy (as typically done in several European countries) or ovariohysterectomy (i.e., spaying as typically done in North America). Gonadectomy prevents subsequent uterine disease and reduces the incidence of mammary tumors in dogs, especially when performed before the first estrus (Concannon, 1995a; Concannon, 1995b; Concannon and Meyers-Wallen, 1991). Nevertheless, gonadectomy is proscribed in some countries as an unnecessary surgical insult to the animal.

STEROID CONTRACEPTIVE MECHANISM OF ACTION

Progestins

When progestins are given by serial administration or depot injection to bitches, the result is an artificial luteal phase that mimics many of the effects of the progesterone secreted during the 2-month long luteal phase that normally follows ovulation in the ovarian cycle. Likewise in cats it mimics the 20- to 40-day luteal phase that follows sterile mating or spontaneous ovulation. Many of the biologic effects of progesterone, and by extension synthetic progestins, are considered to contribute to their contraceptive action. These include an antigonadotropic action potentially resulting in lowered luteinizing hormone (LH) and follicle-stimulating hormone (FSH) concentrations; an antiestrogen action achieved by reducing the concentrations of intracellular estrogen receptors in many tissues, including those regulating gonadotropin secretion; and progestational actions on the reproductive tract occurring out of the normal sequence of the ovarian cycle, resulting in altered endometrial growth and secretion, altered cervical secretion, reduced sperm transport, and altered uterine-tube motility. In addition, progesterone and progestins can have an antiovulatory effect by depressing the preovulatory surge release of gonadotropins (LH and FSH) from the pituitary, the normal stimulus for ovulation. In dogs as in many laboratory animal species, progesterone or progestin administration at or immediately after the follicular phase peak in estrogen can facilitate and advance the preovulatory LH surge and ovulation (unpublished observations). But, when administered beginning several days or more before the peak in estrogen would have occurred, progestins typically prevent the LH surge, possibly by interfering with hypothalamic and pituitary responses to estrogen.

However, none of these actions provides an explanation of how the typical clinical administration of a progestin during anestrus causes an apparent prolongation of anestrus and prevents and delays the occurrence of a new ovarian follicular phase or an associated proestrus. Long-term progestin administration in bitches not only does not lower the systemic concentrations of LH compared to those typically observed during most of normal anestrus but may actually result in a small increase in basal LH (Colon et al., 1993; Concannon et al., 1980). Such an increase possibly may occur by partially interfering with the normal negative feedback effects of estrogen.

The negative feedback effect of progesterone during normal ovarian cycles appears to involve effects on hypothalamic neurons that regulate pulsatile GnRH release. It results in a decrease in GnRH and thus LH and FSH pulsatility and prevents the normal increase in gonadotropin pulsatility that would stimulate the next follicular phase. The same appears to be the case in dogs and probably cats subjected to contraceptive progestin treatment. The progestin prevents the increase in gonadotropin pulsatility normally required to initiate the next estrus cycle. Why in both species the effect is so prolonged following withdrawal of progestin is not understood, but it is similar to what is observed during the normal ovarian cycle, especially in dogs. In the bitch proestrus does not occur until after many weeks or months of an obligate anestrus following the end of the 7- to 10-week luteal phase and the decline in progesterone concentrations to nearly nondetectable levels (Concannon et al., 1993). Likewise in cats the 6- to 8-week luteal phase caused by a spontaneous or induced ovulation not resulting in pregnancy is followed by several weeks of anestrus and low progesterone concentrations before the next proestrus. This obligate anestrus period in dogs, cats, and other carnivores may be an evolutionary adaptation associated with being a monoestrous and/or seasonally breeding species. In both species contraceptive progestin treatment mimics a luteal phase and postpones or reestablishes the onset of anestrus.

Androgens

The contraceptive cycle–postponing effects of androgens, like those of progesterone, appear to primarily involve a negative feedback effect at the level of the hypothalamus and possibly the pituitary. Testosterone is the natural hormone produced by the testes, is secreted by the interstitial cells nested between seminiferous tubules, and is required in high concentrations locally within the tubules for normal spermatogenesis to occur. Circulating serum testosterone in males has a negative feedback action on gonadotropin secretion, reducing both LH and FSH concentrations. The contraceptive and other effects of androgens in females may be exactly the same as in males by binding to androgen receptors or may involve cross talk with other steroid receptors. Androgen receptors have been observed in estrogen target tissues, and androgen binging can result in reduced responsiveness to estrogen. The cycle-inhibiting effect of androgens may be different from that achieved by progesterone in terms of duration of effect following hormone withdrawal. Following withdrawal, androgen therapy especially is reportedly often followed by rapid return to estrus within a few weeks, whereas progestin therapy is followed by many weeks or months of anestrus (England, 1998). However, some androgen therapy such as mibolerone typically has required 2 to 3 months for return to estrus, with a range of 1 to 7 months. In addition, termination of long-term androgen use in bitches, especially with testosterone, can also result in a prolonged or even permanent posttreatment anestrus, as observed in some racing greyhound bitches.

SIDE EFFECTS OF CONTRACEPTIVE STEROIDS

Most, if not all, contraceptive progestins have been observed to result in both predictable and understandable side effects and less predictable and less understandable side effects. Undesirable side effects can occur from excessive dosing, prolonged exposure to lower doses, or an idiosyncratic sensitivity and responsiveness of some bitches to a particular regimen. These side effects have included uterine hyperstimulation, development of mammary tumors, and diabetes mellitus in both dogs and cats and gallbladder disease, growth hormone hypersecretion, and acromegaly in dogs (Concannon et al. 1980; Concannon, 1983). Stimulation of the endometrium can result in mucometra, cystic endometrial hyperplasia, and eventually pyometra. Uterine effects may be more pronounced when progestin is administered during or after stimulation by endogenous estrogen during proestrus and estrus or during the natural luteal phase. The occurrence of diabetes appears to involve insulin resistance possibly as a direct effect of the progestin. In dogs the insulin resistance is also related to increased serum growth hormone. Progestin-induced growth hormone secretion can result in signs of acromegaly of varying severity and appears to be related to a spontaneous phenomenon reported in older intact bitches. In the latter, natural luteal phase elevations in progesterone can result in waxing and then waning elevations in growth hormone, which in turn cause transient symptoms of acromegaly. Progestin-induced increased serum growth hormone concentrations appear to result from progestin-stimulated secretion of growth hormone by mammary tissue (Mol et al., 1996), although there is an increase in pituitary acidophils as well (El Etreby, 1979). Reduced adrenal size and reduced concentrations of cortisol also have been observed with high doses of progestin.

Side effects encountered with androgenic contraceptives are those expected for all androgens, including testosterone, and include increased muscle mass and strength, aggression, and clitoral hypertrophy. Anal gland inspissations and excessive lacrimation have been noted with at least one androgen, mibolerone (Sokolowski, 1978). Both androgens and progestins can result in masculinization of female fetuses if administered to pregnant bitches in error (Concannon and Meyers-Wallen, 1991).

PROGESTIN PRODUCTS AND APPLICATIONS

Megestrol Acetate Tablets

Megestrol acetate is marketed in North America as Ovaban tablets (Schering) for the prevention and postponement of proestrus and estrus in anestrus bitches and for the curtailment of proestrus and prevention of ovulation and estrus in early proestrus bitches. The product is marketed in bottles of 5- or 20-mg tablets for oral administration. The recommended dosage is 0.55 mg/kg/day (or 0.25 mg/lb/day) for 32 days in anestrus bitches. Higher dosages of 2.2 mg/kg/day (or 1 mg/lb/day) for 8 days are given to bitches already in early proestrus. The indication is for use in adult bitches for up to two successive cycles, with no indication for use in cats. In some other countries, including the United Kingdom, there is an indication for the use of megestrol acetate in pubertal dogs as well as adults. In some instances there is also an indication for use in cats. Diabetes mellitus, mammary tumors, uterine disease, and liver disease are all contraindications to the use of megestrol acetate, as is pregnancy. Bitches with an unknown or ill-defined reproductive history should be confirmed to be in anestrus by vaginal cytology and progesterone assay before treatment. Administration during pregnancy can result in masculinization of female fetuses. It is recommended that treatment should not be repeated beyond two successive cycles without allowing an intervening normal cycle.

Administration during anestrus should be initiated 1 to 2 weeks or more before the next expected proestrus. If initiated too late in anestrus, a spontaneous proestrus may occur and require changing to the higher, proestrus-regimen dosing. If treatment is started immediately before the onset of proestrus, the subsequent proestrus may occur a few weeks after withdrawal. If megestrol acetate is initiated too early in anestrus, there may be no apparent postponement of the next cycle. The next proestrus typically occurs 4 to 6 months after treatment, with a range of 1 to 7 months (Burke and Reynolds, 1975). The advantages of the oral formulation are ease of administration and administration by the owner; concerns include compliance by the owner and potential for underdosing or overdosing. The bitch's body weight should be determined with exactitude, and the precise number of tablets or partial tablets of a specific formulation to be administered each day should be provided with written instructions.

Administration of megestrol acetate in early proestrus should begin within 3 days of proestrus onset. Client education as to the signs of early proestrus is important. A bitch with a normal proestrus usually lasting less than 4 days or longer than 20 days is reportedly not a good candidate for Ovaban treatment during proestrus (Harding, 1981). Early proestrus status can be confirmed by vaginal cytology showing less than 50% superficial cells, increasing rather than decreasing vulval turgidity, and serum progesterone concentrations less than 0.5 ng/ml. Proestrus treatment with megestrol acetate should be combined with isolation of the bitch from males for 3 to 8 days and until the end of serosanguineous discharge, following the recommendation of the manufacturer. The suppression of proestrus symptoms occurs by 3 to 8 days after initiation of treatment. The subsequent proestrus is expected in 4 to 6 months but ranged from 1 to 7 months in clinical trials. Administration too late in proestrus can likely result in induction of ovulation, failure to prevent ovulation, and/or the occurrence of estrus.

Megestrol acetate is currently the only cycle preventive or estrus preventive marketed for dogs in the United States and is approved for use in two successive cycles. No product is marketed for cats in the United States.

In the United Kingdom similar dosages of megestrol acetate (Ovarid, Malinckrodt Veterinary) are recommended, including 0.5 mg/kg/day for 40 days in anestrus, 2 mg/kg/day for 8 days in early proestrus. However, when used in a pubertal proestrus, in bitches with a history of pseudopregnancy, or in bitches housed with other bitches and susceptible to pheromone effects, the recommendation has been to use a dose of 2 mg/kg for 4 days and then 0.5 mg/kg for 16 days. It is important that the onset of proestrus be accurately determined when it is used during proestrus, especially in first-cycle bitches (Bigbee and Hennessy, 1977). The treatment of anestrus bitches also includes the option to continue treating with lower doses of 0.2 mg/kg twice weekly for up to 4 months after the initial 40 days of treatment but then allowing a normal estrus to occur before retreating. Or the 40-day regimen can be followed with an early proestrus treatment at the next cycle.

In other countries generic megestrol acetate is marketed under many brand names for use in dogs and/or cats in tablets of various content (5, 10, or 20 mg), sometimes of a single content (10 mg). The 10-mg tablets can make it difficult to accurately dose smaller animals. The drug should be administered according to the manufacturer's recommendation unless there is reason to assume that a lower dose or shorter period of treatment will be effective based on recommendations of other manufacturers or review articles. Side effects in dogs most frequently mentioned by manufacturers include increased appetite and weight gain, decreased aggression, increased docility, and mammary enlargement. Megestrol acetate tablets marketed as human drugs may also be encountered (Megace, Bristol-Meyers Squibb).

Megestrol acetate at the higher proestrus dose has also been proposed and used to prevent the induction of proestrus at the onset of a treatment with a GnRH-agonist subcutaneous implant administered for long-term estrus suppression (Verstegen, Onclin, and Boisrame, 2001).

Megestrol Acetate in Cats

Ovaban is not indicated for use in cats as marketed in the United States. The drug was reported to prevent estrus in cats when administered at 5 mg/cat for 3 days followed by doses of 2.5 or 5 mg/cat once weekly, depending on size, for 10 weeks (Houdeshell and Hennessey, 1977). In the United Kingdom megestrol acetate has been marketed with an indication for long-term prevention of estrus cycles in cats, using 2.5 mg/cat weekly for up to 18 months. Presumably the drug should be initiated in interestrus or late in seasonal anestrus in preference to treating in proestrus or estrus to reduce the risk of uterine complications. Potential side effects include uterine disease; diabetes; adrenal suppression; and mammary complications, including mammary enlargement and mammary tumors. In countries where its use in cats is extralabel, a signed release should be obtained.

Medroxyprogesterone Acetate Injections

A depot injectable formulation of MPA was marketed as a dog contraceptive (Promone) in North America several decades ago but was removed from the market because of a high incidence of uterine disease. Currently an injectable depot formulation of MPA is marketed as a human contraceptive product (Depo-Provera) and has been administered to bitches by owners and in animals imported from Europe. Injectable depot MPA is widely marketed as a veterinary drug in Europe and other locales under several trade names (Promone-E, Pharmacia-Upjohn; Perlutex Injection, Leo Laboratories; Supprestal, Vetoquinol) with an indication for prevention of ovarian cycles in bitches during anestrus and/or in cats. Various regimens for dosage and injection intervals have been recommended for bitches; they include 2.5 to 3 mg/kg every 5 months and 50 mg/bitch every 6 months. Side effects appear to be dose dependent, and dosing on a body-weight basis would be more appropriate than dosing on a per animal basis. Published dose-response studies in dogs have typically involved nonclinical, high doses in comparison to doses assumed to be near the minimal effective dose, as part of toxicity testing for human use. Side effects commonly seen with the higher doses or long-term treatment with lower doses include cystic endometrial hyperplasia, pyometra, acromegaly, gallbladder calculi and mucosal hyperplasia, and mammary tumors (Concannon et al., 1980). The mammary tumors were mostly benign, but adenocarcinomas have been observed. Development of diabetes also has been reported. Injection doses considered to be near the minimal effective dose and clinically more appropriate than higher doses are 2 mg/kg every 3 months and 2.5 mg/kg every 5 months. MPA has also been used in cats. Side effects in cats include an increased incidence of mammary adenocarcinoma (Hernandez, Fernandez, and Gage, 1975) and diabetes. An MPA dose that has been used in cats is 2 mg/kg injected every 5 months. If used in dogs, depot MPA should only be administered during confirmed anestrus. Administration during midproestrus or late proestrus (or early estrus) can result in ovulation, in pregnancy and possibly failure of parturition, in pyometra, or in pseudopregnancy. Directions by some marketers of MPA to treat animals are based on a single dose per animal or on doses for a limited number of body-weight ranges and should be replaced by doses based on body weight. Directions to use doses greater than those mentioned previously likewise would seem inappropriate, although there is some anecdotal evidence that the same progestin from different manufacturers may have different biopotencies per unit of product weight.

Proligestone Injections

Proligestone is available as a depot injectable progestin in Europe (Delvosteron, Intervet; Covinan, Intervet) and some other locations, with indications for estrus prevention in female dogs, cats, and ferrets. It is not marketed in North America. Doses of 10 to 33 mg/kg, varying inversely with body weight and including 17.5 mg/kg for 20-kg dogs and 10 mg/kg/day for all bitches 60 kg and larger, are given to bitches at 0, 3 and 7 months of treatment and subsequently at 5-month intervals. There is also an indication for its administration during proestrus to prevent ovulation and estrus. Initial studies suggested that proligestone treatment need not be restricted to any stage of the cycle and did not increase the incidence of mammary tumors or uterine disease (Concannon, 1995a; Hegstad and Johnston, 1989). However, more recently various reports and anecdotal evidence have suggested that uterine disease, including pyometra, mammary tumors, and acromegaly, may be side effects of proligestone, as with other progestins, and that administration is best initiated during anestrus with an appreciation of potential occurrences of side effects similar to those observed with other progestins (Mol et al., 1996; Knottenbelt and Herrtage, 2002).

Other Progestin Formulations

Oral formulations of MPA are marketed as human drugs in the United States (Provera, Pharmacia Upjohn; Farlutal, Pharmacia Upjohn) and also as veterinary drugs in other countries (Perlutex Vet Tablets, Leo Laboratories). Oral MPA is marketed in the United Kingdom with an indication for use in cats (Perlutex). A suggested dosing regimen in dogs is reported to be 10 mg/bitch for 4 days and then 5 mg/bitch for 12 days, doubling the doses for bitches weighing over 15 kg (England, 1998). As with any drug, dosing on a body-weight basis could more appropriately be done by providing a dose per kilogram of body weight or by providing doses for five different body-weight ranges.

Steroid Implants

Subcutaneous Silastic (Dow Corning) implants that release a progestin have been used experimentally, especially for the contraception of exotic carnivores in zoos. Such implants can have a functional life of up to several years. Steroids that have been incorporated into such implants have included progesterone, melengestrol acetate, megestrol acetate, and levonorgestrel (Baldwin et al., 1994; Concannon, 1995; Concannon and Meyers-Wallen, 1991). None are marketed commercially. Recently a Silastic implant formulated to steadily release natural progesterone in low doses was reported to have contraceptive efficacy without side effects in small and large domestic bitches and in cats over a 4-year treatment period, with treatment initiated during anestrus in all cases (Verstegen Onclin, and Boisrame, 2004). However, plans for commercial development have not been reported.

ANDROGEN PRODUCTS

Natural androgens, including testosterone, and synthetic androgens are by definition all masculinizing and anabolic steroids, and effects are dose dependent. None are marketed with an indication for prevention of ovarian cycles in small animals in the United States, and none can be considered to be recommended or appropriate. Several are marketed in Europe and elsewhere with such indications.

Mibolerone

The androgen mibolerone, a specific androgen receptor agonist, until recently was marketed in the United States for cycle prevention in dogs (Concannon and Meyers-Wallen, 1991). The liquid formulation for oral administration was recommended at a dosage of 30, 60, 120 or 180 mcg/day continuously for up to 2 years, with the dose depending on body weight (<12, 12 to 23, 23 to 45, or <45 kg, respectively) and all Alsatians or Alsatian-derived bitches receiving the highest dosage (Sokolowski, 1978). Administration initiated later than 1 month before the next expected estrus could result in failure to prevent proestrus. It was never marketed for use in cats because of potential effects on the clitoris, liver, and thyroid. Mibolerone is no longer marketed for veterinary use in North America, presumably because it has been implicated frequently as a drug abused by athletes to enhance strength. Like all androgens, mibolerone has anabolic effects on skeletal muscle and also had become a favored contraceptive regimen in working dogs and racing sled dogs. It is listed as a Controlled Substance in the legislation of several states.

Mibolerone liquid (100 mcg/ml) for oral administration is available from some veterinary compounding pharmacies at a cost approximating $100 per 5000 to 60,000 mcg, making the cost not unreasonable for small and medium-sized bitches. Consideration should be given to confirmation of anestrus status before treatment initiation, potential masculinization of fetuses in pregnant bitches, possible increased incidence in ovarian fibromas with long-term use, and potential for anal gland inspissation with overdosage. Another extralabel use of mibolerone is to postpone estrus briefly (i.e., for 3 to 6 months in bitches with a history of abnormally short estrus cycles).

Testosterone

Testosterone in various chemical states and formulations and several other androgens are marketed as anabolic steroids for use in human geriatric, surgical, and anemia patients, among others, and are also subject to abuse. Testosterone particularly has been used by animal owners to effect cycle prevention and contraception in dogs used in sporting events, including sled dogs and racing greyhounds. In greyhounds weekly intramuscular injections of testosterone propionate at 110 mg/dog have been used to prevent ovarian cycles (Gannon, 1976). Oral administration of 25 mg of methyl testosterone once weekly for up to 5 years has also been used in greyhounds (Burke, 1982). Masculinizing and anabolic side effects are common. Permanent or prolonged anestrus may be a complication after treatment. The extent to which anabolic steroids are used in sporting dogs is not known. Androgen use should be considered as a possible complication in racing bitches with clitoral hypertrophy or anal gland inspissation.

In Europe available androgen products used for pet contraception include methyl testosterone and mesterolone tablets for oral administration and injectable solutions of testosterone propionate, testosterone phenylpropionate, and mixtures of testosterone esters. As England (1998) reviewed, the most common use of androgens as a cycle preventive administered during anestrus is the depot injection of mixed testosterone esters (25 mg/kg), typically every 4 to 6 weeks, often supplemented with oral dosages of methyl testosterone at 0.25 to 0.50 mg/kg.

GONADOTROPIN-RELEASING HORMONE–AGONIST IMPLANTS

GnRH-agonist (deslorelin)-releasing implants that result in the down-regulation of LH and FISH secretion and suppression of gonadal function in male dogs are currently marketed in Australia and New Zealand for use in male dogs only and are scheduled for marketing in Europe in the near future. The GnRH agonist in the circulation binds to GnRH receptors on the pituitary cells and, after an initial transient phase of stimulation of LH and FSH release, the agonist down-regulates gonadotrope cell function and chronically prevents release of gonadotropins in amounts needed to support normal gonadal function.

The application of this same technology for chronic contraception in female dogs and cats is likely to see approval in some countries within the next few years. Continuous treatment with down-regulating (i.e., desensitizing) doses of a GnRH-agonist initiated in young (3.5 to 5 months) prepubertal bitches has been shown to be 100% effective in suppressing ovarian cycles throughout treatments of 1 year and longer. It is without any obvious side effects and allows for a return to a normal puberty (albeit at an adult age) and fertility following implant removal (Rubion et al., 2006; Trigg et al., 2001; Vickery et al., 1989; Concannon, Montanez, and Frank, 1988). In adult bitches and in prepubertal bitches 7 months of age or older, the same treatment is equally effective long term and likewise reversible, except that there is typically an initial ovarian-stimulation response that often results in a proestrus and estrus during the first 2 weeks after treatment onset. The induced cycle involves increased estrogen secretion in response to the initial stimulation of LH and FSH release and can result in a spontaneous ovulation-inducting LH surge and fertile ovulation. However, pregnancies that result from breeding at the induced estrus typically fail to proceed much beyond implantation because of abnormal luteal function that occurs during continued GnRH-agonist administration. Interestingly, the same technology, with discontinuation of treatment following estrus induction and mating in adult bitches, has been used experimentally to synchronize pregnancies and treat prolonged anestrus in research dogs.

Clinical trials on two commercial long-term GnRH-agonist implant formulations in female dogs are being conducted in the expectation of gaining marketing approval for estrus suppression in bitches. These products include (1) a revised formulation of the biodegradable deslorelin-releasing implant currently marked for male dogs in Australia (Suprelorin, Peptech Animal Health), and (2) a nonbiodegradable azagly-nafarelin releasing implant (Gonazon CR, Intervet). Single Gonazon implants administered once to prepubertal bitches at 4 to 5 months of age prevented puberty throughout the 12-month treatment, and normal estrus occurred at variable times following implant removal. Such products are likely to gain marketing approval for use in bitches in several countries because of the lack of side effects and the large margin of safety shown for these and a variety of other GnRH-agonists developed for human use. Interestingly, Gonazon-induced suppression of puberty and the resulting delay in puberty onset to 18 months of age and older had no effect on growth or body weight measured at 22 months of age when compared to untreated control bitches (Rubion et al., 2006). The investigators speculate that perhaps weight gains sometimes associated with surgical spaying are less likely to occur with the GnRH-agonist mode of contraception.

The undesirable GnRH-agonist side effect of estrus induction in adult bitches is typically not seen when bitches are treated during early or midmetestrus (diestrus) and when progesterone is above 5 ng/ml. Some reports suggest that the estrus induction effect can be suppressed or inhibited by pretreatment with megestrol acetate at 2 mg/kg but not 1 mg/kg daily for 2 weeks (but not 1 week) before and 1 week after initiation of agonist treatment (Verstegen, Onclin, and Boisrame, 2001).

THE FUTURE OF SMALL ANIMAL CONTRACEPTION

Advances in methods to terminate pregnancy, including the use of progesterone antagonists and moderate doses of prostaglandin $F_{2\alpha}$ in combination with moderate doses of dopamine agonists have occurred within the last several years. Similar advances in the clinically applicable use of new drugs or technologies for long-term or permanent inhibition of ovarian cycles have not emerged except for the previously mentioned use of GnRH-agonist implants for suppressing LH and FSH secretion and thereby preventing recurrence of ovarian cycles. Nevertheless, several alternative technologies are being tested currently, including immunization against GnRH (Singh, 1985; Jung et al., 2005) or ovarian zona pellucida proteins (Srivastava et al. 2002; Mahi-Brown et al., 1985) and the administration of GnRH (or other reproductive hormones) conjugated to cytotoxins and thus targeting the destruction of pituitary gonadotroph cells (or other cell types) as cells required for normal cycles and/or fertility (Qi et al., 2004).

In the near term in the United States the only option for pharmacologic prevention of ovarian cycles in small animals while following the indicated use of the approved product(s) involves the oral administration of megestrol acetate to bitches in doses and durations appropriate for either anestrus bitches or for bitches already in proestrus. The use of megestrol acetate in cats, as indicated for some European formulations of the same drug, is an extralabel use in North America and should only be done in conjunction with a release-and-consent document signed by the cat owner. In other countries there can often be a greater choice, including one or more depot injectable progestins, one or more oral formulations with indications and dosages recommended for both dogs and cats, and in the near future GnRH-agonist–releasing implants for use in female and male dogs and cats. However, in cases involving steroids the veterinary practitioner should determine the time of the cycle for administration and calculate the appropriate dose on a body-weight basis by using all information available from the research and review literature and from other manufacturers. The use of cycle-suppressing hormone therapy should be proposed only for animals intended for breeding within 1 to 3 years. Animals not intended for breeding are best managed by surgical sterilization.

References and Suggested Reading

Baldwin CJ et al: The contraceptive effects of levonorgestrel in the domestic cat lab, *Anim Sci* 44:261, 1994.

Bigbee HG, Hennessy PW: Megesterol acetate for postponing estrus in first heat bitches, *Vet Med Small Anim Clin* 72:1727, 1977.

Burke TJ: Pharmacologic control of estrus in bitch and queen, *Vet Clin North Am Small Anim Pract* 12:79, 1982.

Burke TJ, Reynolds HA Jr: Megestrol acetate for estrus postponement in the bitch, *J Am Vet Med Assoc* 167:285, 1975.

Colon J et al: Effects of contraceptive doses of the progestagen megestrol acetate on LH and FSH secretion in female dogs, *J Reprod Fertil* 47(suppl):519, 1993(abstract).

Concannon PW: Reproductive physiology and endocrine patterns of the bitch. In Kirk RW, editor: *Current veterinary therapy, small animal practice VIII*, Philadelphia, 1983, Saunders, p 886.

Concannon P: Reproductive endocrinology, contraception and pregnancy termination in dogs. In Ettinger S, Feldman E, editors: *Textbook of veterinary internal medicine*, Philadelphia, 1995a, Saunders, p 1625.

Concannon PW: Contraception in the dog. In *The veterinary annual*, Oxford, UK, 1995b, Blackwell Scientific, p 177.

Concannon PW, Meyers-Wallen VN: Current and proposed methods for contraception and termination of pregnancy in dogs and cats, *J Am Vet Med Assoc* 198:1214, 1991.

Concannon PW, Montanez A, Frank D: Suppression of LH secretion by constant infusion of GnRH agonist in ovariectomized dogs and prolonged contraception of prepubertal bitches by constant subcutaneous administration of GnRH-agonist, Proceedings of the 11th International Congress on Animal Reproduction and Artificial Insemination, 1988, vol 4 p 427.

Concannon PW et al: Growth hormone, prolactin and cortisol in dogs developing mammary nodules and an acromegaly-like appearance during treatment with medroxyprogesterone acetate, *Endocrinology* 106(4):1173, 1980.

Concannon PW et al: Synchronous delayed oestrus in beagle bitches given infusions of GnRH superagonist following withdrawal of progesterone implants, *J Reprod Fertil* 47(suppl):522, 1993.

El Etreby MF: Effect of cyproterone acetate, levonorgestrel and progesterone on adrenal glands and reproductive organs in the beagle bitch, *Cell Tissue Res* 200:229, 1979.

England G: Pharmacological control of reproduction in the bitch. In Simpson G, England GE, Harvey MJ, editors: *Manual of small animal reproduction and neonatology*, Birmingham, UK, 1998, British Small Animal Association, p 198.

Gannon J: Clinical aspects of the oestrus cycle in the greyhound, *Racing Greyhound* 1:12, 1976.

Harding RB: The use of megestrol acetate in oestrus control in dogs, *Post Acad Onderstepoort* 13:30, 1981.

Hegstad RL, Johnston SD: Use of a rapid qualitative ELISA technique (Biometallics, Inc) to determine serum progesterone concentrations in the bitch, *Theriogenology* 277, 1989.

Hernandez FJ, Fernandez BB, Gage PA: Feline mammary carcinoma and progestogens. *Feline Pract* 5:45, 1975.

Houdeshell JW, Hennessey PW: Megestrol acetate for control of estrus in the cat, *Vet Med Small Anim Clin* 72:1727, 1977.

Jung MJ et al: Induction of castration by immunization of male dogs with recombinant gonadotropin-releasing hormone (GnRH)–canine distemper virus (CDV) T helper cell epitope p35, *J Vet Sci* 6:21, 2005.

Knottenbelt CM, Herrtage ME: Use of proligestone in the management of three German shepherd dogs with pituitary dwarfism, *J Small Anim Pract* 43:164, 2002.

Mahi-Brown CA et al: Fertility control in the bitch by active immunization with porcine zonae pellucidae: use of different adjuvants and patterns of estradiol and progesterone level in estrous cycles, *Biol Reprod* 32:761, 1985.

Mol JA et al: New insights in the molecular mechanism of progestin-induced proliferation of mammary epithelium: induction of the local biosynthesis of growth hormone (GH) in the mammary glands of dogs, cats and humans, *J Steroid Biochem Mol Biol* 57(1):67, 1996.

Qi L et al: Binding and cytotoxicity of conjugated and recombinant fusion proteins targeted to the gonadotropin-releasing hormone receptor, *Cancer Res* 64:2090, 2004.

Rubion S et al: Treatment with a subcutaneous GnRH agonist containing controlled release device reversibly prevents puberty in bit *Theriogenology* 66:1651, 2006.

Singh V: Active immunization of female dogs against luteinizing hormone–releasing hormone (LHRH) and its effects on ovarian steroids and estrus suppression, *Indian J Exp Biol* 23:667, 1985.

Sokolowski JH: The evaluation of efficacy of mibolerone for estrus prevention in the bitch, *Proc Cheque Canine Contraception* B 24, 1978.

Srivastava N et al: Evaluation of the immunocontraceptive potential of *Escherichia coli*–expressed recombinant dog ZP2 and ZP3 in a homologous animal model, *Reproduction* 123:847, 2002.

Trigg TE et al: Use of a GnRH analogue implant to produce reversible long-term suppression of reproductive function in male and female domestic dogs, *J Reprod Fertil* 57(suppl):255, 2001.

Verstegen, J, Onclin, K, and Boisrame, B: Contraception of dogs and cats using a silastic-based progestin implant: an efficient alternative to immunocontraception, Abstract, Progam of the Fifth International Symposium of Canine Feline Reproduction, Sao Paulo, Brazil, p 58, 2004.

Vickery BH et al: Use of potent LHRH analogues for chronic contraception and pregnancy termination in dogs, *J Reprod Fertil* 39(suppl):175, 1989.

Wright PJ et al: Suppression of the oestrous responses of bitches to the GnRH analogue deslorelin by progestin, *J Reprod Fertil* 57(suppl):263, 2001.

CHAPTER 223

Canine Pregnancy Termination

BRUCE E. EILTS, *Baton Rouge, Louisiana*

If a perfect pregnancy termination drug existed, it could be given at any stage of estrus or pregnancy, it would be 100% effective, it would cause no vaginal discharge, it would have no side effects, it would not impair future fertility, it would be readily available, and it would be inexpensive. Unfortunately such a drug does not yet exist. In cases in which the bitch is not a valuable breeding animal the client should be counseled that the best option to terminate the pregnancy and prevent future pregnancies is ovariohysterectomy. The drugs available for pregnancy terminations are discussed under the general categories of those that can be used during estrus and those that can be used after pregnancy is confirmed. A comprehensive list of drugs to terminate pregnancy is not presented; however, the drugs most commonly available in the United States are discussed.

DRUGS USED DURING ESTRUS

The only drugs available to terminate pregnancy during estrus are the estrogens. The action of estrogens is not completely known; however, it is believed that they block ova transport or prevent implantation. The use of estrogens for mismate management is cited in many texts and by many academicians as being unsafe to the extent of being malpractice; however, little published data substantiate these statements. Estrogens should be used only during estrus because their use during diestrus significantly increases the chance of inducing a pyometra. A vaginal cytology examination having 90% to 100% cornified cells shows that the bitch is truly in estrus; whereas, if the cells are not cornified, the bitch is not in estrus. Since there are potential side effects such as prolonged estrus, pyometra, and aplastic anemia (pancytopenia), it should be documented that the bitch was actually bred based on owner observation of a mating or laboratory identification or the presence of sperm cells in a vaginal swab. Sperm cells can be identified in 100% of bitches mated within 24 hours and 75% of bitches mated within 48 hours by placing the tip of the vaginal cytology swab into a tube containing 0.5 ml saline for 10 minutes, squeezing the swab dry into a tube and centrifuging the fluid at 2000 × g for 10 minutes, and finally staining the sediment (Whitacre et al., 1992).

Estradiol cypionate (ECP, Pharmacia) was shown to have 100% efficacy and no side effects during the study period when administered at a dose of 44 mcg/kg intramuscularly one time during estrus; however, a 25% (1/4) incidence of pyometra was seen when administered during diestrus (Bowen et al., 1985). Estradiol benzoate (Oestradiol Benzoate, Intervet) at a dose of 0.01 mg/kg

intramuscularly at 3 and 5 days (and occasionally 7 days) after mating in 358 bitches resulted in only 4.5% (16/358) of the bitches actually whelping; in none of the bitches was bone marrow aplasia reported. The 7.3% incidence of pyometra reported was not different from the normal prevalence reported as 2% to 10% (Sutton, Geary, and Bergman, 1997). Administration of diethyl stilbestrol is not effective as a mismate therapy (Bowen et al., 1985).

I do not encourage estrogen use routinely because alternative treatments after the bitch is diagnosed pregnant are probably better; however, their use in not unconditionally condemned as malpractice.

DRUGS USED DURING CONFIRMED PREGNANCY

If the bitch is mated or thought to have been mated, it is best to wait and perform a pregnancy diagnosis before proceeding to terminate pregnancy. Even though conception rates in controlled breeding situations resulted in a pregnancy rate of about 90% when only a single mating was allowed on any day of estrus (up to the last 2 days of estrus) (Holst and Phemister, 1974), only 38% of bitches presented for mismate may actually be pregnant (Feldman et al., 1993). A pregnancy examination should be performed at least 30 to 40 days after the last possible breeding to minimize false-negative diagnoses caused by errors in calculating the gestation duration from a mating that occurred early in estrus. Only if a bitch is pregnant should therapy be instituted. Drugs that terminate pregnancy can cause luteal demise by direct luteolytic action, inhibiting prolactin synthesis, acting as a progesterone inhibitor, or unknown mechanisms.

Prostaglandins work by lysing the corpora lutea. The natural $PGF_{2\alpha}$ (Lutalyse, Pharmacia) given at a dose of 0.1 to 0.25 mg/kg BID or TID subcutaneously is very effective at terminating pregnancy. A protocol found to have the fewest side effects is $PGF_{2\alpha}$ administered at a dose of 0.1 mg/kg every 8 hours subcutaneously for 2 days and then 0.2 mg/kg every 8 hours subcutaneously until abortion is complete (Feldman et al., 1993). Abortion is usually complete within 9 days, but some bitches abort fetuses and still have live fetuses after 9 days. It is extremely important to continue the treatments until abortion is complete. Side effects include vomiting, diarrhea, and possibly circulatory collapse. The side effects usually subside within 20 minutes, but the bitch should be monitored carefully during this time. To minimize caloric loss, bitches should be fed at least 1 hour after treatment. To shorten the treatment period required to induce abortion with natural prostaglandin, a combination of prostaglandin at a dose of 0.1 mg/kg TID subcutaneously for 2 days and then at a dose of 0.2 mg/kg TID subcutaneously to effect was administered with misoprostol (Cytolec, Pharmacia) at a dose of 1 to 3 mcg/kg SID deposited into the cranial vaginal vault. The mean time to complete abortion using this combination was 5 days compared to a mean of 7 days for prostaglandin alone (Davidson, Nelson, and Feldman, 1997).

Synthetic prostaglandins are more potent and have fewer side effects than natural prostaglandins. Cloprostenol and fluprostenol (Equimate, Bayer) are both effective for inducing abortion (Jackson, Furr, and Hutchinson, 1982; Shille, Dorsey, and Thatcher, 1984). Cloprostenol (Estrumate, Schering-Plough) at a dose of 1 to 2.5 mcg/kg SID subcutaneously for 4 to 5 days was 100% effective at inducing abortion after a 4- to 7-day treatment regimen, and the side effects were noted to be minimal to none at a 1-mcg/kg SID subcutaneous dose (Verstgen, 2000). Once-daily treatments provide an advantage over the every-8-hour treatments required when using the natural prostaglandin. Hospitalization and/or frequent injections add greatly to the client cost when using prostaglandins as abortifacients.

The dopaminergic drugs are prolactin inhibitors. Prolactin inhibitors currently available include bromocriptine and cabergoline. Bromocriptine (Parlodel, Sandoz) administered at a dose of 62.5 mcg/kg BID orally to dogs at 43 to 45 days after ovulation resulted in only two of four bitches aborting; side effects included emesis and loose stools (Wichtel et al., 1990). Because the dose is so low and the tablets contain so much active drug, the bromocriptine tablets can be crushed and dissolved in water to ease dosing. Cabergoline (Dostinex, Pharmacia) at a dose of 1.65 mcg/kg SID subcutaneously for 5 to 6 days at 25 to 40 days after the first mating resulted in abortion for all (5/5) bitches greater than 40 days' gestation but only for 50% (1/4 at 25 days and 4/6 at 30 days) of those less than 40 days (Onclin et al., 1993). Side effects were minimal, and bitches that aborted were bred successfully after treatment. Only an oral 0.5-mg tablet of cabergoline is available in the United States; when given at a dose of 160 mcg orally to a 32-kg German shepherd dog after 40 days of gestation, it resulted in abortion after 7 days with no side effects (Arbeiter and Flatscher, 1996). Although cabergoline is not very expensive for each dose, it may be difficult to administer because the tablets are 0.5 mg and the dose for a 10-kg dog is only 0.05 mg. An oral solution can be made to dissolve and dilute the tablets. Even though each dose of cabergoline may be only about $1.80, an initial investment of around $145 is necessary to purchase the minimum package.

In an effort to reduce the side effects and increase the efficacy of prostaglandins and prolactin inhibitors, a combination of the two has been used. Cloprostenol at a dose of 1 or 2.5 mcg/kg SID subcutaneously in combination with cabergoline at a dose of 1.65 mcg/kg SID subcutaneously for 5 days from midgestation induced abortion with no adverse side effects at the low dose (Onclin, Silva, and Verstegen, 1995). Cabergoline at a dose of 5 mcg/kg SID orally 1 hour after cloprostenol at a dose of 1 mcg/kg every 48 hours subcutaneously caused fetal death with no side effects after a mean of three injections (9 days) when started 25 days after the luteinizing hormone peak (Onclin and Verstegen, 1996). Treatments of cabergoline at a dose of 5 mcg/kg SID orally for 10 days combined with either a single cloprostenol injection of 2.5 mcg/kg subcutaneously at the start of the treatment or two doses of 1 mcg/kg subcutaneously at the start of the treatment and 4 days later were successful at inducing resorption. Similarly bromocriptine administered at a dose of 30 mcg/kg TID orally for 10 days plus either a single dose of 2.5 mcg/kg subcutaneously of cloprostenol or two doses subcutaneously of 1 mcg/kg cloprostenol was also successful at inducing resorption (Onclin and Verstegen, 1999). All bitches in the aforementioned study became pregnant during the subsequent estrus cycle, which occurred sooner than normally anticipated.

The antiprogesterone compound mifepristone, more commonly known as RU486 or RU 38486 for its use in preventing human pregnancies, administered at a dose of 2.5 mg/kg BID orally for 4.5 days starting at day 32 of gestation resulted in 100% (5/5) of the bitches having pregnancy loss around 3 days after treatment initiation, with no side effects (Concannon, Yeager, and Concannon, 1990). Doses as low as 8.3 mg/kg and up to 20 mg/kg SID orally for one or two treatments resulted in abortion within 2 to 11 days at days 35 to 39 of pregnancy (Linde-Forsberg, Kindahl, and Madej, 1992). Mifepristone (Mifeprex, Danco) is only available as a human-labeled 200-mg tablet in the United States and can cost as much $90 a dose for a 10-kg dog; an initial purchase of $270 is required to purchase a package of the drug. Aglipristone (Alizine, Virbac) is another progesterone blocker that is available in France, Norway, and Sweden but not in the United States to terminate pregnancy in the bitch. Two doses of 0.33 ml/kg SID subcutaneously for 2 days caused uncomplicated abortions within 14 days in 94.4% (117/124) of bitches after 26 days of pregnancy (Fieni et al., 2001). A brown mucoid vaginal discharge was seen 24 hours before fetal expulsion, and other side effects included slight depression, transitory anorexia, and mammary gland congestion.

Although the mechanism of action is not completely known, dexamethasone was effective at inducing fetal resorption from midgestation with the use of a 9.5-day dosage schedule as follows: 0.2 mg/kg orally BID for 7 days, 0.16 mg/kg orally on the morning of the eighth day, 0.12 mg/kg orally in the evening of the eighth day, 0.08 mg/kg orally in the morning of the ninth day, 0.04 mg/kg orally in the evening of the ninth day, and 0.02 mg/kg orally the morning of the tenth day. Pregnancies less than 40 days generally had no fetuses expelled, and the majority had no external signs of pregnancy loss except for a mild vaginal discharge seen in about 34% (26/75) of the bitches that resorbed fetuses (Zone et al., 1995; Wanke et al., 1997). Abortion or resorption generally was complete 10 to 23 days after the treatment started (Wanke et al., 1997). The main side effects of dexamethasone treatment included anorexia; polydipsia; and polyuria, which usually began around 2 to 3 days after treatment started, was greatest 4 to 5 days later, and then subsided 3 to 4 days after the termination of treatment. Successful pregnancies were obtained in 18 of 20 bitches bred during the first estrus after treatment and 2 of 2 on the second estrus. At my institution an oral dose of 0.2 mg/kg BID until fetal resorption occurs is used, with no tapering of the dose. I have observed no more than the anticipated normal side effects from not tapering the dose. Dexamethasone eliminates most of the side effects seen with other drugs and avoids the requirement for hospitalization or office visits for injections. Since dexamethasone is inexpensive, readily available, can be administered easily by clients, is effective, and has few side effects, it is my choice for terminating pregnancy in the bitch.

Several other drugs have been used to terminate pregnancy in the bitch, including tamoxifen citrate (Taxol, Bristol-Meyers Squibb), which acts as an estrogen; epostane, which inhibits steroid synthesis by inhibition of 3β hydroxysteroid dehydrogenase; and Δ5-4 isomerase and isoquinolones L-12717 (Lotifren). These are either not efficacious or not available in the United States.

References and Suggested Reading

Arbeiter K, Flatscher C: Induction of abortion in the bitch using cabergoline (Galastop), *Kleintierprax* 41:747, 1996.

Bowen RA et al: Efficacy and toxicity of estrogens commonly used to terminate canine pregnancy, *J Am Vet Med Assoc* 186:783, 1985.

Concannon PW, Yeager A, Concannon PW: Termination of pregnancy and induction of premature luteolysis by the antiprogestagen, mifepristone in dogs, *J Reprod Fertil* 88: 99, 1990.

Davidson AP, Nelson RW, Feldman EC: Induction of abortion in 9 bitches with intravaginal misoprostol and parenteral $PGF_{2\alpha}$, *J Vet Intern Med* 11:123, 1997.

Feldman EC et al: Prostaglandin induction of abortion in pregnant bitches after misalliance, *J Am Vet Med Assoc* 202:1855, 1993.

Fieni F et al: Clinical use of anti-progestins in the bitch. In Concannon PW, England G, Verstegen J, editors: *Recent advances in small animal reproduction*, Ithaca, 2001, p A1219.0201.

Holst PA, Phemister RD: Onset of diestrus in the beagle bitch: definition and significance, *Am J Vet Res* 35:401, 1974.

Jackson PS, Furr BJA, Hutchinson FG: A preliminary study of pregnancy termination in the bitch with slow-release formulations of prostaglandin analogues, *J Small Anim Pract* 23:287, 1982.

Linde-Forsberg C, Kindahl H, Madej A: Termination of mid-term pregnancy in the dog with oral RU 486, *J Small Anim Pract* 33:331, 1992, available at http://www.ivis.org/advances/Concannon/fieni/chapterfrm.asp.

Onclin K, Verstegen JP: Practical use of a combination of a dopamine agonist and a synthetic prostaglandin analogue to terminate unwanted pregnancy in dogs, *J Small Anim Pract* 37:211, 1996.

Onclin K, Verstegen JP: Comparisons of different combinations of analogues of $PGF_{2\alpha}$ and dopamine agonists for the termination of pregnancy in dogs, *Vet Rec* 144:416, 1999.

Onclin K, Silva LDM, Verstegen JP: Termination of unwanted pregnancy in dogs with the dopamine agonist, cabergoline, in combination with a synthetic analog of PGF2Alpha, either cloprostenol or alphaprostol, *Theriogenology* 43:813, 1995.

Onclin K et al: Luteotrophic action of prolactin in dogs and the effects of a dopamine agonist, cabergoline, *J Reprod Fertil* 47(suppl):403, 1993.

Shille VM, Dorsey D, Thatcher MJ: Induction of abortion in the bitch with a synthetic prostaglandin analog, *Am J Vet Res* 45:1295, 1984.

Sutton DJ, Geary MR, Bergman JGHE: Prevention of pregnancy in bitches following unwanted mating—a clinical trial using low-dose estradiol benzoate, *J Reprod Fertil* 51(suppl):239, 1997.

Verstgen JP: Overview of mismating for the bitch. In Bonagura JD, editor: *Current veterinary therapy XIII (small animal practice)*, Philadelphia, 2000, Saunders, p 947.

Wanke M et al: Clinical use of dexamethasone for termination of unwanted pregnancy in dogs, *J Reprod Fertil* 51(suppl):233, 1997.

Whitacre MD et al: Detection of intravaginal spermatozoa after natural mating in the bitch, *Vet Clin Pathol* 21:85, 1992.

Wichtel JJ et al: Comparison of the effects of $PGF_{2\alpha}$ and bromocriptine in pregnant beagle bitches, *Theriogenology* 33:829, 1990.

Zone M et al: Termination of pregnancy in dogs by oral administration of dexamethasone, *Theriogenology* 43:487, 1995.

CHAPTER 224

Inherited Disorders of the Reproductive Tract in Dogs and Cats

VICKI N. MEYERS-WALLEN, *Ithaca, New York*

NORMAL SEXUAL DEVELOPMENT

Normal sexual development depends on successful completion of three consecutive steps: (1) establishment of chromosomal sex, (2) development of gonadal sex, and (3) development of phenotypic sex. *Chromosomal sex*, which corresponds to genetic sex in normal animals, is established at fertilization. The zygote receives either two X chromosomes or an X and a Y chromosome and maintains this chromosomal constitution in all cells by mitotic division. Morphology of early XX and XY embryos is sexually indifferent. Both have a genital ridge, from which the testis or ovary will develop. They also have müllerian and wolffian ducts, a urogenital sinus, a genital tubercle, and genital swellings, from which the internal and external genitalia will arise (Fig. 224-1). Differentiation of the genital ridge into a testis or an ovary defines gonadal sex and marks the end of the sexually indifferent stage. Although several genes undoubtedly are necessary for normal development through the sexually indifferent stage, genes that determine gonadal sex have a pivotal role in sexual development.

Gonadal sex is normally determined by sex chromosome constitution: presence of the Y chromosome results in testis development, whereas its absence results in ovarian development. The sex-determining region Y gene, *Sry*, is normally located on the Y chromosome. This gene encodes the testis-determining factor and is the genetic signal for initiating testis differentiation in the genital ridge (reviewed in Goodfellow and Lovell-Badge, 1993). *Sry* is distinctly different from the gene for H-Y antigen, which is no longer thought to have a role in testis induction. Transgenic experiments in mice have demonstrated that *Sry* is the only Y-linked gene needed for testis induction (Koopman et al, 1991), and other evidence supports this theory (reviewed in Goodfellow and Lovell-Badge, 1993). In the absence of the Y chromosome and *Sry*, the genital ridge normally becomes an ovary. Although several genes have been identified as having roles in ovarian differentiation, none has yet been shown to have a role analogous to that of *Sry* in testis induction. However, ovarian induction is not a passive process, as it is now recognized that both testis-promoting and ovary-promoting signaling pathways are responsible for gonadal sex determination (DiNapoli and Capel, 2008).

Phenotypic sex is normally controlled by gonadal sex. If the genital ridges are removed from XX or XY embryos before gonadal differentiation occurs, a female phenotype develops. This indicates that the embryo is programmed to develop as a female and must be diverted from this pathway to develop as a male. The critical diverting step is testis development. The testis secretes two substances that act within an embryonic critical period to induce masculinization: (1) müllerian inhibiting substance (MIS), which causes the müllerian ducts to regress, and (2) testosterone, which stimulates formation of the vasa deferentia and epididymides from the wolffian ducts (see Fig. 224-1). In the external genitalia, testosterone (T) is converted to dihydrotestosterone (DHT) by the enzyme 5α-reductase. Dihydrotestosterone stimulates formation of the prostate and male urethra, penis, and scrotum from the urogenital sinus, genital tubercle, and genital swellings, respectively (see Fig. 224-1). Descent of the testes into the scrotum completes the male external genitalia, but the genetic and hormonal control of this process is incompletely understood. Testosterone and insulin-like 3 factor (*Insl3*), both secreted by Leydig cells, are required for testis descent, but other, unknown factors are also likely to be involved (Tomboc et al, 2002). In the absence of a testis and its masculinizing hormones, female genitalia develop (see Fig. 224-1).

DIAGNOSIS OF DISORDERS OF SEXUAL DEVELOPMENT

Intersex is a general term used to describe an animal with ambiguous genitalia. However, it is nonspecific, in that ambiguous genitalia can arise from an abnormality at any step in sexual development. Disorders in sexual differentiation can be classified by the initial step at which development differs from normal, thus falling into three general categories: abnormalities of chromosomal sex, gonadal sex, and phenotypic sex (Table 224-1). A more precise diagnosis, which defines the disorder according to its etiology, should be made when such information can be obtained. In the near future, for example, these disorders are likely to be defined by the specific gene mutation that is responsible for the defect.

The diagnostic plan should include investigation of chromosomal sex by direct examination of the chromosomes and construction of a karyotype. The presence or absence of the *Sry* gene in dogs can also be examined by molecular assays, such as polymerase chain reaction (see XX sex reversal later). Gonadal sex is best determined by histology and may require serial gonadal sections for identification of the ovotestes. A concise description of the internal and external

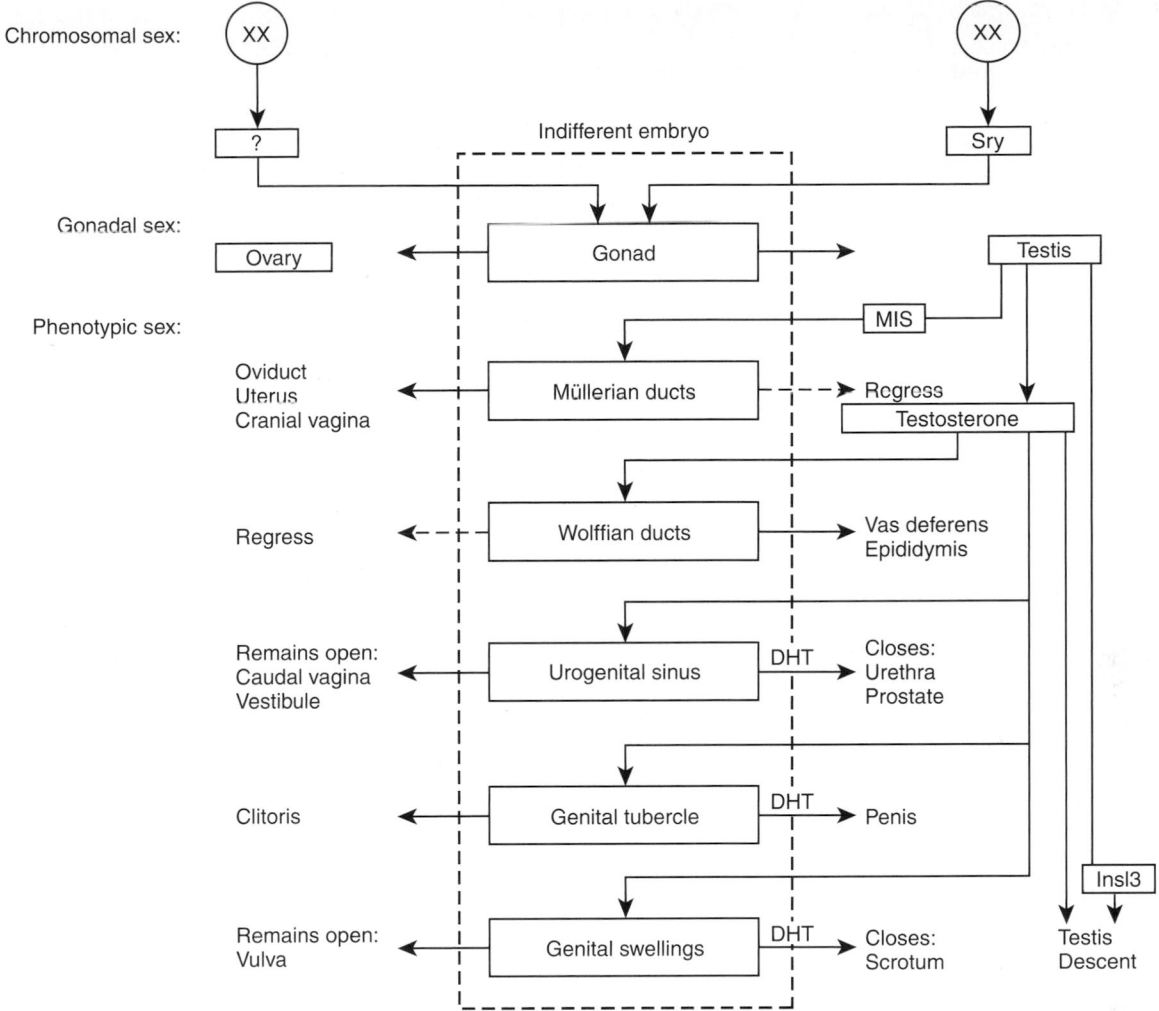

Fig 224-1 Normal sexual development. (Modified from Morrow DA: Current therapy in theriogenology, ed 2, Philadelphia, 1986, Saunders, with permission.)

genitalia is necessary for defining phenotypic sex. Assays of peripheral hormones may be helpful, but gonadotropin-releasing hormone (GnRH) or human chorionic gonadotropin (hCG) stimulation tests are necessary in many cases, particularly those in which peripheral androgen concentrations are of concern (Shille and Olson, 1989).

Abnormalities of Chromosomal Sex

Many disorders of sexual differentiation have been reported in which the primary cause was an abnormality in the number or structure of the sex chromosomes (reviewed in Meyers-Wallen and Patterson 1989a). To summarize, animals with abnormalities in sex chromosome number, such as those with XXY and XO syndromes, generally have underdeveloped genitalia and are sterile but are unambiguously male or female in phenotype (see Table 224-1). The gonadal sex of chimeras and mosaics depends on the distribution of XX and XY cells within the genital ridge. Phenotypic sex is then determined by the presence and amount of functional testicular tissue in the gonad. Abnormalities in chromosomal sex are usually due to chance events, such as errors in chromosome segregation or fusion of zygotes. Therefore, familial aggregation of affected individuals is not expected.

Abnormalities of Gonadal Sex

In this category, there is disagreement between the chromosomal sex and the gonadal sex of the individual. These animals are termed *sex-reversed*. In XX sex reversal, the chromosome constitution is XX but the individual develops testicular tissue in the gonad (testis or ovotestis). This has been reported in dogs, but not in cats.

XX Sex Reversal

Dogs affected with XX sex reversal have a 78,XX chromosome constitution and varying amounts of testicular tissue in the gonad. Affected dogs are termed either *XX true hermaphrodites*, which have at least one ovotestis, or *XX males*, which have bilateral testes (see Table 224-1). Both phenotypes can appear in the same family. Phenotypic masculinization is dependent on the amount of testicular tissue in the affected individual. Thus, XX true hermaphrodites may have normal female external genitalia or have an enlarged clitoris with an os clitoris that resembles a penis or have any phenotype in between. XX males generally have a caudally displaced prepuce and a penis with hypospadias and are bilaterally cryptorchid. XX sex reversal has been reported as a familial disorder in the English cocker spaniel, beagle,

Table 224-1

Main Features of Selected Disorders of Sexual Development*

Abnormality of	Karyotype	Gonad	Müllerian Duct Derivates	Wolffian Duct Derivatives	External Genitalia	Diagnosis
Chromosomal sex	XXY	Testis	None	Epididymis, vas deferens	Male	XXY syndrome
	X0	Streak gonad	Uterus, oviduct vagina	None	Female	X0 syndrome
	XX/XY	Ovary or ovotestis or testis	Varies depending on amount of functional testis		Female or ambiguous or male	Chimera
Gonadal sex	XX	Testis	Uterus	Epididymis, +/− vas deferens	Cryptorchid, hypospadias, displaced prepuce	XX sex reversal (Sry-negative): XX male
	XX	Ovotestis	Uterus ± oviduct	+/− epididymis	Female or enlarged clitoris	XX true hermaphrodite
Phenotypic sex						
Female pseuohermaphrodite	XX	Ovary	Uterus, oviduct	+/− epididymis	Ambiguous or male	Exogenous androgen or progestagen
Male pseuohermaphrodite	XY	Testis	Uterus, oviduct	Epididymis, vas deferens	Male +/− cryptorchid	Persistent Mullerian duct syndrome
	XY	Testis	None	None	Female	Complete Tfm
	XY	Testis	None	+/− epididymis +/− vas deferens	Ambiguous or Female	Incomplete Tfm

*Examples are disorders reported in dogs or cats.

weimaraner, Kerry blue terrier, Chinese pug (reviewed in Meyers-Wallen and Patterson, 1989a), and German short-haired pointer (Meyers-Wallen et al., 1995b). It is likely to be inherited in all of these breeds, but the mode of inheritance has not been determined. In the American cocker spaniel, XX sex reversal is inherited as an autosomal recessive trait (Meyers-Wallen and Patterson, 1988). Sry-negative XX sex reversal has also been reported in a number of other dog breeds (Meyers-Wallen et al., 1999; Melniczek et al., 1999; De Lorenzi et al., 2008).

Diagnosis of XX sex reversal classically depends on confirmation of a 78,XX chromosome constitution and the presence of at least one ovotestis or testis. Whereas elevation in peripheral T concentrations in response to GnRH or hCG stimulation strongly suggests that testicular tissue is present, it is not diagnostic (Shille and Olson, 1989). The inability to provoke T elevation by a stimulation test does rule out the diagnosis of XX sex reversal. Histologic demonstration of testicular tissue in at least one gonad in a 78,XX dog is necessary for a definitive diagnosis. To define the etiology of XX sex reversal more precisely and aid in genetic counseling, the diagnostic work-up should include a molecular test for the presence or absence of Sry. For example, in most humans with XX sex reversal, a Y chromosome is not detectable in the karyotype, yet the Sry gene is present, as demonstrated by molecular techniques such as PCR. These Sry-positive XX individuals have received an Sry translocation from the parent. That is, the Sry gene has been transferred from the Y to another chromosome through abnormal crossing over, probably during gamete formation. Therefore only one affected individual with Sry-positive XX sex reversal usually occurs within a family. Sry-positive XX sex reversal has not been reported in the dog. In addition to dogs

(Meyers-Wallen et al., 1995a, 1995b), Sry-negative XX sex reversal has been reported in humans (reviewed in Sarafoglou and Ostrer, 2000), goats (Pailhoux et al., 2001), pigs (Pailhoux et al., 1994), horses (Buoen et al., 2000; Meyers-Wallen et al., 1997) and llamas (Drew et al., 1999; Wilker et al., 1994). There is no Sry translocation detectable in these affected individuals, because the Sry gene is truly absent. Causative mutations have been identified only in humans and goats. In one human XX male, a Sox9 duplication was identified (Huang et al., 1999), which was proposed to cause Sox9 overexpression, as in transgenic mouse models of this disorder (Bishop et al., 2000). Recently mutations in R-spondin1 (Rspo1) were identified as the cause of XX males in one human family (Parma et al., 2006). Subsequently, a different Rspo1 mutation was identified in an XX true hermaphrodite in a another family (Tomaselli et al., 2008). In polled goats, the causative defect is a deletion that removes the regulatory region for at least three genes. However, mutations in the homologous region have not been associated with sex reversal in other mammals, including dogs (Kothapalli et al., 2003; Pujar et al., 2007).

This form of canine sex reversal has been studied most extensively in a pedigree derived from the American cocker spaniel, in which an autosomal recessive mode of inheritance was identified through experimental matings (Meyers-Wallen and Patterson, 1988). A genome-wide linkage analysis in this model pedigree identified linkage to CFA29 (Pujar et al., 2007). Neither Sox9 nor Rspo1 is located in this region, and a candidate gene has not been identified. The causative mutation is likely to be the same in American and English cocker spaniels, because they share recent common ancestry. It is unclear whether the same gene locus is responsible in other breeds (De Lorenzi et al., 2008).

XX males are sterile, as are most XX true hermaphrodites. Treatment of XX true hermaphrodite and XX male dogs is limited to surgical removal of the gonads and uterus and, if the dog is uncomfortable, excision of the enlarged clitoris and os clitoris. During breeding studies in the American cocker spaniel, some XX true hermaphrodites had estrous cycles and a few produced offspring. Nevertheless, the mating of affected dogs of any breed is strongly discouraged, as it will increase the frequency of the causative mutation within the breed. Similarly, parents of affected dogs should not be bred. As the causative mutation is unknown, a laboratory test for detecting carriers or affected dogs is not available. Currently there is no practical method of determining which siblings of affected dogs carry the causative mutation.

Abnormalities of Phenotypic Sex

The chromosomal and gonadal sex are in agreement in these animals, yet the internal or external genitalia are ambiguous. Affected individuals are generally termed either *male* or *female pseudohermaphrodites* (see Table 224-1).

Female Pseudohermaphroditism
Female pseudohermaphrodites have an XX chromosome constitution and bilateral ovaries. Development of ambiguous genitalia is due to the presence of exogenous or endogenous androgens during development (Meyers-Wallen and Patterson, 1989a). The canine cases were XX individuals with bilateral ovaries and phenotypic masculinization ranging from mild clitoral enlargement to nearly normal male external genitalia with an internal prostate. An iatrogenic cause was known in some cases: either an androgen or a progestagen had been administered during gestation. The presenting signs were related to bleeding at the onset of proestrus, urinary incontinence, or uterine infection.

Although adrenal enzyme defects (adrenogenital syndromes) are a common cause of female pseudohermaphroditism in humans, they are apparently rare in dogs and cats. However, excess adrenal androgen production due to 11 beta-hydroxylase deficiency has been reported in a calico cat that presented with male external genitalia, but no testes palpable in the scrotum (Knighton, 2004). Internal genitalia consisted of ovaries, bicornuate uterus, and oviducts, and the karyotype was that of a normal female (38,XX). Clinical signs included polydipsia, polyuria, and inappropriate urination. After ovariohysterectomy, penile spines persisted and peripheral testosterone concentrations were in the normal range of an intact male.

Diagnosis of female pseudohermaphrodites depends on confirmation of an XX chromosome constitution and ovaries. Before the gonads are removed, the diagnostic work-up could include tests for investigating endogenous androgen production (Shille and Olson, 1989). Elevation of serum T in response to GnRH or hCG would suggest testicular androgen production. Along with an XX chromosome constitution, this result would suggest a diagnosis of XX sex reversal (see earlier), and not female pseudohermaphroditism. Gonadal histology is necessary for distinguishing the difference. Abnormal elevation of serum androgens in response to adrenocorticotropic hormone stimulation would suggest adrenal androgen production, such as in the human adrenogenital syndromes. If no evidence of endogenous androgen production is found, historical confirmation of exogenous androgen exposure should be sought.

Ovariohysterectomy, with gonadal histopathology, is recommended for female pseudohermaphrodites. However, when urinary abnormalities are present, contrast studies are recommended before surgery to determine whether additional surgical treatment is necessary. As the most common cause is iatrogenic androgen administration, prevention may be best achieved by avoidance of steroid administration, such as androgens or progestagens, during gestation. Because the canine internal and external genitalia normally develop between gestational days 34 and 46, counting from the serum luteinizing hormone peak of the dam (Meyers-Wallen et al, 1991, 1993), it would be prudent to avoid steroid administration during this period.

Male Pseudohermaphroditism
A male pseudohermaphrodite has an XY chromosome constitution and testes, yet has female internal or external genitalia to some degree (see Table 224-1). Obviously this definition excludes XX males, in which chromosomal and gonadal sex do not agree (see XX sex reversal earlier). Two etiologically distinct categories of male pseudohermaphroditism are recognized: (1) failure of müllerian duct regression (as in persistent müllerian duct syndrome) and (2) failure of androgen-dependent masculinization (including defects in androgen synthesis, 5α reductase, or the androgen receptor).

Persistent Müllerian duct syndrome. Persistent müllerian duct syndrome (PMDS) has been reported in the miniature schnauzer in the United States and the basset hound in the Netherlands and may also occur in the Persian cat (reviewed in Meyers-Wallen and Patterson, 1989a). Affected miniature schnauzers are XY males with bilateral testes and normal androgen-dependent masculinization of the internal and external genitalia. However, they also have bilateral oviducts, a complete uterus with cervix, and the cranial portion of the vagina. Approximately half of affected dogs have unilateral or bilateral cryptorchidism, while the remaining half have normally descended testes. Therefore affected males may not be detected by physical examination alone. Affected males are frequently detected when clinical signs related to pyometra, urinary tract infection, prostate infection, or neoplasia in cryptorchid testes arise.

Diagnosis of PMDS depends on confirmation of an XY chromosome constitution, bilateral testes, and the presence of all müllerian duct derivatives (see Table 224-1). Treatment is limited to castration and hysterectomy. The uterine body terminates in a small cervix and cranial vagina at the craniodorsal aspect of the prostate gland. In some cases, there is a short, small-diameter communication between the cranial vaginal portion and the prostatic urethra, which may allow ascending infection to the uterus. During hysterectomy, care should be taken to remove as much of the vaginal portion as possible.

Prevention is limited to removing affected and carrier dogs from the breeding population. In the miniature schnauzer, PMDS is inherited as an autosomal recessive trait (Meyers-Wallen et al, 1989c). Although both females and males can be carriers, only homozygous males express the affected phenotype. Affected dogs with scrotal testes are usually fertile, but breeding of such dogs is strongly discouraged. Affected dogs will transmit the PMDS trait to all of their offspring, producing only carriers or affected dogs. The etiology of this defect is unknown. Affected dogs produce biologically active MIS during the embryonic critical period for müllerian duct regression (Meyers-Wallen et al, 1989c, 1993). Therefore, it is suspected that the müllerian ducts are insensitive to MIS, possibly because of a receptor defect.

Defects in Androgen-Dependent Masculinization. Affected animals in this category are XY males that have bilateral testes and normal regression of the müllerian duct system. However, genitalia that require androgens for masculinization fail to develop normally (see Table 224-1). Inherited defects of this type generally affect both prenatal and postnatal male development. Failure of androgen-dependent masculinization can range from mild (incomplete failure) to severe (complete failure). The primary defect causing these phenotypes may lie in (1) androgen production, (2) conversion of T to DHT, or (3) androgen reception at the target organ level. Defects in androgen production have not been documented in the dog or cat. The terms *androgen resistance* and *androgen insensitivity* refer to syndromes in which androgen production is normal but there is still failure of masculinization. These include defects in the 5α-reductase enzyme and the androgen receptor. Defects in 5α-reductase affect conversion of T to DHT and have not been reported in dogs and cats. The term *testicular feminization* is reserved for androgen receptor defects. In the testicular feminization syndromes, both T- and DHT-dependent masculinization can be affected, resulting in either complete or partial failure of masculinization (see Table 224-1). Defects of this type have been reported in dogs and cats.

Hypospadias. Hypospadias is an abnormality in location of the urinary orifice caused by incomplete masculinization of the urogenital sinus during formation of the male urethra. As a result, the urethral opening may be located anywhere along the embryologic course of the urogenital sinus to the genital tubercle. Hypospadias has been reported as a familial defect in some dog breeds, particularly in the Boston terrier, whereas teratogen-induced hypospadias has been reported in other species (see *CVT X*, p. 1267, reviewed in Meyers-Wallen and Patterson, 1989a). The initial differential diagnosis may include inherited defects such as XX sex reversal, particularly when hypospadias is accompanied by scrotal abnormalities or a uterus. A diagnostic plan that includes investigation of chromosomal and gonadal sex will lead to appropriate diagnosis and genetic counseling. Surgical correction of this defect is usually unnecessary, because hypospadias does not usually cause urinary difficulties. Affected dogs with mild hypospadias may be able to breed normally. However, when the etiology of hypospadias is unknown, it is recommended that affected dogs be removed from the breeding program to prevent further dissemination of familial hypospadias.

Testicular feminization syndromes. Testicular feminization syndromes are caused by mutations in the X-linked androgen receptor gene. Affected individuals are XY males with bilateral testes (see Table 224-1). Müllerian duct derivatives are absent, as expected for a male. However, there is either complete or partial failure of androgen-dependent masculinization, depending on whether the androgen receptor is nonfunctional or partially functional. Although T production and conversion to DHT are normal, the target organs are unable to respond appropriately.

In complete testicular feminization, the androgen receptor is completely nonfunctional and androgen-dependent masculinization is entirely absent. Affected males often present as females that fail to cycle and are sterile. A defect of this type has been reported in a domestic shorthaired cat (Meyers-Wallen et al., 1989b). Bilateral abdominal testes were present, but there were no epididymides nor vasa deferentia. The uterus was absent as expected, because MIS production and response is unaffected. The external genitalia were phenotypically female. High-affinity binding of DHT was virtually undetectable in cultured genital fibroblasts, confirming receptor malfunction.

In humans, incomplete testicular feminization syndromes are caused by different mutations of the androgen receptor gene that produce varying degrees of masculinization. The spectrum caused by these defects ranges from individuals with ambiguous genitalia to phenotypic males that are infertile. The author has observed a number of cats that probably have incomplete testicular feminization syndromes. They were XY and had bilateral testes within a bifid scrotum. The external genitalia resemble that of a female, in that there is a vulva-like genital opening with a female urethral orifice and a blind-ending vagina. There are severe perineal hypospadias, and the penis resembles a clitoris, yet develops spines. Studies in one cat indicated that neither T nor DHT was deficient (Meyers-Wallen and Patterson, 1989a). Although androgen-receptor assays were not performed, this suggests that the partial masculinization was due to an androgen-receptor defect in which the receptor was partially functional.

A similar case has been described in a mixed breed dog (Peter et al., 1993). In this XY male with bilateral testes in a bifid scrotum, the testes appeared as swellings on each side of a vulva that opened into a blind vaginal pouch. Peripheral T and DHT concentrations were normal after hCG stimulation. Epididymides were present adjacent to the testes, indicating that T-dependent masculinization was unimpaired during embryonic development. High-affinity binding of DHT was undetectable in cultured genital fibroblasts. These data suggest that DHT binding was abnormal but T binding was not. Both T and DHT bind to the same androgen receptor, which is encoded by a single gene. Nevertheless, there is pharmacologic evidence that the androgen receptor can exhibit different binding affinity preference for DHT relative to T in adult canine tissues (Summerfield et al., 1995). Therefore it is possible that a mutation in the androgen receptor could affect DHT-dependent masculinization but not T-dependent masculinization, as the findings in this case would suggest.

Diagnosis of a testicular feminization syndrome is dependent on demonstration of an XY chromosome constitution, bilateral testes, and abnormal androgen binding in androgen-responsive tissues. GnRH/hCG stimulation tests in the intact animal will confirm that peripheral androgens are present (Shille and Olson, 1989), providing further evidence for androgen resistance. In the future, when the range of canine and feline androgen receptor mutations has been documented as in humans, it should be possible to diagnose these defects at the level of the androgen receptor gene. Castration is the recommended treatment for affected dogs and cats. Prevention is limited to genetic counseling regarding the X-linked inheritance of this disorder. Carrier females are fertile. Of their offspring, 50% of the males are expected to be affected, whereas 50% of the females are expected to be carriers. However 50% of the male offspring will not receive the X chromosome bearing the testicular feminization mutation. These males should have normal genitalia and can be used in a breeding program.

Cryptorchidism. Cryptorchidism is included here somewhat arbitrarily because the underlying mechanisms for abnormal testis descent are incompletely understood. Cryptorchidism is associated with other defects in sexual development, as mentioned earlier, but can also appear as the only defect of the reproductive system, which is referred to here as isolated cryptorchidism. As previously reviewed (Meyers-Wallen and Patterson, 1989a), isolated cryptorchidism is the most common disorder of the reproductive tract reported in dogs. A diagnosis of cryptorchidism is warranted if both testes are not palpable within the scrotum at 8 weeks of age because the testes normally descend by 10 days after birth. Although canine testis descent later than 10 days is anecdotally known to most veterinarians, the frequency of such delayed descent is unknown. In one study (Dunn et al., 1968), pups with cryptorchidism were examined every 2 weeks from 6 to 14 weeks of age, then again at 6 and 12 months of age. They observed that 24.6% of cryptorchid testes descended by 6 months of age, with the majority descending by 14 weeks of age. Testis descent after 6 months of age was not observed in any case monitored. There is evidence in humans and mice that delayed testis descent is a variation of cryptorchidism rather than a variation of normal. For example, delayed testis descent was observed in humans with heterozygous *Insl3* mutations (Tomboc et al., 2002).

Dogs with bilateral cryptorchidism are sterile, whereas those with unilateral cryptorchidism can be fertile. However, the recommended treatment for both is bilateral castration. First, there is an increased risk of Sertoli cell tumor in cryptorchid testes. Second, isolated cryptorchidism is clearly a familial trait in several breeds and is likely to be inherited in dogs, as it is in other mammals. Although mutations in *Insl3* and its receptor have been identified to cause cryptorchidism in mice and humans, mutations in these genes have not been identified in cryptorchid dogs. Furthermore, mutations in those genes account for a small number of human cases (1.4%, Tomboc et al., 2002), indicating that additional genes are likely to play a role in cryptorchidism.

Although the genetics of this disorder in dogs are incompletely characterized, there are enough data to allow genetic counseling. Inheritance of isolated cryptorchidism as a sex-limited recessive trait is consistent with available data. Using this model, the first recommendation is that affected dogs be removed from the breeding population. The second recommendation is that both the father and mother of affected dogs should be considered to be carriers. Some full siblings of the affected dog will also be carriers. In other species in which cryptorchidism occurs as a simple (single-gene) recessive trait, a reduction in the frequency of affected animals was obtained in a few generations by removing carrier parents and affected males from the breeding population. This is probably the minimum program that should be pursued in dogs. It may also be necessary to remove siblings of affected dogs from the breeding program. Although medical regimens have been suggested to induce testicular descent in cryptorchid dogs, there are no published reports to confirm that these are more successful than no treatment, in which 24.6% of cryptorchid testes could descend by 6 months of age. Furthermore, even if delayed testis descent occurs, the genes responsible for cryptorchidism remain unchanged and will be transmitted to the offspring.

It is recommended that cryptorchid dogs and those with late testicular descent be removed from the breeding program to reduce the gene frequency of these disorders in the breed.

References and Suggested Reading

Bishop CE et al: A transgenic insertion upstream of *SOX9* is associated with dominant XX sex reversal in the mouse, *Nat Genet* 26:490, 2000.

Buoen LC et al: *SRY*-negative, XX intersex horses: the need for pedigree studies to examine the mode of inheritance of the condition, *Equine Vet J* 32:78, 2000.

De Lorenzi L et al: Mutations in the *RSPO1* coding region are not the main cause of canine *Sry*-negative sex reversal in several breeds, *Sexual Development*, 2008 (in press).

DiNapoli L, Capel B: SRY and the standoff in sex determination, *Molec Endocrinol* 22:1, 2008.

Drew ML et al: Presumptive *SRY*-negative XX sex reversal in a llama with multiple congenital anomalies, *J Am Vet Med Assoc* 215:1134, 1999.

Dunn ML, Foster WJ, and Goddard KM: Cryptorchidism in dogs: a clinical survey, *Anim Hosp* 4:180, 1968.

Goodfellow PN, Lovell-Badge R: SRY and sex determination in mammals, *Annu Rev Genet* 27:71, 1993.

Huang B et al: Autosomal XX sex reversal caused by duplication of *SOX9*, *Am J Med Genet* 87:349, 1999.

Knighton E: Congenital adrenal hyperplasia secondary to 11 beta-hydroxylase deficiency in a domestic cat, *J Am Vet Med Assoc* 225:238, 2004.

Koopman P et al: Male development of chromosomally female mice transgenic for *Sry*, *Nature (London)* 351:117, 1991.

Kothapalli K et al: Exclusion of PISRT1 as a candidate locus for canine *SRY*-negative XX sex reversal, *Anim Genet* 34:467, 2003.

Melniczek JR: *Sry*-negative XX sex reversal in a family of Norwegian elkhounds, *J Vet Intern Med* 13:564, 1999.

Meyers-Wallen VN, Patterson DF: XX sex reversal in the American cocker spaniel dog: phenotypic expression and inheritance, *Hum Genet* 80:23, 1988.

Meyers-Wallen VN, Patterson DF: Disorders of sexual development in the dog. In Kirk RW, Bonagura JD, eds: *Current veterinary therapy: small animal practice, X*, Philadelphia, 1989a, Saunders, p 1261.

Meyers-Wallen VN et al: Testicular feminization in a cat, *J Am Vet Med Assoc* 195:631, 1989b.

Meyers-Wallen VN et al: Mullerian inhibiting substance is present in testes of dogs with persistent mullerian duct syndrome, *Biol Reprod* 41:881, 1989c.

Meyers-Wallen VN et al: The critical period for mullerian duct regression in the dog embryo, *Biol Reprod* 45:626, 1991.

Meyers-Wallen VN et al: Mullerian inhibiting substance is present in embryonic testes of dogs with persistent mullerian duct syndrome, *Biol Reprod* 48:141, 1993.

Meyers-Wallen VN et al: *Sry*-negative XX sex reversal in the American cocker spaniel dog, *Mol Reprod Dev* 41:300, 1995a.

Meyers-Wallen VN et al: *Sry*-negative XX sex reversal in the German shorthaired pointer dog, *J Hered* 86: 369, 1995b.

Meyers-Wallen VN et al: *SRY*-negative XX true hermaphroditism in a Pasa Fino horse, *Equine Vet J* 29:404, 1997.

Meyers-Wallen VN et al: *SRY*-negative XX sex reversal in purebred dogs, *Molec Reprod Dev* 53:266, 1999.

Pailhoux E et al: Genetic analysis of 38,XX males with genital ambiguities and true hermaphrodites in pigs, *Anim Genet* 25:299, 1994.

Pailhoux E et al: A 11.7-kb deletion triggers intersexuality and polledness in goats, *Nat Genet* 29:453, 2001.

Parma P et al: R-spondin is essential in sex determination, skin differentiation and malignancy, *Nat Genet* 38:1304, 2006.

Peter AT, Markwelder, Asem EK: Phenotypic feminization in a genetic male dog caused by nonfunctional androgen receptors, *Theriogenology* 40:1093, 1993.

Pujar S et al: Linkage to CFA29 detected in a genome wide linkage screen of a canine pedigree segregating *Sry*-negative XX sex reversal, *J Hered* 98:438, 2007.

Sarafoglou K, Ostrer H: Familial sex reversal: a review, *J Clin Endocrinol Metab* 2:483, 2000.

Shille VM, Olson PN: Dynamic testing in reproductive endocrinology. In Kirk RW, Bonagura JD, eds: *Current veterinary therapy: small animal practice*, Philadelphia, 1989, Saunders, p 1282.

Summerfield AE et al: Tissue-specific pharmacology of testosterone and 5-alpha-dihydrotestosterone analogues: characterization of a novel canine liver androgen-binding protein, *Mol Pharmacol* 47:1080, 1995.

Tomaselli S et al: Syndromic true hermaphroditism due to an R-spondin1 (*RSPO1*) homozygous mutation, *Hum Mutat* 29:220, 2008.

Tomboc M et al: Insulin-like 3/Relaxin-like factor gene mutations are associated with cryptorchidism, *Clin Endocr Metab* 85:4013, 2002.

Wilker CE et al: XX sex reversal in a llama, *J Am Vet Med Assoc* 204:112, 1994.

CHAPTER 225

Ovarian Remnant Syndrome in Cats

MARGARET V. ROOT KUSTRITZ, *St. Paul, Minnesota*

Ovarian remnant syndrome (ORS) is a complication of ovariohysterectomy, defined as appearance of estrous behavior in an ovariohysterectomized female cat. Onset of estrous behavior may occur weeks to years after ovariohysterectomy and assumes normal cyclicity once it begins. The only other differential for estrous behavior in an ovariohysterectomized animal is secretion of sex hormones from the adrenal gland; this is extremely uncommon and would not be likely to be cyclic.

One possible cause of ORS is surgeon error. It has been demonstrated that pieces of ovarian tissue left free floating in the abdomen or sutured to the mesentery can revascularize and become functional (DeNardo et al., 2001; Shemwell and Weed, 1970). However, the relative ease of ovariohysterectomy in the cat is at odds with the apparent incidence of the disorder; true incidence is unknown. Another possible cause of ORS is presence of an accessory piece of ovary, located well away from the main ovary in the ovarian ligament, which becomes functional after removal of the main ovary. At present there is no technique allowing definitive differentiation of the possible causes.

Diagnosis requires demonstration of estrogen secretion followed by progesterone secretion after induction of luteinization. The following diagnostic plan is definitive for ORS since only ovarian tissue can secrete estrogen and then be induced to secrete progesterone.

1. See the queen when the owner perceives her to be in estrus.
2. Collect a vaginal cytology specimen. Cornified cytology is indicative of estrogen secretion. Presence of ovarian follicle is inferred. Measurement of estrogen in serum is not recommended because estrogen is not present in high enough concentrations to allow accurate assay in all cases and because serum estradiol concentrations have not been demonstrated to be well correlated with behavioral and cytologic estrus (Wallace, 1991).
3. Administer either gonadotropin-releasing hormone 50 mcg intramuscularly or human chorionic gonadotropin 500 units intramuscularly when the putative follicle is present to induce luteinization.
4. Draw blood for measurement of progesterone in serum 2 to 3 weeks later. Concentration of more than 2 ng/ml is indicative of luteal function.
5. Perform exploratory laparotomy.

Surgery is the recommended therapy in all cases. There are no estrus-suppressing drugs available for use in cats that are safe or approved in the United States. Surgery should be performed when there is a structure on the remnant that makes it easy to see (i.e., either a follicle or a corpus luteum). I prefer to perform surgery when luteal tissue is present on the remnant, since the cat bleeds less under the influence of progesterone than under the influence of estrogen and since luteal tissue persists for several weeks after its induction. Remnants may be unilateral or bilateral; they are reported to be bilateral in 27% to 48% of cases (Miller, 1995; Wallace, 1991). Ovarian remnants most commonly are found at the ovarian pedicles, but I am aware of anecdotal and published reports of ovarian remnants found in the omentum, in the subcutaneous space at the linea alba, adhered to the kidney capsule, and on the dorsal body wall. If no obvious remnant is visible, scar tissue at the pedicles should be removed since the remnant may be within this tissue. Any excised tissue should be submitted for histopathology; occasionally ovarian remnants contain neoplastic tissue (Root Kustritz and Rudolph, 2001; Wallace, 1991).

References and Suggested Reading

DeNardo GA et al: Ovarian remnant syndrome: revascularization of free-floating ovarian tissue in the feline abdominal cavity, *J Am Anim Hosp Assoc* 37:290, 2001.

England GCW: Confirmation of ovarian remnant syndrome in the queen using hCG administration, *Vet Rec* 141:309, 1997.

Miller DM: Ovarian remnant syndrome in dogs and cats: 46 cases (1988-1992), *J Vet Diag Invest* 7:572, 1995.

Root Kustritz MV, Rudolph KD: Theriogenology question of the month: Ovarian teratoma as an ovarian remnant in a cat, *J Am Vet Med Assoc* 219:1065, 2001.

Shemwell RE, Weed JC: Ovarian remnant syndrome, *Obstet Gynecol* 36:299, 1970.

Wallace MS: The ovarian remnant syndrome in the bitch and queen, *Vet Clin North Am* 21:501, 1991.

CHAPTER 226

Pregnancy Loss in the Queen

CLAUDIA J. BALDWIN, *Ames, Iowa*

PREGNANCY LOSS

Confirmation of Pregnancy

Breeding of a fertile queen and tom should result in attainment of pregnancy 70% of the time. Failure to ovulate can be ruled out by measuring serum or plasma progesterone. Pregnancy may be confirmed as early as 2 weeks after breeding. Uterine segmental swellings associated with gestation sacs, fetal poles, heartbeat, and fetal membranes may be seen as early as days 11, 15, 16, and 21, respectively, using ultrasound imaging (Davidson, Nyland, and Tsutsui, 1986). Abdominal palpation may be performed to identify uterine sacculations by day 21, or earlier in cooperative queens, but confirmation of viable fetuses is not possible.

Queens presented during the later phase of expected pregnancy may be subjected to abdominal palpation, abdominal and uterine ultrasound evaluation, and possibly radiographic examination. Uterine segmental swellings may remain easily palpable up until day 35 of gestation, at which time the uterus becomes uniformly enlarged. During the last 7 to 14 days of gestation, the fetuses may be assessed by palpation for movement. Ultrasound evaluation during the later phases of gestation allows more complete assessment of fetal development and heart activity. Radiographic evaluation for presence of developing kittens is best done after day 45. Morphology and development of kittens can be assessed using standards that are widely published. Unfortunately

the majority of queens presented for pregnancy loss will not have had pregnancy diagnosis performed.

A final form of pregnancy loss is the stillborn. This is a well-recognized and much easier event to confirm. It has been reported that stillbirths may occur on an average of 13% of total kitten births.

Historical and Clinicopathologic Findings of Pregnancy Loss

When a queen is presented for failure to produce kittens or for abortion, a careful history should be taken to assess the individual queen and the population. Health maintenance such as vaccination history/protocols, deworming, and serologic tests for feline leukemia virus (FeLV) and feline immunodeficiency virus (FIV) is queried. Dietary management is explored in detail. Breeding dates, the tom used, and the relationship of the tom to the queen are pertinent issues. Past reproductive history and relation to others in the colony are also important. Active and historical illnesses of the queen and the colony are explored. Medications prescribed or used are recorded. Questions are asked about housing of the queen and the typical housing practices of the breeding facility such as sequestration of third-trimester queens, sequestration of the queens and kittens, and other isolation procedures.

The history related to the pregnancy loss may vary considerably. In the event of failure to produce kittens at the time of expected term pregnancy, there may be no additional history. Other historical findings might include a decrease in abdominal size, weight loss, anorexia, or gastrointestinal signs. When abortion has been observed or is threatened based on characteristic signs of parturition, owners should be questioned about fetal material presented, viability of fetuses, and placentas. The owner may simply have noticed a vaginal discharge that is mucoid, greenish, or serosanguineous. Alternatively the client may present a queen that has produced one or more stillborn kittens.

Physical examination of the queen should be complete, with careful assessment of all body systems by means of observation, auscultation, and palpation. Examination of the reproductive system should include vaginal inspection for discharge or presence of a fetus and uterine palpation. Mammary glands are inspected for development and presence of colostrum or milk. Neonatal, fetal, and placental materials are inspected and handled carefully for further evaluation (e.g., bacterial culture, viral studies, karyotyping). Abnormalities are noted and investigated.

Diagnostic tests may be indicated to ascertain the general health of the queen. Abnormalities in hematology, serum biochemistries, and urinalysis may reflect underlying disease. Assessment of FeLV and FIV status is indicated if not yet performed and reassessed if the colony is not closed. It should be mentioned that a queen develops a dilutional anemia during gestation. Hematologic parameters (red blood cell count, hematocrit, and hemoglobin), along with a decrease in serum protein concentrations, reach a nadir by 8 weeks of gestation and quickly return to normal after queening. Additional diagnostics used to assess pregnancy status include imaging via ultrasound or radiology. Other indicated diagnostics depend on history and physical examination findings.

Confirmation of early embryonic loss before nidation is not possible currently in clinical practice. Early in gestation anechoic gestational sacs may be present, which over time fail to exhibit evidence of fetal structures, suggesting failure of successful nidation or early fetal death. Later in gestation characteristics of fetal death are typified by a variety of findings such as smaller-sized fetus, abnormal placentation, and absence of heartbeat. Fetal resorptions may be seen as focal thickening of the uterus (Yeager and Concannon, 1995). Fetal losses during the pregnancy may be complete or partial; thus as much of the uterus as possible should be scanned. If remaining viable fetuses are identified by ultrasound imaging, prediction of day of parturition may be possible (Beck, Baldwin, and Bosu, 1990). Radiographic imaging may be used to assess presence and location of remaining fetuses, morphologic developmental stage, and signs of fetal death.

DIAGNOSIS AND TREATMENT OF DISORDERS ASSOCIATED WITH PREGNANCY LOSS

There are numerous differential diagnoses for pregnancy loss. The first goal should be to rule out normal pregnancy. Using history, physical examination findings, and imaging, this can be done successfully. On occasion a queen may be presented with a mucoid vaginal discharge near the expected date of parturition. Cytology of this fluid may reveal mucous and nondegenerate neutrophils without intracellular bacteria. This can be a normal finding. If normal pregnancy is suspected based on examination and testing, the owner should be instructed to isolate and observe the queen. If the queen is thought to have entered stage II of parturition, as evidenced by active straining and normal-sized kittens, the clinician must determine whether normal delivery can occur. If the queen has been presented with one or more stillborn full-term kittens, it is necessary to determine if they might be the result of dystocia and if other fetuses are present. When there is no evidence of pregnancy or if uterine changes suggest disease or mummified or resorbed fetuses or placentation sites in an otherwise healthy young queen, the owner should be counseled. Optimal breeding protocols are discussed, and the client advised to confirm pregnancy after the next breeding. Older queens may benefit from a battery of diagnostic tests (e.g., complete blood count, serum biochemistries, urinalysis, measurement of thyroid hormone [total T_4]) along with ultrasound investigation of the reproductive tract.

Differential Diagnostic Approach to Pregnancy Loss in the Queen

One cannot follow a single differential diagnostic scheme when working through a case of pregnancy loss. Pregnancy loss may be caused by a maternal disorder that has resulted in death of the developing embryo or fetus. This may be caused by disease of a single organ system or one that is multisystemic. Pregnancy loss may also be caused by fetal disorders that cannot be attributed solely to the queen (Box 226-1).

Maternal System Disorders

Maternal system causes of pregnancy loss include both overt and occult disorders. A careful history and clinical evaluation should help identify underlying disease (e.g., renal, cardiac, endocrine, respiratory). Renal disease should be suspected in cats with small kidneys or large and irregular kidneys. Cardiac

---

Box 226-1

Categories of Pregnancy Loss in the Queen

Maternal System Disorders
- Renal
- Cardiac
- Endocrine
- Reproductive

Maternal Polysystemic Disorders
- Metabolic
- Neoplastic
- Nutritional
- Inflammatory
- Toxicity
- Trauma

Fetal Disorders
- Developmental
- Genetic/chromosome error

disease should be suspected in cats with murmurs, gallop or irregular rhythms, or poor perfusion or pulse quality. Development of pancreatic disorders, in particular diabetes mellitus, should be suspected in queens with recent onset of polyuria, polydipsia, and weight loss. Each of these systems is of particular interest in purebred cats because polycystic kidney disease, hypertrophic cardiomyopathy, and diabetes mellitus have been associated with the Persian/Himalayan, the Maine coon cat, and the Burmese lines in Australia, respectively. Significant dysfunction of these organ systems could lead to pregnancy complication and loss, as has been documented in studies of Maine coon cats with hypertrophic cardiomyopathy. Other nonbreed-associated congenital or developmental diseases may compromise maintenance of pregnancy. Treatment of these depends on the disease identified.

Primary uterine disease of an inflammatory or infectious nature may be responsible for pregnancy loss or may mimic pregnancy (Fig. 226-1). Inflammatory lesions in the form of cystic endometrial hyperplasia, metritis, or pyometra may be encountered. These may be segmental, likely associated with sites of fetal resorption, or the lesions may be more diffuse, involving one horn or the entire uterus. Clinical signs may be inapparent even when the pathology is sufficient to prohibit nidation and support of pregnancy. In other cases abdominal distention may be the notable sign. When the cervix is open, a vaginal discharge may be present, usually characterized as purulent to serosanguineous. Cytologically either discharge would show an abundance of degenerate neutrophils with intracellular bacteria, suggestive of a septic condition. Numerous bacteria, including normal vaginal flora (e.g., *Escherichia coli*, *Staphylococcus* spp., *Streptococcus* spp., *Mycoplasma* spp.), and pathogens such as *Brucella* spp., *Coxiella burnetii*, and *Salmonella* spp. have been associated with pregnancy loss in the queen. More severe clinicopathologic signs include anorexia, fever, dehydration, polydipsia, collapse, and shock, with leukopenia or leukocytosis and azotemia.

Ultrasound examination of the uterus should assist in diagnosis. Segmental areas of inflammation may not compromise the pregnancy. Metritis or pyometra, with or without pregnancy, requires antibiotics and possibly

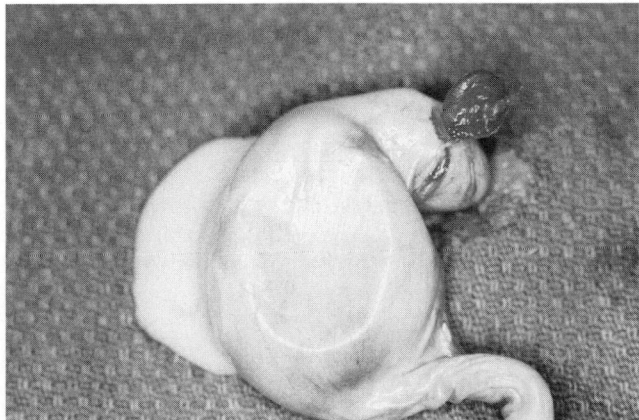

Fig. 226-1 Photograph of segmental pyometra in a queen that could have been mistaken for normal segmental swelling of the uterus caused by pregnancy. Ovarian pedicle is located in the upper right of the photograph.

intravenous fluid therapy. Additional therapy may include prostaglandin administration in the stable queen or hysterotomy to evacuate the uterine contents when reproductive potential of the queen is important. Alternatively ovariohysterectomy may be the best option (Johnston, Root Kustritz, and Olson, 2001b).

Dystocia must be considered as a cause of pregnancy loss in the queen. There is an increased incidence of dystocia in the purebred cat, and there may be a higher incidence in brachiocephalic and dolichocephalic breeds. Dystocia is often of maternal rather than fetal origin. The queen produces a litter over a highly variable period, although many deliver within hours. After onset of stage II labor, with active straining by the queen the first kitten should be produced within 2 hours, and intervals of straining between kittens should last no longer than 1 hour. If the queen has not been monitored closely, fetal death may occur. When a queen is presented for failure to produce kittens, care should be taken to document the days the queen was bred and previous queen and family history of breeding and problems. Clinical signs related to dystocia may vary. Careful physical examination followed by diagnostic imaging should reveal the presence and size of fetuses. Movement of the kittens on palpation or during ultrasound examination, along with heartbeats, confirms viability. Management of dystocia is based on size of the fetuses and condition of the queen. Medical management may be attempted with oxytocin, provided obstructions to the pelvic canal or oversized and malpositioned fetuses have been ruled out. Once medical management is begun, the queen should be monitored closely, and prompt surgical intervention undertaken if labor is unproductive. There is concern that repeated injections of oxytocin may cause premature separation of the placenta and subsequent death of remaining fetuses.

Other causes of pregnancy loss include uterine torsion and extrauterine mummified fetuses. Clinical signs of uterine torsion can include straining, resembling stage II of parturition; or the queen may present ill with depression, anorexia, and abdominal pain. More severe signs include hypothermia, tachycardia, shock, or collapse. Diagnostic evaluation ideally includes ultrasound imaging that might reveal altered blood flow or congestion. Definitive diagnosis can be made at exploratory surgery. Ovariohysterectomy is the treatment of choice, along with supportive therapy. Extrauterine mummified fetuses, also described as ectopic pregnancy, have been reported frequently in the cat. This condition is a potential cause of pregnancy loss in the queen but is usually an incidental finding. Most commonly the introduction of mummies into the abdomen follows damage to the uterine wall. Treatment for these usually sterile mummies is surgical removal. Careful evaluation of the uterus is advised in the breeding queen to identify uterine scars and anatomic changes that might preclude successful pregnancy or queening in the future.

Failure to maintain pregnancy may stem from insufficient production of progesterone. This should be suspected in the queen that suffers from repeated pregnancy loss. Although this physiologic disorder could occur at any stage of gestation, some theriogenologists suspect that it explains the high incidence of abortion around day 40 or later of gestation in otherwise healthy queens. A history of repeated abortions in a healthy queen would warrant frequent monitoring and administration of supplemental progesterone (Johnston, Root Kustritz, and Olson, 2001a). However, progesterone therapy can be problematic since it promotes an environment attractive to bacteria and may cause masculinization of female fetuses.

Maternal Polysystemic Disorders: The DAMNITT Approach

It is often helpful to approach differential diagnoses in a systematic way. The *D*egenerative, *A*llergic, *M*etabolic, *N*eoplastic, *I*atrogenic, *T*oxic, *T*raumatic (DAMNITT) scheme has been used for many years in medicine to categorize etiologic diagnoses as: Degenerative, developmental; Allergic, autoimmune (immune-mediated); Metabolic; Neoplastic, nutritional; Iatrogenic, ischemic, idiopathic, inflammatory: infectious, noninfectious, or immune-mediated; Toxic; or Traumatic. Box 226-2 puts this diagnostic approach to use when considering potential causes of pregnancy loss in the queen.

Metabolic

Metabolic disorders can occur in any breed or at any age. Effects of these disorders, if widespread or severe, could threaten the queen's ability to reproduce. A thorough history and physical examination are extremely helpful in diagnosis, along with appropriate diagnostic tests. As presented earlier in the section on Maternal System Disorders, Burmese cats are overrepresented in the population of cats diagnosed with diabetes mellitus in Australia. This is a prime example of breed preponderance of disease that should be considered under metabolic disease. A good example of age predisposition to disease is hyperthyroidism. Older breeding queens (6 years or older) should be assessed for thyroid status before breeding and again if reproductive failure occurs.

Neoplastic

Neoplastic disease that might occur in a breeding queen could certainly lead to pregnancy loss. Neoplasms not only cause dysfunction of the organs involved, but also promote metabolic changes and possibly fever. These events threaten the affected queen and may impact reproductive performance.

Nutrition

Nutrition is extremely important to reproductive health. The cat is a carnivore and depends on ingestion of meat-based foods to maintain health. Ingestion of taurine is mandatory and is available only in meat. Taurine-deficient rations (<200 ppm of diet) fed to queens for at least 6 months before breeding resulted in decreased reproductive performance, including resorption, abortion, and stillbirths. These effects persisted after feeding a diet with normal amounts of taurine for 6 months (Sturman, 1991). Other work has indicated that restriction results in a postovulatory defect within the first 10 days after implantation (Dieter et al., 1993). Effects on the queens and the live-born kittens were also apparent in these and similar studies. When taking the medical history from clients, careful questioning is necessary. There are many "natural foods," including vegetable-based diets, that are marketed as premium line but may not provide needed nutrition. Education of the client about taurine deficiency and appropriate dietary intake must be ongoing. In my practice discussions of diet are repeated with cat owners and breeders alike.

Inflammatory/Infectious

A number of inflammatory/infectious agents have been incriminated in pregnancy loss in the queen. In addition to those described in the section on Maternal System Disorders involving the uterus and those listed in Box 226-2, one specifically should consider *Brucella* spp. and *Salmonella*. Moreover newly recognized infectious causes are being recognized, through both traditional and emerging diagnostic techniques. The agents most clearly documented are presented in the following paragraphs.

Viral infections, including feline herpesvirus (FHV), calicivirus, feline leukemia, FIV, and feline coronavirus infection may impair reproductive performance in queens and cause fetal death and abortion (see Chapter 224).

Toxoplasma gondii, a protozoan, can also cause pregnancy loss. Infection induced in pregnant queens can cause placentitis and resultant infection in the fetus. Stillborns have been documented. The presence of tachyzoites in stillborn tissues is diagnostic. Clinical signs of toxoplasmosis in the queen are variable. A tentative diagnosis may be made with compatible clinical signs and careful interpretation of serologic titers (both immunoglobulin [Ig]G and IgM). Therapy of toxoplasmosis is described elsewhere in this volume.

Coxiella burnetii, a bacterium known to cause Q fever, has been documented as a cause of abortion in the cat. The cat may not show any signs of disease other than abortion. Infection may occur by tick bites or by ingestion or inhalation. This disease is also important because of the public health aspects. There are numerous reports of people contracting Q fever after exposure to queens (or bitches) during abortion or parturition. Aerosols or fomites are believed to be the route of transmission. Diagnostic tests include antibody tests on serum measured by complement fixation, enzyme-linked immunosorbent assay (ELISA), or fluorescent antibody (FA).

Box 226-2

Maternal Polysystemic Disorders Implicated in Pregnancy Loss in the Queen

- Metabolic
- Neoplastic
- Nutritional
  - Taurine-deficient diets
- Inflammatory/Infectious
  - Upper respiratory disease pathogens
  - Feline leukemia virus
  - Feline immunodeficiency virus
- Feline infectious peritonitis
- Parvovirus
- *Toxoplasma gondii*
  - *Coxiella burnetii*
- Toxicity
- Traumatic

Other infectious agents can threaten pregnancy, especially when they endanger the life of the queen. However, in my experience predictions are not always accurate. An example of this would be a multiparous queen that presented with symptomatic pulmonary blastomycosis and was treated with itraconazole. Any intervention to end the pregnancy was considered too dangerous. Despite the poor prognosis, the queen delivered a live healthy singlet kitten several days after release from the hospital.

Toxicity

Some drugs are known to be teratogenic or to cause pregnancy loss in the queen. Administration of griseofulvin is widely known to produce defects (head, brain, palate, and skeleton) in the developing fetus. Prednisone, a drug that might be needed during pregnancy (e.g., for treatment of asthma, head trauma), can induce premature parturition. It has also been linked to abnormalities in the palate and limbs. Alkylating agents such as cyclophosphamide are embryotoxic in rodents. In general owners should be aware of the known or potential effects of drugs on the pregnancy before administration or prescription.

Trauma

Physical trauma can certainly threaten gestation. In my experience severe trauma such as the queen being hit by a car can produce abortion. This might be because of blunt abdominal trauma, but it can be seen without evidence of this, likely as a result of the physiologic stress imposed by the event. It is also believed that environmental stress can cause pregnancy loss in the queen, possibly from hormonal stress responses, although to my knowledge it has not been documented.

Fetal Disorders

Fetal defects can occur secondary to exposure to a pathogen or substance during a critical phase of development. The magnitude of the defect dictates whether fetal death will occur (Fig. 226-2). It is not uncommon for only some kittens in a litter to display defects. The cause of the disorder may never be detected. Fetal lesions may also relate to chromosomal defects. Lethal gene combinations are known to occur in some feline breeds when bred for particular physical char-

acteristics. Karyotypes can be investigated by submitting an ear tip from an affected fetus for analysis. Inborn errors of metabolism may also cause pregnancy loss. Urine submission to a genetics laboratory may be useful for confirmation.

THERAPY AND MANAGEMENT

Analysis of the pedigree and screening of breeds with inherited or prevalent organ system disease or dysfunction (e.g., cardiac and renal) before breeding is highly suggested. Maternal disease should be assessed, and appropriate diagnostic tests should follow if abnormalities are found. A mandatory test in my practice is an ELISA for FeLV and FIV.

The queen that is pregnant or one with a threatened loss of pregnancy should be isolated. Sometimes it is necessary to hospitalize the queen, but the addition of this stress must be weighed against the advantages of easier monitoring. In the event of an ongoing or threatened abortion, it is unlikely that medical management will halt the process.

General supportive care (e.g., maintaining adequate hydration by delivery of intravenous fluids) should be offered if it is thought to be of benefit. Treatment of specific diseases may be necessary. The veterinarian should always discuss the potential effect of treatments on the gestating fetuses. The owner will then need to decide whether the queen or the litter is of greatest value. In general I do not attempt to disrupt a pregnancy when treating a specific medical condition since this may threaten the queen more than abortion or parturition. When viral disease is highly suspected, treatment with antiviral drugs might be considered. These drugs have been studied primarily in association with FeLV, FIV, and FHV-1 infection. I am not aware of any studies that assess their effect on pregnancy in the queen.

For future breedings serial ultrasound examinations may be useful if a cause for pregnancy loss has not been identified. Measurement of progesterone concentrations may also be advisable. Use of a different tom, not closely related to the last, is usually recommended. On occasion a repeat breeding is necessary to determine if results of the unsuccessful pregnancy can be duplicated. Recently a gene for miscarriage has been reported in mice. With the feline genome having been sequenced, much more will soon be learned about the genetic basis of specific medical conditions. A mutation has been identified for autosomal dominant polycystic kidney disease (PKD 1) and the breeds affected have expanded. As no homozygous cats have been identified, it is thought that this mutation will result in embryonic death (Lyons et al., 2004). In many Maine coon cats, hypertrophic cardiomyopathy is now known to be an autosomal dominant, single gene defect, with studies of other breeds occurring as well. More recently, 20,285 putative genes in the cat genome have been identified using the genomes of other mammalian species (human, chimpanzee, mouse, rat, dog, and cow) (Pontius, 2007). Genetic testing is now a reality.

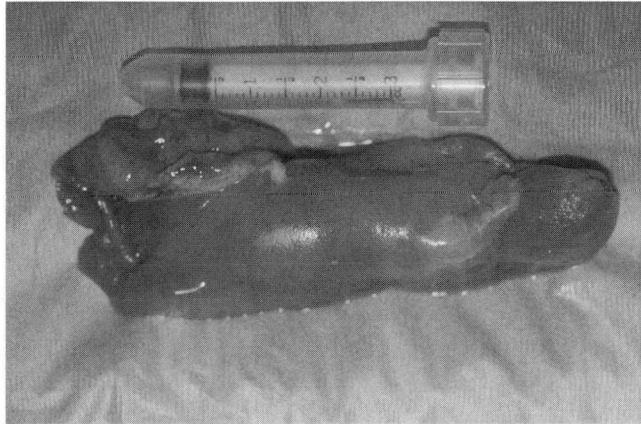

Fig. 226-2 Photograph of a kitten delivered vaginally near term. This kitten was affected by hydrops fetalis, or anasarca.

References and Suggested Reading

Beck KA, Baldwin CJ, Bosu WTK: Ultrasound prediction of parturition in queens, *Vet Radiol* 31:32, 1990.

Davidson AP, Nyland TG, Tsutsui T: Pregnancy diagnosis with ultrasound in the domestic cat, *Vet Radiol* 27:109, 1986.

Dieter JA et al: Pregnancy failure in cats associated with long-term dietary taurine insufficiency, *J Reprod Fertil* 47(suppl):457, 1993.

Johnston SD, Root Kustritz MV, Olson NS: Feline pregnancy. In Johnston SD, Kustritz MV, Olson NS, editors: *Canine and feline theriogenology*, Philadelphia, 2001a, Saunders, p 421.

Johnston SD, Root Kustritz MV, Olson NS: Disorders of feline uterus and uterine tubes (oviducts): feline pregnancy. In Johnston SD, Kustritz MV, Olson NS, editors: *Canine and feline theriogenology*, Philadelphia, 2001b, Saunders, p 463.

Lyons LA et al: Feline polycystic kidney disease mutation identified in PKD1, *J Am Soc Nephrol* 15:2548, 2004.

Pontius JU et al: Initial sequence and comparative analysis of the cat genome, *Genome Res* 17:1675, 2007.

Sturman JA: Dietary taurine and feline reproduction and development, *J Nutr* 121:S166, 1991.

Yeager AE, Concannon PW: Ultrasonography of the reproductive tract of the female dog and cat. In Bonagura *Current veterinary therapy XII (small animal practice)*, Philadelphia, 1995, Saunders, 1995, p 1040.

CHAPTER 227

Medical Treatment of Benign Prostatic Hypertrophy and Prostatitis in Dogs

KAITKANOKE SIRINARUMITR, *Bangkok, Thailand*

The prostate is the major accessory sex gland in the male dog. It is an encapsulated, bilobed, and bilaterally symmetric ovoid gland that is located caudal to the bladder and circling the proximal urethra. The canine prostate is composed of glandular acini and stromal components. Prostatic fluid is secreted from the glandular acini and excreted through the prostatic duct and prostatic urethra during ejaculation. The normal canine prostate continues to grow from birth to approximately 2 years of age. After 2 years of age the gland is maintained with no further normal growth. The Doberman pinscher and the German shepherd are breeds most frequently identified with prostatic diseases.

BENIGN PROSTATIC HYPERTROPHY

Benign prostatic hypertrophy (BPH) is a spontaneous and age-related condition in men and intact dogs. More than 80% of intact dogs over 5 years of age have either gross or microscopic evidence of BPH. The prostate gland of dogs with BPH is symmetrically enlarged and of moderately firm texture when examined by rectal palpation (Krawiec, 1994). Dogs with BPH are predisposed to prostatic cysts, infection, and prostatic abscessation; and the enlarged prostate may compress the descending colon and/or rectum (Johnston et al., 2001). In dogs older than 5 years of age, the overall rate of cell growth, which is modulated by estrogen and dihydrotestosterone (DHT), outpaces the rate of cell death, which is modulated by apoptosis, leading to a gradual increase in prostate size.

Pathogenesis of BPH

The pathogenesis of BPH is not completely known. Testosterone, DHT, estradiol, and some growth factors such as epidermal growth factor, transforming growth factor, keratinocyte growth factor. and basic growth factor are involved in prostatic growth (Lee, Kozlowski, and Grayhack, 1995). DHT, a form of testosterone metabolized by 5α-reductase enzyme, is a major hormone involved in prostatic enlargement; it enhances growth of both stromal and glandular components (Sirinarumitr et al., 2001). The uptake of DHT by prostatic cells is stimulated by estradiol. Prostatic DHT concentration in dogs with BPH was reported to be approximately two to four times greater than in normal intact male dogs. However, plasma and prostatic testosterone concentration of dogs with BPH were in the normal range.

Diagnosis of BPH

The diagnosis of BPH is based on detection of prostate enlargement without any other prostatic diseases, and affected dogs may or may not show clinical signs of BPH. Prostatic enlargement is diagnosed when prostatic diameter on the lateral radiograph exceeds 70% of the distance between the sacral promontory and the pubis (Weichselbaum et al., 1995). Clinical signs of dogs with BPH include constipation, sanguineous discharge dripping from the tip of penis, blood in the urine or semen, and difficult urination. Straining to defecate may result in perineal hernias. Clinical signs of BPH in Scottish terriers may be more severe than in other breeds. Digital rectal examination reveals a symmetrically large and firm prostate with no sign of pain during examination (Sirinarumitr et al., 2001). A dog with BPH with a large prostatic cyst may have an asymmetric lobe. Ultrasonographically the prostate gland is usually symmetrically enlarged with parenchyma that is homogenous in echogenicity and either with or without cavitating cystic lesions (Weichselbaum et al., 1995). A prostatic cyst is usually visible as a discrete, hypoechoic lesion within the parenchyma. The volume of prostatic tissue can be predicted using the formula:

$$(1/2.6 [L \times W \times D]) + 1.8$$

where L = the greatest craniocaudal, W = transverse dimension, and D = the dorsoventral length of the prostate measured by ultrasonography (Kamolpatana, Johnston, and Johnston, 2000). Prostatic volume in the dog with BPH is usually greater than 10 ml and is generally 2 to 6.5 times greater than that of normal dogs of similar weight (Sirinarumitr et al., 2001). Bacterial culture of prostatic fluid collected either by ejaculation or prostatic massage in the dog with BPH should yield less than 10^4 colony-forming units (CFUs) of aerobic bacteria per milliliter and no anaerobic bacteria, *Mycoplasma* spp., or *Ureaplasma* spp. Inflammatory cells should not be seen in the seminal fluid sediment. The complete blood count in dogs with BPH is usually normal (Sirinarumitr et al., 2001).

Medical Treatment of BPH

The treatment objectives in dogs with BPH are to decrease the size of the prostate gland and to alleviate signs related to BPH. Castration is recommended for BPH in most dogs. Medical treatment is indicated for breeding dogs or in cases in which the risk of anesthesia or surgery is high.

Finasteride (Proscar, Merck) 5-mg/tablet, at a dose of 0.1 to 0.5 mg/kg (or 1 tablet/dog weighing between 1 and 50 kg) every 24 hours orally is the recommended drug for BPH treatment in dogs (Sirinarumitr et al., 2001). Finasteride is a 5α-reductase inhibitor and blocks production of DHT from testosterone (Kamolpatana et al., 1998). The prostate in dogs with BPH treated with finasteride creates involution of the gland via programmed cell death (apoptosis) rather than necrosis; thus there is no associated inflammatory process (Sirinarumitr et al., 2002). Finasteride significantly decreases prostatic volume and serum DHT concentration by 40% to 50% but does not adversely affect semen quality, libido, or serum testosterone in dogs with BPH. The only effect of finasteride on semen quality is a decrease in semen volume. Clinical signs related to BPH such as constipation or blood in semen abate within 1 to 4 weeks after the onset of finasteride treatment and no other adverse effects have been reported (Sirinarumitr et al., 2001). Both during and after finasteride treatment, dogs with BPH have successfully bred to bitches that subsequently underwent normal pregnancy, gestation duration, and litter size (Ouada and Verstegen, 1997; Sirinarumitr et al., 2001). Dogs with BPH should receive finasteride treatment for 1 to 4 months. Prostate size and clinical signs are significantly decreased at the end of 1 month of treatment in most dogs.

Diethylstilbestrol (0.2 to 1 mg/dog orally [PO] every 2 to 3 days for 3 to 4 weeks) has been reported to reduce the prostatic size. However, the potential side effects of estrogen treatment in dogs include bone marrow suppression with resultant anemia, thrombocytopenia, or pancytopenia. Repeated administration of high doses of estrogen may incite growth of fibromuscular stroma and induce squamous metaplasia of the prostate.

Medroxyprogesterone acetate (3 mg/kg, with a minimum dose of 50 mg, in two subcutaneous injections 4 weeks apart) (Bamberg-Thalen and Linde-Forsberg, 1993) and megestrol acetate (0.55 mg/kg/day PO for 4 weeks) represent other reported medical treatments for BPH in dogs. Approximately 50% of treated dogs showed decreased prostatic size. Potential side effects of medroxyprogesterone acetate treatment included increased appetite, hypothyroidism, diabetes mellitus, testicular degeneration, and decreased serum concentration of testosterone. Flutamide, an antiandrogen (5 mg/kg q24h PO) significantly decreases prostate size, as determined by ultrasonography, within 10 days of treatment. Libido and sperm production were unchanged in male dogs treated with flutamide for 1 year; however, a course of flutamide treatment is expensive (Barsenti and Finco, 1995). Win 49596, an androgen receptor antagonist, and FRI46687, a steroid 5α-reductase inhibitor, also reportedly decreased prostatic size in research dogs. However, neither drug is available commercially.

PROSTATITIS

Bacterial prostatitis is a very common prostate disease in sexually intact male dogs. Most dogs with prostatitis are over 5 years old. The disease can be either acute or chronic in course. Prostatitis is usually caused by ascending infection of normal (aerobic) urethral bacteria into the hypertrophied gland. Dogs with prostatitis may progress to prostatic abscessation. Prostatitis is predisposed by prostatic diseases such as BPH, prostatic cyst, or prostatic neoplasia. *Escherichia coli*, the most common organism, is found in 70% of dogs with prostatitis, followed by *Staphylococcus* spp., *Streptococcus* spp., *Klebsiella* spp., *Proteus* spp., *Mycoplasma* spp., *Pseudomonas* spp., *Enterobacter* spp., *Pasteurella* spp., and *Hemophilus* spp. (Johnston et al., 2000). Infection with anaerobic bacteria or fungi also has been reported.

Clinical Signs

Clinical Signs of Acute Prostatitis

Clinical signs in dogs with acute prostatitis include fever, pain, depression, straining to urinate or defecate, a "stiff-legged" gait, hematuria, and pollakiuria. There may be edema of the scrotum, prepuce, or hind limb. Dogs with acute prostatitis usually show signs of pain during digital rectal examination of the prostate. The prostate is generally symmetric to palpation. Asymmetric enlargement of a lobe may be found in prostatitis abscessation. The gland may have a fluctuant swelling or be firm on rectal examination. Dogs with prostatic abscessation may show signs of septicemia (Johnston et al., 2001).

Clinical Signs of Chronic Prostatitis

Dogs with chronic prostatitis may be infertile and have signs of poor semen quality such as a decrease in percentage motility, although morphologically normal sperm may be evident. If prostatic contraction is painful, dogs may show decreased libido. Chronic prostatitis dogs may show signs of lower urinary tract disease. Prostatic character on digital rectal examination is symmetric, and dogs may or may not show sign of pain during rectal examination (Krawiec, 1994).

Diagnosis of Prostatitis

Prostatitis is suspected based on a history of constitutional illness, clinical signs, results of complete general physical examination, digital rectal examination of the prostate, hematology, and urinalysis. The condition is verified and staged by quantitative bacterial urine, seminal or prostatic fluid culture, cytologic examination of ejaculated semen or prostatic fluid, abdominal radiography, and either retrograde urethrocystography or prostatic ultrasonography. Complete blood count in dogs with prostatitis shows regenerative leukocytosis. Urine may contain blood, bacteria, or leukocytes. Prostatic fluid collected by ejaculation or prostatic massage contains significant numbers of inflammatory cells, and quantitative culture of prostatic fluid contains bacteria greater than 10,000 CFUs/ml (Johnston et al., 2001). Prostatic abscesses detected by ultrasonography are visible as discrete hypoechoic or anechoic lesions with or without distant enhancement. Prostatic abscess or cyst cannot be differentiated solely by using ultrasound.

Treatment of Prostatitis

Treatment strategies for canine prostatitis center on an appropriate antimicrobial therapy with other supportive treatments. The clinician may consider a combination treatment to decrease prostatomegaly caused by BPH; either antiandrogen (finasteride) or castration is appropriate. Antimicrobial therapy is based on the result of sensitivity of bacteria cultured from prostatic fluid collected by ejaculation or prostatic massage. The antimicrobial drug should diffuse into prostatic fluid. Antimicrobial drug for prostatitis treatment should have high lipid solubility, low protein binding in plasma, and low pK_a allowing diffusion of the nonionized form of the drug across the lipid prostatic membrane (Dorfman and Barsenti, 1995). Antimicrobial drugs that are highly lipid soluble include trimethoprim-sulfa, chloramphenicol, and the fluoroquinolones enrofloxacin and ciprofloxacin. These drugs are all effective against aerobic bacterial infection (Johnston et al., 2001; Dorfman and Barsenti, 1995). Fluoroquinolones are also effective against *Mycoplasma* spp. infection, and chloramphenicol is effective against anaerobic infection. Treatment with a specific antimicrobial drug should be continued for at least 4 to 6 weeks. Before treatment the size of prostate or abscess should be measured and recorded. Complete blood count, blood chemistry profiles, and prostatic ultrasonography should be evaluated before and 2 to 3 weeks after antimicrobial therapy and again once antibiotic is withdrawn. If the selected antibiotic is appropriate, clinical signs are relieved, prostatic abscessation is reduced in size or eliminated, and total white blood cell count is decreased. Prostatic fluid should be recultured at 7 to 10 days and again at 30 days once antibiotic treatment is concluded to ensure clearance of the bacterial infection. Some dogs with prostatitis may require antibiotic therapy of more than 2 months. Adverse effects or toxicities of chronic antibiotic therapy should be considered by the attending veterinarian. A combination treatment of a selective antibiotic and antiandrogen (finasteride) therapy is more successful for treating prostatitis than antibiotic treatment alone. Castration should be considered in canine prostatitis, especially if the disorder is recurrent or when an intact male is not a breeding dog. Before castration, prostatitis dogs should be retreated with antibiotics until signs of prostatitis are resolved.

I have not found surgical or needle drainage of prostatic abscesses to be necessary. Long-term antibiotic therapy (up to 4 months) and antiandrogenic treatment may be necessary to achieve medical resolution. Prostatic ultrasonography and complete blood count should be performed every 2 to 4 weeks to monitor resolution of the abscess, and treatment should continue until the abscess is no longer visible ultrasonographically. After resolution of the prostatic abscess, castration or finasteride treatment should be used to further decrease prostate size and likelihood of recurrence.

References and Suggested Reading

Bamberg-Thalen B, Linde-Forsberg C: Treatment of canine benign prostatic hyperplasia with medroxyprogesterone acetate, *J Am Anim Hosp Assoc* 29:211, 1993.

Barsenti JA, Finco DR: Medical management of canine prostate hyperplasia. In Bonagura JD, Kirk RW, editors: *Kirk's current veterinary therapy XII (small animal practice)*, Philadelphia, 1995, Saunders, p 1033.

Dorfman M, Barsenti JA: CVT update treatment of canine bacterial prostatitis. In Kirk RW, Bonagura JD, editors: *Kirk's current veterinary therapy XII (small animal practice)*, Philadelphia, 1995, Saunders, p. 1029.

Johnston SD et al: Prostatic disorders in the dog, *Anim Reprod Sci* 60:405, 2000.

Johnston SD, Root Kustritz MVR, Olson PNS: Disorders of the canine prostate. In *Canine and feline theriogenology*. Philadelphia, 2001, Saunders, p 337.

Kamolpatana K et al: Effect of finasteride on serum concentrations of dihydrotestosterone and testosterone in three clinically normal sexually intact adult male dogs, *Am J Vet Res* 59:762, 1998.

Kamolpatana K, Johnston GR, Johnston SD: Determination of canine prostatic volume using transabdominal ultrasonography, *Vet Radiol Ultrasound* 41:73, 2000.

Lee C, Kozlowski JM, Grayhack JT: Etiology of benign prostatic hyperplasia, *Urol Clin North Am* 22:237, 1995

Krawiec DR: Canine prostate disease, *J Am Vet Med Assoc* 204:1561, 1994.

Ouada I, Verstegen M: Effects of finasteride (Proscar MSD) on seminal composition, prostate function and fertility in male dogs, *J Reprod Fertil* 51 (suppl):139, 1997.

Sirinarumitr K et al: Effects of finasteride on size of the prostate gland and semen quality in dogs with prostatic hypertrophy, *J Am Vet Med Assoc* 218:1275, 2001.

Sirinarumitr K et al: Finasteride-induced prostatic involution by apoptosis in dogs with benign prostatic hypertrophy, *Am J Vet Res* 63:495, 2002.

Weichselbaum RE et al: Imaging the reproductive tract in the male dog. In Kirk RW, Bonagura JD, editors: *Current veterinary therapy XII*, Philadelphia, 1995, Saunders, p 1052.

CHAPTER 228

Aspermia/Oligozoospermia Caused by Retrograde Ejaculation in the Dog

STEFANO ROMAGNOLI, *Legnaro, Italy*
GIOVANNI MAJOLINO, *Collecchio, Italy*

A retrograde flow of small quantities of spermatozoa into the bladder is a normal event. This may occur during ejaculation, as well as during sexual rest, and has been documented in many species, including bull, ram, cat, dog, and humans (Dooley et al., 1986, 1990, 1991; Pineda and Dooley, 1991). Since testicular sperm production is a continuous event, sperm leave the testis at a constant rate and move through the caput and corpus epididymis as a result of rhythmic contractions of the smooth-muscle epididymal wall. Although the cauda epididymis is normally quiescent, occasional smooth-muscle contractions at this level promote voiding of spermatozoa and epididymal fluids into the urethra during periods of sexual rest, which explains the common finding of spermatozoa in the urine sediment of both humans and domestic male animals (Doxey, 1983; Bush, 1991). In dogs examination of the urine sediment has been suggested as a way of establishing that spermatogenesis is occurring (Ferguson and Renton, 1987).

A retrograde flow of large quantities of spermatozoa back into the bladder is an abnormal event, which may occur during ejaculation as a result of a partial or complete absence of bladder neck contraction during semen expulsion. When this happens, the bladder becomes the least resistant pathway for seminal fluids coming from the urethra. The ejaculate is scant or absent, and spermatozoa can be retrieved in large quantities from the bladder. Following erection and pelvic thrusting, a normal dog produces an ejaculate composed of 0.5 to 2.5 ml of presperm and sperm-rich fraction and 4 to 45 ml of prostatic fluid fraction, depending on testicular volume. A complete lack of ejaculate or production of minute quantities of ejaculate may indicate that semen was totally or almost totally diverted from its normal ejaculatory path and flowed into the bladder. Retrograde ejaculation is defined as a retrograde flow of the majority of or all the semen into the bladder, resulting in no semen (aspermia) or minute quantities of semen (oligozoospermia) being ejaculated antegradely.

Aspermia in the dog may be caused by sexual immaturity, pain, psychologic factors, drug therapy, diseases of the reproductive tract such as *Brucella canis* and *Pseudomonas aeruginosa* infection (George, Duncan, and Carmichael, 1979; Janza et al., 1988, Johnston, Root Kustrizt, and Olson, 2001), or sympathetic neuropathy either idiopathic or secondary to diabetes mellitus or spinal cord injury. Oligozoospermia in the dog may be idiopathic or caused by season; unilateral Sertoli cell tumor; prostate disease, orchitis and epididymitis caused by *B. canis*, *E. coli* mycoplasma, and other aerobic organisms; immune-mediated orchitis; or use of drugs such as steroids, chemotherapeutic agents, ketoconazole, and gonadotropin-releasing hormone agonists/antagonists (Jonhston, Root Kustrizt, and Olson, 2001). An oligozoospermic ejaculate is characterized by a low number of spermatozoa diluted in a very small quantity or in a normal quantity of prostatic fluid. However, presence of a normal quantity of prostatic fluid in the ejaculate generally rules out failure of bladder neck closure. Therefore retrograde ejaculation should be suspected whenever an aspermic or oligozoospermic (0.1 to 0.3 ml total volume) ejaculate is produced following normal erection and pelvic thrusting.

ANTEGRADE EJACULATION

The ejaculatory process consists of three distinct events: *seminal emission* (the deposition of seminal fluid originating from the vasa deferentia and the prostate into the prostatic urethra), *bladder neck closure* (caused by contraction of the dorsal segment of the bladder neck), and *seminal expulsion* or *ejaculation* (the passage of seminal fluids through the urethra followed by their expulsion through the external urethral orifice). Once erection is achieved, peristaltic contractions in the epididymis and vas deferens caused or increased by oxytocin start to convey spermatozoa and seminal plasma into the prostatic urethra, causing an increase in urethral pressure. Such an increase (helped by contraction of the smooth muscle cell component of prostatic lobules) forces prostatic fluid into the prostatic urethra (Shafik et al., 2006), which in the adult male dog has a rich elastic layer in the submucosa and is almost devoid of smooth muscle (Cullen, Fletcher, and Bradley, 1981). Further increase in intraurethral pressure occurs when the erectile tissue of the urethra expands, thereby reducing the urethral lumen. When the intraluminal pressure of the vasa deferentia and prostatic urethra reaches maximum, a relaxation of the striated musculature of the pelvic urethra occurs, which allows expulsion of seminal fluid outside through the pelvic and penile urethra (Hovell et al., 1969). Seminal emission is powered by recoil of elastic fibers in the prostatic urethra (Cullen, Fletcher, and Bradley, 1981). At this point a striated urethral muscle peristaltic wave cycle sets in motion, which completes the ejaculatory process.

The bladder neck plays an important role during seminal emission and seminal expulsion, preventing a retrograde flow of semen into the urinary bladder. During the ejaculatory process the canine bladder neck shows periods of intense contractile activity followed by phases of relaxation (Koraitim et al., 1977); the duration of each relaxation phase decreases gradually until a continuous contractile momentum of the dorsal segment of the bladder neck (the ventral segment of the canine bladder neck is mainly concerned with continence and voiding) occurs toward the end of the ejaculatory process. When the dorsal segment of the bladder neck is relaxed (during sexual rest and in-between urethral muscle peristaltic contractions early in the ejaculatory process), semen may flow back into the urinary bladder following the least resistant pathway. If the bladder neck contracts at ejaculation, the urethra becomes the least resistant pathway through which semen is propelled outside.

The ejaculatory process is coordinated by sympathetic and parasympathetic neural activity. The brain facilitates or inhibits sexual function by mediating and integrating reproductive motivation and reproductive behavior with other types of social behavior, whereas the spinal cord integrates visceral and somatic stimuli, evoking the reflexes of erection and ejaculation (Hart, 1974). Spinal reflexes occurring during the ejaculatory process in the dog are listed in Box 228-1.

Rationale for Treatment of Retrograde Ejaculation

The fact that the canine vas deferens, epididymis, prostate, and bladder neck are primarily under sympathetic nervous system control gives to sympathomimetic agents a pivotal role in the pharmacologic treatment of retrograde ejaculation. Following administration of sympa-

---

Box 228-1

Spinal Reflexes Occurring in the Dog During the Ejaculatory Process

Type 1: A very intense ejaculatory reflex occurring soon after intromission and lasting 15-30 seconds characterized by pelvic thrusting, alternate stepping of the hind legs, rapid engorgement of the erectile penile tissue, and expulsion of the sperm-rich fraction of semen.

Type 2: A less intense ejaculatory reflex lasting 10-45 minutes characterized by rhythmic contractions of the bulbospongiosus muscle and ejaculation of prostatic fluid accompanied by rhythmic contractions of the anal sphincter.

Type 3: Pelvic thrusting provoked by manual stimulation of the glans penis, often accompanied by partial erection without ejaculation.

Type 4: Lordosis and strong extension of the hind legs when the distal end of the penis is touched.

From Hart BL: *Vet Clin North Am Small Anim Pract* 4:557, 1974.

---

thomimetic drugs, the canine epididymal and prostatic tissue displays phases of rhythmic contractions (Arver and Sjostrand, 1982; Noguchi et al., 2008). Contraction and relaxation of the vas deferens are mediated by α- and β-adrenoceptors, respectively (Trachte, 1987; Noguchi et al., 2008). The use of an α-adrenoceptor agonist together with a β-adrenoceptor antagonist has been proposed to increase spermatozoal output in the dog (Rath, 1983). Administration of xylazine (an α_2-adrenoceptor agonist) in the dog increases contractility of the vas deferens and epididymis and decreases urethral pressure, inducing nonejaculatory displacement of canine spermatozoa in the bladder (Dooley et al., 1990). Selective α_2-adrenoceptor antagonists such as yohimbine or rauwolscine have a stimulatory effect on ejaculation in dogs when administered at low doses (both drugs have been used at 0.01 to 0.1 mg/kg intraperitoneally); when used at this dose, yohimbine can prevent in the dog the decrease in the amount of ejaculate produced by repeated semen collections (up to eight times a day), whereas a high dose (1 mg/kg) decreases the amount of ejaculate produced (Yonezawa et al., 1990).

The canine bladder neck has a rich cholinergic and adrenergic innervation. Cholinergic stimulation produces gradual contraction of the neck, as well as of the whole bladder (occurring during micturition); whereas adrenergic stimulation occurring at ejaculation causes contraction of the neck and relaxation of the body of the bladder (Raezer et al., 1973). Administration of the α-adrenoceptor antagonist phentolamine 5 to 10 minutes before semen collection may increase the retrograde flow of canine spermatozoa into the bladder up to 2.5% of the total ejaculate (Schnee, 1985). Administration of the β-receptor agonist clenbuterol before semen collection increased the number of spermatozoa found in the bladder of two of three dogs, whereas administration of the α-receptor agonist midodrine was able to counteract the effect of clenbuterol (Hahmann, 1988).

Sympathomimetic agents such as ephedrine, pseudoephedrine hydrochloride, phenylpropanolamine, and imipramine are generally used (alone or in combination) to treat human retrograde ejaculation (Lipshultz, McConnel, and Benson, 1981; Lange et al., 1983). Treatment protocols using sympathomimetic drugs reported in the dog include phenylpropanolamine (3 mg/kg orally [PO] twice daily) and pseudoephedrine hydrochloride (3 to 5 mg/kg PO three times daily or 3 and 1 hours before breeding/semen collection) (Romagnoli et al., 1992; Root, Johnston, and Olson, 1994; Johnston, Root Kustrizt, and Olson, 2001).

Success of treatment depends on etiology. Retrograde ejaculation can be the result of *anatomic causes* (iatrogenic defects following bladder or prostate surgery), *neuropathic causes* (diabetes; prolonged treatment with ganglionic or adrenergic blocking drugs such as methyldopa, phenoxybenzamine, guanethidine, reserpine and phentolamine; or following retroperitoneal lymph node dissection for testicular cancer) or *psychologic factors* (pain, fear of new environment, uneasiness when a manual semen collection is attempted for the first time, or lack of interest in the bitch). Treatment of retrograde ejaculation from anatomic causes generally is unsuccessful. Humans with lack of antegrade ejaculation caused by diabetes or retroperitoneal lymph node dissection for testicular cancer are treated successfully with sympathomimetic drugs; whereas in the case of chronic therapy with ganglionic or adrenergic blocking drugs, cessation of treatment reestablishes an antegrade ejaculation. In men the use of drugs influencing libido such as human chorionic gonadotropin is reported as effective in the case of retrograde ejaculation caused by psychologic factors (Lipshultz, McConnel, and Benson, 1981).

Incidence of Retrograde Ejaculation in the Dog

In the dog retrograde ejaculation has been observed by researchers while doing experiments on male reproductive physiology (Ferguson and Renton, 1987; Dooley et al., 1990; Pineda and Dooley, 1991; Dooley et al., 1991). In addition, spontaneous (nondrug-induced) retrograde ejaculation causing aspermia has been reported in a 4-year old German shepherd (Meinecke, 1976) and in a 7-year English cocker spaniel (Romagnoli et al., 1992), and oligozoospermia has been reported in a 19-month-old Labrador retriever (Root, Johnston, and Olson, 1994). The German shepherd had never fathered a litter of pups before referral, and its libido was normal; it showed a complete lack of ejaculate, and a high number of 30% progressively motile sperm were found in the bladder following an attempt at semen collection. Pharmacologic treatment was not attempted in this dog (Meinecke, 1976).

The English cocker spaniel had previously fathered two litters of six and five puppies and had been treated with megestrol acetate because of behavioral problems for about 8 months, during which time it progressively lost his libido. Several months following cessation of therapy the dog was examined for breeding soundness because of infertility. Its blood glycemia and libido were normal; but on semen collection performed various times over a 2-month period it consistently failed to produce any ejaculate, whereas large numbers of 50% to 70% motile spermatozoa were retrieved in voided urine samples (Fig. 228-1). Oral pseudoephedrine

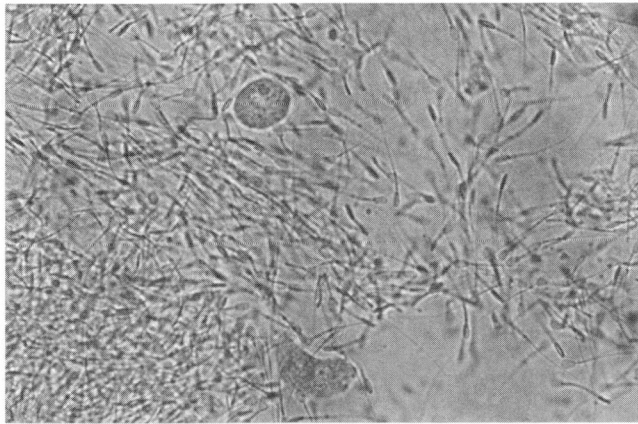

Fig. 228-1 Smear of the sediment of a voided urine sample of a 7-year-old English cocker spaniel dog following an aspermic ejaculation. A cross-sectioned hyaline cylinder can be observed in the upper half of the picture (Harris-Schorr, 400×).

failed to induce an antegrade ejaculation when administered at a dose of 5mg/kg three times at 8-hour intervals, whereas a normal antegrade ejaculation was obtained when pseudoephedrine was administered at a dose of 3mg/kg 3 and 2 hours before semen collection. During this time the dog produced a litter of three normal pups using semen collected with a pseudoephedrine pretreatment, and several months later it regained its capability to ejaculate antegradely without pseudoephedrine pretreatment (Romagnoli et al., 1992).

The Labrador retriever had bred two bitches, neither of which had produced a litter. On semen collection with an estrous teaser bitch it ejaculated 1ml of semen containing 1 million spermatozoa with 50% progressive motility. Hypothyroidism was diagnosed based on decreased resting serum levels of triiodothyronine and thyroxine. On treatment with pseudoephedrine hydrochloride at the dose of 4mg/kg given orally 1 and 3 hours before semen collection, the dog produced 1.5ml of semen with 250 million spermatozoa with 60% to 70% progressive motility. One month later the hypothyroidism had been solved, but the dog would ejaculate normally only following a pseudoephedrine treatment. This dosage allowed collection of a good-quality semen sample with which a litter of 5 puppies was produced. A cause-and-effect relationship between hypothyroidism and retrograde ejaculation could not be established in this case (Root, Johnston, and Olson, 1994).

We have observed retrograde ejaculation causing oligozoospermia in one English setter and aspermia in one German shepherd (data not published). An 8-year-old previously fertile English setter was referred with a history of infertility observed over the last 2 years. On the first two semen collections with estrous teaser bitches the dog showed good libido, displaying pelvic thrusting, alternate stepping on the hind limbs, and anal contractions and lordosis but produced only 0.0 and 0.1ml of semen (the latter with 70% progressively motile spermatozoa), respectively. A 15-ml voided urine sample collected at the second semen evaluation showed a total count of 45 million 70% progressively motile spermatozoa. The dog was treated with pseudoephedrine at the dose of 5mg/kg 4, 1, and 0.5 hours before semen collection and produced on two different occasions 1 week apart 0.3 and 1ml of normal semen with 70% progressively motile spermatozoa, respectively; the owner was instructed to administer pseudoephedrine at home using this dosage before natural breeding, and the dog produced a normal litter. A 4-year-old German shepherd was referred for having never produced a litter of puppies. The referring veterinarian had attempted semen collection on two different occasions, always in the presence of estrous teaser bitches: on both instances the dog showed normal libido, pelvic thrusting, alternate stepping of the hind limb, and anal contractions but produced no ejaculate; a voided urine sample collected at the second semen evaluation performed by the referring veterinarian showed a low concentration of dead spermatozoa. When semen was collected subsequently in the presence of an estrous bitch, the dog again showed a normal libido and produced no semen; a voided urine sample showed large numbers of live and progressively normal spermatozoa. The owner was instructed to administer pseudoephedrine before a natural breeding at home, but the dog died of trauma shortly thereafter.

Clinical Considerations for Diagnosis and Treatment

When performing a breeding soundness evaluation in the dog, it is important to carefully observe behavior during semen collection or natural breeding. A normal dog in a comfortable environment consistently displays types 1 and 2 spinal reflexes, indicative of ejaculation such as pelvic thrusting and alternate stepping on the hind legs, followed by rhythmic anal contractions. Pelvic thrusting is generally displayed both during natural breeding and semen collection, whereas alternate stepping on the hind legs is often observed only during natural breeding. If rhythmic contractions of the anal sphincter (indicating contractions of bulbospongiosus muscle causing ejaculation of prostatic fluid) are not preceded by pelvic thrusting, ejaculation may be incomplete (only prostatic fluid) or absent. If both types 1 and 2 spinal reflexes are displayed and no semen is collected or no spermatozoa are observed in a vaginal smear following breeding, evaluation of a voided/cystocentesis urine sample looking for large numbers of live, normal spermatozoa is warranted.

Although considered a rare event, retrograde ejaculation in the dog could be more frequent than expected. Inadequate penile manipulation during canine semen collection may increase the percentage of retrograde flowing spermatozoa from 0% to 60% (Schnee, 1985). Also, lack of interest in the bitch or fear of a new environment could be responsible for lack of or insufficient spinal reflexes, leading to insufficient activation of the sympathetic system, thereby causing retrograde ejaculation. The role of diabetes mellitus, urinary/prostatic surgery, or retroperitoneal lymph node dissection in the pathogenesis of canine retrograde ejaculation has not been investigated. When diagnosing oligozoospermia (with minute quantities of semen) or aspermia, clinicians should rule out retrograde ejaculation by collecting a voided/cystocentesis urine sample and looking for large numbers of live, normal spermatozoa.

Human spermatozoa ejaculated retrogradely into the bladder can be retrieved and used for artificial insemination provided that the urinary environment is alkaline (pH >7.0) and with a low osmolality (200 to 300 mOsm/kg of water). This is achieved by having the man drink large amounts of water and take sodium bicarbonate on the day before and the day of semen collection. Voided or catheterized urine is centrifuged at 300 to 500 g, the sperm pellet resuspended in a semen extender, and inseminated. Although such a procedure has been attempted in the dog without success (Post et al., 1992), more clinical research is needed on this topic.

Sympathomimetic agents deserve more attention from clinicians because of their specific action on sperm production and output in the dog. Yohimbine appears to be able to increase sperm output in the dog, a claim that, if substantiated by clinical reports, could open new interesting avenues for the treatment of oligozoospermic dogs. In the treatment of human retrograde ejaculation the use of some of the sympathomimetic agents is characterized by development of tachyphylaxis (caused by depletion of norepinephrine stores at the terminal nerve endings), a feature that is less common when using the α-sympathomimetic drug phenylpropanolamine. The occurrence of tachyphylaxis following treatment with sympathomimetic drugs has not been extensively studied in small animals; however, tachyphylaxis due to ephedrine and phenylpropanolamine is reported to occur in the cat and dog, respectively (Cowan et al., 1963; Weiss and Ellis, 1994). Adverse effects of sympathomimetics on heart rhythm and blood pressure should be appreciated.

References and Suggested Reading

Arver S, Sjostrand NO: Functions of adrenergic cholinergic nerves in canine effectors of seminal emission, *Acta Physiol Scand* 115:67, 1982.

Bush BM: Urinalysis. In Bush BM: *Interpretation of laboratory results for small animal clinicians*, Blackwell Scientific Publications, 1991, Oxford, p 411.

Cowan FF, Koppanyi T, Maengwyn-Davies GD: Tachyphylaxis. III. Ephedrine, *J Pharm Sci* 52(9):878, 1963.

Cullen WG, Fletcher T, Bradley WE: Histology of the canine urethra. II. Morphometry of the male pelvic urethra, *Anat Rec* 199:187, 1981.

Dooley MP: Evidence for retrograde flow of spermatozoa into the urinary bladder of bulls during electroejaculation, *Theriogenology* 26:101, 1986.

Dooley MP et al: Retrograde flow of spermatozoa into the urinary bladder of cats during ejaculation or after sedation with xylazine, *Am J Vet Res* 51:1574, 1990.

Dooley MP et al: Retrograde flow of spermatozoa into the urinary bladder of dogs during electroejaculation, collection of semen with an artificial vagina, and mating, *Am J Vet Res* 52:687, 1991.

Doxey DL: The urinary system. In Doxey DL: *Clinical Pathology and Diagnostic Procedures*, ed 2, London, 1983, Baillière Tindall p 131.

Ferguson JM, Renton JP: Observation on the presence of spermatozoa in canine urine, *J Small Animal Pract* 29: 691, 1987.

George LW, Duncan JR, Carmichael LE: Semen examination in dogs with canine brucellosis, *Am J Vet Res* 40:1589, 1979.

Hahmann C: *Investigations upon the influence of the alpha- and/or beta-sympathomimetic drugs norepinephrine, midodrine, and clenbuterol on mating behaviour and ejaculation of healthy beagles*, Thesis, Tierarztliche Hochschule, Hannover, Germany, 1988.

Hart BL: Physiology of sexual function, *Vet Clin North Am Small Anim Pract* 4:557, 1974.

Janza F et al: Aetiological studies and therapy of genital infections in male dogs, *Magyar Allatorvosok Lapja* 43:733, 1988.

Johnston SD, Root Kustrizt MV, Olson PN: Clinical approach to infertility in the male dog. In Johnston SD, Root-Kustritz MV, Olson PNS: *Canine and feline theriogenology*, Philadelphia, 2001, Saunders, p 370.

Koraitim M et al: Dynamic activity of bladder neck and external sphincter in ejaculation: electromyographic study in dogs, *Urology* 10:130, 1977.

Lange H et al: Return of fertility after treatment for nonseminomatous testicular cancer: changing concepts, *J Urol* 129:1131, 1983.

Lipshultz LI, McConnel J, Benson GS: Current concepts of the mechanisms of ejaculation, *J Reprod Med* 26:499, 1981.

Meinecke B: Retrograde ejaculation in the dog, *Zuchthygiene* 11:122, 1976.

Noguchi Y et al: In vivo study on the effects of a1-adrenoceptor antagonists on intraurethral pressure in the prostatic urethra and intraluminal pressure in the vas deferens in male dogs, *Eur J Pharmacol* 580:256, 2008.

Pineda MH, Dooley MP: Effect of method of seminal collection on the retrograde flow of spermatozoa into the urinary bladder of rams, *Am J Vet Res* 52:307, 1991.

Post K et al: Retrograde ejaculation in a Shetland sheepdog, *Can Vet J* 33:53, 1992.

Raezer DM et al: Autonomic innervation of the canine urinary bladder, *Urology* 2:211, 1973.

Romagnoli S et al: Retrograde ejaculation in the dog, Proceedings of the XVII Congress World Small Animal Veterinary Association, Rome, 1992, p 1435.

Root MV, Johnston SD, Olson PN: Concurrent retrograde ejaculation and hypothyroidism in a dog: case report, *Theriogenology* 41:593, 1994.

Schnee CM: Studies on the induction of retrograde ejaculation by alpha-receptor blockade and incorrect semen collection proce-

dure in the dog, Thesis, Tierärztliche Hochschule, Hannover, Germany, 1985.

Shafik A et al: Contractile activity of the prostate at ejaculation: an electrophysiologic study, *Urology* 67(4):793, 2006.

Vick J, Weiss L, Ellis S: Cardiovascular studies of phenylpropanolamine, *Arch Int Pharmacodyn Ther* 327(1):134, 1994.

Yonezawa A : Diminution of ejaculatory capacity induced by frequent ejaculation in dogs: prevention and reversal by yohimbine, *Andrologia* 23:71, 1990.

CHAPTER 229

Intermittent Erection of the Penis in Castrated Male Dogs

MARGARET V. ROOT KUSTRITZ, *St. Paul, Minnesota*

Intermittent erection of the penis in castrated male dogs primarily is a behavioral problem. It should be differentiated from paraphimosis, which is inability of the male to replace the nonerect penis in the prepuce, and priapism, which is persistent erection of the penis.

Erection is a nonhormonal event, mediated neurologically by the parasympathetic nervous system via the pelvic nerve and psychogenically by cerebral centers that augment neurologic activity. Therefore intermittent erection of the penis may occur in any male dog, regardless of sexual status, age, or history of sexual activity.

Onset of intermittent erection of the penis is variable. Some dogs exhibit this behavior throughout their lives, whereas others may show no such behavior until years after castration. Clinical signs vary from apparent inattention to the erect penis, to occasional licking of the erect penis, to apparent pain with frantic licking and biting at the erect penis and prepuce.

Physical examination reveals a penis that is readily extruded and replaced within the prepuce and that has no visible lesions or inflammation other than that caused by self-trauma. In one report of six intact male dogs with idiopathic chronic penile protrusion, all had drying or mild erythema of the tip of the penis and no other clinical signs (Papazoglou, 2001).

Treatment is geared toward eliminating any situation causing sexual arousal or excitement that can be correlated with episodes of penile erection. In many cases there is no identifiable underlying cause, and ignoring the behavior may be the best behavioral therapy. Owners tend to overreact to penile erection, giving the dog a large positive reinforcement whenever it occurs. Tranquilizers or antipsychotic drugs may be beneficial in dogs that damage the penis or prepuce from frantic licking and biting. Progestogens may be beneficial, perhaps because of their anxiolytic and antiinflammatory properties. Examples include megestrol acetate (Ovaban, Schering-Plough; 0.5 mg/kg once daily orally [PO] for a maximum of 30 days or 2 mg/kg once daily PO for 8 days), medroxyprogesterone acetate (2.5 mg/kg subcutaneously [SQ] every 5 months for a maximum total length of 1 year of treatment), and proligestone (10 mg/kg SQ for a maximum of four injections with a 3-month interval between the first two injections, a 4-month interval between the second and third, and a 5-month interval between the third and fourth). Side effects of progestogen therapy include polyphagia and depression, as well as predisposition to diabetes mellitus and perhaps mammary neoplasia.

References and Suggested Reading

Papazoglou LG: Idiopathic chronic penile protrusion in the dog: a report of six cases, *J Small Anim Pract* 42:510, 2001.

Root Kustritz MV: Disorders of the canine penis, *Vet Clin North Am* 31:247, 2001.

CHAPTER 230

Methods and Availability of Tests for Hereditary Disorders of Dogs

EDWARD E. (NED) PATTERSON, *St. Paul, Minnesota*

Study of the biochemical and physiologic bases of canine heritable disorders over the last 10 to 20 years has identified mutations responsible for a number of diseases. The progress of the canine genome maps and the recent publication of the canine genome sequence (Lindblad-Toh et al., 2005), coupled with comparative data from human genome research, have led to the recent discovery of the molecular basis of additional canine inherited disorders. There are now more than 370 recognized inherited diseases in dogs (Patterson, 2000), but in many the biochemical or molecular basis is not yet identified. With additional research and emerging technologies, the number of available tests will grow exponentially in the near future. A working knowledge of the basic methods and availability of such tests will increasingly be an important part of the knowledge base of the small animal veterinarian. Biochemical, direct mutation, and genetic linkage tests are the three major categories of inherited disease diagnostic tests.

SCIENTIFIC BASIS OF THE TESTS

At present, there is no standardization of the basis, methods, techniques, or quality control of inherited disease testing for small animals. In addition, there is no oversight or accreditation of animal genetic testing laboratories and companies. There is a need for regulations and guidelines for small animal genetic testing. Until these are enacted, veterinarians submitting samples for canine genetic disease testing need to evaluate each test individually to determine its accuracy and reliability. A basic knowledge of the methods of the test and an evidence-based approach to its evaluation are important to guide decisions about when to use a specific test. Criteria for molecular genetic testing should be similar to those for any diagnostic medical test. Within a reasonable amount of time after development, the data and results of the test should be published in a peer-reviewed scientific journal. Ideally the test should be verified independently by an outside group. Any test that has not had peer-reviewed scrutiny should be used cautiously. Short of a peer-reviewed publication, all available evidence and data should be very critically evaluated. For some of the currently available tests, only patent information is available at this time, and this information can be reviewed through the U.S. patent website (www.uspto.gov/main/patents.htm). In some cases companies offering tests are awaiting resolution of intellectual property issues.

BIOCHEMICAL TESTS

Biochemical tests for inherited disorders in dogs have been available for many years and will continue to play a very important role in diagnosis of inherited disorders in which the chromosomal location or gene for the defect has not yet been identified. Most biochemical tests require only a simple blood or urine sample. Biochemical tests are also necessary to help evaluate newly developed molecular genetic tests, especially those lacking documentation or presenting controversy. Examples of some of the currently available biochemical tests include those for mucopolysaccharidosis, Fanconi syndrome, erythrocyte osmotic fragility, methylmalonic aciduria, cystinuria, urinary acids, urinary amino acids, urinary carbohydrates, urinary glycosaminoglycans, urinary oligosaccharides, and other inborn errors of metabolism performed at the University of Pennsylvania School of Veterinary Medicine (PennGen) (Table 230-1). Factor assay tests for von Willebrand disease and other inherited coagulopathies are performed at a number of veterinary diagnostic laboratories. In many cases biochemical tests are the best estimate of the genetic status of an individual (affected, carrier, or clear). However, test results can fall into overlapping categories, causing problems with classification and definition.

DEOXYRIBONUCLEIC ACID–BASED TESTS

The dog has 39 chromosome pairs, with one of each pair inherited from each parent. There is complimentary base pairing of adenine-thymine and cytosine-guanine nucleotide representing the building blocks of deoxyribonucleic acid (DNA). Restriction enzymes cut DNA at specific, short sequences of DNA. There are many genetic markers that do not code for messenger ribonucleic acid or proteins (noncoding markers). These markers are interspersed throughout all chromosomes, and there are a number of noncoding markers near every gene. The markers tend to be variable among individuals because changes in the nucleotides do not have any known functional effect. Many of the markers currently used in canine genetic studies are repeats of nucleotides (e.g., CA repeated 10 to 30 times). The resulting different lengths of DNA can be detected on a gel because the fragments migrate in an electrical field in inverse proportion to their size. The different lengths of the marker are called different alleles, just as different blood types represent different alleles of a coding gene. Single nucleotide polymorphisms (SNPs)

Table **230-1**

List of Some Laboratories and Companies Offering Canine Genetic Testing in the United States and United Kingdom

Name	Phone	Website
Animal Health Trust (AHT) UK	44-08700-509144	www.aht.org.uk
OptiGen LLC (Ithaca, NY)	607-257-0301	www.optigen.com
PennGen (U. of Pennsylvania)	215-898-3375	www.vet.upenn.edu/penngen
U. of California, Davis, Veterinary Genetics Laboratory	530-752-2211	www.vgl.ucdavis.edu
VetGen LLC (Ann Arbor, MI)	800-483-8436	www.vetgen.com

have another type of genetic marker, and canine SNP arrays that can genotype thousands of SNP markers for one individual are just becoming commercially available.

A genetic marker can be strongly associated or linked with a disease gene if it is very close to a gene and the marker has more than one allele. The farther a marker is from a gene on the same chromosome, the more likely recombination is to have occurred during meiosis. The percentage of time a marker and gene have recombination between them is termed the *recombination fraction*. For a marker to be potentially useful as a screening genetic test, there generally needs to be a recombination fraction of 5% or less. Fig. 230-1 illustrates marker and gene linkage and recombination. Understanding that a marker allele is linked to a disease is probably the most difficult concept preventing an understanding of published chromosomal locations of causative genes and molecular genetic disease testing.

Direct mutation tests detect DNA sequence differences in the specific causative gene. A genetic marker test detects a marker allele linked with a mutation in a nearby, unknown gene. For either type of molecular genetic test only a small DNA sample obtained from a special cheek swab kit or an ethylenediaminetetraacetic acid whole-blood sample is needed. Instructions for the type of sample are easily found on the laboratory website or via phone contact. These tests can be performed at any age after weaning and need be done only once in a lifetime. Laboratories should always run positive and negative controls for all

molecular genetic tests to ensure accuracy and reliability. A list of the major canine molecular genetic testing laboratories can be found in Table 230-1. This is not an inclusive list since new laboratories are frequently established. Cost for molecular genetic tests currently range from about $40 to $260 for a single test on one individual.

Direct Mutation Tests

The testing procedure for a direct mutation test is straightforward and relatively simple. Depending on the exact mutation, there are several different detection methods. For many of the tests the specific DNA in the area of the specific known mutation is polymerase chain reaction (PCR) amplified and then cut with a restriction enzyme that differentially cuts or does not cut the normal and mutated sequences. The restriction enzyme products are then size separated on a gel, and the different-sized products can be categorized into normal, heterozygous (carrier for a recessive disease or affected for a dominant disease), and homozygous-affected categories. See Fig. 230-2 for a hypothetic example that illustrates direct mutation testing for a recessive disease. It is very important to realize that each specific test checks for only one mutation in the gene. Table 230-2 contains a list of the direct mutation tests that are currently available.

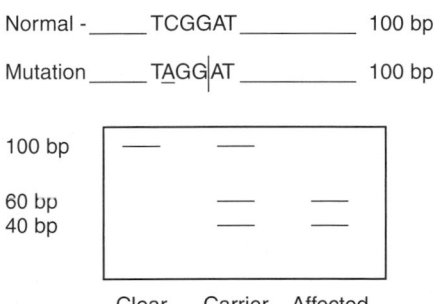

Fig. 230-2 Gel electrophoresis results for a hypothetic direct mutation test for a recessive disease. The normal and mutation polymerase chain reaction sequence products are both 100 base pairs (bp) long. They differ in a C to A substitution in the second nucleotide shown. A restriction enzyme cuts the mutation sequence between the G and A into a 60- and a 40-base pair fragment, but does not cut the normal product. The fragments are size separated and visualized on a gel. The results unequivocally categorize individuals into clear, carrier, or affected for this one specific mutation. This does not test for other mutations in the same gene. Laboratories should always run positive and negative controls for all molecular genetic tests.

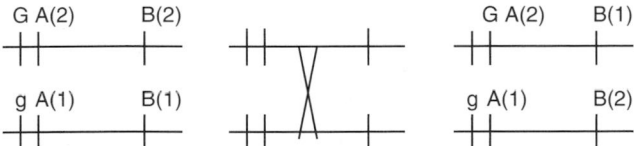

Fig. 230-1 Genetic linkage of a marker A and gene G, and recombination between G and marker B. The left portion shows two homologous chromosomes with gene G and markers A and B. G refers to the normal gene allele and g refers to the mutated gene allele. A(2) is marker A allele 2, and A(1) is marker a allele 1. The left side shows the A(1) and B(1) marker alleles linked with the mutation g. The middle shows a recombination event during meiosis, and the right side shows that marker A, which is very close to the gene, still has allele A(1) linked with the mutation g. However, marker B now has changed to allele B(2) linked with mutation g as a result of the recombination event. A marker must be very close to the gene with a low recombination frequency and with specific population dynamics of the alleles to be a reliable screening test.

Table 230-2

List of Some Direct Mutation Tests for Canine Inherited Disorders

Disease	Breed(s)	Inheritance	Laboratory	Basis
Canine leukocyte	Irish setter	AR	OptiGen	PBL
Adhesion deficiency	Irish setter	AR	AHT	PBL
Canine multifocal retinopathy	Bullmastiffs	AR?	OptiGen	NDY
	Coton de Tulear	AR?	OptiGen	NDY
	Great Pyrennes	AR?	OptiGen	NDY
Cataracts	Staffordshire bull terrier	AR	AHT	NDY
Ceroid lipofuscinosis	Border collie	AR	AHT	PBL
Ceroid lipofuscinosis	American bulldog	AR	U of MO	PBL
	Dachshund	AR	U of MO	PBL
	English setter	AR	U of MO	PBL
Collie eye anomaly	Australian shepherd	AR	OptiGen	Patent pending
	Border collie	AR	OptiGen	Patent pending
	Rough collie	AR	OptiGen	Patent pending
	Shetland sheepdog	AR	OptiGen	Patent pending
	Smooth collie	AR	OptiGen	Patent pending
Cone degeneration	German shorthaired pointer	AR	OptiGen	NDY
Congenital stationary night blindness	Briard	AR	OptiGen	PBL
	Briard	AR	AHT	PBL
Copper toxicosis	Bedlington terrier	AR	AHT	PBL
in combo with marker test (at VetGen)	Bedlington terrier	AR	VetGen	PBL
Cystinuria	Newfoundland	AR	Penn	PBL
	Newfoundland	AR	OptiGen	PBL
	Newfoundland	AR	VetGen	PBL
Familial nephropathy (hereditary nephritis)	English cocker spaniel	AR	OptiGen	PBL
Factor VII deficiency	Beagle	AR	Penn	PBL
	Scottish deerhound	AR	Penn	PBL
Factor XI deficiency	Kerry blue terrier	AD(P)?	Penn	NDY
Fucosidosis	English springer spaniel	AR	Penn	PBL
	English springer spaniel	AR	AHT	PBL
Glanzmann's thrombasthenia (I)	Great Pyrenees	AR	Auburn	PBL
	Otter hound	AR	Auburn	PBL
Hemophilia B	German wirehaired pointer	XL	Cornell	PBL
Ivermectin toxicity	Australian shepherd	AR	Wash State	PBL
	Collie	AR	Wash State	PBL
	Long-haired whippes	AR	Wash State	PBL
	Old English sheepdogs	AR	Wash State	PBL
	Sheepdogs (shelties)	AR	Wash State	PBL
L-2-hydroxyl glutaric aciduria	Staffordshire bull terriers	AR	AHT	PBL
Mucopolysaccharidosis IIIB	Schipperke	AR	Penn	PBL
Mucopolysaccharidosis VI	Miniature pinscher	AR	Penn	PBL
Mucopolysaccharidosis VII	German shepherd	AR	Penn	PBL
Myotonia congenita	Miniature schnauzer	AR	Penn	PBL
	Miniature schnauzer	AR	OptiGen	PBL
Narcolepsy	Dachshund	AR	OptiGen	PBL
	Doberman pinscher	AR	OptiGen	PBL
	Labrador retriever	AR	OptiGen	PBL
Neonatal encephalopathy	Standard poodle	AR	U of MO	PBL
Phosphofructokinase deficiency	American cocker spaniel	AR	OptiGen	PBL
	American cocker spaniel	AR	Penn	PBL
	American cocker spaniel	AR	VetGen	PBL
	English springer spaniel	AR	OptiGen	PBL
	English springer spaniel	AR	Penn	PBL
	English springer spaniel	AR	VetGen	PBL
	English springer spaniel	AR	AHT	PBL
Progressive retinal atrophy (PRA) type A	Miniature schnauzer	AD(P)	OptiGen	NDY
Progressive retinal atrophy—dominant	Bullmastiff	AD	OptiGen	PBL
	Old English mastiff	AD	OptiGen	PBL

Table **230-2**—Cont'd

List of Some Direct Mutation Tests for Canine Inherited Disorders

Disease	Breed(s)	Inheritance	Laboratory	Basis
Progressive retinal atrophy—X-linked	Siberian husky	XL	OptiGen	PBL
	Samoyed	XL	OptiGen	PBL
Progressive retinal atrophy (Rcd3)	Cardigan Welsh corgi	AR	OptiGen	PBL
Pyruvate kinase deficiency	Basenji	AR	OptiGen	PBL
	Basenji	AR	Penn	PBL
	Basenji	AR	Vetgen	PBL
	Basenji	AR	AHT	PBL
	Beagle	AR	Penn	PBL
	Cairn terrier	AR	Penn	PBL
	Dachshund	AR	Penn	PBL
	Eskimo	AR	Penn	PBL
	West Highland white terrier	AR	Penn	PBL
	West Highland white terrier	AR	AHT	PBL
Rod cone dysplasia -1 (Rcd1)	Irish setter	AR	OptiGen	PBL
	Irish setter	AR	VetGen	PBL
	Irish setter	AR	AHT	PBL
Rod cone dysplasia -1 (Rcd1a)	Sloughi	AR	OptiGen	PBL
	Sloughi	AR	AHT	PBL
Rod cone dysplasia-3 (form of PRA)	Cardigan Welsh terrier	AR	OptiGen	PBL
Progressive rod cone degeneration (PRCD)	American Eskimo	AR	OptiGen	Patent
	Australian cattle dog	AR	OptiGen	Patent
	Australian shepherd	AR	OptiGen	Patent
	Chesapeake Bay retriever	AR	OptiGen	Patent
	Chinese crested	AR	OptiGen	Patent
	English cocker spaniel	AR	OptiGen	Patent
	Labrador retriever	AR	OptiGen	Patent
	Nova Scotia duck TR	AR	OptiGen	Patent
	Miniature and toy poodle	AR	OptiGen	Patent
	Portuguese water dog	AR	OptiGen	Patent
Severe combined immunodeficiency	Bassett hound	XL	Penn	PBL
	West Highland white terrier	XL	Penn	PBL
	Cardigan Welsh corgi	XL	Penn	PBL
von Willebrand disease type I	Bernese mountain dog	AR?	VetGen	Patent
	Doberman pinscher	AR?	VetGen	Patent
	German pinscher	AR?	VetGen	Patent
	Kerry blue terrier	AR?	VetGen	Patent
	Manchester terrier	AR?	VetGen	Patent
	Papillon	AR?	VetGen	Patent
	Pembroke Welsh corgi	AR?	VetGen	Patent
	Poodle (all varieties)	AR?	VetGen	Patent
von Willebrand disease type II	German shorthaired pointer	AR	VetGen	PBL
von Willebrand disease type III	Scottish terrier	AR	VetGen	PBL
	Shetland sheepdog	AR	VetGen	Patent

AD, Autosomal-dominant; *AD(P)*, autosomal-dominant with partial penetrance; *AR*, autosomal-recessive; *NDY*, no data yet: no publicly available data at present to my knowledge beyond that indicated on the website; *patent*, patent which can be viewed on U.S. patent website; *PBL*, peer-reviewed publication; *Un*, unknown; *XL*, X-linked–recessive.

Direct mutation tests can be virtually 100% accurate if there is a strong founder effect within the breed, but another mutation in the same gene or a different gene causing the disease is always a possibility in some percentage of the cases. (All information in this table is deemed reliable at the time of writing, but I do not guarantee its accuracy or completeness; see the individual laboratory for full details).

Once a causative mutation for an inherited disorder has been well documented, a direct mutation test can be nearly 100% accurate if the disease in the breed has been passed on by a popular breeding animal. Many genetic diseases in the dog are recessive because of this founder effect (Ostrande, Galibert, and Patterson, 2000). In humans with recessive diseases, affected individuals often are compound heterozygotes (i.e., they have two different mutations of the same gene causing the disease). On the other hand, affected dogs often have two identical copies of the same mutation passed on from the founding individual through both their sire and dam lines. If the founder effect is very strong within a breed for a particular disease and no other similar forms of the disease are caused by a different mutation in the same gene or other genes, a direct mutation test is highly accurate. However, one must always consider the possibility of a new (de novo) mutation occurring in the same gene. These are different from the primary mutation within that breed and create the possibility of heterogeneity of an identical-appearing disorder caused by a different gene. Among breeds the specific mutations are sometimes exactly the same, as in some instances of type 1 von Willebrand's disease. Other times the mutations are breed specific as with the three different mutations for narcolepsy in the hypocretin receptor gene of Doberman pinschers, Labrador retrievers, and dachshunds (Hungs et al., 2001).

Genetic Linkage Tests

A genetic linkage test is based on linkage between a genetic marker allele and a disease. There are two major ways to prove linkage. The first is a family linkage study in which marker alleles are tracked through generations of affected families in a breed to determine if the marker allele cosegregates with the disease. When statistically significant linkage is found through a significant log of odds score of 3 or greater, this is direct evidence of the causative mutation residing on the chromosomal segment containing the marker. The other major method of showing association between marker allele and a disease is by a linkage association study, which is done by testing markers on a group of affected individuals versus a matched group of normal control individuals. A statistically significant association by chi square or other statistical analysis can identify chromosomal regions that potentially contain the causative gene for an inherited disorder. This type of association of a marker allele and disease is termed *linkage disequilibrium* (Mostoskey et al., 2000) and indicates that one allele of a marker is associated with a disease far more often than would be expected if the marker allele frequencies were in Hardy-Weinberg equilibrium.

Statistical association in linkage studies is not necessarily direct evidence that a gene is in a chromosomal segment close to the marker. There is always the possibility of confounding variables and false positives. If the association is true, evidence from linkage association studies should be verifiable through family linkage studies. Positive association studies are insufficient evidence for validating a marker linkage test. A genetic linkage test should be used for individuals only when it has been proven through family analysis and strong association in the breed population. See Fig. 230-3 for a hypothetic example of a genetic linkage test done on a family.

Genetic linkage tests are never 100% accurate for all individuals in a breed; therefore they should be considered screening tests only. As previously discussed, depending on population dynamics and other factors, a direct mutation test can sometimes be very close to 100% accurate and therefore is considered the definitive test. The accuracy of the genetic linkage test depends on the recombination fraction between the marker and the gene and the population dynamics of the breed. One specific allele of the linked marker is most often associated with the mutation because of a popular founding individual. However, often a few individuals have the same specific allele but do not have the mutation because of a previous recombination between the marker and the gene. This false association also can be caused by population dynamics in which some family lines always hold the same specific marker allele yet not associated with the mutated gene. A sensitivity, specificity, positive predictive value and a negative predictive value can be calculated from sufficient data for a genetic marker test. A currently available genetic linkage test for copper toxicosis is listed Table 230-3.

Genetic linkage tests generally are often temporary screening tests because, once a linked marker is documented, the genetic mutation is likely to be identified by positional cloning. An example of this is copper toxicosis in Bedlington terriers for which a linked marker and corresponding marker test were identified in 1997 (Yuzbasiyan-Gurkan et al., 1997). The genetic linkage test was verified in a larger population shortly thereafter (Rothuizen et al., 1999), and a number of years later the putative mutation was identified (van de Sluis et al., 2002).

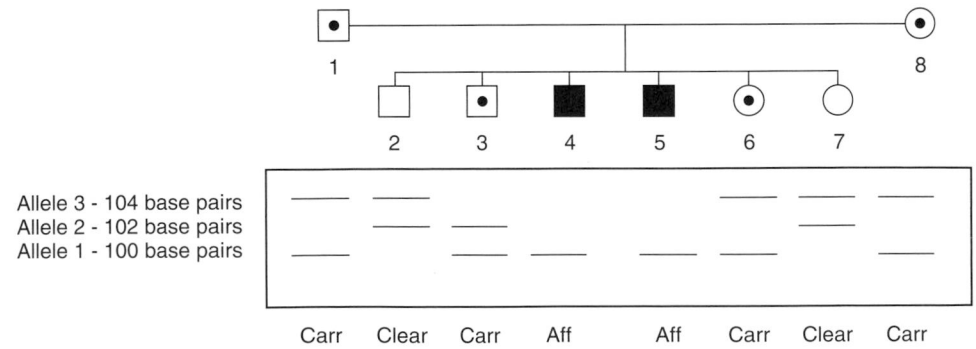

Fig. 230-3   Gel electrophoresis results for a hypothetic genetic linkage test in a family. Marker A has three alleles that vary in size by two base pairs in size of a dinucleotide marker repeat such as CA. The marker is closely linked to the gene defect, with allele 1 usually being associated with the disease allele and alleles 2 and 3 usually being associated with the normal gene allele. The alleles from each individual can be separated and visualized on a gel by electrophoresis. Squares are males and circles are females. Individuals 1 and 8 are the parents and are both carriers. Individuals 4 and 5 are both affected and have two of the 1 alleles (only one band is visualized because the 1 alleles from each parent are the same size). The status indicated below each set of gel band for each individual is the most likely genetic status (Clear = likely clear, Carr = likely carrier, Aff = likely affected) for a hypothetic recessive disease. Genetic linkage tests are never 100% accurate because of recombination events and/or population dynamics, but they can be good screening tests if there is a low recombination frequency and a strong founder effect. Eventually the actual mutation should be able to be identified, and a direct gene test developed. Laboratories should always run positive and negative controls for all molecular genetic tests.

Table **230-3**

Genetic Linkage Test for Canine Inherited Disorder

Disease	Breed(s)	Inheritance	Laboratory	Basis
Copper toxicosis	Bedlington Terrier	AR	Vetgen	PBL

AR, Autosomal-recessive; *PBL,* peer-reviewed publication. For complete laboratory details see Table 230-1. Genetic linkage tests are never 100% accurate and should be used as screening test only until the mutation is identified.

FUTURE TEST DEVELOPMENT, OTHER SERVICES, AND UPDATED TEST LISTS

The field of canine molecular genetics is evolving at a fast pace; therefore the list of available tests and services is also changing rapidly. Individual results for a direct mutation test generally have a straightforward interpretation. If direct mutation test results will be used in a breeding program or if results of a genetic linkage test are currently used, a canine geneticist should be consulted for genetic counseling. Many of the listed laboratories (see Table 230-1) and some other laboratories offer additional services such as individual DNA identification, parentage testing, DNA storage, coat color genetic testing, and/or karyotyping.

The principles and details outlined here apply equally well to testing for inherited disorders of cats. Updated lists of the available tests for dogs can be found at the website for the American Kennel Club Canine Health Foundation: http://www.akcchf.org/research/genetic_tests.pdf.

References and Suggested Reading

Giger U: Clinical genetics. In Ettinger SF, Feldman EC, editors: *The textbook of veterinary internal medicine,* Philadelphia, 2000, Saunders, p 2.

Hungs M et al: Identification and functional analysis of mutations in the hypocretin (orexin) genes of narcoleptic canines, *Genome Res* 11(4):531, 2001.

Lindblad-Toh K et al: Genome sequence, comparative analysis and haplotype structure of the domestic dog, *Nature* 438(7069): 803, 2005.

Metallinos DL: Canine molecular genetic testing. In Davidson AP, editor: *Vet Clin North Am Small Anim Pract* 31(2):421, 2001.

Mostosky UV et al: Canine molecular genetic diseases, *Compend Contin Educ* 22(5):480, 2000.

Ostrander EA, Galibert F, Patterson DF: Canine genetics comes of age, *Trends Genet* 16(3):117-124, 2000.

Patterson DF: Companion animal medicine in the age of medical genetics, *J Vet Intern Med* 14(1):1, 2000.

Rothuizen J et al: Diagnostic value of a microsatellite DNA marker for copper toxicosis in West-European Bedlington terriers and incidence of the disease, *Anim Genet* 30(3):190, 1999.

van de Sluis B et al: Identification of a new copper metabolism gene by positional cloning in a purebred dog population, *Hum Mol Genet* 15;11(2):165, 2002.

Yuzbasiyan-Gurkan V et al: Linkage of a microsatellite marker to the canine copper toxicosis locus in Bedlington terriers, *Am J Vet Res* 58(1):23, 1997.

SECTION XI

Neurologic and Musculoskeletal Diseases

Rodney S. Bagley

CHAPTER 231
Treatment of Status Epilepticus

MICHAEL PODELL, *Northbrook, Illinois*

Status epilepticus (SE) is a life-threatening neurologic emergency characterized by prolonged seizure activity. SE has been defined as an epileptic seizure or sequence of recurrent seizures persisting for at least 30 minutes during which the patient does not regain normal consciousness (Drislane, 2005). A stricter criterion includes the presence of electrical seizure activity for at least 30 minutes' duration, even if consciousness is not impaired. However, data from human patients indicate that seizures lasting for at least 10 minutes are unlikely to stop on their own without pharmacologic intervention (DeLorenzo et al., 1999). Many epileptic dogs and cats exhibit recurrent generalized epileptic seizures within a 24-hour period, termed *cluster seizures*. Since little information is available on the electrical activity of the brain of these patients during these events, coupled with the fact that many of these cluster seizures are intermixed with difficult-to-observe partial seizures and abnormal behavior, it is possible that many of these affected animals are exhibiting a form of SE unique to this species. Failure to control these seizures can not only be a life-threatening event, but also may also contribute to poor long-term seizure control (Kwan, 2000).

INITIAL APPROACH AND DIAGNOSIS

The cause of SE is often related to whether previous epilepsy has been diagnosed. In general there has been no definitive evidence correlating SE to specific etiology. A higher proportion of dogs with previous seizures in the age range of 1 to 5 have idiopathic epilepsy. Approximately 25% of the SE cases in one study were idiopathic in nature (Bateman and Parent, 1999). Many of these animals develop SE or cluster seizures because of inadequate antiepileptic drug (AED) therapy, drug tolerance, or recent changes in therapy (Saito et al., 2001). In contrast, dogs with new onset of seizure activity that are younger than 1 year or older than 7 years are more likely to have symptomatic epilepsy as a result of a predisposing underlying brain disease. Younger animals are more susceptible to toxicity, metabolic encephalopathies (e.g., portosystemic shunts), and encephalitic diseases as a cause for seizures. However, older cats and dogs are more likely to suffer from underlying brain neoplasm, cerebrovascular disease, and metabolic encephalopathy from advancing renal or liver disease.

Immediate diagnostic testing should revolve around the current physiologic status of the seizing animal. Basic cardiopulmonary resuscitation requirements of ensuring that there is an open airway with adequate blood oxygenation with a pulse oximeter and/or blood gas and providing fluid support to maintain normal blood pressure is critical. Minimal STAT testing includes analysis of blood glucose, electrolytes (sodium, potassium, calcium, chloride), and packed cell volume and total plasma protein. Optimal STAT testing includes a complete blood count, serum chemistry panel (to include creatine phosphokinase), blood gas analysis, and existing AED serum concentrations. However, the latter tests typically are unavailable to most emergency clinics. Serum should be collected in a nonserum separator tube at the time of admission for future submission of AED serum concentrations.

Delayed or advanced diagnostic testing entails determination of the underlying cause for the seizures, as well as evaluation of existing serum AED levels as applicable. These tests include thoracic and abdominal radiographs, possible abdominal ultrasound, and any follow-up biochemical testing as indicated by the initial laboratory testing. Advanced imaging of the brain (i.e., magnetic resonance imaging scan) is strongly recommended for any new-onset seizure dog over the age of 7 years and for any cat proven not to have a metabolic disease. Collection of cerebrospinal fluid typically depends on results of the imaging. Results of neuroimaging can be abnormal as a consequence of SE in a high proportion of dogs (Platt and Haag, 2002)

TREATMENT

The goals of treating SE are simple: *stop* the seizures, *protect* the brain from further damage, and allow full *recovery* from the episode of SE. The longer an animal seizes, the greater the chances are that neuronal injury will occur. Brain damage in the epileptic patient begins at the subcellular level, progresses to the cellular level, and over time will result in overt pathologic changes to the brain that may lead to permanent changes in brain function. With the onset of a seizure, several mechanisms occurring simultaneously can lead to neuronal death. Understanding the effect of these changes on the brain is important when planning proper emergency seizure therapy. Several factors lead to direct cytotoxicity, including hypoxemia, ischemia, and excitotoxicity. Excitotoxicity is caused by an excessive activation of glutamate receptors, an excitatory neurotransmitter, resulting in an excessive and prolonged influx of intracellular calcium that disrupts the normal metabolic activity of the cell. Thus the acute pathogenesis of brain injury during seizures dictates therapy designed to stop the ictal event, reduce intracranial pressure by decreasing cerebral edema, and provide the care to support neuronal metabolic activity. Cerebral edema and hippocampal necrosis have been identified in cats with prolonged seizure activity, suggesting that rapid-onset cytotoxicity may occur as compared to dogs (Fatzer et al., 2000).

Management of SE is most effective when a preestablished protocol is followed. Although individual variations in treatment protocols exist in both human and veterinary medicine, the key to a successful outcome is threefold: (1) Establish physiologic supportive care; (2) provide effective and immediate-acting AED therapy; and (3) institute AED therapy that will maintain prolonged antiepileptic action (Podell, 1996). Specific AED therapy revolves around the ability of the drug to rapidly enter the brain, provide effective and immediate seizure cessation, possess no-to-minimal adverse systemic or neurologic effects, and be retained in the brain to prevent future seizures. The protocols listed in Fig. 231-1 provide a sequential plan of action starting from initial care through complete anesthesia for the dog and cat.

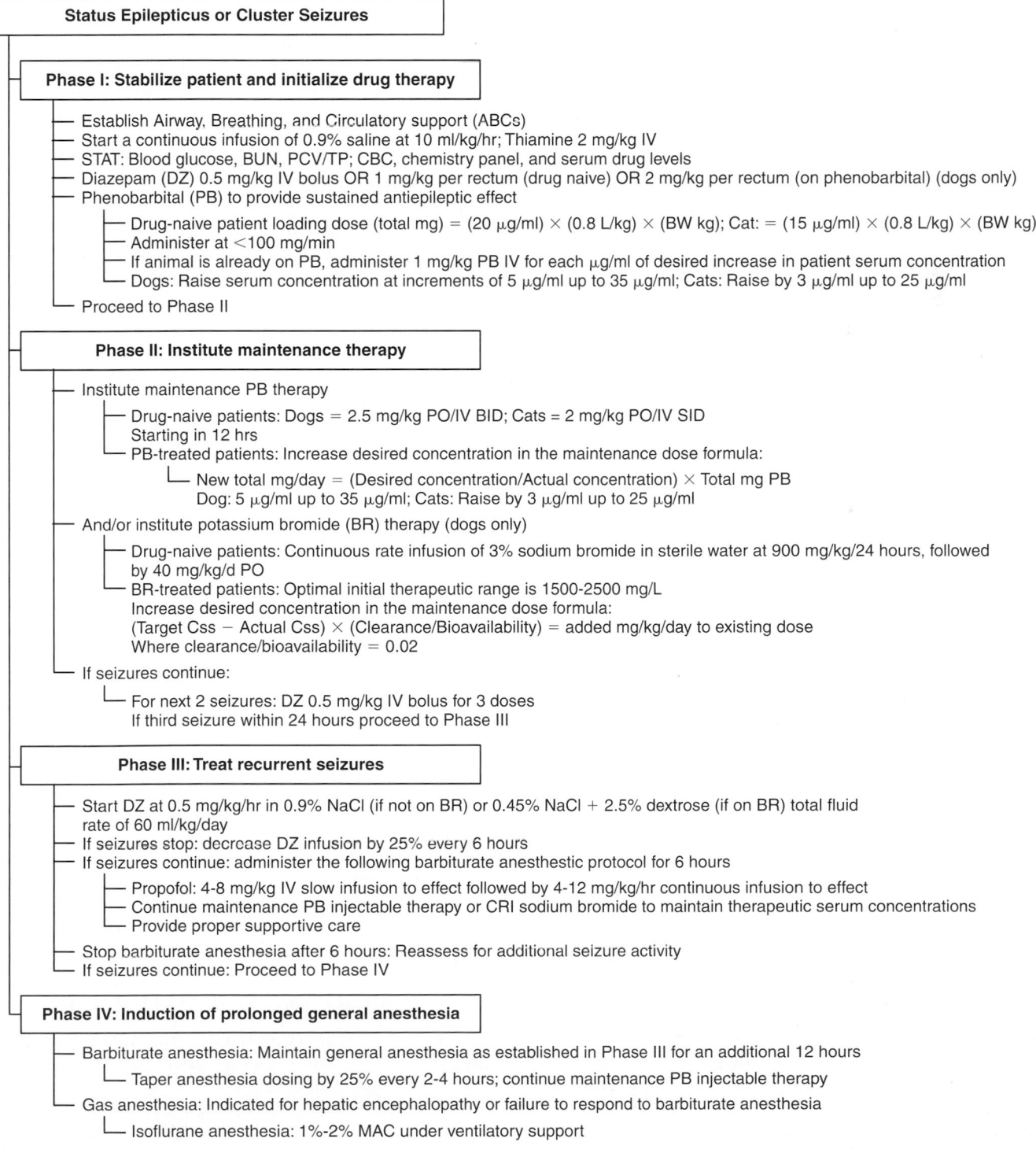

Status Epilepticus or Cluster Seizures

Phase I: Stabilize patient and initialize drug therapy

- Establish Airway, Breathing, and Circulatory support (ABCs)
- Start a continuous infusion of 0.9% saline at 10 ml/kg/hr; Thiamine 2 mg/kg IV
- STAT: Blood glucose, BUN, PCV/TP; CBC, chemistry panel, and serum drug levels
- Diazepam (DZ) 0.5 mg/kg IV bolus OR 1 mg/kg per rectum (drug naive) OR 2 mg/kg per rectum (on phenobarbital) (dogs only)
- Phenobarbital (PB) to provide sustained antiepileptic effect
  - Drug-naive patient loading dose (total mg) = (20 μg/ml) × (0.8 L/kg) × (BW kg); Cat: = (15 μg/ml) × (0.8 L/kg) × (BW kg)
  - Administer at <100 mg/min
  - If animal is already on PB, administer 1 mg/kg PB IV for each μg/ml of desired increase in patient serum concentration
  - Dogs: Raise serum concentration at increments of 5 μg/ml up to 35 μg/ml; Cats: Raise by 3 μg/ml up to 25 μg/ml
- Proceed to Phase II

Phase II: Institute maintenance therapy

- Institute maintenance PB therapy
  - Drug-naive patients: Dogs = 2.5 mg/kg PO/IV BID; Cats = 2 mg/kg PO/IV SID
  - Starting in 12 hrs
  - PB-treated patients: Increase desired concentration in the maintenance dose formula:
    - New total mg/day = (Desired concentration/Actual concentration) × Total mg PB
    - Dog: 5 μg/ml up to 35 μg/ml; Cats: Raise by 3 μg/ml up to 25 μg/ml
- And/or institute potassium bromide (BR) therapy (dogs only)
  - Drug-naive patients: Continuous rate infusion of 3% sodium bromide in sterile water at 900 mg/kg/24 hours, followed by 40 mg/kg/d PO
  - BR-treated patients: Optimal initial therapeutic range is 1500-2500 mg/L
    Increase desired concentration in the maintenance dose formula:
    (Target Css − Actual Css) × (Clearance/Bioavailability) = added mg/kg/day to existing dose
    Where clearance/bioavailability = 0.02
- If seizures continue:
  - For next 2 seizures: DZ 0.5 mg/kg IV bolus for 3 doses
    If third seizure within 24 hours proceed to Phase III

Phase III: Treat recurrent seizures

- Start DZ at 0.5 mg/kg/hr in 0.9% NaCl (if not on BR) or 0.45% NaCl + 2.5% dextrose (if on BR) total fluid rate of 60 ml/kg/day
- If seizures stop: decrease DZ infusion by 25% every 6 hours
- If seizures continue: administer the following barbiturate anesthestic protocol for 6 hours
  - Propofol: 4-8 mg/kg IV slow infusion to effect followed by 4-12 mg/kg/hr continuous infusion to effect
  - Continue maintenance PB injectable therapy or CRI sodium bromide to maintain therapeutic serum concentrations
  - Provide proper supportive care
- Stop barbiturate anesthesia after 6 hours: Reassess for additional seizure activity
- If seizures continue: Proceed to Phase IV

Phase IV: Induction of prolonged general anesthesia

- Barbiturate anesthesia: Maintain general anesthesia as established in Phase III for an additional 12 hours
  - Taper anesthesia dosing by 25% every 2-4 hours; continue maintenance PB injectable therapy
- Gas anesthesia: Indicated for hepatic encephalopathy or failure to respond to barbiturate anesthesia
  - Isoflurane anesthesia: 1%-2% MAC under ventilatory support

Fig. 231-1 Medical management of status epilepticus in the dog and cat.

The majority of animals that present for SE have experienced or are actively suffering from generalized seizure activity. Immediate cessation of seizure activity is the primary treatment goal (see Fig. ##-1). Administration of benzodiazepine therapy is the most effective method to rapidly stop electrical epileptic seizure activity. Administration of diazepam per rectum at 1 mg/kg in drug-naïve dogs or 2 mg/kg in dogs on phenobarbital (PB) provides a rapid method of initiation of drug therapy that is especially helpful before intravenous catheter placement and diazepam intravenous therapy (0.5 mg/kg intravenously [IV]). The benefit of rectal administration in cats has not been well documented. Higher doses of diazepam are not recommended because the risk of respiratory depression outweighs any further anticonvulsant benefit. Midazolam (0.3 mg/kg IV) and lorazepam (0.2 mg/kg IV) are alternative benzodiazepine therapies with proven prolonged anticonvulsant benefit in people but are more expensive and unproven in canine or feline SE.

All cases of SE are treated as "trauma" patients. It is essential to maintain a patent airway, support proper breathing patterns and oxygenation, and provide circulatory support. Stabilizing the patient and reversing the physiologic sequelae of prolonged or recurrent seizure activity within the first 30 minutes of SE are critical since dogs develop arterial hypertension, increased cerebral blood flow, hypoxemia, hypercarbemia, hyperglycemia, and lactic acidosis. Subsequent changes may include arterial hypotension, decrease in blood pH, pyrexia, hyperkalemia, myoglobinuria, and hypoglycemia. The combination of circulatory collapse, organ hypoperfusion, and energy depletion can lead to severe, irreversible organ failure (renal, cardiac, hepatic). Thiamine (2 mg/kg IV) should be administered since this B vitamin is an important cofactor for cerebral aerobic glycolytic metabolism. Dextrose-containing solutions should *not* be administered unless hypoglycemia is documented. Hyperglycemia in the face of reduced oxidative phosphorylation in the brain results in central nervous system lactic acidosis and resultant neuronal necrosis. Mannitol at 1 g/kg IV over a 15-minute period along with low-steroid therapy (dexamethasone SP 0.25 mg/kg IV) is recommended to treat for cerebral edema.

Following initial diazepam therapy, institution of a maintenance therapy is critical to prevent seizure recurrence. PB therapy is the current drug of choice because of its ability to provide a rapid intravenous loading dose, its efficacy to suppress seizure activity, a long elimination half-life, and cost effectiveness. An initial PB dose of 16 mg/kg and 12 mg/kg IV given at a rate of 100 mg/minute will provide a serum concentration of 20 mcg/ml and 15 mcg/ml in drug-naïve dogs and cats, respectively. For previously treated dogs the goal is to raise the PB serum concentration by 5 mcg/ml by using either STAT laboratory testing or the most recent PB serum concentration, to a maximum of 35 mcg/ml. PB has a more prolonged elimination half-life in the cat; therefore sedative effects may be prevalent (Parent and Quesnel, 1996). Thus the initial therapeutic range is lower, typically between 10 and 20 mcg/ml, and dosing is highly individualized. Most cats can be treated with a maintenance dosage of 1 to 2 mg/kg/day, with once daily dosing initially at night.

The author recommends bromide (BR) loading therapy in dogs with suspected or documented hepatic disease or cases refractory to PB therapy. I prefer intravenous loading of sodium BR over oral or rectal loading techniques because this protocol provides a more predictable rise in bromide serum concentration without the risk for adverse gastrointestinal problems. A 3% sterile sodium BR solution is prepared by diluting 30 g of gas-sterilized sodium BR salt into 1 L of sterile water and administered through a 40-μm filter at a dose of 900 mg/kg/24 hours to achieve a serum BR concentration of 2000 mg/L at the end of the loading period. Potassium BR is then dosed at 40 mg/kg PO every 24 hours. There is a potential for enhanced sedation with this treatment that typically resolves within several days. BR therapy in cats is *not* recommended as a standard therapy because of the relatively high prevalence of adverse respiratory problems (Boothe, 2002). Cats can develop cough and more severe respiratory signs suggestive of an allergic asthmatic disease.

Levetiracetam (Keppra) is the S-enantiomer of the ethyl analogue of piracetam that binds to SV2A, a synaptic vesicle protein, which correlates to anticonvulsant potency. The drug is well absorbed without hepatic metabolism, has minimal protein binding, is available as a parenteral formulation, and has minimal adverse effects. An initial loading dose of 60 mg/kg IV over 30 minutes is recommended, followed by an oral maintenance dose of 20 mg/kg every 8 to 12 hours, as levetiracetam has a relatively short elimination half-life of 4 to 8 hours in dogs. No pharmacokinetic data could be found for cats. Although levetiracetam is considerably more expensive than bromide therapy, I have found it to be an effective alternative to bromide loading without the potential for posttreatment sedation.

Recurrent seizure activity beyond this initial therapy is treated with continuous rate infusion (CRI) of diazepam (see Fig. 231-1). A gradual taper of 25% every 6 hours is recommended to avoid potential withdrawal-induced seizure activity. Longer-term barbiturate CRI is the next level of treatment for breakthrough seizure activity. Propofol is recommended because of the short-elimination half-life and subsequent ability for rapid awakening. The initial induction dose is 4 to 8 mg/kg IV to effect followed by a CRI of 8 to 12 mg/kg/hour. Higher doses of propofol are typically needed to achieve optimal treatment with burst suppression and absence of epileptic activity on electroencephalogram monitoring in people and dogs. Barbiturate CRI treatment is recommended for an initial 6-hour period before cessation. Induction of prolonged general anesthesia with CRI barbiturate is instituted for 24 hours if breakthrough seizures occur. Isoflurane general anesthesia is the last treatment phase and typically is reserved for patients with recurrent seizure activity or dogs with hepatic disease.

MONITORING AND SUPPORTIVE CARE

Generalized convulsive SE is a dynamic condition, with a progressive diminution of convulsive activity as the seizures continue. Thus observation alone may be an inadequate method of determining seizure control. Monitoring of electroencephalographic activity has been instituted to ensure that complete cessation of all electrical epileptic activity has been achieved. Improvements in seizure control and eventual outcome can be related to the ability to determine cessation of all epileptic brain activity. Other parameters to monitor include heart rate, blood pressure, respiratory rate, pulse oximetry, and serial neurologic examinations. Rectal temperature should be closely monitored during the first hour. Animals should be cooled with ice and cold water if rectal temperature is 104°F or higher. Cooling should stop when rectal temperature is 102°F to prevent rebound hypothermia. Endotracheal intubation and assisted ventilation may be required in patients on barbiturate CRI with induced general anesthesia.

In conclusion, SE is a serious, life-threatening disorder that requires rapid medical intervention. Recurrence of seizure activity is often the result of failure to maintain continuous therapeutic serum AED levels for sufficient periods of time to suppress epileptic activity. Successful treatment requires early recognition and intervention and the use of a standardized treatment protocol. A preemptive treatment protocol as presented here allows patients to benefit not only from the initial relief from current seizure activity but also from potential overall improvement in long-term seizure control.

References and Suggested Reading

Bateman SW, Parent JM: Clinical findings, treatment, and outcome of dogs with status epilepticus or cluster seizures: 156 cases (1990-1995), *J Am Vet Med Assoc* 215:1463, 1999.

Boothe DM, George KL: Disposition and clinical use of bromide in cats, *J Am Vet Med Assoc* 221:1131, 2002.

DeLorenzo RJ et al: Comparison of status epilepticus with prolonged seizure episodes lasting from 10 to 29 minutes, *Epilepsia* 40:164, 1999.

Drislane FW: *Types of status epilepticus: definitions and classification.* In *Status epilepticus: a clinical perspective,* 2005, Humana Press, Totowa, NJ, p 11.

Fatzer F et al: Necrosis of hippocampus and piriform lobe in 38 domestic cats with seizures: a retrospective study on clinical and pathologic findings, *J Vet Intern Med* 14:100, 2000.

Kwan P et al: Early identification of refractory epilepsy, *N Engl J Med* 342:314, 2000.

March PA, Podell M, Sams RA: Pharmacokinetics and toxicity of bromide following high-dose oral potassium bromide administration in healthy Beagles, *J Vet Pharmacol Ther* 25:425, 2002.

Parent JM, Quesnel AD: Seizures in cats, *Vet Clin North Am Small Anim Pract* 26:811, 1996.

Platt SR, Haag M: Canine status epilepticus: a retrospective study of 50 cases, *J Small Anim Pract* 43:151, 2002.

Podell M: The use of diazepam per rectum at home for the acute management of cluster seizures in dogs, *J Vet Intern Med* 8:68, 1995.

Podell M: Seizures in dogs, *Vet Clin North Am Small Anim Pract* 26:779, 1996.

Saito M et al: .Risk factors for development of status epilepticus in dogs with idiopathic epilepsy and effects of status epilepticus on outcome and survival time: 32 cases, *J Am Vet Med Assoc* 219: 618, 2001.

CHAPTER 232

New Maintenance Anticonvulsant Therapies for Dogs and Cats

CURTIS W. DEWEY, *Ithaca, New York*

Over the last 15 years the paradigm for treating dogs and cats with seizure disorders has changed, coincident with the introduction of several new anticonvulsant drugs. Although phenobarbital (dogs and cats) and bromide (dogs) remain valuable first-choice anticonvulsant drug choices for pets with seizure disorders, a number of alternative drugs can be used as either adjunctive (i.e., for refractory seizures) or sole therapeutic options. The major impediments to widespread use of these newer anticonvulsant drugs are principally increased cost compared with phenobarbital and bromide and clinical unfamiliarity with their usage. Since several of these drugs (gabapentin, zonisamide, levetiracetam) are now available in generic forms, cost is now less of a concern. Information is available concerning several newer anticonvulsant drugs for canine use. Unfortunately much of the information regarding new anticonvulsant therapy for cats remains largely anecdotal. Despite this limitation, there is sound clinical evidence supporting the use of levetiracetam in cats as an add-on drug for patients that are refractory to phenobarbital therapy. This chapter summarizes some of these newer anticonvulsant drugs with recommendations based on published literature and my own clinical experience. Additionally, the next generation of some of these compounds is discussed briefly.

GABAPENTIN

Gabapentin, a structural analog of γ-aminobutyric acid (GABA), probably exerts its antiseizure effects via inhibition of voltage-gated calcium channels in the brain. Gabapentin is well absorbed in both dogs and people, with peak serum concentrations occurring within 1 to 3 hours after ingestion. In dogs 30% to 40% of the orally administered dose of gabapentin undergoes hepatic metabolism to N-methyl-gabapentin. Despite undergoing some hepatic metabolism in dogs, there is no appreciable induction of hepatic microsomal enzymes in this species. The half-life of elimination for gabapentin in dogs is between 3 and 4 hours. Because of its short half-life in dogs, gabapentin probably needs to be administered at least every 8 hours and possibly every 6 hours to maintain serum gabapentin concentrations within the therapeutic range. The potential need for every-6-hour dosing can make it difficult for some pet owners to administer gabapentin consistently.

The recommended *daily* dosage range of gabapentin for dogs is 25 to 60 mg/kg of body weight, *divided*, every 6 to 8 hours. I recommend an initial dose regimen of 10 mg/kg of body weight every 8 hours. The suspected therapeutic plasma concentration for dogs is 4 to 16 mg/L. Gabapentin concentrations are seldom measured in dogs.

Efficacy of gabapentin in dogs has been evaluated in some small studies. In one prospective study evaluating gabapentin as an add-on therapy for dogs with refractory seizure activity, there was no significant decrease in overall seizure activity over a 4-month evaluation period. Despite this, 3 of 17 dogs became seizure free, and 4 others experienced a 50% or more reduction in seizure frequency during the evaluation period. In a similar study evaluating 11 dogs, an overall significant reduction in seizure frequency was found, and 6 dogs experienced a 50% or more reduction in seizure frequency. Sedation and pelvic limb ataxia were the only reported side effects in these two studies. In my experience gabapentin is occasionally helpful as an anticonvulsant drug in dogs. In humans gabapentin appears to be much more effective in the treatment of focal seizure disorders than in that of generalized seizures.

Long-term canine toxicity trials for gabapentin have not been reported. However, the drug seems to be very well tolerated in this species, usually with little to no side effects. Sedation does not appear to be a major problem. However, I have had many clients report that their dogs experienced mild sedation or mild polyphagia and weight gain associated with gabapentin use.

Only anecdotal information is available regarding gabapentin use in cats. An oral dose of 5 to 10 mg/kg of body weight every 8 to 12 hours has been suggested but is not based on any published data. To my knowledge there is no information regarding either the safety or efficacy of chronic gabapentin administration to cats.

A new gabapentin analog, pregabalin, has recently been approved for human use. Pregabalin has an increased affinity for the α2δ-subunit of voltage-gated calcium channels compared with gabapentin and is purportedly more effective in people than its predecessor as both an anticonvulsant and a pain-relieving drug. My colleagues and I have recently investigated the pharmacokinetics of pregabalin in normal dogs. In addition, we have preliminary data regarding the efficacy of pregabalin in dogs with refractory epilepsy. Pregabalin has a favorable pharmacokinetic profile in dogs and appears to be an effective add-on anticonvulsant drug, based on a limited number of cases.

FELBAMATE

Felbamate is a dicarbamate drug that has demonstrated efficacy for both focal (partial) and generalized seizures in experimental animal studies and human clinical trials. Proposed mechanisms of action include blocking of N-methyl-D-aspartate (NMDA)–mediated neuronal excitation, potentiation of GABA-mediated neuronal inhibition, and inhibition of voltage-sensitive neuronal sodium and calcium channels. Felbamate may also offer some protection to neurons from hypoxic/ischemic damage.

Approximately 70% of the orally administered dose of felbamate in dogs is excreted in the urine unchanged; the remainder undergoes hepatic metabolism. The half-life of felbamate in adult dogs is typically between 5 and 6 hours (range 4 to 8 hours). Felbamate is well absorbed after oral administration in adult dogs, but bioavailability in puppies may be only 30% that of adults. The half-life of elimination in puppies has also been shown to be much shorter than in adult dogs (approximately 2.5 hours). For adult dogs I recommend an initial felbamate dosage regimen of 15 mg/kg of body weight every 8 hours. Felbamate has a wide margin of safety in dogs, with serious toxic effects usually not apparent below a daily dose of 300 mg per kilogram of body weight per day. If the initial dose of felbamate is ineffective, the dose is increased by 15-mg/kg increments every 2 weeks until efficacy is achieved, unacceptable side effects are evident, or the drug becomes cost prohibitive. The therapeutic range for serum felbamate concentration in dogs is believed to be similar to that in people (20 to 100 mcg/ml). Typically serum felbamate assays are costly. In addition, the wide therapeutic range and low toxicity potential of felbamate make routine serum drug monitoring of questionable clinical value. I do not routinely check felbamate levels in dogs.

The limited published material regarding clinical efficacy of felbamate is similar to my experience. In one report of refractory epileptic dogs, 12 of 16 patients experienced a reduction of seizure frequency following initiation of felbamate therapy. In another report of six dogs with suspected focal seizure activity, all dogs experienced a substantial reduction in seizure frequency when felbamate was used as a sole anticonvulsant drug; two of these dogs became seizure free.

I have used felbamate extensively in the treatment of dogs with seizure disorders. Felbamate appears to be very effective both as an add-on therapy and as a sole anticonvulsant agent for patients with focal and generalized seizures. Because of its lack of sedation, felbamate is particularly useful as monotherapy in dogs exhibiting obtunded mental status as a result of their underlying neurologic disease (e.g., brain tumor, cerebral infarct). I have found side effects from felbamate to be very infrequent, especially when it is used as a sole anticonvulsant drug. Hepatic dysfunction associated with felbamate use tends to resolve following discontinuation of the drug. In dogs with evidence of preexisting hepatic disease, felbamate should be avoided. Because of the potential for hepatotoxicity, it is recommended that serum biochemistry analysis be performed every 6 months for dogs receiving felbamate, especially if given concurrently with phenobarbital. It may also be advisable to evaluate complete blood counts every few months in the unlikely event that a blood dyscrasia develops.

Side effects are infrequently observed with felbamate use in dogs. Unlike other anticonvulsants, felbamate does not cause sedation. Because felbamate does undergo some hepatic metabolism, liver dysfunction is a potential side effect. In one study 4 of 12 dogs receiving felbamate as an add-on therapy developed liver disease; however, each of these dogs was also receiving high doses of phenobarbital. In humans felbamate has been shown to increase serum phenobarbital concentrations in some patients receiving combination therapy. It is unclear whether felbamate, phenobarbital, or the combination of the two drugs is responsible for the reported hepatotoxicity in dogs. In humans serious hepatotoxicity is rarely associated with felbamate use and usually occurs in patients concurrently receiving other anticonvulsant drugs. Aplastic anemia (caused by bone marrow suppression) has been reported to occur in people receiving felbamate at a rate of 10/100,000 patients; this uncommon and severe side effect is also usually encountered with patients receiving combination anticonvulsant drug therapy. Fortunately this does not appear to occur in dogs. However, in one report, reversible bone marrow suppression was suspected in two dogs receiving felbamate; one dog developed mild thrombocytopenia, the other mild leukopenia. Both of these abnormalities resolved following discontinuation of the drug. One patient in this report developed bilateral keratoconjunctivitis sicca (KCS); it is unknown whether this was related to felbamate use, though I have encountered several patients on felbamate that developed KCS. Generalized tremor activity in small-breed dogs receiving high doses of felbamate has also been reported as a rarely encountered side effect.

To my knowledge there is no clinical information regarding the use of felbamate in cats. Because of the potential for felbamate-associated hepatotoxicity and blood dyscrasias in dogs, felbamate is not likely to become a viable anticonvulsant option for cats.

Because of the problems of hepatoxicity and blood dyscrasias occasionally associated with felbamate use in people, a new derivative of the drug—fluorofelbamate—has been developed and is undergoing clinical trials for human use. In experimental animal epilepsy models fluorofelbamate has been shown to have equal or superior anticonvulsant potency in comparison with felbamate. A reactive aldehyde intermediate that is formed from felbamate metabolism has been linked to the hepatic and hematologic side effects of this drug. This toxic intermediate is not produced from metabolism of fluorofelbamate.

LEVETIRACETAM

Levetiracetam is a new piracetam anticonvulsant drug that has demonstrated efficacy in the treatment of focal and generalized seizure disorders in people, as well as in several experimental animal models. Although generally recommended as an add-on anticonvulsant drug, levetiracetam has been used successfully as monotherapy in people. In humans with refractory epilepsy, levetiracetam has manifested antiseizure effects within the first day of treatment. The mechanism of action for the anti-convulsant effects of levetiracetam is not entirely clear, but appears to be related to its binding with a specific synaptic vesicle protein (SV2A) in the brain. Unlike other anticonvulsant drugs, levetiracetam does not appear to directly affect common neurotransmitter pathways (e.g., GABA, NMDA) or ion channels (e.g., sodium, T-type calcium). Levetiracetam has demonstrated neuroprotective properties and may ameliorate seizure-induced brain damage. Levetiracetam has also been reported to have an "anti-kindling" effect, which may diminish the likelihood of increasing seizure frequency over time. Orally administered levetiracetam is approximately 100% bioavailable in dogs, with a serum half-life of 3 to 4 hours. Levetiracetam appears to exert an anticonvulsive effect that persists longer than its presence in the bloodstream would suggest. In dogs approximately 70% to 90% of the administered dose of levetiracetam is excreted unchanged in the urine; the remainder is hydrolyzed in the serum and other organs. There does not appear to be any appreciable hepatic metabolism of levetiracetam in either humans or dogs. The effective serum levetiracetam concentration in people is 5 to 45 mcg/ml. Because there is no clear relationship between serum drug concentration and efficacy for levetiracetam and since the drug has an extremely high margin of safety, routine therapeutic drug monitoring is not typically recommended for this drug in humans.

I have used levetiracetam in dogs as an add-on therapy with favorable results. In a recent report use of levetiracetam as an add-on drug in epileptic dogs was associated with a significant reduction (54%) in seizure frequency, with no apparent side effects. Because of its paucity of side effects and lack of hepatic metabolism, levetiracetam also presents an attractive anticonvulsant choice for patients with hepatic dysfunction. It has recently been suggested that some dogs that initially improve with levetiracetam therapy may return to baseline seizure frequency over a 4- to 8-month period (the "honeymoon effect").

I recommend an initial dosing schedule of 20 mg/kg of body weight every 8 hours based on both pharmacokinetic data and clinical experience. This dose can be increased by 20-mg/kg increments until efficacy is achieved, side effects become apparent, or the drug becomes cost prohibitive. At present, I recommend therapeutic blood monitoring of levetiracetam in dogs and cats, both for purposes of establishing a therapeutic range of the drug for these species, and for individual therapeutic decision making.

Long-term toxicity data for levetiracetam in dogs confirm that the drug is extremely safe. In one study dogs were administered oral levetiracetam at doses up to 1200 mg/kg/day for 1 year. One of eight dogs receiving 300 mg/kg/day developed a stiff/unsteady gait. Other side effects (salivation, vomiting) were confined to dogs receiving 1200 mg/kg/day. There were no treatment-related mortalities or histopathologic abnormalities.

My colleagues I and have prospectively investigated the use of oral levetiracetam as an add-on anticonvulsant therapy for epileptic cats refractory to phenobarbital. Levetiracetam appears to be very well tolerated in this species, usually with no apparent side effects. The half-life of elimination is approximately 3 hours after oral administration. A dose of 20 mg/kg PO every 8 hours typically achieves a serum drug level within the therapeutic range reported for people. Two of 12 cats experienced transient inappetance and lethargy that resolved without dose adjustment within 2 weeks. Although there is some degree of variability among cats, the mean reduction of seizure frequency in cats receiving levetiracetam as an add-on drug is approximately 68%; this was found to be statistically significant when compared to the prelevetiracetam time period. In addition, 7 of 10 cats evaluated for seizure frequency reduction were responders (i.e., reduction of seizure frequency of 50% or more), with a mean reduction of seizures of 92%. I consider levetiracetam to be the preferred add-on anticonvulsant drug for cats receiving phenobarbital because of lack of serious side effects and evidence of efficacy.

Intravenous levetiracetam has shown promise as a treatment for experimental status epilepticus in a rat model. In this study intravenous levetiracetam and diazepam appeared to potentiate the anticonvulsant effect of one another. Intravenous levetiracetam seems well tolerated in dogs, even at doses as high as 400 mg/kg of body weight. I have had limited but positive clinical experience using intravenous levetiracetam in dogs. Currently the pharmacokinetics of intravenous levetiracetam in normal dogs is under investigation.

Since the discovery of levetiracetam's unique binding site in the brain, two related anticonvulsant drugs—brivaracetam and seletracetam—with higher affinity than levetiracetam for the SV2A receptor have been developed. These drugs have been demonstrated to have improved anticonvulsant activity over levetiracetam in experimental animal seizure models and currently are being evaluated in human clinical epilepsy trials.

ZONISAMIDE

Zonisamide is a sulfonamide-based anticonvulsant drug recently approved for human use; it has demonstrated efficacy in the treatment of both focal and generalized seizures in people with minimal side effects. Suspected anticonvulsant mechanisms of action include blockage of T-type calcium and voltage-gated sodium channels in the brain, facilitation of dopaminergic and serotonergic neurotransmission in the central nervous system, scavenging free radical species, enhancing actions of GABA in the brain, inhibition of glutamate-mediated neuronal excitation in the brain, and inhibition of carbonic anhydrase activity. Zonisamide is metabolized primarily by hepatic microsomal enzymes, and the half-life in dogs is approximately 15 hours. In humans it has been shown that the elimination half-life of zonisamide is dramatically shorter in patients already receiving drugs that stimulate hepatic microsomal enzymes than in patients who are not receiving such drugs. A similar phenomenon appears to occur in dogs. When used as an add-on therapy for dogs already receiving drugs requiring hepatic metabolism (e.g., phenobarbital), I recommend an initial oral zonisamide dosage schedule of 10 mg/kg of body weight every 12 hours. This dosage regimen has been shown to maintain canine serum zonisamide concentrations within the therapeutic range reported for people (10 to 40 mcg/ml) when used as an add-on therapy. For dogs not concurrently receiving drugs that induce hepatic microsomal enzymes, it is recommended to start zonisamide at a dosage of 5 mg/kg of body weight every 12 hours. I generally check trough serum zonisamide concentrations after approximately 1 week of zonisamide treatment. Zonisamide has a high margin of safety in dogs. In one study minimal side effects occurred in beagles administered daily zonisamide doses up to 75 mg/kg of body weight per day for 1 year.

In one study zonisamide was found to decrease seizure frequency by at least 50% in 7 of 12 dogs with refractory idiopathic epilepsy. In this responder group the mean reduction in seizure frequency was 81.3%. In six of the seven responder dogs phenobarbital was able to be reduced by an average of 92.2%. Mild side effects (e.g., transient sedation, ataxia, vomiting) occurred in six dogs (50%); none of the side effects was considered severe enough to discontinue zonisamide therapy. In a more recent, similarly designed study, 9 of 11 refractory epileptic dogs treated with zonisamide were responders, with a median seizure reduction of 92.9%; transient ataxia and sedation occurred in six dogs.

Zonisamide has been shown to be very effective as a sole anticonvulsant drug in people. I have used zonisamide as a sole anticonvulsant drug in a large number of dogs. These have been primarily small-breed patients whose owners wished to avoid side effects associated with phenobarbital and bromide use. Zonisamide appears to be effective as a sole anticonvulsant therapy, with few- to–no apparent side effects in dogs.

I have treated two epileptic cats with zonisamide as an add-on to phenobarbital therapy. One cat became anorexic, necessitating drug discontinuation. The other cat experienced a substantial reduction in seizure frequency. This cat also had no side effects or blood work abnormalities attributable to zonisamide therapy after approximately 1 year of administration. Further data are needed regarding the use of zonisamide in cats before it can be recommended for use in this species.

References and Suggested Reading

Bailey KS et al: Levetiracetam as an adjunct to phenobarbital treatment in cats with suspected idiopathic epilepsy, 232: 867, 2008.

Bialer M: New antiepileptic drugs that are second generation to existing antiepileptic drugs, *Expert Opin Investig Drugs* 15:637, 2006.

Dewey CW: Anticonvulsant therapy in dogs and cats, *Vet Clin Small Anim* 36:1107, 2006.

Dewey CW et al: Pregabalin therapy for refractory idiopathic epilepsy in dogs, *J Vet Intern Med* (abstract in press), 2008.

Dewey CW et al: Zonisamide therapy for refractory idiopathic epilepsy in dogs, *J Am Anim Hosp Assoc* 40:285, 2004.

Govendir M, Perkins M, Malik R: Improving seizure control in dogs with refractory epilepsy using gabapentin as an adjunctive agent, *Aust Vet J* 83:602, 2005.

Mazarati AM, Sofia RD, Wasterlain CG: Anticonvulsant and antiepileptogenic effects of fluorofelbamate in experimental status epilepticus, *Seizure* 11:423, 2002.

Ramael S et al: Levetiracetam intravenous infusion: a randomized, placebo-controlled safety and pharmacokinetic study, *Epilepsia* 47:1128, 2006.

Salazar V et al: Pharmacokinetics of single-dose oral pregabalin adminstration in normal dogs, *J Vet Intern Med* (abstract in press), 2008.

Vartanian MG et al: Activity profile of pregabalin in rodent models of epilepsy and ataxia, *Epilepsy Res* 68:189, 2006.

Volk HA et al: The short and long term efficacy and tolerability of levetiracetam in pharmacoresistant epileptic dogs (abstract), *J Vet Intern Med* 21:592, 2007.

Von Klopman T et al: Prospective study of zonisamide therapy for refractory idiopathic epilepsy in dogs, *J Small Anim Pract*, 48:134, 2007.

CHAPTER 233

Treatment of Primary Central Nervous System Inflammation (Encephalitis and Meningitis)

ANDREA TIPOLD, *Hannover, Germany*

TREATMENT OF CENTRAL NERVOUS SYSTEM INFLAMMATION

Central nervous system (CNS) inflammatory lesions are an important group of disorders in all animal species and a challenge for the veterinarian. In our referral clinic this group of diseases accounts for about 10% of all neurologic cases in small animals. Besides causing severe neurologic impairment, several of these diseases are zoonoses. There are a large number of disorders in this category of inflammatory disease of both known and idiopathic etiology. Examples of meningoencephalomyelitides of known cause include canine distemper encephalitis, feline infectious peritonitis (FIP), central European tick-borne encephalitis, rabies, pseudorabies, canine herpesvirus encephalitis, West Nile virus infection, encephalomalacia caused by canine parvovirus, encephalitis caused by canine parainfluenza virus, and postvaccinal encephalitis after distemper or rabies vaccination. Besides viral infections, protozoal encephalomyelitis, bacterial meningoencephalitis, and mycotic infections of the CNS are causes of neurologic signs. In addition, a variety of meningoencephalomyelitides of unknown etiology are encountered. These include diseases with suspected viral etiology such as periventricular encephalitis; granulomatous meningoencephalomyelitis (GME); steroid-responsive meningitis-arteritis (SRMA); necrotizing meningoencephalitis of pugs, Maltese, and Yorkshire terriers; eosinophilic meningoencephalomyelitis; and a variety of inflammatory conditions of unknown origin, which are not even classified by histopathology. Because of this wide range of inflammatory conditions, it is not surprising that distinguishing the cause of meningoencephalomyelitides remains a diagnostic and therapeutic challenge for the clinician, even with newly developed techniques such as magnetic resonance imaging (MRI) and polymerase chain reactions (PCRs).

Before a treatment plan can be established, the diagnostic workup of such lesions has to be performed. Inflammatory lesions are not associated with classical clinical signs. Depending on which part of the CNS is affected, the clinical signs may vary from spinal cord to intracranial signs; in some cases the nerve roots and muscles are also involved. Some diseases have a different clinical picture, depending on the age of the patient. In this chapter the workup of CNS inflammation is discussed briefly, followed by the appropriate treatment, depending on the etiology of the disease.

CLINICAL SIGNS

The presence of multifocal signs, often considered the hallmark clinical feature of this group of diseases, is only noticed in about on-third of affected dogs. Other cases are presented with signs suggestive of a focal lesion in a region of the brain or the spinal cord. Signalment, history, and extraneural signs contribute, to a limited degree, to establishing a specific diagnosis. In breed-specific encephalitides the signalment can give a certain hint (pugs and Maltese, Yorkshire terriers, greyhounds, Chihuahua, Shih Tzu). The presence of extraneural signs in dogs with focal lesions may be helpful in establishing a presumptive diagnosis of meningoencephalomyelitis. A typical extraneural sign, which is found only in dogs with distemper—in about 20% of cases—is hyperkeratosis of the foot pad or the nose. Dogs with distemper may also develop rapid cachexia. An elevated body temperature may be seen in dogs with different encephalitides, mostly after bacterial infection, and in dogs with SRMA.

In many cases the localization of the lesion is of little help in establishing a diagnosis since a large variety of neurologic signs are associated with different inflammatory diseases. Certain signs occur more often with certain diseases (e.g., myoclonus, involuntary rhythmic jerking of single muscles or muscle groups, has been considered to be nearly pathognomonic for distemper). However, myoclonus may also occur in non-distemper meningoencephalomyelitis (albeit less frequently). In the acute form of SRMA typical clinical symptoms are cervical rigidity and neck pain. In pug encephalitis the most consistent sign is the occurrence of focal or generalized seizures. In Yorkshire terriers signs of encephalitis are referrable to brainstem injury (abnormal mental status, multiple cranial nerve deficits, and gait abnormalities). Hydrocephalus with periventricular encephalitis occurs in puppies between 2 and 6 months of age. These puppies develop acute neurologic signs with a rapid skull enlargement. Neurologic signs include forebrain signs such as behavioral changes and central blindness.

CLINICAL PATHOLOGY

Clinical pathology tests, especially analysis of cerebrospinal fluid (CSF), provide the principal information needed for diagnosis of inflammatory CNS diseases. The CSF cell count, cytology, and demonstration of a high immunoglobulin-G (IgG) index are pivotal to establishing the diagnosis of inflammatory disease. The IgG index helps to identify intrathecal IgG-production calculating IgG and albumin in CSF and serum. In addition, CSF examination may help to differentiate some diseases. For example, a high IgA concentration in serum and CSF is common in dogs with SRMA. Pleocytosis with predominantly lymphocytes and plasma cells is found in viral infections and during the chronic phase of SRMA, in GME, and in breed-specific necrotizing encephalitis. A predominantly neutrophilic pleocytosis is characteristic of bacterial infections and the acute stage of SRMA. A mixed cell population is frequently seen in protozoal diseases, FIP, chronic bacterial infections, necrotic lesions, and GME. Eosinophils are found in the rare eosinophilic encephalitis of unknown origin; in protozoal, parasitic, and mycotic infections; and also occasionally in GME and FIP.

OTHER SPECIAL EXAMINATIONS

Ancillary diagnostic tests contribute to the diagnoses of meningoencephalomyelitides to varying degrees. Electroencephalography is helpful for detecting an ongoing irritating process, and electromyography can help identify lower motor neuron lesions.

Imaging techniques are useful for excluding diseases other than inflammation or for finding extraneural primary lesions such as in bacterial encephalitis, which is usually the result of hematogenous dissemination of bacteria or spreading of an inflammation in the cranium (e.g., otitis media/interna or sinusitis) or the vertebral column (e.g., diskospondylitis, biting wounds). In addition, imaging may uncover secondary CNS changes such as hydrocephalus secondary to an inflammatory process related to CSF flow obstruction or defective absorption. When computed tomography (CT) demonstrates contrast enhancement of multifocal lesions, the suspicion of an inflammatory disease is raised. MRI provides the advantage of better visualization of soft-tissue (brain and spinal cord). This facilitates the discovery of inflammatory CNS lesions per se. Inflammatory CNS disease is suggested by the presence of multifocal, hyperintense lesions in T2-weighted images, which appear more or less hypointense in T1-weighted images and are enhanced by contrast. However, even with MRI techniques, different encephalitides cannot be distinguished with certainty, and some neoplasms create the same appearance. In addition, single granulomas may mimic a neoplastic lesion. MRI has also revealed hyperintensity in T2-weighted images and contrast enhancement in areas of myelin swelling and demyelination in acute canine distemper virus infection without the presence of inflammatory lesions.

Thus biopsy sampling is highly recommended to obtain an exact diagnosis, especially in inflammatory lesions of unknown origin. Refinement of future therapies of brainstem inflammation will require definitive diagnosis including results of a biopsy sample. In the clinical workup without histopathologic examination, a diagnosis of a specific inflammatory/infectious disease must be based mainly on a combination of clinical, laboratory, imaging, and CSF findings.

Bacterial Infection

Many dogs with bacterial encephalitis can be diagnosed with high probability on the basis of severe CSF changes with neutrophilic pleocytosis and rapid deterioration. With the aid of imaging techniques, extraneural lesions such as sinusitis or otitis media may be detected as predisposing causes. Microbiologic examinations of the CSF (culture, PCR) might identify a specific agent, but this is uncommonly found. A rapid diagnostic workup is necessary to start treatment before the CNS tissue is destroyed irreparably.

Viral Encephalitis

A sizable proportion of dogs with distemper can be diagnosed based on a combination of their young age, hyperkeratosis, lymphopenia, myoclonus, normal or moderately abnormal CSF with mononuclear pleocytosis, and positive antigen detection (PCR or immunocytochemistry) in the CSF. Postvaccinal distemper encephalitis can be suspected on the basis of the temporal association of these signs and vaccination.

Parasitic Infection

Lower motor neuron spinal cord signs in a puppy with severe muscle involvement, spastic hind limbs, high CK activity, and eosinophilia can be diagnosed as a likely protozoal infection. Muscle biopsies also might be helpful in these cases, and parasites might be seen histopathologically. In adult dogs with multifocal signs and suspicion of a granulomatous lesion, MRI findings, a positive PCR for *neospora caninum* and high antibody titers directed against this microorganism all support the diagnosis of neosporosis.

Inflammatory Lesions of Unknown Origin

The findings in a young dog of acute fever, cervical hyperesthesia, neutrophilia, and massive pleocytosis with neutrophils in the CSF are characteristic of SRMA. In about 90% of cases a combined elevation of IgA in CSF and serum is detected. Contrast enhancement in MRI might be evident within the meninges.

Pug encephalitis probably can be diagnosed with reasonable certainty on the basis of breed, history, and occurrence of seizures. In breed-specific encephalitides, imaging techniques showing the presence of necrotic lesions are helpful.

Unfortunately, these "typical" cases account for less than half of all dogs with inflammatory/infectious diseases of the CNS. In the remaining dogs the differential diagnosis is a challenge, especially in adult and older dogs. It may be difficult to distinguish GME from inflammatory disease caused by distemper unless high numbers of neutrophils are present in the CSF. In this case, the diagnosis of GME will also need to be differentiated from chronic protracted steroid responsive meningitis-arteritis (SRMA); as both diseases increase CSF cell counts and are also steroid responsive. If a purely mononuclear pleocytosis is present, all relevant viral diseases must be considered in the differential diagnosis. MRI is helpful in cases of suspect GME, particularly if multifocal contrast-enhancing lesions are seen.

In summary, in typical cases of inflammatory disease of the CNS, the diagnosis will be made according to the following diagnostic scheme:

- Clinical examination: extraneural signs
- Neurologic examination: multifocal lesions
- Blood and urine examinations
- Imaging techniques (extraneural lesions)
- CSF examination (protein content, total and differential cell count)
- MRI, ev. CT scan (multifocal contrast-enhancing lesions)
- Antigen determination
- Antibodies (only with follow-up examination and rising titers).

Obviously a number of these studies require general anesthesia and careful planning. In many cases referral to a specialist with capability for advanced diagnostics is needed and should not be delayed less the patient deteriorate during a course of empiric therapy.

TREATMENT

Bacterial Infection

In bacterial meningoencephalitis extraneural lesions should be sought and treated appropriately (e.g., surgery). In the acute phase of encephalitis steroid treatment can be given once at the beginning (e.g., dexamethasone 0.15 mg/kg intravenously [IV], subcutaneously [SC], PO). Some authors state that there is an advantage when steroids are given before antibiotic treatment is started to reduce high intracranial pressure and brain edema (15 to 20 minutes before starting antibiotics) (Messer et al., 2006). This concept has been extrapolated from experiments on rabbits or is described for treatment of bacterial meningoencephalitis in humans (van de Beek et al., 2007). In small animals large studies are missing, and only case reports support this notion. In addition, steroid treatment is still under debate; for example, delayed steroid treatment 12 to 24 hours after the application of antibiotics shows no beneficial effect. Glucocorticoid treatment before diagnostic workup is contraindicated. Antibiotics should be started directly once the diagnosis is strongly suspected. Ideally antimicrobials are chosen after susceptibility testing. Since there is no time to wait for sensitivity testing or isolation of the microorganism, treatment has to be started empirically. Drugs prescribed should either have a good penetration through the blood-brain barrier or demonstrate efficacy against bacteria commonly found in the hospital setting. For gram-positive bacteria ampicillin (5 to 22 mg/kg q6h IV), cephalosporins (cephalexin 20 mg/kg q8h PO), trimethoprim-sulfonamide (15 to 20 mg/kg q8–12h IV or PO) and minocycline (5 to 12 mg/kg q12h IV or PO) are recommended. For gram-negative bacteria, in addition to the drugs mentioned previously, metronidazole (10 to 15 mg/kg q8h PO), chloramphenicol (40 to 50 mg/kg q6–8h PO) and gentamycin (2 mg/kg q8h IV, intramuscularly [IM]) can be applied. During bacterial encephalitis the blood-brain barrier permeability is increased, which increases the delivery of antibacterial drugs. Since it will not known which bacteria are causing the disease

initially, a combination of drugs such as cephalosporins-metronidazole or ampicillin-chloramphenicol is frequently recommended. In addition, supportive treatment such as fluid therapy in dehydrated patients, external cooling for hyperthermia, or analgesia in animals with hyperesthesia is initiated. Pharmacologic treatment of fever is only recommended in cases with extremely high body temperatures. Decrease in the body temperature is a useful indicator for successful antimicrobial treatment. Seizures are treated with phenobarbital.

Viral Encephalitis

Currently there are no specific antiviral treatments for viral encephalitis. Therefore treatment in viral encephalitis mainly has to be supportive. Secondary bacterial infections are treated with antimicrobial drugs and nonspecific supportive therapy such as fluid therapy and administration of B-vitamins can be considered. Extraneural signs are treated with supportive therapy and good nursing care. Seizures are treated with phenobarbital. Some studies have been performed using immunomodulators such as feline interferon-ω; however, no controlled studies have proven efficacy in vivo.

Parasitic Infection

Treatment of toxoplasmosis and neosporosis should start early in the course of the disease and last for 4 to 8 weeks. Information regarding the efficacy of such treatment efforts is limited. Adult dogs seem to respond better than puppies with muscle contraction. In case of muscular involvement clindamycin (15 to 22 mg/kg q12h PO, SC) is recommended. When the CNS is affected, trimethoprim-sulfonamide (15 to 20 mg/kg q12h PO) is given. A combination of both drugs is useful. Vitamin B substitution should be considered (folic acid at 1 mg/day or Brewer's yeast 100 mg/kg q24h PO). In addition, pyrimethamine (for *neospora* with trimethoprim-sulfonamide 1 mg/kg q24h PO for 28 days) can be given in dogs, with consideration of potentially severe side effects such as anorexia, vomiting, depression, and bone marrow depression. Monitoring of CBC and platelet counts is recommended if pyrimethamine is administered.

Mycotic Infection

Antifungal drugs are used to treat systemic mycoses. The prognosis for mycotic involvement of the CNS is poor, but treatment should be initiated because it can be curative in immunocompetent animals. In immunocompromised animals infection may persist. Long-term treatment for 1 to 9 months or longer is necessary. CNS involvement by cryptococcosis is treated in cats and dogs with amphotericin B (0.5 mg/kg 3 times/week IV, SC), ketoconazole (dogs: 5 to 15 mg/kg q12h PO; cats: 50 mg total q24h PO or q48h if toxicity occurs), itraconazole (dogs: 10 mg/kg q24h PO; cats: 10 to 20 mg/kg q24h PO), or fluconazole (dogs and cats: 5 to 15 mg/kg q12–24h PO). It is advisable to consult a specialist when considering therapeutic options. In general, cats with CNS involvement seem to show a better recovery if treated with a combination of amphotericin B and fluconazole. For most dogs the administration of amphotericin B is recommended; itraconazole is given as maintenance therapy after an initial treatment with amphotericin B. In dogs with extradural granuloma, surgical removal of the lesions might support medical treatment. Treatment of fungal infections remains a challenge for the veterinarian. Individual treatment schedules must be constructed for each patient, considering toxic side effects of medication, costs, and other underlying diseases such as feline leukemia virus infection in cats.

Inflammatory Lesions of Unknown Origin

Steroid-Responsive Meningitis-Arteritis

Treatment of SRMA is centered on antiinflammatory therapy. If initial signs are mild and neutrophilic pleocytosis is not higher than 100 cells/μl in CSF, nonsteroidal antiinflammatory drugs might be used if the animal is carefully monitored. After the first relapse, when symptoms become worse, or when CSF analysis shows a massive pleocytosis, long-term treatment with prednisolone for at least 6 months must be initiated. The dosage is adjusted based on careful monitoring of clinical signs and adverse effects. Prednisolone is given initially at a dosage of 4 mg/kg q24h PO for 1 or 2 days; thereafter the dosage is 2 mg/kg q24h for about 1 to 2 weeks followed by 1 mg/kg q24h. The dogs are reexamined, including a CSF tap and blood profile, every 4 to 6 weeks after beginning therapy. As soon as the neurologic examination and CSF are found to be normal, the steroid dosage can be reduced to half of the previous until a dosage of 0.5 mg/kg q48h or q72h is reached. If pleocytosis persists, the same dosage should be continued. After about 6 months of therapy, if the patient appears clinically normal and demonstrates a normal CSF tap and blood profile for two consecutive examinations, the treatment is stopped. In long-standing cases, the same regimen is started from the beginning. If the dog does not respond sufficiently to therapy with prednisolone alone, immunosuppressive drugs such as azathioprine may be used in combination with steroids. It appears useful to azathioprine treatment every other day with steroids, with both drugs given every other day. Azathioprine may be prescribed at a dosage of 1.5 to 2 mg/kg q48h PO. Since neutrophils are an important cell population in SRMA, prednisolone is still a useful drug because of its broad-spectrum ability to suppress inflammation.

Often antibiotics are administered at the onset of treatment for SRMA because a bacterial infection cannot be excluded without analysis and culture of the CSF. Furthermore, protection against ulceration in the gastrointestinal tract should always be considered with long-term corticosteroid treatment. Owners should be advised that therapy with high doses of corticosteroids can lead to serious complications; treatment is not tolerated in about 5% of the dogs. In addition to serious complications, nonlifethreatening side effects such as polyuria, polydispia, polyphagia, and weight gain are observed. Therefore individual management and monitoring of patients are the most important factors to provide successful patient management.

Pug Dog Encephalitis/Breed Specific Encephalitides

There is no treatment for this disease. Glucocorticoids do not alter the course of this necrotizing encephalitis in confirmed cases, and antiepileptic drugs are often ineffective in controlling seizures.

GME/Encephalitis of Unknown Origin

It is difficult to definitively diagnose GME without histopathology. Since obtaining a brain biopsy is not always possible, both GME and encephalitis of unknown origin should be considered as potential causes of CNS inflammation. These are discussed together.

Only a few treatment studies are available for management of GME, and a definitive diagnosis was often unavailable for the reported cases. Therefore our current knowledge of therapy relates to treatment of the so-called *encephalitis of unknown origin* or of dogs with presumptive antemortem diagnosis of GME.

There is no specific therapy for GME, although improvement has been observed following administration of glucocorticosteroid or other immunosuppressive drugs. Glucocorticoid treatment frequently provides only temporary improvement, and side effects can limit usefulness. Typical dosages include prednisone or prednisolone 0.25 to 2 mg/kg q12–24h PO or dexamethasone 0.2 to 0.4 mg/kg q24h PO, IM, SC, depending on clinical improvement and side effects. Additional medications such as cytosine arabinoside (100 mg/m² q24h IV, SC [Zarfoss et al., 2006]); cyclosporine (3 to 6 mg/kg q12h PO [Adamo and O'Brien, 2004]) or procarbazine (25 to 50 mg/m² q24h PO [Coates et al, 2007]) may be considered as adjunctive treatments or treatment on their own. With this array of choices, it is useful to consult a neurologist for additional perspective when treating these patients.

CSF reexaminations and clinical monitoring, including regular blood examinations, are necessary. In case of myelosuppression from procarbazine, some authors recommend reducing the dosage by 50% or discontinuing therapy, depending on the severity of adverse effects (Coates et al., 2007). Azathioprine may be given at a dosage of 2 mg/kg q24–48h PO in addition to glucocorticosteroids, allowing for reduction in the amount of these drugs in case of severe side effects. In my experience it seems useful to alternate azathioprine treatment every other day with corticosteroids as discussed previously in this chapter. Radiation therapy is thought to have some efficacy in dogs with focal GME. Controlled multicenter studies should be conducted to learn more about the nature of this group of diseases and their treatment.

References and Suggested Reading

Adamo FP, O'Brien RT: Use of cyclosporine to treat granulomatous meningoencephalitis in three dogs, *J Am Vet Med Assoc* 225:1211, 2004.

Coates JR et al: Procarbazine as adjunctive therapy for treatment of dogs with presumptive antemortem diagnosis of granulomatous meningoencephalomyelitis: 21 cases (1998-2004), *J Vet Intern Med* 21:100, 2007.

Irving G, Chrisman C: Long-term outcome of five cases of corticosteroid-responsive meningomyelitis, *J Am Anim Hosp Assoc* 26:324, 1990.

Meric SM, Perman V, Hardy RM: Corticosteroid-responsive meningitis in ten dogs, *J Am Anim Hosp Assoc* 21:677, 1985.

Messer JS et al: Meningoencephalomyelitis caused by Pasteurella multocida in a cat, *J Vet Intern Med* 20:1033, 2006.

Plumb DC: *Plumb's veterinary drug handbook,* ed 5, Ames, 2005, Blackwell Scientific.

Tipold A: Diagnosis of inflammatory and infectious diseases of the central nervous system in dogs: a retrospective study, *J Vet Intern Med* 9:304, 1995.

Tipold A, Jaggy A: Steroid-responsive meningitis-arteritis in dogs: long-term study of 32 cases, *J Small Anim Pract* 35:311, 1994.

Tipold A, Vandevelde M: Neurologic diseases of suspected infectious origin and prion disease. In Greene CE: *Infectious diseases of the dog and cat,* ed 3, Philadelphia, 2006, Saunders, p 795.

Van de Beek D et al: Corticosteroids in acute bacterial meningitis, *Cochrane Database Syst Rev* CD004405, 2007.

Zarfoss M et al: Combined cytosine arabinoside and prednisolone therapy for meningoencephalitis of unknown etiology in 10 dogs, *J Small Anim Pract* 47:588, 2006.

CHAPTER 234

Treatment of Cerebrovascular Disease

LAURENT S. GAROSI, *Higham Gobion, England*
SIMON R. PLATT, *Athens, Georgia*

CEREBROVASCULAR ACCIDENT (OR STROKE)

There has been a good deal of confusion in the veterinary literature regarding the terms *cerebrovascular disease, cerebrovascular accident,* and *stroke.* Cerebrovascular disease refers to any abnormality of the brain caused by a pathologic process compromising blood supply. Pathologic processes that may result in cerebrovascular disease include occlusion of the lumen by a thrombus or embolus, rupture of a blood vessel wall, a lesion or altered permeability of the vessel wall, and increased viscosity or other changes in the quality of the blood. Stroke or cerebrovascular accident (CVA) is the most common clinical presentation of cerebrovascular disease and is defined as a sudden onset of nonprogressive focal brain signs secondary to cerebrovascular disease. By convention these signs must persist for more than 24 hours to qualify for the diagnosis of stroke, which is usually associated with permanent damage to the brain. If the clinical signs resolve within 24 hours, the episode is called a *transient ischemic attack.* From a pathologic point of view, a CVA falls into one or two broad categories: 1) ischemia with or without infarction secondary to obstructed blood vessels, or 2) hemorrhage caused by rupture of the blood vessel wall.

Ischemic Stroke

With limited stores the brain relies on a permanent supply of glucose and oxygen to maintain ionic pump function.

When perfusion pressure falls to critical levels, ischemia develops, progressing to infarction if hypoperfusion persists long enough. An infarct is an area of compromised or necrotic brain parenchyma caused by a focal occlusion of one or more blood vessels. It may be caused by either vascular obstruction that develops within the affected vessels (thrombosis) or obstructive material that originates from another vascular bed and travels to the brain (thromboembolism). Depending on the size of vessel involved, infarcts can be the consequence of small-vessel disease (i.e., superficial or deep perforating artery), which gives rise to a lacunar infarct; or large-vessel disease (a major artery of the brain or its main branches), which gives rise to a territorial infarct. Two distinct regions can be distinguished: the core where ischemia is severe and infarction develops rapidly; and the penumbra that surrounds the core and demonstrates a less severe reductions of cerebral blood flow (CBF), allowing longer durations of ischemic stress to be tolerated. The relative volume of pathology within these two regions changes as the infarct evolves. The factors favoring evolution of the penumbra to irreversible brain injury are multiple and complex. The time window during which the penumbra is no longer viable depends on the degree of blood flow reduction, the region of the brain involved, and the individual. In the penumbra neurons are still viable but at risk of becoming irreversibly injured. Penumbra tissue has the potential for recovery and therefore is the target for interventional therapy in acute ischemic stroke.

Ischemic strokes have been reported infrequently in veterinary publications when compared with human medical literature. Most reports have been based on post-mortem results in dogs that either died or were euthanized as a result of the severity of the ischemic stroke and/or the suspected underlying cause of the stroke. This retrospective reporting may affect the prevalence and type of underlying causes identified in canine CVA, because only the most severely cases are likely to be reported. In a similar vein, dogs in which infarction occurred secondarily to a disease with a poor prognosis would also die or be euthanized. Suspected underlying causes identified in histopathologically confirmed cases included septic thromboemboli, atherosclerosis associated with primary hypothyroidism, migrating parasite or parasitic emboli (*Dirofilaria immitis*), embolic metastatic tumor cells, intravascular lymphoma, and fibrocartilaginous embolism. In our magnetic resonance imaging (MRI)–based study a concurrent medical condition was detected in just over 50% of dogs affected by brain infarcts. Hypertension was documented in 30% of dogs. Of these dogs, chronic kidney disease and hyperadrenocorticism were the most commonly suspected underlying causes for the hypertension. No underlying cause could be identified antemortem in nearly half of the dogs. An infarct of unknown origin is called cryptogenic. No age, sex, or breed predisposition was identified. However, cavalier King Charles spaniels and greyhounds appeared overrepresented.

Hemorrhagic Stroke

In hemorrhagic stroke blood leaks from the vessel directly into the brain, forming a hematoma within the brain parenchyma or into the subarachnoid space. The mass of clotted blood causes physical disruption of the tissue and pressure on the surrounding brain. This alters central nervous system volume/pressure relationships with the possibility of increasing intracranial pressure (ICP) and decreasing CBF. In contrast to the high incidence in humans, intracerebral hemorrhage resulting from spontaneous rupture of vessels is considered rare in dogs. Secondary hemorrhage in dogs has been associated with rupture of congenital vascular abnormalities, primary and secondary brain tumors, inflammatory disease of the arteries and veins, intravascular lymphoma, brain infarction (hemorrhagic infarction), or impaired coagulation. Nontraumatic subarachnoid hemorrhage has been reported in dogs but remains very rare. This is in contrast to humans patients in whom aneurysmal rupture of blood vessels is the most common underlying cause of hemorrhagic stroke.

CLINICAL PRESENTATION

In all forms of stroke the denominative feature is the temporal profile of neurologic events. The abruptness with which the neurologic deficits develop is highly suggestive that the disorder is vascular. This is then followed by an arrest and then regression of the neurologic deficit in all except fatal strokes. Worsening of edema (associated with the secondary injury phenomenon) can result in progression of neurologic signs for a short period of 24 to 72 hours. Intracranial hemorrhage can be an exception to this description, presenting with a more progressive onset over a very short period of time. Clinical signs usually regress after 24 to 72 hours; this is attributable to diminution of the mass effect caused by hemorrhage with subsequent reorganization or to edema resorption. Neurologic deficits usually refer to a focal anatomic diagnosis and depend on the neurolocalization of the vascular insult (telencephalon, thalamus, midbrain, pons, medulla, cerebellum). Infarction of an individual brain region is associated with specific clinical signs that reflect the loss of function of that specific region. With hemorrhagic stroke the total clinical picture is different because the hemorrhage usually involves the territory of more than one artery, and pressure effects cause secondary signs. Neurologic signs are largely related to increasing ICP, which gives rise to nonspecific signs of forebrain or brainstem disease. Fundus examination is important and may reveal findings such as tortuous vessels (suggestive of systemic hypertension), hemorrhage (suggestive of coagulopathy or systemic hypertension), or papilledema (suggestive of elevated ICP).

Imaging studies of the brain (computed tomography, conventional and functional MRI) are necessary to confirm the suspicion of stroke, define the vascular territory involved and the extent of the lesion, and distinguish between ischemic and hemorrhagic stroke. Imaging studies are also necessary to rule out other causes of neurologic deficit such as tumor, head trauma, and encephalitis. (See References and Suggested Reading for more details.)

Ancillary diagnostic tests in ischemic stroke should focus on evaluating the animal for hypertension (and underlying causes), endocrine disease (hyperadrenocorticism, hypothyroidism, hyperthyroidism, diabetes mellitus), kidney disease (especially protein-losing nephropathy), heart disease (a greater risk factor in cats with cardiomyopathy), and metastatic disease. In cases of ischemic strokes, D-dimer assays and antithrombin III evaluation should be routinely included in the screening tests for thromboembolic disease as a possible cause of ischemic stroke. D-dimer is considered to be more useful test for detecting thromboembolic disease in dogs when compared to traditional tests currently in use (platelet count and clotting times). In cases of hemorrhagic stroke, diagnostic tests should be targeted to screen the animal for a coagulation disorder (and underlying causes), hypertension (and underlying causes), and metastatic disease (particularly hemangiosarcoma).

TREATMENT AND PROGNOSIS OF STROKE

Once the diagnosis of a stroke has been made, any potential underlying disease should be identified and treated accordingly. Generally treatment of these patients aims to provide supportive care, maintain adequate tissue oxygenation, and manage neurologic and nonneurologic complications. Nursing management of a recumbent dog is vital to the success of more specific therapies. Such management includes prevention of decubital ulceration, aspiration pneumonia, and urine scald, in addition to physical therapy and enteral nutrition provision. More specific therapies are aimed at preventing further neurologic deterioration.

Treatment of Ischemic Stroke

Treatment of an ischemic stroke revolves around three principles: monitoring and correcting basic physiologic variables (e.g., oxygen level, fluid balance, blood pressure, body temperature), inhibiting the biochemical and metabolic cascades subsequent to ischemia to prevent neuronal death (the concept of neuroprotection), and restoring or improving CBF by thrombolysis in the presence of a thrombus. The potentially salvageable portion of the ischemic zone (ischemic penumbra) is the presumed therapeutic target for both thrombolytic and neuroprotective stroke therapy. The time period during which injury may be reversible is called the therapeutic window. It is estimated that this "window of opportunity" is approximately 6 hours before irreversible neurologic damage occurs. Fortunately the vast majority of ischemic stroke patients have no major difficulty maintaining their airways, breathing efforts, or circulatory competence early in their clinical course.

There is some controversy surrounding the management of hypertension in the setting of an ongoing acute ischemic stroke. While a potential risk factor for a CVA, hypertension also can develop as a physiologic response to a stroke to ensure an adequate cerebral perfusion pressure (CPP) in the penumbra of the infarct. Elevated blood pressure can persist for up to 72 hours after the onset of injury. Maintenance of systemic arterial blood pressure within the physiologic range is essential, and aggressive lowering of blood pressure should be avoided during the acute stages unless the patient is at a high risk of end-stage organ damage (systolic blood pressures remaining above 180 mm Hg). In such cases hypertension often can be controlled with an angiotensin-converting enzyme inhibitor such as enalapril (0.25 to 0.5 mg/kg BID) or benazepril (0.25 to 0.5 mg/kg BID) and/or calcium channel blockers such as amlodipine (0.1 to 0.25 mg/kg once or twice daily). Amlodipine is more effective in severe hypertension.

There is no evidence that glucocorticoid treatment provides any beneficial neuroprotection in stroke. Aside from the lack of proven benefit in veterinary stroke patients, the use of glucocorticoids may increase the risk of gastrointestinal complications and infection. Treatment strategies for ischemic stroke considered in humans using other neuroprotective agents (N-methyl-D-aspartate [NMDA] antagonists, Ca^{2+} channel blockers, sodium channel modulators) or antiplatelets and thrombolytic therapy remain to be evaluated clinically in dogs. Although these neuroprotective agents have resulted in a dramatic decrease in the size of stroke lesion in experimental animal models, they have either failed to prove their efficacy in clinical trials or are awaiting further investigation. At the time of writing, there are no definitive data in humans or animals to confirm a significant improvement in clinical outcome in patients with acute ischemic stroke treated with unfractionated heparin as anticoagulant therapy. Despite conflicting results regarding its efficacy, intravenous recombinant tissue plasminogen activator (tPA) is

sometimes used in human ischemic stroke patients if it can be given within the first 3 hours. This critical time window makes the use of thrombolytic treatment unrealistic in veterinary neurology. Furthermore, this type of treatment carries a significant risk of intracranial hemorrhage following treatment. Antiplatelet therapy with low-dose aspirin (0.5 mg/kg PO SID) or perhaps clopidogrel can be used prophylactically to prevent clot formation in proven cardiac sources of an embolus.

Treatment of Hemorrhagic Stroke

The medical management of dogs with intracranial hemorrhage commonly includes stabilization of the patient (airway protection, monitoring and correction of vital signs); assessment and monitoring of the neurologic status; determination and treatment of potential underlying causes of the hemorrhage; and assessment for the need for specific treatment measures, including management of raised ICP. The risk of neurologic deterioration and cardiovascular instability is highest during the first 24 hours after the onset of an intracranial hemorrhage as the space-occupying lesion slowly expands and cerebral vasogenic edema develops. Therefore careful monitoring, including assessment of vital parameters (e.g., oxygen levels, fluid balance, blood pressure, body temperature) and neurologic status, is essential during this initial period. Unfortunately clinical signs of raised ICP are often delayed, inconsistent, and nonspecific. The size of an intracranial hematoma can be difficult to estimate from the neurologic examination alone. ICP monitoring systems are used frequently in human hospitals, but their use is very limited in veterinary hospitals. As a hematoma develops initially, ICP may be maintained at a constant as a result of a system of compensation. Within the closed space of the skull a change in the volume of one intracranial constituent (brain tissue, arterial blood, venous blood, or cerebrospinal fluid) is balanced by a compensatory change in another incompressible constituent. This is the Monroe-Kellie doctrine, which explains why some animals with large intracranial bleeds develop substantial increases in ICP at the time of herniation. The exhaustion of the compensating mechanisms for an intracranial space-occupying lesion implies that any further increase in the volume of the hematoma will produce a massive rise in ICP, and clinically this can be associated with herniation. Because of mechanical autoregulation, CBF remains constant, even though the CPP may vary between 40 and 120 mm Hg. The normal autoregulation of CBF may be impaired following a CVA, causing blood flow to damaged regions to become directly dependent on systemic blood pressure. Such animals may be unable to compensate for reductions in mean arterial blood pressure, causing decreased CPP in the presence of increased ICP. This emphasizes the importance of maintaining systemic blood pressure. In these circumstances systemic hypotension can result in inadequate perfusion of the brain, which leads to cerebral ischemic and secondary neuronal injury. Hypovolemia should be recognized and treated with volume expansion using crystalloids, colloids, or hypertonic saline. Central venous pressure monitoring can be useful as an aid to assessing the effectiveness of volume resuscitation, assuming cardiac function is otherwise normal. The use of glucose-containing solutions is discouraged since hyperglycemia has been shown to correlate with poor outcome in human stroke patient. As such, blood glucose should be monitored from the time of presentation. However, moderate levels of hypertension should not be treated because systemic hypertension may be secondary to the intense reflex sympathetic response to intracranial hypertension, which is a compensatory mechanism to maintain cerebral perfusion. As for ischemic stroke, attempts to lower and normalize the blood pressure should be reserved for animals at a high risk of end-stage organ damage (systolic blood pressures remaining above 180 mm Hg) and/or animals with severe ocular manifestations of hypertension such as retinal detachment or intraocular hemorrhage. Treatment recommendations for lowering blood pressure are detailed in the preceding section on treatment of ischemic stroke.

There is no evidence in humans to support the routine use of oxygen for the treatment of hemorrhagic stroke in the absence of hypoxia. In a rapidly deteriorating animal hyperventilation can be used temporarily to reduce ICP. The aim of hyperventilation is to reduce cerebral blood volume and hence ICP by causing a hypocapnic vasoconstriction. However, excessive hyperventilation can be accompanied by a reduction in global cerebral blood flow, which may drop below ischemic thresholds; therefore it is not a recommended therapy unless the Pa_{CO_2} can be closely monitored with capnography or arterial blood gas analysis.

Mannitol has been used traditionally to treat intracranial hypertension associated with pathologies such as head trauma, brain tumors, or encephalitis. There is insubstantial evidence to suggest that mannitol exacerbates intracranial hemorrhage; therefore osmotic diuretics are used routinely in the control of ICP in human patients with known intracranial hemorrhage. Mannitol therapy (0.25 to 1 g/kg intravenously over 10 to 20 minutes up to every 8 hours) may be initiated to treat suspected elevated ICP secondary to hemorrhagic stroke. The main effect of mannitol is to enhance CBF by reducing blood viscosity. Surgical evacuation of the hematoma can be used in dogs with large hematomas (mostly subarachnoid) and a deteriorating neurologic status.

PROGNOSIS

The prognosis for ischemic or hemorrhagic stroke depends overall on the initial severity of the neurologic deficit, the initial response to supportive care, and the severity of the underlying cause if one has been identified. Fortunately most cases of ischemic stroke recover within several weeks with only supportive care. In a recent retrospective study of 33 dogs with MRI or necropsy evidence of brain infarction, there was no association between the region of the brain involved (telencephalic, thalamic/midbrain, cerebellum), the type of infarction (territorial or lacunar), and the outcome. However, dogs with a concurrent medical condition had a significantly shorter survival time than those with no identifiable medical condition. Dogs with a concurrent medical condition also were significantly more likely to suffer from recurrent neurologic signs caused by subsequent infarcts.

References and Suggested Reading

Garosi LS, McConnell JF: Brain infarct in dog and human: a comparative review, *J Small Anim Pract* 46:521, 2005.

Garosi LS et al: Results of diagnostic investigations and long-term outcome of 33 dogs with brain infarction (2000-2004), *J Vet Intern Med* 19:725, 2005.

Garosi LS et al: Clinical and topographical magnetic resonance characteristics of suspected brain infarctions in 40 dogs, *J Vet Intern Med* 20:311, 2006.

Hillock SM et al: Vascular encephalopathies in dogs: diagnosis, treatment, and prognosis, *Compend Contin Educ Pract Vet* 28:208, 2006.

McConnell JF, Garosi LS, Platt SR: MRI findings of presumed cerebellar cerebrovascular accident in twelve dogs, *Vet Radiol Ultrasound* 46:1, 2005.

Platt SR, Garosi LS: Canine cerebrovascular disease: do dogs have strokes? *J Am Anim Hosp Assoc* 39:337, 2003.

CHAPTER 235

Treatment of Intracranial Tumors

JILL NARAK, *Auburn, Alabama*
TODD W. AXLUND, *Akron, Ohio*
ANNETTE N. SMITH, *Auburn, Alabama*

Intracranial tumors cause a devastating clinical picture, with signs that may include seizures, behavior changes, proprioceptive deficits, altered mentation, vestibular disease, and other cranial nerve abnormalities. Clinical signs are caused by the destruction of normal brain tissue that accompanies tumors; but patients also deteriorate because of secondary effects, including peritumoral edema and hemorrhage, leading to increased intracranial pressure and potentially brain herniation. Intracranial neoplasia affecting dogs and cats can arise from primary or secondary sources. Primary tumors arise directly from intracranial structures and include meningioma, glial tumors, neuroepithelial tumors, neural tumors, pituitary gland tumors, pineal gland tumors, and germ cell tumors. Secondary tumors arise from extracranial structures and include extension of nasal or skull tumors and metastatic neoplasia.

All intracranial tumors carry a poor prognosis; however, it is often difficult to discuss prognoses because treatment is sometimes initiated without a definitive diagnosis. Definitive treatment relies on an accurate histopathologic tumor diagnosis, although correlations between tumor appearance on magnetic resonance imaging (MRI) and histopathologic diagnoses have been reported (Kraft et al., 1997; Snyder et al., 2006). The patient's prognosis is related to tumor biologic behavior, as well as severity and progression of clinical signs. Without treatment intracranial tumors offer a grave prognosis.

DEFINITIVE THERAPIES

Definitive treatments include surgical excision, irradiation, and chemotherapy. These therapies aim to reduce or eradicate the tumor mass and decrease its secondary effects such as peritumoral edema, hemorrhage, and intracranial hypertension.

Surgical Excision

Surgical Approaches and Considerations

Surgical removal of an intracranial tumor achieves many treatment goals, including decompression and reduction of intracranial pressure and obtaining a histopathologic diagnosis, which allows for prognostication and additional treatment planning in the case of subtotal resection. Surgical approaches include rostrotentorial, caudotentorial, transfrontal, and suboccipital craniotomies or craniectomies; combinations of these approaches may be used. The tumor size, degree of invasiveness, and location determine whether or not surgical removal is a viable option; and it guides the neurosurgeon's choice of approach. Intraaxial tumors, which are located within the brain parenchyma, are more difficult to remove compared with extraaxial tumors. In addition, approaches to the caudal fossa are difficult and seldom attempted because of the possibility of inducing iatrogenic trauma to the brainstem and causing severe clinical signs in the patient.

In most cases the goal of surgery is removal of the entire mass. Tumor removal can be achieved using a combination of sharp and blunt dissection, or an ultrasonic aspirator can be used. Adequate dissection can be difficult because many tumors are not well delineated from normal tissue, and adjacent normal brain tissue may be compromised because of peritumoral edema or hemorrhage.

The dura mater must be incised or removed to obtain adequate visualization of the underlying brain structures. The defect can be closed using a graft (synthetic or fascial), or it may be left open. In dogs and cats cerebrospinal fluid (CSF) does not typically cause complications when leaked into the surrounding tissues (Niebauer, Dayrell-Hart, and Speciale, 1991). To protect the underlying brain, the skull defect is usually replaced when using a transfrontal or radical rostrotentorial approach; replacement is not necessary when using other approaches.

To assess the completeness of resection, the neurosurgeon can check the gross surgical margins intraoperatively using a sterile ultrasound technique or after surgery using MRI. If necessary, the surgeon can reoperate immediately to remove more tumor tissue or address life-threatening postoperative hemorrhage or cerebral swelling. Microscopic surgical margins can be assessed intraoperatively by histopathology using cryosectioned biopsy samples.

A tissue diagnosis may also be obtained using the less invasive computed tomography (CT)– guided biopsy; stereotactic or freehand CT-guided biopsy may be performed. Both techniques may induce iatrogenic hemorrhage; and, if necessary, a craniotomy will need to be performed to manage hemostasis.

Anesthetic Considerations

Intracranial tumor patients typically are older animals, and concurrent disease may be present. Preanesthetic screening, including complete blood count (CBC), serum biochemistry profile, urinalysis, thoracic radiography, and abdominal ultrasound, is indicated both to ensure the general health of the patient and to identify metastatic or other systemic disease, which could change the management approach.

In addition, these patients often have elevated intracranial pressure; thus the anesthetist should take measures to avoid or reduce intracranial hypertension, including maintaining normotension (systolic blood pressure 110 to 160 mm Hg or mean arterial pressure 80 to 110 mm Hg), eucarbia (35 to 45 mm Hg), and analgesia. Inhalant anesthetics increase cerebral blood flow, which can lead to or potentiate intracranial hypertension; injectable anesthetics such as propofol and fentanyl can be used to decrease the requirement of inhalant anesthetics. Diuretics and glucocorticoids may be given to decrease brain edema (Table 235-1). Intracranial surgery can be associated with intraoperative hemorrhage; thus one should be prepared for a blood transfusion. After surgery the patient should be allowed to recover gradually from anesthesia. It is critically important to avoid excitement on recovery, and additional sedation may be required. Analgesia should be continued and titrated to the patient's needs.

Intraoperative and Postoperative Considerations

Intraoperative complications include hemorrhage and hypotension, intracranial hypertension, and air embolism. Postoperative infection may be of concern after transfrontal craniotomy because the approach involves incision through the contaminated frontal sinus. However, postoperative infection is not a typical complication associated with intracranial surgery, possibly because of the routine use of perioperative antibiotics (see Table 235-1). Intracranial hypertension is a concern following surgery, and patient positioning can aid in keeping intracranial pressure in the normal range. Intracranial pressure can be measured directly, or it can be monitored indirectly by observing for changes associated with intracranial hypertension, including the Cushing's response (systemic hypertension with bradycardia) and changes in pupil size and symmetry. The patient's head should be elevated (approximately 30 degrees), jugular occlusion should be avoided (e.g., no jugular venipuncture or neck leads), and pain and excitement should be prevented. If necessary, diuretics and/or glucocorticoids can be continued in the postoperative period. If the patient is recumbent, urinary catheterization may be necessary. Care should be taken to keep the patient clean and dry, and appropriate bedding with frequent rotation or placement in a sling to prevent the formation of decubital ulcers is required. To avoid aspiration pneumonia the patient should be given nothing per os for 24 hours postoperatively. Nutritional and intravenous fluid support is indicated in a patient who cannot maintain adequate nutrition orally.

Meningioma

Meningiomas are usually easily accessible to the neurosurgeon since they are often extraaxial masses. However, meningiomas located along the brainstem or those located on the falx cerebri or tentorium cerebelli or along the lateral ventricles may be more difficult to access.

Surgical removal of feline meningiomas may be curative since the entire mass can often be removed in total; surgical excision is the treatment of choice for feline

Table 235-1

Medications Used in the Treatment of Intracranial Tumors

Drug	Dose	Use/Indication
Carmustine	50 mg/ml q6wk IV (over 15-20 min)	Nitrosurea chemotherapeutic agent; may be used to treat meningioma and glioma
Cefazolin	22 mg/kg q90min IV	Perioperative antibiotic
Cytosine arabinoside	20-100 mg/m² q1wk intrathecally	Chemotherapeutic agent, used to treat CNS lymphoma
Diazepam and midazolam	0.5 mg/kg as needed IV; or 2 mg/kg as needed per rectum	Anticonvulsant used in emergency management of status epilepticus or cluster seizures
Dimenhydrinate	Dog: 25-50 mg 8-24h PO Cat: 12.5 mg q8-24h PO	Antihistamine (antiemetic used for vestibular disease)
Hydroxyurea	20 mg/kg q24h PO	Chemotherapeutic agent; may be used to treat meningioma
Lomustine	Dog: 60-90 mg/m² q3-6wk PO Cat: 50-60 mg/m² q6wk PO	Nitrosurea chemotherapeutic agent; may be used to treat meningioma and glioma
Mannitol	0.5-1 g/kg q4h or as needed IV	Osmotic diuretic used to decrease brain edema and lower intracranial pressure
Meclizine	25 mg/dog and 12.5 mg/cat q24h PO	Antihistamine (antiemetic used for vestibular disease)
Methylprednisolone sodium succinate	30 mg/kg once IV; or 100 mg/kg given over 24 hours IV	Glucocorticoid used to decrease peritumoral brain edema and lower intracranial pressure
7.5% NaCl	5-20 ml/kg as needed IV	Osmotic diuretic used to decrease brain edema and lower intracranial pressure
Phenobarbital	Loading dose: 5 mg/kg as needed IV (up to 20 mg/kg total) Maintenance dosage: 2-3 mg/kg q12h PO	Anticonvulsant
Potassium bromide	Loading dose: 70 mg/kg q12h PO Maintenance dosage: 20 mg/kg q12h PO	Anticonvulsant
Prednisone	0.5-1 mg/kg q12h PO	Glucocorticoid used for supportive therapy of intracranial tumors

CNS, Central nervous system; *IV,* intravenously; *PO,* orally.

Table 235-2

Comparison of Median Survival Times in Dogs and Cats With Intracranial Tumors Treated With Surgical Excision And Irradiation*

Authors	Tumor Type	Number of Patients	Treatment Type	Median Survival Time (Days)
Troxel et al.	Meningioma	34 cats	Surgical excision	685
Greco et al.	Meningioma	17 dogs	Surgical excision	1254
Axlund et al.	Meningioma	14 dogs	Surgical excision	210
	Meningioma	12 dogs	Surgical excision followed by irradiation	495
Brearley et al.	Extraaxial tumors	41 dogs	Irradiation	347
	Intraaxial tumors	34 dogs	Irradiation	282
	Pituitary tumors	8 dogs	Irradiation	147

*Determined by the Kaplan-Meier Product Limit Method.

meningiomas. Troxel and associates (2003) reported that cats treated with surgical removal of meningiomas had a significantly longer survival time than cats treated by any other modality (Table 235-2). Niebauer, Dayrell-Hart, and Speciale (1991) reported that 50% of cats were alive 2 years after surgery.

Canine meningiomas are more difficult to remove totally. Histologically these tumors tend to be more aggressive and invasive than the feline form. Thus surgical removal often leaves behind microscopic disease and should be followed with radiation therapy or chemotherapy. Greco and colleagues (2006) reported that histopathologic tumor subtype influenced prognosis: transitional and meningothelial meningiomas yielded higher median survival times than fibroblastic, anaplastic, and psammomatous meningiomas. Théon and associates (2000) found that a high tumor proliferative index, noted on immunohistochemical analysis of histologic tumor sections, was a significant prognostic indicator for tumor progression in dogs with meningioma.

Glioma

Surgical removal can be helpful to debulk and histopathologically diagnose gliomas. However, gliomas are invasive tumors, and it is difficult to obtain clean margins. These tumors are typically highly vascular; and, because of their deep location, surgical resection may cause damage to normal brain parenchyma. Their location may also make them difficult to visualize at surgery; intraoperative ultrasound may be useful to delineate tumor margins. For these reasons surgical removal of gliomas is usually followed with radiation therapy.

Others

Pituitary microadenomas may be amenable to surgical removal, but macroadenomas typically are too large for excision. Radiation therapy is the treatment of choice for these tumors, although the prognosis is worse if neurologic signs are present. The pituitary height-to-brain area ratio is used to discriminate between pituitary microadenoma and macroadenoma and to determine ease of surgical removal. Traditionally a macroadenoma may be defined as a pituitary gland that is greater than 1 cm in height, although Meij and associates (1998) describe that in veterinary medicine a pituitary macroadenoma is defined when the pituitary

height-to-brain ratio is greater than 0.31. Techniques described for pituitary microadenoma removal include the transsphenoidal and ventral paramedian approaches.

Neuroepithelial tumors such as choroid plexus papillomas and ependymomas may be removed surgically; however, they are often located in difficult locations (in the ventricular system). As a result of their location, obstructive hydrocephalus may occur and exacerbate clinical signs. To relieve hydrocephalus, a viable option is the placement of a ventriculoperitoneal shunt; this procedure may or may not be combined with tumor removal.

Radiation Therapy

Radiation therapy (see Chapter 67) may be used as adjunct treatment to surgical excision; in fact, it may be most efficacious when combined with surgical tumor removal (see Table 235-2). Radiation therapy can also be used as sole therapy for intracranial tumors. Because of the potential morbidity associated with surgical removal of brainstem masses, the use of radiation as sole therapy is the treatment of choice for these tumors. The use of radiation as sole therapy is justified if surgical expertise is not available; however, radiation therapy also often requires referral to a specialty referral center. Megavoltage radiation is recommended, but orthovoltage has also been used. Radiation oncologists base treatment planning on the known or suspected tumor type and location, keeping in mind the acute and late side effects that may be induced by radiation therapy.

The goal of radiation therapy is to deliver a tumoricidal dose of radiation while sparing normal brain tissue. High doses of radiation improve control of brain tumors but put the patient at risk for radiation-induced brain necrosis; thus the risk-to-benefit ratio needs to be considered for each patient. Radiation-induced brain damage is the result of focal necrosis and local hemorrhage. Fractionation is a strategy used to avoid radiation-induced brain necrosis. This approach relies on the ability of normal tissue to repair itself between doses of radiation. Tumor cells have lost this ability for repair; thus the radiation doses are lethal to the tumor mass. Typical fractionation schedules call for three to five anesthetic episodes per week, which can be stressful to the typical geriatric brain tumor patient. Ideally, to avoid radiation-induced brain necrosis, treatments are delivered in fractions of less than 300 cGy to reach a total dose of 45 to 50 Gy.

Therapy may fail as a result of tumor recurrence or radiation-induced brain necrosis. Advanced imaging cannot distinguish between these processes, and both present with similar clinical signs; it can be difficult to know if a patient is deteriorating as a result of tumor progression or brain necrosis. A severe and rapid neurologic decline may be the result of radiation-induced brain necrosis, compared to a slowly progressive decline in neurologic status, which may represent tumor regrowth (Brearley et al., 1999). Ultimately though, this differentiation can be made only on postmortem examination. Brain is a late responding tissue; thus these radiation side effects may not be noted until months to years after treatment, and Spugnini and associates (2000) reported that only 5% to 20% of brain tumor patients survive to be at risk for these effects. Another late side effect to consider is new tumor growth induced by radiation, as noted in one report by Théon et al. (2000).

Acute side effects of radiation therapy in the brain can be seen weeks to months after therapy and include transient demyelination, which usually responds to anti-inflammatory doses of corticosteroids (see Table 235-1). Other acute side effects of radiation therapy depend on the treatment portal used and may include keratoconjunctivitis, corneal ulcers, mucositis, otitis externa, and dermatitis. Although these effects are not life threatening, they may cause debilitation in the short term and require appropriate management.

Stereotactic radiosurgery is a technique allowing for the precise delivery of radiation to the tumor while sparing adjacent normal brain tissue. Only one anesthetic episode is required because a sufficient dose of radiation is delivered to the tumor at once while only a fraction of that dose is delivered to normal brain tissue. This technique can be used for tumors of relatively small diameter and requires referral to an adequately equipped specialty center. Other techniques such as boron neutron capture therapy and brachytherapy have been attempted to deliver a precise dose of radiation to the tumor tissue.

Chemotherapy

Chemotherapy has been largely ineffectual in the treatment of brain tumors, but certain therapeutics deserve consideration. The blood-brain barrier is impermeable to large, hydrophilic compounds; most drugs are unable to penetrate the blood-brain barrier and therefore are unable to exert their tumoricidal effects on brain tumors. However, in the face of significant pathology, the blood-brain barrier may not be completely impenetrable, and some drug therapy may have limited success. To increase effectiveness of a chemotherapeutic drug, agents that increase blood-brain barrier permeability may be given (e.g., mannitol); however, this technique may also increase the toxic side effects of a chemotherapeutic drug and is generally not advised. To obtain maximum delivery into the central nervous system (CNS), agents can be directly injected into the subarachnoid space (intrathecal injection). Intratumoral injections of chemotherapy have been tried in humans and may be useful in delivering a precise dose of chemotherapy directly into the brain tumor; however, this is an invasive technique. Certain tumors are considered to be relatively chemoresponsive (e.g., CNS lymphoma, medulloblastoma, oligodendroglioma), but chemotherapy may be considered for any patient with an intracranial tumor. Lymphoma of the CNS is considered to be nonsurgical and is instead treated with systemic and intrathecal chemotherapy. Chemotherapy is also used in the face of metastatic brain neoplasia; the protocol used depends on the primary tumor. Surgical debulking and radiation therapy may not be advised in the face of metastatic brain neoplasia because of the poor prognosis; however, these modalities can be offered as palliative therapy. Standard protocols for chemotherapy in the face of intracranial tumors have not been developed, but certain chemotherapeutics are discussed here.

Nitrosureas

Nitrosureas are highly lipophilic and obtain rapid passage across the blood-brain barrier. Lomustine (CeeNu, Bristol Labs Oncology) and carmustine (BiCNU, Bristol-Myers Squibb) are used as adjunct therapy for brain tumors (see Table 235-1). These agents have been used to treat glioma and meningioma with varying success. Side effects of the nitrosureas include myelosuppression; thus CBCs should be monitored weekly, beginning after the first week of treatment. Maximum myelosuppression may not occur until 4 to 6 weeks after treatment, and the effects (neutropenia and thrombocytopenia) may be cumulative. If the patient becomes neutropenic at $<1000 \times 10^3/\mu l$ but appears to be otherwise healthy, broad-spectrum oral antibiotics may be advised; if a patient is neutropenic at $<1000 \times 10^3/\mu l$ and displays signs of sepsis or systemic illness (lethargy, vomiting, diarrhea, or fever), the patient should be hospitalized and placed on broad-spectrum intravenous antibiotics while monitoring for progression of sepsis. Lomustine can also cause hepatotoxicity and nephrotoxicity; thus it is important to monitor serial serum biochemistry profiles. If evidence of toxicity is present, hepatic and renal function tests and/or abdominal ultrasound should be performed. It is important to note that the same hepatic microsomal enzymes induced by phenobarbital are necessary for generating the antineoplastic metabolites of lomustine; thus, before being treated with lomustine, the patient may need to be switched from phenobarbital to a different anticonvulsant such as potassium bromide.

Hydroxyurea

Hydroxyurea is a chemotherapeutic agent that also crosses the blood-brain barrier and may be useful in the treatment of intracranial tumors (see Table 235-1). Hydroxyurea has shown promise in treating humans with unresectable or recurrent meningioma, but there is no evidence demonstrating its efficacy in dogs or cats. The most serious side effect of hydroxyurea is myelosuppression; serial CBCs should be monitored.

Cytosine Arabinoside

Intrathecal delivery of cytosine arabinoside (Cytosar, Pharmacia & Upjohn) has been used in the treatment of CNS lymphoma when malignant cells are found in the CSF. Cytosine arabinoside may be delivered intrathecally (see Table 235-1). The chemotherapy is given 1 week beyond an atypical lymphocyte-free CSF tap; three to six treatments are usually necessary. Intrathecal delivery of chemotherapy requires general anesthesia and the technical expertise to perform a CSF tap. Systemic chemotherapy is recommended in conjunction with intrathecal chemotherapy; protocols are discussed elsewhere. Response to treatment is usually weeks to months.

Others

The combination of procarbazine, lomustine, and vincristine has been used to treat certain types of human glioma. Temozolamide is an alkylating agent that has also been used with varying success in humans with glioma. Methotrexate has been used intrathecally to treat humans with CNS lymphoma. Studies need to be performed in veterinary medicine to address the efficacy of these drugs.

SUPPORTIVE THERAPIES

The goals of supportive therapy include seizure control and reduction in intracranial pressure, and these therapeutics are often instituted regardless of whether or not definitive therapies are undertaken. When used in combination with definitive therapy such as surgery or radiation, these treatments aid in reducing the patients' clinical signs in the short term while waiting for definitive treatments to take effect. Supportive therapies can be used as the sole means of treatment, but owners should be made aware that the patient's prognosis is poor; these therapies treat only the symptoms of the intracranial tumor and do not affect the tumor itself. The use of supportive therapies as the sole means of therapy is short-lived because eventually the tumor mass enlarges and exacerbates the patient's clinical signs. However, supportive care can extend a patient's life in the short term and temporarily alleviate clinical signs associated with the intracranial tumor.

Treatment of Intracranial Hypertension

Intracranial hypertension can develop as a result of the presence of a brain tumor or because of its secondary effects such as edema and hemorrhage. Left untreated, intracranial hypertension can cause brain herniation and death. Intravenous fluid support is given to maintain normotension and support blood flow to the brain since cerebral perfusion pressure relies on adequate mean arterial blood pressure. Methylprednisolone sodium succinate (Solu-Medrol, Pfizer) is a glucocorticoid effective at decreasing peritumoral edema (see Table 235-1). Diuretics may also be given to decrease brain edema. Mannitol and hypertonic saline are osmotic diuretics effective at decreasing intracranial pressure (see Table 235-1). It is important to monitor the patient's hydration status when using diuretics since therapy can lead to hypovolemia and hypotension, which can exacerbate cerebral ischemia caused by hypoxia.

Anticonvulsants

Phenobarbital and potassium bromide are the typical first-line anticonvulsants used in veterinary patients (Table 235-1). Serum phenobarbital concentrations should be measured 2 weeks after initiating maintenance therapy; the therapeutic range is 15 to 45 mcg/ml when used as monotherapy. High levels of phenobarbital may be associated with hepatotoxicity. Increased alkaline phosphatase may be noted on a serum biochemistry profile, although this is associated with hepatic enzyme induction rather than hepatotoxicity. Bone marrow hypoplasia is an uncommon side effect of phenobarbital therapy. Additional side effects include polydipsia and polyuria, polyphagia, sedation, ataxia, and paraparesis. These side effects often resolve within 1 to 2 weeks of initiating therapy. Patients on phenobarbital therapy should have serial serum biochemistry profiles measured, along with regular monitoring of serum phenobarbital concentration to aid in dose adjustments if needed.

Potassium bromide can be used as sole therapy, or it may be added to phenobarbital therapy in refractory cases. Because it takes a long time to reach steady state, patients are usually given a loading dose for 5 days, and a maintenance dosage is given thereafter. Serum concentrations of potassium bromide should be measured in 3 weeks, and the dosage adjusted accordingly. Side effects of potassium bromide are similar to those of phenobarbital. Potassium bromide is not known to cause hepatotoxicity, although it may be associated with pancreatitis. Potassium bromide is not recommended for use in cats since it may be associated with the development of inflammatory pneumonitis. It is important to keep the salt content of the patient's diet consistent while on bromide therapy since increased dietary chloride can reduce the serum levels of bromide and affect seizure control.

The appearance of cluster seizures or status epilepticus is an emergency, and treatment includes the administration of diazepam (Valium, Roche) or midazolam (Versed, Roche). Phenobarbital may be given as a loading dose (see Table 235-1). If these anticonvulsants cannot control the patient's seizures, anesthetics such as pentobarbital, propofol, and gas anesthesia should be considered, realizing that the patient may require ventilatory support.

Corticosteroids

Glucocorticoids may be given to reduce peritumoral edema and decrease CSF production. An antiinflammatory dose of prednisone is recommended (see Table 235-1). This dose can be adjusted based on the patient's response to therapy.

Antihistamines

Meclizine and dimenhydrinate are antihistamines with antiemetic effects, which are useful to alleviate nausea in patients with vestibular disease (see Table 235-1).

Emerging molecular therapies such as immunotherapy, gene therapy, and oncolytic viral therapy have been used with varying success in humans, and these areas may represent direction for future research in brain tumors of veterinary patients.

References and Suggested Reading

Axlund TW, McGlasson ML, Smith AN: Surgery alone or in combination with radiation therapy for treatment of intracranial meningiomas in dogs: 31 cases (1989-2002), *J Am Vet Med Assoc* 221:1597, 2002.

Brearley MJ et al: Hypofractionated radiation therapy of brain masses in dogs: a retrospective analysis of survival of 83 cases (1991-1996), *J Vet Intern Med* 13:408, 1999.

Greco JJ et al: Evaluation of intracranial meningioma resection with a surgical aspirator in dogs: 17 cases (1996-2004), *J Am Vet Med Assoc* 229:394, 2006.

Kraft SL et al: Retrospective review of 50 canine intracranial tumors evaluated by magnetic resonance imaging, *J Vet Intern Med* 11:218, 1997.

Meij BP et al: Results of transsphenoidal hypophysectomy in 52 dogs with pituitary-dependent hyperadrenocorticism, *Vet Surg* 27:246, 1998.

Niebauer GW, Dayrell-Hart BL, Speciale J: Evaluation of craniotomy in dogs and cats, *J Am Vet Med Assoc* 198:89, 1991.

Snyder JM et al: Canine intracranial primary neoplasia: 173 cases (1986-2003), *J Vet Intern Med* 20:669, 2006.

Spugnini EP et al: Primary irradiation of canine intracranial masses, *Vet Radiol Ultrasound* 41:377, 2000.

Théon AP et al: Influence of tumor cell proliferation and sex-hormone receptors on effectiveness of radiation therapy for dogs with incompletely resected meningiomas, *J Am Vet Med Assoc* 216:701, 2000.

Troxel MT et al: Feline intracranial neoplasia: retrospective review of 160 cases (1985-2001), *J Vet Intern Med* 17:850, 2003.

CHAPTER 236

Diagnosis and Treatment of Atlantoaxial Subluxation

BEVERLY K. STURGES, *Davis, California*

Atlantoaxial (AA) instability with subluxation of C2 relative to C1 is a frequent cause of cervical pain and/or myelopathy in toy and miniature breeds of dogs. On rare occasions large breeds of dogs, as well as cats, may also be affected. Because AA subluxation is a potentially life-threatening problem, it is important to recognize when AA instability *may* be present so that the patient is handled appropriately. This will prevent exacerbation of the clinical signs until a definitive diagnosis is made and appropriate treatment is instituted.

GENERAL CONSIDERATIONS: ANATOMY AND PHYSIOLOGY

The atlas (C1) and axis (C2) form a pivotal joint that allows free movement of the head about the longitudinal axis of the spine. Most of the rotational movement centers around the dens, a bony process projecting from the rostral aspect of the body of the axis, which is held in position relative to the atlas by several ligaments (Figs. 236-1 and 236-2):

- The *apical and alar ligaments* leave the apex of the dens in three sections: the middle one, forming the

apical ligament, goes straight forward and attaches to the ventral border of the foramen magnum; the lateral sections, forming the alar ligaments, attach to the skull medial to the occipital condyles.

- The *transverse atlantal ligament* is a strong ligament that crosses over the top of the dens and connects one side of the ventral arch of C1 to the other. It is particularly important to AA joint stability since this ligament holds the dens firmly against the ventral aspect of the atlas.
- The *dorsal AA membrane* is a fibrous extension of the joint capsule running between the arch of the atlas and the spinous process of the axis. It adds support, limiting the amount of dorsoventral movement between C1 and C2.

The atlas articulates rostrally with the occipital condyles of the skull and forms a joint of which the main movements are flexion and extension of the head, the "yes" joint. Caudally the atlas articulates with the axis allowing lateral (and rotational) movement of the head, the "no" joint. Working together, these two joints allow free motion of the head in all directions. The large nuchal ligament, which attaches the spinous process of C2 with

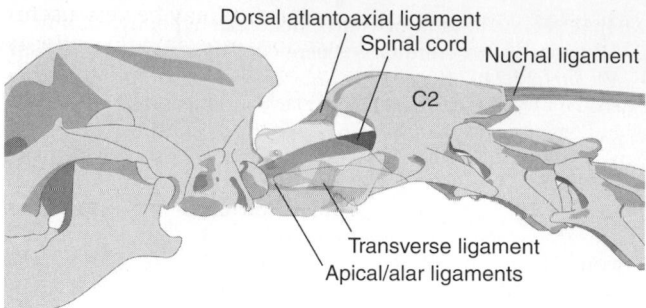

Fig. 236-1 Normal atlantoaxial joint, lateral view. Note the relationships of the ligamentous and bony structures of the AA joint that allow for normal head movement without injury to neural structures.

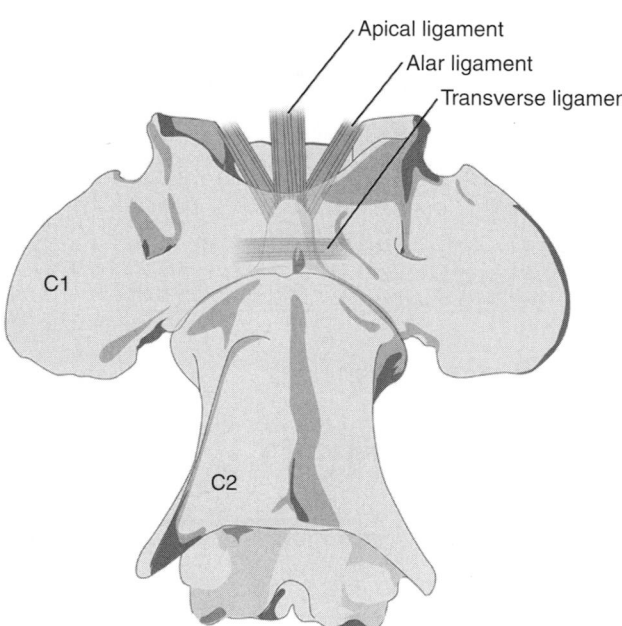

Fig. 236-2 Normal atlantoaxial joint, ventrodorsal view. The apical and alar ligaments attach the dens to the occipital bones of the skull while the transverse ligament crosses over the top of the dens, keeping it firmly in place against the ventral aspect of the atlas.

those of T1 and T2, functions in suspension of the head by forming a fulcrum at the AA joint (see Fig. 236-1).

PATHOPHYSIOLOGY

Instability of the AA region allows excessive flexion of the joint, which may result in subluxation, traumatic spinal cord injury, and compression. This usually occurs secondary to congenital or developmental abnormalities of the bones or ligaments of the AA joint, traumatic injury to the joint, or a combination of both. In many instances the abnormalities present are associated with the dens and include agenesis/hypoplasia of the dens, dorsal angulation of the dens, and fracture or avulsion of the dens with the axis. Absence or rupture of associated AA ligaments often contributes to the instability caused by congenital anomalies in the region. Traumatic rupture of the AA ligaments without associated anomalies of the AA joint also

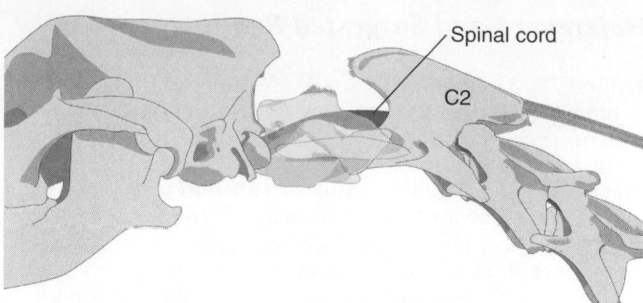

Fig. 236-3 Atlantoaxial subluxation, lateral view. Subluxation of the axis (C2) relative to the axis causes traumatic injury and compression of the cranial spinal cord, Associated hemorrhage and edema may extend rostrally to affect brainstem function.

can occur, resulting in instability and spinal cord injury. Dorsal displacement of the cranial portion of the body of the axis into the vertebral canal, acutely or chronically, causes compression, edema, and inflammation of the spinal cord that may extend cranially into the caudal brainstem (Fig. 236-3).

DIAGNOSIS

Clinical Presentation

Malformations of the AA joint occur most frequently in toy and miniature breeds of dogs especially Chihuahuas, Yorkshire terriers, toy and miniature poodles, Pomeranians, Japanese chins, and Maltese. Clinical signs of a C1-C5 myelopathy and/or cervical pain occur and may be acute or chronic at onset and progressive, nonprogressive, or intermittent in nature. Often the signs occur secondary to mild trauma such as jumping off furniture or roughhousing with other dogs. Reportedly signs usually occur within the first year of life; however, at my institution the majority of cases have occurred in dogs older than a year, including middle- to older-age animals. Severity varies from mild to profound cervical pain to tetraparesis, respiratory paralysis, and caudal brainstem signs (e.g., hypoventilation, vestibular syndrome). Traumatic AA instability, with or without an underlying congenital malformation, is usually the cause of AA subluxation in larger-breed dogs (>10 kg).

Occasionally dogs with AA instability may present with a history of seizure-like signs occurring intermittently with or without transient apnea and paresis. Episodes are usually related to a mild traumatic incident and commonly occur with malformations of the dens, specifically agenesis or dorsal angulation of the dens.

Differential diagnoses for dogs with this clinical presentation should include intervertebral disk disease, cervical trauma/spinal fracture, infectious/inflammatory disease (e.g., granulomatous meningoencephalitis [GME], other craniospinal anomalies (e.g., syringomyelia, Chiari-like malformation), and neoplasia (cervical spine or brain). Although the history, signalment, and clinical signs of AA subluxation may be indistinguishable from other common diseases such as GME, disk disease, and Chiari-like malformation/syringomyelia, a diagnosis of instability at the AA joint should be considered significant and treated promptly.

Radiography

Plain cervical radiography usually provides the diagnosis in most instances. Because it is essential that positioning be accurate when evaluating the AA region of the cervical spine, general anesthesia is necessary. It is easy to misdiagnose AA subluxation on imperfectly positioned radiographs or where the beam is not centered on C1-C2. Care must be taken when manipulating an animal suspected of having AA instability during intubation, handling under anesthesia, and radiography since flexion of the animal's neck may result in further spinal cord compression. Placing a Robert Jones–style bandage on the patient before anesthetizing with the head in mild extension provides support and comfort for the animal and serves as a safeguard for keeping the AA joint in extension. Radiographically the body of the axis is displaced dorsally and cranially into the vertebral canal, and the distance between the dorsal arch of the atlas and spinous process of the axis is increased (Fig. 236-4). If lateral views are not diagnostic, slight flexion of the head may be necessary to demonstrate subluxation or instability of the AA joint. Abnormalities of the dens may be seen clearly on oblique lateral views in which the wings of the atlas are not superimposed on the dens and/or ventrodorsal views.

Advanced Imaging

Myelography and/or computed tomography (CT) may be required to confirm that subluxation is present, to further delineate regional problems when multiple congenital anomalies are present, and/or to rule out other differential diagnoses in the same region of localization (e.g., disk disease). Lumbar puncture should be done since cisternal puncture for cerebrospinal fluid (CSF) sampling or myelography is not recommended in dogs with AA subluxation on the differential list. In most cases plain radiography with or without myelography or CT-myelography is sufficient to diagnose AA instability/subluxation.

Magnetic resonance imaging (MRI) may be very useful in the diagnosis of AA subluxation, especially in patients with clinical signs of brain or brainstem disease, as well as cervical pain and myelopathy. The extent of the parenchymal injury to the cervical cord or caudal brainstem is best visualized on MRI. Typically a region of hyperintensity on T2W images is visible in the cranial cervical spinal cord, caudal brainstem, or both locations on MRI. In addition, MRI is useful for ruling out the presence of concurrent diseases with clinical signs localizing to the same region and for identifying underlying disease that may influence long-term prognosis. For example, cavalier King Charles spaniels with signs of cervical pain and myelopathy should be evaluated for the presence of Chiari-like malformation and syringomyelia as well as AA instability. Collection of CSF is recommended in cases in which the diagnosis is not straightforward on imaging, especially in breeds of dogs typically prone to inflammatory disease (e.g., GME) of the brain.

TREATMENT

Patients with cervical pain only or minimal neurologic deficits may respond well to splinting of the head and neck in mild extension and strict cage rest for at least 6 weeks. However, clinical signs often recur once normal activity resumes. Surgical decompression and stabilization is indicated in cases with moderate-to-severe neurologic deficits or intense pain or those that are unresponsive to nonsurgical treatment. Surgery is also recommended when angulation of the dens results in spinal cord injury. Animals less than 6 months of age are best treated conservatively, if possible, to allow for more complete mineralization of bone and closure of vertebral physes before attempting surgical stabilization. Certainly conservative treatment should be attempted in situations in which financial constraints do not allow surgical repair to be done.

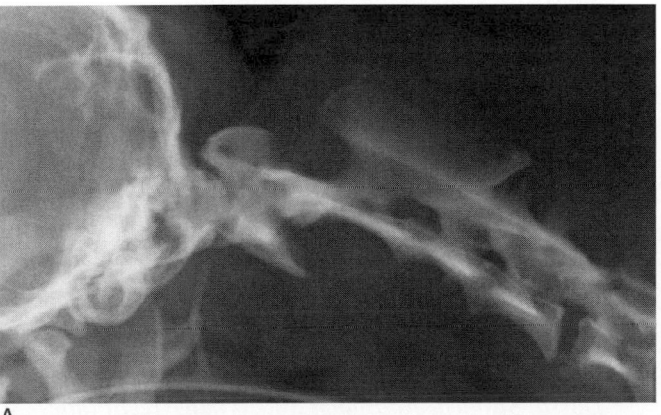
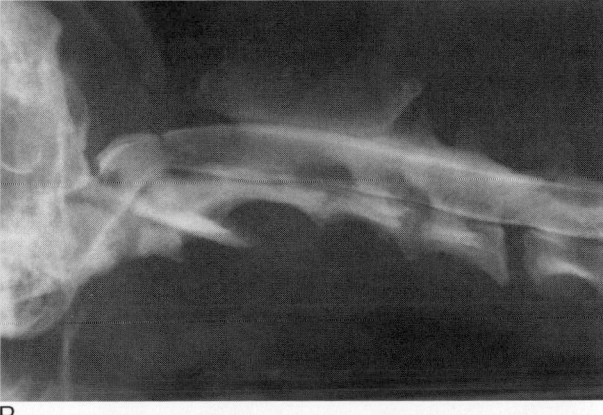

A   B

Fig. 236-4 **A,** Plain lateral radiograph of a 3-year-old Miniature Poodle with atlantoaxial subluxation. With the head in a neutral position, there is increased space between the arch of C1 and the spinous process of C2, and the cranial aspect of C2 is luxated into the vertebral canal. This dog had several congenital abnormalities, including agenesis of the dens, an associated lack of normal atlantoaxial ligaments and block vertebrae from C2 to C4. **B,** Lateral myelogram of the same dog. The head is now positioned in extension in an effort to relieve compression on the spinal cord. Usually this will allow C1-2 to assume a more normal relationship (thus confirming atlantoaxial instability is present). Due to the chronicity of the problem in this dog and associated formation of fibrous tissue, external reduction of the subluxation was minimal.

Nonsurgical Treatment

Cage confinement, immobilization of the AA region with or without nonsteroidal antiinflammatory drugs (NSAIDs), often results in clinical improvement. Splinting allows for formation of fibrous tissues and healing of ligamentous structures to re-stabilize the AA joint. Ideally it should extend from the mandible to the sternum, incorporating the head in mild extension in an attempt to immobilize the AA joint as much as possible. Casting materials, thermoplastic, or malleable metals may be used to form the splint, which should then be well padded before applying to the patient. Some patients do not tolerate this degree of immobilization well. Toy breeds, especially immature animals, may even experience difficulties eating, walking, and supporting the cranial half of the body. In lieu of this type of splinting, a shorter, Robert Jones–style bandage may be used that incorporates the head (including the caudal aspect of the mandible) down to the caudal cervical region. This is generally tolerable to the patient, keeps the head in mild extension, is easily supported, and appears to be effective, especially in very small dogs (Fig. 236-5). Splints and bandages of any kind should be checked regularly for any signs of complication, including otitis, facial, and corneal excoriations and dermatitis. Bandages are typically left on for a period of 4 to 8 weeks and then removed. The animal is allowed a gradual return to normal activity. If clinical signs of AA instability return, nonsurgical treatment may be reinstituted; however, surgical repair is strongly recommended at this point. Clients often become distraught with repeated episodes of pain/myelopathy and are usually amenable to more definitive treatment with surgery after the first episode.

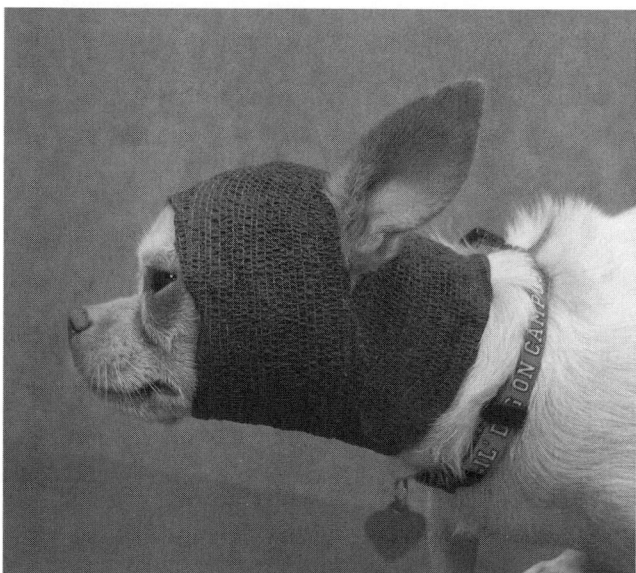

Fig. 236-5 Supportive bandage for atlantoaxial instability. This Robert Jones–style bandage is useful for providing support to the atlantoaxial joint and maintaining the head in mild extension, thus protecting the spinal cord from further injury. The bandage extends from mid-mandible to the level of C6 and should be loose enough to be comfortable and not cause compression of the jugular veins.

Surgical Treatment

Surgery is indicated for most dogs and cats with clinical signs of AA subluxation. Stabilization of the joint usually results in immediate relief of pain and improved neurologic status, even in the most severely affected animals. Many methods of repair have been described in the veterinary literature. In most circumstances dorsal repairs have largely been replaced by ventral fusion techniques. Stabilization of the AA joint reduces the lateral and rotational mobility of the patient's head, although this is usually well tolerated physically by the animal. The "domino" effect, which is frequently of concern with fusion of vertebrae in the caudal cervical spine, does not appear to be a problem at C1–2.

Ventral Surgical Approach and Technique
Ventral fixation of the AA joint is preferred since these techniques provide direct access to the AA joint. This allows the surgeon to reduce the subluxation and decompress the spinal cord, perform an odontectomy if indicated, and promote arthrodesis between C1 and C2 by removing the articular cartilage and placing a bone graft. However, ventral approaches are technically difficult for many reasons, and complications may occur as a result of:

- Bones that are usually very small, often malformed, and easily fractured during reduction and implant placement.
- Vertebral movement and/or incorrect positioning of implant during placement, causing further injury to the spinal cord and possible paralysis, ventilatory failure, or death.
- Trauma to vital soft tissue structures in the area (e.g., vagosympathetic trunk, carotid artery, trachea, brainstem).

Many ventral techniques for surgical management of AA instability in dogs have been reported (Sharp, 2005; Platt, Chambers, and Cross, 2004; Sanders et al., 2004; Schulz, Waldron, and Fahie, 1997; McCarthy, Lewis, and Hosgood, 1995). In each of these the patient is positioned in dorsal recumbency with the neck in extension, similar to positioning for ventral slot procedures. Usually one or more of a combination of pins, screws, and bone cement is used to immobilize the joint, whereas bony fusion at the site is promoted by the placement of a bone graft into the AA joint (Fig. 236-6). Postoperative care is usually minimal, with pain medications needed for the first 24 to 36 hours and NSAIDs used to treat associated inflammation as needed. Improvement in the neurologic status and the pain score of the patient is usually seen immediately following surgery. Restricted activity or cage confinement is recommended for the first 4 to 6 weeks.

Dorsal Surgical Approach and Wiring Technique
Dorsal repairs of the AA joint were the earliest techniques described for immobilization (McCarthy et al., 1995). However, since fusion of the joint is not achieved, these should be considered palliative procedures only and are not recommended as the first choice for treatment of AA subluxation. The dorsal wiring/suturing technique is the most common (dorsal) method still in use. The

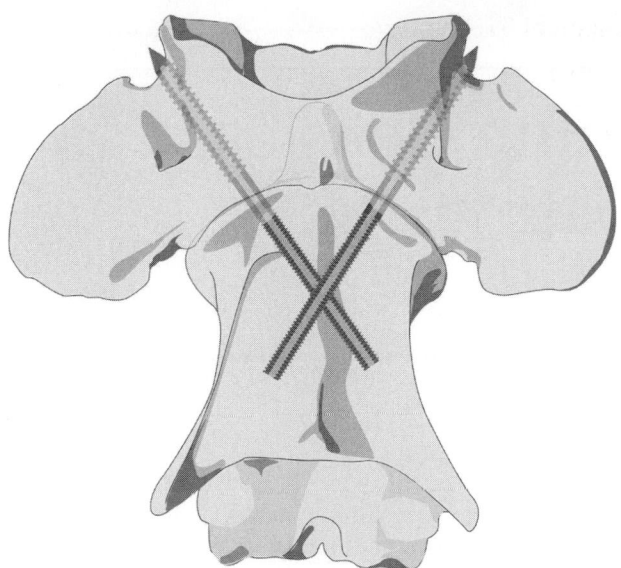

Fig. 236-6 Ventral surgical repair technique of the atlanto-axial joint, ventrodorsal view. In addition to the positive-profile threaded transarticular pins illustrated here, a cancellous bone graft is placed intraarticularly to promote arthrodesis. Larger dogs may require additional pins/screws be placed into C1 and C2 to add more stability until bony fusion occurs.

approach is easy technically, but correct placement of the wire/suture may be difficult and associated with several potential complications:

- Further injury to the spinal cord may occur during wire placement.
- Disruption of internal vertebral venous sinus may cause significant hemorrhage and/or hematoma formation within the vertebral canal, exacerbating clinical signs.
- Wire/suture may cut through the lamina of C1, especially in the soft bones of immature dogs.

Postoperative placement of a splint or bandage is recommended for 6 weeks to keep the AA joint as immobilized as possible until scar tissue forms.

PROGNOSIS

The prognosis for animals with AA subluxation varies, depending on the chronicity and severity of the spinal cord injury that occurs. Generally speaking, long-term outcome is very good to excellent for animals treated surgically that have clinical signs of pain with or without mild to moderate neurologic deficits. Animals presenting with severe tetraparesis/tetraplegia and respiratory distress, especially with a chronic history, have a guarded prognosis for good recovery of neurologic function (Beaver et al., 2000; Knipe et al., 2002). Reported success rates of ventral surgical techniques vary from 79% to 92% for a good-to-excellent outcome (Schulz, Waldron, and Fahie, 1997; Beaver et al., 2000; Sanders et al., 2004; Platt, Chambers, and Cross, 2004; Knipe et al., 2002), with no one method overtly superior with respect to long-term survival. The experience and comfort level of the surgeon in performing surgery in the AA region is likely one of most important influences on the overall outcome of patients with atlantoaxial disease.

A study that followed the long-term outcome of dogs treated nonsurgically found that dogs with an acute onset of clinical signs and no prior history of signs of AA instability had a good outcome about 60% of the time, regardless of the severity of the presenting neurologic status (Havig et al., 2005). However, dogs treated nonsurgically that had clinical signs for longer than 30 days were significantly more likely to have a poor final outcome.

It is emphasized that *the presence of pain perception is of little prognostic value in animals with AA subluxation* because severity of compression required for loss of deep pain at this level of the spinal cord usually causes respiratory paralysis and death.

References and Suggested Reading

Beaver DP et al: Risk factors affecting the outcome of surgery for atlantoaxial subluxation in dogs: 46 cases (1978-1998), *J Am Vet Med Assoc* 216:7, 1104, 2000.

Havig ME et al: Evaluation of nonsurgical treatment of atlantoaxial subluxation in dogs: 19 cases (1992-2001), *J Am Vet Med Assoc* 222:2, 257, 2005.

Knipe MF et al: Atlantoaxial instability in 17 dogs, 20th Annual ACVIM Forum Abstract, Dallas, Texas, May 29-June 1, 2002.

McCarthy RJ, Lewis, DD, Hosgood G: Atlantoaxial subluxation in dogs, *Compend Cont Educ Pract Vet* 17:2, 215, 1995.

Platt SR, Chambers JN, Cross A: A modified ventral fixation for surgical management of atlantoaxial subluxation, *Vet Surg* 33:349, 2004.

Sanders SG et al: Outcomes and complications associated with ventral screws, pins, and polymethyl methacrylate for atlantoaxial instability in 12 dogs, *J Am Anim Hosp Assoc* 40:204, 2004.

Schulz KS, Waldron DR, Fahie M: Application of ventral pins and polymethylmethacrylate for the management of atlantoaxial instability: results in nine dogs, *Vet Surg* 33:317, 1997.

Sharp NJH: Atlantoaxial subluxation. In Sharp NJH, Wheeler SJ, editors: *Diagnosis and surgery of small animal spinal disorders*, St Louis, 2005, Elsevier, p 161.

CHAPTER 237

Treatment of Canine Cervical Spondylomyelopathy: A Critical Review

ANNIE V. CHEN, *Pullman, Washington*

RODNEY S. BAGLEY, *Pullman, Washington*

Cervical spondylomyelopathy (CSM) is a neurologic condition that affects large-breed dogs, particularly Great Danes and Doberman pinschers. Numerous medical and surgical treatments have been attempted; however, the most appropriate treatment still remains controversial. Reasons for such controversy arise from the complexity of this disease process and the incomplete understanding of its pathogenesis. Opinions vary as to the etiology, diagnosis, and treatment of this disease; consequently it has acquired several names. Diagnostic descriptors include wobbler syndrome, cervical spondylopathy, cervical vertebral instability, cervical vertebral malformation-malarticulation, and cervical spondylolisthesis.

ETIOLOGY AND PATHOPHYSIOLOGY

The etiology of CSM is likely multifactorial and has been speculated to be caused by nutritional, traumatic, or genetic factors. The fact that large-breed dogs are most commonly affected heightens the suspicion that breeds with long necks and heavy heads create increased physical stress on the cervical spine and therefore predispose these breeds to this disease. In addition, rapid growth in large-breed dogs can adversely affect the development of the cervical spine, contributing to vertebral canal stenosis, vertebral body malformation, vertebral subluxation, and vertebral instability. Pedigrees have also been reviewed in both Great Danes and Doberman pinschers that suggest a genetic contribution to this disease. Regardless of the etiology, this disease becomes clinically significant when it leads to compression of the spinal cord and/or instability of the spine.

There are two major types of compressive lesions encountered with CSM: osseous and primary soft-tissue abnormalities. Osseous compression (bony stenosis) is typically seen in young, immature dogs, particularly large or giant breeds such as Great Danes. These dogs may have congenital malformations of the cervical vertebrae (articular facet, pedicle, vertebral arches) that then lead to a narrowed vertebral canal. Multiple vertebral sites are usually involved, although focal osseous malformation is also possible. The degree of osseous compression can change with flexion or extension of the neck. These abnormalities may result in either dynamic or static compressive lesions.

Soft-tissue compression can be dorsal, lateral, or ventral but is most often dorsal or lateral in these young, large- or giant-breed dogs. Types of dorsolateral soft-tissue compression include ligamentum flavum (interarcuate ligament) hypertrophy, joint capsule proliferation, and synovial cyst formation.

Ventral soft-tissue compression typically is related to intervertebral disk degeneration with protrusion of the annulus fibrosus. This is most commonly seen in older adult dogs, particularly Doberman pinschers. Subluxation or "tipping" of the cranial aspect of the vertebral body dorsally into the spinal canal can also result secondary to the degenerative disk. It is important to recognize that not all radiographically apparent vertebral "tipping" leads to spinal cord compression and clinical deficits. Doberman pinschers are most commonly affected at the C6-7 intervertebral disk space and to a lesser extent at C5-6 and C4-5. This type of compression can also be dynamic with alleviation of the ventral spinal cord compression on flexion of the neck.

MEDICAL TREATMENT AND PROGNOSIS

Traditionally medical management of CSM has consisted of cage confinement, restricted activity, external support braces or bandages, pain medication, muscle relaxants, and/or antiinflammatory drugs such as corticosteroids or nonsteroidal antiinflammatory drugs. Although each of these treatments have been perpetuated in the veterinary literature, the available evidence to support the success of these treatments is mostly anecdotal.

Results of medical management of CSM have varied in the literature. Interpretation of reported results is complicated by the fact that documentation of the natural course of this disease in a large group of similarly affected dogs has not been performed. Since this overall pattern of disease with an associated prognosis is not established, assessment of treatment options becomes difficult without a well-defined, prospective, randomized study. Therefore reported outcomes of medical management are difficult to interpret. It is also important to realize that cases treated successfully in private practice with medical therapy may not form part of the literature. Therefore it is possible that the success rate with medical management is higher than reported.

Denny, Gibbs, and Gaskell (1977) retrospectively reviewed 25 large-breed dogs, primarily Great Danes, with CSM that had restricted exercise as the treatment. Nineteen dogs (75%) were euthanized for their neurologic disease, one dog recovered after a few months and remained normal for 3 years, one dog slightly improved at 1 year follow-up, one dog showed no change at 1 year follow-up, and three dogs were lost to follow-up. Duration to euthanasia ranged from 2 weeks to 5 years with a median of 4 months.

Overall, medical treatment may be effective for dogs with less severe clinical signs of CSM, although this has not been evaluated objectively. Typically surgery is performed in dogs that present with severe neurologic deficits, are unresponsive to medical management, or show signs of progressive disease.

SURGICAL TREATMENT AND PROGNOSIS

Surgical treatment of CSM has been used since the 1970s. Despite various case studies describing and evaluating different surgical techniques, there is no strong evidence (double-blinded, placebo-controlled, randomized, multicenter study) that shows one surgical procedure to be superior over the others or in some instances better than nonsurgical management. To further complicate the assessment of treatment responses, identification of the unique patient factors that may make one therapy more or less effective for an individual patient is currently unestablished. Therefore information reported historically about surgical treatment of this disease is primarily descriptive.

One of the earliest published reports on surgical treatment for CSM in Doberman pinschers was described by Mason in 1977. Cervical spondylomyelopathy was diagnosed based on clinical signs and radiographic changes without or in some instances with myelography. The results of the radiographic changes in relationship to the age of the dog suggested that intervertebral instability was the primary lesion and that degenerative changes to the disk and proliferative changes to the vertebrae were secondary to excessive mobility and abnormal forces. Twenty-five Doberman pinchers had fenestration of the intervertebral disks with a Bard Parker No. 11 blade and the removal of the nucleus with a small spatula from C2-T1. The proposed theory behind this procedure was that, with the removal of the nucleus, the intervertebral disk space would collapse and form fibrosis, which would increase the stability of the cervical spine. Treatment was considered effective if alleviation of clinical signs were noted. The author concluded that treatment by fenestration was effective in cases that showed only vertebral instability (younger dogs) and much less effective in older dogs (>2.5 years old) with associated degenerative changes. How the author determined vertebral instability was not clearly defined in this report.

In 1977 Denny, Gibbs, and Gaskell published data from 10 large-breed dogs with CSM that were treated surgically. Clinical diagnosis was supported by radiographic demonstration of cervical vertebral abnormality. The principal radiologic sign of intervertebral instability was dorsal displacement of the cranial margin of a vertebral body with respect to the caudal margin of the vertebra cranial to it. The affected vertebrae were stabilized by screw fixation of the vertebral bodies across the intervertebral disk space in eight dogs (Gage and Horelein, 1973), by plate fixation of the vertebral bodies in one dog, and by screw fixation of the laminar articular facets in one dog (Parker et al., 1973). Bone grafts were used in nine dogs to help promote early spinal fusion. Dorsal laminectomy was carried out in conjunction with stabilization in one dog. Six dogs (60%) improved at various follow-up times, one had no improvement, and three showed a transient improvement followed by deterioration and were euthanized.

Ventral decompression was evaluated as a treatment for cervical disk protrusion in large- and giant-breed dogs by Chambers and colleagues (1982). Twelve dogs, the majority of them Doberman pinschers (9/12), diagnosed with caudal cervical disk herniation (soft-tissue compression) with radiographs and myelograms underwent ventral decompression with the removal of the dorsal annulus, dorsal longitudinal ligament, and herniated disk material (full-thickness ventral slot) (Gilpin, 1976). After a follow-up period averaging 16 months after surgery, six dogs (50%) were neurologically normal, and six dogs (50%) were functional pets with minor residual proprioceptive deficits. These authors concluded that ventral decompression alone is a satisfactory treatment for dogs with caudal cervical disk herniation without coincidental instability. It is important to note that dogs with radiographic evidence of vertebral instability (vertebral subluxation, misshapen vertebrae, spinal canal stenosis, spondylosis deformans, or proliferation of the articular facets) were excluded from this study.

Fenestration for treatment of degenerative disk disease in the caudal cervical region of large-breed dogs was evaluated by Lincoln and Pettit in 1985. Fifteen of the seventeen dogs were Doberman pinschers. Disk disease was diagnosed based on survey radiographs and myelograms. Fenestration of multiple caudal cervical disks was performed using a No. 11 scalpel blade, and disk material was removed using curettes and rongeurs. Four dogs (24%) had complete remission of clinical signs; seven dogs (41%) showed persistence or return of pain, ataxia, or dysmetria but without further progression; and six dogs (35%) had deterioration of clinical signs after surgery. In general, dogs with spinal cord compression that was not relieved by flexion or traction of the neck on the stress myelograms and those with spinal canals of smaller diameter became progressively worse after fenestration. The authors concluded that disk fenestration may not resolve a problem caused by a compressive degenerative disk since the dorsal part of the annulus fibrosus remains and may even be pushed into the spinal canal after fenestration. This was confirmed on two postmortem examinations.

In 1986 Chambers, Oliver, and Björling published a retrospective study on 27 CSM-affected Doberman pinschers that underwent full-thickness ventral slot for decompression of the spinal cord. Myelograms were used to identify the site(s) of compression. The types of compression present were not clarified by the authors. There were no deaths during surgery or in the immediate postoperative period. Within a few months of surgery 9 of the 27 dogs

(33%) either died or were euthanized because of postoperative complications or persistent or progressive neurologic deficits. Six dogs were necropsied, and residual spinal cord compression was found at a previous surgical site. The remaining dogs (67%) were either normal or had minimal residual deficits. The follow-up period varied from 6 months to 4 years. The authors concluded that this surgical technique was very challenging to perform and had a high percentage of failures.

A distracted cervical spinal fusion technique using an autogenous bone graft from the iliac crest, 4-mm cancellous bone screws, and polymethyl methacrylate (PMMA) was described by Ellison, Seim, and Clemmons in 1988. Ten CSM-affected Doberman pinschers had evidence of dynamic soft-tissue spinal cord compression on the stress myelograms. Dogs with disk herniation that did not flatten with traction views were not candidates for this surgery. A partial-thickness ventral slot was performed up to the level of the dorsal portion of the annulus fibrosus and the dorsal longitudinal ligament. Gentle traction was placed on the neck, and the proper-size bone graft was placed in the slot using a pin tap. Partially threaded 4-mm -diameter cancellous bone screws were initiated on midline and angled 30 degrees away from perpendicular. Two diverging screws were placed in each of the adjacent vertebrae, and PMMA was used to cover the ventral aspect of the screws. After surgery, eight dogs (80%) had either improved neurologic status or elimination of cervical pain. Implant loosening was seen in three dogs, and two of them were euthanized because of lack of neurologic improvement. Evidence of bony cervical fusion was seen on radiographs during a 9- to 24-week period in six of the eight surviving dogs. The authors concluded that this was a valid surgical procedure for treatment of CSM in dogs when the compressive lesion is limited to one cervical intervertebral disk space.

In 1989 Bruecker, Seim, and Withrow retrospectively evaluated three surgical methods for the treatment of CSM caused by chronic degenerative disk disease in 64 dogs, of which 48 were Doberman pinschers. Twenty dogs had full-thickness ventral slot exposing the spinal cord. Seven dogs had partial-thickness ventral slot, linear traction, bone graft, and interbody screw placement. Thirty-seven dogs had partial-thickness ventral slot, linear traction, bone graft, and placement of the plastic plate on the ventral aspect of the vertebral bodies. Interbody screw stabilization was ineffective because of an unacceptably high rate of implant failure. Full-thickness ventral slot or plastic plate stabilization was an effective treatment for CSM patients with mild-to-moderate neurologic deficits. Dogs with severe neurologic deficits (weakly ambulatory to nonambulatory tetraparesis) had variable success rates and prolonged recovery periods. Follow-up time ranged from 3 to 50 months with a mean of 20 months. A second compressive lesion developing at an adjacent intervertebral space (known as domino lesion) was seen with all three surgical methods.

In 1990 McKee and colleagues prospectively evaluated a vertebral distraction-fusion technique using a transvertebral screw and two interbody washers. Seventeen Doberman pinschers and three Great Danes were included in this study. A diagnosis of CSM was made based on stress myelography. All dogs had evidence of spinal cord compression at C6-7, and six dogs also had spinal cord compression at C5-6. Spinal cord compression was associated with the dorsal protrusion of the annulus fibrosus. Traction on the cervical spine reduced the degree of compression in 23 of the 26 protrusions. Double washers were used at 24 sites, and a single washer was used at two sites of cord compression because of inability to distract the affected disk spaces sufficiently. Fifteen dogs were radiographed 6 months following surgery; they all showed evidence of vertebral end-plate resorption and new bone production ventrally around the implants. Ten dogs radiographed 18 months following surgery showed bone production around the implants, which the authors concluded to be vertebral bony fusion. Seventeen dogs (85%) improved following surgery, one died in the early postoperative period as a result of a gastric dilation and volvulus, and two were destroyed because of fracture of the ventral spinous process of C6.

A modified distraction-stabilization technique using an interbody PMMA plug in dogs with CSM was described by Dixon, Tomlinson, and Kraus in 1996. Eighteen Doberman pinchers, two German shepherds, one Great Dane, and one rottweiler underwent this surgical procedure. Diagnosis of CSM was made on the basis of history, clinical signs, and myelographic confirmation of a dynamic compressive cervical lesion. The predominant component of the compressive lesion was ventral to the cord as a result of a protruded dorsal annulus. A partial-thickness ventral slot was performed, and approximately 3 to 5 mm of dorsal annulus and bony end plates was left intact. Linear distraction was applied using blunted Gelpi retractors and laminectomy spreaders. PMMA anchor holes were drilled into the vertebral end plates using a pneumatic drill. PMMA was placed into the prepared disk space while traction was maintained. After PMMA hardened, the traction device was removed, and cancellous bone graft was placed along the ventral aspect of the exposed vertebral bodies. This technique was used for two adjacent disk spaces in nine dogs and in a single disk space in thirteen dogs. Nineteen dogs (86%) were considered successes long term, with 50% of the dogs returning to normal neurologic function. Two dogs (9%) were considered failures. The two failures were both nonambulatory before surgery. Follow-up time ranged from 3 to 60 months with a median of 18 months. Criteria for success and failure were defined by the authors. Major complications with this procedure were not observed. This procedure was not recommended in dogs with static ventral spinal cord compressions.

In 1998 Rusbridge and colleagues compared two surgical techniques for the management of CSM in Doberman pinchers: full-thickness ventral slot (Swaim, 1973) versus vertebral distraction and stabilization using the screw and washer technique (McKee et al., 1990). Twenty-eight Doberman pinchers were retrospectively included in the study. Immediately following the ventral slot procedure, 6 of 14 dogs (43%) deteriorated neurologically. This neurologic deterioration was suspected to be caused by iatrogenic injury during surgery or reperfusion injury after decompression of the spinal cord. At 6 months after surgery, 13 of 14 of the ventral slot dogs and 12 of 14 of the screw and washer dogs had satisfactory outcomes. At 1 year after surgery the recurrence rate was zero for the ventral slot procedure and 5 of 14 (36%) for the screw and washer technique. At 2 years after surgery, 4 of 14 (29%) of the ventral slot dogs had deteriorated compared to 7 of 14 (50%) of the screw and washer dogs. When clarified, the cause of the deterioration was the result of either a domino disk lesion or dorsal displacement of the screw and washer secondary to vertebral end-plate collapse. The authors concluded that both procedures have satisfactory short-term results. The ventral slot procedure was more time consuming and had more immediate postoperative deterioration. However, recurrence of clinical signs more likely was seen after the screw and washer technique.

In 1998 Queen and colleagues questioned the need for distraction in dogs with disk-associated CSM. Because of the increased risk of vertebral collapse secondary to the distraction reported in the literature, the authors described a technique of vertebral body fusion without distraction, using two position screws (for short-term stability) and a partial-thickness ventral slot filled with cancellous bone graft (to promote fusion for long-term stability). Seventeen Doberman pinchers were diagnosed with CSM based on radiography and myelography. A partial-thickness ventral slot was performed at C6-7, two cortical bone screws were placed parallel to each other across the disk space, and cancellous bone graft taken from the proximal humerus was placed into and around the slot. Follow-up interval ranged from 3 weeks to 35 months. One dog was lost to follow-up. Thirteen of 16 cases (81%) neurologically improved within the first 3 months after surgery. Three cases (19%) were euthanized after surgery because of neurologic deterioration as a result of incorrect screw placement of one of the screws. The authors hypothesized that increased vertebral stability is the major contributor to long-term clinical improvement by allowing atrophy of the intervertebral soft tissues and/or by eliminating any dynamic component of this disease.

The intervertebral metal washer technique for the management of CSM-associated intervertebral disk protrusions was reevaluated by McKee, Butterworth, and Scott in 1999. Seventy-eight cases were reviewed retrospectively. Myelography demonstrated traction-responsive cervical spinal cord compression. Fifty lesions were evaluated myelographically on immediate postoperative radiographs. Of these, 32 spinal cord compressions had been eliminated, and 18 had been reduced. Within 6 months of surgery, euthanasia was performed in nine dogs (12%) because of neurologic deterioration, and 15 dogs (19%) had varying degrees of neck pain. Vertebral end-plate fracture was considered a key factor in these 24 cases. Sixty-five of the 78 cases were studied long term with a median follow-up time of 32 months. Sixty-three of the 65 cases (97%) improved after surgery. However, neurologic deterioration eventually occurred in 17 of the 65 cases (26%). Myelographic evaluation in 8 of the 17 cases revealed additional disk protrusions with no evidence of cord compression at previous surgery sites. These additional disk protrusions were suspected to be domino lesions. The authors concluded that, although the intervertebral washer technique had low perioperative morbidity and was effective in eliminating or reducing spinal

cord compression, the unpredictable nature of vertebral end-plate fracture remained a significant concern.

In 2001 Lipsitz and colleagues evaluated the continuous dorsal laminectomy technique in 14 large-breed dogs with CSM. All dogs were ambulatory at the time of presentation. Spinal cord compression as a result of the hypertrophy of the interarcuate ligament, hypertrophy and soft-tissue proliferation associated with the articular processes, and synovial cysts were identified using magnetic resonance imaging. These changes were all confirmed at surgery. The follow-up period ranged from 2 months to 2 years. Eleven dogs (79%) had an excellent outcome based on resolution of clinical signs as defined by recheck examination and owner telephone consultation. Three dogs had a poor outcome: one died after surgery from cardiac arrhythmias, one deteriorated neurologically after an epileptic event, and one sustained iatrogenic spinal cord injury during surgery but was improving 2 months later. The authors concluded that a dorsal laminectomy can be performed at multiple levels in CSM-affected dogs with lesions at multiple sites.

A retrospective study was performed by De Risio et al. in 2002 to evaluate the postoperative morbidity and long-term outcome of CSM-affected dogs after dorsal laminectomy. Twenty dogs were included in this study; seven were Great Danes, and six were Doberman pinchers. Myelography and/or computed tomography was used for the diagnosis of CSM. The dynamic nature of the disease was not evaluated in all dogs. Sites of spinal cord compression varied from 1 to 4 and were osseous and/or soft tissue in nature. All dogs had dorsal laminectomy at the site(s) of spinal cord compression. Neurologic status worsened in fourteen dogs (70%) 2 days after surgery but improved in all but one dog over long-term follow-up of 7 months to 9 years. Nineteen dogs (95%) were clinically improved according to owners and referring veterinarians after surgery. Mean time to optimal recovery was 3.6 months. However, recurrence of clinical signs was seen in six dogs (30%). The authors concluded that, although most dogs worsen neurologically in the immediate postoperative period after a dorsal laminectomy, this deterioration was usually transient, and the average time to reach optimal neurologic status was similar to the recovery time for other cervical spinal cord surgery.

OBSERVATIONS AND CONCLUSIONS

Although the literature contributes to our knowledge of CSM in dogs, there are limitations to these studies. When reviewing the literature critically, variable details on the rate of onset, duration of neurologic signs, severity of neurologic dysfunction, diagnostic work-up, and clinical follow-up make comparison of these surgical techniques difficult. For example, different patient inclusion criteria were used between studies. Although all dogs had some form of CSM, certain studies only evaluated specific breeds of dogs, assessed only traction-responsive (dynamic) lesions, excluded dogs with osseous lesions, or never made a distinction between dynamic and static lesions. The majority of the studies focused primarily on traction-responsive, disk-associated soft-tissue compressions. There were fewer studies on the surgical treatment of the osseous form of CSM. This exclusion ultimately creates a bias and makes interpretation of the results challenging. In addition, the definition of long-term follow-up differed among studies. Even within a study itself, the follow-up times varied between weeks and years, making the reported long-term outcome and recurrence rate somewhat unreliable. Follow-up methods also were variable in that some were performed by veterinarians whereas others were based on client surveys or telephone interviews. Finally, the surgical approach and technique can differ significantly among surgeons. For example, a ventral slot can be made at different widths and lengths and can be of full or partial thickness. Distraction also can be variable since the optimal degree of distraction is unknown. Therefore, depending on what was actually performed and the surgical skills of the surgeon, the outcomes and potential risks can vary tremendously, even with a specific procedure.

In general, surgical techniques for CSM have focused on decompression, stabilization, or both. Decompression can be either direct or indirect. Direct decompression typically is done through a ventral slot or dorsal laminectomy. Indirect decompression uses bone plates, pins, screws, or PMMA to maintain vertebral distraction. Using surgical implants can also eliminate vertebral instability at least in the short term while the vertebrae fuse. Additional procedures such as disk fenestration and bone grafting have also been described. Bone grafts often are used in conjunction with distraction techniques for the purpose of promoting bony fusion. All of these techniques can be useful, but there is no single surgical technique that can be applied effectively to all forms of CSM.

Therefore the *choice of surgical technique depends on a number of factors*: the location of the compression (ventral, lateral or dorsal) to the spinal cord, the type of compression (soft versus osseous), the number of disk spaces involved (single versus multiple sites), and whether or not the lesion is traction responsive (dynamic versus static). In general, decompression of a dorsal or lateral, osseous or soft-tissue compression (interarcuate hypertrophy, joint capsule proliferation, extradural synovial cyst) requires a dorsal laminectomy. Some surgeons may also advocate stabilization, hoping for regression of osseous and soft-tissue proliferation over time. The ventral, soft-tissue, traction-nonresponsive (static) lesion requires direct decompression through a ventral slot. Surgical treatment for the ventral, soft-tissue, traction-responsive (dynamic) lesion is most controversial. Both direct and indirect decompressions have been described. Whether or not stabilization of the affected vertebrae is necessary still remains in question.

Initially instability was proposed in the pathogenesis of CSM because of malalignment of the caudal cervical vertebrae on radiographs during flexion and extension. This idea has been perpetuated over time and has not been evaluated objectively. Although there are case studies that advocate the importance of stabilization for the treatment of CSM, there are also studies that have had comparable postoperative results without stabilization. Some surgeons argue that stabilization should be performed in all forms of CSM (dynamic and static) because increased vertebral stability can result in intervertebral disk atrophy and osseous regression, which can lead to eventual absence of spinal cord compression. However, other surgeons argue against stabilization because of the reported implant failure or domino lesions. Whether or not instability can be proven in CSM-affected dogs becomes the important question. It is possible that some CSM-affected dogs have underlying instability whereas others don't, which then makes this distinction important before surgery. Also, some clinicians propose that CSM-affected dogs may have instability during the early stages of disease but can actually restabilize as the intervertebral disk degenerates further. Dynamic imaging studies such as stress myelography or magnetic resonance imaging may help identify instability, but microinstability is not detectable with such modalities. The clinician is often left with deciding whether or not stabilization is appropriate based on an educated guess as to the degree of spinal instability. Typically a significant dynamic lesion suggests that surgical therapy should involve stabilization of the vertebrae. The goal of stabilization may be to treat instability in the short term, but long-term stability requires bony fusion, or the implants can fail. Whether spinal fusion ever occurs and to what extent in the stabilized patient remains unclear. Bony proliferation on radiographic follow-up may suggest bony fusion and stabilization, but no concurrent histopathologic and biomechanical studies have proven this to be true.

Risks of the surgical procedure should also be taken into consideration when choosing the appropriate surgical technique. Dorsal laminectomy and ventral slot have been associated with a higher level of postoperative morbidity in some studies. This morbidity may be due to the result of iatrogenic injury to the spinal cord, an acute increase in vertebral instability caused by the removal of surrounding stabilizing structures, or hypothesized reperfusion injury to the spinal cord after decompression. Reported morbidity is variable and most likely the result of differences in surgical approach and technique among surgeons. Indirect decompression (distraction) can also lead to catastrophic consequences. Distraction is often lost over time because of bone resorption on either side of implant. This can be clinically inconsequential, but this implant/end-plate failure can result in significant vertebral instability, vertebral collapse, and end-plate fracture in some dogs.

In addition, *recurrence rates* have been documented for most surgical techniques in the literature. In general, reported recurrence rate after CSM surgery in the dog is between 10% and 40%. Recurrence of clinical signs can be caused by progression of previously identified disease or secondary to domino lesions. It has been suggested that intervertebral immobilization promoted by distraction/stabilization techniques may predispose degeneration of the neighboring intervertebral disk spaces, resulting in domino lesions. It is also possible that the degeneration of the neighboring disks is part of the natural course of CSM and is unrelated to the immobilization of the spine. Overall, recurrence rates need to be interpreted carefully because of the differences in follow-up times, follow-up methods, and surgical skills of the surgeons.

The lack of knowledge of the natural history of canine cervical spondylomyelopathy makes treatment recommendation for this disease difficult. It is known anecdotally that some dogs can respond to medical management alone whereas others require surgical intervention or both. However, the dilemma in veterinary medicine centers around the lack of solid evidence in our literature. With the reported variation across published studies, interpretation of the results is challenging. For clinicians to better understand the natural history of CSM and make appropriate recommendations for treatment will require double-blinded, placebo-controlled, randomized, large sample–size studies. Until that time, definitive recommendations cannot be made, and the clinician should try to appreciate the complex nature of this disorder so to best counsel the client.

References and Suggested Reading

Bruecker KA, Seim HB, Withrow SJ: Clinical evaluation of three surgical methods for treatment of caudal cervical spondylomyelopathy of dogs, *Vet Surg* 18:197, 1989.

Chambers JN et al: Ventral decompression for caudal cervical disk herniation in large- and giant-breed dogs, *J Am Vet Med Assoc* 180:410, 1982.

Chambers JN, Oliver JE, Björling DE: Update on ventral decompression for caudal cervical disk herniation in Doberman pinchers, *J Am Anim Hosp Assoc* 22:775, 1986.

Da Costa RC et al: Morphologic and morphometric magnetic resonance imaging features of Doberman pinchers with and without clinical signs of cervical spondylomyelopathy, *Am J Vet Res* 67:1601, 2006.

Denny HR, Gibbs C, Gaskell CJ: Cervical spondylopathy in the dog—a review of thirty-five cases, *J Small Anim Pract* 18:117, 1977.

De Risio L et al: Dorsal laminectomy for caudal cervical spondylomyelopathy: postoperative recovery and long-term follow-up in 20 dogs, *Vet Surg* 31:418, 2002.

Dixon BC, Tomlinson, JL, Kraus KH: Modified distraction-stabilization technique using an interbody polymethyl methacrylate plug in dogs with caudal cervical spondylomyelopathy, *J Am Vet Med Assoc* 208:61, 1996.

Ellison GW, Seim HB, Clemmons RM: Distracted cervical spinal fusion for management of caudal cervical spondylomyelopathy in large-breed dogs, *J Am Vet Med Assoc* 193:447, 1988.

Gage ED, Horelein BF: Surgical repair of cervical subluxation and spondylithesis in the dog, *Anim Hosp Assoc* 9:385, 1973.

Gilpin GN: Evaluation of three techniques of ventral decompression of the cervical spinal cord in the dog, *J Am Vet Med Assoc* 168:325, 1976.

Jeffery ND, McKee WM: Surgery for disc-associated wobbler syndrome in the dog—an examination of the controversy, *J Small Anim Pract* 42:574, 2001.

Lincoln JD, Pettit GD: Evaluation of fenestration for treatment of degenerative disc disease in the caudal cervical region of large dogs, *Vet Surg* 14:240, 1985.

Lipsitz D AE et al: Magnetic resonance imaging features of cervical stenotic myelopathy in 21 dogs, *Vet Radiol Ultrasound* 42:20, 2001.

Mason TA: Cervical vertebral instability in the Doberman, *Aust Vet J* 53:440, 1977.

McKee WM, Butterworth SJ, Scott HW: Management of cervical spondylopathy–associated intervertebral disc protrusions using metal washers in 78 dogs, *J Small Anim Pract* 40:465, 1999.

McKee WM et al: Vertebral distraction-fusion for cervical spondylopathy using a screw and double washer technique, *J Small Anim Pract* 31:21, 1990.

Parker AJ et al: Cervical vertebral instability in the dog, *J Am Vet Med Assoc* 163:71, 1973.

Queen JP et al: Management of disc-associated wobbler syndrome with a partial slot fenestration and position screw technique, *J Small Anim Pract* 39:131, 1998.

Rusbridge C et al: Comparison of two surgical techniques for the management of cervical spondylomyelopathy in Dobermans, *J Small Anim Pract* 39:425, 1998.

Swaim SF: Ventral decompression of the cervical spinal cord of the dog, *J Am Vet Med Assoc* 162:276, 1973.

CHAPTER 238

Treatment of Degenerative Lumbosacral Stenosis

DANIEL G. HICKS, *Pullman, Washington*
RODNEY S. BAGLEY, *Pullman, Washington*

A degenerative condition of the lumbosacral (LS) joint causing radiculopathy is encountered regularly in dogs. Despite the common occurrence of this disorder, details of pathophysiology, diagnosis, and appropriate treatment are still debated. In addition, most reports detailing diagnosis and treatment are retrospective in nature, without a standard of diagnosis. Because of the complex pathophysiology involved, grouping dogs into a single disease that involves degeneration of the LS articulation may not be reasonable. These and other factors contribute to the debate about which therapy is most effective.

The LS region is comprised of the vertebral bodies of the caudal lumbar and sacral spine, facet joints and synovial joint capsules, the intervertebral disk elements of the L7-S1 disk, ligamentum flavum, intervertebral foramina, paraspinal musculature, other associated supporting structures, and terminal spinal nerves. Additional musculoskeletal elements of the pelvic limbs may biomechanically influence events in the LS region. These include the LS articulation, pelvis, sacroiliac, and coxofemoral structures. Concentrating purely on the neural elements, any abnormality that causes static or dynamic compression of neural elements in this region can lead to radiculopathy. Since one of the most common clinical features of LS disease process is pain, any of the aforementioned anatomic elements may contribute to this clinical sign.

TERMINOLOGY

Before attempting to determine if a treatment is effective, it is paramount that the disease under treatment be identified specifically and its pathophysiology understood. As stated above, multiple pathologic processes may affect the LS region in dogs and cats causing similar clinical signs. Neoplasia, diskospondylitis, fracture/luxations, meningitis, and vascular-based spinal disease could mimic degenerative LS stenosis (DLSS). In the past, these diverse disease processes have been grouped under the same general term of "LS disease" (Berzon and Dueland, 1979; Mayhew et al., 2002). Inappropriate conclusions about diagnosis, treatment, and prognosis of DLSS could be drawn from such reports, when the actual cause of the LS diseases was not established. Furthermore, terms such as *cauda equina syndrome, LS disease, LS stenosis,* and *degenerative LS stenosis* all have been used to imply a more generic description of clinical signs reflective of an abnormality within the LS region. For this discussion DLSS will be used to describe a degenerative process of the LS region and exclude other potential etiologies of LS disease. This degeneration may occur spontaneously or may be the result of excessive or repeated "wear and tear" of this region.

PATHOPHYSIOLOGY

Degenerative LS stenosis implies that the spinal nerves coursing through the terminal spinal canal or associated intervertebral foramina are pathologically altered, usually by some form of compression or impingement. The extent of radiculopathy leads to a wide spectrum of clinical manifestation, including pain and nervous system dysfunction. Neural element compression is caused by intervertebral disk degeneration (protrusion of dorsal annulus fibrosus), proliferation of the ligamentum flavum or synovial joint capsule, vertebral joint osteophytosis, intermittent claudication, and LS spondylosis (De Risio et al., 2001; Shulman and Lippincott, 1988; Berzon and Dueland, 1979). Chronic repetitive motion of the LS joint leads to accelerated degeneration in some dogs and cats. In addition, compression of neural elements may be dynamic and influenced by the position of the spine, pelvis, and limbs. Flexed compared to extended radiography and magnetic resonance imaging have demonstrated position-dependent changes in the vertebral conformation and neural element compression (Oliver, Selcer, and Simpson, 1978; Schmid and Lang, 1993; Hicks et al., 2006). Whether LS joint degeneration leads to clinically apparent disease is potentially the result of numerous pathologic variables. Malarticulation, malformation, osteochondrosis dissecans, transitional vertebra, congenital malformation or stenosis, and long-term high motion of this joint complex are usually suspected to be components of this disease process. Breed predispositions may reflect inherent genetic or congenital conformational attributes or represent dogs more commonly selected as working dogs.

Complexities in the pathophysiology of DLSS may result in different clinical manifestations. These clinical features can include LS pain, reduced activity, unwillingness to climb stairs or jump, reluctance to sit, fecal or urinary incontinence, changes in tail carriage, kyphotic posturing, a stiff, stilted, or lame pelvic limb gait, pain on tail manipulation, or pain on direct LS palpation (external or per rectum) (Shulman and Lippincott, 1988; Oliver, Selcer, and Simpson, 1978; Scharf et al., 2004). Paraparesis or monoparesis also may be present. Spinal reflex abnormalities include decreased withdrawal, decreased anal tone, and decreased bulbocavernosus reflex. The patellar reflex is not reduced but can appear increased (pseudohyperreflexic) or normal. Decreased tail tone and muscle atrophy (especially the sciatic nerve–dependent muscles) may also be present. Attention should be given to the symmetry of muscle tone and size (particularly the cranial tibial muscles) between pelvic limbs. Incontinence or perineal hypalgesia may be noted, reflecting pudendal nerve dysfunction. Occasionally self-mutilation is noted, likely resulting from a local paresthesia (Mayhew et al., 2002).

DIAGNOSIS

Diagnosis of DLSS can be challenging considering the various pathophysiologic changes. Moreover, historically-used diagnostic tests were not specific or always accurate. Lacking standardized criteria for diagnosis of DLSS, universal agreement on the diagnosis is difficult and it follows that comparisons of treatments may not be possible.

Magnetic resonance imaging has become the "gold-standard" in evaluating the anatomic components of the central nervous system; however, it may have limitations for diagnosis of DLSS (De Risio, Thomas, and Sharp, 2000; Adams et al., 1995; Karkkainen, Punto, and Tulamo, 1993; Chambers et al., 1997). In addition, the LS joint can be imaged in different positions (extension, neutral, and flexion) to assess changes in neural element compression. Findings consistent with DLSS include degeneration of the L7-S1 intervertebral disk (loss of signal intensity of the nucleus pulposus on T2-weighted images); spinal canal narrowing caused by protrusion of the dorsal annulus fibrosus; extrusion of the nucleus pulposus; hypertrophy of the dorsal longitudinal ligament, interarcuate ligament, and/or synovial joint capsules (facet joints); synovial cysts; osteophytosis of the facet joints; and loss of epidural fat in the LS region (Jones, Banfield, and Ward, 2000; Rossi et al., 2004). It is important to note that abnormal imaging findings may occur in some dogs without obvious associated clinical signs. In the absence of such signs, pathologic imaging alterations in the LS region could lead to over diagnosis of DLSS (DeRisio, Thomas, and Sharp, 2000; Mayhew et al., 2002).

TREATMENT

Historically both medical and surgical options have been used as treatment of DLSS. Current treatment recommendations for this disease often are based on historical precedent, anecdotal communication, and retrospective studies. No standardized, blinded, randomized, and controlled clinical trials have been published regarding treatment of this condition.

Historically dogs with less severe clinical signs or those with contraindications for surgery receive medical treatment alone, resulting in inherent bias in patient selection. Severely affected dogs such as those with fecal or urinary incontinence or marked sensory or motor deficits or those that do not respond to medical management are surgical candidates, resulting in a similar treatment bias (Chambers, 1989). Multiple surgical techniques have been used to (1) decompress LS neural elements, and/or (2) distract and fuse the LS joint (Auger et al., 2000; Berzon and Dueland, 1979; Schmid and Lang, 1993; Sharp and Wheeler, 2005; Slocum and Devine, 1986). Evidence favoring either of these techniques has not been firmly established.

Dorsal laminectomy, partial diskectomy, foraminotomy, and facetectomy have been used for neural element decompression (Chambers, Selcer, and Oliver, 1988; Danielsson and Sjöstrom, 1999; Lorraine et al., 2003; Tarvin and Prata, 1980). One study of 26 dogs with presumptive DLSS reported clinical improvement in all dogs after dorsal laminectomy and excision of hypertrophied tissue (Chambers, Selcer, and Oliver, 1988). Another retrospective study evaluated 69 dogs after dorsal laminectomy to treat suspected DLSS. Fifty-four of the 69 dogs improved after surgery according to reevaluation either by the veterinary specialists or the referring veterinarian or telephone interviews with the owner (De Risio et al., 2001). An investigation of 26 military working dogs treated with decompressive surgery was also reported. Surgeries were dissimilar and included laminectomy alone or laminectomy in combination with facetectomy, foraminotomy, diskectomy, or distraction/fusion. Six of these dogs did not return to function, 9 improved, and 11 returned to normal (Lorraine et al., 2003). Overall, dogs more severely affected neurologically before surgery tended to have a poorer prognosis. A larger study of 131 dogs diagnosed with DLSS based on clinical signs, history, and radiography had a dorsal laminectomy with or without a foraminotomy. Telephone interviews with clients reported that all dogs improved after surgery; 103 reportedly became normal, and 28 were less clinically affected (Danielsson and Sjöstrom, 1999). Dorsal laminectomy has also been reported as a possible treatment of DLSS in cats (Hurov, 1985).

Distraction and fusion of the LS joint without laminectomy has also reportedly been used to treat dogs with DLSS (Auger et al., 2000; Slocum and Devine, 1986; Watt, 1991). Fourteen dogs with suspected DLSS were evaluated clinically after distraction, and LS joint fusion was performed without laminectomy. Improvements were seen in all cases 2 months after surgery (Slocum and Devine, 1986).

OBSERVATIONS AND CONCLUSION

The reported efficacy of surgical interventions must be interpreted carefully and with knowledge of the variability in clinical diagnosis, treatment selection criteria, treatment modalities, and follow-up assessments. Scientific reports regarding treatment of DLSS have tended to be primarily retrospective studies with diagnostic standards inconsistent among investigators. Retrospective studies by nature are insufficient to evaluate most treatments since these are not randomized, blinded, or multicenter and it is difficult to eliminate bias from the results. As stated above, differences in the criteria for diagnosis are also pivotal, as inaccuracy of survey or contrast radiography for demonstrating neural compression will alter the patient entry criteria. Surgery as the standard of diagnosis is also misleading because of the difficulty in assessing the degree of compression at surgery. In addition, surgeon bias is possible as a result of the unfavorable connotation associated with negative surgical findings.

We recognize that specific surgical treatment recommendations for DLSS are poorly supported. However, we currently use a combination of decompression, distraction, and fusion. Removal of the ligamentum flavum is performed to allow exploration of the nerve roots. Proliferative tissue is excised, and the LS intervertebral foramina are explored. A partial diskectomy is also performed when possible. Distraction of the LS joint is achieved using modified Gelphi's or a lamina spreader. Once reduction of the facet joints is achieved with distraction, cortical screws are placed transarticularly in both facet joints to maintain distraction.

The imaging modalities currently used in veterinary medicine have improved the knowledge of DLSS. Important future considerations should be toward establishing universally agreed diagnostic criteria and scientifically accepted evidence for treatment efficacy. Although veterinary surgeons have described various techniques used to treat DLSS, it is unclear what extent surgery has on outcome. Prospective case-controlled studies with random allocation of treatments is needed.

References and Suggested Reading

Adams W et al: MRI of the caudal lumbar and lumbosacral spine in 13 dog, *Vet Radiol Ultrasound* 36:3, 1995.

Auger J et al: Surgical treatment of lumbosacral instability caused by diskospondylitis in four dogs, *Vet Surg* 29:70, 2000.

Barthez P, Morgan J, Lipsitz D: Discography and epidurography for evaluation of the lumbosacral junction in dogs with cauda equina syndrome, *Vet Radiol Ultrasound* 35(3):152, 1994.

Berzon JL, Dueland R: Caudal equina syndrome: pathophysiology and report of seven cases, *J Am Anim Hosp Assoc* 5: 635, 1979.

Chambers JN, Selcer BA, Oliver JE: Results of treatment of degenerative LS stenosis in dogs by exploration and excision, *Vet Comp Orthop Traumatol* 3:130, 1988.

Chambers JN: Optimal treatment for degenerative lumbosacral stenosis: surgical exploration and excision of tissue, *Vet Med Rep* 1: 248, 1989.

Chambers J et al: Diagnosis of lateralized lumbosacral disk herniation with MRI, *J Am Anim Hosp Assoc* 33:296, 1997.

Danielsson F, Sjöstrom L: Surgical treatment of degenerative lumbosacral stenosis in dogs, *Vet Surg* 28:91, 1999.

DeRisio LD, Thomas WB, Sharp NJH.: Degenerative lumbosacral stenosis, *Vet Clin North Am Small Anim Pract* 30:111, 2000.

De Risio L et al: Predictors of outcome after dorsal decompressive laminectomy for degenerative lumbosacral stenosis in dogs: 69 cases (1987-1997), *J Am Vet Med Assoc* 219:624, 2001.

Hicks DH et al: Positional magnetic resonance imaging of the lumbosacral region in dogs with degenerative lumbosacral stenosis, Proceedings of the 24th ACVIM Forum, Louisville, Ky, 2006, p 782.

Hurov L: Laminectomy for treatment of cauda equina syndrome in a cat, *J Am Vet Med Assoc* 186:504, 1985.

Janssens LAA, Moens Y: Lumbosacral degenerative stenosis in the dog, *Vet Comp Orthop Traumatol* 13:97, 2000.

Jones J, Banfield C, Ward D: Association between postoperative outcome and results of magnetic resonance imaging and computed tomography in working dogs with degenerative lumbosacral stenosis, *J Am Vet Med Assoc* 216:1769, 2000.

Jones J et al: Evaluation of canine lumbosacral stenosis using intravenous contrast-enhanced computed tomography, *Vet Radiol Ultrasound* 40:108, 1999.

Karkkainen M, Punto LU, Tulamo RM: Magnetic resonance imaging of canine degenerative lumbar spine diseases, *Vet Radiol Ultrasound* 34:399, 1993.

Lorraine LL et al: Lumbosacral stenosis in 29 military working dogs: epidemiologic findings and outcome after surgical intervention, *Vet Surg* 32:21, 2003.

Mayhew PD et al: Association of cauda equine cauda equina compression on magnetic resonance images and clinical signs in dogs with degenerative lumbosacral stenosis, *J Am Anim Hosp Assoc* 38:555, 2002.

Ness MG: Degenerative lumbosacral stenosis in the dog: a review of 30 cases, *J Small Anim Pract* 35:185, 1994.

Oliver J, Selcer R, Simpson S: Cauda equina compression from lumbosacral malarticulation and malformation in the dog, *J Am Vet Med Assoc* 978:207, 1978.

Rossi F et al: Magnetic resonance imaging of articular process joint geometry and intervertebral disk degeneration in the caudal lumbar spine of dogs with clinical signs of cauda equina compression, *Vet Radiol ultrasound* 45(5):381, 2004.

Scharf G et al: The lumbosacral junction in working German shepherd dogs—neurological and radiological evaluation, *J Vet Med* 51:27, 2004.

Schmid V, Lang J: Measurements on the lumbosacral junction in normal dogs and those with cauda equina compression, *J Small Anim Pract* 34:437, 1993.

Sharp NJH, Wheeler SJ: Lumbosacral disease. In Sharp NJH, editor: *Small animal spinal disorders: diagnosis and surgery*, ed 2, Philadelphia, 2005, Elsevier Mosby, p 181.

Shulman AJ, Lippincott CL: Canine cauda equina syndrome, *Comp Small Animal* 10:835, 1988.

Sisson A et al: Diagnosis of cauda equina abnormalities by using electromyography, discography, and epidurography in dogs, *J Vet Intern Med* 6:253, 1992.

Slocum B, Devine T: L7-S1 fixation-fusion for treatment of cauda equinae compression in the dog, *J Am Vet Med Assoc* 188:31, 1986.

Steffen FS, Berger M, Morgan JP: Asymmetrical, transitional, lumbosacral vertebral segments in six dogs: a characteristic spinal syndrome, *J Am Anim Hosp Assoc* 40:338, 2004.

Tarvin G, Prata RG: Lumbosacral stenosis in the dogs, *J Am Vet Med Assoc* 77:154, 1980.

Watt PR: Degenerative lumbosacral stenosis in 18 dogs, *J Sm Anim Pract* 32:125, 1991.

CHAPTER 239

Vestibular Disease of Dogs and Cats

RODNEY S. BAGLEY, *Pullman, Washington*

Disease of the vestibular system results in some of the most dramatic clinical presentations seen in clinical neurology. The vestibular system is largely responsible for keeping the animal oriented with respect to gravity. Therefore vestibular dysfunction is reflected in malpositioning of the body, including the head, limbs, and eyes. Falling, incoordination, head tilting, nystagmus, and ataxia result. This chapter reviews the more common disease processes affecting the vestibular system of dogs and cats.

ANATOMY

The anatomic components of the vestibular system have been reviewed (deLahunta, 1983). Simplistically, the vestibular system is made up of receptor organs within the ear. These receptor organs sense the static position and movement of the head in relation to the ground (gravity). For integration of static posture, small, weighted bodies (statconia) of the vestibular receptors (macula utriculi and sacculi) within the inner ear are acted on by gravity. Statconia lie within a gelatinous covering. Cilia from the vestibular receptor cells protrude into this gelatinous covering. The force exerted on these statconia results in deflection of the ciliated receptor, thus providing positional information that is integrated centrally.

For detection of head motion, movement of fluid (endolymph) in small tubular structures (semicircular canals) results in motion of cilia on additional receptor cells within terminal dilations (crista ampullaris). This movement of cilia excites the receptor cell that conveys this information through the vestibular nerve to the central components of the vestibular system. Thus the vestibular receptors collect information regarding the movement of the head in space.

Nerve fibers coursing from these peripheral receptors form the vestibular nerve proper. The nerve itself is relatively short. Nerve fibers can then terminate in the vestibular nuclei or within parts of the cerebellum (flocculonodular lobe) associated with vestibular functions, providing the anatomic reason that vestibular-type signs can be seen with cerebellar diseases.

CLINICAL SIGNS OF VESTIBULAR DISEASE

Clinical signs of vestibular dysfunction reflect abnormal orientation of the head, limbs, and eyes. A head tilt, nystagmus, and ataxia are common, regardless of whether the disease involves the peripheral receptors (peripheral vestibular disease) or the central nuclei, cerebellum, or projection pathways (central vestibular disease). However, the head is usually tilted in the direction of the lesion. With lesions of the caudal cerebellar peduncle, the head is often tilted away from the side of the lesion. An associated ipsilateral hemiparesis is often helpful in lesion localization as to the side of the lesion.

Nystagmus, a characteristic eye movement with a quick and slow phase, is commonly associated with vestibular dysfunction. Nystagmus can be induced normally (oculovestibular response) by turning the head from side to side. The fast phase of eye movement is in the direction that the head is moved. This slow drift and quick reset during sideways movement of the head is normal. In animals with bilateral vestibular disease, the oculovestibular response is absent. When the vestibular system is dysfunctional, the eyes have a tendency to spontaneously drift in the direction of the lesion (slow phase), and through a brainstem reset mechanism the eyes are quickly returned to their initial location (fast phase).

Abnormal nystagmus can occur spontaneously (present at rest) or with abnormal head positions (i.e., positional nystagmus). This latter nystagmus is only present when the head is placed into an abnormal orientation by the examiner. A positional nystagmus is most easily elicited by placing the animal upside down on its back. The direction of the nystagmus is described in relation to the horizontal axis through the palpebral fissure. With a horizontal nystagmus, eye movement is in the direction of this axis. A vertical nystagmus is in the direction perpendicular to this axis. With a rotatory nystagmus, the eye moves around the axis in either a clockwise or counterclockwise direction.

By convention, the direction of the nystagmus is described according to the direction of its fast phase. This can be confusing because the lesion is present on the side of the slow phase of the nystagmus. With peripheral lesions the fast phase of the nystagmus is directed away from the side of lesion. With central lesions the direction of the slow phase in relation to the side of the lesion can vary.

The vestibular system affects limb movement, normally being facilitatory to ipsilateral limb extension. A lack of vestibular input can result in ataxia or falling and rolling. The laterally recumbent animal prefers to lie on the side of the body with the lesion. The ipsilateral limb often has decreased extensor tone, with the opposite side limbs having increased extensor tone. The animal may circle, usually toward the side of the lesion. Central lesions that affect the vestibular system often involve ascending and descending motor and sensory pathways to the limb. Therefore paresis is common. Because the vestibular influence over limb function is ipsilateral, a brainstem lesion affects the limbs on the same side of the body as the lesion.

Normal vestibular control is also important for maintaining the eye in a normal position within the orbit. Vestibular information is projected through the medial longitudinal fasciculus to cranial nerves III, IV, and VI. If the vestibular input is abnormal, an abnormal eye position (strabismus) may be seen when the examiner moves the head into an aberrant position. This is most readily seen as the animal's head is extended dorsally. When viewed from above, a ventral or ventrolateral strabismus is present in the eye on the affected side. The dorsal sclera of this affected eye is more exposed than in the unaffected eye.

Vomiting and nausea are common in humans with vestibular disease and are more often associated with peripheral vestibular disease. Vomiting is also recognized in animals, more often with acute vestibular dysfunction. Nausea is difficult to assess in animals but may contribute to the anorexia often seen with acute vestibular dysfunction.

NEUROANATOMIC LOCALIZATION

Differentiation as to whether the lesion is central (within the brainstem) or peripheral (within CN VIII proper or its peripheral receptors) is important for selection of appropriate diagnostic tests (Table 239-1). The presence of certain clinical signs is associated with a central vestibular lesion. However, if these signs are not present, a central lesion cannot be excluded. A head tilt, horizontal or rotatory nystagmus, and ataxia can occur with both peripheral and central vestibular disease. A positional vertical nystagmus and limb paresis are the most consistent signs of central vestibular disease. With unilateral central vestibular lesions, hemiparesis may be seen ipsilateral to the lesion. Occasionally a hemiparesis is present on the side of the body opposite from the direction of the head tilt (paradoxical vestibular syndrome). In this situation the lesion occurs on the side of the body ipsilateral to the hemiparesis.

In dogs with bilateral peripheral vestibular abnormalities, no oculovestibular response is elicited on head movement. The animal often has a wide-based stance. The head is held closer to the ground and may be swung in wide excursions from side to side.

Once the lesion has been localized, appropriate differential diagnoses can be formulated. Unfortunately intracranial lesions occasionally result in signs indicative of a peripheral lesion. Conversely, animals with acute, severe peripheral vestibular dysfunction may be so incapacitated that accurate interpretation of neurologic examination findings may not be possible. Because of these nuances, if the examiner is unsure of location of the lesion, an evaluation for central vestibular disease should occur concurrently with an evaluation for peripheral disease.

PERIPHERAL VESTIBULAR DISEASES

Idiopathic peripheral vestibular disease occurs in both dogs and cats (Schunk, 1990). Older dogs (canine geriatric vestibular disease) and young to middle-aged cats are most commonly affected. Cats in the northeast are commonly affected in late summer and early fall. No cause is defined. In the southeast a similar syndrome is suspected to be caused in cats from eating the tail of the blue tail lizard.

Clinical signs are of an acute peripheral vestibular disorder with nystagmus (horizontal or rotary), head tilt (toward the side of the lesion), rolling, and falling. No other neurologic signs are seen. Initially clinical signs are severe. If Horner's syndrome or facial nerve paresis is also present, other differentials should be considered. Differential diagnosis of peripheral vestibular disease include otitis interna in dogs and cats, middle ear polyps in cats, and neoplasia (squamous cell carcinoma of the middle ear) in both species. Otoscopic examination, bulla radiographs, and other advanced imaging studies (computed tomography [CT], magnetic resonance imaging [MRI]) are normal.

Clinical signs of idiopathic vestibular disease usually improve dramatically in 1 to 2 weeks. The nystagmus usually resolves quickly (within the first few days). Improvements in posture and walking occur within 5 to 7 days, whereas a mild head tilt may remain persistent. Although most animals compensate well, some may have episodic ataxia when performing tasks such as jumping up on furniture. No treatment has proved beneficial, and recurrence is possible.

Otitis media/interna is a common cause of vestibular dysfunction (Kirk and Bonagura, 1995, p. 1128). Most often this is the result of a bacterial infection, from either inward extension from the external ear or migration from the pharynx via the auditory tube. Less commonly infection stems from hematogenous spread. Foreign bodies such as grass awn migration may predispose to severe ear infections.

Clinical signs may reflect primary ear, vestibular, or auditory dysfunction. A painful external ear and/or pain

Table 239-1

Differentiation of Peripheral Versus Central Vestibular Disease

Clinical Sign	Central	Peripheral
Nystagmus		
Spontaneous	Horizontal	Horizontal
	Rotatory	Rotatory
	Vertical	
Positional	*Changing*	Constant
Head tilt	Present	Present
Cranial nerve deficits	*Any other than VII*	VII
Horner's syndrome	±	±
Conscious proprioceptive abnormalities	*Present*	Absent

Italics indicate clinical signs more often associated with central disease.

on opening the mouth are often present. It has been suggested that as many as 50% of animals with otitis media/interna have associated facial nerve involvement. Otoscopic examination should be used to examine the tympanic membrane. This may be difficult in animals with severe otitis externa before cleansing. The tympanic membrane is often discolored (hyperemic), opaque, and bulging outward with middle ear disease. Clear-to-yellow fluid may be seen behind the membrane. Diagnosis may also be supported by bulla radiographs or advanced imaging studies (Remedios, Fowler, and Pharr, 1991) (Fig. 239-1). Definitive diagnosis is made through culture of the organism via a myringotomy or at surgical exploration.

Tumors of the ear more often occur in older animals. Squamous cell carcinoma and adenocarcinoma are most common. Inflammatory polyps occur in cats. Tumors that extend through the tympanic membrane may be seen during otoscopic examination (Fig. 239-2). Skull radiographs or advanced imaging is necessary to assess the middle and inner ear. However, abnormalities seen with these studies are not always definitive for neoplasia, and tissue diagnosis at surgery is often necessary for accurate assessment. Destruction (lysis) of the bone of the bulla is associated more often with neoplasia than with inflammation. Treatment options include surgical resection/debulking, radiation, and chemotherapies.

Congenital peripheral vestibular disease is seen in German shepherds, Doberman pinschers, English cocker spaniels, and Siamese and Burmese cats. Although often this is an idiopathic condition, congenital peripheral vestibular disease has been associated with lymphocytic labyrinthitis in young Doberman pinschers (Forbes and Cook, 1991). Bilateral congenital vestibular disease is

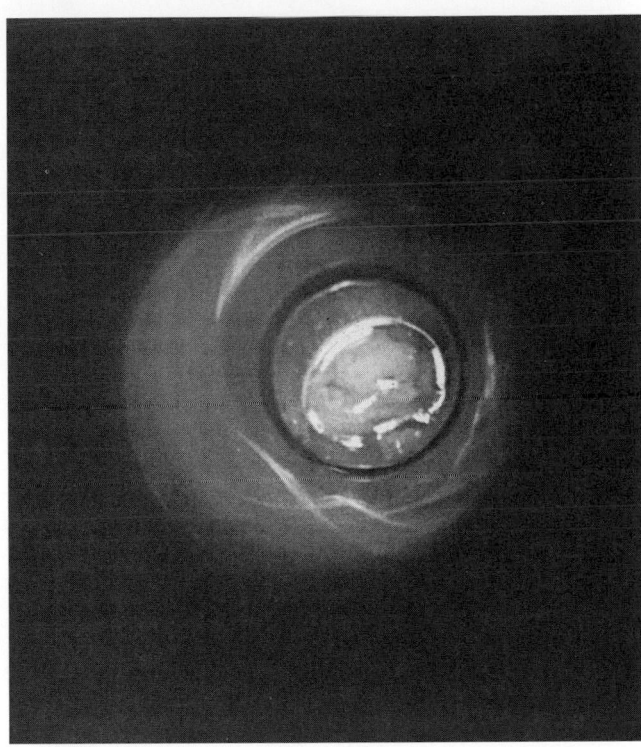

Fig. 239-2 Otoscopic view of the external ear of a dog with a head tilt. A clear fluid is overlying a mass. Histologic diagnosis was inflammatory polyp.

seen in beagles and Akitas. Clinical signs include head tilt, ataxia, and, in some, deafness. Signs may remain persistent throughout life or may improve spontaneously. There is no treatment.

Metronidazole toxicity may result in central vestibular signs in both dogs and cats (Dow et al., 1989; Saxon and Magne, 1993). Usually this is associated with high doses of the drug. However, since metronidazole is metabolized by the liver, toxic serum levels can occur with appropriate doses in animals with liver dysfunction. Ataxia is usually the initial clinical sign, progressing to nystagmus and more severe vestibular dysfunction. Clinical signs often reflect central vestibular dysfunction, and morphologic lesions have been found in the brainstem of affected dogs. Serum concentrations of metronidazole will be in the toxic range if measured soon after clinical signs begin. If there is a delay in collecting blood for drug concentrations after the initiation of clinical signs, serum concentrations of metronidazole may be decreased into the normal range even as the clinical signs remain persistent.

Diazepan is often a helpful treatment for metronidazole toxicity. Discontinuation of the drug is imperative. If clinical signs are initially severe, some dogs may die. Other dogs recover completely, usually over 1 to 2 weeks.

Aminoglycosides administered either systemically or topically may cause deafness and vestibular signs (Mansfield, 1990). Streptomycin and gentamicin have the most pronounced effects on the vestibular receptors; whereas neomycin, kanamycin, and amikacin preferentially damage auditory receptors. Chlorhexidine solution used to clean the external ear may result in vestibular abnormalities.

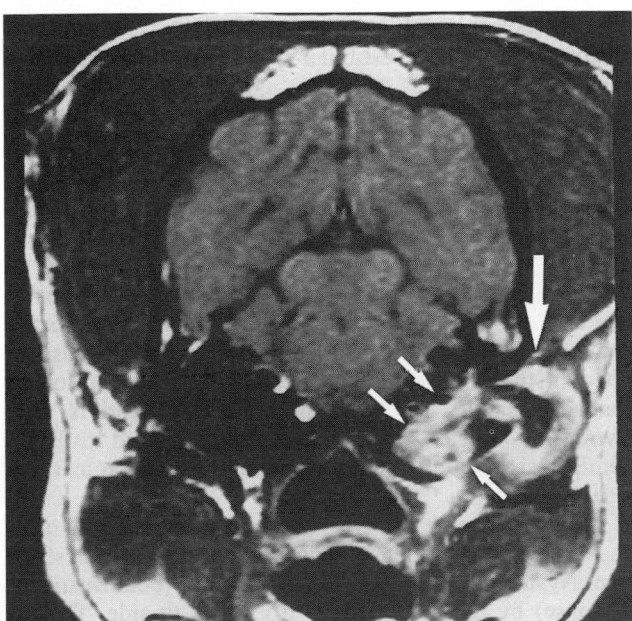

Fig. 239-1 Transaxial, contrast-enhanced T_1-weighted magnetic resonance image of a dog with otitis externa. Note the contrast enhancing lesion within the right bulla *(small arrows)*. The external ear canal is also enhanced *(large arrow)*. Histologic diagnosis was chronic infection caused by grass and foreign body migration.

Other idiopathic or inflammatory neuropathies may affect the vestibular nerve. Overall these diseases are poorly described and difficult to diagnose definitively. Similarly, a possible relationship exists between some metabolic diseases such as hypothyroidism and a vestibular neuropathy. However, a cause-and-effect relationship is not always established.

CENTRAL VESTIBULAR DISEASES

Tumors of the infratentorial space such as meningiomas and choroid plexus tumors may cause vestibular signs from infiltration or compression of the vestibular nerve (Fig. 239-3). Meningiomas may form a mass or grow in a sheetlike configuration ("en plaque"). Choroid plexus tumors arise around the fourth ventricle, often at the level of the lateral apertures. Diagnosis of an intracranial mass is made with advanced imaging studies. Lesions and associated brain structures are often better seen with MRI versus CT because beam-hardening artifact with the latter commonly obscures structural detail in this area. Surgical debulking or resection of these tumors is ideal but is often hindered by lack of surgical exposure and intimate association with vital brain structures. Radiation may provide some benefit by slowing tumor growth. However, choroid plexus tumors are relatively radiation resistant.

Thiamine deficiency is the most common nutritional deficiency affecting the central nervous system (CNS). This deficiency most often affects cats and results in lesions in the oculomotor and vestibular nuclei, the caudal colliculus, and lateral geniculate. The earliest clinical sign is vestibular ataxia, progressing to seizures with ventral neck flexion and dilated, nonresponsive pupils. Treatment is administration of thiamine, either parenterally or intravenously.

Inflammatory disease can affect the brainstem as well as other areas of the nervous system. These include both infectious and noninfectious etiologies. The incidence of infectious diseases associated with meningitis varies with geographic location. Most meningitis syndromes (60%) in small animals do not have a definable infectious cause. Infectious agents causing brain disease include viruses (distemper, parvovirus, parainfluenza, herpes, feline infectious peritonitis, pseudorabies, rabies), bacteria, rickettsia (Rocky Mountain spotted fever, *Ehrlichia*), spirochetes (Lyme disease, leptospirosis), fungi (blastomycosis, histoplasmosis, cryptococcosis, coccidioidomycosis, aspergillosis), protozoa (toxoplasmosis, neosporosis), and unclassified organisms (prototothecosis).

Specifically, the rickettsia associated with Rocky Mountain spotted fever commonly involves the brainstem, particularly the vestibular system (Greene et al., 1985). Usually there is a history of systemic illness (most often with thrombocytopenia) 5 to 10 days before development of neurologic signs. As the animal's fever is decreasing, neurologic signs appear. There is no mass lesion present on intracranial advanced imaging studies. Occasionally increased contrast enhancement is noted in the choroid plexus area in affected dogs. This must be differentiated from the degree of contrast enhancement normally seen in these structures. Cerebrospinal fluid (CSF) usually contains milder increases in nucleated cells (<50 nucleated cells/μl; normal <5 nucleated cells/μl) and milder increases in protein concentration (<50 mg/dl; normal <25 mg/dl). Diagnosis is supported by increasing serum titers to the organism, but results often are available after the disease has progressed. Prognosis depends primarily on the severity of clinical signs before treatment. Dogs that are severely obtunded before treatment are less likely to recover. Therefore dogs with clinical features of vestibular disease after a systemic febrile illness associated with thrombocytopenia should be treated with tetracycline or doxycycline before establishing a definitive diagnosis with titers.

Brainstem trauma usually occurs secondary to being hit by a car. Brainstem function can be assessed by evaluation of cranial nerve function, particularly the oculovestibular response. Occasionally dogs have brainstem signs with cranial cervical lesions; therefore manipulation for the oculovestibular response should be made only after assessing for unstable cervical fracture or luxations. An otoscopic examination also may reveal hemorrhage in the ear canals.

Diagnosis is supported by a history of a witnessed traumatic event. Skull fractures may be seen with skull radiography. Advanced imaging studies are used to assess for

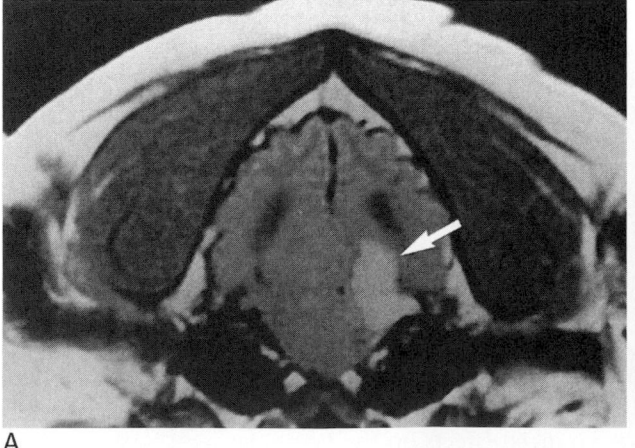
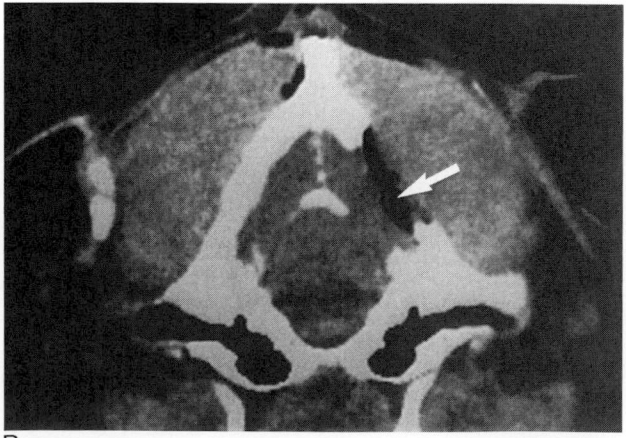

A   B

Fig. 239-3   Preoperative, T_1-weighted contrast-enhanced magnetic resonance image **(A)** of a dog with a right head tilt. There is a contrast-enhancing mass in the right cerebellopontine angle *(arrow)*. **B,** Postoperative, contrast-enhanced computed tomography image (3B) at approximately the same level showing resection of the mass *(arrow)*. Histologic diagnosis was a meningioma.

intracranial hemorrhage and edema. With acute trauma (within the first 12 hours), CT may be better at delineating intracranial hemorrhage. Treatment centers around recognizing and treating the pathophysiologic sequelae to brain trauma such as brain edema. Occasionally surgical removal of debris or hemorrhage is necessary to stabilize intracranial pressure.

Vascular diseases that involve the central vestibular areas and associated cerebellum are uncommon. However, with the advent of advanced imaging studies, antemortem diagnosis should be improved.

DIAGNOSTIC TESTING

If a lesion is suspected to involve the central vestibular structures (forebrain, brainstem, or cerebellum) in small animals, an advanced imaging study such as CT or MRI is used to assess the structural integrity of these areas. These studies are noninvasive but do require anesthesia in all but the comatose animal. Survey radiographs of the skull are useful in instances of skull fracture or middle ear (bulla) disease; however, they do not allow for assessment of nervous system parenchyma. If peripheral disease is suspected, a thorough otoscopic examination, preferably while the animal is anesthetized, is mandatory.

CSF analysis is helpful primarily to determine the presence of inflammatory diseases. In general, collection of spinal fluid caudal to the level of the lesion is most accurate for diagnosis. Fluid is analyzed for cellularity, protein content, and cell morphology. Although CSF analysis is often helpful in determining the presence of nervous system disease, used alone it does not often lead toward a specific etiologic diagnosis. Titers to specific infectious agents can be measured in CSF to assess for intrathecal production of antibody. However, in the presence of blood-brain barrier breakdown, antibodies may nonspecifically cross into the CSF from the systemic circulation. In this instance correlation of the CSF to serum titer may be necessary. An increased antibody titer in the CSF relative to the serum antibody titer suggests local production of antibodies within the CNS, suggestive of actual CNS infection. Protein electrophoresis on CSF can give additional information concerning integrity of the blood-brain barrier and local production of immunoglobulins.

Recording the brainstem auditory potential (BAEP or BAER) may be helpful in determining the presence of intact hearing pathways and may also provide some information about the integrity of central (brainstem) projection pathways associated with hearing (Steiss, Cox, and Hathcock, 1994; Fischer and Obermaier, 1994).

Surgical biopsy is often necessary for definitive antemortem diagnosis of structural intracranial disease. This is more difficult in the infratentorial space because surgical exposure, especially of ventrally located lesions, is often incomplete. Surgical exposure of lesions at the cerebellopontine angle area may be increased by occlusion of the overlying transverse sinus. The limited access to this area often hinders complete lesion resection.

For lesions of the ear canal and bulla, lateral ear canal resection and bulla osteotomy, respectively or in combination, are useful for biopsy, lesion resection, and drainage of infected tissue. If these procedures are performed for ear exploration in animals without vestibular signs, head tilts, ataxia, and nystagmus may result from damage of the vestibular structures during the surgical procedure itself.

TREATMENT

Specific treatments can best be recommended after a definitive diagnosis is made. If intracranial tumors are diagnosed, specific treatments such as surgical debulking/resection and radiation therapy may be helpful. With primary inflammatory diseases the etiologic organism should be determined, if possible, and specific treatments directed toward killing the organism. With Rocky Mountain spotted fever, tetracycline and doxycycline can eliminate the vestibular signs (Kirk and Bonagura, 1995, p. 293). With toxoplasmosis a combination of clindamycin and trimethoprim/sulfadiazine often improves or eliminates clinical signs. Noninfectious, inflammatory CNS disease will be responsive to corticosteroids initially. Granulomatous meningoencephalitis has also been treated with radiation.

Nonspecific treatments include protecting the eyes from damage, especially if there is an associated facial nerve deficit or if the animal is lateral recumbent and rolling into the ground. Antihistamines (Kirk and Bonagura, 1995, p. 48) such as diphenhydramine (1 to 2 mg/kg PO or IV every 12 to 24 hours) have been useful in decreasing anxiety, anorexia, and in some instances the severity of the associated head tilt and nystagmus.

References and Suggested Reading

deLahunta A: *Veterinary neuroanatomy and clinical neurology,* ed 2, Philadelphia, 1983, Saunders.

Dow SW et al: Central nervous system toxicosis associated with metronidazole treatment of dogs: five cases (1984-1987), *J Am Vet Med Assoc* 3:365, 1989.

Fischer A, Obermaier G: Brainstem auditory-evoked potentials and neuropathologic correlates in 26 dogs with brain tumor, *J Vet Intern Med* 8:363, 1994.

Forbes S, Cook JR Jr: Congenital peripheral vestibular disease attributed to lymphocytic labyrinthitis in two related litters of Doberman pinscher pups, *J Am Vet Med Assoc* 198:447, 1991.

Greene CE et al: Rocky Mountain spotted fever in dogs and its differentiation from canine ehrlichiosis, *J Am Vet Med Assoc* 186:465, 1985.

Kirk RW, Bonagura JD, editors: *Kirk's current veterinary therapy XII (small animal practice),* ed XII, Philadelphia, 1995, Saunders.

Mansfield PD: Ototoxicity in dogs and cats, *Compend Contin Educ* 12:331, 1990.

Remedios AM, Fowler JD, Pharr JW: A comparison of radiographic versus surgical diagnosis of otitis media, *J Am Anim Hosp Assoc* 27:183, 1991.

Saxon B, Magne ML: Reversible central nervous system toxicosis associated with metronidazole therapy in three cats, *Prog Vet Neurol* 4:25, 1993.

Schunk KL: Disease of the vestibular system, *Prog Vet Neurol* 1:247, 1990.

Steiss JE, Cox NR, Hathcock JT: Brain stem auditory-evoked response abnormalities in 14 dogs with confirmed central nervous system lesions, *J Vet Intern Med* 8:293, 1994.

CHAPTER 240

Treatment of Canine Chiari-Like Malformation and Syringomyelia

CLARE RUSBRIDGE, *London, England*
CURTIS W. DEWEY, *Ithaca, New York*

Chiari-like malformation (CM) is a condition characterized by a mismatch between the caudal fossa (skull) volume and its contents, the cerebellum and brainstem. The neural structures are displaced into the foramen magnum, obstructing cerebrospinal fluid (CSF) movement. A consequence of this is syringomyelia (SM) in which fluid-filled cavities develop within the spinal cord (Fig. 240-1). The primary clinical sign of CM/SM is pain, caused either by obstruction of the CSF pulse pressure and/or a neuropathic pain syndrome resulting from damage to the spinal cord dorsal horn. This disease has also been referred to as *occipital hypoplasia* and *caudal occipital malformation syndrome* (COMS) (Dewey et al., 2005). CM/SM is sometimes erroneously confused with *Arnold Chiari malformation* (cerebellar and medulla herniation associated with myelomeningocele) and *occipital dysplasia* (incomplete ossification of the supraoccipital bone).

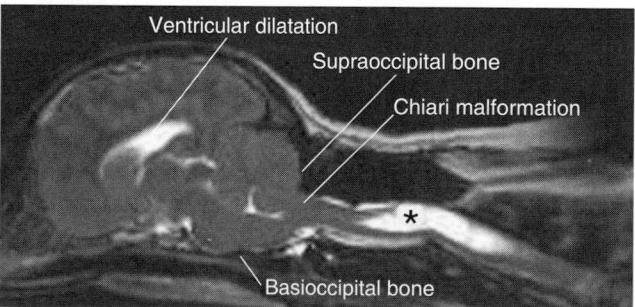

Fig. 240-1 Midsagittal T2-weighted MRI of the brain and upper cervical spinal cord from a 3-year-old female CKCS with syringomyelia *(asterisks)* that first developed signs of pain at 1.7 years old. Clinical signs included shoulder scratching at exercise and when excited. She would not tolerate her right ear to shoulder area to be touched or groomed. She frequently screamed, and she became distressed whenever her owners tried to exercise her. She also had a mild pelvic limb weakness. She was managed with a foramen magnum decompression and despite persistence of the syrinx made a satisfactory postoperative recovery that was maintained for 1.8 years. Following this deterioration she was managed medically for a further 3.8 years and currently is 7 years old.

PATHOGENESIS

The pathogenesis of canine CM/SM is not fully understood. An important contributory factor is thought to be an inadequate small caudal fossa volume that early observations suggested is caused by a relatively short basioccipital bone (i.e., an inappropriately short skull base) (see Fig. 240-1). However, it is likely there are other unidentified anatomic or environmental factors. Studies comparing intracranial dimensions did not demonstrate a significant difference between the size of the caudal fossa in cavalier King Charles spaniels (CKCSs) with and without SM (Carruthers et al., 2006; Cerda-Gonzalez, Olby, and Pease, 2006).

The precise pathogenetic mechanism of development of SM is much debated (reviewed by Rusbridge, Greitz, and Iskandar, 2006; Greitz, 2006), although there is increasing agreement that the syrinx fluid is not CSF but most likely extracellular fluid that accumulates within the central canal or spinal cord substance as a consequence of abnormal pressure differentials between the spinal cord and subarachnoid space (Levine, 2004; Greitz, 2006). Early proposals for the pathogenesis of SM such as the *water-hammer* and *suck effect* theory now seem unlikely because these rely on the presence of a connection between the fourth ventricle and central canal in addition to a lower pressure system within the syrinx relative to the ventricle and subarachnoid space. The *intramedullary pulse pressure* theory of SM postulates that the obstruction of CSF flow results in relative increase in intrathecal pressure and decrease in subarachnoid pressure, the consequence of which is repeated mechanical distention of the spinal cord. This in turn results in dilation of the central canal and accumulation of extracellular fluid, which eventually coalesces into cavities (Fig. 240-2).

Incidence

The CKCS is overwhelmingly overrepresented for cases of CM/SM. An estimated 95% of the population have CM, and as many as 50% have CM/SM, with the proportion of affected dogs increasing with age. There is no color or sex predisposition. Since a shortened skull is a risk factor, any breed with a degree of brachycephalism

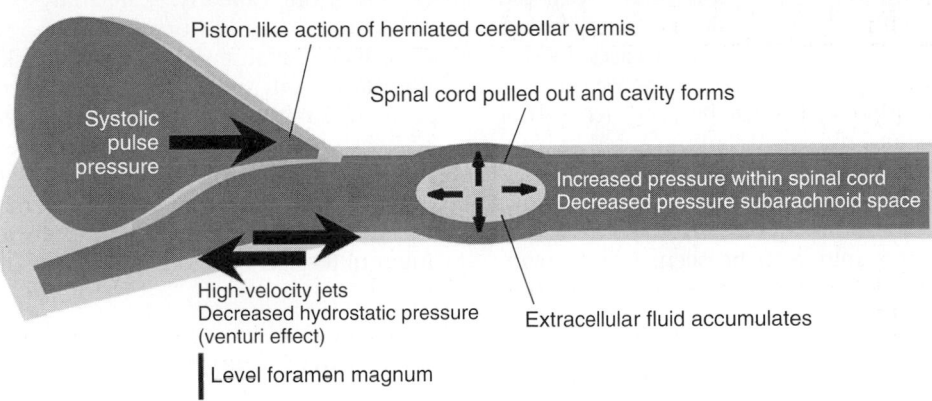

Piston-like action of herniated cerebellar vermis

Spinal cord pulled out and cavity forms

Systolic pulse pressure

Increased pressure within spinal cord
Decreased pressure subarachnoid space

High-velocity jets
Decreased hydrostatic pressure
(venturi effect)

Extracellular fluid accumulates

Level foramen magnum

Fig. 240-2 The intramedullary pulse pressure theory of syringomyelia. Chiari malformation and obstruction of the foramen magnum prevent transmission of the systolic CSF pulse pressure wave to the distal CSF spaces. The pulse pressure is instead transmitted and reflected into the spinal cord tissues, resulting in a relative increase in intrathecal pressure and decrease in subarachnoid pressure. In addition, because of the partial obstruction, the CSF displaced by each systole is forced through the narrower opening, resulting in high-velocity jets of CSF ventrally within the foramen magnum. These high-velocity jets decrease the hydrostatic pressure in the subarachnoid space (Venturi effect / Bernoulli theorem). The changes in pressure have a "suction effect" on the spinal cord. Repeated spinal cord distention results in extracellular fluid accumulation and eventually syringomyelia.

and/or miniaturization could potentially be predisposed to CM/SM. To date the condition has been also reported in King Charles spaniels, Brussels griffons, Yorkshire terriers, Maltese terriers, Chihuahuas, miniature dachshunds, miniature/toy poodles, bichon frise, pugs, Shih Tzus, Pomeranians, Staffordshire bull terriers, a Boston terrier, French bulldogs, a Pekingese, and a miniature pinscher. Recent studies suggest that 35% of SM-affected dogs have clinical signs of the condition. The youngest reported dogs with SM have been 12 weeks old. Dogs may be presented at any age, although the majority of dogs (approximately 45%) develop first signs of the disease within the first year of life and approximately 40% of cases have first signs between 1 and 4 years old. As many as 15% develop signs as mature dogs, with the oldest reported case first developing signs of disease at age 6.8 years. Because of the vague nature of signs in some cases and lack of awareness about the disease, there is often a considerable time period (mean 1.6 years) between the onset of signs and confirmation of a diagnosis.

Clinical Signs

The most important and consistent clinical sign of CM/SM is pain; however, this may be difficult to localize on clinical examination and, because it is often intermittent, may be dismissed by owners or veterinarians. Therefore historical signs of pain should be considered seriously in predisposed breeds. Owners may describe postural pain; for example, affected dogs may suddenly scream and/or lie with the head on the ground between the paws after jumping up or during excitement. It is also common to sleep with the head in unusual positions (e.g., elevated). Discomfort often appears worse in the evening and early morning or when the dog is excited and can be associated with defecation or may vary with weather conditions. Some of the signs of SM such as posture-related pain could be explained by obstruction to CSF flow, but

SM also results in a neuropathic pain syndrome probably caused by damage to the spinal cord dorsal horn. Affected dogs behave as if they experience allodynia (i.e., pain arising in response to a nonnoxious stimulus); for example, they appear to dislike touch to certain areas of the skin (ear, neck, forelimb, or sternum) and may be unable to tolerate grooming or a neck collar. Pain is positively correlated with syrinx width (Fig. 240-3); that is, dogs with a wider syrinx are more likely to experience discomfort, and dogs with a narrow syrinx may be asymptomatic, especially if the syrinx is symmetric and not deviated into the dorsal horn. A dog with a wide syrinx may also scratch, typically on one side only, while it is walking and often without making skin contact; such behavior is often referred to as an *air guitar* or *phantom* scratching. This sign is highly suggestive of dysesthesia (i.e., a spontaneous or evoked unpleasant abnormal sensation). Humans with SM-associated dysesthesia describe painful, burning itching and/or an intense sensation suggesting insects crawling on the skin.

Dogs with a wide syrinx are also more likely to have scoliosis. This is likely to relate to damage to the dorsal grey column and a unilateral loss of proprioceptive information.

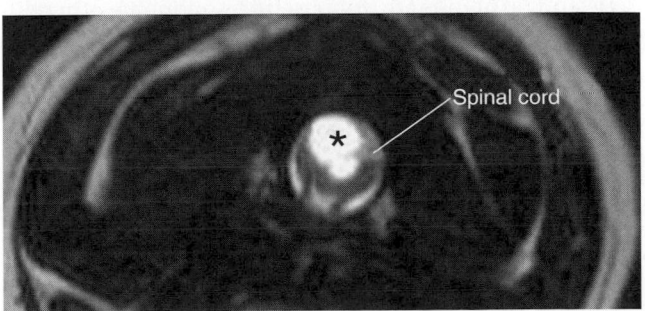

Spinal cord

Fig. 240-3 T2-weighted transverse image through a wide syrinx *(asterisk)* demonstrating the asymmetric involvement of the right dorsal horn.

Scoliosis is more common in dogs less than 1 year old and may be the first clinical signs of SM, appearing before signs of neuropathic pain develop. In many cases the scoliosis slowly resolves despite persistence of the syrinx.

SM may result in other neurologic deficits such as thoracic limb weakness and muscle atrophy (caused by ventral horn cell damage) and pelvic limb ataxia and weakness (caused by white matter damage or involvement of the lumbar spinal cord by the syrinx). Seizures, facial nerve paralysis, and deafness may also be seen; however, no direct relationship has been proven, and this association may be circumstantial.

CM alone appears to cause facial pain in some dogs, with owners describing ear and facial rubbing/scratching. It has been proposed that CM and direct compression of the medulla can result in a disorder of sensory processing and a pain syndrome (Thimineur et al., 2002). In this circumstance it can be difficult to be certain that the CM, as apposed to ear, oral or skin disease, is the cause of the distress, especially since CM is a common incidental finding in the CKCS breed.

Clinical Course

Progression of disease is variable. Some dogs remain stable or deteriorate minimally over years. Other affected dogs can be severely disabled by pain and neurologic deficits within 6 months of the first observed signs.

Diagnosis

Magnetic resonance imaging (MRI) is essential for diagnosis and determining the cause of SM (see Fig. 240-1). With CM/SM the cerebellum and medulla extend into or through the foramen magnum, which is occluded with little or no CSF around the neural structures. The size of the cerebellar herniation is not correlated with severity. Typically there is ventricular dilation. SM is indicated by fluid-containing cavities within the spinal cord. The upper cervical and thoracic segments typically are most severely affected. The shape of the cavity may be complex with septation (i.e., haustra) and generally involves a portion of the central canal at some level. Maximum syrinx width is the strongest predictor of pain, scratching behavior, and scoliosis; 95% of CKCSs with a maximum syrinx width of 0.64 cm or more will have associated clinical signs.

Laboratory tests such as hematology, serum biochemistry, and urinalysis are only useful to eliminate other differentials or to establish that there is no reason to preclude surgical or medical management. Radiographs have limited value. In severe cases cervical images may suggest widening of the vertebral canal, especially in the C2 region, and/or scoliosis. Flexed and extended images of the neck can be used to rule out vertebral abnormalities such as atlantoaxial subluxation and to indicate the likelihood of intervertebral disk disease. Ultrasonography through the cisterna magnum may confirm cerebellar vermis herniation; however, since CM is so common in the CKCS, this information has limited value. Likewise a syrinx may be identified if within the cranial cervical segment; however, failure to detect a syrinx does not eliminate the possibility

of one more caudally. CSF analysis may be useful to rule out inflammatory diseases. Sampling requires experience because there is a high risk of inaccurate needle placement. Myelography is contraindicated for the same reason. CM/SM does not appear to increase risk of anesthesia. Preliminary data suggest that asymmetric brainstem auditory evoked-response (BAER) test results are predictive of the presence of CM in mature CKCSs; whether or not this test will have wide use as a screening tool for early diagnosis of the disorder is unknown at this time.

Differential Diagnosis

The most important differential diagnoses are other causes of pain and spinal cord dysfunction such as intervertebral disk disease, CNS inflammatory diseases such as granulomatous meningoencephalomyelitis, vertebral abnormities such as atlantoaxial subluxation, neoplasia, and diskospondylitis. When scratching or facial/ear rubbing is the predominant clinical sign, ear and skin disease should be ruled out. The scratching behavior for SM is classically to one distinct area. It is a common *incidental* finding for CKCSs to have a mucoid material in one or both tympanic bullae, and in most cases this is not associated with clinical signs. Some dogs with scoliosis appear to have a head tilt, which could be confused with vestibular dysfunction. If in doubt, cervical radiographs can confirm scoliosis.

Treatment and Prognosis

The main treatment objective is pain relief. The most common surgical management is cranial cervical decompression (also described as foramen magnum or suboccipital decompression) establishing a CSF pathway via the removal of part of the supraoccipital bone and dorsal arch of C1 (Fig. 240-4). This may be combined with a durotomy (incision of the dura with or without incision of subarachnoid meninges) with or without patching with a suitable graft material such as biocompatible collagen matrix (Vet BioSIST, Cook/Global Veterinary Products). Cranial cervical decompression surgery is successful in reducing pain and improving neurologic deficits in approximately 80% of cases, and approximately 45% of cases may still have a satisfactory quality of life 2 years after surgery (Rusbridge, 2007). However, surgery may not adequately address the factors leading to SM, and the syrinx appears persistent. The clinical improvement is probably attributable to improvement in CSF flow through the foramen magnum. In some cases scarring and fibrous tissue adhesions over the foramen magnum seem to result in reobstruction, and as many as 50% of cases can eventually deteriorate (Rusbridge, 2007). This can be as early as 2 months after surgery. Recently a cranioplasty procedure used in human cranial cervical decompression surgery to decrease the incidence of postoperative compressive scar tissue formation has been adapted for use in dogs. The procedure entails placement of a plate constructed of titanium mesh and polymethylmethacrylate on preplaced titanium screws bordering the occipital bone defect (Fig. 240-5). Although results are preliminary (based on

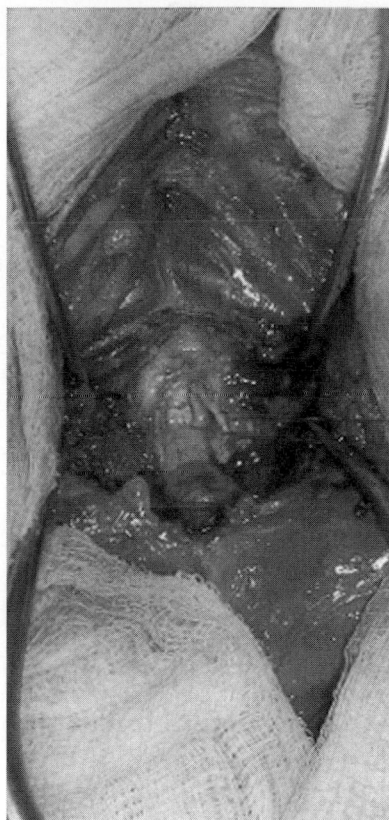

Fig. 240-4   Cranial cervical decompression. The dura and arachnoid meninges have been incised and are supported by a stay suture. The spinal cord and the cerebellar vermis can be visualized though the meningeal defect. The dog's head is at the top of the picture.

21 dogs to date), the procedure is well tolerated and may have decreased the need for reoperation because of excessive postoperative scar tissue formation (Dewey et al., 2006). An alternative method of managing SM is direct shunting of the cavity. In humans this is not a preferred technique for management of CM/SM because long-term outcome is poor as a result of shunt obstruction and/or spinal cord tethering. However, the short-term results are reasonable, with syrinx collapse occurring in a majority of human cases. There has been a single report of syringosubarachnoid shunting in a dog using an equine ocular lavage tube (Cook/Global Veterinary Products). However, postoperative MRI revealed that SM was still prominent although there was a clinical improvement in the dog (Skerritt and Hughes, 1998).

Because of the persistence of SM and/or spinal cord dorsal horn damage, it is likely that the postoperative patient will also require continuing medical management for pain relief; in some patients medical management alone is chosen because of financial reasons or owner preference. Three main drug categories are used for treatment of CM/SM: drugs that reduce CSF production; analgesics; and corticosteroids (Fig. 240-6). If the dog's history suggests postural pain or discomfort relating to obstruction of CSF flow, a trial of a drug that reduces CSF pressure (e.g., furosemide, cimetidine, or omeprazole) is appropriate. These drugs also can be useful when it is difficult to determine if the cause of discomfort is CM versus, for example, ear disease. CSF pressure–reducing drugs may be sufficient to control signs in some dogs, but additional analgesics are likely to be necessary for an individual with a wide syrinx. In this circumstance we suggest that nonsteroidal antiinflammatory drugs are the medication of first choice partly because there are several licensed products. However, for dogs with signs of neuropathic pain (i.e., allodynia and scratching behavior [suspected dysesthesia]), a drug that is active in the dorsal horn is more likely to be effective. Because gabapentin has established use in veterinary medicine, we suggest that this is the drug of first choice, but amitriptyline or pregabalin may also be suitable. Corticosteroids are an option if pain persists or when available finances prohibit the use of other drugs. Because the mechanisms of development of neuropathic pain are multifactorial, appropriate polypharmacy is likely to be more effective than treatment with

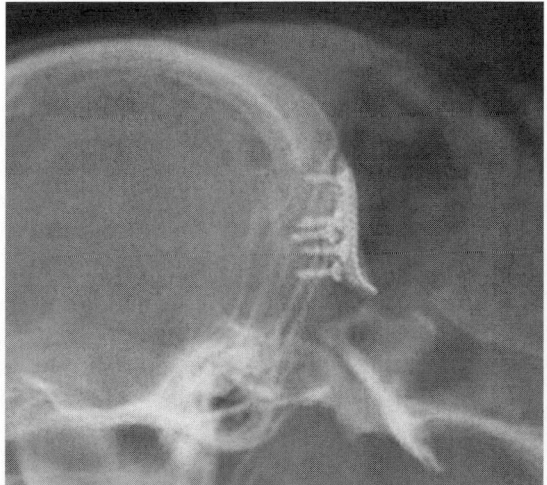
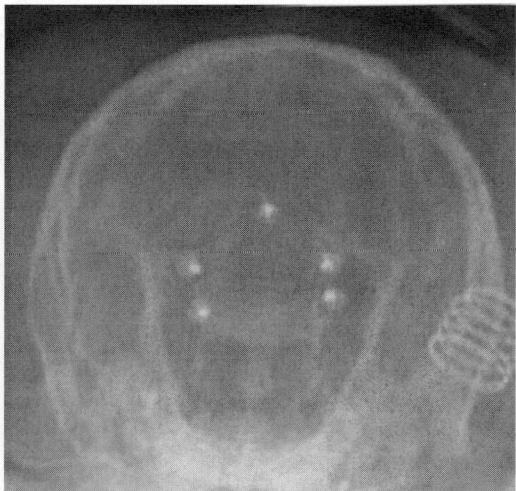

Fig. 240-5   Postoperative images following cranioplasty demonstrating surgical placement of a titanium mesh/polymethylacrylate plate on preplaced titanium screws at the border of the occipital bone defect.

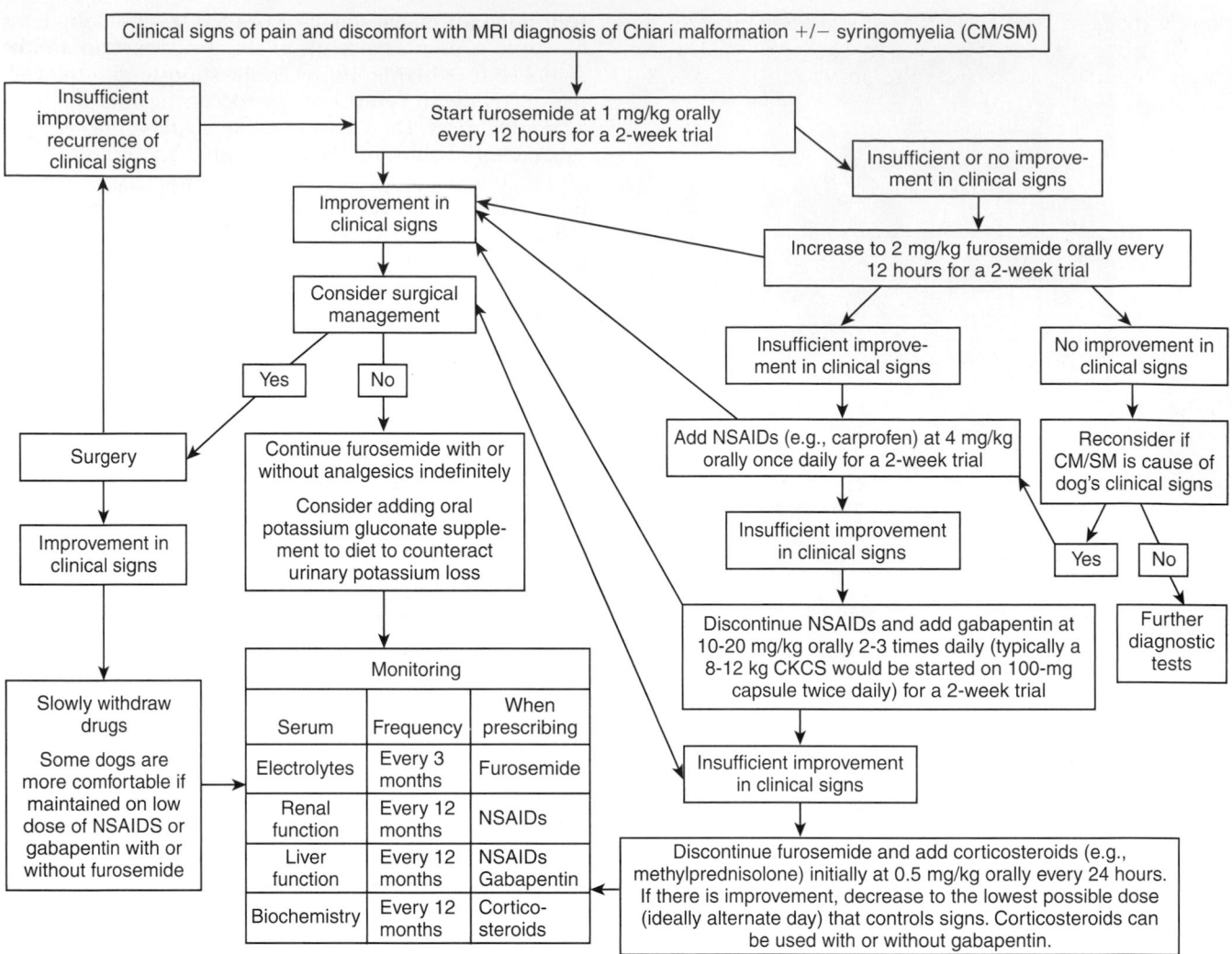

Fig. 240-6 Treatment algorithm for the management of Chiari malformation with or without syringomyelia in the dog. (From Rusbridge C et al: Current concepts in pathogenesis, diagnosis, and treatment, *J Vet Intern Med* 20:469, 2006.)

single agents. Anecdotally acupuncture and alphasonic treatments have been reported to be useful adjunctive therapy in some cases. The dog's activity need not be restricted, but the owner should understand that the dog may avoid some activities and grooming may not be tolerated. Simple actions (e.g., raising the food bowl and removing neck collars) can also help.

Prognosis for CM/SM managed medically is guarded, especially for dogs with a wide syrinx or with first clinical signs before 4 years of age. Study of a small case series (14 CKCSs) managed conservatively for neuropathic pain suggested that 36% were eventually euthanatized as a consequence of uncontrolled pain. However, 43% of the group survived to be older than 9 years of age (average life expectancy for a CKCS is 10.7 years). Most dogs retain the ability to walk, although some may be significantly tetraparetic and ataxic.

Genetics and Breeding Recommendations

CM/SM in the CKCS can be traced back to two United Kingdom bitches from the post–World War II era, which were foundational dogs for the modern breed "created"

from the shorter-nosed King Charles spaniel. A CKCS genome scan is currently underway with the hope of identifying the causal genes. The mode of inheritance, including the number, identity, and relative contribution of the causative genes, is not yet determined; however, preliminary results from the genome have suggested some interesting regions that warrant further investigation. However, because of the ubiquity of the condition within the CKCS breed, this is a complex task, and focus is now centering on comparison with sporadic cases in other breeds. The etiology of both conditions could be further complicated by variable penetrance of the various genotypes and the involvement of environmental factors. Current breeding recommendations for CKCSs concentrate on removal of dogs with early-onset SM (i.e., within the first 2.5 years of life) from the breeding pool (for precise recommendations and grading system). This involves MRI screening of potential breeding stock and therefore is a costly process. The aim of current breeding recommendations is to limit the number of severely affected dogs rather than eliminate the disease from the CKCS population. Because of the number of affected dogs, there is a danger that very restrictive breeding practices will further narrow the gene pool and other diseases will emerge. It should also be borne in mind that absence of SM in a young dog does not exclude the possibility that it will develop with time.

References and Further Reading

Carruthers H et al: Association between cervical and intracranial dimensions and SM in the cavalier King Charles spaniel. In Rusbridge C: *Chiari-like malformation and syringomyelia in the cavalier King Charles spaniel,* 82, 2006.

Cerda-Gonzalez S, Olby NJ, Pease TP: Morphology of the caudal fossa in cavalier King Charles spaniels, *J Vet Intern Med* 20: 736, 2006.

Dewey CW et al: Foramen magnum decompression for treatment of caudal occipital malformation syndrome in dogs, *J Am Vet Med Assoc* 227:1270, 2005.

Dewey CW et al: Foramen magnum decompression with cranioplasty for treatment of caudal occipital malformation syndrome in dogs, *J Vet Intern Med* 20:783, 2006.

Greitz D: Unravelling the riddle of syringomyelia, *Neurosurg Rev* 29:251, 2006.

Levine DN: The pathogenesis of syringomyelia associated with lesions at the foramen magnum: a critical review of existing theories and proposal of a new hypothesis, *J Neurol Sci* 220:3, 2004.

Lillington K: http://www.cavaliertalk.com/SM.

Rusbridge C: Chiari-like malformation with syringomyelia in the cavalier King Charles spaniel: long-term follow up after surgical management, *Vet Surg* 36:396, 2007.

Rusbridge C, Greitz D, Iskandar BJ: Syringomyelia: current concepts in pathogenesis, diagnosis, and treatment, *J Vet Intern Med* 20:469, 2006.

Rusbridge C, Jeffery NJ: Pathophysiology and treatment of neuropathic pain associated with syringomyelia, *Vet J* 175:164, 2008.

Rusbridge C, Knowler SP: Inheritance of occipital bone hypoplasia (Chiari type I malformation) in cavalier King Charles spaniels, *J Vet Intern Med* 18:673, 2004.

Skerritt GC, Hughes D: A syndrome of syringomyelia in the cavalier King Charles spaniel and its treatment by syringo-subarachnoid shunting. In Proceedings from the 12th Annual Symposium of the European Society of Veterinary Neurology, Vienna, 1998, p 23.

Smith SR: *For the love of ollie,* a story of compassion and courage, Trimatrix Management Consulting Inc, 2047 Pen Street, Oakville, Ontario, Canada, available though http://www.fortheloveoffollie.com, 2006.

Thimineur M et al: Functional abnormalities of the cervical cord and lower medulla and their effect on pain: observations in chronic pain patients with incidental mild Chiari I malformation and moderate to severe cervical cord compression, *Clin J Pain* 18:171, 2002.

CHAPTER 241

Treatment of Autoimmune Myasthenia Gravis

G. DIANE SHELTON, *La Jolla, California*

The name *myasthenia gravis* (MG) was originally given to a human disease that was frequently fatal. As recently as 30 years ago, 25% of patients died of this disease. Canine MG has also been associated with a high death rate and, in many older textbooks of veterinary medicine, a poor prognosis for recovery. We now know that, with early recognition of the disease, a correct diagnosis, and appropriate treatment, the prognosis for a relatively normal quality of life and life span is favorable in both human and canine MG.

Canine MG is the most common neuromuscular disease diagnosed in my laboratory. Feline autoimmune MG occurs much less frequently but has a higher incidence of a cranial mediastinal mass (25.7%) than canine MG (3.4%). The spectrum of clinical presentations in both species is broad and variable; thus autoimmune MG should be high on the list of differential diagnoses for any dog or cat presenting with focal or generalized neuromuscular weakness, megaesophagus, or dysphagia. In-depth discussions of the diversity of clinical presentations in canine and feline MG are in the literature (Shelton and Lindstrom, 2001; Dewey 1997; Shelton, Schule, and Kass, 1997; Shelton, Ho, and Kass, 2000; Shelton, 2002).

The onset of clinical signs commonly is acute in nature, occurring only a few days to a few weeks before presentation. Ideally a serum sample should be collected for acetylcholine receptor (AChR) antibody testing, and the diagnosis confirmed before initiation of therapy. The gold standard for the diagnosis of autoimmune MG continues to be the demonstration of autoantibodies against muscle AChRs by immunoprecipitation radioimmunoassay. The assay is specific and sensitive and documents an autoimmune response against muscle AChRs. Although seronegative MG occurs in approximately 2% of dogs with generalized MG, false-positive results are rare. The edrophonium chloride challenge (Tensilon, Enlon, 0.1 to 0.2 mg/kg in dogs and 0.25 to 0.5 mg/kg in cats intravenously) should also be performed since a dramatic positive test would give a presumptive diagnosis of MG and allow initiation of therapy before serologic confirmation. A negative edrophonium chloride challenge should not eliminate a diagnosis of MG. In addition, a subjective improvement in muscle strength may be found with other neuromuscular diseases; thus, unless the response is dramatic, the edrophonium chloride challenge test should not be used alone to confirm a diagnosis. Because of the propensity of dogs with MG to develop aspiration pneumonia, autoimmune MG is one disease in which a delay in obtaining a diagnosis or assuming the wrong diagnosis can result in a fatal outcome.

No single treatment regimen is ideal for all cases of MG. Choices must be made among the therapeutic options, with the goal of obtaining the best result while keeping the risks and side effects as low as possible. Each case needs an individual treatment plan, which may have to be changed from time to time as determined by the stage of the disease and response to treatments. For discussion of available treatments, autoimmune MG will be divided into focal (group 1), generalized (group 2), acute fulminating (group 3), and paraneoplastic (group 4) forms. Unlike human MG in which treatments are usually life-long, dogs with MG routinely go into spontaneous remission, if they survive the initial month following onset of clinical signs and do not have a thymoma (Shelton and Lindstrom, 2001).

SUPPORTIVE CARE

General supportive care and dedicated owners are integral parts of treatment for all groups of MG patients. The owners should be advised that treatment for MG may be for as short as a few months or need to be continued for several months to a couple of years, depending on the severity of disease. Differentiation of vomiting from regurgitation and recognition of esophageal dilation or pharyngeal weakness are critical. As in any dog with esophageal dilation, altered feeding procedures, including elevation of food and water or placement of a gastrostomy tube, should be used to facilitate adequate hydration, nutrition, and drug delivery. If there is a delay in recognition of megaesophagus, inadequate nutrition and poor hydration may occur, which could worsen the clinical status of the animal. Nutritional support can be expected to decrease morbidity and improve immune status. Aspiration pneumonia should be treated aggressively (see Chapter 149). In cases of acute fulminating MG, referral of patients to centers with intensive care facilities is optimal.

Cholinesterase Inhibitors

Cholinesterase inhibitors are the cornerstone of treatment for MG and are advised for all patient groups. These drugs result in improved muscle strength by decreasing the hydrolysis of acetylcholine (ACh) at the neuromuscular junction. This allows for a greater number of ACh molecules to bind to and activate AChRs on the postsynaptic membrane, prolongs the action of ACh, and enhances neuromuscular transmission. Cholinesterase inhibitors do not treat the underlying aberrant immune response and thus do not modify the course of the disease, but they do control the clinical signs. In the case of canine nonthymomatous MG, this is not a problem, since the natural course of disease is to go into remission in the absence of immunosuppression. If an optimal response to therapy is obtained and there is return of normal limb muscle strength and decreased or resolved regurgitation, supportive care and management of megaesophagus, anticholinestersase drugs, and time may be all that is required.

Pyridostigmine bromide (Mestinon, 1 to 3 mg/kg PO q8-12h) and neostigmine bromide (Prostigmin, 2 mg/kg/day administered orally in divided doses to effect) are the most commonly used cholinesterase inhibitors; the former is preferred in most clinical situations because of its longer duration of action and fewer cholinergic side effects. The dosage must be adjusted individually for each animal, depending on the response to the drug and tolerance of the side effects. Pyridostigmine bromide is available in syrup, tablet, and time-released forms. The syrup form may be optimal for dosing in smaller breeds of dogs but should be diluted 50:50 in water before use because gastric irritation may result if it is given straight. For critical animals in which oral dosing is not possible, constant rate infusion of pyridostigmine bromide (0.01 to 0.03 mg/kg/hour) may be used until oral feedings are resumed or a feeding tube is placed. For dosing in cats, pyridostigmine bromide (0.1 to 0.25 mg/kg q24h) has been recommended.

Side effects of cholinesterase inhibitors result from excessive cholinergic stimulation following the accumulation of ACh at muscarinic receptors of smooth muscle, autonomic glands, the central nervous system, and nicotinic receptors of skeletal muscle. Bradycardia, which results from excessive vagal activity, is seen almost exclusively after parenteral injections of ACh inhibitors. Gastrointestinal side effects may occur after administration by any route and include nausea, vomiting, abdominal cramping, loose stools, or overt diarrhea. Increased bronchial and oral secretions may be a problem if dysphagia is present. Adverse effects may be reduced by administering small doses of atropine or having the animal take medication after meals when feasible.

Overtreatment with cholinesterase inhibitors can result in excessive accumulation of ACh at the neuromuscular junction, with worsening of weakness as a result of depolarization or desensitization of the postsynaptic membrane. Any increase in anticholinesterase medication that does not produce clear-cut improvement in muscle strength should be promptly reversed.

Corticosteroids

If myasthenic animals cannot be managed successfully with supportive care and cholinesterase inhibitors alone, corticosteroids may be added carefully. Corticosteroids have been shown to be of benefit in human MG and may improve the long-term prognosis in some cases of canine MG. However, the side effects may be life threatening. Glucocorticoids result in polydypsia and polyphagia in an animal that may have difficulty swallowing or is regurgitating. In addition, there is an increased susceptibility to infection. Increased weakness often occurs early in the course of steroid treatment, requiring hospitalization and sometimes intensive medical care with respiratory support. To prevent the initial steroid-induced weakness, low-dose prednisone therapy has been recommended in mild and moderately affected human myasthenic patients. I have also recommended a similar therapeutic approach for myasthenic dogs in groups 1 and 2. Antiinflammatory dosages (0.5 mg/kg PO q24h), not immunosuppressive dosages, of corticosteroids are suggested. Relative contraindications for corticosteroid therapy include severe obesity, diabetes mellitus, uncontrolled hypertension, gastrointestinal ulcerations, and ongoing infections or aspiration pneumonia.

Although myasthenic cats can be treated successfully with anticholinesterase drugs, it is my impression that cats generally respond better to corticosteroid therapy. Unlike the case in dogs, exacerbation of muscle weakness and other unwanted side effects may not occur as frequently in myasthenic cats treated with high doses of corticosteroids.

Immunosuppressive Drugs

Other immunosuppressive drugs have not been studied adequately in canine and feline MG, and there are only a few case reports suggesting effectiveness. Clearly, controlled clinical trials are warranted. Since most cases of canine or feline MG can be managed successfully with anticholinesterase drugs alone or in combination with prednisone, most of these immunosuppressive drugs should be reserved for severe, nonresponsive forms of MG. Disadvantages of these agents are the time it takes for improvement to begin, the side effects, the expense, and the need for chronic administration (Kent, 2004).

Azathioprine

Azathioprine is the most frequently used immunosuppressive agent in MG after prednisolone. Side effects are related to gastrointestinal and myelosuppressive toxicity. A complete blood cell count should be performed 7 to 10 days after initiation of therapy and monthly thereafter. Azathioprine may be used as an alternative to prednisone when the latter drug is relatively contraindicated and when a less rapid response to therapy is acceptable. Azathioprine may also be used for its "steroid-sparing" effects in patients who have developed unacceptable side effects to prednisone, when it has not been possible to reduce the dose of prednisone to acceptable levels, or when the response to prednisone has not been satisfactory. The recommended dosage is 1.1 to 2.2 mg/kg PO every 24 hours or every other day. Since azathioprine can result in neuromuscular blockade in cats, its use is not recommended.

Cyclophosphamide

Cyclophosphamide can cause severe leukopenia, specifically neutropenia, and routine complete blood counts should be performed every 7 to 10 days after administration. Gastrointestinal disturbances can also occur. Sterile hemorrhagic cystitis is another serious side effect of cyclophosphamide, which can occur not only with prolonged administration but after a single dose. This drug has not been evaluated in canine MG, and, given the serious side effects, the risks do not outweigh the benefits.

Cyclosporine

Cyclosporine has been used in a variety of immune-mediated diseases in the dog but has not been evaluated specifically for the treatment of MG. In human MG cyclosporine is used in patients who are candidates for immunosuppression but who cannot take or who have not responded satisfactorily to azathioprine. It has been used as the primary immunosuppressant in human MG and with prednisone, which permits use of lower corticosteroid doses. The maximum response is usually seen within 3 to 4 months. Suggested dosage ranges for canine immune-mediated diseases are from 5 to 10 mg/kg/day divided into two doses. Side effects include vomiting, diarrhea, weight loss, gingival hyperplasia, and involuntary shaking. Although it is nephrotoxic, dogs seem relatively resistant to this side effect.

Mycophenolate Mofetil

Although mycophenolate mofetil (MMF) has been widely used in human medicine, reports in veterinary medicine have been limited to its use in a case of immune-mediated glomerulonephritis and in a dog with MG. At a dosage of 20 mg/kg every 12 hours gastrointestinal signs may be observed, including vomiting, diarrhea, and anorexia, which are dosage related. For this reason, in patients with MG a 50% reduction in MMF dosage should be made once significant improvement or resolution of clinical signs is noted.

Thymectomy

Most human neurologists recommend thymectomy in their MG patients, although no controlled clinical trial has proven this to be of significant benefit. In human patients there is a high incidence of thymic hyperplasia, which in my experience has only rarely been identified in canine or feline myasthenic patients. In canine and feline MG thymectomy should be reserved for cases of confirmed MG and a cranial mediastinal mass (group 4: paraneoplastic MG). It is my opinion that all animals with a cranial mediastinal mass should be tested for MG before surgical removal. Weakness may become clinical after the surgery, and knowing the antibody status before surgery should aid in therapeutic management. If a cranial mediastinal mass can be removed completely, the AChR antibody titer should return to the reference range, and clinical signs of MG should resolve. If the mass cannot be removed completely, the antibody titer would remain positive, and treatment for MG would need to be continued. Specific treatments would be similar to that of either group 2 (preceding paragraphs) or group 3 (following paragraphs).

Acute Fulminating Myasthenia Gravis

Management of acute, severe generalized MG (group 3: acute fulminating MG) can be difficult and ideally should be performed in intensive care facilities (King and Vite, 1998). In humans expensive short-term treatment modalities such as plasma exchange (plasmapheresis) and intravenous immunoglobulin are commonly used; however, because of the expense and technical difficulty of performing these therapies, they are not commonly used in veterinary medicine. Ventilatory support and placement of a feeding tube are usually required. Respiratory failure, either from ventilatory failure caused by weakness in the intercostal muscles or diaphragm or by severe aspiration pneumonia, may be the most common cause of death in dogs with acute fulminating myasthenic crisis. If possible, cultures should be obtained from the respiratory tract by tracheal wash, and broad-spectrum intravenous antibiotics should be instituted immediately. Aminoglycosides and ampicillin should be avoided because of possible detrimental effects on neuromuscular transmission.

For critical animals in which oral medication is not possible, a constant rate infusion of pyridostigmine bromide (0.01 to 0.03 mg/kg/hour) may be used until oral feedings are resumed. Alternatively anticholinesterase therapy can be administered through a feeding tube.

Myasthenic crisis may be precipitated by concurrent infection or high doses of daily prednisone. Corticosteroids should be avoided initially in patients with overwhelming aspiration pneumonia. Once an infection has been controlled, corticosteroids or other immunosuppressive agents such as azathioprine, cyclosporine, or mycophenolate can be added to the regimen, if necessary. High-dose intravenous methylprednisolone sodium succinate therapy may be of benefit in severe cases of MG without worsening of muscle weakness. In one study of 15 human patients, 2g of methylprednisolone sodium succinate was given intravenously every 5 days for a total of 15 days. Satisfactory improvement without exacerbation of muscle weakness occurred in 10 of 15 patients (Arsura et al., 1985).

MONITORING THE COURSE OF AUTOIMMUNE MYASTHENIA GRAVIS

Although a positive AChR antibody titer is diagnostic of autoimmune MG, there is a poor correlation between the severity of the disease and the antibody concentration. However, in the absence of immunosuppression, determination of serial AChR antibody titers in an individual animal is a good indicator of disease status and should help determine duration of treatment. As long as the AChR antibody titer remains positive, treatment should be continued. In my laboratory there has been an excellent correlation between resolution of clinical signs, including megaesophagus, and return of AChR antibody titers to within the reference range. Monitoring the AChR antibody titer is also suggested in paraneoplastic MG since it gives a good indication as to whether a cranial mediastinal mass has been completely removed. In most cases of canine autoimmune MG, once remission has occurred, recurrence of MG has been rare. Do not misinterpret a therapeutically induced decrease in AChR antibody titer and absence of clinical signs while the dog is on immunosuppressive therapy as a remission. In these cases clinical signs can return once the dosage of immunosuppressive drug is decreased. The natural course of autoimmune

MG in cats has not been determined, although it is my impression that spontaneous remissions are not as common as in dogs.

With an accurate diagnosis and early treatment, autoimmune MG is a treatable disease. Since there is a genetic predisposition to autoimmune diseases, including MG, it is recommended that myasthenic animals not be bred. Myasthenic female dogs and cats should be spayed as soon as possible after MG is under control because heat cycles and pregnancy can exacerbate active MG. Finally, vaccinations during active MG should be avoided because general immune stimulation can result in exacerbations of weakness and elevations of the AChR antibody titer (Shelton and Lindstrom, 2001; Shelton unpublished). Whether or not vaccinations can trigger MG is still an unresolved question.

References and Suggested Reading

Arsura E et al: High-dose intravenous methylprednisolone in myasthenia gravis, *Arch Neurol* 42:1149, 1985.

Dewey CW et al: Clinical forms of acquired myasthenia gravis in dogs: 25 cases (1998-1995), *J Vet Intern Med* 11:50, 1997.

Ducoté JM, Dewey CW, Coates JR: Clinical forms of acquired myasthenia gravis in cats, *Compend Contin Educ Pract Vet* 21:440, 1999.

Kent M: Therapeutic options for neuromuscular diseases, *Vet Clin North Am Small Anim Pract* 34:1525, 2004.

King LG, Vite CH: Acute fulminating myasthenia gravis in five dogs, *J Am Vet Med Assoc* 212:830, 1998.

Shelton GD: Myasthenia gravis and disorders of neuromuscular transmission, *Vet Clin North Am Small Anim Pract* 32:189, 2002.

Shelton GD et al: Acquired myasthenia gravis: selective involvement of esophageal, pharyngeal, and facial muscles, *J Vet Intern Med* 4:281, 1990.

Shelton GD, Lindstrom JM: Spontaneous remission in canine myasthenia gravis: implications for assessing human MG therapies, *Neurology* 57:2139, 2001.

Shelton GD, Schule A, Kass PH: Risk factors for acquired myasthenia gravis in dogs: 1154 cases (1991-1995), *J Am Vet Med Assoc* 211:1428, 1997.

Shelton GD, Ho M, Kass PH: Risk factors for acquired myasthenia gravis in cats: 105 cases (1986-1998), *J Am Vet Med Assoc* 216:55, 2000.

CHAPTER **242**

Treatment of Myopathies and Neuropathies

G. DIANE SHELTON, *La Jolla, California*

Neuromuscular diseases can be difficult diagnostic challenges with only a limited number of available therapeutic options. However, the most common diseases affecting muscle and peripheral nerve are treatable if a correct diagnosis is reached before irreversible pathologic changes occur. For other neuromuscular diseases, particularly the inherited myopathies and neuropathies, no therapeutic options are currently available. The old dictum of "to help, or at least to do no harm" (Hippocrates) is particularly true for this group of diseases. Treatment trials with corticosteroids before performing at least the minimum necessary diagnostics can delay or impair the ability to reach a correct diagnosis, delay initiation of specific therapies, and possibly result in irreversible contractures or even death of the animal. Further, glucocorticoids result in a polydypsic and polyphagic animal with an increased susceptibility to infection.

The first important step is to obtain an accurate neuroanatomic localization (Glass and Kent, 2002). Neuromuscular diseases are disorders of the motor unit and as such affect neuronal cell bodies in the ventral gray matter (ventral horn) of the spinal cord (motor neuron disease), peripheral nerve (neuropathies), neuromuscular junction (disorders of neuromuscular transmission), and muscle (myopathies). A careful neurologic examination is critical. If the wrong anatomic localization is made, an incorrect diagnostic pathway would be chosen, and valuable time wasted. An incorrect diagnosis leading to inappropriate treatments could result in severe debilitation or may be life threatening.

Once clinical signs have been localized to the neuromuscular system, specific laboratory testing should be performed to reach an accurate diagnosis. A minimum database for neuromuscular diseases should include a complete blood cell count; serum chemistry profile, including creatine kinase (CK) and electrolytes; thyroid screen; urinalysis; and in most cases the acetylcholine receptor antibody titer for myasthenia gravis. Electrodiagnostic testing, including electromyography and measurement of sensory and motor nerve conduction velocity, provides important information regarding the distribution and nature of the disorder but requires specialized equipment and expertise (Cuddon, 2002). Cerebrospinal fluid analysis may be beneficial in disorders of nerve roots such as acute polyradiculoneuritis and protozoal diseases. The definitive diagnosis ultimately requires histopathologic evaluation of appropriately collected and processed muscle and peripheral nerve biopsies (Dickenson and LeCouteur, 2002). Although a specific diagnosis may not be reached in all cases, information regarding the underlying pathologic process can guide empiric therapy.

Treatment of the most common inflammatory (masticatory muscle myositis, infectious myositis) and noninflammatory (endocrine and exogenous corticosteroid-induced) myopathies, the less common noninflammatory myopathies (inherited myopathies), and the neuropathies are described in this chapter. Specific treatments for the various clinical forms of myasthenia gravis are covered in a separate chapter.

TREATMENT OF INFLAMMATORY MYOPATHIES

The inflammatory myopathies, including the immune-mediated forms (masticatory muscle myositis, polymyositis, extraocular myositis, and dermatomyositis) and those associated with infectious diseases (particularly the protozoal diseases *Toxoplasma gondii, Neospora caninum,* and *Hepatozoon americanum*) are relatively common in dogs. Myositis associated with neoplasia as a paraneoplastic or preneoplastic process occurs less commonly. Inflammatory myopathies occur rarely in cats as a paraneoplastic syndrome (thymoma) or associated with feline immunodeficiency virus (FIV) or feline leukemia virus (FeLV) infection. In my experience, purely immune-mediated inflammatory myopathies are uncommon in cats. Following a histologic diagnosis of an inflammatory myopathy, infectious diseases should be ruled out by serology, and screening for neoplasia should be initiated. If negative, an immune-mediated cause is likely.

Masticatory Muscle Myositis

Masticatory muscle myositis (MMM) is the most common inflammatory myopathy occurring in dogs and rarely in cats. In MMM clinical signs are restricted to the muscles of mastication without involvement of the limb muscles or other muscle groups. MMM has been recognized in most breeds of dogs and can begin as early as 3 months of age. Although MMM is a bilateral disease, clinical signs can appear unilateral, with one side more markedly affected than the other. A particularly severe, breed-associated form of MMM has recently been identified in young cavalier King Charles spaniels. In the acute form of MMM pain and swelling of the masticatory muscles and trismus are common clinical findings. Typically the jaws cannot be opened, even under anesthesia. The cause of this inability to the open the jaw in the acute stage has not been identified, and fibrosis is not obvious in muscle biopsy specimens. In the chronic stage there is atrophy of the masticatory muscles in the presence or absence of jaw pain or mobility. In end-stage MMM, atrophy is severe, and the jaw may not open greater than a couple of centimeters. In muscle biopsy specimens of end-stage disease, there is severe loss of muscle mass and replacement with fibrous tissue. MMM is very corticosteroid responsive in the acute stages and moderately so in the chronic stages. Once end-stage MMM is present, there is typically only minimal, if any, response to corticosteroids.

Because of the propensity for fibrosis, an early and accurate diagnosis is critical to a positive clinical outcome. The serum CK concentration is usually normal or only mildly elevated. Although a serologic assay currently is available for the diagnosis of MMM (demonstration of 2M antibodies by either immunohistochemistry or enzyme-linked immunosorbent assay), a biopsy of the temporalis muscle is also recommended for determination of the severity of the disease and long-term prognosis. Previous corticosteroid therapy at immunosuppressive dosages for greater than 7 to 10 days can lower antibody titers with negative results. In addition, cases with chronic, end-stage MMM can be negative for antibodies against type 2M fibers because most fibers of this type have been destroyed, removing the antigenic stimulus. If a biopsy is collected, care must be taken that the correct muscle is sampled. A common mistake is to biopsy the frontalis and not the temporalis muscle. The frontalis muscle lies directly under the skin and is not part of the masticatory muscle group. A biopsy from the frontalis muscle will not be diagnostic. Instructions for collection of an appropriate temporalis muscle biopsy specimen are given in a review of MMM by Melmed and colleagues (2004).

Following confirmation of the diagnosis of MMM, immunosuppressive therapy with prednisone should be initiated at 1 to 2 mg/kg PO every 12 hours. Treatment should be continued until the CK concentration (if elevated) has returned to the normal range, jaw mobility has returned to normal, and clinically evident jaw pain has resolved. Prednisone dosage then should be decreased gradually to the lowest alternate-day dose that will keep the dog free of clinical signs and continued for a period of at least 4 to 6 months. Relapses are common if treatment is stopped too soon. The most frequent causes of a poor clinical outcome are a delay in initiating appropriate treatment, inappropriate dosages of corticosteroids, and treatment for too short a period of time. If prednisone is poorly tolerated, other immunosuppressive drugs such as azathioprine may be used to reduce the glucocorticoid dosages. There are no controlled clinical trials detailing the efficacy of any therapeutic regimen in the treatment of canine inflammatory myopathies; thus recommendations for other agents, including cyclosporine, mycophenolate mofetil, and intravenous immunoglobulin, cannot be given.

In end-stage masticatory muscle myositis, fibrosis may be severe, and the jaw only opened a few centimeters, if that. In these cases resolution of clinical signs with corticosteroid therapy should not be expected. Maintenance of hydration and adequate nutrition may be problematic, and dogs may present with generalized muscle wasting from malnourishment related to the lack of food intake. Under no circumstances should the jaw be opened forcibly, even under sedation or anesthesia, because a jaw fracture may result. Surgical procedures such as mandibular symphysiotomy or partial mandibulectomy or hemimandibulectomy may allow tongue movement for lapping food and water.

Polymyositis

Polymyositis (PM) is an immune-mediated inflammatory myopathy that can affect all muscle groups, including the masticatory muscles; the limb muscles; and the esophageal, pharyngeal, and laryngeal muscles. PM can occur alone or as part of a generalized autoimmune disorder such as systemic lupus erythematosus. The serum CK concentration may be normal or mildly to moderately elevated, depending on the degree of muscle damage and distribution of cellular infiltrates. The 2M antibody titer is negative is most cases, even with clinical involvement of the masticatory muscles. Clinical signs may include a stiff, stilted gait; muscle atrophy; variable myalgia; regurgitation and dysphagia; and contractures in chronic cases. The diagnosis of PM is confirmed by muscle biopsy. Biopsies should be collected from more than one muscle since cellular infiltrates can have a patchy distribution and be missed on individual biopsy specimens. The large proximal limb muscles such as the vastus lateralis or biceps femoris from the pelvic limb and the triceps muscle from the thoracic limb are suggested. Once a diagnosis of an inflammatory myopathy has been histologically confirmed and infectious agents have been ruled out, immunosuppressive therapy should be initiated as for MMM. The serum CK concentration should be monitored, as well as resolution of clinical signs. Periodic screening for an underlying neoplasia is also suggested, particularly in the boxer breed (Evans, Levesque, and Shelton, 2004).

Extraocular Muscle Myositis

A focal, presumed immune-mediated inflammatory myopathy, extraocular myositis (EOM), selectively affects the extraocular muscles while sparing the masticatory and limb muscles. The clinical presentation is for bilateral exophthalmos in the acute stage or a restrictive strabismus in the chronic stage. The serum CK concentration is normal, and 2M antibodies are negative. A presumptive diagnosis of EOM can be made by clinical presentation, a negative 2M antibody test, and demonstration of swollen extraocular muscles by orbital ultrasound or magnetic resonance imaging examinations. In the acute stage resolution of clinical signs with immunosuppressive dosages of corticosteroids can be rapid. In chronic stages of EOM with fibrosis of the extraocular muscles, a favorable response to immunosuppression should not be expected.

Restrictive strabismus may result in cases with inappropriate or delayed treatments.

Dermatomyositis

Canine dermatomyositis (DM) is a familial, immune-mediated inflammatory disease of striated muscle, skin, and microvasculature in young collies, Shetland sheepdogs (shelties), and collie-crossbred dogs, but it can occur rarely in other breeds. In familial DM the clinical diagnosis is based on classic skin changes and myositis in a collie or sheltie. The onset of clinical signs is typically within the first 6 months of life. Clinical signs of myositis develop after the dermatitis and correlate approximately in severity to the degree of dermatitis. Serum CK usually is only mildly elevated. A specific diagnosis is made by skin and muscle biopsy examinations. Unlike PM, in DM the temporalis and distal limb muscles (such as the cranial tibial muscle) are more markedly affected. Treatment involves immunosuppression as in MMM and PM and symptomatic relief of skin lesions, including avoidance of sunlight, treatment of underlying pyoderma, and vitamin E (400 units q24h PO).

Inflammatory Myopathies Secondary to Infectious Agents

In my laboratory the most common cause of infectious myositis in dogs is the protozoal organism *N. caninum*. Young dogs infected with *N. caninum* can present clinically with rigid pelvic limb hyperextension, muscle atrophy resulting from myositis, and concurrent polyradiculoneuritis. In older dogs infection can cause either an inflammatory or a necrotizing myopathy. Infection with *T. gondii* is considered more common in cats, with clinical signs predominantly related to the central nervous system, respiratory system, and gastrointestinal system. Although parasite cysts may be identified in muscle biopsies from cats with neuromuscular diseases, an inflammatory myopathy with cellular reactions around the cysts is a rare finding. Although a presumptive diagnosis is based on positive immunoglobulin (Ig)G or IgM antibody titers, the definitive diagnosis depends on demonstration of the organism within muscle or other tissue by immunohistochemical or molecular methods. A combination treatment of clindamycin (10 mg/kg q8h PO) and trimethoprim-sulfa (15 mg/kg q12h PO) for 4 weeks has been suggested for canine neosporosis. Clindamycin (25 to 50 mg/kg q8-12h) is the treatment of choice for feline toxoplasmosis.

Infection with other protozoal organisms may cause myositis in dogs, including *H. americanum* in the southern region of the United States and *Leishmania infantum* in the Mediterranean area. *Trypanosoma cruzi* may affect the myocardium and skeletal muscle of dogs in the temperate to tropical regions of the world. Although bacterial and rickettsial infectious diseases are common in the dog and cat, reports of an associated myositis are infrequent. Viral-related inflammatory myopathies are well documented in people, with retroviruses and enteroviruses most commonly implicated. Inflammatory myopathies and neuropathies have been identified in my laboratory in FeLV- and FIV-infected cats. For more in-depth discussions of infectious causes of neuromuscular diseases and appropriate antimicrobials, references by Podell (2002) and Kent (2004) are suggested.

TREATMENT OF NONINFLAMMATORY MYOPATHIES

The largest group of treatable noninflammatory myopathies encountered in clinical practice are associated with endocrine disorders such as hypothyroidism, hyperthyroidism, and Cushing's syndrome or secondary to chronic corticosteroid therapy (the so-called *steroid myopathy*). The presence of weakness, stiffness, reluctance to move, muscle wasting, and myalgia may be the first indications of an underlying endocrine disorder in the absence of classical clinical signs.

Hypothyroid Myopathy

In newly diagnosed human hypothyroid patients, as many as 38% have clinical muscular weakness, and 80% have complaints suggestive of muscle dysfunction. The incidence of myopathic signs in canine hypothyroidism is not known but may be similar. The serum CK concentration may be normal or mildly elevated. A diagnosis of hypothyroidism can be highly suspected from histochemical evaluation of a muscle biopsy specimen and confirmed with laboratory testing, including measurement of endogenous canine thyroid-stimulating hormone and serum-free thyroxine levels by dialysis. The prognosis for recovery in hypothyroid myopathy is excellent and rapid once the dog is restored to a euthyroid state.

Hyperthyroid Myopathy

Muscle weakness and tremors may occur in feline hyperthyroidism. The serum CK may be markedly elevated, but muscle biopsies are usually normal. Resolution of clinical weakness rapidly follows correction of electrolyte abnormalities and a return to a euthyroid state. A side effect of the antithyroid drug methimazole is the development of muscle weakness approximately 2 to 4 months after initiation of therapy, with a positive acetylcholine receptor antibody titer diagnostic of acquired myasthenia gravis. Clinical signs of myasthenia resolve, and the acetylcholine receptor antibody titer returns to the normal range after cessation of the drug.

Cushing's Myopathy and Myotonia

Muscle wasting, weakness, gait abnormalities, and in some cases myotonia may be found in older dogs with Cushing's syndrome. Muscle stiffness and lameness may be an early clinical indicator of an underlying endocrinopathy. Although laboratory testing can confirm hyperadrenocorticism, type 2 fiber atrophy and excessive lipid accumulation are commonly found on histochemical examination of muscle biopsy specimens, consistent with this disease. Although not thoroughly studied, peripheral neuropathy may also be associated with Cushing's syndrome. Clinical signs of myopathic weakness in the absence of myotonia should resolve following specific treatment. Muscle rigidity associated with myotonia is not as responsive to therapy, and deficits can persist.

Steroid Myopathy

Profound muscle weakness and atrophy can occur following chronic exogenous corticosteroid therapy in dogs. The masticatory muscles are usually the most severely affected; however, weakness and atrophy may affect the whole body musculature. As in the myopathy associated with Cushing's syndrome, prominent atrophy of type 2 fibers is a classic histologic change in muscle biopsy specimens. The fluorinated corticosteroids such as triamcinolone, betamethasone, and dexamethasone have been reported to have the most myopathic potential; thus conversion to a nonfluorinated steroid preparation with alternate-day treatment is recommended. Addition of another immunosuppressive agent that would allow lowering the dosage of corticosteroids is also suggested. Improvement usually follows but can take several weeks. Nutritional supplements may also be of benefit (see Nutritional Supplements at the end of this chapter).

Myopathies Associated with Inherited Diseases

Most of the inherited myopathies, including the muscular dystrophies (Shelton and Engvall, 2002) and other degenerative muscle diseases, occur in purebred dogs and cats less than 1 year of age. In some cases gait abnormalities and small stature may be first noticed at the time of ambulation. The breed of an affected animal is one of the most useful distinguishing diagnostic criteria of inherited diseases (Compendia of Inherited Diseases, see Fyfe, 2002). For the majority of these diseases there is no cure, and treatment options are mainly supportive. An accurate pathologic diagnosis is of particular importance to breeding programs because the goal is development of reliable molecular testing procedures for identification of carrier animals. Obtaining a specific diagnosis of these diseases is also important because inherited diseases constitute a significant proportion of diseases that cause poor quality of life or death in all breeds of dogs and cats.

TREATMENT OF PERIPHERAL NEUROPATHIES

Peripheral neuropathy remains a challenging area with regard to recognition, diagnosis, and therapy. Most often the cause of a peripheral neuropathy remains elusive despite extensive biochemical, toxicologic and electrophysiologic, histochemical, histopathologic, and electron microscopic studies of muscle and nerve biopsies. This is partly because of the limited number of ways in which peripheral nerves react to disease. Even though a specific cause may not be identified, evaluation of peripheral nerve biopsies in plastic sections can provide valuable information regarding disease severity and presence or absence of regeneration.

Neuropathies Associated With Endocrine Diseases

Neuropathies associated with endocrine diseases are relatively common with treatment based on the primary endocrinopathy. Diabetes mellitus can cause both a sensory and motor neuropathy in cats with clinical signs of a plantigrade, and in some cases palmigrade, stance. Resolution of clinical signs usually follows adequate glycemic control; however, residual deficits may occur in chronic, poorly controlled cats. Weakness and muscle atrophy consistent with neuropathy may also occur in diabetic dogs, although most cases are complicated by hypothyroidism or Cushing's syndrome. Hypothyroidism in dogs may be associated with peripheral neuropathy, although the mechanisms are poorly understood. Following hormone replacement, gradual improvement in neurologic signs should result; however, this may take several months. Neuropathy is also a rare complication of pancreatic β-cell (adeno)carcinoma. Although clinical signs of neuropathy may improve following surgical intervention, the prognosis for complete remission from an insulinoma and the accompanying peripheral neuropathy is poor.

Nutritional and Toxic Causes of Polyneuropathy

Although nutritional and toxic causes of polyneuropathy are not common or well documented in veterinary medicine, they may be treatable; thus the owner should be questioned carefully about diet, dietary supplements, and any previous drug therapies. Review of the health history and a through physical examination should also be performed for identification of an underlying gastrointestinal disease that could impair absorption. In my laboratory neuropathies have been identified in dogs associated with a several-year history of a raw fish diet and vitamin B deficiency (http://vetneuromuscular.ucsd.edu, March 2001 Case of the Month), chronic treatment with metronidazole (March 2002 Case of the Month), and a several-week history of nitrofurantoin treatment for chronic urinary tract infections (September 2001 Case of the Month). Although not fully documented in the veterinary literature, vitamin B_1 deficiency and toxic neuropathies associated with metronidazole and nitrofurantoin treatments are described in the human literature.

Neuropathies and Neoplastic Disorders

Lymphoma is the most common tumor of nonneural origin that affects the peripheral nervous system (PNS). Neoplastic cells, particularly in cats, can infiltrate the nerve and nerve roots, resulting in clinical signs of polyneuropathy in addition to signs of multicentric lymphoma. The diagnosis is confirmed by electrodiagnostic testing and demonstration of neoplastic cells within a peripheral nerve biopsy. Chemotherapy should be aimed at treating the underlying neoplasia. Chemotherapeutic drugs such as vincristine and cisplatin used in the treatment of lymphoma and solid tumors respectively may themselves cause peripheral neuropathy. Malignant peripheral nerve sheath tumors are the most common primary nerve tumor affecting the PNS. Although surgical excision and amputation are described, the prognosis is poor because recurrence is common with extension into the vertebral canal or thorax.

Inflammatory and Immune-Mediated Neuropathies

Organisms such as *T. gondii* and *N. caninum* can cause inflammatory and degenerative changes in peripheral nerves and nerve roots, as well as muscle. Diagnosis and treatment are as stated previously. Acute canine polyradiculoneuritis (coonhound paralysis, ACP) is one of the most commonly recognized canine peripheral neuropathies, characterized by lymphocytic radiculitis and demyelination of the ventral, and less commonly dorsal, nerve roots. Ascending tetraparesis or tetraplegia occurring over 1 to 2 days is characteristic of this disease. Treatment is supportive and includes physical therapy and bladder evacuation. Corticosteroids should not be used in dogs with ACP because they do not improve clinical signs or shorten the course of the disease and may in fact exacerbate the disease and reduce survival rate.

Chronic (relapsing) demyelinating polyradiculoneuritis refers to a group of chronic, progressive, or relapsing motor and sensory peripheral neuropathies that are associated with inflammatory changes in the spinal nerve roots, as well as in the cranial nerves and more peripheral regions of appendicular nerves. An autoimmune attack against peripheral nerve myelin is suspected. A definitive diagnosis of the pathologic nature of the neuropathy and the severity and distribution is achieved by electrophysiologic evaluation and muscle and peripheral nerve biopsies. Because of the suspected immune-mediated nature of this group of neuropathies, immunosuppression with prednisone (1 to 1.5 mg/kg q12h) has been recommended. Even with therapy, the long-term prognosis is guarded since relapses are common and the disease is progressive over months to years.

Cellular infiltrates may invade the most distal intramuscular nerve branches and be evident within muscle biopsies, particularly in cats. Although studies of this disorder are still in progress, this neuropathy appears to be steroid responsive, with complete resolution of clinical signs following corticosteroid therapy.

Chronic Axonal Degeneration

Chronic, slowly progressive, idiopathic axonal degeneration affects middle-age–to–older large-breed dogs. Clinical presentation is for progressive paraparesis or tetraparesis. Laryngeal paralysis may be an early clinical sign of a generalized peripheral neuropathy. A typical scenario is onset of peripheral weakness several months following laryngeal tie-back surgery, or weakness and atrophy of the distal limb muscles may be present at the time of surgery. All diagnostic evaluations (biochemical, endocrine, or metabolic screening, as well as radiography and ultrasonography) are normal. Diagnosis is based on electrodiagnostic testing and muscle and peripheral nerve biopsy. Peripheral nerve biopsy is of particular importance in these cases because the extent of nerve fiber loss or endo-neurial fibrosis and the presence or absence of regeneration are important in determining the course of disease and long-term prognosis. At this time no proven successful therapeutic options are available. Physical therapy and nutritional supplements are suggested in the following paragraphs.

ADJUNCTIVE THERAPY

Unless indicated by obvious cellular infiltrates within muscle and peripheral nerve biopsies or an inflammatory cerebrospinal fluid, treatment trials with glucocorticoids in the absence of a specific diagnosis can do more harm than good. Corticosteroids are catabolic in nature and thus could worsen muscle mass and weakness. Suggested supportive therapies for myopathies or neuropathies without a specific underlying cause include physical therapy and nutritional supplementation.

Physical Therapy

Inactivity can further diminish muscle mass in cases of neuromuscular diseases, and weakness may be aggravated by contractures. Mild exercise may prevent some of the atrophy induced by glucocorticoid treatments or hyper-adrenocorticism; thus walking should be encouraged. Passive range-of-motion exercises positively influence reinnervation and the sprouting process in denervated muscle and may be of therapeutic value.

Nutritional Supplements

Nutritional supplements may be beneficial when a specific diagnosis is not identified or used in conjunction with corticosteroids in inflammatory myopathies or neuropathies to counteract the side effects of additional muscle atrophy and weakness. Although controlled studies have not yet been performed, various vitamins and nutritional supplements have been advocated for patients with neuromuscular diseases. The goal is to increase muscle mass and strength by anabolic agents, exercise, and physical therapy rather than worsen muscle weakness and atrophy by inactivity and harmful drugs. I recommend L-carnitine (100 mg/kg q24h), coenzyme Q_{10} (4 mg/kg q24h), and supplementation with B vitamins. This therapy should not be harmful and may help improve muscle strength. Several different muscle diseases are associated with low muscle carnitine concentrations (Shelton, unpublished data), and dramatic improvement may result in some cases. The owners should be informed that in most cases this is not a cure, but, most important, it cannot be harmful. The metabolic benefits of L-carnitine include transportation of fatty acids into the mitochondria for energy generation and the urinary excretion of abnormal metabolites. Coenzyme Q_{10} functions as a cofactor in several enzyme systems related to energy conversion (electron transport) and is a vital catalyst to energy production at the cellular level. It is also a free radical scavenger. For degenerative peripheral nerve diseases, acetyl-L-carnitine may be more beneficial than the L-carnitine form. Clearly controlled clinical trials are necessary to document the efficacy of these treatments of neuromuscular diseases.

References and Suggested Reading

Cuddon P: Electrophysiology in neuromuscular disease, *Vet Clin North Am Small Anim Pract* 32:31, 2002.

Dickinson PJ, LeCouteur RA: Muscle and nerve biopsy, *Vet Clin North Am Small Anim Pract* 32:63, 2002.

Evans J, Levesque D, Shelton GD: Canine inflammatory myopathies: a clinicopathologic review of 200 cases, *J Vet Intern Med* 18:679, 2004.

Fyfe JC: Molecular diagnosis of inherited neuromuscular disease, *Vet Clin North Am Small Anim Pract* 32:287, 2002.

Glass EN, Kent M: The clinical examination for neuromuscular disease, *Vet Clin North Am Small Anim Pract* 32:1, 2002.

Kent M: Therapeutic options for neuromuscular diseases, *Vet Clin North Am Small Anim Pract* 34:1525, 2004.

Melmed C : Masticatory muscle myositis: pathogenesis, diagnosis, and treatment, *Compend Cont Educ Pract Vet* 26:590, 2004.

Platt SR: Neuromuscular complications in endocrine and metabolic disorders, *Vet Clin North Am Small Anim Pract* 32:125, 2002.

Podell M: Inflammatory myopathies, *Vet Clin North Am Small Anim Pract* 32:147, 2002.

Shelton GD, Engvall E: Muscular dystrophies and other inherited myopathies, *Vet Clin North Am Small Anim Pract* 32:103, 2002.

CHAPTER 243

Treatment of Supraspinatus Tendon Disorders in Dogs

BOEL A. FRANSSON, *Pullman, Washington*

Forelimb lameness in adult dogs is generally considered one of the most frustrating orthopedic problems facing veterinarians. Well-described disorders in small animal orthopedics such as biceps tendonitis or nerve sheath tumors may be difficult to diagnose. Add to that the likelihood that many causes of forelimb lameness remain undescribed in veterinary medicine, and it is understandable that inability to reach a final diagnosis in cases with forelimb lameness is more common than in hind limb lameness.

Successful treatment of forelimb lameness in dogs requires an accurate diagnosis of the underlying problem. Traditionally lameness elicited from nonosseous disorders of the extraarticular shoulder region have been particularly difficult to diagnose since radiographic examination is an insensitive detector of soft-tissue abnormalities and direct visualization via arthroscopy is not possible. Increasing access to more advanced imaging technology is expanding our abilities to recognize disorders of structures such as the supraspinatus tendon. The main abnormality of the supraspinatus tendon previously recognized has been mineralization (calcification) of the tendon insertion. Magnetic resonance imaging (MRI) provides high resolution delineation of soft tissues in three dimensions. In addition, by using several image sequences, MRI may provide some information about the characteristics of abnormalities seen (e.g., fluid content, fat content, vascular supply). With MRI becoming increasingly available to the practicing clinician, it is reasonable to believe that the veterinary community will see emerging diagnoses that will require novel treatments. Overuse tendinopathy (tendinosis) of the supraspinatus tendon is one such recently described diagnosis that has been demonstrated to occur in dogs. Diagnosis and management of the two supraspinatus disorders described to date in dogs are discussed.

SUPRASPINATOUS TENDON ANATOMY

The supraspinatus muscle in dogs arises from and is located in the supraspinous fossa of the scapula. The muscle curves around the neck of the scapula and ends in a short, approximately 9-mm thick (in dogs 19 to 28 kg) tendon on the craniomedial aspect of the major tubercle of the humerus. The supraspinatus muscle is innervated by the suprascapular nerve, and the action of this musculotendinous unit is to extend the shoulder joint and advance the limb forward. The supraspinatus tendon of insertion lies immediately craniomedial to the bicipital tendon in the intertubercular groove (Fig. 243-1). These two tendons are separated by the bicipital tendon sheath (an extension of the shoulder joint capsule) and, at the distal half of the greater tubercle, also the transverse humeral ligament.

An area of diminished or absent vascularization ("critical zone") is located in the part of the supraspinatous tendon immediately adjacent to the greater tubercle. This hypovascularization, which is also seen in humans, has been suggested to be a cause for supraspinatus tendon degeneration. Similar to that of most normal tendons, the collagen composition of the supraspinatus tendon consists primarily of type I collagen. However, in the insertion area of the canine supraspinatous tendon a significant amount of type III collagen has been demonstrated. Type III collagen is usually part of the early phase of wound repair and tends to be replaced with type I as the mechanical strength of the wound returns to normal. This differential collagen composition of the supraspinatous tendon may indicate that the insertion region is subjected to different stress than other tendons and may contribute to formation of degenerative changes.

SUPRASPINATUS TENDON MINERALIZATION

A calcifying tendinopathy of the supraspinatus tendon was first described in dogs by Flo and Middleton (1990). However, this abnormality may also represent an incidental finding in dogs, and a major difficulty in the diagnostic workup of this disorder is to rule out any other possible source of lameness.

Histopathologic examination of tissue resected in dogs with mineralization of supraspinatus tendon reveals fibrocartilaginous metaplasia with dystrophic mineralization of the tendon. Collagen bundles are often arranged haphazardly, and collagen fibers are separated by a myxomatous matrix, which can be verified by Alcian blue staining. There are no or minimal inflammatory changes.

Medium- to large-breed adult dogs are affected most commonly, and the lameness tends to show an insidious onset resulting in an intermittent or progressive weight-bearing forelimb lameness worsening during or after exercise. The lameness has often been present for several months by the time of diagnosis.

On physical examination many dogs show pain or resistance to movement during shoulder flexion. Less often pain is elicited by deep palpation with pressure focused

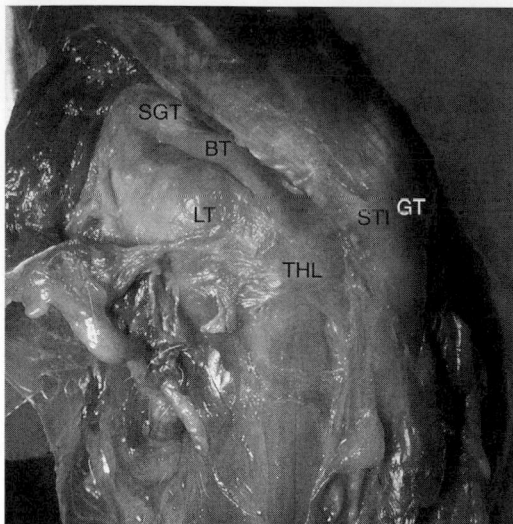

Fig. 243-1 Cranial-to-caudal view of the left shoulder. The pectoral muscle insertion is transected to expose the musculotendinous junction of the biceps. *BT*, Biceps tendon; *GT*, greater tubercle (laterally); *LT*, lesser tubercle (medially); *SGT*, supraglenoid tubercle; *STI*, the center of the supraspinatus tendon insertion; *THL*, transverse humeral ligament.

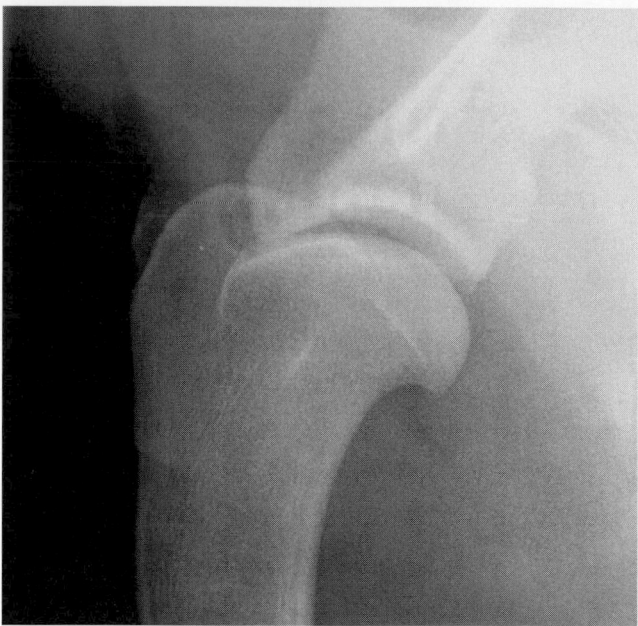

Fig. 243-2 Lateral view of the shoulder of a dog with mineralization of the supraspinatus tendon of insertion. The mineralization is visible in the tendon insertion immediately cranial to the greater tubercle.

over the craniomedial aspect of the greater tubercle. In some cases pain cannot be elicited by shoulder manipulation or digital palpation of the tendon. In general, the mineralizations are not large enough to be palpated.

During physical examination attention must be paid to any other possible source of lameness. Shoulder or elbow joint dysplasia or osteoarthritis, osteosarcoma of the proximal humerus, bicipital tenosynovitis, cervical intervertebral disk disease, and brachial plexus nerve sheath tumors, among other disorders, may all show lameness with similar characteristics as elicited from supraspinatus tendon mineralization. Bicipital tendon pain elicited by digital palpation in dogs with concurrent mineralization of the supraspinatus tendon may present a problem.

Diagnosis of supraspinatus mineralization can be confirmed by radiographic examination, but one must bear in mind that radiographic diagnosis does not confirm that lameness stems from this abnormality. A lateral view of the shoulder joint often shows the mineralization (Fig. 243-2). However, the mineralization might be obscure as a result of superimposition of the greater tubercle. Commonly bilateral radiographic changes are seen despite unilateral lameness.

To demonstrate that the mineralization is located in the plane of the supraspinatus tendon, a cranioproximal to craniodistal radiographic view (Fig. 243-3) of the shoulder joint is necessary. This view is obtained by placing the dog in sternal recumbency with the cassette placed on top of the forearm with the elbow flexed. The radiographic tube is positioned in a proximal-to-distal orientation directly over the scapulohumeral joint. To facilitate positioning of the tube the head of the dog has to be pulled to the contralateral side. A traditional craniocaudal projection usually adds little information and is not necessary.

With MRI there is often a hyperintense signal within the tendon on T2-weighted and fat-suppressed images, indicating increased fluid content in the part of the biceps tendon that is immediately adjacent to the mineralization in the supraspinatus tendon. We suspect that the mineralized supraspinatus tendon may cause mechanical irritation of the bicipital tendon sheath or tendon. However, ruling out bicipital tenosynovitis as the primary source of the lameness in these cases may prove difficult. Careful palpation of the intertubercular groove, with digital pressure applied on the biceps tendon while avoiding placing pressure on the slightly more laterally located

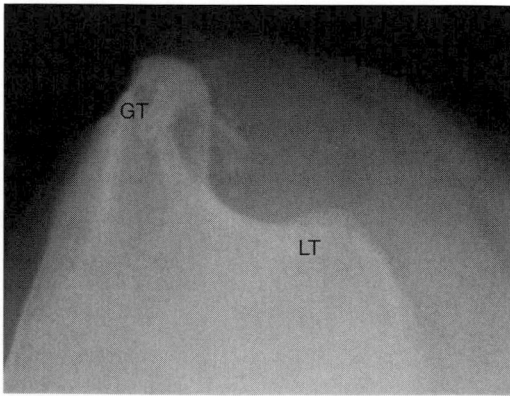

Fig. 243-3 Cranioproximal-to-craniodistal radiographic view of the canine shoulder in Fig. 243-2. The biceps tendon is located in the intertubercular groove between the greater (GT) and lesser (LT) tubercles, but it is not visible on the radiograph. The mineralizations medial to the greater tubercle were all located in the supraspinatus tendon in this case.

supraspinatus tendon, may distinguish pain elicited from the biceps tendon but will not reveal which of the problems is the primary cause of pain. Direct visualization of the biceps tendon through arthroscopy can help rule out primary biceps tenosynovitis.

Treatment

Rest and nonsteroidal antiinflammatory drugs (NSAIDs) have been reported to improve the lameness in a small number of dogs (Laitinen and Flo, 2000). These dogs had lameness of short duration (2 months or less), and the recovery time ranged from 2 to 8 weeks.

In dogs that are unresponsive to conservative management, surgery has been reported to improve lameness dramatically. Surgery consists of a 4- to 7-cm long cranial skin incision centered over the greater tubercle. The deeper dissection involves the brachiocephalic muscle, the fibers of which are divided longitudinally to gain access to the supraspinatus tendon of insertion. Longitudinal incisions in the tendon reveal the mineralized material that is removed. Closure is made in layers with absorbable or nonabsorbable suture material. Time to recovery after surgery seems to be highly variable with a median of 8 to 12 weeks. However, some dogs require 24 weeks before the end result of the treatment is reached.

Extracorporeal shock wave therapy has been reported to improve lameness associated with supraspinatus mineralization in two dogs (Danova and Muir, 2003). The single noninvasive treatment was carried out under sedation only. The long-term outcome of this novel treatment is unknown because the follow ups were very short (3 to 7 weeks).

SUPRASPINATUS TENDINOSIS

Chronic degenerative tendinopathy, tendinosis, is commonly seen in the common calcaneal (Achilles), patellar, and supraspinatus tendons in humans. Although the etiology is unknown, overuse injury has been suggested and supported by findings of experimental animal models. The disorder is characterized by persistent activity-related pain and swelling localized to the affected tendon.

A disorder of the supraspinatus tendon in a dog very similar to human tendinosis was recently reported from our institution, and this abnormality has subsequently been demonstrated in several other cases at our hospital and at other institutions. Histopathologic changes have shown disorganized collagen fibers that lack reflectivity under polarized light and a prominent myxomatous degeneration without calcification or inflammatory changes. It seems likely that the lack of radiographic changes associated with this disorder has prevented confirmation of the diagnosis previously. With the current, more frequent use of advanced imaging, soft-tissue changes such as tendinosis are easier to demonstrate.

Signalment and clinical features of dogs with tendinosis are strikingly similar to those of supraspinatus mineralization. Adult medium- to large-breed dogs, usually with a very active lifestyle, appear to be affected most frequently. In a majority of cases the lameness has been long-standing, intermittent to continuous, and nonresponsive to NSAID treatment. Despite the fact that most dogs show bilateral changes, the lameness is usually unilateral. Palpation of the tendon does not elicit a strong pain response, but some discomfort or pain is usually noted on shoulder flexion.

Application of MRI has aided diagnosis. The most consistent finding is an increased mass of the supraspinatus tendon of insertion, with hyperintense signal on T2-weighted and short tau inversion recovery (STIR) images. A curious finding in many dogs is that the increased mass of the supraspinatus tendon appears to displace the biceps tendon medially. Sometimes this is associated with a focal increase in signal intensity on T2-weighted and STIR images in the biceps tendon located at the point of maximum contact between the tendons. We suspect that the increased mass of the supraspinatus tendon mechanically interferes with the biceps tendon and its related structures, leading to focal irritation or degeneration and possibly pain. The chronic irritation may lead to secondary changes in the biceps tendon itself or in structures such as the transverse humeral ligament, which restricts the medial translation of the biceps tendon induced by the increased supraspinatus tendon volume. Definitive diagnosis is confirmed by histopathologic examination.

Treatment

Long-term outcome of surgery has only been reported in one dog at present. After surgical resection of the degenerated part of the tendon and thus decompression of the biceps tendon, the dog rapidly improved, and the lameness of 5 months' duration remained resolved 2 years after surgery. Further data are needed to predict to refine the prognosis and outcomes for this disorder.

In humans continuous rest of 3 to 6 months has been suggested to combat collagen breakdown and promote recovery from chronic tendinosis. Surgery has been considered a last resort for humans with tendinosis. However, secondary changes in the biceps tendon have not been noted in humans, probably because of the difference in anatomy, leading to a lack of interference between the two tendons.

At our institution surgery is the recommended treatment in dogs to prevent degeneration of the biceps tendon and also to establish diagnosis. At the time of surgical exploration of the supraspinatus tendon, arthroscopy of the ipsilateral shoulder joint is generally performed to confirm that coinciding shoulder disorders are not present. If the transverse humeral ligament appears thickened or fibrotic based on MRI and direct visual examination, transection of this structure is considered in an attempt to minimize irritation and/or ischemia of the biceps tendon.

Histopathologic examination has not demonstrated inflammatory changes associated with this disorder. Therefore antiinflammatory NSAIDs are prescribed only to minimize the inflammation and discomfort associated with surgery (i.e., 5 to 7 days). There appears to be no advantage in using corticosteroids locally or systemically for this disorder; in humans, corticosteroids are contraindicated because they inhibit collagen repair. Adjunctive therapy that has included laser treatment, high-voltage galvanic stimulation, application of load-decreasing devices, and strengthening exercises have been described for supraspinatus tendinosis in affected people.

Are the Two Disorders One?

Signalment and clinical presentation in both of the disorders described in this chapter are strikingly similar. In addition, the location of pathologic changes and the histopathologic findings are very similar, with the only notable difference being lack of mineralization in cases with tendinosis. It is possible that both disorders represent the same disease process, with an individual variation of the propensity for hydroxyapatite crystal deposition leading to variable mineralization. Hereditary, traumatic, metabolic, neurologic, degenerative, and vascular factors have all been suggested as underlying reasons for hydroxyapatite crystal deposition in human paraarticular tissues. Future research, including larger clinical studies, may

shed more light on the pathophysiology of canine degenerative disorders of the supraspinatus tendon.

References

Danova NA, Muir P: Extracorporeal shock wave therapy for supraspinatus calcifying tendinopathy in two dogs, *Vet Rec* 152:208, 2003.

Flo GL, Middleton D: Mineralization of the supraspinatus tendon in dogs, *J Am Vet Med Assoc* 197:95, 1990.

Fransson BA, Gavin PL, Lahmers KK: Supraspinatus tendinosis associated with biceps brachii tendon displacement in a dog, *J Am Vet Med Assoc* 227:1429, 2005.

Laitinen OM, Flo GL: Mineralization of the supraspinatus tendon in dogs: a long-term follow-up, *J Am Anim Hosp Assoc* 36:262, 2000.

Piermattei DL, Flo GL: The shoulder joint. In Piermattei DL, Flo GL, editors: *Brinker, Piermattei, and Flo's handbook of small animal orthopedics and fracture repair,* ed 3, Philadelphia, 1997, Saunders, p 228.

CHAPTER **244**

Medical Treatment of Coxofemoral Joint Disease

DENIS J. MARCELLIN-LITTLE, *Raleigh, North Carolina*

The diseases of the hip joint in dogs include hip dysplasia, Legg-Perthes disease, and osteoarthritis (OA). Canine hip dysplasia is a ubiquitous disease affecting most if not all dog breeds. Hip dysplasia is considered to be the most common orthopedic disease. In two recent scientific reports hip dysplasia was present in more than 40% of golden retrievers, Labrador retrievers, or rottweilers (Paster et al., 2005; Smith et al., 2006). Although canine hip dysplasia has been the core of several hundred scientific publications, the majority of these publications are linked to the genetic basis of the disease and its surgical management. Only a handful of articles cover the conservative management of the disease, with, to our knowledge, only one study having assessed prospectively its long-term clinical signs and progression (Smith et al., 2006). As a consequence, most of the recommendations included in this article are extrapolated from anecdotal reports, clinical experience, research models, or clinical studies in humans.

Development of OA in the canine hip joint most often results from hip dysplasia, but may also result from fractures of the acetabulum, femoral head, or femoral neck. Most acetabular fractures result from motor vehicle accidents. OA was present in 9 of 10 (90%) and 11 of 14 (79%) hip joints after acetabular fracture repair in two reports by Anson (1988) and Lewis (1989). Another report identified OA in all 15 caudal acetabular fractures managed without surgery (Boudrieau and Kleine, 1988). Most femoral head fractures are physeal fractures of the capital physis of the femur. Their surgical repair may lead to hip OA.

Hip dysplasia is an inherited developmental condition involving a lack of fit between the femoral head and acetabulum, invariably leading to OA (Lust, 1997). When present, hip dysplasia is most often bilateral. The clinical signs of hip dysplasia are most often described as acute in skeletally immature or young adult dogs and chronic in older dogs. Acute clinical signs tend to reflect acute pain: a potentially severe, often unilateral lameness. They generally appear between 4 and 8 months of age. Affected dogs may show a reluctance to perform propulsive activities, including jumping, climbing steps or stairs, galloping, or walking for extended periods of time; or they may exhibit behavioral changes, including reluctance to play, introversion, or showing aggressive tendencies. The chronic clinical signs of hip dysplasia include exercise intolerance, a reluctance to jump up and climb steps or stairs, and a bunny-hopping gait anomaly at a gallop.

Surprisingly, little has been written about the specific body changes present in dogs with chronic hip dysplasia (Barr et al., 1987; Johnston, 1992; Remedios and Fries, 1995; Read, 2000). Dogs with hip dysplasia have pain arising from their femoral and acetabular joint surfaces and hip joint capsule, particularly when moving at higher speed and during extension of the hip joints. Over time dysplastic dogs tend to lose hip extension but do not appear to lose hip flexion. Dogs lose joint motion because of the development of large osteophytes and enthesophytes on the caudal and ventral aspects of the acetabulum and on the femoral neck and caudal aspect of the greater trochanter. Pain response during hip joint flexion, subjectively, is very unusual and may be the consequence of other problems such as a septic arthritis, a bone tumor, or another problem. Most dysplastic dogs lose muscle mass in their pelvic limbs. Some may displace their center of gravity forward by flexing their spine, shoulder, and elbow joints. Overall the clinical signs of hip dysplasia vary widely among affected dogs. Some have very discrete signs that may appear after long periods of strenuous exercise; others have a severe disability and are unable to trot, gallop, or jump.

Little is known about the relationship of specific aspects of hip joint disease (i.e., dorsal subluxation, dorsal luxation, cartilage wear, dorsal rim wear, joint capsule thickening, osteophyte production, and the presence of joint mice) and the type and severity of clinical signs. Surprisingly, dorsal hip luxation is sometimes diagnosed in dogs with relatively mild clinical signs of dysplasia. Other dogs without luxation have significantly more hip pain. Also surprisingly, the size and location of osteophytes do not appear to correlate well with clinical signs of hip dysplasia. Clinical signs also appear to be linked to dog size: larger dogs are less likely to be nonweight bearing or to present with severe limb disuse than smaller dogs.

The management of hip dysplasia may involve surgery. Surgery may be performed early in life to positively influence the developing pelvis and hip joint or later in life to limit the pain and disability resulting from hip OA. Many patients with hip dysplasia are managed conservatively without surgery. Because hip dysplasia is a lifelong, progressive disease that impacts the daily activities of affected animals, it is critical for veterinarians to establish long-term, sustainable management programs for their patients. These programs must also be multifaceted because managing OA involves several objectives: decreasing pain, maintaining cardiovascular fitness, maintaining or increasing muscle strength, restoring or maintaining joint mobility, maintaining proprioception, optimizing weight, and adapting the home and environment.

OPTIMIZING SKELETAL DEVELOPMENT

Screening for Hip Laxity and Subluxation

Because of the high incidence of hip dysplasia in many breeds, particularly in large breeds with thick subcutaneous tissues and relatively modest muscle development (e.g., Saint Bernard, Bernese mountain dog, and mastiffs), it is indicated to screen breeds at risk for the presence of predisposing factors to hip dysplasia early in life. Since hip subluxation appears to be the key predisposing factor to dysplasia, the hip joints should be screened for the presence of hip subluxation at a young age. Hip subluxation may be reliably detected at 16 weeks of age using stress (distraction) radiography and, to a lesser extent, palpation. Palpation may be performed with the dog awake or under sedation. Palpation is ideally performed with the patient in lateral recumbency with the hip joint held in a position similar to a standing position. A flat hand may be placed on the proximal and medial aspect of the thigh, and abaxial pressure may be placed on that thigh. Abaxial displacement of the femur in relation to the pelvis may be palpated by feeling the relative position of the greater trochanter and the ischial tuberosity (Bardens sign). Also on palpation, preferably with the dog in dorsal recumbency, a reduction of the femoral head in the acetabulum may be felt by placing the hip in a position similar to a standing position and slowly abducting the femur. If the hip joint is subluxated initially and returns in a reduced position, a clunking sound will be heard during hip reduction (Ortolani sign). The angle at which the Ortolani sign occurs is a reflection of potential wear of the dorsal acetabular rim; more severe wear is expected with higher angles.

When the femur is slowly adducted toward a standing position, a more subtle displacement may be felt as the hip joint subluxates again (Barlow sign).

As for the reduction angles, higher subluxation angles indicate more severe dorsal rim wear. The feel of the Ortolani sign and subluxation may be smooth and crisp in hip joints with minor damage or rough and subtle in hip joints with cartilage and dorsal acetabular rim damage. We often see 20- to 40-degree differences between the angle of reduction and the angle of subluxation. A positive angle indicates abduction; a negative angle indicates adduction. Dogs with hip laxity without dorsal rim damage often have angles of reduction around 20 degrees and angles of subluxation around –20 degrees. Dogs with severe dorsal rim damage often have angles of reduction around 45 degrees and angles of subluxation around 20 degrees. Subjectively it appears that higher reduction and subluxation angles are more a factor of dorsal rim wear than of pure joint laxity. A dog with low reduction and negative subluxation angles may be able to maintain its hip joint reduced or intermittently reduce its hip joint during locomotion by slightly abducting its femur, in the same way that a dog with patellar luxation may relocate its patella. This may be observed at a walk or trot. With time, most dogs with hip subluxation will develop dorsal rim wear, and the positive Ortolani sign will disappear because of permanent dorsal hip subluxation. The age at which the Ortolani sign disappears in dysplastic dogs has not been scientifically assessed to our knowledge. Clinically most Ortolani signs disappear by 18 months of age. Most but not all dogs with positive Ortolani signs will develop hip dysplasia during the first few years of their adult life.

The laxity present in hip joints may be measured reliably at 16 weeks of age and later using stress radiography. Although multiple radiographic assessment methods are available, the PennHIP method is the most accurate method used to assess the presence of hip laxity. A PennHIP evaluation includes a distraction view that quantifies the degree of abaxial displacement of the femoral head in relation to the acetabulum during a maneuver resembling the Bardens sign. Reliable hip distraction is achieved using foam-covered adjustable acrylic tubes. The distraction index (DI) is the distance separating the centers of the acetabulum and femoral head during distraction divided by the radius of the femoral head. Dogs with low DI (<0.30) are very unlikely to develop hip dysplasia. Dogs with higher DI (>0.70) are very likely to develop hip dysplasia. Some dog breeds are more laxity tolerant than other breeds; for example, in a study involving 3729 German shepherds and 6278 Labrador retrievers older than 24 months, the likelihood of having hip OA in dogs with a DI of 0.6 was approximately 58% for German shepherds compared to approximately 16% for Labrador retrievers. This shows that joint laxity is not the sole factor leading to the development of hip arthritis and suggests that differences in anatomy and joint mechanics play an important role in the development of hip dysplasia (Smith et al., 2001). In a report assessing 459 clinically normal dogs, palpation was at best moderately correlated with radiographic measures of joint laxity, indicating the need to combine palpation with stress radiography when screening dogs for hip laxity (Puerto et al., 1999).

Optimizing Growth

Within litters both the severity and rate of progression of hip dysplasia are increased in larger dogs compared to smaller dogs and in dogs receiving calcium or phosphorus oversupplementation. Also, severity and rate of progression of hip dysplasia are decreased in dogs with slight (i.e., 25%) caloric restrictions during growth compared to dogs eating *ad libitum*. Protein amounts in the food do not appear to impact skeletal growth directly but may impact it indirectly if skeletally immature dogs are fed a low-protein diet; the need to eat more food to fulfill their protein needs will increase their energy/caloric consumption, increasing their risk of developing hip dysplasia.

Twice-weekly administration of polysulfated glycosaminoglycans between 6 weeks and 8 months of age has lead to less subluxation and indicated a trend toward less cartilage damage for pups predisposed to the development of hip dysplasia in one prospective study (Lust et al., 1992).

Minimizing Joint Pain

When hip dysplasia is detected in an adult dog, conservative management options are aimed at minimizing pain; optimizing living conditions; maintaining cardiovascular fitness, muscular strength and endurance, and joint motion; and, if deemed necessary, providing ambulation assistance.

Minimizing joint pain is a major aspect of the conservative management of hip dysplasia. It is achieved by optimizing the living conditions of patients, tailoring their activities, encouraging weight loss, giving pain medications, and food supplementation. Little is known about the impact of living conditions on the clinical signs of hip dysplasia in dogs. The general clinical signs of OA in humans include periods of relative calm and periods of sudden exacerbation of signs (flares or flare-ups). With time flares become more frequent and more severe and tend to last longer. In dogs with hip dysplasia, flares seem to result from excessive activity in unfit dogs (the weekend warrior syndrome) or from events that place excessive stress on arthritic joints such as jumping or stepping in a hole. Flares may last several hours to several weeks. Determining if an arthritic joint has flared is an important part of the initial assessment of all OA patients because treatment goals and methods differ. A flare is likely to be present in dogs with clinical signs that are significantly more severe than they were in preceding weeks. It is very common to first examine arthritic dogs at the time of a flare because the sudden increase in severity of their clinical signs gives owners a clear incentive for presentation to a veterinarian. A sudden loss of performance (e.g., inability to climb steps or into a motor vehicle, exercise intolerance) is often the result of a chronic, progressive loss of strength and fitness secondary to OA and aging, a change in the status of an arthritic joint (i.e., a subluxated hip joint becomes luxated), or the presence of a flare. Irreversible decisions such as surgery or euthanasia are ill-advised during flares because patients may appear overly affected and often are demonstrating dramatically decreased mobility. Instead the focus should be on comprehensive pain management and rest. Between flares owners should avoid strenuous activities that lead to an increase in clinical signs of OA and promote activities that do not. Potentially strenuous activities include jumping up, chasing, retrieving, and playing with other dogs. Unfortunately these activities are often chosen by owners because dogs love them, because they are easy to perform, and because they require minimal to no owner participation.

Changes in temperature (cold wave), humidity, and barometric pressure (decrease in pressure) have been reported to influence the pain perceived from arthritic joints in humans. To minimize the potential impact of weather conditions on arthritic dogs, it may be beneficial to make sure that they are housed in a weather-controlled environment. Minimizing slipping and falling may benefit them as well and may be achieved by improving the traction of walking surfaces and avoiding activities requiring sudden changes in direction or speed. In dogs with severe OA ambulation assistance may be provided by a step-in sling or harness. Neoprene harnesses with hook and loop fasteners are popular because they are ergonomic, relatively soft, durable, and washable. For large, heavy, or independent dogs with locomotion difficulties, an ambulation cart may provide effective ambulation assistance. In most instances, when pain and weakness are limited to the pelvic region, a two-wheel cart is used.

When dogs have problems involving all four limbs, a four-wheel (quad) cart may be used. The cart supports the pelvic region during outdoor activity. Some, but not all dogs, learn to negotiate door frames and may use their cart indoors. Because arthritic dogs maintain normal motor function during activity, we have the subjective impression that neoprene slings may be the optimal support material for the pelvis of arthritic dogs. On the other hand, neurologically compromised dogs that have abnormal pelvic motor function may ambulate more effectively with rigid pelvic resting surfaces (foam-covered aluminum rings).

Without appropriate pain relief, strengthening and maintaining joint mobility is rarely accomplished. Relief is achieved by interfering with the *peripheral* (tissue inflammation and damage) and *central* (neuropathic; involving the central nervous system) aspects of pain. Managing the peripheral component of OA pain hinges on pharmacologic treatment, specifically nonsteroidal antiinflammatory drugs (NSAIDs) that decrease the transduction and transmission of noxious stimuli in affected tissues and peripheral nerves. NSAID administration in dogs may lead to dramatic improvement in limb use and overall function. Several NSAIDs are approved for chronic use in the United States and other countries. Several scientific reports, often used as supporting studies for drug approval, have shown that NSAID administration has led to an increase in the peak vertical force and vertical impulse placed on the pelvic limbs of arthritic dogs. There is no published peer-reviewed study that has compared the commercially available NSAIDs using a blinded, prospective, randomized, crossover design. Despite the absence of such data, it is clear that NSAIDs have a significant positive impact on the comfort and mobility of dysplastic dogs. The relative occurrence and seriousness of side effects after administration of various NSAIDs in dogs has not been evaluated scientifically. All NSAIDs have infrequent but potentially serious side effects and should be used cautiously in dogs, particularly in patients with compromised liver or renal functions, hypovolemic patients, and patients with gastrointestinal disease or congestive heart failure. This is particularly relevant since many arthritic dogs show an increase in clinical signs later in life when liver, renal, cardiovascular, and gastrointestinal problems are more likely to be present. Periodic enzymatic and liver function screening is recommended in dogs receiving NSAIDs. Although there is no consensus on the frequency of these screenings, it seems reasonable to perform them before the administration of NSAIDs, after a few weeks of NSAID administration, and if clinical signs arise. As in all forms of chronic pain, peripheral sensitization and spinal cord wind-up occur with chronic hip dysplasia. Multimodal drug and nondrug therapy has been recommended to manage this chronic pain. This includes the use of pain medications that are adjunctive or alternative to NSAIDs. Adjunctive drugs may be considered for NSAID-intolerant dogs or for dogs with clinical signs that are only partially improved during NSAID therapy. The scientific information supporting these alternative medications is scant, but clinical research in that area is active. Tramadol, a synthetic morphine analog, is seemingly the most commonly used adjunctive drug for chronic hip pain. Other emerging drugs used in the multimodal drug management of OA include the γ-aminobutyric acid analog drug gabapentin and the antiviral drug amantadine (Lascelles et al., 2008).

In addition, subjectively, dogs with severe arthritic flares may benefit from continuous-rate intravenous infusion of a combination of an α-2 adrenergic agonist (medetomidine), sodium channel blockers (lidocaine and N-methyl D-aspartate receptor antagonists (ketamine, amantadine).

Nutritional supplementation has long been used to potentially decrease the pain associated with arthritic pain in humans, most often through the use of compounded herbs and vegetables such as in traditional Chinese and Indian Ayurvedic medicine. More than 30 herbs or compounds have shown some level of pain relief in prospective randomized trials involving humans with OA. In Western medicine the attention has focused mainly on the use of glucosamine, chondroitin sulphate, and polyunsaturated (omega-3) fatty acids for the management of arthritic joint pain, with several well-structured studies documenting their benefits. By comparison, little is known about the benefits of nutritional supplements in arthritic dogs. However, several clinical trials have documented the benefits of a diet containing glucosamine, chondroitin, and eicosapentaenoic acid (EPA), an omega-3 fatty acid, on the clinical signs of hip dysplasia in dogs. Several reports have documented the antiinflammatory or anticatabolic effects of omega-3 fatty acids, glucosamine, or chondroitin on human and canine chondrocytes in vitro. Increasing the nutritional intake of EPA has been shown to decrease osteoarthritic pain, probably by decreasing arachidonic acid concentrations and increasing EPA concentrations in the cell membranes of canine chondrocytes. Green-lipped mussel supplements also appear to alleviate the clinical signs of OA in dogs. Our current body of knowledge suggests that the most reasonable drug administration and nutritional plans for arthritic dogs would be to keep them free of clinical signs by using NSAIDs, omega-3 fatty acids, glucosamine, and chondroitin sulphate and by potentially adding adjunctive drugs (if deemed necessary based on the clinical signs or as an alternative to NSAIDs if clinical signs of intolerance are present).

Nonpharmacologic, antiinflammatory options for peripheral pain management include cold therapy (icing) and massage. Icing provides direct pain relief by decreasing nerve conduction velocity. It also provides secondary pain relief by decreasing edema (itself a source of pain) and decreasing the overactivity of catabolic enzymes in osteoarthritic cartilage. Icing is a good consideration for osteoarthritic pets with flares. It may also help after a period of exercise or before bedtime. Ice cubes or frozen vegetables are not recommended because they have large air pockets that decrease cold conduction. Ice bags (filled with ice chips or crushed ice) or cold packs provide more effective cold delivery. Most cold packs reach therapeutic temperatures after 2 hours in a freezer. For long-haired patients, place and hold an ice bag or cold pack directly on the pet's arthritic joint or joints and secure it with a self-adhesive band. A pillowcase may be used between the cold pack or bag and the skin in patients with short or no hair. Some cold packs have a built-in self-adhesive band. A neoprene sleeve may also be used to secure a cold pack or bag. Icing may last for 10 to 15 minutes. Most patients tolerate the treatment. The person applying the ice should make sure the patient is not uncomfortable and that the skin surface feels cold to the touch after icing is complete.

The short- and long-term effects of massage on companion animals are not known. Massage may decrease myofascial pain and muscle tension. Nonpharmacologic options for central pain management include low-level heating; massage; and possibly acupuncture, acupressure, and electroacupuncture. These methods primarily stimulate Aβ sensory fibers with conduction velocities that are more rapid (30 to 70 m/sec) than Aδ (12 to 30 m/sec) and C fibers (0.5 to 3 m/sec).

Heat is widely considered to impact OA patients in pain positively. The use of heat is twofold. Low-level heat (elevation of tissue temperature by 1°C to 2°C) relieves pain through the stimulation of nonnociceptive Aβ sensory fibers, as well as the vasodilation and normalization of blood flow. This low-level tissue relaxation may be achieved by keeping osteoarthritic patients in relatively dry and warm temperatures throughout the day (e.g., sleeping in heated indoor environments or providing heated beds). More intense heat (elevation of tissue temperature by 3°C to 4°C) is used to increase the effectiveness of stretching while minimizing tissue damage. Intense heating is most often applied by a health care professional using a hot pack that is heated by a Hydrocollator or microwave oven. Four layers of dry towels are generally placed between a hot pack and the skin, and heat is generally applied for 15 to 20 minutes. Caution must be used when placing a hot pack on a dog because burns can occur. Initially the packs may not appear excessively hot to the touch, but they can induce thermal damage after several minutes of contact. Therefore it's important to check for excessive redness, skin swelling, or blistering every few minutes during intense-heat therapy.

Maintaining Fitness and Limb Strength

Adult arthritic patients often present with excessive body weight. Although weight loss in dogs is an area that has received much increased attention in recent years, little scientific information regarding the effectiveness of various weight loss plans on overweight and arthritic dogs has been published. Weight loss of 11% to 18% body weight had a clearly beneficial effect on lameness score at a walk and trot in a report involving nine overweight arthritic dogs (Impellizeri et al., 2000). The lifelong benefits of having a lighter body weight on OA, NSAID use, and longevity have been clearly documented in the Labrador retriever lifelong study mentioned previously (Smith et al., 2006). In that study, compared to their overweight counterparts, the lighter dogs required half the NSAIDs over their lifetime and lived 1.8 years longer. However, for both groups lack of mobility late in life because of OA was the dominant cause of euthanasia (Lawler et al., 2005). This study proved that OA progressed more slowly and was more easily controlled in lighter dogs. Similarly, OA was a major reason for euthanasia of military working dogs. Weekly weight loss rates of 1% to 2% body weight are recommended for overweight dogs. This may

be achieved by feeding an amount approximately equivalent to 60% of the calories needed to maintain current body weight.

Muscle strength has been shown to decrease in humans with OA potentially as a result of limb disuse and the reflex inhibition of the contraction of muscles adjacent to arthritic joints. This loss of strength is both quantitative (caused by a loss of muscle mass) and qualitative (caused by a loss of muscle performance). Loss of strength has not been assessed in arthritic dogs to our knowledge. However, loss of muscle mass is universally reported in dogs with chronic hip dysplasia. Maintaining muscle strength is achieved through active exercises with few exceptions. These exceptions include neuromuscular electrical stimulation and active range-of-motion therapy. Neuromuscular electrical stimulation may be considered in arthritic dogs with severe loss of muscle strength who cannot exercise successfully because of severe pain or limb disuse. However, as a general rule it is simpler and more effective to use adapted therapeutic exercises for arthritic patients (Table 244-1).

Cardiovascular fitness and muscle endurance have been poorly described in dogs. Based on the anticipated impact of OA in dogs, it appears reasonable to maintain a good cardiovascular fitness and muscle endurance through regular aerobic physical activities. The building of muscle endurance requires repeated motion over several minutes. Such endurance building is unlikely to be achieved through self-driven activities in areas with limited space such as leaving a dog unattended in an average fenced-in backyard.

As mentioned previously, little is known about the impact of hip arthritis on joint motion; dysplastic hip joints seemingly lose extension but not flexion. A loss of hip extension of 30 degrees or more likely will lead to the dog's inability to gallop, trot, jump up, or climb steps or stairs. Therefore it appears beneficial to assess joint motion in dogs with chronic hip dysplasia. Since it is much easier to maintain joint motion than to regain it when lost, it seems reasonable to recommend intermittent physical activity

---

Table 244-1

Therapeutic Exercises Potentially Included in the Management of Canine Hip Dysplasia

Purpose	Possible Therapeutic Exercises
Increasing limb strength	Daily walk or trot longer than 10 minutes; tunnel-walk repetitions; sit-to-stand and stand-to-sit repetitions
Increasing core strength	Daily walk or trot longer than 10 minutes; swimming
Increasing cardiovascular fitness	Daily walk or trot longer than 10 minutes
Stretching pelvic limbs	Climbing up slopes, hills, and stairs; low jumps
Increasing proprioception	Daily walk or trot longer than 10 minutes; walk on soft surfaces: sand, mulch, gravel, leaves, grass; teeter-totter or pole weaving

that leads to enhanced hip joint extension (compared to a walk on a flat surface) without creating significant clinical signs. These activities may include walking uphill or dancing backward (Weigel et al., 2005). If regaining joint motion is deemed important, a stretching program may be implemented. Stretching is more effective when tissues are heated immediately before and during the stretching session. We empirically recommend performing 10 to 15 repetitions of 20- to 40-second-long sustained stretches during each session. Sessions may be performed two to three times per day. With chronic loss of motion, a gain of 3 to 5 degrees of joint motion per week is anticipated.

Although little is known about the negative impact of naturally occurring OA on proprioception in dogs, there is clear evidence that osteoarthritis progresses rapidly in patients with joint injuries that have sensory deficits. In older humans with decreased proprioception, balance exercises readily improve proprioception. In dogs with OA it is logical to dedicate a small portion of exercise programs to exercises requiring rapid and unpredictable side-to-side weight shifts and to a lesser extent front-to-back and back-to-front weight shifts. These exercises may include walking on soft or irregular surfaces and gentle agility exercises, including pole weaving and walking on a teeter-totter, dog walk, or over low rails.

Choosing a Treatment Program

Dysplastic dogs with minor locomotion problems will have a treatment program focused on decreasing pain, maintaining limb and core strength, stretching affected joints, and stimulating proprioception. Pain management is generally achieved with simple pharmacologic steps, rest, and exercise supervision and customization. Pharmacologic and other forms of pain relief may be intermittent as long as dogs adhere to a long-term exercise program.

Because OA screening is not done routinely in dogs, OA is most often discovered in its later stages. Losing mobility because of severe OA is common in large-breed dogs. For patients with severe OA, it is critically important to implement all possible support strategies to decrease the impact of the disease on the dog's well-being and mobility. These may include multimodal pharmacologic management, ice, heat, massage, acupuncture, acupressure, electroacupuncture, transcutaneous electrical nerve stimulation, and rest. Once pain is managed, it is important to initiate an initially conservative and subsequently progressive exercise program. Patients with severe OA may need temporary or permanent ambulation assistance. Slings are the most common and cost-effective

ambulation assistance devices. Severely impaired dogs may benefit from an ambulation cart. Overall a management program for companion animals with OA should be simple and logical. Managing pain is the first priority for all patients. The program must then address the most critical aspects of each patient's unique situation and over time improve the patient's mobility, strength, proprioception and, above all, quality of life.

References and Suggested Reading

Barr ARS et al: Clinical hip dysplasia in growing dogs: the long-term results of conservative management, *J Small Anim Pract* 28:243, 1987.

Boudrieau RJ, Kleine LJ: Nonsurgically managed caudal acetabular fractures in dogs: 15 cases (1979-1984), *J Am Vet Med Assoc* 193:701, 1988.

Impellizeri JA et al: Effect of weight reduction on clinical signs of lameness in dogs with hip osteoarthritis, *J Am Vet Med Assoc* 216(7):1089, 2000.

Johnston SA: Conservative and medical management of hip dysplasia, *Vet Clin North Am Small Anim Pract* 22(3):595, 1992.

Lascelles BDX et al: Amantadine in a multimodal analgesic regimen for alleviation of refractory osteoarthritis pain in dogs, *J Vet Intern Med* 22:53, 2008.

Lawler DF et al: Influence of lifetime food restriction on causes, time, and predictors of death in dogs, *J Am Vet Med Assoc* 226(2):225, 2005.

Lust G: An overview of the pathogenesis of canine hip dysplasia, *J Am Vet Med Assoc* 210(10):1443, 1997.

Lust G et al: Effects of intramuscular administration of glycosaminoglycan polysulfates on signs of incipient hip dysplasia in growing pups, *Am J Vet Res* 53(10):183, 1992.

Paster ER et al: Estimates of prevalence of hip dysplasia in golden retrievers and rottweilers and the influence of bias on published prevalence figures, *J Am Vet Med Assoc* 226(3):387, 2005.

Puerto DA et al: Relationships between results of the Ortolani method of hip joint palpation and distraction index, Norberg angle, and hip score in dogs, *J Am Vet Med Assoc* 214(4):497, 1999.

Read RA: Conservative management of juvenile canine hip dysplasia, *Aust Vet J* 78(12):818, 2000.

Remedios AM, Fries CL: Treatment of canine hip dysplasia: a review, *Can Vet J* 36(8):503, 1995.

Smith GK et al: Evaluation of risk factors for degenerative joint disease associated with hip dysplasia in German shepherd dogs, golden retrievers, Labrador retrievers, and rottweilers, *J Am Vet Med Assoc* 219(12):1719, 2001.

Smith GK et al: Lifelong diet restriction and radiographic evidence of osteoarthritis of the hip joint in dogs, *J Am Vet Med Assoc* 229(5):690, 2006.

Weigel JP et al: Biomechanics of rehabilitation, *Vet Clin North Am Small Anim Pract* 35:1255, 2005.

CHAPTER 245

Treatment of Animals With Spinal and Musculoskeletal Pain

JOAN R. COATES, *Columbia, Missouri*

Pain is a complex yet continually evolving issue in both human and veterinary medicine. In animals, pain has been defined as "an aversive sensory and emotional experience (a perception), which elicits protective motor actions, results in learned avoidance, and may modify species-specific traits of behavior, including social behavior." (Kitchell, 1987). According to the American Veterinary Medical Association guidelines in recent years, pain management has become an important part of any standard of care when treating our veterinary patients (Colloquium, 1987). Understanding underlying mechanisms of specific pain types (Table 245-1) will assist with the diagnostic approach and establishment of appropriate pharmacologic and clinical interventions for pain management.

CLINICAL ASPECTS OF PAIN INFLUENCING TREATMENT

Pathologic states of clinical pain can be classified as inflammatory pain or neuropathic pain (Muir and Woolf, 2001). Tissue damage or inflammation produces pain through stimulation of nociceptors that are sensitive to mechanical, thermal, and chemical stimuli. Neuropathic pain occurs with injury to neural tissue and represents abnormalities in transmission and somatosensory processing in the peripheral or central nervous system. Some disease processes encompass both nociceptive/inflammatory and neuropathic pain mechanisms. Cancers can infiltrate and compress neural tissue and pain-sensitive structures or cause unlocalizable pain through paraneoplastic effects (Ogilvie and Moore, 2006). Pain associated with chemotherapy and radiation may result from induced axonal injury and vascular compromise.

Pain can be characterized by a careful history to obtain mode of onset and temporal evolution (Table 245-2). Pain in humans is classified based on duration as acute or chronic (Kitchell, 1987). Acute monophasic pain often has an obvious underlying pathologic process that requires immediate clinical intervention to provide relief. Pain is classified as chronic if it exists for more than 6 months. Chronic pain associated with nonprogressive or slowly progressive disease is characteristic of musculoskeletal and neuropathic pain syndromes. The underlying disease process may be apparent, but the associated pain often requires pharmacologic and physical therapies. Pain also is characterized based on site of origin (Kitchell, 1987). It is important to identify factors that exacerbate or relieve the pain. Previous therapy also may influence the disease course.

In human medicine the patient has the ability to record the intensity of pain. Pain intensity in animals is measured using physiologic data and behavioral observation (Conzemius and Hill, 1999; Lorenz and Kornegay, 2004). Examples of physiologic data include heart and respiratory rates; blood pressure; and serum concentrations of cortisol, glucose, and norepinephrine (Holton et al 1998a). Lack of validated diagnostic techniques and pain-scoring systems in veterinary medicine compound the difficulty to reliably assess behaviors associated with pain. Despite establishment of accuracy, significant variability exists among trained observers when using pain-rating scales in veterinary medicine (Holton et al 1998b). Survey instruments for measuring pain are being developed to allow consistency and objectivity of responses for monitoring pain and effects of therapeutic interventions: www.gla.ac.uk/vet/research/cascience/painandwelfare/cmps.htm.

Differential Diagnosis

Determining the underlying cause for inflammatory and neuropathic pain can help guide appropriate treatment strategies and pain management. The neurologic and orthopedic examinations assist with establishment of differential diagnosis. Disorders of chronic onset and neuropathic pain can be more difficult to manage than those of acute onset and inflammatory pain. Spinal and musculoskeletal pain occur in diseases or disorders associated with compression, inflammation, or trauma of pain-sensitive tissues (Table 245-3)(Lorenz and Kornegay, 2004; Platt, 2004).

TREATMENT OF CLINICAL PAIN

Pain management includes determining the cause to the fullest extent and instituting a treatment plan that has established safety and efficacy. An effective treatment plan provides acceptable analgesia with few side effects. In veterinary medicine this may include clinical interventions and pharmacologic and rehabilitative approaches singly or in combination. Currently multicenter, randomized, controlled studies are lacking for management of clinical pain in veterinary medicine. Thus guidelines for pain management often are empirically based. Goals are to reduce pain and improve function as much as possible. Efficacy, tolerability, cost, and safety need consideration with any type of pharmacologic therapy. Routes of administration may factor into effective pain control. Different routes of administration include oral, parenteral (intravenous, intramuscular, subcutaneous), epidural, transdermal, transmucosal, and local nerve blocks (Ogilvie and Moore, 2006). Considerations should also be given for short- and long-term therapeutic regimens (also see Chapter 2).

Identification of mechanisms underlying signal transduction and transmission and processing of painful stimuli has led to the development of drugs that target chemical mediators of pain (Muir and Woolf, 2001). Steroidal and nonsteroidal antiinflammatory drugs (NSAIDs) are effective for inflammation; opioids and α-2 agonists modulate excitatory and inhibitory neuronal

Table 245-1

Nomenclature Used for Description of Pain

Term	Definition
Dysesthesia*	Any abnormal sensation described as unpleasant by patient
Hyperalgesia	Exaggerated pain response from a normally painful stimulus
Hyperpathia	Abnormally painful and exaggerated reaction to a painful stimulus
Hyperesthesia (hypesthesia)	Exaggerated perception of touch stimulus
Allodynia*	Abnormal perception of pain from a normally nonpainful mechanical or thermal stimulus (delay in perception)
Hypoalgesia (hypalgesia)	Decreased sensitivity and raised threshold to painful stimuli
Anesthesia	Reduced perception of all sensation
Analgesia	Reduced perception of pain stimulus
Paresthesia*	Spontaneous abnormal sensation that is not unpleasant
Causalgia*	Burning pain in distribution of one or more peripheral nerves

*Symptoms used to describe pain in humans but difficult to recognize as clinical signs in animals.

Table 245-2

Clinical Characteristics of Pain

Characteristics	Descriptors
Location	*Nociceptive* (musculoskeletal—axial and appendicular; muscles), *neuropathic*
Distribution	Focal, multifocal, diffuse, referred
Mode of onset	Acute (hours to days), chronic (weeks to >3 months)
Temporal evolution	Static, progressive, intermittent, recurrent
Severity	Mild, moderate, severe
Associated behaviors	Vocalization; rubbing, chewing, biting affected area; stiff and stilted gait; guarding; reluctance to move, jump, or climb stairs; unwilling to drink or eat from bowl; attitude change (depression, aggression); unable to obtain resting position or restlessness; anorexia; autonomic signs
Relieving factors	Specific postures and exercise may relieve joint pain, limit movements/activity, therapeutics
Provoking factors	Palpation, specific movements/activities, exercise

Table 245-3

Differentials for Clinical Pain Associated With the Musculoskeletal System

Differential Category	Nociceptive/Inflammatory Pain	Neuropathic Pain
Degenerative	Degenerative joint disease (axial and appendicular skeleton)	IVDD (types I and II), caudal cervical spondylomyelopathy, degenerative lumbosacral syndrome, paraspinal cysts
Anomalous	Axial/appendicular skeletal malformation	Spinal malformation, caudal occipital malformation syndrome (Chiari-like malformation), syringohydromyelia, atlantoaxial instability
Metabolic	Hyperparathyroidism	Hyperparathyroidism
Neoplastic	Primary and metastatic neoplasms of bone, joint, muscle, spine, meninges	Malignant nerve sheath tumor, brain tumor, extradural, intradural/extramedullary, intramedullary (less likely) spinal cord tumors, vertebral/skull tumors, metastatic tumors, paraneoplastic
Nutritional	Hypervitaminosis A	
Inflammatory (infectious/noninfectious)	Osteoarthritis, osteomyelitis, hypertrophic osteodystrophy, infectious and noninfectious meningitis, diskospondylitis, spinal empyema	Meningitis, spinal empyema
Immune	Osteoarthritis, myositis, systemic lupus erythema, rheumatoid disease	Chronic osteoarthritis
Idiopathic		Spinal arachnoid diverticulum
Traumatic	Fracture, type I IVDD	Spinal fracture, type I IVDD extrusion, neuroma, nerve avulsion, syrinx
Vascular	Osteonecrosis	Ischemic neuromyopathy, extradural hemorrhage

IVDD, Intervertebral disk disease.

activity; and local anesthetics suppress electrical impulses (Table 245-4). Nonopioid drugs act at the nociceptor level and alter transduction processes of pain. Opioids alter transmission and perception of pain in the central nervous system. Various pharmacologic regimens most often are based on complementary mechanisms of action that need to be combined in a rational fashion (Muir and Woolf, 2001). For chronic pain combination therapy or multimodality therapies may be more effective than a single agent. NSAIDs appear to have synergistic effects with opioids and may allow for lower dosage of both (Muir and Woolf, 2001; Mathews, 2002).

Nonopioid Analgesics

Glucocorticoids

Inflammatory pain can be alleviated through antiinflammatory actions of glucocorticoids by inducing lymphopenia, reducing differentiation and proliferation of lymphocytes, disrupting cytokine function and intercellular

Table 245-4

Common Drugs Used for Pain Management in Dogs And Cats

Generic Name	Proprietary Name (Company)	Dosage for Dogs	Dosage for Cats
Glucocorticoids			
Prednisone, prednisolone	Generic	0.5-1 mg/kg q12-24h PO	0.5-1 mg/kg or higher q12-24h, PO (prednisolone)
Dexamethasone	Generic	0.07-0.15 mg/kg q12-24h, IV, IM, PO	0.07-0.15 mg/kg q12-24h IV, IM, PO
Nonsteroidal Antiinflammatory Drugs			
Aspirin	Generic	10-25 mg/kg q12h PO	10 mg/kg q48h PO
Etodolac	Etogesic (Fort Dodge Animal Health)	10-15 mg/kg q24h PO	Not used
Carprofen	Rimadyl (Pfizer Animal Health)	2-2.2 mg/kg q12h PO	2-2.2 mg/kg q12h PO (extra-label use)
Ketoprofen	Orudis KT (White-Hall Robins)	1-2 mg/kg q24h PO (extra label use)	1-2 mg/kg q24h PO (extra label use)
Meloxicam	Metacam (Boehringer Ingelheim Vetmedica)	0.1-0.2 mg/kg q24h PO	0.1-0.2 mg/kg q24h for 1-2 days; then 0.025 mg/kg 2-3 times/week PO (extra-label use)
Deracoxib	Deramaxx (Novartis Animal Health)	1-2 mg/kg q24h PO	Not used
Tepoxalin	Zubrin (Schering-Plough Animal Health)	10 mg/kg q24h PO	Not used
Firocoxib	Previcox (Merial)	5 mg/kg q24h PO	Not used
Opioids			
Fentanyl Citrate	Sublimaze (Taylor), Duragesic (Janssen), generic	5 mcg/kg/h CRI 5-10 mcg/kg q2h IV, IM, SQ; 50 mcg/ 10-20 kg q3-5 days, transdermal	2 mcg/kg/h IV CRI 5-10 mcg/kg q2h IV, IM, SQ; 50 mcg q3-5 days, transdermal
Hydromorphone	Dilaudid (Abbott); generic	0.1-0.2 mg/kg q4-6h IV, IM	0.1-0.2 mg/kg q4-6h IV, IM
Morphine	Generic	0.1-1 mg/kg q4h IV, IM, SQ; q8h PO	0.05-0.1 mg/kg q3-6h IM, SQ
Oxymorphone	Numorphan (Endo Labs)	0.1-0.2 mg/kg initial; redose with ½ dose q1-2h IV, IM, SQ	0.1-0.2 mg/kg initial; redose with ½ dose q1-2h IV, IM, SQ
Buprenorphine	Buprenex (Reckitt Benkhiser)	0.005-0.02 mg/kg q4-8h IV, IM, SQ	0.005-0.02 mg/kg q4-8h IV, IM
Butorphanol	Torbugesic (Fort Dodge)	1-4 mg/kg q2-4h, IV, IM, SQ; q6h PO	1.5 mg/kg q2-6h IV, SQ; q4-8h PO
α-2 Agonists			
Medetomidine	Domitor (Pfizer)	5-10 mcg/kg IM or SQ; 1-4 mcg/kg IV	5-10 mcg/kg IM or SQ; 1-4 mcg/kg IV
Xylazine	Rompun (Miles); Generic	0.1-0.5 mg/kg q12h IV, IM, SQ	0.1-0.5 mg/kg q12h IV, IM, SQ
Local (Epidural) Anesthetics			
Bupivacaine	Marcaine (Abbott)	1 ml/10 cm	1 ml/10 cm
Lidocaine	Generic	4.4 mg/kg	4.4 mg/kg
Mepivacaine	Carbocaine (Abbott)	0.5 ml q30sec until absent reflex; not exceeding 8 mg/kg	0.5 ml q30sec until absent reflex; not exceeding 8 mg/kg
Other Drugs			
Tramadol	Ultram (Ortho-McNeil); generic	2-4 mg/kg q6-12h PO	2 mg/kg q12h PO
Amitriptyline	Elavil (Zeneca)	1-4 mg/kg q24h PO	2-4 mg/cat/day PO
Gabapentin	Neurontin (Pfizer); Generic	3-10 mg/kg q8-24h PO	3-10 mg/kg PO q8-24h PO

CRI, Continuous rate infusion; *IM,* intramuscular; *IV,* intravenous.

trafficking among leukocytes, and inhibiting macrophage functions. These mechanisms of action suppress aspects of the inflammatory response by reduction of cell numbers, phagocytosis, migration, and antigen presenting and processing. Glucocorticoids also inhibit phospholipase activity, which converts membrane-released phospholipids to arachidonic acid.

Specific disease processes vary widely in optimal corticosteroid usage (Platt, Abramson, and Garosi, 2005). It is important to obtain a confirmatory diagnosis before glucocorticoid usage. Initial rapid improvements without a differential diagnosis can be misleading. Unsupervised chronic use of corticosteroids without monitoring can lead to deleterious side effects (Behrend and Kemppainen, 1997). Protocols with high-dose regimens should not be combined with antiinflammatory regimens. For compressive spinal cord disease, dexamethasone and prednisone have been administered at antiinflammatory doses to control inflammatory response and pain and to reduce spinal cord edema. Concurrently strict cage rest is important to prevent excessive activity in animals with spinal disease. Only a short-term antiinflammatory regimen of prednisone is recommended. Immunosuppressive regimens are used for immune-mediated causes of musculoskeletal disease. Gradual taper is instituted according to the patient's overall condition.

Nonsteroidal Antiinflammatory Drugs

NSAIDs are most often used for treatment of pain associated with inflammatory conditions but may also be useful in noninflammatory conditions and chronic pain. The antiinflammatory properties of NSAIDs are caused primarily by inhibition of cyclooxygenase (COX) isoenzymes 1 and 2 that synthesize prostanoids from arachidonic acid (Fig. 245-1) COX-1 is constitutive; whereas COX-2 is induced by growth factors, cytokines, and tumor promoters. COX-2 ultimately is synthesized by macrophages and inflammatory cells in the presence of tissue injury and inflammation. Secondary increases in prostanoids amplify nociceptive input and transmission in the peripheral and central nervous systems. COX-2 is involved to a greater degree than COX-1 in pain transmission after tissue injury (Curry, Cogar, and Cook, 2005; Mathews, 2002). Arachidonic acid also is metabolized by lipoxygenase to leukotrienes, which participate as inflammatory mediators (see Fig. 245-1).

Common subclasses of NSAIDs used in dogs and cats include salicylates (aspirin), propionates, indoles, and fenamates. Some NSAIDs have both COX-1 and COX-2 inhibitory effects (aspirin, ketoprofen, etolac), whereas others selectively inhibit COX-2 or are COX-1 sparing (carprofen, meloxicam, deracoxib, tepoxalin, firocoxib) (Curry, Cogar, and Cook, 2005) (see Fig. 245-1). Since COX-2 appears to play a significant role in nociceptive transmission, drugs that spare COX-1 should be sufficient, with fewer adverse effects in pain management. Inhibition of COX isoenzymes may cause arachidonic acid metabolites to enter the lipoxygenase pathway and increase the inflammatory effects of leukotrienes. Some NSAIDs have been shown to inhibit both COX and lipoxygenase (ketoprofen and tepoxalin). Most NSAIDs undergo hepatic metabolism and are eliminated through the enterohepatic circulation or by renal clearance. Adverse reactions associated with NSAIDs occur in the gastrointestinal tract, liver, and kidney. Other side effects may include coagulopathy, inhibition of healing, and altered bone formation. The plethora of different NSAIDs (see Table 245-4) available for use in dogs and cats provides the practitioner with a choice for the most appropriate NSAID that best complements pain management while minimizing patient side effects (Curry, Cogar, and Cook, 2005). Response to a specific NSAID may vary with each individual patient and the type of pain (Mathews, 2002). If one NSAID does not appear to remedy the pain, an alternative NSAID or adjunctive use of a different class of

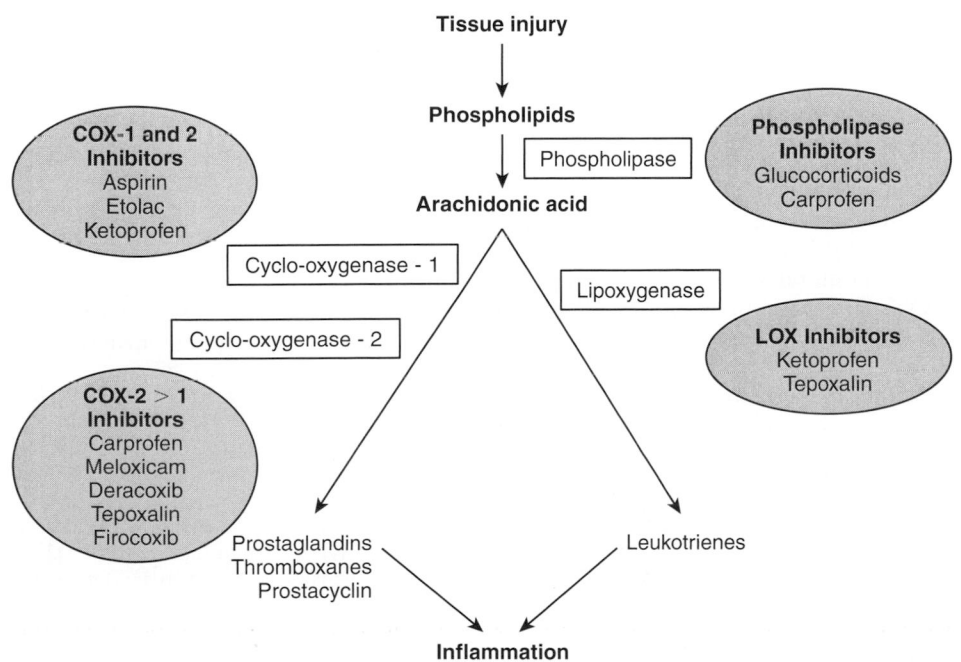

Fig. 245-1 Schematic depicting pharmacologic inhibitors of arachidonic acid metabolism and the cyclooxygenase (COX) and lipoxygenase (LOX) pathways.

analgesic needs consideration. Concurrent use of other NSAIDs or glucocorticoids should be avoided. A "washout" period (48 to 72 hours) should be allowed before administering a different NSAID.

Opioid Analgesics

Opioid analgesics are classified into various groups based on their pharmacologic activity, potency, and clinical use. Type and dosage of opioid selection varies, depending on severity of pain (see Table 245-4). Opioid analgesics modify pain perception and behavioral reactions and relieve anxiety and distress. Pharmacologic dosages of opiates supplement the natural activity of endogenous opiates and suppress neurons in the spine and medulla that transmit pain (Jenkins, 1987). Effectiveness of pharmacologic opiates may vary with route of administration: parenteral, epidural, rectal, oral, and transdermal (fentanyl patch). Direct delivery of opioids to the spinal cord (epidural anesthesia) is used to produce effective anesthesia for surgical procedures. Opioids are more effective for postsurgical and traumatic pain (Chapter 2) and considered less effective for neuropathic pain (Lorenz and Kornegay, 2004; Muir and Woolf, 2001). Opioids that are pure agonists may provide more effective pain control than agonist-antagonist opioids. Tolerance to opiate effects may develop during repeated and chronic administration. Side effects may include altered consciousness, including dysphoria and respiratory depression.

Other Pharmacologic Therapies

α-2 Agonists such as xylazine and medetomidine are centrally acting and possess sedative, muscle relaxant, and analgesic properties (see Table 245-4). Analgesic effects are enhanced when used in combination with opioids. In humans the mainstay for chronic treatment of neuropathic pain is tricyclic antidepressants and anticonvulsants (Truini and Cruccu, 2006). Analgesic actions of antidepressant drugs are most likely related to effects on endogenous pain-modulating pathways (Muir and Woolf, 2001). The anticonvulsant gabapentin has been extensively investigated and proven to be effective for a variety of neuropathic pains. The mechanism of action is unclear. Gabapentin is an analog of γ-aminobutyric acid, the major inhibitory neurotransmitter in the central nervous system. Gabapentin may alter voltage-sensitive ion channels. Unlike many analgesics, gabapentin is minimally metabolized by the liver and eliminated by renal clearance. In veterinary patients gabapentin has been used empirically for management of refractory neuropathic pain. Muscle relaxants (e.g., diazepam, methocarbamol) can be administered for musculoskeletal pains that cause muscle spasm.

Physical Therapy

Physical therapy during recovery from orthopedic and neurologic disorders is important not only for strengthening and increasing flexibility but also for pain reduction (Sherman and Olby, 2004). Physical therapy in recumbent patients begins with passive range of motion (ROM). Joints of limbs are extended and flexed through normal ROM 5 to 10 minutes several times a day. Active ROM includes swimming and standing exercises. Water buoyancy aids in rehabilitation of weak muscles and painful joints by minimizing the amount of weight-bearing on the joint while generating the gait cycle. As the patient begins to ambulate without assistance, therapeutic exercising includes standing and more dynamic ambulation activities, which serve to enhance ROM, muscle strength, balance, and overall daily function. Static and mechanical forms of stretching techniques are performed in conjunction with ROM exercises to prevent fibrosis and contracture of joints and muscles. Other modalities of physical therapy and supplemental therapies that complement mobility therapies include thermal, electrical stimulation, massage, ultrasonographic, acupuncture, and weight loss. Rehabilitation protocols are individually tailored to meet patient's needs during the recovery process.

Surgical Intervention in Spinal Pain

Patients with compressive myelopathy or radiculopathy often require decompressive and/or stabilization procedures (See Chapters 237 and 238). Outcomes in dogs with a rapid onset and defined compressive cause of myelopathy often are favorable (Olby et al., 2003). Long-term outcome of surgery in dogs with chronic-onset compressive or destabilizing myelopathy remains unknown. In humans electrical stimulation or neuroablative surgical procedures have been used to treat central pain with limited success.

References

Behrend EN, Kemppainen RJ: Glucocorticoid therapy: pharmacology, indications, and complications, *Vet Clin North Am Small Anim Pract* 27:187, 1997.

Colloquium on recognition and alleviation of animal pain and distress, *J Am Vet Med Assoc* 191:1184, 1987.

Conzemius MG, Hill CM: Correlation between subjective and objective measures used to determine severity of postoperative pain in dogs, *J Am Vet Med Assoc* 210:1619, 1999.

Curry SL, Cogar SM, Cook JL: Nonsteroidal antiinflammatory drugs: a review, *J Am Anim Hosp Assoc* 41:298, 2005.

Holton LL et al: Relationship between physiological factors and clinical pain in dogs scored using a numerical scale, *J Small Anim Pract* 39:469, 1998a.

Holton LL et al: Comparison of three methods used for assessment of pain in dogs, *J Am Vet Med Assoc* 212:61, 1998b.

Jenkins WL: Pharmacologic aspects of analgesic drugs in animals: an overview, *J Am Vet Med Assoc* 191:1231, 1987.

Kitchell RL: Problems in defining pain and peripheral mechanisms of pain, *J Am Vet Med Assoc* 191:1195, 1987.

Lorenz MD, Kornegay JN: Pain. In Lorenz MD, Kornegay JN, editors: Handbook of veterinary neurology, St Louis, Elsevier, 2004, p 345.

Mathews KA: Non-steroidal anti-inflammatory analgesics: a review of current practice, *J Vet Emerg Crit Care* 12:89, 2002.

Muir WW, Woolf CJ: Mechanisms of pain and their therapeutic implications *J Am Vet Med Assoc* 219:1346, 2001.

Ogilvie GK, Moore AS: Oncologic pain in dogs: prevention and treatment, *Compend Contin Educ Pract Vet* 28:776, 2006.

Olby N et al: Long-term functional outcome of dogs with severe injuries of the thoracolumbar spinal cord: 87 cases (1996-2001), *J Am Vet Med Assoc* 222:762, 2003.

Platt SR: Neck and back pain. In Platt SR, Olby NJ, editors: *BSAVA Manual of canine and feline neurology*, Gloucester, 2004, BSAVA, p 202.

Platt SR, Abramson CJ, Garosi LS: Administering corticosteroids in neurologic diseases, *Compend Contin Educ Pract Vet* 27:210, 2005.

Sherman J, Olby NJ: Nursing and rehabilitation of the neurological patient. In Platt SR, Olby NJ, editors: *BSAVA Manual of canine and feline neurology*, Gloucester, 2004, BSAVA, p 394.

Truini A, Cruccu G: Pathophysiologic mechanisms of neuropathic pain, *Neurol Sci* 27:S179, 2006.

CHAPTER 246

Physical Therapy and Rehabilitation of Neurologic Patients

DARRYL L. MILLIS, *Knoxville, Tennessee*

Physical rehabilitation is an important part of therapy for patients with neurologic conditions. Rehabilitation may be used in a variety of situations, including medical and postsurgical neurologic conditions, peripheral nerve conditions, and neuromuscular disorders. Both upper and lower motor neuron conditions may benefit from rehabilitation. It is important to realize that physical rehabilitation should be used in conjunction with other standard treatments such as decompressive surgery of an intervertebral disk herniation rather than as the primary treatment. The specific rehabilitation plan should be based on the type and severity of the neurologic condition and the specific needs of the patient. In general, maintaining joint function and range of motion, improving balance and proprioception, preserving or increasing muscle strength, and improving overall function are goals for the neurologic patient. Rehabilitation may increase the rate of recovery in patients that are expected to recover eventually from their neurologic condition. In patients with progressive neurologic conditions such as degenerative myelopathy, rehabilitation may retard deterioration of the patient.

JOINT FUNCTION AND PASSIVE RANGE OF MOTION

Placing each joint through a normal range of motion helps to maintain joint health in patients with neurologic deficits. Reduced or unopposed muscle tone of either the flexor or extensor muscles may result in contracture of the joints of the limb if a complete range of motion is not achieved at least daily. Passive range of motion (PROM) should be performed with the patient lying in lateral recumbency on a well-padded area, and the uppermost limbs put through gentle flexion and extension of each joint within the patient's comfortable range of motion. Each joint should be moved through 15 to 20 cycles. As the animal progresses, the entire limb may be put through an exaggerated gait movement, called *range of motion through functional patterns or bicycling*. These movements should be performed for 15 to 20 repetitions. The patient is then repositioned with the other side down, and the exercises are repeated on the other limbs. These exercises should be performed two to four times per day until the patient is able to ambulate or has reached a recovery plateau.

PROM may be combined with stretching in joints that have already lost some range of motion. The affected joint and adjacent muscles should be prewarmed with a warm pack, massage, or both. PROM should be applied to the joint, and on reaching the respective end point of flexion and extension the therapist should exert a gentle stretch for 15 seconds to maintain the joint at the upper limits of flexion or extension, being careful not to induce unnecessary discomfort.

In patients with limited voluntary movement, eliciting a flexor reflex of the forelimb or hind limb results in some muscle contraction, joint motion, and sensory input to the limb and spinal cord. As the limb retracts, additional strengthening may be achieved by providing resistance to limb motion. In patients with poor-to-absent pain perception, caution must be used in eliciting the flexor reflex to avoid damage to the skin and other soft tissues of the toes.

INITIAL STRENGTH, BALANCE, AND PROPRIOCEPTION EXERCISES FOR THE NEUROLOGIC PATIENT

A variety of exercises help to improve strength, balance, and coordination. These exercises are especially useful in patients that have voluntary movement with varying degrees of proprioceptive deficits.

Standing Exercises

The most basic coordination exercise is the standing exercise. It entails having the patient in a standing position with all four limbs placed in a square, symmetric position on the ground with support of the body provided by a sling or other assistive device. As the patient begins to weaken and collapse to the ground, the therapist lifts the dog back into a square standing position. Initially standing exercises are performed for 1 to 3 minutes, with the goal of standing unassisted for 5 minutes. At this point the patient likely has adequate strength and stamina to begin other exercises. Standing in water is also an excellent exercise because the buoyancy of the water helps to support the body while the dog actively tries to stand and move the limbs. Exercise in water must always be attended to prevent drowning! When an animal is able to stand (independently or with some assistance), activities to improve balance may begin. These exercises should be conducted on a nonslip surface to reduce the risk of falling.

Weight Shifting

While the animal is standing, a treat or ball may be used to encourage weight shifting. The therapist should move the treat or ball, allowing the dog to move its head and follow the treat up and down and side to side. He or she should start with small movements and progress to larger, more challenging movements. The movement of the head causes the dog's center of gravity to shift, and the dog must shift its weight to maintain its balance.

The handler may also disturb the animal's balance by gently pushing it at the hips or shoulder. The goal is to disturb its balance just enough so the animal can recover, being careful not to push too hard. Some dogs become conditioned to this activity and shift their weight toward the therapist to prevent being pushed toward the affected side. In this case a rebound weight shift may be effective, with the therapist gently pushing the animal toward the affected side. When the animal shifts its weight to resist, the therapist suddenly releases pressure and simultaneously pushes gently toward the unaffected side. This results in a sudden unbalancing; the animal initially shifts its weight toward the unaffected side, but to keep from falling it shifts its weight back to the affected side. Additional challenges may be added by slowly moving a supporting towel back and forth to force the dog to shift its weight. A limb may also be lifted off the ground. This requires the patient to adjust and redistribute its weight to the remaining three limbs. This exercise may be performed on each limb on an alternating basis. Weight shifts may also be performed during walking. As the animal is walked, the handler gently bumps or pushes the animal to one side. Caution should be exercised to avoid falls and injury.

Assisted Ambulation/Gait Training

If a dog is unable to walk independently, a sling, towel, harness, or canine cart may be used to support the animal as needed. Encourage the dog to move slowly, allowing time for it to advance the limbs as independently as possible. It may be necessary to manually assist the dog in the sequencing and placement of the limbs. The emphasis is on weight bearing with each and every step, encouraging a slow gait so that neuromuscular coordination and muscle strengthening may occur. Walking in water is beneficial because the animal's weight is partially supported and the limbs typically move at a slower speed than land-based walking. Supported swimming can also provide benefits in patients with severe neurologic conditions; in some cases animals generate some limb movement, even if in an uncoordinated fashion, allowing strengthening and neuromuscular reeducation.

ADVANCED STRENGTH, BALANCE, AND PROPRIOCEPTION EXERCISES FOR THE NEUROLOGIC PATIENT

A platform may be used to rock the dog forward and backward and side to side. A human Biomechanical Ankle Platform System board may be used to help the animal practice proprioceptive positioning on just the forelimbs or the hind limbs. If the goal is to have the animal exercise using all four limbs, a specially made platform must be used that accommodates quadrupeds. It is important to provide support to allow the animal to shift its weight and exercise its proprioceptive mechanism.

Several commercial or homemade objects may also be used for this purpose. Balance balls or rolls are large-diameter exercise round or elongated balls that the patient can be placed on and supported to improve balance, coordination, and strength. The forelimbs are placed on the ball and supported by the handler, requiring the dog to maintain static balance of the caudal trunk and rear limbs. Dynamic balance may also be challenged as the ball or roll is slowly moved forward, backward, and side to side, challenging the rear legs to maintain balance while movement occurs. To address the cranial trunk and forelimbs, the rear limbs are placed over the ball as the forelimbs are asked to balance the body weight during both stance and gentle movements. A balance board is a rectangular piece of plywood with a narrow rod running longitudinally or transversely along the bottom. The board tips in a lateral or cranial-caudal direction, respectively, when the patient stands on it. Cavaletti rails are horizontal poles that are elevated such that the patient must pick its limbs up to step over the poles. Having the patient walk across or stand on a foam mattress or trampoline may also be used to improve balance and coordination.

Balancing and coordination activities may be incorporated into regular walking activities. Altering the texture of the ground challenges the animal's functional walking proprioceptive ability. Standing or walking on foam-rubber mattresses, air mattresses, and trampolines allows the animal to negotiate various surfaces. The patient may also spend part of its walk negotiating cavaletti rails, which challenges the patient's ability to negotiate obstacles of different heights. These exercises should be continued until the patient has a normal or very near–normal gait.

In addition to walking over regular surfaces and surfaces of differing textures, dogs may be walked on the ground or on an underwater treadmill. Walking on a treadmill provides additional challenges to proprioception and is valuable in rehabilitation of human stroke patients. Walking on an underwater treadmill allows support of the patient's body weight, and the water provides resistance of movement and muscle strengthening. Other strengthening activities include sit-to-stand exercises, walking with weights strapped on the limbs, or placing elastic bands around the distal limb with the therapist providing gentle resistance during motion.

ASSISTIVE DEVICES

Assistive devices provide increased independence for the pet, give support to a weak or nonfunctioning body part, and help the handler maintain proper body mechanics while performing therapy. These devices can also help to protect the feet during walking to prevent ulcers from forming. They are available in a variety of forms, including slings, two-wheeled and four-wheeled carts, boots, and prosthetics.

Boots are an excellent way to protect the feet when an animal with neurologic deficits is knuckling or turning its feet over and walking on the dorsum of the foot. Animals with poor proprioception are unaware of the placement of their distal limbs and tend to walk on the dorsum of their paws or drag the nails when walking. Boots act as socklike coverings that are securely fastened by Velcro straps at the top. Most have a rubber sole to prevent slipping and are machine washable. It is important to remove the boots periodically (several times daily) to assess skin condition, especially in neurologically impaired patients, and, if possible, to increase weight bearing and proprioception through the bottom of the pads when performing therapeutic exercise. If not fitted properly, boots can interrupt circulation, become cumbersome and impede gait patterns or strides, and potentially cause more problems if the animal stumbles and falls. Proper fit is essential, and appropriate client education instructions for skin care and rehabilitative exercises must be communicated to the owner.

When choosing the proper boot, the handler should ascertain that it is washable, waterproof or water resistant, and constructed of durable material that will not wear down quickly. The bottom surface should have a nonskid material that prevents slipping. Old socks may also be used to help provide padding; however, caution must be exercised if the top is secured with tape to avoid cutting off circulation.

Slings come in a variety of shapes and sizes. Some products may be strapped around the belly or fitted for the forelimbs, hind limbs, or both. Slings should have long handheld straps attached to allow proper body mechanics to avoid personal injury to the handler when supporting the pet. These devices aid in transitioning a recumbent animal to a standing position and are especially useful for larger dogs. A sling can also assist with ambulation and prevent falls on slippery floors, especially after surgery, thereby avoiding further injury to the animal. Support slings are also available for forelimb assistance.

Slings are available in a variety of sizes to provide the best fit. It is important to select a properly sized sling for safety and comfort of the patient. The sling used for the forelimbs should not obstruct respiration, and urine flow should not be compromised with hind limb slings in male dogs. A sling should have a soft lining against the animal's skin to avoid irritation and sores, and the material should be washable. The sling must not be too thin, especially around the groin and belly region, to avoid excessive pressure and development of sores. Slings are also useful during the later phases of rehabilitation for supporting standing during therapeutic exercises such as repeated sit to stands. When documenting patient progress, the amount of assistance given through sling support can be rated as minimum, moderate, or maximum assistance.

Carts, or canine wheelchairs, provide support, allow independence for the animal, and help prevent the deleterious effects of recumbency. Two- or four-wheeled carts are available for disabled paraplegic or quadriplegic patients. Carts should not be used too early in the course of rehabilitation because dogs may become too dependent on their support. They should be fitted properly according to manufacturers' recommendations. Animals should be supervised at all times when in a cart so that they do not fall down stairs or tip over, and dogs should not be placed in the cart for long periods of time to prevent fatigue. Skin condition should be assessed daily to be certain that no areas of tissue breakdown occur.

MANAGING THE RECUMBENT PATIENT

Some conditions require a lengthy recovery, and animals initially may be recumbent. During this critical time, it is especially important to provide intensive nursing care to avoid serious complications.

Recumbent patients should be placed on a padded bed. An absorbent pad should be placed under the animal if incontinence is an issue. For patients that urinate frequently, it may be necessary to have the animal on an elevated grate that will not allow urine to pool under the patient. Appropriate bladder management must be performed carefully, balancing evacuation of the bladder with minimum trauma while expressing the bladder. Appropriate pharmacologic intervention may be useful to minimize urine retention (see Chapter 207). Animals recumbent for a very long time are at risk for developing decubital ulcers. Dogs with thin skin and prominent bony protuberances such as greyhounds and whippets are especially prone to developing decubital ulcers. Preventing ulcers is far superior to treating them. Therefore the skin should be assessed each day for redness or other evidence of skin breakdown. Patients should be kept on a soft padded bed and turned every 4 to 6 hours. If redness or irritation of skin is noted, a "donut" may be made to help distribute pressure away from the area.

The environment should be comfortable for the patient. The animal should be moved from a cold, damp environment to a warm, dry inside environment. A soft, well-padded bed or waterbed should be offered. A circulating warm-water blanket may reduce morning stiffness, but an electric heating pad that cycles on and off should be avoided because it may cause burns if the patient cannot get away from it if it is too hot. Consideration should be given to the activities of other pets in the household, because they may be a source of irritation to dogs recovering from neurologic conditions. Changes should be made to minimize climbing stairs. Commercial ramps or steps are available to help patients get into cars or on furniture.

REHABILITATION CONSIDERATIONS IN PATIENTS WITH SPECIFIC CONDITIONS

Intervertebral Disk Disease

Canine patients with intervertebral disk disease are presented with a variety of clinical manifestations. Most have thoracolumbar disk disease, although cervical disk disease is also common. Most dogs have upper motor neuron signs, although lower motor neuron signs may be present in some cases. Finally, consideration must be given to whether a patient has had surgical intervention or if conservative therapy has been initiated. Rehabilitation efforts should be directed to correct decreased or absent superficial or deep pain, decreased or absent motor function, ataxia and proprioceptive deficits, muscle atrophy of variable severity, and tense back and limb muscles.

In most cases it is contraindicated to perform any type of active exercise in animals with acute back pain and neurologic deficits that are managed conservatively because the annulus fibrosis is weak and exercise may worsen the condition. These dogs require strict cage rest until the annulus

---

Box 246-1

Sample Rehabilitation Program for Dogs With Intervertebral Disk Disease

Step 1: Immediately After Surgery to Supporting Weight
- Cryotherapy of the incision site and underlying tissues to reduce inflammation and swelling of the surgical area for 20-30 minutes TID
- Passive range of motion (PROM) to all joints of the affected limbs, 20 repetitions BID-TID
- Massage of the limb muscles in cases with upper motor neuron lesions; tapotement of the muscles may be beneficial to help maintain muscle tone in cases with lower motor neuron lesions
- Neuromuscular electrical stimulation to the affected muscles is helpful to attenuate muscle atrophy if lower motor neuron signs are present
- Standing exercises instituted the day after surgery to encourage neuromuscular reeducation of the muscles responsible for maintaining normal standing posture and to strengthen muscles to allow weight bearing and ambulation
- Nursing care instituted to recumbent dogs
- Use of assistive devices such as slings for body support and protective boots to help protect feet from injury and to position the foot in a more natural standing position

Step 2: Supporting Weight to Initial Motor Function
- PROM and standing exercises continued
- Standing in water and assisted swimming begun to encourage early motor function
- Weight-shifting exercises in a standing position
- Assisted walking with support

Step 3: Initial Motor Function to Good Motor Function With Proprioceptive Deficits
- Swimming
- Ground treadmill walking with the therapist positioned to assist gait and correct placement of the foot when it is advanced and to help with gait training

- Balancing activities such as a balance board, weight shifts, standing on a physioroll while it is rocked back and forth; varying the speed of ambulation, incorporating "zig-zags" figure eights, circles to the right and left when walking; walking on trampolines or other unstable surfaces

Step 4: Good Motor Function With Proprioceptive Deficits to Near-Normal Gait
- Swimming and treadmill walking continued, with increased speed and length of treadmill walking to help challenge patients to achieve a higher level of functioning
- Stair climbing and sit-to-stand exercises may be added for proprioceptive and strength training
- Balancing activities continued as in step 3
- Walking over raised cavaletti rails
- Jogging may be added as the patient regains proprioceptive functioning

Step 5: Near Normal To Normal Gait
- Activities in previous steps may be continued
- The length of time spent swimming is increased to improve endurance and strength
- Jogging on the treadmill and jogging up and down small stairs may be added to encourage proprioceptive challenges at higher speeds
- Walking over raised cavaletti rails is continued; and, if the patient is able, it may negotiate the rails while jogging
- Playing ball is added as the patient nears return to a normal gait

heals sufficiently to withstand the additional stress of mild activity. Massage, transcutaneous electrical nerve stimulation, and PROM of joints may be administered. After 3 to 6 weeks whirlpool therapy may be used cautiously in patients carefully supported in a sling. Progressive strengthening may be achieved with deep-water aquatic therapy, proprioception exercises on therapy balls or rolls, assisted walking, and dry and underwater treadmill activity.

Postoperative physical rehabilitation is an integral part of the overall care of patients having decompressive surgery and is provided in a stepwise fashion, with activities based on the stage of recovery (Box 246-1).

Degenerative Myelopathy

Although degenerative myelopathy is a progressive condition with no known cure, one study indicated that dogs that received intensive physical rehabilitation had a longer mean survival time (255 days) compared with dogs with moderate (130 days) or no (55 days) therapy (Kathmann et al, 2006). Moreover, affected dogs receiving physical rehabilitation remained ambulatory longer than animals that did not receive physical treatment. A sample rehabilitation program is outlined in Box 246-2.

Box 246-2

Sample Rehabilitation Program for Dogs With Degenerative Myelopathy*

Active Exercises
- Slow leash walking 5-10 minutes at least five times/day
  - If knuckling, place protective boots or use an elastic band around the foot to allow the therapist to correct the position of the paw with each step
  - Short, frequent exercise periods are preferred to long exercise periods
  - A rolled towel may be taped to the middle of a sling to maintain the hind limbs in a normal position or in slight abduction if the dog has a tendency to adduct the limbs while walking
- Sit-to-stand exercise if the dog is able
- Assistance with a sling if needed or sit-to-stand from an elevated position or in water
- Weight-shifting exercises while standing
- Walking on different surfaces
- Stair climbing, walking uphill

Passive Exercises
- Passive range of motion of each joint of both hind limbs three times/day, 20 repetitions for each joint
- Massage of the paravertebral muscles and limbs, starting distally and working to proximal three times/day
- Hydrotherapy
- If available, walking on underwater treadmill; otherwise, swimming or walking in water, depending on dog's ability at least once a week, 5-20 minutes
  - The type, length, and intensity of the exercise should be adapted to the dog's condition
  - Assistance with a sling is provided as needed
  - Weight shifting while standing in water is encouraged, especially in the later stages

*Modified from Kathmann et al., 2006.

Peripheral Nerve Injury

Currently there are no accurate clinical indicators of whether a peripheral nerve injury will recover and, if so, the degree of recovery that will occur. If a degree of function does return, the functional status of the affected limb will depend on the degree of muscle atrophy that occurs during the period of nerve regeneration and contracture of joints. Muscle atrophy associated with nerve injury is a combination of disuse and degeneration. The ability of the patient to regain functional use of a limb depends on a number of factors, including the severity of nerve injury; the distance through which the nerve must regenerate; the age of the patient; and other associated tendon, soft-tissue and bony damage. Electrical stimulation of denervated muscle during the period of nerve regeneration may help to maintain the integrity of the muscle fibers and their potential functional capacity. Studies have indicated a beneficial effect of electrical stimulation on denervated muscles, with improved morphology and functional capacity of the reinnervated stimulated muscles when compared with nonstimulated controls (Williams, 1996). In addition to electrical stimulation of muscles, it is also important to perform PROM and stretching to help prevent contracture of joints, especially of the digits, as a result of unopposed muscle tone in some peripheral nerve injuries. These exercises must be performed several times daily throughout the recovery period to avoid pathologic shortening of muscle-tendon units and fibrosis of joint capsules. Stimulation of the flexor reflex, standing exercises, aquatic activity, and other weigh-bearing exercises may be performed as the patient progresses.

References and Suggested Reading

Bochstahler B: Neurological diseases. In Bockstahler B, Levine D, Millis DL, editors: *Essential facts of physiotherapy in dogs and cats,* Babenhausen, Germany, 2004, VetVerlag, p 227.

Hamilton S et al: Therapeutic exercises. In Millis DL, Levine D, Taylor RA, editors: *Canine rehabilitation and physical therapy,* Philadelphia, 2004, Elsevier, p 244.

Kathmann I et al: Daily controlled physiotherapy increases survival time in dogs with suspected degenerative myelopathy, *J Vet Intern Med* 20:927, 2006.

Levine D, Ritenberry L, Millis DL: Aquatic therapy. In Millis DL, Levine D, Taylor RA, editors: *Canine rehabilitation and physical therapy,* Philadelphia, 2004, Elsevier, p 264.

Millis DL, Lewelling A, Hamilton S: Range of motion and stretching exercises. In Millis DL, Levine D, Taylor RA, editors: *Canine rehabilitation and physical therapy,* Philadelphia, 2004, Elsevier, p 228.

Olby N, Halling K, Glick T: Rehabilitation for the neurological patient, *Vet Clin North Am Small Anim Pract* 2005.

Shealy P, Thomas WB, Immel L: Neurologic conditions and physical rehabilitation of the neurologic patient. In Millis DL, Levine D, Taylor RA, editors: *Canine rehabilitation and physical therapy,* Philadelphia, 2004, Elsevier, p 388.

Williams HB: The value of continuous electrical muscle stimulation using a completely implantable system in the preservation of muscle function following motor nerve injury and repair: an experimental study, *Microsurgery* 17:598, 1996.

CHAPTER 247

Hypokalemic Myopathy in Cats

BOYD R. JONES, *Dublin, Ireland*

Hypokalemia results from one of the following: reduced potassium intake, increased potassium entry into the cells, or increased potassium loss from the body. Of these causes in cats, renal potassium loss is the most important, especially if such loss is associated with inadequate intake. In healthy cats the daily potassium intake should equal daily loss. Potassium maintains the intracellular fluid volume and normal membrane potential. If the ratio between intracellular and extracellular potassium is altered significantly, the muscle membrane potential of excitatory tissue such as nerve and muscle is affected. Hypokalemia significantly affects muscle membrane activity and muscle function and can, if severe, result in rhabdomyolysis. As potassium is depleted, a progressive increase in the muscle cell resting transmembrane potential (hyperpolarization) results so that the myocyte becomes increasingly refractory to electrical stimulation. Eventually, however, the muscle cell membrane suddenly becomes permeable to sodium ions, and the resulting sudden membrane hypopolarization induces rapid, severe weakness. If the potassium deficit is not corrected, the muscular dysfunction may progress to paralysis. The increase in intracellular sodium (and chloride) often exceeds the degree of potassium depletion that predisposes to rhabdomyolysis by osmotic expansion of the cell (Fettman, 1989). Additional factors that may contribute to the myopathy and rhabdomyolysis are a reduction in muscle blood flow that occurs with exercise and altered muscle carbohydrate metabolism (Fettman, 1989).

There have been numerous reports of polymyopathy in cats associated with a variety of different causes of hypokalemia (Box 247-1). Of these causes, cats with chronic renal failure and Burmese kittens that develop hypokalemia associated with disturbances in the intracellular and extracellular balance of potassium show the most severe myopathic signs. The syndrome in Burmese kittens (2 to 6 months of age) bears many similarities to hypokalemic periodic paralysis in humans, a condition that is thought to be related to a calcium channel disorder. The condition has a familial and inherited basis (putative autosomal-recessive), with affected kittens being produced in specific lines of this breed.

In the acquired disease dietary factors appear to contribute significantly to the development of hypokalemia and subsequent myopathy; potassium-depleted diets, acidifying diets, magnesium-restricted diets, and high-protein diets have been incriminated. In recent years pet food manufacturers have ensured that appropriate concentrations of minerals are added and that the formulation of diets for cats is not overacidifying. Primary hyperaldosteronism (Conn's syndrome) caused by a functional tumor of the zona glomerulosa of the adrenal glands has been reported more frequently in aged cats. Both benign adenoma and adenocarcinoma have been found (Shiel and Mooney, 2007).

CLINICAL SIGNS

Whatever the cause of hypokalemia, the clinical signs shown by the affected cats are similar. The clinical signs may be transient or persistent. The earliest sign of severe potassium depletion is muscle dysfunction. There is generalized muscle weakness with persistent ventroflexion of the neck, with the head being tucked into the sternum (Fig. 247-1). The cats are intolerant of exercise; and some walk with an awkward, stiff, stilted gait. There may be exertional muscle tremor followed by sudden fatigue and collapse. Severely affected cats are reluctant to move, and some owners report that their cat showed lethargy and tiredness for some months before a severe episode occurred. Some cats show pain when their muscles are palpated. The clinical course in Burmese kittens is much more transient, with moderate-to-severe episodes followed by improvement (with or without treatment)

Box 247-1

Some Conditions Associated With Hypokalemia in Cats

- Acidified diets
- Chronic renal failure
- Chronic vomiting /diarrhea
- Diet—Potassium deficient or prolonged anorexia
- Diuretic therapy (furosemide)
- Fluid administration (plasma dilution and volume-induced diuresis)
- Hepatic disease
- Hyperaldosteronism (Conn's syndrome) caused by an adrenocortical tumor
- Idiopathic (Burmese breed)
- Infectious disease
- Insulin overdose
- Metabolic acidosis
- Metabolic alkalosis
- Potassium deficiency
- Renal tubular acidosis
- Systemic diseases
- Thyrotoxicosis

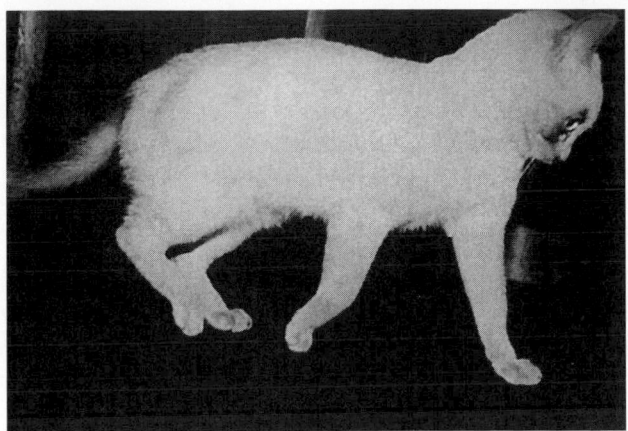

Fig. 247-1 A 9-month-old Burmese cat with hypokalemia and ventroflexion of the head.

and relapse. Postural reactions and spinal reflexes are normal.

Cats with advanced potassium depletion may show other signs, including poor body condition with weight loss; a poor, unkempt hair coat; and polydipsia and polyuria. These latter signs are mostly present in cats in which concurrent chronic renal failure is present.

Cats with Conn's syndrome may have concurrent hypertension with hypertensive cardiac, ocular, or neurological signs, or they may be asymptomatic.

DIAGNOSIS

The history, clinical findings, and breed (Burmese) provide a high index of suspicion of hypokalemia and the likely cause of potassium depletion.

The presence of low serum potassium, usually less than 3 mmol/L, confirms the diagnosis of hypokalemia; however, clinical signs occasionally can develop in cats with higher serum potassium values. Furthermore, serum potassium concentrations can increase after cage confinement or hospitalization because the myopathy and clinical signs are frequently precipitated or exacerbated by exercise. The low serum potassium concentration is frequently accompanied by increased serum activity (5,000 to 10,000 units/L) of serum creatine kinase (CK). The CK is released only when the concentration of potassium in muscle is very low. In affected Burmese kittens serum CK values can be very elevated (>50,000 units/L).

Other biochemical abnormalities that have been observed in hypokalemic cats include azotemia, hypercholesterolemia, hyperchloridemia, hyperglycemia, and elevated serum creatinine. Such findings are frequently associated with concurrent renal dysfunction.

Elevation of blood pressure in conjunction with hypokalemia may suggest primary hyperaldosteronism. In such cases, ultrasonography of the adrenal glands is recommended and may detect unilateral adrenal enlargement, with or without local invasion or metastasis, if an aldosterone-secreting tumor is present.

Determination of the fractional excretion of potassium as ascertained by the formula that follows may help differentiate renal and nonrenal sources of potassium loss. The FE_{K^+} should be less than 5% in a healthy cat with normal renal function and a potassium-depleted cat with normal renal function (e.g., in Burmese kittens with idiopathic hypokalemia). An FE_{K^+} of greater than 10% to 15% indicates significant renal potassium loss. Urinary loss may be determined more accurately by measuring the 24-hour urinary potassium loss.

$$FE_{K^+} (\%) = \frac{UK^+}{PK^+} \times \frac{PCr}{UCr} \times 100$$

where P = plasma, U = urine, Cr = creatinine, and K^+ = potassium.

The differential diagnosis of hypokalemic myopathy includes polyneuropathy, myasthenia gravis, organophosphate toxicity, thiamine deficiency, other electrolyte abnormalities, primary myopathies, tick paralysis, and snake bite.

Diffuse electromyographic abnormalities are sometimes present (e.g., positive sharp waves may be recorded). Muscle biopsy specimens are mostly normal on light microscopy, but mild myofiber necrosis is observed occasionally.

TREATMENT

The goal of treatment of the cat with hypokalemia and myopathic signs is to restore the serum potassium concentration to and maintain it in the reference range without causing the toxic side effects of potassium therapy. The clinical signs of muscle weakness are reversible, and the response to potassium supplementation is rapid. If potassium depletion is severe, potassium supplementation should be administered both orally and intravenously according to the dosage and administration rates detailed in Table 247-1. Intravenous potassium supplementation should not exceed 0.5 mmol(mEq)/kg/hr; otherwise cardiac dysrhythmias or asystole may occur. Electrocardiographic monitoring during therapy should be considered, and administration stopped if

Table **247-1**

Intravenous Potassium Administration*

Serum Potassium (mmol/L)	Potassium Chloride Added to Fluids[†]	Maximum Volume Infusion Rate (ml/kg/hr) [‡]
3.6-5.0	20	25
3.1-3.5	30	17
2.6-3.0	40	12
2.1-2.5	60	8
<2.0	80	6

*Includes quantity and rate of administration not to exceed 0.5 mmol of potassium per liter per hour.
[†]mmol (mEq) of potassium per liter of crystalloid fluid; sufficient KCl should be added to achieve this concentration per liter.
[‡]Infusion rate of crystalloid (e.g., lactated Ringer's solution) containing supplemental KCl.
Note: Never inject KCl solutions intravenously.

dysrhythmias occur. It should be noted that in some cats the serum potassium may actually decline with intravenous fluid therapy, and frequent determinations should be made.

Once acute potassium depletion is corrected, oral treatment should be continued (see following paragraphs). If the cat is not severely affected, oral potassium supplementation is safe and effective for correcting clinical signs.

Potassium gluconate solution (Kaon Elixir, Adria Laboratories), tablets, or powder (Tumil K, Daniels Pharmaceuticals) can be administered in food. Potassium chloride is not an appropriate oral form of potassium because it can contribute to metabolic acidosis. A dosage rate of 2 to 4 mmol/cat/day orally is a safe and usually effective starting dosage. The serum potassium concentration should be rechecked every 10 to 14 days until serum values are stable in the reference range.

The link between renal disease and potassium depletion is well established; and, importantly, there is evidence that oral potassium supplementation will improve or stabilize the remaining renal function. Potassium depletion can contribute to ongoing renal damage; therefore cats with chronic renal failure should receive daily oral potassium supplementation (2 to 4 mmol/cat/day orally). Burmese kittens with transient periodic hypokalemia also benefit from daily oral supplementation.

If a diagnosis of hypokalemia is correct, the response to intravenous or oral potassium therapy is usually favorable and rapid (2 to 5 days). However, complete recovery of normal muscle strength in cats with myopathy can take up to several weeks. The prognosis is favorable with most affected cats, especially Burmese kittens, but the severity of the renal disease may alter that prognosis in some cats. In cats with Conn's syndrome the prognosis depends on identification and effective surgical treatment of the adrenal tumor. Preoperative stabilization of the hypokalemia and hypertension (if present) is required and important for optimal management. Concurrent therapy with spironolactone (2-4 mg PO q24h) and amlodopine (0.625-1.25 mg/cat, q24h) is recommended.

References and Suggested Reading

Dow SW et al: Hypokalemia in cats: 186 cases (1984-87), *J Am Vet Med Assoc* 194:1604, 1989.

Fettman MJ: Feline kaliopenic polymyopathy/nephropathy syndrome, *Vet Clin North Am Small Anim Pract* 19:415, 1989.

Mardell F, Sparkes A: Investigation of feline hypokalaemia, *BSAVA Manual Canine and Feline Endocrinology* ed 3, BSAVA, 2004, p 43.

Shiel R, Mooney CT: Diagnosis and management of primary aldosteronism in cats, *In Practice* 29:194, 2007.

SECTION XII

Ophthalmic Diseases

David J. Maggs

VOLUME XIII CONTENT ON EVOLVE: http://evolve.elsevier.com/Bonagura/Kirks/

CHAPTER 248

Pearls of the Ophthalmic Examination

DAVID J. MAGGS, *Davis, California*

Although signalment and historical data often provide essential clues to ocular diagnoses, ready visualization of almost all parts of the eye means that nothing can replace a complete examination. Fortunately a thorough ophthalmic examination is performed with just five requirements, five skills, and minimal equipment.

There are five essential requirements for a thorough ophthalmic examination:

1. Patient and veterinarian at eye level with each other
2. Dim ambient light
3. A bright and focal light source
4. A source of magnification
5. An orderly and complete approach

To minimize the extent to which the eyelids and orbital structures obscure the ocular structures, the patient should always be placed at eye level with the examining veterinarian. This is usually achieved simply by placing the patient on the examination table, which also limits patient movement. Having an assistant rather than the owner restrain the pet further reduces movement and is especially important when a detailed examination with magnification is performed. Since many structures within the normal eye are transparent, they are best examined in a darkened room using a very focal light source. This combination maximizes reflections, which are useful for examining ocular surfaces and enhance the examiner's ability to direct the light and their attention into the darker interior of the globe. Many ocular abnormalities are small and will be missed without a source of magnification and a bright light source. This combination can best be achieved in practice using an Optivisor head loupe and Finoff (Welch-Allyn) transilluminator. A readily available alternative is the otoscope used without the plastic cone. This provides a focal light source and approximately 2× to 3× magnification. Slit-lamp biomicroscopes are used by ophthalmologists and some general practitioners and maximize the combination of magnification and focal light source. By focusing the light to a narrow slit, an optical section provides microscopic detail in transparent ocular media such as the tear film, cornea, aqueous, lens, and vitreous.

The ophthalmic examination should be carried out in a repeatable and sequential manner to ensure that nothing is overlooked. A prepared examination sheet reminds the practitioner to perform all necessary tests in the correct sequence and permits lesions to be drawn. The examination begins by examining the patient from a distance for behavioral evidence of vision loss. The patient's head and periocular tissues should then be more closely examined for facial symmetry, globe position and movement, periocular discharge, and overt ocular abnormalities. Brief but complete testing of the cranial nerves involved in normal ocular function follows. This should include tests of the menace response, palpebral reflex, pupillary light reflex, and dazzle reflex. More detailed examination of each eye is then performed.

Examining the unaffected eye before the affected eye in animals with unilateral disease ensures that the normal eye is not forgotten and provides information on each patient's normal ocular appearance.

Mastering the following five skills will provide all of the essential information from the anterior and posterior segments of the eye:

1. Retroillumination
2. Transillumination (or focal illumination)
3. Tonometry (measurement of intraocular pressure)
4. Assessment of aqueous flare
5. Fundic examination

Retroillumination is a simple but extremely useful technique for assessment of pupils and all parts of the transparent ocular media (tear film, cornea, aqueous, lens, and vitreous). A focal light source such as a Finoff transilluminator is held close to the examiner's eye and directed over the bridge of the patient's nose from at least arm's length (Fig. 248-1). Alternatively the direct ophthalmoscope can be held up against the examiner's eye (as for the fundic examination, see skill 5) but about arm's length from the patient. Either technique will elicit the fundic reflection, which is usually gold or green in tapetal animals or red in atapetal individuals. Because the examination is done at arm's length, each eye can be illuminated equally, and the fundic reflex can be used to assess and compare equality of pupil size and shape. In addition, opacities in any of the clear ocular media (e.g., corneal blood vessels, cataracts, vitreous debris) will obstruct the fundic reflection and are noted as black "shadows" against the fundic reflection. These opacities should be noted for subsequent and more detailed examination, with retroillumination repeated from close to the patient following pupil dilation. They should also be examined using transillumination and a source of magnification. Retroillumination is particularly useful for differentiating nuclear sclerosis from cataract.

Transillumination (sometimes called *focal illumination*) is then used to sequentially examine all ocular structures in front of and including the lens (the "anterior segment"). A focal light source should be directed at the eye from

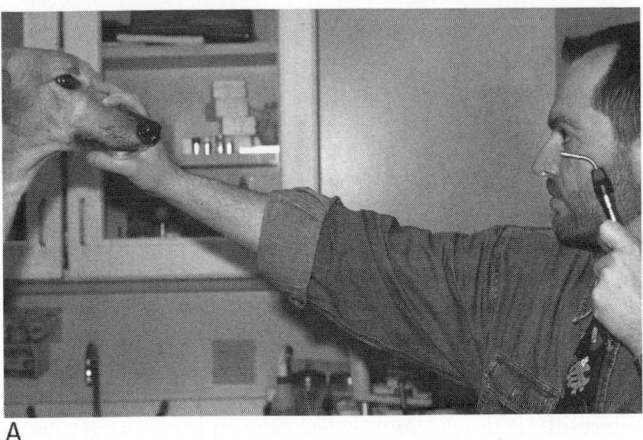
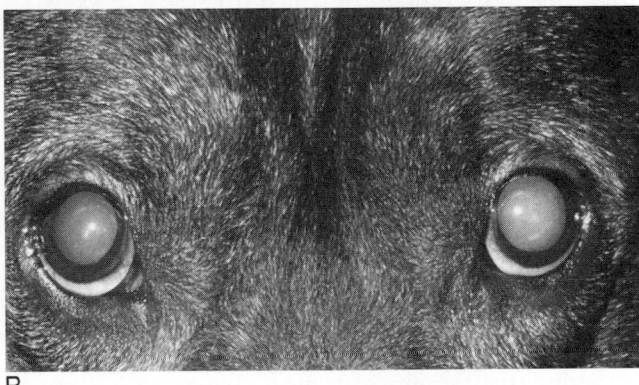

Fig. 248-1 Retroillumination. A Finoff transilluminator is held close to the examiner's eye and directed over the bridge of the patient's nose from at least arm's length **(A).** The reflection from the animal's fundus is used to judge pupil size and the clarity of the ocular media. **B,** This patient has nuclear sclerosis visible as a subtle ring inside the pupil. (From Maggs DJ et al: Slatter's fundamentals of veterinary ophthalmology, ed 4, 2008, St. Louis, Saunders.)

many angles while the examiner simultaneously varies the viewing angle (Fig. 248-2). Varying the viewing and lighting angles relative to each other permits the examiner to use parallax, reflections, perspective, and shadows to gain valuable information regarding lesion depth. This technique is particularly useful for examining the anterior chamber since changes within this chamber can be more easily differentiated from corneal, iridal, or lenticular changes when viewed transversely. In cats the corneal curvature and anterior chamber depth are so great that limited visualization of the iridocorneal angle is also possible.

The importance of a sequential anterior segment examination cannot be overstated. An obvious method is to begin at the front and progress to the back of the eye while simultaneously moving from peripheral to axial. This ensures that the eyelids (including periocular skin, eyelid margin, and cilia), conjunctiva (third eyelid, bulbar, and palpebral conjunctival surfaces, as well as nasolacrimal puncta), sclera, cornea (including the limbus and tear film), anterior chamber, iris, pupil, and lens

are examined completely. Anterior segment examination should be initiated before dilation so that the iris face is easily examined; however, complete examination of the lens requires full dilation. The complete anterior segment should be examined using transillumination and a source of magnification such as the Optivisor, otoscope head, or a slit-lamp biomicroscope. Following pupil dilation, retroillumination can be repeated from close to the patient and with a source of magnification so that lesions in the clear ocular media can be both backlit and magnified without the pupil constricting. The otoscope head is particularly useful for this because the examiner can alter the viewing angle until the lesion is either backlit by the tapetal reflection dorsally or viewed against the dull nontapetal area of the fundus ventrally while illuminated from in front. In both cases the otoscope head is moved in or out from the eye until the lesion is in crisp focus and under full magnification against the chosen background.

Tonometry is the measurement of intraocular pressure (IOP) and is essential for differentiation of the two major vision-threatening conditions in which red eye is the

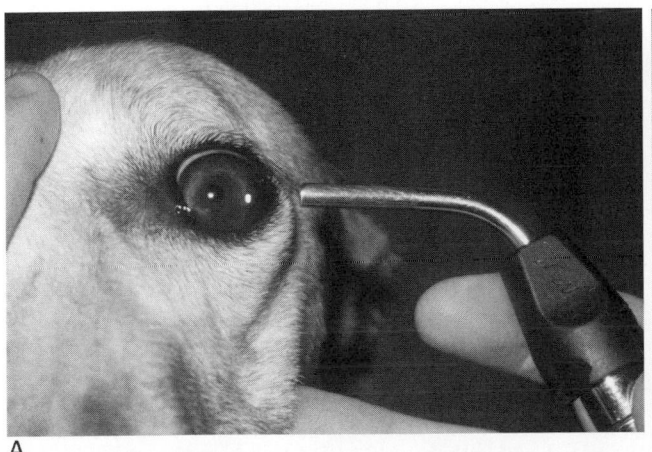
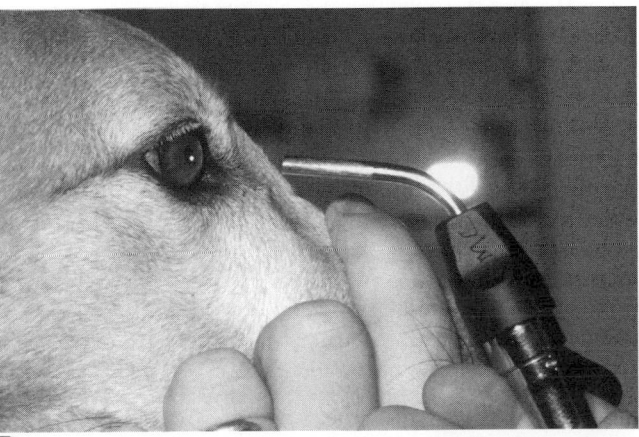

Fig. 248-2 Transillumination. A focal light source is directed at the eye from many angles while the examiner simultaneously varies the viewing angle. Varying the viewing and lighting angles relative to each other permits the examiner to use parallax, reflections, perspective, and shadows to gain valuable information regarding lesion depth.

hallmark feature: uveitis and glaucoma (see Chapters 263 and 264). Digital tonometry, in which the IOP is crudely assessed by compressing the globe against the orbital rim, is completely unreliable. The Schiøtz tonometer is reliable but awkward to use and requires conversion tables to convert the scale reading to the standard unit of IOP (millimeters of mercury). The availability of easily used and reasonably priced applanation tonometers such as the Tonopen has made measurement of IOP easier in all species, particularly cats. Unlike the Schiøtz tonometer, the Tonopen measures IOP directly and does not require any conversion. It can also be held horizontally and therefore allows measurements to be performed with the patient's head held in a normal, relaxed position. Finally, it has a small probe that permits easy measurement of IOP in even the smallest feline and pediatric canine eyes.

The Tonopen comes with an excellent instructional video and manual; however, the following tips may help the veterinarian achieve optimal results. A drop of topical anesthetic is applied to the cornea. A disposable cover is placed over the Tonopen tip; and the pen is turned on with firm, somewhat protracted pressure on the large black button about one third down the shaft. The equipment should be periodically calibrated according to the manufacturer's directions. Correct patient restraint is essential. The patient should be lightly restrained so as to not artificially raise IOP. In particular, direct pressure on the jugular veins by the holder or by a collar should be avoided. Similarly, no pressure should be exerted on the globe itself via the eyelids. This is best achieved by having an assistant (not the owner) restrain the patient's head, holding the angle of the mandible and the occiput. The Tonopen is then held in the dominant hand, and the patient's eyelids are gently parted using the nondominant hand so that pressure is applied to the underlying orbital rim, not the globe. The hand holding the Tonopen should then be rested onto the hand holding the eyelids or onto the patient's head itself. Very small, rapid (almost tremorlike) movements of the Tonopen away from and back toward the cornea such that the cornea is very lightly "blotted" with the Tonopen tip will enhance the reliability and reproducibility of the readings while reducing the number of readings necessary. Particular attention should be paid to the "approach angle" of the Tonopen tip to the cornea. The flat surface of the tip should be exactly parallel to the corneal surface. This is best achieved by viewing the interface between the cornea and the tip from the side. Said another way, the Tonopen itself should approach the globe as close to perpendicular to the corneal surface as possible. Therefore, because of corneal curvature, the approach angle must be changed dramatically if any area other than the central cornea is used or if the patient's globe moves.

Each time the cornea is appropriately "blotted" with the probe, an electronic tone will advise the operator that a reading has been obtained. When a suitable number of readings have been obtained, a tone of a different pitch will sound, and no further readings can be obtained without restarting the Tonopen using the large black button again. The number of readings required to achieve an average varies, depending on how disparate the readings are from each other and from the normal physiologic range.

A small digital screen displays the IOP in mm Hg and provides an estimate of the "reliability" (coefficient of variance) of the result. This appears as a small bar above one of four percentage readings. This bar should be above the 5% mark, or tonometry should be repeated for that eye. Across large populations, normal canine and feline IOP is reported as approximately 10 to 20 mm Hg. However, variation is noted between individuals, technique, and time of day. Therefore comparison of IOP between right and left eyes is critical to interpretation of results. A good rule of thumb is that IOP should not vary between eyes of the same patient by more than 20%.

Aqueous flare is a pathognomonic sign of uveitis and is the result of breakdown of the blood-ocular barrier, with subsequent leakage of plasma proteins into the anterior chamber where, with special technique, they can be seen. Aqueous flare is best detected using a very focal, intense light source in a totally darkened room. The passage taken by the beam of light is viewed from an angle. In the normal eye a focal reflection is seen where the light strikes the cornea. The beam is then invisible as it traverses the almost protein- and cell-free aqueous humor in the anterior chamber. Because of presence of lens proteins, the light beam becomes visible again as a focal reflection on the anterior lens capsule and then as a diffuse beam through the body of the normal lens. If uveitis has allowed leakage of serum proteins into the anterior chamber, these proteins will cause a scattering of the light as it passes through the aqueous (Fig. 248-3). This is called *aqueous flare* and is seen as a beam of light traversing the anterior chamber and joining the focal reflections on the corneal surface and the anterior lens capsule or iris. A slit lamp provides ideal conditions for detecting aqueous flare; however, the beam produced by the smallest circular aperture on the direct ophthalmoscope, at brightest illumination, in a completely darkened room, held as closely as possible to the cornea, and viewed transversely will also provide excellent results. The slit beam on the direct ophthalmoscope is not as intense as the small circular aperture and does not provide as many "edges" of light against which flare can be appreciated most easily. Aqueous flare is best

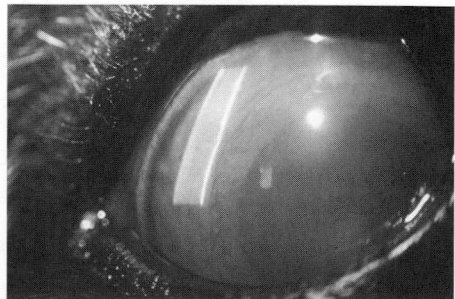

Fig. 248-3   Aqueous flare is present in this dog with anterior uveitis. A very focal, intense beam of light is directed across the anterior chamber and viewed transversely with magnification in a totally darkened room. Leakage of serum proteins into the anterior chamber causes scattering of the light as it passes through the aqueous between the cornea and iris.

seen against a black "backdrop," which in the eye is the pupil. Therefore assessment of flare is sometimes easier after complete pupil dilation. Combined assessment of IOP and aqueous flare should be performed whenever glaucoma or uveitis is suspected because of the frequency with which these conditions coexist.

Fundic examination is probably the greatest challenge in the ophthalmic examination. Fortunately anterior segment abnormalities tend to outnumber fundic abnormalities in general practice. However, funduscopy is critical in the assessment of animals presenting with visual disturbance, pupil abnormalities, or systemic disease. Traditionally there have been two methods for viewing the fundus: indirect and direct ophthalmoscopy. Recently Welch-Allyn and Keeler have both introduced new ophthalmoscopes (the Panoptic and the Wide-Angle Twin Mag, respectively) that combine some of the best features of both methods. Regardless of which method is used, funduscopy requires full pupil dilation. This is best achieved by examining the patient at least 15 minutes after topical application of a single drop of tropicamide.

THE DIRECT OPHTHALMOSCOPE

This instrument hangs on the walls of most veterinary examination rooms the world over and yet is not the best method for examining the fundus. It is used by turning the lens power to "0", selecting the largest circle of light that it emits, turning the light to almost full brightness, turning the room lights off or to a dim setting, and resting the brow rest of the ophthalmoscope against the operator's brow. Ideally the operator's right eye should be used for examining the patient's right eye and vice versa; although some people have trouble using their nondominant eye. The examiner should hold the animal's eyes open while an assistant holds the head steady and begin viewing at arm's length from the patient and move around until a bright tapetal reflection is obtained (as for retroillumination). The examiner should then slowly approach the animal, while always aiming at the tapetal reflection of the eye to be examined. Good focus in a normal patient should be reached within just a few centimeters of the eye. Therefore it is sometimes useful to extend the index finger of the hand holding the ophthalmoscope and rest the finger against the patient's cheek.

The direct ophthalmoscope presents a highly magnified, upright image of a very small region of the patient's fundus. In compliant human patients this instrument can then be used to slowly and sequentially examine the whole fundus in minute detail. However, in veterinary patients this small field of view frequently means that areas of the fundus, particularly peripherally, are never examined and that one area of the retina cannot be compared readily to another region.

THE INDIRECT OPHTHALMOSCOPE

Because of the large field of view achieved with indirect ophthalmoscopy, this is the preferred method for examining the dog or cat fundus. This larger field of view permits the examiner to compare regions of the fundus against each other so that focal areas of subtle pathology may be detected by comparison with neighboring normal areas. It also makes a complete examination of the whole fundus more likely and easier than when performed with direct ophthalmoscopy. The perceived downfalls are that the image is less magnified; however, this can be countered by moving closer to the patient while performing indirect ophthalmoscopy or by a subsequent (more magnified) examination of any "suspect" areas using the direct ophthalmoscope. Another difficulty for beginning ophthalmoscopists is that indirect ophthalmoscopy produces an inverted view. This makes navigation around the fundus and correct anatomic localization of lesions a little more difficult at first, but this disadvantage can be readily overcome with practice. A Volk 20D or 2.2 Pan Retinal indirect lens is ideal for examining the small animal fundus.

MONOCULAR INDIRECT OPHTHALMOSCOPES

Monocular indirect ophthalmoscopes have been introduced that fit to common existing battery handsets in practice, are reasonably easily mastered, and produce a view of the fundus with many of the best features of those produced using direct and indirect ophthalmoscopy. The image is upright and moderately magnified and includes more of the fundus than is possible with the direct ophthalmoscope but less than that provided by the indirect ophthalmoscope.

OTHER DIAGNOSTIC TECHNIQUES IN VETERINARY OPHTHALMOLOGY

Unlike assessment of other less accessible organs, visual examination of the eyes frequently provides all of the clues necessary to reach a clinical diagnosis. However, ancillary tests can provide valuable information in specific disease conditions.

The Schirmer tear test (STT) records basal and reflex tearing as number of millimeters of wetting of a strip of absorbent paper placed in the lateral aspect of the ventral conjunctival fornix for 1 minute. The lateral aspect is used to ensure that the strip lightly abrades the cornea and produces reflex tearing. If the strip is placed more medially, it may be prevented from touching the cornea by the third eyelid. The STT should be performed before application of any topical solutions, particularly anesthetic drops. General anesthesia and sedation also cause a temporary depression of normal tearing (for at least 48 hours). Normal STT values for dogs are well established; an STT reading of more than 15 mm in 60 seconds is considered normal. Wetting of less than 10 mm in 60 seconds is abnormal and is usually associated with evidence of keratoconjunctivitis. Wetting of 10 to 15 mm in 60 seconds represents a "gray zone" and warrants careful assessment and sometimes reassessment in light of clinical signs. The range of reported STT values in normal cats (3 to 32 mm; mean = 17 mm in 60 seconds) is much wider and more difficult to interpret than in dogs. However, experience suggests that lower readings than the reported mean can frequently be expected in completely normal cats. This is probably because of autonomic control of tear secretion and short-term alterations in tear flow as a result of stress in the examination room.

Feline STT values should still be recorded and interpreted in conjunction with clinical signs.

Application of fluorescein dye to the cornea can yield a large amount of information. A few drops of irrigation solution are trickled over a strip impregnated with fluorescein to liberate dye onto the cornea. Care should be taken not to touch the strip onto the cornea. Excess dye is then rinsed from the corneal surface, and the eye examined with either white or cobalt blue light. This simple, water-soluble dye has great affinity for the hydrophilic corneal stroma but is not absorbed by epithelial cells or Descemet's membrane. Therefore its most common use is identification and characterization of corneal ulcers. Excitement of the fluorescent dye with a cobalt blue light can assist with identification of minor lesions; however, excessive dye must be adequately rinsed from the cornea to avoid overinterpretation of normal pooling. Small, "scuffed" areas of corneal epithelium are occasionally seen following the STT.

Passage of dye down the nasolacrimal duct is referred to as the *Jones test* and is used to assess functional and anatomic patency of the nasolacrimal apparatus. *Seidel's test* also uses fluorescein stain. This test is used to assess integrity of the cornea following suspected penetrating trauma or ulceration and to guide decisions regarding management of such wounds. In Seidel's test the excessive dye is not rinsed from the cornea and the surface is examined with a cobalt blue light and magnification for possible perforation. Leakage of aqueous humor will cause small rivulets to form in the fluorescein dye pooled on the corneal surface.

Rose bengal stain is retained by devitalized corneal or conjunctival epithelial cells. Recent studies have suggested that even changes in amount or quality of some normal tear film components such as mucin and albumin can cause otherwise viable epithelial cells to retain rose bengal stain. Therefore its clinical utility is detection of subtle epithelial abnormalities as seen in keratoconjunctivitis sicca ("dry eye") or the dendritic ulcers that are pathognomonic for canine and feline herpesvirus keratitis. Rose bengal and fluorescein stains may affect culture and virologic results and should be applied following collection of microbiologic samples. Rose bengal is also epitheliotoxic and may cause discomfort in some animals; therefore it should be reserved for cases in which it may provide useful additional information.

Retropulsion of the globe is a simple but useful method for investigating orbital disease. It is performed by applying gentle digital pressure to both globes in a posterior direction through closed lids. The resistance to retropulsion and the resilience with which the globes "spring" back against the retropulsive force are subjectively assessed. Retropulsion of the globe in a variety of directions may further localize orbital masses or outline smaller masses that would be missed by direct caudal retropulsion only.

Cannulation of the nasolacrimal puncta and gentle flushing with saline can be readily performed in most conscious dogs following application of a topical ophthalmic anesthetic. However, it is particularly challenging in cats without sedation or general anesthesia. A ¾-inch, 22- or 24-gauge Teflon intravenous catheter without the stilette is easy to use and usually well tolerated; however, more rigid, specialized metal cannulae are also available. The inferior or superior punctum is identified and cannulated. Gentle injection of saline through one punctum should elicit flow from the other in the same eye without any resistance. Following assessment of patency between the superior and inferior puncta, gentle digital obstruction of the noncannulated punctum should cause passage of the solution through the nasolacrimal duct and out the ipsilateral nostril. Frequently in cats and brachycephalic dogs, the nasolacrimal ducts open caudally enough in the nose that flush solutions are not evident at the external nares but exit into the nasopharynx and then the oral cavity. Inclusion of a small amount of fluorescein in the flush solution and observation of the nares and oral cavity with a cobalt blue light source may assist with identification of patency. Fluorescein should be avoided if culture or cytology of nasolacrimal fluid is intended.

Cytology, aspirates, and biopsies can be harvested relatively easily from ocular tissues, sometimes without sedation. Scraping or aspirate samples from the eyelid are collected using the same procedures as elsewhere on skin; however, particular care is taken not to damage the eyelid margin and to direct the instruments used away from the globe. Scrapings from the cornea or conjunctiva are performed following several applications of topical anesthesia and using either a Kimura platinum spatula or the dull, handle-end of a scalpel blade. Cytology specimens are spread gently onto glass slides and stained with Diff Quik and/or Gram stains. Conjunctival "snip biopsies" can usually be harvested following application of topical anesthetic and without sedation. A small section of conjunctiva is gently "tented up" with fine forceps and resected with small tenotomy scissors (see Fig. 260-3). Minimal and careful handling is essential to avoid artifactitious disruption of this delicate tissue before histologic interpretation. Corneal biopsies are usually gathered by lamellar keratectomy and require general anesthesia, magnification, and sometimes neuromuscular blockade and therefore are more commonly collected by those with specialty training.

Imaging techniques for the globe and orbit are becoming more widely available. These are particularly useful when opacity of the ocular media (cornea, lens, aqueous humor, or vitreous) prohibits detailed examination of intraocular structures and for diagnosis of orbital disease. Ultrasonographic assessment has proved particularly useful. A 7.5- to 10-MHz (or preferably 12 to 20 MHz) probe is required. Examination of a conscious patient following application of topical anesthetic is preferred since sedation tends to cause ventral rolling of the eyeball and enophthalmos, which make obtaining adequate images difficult. Transcorneal or transpalpebral approaches are used most commonly; however, a temporal approach has been described for retrobulbar examination. Sterile coupling gel is applied to the cornea or lids, and the probe is applied with gentle pressure sufficient to ensure a clear image. Particular care should be taken if corneal perforation is imminent.

Radiographic assessment is particularly useful for diagnosis of orbital fractures, assessment of bony involvement when invasive tumors are suspected, or identification of radiopaque foreign bodies, particularly gunshot injuries.

Magnetic resonance imaging and computed tomography scanning provide valuable information regarding extent and character of orbital disease and also provide surprisingly good intraocular definition.

Gonioscopy is examination of the iridocorneal angle (ICA). In dogs a small plastic corneal lens is required. In cats (because of their large corneas and degree of corneal curvature), magnification and a focal light source (i.e., an otoscope head) will provide some assessment of this area. However, this should still be supplemented with a gonioscopic lens before a final assessment is made. The clinician should focus initially on the iris and then follow it out peripherally until the ICA and pectinate ligaments come into view. These are usually long and relatively straight (especially in cats) and should have large spaces between them. They are usually pigmented to the same degree as the iris. Examination of the ICA provides essential information for diagnosis and prognosis of glaucoma and uveitis. Although this technique is learned relatively easily, familiarity with angle anatomy and interpretation of abnormal findings require practice.

Anterior chamber, vitreous, and subretinal aspirates are sometimes used in the assessment of uveitis or intraocular masses if less invasive techniques have not yielded a diagnosis. Samples gathered in this fashion can be examined serologically or cytologically or submitted for PCR culture and sensitivity testing. Due to the risk of irreversible globe damage during these procedures, they are best performed by ophthalmologists.

The electroretinogram is a measure of retinal electrical activity in response to stimulation with light. It is a routine part of assessment of patients before cataract surgery and may also be used to differentiate blindness resulting from retinal and optic nerve or central neurologic disease. The specialized equipment needed and knowledge of the technique limit this study to specialist ophthalmology practices.

CHAPTER 249

Ocular Pharmacology

DANIEL A. WARD, *Knoxville, Tennessee*

Ocular disease represents a considerable segment of most small animal veterinary practices. The majority of ocular disease in small animals is addressed by pharmacologic management, either alone or in conjunction with surgery. Therefore it is beneficial to most small animal veterinarians to have an understanding of ocular pharmacology. The goal of this chapter is to provide such a foundation.

When making decisions regarding medical management of ocular disease, one must first consider which tissue within the eye is the target of therapy. It is a mistake to consider the eye as a homogenous tissue. Rather, the eye should be considered a heterogeneous structure containing a number of substructures as potential therapeutic targets, including the lids, conjunctiva, corneal epithelium, corneal stroma, anterior uvea (consisting of the iris and ciliary body), iridocorneal angle, lens, vitreous, choroid, retina, sclera, and orbital tissue (which includes fat, muscle tissue, nervous tissue, vasculature, and bone). The reason for this separation is that there are a number of ways of delivering medication to the eye and different ocular targets are best reached by different routes.

OCULAR SURFACE

Topical application of medication is generally the preferred route of administration for ocular surface disease, which includes disorders of the conjunctiva and corneal epithelium (e.g., conjunctivitis and superficial keratitis). Because topical agents can be applied directly to the ocular surface, very high drug concentrations can be achieved in these tissues.

At the same time, several precorneal factors exact constraints on achieving high concentrations at the ocular surface following topical delivery. For example, the volume of a typical eyedrop is approximately 50 μl. But the tear film of a normal canine eye can contain approximately only 10 μl, meaning that 80% of the applied drop is immediately lost through nasolacrimal drainage or spillage onto the face. In addition, a topically applied drop is immediately diluted by the tears present on the ocular surface at the moment of application. When the eye is painful (as is usually the case with ocular disorders), lacrimation in response to the pain can be substantial, making the dilutional effect even greater. Further dilution occurs as a result of reflex lacrimation that occurs when the eyedrop makes contact with the ocular surface. Nasolacrimal drainage offers a constant and substantial sump for draining drug away from the ocular surface, and it is increased when the eye is painful because of an increased blink rate (in humans, each blink forces $2\,\mu l$ of tears into the nasolacrimal duct). Taken together, these volume limitations, dilution, and tear drainage dictate that only about 1% to 7% of any eyedrop applied to the eye is actually available to ocular tissues and that peak effects are relatively fixed at 20 to 60 minutes following application. The extent of these losses will vary somewhat based on the physicochemical properties of the drug under consideration, but ocular pharmacokinetic research has shown that these parameters hold true for almost all topically applied drops.

There are several strategies for maximizing bioavailability to the ocular surface. Increasing viscosity by using viscous solutions or ointments as drug vehicles extends contact time and reduces the effects of dilution and nasolacrimal drainage. For example, addition of viscous polymers such as polyvinylpyrrolidone or hydroxypropyl methylcellulose to eyedrops may increase bioavailability by 50% to 100%, primarily by reducing the dilutional effect. Simple ointments (drug dissolved or suspended in long-chain hydrocarbon oil) and compound ointments (drug incorporated in biphasic dispersion of water–in–oil or oil-in-water) also increase availability to the ocular surface. These agents probably create a drug reservoir that retards nasolacrimal drainage, which in turn tends to enhance both the maximal attainable tear film concentration and the duration of therapeutic effect. However, it should be noted that these parameters are highly dependent on the physicochemical composition of the drug in question. For example, in rabbit studies of ointment and solution formulations of the hydrophilic antiglaucoma agent pilocarpine and lipophilic corticosteroid fluorometholone, the ointment form of both agents increased the maximal attainable concentration twofold to threefold compared to the solution form. However, duration of action was significantly prolonged (by approximately threefold) only with the ointment formulation of fluorometholone.

Occlusion of the nasolacrimal puncta following eyedrop administration is sometimes advocated in humans as a means of increasing concentrations and prolonging duration of action. However, tear film concentration of most eyedrops falls by only about 10% per minute; thus punctal occlusion would have to be maintained for several minutes to have an appreciable effect on duration. A simpler alternative may be to repeat instillation once or twice at 5- to 10-minute intervals. We have observed the benefit of this strategy with the antiglaucoma eyedrop apraclonidine, in which administration of a single drop has virtually no effect on intraocular pressure in dogs, yet application of 2 drops 5 minutes apart reduces intraocular pressure by 30%.

In the foregoing discussion of topical drug application for ocular surface disease, it is implied that drops or ointments are applied at regular intervals—so-called *"pulsed delivery."* Despite the strategies mentioned previously to improve drug concentration in the tear film, pulsed therapy will always be associated with concentration peaks and nadirs, with nadirs generally falling into the subtherapeutic range for at least a portion of each interdosing interval. Variation in concentration can be reduced by nonpulsed delivery techniques. Although not commonly used in small animal practice, such techniques include constant rate pump systems that can be attached to subpalpebral lavage systems, biodegradable drug delivery devices, and application of hydrophilic soft contact lenses soaked in medication.

Apart from enhanced drug concentration, topical delivery to treat ocular surface disorders is desirable because systemic side effects are reduced compared to systemic administration. There are certainly exceptions to this general rule. For example, topical β-blockers used in the treatment of glaucoma can cause bradycardia and bronchospasm, especially in smaller patients. Topically applied corticosteroids given at concentrations and frequencies often used clinically commonly induce polydipsia or polyuria, suppression of the pituitary-adrenal axis, and hepatic vacuolar changes. But in general, untoward systemic side effects are less frequent with topical than with systemic administration.

Corneal surface disease is sometimes treated with subconjunctival injection. In this technique a small depot of drug (usually either a corticosteroid or antibiotic) is injected beneath the bulbar conjunctiva 4 to 6 mm posterior to the limbus. The disposition of an agent delivered in this way varies; some regurgitates through the conjunctival puncture to bathe the cornea (at which point it essentially behaves as a continuously applied topical drop), some enters the systemic circulation, and some diffuses directly into and possibly through the sclera. For treatment of ocular surface disorders, the regurgitated fraction is probably the most important. In general, drugs given by this route have a longer duration of action than topically applied drops. Repositol corticosteroids (e.g., methylprednisolone acetate and triamcinolone acetonide) may provide 3 to 4 weeks of antiinflammatory activity following a single injection. The principle drawback to subconjunctival injection is that, should a complication arise necessitating discontinuation of the agent (e.g., a dog with chronic superficial keratoconjunctivitis or "pannus" that develops a corneal ulcer), it may be difficult or impossible to remove. Recommended subconjunctival drug doses are listed in Table 249-1.

CORNEAL STROMA AND ANTERIOR UVEA

Delivery of drug to the corneal stroma and anterior uveal tissues by topical application is hindered by the same precorneal factors addressed previously. However, treatment of these tissues is further hindered by the corneal epithelial barrier, which severely limits passage of all but the most lipophilic compounds. For example, most topical antibiotics are hydrophilic and reach low concentrations in the corneal stroma. Therefore treatment of bacterial stromal abscesses in which the stroma is infected but the overlying epithelium is intact may be difficult because most commonly available topical agents will not reach the site of infection in appreciable concentrations. To overcome this problem, the clinician can periodically denude the epithelium overlying the abscess, or alternatively

Table **249-1**

Subconjunctival Drug Dosages

Drug	Dosage (milligrams)*
Antibiotics	
Amikacin	25
Cefazolin	100
Gentamycin	20
Kanamycin	20
Oxacillin	50
Tobramycin	20
Vancomycin	25
Corticosteroids	
Betamethasone	1
Dexamethasone	1
Methylprednisolone	5
Triamcinolone	5
Mydriatics	
Atropine	1

*Administered volume should not exceed 0.5 ml in dogs or cats and should not exceed systemic dose in exotic animals.

coapply the epitheliotoxic topical anesthetic proparacaine at the same time the antibiotic is applied. Another approach is the use of topical formulations of chloramphenicol. As an amphipathic agent, it can take on either polar or nonpolar characteristics, depending on its local microenvironment. It is thus capable of superior corneal epithelial penetration, and we have successfully treated a number of refractory bacterial stromal abscesses by simply switching antibiotic therapy from a more hydrophilic agent (such as an aminoglycoside) to chloramphenicol. However, it bears emphasis that this approach is only useful if the offending organism is sensitive to chloramphenicol. Also, it is important to recall that chloramphenicol is a bacteriostatic antibiotic and bactericidal agents are preferred for corneal infections when practicable.

Topical corticosteroids are often used in the treatment of inflammation of the deep corneal stroma and anterior uvea. Tremendous differences exist among topical corticosteroids with respect to both potency and corneal epithelial penetrability. For example, it is generally accepted that dexamethasone is a more potent steroid base than prednisolone. But most dexamethasone products are formulated as sodium phosphate salts, which are highly polar and penetrate corneal epithelium poorly. Therefore these products are very effective for treatment of ocular surface inflammation but less so for anterior uveitis. By contrast, the acetate salt of prednisolone is very lipophilic and penetrates the corneal epithelium quite well. Therefore it is generally more effective than dexamethasone sodium phosphate for treatment of anterior uveitis.

For some agents it is possible to enhance drug delivery through the corneal epithelium by formulating a prodrug with superior lipid solubility that is then metabolized by corneal stromal enzymes once the epithelial barrier has been breached. Examples of such drugs include the mydriatic phenylephrine oxazolidine (which is metabolized to phenylephrine) and the antiglaucoma agents dipivefrin (metabolized to epinephrine) and latanoprost (metabolized to prostaglandin $F_{2\alpha}$).

Even assuming adequate corneal epithelial penetration, deep corneal stromal and anterior uveal drug concentration following topical delivery may be further complicated by enzymatic degradation, dilution and washout by aqueous humor, protein binding, and (for uveal delivery) binding to melanin.

Although a number of enzyme systems such as catechol O-methyltransferase, monoamine oxidase, and glucuronide transferase are present within corneal stroma, it is generally not considered a major site of topical drug degradation. Rather, these enzyme systems are exploited in the pharmaceutical formulation of agents to enhance corneal epithelial penetration (as are the lipophilic prodrugs mentioned previously) or to reduce systemic absorption or duration of action. Agents using the latter mechanism are termed "soft drugs." Examples include an analog of atropine, which retains the mydriatic potency of atropine but has a much shorter duration of effect on the diseased eye and no effect on the fellow eye, and "soft" steroids such as loteprednol etabonate, which retain ocular antiinflammatory activity but have fewer ocular and systemic side effects.

Dilution and washout of topically applied drugs destined for the anterior uveal tissues is predictable but unavoidable. The drugs most commonly used to target these tissues are steroidal and nonsteroidal antiinflammatory agents, antiglaucoma medications, and drugs that alter pupil size. The precorneal effects and corneal epithelial barrier mechanisms discussed previously, as well as dilution and washout within aqueous humor, do limit uveal concentrations attainable with these agents. Despite this, topical delivery is still generally preferred because systemic delivery of these drugs must surmount the even more formidable blood-aqueous humor barrier. In the normal dog eye aqueous humor is replenished at the rate of approximately 1% per minute, meaning that the entire aqueous humor volume is replenished approximately once every 100 minutes. Yet most compounds active within the anterior uvea retain activity for far longer (i.e., there is a pharmacokinetic-pharmacodynamic dissociation). This phenomenon can variously be explained by pharmaceutical formulations that prolong the residence time of the drug on the ocular surface, the presence of bioactive metabolites, binding to, and subsequent metered release from, ocular proteins and melanin, and activity through second messenger systems.

Protein and melanin binding can be beneficial or detrimental to the anterior uveal activity of a drug following topical application. For example, most nonsteroidal antiinflammatory drugs are highly protein bound (e.g., >99% for flurbiprofen), yet only free drug has antiinflammatory efficacy; thus relatively high anterior segment concentrations must be achieved to retain antiinflammatory efficacy. Similarly, many mydriatic agents and antiglaucoma β-blockers are avidly bound by melanin. Once saturated, they may be released slowly and provide a sustained duration of activity.

As with treatment of ocular surface diseases, disorders of the corneal stroma and anterior uveal tissues are sometimes treated by subconjunctival injection. The route by which these drugs ultimately enter these tissues (transcorneal, transscleral, or from the systemic circulation) varies greatly, depending on the drug in question. In general, higher concentrations are achieved with subconjunctival injection than with topical application.

LENS

The lens is almost never a target of drug delivery, although this may change with development of aldose reductase inhibitors to treat diabetic cataracts. Presently the primary concern regarding drug delivery to the lens is unintended drug accumulation within the lens and subsequent cataract formation. For most drugs studied, accumulation in the lens fortunately does not occur, probably because of anatomic features of the lens itself. The presence of an anterior layer of epithelium and densely packed lens fibers subjacent to the epithelium make the lens a very nonporous structure that likely resists movement of hydrophilic compounds.

VITREOUS

The primary indication for drug delivery to the vitreous is infectious endophthalmitis. Topical delivery of antibiotics to the vitreous body is ineffective because not only must the antibiotics survive passage through and dilution within the tear film, cornea, and aqueous humor in adequate concentrations and avoid uveal melanin binding, they must also traverse the relatively closed lens-iris diaphragm. Higher vitreal concentrations are achieved with systemic delivery or intravitreal injection.

Systemically administered drugs enter the vitreous by way of the ciliary, retinal, or choroidal circulation, although passage via these routes is limited by the blood-aqueous humor and blood-retinal barriers. In addition, once a drug has reached the peripheral vitreous by one of these routes, further migration throughout the vitreous is slow and inconsistent, regardless of the physicochemical properties of the drug, and significant accumulation often does not occur. The only reliable way of achieving homogenous drug distribution within the vitreous is via intravitreal injection. The technique is straightforward with adequate training and assuming important safeguards are taken. The patient is anesthetized with a short-acting general anesthetic, the ocular surface is sterilized with dilute (1:10) povidone-iodine (Betadine) solution, the limbus is grasped with a small-toothed forceps, and a 22-gauge needle with syringe attached is inserted into the globe 8 mm posterior to the limbus. To avoid inadvertent rupture of the posterior lens capsule and globe-threatening uveitis, the needle must be directed toward the center of the vitreous body, *not* the center of the globe itself. Careful attention must be paid to the volume and amount of agent injected because many drugs (especially antimicrobial agents) have a dose-dependent propensity for retinal toxicity. Recommended intravitreal dosages are listed in Table 249-2.

CHOROID AND RETINA

Many disorders of the canine posterior segment are developmental or degenerative and are not as yet amenable to medical therapy. The most commonly encountered conditions that are effectively managed medically are bacterial and fungal infections and some vascular disorders. Because they tend to affect both the choroid and the retina, these structures are considered together.

As with the vitreous, topical delivery of drugs invariably fails to reach therapeutic concentrations in the retina. Better concentrations are generally achieved with systemic administration and in some instances posterior subconjunctival administration. Following systemic administration in normal dogs, high drug concentrations are generally achievable in choroidal tissue because of the permeability of the choroidal vasculature. However, movement of drugs from choroidal tissue into the retina is hindered by the "outer" blood-retinal barrier composed of tight junctions between adjacent retinal pigment epithelial cells. Similarly, systemically administered agents are restricted from entering retinal tissue from the retinal vasculature because of tight junctions between adjacent retinal vascular endothelial cells (the "inner blood-retinal barrier"). However, in most circumstances in which drugs need to be delivered to retinal tissue (e.g., an antifungal agent in a patient with chorioretinal blastomycosis), these barriers are dysfunctional secondary to inflammation, and drug entry is facilitated.

Retrobulbar injection has been used successfully in the treatment of chorioretinal disease in experimental animals and is occasionally advocated for clinical use in humans, but this route is not commonly used in the treatment of chorioretinal disease in domestic animals.

EYELIDS AND ORBIT

In general, eyelid and orbital diseases can be viewed as integumentary and deep soft-tissue disorders, respectively. As such, they are usually treated with systemically administered drugs. Management of disorders of the eyelid margin (such as meibomian gland infection) may be supplemented by direct application of ophthalmic ointments. In rare instances orbital diseases are treated by retrobulbar injection.

Table 249-2

Intravitreal Antibiotic Dosages

Antibiotic	Dosage (micrograms)*
Amikacin	400
Cefazolin	2250
Gentamycin	100
Kanamycin	500
Oxacillin	500
Tobramycin	100
Vancomycin	1000

*Administered volume should not exceed 20 microliters in dogs or cats and should not exceed systemic dose in exotic animals.

References and Suggested Reading

Maurice DM, Mishima S: Ocular pharmacokinetics In Sears ML, editor: *Pharmacology of the eye*, New York, 1984, Springer-Verlag, p 19.

Mishima S: Clinical pharmacokinetics of the eye, *Invest Ophthalmol Vis Sci* 21:504, 1981.

Schoenwald RD: Ocular pharmacokinetics. In Zimmerman TJ, editor: *Textbook of ocular pharmacology*, Philadelphia, 1997, Lippincott-Raven, p 119.

CHAPTER **250**

Ocular Immunotherapy

STEVEN R. HOLLINGSWORTH, *Davis, California*

Owing to the fragility of intraocular structures and the need to maintain transparent optical media, control of ocular immunologic responses is arguably the most important aspect of ocular therapeutics. Over the last 25 years, an impressive array of medications has become available for this purpose. Although all of these agents have in common the ability to modulate the immune response of the eye, they are significantly different with regard to mode of action, site of action, route of administration, penetrability, and side effects. Proper management of ophthalmic disease requires a thorough understanding of these characteristics to select the most appropriate treatment for a specific patient.

Ocular immunotherapeutic agents may be administered by three routes: topically, subconjunctivally, or systemically (also see Chapter 249). Topical medications have the advantage of achieving high ocular tissue levels without significant systemic drug exposure. However, they are effective only against conditions involving the conjunctiva, cornea, nasolacrimal drainage apparatus, and (for some drugs) anterior uvea. Because of the biphasic anatomic character of the cornea, bipolar acetate and alcohol preparations enjoy far greater penetration than phosphate formulations and are preferred for use with intraocular conditions. Effect of topical medications can be enhanced by increasing the frequency of application.

The subconjunctival route is used under conditions in which an immediate high level of drug delivery to the anterior segment is desired and/or in situations in which frequent topical administration is not possible. The specific formulation of the drug determines the rapidity of its effect and duration of action. Because the lipophilic epithelial barrier is partially bypassed by subconjunctival delivery, water-soluble phosphate preparations are rapidly absorbed but have a short duration of action. Conversely, acetate-based preparations are slowly absorbed but remain active for a longer period of time. Among the immunotherapeutic class of drugs, only corticosteroids are delivered via this route.

Systemically administered medications are necessary to treat diseases involving the eyelids, posterior segment, and orbit and can be a useful adjunct in anterior uveitis. These drugs as a class carry the potential of adverse systemic sequelae, including immunosuppression, gastrointestinal ulceration, and steroid-induced hepatopathy.

Ocular inflammation is initiated by noxious stimuli that trigger the release of arachidonic acid from the cell membrane by the action of phospholipase A_2. Arachidonic acid is subsequently acted on by two classes of enzymes—lipoxygenase and cyclooxygenase (COX)—to produce various inflammatory mediators known collectively as the eicosanoids. The lipoxygenase pathway produces leukotrienes, which are powerful chemotactic agents. The primary end products of the cyclooxygenase pathway are prostaglandins, which cause miosis, increased vascular permeability, and diminished platelet aggregation and compromise of the blood aqueous barrier. The COX enzymes are further subdivided into COX-1 and COX-2 isoenzymes. COX-1 is sometimes referred to as the constitutive form because its end products facilitate normal physiologic functions such as gastric mucosal protection, renal perfusion, and platelet aggregation. The COX-2 isoenzyme is known as the inflammatory form because it is released in response to noxious stimuli and results in products that mediate inflammation.

In addition to the inflammatory cascade described in the previous paragraph, the eye is the target organ for a number of relatively common disorders that are characterized by self-perpetuating autoimmune inflammation. Chief among these conditions are keratoconjunctivitis sicca (KCS), chronic superficial keratitis ("pannus"), and uveodermatologic syndrome (or VKH-like syndrome). The clinical signs associated with these syndromes are discussed elsewhere. Although the pathophysiology of these conditions is complex, each is fundamentally fueled by the activation of local T lymphocytes, which leads to recruitment of additional T lymphocytes, and elaboration of interleukin and other proinflammatory agents.

To address these processes, several immunosuppressive medications have been developed that act directly on T lymphocytes.

CORTICOSTEROIDS

Corticosteroids are the most frequently used ophthalmic antiinflammatory agents and are efficacious against surface and intraocular conditions. Corticosteroids exert their antiinflammatory effect by causing upregulation of lipocortin, a protein that inhibits phospholipase A_2 and thus decreases the release of arachidonic acid. For this reason, corticosteroids suppress the formation of eicosanoids from both branches of the inflammatory pathway. Corticosteroids may be administered topically, subconjunctivally, or systemically. Specific formulations, routes of administration, and dosages are summarized in Table 250-1.

Topical Agents

Topical preparations vary in their innate potency, their ability to penetrate an intact cornea, and therefore their ability to influence intraocular inflammation. Because they suppress the local immune response, inhibit corneal healing, and potentiate proteases and collagenases, topical steroids are *absolutely contraindicated in the presence of corneal ulceration*. Although topically applied medications generally are not associated with significant systemic side effects, chronic use of topical corticosteroids has been demonstrated to cause adrenal suppression and interfere with regulation of diabetes mellitus (Murphy, Feldman, and Bellhorn, 1990).

Prednisolone is a moderately potent corticosteroid. For topical application it is commercially available as a 0.125% or 1% sodium phosphate solution or acetate suspension. The acetate preparation has excellent ocular penetration and at the 1% concentration is frequently the drug of choice for anterior uveitis. Dexamethasone is a highly potent corticosteroid. It is available at a concentration of 0.1% in a suspension or sodium phosphate formulation either alone or in combination with neomycin and/or polymyxin B. Because dexamethasone is available in all of these forms, it is important to know the specific formulation of an individual product before selecting it for use. For example, all of these products are excellent choices for surface conditions such as conjunctivitis, keratitis, and dacryocystitis; whereas for anterior uveitis the suspension formulation is preferred over sodium phosphate preparations because of better corneal penetration. Hydrocortisone is available for topical use combined with neomycin, polymyxin B, and usually bacitracin. Because it is significantly less potent than dexamethasone or prednisolone, its only use is the treatment of mild conjunctivitis in dogs.

Subconjunctival Agents

Corticosteroids may be administered by subconjunctival injection of a solution or suspension under the bulbar conjunctiva to treat anterior segment inflammation. Because frequent topical administration of medications

Table **250-1**

Corticosteroid Agents

	Formulations	Dose*
Topical Medications		
Prednisolone	0.125% or 1% acetate suspension or sodium phosphate solution	q2-48 h, depending on severity of inflammation; usually BID to QID
Dexamethasone	0.1% suspension or ointment alone or with neomycin and polymyxin; 0.1% sodium phosphate solution or ointment	q2-48 h, depending on severity of inflammation; usually BID to QID
Hydrocortisone	1% suspension or ointment usually with neomycin and polymyxin ± bacitracin	q2-48 h, depending on severity of inflammation; usually BID to QID
Subconjunctival Medications		
Triamcinolone acetonide	2, 3, 6, 10 or 40 mg/ml injectable suspension	3-15 mg
Dexamethasone or dexamethasone sodium phosphate	2, 4, or 10 mg/ml injectable solution	0.5-1 mg
Betamethasone acetate or betamethasone sodium phosphate	3 or 6 mg/ml injectable solution	1-3 mg
Systemic Medications		
Prednisolone or prednisolone acetate or sodium succinate	5- to 20-mg tablets; 3 mg/ml oral suspension; 1 or 5 mg/ml oral syrup; 25, 50, or 100 mg/ml injectable	0.5-2 mg/kg/day PO; 2 to 4 mg/kg IM or IV
Dexamethasone or dexamethasone sodium phosphate, acetate or sodium succinate	0.25- to 4-mg tablets; 2, 4, or 10 mg/ml injectable	0.1 mg/kg/day PO; 0.2 mg/kg IM or IV
Prednisone	1- to 50-mg tablets; 1- to 5-mg/ml oral suspension	0.5-2 mg/kg/day PO

*Doses listed are those initially recommended for immunotherapy. These doses should be tapered as rapidly as clinical improvement permits.
IM, Intramuscularly; *IV,* intravenously.

results in drug concentrations superior to those achieved by subconjunctival injection, the primary indication for subconjunctival injections is a situation in which instillation of topical medication is problematic. Subconjunctival injections are administered after application of a topical anesthetic. The dorsolateral aspect of the bulbar conjunctiva is grasped approximately 4 to 5 mm from the limbus with fine-tissue forceps and gently elevated. Using a 25- or 27-gauge needle and a tuberculin syringe, 0.25 to 0.5 ml of drug is injected under the conjunctiva. Products intended for topical application are *not* appropriate for injection by this or any other route because of irritation caused by the preservatives in these preparations. Common corticosteroid products used for subconjunctival injections include triamcinolone, dexamethasone, and betamethasone. Triamcinolone and betamethasone are commercially available in an acetate formulation; therefore they have a longer duration of action, usually 2 to 3 weeks. Methylprednisolone acetate should be avoided for subconjunctival injection because of its tendency to form painful, granulomatous plaques. Other major disadvantages of this route of administration are the danger of globe perforation and the possibility of needing to remove the drug depot because of a change in the patient's condition.

Systemic Agents

Systemic corticosteroids are indicated in the treatment of inflammatory processes involving the eyelids, anterior uvea, choroid, optic nerve, and orbit. In addition to reaching ocular and periocular structures not reached by topical mediations, systemically administered corticosteroids can also be used under conditions such as corneal ulceration. Prednisone, prednisolone, and dexamethasone are the most commonly administered systemic corticosteroids and are available in oral or injectable forms. The adverse side effects of systemic corticosteroid administration include polyuria, polydipsia, and iatrogenic endocrinopathies.

NONSTEROIDAL ANTIINFLAMMATORY DRUGS

Nonsteroidal antiinflammatory drugs (NSAIDs) exert their effect by disrupting the COX branch of the arachidonic acid inflammatory cascade and thereby preventing prostaglandin formation. Because prostaglandins are responsible for many of the changes and clinical signs associated with anterior uveitis, they are frequently used for treatment of this malady. They are especially useful because they can be applied topically in instances such as corneal ulceration or diabetes mellitus in which topical administration of corticosteroids is contraindicated. In addition, NSAIDs frequently are used before cataract surgery to prevent miosis during surgery. NSAIDs are available for both topical and systemic use. Although systemic administration of both NSAIDs and corticosteroids is unwise, they may be used together in all other combinations of routes (i.e., one systemically and one topically or both topically). Specific formulations, routes of administration, and dosages for commonly used NSAIDs are summarized in Table 250-2.

Topical Agents

Four topical NSAIDs are currently commercially available in the United States: flurbiprofen, diclofenac, ketorolac, and suprofen. Flurbiprofen is available as a 0.03% solution and is primarily used to treat anterior uveitis. Flurbiprofen has been demonstrated to decrease aqueous outflow in dogs and therefore to contribute to an increase in intraocular pressure. Furthermore, this effect is more

---

Table **250-2**

Nonsteroidal Antiinflammatory Agents

	Formulations	Dose
Topical Medications		
Flurbiprofen	0.03% solution	BID to QID, depending on severity of inflammation
Suprofen	1% solution	BID to QID, depending on severity of inflammation
Diclofenac	0.1% solution	BID to QID, depending on severity of inflammation
Ketorolac	0.5% solution	BID to QID, depending on severity of inflammation
Systemic Medications		
Carprofen (dogs and cats)	25-, 75-, or 100-mg caplets or tablets; 50 mg/ml injectable	4.4 mg/kg/day PO or SQ initially, then 2.2 mg/kg/day
Meloxicam (dogs and cats)	1.5 mg/ml oral suspension, 7.5- or 15-mg tablets; 5 mg/ml injectable	0.2 mg/kg PO, SQ, or IV initially, then 0.1 mg/kg/day
Deracoxib (dogs)	25- or 100-mg chewable tablets	1 to 2 mg/kg/day PO
Etodolac (dogs)	150- or 300-mg tablets	5 to 15 mg/kg/day
Ketoprofen (dogs and cats)	50-, 75-, 100-, or 200-mg capsules, 12.5-mg tablets; 100 mg/ml injectable	2 mg/kg/day initially, then 1 mg/kg/day
Ketorolac	0.5% solution	BID to QID, depending on severity of inflammation

pronounced in eyes with anterior uveitis. Because of this, *intraocular pressures should be monitored* in patients with anterior uveitis and those being treated with flurbiprofen. Similar to topical corticosteroids, flurbiprofen has been demonstrated to inhibit corneal wound healing and exacerbate herpetic keratoconjunctivitis in cats. However, flurbiprofen does not potentiate other corneal infectious agents as corticosteroids do and may be used in the presence of uncomplicated (noninfected) corneal ulcers.

Along with flurbiprofen, diclofenac is routinely used in veterinary medicine. It is available as a 0.1% solution. Numerous studies and personal experience indicate that it is a more potent intraocular antiinflammatory agent than flurbiprofen and probably comparable to prednisolone acetate. Suprofen is available as a 1% solution and is closely related to flurbiprofen. Ketorolac is commercially available as a 0.5% solution. It is most commonly used to treat allergic conjunctivitis in humans. Although not widely used in veterinary medicine, it does not appear to cause an increase in intraocular pressure as flurbiprofen does.

Systemic Agents

The primary ocular indications for most NSAIDs approved for veterinary use are perioperative analgesia in dogs. Although they may be administered orally or parentally to treat anterior uveitis, only carprofen has been specifically demonstrated to be beneficial against this condition in small animals. Anorexia, vomiting, diarrhea, melena, gastric ulcers; hepatotoxicity, renal disease, and blood dyscrasias are the most frequently reported adverse effects of systemically administered NSAIDs. Caution is especially warranted with concomitant use of systemically administered corticosteroids because of the possibility of exacerbating hemorrhagic gastrointestinal problems.

Carprofen is the most frequently administered systemic NSAID in small animal practice and is a COX-2–specific inhibitor. It is available in injectable and oral forms. When given preemptively, it reduces aqueous flare in dogs with experimentally induced anterior uveitis. This has led to its common use as a treatment for this condition. In general, carprofen can be safely used in cats, but careful dose selection and patient monitoring are advisable because severe gastrointestinal side effects have been reported.

Several systemically administered NSAIDs such as meloxicam, deracoxib, etodolac, and ketoprofen have become available in the last few years. Meloxicam and deracoxib are COX-2–preferential or COX-2–specific inhibitors. The primary ocular indication for all of these medications in small animal patients is anterior uveitis, although their efficacy has not been experimentally demonstrated. Etodolac has been associated with causing severe and irreversible decrease in tear production in dogs; thus tear production should be monitored before and during treatment with this product (Klauss et al., 2003). Ketoprofen is approved for use in horses in the United States but has been successfully used in cats and dogs. It is a nonspecific COX inhibitor.

T CELL INHIBITORS

T cell inhibitors are indicated for autoimmune conditions characterized by T lymphocyte elaboration of proinflammatory proteins. Specific formulations, routes of administration, and dosages are summarized in Table 250-3.

Topical Agents

Cyclosporine A (CsA) is the most commonly used topical T cell inhibitor for ophthalmic conditions. CsA inhibits the action of T lymphocytes in two ways. First, CsA enters T lymphocytes and blocks transcription of ribonucleic acid, which is necessary for production of interleukin-2. Second, CsA obstructs interleukin receptors on the T lymphocyte surface. In treating ophthalmic disease CsA is virtually always administered topically. It is very lipophilic and accumulates in high levels in the anterior cornea, conjunctiva, sclera, and lacrimal tissues. Because of this, CsA has been the drug of choice for KCS in dogs and is a mainstay treatment of canine chronic superficial keratoconjunctivitis ("pannus"). However, CsA penetrates into the eye poorly and is not appropriate for anterior uveal disease. Unlike topical corticosteroids, chronic use of CsA does not appear to cause significant systemic problems. It is commercially available as a 0.2% ointment and also via compounding pharmacies as a 1% or 2% suspension in various oils. When monitoring response to therapy, it is important to remember that CsA often requires 4 to 6 weeks to fully exert its effect.

Tacrolimus has a mode of action very similar to that of CsA; however, it is estimated to be 10 to 100 times more potent than CsA in vitro. Tacrolimus has been used systemically in both human and veterinary medicine for organ transplant patients, but its use has been limited because of concerns about multisystem adverse side effects. It is approved for use in an ointment form for

Table 250-3

T Cell Inhibitory Agents

	Formulations	Dose
Topical Medications		
Cyclosporine A	0.2% ointment, 1% or 2% suspension in oil	Typically BID; titrate based on severity of clinical signs
Tacrolimus	0.02% ointment or solution	Typically BID; titrate based on severity of clinical signs
Systemic Medication		
Azathioprine (dogs)	50-mg tablets	2 mg/kg/day PO 1 to 2 weeks, then taper

treatment of atopic dermatitis in humans. Although not commercially available, tacrolimus can be obtained as a 0.02% ointment or solution from compounding pharmacies for topical ophthalmic use. In one recent study 0.02% tacrolimus suspension administered twice daily was effective in significantly increasing tear production in dogs with KCS, even in patients that had not responded well to topically applied CsA (Berdoulay, English, and Nadelstein, 2005). Its use against other surface inflammatory conditions has not been investigated.

Systemic Agent

Azathioprine is a systemic immunosuppressive drug that exerts cytotoxic effects on helper T lymphocytes. Its most common use in veterinary ophthalmology is the treatment of nodular granulomatous episclerokeratitis (NGE) or uveodermatologic syndrome, where it is often combined with topical and/or systemic corticosteroids. Azathioprine is available as a tablet or injection. Bone marrow suppression is the most common side effect and is especially severe in cats. For this reason, azathioprine is usually not recommended for feline patients. Hepatotoxicity, gastrointestinal upset, and pancreatitis have also been associated with azathioprine use in dogs. Because of the potential severity of these side effects, complete blood counts and serum chemistry analysis are necessary before therapy, about 14 days after initiation of therapy, and then every 2 to 3 months during therapy.

References and Suggested Reading

Berdoulay A, English RV, Nadelstein B: Effect of topical 0.02% tacrolimus aqueous suspension on tear production in dogs with keratoconjunctivitis sicca, *Vet Ophthalmol* 8:225, 2005.

Gilger BC, Allen JB: Cyclosporine A in veterinary ophthalmology, *Vet Ophthalmol* 1:181, 1998.

Giuliano EA: Nonsteroidal anti-inflammatory drugs in veterinary ophthalmology, *Vet Clin North Am Small Anim Pract* 34:707, 2004.

Holmberg BJ, Maggs DJ: The use of corticosteroids to treat ocular inflammation, *Vet Clin North Am Small Anim Pract* 34:693, 2004.

Klauss G et al: Canine keratoconjunctivitis sicca associated with etodolac administration, *Vet Ophthalmol* 6:361, 2003.

Millichamp NJ, Dziezyc J: Mediators of ocular inflammation, *Prog Vet Comp Ophthalmol* 1:41, 1991.

Moore CP: Immunomodulating agents, *Vet Clin North Am Small Anim Pract* 34:725, 2004.

Murphy CJ, Feldman E, Bellhorn R: Iatrogenic Cushing's syndrome in a dog caused by topical ophthalmic medications, *J Am Anim Hosp Assoc* 26:640, 1990.

Regnier A: Antimicrobials, anti-inflammatory agents, and antiglaucoma drugs. In Gelatt KN, editor: *Veterinary ophthalmology*, ed 3, Philadelphia, 1999, Lippincott Williams & Wilkins, p 308.

CHAPTER **251**

Ocular Neoplasia

BRADFORD J. HOLMBERG, *Stockholm, New Jersey*
MICHAEL S. KENT, *Davis, California*

Neoplasia of the eye and its associated support structures is not uncommon. Early detection and discrimination between benign and malignant tumors are necessary to determine the prognosis for ocular health, as well as for patient survival. The purpose of this chapter is to summarize the appearance, diagnosis, clinical behavior, and treatment of common ophthalmic neoplasms.

ORBITAL NEOPLASIA

Orbital neoplasia is rare in dogs and cats, accounting for less than 4% of all reported neoplasms. The most common presenting clinical sign is exophthalmos, or anterior protrusion of the globe. Other accompanying clinical signs may include strabismus or globe displacement (typically away from the location of the tumor), protrusion of the third eyelid, epiphora, and exposure keratitis. Decreased retropulsion of the globe is consistent with a retrobulbar, space-occupying mass. Differentiation between orbital inflammation and neoplasia is critical for both treatment and prognosis and is discussed in detail elsewhere (see Section XII on Evolve). Orbital neoplasia is usually slowly progressive and nonpainful (unless significant inflammation or bone destruction is associated with the tumor) and tends to affect older dogs (mean age of 8 years) and cats (mean age of 12.5 years).

Diagnosis of an orbital neoplasm is aided by diagnostic imaging techniques. Orbital ultrasonography is frequently inadequate. Computed tomography (CT) is very useful with osseous tumors or those affecting the bone (Fig. 251-1), whereas magnetic resonance imaging (MRI) is the imaging modality of choice when a soft-tissue mass is suspected. Ultrasonography is valuable for guidance of a fine-needle aspiration or nonsurgical biopsy of orbital masses since it allows visualization of the globe and mass and minimizes inadvertent globe puncture.

Approximately 75% to 91% of orbital neoplasms in dogs and 88% in cats are malignant. In dogs these tumors tend to be primary neoplasms, with osteosarcoma, multilobular osteosarcoma, and fibrosarcoma most frequently diagnosed. Secondary tumors in the orbit are much less common; but when present they usually arise from adjacent structures, including the nose, sinuses, oral cavity, and orbital glands. Nasal adenocarcinoma is the most common secondary orbital neoplasm in dogs. Cats do not follow this trend. Although primary orbital melanoma and squamous cell carcinoma have been reported in the cat, they are more likely to have secondary tumor involvement in the orbit, including fibrosarcoma, undifferentiated sarcoma, adenocarcinoma, and lymphoma. Only 14% of orbital neoplasia in cats is primary and, when present, usually represents squamous cell carcinoma, which may invade bone.

Because of the malignant behavior of most orbital neoplasms in dogs and cats, prognosis is poor. Determination of the prognosis in dogs is improved through either CT or radiography. However, skull radiographs are much less sensitive in identifying bone invasion. The presence of osteolysis of any of the orbital bones carries a worse prognosis. Mean survival time in dogs with osteolysis was 5.1 months versus 18.6 months for those without osteolysis. Considering all orbital tumors, approximately 50% of dogs were dead within 6 months, 1-year survival rate was 19%, and mean survival time was 10 months. The prognosis for cats with orbital neoplasia is grave, with survival times at only 1 to 2 months following diagnosis. An exception is nasal lymphoma, for which a median survival of 2 years has been reported with radiation therapy.

Because of the high morbidity associated with orbital neoplasia, treatment must be aggressive and initiated relatively early in the course of disease. When possible, surgical excision of primary tumors via orbitectomy or orbitotomy is the treatment of choice and may be curative. However, the extensive nature of the mass and proximity to the brain usually make surgery difficult or contraindicated. Imaging with either CT or MRI helps to determine if surgery is feasible and to plan the extent of surgery. Tissue margins should be inked for submission to a pathologist. If evaluation of the surgical margin reveals that residual tumor has been left behind, either additional surgery or possibly radiation therapy is in order to obtain better local control of the tumor.

ADNEXAL NEOPLASIA

Neoplasia of the eyelids is observed frequently in dogs but rarely in cats. Adnexal tumors may involve the palpebral skin with or without affecting the eyelid margin. Depending on the location of the mass, eyelid function may be disrupted, resulting in loss of the normal tear film and signs associated with exposure keratitis. In addition, if the mass contacts the cornea, it may irritate the surface and potentially result in corneal ulceration. Fortunately approximately 90% of eyelid neoplasms in dogs are benign, with meibomian adenomas, melanomas, and papillomas most common. Although 25% of these masses appear malignant on histologic evaluation, metastasis is rarely reported. Older, purebred dogs are commonly affected. Diagnosis of these masses is usually made based on clinical appearance, although a fine-needle aspirate or biopsy can be performed for larger or atypical-appearing masses. Treatment is surgical. The mass may be removed by a wedge resection, carbon dioxide laser, or a combination of sharp dissection and cryotherapy. Recurrence is uncommon but may occur if excision is not complete. Growth of new masses at different sites along the eyelids is common and should not be considered as recurrences. Less common adnexal neoplasms include histiocytoma, malignant melanoma, adenocarcinoma, basal cell carcinoma, mast cell tumor, squamous cell carcinoma, and hemangiosarcoma. Of these, malignant melanoma and mast cell tumors are reported to metastasize. Treatment involves wide surgical excision using an appropriate blepharoplastic technique, with ancillary therapy as dictated by the size and type of tumor. Prognosis varies significantly, depending on the type of tumor. Systemic staging of patients with malignant melanoma or mast cell tumors should be completed. Adjuvant therapy with

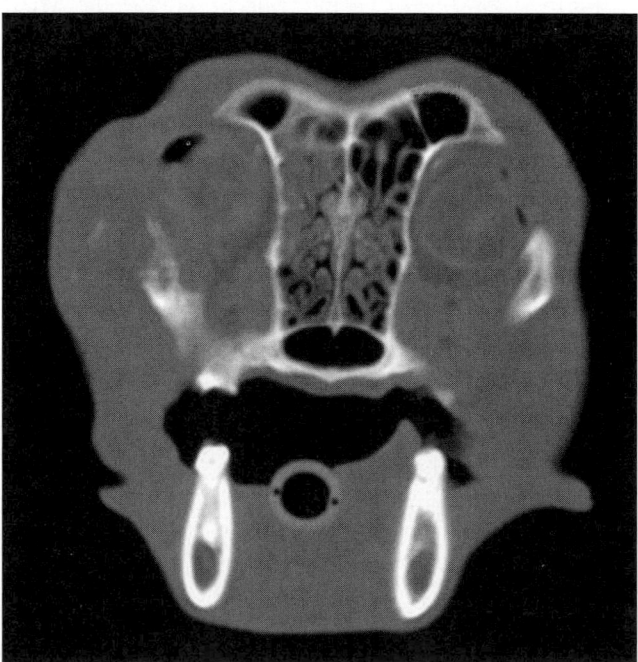

Fig. 251-1 Axial computed tomography (CT) image of an orbital osteosarcoma in a dog that presented with conjunctivitis and swelling along the left zygomatic arch. The CT reveals osteolysis along with marked periosteal reaction of the orbital bones.

carboplatin for malignant melanoma and with lomustine (CCNU) and/or vinblastine along with prednisone can be used to treat possible metastasis of mast cell tumors (see Chapter 65).

Squamous cell carcinoma is the most common eyelid tumor in cats. Most affected cats are older and lack periocular pigmentation. These tumors are suspected to be associated with ultraviolet light exposure. Cats are presented with either a proliferative pink-to-white mass with a "cobblestoned" surface or an ulcerative lesion that destroys the eyelid margin (Fig. 251-2). This tumor is frequently mistaken as bacterial or traumatic blepharitis or as an eosinophilic granuloma; therefore appropriate treatment is often delayed, resulting in large tumors that are difficult to manage. The presence of an ulcerated mass on the eyelid always warrants further examination, including cytology and/or biopsy. Adnexal squamous cell carcinoma has the potential to invade the orbit or to metastasize to regional lymph nodes, both of which carry a poor prognosis. However, early surgical excision, sometimes with adjunctive therapy, may be curative. Superficial squamous cell carcinoma of the eyelid margin may be responsive to strontium-90 β-therapy. Other palpebral neoplasms in cats include mast cell tumor, basal cell carcinoma, fibrosarcoma, spindle cell sarcoma, and apocrine hidrocystoma. Although these masses can be expansile and disrupt the eyelid margin, they tend not to metastasize. Recurrence is common without complete excision.

The biologic behavior of mast cell tumors on the eyelids of cats and dogs is poorly defined, although metastasis has been confirmed in several clinical cases.

SURFACE OCULAR NEOPLASIA

Of all ocular neoplasia, tumors of the conjunctiva, third eyelid, and cornea are the least common. Dermoids are congenital tumors derived from ectoderm and mesoderm. They usual involve the lateral limbus but may also affect the eyelid margin or third eyelid. They have the characteristic appearance of haired skin. Breeds most commonly affected include the dalmatian, dachshund, Doberman, German shepherd, and Saint Bernard dogs and Burmese cats. Although benign, they may become irritating locally and therefore should be removed by superficial keratectomy and conjunctivectomy. Excision is curative provided all hair follicles are removed. Another benign tumor frequently arising at the dorsolateral limbus of dogs and cats is the epibulbar or limbal melanocytoma. German shepherds and Labrador retrievers are predisposed. In both cats and dogs these tumors can be locally expansile, potentially extending through the corneal stroma and entering the anterior chamber. In young dogs these tumors progress more rapidly and require removal using partial- to full-thickness keratectomy/sclerectomy. Adjunctive therapy following partial keratectomy has included cryotherapy, β-irradiation, and laser photoablation. Although strontium-90 radiotherapy used as adjuvant treatment is effective, with only one reported recurrence in a series of 30 dogs, acute and late side effects, including corneal scarring, corneal vascularization, conjunctivitis, lipid keratopathy, localized bullous keratopathy, deep scleral thinning, and scleral perforation were seen in 63% of cases. Metastasis has not been reported in dogs or cats. Before diagnosing a pigmented mass at the limbus as a limbal melanocytoma, a thorough ophthalmic examination is recommended to ensure that the mass does not represent extrascleral extension of an intraocular melanoma, which may carry a more serious prognosis.

Conjunctival neoplasia is quite rare in dogs and cats. Reported tumors include hemangioma, hemangiosarcoma, mast cell tumor, lymphoma (primary or metastatic), squamous cell carcinoma, and papilloma. Complete excision with or without adjunctive therapy is usually curative. Two exceptions include malignant melanoma in both the dog and cat and systemic histiocytosis in the dog. Conjunctival melanoma appears as a raised, irregular, melanotic mass on the bulbar, third eyelid, or palpebral conjunctiva (Fig. 251-3). Although usually small in size, they can be locally aggressive and invasive. Metastasis to the regional lymph nodes (cats) and the orbit, pulmonary parenchyma, and liver (dogs) has been reported. Treatment includes surgery, but other

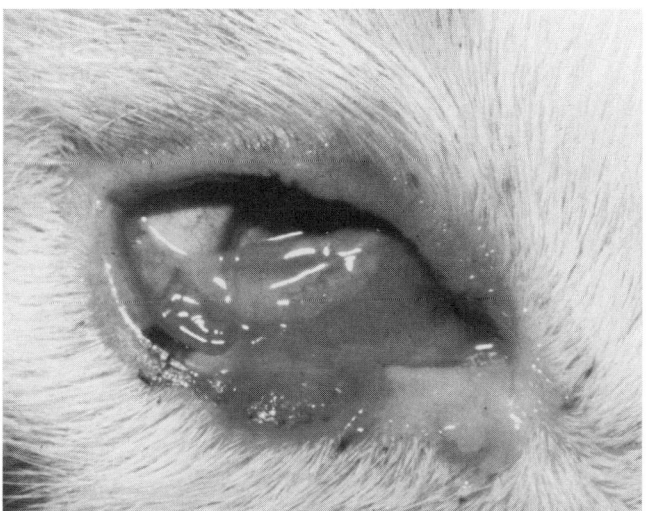

Fig. 251-2 Squamous cell carcinoma of the central aspect of the lower eyelid of a cat. Note the ulcerated appearance and local destruction of the eyelid margin.

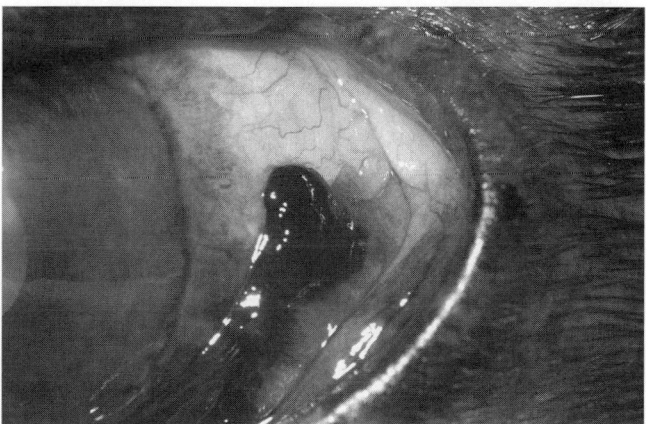

Fig. 251-3 Raised melanotic mass along the lateral bulbar conjunctiva of a dog. Biopsy was consistent with a melanoma.

local therapy such as irradiation with strontium-90 should be considered since clean surgical margins have rarely been obtained in reported clinical cases.

Malignant histiocytosis has a predilection for Bernese mountain dogs. Frequently affected dogs demonstrate severe chemosis secondary to a subconjunctival infiltrate. Exophthalmos, episcleral nodule formation, corneal edema, uveitis, and retinal detachment may also be present. The signalment and clinical signs are suggestive of the diagnosis, and it is confirmed by biopsy of the subconjunctiva. Although the ocular signs may appear first, the systemic nature of this disease and its poor response to medical therapy usually result in euthanasia. However, a recent report has indicated that treatment with lomustine may be effective at helping control this disease.

Neoplasia of the third eyelid or nictitating membrane is uncommon. Depending on the extent and location of the mass, the clinical appearance varies. Large masses at the base of the third eyelid, particularly those affecting the gland of the third eyelid, tend to result in third eyelid protrusion and exophthalmos with or without lateral displacement of the globe. By contrast, large masses on the anterior face of the third eyelid tend to cause enophthalmos. Discrete tumors on the surface or leading edge of the third eyelid are usually easily recognized by their altered color and contour. Retropulsion of the globe allows examination of almost the entire third eyelid (except for the orbital aspect) and greatly facilitates diagnosis of a third eyelid tumor. The behavior of third eyelid neoplasms differs significantly between dogs and cats, with most neoplasms benign in dogs but malignant in cats.

Adenocarcinoma of the gland of the third eyelid is the most common third eyelid tumor in dogs. Over 50% of these tumors recur without complete excision but rarely metastasize. Therefore removal of the entire third eyelid is recommended and frequently achieves a cure. Other reported third eyelid tumors in dogs include hemangiosarcoma, lobular adenoma, and squamous cell carcinoma. Surgical excision with or without ancillary therapy has been effective. Melanoma of the third eyelid in dogs is not benign and behaves similarly to conjunctival melanomas previously described.

As for the upper and lower eyelids, squamous cell carcinoma is the most common neoplasm of the third eyelid of cats. Treatment and success of therapy depend on extent of tumor involvement. Tumors that only involve the third eyelid can be managed successfully by complete excision of the third eyelid. However, because metastasis to the orbit is possible, staging should be completed before surgery. Unlike dogs, feline third eyelid adenocarcinomas have been demonstrated to metastasize to the lungs, liver, and kidneys. Other reported malignant (primary or secondary) third eyelid tumors in cats include fibrosarcoma and lymphoma. Presence of third eyelid neoplasia in cats warrants a complete systemic workup, including three-view thoracic radiographs and abdominal ultrasound, since most tumors are invasive and have the potential to metastasize. One exception is hemangiosarcoma, which appears to behave in a benign fashion and for which surgical removal is usually curative.

INTRAOCULAR NEOPLASIA

Intraocular tumors in dogs and cats occur sporadically and are usually secondary findings on the clinical examination. Animals may present with glaucoma, hyphema, corneal edema, buphthalmos, dyscoria, uveitis, retinal detachment, and/or blindness. Observation of a change in contour of the iris surface or alteration in iris color may be early signs of an intraocular mass (Fig. 251-4). In both dogs and cats anterior uveal melanoma is unquestionably the most frequently diagnosed intraocular neoplasm. The appearance and behavior of this tumor differs dramatically between species. In dogs these tumors are usually solitary, nodular, darkly pigmented, and benign. Most affected dogs are older, with golden and Labrador retrievers, boxers, and German shepherds predisposed. Eighty-two percent of intraocular melanomas in dogs are benign, with a 0% metastasis rate. The rest (18%) are considered malignant melanomas based on histologic appearance and mitotic index. However, biologically most canine intraocular melanomas behave in a benign fashion, with a metastatic potential of only 4% to 6%. Systemic staging, including three-view thoracic radiographs and abdominal ultrasound, are warranted in patients having tumors with a high mitotic index or other indicators of malignancy. Treatment is based on the size of the tumor and presence of complicating secondary factors. Some focal tumors can be ablated or reduced in size using a diode laser. Larger tumors or those compromising the overall health of the eye are treated by enucleation. In cases of malignant melanoma with evidence of metastasis, systemic chemotherapy with an agent such as carboplatin may be considered.

Anterior uveal melanomas in cats carry a worse prognosis than those in dogs. The majority of these tumors are considered malignant, although the time or stage at which they metastasize is unknown and controversial. Cats usually present with focal- to-multifocal areas of iris hyperpigmentation known as *nevi* or *freckles*. The masses are usually not raised but may take on a velvety appearance (Fig. 251-5). Diagnosis is made based on clinical appearance, and the owner should be informed of the

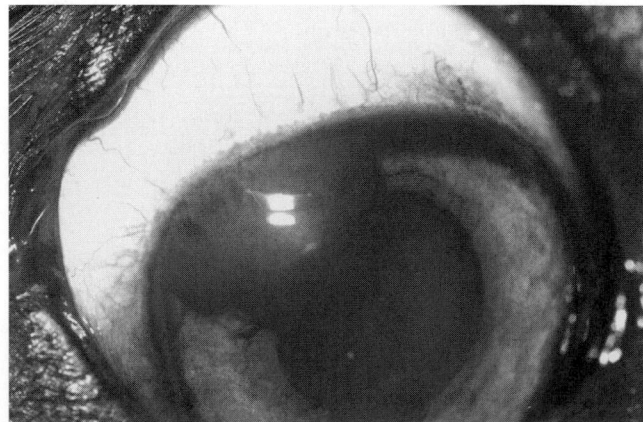

Fig. 251-4 Intraocular melanoma in a dog presenting as a focal, raised, pigmented mass arising from the surface of the iris and resulting in dyscoria.

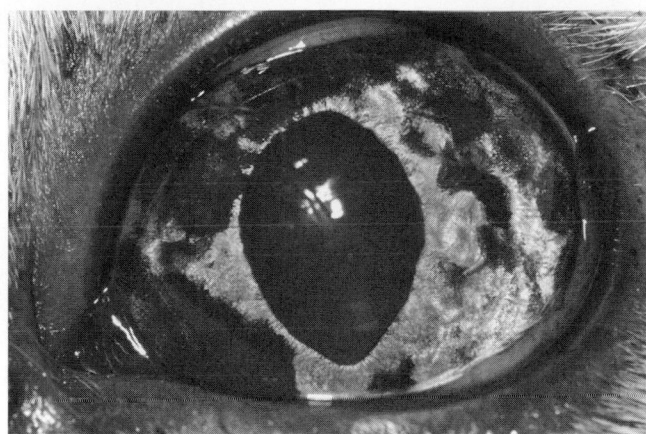

Fig. 251-5 Diffuse iris melanoma in a cat. Note the lack of a defined mass, but instead multifocal areas of iridal hyperpigmentation. Mild dyscoria is present, potentially indicating aggressive tumor involvement.

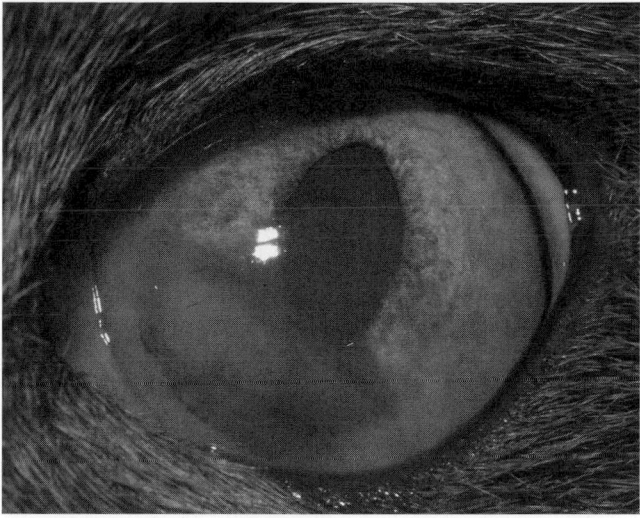

Fig. 251-6 Large fibrinohemorrhagic clot within the anterior chamber of a cat with multicentric lymphoma. Numerous neoplastic lymphoblasts were identified during cytologic evaluation of an aqueous humor aspirate.

metastatic potential. Two-year survival rates for cats with tumor in the iris only were 100%. However, microscopic evidence of extension to involve the ciliary body reduced this to 80%, and with scleral involvement the 2-year survival rate was 20%. Treatment is enucleation, preferably early to prevent metastasis. Clinical signs that suggest that the tumor is aggressive and that enucleation should be performed include dyscoria, glaucoma, uveitis, and the presence of free-floating tumor cells within the aqueous humor.

Other primary intraocular tumors in dogs include ciliary body adenocarcinoma and medulloepithelioma. Iridociliary adenocarcinomas, despite their histologic description, tend to be biologically benign and have a predilection for golden and Labrador retrievers. Medulloepitheliomas are embryologic neuroepithelial tumors usually arising in the ciliary body of young dogs. Although both of these tumors are benign, they are locally invasive and destructive and usually require enucleation.

Cats that receive penetrating trauma to the eye, especially if lens capsule rupture has occurred, are predisposed to the development of posttraumatic sarcoma. The origin of this tumor is debatable, although some tumors express collage type IV and crystalline α-A, which is consistent with a lens capsule epithelium origin. These tumors are extremely aggressive and destructive, rarely respecting the scleral boundaries. Unfortunately, by the time the tumor has been detected, extraocular extension usually has occurred. The tumor frequently courses along the optic nerve toward the brain, resulting in a mortality rate of over 90%. Treatment is effective only if there is early detection followed by early enucleation. For this reason blind eyes of cats that have experienced trauma should always be removed as early as possible.

Although almost any neoplasm can metastasize to the eye, the most common secondary intraocular tumor in dogs and cats is lymphoma. Most animals initially present with anterior uveitis with notable cellular exudate in the anterior chamber (hypopyon). Cats may have obvious iridal nodule formation or clusters of fibrinohemorrhagic debris in the anterior chamber (Fig. 251-6). Although there

are many causes of uveitis in dogs and cats (see Chapter 262), these patients are excellent examples of why a thorough diagnostic investigation of all patients with uveitis is warranted. If lymphoma is identified as the cause of uveitis in these patients, not only can specific rather than empiric therapy be initiated, but there is a greater opportunity to extend the patient's quality and length of life. If a thorough systemic diagnostic investigation does not yield an etiologic diagnosis in a patient with uveitis suspected to be caused by lymphoma, aqueocentesis is indicated. Treatment for intraocular lymphoma includes topical application of 1% prednisolone acetate ophthalmic suspension, which will decrease the uveitis, along with systemic chemotherapy with a "'CHOP-based" protocol (see Chapters 65 and 72), which often result in remission and resolution of ocular and extraocular clinical signs. Most cases of ocular lymphoma respond very favorably to topical and systemic therapy, if secondary sequela (glaucoma, iris bombé, cataract, retinal detachment) do not occur. Median survival times for dogs and cats with multicentric lymphoma treated with chemotherapy are reported to be about 1 year and 6 months, respectively. Secondary (metastatic) intraocular tumors other than lymphoma do not usually respond to medical therapy, and secondary complications typically ensue. Symptomatic therapy with antiinflammatory and antiglaucoma medications to improve ocular comfort typically is necessary. Surgery (enucleation) is palliative but is rarely performed because of the patient's overall systemic health.

Suggested Reading

Calia CM et al: The use of computed tomography scan for the evaluation of orbital disease in cats and dogs, *Vet Comp Ophthalmol* 4:24, 1997.

Donaldson D, Sansom J, Adams V: Canine limbal melanoma: 30 cases (1992-2004). Part 2: Treatment with lamellar resection and adjunctive strontium-90 β plesiotherapy—efficacy and morbidity, *Vet Ophthalmol* 9:179, 2006.

Dubielzig RR: Ocular neoplasia in small animals, *Vet Clin North Am Small Anim Pract* 20:837, 1990.

Gilger BC et al: Orbital neoplasms in cats: 21 cases (1974-1990), *J Am Vet Med Assoc* 201:1083, 1992.

Guiliano EA et al: A matched observational study of canine survival with primary intraocular melanocytic neoplasia, *Vet Ophthalmol* 2:185, 1999.

Gwin RM, Gelatt KN, Williams LW: Ophthalmic neoplasms in the dog, *J Am Anim Hosp Assoc* 18:853, 1982.

Hendrix DV, Gelatt KN: Diagnosis, treatment, and outcome of orbital neoplasia in dogs: a retrospective study of 44 cases, *J Small Anim Pract* 41:105, 2000.

Kalishman JB et al: A matched observational study of survival in cats with enucleation due to diffuse iris melanoma, *Vet Ophthalmol* 1:25, 1998.

Kern TJ: Orbital neoplasia in 23 dogs, *J Am Vet Med Assoc* 186:489, 1985.

Krehbiel JD, Langham RF: Eyelid neoplasms of dogs, *Am J Vet Res* 36:115, 1975.

Morgan RV, Daniel GB, Donnell RL: Magnetic resonance imaging of the normal eye and orbit of the dog and cat, *Vet Radiol Ultrasound* 35:102, 1994.

Mughannam AJ, Hacker DV, Spangler WL: Conjunctival vascular tumors in six dogs, *Vet Comp Ophthalmol* 7:5659, 1997.

Peiffer RL: Primary intraocular tumors in the dog. Part I, *Mod Vet Pract* 60:383, 1979.

Wilcock BP, Peiffer RL: Morphology and behavior of primary ocular melanomas in 91 dogs, *Vet Pathol* 23;418, 1986.

Willis AM, Wilkie DA: Ocular oncology, *Clin Tech Small Anim Pract* 16:77, 2001.

CHAPTER 252

Corneal Colors As a Diagnostic Aid

DAVID J. MAGGS, *Davis, California*

The cornea is optically transparent; it is the major refractive structure of the eye, richly innervated, and the ocular structure most obvious to the owner. As such it is a physiologically fragile, visually critical, highly sensitive, and easily observed ophthalmic tissue and therefore frequently is the reason for presentation of a small animal to a veterinarian. For this reason, correctly interpreting corneal pathology is critical for diagnosing not only corneal disease but many other ocular and some systemic diseases. Fortunately corneal pathology is frequently visible as a characteristic corneal color change or loss of corneal clarity. Common pathologic responses within the cornea include vascularization, edema, scarring, lipid and/or mineral deposition, pigmentation, and inflammatory cell infiltration. These changes frequently are seen in various combinations. Each of these pathologic changes is associated with a defining color change. Because some of the colors are similar, an appreciation for the "texture" or other character of these changes is also important. Learning to recognize and interpret these color changes and the mechanisms responsible for them provides a simple and logical approach to diagnosis of all corneal and some intraocular diseases. Such understanding also facilitates selection of appropriate diagnostic tests. This chapter is designed to assist the general practitioner in the interpretation of corneal color changes.

RED AND LINEAR

Corneal vascularization causes a red discoloration of the cornea and is a nonspecific indication of chronic inflammatory disease. However, distribution of corneal blood vessels provides valuable information regarding location and depth of the inciting cause (i.e., blood vessels reveal not *what* the inciting cause is but *where* it is). Therefore differentiation of deep from superficial corneal vascularization is critical for selection of further diagnostic steps and for differentiation of vision-threatening intraocular disease from irritating surface ocular disease (Fig. 252-1). Superficial corneal vessels arise from the conjunctiva at the limbus. They tend to be fine, branch dichotomously to form "tree-shaped" patterns on the cornea, and can be seen crossing the limbus (Fig. 252-2). Superficial vessels reflect surface ocular disease caused by inadequate protection (from the eyelids or tear film) or excessive frictional irritation of the corneal surface (by an exogenous or endogenous influence). Although a large list of potential causes should be considered, the diagnostic testing required to

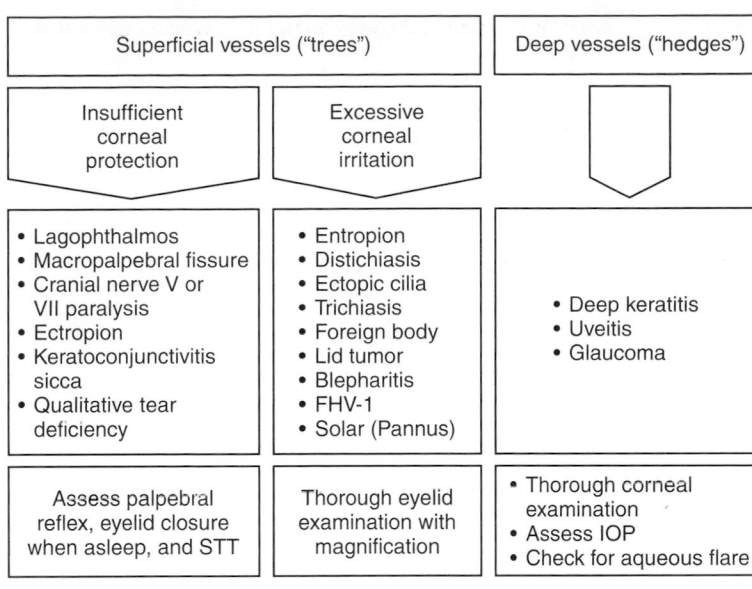

Fig. 252-1 Causes of and diagnostic steps for corneal vascularization, which causes red "linear" discoloration of the cornea. *CN,* Cranial nerve; *KCS,* keratoconjunctivitis sicca; *FHV-1,* feline herpesvirus type 1; *STT,* Schirmer's tear test; *IOP,* intraocular pressure.

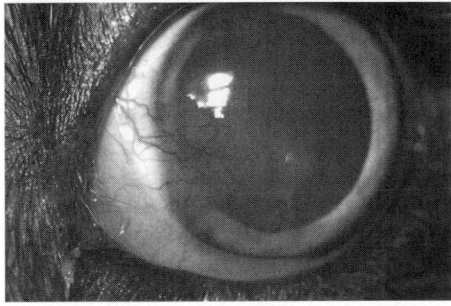

Fig. 252-2 Superficial corneal vessels. Note that they cross the limbus, branch, and appear "tree-like." They indicate superficial or "surface" corneal disease. (Courtesy University of California Davis Veterinary Ophthalmology Service.)

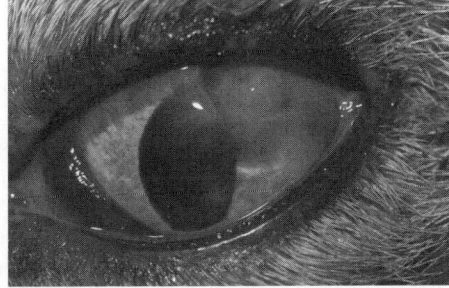

Fig. 252-3 Deep corneal (stromal) vessels in a cat with a deep ulcer. Note that the blood vessels do not cross the limbus or branch and appear more "hedge-like." They indicate deep corneal (stromal) or intraocular disease. Note also the stromal white blood cells within the ulcer bed producing a yellow-green discoloration. (Courtesy University of California Davis Veterinary Ophthalmology Service.)

differentiate these is simple (see Fig. 252-1). Deep corneal vessels arise from perilimbal ciliary and scleral vessels; tend to be darker, shorter, and straighter; and tend not to branch overtly (Fig. 252-3). They cannot be seen crossing the limbus but instead arise from under the scleral shelf. They form a "hedge-shaped" pattern on the cornea. They are characteristic of serious, vision-threatening diseases such as deep keratitis, uveitis, or glaucoma, which require similarly straightforward tests but different from those suggested by superficial corneal vessels (see Fig. 252-1).

BLUE AND "FLUFFY"

Corneal edema is usually evident as a bluish discoloration of the cornea, often in a "fluffy" or "ground glass" pattern (Fig. 252-4). Although the edema accumulates in the collagenous corneal stroma, it occurs as a result of dysfunction of one or both of the cell layers responsible for corneal deturgescence—the epithelium or endothelium. Application of fluorescein stain and careful attention to the severity and area of edema will suggest which cell

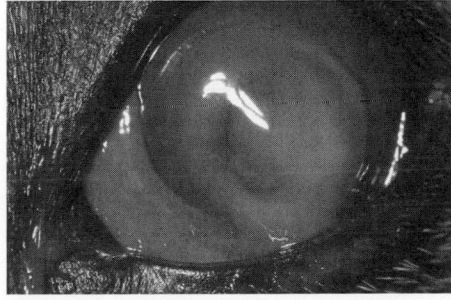

Fig. 252-4 Corneal edema causes a blue and "fluffy" corneal discoloration. This dog has a deep and malacic ("melting") ulcer. (Courtesy University of California Davis Veterinary Ophthalmology Service.)

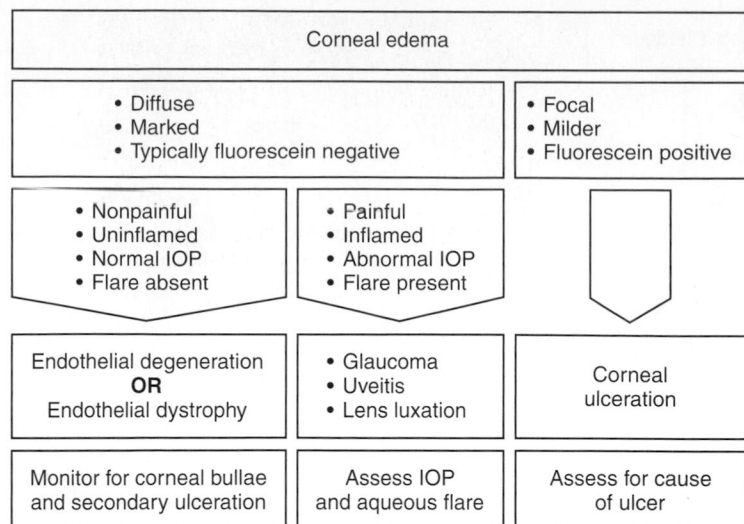

Fig. 252-5 Causes of and diagnostic steps for corneal edema. *IOP,* Intraocular pressure.

layer is more likely dysfunctional (Fig. 252-5). Epithelial loss (corneal ulceration) produces more focal and milder edema in close spatial association with a fluorescein-positive area of cornea. Endothelial decompensation tends to produce more severe and diffuse corneal edema because endothelium has the more important role in maintaining deturgescence. Endothelial dysfunction may occur as a primary event, especially in dogs. Primary endothelial dystrophy is relatively common in Boston terriers and Chihuahuas, whereas senile endothelial degeneration might be suspected in older dogs of any breed. Unless ulceration occurs secondary to corneal bullae (blister) formation, these primary endothelial diseases are characteristically nonpainful, and the cornea does not retain fluorescein. Secondary endothelial decompensation occurs in dogs and cats with uveitis, glaucoma, anterior lens luxation, or scleritis and is associated with ocular pain, inflammation, and other specific abnormalities. Because domestic (outbred) cats are less prone to primary inherited disease and the feline endothelium seems more resistant to senile changes, diffuse corneal edema in cats is usually secondary to these more serious intraocular diseases and warrants urgent and complete examination. An exceptional disease that seems peculiar to cats in which corneal edema is the major sign is feline acute bullous keratopathy. This tends to occur in younger cats without any recognized predisposing cause or history. The onset of massive stromal edema and sometimes rupture can occur within hours! The pathogenesis is proposed to involve the stroma itself rather than the endothelium. Treatment involves emergency conjunctival grafting.

GRAY AND WISPY

Corneal scars are caused by derangement of the usual highly regular array of stromal collagen. The scattering of light this induces causes gray, wispy discolorations in an uninflamed cornea (Fig. 252-6). These lesions do not retain fluorescein stain. Scars are by definition inactive and require no further treatment. Presence of inflammatory signs such as vascularization or cellular infiltrates in association with scarring suggests continuing active inflammation.

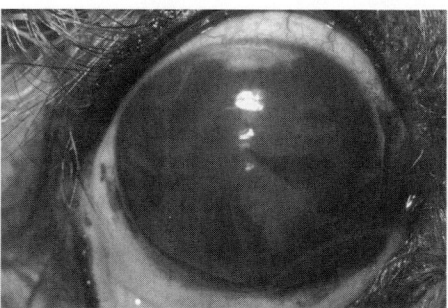

Fig. 252-6 Corneal fibrosis (scarring) evident as a generalized gray and "wispy" discoloration of the cornea. There are also superficial corneal blood vessels and corneal melanosis present. (Courtesy University of California Davis Veterinary Ophthalmology Service.)

WHITE AND "SPARKLY" OR "CREAMY"

Subepithelial accumulation of lipid and/or mineral in the anterior stroma appears as sparkly, crystalline, or more coalescing creamy or shiny areas of white discoloration. These accumulations frequently contain cholesterol and/or calcium; however, varying combinations of lipids and minerals are possible. The clinician's major goal following identification of this characteristic change is to determine if the lipid/mineral accumulation represents a primary or secondary disease (Fig. 252-7). Corneal lipid dystrophy describes a primary inherited, but not necessarily congenital, condition that occurs in many dog breeds but rarely in cats. Corneal lipid dystrophy is usually bilateral and approximately symmetric, with lipid usually deposited in the central or paracentral cornea, often in a circular or elliptical shape (Fig. 252-8). Because the lipid deposits typically are subepithelial, the cornea is usually negative to fluorescein stain retention and patients appear nonpainful. However, occasionally the overlying epithelium ulcerates. The disease may be slowly progressive but has minimal effect on vision and requires no therapy. Commonly affected breeds include the Siberian husky, Samoyed, bichon frise, and cavalier King Charles spaniel.

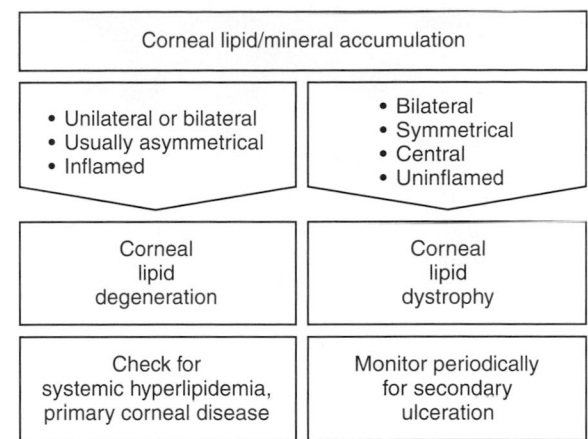

Corneal lipid/mineral accumulation

- Unilateral or bilateral
- Usually asymmetrical
- Inflamed

- Bilateral
- Symmetrical
- Central
- Uninflamed

Corneal lipid degeneration

Corneal lipid dystrophy

Check for systemic hyperlipidemia, primary corneal disease

Monitor periodically for secondary ulceration

Fig. 252-7 Causes of and diagnostic steps for corneal accumulation of lipid and/or mineral, which causes white "creamy" or "sparkly" discoloration of the cornea.

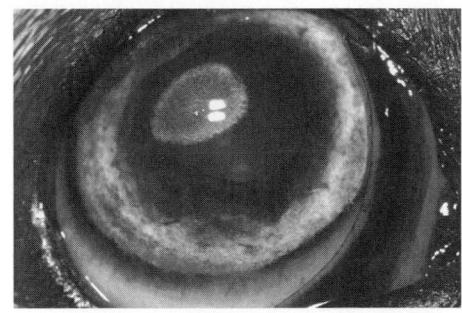

Fig. 252-8 Corneal lipid dystrophy. The other eye of this dog was similarly affected. (Courtesy University of California Davis Veterinary Ophthalmology Service.)

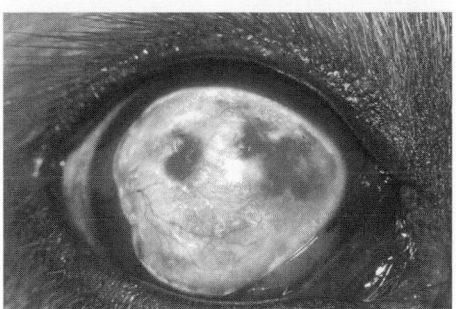

Fig. 252-9 Corneal lipid degeneration in a dog. Note the cream-to-sparkly white discoloration with associated corneal vascularization. (Courtesy University of California Davis Veterinary Ophthalmology Service.)

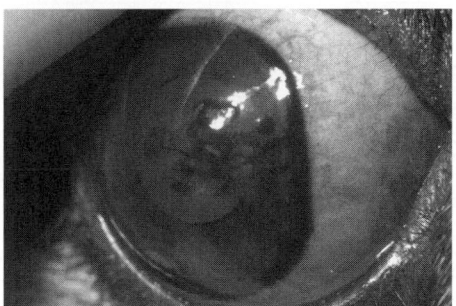

Fig. 252-10 Corneal melanosis in a dog. Note the superficial corneal blood vessels, which are a common finding with corneal melanin since they share the same mechanism. (Courtesy University of California Davis Veterinary Ophthalmology Service.)

Alternatively, lipid may accumulate secondary to corneal inflammation or injury in dogs or rarely cats. In these cases it is termed corneal degeneration, is usually unilateral, and frequently is associated with inflammation evident as coincident corneal edema or vascularization (Fig. 252-9). These lesions are frequently seen in animals with chronic uveitis, especially with long-term corticosteroid use. Typically there will be a history of ocular trauma, often with ulceration that healed with vascularization and subsequent lipid deposition. However, some animals deposit lipid in their cornea without evidence of prior trauma. These animals usually develop a sparkly-to-creamy, sometimes vascularized band of perilimbal corneal lipid as a result of elevated serum lipid. Investigation of common causes of systemic hyperlipidemia such as hypothyroidism, diabetes mellitus, hyperadrenocorticism, or primary hyperlipidemia is essential in such animals. Serum triglycerides and cholesterol should both be measured.

BLACK AND GEOGRAPHIC ("MAP-SHAPED")

Corneal pigmentation causes an obvious black discoloration of the superficial (epithelial and anterior stromal) cornea. In dogs the pigment is melanin and tends to encroach insidiously from the limbus (Fig. 252-10). Heavily pigmented dogs, especially Pekingese, pugs, and chow-chows, seem to be more prone to this change (sometimes called "pigmentary keratitis"). In sharp contrast, black discoloration of the feline cornea is rarely caused by melanin. Instead the feline corneal pigment is soluble and appears to originate from or be spread in the tear film. It may also cause black tear staining of the periocular skin and can be deposited in the corneal stroma. In the latter case it is usually associated with an area of necrotic, sequestered stromal collagen and is called a "corneal sequestrum" (Fig. 252-11). Regardless of pigment type or species affected, corneal pigmentation (like the superficial corneal blood vessels that often accompany it) is a sign of chronic irritation. Like corneal vascularization, pigmentation of the cornea provides no information regarding nature of the specific irritant but does accurately direct attention to the location of the irritation (Fig. 252-12).

TAN AND "GREASY"

Fibrin and white blood cells are commonly seen together and appear as a tannish-gray corneal discoloration. They appear in two common locations, each with characteristic appearance. Keratic precipitates (KPs) are multiple,

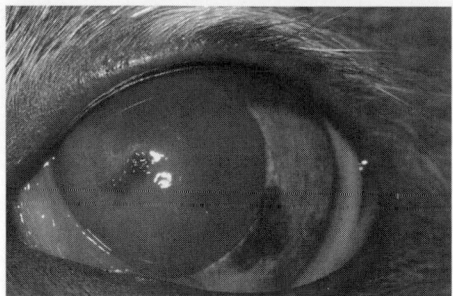

Fig. 252-11 Corneal sequestrum in a cat with feline herpesvirus. Sequestra can vary from amber to dark black and are caused by a soluble pigment. (Courtesy University of California Davis Veterinary Ophthalmology Service.)

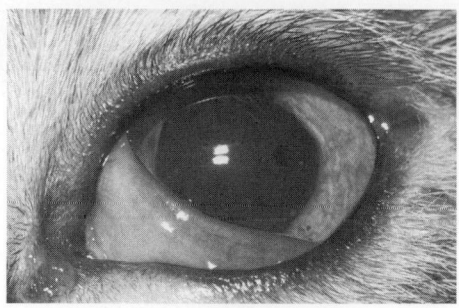

Fig. 252-13 Keratic precipitates are present on the corneal endothelium of this cat with anterior uveitis. The larger darker discolorations are small clumps of hemorrhage (hyphema). (Courtesy University of California Davis Veterinary Ophthalmology Service.)

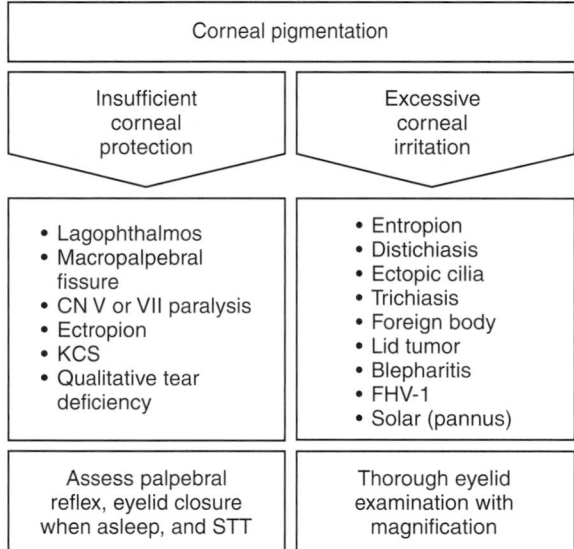

```
                  Corneal pigmentation

   Insufficient                   Excessive
    corneal                        corneal
   protection                     irritation

• Lagophthalmos              • Entropion
• Macropalpebral             • Distichiasis
  fissure                    • Ectopic cilia
• CN V or VII paralysis      • Trichiasis
• Ectropion                  • Foreign body
• KCS                        • Lid tumor
• Qualitative tear           • Blepharitis
  deficiency                 • FHV-1
                             • Solar (pannus)

  Assess palpebral            Thorough eyelid
 reflex, eyelid closure      examination with
 when asleep, and STT          magnification
```

Fig. 252-12 Causes of and diagnostic steps for corneal pigmentation (melanosis or sequestration), which causes a black geographic discoloration of the cornea. *CN,* Cranial nerve; *KCS,* keratoconjunctivitis sicca; *FHV-1,* feline herpesvirus type 1; *STT,* Schirmer's tear test.

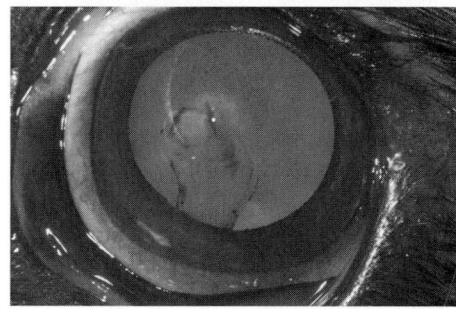

Fig. 252-14 This dog has a ruptured cornea. This is visible as a greasy tan area axially backlit (retroilluminated) here by the tapetal reflection. There is some surrounding (bluish) corneal edema, intraocular hemorrhage (hyphema), and some iris melanin remnants against the anterior lens capsule. This was the result of a cat claw injury. (Courtesy University of California Davis Veterinary Ophthalmology Service.)

clumped accumulations of inflammatory cells and fibrin on the inner corneal (endothelial) surface (Fig. 252-13). They have a greasy appearance, sometimes termed *mutton fat,* and tend to be deposited most densely on the ventral cornea. KPs are a pathognomonic sign of uveitis, and the causes of uveitis should be thoroughly investigated (see Chapter 262). A ruptured globe with prolapsed uvea (a "staphyloma") will also produce a greasy tan discoloration of the usually central cornea (Fig. 252-14). This indicates ulcerative or traumatic perforation. The surrounding corneal health is usually poor (e.g., malacic, edematous, vascularized, infiltrated with white blood cells). The protruding uvea (iris) is coated in a layer of fibrin and inflammatory cells and therefore has a tannish-brown appearance. A staphyloma frequently appears as a raised area in the center of an otherwise deep ulcer.

YELLOW-GREEN

Inflammatory cell infiltration of the corneal stroma is termed *stromal keratitis* or (when the epithelium is intact) a *stromal abscess.* These conditions cause a yellow-green discoloration characteristic of pus elsewhere in the body (see Fig. 252-3). This usually occurs in response to an infectious etiology; however, nonseptic infiltration of the cornea can occur. Inflammatory cells originate from the tear film, limbus, and sometimes the uveal tract and can accumulate within the cornea surprisingly quickly, indicating a potent chemotactic stimulus. This is most often caused by an infection, blunt trauma (corneal contusion), or an intracorneal foreign body. Therefore corneal cytology along with culture and sensitivity testing should be performed, and broad-spectrum antibiotic therapy initiated promptly. Frequent reexamination of the cornea is essential because liberation of lytic enzymes by the inflammatory cells (and any associated bacteria) can cause rapid collagenolysis or corneal "melting."

Table **252-1**

Recommended Diagnostic Tests Based on Corneal Color Changes

Color	Histology	Mechanism	Recommended Tests
Red	Blood vessels	Chronic irritation	Fluorescein stain, STT, palpebral and corneal reflexes
"Fluffy" blue	Stromal edema	Endothelial or epithelial dysfunction	Fluorescein stain, IOP, flare, check for lens luxation
"Wispy" gray	Stromal scar	Previous (inactive) inflammation	Fluorescein stain
"Sparkly" white	Lipid/mineral accumulation	Dystrophy, degeneration, or hyperlipidemia	Fluorescein stain, systemic lipid analyses
Black	Pigmentation	Chronic irritation	Fluorescein stain, STT Palpebral and corneal reflexes
"Punctate" tan	KPs or staphyloma	Uveitis	IOP, flare, systemic disease testing
Yellow-green	Inflammatory cell infiltration	Inflammation (usually septic)	Fluorescein stain, cytology, culture and sensitivity testing, PCR

IOP, Intraocular pressure; *PCR,* polymerase chain reaction; *STT,* Schirmer's tear test.

DIAGNOSTIC TESTING FOR CORNEAL DISEASE

Knowledge of the mechanisms by which these seven corneal color changes occur can be used to direct diagnostic testing as suggested in Table 252-1. The most commonly used tests for investigation of corneal pathology are Schirmer's tear test, fluorescein and/or rose bengal staining, tonometry, assessment of aqueous flare, and corneal cytologic and microbiologic assessment (see Chapter 248). Histopathologic examination of keratectomy samples may be required to confirm a diagnosis in some cases of proliferative or inflammatory corneal disease.

CHAPTER **253**

Differential Diagnosis of Blindness

HOLLY L. HAMILTON, *Loveland, Colorado*
SUSAN A. MCLAUGHLIN, *West Lafayette, Indiana*

Blindness can result from lesions that interfere with the formation of the image by the retina, transmission of the image to the visual cortex, or interpretation of the image by the visual cortex. Numerous diseases can cause bilateral loss of vision. The usual approach to such patients involves confirmation and characterization of the visual impairment, anatomic localization of the cause, and appropriate diagnostic testing.

CONFIRMATION OF BLINDNESS

Diagnostic confirmation of blindness is the essential first step. This can be achieved by watching the animal navigate in the examination room or by setting up an obstacle course. Evaluation should be performed in both bright and dim lighting. Some animals, particularly cats, will not attempt to walk in an unfamiliar environment. Observing the animal's response to noiseless objects such as cotton balls dropped across its visual field works well with animals that will not ambulate. The menace response (a threatening gesture such as a hand moving towards one eye) can be used to assess vision and should elicit rapid eyelid closure, provided that the facial nerve (CN VII) is intact. Care must be taken when testing the menace response not to stimulate the trigeminal nerve by touching the animal or by creating air currents since such stimuli can induce a palpebral reflex (via CN V and CN VII). A Plexiglas shield or vertical hand movements prevent air currents when testing the menace response. The visual placing reaction may also be used to assess vision. The animal is held without restricting the forelegs and advanced toward a table. If the animal sees the table, it will reach out towards the table edge using the front legs.

Pupillary Light Reflex

The pupillary light reflex (PLR) provides valuable information about visual pathways but does not test vision. The PLR should be evaluated in a darkened room with a bright, focal light source. The direct (constriction of the stimulated pupil) and consensual (constriction of the unstimulated pupil) PLR should be evaluated. Absence of a direct and consensual PLR in a blind animal is consistent with (but not pathognomonic for) a lesion in the subcortical visual pathway, which includes the retina, optic nerve, optic chiasm, and optic tract. However, abnormal direct and consensual PLRs also can occur (with or without blindness) as a result of bilateral dysfunction of the efferent pathway such as synechia (iris adhered to lens or cornea), iris atrophy, topical mydriatic application, or oculomotor nerve (CN III) deficits. A frightened or nervous animal may have notably reduced PLRs because of stimulation of the iris dilator muscle by the sympathetic nervous system. Therefore, when a reduced or absent PLR is encountered, it should be reassessed later in the examination once the animal becomes more accustomed to the surroundings. Bilateral lesions in the lateral geniculate nucleus, optic radiation, or visual cortex, often referred to as central or intracranial blindness, cause loss of sight without affecting the PLR. The presence of a PLR also does not absolutely exclude blindness secondary to retinal disease. Some cases of retinal degeneration or retinal detachment are severe enough to cause blindness but not completely prohibit a PLR.

In this chapter the causes of blindness are grouped according to the affected region of the visual pathway. Disorders are discussed in the order in which they would typically be encountered during an ophthalmic examination. When blindness is confirmed in a patient without ocular abnormalities, additional diagnostic tests are required. In addition, even if an ocular cause of blindness is identified, most ophthalmic lesions are not pathognomonic for a specific etiologic agent, and additional diagnostic tests will be needed to identify the cause.

DIAGNOSTIC TESTING

Electroretinography detects and quantifies a mass retinal response to photic stimuli. The electroretinogram (ERG) primarily evaluates the outer retinal layers (especially the photoreceptors), and is severely diminished or absent with blindness caused by retinal disease (e.g., sudden acquired retinal degeneration or end-stage progressive retinal atrophy). The ERG may be normal in early glaucoma because glaucoma affects the ganglion cell and nerve fiber layers of the inner retina before the photoreceptors. An ERG can be performed in an awake or anes-

thetized animal but does require special equipment and thus is typically available only at referral centers. The ERG waveform and amplitude is affected by anesthesia, breed, age, equipment, and technique.

Visual-evoked potentials (VEPs) are used to evaluate electrical potentials in postretinal visual pathways, including the visual cortex in response to light stimulation of the eye. The potentials are recorded by scalp electrodes. The VEP is not as frequently used or as standardized as the ERG, but it can be useful in cases of blindness caused by lesions in the optic nerve, visual tracts, or visual cortex.

Ocular ultrasound is useful for evaluation of the globe in cases of opacification of the ocular media and may aid in identification of retinal detachment or intraocular mass lesions. In most animals this can be performed without sedation, using only topical anesthesia. Ultrasound is also useful for evaluation of orbital contents, especially the optic nerve, but computed tomography or magnetic resonance imaging (MRI) provide superior information regarding this structure.

When exudate within the vitreous or aqueous humor may yield potential cytologic or serologic clues, samples may be collected by centesis under general anesthesia. *Vitreous centesis* is performed using a 20- to 23-gauge needle inserted 6 to 8 mm posterior to the limbus and directed toward the posterior pole. Aspiration is performed in a slow, controlled manner, and 0.1 to 0.2 ml of vitreous should be aspirated for cytology and bacterial and fungal culture. There is some risk of hemorrhage and retinal detachment; thus this is usually performed by experienced personnel when less invasive techniques have failed to identify a cause or in permanently blind eyes. In young, normal animals, the vitreous is gel-like and difficult to aspirate. In patients with posterior segment inflammation, the vitreous becomes more liquefied and easier to aspirate. In patients with anterior segment disease, aqueous humor can be attained in a similar manner but via a limbal entry point. *Aqueous centesis* is most likely to yield positive results with cytologic evaluation in cases of suspected intraocular lymphosarcoma or in evaluation for intraocular antibody production against infectious agents such as *Toxoplasma gondii* (see Chapter 262).

OPACITY OF THE OCULAR MEDIA

The clear ocular media include the cornea, aqueous humor, lens, and vitreous. These structures are transparent to allow passage of light and image formation by the retina. Mild opacification of the ocular media results in blurred vision, and significant opacification results in blindness.

Corneal Opacification

Blindness secondary to corneal disease occurs only with bilateral, severe, diffuse corneal lesions. Typically these are severe enough to obscure the clinician's evaluation of intraocular structures. Causes of corneal opacification include infiltration of the cornea with melanin, edema, blood vessels, or inflammatory or neoplastic cells or misalignment of corneal collagen fibers (scarring). Corneal melanosis resulting from eyelid abnormalities (entropion, ectropion, lagophthalmos, facial nerve paralysis), keratoconjunctivitis sicca, and chronic superficial keratitis ("pannus") can result in blindness. Diffuse, severe corneal edema can occur secondary to corneal endothelial dystrophy, endothelial degeneration, endotheliitis, glaucoma, or anterior uveitis. Symblepharon (conjunctiva adhered to cornea) and inherited corneal dystrophy can also cause corneal opacification.

Aqueous Humor Opacification

Opacification of the aqueous humor typically results from accumulation of red blood cells (hyphema), white blood cells (hypopyon), lipid, or fibrin clots. These typically gravitate ventrally and only partially affect vision. However, if the anterior chamber is diffusely and severely affected to the extent that the iris and other intraocular structures are obscured, blindness may result. Hyphema occurs secondary to coagulopathies (factor deficiencies, warfarin toxicosis, immune-mediated thrombocytopenia), infectious diseases (ehrlichiosis, rickettsiosis), trauma, neoplasia, systemic hypertension, or retinal detachment. Hypopyon results from immune-mediated, neoplastic (lymphosarcoma), or infectious (blastomycosis, cryptococcosis, histoplasmosis, coccidioidomycosis, toxoplasmosis, feline infectious peritonitis, protothecosis, brucellosis, bacterial septicemia) diseases. Lipemic aqueous occurs in patients with hyperlipidemia (serum cholesterol and/or triglycerides) and concurrent blood-aqueous barrier disruption (uveitis). Hypertriglyceridemia can be primary or secondary to diabetes mellitus, hyperadrenocorticism, or hypothyroidism. A complete physical examination is indicated in any patient with opacification of the anterior chamber. Any enlarged lymph nodes, subcutaneous masses, or draining skin tracts should be aspirated for cytologic evaluation. A complete blood count, serum biochemistry profile, urinalysis, thoracic and abdominal imaging, serologic assessment for relevant infectious agents, and assessment of coagulation may also be beneficial.

Lens Opacification

Cataracts are a frequent cause of blindness in dogs, and the majority are inherited. Cataracts also can occur secondary to diabetes mellitus, retinal degeneration, hypocalcemia, trauma, nutritional deficiencies, electric shock, chronic uveitis, or lens luxation. Cataracts are uncommon in cats, but, when they occur, they are most commonly the result of uveitis or lens luxation. For a cataract to be the cause of blindness, the entire lens must be involved, and the cataract must be dense enough to prevent ophthalmoscopic evaluation of the ocular fundus. Cataracts alone do not interfere with the PLR. Therefore, if the PLR is abnormal, a retinal optic nerve, optic tract, CN III, or iridal lesion must also be present. Cataracts must be differentiated from nuclear (lenticular) sclerosis, which is a normal aging change. The cloudy appearance of the lens in nuclear sclerosis is caused by increased density of lens fibers, particularly within the nucleus, causing partial reflection of light. Unlike with cataracts, in patients with nuclear sclerosis the ocular fundus is visible by direct or indirect ophthalmoscopy. Dilation of the pupil with tropicamide is essential for a complete lens examination and will facilitate differentiation between cataracts and nuclear sclerosis.

Vitreous Opacification

Blindness due to opacification of the vitreous can occur secondary to persistent hyperplastic primary vitreous (PHPV), which is a congenital abnormality caused by failed regression of the hyaloid vessel within the primary vitreous. This alone does not cause blindness, but PHPV usually is associated with persistence of embryologic remnants on the posterior lens capsule (persistent tunica vasculosa lentis) and/or vitreous hemorrhage. Leukocoria ("white pupil") results from fibrovascular plaque formation immediately behind the posterior lens capsule. PHPV is inherited in the Doberman pinscher and Staffordshire bull terrier and occurs sporadically in other breeds.

Severe, diffuse hemorrhage or cellular infiltrate into the vitreous can result in blindness. The vitreous is avascular and contains very few cells; thus inflammation and hemorrhage result from disease in adjacent tissues (ciliary body, retina, choroid, or optic nerve). Vitreous hemorrhage can occur with iritis/pars planitis (intermediate uveitis) (see Chapter 262), systemic hypertension (see Chapter 159), retinal detachment (see Chapter 264), intraocular neoplasia (see Chapter 251), blood dyscrasias, and trauma. Vitreous centesis for cytology and bacterial and fungal culture are indicated in cases of inflammatory cell infiltrate if less invasive methods do not identify a cause.

RETINAL DISEASE

Chorioretinitis

The retina is in close approximation to the underlying choroid; thus retinitis frequently occurs secondary to inflammation of the choroid and therefore is referred to as chorioretinitis. Bilateral, diffuse, severe chorioretinitis causes blindness with a significantly reduced or absent PLR. Chorioretinitis is characterized by the presence of hazy, grayish-white, sometimes raised lesions within the ocular fundus. These will appear hyporeflective in the tapetal fundus. In severe cases there may be partial or complete retinal detachment. Potential causes include systemic mycoses (*Blastomyces dermatitidis, Cryptococcus neoformans, Histoplasma capsulatum, Coccidioides immitis, Aspergillus sp., Fusarium sp.*), *Ehrlichia canis, Rickettsia rickettsii*, canine distemper virus, *T. gondii*, feline infectious peritonitis virus, protothecosis, *Brucella canis*, bacterial septicemia, intraocular larval migrans, and neoplasia. There may be concurrent anterior uveitis. Diagnostic measures include those discussed for opacification of the aqueous humor. In addition, vitreous centesis for cytology and bacterial and fungal culture is indicated if detection of the etiologic agent is not possible by less invasive methods.

Retinal Detachment

Retinal detachment typically occurs between the retinal pigmented epithelium (RPE) and the photoreceptors (rods and cones) and is therefore sometimes termed retinal separation. It must be bilateral and marked to cause blindness. The three mechanisms and common causes for retinal detachment are more fully discussed in Chapter 264. All patients with retinal detachment should undergo a complete physical examination and diagnostic testing as dictated by clinical findings.

Retinal Degeneration

Retinal degeneration is a common cause of blindness in dogs and cats. The typical ophthalmoscopic appearance of retinal degeneration is retinal vascular attenuation, diffuse tapetal hyperreflectivity, optic nerve pallor, and mottling of the nontapetal fundus. If the retina is not diffusely affected but has focal or multifocal hyperreflective tapetal or depigmented nontapetal lesions, there may be another cause for the blindness, and further evaluation is needed. Animals with blindness caused by retinal degeneration have a diminished or extinguished ERG.

Progressive retinal atrophy (PRA) refers to a group of inherited retinal diseases, including photoreceptor dysplasias and photoreceptor degenerations. PRA is much more common in dogs than in cats. In most forms of PRA the rods are affected earlier in the course of the disease than the cones, and the first clinical sign is decreased night vision (nyctalopia). The disease progresses to complete blindness in all light levels as the cones become affected. The age of onset and rate of progression of PRA vary by breed. The progression of vision loss can be very gradual such that the pet compensates extremely well and can be so gradual that owners may not detect vision loss until the animal is taken to a strange environment. As a result, these patients are occasionally presented for assessment of apparent acute blindness. Central progressive retinal atrophy (CPRA) is an uncommon disorder in dogs in the United States. CPRA is an RPE dystrophy with secondary retinal degeneration and thus appears as multifocal accumulations of pigment surrounded by hyperreflectivity. CPRA does not always lead to complete blindness.

Sudden acquired retinal degeneration (SARD) results in permanent blindness of acute onset and is seen only in adult dogs. In most cases the PLR is severely reduced or absent at the onset of blindness, but the retina and optic nerve appear ophthalmoscopically normal. SARD is confirmed by ERG, which is extinguished. The cause of SARD is unknown. Overweight female dogs of any breed, dachshunds, and miniature schnauzers are overrepresented. Many dogs with SARD have a history of polyuria, polydipsia, and increased appetite (van der Woedt et al., 1991). These signs are temporary in 80% of dogs. Several weeks to months after the onset of blindness, clinical signs typical of retinal degeneration develop and are indistinguishable from other causes of end-stage retinal degeneration. Histologically the photoreceptors show severe degeneration without inflammatory changes immediately after the onset of blindness, with rods and cones equally affected.

Retinal degeneration in cats has been associated with oral and parenteral administration of enrofloxacin (Wiebe et al., 2002). These cats have increased tapetal reflectivity, retinal vascular attenuation, and extinguished ERGs. Most cats are presented with acute blindness and pupil dilation (Gelatt et al., 2001). Onset or severity of disease may be dose related. Some cats regain partial vision, but in most the retinal degeneration persists or progresses. Other causes of retinal degeneration in cats include taurine deficiency in cats, vitamin E deficiency in dogs, and glaucoma in both species. End-stage glaucoma causes diffuse retinal degeneration, and there is concurrent optic nerve cupping and usually buphthalmos.

OPTIC NERVE DISEASE

Bilateral lesions of the optic nerves interfere with transmission of the image to the visual cortex and result in blindness and an absent PLR.

Optic Neuritis

Inflammation of the optic nerves (optic neuritis) can be caused by infectious agents (canine distemper virus, *T. gondii*, *B. dermatitidis*, *C. neoformans*, *H. capsulatum*, feline infectious peritonitis virus), granulomatous meningoencephalitis (GME), neoplasia, trauma, and idiopathic causes. In patients with optic neuritis, a swollen, indistinct optic disc with or without hemorrhage and exudation is seen funduscopically. The peripapillary retina may also be involved, with retinal edema, exudation, hemorrhage, and/or detachment all possible. Optic neuritis must be differentiated from papilledema in which the optic nerve head is swollen but without evidence of exudation, hemorrhage, blindness, or PLR deficits. Optic neuritis posterior to the globe (retrobulbar optic neuritis) results in blindness with a normal fundic examination. Patients with retrobulbar optic neuritis must be differentiated from those with SARD. This can be achieved simply and inexpensively by an ERG, which will be normal with optic nerve disease but extinguished with SARD. Patients with optic neuritis should undergo thorough physical and neurologic examinations. Diagnostic testing should then include assessment of a complete blood count, serum biochemistry panel, urinalysis, appropriate serologic testing, aspiration of lymph nodes if enlarged, thoracic and abdominal imaging if indicated, and MRI of the central nervous system with cerebrospinal fluid analysis.

Optic Nerve Atrophy

Optic nerve atrophy is apparent funduscopically because the optic nerve head is small, pale or, more chronically, darkly pigmented, depressed, and avascular. There is often associated peripapillary retinal degeneration evident as peripapillary tapetal hyper-reflectivity. Retinal vessels may or may not be severely affected, depending on the underlying cause. The PLR will be severely diminished or absent. Causes of optic nerve atrophy include previous optic neuritis, trauma, retrobulbar inflammation or compression, glaucoma, and end-stage retinal degeneration.

Congenital Optic Nerve Anomalies

Optic nerve hypoplasia is a congenital cause of blindness in which patients have a small (but otherwise normal) optic nerve head and an otherwise normal fundus. This should be differentiated from optic nerve atrophy in which the optic nerve head is not only small but altered and the peripapillary retina is degenerate. Optic nerve coloboma is a congenital notchlike defect of the optic nerve. Extensive colobomas can cause blindness and predispose to retinal detachment. Optic nerve colobomas can be a component of collie eye anomaly and are also frequently found in animals with microphthalmos and merle coat coloring.

INTRACRANIAL CAUSES OF BLINDNESS

The visual pathway has a long intracranial course. Lesions in the optic chiasm, optic tracts, and optic radiations result in failed transmission of the visual image. Lesions in the visual cortex result in failed interpretation (cognition) of the image. Lesions of the optic chiasm or bilateral optic tract lesions result in blindness with an abnormal PLR. Lesions posterior to the site where fibers responsible for the PLR branch from those responsible for vision (i.e., lesions of the lateral geniculate nucleus, optic radiation, or visual cortex) result in blindness with a normal PLR. Animals with blindness caused by intracranial disease typically have a normal fundic examination unless there is retrograde degeneration of the optic nerves. They will also have a normal ERG. Causes of intracranial blindness include neoplasia, GME, infectious agents (canine distemper virus, systemic mycoses, *T. gondii*, feline infec-tious peritonitis virus), trauma, feline cerebral infarction, obstructive hydrocephalus, various storage diseases, and hypoxemia. Affected animals, especially those with chiasmal lesions, do not always show additional central nervous system signs. In a retrospective study the majority of dogs with blindness secondary to neoplasia of the optic chiasm did not have other CNS signs (Davidson et al., 1991).

References and Suggested Reading

Davidson MG: Acute blindness associated with intracranial tumors in dogs and cats: eight cases (1984-1989), *J Am Vet Med Assoc* 199:755, 1991.

Gelatt KN: Enrofloxacin-associated retinal degeneration in cats, *Vet Ophthalmol* 4:99, 231, 2001.

Hendrix DV: Clinical signs, concurrent diseases, and risk factors associated with retinal detachment in dogs, *Prog Vet Comp Ophthalmol* 3:87, 1993.

Martin CL: Evaluation of patients with decreased vision or blindness, *Clin Tech Small Anim Pract* 16:62, 2001.

McLaughlin SA, Hamilton HL: Acute vision loss. In Ettinger SJ, Feldman EC, editors: *Textbook of Veterinary Internal Medicine*, ed 5, Philadelphia, 2000, Saunders, p 17.

Millichamp NJ: Retinal degeneration in the dog and cat, *Vet Clin North Am Small Anim Pract* 20:799, 1990.

Narfstrom, K Ekesten, B: Diseases of the canine ocular fundus. In Gelatt KN, editor: *Veterinary ophthalmology*, ed 3, Philadelphia, 1999, Lippincott Williams & Wilkins, p 869.

van der Woerdt A, Nasisse MP, Davidson MG: Sudden acquired retinal degeneration in the dog: clinical and laboratory findings in 36 cases, *Prog Vet Comp Ophthalmol* 1:11, 1991.

Wiebe V, Hamilton P: Fluoroquinolone-induced retinal degeneration in cats, *J Am Vet Med Assoc* 221:1568, 2002.

CHAPTER 254

Differential Diagnosis of Anisocoria

NANCY B. COTTRILL, *Woburn, Massachusetts*

Anisocoria, or different-size pupils, is abnormal. The clinician's role is to determine which pupil is abnormal and whether the underlying cause is ophthalmic or neurologic. This chapter is intended to provide a logical guide to address frequent owner concerns: What is wrong? What caused it? How is it treated? Will it get better? These goals are best achieved by first examining the eye with the normal pupil, the pupillary light reflexes (PLRs), and then the eye with the abnormal pupil. Identification of lesions will enable a short list of potential causes to be assessed. Once the cause is known, a prognosis can be given.

There are two types of anisocoria: static and dynamic. Static anisocoria refers to unequal pupils when both eyes are receiving equal illumination. In a patient with dynamic anisocoria, the difference in pupil size depends on one pupil being stimulated. Some degree of dynamic anisocoria is normal because of incomplete decussation of afferent (optic nerve) fibers at two locations: the optic chiasm and the pretectal nucleus. At the optic chiasm nerve fibers cross to the contralateral side, whereas at the pretectal nucleus nerve fibers cross back to the original (ipsilateral) stimulated side. Although pupils of both eyes react to light when it is directed at only one eye, the iris sphincter muscle of the directly stimulated eye receives more efferent impulses than the nonstimulated eye. Therefore it is normal for the pupil receiving direct stimulation to be smaller than the fellow (nonstimulated) pupil. This is termed physiologic dynamic anisocoria and does not indicate pathology.

In all patients in which anisocoria is diagnosed, a thorough medical history not restricted to ophthalmic or neurologic inquiries is essential. Standard questions should be posed regarding past medical history, current medications, current medical conditions, and physical signs. The owner should be asked about any trauma or an absence of the pet from its environment for a period of time, as well as prior treatment by either the owner or a previous veterinarian. Occasionally a veterinarian will use atropine in the examination room as a diagnostic tool instead of a more appropriate short-acting, dilating agent such as tropicamide. Alternatively owners may try home remedies, which can include medications used for a previous condition that may alter the pupil size. Because pupil dilation as a result of a single application of atropine may last 2 weeks in the uninflamed eye, this can confuse the diagnosis and confound diagnostic efforts.

A complete ophthalmic examination, including tonometry (measurement of intraocular pressure [IOP]) should always be done. Other ophthalmic diagnostic tests such as application of fluorescein stain or measurement of a Schirmer's tear test should be done if indicated. Finally, a physical examination is done. Recording all examination findings is essential (Fig. 254-1). This activity is helpful in that it commits the examiner to a decision about the observations. It is also invaluable in compiling the information for review before making a decision regarding the etiology of the anisocoria.

ANATOMY OF THE PUPILLARY LIGHT REFLEX

Pupil size (and, in the cat, pupil shape) is determined by the balance between parasympathetic and sympathetic innervation of the iris. Although emotional and other nonneuroophthalmic factors can affect this, pupil size depends in large part on the amount of light illuminating the retina and the afferent and efferent pathways of the PLR. Therefore an understanding of the anatomy of the PLR is essential (Fig. 254-2).

The afferent arm of the PLR consists of the retina, optic nerve, optic chiasm, and optic tract. Nerve fibers originating in the medial retina decussate to the opposite optic tract, whereas fibers from the lateral retina remain in the ipsilateral tract. In the dog approximately 75% of the optic nerve fibers decussate to the contralateral optic tract. In the cat approximately 65% of the optic nerve fibers decussate. The optic tract includes both sensory visual fibers and pupillomotor fibers, which differ according to their destination. This fact is used to aid localization of lesions by noting the presence or absence of vision and PLR in each eye. The pupillomotor fibers progress to the pretectal nucleus, and from there the majority of these

	OD	OS
Vision	−	+
Pupillary light reflexes		
Direct	−	+
Consensual	+	−

Fig. 254-1 Grid to record visual status and pupillary light reflexes (PLRs). Entry variables include +, normal; −, absent; *l*, incomplete: *M*, minimal. The latter two variables are used to designate degrees of constriction in the PLRs (e.g., the "incomplete" designation may be used in cases of iris atrophy). The example in the chart depicts the responses of a lesion of the right retina or prechiasmal optic nerve.

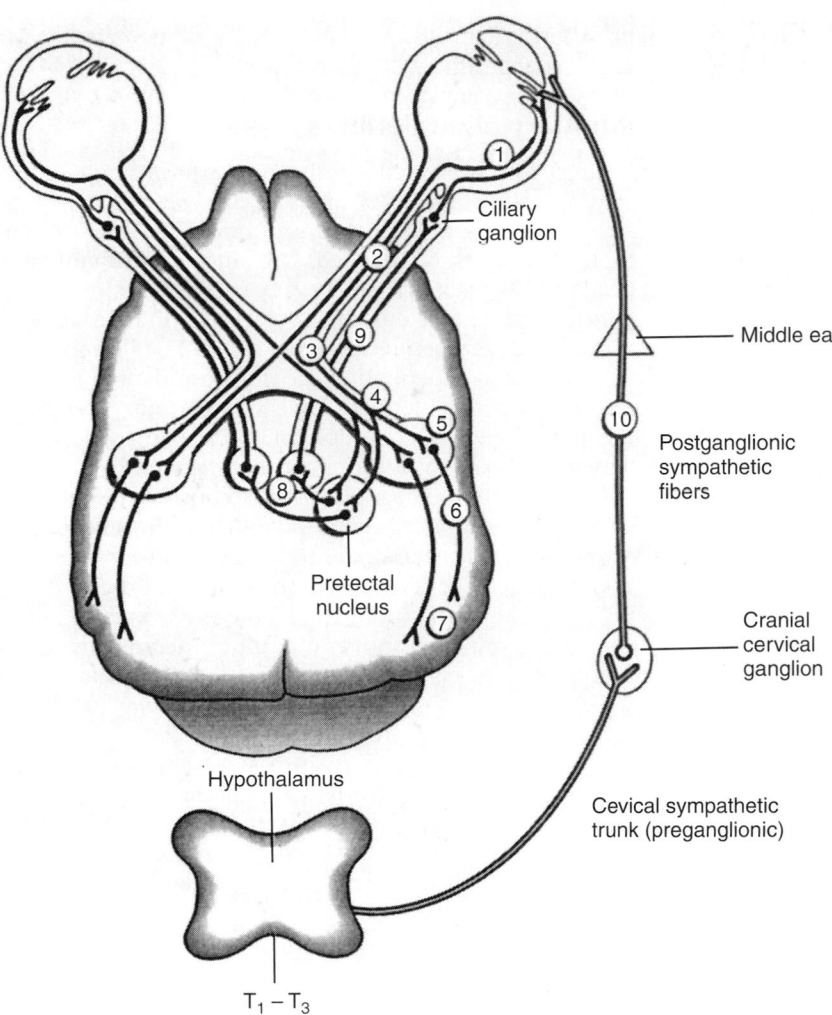

Fig. 254-2 Pathways for vision, the papillary light reflex, and the sympathetic pathway affecting the eye. Numbers correspond to structures, as lesion sites, in Table 254-1. (Modified and redrawn from Oliver JE, Lorenz MD, Kornegay JN: Blindness, anisocoria, and abnormal eye movements. In *Handbook of veterinary neurology*, ed 3, Philadelphia, 1997, Saunders, p 275, with permission.)

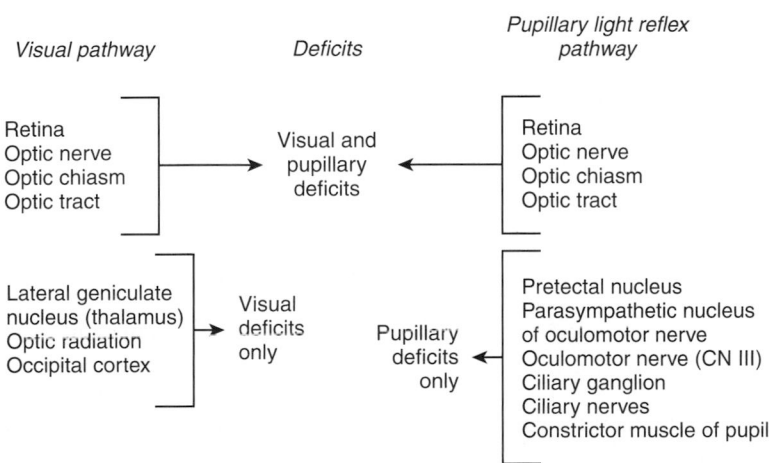

Fig. 254-3 Deficits from lesions of the visual and pupillary light reflex pathways. (From Oliver JE, Lorenz MD, Kornegay JN, editors: Blindness, anisocoria, and abnormal eye movements. In *Handbook of veterinary neurology*, ed 3, Philadelphia, 1997, Saunders, p 274, with permission.)

fibers decussate to the parasympathetic nucleus of the oculomotor nerve (once known as the Edinger-Westphal nucleus) on the contralateral side. This second decussation marks a return to the side of the originating impulse. By contrast, the visual fibers proceed sequentially to the lateral geniculate nucleus, the optic radiation, and the occipital cortex. Therefore lesions that cause anisocoria and affect both PLRs *and* vision can be localized to the retina, optic nerve, optic chiasm, or optic tract (Fig. 254-3). By contrast, lesions affecting vision, but not PLRs, are located in the lateral geniculate nucleus, optic radiation, or occipital cortex.

The efferent arm of the PLR consists of parasympathetic fibers in the oculomotor nerve (CN III) that travel to the ciliary ganglion, ciliary nerves, and finally the iris sphincter muscle. There are distinct differences in composition of the canine and feline postganglionic fibers (ciliary nerves). In the dog there are five to eight short ciliary nerves that have both sympathetic and parasympathetic efferent fibers and are considered "mixed." Therefore a lesion of the ciliary nerve in the dog results in a circular, midrange pupil because both parasympathetic and sympathetic fibers are lost. By contrast, the cat has only two short ciliary nerves that are solely parasympathetic. These nerves are named the nasal (medial) and malar (lateral) nerves. Therefore lesions involving these nerves cause more dramatic pupil dilation than in the dog because sympathetic function is still present and now unopposed. If only the medial or lateral branches are damaged, dyscoria (altered pupil shape) results in addition to anisocoria. For example, a lesion of the medial short ciliary nerve on the right eye will result in a D-shaped pupil, whereas a lesion of the lateral short ciliary nerve on the same eye will result in a reverse D-shaped pupil.

The sympathetic fibers largely innervate the iris dilator muscle. The three-neuron pathway that the sympathetic axons traverse is more complex. The central fibers originate in the hypothalamus and exit the brain with the tectotegmentospinal tract. The preganglionic cell bodies lie in spinal cord segments T1 to T3 and issue fibers with the spinal nerve ventral roots. These pass via the thoracic and cervical sympathetic trunk to terminate in the cranial cervical ganglion, caudal and medial to the tympanic bulla. Postganglionic fibers then exit the ganglion and pass via the cavernous sinus into the periorbita, nasociliary nerve, long ciliary nerve, ciliary body, and finally the iris dilator muscle.

THE OPHTHALMIC EXAMINATION

Observation of Facial Symmetry and Assessment of Cranial Nerves

A crucial part of the neuroophthalmic examination is observation of the carriage of the head and assessment of facial and ocular symmetry. It is quite easy to miss neurologic lesions by focusing on only the apparently affected eye in your assessment of anisocoria. For example, Horner's syndrome is most often recognized during the initial observation of facial symmetry. Cranial nerves other than the optic (CN II) and oculomotor (CN III) should also be assessed as part of the routine ophthalmic examination for a patient with anisocoria.

Visual Status

It is important to determine the visual status of each eye *before* checking the PLRs. The menace response is usually more notable during the initial part of the examination, before the pet has been subjected to bright lights shone in its eyes but after it is relatively calm on the table. A properly performed menace test, done without creating air currents or noise, is a helpful test of vision. However, observing an animal "track" cotton balls dropped in front of it while shielding one eye is perhaps a more reliable test of visual function. Brightly colored soft balls sold as kitten toys provide better contrast against the background of a white wall or clinician's white coat than a white cotton

ball. Maze tests and visual placing are additional tests of vision. Findings should be recorded (see Fig. 254-1).

Pupillary Light Reflexes

A direct PLR is elicited by directing a *bright* light source into the pupil. Ideally a focused, 3.5-volt halogen light source such as a Finoff transilluminator (Welch-Allyn, Skaneateles Falls, NY) is used. The Finoff transilluminator head can be attached to the battery handle used for a direct ophthalmoscope or otoscope. An excellent alternative to this is a halogen penlight (Welch-Allyn).The illumination from an ordinary penlight is too diffuse and often too dim to produce a reliable PLR. A weak light source decreases the amplitude and duration of pupil constriction and may induce a delay before pupil constriction begins. The light source should produce light of consistent brightness so that the examiner becomes familiar with the expected response in the examination room. Pupillary constriction on direct light stimulation is known as the direct PLR. Pupil constriction in the fellow eye is known as the consensual response and, as a result of incomplete decussation of fibers, is usually not quite as complete as the direct response (so-called *physiologic dynamic anisocoria*). If the PLR is incomplete, the light should be redirected to another part of the fundus since areas of the retina may have different light sensitivities, especially with focal or regional pathology of the afferent pathway; particularly the retina. It is easiest to see the direct and consensual PLRs by gently retracting both upper eyelids and directing the light into the eye being tested while an assistant holds the pet. The clinician can easily look at the consensual pupil while still directing the light into the other eye. Normal findings when performing PLRs include equal pupil size and shape in diffuse light, pupils that dilate almost maximally and equally in the dark, and brisk direct and consensual PLRs in both eyes with expected physiologic dynamic anisocoria. Direct and consensual PLRs should be assessed in ambient light first, with findings recorded as normal, absent, incomplete, or minimal (see Fig. 254-1). Committing to a response and some qualifying information about the response is valuable.

Swinging Flashlight Test

The swinging flashlight test is used to assess and compare the function of the retina and the prechiasmal optic nerve in one eye versus the other. A bright light is directed into one eye for a few seconds and then redirected into the fellow eye. The normal response is for the first pupil to fully constrict. Sometimes slight dilation occurs after full pupil constriction in a normal eye as a result of adaptation of the retina to the light stimulus. This is known as *pupillary escape*. As the light is swung to illuminate the second eye, the pupil should constrict a little further (or already be fully constricted as a result of the consensual PLR). An abnormal swinging flashlight test is noted when the pupil of the second eye dilates as the light is directed into it. This is known as a positive swinging flashlight test (or the Marcus Gunn sign) and is a hallmark of a lesion in the retina or prechiasmal optic nerve of the eye that dilates when illuminated.

Dark Adaptation Test and Retroillumination

Once these initial tests are completed, the lights should be turned off to allow the patient's and examiner's eyes to adapt to the darkness for approximately 2 minutes. The examiner should then stand back at arm's length from the patient with the light source set to emit bright illumination and centered between the *examiner's* eyes. This will permit the examiner to assess the tapetal reflex obtained simultaneously from both of the patient's eyes. In particular, the degree and symmetry of pupil dilation should be assessed since some causes of anisocoria are associated with more marked pupil asymmetry in dim than in bright ambient light. The examiner should repeat assessment of PLRs and the swinging flashlight test in the dark because differences are more marked after dark adaptation.

Completion of the Ophthalmic Examination

After vision testing, PLRs, retroillumination, and the swinging flashlight are assessed, a thorough ocular examination, including tonometry and assessment of aqueous flare, should be completed to identify or eliminate ophthalmic causes of anisocoria (see Chapter 248). This approach will allow the clinician to identify and confirm the presence of anisocoria, recognize the abnormal pupil, and begin consideration of causes under the broad mechanistic headings of "nonneurologic" (further divided into ophthalmic or pharmacologic causes) versus "neurologic" (further divided into afferent or efferent lesions).

NONNEUROLOGIC CAUSES OF ANISOCORIA

Ophthalmic Causes of Anisocoria

Ophthalmic causes of anisocoria can be divided into conditions that cause miosis (a constricted pupil) or those that cause mydriasis (a dilated pupil).

Conditions That Cause Miosis

Anterior uveitis (see Chapter 262) may cause miosis. Other signs that are variably present in patients with uveitis include corneal edema, "cloudiness" of the anterior chamber resulting from an increase in the protein content of the aqueous humor (aqueous flare), hyperemic conjunctival or episcleral vessels, and low IOP. PLRs may be sluggish or difficult to see because of extreme miosis. Severe or chronic uveitis may also cause posterior synechiae (adhesions between the iris and the anterior lens capsule) to form. Synechiae typically also cause dyscoria, and PLRs may be slow or absent, depending on the extent of the adhesions. Posterior synechiae may also form while the pupil is dilated and therefore need not always be associated with miosis. Corneal irritation, especially ulcers and lacerations, causes a reflex miosis mediated by the trigeminal nerve called the *axonal reflex*. These conditions are easily recognized by focal corneal edema, plus or minus a corneal stromal defect, and corneal retention of fluorescein dye. Therefore it is wise to apply fluorescein stain to all eyes with miosis as a presenting sign.

Conditions That Cause Mydriasis

Iris atrophy is a normal aging change resulting in an irregular or scallop-edged pupil, as well as transillumination defects in the iris caused by atrophy of the iris musculature. These defects are seen during retroillumination (i.e., by directing a light toward the fundus and observing light reflected from the tapetum through the pupil). In animals with iris atrophy, light can be seen through the body of the iris. Iris atrophy is more common in poodles and Siamese cats. Because the atrophy involves the iris muscles, PLRs typically are altered. Initial pupillary constriction may be normal or minimal; however, constriction is incomplete. Iris atrophy is usually bilateral, but not always symmetric, and such unevenness can produce anisocoria.

Iris hypoplasia is a congenital defect in iris stroma density visible as an area of irregular pigmentation. These areas typically appear dark because of increased visibility of the melanotic posterior pigmented epithelium of the iris, resulting from stromal thinning. The pupil margin may also be irregular and scalloped, and transillumination defects may be seen. Pupillary constriction characteristics are similar to those seen in patients with iris atrophy.

The pupil of glaucomatous eyes may be mydriatic. Other signs include episcleral congestion, generalized corneal edema, and IOP above normal. PLRs are often slow or absent. Visual deficits are also present if the IOP is markedly or chronically elevated. Iris tumors such as melanomas may cause mydriasis if they infiltrate the iridal musculature and impede its function. They may also produce mydriasis if they cause secondary glaucoma. Severe blunt ocular trauma can damage iridal sphincter fibers, with resultant iridoplegia.

Unilateral retinal disease can cause mydriasis, although the anisocoria tends to be relatively subtle (especially in dim ambient light) because decussation of afferent fibers causes stimulation of the iris of the affected eye via the contralateral retina. However, direct and consensual PLRs are typically slow or absent, and the swinging flashlight test should be positive. Visual deficits are usually present. In addition, visual deficits are usually present but may or may not be noted by owners since pets typically compensate well for unilateral vision loss. Fundic examination will reveal the cause of unilateral retinal causes of mydriasis. Perhaps the most common cause of unilateral retinal disease is retinal detachment, which has the ophthalmoscopic appearance of an undulating veil containing blood vessels coming toward the observer (see Chapter 264). Severe chorioretinitis that affects a large area in one eye or one eye more than the other can cause unilateral mydriasis. Areas of active chorioretinitis have a dull tapetal reflex, are often gray, and have indistinct edges. Unilateral optic neuritis and optic nerve neoplasia can also produce mydriasis and vision loss. Although there are multiple known causes of optic neuritis, many cases are idiopathic. The most common optic nerve tumor in the dog is a meningioma. Optic nerve causes of mydriasis usually produce ophthalmoscopically visible changes, but only the retrobulbar portion of the nerve may be affected, in which case the intraocular portion of the nerve may have a normal appearance. Orbital neoplasia, cellulitis, or retrobulbar abscess should also be considered in patients with unilateral loss of vision, altered PLRs, and a positive swinging flashlight test. These patients should be assessed for evidence (sometimes subtle) of exophthalmos or decreased retropulsion.

Pharmacologic Causes of Anisocoria

Pharmacologic causes of anisocoria can be divided into drugs that produce miosis and those that produce mydriasis. Miosis is most often caused by administration of agents used for management of glaucoma. These include pilocarpine, demecarium bromide, or any of the new synthetic prostaglandins such as latanoprost. Mydriasis can be caused by administration of tropicamide or atropine, ocular contact with jimsonweed (*Datura stramonium*) or other toxic plants, or topical administration of collyria or ocular decongestants containing phenylephrine. The likelihood of exposure to pharmacologic agents that alter pupil size should be specifically elicited when the patient history is obtained.

NEUROLOGIC CAUSES OF ANISOCORIA

Afferent Versus Efferent Pupillary Defects

Neurologic causes of anisocoria should be neuroanatomically localized as afferent or efferent. Although a complete ophthalmic examination and history of exposure to pharmacologic agents are essential, monitoring the change in anisocoria during dark adaptation will greatly assist with localization.

Afferent Lesion Characteristics

Anisocoria caused by an afferent arm lesion is abolished (or sometimes reduced) as both pupils dilate in the dark.

This is because the stimulus producing the anisocoria (light causing constriction of the normal pupil but inadequate constriction of the abnormal pupil) is eliminated. Thus anisocoria caused by afferent lesions is less prominent in dim ambient light and more prominent in bright light. In addition, afferent lesions cause abnormal PLRs in *both* the abnormal and the normal pupil (Table 254-1; see Fig. 254-2). If the pupils remain unequal or do not dilate completely in the dark, the lesion must be in the sympathetic efferent arm or be ophthalmic or pharmacologic in origin.

Efferent Lesion Characteristics

Signs of lesions involving the efferent arm of the PLR produce some dramatically different signs, depending on:

- Whether they affect the parasympathetic or sympathetic neurons of the efferent arm.
- Whether they affect the central (for the sympathetic supply) or preganglionic or postganglionic (for both parasympathetic and sympathetic supplies) neurons.
- Whether the patient is feline or canine.
- The intensity of the ambient light in which the examination is conducted.

These differences are discussed more fully in the following paragraphs. However, efferent lesions of any type or site do not cause visual deficits in either species (see Table 254-1 and Fig. 254-2).

Afferent Lesions

Unilateral Retinal or Prechiasmal Optic Nerve Lesions
Patients with unilateral retinal or prechiasmal lesions have mydriasis (usually subtle) and a slow or absent

Table 254-1

Signs of Lesions in the Visual Pathways*

Complete Lesion on Right Side	VISION		RESTING PUPIL		PUPILLARY LIGHT REFLEX	
	Right Eye	Left Eye	Right Eye	Left Eye	Light in Right Eye	Light in Left Eye
1. Retina or optic nerve	Absent	Normal	Slightly dilated	Normal	No response	Both constrict
2. Orbit (CN II, III)	Absent	Normal	Dilated	Normal	No response	Left constricts
3. Optic chiasm (bilateral)†	Absent	Absent	Dilated	Dilated	No response	No Response
4. Optic tract	Normal	Absent‡	Normal or slightly miotic	Normal or slightly dilated	Both constrict	Both constrict
5. Lateral geniculate nucleus	Normal	Absent‡	Normal	Normal	Both constrict	Both constrict
6. Optic radiation	Normal	Absent‡	Normal	Normal	Both constrict	Both constrict
7. Occipital cortex	Normal	Absent‡	Normal	Normal	Both constrict	Both constrict
8. Parasympathetic nucleus of CN III (bilateral)†	Normal	Normal	Dilated	Dilated	No response	No response
9. Oculomotor nerve	Normal	Normal	Dilated	Normal	Left constricts	Left constricts
10. Sympathetic nerve	Normal	Normal	Constricted	Normal	Both constrict	Both constrict

*Numbers correspond to structures, as lesion sites, in Fig. 254-2.
†Unilateral lesions of these structures are rare.
‡Possibly loss of sight in left visual field with partial sparing of right visual field.

direct PLR on the affected side but a normal consensual PLR from the unaffected to the affected eye. They also have visual deficits on the affected side and a pathognomonic positive swinging flashlight test. The last feature is pathognomonic for lesions at these sites. The fundus should be examined for presence of retinal or optic nerve head pathology. If the fundic examination is normal, an electroretinogram (ERG) can be done to localize the lesion further. If the ERG is normal (i.e., the retina is functioning) and the optic nerve head is funduscopically normal, the retrobulbar (but prechiasmal) optic nerve is affected.

Unilateral Optic Tract Lesions

Patients with unilateral optic tract lesions have a mydriatic pupil (usually subtle) in the eye contralateral to the affected optic tract, regardless of which eye is receiving the light stimulus, visual deficits, and a negative swinging flashlight test. Unlike prechiasmal lesions, the pupil *contralateral* to the lesion is affected in postchiasmal lesions because of decussation. Because the majority (75% in dogs, 65% in cats) of CN II fibers in each optic tract decussate from the contralateral optic nerve, the pretectal nucleus on the affected side no longer receives that input, no impulses progress to decussate a second time to the contralateral parasympathetic nucleus of CN III, and stimulation of the oculomotor nerve on the contralateral side does not ensue. The eye contralateral to the optic tract lesion also will have a partial visual deficit because the majority of the optic tract is composed of fibers from the medial retina of the contralateral eye.

Optic Chiasm Lesions

Chiasm lesions rarely cause anisocoria; rather they usually cause bilateral mydriatic pupils, absent PLRs, and vision loss.

Efferent Lesions

Parasympathetic Efferent Lesions

In dogs the preganglionic efferent nerves are purely parasympathetic, but the postganglionic nerves are mixed. In cats both nerves are purely parasympathetic over their whole course. Therefore lesion site and species affected cause notable differences in the pupillary signs seen.

Lesions of the nucleus of CN III, the preganglionic fibers, or the ganglion itself produce similar signs in dogs and cats. There will be diminished or absent PLRs on the affected side to both direct and indirect light, normal direct and consensual PLRs on the unaffected side, normal vision, and equally and maximally dilated pupils in the dark.

In cats lesions of the ganglion or postganglionic nerves cause signs identical to those of preganglionic lesions because only parasympathetic fibers are affected. However, pupil shape also will differ if only one of the two postganglionic short ciliary nerves is affected (as discussed earlier in "Anatomy of the PLR"). By contrast, ganglionic or postganglionic lesions in the dog cause anisocoria after dark adaptation, with the smaller pupil being ipsilateral

to the lesion because the mixed nature of these nerves in the dog means that lesions affect the ability of the pupil to constrict and dilate.

Pupil changes induced by dysfunction of the autonomic components of CN III are termed internal ophthalmoplegia. This differentiates them from external ophthalmoplegia, which occurs following damage to the oculomotor fibers that also run in CN III and which is manifest as ptosis (drooping of the upper lid) and lateral strabismus. Dogs and cats can experience internal ophthalmoplegia without concurrent external ophthalmoplegia because the parasympathetic fibers are superficial and medial to the oculomotor fibers of CN III and therefore are more susceptible to injury than the oculomotor fibers. Internal ophthalmoplegia may be the result of trauma from proptosis; retrobulbar disease such as abscess, cellulitis, hemorrhage, or orbital or optic nerve neoplasm; or midbrain lesions.

Pharmacologic Localization of Parasympathetic Lesions

Pharmacologic testing may be used to confirm presence of a lesion in the efferent arm of the PLR, rule out pharmacologic blockade and iridal disease, and localize the lesion as preganglionic or postganglionic. A lesion in the ganglion or postganglionic fibers causes *denervation hypersensitivity* to what would normally be an ineffective concentration of a topically administered parasympathomimetic drug. The first agent used in localizing a lesion in the parasympathetic efferent pathway is an indirect-acting parasympathomimetic such as 0.5% physostigmine. The desired response is miosis. The pupil of an eye with a central or preganglionic lesion will constrict sooner than one with normal parasympathetic innervation. The pupil of an eye with a lesion in the ciliary ganglion or postganglionic fibers will not constrict. Application of dilute pilocarpine (< 0.2%) is perhaps the most useful test for the general practitioner. Denervation hypersensitivity will cause the affected pupil to constrict sooner and more completely and to maintain the constriction longer in response to this low concentration of a direct-acting parasympathomimetic than the pupil in the normal eye. Application of a more concentrated direct-acting parasympathomimetic agent such as 2% pilocarpine can be used to simply confirm the presence of an efferent arm lesion (and to rule out mechanical obstruction such as synechia, iris atrophy, or pharmacologic mydriasis). However, this will not define the lesion location.

Sympathetic Efferent Lesions

The loss of sympathetic tone to the eye is commonly known as Horner's syndrome (HS). Signs of HS are always ipsilateral to the lesion and include miosis, ptosis, protrusion of the third eyelid, and enophthalmos. Miosis may remain after the other signs have disappeared. About 50% of canine cases and 42% of feline cases of HS are idiopathic (Kern, Aromando, and Erb, 1989). However, the patient should be investigated for commonly identified causes of HS in small animals such as trauma to the head, neck, or chest; brachial plexus root avulsion;

intracranial, mediastinal, or intrathoracic neoplasia; otitis media/interna; and injury to the ear during cleaning. Dogs that are tethered outside and repeatedly lunge at the end of the tether are at risk for neck trauma and HS. Golden retrievers and collies are suggested to be predisposed. Most idiopathic cases of HS will resolve in 4 to 16 weeks.

Pharmacologic Localization of Sympathetic Efferent Lesions

As with parasympathetic lesions, pharmacologic testing may be used to confirm presence of a sympathetic lesion in the efferent arm of the PLR, rule out pharmacologic blockade and iridal disease, and further localize the lesion. The same principles of denervation hypersensitivity apply (i.e., lesions of the ganglion or postganglionic neuron cause hypersensitivity); however, in this case mydriasis is the desired response. Ideally the first step is to instill an indirect-acting sympathomimetic such as 1% hydroxyamphetamine into both eyes; however, this drug is difficult to obtain commercially. When it is applied topically, the affected pupil will dilate if the lesion is central or preganglionic, whereas no or little dilation will occur if the lesion is postganglionic. An easier way to confirm the diagnosis of HS is to instill a dilute direct-acting sympathomimetic such as 1% phenylephrine into each eye. Both eyes should be reassessed every 10 minutes until pupil dilation has occurred in the affected eye or until 40 minutes have passed. The denervated (hypersensitive) pupil reacts by dilating before or in the absence of pupillary dilation in the unaffected eye. The other signs of HS may also diminish during this pharmacologic challenge. Some authors suggest that, if mydriasis occurs before 20 minutes, the lesion is postganglionic; and, if it occurs between 20 and 45 minutes, it is likely preganglionic. The phenylephrine test alone does not allow discrimination between a preganglionic and central lesion.

Spastic Pupil Syndrome

This syndrome occurs only in cats and is characterized by static anisocoria (at the time of examination), failure to dilate after dark adaptation, normal vision, and no ocular abnormalities. The curious feature of this syndrome is that the degree of anisocoria and the relative size of the pupils can change from day to day (i.e., the anisocoria can be caused by a relative miosis or mydriasis, and this can change). There may even be intervals when the pupils are normal. Most cats with this syndrome are determined to have positive feline leukemia virus tests.

References and Suggested Reading

Bercovitch M, Krohne S, Lindley D: A diagnostic approach to anisocoria, *Compendium* 17:661, 1995.

Boydell P: Idiopathic horner syndrome in the golden retriever, *J Neuroophthalmol* 20(4):288, 2000.

Collins BK: Disorders of the pupil. In August JR, editor: *Consultations in feline internal medicine* 2, Philadelphia, 1994, Saunders, p 421.

Herrera DH, Suraniti AP, Kojusner NF: Idiopathic Horner's syndrome in collie dogs, *Vet Comp Ophthalmol* 1(1):17, 1998.

Kern TJ, Aromando MS, Erb HN: Horner's syndrome in dogs and cats: 100 cases (1975-1985), *J Am Vet Med Assoc* 195:369, 1989.

Kornegay JN, Lorenz MD: Blindness, anisocoria, and abnormal eye movements. In Kornegay JN, Lorenz MD: *Handbook of veterinary neurology*, St. Louis, 2004, Saunders, p 283.

Larocca RD: Unilateral external and internal ophthalmoplegia caused by intracranial meningioma in a dog, *Vet Ophthalmol* 3(1):3, 2000.

Morgan RV, Zanotti SW: Horner's syndrome in dogs and cats: 49 cases (1980-1986), *J Am Vet Med Assoc* 194:1096, 1989.

Neer TM, Carter JD: Anisocoria in dogs and cats: ocular and neurologic causes, *Compend Contin Educ Pract Vet* 9:817, 1987.

Scagliotti R: Comparative Neuro-Ophthalmology. In Gelatt KN: *Essentials of veterinary ophthalmology*, Philadelphia, 2000, Lippincott Williams & Wilkins, p 439.

CHAPTER 255

Differential Diagnosis of the Red Eye

DIANE V.H. HENDRIX, *Knoxville, Tennessee*

Red eye is perhaps the most common clinical sign observed by pet owners when ocular disease is present. However, knowledge that a patient has a red eye does not give any specific indication as to type or severity of disease or prognosis. This requires the gathering of a complete history, performance of a through ophthalmic examination, and diagnostic testing. First, one must localize the source of the redness noted by the owner. Ocular redness may be focal or generalized. It may involve the adnexa, exterior of the globe, or the interior of the globe. Redness of the adnexa or exterior of the globe may involve the conjunctiva, the third eyelid, the episcleral region, or the cornea. Redness from within the globe may be caused by hemorrhage in the anterior chamber or vitreous, retinal detachment, or neovascularization of the iris. Despite the diversity of causes, ocular redness may be the only obvious sign present in blinding diseases such as glaucoma and anterior uveitis and thus should always be thoroughly investigated. The purpose of this chapter is to introduce the causes of and diagnostic approach for a red eye. The reader is referred to other chapters devoted to specific ocular diseases for information regarding ocular diagnoses introduced in this chapter.

LOCALIZING THE SOURCE OF THE REDNESS

When an animal has a red eye, it is imperative that the precise anatomic location of the redness be determined since this will aid in determining the etiology (Fig. 255-1). The redness may be focal or generalized, involve surface or intraocular structures, and be superficial or deep. The most important aspect of localizing ocular redness is differentiating conjunctival vessels from episcleral vessels; this will permit differentiation of irritating surface eye disease such as conjunctivitis from potentially blinding intraocular disease such as glaucoma or uveitis. If an eye with a blinding disease such as glaucoma or anterior uveitis were treated as if only conjunctivitis were present, vision loss would be likely. Ocular redness associated with conjunctivitis involves the capillaries of the conjunctiva. These superficial blood vessels blanch more rapidly with topical application of dilute (1%) phenylephrine or epinephrine than deeper episcleral vessels. Conjunctival vessels are also more mobile in comparison to episcleral vessels. Vascular mobility can be determined by moving the bulbar conjunctiva by sliding the eyelid over the globe using gentle digital pressure; or a moistened cotton-tipped applicator can be used to lightly slide the conjunctiva over the sclera after topical anesthetic has been instilled. If the engorged vessels are easily moved with either of these techniques, they are conjunctival vessels.

Surface redness associated with intraocular disease tends to involve the episcleral vessels. The episcleral vessels are larger and less mobile than conjunctival vessels. In addition, these vessels do not blanch quickly following topical application of dilute epinephrine or phenylephrine. They may radiate caudally from the limbus as is seen frequently with glaucoma, or they may primarily involve the perilimbal region as is seen commonly with anterior uveitis.

The eye may also appear red if chronic corneal disease has led to corneal vascularization or corneal granulation tissue. In addition, blood in the anterior chamber (hyphema) may make the cornea appear red and completely obscure the iris and pupil. Vitreous hemorrhage can also cause the eye to appear red; however, this must be distinguished from the normal red fundic reflection in dogs and cats with a subalbinotic fundus. Finally, a retinal detachment may cause reddening of the eye because of retinal blood vessels visible against the posterior aspect of the lens.

Once the source of redness has been localized, a complete ocular examination should be performed to diagnose the current disease process, establish a prognosis, and determine appropriate treatment. Pupillary light reflexes; menace response; Schirmer's tear test; intraocular pressure; fluorescein staining of the cornea; examination for aqueous flare; and complete examination of the eyelids, cornea, iris, lens, vitreous, and fundus should be done (see Chapter 248).

Focal Redness

Focal redness is usually caused by subconjunctival hemorrhage or a mass. Trauma resulting from a dog fight or excess pressure applied around the neck by a collar is the most common cause of subconjunctival hemorrhage. Although the hemorrhage may appear severe, no treatment is necessary provided that the remainder of the examination is normal. If there is no historical trauma, the possibility of a systemic bleeding disorder caused by vasculitis or coagulopathy should be investigated. Prolapse of the gland of the third eyelid ("cherry eye") is the most common cause of a red mass on the eye. The prolapsed gland should be replaced by either burying the gland using the pocket technique or tacking the gland to the orbital rim. Neoplasia of the conjunctiva is rare but

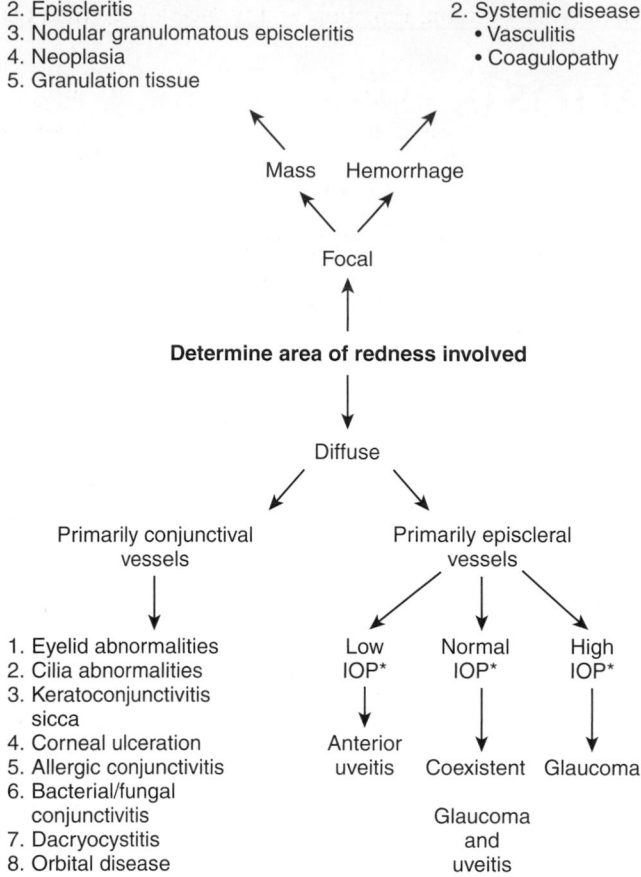

1. Prolapse of the gland of the third eyelid
2. Episcleritis
3. Nodular granulomatous episcleritis
4. Neoplasia
5. Granulation tissue

1. Trauma
2. Systemic disease
   • Vasculitis
   • Coagulopathy

Mass   Hemorrhage

Focal

Determine area of redness involved

Diffuse

Primarily conjunctival vessels

Primarily episcleral vessels

1. Eyelid abnormalities
2. Cilia abnormalities
3. Keratoconjunctivitis sicca
4. Corneal ulceration
5. Allergic conjunctivitis
6. Bacterial/fungal conjunctivitis
7. Dacryocystitis
8. Orbital disease

Low IOP*   Normal IOP*   High IOP*

Anterior uveitis   Coexistent   Glaucoma

Glaucoma and uveitis

*IOP = intraocular pressure

Fig. 255-1 Algorithm for determining the cause of a red eye in dogs or cats.

does occur; biopsy of any questionable mass is indicated (see Chapter 251). Episcleritis and nodular granulomatous episcleritis are inflammatory diseases that produce focal red-to-tan masses, most commonly at the lateral limbus (see Chapter 259).

Generalized Redness

Conjunctival Redness (Conjunctival Hyperemia)

Localization of redness to the conjunctiva is consistent with a clinical diagnosis of conjunctivitis. However, there are many causes of conjunctivitis in dogs and cats (see Section XII on Evolve). More important, dogs and cats with potentially blinding intraocular disease such as anterior uveitis and glaucoma often have conjunctival hyperemia, usually in conjunction with sometimes subtle episcleral injection. Therefore a diagnosis of conjunctival hyperemia or episcleral injection is not mutually exclusive, and the presence of conjunctival hyperemia should stimulate very thorough investigation to prove or disprove the presence of episcleral hyperemia. In the case of episcleral injection with conjunctival hyperemia, the intraocular disease is the primary threat, and with its treatment the conjunctival hyperemia will resolve. Complete ophthalmic examination of a dog or cat with

isolated conjunctivitis should reveal negative retention of fluorescein stain, normal intraocular pressures, and normal pupillary light responses.

Conjunctivitis. Although conjunctivitis literally means inflammation of the conjunctiva and conjunctival hyperemia refers to dilation or congestion of the conjunctival capillaries, the terms are often used interchangeably. Unfortunately "conjunctivitis" usually creates thoughts of mild, nonthreatening vision disease. However, there are many causes of conjunctivitis, some of which (such as corneal ulceration or keratoconjunctivitis sicca [KCS]) can be blinding. Although there is some overlap, causes of feline and canine conjunctivitis tend to differ. Generally conjunctivitis in cats should be considered infectious; therefore treatment with steroids is often contraindicated (see Chapter 257); whereas primary conjunctival pathogens of the dog are very uncommon (see Section XII on Evolve).

In dogs KCS is a common cause of conjunctivitis, and it is the most common primary cause of bacterial conjunctivitis in dogs. Clinical signs of KCS include a mucoid-to-mucopurulent discharge; conjunctivitis; and a dull cornea that may be ulcerated, pigmented, or vascularized. Because of the high incidence of this disease in dogs, a Schirmer's tear test should be done on all dogs with conjunctivitis. A result below 10mm/min of wetting is diagnostic for KCS. A result of 10 to 14mm/minute of wetting is suggestive of KCS, and treatment should be based on clinical signs or the results of a retest at a later date. Treatment for KCS includes replacing the tears with an artificial tear ointment, resolving secondary bacterial infections with a broad-spectrum antibiotic, and increasing tear production with topical cyclosporine or tacrolimus (see Chapter 249 and Section XII on Evolve).

Mechanical irritation is a common cause of conjunctival hyperemia in the dog. Distichia, ectopic cilia, trichiasis, entropion, and ectropion are all common etiologies. Conjunctival hyperemia, epiphora, or a mucoid discharge and corneal disease may be seen. A complete ocular examination is warranted because occasionally the most apparent abnormality such as distichia, trichiasis, or ectropion may not be the only cause of the conjunctivitis. When it has been determined that an eyelid/eyelash abnormality is causing the ocular signs, the appropriate surgical therapy should be undertaken.

Allergic conjunctivitis associated with atopy is often seasonal. Clinical signs are usually restricted to conjunctival hyperemia and epiphora. Control of the atopy in conjunction with a topical antihistamine often resolves clinical signs. Follicular conjunctivitis also is thought to be caused by local antigen exposure and usually affects young large-breed dogs. Ocular examination reveals an abundance of lymphoid follicle formation, conjunctival hyperemia, and epiphora. The follicles most commonly occur on the bulbar side of the third eyelid but may also occur on the palpebral side or another conjunctival surface. Cytologic examination of scrapings of the follicles reveals numerous lymphocytes. Topical application of a corticosteroid will frequently bring relief. Allergic and follicular conjunctivitis caused by antigen exposure occurs much less commonly in cats than dogs; infections such as those due to *Chlamydophila felis* are more common causes of conjunctivitis in cats.

Canine distemper virus frequently causes conjunctivitis with epiphora or a mucoid-to-purulent discharge. KCS, corneal ulceration, chorioretinitis, and optic neuritis may also be present in association with systemic signs. Cytologic evaluations of conjunctival scrapings from the gland of the third eyelid may reveal cytoplasmic inclusion bodies, but they are rarely seen. Direct or indirect immunofluorescent antibody testing of the conjunctival scrapings may also be diagnostic. Fluorescein stain interferes with immunofluorescent antibody testing; therefore samples should be acquired before using fluorescein stain. Treatment with topical antibiotics to prevent secondary bacterial infections and treatment with tear replacement ointments may be indicated.

Primary bacterial conjunctivitis is very rare in the dog. *Staphylococcus* sp. is usually the offending bacteria. Dogs with bacterial conjunctivitis have a purulent ocular discharge with or without swollen eyelid margins. Cytology, culture, and nasolacrimal duct flush (to rule out dacryocystitis) should be done. Ophthalmic antibiotics are usually indicated. Systemic antibiotics are necessary if the eyelids are involved or if dacryocystitis is present. The choice of antibiotic should be based on culture and sensitivity results. If a complete and rapid response does not occur with treatment, the patient should be reevaluated.

Conjunctivitis in cats is almost exclusively infectious in nature. The most common agents are feline herpesvirus I (FHV-1; also known as feline rhinotracheitis virus) and *C. felis*. Primary infection with FHV-1 is manifest by sneezing and ocular and nasal discharge in young cats. Their conjunctivitis is characterized by conjunctival hyperemia and some chemosis. Serous ocular discharge later becomes mucoid to mucopurulent. Most cases spontaneously resolve in 10 to 14 days; however, most cats become latently infected. A percentage of adult cats then will show unilateral ocular disease without upper respiratory signs. In these adults the disease is more likely to be chronic or recurrent. Fluorescent antibody techniques, virus isolation, and polymerase chain reaction may aid in diagnosis in acute infections (see Chapter 258 and Section XII on Evolve).

C. felis (formerly *Chlamydia psittaci)* is a common cause of conjunctivitis in cats. The disease is unilateral initially and becomes bilateral. Clinically chemosis and a serous ocular discharge are seen. Cytology may reveal intracytoplasmic inclusion bodies, or fluorescent antibody testing may be of benefit. Topically applied oxytetracycline or erythromycin are effective; however, systemically administered doxycycline or azithromycin may be preferred (see Chapter 257). *Mycoplasma* spp. have been associated with conjunctivitis in cats; however, they also can frequently be cultured from normal cats. Clinical signs include unilateral or bilateral epiphora, papillary hypertrophy of the conjunctiva, chemosis, and pseudomembrane formation. Treatment with ophthalmic oxytetracycline administered four times daily is generally effective.

Occasionally a dog or cat is seen following exposure to a chemical irritant. In these cases corneal ulceration is likely, and fluorescein staining is essential. The cornea and conjunctiva (including the fornices) should be flushed copiously with sterile saline. Treatment with a broad-spectrum antibiotic ointment for lubrication and to prevent bacterial infection of any ulcerated surfaces is recommended.

Clinical signs of corneal ulceration include blepharospasm; conjunctival hyperemia; photophobia; an uneven corneal surface; vascularization of the cornea; and sometimes aqueous flare and miosis. Fluorescein stain retention in the region of ulceration is diagnostic. The primary cause of the corneal ulcer must always be determined by doing a complete ophthalmic examination. Most corneal ulcers will heal rapidly when the cause is removed and when treated with a topical broad-spectrum antibiotic and a parasympatholytic drug such as ophthalmic atropine. If the ulcer is deep or rapidly progressing, culture and placement of a conjunctival graft may be required (see Section XII on Evolve).

Orbital disease causes secondary conjunctival hyperemia caused by inflammation, exposure, and decreased venous return; therefore reddened eyes should be retropulsed. If exophthalmos is present or the affected globe is difficult to retropulse, orbital disease should be suspected (see Section XII on Evolve).

Episcleral Redness

Anterior uveitis. The episcleral redness associated with anterior uveitis is often localized to a somewhat circumferential region behind the limbus and is referred to as *ciliary flush*. Clinical signs of anterior uveitis include miosis, resistance to pupillary dilation with mydriatic agents, anterior or posterior synechia, a darkened iris, and decreased intraocular pressure. The presence of circulating blood components in the anterior chamber (aqueous flare, hypopyon, keratic precipitates, hyphema) is pathognomonic for anterior uveitis. To detect aqueous flare, the smallest white light spot on the direct ophthalmoscope is focused on the cornea. If aqueous flare is present, the light will be scattered, and a continuous beam of light will extend from the cornea to the lens. Low levels of aqueous flare are best detected in a completely dark room. A slightly miotic pupil is more noticeable in a darkened room as well (see Chapter 248).

Anterior uveitis has a multitude of etiologies (see Chapter 262); patients warrant a thorough general physical examination and often systemic disease testing. The goals of treatment of anterior uveitis are to decrease inflammation and prevent sequelae such as synechia, cataract formation, iris bombé, secondary glaucoma, and blindness. Pending an etiologic diagnosis, the eye should be treated topically with parasympatholytic drugs such as atropine (1% ophthalmic solution or ointment) or tropicamide (1% ophthalmic solution). These drugs dilate the pupil, thereby decreasing the iris-to-lens contact and preventing or decreasing the severity of posterior synechia formation, and decrease pain by paralyzing the ciliary body muscle. Topically applied corticosteroids that penetrate an intact corneal epithelium such as prednisolone acetate or dexamethasone are used to decrease inflammation. Hydrocortisone will not penetrate into the anterior chamber and should not be used. Corticosteroids are contraindicated when a corneal ulcer is present. Topical ophthalmic nonsteroidal antiinflammatory drugs may also be used; however, they are not as efficacious as steroids alone.

However, topical ophthalmic nonsteroidal antiinflammatory drugs may be used in the presence of noninfected corneal ulcers; they do not affect diabetic management as corticosteroids do and can have synergistic effects with topical corticosteroids in refractory inflammation.

Hyphema. Hyphema refers to the presence of free blood in the anterior chamber. Often these patients also have episcleral injection. There are many causes of hyphema, and observation of this sign should trigger further examination and diagnostic investigation. A single episode of hemorrhage such as that caused by trauma generally resolves quickly. Recurrent bleeding such as that seen secondary to a retinal detachment, an intraocular tumor, chronic uveitis, vasculitis, systemic hypertension, or coagulopathy may lead to secondary glaucoma or synechia formation. If evaluation of the retina is not possible because of the hyphema, ocular ultrasonography may delineate a retinal detachment. Pending diagnosis, topical prednisolone acetate should be initiated, provided the cornea is not ulcerated. Intraocular pressure should be evaluated periodically and treated appropriately if secondary glaucoma develops.

Glaucoma. Glaucoma is frequently overlooked as a cause of a red eye. One reason for this is that early glaucoma (intraocular pressure <35 mm Hg) often causes only conjunctival hyperemia with or without epiphora and with no other clinical signs. These dogs are frequently treated for "conjunctivitis" when they actually have episcleral injection. Later, when pressures are extremely elevated, many other clinical signs such as pain, corneal edema, mydriasis, blindness, optic nerve cupping, retinal degeneration, buphthalmos, and lens subluxation are also often present. Another frequent reason glaucoma is overlooked is failure to assess intraocular pressure. Tonometry should be performed on all dogs and cats that have a red eye unless a descemetocele is present or the globe is ruptured. Breed predisposition should heighten suspicion of glaucoma (see Chapter 263).

References and Suggested Reading

Gelatt KN, editor: *Veterinary ophthalmology*, ed 4, Ames, Ia, 2007, Blackwell.

Martin CL: *Ophthalmic diseases in veterinary medicine*, London, 2005, Manson.

Slatter D: *Fundamentals of veterinary ophthalmology*, ed 3, Philadelphia, 2001, Saunders.

CHAPTER **256**

Diseases of the Eyelids and Periocular Skin

CATHERINE A. OUTERBRIDGE, *Davis, California*
STEVEN R. HOLLINGSWORTH, *Davis, California*

The eyelids and periocular skin can be affected by a large variety of dermatologic diseases. Inflammation of the eyelids is called *blepharitis,* and many affected animals also have dermatitis elsewhere. In addition, the eyelid margin is a mucocutaneous junction, and the skin diseases that target mucocutaneous junctions often involve the eyelids. This chapter considers some of the more commonly seen medical conditions that can affect the eyelids or periocular skin of dogs and cats.

INFECTIOUS BLEPHARITIS

Bacterial Blepharitis

The most common reason for bacterial blepharitis relates to infections caused by *Staphylococcus* spp. Bacterial infection of eyelids is often secondary to another condition that alters the cutaneous microenvironment and favors bacterial colonization. Hypersensitivity or allergic reactions (e.g., atopic dermatitis or cutaneous adverse food reactions), can cause the animal to self-traumatize the area. Facial fold pyoderma occurs in certain breeds, particularly those that are brachycephalic. If the folds are close to the eyelids, moisture accumulation and bacterial colonization may occur within the skinfolds and extend to the eyelids. Mucocutaneous pyoderma can also develop secondary to a "drainage board" effect at the medial canthi in dogs with chronic epiphora.

Clinical signs of bacterial blepharitis include erythema, swelling, depigmentation, alopecia, and variable degrees of ulceration and crusting. There may be pruritus, particularly if bacterial blepharitis is secondary to underlying allergic disease. There may also be concurrent mucopurulent ocular discharge. Treatment should include appropriate systemic and topical antibiotics and identification of any underlying predisposing skin or ophthalmic disease. In some dogs, surgical removal of facial skin folds may be beneficial or curative.

Bacterial infection of the various glands within the eyelid is termed *hordeolum*. Such infections, usually *Staphylococcus* spp. are thought to originate from the ocular surface flora. Infection of the glands of Zeis or Moll is termed *external hordeolum* or *stye*. Similar involvement of the meibomian glands is referred to as *internal hordeolum*. Both conditions are more frequently seen in young dogs and may represent immune deficiency during the juvenile period. The clinical presentation of both conditions is similar, consisting of swollen, inflamed, and painful eyelid margins. The course is often self-limiting but may be shortened with application of hot compresses along with administration of broad-spectrum topical ophthalmic and systemic antibiotics.

A chalazion results when meibomian secretions thicken, obstruct the duct, and cause the buildup of secretory material in the gland. This eventually leads to glandular rupture and lipogranuloma formation. Clinically chalazia present as firm, noninflamed nodules within the eyelid. When viewed through the palpebral conjunctiva, they appear as aggregates of yellow material. Treatment involves incision of the overlying palpebral conjunctiva and curettage of the granulomatous material. Postoperative treatment is topical application of an ophthalmic antibiotic-steroid ointment for 7 to 14 days.

Fungal Blepharitis

The most common fungal organisms identified in the dog or cat with dermatophytosis are *Microsporum canis, Microsporum gypseum,* and *Trichophyton mentagrophytes*. These fungal organisms are adapted to colonize hair and cornified layers of the skin, where they digest keratin protein. Most animals must come in contact with a minimum infective dose of dermatophyte spores for infection to become established. This dose varies related to the individual animal's overall health and immunologic status.

Dermatophytosis in dogs often results in localized lesions, most commonly affecting the face, feet, or tail. Dogs are often presented with the classical circular alopecia with scale, crust, and follicular papules. A kerion is a localized inflammatory lesion secondary to a dermatophyte infection and presents clinically as a well-circumscribed nodular lesion of furunculosis, often located on the face or distal extremity. Dermatophyte lesions in cats are more pleomorphic. Classic lesions include one or more areas of partial alopecia, with scaling and crusting most commonly noted on the head or forelimbs. Dermatophytosis can also result in lesions that resemble miliary dermatitis.

The clinical appearance of skin lesions is unreliable as the sole criterion for diagnosis of dermatophytosis, and additional tests are required. A Wood's lamp examination can be helpful in some cases but is unreliable as only 50% of *M. canis* infections fluoresce, and most other dermatophyte species do not react at all. Definitive diagnosis of dermatophytosis is grounded in culture and identification of the organism. Culture samples can be obtained from hairs plucked from suspicious lesions based on clinical appearance or from fluorescence positive areas as observed with a Wood's lamp.

Topical therapy has long been advocated for the treatment of dermatophytosis. However, numerous studies have shown that topical therapies alone are less effective than systemic therapy. Lime sulfur and enilconazole are the two most effective antifungal topical therapies. Systemic antifungal therapy has been demonstrated to decrease both the duration and severity of dermatophytosis. Itraconazole (10 mg/kg) is now the preferred recommended systemic therapy for treatment of dermatophytosis. Ketoconazole (10 mg/kg), fluconazole, griseofulvin, and terbinafine are other antifungal agents with activity against dermatophytes.

Malassezia pachydermatis is a normal commensal inhabitant of the skin and external ear canal in dogs and cats. The organism may cause dermatitis as a result of inflammatory or hypersensitivity reactions to yeast antigens by the host. Most dogs with *Malassezia* dermatitis have concurrent dermatoses. Dogs with allergic dermatitis often have increased numbers of *Malassezia* colonizing their skin, and, when treated appropriately with antifungal therapies, both the overall appearance of the skin and the degree of pruritus will improve. About 40% of allergic dogs with *Malassezia* dermatitis also have concurrent superficial pyoderma. The diagnosis of generalized *Malassezia* infection in a cat is strongly linked to concurrent serious systemic disease: diabetes mellitus, positive retroviral status, and internal neoplasia. *Malassezia* dermatitis is diagnosed on the basis of cytologic documentation of increased numbers of the yeast organism. Topical treatment (miconazole, ketoconazole) may be effective, but in chronic or generalized cases systemic therapy with 5 mg/kg of ketoconazole, fluconazole, or itraconazole daily may be necessary. Griseofulvin has no activity against *Malassezia*.

Parasitic Blepharitis

Parasitic blepharitis is most commonly caused by infestation with *Demodex* mites. *Demodex canis* is the most commonly identified *demodex* mite in the dog, but there is also a long-bodied mite, *D. injai,* and an unnamed short-bodied mite. The most common form of demodicosis is localized disease, which is most commonly seen in animals younger than 10 months of age. Clinically dogs are presented with focal areas of alopecia, erythema, and scaling, often involving the face and feet. Generalized demodicosis covers larger areas of the body and is more common in certain breeds such as the Staffordshire terrier, Chinese shar-pei, English bulldog, Boston terrier, boxer, and pug. Clinically there can be marked areas of alopecia and erythema. Complete alopecia of the eyelids and periocular regions develop in some dogs. A cause for generalized demodicosis in adult dogs, such as immunosuppression resulting from underlying disease or a history of chronic corticosteroid use, is found in about 50% of cases. Concurrent bacterial folliculitis or deep pyoderma is almost always present in generalized demodicosis and should be treated appropriately. Feline generalized demodicosis with *D. cati* is also often associated with underlying systemic disease. *D. gatoi* is a short-bodied mite that lives in the stratum corneum and can be a cause of contagious pruritus in cats.

Diagnosis of demodicosis is based on identification of the mite on deep skin scrapings or hair pluckings. Multiple life stages and eggs may also be identified. For localized demodicosis no treatment is needed; it will resolve spontaneously as the dog matures. Dogs with generalized disease should be spayed because the disease may be exacerbated by estrus, and it is a heritable trait. Generalized demodicosis can be treated with total body dips with Amitraz, which is the only licensed therapy for canine demodicosis. "Off-label" systemic therapy with ivermectin (0.4 to 0.6 mg/kg daily) or milbemycin (1 to 2 mg/kg daily) is effective for generalized demodicosis (ensure the patient is heartworm microfilaria negative). Ivermectin should never be used in breeds known or suspected to be sensitive to this drug. Dogs can be tested for carriage of the multidrug resistance gene (MDR-1) that conveys sensitivity to ivermectin toxicity. Regardless of which treatment is used, therapy should be continued for 1 month past the second consecutive monthly skin scraping in which mites are not detected.

Feline Herpetic Ulcerative Dermatitis

Feline herpesvirus-1 (FHV-1) is a common pathogen of domestic cats worldwide that is associated with acute and chronic rhinitis, numerous ocular diseases, stomatitis, and ulcerative facial and nasal dermatitis. Cats with herpetic dermatitis develop ulcerative skin lesions most commonly on the dorsal muzzle and nasal planum, but lesions can involve the medial canthus and periocular regions. Pruritus is variable. Cats may not have any other concurrent signs of FHV-1 infection.

Diagnosis is based on compatible histopathology from skin biopsies of representative lesions. The presence of intranuclear viral inclusions in cells obtained from the face of a cat with marked ulcerative dermatitis is diagnostic. Eosinophilic inflammation also may be evident in affected tissues. If viral inclusions are not found, polymerase chain reaction (PCR) for FHV-1 can be performed on formalin fixed tissue samples taken from skin biopsies. In one study a negative PCR result held a 100% negative predictive value.

Treatments for herpetic ulcerative dermatitis can include subcutaneous interferon-α at 1 million units/m² or systemic antiviral drugs such as famciclovir. Secondary bacterial dermatitis may develop; thus appropriate systemic antibiotics may be warranted initially.

ALLERGIC BLEPHARITIS

Causes of allergic eyelid disease include atopy and food allergy. Immune-mediated skin disorders can also affect the eyelids (see later in this chapter).

Atopic Dermatitis

Atopic dermatitis is a pruritic, inflammatory, allergic skin disease in genetically predisposed animals. The prevalence of canine atopic dermatitis has been estimated to be up to 10%. Breeds predisposed to atopic dermatitis tend to vary geographically. In general, boxers, retrievers, and terrier breeds are overrepresented for this disease. Most dogs show clinical signs of atopic dermatitis between 1 and 3 years of age, and initially the clinical signs are often seasonal. The most common clinical manifestation is pruritus, particularly involving the face, including ears, feet, axillae, and ventrum. Dogs self-traumatize pruritic areas, resulting in lesions of alopecia, erythema, and excoriations. Lichenification and hyperpigmentation can develop in chronic lesions.

Atopic dermatitis is diagnosed on the basis of appropriate signalment, history, and clinical findings and the exclusion of all other causes of pruritic skin disease. Treatment is aimed at decreasing the individual dog's pruritic threshold. This often involves the elimination of any secondary bacterial and *Malassezia* infections; identification of any other concurrent allergic skin diseases; and judicious and prudent use of antihistamines, corticosteroids (topical and systemic), allergen-specific immunotherapy, or cyclosporine in various combinations. Details are discussed more fully throughout Section 5 of this volume.

Cutaneous Adverse Food Reaction (Food Allergy)

A cutaneous adverse food reaction (food allergy) is presumed to be a hypersensitivity reaction to ingested allergens. Food allergy occurs in both dogs and cats, and clinically affected animals demonstrate nonseasonal pruritus that results in lesions caused by self-trauma that include erosions, ulcerations, excoriations with varying degrees of alopecia, lichenification, and hyperpigmentation or erythema. The face, ears, extremities (feet), and ventrum are most commonly affected. Otitis externa is also a common feature of canine food allergy.

Food allergy is diagnosed by compatible history and clinical signs and confirmation of improvement on a strict elimination diet trial using a novel protein diet and relapse on challenge provocation with the original diet (see Section XII on Evolve).

METABOLIC/NUTRITIONAL BLEPHARITIS

Zinc-Responsive Dermatosis

Zinc-responsive dermatosis is a metabolic skin disease that often affects the periocular region in affected dogs. Arctic breeds such as Siberian huskies and Alaskan malamutes are most commonly affected, but it can be observed in other breeds. Two syndromes of zinc-responsive dermatosis are recognized in dogs. Syndrome I has been identified in Siberian huskies, Alaskan malamutes, and occasionally other breeds. These dogs are speculated to have a genetic defect in the intestinal absorption or metabolism of zinc. Dogs with this disease manifest signs even when fed well-balanced diets. Syndrome II occurs in rapidly growing puppies that are often being fed a poor-quality dog food or are being oversupplemented with calcium. These juvenile dogs are thought to have a relative zinc deficiency caused by a combination of low zinc intake and the zinc-binding effects of calcium or phytate in the diet. Dogs affected by syndrome I typically present with scaling, crusting, and alopecia of the mucocutaneous junctions, elbows, and footpad margins. Dogs affected by syndrome II are young large-breed dogs that have generalized crusting, plaques with extensive crusting, and fissuring of the footpads. Diagnosis is based on appropriate signalment and dietary history, typical cutaneous lesions, and histopathology of skin biopsies that reveal marked follicular and epidermal parakeratotic hyperkeratosis.

Many dogs with syndrome II respond simply to feeding a better-quality diet. Other dogs with syndrome II and all dogs with syndrome I require zinc supplementation with 2 to 3 mg/kg of elemental zinc in the form of zinc sulfate, zinc gluconate, or zinc methionine. To date, differences in clinical response have not appeared to depend on which zinc salt is used. Affected female dogs often respond to lower dosages of zinc after being spayed. Clinical signs typically improve within 4 to 6 weeks. Response to zinc supplementation is dramatic in syndrome II zinc deficiency, and therapy is not needed once the dog has reached maturity. Dogs with syndrome I zinc deficiency require ongoing therapy.

Superficial Necrolytic Dermatitis

Superficial necrolytic dermatitis (SND) (or hepatocutaneous disease) is an uncommon skin disease. However, it is being reported with increasing frequency in older dogs, and there have been recent rare reports in cats. Males appear overrepresented in several studies, and the mean age of affected dogs was 10 years. Some dogs with SND have elevated serum glucagon levels, and in a minority of dogs with SND a glucagon-secreting pancreatic tumor has been identified. However, most dogs with SND have a characteristic metabolic hepatopathy. It is unclear at this time what metabolic pathways may be linking liver or pancreatic disease with these skin lesions.

Cutaneous lesions include erythema, crusting, exudation, ulceration, and alopecia of the face (often periocular and perioral regions), genitalia, and pressure points on the trunk and limbs. There is also a marked hyperkeratosis, fissuring, and ulceration of the footpads that is very suggestive clinically. Secondary cutaneous infection with bacteria, yeast, or dermatophytes can also be present; particularly involving the feet. The skin disease may precede any systemic signs. Common clinical signs include development of characteristic skin lesions, lameness secondary to footpad lesions, inappetence, weight loss, polydipsia, and polyuria. The polydipsia and polyuria typically are associated with concurrent diabetes mellitus, which is present in up to 30% of dogs with SND.

Histopathologic findings of a marked parakeratotic epidermis with striking intercellular and intracellular edema in the upper epidermis and hyperplastic basal cells create the so-called "red, white, and blue" lesion that is considered diagnostic for this disease. Elevation of liver enzymes and hypoalbuminemia are common clinicopathologic changes. Glucosuria and hyperglycemia may be documented if diabetes mellitus is present. Abdominal ultrasound often reveals a very characteristic honeycombed pattern to the liver, consisting of variable-size hypoechoic regions surrounded by hyperechoic borders. Grossly livers of affected dogs appear cirrhotic. However, a vacuolar hepatopathy with minimal fibrosis (inconsistent with cirrhosis) is histologically evident in most affected dogs. Many dogs with SND have dramatic reductions in the plasma amino acid concentrations. The hypoaminoacidemia most likely reflects increased hepatic catabolism of amino acids.

Prognosis is poor, with mean survival times of 3 months. However, some dogs have been managed for over a year. Palliative therapy with intravenous and oral amino acid supplementation, often with concurrent oral supplementation with zinc and essential fatty acids, has improved cutaneous lesions in some dogs. Secondary skin infections should also be treated. If present, diabetes mellitus requires appropriate management. Removal of a glucagonoma has been reported to result in resolution of lesions in one dog.

IMMUNE-MEDIATED BLEPHARITIS

Pemphigus Foliaceus

Pemphigus foliaceus (PF) is often considered the most common of the autoimmune skin diseases in the dog. The Akita, bearded collie, chow-chow, Newfoundland, Schipperke, and Doberman pinscher are predisposed to this disease. The English springer spaniel, Chinese shar-pei, and collie also appear to be at increased risk of developing PF. Mean age of affected animals is between 4 and 5 years; but dogs of any age, breed, or sex can develop PF. Three forms are suggested to occur in the dog; these are differentiated by historical information. Spontaneous PF is most common. Drug-induced PF is clinically indistinguishable from spontaneous PF. Therefore obtaining a drug history (particularly any previous antibiotic administration) is critical for all patients with PF. Some cases of PF may occur in patients with a history of chronic, ongoing inflammatory skin disease such as allergic dermatitis. This is important to consider in chronic dermatologic patients that develop atypical or more severe lesions than previous episodes.

Clinically PF is a pustular and crusting disease that often involves the face and head. Most common affected sites include dorsal muzzle, nasal planum, pinnae, periocular skin, and paw pads. Nasal planum and haired dorsal muzzle typically are affected concurrently. Truncal lesions are often diffuse, and paw pad lesions vary considerably in their severity. Intraoral lesions are never a feature of PF. If present, pustules are often large but may quickly progress to adherent crusts. Lesions may occur in "waves" so that the disease may seem to wax and wane in severity. If present, pustules should be biopsied. Older crusted lesions that are no longer tightly adherent often are not diagnostic. Histologically subcorneal pustules containing acantholytic cells often span multiple hair follicles. Pustules with acantholysis can also involve follicular epidermis. Neutrophils predominate within the pustules.

In humans Desmoglein 1 (Dsg 1) is the primary targeted autoantigen in PF. Dsg 1 is an integral protein component of the desmosomes in the superficial layers of the epidermis. Desmosomes are responsible for intercellular cohesion, and, when these structures are damaged, acantholysis results. Until recently Dsg 1 was also believed to be the primary autoantigen in PF in the dog. However, recent evidence suggests that other proteins composing the desmosome may be more common autoantigens targeted in canine PF.

PF should be considered when a dog presents with acquired pustular/crusting disease that is generalized or strongly facial or fails to respond to antibiotics. Differential diagnoses include superficial bacterial folliculitis, superficial pustular dermatophytosis, demodicosis, sebaceous adenitis, and epitheliotropic T cell lymphoma.

Prognosis for PF is generally fair. However, a recent retrospective study found that 50% of dogs diagnosed with PF were euthanized within 1 year of diagnosis; usually as a result of complications from immunosuppressive drug therapy. Dogs that were initially concurrently treated with staphicidal antibiotics tended to have a better prognosis. Prednisone or prednisolone monotherapy rarely maintains remission of PF as dosages are decreased. Therefore concurrent use of azathioprine or chlorambucil is recommended to spare the adverse effects of corticosteroids. A small percentage of dogs with PF can be managed with combination therapy with tetracycline and niacinamide. Focally affected areas sometimes can respond to topical immunosuppressive therapy.

Pemphigus Erythematosus

Pemphigus erythematosus (PE) is a very rare, crusting autoimmune skin disease. It is considered to be a more benign form of PF or a crossover between PF and systemic lupus erythematosus (SLE). The collie and the German shepherd may be breeds at increased risk. Lesions have been proven to be aggravated by light exposure.

Lesions are confined to the face and include crusting, alopecia, and erosions of the dorsal muzzle, pinnae, and periocular areas. The nasal planum is often involved with depigmentation, crusting, and erosions. Biopsies of intact pustules or adherent crusts are most diagnostic. Histologically subcorneal pustules with acantholytic cells (as seen in PF) are present with concurrent interface dermatitis with basal cell damage (as seen in lupus erythematosus). A definitive diagnosis requires immunologic confirmation via immunohistochemistry or immunofluorescence and a positive antinuclear antibody (ANA) test. Differential considerations include facially predominant PF, discoid lupus erythematosus (DLE), superficial pustular dermatophytosis, epitheliotropic T cell lymphoma, uveodermatologic (or Vogt-Koyanagi-Harada–like) syndrome, and SLE.

Systemic Lupus Erythematosus

Skin lesions may be present in fewer than 20% of cases of canine SLE. The cutaneous lesions are pleomorphic, with erythema, scaling, crusting, depigmentation, and ulceration that often involve face, ears, and distal extremities. Panniculitis and oral ulcerations have also been seen. SLE is a progressive disease, and evidence of immunologic involvement in multiple organ systems may not always be evident on the initial presentation.

Biopsies should be taken of intact epidermis. The classic histologic lesion of SLE is an interface dermatitis.

Immunohistochemistry reveals a band of positive fluorescence at the basement membrane zone. Polyarthritis, protein-losing nephropathy, neutropenia, thrombocytopenia, hemolytic anemia, and polymyositis all have been reported in association with SLE. A thorough systemic evaluation, including a complete blood cell count, serum biochemistry, urinalysis, urine protein-to-creatinine ratio, antinuclear antibody test (ANA), arthrocentesis, and cytologic evaluation of joint fluid is warranted in patients suspected of having SLE. Most patients with SLE have an elevated ANA, although this may not always be present. Immunosuppressive therapy is required.

Erythema Multiforme

Erythema multiforme (EM) is an uncommon, acute eruption of the skin and mucous membranes characterized by erythematous macules and papules, crusting, vesicles, ulcers, and urticarial plaques. Annular target lesions with central pallor may be present. Lesions are seen on the trunk, groin, axillae, ears, mucocutaneous junctions, and oral mucosa. Histologically individual cell necrosis of keratinocytes—with or without satellitosis—is the most common lesion in EM. EM likely reflects a multifactorial etiology in which drugs, infection, or neoplasia may be triggers of the skin lesions. In about 50% of canine cases an underlying trigger cannot be found. Drug-induced EM minor is often self-limiting once medications are stopped. Severe generalized mucocutaneous EM (EM major) often requires aggressive supportive care, removal of underlying triggers, and immuno-suppressive therapy.

IATROGENIC BLEPHARITIS

Adverse reaction to topical medications can result in marked eyelid inflammation, with resultant alopecia, erythema, crusting, erosions, and ulcerations. Neomycin is one of the most common topical medications to cause an adverse reaction. If ophthalmic medications cause an adverse reaction, lesions will likely involve the eyelid and possibly the medial canthus owing to a drainage effect. Diagnosis is based on compatible history of use of topical medication. If adverse topical reaction is suspected, all topical medication should be discontinued, and the affected area cleaned. If the inflammatory reaction is severe, systemic or topical corticosteroids may be required.

Self-trauma can result in marked inflammation, with lesions of alopecia, excoriations, and crusting. Affected animals need to be evaluated for secondary infections with bacteria or yeast, evidence of demodicosis, and the possibility of allergic dermatitis.

PIGMENTARY CHANGES INVOLVING THE EYELID

A number of diseases can result in hyperpigmentation or a loss of pigmentation of the cutaneous regions around the eyes.

Lentigo simplex of orange cats is a cosmetic dermatologic condition in which intraepidermal melanocyte proliferation occurs, resulting in hypermelanosis in a macular pattern. The lentigines are well-demarcated black macules that occur most commonly along lip margins, nasal planum, and eyelid margins and increase in size and number. Diagnosis is based on compatible signalment and clinical presentation. No treatment is necessary.

Vitiligo is an acquired immunologic loss of melanocytes that results in patchy or macular hypopigmentation. Belgian Tervurens, rottweilers, and German shepherds are predisposed. Lesions of leukotrichia or leukoderma are typically seen on the nasal planum, lip margins, eyelid margins, dorsal muzzle, and paw pads. Diagnosis is based on compatible history and clinical lesions and histopathology. The disease may wax and wane and, because it is asymptomatic except for esthetic concerns, no therapy is warranted.

Uveodermatologic (or Vogt-Koyanagi-Harada–like) Syndrome

Uveodermatologic syndrome is an uncommon canine immunologic disease that results in granulomatous uveitis and symmetric depigmenting facial skin lesions. Akitas and arctic breeds are at increased risk for the development of uveodermatologic syndrome. Characteristic lesions of leukoderma and leukotrichia with variable erythema and crusting involve the nasal planum, lips, eyelids, and periocular regions.

Diagnosis is based on appropriate signalment, clinical signs, and characteristic histopathology of representative skin biopsies. Treatment requires systemic immunosuppression for therapy of the dermatitis and uveitis, which is often blinding because of retinal detachment or development of secondary glaucoma (see Chapter 262).

Epitheliotropic T cell lymphoma can result in depigmentation often involving mucocutaneous junctions such as the eyelids, nasal planum, and lip margins. It is discussed more fully later in the chapter.

NEOPLASTIC BLEPHARITIS

Meibomian Gland Adenoma

Meibomian gland adenoma is the most common adnexal neoplasm in dogs. These neoplasms are almost always benign, with malignancy being manifested only by rapid local growth, not by adjacent tissue invasion or distant metastasis. Although studies have not demonstrated a consistent breed predisposition, occurrence of this neoplasm is definitely associated with advancing age. The clinical signs consist of a nodular swelling within the eyelid and a papilloma-like growth extending through the duct opening at the eyelid margin. The neoplasm itself typically does not cause discomfort or significant inflammation but is problematic because of its proximity to the cornea. Signalment and clinical appearance allow for a tentative diagnosis that is subsequently confirmed with histopathology. Numerous effective treatment options are available, including wedge resection, laser ablation, or debulking and curettage with adjunctive cryotherapy.

Papillomas

Papillomas also are a relatively common eyelid neoplasm in dogs. Unlike meibomian adenomas, these are found in young dogs. They are almost always self-limiting, and treatment is rarely indicated.

Squamous Cell Carcinoma

Squamous cell carcinoma (SCC) is the most common adnexal neoplasm in cats, although adnexal tumors are far less frequently observed than in dogs. Metastasis is a potential problem but usually occurs only late in the disease course. However, the neoplasm can be locally aggressive, and spread to regional lymph nodes is not uncommon. White-haired coats and actinic radiation are thought to be involved in the pathogenesis. Common clinical presentation is an ulcerative, crusty lesion along the margin of the lower eyelid. Surgical excision, radiation therapy, and cryotherapy all are effective. SCC or actinic dermatitis occurs in areas that are poorly pigmented and in animals with a history of solar exposure. Lesions are initially erythematous, with crusting that progresses to ulceration. Eyelid margins, nasal planum, dorsal muzzle, and pinnal extremities in white animals are the most common sites for lesions.

Lymphosarcoma

Both dogs and cats can have adnexal manifestation of *lymphoma*, which is characterized by diffuse chemosis and conjunctival hyperemia. Although lymphoma is usually accompanied by other ocular or nonocular signs, conjunctival biopsy can be helpful in providing a diagnosis when it is affected.

Epitheliotrophic T cell lymphoma often results in pigment loss with erythema around mucocutaneous junctions such as the eyelid, lip, or philtrum. Other cutaneous lesions can include exfoliative erythroderma and nodular or ulcerative lesions. Diagnosis is made by histopathology sometimes with immunohistochemistry of representative skin biopsies. Systemic therapy with lomustine or retinoids appears to offer the best clinical response.

Mast Cell Tumors

Mast cell tumors also can affect both dogs and cats. These tumors usually appear as noninflamed nodules within or under the eyelid skin. They are usually benign in this location. Diagnosis is by fine-needle aspirate or biopsy. Treatment options include surgical excision and radiation therapy.

MISCELLANEOUS EYELID DISEASES

Juvenile Sterile Granulomatous Dermatitis and Lymphadenitis/Juvenile Cellulitis ("Puppy Strangles")

This disease is seen almost exclusively in puppies. Dachshunds, golden retrievers, and Labrador retrievers seem to be predisposed. The initial clinical sign is acute onset of facial swelling affecting the eyelids, muzzle, and lips. This develops into lesions of erythematous papules, pustules, and nodules that rupture and form crusts or fistulae. These lesions most commonly develop in the periocular regions, dorsal muzzle, and pinnae. Concurrent lymphadenopathy, lethargy, and fever are common. The disease is very characteristic in its clinical appearance, but *generalized demodicosis* and *primary bacterial infection* need to be ruled out with appropriate cytologic sampling. Histopathology of representative skin biopsies may be necessary to make a definitive diagnosis in early lesions. Affected puppies respond quickly to immunosuppressive doses of glucocorticoids, suggesting some underlying immune dysfunction.

Canine Reactive Histiocytosis

Canine reactive histiocytosis occurs as either a cutaneous or systemic form. Both forms target the skin and subcutaneous tissue; but in the systemic form lymph nodes, conjunctiva, sclera, nasal planum/nares, lungs, spleen, and bone marrow also can be involved. Often skin lesions are multiple, nonpruritic, cutaneous papules, plaques, or nodules that may be alopecic and can ulcerate. Lesions occur most commonly on the head, neck, dorsum, perineum, extremities, and scrotum.

Diagnosis is based on histopathology from skin biopsies of representative lesions. Treatment involves immunosuppressive drugs. Cyclosporine and leflunomide have generated the best clinical response in this disease.

Entropion

Entropion is defined as a rolling in of the eyelid margin that subsequently leads to contact of the eyelid skin with the ocular surface. Entropion is often classified as breed related, spastic, or cicatricial. Breed-related entropion is usually apparent as soon as eyelid margins "open" at about 10 to 14 days postpartum and most frequently seen in dogs. Different breeds often exhibit entropion in different eyelid locations. Midsize-to-large breeds most often have entropion of the lateral aspect of the lower eyelid. Small and toy breeds demonstrate entropion of the medial aspect of the lower lid. All aspects of both eyelid margins are usually involved in shar-peis. Clinical signs of entropion are blepharospasm, epiphora, and wetting of the eyelid skin in the affected areas and corneal ulceration, vascularization, and/or melanosis if the eyelid skin is in contact with the cornea. The appropriate correction is determined by the age of the patient and the eyelid area involved. Dogs under 1 year of age should not have permanent surgical repairs. Such adolescent patients are managed with topical lubricants or eyelid-tacking procedures until they are old enough for surgery. The most commonly used surgical repair of entropion is the Hotz-Celsus technique.

Spastic entropion occurs as a result of ocular surface pain and may or may not be associated with other types of entropion. Because of the potential of spastic entropion, all patients diagnosed with entropion should be further evaluated after the instillation of a topical anesthetic such as proparacaine.

Cicatricial entropion is secondary to eyelid laceration or other injury. In some instances the fibrotic tissue responsible can be identified and excised. Alternatively, a "V-to-Y" surgical technique may prove beneficial.

Ectropion

Ectropion results when the lower eyelid loses contact with the ocular surface. Most instances are breed related in dogs, although this condition can be caused by old age and weakening of the orbicularis oculi muscle. Breeds with "droopy" eyes such as cocker spaniels, bloodhounds, Saint Bernards, and mastiffs are commonly affected. Frequently the only sign associated with ectropion is a mild mucoid discharge and conjunctivitis. If the condition is severe enough, exposure keratitis can result, with accompanying blepharospasm, corneal ulceration, vascularization, and melanosis.

Usually no treatment is indicated for ectropion. In mild cases topical lubricants or antibiotic-steroid combination preparations may be used symptomatically. If corneal lesions are present, a laterally placed wedge resection may be used to "tighten" the lower eyelid.

Distichiasis

The meibomian glands are modified hair follicles. In *distichiasis* some glands fail to differentiate, and the resultant cilium emerges from the ductal opening. This condition occurs in both dogs and cats and is common in some canine breeds, including American cocker spaniels and golden retrievers. Although distichiasis usually does not produce clinical signs, it can lead to blepharospasm, epiphora, and rarely corneal ulceration. Because distichiasis is usually innocuous, manual epilation is advised to confirm that distichia cilia are actually responsible for the patient's clinical signs before more aggressive therapeutic measures are undertaken. When necessary, distichiasis is treated by epilation with cryotherapy.

A variant of distichiasis is *ectopic cilia*. With this condition the undifferentiated meibomian gland gives rise to a cilium that protrudes through the palpebral conjunctiva. Such cilia usually are located approximately centrally in the upper eyelid and may not emerge from the conjunctiva until about 1 year of age. Once they come in contact with the ocular surface, they cause an acute onset of marked blepharospasm and epiphora. They may also cause vertically linear, superficial corneal ulceration. Treatment of ectopic cilia is surgical excision of the palpebral conjunctiva containing the offending cilia and cryotherapy.

Trichiasis

Trichiasis occurs when facial hairs from normal locations come in contact with the ocular surface. It is most commonly seen in small, brachycephalic dog breeds. These hairs often "wick" tears onto the face in the medial canthal region but rarely lead to significant irritation. If they are deemed to be problematic, they can be removed with cryotherapy.

CHAPTER 257

Feline Chlamydiosis

JANE E. SYKES, *Davis, California*

Although *Chlamydophila felis* (formerly *Chlamydia psittaci*) was once known as the organism responsible for feline pneumonitis, it is now recognized largely as a conjunctival pathogen. In fact, *C. felis* and feline herpesvirus type 1 (FHV-1) are believed to be responsible for the vast majority of feline cases of conjunctivitis. Despite this prevalence, recent information suggests that chlamydial organisms other than *C. felis* may cause ocular disease in cats and that *C. felis* can be found at sites other than the eye. Perhaps this explains why topical ocular therapy alone is often unsuccessful in satisfactorily resolving clinical signs of chlamydiosis in feline patients. This chapter presents a review of feline chlamydiosis, emphasizing diagnosis of ocular signs and therapy. For diagnosis and treatment of FHV-1, see Chapter 258 and Section XII on Evolve.

Chlamydiae are obligate intracellular bacteria. The chlamydial developmental cycle involves an alternation between the predominantly extracellular, infectious elementary body (EB), measuring 0.3 μm in diameter, and the intracellular, metabolically active reticulate body (RB), measuring 0.5 to 1.5 μm in diameter. For most chlamydiae the RB divide within an intracellular vacuole called an *inclusion*. The RBs then reorganize into EBs, which are subsequently released from the host cell and may enter a new, uninfected host cell, where they reorganize into RBs. Chlamydial EBs survive only a few days at room temperature. They are easily inactivated with lipid solvents and detergents.

Until recently only one chlamydial organism had been identified in cats, *C. felis* (previously *C. psittaci* var. *felis*). Other chlamydial organisms recently implicated as possible causes of feline conjunctivitis have been shown to belong to the family Parachlamydiaceae, a group of organisms (endocytobionts) that reside within free-living amoebae (Von Bomhard et al., 2003). *Neochlamydia hartmannellae* is found within *Hartmannella vermiformis*, the most common amoeba found within potable water supplies in the United States and a suspected cause of amoebic keratitis in man. The importance of *N. hartmannellae* as a causative agent of feline conjunctivitis and possibly keratitis has not been elucidated.

PATHOGENESIS

C. felis appears to have a predilection for conjunctival epithelial cells. Natural transmission presumably occurs by close contact with other infected cats and their aerosols and via fomites. It is unclear whether venereal transmission occurs in cats. The incubation period is approximately 3 to 5 days.

Infections caused by chlamydiae tend to follow a chronic, insidious course, often progressing through asymptomatic stages; this may be because of chlamydial persistence within tissues. Human chlamydial infections lasting over a decade have been reported, and *C. felis* has been isolated from the conjunctiva in cats for up to 215 days after experimental infection (Wills, 1986). Most cats cease conjunctival shedding at approximately 60 days after infection, although cats may continue to harbor persistent chlamydiae (O'Dair et al., 1994). Prolonged rectal and vaginal excretion by cats with chlamydial conjunctivitis has been documented, suggesting that the intestinal and reproductive tracts may be sites of persistent infection (Wills, 1986). *C. felis* has also been found in the lung, spleen, liver, kidney, and peritoneum of cats, although the significance of infection at these sites is not clear. Hematogenous dissemination has been documented (TerWee et al., 1998) and may explain the presence of this agent at such sites. Regardless, the systemic nature of chlamydial explains why topical ophthalmic application of appropriate antibiotics does not eliminate infection.

Chlamydial disease may be complicated by coinfection with other microorganisms such as feline calicivirus (FCV) or FHV-1. Cats with concurrent FCV infection often have signs such as oral ulceration in addition to conjunctivitis. The concurrent presence of FHV-1 should be considered in cats with keratitis that test positive for *C. felis*. Both *Mycoplasma* spp. and *Bordetella bronchiseptica* can also complicate *C. felis* infections. Coinfections with feline immunodeficiency virus prolong the duration of conjunctivitis and chlamydial shedding (O'Dair et al, 1994). Other bacteria can also act as secondary invaders and worsen disease.

CLINICAL SIGNS

Although previously referred to as the "feline pneumonitis agent," *C. felis* is primarily a conjunctival pathogen capable of causing acute or chronic conjunctivitis with blepharospasm, chemosis, conjunctival hyperemia, and serous-to-mucopurulent ocular discharge. Transient fever, inappetence, and weight loss may occur shortly after infection, although most cats remain well and continue to eat. Clinical signs improve after a few weeks, but mild conjunctivitis often persists for months. Nasal discharge and sneezing may occur in some cats; however, presence of these signs without concurrent ocular involvement is highly unlikely to be associated with *C. felis* infection. The conjunctivitis is typically associated with a neutrophilic infiltrate. *C. felis* has been isolated from cats with neonatal conjunctivitis, although most kittens appear to be protected by maternally derived antibody.

C. felis infection alone is not a confirmed cause of keratitis, in contrast to chlamydial infections of other species. Non-*C. felis* chlamydiae such as *N. hartmannellae* do not appear to be more likely than *C. felis* to cause keratitis, despite the association between keratitis and infection with the amoeba *H. vermiformis* in humans. The ability of chlamydiae to cause corneal disease may also depend on strain and/or host factors.

EPIDEMIOLOGY

The prevalence of *C. felis* in cats with upper respiratory tract disease URTD as determined using culture has ranged from 23% to 31%. Studies using polymerase chain reaction (PCR) on conjunctival swabs from cats with ocular signs or signs of URTD have resulted in prevalence estimates of 12% to 20%. In the study in which novel feline chlamydiae were detected, an additional 88 of 226 cats (39%) had deoxyribonucleic acid evidence of non-*C. felis* chlamydial infection (Von Bomhard et al., 2003).

Cats less than 1 year of age are most likely to be infected with *C. felis*. Cats older than 5 years of age are least likely to be infected with *C. felis*. In contrast, the prevalence of infection with non–*C. felis* chlamydiae was higher (54%) in cats older than 10 years old than in cats less than 1 year old (30%). Chlamydial infection does not appear to have a strong breed or sex predilection.

The prevalence of *C. felis* in clinically normal cats is low; in studies using PCR less than 5% of cats are without clinical signs. Persistent chlamydial shedding after resolution of clinical signs may explain positive results in some normal cats. In contrast, the prevalence of non-*C. felis* chlamydial infection in asymptomatic cats was higher (6 of 30) (20%) (Von Bomhard et al., 2003). This was not significantly different from that in cats with ocular disease; thus further investigation of the importance of these organisms as causes of conjunctivitis in cats is required.

ZOONOTIC POTENTIAL

There is weak evidence that *C. felis* infection may be associated with conjunctivitis in humans. The most convincing evidence was documented recently, when a chlamydial organism was isolated from a human immunodeficiency virus–positive man with chronic conjunctivitis who had recently acquired a stray queen and its kittens (Hartley et al., 2001). Molecular evidence of *C. felis* infection has been detected in a small percentage of humans with respiratory tract disease (Corsaro et al., 2002), and recent serologic evidence also suggested that, although uncommon, *C. felis* may be a causative agent of community-acquired pneumonia (Marrie et al., 2003). If *C. felis* is zoonotic, maintenance of hygienic conditions and prompt treatment of affected cats are recommended to prevent human disease, although further investigation of the zoonotic potential of this organism is needed. Adherence to guidelines designed to protect immunodeficient people from health risks related to pet ownership should also minimize the risk of infection by *C. felis* (Greene and Levy, 2006).

DIAGNOSIS

Chlamydial infection must be differentiated from other infectious and noninfectious causes of feline conjunctivitis. Examination of Giemsa-stained conjunctival smears for chlamydial inclusions is not considered a reliable means of diagnosing feline chlamydial infection. Inclusions are often visible early in the course of infection only, if at all. Melanin granules or topical medication inclusions ("blue bodies") may be confused with chlamydial inclusions (Streeten and Streeten, 1985).

Cell culture uses fluorescent antibodies to detect intracytoplasmic chlamydial inclusions following inoculation of cell monolayers. Special chlamydial transport media containing appropriate antimicrobials are required to preserve chlamydial viability, which can be obtained from the laboratory. Isolation in cell culture is technically demanding, time-consuming, and expensive. Transportation and storage problems can affect the sensitivity of cell culture, and some samples may be toxic for cell culture monolayers. The sensitivity of culture may vary between laboratories, depending on equipment and technical expertise.

Diagnostic PCR assays are more rapid, less expensive, and in many cases more sensitive than traditional techniques such as culture. They are now used routinely for diagnosis of human chlamydial infections, and assays for *C. felis* are becoming increasingly available. With proper sample collection and storage, PCR has good sensitivity and specificity. Fluorescence-based real-time PCR assays permit quantification of organism load and may be less prone to contamination than conventional PCR (Dean et al., 2005). Samples for all PCR assays can be collected from the conjunctival sac using a saline-moistened cotton swab. Veterinarians collecting samples for PCR should contact the laboratory for sample collection and handling guidelines to minimize contamination occurring outside the laboratory and should ensure that the laboratory includes both a positive and a negative control that are subjected to the extraction process on every run.

Currently testing for chlamydiae other than *C. felis* such as *N. hartmannellae* requires broad-spectrum chlamydial PCR, which is only available in certain research laboratories. Further information on the association of these organisms with disease will be required before routine testing in cats with conjunctivitis can be recommended.

TREATMENT

Chlamydiae are susceptible to tetracyclines, erythromycin, rifampin, fluoroquinolones, and the azalide azithromycin. In contrast to popular belief, sulfonamides and chloramphenicol are ineffective against *C. felis*. Systemic antimicrobial therapy is essential because of the systemic nature of infection. Doxycycline is the treatment of choice and appears to be superior to azithromycin, even when azithromycin is administered daily (Owen et al., 2003). Rapid clinical improvement and elimination of the organism occur within 7 days of beginning treatment. In research colonies *C. felis* infection has been cleared effectively using systemic doxycycline alone for 3 weeks (5 mg/kg every 12 hours) (Sykes, Studdert, and Browning, 1999). However, in a recent study, treatment for 7, 14, and then 21 days with doxycycline (10 mg/kg every 24 hours PO) did not eliminate infection in all cats, leading to the recommendation that all cats be treated for 4 weeks with doxycycline (Dean et al., 2005). Recrudescence was noted as long as 35 days after discontinuation of therapy, suggesting that cats be retested for up to 1 month before concluding that infection had been eliminated. In some cases periods of treatment longer than 3 weeks have also been necessary to eliminate natural infections with *C. felis*. A minimum of 6 to 8 weeks of treatment, especially for cattery cats, has also been suggested. Regardless of the treatment course chosen, continuation of therapy for 2 weeks after resolution of clinical signs is probably warranted.

It is possible that in chronic infections the organism may be more difficult to eliminate. However, recurring cases often involve large numbers of cats and poor compliance. All cats must be treated with the full course of antimicrobials, and proper hygiene and quarantine must be maintained. This may be difficult to achieve when a problem exists in a large cat population. Concurrent infection with organisms such as FHV-1 and FCV may also be a problem, and affected animals often show an initial response to antimicrobial therapy because of resolution of secondary bacterial infections. Use of a solution comprising 1 part bleach and 32 parts detergent is recommended for general disinfection when FCV infection remains a possibility.

There is a risk of permanent teeth discoloration in kittens if tetracyclines are used in pregnant queens in the last 2 to 3 weeks of pregnancy or in kittens in the first few months of life. Doxycycline has reduced calcium-binding avidity compared with other tetracyclines, and there is little evidence to suggest that teeth discoloration occurs in kittens given doxycycline. To minimize the risk of doxycycline-induced esophagitis (and the more severe complication of esophageal stricture), doxycycline suspension should be administered, or a water bolus should be administered by syringe after tablet administration. Although penicillin is only considered inhibitory, a 4-week course of amoxicillin–clavulanic acid eliminated *C. felis* in experimentally infected cats, with no recurrence 6 months after discontinuing therapy (Sturgess et al., 2001). This may be a safe alternative to tetracyclines for the treatment of chlamydiosis in young kittens.

VACCINATION AND IMMUNITY

Although immunity to chlamydial infection is generally weak or short-lived, an apparent age-related resistance of cats to *C. felis* infection suggests that some form of protective immunity must develop eventually. Both humoral and cell-mediated immunity appear essential for resolution of infection. Most kittens acquiring colostrum from previously exposed queens appear to be protected by maternally derived antibody until 2 to 3 months of age.

Both modified-live and inactivated cell culture vaccines have been used in the United States, either alone or in combination with feline panleukopenia, FCV, and FHV-1 components. Atypical reactions to *C. felis* vaccines such as fever, lethargy, anorexia, and lameness 7 to 21 days after vaccination have been reported in a small percentage of vaccinated cats. The chlamydial vaccine does not prevent infection or clinical signs, although the latter are generally reduced in severity. Vaccines may be of some benefit as part of a control program in catteries with endemic chlamydiosis.

References

Corsaro D et al: New parachlamydial 16S rDNA phenotypes detected in human clinical samples, *Res Microbiol* 513(9):563, 2002.

Dean R et al: Use of quantitative real-time PCR to monitor the response of *Chlamydophila felis* infection to doxycycline treatment, *J Clin Microbiol* 43:1858, 2005.

Greene CE, Levy JK: Immunocompromised people and shared human and animal infections: zoonoses, sapronoses, and anthroponoses. in Greene CE, editor: *Infectious diseases of the dog and cat*, ed 3, St Louis, 2006, Saunders Elsevier, p 1051.

Hartley JC et al: Conjunctivitis due to *Chlamydophila felis* (*Chlamydia psittaci* feline pneumonitis agent) acquired from a cat: case report with molecular characterization of isolates from the patient and cat, *J Infect* 43:7, 2001.

Marrie TJ et al: *Chlamydia* species as a cause of community-acquired pneumonia in Canada, *Eur Respir J* 21(5):779, 2003.

O'Dair HA et al: Clinical aspects of *Chlamydia psittaci* infection in cats infected with feline immunodeficiency virus, *Vet Rec* 134:365, 1994.

Owen WM et al: Efficacy of azithromycin for the treatment of feline chlamydophilosis, *J Feline Med Surg* 5(6):305, 2003.

Streeten BW, Streeten EA: "Blue-body" epithelial cell inclusions in conjunctivitis, *Ophthalmology* 92:573, 1985.

Sykes JE, Studdert VP, Browning GF: Polymerase chain reaction detection of *Chlamydia psittaci* in untreated and doxycycline-treated experimentally infected cats, *J Vet Intern Med* 13:146, 1999.

Sturgess CP et al: Controlled study of the efficacy of clavulanic acid–potentiated amoxicillin in the treatment of *Chlamydia psittaci* in cats, *Vet Rec* 149:73, 2001.

TerWee J et al: Characterization of the systemic disease and ocular signs induced by experimental infection with Chlamydia psittaci in cats, *Vet Microbiol* 59:259, 1998.

Von Bomhard W et al: Detection of novel chlamydiae in cats with ocular disease, *Am J Vet Res* 64:1421, 2003.

Wills JM: Chlamydial infection in the cat, PhD thesis, 1986, University of Bristol.

CHAPTER 258

Antiviral Therapy for Feline Herpesvirus

DAVID J. MAGGS, *Davis, California*

A large variety of antiviral agents are available for oral or topical treatment of cats infected with feline herpesvirus type 1 (FHV-1). Some general comments regarding these therapies follow. Knowledge of these general principles can be used to better understand antiviral pharmacology and thereby guide therapy of cats infected with FHV-1.

- No antiviral agent has been developed for FHV-1, although many have been tested for efficacy against this virus. Agents highly effective against closely related human herpesviruses are not necessarily or predictably effective against FHV-1, and all should be tested in vitro before they are administered to cats. In vitro potency is described as the drug concentration at which viral replication is suppressed by 50% (or IC_{50}). Therefore a more potent drug will have a lower IC_{50}.
- No antiviral agent has been developed for cats, although some have been tested for safety in this species. Agents with a reasonable safety profile in humans are not always or predictably nontoxic when administered to cats, and all require safety and efficacy testing in vivo.
- Many antiviral agents require host metabolism before achieving their active form. These agents are not reliably or predictably metabolized by cats, and pharmacokinetic studies in cats are required.
- Antiviral agents tend to be more toxic than do antibacterial agents since viruses are obligate intracellular organisms and co-opt or have close analogs of the host's cellular "machinery." This limits many antiviral agents to topical (ophthalmic) rather than systemic use.
- All antiviral agents currently used for cats infected with FHV-1 are virostatic. Therefore they typically require frequent administration to be effective.

The following antiviral agents have been studied to varying degrees for their efficacy against FHV-1, their pharmacokinetics in cats, and/or their safety and efficacy in treating cats infected with FHV-1.

IDOXURIDINE

Idoxuridine is a thymidine analog originally developed for treatment of humans infected with herpes simplex virus (HSV) type 1. Following intracellular phosphorylation, it competes with thymidine for incorporation into viral deoxyribonucleic acid (DNA), rendering the resultant virus incapable of replication. However, apparently it does this less effectively in FHV-1 than in HSV-1, with its reported IC_{50} ranging from 4.3 to 6.8 µM. Idoxuridine is a nonspecific inhibitor of DNA synthesis, affecting any process requiring thymidine. Therefore host cells are similarly affected, systemic therapy is not possible, and corneal toxicity can occur. It has been used as a topical (ophthalmic) 0.1% solution or 0.5% ointment. This drug is reasonably well tolerated by most cats and seems efficacious in many. It is no longer available commercially in the United States but can be obtained from a compounding pharmacist. It should be applied to the affected eye five to six times daily.

VIDARABINE

Vidarabine is an adenosine analog that, following triphosphorylation, appears to affect viral DNA synthesis by interfering with DNA polymerase. However, like idoxuridine, vidarabine is nonselective in its effect and thus is associated with notable host toxicity if administered systemically. Because it affects a viral replication step different from that targeted by idoxuridine, vidarabine may be effective in patients with a disease that seems resistant to idoxuridine. As a 3% ophthalmic ointment, vidarabine often appears to be better tolerated than many of the antiviral solutions. The reported IC_{50} for FHV-1 is 21.4 µM. Where it is not available commercially, it can be obtained from a compounding pharmacist. Like idoxuridine, it should be applied to the affected eye five to six times daily.

TRIFLURIDINE

Trifluridine (or trifluorothymidine) is a nucleoside analog of thymidine. Its specific mechanism of action against HSV-1 (for which it was developed) is incompletely understood and has not been studied in FHV-1. Following intracellular phosphorylation it reduces DNA synthesis via inhibition of thymidylate synthetase. Trifluridine is too toxic to be administered systemically, but topical administration is considered one of the most effective treatments for HSV-1 keratitis. This is in part because of its superior corneal epithelial penetration. It is also one of the more potent antiviral drugs for FHV-1, with a reported IC_{50} of 0.67 µM. It is available commercially in the United States as a 1% ophthalmic solution that should be applied to the affected eye five to six times daily. Unfortunately it is expensive and is often not well tolerated by cats, presumably because of a stinging reaction reported in humans.

ACYCLOVIR

Acyclovir is the prototype of a group of antiviral drugs known as acyclic nucleoside analogs. Members of this group of antiviral agents all require three phosphorylation steps for activation. The first of these steps must be catalyzed by a viral enzyme, thymidine kinase. This property increases their safety and permits them to be administered systemically to humans. However, the activity of this enzyme in FHV-1 has not been verified. The second and third phosphorylation steps must be performed by host enzymes, which may not be present in cats or may not be as effective in cats as they are in humans. This knowledge helps explain why antiviral agents developed for humans infected with HSV-1 may not be safe or effective when administered to cats infected with FHV-1. The IC_{50} reported for acyclovir against FHV-1 ranges from 57.9 to 248.7 μM, which is much higher than that reported for HSV-1. In addition to relatively low antiviral potency against FHV-1, acyclovir has poor bioavailability and is potentially toxic when administered systemically to cats. Oral administration of 50 mg/kg of acyclovir to cats was associated with peak plasma levels of only 33 μM (approximately one third the IC_{50} for this virus). Common signs of toxicity are referable to bone marrow suppression.

However, acyclovir is also available as a 3% ophthalmic ointment in some countries. In one study in which a 0.5% ointment was used five times daily, the median time to resolution of clinical signs was 10 days. Cats treated only three times daily took approximately twice as long to resolve and did so only once therapy was increased to five times daily. Taken together, these data suggest that very frequent topical application of acyclovir may produce concentrations at the corneal surface that exceed the reported IC_{50} for this virus but are not associated with toxicity. There are also in vitro data suggesting that interferon exerts a synergistic effect with acyclovir that could permit an approximately eightfold reduction in acyclovir dosage. In vivo investigation and validation of these data are needed.

VALACYCLOVIR

Valacyclovir is an acyclic nucleoside analog and a prodrug of acyclovir, which in humans and cats is more efficiently absorbed from the gastrointestinal tract compared with acyclovir and is converted to acyclovir by a hepatic hydrolase. Its safety and efficacy have been studied in cats. Plasma concentrations of acyclovir that surpass the IC_{50} for FHV-1 can be achieved after oral administration of this drug. However, in cats experimentally infected with FHV-1, valacyclovir induced fatal hepatic and renal necrosis, along with bone marrow suppression, and did not reduce viral shedding or clinical disease severity. Therefore, despite its superior pharmacokinetics, valacyclovir should not be used in cats.

GANCICLOVIR

Ganciclovir is another acyclic nucleoside analog that also requires triphosphorylation to achieve its active form. Like acyclovir, the first phosphorylation step is mediated by viral thymidine kinase. Despite these similarities, it appears to be approximately tenfold more effective against FHV-1 compared with acyclovir, with its IC_{50} ranging from 5.2 to 12.5 μM. It is available for systemic (intravenous or oral) and intravitreal administration in humans, where it is associated with greater toxicity than acyclovir. Toxicity is typically evident as bone marrow suppression. There are no reports of its safety or efficacy in cats.

PENCICLOVIR

Penciclovir is a nucleoside deoxyguanosine analog with a mechanism of action similar to that of acyclovir and potent antiviral activity for a number of human herpesviruses. It too requires viral and cellular phosphorylation and yet has a relatively low IC_{50} for FHV-1 (13.9 μM). It is available as a dermatologic cream for humans that should not be applied to the eye. Although there are some data regarding administration of famciclovir to cats (which is converted to penciclovir), in vivo studies of safety or efficacy of penciclovir in cats are lacking, and at this time its use in cats cannot be recommended.

FAMCICLOVIR

Famciclovir is a prodrug of penciclovir; however metabolism of famciclovir to penciclovir in humans is complex and requires di-deacetylation, predominantly in the blood, and subsequent oxidation to penciclovir by aldehyde oxidase in the liver. Unfortunately hepatic aldehyde oxidase activity is nearly absent in cats. This necessitates cautious extrapolation to cats of data generated in humans. In fact, a recent study of famciclovir in normal cats suggests that the pharmacokinetics of this drug are extremely complex and likely result from nonlinear famciclovir absorption, metabolism, or a combination of the two. Despite this, some early evidence (Thomasy et al., 2007) and anecdotal reports suggest that famciclovir is most effective in some cats with suspected herpetic disease. Further studies of the pharmacokinetics, safety, and efficacy of this drug are required before dosage rates and frequency can be recommended.

CIDOFOVIR

Cidofovir is a relatively new cytosine analog that requires two host-mediated phosphorylation steps without virally mediated phosphorylation. Its safety arises from its relatively high affinity for viral DNA polymerase compared with human DNA polymerase. The IC_{50} reported for FHV-1 ranges from 11 to 21.5 μM. It is available in injectable form in the United States and is administered intravenously to humans infected with herpesviruses, principally cytomegalovirus. This drug has also been topically applied as a 0.5% or 1% solution in experimental animal models of human herpetic keratoconjunctivitis and found to be as effective when administered only twice daily as trifluridine was when administered four to nine times daily. This is believed to be because of the long tissue half-lives of the metabolites of this drug. Clearly an antiviral drug that could be applied less frequently than the presently available agents would offer marked advantages in veterinary ophthalmology. The efficacy of a 0.5% solution applied topically twice daily to cats experimentally infected with FHV-1 was associated with reduced viral shedding and clinical disease in a recent study (Fontenelle et al., 2008). There are occasional reports of its experimental topical use in humans associated with stenosis of the nasolacrimal drainage system components; as yet it is not available commercially as an ophthalmic agent in humans. Therefore at this stage there are insufficient data to support its long-term safety as a topical agent in cats.

SUMMARY

Currently over 40 antiviral compounds are licensed for clinical use or in advanced clinical trials in humans. In vitro studies have now demonstrated that a subset of these drugs also have sufficient efficacy against FHV-1 to warrant further clinical investigation. However, the more severe and more frequent occurrence of toxicity associated with antiviral drugs, along with the fact that many require host metabolism to activate them, means that very careful and thorough in vivo testing of these drugs in normal cats and cats infected with FHV-1 is necessary to assess their pharmacokinetics and efficacy, respectively. Reliance on data generated when these drugs were administered to a different species, via a different route, and for treatment of a different virus is unwise.

Suggested Reading

Fontenelle JP et al: Effect of topical ophthalmic application of cidofovir on experimentally induced primary ocular feline herpesvirus-1 infection in cats, *Am J Vet Res* 69(2):289, 2008.

Maggs DJ, Clarke HE: In vitro efficacy of ganciclovir, cidofovir, penciclovir, foscarnet, idoxuridine, and acyclovir against feline herpesvirus type 1, *Am J Vet Res* 65(4):399, 2004.

Maggs DJ: Update on pathogenesis, diagnosis, and treatment of feline herpesvirus type 1 (FHV-1), *Clin Tech Small Anim Pract* 20:94, 2005.

Nasisse MP et al: In vitro susceptibility of feline herpesvirus-1 to vidarabine, idoxuridine, trifluridine, acyclovir, or bromovinyl-deoxyuridine, *Am J Vet Res* 50:158, 1989.

Nasisse MP et al: Efficacy of valacyclovir in acute, feline herpesvirus 1 (FHV-1) infection, 26:140, 1995.

Owens JG et al: Pharmacokinetics of acyclovir in the cat, *J Vet Pharmacol Ther* 19:488, 1996.

Thomasy SM et al: Pharmacokinetics and safety of penciclovir following oral administration of famciclovir to cats, *Am J Vet Res* 68(11):1252, 2007.

CHAPTER 259

Episcleritis and Scleritis in Dogs

ANNA R. DEYKIN, *Queensland, Australia*

Primary inflammatory diseases of the sclera and episclera are relatively uncommon but important conditions in canine practice. The pathophysiology of these diseases is poorly understood, and nomenclature can be confusing. These diseases often present as a "red eye" and can be similar to many other ocular conditions. In dogs, unlike in humans, these diseases do not appear to be associated with any systemic disease.

ANATOMY

The sclera, along with the cornea, forms the outer fibrous tunic of the eye. This dense connective tissue layer is composed of collagen fibers arranged in bundles, elastic fibers, and blood vessels. It merges with the cornea at an area called the limbus. The episclera is a thin collagenous, vascular membrane between the sclera and the overlying Tenon's capsule and conjunctiva. It begins at the limbus and extends posteriorly to the insertions of the extraocular muscles. The episclera is considered part of the sclera.

Tenon's capsule is a dense connective tissue layer that attaches anteriorly near the limbus and blends posteriorly with the fascia of the extraocular muscles. It has also been referred to as the superficial episclera.

Episcleritis

Clinically episcleritis seems to be a much more common entity than scleritis. Although inflammation of the episclera may have several clinical appearances, affected patients tend to have nonpainful eyes. The lesion may be simple (or diffuse) or nodular (or proliferative).

Simple Episcleritis

This is seen as a diffuse area of inflammation, affecting a sector or larger area of the episclera. The episcleral vessels become engorged, and the affected area is thickened. These changes begin at the limbus, extending back to near the insertions of the extraocular muscles. It is this thickened or raised area that helps differentiate simple episcleritis from other causes of a red eye such as glaucoma and uveitis. There may be perilimbal corneal edema and some superficial corneal vascularization. The exposed area of episclera at the lateral canthus is the most commonly affected area.

Nodular Episcleritis

Many descriptive labels have been given to nodular inflammatory disease of the episclera, including fibrous histiocytoma, nodular fasciitis, nodular granulomatous episclerokeratitis (NGE), and proliferative keratoconjunctivitis. These terms seem to apply to possibly the same or similar conditions in which the lesion is proliferative or nodular. Most of these episcleral lesions present as slowly progressive pink nodules located on or near the limbus and sometimes infiltrating the cornea. Most of the published literature refers to these lesions in the collie breed. Collies seem to be the most commonly affected breed in the United States, but in other countries this breed predisposition does not seem so overt.

Through common usage, the term *NGE* is now used for nodular episcleritis in the collie breed, which may be different from nodular episcleritis in other breeds. NGE in the collie tends to manifest as multiple nodules affecting both eyes. The nodules tend to be on the lateral limbus and usually extend onto and into the cornea. When the lesions involve the cornea, an arc of lipid infiltrate may be seen in the cornea adjacent to the lesion. The third eyelid also may be involved. In other breeds lesions are usually singular without third eyelid involvement and may be more correctly referred to as nodular episcleritis. Inflammatory episcleral disease is thought to be immune mediated in most cases. There is no other concurrent ocular or systemic disease. Intraocular pressure is normal, and there is no coincident uveitis or ocular discharge.

The inflammatory process in patients with either episcleral or scleral involvement is consistently characterized as chronic granulomatous inflammation, with the main cell types being histiocytes, lymphocytes, and plasma cells. Abundant reticulin fiber formation is seen. This suggests a chronic reaction to a persistent antigen. However, no organisms have been identified in any cases of canine episcleritis or scleritis, and the inflammatory response may be directed toward degenerating collagen. In episcleritis the inflammatory reaction is limited to just the episclera, with anterior extension into the cornea seen in some cases. With scleritis inflammation involves the full scleral thickness. Simple episcleritis is characterized by nongranulomatous inflammation with lymphocytic and plasma cell infiltrates.

Diagnosis of Episcleral Inflammatory Disease

Despite the highly suggestive clinical appearance, biopsy is usually recommended to confirm a diagnosis of NGE, nodular episcleritis, or simple episcleritis. Other causes of red eye need to be ruled out by performing a thorough ophthalmic examination, including tonometry (see Chapter 255). Biopsy should then be performed to differentiate nodular episcleral disease from neoplastic disease such as squamous cell carcinoma or lymphoma and causes of granulation tissue formation such as trauma or a foreign body.

Treatment of Episcleral Inflammatory Disease

Topically or systemically administered immunomodulatory treatment can be used in patients with episcleritis (see also Chapter 250). Both routes may be needed in the initial stages of treatment. Once the clinical signs are controlled with concurrent therapy, systemic treatment may be withdrawn. This approach may minimize systemic effects of antiinflammatory and immunosuppressive medications. Simple episcleritis is often a monophasic disease, and ongoing treatment may not be required. The nodular forms of the disease may respond well to treatment, but recurrences are commonly reported (Table 259-1).

Table 259-1

Drugs Used To Treat Episcleritis

Drug	Dose	Comments
1% Prednisolone acetate ophthalmic drops	1 drop q6h; then reduce to minimum dose possible	May be sufficient for simple episcleritis and mild nodular episcleral disease
0.1% Dexamethasone ophthalmic drops	1 drop q6h; then reduce to minimum dose possible	May be sufficient for simple episcleritis and mild nodular episcleral disease
Cyclosporine 0.2% ointment; 1% or 2% suspension	Small amount q12h	Useful for nodular episcleral disease in combination with topical and/or systemic corticosteroids
Prednisolone	1-2 mg/kg/day PO; then reduce to minimum dose	Possibly the most effective treatment for all types of episcleral and scleral disease
Azathioprine	2 mg/kg q24h; then reduce to 1 mg/kg and taper further to every other day or twice weekly	Effective treatment for NGE but can have side effects
Useful for dogs that cannot tolerate corticosteroids
Tetracycline	Over 10 kg: 500 mg q8h
Under 10 kg: 250 mg q8h	Useful treatment combination with very few side effects long term; may take a long time (6 weeks) for clinical response
Niacinamide	Over 10 kg: 500 mg q8h
Under 10 kg: 250 mg q8h	
Triamcinolone acetonide, 6 mg/ml	0.1-0.2 ml intralesionally	Medium-acting corticosteroid
Methylprednisolone acetate, 20 mg/ml	0.1-0.2 ml intralesionally	Long-acting corticosteroid; may see granuloma formation at injection site
Doxycycline	2.5 mg/kg q12h	

Corticosteroids are commonly used in the treatment of all forms of episcleritis and may be given topically, systemically or intralesionally. Simple episcleritis may respond to topical corticosteroids alone. Nodular forms of episcleritis may also respond to topical corticosteroids but often require systemic treatment concurrently. Surgical debulking and intralesional corticosteroids may have a role in refractory cases. Topical medications used include 1% prednisolone acetate suspension or 0.1% dexamethasone suspension. Treatment may need to be as frequent as every 6 hours initially. Depending on response, systemic corticosteroids such as prednisolone may also be used, initially at a dose of 1 to 2 mg/kg every 24 hours. Intralesional corticosteroids can be useful in the treatment of localized or nodular disease. Methylprednisolone acetate or triamcinolone acetonide can be injected directly into or just adjacent to the lesion using a 27- to 30-gauge needle. This can usually be done with topical anesthesia, with or without sedation.

Topical cyclosporine therapy may also be useful in episcleritis, often in combination with topical or systemic corticosteroids. Cyclosporine is an immunosuppressive agent that inhibits T lymphocyte activation. It is available commercially for veterinary topical use as a 0.2% ointment or can be compounded as 1% or 2% suspensions suitable for topical ophthalmic use.

Azathioprine has been reported to be an effective treatment of NGE in collies. Azathioprine is an immunosuppressive drug that affects rapidly dividing cells and also inhibits T cell function. It should be used with caution since it can have severe side effects such as myelosuppression and hepatotoxicosis. Complete blood counts and serum biochemistry panels should be monitored approximately every 2 weeks during therapy, and treatment stopped if white blood cell counts start to fall. The recommended dosage of azathioprine is 2 mg/kg every 24 hours until the lesions have regressed and then reducing to 1 mg/kg every 24 hours and tapering to every second day or once weekly. Therapy has been discontinued in some cases with no recurrence. Because of the risk of serious side effects and the need for constant monitoring, azathioprine is usually only used in cases that have failed to respond to topical medications or systemic or intralesional corticosteroids. It may also be used in dogs that cannot tolerate corticosteroids.

More recently the use of tetracycline and niacinamide has been reported in the treatment of granulomatous inflammatory skin disease; this may be an important treatment regime in cases of episcleral disease in which the side effects of corticosteroids and azathioprine are a problem. The recommended dosage is 500 mg of tetracycline every 8 hours and 500 mg of niacinamide every 8 hours for dogs over 10 kg. For dogs under 10 kg, the dose is 250 mg of each drug at the same dosage frequency. Doxycycline can be used instead of tetracycline. Recommended dose is 2.5 mg/kg q12h. Treatment usually has to be continued for at least 6 weeks before a clinical response may be seen. This regimen has fewer side effects, especially if long-term therapy is needed.

Cryosurgery has been described for the treatment of NGE in collies, usually after surgical debulking.

Scleritis

Scleritis is seen less commonly than episcleritis in dogs. It can be a difficult disease to recognize clinically since it may resemble other ocular inflammatory diseases and often involves concurrent inflammation of adjacent structures. As with episcleritis, the nomenclature surrounding this disease has been confusing. Traditionally scleritis in humans and dogs has been divided into nonnecrotizing and necrotizing forms. Nonnecrotizing scleritis is seen more commonly than necrotizing scleritis in dogs. The term *nonnecrotizing scleritis* has been used to refer to nodular episcleritis. Scleritis in humans is often associated with systemic autoimmune disorders. Although necrotizing scleritis in dogs was associated with seropositivity to *Ehrlichia canis*, in general concurrent systemic disease has not been identified readily in dogs with scleritis.

The anterior sclera is more commonly affected, but inflammation can extend caudally where it is less easily visualized. The granulomatous inflammatory infiltrate tends to be full thickness; therefore secondary nongranulomatous inflammation of the subjacent anterior uvea, choroid, or retina occurs in many cases. Pain is usually associated with scleritis because of the presence of sensory nerve endings in the sclera where the extraocular muscles attach.

Treatment of Scleritis

Topical corticosteroids may have limited value in scleritis, especially when it is more diffuse and affects more than just the anterior sclera. Systemic corticosteroids and azathioprine, as described for episcleritis, may be more useful. Scleritis is generally more difficult to treat than inflammatory episcleral disease, and relapse is more likely.

Bibliography

Deykin AR, Guandalini A, Ratto A: A retrospective histopathologic study of primary episcleral and scleral inflammatory disease in dogs, *Vet Comp Ophthalmol* 7:245, 1997.

Latimer CA et al: Azathioprine in the management of fibrous histiocytoma in two dogs, *J Am Anim Hosp Assoc* 19:155, 1983.

Paulsen ME: Nodular granulomatous episclerokeratitis in dogs: 19 cases (1973-1985), *J Am Vet Med Assoc* 190:1581, 1987.

Ramsey DT: The sclera, episclera and corneoscleral limbus. In Petersen-Jones S, Crispin S. editors: *BSAVA Manual of small animal ophthalmology*, ed 2, 2002, British SA Veterinary Association, Gloucester, United Kingdom.

Rothstein E, Scott DW, Riis RC: Tetracycline and niacinamide for the treatment of a sterile pyogranulomatous/granuloma syndrome in a dog, *J Am Aim Hosp Assoc* 33:540, 1997.

Wheeler CA, Blanchard GL, Davidson H: Cryosurgery for the treatment of recurrent proliferative keratoconjunctivitis in 5 dogs, *J Am Vet Med Assoc* 195:354, 1989.

CHAPTER 260

Qualitative Tear Film Disturbances of Dogs and Cats

CHRISTINE C. LIM, *Davis, California*

Patients with chronic keratitis and/or conjunctivitis are seen commonly in small animal practice. Many such patients do not have a clinically obvious cause of their signs, as examination of the eyelids reveals no conformational or functional defects and Schirmer's tear test (STT) values fall within limits of normal. Chronic keratoconjunctivitis in these patients may result, at least in part, from deficiencies in components of the tear film other than the aqueous fraction. Such disorders are the focus of this chapter. For more information on aqueous deficiency of the tear film, see Section XII on Evolve.

ANATOMY AND PHYSIOLOGY

The precorneal tear film is a trilaminar structure approximately 7 to 10 μm thick. In addition to the abundant middle aqueous layer, there is an outer lipid layer and an inner mucin layer. Although often forgotten, both of these layers are crucial for optical clarity and surface ocular health. Although tears are responsible for both conjunctival and corneal surface health, the lack of blood supply of the cornea makes effects of tear deficiency more notable there than on the conjunctiva; however, conjunctival effects remain important. Alteration of amount or quality of the lipid or mucin layer is referred to as a qualitative tear film abnormality (Fig. 260-1).

The lipid layer comprises the outermost 0.1 μm of the precorneal tear film and is composed of a mixture of polar and nonpolar lipids. The feline lipid layer resembles that of humans, being thinner than that of the dog. The meibomian or tarsal glands, located within the eyelids, produce this layer of the tear film. The meibomian gland openings can be seen along the eyelid margins and should always be assessed during routine ophthalmic examination. Tear film lipid, or meibum, occurs as a liquid at body temperature, allowing it to be spread across the surface of the precorneal tear film with eyelid movement. The main function of this layer is to minimize evaporation of the precorneal tear film between blinks. Meibum also decreases surface tension of the tear film, thereby maintaining tear film stability and a smooth, optically clear surface.

The innermost 1-2 μm of the precorneal tear film is composed of mucins. The majority of the ocular mucins are secreted by the conjunctival goblet cells; however, a lesser contribution is also made by the epithelial cells of the conjunctiva and cornea. Although goblet cells are located throughout the conjunctiva, these cells are particularly concentrated within the ventromedial conjunctival fornices. Along with meibum, mucin plays an integral role in maintaining tear film stability by decreasing the surface tension of the tear film. Mucin also binds tear film contaminants such as particulate matter and bacteria and aids in maintaining an optically smooth surface by filling irregularities of the corneal epithelial surface. The viscous nature of mucin also promotes adherence of the hydrophilic tear film to the hydrophobic corneal epithelium.

PATHOPHYSIOLOGY

Because of contributions from the lipid and mucin layers, the tear film maintains itself as a continuous film over the cornea. During each blink fresh meibum and mucin are spread across the surface of the globe. At the same time, contaminants from the precorneal tear film are drawn into the lacrimal drainage apparatus. However, if the eyelids remain open for a prolonged period of time, a combination of tear film thinning and increased tear film contamination results in breaks within the tear film, leaving dry spots on the corneal surface. Rapid evaporation of the tear film in turn establishes an osmotic gradient that further dries and damages the corneal surface. The time between eyelid opening and the first appearance of a dry spot within the precorneal tear film is referred to as the tear film breakup time (TFBUT). In health, blinking generally occurs before the breakup of the tear film.

Clinical disease occurs when TFBUT is shorter than the time between blinks. Shortened TFBUT results from abnormalities in either the lipid or mucin portion of the tear film, which destabilizes the tear film, thereby causing breaks within the tear film and the formation of dry spots on the corneal surface. These qualitative tear film abnormalities may either predispose to or result from other disease processes. Regardless, because the tear film may be considered an extension of the cornea and conjunctiva, alterations of the tear components often induce corneal and conjunctival damage. Keratitis may manifest clinically with any combination of superficial corneal vascularization, edema, fibrosis, or melanosis. Corneal ulcers, particularly indolent ulcers, may also be present (see Section XII on Evolve). Conjunctival hyperemia is usually present and may be accompanied by chemosis. Affected animals show varying degrees of blepharospasm and, ironically, lacrimation.

Although qualitative tear film abnormalities may occur in any patient, some conditions predispose to these problems. A high incidence of qualitative tear film abnormalities has been documented in diabetic dogs. In humans

1193

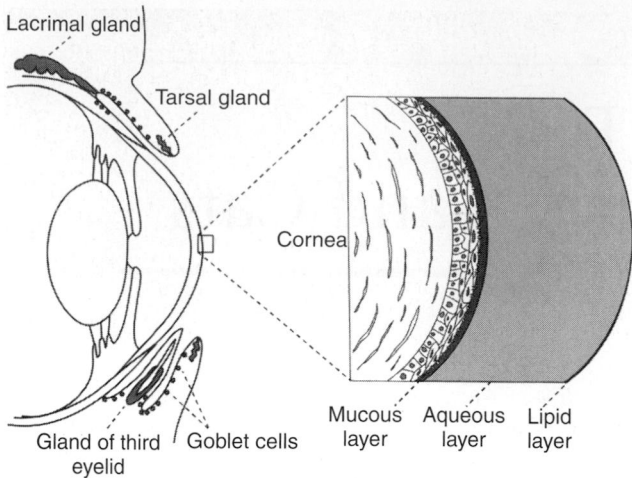

Fig. 260-1 Ultrastructure of the preocular tear film of dogs and cats and the various sites of production, including the goblet cells, lacrimal gland, gland of the third eyelid, tarsal (meibomian) glands. (From Grahn BH, Storey ES: Lacrimostimulants and lacrimomimetics. In *Veterinary Clinics of North America: Small Animal Practice,* May 2004, Vol 34, Issue 3, Fig 1, p. 740.)

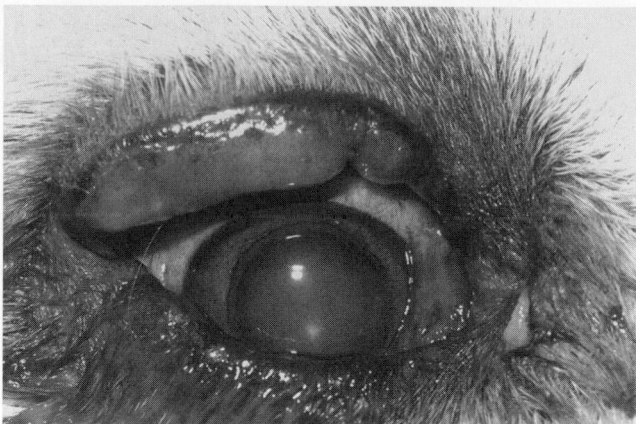

Fig. 260-2 Photograph of the right eye of an 11-year-old female spayed golden retriever. Note the inflamed, thickened upper eyelid, copious mucoid ocular discharge, and conjunctival hyperemia. (Photograph courtesy the UC Davis Veterinary Ophthalmology Service.)

a higher incidence of tear film abnormalities is documented with increasing age, especially in women. When compared to dolichocephalic and mesocephalic animals, brachycephalic breeds are particularly at high risk for development of qualitative tear film abnormalities. This risk likely relates to breed-related exophthalmia, decreased corneal sensitivity, low blink frequency, lagophthalmos, a relatively thinned tear film, increased contamination of the tear film, and an impaired ability to clear tear film contaminants.

Abnormalities in the Lipid Layer

Although congenital absence of meibomian glands has been documented in humans, it has yet to be documented in veterinary patients. However, depending on its severity, eyelid agenesis may result in a reduced number of meibomian glands.

More commonly lipid abnormalities arise as a consequence of blepharitis, especially if it causes secondary meibomianitis (Fig. 260-2). Bacterial (especially *Staphylococcus* spp.), allergic, mycotic, and parasitic (especially *Demodex* spp.) dermatitis; autoimmune disease (pemphigus); endocrine dermatoses; and eyelid neoplasia all may cause blepharitis and, to varying degrees, meibomianitis. Inflammation of the eyelids and thus the meibomian glands alters the structure of its lipid products such that meibum can become directly toxic to the ocular surface. In addition, meibum becomes a paste rather than a fluid, causing obstruction of the glands, further meibomian gland dysfunction, and inefficient spread of lipid over the tear surface.

Abnormalities in the Mucin Layer

In addition to causing tear film instability, mucin deficiency may lessen the ability of the tear film to trap and remove particulate and microbial contaminants from the ocular surface, thereby predisposing the conjunctiva and cornea to secondary infection. Mucin deficiencies occur spontaneously in dogs and cats. They may also occur secondary to conjunctivitis. Squamous metaplasia and decreased goblet cell counts occur in the presence of inflammatory infiltrates following infection with feline herpesvirus (FHV-1) in cats with corneal sequestrum and dogs with keratoconjunctivitis sicca (KCS). Given the association between inflammatory surface ocular disease and mucin deficiency, animals diagnosed with conjunctivitis should be assessed for concurrent tear film instability.

DIAGNOSTIC TESTING

A number of tests may assist in diagnosing abnormalities of the lipid layer; however, for the most part these examinations have been developed for humans and are not yet commonly used or validated for veterinary patients. Of these diagnostic studies, meibometry shows promise for assessing the lipid layer of the tear film in animals. This test is performed by applying tape to the eyelid margins and evaluating the change in optical density of the tape. Although normal meibometry values have been established for dogs, this technique is not yet readily available for clinical use. Currently, detection of lipid abnormalities relies on clinical examination alone. When blepharitis is present, it is generally evident as edema, hyperemia, maceration, alopecia, or excoriation of the eyelids, often in association with ocular discharge. Inspissated meibum may also be evident at the gland orifices, and digital manipulation often yields further extrusion of this substance. When these clinical signs are present, alterations of the lipid layer can be assumed.

Although lipid abnormalities may be assumed in the presence of blepharitis, mucin deficiencies are less clinically obvious, and further testing is required. Of the many available diagnostic tests for evaluating the mucin layer, the TFBUT is perhaps the most noninvasive and simple to perform. The TFBUT is one of the more repeatable measures of tear film stability and is extremely useful as a screening test for qualitative tear film abnormalities. In the absence of blepharitis (and therefore lipid abnormalities), TFBUT can be considered a measure of the function of the mucin portion of the tear film.

The TFBUT is a diagnostic study that measures the time elapsing between eyelid opening and the appearance of the first dry spot within the tear film. This interval should be assessed in a darkened room. Fluorescein is first instilled into the conjunctival sac, and the eyelids are closed immediately. When the eyelids are opened, timing begins, and the examiner then observes a portion of the corneal surface, usually the dorsolateral aspect, using the cobalt blue light and magnification. Ideally the 16× magnification available with a slit-lamp biomicroscope is used, but magnifying loupes may also be useful. Magnification is essential to observe the expected changes in the tear film. The tear film overlying the cornea initially appears homogenously green. However, when the tear film breaks, black spots appear within this film. Timing ceases at the appearance of the first black spot. Average TFBUTs for normal dogs and cats have been reported as 19.7 ± 5 seconds and 16.7 ± 4.5 seconds, respectively. By comparison, TFBUTs as short as 1 second are seen in cats with mucin deficiency.

Goblet cell enumeration is a more reliable indicator of mucin deficiency than direct measurements of tear mucin content. Conjunctival biopsy for documentation of goblet cell numbers confirms mucin-deficient qualitative tear film disturbances. Because of the predominance of goblet cells within the ventromedial conjunctival fornix, this is the recommended site for conjunctival biopsy. Using local anesthesia, conjunctival biopsy can be performed easily in a conscious patient. After placing a drop of 0.5% proparacaine into the conjunctival fornix, cotton-tipped applicators soaked in 2% lidocaine gel are then held against the intended biopsy site for approximately 1 minute. Care should be taken not to apply excess lidocaine to the cornea because of its toxic effects. Small tissue forceps such as Bishop-Harmon forceps are used to elevate the conjunctiva, and a 2- to 3-mm section of conjunctiva is removed using small scissors such as Stevens tenotomy scissors (Fig. 260-3). The tissue sample should include substantia propria in addition to conjunctival epithelium. Care must be taken when obtaining and handling the sample because excessive manipulations may cause goblet cells to release their contents and become less recognizable. The tissue sample should be placed immediately in 10% formalin for histologic analysis. Goblet cells are quantified by determining the number of goblet cells within a standardized length of epithelial cells. Normal goblet cell ratios appear to be above 0.3 in the dog and 0.6 in the cat.

Once a qualitative tear film abnormality has been diagnosed, an attempt to identify the underlying cause, if any, should always be made. Meticulous examination of the adnexa will identify or rule out contributing eyelid abnormalities. Depending on clinical presentation, patients with blepharitis should be screened for bacterial, mycotic, or parasitic infections; autoimmune, allergic, endocrine, or dermatologic disorders; and neoplasia. Cats with conjunctivitis should be screened for FHV-1, *Chlamydophila felis,* and *Mycoplasma* spp. In dogs specific

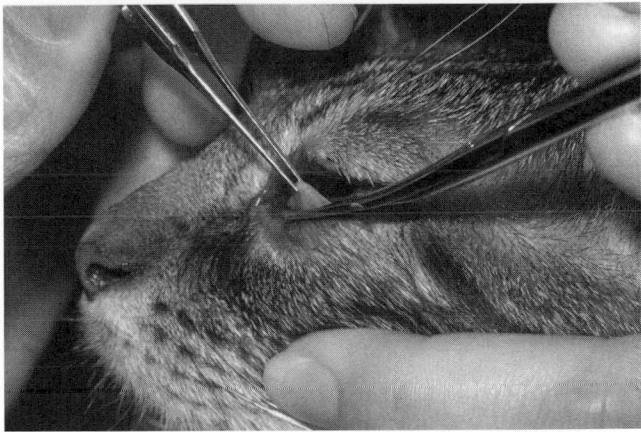

Fig. 260-3 Collection of conjunctiva for biopsy. The conjunctiva of the ventral fornix is tented with small tissue forceps. Tenotomy scissors are used to transect the base of the tented conjunctiva, ensuring adequate sample size. (Courtesy Dr. David J. Maggs.)

differential diagnoses for conjunctivitis include allergic, viral (distemper), fungal (blastomycosis), parasitic (*Thelazia*), rickettsial, or neoplastic causes, along with KCS and pannus.

THERAPY

Treatment for qualitative tear film abnormalities should address the underlying cause for the abnormality, the specific lipid or mucin abnormality, and any disease occurring secondary to the tear film deficiency. Treatment of underlying disease obviously will be tailored to the specific condition. Should secondary ulcerative keratitis be present, antibiotic prophylaxis should be initiated, preferably with a well-tolerated broad-spectrum ophthalmic formulation such as a neomycin–polymyxin B–bacitracin combination applied topically between two and four times daily.

Tear Replacement Products

Treatment of specific lipid or mucin abnormalities relies on the use of tear replacement agents. Many available products differ in their suitability for specific tear film abnormalities. In general, water-soluble formulations are used for mucin deficiencies, whereas ointments are preferred for lipid abnormalities. Lacrimostimulant therapy is not indicated if the aqueous phase is present in adequate amounts. Instead lacrimomimetics, which replace specific portions of the tears, should be used and are complimentary to other topical therapies. Additional considerations are the type or presence of preservative and the specific active ingredients (especially viscosity agents) added to the tear replacement product (see below).

Preservatives are added to all multidose vials to prolong the shelf life of the product. Unfortunately preservatives may induce allergic reactions, and excessive application is toxic to the corneal epithelium, especially if the cornea is already compromised. Patients may differ in their tolerance of ophthalmic products. If one tear substitute is not well accepted, another formulation should be tried. In particular, patients that exhibit signs of irritation after application of preservative-containing solutions should be switched to preservative-free tear substitutes. A preservative-free solution is preferred when corneal and conjunctival disease is moderate to severe or when dose frequency exceeds six times per day. The disadvantage of preservative-free solution lies in its added expense and single-dose packaging.

Viscosity agents are included in tear replacements to increase corneal surface retention time and promote cohesiveness of the tear film. Some common viscosity agents include polyvinyl alcohol, celluloses (methylcellulose, hydroxymethylcellulose), viscoelastics (sodium hyaluronate, chondroitin sulfate), and petrolatum. Of these, 0.1% sodium hyaluronate, high-concentration (1% to 2%) methylcellulose formulations, and polymer formulations (dextran, polyvinylpyrrolidone, polymer 940) demonstrate mucinomimetic properties and have a superior ability to improve tear film stability and wetting of the corneal surface. Therefore these viscosity agents should be included in the treatment regimen when a mucin deficiency has been diagnosed. Petrolatum, lanolin, and mineral oil most closely mimic the lipid layer of the tear film and should be used when lipid abnormalities are present. Generally ocular lubricants containing these materials are formulated as ointments, producing superior corneal retention time. This allows less frequent application (three to four times daily) than ophthalmic solutions (four to six times daily or more). Because of increased corneal contact time, it is recommended that ophthalmic ointments rather than solutions be applied to the eyes at bedtime, especially if the patient sleeps with the eyelids partially open.

Following improvement in clinical signs, tear replacement therapy may be discontinued in some patients. However, some patients require lifelong tear substitution for control of ocular disease.

Cyclosporine

Cyclosporine is an immunomodulator most commonly prescribed for the treatment of KCS. However, in addition to its direct stimulatory effect on the lacrimal gland, cyclosporine also has mucinogenic properties. Therefore, even in absence of aqueous deficiency, cyclosporine should be considered when mucin abnormalities are present. Cyclosporine is available commercially as a 0.2% ophthalmic ointment or may be compounded as suspensions in a variety of oils. Based on observations that the therapeutic effects of cyclosporine decrease over a 12-hour period, the drug is generally administered twice daily. Although therapy for KCS is lifelong (because of the immune-mediated nature of this disease), cyclosporine therapy may be discontinued when used to treat a specific qualitative tear film disorder. Cyclosporine exhibits its maximum mucinogenic effect after 2 weeks of treatment, and may be discontinued 2 weeks after resolution of clinical signs.

Tetracyclines

Tetracycline antibiotics have proven effective in the management of chronic blepharitis, independent of any direct antibacterial effects. Tetracyclines decrease lipase production by ocular flora, thereby decreasing the release from the meibomian glands of lipid degradation products that are toxic to the corneal epithelium. Consequently, these drugs represent another tool for the treatment of tear lipid abnormalities. Tetracyclines are available in topical and oral formulations. Oxytetracycline and tetracycline are constituted as ophthalmic ointments and solutions and are administered three to four times daily, depending on the severity of the blepharitis. In dogs and cats oral tetracycline is generally dosed at 20 mg/kg two to three times daily, and oral doxycycline at 5 to 10 mg/kg one to two times daily. Cats should receive doxycycline as a suspension rather than a tablet because of the risk of esophageal damage, including stricture. Although no specific guidelines are published, therapy should continue for about 1 week beyond the resolution of clinical signs, which can sometimes be as long as 6 to 8 weeks.

Other Treatments

Although medical therapy is the mainstay of treatment for qualitative tear film deficiencies, surgical and supportive measures are also indicated in some cases. For example, the application of warm compresses to inflamed eyelids two to three times daily eases patient discomfort and assists with drainage of inspissated meibum. Gentle removal of any dried ocular discharge with a warm, damp cloth also improves patient comfort and reduces moist blepharitis. Any eyelid abnormalities should be surgically corrected. For example, removal of distichia and ectopic cilia, or a blepharoplasty for correction of entropion, nasal fold trichiasis, or lagophthalmos may remove the underlying cause of many qualitative tear film abnormalities.

Qualitative tear film disorders should be considered in cases of keratoconjunctivitis when the STT is normal and no obvious etiology is evident on ophthalmic examination. Diagnostic testing as described above is relatively simple to perform and can be completed in most general practices. Treatment is aimed at the underlying disease, replacement of the deficient tear film component, and the keratoconjunctivitis arising from the tear film deficiency. Although therapy often can be terminated after resolution of the tear abnormality, many patients require treatment for extended periods of time.

References and Suggested Reading

Cullen CL, Njaa BL, Grahn BH: Ulcerative keratitis associated with qualitative tear film abnormalities, *Vet Ophthalmol* 2:197, 1999.

Grahn BH, Storey ES: Lacrimostimulants and lacrimomimetics, *Vet Clin North Am Small Anim Pract* 34:739, 2004.

Lim CC, Cullen CL: Schirmer tear test values and tear film break-up times in cats with conjunctivitis, *Vet Ophthalmol* 8:305, 2005.

Moore CP, Collier LL: Ocular surface disease associated with loss of conjunctival goblet cells in dogs, *J Am Anim Hosp Assoc* 26:458, 1990.

Ofri R et al: Canine meibometry: Establishing baseline values for meibomian gland secretions in dogs, *Vet J* 174:536, 2007.

Phillips TE, McHugh J, Moore CP: Cyclosporine has a direct effect on the differentiation of a mucin-secreting cell line, *J Cell Physiol* 184:400, 2000.

Shine WJ, McCulley JP, Pandya AG: Minocycline effect on meibomian gland lipids in meibomianitis patients, *Exp Eye Res* 76:417, 2003.

CHAPTER **261**

Nonhealing Corneal Erosions in Dogs

ELLISON BENTLEY, *Madison, Wisconsin*

Nonhealing corneal erosions (or ulcers) in dogs are commonly encountered in general clinical practice and are defined as any corneal erosion that fails to heal in an appropriate amount of time. Most traumatic erosions in dogs are uncomplicated and heal in less than a week with no sequela and minimal scarring. Any erosion that does not follow this simple course or does not exhibit significant improvement in this time period should be considered a nonhealing erosion. Specific disorders may underlie nonhealing erosions. Successful therapy involves directing treatment to the underlying cause. In other cases nonhealing erosions are caused by spontaneous chronic corneal epithelial defects, which generally require specific treatment to bring about healing.

DIAGNOSIS

A patient with an erosion that either fails to heal or enlarges should be examined carefully to determine the underlying cause of impaired wound healing. Numerous factors can delay wound healing, including mechanical trauma from lid masses, entropion, or foreign bodies; secondary infection; corneal exposure caused by paralysis of the lids; exophthalmos; buphthalmos; tear film abnormalities; conformational abnormalities resulting in lagophthalmos; or corneal edema.

Corneal edema may be associated with endothelial dysfunction and loss of the normal regulation of corneal hydration. With chronic corneal stromal edema the epithelial cells lose their firm adhesion to the underlying stroma, and epithelial bullae form (bullous keratopathy), which then rupture, leading to chronic corneal epithelial defects.

Spontaneous chronic corneal epithelial defects (SCCEDs) do not have any obvious underlying cause and occur only in middle-aged dogs, with most studies demonstrating an average age of 8 to 9 years old. In contrast, an underlying cause of a nonhealing erosion can usually be found in dogs less than 5 years of age. SCCEDs are also known as *indolent erosions/ulcers*, boxer ulcers/erosions, persistent corneal erosions, refractory corneal ulcers, nonhealing erosions, and idiopathic corneal erosions. The instigating cause is likely to be superficial trauma, although this is documented infrequently in dogs. Dogs with diabetes mellitus are also predisposed. In SCCEDs the epithelium begins to migrate over the corneal stroma, but the basement membrane is lost, and normal epithelial adhesion complexes do not reform, resulting in delayed wound healing.

Clinically SCCEDs have a characteristic loose rim of epithelium surrounding the corneal defect. This ring is demarcated by a diffuse, less intense ring of fluorescein staining surrounding the defect. SCCEDs are superficial lesions with no loss of stromal substance. Stromal loss indicates a more severe process, is typically infectious, and should be managed accordingly (see Ulcerative Keratitis on Evolve). The degree of blepharospasm, epiphora, and corneal neovascularization varies tremendously in SCCEDs; and central corneal lesions may persist for weeks to months with no vascular response. Vascularization occurs more commonly in peripheral lesions. If corneal edema is present, it is confined to the area of the erosion. Diffuse corneal edema, particularly if present before the onset of the erosions, indicates that the primary problem is likely to be endothelial, with secondary corneal edema and bullous keratopathy. Endothelial degenerations or dystrophies are often bilateral; thus a nonhealing erosion in a patient with corneal edema in both eyes also suggests that bullous keratopathy is the underlying problem rather than SCCEDs. This chapter focuses on SCCEDs and bullous keratopathy; treatment of the other causes of nonhealing erosions is covered in other chapters in this section (and in Section XII on Evolve).

TREATMENT

Spontaneous Chronic Corneal Epithelial Defects

Many treatments have been proposed for patients with SCCEDs, which suggests that no one therapy is ideal. Client education at the onset of treatment is crucial in the successful management of this problem. Clients must understand that multiple treatments may be required and that electing no treatment could result in persistence of the defect and relegate their pet to months of discomfort.

Overall it is important to remember that SCCEDs are by definition nonseptic; therefore frequent application of topical antibiotics is unnecessary. Topical antibiotics should be administered for prophylaxis just two or three times daily. Appropriate broad-spectrum choices for antibiotic therapy are neomycin/polymyxin/gramicidin or gentamicin. Changing antibiotics will not improve healing unless the animal is experiencing a toxic reaction to the antibiotic. Topically applied antibiotics also may delay wound healing. Oral antibiotics typically do not reach the avascular cornea in therapeutic concentrations and are not recommended.

Medical Therapy

A large number of medical therapies for SCCEDs have been suggested. These include drugs such as polysulfated glycosaminoglycans and aprotinin, which decrease proteolytic activity. Doxycycline has been suggested for human use because this drug inhibits matrix metalloproteinases (proteolytic enzymes that degrade components of the basement membrane). However, canine studies suggest that matrix metalloproteinases are not elevated in SCCEDs; therefore doxycycline or other factors that decrease proteolytic activity may not be indicated. Growth factors such as epidermal growth factor and substance P (a neuropeptide found in sensory nerves) have also been used to treat SCCEDs with some success. An antibiotic/chondroitin sulfate combination demonstrated some efficacy, but therapy had to be continued for at least 4 weeks—longer than most other therapies for SCCEDs.

The evidence recommending any topical treatment for canine SCCED is limited. Most canine studies of topical medications have involved small groups of dogs in nonrandomized and uncontrolled clinical trials. Furthermore, most medical treatment studies are isolated, with no further substantiation. Accordingly, interpretation of results is difficult, particularly since most studies included epithelial débridement (see following paragraph), which makes differentiating between resolution caused by drug administration versus epithelial débridement very difficult. Furthermore, many topical therapies have limited to no availability, or the treatment is cost prohibitive, making their widespread use impractical in the private practice setting.

Débridement/Surgical Therapy

Morphologic studies have revealed that distinctive stromal alterations occur in dogs with SCCEDs but not in those undergoing repeated mechanical epithelial débridement, suggesting that stromal alterations likely are intimately involved in the pathophysiology of SCCEDs. Accordingly, treatments that alter the stroma are more successful than medical therapies. A number of procedures may be beneficial, and these are generally performed in the order described in the following paragraphs, with 10 to 14 days separating procedures. Following any of these procedures, the application of a contact lens or creation of a third eyelid flap may improve healing times while also appearing to make patients more comfortable. Epithelial débridement and anterior stromal puncture/grid keratotomy are less invasive and can be repeated multiple times until healing is obtained. Superficial keratectomy is more advanced and can be performed only once. Generally the least invasive approach is taken initially. However, one of the more invasive procedures is not necessarily contraindicated at the first visit, particularly in patients with a protracted history of ulceration.

Epithelial débridement is the least invasive and probably most common treatment for SCCEDs. It is easily performed in conscious patients after application of a topical anesthetic such as proparacaine. Multiple dry, sterile, cotton-tipped applicators are used to gently remove the loose epithelium, starting in the center of the erosion and working toward the corneoscleral limbus in radial motions. The normal attachments of the epithelium to the underlying corneal stroma are extremely strong, and normal corneal epithelium cannot be removed with a cotton-tipped applicator. Therefore débridement should continue until all loose epithelium is removed, which often results in a much larger area of epithelium being removed than originally demonstrated by fluorescein staining. Combining results from various studies suggests a success rate with this technique of approximately 50%.

A more invasive technique involves making either small, superficial punctures or linear scratches in the corneal stroma. Various names and descriptions have been applied to these procedures, including anterior stromal puncture, punctate keratotomy, multiple punctate keratotomy, multifocal superficial punctate keratotomy, and grid keratotomy. It is believed that these punctures create areas for the epithelial cells to penetrate the stromal abnormalities found in patients with SCCEDs. This is supported by the observations of ophthalmologists who developed anterior stromal puncture to treat humans. They noted that recurrent erosions in humans occurred after superficial injury but never after deep injury to the cornea. In my experience anterior stromal puncture results in less scarring and is used preferentially, but these procedures work through the same mechanism and can be grouped together.

To perform an anterior stromal puncture or grid keratotomy, hemostats are used to clamp a 25-gauge needle so that the tip of the needle is barely exposed. This technique allows precise control of the needle and prevents its penetration too far into the corneal stroma. Commercially available anterior stromal puncture needles, with a small curve in the tip of the needle, may also be used (Stromal puncture needle No. 3800, Surgical Specialties Corp.). Before performing the puncture, topical anesthesia is applied, and the loose epithelium is débrided to expose the full extent of the erosion as described previously. Multiple small punctures are then made approximately 0.5 to 1 mm apart across the surface of the defect and into the surrounding, normal-appearing cornea. A grid keratotomy is performed by making lines in a cross-hatched pattern completely across the affected cornea, from normal cornea across the epithelial defect to normal cornea. Combining results from multiple studies suggests a success rate of approximately 80%.

The most invasive procedure for the treatment of SCCEDs is superficial keratectomy. In this technique the affected area is outlined with a corneal trephine, and the abnormal cornea is superficially undermined and removed. Generally the anterior 150μm to 200μm of superficial stroma is removed in this procedure. Care must be taken to débride the loose epithelium to delineate the lesion and ensure that the entire affected area of the cornea is removed. After removal of the abnormal tissue, a contact lens or third eyelid flap can be placed. Unlike the two procedures described previously, superficial keratectomy requires general anesthesia and usually neuromuscular blockade, an operating microscope, and precise microsurgical technique. This procedure should be done by a veterinary ophthalmologist. It probably works by removing the entire area of abnormal superficial stroma, thereby allowing epithelial adhesion. Results from multiple studies suggest a success rate of 100% within 2 to 3 weeks. Although this technique has the highest success rate, it is not often recommended as initial therapy because of the need for referral, the risks associated with general anesthesia, the increased cost, and the increased probability of corneal scarring.

Bullous Keratopathy

Bullous keratopathy is characterized by corneal edema with the formation of large subepithelial bullae. These expose corneal nerves and cause significant pain when they rupture. Medical therapy of bullous keratopathy is often unrewarding. Topical hypertonic agents increase tear film tonicity, which draws excess fluid from the epithelium. As such they may palliate epithelial edema; however, they have no significant effect on stromal edema. The most commonly used ophthalmic hypertonic agent is 5% sodium chloride solution or ointment. Ointment used four times daily appears to be more effective and better tolerated in canine patients with bullous keratopathy. If erosions are present, topical broad-spectrum antibiotics should be used as described for SCCEDs. Contact lenses may relieve pain and discomfort and protect corneal epithelium from mechanical trauma. Contact lenses can be left in place for 2 weeks, and an Elizabethan collar should be placed to facilitate retention.

Surgical therapy provides the most definitive treatment of bullous keratopathy. Goals of therapy are pain relief and visual recovery, if possible. In veterinary medicine pain relief is often the only easily obtainable goal. Thermal cautery is an easy and practical surgical option

for painful bullous keratopathy but usually requires referral. In this process the anterior stroma is denatured by heat. This destroys the abnormal epithelial basement membrane while altering the anterior stroma. Thermal cautery creates a light subepithelial scar that is a barrier to fluid flux. This barrier prevents the formation of bulla and allows the epithelium to reattach. Excessive scar formation often results in decreased vision, but the animals are usually comfortable. If scar formation is minimal, vision can be retained, but owners should be warned that vision might decrease after surgery.

The procedure is performed with the animal under general anesthesia (and sometimes with neuromuscular blockade), using disposable handheld thermal cautery to make small, superficial burns across the affected area after epithelial débridement. A blunt-tipped diathermy probe on its lowest setting may also be used. Several hundred burns may have to be placed. In cases of corneal endothelial degeneration or dystrophy, corneal edema is typically progressive; thus the entire cornea often must be treated to prevent recurrences or new lesions. After surgery a contact lens should be placed, and broad-spectrum topical antibiotics used. Mydriatic agents should be used if the patient appears to be in pain, provided that tear production is normal. After the cornea is epithelialized, topical corticosteroids may be used to decrease scar formation. Skill with microsurgical techniques and a familiarity with working under magnification (preferentially an operating microscope) are required; therefore referral to an ophthalmologist is recommended.

Anterior stromal puncture has been advocated in humans with bullous keratopathy as a means of improving their comfort while awaiting penetrating keratoplasty, which is also the definitive treatment for humans. The punctures penetrate the abnormal basement membrane and anterior stroma, allowing focal epithelial adhesions to occur. One advantage of this procedure is that usually it can be performed in conscious animals using topical anesthesia, which can be an important consideration in elderly patients with endothelial degeneration. Anterior stromal puncture also causes less scarring than thermal cautery but may not be as effective long term since it does not significantly alter the anterior stroma.

Finally, a thin conjunctival flap may also be placed over the cornea in cases of painful bullous keratopathy. Generally thermal cautery is preferred since there is a better chance of retaining vision; however, a thin, partial conjunctival flap may result in decreased edema and retention of vision. This procedure usually requires referral to a veterinary ophthalmologist.

Suggested Reading

Bentley E et al: The effect of chronic corneal epithelial débridement on epithelial and stromal morphology in dogs, *Invest Ophthalmol Vis Sci* 43:2136, 2002.

Bentley E: Spontaneous chronic corneal epithelial defects in dogs: a review, *J Am Anim Hosp Assoc* 41:158, 2005.

Champagne ES, Munger RJ: Multiple punctate keratotomy for the treatment of recurrent epithelial erosions in dogs, *J Am Anim Hosp Assoc* 28:213, 1992.

Michau T et al: Use of thermokeratoplasty for the treatment of ulcerative keratitis and bullous keratopathy secondary to corneal endothelial disease in dogs: 13 cases (1994-2001), *J Am Vet Med Assoc* 222:607, 2003.

Morgan RV, Abrams KL: A comparison of six different therapies of persistent corneal erosions in dogs and cats, *Vet Comp Ophthamoll* 4:38, 1994.

Stanley R, Hardman C, Johnson B: Results of grid keratotomy, superficial keratectomy and débridement for the management of persistent corneal erosions in 92 dogs, *Vet Ophthalmol* 1:233, 1998.

CHAPTER 262

Anterior Uveitis in Dogs and Cats

CYNTHIA C. POWELL, *Fort Collins, Colorado*

Uveitis is a general term describing inflammation of any portion of the uveal tract. Anterior uveitis (inflammation of the iris and ciliary body) and chorioretinitis (inflammation of the choroid and the adjacent retina) are common in cats and dogs. Although uncommon, intermediate uveitis (inflammation centered in the pars plana or junctional area between the posterior-most ciliary body and anterior-most choroid) also occurs. Uveitis results from any injury disrupting the blood-ocular barriers. However, the eye has limited responses to injury; thus uveitis often presents with a similar appearance, regardless of underlying cause. This situation often prompts additional diagnostic steps.

Some of the more common causes of uveitis include trauma, infection, immune-mediated diseases, and neoplasia. After the cause of uveitis is determined, the goals of therapy are to remove the inciting cause, stop inflammation, control pain, and prevent or treat secondary complications, including glaucoma. This main focus of this chapter is anterior uveitis.

ANATOMY AND PHYSIOLOGY

As in other tissues, intraocular inflammation is initiated by local tissue injury (e.g., trauma, infectious agent, antigenic challenge). Damaged tissue and microorganisms release tissue factors that cause vasodilation and changes in vascular permeability, leading to disruption of the blood-ocular barrier. Inflammatory mediators are also released by damaged tissue and cause leukocyte activation and migration. The globe has no lymphatic drainage; thus antigens from degraded organisms are transported via the bloodstream to the spleen or other lymphoid tissue, where they activate antigen-specific T and B lymphocytes.

Immunocompetent T and B lymphocytes then migrate back to the eye and reside in the uveal tract. Elimination of the inciting antigen and production of inhibitory cytokines by T and B lymphocytes help to turn off the ocular immune response. Chronic inflammation results if the inciting antigen cannot be removed completely or the immune response is not appropriately damped.

CLINICAL MANIFESTATIONS

The clinical signs of anterior uveitis in the dog and cat vary, depending on location, duration, and severity of inflammation. Hyperemia or "injection" of conjunctival and episcleral vessels and leakage of intravascular constituents into the anterior chamber are hallmarks of anterior uveitis. Increased protein concentration in the aqueous humor results from disruption of the blood-ocular barrier and is visible to the examiner as *aqueous flare*. Aqueous flare sometimes can be subtle and difficult to detect (see Chapter 248). However, once there is notable exudation of protein (especially if accompanied by white or red blood cells), the anterior chamber appears more obviously cloudy. When corneal edema is present, it also contributes to cloudiness. Inflammatory cells in the aqueous humor may be deposited on the corneal endothelium as keratic precipitates (KPs) (Fig. 262-1). Normal convection currents within the aqueous humor cause KPs to be located primarily on the ventral half of the cornea. KPs vary in size and may persist for some time after resolution of uveitis.

The iris undergoes many changes in patients with anterior uveitis. Prostaglandin release results in miosis by directly inciting spasm of the iris sphincter muscle. However, miosis may be very mild or absent when uveitis

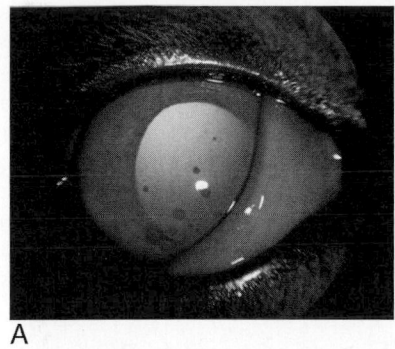
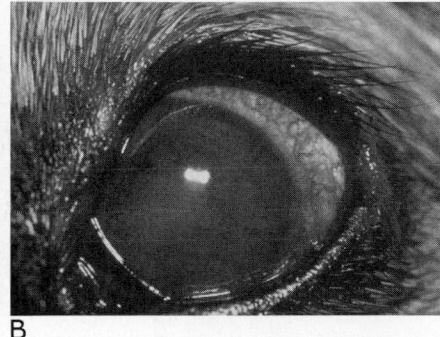

Fig. 262-1   A, Feline eye with anterior uveitis of unknown origin. Many large keratic precipitates (KPs) can be seen primarily located on the ventral half of the cornea. KPs are pathognomonic for anterior uveitis. This photograph was taken using retroillumination from the tapetal reflection, causing the KPs to appear dark. **B,** Canine eye with anterior uveitis of unknown origin. Numerous small KPs cover the ventral and central cornea, making it difficult to see into the anterior chamber. There is also marked episcleral injection and some corneal neovascularization, which, although highly suggestive of anterior uveitis, are not pathognomonic.

is chronic. Subtle sphincter muscle spasm is not evident as miosis but results in an eye that is unresponsive or poorly responsive to tropicamide or other mydriatics. Inflammation also causes ciliary muscle spasm, a major contributor to ocular pain. Iritis, manifested by iris vasodilation and increased iris vessel permeability, often causes a subtle-to-pronounced iris color change. On close examination dilated iris vessels may be obvious (Fig. 262-2), and the iris may appear swollen or "muddy" with loss in tissue architecture or detail. As anterior uveitis becomes more chronic, the iris may form posterior synechia (adhesions to the anterior lens capsule), giving the pupil an irregular shape *(dyscoria)* and impairing its ability to respond to light or dilating agents (Fig. 262-3). If posterior synechia involve the entire pupil margin, aqueous humor cannot move from the posterior chamber (between the iris and lens) to the anterior chamber. In this situation aqueous humor accumulates behind the iris, causing it to billow forward, a condition known as *iris bombé* (see Fig. 262-3). Peripheral anterior synechia (adhesions of the iris root to the cornea) can also form as a result of iris bombé or iris swelling and inflammation.

Intraocular pressure (IOP) can be quite variable in patients with anterior uveitis. Generally aqueous humor formation is impaired, and IOP is lowered when the ciliary body is inflamed. However, anterior uveitis can predispose to development of secondary glaucoma via a number of mechanisms. Inflammatory cells, iris swelling, and peripheral anterior synechia can impair aqueous outflow directly, contributing to the development of secondary glaucoma. In addition, iris bombé prohibits access of the aqueous humor to the anterior chamber and filtration angle, and the forward bowing of the iris obstructs the angle itself. Therefore IOP typically is low in acute uveitis. However, as aqueous humor outflow is impaired by any of these mechanisms, IOP begins to move into the normal range and continues to increase as secondary glaucoma develops.

Pars planitis (or *intermediate uveitis*) causes exudation of inflammatory cells from the pars plana behind the ciliary processes and just anterior to the peripheral retina. These white blood cells accumulate in the peripheral anterior vitreous as white, punctate infiltrates (Fig. 262-4). This so-called *snow-banking* usually requires pupil dilation for detection.

Posterior uveitis is inflammation of the posterior uvea or choroid. Because of their close apposition, retinal inflammation often accompanies inflammation of the choroid; together the syndrome is known as *chorioretinitis*. As with anterior uveitis, the signs of chorioretinitis are related to breakdown of the blood-ocular barrier. In the posterior segment the barrier is contributed to by the retinal blood vessels and the retinal pigment epithelium. Increased permeability of this barrier allows components of the blood to enter the subretinal space and retina. Clinically

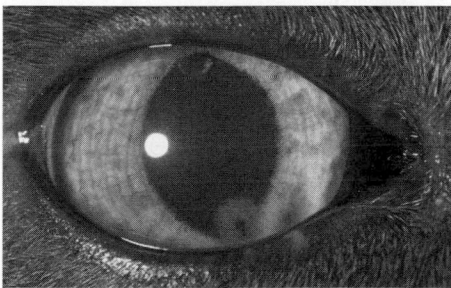

Fig. 262-2   Feline eye with anterior uveitis of unknown origin. The iris is swollen, and the iris vasculature injected. A fibrinous clot can also be seen in the ventral anterior chamber.

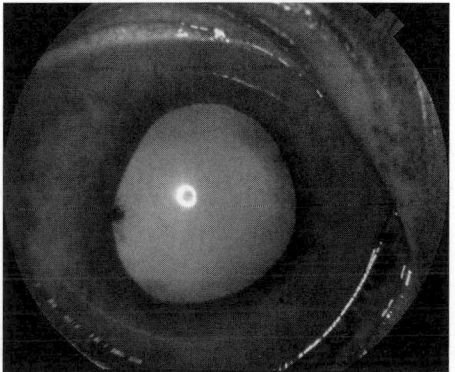

Fig. 262-3   Canine eye with chronic anterior uveitis secondary to uveodermatologic syndrome. The cornea has peripheral neovascularization. The pupil has an irregular shape (dyscoria), there is melanotic debris on the anterior lens capsule (both caused by posterior synechia), and there is iris bombé.

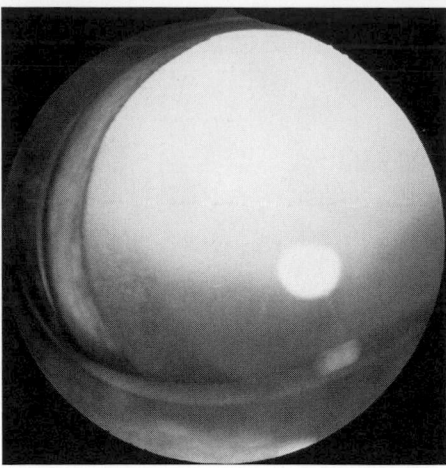

Fig. 262-4 Feline eye with pars planitis or intermediate uveitis. Cellular debris can be seen collecting in a generally cloudy vitreous behind the lens, just inside the dilated pupil. The vitreous cloudiness is caused by inflammatory cells accumulating around the ciliary body *(snow-banking)* and is evidence of pars planitis.

retinal and subretinal edema, exudation, and hemorrhage can be detected (see Chapter 264). Since the retina and subretinal space overlie the tapetum, tapetal reflectivity is diminished or obscured by areas of active chorioretinitis (Fig. 262-5). Severe chorioretinitis can lead to partial or complete retinal detachment, decreased vision, and blindness. Inflammation of both the anterior and posterior uvea is termed *panuveitis*.

DIAGNOSIS

Common causes of anterior uveitis in the dog and cat are summarized in Box 262-1. Anterior uveitis is often associated with systemic diseases, some of which are quite serious. Causes of anterior uveitis unrelated to systemic disease, such as blunt or sharp trauma to the globe, keratitis, and lens-induced uveitis, are often diagnosed simply by obtaining a good history and performing a complete ocular examination. If a systemic disease is suspected as the cause of uveitis, a general physical examination and assessment of a complete blood count, serum chemistry panel, and urinalysis are indicated. The need for imaging studies, ocular ultrasound, and serologic or microbiologic assays is based on results of the physical examination, initial laboratory tests, and clinical suspicion. Diagnosing the cause of uveitis may require examination of either aqueous or vitreous humor. These two ocular fluids can be assessed by cytology, culture and sensitivity, polymerase chain reaction (PCR), and determination of antibody content.

Anterior Chamber Paracentesis

General anesthesia is required for this procedure. Supplies needed to perform paracentesis include a 25- or 27- gauge needle on a 1- or 3-ml syringe, small rat-toothed forceps, adequate lighting, and magnification. The bulbar conjunctiva and cornea are gently flushed with a 1:20 solution of povidone-iodine diluted in sterile saline. (Do *not* use povidone-iodine or Betadine scrub!) Grasp the globe at the limbus with forceps. The dorsolateral limbus is usually the easiest to access. The needle should enter the eye adjacent to the forceps at the limbus and parallel to the iris plane (Fig. 262-6). Care should be taken to keep the needle bevel up and the tip away from the iris and lens. Up to 0.3 ml of aqueous humor can usually be removed slowly without collapsing the anterior chamber. After withdrawing the needle, gentle pressure is applied to the centesis site using a moistened cotton swab. Samples of aqueous humor can be dropped directly onto a swab for culture and sensitivity or stored in a sterile container (such as a red top) for antigen or antibody determination. Cytology is best done on samples stored in a 1.5-ml draw ethylenediaminetetraacetic acid–containing tube, concentrated by centrifugation, and stained with Diff-Quik or Wright's stain. PCR may require a special transport medium. The performing laboratory should be contacted for appropriate handling procedures. Mild hyphema is the most common complication of aqueous humor paracentesis. Serious complications are rare if care is taken to avoid contact with the iris or lens.

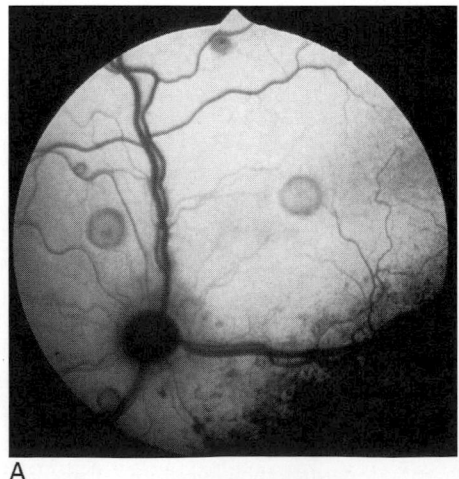
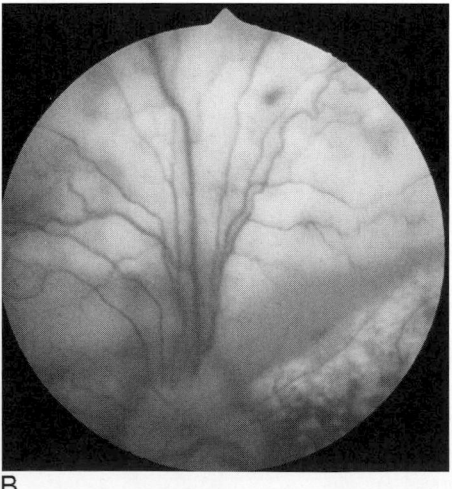

A   B

Fig. 262-5 **A,** Feline ocular fundus. The round gray lesions are areas of chorioretinitis caused by systemic cryptococcosis. **B,** Canine ocular fundus; chorioretinitis of unknown origin. The tapetal reflection is partially obscured by fluid and cells beneath and within the retina. Much of the dorsal half of the retina is detached.

Box 262-1

Causes of Anterior Uveitis in Cats and Dogs

Systemic Infection

Bacterial
Bacteremia or septicemia (e.g., pyometra, abscess) (d,c)
Brucellosis (d)
Bartonellosis (d,c)
Leptospirosis (d)
Borreliosis (Lyme disease) (d)
Rickettsial diseases
Ehrlichiosis (d,c)
Rocky Mountain spotted fever (d)

Viral
Canine adenovirus-1 (d)
Feline leukemia virus (c)
Feline immunodeficiency virus (c)
Feline infectious peritonitis (c)

Mycotic
Blastomycosis (d,c)
Histoplasmosis (d,c)
Coccidiomycosis (d,c)
Cryptomycosis (d,c)
Aspergillosis (d)

Algal
Prototothecosis (d)

Parasitic
Aberrant nematode larval migration
Toxocara (ocular larval migrans) (d,c)
Dirofilaria larvae (d)
Others

Protozoan
Toxoplasmosis (d,c)—primarily cats
Leishmaniasis (d,c)

Immune-Mediated Uveitis
Lens-induced uveitis (d,c)
Canine adenovirus vaccine (CAV-1 or CAV-2) reaction (d)
Uveodermatologic syndrome (d)— primarily Akita and Arctic breeds of dogs
Pigmentary uveitis (d) primarily golden retrievers
Idiopathic anterior uveitis (d,c)

Neoplasia
Primary (d,c)
Metastatic—lymphoma most common (d,c)

Metabolic
Diabetes mellitus—primarily through cataract and lens-induced uveitis (d)
Hyperlipidemia (d)

Trauma
Blunt or sharp trauma to the globe

Miscellaneous causes of blood-eye barrier disruption
Hyperviscosity syndrome (d,c)
Hypertension (d,c)
Scleritis (d)
Ulcerative keratitis (d,c)

c, Cat; *d,* dog.

Vitreous Paracentesis

Vitreous paracentesis is only considered when other methods of diagnosis have been unrewarding or if a large vitreous mass or subretinal exudate is found during ophthalmoscopic or ultrasonographic examination of the globe. Because of the potential for severe intraocular hemorrhage, retinal tears, retinal detachment, and blindness, this should be performed by trained clinicians or reserved for blind or nearly blind eyes. In patients with a blind and painful eye, enucleation is more likely to yield a diagnosis and is also therapeutic. General anesthesia is required for vitreous paracentesis. Before aspiration, the bulbar conjunctiva is cleaned gently with 1:20 povidone-iodine and sterile saline solution to remove all mucus and debris. The dorsolateral globe is grasped 6 to 7 mm behind the limbus with small, toothed forceps. Vitreous is viscous and can be difficult to aspirate; thus a 3-ml syringe is needed for adequate suction. Aspiration through a 25-gauge needle can be attempted first, but a 22-gauge needle often is needed to obtain a sample sufficient for analysis. The needle should be aimed toward the center of the globe and should be introduced into the eye 7 to 9 mm posterior to the limbus, adjacent to the forceps for maximal stabilization (Fig. 262-7). If a mass is present, the needle can be guided via ultrasound into the mass for aspiration. If the ocular media are clear, the needle can be guided by direct visualization, using indirect ophthalmoscopy. Care should be taken not to advance the needle across the globe into the retina and choroid opposite the site of entry. Slightly altering the

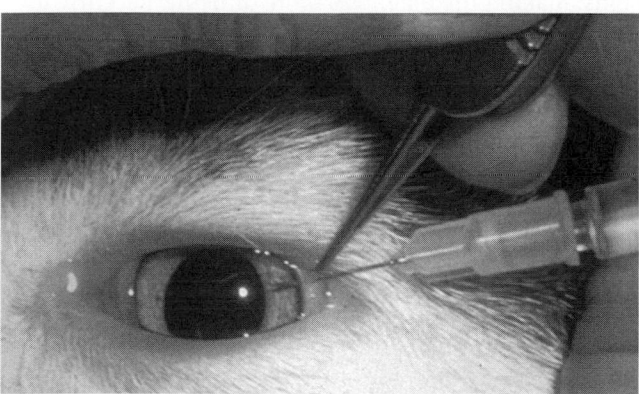

Fig. 262-6 Anterior chamber centesis. The needle enters the eye at the limbus on a plane parallel with the iris and with bevel up to avoid aspiration of the iris into the needle tip.

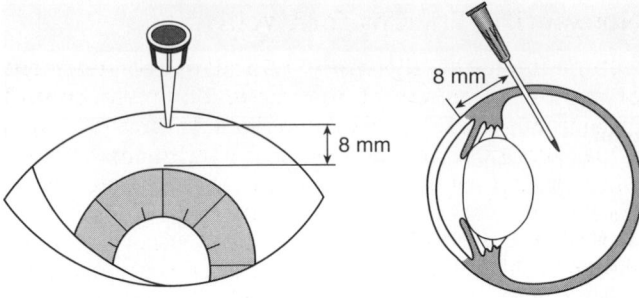

Fig. 262-7 Diagram of vitreous paracentesis. The needle enters the eye 7 to 9 mm behind the dorsolateral limbus and is directed toward the center of the vitreous.

needle position may help if there is difficulty in aspirating fluid. If bacterial endophthalmitis is suspected and a vitreous injection of antibiotic is planned, the syringe should be removed from the needle hub, leaving the needle in place for injection. Vitreous samples should be handled in the same manner as aqueous humor samples for culture, cytology, and PCR assays.

CAUSES

Infectious causes of anterior uveitis are common in dogs and cats. Outdoor cats with anterior uveitis should be tested routinely for *Toxoplasma gondii*, feline leukemia virus (FeLV), and feline immunodeficiency virus (FIV); and cats reared in a cattery or less than 2 years of age should be screened routinely for coronavirus. Although the appearance of uveitis cannot be used to distinguish one cause from another, large KPs (see Fig. 262-1) are more likely to be associated with diseases causing granulomatous inflammation such as feline infectious peritonitis (FIP) or toxoplasmosis; and pars planitis is more likely to be associated with FIV or toxoplasmosis. Ocular lesions of anterior and/or posterior uveitis are most often seen with the noneffusive or "dry" form of FIP. Although a definitive diagnosis of ocular toxoplasmosis is difficult to make and confirm, treatment with an anti-*Toxoplasma* drug is justified when other causes of uveitis have been ruled out and there is serologic evidence of recent or active infection, intraocular *T. gondii* antibody production (particularly immunoglobulin M), or presence of *T. gondii* deoxyribonucleic acid in aqueous humor. Ocular disease does not occur with FeLV infection except by its association with the development of lymphosarcoma or by immune suppression and increased susceptibility to other infectious diseases such as *T. gondii* and systemic mycoses. Clinically cats infected with FIV may develop anterior uveitis, pars planitis, or glaucoma. Screening and treatment for *Bartonella* spp. should be done in cats when other causes of uveitis have been ruled out. Many healthy cats have positive serologic titers for *Bartonella* spp. Cats with uveitis were actually less likely to have a positive *Bartonella* titer.

Ocular signs of systemic mycoses occur in both dogs and cats. Systemic mycoses primarily cause granulomatous chorioretinitis. Anterior uveitis is usually secondary to severe posterior segment infection and inflammation. Blastomycosis and histoplasmosis are found most often in the southern and midwestern United States, and coccidiomycosis in the southwestern United States. Cryptococcosis is found throughout the United States and is the most common mycotic organism to infect cats. *Prototheca* spp. are soil algae that infrequently cause systemic disease in dogs and can cause ocular signs of granulomatous chorioretinitis and anterior uveitis, which are similar to those of systemic mycoses.

Typically, depending on their location and travel history, dogs with anterior uveitis are screened for systemic mycoses, rickettsial diseases, brucellosis, and borreliosis. Rocky Mountain spotted fever (*Rickettsia rickettsii*), and ehrlichiosis (*Ehrlichia* spp.) are found throughout most of the United States but especially in the southeast and southwest. Ocular signs of rickettsial disease are common and can include both anterior and posterior segment inflammation and ocular hemorrhage, including hyphema and retinal hemorrhage. Brucellosis in dogs generally manifests as reproductive disease; but the organism can localize in bone, spleen, kidney, meninges, or the uveal tract. Clinical signs related to ocular involvement include anterior and posterior uveitis, keratitis, and optic neuritis. Lyme borreliosis is most prominent in the northeastern and midwestern United States. Although uncommon, ocular signs of anterior uveitis and chorioretinitis have been reported in dogs with borreliosis.

In spite of aggressive diagnostic testing, a specific cause will not be found in many patients with uveitis, and the cause is often considered to be immune-mediated. In these patients infectious causes still must be considered and ruled out before treatment because therapy requires systemic immune suppression. There are some immune-mediated forms of uveitis in which the offending antigen is recognized. For example, leakage of lens proteins as occurs with mature-to-hypermature cataracts or with traumatic lens capsule rupture elicits an autoimmune response and lens-induced uveitis. Likewise, anterior and posterior uveitis accompanied by poliosis and vitiligo in dogs is highly suggestive of uveodermatologic syndrome, an immune-mediated disease targeting melanin or melanocytes (see Fig. 262-3; Fig. 262-8). However, ocular signs often occur before dermatologic signs, making the diagnosis more difficult. Recently uveitis associated with iris and ciliary body cysts has also been recognized. Golden retrievers are affected most frequently. The hallmark of this disease is the appearance of pigment on the anterior lens capsule associated with clinical signs of chronic anterior uveitis (Fig. 262-9). The disease is presumed to be inherited and immune mediated. The prognosis is guarded, and many patients lose vision as a result of secondary glaucoma despite treatment.

Lymphosarcoma is the most common neoplasm associated with anterior uveitis in both dogs and cats, although many other tumor types have been reported. Lymphosarcoma can appear as a masslike lesion, or it can diffusely infiltrate the iris. When diffuse, lymphosarcoma appears very similar to other causes of anterior uveitis.

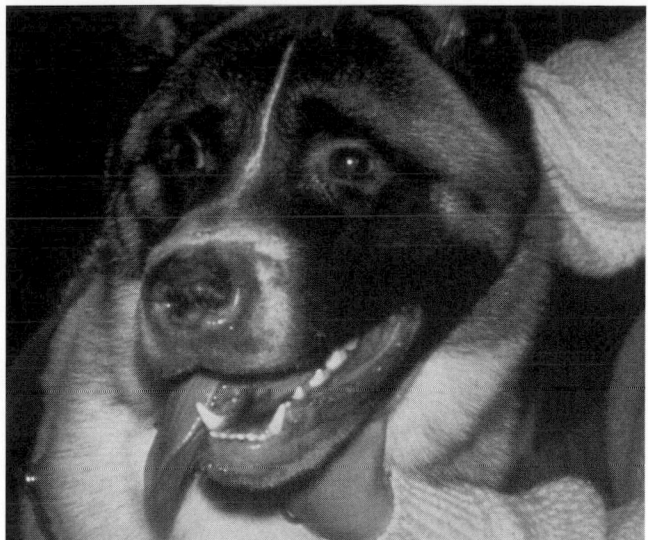

Fig. 262-8 Dog with uveodermatologic syndrome, which is a severe cause of immune-mediated panuveitis in which melanocytes are targeted. There is pigment loss in the skin (vitiligo) and hair (poliosis), especially around the eyes and nose.

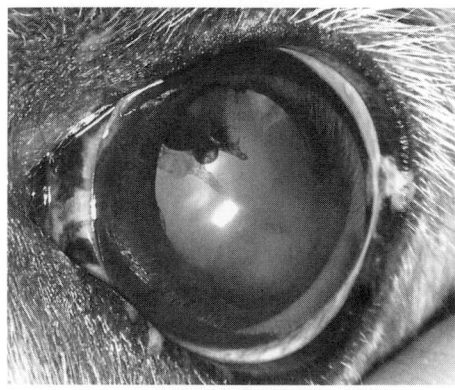

Fig. 262-9 Golden retriever with pigmentary uveitis. A large cyst can be seen in the ventral anterior chamber. Dorsolaterally there is a blood-filled ciliary body cyst adjacent to pigment streaks on the anterior lens capsule.

GENERAL PRINCIPLES OF TREATMENT FOR UVEITIS

The primary treatment goals for uveitis are to stop inflammation, prevent or control the ocular complications of uveitis, and relieve pain. Specific and nonspecific therapies are involved in treatment of uveitis. Specific therapies are used for infectious agents (e.g., bacteria, protozoa, fungi, neoplasia) or other contributors to inflammation (e.g., foreign body, corneal ulcer, luxated lens) identified through the examination and diagnostic evaluation. Nonspecific therapy includes decreasing the ocular inflammatory response with antiinflammatory drugs, mydriasis to prevent synechia formation, and cycloplegia to decrease pain. Ocular hypotensive therapy is also instituted when there is evidence of secondary glaucoma resulting from decreased aqueous humor outflow (see Chapter 263).

Nonspecific Therapy for Uveitis

Antiinflammatory therapy is critical in the treatment of uveitis, regardless of the cause. Failure to control inflammation can lead to anterior and posterior synechia, glaucoma, cataracts, retinal detachment, vitreous degeneration, optic nerve atrophy, and retinal degeneration. Glucocorticoids and nonsteroidal antiinflammatory drugs (NSAIDs) are commonly used to control inflammation. Glucocorticoids can be administered topically, subconjunctivally, or systemically. Anterior uveitis is usually treated topically a minimum of every 4 to 6 hours and as frequently as every 2 hours, depending on the severity of inflammation. Aggressive treatment is continued until the inflammation is controlled; then the frequency of administration should be slowly tapered. If inflammation is not controlled or if frequent treatments are not possible, supplementation with oral glucocorticoids should be considered. Topical preparations with the best potency and corneal penetration are prednisolone acetate suspension (1%) and dexamethasone solution (0.1%) or ointment (0.05%). Topical glucocorticoids are contraindicated in the presence of corneal ulceration because they inhibit wound healing and augment collagenase activity in the cornea. Systemic administration of glucocorticoids has minimal corneal effects unless the cornea is heavily vascularized; therefore this therapy can be given if both corneal ulceration and anterior uveitis are present.

Ocular release of prostaglandins can cause disruption of the blood-ocular barrier and uveitis. NSAIDs decrease inflammation by inhibiting cyclooxygenase, resulting in decreased production of prostaglandins. Unlike glucocorticoids, NSAIDs do not inhibit the lipoxygenase inflammatory pathway. Therefore glucocorticoids tend to control uveitis more potently, and NSAIDs should be considered primarily when glucocorticoids are contraindicated. Frequently used topical ophthalmic NSAIDs include diclofenac 0.1%, flurbiprofen 0.03%, suprofen 1%, and ketorolac 0.5%. Ocular hemorrhage caused by inhibited platelet aggregation can be a potential complication of their use. Topical NSAIDs may complicate bacterial corneal infections and are not recommended when corneal infection is present.

Systemically administered drugs are necessary to treat posterior uveitis because therapeutic concentrations cannot be attained in the retina and choroid with topical drugs. Because glucocorticoids suppress the immune response, they should be used systemically with caution (if at all) when an infectious agent is suspected. If used during infection, concurrent treatment with an effective antimicrobial is essential. Glucocorticoid preparations, dosages, and routes of administration can be found in Table 262-1. Systemic NSAIDs can also be used in dogs and cats, with careful attention to dose, frequency of administration, and possible side effects. Use of systemic NSAIDs in cats has been associated with potentially serious side effects, including bone marrow suppression, gastrointestinal ulceration, hemorrhage, vomiting, and diarrhea. Gastrointestinal side effects, including melena, vomiting, diarrhea, hematemesis, and gastrointestinal ulceration, have been reported in dogs.

Table **262-1**

Drugs Commonly Used for the Treatment of Uveitis in Cats and Dogs

Drug	Route of Administration Treatment Regimen
Topical Glucocorticoid	
Prednisolone acetate 1% (suspension)	q1-12 h
Dexamethasone sodium phosphate 0.1% (solution), 0.05% (ointment)	q1-12 h
Topical NSAID	
Diclofenac 0.1% (solution)	q6-12 h
Flurbiprofen 0.03% (solution)	q6-12 h
Suprofen 1% (solution)	q6-12 h
Ketorolac 0.5% (solution)	q6-12 h
Topical Mydriatic/Cycloplegic (parasympatholytic)	
Atropine sulfate 0.5%, 1% (solution and ointment)	q8-24 h
Tropicamide 0.5%, 1% (solution)	q6-12 h
Topical Mydriatic (sympathomimetic)	
Phenylephrine hydrochloride 2.5%, 10% (solution)	In conjunction with parasympatholytic
Systemic Glucocorticoid	
Prednisolone 5-mg tablet or Prednisone 5-mg, 20-mg tablet	0.5 to 2.2 mg/kg q12-24 h (Higher dosages for initial therapy of severe inflammation)
Systemic NSAID	
Acetylsalicylic acid 80-mg tablet	Cat: 10-20 mg/kg q48-72 h PO
	Dog: 10 mg/kg q12 h PO
Ketoprofen 12.5-mg tablet	Cat: ≤2 mg/kg PO once, ≤1 mg/kg q24 h
	Dog: ≤2 mg/kg PO once, ≤1 mg/kg q24 h
Meloxicam 1.5 mg/ml	Cat: 0.2 mg/kg PO initially, followed by 0.1 mg/kg PO (in food) q24 h × 2 days, then 0.025 mg/kg two to three times a week
	Dog: 0.2 mg/kg PO initially followed by 0.1 mg/kg PO (in food) once daily
Carprofen 25-mg, 75-mg, 100-mg tablet	Dog: 2.2 mg/kg q12-24 h
Deracoxib 25-mg, 100-mg tablet	Dog: 1-2 mg/kg PO q24 h or 3-4 mg/kg PO q24 h (do not exceed 7 days' therapy at this dose)
Subconjunctival Glucocorticoid	
Methylprednisolone acetate	4 mg/eye
Betamethasone	0.75 mg/eye
Triamcinolone	4 mg/eye

NSAID, Nonsteroidal antiinflammatory; *PO,* orally.

Subconjunctivally administered glucocorticoids have been used to supplement topical or systemic therapy in cases of severe ocular inflammation or in patients in which frequent topical treatment is not possible. Commonly used subconjunctival preparations are long acting and give a constant source of drug release for a 2- to 4-week period. A disadvantage to their use is the inability to withdraw the medication if complications such as corneal ulceration arise. Drugs injected subconjunctivally enter the eye through the sclera and, following leakage back out the injection site, through the cornea. Therefore subconjunctival glucocorticoids are contraindicated with corneal ulceration and should be used with extreme caution in dogs prone to development of corneal ulcers, such as brachycephalic breeds. Topical and subconjunctival glucocorticoid use may also result in reactivation of feline herpesvirus-1 (FHV-1) in carrier cats with previous episodes of viral keratitis or conjunctivitis. Therefore it is best not to administer subconjunctival glucocorticoid to cats suspected to have recurrent FHV-1–related ocular disease.

Cycloplegic drugs relieve pain associated with anterior uveitis by relaxing the ciliary body muscle spasm. These agents also cause mydriasis, which can prevent or break down posterior synechia by decreasing iris-lens contact. Cycloplegia and mydriasis can be accomplished by using a parasympatholytic agent. Topical 1% atropine sulfate ointment is used most commonly because the ocular solution is more likely to reach the mouth via the nasolacrimal duct and cause profuse salivation because of its bitter taste, especially in cats. The duration and frequency of application depend on the severity of ocular inflammation. Very mild inflammation is usually treated only once daily, severe inflammation may require treatment up to three to four times daily to maintain iris dilation. Because parasympatholytic agents can decrease tear production, they are best applied "to effect" (i.e., in sufficiently frequently to maintain pupil dilation). The addition of a sympathomimetic may help to achieve mydriasis when synechia have already formed but does not provide the analgesic effect associated with cycloplegia.

PROGNOSIS

The fate of an eye with anterior uveitis rests on a number of factors. Inflammation that can be brought under control very quickly may not leave any evidence of previous uveitis. Consequences of long-standing inflammation can include impaired vision, blindness, or marked ocular pain. Iris inflammation and swelling, inflammatory cells and debris, and iris bombé secondary to posterior synechia all can contribute to obstruction of the iridocorneal angle, resulting in secondary glaucoma. Chronic uveitis can also stimulate the growth of a fibrovascular membrane across the iris, pupil, and iridocorneal angle, which can lead to glaucoma. Secondary glaucoma is very common with anterior uveitis; thus IOP measurements are an integral part of management. Other sequelae to chronic anterior uveitis are development of cataract and retinal inflammation and degeneration. Whether vision-threatening changes occur depends on the severity and chronicity of the inflammation, as well as the cause, timeliness, and appropriateness of therapy and the response to it.

Suggested Reading

Brightman AH, Ogilvie GK, Tompkins M: Ocular disease in FeLV-positive cats: 11 cases (1981-1986), *J Am Vet Med Assoc* 198(6):1049, 1991.

Collins BK, Moore CP: Diseases and surgery of the canine anterior uvea. In Gelatt KN, editor: *Veterinary ophthalmology*, Philadelphia, 1999, Lippincott Williams & Wilkins, p 755.

Davidson MG et al: Feline anterior uveitis: a study of 53 cases, *J Am Anim Hosp Assoc* 27(1):77, 1991.

English RV et al: Intraocular disease associated with feline immunodeficiency virus infection in cats, *J Am Vet Med Assoc* 196(7):1116, 1990.

Giuilano EA: Nonsteroidal antiinflammatory drugs in veterinary ophthalmology, *Vet Clin North Am: Small Anim Pract* 34(3):707, 2004.

Lappin MR, Black JC: *Bartonella* spp. infection as a possible cause of uveitis in a cat, *J Am Vet Med Assoc* 214(8):1205, 1999.

Massa KL et al: Causes of uveitis in dogs: 102 cases (1989-2000), *Vet Ophthalmol* 5(2):93, 2002.

Martin CL, Stiles J: Ocular infections. In Greene CE, editor: *Infectious diseases of the dog and cat*, Philadelphia, 1998, Saunders, p 658.

Powell CC, Lappin MR: Causes of feline uveitis, *Compend Contin Educ Pract Vet* 23(2):128, 2001.

Sapienza JS, Simo FJ, Prades-Sapienza A: Golden retriever uveitis: 75 cases (1994-1999), *Vet Ophthalmol* 3:241, 2000.

Wilkie DA: Control of ocular inflammation, *Vet Clin North Am: Small Anim Pract* 20(3):693, 1990.

CHAPTER **263**

Feline Glaucoma

PAUL E. MILLER, *Madison, Wisconsin*

Glaucoma is a group of disorders united by a common theme in which intraocular pressure (IOP) is too high to permit the optic nerve, and perhaps the retina, to function normally. Ultimately this results in partial or complete loss of vision. The IOP threshold at which vision loss occurs varies considerably from individual to individual, but in general most cats do not tolerate IOP in excess of 25 to 27 mm Hg for very long, and in some animals visual impairment occurs well before this level. The chance of vision loss is directly related to both the magnitude and duration of the increased IOP. For example, a gradual increase in IOP of a few millimeters of mercury may be tolerated for months without overt visual impairment, whereas sudden marked rises (to 50 to 60 mm Hg) often result in irreversible blindness in a matter of hours to days. In some animals vision may continue to be lost because of glaucoma even after IOP has returned to normal.

ANATOMY AND PHYSIOLOGY

A stable IOP requires that aqueous humor production match aqueous humor outflow. Thirty percent of aqueous humor is produced by passive diffusion; the remaining 70% is made by several active, energy-dependent processes, one of which involves the enzyme carbonic anhydrase. The rate of passive diffusion varies inversely with IOP, thereby creating a mechanism for balancing production and outflow. However, active secretion continues at roughly the same rate even if IOP is elevated since it is the major source of nutrition for the eye and the only alternative of the eye is to "starve." Aqueous humor exits the eye via either the conventional pathway (97% in cats) or the uveoscleral pathway (3% in cats). In conventional outflow aqueous humor, which is formed at the tips of the ciliary processes, enters the posterior chamber between the iris and lens, passes through the pupil into the anterior chamber, flows between the strands of the pectinate ligament of the iridocorneal (drainage) angle into the trabecular meshwork, and then drains into the episcleral veins and the systemic circulation. In the uveoscleral pathway aqueous humor percolates through the ciliary body interstitium and ultimately "leaks" through the sclera into the orbit, where it is picked up by orbital lymphatic vessels.

GLAUCOMA CLASSIFICATION

Glaucoma is almost invariably caused by impairments in the aqueous humor outflow pathways that exceed the compensatory abilities of the passive production system. One of the most useful ways of classifying glaucoma, then, is by the location of the impediment (block) to outflow (Box 263–1). Cats with long-standing glaucoma often have multiple obstructions to outflow, explaining in part the difficulty in treating advanced glaucoma in this species. However, understanding the location of these blocks forms the basis for creating a rationale treatment plan that is tailored for each individual.

Other ways of classifying glaucoma include whether the inciting cause is primary or secondary, whether the iridocorneal (drainage) angle is open or closed, and by disease duration. *Primary glaucoma* refers to glaucoma that has no consistent, obvious association with another ocular or systemic disorder. Although uncommon in cats, primary glaucoma is typically bilateral, has a strong breed association, is probably genetic, and may or may not be congenital in onset. *Secondary glaucoma* is associated with another ocular or systemic disorder (e.g., chronic uveitis, intraocular neoplasia) that alters aqueous humor dynamics. Secondary glaucoma may be unilateral or bilateral, may or may not be inherited, and typically is seen in adult cats. These two major categories are further subdivided by whether the drainage angle is *open* or *closed*. Although the latter distinction is best made with a specialized goniolens, it is possible to see a portion of the feline drainage angle with an indirect ophthalmoscope and condensing lens held at an extreme angle to the eye so that the iridocorneal junction is the focal point of the lens instead of the retina.

EPIDEMIOLOGY

According to data collected by the Veterinary Medical Data Base, 1 in 367 (0.3%) of cats presenting to University Teaching Hospitals had a diagnosis of glaucoma. However, this referral population estimate may be low since a study that prospectively screened cats 7 years of age or older in a feline exclusive private practice found that 0.9% of cats (1 in 108) had abnormally high IOP (Kroll et al., 2001). In both of these populations and in several other case series of cats with glaucoma, glaucoma was secondary 95% to

---

Box 263-1

Classification of Glaucoma by Location of the Barrier to Aqueous Humor Outflow

1. Posttrabecular meshwork forms
   a. Episcleral vein obstructions
   b. Scleral outlet channel obstructions
   c. Angular aqueous plexus obstructions
2. Trabecular meshwork obstructions
   a. Primary open-angle glaucoma
      (1) Adult-onset
      (2) Primary juvenile-onset open-angle glaucoma
   b. Secondary obstructions of a conformationally open angle
      (1) Pretrabecular forms: preiridal fibrovascular membranes
      (2) Trabecular forms: material within the meshwork
         • Vitreous
         • Plasma proteins
         • Neoplastic cells
         • Red blood cells (intact or ghost)
         • Pigment
         • Epithelial down-growth
3. Block at the level of the angle
   a. Primary angle-closure glaucoma
   b. Secondary angle-closure glaucomas
      (1) Anterior "pulling" (e.g., peripheral anterior synechia)
      (2) Posterior "pushing" ± pupillary block
4. Block at the level of the iris (pupillary block)
   a. Relative pupillary block caused by iris-lens apposition
   b. Posterior synechia/iris bombé (absolute block)
   c. Lens within pupil aperture: luxations, intumescent lens
   d. Vitreous within pupil aperture
5. Block at the level of the ciliary body
   a. Plateau iris: large or anteriorly rotated ciliary processes
   b. Iris-ciliary body cysts
6. Block at the level of the lens
   a. Phacomorphic glaucoma (swollen lens)
7. Block at the level of the vitreous (malignant glaucoma)
   Components may include:
   a. Previous acute or chronic angle closure
   b. Anterior chamber shallowing
   c. Forward lens movement (zonules intact)
   d. Pupil block by lens or vitreous
   e. Zonular laxity
   f. Anterior rotation/swelling of ciliary body
   g. Expansion of vitreous
   h. Posterior aqueous misdirection into or behind vitreous
   i. Choroidal effusion
8. Combined mechanism: more than one level is affected; often posterior lesions also affect a preceding level
9. Low-tension glaucoma: abnormally flexible lamina cribrosa may deform even at a normal intraocular pressure
10. Idiopathic mechanisms

98% of the time. Uveitis and neoplasia were common causes of secondary glaucoma in retrospective referral center studies, but the most common form of glaucoma in cats 7 years of age or older in the prospective private practice population study was that secondary to misdirection of aqueous humor into the vitreous cavity.

Glaucoma may affect one or both eyes, with secondary glaucoma tending to be unilateral, whereas primary glaucoma is almost invariably bilateral. Most cats affected with glaucoma are older (with the obvious exception of the congenital forms) with an average age of 9.2 ± 4.4 years in one study (Blocker et al., 2001). Several breed predispositions exist. Primary "narrow-to-closed" angle glaucoma was reported in six female Burmese cats aged 7 to 10.5 years, but the classic primary angle-closure glaucoma commonly seen in dogs is very rare to nonexistent in cats. Congenital primary open-angle glaucoma has also been described in a family of Siamese cats. However, the vast majority of cats with glaucoma are domestic shorthairs and longhairs, and any breed of cat is at risk. With the exception of the Burmese report there appears to be no sex predisposition, although there is a trend for uveitis-associated secondary glaucoma to be more common in males since their lifestyle places them at greater risk of exposure to the infectious causes of uveitis (see Chapter 262).

WHAT IS NORMAL FELINE INTRAOCULAR PRESSURE?

Normal feline IOP varies with the time of day (several millimeters of mercury higher at night) and the cat's age. It is also not the same as a dog's normal IOP; values for normal IOP in young adult cats are 20.2 ± 5.5 mm Hg (mean $\pm$ SD). These are higher values than reported in young dogs (16.8 ± 4 mm Hg, Tono-Pen tonometer). A large study of 538 cats (1068 eyes) 7 years of age or older found a mean normal IOP of 12.3 ± 4 mm Hg (Fig. 263-1). Seventy-eight of these cats (154 eyes) were followed over time, and IOP decreased as much as 1.7 mm Hg/year in these cats. The reason for this is unclear, but it may be related to their declining metabolic health and a subsequent reduction in the active secretion of aqueous humor. Therefore normal feline IOP appears to vary with age such that young cats may have a normal upper limit as high as 31 mm Hg, whereas older cats normally do not exceed 21 mm Hg very frequently. Because IOP declines with age in cats, many old cats can have a very low IOP (≤ 7 mm Hg) in the absence of any signs of anterior uveitis.

CLINICAL SIGNS OF FELINE GLAUCOMA

The clinical signs of glaucoma in cats are more subtle than in dogs, at least initially. The acute, congestive form

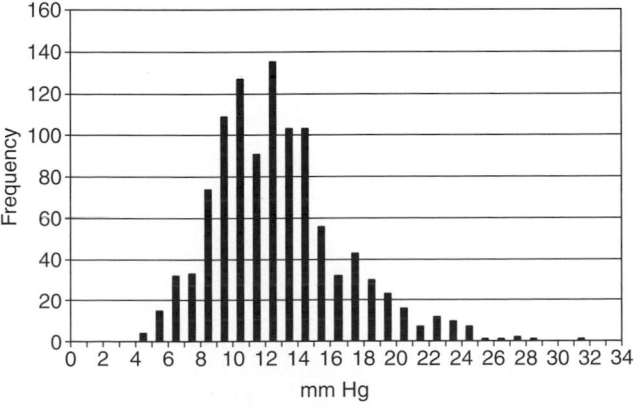

Fig. 263-1 Intraocular pressure (IOP) measurements from 1068 eyes (538 cats) 7 years or older who underwent IOP screening as part of a senior health care profile. (From Kroll MM, Miller, and Rodan: *J Am Vet Med Assoc* 219:1406, 2001.)

of glaucoma seen in dogs in which IOP rises above 50 to 60 mm Hg in a matter of hours is virtually nonexistent in cats. Instead feline glaucoma is often characterized by slow, insidious increases in IOP with minimal, if any, clinical signs until the disease is advanced. In many cats the only externally visible signs are mydriasis (and associated anisocoria), subtle corneal edema, or buphthalmia. Often clinical signs attributable to the primary inciting cause (e.g., uveitis, intraocular neoplasia) are more prominent than the signs attributable to the increased IOP itself. The overt ocular hyperemia and corneal edema that are common in dogs are usually not seen in cats until IOP is quite high. Unfortunately, by the time clinical signs become apparent, irreparable damage to the optic nerve usually has occurred, and 73% of cats with overt signs of glaucoma were blind at initial presentation to a referral center. In contrast, in a private practice setting in which cats 7 years of age or older were screened for glaucoma, a considerably higher percentage of cats retain vision, presumably related to earlier diagnosis. The subtle nature of glaucoma in cats suggests that IOP should be measured in every cat with intraocular disease, anisocoria, mydriasis, or corneal edema (see Chapter 248).

The hallmark of glaucomatous damage and the cause of irreversible vision loss is posterior bowing or "cupping" of the optic disc. As IOP increases, the pores in the sclera through which retinal ganglion cell axons pass (lamina cribrosa) become distorted. Although this distortion is initially quite small and difficult to appreciate clinically, it pinches the nerve fibers at the lamina, disrupting the normal axoplasmic flow of a variety of nutrients and neurotrophic growth factors. Loss of these factors, especially brain-derived neurotrophic growth factor (BDNF), perhaps coupled with impaired blood flow to the optic nerve, causes retinal ganglion cells to die. Clinically apparent optic disc cupping is the result of loss of retinal ganglion cell axons since these are the structures that comprise much of the optic disc. Dying ganglion cells also release excitotoxins such as glutamate, which can then induce adjacent, otherwise normal ganglion cells to undergo apoptosis; and a vicious cycle of cell death is initiated. Therefore, once increased IOP initiates retinal ganglion cell death, the process can become self-perpetuating and continue even if IOP returns to normal. However, this discouraging series of events does allow for the possibility of a variety of novel therapies for glaucoma that extend beyond lowering IOP. Although still experimental, retinal ganglion cell death can be prevented or reduced (in some cases even without reducing IOP) by treatment with a variety of neurotrophic factors, stress proteins, and antiapoptotic compounds.

In humans glaucoma is monitored not only by following IOP but also by carefully determining whether there is progression in the degree of optic disc cupping and measuring the extent of the patient's visual field. However, determining the amount or progression of optic disc cupping in cats is difficult because the normal feline optic disc typically lacks myelin and appears as a circular, dark grey structure that is depressed from the fundus surface. In addition, changes in the appearance of the disc tend to be slowly progressive if the IOP rise is mild to modest. Therefore, when a cat is first diagnosed with glaucoma, it is important to examine the optic disc in detail and to use high magnification on follow-up examinations to assess the depth of the cup and changes in the appearance of the laminar pores (normally visible as small, dark dots in the optic disc), as well as whether there are any changes in the reflectivity of the tissues around the optic disc. The normal feline optic disc may have a partial or complete hyperreflective ring (conus) or hyperpigmented ring around its perimeter. However, a change in these normal variations is very suggestive of ongoing glaucomatous damage. Methods for precisely measuring a cat's visual field as is done in humans do not yet exist, and qualitative assessment of a cat's visual abilities through maze testing or the presence of a menace response provides only a very coarse estimate of the adequacy of therapy.

SCREENING CATS FOR GLAUCOMA

The slow, insidious rise in IOP and relatively paucity of overt clinical signs until vision is substantially impaired in older cats suggests that glaucoma screening may have some value as part of a feline geriatric health profile. False negatives and false positives complicate glaucoma screening, but these can be reduced greatly by good technique (see Chapter 248), following up mild elevations with repeated measurements on another day (before instituting therapy), and performing an ophthalmic examination in conjunction with measuring IOP. Based on a study of 538 cats 7 years of age or older (1068 eyes) screened as part of a routine feline geriatric health profile, an IOP of 28 mm Hg or higher or a difference of 12 mm Hg or more between eyes was found to be highly suggestive of abnormally high IOP. However, only approximately 1% of cats 7 years or older have glaucoma, making screening for this disease a relatively low-yield procedure. Causes of abnormally high IOP in this population were presumed to be aqueous misdirection in four cats and a subluxated cataract in one cat (Kroll et al., 2001).

MEDICAL THERAPY FOR GLAUCOMA IN CATS

Pain relief is a key feature of glaucoma therapy in cats. Mild IOP increases typically are not painful, but increases to 40 mm Hg or greater typically cause humans to complain of headaches that may be of migraine intensity when IOP is higher than 60 mm Hg. Although many cats with glaucoma do not exhibit clinical signs that most owners would associate with pain, careful questioning typically reveals that the cat sleeps more, is less active, hides more, or eats less. Returning IOP into the normal range almost invariably causes the owner to comment that the cat "acts like a new cat," adding further evidence to the notion that cats with IOP above 40 mm Hg do have ocular pain. Lowering IOP is the most effective analgesic in these cats, although short-term use of a variety of systemic analgesics such as oxymorphone (0.05 to 0.1 mg/kg), buprenorphine (0.01 to 0.02 mg/kg), or meloxicam (0.3 mg/kg) may also be helpful.

Ideally medical therapy for glaucoma in cats would identify the exact cause and location(s) of the impediment(s) to aqueous humor outflow and circumvent those blocks. Because of the high frequency of secondary glaucoma in cats (especially uveitis-induced glaucoma), many cats with glaucoma can be controlled with medication alone. However, cats often respond very differently than do other species to many of the commercial antiglaucoma drugs, and no single drug is appropriate for all forms of glaucoma in cats. Five classes of antiglaucoma drugs are available: carbonic anhydrase inhibitors (CAIs), β-adrenergic blockers, β-adrenergic agonists, cholinergics, and prostaglandins (PGs) (Table 263-1).

Carbonic Anhydrase Inhibitors

Inhibition of the enzyme carbonic anhydrase lowers IOP by reducing the active production of aqueous humor. Systemic CAIs such as dichlorphenamide, methazolamide,

Table **263-1**

Common Antiglaucoma Drugs for Use in Cats*

Drug	Class	Route	Frequency	Mechanism
Dorzolamide 2%	Carbonic anhydrate inhibitor (CAI)	Topical	q8h	↓ Production
Brinzolamide 1%	CAI	Topical	q8h	↓ Production
Methazolamide	CAI	Oral	1-2 mg/kg q8-24h	↓ Production
Dichlorphenamide	CAI	Oral	1-2 mg/kg q8-24h	↓ Production
Timolol 0.5%	β-Blocker	Topical	q12h	↓ Production
Betaxolol 0.5%	β-Blocker	Topical	q12h	↓ Production
Epinephrine 1%-2%	β-Adrenergic agonist	Topical	q6-12h	↑ Outflow ↓ Production
Dipivefrin 0.1%	β-Adrenergic agonist	Topical	q6-12h	↑ Outflow ↓ Production
Pilocarpine 2%	Cholinergic	Topical	q6-12h	↓ Outflow
Demecarium bromide 0.125%	Cholinergic (organophosphate)	Topical	q12-24h	↓ Outflow

*Proposed mechanism for reduction of intraocular pressure and suggested feline dosages are indicated. Safety of these compounds is not well studied in cats, and frequency of therapy indicated in this table may not be appropriate for all cats with glaucoma. The commercially available prostaglandin derivatives are ineffective in cats.

and acetazolamide have been used for decades; but their value is limited by their systemic toxicity, which includes metabolic acidosis, panting, hypokalemia, gastrointestinal upset, changes in mentation, and blood dyscrasias. Recently topical CAIs such as 2% dorzolamide (Trusopt, Merck), 2% dorzolamide plus 0.5% timolol (Cosopt, Merck), and 1% brinzolamide (Azopt, Alcon) have become available commercially. These compounds have largely supplanted the systemic CAIs in humans and animals. The main advantage of brinzolamide is that it may be less irritating than dorzolamide. Because almost total inhibition of the enzyme is necessary to lower aqueous humor production, topical CAIs probably need to be administered every 8 hours to be effective. There is little published work with these compounds in cats, but 1% brinzolamide every 12 hours did not lower IOP significantly in normal cats, perhaps because of inadequate dosing frequency. However, dorzolamide 2% every 8 hours markedly lowered IOP in Siamese cats with primary open-angle glaucoma and in cats with feline aqueous humor misdirection syndrome (FAHMS). Drugs in this class are additive to all other antiglaucoma drugs and do not exacerbate anterior uveitis.

β-Adrenergic Blockers

Drugs such as 0.25% to 0.5% timolol maleate (a nonspecific β_1-, β_2- adrenergic antagonist) and 0.5% betaxolol HCL (a cardioselective β_1-adrenergic antagonist) appear to work by reducing aqueous humor production in cats. However, a certain level of adrenergic tone is required for them to be effective; and they do not lower IOP during sleep, which can be problematic given the amount of time cats spend sleeping. Topical nonsteroidal antiinflammatory drugs (NSAIDs) are also experimentally capable of preventing timolol from lowering IOP in cats, suggesting that PGs may also play a role in the mechanism of action of these drugs in cats. Nevertheless, a single topical application of 0.5% timolol maleate reduced IOP 22.3% in the treated eye and 16.3% in the nontreated eye in normal cats. For reasons that are not entirely clear, timolol causes miosis in cats. Topical timolol may also cause bradycardia and worsening of asthma in cats. Although recent work suggests that β_2-receptors are the most prevalent in the cat's anterior segment, betaxolol (which blocks β_1- receptors) may still be of benefit to cats with glaucoma even if it does not lower IOP. Recent work has shown that topically applied betaxolol can reach the retina and optic nerve and that experimentally it improves retinal blood flow and electrical responsiveness in cats with elevated IOP. Because β-adrenergic blockers do not exacerbate uveitis, they are good choices for treating cats with uveitis-induced glaucoma as long as they are not used concurrently with NSAIDs. Drugs in this class are also additive to all classes of antiglaucoma drugs, with the possible exception of the β-adrenergic agonists.

β-Adrenergic Agonists

Drugs such as 1% to 2% epinephrine or its prodrug 0.1% dipivefrin appear to lower IOP in cats by increasing conventional outflow and perhaps by decreasing aqueous humor production. Topical 2% epinephrine HCL every 12 hours for 1 week lowered IOP 27% in normal cats. Drugs in this class may be irritating because they vasoconstrict the ocular surface. Their efficacy tends to decrease with time, and their effect can be partially blocked by topical NSAIDs. They are additive to cholinergics and carbonic anhydrase inhibitors but poorly additive to β-adrenergic blockers. Because they do not exacerbate uveitis and may induce mild pupillary dilation, drugs in this group are good choices for treating cats with uveitis-induced glaucoma. The commercially available α_2-agonist apraclonidine 0.5% (Iopidine, Alcon) is unacceptably toxic to cats.

Cholinergics

Drugs such as 2% pilocarpine (which mimics acetylcholine) or 0.125% demecarium bromide (which inhibits acetylcholinesterase) lower IOP in cats by improving conventional outflow. One application of 2% pilocarpine in normal cats lowered IOP 15.2% in the treated eye and 9.3% in the nontreated eye and reduced pupil diameter 28.5% in the treated eye and 14.2% in the nontreated eye. Like the β-adrenergic agonists, drugs in this class tend to lose efficacy with time, and side effects include ocular irritation. Cholinergics should be used cautiously in uveitis-induced glaucoma because they can exacerbate uveitis and the miosis they create may increase the risk of iris bombé. They are additive to drugs in every other class, although demecarium bromide may inhibit corneal esterases that convert dipivefrin to its active form.

Prostaglandin Derivatives

The IOP-lowering effect of the PG derivatives is highly dependent on subtle variations in the molecule, its concentration, and the species tested. They probably lower IOP by increasing uveoscleral outflow and perhaps by reducing aqueous humor production. Unfortunately in multiple studies the commercially available $PGF_2\alpha$ derivatives such as latanoprost 0.005% (Xalatan, Pfizer), bimatoprost 0.03% (Lumigan, Allergan), unoprostone 0.12% (Rescula, Novartis), and travoprost 0.004% (Travatan, Alcon) do not lower IOP in cats, although they do induce a marked miosis. Although the commercially available PGs are disappointing in cats, this class of drug is promising because experimentally certain PGE_2 and PGA_2 derivatives were well tolerated and highly effective in cats but were discontinued because of lack of efficacy or unacceptable side effects in monkeys or humans.

DRUGS THAT MAY INCREASE INTRAOCULAR PRESSURE IN CATS

Topical 10% phenylephrine (an α_1-adrenergic agonist) that is sometimes used as a mydriatic in cats can inhibit aqueous humor outflow by 67%, which may increase IOP in cats. Another topical mydriatic, tropicamide (an anticholinergic), can markedly increase IOP in both the treated and untreated eye of normal cats (a mean of 3.5 mm Hg, but up to 17 to 18 mm Hg in select individuals) and in cats with primary open-angle glaucoma, even though it dilates the pupil in only the treated eye. Topical

0.1% dexamethasone or 1% prednisolone acetate two to three times a day caused a 4.5–mm Hg gradual increase in IOP in normal cats beginning within 5 to 7 days and reaching peak values within 2 to 3 weeks. IOP returned to baseline values in 6 to 7 days with cessation of therapy. Therefore, when treating cats with uveitis-induced glaucoma, the clinician must weigh the potential increase in IOP caused by use of certain mydriatics or corticosteroids against the potential decreases in IOP caused by the prevention of iris bombé and the reduction of the inflammatory debris from the outflow pathways.

SURGICAL THERAPY FOR FELINE GLAUCOMA

Cats may be less amenable to some of the antiglaucoma surgical procedures than dogs. Often the best results are achieved if the cause of the glaucoma can be addressed directly (e.g., removing a luxated lens that is blocking the pupil, disrupting ciliary cysts that are pushing the peripheral iris into the drainage angle, or breaking down posterior synechia that are creating iris bombé). Placement of an artificial tube (gonio-implant) from the anterior chamber into the subconjunctival space may allow the clinician to bypass an obstructed or closed iridocorneal angle, but frequently these devices do not remain patent in the long-term. If the impediment to aqueous humor outflow cannot be addressed directly, IOP may be lowered by destroying a portion of the ciliary body either by freezing (cyclocryosurgery) or by use of a diode or neodymium:yttrium-aluminum-garnet (Nd:YAG) laser (cyclophotocoagulation). Protocols for treating glaucomatous cats are not well established, but experimentally a 30% reduction in IOP could be achieved in normal cats by transsclerally freezing 12 spots for 1 minute to −80 C or by 80 noncontact Nd:YAG laser applications over 360 degrees 3 mm posterior to the limbus, with a maximum power of 7 to 9 joules and a maximum retrofocus of 3.6 mm. Often IOP tends to creep back up after a cyclodestructive procedure has been performed, necessitating that it be repeated. Cyclodestructive procedures incite considerable uveitis and are probably best reserved for cats with primary glaucoma or nonneoplastic glaucomas when another procedure cannot correct the problem (e.g., removal of a luxated lens). Intravitreous injection of gentamicin to destroy the ciliary body chemically is probably contraindicated in cats because of anecdotal reports of intraocular tumors after this procedure.

If the eye is irreversibly blind and painful, evisceration and placement of an intrascleral prosthesis or enucleation may be considered. Although evisceration and insertion of an intrascleral prosthesis is technically feasible in cats, the cosmetic results achieved with dark-colored spheres are often less successful than in dogs. This has led some to use colored spheres and to tattoo a slit pupil onto the cornea in an effort to improve the final postoperative cosmetic appearance of the eye. Cats tolerate enucleation well, and a silicone sphere may be implanted into the orbit before skin closure to minimize the degree of "sinking in" that typically occurs following removal of the globe. The suggested rejection rate of these spheres in cats, however, may exceed that in dogs.

THERAPY FOR SPECIFIC FORMS OF GLAUCOMA IN CATS

Primary Glaucomas

Primary open-angle glaucoma tends to be congenital in cats and difficult to control medically for very long. In the early stages topical CAIs alone or in combination with a topical β-adrenergic blocker can be used. The addition of a β-adrenergic agonist may also afford an additional reduction in IOP of a few millimeters of mercury. However, surgical therapy usually becomes necessary. A cyclodestructive procedure with or without a gonio-implant may allow vision to be maintained for some time in some of these cats. Fortunately acute primary-angle closure glaucoma is rare in cats. Although there are no data to support any treatment regimen in these patients, it is likely that a cyclodestructive procedure with or without a gonio-implant would be required early in the course of the disease to preserve vision.

Uveitis-Induced Glaucoma

Cats with normal IOP in the face of uveitis are at high risk for developing glaucoma because aqueous humor production (and IOP) is normally low in uveitis. Therefore normal IOP means that the outflow pathways are impaired and that IOP may spike upward as the uveitis is controlled. Uveitis that is severe enough to result in glaucoma merits thorough diagnostic investigation for a potential systemic cause unless the cause is obvious (see Chapter 262). If the eye has vision or the potential for vision, rapid and aggressive antiinflammatory therapy with topical corticosteroids (0.1% dexamethasone or 1% prednisolone acetate q4h) is usually indicated if the cornea is not ulcerated. If not contraindicated, antiinflammatory-to-immunosuppressive doses of systemic corticosteroids should also be considered. Topical CAIs, β-adrenergic blockers, or β-adrenergic agonists are reasonable first choices since they do not exacerbate uveitis. In general, atropine or tropicamide is not used unless the impediment to outflow is caused by posterior synechia and it is believed that breaking these down and reestablishing normal flow of aqueous humor through the pupil is possible. Antiglaucoma drugs are tapered slowly as the uveitis resolves and IOP normalizes, although severe cases may require long-term therapy to preserve vision. Enucleation or evisceration with placement of an intrascleral prosthesis (and histopathologic examination of the excised tissue) is reasonable if the eye is irreversibly blind and painful. In general, the prognosis for vision in cats with uveitis-induced glaucoma is guarded.

Neoplasia-Associated Glaucoma

In the majority of patients with glaucoma secondary to intraocular neoplasia, the only viable options are to stage the tumor and then perform enucleation, or if appropriate, systemic chemotherapy. Enucleation, even if only palliative, alleviates ocular pain and may substantially improve the cat's overall quality of life. In some cats with secondary glaucoma caused by intraocular lymphosarcoma, IOP may normalize with a combination of systemic chemotherapy, aggressive use of topical corticosteroids (0.1% dexamethasone or 1% prednisolone acetate four to six times daily), and a topical CAI or a β-adrenergic blocker. If the tumor is confined to the eye, drugs that increase outflow via the traditional pathway (e.g., cholinergics and β-adrenergic agonists) probably should be used cautiously since they may facilitate neoplastic cells leaving the globe.

Glaucoma Secondary to Anterior Lens Luxation

The relationship between glaucoma, lens luxation, and uveitis in cats is often complicated; and any one of these three disorders may be primary and result in the other two disorders. Often it is difficult, if not impossible, to determine the exact sequence of events, especially in patients seen for the first time in the late stages of the disease; but ideally the temporal relationship between these three disorders would be established in each patient since therapy tends to be different in each scenario. If the eye is irreversibly blind, enucleation or evisceration with placement of an intrascleral prosthesis (and histopathologic examination of the excised tissue) is probably the best therapy. If the eye has the potential for vision, removal of the lens should be considered if it is in the anterior chamber, although glaucoma may persist after surgery if the drainage angle is also impaired. In addition, diagnostic investigation of potential systemic causes of anterior uveitis should be considered if the cause of the uveitis is not readily apparent. If the lens is in the posterior chamber or vitreous, it may be possible to trap it there with a strong miotic such as the organophosphate demecarium bromide (0.125% q12–24 h). However, this drug can exacerbate uveitis, and often it does not control the pupil well enough to prevent the lens from entering the anterior chamber and subsequently increasing IOP.

Glaucoma Associated With Hyphema

This form of glaucoma is relatively uncommon in cats and is most frequently associated with massive intraocular hemorrhage caused by systemic hypertension, lymphosarcoma, severe ocular trauma, and rarely blood dyscrasias. Therapy is somewhat controversial but is directed toward identifying the underlying cause of the bleeding and treating that directly. Topical antiglaucoma drugs that do not exacerbate uveitis (CAIs, β-adrenergic agonists) and topical corticosteroids (0.1% dexamethasone or 1% prednisolone acetate) are good first choices. Topical β-adrenergic blockers may also be used, although the miosis these drugs induce may increase the chance of iris bombé. Atropine and tropicamide should be used with caution if glaucoma is present. Persistent or recurrent intraocular bleeding warrants systemic diagnostic testing and ultrasonographic evaluation of the eye to rule out an underlying cause such as retinal detachment, hypertension, coagulopathies, or intraocular tumor. Surgical evacuation of blood from the anterior chamber is usually of very limited value.

FELINE AQUEOUS HUMOR MISDIRECTION SYNDROME

This recently described entity affects up to 1% of cats 7 years of age or older and may be the most common form of feline glaucoma in a general private practice setting. Most cats are older (mean age 11.7 years, range 4 to 16 years), and females are predisposed. The hallmark of FAHMS is a uniformly shallow anterior chamber without trembling of the iris/lens or other evidence of lens luxation. The most common presenting clinical signs include anisocoria, bilateral mydriasis, a shallow anterior chamber, incipient cataracts, or impaired vision in one or both eyes (Figs. 263-2 and 263-3). There is no apparent pain unless IOP is significantly elevated, and many owners do not appreciate that anything is wrong until the disease is advanced. Initial IOP varies with the degree of anterior chamber shallowing, and in one case series it was 20 mm Hg or higher in 32/40 eyes, with a range of 12 to 58 mm Hg. Increases in IOP tend to be slow and insidious, and not all affected cats have glaucoma at initial presentation.

The underlying pathophysiology appears to be the misdirection of aqueous humor through presumed microscopic breaks in the membrane forming the anterior face of the vitreous. Blinking may increase IOP in the anterior chamber transiently, and this may be transferred to the posterior chamber and force aqueous humor posteriorly through a small tear in the vitreous face. The tear acts like a one-way valve, allowing aqueous humor to enter but not leave the vitreous. Aqueous may accumulate in a variety of locations within the vitreous (Fig. 263-4) and ultimately displaces the vitreous face anteriorly. This is the first block to aqueous humor leaving the eye. A cascading series of additional impediments to outflow may then occur as (1) the vitreous face is forced between the anterior ciliary body and lens; (2) the lens is pushed anteriorly into greater contact with the posterior surface of the iris; (3) the lens:iris diaphragm moves forward, closing the iridocorneal angle; and (4) the ciliary cleft closes. It is easy to understand why advanced stages of this disorder are difficult to treat effectively.

If the eye has vision and the IOP elevation is relatively mild, there is a reasonable chance that IOP may

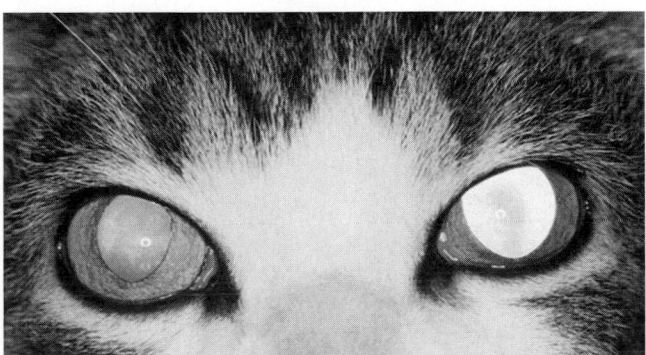

Fig. 263-2 Clinical appearance of a cat with overt feline aqueous humor misdirection syndrome (FAHMS) in the left eye and suspected early FAHMS in the right eye. Both pupils are relatively dilated, but there is anisocoria, with the left pupil larger than the right. (From Czederpiltz JMC et al: *J Am Vet Med Assoc* 227:1476, 2005.)

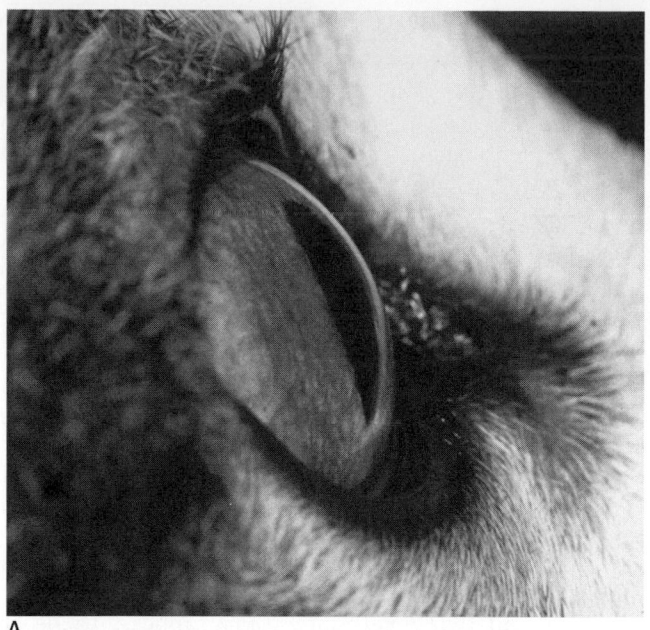

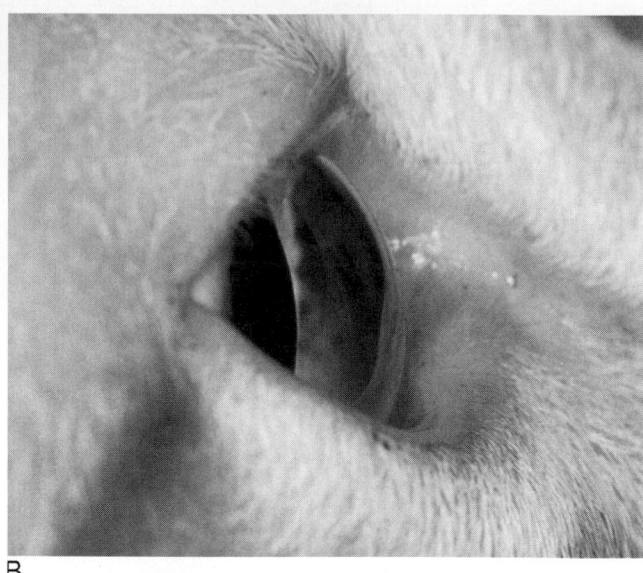

Fig. 263-3   Lateral view of a FAHMS-affected cat **(A)** and normal cat **(B)**. Note the extremely shallow anterior chamber in the FAHMS-affected eye. (From Czederpiltz JMC et al: *J Am Vet Med Assoc* 227:1476, 2005.)

be controlled with a topical CAI for the remainder of the cat's life. Cats that lose vision tend to have very advanced disease at initial presentation or have rapidly progressive disease. Other antiglaucoma drugs besides topical CAIs may also be effective, but miosis can increase the block at the iris:lens interface and rapidly increase IOP to very high levels. If medical therapy is ineffective, anterior vitrectomy and lensectomy may reestablish a more normal outflow pathway, provided more anterior blocks at the iridocorneal angle or ciliary cleft have not occurred.

Suggested Reading

Bhattacherjee P et al: Pharmacological validation of a feline model of steroid-induced ocular hypertension, *Arch Ophthalmol* 117:361, 1999.

Blocker T, Van Der Woerdt A: The feline glaucomas: 82 cases (1995-1999), *Vet Ophthalmol* 4:81, 2001.

Czederpiltz JMC et al: Putative aqueous humor misdirection syndrome as a cause of glaucoma in cats: 32 cases, *J Am Vet Med Assoc* 227:1476, 2005.

Hampson EC, Smith RI, Bernays ME: Primary glaucoma in Burmese cats, *Aust Vet J* 80:672, 2002.

Kroll MM, Miller PE, Rodan R: Intraocular pressure measurements obtained as part of a comprehensive geriatric health examination from cats seven years of age or older, *J Am Vet Med Assoc* 219:1406, 2001.

Miller PE, Picket JP: Comparison of the human and canine Schiøtz tonometry conversion tables in clinically normal cats, *J Am Vet Med Assoc* 201:1017, 1992.

Robertson SA, Taylor PM: Pain management in cats—past, present and future. Part 2: Treatment of pain—clinical pharmacology, *J Feline Med Surg* 6:321, 2004.

Rosenberg LF: Cyclocryotherapy and noncontact Nd:YAG laser cyclophotocoagulation in cats, *Invest Ophthalmol Vis Sci* 37:2029, 1996.

Stadtbaumer K, Kostlin RG, Zahn KJ: Effects of topical 0.5% tropicamide on intraocular pressure in normal cats, *Vet Ophthalmol* 5:107, 2002.

Studer ME, Martin CL, Stiles J: Effects of 0.005% latanoprost solution on intraocular pressure in healthy dogs and cats, *Am J Vet Res* 61:1220, 2000.

Wilcock BP, Peiffer RL, Davidson MG: The causes of glaucoma in cats, *Vet Pathol* 27:35, 1990.

Wilkie DA, Latimer CA: Effects of topical administration of timolol maleate on intraocular pressure and pupil size in cats, *Am J Vet Res* 52:436, 1991.

Fig. 263-4   Proposed concept of ciliovitreolenticular block demonstrating the potential locations where misdirected aqueous humor may collect in the vitreous cavity, including: **(A)** in the anterior peripheral vitreous, **(B)** as lacunae in the central vitreous, **(C)** diffusely throughout the vitreous, and **(D)** between the posterior vitreous and retina. All cause forward displacement of the anterior vitreous face. (From Czederpiltz JMC et al: *J Am Vet Med Assoc* 227:1476, 2005.)

CHAPTER 264

Retinal Detachment

PATRICIA J. SMITH, *Fremont, California*

PATHOGENESIS

A retinal detachment (RD) is a separation of the neurosensory retina from the retinal pigment epithelium (RPE). In the normal eye the vitreous, retina, and lens are connected by various physical and chemical mechanisms. RDs may be caused by at least one of three main mechanisms: exudation (nonrhegmatogenous), associated with retinal tears (rhegmatogenous), or traction pulling on the retina. Complicated RDs are those that involve more than one of the main mechanisms (e.g., a retinal tear or hole that results from a vitreous traction band).

In small animals most RDs are exudative. The subretinal fluid is usually inflammatory but can be serous with diseases such as systemic hypertension or (see Chapters 159 and 197). The subretinal fluid typically results from breakdown of the blood-ocular barrier in the retinal and choroidal vasculature. Because the choroidal vascular bed is much larger than the retinal vascular supply, a large amount of subretinal fluid usually indicates diffuse choroidal involvement; as seen with diseases such as chorioretinitis, systemic hypertension, or hyperviscosity. Initially areas of chorioretinitis appear as variably sized focal or multifocal areas of retinal elevation with indistinct borders. These active areas of chorioretinitis alter the course of the overlying retinal blood vessels and obscure or blur the ophthalmoscopic view of the underlying RPE or tapetum as shown in Fig. 264-1. (For a discussion of the cause of RDs from posterior uveitis, see Chapter 262.)

Rhegmatogenous RD is associated with formation of one or more retinal tears or holes. This type of RD is less common than exudative RD in small animals and occurs more commonly in dogs than in cats. The pathogenesis of rhegmatogenous RD involves the presence of an abnormal retina (i.e., thinned as a result of degeneration, age, or other diseases), which is predisposed to formation of tears or holes, combined with an abnormal vitreous as with vitreous syneresis (liquefaction), traction, or detachment. The vitreous gel is a homogeneous collagen fibril network with hyaluronic acid molecules filling the interfibrillar space. The vitreous is more firmly attached in three locations: the peripheral posterior lens capsule, the vitreous base that overlies the peripheral edge of the retina (the pars plana and ora ciliaris retina), and the margin of the optic nerve. Since the vitreous hydrogel is attached to the lens and retina, perturbations of the vitreous (e.g., inflammation, surgery) or lens can contribute to the development of rhegmatogenous RD by creating retinal traction, which can lead to tear or hole formation. Liquid from the vitreous then moves through the hole or tear into the subretinal space and exacerbates the RD.

ETIOLOGY

Despite the multiple causes of RD, consideration of the type of RD (exudative, traction, or rhegmatogenous), the nature of any subretinal fluid, and whether the detachments are unilateral or bilateral assist with differentiating or prioritizing the likely causes. Although bilateral RD is strongly suggestive of systemic disease or congenital ocular disease, unilateral detachment should not cause these considerations to be disregarded. Serous subretinal fluid with or without hemorrhage is more common with hypertension, hyperviscosity syndromes, and rickettsial disease. When subretinal fluid is opaque as a result of marked cellular infiltrate, causes of exudative disease such as lymphosarcoma, idiopathic inflammatory, uveodermatologic syndrome, and fungal infections should be considered more likely.

Trauma

Penetrating injuries (e.g., dog bites, projectiles) or foreign bodies may result in retinal tears or induce intraocular hemorrhage, inflammation, or vitreous infection with subsequent traction RD. Severe blunt trauma with inflammation and hemorrhage may also cause RD, which may be exudative or rhegmatogenous in nature. However, it is extremely unlikely for a traumatic incident to cause RD in both eyes. The exception is strangulation, which can lead to bilateral exudative (hemorrhagic) RD.

Ocular Anomalies

RD may be associated with severe retinal dysplasia, optic nerve colobomas, vitreous abnormalities, and retinal nonattachment (i.e., developmental failure of the two retinal layers to unite). Animals with RD present at or soon after birth, often having concurrent abnormalities such as microphthalmia or cataracts. Detachment may be unilateral or bilateral.

Later onset genetic anomalies such as cataracts or vitreous degeneration may lead to RD. Rhegmatogenous RD also may occur as a result of vitreous liquefaction or cataract formation, particularly with rapidly forming or hypermature cataracts or when there is lens-induced uveitis. Rhegmatogenous RD may occur as a sequela to cataract surgery (reported incidence 1% to 4%) or lens luxation or subluxation. When an RD is evident but without a history of trauma, cataracts, or lens surgery, a thorough diagnostic workup is indicated to identify predisposing systemic diseases.

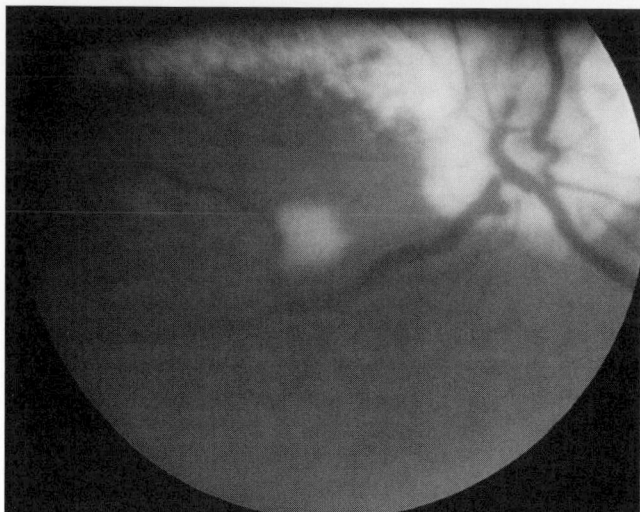

Fig. 264-1 Chorioretinitis in a dog caused by blastomycosis. Small areas of active chorioretinitis are associated with focal, low retinal detachments.

Hypertension/Hyperviscosity

Systemic hypertension (most often related to renal diseases) and hyperviscosity syndromes (caused by severe hyperlipidemia, hyperglobulinemia, or polycythemia) are relatively frequent causes of RD. These diseases typically damage the vasculature of the choroid and retina, creating hemorrhage in the retina and sometimes in the vitreous. Renal failure with secondary hypertension is probably one of the most common causes of bilateral RD in older cats. Hyperthyroidism and pheochromocytoma also should be considered as causes of hypertension, which can lead to bilateral RD.

Neoplasia

The most common neoplastic causes of RD are multiple myeloma (in which hyperproteinemia and hyperviscosity damage retinal and choroidal vasculature) and lymphosarcoma (which may diffusely infiltrate the retina or choroid). Patients with lymphosarcoma also may present with retinal hemorrhage with or without detachment and anterior uveitis. Each of these neoplasms is likely to affect both eyes. Large neoplastic masses (e.g., ciliary body iridal tumors) or metastatic lesions may induce traction RDs. If neoplastic tissue is subretinal or choroidal, exudative RD is more likely to be unilateral.

Chorioretinitis/Retinochoroiditis

Retinochoroiditis is used to imply that retinal tissue was inflamed primarily with secondary choroidal inflammation, whereas the inverse is true for the term *chorioretinitis*. Retinitis or chorioretinitis may cause focal or multifocal RDs. As discussed previously, small areas of inflammation are technically RDs, but this type of lesion is best termed *chorioretinitis* (see Chapter 262). When choroidal inflammation is severe and diffuse, large segmental or complete RDs may occur. In the dog chorioretinitis with RD may be caused by bacteremia or septicemia (e.g., leptospirosis, brucellosis, bartonellosis), rickettsial agents (ehrlichiosis,

Rocky Mountain spotted fever agent), fungal organisms (aspergillosis, blastomycosis, coccidioidomycosis, histoplasmosis, cryptococcosis), algae (geotrichosis, prototheccosis), and rarely today canine distemper virus. Parasitic inflammation of the choroid and retina is more likely to cause smaller areas of detachments (i.e., multifocal chorioretinitis). Causes include ocular larval migrans (from strongyles, ascarid, *Baylisascaris* larvae), toxoplasmosis, leishmaniasis, neospora, and possibly *Babesia*. In cats infection with feline leukemia and/or immunodeficiency viruses may indirectly cause chorioretinitis-related development of lymphosarcoma or an opportunistic infection such as toxoplasmosis. Feline infectious peritonitis virus is a more common cause of small-to-large areas of chorioretinitis and possibly RD As in dogs, any systemic bacterial, parasitic, or fungal infection can cause areas of chorioretinitis or diffuse RD.

Immune-Mediated Disease

Immune-mediated disease can cause vasculitis with or without choroidal inflammation; this can lead to exudative RD or chorioretinitis. In dogs systemic lupus erythematous and uveodermatologic syndrome may result in exudative detachment. Uveodermatologic syndrome is an autoimmune disease directed against melanin. The uvea of pigmented eyes is targeted, resulting in severe anterior and posterior uveitis and RDs. Pigmented cells in the skin are also injured such that affected animals can have mucocutaneous (and later diffuse) dermatitis with eventual depigmentation. I see uveodermatologic syndrome more commonly in arctic breeds such as Akitas, Siberian huskies, and chow-chows, but it also has been reported in other breeds. Granulomatous meningoencephalitis may also cause RD, usually in the peripapillary region and in association with optic neuritis and other signs of central nervous system disease. Idiopathic RD is diagnosed after thorough investigation rules out all other etiologies and the ophthalmic history and examination rule out retinal tears. I diagnose this type of detachment in dogs (especially giant breeds) but rarely in cats. Idiosyncratic reactions to drugs (i.e., trimethoprim-sulfa in dogs, griseofulvin in cats) and ethylene glycol toxicity in dogs may induce RD and multifocal chorioretinitis. There have been isolated reports of retinal diseases in cats from periarteritis nodosa and systemic lupus erythematosus.

DIAGNOSIS

A thorough history should determine if any of the following might be relevant: trauma, swimming in ponds (*Prototheca*), feeding of raw fish (salmon poisoning) or mammalian carcasses (*Salmonella*, parasites), exposure to ticks, or travel history to areas endemic for some of the aforementioned infectious diseases. A complete general physical examination should be undertaken. A thorough ophthalmic examination should be conducted with special attention to intraocular pressure, pupillary light reflexes and menace responses, aqueous flare, lens changes, and indirect and direct ophthalmoscopy of the retina. A systematic approach enables the clinician to diagnose chorioretinitis, RD, and possibly panuveitis if anterior uveitis is present (see Chapter 248).

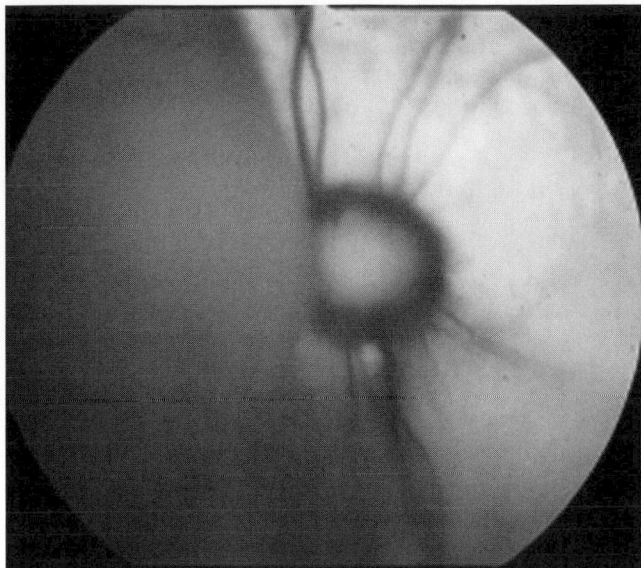

Fig. 264-2 Serous retinal detachment in a cat with hypertensive retinopathy. On fundic examination areas of retinal detachment may be elevated to different degrees. The examiner should note that vessels and the optic nerve are in different planes of focus. The subretinal fluid is transudative (more translucent) in this cat; thus the tapetal color is still visible. Serous retinal fluid is also commonly seen with vasculitis and immune-mediated retinal detachments.

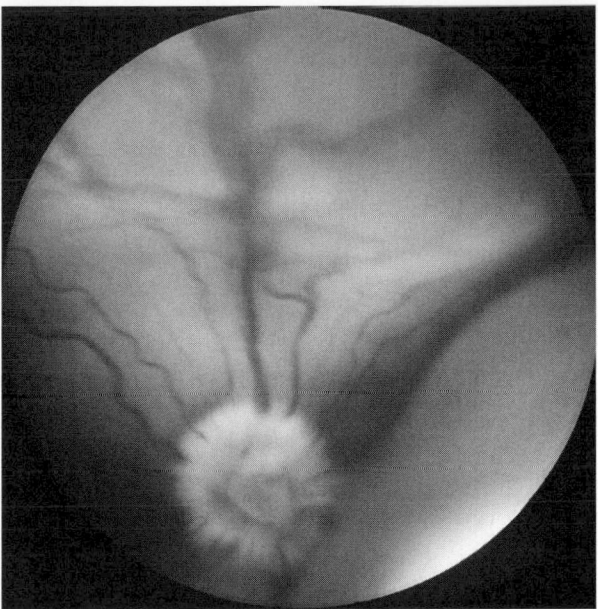

Fig. 264-3 Exudative retinal detachment in a dog. This type of subretinal fluid is more commonly seen with infectious or neoplastic diseases. The exudative fluid obscures view of the normal tapetal and nontapetal colors. This type of subretinal fluid is more detrimental to retinal health than is serous fluid. Even if the etiology is identified and treated, the retina often degenerates quickly so that visual recovery is unlikely even if reattachment occurs.

When a large RD is present, the pupillary light reflex is absent or reduced in the affected eye. With retinal elevation the retinal blood vessels are in focus at a different plane than the optic nerve. If the retina is markedly elevated, a membrane with blood vessels may be visible through the pupil during anterior segment examination. With serous subretinal fluid the underlying RPE, or in subalbinotic animals the choroidal vasculature, is not clearly visualized in the nontapetal region; and a similar dulling of the tapetal region occurs (Fig. 264-2). With severe exudation, a turbid subretinal fluid obscures the view of the normal tapetum and nontapetum (Fig. 264-3). Rhegmatogenous RD may reveal a visible retinal tear or break (Fig. 264-4). If opacification of the cornea, aqueous, lens, or vitreous caused by anterior uveitis or cataract prevents visualization of the retina, ocular ultrasonography can be used to diagnose RD.

If systemic disease is suspected, a complete blood count, serum biochemistry panel, and urinalysis are important initial tests. The results of these tests may point toward an etiology and direct additional tests. For example, if an animal with RD has marked hyperglobulinemia, protein electrophoresis, radiographs of the limbs and spine, and documentation of Bence-Jones proteinuria should be performed, which might lead to a diagnosis of multiple myeloma. Serologic, enzyme-linked immunosorbent assay or polymerase chain reaction–based tests for infective agents may be useful in some cases. Cats should be evaluated for feline immunodeficiency virus and feline leukemia virus infection. Blood pressure should be measured in cases of serous RDs with or without hemorrhage, especially if renal disease or hyperthyroidism is evident.

Repeated blood pressure measurements should be performed if initial blood pressure is normal but hypertension is still suspected, especially in cases of bilateral disease. Additional tests that might be pursued include coagulation profile and cultures and cytology of ocular or body fluids. A dog with panuveitis and mucocutaneous lesions (especially

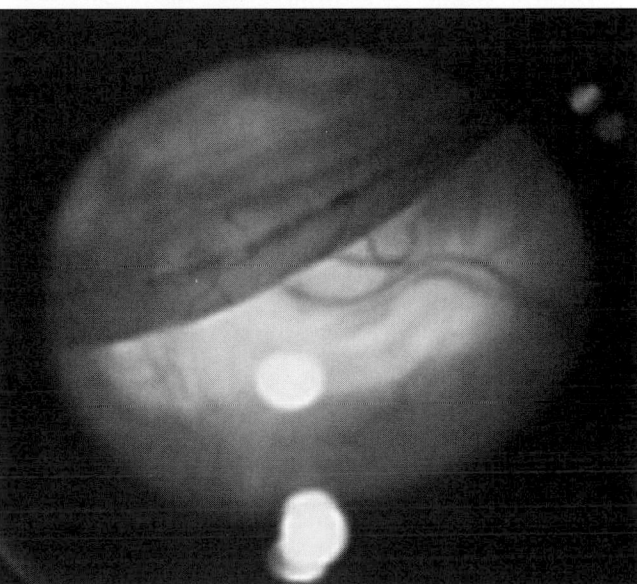

Fig. 264- 4 Rhegmatogenous retinal detachment in a dog that had previously undergone cataract surgery. The edge of the torn retina can be visualized through the pupil in this case. This type of retinal detachment should be treated surgically.

if depigmentation is prevalent) should have the skin lesions biopsied, especially of susceptible breeds (Akita, chow-chow, Samoyed). An antinuclear antibody test may be performed if lupus erythematosus is suspected.

Thoracic radiography is a useful screening test to search for lymphadenopathy, metastatic disease, or infiltrates consistent with infectious agents. Cardiac ultrasound may be indicated in cats with hypertensive retinopathy. Abdominal ultrasound also can add information that may help with the diagnosis if it reveals abnormalities in the organs or peritoneal space such as adrenal masses or lymphadenopathy. Abdominal radiographs may be useful; but abdominal ultrasound is superior for evaluation of the kidneys, adrenal glands, and other organs.

Analysis of cerebrospinal fluid is indicated if signs of central nervous system disease or optic neuritis are present. Vitreocentesis or subretinal fluid aspiration can be performed if other diagnostic tests have failed to yield an etiologic agent and an infectious agent or neoplastic disease is suspected. However, vitreocentesis can aggravate intraocular inflammation or induce vitreous hemorrhage, decreasing the chance of retinal reattachment and restoration of vision. Thus the pros and cons of this procedure should be discussed with the owner. If an eye is irreversibly blind and painful, enucleation with subsequent histopathologic examination may yield a diagnosis.

TREATMENT

Exudative Retinal Detachment

Exudative RD is treated medically by identifying and treating the underlying cause. This may include antimicrobial therapy for bacterial or antifungals for fungal-related infections. In deep organ or bone infection or when abscesses are present, surgical intervention may also be indicated. If systemic hypertension is the cause of an RD, appropriate antihypertensive therapy should be used. Amlodipine is generally the most effective drug for treatment of severe hypertension in cats and dogs (see Chapters 159 and 197). If neoplastic disease is amenable to chemotherapy, it should be treated appropriately.

Resolution of the underlying cause of RD sometimes leads to spontaneous retinal reattachment, especially if the fluid is relatively serous. However, if an inflammatory cause is diagnosed or there is severe chorioretinal inflammation (with a cellular subretinal fluid), it may be necessary to use systemic corticosteroid treatment in conjunction with treatment of the primary disease. The longer a retina is detached and the more turbid the subretinal fluid, the faster the retina degenerates, with consequences of irreversible blindness or vision loss. Systemic steroid use can hasten reattachment; however, it is extremely important to eliminate or concurrently treat diseases such as a systemic mycosis since infections may be exacerbated by systemic steroid administration. If the patient appears to be irreversibly blind and especially if secondary glaucoma is present, enucleation or evisceration may be the best course to minimize systemic steroid use until the definitive cause is determined.

Systemic corticosteroids are the treatment of choice for idiopathic or immune-mediated exudative RD such as that caused by uveodermatologic syndrome. I prescribe prednisone (1.1mg/kg orally [PO] q12h for 3 to 7 days); then, if the retina is beginning to reattach, I begin tapering the dose slowly while watching for signs of recurrent inflammation or detachment. If corticosteroid treatment does not rapidly improve the RD, adjunctive immunosuppressive agents such as azathioprine or cyclosporine may be added to the treatment regimen. Side effects such as bone marrow suppression, hepatopathy, and renal toxicity should be monitored closely when these drugs are used. In cases of hypertensive retinopathy I rarely use systemic corticosteroids unless there is a severe uveitis or vitritis secondary to intraocular hemorrhage. These can be difficult cases to manage, and referral to an ophthalmologist should be strongly considered for diagnosis and treatment of any vision-threatening ophthalmic diseases, including RD.

Rhegmatogenous (Nonexudative) Retinal Detachments

In contrast to exudative RD, rhegmatogenous RD or traction RD represent surgical conditions, and these patients should be referred promptly to an ophthalmologist for diagnosis and treatment. This type of detachment is treated by identifying and then sealing all retinal tears or holes. Small detachments may be stabilized by performing a barrier laser retinopexy around the border of the detachment and at the periphery of the retina. Large or complete detachments with giant retinal tears, several holes, or vitreous problems must be repaired surgically. Surgery involves a pars plana vitrectomy, retinal reattachment, laser retinopexy, and typically tamponade with silicone oil to replace the vitreous. Unfortunately not all patients are good candidates for this surgery. Surgical repair requires protracted general anesthesia and extensive postoperative monitoring and is very costly. Depending on the individual eye, the anatomic success rate may be as high as 90%; however, this does not always correlate with a functional success of vision recovery.

PROGNOSIS

The prognosis for a dog or cat with an RD directly relates to the etiology. If there is a life-threatening systemic disease, the prognosis for life is often poor. If there is no life-threatening disease, an animal may become blind or visually impaired or might lose a painful eye but subsequently may live a well-adjusted life. In patients presented with RD and visual impairment, prognosis is guarded. Recovery of vision relates to the promptness of diagnosis and treatment. If the underlying condition can be identified rapidly and treated, the retina may reattach, and some vision may return. However, up to 80% of the retinal nutrition and oxygen supply is derived from the choroidal vasculature. Therefore, as soon as the retina separates from the choroid and RPE, retinal degeneration begins. The nature of the subretinal fluid, duration of detachment, and height of detachment influence the degree and rapidity of retinal degeneration. Blood or dense exudative subretinal fluid (i.e., systemic mycoses), prolonged RD, and very elevated (bullous) detachment all hasten retinal degeneration and negatively affect visual recovery. Animals with small or partial RD or smaller and/or multifocal areas of chorioretinitis have a fair-to-good prognosis for maintaining some vision if the cause is identified quickly and treated appropriately.

Suggested Reading

Hakansan N, Forrester SD: Uveitis in the dog and cat, *Vet Clin North Am Small Anim Pract* 20(3):715, 1990.

Hendrix DV et al: Clinical signs, concurrent disease, and risk factors associated with retinal detachments in dogs, *Prog Vet Comp Ophthalmol* 3:87, 1993.

Martin CL: Ocular manifestations of systemic disease: the dog. In Gelatt KN, editor: *Veterinary ophthalmology*, ed 3, Philadelphia, 1999, Lippincott Williams & Wilkins, p 1401.

Narfstrom K, Ekesten B: Diseases of the canine ocular fundus. In Gelatt KN, editor: *Veterinary ophthalmology*, ed 3, Philadelphia, 1999, Lippincott Williams & Wilkins, p 869.

Smith PJ: Vitreous and retina. In Slatter D, editor: *Textbook of small animal surgery*, ed 3, Philadelphia, 2003, Saunders, p 1418.

Stiles J: Ocular manifestations of systemic disease: the cat. In Gelatt KN, editor: *Veterinary ophthalmology*, ed 3, Philadelphia,1999, Lippincott Williams & Wilkins, p 1448.

Vainisi SJ, Wolfer JC: Canine retinal surgery, *Vet Ophthalmol* 5:291, 2004.

Wilkie DA: Control of ocular inflammation, *Vet Clin North Am Small Anim Pract* 20(3):693,199, 1990.

SECTION XIII

Infectious Diseases

Rance K. Sellon

VOLUME XIII CONTENT ON EVOLVE: http://evolve.elsevier.com/Bonagura/Kirks/

Bacterial Resistance

Canine Hepatozoonosis

Ocular Manifestations of Systemic
    Diseases

The Rabies Pandemic

Ticks as Vectors of Companion Animal
    Disease

Why Are Infectious Diseases Emerging?

CHAPTER 265

Hospital-Acquired Bacterial Infections

SCOTT P. SHAW, *North Grafton, Massachusetts*

Hospital-acquired infections (HAIs) are well recognized as a serious source of morbidity and mortality in people. There is a vast and rapidly growing body of knowledge pertaining to HAIs in human patients, but information relating to veterinary HAIs is much more limited. There are several individual case reports of epidemic outbreaks within individual hospitals, but there is little published information on the role endemic hospital infections play in veterinary medicine. Currently there is no evidence-based information that can be used by veterinarians to guide infection-control decisions. Instead recommendations must be made based on the small amount of available veterinary research and extrapolation from the human literature.

HAIs are defined as infections that were neither present nor incubating at the time of hospital admission. Typically these infections develop more than 48 hours after admission because of the incubation period of most hospital-acquired pathogens. Hospital-acquired infections can develop up to 30 days after hospitalization or even a year later if an implant was placed. Although HAIs in veterinary hospitals could reflect pathogens of various types, especially bacterial and viral, bacterial infections are the focus of chapter.

EPIDEMIC VERSUS ENDEMIC INFECTIONS

Epidemic infections result from the infection or contamination of an individual source with a potential pathogen. This point source then results in the infection of one or more other individuals. Examples of epidemic infections reported in veterinary medicine include the infection of feline blood with *Serratia marcesans* from contaminated saline flush and *Salmonella krefeld* infection in numerous small animal patients, which was traced back to a caregiver who was an asymptomatic carrier.

Endemic infections are infections that occur regularly at a low or moderate frequency. These infections differ from epidemic infections in that they are not caused by a single point source. Instead, these infections result from a patient's endogenous flora, which is able to establish an infection because of a combination of debilitation from underlying illness, breaches in normal anatomic barriers (intravenous catheters, endotracheal intubation, surgical incisions), or placement of surgical implants. Endemic infections are much more difficult to eliminate since they do not result from a discrete identifiable source but represent the interplay of numerous risk factors, some of which can be mitigated and some of which cannot.

It is estimated that only 5% of all HAIs in humans represent epidemic outbreaks. The remaining 95% of infections are endemic in origin. Epidemic infections are more likely to be published and receive attention from the general public. As a result, their relative importance tends to be overemphasized. Although not investigated, a similar distribution likely occurs in veterinary patients.

PATHOGENESIS OF ENDEMIC INFECTIONS

Understanding the pathogenesis of endemic infections is essential to devise effective control strategies. During the course of illness the normal nonpathogenic flora of the oropharynx, gastrointestinal tract, and occasionally the skin can be replaced by potential pathogens. The basis for these changes in flora is multifactorial. A number of defense mechanisms such as secretion of immunoglobulin (Ig)A antibodies into the oral cavity and respiratory and gastrointestinal tracts, the integrity of the gastrointestinal mucosal barrier, and the presence of normal flora in the oral cavity and gastrointestinal tract protect against colonization by pathogenic bacteria. Critical illness has been shown to decrease IgA secretion, which predisposes the patient to colonization by pathogenic bacteria. In addition, a large number of intensive care unit (ICU) patients receive antimicrobial therapy that disrupts the normal flora to an even greater degree and opens a previously occupied ecologic niche for colonization by pathogens, including some with marked resistance to antimicrobials.

From where do the pathogens that cause HAIs originate? Historically the environment has been implicated as the reservoir for the microbes that cause HAIs. Much time and effort is spent cleaning and culturing the environment in an effort to remove these pathogens, an approach that is still used in some veterinary hospitals. Recently bacterial contamination of multidose drug vials in a veterinary clinic has been demonstrated; although HAIs associated with use of these vials were not the focus of this study, the findings should give users of such vials reason for concern. However, over the last 20 years the focus of infection control in human hospitals has shifted from the environment to the patients and to a lesser extent the staff because the reality is that the major reservoir for potential pathogens in the health care setting is the patient. In most cases positive environmental cultures represent transient contamination of the environment by patients. The pathogens that cause HAIs are transferred from patient to patient, generally on the hands of caregivers. Once a pathogen is transferred to a patient, colonization is likely for the reasons discussed here.

Reducing the Incidence of Endemic Hospital-Acquired Infections Through Surveillance

An active surveillance program is essential for rapidly recognizing epidemic outbreaks and understanding the incidence of endemic infections. A surveillance program can be relatively simple or complex, depending on the depth of knowledge desired and the personnel and financial resources available. In addition, it has been shown that hospitals with active surveillance programs have a higher rate of adherence to infection control policies. This may be because of a Hawthorne effect (i.e., individuals who know they are being observed behave differently from those who are not aware of the observation).

In addition to observing for the occurrence of HAIs, other information, referred to as denominator data, must be collected to accurately quantify the risk. Examples of denominator data include hospital admissions, catheter days, hospital days, and ventilator days. For example, if in the month of January 10 HAIs were identified and in the month of July 15 HAIs were identified, the initial conclusion would be that patients in July were more likely to develop an HAI than those in January. However, if one looked at the denominator data (1000 admissions in January, 1500 admissions in July) the conclusion would be that the incidence of HAIs in both months was identical (i.e., 1 HAI/100 hospital admissions).

Before beginning any surveillance program, it is important to identify the goals to be achieved. Goals of surveillance programs could include reducing infection rates, establishing baseline endemic rates, identifying outbreaks, persuading personnel to adopt preventive behaviors, evaluating control measures, and defending litigation. Collecting only as much data as required to achieve the goals of the surveillance program can protect the investigator from becoming buried with data and having trouble reaching any useful conclusions.

A number of surveillance measures can be readily used in veterinary practices; each has advantages and disadvantages. Some of the different surveillance programs that could be considered for use in small animal practices are passive surveillance, review of culture results, contact with clinicians and owners, daily medical record review, and environmental cultures.

Passive Surveillance

Passive surveillance is the easiest form to implement, but it tends to provide the least amount of useful data. Examples of passive surveillance include regular review of professional and discharge reports or having staff members generate a form every time an HAI is identified. The biggest limitation of passive surveillance is that it relies on staff members to accurately identify HAIs. Numerous studies in humans, as well as a study conducted in our hospital, have shown that untrained staff missed as many as 50% of the HAIs identified by infection control practitioners.

Review of Culture and Sensitivity

Routine review of culture and sensitivity results can provide a wealth of information. This surveillance method is particularly helpful in identifying epidemic outbreaks. By placing culture and sensitivity results in a spreadsheet or database, organisms with similar resistance patterns can be identified, and the possibility of an epidemic outbreak investigated. This method is also helpful for the identification of potentially important pathogens such as methicillin-resistant *Staphylococcus aureus* or vancomycin-resistant *Enterococcus*. Several commercially available programs are designed for this purpose. Some of these programs can download data directly from existing databases, whereas others require manual input.

Relying solely on culture and sensitivity results to guide infection control practices results in a gross underestimation of HAIs. In our hospital only 50% to 60% of patients that develop an HAI have an appropriate culture submitted. If we were to rely solely on these data, we would greatly underestimate the incidence of important infections such as pneumonia and surgical site infections.

Regular Contact

Regular contact with doctors or owners requires the infection control practitioner to regularly interface with the staff, owners, or both. It is superior to purely passive surveillance, but it is limited by the need of an untrained individual (the owner) to identify the presence or absence of infection.

Daily Medical Record Review

A daily medical record review provides the most surveillance information but is the most labor intensive. It requires that every patient in the hospital be surveyed on a daily basis. This approach can be used successfully to establish baseline endemic infection rates. Information gained can then be used to guide future infection control decisions.

Environmental Cultures

Historically a large of amount of time and money was spent on *environmental cultures*. Now that there is a greater understanding of HAIs, the role of environmental cultures in surveillance programs has been greatly reduced, and routine environmental cultures are no longer recommended. Generally the only time an environmental culture should be considered is in the presence of an outbreak that could be environmental in origin. Endemic infections almost never have an environmental reservoir.

Reducing Hospital-Acquired Infection by Hand Washing

There is significant evidence, dating back to Ignaz Semmelweis in 1847, that hand washing reduces the incidence of HAIs. More recently it has been shown that alcohol-based antiseptics are superior to soap and water. Perhaps the most amazing fact is that compliance with hand washing in human hospitals generally ranges from 30% to 50%. The use of antiseptic hand wash is the single intervention most likely to reduce the incidence of HAIs. For hand washing to be most effective, hands should be disinfected immediately before and after patient contact *and* before any contact with other patients or the environment.

A single patient interaction may require a caregiver to wash his or her hands multiple times.

Convincing people about the importance of hand washing and then training them so that hand washing becomes second nature are difficult. A first step in achieving hand washing compliance involves selecting the hand cleaning product(s) that will be made available to clinical staff. Numerous products are Food and Drug Administration–approved for this purpose. At Tuft's University, we have found an alcohol-based hand foam to be the most readily accepted. The second step in achieving compliance is making hand antisepsis convenient. Dispensers should be placed in as many locations as possible. Finally, a staff education program should be implemented. Education can be made more effective if there is a reward for changing behavior. This can be anything from a party for the department with the highest compliance to individual rewards (i.e., movie tickets) randomly distributed when an individual is observed following proper hand antisepsis. An educational campaign is not a one-time event. Without continued reminders, staff behavior will deteriorate. Thus ongoing educational campaigns should be implemented.

Recommendations for Specific Infection Types

Most HAIs fall into one of the following categories: (1) pneumonia, (2) surgical site infections (SSIs), (3) catheter-related infections (CRIs), and (4) urinary tract infections (UTIs). Since these four categories represent the vast majority of HAIs, most measures are focused on preventing these infections. As discussed previously, the most important step in preventing HAIs is the prevention of colonization.

Pneumonia
Pneumonia is not the most common HAI in veterinary patients, but it causes greater morbidity and mortality than other HAIs. Risk factors for the development of pneumonia in veterinary patients are not well studied. In humans numerous potential risk factors have been identified, including endotracheal intubation, positive-pressure ventilation, neurologic injury/surgery, use of H_2 blockers, nasogastric tube placement, propofol use, and sedation. Many of these risk factors create breaches in defense mechanisms that normally prevent aspiration of potentially infectious material or allow bacterial colonization of sites not normally colonized (e.g., the stomach with increases in pH brought about by treatment with H_2 blockers). Such breaches, especially when combined with colonization of the oropharynx by pathogenic bacteria, greatly increase the risk of gross or microaspiration, either of which can lead to the development of pneumonia.

Surgical Site Infections
SSIs are probably the best studied of the veterinary HAIs. Duration of anesthesia, degree of wound contamination, surgical technique, and appropriate antimicrobial prophylaxis, either alone or in combination, represent the most significant risk factors. Length of anesthesia greater than 90 to 120 minutes is associated with significantly higher SSI rates.

Appropriate antimicrobial prophylaxis is essential to prevent SSIs and involves administration of antibiotics so that blood levels are at their peak at the time of the first incision. For example, if cefazolin is used for SSI prophylaxis, it should be given no more than 1 hour and no less than 15 minutes before the start of surgery (not anesthesia) and be redosed every 2 hours. Continuation of prophylaxis for more than 24 hours in wounds that are not infected is not associated with a lower rate of SSIs.

One of the most effective controls of SSIs in humans is using prospective surveillance to determine the rate of SSIs for the surgery department as a whole and reporting individual surgeon SSI rates to each surgeon. This necessitates a high degree of confidentiality since each surgeon should be supplied with his or her SSI rate, as well the SSI rate of the department, without being informed of other surgeons' SSI rates. This approach is thought to encourage self-policing by the surgical staff and should not be viewed as a witch hunt. It should be remembered that the surgeon who routinely fixes open fractures will have a higher SSI rate than one who does mainly spays and neuters.

Catheter-Related Infections
CRIs are thought to occur most frequently from contamination of the catheter at the time of placement. They may also occur because of migration of bacteria along the catheter or from contamination of the catheter tip by systemic bacteremia. It has been my experience that most CRIs represent simple vasculitis in the area of the skin/catheter interface and that the vast majority of these cases resolve spontaneously on catheter removal. True catheter-related bloodstream infections are thought to be rare in veterinary medicine. Prevention of CRIs should focus on appropriate catheter placement and maintenance. Unfortunately there is little research into the best way to place and manage intravenous catheters in veterinary patients.

Urinary Tract Infections
UTI are the most common HAIs in both animals and humans but are associated with the least morbidity and mortality. It is important to distinguish between colonization and contamination when making the diagnosis of UTI. Intermittent catheterization has been shown to be superior to use of indwelling catheters in humans, but no studies have examined this approach in veterinary patients. Control of UTIs should focus on minimizing urinary catheter use and adhering to sterile technique during placement and maintenance. Antimicrobial prophylaxis does not prevent the development of UTIs but rather guarantees that the infection will be resistant to the antimicrobial used and thus should be avoided. In general culturing the urinary catheter tip is not recommended since positive growth frequently represents catheter colonization rather than true infection.

TREATMENT OF HOSPITAL-ACQUIRED INFECTIONS

The clinical importance of many HAIs, particularly those seen in ICU patients, is multidrug resistance. The most likely pathogens and their antibiogram vary between hospitals. It is important to have an understanding of the likely pathogens in an individual hospital since early, appropriate therapy is the key for a successful outcome.

References and Suggested Reading

Bennet JV, Brachman PS: *Hospital infections*, ed 4, Philadelphia, 1998, Lippincott-Raven.

Brown DC et al: Epidemiologic evaluation of postoperative wound infections in dogs and cats, *J Am Vet Med Assoc* 210: 1302, 1997.

Cooke CL et al: Enrofloxacin resistance in Escherichia coli isolated from dogs with urinary tract infections, *J Am Vet Med Assoc* 220:190, 2002.

Eugster E et al: A prospective study of postoperative surgical site infections in dogs and cats, *Vet Surg* 33:542, 2004.

Mayhall CG: *Hospital epidemiology and infection control*, ed 3, Philadelphia, 2004, Lippincott Williams & Wilkins.

Ogeer-Gyles JS, Mathews KA, Boerlin P: Nosocomial infections and antimicrobial resistance in critical care medicine, *J Vet Emerg Crit Care* 16:1, 2005.

Sabino CV, Weese JS: Contamination of multiple-dose vials in a veterinary hospital, *Can Vet J* 47:779, 2006.

CHAPTER 266

Rational Empiric Antimicrobial Therapy

PATRICIA M. DOWLING, *Saskatoon, Saskatchewan, Canada*

Concerns regarding bacterial resistance to antimicrobials are increasing the awareness of rational use in human and veterinary medicine. Effective empiric antimicrobial therapy requires matching the likely pathogen(s) to the antimicrobial drugs that should have sufficient activity against them (Table 266-1). A successful empiric antimicrobial dosage regimen depends on both a measure of drug exposure (pharmacokinetics [PK]) and a measure of the potency of the drug against the infecting organism (pharmacodynamics [PD]). New information is rapidly emerging regarding the PK/PD relationships that determine antimicrobial efficacy in both human and veterinary patients. The PK parameters used in drug dosage design are the area under the plasma concentration versus time curve (AUC) from 0 to 24 hours, the maximum plasma concentration (Cmax), and the time the antimicrobial concentration exceeds a defined PD threshold (T). The most commonly used PD parameter is the bacterial minimum inhibitory concentration (MIC). In relating the PK and PD parameters to clinical efficacy, antimicrobial drug action is classified as either concentration dependent or time dependent.

CONCENTRATION-DEPENDENT ANTIMICROBIALS

For concentration-dependent antimicrobials, high plasma concentrations relative to the MIC of the pathogen (Cmax: MIC) and the area under the plasma concentration–time curve that is above the bacterial MIC during the dosage interval (area under the inhibitory curve [AUC_{0-24hr}:MIC]) are the major determinants of clinical efficacy. These drugs also have prolonged postantibiotic effects, thereby allowing once-a-day dosing while maintaining maximum clinical efficacy. For fluoroquinolones (enrofloxacin, orbifloxacin, difloxacin, marbofloxacin), clinical efficacy is associated with achieving either an AUC_{0-24hr}:MIC >125 or a Cmax:MIC >10. For aminoglycosides (gentamicin, amikacin), achieving a Cmax:MIC >10 is considered optimal for efficacy. Other antimicrobials that appear to have concentration-dependent activity include metronidazole (Cmax:MIC >10 to 25) and azithromycin (AUC_{0-24hr}: MIC>25). For some pathogens such as *Pseudomonas aeruginosa*, achieving the optimum PK/PD ratios may be impossible with label or even higher-than-label dosages. In such cases underdosing is not only ineffective and but contributes to antimicrobial resistance.

TIME-DEPENDENT ANTIMICROBIALS

For time-dependent antimicrobials the time during which the antimicrobial concentration exceeds the MIC of the pathogen determines clinical efficacy (T>MIC). How much above the MIC and for what percentage of the dosing interval concentrations should be above the MIC is still debated and is likely specific for individual bacteria-drug combinations. Typically, exceeding the MIC by one to five multiples for between 40% and 100% of the dosage interval is appropriate for time-dependent bactericidal

Table 266-1

Suggested First-Choice Antimicrobials Based on the Site of Infection

Site of Infection	First-Choice Antimicrobials
Urinary tract	Amoxicillin/ampicillin
	Amoxicillin/clavulanic acid
	Cephalexin/cefadroxil
	Nitrofurantoin
	Tetracycline/doxycycline
Pyoderma	Cephalexin/cefadroxil
	Amoxicillin/clavulanic acid
	Cloxacillin/dicloxacillin/oxacillin
	Clindamycin/lincomycin/erythromycin
Upper respiratory tract	Amoxicillin/clavulanic acid
	Azithromycin
	Doxycycline
Lower respiratory tract	Amoxicillin/clavulanic acid ± fluoroquinolone* or aminoglycoside[†]
	Cephalosporin ± fluoroquinolone* or aminoglycoside[†]
	Clindamycin ± fluoroquinolone*
	Chloramphenicol
	Tetracycline/doxycycline
	Azithromycin
Surgical prophylaxis	Potassium penicillin G
	Cefazolin
Musculoskeletal	Cephalosporin
Septic arthritis, tenosynovitis, osteomyelitis	Clindamycin
	Amoxicillin/clavulanic acid
	Fluoroquinolone*
	Aminoglycoside[†]
Septicemia/bacteremia	Cephalosporin
	Cephalosporin/penicillin + enrofloxacin
	Cephalosporin/penicillin + aminoglycosides[†]
	Cefoxitin

*Fluoroquinolones include enrofloxacin, difloxacin, orbifloxacin, and marbofloxacin.
[†]Aminoglycosides include amikacin and gentamicin. In orthopedic infections these drugs can be used in local therapy to avoid toxicity.

antimicrobials. The T>MIC should be closer to 100% for bacteriostatic antimicrobials and for patients that are immunosuppressed; thus these drugs typically require frequent dosing or constant-rate infusions for appropriate therapy. In sequestered infections penetration of the antimicrobial to the site of infection may require high plasma concentrations to achieve a sufficient concentration gradient. In such cases the AUC_{0-24hr}:MIC and/or Cmax:MIC may also be important in determining efficacy of otherwise time-dependent antimicrobials. The penicillins, cephalosporins, most macrolides and lincosamides, tetracyclines, chloramphenicol, and the potentiated sulfonamides are considered time-dependent antimicrobials.

GUIDELINES FOR SPECIFIC TISSUES

Urinary Tract Infections

Bacterial urinary tract infection (UTI) results from normal skin and gastrointestinal tract flora ascending the urinary tract and overcoming the normal urinary tract defenses that prevent colonization. Large retrospective studies have documented the most common uropathogens in dogs and cats, with *Escherichia coli* representing the single most common isolate from both acute and recurrent UTIs. Gram stain and pH of a urine sample help direct empiric antimicrobial therapy. If the urine is persistently alkaline, suspect a urease-producing pathogen such as *Staphylococcus* spp. if gram-positive cocci are seen or *Proteus* spp. if gram-negative rods are seen. If the urine is acidic, the most likely pathogens are *E. coli* if gram-negative rods are seen and *Enterococcus* spp. if gram-positive cocci are seen. Initial treatment of uncomplicated UTIs is straightforward since most antimicrobials undergo renal elimination to a great extent; thus urine concentrations may be up to 100 times peak plasma concentrations. All of the first-choice treatments are time-dependent antimicrobials; thus frequent dosing is important for efficacy. Amoxicillin or ampicillin has excellent activity against staphylococci, streptococci, enterococci, and *Proteus* spp. and may achieve high enough urinary concentrations to be effective against *E. coli* and *Klebsiella* spp. if dosed frequently. Amoxicillin/clavulanic acid has excellent bactericidal activity against β-lactamase–producing staphylococci, *E. coli,* and *Klebsiella* spp. However, clavulanic acid undergoes some hepatic metabolism and excretion; thus the efficacy of amoxicillin/clavulanic acid may be caused primarily by high concentrations of amoxicillin achieved in urine.

First-generation cephalosporins such as cephalexin or cefadroxil have greater stability to β-lactamases than penicillins and thus have greater activity against staphylococci and gram-negative bacteria. They have excellent activity against staphylococci, streptococci, *E. coli, Proteus* spp., and *Klebsiella* spp. *Pseudomonas* spp., enterococci, and *Enterobacter* spp. are resistant; and the use of cephalosporins predisposes patients to nosocomial enterococcal infections. Nitrofurantoin is an old antimicrobial still used in human medicine only for UTIs since therapeutic concentrations are not attained in plasma or tissues. It is a good first-line treatment for UTIs caused by *E. coli*, enterococci, staphylococci, *Klebsiella* spp., and *Enterobacter* spp.; but it must be dosed every 8 hours, making client compliance difficult.

Tetracyclines are broad-spectrum antimicrobials; but, because of plasmid-mediated resistance, staphylococci, enterococci, *Enterobacter* spp., *E. coli, Klebsiella* spp., and *Proteus* spp. have variable susceptibility. However, the tetracyclines are excreted unchanged in the urine; thus high urinary concentrations may result in therapeutic efficacy despite susceptibility test results that indicate resistance. Doxycycline is a very lipid soluble tetracycline that is better tolerated in cats and achieves therapeutic concentrations in the prostatic and renal tissues. Because of biliary elimination, doxycycline was thought not to be useful for uncomplicated UTIs, but a recent study demonstrated that effective concentrations are achieved in the urine of dogs and cats (Wilson et al., 2006). The combinations of trimethoprim or ormetoprim with a sulfonamide are synergistic and bactericidal against staphylococci, streptococci, *E. coli*, and *Proteus* spp. Activity against enterococci and *Klebsiella* spp. is variable, and *Pseudomonas* spp. are resistant. Although their spectrum of activity makes the potentiated sulfonamides rational first-line treatment choices, they are associated with a number of side effects that discourage more frequent selection.

Enrofloxacin, orbifloxacin, difloxacin, and marbofloxacin are all fluoroquinolones approved for UTIs in the dog, and some are approved in the cat, but all are used in cats. All fluoroquinolones have excellent activity against staphylococci and gram-negative bacteria but have variable activity against streptococci and enterococci. They are the only orally administered antimicrobials with efficacy against *Pseudomonas* spp. The therapeutic advantage of these drugs is their gram-negative antimicrobial activity, their excellent penetration into the prostate gland, and their activity in infected tissues; their concentration-dependent killing allows for once-a-day dosing. However, it is inappropriate to use these important antimicrobials as first-line treatment of uncomplicated UTIs. Their use should be reserved for complicated UTIs such as cases of pyelonephritis that involve gram-negative bacteria and for UTIs in intact male dogs in which prostatic involvement is likely.

Pyoderma

Pyoderma is a common bacterial skin disease of dogs caused by *Staphylococcus intermedius*. *S. intermedius* is normal skin flora and colonizes the upper respiratory tract, the oral cavity, the anal region, and the external ear canal. Most canine staphylococci produce slime that allows the bacteria to adhere to cells; and they contain protein A, which activates the complement cascade and incites inflammation. *E. coli*, *Proteus* spp., and *Pseudomonas* spp. can transiently colonize the skin and occasionally may become involved in pyoderma secondary to the staphylococcal infection. Treatment of the primary staphylococcal infection is usually sufficient to resolve these secondary infections.

Effective treatment of pyoderma requires systemically administered antimicrobials and topically applied antibacterial agents, along with specific treatment of any underlying causes. Appropriate empiric antimicrobials must be resistant to β-lactamase produced by staphylococci. *S. intermedius* typically does not demonstrate antimicrobial resistance because it does not readily retain antimicrobial resistance plasmids. Resistance patterns are predictable when there has been no prior antimicrobial exposure. First-generation cephalosporins such as cephalexin or cefadroxil are the usual first-line treatment choices for staphylococcal pyoderma. Dosage regimens that target T>MIC for 40% to 50% of the dosing interval are efficacious. Cefpodoxime proxetil, a third-generation cephalosporin, is attractive for use because of its once-daily dosing schedule but should be reserved for infections more serious than superficial pyoderma. The antistaphylococcal penicillins (cloxacillin, dicloxacillin, and oxacillin) are excellent for first-choice therapy of pyoderma. However, because of their limited spectrum of activity, these drugs are not usually on stock in a veterinary clinic, but they can be prescribed easily from a human pharmacy. Because of poor oral bioavailability and rapid renal elimination, they

must be dosed every 6 hours, making client compliance difficult. The macrolides and lincosamides are reasonable choices for first-time treatment of pyoderma, but recurrent infections are likely to be resistant. Erythromycin is associated with a high incidence of gastrointestinal upset in dogs. This can be avoided by using enteric-coated tablets, administering with food, prescribing antiemetics for the first 2 to 3 days of therapy, and initiating therapy with a lower dose. This treatment regimen is too complicated and inconvenient for most clients, and most clinicians prefer to use antimicrobials that do not routinely induce vomiting. Lincomycin has the same activity as erythromycin and does not cause gastrointestinal upset. Clindamycin is very active against *Staphylococcus* spp. and anaerobic bacteria. It distributes well into tissues and is active in purulent material. Trimethoprim or ormetoprim combined with a sulfonamide are effective in most cases of superficial pyoderma, but the risks of adverse effects such as keratoconjunctivitis sicca and polysystemic drug reactions limit their use.

Mupirocin is a topical therapy for localized pyoderma. It has excellent activity against gram-positive cocci, is not absorbed systemically, and is chemically unrelated to other antimicrobials. It is well tolerated in cats for the treatment of feline acne. Mupirocin ointment penetrates well into granulomatous lesions such as interdigital abscesses. Owners can decrease the relapse rate and severity of recurrent pyoderma if they immediately apply mupirocin every 12 hours when they first notice early lesions developing.

For most cases of pyoderma 3 to 6 weeks of therapy are required for a clinical cure; and some dogs require chronic low-dose or pulse-dose therapy with amoxicillin/clavulanic acid, cloxacillin, or a cephalosporin for control of recurrent pyodermas. Enrofloxacin, difloxacin, marbofloxacin, and orbifloxacin are first choices only for antimicrobial therapy of deep pyodermas and short-term therapy of recurrent pyoderma when resistance has developed. They have excellent activity against *S. intermedius*, *Pseudomonas* spp., and *Proteus* spp., the organisms most likely to be involved in refractory cases. Fluoroquinolones have ideal pharmacokinetic properties; they accumulate in leukocytes and retain activity in necrotic and purulent debris. Since they are concentration-dependent killers, high-dose once-daily administration is ideal and increases client compliance with the treatment regimen. Fluoroquinolone therapy should be avoided for chronic low-dose or pulse-dose therapy because chromosomal-mediated resistance occurs with chronic exposure.

Respiratory Tract Infections

Upper Respiratory Tract

Primary bacterial infection of the upper respiratory tract is uncommon, but almost all dogs and cats with a mucopurulent or purulent nasal discharge have some bacterial component to their disease. *Bordetella bronchiseptica* can cause primary upper respiratory tract (URT) infections in dogs; whereas *B. bronchiseptica*, *Mycoplasma* spp., and *Chlamydophila felis* cause primary URT infections in the cat. Most cases of bacterial rhinitis are secondary to other diseases and caused by the variety of normal flora found in the nasal passages; culture and susceptibility test results are difficult to interpret. Treating the bacterial infection without correcting the underlying cause is very unrewarding and encourages emergence of antimicrobial-resistant pathogens such as *P. aeruginosa*. Chronic URT infection may lead to sinus osteomyelitis. Empiric therapy for URT infections in dogs and cats includes amoxicillin/clavulanate, cephalexin or cefadroxil, or drugs with efficacy against *Mycoplasma* spp. and *C. felis* such as doxycycline, azithromycin, or a fluoroquinolone. Doxycycline is considered the most effective therapy for chlamydiosis, but clinical signs improve with any of these therapies, and cats frequently remain polymerase chain reaction or immunofluorescent antibody test positive. Doxycycline is often avoided in young animals because of fears of causing dental damage. Even in children, doxycycline is the least likely of the tetracyclines to cause dental damage, and there are no published reports of dental abnormalities from the use of doxycycline in puppies and kittens. However, oral administration to cats is associated with esophageal damage that can lead to stricture; thus administration of tablets or capsules should be followed with food or water to ensure passage into the stomach. Fluoroquinolones should be reserved for serious infections based on of culture and susceptibility testing. Enrofloxacin should be avoided in cats because of the potential for retinal damage. Tetracycline, chloramphenicol, or erythromycin ophthalmic ointments can be used to treat concurrent conjunctivitis. With chronic infections in dogs or cats, drugs that penetrate bone and target anaerobic bacteria such as amoxicillin/clavulanic acid, clindamycin, or cephalexin or cefadroxil should be chosen.

Lower Respiratory Tract
Bacterial pneumonia in dogs and cats is usually secondary to some pathologic process that disrupts normal pulmonary defence mechanisms. Treatment choices are dictated by the specific etiology and the clinical status of the patient. In dogs with community-acquired bacterial infections the likely causative pathogens are *B. bronchiseptica*, *Mycoplasma* spp., *Streptococcus zooepidemicus*, *Pasteurella* spp., and *E. coli*. In cats the pathogens are similar, with the addition of *C. felis*. In previously ill animals or animals with hospital-acquired illness, *E. coli*, *Klebsiella* spp., *Pasteurella* spp., streptococci, staphylococci, anaerobes, *B. bronchiseptica*, *Pseudomonas* spp., and *Mycoplasma* spp. are frequently involved; and more than one bacterial pathogen is commonly isolated. The unpredictable antimicrobial susceptibility of *E. coli* and other gram-negative bacteria makes it difficult to choose antimicrobial therapy without susceptibility testing, thus sampling the lower respiratory tract for culture and sensitivity and cytology is strongly recommended. The critically ill patient should be started on a broad-spectrum, parenteral antimicrobial regimen as soon as possible until results of definitive cultures are obtained. Gram-negative rods frequently are susceptible to potentiated sulfonamides, gentamicin, chloramphenicol, cefpodoxime proxetil,

and the fluoroquinolones (enrofloxacin, orbifloxacin, difloxacin, marbofloxacin). *B. bronchiseptica* typically is susceptible to amoxicillin-clavulanic acid, tetracyclines, or azithromycin; but some isolates are resistant to the fluoroquinolones. Gram-positive cocci are frequently susceptible to amoxicillin/clavulanic acid, chloramphenicol, cephalosporins, or azithromycin. Aminoglycosides or enrofloxacin can be administered concurrently with parenteral formulations of penicillins or cephalosporins for broad-spectrum treatment of seriously ill patients. Clindamycin or metronidazole can be added to provide activity against β-lactamase–producing *Bacteroides fragilis*.

Musculoskeletal Infections

Prophylactic Antimicrobials
Veterinary surgeons routinely use prophylactic antimicrobials in surgical patients undergoing orthopedic procedures, but little evidence from clinical trials demonstrates the efficacy of this practice. In humans undergoing clean bone surgery, antimicrobials are administered intravenously from 30 minutes before skin incision to no longer than 24 hours after the operation. Cefazolin typically is the prophylactic antimicrobial therapy of choice in small animal practice. However, in the only published veterinary trial of prophylactic antimicrobial therapy in dogs undergoing elective orthopedic surgery, prophylaxis decreased the postoperative infection rate, but potassium penicillin G was as efficacious as cefazolin (Whittem et al., 1999). Prophylactic antimicrobial therapy should be followed by close observation and treatment with appropriate antimicrobials and surgery if postoperative infection is diagnosed.

Septic Arthritis, Tenosynovitis, Osteomyelitis
Because of the variety of pathogens involved in musculoskeletal infections, appropriate samples must be submitted for culture and susceptibility testing. Aggressive antimicrobial therapy should be initiated as soon as there is sufficient evidence of infection because of the devastating consequences of bone, joint, or tendon sheath infections. While awaiting culture results, initial antimicrobial selection can be chosen based on clinical case characteristics. In adult dogs and cats, septic arthritis and tenosynovitis commonly result from wounds or iatrogenic contamination with bacteria. In wounds a variety of gram-positive and gram-negative bacteria typically are present, whereas *Staphylococcus aureus* and *S. intermedius* are the usual isolates from iatrogenic infections, with methicillin-resistant *S. aureus* increasingly reported from veterinary cases. Osteomyelitis in dogs and cats is most commonly caused by *S. intermedius*. Polymicrobial infections are common in small animals and may include mixtures of streptococci, enterococci, Enterobacteriaceae (*E. coli*, *Klebsiella* spp., *Pseudomonas* spp.) and anaerobic bacteria. Cat fight abscesses typically are caused by *Pasteurella multocida*. *Pseudomonas* spp. often colonize devitalized tissues such as those occurring with "big dog–little dog" degloving injuries. For most bone and joint infections caused by β-lactamase–producing staphylococci,

cephalosporins (cefazolin, cephalexin, cefpodoxime proxetil), clindamycin, or amoxicillin-clavulanic acid are effective. Clindamycin and metronidazole are used for anaerobic infections. The aminoglycosides (amikacin, gentamicin) and fluoroquinolones (enrofloxacin, orbifloxacin, difloxacin, marbofloxacin) typically have good activity against staphylococci and excellent activity against gram-negative pathogens. Although amikacin usually has good activity against *Pseudomonas* spp., it has poor activity against streptococci compared to gentamicin. Because nephrotoxicity and ototoxicity are related to duration of treatment, the aminoglycosides are often reserved for treatment of musculoskeletal infections by local delivery techniques. The excellent broad-spectrum antimicrobial activity, good safety profiles, and availability of injectable (enrofloxacin) and oral formulations of fluoroquinolones make them popular choices for treatment of musculoskeletal infections. The newer human macrolide antimicrobials (azithromycin, clarithromycin) may also be efficacious for musculoskeletal infections and have good safety profiles in dogs and cats.

Septicemia/Bacteremia

Septicemia is common in critically ill canine and feline patients, and the majority that are septicemic have positive blood cultures for bacteria. In dogs gram-negative bacteria (especially *E. coli*) are most common, followed by gram-positive cocci and anaerobes. Polymicrobial infections are also common and usually involve gram-negative enterics and anaerobes. Bacteria cultured from cats are primarily gram-negative enterics or anaerobes. Therefore it is common to use intravenous β-lactam/aminoglycoside or β-lactam/enrofloxacin combinations for initial therapy of septic dogs and cats. The concentration-dependent drugs are administered once daily, but the time-dependent β-lactam drugs must be administered either by constant rate infusion or at least every 6 hours. Cefoxitin is a second-generation cephalosporin with good activity against anaerobes and gram-negative enterics that can be used in septic dogs and cats. Imipenem, meropenem, and vancomycin occasionally are used to treat resistant infections in severely ill dogs and cats; but because of their importance in human medicine their use should not be routine in veterinary patients.

References and Suggested Reading

Giguere S et al: *Antimicrobial therapy in veterinary medicine*, ed 4, Ames, 2006, Iowa State University Press.

McKellar QA, Sanchez Bruni SF, Jones DG: Pharmacokinetic/pharmacodynamic relationships of antimicrobial drugs used in veterinary medicine, *J Vet Pharmacol Ther* 27:503, 2004.

Wilson BJ et al: Susceptibility of bacteria from feline and canine urinary tract infections to doxycycline and tetracycline concentrations attained in urine four hours after oral dosage, *Aust Vet J* 84:8, 2006.

Whittem TL et al: Effect of perioperative prophylactic antimicrobial treatment in dogs undergoing elective orthopedic surgery, *J Am Vet Med Assoc* 215:212, 1999.

CHAPTER 267

Rational Use of Glucocorticoids in Infectious Disease

ADAM MORDECAI, *Buffalo Grove, Illinois*
RANCE K. SELLON, *Pullman, Washington*

Evidence supporting the use of glucocorticoids in the face of infections in small animal patients is based on anecdotal or retrospective reports. Few prospective controlled studies have critically evaluated the benefits or consequences of glucocorticoid use in this setting. Frequently cited reasons for administration of glucocorticoids in treating infectious disease include suppression of harmful inflammatory or immune responses and suppression of presumed secondary immune-mediated processes. Despite the fact that there is little scientific evidence that supports their use, glucocorticoids are frequently suggested for patients with infectious disease. The aim of this chapter is to review the use of glucocorticoids for infections and to offer guidelines for their use. This chapter does not specifically address the use of glucocorticoids, either topical or systemic, in patients with ocular infections or ocular manifestations of infectious disease, although they are used frequently (see Section XII).

MECHANISM OF ACTION

The mechanisms by which glucocorticoids mediate antiinflammatory activity are not understood completely (also see Chapter 89). Glucocorticoids first diffuse across the plasma membrane and bind to specific glucocorticoid receptors in the cytoplasm. The steroid-receptor complex then exerts a variety of effects. The complex can inactivate proinflammatory transcription factors and increase the production of proteins that inhibit cytokine production. Glucocorticoids can also mediate their actions through nontranscriptional means such as decreasing the half-life of messenger ribonucleic acid for inflammatory cytokines. Glucocorticoids attenuate inflammation by inducing lipocortin-1, which directly inhibits phospholipase A_2, an enzyme that is responsible for production of inflammatory prostaglandins, leukotrienes, and eicosanoids. Through these and other mechanisms inflammation and immune function can be altered or suppressed by glucocorticoids. Both the cellular and humoral arms of the immune system can be affected; however, the cellular response is thought to be most compromised. Poor cellular immune responses could enhance the pathogenic potential of some infectious organisms, prevent cell-mediated clearance of organisms, and perpetuate inflammation secondary to persistence of organisms and activation of other inflammatory pathways. Glucocorticoids are commonly thought to decrease phagocytic and oxidative functions of phagocytic cells in a dose-dependent manner, thereby compromising the ability to kill ingested organisms. It is these general properties that not only support the use of glucocorticoids in patients with infectious disease but also raise concerns about the potential side effects and complications associated with their use.

GLUCOCORTICOIDS IN HUMANS WITH INFECTIOUS DISEASE

A survey of the human literature on the use of glucocorticoids as adjunctive treatment for infectious disease puts into perspective many of the uncertainties. Conclusions regarding the benefits of glucocorticoids given to humans with infectious disease vary, depending on the infectious agent studied, the age of the patient group studied, the dose and/or duration of glucocorticoid therapy, the parameters assessed (e.g., immunologic or infectious agent parameters such as cytokine levels or quantity of infectious agent detected), the presence of other infectious agents, and by extension, perhaps, of other concurrent diseases. Human immunodeficiency virus-1 imposes its own perturbations on immune and inflammatory responses. Many of the case reports either involve small numbers of patients or lack appropriate controls. To illustrate, placebo-controlled studies of children with viral respiratory infection treated with glucocorticoids found benefit when treated with several days of prednisone but no benefit in studies in which a single dose of dexamethasone was given at admission. Glucocorticoids have also been shown to be of benefit in humans with peritonsillar abscesses and to improve survival with mycobacterial meningitis, but they do not prevent postrecovery disability. Interestingly, one study of glucocorticoid treatment of humans with mycobacterial meningitis suggests that the clinical benefits may be from mechanisms other than antiinflammatory or immune modulation after finding no difference in a number of inflammatory and immunologic parameters in placebo- and glucocorticoid- treated groups. Low doses of glucocorticoids generally are accepted as beneficial in people with sepsis, whereas high doses appear to offer no benefit.

GLUCOCORTICOIDS IN SMALL ANIMALS WITH INFECTIOUS DISEASE

Respiratory Infections

It has been proposed that antiinflammatory doses of glucocorticoids for 5 to 7 days may be effective in ameliorating cough associated with uncomplicated infectious tracheobronchitis but do not significantly shorten the clinical course of disease. It is commonly recognized that following initial administration of antifungal agents to patients with fungal pneumonia (i.e., blastomycosis and histoplasmosis) respiratory signs can worsen as a consequence of heightened inflammation associated with fungal death. Glucocorticoids are thought to prevent treatment-induced inflammation from occurring; however, as yet there are no studies showing this benefit. In a retrospective study of chronic histoplasmosis in dogs (Schulman, et al., 1999), clinical signs of coughing from airway obstruction associated with hilar lymphadenomegaly resolved more quickly when treated with immunosuppressive dosages (2 to 4 mg/kg/day) of prednisone alone or prednisone and antifungal drugs compared to those in dogs treated with antifungal chemotherapy alone (less than 3 weeks compared to approximately 9 weeks). In this study the glucocorticoid-treated dogs did not show evidence of dissemination of disease.

Central Nervous System Infections

In central nervous system (CNS) infections inflammatory mediators and toxic factors produced by the immune system may be more responsible for CNS damage than the primary pathogen. The treatment of bacterial organisms can result in their lysis and release of inflammatory cell wall components, including lipopolysaccharides and outer membrane vesicles. As yet there are no controlled studies addressing the use of glucocorticoids in dogs or cats with infectious meningitis, but anecdotal experience, case reports, and the human literature suggest a potential benefit. At our institution patients suspected to have CNS infection based on cerebral spinal fluid (CSF) pleocytosis, elevated CSF protein content, and/or consistent magnetic resonance imaging findings are treated with a broad-spectrum antiinflammatory protocol (trimethoprim sulfa, 15 mg/kg BID; clindamycin, 12.5 mg/kg BID; prednisone, 0.5 mg/kg BID) while awaiting more definitive results, including bacterial culture and viral and protozoal titers. Diagnostic testing should always be performed before any treatment since it may affect CSF analysis and culture results. In addition, glucocorticoids may attenuate the increased blood-brain barrier permeability that results from inflammation, thereby theoretically reducing antimicrobial penetration into the CSF. Clinical studies in small animals with bacterial meningitis that address antibiotic penetration in the face of glucocorticoids are lacking, and long-term consequences of glucocorticoid therapy for infectious meningitis have not been established.

Disseminated/Miscellaneous Infections

Glucocorticoids are used frequently in conjunction with antimicrobials for hemolytic anemia or thrombocytopenia while awaiting results to differentiate a primary immune-mediated hemolytic process from hemolytic disease secondary to an infectious organism such as *Babesia* spp. or *Mycoplasma* spp. Common belief holds that immune-mediated destruction contributes to anemia or thrombocytopenia with these infections and the addition of glucocorticoids may decrease this damage, but there are no controlled studies demonstrating proof of efficacy. In one study glucocorticoid-treated dogs infected by *Rickettsia rickettsii*–induced Rocky Mountain spotted fever (RMSF) did not show evidence of dissemination of disease (Breitschwerdt, et al., 1997). Because treatment with antimicrobials for RMSF is often effective for improving clinical signs within 1 to 2 days of initiating therapy, the need to use glucocorticoids should be based on a case-by-case basis and is not recommended for routine treatment.

Of the many canine and feline infectious diseases, treatment of cats with feline infectious peritonitis (FIP) with glucocorticoids would be a logical application of the drugs, given the key role that immunopathogenesis plays in the clinical disease. Glucocorticoids are often recommended for FIP, despite clinical studies failing to demonstrate the benefits of glucocorticoids. One study has suggested the benefit of concurrent use of recombinant feline interferon and glucocorticoid administration to cats with FIP, but the report included no controls, and the diagnosis of FIP was not confirmed in all cases (Ishida, et al., 2004). Treatment of other systemic infections with glucocorticoids, including *Mycoplasma haemofelis*, and *Babesia canis*, has no support in controlled clinical studies, although glucocorticoids are commonly used in the treatment of patients infected with these organisms.

Juvenile cellulitis (puppy strangles) is a syndrome of facial swelling, lymphadenopathy, deep pyoderma of the head and face, fever, polyarthritis, anorexia, and depression. The disease is seen most often in young dogs and is attributed to immune-mediated responses to bacterial antigens. Affected patients usually respond to antimicrobials and immunosuppressive doses of glucocorticoids, and available literature provides reasonable (although not case-controlled) evidence for the use of immunosuppressive doses of glucocorticoids in the management of this disease. The disease may recur if corticosteroid therapy is tapered too quickly; thus a slower tapering protocol may be required.

Sepsis/Systemic Inflammatory Response Syndrome/Acute Respiratory Distress Syndrome/Relative Adrenal Insufficiency

Systemic inflammatory response syndrome (SIRS) is a term used to describe the clinical consequences of severe systemic inflammation. Severe systemic inflammation can result in secondary conditions such as disseminated intravascular coagulopathy, acute respiratory distress syndrome (ARDS), and multiple organ dysfunction syndrome. Dysregulated systemic inflammation is a major contributor to the morbidity and mortality in sepsis and ARDS. Relative adrenal insufficiency (RAI) is defined as a usually transient lack of response to endogenous or exogenous adrenocorticotropic hormone (ACTH) and occurs in patients with widespread systemic inflammation (also see Chapter 50). Suspicion of RAI is often based on poor systemic pressures despite appropriate hydration (central venous pressures ranging between 5 and 10 cm of water) and vasopressor (dobutamine, norepinephrine) dependency. RAI occurs with relative frequency in human septic SIRS patients and has been described recently in septic dogs (Burkitt, et al., 2007). Human studies have demonstrated that a short course of physiologic doses of glucocorticoids improves clinical outcomes in patients with sepsis. It is likely that future studies will show similar benefits for dogs with sepsis and RAI.

CONSIDERATIONS FOR GLUCOCORTICOID USE

Prednisone and prednisolone are ideal glucocorticoids for use in patients with infectious disease because of their short duration of activity (12 to 36 hours). Prednisolone sodium succinate (Solu-Delta-Cortef, Pfizer Animal Health) or methylprednisolone sodium succinate (Solu-Medrol, Upjohn) are parenteral formulations that may be used if patients are unable to take oral formulations. Dexamethasone would be an additional alternative for these patients, but its activity is approximately 48 hours, making it perhaps a less ideal first choice. Given its long storage life and because it is relatively inexpensive compared to other glucocorticoids, practitioners may elect to use dexamethasone. Depot formulations such as methyl-prednisolone acetate (Depo-Medrol, Upjohn) are not recommended because of their long duration of activity.

Dosage

Systematic evaluation of glucocorticoid dosages in small animal infectious disease patients has not been performed. Typical therapeutic ranges (Table 267-1) to achieve either antiinflammatory or immunosuppressive effects have been suggested. Ideally therapy with glucocorticoids should be initiated at the lowest doses needed to obtain the desired clinical response. Clinicians should be aware of the relative potencies of the commonly used glucocorticoids (Table 267-2) when selecting a glucocorticoid and dose.

Duration of Glucocorticoid Treatment

If the correct underlying cause has been identified and antiinfective treatment is effective, clinical improvement usually occurs within days. It is our recommendation that concurrent glucocorticoid therapy should last only as long as needed to achieve and maintain the desired clinical response—in some patients that period may be days, in others weeks. The decision to stop glucocorticoid therapy depends on the patient's clinical status, clinician preference, and potential for clinical relapse or deterioration.

Common belief holds that glucocorticoid tapering is needed to prevent signs of iatrogenic hypoadrenocorticism. It is our view that tapering is better suited to identify early relapse or recurrence of the syndrome requiring glucocorticoid therapy. If the need arises to acutely stop glucocorticoids, theoretically a clinician should immediately be able to reduce the amount given to a physiologic dose and prevent clinical signs associated with iatrogenic hypoadrenocorticism. Our argument is based on the fact that dogs with glucocorticoid deficiency from spontaneous hypoadrenocorticism fare well with prednisone given at physiologic or slightly higher doses (0.2 to 0.4 mg/kg/day). If the reduction in dose is well tolerated, a brief period of alternate-day therapy should allow return of normal adrenal function. The time period for return of normal adrenal function depends on many variables, including dose, formulation, duration of therapy, and variation in patient response preventing any absolute recommendations. In general, longer durations of therapy with higher doses or use of formulations with greater duration of activity may require a longer period of dose reduction for return of normal adrenal function. Periodic testing in the form of drug cessation trials or ACTH stimulation may be required if iatrogenic hypoadrenocorticism is suspected. A period of dose reduction should also be considered when treating patients concurrently with glucocorticoids and ketoconazole for systemic fungal infections since ketoconazole impairs adrenal glucocorticoid synthesis and could lead to transient iatrogenic hypoadrenocorticism.

Adverse Effects of Glucocorticoids With Infectious Disease

Apart from the usual side effects of glucocorticoids, there is virtually no information on small animal patients that addresses adverse effects of glucocorticoids when given concurrently with antiinfective therapy. The potential for immunosuppression and exacerbation of existing infection or development of additional infections is a valid concern, yet it seldom seems to be recognized clinically. Perhaps it is more important that the clinician not be lulled into a false sense of security regarding apparent positive responses in patients with infections also treated with glucocorticoids. A patient could improve initially because of antiinflammatory properties and yet worsen with time because of decreased immunologic clearance of infectious organisms and progressive infection, particularly if antiinfective therapy is ineffective. Theoretically

Table 267-1

Glucocorticoid Dosing Recommendations (mg/kg/day)

Glucocorticoid	Physiologic Replacement	Antiinflammatory	Immune Suppression
Hydrocortisone	0.5-1.0	2.5-5	Not used
Prednisone	0.1-0.2	0.5-1	2-4 (dog); 4-8 (cat)
Dexamethasone	0.02-0.04	0.1-0.2	0.4-0.8

Table 267-2

Relative Glucocorticoid Potency of Formulations Likely To Be Used in Patients With Infectious Disease

Glucocorticoid	Potency Relative to Hydrocortisone
Hydrocortisone	1
Prednisone/prednisolone	5
Dexamethasone	25

supraphysiologic doses of glucocorticoids could inhibit the inflammation that is necessary for wound repair and retard healing. When adverse effects are suspected secondary to immunosuppression (worsening of disease), rapid reduction of glucocorticoid doses as suggested previously may be required.

The etiologic agents of some infections such as endocarditis may be hard to confirm despite appropriate testing (blood cultures, urine cultures). Treatment with glucocorticoids may increase the chance of recovery of an organism such as *Bartonella* (Dr. Ed Breitschwerdt, personal communication) but glucocorticoids are not advised for that specific intent.

GUIDELINES FOR USE OF GLUCOCORTICOIDS WITH INFECTIONS

We believe that some patients with infections benefit from treatment with antiinflammatory or occasionally higher doses of glucocorticoids. We suspect that this view is held by many other clinicians despite the absence of rigorous evaluation of glucocorticoid use in small animal infections. When using glucocorticoids in patients with infectious disease, whenever possible we try to adhere to the following guidelines:

- Diagnostic studies to identify the specific cause of infection should be completed before the administration of glucocorticoids.
- Glucocorticoid treatment should be implemented after or at the same time as antiinfective therapy.
- The decision to administer glucocorticoids to patients with an infection should be made on a case-by-case basis that weighs the patient's clinical status and relative benefits against the potential risks of complications and adverse effects.
- Glucocorticoid administration should not form a blanket approach to treatment of a given infectious agent.
- Doses of glucocorticoids should be appropriate for the goal of therapy (e.g., antiinflammatory, immunosuppressive, or physiologic replacement for patients with RAI).

- Administration of glucocorticoids with short or intermediate duration of activity (e.g., prednisone) is preferred to glucocorticoids with longer durations of antiinflammatory or immunosuppressive activity; depot forms of glucocorticoids are not advised.
- Glucocorticoids should be administered at the lowest dosages and for no longer than needed to achieve and maintain desired clinical responses.
- Patients treated with glucocorticoids should be assessed regularly and carefully for complications of therapy, particularly progressive infection. Because glucocorticoid administration can attenuate the very patient responses that alert clinicians to the existence of problems (e.g., fever, pain) that could otherwise suggest clinical deterioration in patients not receiving glucocorticoids, enhanced attention is warranted.
- In some patients receiving glucocorticoids concurrently with antiinfective therapy (e.g., those with systemic fungal infections), the duration of the antiinfective treatment period should be extended.
- Owners should be advised of the potential risks associated with a treatment approach (glucocorticoids for infection) that lacks support of appropriately performed clinical studies.

In summary, predominately anecdotal evidence supports the administration of glucocorticoids to some dogs and cats with infectious disease. Definitive studies that examine the benefits or complications of its use are needed to better characterize the indications and contraindications to the administration of glucocorticoids to such patients.

Suggested Reading

Breitschwerdt EB et al: Prednisolone at anti-inflammatory or immunosuppressive dosages in conjunction with doxycycline does not potentiate the severity of *Rickettsia rickettsii* infection in dogs, *Antimicrob Agents Chemother* 41:141, 1997.

Burkitt JM et al: Relative adrenal insufficiency in dogs with sepsis *J Vet Intern Med* 21:226, 2007.

Ishida T et al: Use of recombinant feline interferon and glucocorticoid in the treatment of feline infectious peritonitis, *J Feline Med Surg* 6:107, 2004.

Minneci PC et al: Meta-analysis: the effect of steroids on survival and shock during sepsis depends on the dose, *Ann Intern Med* 141:47, 2004.

Schulman RL, McKiernan BC, Schaeffer DJ: Use of corticosteroids for treating dogs with airway obstruction secondary to hilar lymphadenopathy caused by chronic histoplasmosis: 16 cases, (1979-1997), *J Am Vet Med Assoc* 214:1345, 1999.

Simmons CP et al: The clinical benefit of adjunctive dexamethasone in tuberculous meningitis is not associated with measurable attenuation of peripheral or local immune responses, *J Immunol* 175:579, 2005.

White SD et al: Juvenile cellulitis in dogs: 15 cases (1979-1988), *J Am Vet Med Assoc* 195:1609, 1989.

CHAPTER 268

Canine Brucellosis

AUTUMN P. DAVIDSON, *Davis, California*

Brucellosis is the primary contagious infectious venereal disease of concern in canine reproduction. *Brucella canis* causes reproductive failure in both the male and female dog. Screening for *B. canis* is an important part of the prebreeding evaluation of any dog and should be included in the initial diagnostic approach to any case of canine abortion or apparent infertility. Because the incidence of canine brucellosis is low in many parts of the country, breeder compliance with regular testing can wane, making continued veterinary vigilance important.

ETIOLOGY AND MICROBIOLOGY

Canine brucellosis is caused by *B. canis*, a small, gram-negative, nonspore forming aerobic coccobacillus. *Brucella abortus*, *Brucella melitensis,* and *Brucella suis* have occasionally caused canine infections but are comparatively very rare. Transmission occurs through direct exposure to bodily fluids (semen, lochia, aborted fetuses/placentas, milk, and less commonly urine containing semen) containing an infectious dose of organism. A large amount of organism is shed in the vulvar discharge of bitches 4 to 6 weeks after abortion. The highest concentration of organism is shed in the semen of infected dogs 2 to 3 months after infection, with lesser amounts shed for years. Urine can serve as a contaminated vehicle because of the proximity of the urinary and genital tracts in the dog. Milk also can serve as a vehicle for shedding. Therefore transmission is primarily venereal and oral (i.e., through the mucous membranes); the latter is associated with the ingestion of infectious materials. Urine and indirect mucous membrane contact are not important routes of transmission. The aerosol route is only important if kennel conditions are very crowded. *B. canis* is short lived outside the dog and is readily inactivated by common disinfectants such as 1% sodium hypochlorite, 70% ethanol, iodine/alcohol solutions, glutaraldehyde, and formaldehyde.

Brucella organisms attach to and penetrate the mucous membranes; virulence is proportional to the infectious dose. After replication in regional lymph nodes, bacteremia occurs within 7 to 30 days after exposure with subsequent transportation to monocyte/macrophage series cells, prostate, uterus, and placenta; *B. canis* has a predilection for steroid-dependent (reproductive) tissues. It survives facultatively within monocytes and macrophages. *Brucella* organisms are able to survive and multiply in monocyte/macrophage cells because they inhibit the bactericidal myeloperoxidase-peroxide-halide system by releasing 5′-guanosine and adenine. Early in infection polymorphonuclear cells and macrophages are relatively ineffectual in killing *B. canis* intracellularly.

Brucella organisms can be identified in the rough endoplastic reticulum of placental trophoblastic giant cells in an infected bitch's gravid uterus. Severe necrotizing placentitis with infarction of the labyrinth region, coagulation necrosis of the chorionic villi, and necrotizing arteritis result in fetal death. The organism can be found in the gastric contents of the aborted fetuses. Necrotizing vasculitis causing granulomatous lesions results in epididymal and subsequent testicular and prostatic pathology.

EPIZOOTIOLOGY

Members of the Canidae family are the natural hosts of *B. canis*; and any mature, reproductively active breed of dog is susceptible to infection. Canine brucellosis occurs most commonly as an outbreak in a large commercial kennel and less commonly in privately owned dogs. Outbreaks of canine brucellosis traditionally have geographic orientation, with increased incidence seen in the southernmost states of the United States and more commonly in Mexico, Central and South America, The People's Republic of China, and Japan. The incidence in Europe has been low. The increased practice and success of canine semen processing for exportation (chilling and cryopreservation) for the purpose of artificial insemination now makes canine brucellosis a concern worldwide since direct mucosal contact among dogs is no longer necessary for transmission.

Humans can become infected with *B. canis,* although apparently rarely. Approximately 40 cases of human infection have been reported in several countries; however, the actual number is unknown since human cases are rarely diagnosed or, if diagnosed, reported. Transmission to humans most commonly occurs through contact with semen from an infected dog, vulvar discharge from an infected bitch, aborted fetuses or placentas, or direct accidental laboratory exposure.

CLINICAL SIGNS

Canine brucellosis has high morbidity but low mortality. The clinical systemic signs are often subtle and can include suboptimal athletic performance, lumbar pain, lameness, weight loss, and lethargy.

The primary clinical sign of brucellosis in the bitch is pregnancy loss, which can occur early (day 20) in gestation, resulting in fetal resorption, or more commonly (approximately 75% of cases) later in gestation (generally 45 to 59 days), resulting in abortion. Bitches with pregnancy loss early in gestation can appear to be infertile unless early ultrasonographic pregnancy evaluation is performed. Nongravid bitches can be asymptomatic or can show regional lymphadenopathy (pharyngeal if orally acquired, inguinal and pelvic if venereally acquired).

The primary acute clinical signs of brucellosis in the male dog reflect disease of the portions of the reproductive tract participating in the maturation, transport, and storage of spermatozoa. Epididymitis is common, with associated orchitis, scrotal dermatitis, and resultant deterioration of semen quality and fertility. Chronically testicular atrophy and infertility can occur. The organism can be found in the prostate gland and urine. Antisperm antibodies develop in association with brucellosis-induced epididymal granulomas and further contribute to infertility. Diminished sperm counts (oligospermia), poor sperm motility (asthenospermia), and increased morphologic abnormalities (teratospermia) are characteristic of semen in a *Brucella*-infected dog. Detached sperm heads, proximal and distal cytoplasmic droplets, and acrosomal deformities are the most common morphologic abnormalities. Sperm head-to-head agglutination suggests the presence of antisperm antibodies. Pyospermia develops 3 to 4 months after infection. An absence of sperm in the ejaculate (azoospermia) can also result.

Chronic infections in either sex can result in uveitis, granulomatous splenitis, discospondylitis, granulomatous dermatitis, meningoencephalitis, and nephritis. Bacteremia can persist for years, and asymptomatic dogs can remain infectious for long intervals.

Spontaneous recovery can occur 1 to 5 years after infection but is difficult to document. Bitches can produce normal litters subsequent to multiple abortions but can remain infectious to their offspring. Dogs may remain infertile because of irreparable damage to the spermatogenic apparatus.

DIAGNOSIS

Serology, blood or tissue culture, histopathology, and polymerase chain reaction (PCR) techniques are appropriate for the diagnosis of canine brucellosis. Common screening serologic tests include the rapid slide agglutination test (RSAT), which uses *B. ovis* as the antigen; the semiquantitative 2-mercaptoethanol modified RSAT, which substitutes *B. canis* as the antigen for increased (but not perfect) specificity; the semiquantitative tube agglutination test, in which a titer of 1:200 or greater correlates well with positive blood culture; the indirect fluorescent antibody; the cell wall agar gel immunodiffusion (AGIDcwa); the cytoplasmic agar gel immunodiffusion (AGIDcpa); and the enzyme-linked immunosorbent assay. AGID testing requires trained personnel and special media. Positive serologic results are detected in most dogs within 8 to 12 weeks of infection. Because incubation periods can vary from 2 to 12 weeks, there can be a window of time in which an infected individual may elude serologic diagnosis.

Correct interpretation of serologic results is critical to making an accurate diagnosis. Screening serology is sensitive but not specific: a high rate of false positives occurs because surface antigens of *B. canis* cross-react strongly with antibodies to several other nonpathogenic bacterial species. False-positive rates can be as high as 50% to 60% because of cross-reacting antibodies to *Bordetella* spp.,

Pseudomonas spp., *Moraxella* spp., and *B. ovis*. For patients with positive results on a screening serologic test, confirmatory testing (see following paragraphs) is needed because of the high incidence of false positives. For this reason screening tests are recommended at least 1 month before a planned breeding to give time for more accurate confirmatory testing if the initial screening test is positive. False-negative results with screening serologic tests are very rare. A false negative can occur if a recently infected dog or bitch is less than 8 to 12 weeks postinfective exposure and seroconversion has not yet occurred. Otherwise a negative test is usually indicative of a truly negative dog.

Despite improvements in serologic diagnostic methods, confirmatory blood cultures have classically been indicated when the disease is suspected. *B. canis* is readily isolated from the blood of bacteremic individuals for several months after infection. A positive *B. canis* culture establishes a definitive diagnosis and has been advocated as the best diagnostic test in the first 2 months of the disease; however, dogs can become abacteremic after 27 to 64 months.

B. canis is an aerobe; but, unlike other *Brucella* spp., the addition of CO_2 (5% to 10%) may be inhibitory. Multiplication is slow at the optimum temperature of $37° C$, and enriched medium (tryptose or trypticase soy media) is needed to support adequate growth. *Brucella* colonies become visible on suitable solid media in 2 to 3 days. A culture can be identified as belonging to the genus *Brucella* on the basis of colony morphology, staining, and slide agglutination with anti-*Brucella* serum. Further classification is best done in a specialized laboratory (Carmichael and Joubert, 1998). In the United States the New York State Diagnostic Laboratory at Cornell University, the Tifton Veterinary Diagnostic and Investigational Laboratory in Georgia, and the University of Florida are recognized as reliable laboratories for definitive testing made necessary by initial positive *B. canis* screening tests in dogs intended for breeding, for clinically affected dogs undergoing evaluation for infertility or abortion, or when outbreaks are under clinical management.

Recently a report of successful PCR identification of *B. canis* in semen from dogs failing to have organisms microbiologically identified suggests that PCR-based assays may be the most sensitive method of testing. Thus PCR testing could be considered as part of the male dog prebreeding evaluation, especially in cases in which management of an outbreak is the concern (Keid et al., 2007).

Brucellosis may be a reportable disease in either the dog or human in certain jurisdictions. Agglutinating antibodies are not protective in the dog.

THERAPY

Infected dogs and bitches should be removed from breeding programs and neutered to minimize transmission potential. Historically antibiotic therapy has not been rewarding, likely because the organism is intracellular and bacteremia periodic. Antibiotic therapy may reduce antibody titers without clearing the infection. Relapses are common. Combination therapy with tetracyclines (doxycycline or minocycline 25 mg/kg BID orally [PO] for

4 weeks) and dihydrostreptomycin (10 to 20 mg/kg BID intramuscularly [IM] or subcutaneously [SC] for 2 weeks, week 1 and 4) or an aminoglycoside (gentamicin 2.5 mg/kg BID IM or SC for 2 weeks, week 1 and 4) has been advocated as most successful; but unavailability, nephrotoxicity, parenteral therapy requirements, and expense remain problematic (Greene and Carmichael, 2006).

Recently one study reported an encouraging outcome of therapy with enrofloxacin (5 mg/kg BID PO for 4 weeks) in a small group of infected dogs and bitches (Wanke, Delpino, and Balth, 2006). Enrofloxacin was not completely efficacious in eliminating *B. canis*, but it maintained fertility and avoided the recurrence of abortions, transmission of the disease to subsequently whelped puppies, and dissemination of microorganisms during parturition.

PREVENTION

Attempts to develop an appropriate vaccination capable of inducing immunity yet not provoking serologic responses that interfere with the diagnosis have not been successful. Presently the development of a vaccination is considered undesirable since the *Brucella* vaccinations evaluated to date have offered only moderate protection and immunized dogs have developed antibodies confounding the serodiagnosis.

Prevention of infection and elimination of infected dogs should be the principal control strategy in kennels. Prevention requires annual testing of all breeding stock and the testing of all dogs to be introduced into a kennel. Ideally two negative screening tests should be obtained at least a month apart before a dog or bitch is introduced into a breeding facility. Confirmed positive dogs should be isolated (euthanasia is advised by many authors),

neutered, treated, and tested monthly (AGID, culture, or PCR) until two consecutive negative tests occur, recognizing that occult infection can still be present.

Private breeders should require screening tests of all bitches presented for breeding and negative results on confirmatory tests if positive results occur during screening before accepting a bitch into their kennel. Stud dogs should be screened appropriately at least annually. Because of the potential for oral transmission, screening of maiden dogs and bitches before breeding is also recommended.

References and Suggested Reading

Barr SC et al: *Brucella suis* biotype 1 infection in a dog, *J Am Vet Med Assoc* 189(6):686, 1986.

Carmichael LE, Joubert JC: Transmission of *Brucella canis* by contact exposure, *Cornell Vet* 78:63, 1998.

Greene CE, Carmichael LE: Canine brucellosis. In Greene CE, editor: *Infectious diseases of the dog and cat*, ed 3, Philadelphia, 2006, Saunders, p 369.

Hollet RB: Canine brucellosis outbreaks and compliance, *Theriogenology* 66(3):75, 2006.

Johnson CA, Walker RD: Clinical signs and diagnosis of *Brucella canis* infection, *Compend Contin Educ Pract Vet* 14:763, 1992.

Keid LB et al: A polymerase chain reaction for the detection of *Brucella canis* in semen of naturally infected dogs, *Theriogenology* 67(7):1203, 2007.

Shin SJ, Carmichael LE: Canine brucellosis caused by *Brucella canis*. In Carmichael L, editor: *Recent advances in canine infectious diseases*, Ithaca NY, 1999, International Veterinary Information Service.

Wanke MM, Delpino MV, Balth PC: Use of enrofloxacin in the treatment of canine brucellosis in a dog kennel (clinical trial), *Theriogenology* 66(7):1573, 2006.

CHAPTER 269

Leptospirosis

KENNETH R. HARKIN, *Manhattan, Kansas*

Canine leptospirosis has been considered a reemerging infection in the United States beginning in the mid-1990s. Similarly, leptospirosis is considered the most globally widespread zoonotic disease, with recent increases in human cases acquired in all settings. Beginning in 2003 and continuing through 2005, an outbreak of canine leptospirosis in Colorado emphasized the need for continued vigilance in recognizing clinical leptospirosis, even in areas where the disease is considered rare. The purpose of this chapter is to present updated information on leptospirosis and discussions of controversial aspects rather than provide a comprehensive overview of the disease.

EPIDEMIOLOGY

Leptospirosis is maintained in domestic and wildlife reservoir hosts in which renal colonization occurs. Leptospiruria results in contamination of surface water, which can include not only lakes, rivers, ponds, and streams but also muddy fields, water bowls, birdbaths, and other stagnant water sources. The prolonged phase of renal colonization and leptospiruria in maintenance hosts, particularly burrowing rodents, is responsible for survival and transmission of the organism in even inhospitable desert environments. Peridomestic wildlife reservoirs, including raccoons, opossums, voles, rats, and other rodents, are the most important in the transmission of disease to dogs in suburban and urban areas, particularly for serovar Grippotyphosa. Endemic infections in cattle and swine herds, along with wildlife, are important in disease transmission to dogs in rural environments.

Based on serologic surveys, Grippotyphosa appears to be the most prevalent infecting serovar of dogs in the United States, although a retrospective study identified Pomona and Bratislava as the most prevalent serovars infecting dogs in northern California, with no significant number of Grippotyphosa infections. Another recent serologic survey (Moore et al., 2006) suggested that serovar Autumnalis was now most prevalent, at least for exposure. However, there are questions as to the relevance of titers to serovar Autumnalis. In a recent study (Barr et al., 2005) dogs that were vaccinated with a leptospirosis vaccine containing serovars Grippotyphosa and Pomona developed elevated titers to serovar Autumnalis without concomitant equivalent increases in titers to serovar Grippotyphosa. The rise in serologically documented cases of Autumnalis correlates with the inclusion of serovars Grippotyphosa and Pomona in the leptospirosis vaccine, and the seropositivity to Autumnalis correlates strongest to serovar Pomona. These findings support the possibility that the increase in positive titers to serovar Autumnalis is a reflection of vaccination and not a true increase in Autumnalis infection rates.

A number of retrospective studies have consistently shown that the vast majority of cases ($\approx$80%) are diagnosed between July and December and most are in dogs in suburban and rural environments. Large-breed dogs are more commonly affected, likely because of the tendency for them to be outside and participating in activities that increase their exposure; and there is a possible breed predisposition in the German shepherd. The potential predisposition for German shepherds has been identified in a number of studies (Ward et al., 2002). A possible explanation for this breed predisposition is suggested by an investigation of human triathletes who contracted leptospirosis in Illinois and Wisconsin. That study documented that humans with the major histocompatibility (MHC) phenotype HLA DQ6 were at greater risk of infection than individuals who did not carry the phenotype. It is also possible that the predisposition for German shepherds is associated with immunoglobulin A deficiency, a relatively common problem in the breed and not a specific MHC phenotype.

DISEASE SYNDROMES

Acute renal failure is the most commonly recognized disease syndrome in dogs, accounting for more than 90% of reported cases. These dogs often present with anorexia, depression, and vomiting and may also demonstrate arthralgia or myalgia, icterus, polyuria and polydipsia, dyspnea from pulmonary hemorrhage or pneumonitis, and oculonasal discharge. Uveitis may be subtle and is present in a large number of dogs with acute renal failure from leptospirosis. Uveitis goes unrecognized in most dogs, particularly when a qualified ophthalmologist is not available for consultation.

Hepatic failure occurs concurrently in 10% to 20% of dogs with acute renal failure but may also be present independently. These dogs typically have moderate-to-marked elevations in serum alanine transaminase (ALT), serum alkaline phosphatase (ALP), and bilirubin, although ALP elevations are typically higher than ALT elevations. Polyuria and polydipsia may occur in the absence of azotemia or any other laboratory abnormalities, and dogs may appear relatively healthy despite their profound polyuria. Urine specific gravity in these dogs is often hyposthenuric, and the urine sediment is usually inactive. The profound polyuria is often misdiagnosed as central diabetes insipidus. Marked fever (often in excess of 40°C) of 2 to 4 days' duration in the absence of clinicopathologic abnormalities often occurs days to weeks before the onset of nonazotemic polyuria and polydipsia. Less commonly seen syndromes include intestinal intussusceptions, pleural and pericardial effusion, transverse myelitis, and meningitis.

OUTER MEMBRANE PROTEINS

The outer membrane proteins (OMPs) of pathogenic leptospires play a critical role in pathogenicity and development of the host immune response. Antibodies produced to specific proteins are currently under investigation as diagnostic markers, opening up the possibility of commercial diagnostic tests that do not rely on maintenance of stock cultures of leptospires. The expression of certain OMPs is down-regulated in infection, suggesting that they play a role in survival of the organism outside of the host, but would have no usefulness in vaccine development or serodiagnosis. However, the expression of other OMPs is up-regulated during infection, and these OMPs are potential candidates for vaccine development and diagnostic tests.

LipL32, which may be a hemolysin, is the major OMP of pathogenic leptospires and is expressed both in vitro and in vivo. Its expression is conserved in pathogenic leptospires, and antibodies to LipL32 are consistently identified in sera from infected patients. Although it is immunogenic, LipL32 does not appear to confer protective immunity independently of other OMPs. The transmembrane protein OmpL1 and lipoprotein LipL41 are also conservatively expressed in pathogenic leptospires during infection. Independently they do not confer immunity, but when combined they have a synergistic effect that provides protective immunity. Lig A and Lig B are immunoglobulin-like proteins that can confer protective immunity independently, are up-regulated during infection, and have great promise as vaccine candidates. Their role in pathogenicity is unclear, but leptospires that lose their Lig proteins and *lig* ribonucleic acid transcript expression lose their virulence.

DIAGNOSIS

Leptospirosis should be considered as one of the primary differential diagnoses for any dog that presents with acute renal failure for which the cause is not immediately identified (e.g., ethylene glycol poisoning, pyelonephritis, or aminoglycoside administration). In addition, for any of the previously described disease syndromes of leptospirosis, failure to consider leptospirosis will result in a failure to diagnose.

The microscopic agglutination test (MAT) remains the gold standard for the diagnosis of leptospirosis. Most veterinary diagnostic laboratories in the United States evaluate for antibodies against serovars Canicola, Icterohaemorrhagiae, Grippotyphosa, Pomona, and Hardjo; many also include Bratislava and a few include Autumnalis. Titers of at least 1:800 are supportive of a diagnosis when compatible clinical findings are present, but documentation of a fourfold rising titer over a 2- to 4-week interval is preferred to confirm the diagnosis. When a 2-week convalescent titer is not convincing, a 4-week titer is recommended for confirmation of infection. Identification of

the infecting serovar is not important for therapy but may have epidemiologic significance, especially during outbreaks of disease.

Interpretation of the MAT can be complicated by cross-reactivity, often resulting in equivalently elevated titers to multiple serovars, although the infecting serovar usually provokes the most persistently elevated titer over time. Coinfection with multiple serovars has not been documented. Prior vaccination may also complicate the interpretation of titers obtained by the MAT. Dogs that have been vaccinated recently may have titers as high as 1:3200. Although vaccinal titers often wane within 3 to 4 months, some dogs may have persistently elevated titers. As discussed previously, dogs that have been vaccinated may have elevated titers to nonvaccinal serovars, further complicating the diagnosis. In some cases of leptospirosis dogs may not develop a titer, either because the infecting serovar is not included on the MAT panel or the dog just does not develop an appropriate antibody response. Other diagnostic tests may be necessary in these instances.

The polymerase chain reaction (PCR) assay has promise in the diagnosis of leptospirosis and is available at a number of veterinary diagnostic laboratories. The diagnostic sample of choice is urine (a minimum of 3 to 6 ml is recommended), which can be obtained by free catch, catheterization, or cystocentesis. Other samples (e.g., aqueous humor, fresh kidney or liver, semen, blood, or cerebrospinal fluid) can be evaluated by PCR but are not submitted routinely. There is no appreciable degradation of leptospiral deoxyribonucleic acid (DNA) when the sample is held at room temperature for 72 hours; but, because of the possibility of shipping delays and seasonal high temperatures, the sample should be sent by next-day or 2-day carrier with an ice pack. A positive result indicates that leptospiral DNA was identified in the sample, supporting the diagnosis of leptospirosis. The immune system is efficient at rapidly removing dead leptospires from the kidney; thus, even though it is possible that the PCR is identifying dead leptospires, it is more likely that the sample contains live leptospires. Although the possibility of false-positive results exists from sample contamination, this is an unlikely event in most laboratories. The PCR has the advantage of sensitivity, becoming positive before seroconversion in some dogs, a finding that was confirmed in humans when various tests for the diagnosis of leptospirosis were compared, although most dogs are positive by both serology and PCR when evaluated. Dogs with leptospirosis may have a negative PCR if the number of leptospires in the sample is below the limit of detection of the test, if PCR is performed before establishment of leptospiruria, or if the patient had been treated with appropriate antibiotic therapy before testing. Dogs that are initially PCR positive in the urine will usually still be positive if tested 3 days after initiating intravenous ampicillin therapy. Unlike the MAT, the PCR fails to identify the infecting serovar but is specific for pathogenic leptospires.

Fluorescent-antibody (FA) testing, aimed at identifying the leptospiral organism in urine or tissue, is available at some veterinary diagnostic laboratories. Although the sensitivity of FA testing is better than dark-field microscopic evaluation of urine or silver staining of tissue, its sensitivity does not match that of PCR. Likewise, nonspecific binding of the antibody may result in false-positive results.

A number of diagnostic tests, including dark-field microscopy (low sensitivity), silver staining of tissues (low sensitivity and specificity), and culture (low sensitivity, requires special media) have very little use to most veterinarians. I recommend the combination of the MAT and PCR for optimizing the diagnosis of leptospirosis.

THERAPY

There are two main components of therapy for leptospirosis: supportive and specific. Supportive therapy for dogs with acute renal failure from leptospirosis traditionally centers on fluid therapy. Polyuric renal failure is more common than oliguric or anuric renal failure, simplifying fluid management. When oliguric or anuric renal failure ensues, management of fluid therapy becomes more complex. Both hemodialysis and peritoneal dialysis have been used successfully in the management of oliguric and anuric renal failure caused by leptospirosis.

The cornerstone of specific therapy is the administration of an appropriate antibiotic. Traditionally ampicillin is used initially in the dog acutely ill with leptospirosis. Recommended ampicillin dosages range from 22 to 40 mg/kg intravenously every 6 to 8 hours, although 25 mg/kg intravenously every 8 hours appears safe and effective. Ampicillin should eliminate the leptospiremic phase but does not eliminate the organism from the renal tubules. The recommendation to continue amoxicillin once oral administration can be tolerated appears rooted in the past treatment standard of penicillin therapy for 2 weeks followed by 2 weeks of dihydrostreptomycin. Dihydrostreptomycin therapy was directed at eliminating the leptospiruric phase but was delayed until full recovery from renal failure was achieved.

Doxycycline eliminates all phases of leptospiral infection and does not carry the nephrotoxic potential seen with other tetracyclines. Although it would be appropriate to administer doxycycline intravenously from the point of initial diagnosis, I still prefer to administer ampicillin initially in acutely ill dogs and then transition to doxycycline at 5 mg/kg orally every 12 hours as soon as oral medications can be tolerated. A treatment course with doxycycline of 3 to 4 weeks is recommended. Dogs with leptospirosis that are not vomiting can be administered doxycycline orally as the first-line of therapy.

Ciprofloxacin has been shown to be effective in the treatment of leptospirosis (improved survival versus the untreated group), and it is suspected that other fluoroquinolones would be equally effective. However, ofloxacin was ineffective in eliminating renal infection in a hamster model of leptospirosis; thus fluoroquinolones may not be an acceptable substitute for doxycycline. The ability of the fluoroquinolones to cross the blood-brain barrier may make them attractive for parenteral use when uveitis or meningitis is present. Although most dogs stop shedding leptospires in the urine soon after beginning doxycycline therapy, I have followed three dogs that remained PCR positive for leptospires in the urine for prolonged periods (>60 days) and became PCR negative only after the administration of enrofloxacin at 5 mg/kg orally every 12 hours.

In specific situations the use of corticosteroids (dexamethasone, 0.25 mg/kg intravenously [IV] q12h; or prednisone, 2 mg/kg orally [PO] q24h) may be indicated in the management of leptospirosis. Although thrombocytopenia is typically mild (80,000 to 120,000/μL), in the rare case that develops severe thrombocytopenia (<20,000/μL) with bleeding corticosteroid administration is indicated. Severe thrombocytopenia is a consequence of Kupffer cell phagocytosis and not disseminated intravascular coagulation. In addition, when the serum creatinine continues to climb for more than 10 days despite appropriate fluid therapy and in the presence of polyuria, corticosteroid therapy may help resolve renal parenchymal inflammation and swelling, which may be self-perpetuating despite appropriate leptospirocidal therapy.

PREVENTION

The primary reasons for promoting leptospirosis vaccinations in dogs are minimizing mortality from severe leptospirosis and preventing zoonotic disease. Based on a number of retrospective clinical studies on canine leptospirosis, the overall mortality rate (failure to leave the hospital after acute onset disease) is approximately 20%. A smaller number of dogs develop chronic renal failure, which ultimately results in a shortened life span. Not every dog with environmental exposure to leptospires develops clinical disease (dependent on strain pathogenicity, size of inoculum, previous exposure), but one cannot predict which dogs will fall ill and which ones will die. In my experience German shepherds tend to be at the greatest risk of developing the worst clinical syndromes and have the gravest prognosis. A recent study suggested that serovar Pomona infections were more likely to result in mortality than other serovars.

It is a long-held belief that a humoral immune response and the presence of antibodies at the time of a challenge are responsible for clearing/preventing infection from leptospirosis. This belief has created controversy in recommendations of annual versus semiannual vaccinations since it is well documented that in most animals vaccine titers do not persist for more than 3 to 4 months. However, this paradigm has been challenged. In a recent study (Klaasen et al., 2003) dogs given two vaccines 4 weeks apart were protected from infection with leptospirosis when challenged at 5, 27, or 56 weeks (three different groups of dogs), even though titers were low or not measurable in the vaccinated dogs at 56 weeks. This study demonstrated that anamnestic responses and cell-mediated immunity may be more important than previously considered. This concept has been more conclusively demonstrated in cattle vaccinated with the *Leptospira borgpetersenii* serovar Hardjo bacterin, in which a sustained Th1 or cell-mediated immune response was the critical factor for inducing protective immunity.

Another controversy regarding leptospirosis vaccinations is the concern for vaccine reactions. At one time reactions to leptospirosis vaccines were more common and were related to production of the bacterin in protein-rich media. Studies in the early 1980s showed that leptospires grown in protein-free medium were equally immunogenic, and this has become the standard for all vaccine manufacturers. There are no studies that show that the leptospirosis component used in vaccines today is responsible for vaccine reactions that are seen in dogs. It is my opinion that antigen load is the critical issue in vaccine reactions, not the leptospirosis component. I suggest that leptospirosis vaccinations be given at a separate time from other vaccinations, if for no other reason than to document which vaccine is responsible for the reaction.

Several authors have cited a report by Feigin et al. (1973) as proof that vaccination for leptospirosis does not prevent the renal carrier state, thus questioning the need for vaccination as part of zoonosis prevention. The report by Feigin et al. (1973) is a fascinating account of human infections in a St. Louis neighborhood, but it does not establish that dogs were responsible for the leptospirosis in the humans. Several studies have documented that vaccinations protect against renal carriage in dogs (Broughton and Scarnell, 1985; Klaasen et al., 2003; Schreiber et al., 2005). Most evidence supports the position that vaccination does dramatically reduce the renal carrier state and has potential value in preventing zoonotic spread.

References and Suggested Reading

Adin CA, Cowgill LD: Treatment and outcome of dogs with leptospirosis: 36 cases (1990-1998), *J Am Vet Med Assoc* 216:371, 2000.

Barr SC et al: Serologic responses of dogs given a commercial vaccine against *Leptospira interrogans* serovar pomona and *Leptospira kirschneri* serovar grippotyphosa, *Am J Vet Res* 66:1780, 2005.

Boutilier P, Carr A, Schulman RL: Leptospirosis in dogs: a serologic survey and case series 1996-2001, *Vet Ther* 4:178, 2003.

Broughton ES, Scarnell: Prevention of renal carriage of leptospirosis in dogs by vaccination, *Vet Rec* 117:307, 1985.

Cullen PA, Haake DA, Adler B: Outer membrane proteins of pathogenic spirochetes, *FEMS Microbiol Rev* 28:291, 2004.

Feigin RD et al: Human leptospirosis from immunized dogs, *Ann Intern Med* 79:777, 1973.

Goldstein RE et al: Influence of infecting serogroup on clinical features of leptospirosis in dogs, *J Vet Intern Med* 20:489, 2006.

Harkin KR, Roshto YM, Sullivan JT: Clinical application of a polymerase chain reaction assay for diagnosis of leptospirosis in dogs, *J Am Vet Med Assoc* 222:1224, 2003.

Klaasen HLBM et al: Duration of immunity in dogs vaccinated against leptospirosis with a bivalent inactivated vaccine, *Vet Microbiol* 95:121, 2003.

Levett PN: Leptospirosis, *Clin Microbiol Rev* 14:296, 2001.

Moore GE et al: Canine leptospirosis, United States, 2002-2004, *Emerg Infect Dis* 12:501, 2006.

Schreiber P et al: Prevention of renal infection and urinary shedding in dogs by a *Leptospira* vaccination, *Vet Microbiol* 108:113, 2005.

Shalit I, Barnea A, Shahar A: Efficacy of ciprofloxacin against *Leptospira interrogans* serogroup icterohemorrhagiae, *Antimicrob Agents Chemother* 33:788, 1989.

Truccolo J et al: Quantitative PCR assay to evaluate ampicillin, ofloxacin, and doxycycline for the treatment of experimental leptospirosis, *Antimicrob Agents Chemother* 46:848, 2002.

Ward MP, Glickman LT, Guptill LE: Prevalence of and risk factors for leptospirosis among dogs in the United States and Canada: 677 cases (1970-1998), *J Am Vet Med Assoc* 220:53, 2002.

Ward MP et al: Serovar-specific prevalence and risk factors for leptospirosis among dogs: 90 cases (1997-2002), *J Am Vet Med Assoc* 224:1958, 2004.

Yang HL et al: Thrombocytopenia in the experimental leptospirosis of guinea pig is not related to disseminated intravascular coagulation, *BMC Infect Dis* 6:19, 2006.

CHAPTER 270

Bartonellosis

EDWARD B. BREITSCHWERDT, *Raleigh, North Carolina*

The genus *Bartonella* currently is comprised of at least 20 species and subspecies of vector-transmitted, fastidious, gram-negative bacteria, which are highly adapted to one or more mammalian reservoir hosts (Breitschwerdt and Kordick, 2000; Boulouis et al., 2005). On an evolutionary basis *Bartonella vinsonii* ssp. *berkhoffii* has evolved to cause potentially persistent intravascular infection in dogs and wild canines, including coyotes and foxes. In contrast, *Bartonella henselae* and *Bartonella clarridgeiae* have evolved to cause persistent intravascular infection in domestic cats and wild felid species.

Numerous domestic and wild animals, including bovine, canine, feline, human, and rodent species, can serve as chronically infected reservoir hosts for various *Bartonella* spp. (Breitschwerdt and Kordick, 2000; Boulouis et al., 2005). In addition to the large number of documented reservoir hosts, an increasing number of arthropod vectors, including biting flies, fleas, keds, lice, sandflies, and ticks, have been implicated in the transmission of *Bartonella* spp. (Boulouis et al., 2005; Chomel et al., 2006), although the mode of transmission of any *Bartonella* spp. to domestic or wild canines has not been proven through experimentally controlled vector transmission studies. Epidemiologic evidence and experimental flea transmission studies support an important role for fleas (*Ctenocephalides felis*) in the transmission of *B. henselae* and *B. clarridgeiae* among cats (Boulouis et al., 2005; Chomel et al., 2006). Three other *Bartonella* spp. (*Bartonella koehlarae*, *Bartonella bovis*, and *Bartonella quintana*) have been isolated from cat blood, but the modes of transmission and the reservoir potential of these species in felids have not been definitively established. Epidemiologic evidence supports a role for *Rhipicephalus sanguineus* and perhaps other tick species in the transmission of *B. vinsonii* ssp. *berkhoffii* to dogs. Considering the diversity of *Bartonella* ssp., the large number of reservoir hosts and the spectrum of arthropod vectors, and the clinical and diagnostic challenges posed by *Bartonella* spp., transmission in nature may be much more complex than is currently appreciated in human and veterinary medicine.

Once an animal is infected by a bite, scratch, or arthropod, *Bartonella* spp. localize to erythrocytes and endothelial cells, which provide a potentially unique strategy for bacterial persistence within the bloodstream of reservoir or nonreservoir species (Boulouis et al., 2005). In vitro infection of human CD34+ progenitor cells with *B. henselae* suggests that these bacteria are capable of infecting bone marrow progenitor cells, which may contribute to ongoing erythrocytic infection and perhaps bone marrow dysplasia (Mandle et al., 2005). Infection of bone marrow progenitor cells followed by nonhemolytic intracellular colonization of erythrocytes would preserve *Bartonella* organisms for efficient vector transmission, protect *Bartonella* from the host immune response, facilitate widespread vascular dispersion throughout the tissues of the body, and potentially contribute to decreased antimicrobial efficacy.

In general, persistent bacteremia in a reservoir host does not induce obvious signs of disease or overt pathology. However, immunosuppression (drug or retroviral induced), co-infection with other vector-borne or non-vector-borne pathogens, and preexisting heart valve malformation or injury are factors that facilitate the development of pathology (endocarditis) in animals or humans infected with a reservoir-adapted *Bartonella* spp. Alternatively, when a *Bartonella* spp. is transmitted from a reservoir host (a seemingly well-adapted immunologic association) to a nonreservoir host (a poorly adapted association) by a cat scratch, animal bite, or arthropod vector, infection can result in a seemingly diverse spectrum of clinical and pathologic abnormalities, potentially including polyarthritis, endocarditis, and meningoencephalitis. In humans *Bartonella*-induced disease manifestations can include fever of unknown origin, endocarditis, lymphadenopathy (cat scratch disease [CSD]), granulomatous hepatitis, encephalitis, bacillary angiomatosis, and peliosis hepatis, particularly in immunocompromised individuals (Boulouis et al., 2005; Chomel et al., 2006). Cats are an important zoonotic reservoir host for human infection (CSD), whereas the extent to which dogs and other domestic or wild animals serve as a reservoir for human infection is less well understood.

FELINE BARTONELLOSIS AND CAT SCRATCH DISEASE

The annual number of CSD cases in the United States has been estimated to be between 22,000 and 24,000, with about 2000 cases/year requiring hospitalization (Chomel et al., 2006). Because of large domestic and feral cat populations, thousands of cases may occur annually in Europe and other parts of the world. For nearly a century regional lymphadenopathy has been associated with animal contact, particularly cat scratches. Although historically numerous microorganisms were implicated as the cause of CSD, *B. henselae* is the predominant if not the sole cause of CSD. *B. clarridgeiae*, *B. quintana* and *Afipia felis* are other potential causes of a CSD-like illness in humans (Breitschwerdt and Kordick, 2000, Chomel et al., 2006). In 1992 Regnery and colleagues at the Centers for Disease Control identified seroreactivity to *B. henselae* antigens in 88% of 41 patients with suspected CSD compared to 3% of healthy controls. Subsequently *B. henselae* deoxyribonucleic acid (DNA) was amplified from lymph node samples of 21 of 25 (84%) patients with suspected CSD using a polymerase chain reaction (PCR) assay. When blood was cultured from cats that had induced CSD in a person, 90% of the cats were found to be bacteremic (Breitschwerdt and Kordick, 2000).

Historically atypical manifestations of CSD in humans have included tonsillitis, encephalitis, cerebral arteritis, arthritis, transverse myelitis, granulomatous hepatitis and/or splenitis, osteolysis, pneumonia, pleural effusion, and thrombocytopenic purpura (Boulouis et al., 2005; Chomel et al., 2006). With the recent identification of *B. henselae* as the causative agent of CSD and the improved availability of culture, serology, and PCR for diagnosis, there are an increasing number of reports of human bartonellosis that historically would have been classified as "atypical CSD." Previously *Bartonella* infection would not have been considered as a differential diagnosis by physicians in patients lacking a history of lymphadenopathy and a cat scratch. Dog bites are a frequent cause of emergency room presentations in the United States and may well represent an underrecognized source of *Bartonella* transmission to humans. Animal bites and scratches can pose a major risk for *Bartonella* transmission to veterinary professionals (Chomel et al., 2006). Avoiding bites, scratches, and contact with saliva and quickly washing any animal-induced wound with copious quantities of water should be emphasized in veterinary practices and elsewhere.

The extent to which members of the genus *Bartonella* are pathogenic for cats remains to be definitively determined. *B. henselae* and *B. clarridgeiae* bacteremia can be documented in 25% to 41% of healthy cats in flea-endemic regions (Chomel et al., 2006). Prevalence of infection varies considerably among cat populations (stray or pets) with an increasing gradient from cold climates (0% in Norway) to warm and humid climates (68% in the Philippines). Cats are usually bacteremic for weeks to months, but some cats have been reported to be bacteremic for more than a year. Young cats (≤1 year) are more likely than older cats to be bacteremic, and stray cats are more likely to be bacteremic than pet cats. Self-limiting febrile illness of 48 to 72 hours' duration, mild-to-moderate transient anemia, and transient neurologic dysfunction were observed in cats experimentally infected with *B. henselae* by blood transfusion (Breitschwerdt and Kordick, 2000). Self-limiting fever can occur in naturally infected bacteremic cats following stressors such as surgical procedures. Although unproven, clinical and research findings would suggest that disease manifestations that are transient in nature and resolve spontaneously without antimicrobial treatment can develop in bacteremic cats.

It is obvious that the long-standing evolutionary adaptation between *B. henselae*, flea vectors, and cats as reservoir-adapted hosts supports a minor pathogenic role for these organisms in acute feline illnesses. The extent to which cats with long-standing intravascular infection develop chronic disease manifestations or the extent to which *Bartonella* infection acts as a cofactor in conjunction with other viruses, bacteria, and protozoa is unknown. Because of the high percentage of chronically bacteremic healthy cats in the United States, establishing a cause-and-effect relationship between disease manifestations and bacteremia in cats has proved challenging. Epidemiologic studies suggest that fever, lymphadenopathy, stomatitis and gingivitis, kidney disease, and lower urinary tract disease are significantly associated with *B. henselae* seroreactivity (Breitschwerdt and Kordick, 2000; Chomel et al., 2006). Rare cases of uveitis and endocarditis have been associated with *B. henselae* infection in cats (Breitschwerdt and Kordick, 2000; Chomel et al., 2006). In experimentally infected cats fever, lymphadenopathy, mild neurologic signs, and reproductive disorders have been reported. Gross necropsy results are unremarkable; however, histopathologic lesions can include peripheral lymph node hyperplasia, splenic follicular hyperplasia, lymphocytic cholangitis/pericholangitis, lymphocytic hepatitis, lymphoplasmacytic myocarditis, and interstitial lymphocytic nephritis. Collectively these findings would indicate that antibiotic treatment should be attempted in seroreactive or bacteremic (culture or PCR+) cats with these or other nonspecific disease manifestations. However, because of the high prevalence of infection in certain cat populations, antibiotics are not routinely recommended for healthy seroreactive or bacteremic cats in flea-endemic areas. There is no evidence that most antibiotics used to treat *Bartonella* infection in cats are curative, and reinfection caused by continued flea infestation would be likely. Therefore rigorous efforts to eliminate and prevent future flea infestations in cats is recommended as a means to decrease the potential of *Bartonella* transmission to humans and to decrease the opportunity for ongoing infection with different *Bartonella* spp. or strain types in cats. Cats experimentally infected with *B. henselae* by blood transfusion do not develop protective immunity following homologous or heterologous challenge; therefore prior infection may not result in protective immunity on subsequent challenge with the same or a different *B. henselae* strain. Cross-species protection does not occur (Boulouis et al., 2005).

CANINE BARTONELLOSIS

Historically *B. vinsonii* ssp. *berkhoffii* has been considered the most frequent *Bartonella* spp. that infects and causes disease in dogs (Boulouis et al., 2005; Chomel et al., 2006). However, this conclusion may not be accurate since culture is an insensitive means of *Bartonella* isolation, sera from dogs have not been systematically screened against a large panel of *Bartonella* spp. antigens, and minimal PCR testing has been performed on tissues from naturally infected dogs. Serologic studies from Hawaii, the United Kingdom, Japan, and the southeastern United States identified *B. henselae* prevalences of 6.5% (2/31 dogs), 3% (3/100 dogs), 7.7% (4/52 dogs), and 27% (82/301 dogs), respectively.

The spectrum of disease induced by *Bartonella* infection in dogs currently is unknown (Boulouis et al., 2005; Chomel et al., 2006). Similar to humans, dogs can be infected with several *Bartonella* spp., including *B. vinsonii* ssp. *berkhoffii*, *B. quintana*, *B. clarridgeiae*, *Bartonella elizabethae*, *Bartonella washoensi*, and *Bartonella bovis*. Endocarditis caused by *B. vinsonii* ssp. *berkhoffii* represents the most thoroughly established disease association

(Breitschwerdt et al., 1999; Chomel et al., 2006). *Bartonella* endocarditis occurs in large-breed dogs with a high predilection for aortic valve involvement. In some dogs intermittent lameness, bone pain, epistaxis, or fever of unknown origin can precede the diagnosis of endocarditis by several months; whereas other dogs present with an acute history of cardiopulmonary decompensation. Cardiac arrhythmias secondary to myocarditis can be detected in dogs without echocardiographic evidence of endocarditis. Infection with *B. henselae* or *B. vinsonii* ssp. *berkhoffii* alone or in conjunction with *Ehrlichia canis* may cause epistaxis in dogs (Breitschwerdt et al., 2005). Based on serologic evidence, *B. vinsonii* ssp. *berkhoffii*, *B. henselae*, or other *Bartonella* spp. appear to contribute to the development of dermatologic lesions indicative of a cutaneous vasculitis, anterior uveitis, polyarthritis, meningoencephalitis, immune-mediated thrombocytopenia (ITP), or immune-mediated hemolytic anemia (IMHA) in dogs (Breitschwerdt et al., 2004; Goodman and Breitschwerdt, 2005; Chomel et al., 2006). Experimentally infection with *B. vinsonii* ssp. *berkhoffii* induces several alterations in immune regulation and immune function (Breitschwerdt and Kordick, 2000). Antinuclear antibodies have been detected in the serum of dogs infected with *B. vinsonii* ssp. *berkhoffii* or *E. canis* or coinfected with both organisms, which appears to be relatively common, depending on geographic location (Breitschwerdt and Kordick, 2000; Smith, Tompkins, and Breitschwerdt, 2004). Detection of ITP, IMHA, and polyarthritis in a dog in conjunction with finding antinuclear antibodies would be consistent with a diagnosis of systemic lupus erythematosus (SLE). In dogs with a tentative diagnosis of SLE, ruling out infection with a *Bartonella* spp. should be considered.

Although the pathogenicity of all *Bartonella* spp. in dogs remains poorly characterized, it is becoming increasingly clear that species other than *B. vinsonii* ssp. *berkhoffii* can cause disease in dogs. It appears that *B. henselae* can contribute to the development of granulomatous lesions in dogs since organism-specific DNA sequences have been amplified from dogs with peliosis hepatis, granulomatous hepatitis, systemic granulomatous disease with sialoadenitis, and granulomatous lymphadenitis. *B. clarridgeiae* DNA has been amplified and sequenced from the liver of a Doberman pinscher with copper storage disease and from the aortic valve of a dog with vegetative valvular endocarditis. *B. elizabethae*, a species that infects rodents, was PCR amplified and sequenced from an ethylenediaminetetraacetic acid blood sample obtained from a dog that had experienced chronic weight loss culminating in sudden unexplained death. Recently *B. quintana* has been isolated from the blood or heart valves of dogs with endocarditis. These observations indicate that, although presumably infrequent, *Bartonella* spp. that commonly infect cats or rodents and are known to be transmitted by fleas among reservoir hosts may infect dogs and cause serious disease manifestations such as endocarditis or myocarditis. Circumstantial evidence suggests that cats may transmit *Bartonella* spp. to dogs by way of a scratch or bite, as occurs with human CSD.

Following natural infection, *Bartonella* spp. can be found by PCR in the lymph nodes of healthy or sick dogs. *Bartonella*-induced granulomatous lymphadenitis involving the left submandibular lymph node was diagnosed in a dog on the basis of seroreactivity to *B. vinsonii* ssp. *berkhoffii* antigens, visualization of Warthin-Starry silver staining bacteria within the lymph node, and PCR amplification followed by southern blot hybridization (Pappalardo et al., 2000). Seven days before enlargement of the lymph node, the owners removed an engorged tick from the dog's left ear. Although *Bartonella* spp. DNA can be amplified by PCR from ticks and although there have been no transmission studies to prove vector competence, this case in conjunction with other epidemiologic evidence suggests that ticks can transmit *Bartonella* spp. to dogs and potentially to humans (Chomel et al., 2006). *B. henselae* DNA has also been amplified and sequenced from the lymph nodes of dogs with generalized granulomatous lymphadenopathy.

DIAGNOSIS OF CANINE AND FELINE BARTONELLOSIS

Seroconversion could be used to confirm acute *Bartonella* infection in a cat or a dog. Seroconversion has been documented in humans with acute cat scratch disease and in cats and dogs following experimental infection. Because acute and convalescent samples are rarely submitted for diagnostic testing, seroconversion has not been reported in a naturally infected cat or dog with an acute illness. The kinetics of the serologic response to *B. henselae* antigens in chronically infected experimental cats is highly variable in degree and duration, and the presence or absence of antibodies does not always correlate with the detection of bacteremia. Although providing useful epidemiologic data, serologic test results from a cat may be of limited clinical use for several reasons. *B. henselae*–specific antibodies are not detectable in some bacteremic cats, and *Bartonella* cannot be cultured from some *B. henselae*–seroreactive cats. Negative blood cultures obtained from *B. henselae*–seroreactive cats may reflect a low level bacteremia or the timing of the blood culture, since experimentally infected cats experience a relapsing pattern of bacteremia (Breitschwerdt and Kordick, 2000). Numerous naturally infected cats are persistently bacteremic, generally in conjunction with low antibody titers. High *B. henselae* antibody titers in cats generally correlate with positive blood cultures. The extent of serologic cross-reactivity to *Bartonella* spp. requires additional clarification since both cats and dogs can be coinfected with more than one *Bartonella* spp. Although serology can provide very useful diagnostic information, test results must be interpreted in conjunction with other clinical data.

Ideally the diagnosis of *Bartonella* infection should be confirmed by culturing the organism from blood, lymph node, or heart valve or by amplifying organism-specific DNA sequences from tissues using PCR. Unfortunately this diagnostic objective is complicated by a number of factors. Because of a relatively high level of bacteria in cat blood, successful isolation of *B. henselae* or *B. clarridgeiae* from the blood of an infected cat is relatively easy to achieve compared to the difficulty of isolating of any *Bartonella* spp. from the blood or tissues of an infected dog. Because of the large number of cats that are chronically infected with *B. henselae* in flea-endemic regions, culture or PCR amplification of *Bartonella* DNA would confirm infection but would not confirm that *B. henselae* is the cause of clinical or hematologic abnormalities or a specific disease entity in a sick cat. Because conventional isolation techniques have lacked sensitivity, canine bartonellosis is most frequently diagnosed by PCR amplification of organism-specific DNA sequences and/or through serologic testing. In sick dogs detection of *B. henselae,* and more particularly *B. vinsonii* ssp. *berkhoffii,* antibodies should be considered diagnostically relevant to the patient's illness until more data are available to change this assessment. Recently the development of a more sensitive isolation approach using *Bartonella* α-*Proteobacteria* growth medium (BAPGM) followed by PCR has greatly facilitated the molecular detection or isolation of *Bartonella* spp. from the blood of sick or healthy animals and humans. Similar to cats, it appears that dogs can be infected with a *Bartonella* spp. without mounting a diagnostic antibody response. Because very few *Bartonella* organisms are found in sick dog blood samples, combining a more sensitive culture approach with a highly sensitive and specific PCR assay greatly facilitates the detection of active infection in dogs.

TREATMENT OF *BARTONELLA* INFECTIONS

Because of disparate results among human studies and an overall lack of microbiologic data derived from clinical therapeutic trials in animals, numerous issues related to treatment of *Bartonella* infection remain controversial. In contrast to the apparent lack of response to antimicrobial treatment in human CSD patients, bacillary angiomatosis, parenchymal bacillary peliosis, and acute *Bartonella* bacteremia appear to respond to antimicrobial treatment, even in immunocompromised individuals (Boulouis et al., 2005; Chomel et al., 2006). Doxycycline, erythromycin, and rifampin are recommended antibiotics; but clinical improvement has been reported following the use of penicillin, gentamicin, ceftriaxone, ciprofloxacin, and azithromycin. Treatment for 2 weeks in immunocompetent humans and 6 weeks in immunocompromised humans is generally recommended. Relapses associated with bacteremia have been reported in immunocompromised humans despite treatment for 6 weeks. Antimicrobial efficacy has not been established for any antibiotic for eliminating *B. henselae* bacteremia in cats or dogs. Incomplete treatment responses have been reported in experimentally infected cats treated for 2 or 4 weeks with doxycycline or enrofloxacin (Kordick et al., 1997).

HUMAN HEALTH IMPLICATIONS

Based on the annual increase in publications related to *Bartonella* infections in animals and humans during the past decade, it is obvious that members of this genus are gaining increased international scrutiny by physicians and veterinarians. When examining data generated in specific healthy or sick animal populations, it will be important to recognize the exceptional evolutionary adaptation of these microorganisms, which allows them to induce persistent blood-borne infections in both animals and humans. Efficient adaptation to blood and endothelial cells has complicated efforts to detect and define disease causation in association with intravascular

Bartonella infection. As animals function as reservoirs for various *Bartonella* spp., blood-borne infection facilitates a continued transmission cycle via arthropod or animal bites or scratches (Chomel et al., 2006). Animal contact, which in many instances occurs to a wide spectrum of domestic and wild animal species, is an obvious consequence of the daily activities of veterinarians, veterinary technicians, animal health researchers, ranchers, wildlife biologists, and many other individuals in our society. Recently *B. henselae* or *B. vinsonii* ssp. *berkhoffii* infection has been documented in our laboratory in blood samples from humans with extensive arthropod and animal contact. The potential clinical relevance of detecting *Bartonella* spp. in the blood of humans with occupational animal contact remains to be determined. Despite frequent occupational exposure to animals, it is important to acknowledge that most veterinary professionals, ranchers, and wildlife biologists participate in a diversity of outdoor recreational and occupational activities that also increase the opportunity for *Bartonella* transmission by biting arthropods. Therefore the source of infection in these individuals cannot be clearly established.

LEGAL IMPLICATIONS

Except for *Homo sapiens,* veterinarians are responsible for the medical care and general well-being of all of the animal species on this planet. In regard to zoonotic disease transmission, veterinarians play a pivotal role in the public health infrastructure of our nation. Additional prospective studies are necessary to characterize the risk of human *Bartonella* infection following a cat or dog bite and whether these infections are always self-limiting. Despite the long, natural evolutionary history of *Bartonella* and mammals, the legal implications of *Bartonella* transmission from pets to humans in our modern society may create both complications and opportunities for the veterinary profession. Although recent research findings have substantially improved our understanding of the clinical, microbiologic, and zoonotic aspects of diseases caused by *Bartonella* spp., the exact mode of transmission; the relative role of various insect vectors such as biting flies, fleas, lice and ticks; the identification of new reservoir hosts; and the spectrum of animal and human illnesses caused by these organisms remain largely undetermined. The pathogenic potential of these organisms appears to be of considerable importance in dogs and immunocompromised and immunocompetent humans.

References and Suggested Reading

Boulouis H-J et al: Factors associated with the rapid emergence of zoonotic *Bartonella* infections, *Vet Res* 36:383, 2005.

Breitschwerdt EB, Kordick DL: *Bartonella* infection in animals: carriership, reservoir potential, pathogenicity, and zoonotic potential for human infection, *Clin Microbiol Rev* 13:428, 2000.

Breitschwerdt EB et al: *Bartonella vinsonii* subsp. *berkhoffii* and related members of the alpha subdivision of the *Proteobacteria* in dogs with cardiac arrhythmias, endocarditis, or myocarditis, *J Clin Microbiol* 37:3618, 1999.

Breitschwerdt EB et al: Clinicopathologic abnormalities and treatment response in 24 dogs seroreactive to *Bartonella vinsonii (berkhoffii)* antigens, *J Am Anim Hosp Assoc* 40:92; 2004.

Breitschwerdt EB et al: *Bartonella* species as a potential cause of epistaxis in dogs, *J Clin Microbiol* 43:2529; 2005.

Breitschwerdt EB et al: *Bartonella* species in blood of immuno-competent persons with animal and arthropod contact, *Emerg Infect Dis* 13:938, 2007.

Chomel BB et al: *Bartonella* spp. in pets and effect on human health, *Emerg Infect Dis* 12:389, 2006.

Duncan AW, Maggi RG, Breitschwerdt EB: A combined approach for the enhanced detection and isolation of *Bartonella* species in dog blood samples: pre-enrichment culture followed by PCR and subculture onto agar plates, *J Microbiol Meth* 69:273, 2007.

Goodman RA, Breitschwerdt EB: Clinicopathological findings in dogs seroreactive to *Bartonella henselae* antigens, *Am J Vet Res* 66:2060; 2005.

Kordick DL, Papich MG, Breitschwerdt EB: Efficacy of enro-floxacin or doxycycline for treatment of *Bartonella henselae* or *Bartonella clarridgeiae* infection in cats, *Antimicrob Agents Chemother* 41:2448, 1997.

Mandle T et al: Infection of human CD34+ progenitor cells with *Bartonella henselae* results in intraerythrocytic presence of B. henselae, *Blood* 106:1215, 2005.

Pappalardo BL et al: Granulomatous disease associated with *Bartonella* infection in 2 dogs,. *J Vet Intern Med* 14:37, 2000.

Smith BE, Tompkins MB, Breitschwerdt EB: Antinuclear antibodies can be detected in dog sera reactive to *Bartonella vinsonii* subsp. *berkhoffii*, *Ehrlichia canis*, or *Leishmania infantum* antigens, *J Vet Intern Med* 18:47; 2004.

CHAPTER 271

Canine and Feline Hemotropic Mycoplasmosis

SÉVERINE TASKER, *Bristol, England, United Kingdom*

Feline and canine hemotropic mycoplasmas (hemo-plasmas) are small bacteria that reside on the surface of red blood cells and can mediate hemolytic anemia in their host. Initially the hemoplasmas, including members of the genus *Haemobartonella*, were classified as rickettsial organisms, but gene sequencing analysis and phylogenetic studies have resulted in their reclassification within the genus *Mycoplasma*. *Haemobartonella felis* is now named *Mycoplasma haemofelis*, whereas *Haemobartonella canis* is called *Mycoplasma haemocanis*, and these organisms are collectively known as the hemoplasmas. Molecular studies have also confirmed the existence of additional feline and canine hemoplasmas. These species differ in pathogenicity, and an understanding of their characteristics is important to enable the veterinary clinician to manage cases appropriately.

EXISTENCE OF MULTIPLE SPECIES

M. haemofelis infection is often associated with the development of acute hemolytic anemia in cats. Two additional feline haemoplasma species have now been reported: 'Candidatus M. haemominutum' and 'Candidatus M. turicensis.' 'Candidatus M. haemominu-tum' is less pathogenic than *M. haemofelis* but can induce

anemia in some circumstances. 'Candidatus M. turi-censis' has only recently been discovered and limited reports suggest that it can induce mild-to-severe anemia. Splenectomy is not necessarily required for these agents to induce disease in their feline hosts, although immu-nocompromise may play a role in allowing 'Candidatus M. haemominutum' and 'Candidatus M. turicensis' to cause disease.

M. haemocanis infection usually results in hemolytic anemia only in splenectomized or immunocompromised dogs. A new canine hemoplasma, 'Candidatus M. haema-toparvum,' has recently been described in association with anemia in a dog that had been splenectomized and was immunosuppressed (Sykes et al., 2004).

Phylogenetic studies have shown that, although *M. haemofelis* and *M. haemocanis* are distinct species, they are closely related. 'Candidatus M. haemominutum' and 'Candidatus M. haematoparvum' are also closely related. Some have referred to *M. haemofelis* and *M. haemoca-nis* as *large* forms of hemoplasma, whereas 'Candidatus M. haemominutum' and 'Candidatus M. haematopar-vum' are sometimes called *small* forms since the size of the former species, when seen cytologically, may be larger than the latter, although variation does exist. Interestingly, 'Candidatus M. turicensis' has not been definitively identified cytologically; thus the morphologic appearance of this species has not been described. In phylogenetic analysis 'Candidatus M. turicensis' does not group with the previously described feline and canine hemoplasma spp.; instead it groups with rodent hemoplasma species.

PREVALENCE OF INFECTION

Prevalence studies for feline hemoplasma species have now been performed worldwide. 'Candidatus M. haemominutum' is most common, being identified in 10% to 32.1% of cats sampled in different studies. M. haemofelis and 'Candidatus M. turicensis' infections are less common with rates varying from 1.4% to 6.4% and 1.3% to 26%, respectively. The nature of the cats sampled for these different studies has varied enormously, from healthy cats to cats suspected of having hemoplasmosis, possibly explaining some of the variation in the results obtained. In addition, geographic variation appears to exist, with warmer countries having a higher prevalence of infection. Of additional note is that infection with 'Candidatus M. turicensis' is often associated with coinfection with either and occasionally both of the two other feline hemoplasma species, particularly 'Candidatus M. haemominutum.' Further studies are required to determine the prevalence of canine hemoplasmas, but some work suggests that infection with 'Candidatus M. haematoparvum' is more common than that with M. haemocanis, although a recent Swiss study documented the reverse (Wengi et al., 2008). In another study kenneled dogs were found to have a higher prevalence of infection with M. haemocanis than pet dogs (Kemming et al., 2004).

PATHOGENICITY

Hemoplasma infections induce anemia by causing hemolysis, which is primarily extravascular in nature, although intravascular hemolysis has also been reported. In addition, sequestration of infected red blood cells within the spleen may also result in a reduction in packed cell volume (PCV). An increase in osmotic fragility has been reported in cats infected with M. haemofelis and 'Candidatus M. turicensis.' Differences in pathogenicity exist among hemoplasma species.

'Candidatus M. haemominutum'

Experimental 'Candidatus M. haemominutum' infection of cats does not usually lead to significant clinical signs or anemia, although a fall in erythrocyte parameters can occur. A significant anemia has been seen following 'Candidatus M. haemominutum' infection in retrovirus-infected (combined feline leukemia virus [FeLV] and feline immunodeficiency virus [FIV] or FeLV alone) cats (George et al., 2002), although a recent study failed to document potentiation of anemia in chronically infected asymptomatic FIV cats (Tasker et al., 2006). Most studies in naturally infected cats have failed to find an association between 'Candidatus M. haemominutum' infection and anemia. 'Candidatus M. haemominutum' associated anemia has also been reported in a cat undergoing chemotherapy for lymphoma (De Lorimier and Messick, 2004).

An association between 'Candidatus M. haemominutum' and renal insufficiency has also been suggested (Willi et al., 2006a), although this causal association may be coincidental in that older cats are more likely to be 'Candidatus M. haemominutum' infected and have chronic renal insufficiency.

Mycoplasma haemofelis

Experimental infection with M. haemofelis often results in a severe hemolytic anemia, although the severity of anemia varies considerably. Some studies of naturally infected cats have found an association between anemia and M. haemofelis infection, but others have not. It has been hypothesized that acute infection with M. haemofelis can result in severe hemolytic anemia but that chronically infected cats are not anemic (Willi et al., 2006a).

'Candidatus M. turicensis'

Experimental studies with 'Candidatus M. turicensis' are limited in number, but this organism has been shown to induce moderate-to-severe anemia in two cats, being more severe in a cat given methylprednisolone acetate to induce immunosuppression. Difficulties exist in assigning clinical signs solely to 'Candidatus M. turicensis' infection in naturally infected cats since many 'Candidatus M. turicensis' infected cats are coinfected with other feline hemoplasmas. Cats coinfected with either 'Candidatus M. turicensis' and 'Candidatus M. haemominutum' or 'Candidatus M. turicensis' and M. haemofelis have significantly lower PCVs than hemoplasma-free cats, whereas those infected with 'Candidatus M. turicensis' alone do not (Willi et al., 2006b). In addition, cats naturally infected with 'Candidatus M. turicensis' often have concurrent diseases. Therefore it is possible that immunosuppression or stress influences the pathogenic potential of this species.

Canine Hemoplasmas

Studies regarding the pathogenicity of canine hemoplasmas are sparse. As mentioned previously, infection usually only results in hemolytic anemia in splenectomized or immunocompromised dogs, and asymptomatic latent M. haemocanis infections can be reactivated following splenectomy.

CLINICAL PRESENTATION

The clinical disease that follows hemoplasma infection is influenced by the species of hemoplasma involved, whether there is acute or chronic infection, and whether concurrent disease or immunosuppression is present. Common clinical signs seen in cats and dogs affected by hemoplasma infection include dehydration, anorexia, lethargy, weight loss, depression and intermittent pyrexia, and anemia. Splenomegaly may also be evident.

CLINICAL PATHOLOGY

Pathogenic hemoplasma infection typically causes a regenerative anemia that is macrocytic and hypochromic in nature, although pronounced reticulocytosis is not always evident. Normoblasts may be present. Positive Coombs' tests, particularly with cold agglutinins, and autoagglutination have been reported in acute hemoplasmosis, indicating the presence of erythrocyte-bound antibodies. Spherocytes may also be evident in canine infections. Icterus is seen occasionally but is uncommon.

The influence of retroviral status on feline hemoplasmosis is not fully understood. Some studies have found that FeLV and/or FIV infection is associated with an increased risk of coinfection with 'Candidatus M. haemominutum' and M. haemofelis. Therefore it seems prudent to perform FeLV and FIV testing in hemoplasma-infected cats, especially if the retroviral status of the cat is not known.

CARRIER STATUS

Long-term carrier status can occur with hemoplasma infection. Our experience at the University of Bristol suggests that this is particularly common with 'Candidatus M. haemominutum' infection, although suspected clearance of infection has been reported by others with and without antibiotic treatment (Willi et al., 2006a). We have observed that a large proportion of M. haemofelis–infected cats spontaneously clear infection from peripheral blood a few months following acute infection; this has also been reported for 'Candidatus M. turicensis.' However, generalized statements regarding long-term carrier status cannot be made since great variation exists, likely because of differences in the host-organism interaction and hemoplasma isolates. Carrier cats are often asymptomatic, but reactivation of infection can occur and may result in clinical disease (Foley et al., 1998); this is uncommon in our experience.

Little work has been done regarding the time course of carrier status with canine hemoplasmas, but asymptomatic carrier dogs infected with 'Candidatus M. haematoparvum' and M. haemocanis are thought to exist (Kemming et al., 2004; Kenny et al., 2004).

DIAGNOSIS

Examination of Blood Smears

Diagnosis of hemoplasma infection used to rely on cytologic examination of blood smears, but this method has extremely poor sensitivity and variable specificity. Although organisms sometimes may be visible for a short period during peak parasitemia after acute infection, cytology is too insensitive to be relied on for making a diagnosis of hemoplasmosis; thus the polymerase chain reaction (PCR) has emerged as the diagnostic test of choice.

Polymerase Chain Reaction

When designed and executed properly, PCR is extremely sensitive and specific for the diagnosis of hemoplasma infection. It is extremely important that a reputable laboratory carry out the PCR and that the sensitivity and specificity and quality assurance of the PCR assays used be communicated by commercial laboratories so reliability can be evaluated by the practicing veterinarian.

Conventional non-quantitative PCRs can be designed to detect and distinguish all of the feline and canine hemoplasmas. Real-time quantitative PCRs additionally quantify the amount of hemoplasma deoxyribonucleic acid (DNA) present within blood samples (Tasker et al., 2003). Quantification of the amount of hemoplasma DNA present in a sample may help determine the significance of infection and monitor response to treatment. However, it has been shown that organism numbers in some cats infected with M. haemofelis fluctuate markedly and spontaneously, sometimes occurring in regular cycles of increases and decreases in copy number over a long period of time (months), complicating interpretation of quantitative data for this species.

Cats can become PCR-negative during effective antibiotic treatment, but it may take several days or even weeks for the hemoplasma levels to fall below the sensitivity of the PCR (Fig. 271-1). However, it has been found that cats can become PCR positive again after antibiotic treatment is stopped, possibly because of the release of organisms back into the blood from sites of sequestration in the body. Thus a single negative PCR result cannot be taken as evidence of clearance of hemoplasma infection. Obtaining several sequential negative PCR results increases the likelihood that elimination has occurred.

TREATMENT

Antibiotic therapy

Tetracycline derivatives are most commonly used to treat hemoplasma infections, with doxycycline (10 mg/kg q24h orally [PO]) the preferred drug. Although controlled studies have been performed only for M. haemofelis, based on observations of individual cases doxycycline also has activity against most isolates of the other feline hemoplasmas, as well as the canine hemoplasmas. Esophageal strictures secondary to oral doxycycline treatment have been reported in cats; thus it is recommended that dosing be followed by the administration of water by syringe or food to encourage passage of the drug into the stomach.

Fluoroquinolones can also be effective in treating hemoplasmosis. Enrofloxacin (5 mg/kg q24h PO) successfully treated M. haemofelis infection in controlled studies. Diffuse retinal degeneration and acute blindness have been reported following enrofloxacin treatment in cats, although this is said to be rare. Marbofloxacin (2 to 5.5 mg/kg q24h PO) has also been effective in reducing M. haemofelis and 'Candidatus M. haemominutum' organism numbers in the blood of cats treated in controlled studies using a dosage of 2 mg/kg every 24 hours orally, although the fall in 'Candidatus M. haemominutum' organism numbers was less pronounced than that of M. haemofelis.

Unfortunately there is as yet no treatment regimen described that consistently eliminates hemoplasma. Although these treatments effectively treat clinical disease in most cases, they do not always induce consistently negative PCR results (see Fig. 271-1). Work evaluating field cases of hemoplasmosis suggests that different hemoplasma isolates may respond differently to antibiotic treatment regimens. There may be a role for the use of imidocarb dipropionate (5 mg/kg intramuscularly [IM] q14days) in refractory hemoplasma cases, but controlled studies evaluating its efficacy are lacking.

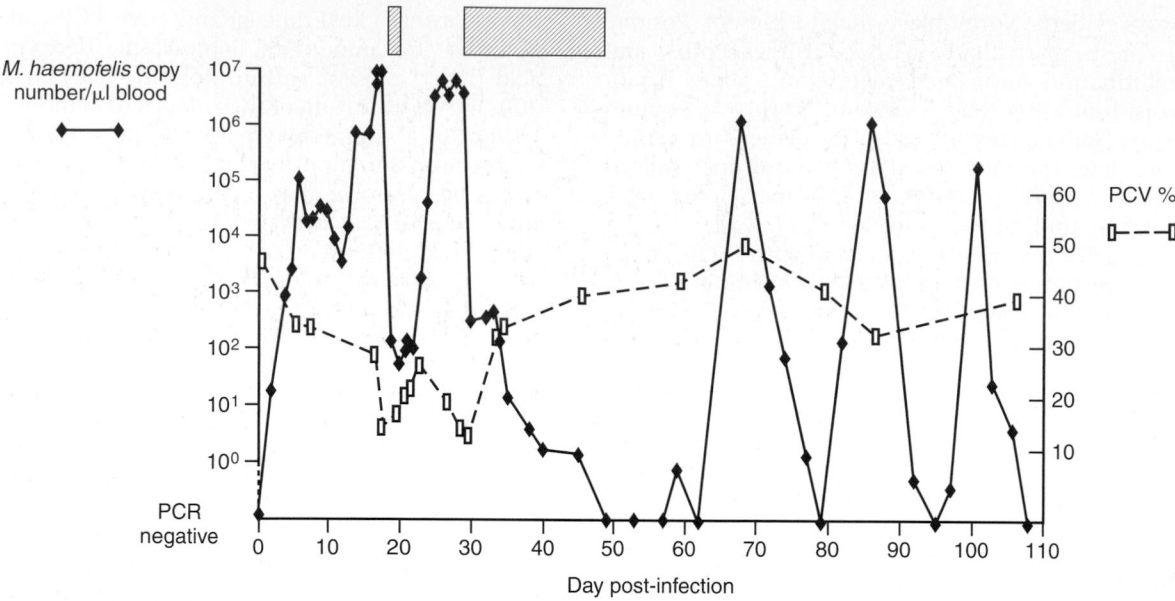

Fig. 271-1 Graph illustrating outcome of infection with *M. haemofelis* during periods with and without antibiotic therapy. The left y-axis represents *M. haemofelis* copy number *(solid line)* that is broadly equivalent to *M. haemofelis* organism number per microliter of blood. The x-axis represents day post-infection with *M. haemofelis* inoculated intravenously on day 0. The right y-axis represents packed cell volume (PCV) *(dashed line)*, the normal reference range being 25% to 45%. The hatched boxes represent those times during which doxycycline antibiotic was administered at a dosage rate of 10 mg/kg q24h orally. The graph shows the increase in *M. haemofelis* copy number over time following initial infection. Doxycycline treatment (initially for only 2 days, and then for a 21-day period) was associated with a corresponding fall in *M. haemofelis* copy number. Although three negative *M. haemofelis* polymerase chain reaction (PCR) results were obtained at the end of, and after, the 21-day doxycycline treatment period (days 49, 53 and 56 after infection), these did not represent clearance of infection since *M. haemofelis* PCR then became positive again, with apparent cycling of *M. haemofelis* copy number over the following 45 days. Therefore a single negative PCR results does not confirm elimination of infection.

Corticosteroid Treatment

The anemia induced by feline hemoplasma infection is in part immune mediated; thus corticosteroids have been recommended as treatment in addition to antibiotics, although studies have not evaluated their effectiveness. The use of corticosteroids (prednisolone, 2 to 4 mg/kg/day PO) may be indicated in cases that are Coombs' positive or in which an inadequate response is seen to antibiotics. However, we have observed clinically ill cats, including ones that are Coombs' positive, respond to antibiotic treatment alone without the need for corticosteroids.

Other Treatment

Supportive care also may be required, notably correction of dehydration with fluid therapy and blood transfusion if the anemia is very severe. Although the mode of transmission of hemoplasma infection in field cases has not been confirmed, transmission by fleas and ticks has been implicated in several studies; thus ectoparasite treatment should also be instigated.

References and Suggested Reading

De Lorimier LP, Messick JB: Anemia associated with 'Candidatus Mycoplasma haemominutum' in a feline leukemia virus-negative cat with lymphoma, *J Am Animal Hosp Assoc* 40:423, 2004.

Foley JE et al: Molecular, clinical, and pathologic comparison of two distinct strains of *Haemobartonella felis* in domestic cats, *Am J Vet Res* 59:1581, 1998.

George JW et al: Effect of preexisting FeLV infection or FeLV and feline immunodeficiency virus coinfection on pathogenicity of the small variant of *Haemobartonella felis* in cats, *Am J Vet Res* 63:1172, 2002.

Kemming GI et al: Mycoplasma haemocanis infection—a kennel disease? *Comp Med* 54:404, 2004.

Kenny MJ et al: Demonstration of two distinct hemotropic mycoplasmas in French dogs, *J Clin Microbiol* 42:5397, 2004.

Sykes JE et al: 'Candidatus Mycoplasma haematoparvum' sp.nov., a novel small haemotropic mycoplasma from a dog, *Int J Syst Evol Microbiol* 55:27, 2004.

Tasker S et al: Use of real-time PCR to detect and quantify *Mycoplasma haemofelis* and 'Candidatus Mycoplasma haemominutum' DNA, *J Clin Microbiol* 41:439, 2003.

Tasker S et al: Effect of chronic FIV infection, and efficacy of marbofloxacin treatment, on 'Candidatus Mycoplasma haemominutum' infection, *Microbes Infect* 8:653, 2006.

Tasker S et al: Effect of chronic FIV infection, and efficacy of marbofloxacin treatment, on 'Candidatus Mycoplasma haemominutum' infection, *Microbes Infect* 8:653, 2006.

Wengi N et al: Real-time PCR-based prevalence study, infection followup and molecular characterization of canine hemotropic mycoplasmas, *Vet Microbiol* 126:132, 2008.

Willi B et al: Prevalence, risk factor analysis, and follow-up of infections caused by three feline hemoplasma species in cats in Switzerland, *J Clin Microbiol* 44:961, 2006a.

Willi B et al: Phylogenetic and risk factor analysis for 'Candidatus Mycoplasma turicensis' in United Kingdom, Australian and South African pet cats, *J Clin Microbiol* 44:4430, 2006b.

CHAPTER 272

Canine Anaplasma Infection

LEAH A. COHN, *Columbia, Missouri*
STEPHANIE J. KOTTLER, *Columbia, Missouri*

Two species of *Anaplasma* can cause disease in dogs: *Anaplasma platys* and *Anaplasma phagocytophilum*. Infection with *A. platys* leads to infectious cyclic thrombocytopenia. Infection with *A. phagocytophilum* leads to a distinct clinical illness often referred to simply as canine anaplasmosis.

THE ORGANISMS

Each with a worldwide distribution, both *A. platys* and *A. phagocytophilum* are small, obligate intracellular bacteria that replicate in membrane-bound vacuoles of eukaryotic cells. *A. platys* replicates within canine thrombocytes. *A. phagocytophilum* resides in granulocytic white blood cells, primarily neutrophils, but occasionally in eosinophils as well. Known primarily as a pathogen of dogs, inclusions purported to be those of *A. platys* have also been identified in cats. Compared to related organisms, *A. phagocytophilum* is fairly promiscuous in its ability to infect different animal species. The organism may cause disease in a variety of species, including dogs, cats, horses (equine granulocytic "ehrlichiosis"), small ruminants (tick fever), and humans (human granulocytic "ehrlichiosis").

Until recently both *A. platys* and *A. phagocytophilum* were considered species within the genus *Ehrlichia*. Based on classification schemes that use sequence homology of 16S ribosomal ribonucleic acid genes to determine the genetic relation of various organisms and group them taxonomically, some *Ehrlichia*-related organisms were moved from the family Rickettsiaceae into the family Anaplasmataceae. Further, several organisms formerly considered members of the genus *Ehrlichia* were moved to more appropriate genus groups. These included *A. platys* (formerly *Ehrlichia platys*) and several other organisms (*Ehrlichia equi, Ehrlichia phagocytophila*, and the human granulocytic ehrlichial agent) that were moved and consolidated into the new species *A. phagocytophilum* (Dumler, 2001). Before sophisticated molecular tools became available, these organisms were grouped taxonomically by morphology, cellular tropism, host species, or other parameters.

DISEASE TRANSMISSION

Ticks are believed to be the primary vectors of transmission for canine *Anaplasma* infection. Although *A. platys* has been isolated from several species of tick, including *Rhipicephalus sanguineus*, vector competence has not been demonstrated for any tick. *Ixodid* ticks are vectors for transmission of *A. phagocytophilum*. The organism is acquired by the tick during feeding and later passed to a new host through salivary secretions; a minimum feeding time of 24 hours is required for successful transmission of *A. phagocytophilum*. Different species of *Ixodid* ticks serve as vectors in different parts of the world. In Europe *Ixodes ricinus* is the primary vector tick, whereas *Ixodes scapularis* (black-legged or deer tick) is the vector in the upper Midwestern, mid-Atlantic, and northeastern parts of the United States, and *Ixodes pacificus* (western black-legged tick) serves the same role in northern California and the Oregon and Washington coastal regions. Reservoir hosts for *A. phagocytophilum* include white-tailed deer, gray squirrel, white-footed mouse, raccoons, and other rodents. Because of the feeding cycle of *Ixodid* ticks, infection with *A. phagocytophilum* occurs most frequently in the spring to early summer and then again in the fall of the year. Although perinatal transmission of *A. phagocytophilum* has been reported in humans, it is likely at most a minor means of transmission in domestic animals. Infection with either organism also can be acquired iatrogenically via administration of contaminated blood products. Although humans can be infected with *A. phagocytophilum*, there is no evidence of transmission directly from dogs (or cats) to humans.

CLINICAL DISEASE

Infectious Canine Thrombocytopenia

Clinical signs of infection begin within 1 to 2 weeks of experimental inoculation with *A. platys*. Platelet counts drop markedly within a few days and can increase just as rapidly. Thrombocytopenia and recovery occur cyclically at 1- to 2-week intervals. Typically the severity of thrombocytopenia gradually lessens with each subsequent cycle. There seem to be differences in disease severity in different regions of the world. Although clinical signs related to thrombocytopenia (e.g., epistaxis, petechiae) have been reported occasionally, most dogs infected with the strains found in the United States remain well, and infection with *A. platys* is often discovered incidentally. In fact, epidemiologic studies suggest that the prevalence of infection is far greater than might be suspected based on incidence of clinical illness. More pathogenic strains may occur in other parts of the world. Bleeding tendencies, fever, lethargy, weight loss, lymphadenomegaly, and other manifestations of a more severe illness are reported in infected dogs from Greece and Israel. Although strains of *A. platys* outside the United States may be more virulent, it is also possible that coinfection with other pathogens contributes to the more severe clinical disease manifestations in these dogs.

Canine Anaplasmosis, or Granulocytic Anaplasmosis

There is not yet a clear clinical picture of a typical *A. phagocytophilum* infection in dogs. Few experimental infection studies have been carried out in dogs (Egenvall et al.,1998; Lilliehöök, Egenvall, and Tvedten, 1998), and reports of naturally occurring infection may be confounded by lack of a definitive diagnosis or exclusion of coinfection. Until recently infection with *A. phagocytophilum* (then known as *E. equi*) was one of two causes of canine "granulocytic ehrlichiosis." *Ehrlichia ewingii*, the other cause of granulocytic ehrlichiosis in dogs from the central Midwest and southeastern United States, forms granulocytic morulae that are indistinguishable from those of *A. phagocytophilum.* Dogs infected with *E. ewingii* typically experience an acute illness very similar to that described for dogs infected with *A. phagocytophilum.* Except for crude geography (e.g., a dog from Missouri would be assumed to have *E. ewingii,* whereas a dog from Minnesota would be assumed to have *A. phagocytophilum*), these two infections were seldom differentiated until recently. Therefore retrospective and clinical reports of granulocytic ehrlichiosis might reflect infection with either *A. phagocytophilum* or *E. ewingii.*

To further obfuscate the disease manifestations of *A. phagocytophilum* infection, coinfection with multiple tick-borne pathogens may be common. Both *I. scapularis* and *I. pacificus* serve as transmission vectors for pathogens other than *A. phagocytophilum,* including *Borrelia burgdorferi* (the causative agent of Lyme disease). Based on recent evidence, coinfection with *A. phagocytophilum* and *B. burgdorferi* is common in endemic regions. In addition, sick dogs from such endemic regions were more likely to have coinfections with both *A. phagocytophilum* and *B. burgdorferi* than to have either infection alone. Because clinical signs might be related to coinfection or even to *B. burgdorferi,* descriptions of the clinical syndrome resulting from *A. phagocytophilum* infection must be considered suspect unless the infected dogs are tested for both pathogens.

It is likely that infection can either remain subclinical or result in acute disease manifestations. Clinical signs associated with *A. phagocytophilum* infection are often nonspecific and most commonly include fever, lethargy, and anorexia. Although polyarthritis occurs, it seems to be a more consistent finding during infection with *E. ewingii* than with *A. phagocytophilum.* Most dogs diagnosed with *A. phagocytophilum* infection have musculoskeletal pain, but clearly defined joint pain may or may not be present. Other reported signs include splenomegaly, hepatomegaly, central nervous system signs (e.g., ataxia, seizures), and lymphadenomegaly. Gastrointestinal and respiratory tract signs are rare. To date chronic complications commonly attributed to *E. canis* infection have not been described for *A. phagocytophilum.* With the recent advent of in-clinic diagnostic tests to confirm infection with *A. phagocytophilum* (see following section on Diagnosis), it is likely that a much better–defined understanding of the clinical disease will soon be available.

DIAGNOSIS

Although identification of morulae (elementary or inclusion bodies) on microscopic examination of canine blood smears can be suggestive of infection with *Anaplasma,* it is at best an insensitive and nonspecific diagnostic tool. On Romanowsky-type (e.g., Giemsa, Diff-Quik) stained peripheral blood smears, morulae of *A. platys* appear as basophilic (blue) inclusion bodies within platelets. It can be difficult to differentiate between *A. platys* inclusion bodies and dense platelet granules via light microscopy. Although inclusions can be found as soon as 1 to 2 weeks after experimental inoculation, it may be extremely difficult to find infected platelets during periods of thrombocytopenia. Morulae can be seen within the cytoplasm of granulocytes from 4 to 18 days after infection with *A. phagocytophilum.* Although most dogs with clinical infection attributed to *A. phagocytophilum* in the recorded veterinary literature were recognized because of observed granulocytic morulae, morulae are not uniformly present during infection. Thus absence of morulae cannot be used to rule out anaplasmosis. Even when granulocytic morulae are visualized, the appearance of *A. phagocytophilum* and *E. ewingii* is identical; thus microscopic visualization of morulae alone cannot confirm infection (Fig. 272-1).

There are no other specific findings on routine blood tests from infected dogs. The most common clinicopathologic abnormality identified during infection with either *A. phagocytophilum* or *A. platys* is thrombocytopenia, which may range in severity from mild to marked. Occasionally dogs with either infection may present with platelet counts within the reference range. Lymphopenia, eosinopenia, neutrophilia, and normocytic normochromic anemia have also been described inconsistently in infected dogs. Rarely *A. phagocytophilum* has been associated with apparent hemolytic anemia and severe thrombocytopenia. Biochemical changes may include hypoalbuminemia and mild-to-moderate increases in alkaline phosphatase activity.

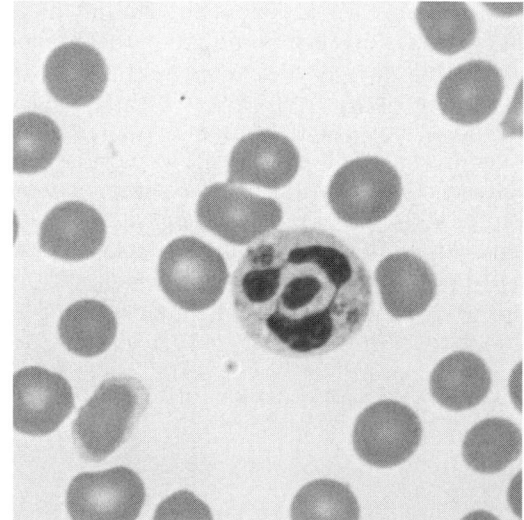

Fig. 272-1 Granulocytic inclusion (i.e., morula) in the neutrophil of a dog. The microscopic appearance of inclusions resulting from infection with *Anaplasma phagocytophilum* are indistinguishable from those resulting from infection with *Ehrlichia ewingii.* (Wright-Giemsa stain, ×1000.) (Image courtesy Dr. Linda Berent, University of Missouri–Veterinary Medical Diagnostic Laboratory.)

A variety of serologic tests have been used to look for antibodies to these pathogenic organisms. There seems to be little serologic cross-reactivity between *E. canis* and *A. phagocytophilum* and essentially no cross-reactivity between *E. canis* and *A. platys*. On the other hand, considerable serologic cross-reactivity is found between the two types of *Anaplasma* infections. Commercial indirect fluorescent antibody tests for one pathogen may provide positive test results when the dog has been exposed to the other pathogen. Because canine granulocytic anaplasmosis is an acute illness, either seroconversion or a four-fold increase in convalescent titers obtained 7 to 21 days after acute titers is required to document active infection (Lester et al., 2005). If chronic *A. platys* infection is detected via positive serology, there may not be a significant rise in titer. Recently a commercial enzyme-linked immunosorbent assay that detects the presence of antibodies to *A. phagocytophilum*, *B. burgdorferi*, *E. canis*, and *Dirofilaria immitis* has been marketed (Snap 4Dx IDEXX Laboratories). Reported sensitivity and specificity of the test for *A. phagocytophilum* is 99.4% and 100%, respectively. Apparently infection with *A. platys* results in a positive test result using this in-clinic diagnostic tool.

Serology documents the dog's antibody response to infection; however, other methods of diagnosis rely on identification of the organism. Visualization of morulae has already been described. Assays based on amplification of nucleic acid sequences (i.e., polymerase chain reaction [PCR]) have been used to identify infected dogs. As with all PCR assays, appropriate primer selection is crucial. Primer sequences can be more or less specific; some detect any of several *Anaplasma* or *Ehrlichia* spp., whereas others are specific for a single species. It is incumbent on the veterinary practitioner to use only a reputable laboratory and to understand what will be detected by the primers used in that laboratory.

THERAPY/PREVENTION

Tetracyclines are the mainstay of treatment for both *A. phagocytophilum* and *A. platys* infection. Doxycycline (5 to 10 mg/kg orally [PO] q12–24h) is recommended. Response to treatment is usually rapid, occurring within 24 to 48 hours. The optimum duration of therapy is unknown, but recommendations range from 10 to 28 days. Persistent infection with *A. phagocytophilum* has been documented experimentally after a short course of therapy, and relapses are noted anecdotally. We recommend a full 28-day course of antibiotic treatment. In most treated dogs serum antibodies revert to low or negative concentrations

within 7 to 8 months after treatment. Lack of rapid clinical response should prompt investigation of other disease processes, including *B. burgdorferi*.

Currently there are no vaccines to prevent either of these infections. In addition, recovered animals seem to be susceptible to reinfection with *A. phagocytophilum*. For now, prevention consists of adequate tick control. Environmental controls can minimize tick exposure but do not completely eliminate the acquisition of new ticks. Chemical methods of tick control usually are warranted. Typical choices include amitraz-impregnated collars, fipronil spray or spot-on formulations, and permethrin spray and spot-on formulations. (Dryden and Payne, 2004) Routine home examinations should be encouraged not only to identify and remove individual ticks but to determine if other aspects of tick prevention are working adequately. The role of routine annual screening for canine *Anaplasma* infection remains to be determined.

References and Suggested Reading

Bexfield NH, Villiers EJ, Herrtage ME: Immune-mediated haemolytic anaemia and thrombocytopenia associated with *Anaplasma phago cytophilum* in a dog, *J Small Anim Pract* 46:543, 2005.

Bradfield JF, Vore SJ, Pryor WH, Jr: *Ehrlichia platys* infection in dogs, *Lab Anim Sci* 46:565. 1996.

Cohn LA: Ehrlichiosis and related infections, *Vet Clin North Am Small Anim Pract* 33:863, 2003.

Dryden MW, Payne PA: Biology and control of ticks infesting dogs and cats in North America, *Vet Ther* 5:139. 2004.

Dumler JS, Barbet AF, Bekker CP: Reorganization of genera in the families Rickettsiaceae and Anaplasmataceae in the order Rickettsiales: unification of some species of *Ehrlichia* with *Anaplasma*, *Cowdria* with *Ehrlichia* and *Ehrlichia* with *Neorickettsia*, descriptions of six new species combinations and designation of *Ehrlichia equi* and 'HGE agent' as subjective synonyms of *Ehrlichia phagocytophila*, *Int J Syst Evol Microbiol* 51:2145, 2001.

Egenvall A et al: Early manifestations of granulocytic ehrlichiosis in dogs inoculated experimentally with a Swedish *Ehrlichia* species isolate, *Vet Rec* 143:412. 1998.

Lester SJ et al: *Anaplasma phagocytophilum* infection (granulocytic anaplasmosis) in a dog from Vancouver Island, *Can Vet J* 46:825, 2005.

Lilliehöök I, Egenvall A, Tvedten HW: Hematopathology in dogs experimentally infected with a Swedish granulocytic *Ehrlichia* species, *Vet Clin Pathol* 27:116. 1998.

McQuiston JH, McCall CL, Nicholson WL: Ehrlichiosis and related infections, *J Am Vet Med Assoc* 223:1750, 2003.

CHAPTER 273

American Leishmaniasis

GREGORY C. TROY, *Blacksburg, Virginia*

North American canine visceral leishmaniasis (CVL) is caused by the protozoan parasite *Leishmania infantum* which is of the MON-1 zymodeme, the primary zymodeme of *Leishmania* endemic to southern Europe (Baneth, 2006; Ferrer, 1992). Autochthonous CVL was first recognized in North America in the early 1980s. Cases of autochthonous CVL are reported in individual dogs from Texas, Maryland, Oklahoma, and North Carolina and in kennels located in Michigan, Alabama, and Virginia (Schantz et al., 2005). Before 2000 most cases in the United States were identified in dogs with travel histories to geographic regions of the world with endemic leishmaniasis (Schantz et al., 2005). Since 2001 this disease has been recognized in 21 states and in two Canadian provinces and is now considered well established in certain canine populations in North America (Gaskin et al, 2002; Schantz et al., 2005).

EPIDEMIOLOGY

CVL is considered a worldwide zoonotic disease. Domestic and wild canids are important reservoir hosts for human visceral leishmaniasis in geographic regions of the world where it is endemic. Ownership of infected dogs in endemic areas is considered a risk factor for human visceral leishmaniasis. In North America risk to humans from infected dogs has not been established because individuals that worked intimately with dogs have not been infected.

The primary mode of transmission of the North American isolate of *Leishmania infantum* is not definitively known at this time (Breitschwerdt and Schantz, 2006; Schantz et al., 2005; Rosypal, Zajac, and Lindsay, 2003). Phlebotomine sandflies of the genus *Lutzomyia* are present in North America, but only *Lutzomyia shannoni* is considered a possible competent insect reservoir (Baneth, 2006; Rosypal, Zajac, and Lindsay, 2003). In kennel situations older dogs and dogs that travel to the southern United States appear more likely to become infected with *L. infantum*, implying that different insect vectors or different modes of transmission play a role in maintenance of infection. Transmission of CVL has occurred by use of whole and packed red cell blood transfusions and by direct and transplacental routes. Experimental infection in mice and dogs with *L infantum* (strain—*L. infantum* Virginia Tech–1; LIVT-1) has shown low levels of vertical and sexual transmission. These findings provide a plausible explanation for transmission of CVL in kennel situations resulting in low-grade maintenance of infection; these modes of transmission of *L. infantum* may play a

more significant role in North American CVL than in other worldwide geographic regions with CVL.

Leishmania organisms reside intracellularly within macrophages in mammals and as extracellular promastigotes in their insect vector. The promastigote is the infective stage of the parasite, which, when injected into the skin of the dog, is transformed into amastigotes. Amastigote multiplication occurs in macrophages by binary fission within cutaneous, subcutaneous, and visceral tissues.

CLINICAL ASPECTS

The predominant clinical presentation of CVL is a generalized, chronic, debilitating systemic disease process affecting cutaneous and visceral tissues. In humans the disease is divided into three different forms, depending on clinical presentation and the propensity of the infecting species to affect certain tissues. These forms are cutaneous, mucocutaneous, or visceral forms. In dogs cutaneous lesions imply concurrent visceral involvement.

In naturally occurring and experimental canine leishmanial infections, a high percentage of dogs become infected, but a smaller percentage of dogs show overt clinical manifestations of disease. In a recent longitudinal study in dogs conducted over three transmission seasons in Italy, the number of dogs infected with *L. infantum* increased sequentially from 27% to approximately 97% of the dogs by the end of the third transmission season (Oliva et al., 2006). Zero percentage, 16%, and 53% of dogs had compatible clinical signs of leishmaniasis at the end of each year of the 3-year study (Oliva et al., 2006). Most dogs exhibit serologic conversion within 6 to 7 months after exposure. In an experimental study in beagles infected with the LIVT-1 strain and followed for 2 years, seroconversion (indirect immunofluorescent antibody test [IFAT]) occurred at 6 months and persisted for the duration of observation with minor fluctuations in reciprocal serologic titers.

Clinical manifestations described in dogs with CVL in the United States are variable and appear dependent on the phase of disease and state of immunity in the animal, but they are similar to dogs with CVL from other geographic locations. Genetic susceptibility in certain breeds of dogs also plays a role in infection. In an experimental study clinical manifestations were more notable in dogs administered a higher dose of *L. infantum* organisms. Common clinical and historical findings included lethargy, exercise intolerance, weight loss, inappetence, and lameness. Physical abnormalities included weight loss; generalized lymphadenopathy; and periocular, facial, and auricular dermatitis with exfoliation and development of cutaneous ulcers over boney protuberances, with extension to the trunk and extremities. Onychogryphosis was not observed. Ocular discharge was notable and resulted from keratoconjunctivitis, with no evidence of uveitis or panophthalmitis. Acute polyarthritis was evident in three of four experimentally infected beagles with the LIVT-1 strain and was characterized by purulent exudative synovitis. Administration of nonsteroidal antiinflammatory drugs (NSAIDs) resulted in clinical resolution of lameness within a short time in all dogs. Only one dog required long- term therapy with NSAIDs. Culture of *Leishmania* was attempted from joint effusions but was negative for growth on all occasions.

DIAGNOSIS

A diagnosis of leishmaniasis should be suspected in dogs exhibiting chronic skin lesions, ocular discharge, generalized lymphadenopathy, splenomegaly, and weight loss. Laboratory abnormalities that should heighten clinical suspicion of leishmaniasis include mild nonregenerative anemia, thrombocytopenia, hyperproteinemia, hypergammaglobulinemia, hypoalbuminemia, azotemia, and proteinuria.

A definitive diagnosis of leishmaniasis can be made when amastigotes are observed in tissue samples or by growth of the organism in culture. Splenic, lymph node, and bone marrow aspirates and imprints from skin lesions are commonly used in suspected animals in attempts to identify the organism. Microscopic detection rates of amastigotes range from 20% to 60% and depend on the quality of samples and preparations and time allotted to evaluate samples. In one study of beagles experimentally infected with *Leishmania chagasi* (Rosypal et al., 2005), organisms were identified more frequently in aspirates of bone marrow than lymph node aspirates; two positive control dogs infected for longer than 3 years had cytologically detectable amastigotes for approximately 2 years. However, in another study of beagles infected with the LIVT-1 strain, culture of lymph node aspirates was positive more often than bone marrow culture. The IFAT is considered the standard to which other serologic methods are compared and is useful for evaluating suspected infected dogs (Schantz et al., 2005). A titer of 1:64 is usually considered positive. Titers can fluctuate during the course of the disease, and dogs with titers of 1:64 should be evaluated more comprehensively. Other serologic methods to evaluate suspect dogs include complement fixation, direct agglutination, indirect hemagglutination, antigen specific enzyme-linked immunosorbent assay, Western blot, rK39 (see following paragraph), and an antigen dipstick immunoassay.

A variety of polymerase chain reaction (PCR) strategies (single, nested, real-time) have been used to demonstrate *Leishmania* deoxyribonucleic acid (DNA). PCR using primers that amplify a conserved minicircle region of the kinetoplast (extranuclear DNA structure of parasitic flagellates) that is common to all *Leishmania* spp. is available at several diagnostic laboratories. The sensitivity of PCR testing on blood, bone marrow, and lymph node aspirates is appropriately 90% to 95% and is higher on bone marrow and lymph node samples than on blood (Baneth, 2006; Breitschwerdt and Schantz, 2006). Differences in sensitivities among PCR assays appear to be caused by different levels of parasitemia present in tissues. PCR test results also support the observation that there are fewer symptomatic dogs than the number of dogs exposed and infected. A recombinant antigen immunoassay (rK39) is a more rapid testing method with fewer technical limitations than IFAT or PCR testing (Scalone et al., 2002). This recombinant antigen is a repetitive immunodominant epitope that mimics a kinesin-related protein that is highly conserved among viscerotropic *Leishmania* spp. This immunoassay has an excellent correlation to the IFAT. In an experimental study the rK39 assay detected 90% of infected dogs (Rosypal et al., 2005). In addition, the rK39 test does not cross-react with antibodies to *Trypanosoma cruzi*, which is a problem with the IFAT test in areas where this parasite may be endemic. The rK39 assay is commercially available (Kalazar Detect Rapid Test, InBios International, Ltd.).

TREATMENT AND PREVENTION

Treatment of infected dogs in the United States is controversial at this time because of lack of effective chemotherapeutics that result in parasitic cures, with the resultant persistently infected dogs potentially increasing the risk of human transmission. Pentavalent antimonials are the primary drugs used in treatment regimens. Meglumine antimoniate (Glucantime, Merial) (100 mg/kg intravenously [IV], subcutaneously [SQ] q24h for 3 to 4 weeks) and sodium stibogluconate (Pentostam, Wellcome Foundation Ltd.) (30 to 50 mg/kg IV, SQ, q24h for 3 to 4 weeks) are parenteral drugs requiring daily administration. Only sodium stibogluconate is available in the United States through the Centers for Disease Control and Prevention. Side effects of these drugs, including vomiting, diarrhea, muscle pain/fibrosis, abscessation, thrombophlebitis, and renal failure, are common and can be severe. Allopurinol (20 mg/kg orally [PO] q12 or 24h), a xanthine oxidase inhibitor, can be used concurrently with the pentavalent antimonials and as a maintenance drug. Dogs treated with meglumine antimoniate and allopurinol had prolonged survival times (>4 years) with fewer relapses (Slappedel and Teske, 1999). Treatment of dogs with these compounds requires frequent monitoring, especially of renal function because of potential nephrotoxicity in dogs that frequently already have renal disease. Additional drugs that show some effectiveness in treatment of leishmaniasis are amphotericin B (desoxycholate, lipid emulsion and liposomal preparations), miltefosine, pentamidine, and aminosidine (Noli and Auxiliz, 2005). Parasitic cures are uncommon with these products, but clinical improvements do result. A recent in vitro study with marbofloxacin could hold promise for a less toxic treatment of leishmaniasis.

Until a definitive mode of transmission is identified in North America, dogs should not be held under crowded conditions, and effective topical insecticides should be used to minimize exposure to possible insect vectors. A commercial vaccine against canine visceral leishmaniasis has been licensed in Brazil and contains the Fucose-Mannose-ligand antigen of *Leishmania donovani* (Nogueira, 2005). This product has proven effective in reducing infection rates in dogs and humans where visceral leishmaniasis is endemic (Leishmune[R], Fort Dodge Saude Animal Ltd.).

References and Suggested Reading

Baneth G: Leishmaniases. In: Greene CE, editor, *Infectious diseases of the dog and cat*, ed 3, St. Louis, 2006, Saunders p.685.

Breitschwerdt EB, Schantz P: Canine visceral leishmaniasis in North America. In Greene CE, editor: *Infectious diseases of the dog and cat*, ed 3, St Louis, 2006, Saunders, p 696.

Ferrer L: Leishmaniasis. In Kirk RW, Bonagura JD, editors: *Current veterinary therapy XI (small animal practice)*, Philadelphia, 1992, Saunders, p 266.

Gaskin AA et al: Visceral leishmaniasis in a New York foxhound kennel, *J Vet Intern Med* 16:34, 2002.

Nogueira FS et al: Leishmune[R] vaccine blocks the transmission of canine visceral leishmaniasis: absences of *Leishmania* parasites in blood, skin and lymph nodes of vaccinated exposed dogs, *Vaccine* 23:4805, 2005.

Noli C, Auxiliz ST: Review: treatment of canine Old World visceral leishmaniasis: a systemic review, *Vet Dermatol* 16:213, 2005.

Oliva G et al: Incidence and time course of *Leishmania infantum* infections examined by parasitological, serologic, and nested-PCR techniques in a cohort of naïve dogs exposed to three consecutive transmission seasons, *J Clin Microbiol* 44:1318, 2006.

Rosypal AC, Zajac AM, Lindsay DS: Canine visceral leishmaniasis and its emergence in the United States, *Vet Clin N Am Sm Anim Pract* 33:921, 2003.

Rosypal AC et al: Utility of diagnostic tests used in diagnosis of infection in dogs experimentally inoculated with a North American isolate of *Leishmania infantum*, *J Vet Intern Med* 19:802, 2005.

Schantz et al: Autochthonous visceral leishmaniasis in dogs in North America, *J Am Vet Med Assoc* 226:1316, 2005.

Scalone A et al: Evaluation of the *Leishmania* recombinant K39 antigen as a diagnostic marker for canine leishmaniasis and validation of a standardized enzyme-linked immunosorbent assay, *Vet Parasitol* 104:275, 2002.

Slappedel RJ, Teske E: A review of canine leishmaniasis presenting outside endemic areas, Proceedings of the International Canine Leishmaniosis Forum, Barcelona, Spain,1999, p 54.

CHAPTER 274

Toxoplasmosis

MICHAEL R. LAPPIN, *Fort Collins, Colorado*

Familiarity with *Toxoplasma gondii* is important for all small animal practitioners because of pet ownership issues, as well as the occasional association of *T. gondii* with clinical illness in cats and dogs. The life cycle, diagnosis, treatment, and prevention of feline and canine toxoplasmosis has been reviewed extensively over the years (Dubey and Lappin, 2006). In addition, the American Association of Feline Practitioners and the Centers for Disease Control and Prevention have provided information concerning cat ownership as it relates to *T. gondii* and other infectious agents (Brown et al., 2003; Kaplan, Massur, and Holmes, 2002).* This chapter emphasizes some of the most important points about this disease and provides recently published information concerning the zoonotic and clinical considerations for this protozoan.

AGENT AND EPIDEMIOLOGY

T. gondii is one of the most prevalent parasites infecting warm-blooded vertebrates; a recent survey of clinically ill cats in the United States showed an overall seroprevalence rate of 31.6% (Vollaire, Radecki, and Lappin, 2005). Approximately 20% of dogs in the United States are seropositive for *T. gondii* antibodies. Only cats complete the coccidian life cycle and pass environmentally resistant oocysts in feces. Dogs do not produce *T. gondii* oocysts like cats but can mechanically transmit oocysts after ingesting feline feces. *Sporozoites* develop in oocysts after 1 to 5 days of exposure to oxygen and appropriate environmental temperature and humidity. Thus, to lessen the potential of exposure to *T. gondii* for veterinary staff members in the laboratory, fresh feces should be used for fecal flotation, or the feces should be stored refrigerated until examined. *Tachyzoites* are the rapidly dividing stage of the organism; they disseminate in blood or lymph during active infection and replicate rapidly intracellularly until the cell is destroyed. Tachyzoites can be detected

---

*www.aafponline.org/resources/guidelines/ZooFinal2003.pdf
www.cdc.gov/ncidod/dpd/parasites/toxoplasmosis/default.htm

in blood, aspirates, and effusions in some dogs or cats with disseminated disease. *Bradyzoites* are the slowly dividing, persistent tissue stage that form in the extraintestinal tissues of infected hosts as immune responses attenuate tachyzoite replication. Bradyzoites form readily in the central nervous system (CNS), muscles, and visceral organs. *T. gondii* bradyzoites can be the source of reactivated acute infection (e.g., during immune suppression by feline immunodeficiency virus [FIV] or high-dose cyclosporine therapy), or they may be associated with some chronic disease manifestations (e.g., uveitis). Infection of warm-blooded vertebrates occurs following ingestion of any of these three life stages of the organism or transplacentally. Cats infected by ingesting *T. gondii* bradyzoites during carnivorous feeding shed oocysts in feces from 3 to 21 days. Fewer numbers of oocysts are shed for longer time periods if sporulated oocysts are ingested. Sporulated oocysts can survive in the environment for months to years and are resistant to most disinfectants. For dogs, cats, and humans it is believed that bradyzoites persist in tissues for the life of the host, regardless of whether drugs with presumed *T. gondii* activity are administered.

CLINICAL FEATURES OF FELINE INFECTION

Approximately 10% to 20% of cats that are experimentally inoculated with *T. gondii* tissue cysts develop self-limiting small bowel diarrhea for 1 to 2 weeks; this is presumed to be caused by local replication of the organism during the intestinal phase of infection. However, detection of *T. gondii* oocysts in feces is rarely reported in studies of client-owned cats with diarrhea, in part because of the short oocyst shedding period. Although *T. gondii* enteroepithelial stages were found in intestinal tissues from two cats with inflammatory bowel disease that responded to anti- *T. gondii* drugs, it is my experience that chronic gastrointestinal disease in cats from toxoplasmosis is uncommon.

Fatal toxoplasmosis can develop during acute dissemination and intracellular replication of tachyzoites; hepatic, pulmonary, CNS, and pancreatic tissues are commonly involved (Dubey and Lappin, 2006). Transplacentally or lactationally infected kittens develop the most severe signs of extraintestinal toxoplasmosis and generally die of pulmonary or hepatic disease. Common clinical findings in cats with disseminated toxoplasmosis include depression, anorexia, fever followed by hypothermia, peritoneal effusion, icterus, and dyspnea. If a host with chronic toxoplasmosis is immunosuppressed, bradyzoites in tissue cysts can replicate rapidly and disseminate again as tachyzoites; this is common in humans with acquired immune deficiency syndrome (AIDS). Disseminated toxoplasmosis has been documented in cats concurrently infected with feline leukemia virus (FeLV), FIV, and feline infectious peritonitis virus. Commonly used clinical doses of glucocorticoids do not appear to predispose to activated toxoplasmosis. However, administration of cyclosporine to cats or dogs with renal transplantations or dermatologic disease has been associated with fatal disseminated toxoplasmosis (Bernstein et al., 1999; Last et al., 2004; Barrs, Martin, and Beatty, 2006).

Chronic toxoplasmosis with vague and recurrent clinical signs of disease appears to occur in some cats. *T. gondii* infection should be on the differential diagnoses list for cats with anterior or posterior uveitis, fever, muscle hyperesthesia, weight loss, anorexia, seizures, ataxia, icterus, diarrhea, or pancreatitis.

Based on results of *T. gondii*–specific aqueous humor antibody and polymerase chain reaction (PCR) studies, toxoplasmosis appears to be one of the most common infectious causes of uveitis in cats. It is unknown why the majority of cats infected with *T. gondii* are subclinically affected and other cats develop clinical signs of disease. Similar to what is reported in humans, kittens infected with *T. gondii* transplacentally or lactationally commonly develop ocular disease. Immune complex formation and deposition in tissues and delayed hypersensitivity reactions may be involved in chronic clinical toxoplasmosis. Since none of the anti-*Toxoplasma* drugs totally clear the body of the organism, recurrence of disease is common. This fact should be made clear to owners in discharge instructions, and the communication noted in the medical record.

CLINICAL FEATURES OF CANINE INFECTION

Before 1988 many dogs diagnosed with toxoplasmosis based on histologic evaluation were truly infected with *Neospora caninum*. However, *T. gondii* infection frequently occurs in dogs and rarely can be associated with clinical disease. The most common syndromes associated with disseminated toxoplasmosis in dogs have involved the respiratory, gastrointestinal, or neuromuscular systems, resulting in fever, vomiting, diarrhea, dyspnea, and icterus. Disseminated toxoplasmosis is most common in immunosuppressed dogs such as those with canine distemper virus infection or those receiving cyclosporine to prevent rejection of a renal transplant.

Neurologic signs depend on the location of the primary lesions and include ataxia, seizures, tremors, cranial nerve deficits, paresis, and paralysis. Dogs with myositis present with weakness, stiff gait, or muscle wasting. Rapid progression to tetraparesis and paralysis with lower motor neuron dysfunction can occur. Myocardial infection resulting in ventricular arrhythmias occurs in some infected dogs. Retinitis, anterior uveitis, iridocyclitis, and optic neuritis occur in some dogs with toxoplasmosis but for unknown reasons seem to be less common than in the cat.

CLINICAL DIAGNOSIS

Cats and dogs with clinical toxoplasmosis can have a variety of clinicopathologic and radiographic abnormalities, but none of the findings alone can be used to document the disease. Nonregenerative anemia, neutrophilic leukocytosis, lymphocytosis, monocytosis, neutropenia, eosinophilia, proteinuria, bilirubinuria, and increases in serum globulins and bilirubin concentration can be seen. In addition, increased activities of creatinine kinase, alanine aminotransferase, alkaline phosphatase, and lipase occur in some affected animals.

Pulmonary toxoplasmosis most commonly causes diffuse interstitial-to-patchy alveolar patterns or pleural effusion. Cerebrospinal fluid (CSF) protein concentrations and cell counts are often higher than normal; the predominant white blood cells in CSF are small mononuclear cells and neutrophils. The detection of these abnormalities should direct the clinician to perform additional, more specific *T. gondii* tests, particularly if there is a high likelihood of exposure to sporulated oocysts or uncooked meat or there is historic or other evidence of immunodeficiency.

The antemortem definitive diagnosis of toxoplasmosis can be made if the organism or its deoxyribonucleic acid (DNA) is demonstrated; this is most likely to be achieved in cats or dogs with acute disseminated disease. Tachyzoites or bradyzoites have been detected in tissues, effusions, bronchoalveolar lavage fluids, aqueous humor, or CSF. Detection of *T. gondii* organisms is unlikely in cats or dogs with chronic disease manifestations. *T. gondii* DNA can be amplified from tissues and fluids; thus PCR detection is considered more sensitive and specific than cytologic or histopathologic detection of the organism. Multiple laboratories offer PCR assays that can amplify DNA of *T. gondii* and *N. caninum* (dogs); these assays should be considered if *T. gondii* or *N. caninum* is suspected but are not documented cytologically. Tissues, fluids, or aspirates for *T. gondii* PCR testing can be maintained frozen until assayed because the DNA is very stable. *T. gondii* PCR assays seem to be less sensitive if performed on formalin-fixed samples; thus use of fresh tissue is preferred. Immunohistochemistry can also be performed on tissues to document the presence of *T. gondii* and to differentiate *T. gondii* from *N. caninum*.

Detection of 10 × 12 micrometer diameter oocysts in feces in cats with diarrhea suggests toxoplasmosis but is not definitive since *Besnoitia* and *Hammondia* infections of cats produce morphologically similar oocysts. In these cases *T. gondii* serology should be performed, and, if the primary infection is *T. gondii,* seroconversion should be documented within 2 to 3 weeks. In dogs *N. caninum* oocysts are morphologically similar to *T. gondii* oocysts. These dogs can be screened for *N. caninum* and *T. gondii* antibodies in 2 to 3 weeks to determine the organism that was associated with the infection.

A multitude of tests for detection of *T. gondii*–specific antibodies (immunoglobulin [Ig]M, IgG, IgA), antigens, and immune complexes have been evaluated (Dubey and Lappin, 2006). Unfortunately test results can be positive in healthy animals, as well as those with clinical signs of toxoplasmosis; thus it is impossible to make an antemortem diagnosis of clinical toxoplasmosis based on results of these tests alone. Of the serum tests, IgM titers correlate best with clinical toxoplasmosis since this antibody class is rarely detected in serum of healthy animals; thus many laboratories offer IgM and IgG test results separately. The antemortem diagnosis of clinical toxoplasmosis can tentatively be based on the combination of (1) clinical signs of disease referable to toxoplasmosis; (2) demonstration of antibodies in serum, which documents exposure to *T. gondii*; (3) demonstration of an IgM titer >1:64 or a fourfold or greater increase in IgG titer, which suggests recent or active infection;

(4) exclusion of other common causes of the clinical syndrome; and (5) positive response to appropriate treatment. In dogs gneosporosis and toxoplasmosis appear clinically similar; thus I frequently combine *T. gondii* and *N. caninum* serologic tests in my diagnostic workup of suspect patients.

Some cats and dogs with clinical toxoplasmosis will have reached their maximal IgG titer or will have undergone antibody class shift from IgM to IgG by the time they are serologically evaluated; thus failure to document an increasing IgG titer or a positive IgM titer does not exclude the diagnosis of toxoplasmosis. This problem is most common in cats and dogs with chronic disease manifestations. Some healthy cats and dogs have extremely high serum antibody titers, and some clinically ill cats and dogs have low serum antibody titers, thus the magnitude of titer is relatively unimportant in the clinical diagnosis of toxoplasmosis. Because the organism cannot be cleared from the body, most cats and dogs will be antibody-positive for life; thus there is no clinical use in repeating serum antibody titers after disease manifestations have resolved.

The combination of *T. gondii*–specific antibody detection in aqueous humor or CSF and organism DNA amplification by PCR is the most accurate way to diagnose ocular or CNS toxoplasmosis in cats. *T. gondii*–specific IgA, IgG, and DNA can be detected in aqueous humor and CSF of both normal and clinically ill cats; however, *T. gondii*–specific IgM has only been detected in the aqueous humor or CSF of clinically ill cats and so may be the best indicator of clinical disease (Lappin MR, Unpublished data). My laboratory has rarely amplified *T. gondii* DNA or shown *T. gondii* antibody production in aqueous humor or CSF from dogs. CNS toxoplasmosis and neosporosis can appear clinically similar in dogs; thus I frequently combine PCR testing for both organisms on CSF samples from dogs with inflammatory CNS disease.

T. gondii antigens or DNA can be detected in the blood of healthy cats; the source of the organism is likely bradyzoites from tissue cysts. Since *T. gondii* DNA can be detected in blood of healthy cats, positive PCR results do not always correlate to clinical disease. Whether parasitemia can be documented in more dogs with toxoplasmosis than healthy dogs is currently unknown.

THERAPY

Supportive care should be instituted as needed. I have used clindamycin hydrochloride administered at 10 to 12 mg/kg orally every 12 hours for 4 weeks or trimethoprim-sulfonamide combination administered at 15 mg/kg orally every 12 hours for 4 weeks most frequently for the treatment of clinical feline or canine toxoplasmosis. These two drugs can also be used in combination. Trimethoprim sulfa is likely to penetrate an intact blood-brain barrier better than clindamycin and thus should be considered for CNS toxoplasmosis, particularly if there is a poor response to clindamycin in the first 7 days of therapy. Azithromycin administered at 7.5 mg/kg orally every 12 hours has been used successfully in a limited number of cats and dogs, but the optimal interval or duration of this expensive drug is unknown. Recently a case of azithromycin-resistant, clindamycin-responsive pulmonic toxoplasmosis in a dog was documented (Lappin MR, unpublished data). It is likely that, just like bacteria, different *T. gondii* isolates have different antimicrobial susceptibilities; thus, if the first drug attempted fails, an alternate drug should be attempted if the organism is still high on the differential list. Pyrimethamine combined with sulfa drugs is effective for the treatment of human toxoplasmosis but commonly results in toxicity in cats; thus I never use the drug for this purpose.

Cats or dogs with systemic clinical signs of toxoplasmosis combined with uveitis should be treated with anti-*Toxoplasma* drugs in combination with topical, oral, or parenteral corticosteroids to avoid secondary glaucoma and lens luxations. Prednisolone acetate (1% solution) applied topically to the eye three to four times daily is generally sufficient. *T. gondii*–seropositive cats or dogs with uveitis that are otherwise normal can be treated with topical glucocorticoids alone unless uveitis is recurrent or persistent. In the latter situation it may be beneficial to administer a drug with anti–*T. gondii* activity.

Clinical signs not involving the eyes or the CNS usually begin to resolve within the first 2 to 3 days of clindamycin or trimethoprim-sulfonamide administration; ocular and CNS toxoplasmosis respond more slowly to therapy. If fever or muscle hyperesthesia is not lessening after 3 days of treatment, other causes should be considered, or an alternate anti-*Toxoplasma* drug prescribed. Recurrence of clinical signs may be more common in cats treated for less than 4 weeks. In cases of pulmonary toxoplasmosis, total resolution of radiographic abnormalities may not occur for several weeks. The prognosis is usually poor for cats or dogs with hepatic or pulmonary disease resulting from organism replication, particularly in those that are immunocompromised.

It is currently unknown whether there is benefit to testing cats or dogs for *T. gondii* infection and treating the seropositive animals before administering cyclosporine therapy for other clinical diseases. If cyclosporine is to be used, it seems prudent to use the lowest dose possible and to attempt to avoid exposure to *T. gondii* by restricting hunting activity and feeding processed foods.

ZOONOTIC ASPECTS AND PREVENTION

T. gondii is an important zoonotic agent. Primary infection of mothers during gestation can lead to clinical toxoplasmosis in the fetus; stillbirth, CNS disease, and ocular disease are common clinical manifestations. Primary infection in immunocompetent individuals results in self-limiting fever, malaise, and lymphadenopathy. As T-helper cells counts decline, approximately 10% of humans with AIDS develop toxoplasmic encephalitis from activation of bradyzoites in tissue cysts. *T. gondii* is known to alter behavior of prey species, which may benefit the organism by allowing the feline definitive host to more easily ingest the parasite and continue the life cycle. Interestingly there have also been a number of papers suggesting that chronic *T. gondii* infection of humans may result in a variety of CNS diseases, including behavior changes and schizophrenia (Flegr, 2007; Webster, 2007). However, to date none of the work has documented a definitive link

to toxoplasmosis; and, because *T. gondii* infection can be acquired in several ways, there is no reason to relinquish a personal cat for this concern.

Humans most commonly acquire toxoplasmosis by ingesting sporulated oocysts or tissue cysts or transplacentally. To prevent toxoplasmosis, humans should avoid eating undercooked meats or ingesting sporulated oocysts. Although owning a pet cat has been associated epidemiologically with acquiring toxoplasmosis in some studies, the majority of work suggests that touching individual cats is probably not a common way to acquire toxoplasmosis for the following reasons: (1) cats generally only shed oocysts for days to several weeks following primary inoculation; (2) repeat oocyst shedding is rare, even in cats receiving glucocorticoids or cyclosporine or in those infected with FIV or FeLV; (3) cats with toxoplasmosis inoculated with tissue cysts 16 months after primary inoculation did not shed oocysts; (4) cats are very fastidious and usually do not allow feces to remain on their skin for time periods long enough to lead to oocyst sporulation (the organism was not isolated from the fur of cats shedding millions of oocysts 7 days previously); (5) increased risk of acquired toxoplasmosis was not associated with cat ownership in studies of veterinary health care providers or humans with AIDS. However, since some cats will repeat oocyst shedding when exposed a second time, feces should always be handled carefully. If a fecal sample from a cat is shown to contain oocysts measuring 10 × 12 microns, it should be assumed that the organism is *T. gondii*. The feces should be collected daily until the oocyst shedding period is complete; administration of clindamycin (25 to 50 mg/kg divided q12h orally [PO]) or sulfonamides (100 mg/kg divided q12h, PO) can reduce levels of oocyst shedding.

Box 274-1

Guidelines for Cat Owners To Avoid Acquiring Toxoplasmosis

- Wash hands after handling cats, especially if you are pregnant or immunocompromised.
- Remove fecal material from the home environment daily.
- If possible, do not have immunocompromised humans clean the litter box. If immunocompromised humans must clean the litter box, they should wear gloves and wash hands thoroughly when finished.
- Use litter box liners and periodically clean the litter box with scalding water and detergent.
- Wear gloves when gardening and wash hands thoroughly when finished.
- Cover children's sandboxes when not in use to lessen fecal contamination by outdoor cats.
- Only feed cats cooked or commercially processed food.
- Control potential transport hosts such as flies and cockroaches that may bring the organism into the home.
- Filter or boil water from sources in the environment.
- Housing cats indoors may lessen their exposure.
- Cook meat for human consumption to 80° C for 15 minutes minimum (medium-well).
- Wear gloves when handling meat and wash hands thoroughly with soap and water when finished.

Since humans are not commonly infected with *T. gondii* from contact with individual cats, testing healthy cats for toxoplasmosis is not recommended (Brown et al., 2003). Fecal examination is an adequate procedure to determine when cats are actively shedding oocysts but cannot predict when a cat has shed oocysts in the past. There is no serologic assay that accurately predicts when a cat shed *T. gondii* oocysts in the past, and most cats that are shedding oocysts are seronegative. Most seropositive cats have completed the oocyst shedding period and are unlikely to repeat shedding; most seronegative cats would shed the organism if infected. If owners are concerned that they may have acquired toxoplasmosis, they should see their doctor for testing. Common sense practices should also be followed (Box 274-1).

References and Suggested Reading

Barrs VR, Martin P, Beatty JA: Antemortem diagnosis and treatment of toxoplasmosis in two cats on cyclosporine therapy, *Aust Vet J* 84:30, 2006.

Bernstein L et al: Acute toxoplasmosis following renal transplantation in three cats and a dog, *J Am Vet Med Assoc* 215:1123, 1999.

Brown RR et al: Feline zoonoses guidelines from the American Association of Feline Practitioners, *Compend Contin Educ Pract Vet* 25:936, 2003.

Dubey JP, Lappin MR: Toxoplasmosis and neosporosis. In Greene CE, editor: *Infectious diseases of the dog and cat*, ed 3, St Louis, 2006, Saunders, 2006, p 754.

Flegr J: Effects of *Toxoplasma* on human behavior, *Schizophr Bull* 2007.

Kaplan JE, Massur H, Holmes KK: Guidelines for preventing opportunistic infections among HIV-infected persons, *MMWR* 51(RR08):1, 2002.

Last RD et al: A case of fatal systemic toxoplasmosis in a cat being treated with cyclosporine A for feline atopy 15:194, 2004.

Lindsay DS, Blagburn DL, Dubey JP: Feline toxoplasmosis and the importance of the *Toxoplasma gondii* oocyst, *Compend Contin Educ Pract Vet* 19:448, 1997.

Vollaire MR, Radecki SV, Lappin MR: Seroprevalence of *Toxoplasma gondii* antibodies in clinically ill cats of the United States, *Am J Vet Res* 66:874, 2005.

Webster JP: The effect of *Toxoplasma gondii* on animal behavior: playing cat and mouse, *Schizophr Bull* 2007.

CHAPTER 275

Pneumocystosis

REMO LOBETTI, *Bryanston, South Africa*

*P*neumocystis carinii is a saprophyte of low virulence that primarily occurs in the mammalian lung. Clinical pneumonia has been reported to occur spontaneously in dogs associated with a suspected immunodeficiency. Airborne transmission is suspected because healthy animals become infected when they are housed with infected animals. It is presumed that the organism may have a dormant life stage in the environment. The taxonomy of *P. carinii* is uncertain. It has been classified as a unicellular protozoan belonging to the phylum Sarcomastigophora, subphylum Sarcodina. However, its reproductive behavior is similar to that of yeast cells. On the other hand, phylogenetic classification based on 16S-like ribosomal ribonucleic acid sequences indicates that *P. carinii* is most closely related to fungi of the class Ascomycetes, yet it behaves like a protozoan because it is sensitive to drugs used to treat protozoan infections.

The morphology of *P. carinii* and the histopathology of the lesions produced by both human and animal isolates throughout the world are similar. Only a single species name has been assigned to the genus *Pneumocystis*, but antigenic differences suggest that several strains may exist. Although currently controversial, four species have been described: two species that infect dogs and rats, *P. carinii* and *Pneumocystis wakefieldiae*; one species, *Pneumocystis murina*, which infects mice; and *Pneumocystis jirvecii*, which infects humans. Biologic differences among isolates from different hosts are suggested by the relative difficulty of experimental interspecies transmission.

EPIDEMIOLOGY

P. carinii appears to be maintained in nature by transmission from infected to susceptible animals within a species. The primary mode of spread is thought to be airborne droplet transmission between hosts. The contagious nature of pneumocystosis is suggested by the epidemic spread that has occurred in institutionalized humans. Sporadic case reports may represent an activation of latent infection by stress, crowding, and immunosuppressive therapy during hospitalization of latent carriers. Clinical disease also has been experimentally activated after cortisone therapy, cytotoxic chemotherapy, and irradiation. A higher prevalence of infection has been found in dogs with canine distemper compared with a corresponding control population.

The entire life cycle of *P. carinii* is completed within the alveolar spaces, where organisms adhere in clusters to the pneumocytes. Two main forms, the trophozoite and cyst, are found. Although *Pneumocystis* infections are usually limited to the lung, in humans and in a single dog organisms have been reported in extrapulmonary sites. Severe immunodeficiency states in humans such as acquired immune deficiency syndrome (AIDS) can be associated with lymphatic or hematogenous dissemination of the organisms from the lungs to other tissues. Transmission of infection to an offspring may occur via aspiration of amniotic fluid contaminated by placental infection.

PATHOGENESIS

Pneumocystis can be inhaled from the environment and can colonize the lower respiratory tract of clinically healthy mammals; however, organisms rarely multiply to large numbers in the lungs of clinically healthy hosts. In conditions in which there is impaired host resistance or preexisting pulmonary disease, proliferation of organisms can occur. Alveolocapillary blockage and decreased gaseous exchange result secondary to the overgrowth and clustering of *P. carinii* within the alveolar spaces. Intraalveolar organisms are often accompanied by thickening of alveolar septa, but organisms seldom invade the pulmonary parenchyma and are rarely found in alveolar macrophages. The inflammatory response that the organism provokes contributes to the pulmonary alveolar damage and clinical pathophysiology.

CLINICAL FINDINGS

Most reported canine cases have been in miniature dachshunds younger than 1 year, although cases of pneumocystosis have been reported in a Shetland sheepdog, a Yorkshire terrier, and cavalier King Charles spaniels. The syndrome of common variable immunodeficiency, in which there is absence of B cells resulting in little or no antibody production in association with defective T cells, appears to occur in affected miniature dachshunds and is likely a risk factor for clinical disease in these dogs.

The typical clinical history in dogs with pneumocystosis is that of gradual weight loss and variable polypnea progressing over a period of time. Weight loss, which occurs in spite of a good appetite in most dogs, may be associated with diarrhea and occasional vomiting. Coughing is not always present, but exercise intolerance is present consistently. Infected animals may show some response to antibiotic or cortisone therapy.

Affected dogs generally remain relatively alert and afebrile. Abnormalities on clinical examination include polypnea, tachycardia, and pulmonary crackles on thoracic auscultation. Animals are usually in poor condition, cachectic, and often show dermatologic changes such as superficial bacterial pyoderma and demodicosis. Although the mucous membranes generally are of normal color, in severely affected animals they may be cyanotic.

DIAGNOSIS

Hematologic abnormalities are usually nonspecific, with neutrophilic leukocytosis and left shift seen most consistently; eosinophilia and monocytosis occur less frequently. The white cell response often appears inadequate in light of the pulmonary changes. Polycythemia may occur secondary to arterial hypoxemia from impaired gaseous exchange. Thrombocytosis is often also present. Serum proteins are usually normal with a low-to–low normal globulin level, which correlates with low γ-globulin levels on serum protein electrophoresis. Decreased lymphocyte function and low levels of serum immunoglobulin (Ig)A, IgG, and IgM have been reported. Arterial hypoxemia, hypocapnia, and alkalemia indicate an uncompensated respiratory alkalosis. The P_aO_2 is often lower than would be expected from the clinical signs and thoracic radiographs.

Findings on survey thoracic radiography include diffuse, bilaterally symmetric, alveolar-to-interstitial lung disease. Solitary lesions, unilateral involvement, cavitary lesions, spontaneous pneumothorax, or lobar infiltrate occasionally may be present. Tracheal elevation, right-sided heart enlargement, and pulmonary arterial enlargement reflect cor pulmonale secondary to the chronic pulmonary disease.

The diagnosis of pneumocystosis requires direct demonstration of *P. carinii* in either lung biopsy specimens or respiratory fluids. Transtracheal or endotracheal washings and oropharyngeal secretions may contain organisms, with transtracheal aspirates being very effective in identifying organisms in dogs. Samples for cytology may be obtained by endobronchial brushing and transbronchoscopic biopsy, but these procedures require special endoscopic equipment and involve the risks of general anesthesia. Transtracheal or endotracheal lavage and percutaneous transthoracic needle aspiration are more available to practitioners and have been shown to have a good correlation with transbronchoscopic biopsy findings in confirming a diagnosis. None of the cytologic techniques are as reliable or as definitive as lung biopsy for documenting active pneumocystosis. Unfortunately lung biopsy has the greatest risk of complications such as hemorrhage, secondary infection, pneumothorax, and death from anesthesia. Antimicrobial therapy can begin 24 to 48 hours before specimen collection in a patient suspected of having pneumocystosis without hindering the identification of organisms in the sample. Diff-Quik (a modified Giemsa stain) can be used as a fast and inexpensive screening stain after which negative results can be confirmed with more sensitive staining such as methenamine silver for cysts or with Giemsa for nuclei of intracystic sporozoites and trophozoites.

Other diagnostic tests that have been used include direct or indirect fluorescent antibody test for detecting organisms in tracheal aspirates and immunoperoxidase stains for impression smears and formalin-fixed, paraffin-embedded lung sections. The polymerase chain reaction has been effective in the detection of organisms in bronchoalveolar lavage specimens from humans and lung tissue from dogs. In humans serologic tests have been developed; however, their diagnostic value is uncertain since antigenemia is found in up to 15% of clinically normal humans.

THERAPY

Specific therapy is most beneficial in cases in which the disease has been diagnosed during the early stages. Although a number of drugs have been used in the treatment of *P. carinii*, the two drugs that have been used successfully to treat pneumocystosis are pentamidine isethionate and the combination of trimethoprim and sulfamethoxazole, the latter being the most effective in the dog.

Pentamidine isethionate is an aromatic diamidine used in humans. Its major side effects include impaired renal function, hepatic dysfunction, hypoglycemia, hypotension, hypocalcemia, urticaria, and hematologic disorders. Intramuscular administration of this drug has been successful in treating a dog with pneumocystosis, with the only side effect being localized pain at the injection site. Pentamidine has also been used at a reduced dosage in combination with sulfonamides to lower its toxic side effects. Other aromatic diamidines such as diminazene, imidocarb, and amicarbalide have been more effective than pentamidine in treating experimental *P. carinii* pneumonia.

The combination of trimethoprim and sulfamethoxazole has been found to be more effective and less toxic than pentamidine in treating and preventing *Pneumocystis* pneumonia in immunosuppressed humans. A dosage of 15 mg/kg TID or 30 mg/kg BID for 3 weeks has been used successfully in miniature dachshunds with pneumocystosis. Folic acid supplementation should be given if side effects such as leukopenia and anemia are observed or if long-term therapy is required.

Atovaquone is another drug licensed for the treatment of humans with pneumocystosis. It is not as effective as pentamidine or trimethoprim-sulfamethoxazole but has a reported lower toxicity. Bioavailability is increased when the drug is given with food with a high fat content.

Combination therapy using clindamycin and primaquine has also been effective both in vivo and in vitro, but neither drug is effective alone. Dapsone and trimethoprim or pyrimethamine in combination have been effective in experimental animals and clinical trials in immunosuppressed humans with pneumocystosis. Trimetrexate, a lipid-soluble antifolate, has been given concomitantly with leucovorin to humans with *Pneumocystis* pneumonia and AIDS. As with most of the other drugs, neutropenia with or without thrombocytopenia has been the main

side effect. In experimentally infected animals *P. carinii* is resistant to imidazole antifungal drugs, but the anthelmintics benzimidazole and albendazole have been shown to have some effect.

Supportive care is essential for any patient with pneumocystosis. Oxygen therapy administered by cage, mask, or intubation is needed (Chapter 137); and ventilatory assistance may also be required (Chapter 138). Bronchodilators may help reduce airway resistance. If a patient is receiving immunosuppressive agents, they should be discontinued temporarily; however, antiinflammatory drugs may be indicated. In humans the successful treatment of pneumocystosis results in additional pulmonary dysfunction and a decline in arterial oxygen related to the inflammatory reaction to dying organisms, and the administration of antiinflammatory doses of cortisone has been shown to improve pulmonary function and survival. Nonspecific immunostimulants such as cimetidine and levamisole have been given adjunctively to treat affected miniature dachshunds, but in all probability they have limited effect.

Once a diagnosis of pneumocystosis is made, it is very important that a predisposing immune deficiency state be investigated. In humans prophylactic treatment with trimethoprim-sulfamethoxazole drugs has been used in hospitalized patients who are receiving irradiation or immunosuppressive agents or who have immunodeficiencies and debilitating diseases. Similar precautions are deemed not warranted for pets because pneumocystosis has not been recognized with similar frequency in such instances.

References and Suggested Reading

Beard CB et al: Genetic variation in *Pneumocystis carinii* isolates from different geographic regions: implications for transmission, *Emerg Infect Dis* 6:265, 2000.

Cabanes FJ et al: *Pneumocystis carinii* pneumonia in a Yorkshire terrier dog, *Med Mycol* 38:451, 2000.

Greene CE, Chandler F, Lobetti RG: Pneumocystosis. In Greene CE, editor: *Infectious diseases of the dog and cat*, ed 3, St Louis, 2005, Saunders, p 651.

Kirberger RM, Lobetti RG: Radiographic aspects of *Pneumocystis carinii* pneumonia in the miniature dachshund, *Vet Radiol Ultrasound* 39:313, 1998.

Kovacs JA et al: New insights into transmission, diagnosis, and drug treatment of *Pneumocystis carinii* pneumonia, *J Am Med Assoc* 286:2450, 2001.

Lobetti R: Common variable immunodeficiency in miniature dachshunds affected with *Pneumocystis carinii* pneumonia, *J Vet Diagn Invest* 12:39, 2000.

Lobetti R: *Pneumocystis carinii* infection in miniature dachshunds, *Compend Contin Educ Pract Vet* 23:320, 2001.

Watson PJ et al: Immunoglobulin deficiency in cavalier King Charles spaniels with *Pneumocystis* pneumonia, *J Vet Intern Med* 20:523, 2006.

Sukura A, Saari S, Jarvinen A: *Pneumocystis carinii* pneumonia in dogs: a diagnostic challenge, *J Vet Diagn Invest* 8:124, 1996.

CHAPTER 276

Feline Cytauxzoonosis

J. PAUL WOODS, *Guelph, Ontario, Canada*

Cytauxzoon felis is an emerging tick-transmitted intracellular protozoon in wild and domestic cats. In domestic cats this microorganism causes severe disease characterized by hemolytic anemia and circulatory impairment with high mortality. The genus *Cytauxzoon* belongs to the subphylum Apicomplexa, order Piroplasmidae, family Theileriidae, which are parasites of mammals. *Cytauxzoon* exist in two distinct tissue forms: an erythrocyte phase (piroplasm) (Fig. 276-1) and a tissue phase (schizont) (Fig. 276-2). The genus *Cytauxzoon* was designated for species reported initially in African ungulates in which the tissue phase develops in mononuclear phagocytes lining the blood vessels of numerous organs, whereas the genus *Theileria* invades lymphocytes during the schizogenous phase. *Cytauxzoon* are closely related to the genus *Babesia*; however, *Babesia* spp. have an erythrocyte stage exclusively without a tissue phase.

EPIDEMIOLOGY

C. felis was first recognized in 1976 in Missouri. It has now been reported in the south central, southeastern, mid-Atlantic, and Gulf coast states of the United States. The pattern of geographic distribution is probably affected by the availability of both reservoir hosts (wild bobcats) and arthropod vectors (*Dermacentor variabilis*). The natural life cycle of *C. felis* is not completely understood. The cat was presumed to be an accidental terminal host with a predominant rapidly fatal disease, but recent findings of asymptomatic infected cats have led to the possibility of cats serving as an additional reservoir for *C. felis*. In contrast, bobcats (*Lynx rufus*) are the presumed reservoir hosts, acting as persistent carriers of the organism and usually developing only mild or subclinical infection. However, there is a paucity of information on blood parasites of free-ranging cats, and *Cytauxzoon* has only been reported in bobcats since 1982; thus questions remain as to whether this is a new disease of felids or only a newly identified disease. Mountain lions (*Felis concolor*) from Florida and Texas also have been reported to carry the organism. There has been a correlation of disease with tick interchange among wild and domestic felids, with ticks presumably transmitting the organism between cats by feeding. The only tick demonstrated experimentally to be a competent vector for *Cytauxzoon* is *D. variabilis* (American dog tick). Transtadial transmission occurs in ticks, but transovarial transmission has not been demonstrated. However, cytauxzoonosis may be more widespread than previously recognized because cytauxzoonosis-like diseases have been reported in domestic cats in Zimbabwe and Spain, in Pallas' cats (*Otocolobus manul*) from Mongolia, and in a lion (*Panthera leo*) in Brazil. Experimental studies have revealed no zoonotic or agricultural risk for *C. felis*.

Feline cytauxzoonosis is highly seasonal, occurring in spring to early fall, with the highest incidence in early spring to early summer, which correlates with tick activity. Outdoor cats with access to wooded environments are at greatest risk of infection, presumably because of increased exposure to tick vectors. Within endemic areas there is a large variability in incidence of disease between relatively short distances. In fact, there are hyperendemic foci as suggested by detection of infection in more than one cat in multicat households, a phenomenon likely the result of common exposure to tick populations rather than direct cat-to-cat transmission. Cytauxzoonosis has been most commonly reported in middle-aged cats, but it can occur in cats of any age, with no sex or breed predilections. A recent report suggested young male cats to be at higher risk. A recent study screening for *C. felis* in feral cats in the southeastern United States reported a prevalence of 0.3% with an estimated prevalence range of 0% to 0.8%.

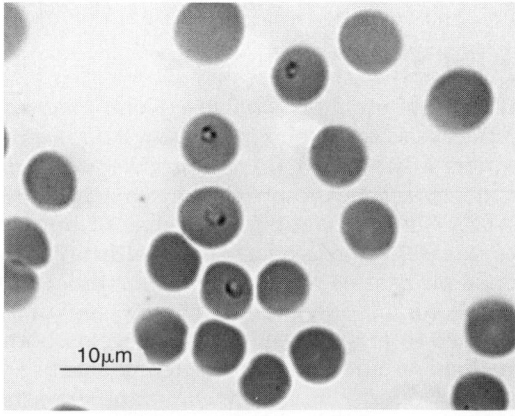

Fig. 276-1 Peripheral blood from a cat with cytauxzoonosis. Four piroplasms are present within erythrocytes. Two of the piroplasms *(top)* each contain two nuclear areas. Two of the erythrocytes *(bottom)* contain small particulate stain precipitate that must be differentiated from organisms (Wright-Giemsa stain). (From Meinkoth J, Kocan AA: Feline cytauxzoonosis, *Vet Clin Small Anim* 35:89, 2005, with permission.)

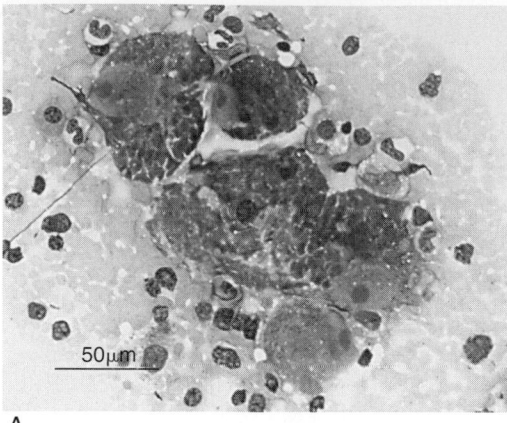

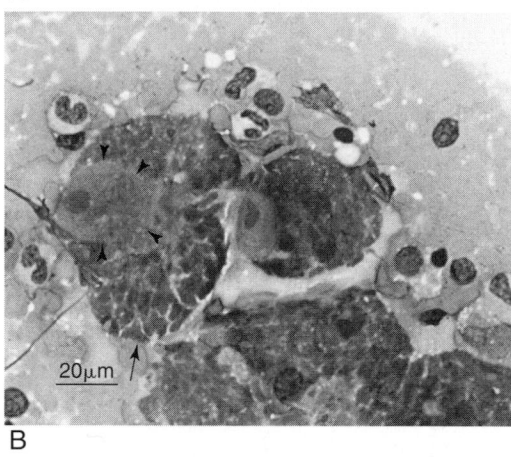

Fig. 276-2   A, Impression smear of spleen from a cat with cytauxzoonosis. Five large schizon-containing macrophages are present. Scattered myeloid cells and plasma cells are also present. **B,** Higher magnification of the area shown in **A.** The nucleus of a host cell is outlined by arrowheads. The host cell nucleus contains a greatly enlarged nucleolus. The schizont completely fills the cells' cytoplasm, often being indistinct. In portions of the cells multiple merozoites are seen forming within the schizont, giving the cytoplasm a "packeted" appearance *(arrow)* (Wright-Giemsa stain). (From Meinkoth J, Kocan AA: Feline cytauxzoonosis, *Vet Clin Small Anim* 35:89, 2005, with permission.)

PATHOGENESIS

The limited information available from investigations of *C. felis* reveals a complex pathogenesis. Experimental studies demonstrate that the clinical disease in domestic cats depends on exposure to the schizogenous tissue phase of *C. felis*. Inoculation with schizont homogenate induces disease, whereas inoculation with only erythrocyte-phase piroplasms results in only erythroparasitemia without schizont development or clinical signs of disease. Cats exposed to infected *D. variabilis* develop both schizogenous phases and erythroparasitemia and become ill with cytauxzoonosis. Piroplasms cannot progress through their natural life cycle without passing through the tick host. Thus the ticks are not just mechanical vectors but are also necessary to complete the *C. felis* life cycle. In ticks, transtadial but not transovarial transmission has been demonstrated. Oral and contact exposure does not result in disease; therefore close contact between cats without tick vectors does not pose a risk for disease transmission.

After infection the organism undergoes schizogony, an asexual reproductive phase, in mononuclear phagocytic cells associated with vessels of almost every organ. As the schizonts (see Fig. 276-2) undergo schizogony and binary fission, macrophages lining the blood vessels enlarge tremendously and occlude venules in liver, spleen, lung, and lymph nodes, resulting in a thrombus-like mechanical obstruction of blood flow and tissue hypoxia. The schizont is associated with clinical disease; the greater the schizont burden, the more severe the clinical illness. Domestic cats have extensive schizont burdens, whereas mildly affected bobcats have a limited and transient schizogenous phase. The tissue phase is also suspected to release toxic, pyrogenic, and vasoactive products that contribute to clinical manifestations. The schizogenous tissue phase, detectable by 12 days after infection, is responsible for the venous congestion, thrombotic disease, and organ failure that lead to death in most cats within 3 weeks of infection.

Schizonts develop merozoites that are released when infected macrophages rupture. Merozoites undergo endocytosis by erythrocytes, giving rise to late-stage erythroparasitemia, recognized as piroplasms (see Fig. 276-1) as the disease progresses. Although graphic, the piroplasm itself is relatively innocuous; however, it may induce erythrocyte destruction and erythrophagocytosis. Cats exposed to just piroplasms remain parasitemic (piroplasms may decrease to a low level) but do not develop protective immunity. In experimental studies of infection a few cats (≈4 out of >500 cats) did survive infection from exposure to schizonts. In contrast to the piroplasm-exposed cats, these cats developed protective immunity.

CLINICAL MANIFESTATIONS

Cytauxzoonosis follows an acute course, with the stage of disease determining the presenting clinical signs. In natural infections the prepatent period is between 2 to 3 weeks, with the onset of clinical disease occurring 1 to 3 weeks after infection. The clinical signs are initially nonspecific, consisting of depression, dehydration, and anorexia followed by fever (as high as 40 to 41.6°C [107°F]), icterus, anemia, dark urine, tachycardia, splenomegaly, variable hepatomegaly, reluctance to move, and vocalizing with generalized pain. In late stages the cats are terminally moribund and dyspneic, and after fever peaks the body temperature may subside to normal or frequently become subnormal (24 to 48 hours before death). Miscellaneous neurologic signs observed in some cats have included ataxia, nystagmus, seizures, tetany, aggression, and coma. Typically the course of disease is rapid, and cats usually die within 7 days after the onset of clinical signs. However, some cats survive infection and may remain asymptomatic carriers for months to years.

LABORATORY AND PATHOLOGIC FINDINGS

In cats infected with cytauxzoonosis a complete blood count may reveal any combination of cytopenias. Anemia, probably caused by erythrophagocytosis and characterized as normocytic, normochromic, and nonregenerative, is common. In contrast to anemia associated with infection from other hemoparasites, the absence of regenerative responses may be because the acute course of the disease gives insufficient time for a regenerative response or because of bone marrow suppression from inflammatory disease. Leukopenia consisting of neutropenia with toxic changes is common. Thrombocytopenia may result from increased consumption. Activated partial thromboplastin time and partial thromboplastin time have been prolonged in some cats.

Red blood cells (RBCs) stained with Wright, Giemsa, or other Romanovsky stains may demonstrate piroplasms (see Fig. 276-1), the erythrocytic phase of *C. felis*. The piroplasms consist of a dark purple, eccentric nucleus within a pale light blue or nearly colorless cytoplasm. There are usually one to two organisms per RBC, but there can be as many as four. The piroplasms are pleomorphic, classically appearing as 1- to 2-µm–diameter "signet ring" (round to oval with a single peripherally located nucleus). They can also be elongated with a bipolar nucleus ("safety pin"), comma-shaped, linear, or tetrad ("Maltese cross"). The piroplasms are located intracellularly, in contrast to the epicellular location of *Mycoplasma hemofelis*. Piroplasms appear late in the course of disease and may be absent or in very low numbers on initial examination in up to 50% of cases. The proportion of affected RBCs with observable piroplasms is generally low (<1%), and often they are not present at the time of death; however, occasionally infected cats have parasitemia as high as 25%. Piroplasms can be at greatest number at the peripheral and distal edges of blood films.

Biochemical changes found consistently are hyperbilirubinemia and hypoalbuminemia, particularly late in the course of the disease. Other more variable and nonspecific changes can include prerenal azotemia, elevated liver enzymes, hyperglycemia, and electrolyte and acid-base disturbances. Bilirubinuria is common. Diagnostic imaging may reveal splenomegaly, hepatomegaly, effusions, and bronchointerstitial pulmonary pattern. Bone marrow examination may show depletion of mature myeloid cells, toxic change, erythrophagocytosis, and schizont-laden macrophages. Erythrophagocytosis and schizont-laden macrophages are also prominent in smears and histologic sections of spleen (see Fig. 276-2), lymph node, liver, and bone marrow.

Postmortem findings indicate a rapid course of disease with good body condition; pallor; icterus; splenomegaly; lymphadenomegaly; and congested, edematous lungs. There can be petechial and ecchymotic hemorrhages in many tissues, including lungs, urinary bladder, kidneys, heart, and meninges. Abdominal veins may be distended and pleural, pericardial, and peritoneal effusions may be present. Histologic examination reveals characteristic large schizont-laden macrophages within the lumens of small vessels of many organs, including the lungs, spleen, liver, kidneys, lymph nodes, bone marrow, heart, and brain. There is minimal inflammatory reaction in the tissues.

DIAGNOSIS

Initial suspicion of feline cytauxzoonosis is based on compatible clinical signs and laboratory findings of acute-onset fever, depression, icterus, anemia, and hepatosplenomegaly in a free-roaming cat with exposure to ticks in an endemic area. Definitive diagnosis requires identification of the organism. Blood smear examination may identify piroplasms (see Fig. 276-1); however, disease from the schizogenous phase may precede detectable erythroparasitemia. Also, levels of piroplasms may be low; therefore the laboratory should be alerted to the clinical suspicion for *C. felis* so that specific attention is directed at the RBCs for organisms. Dramatic increases in the number of piroplasms can occur within 24 hours; thus a negative smear should be reevaluated when there is clinical suspicion for *C. felis*. The small pleomorphic piroplasms must be differentiated from *M. hemofelis*, nuclear remnants (Howell-Jolly bodies), artifact (stain precipitates, refractile artifacts, water), and *Babesia felis*. Diagnosis can be difficult and may require a well-made thin blood smear that is thoroughly air dried before staining. Diagnosis should not be based on identification of one presumed organism.

Occasionally macrophages containing schizonts are found on the feathered edge of Wright-stained smears of blood and bone marrow. If parasitemia is not observed, fine-needle aspirates or impression smears of tissues, including lymph nodes, spleen, liver, bone marrow or lung, may identify schizogenous forms of *C. felis*. These organs typically are heavily infiltrated with greatly enlarged schizont-parasitized macrophages (see Fig. 276-2). Similarly postmortem examination reveals characteristic histopathologic findings of *C. felis*. Recently a polymerase chain reaction test to detect subunit ribosomal ribonucleic acid of *C. felis* has become available to confirm the presence of *C. felis*.

THERAPY AND PREVENTION

Feline cytauzoonosis has a grave prognosis, with virtually 100% mortality occurring soon after illness in experimental and natural infections despite various antimicrobial and supportive therapies. However, there have been recent reports of some cats surviving clinical disease and recovering to an asymptomatic erythroparasitic state (some for >6 years). Unfortunately investigations of the survivor cats have not elucidated if survival was caused by therapeutic management, the survivor cats' innate immunity, detection of previously unrecognized carriers, atypical route of infection (e.g., bite wound) resulting in asymptomatic parasitemia, or a less virulent form of *C. felis*.

Although no definitive antiprotozoal therapy has been proven consistently effective, cats present in severe distress, requiring immediate aggressive supportive therapy. The goal of therapy is to sustain the cat to gain time for its innate defenses to battle the infection and/or for investigational antiprotozoal therapy. Depending on the cat's condition, treatment can involve intravenous fluid therapy to rehydrate and correct metabolic imbalances, prophylactic antibiotics for secondary bacterial infection, heparin (100 to 150 U/kg subcutaneously [SQ] q8h) to minimize thrombus formation and development of disseminated intravascular coagulation, and blood products as needed for anemia.

Administration of definitive antiprotozoal treatments to infected cats is controversial because of drug toxicity, the lack of availability and approval, and mostly the paucity of evidence supporting clinical efficacy. Therapies that have been unsuccessful include parvaquone, buparvaquone, sodium thiacetarsemide, and tetracycline. Therapies that have reported inconsistent success are imidocarb dipropionate (Imizol, Schering Plough Animal Health) at a dosage of 2 to 4 mg/kg every 7 days intramuscularly pretreated with glycopyrrolate (0.005 to 0.01 mg/kg intramuscularly [IM] or SQ); atovaquone (Mepron, GlaxoSmithKline) at a dosage of 15 mg/kg every 8 hours orally for 10 days combined with azithromycin (Zithromax, Pfizer) at a dosage of 10 mg/kg every 24 hours orally for 10 days. Although unavailable in North America, another therapy is diminazene aceturate (Berenil, Intervet) at a dosage of 2 mg/kg every 7 days intramuscularly. Although at present a vaccine is not available, one of the surviving experimental cats was resistant to subsequent challenge with lethal doses of *C. felis*, suggesting that it may be possible to vaccinate cats against *C. felis*.

Until better therapy is developed, prevention of infection is paramount. Transmission cannot occur directly from cat to cat; therefore prevention involves minimizing chances of infection from the tick vector by indoor confinement during tick season, avoidance of rural wooded areas, and ectoparasite control (e.g., pyrethrins, fipronil). It is unknown how long a tick must be attached to transmit the disease. Feline blood donors should be screened and free of ectoparasites (ideally kept indoors). Transfusions from recovered cats do not result in illness even if piroplasm-containing erythrocytes are transfused; however, recently infected cats can transmit schizont-containing circulating monocytes, which can cause disease.

Despite its geographic restrictions, feline cytauxzoonosis is more widespread then previously reported. Recently cases have been recognized in new regions and with increased frequency in previous endemic areas. This change could be the result of changes in distribution, prevalence, or transmission of infected ticks or infected reservoir animals. Concomitantly there has been an increase in recognition and diagnosis by veterinarians. Because of the potential dangers of spread by importation, veterinarians outside endemic areas need to be cognizant of feline cytauxzoonosis and aware of the potential concern for domestic and exotic cats in areas with appropriate reservoirs and tick vectors.

Suggested Reading

Birkenheuer AJ et al: Development and evaluation of a PCR assay for the detection of *Cytauxzoon felis* DNA in feline blood samples, *Vet Parasitol* 137:144, 2006.

Bondy PJ, Cohn LA, Kerl ME: Feline cytauxzoonosis, *Compend Contin Educ Pract Vet* 27:69, 2005.

Greene CE et al: Administration of diminazene aceturate or imidocarb dipropionate for treatment of cytauxzoonosis in cats, *J Am Vet Med Assoc* 215:497, 1999.

Haber MD et al: The detection of *Cytauxzoon felis* in apparently healthy free-roaming cats in the USA, *Vet Parasitol* 146:316, 2007.

Meinkoth J et al: Cats surviving natural infection with *Cytauxzoon felis*: 18 cases (1997–1998), *J Vet Intern Med* 14:521, 2000.

Meinkoth J, Kocan AA: Feline cytauxzoonosis, *Vet Clin Small Anim* 35:89, 2005.

CHAPTER 277

Systemic Fungal Infections

RANCE K. SELLON, *Pullman, Washington*
ALFRED M. LEGENDRE, *Knoxville, Tennessee*

The systemic fungal infections are a collection of well-known and well-described conditions causing clinical signs of multisystemic disease. Most discussions of systemic fungal infections focus on four organisms: *Blastomyces dermatitidis*, *Coccidioides immitis*, *Histoplasma capsulatum*, and *Cryptococcus neoformans*. Most of the information about the pathology and pathophysiology of these infections has been well described in other texts and will not be repeated. This chapter summarizes important findings about the epidemiology of infection, spectrum of clinical disease, and diagnostic developments published in the recent veterinary medical literature. Finally, therapeutic approaches are described for the common systemic mycotic infections.

EPIDEMIOLOGY

In the United States the principal endemic areas of infection for each of the systemic fungal organisms remain constant (Table 277-1). However, some systemic fungal infections have occurred in patients living in areas outside the typical foci of endemic fungal infection. In one report two cats that had not traveled outside of California had confirmed histoplasmosis. The cats lived in an area where there had been recent soil disruption. Interestingly, both of the cats in this report were noted to be completely indoor cats. An outbreak of cryptococcosis on Vancouver Island, BC, Canada saw a spike in disease of both humans and animals (Kidd et al., 2004). In contrast to infection with *C. neoformans*, affected patients were infected with *Cryptococcus gattii*, a species of *Cryptococcus* more prevalent in Australia. Blastomycosis has been documented recently in humans living in Colorado who were working with prairie dogs, potentially extending the distribution of this organism westward.

Although animals that go outdoors are at the greatest risk of exposure to infection, animals that are exclusively indoors have also contracted systemic fungal infections. In addition to the cats with acquired histoplasmosis, blastomycosis has been documented in strictly indoor cats. In humans acquisition of systemic fungal infection (histoplasmosis) has been linked to air-handling systems that channel infectious organisms into buildings (Luby et al., 2005) and a similar means may operate to cause infection in indoor animals. As with the California cats, disruption of soil or ground surface has been associated with infection in humans in nearby buildings.

The clinician's assessment of risk of infection/exposure should consider the possibility of infection in nontraditional areas. Understanding the widening geographic distributions that have emerged in humans could also serve as a sentinel warning for veterinarians in such areas.

Additional studies have explored the risk factors for canine infection with *C. immitis*. Dogs that spent a lot of time outdoors, that roamed over a large surface area, and that spent time walking across the desert had a greater risk of *C. immitis* infection than mainly indoor dogs or dogs that walked on sidewalks. (Butkiewicz et al., 2005). Many dogs in an endemic area become infected with *C. immitis* (as determined by development of *C. immitis* antibodies), but few actually develop clinical disease.

CLINICAL DISEASE

The spectrum of clinical disease caused by the systemic fungal organisms is well known to clinicians that practice in endemic areas; each of the organisms has a predilection for certain organ systems, and the disease typically reflects affected organs. Common to most of the systemic fungal organisms are respiratory disease, bone infection, central nervous system infection (including eyes), lymph node involvement, and skin lesions (Table 277-2). An additional presentation for coccidioidomycosis is pericardial effusion. In 17 dogs with *C. immitis*– induced pericardial disease, affected dogs had clinical signs typical of pericardial disease and right heart failure: abdominal effusion, muffled heart sounds, poor pulse quality, tachypnea, and jugular pulses (Heinritz, et al., 2005). Cardiac ultrasound examinations documented the presence of pericardial effusion and thickened pericardium in most of the dogs. Subtotal pericardectomy was associated with resolution of clinical signs of right heart failure but was also associated with high (23.5%) perioperative mortality; however, the exact cause of death was established in few of the dogs. There was pyogranulomatous pericarditis in all dogs, and there were *C. immitis* spherules in a majority of dogs. In addition to surgical treatment, dogs with pericardial coccidioidomycosis were also treated with antifungal drugs.

Cardiovascular disease is uncommon in dogs with blastomycosis, but there was a report of eight dogs with cardiovascular blastomycosis (Schmiedt, et al., 2006). Affected dogs had clinical signs typical of blastomycosis, including fever and signs of respiratory disease that reflected fungal pneumonia (lethargy, cough, dyspnea). Some dogs had syncope and cardiac arrhythmias, including atrioventricular blocks. Most had echocardiographic abnormalities that varied from mass-like lesions to evidence of pulmonary hypertension and associated right-sided cardiomegaly.

Table 277-1

Usual Geographic Distribution of the Systemic Fungal Infections

Organism	Geographic Distribution
Coccidioides immitis	Southwestern United States, especially California and Arizona; Mexico; Central America; South America
Histoplasma capsulatum	United States primarily east of the Mississippi river; Central America; South America
Blastomyces dermatitidis	Ohio, Missouri and Mississippi river drainages; mid-Atlantic states (Georgia, South Carolina, North Carolina, Virginia, Maryland); Canada (Ontario, Manitoba, Quebec)
Cryptococcus neoformans	Worldwide
Cryptococcus gattii	Tropical and subtropical regions worldwide; Vancouver Island and Vancouver, British Columbia, Canada

Necropsy lesions included myocardial blastomycosis, blastomycosis-induced epicarditis or pericarditis, infection of the adventitia of the aorta, and inflammation and fibrosis of the atrioventricular nodal region. Typical blastomycosis lesions were found in other organs. Although the authors speculated that cardiac involvement in dogs with blastomycosis is likely more widespread than recognized in this retrospective study, it still appears to be uncommon. Nevertheless, blastomycosis should be suspected in dogs with clinical signs of myocardial or conduction system disease.

Blastomycosis is an uncommon disease in cats compared to dogs, but the spectrum of clinical disease in eight cats with blastomycosis resembled the disease in dogs (Gilor, et al., 2006). Fever, lethargy, anorexia, and

Table 277-2

Systems Commonly Affected in Patients With Systemic Fungal Infections*

Organism	Organ Systems
Coccidioides immitis	Respiratory tract, skeleton, skin, pericardium
Histoplasma capsulatum	Respiratory tract, liver, spleen, gastrointestinal tract (dog), skeleton, eyes
Blastomyces dermatitidis	Respiratory tract, bone, lymph nodes, eyes, brain, skin/subcutaneous tissue, external nares
Cryptococcus neoformans; C. gattii	Nasal cavity, skin, eyes, central nervous system, lymph nodes

*In any given patient, dissemination to other organs is possible.

weight loss were common clinical complaints. Cats with blastomycosis had skin and respiratory tract disease (dyspnea, tachypnea, cough). Skin lesions were primarily nonulcerated dermal masses; in contrast to cutaneous blastomycosis in dogs, in which draining lesions are common, the cutaneous lesions in these cats were not draining. Peripheral lymph node enlargement was not seen in any of the cats. Chorioretinitis and central nervous system disease were also observed. Results of complete blood count and serum biochemical profile were nonspecific in the cats of the study. Thoracic radiographs of affected cats demonstrated nodular interstitial-to-alveolar patterns and consolidation. Involvement of the right cranial lung lobe was common, and diffuse bronchial patterns were also frequently observed. As is true with dogs, antemortem diagnosis of blastomycosis in the cats of this study was accomplished by cytologic identification of organisms obtained from aspirates/imprints (skin, lungs, spleen) or lavage of the respiratory tract.

DIAGNOSIS

The definitive diagnosis of all of the systemic fungal infections is established by demonstration of organisms in samples obtained for cytologic or histopathologic examination. With the exception of cryptococcosis, for which serologic assays detect capsular antigen, diagnosis of the other fungal infections based on serologic assays has remained problematic, typically because of low sensitivity and/or specificity of assays that detect antibody. Radioimmunoassays that detect antibody to the WI-1 antigen, the major surface protein of B. dermatitidis, have proven more sensitive and specific than assays that detect antibody to B. dermatitidis antigen A. However, the radioimmunoassay is not yet available commercially.

Other developments in the diagnosis of the systemic fungal infections by serologic assays in humans have seen initial translation to veterinary medicine. Diagnosis of canine blastomycosis by detection of specific antigen in serum or urine is promising (Spector et al., 2006). The urine antigen assay is more sensitive than the serum assay. The sensitivity and specificity of the urine assay was 93% and 98%, respectively, when evaluating known positive and negative samples. The assay may also have application in determining duration of treatment, but further studies are needed. Additional information on this assay can be found at www.miravistalabs.com. There is cross-reactivity between the Histoplasma and Blastomyces organisms. There is also an antigen assay for histoplasmosis, but no studies have been published yet on its application in dogs and cats. These antigen assays are currently available.

The work by Shubitz and associates (2005) indicated that, because of overlap in titers between subclinically and clinically infected dogs, serologic titers alone are insufficient to establish a definitive diagnosis of coccidioidomycosis. Thus the diagnosis of this infection requires that additional supportive information (physical examination abnormalities, laboratory abnormalities, radiographic imaging, cytology, and histology) be obtained to establish a clinical diagnosis.

Table **277-3**	

Therapeutic Suggestions for the Systemic Fungal Infections*

Organism	Treatment Recommendations[†‡]
Coccidioides immitis	Ketoconazole[§] 10 mg/kg PO q12h or fluconazole 10 mg/kg PO q12h
Histoplasma capsulatum	Itraconazole[§] 5-10 mg/kg PO q12-24h
	Amphotericin B 0.5 mg/kg IV q48h for gastrointestinal infection
Blastomyces dermatitidis	Dogs: itraconazole 5 mg/kg PO q24h
	Cats: itraconazole 10 mg/kg PO daily
Cryptococcus neoformans;	Cat: itraconazole 50-100 mg/cat daily; terbinafine 10 mg/kg/day for cats that develop resistance to azoles
C. gattii	Dog: optimal therapy not established, but itraconazole 10 mg/kg/day or amphotericin B 1 mg/kg intravenously three times weekly is suggested

*Initial suggestions only; for more comprehensive treatment information, consult Bonagura JD, editor: *Kirk's current veterinary therapy XIII (small animal practice),* ed XIII, Philadelphia, 2000; or relevant chapters in Greene CE, editor: *Infectious diseases of the dog and cat,* ed 3, Philadelphia, 2006, Saunders Elsevier.
[†]If unfamiliar with drugs or their administration, please consult a veterinary formulary or other suggested readings.
[‡]Duration of therapy for most is a minimum of 60 to 90 days, or at least 30 days beyond resolution of all clinical signs. *C. immitis* infections may require longer treatment periods.
[§]Give with food to increase absorption.

TREATMENT

A number of newer antifungal drugs have been developed and proven efficacious in the treatment of the systemic fungal infections in humans. Many belong to the azole class of drugs that includes itraconazole and ketoconazole. Some of the newer azoles used in humans include voriconazole, posaconazole, and ravuconazole. Although such drugs have proven to be of benefit in humans with fungal infections refractory to therapy with the older azoles such as itraconazole, ketoconazole, and fluconazole, there are no published investigations in small animal patients. A common feature of these drugs is the high cost for these agents. Currently accepted recommendations for the treatment of the various systemic fungal infections are summarized in Table 277-3.

References and Suggested Reading

Butkiewicz CD, Shubitz LF, Dial SM: Risk factors associated with *Coccidioides* infection in dogs, *J Am Vet Med Assoc* 226:1851, 2005.

Gilor C et al: Clinical aspects of natural infection with *Blastomyces dermatitidis* in cats: 8 cases (1991-2005), *J Am Vet Med Assoc* 229(1):96, 2006.

Heinritz CK et al: Subtotal pericardectomy and epicardial excision for treatment of coccidioidomycosis-induced effusive-constrictive pericarditis in dogs: 17 cases (1999-2003), *J Am Vet Med Assoc* 227:435, 2005.

Kidd SE et al: A rare genotype of *Cryptococcus gattii* caused the cryptococcosis outbreak on Vancouver Island (British Columbia, Canada), *Proc Natl Acad Sci USA* 101(49):17258, 2004.

Luby JP et al: Recurrent exposure to *Histoplasma capsulatum* in modern air-conditioned buildings, *Clin Infect Dis* 41:170, 2005.

Schmiedt C et al: Cardiovascular involvement in 8 dogs with *Blastomyces dermatitidis* infection, *J Vet Intern Med* 20:1351, 2006.

Shubitz LF et al: Incidence of *Coccidioides* infection among dogs residing in a region in which the organism is endemic, *J Am Vet Med Assoc* 226:1846, 2005.

Spector D et al: Antigen testing for the diagnosis of blastomycosis, *J Vet Intern Med* 20:711, 2006.

CHAPTER 278

Pythiosis and Lagenidiosis

AMY M. GROOTERS, *Baton Rouge, Louisiana*

*P*ythium insidiosum and *Lagenidium* spp., the causative agents of pythiosis and lagenidiosis, are pathogenic "water molds" in the class Oomycetes. Although they are often grouped with fungi because they grow on mycologic media and produce hyphal structures in tissue, they differ from true fungi in producing motile, flagellate zoospores; having cell walls that lack chitin; and having cell membranes that generally lack ergosterol. Both pythiosis and lagenidiosis cause lesions characterized by eosinophilic and pyogranulomatous inflammation associated with broad, irregularly branching, sparsely septate hyphae; and as a result they are often confused with zygomycosis (infections caused by true fungi in the class Zygomycetes, which produce similar lesions). Although the clinical syndromes associated with *P. insidiosum* infection have been described for many decades, *Lagenidium* spp. have only been recognized as mammalian pathogens since 1999.

PYTHIOSIS

P. insidiosum infection is a devastating and often fatal cause of gastrointestinal or cutaneous lesions in dogs and cats. In small animal patients, pythiosis is encountered most often in the southeastern United States but has also been identified in animals living in New Jersey, Virginia, Kentucky, southern Illinois, Indiana, Oklahoma, Missouri, Kansas, Arizona, California, and the Cayman Islands. Young large-breed dogs (especially outdoor working breeds such as Labrador retrievers) are most often infected. In cats specific breed and sex predilections have not been observed in the few cases that have been reported to date. However, the development of cutaneous pythiosis in very young animals appears to occur more often in cats than in dogs. Of 27 cats with cutaneous pythiosis diagnosed through my laboratory in the past 8 years, 11 were less than 1 year old, with an age range of 4 months to 9 years.

The infective form of *P. insidiosum* is thought to be the motile biflagellate zoospore, which is released into aquatic environments and likely causes infection by encysting in damaged skin or gastrointestinal mucosa. Many dogs with pythiosis have a history of recurrent exposure to warm freshwater habitats. However, disease is also identified regularly in suburban house dogs with no history of access to lakes or ponds. Affected animals typically are immunocompetent and otherwise healthy.

Clinical Findings

Gastrointestinal Pythiosis

In dogs gastrointestinal pythiosis typically results in severe, segmental transmural thickening of the stomach, small intestine, colon, rectum, or rarely the esophagus. The gastric outflow area, proximal duodenum, and ileocolic junction are the most frequently affected locations; and it is not unusual to find two or more segmental lesions in the same patient. Mesenteric lymphadenopathy is common but most often represents reactive hyperplasia rather than infection. Involvement of the mesenteric root may cause severe enlargement of mesenteric lymph nodes, which are typically embedded in a single large, firm granulomatous mass that is palpable in the midabdomen. Extension of disease into mesenteric vessels may result in bowel ischemia, infarction, perforation, or acute hemoabdomen. In addition, infection in gastrointestinal tissues may extend into contiguous organs such as pancreas and uterus. Gastrointestinal pythiosis is rare in cats but was recently described in two young adult male cats with focal intestinal lesions that were amenable to surgical resection (Rakich, Grooters, and Tang, 2005).

Clinical signs associated with gastrointestinal pythiosis include weight loss, vomiting, diarrhea, and hematochezia. Physical examination often reveals a very thin body condition and a palpable abdominal mass. Signs of systemic illness such as lethargy or depression typically are not present unless intestinal obstruction, infarction, or perforation occurs. Laboratory abnormalities that may be associated with pythiosis include eosinophilia, anemia, hyperglobulinemia, hypoalbuminemia, and rarely hypercalcemia. Abdominal radiography and sonography usually reveal severe segmental thickening of the gastrointestinal tract, an abdominal mass, and/or mesenteric lymphadenopathy.

Cutaneous Pythiosis

Cutaneous pythiosis in dogs typically causes nonhealing wounds and invasive masses that contain ulcerated nodules and draining tracts, most often involving the extremities, tail head, ventral neck, or perineum. In contrast to gastrointestinal pythiosis, regional lymphadenopathy in dogs with cutaneous pythiosis usually reflects extension or postsurgical recurrence of infection rather than just reactive inflammation. Cutaneous and gastrointestinal lesions are rarely encountered together in the same patient.

Cats with pythiosis most often present with nasopharyngeal lesions; invasive subcutaneous masses in the periorbital, tail head, or inguinal regions; or draining nodular lesions or ulcerated plaquelike lesions on the extremities, sometimes centered on the digits or footpad. In contrast to dogs, cats with pythiosis often have firm, nodular, subcutaneous lesions without overlying cutaneous lesions or alopecia.

Diagnosis

Cytology and Histopathology

In dogs with pythiosis pyogranulomatous and eosinophilic inflammation is often apparent on cytologic evaluation of exudate from draining tracts, impression smears made from ulcerated skin lesions, or fine-needle aspirates of enlarged lymph nodes or thickened gastrointestinal tissues. Hyphae are observed occasionally, and their morphologic appearance (broad, rarely septate with tapered, rounded ends) in conjunction with a typical inflammatory response can provide a tentative diagnosis of pythiosis, lagenidiosis, or zygomycosis. Microscopic examination of macerated tissue that has been digested in 10% potassium hydroxide may be more likely to reveal hyphal elements than other cytologic specimens.

Histologically pythiosis is characterized by eosinophilic pyogranulomatous inflammation. Affected tissues contain multiple foci of necrosis surrounded and infiltrated by neutrophils, eosinophils, and macrophages. In addition, discrete granulomas composed of epithelioid macrophages, plasma cells, multinucleate giant cells; and fewer neutrophils and eosinophils are often observed. Organisms typically are found within areas of necrosis or at the center of granulomas. Vasculitis is present occasionally. In gastrointestinal pythiosis inflammation centers on the submucosal and muscular layers rather than the mucosa and lamina propria. Therefore the diagnosis of pythiosis may be missed on endoscopic biopsies that fail to reach deeper tissues. Similarly, disease in animals with cutaneous pythiosis typically is found in the deep dermis and subcutis, necessitating deep wedge biopsies rather than punch biopsies for optimal evaluation. *P. insidiosum* hyphae are not visualized routinely on H&E-stained sections but may be identified as clear spaces surrounded by a narrow band of eosinophilic material. Hyphae are readily visualized in sections stained with Gomori's methenamine silver (GMS) but usually do not stain well with periodic acid–Schiff (PAS). *Pythium* hyphae are broad (mean, 4 μm; range, 2 to 7 μm), infrequently septate, and occasionally branching (usually at right angles).

Culture

Isolation of *P. insidiosum* from infected tissues is not difficult when appropriate sample handling and culture techniques are used. For best results room temperature (i.e., not refrigerated) tissue samples should be wrapped in a saline-moistened gauze sponge and shipped at ambient temperature to arrive at the laboratory within 24 hours. Small pieces of fresh, nonmacerated tissue should be placed directly on the surface of vegetable extract agar supplemented with streptomycin and ampicillin (or an alternative selective medium) and incubated at 37° C. Growth typically is observed within 12 to 24 hours. Isolation of *P. insidiosum* from swabs of exudate collected from draining skin lesions is generally unsuccessful. Identification of *P. insidiosum* should be based on morphologic features; growth at 37° C; production of motile, biflagellate zoospores; and, if possible, species-specific polymerase chain reaction (PCR) amplification (Grooters and Gee, 2002) or ribosomal ribonucleic acid (rRNA) gene sequencing. Although production of zoospores is an important supporting feature for the identification of pathogenic Oomycetes, it is not specific for *P. insidiosum*. Species-specific PCR amplification can also be used to identify *P. insidiosum* deoxyribonucleic acid (DNA) in fresh, frozen, or paraffin-embedded tissues.

Serology

A highly sensitive and specific enzyme-linked immunosorbent assay (ELISA) for the detection of anti–*P. insidiosum* antibodies in dogs and cats is currently available through my laboratory (Grooters et al., 2002a). In addition to providing a means for early, noninvasive diagnosis, this assay is also very useful for monitoring response to therapy. Following complete surgical resection of infected tissues, a dramatic decrease in antibody levels is typically detected within 2 to 3 months. In contrast, antibody levels remain high in animals that go on to develop clinical recurrence following surgical treatment. In animals treated medically antibody levels change much more slowly, but I have observed significant decreases coincident with clinical improvement within 3 to 4 months of initiating medical therapy for nonresectable disease.

Immunohistochemistry

Several different immunohistochemical techniques have been used previously to confirm the diagnosis of pythiosis. However, the specificity of the antibodies used in these assays has not always been well established. A more recently developed polyclonal anti-*P. insidiosum* antibody raised in chickens and adsorbed with *Lagenidium* and *Conidiobolus* hyphae appears to be highly specific for the immunohistochemical detection of *P. insidiosum* hyphae in tissues. Immunohistochemical staining of tissues for diagnostic purposes using this antibody is available through the author's laboratory.

Therapy

Aggressive surgical resection of all infected tissues is the treatment of choice for pythiosis. In animals with cutaneous lesions confined to a single distal extremity, amputation should be recommended. In patients with gastrointestinal pythiosis segmental lesions should be resected with 3- to 4-cm margins whenever possible. Despite the fact that mesenteric lymphadenopathy is almost always present, *P. insidiosum* hyphae typically are absent in enlarged mesenteric nodes. Therefore the presence of nonresectable mesenteric lymphadenopathy should *not* dissuade the surgeon from pursuing complete resection of a segmental bowel lesion. However, enlarged regional lymph nodes should always be biopsied for prognostic information. Unfortunately most dogs with gastrointestinal pythiosis are not presented to a veterinarian until late in the course of disease, when complete excision is impossible. In addition, the anatomic location of the lesion may prevent complete surgical excision when the esophagus, gastric outflow tract, rectum, or mesenteric root is involved.

Local postoperative recurrence of pythiosis is common (especially when wide surgical margins cannot be achieved) and can occur either at the site of resection or in regional lymph nodes. For this reason medical therapy with itraconazole (10 mg/kg q24h orally [PO]) and terbinafine (5 to 10 mg/kg q24h PO) is recommended for at least 2 to 3 months after surgery. To monitor for recurrence, ELISA serology should be performed before (or within 7 days of) and 2 to 3 months after surgery. In animals that have had a complete surgical resection and have no recurrence of disease, serum antibody levels drop 50% or more within 3 months of surgery. If this occurs, medical therapy can be discontinued, with optional subsequent reevaluation of serum antibody levels in 2 to 3 months. In my experience surgery is curative in a majority of animals with a distal limb lesion treated with amputation or with a midjejunal lesion that the surgeon believes was completely resected with good margins.

Medical therapy for nonresectable pythiosis is typically unrewarding, likely because ergosterol (the target for most currently available antifungal drugs) is generally lacking in the Oomycete cell membrane. Despite this fact, I have observed clinical and serologic cures in a number of patients treated with a combination of itraconazole (10 mg/kg q24h PO) and terbinafine (5 to 10 mg/kg q24h PO). Although the percentage of animals responding is still quite low (<15%), the combination protocol appears to be superior to itraconazole or amphotericin B alone.

LAGENIDIOSIS

The majority of species in the genus *Lagenidium* are pathogens of insects, crustaceans, algae, and nematodes. The most well-studied species, *Lagenidium giganteum*, is a mosquito larval pathogen that is an Environmental Protection Agency–approved biologic pesticide used for control of mosquito populations. Two morphologically and molecularly distinct species of *Lagenidium* have been isolated from dogs with cutaneous lesions. The first of these species causes uniformly fatal dermatologic and disseminated disease in dogs in the southeastern United States (Grooters et al, 2003). The second pathogenic *Lagenidium* spp. is less common than the first and in dogs is a cause of chronic ulcerative nodular dermatopathy that has a prolonged course and does not appear to extend past local tissues. Although strong antigenic and molecular similarities suggest that the first canine pathogenic *Lagenidium* spp. is closely related to *L. giganteum*, differences in their morphologic and in vitro growth characteristics suggest that they are likely distinct species. Little is currently known about the life cycles of the canine pathogenic *Lagenidium* spp.; however, sporulation and infectivity for these pathogens is likely similar to that associated with *P. insidiosum* and *L. giganteum*. Therefore they would be expected to cause infection via motile aquatic zoospores that adhere to and encyst in damaged tissues.

The epidemiologic features of lagenidiosis that have been identified thus far are similar in many respects to those that have been associated previously with cutaneous pythiosis. Affected animals are typically young to middle-aged dogs living in the southeastern United States. Although most of these dogs have lived in Florida or Louisiana, cases in Texas, Tennessee, Alabama, Georgia, South Carolina, Maryland, Virginia, Indiana, and Illinois have been identified. A number of infected dogs have had frequent exposure to lakes or ponds. None of the affected animals have had historical evidence of immunocompromise or were treated with immunosuppressive therapy before developing the infection. To date lagenidiosis has not been identified in cats.

Clinical Findings

Dogs with *Lagenidium* infection typically are presented for evaluation of progressive cutaneous or subcutaneous lesions (often multifocal) involving the extremities,

mammary region, perineum, or trunk. Grossly these lesions appear as firm dermal or subcutaneous nodules or as ulcerated, thickened, edematous areas of deep cellulitis with regions of necrosis and numerous draining tracts. Hypercalcemia has been associated with *Lagenidium* infection in one dog with cutaneous lesions on all four limbs and severe infection and enlargement of popliteal, inguinal, and prescapular lymph nodes. Similar to the clinical course associated with cutaneous pythiosis, skin lesions in dogs with lagenidiosis tend to be progressive, locally invasive, and poorly responsive to medical therapy.

In dogs infected with the more aggressive species of *Lagenidium*, regional lymphadenopathy is often present and may occur in the absence of obvious cutaneous lesions. Unlike dogs with cutaneous pythiosis, these dogs typically have occult lesions in the thorax or abdomen, including involvement of the great vessels, sublumbar and/or inguinal lymph nodes, lung, pulmonary hilus, and cranial mediastinum. Animals with great vessel or sublumbar lymph node involvement typically have cutaneous or subcutaneous lesions on the hind limbs and often develop hind limb edema. Sudden death caused by great vessel rupture and associated hemoabdomen may occur in these patients.

In dogs infected with the less aggressive species of *Lagenidium*, lesions tend to be locally invasive but rarely extend beyond cutaneous and subcutaneous tissues. Distant lesions in the chest and abdomen have not been identified, and the clinical course appears to be chronic and slowly progressive, with some patients having lesions that progress slowly or are somewhat stable for more than 2 years.

Diagnosis

Because of its clinical, epidemiologic, and histologic similarities to pythiosis, lagenidiosis is often misdiagnosed as pythiosis during routine histologic evaluation. In addition, since many pathologists are more familiar with the Zygomycetes than the Oomycetes, lagenidiosis may also be misdiagnosed as zygomycosis. Although there are subtle differences in hyphal size, morphology, and distribution among these three infections, histologic lesions associated with lagenidiosis are still often labeled as *suspected pythiosis* or *suspected zygomycosis* during routine evaluation. For this reason clinicians should always attempt to follow a suspected histologic diagnosis with serology, culture, immunohistochemical, or molecular confirmation.

Cytology and Histopathology

Cytologic examination of lymph node aspirates or impression smears of draining exudate from dogs with lagenidiosis may reveal pyogranulomatous to eosinophilic inflammation with or without broad, poorly septate hyphal elements. The histologic features of lagenidiosis are similar to those associated with pythiosis and zygomycosis and are characterized by pyogranulomatous and eosinophilic inflammation associated with broad, irregularly branching, infrequently septate hyphae. Multinucleated giant cells and plasma cells commonly are present. In contrast to *P. insidiosum*, *Lagenidium* spp. hyphae are often visible on H&E-stained sections. On GMS-stained sections numerous broad, thick-walled, irregularly septate hyphae are easily recognized. *Lagenidium* hyphae typically vary greatly in size but in general are larger than *P. insidiosum* hyphae, ranging from 7 to 25 μm in diameter, with an average of 12 μm for the more aggressive species and 7.5 μm for the less aggressive species. In some sections hyphae appear as round or bulbous structures, and occasionally right angle branching is observed. A scant-to-thin eosinophilic sleeve may be noted around the hyphae.

Serology

Immunoblot serology for the detection of anti-*Lagenidium* antibodies in canine serum can provide a presumptive diagnosis of lagenidiosis but must be interpreted in conjunction with results of serologic testing for *P. insidiosum* infection because of the potential for cross-reactivity in serum from dogs with pythiosis. In addition, I have observed nonspecific anti-*Lagenidium* seroreactivity in dogs with other fungal or nonfungal infections, including histoplasmosis and severe pyoderma. Therefore serology alone cannot be used as a basis for the diagnosis of lagenidiosis. However, in the presence of histologic evidence of oomycosis or zygomycosis and the absence of anti-*P. insidiosum* seroreactivity, the identification of anti-*Lagenidium* seroreactivity on immunoblot analysis strongly suggests lagenidiosis. Unfortunately serology is not helpful in differentiating between the two canine pathogenic species of *Lagenidium*.

Culture

The diagnosis of lagenidiosis is best made by culture, which not only provides a definitive diagnosis but is also the only tool currently available for differentiating between the two pathogenic species, which is essential for determining prognosis. Isolation techniques for *Lagenidium* spp. are similar to those described for *P. insidiosum* but with peptone-yeast-glucose agar. For best results small pieces of fresh, nonmacerated tissue should be placed directly on the surface of the agar and incubated at 37°C. Growth typically is observed within 24 to 48 hours. Identification of *Lagenidium* spp. isolates based on morphologic characteristics is more difficult than identification of *P. insidiosum* because zoospores are not as easily produced and because sexual reproductive structures have not yet been identified. Because of the current limitations associated with morphologic characterization, definitive identification of *Lagenidium* spp. should be based on rRNA gene sequencing or genus-specific PCR amplification. This same PCR assay can also be used for the detection of *Lagenidium* DNA in infected tissue samples (Znajda, Grooters, and Marsella, 2002).

Therapy

As with pythiosis, aggressive surgical resection of infected tissues is the treatment of choice for lagenidiosis. When lesions are limited to a single distal extremity, amputation is recommended. In patients with cutaneous lesions in other areas of the body, the surgeon should pursue aggressive resection with wide margins. Since dogs infected with the more aggressive species of *Lagenidium* often have occult systemic lesions, radiographic imaging of the chest and abdomen and sonographic imaging of the abdomen are recommended to determine the extent of disease before attempting surgical resection of cutaneous lesions. Unfortunately the vast majority of dogs infected with this pathogen have nonresectable disease in regional lymph nodes or distant sites by the time the initial diagnosis is made, making the prognosis for these dogs generally grave. In dogs infected with the less aggressive species, surgery that achieves 3-cm margins is often curative. As with pythiosis, medical therapy for lagenidiosis is usually ineffective. However, a combination of itraconazole (10 mg/kg q24h PO) and terbinafine (5 to 10 mg/kg q24h PO) along with repeated aggressive surgical resection was effective in resolving *Lagenidium* infection in one dog with recurrent multifocal cutaneous lesions.

References and Suggested Reading

Bissonnette KW et al: Nasal and retrobulbar mass in a cat caused by *Pythium insidiosum*, *J Med Vet Mycol* 29:39, 1991.

Foil CSO et al: A report of subcutaneous pythiosis in five dogs and a review of the etiologic agent *Pythium* spp, *J Am Anim Hosp Assoc* 20:959, 1984.

Grooters AM: Pythiosis, lagenidiosis, and zygomycosis in small animals, *Vet Clin North Am Small Anim Pract* 33:695, 2003.

Grooters AM, Gee MK: Development of a nested PCR assay for the detection and identification of *Pythium insidiosum*, *J Vet Intern Med* 16:147, 2002.

Grooters AM et al: Development and evaluation of an enzyme-linked immunosorbent assay for the serodiagnosis of pythiosis in dogs, *J Vet Intern Med* 16:142, 2002a.

Grooters AM et al: Evaluation of microbial culture techniques for the isolation of *Pythium insidiosum* from equine tissues, *J Vet Diagn Invest* 14:288, 2002b.

Grooters AM et al: Clinicopathologic findings associated with *Lagenidium* spp infection in six dogs: initial description of an emerging oomycosis, *J Vet Intern Med* 17:637, 2003.

Rakich PM, Grooters AM, Tang KN: Gastrointestinal pythiosis in two cats, *J Vet Diagn Invest* 17:262, 2005.

Thomas RC, Lewis DT: Pythiosis in dogs and cats, *Compend Contin Educ Pract Vet* 20:63, 1998.

Znajda NR, Grooters AM, Marsella R: PCR-based detection of *Pythium* and *Lagenidium* DNA in frozen and ethanol-fixed animal tissues, *Vet Dermatol* 13:187, 2002.

CHAPTER 279

Canine Vaccination Guidelines

RICHARD B. FORD, *Raleigh, North Carolina*

In 2006 the American Animal Hospital Association (AAHA) Canine Vaccine Task Force reconvened to address updates regarding existing vaccines and to review data on new vaccines that have entered the marketplace since the last publication of these recommendations in April 2003. Today the complete text, including references, of the 2006 AAHA Canine Vaccine Guidelines (amended February 2007) is available without restriction at www.aahanet.org (search: Resources/References).

One of the principle reasons stimulating the publication of Guidelines on canine vaccination is the proliferation of licensed vaccines over the past two decades. In the United States alone there are now at least 80 proprietary canine vaccines that include one or a combination of over 25 different antigen types. It is inappropriate to assume that every dog (and every cat) should be inoculated annually against each of the infections for which a vaccine is licensed. Vaccines clearly represent one of the best health care values for animals. Yet, despite the obvious benefits associated with vaccination, there are also risks. Therefore it is the responsibility of veterinarians to acknowledge the fact that vaccination requires a medical decision based on reasonable knowledge of the patient's risk for exposure, life style, and stage of life.

HIGHLIGHTS OF THE 2006 AAHA CANINE VACCINE GUIDELINES

It should be emphasized that the 2006 AAHA Canine Vaccine Guidelines are *recommendations* for the selection and use of canine vaccines in clinical practice. Although the Guidelines represent the most current interpretations of available science, they are not to be construed as dictating an exclusive protocol, course of treatment, or procedure. The decision to implement any part of the published Guidelines is optional. However, the revised Guidelines include information of importance to all practitioners who administer vaccines to dogs. Part 1 of the 2006 Guidelines, entitled Canine Vaccination in the General Veterinary Practice, addresses vaccination recommendations for puppies and adult dogs. These recommendations are summarized in Tables 279-1 and 279-2. Additional topics presented in Part 1 include technologic developments in canine vaccines, vaccine licensing requirements, the role of serologic testing (antibody titers) to assess immunity following vaccination, adverse event recognition and reporting, and medicolegal aspects of vaccination. Recommendations for documenting vaccine administration in the medical record are also addressed. Part 2 of the 2006 Guidelines is new and specifically addresses recommendations for administering vaccines to shelter-housed dogs. Part 2 will be of particular value to veterinarians who advise shelters on vaccination procedures.

Core Vaccines

Core vaccines are those deemed most important to patient health based on factors related to exposure risk (e.g., parvovirus), severity of disease (e.g., distemper), and transmissibility to humans (e.g., rabies). The Task Force has designated canine distemper virus (CDV), canine parvovirus (CPV), canine adenovirus-2 (CAV-2) (for its ability to protect against canine hepatitis [CAV-1]), and rabies vaccines as core. When feasible, modified-live virus (MLV) vaccines are recommended over killed vaccines. New information on the recombinant canine distemper vaccine has resulted in reclassification of this product as a core vaccine having efficacy that is comparable to MLV distemper vaccines. In addition, the recombinant CDV has been shown to immunize puppies (7 to 9 weeks of age) despite the presence of maternal antibody (Pando et al., 2007). There is no killed CDV vaccine. Killed rabies vaccines, designated 1-year or 3-year vaccines, are the only types available for administration to dogs within the United States and most other countries. The AAHA Canine Vaccine Guidelines on rabies vaccination do not replace or supersede state and/or local statutes.

As outlined in the 2003 AAHA Canine Vaccine Guidelines, a minimum of three doses of core vaccines (CDV, CPV, and CAV-2) should be administered to puppies between 6 and 16 weeks of age. It is emphasized that the final dose be administered at 14 to 16 weeks of age. A subsequent inoculation of the core vaccines should be administered 1 year following administration of the last dose of vaccine in the initial puppy series. Subsequently a single dose (booster) is recommended every 3 years thereafter. Triennial vaccine recommendations apply to *all* of the core vaccines, regardless of manufacturer. Challenge studies involving the MLV core vaccines (CDV, CPV, and CAV-2) have been conducted independently of the manufacturers and have documented the ability of all commercially licensed vaccines to protect dogs against virus challenge for a minimum of 5 years. There is no legal mandate requiring veterinarians to administer a vaccine licensed as a "3-year vaccine" to comply with the AAHA Canine Vaccine Guidelines. A recent study on the duration of immunity derived from vaccination of dogs with the recombinant CDV vaccine also supports a triennial booster recommendation in adult dogs.

Table 279-1

Core Canine Vaccines and Recommendations for Administration

Core Vaccines	Primary Puppy Series (≤16 weeks)	Primary Adult Series (>16 weeks)	Booster Interval
Distemper Recombinant or modified-live **Parvovirus** Modified-live **Adenovirus-2** Modified-live	Administer one dose at 6-8 weeks of age and then every 3-4 weeks until 14-16 weeks of age.	Administer two doses 3-4 weeks apart.	Administer one dose 1 year following completion of the initial series and then every 3 years thereafter.
Rabies Killed-1 Year Killed-3 Year	Administer one dose at 12-16 weeks of age.	Administer one dose.	Administer one dose 1 year following administration of the first dose and then every 3 years thereafter.

NOTE: Requirements for canine rabies vaccination are established by state and/or local statutes and may differ from the recommendations listed here.

Table 279-2

Noncore Canine Vaccines and Recommendations for Administration

Noncore (Optional) Vaccines	Primary Puppy Series (≤16 weeks)	Primary Adult Series (>16 weeks)	Booster Interval
***Bordetella bronchiseptica* +** **Parainfluenza** Avirulent-live (intranasal administration ONLY)	A single dose is recommended by the manufacturers and may be given as early as 3-4 weeks of age. Two doses 2-4 weeks apart are suggested for best results. May be given as early as 3-4 weeks of age.	A single dose	Annually; animals in a high risk/exposure environment may benefit from a booster if longer than 6 months since the previous dose.
Bordetella bronchiseptica Killed, or antigen extract	Administer two doses 2-4 weeks apart beginning as early as 8 weeks of age.	Administer two doses 2-4 weeks apart.	Annually; animals in a high risk/exposure environment may benefit from a booster if longer than 6 months since the previous dose.
Leptospira interrogans (Serovars: canicola, icterohaemorrhagiae, pomona, grippotyphosa) Various two-way and four-way combinations are available. Killed bacterin	Administer two doses 2-4 weeks apart beginning as early as 12 weeks of age. (Vaccination of dogs less than 12 weeks of age is generally not recommended.)	Administer two doses, 2 to 4 weeks apart.	Annual booster is recommended for dogs with a defined risk of exposure. Vaccination is *not* recommended for all dogs. Exposure risk should be considered before recommending.
Lyme borreliosis Recombinant or killed bacterin	Administer two doses 2-4 weeks apart beginning as early as 12 weeks of age.	Administer two doses 2-4 weeks apart.	Annual booster is recommended for dogs with a defined risk of exposure. Vaccination is not recommended for all dogs.

NOTE: Unless indicated, all vaccines may be administered by the subcutaneous route.

Noncore or Optional Vaccines

All dogs do not share equal risk of exposure to infectious agents. Principle variables affecting exposure risk include age, breed, health status, life style, geographic location, and travel history. Vaccines classified as noncore are those that a veterinarian may recommend or *not* recommend based on a reasonable assessment of risk in the individual patient. The 2006 AAHA Canine Vaccine Guidelines have classified the following vaccines as noncore: distemper-measles, all *Bordetella bronchiseptica* vaccines, parainfluenza virus, *Borrelia burgdorferi* (Lyme borreliosis), and *Leptospira interrogans* (all four serovars). The frequency of administration for noncore vaccines differs depending on the antigen type (avirulent live [topical] versus killed [parenteral]) and the manufacture's recommendation. When noncore vaccines are indicated for administration in adult dogs, annual administration generally is recommended. Because of the variation among individual products, veterinarians should be familiar with dosing, frequency, and administration requirements of the individual vaccine product selected. Veterinarians are also urged to consult the "Comments and Recommendations" section listed in the summary table of the full text version of the Guidelines (Part 1) to review specific recommendations on administering a particular vaccine type.

Conditionally Licensed Vaccines

Two new canine vaccines, conditionally licensed by the U.S. Department of Agriculture (USDA), are available throughout the United States: *Crotalus atrox* toxoid (western diamondback rattlesnake vaccine) and *Porphyromonas* spp. vaccine (an aid in the prevention of periodontitis). Neither of these vaccines has been subjected to conventional challenge studies. Although a reasonable expectation of efficacy exists, there is currently minimal field validation of efficacy. The AAHA Canine Vaccine Task Force elected not to categorize these vaccines as core, noncore, or "not recommended." Veterinarians considering the use of either of these products are encouraged to review the product literature and, when feasible, the experience offered by colleagues who have experience with the individual product.

Vaccines Not Recommended for Routine Administration

Several vaccine types have been classified by the AAHA Canine Vaccine Task Force as "not recommended." Reasons for assigning such a classification to a particular vaccine include such factors as lack of vaccine efficacy, diminished efficacy compared to alternative antigen types (e.g., killed virus vaccines are expected to be less efficacious than MLV vaccines), and safety. Vaccines classified as "not recommended" are: CAV-1, *Giardia lamblia*, coronavirus (killed virus and MLV), killed CPV, killed CAV-2, and topical (MLV) CAV-2. Each of these vaccines is currently licensed by the USDA and may be selected for administration to dogs at the discretion of the clinician. Veterinarians are encouraged to consult the full text of the 2006 Canine Vaccine Guidelines for additional discussion behind the reason an individual vaccine was given this classification.

GUIDELINES FOR SHELTER-HOUSED DOGS

The frequent introduction of healthy and sick dogs, seasonal variation in population density, and variable risk of exposure among shelter populations make it impractical to define specific "core" vaccine recommendations that will serve all facilities comparably. Only vaccines that are expected to demonstrate a clear benefit against common

and high-threat shelter infections are recommended. The AAHA Canine Vaccine Task Force recognizes the need for individual shelters to tailor vaccination requirements in a manner that is consistent with exposure risk and financial constraints of the individual facility. Because of the high exposure risk faced by shelter-housed dogs, vaccination recommendations made within this section of guidelines are considerably more aggressive than those recommended in general practice.

All dogs should be inoculated with CDV, CPV, and CAV-2 vaccine at the time of entry into the facility. Delaying vaccination by even a few hours could pose significantly increased risk of infection for individual dogs, especially puppies. Vaccines should be MLV; alternatively a recombinant vaccine may be used interchangeably with MLV vaccine for CDV. The recombinant CDV vaccine has the added advantage of immunizing puppies as young as 8 weeks of age even in the presence of passively acquired maternal antibody. With the exception of rabies, killed virus vaccines should not be used in animal shelter vaccination program. When feasible, a single dose of intranasal *B. bronchiseptica* (avirulent live) combined with parainfluenza virus is preferred and should also be administered at the time of entry into the facility. Vaccination is recommended as early as 4 weeks of age (3 weeks of age for intranasal *B. bronchiseptica*), particularly when infection rates within the facility are considered to be high. Vaccines for CDV, CPV, and CAV-2 are repeated every 2 weeks until 16 weeks of age. Dogs over 16 weeks of age should receive a second dose 2 weeks later if still in the facility. A 1-year rabies vaccine is recommended at the time of release from the shelter. Several options for alternative protocols are included in the Guidelines. Individuals seeking detailed information on recommendations for vaccinating shelter-housed dogs should refer to Part 2 of the AAHA Canine Vaccine Guidelines (www.aahanet.org).

Suggested Reading

Böhm M et al: Serum antibody titres to canine parvovirus, adenovirus, and distemper, *Vet Rec* 154:457, 2004.

Carmichael LE: Canine viral vaccines at a turning point: a personal perspective. In Schultz RD, editor: *Advances in veterinary medicine 41: veterinary vaccines and diagnostics*, San Diego, 1999, Academic Press, p 289.

Greene CE, Schultz RD: Immunoprophylaxis. In Greene CE, editor: *Infectious diseases of the dog and cat*, ed 3, St. Louis, 2006, Saunders-Elsevier, p 1068.

Klingborg DJ et al: AVMA Council on Biologic and Therapeutic Agents' report on cat and dog vaccines, *J Am Vet Med Assoc* 221(10):1401, 2002.

Mouzin DE et al: Duration of immunity in dogs after vaccination or naturally acquired infection, *J Am Vet Med Assoc* 224:55, 2004.

Pardo MC, Bauman JE, Mackowiak M: Protection of dogs against canine distemper by vaccination with a canarypox virus recombinant expressing canine distemper virus fusion and hemagglutinin glycoproteins, *Am J Vet Res* 58:833, 1997.

Pardo MC et al: Immunization of puppies in the presence of maternally derived antibodies against canine distemper virus, *J Comp Path* 137:572, 2007.

CHAPTER 280

Feline Vaccination Guidelines

RICHARD B. FORD, *Raleigh, North Carolina*

In November 2006 the American Association of Feline Practitioners (AAFP) published the latest report of the Feline Vaccine Advisory Panel outlining current feline vaccination recommendations (Richards et al, 2006). This was the first update published since 2000 and provided considerable new information on feline vaccines and vaccination practices. Whether or not an individual veterinarian intends to incorporate the 2006 feline vaccination recommendations into his or her practice, the current document is worthy of review and consideration. In addition to basic recommendations on vaccine administration, the report includes critical information on the selection and use of feline vaccines in practice. As more feline vaccines are introduced, veterinarians have the increasingly complex task of ensuring that individual patients are vaccinated against diseases that pose a *realistic* threat to the individual animal's health yet avoid the risk of adverse reactions associated with vaccination.

There can be little argument that routine vaccination programs remain an exceptional health care value for pets today. Yet the proliferation of new vaccines and new vaccine technology give emphasis to the fact that all vaccines are not necessarily alike. Likewise all cats do not share the same level of risk for exposure to infectious pathogens. It is the objective of the AAFP Feline Vaccine Advisory Panel to develop a document that will facilitate the efforts of practitioners in developing rational vaccination protocols for feline patients. As written, the Advisory Panel's report is not intended to represent a universal protocol applicable for all cats, nor is it intended to represent the standard of care by which all cats must be vaccinated. Although certainly there is no requirement for individual practices to implement the recommendations in the report, this document does contain important, relevant information pertaining to the routine selection and use of feline vaccines in clinical practice. The entire report is available at www.aafponline.org, (search: Practice Guidelines).

HIGHLIGHTS OF THE 2006 AAFP FELINE VACCINE GUIDELINES

The 2006 Report of the AAFP Feline Vaccine Advisory Panel is the most comprehensive review of feline vaccines and vaccination programs yet published. The report is comprehensive and includes 14 separate sections that address topics such as basic vaccine immunology, the types of vaccines available today, and recommendations on routes of vaccine administration. The report also includes a number of special considerations that pertain directly to the administration of vaccines in cats such as age, breed, and vaccination intervals. Additional special considerations include administration of vaccine to cattery cats, lactating queens, sick cats, retrovirus-infected cats, cats receiving corticosteroids, and cats having a prior history of vaccine-associated adverse reactions (events). Updated information on controversial topics such as the extended duration of immunity for the feline (core vaccines) and the triennial booster recommendations is also presented. Of importance to all practitioners is the section on legal considerations, which centers on liability associated with vaccinating cats. Topics on vaccine standards of care and informed consent are also presented.

The section on vaccine adverse events, also called adverse reactions, highlights the exceptional safety record of vaccines yet outlines concerns over the lack of available data for the types of reactions that are believed to occur. Much of the discussion addresses vaccine-associated fibrosarcomas, perhaps the single most important vaccine adverse event that occurs in companion animal medicine. Veterinarians in the United States are encouraged to report feline vaccine adverse events, known or suspected, to the Center for Veterinary Biologics (CVB, www.aphis.usda.gov/vs/cvb) online and to the vaccine manufacturer (manufacturers are required to forward reports to the CVB).

One noteworthy addition to the report is the section on vaccination of shelter-housed cats. This section complements information found in the 2006 American Animal Hospital Association (AAHA) Canine Vaccine Guidelines, which is available on the AAHA website available at www.aahanet.org (also see Chapter 279). Furthermore, new recommendations on the vaccination of cats in trap-neuter-return programs and kitten socialization classes are included. The report also includes six appendices that focus on issues ranging from vaccination site recommendations to vaccine handling and storage requirements.

Core Vaccines

For several years the primary vaccination series for kittens has been a single dose administered at 9 and 12 weeks of age. The current guidelines, however, recommend that the first dose of core vaccines (feline parvovirus [panleukopenia virus], herpesvirus-1, and calicivirus) be administered as early as 6 weeks of age and then every 3 to 4 weeks until 16 weeks of age. This should be followed by a booster at 1 year of age and every 3 years thereafter. A rabies vaccine, also recommended as core for all cats, can be administered as a single dose as early as 12 weeks of age; a booster is administered 1 year later. State or local rabies ordinances that dictate different requirements have precedence over any recommendations published in the 2006 AAFP Feline Vaccine Advisory Panel Report (Tables 280-1 and 280-2).

Table 280-1

Core Feline Vaccines and Recommendations for Administration

Core Vaccines	Primary Kitten Series (≦16 weeks)	Primary Adult Series (>16 weeks)	Booster Interval
Parvovirus (Panleukopenia) **Herpesvirus-1 and calicivirus** Modified-live (nonadjuvanted) or killed (adjuvanted) (subcutaneous or intranasal administration)	Administer one dose as early as 6 weeks of age and then every 3-4 weeks until 16 weeks of age.	Administer two doses 3-4 weeks apart.	Administer one dose 1 year following completion of the initial series and then every 3 years thereafter. NOTE: It is still appropriate to recommend annual booster against feline herpesvirus-1 and feline calicivirus for cats housed in high risk environments.
Rabies Recombinant (nonadjuvanted)	Administer one dose at 12-16 weeks of age.	Administer one dose.	Annually
Rabies Killed: 1 year Killed: 3 year (adjuvanted)	Administer one dose at 12-16 weeks of age.	Administer one dose.	Administer one dose 1 year following administration of the first dose and then every 3 years thereafter.

NOTE: Requirements for feline rabies vaccination are established by state and/or local statutes and may differ from the recommendations listed here.

Table 280-2

Noncore Feline Vaccines and Recommendations for Administration

Noncore (Optional) Vaccines	Primary Kitten Series (≦16 weeks)	Primary Adult Series (>16 weeks)	Booster Interval
Feline Leukemia Recombinant (nonadjuvanted) (transdermal administration *only*)	Administer two doses 3-4 weeks apart beginning as early as 12 weeks of age.	Administer two doses 3-4 weeks apart.	Annual booster; booster vaccination is *not* recommended for all cats. Exposure risk should be considered before recommending.
Feline Leukemia Killed (adjuvanted)	Administer two dose 3-4 weeks apart beginning as early as 12 weeks of age.	Administer two doses 3-4 weeks apart.	Annual booster; booster vaccination is *not* recommended for all cats. Exposure risk should be considered before recommending.
Chlamydophila felis Avirulent live (nonadjuvanted)	Administer two doses 3-4 weeks apart beginning as early as 12 weeks of age.	Administer two doses 3-4 weeks apart.	Annual booster; booster vaccination is *not* recommended for all cats. Exposure risk should be considered before recommending.
Chlamydophila felis Killed (adjuvanted)	Administer two doses 3-4 weeks apart beginning as early as 12 weeks of age.	Administer two doses 3-4 weeks apart.	Annual booster; booster vaccination is *not* recommended for all cats. Exposure risk should be considered before recommending.
Feline Immunodeficiency Virus Killed (adjuvanted)	Administration of three initial doses is required. Beginning as early as 8 weeks of age, administer two additional doses 2-3 weeks apart.	Administration of three initial doses is required. Each dose should be administered 2-3 weeks apart.	Annual booster; booster vaccination is *not* recommended for all cats. Exposure risk should be considered before recommending. NOTE: A single dose of feline immunodeficiency virus (FIV) vaccine can result in a false-positive test result on all commercial FIV tests for at least 1 year.
Bordetella bronchiseptica Avirulent live (nonadjuvanted) (intranasal *only*)	Administer a single dose as early as 8 weeks of age.	Administer a single dose.	Administer annually, but only in cats with established risk of exposure.

NOTE: Routine vaccination of cats against feline infectious peritonitis virus and *Giardia lamblia* is *not generally recommended*. Unless otherwise stipulated, all feline vaccines should be administered by the subcutaneous route.

Feline Leukemia Virus Vaccine

Feline leukemia virus (FeLV) vaccine continues to be listed as noncore. However, since kittens are more likely than adults to become persistently viremic following exposure, the Advisory Panel highly recommends that all kittens receive a two-dose primary series, beginning as early as 8 weeks of age, and a booster 1 year after completion of the initial series. There are no published studies documenting vaccine duration of immunity beyond 1 year. Therefore adults deemed to be at sustained risk of exposure (e.g., outdoor cats) should be vaccinated annually. Documentation of a negative FeLV (antigen) test is recommended before administration of the FeLV vaccine.

Vaccination of Retrovirus-Positive Cats

Studies evaluating the ability of FeLV- and feline immunodeficiency virus (FIV)–infected cats to mount a protective immune response subsequent to vaccination vary. However, it is the recommendation of the Advisory Panel that feline core vaccines should be administered to healthy, retrovirus-positive cats. It is left to the discretion of the clinician whether the risk of exposure in an individual cat justifies vaccine administration. There is no known therapeutic value in administering either an FeLV or FIV vaccine to a retrovirus-infected cat.

Adjuvanted versus Nonadjuvanted Feline Vaccine

Based on the finding of several published studies, the association between adjuvanted vaccine use and the development of vaccine-associated fibrosarcomas is deemed to be sufficiently compelling that the Advisory Panel recommends that "veterinarians use less inflammatory products whenever possible." Avoiding adjuvanted vaccines is not a guarantee that an individual cat will never develop cancer at an injection site; however, simply recommending that injectable vaccines be administered as low (distal) on the leg as feasible to facilitate amputation remains an impractical solution to the vaccine-associated sarcoma problem. At this writing, all feline killed virus and killed bacterial vaccines contain adjuvant. Modified-live virus, avirulent live bacteria (e.g., intranasal administration), and recombinant vaccines do not contain adjuvant.

Vaccination Against Feline Immunodeficiency Virus

Particularly important is the fact that a single dose of the FIV vaccine can result in the production of antibodies that cause (false)-positive test results on all commercially available FIV tests. Vaccine-induced antibodies can also be passed from queen to kittens via colostrum and interfere with testing beyond the age of weaning. FIV test interference in adult vaccinated cats has been shown to persist for at least 1 year. In kittens test interference derived from ingestion of colostrum appears to wane by 12 weeks of age. Cats receiving the current FIV vaccine should be permanently identified (e.g., microchip).

Vaccines Not Recommended for Routine Administration

Consistent with recommendations published in 2000, the Advisory Panel continues to stipulate that vaccination of cats against feline coronavirus (FCoV), to prevent feline infectious peritonitis (FIP) infection, and *Giardia lamblia* is "not generally recommended." Although considerable controversy surrounds the ability of the FIP vaccine to protect cats from infection, most studies have shown little or no benefit from routine inoculation. The *G. lamblia* vaccine contains chemically inactivated (killed) trophozoites and an adjuvant. In independent studies administration of this vaccine did not lessen cyst shedding in experimentally infected cats when compared with control cats.

Virulent Systemic Feline Calicivirus Vaccine

In January 2007 a killed, adjuvanted vaccine was licensed in the United States as an aid in preventing infection with virulent systemic feline calicivirus (VS-FCV). Earlier a bivalent, killed (nonadjuvanted) calicivirus vaccine was licensed in the United Kingdom. Neither of these vaccines was addressed is the 2006 Advisory Panel Report. An amendment to the report addressing recommendations on the use of the VS-FCV vaccine is expected later in 2008. VS-FCV is a highly contagious, severe infection that occurs predominantly in adult cats; most reports involve cats residing in shelters. At least one outbreak has been documented in a veterinary hospital housing shelter cats. However, in the last decade fewer than 10 outbreaks have been documented in the United States and United Kingdom combined. Vaccine efficacy has been demonstrated in cats experimentally challenged with a calicivirus strain that was homologous with the virus strain used in the vaccine. However, the literature currently does not support the ability of a single VS-FCV strain to provide cross-protection against VS-FCVs that may be encountered in cats in future outbreaks. This vaccine is neither a replacement for nor an alternative to the combined calicivirus vaccine plus feline herpesvirus-1 administered to cats for the prevention of viral upper respiratory infections.

VACCINATION OF SHELTER-HOUSED CATS

Vaccination of cats presented to and maintained in a shelter-type environment presents a number of unique and challenging issues to veterinarians attempting to manage morbidity and limit mortality associated with contagious infectious diseases, particularly panleukopenia, herpesvirus-1, and calicivirus infection. In general, the Advisory Panel recommends that all cats receive vaccine against panleukopenia, herpesvirus-1, and calicivirus on entry to the facility; a 1-year rabies vaccine is administered at the time of release. There are no indications for administration of FeLV, FIV, *G. lamblia*, and *Bordetella bronchiseptica* vaccine in the shelter environment. One exception for consideration includes vaccination of kittens against FeLV when housing requirements dictate that unrelated kittens be housed together. For specific recommendations on individual vaccines, the full text of the 2006 Feline Vaccine Guidelines should be consulted.

References and Suggested Reading

Gaskell RM et al: Veterinary Products Committee (VPC) Working Group Report of Feline and Canine Vaccination. Final Report to the VPC, London, 2002, Dept Environmental, Food and Rural Affairs (Monograph).

Greene CE, Schultz RD: Immunoprophylaxis. In Greene CE, editor: *Infectious diseases of the dog and cat*, ed 3, St Louis, 2006, Saunders, p 1069.

Lappin MR: Use of serologic tests to predict resistance to feline herpesvirus-1, feline calicivirus, and feline parvovirus infection in cats, *J Am Vet Med Assoc* 220:38, 2002.

Meyer EK: Vaccine-associated adverse events, *Vet Clin North Am Small Anim Pract* 31:493, 2001.

Mouzin DE: Duration of serologic response to three viral antigens in cats, *J Am Vet Med Assoc* 224:61, 2004.

Richards JR et al: The 2006 American Association of Feline Practitioners Feline Advisory Panel Report, *J Am Vet Med Assoc* 229(9):1405, 2006.

Scott FW, Geissinge CM: Long-term immunity in cats vaccinated with an inactivated trivalent vaccine, *Am J Vet Res* 60:652, 1999.

CHAPTER 281

Feline Leukemia Virus and Feline Immunodeficiency Virus

KATRIN HARTMANN, *Munich, Germany*

The three feline retroviruses, feline immunodeficiency virus (FIV), feline leukemia virus (FeLV), and feline foamy virus (FeFV), are global and widespread. Although all three viruses are in the family Retroviridae, they differ in their potential to cause disease. FeFV (previously known as feline syncytium-forming virus, FeSFV), a spumavirus, is not associated with disease; thus routine testing is not performed.

FIV, a lentivirus that shares many properties with human immunodeficiency virus (HIV), can cause an acquired immune deficiency syndrome in cats, with increased risk for opportunistic infections, neurologic diseases, and tumors. In most naturally infected cats FIV infection does not cause a severe clinical syndrome, and with proper care FIV-infected cats can live many years. Many in fact die at an older age from causes completely unrelated to FIV infection. In a study of naturally FIV-infected cats, the rate of progression was variable, with death occurring in about 18% of infected cats within the first 2 years of observation (about 5 years after the estimated time of infection). An additional 18% developed increasingly severe disease, but more than 50% remained clinically asymptomatic during the 2 years of observation (Levy et al., 2000). FIV infection has little impact on a cat population, and does not reduce the number of cats in a household. Thus overall survival time is not necessarily shorter than in uninfected cats, and quality of life is usually fairly high over an extended period of time.

FeLV, an oncornavirus, is the most pathogenic of the three viruses. Historically it was considered to account for more disease-related deaths and clinical syndromes than any other single infectious agent in cats. More recently the prevalence and consequently the importance of FeLV as a pathogen in cats have been decreasing, mainly because of testing and eradication programs and the relatively common use of FeLV vaccines. The death rate of persistently viremic cats in multicat households is approximately 50% in 2 years and 80% in 3 years but is lower in cats kept strictly indoors in single-cat households. Despite the fact that persistent FeLV viremia is associated with a decrease in life expectancy, many owners elect to provide treatment for the clinical syndromes that accompany infection. With proper care, many FeLV-infected cats kept indoors only may live for many years with good quality of life.

A decision for treatment or for euthanasia of a cat should never be based solely on the presence of a retrovirus infection. FIV- and FeLV-infected cats are subject to the same diseases that befall cats free of those infections, and illness in a given cat may not be related to the retrovirus infection at all. However, in all cats, healthy or sick, FIV and FeLV status should be known because retrovirus infection impacts health status and long-term patient management.

MANAGEMENT OF RETROVIRUS-INFECTED MULTICAT HOUSEHOLDS

When a cat in a multicat household is diagnosed with a retrovirus infection, all cats in that household should be tested to determine their virus status. If positive and negative cats are identified within the same household, the owner must be informed of the potential danger to uninfected cats and told that the best method of preventing spread of infection is to isolate the infected individuals and prevent them from interacting with housemates. However, despite this admonition, the overall risk of transmission between these cats is not very high for either infection.

FIV transmission in households with a stable social cat environment is rare because FIV is mainly transmitted through biting and fighting; if no fights occur, FIV will not be transmitted. In long-term studies of households with FIV-infected cats, few additional cats became FIV positive over time; in some households no transmission occurred over many years. All cats in these households should be neutered, and it is crucial not to introduce a new cat into the household since this might lead to fights and to transmission, even between cats that have lived together peacefully for a long time.

The benefit of FIV vaccination of FIV-negative cats in households with an FIV-positive cat is controversial (see Chapter 280). The vaccine currently available has not been tested under these conditions. Usually the FIV subtype of the infected cat is unknown, and cross-protection by the vaccine against some FIV subtypes (e.g., the frequently found subtype B) is uncertain. Because the vaccine contains whole virus, cats respond to vaccination by producing antibodies that are indistinguishable from those produced during natural infection. Therefore *all vaccinated cats will be antibody positive*, and assessment of their true infection status can be difficult. Ideally, before vaccination is considered the veterinarian should ensure that the virus in the infected cat can be detected by polymerase chain reaction (which is only possible in 50% to 80% of cases). Only if the virus strain of the infected cat is detectable by PCR will it be possible to later identify another cat in the household that might become infected despite vaccination.

If an FeLV-infected cat has lived for some time in an otherwise FeLV-negative household, the other cats that have been together with the FeLV-infected cat will already have been infected. Thus, these cats are most likely immune to new infection, and an owner may elect to keep all of the cats together. However, studies in cluster households have shown that virus-neutralizing antibodies do not persist for life; thus a previously immune cat may become viremic. This may be the result of new infection or reactivation of a long-persisting latent infection. The risk of infection in adult FeLV-negative cats is approximately 10% to 15% if they have lived with a viremic cat for several months. If owners refuse to separate housemates, the *uninfected cats should receive FeLV vaccination* to enhance their natural level of immunity. However, owners should be informed that vaccination does not provide sufficient levels of protection in these environments of high viral exposure. If the household is closed to new cats, the FeLV-negative cats tend to outlive the infected cats.

MANAGEMENT OF INDIVIDUAL RETROVIRUS-INFECTED CATS

The most important life-prolonging advice the veterinarian can advance to owners of retrovirus-infected cats is "keep the cats strictly indoors". This not only avoids spread to other cats in the neighborhood, but also prevents exposure of the immunosuppressed, retrovirus-infected cat to infectious agents carried by other animals. In FIV-infected cats, secondary infections not only cause clinical signs but also may lead to progression of the FIV infection itself. This is probably not the case in FeLV infection in which the retroviral infection itself it more pathogenic and progresses relatively independently of cofactors.

"Routine vaccination" of retrovirus-infected cats is subject to much discussion. It is the recommendation of an Advisory Panel on Feline vaccination that feline core vaccines should be administered to healthy, retrovirus-positive cats at risk (see Chapter 280 for details). The author's recommendations follow.

While there is no scientific proof that retrovirus-infected cats are at increased risk from modified-life virus (MLV) vaccines, inactivated vaccines are recommended out of concern that MLV vaccines given to immune-suppressed animals may regain pathogenicity. FIV-infected cats are susceptible to secondary infection (thus regular vaccination would seem indicated). Studies have shown that healthy FIV-infected cats are able to mount appropriate levels of protective neutralizing antibodies after vaccination. However, it is the author's opinion that vaccines should not be given to FIV-infected cats, if strictly kept indoors because not only immune suppression, but also immune stimulation, can lead to progression of FIV infection by altering the balance between the immune system and the virus. Stimulation of FIV-infected lymphocytes is known to promote virus production in vitro. In vivo vaccination of chronically infected FIV-infected cats with a synthetic peptide was associated with a decrease in the CD4/CD8 ratio. Thus the potential tradeoff to protection from infection with vaccination is progression of FIV infection secondary to increased virus production. If FIV-infected cats are kept strictly indoors, the risk of secondary infections is lower than the possible adverse effects of vaccination. It should be noted that in some countries or states legal requirements for rabies vaccination may supersede these issues.

The author, however, agrees with the recommendation that FeLV-infected cats should be administered routine vaccinations. In studies of immune response to rabies vaccination, it was demonstrated that FeLV-infected cats may not be able to mount adequate immune responses. Therefore protection in an FeLV-infected cat after vaccination is not comparable to that in a healthy cat, and more frequent vaccinations than usually recommended must be considered (e.g., every 6 months), especially in cats that are allowed to go outside in areas with high rabies prevalence.

Retrovirus-infected cats should have veterinary evaluations at least semiannually to promptly detect changes in health status. A complete blood count (CBC), biochemistry profile, and urinalysis should be performed at least annually

(CBC every 6 months in FeLV-infected cats to detect anemia or other cytopenias associated with FeLV infection). Intact male and female retrovirus-infected cats should be neutered to reduce stress associated with estrus and mating behavior and the desire to roam outside the house or interact aggressively. Surgery is generally well tolerated by asymptomatic retrovirus-infected cats, but perioperative antibiotic administration should be used for all surgeries and dental procedures. Since the viruses live for only minutes outside of the host and are susceptible to all disinfectants (including common soap), simple precautions and routine cleaning procedures will prevent transmission in the hospital. Retrovirus-infected cats can be housed in the same ward as other hospitalized patients; however, they should be housed in individual cages. They may be immune suppressed and should be kept away from cats with other infectious diseases. Under no circumstances should they be placed in a "contagious disease ward" with cats suffering from infections such as viral respiratory disease.

If retrovirus-infected cats are sick, prompt and accurate identification of the secondary illness is essential to allow early therapeutic intervention and a successful treatment outcome. Therefore more intensive diagnostic testing should proceed earlier in the course of illness than might be recommended for uninfected cats. Many cats with retrovirus infection respond as well as uninfected cats to appropriate medications, although a longer or more aggressive course of therapy (e.g., antibiotics) may be needed. Corticosteroids or other immune-suppressive or bone marrow–suppressive drugs should be avoided. Griseofulvin has been shown to cause bone marrow suppression in FIV-infected cats and should not be used.

Recombinant human granulocyte colony-stimulation factor (rHuG-CSF; Filgastrim) is contraindicated in neutropenic FIV-infected cats. Although it increases neutrophil counts, treatment can also lead to a significant increase in viral load in peripheral blood mononuclear cells by enhancing infection of lymphocytes or increasing expression of FIV by infected lymphocytes. Until data in FeLV-infected cats are available, rHuG-CSF therapy also cannot be recommended.

Recombinant human erythropoietin (rHuEPO) may be effective in cats with nonregenerative anemia. FIV-infected cats treated with HuEPO (100 units/kg subcutaneously [SQ] q48h) showed a gradual increase in red and white blood cell counts, and increases in viral loads were not observed; thus rHuEPO appears to be safe in FIV-infected cats. No studies are available for FeLV-infected cats, but the author assumes rHuEPO will have the same positive effects.

Recombinant human insulin-like growth factor-1 (rHuIGF-1) can induce thymic growth and stimulate T cell function. Treatment with rHuIGF-1 resulted in a significant increase in thymus size and thymic cortical regeneration replenishing the peripheral T cell pool in experimentally FIV-infected cats. It could be considered in young FIV-infected cats as supportive treatment, but there are no field studies so far to show its effect in naturally FIV-infected cats. Its usefulness in FeLV infection is also unknown.

IMMUNE MODULATOR THERAPY

Immune modulators or interferon inducers are widely used in retrovirus-infected cats, especially FeLV-infected cats (Table 282-1). Although reports of uncontrolled studies frequently suggest sometimes dramatic clinical improvement, these effects generally have not been reproduced in properly controlled studies. It has been suggested that these agents may benefit infected animals by restoring compromised immune function, thereby allowing the patient to control viral burden and recover from the disease. Most reports in the veterinary literature are difficult to interpret because of vague diagnostic criteria, lack of clinical staging or follow-up, small numbers of cats studied, absence of a placebo-treated control group, the natural variability of the course of disease, and the fact that additional supportive treatments were administered. Especially the homeopathic remedies have not been sufficiently evaluated in feline retrovirus infections and these drugs cannot be recommended.

In FeLV-infected cats every immune modulator therapy should be considered very carefully. There is no conclusive evidence from controlled studies that immune modulators or alternative drugs have any beneficial effects on health or survival of asymptomatic or symptomatic FIV-infected cats. As suggested previously, nonspecific stimulation of the immune system might even be contraindicated in FIV infection because it can lead to an increase in virus replication caused by activation of latently infected lymphocytes and macrophages. Thus nonspecific immunomodulators with unknown effects are not recommended in FIV-infected cats.

A number of immune modulators have been used against FeLV infection. Pind-avi (parapox virus avis) and pind-orf (parapox virus ovis) are inactivated poxviruses that belong to the so-called *paramunity inducers*. Their suggested mode of action is primarily induction of interferons and activation of natural killer cells. These compounds caused a sensation in Germany when it was published that their administration resulted in a cure of 80% to 100% of FeLV-infected cats, even those in moribund condition. Paramunity inducers (1 ml SQ twice a week for 6 weeks) quickly became the most commonly used treatment for FeLV infection in Europe. However, two placebo-controlled, double-blind trials (including 120 and 30 cats, respectively) using the same treatment protocol in naturally FeLV-infected cats under controlled conditions failed to reproduce these striking results. There were no significant differences between the cats treated with paramunity inducers and placebo-treated cats in the number of cats that terminated viremia or in any clinical, laboratory, immunologic, or virologic parameter investigated (Hartmann et al., 1998). These studies demonstrate the importance of sufficiently controlled clinical trials in the assessment of novel therapies for feline retrovirus infections.

Acemannan, a water-soluble, long-chain complex carbohydrate polymer derived from the aloe vera plant, is thought to be taken up by macrophages, stimulating them to release cytokines, which in turn stimulate cell-mediated immune responses, including cytotoxicity. In one uncontrolled trial, 50 cats with natural FeLV infection were treated with acemannan (2 mg/kg intraperitoneally [IP] once a week for 6 weeks). After 12 weeks 71% of the cats were known to be alive, all cats remained FeLV antigen positive, and no significant change was noted in their clinical signs or hematologic parameters. There was no control group; thus assessment of the results is difficult (Sheets et al., 1991).

Table 281-1

Treatment Options for Retrovirus-Infected Cats

Drug		Efficacy in vitro?	Controlled Studies in vivo?	Efficacy in vivo?	Author Opinion on Use
Antiviral Drugs					
Zidovudine	FIV	Yes	Yes	Yes	Effective in some cats
	FeLV	Yes	Yes	No	Not effective in field cats
Stavudine	FIV	Yes	No	n.d.	Possibly effective
	FeLV	n.d.	No	n.d.	Possibly effective
Didanosine	FIV	Yes	No	n.d.	Possibly effective
	FeLV	Yes	No	n.d.	Possibly effective
Zalcitabine	FIV	Yes	No	n.d.	Toxic in high dosages
	FeLV	Yes	Yes	No	Toxic in high dosages
Lamivudine	FIV	Yes	Yes	No	Toxic in high dosages
	FeLV	No	No	n.d.	Toxic in high dosages
Ribavirin	FIV	Yes	No	n.d.	Toxic in cats
	FeLV	Yes	No	n.d.	Toxic in cats
Foscarnet	FIV	Yes	No	n.d.	Toxic
	FeLV	Yes	No	n.d.	Toxic
Suramin	FIV	n.d.	No	n.d.	Likely ineffective
	FeLV	n.d.	No	n.d.	Likely ineffective
T20	FIV	No	No	No	Ineffective
	FeLV	n.d.	No	n.d.	Likely ineffective
AMD3100	FIV	Yes	Yes	Yes	Some effect in field cat
	FeLV	n.d.	No	n.d.	Likely ineffective
Lactoferrin	FIV	n.d.	Yes	±	Possibly effective in stomatitis
	FeLV	n.d.	No	n.d.	Possibly effective in stomatitis
Human interferon-α	FIV	Yes	No	n.d.	Likely ineffective
subcutaneous high dose	FeLV	Yes	Yes	No	Ineffective
oral low dose	FIV	Yes	No	±	Improved survival
	FeLV	Yes	Yes	No	Ineffective
Feline interferon-ω	FIV	Yes	Yes	No	Ineffective
	FeLV	Yes	Yes	±	Improved survival
Immune Modulators					
Polyriboinosinic-	FIV	n.d.	No	n.d.	Contraindicated
polyribocytidylic acid	FeLV	n.d.	No	n.d.	Likely ineffective
Pind-avi/Pind-orf	FIV	n.d.	No	n.d.	Contraindicated
	FeLV	n.d.	Yes	No	Ineffective
Acemannan	FIV	n.d.	No	n.d.	Contraindicated
	FeLV	n.d.	No	n.d.	Likely ineffective
Staphylococcus protein A	FIV	n.d.	No	n.d.	Contraindicated
	FeLV	n.d.	Yes	±	Possibly effective
Propionibacterium acnes	FIV	n.d.	No	n.d.	Contraindicated
	FeLV	n.d.	No	n.d.	Likely ineffective
Bacille Calmette-Guérin (BCG)	FIV	n.d.	No	n.d.	Contraindicated
	FeLV	n.d.	Yes	No	Ineffective
Serratia marcescens	FIV	n.d.	No	n.d.	Contraindicated
	FeLV	n.d.	Yes	No	Ineffective
Levamisole	FIV	n.d.	No	n.d.	Contraindicated
	FeLV	n.d.	No	n.d.	Likely ineffective
Diethylcarbamazine	FIV	n.d.	No	n.d.	Contraindicated
	FeLV	n.d.	Yes	No	Ineffective
Nosodes	FIV	n.d.	No	n.d.	Contraindicated
	FeLV	n.d.	No	n.d.	Likely ineffective

FeLV, Feline leukemia virus; *FIV,* feline immunodeficiency virus; *n.d.,* not determined; ±, some effect.

Staphylococcus protein A (SPA), a bacterial polypeptide purified from cell walls of *Staphylococcus aureus* Cowan I, can bind to the Fc portion of certain immunoglobulin G subclasses by a nonimmunologic mechanism without disturbing antigen binding and may combine with immune complexes; stimulate complement activation; and induce T cell activation, stimulation of natural killer cells, and interferon production. A variety of SPA sources and treatments have been used in FeLV-infected cats. In some studies a high rate of tumor remission and conversion to

FeLV-negative status was observed; in others responses were less dramatic and short lived. However, in an experimental study that included kittens with experimental FeLV infection, SPA treatment neither reversed anemia nor improved humoral immune function. In a placebo-controlled study, treatment of ill client-owned FeLV-infected cats with SPA (10 mcg/kg twice weekly for up to 10 weeks) did not cause a statistically significant difference in FeLV status, survival time, or clinical and hematologic parameters when compared with a placebo-treated control group; but it did result in significant improvement in the owners' subjective impression of the health of their pets (McCaw et al., 2001).

Propionibacterium acnes, formerly *Corynebacterium parvum*, is a killed bacterial product that stimulates macrophages and the release of various cytokines and interferons and enhances T cell and natural killer cell activity in mice. It has been used in FeLV-infected cats (0.2 mg/cat intravenously [IV] twice a week and then once a week for at least 6 weeks), but no prospective studies have been performed, and anecdotal reports note that about 50% of the treated cats improved. A number of other immunostimulants, including a cell wall extract of a nonpathogenic strain of *Mycobacterium bovis* (Bacille Calmette-Guérin), extracts of *Serratia marcescens*, levamisole, and diethylcarbamazine, have not shown any efficacy in altering virus production or immune function in properly performed (controlled) studies despite in vitro evidence of immunomodulatory effects.

ANTIVIRAL CHEMOTHERAPY

Most antivirals used in cats are licensed for humans and are intended specifically for treatment of HIV infection. Some can be used to treat FIV infection because most enzymes of FIV and HIV have similar sensitivities to various inhibitors. However, few controlled studies have been performed to support their use in cats. Nucleoside analogs are usually less effective against FeLV when compared to FIV because FeLV is not as closely related to HIV.

Zidovudine, 3'-azido-2',3'-dideoxythymidine (AZT), is a nucleoside analog (thymidine derivative) that blocks the reverse transcriptase of retroviruses and inhibits new infections of cells. AZT can inhibit FIV replication in vitro and in vivo, reduce plasma virus load, improve the immunologic and clinical status of FIV-infected cats, increase quality of life, and prolongs life expectancy. In a placebo-controlled trial, AZT improved stomatitis in naturally infected cats. It should be used at a dosage of 5 to 10 mg/kg every 12 hours orally or subcutaneously. The higher dose should be used carefully since side effects can develop. For subcutaneous injection the lyophilized product should be diluted in isotonic NaCl solution to prevent local irritation. For oral application syrup or gelatin capsules (with dosage individualized for the cat) can be used. During treatment a CBC should be performed regularly (weekly for the first month) because nonregenerative anemia is a common side effect, especially if the higher dosage is used. If blood values are stable after the first month, a monthly check is sufficient. Cats with bone marrow suppression should not be treated with AZT. Studies in which FIV-infected cats were treated for 2 years showed that AZT is well tolerated. Some cats may develop a mild decrease of hematocrit initially in the first 3 weeks that resolves

even if treatment is continued. If hematocrit drops below 20%, discontinuation is recommended, and anemia usually resolves within a few days. Unfortunately, as in HIV, AZT-resistant mutants of FIV can arise as early as 6 months after initiation of treatment. AZT is also effective against FeLV in vitro. When treated less than 1 week after experimental inoculation, cats were protected from FeLV bone marrow infection and persistent viremia. However, in a study with naturally FeLV-infected cats, 6 weeks of treatment with AZT did not lead to a statistically significant improvement of clinical, laboratory, immunologic, or virologic parameters. In general, therapeutic efficacy of AZT in FeLV-infected cats seems to be less promising than in cats infected with FIV. It should be used only at low dosage (5 mg/kg orally [PO] or SQ q12h) in FeLV-infected cats because of its bone marrow–suppressive effects.

Several other nucleoside analogs with a similar mode of action to that of AZT and licensed for treatment of HIV-infected patients have activity against feline retroviruses. The in vitro and in vivo activity of these drugs against FIV and FeLV is summarized in Table 286-1.

Foscarnet is a pyrophosphate analog that reversibly inhibits virus-specific deoxyribonucleic acid (DNA) and ribonucleic acid (RNA) polymerase and reverse transcriptase by binding to the enzymes at a site distinct from that of nucleoside analogs. It has a wide spectrum of activity against DNA and RNA viruses. In vitro foscarnet has activity against FIV and FeLV, but no reliable data exist on its in vivo efficacy in cats, and its use in cats is limited because of toxicity. It is nephrotoxic and myelosuppressive and chelates cations such as calcium, so that hypocalcemia, hypomagnesemia, and hypokalemia may develop. Foscarnet is toxic to epithelial cells and mucous membranes, leading to severe gastrointestinal side effects and ulceration of genital epithelium.

Suramin, a sulfated naphthylamine, has been used primarily as an antiparasitic. It is also effective against several viruses through inhibition of reverse transcriptase by interacting with the template-primer binding site of the enzyme that is necessary for DNA prolongation. However, it is also associated with severe side effects, including nausea and anaphylactic shock (during administration), peripheral neuritis, agranulocytosis, hemolytic anemia, and destruction of the adrenal cortex. No reliable studies exist to show its effect against FIV. Suramin was used to treat FeLV-infected cats, although only a limited number of cats were studied. FeLV-related anemia improved in these cats, and serum viral infectivity ceased transiently. However, because these studies were not controlled, results must be interpreted carefully, and the severe side effects limit its use in cat patients.

T20 is a new anti-HIV drug that inhibits virus entry by inhibiting fusion of the virus with the cell membrane. It has been tested against several retroviruses, including FIV, but showed minimal antiviral effect likely because of insufficient sequence homology of the primary amino acid sequence of HIV and FIV in the critical regions. It has not been tested against FeLV but is likely ineffective. AMD3100 belongs to the new class of bicyclams that act as selective antagonists of the chemokine receptor CXCR4. CXCR4 is the main coreceptor for T cell–line-adapted HIV strains, and blocking the CXCR4 receptor leads to inhibition of virus entry. FIV also uses CXCR4 for virus entry, and a high degree of homology exists between the human and feline CXCR4. AMD3100 is not licensed as an antiviral compound but as a stem cell activator for patients that undergo bone marrow transplantation. It is effective against FIV in vitro; and in a placebo-controlled double-blind study in which 40 naturally FIV-infected cats were treated with AMD 3100 (0.5 mg/kg q12h SQ for 6 weeks) it caused a statistically significant improvement in clinical signs and decreased the proviral load in FIV-infected cats without side effects. AMD3100 has not been tested against FeLV but is likely ineffective because FeLV uses different receptors for virus entry into the cell.

Lactoferrin is a mammalian iron-binding glycoprotein that has antibacterial, antifungal, antiprotozoal, and antiviral properties. Antiviral activity may occur as a result of lactoferrin interaction with the viral receptors on the cell surface or by direct neutralization or inhibition of the viral particle. Lactoferrin is produced by mucosal epithelial cells of many mammalian species and is present in secretions such as tears, milk, saliva, seminal or vaginal fluids, and low concentrations in plasma. Side effects are not described. Lactoferrin had some effect in cats with stomatitis, and it may be an option for treatment of FIV- and FeLV-related stomatitis.

Human interferon-α has immune-modulatory effects but also acts as a true antiviral compound by inducing a general antiviral state of cells that protects them against virus replication (also see Chapter 85). Two common treatment regimens are used in cats: subcutaneous injection of high-dose interferon (10^4 to 10^6 units/kg q24h), or oral application of a low-dose treatment (1 to 50 units/kg q24h). Measurable serum levels can be obtained when given subcutaneously, but using this regimen it becomes ineffective after 3 to 7 weeks because of development of neutralizing antibodies. Human interferon-α given orally is not absorbed but is destroyed in the gastrointestinal tract; no measurable serum levels develop. The only way oral interferon may have an effect is by stimulation of the local lymphoid tissue in the oral cavity. In murine studies it was shown that subcutaneous administration of interferon-α had an antiviral effect, whereas oral administration only caused immunomodulation. In a recent study a positive effect on the survival of FIV-infected cats could be demonstrated using low-dose oral human interferon-α. Human interferon-α inhibits FeLV replication in vitro and has been used in several studies in FeLV-infected cats. Treatment with high dosages of subcutaneous human interferon-α (1.6×10^4 and 1.6×10^6 units/kg SQ) in experimentally FeLV-infected cats with high levels of persistent antigenemia resulted in significant decreases in circulating FeLV p27 antigen. However, as a result of anti-interferon-α antibody development, cats became refractory to therapy after 3 or 7 weeks. In a study of naturally FeLV-infected cats, high-dose subcutaneous treatment with human interferon-α (1×10^5 units/kg SQ q24h for 6 weeks) did not lead to a statistically significant improvement of clinical, laboratory, immunologic, or virologic parameters. In an experimental placebo-controlled study, low-dose oral interferon-α (0.5 units/cat or 5 units/cat PO) did not lead to a difference in the development of viremia when treatment started directly after challenge, although treated cats had significantly fewer clinical signs and longer survival times when compared to the placebo group (with a

better response using 0.5 units/cat). In a recent placebo-controlled study including ill client-owned FeLV-infected cats that were treated with low-dose oral interferon-α (30 units/cat q24h for 7 consecutive days on a 1-week-on/1-week-off schedule), there were no statistically significant differences in FeLV status, survival time, clinical or hematologic parameters or subjective improvement in the owners' impression of clinical signs.

Feline interferon-ω recently was licensed for use in veterinary medicine in some European countries and Japan. Interferons are species-specific; therefore feline interferon-ω can be used for prolonged periods without antibody development. No side effects have been reported in cats. Feline interferon-ω is active against FIV in vitro, but to date only one study has been performed in field cats, and the study did not show significant changes in survival rate when compared to a placebo group. Feline interferon-ω also inhibits FeLV replication in vitro. In a placebo-controlled field study, 48 cats with FeLV infection were treated with interferon-ω (10^6 units/kg SQ q24h on 5 consecutive days repeated three times with several weeks between treatments). A statistically significant difference was found in the survival time of treated versus untreated cats (De Mari et al., 2004). However, no virologic parameters were measured during the study to support the hypothesis that the interferon actually had an anti-FeLV effect rather than an inhibition of secondary infections, and further studies are needed. A summary of reported experimental treatments is found in Table 286-1.

References and Suggested Reading

Arai M et al: The use of human hematopoietic growth factors (rhGM-CSF and rhEPO) as a supportive therapy for FIV-infected cats, *Vet Immunol Immunopathol* 77:71, 2000.

De Mari K et al: Therapeutic effects of recombinant feline interferon-omega on feline leukemia virus (FeLV)–infected and FeLV/feline immunodeficiency virus (FIV)–coinfected symptomatic cats, *J Vet Intern Med* 18:477, 2004.

Hartmann K: Feline leukemia virus infection. In Greene CE, editor: *Infectious diseases of the dog and cat*, St Louis, 2006a, Elsevier Saunders, p 105.

Hartmann K: Antiviral and immunomodulatory chemotherapy. In Greene CE, editor: *Infectious diseases of the dog and cat*, St, Louis, 2006b, Elsevier Saunders, p 10.

Hartmann K et al: Treatment of feline leukemia virus-infected cats with paramunity inducer, *Vet Immunol Immunopathol* 65:267, 1998.

Hartmann K, Donath A, Kraft W: AZT in the treatment of feline immunodeficiency virus infection, *Feline Pract* 5:16; 6:13, 1995.

Levy JK: CVT update: feline immunodeficiency virus. In Bonagura JD, editor: *Kirk's current veterinary therapy XIII small animal practice*, Philadelphia, 2000, Saunders, p 284.

Levy J et al: 2001 Report of the American Association of Feline Practitioners and Academy of Feline Medicine Advisory Panel on feline retrovirus testing and management, *J Feline Med Surg* 5:3, 2003.

McCaw DL et al: Immunomodulation therapy for feline leukemia virus infection, *J Am Anim Hosp Assoc* 37:356, 2001.

Sellon RK, Hartmann K: Feline immunodeficiency virus infection. In Greene CE, editor: *Infectious diseases of the dog and cat*, St Louis, 2006, Elsevier Saunders, p 131.

Sheets MA et al: Studies of the effect of acemannan on retrovirus infections: clinical stabilization of feline virus–infected cats, *Mol Biother* 3:41, 1991.

CHAPTER 282

Feline Calicivirus Infection

JANE E. SYKES, *Davis, California*

Feline calicivirus (FCV) is a common cause of feline upper respiratory tract disease (URTD), accounting for anywhere between 20% and 53% of cases. Infection may be manifested by fever, conjunctivitis, rhinitis, oral ulcerations, and/or chronic stomatitis, although occasionally skin ulcerations, lameness, and pneumonia may occur. The severity and signs of illness depend on the strain of FCV involved, the infecting dose, and the degree of host immunity.

FCV is a nonenveloped, single-stranded ribonucleic acid (RNA) virus with a spheric capsid studded with cup-shaped depressions. Like other RNA viruses, the genome of FCV continually undergoes rapid mutation with minimal rates of repair, increasing the diversity of strains over time.

Cats that recover from URTD may develop a persistent oropharyngeal infection with continuous shedding of virus from this site, although the magnitude of shedding varies over time and among individual cats. In many cats shedding terminates weeks to months after infection, but in a few cats shedding is lifelong. Some cats appear never to shed virus. Because of the carrier state, the prevalence of FCV infection in the general cat population is high, ranging from 8% to 47%, depending on the density of the cat population sampled. A single cat may be infected with multiple variants of FCV at the same time, each derived from the original infecting strain as a result of genetic mutation, drift, and selection pressures (Radford et al., 1998).

URTD caused by FCV is a problem especially in cats residing in multiple-cat households and breeding and boarding catteries. Although the introduction of vaccines targeting FCV in the mid 1970s may have reduced the severity of clinical signs, the vaccines do not prevent infection or persistent shedding of FCV, and outbreaks of URTD still occur, even in well-vaccinated cat populations. Vaccine virus itself may be shed from the oropharynx, and virus closely related to the F9 vaccine strain has been detected in cat colonies that are chronically shedding FCV. There has been some concern that vaccine pressure may have led to selection of FCV strains that have poor cross-reactivity with the vaccine strain F9, and incorporation of additional strains into vaccines has been proposed (Dawson et al., 1993).

Over the last 5 years several highly virulent strains of FCV have been isolated from outbreaks of a systemic, febrile illness in North American cats. This condition was described initially in northern California (Pedersen et al., 2000) and subsequently in several other American states (Rong et al., 2006). Most recently it has been described in the United Kingdom (Coyne et al., 2006). The disease has been termed *FCV-associated virulent systemic disease (VSD)*, and in some outbreaks has been associated with mortalities of up to 67%. Furthermore, vaccination with currently available FCV vaccines apparently has not been protective. The purpose of this chapter is to discuss the clinical signs, epidemiology, diagnosis, control, and treatment of FCV infections, with particular emphasis on the recently reported outbreaks of VSD.

EPIDEMIOLOGY

Infection with FCV may be acquired by direct contact with an acutely infected cat, organisms persisting within the environment, or a carrier cat. FCV is shed primarily in oral, nasal, and ocular secretions and can also be found in blood, urine, and feces of infected cats. Transmission over distances of about 4 feet may occur via droplets generated by sneezing cats.

FCV-associated VSD was first described in northern California in 1998 (Pedersen et al., 2000). Death occurred in 33% to 50% of infected cats, and this strain was highly contagious, spreading via contaminated fomites despite implementation of aggressive disinfection measures. A novel FCV strain, FCV-Ari, was isolated from affected cats. Laboratory cats experimentally infected with FCV-Ari developed a disease syndrome identical to that seen in naturally infected cats. Since FCV-Ari was described, at least five additional outbreaks have been recognized in Pennsylvania, Massachusetts, Tennessee, Nevada, and southern California; and in 2003 an outbreak of systemic caliciviral disease occurred in Staffordshire, England (Coyne et al., 2006). FCV-Kaos, a genetically distinct strain from FCV-Ari, was isolated from cats in the southern California outbreak (Hurley et al., 2004), and the strains isolated in the Massachusetts (FCV-Diva) and United Kingdom (UKOS) outbreaks also have been genetically distinct. This may suggest that the mutation(s) associated with VSD are different in each case or that these mutations occurred in a part of the FCV genome that was not sequenced.

In the majority of outbreaks a hospitalized shelter cat appeared to be the source of infection. Three outbreaks involved a single veterinary hospital, one spread to a veterinary research facility in the course of the outbreak investigation, and the largest reported outbreak affected 54 cats in three veterinary practices and a rescue group in the west Los Angeles area from June to August, 2002 (Hurley et al., 2004). The spread of this southern California outbreak was attributed to the travel of clients and staff between multiple practices located within a 1-mile radius. With the exception of the United Kingdom outbreak, which involved two neighboring households, spread of disease was limited to the affected clinic(s) or shelter, with no spread within the community reported. Otherwise healthy, adult, vaccinated cats were affected predominantly, whereas kittens tended to show less severe signs. In all cases the outbreaks resolved within approximately 2 months. Two outbreaks occurred in the spring, three in the summer, and two in the fall. No outbreak has yet been reported in winter, a time when the kitten population is lowest, reflecting the possible role of kittens in the generation and transmission of virulent FCV strains.

Transmission of the virulent FCV strains occurs readily through fomite transmission via veterinary hospital staff and pet owners, by movement of clinically and subclinically infected cats between clinics and private homes, and by indirect contact of outpatients with subclinically infected inpatients.

An epidemiologic analysis of the outbreak that occurred in southern California showed that adult cats (>1 year old) were at significantly higher risk than kittens (<6 months old) for severe disease or death (odds ratio 9.56, $p < 0.001$) (Hurley et al., 2004). No sex or breed predilection was noted. The attack rate for cats hospitalized for ≥12 hours concurrently with an infected cat or from the same household as a case cat was 94%. In one study four kittens orally immunized with the current vaccine strain (F9) experienced less severe clinical signs when experimentally infected with FCV-Ari, but vaccination did not appear to prevent severe disease or death in the FCV-Kaos outbreak (Pedersen et al., 2000). The surviving cats in the United Kingdom outbreak had been vaccinated more recently than the nonsurvivors (Coyne et al., 2006).

As with other FCV infections, cats infected with highly virulent strains may shed virus for months after infection (Hurley et al., 2004). Despite these observations, there has been no report of transmission of the VSD from recovered cats. Loss of the virulence-enhancing mutation(s) may have occurred during passage in these cats; alternatively, implementation of effective control measures may have played a role in outbreak resolution.

CLINICAL SIGNS

Acute URTD caused by FCV occurs after an incubation period of 2 to 10 days. Typical signs of URTD include serous or mucopurulent nasal and ocular discharge, sneezing, conjunctival hyperemia, blepharospasm, and chemosis. Depression, anorexia, hypersalivation, and pyrexia also may be seen; and occasionally pneumonia may develop with coughing and dyspnea. Lameness, which may reflect polyarthritis, can be seen in infected cats. Ulcerative glossitis develops in some affected cats, and a small proportion of FCV carriers develop chronic lymphoplasmacytic or ulceroproliferative stomatitis, which may be refractory to treatment.

Cats exposed to FCV strains causing VSD have developed signs 1 to 5 days after exposure to affected cats. The incubation period has been longer (up to 12 days) for some cats exposed in the home environment (Hurley et al., 2004). Affected cats frequently show signs typical of caliciviral URTD, including anorexia, oral ulceration, and nasal and/or ocular discharge; these signs are often severe.

Pyrexia is present in most cases and may be profound, often exceeding 105° F. Distinctive clinical signs of VSD include peripheral edema with or without alopecia, crusting, and ulceration. Edema is most commonly noted on the head and limbs; and crusting and ulceration, if present, are most prominent on the nose, lips, pinnae, periocular skin, and distal limbs. Some cats may be reluctant to walk. Severe respiratory distress, sometimes caused by pulmonary edema or pleural effusion, develops in some cats. Dysphonia was reported in several cats in the United Kingdom outbreak. Icterus has been noted in many cats, and the presence of jaundice and dyspnea has been associated with a poor prognosis. Involvement of the gastrointestinal tract, including the liver and pancreas, may be associated with signs of vomiting and/or diarrhea. Rarely epistaxis and hematochezia have been noted. Peracutely affected cats may die suddenly with few preceding signs except fever. Overall mortality in the VSD cases has been approximately 50%.

DIAGNOSIS

The clinical signs resulting from uncomplicated FCV infection can result from infection with other agents, especially feline herpesvirus 1 but also bacterial pathogens such as *Chlamydophila felis* and *Bordetella bronchiseptica*. Thus clinical signs alone are not useful for establishment of a definitive diagnosis, although the presence of severe oral ulcerations and/or lameness may be suggestive of FCV infection. Mixed-pathogen infections are common in cattery situations, further complicating diagnosis. Cats presenting with signs of epistaxis, unilateral nasal discharge, facial deformity, fundic abnormalities, or marked submandibular lymphadenopathy should receive a thorough workup to rule out other causes of URTD such as neoplasia, nasopharyngeal polyps, coagulopathy, foreign bodies, dental disease, and cryptococcosis. Although clinical signs of VSD are more characteristic, conditions such as cryptococcosis, feline infectious peritonitis, and immune-mediated vasculitides represent possible differential diagnoses.

Clinicopathologic abnormalities resulting from infection with less virulent FCV strains are generally nonspecific. Hyperglobulinemia may be noted in cats with chronic stomatitis. In contrast, infection with highly virulent strains may result in clinicopathologic abnormalities, reflecting damage to multiple organ systems (Hurley et al., 2004). Frequently reported serum chemistry profile abnormalities include mild-to-moderate hyperbilirubinemia, hypoalbuminemia, hyperglycemia, elevated creatine phosphokinase and aspartate aminotransferase activity, and mildly elevated alanine aminotransferase activity. Abnormalities on the complete blood count have included lymphopenia, mild-to-moderate neutrophilia, and mild anemia.

Necropsy findings in VSD cases are variable. In addition to icterus, cutaneous edema, and ulceration, which are apparent grossly, the most common pathology finding has been individual or centrilobular hepatocellular necrosis (Coyne et al., 2006; Pesavento et al., 2004). Other reported abnormalities have included acute bronchointerstitial pneumonia, pancreatic necrosis and saponification of peripancreatic fat, splenic and lymphoid necrosis, and free pleural and abdominal fluid. Intestinal crypt lesions were reported in four experimentally infected and one naturally infected cat (Hurley et al., 2004; Pedersen et al., 2000). Gastrointestinal ulceration has been reported occasionally. Viral antigen has been detected in both endothelial and epithelial cells in affected tissues, with epithelial cell cytolysis and associated systemic vascular compromise (Pesavento et al., 2004). Ideally a full necropsy should be performed whenever VSD is suspected. At minimum, tissues to examine include skin (particularly footpads, nasal planum, and any areas of ulceration), tongue, lung, liver, spleen, gastrointestinal tract, pancreas, and lymph nodes.

Attempts to make a specific diagnosis in cases of URTD are especially encouraged in cattery situations because knowledge of the causative organism can assist with management strategies. Diagnostic evaluation is also recommended for individual cats that do not respond to conventional symptomatic treatment or those that experience recurrent episodes of URTD. Because of the communicability and high mortality associated with highly virulent FCV infection, microbiologic testing is essential for cats suspected to have VSD, and suspect cats should be treated and handled immediately as if they were infected with hypervirulent FCV.

The most reliable microbiologic assay for FCV is virus isolation from nasal, conjunctival, and/or oropharyngeal swabs after inoculation of cell monolayers grown in the laboratory. Oropharyngeal swabs are most likely to yield a diagnosis; although, if possible, collection of nasal and conjunctival swabs, in addition to oropharyngeal swabs, increases the chance of obtaining a positive result. Swabs should be transported on ice in a viral transport medium containing antibiotics to prevent bacterial overgrowth; commercial swabs are available for this purpose.

Virus isolation from oropharyngeal swabs collected from acute cases of VSD or tissue samples obtained at necropsy has had high sensitivity (>90%). Positive culture results were also obtained on serum samples from acutely ill cats, although the sensitivity was lower than with culture from oropharyngeal swabs. Sensitivity of viral culture on oropharyngeal swabs decreases rapidly in recovering cats, and a single negative swab taken more than a week after onset of clinical signs does not rule out infection with FCV. At least two to three negative cultures should be obtained at weekly intervals before concluding that virus shedding is likely to have terminated.

In general, serology is not recommended for routine diagnosis of FCV infections. Because of widespread exposure to FCV, acute and convalescent phase samples are required to demonstrate recent infection. Titers induced by vaccination can confound diagnosis; and, because of the large numbers of FCV strains, titers may vary, depending on the degree of homology between the infecting virus and the FCV strain used in the assay. Nevertheless, in the case of FCV strains causing VSD, serology using virus neutralization has been sensitive and specific and was useful for investigation and control of the southern California outbreak (Hurley et al., 2004). There was no cross-neutralization between the vaccine (F9) strain and FCV-Kaos or FCV-Ari; thus identification of unexposed cats even in the face of recent vaccination may be possible. Whether this will be true for other hypervirulent strains (and thus for other outbreaks) awaits further investigation.

Amplification of FCV nucleic acid using the reverse-transcriptase polymerase chain reaction (RT-PCR) represents another diagnostic assay that may be considered for diagnosis. Compared with those for deoxyribonucleic acid viruses such as feline herpesvirus 1, PCR-based assays for FCV are less reliable because of the difficulty in designing assays that amplify nucleic acid from a variety of different strains and the susceptibility of viral RNA to rapid degradation by RNase enzymes in the environment. False-positive results associated with contamination can occur during sample collection or in the laboratory. Current PCR-based assays for FCV are generally only available in research laboratories, and quality control may vary from laboratory to laboratory and even between individual staff members working in the same laboratory. Therefore the results of PCR-based testing should be interpreted with caution. In the southern California outbreak of VSD, all isolates recovered in culture were successfully amplified using RT-PCR (Hurley et al., 2004).

Regardless of the method used to detect FCV infection, the results of diagnostic testing should always be interpreted in the light of clinical signs because asymptomatic cats may shed FCV. The same applies for FCV strains associated with VSD; because there have been no consistent molecular differences identified between highly virulent strains and other strains of FCV, it is not possible to identify an isolate as a VSD strain using molecular typing methods. Positive identification of an outbreak requires that a molecularly distinct strain of FCV be isolated and sequenced from at least two affected cats in association with the appearance of consistent clinical signs. Once an outbreak has been identified in this manner, nucleic acid sequencing may be useful for determining whether additional FCV isolates obtained in the outbreak have the potential to cause VSD (because of their relation to the original isolates) or whether they represent unrelated field FCV or vaccine strains. Because subclinically infected cats are capable of transmitting VSD, all exposed cats, whether symptomatic or not, should be checked by viral culture or RT-PCR before being introduced to naïve cats.

TREATMENT

Treatment of disease resulting from FCV infection is symptomatic. Broad-spectrum antimicrobials (e.g., amoxicillin, 22 mg/kg orally [PO] q12h; or doxycycline, 10 mg/kg PO q24h) may be required to counteract secondary bacterial infection. Fluid and nutritional support is essential in severe cases, and airway humidification should also be considered. Placement of esophagostomy or gastrostomy tubes allows enteral nutrition of cats with inappetence. Oxygen may be required for cats with pneumonia.

In addition to the treatments described in the previous paragraph, cats with VSD should be placed in isolation and treated aggressively with colloid-containing fluids such as Hetastarch (Hespan, Baxter; Deerfield, IL). A variety of different treatments have been tried, including a wide range of broad-spectrum antibiotics and oral interferon-α. Glucocorticoids at immunosuppressive doses

(1 mg/kg PO q12h) have also been used. In the outbreak in southern California five severely affected cats were treated with dexamethasone (in addition to other supportive treatments) and survived; one cat that was treated with prednisone died, but the remaining cats that died did not receive glucocorticoids (Hurley and Sykes, 2003). One cat in the northern California outbreak lived following glucocorticoid treatment; the remainder were not treated with steroids.

RECOMMENDATIONS FOR CONTROL

Although outbreaks can be devastating within an affected clinic or shelter, VSD remains extremely uncommon. Quick recognition and implementation of effective control measures, including proper disinfection, quarantine, and testing procedures, will further reduce the impact of this disease.

Recognizing that VSD may be spread even by mildly symptomatic cats (especially kittens), veterinarians should exercise careful infectious disease control whenever dealing with a cat with URTD. FCV is reliably inactivated by sodium hypochlorite (in the absence of organic matter and with adequate contact time) but not by other compounds commonly used for disinfection in veterinary hospitals such as chlorhexidine or quaternary ammonium compounds. Therefore routine decontamination after exposure to a cat with upper respiratory infection should be to clean with a detergent solution and then disinfect with 5% sodium hypochlorite diluted with water to 1:32 (½ cup of 5% bleach per gallon of water). In the absence of effective disinfection, FCVs reportedly can persist in a dried state at room temperature (20° C) for up to 28 days (Doultree et al., 1999). Therefore effective cleaning and quarantine are crucial. Specific control measures recommended when VSD is diagnosed or strongly suspected include strict isolation of suspect cases, isolation of exposed cats for at least 2 weeks after exposure, ensuring that exposed or infected cats are not shedding virus before release into environments containing naïve cats, and thorough disinfection with 5% bleach solution or heat sterilization. Carpeted areas/homes should be steam cleaned and closed to cats for a minimum of 4 weeks. Clinics in which disease continues to spread despite instituting these precautions should consider closing to cat admissions for 1 to 2 weeks. If recently vaccinated cats are less severely affected in any outbreak, vaccination of naïve cats with a modified-live vaccine at least 1 to 2 weeks before potential exposure may be helpful, although it should be recognized that vaccination with a modified-live vaccine may result in positive test results using virus isolation.

References and Suggested Reading

Coyne KP et al: Lethal outbreak of disease associated with feline calicivirus infection in cats, *Vet Rec* 158(16):544, 2006.

Dawson S et al: Typing of feline calicivirus isolates from different clinical groups by virus neutralisation tests, *Vet Rec* 133(1):13, 1993.

Doultree JC et al: Inactivation of feline calicivirus, a Norwalk virus surrogate, *J Hosp Infect* 41(1):51, 1999.

Hurley K, Sykes JE: Update on feline calicivirus: new trends, *Vet Clin North Am Small Anim Pract* 33(4):759, 2003.

Hurley K et al: An outbreak of virulent systemic feline calicivirus disease, *J Am Vet Med Assoc* 224(2):241, 2004.

Pedersen NC et al: An isolated epizootic of hemorrhagic-like fever in cats caused by a novel and highly virulent strain of feline calicivirus, *Vet Microbiol* 73(4):281, 2000.

Pesavento PA et al: Pathologic, immunohistochemical, and electron microscopic findings in naturally occurring virulent systemic feline calicivirus infection in cats, *Vet Pathol* 41(3):257, 2004.

Radford AD et al: Quasispecies evolution of a hypervariable region of the feline calicivirus capsid gene in cell culture and in persistently infected cats, *J Gen Virol* 79(pt 1):1, 1998.

Rong S et al: Characterization of a highly virulent feline calicivirus and attenuation of this virus, *Virus Res* 122(1-2):95, 2006.

CHAPTER 283

Babesiosis

ADAM J. BIRKENHEUER, *Raleigh, North Carolina*

One of the earliest descriptions of intraerythrocytic parasites in dogs with signs consistent with babesiosis was made in 1896, and the first documented case of canine babesiosis in the United States was reported in 1934. Initially there were only two species of *Babesia* believed to infect dogs; however, at the time of this writing, there are at least nine genetically unique piroplasma that have been identified in the blood of dogs (Table 283-1).

EPIZOOTIOLOGY

Piroplasma are intraerythrocytic protozoan parasites of the phylum Apicomplexa that are frequently transmitted by ticks. Piroplasma include organisms in the families Babesiidae and Theileridae. *Babesia* spp. are distinguished from *Theileria* spp. by the absence of any preerythrocytic stage in the mammalian host. In contrast, *Theileria* spp. first infect leukocytes (typically lymphocytes) before the organisms infect erythrocytes. Babesiosis was the first documented tick-transmitted infection, demonstrated by Smith and Kilbourne in 1888. They demonstrated that "Texas fever" was transmitted by ticks in cattle and that the causative agent was believed to be either *Babesia bigemina* or *Babesia bovis*. Over 100 species of *Babesia* have since been described, and with the advent of molecular techniques such as the polymerase chain reaction (PCR) many new species and genotypes are identified each year. Although many vertebrate species can be infected with two or more of the known *Babesia* spp., this chapter focuses on canine piroplasmosis.

TRANSMISSION AND RISK FACTORS

The primary route of transmission for piroplasma is believed to be via a tick vector. The known or suspected tick vectors for each piroplasma are listed in Table 283-1. The recent emergence of some piroplasma such as *Babesia gibsoni* is likely to be associated with nontick-associated routes of transmission. In North America the majority of *B. gibsoni* transmission appears to be among American pit bull terriers and is associated with transplacental infection and direct inoculation via dog bites. Cases of *B. gibsoni* in dogs that were not of this breed were frequently bitten by an American Pit Bull terrier or received a transfusion with blood donated by a dog of that breed. However, more *B. gibsoni* cases are being identified in other canine breeds within the United States, without these exposure to these known risk factors. Breed associations and risk factors for infection are listed in Table 283-1.

CLINICAL DISEASE

The disease manifestations of canine piroplasma infection are highly variable. Multiple factors are responsible for the differences in pathogenicity, including the genotype/species of piroplasm, individual host immune responses, and age and possibly breed of the host. Classic canine piroplasmosis is characterized by anemia, thrombocytopenia, hyperglobulinemia, fever that may wax and wane, and splenomegaly. These findings are fairly consistent in most cases regardless of geographic region, genotype of piroplasm, or host. Hemoglobinemia is a relatively rare finding in dogs in North America and is most commonly documented in dogs in South Africa. In at least one study 85% of dogs with piroplasmosis had Coombs'-positive test results. Thus piroplasmosis should be considered as a differential diagnosis for all dogs presenting with immune-mediated hemolytic anemia (IMHA) and or thrombocytopenia. In highly endemic areas, for dogs with a history of known risk factors for piroplasmosis or for dogs of a breed known to be at high risk for piroplasmosis, empiric antiprotozoal therapy (see following paragraphs) should be started immediately after samples are obtained for specific testing.

There are no pathognomonic biochemical or urinalysis findings in dogs with piroplasmosis. The most consistent biochemical findings include hyperglobulinemia and less commonly hyperbilirubinemia with mildly increased liver enzymes. Some dogs present for pigmenturia consisting most commonly of bilirubin and occasionally hemoglobin.

There are recognized differences in the virulence of the different species/genotypes of piroplasms that infect dogs (see Table 283-1). *Babesia canis rossi*, which has only been documented in southern Africa, is considered highly virulent and has been associated with severe disease manifestations such as disseminated intravascular coagulation, central nervous system signs and hypoglycemia, and in some cases death. *Babesia canis vogeli* has a nearly worldwide distribution and is typically considered the least virulent. *Babesia canis canis* is considered to have virulence intermediate to *B. canis rossi* and *B. canis vogeli* and is recognized primarily in Europe, with the majority of cases having been reported in France. *B. gibsoni* is a small piroplasm (1 to 3 μm) that is rapidly emerging and seems to now have a nearly worldwide distribution. *B. gibsoni* is considered a moderately virulent piroplasma. A *Babesia microti*–like parasite, formerly referred to as *Theileria annae*, has been recently recognized in Spain. In addition to the classic signs associated with piroplasmosis, this organism has been associated with renal failure and proteinuria,

Table 283-1

Overview of Canine Piroplasmosis

Genotype/Species	Distribution	Vector	Risk Factors	Virulence	Treatment	Parasite Clearance With Treatment
Babesia canis vogeli	Worldwide	*Rhipicephalus sanguineus*	Greyhounds, ticks, blood transfusion	+	Imidocarb dipropionate (6.6 mg/kg IM q2 weeks)	Y
Babesia canis rossi	South Africa	*Haemaphysalis leachi*	Ticks	+++	Imidocarb dipropionate (6.6 mg/kg IM q2 weeks)	Y
Babesia canis canis	Europe	*Dermacentor reticulates*	Ticks	++	Imidocarb dipropionate (6.6 mg/kg IM q2 weeks)	Y
Babesia gibsoni	Worldwide	*Haemaphysalis* spp., others?	American pit bull terriers, dog bites, ticks, blood transfusion	++	Atovaquone (13.3 mg/kg PO TID w/ a fatty meal) and Azithromycin (10 mg/kg PO q24h) simultaneously for 10 days	Likely in 85% of cases
Babesia microti-like (*Theileria annae*)	Spain	*Ixodes hexagonus?*	Ticks	+++	?	?
Babesia conradae	California	?	?	+++	? Atovaquone (13.3 mg/kg PO TID w/ a fatty meal) and azithromycin (10 mg/kg PO q24h) simultaneously for 10 days?	?
Babesia spp. (UK)	United Kingdom only?	?	?	++?	?	?
Babesia spp. (Coco)	United States only?	?	Neoplasia, splenectomy	+?	Imidocarb dipropionate (6.6 mg/kg IM q2 weeks)	Likely
Theileria equi	Europe only?	?	?	?	?	?

IM, Intramuscularly; *PO*, orally; *TID*, three times a day; *Y*, yes; *?*, unknown or not studied; +, mild; ++, moderate; +++, severe.

presumably caused by glomerular disease. *Babesia conradae*, originally believed to be *B. gibsoni*, is a highly virulent parasite and is associated with high mortality rates. It is important to note that all species have caused severe disease manifestations in individual patients; thus the guidelines for virulence may not be strictly clinically relevant. However, it is important that the clinician accurately identify the species/genotype infecting the individual patient because the prognosis and treatment for each species can vary.

"Atypical" presentations of canine piroplasma infection appear to be becoming more common. The most common atypical presentations include thrombocytopenia and hyperglobulinemia without anemia, thrombocytopenia alone, hyperglobulinemia alone, and the complete absence of hematologic or biochemical abnormalities. The reasons behind these atypical presentations are not clearly understood, but possible causes include parasite adaptations to canine hosts resulting in decreased virulence, increased clinician vigilance and willingness to test, spontaneous recovery, and alternative routes of transmission that may be associated with decreased virulence (direct inoculation or transplacental transmission).

DIAGNOSIS

The diagnosis of piroplasmosis in the clinical setting can be quite challenging. Several factors can increase the clinician's index of suspicion such as breed (greyhounds have increased prevalence of *B. canis vogeli*, and American Pit Bull terriers have increased prevalence of *B. gibsoni* infections), history of a dog bite, blood transfusion, or tick attachment. Three basic methods are available to diagnose piroplasmosis: light microscopy, serology, and nucleic acid–based detection methods. Unfortunately the clinical sensitivity and specificity of most of the available tests are unknown; but clinical experience, case series and reports, and limited studies performed on experimentally infected dogs have demonstrated that all modalities can have either false-positive or false-negative results.

When performed by an experienced reader, light microscopy is highly specific for the presence of piroplasmosis, but, because of the relatively low limit of detection (0.001% parasitemias), the sensitivity is poor; thus it is not recommended as a sole screening test. In addition, several species/genotypes are virtually indistinguishable by light microscopy, making accurate identification to the species/genotype level nearly impossible. Serologic detection of antipiroplasma antibodies, which is almost always performed in commercial laboratories by the use of indirect fluorescent antibody (IFA) assays, is considered to be fairly sensitive as a screening test. Since serology only provides indirect evidence of infection and is well documented to have false-negative results in some clinical cases, it is the responsibility of the clinician to interpret the results in light of the clinical presentation and the response to treatment. Despite the fact that IFA assays are available for several different genotypes, the ability of these assays to accurately differentiate the species/genotype actually causing a given infection is relatively poor (i.e., the highest titer does not always correlate to which species is present). It is for these reasons that nucleic acid based testing is quickly becoming an important component to the diagnosis of canine babesiosis.

PCR assays are the primary molecular method used by commercial diagnostic laboratories. PCR is generally accepted to have increased sensitivity compared to light microscopy, and in some cases the limit of detection is 1300 times lower. The overall sensitivity of one assay for the diagnosis of chronic *B. gibsoni* infections was 90% over three different testing periods. The assay detected infection in 100% of studied dogs when two consecutive tests were performed. Although this improved sensitivity is important, it is the exquisite specificity of PCR (>99.9% when the proper controls are used) that give it outstanding clinical usefulness. A positive result from a reputable laboratory is consistent with infection and should identify the specific species/genotype so appropriate therapeutic decisions can be made. The major clinical concern for PCR assays is the lack of assay standardization among laboratories and the marked variability in sensitivity and specificity (differences of limits of detection ≥1000 fold) with different assay design, reaction protocols, controls, and reagents. Therefore it is critical that clinicians contact individual laboratories and get specific information about each assay and the controls used for proper interpretation of test results. Ultimately in some cases a multifaceted approach that includes microscopy, serology, and PCR may be necessary to maximize the chances of diagnosing piroplasma infections.

TREATMENT AND PREVENTION

Significant improvements in the availability and types of treatments for canine babesiosis have been made. In highly endemic areas or in breeds with increased risk of infection, therapy should be started as soon as possible and is often administered empirically based on clinical suspicion. Specific therapies for canine piroplasmosis are presented in Table 283-1. Based on our clinical experience, treatment with atovaquone (Mepron, GlaxoSmithKline) and azithromycin is effective and capable of clearing *B. canis vogeli* infections but is

considerably more expensive than imidocarb dipropionate (Imizol, Schering-Plough). A combination formulation of atovaquone with proguanil hydrochloride (Malarone, GlaxoSmithKline) is less expensive, but it is poorly tolerated by dogs, with substantial vomiting as an adverse effect. Imidocarb and the less widely available diminazene aceturate are both capable of inducing remission of clinical signs in dogs with *B. gibsoni* infection, but neither treatment is successful at clearing the infection. Their use in *B. gibsoni* infections is warranted when atovaquone and azithromycin are unavailable or the cost of treatment is prohibitive.

The clinical signs associated with piroplasmosis typically begin to improve within 1 week of beginning specific therapy. If patients are not responding to specific therapy, secondary treatments should be administered, or alternative diagnoses should be considered. Since the anemia and thrombocytopenia associated with piroplasmosis are often immune mediated, immunosuppressive therapy is frequently considered as an adjunctive therapy. If piroplasmosis is highly suspected or definitively identified, I recommend only supportive care and antiprotozoal therapy. It is my experience that prolonged immunosuppressive therapy (i.e., weeks to months) or splenectomy before treatment with specific antiprotozoal drugs substantially reduces the ability to clear the parasitemias and subsequently is associated with a worse prognosis because of relapsing disease. In addition, many dogs with secondary IMHA and immune mediated thrombocytopenia purpura have responded to antiprotozoal drugs alone and have not required additional treatments. Clinical signs should resolve in most cases within 5 to 7 days of beginning antiprotozoal treatment. If immunosuppressive treatment must be instituted, prednisone alone (2 mg/kg/day) is usually sufficient and can be tapered more quickly (every 2 weeks versus every 3 to 4 weeks) compared to protocols for the treatment of idiopathic IMHA. Follow-up testing should consist of at least two consecutive negative PCR tests approximately 30 days apart.

The best approach to the prevention of piroplasmosis has not been established, but several logical strategies have been proposed. In France a vaccine composed of an adjuvant and soluble antigens collected from supernatants of *B. canis* cultures is available. This vaccine induces partial protection (i.e., less severe clinical disease) but does not prevent infection and has only been demonstrated to be efficacious against *B. canis*. The avoidance of risk factors (see Table 283-1) is likely to result in reduced infection rates. The use of topical acaricides is likely to result in reduced infection rates, assuming that the agents either repel ticks or actually block the transmission. To date there are no data evaluating the efficacy of topical acaricides for the prevention of piroplasmosis, but their use in highly endemic areas is probably warranted based at least on the theoretic advantages. Finally, blood donors should be screened aggressively for the presence of piroplasma infections before their entry into a donor program and periodically if they have potentially been infected between screening and donation (e.g., ticks, volunteer donors that are indoor/outdoor).

Suggested Reading

Birkenheuer AJ et al: Geographic distribution of babesiosis among dogs in the United States and association with dog bites: 150 cases (2000-2003), *J Am Vet Med Assoc* 227:942, 2005.

Birkenheuer AJ, Levy MG, Breitschwerdt EB: Efficacy of combined atovaquone and azithromycin for therapy of chronic Babesia gibsoni (Asian genotype) infections in dogs, *J Vet Intern Med*18:494, 2004.

Boozer AL, Macintire DK: Canine babesiosis, *Vet Clin North Am Small Anim Pract* 33:885, 2003.

Bourdoiseau G: Canine babesiosis in France, *Vet Parasitol* 138:118, 2006.

Jacobson LS: The South African form of severe and complicated canine babesiosis: clinical advances 1994-2004, *Vet Parasitol* 138:126, 2006.

CHAPTER **284**

Canine Influenza

GABRIELE A. LANDOLT, *Fort Collins, Colorado*
KATHARINE F. LUNN, *Fort Collins, Colorado*

Influenza is a well-known and highly contagious disease that has burdened humans, poultry, horses, and pigs since ancient times. Before 2004 dogs were not commonly regarded as hosts for influenza A viruses. Since then canine influenza has been recognized as a recently emerged respiratory pathogen in dogs in the United States. First isolated from racing greyhounds in Florida, the virus has since spilled over into the nongreyhound dog population and has caused outbreaks of respiratory disease throughout the United States.

ETIOLOGY

Canine influenza is primarily a respiratory disease caused by an influenza A virus. Influenza A viruses are members of the family Orthomyxoviridae and are enveloped viruses with segmented, single-stranded, negative-sense ribonucleic acid genomes. Based on antigenic properties of the two major envelope glycoproteins, hemagglutinin (HA) and neuraminidase (NA), influenza A viruses are further classified into 16 HA (H1-H16) and 9 NA (N1-N9) subtypes. The viruses exhibit only partial restriction of their host range, and occasionally influenza viruses or their genes are transferred between species. Undoubtedly the most prominent examples of direct transmission of influenza viruses among species are the recent infections of humans and cats with the highly pathogenic avian H5N1 viruses ("bird flu"). Yet, although cross-species transmission of influenza viruses may occur relatively frequently, these transmission events tend to be self-limiting; and the

newly introduced viruses are only rarely maintained in the new host species. One of the few notable exceptions to this scenario is the recent transmission of an equine-lineage H3N8 virus to dogs in the United States, with apparent maintenance of the virus within the dog population. In the spring of 2004, 22 racing greyhounds housed at a training facility in Florida suffered from a severe respiratory illness that was characterized by cough and high fever. Eight of the affected dogs died from hemorrhagic pneumonia, and influenza A virus was recovered from the lung tissue of one animal. Sequence analysis of the viral genome revealed that the canine isolate was closely related to, and had evolved from, a contemporary equine H3N8 influenza virus. Over the course of that same year, outbreaks of influenza occurred at 14 greyhound racetracks in six states, and by 2005 the virus had spilled over into the nongreyhound dog population.

Recent reports from researchers in the United Kingdom provide data supporting two additional independent incidents in which equine influenza viruses have been transmitted to dogs. When alerted to the canine influenza outbreak in the United States, researchers in the United Kingdom reanalyzed outbreaks of respiratory illness in foxhounds that had occurred in 2002 and 2003 and found evidence indicating that two distinct strains of equine influenza were the causative agents. Yet, in contrast to the apparent maintenance of the virus in the canine population in the United States, both equine-to-canine transmission events in the United Kingdom appear to have been self-limiting.

EPIDEMIOLOGY AND DISEASE TRANSMISSION

Canine influenza virus infection has as of now been documented in the United States in at least 26 states and the District of Columbia. Because this disease has recently emerged in the dog population, there is little natural immunity to influenza virus infection; and all dogs are potentially susceptible, regardless of age, breed, sex, or vaccination status. Disease is most likely to occur in dogs that are housed in groups (e.g., in shelters, boarding or breeding kennels, canine day-care centers, or veterinary clinics). When canine influenza virus is introduced to a group of susceptible dogs, infection spreads rapidly, usually resulting in a significant outbreak of respiratory disease. These outbreaks are characterized by disease in all ages of dogs, regardless of vaccination status, with morbidity rates as high as 80% to 90%. Mortality rates are lower and most likely to be 5% or less.

Canine influenza virus is shed in respiratory secretions and is highly contagious. Virus may be spread by direct dog-to-dog contact or by airborne transmission through droplets or aerosols generated by coughing or sneezing. It is likely that airborne spread of virus can occur over several feet, and the virus may survive for up to 48 hours in the environment. Fomites also play an important role in the transmission of canine influenza virus, with spread occurring through contact with infected bedding, feeding, or grooming equipment and even the clothing of personnel working with infected dogs.

The time from exposure to canine influenza virus to onset of clinical signs is approximately 2 to 4 days. Viral shedding begins as soon as 2 days after exposure, peaks at 2 to 4 days, and may persist for 7 to 10 days. Thus dogs with canine influenza may shed virus before the development of clinical signs or very early in the course of disease. This has significant implications for both diagnosis and disease control. It is also important to note that infected dogs are unlikely to be shedding virus by 10 to 14 days after infection.

There is no true carrier state for canine influenza virus infection; however, as many as 10% to 20% of infected dogs may shed virus with no apparent clinical signs. Therefore dogs that have been in contact with influenza suspects should also be regarded as potentially infectious to other dogs for 10 to 14 days after possible exposure.

CLINICAL SIGNS AND DIFFERENTIAL DIAGNOSIS

The most common clinical sign of canine influenza virus infection is a cough. The cough is typically soft and moist but may be harsh or dry. It may persist for several days or even weeks. Affected dogs may also have a serous or purulent nasal discharge. Fever may be noted in the early stages of infection and is usually transient. The signs of canine influenza virus infection are clinically indistinguishable from those of infection with other respiratory pathogens such as *Bordetella bronchiseptica*, adenovirus, or parainfluenza virus (See Chapter 147). However, when compared to kennel cough or more classic canine infectious tracheobronchitis, an outbreak of canine influenza typically involves a much larger percentage of susceptible dogs, and disease is seen in animals that have been vaccinated against other respiratory pathogens. It is also important to remember that coinfections may occur with canine influenza virus and other kennel cough organisms.

A small percentage of dogs exposed to canine influenza virus develop a more severe form of disease characterized by persistent fever, lethargy, dyspnea, and signs of bronchopneumonia. This form of the disease may be fatal; however, it is much less common than the milder form of disease and probably accounts for fewer than 10% of cases. The initial report of influenza virus infection in racing greyhounds described a peracute hemorrhagic pneumonia with a case fatality rate of 36%. Fortunately it appears that this is an uncommon manifestation of the disease in other dog populations.

DIAGNOSIS

The laboratory diagnosis of canine influenza is based on the culture of the etiologic agent (virus isolation), the demonstration of the viral nucleic acid (polymerase chain reaction [PCR]–based assays) or viral antigen in nasal or pharyngeal swab samples (e.g., detection of antigen by immunofluorescence, enzyme-linked immunosorbent assay [ELISA], or immunoperoxidase), or the detection of virus-specific antibodies (serology). Each of these methods has both merits and disadvantages; therefore it may be necessary to combine several diagnostic tools to identify canine influenza virus accurately and rapidly. Moreover, the timing of sample collection relative to the onset of clinical signs is critical in regard to appropriate test selection. For instance, virus shedding in nasal secretions is heaviest within the first few days after infection. Therefore nasal or pharyngeal swab samples submitted for virus isolation, nucleic acid, or antigen detection should be collected early in the course of disease (i.e., within the first 24 to 48 hours after onset of clinical signs). In contrast, since insufficient time has passed to allow for production of a detectable antibody response, serologic testing often may produce a negative result in the first few days after infection.

Virus Isolation

Although virus isolation from clinical samples is critical for epidemiologic investigation and for future vaccine production, this technique may have limited value for diagnostic purposes. Virus isolation can take a minimum of 2 to 3 days; and the success of this technique for detection of infectious virus is influenced by virus strain, amount of viable virus present in the sample, and sample collection and storage techniques. Moreover, if the amount of virus shed is low, several serial passages may be required before sufficiently high viral titers are reached to allow detection using conventional hemagglutination assays. For sample collection, a short polyester-tipped swab should be used for the collection of secretions on the nasal mucosa. Cotton-tipped swabs should be avoided since influenza virus has been found to adhere to the cotton fibers, thus decreasing the chances of virus recovery. Optimally the swab should be placed in sterile viral transport medium (often available from a diagnostic laboratory) and kept on ice or refrigerated until further analysis.

Antigen Detection

The most important advantages of diagnostic tests aimed at the detection of viral antigen over traditional virus isolation are the faster turnaround time and the ability to detect virions that have lost their infectivity. Immunofluorescence uses influenza-specific fluorochrome-labeled antibodies to detect virus-infected cells. The technique is highly sensitive and can be used to detect viral antigen in a broad range of clinical samples such as frozen tissue sections, tissue imprints, cells obtained from nasal scrapings, tracheal washes, and bronchoalveolar lavage fluid. Commercially available antigen-capture ELISA assays originally were developed for the rapid, on-site detection of human influenza A viruses (e.g., Flu OIA assay, Biostar; Directigen Flu-A assay, Becton Dickinson Microbiology Systems). The tests have been designed to detect the human influenza A virus nucleoprotein. Because the viral nucleoprotein is highly conserved among influenza A viruses of different subtypes and lineages, these assays have also been used to detect influenza infection in other species. For example, these rapid stall-side tests have been evaluated for the detection of influenza virus in horses and have been found to perform with high specificity and reasonable sensitivity. Similarly, recent studies conducted in dogs suggest that the commercial ELISA-based tests perform with a sensitivity similar to that of traditional virus isolation.

Polymerase-Chain Reaction–Based Assays

Several diagnostic laboratories offer PCR-based tests (conventional and/or real-time PCR) for the diagnosis of canine influenza virus infection. PCR-based assays are extremely sensitive and theoretically can detect a single copy of the target nucleic acid in a sample. However, because of the high sensitivity of the assay, the greatest challenge facing the diagnostic application of PCR is the production of false-positive results. Nonetheless, PCR-based testing offers a more sensitive tool for the diagnosis of canine influenza than conventional techniques such as virus isolation or immunoassays. Real-time PCR assays are being used with increasing frequency in veterinary diagnostic laboratories. In contrast to conventional PCR methods, real-time PCR does not require post-PCR processing steps (e.g., gel electrophoresis and determination of fragment size) and therefore can generate results within 4 to 5 hours. By using a target-specific fluorescent probe, real-time PCR can also be used for quantification of virus and can be and has been used in routine diagnostic settings.

Antibody Detection

Detection of virus-specific antibodies has been and continues to be an important tool in the diagnosis of canine influenza. Because most serologic assays are relatively easy to perform and cost-effective and large numbers of samples can be tested simultaneously, serologic testing is particularly useful in large-scale population surveillance. However, although it is useful, there are several limitations to serologic testing. Although the presence of antibody indicates exposure to antigen, it does not necessarily signify active infection or disease. Furthermore, antibody is not always detected in the presence of active infection. Experimental data obtained from dogs infected with canine influenza virus indicate that measurable antibody titers typically develop 7 or more days after infection. Therefore antibody may not be present during the first week of active infection, which is the period that is often most critical for disease management in settings where large numbers of dogs are housed together.

THERAPY

In the majority of affected dogs canine influenza is a self-limiting respiratory disease that does not require medical therapy. Secondary bacterial infections may complicate canine influenza and may manifest as purulent nasal discharge, persistent fever, or signs of pneumonia. These complications should be managed with antibiotic therapy. For dogs with bronchopneumonia, ideally antibiotic choices should be based on the results of culture and antibiotic sensitivity testing of samples obtained by transoral or transtracheal washes or bronchoalveolar lavage. If culture and sensitivity testing cannot be performed, broad-spectrum antibiotics that achieve adequate concentrations in the respiratory tract should be selected. Depending on the severity of the disease, dogs with pneumonia may also benefit from intravenous fluid therapy, nutritional support, oxygen therapy, nebulization, and coupage (Chapter 149).

Antiviral drugs such as oseltamivir (Tamiflu, Roche) are not recommended in the management of canine influenza. The dose, duration, safety, and efficacy of this therapy are all currently unknown in dogs. In addition, these medications should be reserved as a vital defense for the protection of human health.

DISEASE CONTROL

Canine influenza should be considered in the differential diagnosis of any dog with acute cough, fever, or nasal discharge. This is particularly important if the dog has a recent history of exposure to other dogs such as at a canine day-care center, shelter, or boarding facility. Dogs that are considered to be influenza suspects should be separated from other dogs when presented to a veterinary clinic. Veterinary staff should wear a disposable gown, gloves, and shoe covers when working with influenza suspects; examination room surfaces and tables and any in-contact equipment should be disinfected when the patient leaves the hospital. If an influenza suspect requires hospitalization (e.g., for the management of pneumonia), the patient should be placed in an isolation facility to reduce the risk of disease transmission to other hospitalized patients. Again, disposable protective clothing should be worn when handling the patient, and care must be taken to avoid spread of virus by fomites. When determining the need for isolation of influenza suspects, it should be remembered that shedding of infectious virus ceases by 10 to14 days after infection and that exposed dogs may shed virus before the onset of clinical signs.

If a dedicated isolation facility is not available in the veterinary hospital, strict barrier nursing precautions must be used in the management of hospitalized influenza suspects. These precautions include the use of dedicated or disposable protective clothing when working with the patient; maximum physical separation from other dogs in the same room; disinfection of all in-contact items such as food and water bowls, medical equipment, and bedding; the use of disinfectant foot baths or foot mats; and rigorous hand washing between patients. If staffing levels allow, personnel caring for influenza suspects should avoid contact with other hospitalized patients.

When influenza outbreaks occur in groups of dogs, it is important to separate exposed or infected dogs from unexposed dogs. Because the infection spreads rapidly and virus shedding can precede the onset of clinical signs, all dogs present in a facility should be considered infected at the time of diagnosis. These animals should subsequently have no direct or indirect contact with unexposed dogs for 14 days. In addition to physical separation of exposed or infected dogs from unexposed susceptible dogs, it is important to avoid transmission by fomites such as clothing and equipment used by animal care personnel. If possible, exposed or infected dogs and unexposed susceptible dogs should be maintained in areas with separate air supplies and managed by separate teams of staff. However, these measures may not be possible in all facilities.

Canine influenza virus is inactivated by many detergents and disinfectants. Hand washing with soap between patients reduces the spread of infection, and surfaces should be decontaminated by cleaning followed by disinfection. Cleaning is necessary to remove organic debris that may inhibit or inactivate disinfectants. Bleach, alcohol, quaternary ammonium compounds, and oxidizing agents are all effective for the inactivation of canine influenza virus.

PREVENTION

Although a number of manufacturers are in the process of developing vaccines, at this time there are no licensed canine influenza vaccines on the market. Therefore the two main principles used in controlling canine influenza infection and disease are the reduction in the spread of virus between dogs and the prevention of secondary complications. Under optimal circumstances dogs should be isolated for up to 4 weeks before introduction into a disease-free population. During this isolation period no clinical signs should be detected, and no new

animals should be introduced into the isolation facility. Since these criteria may be too stringent for most animal facilities such as humane shelters and boarding kennels, 2 weeks of full isolation may constitute an acceptable compromise. Other management procedures such as segregating dogs in separate rooms can be valuable since segregation may allow for containment of disease outbreaks. As outlined previously, sharing of feeding, grooming, and cleaning equipment also increases the risk of disease spread.

PUBLIC HEALTH CONSIDERATIONS

As discussed in the introduction, influenza A viruses occasionally are transmitted directly from one host species to another. Yet in many instances these transmission events are self-limiting, and the introduced viruses are only rarely maintained in the new host species. Moreover, a number of influenza virus lineages are rarely detected in animals other than their typical host. For example, although the susceptibility of human volunteers to infection with H3 equine-lineage viruses has been demonstrated, there is no evidence that horse-to-human or human-to-horse transmission routinely occurs under natural conditions. Similarly, there is no evidence at this time that canine-to-human transmission of influenza takes place. However, given the plasticity of the influenza virus genome, it is possible that at some time in the future the canine viruses may acquire the capability to infect another host species. This emphasizes the central role of the veterinarian in the control of canine influenza because only by continuing to sample animals with influenza-like illness and submitting these samples for virus isolation, antigenic, and genetic analyses will veterinarians be able to assess the extent of genetic evolution and to gauge the risks posed to other species by the canine H3N8 viruses.

References and Suggested Reading

Crawford PC et al: Transmission of equine influenza virus to dogs, *Science* 310:482, 2005.
Newton R et al: Canine influenza virus: cross-species transmission from horses, *Vet Rec* 161:142, 2007.
Smith KC et al: Canine influenza virus, *Vet Rec* 157:599, 2005.
Webster RG et al: Evolution and ecology of influenza A viruses, *Microbiol Rev* 56:152, 1992.
Yoon K-J et al: Influenza virus infection in racing greyhounds, *Emerg Infect Dis* 11:1974, 2005.
http://diaglab.vet.cornell.edu/issues/civ-stat.asp: Test summary for canine influenza virus in dogs not affiliated with greyhound racetracks.

CHAPTER 285

Feline Infectious Peritonitis: Therapy and Prevention

DIANE D. ADDIE, *Etchebar, France*
TAKUO ISHIDA, *Tokyo, Japan*

Feline infectious peritonitis (FIP) has been considered an incurable disease, and a diagnosis of FIP usually resulted in euthanasia. Recent advances in the understanding of FIP pathogenesis and novel diagnostic tests now enable earlier and more accurate diagnosis of FIP. With the recent introduction of recombinant *feline interferon ω* (rFeIFN-ω), there is hope for an effective treatment regimen in some cases.

The first step in FIP treatment is establishing an accurate diagnosis. Despite many manufacturers' claims that their tests are FIP tests, currently there is no specific FIP test. Existing tests actually detect feline coronavirus (FCoV) antibodies or viral RNA. Only histopathology can diagnose FIP unequivocally. This is because the majority of cats that become infected with feline coronavirus (FCoV) do *not* develop FIP (Fig. 285-1); therefore *no healthy FCoV-infected cat should ever be said to have FIP*. The problem for clinicians is distinguishing look-alike conditions from FIP in the FCoV-infected cat. Details of how to do this and further information can be found on catvirus.com or other literature sources.

PATHOGENESIS

Cats become infected with FCoV orally, usually indirectly, by contact with FCoV-contaminated cat litter. FCoV is highly infectious, and in a multicat household over 90% of cats will seroconvert. Virus is shed in the feces from 2 days after infection, and cats seroconvert 18 to 21 days after infection. Initial infection may be clinically inapparent or accompanied by transient upper respiratory tract signs or diarrhea, which may be mild but can occasionally be extremely severe. Most cats clear the virus after 2 to 3 months of fecal shedding, although some cats are persistently infected. The mechanism for viral clearance is not wholly understood. Chronic carrier cats are usually healthy, although one of the authors (DA) has observed some cats develop chronic large intestinal diarrhea in older age.

FCoV antibody titers in infected cats that do not develop FIP tend to decrease to zero over time (Addie and Jarrett, 2001). Increasing FCoV antibody titer in a healthy cat usually is followed by a decrease to zero over several months (Addie and Jarrett, 2001). However, in the experience of one of the authors (TI), if accompanied by polyclonal gammopathy and rising α_1-acid glycoprotein (AGP) levels, rising antibody titers occasionally may be associated with FIP.

FIP is a misnomer since many cats do not present with peritonitis. The histopathologic lesion of FIP is a phlebitis or perivascular pyogranuloma. Recent developments in understanding the pathogenesis of FIP are useful in understanding how clinical signs develop and for devising new strategies for therapy. Using immunohistochemistry FCoV has been found within monocytes adhering to blood vessel walls and extravasating to adjacent tissues (Kipar et al., 2005). This is a key event in the development of FIP since FCoV-infected macrophages release a number of cytokines that drive the clinical disease. Interleukin-6 (IL-6) stimulates B lymphocytes to differentiate into plasma cells, and high IL-6 levels found in cats with FIP are the likely cause of hypergammaglobulinemia. In early infection IL-6 stimulates hepatocytes to release acute-phase proteins, including AGP and high AGP levels can be used to aid in the diagnosis of FIP. A rise in AGP levels was found not only in cats that develop FIP but also transiently in cats in contact with a sick FIP cat (Giordano et al., 2004), leading to speculation that the early AGP response could, in fact, be protective against FIP development (Addie, 2004).

Why one cat develops FIP while other infected in-contact cats remain healthy is unknown. Some laboratory strains are exceptionally virulent, causing FIP in almost every cat infected with them; these have been called *FIPVs*. There are also biotypes with far less virulence, commonly called *feline enteric coronaviruses (FECVs)*. These laboratory strains have varying ability to replicate in monocytes, and it has been assumed that the occurrence of FIP was related solely to the virulence of the strain of virus infecting the cat. However, a recent study has shown that monocytes of different cats support FCoV replication to varying extents (Dewerchin, Cornelissen, and Nauwynck, 2005) and that some cat's monocytes do not support viral replication at all, which could be an explanation for the occurrence of FCoV-resistant cats previously reported by Addie and Jarrett (2001). The "internal mutation theory" (i.e., that FECVs must mutate to FIPVs for FIP to arise) has been questioned after sequence analysis of the entire genome of viruses found both in the gut and systemically in a cat that died of FIP were found to be identical (Dye and Siddell, 2007). The recent advent of quantitative (or real-time) polymerase chain reaction will enable the role of viral load in FIP development to be investigated more fully.

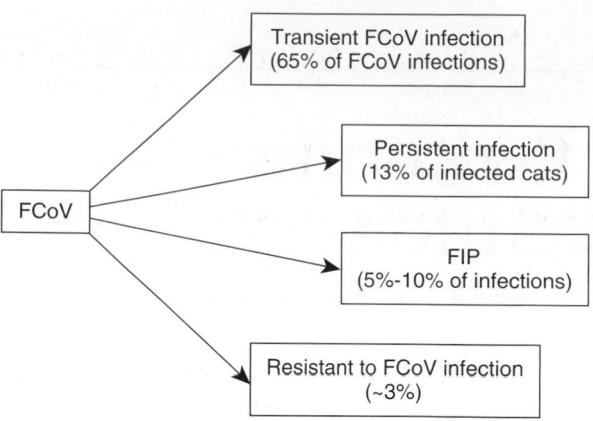

Fig. 285-1 Potential outcomes of feline coronavirus infection. (The percentages are approximate and do not add up to 100% because not all of the cats in the study had sufficient samples taken for their status to be defined [Addie and Jarrett, 2001]).

THERAPY

Current Therapies

Clinical FIP is caused by the cat's inflammatory and immune-mediated response to FCoV. Therapy is aimed at suppressing that inflammatory and immune-mediated response, usually with corticosteroids. One problem with corticosteroid therapy is that it suppresses the immune response nonselectively, suppressing both cell-mediated and humoral immune responses. It is likely that one would wish to support cell-mediated responses while suppressing humoral responses, at least in effusive FIP. It is possible that in noneffusive FIP both cell-mediated and humoral responses should be suppressed.

Until recently FIP was almost 100% fatal. However, two publications have reported cure or remission in some cats.

Administration of a thromboxane synthetase inhibitor with prednisolone reportedly cured one cat and gave remission for 8 months in a second effusive FIP (Watari et al., 1998). However, one of the authors (TI) has been unable to reproduce this result. Use of rFeIFN-ω (Virbagen-ω, Virbac) and prednisolone resulted in recovery in 4 of 12 cats and remission of 4 and 5 months in two others (Ishida et al., 2004). However, a second study evaluating rFeIFN-ω therapy was unable to show an effect on survival time or quality of life in cats with FIP (Ritz, Egberink and Hartman, 2007).

IFN-ω is a monomeric glycoprotein distantly related in structure to IFN-α and IFN-β but unrelated to IFN-γ. It has antiviral properties, stimulates natural killer cell activity, and enhances expression of major histocompatibility complex class I (but not class II) antigens. Although effusive and noneffusive FIP are not distinct diseases but rather gradations of the same process.

The use of interferons for the treatment of cats infected with FIP is controversial, though the authors believe such therapy is warranted considering the relative lack of therapeutic options. Both negative treatment studies (Ritz, Egberink, and Hartmann, 2007) and positive treatment studies (Ishida et al., 2004) have been published. Our treatment approach to the cat with an effusive or noneffusive form of FIP infection is outlined in Box 285-1. Only over time and with additional studies will the effectiveness of rFeIFN-ω or other therapies in the treatment of FIP become evident.

Possible Future Therapies

A number of other drugs also have theoretic application in the treatment of cats with FIP and are offered in Table 285-1. Most have never been used to treat FIP or have been used in only a few cats; thus the reader should exercise appropriate caution when choosing patients to receive these unproven drugs.

Box 285-1

Treatment Protocols Used for Effusive and Noneffusive Feline Infectious Peritonitis

EFFUSIVE

Glucocorticoids

Dexamethasone 1 mg/kg intrathoracic, intraperitoneal or intravenous once followed by:

- Prednisolone sliding dose; 4 mg/kg q24h for 10-14 days, reducing to 2 mg/kg q24h for 10-14 days, then 1 mg/kg q24h for 10-14 days, then 0.5 mg/kg q24h for 10-14 days, then 0.25 mg/kg q24h for 10-14 days, then 0.25 mg/kg q48h and so on, ceasing after complete remission of clinical signs; if, at any point, the cat's condition regresses, go back to the previous dose

Feline interferon-ω

1 million units(MU)/kg subcutaneously q48h, reducing to once weekly if remission occurs

Broad-spectrum antibiotics

NONEFFUSIVE

Glucocorticoids

Prednisolone sliding dose as for effusive feline infectious peritonitis (FIP); with FIP-related uveitis topical corticosteroids should be used.

Feline interferon-ω

50,000 units per cat PO q24h until acid glycoproteins, serum amyloid A, globulins, hematocrit, lymphocyte count, and clinical signs return to normal.

Diluting feline interferon-ω

Feline interferon (IFN)-ω (Virbagen Omega, Virbac) comes in vials of 10 MU. It is reconstituted with 1 ml of diluent. Ten aliquots of 0.1 ml (1 MU per syringe) are prepared in insulin syringes. Nine syringes out of 10 are kept in the freezer (can be stored up to 6 months). The tenth syringe is diluted with 19.9 ml of sterile 0.9% saline solution to obtain 20 ml of solution containing a total of 1 MU (50,000 U/ml) of feline IFN-ω. This syringe is stored in the refrigerator at +4° C, where it will last up to 3 weeks (do not freeze diluted IFN-ω because it is unstable). Dosage: 1 ml of this diluted solution (containing 0.05 MU) orally daily, using the syringe without the needle.

Table 285-1

Potential Future Drugs for the Treatment of Feline Infectious Peritonitis*

Potential Treatment	Suggested Mode of Action	Suggested Dosage	Comments
Ozagrel hydrochloride	Thromboxane synthetase inhibitors	5-10 mg/kg twice a day	Cured one cat and gave remission for 8 months in a second effusive feline infectious peritonitis (FIP); no cures in a second study (Ishida, unpublished)
Infliximab (Remicade, Centocor)	Monoclonal antibody against tumor necrosis factor (TNF)-α	Unknown	Use in effusive and noneffusive FIP; increases risk of bacterial infections
Etanercept (Enbrel, Immunex Corp.)	Soluble p75 TNF-α receptor coupled to Fc portion of immunoglobulin G	Unknown	Use in effusive and noneffusive FIP; increases risk of bacterial infections
Dehydroepiandrosterone (DHEA)	Down-regulates endothelial adhesion molecules and reduces neutrophil extravasation		Use in effusive but not in noneffusive FIP
16α-Bromo-epiandrosterone (epiBr)	Synthetic derivative of DHEA	40 mg/cat/day	Use in effusive but not innoneffusive FIP
Cimetidine	Stimulates cell-mediated immunity and reverses lymphopenia	50 mg once a day	Safe; may be more useful in effusive than noneffusive FIP
Thalidomide	Antiinflammatory and pushes immune response from Th2 to Th1	50-100 mg once a day in the evening	Safe but difficult to source
Salvianolic acid B	Matrix metalloproteinase 9 inhibitor	10 mg/kg once a day	Likely to be more useful in effusive than noneffusive FIP
Tropisetron	5-hydroxytryptamine (3) receptor antagonist	300 mcg/kg once a day	
Coronavirus 3C–like protease inhibitors	Anticoronavirus drug	Intravenous administration likely	Not yet available

*NOTE: Listed in Table 285-1 are potential theoretic treatments for cats with FIP that are lacking published clinical or research studies. The reader should exercise appropriate caution in use of these unproven drugs.

PREVENTION OF FELINE INFECTIOUS PERITONITIS AND FELINE CORONAVIRUS INFECTION

There is no single, easy method to prevent FIP; a combination of the techniques discussed in the following paragraphs is most effective. Obviously, if cats do not become infected with FCoV, FIP will not develop.

Prevention of Feline Infectious Peritonitis by Vaccination

The one commercially available FIP vaccine, a temperature-sensitive mutant (Primucell, Pfizer) that only replicates in the cooler nasal mucosa of cats, has been beset by controversy (also see Chapter 280). Basically there are two questions: is it effective, and does it cause antibody-dependent enhancement of disease?

In an independent study in Switzerland, cats entering a rescue cattery were vaccinated with Primucell. There was no difference in mortality rates from FIP between vaccinated and unvaccinated cats in the first 150 days after vaccination (Fehr et al., 1995, 1997). However, after 150 days there was a marked reduction in the number of cats succumbing to FIP in the vaccinated but not the control group. When the investigators returned to stored blood samples from the cats that developed FIP, they found

that these cats were already viremic at the time of vaccination (Fehr et al., 1997) (i.e., they were incubating FIP at the time of vaccination). Only FCoV-naive cats can be prevented from developing FIP by vaccination.

From this study it is possible to suggest certain vaccine guidelines:

- All cats going into rescue and boarding catteries should be vaccinated against FIP.
- Cat breeders should maintain their kittens FCoV-free until FIP vaccination is possible (current recommendation is that vaccination commences at 16 weeks of age).

Another point sometimes made in relation to the efficacy of Primucell vaccine is that it is derived from a type II FCoV, the strain DF2. There are two types of FCoV: type I, which is wholly feline; and type II, which is a recombinant virus with much of the viral spike protein being derived from canine coronavirus. The majority of field strains of FCoV are type I. In the study mentioned previously, it is likely that most of the FCoVs the cats naturally encountered in the rescue shelter were type I since a recent study showed that type I is the most prevalent type in Switzerland (Kummrow et al., 2005). Thus, although unproven, the vaccine is likely to be equally effective against types I and II FCoV.

Antibody-dependent enhanced (ADE) FIP is a phenomenon in which vaccination contributes to disease pathogenesis. ADE FIP is the reason why most experimental FIP vaccines have failed (i.e., more vaccinated cats than unvaccinated cats developed FIP, and they did so more quickly and with worse clinical and pathologic features than unvaccinated cats). In two laboratory experiments in which Primucell appeared to cause ADE, a highly virulent laboratory strain of FCoV was used in the challenge (McArdle et al., 1995; Scott, Olsen, and Corapi, 1995). In contrast, in two field trials with Primucell the vaccine was protective (Fehr et al., 1995, 1997; Postorino-Reeves, 1995). One recommendation of the Second International Feline Coronavirus and Feline Infectious Peritonitis Symposium workshop was that the 79–1146 strain of FCoV not be used in vaccine challenge experiments since it is too virulent to give an accurate representation of how the vaccine would perform in field conditions (Addie et al., 2004).

Prevention of Feline Coronavirus Infection and Feline Infectious Peritonitis by Hygiene and Quarantine

FIP vaccination is not 100% protective; thus it is preferable that cats never be exposed to FCoV infection. This is especially true for cat breeders and their kittens since kittens cannot be vaccinated before 16 weeks of age but they are susceptible to infection after 5 to 6 weeks of age. Indeed, in large catteries virus load may even overcome maternally derived antibody to cause infection in kittens as young as 2 weeks (Addie et al., 2004).

FCoV is shed mainly in feces; therefore avoiding FCoV infection centers around litter tray hygiene and limiting contact of FCoV-naive cats with FCoV-contaminated cat litter or fomites. FCoV is killed by many disinfectants, including household bleach. Regular disinfection of litter trays helps to minimize environmental viral load. Provision of adequate numbers of litter trays in multicat households helps ensure that cats do not have to use a soiled tray, and self-cleaning litter trays or nontracking cat litter should be used wherever possible. Regular vacuum cleaning reduces environmental contamination by microscopic particles of infected cat litter.

FCoV infection is maintained in a household or cattery by continual cycles of infection and reinfection (Foley et al., 1997, Addie et al., 2003). Commonly available reverse transcriptase polymerase chain reaction tests can detect FCoV in feces, so that it is possible to establish which cats are shedding FCoV and separate them from cats that are not shedding FCoV. Virus shedding usually continues for 2 to 3 months, although it can be longer. Cats that shed FCoV for 9 months or more are likely to be lifelong carriers of the virus (although one cat stopped shedding virus after 5 years). By repeat testing and separation of shedding from nonshedding cats, it is possible to eliminate FCoV from a multicat pet or breeding household. Quarantine and testing of new-arrival cats prevents FCoV from being (re)introduced into such a household.

Kittens are protected from FCoV infection by maternally derived antibodies until they are between 5 and 6 weeks of age. Thus it is possible to prevent FCoV infection of young kittens by isolating them with their queens from birth onward and removing them to a clean environment when they are 5 to 6 weeks old. For this technique to work, the breeder requires a thorough understanding of barrier nursing techniques. Transplacental transmission of FCoV does not appear to occur.

Many cats with FIP have a history of having recently been stressed (e.g., by a neutering operation). Cats at risk for FIP are easy to identify: they are purebred or have a history of having come from a multicat environment such as a rescue shelter or pet shop. Fifty percent of FIP occurs in cats under 2 years old. It is possible that the development of FIP in these cats could be averted by determining whether or not they are infected (e.g., by testing their feces for FCoV) and delaying elective surgery until the cat has cleared the virus. Cats are at greatest risk of developing FIP soonest after FCoV infection (Addie et al., 1995), and the risk diminishes with time. When there is no choice but to go ahead with surgery, stress can be minimized as much as possible (e.g., by not keeping the cat in a waiting room with dogs). For the reasons outlined previously, it would be prudent to advise clients to avoid stresses such as visits to the boarding cattery until FCoV-infected cats have cleared the virus.

In summary, FIP therapy is still in early stages and likely can only be advanced after a definitive diagnostic test is developed. Therefore all efforts should be directed to preventing FIP by careful cat management (good hygiene, stress reduction, quarantine) and by vaccination.

References and Suggested Reading

Addie DD: Feline coronavirus: that enigmatic little critter, *Vet J* 167:15, 2004.

Addie DD: Feline infectious peritonitis. In de Mari K, ed: *Veterinary interferon handbook,* ed 2, Carros, France, 2008, Virbac Animal Health, p 132.

Addie DD, Jarrett O: A study of naturally occurring feline coronavirus infection in kittens, *Vet Rec* 130:133, 1992.

Addie DD, Jarrett JO: Use of a reverse-transcriptase polymerase chain reaction for monitoring feline coronavirus shedding by healthy cats, *Vet Rec* 148:649, 2001.

Addie DD, Paltrinieri S, Pedersen NC: Recommendations from workshops of the second international feline coronavirus/feline infectious peritonitis symposium, *J Feline Medicine Surgery* 6:125, 2004.

Addie DD et al: The risk of feline infectious peritonitis in cats naturally infected with feline coronavirus, *Am J Vet Res* 56(4):429, 1995a.

Addie DD et al: The risk of typical and antibody-enhanced feline infectious peritonitis among cats from feline coronavirus endemic households, *Feline Pract* 23(3):24, 1995b.

Addie DD et al: Persistence and transmission of natural type I feline coronavirus infection, *J Gen Virol* 84 (Pt 10):2735, 2003.

Dewerchin HL, Cornelissen E, Nauwynck HJ: Replication of feline coronaviruses in peripheral blood monocytes, *Arch Virol* 150:2483, 2005.

Dye C, Siddell SG: Genomic RNA sequence of feline coronavirus strain FCoV F1Je, *J Feline Med Surg* 9(3):202, 2007.

Fehr D et al: Evaluation of the safety and efficacy of a modified live FIPV vaccine under field conditions, *Feline Pract* 23:83, 1995.

Fehr D et al: Placebo-controlled evaluation of a modified life virus vaccine against feline infectious peritonitis: safety and efficacy under field conditions, *Vaccine* 15(10):1101, 1997.

Foley JE et al: Patterns of feline coronavirus infection and fecal shedding from cats in multiple-cat environments, *J Am Vet Med Assoc* 210(9):1307, 1997.

Giordano A et al: Changes in some acute phase protein and immunoglobulin concentrations in cats affected by feline infectious peritonitis (FIP) or exposed to feline coronavirus infection, *Vet J* 167:38, 2004.

Ishida T et al: Use of recombinant feline interferon and glucocorticoid in the treatment of feline infectious peritonitis, *J Feline Med Surg* 6(2):107, 2004.

Kipar A et al: Morphologic features and development of granulomatous vasculitis in feline infectious peritonitis, *Vet Pathol* 42:321, 2005.

Kummrow M et al: Feline coronavirus serotypes 1 and 2: seroprevalence and association with disease in Switzerland, *Clin Diagn Lab Immunol* 12:1209, 2005.

McArdle F et al: Independent evaluation of a modified-live FIPV vaccine under experimental conditions (University of Liverpool experience), *Feline Pract* 23:67, 1995.

Postorino-Reeves N: Vaccination against naturally occurring FIP in a single large cat shelter, *Feline Pract* 23:81, 1995.

Ritz S, Egberink H, Hartmann K: Effect of feline interferon-omega on the survival time and quality of life of cats with feline infectious peritonitis. *J Vet Intern Med* 21:1193, 2007.

Scott FW, Olsen CW, Corapi WV: Independent evaluation of a modified live FIPV vaccine under experimental conditions (Cornell experience), *Feline Pract* 23(3):74, 1995.

Watari T et al: Effects of thromboxane synthetase inhibitor on feline infectious peritonitis in cats, *J Vet Med Sci* 60:657, 1998.

Useful Feline Coronavirus/Feline Infectious Peritonitis Websites

www.catvirus.com: FCoV/FIP website with the latest information for veterinary surgeons and information for cat guardians and breeders.

www.felinecoronavirus.com: website for FCoV/FIP symposia news.

www.ncbi.nlm.nih.gov/entrez/query.fcgi?DB=pubmed: National Institutes of Health website with search facility for finding the latest scientific and veterinary publications on FCoV and FIP.

CHAPTER **286**

Control of Viral Diseases in Catteries

DIANE D. ADDIE, *Etchebar, France*

The control of viral disease in catteries will depend largely on the type of cattery. Catteries mainly fall into six distinct types with different feline populations:

1. *Boarding/Quarantine:* Transient population, but mainly vaccinated. Indoor for duration of cattery stay, but possibly free-ranging before then.
2. *Rescue:* Transient population of unknown vaccine status. Indoor for duration of cattery stay, but a mix of free-ranging and indoor housing prior to relinquishment.
3. *Breeding:* Longer term population, closed, but with possible contact with other cats for mating, or at shows. Vaccination and infectious disease screening variable. Usually indoor housing.
4. *Multicat pet household:* Longer term population, free-ranging or indoor housing. Vaccination and infectious disease screening variable.
5. *Veterinary premises:* Transient population of known and unknown infectious disease status.
6. Specific pathogen free (SPF): Closed, indoor population with strictly known vaccination and infectious disease status.

Clearly, the problems encountered within each of the different types of cattery are extremely diverse. In this chapter I will approach the control of the main feline viral diseases, referring only to cattery type when it affects the control of that particular virus. The infections considered in this chapter are listed in Table 286-1. Information on more unusual viral infections, such as Borna virus and Aujeszky's (pseudorabies), are considered in other textbooks (Greene, 2006). Full clinical details, treatment, and diagnosis of viral diseases are omitted in this chapter, except where they affect disease control (for more therapy details, see Section XIII in this volume). The most

Table **286-1**

Viral Transmission and Shedding

Infection	Survival Outside Host	Virus Shedding	Quarantine Time Before Testing	Mode of Transmission	Prevention of Infection
FCV	Days to weeks	Continuous, half-life 75 days	7 days	Direct contact, sneezed droplets	Test all cats before mixing them; excellent hygiene; sneeze barriers
FHV	12-18 hours	Intermittent, lasts 7-14 days	3 weeks	Direct contact, sneezed droplets	Vaccination prevents clinical signs, but not infection; testing reliable if positive result, but since latent infection, negative result not definite
FeLV	Minutes	Continuous	12 weeks	Direct contact essential, transplacental	Test all cats before mixing them; vaccination
FIV	Minutes	Continuous*	12 weeks	Direct contact essential—mainly biting; transplacental rare	Test all cats before mixing them
FCoV/FIP	Up to 7 weeks	Usually continuous	3 weeks (antibody, 1 wk virus)	Indirect, through cat litter/shared litter trays, poop scoops; not transplacental	Test all cats before mixing them; excellent hygiene
Parvovirus	Up to a year	Usually only 24-48 hours, but can be up to 6 weeks	None	Indirect, transplacental	Vaccination; excellent hygiene and disinfection; don't have too many unvaccinated cats/kittens on premises
Feline pox virus		Not infectious to other cats	None	Contact with small rodents	Can't stop cats hunting!
Rabies	Minutes	Continuous	None if adequate antibodies: >0.5 units or 6 months	Biting	Vaccination is effective

FCV, Feline calicivirus; *FCoV,* feline coronavirus; *FeLV,* feline leukemia virus; *FHV,* feline herpesvirus; *FIV,* feline immunodeficiency virus; *FIP,* feline infectious peritonitis.
*Virus load is very low during the long asymptomatic phase.

essential part of infectious disease control in all types of cattery, and for all infectious diseases, is good hygiene, so we will begin with that.

CONTROL OF VIRAL TRANSMISSION BY HYGIENE

The essence of "barrier nursing" is preventing transfer of infection within the cattery. Clean cats/food bowls/litter trays/pens should be dealt with before dirty ones. The cats' food should be distributed before dealing with litter trays or cleaning kennels; ideally there would be different people dealing with the food and the cleaning. Clean litter trays should be put out in the runs first, and then the dirty trays should be picked up; a clean tray should never be touched after a dirty one, and the same poop scoop or litter rake should never be used from one pen to another! The first rule is to deal first with the least-infected area of the surgery or cattery (for example, any kittens or surgery cases), and gradually move up to the most-infected area (locations where there are animals sick with infectious disease or known healthy carriers of infection). It is useful to establish a routine order of tending to the animals in a cattery so that the least-infected

area is always dealt with first. This applies to cleaning of litter trays, feeding, grooming, or even when the cats are petted.

Indirect transmission of viruses can occur on hands, shoes, or clothes when moving about the cattery. Therefore hands should be washed or disinfected before every contact with a cat or kennel. Ideally there should be disinfectant foot baths between each major area of a cattery.

Kittens should have food bowls, litter trays, and litter scoops that are used only for them, and these should be cleaned daily and disinfected/steam cleaned once or twice a week. The beds, dishes, litter trays, and scoops of cats in different areas of the cattery should be color coded so that it is immediately obvious if something is in the wrong place. Thus if a kitten's litter tray had been inadvertently put into the pen of an adult cat, it could be spotted instantly, removed, and disinfected before being returned to the kittens' area.

Cattery design is crucial. Sneeze barriers are essential for the control of airborne viruses in all cattery categories except for the pet household. It is vital that air conditioning pushes the air past the cat straight to the outdoors (i.e., positive pressure rather than negative pressure) or to a virus filter system and not past other cats.

Quarantine is useful to establish whether new cats are incubating disease. For example, feline herpesvirus (FHV) shedding recrudesces following stress, and the biggest stress a cat can face is being rehomed or going to a boarding cattery; thus virus is shed again, with or without accompanying upper respiratory tract signs. The United Kingdom quarantines cats from countries with endemic rabies for up to 6 months to allow them time to display clinical signs of rabies if they were infected. The time required for quarantine depends on which pathogen is the concern (see Table 286-1).

FELINE CALICIVIRUS

Feline calicivirus (FCV) is a ribonucleic acid (RNA) virus. It exists in cats as a quasispecies, continually mutating to evade the neutralizing antibodies of its host (Radford et al., 1998). Vaccination ameliorates clinical signs but doesn't prevent virus shedding and may even promote carrier status. Indeed, 40% of so-called vaccine breakdowns are caused by the vaccinal strain. If a live vaccine is aerosolized or inadvertently spilled onto the cat and the cat licks it off, it can infect the cat; thus catteries that are free of FCV preferably should use killed, or antigen-only, vaccines.

Natural selection has driven field strains of FCV away from older vaccine strains. In cattery situations vaccines containing newer FCV strains should be used to give as broad a protection as possible. FCV strains causing virulent systemic disease (VSD) (Pesavento et al., 2004; Coyne et al., 2006) tend to arise de novo in the cattery situation; therefore there is no benefit in vaccines containing a FCV VSD strain. For situations in which rapid onset of protection is needed, intranasal vaccines should be considered (Radford et al., 2007).

Vaccination alone will not prevent FCV spread in a cattery. SPF and breeding catteries can avoid its introduction completely by testing new cats prior to introduction, provided the test is sensitive enough (virus isolation of an oropharyngeal swab). Reverse transcriptase–polymerase chain reaction [RT-PCR] has to be used with caution because of the high variability of the FCV genome; some tests will give false negative results. Fortunately FCV is shed continuously (as opposed to intermittently).

FCV is shed by 10% of pet cats, 25% of cats at shows, 40% of colony cats, and almost 100% of cats with chronic lymphocytic plasmacytic gingivostomatitis. The half-life of FCV shedding is 75 days; thus there should be 2.5 months between tests of cats to detect when they have stopped shedding FCV.

Cat breeders preferably should use only FCV-negative queens. If this is not possible, maternally derived antibody (MDA) lasts up to 2 to 3 weeks; thus kittens can be weaned early and kept in isolation from infected individuals.

At time of writing, no antiviral drug is effective against FCV.

FELINE HERPESVIRUS

FHV-1 is a deoxyribonucleic acid (DNA) virus, and there is essentially only one serotype (reports of a FHV-2 were never fully scientifically confirmed). Viral persistence in the host cat is completely different from the other flu virus, FCV, in that FHV becomes latent within the trigeminal ganglion of the host. The trigeminal ganglion is an immune-privileged site, and the DNA of the FHV exists in the ganglion without expressing viral proteins. However, if the cat is stressed (e.g., because of rehoming or pregnancy), the virus can re-emerge, travel down the trigeminal nerve, and be shed in the oropharynx and/or the eye. Recrudescence of FHV shedding occurs 7 to 10 days after stress and lasts for 1 to 2 weeks. Vaccination prevents the worst of clinical signs, but does not prevent infection of the cat or the development of latency. It is estimated that 90% of cats have been exposed to FHV and 80% of exposed cats become latently infected for life. Testing for infection is of limited value because negative results may simply mean that the virus was latent at the time of testing.

As with FCV, prevention of FHV depends on factors such as good hygiene. However, the amino acid l-lysine competes with arginine in the formation of the herpesvirus particle, and a dosage of 250 to 500 mg/cat/day may reduce FHV shedding. Breeders attempting to reduce FHV infection of the neonate may stress the queen 3 to 4 weeks before kittening by moving her to a room or chalet on her own so that FHV shedding will have passed by the time the kittens are born. MDA is only protective for up to 2 to 3 weeks; thus the kittens should be weaned early and then kept in total isolation from the adult cats in the household.

Aside from topical preparations for ocular FHV, use of human antiherpesvirus drugs in cats is limited by their poor efficacy against FHV and by their toxicity in the cat (Maggs, 2001).

FELINE LEUKEMIA VIRUS

Feline leukemia virus (FeLV) is an RNA retrovirus. For an RNA virus it is remarkably conserved. The virus has avoided the need to mutate to evade the cat's immune response by switching off the cat's immune response, which is why it causes immunodeficiency. FeLV is a fragile virus, requiring direct contact for transmission. Transplacental transmission occurs.

Infection to viremia takes 3 to 6 weeks, which is why it is important to retest a negative cat suspected of FeLV exposure after 6 to 12 weeks. Following oronasal exposure, FeLV infects local lymph nodes and travels to bone marrow and other lymphoid tissues. It then moves to mucosa, where it is shed mainly in the saliva (although possibly in the tears, urine, feces, and milk as well). The cat has the opportunity to recover at any of these stages of infection, so it is important to retest a healthy cat with a positive FeLV test after an interval of 12 weeks.

After the age of 4 months cats are increasingly able to mount an effective immune response to FeLV. However, this age-related resistance to FeLV can be overwhelmed by high viral doses such as are found in infected multi-cat households in which approximately 40% of cats can be viremic. Cytotoxic T cells appear early in FeLV infection (in a week). Immunity to natural FeLV exposure can be measured by detecting virus-neutralizing antibodies (VNAs), which appear from 6 weeks after infection.

Cats with active FeLV infection have a VNA titer of 0. The immune response to vaccines is not easy to measure commercially.

No FeLV vaccine is 100% effective. Vaccination has a place in free-roaming pet cats but should not be necessary for veterinary surgeries or boarding or rescue catteries (since cats from different backgrounds should not be allowed to mix and FeLV is unlikely to be transmitted indirectly). Neither should breeding or SPF catteries require vaccination, since these cats are usually kept indoors and should have been tested and found to be FeLV negative before being introduced into these catteries.

It is important to use in-house diagnostic tests for FeLV wisely (Table 286-2). Point of care FeLV tests for FeLV p27 antigen should be considered as screening tests; accordingly, a positive result should be confirmed by a more specific test, such as immunofluorescence (IF), virus isolation (VI), or polymerase chain reaction (PCR), which will usually be carried out by a specialist or reference laboratory. The reason for confirmation is that in situations in which the prevalence of FeLV infection is very low, as is the case in many populations of healthy cats, the positive predictive value of an in-house test is relatively low (i.e., the occurrence of false positive results is relatively high). Cats that are persistently viremic will test positive with all of these diagnostic tests. The advantage of immunofluorescence and virus isolation tests is that they definitively detect viremic, virus-excreting cats and can be considered the gold standard for FeLV diagnosis. PCR is very sensitive and detects proviral DNA in leukocytes. However, many, if not all, cats that recover from FeLV infection and lead perfectly healthy lives without excreting virus will also be positive on PCR testing. Quantitative, real time PCR avoids some of this problem in that high virus load is associated with viremia, but it cannot discriminate completely between viremic and nonviremic cats.

FELINE IMMUNODEFICIENCY VIRUS

Feline immunodeficiency virus (FIV) is a fragile RNA retrovirus, easily killed by disinfectants. FIV usually is not transmitted indirectly, except by reusing syringes or operating kits or using dental descalers from cat to cat without sufficient hygiene. It is transmitted mainly by biting and occasionally by sharing food bowls or mutual grooming. It is rarely transmitted transplacentally or in the milk, but it is possible that an FIV-positive queen could infect her kittens when she bites through the umbilical cord or when she grooms them.

Most FIV tests detect antibody, not virus (the major exception being PCR, which detects viral DNA as provirus in the cat's genome). The period from infection to seroconversion takes up to 12 weeks; therefore antibody testing should be 12 weeks after suspected exposure. In-house FIV antibody tests can give false-positive results; thus they should be confirmed by gold standard tests (immunofluorescence, western blotting) (see Table 286-2). In addition, some FIV-infected cats don't have detectable antibody; thus a viral detection test such as PCR of the buffy coat should be used.

Transmission of FIV should not be an issue in most catteries, provided that cats from different backgrounds aren't mixed. The main situation in which FIV is a problem is the multicat pet household (cats can be screened before introduction, but if they are free ranging, they may become infected at any time). At time of writing there is one commercially available FIV vaccine in the United States; it causes positive antibody tests. As in FeLV infection, FIV vaccination won't be required in breeding, SPF, boarding catteries, or veterinary surgeries since there should be no opportunities for transmission in these environments.

Table **286-2**

Use of In-House Feline Leukemia Virus and Feline Immunodeficiency Virus Tests in Different Cattery Types

Type of Cattery	Whether Cats are Tested	Action After Use of In-House Test
Boarding/quarantine	Not usually tested	
Rescue	Sometimes tested	Positive results *must* be confirmed since the cat may be euthanized.
		Negative results from testing a healthy animal are fine but from a sick animal should be confirmed.
Breeding	Always tested	Positive results likely to be false positive if pedigree cat from FeLV- and FIV-negative background; therefore confirm using gold standard test.*
Multicat pet household	Sometimes tested	Isolate cat and retest after 12 weeks. Confirm all positive results.
Veterinary premises	Rarely screened unless symptomatic	If symptomatic, negative results should be confirmed using gold standard test.*
Specific pathogen free	Always screened	Positive results likely to be false positive; therefore confirm using gold standard test.*

FeLV, Feline leukemia virus; *FIV,* feline immunodeficiency virus.
nB: FeLV vaccination does **not** affect in-house test results.
nB: FIV vaccination can cause positive antibody test results. FIV tests will detect maternally derived antibody until around 16 weeks of age in uninfected kittens of FIV-positive queens.
*Gold standard tests for FeLV are virus isolation and immunofluorescence. Gold standard tests for FIV are western blotting and immunofluorescence.

FELINE CORONAVIRUS/FELINE INFECTIOUS PERITONITIS

Feline coronavirus (FCoV) is an extremely infectious virus; over 90% of cats that encounter it seroconvert. FCoV is an RNA virus that mutates frequently. In the literature there are references to feline enteric coronavirus (FECV) as an avirulent FCoV responsible for the large number of seropositive cats in the absence of feline infectious peritonitis (FIP). However, it is now widely recognized that all strains of FCoV have the potential to cause FIP.

There are essentially two types of FCoV: type I is wholly feline; type II FCoVs arise by recombination with canine coronavirus (CCoV), and much of the spike of the type II FCoV is canine. About 90% of field isolates are type I; 10% are type II.

Feline Infectious Peritonitis Prevention and Feline Coronavirus Control

The key to prevention of FIP is to prevent FCoV infection. FCoV infection is perpetuated by a cycle of infection, virus shedding, development of immune response, loss of humoral immunity, and reinfection. In breeding catteries and ordinary pet households, control has been affected by excellent hygiene and by separating immunofluorescent antibody test (IFAT) seropositive and seronegative cats. Cats are tested every 3 to 6 months, and as their antibody titer falls they are put into a seronegative group, which is kept isolated from the seropositive group. Detection of virus is less useful, since cats can shed FCoV intermittently (see following paragraphs). The fewer cats in the cattery (or household), the better the chance of eliminating FCoV. Once a cattery is free of FCoV, all new cats should be antibody-tested negative before introduction.

Cat breeders should antibody test their cats for FCoV annually and only mate positive cats with other positive cats and negative cats with negative cats. Kittens of positive-to-positive cat matings can be prevented from becoming infected by early weaning and isolation.

FCoV is only shed transiently (a few days) in the saliva of a minority of cats. The main source of virus is the feces, and infection is by accidental ingestion of particulate feces (e.g., from grooming paws after using a litter tray or from airborne particles from a litter tray contaminating food). FCoV is a fragile virus, surviving only days outdoors, but it can survive indoors up to 7 weeks in dried feces in cat litter particles. See Chapter 285 and Box 286-1 for recommendations on minimizing exposure to FCoV. FCoV does not generally cross the placenta.

Vaccination

Experimental FIP vaccines have been plagued with the problem of inducing antibody-dependent enhanced disease (i.e., in which vaccinated cats are more likely to die of FIP than unvaccinated cats), and only a single FIP vaccine, Primucell (Pfizer) is commercially available. Primucell is a temperature-sensitive mutant that is instilled intranasally and gives rise to local immunoglobulin A and cell-mediated immunity. Primucell prevents FIP in 50% to 75% of cats that would have otherwise developed it but is ineffective in cats

---

Box **286-1**

Protocol for Minimizing Feline Coronavirus Introduction or Spread in a Cattery*

A. Reduce the numbers of cats in any area.
- Ordinary house owners should keep no more than 6 to 10 cats.
- Cats should be kept in stable groups of up to three or four.
- In rescue facilities cats should be kept singly.
- In an FCoV eradication program cats should be kept in small groups according to their antibody or virus excretion status.
  - Antibody- or virus-negative cats together
  - Antibody- or virus-positive cats together

B. Avoid introducing virus to uninfected cats: antibody or virus testing.
- Incumbent cats should be tested before introducing new cats or breeding.
- Only antibody- or virus-negative cats should be introduced into FCoV-free catteries.
- It is safer to introduce antibody-positive cats than antibody-negative cats into FCoV-infected households, but there is still a risk of FIP in both the newcomer and the incumbent cats.

C. Prevent kitten infection: early weaning and isolation.
- Both cat breeders and rescuers of pregnant cats should follow the protocol outlined in Table 286-2.

D. Reduce fecal contamination of the environment.
- Have adequate numbers of litter trays—at least one tray per cat.
- Litter trays should be declumped at least daily.
- Choose a nontracking cat litter.
- Remove all litter and disinfect litter tray at least once a week.
- Place litter trays away from the food area.
- Vacuum around litter trays regularly.
- Clip fur off hindquarters of long-haired cats.

E. Vaccinate with Primucell.
- If new cats must be introduced into a household with endemic infection, they should receive a full course of Primucell vaccine before introduction.
- When economically possible, rescue catteries should vaccinate all new cats with Primucell.

FCoV, Feline coronavirus.
*Based on recommendations from working groups of the international feline enteric coronavirus and feline infectious peritonitis workshop. (From Pedersen NC, Addie D, Wolf A: Recommendations from working groups of the international feline enteric coronavirus and feline infectious peritonitis workshop, *Feline Pract* 23:108, 1995.)

---

previously exposed to FCoV. Thus in catteries wherein FCoV is endemic (most cat breeders' catteries), Primucell must be used in kittens that have already undergone a special management procedure known as early weaning and isolation so they are FCoV free when vaccinated. In addition, we know that Primucell vaccination does not prevent a cat from shedding FCoV (Addie, unpublished observations).

Feline Coronavirus Prevention in Kittens

Kittens are protected from FCoV infection by MDA, which wanes at around 5 to 6 weeks. This discovery has enabled the breeding of uninfected kittens even in households in which FCoV is endemic and the queen is infected. Essentially the queen is isolated before giving birth in a single room or pen that has been well cleaned. The queen and litter are maintained in isolation with barrier nursing until the kittens are 5 to 6 weeks of age, when the queen is removed and the room thoroughly cleaned again. New clean litter trays are introduced. Detailed information about early weaning and isolation for owners is available on the Internet (www.catvirus.com), and a summary is given in Box 286-2.

Feline Coronavirus Tests

For control of FCoV to work, use of a reliable antibody test is essential. Samples split and sent to five different laboratories in the United States gave five completely different results (Postorino-Reeves, personal communication). The IFAT is the gold standard, but there is a risk of false positive results if antinuclear antibodies are present. IFA gives an antibody titer that is useful for comparison in sequential testing and should contain an internal negative control at each dilution.

RT-PCR detects the RNA of the FCoV. Detection of FCoV RNA in the blood or feces is not diagnostic of FIP, since many healthy animals or animals with non-FIP illness are also positive. Fecal RT-PCR is most useful in FCoV control as part of a series of tests; a single negative or positive test is usually meaningless. Determination of carrier cats requires nine monthly consecutive positive fecal RT-PCR tests (this may change as quantitative RT-PCR becomes more widely available). Determination that a cat has eliminated FCoV infection requires five consecutive negative fecal RT-PCR tests or the return of the cat's antibody titer to less than 10.

Prevention of the Seropositive Cat From Developing Feline Infectious Peritonitis

Approximately 1 cat in 10 infected with FCoV develops FIP. Cats that have FCoV antibodies should not be stressed if at all possible (e.g., they should not be rehomed; neutering or any other operation that is not lifesaving should be delayed). If the owner has to leave the seropositive cat, having a "cat sitter" look after the cats in their own home is preferable to putting the cats into a cattery.

FELINE PARVOVIRUS, FELINE PANLEUKOPENIA, FELINE INFECTIOUS ENTERITIS, CANINE PARVOVIRUS

It is tempting to assume that feline parvovirus (FPV) (feline panleukopenia, feline infectious enteritis) is an infection of the past that has been more or less eradicated by vaccination. However, outbreaks are still ubiquitous wherever there are groups of susceptible cats and often manifest as sudden death or acute illness. FPV is the major cause of death of kittens under 4 months of age in rescue and breeding catteries and pet shops in the United Kingdom (Cave et al, 2002).

Unlike FPV, which has been recognized in cats for at least 100 years, canine parvovirus (CPV) type 2 emerged suddenly in the 1970s. CPV2 was subsequently replaced by antigenically variant viruses (CPV2a and CPV2b), which now coexist in dog populations worldwide. CPV2 isolates did not replicate in cats, but both CPV2a and CPV2b will. In a Japanese study about 10% of the virus isolates from cats with feline enteritis were found to be CPV2a or CPV2b. A third strain, CPV2c, isolated from leopard cats, can also infect domestic cats. Surprisingly, only 30% of parvoviruses from cheetahs and other large cats in zoos were FPV; the others were CPV.

Parvovirus is shed in feces but is also present in other secretions and can survive up to a year in the environment. Transmission of parvoviruses is mainly indirect; transplacental transmission also occurs. Despite the good acceptance of excellent vaccines by the cat-owning community, parvovirus manages to avoid extinction by subclinically infecting susceptible cats and kittens in whom it replicates. These cats shed huge amounts of viral particles for a few days to possibly weeks so that the environment becomes recontaminated. The virus can be transported on shoes or in cats' baskets to contaminate new environments so that even cats kept permanently indoors are not safe from infection. Thus cats in all types of catteries should be vaccinated. Live vaccines should not be used in pregnant queens because the virus can infect unborn kittens.

Attenuated live and inactivated vaccines are available against FPV and protect against both FPV and CPV2a, CPV2b, and CPV2c, but protection of inactivated vaccines is weaker against CPV types than against FPV. Most

---

Box 286-2

Protocol for Prevention of Feline Coronavirus Infection in Kittens

- Prepare kitten room
  - Remove all cats and kittens 1 week before introducing queen.
  - Disinfect room as far as possible using 1:32 dilution of sodium hypochlorite.
  - Dedicate litter trays, food and water bowls to this room and disinfect with sodium hypochlorite.
  - Introduce queen 1-2 weeks before she is due to give birth.
- Practice barrier nursing
  - Deal with the kitten room before tending other cats.
  - Clean hands with disinfectant before going into kitten room.
  - Have shoes and coveralls dedicated to the kitten room.
- Wean and isolate kittens early
  - Test queen for FCoV antibodies either before or after kittening.
  - If queen's antibody titer is greater than zero, the kittens should be removed to another clean room when they are 5-6 weeks old.
  - If the queen has an antibody titer of zero, she can remain with the kittens until they are older.
  - Take care to socialize isolated kittens to accustom them to humans during the 2-7–week-old period.
- Test kittens
  - Test kittens for FCoV antibodies at over 10 weeks of age.

FCoV, Feline coronavirus.

manufacturers recommend vaccination from 8 weeks of age onward, with a second dose at 12 weeks. A booster at 1 year of age is essential to cover cats in which the initial course was ineffective because of the presence of MDA.

MDA can persist until almost 20 weeks of age in kittens, particularly in those born to naturally exposed mothers who have very high antibody titers that interfere with vaccination and leave apparently vaccinated kittens susceptible to FPV. This is a problem in breeding catteries. Annual boosters are recommended by the manufacturer, but other than the first year, vaccination may not be absolutely necessary. There is evidence to suggest that immunity may persist; nine cats that were vaccinated with an inactivated FPV vaccine, kept in isolation, and given no boosters were challenged 7.5 years later and all still appeared to be immune (Scott and Geissinger, 1999).

When colostrum is not available, vaccination of newborn kittens is possible, and neutralizing antibodies appear at 7 to 12 days of age, indicating protection. However, live vaccines should not be used in kittens under 4 weeks of age or in pregnant queens because of the risk of cerebellar hypoplasia. Since FPV may only be shed for a matter of hours (sometimes as little as 36 hours), detection of the virus itself in cat feces is of limited value, and direct detection of FPV in the environment is currently not possible. Antibody testing of the sick cat can be more useful than detection of the virus itself. Antibodies to FPV can be detected by hemagglutination inhibition and enzyme-linked immunosorbent assay tests. For postmortem diagnosis of FPV, three 1-cm sections of different levels of the small intestine (duodenum, jejunum, and ileum) in 10% formol saline should be sent to a laboratory for histopathologic examination.

Advice for Rescue and Breeding Catteries and Pet Shops

Once parvovirus has occurred on the premises, the virus can be present for at least a year. Disinfection is difficult, with parvovirus resisting many disinfectants. Parvovirus is killed by sodium hypochlorite (domestic bleach). Disinfection with sodium hypochlorite (diluted 1:32) can reduce virus dose but will not eliminate the virus from soft furnishings. Since bleach is inactivated by organic material, thorough cleaning beforehand is vital for the success of disinfection. It is important to realize that infection is maintained in premises by subclinical infection of susceptible animals that become infected, produce huge amounts of virus, and then recover. Therefore susceptible animals are at risk if introduced within a year, and any new animals should have had a full course of vaccination, completed at least a week before being introduced.

To establish whether a cattery has parvovirus, some of the breeding animals should be tested for antibodies.

Antibody titers will be much higher in naturally exposed cats than in vaccinated cats. One option to prevent parvovirus is to stop breeding for a year so that no susceptible kittens are introduced.

Kittens are protected from parvovirus by MDA. The time over which antibody wanes can be calculated by halving the mother's antibody titer every 9.5 days of the offspring's life (97% of the queen's titer is found in the kitten). Thus if a queen had an antibody titer of 1024, at 9.5 days old the kitten's titer would be approximately 512, at 19 days 256, at 28.5 days 128, and so on (providing the kitten had suckled colostrum adequately). In this example, the kitten's titer would be 32 at 47.5 days. Thus the kitten should be rehomed to a parvovirus-free environment at that stage and vaccinated when its antibody titer has fallen to less than 10. Further vaccination of adult breeding stock is often pointless since many cats have a very high naturally acquired immunity, but it may be useful to screen all the breeding stock for antibodies and boost any cats that have very low antibody titers using a live vaccine (or inactivated vaccine if the cat is pregnant).

References and Suggested Reading

Cave TA et al: Kitten mortality in the United Kingdom: a retrospective analysis of 274 histopathological examinations (1986-2000), *Vet Rec* 151:497, 2002.

Chandler EA, Gaskell CJ, Gaskell RM, editors: *Feline medicine and therapeutics,* Oxford, Blackwell Science.

Coyne KP et al: Lethal outbreak of disease associated with feline calicivirus infection in cats, *Vet Rec* 158:544, 2006.

Green CE, editor: *Infectious diseases of the dog and cat,* ed 3, Philadelphia, 2006, Saunders.

Maggs DJ: Update on the diagnosis and management of feline herpesvirus-1 infection. In August JR, editor: *Consultations in feline internal medicine,* vol 4, Philadelphia, 2001, Saunders, p 51.

Pesavento PA et al: Pathologic, immunohistochemical, and electron microscopic findings in naturally occurring virulent systemic feline calicivirus infection in cats, *Vet Pathol* 41:257, 2004.

Radford AD et al: Quasispecies evolution of a hypervariable region of the feline calicivirus capsid gene in cell culture and in persistently infected cats, *J Gen Virol* 79:1, 1998.

Radford AD et al: Feline calicivirus, *Vet Res* 38:319, 2007.

Scott FW, Geissinger CM: Long-term immunity in cats vaccinated with an inactivated trivalent vaccine, *Am J Vet Res* 60:652, 1999. Published erratum appears in *Am J Vet Res* 60:763, 1999. Available at http://www.catvirus.com for FCoV.

Websites

Addie DD: www.catvirus.com
www.sheltermedicine.com

APPENDIX I

Table of Common Drugs: Approximate Dosages

MARK G. PAPICH, *Consulting Editor*

Drug Name	Other Names	Formulations Available	Dosage
Acepromazine	PromAce and many generic brands	5-, 10-, and 25-mg tablets and 10-mg/ml injection	Dog: 0.02-0.1 mg/kg IM, SC, IV; 0.56-2.25 mg/kg PO q6-8hr Cat: 0.02-0.1 mg/kg IM, SC, IV; or 1-2 mg/kg PO q8-12hr
Acetaminophen	Tylenol and many generic brands	120-, 160-, 325-, and 500-mg tablets	Dog: 15 mg/kg PO q8hr Cat: Not recommended
Acetaminophen with codeine	Tylenol with codeine and many generic brands	Oral solution and tablets. Many forms (e.g., 300 mg acetaminophen plus either 15, 30, or 60 mg codeine)	Follow dosing recommendations for codeine
Acetazolamide	Diamox	125- and 250-mg tablets	5-10 mg/kg PO q8-12hr (glaucoma) 4-8 mg/kg PO q8-12hr (other diuretic uses)
Acetylcysteine	Mucomyst	20% solution	Antidote: 140 mg/kg (loading dose) then 70 mg/kg IV or PO q4hr for five doses Eye: 2% solution topically q2hr
Acetylsalicylic acid	*See* Aspirin		
ACTH	*See* Corticotropin		
Activated charcoal	*See* Charcoal, activated		
Adequan	*See* Polysulfated glycosaminoglycan (PSGAG)		
Albendazole	Valbazen	113.6-mg/ml suspension and 300-mg/ml paste	25-50 mg/kg PO q12hr for 3 days For *Giardia* use 25 mg/kg q12hr for 2 days
Albuterol	Proventil or Ventolin	2-, 4-, and 5-mg tablets; 2 mg/5 ml syrup	20-50 mcg/kg q6-8hr; up to maximum of 100 mcg/kg q6-8hr PO
Allopurinol	Lopurin, Zyloprim	100- and 300-mg tablets	10 mg/kg q8hr, then reduce to 10 mg/kg q24hr
Aluminum carbonate gel	Basalgel	Capsule (equivalent to 500 mg aluminum hydroxide)	10-30 mg/kg PO q8hr (with meals)
Aluminum hydroxide gel	Amphojel	64-mg/ml oral suspension; 600-mg tablet	10-30 mg/kg PO q8hr (with meals)
Amikacin	Amiglyde-V (veterinary) and Amikin (human)	50- and 250-mg/ml injection	Dog: 15-30 mg/kg IV, SC, IM q24hr Cat: 10-14 mg/kg IV, SC, IM q24hr
Amiodarone	Cordarone	200-mg tablets; 50-mg/ml injection	Dog: Start with 15-mg/kg loading dose, then 10 mg/kg/day thereafter
Aminopentamide	Centrine	0.2-mg tablet; 0.5-mg/ml injection	Dog: 0.01-0.03 mg/kg IM, SC, PO q8-12hr Cat: 0.1 mg/cat IM, SC, PO q8-12hr

Drug Name	Other Names	Formulations Available	Dosage
Aminophylline	Many (generic) (Theophylline is preferred for oral therapy)	100- and 200-mg tablets; 25-mg/ml injection	Dog: 10 mg/kg PO, IM, IV q8hr Cat: 6.6 mg/kg PO q12hr
6-Aminosalicylic acid	See Mesalamine, Olsalazine		
Amitraz	Mitaban	10.6-ml concentrated dip (19.9%)	10.6 ml per 7.5 L water (0.025% solution). Apply three to six topical treatments q2wk. For refractory cases, this dose has been exceeded to produce increased efficacy. Doses that have been used include 0.025%, 0.05%, and 0.1% concentration applied twice per week and 0.125% solution applied to one-half body every day for 4 weeks to 5 months.
Amitriptyline	Elavil	10-, 25-, 50-, 75-, 100-, and 150-mg tablets; 10-mg/ml injection	Dog: 1-2 mg/kg PO q12-24hr (range: 0.25-4 mg/kg q12-24hr) Cat: 2-4 mg/cat/day PO; for cystitis: 2 mg/kg/day (2.5-7.5 mg/cat/day)
Amlodipine besylate	Norvasc	2.5-, 5-, and 10-mg tablets	Dog: 2.5 mg/dog or 0.1 mg/kg PO once daily Cat: 0.625 mg/cat/day PO initially and increase if needed to 1.25 mg/cat/day (average is 0.18 mg/kg)
Ammonium chloride	Generic	Available as crystals	Dog: 100 mg/kg PO q12hr Cat: 800 mg/cat (approximately ⅓ to ¼ tsp) mixed with food daily
Amoxicillin trihydrate	Amoxi-Tabs, Amoxi-drops, Amoxil, and others	50-, 100-, 200-, and 400-mg tablets; 50-mg/ml oral suspension	6.6-20 mg/kg PO q8-12hr
Amoxicillin/clavulanic acid	Clavamox	62.5-, 125-, 250-, and 375-mg tablets; 62.5-mg/ml suspension	Dog: 12.5-25 mg/kg PO q12hr Cat: 62.5 mg/cat PO q12hr; consider administering these doses q8hr for gram-negative infections
Amphotericin B	Fungizone	50-mg injectable vial	0.5 mg/kg IV (slow infusion) q48hr, to a cumulative dose of 4-8 mg/kg
Amphotericin B (Liposomal)	Amphotec, Abelcet, AmBisome		Dog: 2-3 mg/kg IV 3 times/wk for 9-12 treatments for a cumulative dose of 24-27 mg/kg Cat: 1 mg/kg IV 3 times/wk for 12 treatments
Ampicillin	Omnipen, Principen, others	250-, and 500-mg capsules; 125-, 250-, and 500-mg vials of ampicillin sodium	10-20 mg/kg IV, IM, SC q6-8hr (ampicillin sodium) 20-40 mg/kg PO q8hr
Ampicillin + sulbactam	Unasyn	1.5- and 3-gm vials in 2:1 combination for injection	10-20 mg/kg IV, IM q8hr
Ampicillin trihydrate	Polyflex	10- and 25-mg vials for injection	Dog: 10-50 mg/kg SC, IM q24hr Cat: 10-20 mg/kg SC, IM q24hr
Amprolium	Amprol, Corid	9.6% (9.6 gm/dl) oral solution; soluble powder	1.25 gm of 20% amprolium powder to daily feed, or 30 ml of 9.6% amprolium solution to 3.8 L of drinking water for 7 days
Antacid drugs	See Aluminum hydroxide gel, Magnesium hydroxide, and Calcium carbonate		
Apomorphine hydrochloride	Generic	6-mg tablet	0.44 mg/kg IM; 0.05 mg/kg IV; 0.1 mg/kg SC, or instill 0.25 mg in conjunctiva of eye (dissolve 6-mg tablet in 1-2 ml of saline)
Ascorbic acid	Vitamin C	Various forms	100-500 mg/animal/day (diet supplement) or 100 mg/animal q8hr (urine acidification)

Continued

Appendix I—cont'd

Drug Name	Other Names	Formulations Available	Dosage
L-Asparaginase	Elspar	10,000 U per vial for injection	400 U/kg IV, IP, IM weekly; or 10,000 U/m^2 weekly for 3 wk
Aspirin	Many generic and brand names (Bufferin, Ascriptin)	81-mg and 325-mg tablets	Dog: Mild analgesia: 10 mg/kg q12hr Antiinflammatory: 20-25 mg/kg q12hr Antiplatelet: 5-10 mg/kg q24-48hr Cat: 81 mg q48hr PO
Atenolol	Tenormin	25-, 50-, and 100-mg tablets; 25-mg/ml oral suspension; and 0.5-mg/ml ampule for injection	Dog: 6.25-12.5 mg/dog q12hr (or 0.25-1.0 mg/kg q12-24hr) PO Cat: 6.25-12.5 mg/cat q12hr (approximately 3 mg/kg) PO
Atipamezole	Antisedan	5-mg/ml injection	Inject same volume as used for medetomidine
Atracurium	Tracrium	10-mg/ml injection	0.2 mg/kg IV initially, then 0.15 mg/kg q30min (or IV infusion at 4-9 mcg/kg/min)
Atropine	Many generic brands	400-, 500-, and 540-mcg/ml injection; 15-mg/ml injection	0.02-0.04 mg/kg IV, IM, SC q6-8hr 0.2-0.5 mg/kg (as needed) for organophosphate and carbamate toxicosis
Auranofin (triethyl-phosphine gold)	Ridaura	3-mg capsule	0.1-0.2 mg/kg PO q12hr
Aurothioglucose	Solganol	50-mg/ml injection	Dog <10 kg: 1 mg IM first wk, 2 mg IM second wk, 1 mg/kg/wk maintenance Dog >10 kg: 5 mg IM first wk, 10 mg IM second wk, 1 mg/kg/wk maintenance Cat: 0.5-1 mg/cat IM q7 days
Azathioprine	Imuran	50-mg tablet; 10-mg/ml for injection	Dog: 2 mg/kg PO q24hr initially then 0.5-1 mg/kg q48hr Cat (use cautiously): 0.3 mg/kg PO q48hr
Azithromycin	Zithromax	250-mg capsule; and 250- and 600-mg tablets; 20-mg/ml oral suspension	Dog: 10 mg/kg PO q48hr or 3.3 mg/kg once daily Cat: 5-10 mg/kg PO every other day
AZT (azidothymidine)	See Zidovudine		
Bactrim (sulfamethoxazole + trimethoprim)	See Trimethoprim-sulfonamide combinations		
BAL	See Dimercaprol		
Benazepril	Lotensin	5-, 10-, 20-, and 40-mg tablets	Dog: 0.25-0.5 mg/kg PO q24hr Cat: 0.5-1 mg/kg q24hr PO or 2.5 mg/cat/day up to a maximum of 5 mg/cat/day
Betamethasone	Celestone	600-mcg (0.6-mg) tablet; 3-mg/ml sodium phosphate injection	0.1-0.2 mg/kg PO q12-24hr
Bethanechol	Urecholine	5-, 10-, 25-, and 50-mg tablets; 5-mg/ml injection	Dog: 5-15 mg/dog PO q8hr Cat: 1.25-5 mg/cat PO q8hr
Bisacodyl	Dulcolax	5-mg tablet	5 mg/animal PO q8-24hr
Bismuth subsalicylate	Pepto Bismol	Oral suspension: 262 mg/15 ml or 525 mg/ml in extra-strength formulation; 262-mg tablet	1-3 ml/kg/day (in divided doses) PO
Bleomycin	Blenoxane	15-U vials for injection	10 U/m^2 IV or SC for 3 days, then 10 U/m^2 weekly (maximum cumulative dose 200 U/m^2)
Bromide	See Potassium bromide		

Drug Name	Other Names	Formulations Available	Dosage
BSP (Bromsulphalein)	*See* Sulfobromophthalein (BSP)		
Budesonide	Enterocort	3-mg capsule	Dog, cat: 0.125 mg/kg q6-8hr PO; dose interval may be increased to every 12 hr when condition improves
Bunamidine hydrochloride	Scolaban	400-mg tablet	20-50 mg/kg PO
Bupivacaine	Marcaine and generic	2.5- and 5-mg/ml solution injection	1 ml of 0.5% solution per 10 cm for an epidural
Buprenorphine	Temgesic (Vetergesic in the UK)	0.3-mg/ml solution	Dog: 0.006-0.02 mg/kg IV, IM, SC q4-8hr Cat: 0.005-0.01 mg/kg IV, IM q4-8hr Buccal administration in cats: 0.01-0.02 mg/kg q12hr
Buspirone	BuSpar	5- and 10-mg tablets	Dog: 2.5-10 mg/dog PO q12-24hr; or 1 mg/kg q12hr PO Cat: 2.5-5 mg/cat PO q24hr (may be increased to 5-7.5 mg/cat twice daily for some cats)
Busulfan	Myleran	2-mg tablet	3-4 mg/m² PO q24hr
Butorphanol	Torbutrol Torbugesic	1-, 5-, and 10-mg tablets; 0.5- or 10-mg/ml injection	Dog: Antitussive: 0.055 mg/kg SC q6-12hr or 0.55 mg/kg PO Preanesthetic: 0.2-0.4 mg/kg IV, IM, SC (with acepromazine) Analgesic: 0.2-0.4 mg/kg IV, IM, SC q2-4hr or 0.55-1.1 mg/kg PO q6-12hr Cat: Analgesic: 0.2-0.8 mg/kg IV, SC q2-6hr, or 1.5 mg/kg PO q4-8hr
Calcitriol	Rocaltrol, Calcijex	Available as injection (Calcijex) and capsules (Rocaltrol): 0.25- and 0.5-mcg capsules; 1- or 2-mcg/ml injection	Dog: 0.25-0.5 mcg/dog/day or approx. 0.12 mg/kg Cat: 0.25 mcg/cat every other day; or 0.01-0.04 mcg/kg/day
Calcium carbonate	Many brands available: Titralac, Tums, generic	Many tablets or oral suspension (e.g., 650-mg tablet contains 260 mg calcium ion)	For phosphate binder: 60-100 mg/kg/day in divided doses PO For calcium supplementation: 70-180 mg/kg/day added to food
Calcium chloride	Generic	10% (100 mg/ml) solution	0.1-0.3 ml/kg IV (slowly)
Calcium citrate	Citracal (OTC)	950-mg tablet (contains 200 mg calcium ion)	Dog: 20 mg/kg/day added to food Cat: 10-30 mg/kg PO q8hr (with meals)
Calcium disodium EDTA	*See* Edetae calcium disodium		
Calcium gluconate	Kalcinate and generic	10% (100 mg/ml) injection	0.5-1.5 ml/kg IV (slowly)
Calcium lactate	Generic	OTC tablet	Dog: 0.5-2.0 gm/dog/day PO (in divided doses) Cat: 0.2-0.5 gm/cat/day PO (in divided doses)
Captopril	Capoten	25-mg tablet	Dog: 0.5-2 mg/kg PO q8-12hr Cat: 3.12-6.25 mg/cat PO q8hr
Carbenicillin	Geopen, Pyopen	1-, 2-, 5-, 10-, and 30-gm vials for injection	40-50 mg/kg and up to 100 mg/kg IV, IM, SC q6-8hr
Carbenicillin indanyl sodium	Geocillin	500-mg tablet	10 mg/kg PO q8hr
Carbimazole	Neo-mercazole	Available in Europe	Cat: 5 mg/cat PO q8hr (induction), followed by 5 mg/cat PO q12hr
Carboplatin	Paraplatin	50- and 150-mg vial for injection	Dog: 300 mg/m² IV q3-4wk Cat: 200 mg/m² IV q4wk

Continued

Appendix I—cont'd

Drug Name	Other Names	Formulations Available	Dosage
Carprofen	Rimadyl (Zinecarp in the UK) Novox (generic)	25-, 75-, and 100-mg tablets 50 mg/ml solution	Dog: 2.2 mg/kg PO q12hr; or 4.4 mg/kg once daily PO; 2.2 mg/kg q12hr or 4.4 mg/kg once daily SC Cat: Doses not available
Carvedilol	Coreg	3.125-, 6.25-, 12.5-, and 25-mg tablets	Dog: 0.2 to 0.4 mg/kg q12hr PO; titrate dose up to 1.5 mg/kg q12hr PO if needed
Cascara sagrada	Many brands (e.g., Nature's Remedy)	100- and 325-mg tablets	Dog: 1-5 mg/kg day PO Cat: 1-2 mg/cat/day
Castor oil	Generic	Oral liquid (100%)	Dog: 8-30 ml/day PO Cat: 4-10 ml/day PO
Cefadroxil	Cefa-Tabs, Cefa-Drops	50-mg/ml oral suspension; 50-, 100-, 200-, and 1000-mg tablets	Dog: 22-30 mg/kg PO q12hr Cat: 22 mg/kg PO q24hr
Cefazolin sodium	Ancef, Kefzol, and generic	50 and 100 mg/50 ml for injection	20-35 mg/kg IV, IM q8hr For perisurgical use: 22 mg/kg q2hr during surgery
Cefdinir	Omnicef	300-mg capsules; 25-mg/ml oral suspension	Dose not established (human dose is 7 mg/kg PO q12hr)
Cefixime	Suprax	20-mg/ml oral suspension and 200- and 400-mg tablets	10 mg/kg PO q12hr For cystitis: 5 mg/kg PO q12-24hr
Cefotaxime	Claforan	500-mg and 1-, 2-, and 10-gm vials for injection	Dog: 50 mg/kg IV, IM, SC q12hr Cat: 20-80 mg/kg IV, IM q6hr
Cefotetan	Cefotan	1-, 2-, and 10-gm vials for injection	30 mg/kg IV, SC q8hr
Cefovecin	Convenia	80 mg/ml injection	Dog, cat: 8 mg/kg SC once every 14 days
Cefoxitin sodium	Mefoxin	1-, 2-, and 10-gm vials for injection	30 mg/kg IV q6-8hr
Cefpodoxime proxetil	Simplicef	100- and 200-mg tablets; 10- or 20-mg/ml human label suspension	Dog: 5-10 mg/kg PO once daily Cat: Dose not established
Ceftazidime	Fortaz, Ceptaz, Tazicef	0.5-, 1-, 2- and 6-gm vials reconstituted to 280 mg/ml	30 mg/kg IV, IM q6hr
Ceftiofur	Naxcel (ceftiofur sodium); Excenel (ceftiofur HCl)	50-mg/ml injection	2.2-4.4 mg/kg SC q24hr (for urinary tract infections)
Cephalexin	Keflex and generic forms	250- and 500-mg capsules; 250- and 500-mg tablets; 100-mg/ml or 125- and 250-mg/5-ml oral suspension	10-30 mg/kg PO q6-12hr; for pyoderma, 22-35 mg/kg PO q12hr
Cetirizine	Zyrtec	1-mg/ml oral syrup; 5- and 10-mg tablets	Dog: 5-10 mg/dog q12hr, PO, up to a dose of 2 mg/kg q12hr, PO Cat: 5 mg/cat, PO, q24hr
Charcoal, activated	ActaChar, Charcodote, Toxiban, generic	Oral suspension	1-4 gm/kg PO (granules) 6-12 ml/kg (suspension)
Chlorambucil	Leukeran	2-mg tablet	Dog: 2-6 mg/m^2 or 0.1-0.2 mg/kg PO q24hr initially, then q48hr Cat: 0.1-0.2 mg/kg q24hr initially, then q48hr PO
Chloramphenicol and chloramphenicol palmitate	Chloromycetin, generic forms	30-mg/ml oral suspension (palmitate); 250-mg capsule; and 100-, 250-, and 500-mg tablets	Dog: 40-50 mg/kg PO q8hr Cat: 12.5-20 mg/kg PO q12hr
Chlorothiazide	Diuril	250- and 500-mg tablets; 50-mg/ml oral suspension and injection	20-40 mg/kg PO q12hr or IV
Chlorpheniramine maleate	Chlor-Trimeton, Phenetron, and others	4- and 8-mg tablets	Dog: 4-8 mg/dog PO q12hr (up to a maximum of 0.5 mg/kg q12hr) Cat: 2 mg/cat PO q12hr
Chlorpromazine	Thorazine	25-mg/ml injection solution	Dog: 0.5 mg/kg IM, SC q6-8hr (before cancer chemotherapy administer 2 mg/kg SC q3hr) Cat: 0.2-0.4 mg/kg q6-8hr IM, SC

Drug Name	Other Names	Formulations Available	Dosage
Chorionic gonadotropin	*See* Gonadotropin		
Cimetidine	Tagamet (OTC and prescription)	100-, 150-, 200-, and 300-mg tablets and 60-mg/ml injection	10 mg/kg IV, IM, PO q6-8hr (in renal failure administer 2.5-5 mg/kg IV, PO q12hr)
Ciprofloxacin	Cipro and generic	250-, 500-, and 750-mg tablets; 2-mg/ml injection	Dog: 10-20 mg/kg PO, IV q24hr Cat: Not recommended
Cisapride	Must be compounded		Dog: 0.1-0.5 mg/kg PO q8-12hr (doses as high as 0.5-1.0 mg/kg have been used in some dogs) Cat: 2.5-5 mg/cat PO q8-12hr (as high as 1 mg/kg q8hr has been administered to cats)
Cisplatin	Platinol	1-mg/ml injection; 50-mg vials	Dog: 60-70 mg/m^2 q3-4wk (administer fluid for diuresis with therapy) Cat: Not recommended
Clavamox	*See* Amoxicillin-clavulanic acid combination		
Clavulanic acid	*See* Amoxicillin-clavulanic acid combination		
Clemastine	Tavist, Contac 12-hr allergy, and generic	1.34-mg tablet (OTC); 2.64-mg tablet (Rx); 0.134-mg/ml syrup	Dog: 0.05-0.1 mg/kg PO q12hr
Clindamycin	Antirobe, Cleocin, and generic	Oral liquid 25-mg/ml; 25-, 75-, 150-, and 300-mg capsule; and 150-mg/ml injection (Cleocin)	Dog: 11-33 mg/kg q12hr PO; for oral and soft tissue infection: 5.5-33 mg/kg q12hr PO Cat: 11-33 mg/kg q24hr PO for skin and anaerobic infections Toxoplasmosis: 12.5-25 mg/kg PO q12hr for 4 wks
Clofazimine	Lamprene	50- and 100-mg capsules	Cat: 1 mg/kg PO up to a maximum of 4 mg/kg/day
Clomipramine	Anafranil (human label); Clomicalm (veterinary label)	10-, 25-, and 50-mg tablets (human) 5-, 20-, and 80-mg tablets (veterinary)	Dog: 1-2 mg/kg PO q12hr up to a maximum of 3 mg/kg PO q12hr Cat: 1-5 mg/cat PO q12-24hr
Clonazepam	Klonopin	0.5-, 1-, and 2-mg tablets	Dog: 0.5 mg/kg PO q8-12hr Cat: 0.1-0.2 mg/kg q12-24hr PO
Clopidogrel	Plavix	75-mg tablets	Dog: 2-4 mg/kg q24hr PO; give oral loading dose of 10 mg/kg Cat: 19 mg per cat (¼ tablet) q24hr PO
Clorazepate	Tranxene	3.75-, 7.5-, 11.25-, 15-, and 22.5-mg, tablets	Dog: 2 mg/kg PO q12hr Cat: 0.2-0.4 mg/kg q12-24hr PO (up to 0.5-2 mg/kg)
Cloxacillin	Cloxapen, Orbenin, Tegopen	250- and 500-mg capsules; 25-mg/ml oral solution	20-40 mg/kg PO q8hr
Codeine	Generic	15-, 30-, and 60-mg tablets; 5-mg/ml syrup; 3-mg/ml oral solution	Analgesia: 0.5-1 mg/kg PO q4-6hr Antitussive: 0.1-0.3 mg/kg PO q4-6hr
Colchicine	Generic	500- and 600-mcg tablets; 500-mcg/ml ampule injection	0.01-0.03 mg/kg PO q24hr
Colony-stimulating factor	Sargramostim (Leukine) and Filgrastim (Neupogen)	300 mcg/ml (Neupogen) and 250 or 500 mcg/ml (Leukine)	Leukine: 0.25 mg/m^2 q12hr SC or IV infusion Neupogen: 0.005 mg/kg (5 mcg/kg) q24hr SC for 2wk
Corticotropin (ACTH)	Acthar	Gel 80 U/ml	Response test: Collect pre-ACTH sample and inject 2.2 IU/kg IM; collect post-ACTH sample in 2 hr in dogs and at 1 and 2 hr in cats

Continued

Appendix I—cont'd

Drug Name	Other Names	Formulations Available	Dosage
Cosequin	*See* Glucosamine chondroitin sulfate		
Cosyntropin	Cortrosyn	250 mcg per vial (can be stored in freezer for 6 months)	Response test: Dog: Collect pre-ACTH sample and inject 5 mcg/kg IV or IM and collect sample at 30 and 60 min Cat: 0.125 mg IV or IM and collect sample at 30 min and 60 min after IV administration and 30 and 60 min after IM administration
Cyanocobalamin (vitamin B_{12})	Many	100-mcg/ml injection	Dog: 100-200 mcg/day PO Cat: 50-100 mcg/day PO
Cyclophosphamide	Cytoxan, Neosar	25-mg/ml injection; 25- and 50-mg tablets	Dog: Anticancer: 50 mg/m² PO once daily 4 days/wk or 150-300 mg/m² IV and repeat in 21 days Immunosuppressive therapy: 50 mg/m² (approx. 2.2 mg/kg) PO q48hr or 2.2 mg/kg once daily for 4 days/wk Cat: 6.25-12.5 mg/cat once daily 4 days/wk
Cyclosporine (cyclosporin A)	Atopica, Neoral, Optimmune (ophthalmic)	Atopica: 10-, 25-, 50-, and 100-mg capsules Neoral: 25-mg and 100-mg microemulsion capsules; 100-mg/ml oral solution (for microemulsion) Optimmune: 0.2% ointment	Dog: 3-7 mg/kg/day; for atopic dermatitis some dogs are controlled with q48hr dosing Cat: 5 mg/kg PO q24hr
Cyropheptadine	Periactin	4-mg tablet; 2-mg/5-ml syrup	Antihistamine: 1.1 mg/kg PO q8-12hr Appetite stimulant: 2 mg/cat PO
Cytarabine (cytosine arabinoside)	Cytosar-U	100-mg vial	Dog (lymphoma): 100 mg/m² IV, SC once daily or 50 mg/m² twice daily for 4 days Cat: 100 mg/m² once daily for 2 days
Dacarbazine	DTIC	200-mg vial for injection	200 mg/m² IV for 5 days q3wk; or 800-1000 mg/m² IV q3wk
Dalteparin	Fragmin	16 mg/0.2 ml; 32 mg/0.2 ml in prefilled syringes or 64 mg/ml multidose vials for injection	Dog: 100-150 units/kg q8hr SC Cat: 180 units/kg q6hr SC
Danazol	Danocrine	50-, 100-, and 200-mg capsules	5-10 mg/kg PO q12hr
Dantrolene	Dantrium	100-mg capsule and 0.33-mg/ml injection	For prevention of malignant hyperthermia: 2-3 mg/kg IV For muscle relaxation: Dog: 1-5 mg/kg PO q8hr Cat: 0.5-2 mg/kg PO q12hr
Dapsone	Generic	25- and 100-mg tablets	Dog: 1.1 mg/kg PO q8-12hr Cat: Do not use
Darbazine (prochlorperazine + isopropamide)	Darbazine	No. 1, 2, and 3 capsules	Dog, cat: 0.14-0.2 ml/kg SC q12hr Dog 2-7 kg: 1-#1 capsule PO q12hr Dog 7-14 kg: 1-#2 capsule PO q12hr Dog >14 kg: 1-#3 capsule PO q12hr
Deferoxamine	Desferal	500-mg vial for injection	10 mg/kg IV, IM q2hr for two doses; then 10 mg/kg q8hr for 24hr
Deprenyl (L-deprenyl)	*See* Selegiline (Anipryl)		
Deracoxib	Deramaxx	25-, 100-mg tablets	Dog: 3-4 mg/kg q24hr PO for 7 days; or 1-2 mg/kg q24hr PO for long-term use Cat: Dose not established

Drug Name	Other Names	Formulations Available	Dosage
Desmopressin acetate	DDAVP	100-mcg/ml injection and desmopressin acetate nasal solution (0.01% metered spray); 0.1- and 0.2-mg tablets	Diabetes insipidus: 2-4 drops (2 mcg) q12-24hr intranasally or in eye Animal oral dose: 0.05-0.1 mg/dog q12hr PO initially, then increase to 0.1-0.2 mg/dog q12hr as needed von Willebrand's disease treatment: 1 mcg/kg (0.01 ml/kg) SC, IV, diluted in 20 ml of saline administered over 10 min
Desoxycorticosterone pivalate	Percorten-V, DOCP, or DOCA pivalate	25 mg/ml injection	1.5-2.2 mg/kg IM q25days
Dexamethasone (dexamethasone solution and dexamethasone sodium phosphate)	Azium solution in polyethylene glycol. Sodium phosphate forms include Dexaject SP, Dexavet, and Dexasone. Tablets include Decadron and generic	Azium solution, 2 mg/ml. Sodium phosphate forms are 3.33 mg/ml; 0.25-, 0.5-, 0.75-, 1-, 1.5-, 2-, 4-, and 6-mg tablets	Antiinflammatory: 0.07-0.15 mg/kg IV, IM, PO q12-24hr Dexamethasone suppression test: Dog: 0.01 mg/kg IV Cat: 0.1 mg/kg IV Collect sample at 0, 4, and 8 hr
Dexmedetomidine	Dexdomitor	0.5-mg/ml injectable solution	Dog: Sedative and analgesic: 375 mg/m² IV or 500 mg/m² IM Dog: Preanesthetic: 125 mg/m² IM Cat: Sedative and analgesic: 40 mcg/kg IM
Dextran	Dextran 70 Gentran-70	Injectable solution: 250, 500, and 1000 ml	10-20 ml/kg IV to effect
Dextromethorphan	Benylin and others	Available in syrup, capsule, and tablet; many OTC products	0.5-2 mg/kg PO q6-8hr has been reported, but effective dose not established
Dextrose solution 5%	D5W	Fluid solution for IV administration	40-50 ml/kg IV q24hr
Diazepam	Valium and generic	2- and 5-mg tablets; 5-mg/ml solution for injection	Preanesthetic: 0.5 mg/kg IV Status epilepticus: 0.5 mg/kg IV, 1.0 mg/kg rectal; repeat if necessary Appetite stimulant (cat): 0.2 mg/kg IV
Dichlorophen	Vermiplex (*See* Toluene)		
Dichlorphenamide	Daranide	50-mg tablet	3-5 mg/kg PO q8-12hr
Dichlorvos	Task	10- and 25-mg tablets	Dog: 26.4-33 mg/kg PO Cat: 11 mg/kg PO
Dicloxacillin	Dynapen	125-, 250-, and 500-mg capsules; 12.5-mg/ml oral suspension	25 mg/kg IM q6hr Oral doses not absorbed
Diethylcarbamazine (DEC)	Caricide, Filaribits	Chewable tablets; 50-, 60-, 180-, 200-, and 400-mg tablets	Heartworm prophylaxis: 6.6 mg/kg PO q24hr
Diethylstilbestrol (DES)	DES, generic (no longer manufactured in US)	1- and 5-mg tablet; 50-mg/ml injection	Dog: 0.1-1.0 mg/dog PO q24hr Cat: 0.05-0.1 mg/cat PO q24hr
Difloxacin	Dicural	11.4-, 45.4-, and 136-mg tablets	Dog: 5-10 mg/kg/day PO Cat: Safe dose not established
Digoxin	Lanoxin, Cardoxin	0.0625-, 0.125-, 0.25-mg tablets; 0.05- and 0.15-mg/ml elixir	Dog: <20 kg body weight: 0.01 mg/kg q12hr; >20 kg use 0.22 mg/m² PO q12hr (subtract 10% for elixir) Dog: (rapid digitalization): 0.0055- 0.011 mg/kg IV q1hr to effect Cat: 0.008-0.01 mg/kg PO q48hr (approximately ¼ of a 0.125-mg tablet/cat)
Dihydrotachysterol (vitamin D)	Hytakerol, DHT	0.125-mg tablet; 0.5-mg/ml oral liquid	0.01 mg/kg/day PO; for acute treatment administer 0.02 mg/kg initially, then 0.01-0.02 mg/kg PO q24-48hr thereafter

Continued

Appendix I—cont'd

Drug Name	Other Names	Formulations Available	Dosage
Diltiazem	Cardizem, Dilacor	30-, 60-, 90-, and 120-mg tablets; 50-mg/ml injection	Dog: 0.5-1.5 mg/kg PO q8hr, 0.25 mg/kg over 2 min IV (repeat if necessary) Cat: 1.75-2.4 mg/kg PO q8hr For Dilacor XR or Cardizem CD dose is 10 mg/kg PO once daily
Dimenhydrinate	Dramamine (Gravol in Canada)	50-mg tablets; 50-mg/ml injection	Dog: 4-8 mg/kg PO, IM, IV q8hr Cat: 12.5 mg/cat IV, IM, PO q8hr
Dimercaprol (BAL)	BAL in oil	Injection	4 mg/kg IM q4hr
Dinoprost tromethamine	*See* Prostaglandin F$_{2\alpha}$ 5-mg/ml injection		
Dioctyl calcium sulfosuccinate	*See* Docusate calcium		
Dioctyl sodium sulfosuccinate	*See* Docusate sodium		
Diphenhydramine	Benadryl	Available OTC: 2.5-mg/ml elixir; 25- and 50-mg capsules and tablets; 50-mg/ml injection	Dog: 25-50 mg/dog IV, IM, PO q8hr Cat: 2-4 mg/kg q6-8hr PO or 1 mg/kg IM, IV q6-8hr
Diphenoxylate	Lomotil	2.5 mg	Dog: 0.1-0.2 mg/kg PO q8-12hr Cat: 0.05-0.1 mg/kg PO q12hr
Diphenylhydantoin	*See* Phenytoin		
Diphosphonate disodium etidronate	*See* Etidronate disodium		
Dipyridamole	Persantine	25-, 50-, 75-mg tablets; 5-mg/ml injection	4-10 mg/kg PO q24hr
Dirlotapide	Slentrol	5-mg/ml oral oil-based solution	Dog: Start with 0.01 ml/kg/day PO Adjust by doubling the dose in 2 wks. Monthly adjustments to dose should be done on the basis of animal's weight loss. Do not exceed 0.2 ml/kg/day. Cat: Do not administer to cats
Disopyramide	Norpace (Rhythmodan in Canada)	100- and 150-mg capsules (10-mg/ml injection in Canada only)	6-15 mg/kg PO q8hr
Dithiazanine iodide	Dizan	10-, 50-, 100-, and 200-mg tablets	Heartworm: 6.6-11 mg/kg PO q24hr for 7-10 days For other parasites: 22 mg/kg PO
Divalproex sodium	*See* Valproic acid		
Dobutamine	Dobutrex	250-mg/20-ml vial for injection (12.5 mg/ml)	Dog: 5-20 mcg/kg/min IV infusion Cat: 2 mcg/kg/min IV infusion
Docusate calcium	Surfak, Doxidan	60-mg tablet (and many others)	Dog: 50-100 mg/dog PO q12-24hr Cat: 50 mg/cat PO q12-24hr
Docusate sodium	Colace, Doxan, Doss, many OTC brands	50-, and 100-mg capsules; 10-mg/ml liquid	Dog: 50-200 mg/dog PO q8-12hr Cat: 50 mg/cat PO q12-24hr
Dolasetron mesylate	Anzemet	50-, 100-mg tablets; 20-mg/ml injection	Dog, cat: Prevention of nausea and vomiting: 0.6 mg/kg IV or PO q24hr Treating vomiting and nausea: 1.0 mg/kg PO or IV once daily
Domperidone	Motilium	Not available in US	2-5 mg/animal PO
Dopamine	Intropin	40-, 80-, or 160-mg/ml	Dog, cat: 2-10 mcg/kg/min IV infusion
Doxapram	Dopram, Respiram	20-mg/ml injection	5-10 mg/kg IV Neonate: 1-5 mg SC, sublingual, or via umbilical vein

Drug Name	Other Names	Formulations Available	Dosage
Doxorubicin	Adriamycin	2-mg/ml injection	30 mg/m² IV q21 days or >20 kg use 30 mg/m² and <20 kg use 1 mg/kg Cat: 20 mg/m² or approximately 1-1.25 mg/kg IV q3wk
Doxycycline	Vibramycin and generic forms	10-mg/ml oral suspension; 100-mg injection vial; 50- or 100-mg tablets or capsules	3-5 mg/kg PO, IV q12hr or 10 mg/kg PO q24hr For *Rickettsia* in dogs: 5 mg/kg q12hr
Edetate calcium disodium (CaNa₂EDTA)	Calcium disodium versenate	20-mg/ml injection	25 mg/kg SC, IM, IV q6hr for 2-5 days
Edrophonium	Tensilon and others	10-mg/ml injection	Dog: 0.11-0.22 mg/kg IV Cat: 0.25-0.5 mg/cat (total dose) IV
Enalapril	Enacard, Vasotec	2.5-, 5-, 10-, and 20-mg tablets	Dog: 0.5 mg/kg PO q12-24hr Cat: 0.25-0.5 mg/kg PO q12-24hr
Enflurane	Ethrane	Available as solution for inhalation	Induction: 2%-3% Maintenance: 1.5%-3%
Enilconazole	Imaverol, Clina-Farm-EC	10% or 13.8% emulsion	Nasal aspergillosis: 10 mg/kg q12hr instilled into nasal sinus for 14 days (10% solution diluted 50/50 with water) Dermatophytes: Dilute 10% solution to 0.2% and wash lesion with solution four times at 3- to 4-day intervals
Enoxaparin	Lovenox	30 mg/0.3 ml, 40 mg/0.4 ml, 60 mg/0.6 ml, 80 mg/0.8 ml, and 100 mg/1 ml in prefilled syringes for injection	Dog: 0.8 mg/kg SC q6hr Cat: 1.25 mg/kg SC q6hr
Enrofloxacin	Baytril	68-, 22.7-, and 5.7-mg tablets. Taste Tabs are 22.7 and 68 mg; 22.7-mg/ml injection	Dog: 5-20 mg/kg/day PO, IM Cat: 5 mg/kg/day PO (do not exceed dose)
Ephedrine	Many, generic	25- and 50-mg/ml injection	Vasopressor: 0.75 mg/kg, IM, SC; repeat as needed
Epinephrine	Adrenaline and generic forms	1-mg/ml (1:1,000) injection solution	Cardiac arrest: 10-20 mcg/kg IV or 200 mcg/kg intratracheal (may be diluted in saline before administration) Anaphylactic shock: 2.5-5 mcg/kg IV or 50 mcg/kg intratracheal (may be diluted in saline)
Epoetin alpha (Erythropoietin) (r-HuEPO)	Epogen, epoetin alfa (r-HuEPO)	2000-U/ml injection	Doses range from 35 or 50 U/kg three times/wk to 400 U/kg/wk IV, SC (adjust dose to hematocrit of 0.30-0.34) Cat: Start with 100 units/kg three times/wk and adjust dose based on hematocrit
Epsiprantel	Cestex	Coated tablet	Dog: 5.5 mg/kg PO Cat: 2.75 mg/kg PO
Ergocalciferol (vitamin D₂)	Calciferol, Drisdol	400-U tablet (OTC); 50,000-U tablet (1.25 mg); 500,000-U/ml (12.5 mg/ml) injection	500-2000 U/kg/day PO
Erythromycin	Many brands and generic	250- or 500-mg capsule or tablet	Antibacterial dose: 10-20 mg/kg PO q8-12hr Prokinetic dose: 0.5-1.0 mg/kg PO q8hr

Continued

Appendix I—cont'd

Drug Name	Other Names	Formulations Available	Dosage
Esmolol	Brevibloc	10-mg/ml injection	500 mcg/kg IV, which may be given as 0.05-0.1 mg/kg slowly every 5 min or 50-200 mcg/kg/min infusion
Estradiol cypionate (ECP)	ECP, Depo-Estradiol, generic	2-mg/ml injection	Dog: 22-44 mcg/kg IM (total dose not to exceed 1.0 mg) Cat: 250 mcg/cat IM between 40 hr and 5 days of mating
Etidronate disodium	Didronel	200- and 400-mg tablets; 50-mg/ml injection	Dog: 5 mg/kg/day PO Cat: 10 mg/kg/day PO
Etodolac	EtoGesic, veterinary; Lodine, human	150- and 300-mg tablets	Dog: 10-15 mg/kg PO once daily Cat: Dose not established
Etretinate	Tegison	10- and 25-mg capsules	Dog: 1 mg/kg PO, with food/day or for <15 kg 10 mg/dog PO q24hr; >15 kg 10 mg/dog PO q12hr Cat: 2 mg/kg/day
Famotidine	Pepcid	10-mg tablet; 10-mg/ml injection	Dog: 0.1-0.2 mg/kg IM, SC, PO, IV q12hr; or 0.5 mg/kg PO q24hr, or 0.5 mg/kg IM, SC, PO, IV q24hr Cat: 0.2-0.25 mg/kg IM, IV, SC, PO q12-24hr
Felbamate	Felbatol	400- and 600-mg tablets; 120-mg/ml oral flavored suspension	Dog: Start with 15 mg/kg PO q8hr and increase gradually to maximum of 65 mg/kg q8hr
Fenbendazole	Panacur, Safe-Guard	Panacur granules 22.2% (222 mg/gm); 100-mg/ml liquid	50 mg/kg/day PO for 3 days
Fentanyl	Sublimaze, generic	50-mcg/ml injection	0.02-0.04 mg/kg IV, IM, SC q2hr or 0.01 mg/kg IV, IM, SC (with acetylpromazine or diazepam) For analgesia: 0.01 mg/kg IV, IM, SC q2hr
Fentanyl transdermal	Duragesic	25-, 50-, 75-, and 100-mcg/hr patch	Dog: 10-20 kg, 50-mcg/hr patch q72hr Cat: 25-mcg patch every 118hr
Ferrous sulfate	Many OTC brands	Many	Dog: 100-300 mg/dog PO q24hr Cat: 50-100 mg/cat PO q24hr
Finasteride	Proscar	5-mg tablets	Dog (BPH): 5-mg tablet/dog PO q24hr
Firocoxib	Previcox	57- or 227-mg tablets	Dog: 5 mg/kg PO, once daily Cat: 1.5 mg/kg, once; long-term safety in cats has not been determined
Florfenical	Nuflor	300 mg/ml (cattle)	Dog: 20 mg/kg q6hr PO, IM Cat: 22 mg/kg q12hr IM, PO
Fluconazole	Diflucan	50-, 100-, 150-, and 200-mg tablets; 10- or 40-mg/ml oral suspension; 2-mg/ml IV injection	Dog: 10-12 mg/kg day PO For malassezia 5 mg/kg q12hr PO Cat: 50 mg/cat PO q12hr or 50 mg/cat/day PO
Flucytosine	Ancobon	250-mg capsule; 75-mg/ml oral suspension	25-50 mg/kg PO q6-8hr (up to a maximal dose of 100 mg/kg PO q12hr)
Fludrocortisone	Florinef	100-mcg (0.1 mg) tablet	Dog: 0.2-0.8 mg/dog or 0.02 mg/kg PO q24hr (13-23 mcg/kg) Cat: 0.1-0.2 mg/cat PO q24hr
Flumazenil	Romazicon	100-mcg/ml (0.1 mg/ml) injection	0.2 mg (total dose) IV as needed
Flumethasone	Flucort	0.5-mg/ml injection	Dog, cat: Antiinflammatory: 0.15-0.3 mg/kg IV, IM, SC q12-24hr

Drug Name	Other Names	Formulations Available	Dosage
Flunixin meglumine	Banamine	250-mg packet granules; 10- and 50-mg/ml injection	1.1 mg/kg IV, IM, SC once or 1.1 mg/kg/day PO 3 days/wk Ophthalmic: 0.5 mg/kg IV once
5-Fluorouracil	Fluorouracil	50-mg/ml vial	Dog: 150 mg/m^2 IV once/week Cat: Do not use
Fluoxetine	Prozac, Reconcile	8-, 16-, 32-, and 64-mg chewable tablets for dogs. Human formulation is 10- and 20-mg capsules and 4-mg/ml oral solution	Dog: 1-2 mg/kg/day PO q24hr Cat: 0.5-4 mg/cat PO q24hr
Follicle-stimulating hormone (FSM)	See Urofollitropin		
Fomepizole	4-Methylpyrazole, Antizole, and Antizol-vet	5% solution	Dog: 20 mg/kg initially IV, then 15 mg/kg at 12- and 24-hr intervals, then 5 mg/kg at 36hr; repeat q12hr if necessary
Furazolidone	Furoxone	100-mg tablet	4 mg/kg PO q12hr for 7-10 days
Furosemide	Lasix, generic	12.5-, 20-, and 50-mg tablets; 10-mg/ml oral solution; 50-mg/ml injection	Dog: 2-6 mg/kg IV, IM, SC, PO q8-12hr (or as needed) Cat: 1-4 mg/kg IV, IM, SC, PO q8-24hr
Gabapentin	Neurontin	100-, 300-, 400-mg capsules; 100-, 300-, 400-, 600-, 800-mg scored tablets; 50-mg/ml oral solution	Dog, cat: Anticonvulsant dose: 2.5-10 mg/kg q8-12hr PO For analgesia: 10-15 mg/kg q8hr PO
Gemfibrozil	Lopid	300-mg capsules; 600-mg tablets	7.5 mg/kg PO q12hr
Gentamicin	Gentocin	50- and 100-mg/ml solution for injection	Dog: 9-14 mg/kg IV, IM, SC q24hr Cat: 5-8 mg/kg IV, IM, SC q24hr
Glipizide	Glucotrol	5- and 10-mg tablets	Dog: Not recommended Cat: 2.5-7.5 mg/cat PO q12hr. Usual dose is 2.5 mg/cat initially, then increase to 5 mg/cat q12hr
Glucosamine chondroitin sulfate	Cosequin and others	Regular (RS) and double-strength (DS) capsules	Dog: 1-2 RS capsules/day (2-4 capsules of DS for large dogs) Cat: 1 RS capsule/day
Glyburide	Diabeta, Micronase, Glynase	1.25-, 2.5-, and 5-mg tablets	0.2 mg/kg/day PO; or 0.625 mg/cat
Glycerin	Generic	Oral solution	1-2 ml/kg, up to PO q8hr
Glycopyrrolate	Robinul-V	0.2-mg/ml injection	0.005-0.01 mg/kg IV, IM, SC
Gold sodium thiomalate	Myochrysine	10-, 25- and 50-mg/ml injection	1-5 mg IM on first wk, then 2-10 mg IM on second wk, then 1 mg/kg once/wk IM maintenance
Gold therapy	See Aurothioglucose, Gold sodium thiomalate, or Auranofin		
GoLYTELY	See Polyethylene glycol electrolyte solution		
Gonadorelin (GnRH, LHRH)	Factrel	50-mcg/ml injection	Dog: 50-100 mcg/dog/day IM q24-48hr Cat: 25 mcg/cat IM once
Gonadotropin, chorionic (HCG)	Profasi, Pregnyl, generic, A.P.L.	Injection sizes of 5,000, 10,000 and 20,000 U	Dog: 22 U/kg IM q24-48hr or 44 U IM once Cat: 250 U/cat IM once
Gonadotropin-releasing hormone	See Gonadorelin		
Granisetron	Kytril	1-mg/ml injection; 1-mg tablet	0.01 mg/kg (10 mcg/kg) IV
Griseofulvin (microsize)	Fulvicin U/F	125-, 250-, and 500-mg tablets; 25-mg/ml oral suspension; 125-mg/ml oral syrup	50 mg/kg PO q24hr (up to a maximum dose of 110-132 mg/kg/day in divided treatments)
Griseofulvin (ultramicrosize)	Fulvicin P/G, GrisPEG	100-, 125-, 165-, 250-, and 330-mg tablets	30 mg/kg/day in divided treatments PO

Continued

Appendix I—cont'd

Drug Name	Other Names	Formulations Available	Dosage
Growth hormone (hGH, somatrem, somatropin)	Protropin, Humatrope, Nutropin	5- and 10-mg/vial	0.1 U/kg SC, IM three times/wk for 4-6 wks (Usual human pediatric dose is 0.18-0.3 mg/kg/wk)
Guaifenesin	Glyceryl guaiacolate, Guaiphenesin, Mucinex	Tablets: 100-, 200-mg; 600-mg extended-release tablets Oral solution: 20 mg/ml or 40 mg/ml	Dog, cat: Expectorant: 3-5 mg/kg q8hr PO Dog: Anesthetic adjunct: 2.2 ml/kg/hr of a 5% solution IV
Halothane	Fulothane	250-ml bottle	Induction: 3% Maintenance: 0.5%-1.5%
Hemoglobin glutamer	Oxyglobin	13-gm/dl in 125-ml single-dose bags	Dog: One-time dose of 10-30 ml/kg IV at a rate not to exceed 10 ml/kg/hr Cat: One-time dose of 3-5 ml/kg slowly IV
Heparin sodium	Liquaemin (US); Hepalean (Canada)	1,000- and 10,000-U/ml injection	100-200 units/kg IV loading dose; then 100-300 units/kg SC q6-8hr Low-dose prophylaxis (dog and cat): 70 U/kg SC q8-12hr
Hetastarch	Hydroxyethyl starch (HES)	Injectable solution	Dog: 10-20 ml/kg/day IV Cat: 5-10 ml/kg/day IV
Hycodan	*See* Hydrocodone bitartrate		
Hydralazine	Apresoline	10-mg tablet; 20-mg/ml injection	Dog: 0.5 mg/kg (initial dose); titrate to 0.5-2 mg/kg PO q12hr Cat: 2.5 mg/cat PO q12-24hr
Hydrochlorothiazide	HydroDIURIL, and generic	10- and 100-mg/ml oral solution and 25-, 50-, and 100-mg tablets	2-4 mg/kg PO q12hr
Hydrocodone bitartrate	Hycodan	5-mg tablet; 1-mg/ml syrup	Dog: 0.22 mg/kg PO q4-8hr Cat: No dose available
Hydrocortisone	Cortef, and generic	5-, 10-, 20-mg tablets	Replacement therapy: 1-2 mg/kg PO q12hr Antiinflammatory: 2.5-5 mg/kg PO q12hr
Hydrocortisone sodium succinate	Solu-Cortef	Various size vials for injection	Shock: 50-150 mg/kg IV Antiinflammatory: 5 mg/kg IV q12hr
Hydromorphone	Dilaudid, Hydrostat, and generic	1-, 2-, 4-, 10-mg/ml injection Oral forms are available, but there is no assurance of oral absorption in dogs.	0.22 mg/kg IM or SC. Repeat every 4-6 hr, or as needed for pain treatment.
Hydroxyethyl starch (HES)	HES, Hetastarch	Injection	10-20 ml/kg IV to effect
Hydroxyurea	Hydrea	500-mg capsule	Dog: 50 mg/kg PO once daily, 3 days/wk Cat: 25 mg/kg PO once daily, 3 days/wk
Hydroxyzine	Atarax	10-, 25-, and 50-mg tablets; 2-mg/ml oral solution	Dog: 2 mg/kg q12hr PO, IV, IM Cat: Safe dose not established
Ibuprofen	Motrin, Advil, Nuprin	200-, 400-, 600-, and 800-mg tablets	Safe dose not established
Imipenem	Primaxin	250- or 500-mg vials for injection	3-10 mg/kg q6-8hr IV, SC, or IM; usually 5 mg/kg q6-8hr IM, IV, or SC q6-8hr
Imipramine	Tofranil	10-, 25-, and 50-mg tablets	Dog: 2-4 mg/kg PO q12-24hr Cat: 0.5-1.0 mg/kg q12-24hr PO
Indomethacin	Indocin		Safe dose has not been established

Drug Name	Other Names	Formulations Available	Dosage
Insulin, regular crystalline		100-U/ml injection	Ketoacidosis: animals <3 kg, 1 U/animal initially, then 1 U/animal q1hr; animals 3-10 kg, 2 U/animal initially, then 1 U/animal q1hr; animals >10 kg, 0.25 U/kg initially, then 0.1 U/kg IM q1hr
Insulin, NPH isophane, Ultralente, or PZI		100-U/ml injection	Dog <15 kg: 1 U/kg SC q24hr (to effect) Dog >25 kg: 0.5 U/kg SC q24hr (to effect) Cat: PZI or Ultralente initial dose 0.5-1.0 U/kg SC, usually twice/day
Interferon (interferon alpha, HuIFN-alpha)	Roferon	5- and 10-million U/vial	Dog: 2.5 million U/kg IV once daily for 3 days Cat: 1 million U/kg IV once daily for 5 consecutive days at 0, 14, and 60 days
Iodide	See Potassium iodide		
Ipecac syrup	Ipecac	Oral solution: 30-ml bottle	Dog: 3-6 ml/dog PO Cat: 2-6 ml/cat PO
Ipodate	Cholecystographic agent	50-mg capsules	Cat: 15 mg/kg q12hr PO (usually 50 mg/cat q12hr)
Iron	See Ferrous sulfate		
Isoflurane	AErrane	100-ml bottle	Induction: 5% Maintenance: 1.5%-2.5%
Isoproterenol	Isuprel	0.2-mg/ml ampules for injection	10 mcg/kg IM, SC q6hr; or dilute 1 mg in 500 ml of 5% dextrose or Ringer's solution and infuse IV 0.5-1 ml/min (1-2 mcg/min) or to effect
Isosorbide dinitrate	Isordil, Isorbid, Sorbitrate	2.5-, 5-, 10-, 20-, 30-, and 40-mg tablets; 40-mg capsules	2.5-5 mg/animal PO q12hr (or 0.22-1.1 mg/kg PO q12hr)
Isosorbide mononitrate	Monoket	10-, and 20-mg tablets	5 mg/dog PO two dose/day 7 hr apart
Isotretinoin	Accutane	10-, 20-, and 40-mg capsules	Dog: 1-3 mg/kg/day (up to a maximum recommended dose of 3-4 mg/kg/day PO) Cat: Dose not established
Itraconazole	Sporanox	100-mg capsules; 10-mg/ml oral solution	Dog: 2.5 mg/kg PO q12hr or 5 mg/kg PO q24hr For dermatophytes: 3 mg/kg/day PO for 15 days For Malassezia: 5 mg/kg q24hr PO for 2 days, repeated each wk for 3 wks Cat: 1.5-3.0 mg/kg, up to 5 mg/kg PO for 15 days
Ivermectin	Heartguard, Ivomec, Eqvalan liquid	1% (10 mg/ml) injectable solution; 10-mg/ml oral solution; 18.7-mg/ml oral paste; 68-, 136-, and 272-mcg tablets	Heartworm preventative: Dog: 6 mcg/kg PO q30 days Cat: 24 mcg/kg PO q30 days Microfilaricide: 50 mcg/kg PO 2 wks after adulticide therapy Ectoparasite therapy (dog and cat): 200-300 mcg/kg IM, SC, PO Endoparasites (dog and cat): 200-400 mcg/kg SC, PO weekly Demodex therapy: Start with 100 mcg/kg, then, increase to 600 mcg/kg/day PO for 60-120 days

Continued

Appendix I—cont'd

Drug Name	Other Names	Formulations Available	Dosage
Kanamycin	Kantrim	200- and 500-mg/ml injection	10 mg/kg IV, IM, SC q6-8hr; or 20 mg/kg q24hr IV, IM, SC
Kaopectate (kaolin + pectin)	Kaopectate	Oral suspension 12 oz	1-2 ml/kg PO q2-6hr
Ketamine	Ketalar, Ketavet, Vetalar	100-mg/ml injection solution	Dog: 5.5-22 mg/kg IV, IM (recommend adjunctive sedative or tranquilizer treatment) Cat: 2-25 mg/kg IV, IM (recommend adjunctive sedative or tranquilizer treatment)
Ketoconazole	Nizoral	200-mg tablet; 100-mg/ml oral suspension (only available in Canada)	Dog: 10-15 mg/kg PO q8-12hr For *Malassezia canis* infection use 5 mg/kg PO q24hr Hyperadrenocorticism: 15 mg/kg PO q12hr Cat: 5-10 mg/kg PO q8-12hr
Ketoprofen	Orudis-KT (human OTC tablet); Ketofen (veterinary injection)	12.5-mg tablet (OTC); 100-mg/ml injection	Dog, cat: 1 mg/kg PO q24hr for up to 5 days or 2.0 mg/kg IV, IM, SC for one dose
Ketorolac tromethamine	Toradol	10-mg tablet; 15- and 30-mg/ml injection in 10% alcohol	Dog: 0.5 mg/kg PO, IM, IV q12hr for not more than two doses
L-Dopa	*See* Levodopa		
Lactated Ringer's solution	Generic	250-, 500-, and 1,000-ml bags	Maintenance: 55-65 ml/kg/day IV For severe dehydration 50 ml/kg/hr IV or for shock 90 ml/kg IV (dogs) and 60-70 ml/kg IV (cats)
Lactulose	Chronulac, generic	10 gm/15 ml	Constipation: 1 ml/4.5 kg PO q8hr (to effect) Hepatic encephalopathy: Dog: 0.5 ml/kg PO q8hr Cat: 2.5-5 ml/cat PO q8hr
Leucovorin (folinic acid)	Wellcovorin and generic	5-, 10-, 15-, and 25-mg tablets; 3- and 5-mg/ml injection	With methotrexate administration: 3 mg/m² IV, IM, PO Antidote for pyrimethamine toxicosis: 1 mg/kg PO q24hr
Levamisole	Levasole, Tamisol, Ergamisol	0.184-gm bolus; 11.7 gm/13-gm packet; 50-mg tablet (Ergamisol)	Dog (hookworms): 5-8 mg/kg PO once (up to 10 mg/kg PO for 2 days) Microfilaricide: 10 mg/kg PO q24hr for 6-10 days Immunostimulant: 0.5-2 mg/kg PO three times/wk Cat: 4.4 mg/kg once PO For lungworms: 20-40 mg/kg PO q48hr for five treatments
Levetiracetam	Keppra	250-, 500-, 750-mg tablets	Dog: Start with 20 mg/kg q8hr PO; increase gradually as necessary Cat: 30 mg/kg q12hr PO
Levodopa (L-dopa)	Larodopa, L-dopa	100-, 250-, and 500-mg tablets or capsules	Hepatic encephalopathy: 6.8 mg/kg initially then 1.4 mg/kg q6hr
Levothyroxine sodium (T₄)	Soloxine, Thyro-Tabs, Synthroid	0.1- to 0.8-mg tablets (in 0.1-mg increments)	Dog: 18-22 mcg/kg PO q12hr (adjust dose via monitoring) Cat: 10-20 mcg/kg/day PO (adjust dose via monitoring)

Drug Name	Other Names	Formulations Available	Dosage
Lidocaine	Xylocaine and generic brands	5-, 10-, 15-, and 20-mg/ml injection	Antiarrhythmic: Dog: 2-4 mg/kg IV (to a maximum dose of 8 mg/kg over 10-min period); 25-75 mcg/kg/min IV infusion; 6 mg/kg IM q1.5hr Cat: 0.25-0.75 mg/kg IV slowly; or 10-40 mcg/kg/min infusion For epidural (dog and cat): 4.4 mg/kg of 2% solution
Lincomycin	Lincocin	100-, 200-, and 500-mg tablets	15-25 mg/kg PO q12hr For pyoderma: Doses as low as 10 mg/kg q12hr have been used
Linezolid	Zyvox	400- and 600-mg tablets; 20-mg/ml oral suspension; 2-mg/ml injection	Dog, cat: 10 mg/kg q8-12hr PO, IV
Liothyronine (T_3)	Cytomel	60-mcg tablet	4.4 mcg/kg PO q8hr For T_3 suppression test (cats): Collect presample for T_4 and T_3; administer 25 mcg q8hr for seven doses, then collect post samples for T_3 and T_4 after last dose
Lisinopril	Prinivil, Zestril	2.5-, 5-, 10-, 20-, and 40-mg tablets	Dog: 0.5 mg/kg PO q24hr Cat: No dose established
Lithium carbonate	Lithotabs	150-, 300-, and 600-mg capsules; 300-mg tablet; 300-mg/5 ml syrup	Dog: 10 mg/kg PO q12hr Cat: Not recommended
Lomotil	*See* Diphenoxylate		
Lomustine	CCNU, CeeNU	10-, 40-, 100-mg capsules	Dog: 70-90 mg/m², every 4 wks PO For brain tumors: Use 60-90 mg/m² q6-8wk PO Cat: 50-60 mg/m² PO q3-6wk or 10 mg/cat PO every 3 wks
Loperamide	Imodium and generic	2-mg tablet; 0.2-mg/ml oral liquid	Dog: 0.1 mg/kg PO q8-12hr Cat: 0.08-0.16 mg/kg PO q12hr
Lufenuron	Program	45-, 90-, 135-, 204.9-, and 409.8-mg tablets; 135- and 270-mg suspension per unit pack	Dog: 10 mg/kg PO q30 days Cat: 30 mg/kg PO q30 days, 10 mg/kg SC q6mo
Lufenuron + milbemycin oxime	Sentinel tablets and Flavor Tabs	Milbemycin/lufenuron ratio is as follows: 2.3/46-mg tablets; 5.75/115-11.5/230-, and 23/460-mg Flavor Tabs	Administer 1 tablet q30 days; each tablet formulated for size of dog
Luteinizing hormone	*See* Gonadorelin		
L-Lysine	Enisyl-F	250-mg/ml paste	Paste formulation: 1-2 ml/cat, PO, to adult cats (approximately 400 mg/cat) and 1 ml/cat, PO, for kittens
Magnesium citrate	Citroma, Citro-Nesia (Citro-Mag in Canada)	Oral solution	2-4 ml/kg PO
Magnesium hydroxide	Milk of Magnesia	Oral liquid	Antacid: 5-10 ml/kg PO q4-6hr Cathartic: Dog: 15-50 PO ml/kg Cat: 2-6 ml/cat PO q24hr
Magnesium sulfate	Epsom salts	Crystals, many generic preparations	Dog: 8-25 gm/dog PO q24hr; for treating arrhythmias: 0.15-0.3 mEq/kg slowly IV over 5-15 min followed by 0.75-1.0 mEq/kg/day; fluid supplementation: 0.75-1.0 mEq/kg/day Cat: 2-5 gm/cat PO q24hr

Continued

Appendix I—cont'd

Drug Name	Other Names	Formulations Available	Dosage
Mannitol	Osmitrol	5%-25% solution for injection	Diuretic: 1 gm/kg of 5%-25% solution IV to maintain urine flow Glaucoma or central nervous system edema: 0.25-2 gm/kg of 15%-25% solution IV over 30-60 min (repeat in 6 hr if necessary)
Marbofloxacin	Marbocyl, Zeniquim	25-, 50-, 100-, and 200-mg tablets	Dog, cat: 2.75-5.55 mg/kg PO q24hr
Maropitant	Cerenia	10-mg/ml injection; 16-, 24-, 60-, 160-mg tablets	Dog: 1 mg/kg SC once daily for up to 5 days; 2 mg/kg PO once daily for up to 5 days For motion sickness: 8 mg/kg PO once daily for up to 2 days Cat: Dose not established
MCT oil	MCT oil (many sources)	Oral liquid	1-2 ml/kg/day in food
Mebendazole	Telmintic	Each gram of powder contains 40 mg	22 mg/kg (with food) q24hr for 3 days
Meclizine	Antivert, generic	12.5-, 25-, and 50-mg tablets	Dog: 25 mg PO q24hr (for motion sickness, administer 1 hr before traveling) Cat: 12.5 mg PO q24hr
Meclofenamic acid (meclofenamate sodium)	Arquel, Meclomen	50- and 100-mg capsules	Dog: 1 mg/kg/day PO for up to 5 days Cat: Not recommended
Medetomidine	Domitor	1.0-mg/ml injection	750 mcg/m² IV 1,000 mcg/m² IM
Medium-chain triglycerides	*See* MCT oil		
Medroxyprogesterone acetate	Depo-Provera (injection); Provera (tablets)	150- and 400-mg/ml suspension injection; 2.5-, 5-, and 10-mg tablets	1.1-2.2 mg/kg IM q7 days; for behavioral use 10-20 mg/kg SC for prostate 3-5 mg/kg SC, IM
Megestrol acetate	Ovaban	5-mg tablet	Dog: Proestrus: 2 mg/kg PO q24hr for 8 days Anestrus: 0.5 mg/kg PO q24hr for 30 days Behavior: 2-4 mg/kg q24hr for 8 days (reduce dose for maintenance) Cat: Dermatologic therapy or urine spraying: 2.5-5 mg/cat PO q24hr for 1 wk, then reduce to 5 mg once or twice/wk Suppress estrus: 5 mg/cat/day for 3 days, then 2.5-5 mg once/wk for 10 wks
Melarsomine	Immiticide	25-mg/ml injection; after reconstitution retains potency for 24hr	Administer via deep IM injection. Class 1-2 dogs: 2.5 mg/kg/day for 2 consecutive days Class 3 dogs: 2.5 mg/kg once, then in 1 month two additional doses 24 hr apart
Meloxicam	Metacam (veterinary); Mobic (human)	Veterinary: 1.5-mg/ml oral suspension and 5-mg/ml injection Human: 7.5-mg tablets	Dog: 0.2 mg/kg initially PO, then 0.1 mg/kg q24hr PO thereafter; injection 0.1 mg/kg IV or SC Cat: 0.3 mg/kg SC one-time injection; 0.05 mg/kg q24-48hr PO for chronic use
Melphalan	Alkeran	2-mg tablet	1.5 mg/m² (or 0.1-0.2 mg/kg) PO q24hr for 7-10 days (repeat every 3 wks)

Drug Name	Other Names	Formulations Available	Dosage
Meperidine	Demerol	50- and 100-mg tablets; 10-mg/ml syrup; 25-, 50-, 75-, and 100-mg/ml injection	Dog: 5-10 mg/kg IV, IM as often as q2-3hr (or as needed) Cat: 3-5 mg/kg IV, IM q2-4hr (or as needed)
Mepivacaine	Carbocaine-V	2% (20 mg/ml) injection	Variable dose for local infiltration. For epidural: 0.5 ml of 2% solution q30sec until reflexes are absent
6-Mercaptopurine	Purinethol	50-mg tablet	Dog: 50 mg/m^2 PO q24hr Cat: Do not use
Meropenem	Merrem	500 mg in 20-ml vial, or 1-gm vial in 30-ml vial for injection	Dogs, cats: 8.5 mg/kg SC q12hr up to 12 mg/kg SC q12hr or 24 mg/kg IV q12hr
Mesalamine	Asacol, Mesasal, Pentasa	400-mg tablet; 250-mg capsule	Veterinary dose has not been established, the usual human oral dose is 400-500 mg q6-8hr (*also see* Sulfasalazine, Olsalazine)
Metaproterenol	Alupent, Metaprel	10- and 20-mg tablets; 5-mg/ml syrup; inhalers	0.325-0.65 mg/kg PO q4-6hr
Methadone	Methadose and generic	2-mg/ml oral solution; 10- and 20-mg/ml solution for injection; 5-, 10-, 40-mg tablets	Dog: 0.5-2.2 mg/kg IV, SC, IM, or 0.5-1.0 mg/kg IV q3-4hr for analgesia Cat: 0.2-0.5 mg/kg SC or IM, or 0.05-0.1 mg/kg up to 0.2 mg/kg IV q3-4hr for analgesia
Methazolamide	Neptazane	25- and 50-mg tablets	2-3 mg/kg PO q8-12hr
Methenamine hippurate	Hiprex, Urex	1-gm tablet	Dog: 500 mg/dog PO q12hr Cat: 250 mg/cat PO q12hr
Methenamine mandelate	Mandelamine and generic	1-gm tablet; granules for oral solution; 50- and 100-mg/ml oral suspension	10-20 mg/kg PO q8-12hr
Methimazole	Tapazole	5- and 10-mg tablets	Cat: 2.5 mg/cat q12hr PO for 7-14 days then 5-10 mg/cat PO q12hr and adjust by monitoring T$_4$
DL-Methionine	*See* Racemethionine		
Methocarbamol	Robaxin-V	500- and 750-mg tablets; 100-mg/ml injection	44 mg/kg PO q8hr on the first day then 22-44 mg/kg PO q8hr
Methohexital	Brevital	0.5-, 2.5-, and 5-gm vials for injection	3-6 mg/kg IV (give slowly to effect)
Methotrexate	MTX, Mexate, Folex, Rheumatrex, generic	2.5-mg tablet; 2.5- or 25-mg/ml injection	2.5-5 mg/m^2 PO q48hr (dose depends on specific protocol) or Dog: 0.3-0.5 mg/kg IV once/wk Cat: 0.8 mg/kg IV q2-3wk
Methoxamine	Vasoxyl	20-mg/ml injection	200-250 mcg/kg IM or 40-80 mcg/kg IV
Methoxyflurane	Metofane	4-oz bottle for inhalation	Induction: 3% Maintenance: 0.5%-1.5%
Methylene Blue 0.1%	Generic, also called New Methylene Blue	1% solution (10 mg/ml)	1.5 mg/kg IV, slowly
Methylprednisolone	Medrol	1-, 2-, 4-, 8-, 18-, and 32-mg tablets	0.22-0.44 mg/kg PO q12-24hr
Methylprednisolone acetate	Depo-Medrol	20- or 40-mg/ml suspension for injection	Dog: 1 mg/kg (or 20-40 mg/dog) IM q1-3wk Cat: 10-20 mg/cat IM q1-3wk
Methylprednisolone sodium succinate	Solu-Medrol	1- and 2-gm and 125- and 500-mg vials for injection	For emergency use: 30 mg/kg IV and repeat at 15 mg/kg IV in 2-6 hr
4-Methylpyrazole (fomepizole)	5% solution	Antizole, Antizol-Vet (Fomepizole)	*See* Fomepizol for dose

Continued

Appendix I—cont'd

Drug Name	Other Names	Formulations Available	Dosage
Methyltestosterone	Android, generic	10- and 25-mg tablets	Dog: 5-25 mg/dog PO q24-48hr Cat: 2.5-5 mg/cat PO q24-48hr
Metoclopramide	Reglan, Clopra, and others	5- and 10-mg tablets; 1-mg/ml oral solution; 5-mg/ml injection	0.2-0.5 mg/kg IV, IM, PO q6-8hr or IV loading dose at 0.4 mg/kg followed by 0.3 mg/kg/hr IV
Metoprolol tartrate	Lopressor	50- and 100-mg tablets; 1-mg/ml injection	Dog: 5-50 mg/dog (0.5-1.0 mg/kg) PO q8hr Cat: 2-15 mg/cat PO q8hr
Metronidazole and metronidazole benzoate	Flagyl and generic	250- and 500-mg tablets; 50-mg/ml suspension; 5-mg/ml injection; the benzoate form is not available commercially and must be obtained from a compounding pharmacist	For anaerobes: Dog: 15 mg/kg PO q12hr or 12 mg/kg q8hr Cat: 10-25 mg/kg PO q24hr For *Giardia:* Dog: 12-15 mg/kg PO q12hr for 8 days Cat: 17 mg/kg (⅓ tablet/cat) q24hr for 8 days
Mexiletine	Mexitil	150-, 200-, and 250-mg capsules	Dog: 5-8 mg/kg PO q8-12hr (use cautiously) Cat: Do not use
Mibolerone	Cheque-drops	55-mcg/ml oral solution	Dog: 0.45-11.3 kg, 30 mcg; 11.8-22.7 kg, 60 mcg; 23-45.3 kg, 120 mcg; >45.8 kg, 180 mcg; or approximately 2.6-5 mcg/kg/day PO Cat: Safe dose not established
Midazolam	Versed	5-mg/ml injection	Dog: 0.1-0.25 mg/kg IV, IM (or 0.1-0.3 mg/kg/hr IV infusion) Cat: 0.05 mg/kg IV; or 0.3-0.6 mg/kg IV (combine with 3 mg/kg ketamine)
Milbemycin oxime	Interceptor and Interceptor Flavor Tabs	23-, 11.5-, 5.75-, and 2.3-mg tablets	Dog: Microfilaricide; 0.5 mg/kg; Demodex: 2 mg/kg PO q24hr for 60-120 days Heartworm prevention: 0.5 mg/kg PO q30 days Cat: 2 mg/kg q30 days PO
Milk of Magnesia	*See* Magnesium hydroxide		
Mineral oil	Generic	Oral liquid	Dog: 10-50 ml/dog PO q12hr Cat: 10-25 ml/cat PO q12hr
Minocycline	Minocin	50-, 75-, and 100-mg tablets or capsules; 10-mg/ml oral suspension	5-12.5 mg/kg PO q12hr
Misoprostol	Cytotec	0.1-mg (100 mcg), 0.2-mg (200 mcg) tablets	Dog: 2-5 mcg/kg PO q6-8hr; for atopic dermatitis 5 mcg/kg q8hr PO Cat: Dose not established
Mithramycin	*See* Plicamycin (Mithracin)		
Mitotane (*o,p'*-DDD)	Lysodren	500-mg tablet	Dog: For pituitary-dependent hypercorticism: 50 mg/kg/day (in divided doses) PO for 5-10 days, then 50-70 mg/kg/wk PO For adrenal tumor: 50-75 mg/kg day for 10 days, then 75-100 mg/kg/wk PO
Mitoxantrone	Novantrone	2-mg/ml injection	Dog: 6 mg/m^2 IV q21 days Cat: 6.5 mg/m^2 IV q21 days

Drug Name	Other Names	Formulations Available	Dosage
Morphine	Generic	1- and 15-mg/ml injection; 30- and 60-mg delayed-release tablets	Dog: 0.1-1 mg/kg IV, IM, SC (dose is escalated as needed for pain relief) q4-6hr; Dog: 0.5 mg/kg q2hr IV, IM, or CRI 0.2 mg/kg followed by 0.1 mg/kg/hr IV Epidural: 0.1 mg/kg Cat: 0.1 mg/kg q3-6hr IM, SC (or as needed)
Moxidectin	Cydectin	Injection	Dog: Heartworm prevention: 3 mcg/kg Endoparasites: 25-300 mcg/kg Demodex: 400 mcg/kg/day up to 500 mcg/kg/day for 21-22 wks
Moxifloxacin	Avelox	400-mg tablet	10 mg/kg q24hr PO
Mycochrysine	See Gold sodium thiomalate		
Mycophenolate	Cell Cept	250-mg capsule	Dog: 10 mg/kg q8hr PO Cat: No dose established
Naloxone	Narcan	20- or 400-mcg/ml injection	0.01-0.04 mg/kg IV, IM, SC as needed to reverse opiate
Naltrexone	Trexan	50-mg tablet	For behavior problems: 2.2 mg/kg PO q12hr
Nandrolone decanoate	Deca-Durabolin	Nandrolone decanoate injection: 50-, 100-, and 200-mg/ml	Dog: 1-1.5 mg/kg/wk IM Cat: 1 mg/cat/wk IM
Naproxen	Naprosyn, Naxen, Aleve (naproxen sodium)	220-mg tablet (OTC); 25-mg/ml suspension liquid; 250-, 375-, and 500-mg tablets (Rx)	Dog: 5 mg initially, then 2 mg/kg q48hr Cat: Not recommended
Neomycin	Biosal	500-mg bolus; 200-mg/ml oral liquid	10-20 mg/kg PO q6-12hr
Neostigmine bromide and neostigmine methylsulfate	Prostigmin; Stiglyn	15-mg tablet (neostigmine bromide); 0.25- and 0.5-mg/ml injection (neostigmine methylsulfate)	2 mg/kg/day PO (in divided doses, to effect) Injection: Antimyasthenic: 10 mcg/kg IM, SC, as needed Antidote for nondepolarizing neuromuscular block: 40 mcg/kg IM, SC Diagnostic aid for myasthenia gravis: 40 mcg/kg IM or 20 mcg/kg IV
Nifedipine	Adalat, Procardia	10- and 20-mg capsules	Dose not established; in humans, the dose is 10 mg/human three times/day and increased in 10-mg increments to effect
Nitenpyram	Capstar	11.4- or 57-mg tablet	1 mg/kg PO daily as needed to kill fleas
Nitrates	See Nitroglycerin, Isosorbide dinitrate, or Nitroprusside		
Nitrofurantoin	Macrodantin, Furalan, Furatoin, Furadantin, or generic	Macrodantin and generic 25-, 50-, and 100-mg capsules; Furalan, Furatoin, and generic 50- and 100-mg tablets; Furadantin 5-mg/ml oral suspension	10 mg/kg/day divided into four daily treatments, then 1 mg/kg PO at night
Nitroglycerin ointment	Nitrol, Nitro-Bid, Nitrostat	0.5-, 0.8-, 1-, 5-, and 10-mg/ml injection; 2% ointment; transdermal systems (0.2 mg/hr patch)	Dog: 4-12 mg (up to 15 mg) topically q12hr Cat: 2-4 mg topically q12hr (or ¼ inch of ointment per cat)
Nitroprusside	Nitropress	50-mg vial for injection	1-5, up to a maximum of 10 mcg/kg/min IV infusion
Nizatidine	Axid	150- and 300-mg capsules	Dog: 5 mg/kg PO q24hr
Norfloxacin	Noroxin	400-mg tablet	22 mg/kg PO q12hr
o,p'-DDD	See Mitotane (Lysodren)		

Continued

Appendix I—cont'd

Drug Name	Other Names	Formulations Available	Dosage
Olsalazine	Dipentum	500-mg tablet	Dose not established (usual human dose is 500 mg or 5-10 mg/kg PO twice daily)
Omeprazole	Prilosec (formerly Losec), Gastrogard (equine paste)	20-mg capsule	Dog: 20 mg/dog PO once daily (or 0.7 mg/kg q24hr) Cat: 0.5-0.7 mg/kg q24hr PO
Ondansetron	Zofran	4- and 8-mg tablets; 2-mg/ml injection	0.5-1.0 mg/kg IV, PO 30 minutes before administration of cancer drugs
Orbifloxacin	Orbax	5.7-, 22.7-, and 68-mg tablets	2.5-7.5 mg/kg PO once daily
Ormetoprim	See Primor (ormetoprim-sulfadimethoxine)		
Oxacillin	Prostaphlin and generic	250- and 500-mg capsules; 50-mg/ml oral solution	22-40 mg/kg PO q8hr
Oxazepam	Serax	15-mg tablet	Cat: Appetite stimulant: 2.5 mg/cat PO
Oxtriphylline	Choledyl-SA	400- and 600-mg tablet (oral solutions and syrup available in Canada but not US)	Dog: 47 mg/kg (equivalent to 30 mg/kg theophylline) PO q12hr
Oxybutynin chloride	Ditropan	5-mg tablet	Dog: 5 mg/dog PO q6-8hr
Oxymetholone	Anadrol	50-mg tablet	1-5 mg/kg/day PO
Oxymorphone	Numorphan	1.5- and 1-mg/ml injection	Dog, cat: Analgesia: 0.1-0.2 mg/kg IV, SC, IM (as needed), redose with 0.05-0.1 mg/kg q1-2hr Preanesthetic: 0.025-0.05 mg/kg IM, SC
Oxytetracycline	Terramycin	250-mg tablets; 100- and 200-mg/ml injection	7.5-10 mg/kg IV q12hr; 20 mg/kg PO q12hr
Oxytocin	Pitocin and Syntocinon (nasal solution) and generic	10- and 20-U/ml injection; 40-U/ml nasal solution	Dog: 5-20 U/dog SC, IM (repeat every 30 min for primary inertia) Cat: 2.5-3 U/cat SC, IM (repeat every 30 min)
2-PAM	See Pralidoxime chloride		
Pamidronate	Aredia	30-, 60-, 90-mg vials for injection	Dog: 2 mg/kg IV, SC For treatment of cholecalciferol toxicosis: 1.3-2 mg/kg for two treatments
Pancreatic enzyme	See Pancrelipase		
Pancrelipase	Viokase	16,800 U of lipase, 70,000 U of protease, and 70,000 U of amylase per 0.7 gm; also capsules and tablets	Mix 2 tsp powder with food per 20 kg body weight or 1-3 tsp/0.45 kg of food 20 min before feeding
Pancuronium bromide	Pavulon	1- and 2-mg/ml injection	0.1 mg/kg IV or start with 0.01 mg/kg and additional 0.01-mg/kg doses every 30 min
Pantoprazole	Protonix	40-mg tablets, 0.4-mg/ml vials for injection	Dog, cat: 0.5 mg/kg q24hr IV or 0.5-1 mg/kg IV infusion over 24 hr
Paregoric	Corrective mixture	2 mg morphine per 5 ml of paregoric	0.05-0.06 mg/kg PO q12hr
Paroxetine	Paxil	10-, 20-, 30-, and 40-mg tablets	Cat: 1/8 to 1/4 of a 10-mg tablet daily PO
D-Penicillamine	Cuprimine, Depen	125- and 250-mg capsules and 250-mg tablets	10-15 mg/kg PO q12hr
Penicillin G benzathine	Benza-pen and other names	150,000 U/ml, combined with 150,000 U/ml of procaine penicillin G	24,000 U/kg IM q48hr
Penicillin G potassium; penicillin G sodium	Many brands	5- to 20-million unit vials	20,000-40,000 U/kg IV, IM q6-8hr

Drug Name	Other Names	Formulations Available	Dosage
Penicillin G procaine	Generic	300,000 U/ml suspension	20,000-40,000 U/kg IM q12-24hr
Penicillin V	Pen-Vee	250- and 500-mg tablets	10 mg/kg PO q8hr
Pentobarbital	Nembutal and generic	50 mg/ml	25-30 mg/kg IV to effect; or 2-15 mg/kg IV to effect, followed by 0.2-1.0 mg/kg/hr IV
Pentoxifylline	Trental	400-mg tablet	Dog: For use in canine dermatology and for vasculitis, 10 mg/kg PO q12hr and up to 15 mg/kg q8hr Cat: ¼ of 400-mg tab PO, q8-12hr
Pepto Bismol	*See* Bismuth subsalicylate		
Phenobarbital	Luminal and generic	15-, 30-, 60-, and 100-mg tablets; 30-, 60-, 65-, and 130-mg/ml injection; 4-mg/ml oral elixir solution	Dog: 2-8 mg/kg PO q12hr Cat: 2-4 mg/kg PO q12hr Dog and cat: Adjust dose by monitoring plasma concentration Status epilepticus: Administer in increments of 10-20 mg/kg IV (to effect)
Phenoxybenzamine	Dibenzyline	10-mg capsule	Dog: 0.25 mg/kg PO q8-12hr or 0.5 mg/kg q24hr Cat: 2.5 mg/cat q8-12hr or 0.5 mg/cat PO q12hr (in cats, doses as high as 0.5 mg/kg IV have been used to relax urethral smooth muscle)
Phentolamine	Regitine (Rogitine in Canada)	5-mg vial for injection	0.02-0.1 mg/kg IV
Phenylbutazone	Butazolidin and generic	100-, 200-, 400-mg and 1-gm tablets; 200-mg/ml injection	Dog: 15-22 mg/kg PO, IV q8-12hr (44 mg/kg/day) (800 mg/dog maximum) Cat: 6-8 mg/kg IV, PO q12hr
Phenylephrine	Neo-Synephrine	10-mg/ml injection; 1% nasal solution	0.01 mg/kg IV q15min 0.1 mg/kg IM, SC q15min
Phenylpropanolamine	PPA, Propalin, Proin PPA	25-, 50-, and 75-mg tablets and 25-mg/ml liquid	Dog: 1 mg/kg q12hr, PO and increase to 1.5-2.0 mg/kg as needed q8hr PO
Phenytoin	Dilantin	30- and 125-mg/ml oral suspension; 30- and 100-mg capsules; 50-mg/ml injection	Antiepileptic dog: 20-35 mg/kg q8hr Antiarrhythmic: 30 mg/kg PO q8hr or 10 mg/kg IV over 5 min
Physostigmine	Antilirium	1-mg/ml injection	0.02 mg/kg IV q12hr
Phytomenadione	*See* Vitamin K$_i$		
Phytonadione	*See* Vitamin K$_i$		
Pimobendan	Vetmedin	2.5- and 5-mg capsules (Europe and Canada); 1.25-, 2.5-, 5-mg chewable tablets (US)	Dog: 0.05 mg/kg/day in divided treatments q12hr Cat: Dose not established
Piperacillin	Pipracil	2-, 3-, 4-, and 40-gm vials for injection	40 mg/kg IV or IM q6hr
Piperazine	Many	860-mg powder; 140-mg capsule, 170-, 340-, and 800-mg/ml oral solution	44-66 mg/kg PO administered once
Piroxicam	Feldene and generic	10-mg capsule	Dog: 0.3 mg/kg PO q48hr Cat: 0.3 mg/kg q24hr PO
Pitressin (ADH)	*See* Vasopressin, Desmopressin acetate		
Plicamycin (old name is mithramycin)	Mithracin	2.5-mg injection	Dog: Antineoplastic: 25-30 mcg/kg day IV (slow infusion) for 8-10 days Antihypercalcemic: 25 mcg/kg/day IV (slow infusion) over 4 hr Cat: Not recommended

Continued

Appendix I—cont'd

Drug Name	Other Names	Formulations Available	Dosage
Polyethylene glycol electrolyte solution	GoLYTELY	Oral solution	25 ml/kg PO repeat in 2-4 hr PO
Polysulfated glycosami-noglycan (PSGAG)	Adequan Canine	100-mg/ml injection in 5-ml vial (for horses vials are 250 mg/ml)	4.4 mg/kg IM twice weekly for up to 4 wks
Potassium bromide (KBr)	No commercial formulation	Usually prepared as oral solution Must be compounded	Dog and cat: 30-40 mg/kg PO q24hr If administered without phenobarbital, higher doses of up to 40-50 mg/kg may be needed. Adjust doses by monitoring plasma concentrations. Loading doses of 600-800 mg/kg divided over 3-4 days have been administered.
Postassium chloride (KCl)	Generic	Various concentrations for injection (usually 2 mEq/ml); oral suspension and oral solution	0.5 mEq potassium/kg/day; or supplement 10-40 mEq/500 ml of fluids, depending no serum potassium
Postassium citrate	Generic, Urocit-K	5-mEq tablet; some forms are in combination with postassium chloride	0.5 mEq/kg/day PO
Potassium gluconate	Kaon, Tumil-K, generic	2-mEq tablet; 500-mg tablet; Kaon elixir is 20-mg/15-ml elixir	Dog: 0.5 mEq/kg PO q12-24hr Cat: 2-8 mEq/day PO divided twice daily
Postassium iodide			30-100 mg/cat daily (in single or divided doses) for 10-14 days
Pralidoxime chloride (2-PAM)	2-PAM, Protopam Chloride	50-mg/ml injection	20 mg/kg q8-12hr (initial dose) IV slow or IM
Praziquantel	Droncit	23- and 34-mg tablets; 56.8-mg/ml injection	Dog (PO): <6.8 kg, 7.5 mg/kg, once; >6.8 kg, 5 mg/kg, once (IM, SC): <2.3 kg, 7.5 mg/kg, once; 2.7-4.5 kg, 6.3 mg/kg, once; >5 kg, 5 mg/kg, once Cat (PO): <1.8 kg, 6.3 mg/kg, once; >1.8 kg, 5 mg/kg, once (for *Paragonimus* use 25 mg/kg q8hr for 2-3 days) (IM, SC): 5 mg/kg
Prazosin	Minipress	1-, 2-, and 5-mg capsules	0.5- and 2-mg/animal (1 mg/15 kg) PO q8-12hr
Prednisolone	Delta-Cortef and many others	5- and 20-mg tablets	Dog (cat often requires two times dog dose) Antiinflammatory: 0.5-1 mg/kg IV, IM, PO q12-24hr initially, then taper to q48hr Immunosuppressive: 2.2-6.6 mg/kg/day IV, IM, PO initially, then taper to 2-4 mg/kg q48hr Replacement therapy: 0.2-0.3 mg/kg/day PO
Prednisolone sodium succinate	Solu-Delta-Cortef	100- and 200-mg vials for injection (10 and 50 mg/ml)	Shock: 15-30 mg/kg IV (repeat in 4-6 hr) Central nervous system trauma: 15-30 mg/kg IV, taper to 1-2 mg/kg q12hr
Prednisone	Deltasone and generic; Meticorten for injection	1-, 2.5-, 5-, 10-, 20-, 25-, and 50-mg tablets; 1-mg/ml syrup (LiquidPred in 5% alcohol) and 1-mg/ml oral solution (in 5% alcohol); 10- and 40-mg/ml prednisone suspension for injection	Same as prednisolone, except that prednisone is not recommended for cats

Drug Name	Other Names	Formulations Available	Dosage
Primidone	Mylepsin, Neurosyn (Mysoline in Canada)	50- and 250-mg tablets	8-10 mg/kg PO q8-12hr as initial dose, then is adjusted via monitoring to 10-15 mg/kg q8hr
Primor (ormetoprim + sulfadimethoxine)	Primor	Combination tablet (ormetoprim + sulfadimethoxine)	27 mg/kg on first day, followed by 13.5 mg/kg PO q24hr
Procainamide	Pronestyl, generic	250-, 375-, 500-mg tablets or capsules; 100- and 500-mg/ml injection	Dog: 10-30 mg/kg PO q6hr (to a maximum dose of 40 mg/kg), 8-20 mg/kg IV IM; 25-50 mcg/kg/min IV infusion Cat: 3-8 mg/kg IM, PO q6-8hr
Prochlorperazine	Compazine	5-, 10-, and 25-mg tablets (prochlorperazine maleate); 5-mg/ml injection (prochlorperazine edisylate)	0.1-0.5 mg/kg IM, SC q6-8hr
Progesterone, repositol	*See* Medroxyprogesesterone acetate		
Promethazine	Phenergan	6.25- and 25-mg/5-ml syrup; 12.5-,25-, 50-mg tablets; 25- and 50-mg/ml injection	0.2-0.4 mg/kg IV, IM PO q6-8hr (up to a maximum dose of 1 mg/kg)
Propantheline bromide	Pro-Banthine	7.5- and 15-mg tablet	0.25-0.5 mg/kg PO q8-12hr
Propiomazine	Tranvet	5-, 10-mg/ml injection or 20-mg tablet	1.1-4.4 mg/kg q12-24hr PO or 0.1-1.1 mg/kg IM, IV (range of dose depends on degree of sedation needed)
Propofol	Rapinovet and PropoFlo (veterinary); Diprivan (human)	1% (10 mg/ml) injection in 20-ml ampules	6.6 mg/kg IV slowly over 60 seconds; constant-rate IV infusions have been used at 5 mg/kg slowly IV, followed by 100-400 mcg/kg/min IV
Propranolol	Inderal	10-, 20-, 40-, 60-, 80-, and 90-mg tablets; 1-mg/ml injection; 4- and 8-mg/ml oral solution	Dog: 20-60 mcg/kg over 5-10 min IV; 0.2-1 mg/kg PO q8hr (titrate dose to effect) Cat: 0.4-1.2 mg/kg (2.5-5 mg/cat) PO q8hr
Propylthiouracil (PTU)	Generic, Propyl-Thyracil	50- and 100-mg tablets	11 mg/kg PO q12hr
Prostaglandin F2 alpha (dinoprost)	Lutalyse	5-mg/ml solution for injection	Pyometra: Dog: 0.1-0.2 mg/kg SC once daily for 5 days Cat: 0.1-0.25 mg/kg SC once daily for 5 days Abortion: Dog: 0.025-0.05 mg (25-50 mcg)/kg IM q12hr Cat: 0.5-1 mg/kg IM for two injections
Pseudoephedrine	Sudafed and many others (some formulations have been discontinued)	30- and 60-mg tablets; 120-mg capsule; 6-mg/ml syrup	0.2-0.4 mg/kg (or 15-60 mg/dog) PO q8-12hr
Psyllium	Metamucil and others	Available as powder	1 tsp/5-10 kg (added to each meal)
Pyrantel pamoate	Nemex, Strongid	180-mg/ml paste and 50-mg/ml suspension	Dog: 5 mg/kg PO once and repeat in 7-10 days Cat: 20 mg/kg PO once
Pyridostigmine bromide	Mestinon, Regonol	12-mg/ml oral syrup; 60-mg tablet; 5-mg/ml injection	Antimyasthenic: 0.02-0.04 mg/kg IV q2hr or 0.5-3 mg/kg PO q8-12hr Antidote (nondepolarizing muscle relaxant): 0.15-0.3 mg/kg IM, IV
Pyrimethamine	Daraprim, ReBalance (Equine)	25-mg tablet Equine formulation (ReBalance) contains 250 mg sulfadiazine and 12.5 mg pyrimethamine per ml	Dog: 1 mg/kg PO q24hr for 14-21 days (5 days for *Neosporum caninum*) Cat: 0.5-1 mg/kg PO q24hr for 14-28 days

Continued

Appendix I—cont'd

Drug Name	Other Names	Formulations Available	Dosage
Quinidine gluconate	Quiniglute, Duraquin	324-mg tablets; 80-mg/ml injection	Dog: 6-20 mg/kg IM q6hr; 6-20 mg/kg PO q6-8hr (of base)
Quinidine sulfate	Cin-Quin, Quinora	100-, 200-, and 300-mg tablets; 200- and 300-mg capsules; 20-mg/ml injection	Dog: 6-20 mg/kg PO q6-8hr (of base); 5-10 mg/kg IV
Quinidine polygalacturonate	Cardioquin	275-mg tablet	Dog: 6-20 mg/kg PO q6hr (of base) (275 mg quinidine polygalacturonate = 167 mg quinidine base)
Racemethionine (DL-methionine)	Uroeze, MethioForm, and generic. Human forms include Pedameth, Uracid, and generic	500-mg tablets and powders added to animal's food; 75-mg/5 ml pediatric oral solution; 200-mg capsule	Dog: 150-300 mg/kg/day PO Cat: 1-1.5 gm/cat PO (added to food each day)
Ranitidine	Zantac	75-, 150-, and 300-mg tablets; 150- and 300-mg capsules; 25-mg/ml injection	Dog: 2 mg/kg IV, PO q8hr Cat: 2.5 mg/kg IV q12hr, 3.5 mg/kg PO q12hr
Retinoids	See Isotretinoin (Accutane), Retinol (Aquasol-A), or Etretinate (Tegison)		
Retinol	See Vitamin A (Aquasol-A)		
Riboflavin (vitamin B$_2$)	See Vitamin B$_2$		
Rifampin	Rifadin	150- and 300-mg capsules	5-15 mg/kg PO q24hr
Ringer's solution	Generic	250-, 500-, and 1000-ml bags for infusion	55-65 ml/kg/day IV, SC, or IP; 50 ml/kg/hr IV for severe dehydration
Ronidazole	No formulation available; must be compounded	There are no commercial formulations. However, compounding pharmacies have prepared formulations for cats.	Dog: Dose not established Cat: 30-60 mg/kg/day PO for 2 wks
Salicylate	See Aspirin, acetylsalicylic acid		
Selegiline (deprenyl)	Anipryl (also known as deprenyl, and l-deprenyl); human dose form is Eldepryl	2-, 5-, 10-, 15-, and 30-mg tablets	Dog: Begin with 1 mg/kg PO q24hr; If there is no response within 2 months, increase dose to maximum of 2 mg/kg PO q24hr Cat: 0.25-0.5 mg/kg q12-24hr PO
Senna	Senokot	Granules in concentrate, or syrup	Dog: Syrup; 5-10 ml/dog q24hr; Granules: $1/2$ to 1 tsp/dog q24hr PO with food Cat: Syrup: 5 ml/cat q24hr; granules: ½ teaspoon/cat q24hr (with food)
Septra (sulfamethoxazole + trimethoprim)	See Trimethoprim/sulfonamides		
Sildenafil	Viagra	25-, 50-, 100-mg tablets	Dog: 0.5-1 mg/kg q12hr PO; higher dose of 2-3 mg/kg q8hr may be needed in some cases
Silymarin	Silybin, Marin, "milk thistle"	Silymarin tablets are widely available OTC. Commercial veterinary formulations (Marin) also contain zinc and vitamin E in a phosphatidyl-choline complex in tablets for dogs and cats.	30 mg/kg/day PO
Sodium bicarbonate (NaHCO$_3$)	Generic, Baking Soda, Soda Mint	325-, 520-, and 650-mg tablets; injection of various strengths (4.2% to 8.4%), and 1 mEq/ml	Acidosis: 0.5-1 mEq/kg IV Renal failure: 10 mg/kg PO q8-12hr Alkalization of urine: 50 mg/kg PO q8-12hr (1 tsp is approximately 2 gm)

Drug Name	Other Names	Formulations Available	Dosage
Sodium bromide	No commercial form	Must be compounded	Same as potassium bromide, except dose is 15% lower (30 mg/kg potassium bromide is equivalent to 25 mg/kg sodium bromide)
Sodium chloride 0.9%	Generic	500- and 1,000-ml infusion	15-30 ml/kg/hr IV
Sodium chloride 7.5%	Generic	Infusion	2-8 ml/kg IV
Sodium thiomalate	*See* Gold sodium thiomalate		
Somatrem, Somatropin	*See* Growth hormone		
Sotalol	Betapace	80-, 160-, 240-mg tablets	Dog: 1-2 mg/kg PO q12hr (one can start with 40 mg/dog q12hr, then increase to 80 mg if no response) Cat: 1-2 mg/kg PO q12hr
Spironolactone	Aldactone	25-, 50-, and 100-mg tablets	2-4 mg/kg/day (or 1-2 mg/kg PO q12hr)
Stanozolol	Winstrol-V	50-mg/ml injection; 2-mg tablet	Dog: 2 mg/dog (or range of 1-4 mg/dog) PO q12hr; 25-50 mg/dog/wk IM Cat: 1 mg/cat PO q12hr; 25 mg/cat/wk IM
Succimer	Chemet	100-mg capsule	Dog: 10 mg/kg PO q8hr for 5 days, then 10 mg/kg PO q12hr for 2 more wks Cat: 10 mg/kg q8hr for 2 wks
Sucralfate	Carafate (Sulcrate in Canada)	1-gm tablet; 200-mg/ml oral suspension	Dog: 0.5-1 gm/dog PO q8-12hr Cat: 0.25 gm/cat PO q8-12hr
Sufentanil citrate	Sufenta	50-mcg/ml injection	2 mcg/kg IV, up to a maximum dose of 5 mcg/kg
Sulfadiazine	Generic, combined with trimethoprim in Tribrissen	500-mg tablet; trimethoprim-sulfadiazine 30-, 120-, 240-, 480-, and 960-mg tablets	100 mg/kg IV, PO (loading dose), followed by 50 mg/kg IV, PO q12hr (*see also* Trimethoprim)
Sulfadimethoxine	Albon, Bactrovet, and generic	125-, 250-, and 500-mg tablets; 400-mg/ml injection; 50-mg/ml suspension	55 mg/kg PO (loading dose), followed by 27.5 mg/kg PO q12hr (*see also* Primor)
Sulfamethoxazole	Gantanol	50-mg tablet	100 mg/kg PO (loading dose), followed by 50 mg/kg PO q12hr (*see also* Bactrim, Septra)
Sulfasalazine (sulfapyridine + mesalamine)	Azulfidine (Salazopyrin in Canada)	500-mg tablet	Dog: 10-30 mg/kg PO q8-12hr (*see also* Mesalamine, Olsalazine) Cat: 20 mg/kg q12hr PO
Sulfisoxazole	Gantrisin	500-mg tablet; 500-mg/5 ml syrup	50 mg/kg PO q8hr (urinary tract infections)
Tamoxifen	Nolvadex	10- and 20-mg tablets (tamoxifen citrate)	Veterinary dose not established; 10 mg PO q12hr is human dose
Taurine	Generic	Available in powder	Dog: 500 mg PO q12hr Cat: 250 mg/cat PO q12hr
Telezol	*See* Tiletamine-Zolazepam		
Tepoxalin	Zubrin	50-, 100-, 200-mg tablets	Dog: 10-20 mg/kg PO initially, followed by 10 mg/kg q24hr PO thereafter Cat: Safe dose not established
Terbinafine	Lamisil	125-, 250-mg tablets	Dog: *Malassezia* dermatitis: 30 mg/kg/day PO Cat: Dermatophytosis: 30-40 mg/kg PO q24hr
Terbutaline	Brethine, Bricanyl	2.5- and 5-mg tablets; 1-mg/ml injection (equivalent to 0.82 mg/ml)	Dog: 1.25-5 mg/dog PO q8hr Cat: 0.1-0.2 mg/kg PO q12hr (or 0.625 mg/cat, ¼ of 2.5-mg tablet) For acute treatment in cats: 5-10 mcg/kg q4hr SC or IM

Continued

Appendix I—cont'd

Drug Name	Other Names	Formulations Available	Dosage
Testosterone cypionate ester	Andro-Cyp, Andronate, Depo-Testosterone and other forms	100- and 200-mg/ml injection	1-2 mg/kg IM q2-4wk (see also Methyltestosterone)
Testosterone propionate ester	Testex (Malogen in Canada)	100-mg/ml injection	0.5-1 mg/kg 2-3 times/wk IM
Tetracycline	Panmycin	250- and 500-mg capsules; 100-mg/ml suspension	15-20 mg/kg PO q8hr; or 4.4-11 mg/kg IV, IM q8hr
Thenium closylate	Canopar	500-mg tablet	Dog: >4.5 kg: 500 mg PO once, repeat in 2-3 wks 2.5-4.5 kg: 250 mg q12hr for 1 day, repeat in 2-3 wks
Theophylline	Many brands and generic	100-, 125-, 200-, 250-, and 300-mg tablets; 27-mg/5 ml oral solution or elixir; injection in 5% dextrose	Dog: 9 mg/kg PO q6-8hr Cat: 4 mg/kg PO q8-12hr
Theopylline extended-release	Inwood Labs extended release	100-, 200-, 300-, and 400-mg tablets or 125-, 200-, 300-mg capsules	Dog: 10 mg/kg q12hr PO of extended-release tablet or capsule Cat: 20 mg/kg q24-48hr PO extended-release tablet or 25 mg/kg q24-48hr PO extended-release capsule
Thiamine (vitamin B₁)	Bewon and others	250-mcg/5 ml elixir; tablets of various size from 5 mg to 500 mg; 100- and 500-mg/ml injection	Dog: 10-100 mg/dog/day PO or 12.5-50 mg/dog IM or SC/day Cat: 5-30 mg/cat/day PO (up to a maximum dose of 50 mg/cat/day) or 12.5-25 mg/cat IM or SC/day
Thiamylal sodium	No longer available; substitute Thiopental		
Thioguanine (6-TG)	Generic	40-mg tablet	40 mg/m² PO q24hr Cat: 25 mg/m² PO q24hr for 1-5 days, then repeat every 30 days
Thiomalate sodium	See Gold sodium thiomalate		
Thiopental sodium	Pentothal	Various size vials from 250 mg to 10 gm (mix to desired concentration)	Dog: 10-25 mg/kg IV (to effect) Cat: 5-10 mg/kg IV (to effect)
Thiotepa	Generic	15-mg injection (usually in solution of 10 mg/ml)	0.2-0.5 mg/m² weekly, or daily for 5-10 days IM, intracavitary, or intratumor
Thyroid hormone	See Levothyroxine sodium (T₄), or Liothyronine		
Thyrotropin, thyroid-stimulating hormone (TSH)	Thytropar, thyrogen	10-U vial; old forms difficult to obtain; thyrogen is 1000 mcg/vial	Dog: Collect baseline sample, followed by 0.1 U/kg IV (maximum dose is 5 U); collect post-TSH sample at 6 hr Cat: Collect baseline sample, followed by 2.5 U/cat IM and collect a post-TSH sample at 8-12 hr
Ticarcillin	Ticar, Ticillin	Vials containing 1, 3, 6, 20, and 30 gm	33-50 mg/kg IV, IM q4-6hr
Ticarcillin + clavulanate	Timentin	3-gm/vial for injection	Dose according to rate for ticarcillin
Tiletamine + zolazepam	Telazol, Zoletil	50 mg of each component per milliliter	Dog: 6.6-10 mg/kg IM (short term) or 10-13 mg/kg IM (longer procedure) Cat: 10-12 mg/kg IM (minor procedure) or 14-16 mg/kg IM (for surgery)
Tobramycin	Nebcin	40-mg/ml injection	Dog: 9-14 mg/kg IM, IV, SC q24hr Cat: 5-8 mg/kg IM, SC, IV q24hr
Tocainide	Tonocard	400- and 600-mg tablets	Dog: 15-20 mg/kg PO q8hr Cat: No dose established
Toluene	Vermiplex		267 mg/kg PO (of toluene), repeat in 2-4 wk

Drug Name	Other Names	Formulations Available	Dosage
Tramadol hydrochloride	Ultram and generic	Tramadol immediate-release tablets are available in 50-mg tablets	Dog: 5 mg/kg PO q6-8hr Cat: Safe dose not established
Trandolapril	Mavik	1-, 2-, and 4-mg tablets	Not established for dogs; human dose is 1 mg/person/day to start, then increase to 2-4 mg/day
Triamcinolone	Vetalog, Trimtabs, Aristocort, generic	Veterinary (Vetalog) 0.5- and 1.5-mg tablets. Human form: 1-, 2-, 4-, 8-, and 16-mg tablets; 10-mg/ml injection	Antiinflammatory: 0.5-1 mg/kg PO q12-24hr, then taper dose to 0.5-1 PO mg/kg q48hr (however, manufacturer recommends doses of 0.11 to 0.22 mg/kg/day)
Triamcinolone acetonide	Vetalog	2- or 6-mg/ml suspension injection	0.1-0.2 mg/kg IM, SC, repeat in 7-10 days Intralesional: 1.2-1.8 mg, or 1 mg for every cm diameter of tumor q2wk
Triamterene	Dyrenium	50- and 100-mg capsules	1-2 mg/kg PO q12hr
Tribrissen	*See* Trimethoprim-sulfadimethoxine combination		
Trientine hydrochloride	Syprine	250-mg capsule	10-15 mg/kg PO q12hr
Trifluoperazine	Stelazine	10-mg/ml oral solution; 1-, 2-, 5-, and 10-mg tablets; 2-mg/ml injection	0.03 mg/kg IM q12hr
Triflupromazine	Vesprin	10- and 20-mg/ml injection	0.1-0.3 mg/kg IM, PO q8-12hr
Tri-iodothyronine	*See* Liothyronine		
Trilostane	Vetoryl	10-, 30-, 60-, and 120-mg capsules; no formulations approved in US; must be imported	Dog: 3.9-9.2 mg/kg/day PO (most common dose is 6.1 mg/kg/day); adjust dose based on cortisol measurements
Trimeprazine tartrate	Temaril (Panectyl in Canada)	2.5-mg/5 ml syrup; 2.5-mg tablet	0.5 mg/kg PO q12hr
Trimethobenzamide	Tigan and others	100-mg/ml injection; 100- and 250-mg capsules	Dog: 3 mg/kg IM, PO q8hr Cat: Not recommended
Trimethoprim + sulfonamides (sulfadiazine or sulfamethoxazole)	Tribrissen and others	30-, 120-, 240-, 480-, and 960-mg tablets with trimethoprim to sulfa ratio 1:5	15 mg/kg PO q12hr, or 30 mg/kg PO q12-24hr For *Toxoplasma*: 30 mg/kg PO q12hr
Tripelennamine	Pelamine, PBZ	25- and 50-mg tablets; 20-mg/ml injection	1 mg/kg PO q12hr
TSH (thyroid-stimulating hormone)	*See* Thyrotropin		
Tylosin	Tylocine, Tylan, Tylosin tartrate	Available as soluble powder 2.2 gm tylosin per tsp (tablets for dogs in Canada)	Dog, cat: 7-15 mg/kg PO q12-24hr Dog: For colitis: 10-20 mg/kg q8hr with food initially, then increase interval to q12-24hr
Urofollitropin (FSH)	Metrodin	75 U/vial for injection	75 U/day IM for 7 days
Ursodiol (ursodeoxycholate)	Actigall	300-mg capsule, 250-mg tablets	10-15 mg/kg PO q24hr
Valproic acid, divalproex	Depakene (valproic acid); Depakote (divalproex)	125-, 250-, and 500-mg tablets (Depakote); 250-mg capsule; 50-mg/ml syrup (Depakene)	Dog: 60-200 mg/kg PO q8hr; or 25-105 mg/kg/day PO when administered with phenobarbital
Vancomycin	Vancocin, Vancoled	Vials for injection (0.5 to 10 gm)	Dog: 15 mg/kg q6-8hr IV infusion Cat: 12-15 mg/kg q8hr IV infusion
Vasopressin (ADH)	Pitressin	20 U/ml (aqueous)	10 U IV, IM
Verapamil	Calan, Isoptin	40-, 80-, and 120-mg tablet; 2.5-mg/ml injection	Dog: 0.05 mg/kg IV q10-30 min (maximum cumulative dose is 0.15 mg/kg)
Vinblastine	Velban	1-mg/ml injection	2 mg/m^2 IV (slow infusion) once/wk

Continued

Appendix I—cont'd

Drug Name	Other Names	Formulations Available	Dosage
Vincristine	Oncovin, Vincasar, generic	1-mg/ml injection	Antitumor: 0.5-0.7 mg/m² IV (or 0.025-0.05 mg/kg) once/wk For thrombocytopenia: 0.02 mg/kg IV once/wk
Viokase	*See* Pancrelipase		
Vitamin A (retinoids)	Aquasol A	Oral solution: 5000 U (1,500 RE) per 0.1 ml 10,000-, 25,000-, and 50,000-U tablets	625-800 U/kg PO q24hr
Vitamin B₁	*See* Thiamine		
Vitamin B₂ (riboflavin)	Riboflavin	Various-size tablets in increments from 10 to 250 mg	Dog: 10-20 mg/day PO Cat: 5-10 mg/day PO
Vitamin B₁₂ (cyanocobalamin)	Cyanocobalamin	Various-size tablets in increments from 25 to 100 mcg and injections	Dog: 100-200 mcg/day PO Cat: 50-100 mcg/day PO
Vitamin C (ascorbic acid)	*See* Ascorbic acid	Tablets of various sizes and injection	100-500 mg/day
Vitamin D	*See* Dihdyrotachysterol or Ergocalciferol		
Vitamin E (alpha-tocopherol)	Aquasol E, and generic	Wide variety of capsules, tablets, oral solution available (e.g., 1000 units per capsule)	100-400 U PO q12hr (or 400-600 U PO q12hr for immune-mediated skin disease)
Vitamin K₁ (phytonadione, phytomenadione)	AquaMEPHYTON (injection), Mephyton (tablets); Veta-K1 (capsules)	2- or 10-mg/ml injection; 5-mg tablet (Mephyton) 25-mg capsule (Veta-K1)	Short-acting rodenticides: 1 mg/kg/day IM, SC, PO for 10-14 days Long-acting rodenticides: 2.5-5 mg/kg/day and up to 6 wks IM, SC, PO for 3-4 wk Birds: 2.5-5 mg/kg q24hr
Warfarin	Coumadin, generic	1-, 2-, 2.5-, 4-, 5-, 7.5-, and 10-mg tablets	Dog: 0.1-0.2 mg/kg PO q24hr Cat: Thromboembolism: Start with 0.5 mg/cat/day and adjust dose based on clotting time assessment
Xylazine	Rompun and generic	20- and 100-mg/ml injection	Dog: 1.1 mg/kg IV, 2.2 mg/kg IM Cat: 1.1 mg/kg IM (emetic dose is 0.4-0.5 mg/kg IV)
Yohimbine	Yobine	2-mg/ml injection	0.11 mg/kg IV or 0.25-0.5 mg/kg SC, IM
Zidovudine (AZT)	Retrovir	10-mg/ml syrup; 10-mg/ml Injection	Cat: 15 mg/kg PO q12hr to 20 mg/kg q8hr (doses as high as 30 mg/kg/day also have been used)
Zolazepam	*See* Tiletamine-zolazepam combination		
Zonisamide	Zonegram	100-mg capsule	Dog: 3 mg/kg q8hr PO; it has also been administered to dogs at 10 mg/kg q12hr PO Cat: Dose not established

NOTE: Doses listed are for dogs *and* cats, unless otherwise listed. Many of the doses listed are extra-label or are human drugs used in an off-label or extra-label manner. Doses listed are based on best available evidence at the time of table preparation; however, the author cannot ensure efficacy of drugs used according to recommendations in this table. Adverse effects may be possible from drugs listed in this table of which author was not aware at the time of table preparation. Veterinarians using these tables are encouraged to check current literature, product label, and the manufacturer's disclosure for information regarding efficacy and any known adverse effects or contraindications not indentified at the time of preparation of these tables.

IM, Intramuscular; *IV,* intravenous; *OTC,* over-the-counter (without prescription); *PO,* per os (oral); *Rx,* prescription only; *SC,* subcutaneous; *U,* units.

APPENDIX II

Treatment of Parasites

CLIFF MONAHAN, *Columbus, Ohio*

Helminths

Drug(s)	Species	Target Parasites	Route*	Veterinary Formulations
Emodepside/Praziquantel	Feline only	Roundworms, hookworms, *Dipylidium caninum*, *Echinococcus multilocularis*, *Taenia taeniaeformis*	Topical	Profender
Epsiprantel	Canine and feline	*Dipylidium caninum, Taenia* spp.	Oral	Cestex
Febantel/Praziquantel/Pyrantel Pamoate	Canine only	Roundworms, hookworms, *Trichuris vulpis, Dipylidium caninum, Echinococcus granulosus, Taenia pisiformis*	Oral	Drontal Plus
Fenbendazole	Canine	Roundworms, hookworms, *Trichuris vulpis, Giardia intestinalis, Taenia pisiformis*	Oral	Panacur
Imidacloprid/Moxidectin	Canine and feline	Roundworms, hookworms, *Trichuris vulpis* in dogs; *Dirofilaria immitis* prevention	Topical	Advantage Multi
Ivermectin	Canine and feline	Roundworms, hookworms, in cats, *Dirofilaria immitis* prevention in dogs and cats	Oral	Heartgard
Ivermectin/Praziquantel/Pyrantel Pamoate	Canine only	Roundworms, hookworms, *Dipylidium caninum, Echinococcus granulosus, Taenia pisiformis, Dirofilaria immitis* prevention	Oral	Iverhart Max
Ivermectin/Pyrantel Pamoate	Canine only	Roundworms, hookworms, *Dirofilaria immitis* prevention	Oral	Heartgard Plus, Iverhart Plus, TriHeart Plus
Milbemycin Oxime	Canine and feline	Roundworms, *Ancylostoma* spp., *Trichuris vulpis* in dogs; *Dirofilaria immitis* prevention	Oral	Interceptor
Praziquantel	Canine and feline	*Dipylidium caninum, Echinococcus* spp., *Taenia* spp.	Oral injectable	Droncit
Praziquantel/Pyrantel Pamoate	Feline only	Roundworms, hookworms, *Dipylidium caninum*, *Echinococcus multilocularis*, *Taenia taeniaeformis*	Oral	Drontal
Pyrantel Pamoate	Canine and feline	Roundworms and hookworms in dogs and cats	Oral	Nemex
Selamectin	Canine and feline	Roundworms and hookworms in cats; *Dirofilaria immitis* prevention in dogs and cats	Topical	Revolution

Protozoa

Drug(s)	Species	Target Parasite(s)	Route(s) and Frequency of Administration	Veterinary Formulations
Fipronil	Canine and feline	Fleas, lice, mites, ticks	Topical, monthly	Frontline, Frontline Plus
Imidacloprid	Canine and feline	Fleas, lice	Topical, monthly	Advantage
Imidacloprid/Permethrin	Canine only	Fleas, lice, mites, ticks	Topical, monthly	Advantix
Metaflumizone	Feline only	Fleas, lice	Topical, monthly	ProMeris for Cats
Metaflumizone/Amitraz	Canine only	Fleas, lice, mites, ticks	Topical, monthly	ProMeris for Dogs
Nitenpyram	Canine and feline	Fleas	Oral, daily	Capstar
Spinosad	Canine only	Fleas	Oral, monthly	Comfortis

Ectoparasites

Drug(s)	Species	Target Parasite(s)	Route of Administration and Dosages	Veterinary Formulations
Amprolium	Canine	*Isospora* spp.	Oral, 100 mg/kg SID, 7-10 days	Corid
Clindamycin	Canine and feline	*Toxoplasma gondii* (systemic infections)	Oral, 10-15 mg/kg BID, 14-28 days as needed	Antirobe
Doxycycline	Canine and feline	*Toxoplasma gondii* (systemic infections)	Oral 5-10 mg/kg BID, 28 days	Vibramycin
Fenbendazole	Canine and feline	*Giardia intestinalis*	Oral, 50 mg/kg SID, 3 days	Panacur
Imidocarb diproprionate	Canine and reline	*Babesia* spp., *Cytauxzoon felis*	IM or SC, 6.6 mg/kg; repeat in 14 days	Imizol
Metronidazole	Canine and feline	*Giardia intestinalis*	Oral, 25 mg/kg SID, 5 days	Flagyl
Nitazoxanide	Canine and feline	*Giardia intestinalis, Cryptosporidium* spp.	Oral, 100 mg/kg BID, 3 days	Alinia (Human) Navigator (Horses)
Ponazuril	Canine and feline	*Isospora* spp., *Toxoplasma gondii*	Oral, 15 mg/kg SID, 3 days; 30 mg/kg SID, 1 day	Marquis (Horses)
Sulfadiazine and Trimethoprim	Canine and feline	*Isospora* spp., *Toxoplasma gondii* (intestinal infections)	Oral, 30 mg/kg BID, 14 days as needed	Tribrissen
Sulfadimethoxine	Canine and reline	*Isospora* spp., *Toxoplasma gondii* (intestinal infections)	Oral, 50 mg/kg day 1, then 25 mg/kg SID for 14-21 days as needed	Albon

*Follow manufacturer's recommendations for indicated use; see Appendix I, Table of Commonly Used Drugs, for extralabel use.

APPENDIX III

AAFCO Dog and Cat Food Nutrient Profiles

DAVID A. DZANIS, *Santa Clarita, California*

The Association of American Feed Control Officials (AAFCO) is a non-governmental body, but it is composed solely of representatives from agencies within individual states and territories, federal agencies such as the U.S. Food and Drug Administration (FDA), and foreign governments such as Canada. A primary function of AAFCO is the publication of a model feed bill, animal feed regulations, and ingredient definitions, all of which a state may adopt as a part of its own feed laws and regulations. A pet food that bears a "complete and balanced" label claim that does not, in fact, offer adequate nutrition is both misbranded and unsafe. To address this concern, included in the model pet food regulations are means of substantiating nutritional adequacy for complete and balanced dog and cat foods.

One method of substantiating nutritional adequacy requires that the product be formulated so that essential nutrient levels meet a prescribed profile. Historically, AAFCO relied on the publications of the National Research Council (NRC) as its authority with respect to the levels of nutrients that constituted a complete and balanced dog or cat food. However, to address several technical concerns regarding the applicability of the NRC recommendations to the practical formulation of pet foods, they were replaced by the AAFCO Dog and Cat Food Nutrient Profiles (Tables 1 and 2) in the early 1990s.

The profiles are the product of the AAFCO Canine Nutrition Expert (CNE) and Feline Nutritional Expert (FNE) Subcommittees, which met in 1990 and 1991, respectively. Nationally recognized experts from both academia and industry were convened to establish practical profiles based on commonly used ingredients. In addition to this author (at that time representing the FDA), members of the CNE included Dr. Jim Corbin, University of Illinois; Dr. Gail Czarnecki-Maulden, Westreco, Inc.; Dr. Diane Hirakawa, The Iams Company; Dr. Francis Kallfelz, Cornell University; Dr. Mark Morris, Mark Morris Associates; and Dr. Ben Sheffy, Cornell University. Added to the original members of the CNE were two new members on the FNE to bring additional expertise in the field of cat nutrition; Dr. Quinton Rogers, University of California-Davis; and Dr. Angele Thompson, Kal Kan Foods. Mr. Wenell Kerr of Westreco, Inc., also participated to provide statistical support to both subcommittees. The CNE and FNE met once again in 1995 to review and update both the dog and the cat food profiles. At the time of this writing, a new AAFCO expert panel has been convened to review recent data and recommend revision of the profiles where appropriate.

Nutrient levels in the AAFCO Dog and Cat Food Nutrient Profiles are based on the CNE and the FNE members' knowledge of published and unpublished research, as well as their personal expertise and experiences in practical formulation. Much of the scientific data on nutrient requirements are based on studies using purified diets and the presumption of 100% bioavailability. However, since commercial products are composed of nonpurified, complex ingredients, allowances to account for the effects of ingredients, ingredient interactions, and processing on bioavailability were also considered in establishing nutrient levels. Comments on the bioavailability or the effect of processing and ingredient interaction on some nutrients are also added in the footnotes to tables.

In addition to minimum nutrient levels, the AAFCO Dog and Cat Food Nutrient Profiles also set maximum levels of intake of some nutrients. This was done out of concern that the risk of nutrient excess, rather than deficiency, was a concern with some pet foods. Thus maximum limits on the amounts of calcium, phosphorus, magnesium, fat-soluble vitamins, and most trace minerals in dog foods are established. Whereas the list of maximum levels for cat foods is not as extensive as that for dog foods, it should not be inferred that cats are more tolerant of nutrient excesses than dogs. Rather it reflects the paucity of information on the toxic effects of nutrients in cats. Establishing maximum levels arbitrarily might prove worse than no maximum at all. Setting a maximum level implies safety below that level, which the subcommittees could not reasonably ensure.

Replacing the previous "meets or exceeds the NRC recommendations" verbiage, the required label wording for reference to the nutrient profiles is that the product is "... formulated to meet the nutrient levels established by the AAFCO Dog (or Cat) Food Nutrient Profiles for ..." a given life stage. For both dog and cat foods, there are two separate AAFCO profiles: one for growth and reproduction (gestation and lactation), and one for adult maintenance. This allows foods formulated for adult dogs or cats to contain lower amounts of some nutrients, eliminating unnecessary excesses. Products that meet only the adult maintenance profile should include "maintenance" as its given life stage. Since products suitable for the more stringent nutrient requirements of growth and reproduction

Table 1

AAFCO Dog Food Nutrient Profiles*

Nutrient	Units DM Basis	Growth and Reproduction Minimum	Adult Maintenance Minimum	Maximum
Crude protein	%	22.0	18.0	
Arginine	%	0.62	0.51	
Histidine	%	0.22	0.18	
Isoleucine	%	0.45	0.37	
Leucine	%	0.72	0.59	
Lysine	%	0.77	0.63	
Methionine-cystine	%	0.53	0.43	
Phenylalanine-tyrosine	%	0.89	0.73	
Threonine	%	0.58	0.48	
Tryptophan	%	0.20	0.16	
Valine	%	0.48	0.39	
Crude fat[†]	%	8.0	5.0	
Linoleic acid	%	1.0	1.0	
Minerals				
Calcium	%	1.0	0.6	2.5
Phosphorus	%	0.8	0.5	1.6
Ca:P ratio		1:1	1:1	2:1
Potassium	%	0.6	0.6	
Sodium	%	0.3	0.06	
Chloride	%	0.45	0.09	
Magnesium	%	0.04	0.04	0.3
Iron[‡]	mg/kg	80	80	3,000
Copper[§]	mg/kg	7.3	7.3	250
Manganese	mg/kg	5.0	5.0	
Zinc	mg/kg	120	120	1,000
Iodine	mg/kg	1.5	1.5	50
Selenium	mg/kg	0.11	0.11	2
Vitamins and other				
Vitamin A	IU/kg	5,000	5,000	250,000
Vitamin D	IU/kg	500	500	5,000
Vitamin E	IU/kg	50	50	1,000
Thiamine[‖]	mg/kg	1.0	1.0	
Riboflavin	mg/kg	2.2	2.2	
Pantothenic acid	mg/kg	10	10	
Niacin	mg/kg	11.4	11.4	
Pyridoxine	mg/kg	1.0	1.0	
Folic acid	mg/kg	0.18	0.18	
Vitamin B_{12}	mg/kg	0.022	0.022	
Choline	mg/kg	1,200	1,200	

*Presumes an energy density of 3.5 kcal ME/g DM, based on the "modified Atwater" values of 3.5, 8.5, and 3.5 kcal/g for protein, fat, and carbohydrate (nitrogen-free extract, NFE), respectively. Rations greater than 4.0 kcal/g should be corrected for energy density; rations less than 3.5 kcal/g should not be corrected for energy. Rations of low-energy density should not be considered adequate for growth or reproductive needs based on comparison to the profiles alone.
[†]Although a true requirement for fat per se has not been established, the minimum level was based on recognition of fat as a source of essential fatty acids, as a carrier of fat-soluble vitamins, and on the amount needed to enhance palatability and to supply an adequate caloric density.
[‡]Because of very poor bioavailability, iron from carbonate or oxide sources that are added to the diet should not be considered in determining the minimum nutrient level.
[§]Because of very poor bioavailability, copper from oxide sources that are added to the diet should not be considered in determining the minimum nutrient level.
[‖]Because processing may destroy up to 90% of the thiamine in the diet, allowances in formulation should be made to ensure that the minimum nutrient level is met after processing.

are also presumed to be adequate for adult maintenance, products meeting the growth and reproduction profile can list their intended use for either maintenance, growth, gestation and lactation, or "all life stages."

Nutrient levels in the tables are expressed on a dry matter (DM) basis. To accurately compare levels for a pet food as given in the guaranteed analysis portion of a label or elsewhere on an "as fed" basis, the values must first be corrected for moisture content. For most dry pet foods (10% moisture), "as fed" values should be multiplied by 1.1. For 75% moisture canned product, values should be multiplied by 4.0. The profiles are also set at

Table 2

AAFCO Cat Food Nutrient Profiles[*]

Nutrient	Units DM Basis	Growth and Reproduction Minimum	Adult Maintenance Minimum	Maximum
Crude protein	%	30.0	26.0	
Arginine	%	1.25	1.04	
Histidine	%	0.31	0.31	
Isoleucine	%	0.52	0.52	
Leucine	%	1.25	1.25	
Lysine	%	1.20	0.83	
Methionine-cystine	%	1.10	1.10	
Methionine	%	0.62	0.62	1.5
Phenylalanine-tyrosine	%	0.88	0.88	
Phenylalanine	%	0.42	0.42	
Threonine	%	0.73	0.73	
Tryptophan	%	0.25	0.16	
Valine	%	0.62	0.62	
Crude fat[†]	%	9.0	9.0	
Linoleic acid	%	0.5	0.5	
Arachidonic acid	%	0.02	0.02	
Minerals				
Calcium	%	1.0	0.6	
Phosphorus	%	0.8	0.5	
Potassium	%	0.6	0.6	
Sodium	%	0.2	0.2	
Chloride	%	0.3	0.3	
Magnesium[‡]	%	0.08	0.04	
Iron[§]	mg/kg	80	80	
Copper (extruded)[‖]	mg/kg	15	5	
Copper (canned)[‖]	mg/kg	5	5	
Manganese	mg/kg	7.5	7.5	
Zinc	mg/kg	75	75	2,000
Iodine	mg/kg	0.35	0.35	
Selenium	mg/kg	0.1	0.1	
Vitamins and others				
Vitamin A	IU/kg	9,000	5,000	750,000
Vitamin D	IU/kg	750	500	10,000
Vitamin E[¶]	IU/kg	30	30	
Vitamin K[#]	mg/kg	0.1	0.1	
Thiamine[**]	mg/kg	5.0	5.0	
Riboflavin	mg/kg	4.0	4.0	
Pantothenic acid	mg/kg	5.0	5.0	
Niacin	mg/kg	60	60	
Pyridoxine	mg/kg	4.0	4.0	
Folic acid	mg/kg	0.8	0.8	
Biotin[††]	mg/kg	0.07	0.07	
Vitamin B_{12}	mg/kg	0.02	0.02	
Choline[‡‡]	mg/kg	2,400	2,400	
Taurine (extruded)	%	0.10	0.10	
Taurine (canned)	%	0.20	0.20	

[*]Presumes an energy density of 4.0 kcal ME/g DM, based on the "modified Atwater" values of 3.5, 8.5, and 3.5 kcal/g for protein, fat, and carbohydrate (nitrogen-free extract, NFE), respectively. Rations greater than 4.5 kcal/g should be corrected for energy density; rations less than 4.0 kcal/g should not be corrected for energy. Rations of low-energy density should not be considered adequate for growth or reproductive needs based on comparison to the profiles alone.

[†]Although a true requirement for fat per se has not be established, the minimum level was based on recognition of fat as a source of essential fatty acids, as a carrier of fat-soluble vitamins, to enhance palatability, and to supply an adequate caloric density.

[‡]If the mean urine pH of cats fed ad libitum is not below 6.4, the risk of struvite urolithiasis increases as the magnesium content of the diet increases.

[§]Because of very poor bioavailability, iron from carbonate or oxide sources that are added to the diet should not be considered in determining the minimum nutrient level.

[‖]Because of very poor bioavailability, copper from oxide sources that are added to the diet should not be considered in determining the minimum nutrient level.

[¶]Add 10 IU of vitamin E above minimum level per gram of fish oil per kilogram of diet.

[#]Vitamin K does not need to be added unless diet contains more than 25% fish on a dry matter basis.

[**]Because processing may destroy up to 90% of the thiamine in the diet, allowances in formulation should be made to ensure that the minimum nutrient level is met after processing.

[††]Biotin does not need to be added unless diet contains antimicrobial or antivitamin compounds.

[‡‡]Methionine may be used to substitute for choline as a methyl donor at rate of 3.75 parts for 1 part choline by weight when methionine exceeds 0.62%.

presumed energy densities (3.5 kcal ME/g DM for dog foods, 4.0 kcal ME/g DM for cat foods). Since a dog or cat is presumed to eat less of a high-calorie food, the levels of the nutrients must be proportionally higher in order for the animal to meet its needs with lower food intake. Thus products very high in caloric density should also be corrected for energy content before comparisons with the profiles are made.

The AAFCO Dog and Cat Food Nutrient Profiles and accompanying information on using the tables are published annually in the AAFCO Official Publication. Information on AAFCO and how to obtain a copy of the AAFCO Official Publication can be found on its website (http://www.aafco.org) or by writing to: Ms Sharon Krebs, AAFCO Assistant Secretary-Treasurer, P.O. Box 478, Oxford, IN 47971.

Index

Page numbers followed by f indicate figures; t, tables; b, boxes.

Conversion Table of Weight to Body Surface Area (in Square Meters) For Dogs*

kg	m²	kg	m²	kg	m²	kg	m²
0.5	0.06	26.0	0.88	13.0	0.55	39.0	1.15
1.0	0.10	27.0	0.90	14.0	0.58	40.0	1.17
2.0	0.15	28.0	0.92	15.0	0.60	41.0	1.19
3.0	0.20	29.0	0.94	16.0	0.63	42.0	1.21
4.0	0.25	30.0	0.96	17.0	0.66	43.0	1.23
5.0	0.29	31.0	0.99	18.0	0.69	44.0	1.25
6.0	0.33	32.0	1.01	19.0	0.71	45.0	1.26
7.0	0.36	33.0	1.03	20.0	0.74	46.0	1.28
8.0	0.40	34.0	1.05	21.0	0.76	47.0	1.30
9.0	0.43	35.0	1.07	22.0	0.78	48.0	1.32
10.0	0.46	36.0	1.09	23.0	0.81	49.0	1.34
11.0	0.49	37.0	1.11	24.0	0.83	50.0	1.36
12.0	0.52	38.0	1.13	25.0	0.85		

*From Ettinger SJ: Textbook of veterinary internal medicine; Diseases of the dog and cat, ed 2, Philadelphia, Saunders, 1975, p 146.
Although the above chart was compiled for dogs, it can also be used for cats. A formula for more precise values follows:
BSA In m = $(K \times W^{2/3}) \times 10^{-4}$ where m² = square meters, BSA = body surface area, W = weight in gm, and K = constant of 10.1 in dogs and 10.0 in cats.

Système International (SI) Units in Clinical Chemistry

Analyte	Traditional Unit (with examples)	Conversion Factor	SI Unit (with examples)
Alanine aminotransferase	0-40 U/L	1.00	0-40 U/L
Albumin	2.8-4.0 gm/dl	10.0	28-40 gm/L
Alkaline phosphatase	30-150 U/L	1.00	30-150 U/L
Ammonia	10-80 mcg/dl	0.5871	5.9-47.0 µmol/L
Amylase	200-800 U/L	1.00	200-800 U/L
Aspartate aminotransferase	0-40 U/L	1.00	0-40 U/L
Bile acids (total)	0.3-2.3 mcg/ml	2.45	0.74-5.64 µmol/L
Bilirubin	0.1-0.2 mg/dl	17.10	2-4 µmol/L
Calcium	8.8-10.3 mg/dl	0.2495	2.20-2.58 mmol/L
Carbon dioxide	22-28 mEq/L	1.00	22-28 mmol/L
Chloride	95-100 mEq/L	1.00	95-100 mmol/L
Cholesterol	100-265 mg/dl	0.0258	2.58-5.85 mmol/L
Copper	70-140 mcg/dl	0.1574	11.0-22.0 µmol/L
Cortisol	2-10 mcg/dl	27.59	55-280 nmol/L
Creatine kinase	0-130 U/L	1.00	0-130 U/L
Creatinine	0.6-1.2 mg/dl	88.40	50-110 µmol/L
Fibrinogen	200-400 mg/dl	0.01	2.0-4.0 gm/L
Folic acid	3.5-11.0 mcg/L	2.265	7.93-24.92 nmol/L
Glucose	70-110 mg/dl	0.05551	3.9-6.1 mmol/L
Iron	80-180 mcg/dl	0.1791	14-32 µmol/L
Lactate	5-20 mg/dl	0.1110	0.5-2.0 mmol/L
Lead	150 mcg/dl	0.04826	7.2 µmol/L
Lipase Sigma Tietz (37°C)	≤1 ST U/dl	280	≤280 U/L
Lipase Cherry Crandall (30°C)	0-160 U/L	1.00	0-160 U/L
Lipids (total)	400-850 mg/dl	0.01	4.0-8.5 gm/L
Magnesium	1.8-3.0 mg/dl	0.4114	0.80-1.20 mmol/L
Mercury	≤1.0 mcg/dl	49.85	≤50 nmol/L
Osmolality	280-300 mOsm/kg	1.00	280-300 mmol/L
Phosphorus	2.5-5.0 mg/dl	0.3229	0.80-1.6 mmol/L
Potassium	3.5-5.0 mEq/L	1.0	3.5-5.0 mmol/L
Protein (total)	5-8 gm/dl	10.0	50-80 gm/L
Sodium	135-147 mEq/L	1.00	135-147 mmol/L
Testosterone	4.0-8.0 mg/ml	3.467	14.0-28.0 nmol/L
Thyroxine	1-4 mcg/dl	12.87	13-51 nmol/L
Triglyceride	10-500 mg/dl	0.0113	0.11-5.65 mmol/L
Urea nitrogen	10-20 mg/dl	0.3570	3.6-7.1 nmol/L
Uric acid	3.6-7.7 mg/dl	59.44	214-458 µmol/L
Urobilinogen	0-4.0 mg/dl	16.9	0.0-6.8 µmol/L
Vitamin A	90 mcg/dl	0.03491	3.1 µmol/L
Vitamin B$_{12}$	300-700 ng/L	0.738	221-516 pmol/L
Vitamin E	5.0-20.0 mg/L	2.32	11.6-46.4 µmol/L
D-Xylose	30-40 mg/dl	0.06666	2.0-2.71 mmol/L
Zinc	75-120 mcg/dl	0.1530	11.5-18.5 µmol/L

WEIGHT EQUIVALENTS

1 lb = 453.6 g = 4536 kg = 16 oz
1 oz = 28.35 gm
1 kg = 1,000 g = 2.2046 lb
1 gm = 1,000 mg
1 mg = 1,000 mcg = 0.001 gm
1 mcg = 0.001 mg = 0.000001 gm
1 mcg per gm or 1 mg per kg is the same as 1 ppm

VOLUME EQUIVALENTS

Household	Metric
1 drop (gt)	= 0.06 milliliter (ml)
15 drops (gtt)	= 1 ml (1 cc)
1 teaspoon (tsp)	= 5 (4) ml
1 tablespoon (tbs)	= 15 ml
2 tablespoons	= 30 ml
1 ounce (oz)	= 30 ml
1 teacup	= 180 ml (6 oz)
1 glass	= 240 ml (8 oz)
1 measuring cup	= 240 ml (1/2 pint)
2 measuring cups	= 500 ml (1 pint)

PRESSURE EQUIVALENTS

1 cm H_2O	= 0.736 mmHg	= 0.098 kPa
1 mmHg (torr)	= 1.36 cm H_2O	= 0.133 kPa
1 kPa	= 7.5 mmHg	= 10.2 cm H_2O
1 atm	= 760 mmHg	= 1033.6 cm H_2O

Weight-Unit Conversion Factors

Units Given	Units Wanted	For Conversion Multiply by
lb	gm	453.6
lb	kg	0.4536
oz	gm	28.35
kg	lb	2.2046
kg	mg	1,000,000.
kg	gm	1,000.
gm	mg	1,000.
gm	mcg	1,000,000.
mg	mcg	1,000.
mg/gm	mg/lb	453.6
mg/kg	mg/lb	0.4536
mcg/kg	mcg/lb	0.4536
Mcal	kcal	1,000.
kcal/kg	kcal/lb	0.4536
kcal/lb	kcal/kg	2.2046
ppm	mcg/gm	1.
ppm	mg/kg	1.
ppm	mg/lb	0.4536
mg/kg	%	0.0001
ppm	%	0.0001
mg/gm	%	0.1
gm/kg	%	0.1

Conversion Factors

1 milligram	= 1/65 grain	(1/60)
1 gram	= 15.43 grains	(15)
1 kilogram	= 2.20 pounds	(avoirdupois)
	= 2.65 pounds	(Troy)
1 milliliter	= 16.23 minims	(15)
1 liter	= 1.06 quarts	(1+)
	= 33.80 fluid ounces	(34)
1 grain	= 0.065 gm	(60 mg)
1 dram	= 3.9 gm	(4)
1 ounce	= 31.1 gm	(30+)
1 minim	= 0.062 ml	(0.06)
1 fluid dram	= 3.7 ml	(4)
1 fluid ounce	= 29.57 ml	(30)
1 pint	= 473.2 ml	(500−)
1 quart	= 946.4 ml	(1000−)

Figures in parentheses are commonly employed approximate values.

Approximate Equivalents for Degrees Fahrenheit and Celsius*

°F	°C
0	−17.8
32	0
85	29.4
86	30.0
87	30.6
88	31.1
89	31.7
90	32.2
91	32.7
92	33.3
93	33.9
94	34.4
95	35.0
96	35.5
97	36.1
98	36.7
99	37.2
100	37.8
101	38.3
102	38.9
103	39.4
104	40.0
105	40.6
106	41.1
107	41.7
108	42.2
109	42.8
110	43.3
212	100

*Temperature conversion: °Celsius to °Fahrenheit, (°C) (9/5) + 32°;
°Fahrenheit to °Celsius, (°F − 32°) (5/9).

Metric Apothecary

Milligrams	Grains
1 mg	= 1/60 gr
15 mg	= 1/4 gr
30 mg	= 1/2 gr
40 mg	= 2/3 gr
50 mg	= 3/4 gr
60 mg	= 1 gr

Catheter, Wire, and Tubing Size Measurements

Gauge	Approximate External Diameter (mm)	Approximate External Diameter (in)	French Gauge*
29	0.330	0.013	1
22	0.711	0.028	2
18	1.270	0.050	3
17	1.473	0.058	4
16	1.651	0.065	5
14	2.108	0.083	6

Modified from Silverstein/Hopper: Small Animal Critical Care Medicine, 2008, Saunders.
*French Gauge = 3 × External diameter in mm